Drug Information Handbook

2002-2003

10TH ANNIVERSARY EDITION

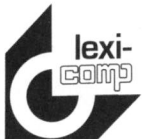

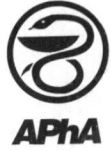

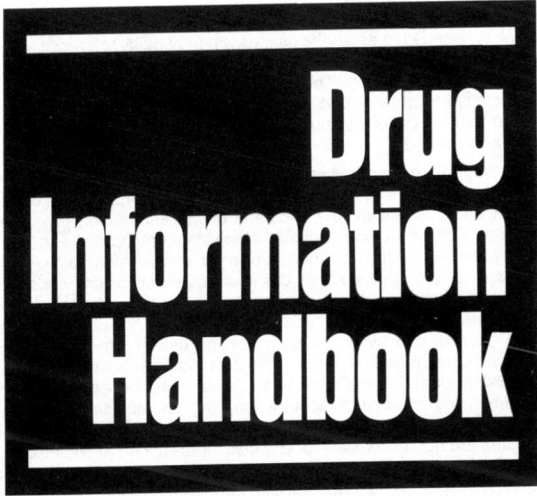

Drug Information Handbook

10th Edition ‖ 2002-2003

Charles F. Lacy, PharmD, FCSHP
Facilitative Officer, Professional Programs
Professor, Pharmacy Practice
Nevada College of Pharmacy
Las Vegas, Nevada

Lora L. Armstrong, PharmD, BCPS
Manager, Clinical Services
Caremark Rx, Inc.
Northbrook, Illinois

Morton P. Goldman, PharmD, BCPS
Assistant Director, Pharmacotherapy Services
Department of Pharmacy
Cleveland Clinic Foundation
Cleveland, Ohio

Leonard L. Lance, RPh, BSPharm
Pharmacist
Lexi-Comp, Inc.
Hudson, Ohio

LEXI-COMP INC
Hudson (Cleveland)

**AMERICAN
PHARMACEUTICAL
ASSOCIATION** APhA

NOTICE

This handbook is intended to serve the user as a handy quick reference and not as a complete drug information resource. It does not include information on every therapeutic agent available. The publication covers commonly used drugs and is specifically designed to present certain important aspects of drug data in a more concise format than is generally found in medical literature or product material supplied by manufacturers.

The nature of drug information is that it is constantly evolving because of ongoing research and clinical experience and is often subject to interpretation. While great care has been taken to ensure the accuracy of the information presented, the reader is advised that the authors, editors, reviewers, contributors, and publishers cannot be responsible for the continued currency of the information or for any errors, omissions, or the application of this information, or for any consequences arising therefrom. Therefore, the author(s) and/or the publisher shall have no liability to any person or entity with regard to claims, loss, or damage caused, or alleged to be caused, directly or indirectly, by the use of information contained herein. Because of the dynamic nature of drug information, readers are advised that decisions regarding drug therapy must be based on the independent judgment of the clinician, changing information about a drug (eg, as reflected in the literature and manufacturer's most current product information), and changing medical practices. The editors are not responsible for any inaccuracy of quotation or for any false or misleading implication that may arise due to the text or due to the quotation of revisions no longer official. Further, the reader/user, herewith, is advised that information shown under the heading **Usual Dosage** is provided only as an indication of the amount of the drug typically given or taken during therapy. Actual dosing amount for any specific drug should be based on an in-depth evaluation of the individual patient's therapy requirement and strong consideration given to such issues as contraindications, warnings, precautions, adverse reactions, along with the interaction of other drugs. The manufacturers most current product information or other standard recognized references should always be consulted for such detailed information prior to drug use.

The editors, authors, and contributors have written this book in their private capacities. No official support or endorsement by any federal agency or pharmaceutical company is intended or inferred.

The publishers have made every effort to trace the copyright holders for borrowed material. If they have inadvertently overlooked any, they will be pleased to make the necessary arrangements at the first opportunity.

If you have any suggestions or questions regarding any information presented in this handbook, please contact our drug information pharmacist at

1-877-837-LEXI (5394)

This manual was produced using the FormuLex™ Program —
a complete publishing service of Lexi-Comp Inc.

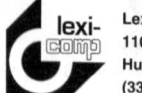

Lexi-Comp Inc
1100 Terex Road
Hudson, Ohio 44236
(330) 650-6506

ISBN 1-59195-016-3 North American
ISBN 1-59195-019-8 International

TABLE OF CONTENTS

ABOUT THE AUTHORS

Charles F. Lacy, PharmD, FCSHP

Dr Lacy is the Facilitative Officer for Clinical Programs and Professor of Pharmacy Practice at the Nevada College of Pharmacy. In his current capacity, Dr Lacy oversees the clinical curriculum, clinical faculty activities, the computer information systems, student experiential programs, pharmacy residency programs, continuing education programs, entrepreneurial activities, and all of the drug information needs for the college. Prior to coming to the Nevada College of Pharmacy, Dr Lacy was the Clinical Coordinator for the Department of Pharmacy at Cedars-Sinai Medical Center. With over 19 years of clinical experience at one of the nation's largest teaching hospitals, he has developed a reputation as an acknowledged expert in drug information and critical care drug therapy.

Dr Lacy received his doctorate from the University of Southern California School of Pharmacy and still works with the University as a member of their alumni board to advance the curriculum of pharmacy students in the Southern California area.

Presently, Dr Lacy holds teaching affiliations with the Nevada College of Pharmacy, the University of Southern California School of Pharmacy, the University of California at San Francisco School of Pharmacy, the University of the Pacific School of Pharmacy, Western University of Health Sciences School of Pharmacy, and the University of Alberta at Edmonton, School of Pharmacy and Health Sciences.

Dr Lacy is an active member of numerous professional associations including the American Society of Health-System Pharmacists (ASHP), the American College of Clinical Pharmacy (ACCP), the American Society of Consultant Pharmacists (ASCP), the American Association of Colleges of Pharmacy (AACP), American Pharmaceutical Association (APhA), the Nevada Pharmacy Alliance (NPA), and the California Society of Hospital Pharmacists (CSHP), through which he has chaired many committees and subcommittees.

Lora L. Armstrong, PharmD, BCPS

Dr Armstrong received her bachelor's degree in pharmacy from Ferris State University and her Doctor of Pharmacy degree from Midwestern University. Dr Armstrong is a Board Certified Pharmacotherapy Specialist (BCPS).

In her current position, Dr Armstrong serves as the senior manager of the Pharmacy and Therapeutics Committee process at Caremark Rx, Inc, Prescription Services Division. Caremark is a prescription benefit management company (PBM). Dr Armstrong is responsible for coordination of the Caremark National Pharmacy & Therapeutics Committee and she chairs the Caremark Pharmacy & Therapeutics Subcommittee. Dr Armstrong is also responsible for coordinating the Caremark Clinical Practice Committee, monitoring the pharmaceutical product pipeline, monitoring drug surveillance, and communicating Pharmacy & Therapeutics Committee Formulary information to Caremark's internal and external customers.

Prior to joining Caremark Rx, Inc, Dr Armstrong served as the Director of Drug Information Services at the University of Chicago Hospitals. She obtained 17 years of experience in a variety of clinical settings including critical care, hematology, oncology, infectious diseases, and clinical pharmacokinetics. Dr Armstrong played an active role in the education and training of medical, pharmacy, and nursing staff. She coordinated the Drug Information Center, the medical center's Adverse Drug Reaction Monitoring Program, and the continuing Education Program for pharmacists. She also maintained the hospital's strict formulary program and was the editor of the University of Chicago Hospitals' *Formulary of Accepted Drugs* and the drug information center's monthly newsletter *Topics in Drug Therapy*.

Dr Armstrong is an active member of the Academy of Managed Care Pharmacy (AMCP), the American Society of Health-Systems Pharmacists (ASHP), the American Pharmaceutical Association (APhA), and the American College of Clinical Pharmacy (ACCP). Dr Armstrong wrote the chapter entitled "Drugs and Hormones Used in Endocrinology" in the 4th edition of the textbook *Endocrinology*. She also serves on the Editorial Advisory Board of the *Drug INFO Line* Newsletter.

Morton P. Goldman, PharmD, BCPS

Dr Goldman received his bachelor's degree in pharmacy from the University of Pittsburgh, College of Pharmacy and his Doctor of Pharmacy degree from the University of Cincinnati, Division of Graduate Studies and Research. He completed his concurrent 2-year hospital pharmacy residency at the VA Medical Center in Cincinnati. Dr Goldman is presently the Assistant Director of Pharmacotherapy Services for the Department of Pharmacy at the Cleveland Clinic Foundation (CCF) after having spent over 4 years at CCF as an Infectious Disease pharmacist and 4 years as Clinical Manager. He holds faculty appointments from Case Western Reserve University, College of Medicine and The University of Toledo, College of Pharmacy. Dr Goldman is a Board-Certified Pharmacotherapy Specialist (BCPS) with added qualifications in infectious diseases.

In his capacity as Assistant Director of Pharmacotherapy Services at CCF, Dr Goldman remains actively involved in patient care and clinical research with the Department of Infectious Disease, as well as the continuing education of the medical and pharmacy staff. He is an editor of CCF's *Guidelines for Antibiotic Use* and participates in their annual Antimicrobial Review retreat. He is a member of the Pharmacy and Therapeutics Committee and many of its subcommittees. Dr Goldman has authored numerous journal articles and lectures locally and nationally on infectious diseases topics and current drug therapies. He is currently a reviewer for the *Annals of Pharmacotherapy* and the *Journal of the American Medical Association*, an editorial board member of the *Journal of Infectious Disease Pharmacotherapy*, and coauthor of the *Infectious Diseases Handbook* and the *Drug Information Handbook for the Allied Health Professional* produced by Lexi-Comp, Inc. He also provides technical support to Lexi-Comp's Clinical Reference Library™ publications.

Dr Goldman is an active member of the Ohio College of Clinical Pharmacy, the Society of Infectious Disease Pharmacists, the American College of Clinical Pharmacy, and the American Society of Health-Systems Pharmacists.

Leonard L. Lance, RPh, BSPharm

Leonard L. (Bud) Lance has been directly involved in the pharmaceutical industry since receiving his bachelor's degree in pharmacy from Ohio Northern University in 1970. Upon graduation from ONU, Mr Lance spent four years as a navy pharmacist in various military assignments and was instrumental in the development and operation of the first whole hospital I.V. admixture program in a military (Portsmouth Naval Hospital) facility.

After completing his military service, he entered the retail pharmacy field and has managed both an independent and a home I.V. franchise pharmacy operation. Since the late 1970s, Mr Lance has focused much of his interest on using computers to improve pharmacy service. The independent pharmacy he worked for was the first retail pharmacy in the State of Ohio to computerize (1977).

His love for computers and pharmacy lead him to Lexi-Comp, Inc. in 1988. He developed Lexi-Comp's first drug database in 1989 and was involved in the editing and publishing of Lexi-Comp's first *Drug Information Handbook* in 1990.

As a result of his strong publishing interest, he presently serves in the capacity of pharmacy editor and technical advisor as well as pharmacy (information) database coordinator for Lexi-Comp. Along with authoring the *Drug Information Handbook for the Allied Health Professional* and *Lippincott Williams & Wilkins Quick Look Drug Book*, he provides technical support to Lexi-Comp's reference publications. Mr Lance also assists approximately 200 major hospitals in producing their own formulary (pharmacy) publications through Lexi-Comp's custom publishing service.

Mr Lance is a member and past president (1984) of the Summit Pharmaceutical Association (SPA). He is also a member of the Ohio Pharmacists Association (OPA), the American Pharmaceutical Association (APhA), and the American Society of Health-System Pharmacists (ASHP).

EDITORIAL ADVISORY PANEL

Thom C. Dumsha, DDS
Associate Professor and Chair
Dental School
University of Maryland at Baltimore
Baltimore, Maryland

Matthew A. Fuller, PharmD, BCPS, BCPP, FASHP
Clinical Pharmacy Specialist, Psychiatry
Cleveland Department of Veterans Affairs Medical Center
Brecksville, Ohio
Associate Clinical Professor of Psychiatry
Clinical Instructor of Psychology
Case Western Reserve University
Cleveland, Ohio
Adjunct Associate Professor of Clinical Pharmacy
University of Toledo
Toledo, Ohio

Mark C. Geraci, PharmD, BCOP
Clinical Specialist
Department of Veterans Affairs
Hines VA Hospital
Hines, Illinois

Jeff Gonzales, PharmD
Critical Care Pharmacy Specialist
Cleveland Clinic Foundation
Cleveland, Ohio

Barbara L. Gracious, MD
Assistant Professor of Psychiatry and Pediatrics
Case Western Reserve University
Director of Child Psychiatry and Training & Education
University Hospitals of Cleveland
Cleveland, Ohio

Larry D. Gray, PhD
TriHealth Clinical Microbiology Laboratory
Bethesda Oak Hospital
Cincinnati, Ohio

James L. Gutmann, DDS
Professor and Director of Graduate Endodontics
The Texas A & M University System
Baylor College of Dentistry
Dallas, Texas

Martin D. Higbee, PharmD, CGP
Associate Professor
Department of Pharmacy Practice and Science
The University of Arizona
Tucson, Arizona

Jane Hurlburt Hodding, PharmD
Director, Pharmacy
Miller Children's Hospital
Long Beach, California

Rebecca T. Horvat, PhD
Assistant Professor of Pathology and Laboratory Medicine
University of Kansas Medical Center
Kansas City, Kansas

Collin A. Hovinga, PharmD
Neuropharmacology Specialist
Cleveland Clinic Foundation
Cleveland, Ohio

Darrell T. Hulisz, PharmD
Department of Family Medicine
Case Western Reserve University
Cleveland, Ohio

Carlos M. Isada, MD
Department of Infectious Disease
Cleveland Clinic Foundation
Cleveland, Ohio

Sana Isa-Pratt, MD
Attending Physician
Department of Medicine
Overlake Hospital
Bellevue, Washington

EDITORIAL ADVISORY PANEL *(Continued)*

Bradley G. Phillips, PharmD, BCPS
Associate Professor
University of Iowa College of Pharmacy
Clinical Pharmacist
Veterans Affairs Medical Center
Iowa City, Iowa

Laura-Lynn Pollack, BSPharm, NARTC
Pharmacist / Health Educator
Victoria, British Columbia

Luis F. Ramirez, MD
Adjunct Associate Professor of Psychiatry
Case Western Reserve University
Cleveland, Ohio

A.J. (Fred) Remillard, PharmD
Assistant Dean, Research and Graduate Affairs
College of Pharmacy and Nutrition
University of Saskatchewan
Saskatoon, Saskatchewan

Martha Sajatovic, MD
Associate Professor of Psychiatry
Case Western Reserve University
Cleveland, Ohio

Todd P. Semla, PharmD
Associate Director, Psychopharmacology Clinical and Research Center
Department of Psychiatry and Behavioral Sciences
Evanston Northwestern Healthcare Medical Group
Evanston, Illinois
Clinical Assistant Professor of Pharmacy Practice in Medicine,
Section of Geriatric Medicine
University of Illinois at Chicago
Chicago, Illinois

Stephen Shalansky, PharmD, FCSHP
Research Coordinator, Pharmacy Department
St Paul's Hospital
Vancouver, British Columbia

Dominic A. Solimando, Jr, MA
Oncology Pharmacist
President, Oncology Pharmacy Services, Inc
Arlington, VA

Virend K. Somers, MD, DPhil
Consultant in Hypertension and in Cardiovascular Disease
Mayo Clinic
Professor
Mayo Medical School
Rochester, MN

Carol K. Taketomo, PharmD
Pharmacy Manager
Children's Hospital of Los Angeles
Los Angeles, California

Beatrice B. Turkoski, RN, PhD
Associate Professor, Graduate Faculty, Advanced Pharmacology
College of Nursing
Kent State University
Kent, Ohio

Anne Marie Whelan, PharmD
College of Pharmacy
Dalhousie University
Halifax, Nova Scotia

Richard L. Wynn, PhD
Professor of Pharmacology
Baltimore College of Dental Surgery
Dental School
University of Maryland at Baltimore
Baltimore, Maryland

PREFACE

Every day, millions of Americans rely on medicines to live longer and healthier, more productive lives. We are fortunate to live in an age where medications are readily available to cure and treat a wide variety of conditions. With the great potential for continued pharmaceutical breakthroughs, new medications will continue to play an important role in improving the health of people the world over. Even as overall healthcare expenditures increase, drug therapies continue to represent a viable option for the treatment of disease.

For patients suffering from heart disease, stroke, cancer, Alzheimer's, AIDS, and many other illnesses, pharmaceutical companies brought more than 32 new treatment options to the market in the year 2001. With the growth of dollars spent by pharmaceutical manufacturers on research and development, the number of new molecular entities being approved and the ever increasing sophistication of these new pharmaceuticals, the practitioner is constantly being challenged to stay abreast of the knowledge base of new medicines. The enormous volume of available literature on pharmacotherapeutics continues to explode which poses a significant challenge for all practitioners in healthcare.

It remains the goal of the authors of the *Drug Information Handbook* to provide you, the user, with the critical information available regarding these new agents in a comprehensive, yet concise compendium, that is easy-to-use and practical to carry. With this explosion of information, it becomes ever more important for a handbook to provide the depth desired and yet be able to stay within the required size constraints of portability. To maintain a balance between depth and practicality, with this 10th edition, we have attempted to transition many fields of drug information into smaller and more compact formats, while retaining the quality and quantity of the information presented. We do hope you find this format useful to your practice and, as always, it is our goal to provide you with a comprehensive collection of drug information that will offer you assistance in your therapeutic decision-making.

— Charles F. Lacy, PharmD, FCSHP

ACKNOWLEDGMENTS

The *Drug Information Handbook* exists in its present form as the result of the concerted efforts of the following individuals: Robert D. Kerscher, publisher and president of Lexi-Comp, Inc; Lynn D. Coppinger, managing editor; Barbara F. Kerscher, production manager; David C. Marcus, director of information systems; Stacy S. Robinson, project manager; Kristin M. Thompson, product manager; Tracey J. Reinecke, graphic designer; and Julian I. Graubart, American Pharmaceutical Association (APhA), Director of Books and Electronic Products.

Special acknowledgment goes to all Lexi-Comp staff for their contributions to this handbook.

Much of the material contained in this book was a result of pharmacy contributors throughout the United States and Canada. Lexi-Comp has assisted many medical institutions to develop hospital-specific formulary manuals that contain clinical drug information as well as dosing. Working with these clinical pharmacists, hospital pharmacy and therapeutics committees, and hospital drug information centers, Lexi-Comp has developed an evolutionary drug database that reflects the practice of pharmacy in these major institutions.

In addition, the authors wish to thank their families, friends, and colleagues who supported them in their efforts to complete this handbook.

In particular, Dr Lacy would like to thank Kevin Landa for his assistance in composition evaluation and Edna M. Chan, RPh, PharmD, a clinical pharmacist at Children's Hospital of Los Angeles for her contribution as an editorial advisor.

DESCRIPTION OF SECTIONS AND FIELDS USED IN THIS HANDBOOK

The *Drug Information Handbook, 10th Edition* is divided into four sections.

The first section is a compilation of introductory text pertinent to the use of this book.

The drug information section of the handbook, in which all drugs are listed alphabetically, details information pertinent to each drug. Extensive cross-referencing is provided by U.S. brand names, Canadian brand names, and synonyms. Many combination monographs have been added to this edition; however, they have been condensed with only brand names and forms available. For more information on these products, see the individual components.

The third section is an invaluable appendix which offers a compilation of tables, guidelines, nomograms, algorithms, and conversion information which can be helpful when considering patient care.

The last section of this handbook contains a Therapeutic Category & Key Word Index which lists all drugs in this handbook in their unique therapeutic class; also listed are controlled substances by their restriction class.

The **Alphabetical Listing of Drugs** is presented in a consistent format and provides the following fields of information:

Generic Name	U.S. adopted name
Pronunciation	Phonetic pronunciation guide
Related Information	Cross-reference to other pertinent drug information found elsewhere in this handbook
U.S. Brand Names	Trade names (manufacturer-specific) found in the United States
Canadian Brand Names	Trade names found in Canada
Synonyms	Other names or accepted abbreviations of the generic drug
Therapeutic Category	Unique systematic classification of medications
Use	Information pertaining to appropriate FDA-approved indications of the drug.
Unlabeled/ Investigational Use	Information pertaining to non-FDA approved and investigational indications of the drug.
Restrictions	The controlled substance classification from the Drug Enforcement Agency (DEA). U.S. schedules are I-V. Schedules vary by country and sometimes state (ie, Massachusetts uses I-VI)
Pregnancy Risk Factor	Five categories established by the FDA to indicate the potential of a systemically absorbed drug for causing birth defects. The pregnancy risk factor as stated by the manufacturer is listed as well as risk factors based on expert analysis (Briggs GG, Freeman RK, and Yaffe SJ, *Drugs in Pregnancy and Lactation*, 5th ed, Baltimore, MD: Williams & Wilkins, 1998.)
Pregnancy/Breast-Feeding Implications	Information pertinent to or associated with the use of the drug as it relates to clinical effects on the fetus, breast-feeding/ lactation, and clinical effects on the infant
Contraindications	Information pertaining to inappropriate use of the drug
Warnings/Precautions	Precautionary considerations, hazardous conditions related to use of the drug, and disease states or patient populations in which the drug should be cautiously used
Adverse Reactions	Side effects are grouped by percentage of incidence (if known) and/or body system; in the interest of saving space, <1% effects are grouped only by percentage
Overdosage/ Toxicology	Comments and/or considerations are offered when appropriate and include signs/symptoms of excess drug and suggested management of the patient

Drug Interactions

Cytochrome P450 Effect	If a drug has demonstrated involvement with cytochrome P450 enzymes, the initial line of this field will identify the drug as an inhibitor, inducer, or substrate of specific isoenzymes (ie, CYP1A2). A summary of this information can also be found in a tabular format within the appendix section of this handbook.
Increased Effect/ Toxicity	Drug combinations that result in an increased or toxic therapeutic effect between the drug listed in the monograph and other drugs or drug classes.
Decreased Effect	Drug combinations that result in a decreased therapeutic effect between the drug listed in the monograph and other drugs or drug classes.
Ethanol/Nutrition/Herb Interactions	Information regarding potential interactions with food, nutritionals, herbal products, vitamins, or ethanol.
Stability	Information regarding storage of product or steps for reconstitution. Provides the time and conditions for which a solution or mixture will maintain full potency. For example, some solutions may require refrigeration after reconstitution while stored at room temperature prior to preparation. Also includes compatibility information. **Note:** Professional judgment of the individual pharmacist in application of this information is imperative. While drug products may exhibit stability over longer durations of time, it may not be appropriate to utilize the drug product due to concerns in sterility.
Mechanism of Action	How the drug works in the body to elicit a response
Pharmacodynamics/ Kinetics	The magnitude of a drug's effect depends on the drug concentration at the site of action. The pharmacodynamics are expressed in terms of onset of action and duration of action. Pharmacokinetics are expressed in terms of absorption, distribution (including appearance in breast milk and crossing of the placenta), protein binding, metabolism, bioavailability, half-life, time to peak serum concentration, and elimination.
Usual Dosage	The amount of the drug to be typically given or taken during therapy for children and adults; also includes any dosing adjustment/comments for renal impairment or hepatic impairment and other suggested dosing adjustments (eg, hematological toxicity)
Dietary Considerations	Includes information on how the medication should be taken relative to meals or food.
Administration	Information regarding the recommended final concentrations, rates of administration for parenteral drugs, or other guidelines when giving the medication
Monitoring Parameters	Laboratory tests and patient physical parameters that should be monitored for safety and efficacy of drug therapy
Reference Range	Therapeutic and toxic serum concentrations listed including peak and trough levels
Test Interactions	Listing of assay interferences when relevant; (B) = Blood; (S) = Serum; (U) = Urine
Patient Information	Specific information pertinent for the patient
Nursing Implications	Includes additional instructions for the administration of the drug and monitoring tips from the nursing perspective
Additional Information	Information about sodium content and/or pertinent information about specific brands
Dosage Forms	Information with regard to form, strength, and availability of the drug
Extemporaneous Preparations	Directions for preparing liquid formulations from solid drug products. May include stability information and references.

FDA PREGNANCY CATEGORIES

Throughout this book there is a field labeled Pregnancy Risk Factor (PRF) and the letter A, B, C, D or X immediately following which signifies a category. The FDA has established these five categories to indicate the potential of a systemically absorbed drug for causing birth defects. The key differentiation among the categories rests upon the reliability of documentation and the risk:benefit ratio. Pregnancy Category X is particularly notable in that if any data exists that may implicate a drug as a teratogen and the risk:benefit ratio is clearly negative, the drug is contraindicated during pregnancy.

These categories are summarized as follows:

A   Controlled studies in pregnant women fail to demonstrate a risk to the fetus in the first trimester with no evidence of risk in later trimesters. The possibility of fetal harm appears remote.

B   Either animal-reproduction studies have not demonstrated a fetal risk but there are no controlled studies in pregnant women, or animal-reproduction studies have shown an adverse effect (other than a decrease in fertility) that was not confirmed in controlled studies in women in the first trimester and there is no evidence of a risk in later trimesters.

C   Either studies in animals have revealed adverse effects on the fetus (teratogenic or embryocidal effects or other) and there are no controlled studies in women, or studies in women and animals are not available. Drugs should be given only if the potential benefits justify the potential risk to the fetus.

D   There is positive evidence of human fetal risk, but the benefits from use in pregnant women may be acceptable despite the risk (eg, if the drug is needed in a life-threatening situation or for a serious disease for which safer drugs cannot be used or are ineffective).

X   Studies in animals or human beings have demonstrated fetal abnormalities or there is evidence of fetal risk based on human experience, or both, and the risk of the use of the drug in pregnant women clearly outweighs any possible benefit. The drug is contraindicated in women who are or may become pregnant.

DRUGS IN PREGNANCY

Analgesics
Acceptable: Acetaminophen, meperidine, methadone
Controversial: Codeine, propoxyphene
Unacceptable: Nonsteroidal anti-inflammatory agents, salicylates, phenazopyridine

Antimicrobials
Acceptable: Penicillins, 1st and 2nd generation cephalosporins, erythromycin (base and EES), clotrimazole, miconazole, nystatin, isoniazid*, lindane, acyclovir, metronidazole
Controversial: 3rd generation cephalosporins, aminoglycosides, nitrofurantoin†
Unacceptable: Erythromycin estolate, chloramphenicol, sulfa, tetracyclines

ENT
Acceptable: Diphenhydramine*, dextromethorphan
Controversial: Pseudoephedrine
Unacceptable: Brompheniramine, cyproheptadine, dimenhydrinate

GI
Acceptable: Trimethobenzamide, antacids*, simethicone, other H_2-blockers, psyllium, bisacodyl, docusate
Controversial: Metoclopramide, prochlorperazine

Neurologic
Controversial: Phenytoin, phenobarbital
Unacceptable: Carbamazepine, valproic acid, ergotamine

Pulmonary
Acceptable: Theophylline, metaproterenol, terbutaline, inhaled steroids
Unacceptable: Epinephrine, oral steroids

Psych
Acceptable: Hydroxyzine*, lithium*, haloperidol
Controversial: Benzodiazepines, tricyclics, phenothiazines

Other
Acceptable: Heparin, insulin
Unacceptable: Warfarin, sulfonylureas

*Do not use in first trimester
†Do not use in third trimester

SAFE WRITING

Health professionals and their support personnel frequently produce handwritten copies of information they see in print; therefore, such information is subjected to even greater possibilities for error or misinterpretation on the part of others. Thus, particular care must be given to how drug names and strengths are expressed when creating written healthcare documents.

The following are a few examples of safe writing rules suggested by the Institute for Safe Medication Practices, Inc.*

1. There should be a space between a number and its units as it is easier to read. There should be no periods after the abbreviations mg or mL.

Correct	Incorrect
10 mg	10mg
100 mg	100mg

2. Never place a decimal and a zero after a whole number (2 mg is correct and 2.0 mg is **incorrect**). If the decimal point is not seen because it falls on a line or because individuals are working from copies where the decimal point is not seen, this causes a tenfold overdose.

3. Just the opposite is true for numbers less than one. Always place a zero before a naked decimal (0.5 mL is correct, .5 mL is **incorrect**).

4. Never abbreviate the word unit. The handwritten U or u, looks like a 0 (zero), and may cause a tenfold overdose error to be made.

5. IU is not a safe abbreviation for international units. The handwritten IU looks like IV. Write out international units or use int. units.

6. Q.D. is not a safe abbreviation for once daily, as when the Q is followed by a sloppy dot, it looks like QID which means four times daily.

7. O.D. is not a safe abbreviation for once daily, as it is properly interpreted as meaning "right eye" and has caused liquid medications such as saturated solution of potassium iodide and Lugol's solution to be administered incorrectly. There is no safe abbreviation for once daily. It must be written out in full.

8. Do not use chemical names such as 6-mercaptopurine or 6-thioguanine, as sixfold overdoses have been given when these were not recognized as chemical names. The proper names of these drugs are mercaptopurine or thioguanine.

9. Do not abbreviate drug names (5FC, 6MP, 5-ASA, MTX, HCTZ, CPZ, PBZ, etc) as they are misinterpreted and cause error.

10. Do not use the apothecary system or symbols.

11. Do not abbreviate microgram as µg; instead use mcg as there is less likelihood of misinterpretation.

12. When writing an outpatient prescription, write a complete prescription. A complete prescription can prevent the prescriber, the pharmacist, and/or the patient from making a mistake and can eliminate the need for further clarification. The legible prescriptions should contain:

    a. patient's full name

    b. for pediatric or geriatric patients: their age (or weight where applicable)

    c. drug name, dosage form and strength; if a drug is new or rarely prescribed, print this information

    d. number or amount to be dispensed

    e. complete instructions for the patient, including the purpose of the medication

    f. when there are recognized contraindications for a prescribed drug, indicate to the pharmacist that you are aware of this fact (ie, when prescribing a potassium salt for a patient receiving an ACE inhibitor, write "K serum level being monitored")

*From "Safe Writing" by Davis NM, PharmD and Cohen MR, MS, Lecturers and Consultants for Safe Medication Practices, 1143 Wright Drive, Huntington Valley, PA 19006. Phone: (215) 947-7566.

FDA NAME DIFFERENTIATION PROJECT THE USE OF TALL-MAN LETTERS

Confusion between similar drug names is an important cause of medication errors. For years, The Institute For Safe Medication Practices (ISMP), has urged generic manufacturers to use a combination of large and small letters as well as bolding (ie, chlorpro**MAZINE** and chlorpro**PAMIDE**) to help distinguish drugs with look-alike names, especially when they share similar strengths. Recently the FDA's Division of Generic Drugs began to issue recommendation letters to manufacturers suggesting this novel way to label their products to help reduce this drug name confusion. Although this project has had marginal success, the method has successfully eliminated problems with products such as diphenhydr**AMINE** and dimenhy**DRINATE**. Hospitals should also follow suit by making similar changes in their own labels, preprinted order forms, computer screens and printouts, and drug storage location labels.

Lexi-Comp Medical Publishing will begin using these "Tall-Man" letters for the drugs suggested by the FDA.

The following is a list of product names and recommended FDA revisions.

Drug Product	Recommended Revision
acetazolamide	aceta**ZOLAMIDE**
acetohexamide	aceto**HEXAMIDE**
bupropion	bu**PROP**ion
buspirone	bus**PIR**one
chlorpromazine	chlorpro**MAZINE**
chlorpropamide	chlorpro**PAMIDE**
clomiphene	clomi**PHENE**
clomipramine	clomi**PRAMINE**
cycloserine	cyclo**SERINE**
cyclosporine	cyclo**SPORINE**
daunorubicin	**DAUNO**rubicin
dimenhydrinate	dimenhy**DRINATE**
diphenhydramine	diphenhydr**AMINE**
dobutamine	**DOBUT**amine
dopamine	**DOP**amine
doxorubicin	**DOXO**rubicin
glipizide	glipi**ZIDE**
glyburide	gly**BURIDE**
hydralazine	hydr**ALAZINE**
hydroxyzine	hydr**OXY**zine
medroxyprogesterone	medroxy**PROGESTER**one
methylprednisolone	methyl**PREDNIS**olone
methyltestosterone	methyl**TESTOSTER**one
nicardipine	ni**CAR**dipine
nifedipine	**NIFE**dipine
prednisolone	predniso**LONE**
prednisone	predni**SONE**
sulfadiazine	sulfa**DIAZINE**
sulfisoxazole	sulfi**SOXAZOLE**
tolazamide	**TOLAZ**amide
tolbutamide	**TOLBUT**amide
vinblastine	vin**BLAS**tine
vincristine	vin**CRIS**tine

Institute for Safe Medication Practices. "New Tall-Man Lettering Will Reduce Mix-Ups Due to Generic Drug Name Confusion," *ISMP Medication Safety Alert*, September 19, 2001. Available at: http://www.ismp.org.

Institute for Safe Medication Practices. "Prescription Mapping, Can Improve Efficiency While Minimizing Errors With Look-Alike Products," *ISMP Medication Safety Alert*, October 6, 1999. Available at: http://www.ismp.org.

U.S. Pharmacopeia, "USP Quality Review: Use Caution-Avoid Confusion," March 2001, No. 76. Available at: http://www.usp.org.

ALPHABETICAL LISTING OF DRUGS

- **A-200™ [OTC]** *see Pyrethrins and Piperonyl Butoxide on page 1160*
- **A200® Lice [OTC]** *see Permethrin on page 1065*
- **A and D™ Ointment [OTC]** *see Vitamin A and Vitamin D on page 1422*

Abacavir *(a BAK a veer)*
Related Information
Antiretroviral Agents Comparison *on page 1488*
Management of Healthcare Worker Exposures to HIV, HBV, HCV *on page 1555*
U.S. Brand Names Ziagen®
Canadian Brand Names Ziagen®
Therapeutic Category Antiretroviral Agent, Nucleoside Reverse Transcriptase Inhibitor (NRTI) [Quanosine Analog]
Use Treatment of HIV infections in combination with other antiretroviral agents
Pregnancy Risk Factor C
Pregnancy/Breast-Feeding Implications It is not known if abacavir crosses the human placenta. Cases of lactic acidosis/hepatic steatosis syndrome have been reported in pregnant women receiving nucleoside analogues. It is not known if pregnancy itself potentiates this known side effect; however, pregnant women may be at increased risk of lactic acidosis and liver damage. Hepatic enzymes and electrolytes should be monitored frequently during the 3rd trimester of pregnancy in women receiving nucleoside analogues. Health professionals are encouraged to contact the antiretroviral pregnancy registry to monitor outcomes of pregnant women exposed to antiretroviral medications (1-800-258-4263).
Contraindications Hypersensitivity to abacavir (or carbovir) or any component of the formulation; do not rechallenge patients who have experienced hypersensitivity to abacavir
Warnings/Precautions Should always be used as a component of a multidrug regimen. Fatal hypersensitivity reactions have occurred. **Patients exhibiting symptoms of fever, skin rash, fatigue, respiratory symptoms (eg, pharyngitis, dyspnea, cough) and GI symptoms (eg, abdominal pain, nausea, vomiting) should discontinue therapy immediately and call for medical attention. Abacavir should be permanently discontinued if hypersensitivity cannot be ruled out, even when other diagnoses are possible. Abacavir SHOULD NOT be restarted because more severe symptoms may occur within hours, including LIFE-THREATENING HYPOTENSION AND DEATH. Fatal hypersensitivity reactions have occurred following the reintroduction of abacavir in patients whose therapy was interrupted (interruption in drug supply, temporary discontinuation while treating other conditions). Reactions occurred within hours. In some cases, signs of hypersensitivity may have been previously present, but attributed to other medical conditions (acute onset respiratory diseases, gastroenteritis, reactions to other medications). If abacavir is restarted following an interruption in therapy, evaluate the patient for previously unsuspected symptoms of hypersensitivity. Do not restart if hypersensitivity is suspected or if hypersensitivity cannot be ruled out. To report these events on abacavir hypersensitivity, a registry has been established (1-800-270-0425).** Use with caution in patients with hepatic dysfunction; prior liver disease, prolonged use, and obesity may be risk factors for development of lactic acidosis and severe hepatomegaly with steatosis.
Adverse Reactions Note: Hypersensitivity reactions, which may be fatal, occur in ~5% of patients (see Warnings/Precautions). Symptoms may include anaphylaxis, fever, rash, fatigue, diarrhea, abdominal pain, respiratory symptoms (eg, pharyngitis, dyspnea, or cough), headache, malaise, lethargy, myalgia, myolysis, arthralgia, edema, paresthesia, nausea and vomiting, mouth ulcerations, conjunctivitis, lymphadenopathy, hepatic failure, and renal failure.

Rates of adverse reactions were defined during combination therapy with lamivudine. Adverse reaction rates attributable to abacavir alone are not available.

Adults:
  Central nervous system: Insomnia (7%)
  Endocrine & metabolic: Hyperglycemia, hypertriglyceridemia (25%)
  Gastrointestinal: Nausea (47%), vomiting (16%), diarrhea (12%), anorexia (11%), pancreatitis
  Neuromuscular & skeletal: Weakness
  Miscellaneous: Elevated transaminases
Children:
  Central nervous system: Fever (19%), headache (16%)
  Dermatologic: Rash (11%)
  Gastrointestinal: Nausea (38%), vomiting (38%), diarrhea (16%), anorexia (9%)
1% to 10%:
  Cardiovascular: Hypotension, cyanosis
  Central nervous system: Headache, dizziness
  Dermatologic: Rash, pruritus
  Gastrointestinal: Nausea, abdominal discomfort
  Genitourinary: Decreased urinary frequency
  Miscellaneous: Hypersensitivity reaction (4.4%)
  <1% (Limited to important or life-threatening): Anaphylactoid reaction, pulmonary hypertension

Drug Interactions
Increased Effect/Toxicity: Ethanol may increase the risk of toxicity. Abacavir increases the blood levels of amprenavir. Abacavir may decrease the serum concentration of methadone in some patients.
Stability Store at room temperature; do not freeze oral solution. Oral solution may be refrigerated.
Mechanism of Action Nucleoside reverse transcriptase inhibitor. Abacavir is a guanosine analogue which is phosphorylated to carbovir triphosphate which interferes with HIV viral RNA dependent DNA polymerase resulting in inhibition of viral replication.
Pharmacodynamics/Kinetics
Distribution: V_d: 0.86 L/kg

Protein binding: 27% to 33%

Metabolism: Hepatic via alcohol dehydrogenase and glucuronyl transferase to inactive carboxylate and glucuronide metabolites

Bioavailability: 83%

Half-life elimination: 1.5 hours

Time to peak: 0.7-1.7 hours

Excretion: Primarily urine (as metabolites, 1.2% as unchanged drug); feces (16% total dose)

Usual Dosage Oral:

Children: 3 months to 16 years: 8 mg/kg body weight twice daily (maximum 300 mg twice daily) in combination with other antiretroviral agents

Adults: 300 mg twice daily in combination with other antiretroviral agents

Administration May be administered with or without food.

Patient Information This is not a cure for HIV infection, nor will it reduce the risk of transmission to others. Long-term effects are not known. You will need frequent blood tests to adjust dosage for maximum therapeutic effect. Take as directed, for full course of therapy; do not discontinue (even if feeling better). You may experience headache or muscle pain or weakness. If you experience any of the following: Fever, skin rash, fatigue, nausea, vomiting, diarrhea, abdominal pain, contact your prescriber IMMEDIATELY. If you are instructed to stop the medication, DO NOT TAKE THIS MEDICATION IN THE FUTURE. Do not restart without specific instructions by your prescriber.

Additional Information A medication guide is available and should be dispensed with each prescription or refill for abacavir. A warning card is also available and patients should be instructed to carry this card with them.

Dosage Forms

Solution, oral, as sulfate: 20 mg/mL (240 mL) [strawberry-banana flavor]

Tablet, as sulfate: 300 mg

Abacavir, Lamivudine, and Zidovudine

(a BAK a veer, la MI vyoo deen, & zye DOE vyoo deen)

U.S. Brand Names Trizivir®

Synonyms Azidothymidine, Abacavir, and Lamivudine; AZT, Abacavir, and Lamivudine; Compound S, Abacavir, and Lamivudine; Lamivudine, Abacavir, and Zidovudine; 3TC, Abacavir, and Zidovudine; ZDV, Abacavir, and Lamivudine; Zidovudine, Abacavir, and Lamivudine

Therapeutic Category Antiretroviral Agent, Reverse Transcriptase Inhibitor (Combination)

Use Treatment of HIV infection (either alone or in combination with other antiretroviral agents) in patients whose regimen would otherwise contain the components of Trizivir® (based on analyses of surrogate markers in controlled studies with abacavir of up to 24 weeks; there have been no clinical trials conducted with Trizivir®)

Pregnancy Risk Factor C

Usual Dosage Adolescents and Adults: Oral: 1 tablet twice daily; **Note:** Not recommended for patients <40 kg

Dosage adjustment in renal impairment: Because lamivudine and zidovudine require dosage adjustment in renal impairment, Trizivir® should not be used in patients with Cl_{cr} ≤50 mL/minute

Elderly: Use with caution

Additional Information Complete prescribing information for this medication should be consulted for additional detail.

Dosage Forms Tablet: Abacavir 300 mg, lamivudine 150 mg, and zidovudine 300 mg

♦ **Abbokinase®** see Urokinase **Not Currently Manufactured** on page 1392

♦ **Abbreviations and Measurements** see page 1452

♦ **ABCD** see Amphotericin B Cholesteryl Sulfate Complex on page 87

Abciximab (ab SIK si mab)

Related Information

Glycoprotein Antagonists on page 1500

U.S. Brand Names ReoPro®

Canadian Brand Names Reopro™

Synonyms C7E3; 7E3

Therapeutic Category Antiplatelet Agent; Glycoprotein IIb/IIIa Inhibitor; Platelet Aggregation Inhibitor

Use Prevention of acute cardiac ischemic complications in patients at high risk for abrupt closure of the treated coronary vessel and patients at risk of restenosis; an adjunct with heparin to prevent cardiac ischemic complications in patients with unstable angina not responding to conventional therapy when a percutaneous coronary intervention is scheduled within 24 hours

Pregnancy Risk Factor C

Pregnancy/Breast-Feeding Implications Clinical effects on the fetus: It is not known whether abciximab can cause fetal harm when administered to a pregnant woman or can affect reproduction capacity

Contraindications Hypersensitivity to abciximab, to murine proteins, or any component of the formulation; active internal hemorrhage or recent (within 6 weeks) clinically significant GI or GU bleeding; history of cerebrovascular accident within 2 years or cerebrovascular accident with significant neurological deficit; clotting abnormalities or administration of oral anticoagulants within 7 days unless prothrombin time (PT) is ≤1.2 times control PT value; thrombocytopenia (<100,000 cells/μL); recent (within 6 weeks) major surgery or trauma; intracranial tumor, arteriovenous malformation, or aneurysm; severe uncontrolled hypertension; history of vasculitis; use of dextran before PTCA or intent to use dextran during PTCA; concomitant use of another parenteral GP IIb/IIIa inhibitor

Warnings/Precautions Administration of abciximab is associated with a significantly increased frequency of major bleeding complications including retroperitoneal bleeding, spontaneous GI or GU bleeding and bleeding at the arterial access site

(Continued)

Abciximab *(Continued)*

Clinical data indicate that the risk of major bleeding due to abciximab therapy may be elevated in the following settings:

Patients weighing <75 kilograms
Elderly patients (>65 years of age)
History of previous gastrointestinal disease
Recent thrombolytic therapy

Increased risk of hemorrhage during or following angioplasty is associated with the following factors; these risks may be additive to that associated with abciximab therapy:

Unsuccessful PTCA
PTCA procedure >70 minutes duration
PTCA performed within 12 hours of symptom onset for acute myocardial infarction

The safety and efficacy of readministering abciximab has not yet been established; administration of abciximab may result in human antichimeric antibody formation that can cause hypersensitivity reactions (including anaphylaxis), thrombocytopenia, or diminished efficacy. Anticoagulation, such as with heparin, may contribute to the risk of bleeding.

Adverse Reactions As with all drugs which may affect hemostasis, bleeding is associated with abciximab. Hemorrhage may occur at virtually any site. Risk is dependent on multiple variables, including the concurrent use of multiple agents which alter hemostasis and patient susceptibility.

>10%:
Cardiovascular: Hypotension (14.4%), chest pain (11.4%)
Gastrointestinal: Nausea (13.6%)
Hematologic: Minor bleeding (4.0% to 16.8%)
Neuromuscular & skeletal: Back pain (17.6%)

1% to 10%:
Cardiovascular: Bradycardia (4.5%), peripheral edema (1.6%)
Central nervous system: Headache (6.45)
Gastrointestinal: Vomiting (7.3%), abdominal pain (3.1%)
Hematologic: Major bleeding (1.1% to 14%), thrombocytopenia: <100,000 cells/mm^3 (2.5% to 5.6%); <50,000 cells/mm^3 (0.4% to 1.7%)
Local: Injection site pain (3.6%)

<1% (Limited to important or life-threatening): Abnormal thinking, allergic reactions/anaphylaxis (possible), AV block, bronchospasm, bullous eruption, coma, confusion, diabetes mellitus, embolism, hyperkalemia, ileus, inflammation, intracranial hemorrhage, myalgia, nodal arrhythmia, pleural effusion, pulmonary embolism, prostatitis, pruritus, stroke, urinary retention, ventricular tachycardia, xerostomia

Overdosage/Toxicology The antiplatelet effects can be quickly reversed with the administration of platelets.

Drug Interactions
Increased Effect/Toxicity: The risk of bleeding is increased when abciximab is given with heparin, other anticoagulants, thrombolytics, or antiplatelet drugs. However, aspirin and heparin were used concurrently in the majority of patients in the major clinical studies of abciximab. Allergic reactions may be increased in patients who have received diagnostic or therapeutic monoclonal antibodies due to the presence of HACA antibodies. Concomitant use of other glycoprotein IIb/IIIa antagonists is contraindicated.

Stability Vials should be stored at 2°C to 8°C, do not freeze; after admixture, the prepared solution is stable for 12 hours; abciximab should be administered in a separate intravenous line; no incompatibilities have been observed with glass bottles or PVC bags

Mechanism of Action Fab antibody fragment of the chimeric human-murine monoclonal antibody 7E3; this agent binds to platelet IIb/IIIa receptors, resulting in steric hindrance, thus inhibiting platelet aggregation

Pharmacodynamics/Kinetics Half-life elimination: ~30 minutes

Usual Dosage I.V.: 0.25 mg/kg bolus administered 10-60 minutes before the start of intervention followed by an infusion of 0.125 mcg/kg/minute (to a maximum of 10 mcg/minute) for 12 hours

Patients with unstable angina not responding to conventional medical therapy and who are planning to undergo percutaneous coronary intervention within 24 hours may be treated with abciximab 0.25 mg/kg intravenous bolus followed by an 18- to 24-hour intravenous infusion of 10 mcg/minute, concluding 1 hour after the percutaneous coronary intervention

Administration Abciximab is intended for coadministration with aspirin postangioplasty and heparin infused and weight adjusted to maintain a therapeutic bleeding time (eg, ACT 300-500 seconds)

Bolus dose: Aseptically withdraw the necessary amount of abciximab (2 mg/mL) for the bolus dose through a 0.22-micron filter into a syringe; the bolus should be administered 10-60 minutes before the procedure

Continuous infusion: Aseptically withdraw 4.5 mL (9 mg) of abciximab for the infusion through a 0.22 micron filter into a syringe; inject this into 250 mL of NS or D$_5$W to make a solution with a final concentration of 35 mcg/mL. Infuse at a rate of 17 mL/hour (10 mcg/minute) for 12 hours via pump; **filter all infusions.**

Monitoring Parameters Prothrombin time, activated partial thromboplastin time, hemoglobin, hematocrit, platelet count, fibrinogen, fibrin split products, transfusion requirements, signs of hypersensitivity reactions, guaiac stools, and Hemastix® urine

Nursing Implications Do not shake the vial; maintain bleeding precautions, avoid unnecessary arterial and venous punctures, use saline or heparin lock for blood drawing, assess sheath insertion site and distal pulses of affected leg every 15 minutes for the first hour and then every 1 hour for the next 6 hours. Arterial access site care is important to prevent bleeding. Care should be taken when attempting vascular access that only the anterior wall of the femoral artery is punctured, avoiding a Seldinger (through and through) technique for obtaining sheath access. Femoral vein sheath placement should be avoided unless needed. While the vascular sheath is in place, patients should be maintained on complete bed rest with the head of the bed at a 30° angle and the affected limb restrained in a straight position.

Observe patient for mental status changes, hemorrhage, assess nose and mouth mucous membranes, puncture sites for oozing, ecchymosis and hematoma formation, and examine urine, stool and emesis for presence of occult or frank blood; gentle care should be provided when removing dressings.

Additional Information
Patients at high risk of closure or restenosis:
Acute evolving myocardial infarction (MI) within 12 hours of onset of symptoms requiring rescue PTCA
Early postinfarction angina or unstable angina with at least 2 episodes of angina associated with EKG changes during previous 24 hours
Non-Q-wave myocardial infarction
Clinical or angiographic characteristic indicating high risk (see "Characteristics of Type A, B, and C Lesions" below)
Unfavorable anatomy (ie, 2 or more Type B lesions) **or**
One or more Type B lesions with diabetes **or**
One or more Type B lesions and a female and over the age of 65 **or**
One Type C lesion
Thrombus score is based upon angiographic evidence

Characteristics of Type A, B, and C Lesions
Type A lesions (minimally complex)
Discrete (length <10 mm)
Concentric
Readily accessible
Nonangulated segment (<45°)
Smooth contour
Little or no calcification
Less than totally occlusive
Not ostial in location
No major side branch involvement
No thrombus
Type B lesions (moderately complex)
Tubular (length 10-20 mm)
Eccentric
Moderate tortuosity of proximal segment
Moderate angulated segment (>45°, <90°)
Irregular contour
Moderate or heavy calcification
Total occlusions <3 months old
Ostial in location
Bifurcation lesions requiring double lead wires
Some thrombus present
Type C lesions (severely complex)
Diffuse (length >20 mm)
Excessive tortuosity of proximal segment
Extremely angulated segments >90°
Total occlusions >3 months old and/or bridging collaterals
Inability to protect major side branches
Degenerated vein grafts with friable lesions

Dosage Forms Injection, solution: 2 mg/mL (5 mL)

♦ **ABC Pack™ (Avelox®)** *see* Moxifloxacin *on page 938*
♦ **Abelcet®** *see* Amphotericin B (Lipid Complex) *on page 90*
♦ **Abenol® (Can)** *see* Acetaminophen *on page 22*
♦ **ABLC** *see* Amphotericin B (Lipid Complex) *on page 90*
♦ **Abreva™ [OTC]** *see* Docosanol *on page 430*
♦ **Absorbine® Antifungal [OTC]** *see* Tolnaftate *on page 1347*
♦ **Absorbine® Jock Itch [OTC]** *see* Tolnaftate *on page 1347*
♦ **Absorbine Jr.® Antifungal [OTC]** *see* Tolnaftate *on page 1347*

Acarbose (AY car bose)
Related Information
Diabetes Mellitus Treatment *on page 1657*
Hypoglycemic Drugs & Thiazolidinedione Information *on page 1502*
U.S. Brand Names Precose®
Canadian Brand Names Prandase®
Therapeutic Category Alpha-Glucosidase Inhibitor; Antidiabetic Agent, Alpha-glucosidase Inhibitor; Hypoglycemic Agent, Oral
Use
Monotherapy, as indicated as an adjunct to diet to lower blood glucose in patients with type 2 diabetes mellitus (noninsulin dependent, NIDDM) whose hyperglycemia cannot be managed on diet alone
Combination with a sulfonylurea, metformin, or insulin in patients with type 2 diabetes mellitus (noninsulin dependent, NIDDM) when diet plus acarbose do not result in adequate glycemic control. The effect of acarbose to enhance glycemic control is additive to that of other hypoglycemic agents when used in combination.
Pregnancy Risk Factor B
Pregnancy/Breast-Feeding Implications Abnormal blood glucose levels are associated with a higher incidence of congenital abnormalities. Insulin is the drug of choice for the control of diabetes mellitus during pregnancy.
Breast-feeding/lactation: It is not known whether acarbose is excreted in human milk
Contraindications Hypersensitivity to acarbose or any component of the formulation; patients with diabetic ketoacidosis or cirrhosis; patients with inflammatory bowel disease, colonic ulceration, partial intestinal obstruction, or in patients predisposed to intestinal obstruction; patients who have chronic intestinal diseases associated with marked disorders of digestion (Continued)

Acarbose (Continued)

or absorption, and in patients who have conditions that may deteriorate as a result of increased gas formation in the intestine

Warnings/Precautions Hypoglycemia: Acarbose may increase the hypoglycemic potential of sulfonylureas. Oral glucose (dextrose) should be used in the treatment of mild to moderate hypoglycemia. Severe hypoglycemia may require the use of either intravenous glucose infusion or glucagon injection.

Elevated serum transaminase levels: Treatment-emergent elevations of serum transaminases (AST and/or ALT) occurred in 15% of acarbose-treated patients in long-term studies. These serum transaminase elevations appear to be dose related. At doses >100 mg 3 times/day, the incidence of serum transaminase elevations greater than 3 times the upper limit of normal was 2-3 times higher in the acarbose group than in the placebo group. These elevations were asymptomatic, reversible, more common in females, and, in general, were not associated with other evidence of liver dysfunction.

When diabetic patients are exposed to stress such as fever, trauma, infection, or surgery, a temporary loss of control of blood glucose may occur. At such times, temporary insulin therapy may be necessary.

Adverse Reactions
>10%:
Gastrointestinal: Abdominal pain (21%) and diarrhea (33%) tend to return to pretreatment levels over time, and the frequency and intensity of flatulence (77%) tend to abate with time
Hepatic: Elevated liver transaminases
<1% (Limited to important or life-threatening): Severe gastrointestinal distress

Overdosage/Toxicology An overdose will not result in hypoglycemia. An overdose may result in transient increases in flatulence, diarrhea, and abdominal discomfort which shortly subside.

Drug Interactions
Increased Effect/Toxicity: Acarbose may increase the risk of hypoglycemia when used with oral hypoglycemics. See Warnings/Precautions.
Decreased Effect: The effect of acarbose is antagonized/decreased by thiazide and related diuretics, corticosteroids, phenothiazines, thyroid products, estrogens, oral contraceptives, phenytoin, nicotinic acid, sympathomimetics, calcium channel-blocking drugs, isoniazid, intestinal adsorbents (eg, charcoal), and digestive enzyme preparations (eg, amylase, pancreatin).

Ethanol/Nutrition/Herb Interactions Ethanol: Limit ethanol.

Stability Store at <25°C (77°F) and protect from moisture

Mechanism of Action Competitive inhibitor of pancreatic α-amylase and intestinal brush border α-glucosidases, resulting in delayed hydrolysis of ingested complex carbohydrates and disaccharides and absorption of glucose; dose-dependent reduction in postprandial serum insulin and glucose peaks; inhibits the metabolism of sucrose to glucose and fructose

Pharmacodynamics/Kinetics
Absorption: <2% as active drug
Metabolism: Exclusively in GI tract, principally by intestinal bacteria and digestive enzymes; 13 metabolites identified
Bioavailability: Low systemic bioavailability of parent compound; acts locally in GI tract
Excretion: Urine (~34%)

Usual Dosage Oral:
Adults: Dosage must be individualized on the basis of effectiveness and tolerance while not exceeding the maximum recommended dose
Initial dose: 25 mg 3 times/day with the first bite of each main meal
Maintenance dose: Should be adjusted at 4- to 8-week intervals based on 1-hour post-prandial glucose levels and tolerance. Dosage may be increased from 25 mg 3 times/day to 50 mg 3 times/day. Some patients may benefit from increasing the dose to 100 mg 3 times/day.
Maintenance dose ranges: 50-100 mg 3 times/day.
Maximum dose:
≤60 kg: 50 mg 3 times/day
>60 kg: 100 mg 3 times/day
Patients receiving sulfonylureas: Acarbose given in combination with a sulfonylurea will cause a further lowering of blood glucose and may increase the hypoglycemic potential of the sulfonylurea. If hypoglycemia occurs, appropriate adjustments in the dosage of these agents should be made.
Dosing adjustment in renal impairment: Cl_{cr} <25 mL/minute: Peak plasma concentrations were 5 times higher and AUCs were 6 times larger than in volunteers with normal renal function; however, long-term clinical trials in diabetic patients with significant renal dysfunction have not been conducted and treatment of these patients with acarbose is not recommended.

Administration Should be administered with the first bite of each main meal.

Monitoring Parameters Postprandial glucose, glycosylated hemoglobin levels, serum transaminase levels should be checked every 3 months during the first year of treatment and periodically thereafter

Patient Information Take acarbose 3 times/day at the start (with the first bite) of each main meal. It is important to continue to adhere to dietary instructions, a regular exercise program, and regular testing of urine and/or blood glucose.

The risk of hypoglycemia, its symptoms and treatment, and conditions that predispose to its development should be well understood by patients and responsible family members. A source of glucose (dextrose) should be readily available to treat symptoms of low blood glucose when taking acarbose in combination with a sulfonylurea or insulin. If side effects occur, they usually develop during the first few weeks of therapy and are most often mild to moderate gastrointestinal effects, such as flatulence, diarrhea, or abdominal discomfort and generally diminish in frequency and intensity with time.

Nursing Implications Administer acarbose 3 times/day at the start (with the first bite) of each main meal. It is important to continue to adhere to dietary instructions, a regular exercise program, and regular testing of urine and/or blood glucose. The risk of hypoglycemia, its symptoms and treatment, and conditions that predispose to its development should be well understood by patients and responsible family members. A source of glucose (dextrose) should be readily available to treat symptoms of low blood glucose when taking acarbose in combination with a sulfonylurea or insulin. If side effects occur, they usually develop during the first few weeks of therapy and are mild to moderate gastrointestinal effects, such as flatulence, diarrhea, or abdominal discomfort and generally diminish in frequency and intensity with time.

Dosage Forms Tablet: 25 mg, 50 mg, 100 mg

♦ **A-Caro-25**® *see Beta-Carotene on page 161*
♦ **Accolate**® *see Zafirlukast on page 1430*
♦ **AccuNeb**™ *see Albuterol on page 41*
♦ **Accupril**® *see Quinapril on page 1166*
♦ **Accuretic**™ *see Quinapril and Hydrochlorothiazide on page 1168*
♦ **Accutane**® *see Isotretinoin on page 753*
♦ **ACE** *see Captopril on page 218*

Acebutolol (a se BYOO toe lole)
Related Information
Beta-Blockers Comparison *on page 1491*

U.S. Brand Names Sectral®
Canadian Brand Names Apo-Acebutolol; Gen-Acebutolol; Monitan®; Novo-Acebutolol; Nu-Acebutolol; Rhotral; Sectral®
Synonyms Acebutolol Hydrochloride
Therapeutic Category Antihypertensive Agent; Beta-Adrenergic Blocker
Use Treatment of hypertension, ventricular arrhythmias, angina
Pregnancy Risk Factor B (manufacturer); D (2nd and 3rd trimesters - expert analysis)
Contraindications Hypersensitivity to beta-blocking agents; uncompensated congestive heart failure; cardiogenic shock; bradycardia or second- and third-degree heart block (except in patients with a functioning artificial pacemaker); sinus node dysfunction; pregnancy (2nd and 3rd trimesters)
Warnings/Precautions Abrupt withdrawal of drug **should be avoided.** May result in an exaggerated cardiac responsiveness such as tachycardia, hypertension, ischemia, angina, myocardial infarction, and sudden death. It is recommended that patients be gradually tapered off beta-blockers (over a 2-week period) rather than via abrupt discontinuation. Although acebutolol primarily blocks beta₁-receptors, high doses can result in beta₂-receptor blockage. Use with caution in diabetic patients. Beta-blockers may impair glucose tolerance, potentiate hypoglycemia, and/or mask symptoms of hypoglycemia in a diabetic patient. Use with caution in bronchospastic lung disease and renal dysfunction (especially the elderly). Beta-blockers with intrinsic sympathomimetic activity do not appear to be of benefit in congestive heart failure and should be avoided. See Usual Dosage - Renal/Hepatic Impairment.

Adverse Reactions
>10%: Central nervous system: Fatigue (11%)
1% to 10%:
 Cardiovascular: Chest pain (2%), edema (2%), bradycardia, hypotension, congestive heart failure
 Central nervous system: Headache (6%), dizziness (6%), insomnia (3%), depression (2%), abnormal dreams (2%), anxiety, hyperesthesia, hypoesthesia, impotence
 Dermatologic: Rash (2%), pruritus
 Gastrointestinal: Constipation (4%), diarrhea (4%), dyspepsia (4%), nausea (4%), flatulence (3%), vomiting, abdominal pain
 Genitourinary: Micturition frequency (3%), dysuria, nocturia, impotence (2%)
 Neuromuscular & skeletal: Arthralgia (2%), myalgia (2%), back pain, joint pain
 Ocular: Abnormal vision (2%), conjunctivitis, dry eyes, eye pain
 Respiratory: Dyspnea (4%), rhinitis (2%), cough (1%), pharyngitis, wheezing
<1% (Limited to important or life-threatening): AV block, exacerbation of pre-existing renal insufficiency, hepatotoxic reaction, impotence, lichen planus, pleurisy, pneumonitis, pulmonary granulomas, systemic lupus erythematosus, urinary retention, ventricular arrhythmias

Potential adverse effects (based on experience with other beta-blocking agents) include reversible mental depression, disorientation, catatonia, short-term memory loss, emotional lability, slightly clouded sensorium, laryngospasm, respiratory distress, allergic reactions, erythematous rash, agranulocytosis, purpura, thrombocytopenia, mesenteric artery thrombosis, ischemic colitis, alopecia, Peyronie's disease, claudication

Overdosage/Toxicology Symptoms include cardiac disturbances, CNS toxicity, bronchospasm, hypoglycemia, and hyperkalemia. The most common cardiac symptoms include hypotension and bradycardia. Atrioventricular block, intraventricular conduction disturbances, cardiogenic shock, and asystole may occur with severe overdose, especially with membrane-depressant drugs (eg, propranolol). CNS effects include convulsions, coma, and respiratory arrest is commonly seen with propranolol and other membrane-depressant and lipid-soluble drugs. Treatment is symptomatic for seizures, hypotension, hyperkalemia and hypoglycemia. Bradycardia and hypotension resistant to atropine, isoproterenol or pacing, may respond to glucagon. Wide QRS defects caused by membrane-depressant poisoning may respond to hypertonic sodium bicarbonate. Repeat-dose charcoal, hemoperfusion, or hemodialysis may be helpful.

Drug Interactions
 Increased Effect/Toxicity: Acebutolol may increase the effects of other drugs which slow AV conduction (digoxin, verapamil, diltiazem), alpha-blockers (prazosin, terazosin), and
(Continued)

Acebutolol *(Continued)*

alpha-adrenergic stimulants (epinephrine, phenylephrine). Acebutolol may mask the tachycardia from hypoglycemia caused by insulin and oral hypoglycemics. In patients receiving concurrent therapy, the risk of hypertensive crisis is increased when either clonidine or the beta-blocker is withdrawn. Reserpine has been shown to enhance the effect of acebutolol. Beta-blockers may increase the action or levels of ethanol, disopyramide, nondepolarizing muscle relaxants, and theophylline although the effects are difficult to predict.

Decreased Effect: Decreased effect of acebutolol with aluminum salts, barbiturates, calcium salts, cholestyramine, colestipol, NSAIDs, penicillins (ampicillin), rifampin, and salicylates due to decreased bioavailability and plasma levels. The effect of sulfonylureas may be decreased by beta-blockers; however, the decreased effect has not been shown with tolbutamide.

Ethanol/Nutrition/Herb Interactions

Food: Peak serum acebutolol levels may be slightly decreased if taken with food.

Herb/Nutraceutical: Avoid dong quai if using for hypertension (has estrogenic activity). avoid yohimbe, ginseng (may worsen hypertension).

Stability Store at room temperature (~25°C/77°F); protect from light and dispense in a light-resistant, tight container

Mechanism of Action Competitively blocks beta$_1$-adrenergic receptors with little or no effect on beta$_2$-receptors except at high doses; exhibits membrane stabilizing and intrinsic sympathomimetic activity

Pharmacodynamics/Kinetics

Onset of action: 1-2 hours

Duration: 12-24 hours

Absorption: Oral: 40%

Protein binding: 5% to 15%

Metabolism: Extensive first-pass effect

Half-life elimination: 6-7 hours

Time to peak: 2-4 hours

Excretion: Feces (~55%); urine (35%)

Usual Dosage Oral:

Adults:

Hypertension: 400-800 mg/day (larger doses may be divided); maximum: 1200 mg/day

Ventricular arrhythmias: Initial: 400 mg/day; maintenance: 600-1200 mg/day in divided doses

Elderly: Initial: 200-400 mg/day; dose reduction due to age related decrease in Cl_{cr} will be necessary; do not exceed 800 mg/day

Dosing adjustment in renal impairment:

Cl_{cr} 25-49 mL/minute/1.73 m^2: Reduce dose by 50%.

Cl_{cr} <25 mL/minute/1.73 m^2: Reduce dose by 75%.

Dosing adjustment in hepatic impairment: Use with caution.

Dietary Considerations May be taken without regard to meals.

Administration To discontinue therapy, taper dose gradually

Monitoring Parameters Blood pressure, orthostatic hypotension, heart rate, CNS effects, EKG

Test Interactions ↑ triglycerides, potassium, uric acid, cholesterol (S), glucose; ↓ HDL, ↑ thyroxine (S)

Patient Information Do not discontinue abruptly; consult pharmacist or physician before taking with other adrenergic drugs (eg, cold medications); notify physician if CHF symptoms become worse or if other side effects occur; take at the same time each day; use with caution while driving or performing tasks requiring alertness; may mask signs of hypoglycemia in diabetics; may be taken without regard to meals

Nursing Implications Advise against abrupt withdrawal; monitor blood pressure, orthostatic hypotension, heart rate, CNS effects, EKG, and CVP

Dosage Forms Capsule, as hydrochloride: 200 mg, 400 mg

♦ **Acebutolol Hydrochloride** *see* Acebutolol *on page 21*

♦ **Aceon**® *see* Perindopril Erbumine *on page 1063*

♦ **Acephen**® **[OTC]** *see* Acetaminophen *on page 22*

Acetaminophen *(a seet a MIN oh fen)*

Related Information

Acetaminophen Toxicity Nomogram *on page 1695*

U.S. Brand Names Acephen® [OTC]; Aspirin Free Anacin® Maximum Strength [OTC]; Cetafen® [OTC]; Cetafen Extra® [OTC]; Feverall® [OTC]; Genapap® [OTC]; Genapap® Children [OTC]; Genapap® Extra Strength [OTC]; Genapap® Infant [OTC]; Genebs® [OTC]; Genebs® Extra Strength [OTC]; Infantaire [OTC]; Liquiprin® for Children [OTC]; Mapap® [OTC]; Mapap® Children's [OTC]; Mapap® Extra Strength [OTC]; Mapap® Infants [OTC]; Redutemp® [OTC]; Silapap® Children's [OTC]; Silapap® Infants [OTC]; Tylenol® [OTC]; Tylenol® Arthritis Pain [OTC]; Tylenol® Children's [OTC]; Tylenol® Extra Strength [OTC]; Tylenol® Infants [OTC]; Tylenol® Junior Strength [OTC]; Tylenol® Sore Throat [OTC]; Valorin [OTC]; Valorin Extra [OTC]

Canadian Brand Names Abenol®; Apo®-Acetaminophen; Atasol®; Pediatrix; Tempra®; Tylenol®

Synonyms APAP; N-Acetyl-P-Aminophenol; Paracetamol

Therapeutic Category Analgesic, Miscellaneous; Antipyretic

Use Treatment of mild to moderate pain and fever; does not have antirheumatic effects (analgesic)

Pregnancy Risk Factor B

Contraindications Hypersensitivity to acetaminophen or any component of the formulation; patients with known G6PD deficiency

Warnings/Precautions May cause severe hepatic toxicity on overdose; use with caution in patients with alcoholic liver disease; chronic daily dosing in adults of 5-8 g of acetaminophen over several weeks or 3-4 g/day of acetaminophen for 1 year have resulted in liver damage

Adverse Reactions <1% (Limited to important or life-threatening): Analgesic nephropathy, anemia, blood dyscrasias (agranulocytosis, thrombocytopenia, neutropenia, pancytopenia, leukopenia), hepatitis, nephrotoxicity with chronic overdose, sterile pyuria

Overdosage/Toxicology Refer to the "Acetaminophen Toxicity Nomogram" *on page 1695* in the Appendix. Symptoms include hepatic necrosis, transient azotemia, renal tubular necrosis with acute toxicity, anemia, and GI disturbances with chronic toxicity. Acetylcysteine 140 mg/kg orally (loading) followed by 70 mg/kg every 4 hours for 17 doses. Therapy should be initiated based upon laboratory analysis suggesting high probability of hepatotoxic potential. Activated charcoal is very effective at binding acetaminophen.

Drug Interactions

Cytochrome P450 Effect: CYP1A2 enzyme substrate (minor), CYP2E1 and 3A3/4 enzyme substrate

Increased Effect/Toxicity: Barbiturates, carbamazepine, hydantoins, isoniazid, rifampin, sulfinpyrazone may increase the hepatotoxic potential of acetaminophen; chronic ethanol abuse increases risk for acetaminophen toxicity; effect of warfarin may be enhanced

Decreased Effect: Barbiturates, carbamazepine, hydantoins, rifampin, sulfinpyrazone may decrease the analgesic effect of acetaminophen; cholestyramine may decrease acetaminophen absorption (separate dosing by at least 1 hour)

Ethanol/Nutrition/Herb Interactions

Ethanol: Excessive intake of ethanol may increase the risk of acetaminophen-induced hepatotoxicity. Avoid ethanol or limit to <3 drinks/day.

Food: May slightly delay absorption of extended-release preparations; rate of absorption may be decreased when given with food high in carbohydrates.

Herb/Nutraceutical: St John's wort may decrease acetaminophen levels.

Mechanism of Action Inhibits the synthesis of prostaglandins in the central nervous system and peripherally blocks pain impulse generation; produces antipyresis from inhibition of hypothalamic heat-regulating center

Pharmacodynamics/Kinetics

Onset of action: <1 hour

Duration: 4-6 hours

Protein binding: 20% to 50%

Metabolism: At normal therapeutic dosages, metabolized hepatically to sulfate and glucuronide metabolites, while a small amount is metabolized by microsomal mixed function oxidases to a highly reactive intermediate (acetylimidoquinone) which is conjugated with glutathione and inactivated; at toxic doses (as little as 4 g daily) glutathione conjugation becomes insufficient to meet the metabolic demand causing an increase in acetylimidoquinone concentration, which is thought to cause hepatic cell necrosis

Half-life elimination:

Neonates: 2-5 hours

Adults: 1-3 hours

Time to peak, serum: Oral: 10-60 minutes; may be delayed in acute overdoses

Excretion: Urine

Usual Dosage Oral, rectal (if fever not controlled with acetaminophen alone, administer with full doses of aspirin on an every 4- to 6-hour schedule, if aspirin is not otherwise contraindicated):

Children <12 years: 10-15 mg/kg/dose every 4-6 hours as needed; do **not** exceed 5 doses (2.6 g) in 24 hours; alternatively, the following age-based doses may be used. See table.

Acetaminophen Dosing

Age	Dosage (mg)	Age	Dosage (mg)
0-3 mo	40	4-5 y	240
4-11 mo	80	6-8 y	320
1-2 y	120	9-10 y	400
2-3 y	160	11 y	480

Adults: 325-650 mg every 4-6 hours or 1000 mg 3-4 times/day; do **not** exceed 4 g/day

Dosing interval in renal impairment:

Cl_{cr} 10-50 mL/minute: Administer every 6 hours

Cl_{cr} <10 mL/minute: Administer every 8 hours (metabolites accumulate)

Hemodialysis: Moderately dialyzable (20% to 50%)

Dosing adjustment/comments in hepatic impairment: Use with caution. Limited, low-dose therapy usually well tolerated in hepatic disease/cirrhosis. However, cases of hepatotoxicity at daily acetaminophen dosages <4 g/day have been reported. Avoid chronic use in hepatic impairment.

Monitoring Parameters Relief of pain or fever

Reference Range

Therapeutic concentration (analgesic/antipyretic): 10-30 µg/mL

Toxic concentration (acute ingestion) with probable hepatotoxicity: >200 µg/mL at 4 hours or 50 µg/mL at 12 hours after ingestion

Nursing Implications

Suppositories: Do not freeze

Suspension, oral: Shake well before pouring a dose

Dosage Forms

Caplet (Genapap® Extra Strength, Genebs® Extra Strength, Tylenol® Extra Strength): 500 mg

Caplet, extended release (Tylenol® Arthritis Pain): 650 mg

Capsule (Mapap® Extra Strength): 500 mg

Elixir: 160 mg/5 mL (5 mL, 10 mL, 20 mL, 120 mL, 240 mL, 500 mL, 3780 mL)

Genapap® Children: 160 mg/5 mL (120 mL) [cherry and grape flavors]

(Continued)

Acetaminophen *(Continued)*

    Silapap® Children's: 160 mg/5 mL (120 mL, 240 mL, 480 mL)

    Gelcap (Genapap® Extra Strength, Tylenol® Extra Strength): 500 mg

    Geltab (Tylenol® Extra Strength): 500 mg

    Liquid, oral: 160 mg/5 mL (120 mL, 240 mL, 480 mL, 3870 mL); 500 mg/15 mL (240 mL)

      Redutemp®: 500 mg/15 mL (120 mL)

      Tylenol® Sore Throat: 500 mg/15 mL (240 mL) [cherry and honey-lemon flavors]

    Solution, oral drops: 100 mg/mL (15 mL, 30 mL) [droppers are marked at 0.4 mL (40 mg) and at 0.8 mL (80 mg)]

      Genapap® Infant: 80 mg/0.8 mL (15 mL)

      Infantaire®, Silapap® Infant's: 80 mg/0.8 mL (15 mL, 30 mL)

      Liquiprin® for Children: 80 mg/0.8 mL (30 mL)

    Suppository, rectal: 80 mg, 120 mg, 325 mg, 650 mg

      Acephen®: 120 mg, 325 mg, 650 mg

      Feverall®: 80 mg, 120 mg, 325 mg

      Mapap®: 120 mg, 650 mg

    Suspension, oral: 160 mg/5 mL (120 mL)

      Mapap® Children's: 160 mg/5 mL (120 mL) [cherry, grape, and bubblegum flavors]

      Tylenol® Children's: 160 mg/5 mL (120 mL, 240 mL) [cherry, grape, and bubblegum flavors]

    Suspension, oral drops: 100 mg/mL (15 mL, 30 mL) [droppers are marked at 0.4 mL (40 mg) and at 0.8 mL (80 mg)]

      Mapap® Infants 80 mg/0.8 mL (15 mL, 30 mL) [cherry flavor]

      Tylenol® Infants: 80 mg/0.8 mL (15 mL, 30 mL) [cherry and grape flavors]

    Syrup, oral: 160 mg/5 mL (120 mL)

    Tablet: 160 mg, 325 mg, 500 mg

      Aspirin Free Anacin® Maximum Strength, Cetafen® Extra Strength, Genapap® Extra Strength, Genebs® Extra Strength, Mapap® Extra Strength, Redutemp®, Tylenol® Extra Strength, Valorin Extra: 500 mg

      Cetafen®, Genapap®, Genebs®, Mapap®, Tylenol®, Valorin: 325 mg

      Mapap®: 160 mg

    Tablet, chewable: 80 mg, 160 mg

      Genapap® Children, Mapap® Children's: 80 mg [contains phenylalanine 3 mg/tablet; fruit and grape flavors]

      Tylenol® Children's: 80 mg [fruit and grape flavors contain phenylalanine 3 mg/tablet; bubblegum flavor contains phenylalanine 6 mg/tablet]

      Tylenol® Junior Strength: 160 mg [contains phenylalanine 6 mg/tablet; fruit and grape flavors]

♦ **Acetaminophen and Chlorpheniramine** *see* Chlorpheniramine and Acetaminophen *on page 279*

Acetaminophen and Codeine *(a seet a MIN oh fen & KOE deen)*

U.S. Brand Names Capital® and Codeine; Phenaphen® With Codeine; Tylenol® With Codeine

Canadian Brand Names Empracet®-30; Empracet®-60; Emtec-30; Lenoltec; Triatec-8; Triatec-8 Strong; Triatec-30; Tylenol® with Codeine

Synonyms Codeine and Acetaminophen

Therapeutic Category Analgesic, Narcotic

Use Relief of mild to moderate pain

Restrictions C-III; C-V

Pregnancy Risk Factor C

Usual Dosage Doses should be adjusted according to severity of pain and response of the patient. Adult doses ≥60 mg codeine fail to give commensurate relief of pain but merely prolong analgesia and are associated with an appreciably increased incidence of side effects.

  Oral:

    Children: Analgesic:

      Codeine: 0.5-1 mg codeine/kg/dose every 4-6 hours

      Acetaminophen: 10-15 mg/kg/dose every 4 hours up to a maximum of 2.6 g/24 hours for children <12 years; **alternatively, the following can be used:**

        3-6 years: 5 mL 3-4 times/day as needed of elixir

        7-12 years: 10 mL 3-4 times/day as needed of elixir

        >12 years: 15 mL every 4 hours as needed of elixir

    Adults:

      Antitussive: Based on codeine (15-30 mg/dose) every 4-6 hours (maximum: 360 mg/24 hours based on codeine component)

      Analgesic: Based on codeine (30-60 mg/dose) every 4-6 hours (maximum: 4000 mg/24 hours based on acetaminophen component)

Dosing adjustment in renal impairment: Refer to individual monographs for Acetaminophen and Codeine

Additional Information Complete prescribing information for this medication should be consulted for additional detail.

Dosage Forms

    Capsule [C-III]: #3 (Phenaphen® With Codeine): Acetaminophen 325 mg and codeine phosphate 30 mg

    Elixir, oral [C-V]: Acetaminophen 120 mg and codeine phosphate 12 mg per 5 mL (5 mL, 10 mL, 12.5 mL, 15 mL, 120 mL, 480 mL, 3840 mL) [contains alcohol 7%]

      Tylenol® with Codeine: Acetaminophen 120 mg and codeine phosphate 12 mg per 5 mL (480 mL) [contains alcohol 7%; cherry flavor]

    Suspension, oral [C-V] (Capital® and Codeine): Acetaminophen 120 mg and codeine phosphate 12 mg per 5 mL [alcohol free; fruit punch flavor]

    Tablet [C-III]:

      #2: Acetaminophen 300 mg and codeine phosphate 15 mg

      #3 (Tylenol® with Codeine): Acetaminophen 300 mg and codeine phosphate 30 mg [contains sodium metabisulfite]

#4 (Tylenol® with Codeine): Acetaminophen 300 mg and codeine phosphate 60 mg [contains sodium metabisulfite]

Acetaminophen and Diphenhydramine
(a seet a MIN oh fen & dye fen HYE dra meen)

U.S. Brand Names Anacin PM Aspirin Free [OTC]; Excedrin® P.M. [OTC]; Goody's PM® Powder; Legatrin PM® [OTC]; Tylenol® PM Extra Strength; Tylenol® Severe Allergy [OTC]

Synonyms Diphenhydramine and Acetaminophen

Therapeutic Category Analgesic, Miscellaneous

Use Aid in the relief of insomnia accompanied by minor pain

Usual Dosage Oral: Adults: 50 mg of diphenhydramine HCl (76 mg diphenhydramine citrate) at bedtime or as directed by physician; do not exceed recommended dosage; not for use in children <12 years of age

Additional Information Complete prescribing information for this medication should be consulted for additional detail.

Dosage Forms
Caplet:
Excedrin® P.M.: Acetaminophen 500 mg and diphenhydramine citrate 38 mg
Legatrin PM®: Acetaminophen 500 mg and diphenhydramine 50 mg
Tylenol® PM Extra Strength: Acetaminophen 500 mg and diphenhydramine 25 mg
Tylenol® Severe Allergy: Acetaminophen 500 mg and diphenhydramine 12.5 mg
Gelcap (Tylenol® PM Extra Strength): Acetaminophen 500 mg and diphenhydramine 25 mg
Geltab:
Excedrin® P.M.: Acetaminophen 500 mg and diphenhydramine citrate 38 mg
Tylenol® PM Extra Strength: Acetaminophen 500 mg and diphenhydramine hydrochloride 25 mg
Powder for oral solution (Goody's PM® Powder): Acetaminophen 500 mg and diphenhydramine citrate 38 mg
Tablet:
Anacin® PM Aspirin-Free, Tylenol® PM Extra Strength: Acetaminophen 500 mg and diphenhydramine hydrochloride 25 mg
Excedrin® P.M.: Acetaminophen 500 mg and diphenhydramine citrate 38 mg

- **Acetaminophen and Hydrocodone** see Hydrocodone and Acetaminophen on page 676
- **Acetaminophen and Oxycodone** see Oxycodone and Acetaminophen on page 1026

Acetaminophen and Phenyltoloxamine
(a seet a MIN oh fen & fen il to LOKS a meen)

U.S. Brand Names Genesec® [OTC]; Percogesic® [OTC]; Phenylgesic® [OTC]

Synonyms Phenyltoloxamine and Acetaminophen

Therapeutic Category Analgesic, Miscellaneous

Use Relief of mild to moderate pain

Pregnancy Risk Factor B

Usual Dosage Oral:
Analgesic: Based on acetaminophen component:
Children: 10-15 mg/kg/dose every 4-6 hours as needed; do **not** exceed 5 doses/24 hours
Adults: 325-650 every 4-6 hours as needed; do **not** exceed 4 g/day

Product labeling:
Percogesic®:
Children 6-12 years: 1 tablet every 4 hours; do **not** exceed 4 tablets/24 hours
Adults: 1-2 tablets every 4 hours; do **not** exceed 8 tablets/24 hours

Additional Information Complete prescribing information for this medication should be consulted for additional detail.

Dosage Forms Tablet: Acetaminophen 325 mg and phenyltoloxamine citrate 30 mg

Acetaminophen and Pseudoephedrine
(a seet a MIN oh fen & soo doe e FED rin)

U.S. Brand Names Children's Tylenol® Sinus [OTC]; Infants Tylenol® Cold [OTC]; Medi-Synal [OTC]; Names Alka-Seltzer Plus® Cold and Sinus [OTC]; Ornex® [OTC]; Ornex® Maximum Strength [OTC]; Sinus-Relief® [OTC]; Sinutab® Sinus Maximum Strength Without Drowsiness [OTC]; Sudafed® Cold and Sinus [OTC]; Sudafed® Sinus Headache [OTC]; Tylenol® Sinus Non-Drowsy [OTC]

Canadian Brand Names Dristan® N.D.; Dristan® N.D., Extra Strength; Sinutab® Non Drowsy; Sudafed® Head Cold and Sinus Extra Strength; Tylenol® Decongestant; Tylenol® Sinus

Synonyms Pseudoephedrine and Acetaminophen

Therapeutic Category Alpha/Beta Agonist; Analgesic, Miscellaneous

Use Relief of mild to moderate pain; relief of congestion

Usual Dosage Oral:
Analgesic: Based on acetaminophen component:
Children: 10-15 mg/kg/dose every 4-6 hours as needed; do **not** exceed 5 doses in 24 hours
Adults: 325-650 mg every 4-6 hours as needed; do **not** exceed 4 g/day
Decongestant: Based on pseudoephedrine component:
Children:
2-6 years: 15 mg every 4 hours; do **not** exceed 90 mg/day
6-12 years: 30 mg every 4 hours; do **not** exceed 180 mg/day
Children >12 years and Adults: 60 mg every 4 hours; do **not** exceed 360 mg/day

Product labeling:
Alka-Seltzer Plus® Cold and Sinus:
Children 6-12 years: 1 dose with water every 4 hours (maximum: 4 doses/24 hours)
Adults: 2 doses with water every 4 hours (maximum: 4 doses/24 hours)
(Continued)

Acetaminophen and Pseudoephedrine *(Continued)*

Children's Tylenol® Sinus: Children:
Liquid:
2-5 years (24-47 lbs): 1 teaspoonful every 4-6 hours (maximum: 4 doses/24 hours)
6-11 years (48-95 lbs): 2 teaspoonfuls every 4-6 hours (maximum: 4 doses/24 hours)
Tablet, chewable:
2-5 years (24-47 lbs): 2 tablets every 4-6 hours (maximum: 4 doses/24 hours)
6-11 years (48-95 lbs): 4 tablets every 4-6 hours (maximum: 4 doses/24 hours)
Sine-Aid® Maximum Strength, Tylenol® Sinus Maximum Strength: Children >12 years and
Adults: 2 doses every 4-6 hours (maximum: 8 doses/24 hours)
Sinutab® Sinus Maximum Strength Without Drowsiness, Tavist® Sinus: Children >12 years
and Adults: 2 doses every 6 hours; (maximum: 8 doses/24 hours)
Additional Information Complete prescribing information for this medication should be
consulted for additional detail.
Dosage Forms
Caplet:
Ornex®: Acetaminophen 325 mg and pseudoephedrine hydrochloride 30 mg
Ornex® Maximum Strength, Sinutab® Sinus Maximum Strength Without Drowsiness,
Sudafed® Sinus Headache, Tylenol® Sinus Non-Drowsy: Acetaminophen 500 mg and
pseudoephedrine hydrochloride 30 mg
Capsule, liquid (Alka-Seltzer Plus® Cold and Sinus, Sudafed® Cold and Sinus): Acetamino-
phen 325 mg and pseudoephedrine hydrochloride 30 mg
Gelcap (Tylenol® Sinus Non-Drowsy): Acetaminophen 500 mg and pseudoephedrine hydro-
chloride 30 mg
Geltab (Tylenol® Sinus Non-Drowsy): Acetaminophen 500 mg and pseudoephedrine hydrochloride 30 mg
Liquid, oral drops (Infants Tylenol® Cold): Acetaminophen 80 mg/0.8 mL and pseudoephedrine 7.5 mg/0.8 mL [bubblegum flavor]
Suspension (Children's Tylenol® Sinus): Acetaminophen 160 mg and pseudoephedrine
hydrochloride 15 mg/5 mL [fruit flavor]
Tablet (Sudafed® Sinus Headache): Acetaminophen 500 mg and pseudoephedrine hydrochloride 30 mg
Tablet, chewable (Children's Tylenol® Sinus): Acetaminophen 80 mg and pseudoephedrine
hydrochloride 7.5 mg [fruit flavor] [contains phenylalanine 5 mg/tablet]

Acetaminophen and Tramadol (a seet a MIN oh fen & TRA ma dole)
U.S. Brand Names Ultracet™
Synonyms APAP and Tramadol; Tramadol Hydrochloride and Acetaminophen
Therapeutic Category Analgesic, Miscellaneous
Use Short-term (≤5 days) management of acute pain
Pregnancy Risk Factor C
Usual Dosage Oral: Adults: Acute pain: Two tablets every 4-6 hours as needed for pain relief
(maximum: 8 tablets/day); treatment should not exceed 5 days
Dosage adjustment in renal impairment: Cl$_{cr}$ <30 mL/minute: Maximum of 2 tablets every
12 hours; treatment should not exceed 5 days
Dosage adjustment in hepatic impairment: Not recommended.
Additional Information Complete prescribing information for this medication should be
consulted for additional detail.
Dosage Forms Tablet: Acetaminophen 325 mg and tramadol hydrochloride 37.5 mg

Acetaminophen, Aspirin, and Caffeine
(a seet a MIN oh fen, AS pir in, & KAF een)
U.S. Brand Names Excedrin® Extra Strength [OTC]; Excedrin® Migraine [OTC]; Genaced
[OTC]; Goody's® Extra Strength Headache Powder [OTC]; Vanquish® Extra Strength Pain
Reliever [OTC]
Synonyms Aspirin, Acetaminophen, and Caffeine; Aspirin, Caffeine and Acetaminophen;
Caffeine, Acetaminophen, and Aspirin; Caffeine, Aspirin, and Acetaminophen
Therapeutic Category Analgesic, Miscellaneous
Use Relief of mild to moderate pain; mild to moderate pain associated with migraine headache
Pregnancy Risk Factor D
Usual Dosage Oral: Adults:
Analgesic:
Based on **acetaminophen** component:
Mild to moderate pain: 325-650 mg every 4-6 hours as needed; do **not** exceed 4 g/day
Mild to moderate pain associated with migraine headache: 500 mg/dose (in combination
with 500 mg aspirin and 130 mg caffeine) every 6 hours while symptoms persist; do
not use for longer than 48 hours
Based on **aspirin** component:
Mild to moderate pain: 325-650 mg every 4-6 hours as needed; do **not** exceed 4 g/day
Mild to moderate pain associated with migraine headache: 500 mg/dose (in combination
with 500 mg acetaminophen and 130 mg caffeine) every 6 hours; do not use for longer
than 48 hours

Product labeling:
Excedrin® Extra Strength, Excedrin® Migraine: Children >12 years and Adults: 2 doses every
6 hours (maximum: 8 doses/24 hours)
Note: When used for migraine, do not use for longer than 48 hours
Goody's® Extra Strength Headache Powder: Children >12 years and Adults: 1 powder,
placed on tongue or dissolved in water, every 4-6 hours (maximum: 4 powders/24 hours)
Goody's® Extra Strength Pain Relief Tablets: Children >12 years and Adults: 2 tablets every
4-6 hours (maximum: 8 tablets/24 hours)
Vanquish® Extra Strength Pain Reliever: Children >12 years and Adults: 2 tablets every 4
hours (maximum: 12 tablets/24 hours)

Additional Information Complete prescribing information for this medication should be consulted for additional detail.

Dosage Forms
Caplet:
Excedrin® Extra Strength: Acetaminophen 250 mg, aspirin 250 mg, and caffeine 65 mg
Vanquish® Extra Strength Pain Reliever: Acetaminophen 194 mg, aspirin 227 mg, and caffeine 33 mg
Geltab (Excedrin® Extra Strength): Acetaminophen 250 mg, aspirin 250 mg, and caffeine 65 mg
Powder (Goody's® Extra Strength Headache Powder): Acetaminophen 260 mg, aspirin 520 mg, and caffeine 32.5 mg
Tablet:
Excedrin® Extra Strength, Excedrin® Migraine, Genaced: Acetaminophen 250 mg, aspirin 250 mg, and caffeine 65 mg

♦ **Acetaminophen, Caffeine, Hydrocodone, Chlorpheniramine, and Phenylephrine** *see* Hydrocodone, Chlorpheniramine, Phenylephrine, Acetaminophen, and Caffeine *on page 682*

Acetaminophen, Chlorpheniramine, and Pseudoephedrine
(a seet a MIN oh fen, klor fen IR a meen, & soo doe e FED rin)
U.S. Brand Names Alka-Seltzer® Plus Cold Liqui-Gels® [OTC]; Children's Tylenol® Cold [OTC]; Comtrex® Allergy-Sinus [OTC]; Sinutab® Sinus Allergy Maximum Strength [OTC]; Thera-Flu® Flu and Cold; Tylenol® Allergy Sinus [OTC]
Canadian Brand Names Sinutab® Sinus & Allergy; Tylenol® Allergy Sinus; Tylenol® Cold
Synonyms Acetaminophen, Pseudoephedrine, and Chlorpheniramine; Chlorpheniramine, Acetaminophen, and Pseudoephedrine; Chlorpheniramine, Pseudoephedrine, and Acetaminophen; Pseudoephedrine, Acetaminophen, and Chlorpheniramine; Pseudoephedrine, Chlorpheniramine, and Acetaminophen
Therapeutic Category Analgesic, Miscellaneous; Antihistamine
Use Temporary relief of sinus symptoms
Pregnancy Risk Factor B
Usual Dosage Oral:
Analgesic: Based on **acetaminophen** component:
Children: 10-15 mg/kg/dose every 4-6 hours as needed; do **not** exceed 5 doses in 24 hours
Adults: 325-650 mg every 4-6 hours as needed; do **not** exceed 4 g/day
Antihistamine: Based on chlorpheniramine maleate component:
Children:
2-6 years: 1 mg every 4-6 hours (maximum: 6 mg/24 hours)
6-12 years: 2 mg every 4-6 hours (maximum: 12 mg/24 hours)
Children >12 years and Adults: 4 mg every 4-6 hours (maximum: 24 mg/24 hours)
Decongestant: Based on **pseudoephedrine** component:
Children:
2-6 years: 15 mg every 4 hours (maximum: 90 mg/24 hours)
6-12 years: 30 mg every 4 hours (maximum: 180 mg/24 hours)
Children >12 years and Adults: 60 mg every 4 hours (maximum: 360 mg/24 hours)

Product labeling:
Alka-Seltzer Plus® Cold Medicine Liqui-Gels®:
Children 6-12 years: 1 softgel every 4 hours with water (maximum: 4 doses/24 hours)
Children >12 years and Adults: 2 softgels every 4 hours with water (maximum: 4 doses/24 hours)
Sinutab® Sinus Allergy Maximum Strength: Children >12 years and Adults: 2 tablets/caplets every 6 hours (maximum: 8 doses/24 hours)
Thera-Flu® Maximum Strength Flu and Cold Medicine for Sore Throat: Children >12 years and Adults: 1 packet dissolved in hot water every 6 hours (maximum: 4 packets/24 hours)
Additional Information Complete prescribing information for this medication should be consulted for additional detail.
Dosage Forms
Caplet (Sinutab® Sinus Allergy Maximum Strength, Tylenol® Allergy Sinus): Acetaminophen 500 mg, chlorpheniramine maleate 2 mg, and pseudoephedrine hydrochloride 30 mg
Capsule, liquid (Alka-Seltzer® Plus Cold Liqui-Gels®): Acetaminophen 325 mg, chlorpheniramine maleate 2 mg, and pseudoephedrine hydrochloride 30 mg
Gelcap (Tylenol® Allergy Sinus): Acetaminophen 500 mg, chlorpheniramine maleate 2 mg, and pseudoephedrine hydrochloride 30 mg
Geltab (Tylenol® Allergy Sinus): Acetaminophen 500 mg, chlorpheniramine maleate 2 mg, and pseudoephedrine hydrochloride 30 mg
Liquid (Children's Tylenol® Cold): Acetaminophen 160 mg, chlorpheniramine maleate 1 mg, and pseudoephedrine hydrochloride 15 mg per 5 mL (120 mL) [grape flavor]
Powder for oral solution [packet] (Thera-Flu® Flu and Cold): Acetaminophen 650 mg, chlorpheniramine maleate 4 mg, and pseudoephedrine hydrochloride 60 mg [lemon flavor]
Tablet (Comtrex® Allergy-Sinus): Acetaminophen 500 mg, chlorpheniramine maleate 2 mg, and pseudoephedrine hydrochloride 30 mg
Tablet, chewable (Children's Tylenol® Cold): Acetaminophen 80 mg, chlorpheniramine maleate 0.5 mg, and pseudoephedrine hydrochloride 7.5 mg [contains phenylalanine 6 mg/tablet; grape flavor]

Acetaminophen, Dextromethorphan, and Pseudoephedrine
(a seet a MIN oh fen, deks troe meth OR fan, & soo doe e FED rin)
U.S. Brand Names Alka-Seltzer® Plus Flu Liqui-Gels® [OTC]; Comtrex® Non-Drowsy Cough and Cold [OTC]; Contac® Severe Cold and Flu/Non-Drowsy [OTC]; Infants' Tylenol® Cold Plus Cough Concentrated Drops [OTC]; Sudafed® Severe Cold [OTC]; Thera-Flu® Non-Drowsy Flu, Cold and Cough [OTC]; Triaminic® Sore Throat Formula [OTC]; Tylenol® Cold Non-Drowsy [OTC]; Tylenol® Flu Non-Drowsy Maximum Strength [OTC]; Vicks® DayQuil® Cold and Flu Non-Drowsy [OTC]
(Continued)

Acetaminophen, Dextromethorphan, and Pseudoephedrine
(Continued)

Canadian Brand Names Contac® Cough, Cold and Flu Day & Night™; Sudafed® Cold & Cough Extra Strength; Tylenol® Cold

Synonyms Dextromethorphan, Acetaminophen, and Pseudoephedrine; Pseudoephedrine, Acetaminophen, and Dextromethorphan; Pseudoephedrine, Dextromethorphan, and Acetaminophen

Therapeutic Category Antihistamine; Antitussive

Use Treatment of mild to moderate pain and fever; symptomatic relief of cough and congestion

Usual Dosage Oral:

Analgesic: Based on acetaminophen component:
Children: 10-15 mg/kg/dose every 4-6 hours as needed; do **not** exceed 5 doses/24 hours
Adults: 325-650 mg every 4-7 hours as needed; do **not** exceed 4 g/day

Cough suppressant: Based on dextromethorphan component:
Children 6-12 years: 15 mg every 6-8 hours; do **not** exceed 60 mg/24 hours
Children >12 years and Adults: 10-20 mg every 4-8 hours **or** 30 mg every 8 hours; do **not** exceed 120 mg/24 hours

Decongestant: Based on pseudoephedrine component:
Children:
2-6 years: 15 mg every 4 hours (maximum: 90 mg/24 hours)
6-12 years: 30 mg every 4 hours (maximum: 180 mg/24 hours)
Children >12 years and Adults: 60 mg every 4 hours (maximum: 360 mg/24 hours)

Product labeling:

Alka-Seltzer Plus® Cold and Flu Liqui-Gels®:
Children 6-12 years: 1 dose every 4 hours (maximum: 4 doses/24 hours)
Children >12 years and Adults: 2 dose every 4 hours (maximum: 4 doses/24 hours)

Infants' Tylenol® Cold Plus Cough Concentrated Drops: Children 2-3 years (24-55 lbs): 2 dropperfuls every 4-6 hours (maximum: 4 doses/24 hours)

Sudafed® Severe Cold, Thera-Flu® Non-Drowsy Maximum Strength (gelcap), Tylenol® Flu Non-Drowsy Maximum Strength: Children >12 years and Adults: 2 doses every 6 hours (maximum: 8 doses/24 hours)

Tylenol® Cold Non-Drowsy:
Children 6-11 years: 1 dose every 6 hours (maximum: 4 doses/24 hours)
Children ≥12 years and Adults: 2 doses every 6 hours (maximum: 8 doses/24 hours)

Thera-Flu® Non-Drowsy Maximum Strength: Children >12 years and Adults: 1 packet dissolved in hot water every 6 hours (maximum: 4 packets/24 hours)

Additional Information Complete prescribing information for this medication should be consulted for additional detail.

Dosage Forms

Caplet:
Contac® Severe Cold and Flu/Non-Drowsy, Sudafed® Severe Cold, Tylenol® Cold Non-Drowsy: Acetaminophen 325 mg, dextromethorphan hydrobromide 15 mg, and pseudoephedrine hydrochloride 30 mg

Comtrex® Non-Drowsy Cough and Cold, Thera-Flu® Non-Drowsy Flu Cold and Cough: Acetaminophen 500 mg, dextromethorphan hydrobromide 15 mg, and pseudoephedrine hydrochloride 30 mg

Capsule, liquid
Alka-Seltzer Plus® Flu Liqui-Gels®: Acetaminophen 325 mg, dextromethorphan hydrobromide 10 mg, and pseudoephedrine hydrochloride 30 mg

Vicks® DayQuil® Cold and Flu Non-Drowsy: Acetaminophen 250 mg, dextromethorphan hydrobromide 10 mg, and pseudoephedrine hydrochloride 30 mg

Gelcap:
Tylenol® Cold Non-Drowsy: Acetaminophen 325 mg dextromethorphan hydrobromide 15 mg, and pseudoephedrine hydrochloride 30 mg

Tylenol® Flu Non-Drowsy Maximum Strength: Acetaminophen 500 mg, dextromethorphan hydrobromide 15 mg, and pseudoephedrine hydrochloride 30 mg

Liquid:
Triaminic® Sore Throat Formula: Acetaminophen 160 mg, dextromethorphan hydrobromide 7.5 mg, and pseudoephedrine hydrochloride 15 mg per 5 mL (120 mL, 240 mL) [grape flavor]

Vicks® DayQuil® Cold and Flu Non-Drowsy: Acetaminophen 325 mg, dextromethorphan hydrobromide 10 mg, and pseudoephedrine hydrochloride 30 mg per 15 mL (175 mL)

Powder for oral solution [packet] (Thera-Flu® Non-Drowsy Flu, Cold and Cough): Acetaminophen 1000 mg, dextromethorphan hydrobromide 30 mg, and pseudoephedrine hydrochloride 60 mg [lemon flavor]

Solution, oral concentrate [drops] (Infants' Tylenol® Cold Plus Cough Concentrated Drops): Acetaminophen 160 mg, dextromethorphan hydrobromide 5 mg, and pseudoephedrine hydrochloride 15 mg per 1.6 mL (15 mL) [1.6 mL = 2 dropperfuls] [cherry flavor]

Tablet (Sudafed® Severe Cold): Acetaminophen 325 mg, dextromethorphan hydrobromide 15 mg, and pseudoephedrine hydrochloride 30 mg

♦ **Acetaminophen, Dichloralphenazone, and Isometheptene** *see* Acetaminophen, Isometheptene, and Dichloralphenazone *on page 28*

Acetaminophen, Isometheptene, and Dichloralphenazone
(a seet a MIN oh fen, eye soe me THEP teen, & dye KLOR al FEN a zone)

U.S. Brand Names Midrin®; Migratine®

Synonyms Acetaminophen, Dichloralphenazone, and Isometheptene; Dichloralphenazone, Acetaminophen, and Isometheptene; Dichloralphenazone, Isometheptene, and Acetaminophen; Isometheptene, Acetaminophen, and Dichloralphenazone; Isometheptene, Dichloralphenazone, and Acetaminophen

Therapeutic Category Antimigraine Agent, Prophylactic

Use Relief of migraine and tension headache

Restrictions C-IV
Pregnancy Risk Factor B
Usual Dosage Adults: Oral:
Migraine headache: 2 capsules to start, followed by 1 capsule every hour until relief is obtained (maximum: 5 capsules/12 hours)
Tension headache: 1-2 capsules every 4 hours (maximum: 8 capsules/24 hours)
Additional Information Complete prescribing information for this medication should be consulted for additional detail.
Dosage Forms Capsule: Acetaminophen 325 mg, isometheptene mucate 65 mg, dichloral-phenazone 100 mg

♦ **Acetaminophen, Pseudoephedrine, and Chlorpheniramine** see Acetaminophen, Chlorpheniramine, and Pseudoephedrine on page 27

♦ **Acetaminophen Toxicity Nomogram** see page 1695

♦ **Acetasol® HC** see Acetic Acid, Propylene Glycol Diacetate, and Hydrocortisone on page 31

AcetaZOLAMIDE (a set a ZOLE a mide)

Related Information
Anticonvulsants by Seizure Type on page 1481
Epilepsy & Seizure Treatment on page 1659
Glaucoma Drug Therapy Comparison on page 1499
Sulfonamide Derivatives on page 1515
U.S. Brand Names Diamox®; Diamox Sequels®
Canadian Brand Names Apo®-Acetazolamide; Diamox®
Therapeutic Category Anticonvulsant; Carbonic Anhydrase Inhibitor; Diuretic, Carbonic Anhydrase Inhibitor
Use Lowers intraocular pressure to treat glaucoma, also as a diuretic, adjunct treatment of refractory seizures and acute altitude sickness; centrencephalic epilepsies (sustained release not recommended for anticonvulsant)
Pregnancy Risk Factor C
Pregnancy/Breast-Feeding Implications
Clinical effects on the fetus: Despite widespread usage, no reports linking the use of acetazolamide with congenital defects have been located
Breast-feeding/lactation: The AAP considers acetazolamide to be **compatible** with breast-feeding
Contraindications Hypersensitivity to acetazolamide, to any component of the formulation, or to sulfonamides; patients with hepatic disease or insufficiency; patients with decreased sodium and/or potassium levels; patients with adrenocortical insufficiency, hyperchloremic acidosis, severe renal disease or dysfunction, or severe pulmonary obstruction; long-term use in noncongestive angle-closure glaucoma
Warnings/Precautions Use in impaired hepatic function may result in coma. Use with caution in patients with respiratory acidosis and diabetes mellitus. Impairment of mental alertness and/or physical coordination may occur. Chemical similarities are present among sulfonamides, sulfonylureas, carbonic anhydrase inhibitors, thiazides, and loop diuretics (except ethacrynic acid). Use in patients with sulfonamide allergy is specifically contraindicated in product labeling, however a risk of cross-reaction exists in patients with allergy to any of these compounds; avoid use when previous reaction has been severe.
I.M. administration is painful because of the alkaline pH of the drug
Drug may cause substantial increase in blood glucose in some diabetic patients; malaise and complaints of tiredness and myalgia are signs of excessive dosing and acidosis in the elderly
Adverse Reactions
>10%:
Central nervous system: Malaise, unusual drowsiness or weakness
Gastrointestinal: Anorexia, weight loss, diarrhea, metallic taste, nausea, vomiting
Genitourinary: Polyuria
Neuromuscular & skeletal: Numbness, tingling, or burning in hands, fingers, feet, toes, mouth, tongue, lips, or anus
1% to 10%:
Central nervous system: Mental depression
Renal: Renal calculi
<1% (Limited to important or life-threatening): Blood dyscrasias, bone marrow suppression, cholestatic jaundice, convulsions, hyperchloremic metabolic acidosis, hyperglycemia, hypokalemia
Overdosage/Toxicology Symptoms include low blood sugar, tingling of lips and tongue, nausea, yawning, confusion, agitation, tachycardia, sweating, convulsions, stupor, and coma. Hypoglycemia should be managed with 50 mL I.V. dextrose 50% followed immediately with a continuous infusion of 10% dextrose in water (administer at a rate sufficient enough to approach a serum glucose level of 100 mg/dL). The use of corticosteroids to treat the hypoglycemia is controversial, however, the addition of 100 mg of hydrocortisone to the dextrose infusion may prove helpful.
Drug Interactions
Increased Effect/Toxicity: Concurrent use with diflunisal may increase the effect of acetazolamide causing a significant decrease in intraocular pressure. Cyclosporine concentrations may be increased by acetazolamide. Salicylate use may result in carbonic anhydrase inhibitor accumulation and toxicity. Acetazolamide-induced hypokalemia may increase the risk of toxicity with digoxin.
Decreased Effect: Use of acetazolamide may increase lithium excretion and alter excretion of other drugs by alkalinization of urine (eg, amphetamines, quinidine, procainamide, methenamine, phenobarbital, salicylates). Primidone serum concentrations may be decreased.
(Continued)

AcetaZOLAMIDE *(Continued)*

Stability

Reconstituted solution may be stored up to 12 hours at room temperature (15°C to 30°C) and for 3 days under refrigeration (2°C to 8°C)

Standard diluent: 500 mg/50 mL D_5W

Minimum volume: 50 mL D_5W

Stability of IVPB solution: 5 days at room temperature (25°C) and 44 days at refrigeration (5°C)

Reconstitute with at least 5 mL sterile water to provide a solution containing not more than 100 mg/mL; further dilution in 50 mL of either D_5W or NS for I.V. infusion administration

Mechanism of Action Reversible inhibition of the enzyme carbonic anhydrase resulting in reduction of hydrogen ion secretion at renal tubule and an increased renal excretion of sodium, potassium, bicarbonate, and water to decrease production of aqueous humor; also inhibits carbonic anhydrase in central nervous system to retard abnormal and excessive discharge from CNS neurons

Pharmacodynamics/Kinetics

Onset of action: Capsule, extended release: 2 hours; I.V.: 2 minutes

Peak effect: Capsule, extended release: 3-6 hours; I.V.: 15 minutes; Tablet: 1-4 hours

Duration: Capsule, extended release: 18-24 hours; I.V.: 4-5 hours; Tablet: 8-12 hours

Distribution: Erythrocytes, kidneys; blood-brain barrier and placenta; distributes into milk (~30% of plasma concentrations)

Protein binding: 95%

Half-life elimination: 2.4-5.8 hours

Excretion: Urine (70% to 100% as unchanged drug)

Usual Dosage Note: I.M. administration is not recommended because of pain secondary to the alkaline pH

Neonates and Infants: Hydrocephalus: To slow the progression of hydrocephalus in neonates and infants who may not be good candidates for surgery, acetazolamide I.V. or oral doses of 5 mg/kg/dose every 6 hours increased by 25 mg/kg/day to a maximum of 100 mg/kg/day, if tolerated, have been used. Furosemide was used in combination with acetazolamide.

Children:

Glaucoma:

Oral: 8-30 mg/kg/day or 300-900 mg/m²/day divided every 8 hours

I.M., I.V.: 20-40 mg/kg/24 hours divided every 6 hours, not to exceed 1 g/day

Edema: Oral, I.M., I.V.: 5 mg/kg or 150 mg/m² once every day

Epilepsy: Oral: 8-30 mg/kg/day in 1-4 divided doses, not to exceed 1 g/day; sustained release capsule is not recommended for treatment of epilepsy

Adults:

Glaucoma:

Chronic simple (open-angle): Oral: 250 mg 1-4 times/day or 500 mg sustained release capsule twice daily

Secondary, acute (closed-angle): I.M., I.V.: 250-500 mg, may repeat in 2-4 hours to a maximum of 1 g/day

Edema: Oral, I.M., I.V.: 250-375 mg once daily

Epilepsy: Oral: 8-30 mg/kg/day in 1-4 divided doses; **sustained release capsule is not recommended for treatment of epilepsy**

Altitude sickness: Oral: 250 mg every 8-12 hours (or 500 mg extended release capsules every 12-24 hours)

Therapy should begin 24-48 hours before and continue during ascent and for at least 48 hours after arrival at the high altitude

Urine alkalinization: Oral: 5 mg/kg/dose repeated 2-3 times over 24 hours

Elderly: Oral: Initial: 250 mg twice daily; use lowest effective dose

Dosing adjustment in renal impairment:

Cl_{cr} 10-50 mL/minute: Administer every 12 hours

Cl_{cr} <10 mL/minute: Avoid use → ineffective

Hemodialysis: Moderately dialyzable (20% to 50%)

Peritoneal dialysis: Supplemental dose is not necessary

Dietary Considerations May be taken with food to decrease GI upset.

Administration

Oral: May cause an alteration in taste, especially carbonated beverages; short-acting tablets may be crushed and suspended in cherry or chocolate syrup to disguise the bitter taste of the drug, do not use fruit juices, alternatively submerge tablet in 10 mL of hot water and add 10 mL honey or syrup

I.V.: Recommended rate of administration: 100-500 mg/minute for I.V. push and 4-8 hours for I.V. infusions

Monitoring Parameters Intraocular pressure, potassium, serum bicarbonate; serum electrolytes, periodic CBC with differential

Test Interactions May cause false-positive results for urinary protein with Albustix®, Labstix®, Albutest®, Bumintest®

Patient Information Report numbness or tingling of extremities to physician; do not crush, chew, or swallow contents of long-acting capsule, but may be opened and sprinkled on soft food; ability to perform tasks requiring mental alertness and/or physical coordination may be impaired; take with food; drug may cause substantial increase in blood glucose in some diabetic patients

Nursing Implications

Oral: Tablet may be crushed and suspended in cherry or chocolate syrup to disguise the bitter taste of the drug

Parenteral: Reconstitute with at least 5 mL sterile water to provide an I.V. solution containing not more than 100 mg/mL; maximum concentration: 100 mg/mL; maximum rate of I.V. infusion: 500 mg/minute

Additional Information Sodium content of 500 mg injection: 47.2 mg (2.05 mEq)

Dosage Forms
Capsule, sustained release (Diamox Sequels®): 500 mg
Injection, powder for reconstitution: 500 mg
Tablet: 125 mg, 250 mg
Diamox®: 250 mg
Extemporaneous Preparations Tablets may be crushed and suspended in cherry, chocolate, raspberry, or other highly flavored carbohydrate syrup in concentrations of 25-100 mg/mL; simple suspensions are stable for 7 days. For solutions with longer stability, see References Parastampuria and Alexander.

Alexander KS, Haribhakti RP, and Parker GA, "Stability of Acetazolamide in Suspension Compounded From Tablets," *Am J Hosp Pharm*, 1991, 48(6):1241-4.
McEvoy G, ed, AHFS Drug Information 96, Bethesda, MD: American Society of Health System Pharmacists, 1996.
Parastampuria J and Gupta VD, "Development of Oral Liquid Dosage Forms of Acetazolamide," *J Pharm Sci*, 1990, 79:385-6.

Acetic Acid (a SEE tik AS id)
U.S. Brand Names Aci-jel®; VōSol®
Synonyms Ethanoic Acid
Therapeutic Category Antibacterial, Otic; Antibacterial, Topical
Use Irrigation of the bladder; treatment of superficial bacterial infections of the external auditory canal and vagina
Pregnancy Risk Factor C
Contraindications Hypersensitivity to acetic acid or any component of the formulation; during transurethral procedures
Warnings/Precautions Not for internal intake or I.V. infusion; topical use or irrigation use only; use of irrigation in patients with mucosal lesions of urinary bladder may cause irritation; systemic acidosis may result from absorption
Adverse Reactions <1% (Limited to important or life-threatening): Hematuria, systemic acidosis, urologic pain
Usual Dosage
Irrigation (note dosage of an irrigating solution depends on the capacity or surface area of the structure being irrigated):
For continuous irrigation of the urinary bladder with 0.25% acetic acid irrigation, the rate of administration will approximate the rate of urine flow; usually 500-1500 mL/24 hours
For periodic irrigation of an indwelling urinary catheter to maintain patency, about 50 mL of 0.25% acetic acid irrigation is required
Otic: Insert saturated wick; keep moist 24 hours; remove wick and instill 5 drops 3-4 times/day
Vaginal: One applicatorful every morning and evening
Administration Not for internal intake or I.V. infusion; topical use or irrigation use only
Nursing Implications For continuous or intermittent irrigation of the urinary bladder, urine pH should be checked at least 4 times/day and the irrigation rate adjusted to maintain a pH of 4.5-5
Dosage Forms
Jelly, vaginal (Aci-jel®): 0.921% [contains oxyquinolone sulfate 0.025%, ricinoleic acid 0.7%, and glycerin 5%] (85 g)
Solution for irrigation: 0.25% (250 mL, 500 mL, 1000 mL)
Solution, otic (VōSol®): 2% [in propylene glycol] (15 mL)

♦ **Acetic Acid and Aluminum Acetate Otic** *see* Aluminum Acetate and Acetic Acid *on page 62*
♦ **Acetic Acid, Hydrocortisone, and Propylene Glycol Diacetate** *see* Acetic Acid, Propylene Glycol Diacetate, and Hydrocortisone *on page 31*

Acetic Acid, Propylene Glycol Diacetate, and Hydrocortisone
(a SEE tik AS id, PRO pa leen GLY kole dye AS e tate, & hye droe KOR ti sone)
U.S. Brand Names Acetasol® HC; VōSol® HC
Canadian Brand Names VōSol® HC
Synonyms Acetic Acid, Hydrocortisone, and Propylene Glycol Diacetate; Hydrocortisone, Acetic Acid, and Propylene Glycol Diacetate; Hydrocortisone, Propylene Glycol Diacetate, and Acetic Acid; Propylene Glycol Diacetate, Acetic Acid, and Hydrocortisone; Propylene Glycol Diacetate, Hydrocortisone, and Acetic Acid
Therapeutic Category Antibiotic/Corticosteroid, Otic
Use Treatment of superficial infections of the external auditory canal caused by organisms susceptible to the action of the antimicrobial, complicated by swelling
Usual Dosage Adults: Instill 4 drops in ear(s) 3-4 times/day
Additional Information Complete prescribing information for this medication should be consulted for additional detail.
Dosage Forms Solution, otic: Acetic acid 2%, propylene glycol diacetate 3%, and hydrocortisone 1% (10 mL)

AcetoHEXAMIDE (a set oh HEKS a mide)
Related Information
Antacid Drug Interactions *on page 1477*
Hypoglycemic Drugs & Thiazolidinedione Information *on page 1502*
Sulfonamide Derivatives *on page 1515*
U.S. Brand Names Dymelor® [DSC]
Therapeutic Category Antidiabetic Agent, Sulfonylurea; Hypoglycemic Agent, Oral; Sulfonylurea Agent
Use Adjunct to diet for the management of mild to moderately severe, stable, type 2 diabetes mellitus (noninsulin dependent, NIDDM)
Pregnancy Risk Factor D
(Continued)

AcetoHEXAMIDE *(Continued)*

Usual Dosage Adults: Oral (elderly patients may be more sensitive and should be started at a lower dosage initially):

Initial: 250 mg/day; increase in increments of 250-500 mg daily at intervals of 5-7 days up to 1.5 g/day. Patients on ≤1 g/day can be controlled with once daily administration. Patients receiving 1.5 g/day usually benefit from twice daily administration before the morning and evening meals. Doses >1.5 g daily are not recommended.

Dosing adjustment in renal impairment: Cl_{cr} <50 mL/minute: Not recommended due to increased potential for developing hypoglycemia

Dosing adjustment in hepatic impairment: Initiate therapy at lower than recommended doses; further dosage adjustment may be necessary because acetohexamide is extensively metabolized but no specific guidelines are available

Additional Information Complete prescribing information for this medication should be consulted for additional detail.

Dosage Forms Tablet: 250 mg, 500 mg

◆ **Acetoxymethylprogesterone** *see* MedroxyPROGESTERone *on page 848*

Acetylcholine (a se teel KOE leen)

U.S. Brand Names Miochol-E®

Canadian Brand Names Miochol®-E

Synonyms Acetylcholine Chloride

Therapeutic Category Cholinergic Agent, Ophthalmic; Ophthalmic Agent, Miotic

Use Produces complete miosis in cataract surgery, keratoplasty, iridectomy and other anterior segment surgery where rapid miosis is required

Pregnancy Risk Factor C

Pregnancy/Breast-Feeding Implications Acetylcholine is used primarily in the eye and there are no reports of its use in pregnancy; because it is ionized at physiologic pH, transplacental passage would not be expected

Contraindications Hypersensitivity to acetylcholine chloride or any component of the formulation; acute iritis and acute inflammatory disease of the anterior chamber

Warnings/Precautions Systemic effects rarely occur but can cause problems for patients with acute cardiac failure, bronchial asthma, peptic ulcer, hyperthyroidism, GI spasm, urinary tract obstruction, and Parkinson's disease; open under aseptic conditions only

Adverse Reactions Frequency not defined.

Cardiovascular: Bradycardia, hypotension

Ocular: Altered vision, transient lenticular opacities

Respiratory: Dyspnea

Overdosage/Toxicology Treatment includes flushing eyes with water or normal saline and supportive measures. If accidentally ingested, induce emesis or perform gastric lavage.

Drug Interactions

Increased Effect/Toxicity: Effect may be prolonged or enhanced in patients receiving tacrine.

Decreased Effect: May be decreased with flurbiprofen and suprofen, ophthalmic.

Stability Prepare solution immediately before use and discard unused portion; acetylcholine solutions are unstable; reconstitute immediately before use

Mechanism of Action Causes contraction of the sphincter muscles of the iris, resulting in miosis and contraction of the ciliary muscle, leading to accommodation spasm

Pharmacodynamics/Kinetics

Onset of action: Rapid

Duration: ~10 minutes

Usual Dosage Adults: Intraocular: 0.5-2 mL of 1% injection (5-20 mg) instilled into anterior chamber before or after securing one or more sutures

Administration Reconstitute immediately before use.

Patient Information May sting on instillation; use caution while driving at night or performing hazardous tasks; do not touch dropper to eye

Nursing Implications Discard any solution that is not used; open under aseptic conditions only

Dosage Forms Powder for intraocular suspension, as chloride: 1:100 [10 mg/mL] (2 mL)

◆ **Acetylcholine Chloride** *see* Acetylcholine *on page 32*

Acetylcysteine (a se teel SIS teen)

U.S. Brand Names Mucomyst®; Mucosil™

Canadian Brand Names Mucomyst®; Parvolex®

Synonyms Acetylcysteine Sodium; Mercapturic Acid; NAC; N-Acetylcysteine; N-Acetyl-L-cysteine

Therapeutic Category Antidote, Acetaminophen; Mucolytic Agent

Use Adjunctive mucolytic therapy in patients with abnormal or viscid mucous secretions in acute and chronic bronchopulmonary diseases; pulmonary complications of surgery and cystic fibrosis; diagnostic bronchial studies; antidote for acute acetaminophen toxicity

Unlabeled/Investigational Use Prevention of radiocontrast-induced renal dysfunction

Pregnancy Risk Factor B

Pregnancy/Breast-Feeding Implications Based on limited reports using acetylcysteine to treat acetaminophen overdose in pregnant women, acetylcysteine has been shown to cross the placenta and may provide protective levels in the fetus.

Contraindications Hypersensitivity to acetylcysteine or any component of the formulation

Warnings/Precautions Since increased bronchial secretions may develop after inhalation, percussion, postural drainage and suctioning should follow; if bronchospasm occurs, administer a bronchodilator; discontinue acetylcysteine if bronchospasm progresses

Adverse Reactions
Inhalation:
>10%:
Stickiness on face after nebulization
Miscellaneous: Unpleasant odor during administration
1% to 10%:
Central nervous system: Drowsiness, chills, fever
Gastrointestinal: Vomiting, nausea, stomatitis
Local: Irritation
Respiratory: Bronchospasm, rhinorrhea, hemoptysis
Miscellaneous: Clamminess
Systemic:
1% to 10%:
Central nervous system: Fever, drowsiness, dizziness (10%; prevention of radiocontrast-induced renal function)
Gastrointestinal: Nausea, vomiting
<1% (Limited to important or life-threatening): Anaphylactoid reaction, bronchospastic allergic reaction, EKG changes (transient)

Overdosage/Toxicology The treatment of acetylcysteine toxicity is usually aimed at reversing anaphylactoid symptoms or controlling nausea and vomiting. The use of epinephrine, antihistamines, and steroids may be beneficial.

Drug Interactions
Decreased Effect: Adsorbed by activated charcoal; clinical significance is minimal, though, once a pure acetaminophen ingestion requiring N-acetylcysteine is established; further charcoal dosing is unnecessary once the appropriate initial charcoal dose is achieved (5-10 g:g acetaminophen)

Stability Store opened vials in the refrigerator, use within 96 hours; dilutions should be freshly prepared and used within 1 hour; light purple color of solution does **not** affect its mucolytic activity

Mechanism of Action Exerts mucolytic action through its free sulfhydryl group which opens up the disulfide bonds in the mucoproteins thus lowering mucous viscosity. The exact mechanism of action in acetaminophen toxicity is unknown; thought to act by providing substrate for conjugation with the toxic metabolite.

Pharmacodynamics/Kinetics
Onset of action: Inhalation: 5-10 minutes
Duration: Inhalation: >1 hour
Distribution: Oral: 0.33-0.47 L/kg
Protein binding, plasma: Oral: 50%
Half-life elimination: Reduced acetylcysteine: 2 hours; Total acetylcysteine: 5.5 hours
Time to peak, plasma: Oral: 1-2 hours

Usual Dosage
Acetaminophen poisoning: Children and Adults: Oral: 140 mg/kg; followed by 17 doses of 70 mg/kg every 4 hours; repeat dose if emesis occurs within 1 hour of administration; therapy should continue until all doses are administered even though the acetaminophen plasma level has dropped below the toxic range
Inhalation: Acetylcysteine 10% and 20% solution (Mucomyst®) (dilute 20% solution with sodium chloride or sterile water for inhalation); 10% solution may be used undiluted
Infants: 1-2 mL of 20% solution or 2-4 mL 10% solution until nebulized given 3-4 times/day
Children: 3-5 mL of 20% solution or 6-10 mL of 10% solution until nebulized given 3-4 times/day
Adolescents: 5-10 mL of 10% to 20% solution until nebulized given 3-4 times/day
Note: Patients should receive an aerosolized bronchodilator 10-15 minutes prior to acetylcysteine
Meconium ileus equivalent: Children and Adults: 100-300 mL of 4% to 10% solution by irrigation or orally
Prevention of radiocontrast-induced renal dysfunction (unlabeled use): Adults: Oral: 600 mg twice daily for 2 days (beginning the day before the procedure); may be given as powder in capsules, some centers use solution (diluted in cola beverage or juice). Hydrate patient with saline concurrently.

Administration For treatment of acetaminophen overdosage, administer orally as a 5% solution
Dilute the 20% solution 1:3 with a cola, orange juice, or other soft drink
Use within 1 hour of preparation; unpleasant odor becomes less noticeable as treatment progresses

Reference Range Determine acetaminophen level as soon as possible, but no sooner than 4 hours after ingestion (to ensure peak levels have been obtained); administer for acetaminophen level >150 µg/mL at 4 hours following ingestion; toxic concentration with probable hepatotoxicity: >200 µg/mL at 4 hours or 50 µg at 12 hours

Patient Information Clear airway by coughing deeply before aerosol treatment

Nursing Implications Assess patient for nausea, vomiting, and skin rash following oral administration for treatment of acetaminophen poisoning; intermittent aerosol treatments are commonly given when patient arises, before meals, and just before retiring at bedtime

Dosage Forms Solution, as sodium: 10% [100 mg/mL] (4 mL, 10 mL, 30 mL); 20% [200 mg/mL] (4 mL, 10 mL, 30 mL, 100 mL)

♦ **Aclovate**® *see Alclometasone on page 43*

Acrivastine and Pseudoephedrine (AK ri vas teen & soo doe e FED rin)

U.S. Brand Names Semprex®-D
Synonyms Pseudoephedrine and Acrivastine
Therapeutic Category Antihistamine, H₁ Blocker; Decongestant
Use Temporary relief of nasal congestion, decongest sinus openings, running nose, itching of nose or throat, and itchy, watery eyes due to hay fever or other upper respiratory allergies
Pregnancy Risk Factor B
Usual Dosage Adults: 1 capsule 3-4 times/day
  Dosing comments in renal impairment: Do not use
Additional Information Complete prescribing information for this medication should be consulted for additional detail.
Dosage Forms Capsule: Acrivastine 8 mg and pseudoephedrine hydrochloride 60 mg

♦ **ACT** *see Dactinomycin on page 356*
♦ **ACT**® **[OTC]** *see Fluoride on page 574*
♦ **Act-A-Med**® **[OTC]** *see Triprolidine and Pseudoephedrine on page 1380*
♦ **Actanol**® **[OTC]** *see Triprolidine and Pseudoephedrine on page 1380*
♦ **Actedril**® **[OTC]** *see Triprolidine and Pseudoephedrine on page 1380*
♦ **ActHIB**® *see Haemophilus b Conjugate Vaccine on page 651*
♦ **Acticin**® *see Permethrin on page 1065*
♦ **Actidose**® **[OTC]** *see Charcoal on page 268*
♦ **Actidose-Aqua**® **[OTC]** *see Charcoal on page 268*
♦ **Actifed**® **[OTC]** *see Triprolidine and Pseudoephedrine on page 1380*
♦ **Actifed**® **Allergy (Night) [OTC]** *see Diphenhydramine and Pseudoephedrine on page 415*
♦ **Actigall**™ *see Ursodiol on page 1393*
♦ **Actimmune**® *see Interferon Gamma-1b on page 737*
♦ **Actinex**® *see Masoprocol on page 840*
♦ **Actinomycin D** *see Dactinomycin on page 356*
♦ **Actiq**® *see Fentanyl on page 551*
♦ **Activase**® *see Alteplase on page 59*
♦ **Activase**® **rt-PA (Can)** *see Alteplase on page 59*
♦ **Activated Carbon** *see Charcoal on page 268*
♦ **Activated Charcoal** *see Charcoal on page 268*
♦ **Activated Ergosterol** *see Ergocalciferol on page 481*
♦ **Activated Protein C, Human, Recombinant** *see Drotrecogin Alfa on page 453*
♦ **Activella**™ *see Estradiol and Norethindrone on page 494*
♦ **Actonel**™ *see Risedronate on page 1199*
♦ **Actos**™ *see Pioglitazone on page 1087*
♦ **Actron**® **[OTC]** *see Ketoprofen on page 763*
♦ **ACU-dyne**® **[OTC]** *see Povidone-Iodine on page 1114*
♦ **Acular**® *see Ketorolac on page 764*
♦ **Acular**® **PF** *see Ketorolac on page 764*
♦ **ACV** *see Acyclovir on page 34*
♦ **Acycloguanosine** *see Acyclovir on page 34*

Acyclovir (ay SYE kloe veer)

Related Information
  Treatment of Sexually Transmitted Diseases *on page 1609*
  USPHA/IDSA Guidelines for the Prevention of Opportunistic Infections in Persons With HIV *on page 1574*
U.S. Brand Names Zovirax®
Canadian Brand Names Apo®-Acyclovir; Avirax™; Nu-Acyclovir; Zovirax®
Synonyms Aciclovir; ACV; Acycloguanosine
Therapeutic Category Antiviral Agent, Nonantiretroviral; Antiviral Agent, Oral; Antiviral Agent, Parenteral; Antiviral Agent, Topical
Use Treatment of initial and prophylaxis of recurrent mucosal and cutaneous herpes simplex (HSV-1 and HSV-2) infections; herpes simplex encephalitis; herpes zoster; genital herpes infection; varicella-zoster infections in healthy, nonpregnant persons >13 years of age, children >12 months of age who have a chronic skin or lung disorder or are receiving long-term aspirin therapy, and immunocompromised patients; for herpes zoster, acyclovir should be started within 72 hours of the appearance of the rash to be effective; acyclovir will not prevent postherpetic neuralgias
Pregnancy Risk Factor B
Contraindications Hypersensitivity to acyclovir, valacyclovir, or any component of the formulation
Warnings/Precautions Use with caution in patients with pre-existing renal disease or in those receiving other nephrotoxic drugs concurrently; maintain adequate urine output during the first 2 hours after I.V. infusion; use with caution in patients with underlying neurologic abnormalities, serious hepatic or electrolyte abnormalities, or substantial hypoxia
Adverse Reactions
  Systemic: Oral:
    1% to 10%:
      Central nervous system: Lightheadedness, headache
      Gastrointestinal: Nausea, vomiting, abdominal pain
  Systemic: Parenteral:
    >10%:
      Central nervous system: Lightheadedness
      Gastrointestinal: Nausea, vomiting, anorexia

Local: Inflammation at injection site or phlebitis

1% to 10%: Renal: Acute renal failure

Topical:

>10%: Mild pain, burning, or stinging

1% to 10%: Itching

All forms: <1% (Limited to important or life-threatening): Aggression, alopecia, anaphylaxis, anemia, angioedema, ataxia, delirium, encephalopathy, erythema multiforme, hallucinations, hepatitis, hyperbilirubinemia, jaundice, leukocytoclastic vasculitis, leukopenia, local tissue necrosis (following extravasation), mental depression, paresthesia, photosensitization, pruritus, psychosis, renal failure, seizures, somnolence, Stevens-Johnson syndrome, thrombocytopenia, thrombocytopenic purpura/hemolytic uremic syndrome (TTP/HUS), toxic epidermal necrolysis, urticaria

Overdosage/Toxicology Symptoms include seizures, somnolence, confusion, elevated serum creatinine, and renal failure. In the event of an overdose, sufficient urine flow must be maintained to avoid drug precipitation within the renal tubules. Hemodialysis has resulted in up to 60% reductions in serum acyclovir levels.

Drug Interactions

Increased Effect/Toxicity: Increased CNS side effects when taken with zidovudine or probenecid.

Ethanol/Nutrition/Herb Interactions Food: Does not appear to affect absorption of acyclovir.

Stability Incompatible with blood products and protein-containing solutions; reconstituted solutions remain stable for 24 hours at room temperature; do not refrigerate reconstituted solutions as they may precipitate; in patients who require fluid restriction, a concentration of up to 10 mg/mL has been infused, however, concentrations >10 mg/mL (usual recommended concentration: <7 mg/mL in D_5W) increase the risk of phlebitis

Mechanism of Action Acyclovir is converted to acyclovir monophosphate by virus-specific thymidine kinase then further converted to acyclovir triphosphate by other cellular enzymes. Acyclovir triphosphate inhibits DNA synthesis and viral replication by competing with deoxyguanosine triphosphate for viral DNA polymerase and being incorporated into viral DNA.

Pharmacodynamics/Kinetics

Absorption: Oral: 15% to 30%

Distribution: Widely (ie, brain, kidney, lungs, liver, spleen, muscle, uterus, vagina, CSF)

Protein binding: <30%

Metabolism: Hepatic (small amounts)

Half-life elimination: Terminal: Neonates: 4 hours; Children 1-12 years: 2-3 hours; Adults: 3 hours

Time to peak, serum: Oral: Within 1.5-2 hours; I.V.: Within 1 hour

Excretion: Urine (30% to 90% as unchanged drug)

Usual Dosage

Dosing weight should be based on the smaller of lean body weight or total body weight

Treatment of herpes simplex virus infections: Children >12 years and Adults:

I.V.:

Mucocutaneous HSV or severe initial herpes genitalis infection: 750 mg/m²/day divided every 8 hours or 5 mg/kg/dose every 8 hours for 5-10 days

HSV encephalitis: 1500 mg/m²/day divided every 8 hours or 10 mg/kg/dose for 10 days

Topical: Nonlife-threatening mucocutaneous HSV in immunocompromised patients: ½" ribbon of ointment for a 4" square surface area every 3 hours (6 times/day) for 7 days

Treatment of genital herpes simplex virus infections: Adults:

Oral: 200 mg every 4 hours while awake (5 times/day) for 10 days if initial episode; for 5 days if recurrence (begin at earliest signs of disease)

Topical: ½" ribbon of ointment for a 4" square surface area every 3 hours (6 times/day) for 7 days

Treatment of varicella-zoster virus (chickenpox) infections:

Oral:

Children: 10-20 mg/kg/dose (up to 800 mg) 4 times/day for 5 days; begin treatment within the first 24 hours of rash onset

Adults: 600-800 mg/dose every 4 hours while awake (5 times/day) for 7-10 days or 1000 mg every 6 hours for 5 days

I.V.: Children and Adults: 1500 mg/m²/day divided every 8 hours or 10 mg/kg/dose every 8 hours for 7 days

Treatment of herpes zoster (shingles) infections:

Oral:

Children (immunocompromised): 250-600 mg/m²/dose 4-5 times/day for 7-10 days

Adults (immunocompromised): 800 mg every 4 hours (5 times/day) for 7-10 days

I.V.:

Children and Adults (immunocompromised): 10 mg/kg/dose or 500 mg/m²/dose every 8 hours

Older Adults (immunocompromised): 7.5 mg/kg/dose every 8 hours

If nephrotoxicity occurs: 5 mg/kg/dose every 8 hours

Prophylaxis in immunocompromised patients:

Varicella zoster or herpes zoster in HIV-positive patients: Adults: Oral: 400 mg every 4 hours (5 times/day) for 7-10 days

Bone marrow transplant recipients: Children and Adults: I.V.:

Allogeneic patients who are HSV seropositive: 150 mg/m²/dose (5 mg/kg) every 12 hours; with clinical symptoms of herpes simplex: 150 mg/m²/dose every 8 hours

Allogeneic patients who are CMV seropositive: 500 mg/m²/dose (10 mg/kg) every 8 hours; for clinically symptomatic CMV infection, consider replacing acyclovir with ganciclovir

Chronic suppressive therapy for recurrent genital herpes simplex virus infections: Adults: 200 mg 3-4 times/day or 400 mg twice daily for up to 12 months, followed by re-evaluation

(Continued)

Acyclovir *(Continued)*

Dosing adjustment in renal impairment:
Oral: HSV/varicella-zoster:
Cl_{cr} 10-25 mL/minute: Administer dose every 8 hours
Cl_{cr} <10 mL/minute: Administer dose every 12 hours
I.V.:
Cl_{cr} 25-50 mL/minute: 5-10 mg/kg/dose: Administer every 12 hours
Cl_{cr} 10-25 mL/minute: 5-10 mg/kg/dose: Administer every 24 hours
Cl_{cr} <10 mL/minute: 2.5-5 mg/kg/dose: Administer every 24 hours
Hemodialysis: Dialyzable (50% to 100%); administer dose postdialysis
Peritoneal dialysis: Dose as for Cl_{cr} <10 mL/minute
Continuous arteriovenous or venovenous hemofiltration effects: Dose as for Cl_{cr} <10 mL/minute

Dietary Considerations May be taken with food.

Administration
Oral: May be administered with food.
I.V.: Avoid rapid infusion; infuse over 1 hour to prevent renal damage; maintain adequate hydration of patient; check for phlebitis and rotate infusion sites

Monitoring Parameters Urinalysis, BUN, serum creatinine, liver enzymes, CBC

Patient Information Patients are contagious only when viral shedding is occurring; recurrences tend to appear within 3 months of original infection; acyclovir is **not** a cure; avoid sexual intercourse when lesions are present; may take with food

Nursing Implications Wear gloves when applying ointment for self-protection

Additional Information Injection formulations: Sodium content of 1 g: 96.6 mg (4.2 mEq)

Dosage Forms
Capsule: 200 mg
Injection, powder for reconstitution, as sodium: 500 mg, 1000 mg
Injection, solution, as sodium [preservative free]: 50 mg/mL (10 mL, 20 mL)
Ointment, topical: 5% (3 g, 15 g)
Suspension, oral: 200 mg/5 mL (480 mL) [banana flavor]
Tablet: 400 mg, 800 mg

- ♦ **Adacel® (Can)** *see* Diphtheria, Tetanus Toxoids, and Acellular Pertussis Vaccine *on page 418*
- ♦ **Adagen™** *see* Pegademase Bovine *on page 1043*
- ♦ **Adalat® CC** *see* NIFEdipine *on page 981*
- ♦ **Adalat® PA (Can)** *see* NIFEdipine *on page 981*
- ♦ **Adalat® XL® (Can)** *see* NIFEdipine *on page 981*
- ♦ **Adamantanamine Hydrochloride** *see* Amantadine *on page 65*

Adapalene *(a DAP a leen)*

U.S. Brand Names Differin®
Canadian Brand Names Differin®
Therapeutic Category Acne Products
Use Treatment of acne vulgaris
Pregnancy Risk Factor C

Pregnancy/Breast-Feeding Implications There are no adequate and well-controlled studies in pregnant women. Use only if benefit outweighs the potential risk to fetus. It is not known whether adapalene is excreted in breast milk. Use caution when administering to a nursing woman.

Contraindications Hypersensitivity to adapalene or any component in the vehicle gel

Warnings/Precautions Use with caution in patients with eczema; avoid excessive exposure to sunlight and sunlamps; avoid contact with abraded skin, mucous membranes, eyes, mouth, angles of the nose

Certain cutaneous signs and symptoms such as erythema, dryness, scaling, burning or pruritus may occur during treatment; these are most likely to occur during the first 2-4 weeks and will usually lessen with continued use

Adverse Reactions
>10%: Dermatologic: Erythema, scaling, dryness, pruritus, burning, pruritus or burning immediately after application
≤1% (Limited to important or life-threatening): Acne flares, conjunctivitis, contact dermatitis, dermatitis, eczema, eyelid edema, skin discoloration, skin irritation, stinging sunburn, rash (topical cream)

Overdosage/Toxicology Toxic signs of an overdose commonly respond to drug discontinuation, and generally return to normal spontaneously within a few days to weeks. When confronted with signs of increased intracranial pressure, treatment with mannitol (0.25 g/kg I.V. up to 1 g/kg/dose repeated every 5 minutes as needed), dexamethasone (1.5 mg/kg I.V. load followed with 0.375 mg/kg every 6 hours for 5 days), and/or hyperventilation should be employed.

Mechanism of Action Retinoid-like compound which is a modulator of cellular differentiation, keratinization and inflammatory processes, all of which represent important features in the pathology of acne vulgaris

Pharmacodynamics/Kinetics
Absorption: Topical: Minimal
Excretion: Bile

Usual Dosage Children >12 years and Adults: Topical: Apply once daily at bedtime; therapeutic results should be noticed after 8-12 weeks of treatment

Patient Information Thoroughly wash hands after applying; avoid hydration of skin immediately before application; minimize exposure to sunlight; avoid washing face more frequently than 2-3 times/day; if severe irritation occurs, discontinue medication temporarily and adjust dose when irritation subsides; avoid using topical preparations with high alcoholic content during treatment period; do not exceed prescribed dose

Nursing Implications Observe for signs of hypersensitivity, blistering, excessive dryness; do not apply to mucous membranes

Dosage Forms
Cream, topical: 0.1% (15 g, 45 g)
Gel, topical: 0.1% (15 g, 45 g) [alcohol free]
Pledget, topical: 0.1% (60s)
Solution, topical: 0.1% (30 mL)

♦ **Adderall®** see Dextroamphetamine and Amphetamine on page 389
♦ **Adderall XR™** see Dextroamphetamine and Amphetamine on page 389
♦ **Adenine Arabinoside** see Vidarabine on page 1414
♦ **Adenocard®** see Adenosine on page 37
♦ **Adenoscan®** see Adenosine on page 37

Adenosine (a DEN oh seen)

Related Information
Adult ACLS Algorithms on page 1632
Antiarrhythmic Drugs Comparison on page 1478
U.S. Brand Names Adenocard®; Adenoscan®
Canadian Brand Names Adenocard®
Synonyms 9-Beta-D-ribofuranosyladenine
Therapeutic Category Antiarrhythmic Agent, Miscellaneous
Use
Adenocard®: Treatment of paroxysmal supraventricular tachycardia (PSVT) including that associated with accessory bypass tracts (Wolff-Parkinson-White syndrome); when clinically advisable, appropriate vagal maneuvers should be attempted prior to adenosine administration; **not effective in atrial flutter, atrial fibrillation, or ventricular tachycardia**
Adenoscan®: Pharmacologic stress agent used in myocardial perfusion thallium-201 scintigraphy

Pregnancy Risk Factor C
Pregnancy/Breast-Feeding Implications Clinical effects on the fetus: Case reports (4) on administration during pregnancy have indicated no adverse effects on fetus or newborn attributable to adenosine
Contraindications Hypersensitivity to adenosine or any component of the formulation; second- or third-degree AV block or sick sinus syndrome (except in patients with a functioning artificial pacemaker), atrial flutter, atrial fibrillation, and ventricular tachycardia (this drug is not effective in converting these arrhythmias to sinus rhythm). The manufacturer states that Adenoscan® should be avoided in patients with known or suspected bronchoconstrictive or bronchospastic lung disease.
Warnings/Precautions Patients with pre-existing S-A nodal dysfunction may experience prolonged sinus pauses after adenosine. There have been reports of atrial fibrillation/flutter in patients with PSVT associated with accessory conduction pathways after adenosine. Adenosine decreases conduction through the AV node and may produce a short-lasting first-, second-, or third-degree heart block. Because of the very short half-life, the effects are generally self-limiting. Rare, prolonged episodes of asystole have been reported, with fatal outcomes in some cases. At the time of conversion to normal sinus rhythm, a variety of new rhythms may appear on the EKG. A limited number of patients with asthma have received adenosine and have not experienced exacerbation of their asthma. Adenosine may cause bronchoconstriction in patients with asthma, and should be used cautiously in patients with obstructive lung disease not associated with bronchoconstriction (eg, emphysema, bronchitis).

Adverse Reactions
>10%:
Cardiovascular: Facial flushing (18%), palpitations, chest pain, hypotension
Central nervous system: Headache
Respiratory: Dyspnea (12%)
Miscellaneous: Diaphoresis
1% to 10%:
Central nervous system: Dizziness
Gastrointestinal: Nausea (3%)
Neuromuscular & skeletal: Paresthesia, numbness
Respiratory: Chest pressure (7%)
<1% (Limited to important or life-threatening): Dizziness, headache, hyperventilation, hypotension, intracranial pressure, lightheadedness
Overdosage/Toxicology Since the half-life of adenosine is <10 seconds, any adverse effects are rapidly self-limiting. Intoxication is usually short-lived since the half-life of the drug is very short. Treatment of prolonged effects requires individualization. Theophylline and other methylxanthines are competitive inhibitors of adenosine and may have a role in reversing its toxic effects.

Drug Interactions
Increased Effect/Toxicity: Dipyridamole potentiates effects of adenosine. Use with carbamazepine may increase heart block.
Decreased Effect: Methylxanthines (eg, caffeine, theophylline) antagonize the effect of adenosine.
Ethanol/Nutrition/Herb Interactions Food: Avoid food or drugs with caffeine. Adenosine's therapeutic effect may be decreased if used concurrently with caffeine.
Stability Do **not** refrigerate, precipitation may occur (may dissolve by warming to room temperature)
Mechanism of Action Slows conduction time through the AV node, interrupting the re-entry pathways through the AV node, restoring normal sinus rhythm
Pharmacodynamics/Kinetics
Onset of action: Rapid
(Continued)

Adenosine *(Continued)*

Duration: Very brief

Metabolism: Blood and tissue to inosine then to adenosine monophosphate (AMP) and hypoxanthine

Half-life elimination: <10 seconds

Usual Dosage

Adenocard®: **Rapid I.V. push (over 1-2 seconds) via peripheral line:**

Neonates: Initial dose: 0.05 mg/kg; if not effective within 2 minutes, increase dose by 0.05 mg/kg increments every 2 minutes to a maximum dose of 0.25 mg/kg or until termination of PSVT

Maximum single dose: 12 mg

Infants and Children: Pediatric advanced life support (PALS): Treatment of SVT: 0.1 mg/kg; if not effective, administer 0.2 mg/kg

Alternatively: Initial dose: 0.05 mg/kg; if not effective within 2 minutes, increase dose by 0.05 mg/kg increments every 2 minutes to a maximum dose of 0.25 mg/kg or until termination of PSVT; medium dose required: 0.15 mg/kg

Maximum single dose: 12 mg

Adults: 6 mg; if not effective within 1-2 minutes, 12 mg may be given; may repeat 12 mg bolus if needed

Maximum single dose: 12 mg

Follow each I.V. bolus of adenosine with normal saline flush

Note: Preliminary results in adults suggest adenosine may be administered via a central line at lower doses (ie, initial adult dose: 3 mg).

Adenoscan®: Continuous I.V. infusion via peripheral line: 140 mcg/kg/minute for 6 minutes using syringe or columetric infusion pump; total dose: 0.84 mg/kg. Thallium-201 is injected at midpoint (3 minutes) of infusion.

Hemodialysis: Significant drug removal is unlikely based on physiochemical characteristics.

Peritoneal dialysis: Significant drug removal is unlikely based on physiochemical characteristics.

Note: Patients who are receiving concomitant theophylline therapy may be less likely to respond to adenosine therapy.

Note: Higher doses may be needed for administration via peripheral versus central vein.

Administration For rapid bolus I.V. use only; administer I.V. push over 1-2 seconds at a peripheral I.V. site as proximal as possible to trunk (not in lower arm, hand, lower leg, or foot); follow each bolus with normal saline flush. **Note:** Preliminary results in adults suggest adenosine may be administered via central line at lower doses (eg, adults initial dose: 3 mg)

Monitoring Parameters EKG monitoring, heart rate, blood pressure

Nursing Implications Be alert for possible exacerbation of asthma in asthmatic patients

Dosage Forms Injection, solution [preservative free]:

Adenocard®: 3 mg/mL (2 mL, 4 mL)

Adenoscan®: 3 mg/mL (20 mL, 30 mL)

- **Agrylin®** *see Anagrelide on page 98*
- **AHF (Human)** *see Antihemophilic Factor (Human) on page 102*
- **AHF (Porcine)** *see Antihemophilic Factor (Porcine) on page 104*
- **AHF (Recombinant)** *see Antihemophilic Factor (Recombinant) on page 105*
- **A-hydroCort®** *see Hydrocortisone on page 682*
- **Akarpine®** *see Pilocarpine on page 1083*
- **AKBeta®** *see Levobunolol on page 788*
- **AK-Cide®** *see Sulfacetamide and Prednisolone on page 1269*
- **AK-Con®** *see Naphazoline on page 957*
- **AK-Dex®** *see Dexamethasone on page 380*
- **AK-Dilate® Ophthalmic** *see Phenylephrine on page 1075*
- **AK-Fluor** *see Fluorescein Sodium on page 573*
- **AK-Nefrin® Ophthalmic** *see Phenylephrine on page 1075*
- **AK-Neo-Dex®** *see Neomycin and Dexamethasone on page 968*
- **AK-Pentolate®** *see Cyclopentolate on page 341*
- **AK-Poly-Bac®** *see Bacitracin and Polymyxin B on page 143*
- **AK-Pred®** *see PrednisoLONE on page 1122*
- **AKPro®** *see Dipivefrin on page 422*
- **AK-Spore® H.C.** *see Bacitracin, Neomycin, Polymyxin B, and Hydrocortisone on page 143*
- **AK-Spore® H.C. Otic** *see Neomycin, Polymyxin B, and Hydrocortisone on page 969*
- **AK-Spore® Ophthalmic Solution** *see Neomycin, Polymyxin B, and Gramicidin on page 969*
- **AK-Sulf®** *see Sulfacetamide on page 1268*
- **AKTob®** *see Tobramycin on page 1340*
- **AK-Tracin®** *see Bacitracin on page 142*
- **AK-Trol®** *see Neomycin, Polymyxin B, and Dexamethasone on page 969*
- **Ala-Cort®** *see Hydrocortisone on page 682*
- **Alamast™** *see Pemirolast on page 1048*
- **Ala-Scalp®** *see Hydrocortisone on page 682*
- **Alatrofloxacin Mesylate** *see Trovafloxacin on page 1384*
- **Albalon®-A Liquifilm (Can)** *see Naphazoline and Antazoline on page 958*
- **Albalon® Liquifilm®** *see Naphazoline on page 957*

Albendazole (al BEN da zole)
U.S. Brand Names Albenza®
Therapeutic Category Anthelmintic
Use Treatment of parenchymal neurocysticercosis and cystic hydatid disease of the liver, lung, and peritoneum; albendazole has activity against *Ascaris lumbricoides* (roundworm), *Ancylostoma duodenale* and *Necator americanus* (hookworms), *Enterobius vermicularis* (pinworm), *Hymenolepis nana* and *Taenia* sp (tapeworms), *Opisthorchis sinensis* and *Opisthorchis viverrini* (liver flukes), *Strongyloides stercoralis* and *Trichuris trichiura* (whipworm); activity has also been shown against the liver fluke *Clonorchis sinensis*, *Giardia lamblia*, *Cysticercus cellulosae*, *Echinococcus granulosus*, *Echinococcus multilocularis*, and *Toxocara* sp.
Pregnancy Risk Factor C
Pregnancy/Breast-Feeding Implications Albendazole has been shown to be teratogenic in laboratory animals and should not be used during pregnancy, if at all possible
Contraindications Hypersensitivity to albendazole or any component of the formulation
Warnings/Precautions Discontinue therapy if LFT elevations are significant; may restart treatment when decreased to pretreatment values. Becoming pregnant within 1 month following therapy is not advised. Corticosteroids should be administered 1-2 days before albendazole therapy in patients with neurocysticercosis to minimize inflammatory reactions and steroid and anticonvulsant therapy should be used concurrently during the first week of therapy for neurocysticercosis to prevent cerebral hypertension. If retinal lesions exist in patients with neurocysticercosis, weigh risk of further retinal damage due to albendazole-induced changes to the retinal lesion vs benefit of disease treatment.
Adverse Reactions
  1% to 10%:
    Central nervous system: Dizziness, headache, vertigo, fever
    Dermatologic: Alopecia (reversible)
    Gastrointestinal: Abdominal pain, nausea, vomiting
    Hepatic: Increased LFTs, jaundice
  <1% (Limited to important or life-threatening): Acute renal failure, eosinophilia, granulocytopenia, increased intracranial pressure, leukopenia, neutropenia, pancytopenia
Drug Interactions
  Cytochrome P450 Effect: CYP1A2 enzyme inhibitor (weak)
  Increased Effect/Toxicity: Albendazole serum levels are increased when taken with dexamethasone, praziquantel.
  Decreased Effect: Cimetidine may increase albendazole metabolism.
Ethanol/Nutrition/Herb Interactions Food: Albendazole serum levels may be increased if taken with a fatty meal (increases the oral bioavailability by 4-5 times).
Mechanism of Action Active metabolite, albendazole, causes selective degeneration of cytoplasmic microtubules in intestinal and tegmental cells of intestinal helminths and larvae; glycogen is depleted, glucose uptake and cholinesterase secretion are impaired, and desecratory substances accumulate intracellulary. ATP production decreases causing energy depletion, immobilization, and worm death.
Pharmacodynamics/Kinetics
  Absorption: <5%; may increase up to 4-5 times when administered with a fatty meal
  Distribution: Well inside hydatid cysts and CSF
  Protein binding: 70%
  (Continued)

39

Albendazole *(Continued)*

Metabolism: Hepatic; extensive first-pass effect; pathways include rapid sulfoxidation (major), hydrolysis, and oxidation

Half-life elimination: 8-12 hours

Time to peak, serum: 2-2.4 hours

Excretion: Urine (<1% as active metabolite); feces

Usual Dosage Oral:

Neurocysticercosis:

<60 kg: 15 mg/kg/day in 2 divided doses (maximum: 800 mg/day) with meals for 8-30 days

≥60 kg: 400 mg twice daily for 8-30 days

Note: Give concurrent anticonvulsant and steroid therapy during first week

Hydatid:

<60 kg: 15 mg/kg/day in 2 divided doses with meals (maximum: 800 mg/day) for three 28-day cycles with 14-day drug-free interval in-between

≥60 kg: 400 mg twice daily for 3 cycles as above

Strongyloidiasis/tapeworm: Children >2 years and Adults: 400 mg/day for 3 days; may repeat in 3 weeks

Giardiasis: Adults: 400 mg/day for 3 days

Hookworm, pinworm, roundworm: Children >2 years and Adults: 400 mg as a single dose; may repeat in 3 weeks

Administration Administer with meals; administer anticonvulsant and steroid therapy during first week of neurocysticercosis therapy

Monitoring Parameters Monitor fecal specimens for ova and parasites for 3 weeks after treatment; if positive, retreat; monitor LFTs, and clinical signs of hepatotoxicity; CBC at start of each 28-day cycle and every 2 weeks during therapy

Patient Information Take with a high fat diet

Dosage Forms Tablet: 200 mg

- ◆ **Albenza®** *see Albendazole on page 39*
- ◆ **Albert® Docusate (Can)** *see Docusate on page 430*
- ◆ **Albert® Glyburide (Can)** *see GlyBURIDE on page 635*
- ◆ **Albert® Oxybutynin (Can)** *see Oxybutynin on page 1023*
- ◆ **Albert® Pentoxifylline (Can)** *see Pentoxifylline on page 1061*
- ◆ **Albumarc®** *see Albumin on page 40*

Albumin *(al BYOO min)*

U.S. Brand Names Albumarc®; Albuminar®; Albutein®; Buminate®; Plasbumin®

Canadian Brand Names Plasbumin®-5; Plasbumin®-25

Synonyms Albumin (Human); Normal Human Serum Albumin (Human); Normal Serum Albumin (Human); Salt Poor Albumin; SPA

Therapeutic Category Blood Product Derivative; Plasma Volume Expander, Colloid

Use Plasma volume expansion and maintenance of cardiac output in the treatment of certain types of shock or impending shock; may be useful for burn patients, ARDS, and cardiopulmonary bypass; other uses considered by some investigators (but not proven) are retroperitoneal surgery, peritonitis, and ascites; unless the condition responsible for hypoproteinemia can be corrected, albumin can provide only symptomatic relief or supportive treatment; nutritional supplementation is not an appropriate indication for albumin

Unlabeled/Investigational Use In cirrhotics, administered with diuretics to help facilitate diuresis; large volume paracentesis; volume expansion in dehydrated, mildly-hypotensive cirrhotics

Pregnancy Risk Factor C

Contraindications Hypersensitivity to albumin or any component of the formulation; patients with severe anemia or cardiac failure; avoid 25% concentration in preterm infants due to risk of idiopathic ventricular hypertrophy

Warnings/Precautions Use with caution in patients with hepatic or renal failure because of added protein load; rapid infusion of albumin solutions may cause vascular overload. All patients should be observed for signs of hypervolemia such as pulmonary edema. Use with caution in those patients for whom sodium restriction is necessary. Rapid infusion may cause hypotension. Due to the ongoing occasional shortage of 5% human albumin, 5% solutions may at times be prepared by diluting 25% human albumin with 0.9% sodium chloride or 5% dextrose in water, however, **do not use sterile water** to dilute albumin solutions, as this has been associated with hypotonic-associated hemolysis.

Adverse Reactions

1% to 10%:

Cardiovascular: Precipitation of congestive heart failure, decreased myocardial contractility

Respiratory: Pulmonary edema, dyspnea

Renal: Salt and water retention

<1% (Limited to important or life-threatening): Hypotension, tachycardia

Overdosage/Toxicology Symptoms include hypervolemia, congestive heart failure, and pulmonary edema.

Stability Do not use solution if it is turbid or contains a deposit; use within 4 hours after opening vial

Mechanism of Action Provides increase in intravascular oncotic pressure and causes mobilization of fluids from interstitial into intravascular space

Usual Dosage I.V.:

5% should be used in hypovolemic patients or intravascularly-depleted patients

25% should be used in patients in whom fluid and sodium intake must be minimized

Dose depends on condition of patient:

Children:

Emergency initial dose: 25 g

Nonemergencies: 25% to 50% of the adult dose

Adults: Usual dose: 25 g; no more than 250 g should be administered within 48 hours

Hypoproteinemia: 0.5-1 g/kg/dose; repeat every 1-2 days as calculated to replace ongoing losses

Hypovolemia: 0.5-1 g/kg/dose; repeat as needed; maximum dose: 6 g/kg/day

Administration Albumin administration must be completed within 6 hours after entering the 5% container, provided that administration is begun within 4 hours of entering the container; rapid infusion may cause vascular overload; albumin is best administered at a rate of 2-4 mL/minute; 25% albumin may be given at a rate of 1 mL/minute

Test Interactions ↑ alkaline phosphatase (S)

Nursing Implications

Albumin administration must be completed within 4 hours after entering container; use 5 micron filter or larger, do **not** administer through 0.22 micron filter

Parenteral: I.V. after initial volume replacement:

5%: Do not exceed 2-4 mL/minute

25%: Do not exceed 1 mL/minute

Observe for signs of hypervolemia, pulmonary edema, and cardiac failure

Additional Information Both 5% and 25% albumin have a sodium concentration of 130-160 mEq/L. There is no risk of hepatitis because albumin is heated to 60°C for 10 hours. Currently, there is no known risk for AIDS.

5% albumin is isotonic; 25% albumin is hypertonic (1500 mOsm/L); dilution of 25% albumin with sterile water can produce hemolysis/renal failure; shelf-life: 3-5 years

Dosage Forms Injection, human: 5% [50 mg/mL] (50 mL, 250 mL, 500 mL, 1000 mL); 25% [250 mg/mL] (20 mL, 50 mL, 100 mL)

♦ **Albuminar**® *see* Albumin *on page 40*

♦ **Albumin (Human)** *see* Albumin *on page 40*

♦ **Albutein**® *see* Albumin *on page 40*

Albuterol (al BYOO ter ole)

Related Information

Antacid Drug Interactions *on page 1477*

Bronchodilators, Comparison of Inhaled Sympathomimetics *on page 1493*

U.S. Brand Names AccuNeb™; Proventil®; Proventil® HFA; Proventil® Repetabs®; Ventolin®; Ventolin® HFA; Ventolin Rotacaps® [DSC]; Volmax®

Canadian Brand Names Alti-Salbutamol; Apo®-Salvent; Novo-Salmol

Synonyms Salbutamol

Therapeutic Category Beta$_2$-Adrenergic Agonist Agent; Bronchodilator; Sympathomimetic

Use Bronchodilator in reversible airway obstruction due to asthma or COPD; prevention of exercise-induced bronchospasm

Pregnancy Risk Factor C

Pregnancy/Breast-Feeding Implications Crosses the placenta; tocolytic effects, fetal tachycardia, fetal hypoglycemia secondary to maternal hyperglycemia with oral or intravenous routes reported. Available evidence suggests safe use during pregnancy. No data on crossing into breast milk or clinical effects on the infant.

Contraindications Hypersensitivity to albuterol, adrenergic amines, or any component of the formulation

Warnings/Precautions Use with caution in patients with hyperthyroidism, diabetes mellitus, or sensitivity to sympathomimetic amines; cardiovascular disorders including coronary insufficiency or hypertension; excessive use may result in tolerance. May cause paradoxical bronchospasm. Increased use may indicate a deterioration of condition and requires a re-evaluation of the patient. Excessive use of inhalers has been associated with fatalities.

Because of its minimal effect on beta$_1$-receptors and its relatively long duration of action, albuterol is a rational choice in the elderly when an inhaled beta agonist is indicated. Oral use should be avoided in the elderly due to adverse effects. All patients should utilize a spacer device when using a metered-dose inhaler; spacers and facemasks should be used in children in children <4 years. Patient response may vary between inhalers that contain chlorofluorocarbons and those which are chlorofluorocarbon-free.

Adverse Reactions Incidence of adverse effects is dependent upon age of patient, dose, and route of administration.

Cardiovascular: Angina, atrial fibrillation, chest discomfort, extrasystoles, flushing, hypertension, palpitations, tachycardia

Central nervous system: CNS stimulation, dizziness, drowsiness, headache, insomnia, irritability, lightheadedness, migraine, nervousness, nightmares, restlessness, sleeplessness, tremor

Dermatologic: Angioedema, erythema multiforme, rash, Stevens-Johnson syndrome, urticaria

Endocrine & metabolic: Hypokalemia

Gastrointestinal: Diarrhea, dry mouth, gastroenteritis, nausea, unusual taste, vomiting, tooth discoloration

Genitourinary: Micturition difficulty

Neuromuscular & skeletal: Muscle cramps, weakness

Otic: Otitis media, vertigo

Respiratory: Asthma exacerbation, bronchospasm, cough, epistaxis, laryngitis, oropharyngeal drying/irritation, oropharyngeal edema

Miscellaneous: Allergic reaction, lymphadenopathy

Overdosage/Toxicology Symptoms include hypertension, tachycardia, angina, and hypokalemia. With hypokalemia and tachyarrhythmias it is prudent to use a cardioselective beta-adrenergic blocker (eg, atenolol or metoprolol). Keep in mind the potential for induction of bronchoconstriction in an asthmatic. Dialysis has not been shown to be of value in the treatment of an overdose with this agent.

Drug Interactions

Increased Effect/Toxicity: When used with inhaled ipratropium, an increased duration of bronchodilation may occur. Cardiovascular effects are potentiated in patients also receiving MAO inhibitors, tricyclic antidepressants, and sympathomimetic agents (eg, (Continued)

Albuterol *(Continued)*

amphetamine, dopamine, dobutamine). Albuterol may increase the risk of malignant arrhythmias with inhaled anesthetics (eg, enflurane, halothane).

Decreased Effect: When used with nonselective beta-adrenergic blockers (eg, propranolol) the effect of albuterol is decreased.

Ethanol/Nutrition/Herb Interactions

Food: Avoid or limit caffeine (may cause CNS stimulation).

Herb/Nutraceutical: Avoid ephedra, yohimbe (may cause CNS stimulation).

Stability

HFA aerosols: Store at 15°C to 25°C (59°F to 77°F)

Ventolin® HFA: Discard after using 200 actuations or 3 months after removal from protective pouch, whichever comes first. Store with mouthpiece down.

Inhalation solution: AccuNeb™: Store at 2°C to 25°C (36°F to 77°F). Do not use if solution changes color or becomes cloudy. Use within 1 week of opening foil pouch.

Nebulization 0.5% solution: Store at 2°C to 30°C (36°F to 86°F). To prepare a 2.5 mg dose, dilute 0.5 mL of solution to a total of 3 mL with normal saline; also compatible with cromolyn or ipratropium nebulizer solutions

Syrup: Store at 2°C to 30°C (36°F to 86°F)

Mechanism of Action Relaxes bronchial smooth muscle by action on beta$_2$-receptors with little effect on heart rate

Pharmacodynamics/Kinetics

Onset of action: Peak effect: Nebulization/oral inhalation: 0.5-2 hours; Oral: 2-3 hours

Duration: Nebulization/oral inhalation: 3-4 hours; Oral: 4-6 hours

Metabolism: Hepatic to an inactive sulfate

Half-life elimination: Inhalation: 3.8 hours; Oral: 3.7-5 hours

Excretion: Urine (30% as unchanged drug)

Usual Dosage

Oral:

Children: Bronchospasm (treatment):

2-6 years: 0.1-0.2 mg/kg/dose 3 times/day; maximum dose not to exceed 12 mg/day (divided doses)

6-12 years: 2 mg/dose 3-4 times/day; maximum dose not to exceed 24 mg/day (divided doses)

Extended release: 4 mg every 12 hours; maximum dose not to exceed 24 mg/day (divided doses)

Children >12 years and Adults: Bronchospasm (treatment): 2-4 mg/dose 3-4 times/day; maximum dose not to exceed 32 mg/day (divided doses)

Extended release: 8 mg every 12 hours; maximum dose not to exceed 32 mg/day (divided doses). A 4 mg dose every 12 hours may be sufficient in some patients, such as adults of low body weight.

Elderly: Bronchospasm (treatment): 2 mg 3-4 times/day; maximum: 8 mg 4 times/day

Inhalation: Children ≥4 years and Adults:

Bronchospasm (treatment):

MDI: 90 mcg/spray: 1-2 inhalations every 4-6 hours; maximum: 12 inhalations/day

Capsule: 200-400 mcg every 4-6 hours

Exercise-induced bronchospasm (prophylaxis):

MDI-CFC aerosol: 2 inhalations 15 minutes before exercising

MDI-HFA aerosol: 2 inhalations 15-30 minutes before exercise

Capsule: 200 mcg 15 minutes before exercise

Nebulization:

Children:

Bronchospasm (treatment): 0.01-0.05 mL/kg of 0.5% solution every 4-6 hours

2-12 years: AccuNeb™: 0.63 mg or 1.25 mg 3-4 times/day, as needed, delivered over 5-15 minutes

Children >40 kg, patients with more severe asthma, or children 11-12 years: May respond better with a 1.25 mg dose

Bronchospasm (acute): 0.01-0.05 mL/kg of 0.5% solution every 4-6 hours; intensive care patients may require more frequent administration; minimum dose: 0.1 mL; maximum dose: 1 mL diluted in 1-2 mL normal saline; continuous nebulized albuterol at 0.3 mg/kg/hour has been used safely in the treatment of severe status asthmaticus in children; continuous nebulized doses of 3 mg/kg/hour ± 2.2 mg/kg/hour in children whose mean age was 20.7 months resulted in no cardiac toxicity; the optimal dosage for continuous nebulization remains to be determined.

Adults:

Bronchospasm (treatment): 2.5 mg, diluted to a total of 3 mL, 3-4 times/day over 5-15 minutes

Bronchospasm (acute) in intensive care patients: 2.5-5 mg every 20 minutes for 3 doses, then 2.5-10 mg every 1-4 hours as needed, **or** 10-15 mg/hour continuously

Hemodialysis: Not removed

Peritoneal dialysis: Significant drug removal is unlikely based on physiochemical characteristics

Dietary Considerations Oral forms should be administered with water 1 hour before or 2 hours after meals.

Administration

Inhalation: MDI: Shake well before use; prime prior to first use, and whenever inhaler has not been used for >2 weeks, by releasing 4 test sprays into the air (away from face)

Oral: Volmax®: Do not crush or chew.

Monitoring Parameters Heart rate, CNS stimulation, asthma symptoms, arterial or capillary blood gases (if patients condition warrants)

Test Interactions ↑ renin (S), ↑ aldosterone (S)

Patient Information Do not exceed recommended dosage; rinse mouth with water following each inhalation to help with dry throat and mouth; follow specific instructions accompanying inhaler; if more than one inhalation is necessary, wait at least 1 full minute between inhalations. May cause nervousness, restlessness, insomnia; if these effects continue after dosage reduction, notify physician; also notify physician if palpitations, tachycardia, chest pain, muscle tremors, dizziness, headache, flushing or if breathing difficulty persists.

Nursing Implications Before using, the inhaler must be shaken well; assess lung sounds, pulse, and blood pressure before administration and during peak of medication; observe patient for wheezing after administration, if this occurs, call physician

Dosage Forms
Aerosol, oral: 90 mcg/dose (17 g) [200 doses]
    Proventil®: 90 mcg/dose (17 g) [200 doses]
    Ventolin®: 90 mcg/dose (6.8 g) [80 doses], (17 g) [200 doses]
Aerosol, oral, as sulfate [chlorofluorocarbon free]:
    Proventil® HFA: 90 mcg/dose (6.7 g) [200 doses]
    Ventolin® HFA: 90 mcg/dose (18 g) [200 doses]
Powder for oral inhalation, as sulfate [capsule] (Ventolin Rotacaps® [DSC]): 200 mcg [to be used with Rotahaler® inhalation device; contains lactose 25 mg]
Solution for oral inhalation, as sulfate: 0.083% (3 mL); 0.5% (20 mL)
    AccuNeb™: 0.63 mg/3 mL (5 vials/pouch); 1.25 mg/3 mL (5 vials/pouch)
    Proventil®: 0.083% (3 mL); 0.5% (20 mL)
Syrup, as sulfate: 2 mg/5 mL (120 mL, 480 mL)
    Ventolin®: 2 mg/5 mL (480 mL) [alcohol and sugar free; strawberry flavor]
Tablet, as sulfate: 2 mg, 4 mg
Tablet, extended release, as sulfate:
    Proventil® Repetabs®: 4 mg
    Volmax®: 4 mg, 8 mg

- **Albuterol and Ipratropium** see Ipratropium and Albuterol on page 741
- **Alcaine®** see Proparacaine on page 1144

Alclometasone (al kloe MET a sone)

Related Information
Corticosteroids Comparison on page 1495

U.S. Brand Names Aclovate®

Synonyms Alclometasone Dipropionate

Therapeutic Category Anti-inflammatory Agent; Corticosteroid, Topical (Low Potency)

Use Treatment of inflammation of corticosteroid-responsive dermatosis (low potency topical corticosteroid)

Pregnancy Risk Factor C

Contraindications Hypersensitivity to alclometasone or any component of the formulation; viral, fungal, or tubercular skin lesions

Warnings/Precautions Adverse systemic effects may occur when used on large areas of the body, denuded areas, for prolonged periods of time, with an occlusive dressing, and/or in infants or small children (not for use in children <1 year of age)

Adverse Reactions Frequency not defined.
Dermatologic: Acne, hypopigmentation, allergic dermatitis, maceration of the skin, skin atrophy, striae, miliaria, telangiectasia
Endocrine & metabolic: HPA suppression, Cushing's syndrome, growth retardation
Local: Burning, itching, irritation, dryness, folliculitis, hypertrichosis
Systemic: HPA axis suppression, Cushing's syndrome, hyperglycemia; these reactions occur more frequently with occlusive dressings
Miscellaneous: Secondary infection

Overdosage/Toxicology Symptoms include cushingoid appearance (systemic), muscle weakness (systemic), osteoporosis (systemic) all with long-term use only. When consumed in excessive quantities for prolonged periods, systemic hypercorticism and adrenal suppression may occur; in those cases, discontinuation and withdrawal of the corticosteroid should be done judiciously.

Stability Store between 2°C and 30°C (36°F and 86°F)

Mechanism of Action Stimulates the synthesis of enzymes needed to decrease inflammation, suppress mitotic activity, and cause vasoconstriction

Usual Dosage Topical: Apply a thin film to the affected area 2-3 times/day. Therapy should be discontinued when control is achieved; if no improvement is seen, reassessment of diagnosis may be necessary.

Patient Information Before applying, gently wash area to reduce risk of infection; apply a thin film to cleansed area and rub in gently and thoroughly until medication vanishes; avoid exposure to sunlight, severe sunburn may occur

Nursing Implications For external use only; do not use on open wounds; apply sparingly to occlusive dressings; should not be used in the presence of open or weeping lesions

Dosage Forms
Cream, as dipropionate: 0.05% (15 g, 45 g, 60 g)
Ointment, topical, as dipropionate: 0.05% (15 g, 45 g, 60 g)

- **Alclometasone Dipropionate** see Alclometasone on page 43
- **Alcomicin® (Can)** see Gentamicin on page 627
- **Alconefrin® Nasal [OTC]** see Phenylephrine on page 1075
- **Aldactazide®** see Hydrochlorothiazide and Spironolactone on page 675
- **Aldactazide 25® (Can)** see Hydrochlorothiazide and Spironolactone on page 675
- **Aldactazide 50® (Can)** see Hydrochlorothiazide and Spironolactone on page 675
- **Aldactone®** see Spironolactone on page 1256
- **Aldara™** see Imiquimod on page 709

Aldesleukin (al des LOO kin)

U.S. Brand Names Proleukin®

Canadian Brand Names Proleukin®

(Continued)

Aldesleukin *(Continued)*

Synonyms Epidermal Thymocyte Activating Factor; ETAF; IL-2; Interleukin-2; Lymphocyte Mitogenic Factor; NSC-373364; T-Cell Growth Factor; TCGF; Thymocyte Stimulating Factor

Therapeutic Category Biological Response Modulator; Interleukin

Use Treatment of metastatic renal cell cancer, melanoma

Unlabeled/Investigational Use Investigational: Multiple myeloma, HIV infection, and AIDS; may be used in conjunction with lymphokine-activated killer (LAK) cells, tumor-infiltrating lymphocyte (TIL) cells, interleukin-1, and interferons; colorectal cancer; non-Hodgkin's lymphoma

Pregnancy Risk Factor C

Pregnancy/Breast-Feeding Implications There are no adequate and well-controlled studies in pregnant women; use during pregnancy only if benefits to the mother outweigh potential risk to the fetus. Contraception is recommended for fertile males or females using this medication. Breast-feeding is not recommended.

Contraindications Hypersensitivity to aldesleukin or any component of the formulation; patients with abnormal thallium stress or pulmonary function tests; patients who have had an organ allograft; retreatment in patients who have experienced sustained ventricular tachycardia (≥5 beats), refractory cardiac rhythm disturbances, recurrent chest pain with EKG changes consistent with angina or myocardial infarction, intubation ≥72 hours, pericardial tamponade, renal dialysis for ≥72 hours, coma or toxic psychosis lasting ≥48 hours, repetitive or refractory seizures, bowel ischemia/perforation, GI bleeding requiring surgery

Warnings/Precautions High-dose IL-2 therapy has been associated with capillary leak syndrome (CLS); CLS results in hypotension and reduced organ perfusion which may be severe and can result in death; therapy should be restricted to patients with normal cardiac and pulmonary functions as defined by thallium stress and formal pulmonary function testing; extreme caution should be used in patients with normal thallium stress tests and pulmonary functions tests who have a history of prior cardiac or pulmonary disease. Patients must have a serum creatinine of ≤1.5 mg/dL prior to treatment.

Adverse effects are frequent and sometimes fatal. May exacerbate pre-existing or initial presentation of autoimmune diseases and inflammatory disorders. Patients should be evaluated and treated for CNS metastases and have a negative scan prior to treatment. Mental status changes (irritability, confusion, depression) can occur and may indicate bacteremia, hypoperfusion, CNS malignancy, or CNS toxicity.

Intensive aldesleukin treatment is associated with impaired neutrophil function (reduced chemotaxis) and with an increased risk of disseminated infection, including sepsis and bacterial endocarditis, in treated patients. Consequently, pre-existing bacterial infections should be adequately treated prior to initiation of therapy. Additionally, all patients with indwelling central lines should receive antibiotic prophylaxis effective against *S. aureus*. Antibiotic prophylaxis which has been associated with a reduced incidence of staphylococcal infections in aldesleukin studies includes the use of oxacillin, nafcillin, ciprofloxacin, or vancomycin.

Standard prophylactic supportive care during high-dose IL-2 treatment includes acetaminophen to relieve constitutional symptoms and an H_2 antagonist to reduce the risk of GI ulceration and/or bleeding.

Adverse Reactions

>10%:

Cardiovascular: Sensory dysfunction, sinus tachycardia, arrhythmias, pulmonary congestion; hypotension (dose-limiting toxicity) which may require vasopressor support and hemodynamic changes resembling those seen in septic shock can be seen within 2 hours of administration; chest pain, acute myocardial infarction, SVT with hypotension has been reported, edema

Central nervous system: Dizziness, pain, fever, chills, cognitive changes, fatigue, malaise, disorientation, somnolence, paranoid delusion, and other behavioral changes; reversible and dose related; however, may continue to worsen for several days even after the infusion is stopped

Dermatologic: Pruritus, erythema, rash, dry skin, exfoliative dermatitis, macular erythema

Gastrointestinal: Nausea, vomiting, weight gain, diarrhea, stomatitis, anorexia, GI bleeding

Hematologic: Anemia, thrombocytopenia, leukopenia, eosinophilia, coagulation disorders

Hepatic: Elevated transaminase and alkaline phosphatase, jaundice

Neuromuscular & skeletal: Weakness, rigors which can be decreased or ameliorated with acetaminophen or a nonsteroidal agent and meperidine

Renal: Oliguria, anuria, proteinuria; renal failure (dose-limiting toxicity) manifested as oliguria noted within 24-48 hours of initiation of therapy; marked fluid retention, azotemia, and increased serum creatinine seen, which may return to baseline within 7 days of discontinuation of therapy; hypophosphatemia

Respiratory: Dyspnea, pulmonary edema

1% to 10%: Cardiovascular: Increase in vascular permeability: Capillary-leak syndrome manifested by severe peripheral edema, ascites, pulmonary infiltration, and pleural effusion; occurs in 2% to 4% of patients and is resolved after therapy ends

<1% (Limited to important or life-threatening): Alopecia, coma, congestive heart failure, pancreatitis, polyuria, seizure

Overdosage/Toxicology Side effects following the use of aldesleukin are dose related. Administration of more than the recommended dose has been associated with a more rapid onset of expected dose-limiting toxicities. Adverse reactions generally will reverse when the drug is stopped, particularly because of its short serum half-life. Provide supportive treatment of any continuing symptoms. Life-threatening toxicities have been ameliorated by the I.V. administration of dexamethasone, which may result in a less than therapeutic effect of aldesleukin.

Drug Interactions

Increased Effect/Toxicity: Aldesleukin may affect central nervous function; therefore, interactions could occur following concomitant administration of psychotropic drugs (eg, narcotics, analgesics, antiemetics, sedatives, tranquilizers).

Concomitant administration of drugs possessing nephrotoxic (eg, aminoglycosides, indomethacin), myelotoxic (eg, cytotoxic chemotherapy), cardiotoxic (eg, doxorubicin), or hepatotoxic (eg, methotrexate, asparaginase) effects with aldesleukin may increase toxicity in these organ systems. The safety and efficacy of aldesleukin in combination with chemotherapies has not been established.

Beta-blockers and other antihypertensives may potentiate the hypotension seen with aldesleukin.

Decreased Effect: Corticosteroids have been shown to decrease toxicity of IL-2, but have not been used since there is concern that they may reduce the efficacy of the lymphokine.

Ethanol/Nutrition/Herb Interactions Ethanol: Avoid ethanol (due to CNS adverse effects)

Stability

Store vials of lyophilized injection in a refrigerator at 2°C to 8°C (36°F to 46°F).

Reconstituted or diluted solution is stable for up to 48 hours at refrigerated and room temperatures 2°C to 25°C (36°F to 77°F); however, since this product contains no preservatives, the reconstituted and diluted solutions should be stored in the refrigerator

Compatible only with D₅W; **Incompatible** with NS

Gently swirl, do not shake.

Note: As with most biological proteins, solutions containing IL-2 should not be filtered; filtration will result in significant loss of bioactivity

Recommendations for aldesleukin dilution: See table.

Final Dilution Concentration (mcg/mL)	Final Dilution Concentration (10⁶ int. units/mL)	Stability
<30	<0.49	Albumin must be added to bag **prior to addition** of aldesleukin at a final concentration of 0.1% (1 mg/mL) albumin; stable at room temperature or at ≥32°C (89°F) for 6 days*†
≥30 to ≤70	≥0.49 to ≤1.1	Stable at room temperature at 6 days without albumin added or at ≥32°C (89°F) for 6 days only if albumin is added (0.1%)*†
70-100	1.2-1.6	Unstable; avoid use
>100-500	1.7-8.2	Stable at room temperature and at ≥32°C (89°F) for 6 days*†

*These solutions do not contain a preservative; use for more than 24 hours may not be advisable.

†Continuous infusion via ambulatory infusion device raises aldesleukin to this temperature.

Mechanism of Action IL-2 promotes proliferation, differentiation, and recruitment of T and B cells, natural killer (NK) cells, and thymocytes; IL-2 also causes cytolytic activity in a subset of lymphocytes and subsequent interactions between the immune system and malignant cells; IL-2 can stimulate lymphokine-activated killer (LAK) cells and tumor-infiltrating lymphocytes (TIL) cells. LAK cells (which are derived from lymphocytes from a patient and incubated in IL-2) have the ability to lyse cells which are resistant to NK cells; TIL cells (which are derived from cancerous tissue from a patient and incubated in IL-2) have been shown to be 50% more effective than LAK cells in experimental studies.

Pharmacodynamics/Kinetics

Distribution: V_d: 4-7 L; primarily in plasma and then in the lymphocytes

Bioavailability: I.M.: 37%

Half-life elimination: Initial: 6-13 minutes; Terminal: 80-120 minutes

Usual Dosage Refer to individual protocols; all orders must be written in million International units (million int. units)

I.V.:

Renal cell carcinoma: 600,000 int. units/kg every 8 hours for a maximum of 14 doses; repeat after 9 days of rest for a total of 28 doses per course. Re-evaluate at 4 weeks. Retreat if needed 7 weeks after hospital discharge from previous course.

Melanoma:

Single-agent use: As in renal cell carcinoma

In combination with cytotoxic agents: 24 million int. units/m² days 12-16 and 19-23

S.C.:

Single-agent doses: 3-18 million int. units/day for 5 days weekly and repeated weekly up to 6 weeks

In combination with interferon:

5 million int. units/m² 3 times/week

1.8 million int. units/m² twice daily 5 days/week for 6 weeks

Dose modification: In high-dose therapy of RCC, see manufacturer's guidelines for holding and restarting therapy; hold or interrupt a dose - DO NOT DOSE REDUCE; or refer to specific protocol.

Retreatment: Patients should be evaluated for response approximately 4 weeks after completion of a course of therapy and again immediately prior to the scheduled start of the next treatment course; additional courses of treatment may be given to patients only if there is some tumor shrinkage or stable disease following the last course and retreatment is not contraindicated. Each treatment course should be separated by a rest period of at least 7 weeks from the date of hospital discharge; tumors have continued to regress up to 12 months following the initiation of therapy

Investigational regimen: S.C.: 11 million int. units (flat dose) daily x 4 days per week for 4 consecutive weeks; repeat every 6 weeks

Administration Administer in D₅W only; incompatible with sodium chloride solutions

Management of symptoms related to vascular leak syndrome:

If actual body weight increases >10% above baseline, or rales or rhonchi are audible:

Administer furosemide at dosage determined by patient response

Administer dopamine hydrochloride 2-4 mcg/kg/minute to maintain renal blood flow and urine output

If patient has dyspnea at rest: Administer supplemental oxygen by face mask

(Continued)

45

Aldesleukin *(Continued)*

If patient has severe respiratory distress: Intubate patient and provide mechanical ventilation; administer ranitidine (as the hydrochloride salt), 50 mg I.V. every 8-12 hours as prophylaxis against stress ulcers

Monitoring Parameters

The following clinical evaluations are recommended for all patients prior to beginning treatment and then daily during drug administration:

Standard hematologic tests including CBC, differential, and platelet counts

Blood chemistries including electrolytes, renal and hepatic function tests

Chest x-rays

Daily monitoring during therapy should include vital signs (temperature, pulse, blood pressure, and respiration rate) and weight; in a patient with a decreased blood pressure, especially <90 mm Hg, constant cardiac monitoring for rhythm should be conducted. If an abnormal complex or rhythm is seen, an EKG should be performed; vital signs in these hypotension patients should be taken hourly and central venous pressure (CVP) checked.

During treatment, pulmonary function should be monitored on a regular basis by clinical examination, assessment of vital signs and pulse oximetry. Patients with dyspnea or clinical signs of respiratory impairment (tachypnea or rales) should be further assessed with arterial blood gas determination. These tests are to be repeated as often as clinically indicated.

Cardiac function is assessed daily by clinical examination and assessment of vital signs. Patients with signs or symptoms of chest pain, murmurs, gallops, irregular rhythm or palpitations should be further assessed with an EKG examination and CPK evaluation. If there is evidence of cardiac ischemia or congestive heart failure, a repeat thallium study should be done.

Nursing Implications

Prior to treatment: Standard hematologic tests, blood chemistries, chest x-rays

During treatment: Pulmonary function, assessment of vital signs and pulse oximetry. Patients with dyspnea or clinical signs of respiratory impairment: Arterial blood gas determination

Additional Information

1 Cetus unit = 6 int. units

1.1 mg = 18×10^6 int. units (or 3×10^6 Cetus units)

1 Roche unit (Teceleukin) = 3 int. units

Reimbursement Hotline: 1-800-775-7533

Professional Services: 1-800-244-7668

Dosage Forms Powder for injection, lyophilized: 22×10^6 int. units [18 million int. units/mL = 1.1 mg/mL when reconstituted]

♦ **Aldomet®** *see* Methyldopa *on page 891*

♦ **Aldoril®** *see* Methyldopa and Hydrochlorothiazide *on page 892*

Alemtuzumab *(ay lem TU zoo mab)*

U.S. Brand Names Campath®

Synonyms Campath-1H; DNA-derived Humanized Monoclonal Antibody; Humanized IgG1 Anti-CD52 Monoclonal Antibody

Therapeutic Category Antineoplastic Agent, Monoclonal Antibody

Use Treatment of B-cell chronic lymphocytic leukemia (B-CLL) in patients treated with alkylating agents and who have failed fludarabine therapy

Unlabeled/Investigational Use Rheumatoid arthritis, graft versus host disease, multiple myeloma

Pregnancy Risk Factor C

Pregnancy/Breast-Feeding Implications Human IgG is known to cross the placental barrier; therefore, alemtuzumab may also cross the barrier and cause fetal B- and T-lymphocyte depletion. Well-controlled human trials have not been done. Use during pregnancy only if the benefit to the mother outweighs the potential risk to the fetus. Excretion in breast milk is unknown; breast-feeding is contraindicated.

Contraindications Known type 1 hypersensitivity or anaphylactic reaction to alemtuzumab or any component of the formulation; hypersensitivity to another monoclonal antibody; active systemic infections; underlying immunodeficiency (eg, seropositive for HIV); single doses >30 mg or cumulative doses >90 mg/week; administration by I.V. push or bolus

Warnings/Precautions Serious infections may occur. Prophylactic therapy against PCP pneumonia and herpes viral infections is recommended. Premedicate with an antihistamine and acetaminophen prior to dosing. Gradual escalation to the recommended maintenance dose is required at initiation and if therapy is interrupted for ≥7 days. Irradiation of any blood products administered during lymphopenia is recommended. Discontinue therapy during serious infection, serious hematologic or other serious toxicity until the event resolves. Permanently discontinue if autoimmune anemia or autoimmune thrombocytopenia occurs. Patients should not be immunized with live, viral vaccines during or recently after treatment. Women of childbearing potential and men of reproductive potential should use effective contraceptive methods during treatment and for a minimum of 6 months following therapy. Safety and efficacy have not been established in pediatric patients.

Adverse Reactions

>10%:

Cardiovascular: Hypotension (15% to 32%, infusion-related), peripheral edema (13%), hypertension (11%), tachycardia/SVT (11%)

Central nervous system: Drug-related fever (83%, infusion-related), fatigue (22% to 34%, infusion-related), headache (13% to 24%), dysthesias (15%), dizziness (12%), neutropenic fever (10%)

Dermatologic: Rash (30% to 40%, infusion-related), urticaria (22% to 30%, infusion-related), pruritus (14% to 24%, infusion-related)

Gastrointestinal: Nausea (47% to 54%), vomiting (33% to 41%), anorexia (20%), diarrhea (13% to 22%, infusion-related), stomatitis/mucositis (14%), abdominal pain (11%)

Hematologic: Lymphopenia, severe neutropenia (64% to 70%), severe anemia (38% to 47%), severe thrombocytopenia (50% to 52%)

Neuromuscular & skeletal: Rigors (89%, infusion-related), skeletal muscle pain (24%), weakness (13%), myalgia (11%)

Respiratory: Dyspnea (17% to 26%, infusion-related), cough (25%), bronchitis/pneumonitis (21%), pharyngitis (12%)

Miscellaneous: Infection (43% including sepsis, pneumonia, opportunistic infections; received PCP pneumonia and herpes prophylaxis); diaphoresis (19%)

1% to 10%:

Cardiovascular: Chest pain (10%)

Central nervous system: Insomnia (10%), malaise (9%), depression (7%), temperature change sensation (5%), somnolence (5%)

Dermatologic: Purpura (8%)

Gastrointestinal: Dyspepsia (10%), constipation (9%)

Hematologic: Pancytopenia/marrow hypoplasia (6%), positive Coombs' test without hemolysis (2%), autoimmune thrombocytopenia (2%), antibodies to alemtuzumab (2%), autoimmune hemolytic anemia (1%)

Neuromuscular & skeletal: Back pain (10%), tremor (7%)

Respiratory: Bronchospasm (9%), epistaxis (7%), rhinitis (7%)

<1% (Limited to important or life-threatening): Acidosis, acute renal failure, agranulocytosis, anaphylactoid reactions, angina pectoris, angioedema, anuria, ascites, asthma, bone marrow aplasia, cardiac arrest, cardiac failure, cerebral hemorrhage, coma, deep vein thrombosis, disseminated intravascular coagulation, gastrointestinal hemorrhage, hemolytic anemia, hemoptysis, hepatic failure, hyperthyroidism, hypoxia, interstitial pneumonitis, intestinal perforation, intracranial hemorrhage, malignant lymphoma, marrow depression, meningitis, myocardial infarction, pancreatitis, paralysis, peptic ulcer, pericarditis, peritonitis, pneumothorax, polymyositis, progressive multifocal leukoencephalopathy, pseudomembranous colitis, pulmonary edema, pulmonary embolism, pulmonary fibrosis, renal dysfunction, respiratory alkalosis, respiratory depression, secondary leukemia, seizure (grand mal), splenic infarction, stridor, subarachnoid hemorrhage, syncope, toxic nephropathy, transformation to aggressive lymphoma, transformation to prolymphocytic leukemia, thrombocythemia, thrombophlebitis, ventricular arrhythmia, ventricular tachycardia

Overdosage/Toxicology Symptoms are likely to be extensions of adverse events (may include respiratory distress, bronchospasm, anuria). Tumor lysis syndrome has been associated with accidental overdose. Treatment is symptom directed and supportive.

Stability Prior to dilution, store at 2°C to 8°C (36°F to 46°F). Do not freeze; protect from direct sunlight. Throw away ampuls that have been frozen. Do not shake ampul prior to use. Withdraw dose into a syringe. Filter with a 5-micron filter prior to dilution. Inject into 100 mL NS or D₅W. Gently invert bag to mix solution. Following dilution, use within 8 hours. Store at room temperature or refrigerate; protect from light. Medications should not be added to the solution or simultaneously infused through the same I.V. line.

Mechanism of Action Recombinant monoclonal antibody binds to CD52, a nonmodulating antigen present on the surface of B and T lymphocytes, a majority of monocytes, macrophages, NK cells and a subpopulation of granulocytes. After binding to leukemic cells, an antibody-dependent lysis occurs.

Pharmacodynamics/Kinetics Half-life elimination: 12 days

Usual Dosage Note: **Dose escalation is required;** usually accomplished in 3-7 days. Do not exceed single doses >30 mg or cumulative doses >90 mg/week. Premedicate with diphenhydramine and acetaminophen 30 minutes before initiation of infusion. Start anti-infective prophylaxis. Discontinue therapy during serious infection, serious hematologic or other serious toxicity until the event resolves. Permanently discontinue if evidence of autoimmune anemia or autoimmune thrombocytopenia occurs.

I.V. infusion: Adults: B-CLL:

Initial: 3 mg/day as a 2-hour infusion; when daily dose is tolerated (eg, infusion-related toxicities at or below Grade 2) increase to 10 mg/day and continue until tolerated; when 10 mg dose tolerated, increase to 30 mg/day

Maintenance: 30 mg/day 3 times/week on alternate days (ie, Monday, Wednesday, Friday) for up to 12 weeks

Dosage adjustment for hematologic toxicity (severe neutropenia or thrombocytopenia, not autoimmune):

First occurrence: ANC <250/μL and/or platelet count ≤25,000/μL: Hold therapy; resume at same dose when ANC ≥500/μL and platelet count ≥50,000/μL. If delay between dosing is ≥7 days, initiate at 3 mg/day and escalate dose as above according to patient tolerance

Second occurrence: ANC <250/μL and/or platelet count ≤25,000/μL: Hold therapy; resume at 10 mg/day when ANC ≥500/μL and platelet count ≥50,000/μL. If delay between dosing is ≥7 days, initiate at 3 mg/day and escalate dose to a maximum of 10 mg/day according to patient tolerance.

Third occurrence: ANC <250/μL and/or platelet count ≤25,000/μL: Permanently discontinue therapy

Patients with a baseline ANC ≤500/μL and/or a baseline platelet count ≤25,000/μL at initiation of therapy: If ANC and/or platelet counts decreased to ≤50% of the baseline value, hold therapy. When ANC and/or platelet count return to baseline, resume therapy. If delay between dosing is ≥7 days, initiate at 3 mg/day and escalate dose as above according to patient tolerance.

Administration Administer by I.V. infusion only over 2 hours. Premedicate with diphenhydramine and acetaminophen 30 minutes before initiation of infusion. Start anti-infective prophylaxis. Other drugs should not be added to or simultaneously infused through the same I.V. line. Do not give I.V. bolus or push.

Monitoring Parameters Vital signs; carefully monitor BP especially in patient with ischemic heart disease or on antihypertensive medications; CBC and platelets weekly (more frequent monitoring needed if any hematologic abnormality occurs); signs and symptoms of infection; CD4+ lymphocyte counts

Test Interactions May interfere with diagnostic serum tests that utilize antibodies.

(Continued)

Alemtuzumab *(Continued)*

Patient Information This medication can only be administered I.V. During infusion, you will be closely monitored. You will need frequent laboratory tests during course of therapy. Do not use any prescription or OTC medications unless approved by your prescriber. Maintain adequate hydration (2-3 L/day unless otherwise instructed) and nutrition (frequent small meals will help). You may experience abdominal pain, mouth sores, nausea, or vomiting (small frequent meals, good mouth care with soft toothbrush or swabs, sucking lozenges or chewing gum, and avoidance of spicy or salty foods may help). Report unresolved gastro-intestinal problems, persistent fever, chills, muscle pain, skin rash, unusual bleeding or bruising, signs of infection (mouth sores, sore throat, white plaques in mouth or perianal area, burning on urination); swelling of extremities; difficulty breathing; chest pain or palpitations; or other persistent adverse reactions. Inform prescriber if you are or intend to be pregnant. Do not breast-feed.

Nursing Implications Monitor closely for infusion reactions. These include hypotension, rigors, fever, shortness of breath, bronchospasm, chills, and/or rash. Patient must be closely monitored during infusion.

Dosage Forms Injection, solution: 10 mg/mL (3 mL)

Alendronate *(a LEN droe nate)*

U.S. Brand Names Fosamax®

Canadian Brand Names Fosamax®

Synonyms Alendronate Sodium

Therapeutic Category Bisphosphonate Derivative

Use Treatment and prevention of osteoporosis in postmenopausal females; treatment of osteoporosis in males; Paget's disease of the bone in patients who are symptomatic, at risk for future complications, or with alkaline phosphatase ≥2 times the upper limit of normal; treatment of glucocorticoid-induced osteoporosis in males and females with low bone mineral density who are receiving a daily dosage ≥7.5 mg of prednisone (or equivalent)

Pregnancy Risk Factor C

Pregnancy/Breast-Feeding Implications Safety and efficacy have not been established in pregnant women. Animal studies have shown delays in delivery and fetal/neonatal death (secondary to hypocalcemia). It is not known if alendronate is excreted in human milk; use caution if administering to a nursing woman.

Contraindications Hypersensitivity to alendronate, other bisphosphonates, or any component of the formulation; hypocalcemia; abnormalities of the esophagus which delay esophageal emptying such as stricture or achalasia; inability to stand or sit upright for at least 30 minutes

Warnings/Precautions Use caution in patients with renal impairment; hypocalcemia must be corrected before therapy initiation; ensure adequate calcium and vitamin D intake. May cause irritation to upper gastrointestinal mucosa. Esophagitis, esophageal ulcers, esophageal erosions, and esophageal stricture (rare) have been reported; risk increases in patients unable to comply with dosing instructions. Use with caution in patients with dysphagia, esophageal disease, gastritis, duodenitis, or ulcers (may worsen underlying condition).

Adverse Reactions Note: Incidence of adverse effects increases significantly in patients treated for Paget's disease at 40 mg/day, mostly GI adverse effects.

>10%: Endocrine & metabolic: Hypocalcemia (transient, mild, 18%); hypophosphatemia (transient, mild, 10%)

1% to 10%:

Central nervous system: Headache (0.2% to 3%)

Gastrointestinal: Abdominal pain (1% to 7%), acid reflux (1% to 5%), dyspepsia (1% to 4%), nausea (1% to 4%), flatulence (0.2% to 4%), diarrhea (0.6% to 3%), constipation (0.3% to 3%), esophageal ulcer (0.1% to 2%), abdominal distension (0.2% to 1%), gastritis (0.2% to 1%), vomiting (0.1% to 1%), dysphagia (0.1% to 1%), gastric ulcer (1%), melena (1%)

Neuromuscular & skeletal: Musculoskeletal pain (0.4% to 4%), muscle cramps (0.2% to 1%)

<1% (Limited to important or life-threatening): Angioedema, duodenal ulcer, esophageal erosions, esophageal stricture, esophagitis, hypersensitivity reactions, oropharyngeal ulceration, rash, taste perversion, urticaria, uveitis

Overdosage/Toxicology Symptoms include hypocalcemia, hypophosphatemia, and upper GI adverse events (upset stomach, heartburn, esophagitis, gastritis or ulcer). Treat with milk or antacids to bind alendronate. Dialysis would not be beneficial.

Drug Interactions

Increased Effect/Toxicity: I.V. ranitidine has been shown to double the bioavailability of alendronate. Estrogen replacement therapy, in combination with alendronate, may enhance the therapeutic effects of both agents on the maintenance of bone mineralization. An increased incidence of adverse GI effects has been noted when >10 mg alendronate is used in patients taking aspirin-containing products.

Decreased Effect: Oral medications (especially those containing multivalent cations, including calcium and antacids): May interfere with alendronate absorption; wait at least 30 minutes after taking alendronate before taking any oral medications

Ethanol/Nutrition/Herb Interactions Food: All food and beverages interfere with absorption. Coadministration with caffeine may reduce alendronate efficacy. Coadministration with dairy products may decrease alendronate absorption. Beverages (especially orange juice and coffee), food, and medications (eg, antacids, calcium, iron, and multivalent cations) may reduce the absorption of alendronate as much as 60%.

Stability Store at room temperature of 15°C to 30°C (59°F to 86°F); keep in well-closed container

Mechanism of Action A bisphosphonate which inhibits bone resorption via actions on osteoclasts or on osteoclast precursors; decreases the rate of bone resorption direction, leading to an indirect decrease in bone formation

Pharmacodynamics/Kinetics
Distribution: 28 L (exclusive of bone)
Protein binding: ~78%
Metabolism: None
Bioavailability: Fasting: Female: 0.7%; Male: 0.6%; reduced to 60% with food or drink
Half-life elimination: Exceeds 10 years
Excretion: Urine; feces (as unabsorbed drug)

Usual Dosage Oral: Alendronate must be taken with a full glass (6-8 oz) of plain water first thing in the morning and ≥30 minutes before the first food, beverage, or other medication of the day. Patients should be instructed to stay upright (not to lie down) for at least 30 minutes **and** until after first food of the day (to reduce esophageal irritation). Patients should receive supplemental calcium and vitamin D if dietary intake is inadequate.

Adults:
  Osteoporosis in postmenopausal females:
    Prophylaxis: 5 mg once daily or 35 mg once weekly
    Treatment: 10 mg once daily or 70 mg once weekly
  Osteoporosis in males: 10 mg once daily
  Paget's disease of bone: 40 mg once daily for 6 months
    Retreatment: Relapses during the 12 months following therapy occurred in 9% of patients who responded to treatment. Specific retreatment data are not available. Retreatment with alendronate may be considered, following a 6-month post-treatment evaluation period, in patients who have relapsed based on increases in serum alkaline phosphatase, which should be measured periodically. Retreatment may also be considered in those who failed to normalize their serum alkaline phosphatase.
    Glucocorticoid-induced osteoporosis: Treatment: 5 mg once daily; a dose of 10 mg once daily should be used in postmenopausal females who are not receiving estrogen. Patients treated with glucocorticoids should receive adequate amounts of calcium and vitamin D.

Elderly: No dosage adjustment is necessary

Dosage adjustment in renal impairment:
  Cl_{cr} 35-60 mL/minute: None necessary
  Cl_{cr} <35 mL/minute: Alendronate is not recommended due to lack of experience

Dosage adjustment in hepatic impairment: None necessary

Dietary Considerations Ensure adequate calcium and vitamin D intake; however, wait at least 30 minutes after taking alendronate before taking any supplement. Must be taken with plain water first thing in the morning and at least 30 minutes before the first food or beverage of the day.

Administration It is imperative to administer alendronate 30-60 minutes before the patient takes any food, drink, or other medications orally to avoid interference with absorption. The patient should take alendronate on an empty stomach with a full glass (8 oz) of **plain water** (not mineral water) and avoid lying down for 30 minutes after swallowing tablet to help delivery to stomach.

Monitoring Parameters Alkaline phosphatase should be periodically measured; serum calcium and phosphorus; monitor pain and fracture rate; hormonal status (male and female) prior to therapy; bone mineral density (should be done prior to initiation of therapy and after 6-12 months of combined glucocorticoid and alendronate treatment)

Reference Range Calcium (total): Adults: 9.0-11.0 mg/dL (2.05-2.54 mmol/L), may slightly decrease with aging; phosphorus: 2.5-4.5 mg/dL (0.81-1.45 mmol/L)

Patient Information Patients should be instructed that the expected benefits of alendronate may only be obtained when each tablet is taken with plain water the first thing in the morning and at least 30 minutes before the first food, beverage, or medication of the day. Also instruct them that waiting >30 minutes will improve alendronate absorption. Even dosing with orange juice or coffee markedly reduces the absorption of alendronate.

Instruct patients to take alendronate with a full glass of water (6-8 oz 180-240 mL) and not to lie down (stay fully upright sitting or standing) for at least 30 minutes following administration to facilitate delivery to the stomach and reduce the potential for esophageal irritation.

Patients should be instructed to take supplemental calcium and vitamin D if dietary intake is inadequate. Consider weight-bearing exercise along with the modification of certain behavioral factors, such as excessive cigarette smoking or alcohol consumption if these factors exist.

Nursing Implications Patients should be instructed that the expected benefits of alendronate may only be obtained when each tablet is administered with plain water the first thing in the morning and at least 30 minutes before the first food, beverage, or medication of the day. Also instruct them that waiting >30 minutes will improve alendronate absorption. Even dosing with orange juice or coffee markedly reduces the absorption of alendronate.

Patients should be instructed to take alendronate with a full glass of water (6-8 oz/180-240 mL); do not allow patient to lie down (keep patient fully upright sitting or standing) for at least 30 minutes following administration **and** until after eating the first food of the day to facilitate delivery to the stomach and reduce the potential for esophageal irritation.

Patients should be instructed to take supplemental calcium and vitamin D if dietary intake is inadequate. Consider weight-bearing exercise along with the modification of certain behavioral factors, such as excessive cigarette smoking or ethanol consumption if these factors exist.

Dosage Forms Tablet, as sodium: 5 mg, 10 mg, 35 mg, 40 mg, 70 mg

Alfentanil (al FEN ta nil)

Related Information
Narcotic Agonists Comparison *on page 1506*

U.S. Brand Names Alfenta®

Canadian Brand Names Alfenta®

Synonyms Alfentanil Hydrochloride

Therapeutic Category Analgesic, Narcotic

Use Analgesic adjunct given by continuous infusion or in incremental doses in maintenance of anesthesia with barbiturate or N_2O or a primary anesthetic agent for the induction of anesthesia in patients undergoing general surgery in which endotracheal intubation and mechanical ventilation are required

Restrictions C-II

Pregnancy Risk Factor C

Contraindications Hypersensitivity to alfentanil hydrochloride, to narcotics, or any component of the formulation; increased intracranial pressure, severe respiratory depression

Warnings/Precautions Use with caution in patients with drug dependence, head injury, acute asthma and respiratory conditions; hypotension has occurred in neonates with respiratory distress syndrome; use caution when administering to patients with bradyarrhythmias; rapid I.V. infusion may result in skeletal muscle and chest wall rigidity, impaired ventilation, or respiratory distress/arrest; inject slowly over 3-5 minutes. Alfentanil may produce more hypotension compared to fentanyl, therefore, be sure to administer slowly and ensure patient has adequate hydration.

Adverse Reactions
>10%:
  Cardiovascular: Bradycardia
  Gastrointestinal: Nausea, vomiting
1% to 10%:
  Cardiovascular: Orthostatic hypotension
  Central nervous system: CNS depression
<1% (Limited to important or life-threatening): Biliary tract spasm, pruritus, respiratory depression, urinary retention

Overdosage/Toxicology Symptoms include miosis, respiratory depression, seizures, and CNS depression. Treatment includes naloxone 2 mg I.V. (0.01 mg/kg for children), with repeat administration as necessary, up to a total of 10 mg. May precipitate withdrawal.

Drug Interactions
  Cytochrome P450 Effect: CYP3A3/4 enzyme substrate
  Increased Effect/Toxicity: Dextroamphetamine may enhance the analgesic effect of morphine and other opiate agonists. CNS depressants (eg, benzodiazepines, barbiturates, phenothiazines, tricyclic antidepressants), erythromycin, reserpine, beta-blockers may increase the toxic effects of alfentanil.
  Decreased Effect: Phenothiazines may antagonize the analgesic effect of opiate agonists

Stability Dilute in D_5W, NS, or LR

Mechanism of Action Binds with stereospecific receptors at many sites within the CNS, increases pain threshold, alters pain perception, inhibits ascending pain pathways; is an ultra short-acting narcotic

Pharmacodynamics/Kinetics
Onset of action: Rapid
Duration: 30-60 minutes (dose dependent)
Distribution: V_d: Newborns, premature: 1 L/kg; Children: 0.163-0.48 L/kg; Adults: 0.46 L/kg
Half-life elimination: Newborns, premature: 5.33-8.75 hours; Children: 40-60 minutes; Adults: 83-97 minutes

Usual Dosage Doses should be titrated to appropriate effects; wide range of doses is dependent upon desired degree of analgesia/anesthesia
Children <12 years: Dose not established

Adults: Dose should be based on ideal body weight as follows (see table):

Alfentanil

Indication	Approx Duration of Anesthesia (min)	Induction Period (Initial Dose) (mcg/kg)	Maintenance Period (Increments/ Infusion)	Total Dose (mcg/kg)	Effects
Incremental injection	≤30	8-20	3-5 mcg/kg or 0.5-1 mcg/kg/min	8-40	Spontaneously breathing or assisted ventilation when required.
	30-60	20-50	5-15 mcg/kg	Up to 75	Assisted or controlled ventilation required. Attenuation of response to laryngoscopy and intubation.
Continuous infusion	>45	50-75	0.5-3 mcg/kg/min average infusion rate 1-1.5 mcg/ kg/min	Dependent on duration of procedure	Assisted or controlled ventilation required. Some attenuation of response to intubation and incision, with intraoperative stability.
Anesthetic induction	>45	130-245	0.5-1.5 mcg/kg/ min or general anesthetic	Dependent on duration of procedure	Assisted or controlled ventilation required. Administer slowly (over 3 minutes). Concentration of inhalation agents reduced by 30% to 50% for initial hour.

Administration Administer I.V. slowly over 3-5 minutes or by I.V. continuous infusion

Monitoring Parameters Respiratory rate, blood pressure, heart rate

Reference Range 100-340 ng/mL (depending upon procedure)

Nursing Implications Monitor patient for CNS, respiratory depression, and urticaria

Additional Information Alfentanil may produce more muscle rigidity compared to fentanyl, therefore, be sure to administer slowly.

Dosage Forms Injection, as hydrochloride [preservative free]: 500 mcg/mL (2 mL, 5 mL, 10 mL, 20 mL)

♦ **Alfentanil Hydrochloride** *see Alfentanil on page 50*

♦ **Alferon® N** *see Interferon Alfa-n3 on page 733*

Alglucerase (al GLOO ser ase)

U.S. Brand Names Ceredase®

Synonyms Glucocerebrosidase

Therapeutic Category Enzyme, Glucocerebrosidase

Use Orphan drug: Replacement therapy for Gaucher's disease (type 1)

Pregnancy Risk Factor C

Contraindications Hypersensitivity to alglucerase or any component of the formulation

Warnings/Precautions Prepared from pooled human placental tissue that may contain the causative agents of some viral diseases

Adverse Reactions

>10%: Local: Discomfort, burning, and edema at the site of injection

<1% (Limited to important or life-threatening): Abdominal discomfort, nausea, vomiting

Overdosage/Toxicology No obvious toxicity was detected after single doses of up to 234 units/kg.

Stability Refrigerate (4°C), do not shake

Mechanism of Action Glucocerebrosidase is an enzyme prepared from human placental tissue. Gaucher's disease is an inherited metabolic disorder caused by the defective activity of beta-glucosidase and the resultant accumulation of glucosyl ceramide laden macrophages in the liver, bone, and spleen; acts by replacing the missing enzyme associated with Gaucher's disease.

Pharmacodynamics/Kinetics Half-life elimination: ~4-20 minutes

Usual Dosage Usually administered as a 20-60 unit/kg I.V. infusion given with a frequency ranging from 3 times/week to once every 2 weeks

Administration Filter during administration

Patient Information Alglucerase should be stored under refrigeration (4°C), solutions should not be shaken

Nursing Implications

Parenteral: Dilute to a final volume of 100 mL or less of normal saline and infuse I.V. over 1-2 hours; an in-line filter should be used; do not shake solution as it denatures the enzyme

Monitor CBC, platelets, liver function tests

Dosage Forms Injection, solution: 10 units/mL (5 mL); 80 units/mL (5 mL)

Alitretinoin (a li TRET i noyn)

U.S. Brand Names Panretin®

Canadian Brand Names Panretin™

Therapeutic Category Antineoplastic Agent, Miscellaneous; Retinoic Acid Derivative

Use Orphan drug: Topical treatment of cutaneous lesions in AIDS-related Kaposi's sarcoma; not indicated when systemic therapy for Kaposi's sarcoma is indicated

Pregnancy Risk Factor D

Pregnancy/Breast-Feeding Implications Potentially teratogenic and/or embryotoxic; limb, craniofacial, or skeletal defects have been observed in animal models. If used during pregnancy or if the patient becomes pregnant while using alitretinoin, the woman should be advised of potential harm to the fetus. Women of childbearing potential should avoid becoming pregnant. Excretion in human breast milk is unknown; women are advised to discontinue breast-feeding prior to using this medication.

Contraindications Hypersensitivity to alitretinoin, other retinoids, or any component of the formulation; pregnancy

Warnings/Precautions May cause fetal harm if absorbed by a woman who is pregnant. Patients with cutaneous T cell lymphoma have a high incidence of treatment-limiting adverse reactions. May be photosensitizing (based on experience with other retinoids); minimize sun or other UV exposure of treated areas. Do not use concurrently with topical products containing DEET (increased toxicity may result). Safety in pediatric patients or geriatric patients has not been established. Occlusive dressing should not be used.

Adverse Reactions

>10%:

Central nervous system: Pain (0% to 34%)

Dermatologic: Rash (25% to 77%), pruritus (8% to 11%)

Neuromuscular & skeletal: Paresthesia (3% to 22%)

5% to 10%:

Cardiovascular: Edema (3% to 8%)

Dermatologic: Exfoliative dermatitis (3% to 9%), skin disorder (0% to 8%)

Overdosage/Toxicology There has been no experience with human overdosage of alitretinoin, and overdose is unlikely following topical application. Treatment is symptomatic and supportive.

Drug Interactions

Increased Effect/Toxicity: Increased toxicity of DEET may occur if products containing this compound are used concurrently with alitretinoin. Due to limited absorption after topical application, interaction with systemic medications is unlikely.

Stability Store at room temperature

Mechanism of Action Binds to retinoid receptors to inhibit growth of Kaposi's sarcoma

Pharmacodynamics/Kinetics Absorption: Not extensive

Usual Dosage Topical: Apply gel twice daily to cutaneous Kaposi's sarcoma lesions

Administration Do not use occlusive dressings

(Continued)

Alitretinoin *(Continued)*

Patient Information For external use only; avoid UV light exposure (sun or sunlamps) of treated areas

Dosage Forms Gel: 0.1% (60 g tube)

♦ **Alkaban-AQ®** *see* VinBLAStine *on page 1415*

♦ **Alka-Mints® [OTC]** *see* Calcium Carbonate *on page 207*

♦ **Alka-Seltzer® Plus Cold Liqui-Gels® [OTC]** *see* Acetaminophen, Chlorpheniramine, and Pseudoephedrine *on page 27*

♦ **Alka-Seltzer® Plus Flu Liqui-Gels® [OTC]** *see* Acetaminophen, Dextromethorphan, and Pseudoephedrine *on page 27*

♦ **Alkeran®** *see* Melphalan *on page 854*

♦ **Allegra®** *see* Fexofenadine *on page 559*

♦ **Allegra-D®** *see* Fexofenadine and Pseudoephedrine *on page 560*

♦ **Allerdryl® (Can)** *see* DiphenhydrAMINE *on page 414*

♦ **Allerest® Maximum Strength [OTC]** *see* Chlorpheniramine and Pseudoephedrine *on page 279*

♦ **Allerfed® [OTC]** *see* Triprolidine and Pseudoephedrine *on page 1380*

♦ **Allerfrim® [OTC]** *see* Triprolidine and Pseudoephedrine *on page 1380*

♦ **Allergen®** *see* Antipyrine and Benzocaine *on page 107*

♦ **AllerMax® [OTC]** *see* DiphenhydrAMINE *on page 414*

♦ **Allernix (Can)** *see* DiphenhydrAMINE *on page 414*

♦ **Allerphed® [OTC]** *see* Triprolidine and Pseudoephedrine *on page 1380*

♦ **Allersol®** *see* Naphazoline *on page 957*

Allopurinol *(al oh PURE i nole)*

Related Information

Antacid Drug Interactions *on page 1477*
Desensitization Protocols *on page 1525*

U.S. Brand Names Aloprim™; Zyloprim®

Canadian Brand Names Apo®-Allopurinol; Zyloprim®

Synonyms Allopurinol Sodium Injection

Therapeutic Category Xanthine Oxidase Inhibitor

Use

Oral: Prevention of attack of gouty arthritis and nephropathy; treatment of secondary hyperuricemia which may occur during treatment of tumors or leukemia; prevention of recurrent calcium oxalate calculi

Orphan drug: I.V.: Management of patients with leukemia, lymphoma, and solid tumor malignancies who are receiving cancer chemotherapy which causes elevations of serum and urinary uric acid levels and who cannot tolerate oral therapy

Pregnancy Risk Factor C

Pregnancy/Breast-Feeding Implications Clinical effects on the fetus: There are few reports describing the use of allopurinol during pregnancy; no adverse fetal outcomes attributable to allopurinol have been reported in humans; use only if potential benefit outweighs the potential risk to the fetus

Contraindications Hypersensitivity to allopurinol or any component of the formulation

Warnings/Precautions Do not use to treat asymptomatic hyperuricemia. Discontinue at first signs of rash; reduce dosage in renal insufficiency, reinstate with caution in patients who have had a previous mild allergic reaction, use with caution in children; monitor liver function and complete blood counts before initiating therapy and periodically during therapy, use with caution in patients taking diuretics concurrently. Risk of skin rash may be increased in patients receiving amoxicillin or ampicillin. The risk of hypersensitivity may be increased in patients receiving thiazides, and possibly ACE inhibitors.

Adverse Reactions The most common adverse reaction to allopurinol is a skin rash (usually maculopapular); however, more severe reactions, including Stevens-Johnson syndrome, have also been reported). While some studies cite an incidence of these reactions as high as >10% of cases (often in association with ampicillin or amoxicillin), the product labeling cites a much lower incidence, reflected below. Allopurinol should be discontinued at the first appearance of a rash or other sign of hypersensitivity.

>1%:
  Dermatologic: Rash (1.5%)
  Gastrointestinal: Nausea (1.3%), vomiting (1.2%)
  Renal: Renal failure/impairment (1.2%)

<1% (Limited to important or life-threatening): Acute tubular necrosis, agranulocytosis, angioedema, aplastic anemia, bronchospasm, cataracts, exfoliative dermatitis, granuloma annulare, granulomatous hepatitis, hypersensitivity syndrome, interstitial nephritis, macular retinitis, nephrolithiasis, neuritis, pancreatitis, paresthesia, peripheral neuropathy, Stevens-Johnson syndrome, toxic epidermal necrolysis, toxic pustuloderma, vasculitis

Overdosage/Toxicology At high dosages, it is a theoretical possibility that oxypurinol stones could be formed but no record of such occurrence in overdose exists. Alkalinization of the urine and forced diuresis can help prevent potential xanthine stone formation.

Drug Interactions

Cytochrome P450 Effect: Hepatic enzyme inhibitor; isoenzyme profile not defined

Increased Effect/Toxicity: Allopurinol may increase the effects of azathioprine, chlorpropamide, mercaptopurine, theophylline, and oral anticoagulants. An increased risk of bone marrow suppression may occur when given with myelosuppressive agents (cyclophosphamide, possibly other alkylating agents). Amoxicillin/ampicillin, ACE inhibitors, and thiazide diuretics have been associated with hypersensitivity reactions when combined with allopurinol (rare), and the incidence of rash may be increased with penicillins (ampicillin, amoxicillin). Urinary acidification with large amounts of vitamin C may increase kidney stone formation.

Decreased Effect: Ethanol decreases effectiveness.

Ethanol/Nutrition/Herb Interactions Ethanol: Avoid ethanol (may decrease effectiveness).

Stability Store intact vials of unreconstituted powder at 15°C to 30°C (59°F to 86°F). Allopurinol sodium for injection should be dissolved with 25 mL of sterile water for injection. Reconstitution should yield a clear, almost colorless solution with no more than a slight opalescence. The initial solution should be diluted to the desired concentration with 0.9% sodium chloride injection or 5% dextrose for injection. **Sodium bicarbonate-containing solutions should not be used.** A final concentration of no greater than 6 mg/mL is recommended. The solution should be stored at 20°C to 25°C (68°F to 77°F) and administration should begin within 10 hours after reconstitution. Do not refrigerate the reconstituted and/or diluted product.

Y-site incompatible: Amikacin, amphotericin B, carmustine, cefotaxime, chlorpromazine, cimetidine, clindamycin, cytarabine, dacarbazine, daunorubicin, diphenhydramine, doxorubicin, doxycycline, droperidol, floxuridine, gentamicin, haloperidol, hydroxyzine, idarubicin, imipenem-cilastatin, mechlorethamine, meperidine, metoclopramide, methylprednisolone sodium succinate, minocycline, nalbuphine, netilmicin, ondansetron, prochlorperazine, promethazine, sodium bicarbonate, streptozocin, tobramycin, vinorelbine

Mechanism of Action Allopurinol inhibits xanthine oxidase, the enzyme responsible for the conversion of hypoxanthine to xanthine to uric acid. Allopurinol is metabolized to oxypurinol which is also an inhibitor of xanthine oxidase; allopurinol acts on purine catabolism, reducing the production of uric acid without disrupting the biosynthesis of vital purines.

Pharmacodynamics/Kinetics

Onset of action: Peak effect: 1-2 weeks

Absorption: Oral: ~80%; Rectal: Poor and erratic

Distribution: V_d: ~1.6 L/kg; V_{ss}: 0.84-0.87 L/kg; enters breast milk

Protein binding: <1%

Metabolism: ~75% to active metabolites, chiefly oxypurinol

Bioavailability: 49% to 53%

Half-life elimination:

Normal renal function: Parent drug: 1-3 hours; Oxypurinol: 18-30 hours

End-stage renal disease: Prolonged

Time to peak, plasma: Oral: 30-120 minutes

Excretion: Urine (76% as oxypurinol, 12% as unchanged drug)

Allopurinol and oxypurinol are dialyzable

Usual Dosage

Oral:

Children ≤10 years: 10 mg/kg/day in 2-3 divided doses **or** 200-300 mg/m²/day in 2-4 divided doses, maximum: 800 mg/24 hours

Alternative: <6 years: 150 mg/day in 3 divided doses; 6-10 years: 300 mg/day in 2-3 divided doses

Children >10 years and Adults: Daily doses >300 mg should be administered in divided doses

Myeloproliferative neoplastic disorders: 600-800 mg/day in 2-3 divided doses for prevention of acute uric acid nephropathy for 2-3 days starting 1-2 days before chemotherapy

Gout: Mild: 200-300 mg/day; Severe: 400-600 mg/day

Elderly: Initial: 100 mg/day, increase until desired uric acid level is obtained

I.V.: Hyperuricemia secondary to chemotherapy: Intravenous daily dose can be given as a single infusion or in equally divided doses at 6-, 8-, or 12-hour intervals. A fluid intake sufficient to yield a daily urinary output of at least 2 L in adults and the maintenance of a neutral or, preferably, slightly alkaline urine are desirable.

Children: Starting dose: 200 mg/m²/day

Adults: 200-400 mg/m²/day (max: 600 mg/day)

Dosing adjustment in renal impairment: Must be adjusted due to accumulation of allopurinol and metabolites:

Oral: Removed by hemodialysis; adult maintenance doses of allopurinol* (mg) based on creatinine clearance (mL/minute): See table.

Adult Maintenance Doses of Allopurinol*

Creatinine Clearance (mL/min)	Maintenance Dose of Allopurinol (mg)
140	400 qd
120	350 qd
100	300 qd
80	250 qd
60	200 qd
40	150 qd
20	100 qd
10	100 q2d
0	100 q3d

*This table is based on a standard maintenance dose of 300 mg of allopurinol per day for a patient with a creatinine clearance of 100 mL/min.

Hemodialysis: Administer dose posthemodialysis or administer 50% supplemental dose

I.V.:

Cl_{cr} 10-20 mL/minute: 200 mg/day

Cl_{cr} 3-10 mL/minute: 100 mg/day

Cl_{cr} <3 mL/minute: 100 mg/day at extended intervals

Dietary Considerations Should administer oral forms after meals with plenty of fluid.

Administration The rate of infusion depends on the volume of the infusion. Whenever possible, therapy should be initiated at 24-48 hours before the start of chemotherapy known to cause tumor lysis (including adrenocorticosteroids). I.V. daily dose can be administered as (Continued)

Allopurinol *(Continued)*

a single infusion or in equally divided doses at 6-, 8-, or 12-hour intervals at the recommended final concentration of ≤6 mg/mL.

Monitoring Parameters CBC, serum uric acid levels, I & O, hepatic and renal function, especially at start of therapy

Reference Range Uric acid, serum: An increase occurs during childhood

Adults:

Male: 3.4-7 mg/dL or slightly more

Female: 2.4-6 mg/dL or slightly more

Values >7 mg/dL are sometimes arbitrarily regarded as hyperuricemia, but there is no sharp line between normals on the one hand, and the serum uric acid of those with clinical gout. Normal ranges cannot be adjusted for purine ingestion, but high purine diet increases uric acid. Uric acid may be increased with body size, exercise, and stress.

Patient Information Take after meals with plenty of fluid (at least 10-12 glasses of fluids per day); discontinue the drug and contact physician at first sign of rash, painful urination, blood in urine, irritation of the eyes, or swelling of the lips or mouth; may cause drowsiness; alcohol decreases effectiveness

Nursing Implications Monitor CBC, serum uric acid levels, I & O, hepatic and renal function, especially at start of therapy

Dosage Forms

Injection, powder for reconstitution, as sodium (Aloprim™): 500 mg

Tablet (Zyloprim®): 100 mg, 300 mg

Extemporaneous Preparations Crush tablets to make a 5 mg/mL suspension in simple syrup; stable 14 days under refrigeration

Nahata MC and Hipple TF, *Pediatric Drug Formulations*, 1st ed, Harvey Whitney Books Co, 1990.

♦ **Allopurinol Sodium Injection** *see Allopurinol on page 52*

♦ **All-*trans*-Retinoic Acid** *see Tretinoin (Oral) on page 1363*

♦ **Almora® (Gluconate)** *see Magnesium Salts (Other) on page 835*

Almotriptan *(al moh TRIP tan)*

Related Information

Antimigraine Drugs Comparison *on page 1485*

U.S. Brand Names Axert™

Synonyms Almotriptan Malate

Therapeutic Category Serotonin 5-HT$_{1D}$ Receptor Agonist

Use Acute treatment of migraine with or without aura

Pregnancy Risk Factor C

Pregnancy/Breast-Feeding Implications There are no adequate, well-controlled studies in pregnant women. Use in pregnancy should be limited to situations where benefit outweighs risk to fetus. Excretion in breast milk unknown; use caution.

Contraindications Hypersensitivity to almotriptan or any component of the formulation; use as prophylactic therapy for migraine; hemiplegic or basilar migraine; cluster headache; known or suspected ischemic heart disease (angina pectoris, MI, documented silent ischemia, coronary artery vasospasm, Prinzmetal's variant angina); peripheral vascular syndromes (including ischemic bowel disease); uncontrolled hypertension; use within 24 hours of another 5-HT$_1$ agonist; use within 24 hours of ergotamine derivative; concurrent administration or within 2 weeks of discontinuing an MAO inhibitor (specifically MAO type A inhibitors)

Warnings/Precautions Almotriptan is indicated only in patients ≥18 years of age with a clear diagnosis of migraine headache. If a patient does not respond to the first dose, the diagnosis of migraine should be reconsidered. Do not give to patients with risk factors for CAD until a cardiovascular evaluation has been performed; if evaluation is satisfactory, the healthcare provider should administer the first dose and cardiovascular status should be periodically re-evaluated. Cardiac events (coronary artery vasospasm, transient ischemia, myocardial infarction, ventricular tachycardia/fibrillation, cardiac arrest, and death), cerebral/subarachnoid hemorrhage, stroke, peripheral vascular ischemia and colonic ischemia have been reported with 5-HT$_1$ agonist administration. Significant elevation in blood pressure, including hypertensive crisis, has also been reported on rare occasions in patients with and without a history of hypertension. Use with caution in liver or renal dysfunction. Safety and efficacy in pediatric patients have not been established.

Adverse Reactions

1% to 10%:

Central nervous system: Headache (>1%), dizziness (>1%), somnolence (>1%)

Gastrointestinal: Nausea (1% to 2%), xerostomia (1%)

Neuromuscular & skeletal: Paresthesia (1%)

<1% (Limited to important or life-threatening): Colitis, coronary artery vasospasm, hypertension, myocardial ischemia, myocardial infarction, neuropathy, rash, syncope, tachycardia, ventricular fibrillation, ventricular tachycardia, vertigo

Overdosage/Toxicology Hypertension or more serious cardiovascular symptoms may occur. Clinical and electrocardiographic monitoring is needed for at least 20 hours even if the patient is asymptomatic. Treatment is symptom directed and supportive.

Drug Interactions

Cytochrome P450 Effect: CYP2D6 and 3A4 enzyme substrate

Increased Effect/Toxicity: Ergot-containing drugs prolong vasospastic reactions; ketoconazole and CYP3A4 inhibitors increase almotriptan serum concentration; select serotonin reuptake inhibitors may increase symptoms of hyper-reflexia, weakness, and incoordination; MAO inhibitors may increase toxicity

Stability Store at 15°C to 30°C (59°F to 86°F).

Mechanism of Action Selective agonist for serotonin (5-HT$_{1B}$, 5-HT$_{1D}$, 5-HT$_{1F}$ receptors) in cranial arteries; causes vasoconstriction and reduce sterile inflammation associated with antidromic neuronal transmission correlating with relief of migraine

Pharmacodynamics/Kinetics
Absorption: Well absorbed
Distribution: V_d: 180-200 L
Protein binding: ~35%
Metabolism: MAO type A oxidative deamination (~27% of dose); via CYP3A4 and 2D6 oxidation (~12% of dose); metabolized to inactive metabolites
Bioavailability: 70%
Half-life elimination: 3-4 hours
Time to peak: 1-3 hours
Excretion: Urine (75%); feces (13%)

Usual Dosage Oral: Adults: Migraine: Initial: 6.25-12.5 mg in a single dose; if the headache returns, repeat the dose after 2 hours; no more than 2 doses in 24-hour period
Note: If the first dose is ineffective, diagnosis needs to be re-evaluated. Safety of treating more than 4 migraines/month has not been established.
Dosage adjustment in renal impairment: Initial: 6.25 mg in a single dose; maximum daily dose: ≤12.5 mg
Dosage adjustment in hepatic impairment: Initial: 6.25 mg in a single dose; maximum daily dose: ≤12.5 mg
Dietary Considerations Food: May be taken without regard to meals
Patient Information This drug is to be used to reduce your migraine not to prevent or reduce the number of attacks. Take exactly as directed. If headache returns or is not fully resolved, the dose may be repeated after 2 hours. Do not use more than two doses in 24 hours. Do not take within 24 hours of other migraine medication without consulting prescriber. You may experience dizziness, fatigue, or drowsiness (use caution when driving or engaging in tasks that require alertness until response to drug is known). Report immediately chest pain, palpitations, feeling of tightness or pressure in chest, jaw, or throat; acute headache or dizziness; muscle cramping, pain, or tremors; skin rash; hallucinations, anxiety, panic; or other adverse reactions. Inform prescriber if you are or intend to be pregnant. Consult prescriber if breast-feeding.
Dosage Forms Tablet, as malate: 6.25 mg, 12.5 mg

- ◆ **Almotriptan Malate** *see Almotriptan on page 54*
- ◆ **Alocril™** *see Nedocromil on page 963*
- ◆ **Aloe Vesta® 2-n-1 Antifungal [OTC]** *see Miconazole on page 908*
- ◆ **Alomide®** *see Lodoxamide on page 813*
- ◆ **Aloprim™** *see Allopurinol on page 52*
- ◆ **Alora®** *see Estradiol on page 491*
- ◆ **Alphagan®** *see Brimonidine on page 183*
- ◆ **Alphagan® P** *see Brimonidine on page 183*
- ◆ **Alphanate®** *see Antihemophilic Factor (Human) on page 102*
- ◆ **AlphaNine® SD** *see Factor IX Complex (Human) on page 539*
- ◆ **Alphatrex®** *see Betamethasone on page 161*

Alprazolam (al PRAY zoe lam)
Related Information
Antacid Drug Interactions *on page 1477*
Benzodiazepines Comparison *on page 1490*
U.S. Brand Names Alprazolam Intensol®; Xanax®
Canadian Brand Names Alti-Alprazolam; Apo®-Alpraz; Gen-Alprazolam; Novo-Alprazol; Nu-Alprax; Xanax®; Xanax TS™
Therapeutic Category Antianxiety Agent; Benzodiazepine
Use Treatment of anxiety disorder (GAD); panic disorder, with or without agoraphobia; anxiety associated with depression
Unlabeled/Investigational Use Anxiety in children
Restrictions C-IV
Pregnancy Risk Factor D
Contraindications Hypersensitivity to alprazolam or any component of the formulation (cross-sensitivity with other benzodiazepines may exist); narrow-angle glaucoma; concurrent use of ketoconazole and itraconazole; pregnancy
Warnings/Precautions Rebound or withdrawal symptoms, including seizures may occur 18 hours to 3 days following abrupt discontinuation or large decreases in dose (more common in patients receiving >4 mg/day or prolonged treatment). Dose reductions or tapering must be approached with extreme caution. Between dose, anxiety may also occur. Use with caution in patients receiving CYP3A4 inhibitors, particularly when these agents are added to therapy. Has weak uricosuric properties, use with caution in renal impairment or predisposition to urate nephropathy. Use with caution in elderly or debilitated patients, patients with hepatic disease (including alcoholics), renal impairment, or obese patients.

Causes CNS depression (dose-related) resulting in sedation, dizziness, confusion, or ataxia, which may impair physical and mental capabilities. Patients must be cautioned about performing tasks that require mental alertness (ie, operating machinery or driving). Use with caution in patients receiving other CNS depressants or psychoactive agents. Effects with other sedative drugs or ethanol may be potentiated. Benzodiazepines have been associated with falls and traumatic injury and should be used with extreme caution in patients who are at risk of these events (especially the elderly). Use with caution in patients with respiratory disease or impaired gag reflex.

Use caution in patients with depression, particularly if suicidal risk may be present. Episodes of mania or hypomania have occurred in depressed patients treated with alprazolam. May cause physical or psychological dependence - use with caution in patients with a history of drug dependence. Acute withdrawal, including seizures, may be precipitated in patients after administration of flumazenil to patients receiving long-term benzodiazepine therapy.

Benzodiazepines have been associated with anterograde amnesia. Paradoxical reactions, including hyperactive or aggressive behavior, have been reported with benzodiazepines, *(Continued)*

Alprazolam (Continued)

particularly in adolescent/pediatric or psychiatric patients. Does not have analgesic, antidepressant, or antipsychotic properties.

Adverse Reactions

>10%:

Central nervous system: Drowsiness, fatigue, ataxia, lightheadedness, memory impairment, dysarthria, irritability

Dermatologic: Rash

Endocrine & metabolic: Decreased libido, menstrual disorders

Gastrointestinal: Xerostomia, decreased salivation, increased or decreased appetite, weight gain/loss

Genitourinary: Micturition difficulties

1% to 10%:

Cardiovascular: Hypotension

Central nervous system: Confusion, dizziness, disinhibition, akathisia, increased libido

Dermatologic: Dermatitis

Gastrointestinal: Increased salivation

Genitourinary: Sexual dysfunction, incontinence

Neuromuscular & skeletal: Rigidity, tremor, muscle cramps

Otic: Tinnitus

Respiratory: Nasal congestion

Overdosage/Toxicology Symptoms include somnolence, confusion, coma, and diminished reflexes. Treatment for benzodiazepine overdose is supportive. Mechanical ventilation is rarely required. Flumazenil has been shown to selectively block the binding of benzodiazepines to CNS receptors, resulting in a reversal of benzodiazepine-induced sedation; however, its use may not alter the course of overdose.

Drug Interactions

Cytochrome P450 Effect: CYP3A3/4 enzyme substrate

Increased Effect/Toxicity: Alprazolam potentiates the CNS depressant effects of narcotic analgesics, barbiturates, phenothiazines, ethanol, antihistamines, MAO inhibitors, sedative-hypnotics, and cyclic antidepressants. Serum levels and/or effects of alprazolam may be increased by inhibitors of CYP3A3/4, including amprenavir, cimetidine, ciprofloxacin, clarithromycin, clozapine, diltiazem, disulfiram, digoxin, erythromycin, ethanol, fluconazole, fluoxetine, fluvoxamine, grapefruit juice, isoniazid, itraconazole, ketoconazole, labetalol, levodopa, loxapine, metoprolol, metronidazole, miconazole, nefazodone, nelfinavir, omeprazole, phenytoin, rifabutin, rifampin, ritonavir, troleandomycin, valproic acid, and verapamil.

Decreased Effect: Carbamazepine, rifampin, rifabutin may enhance the metabolism of alprazolam and decrease its therapeutic effect.

Ethanol/Nutrition/Herb Interactions

Ethanol: Avoid ethanol (may increase CNS depression).

Food: Alprazolam serum concentration is unlikely to be increased by grapefruit juice because of alprazolam's high oral bioavailability.

Herb/Nutraceutical: St John's wort may decrease alprazolam levels. Avoid valerian, St John's wort, kava kava, gotu kola (may increase CNS depression).

Mechanism of Action Binds to stereospecific benzodiazepine receptors on the postsynaptic GABA neuron at several sites within the central nervous system, including the limbic system, reticular formation. Enhancement of the inhibitory effect of GABA on neuronal excitability results by increased neuronal membrane permeability to chloride ions. This shift in chloride ions results in hyperpolarization (a less excitable state) and stabilization.

Pharmacodynamics/Kinetics

Onset of action: Within 1 hour

Duration: 8-24 hours

Distribution: V_d: 0.9-1.2 L/kg; enters breast milk

Protein binding: 80%

Metabolism: Hepatic; major metabolite inactive

Half-life elimination: 12-15 hours

Time to peak, serum: 1-2 hours

Excretion: Urine (as unchanged drug and metabolites)

Usual Dosage Oral:

Children: Anxiety (unlabeled use): Initial: 0.005 mg/kg or 0.125 mg/dose 3 times/day; increase in increments of 0.125-0.25 mg, up to a maximum of 0.02 mg/kg/dose or 0.06 mg/kg/day (0.375-3 mg/day)

Adults:

Anxiety: Effective doses are 0.5-4 mg/day in divided doses; the manufacturer recommends starting at 0.25-0.5 mg 3 times/day; titrate dose upward; maximum: 4 mg/day

Depression: Average dose required: 2.5-3 mg/day in divided doses

Ethanol withdrawal: Usual dose: 2-2.5 mg/day in divided doses

Panic disorder: Many patients obtain relief at 2 mg/day, as much as 10 mg/day may be required

Elderly: Elderly patients may be more sensitive to the effects of alprazolam including ataxia and oversedation. The elderly may also have impaired renal function leading to decreased clearance. The smallest effective dose should be used.

Dosing adjustment in hepatic impairment: Reduce dose by 50% to 60% or avoid in cirrhosis

Note: Treatment >4 months should be re-evaluated to determine the patient's need for the drug

Administration Can be administered sublingually with comparable onset and completeness of absorption.

Monitoring Parameters Respiratory and cardiovascular status

Patient Information Avoid alcohol and other CNS depressants; avoid activities needing good psychomotor coordination until CNS effects are known; drug may cause physical or psychological dependence; avoid abrupt discontinuation after prolonged use

Nursing Implications Assist with ambulation during beginning therapy, raise bed rails and keep room partially illuminated at night; monitor for CNS respiratory depression

Additional Information Not intended for management of anxieties and minor distresses associated with everyday life. Treatment longer than 4 months should be re-evaluated to determine the patient's need for the drug. Patients who become physically dependent on alprazolam tend to have a difficult time discontinuing it; withdrawal symptoms may be severe. To minimize withdrawal symptoms, taper dosage slowly; do not discontinue abruptly. Abrupt discontinuation after sustained use (generally >10 days) may cause withdrawal symptoms.

Dosage Forms
Solution, oral (Alprazolam Intensol®): 1 mg/mL (30 mL)
Tablet (Xanax®): 0.25 mg, 0.5 mg, 1 mg, 2 mg

♦ **Alprazolam Intensol**® *see* Alprazolam *on page 55*

Alprostadil (al PROS ta dill)

U.S. Brand Names Caverject®; Edex®; Muse® Pellet; Prostin VR Pediatric®
Canadian Brand Names Caverject™; Prostin® VR
Synonyms PGE₁; Prostaglandin E₁
Therapeutic Category Prostaglandin

Use Temporary maintenance of patency of ductus arteriosus in neonates with ductal-dependent congenital heart disease until surgery can be performed. These defects include cyanotic (eg, pulmonary atresia, pulmonary stenosis, tricuspid atresia, Fallot's tetralogy, transposition of the great vessels) and acyanotic (eg, interruption of aortic arch, coarctation of aorta, hypoplastic left ventricle) heart disease; diagnosis and treatment of erectile dysfunction of vasculogenic, psychogenic, or neurogenic etiology; adjunct in the diagnosis of erectile dysfunction

Unlabeled/Investigational Use Investigational: Treatment of pulmonary hypertension in infants and children with congenital heart defects with left-to-right shunts

Pregnancy Risk Factor X

Contraindications Hypersensitivity to alprostadil or any component of the formulation; hyaline membrane disease or persistent fetal circulation and when a dominant left-to-right shunt is present; respiratory distress syndrome; conditions predisposing patients to priapism (sickle cell anemia, multiple myeloma, leukemia); patients with anatomical deformation of the penis, penile implants; use in men for whom sexual activity is inadvisable or contraindicated; pregnancy

Warnings/Precautions Use cautiously in neonates with bleeding tendencies; apnea may occur in 10% to 12% of neonates with congenital heart defects, especially in those weighing <2 kg at birth; apnea usually appears during the first hour of drug infusion; when used in erectile dysfunction: priapism may occur; treat immediately to avoid penile tissue damage and permanent loss of potency; discontinue therapy if signs of penile fibrosis develop (penile angulation, cavernosal fibrosis, or Peyronie's disease). When used in erectile dysfunction (Muse®), syncope occurring within 1 hour of administration, has been reported; the potential for drug-drug interactions may occur when Muse® is prescribed concomitantly with antihypertensives.

Adverse Reactions
>10%:
Cardiovascular: Flushing
Central nervous system: Fever
Genitourinary: Penile pain
Respiratory: Apnea
1% to 10%:
Cardiovascular: Bradycardia, hypotension, hypertension, tachycardia, cardiac arrest, edema
Central nervous system: Seizures, headache, dizziness
Endocrine & metabolic: Hypokalemia
Gastrointestinal: Diarrhea
Genitourinary: Priapism, penile fibrosis, penis disorder, penile rash, penile edema
Hematologic: Disseminated intravascular coagulation
Local: Injection site hematoma, injection site bruising
Neuromuscular & skeletal: Back pain
Respiratory: Upper respiratory infection, flu syndrome, sinusitis, nasal congestion, cough
Miscellaneous: Sepsis, localized pain in structures other than the injection site
<1% (Limited to important or life-threatening): Abnormal ejaculation, anemia, balanitis, bleeding, bradypnea, bronchospasm, cerebral bleeding, congestive heart failure, hyperbilirubinemia, penile numbness, penile pruritus and erythema, perineal pain, peritonitis, second degree heart block, shock, supraventricular tachycardia, thrombocytopenia, urethral bleeding, ventricular fibrillation, yeast infection

Overdosage/Toxicology Symptoms of overdose when treating patent ductus arteriosus include apnea, bradycardia, hypotension, and flushing. If hypotension or pyrexia occurs, the infusion rate should be reduced until the symptoms subside, while apnea or bradycardia requires drug discontinuation. If intracavernous overdose occurs, supervise until any systemic effects have resolved or until penile detumescence has occurred.

Drug Interactions
Increased Effect/Toxicity: Risk of hypotension and syncope may be increased with antihypertensives.

Ethanol/Nutrition/Herb Interactions Ethanol: Avoid concurrent use (vasodilating effect).

Stability
Ductus arteriosus: Refrigerate ampuls; protect from freezing; prepare fresh solutions every 24 hours; **compatible** in D₅W, D₁₀W, and NS solutions
Erectile dysfunction: Refrigerate at 2°C to 8°C until dispensed; after dispensing, stable for up to 3 months at or below 25°C; do not freeze; use only the supplied diluent for reconstitution (ie, bacteriostatic/sterile water with benzyl alcohol 0.945%)

Mechanism of Action Causes vasodilation by means of direct effect on vascular and ductus arteriosus smooth muscle; relaxes trabecular smooth muscle by dilation of cavernosal
(Continued)

Alprostadil *(Continued)*

arteries when injected along the penile shaft, allowing blood flow to and entrapment in the lacunar spaces of the penis (ie, corporeal veno-occlusive mechanism)

Pharmacodynamics/Kinetics
Onset of action: Rapid
Duration: <1 hour
Distribution: Insignificant following penile injection
Protein binding, plasma: 81% to albumin
Metabolism: ~75% by oxidation in one pass via lungs
Half-life elimination: 5-10 minutes
Excretion: Urine (90% as metabolites) within 24 hours

Usual Dosage
Patent ductus arteriosus (Prostin VR Pediatric®):
I.V. continuous infusion into a large vein, or alternatively through an umbilical artery catheter placed at the ductal opening: 0.05-0.1 mcg/kg/minute with therapeutic response, rate is reduced to lowest effective dosage; with unsatisfactory response, rate is increased gradually; maintenance: 0.01-0.4 mcg/kg/minute

PGE_1 is usually given at an infusion rate of 0.1 mcg/kg/minute, but it is often possible to reduce the dosage to $\frac{1}{2}$ or even $\frac{1}{10}$ without losing the therapeutic effect. The mixing schedule is as follows. Infusion rates deliver 0.1 mcg/kg/minute: See table.

Alprostadil

Add 1 Ampul (500 mcg) to:	Concentration (mcg/mL)	Infusion Rate	
		mL/min/kg Needed to Infuse 0.1 mcg/kg/min	mL/kg/24 h
250 mL	2	0.05	72
100 mL	5	0.02	28.8
50 mL	10	0.01	14.4
25 mL	20	0.005	7.2

Therapeutic response is indicated by increased pH in those with acidosis or by an increase in oxygenation (pO_2) usually evident within 30 minutes

Erectile dysfunction:
Caverject®, Edex®:
Vasculogenic, psychogenic, or mixed etiology: Individualize dose by careful titration; usual dose: 2.5-60 mcg (doses >60 mcg are not recommended); initiate dosage titration at 2.5 mcg, increasing by 2.5 mcg to a dose of 5 mcg and then in increments of 5-10 mcg depending on the erectile response until the dose produces an erection suitable for intercourse, not lasting >1 hour; if there is absolutely no response to initial 2.5 mcg dose, the second dose may increased to 7.5 mcg, followed by increments of 5-10 mcg

Neurogenic etiology (eg, spinal cord injury): Initiate dosage titration at 1.25 mcg, increasing to a doses of 2.5 mcg and then 5 mcg; increase further in increments 5 mcg until the dose is reached that produces an erection suitable for intercourse, not lasting >1 hour

Note: Patient must stay in the physician's office until complete detumescence occurs; if there is no response, then the next higher dose may be given within 1 hour; if there is still no response, a 1-day interval before giving the next dose is recommended; increasing the dose or concentration in the treatment of impotence results in increasing pain and discomfort

Muse® Pellet: Intraurethral: Administer as needed to achieve an erection; duration of action is about 30-60 minutes; use only two systems per 24-hour period

Elderly: Elderly patients may have a greater frequency of renal dysfunction; lowest effective dose should be used. In clinical studies with Edex®, higher minimally effective doses and a higher rate of lack of effect were noted.

Administration Erectile dysfunction: Use a $\frac{1}{2}$ inch, 27- to 30-gauge needle. Inject into the dorsolateral aspect of the proximal third of the penis, avoiding visible veins; alternate side of the penis for injections.

Monitoring Parameters Arterial pressure, respiratory rate, heart rate, temperature, degree of penile pain, length of erection, signs of infection

Patient Information Store in refrigerator; if self-injecting for the treatment of impotence, dilute with the supplied diluent and use immediately after diluting; see physician at least every 3 months to ensure proper technique and for dosage adjustment.

Alternate sides of the penis with each injection; do not inject more than 3 times/week, allowing at least 24 hours between each dose; dispose of the syringe, needle, and vial properly; discard single-use vials after each use; report moderate to severe penile pain or erections lasting >4 hours to a physician immediately; inform a physician as soon as possible if any new penile pain, nodules, hard tissue or signs of infection develop; the risk of transmission of blood-borne diseases is increased with use of alprostadil injections since a small amount of bleeding at the injection site is possible.

Do not share this medication or needles/syringes; do not drive or operate heavy machinery within 1 hour of administration

Nursing Implications
Ductus arteriosus: Monitor arterial pressure; assess all vital functions; apnea and bradycardia may indicate overdose, stop infusion if occurring; infuse for the shortest time and at the lowest dose that will produce the desired effects. Flushing is usually a result of catheter malposition; central line preferred for I.V. administration.

Erectile dysfunction: Use a $\frac{1}{2}$", 27- to 30-gauge needle; inject into the dorsolateral aspect of the proximal third of the penis, avoiding visible veins; alternate side of the penis for injections; if the patient is going to be self-injecting at home, carefully assess their aseptic technique for injection and knowledge of proper disposal of the syringe, needle and vial; observe for signs of infection, penile fibrosis, and significant pain or priapism

Dosage Forms
Injection:
Caverject®: 5 mcg/mL, 10 mcg/mL, 20 mcg/mL
Edex®: 5 mcg/mL, 10 mcg/mL, 20 mcg/mL, 40 mcg/mL
Prostin VR Pediatric®: 500 mcg/mL (1 mL)
Pellet, urethral (Muse®): 125 mcg, 250 mcg, 500 mcg, 1000 mcg

♦ **Alrex**™ *see Loteprednol on page 824*
♦ **Altace**® *see Ramipril on page 1177*
♦ **Altafed® [OTC]** *see Triprolidine and Pseudoephedrine on page 1380*
♦ **Altamist [OTC]** *see Sodium Chloride on page 1245*

Alteplase (AL te plase)

U.S. Brand Names Activase®; Cathflo™ Activase®
Canadian Brand Names Activase® rt-PA
Synonyms Alteplase, Recombinant; Alteplase, Tissue Plasminogen Activator, Recombinant; tPA
Therapeutic Category Fibrinolytic Agent
Use Management of acute myocardial infarction for the lysis of thrombi in coronary arteries; management of acute massive pulmonary embolism (PE) in adults

Acute myocardial infarction (AMI): Chest pain ≥20 minutes, ≤12-24 hours; S-T elevation ≥0.1 mV in at least two EKG leads
Acute pulmonary embolism (APE): Age ≤75 years: As soon as possible within 5 days of thrombotic event. Documented massive pulmonary embolism by pulmonary angiography or echocardiography or high probability lung scan with clinical shock.
Cathflo™ Activase®: Restoration of central venous catheter function
Unlabeled/Investigational Use Peripheral arterial thrombotic obstruction
Pregnancy Risk Factor C
Contraindications Hypersensitivity to alteplase or any component of the formulation
When used in the treatment of acute MI or PE: Active internal bleeding; history of CVA; recent intracranial or intraspinal surgery or trauma; intracranial neoplasm; arteriovenous malformation or aneurysm; known bleeding diathesis; severe uncontrolled hypertension

When used in the treatment of acute ischemic stroke: Evidence of intracranial hemorrhage or suspicion of subarachnoid hemorrhage on pretreatment evaluation; recent (within 3 months) intracranial or intraspinal surgery; prolonged external cardiac massage; suspected aortic dissection; serious head trauma or previous stroke; history of intracranial hemorrhage; uncontrolled hypertension at time of treatment (eg, >185 mm Hg systolic or >110 mm Hg diastolic); seizure at the onset of stroke; active internal bleeding; intracranial neoplasm; arteriovenous malformation or aneurysm; known bleeding diathesis including but not limited to: current use of anticoagulants or an INR >1.7, administration of heparin within 48 hours preceding the onset of stroke and an elevated aPTT at presentation, platelet count <100,000/mm³.
Other exclusion criteria (NINDS recombinant tPA study) include: Stroke or serious head injury within 3 months, major surgery or serious trauma within 2 weeks, GI or urinary tract hemorrhage within 3 weeks, aggressive treatment required to lower blood pressure, glucose level <50 mg/dL or >400 mg/dL, arterial puncture at a noncompressible site or lumbar puncture within 1 week, clinical presentation suggesting post-MI pericarditis, pregnant or lactating women.
Warnings/Precautions Concurrent heparin anticoagulation may contribute to bleeding. Monitor all potential bleeding sites. Doses >150 mg are associated with increased risk of intracranial hemorrhage. Intramuscular injections and nonessential handling of the patient should be avoided. Venipunctures should be performed carefully and only when necessary. If arterial puncture is necessary, use an upper extremity vessel that can be manually compressed. If serious bleeding occurs then the infusion of alteplase and heparin should be stopped.

For the following conditions the risk of bleeding is higher with use of thrombolytics and should be weighed against the benefits of therapy: recent major surgery (eg, CABG, obstetrical delivery, organ biopsy, previous puncture of noncompressible vessels), cerebrovascular disease, recent gastrointestinal or genitourinary bleeding, recent trauma, hypertension (systolic BP >175 mm Hg and/or diastolic BP >110 mm Hg), high likelihood of left heart thrombus (eg, mitral stenosis with atrial fibrillation), acute pericarditis, subacute bacterial endocarditis, hemostatic defects including ones caused by severe renal or hepatic dysfunction, significant hepatic dysfunction, pregnancy, diabetic hemorrhagic retinopathy or other hemorrhagic ophthalmic conditions, septic thrombophlebitis or occluded AV cannula at seriously infected site, advanced age (eg, >75 years), patients receiving oral anticoagulants, any other condition in which bleeding constitutes a significant hazard or would be particularly difficult to manage because of location.

Coronary thrombolysis may result in reperfusion arrhythmias. In treatment of patients with acute ischemic stroke more than 3 hours after symptom onset is not recommended; treatment of patients with minor neurological deficit or with rapidly improving symptoms is not recommended.

Cathflo™ Activase®: When used to restore catheter function, use Cathflo™ cautiously in those patients with known or suspected catheter infections. Evaluate catheter for other causes of dysfunction before use. Avoid excessive pressure when instilling into catheter. Use of Cathflo™ in children <2 years of age (or weighing <10 kg) has not been adequately evaluated.
Adverse Reactions As with all drugs which may affect hemostasis, bleeding is the major adverse effect associated with alteplase. Hemorrhage may occur at virtually any site. Risk is dependent on multiple variables, including the dosage administered, concurrent use of multiple agents which alter hemostasis, and patient predisposition. Rapid lysis of coronary (Continued)

Alteplase (Continued)

artery thrombi by thrombolytic agents may be associated with reperfusion-related atrial and/ or ventricular arrhythmias. **Note:** Lowest rate of bleeding complications expected with dose used to restore catheter function.

1% to 10%:
Cardiovascular: Hypotension
Central nervous system: Fever
Dermatologic: Bruising (1%)
Gastrointestinal: GI hemorrhage (5%), nausea, vomiting
Genitourinary: GU hemorrhage (4%)
Hematologic: Bleeding (0.5% major, 7% minor: GUSTO trial)
Local: Bleeding at catheter puncture site (15.3%, accelerated administration)

<1% (Limited to important or life-threatening): Allergic reactions: Anaphylaxis, anaphylactoid reactions, laryngeal edema, rash, and urticaria (<0.02%); epistaxis; gingival hemorrhage; intracranial hemorrhage (0.4% to 0.87% when dose is ≤100 mg); pericardial hemorrhage; retroperitoneal hemorrhage

Additional cardiovascular events associated **with use in myocardial infarction:** AV block, cardiogenic shock, heart failure, cardiac arrest, recurrent ischemia/infarction, myocardial rupture, electromechanical dissociation, pericardial effusion, pericarditis, mitral regurgitation, cardiac tamponade, thromboembolism, pulmonary edema, asystole, ventricular tachycardia, bradycardia, ruptured intracranial AV malformation, seizure, hemorrhagic bursitis, cholesterol crystal embolization

Additional events associated **with use in pulmonary embolism:** Pulmonary re-embolization, pulmonary edema, pleural effusion, thromboembolism

Additional events associated **with use in stroke:** Cerebral edema, cerebral herniation, seizure, new ischemic stroke

Overdosage/Toxicology Symptoms include increased incidence of intracranial bleeding.

Drug Interactions

Increased Effect/Toxicity: The potential for hemorrhage with alteplase is increased by oral anticoagulants (warfarin), heparin, low molecular weight heparins, and drugs which affect platelet function (eg, NSAIDs, dipyridamole, ticlopidine, clopidogrel, IIb/IIIa antagonists). Concurrent use with aspirin and heparin may increase the risk of bleeding. However, aspirin and heparin were used concomitantly with alteplase in the majority of patients in clinical studies.

Decreased Effect: Aminocaproic acid (an antifibrinolytic agent) may decrease the effectiveness of thrombolytic therapy. Nitroglycerin may increase the hepatic clearance of alteplase, potentially reducing lytic activity (limited clinical information).

Ethanol/Nutrition/Herb Interactions Herb/Nutraceutical: Avoid cat's claw, dong quai, evening primrose, feverfew, red clover, horse chestnut, garlic, green tea, ginseng, ginkgo (all have additional antiplatelet activity).

Stability

Activase®: The lyophilized product may be stored at room temperature (not to exceed 30°C/ 86°F), or under refrigeration; once reconstituted it must be used within 8 hours. Reconstitution:

50 mg vial: Use accompanying diluent (50 mL sterile water for injection); do not shake; final concentration: 1 mg/mL

100 mg vial: Use transfer set with accompanying diluent (100 mL vial of sterile water for injection); no vacuum is present in 100 mg vial; final concentration: 1 mg/mL Alteplase is **incompatible** with dobutamine, dopamine, heparin, and nitroglycerin infusions; physically **compatible** with lidocaine, metoprolol, and propranolol when administered via Ysite; **compatible** with either D_5W or NS. Standard dose: 100 mg/100 mL 0.9% NaCl (total volume: 200 mL).

Cathflo™ Activase®: Store lyophilized product under refrigeration; protect from excessive exposure to light when stored for extended periods of time. Reconstitution: Add 2.2 mL SWFI to vial; do not shake. Final concentration: 1 mg/mL. Once reconstituted, store at 2°C to 30°C (36°F to 86°F). Do not mix other medications into infusion solution.

Mechanism of Action Initiates local fibrinolysis by binding to fibrin in a thrombus (clot) and converts entrapped plasminogen to plasmin

Pharmacodynamics/Kinetics

Duration: >50% present in plasma cleared ~5 minutes after infusion terminated, ~80% cleared within 10 minutes

Excretion: Clearance: Rapidly from circulating plasma at a rate of 550-650 mL/minute, primarily by the liver; >50% present in plasma is cleared within 5 minutes after the infusion has been terminated, and ~80% is cleared within 10 minutes

Usual Dosage

I.V.:

Coronary artery thrombi: Front loading dose (weight-based):
Patients >67 kg: Total dose: 100 mg over 1.5 hours; infuse 15 mg (30 mL) over 1-2 minutes. Infuse 50 mg (100 mL) over 30 minutes. See "Note."
Patients ≤67 kg: Total dose: 1.25 mg/kg; infuse 15 mg I.V. bolus over 1-2 minutes, then infuse 0.75 mg/kg (not to exceed 50 mg) over next 30 minutes, followed by 0.5 mg/kg over next 60 minutes (not to exceed 35 mg). See "Note."

Note: Concurrently, begin heparin 60 units/kg bolus (maximum: 4000 units) followed by continuous infusion of 12 units/kg/hour (maximum: 1000 units/hour) and adjust to aPTT target of 1.5-2 times the upper limit of control. Infuse remaining 35 mg (70 mL) of alteplase over the next hour.

Acute pulmonary embolism: 100 mg over 2 hours.

Acute ischemic stroke: Doses should be given within the first 3 hours of the onset of symptoms. Load with 0.09 mg/kg as a bolus, followed by 0.81 mg/kg as a continuous infusion over 60 minutes. Maximum total dose should not exceed 90 mg. Heparin should not be started for at least 24 hours after starting alteplase for stroke.

Intracatheter: Central venous catheter clearance: Cathflo™ Activase®:

Patients ≥10 to <30 kg: 110% of the internal lumen volume of the catheter (≤2 mg [1 mg/mL]); retain in catheter for ≤2 hours; may instill a second dose if catheter remains occluded

Patients ≥30 kg: 2 mg (1 mg/mL); retain in catheter for ≤2 hours; may instill a second dose if catheter remains occluded

Intra-arterial: Peripheral arterial thrombotic obstruction (unlabeled use): 0.02-0.1 mg/kg/hour for 1-8 hours

Administration

Activase®:

Bolus dose may be prepared by one of three methods:

1) removal of 15 mL reconstituted (1 mg/mL) solution from vial

2) removal of 15 mL from a port on the infusion line after priming

3) programming an infusion pump to deliver a 15 mL bolus at the initiation of infusion

Remaining dose may be administered as follows:

50 mg vial: Either PVC bag or glass vial and infusion set

100 mg vial: Insert spike end of the infusion set through the same puncture site created by transfer device and infuse from vial

If further dilution is desired, may be diluted in equal volume of 0.9% sodium chloride or D_5W to yield a final concentration of 0.5 mg/mL AD

Cathflo™ Activase®: Intracatheter: Instill dose into occluded catheter. Do not force solution into catheter. After a 30-minute dwell time, assess catheter function by attempting to aspirate blood. If catheter is functional, aspirate 4-5 mL of blood to remove Cathflo™ Activase® and residual clots. Gently irrigate the catheter with NS. If catheter remains nonfunctional, let Cathflo™ Activase® dwell for another 90 minutes (total dwell time: 120 minutes) and reassess function. If catheter function is not restored, a second dose may be instilled.

Monitoring Parameters When using for central venous catheter clearance, assess catheter function by attempting to aspirate blood.

Reference Range

Not routinely measured; literature supports therapeutic levels of 0.52-1.8 µg/mL

Fibrinogen: 200-400 mg/dL

Activated partial thromboplastin time (aPTT): 22.5-38.7 seconds

Prothrombin time (PT): 10.9-12.2 seconds

Nursing Implications Assess for hemorrhage during first hour of treatment

Dosage Forms Injection, powder for reconstitution, recombinant:

Activase®: 50 mg [29 million units]; 100 mg [58 million units]

Cathflo™ Activase®: 2 mg

- **Alteplase, Recombinant** *see Alteplase on page 59*
- **Alteplase, Tissue Plasminogen Activator, Recombinant** *see Alteplase on page 59*
- **ALternaGel® [OTC]** *see Aluminum Hydroxide on page 63*
- **Alti-Alprazolam (Can)** *see Alprazolam on page 55*
- **Alti-Amiloride HCTZ (Can)** *see Amiloride and Hydrochlorothiazide on page 71*
- **Alti-Amiodarone (Can)** *see Amiodarone on page 74*
- **Alti-Azathioprine (Can)** *see Azathioprine on page 136*
- **Alti-Beclomethasone (Can)** *see Beclomethasone on page 149*
- **Alti-Captopril (Can)** *see Captopril on page 218*
- **Alti-Clindamycin (Can)** *see Clindamycin on page 309*
- **Alti-Clobetasol (Can)** *see Clobetasol on page 311*
- **Alti-Clonazepam (Can)** *see Clonazepam on page 316*
- **Alti-Desipramine (Can)** *see Desipramine on page 376*
- **Alti-Diltiazem (Can)** *see Diltiazem on page 409*
- **Alti-Diltiazem CD (Can)** *see Diltiazem on page 409*
- **Alti-Divalproex (Can)** *see Valproic Acid and Derivatives on page 1398*
- **Alti-Doxepin (Can)** *see Doxepin on page 440*
- **Alti-Famotidine (Can)** *see Famotidine on page 543*
- **Alti-Flunisolide (Can)** *see Flunisolide on page 572*
- **Alti-Fluoxetine (Can)** *see Fluoxetine on page 578*
- **Alti-Flurbiprofen (Can)** *see Flurbiprofen on page 585*
- **Alti-Fluvoxamine (Can)** *see Fluvoxamine on page 593*
- **Alti-Ipratropium (Can)** *see Ipratropium on page 740*
- **Alti-Minocycline (Can)** *see Minocycline on page 918*
- **Alti-MPA (Can)** *see MedroxyPROGESTERone on page 848*
- **Altinac™** *see Tretinoin (Topical) on page 1365*
- **Alti-Nadolol (Can)** *see Nadolol on page 948*
- **Alti-Nortriptyline (Can)** *see Nortriptyline on page 996*
- **Alti-Piroxicam (Can)** *see Piroxicam on page 1093*
- **Alti-Prazosin (Can)** *see Prazosin on page 1120*
- **Alti-Ranitidine (Can)** *see Ranitidine on page 1178*
- **Alti-Salbutamol (Can)** *see Albuterol on page 41*
- **Alti-Sotalol (Can)** *see Sotalol on page 1252*
- **Alti-Sulfasalazine® (Can)** *see Sulfasalazine on page 1275*
- **Alti-Terazosin (Can)** *see Terazosin on page 1298*
- **Alti-Ticlopidine (Can)** *see Ticlopidine on page 1331*
- **Alti-Trazodone Apo®-Trazodone (Can)** *see Trazodone on page 1362*
- **Alti-Verapamil (Can)** *see Verapamil on page 1412*

Altretamine (al TRET a meen)

U.S. Brand Names Hexalen®
Canadian Brand Names Hexalen®
Synonyms Hexamethylmelamine; HEXM; HMM; HXM; NSC-13875
Therapeutic Category Antineoplastic Agent, Miscellaneous
Use Palliative treatment of persistent or recurrent ovarian cancer following first-line therapy with a cisplatin- or alkylating agent-based combination
Pregnancy Risk Factor D
Contraindications Hypersensitivity to altretamine or any component of the formulation; pre-existing severe bone marrow suppression or severe neurologic toxicity; pregnancy
Warnings/Precautions The U.S. Food and Drug Administration (FDA) currently recommends that procedures for proper handling and disposal of antineoplastic agents be considered. Peripheral blood counts and neurologic examinations should be done routinely before and after drug therapy. Use with caution in patients previously treated with other myelosuppressive drugs or with pre-existing neurotoxicity; use with caution in patients with renal or hepatic dysfunction; altretamine may be slightly mutagenic.
Adverse Reactions
>10%:
Central nervous system: Peripheral sensory neuropathy, neurotoxicity
Gastrointestinal: Nausea, vomiting
Moderate (30% to 60%)
Hematologic: Anemia, thrombocytopenia, leukopenia
1% to 10%:
Central nervous system: Seizures
Gastrointestinal: Anorexia, diarrhea, stomach cramps
Hepatic: Increased alkaline phosphatase
<1% (Limited to important or life-threatening): Alopecia, hepatotoxicity, myelosuppression, tremor
Overdosage/Toxicology Symptoms include nausea, vomiting, peripheral neuropathy, and severe bone marrow suppression. After decontamination, treatment is supportive.
Drug Interactions
Increased Effect/Toxicity: Altretamine may cause severe orthostatic hypotension when administered with MAO inhibitors. Cimetidine may decrease metabolism of altretamine.
Decreased Effect: Phenobarbital may increase metabolism of altretamine which may decrease the effect.
Ethanol/Nutrition/Herb Interactions Ethanol: Avoid ethanol (due to GI irritation)
Mechanism of Action Although altretamine clinical antitumor spectrum resembles that of alkylating agents, the drug has demonstrated activity in alkylator-resistant patients; probably requires hepatic microsomal mixed-function oxidase enzyme activation to become cytotoxic. The drug selectively inhibits the incorporation of radioactive thymidine and uridine into DNA and RNA, inhibiting DNA and RNA synthesis; metabolized to reactive intermediates which covalently bind to microsomal proteins and DNA. These reactive intermediates can spontaneously degrade to demethylated melamines and formaldehyde which are also cytotoxic.
Pharmacodynamics/Kinetics
Absorption: Well absorbed (75% to 89%)
Distribution: Highly concentrated hepatically and renally; low in other organs
Metabolism: Hepatic; rapid and extensive demethylation
Half-life elimination: 13 hours
Time to peak, plasma: 0.5-3 hours
Excretion: Urine (<1% as unchanged drug)
Usual Dosage Refer to individual protocols. Oral:
Adults: 4-12 mg/kg/day in 3-4 divided doses for 21-90 days
Alternatively: 240-320 mg/m^2/day in 3-4 divided doses for 21 days, repeated every 6 weeks
Alternatively: 260 mg/m^2/day for 14-21 days of a 28-day cycle in 4 divided doses
Alternatively: 150 mg/m^2/day in 3-4 divided doses for 14 days of a 28-day cycle
Temporarily discontinue (for ≥14 days) and subsequently restart at 200 mg/m^2/day if any of the following occurs:
GI intolerance unresponsive to symptom management
WBC <2000/mm^3
granulocyte count <1000/mm^3
platelet count <75,000/mm^3
progressive neurotoxicity
Dietary Considerations Should be taken after meals.
Administration Administer orally; administer total daily dose as 3-4 divided oral doses after meals and at bedtime
Patient Information Report any numbness or tingling in extremities to physician; nausea and vomiting may occur and even begin up to weeks after therapy is stopped
Nursing Implications Advise patient to report any numbness or tingling in extremities to physician; nausea and vomiting may occur and even begin up to weeks after therapy is stopped
Dosage Forms Capsule: 50 mg

♦ **Alu-Cap® [OTC]** see Aluminum Hydroxide on page 63

Aluminum Acetate and Acetic Acid

(a LOO mi num AS e tate & a SEE tik AS id)
U.S. Brand Names Otic Domeboro®
Synonyms Acetic Acid and Aluminum Acetate Otic; Burow's Otic
Therapeutic Category Otic Agent, Anti-infective
Use Treatment of superficial infections of the external auditory canal
Usual Dosage Instill 4-6 drops in ear(s) every 2-3 hours; insert saturated wick, keep moist for 24 hours

Additional Information Complete prescribing information for this medication should be consulted for additional detail.

Aluminum Hydroxide (a LOO mi num hye DROKS ide)

U.S. Brand Names ALternaGel® [OTC]; Alu-Cap® [OTC]; Alu-Tab® [OTC]; Amphojel® [OTC]; Dialume® [OTC]

Canadian Brand Names Amphojel®; Basaljel®

Therapeutic Category Antacid; Antidote, Hyperphosphatemia

Use Treatment of hyperacidity; hyperphosphatemia

Pregnancy Risk Factor C

Pregnancy/Breast-Feeding Implications

Clinical effects on the fetus: No data available; available evidence suggests safe use during pregnancy and breast-feeding

Breast-feeding/lactation: No data available

Contraindications Hypersensitivity to aluminum salts or any component of the formulation

Warnings/Precautions Hypophosphatemia may occur with prolonged administration or large doses; aluminum intoxication and osteomalacia may occur in patients with uremia. Use with caution in patients with congestive heart failure, renal failure, edema, cirrhosis, and low sodium diets, and patients who have recently suffered gastrointestinal hemorrhage; uremic patients not receiving dialysis may develop osteomalacia and osteoporosis due to phosphate depletion.

Elderly, due to disease and/or drug therapy, may be predisposed to constipation and fecal impaction. Careful evaluation of possible drug interactions must be done. When used as an antacid in ulcer treatment, consider buffer capacity (mEq/mL) to calculate dose; consider renal insufficiency as predisposition to aluminum toxicity.

Adverse Reactions

>10%: Gastrointestinal: Constipation, chalky taste, stomach cramps, fecal impaction

1% to 10%: Gastrointestinal: Nausea, vomiting, discoloration of feces (white speckles)

<1% (Limited to important or life-threatening): Hypomagnesemia, hypophosphatemia

Overdosage/Toxicology Aluminum antacids may cause constipation, phosphate depletion, and bezoar or fecalith formation. In patients with renal failure, aluminum may accumulate to toxic levels. Deferoxamine, traditionally used as an iron chelator, has been shown to increase urinary aluminum output. Deferoxamine chelation of aluminum has resulted in improvements of clinical symptoms and bone histology; however, remains an experimental treatment for aluminum poisoning and has a significant potential for adverse effects.

Drug Interactions

Decreased Effect: Aluminum hydroxide decreases the effect of tetracyclines, digoxin, indomethacin, iron salts, isoniazid, allopurinol, benzodiazepines, corticosteroids, penicillamine, phenothiazines, ranitidine, ketoconazole, and itraconazole.

Mechanism of Action Neutralizes hydrochloride in stomach to form Al $(Cl)_3$ salt + H_2O

Usual Dosage Oral:

Peptic ulcer disease (dosages empirical):

Children: 5-15 mL/dose every 3-6 hours or 1 and 3 hours after meals and at bedtime

Adults: 15-45 mL every 3-6 hours or 1 and 3 hours after meals and at bedtime

Prophylaxis against gastrointestinal bleeding:

Infants: 2-5 mL/dose every 1-2 hours

Children: 5-15 mL/dose every 1-2 hours

Adults: 30-60 mL/dose every hour

Titrate to maintain the gastric pH >5

Hyperphosphatemia:

Children: 50-150 mg/kg/24 hours in divided doses every 4-6 hours, titrate dosage to maintain serum phosphorus within normal range

Adults: 500-1800 mg, 3-6 times/day, between meals and at bedtime; best taken with a meal or within 20 minutes of a meal

Antacid: Adults: 30 mL 1 and 3 hours postprandial and at bedtime

Amphojel®: 10 mL suspension or two 300 mg tablets 5-6 times/day between meals and at bedtime

Dietary Considerations Should be taken 1-3 hours after meals.

Monitoring Parameters Monitor phosphorous levels periodically when patient is on chronic therapy

Test Interactions Decreases phosphorus, inorganic (S)

Patient Information Dilute dose in water or juice, shake well; chew tablets thoroughly before swallowing with water; do not take oral drugs within 1-2 hours of administration; notify physician if relief is not obtained or if there are any signs to suggest bleeding from the GI tract

Nursing Implications Used primarily as a phosphate binder; dose should be given within 20 minutes of a meal and followed with water

Dosage Forms

Capsule:

Alu-Cap®: 400 mg

Dialume®: 500 mg

Liquid (ALternaGel®): 600 mg/5 mL

Suspension, oral: 320 mg/5 mL, 450 mg/5 mL, 675 mg/5 mL

Amphojel®: 320 mg/5 mL

Tablet:

Alu-Tab®: 500 mg

Amphojel®: 300 mg, 600 mg

Aluminum Hydroxide and Magnesium Carbonate

(a LOO mi num hye DROKS ide & mag NEE zhum KAR bun nate)

U.S. Brand Names Gaviscon® Extra Strength [OTC]; Gaviscon® Liquid [OTC]

Synonyms Magnesium Carbonate and Aluminum Hydroxide

Therapeutic Category Antacid

Use Temporary relief of symptoms associated with gastric acidity

(Continued)

Aluminum Hydroxide and Magnesium Carbonate *(Continued)*

Usual Dosage Adults: Oral:
Liquid:
    Gaviscon® Regular Strength: 15-30 mL 4 times/day after meals and at bedtime
    Gaviscon® Extra Strength Relief: 15-30 mL 4 times/day after meals
    Tablet (Gaviscon® Extra Strength Relief): Chew 2-4 tablets 4 times/day
Additional Information Complete prescribing information for this medication should be consulted for additional detail.
Dosage Forms
Liquid:
    Gaviscon®: Aluminum hydroxide 31.7 mg and magnesium carbonate 119.3 mg per 5 mL (355 mL) [contains sodium 0.57 mEq/5 mL]
    Gaviscon® Extra Strength: Aluminum hydroxide 84.6 mg and magnesium carbonate 79.1 mg per 5 mL (355 mL) [contains sodium 0.9 mEq/5 mL]
    Tablet, chewable (Gaviscon® Extra Strength): Aluminum hydroxide 160 mg and magnesium carbonate 105 mg [contains sodium 1.3 mEq/tablet]

Aluminum Hydroxide and Magnesium Hydroxide
    (a LOO mi num hye DROKS ide & mag NEE zhum hye DROK side)
U.S. Brand Names Maalox® [OTC]; Maalox® TC (Therapeutic Concentrate) [OTC]
Canadian Brand Names Diovol®; Diovol® Ex; Gelusil®; Gelusil® Extra Strength; Mylanta™; Univol®
Synonyms Magnesium Hydroxide and Aluminum Hydroxide
Therapeutic Category Antacid
Use Antacid, hyperphosphatemia in renal failure
Pregnancy Risk Factor C
Usual Dosage Oral: 5-10 mL 4-6 times/day, between meals and at bedtime; may be used every hour for severe symptoms
    Maalox®: 10-20 mL 4 times/day
Additional Information Complete prescribing information for this medication should be consulted for additional detail.
Dosage Forms
Suspension (Maalox®): Aluminum hydroxide 225 mg and magnesium hydroxide 200 mg per 5 mL (150 mL, 360 mL, 780 mL)
Suspension, high potency (Maalox® TC): Aluminum hydroxide 600 mg and magnesium hydroxide 300 mg per 5 mL (360 mL)

Aluminum Hydroxide and Magnesium Trisilicate
    (a LOO mi num hye DROKS ide & mag NEE zhum trye SIL i kate)
U.S. Brand Names Gaviscon® Tablet [OTC]
Synonyms Magnesium Trisilicate and Aluminum Hydroxide
Therapeutic Category Antacid
Use Temporary relief of hyperacidity
Pregnancy Risk Factor C
Usual Dosage Adults: Oral: Chew 2-4 tablets 4 times/day or as directed by healthcare provider
Additional Information Complete prescribing information for this medication should be consulted for additional detail.
Dosage Forms Tablet, chewable (Gaviscon®): Aluminum hydroxide 80 mg and magnesium trisilicate 20 mg [contains sodium 0.8 mEq/tablet]

Aluminum Hydroxide, Magnesium Hydroxide, and Simethicone
    (a LOO mi num hye DROKS ide, mag NEE zhum hye DROKS ide, & sye METH i kone)
U.S. Brand Names Maalox® Fast Release Liquid [OTC]; Maalox® Max [OTC]; Mylanta® Extra Strength Liquid [OTC]; Mylanta® Liquid [OTC]
Canadian Brand Names Diovol Plus®; Mylanta™ Double Strength; Mylanta™ Extra Strength; Mylanta™ regular Strength
Synonyms Magnesium Hydroxide, Aluminum Hydroxide, and Simethicone; Simethicone, Aluminum Hydroxide, and Magnesium Hydroxide
Therapeutic Category Antacid; Antiflatulent
Use Temporary relief of hyperacidity associated with gas; may also be used for indications associated with other antacids
Pregnancy Risk Factor C
Usual Dosage Adults: 10-20 mL or 2-4 tablets 4-6 times/day between meals and at bedtime; may be used every hour for severe symptoms
Additional Information Complete prescribing information for this medication should be consulted for additional detail.
Dosage Forms Liquid:
Maalox® Fast Release: Aluminum hydroxide 500 mg, magnesium hydroxide 450 mg, and simethicone 40 mg per 5 mL (360 mL, 780 mL)
Maalox® Max: Aluminum hydroxide 400 mg, magnesium hydroxide 400 mg, and simethicone 40 mg per 5 mL (360 mL)
Mylanta®: Aluminum hydroxide 200 mg, magnesium hydroxide 200 mg, and simethicone 20 mg per 5 mL (180 mL, 360 mL, 720 mL) [original, cherry, mint, and lemon flavors]
Mylanta® Extra Strength: Aluminum hydroxide 400 mg, magnesium hydroxide 400 mg, and simethicone 40 mg per 5 mL (180 mL, 360 mL, 720 mL) [original, cherry, and mint flavors]

♦ **Aluminum Sucrose Sulfate, Basic** *see* Sucralfate *on page 1266*

Aluminum Sulfate and Calcium Acetate
    (a LOO mi num SUL fate & KAL see um AS e tate)
U.S. Brand Names Bluboro® [OTC]; Domeboro® [OTC]; Pedi-Boro® [OTC]
Synonyms Calcium Acetate and Aluminum Sulfate

Therapeutic Category Topical Skin Product

Use Astringent wet dressing for relief of inflammatory conditions of the skin and to reduce weeping that may occur in dermatitis

Usual Dosage

Topical: Soak affected area in the solution 2-4 times/day for 15-30 minutes or apply wet dressing soaked in the solution 2-4 times/day for 30-minute treatment periods; rewet dressing with solution every few minutes to keep it moist

Domeboro®:

Wet dressing or compress: Saturate dressing and apply to affected area; saturate cloth every 15-30 minutes; repeat as needed

As a soak: Soak for 15-30 minutes 3 times/day

Additional Information Complete prescribing information for this medication should be consulted for additional detail.

Dosage Forms Aluminum sulfate and calcium acetate form aluminum acetate when mixed:

Powder, for topical solution (Bluboro®, Domeboro®, Pedi-Boro®): 1 packet/16 ounces of water = 1:40 solution = Modified Burow's Solution

Tablet, effervescent, for topical solution (Domeboro®): 1 tablet/12 ounces of water = 1:40 solution = Modified Burow's Solution

♦ **Alupent**® *see* Metaproterenol *on page 872*

♦ **Alu-Tab**® **[OTC]** *see* Aluminum Hydroxide *on page 63*

Amantadine (a MAN ta deen)

Related Information

Community-Acquired Pneumonia in Adults *on page 1603*

Depression *on page 1655*

Parkinson's Agents *on page 1513*

USPHA/IDSA Guidelines for the Prevention of Opportunistic Infections in Persons With HIV *on page 1574*

U.S. Brand Names Symmetrel®

Canadian Brand Names Endantadine®; PMS-Amantadine; Symmetrel®

Synonyms Adamantanamine Hydrochloride; Amantadine Hydrochloride

Therapeutic Category Anti-Parkinson's Agent, Dopamine Agonist; Antiviral Agent, Oral; Dopaminergic Agent (Antiparkinson's); Hyperthermia, Treatment

Use Prophylaxis and treatment of influenza A viral infection; treatment of parkinsonism; treatment of drug-induced extrapyramidal symptoms

Unlabeled/Investigational Use Creutzfeldt-Jakob disease

Pregnancy Risk Factor C

Contraindications Hypersensitivity to amantadine or any component of the formulation

Warnings/Precautions Use with caution in patients with liver disease, a history of recurrent and eczematoid dermatitis, uncontrolled psychosis or severe psychoneurosis, seizures and in those receiving CNS stimulant drugs; reduce dose in renal disease; when treating Parkinson's disease, do not discontinue abruptly. In many patients, the therapeutic benefits of amantadine are limited to a few months. Elderly patients may be more susceptible to the CNS effects (using 2 divided daily doses may minimize this effect). Use with caution in patients with CHF, peripheral edema, or orthostatic hypotension. Avoid in angle closure glaucoma.

Adverse Reactions

1% to 10%:

Cardiovascular: Orthostatic hypotension, peripheral edema

Central nervous system: Insomnia, depression, anxiety, irritability, dizziness, hallucinations, ataxia, headache, somnolence, nervousness, dream abnormality, agitation, fatigue, confusion

Dermatologic: Livedo reticularis

Gastrointestinal: Nausea, anorexia, constipation, diarrhea, xerostomia

Respiratory: Dry nose

<1% (Limited to important or life-threatening): Amnesia, congestive heart failure, convulsions, decreased libido, dyspnea, eczematoid dermatitis, euphoria, hyperkinesis, hypertension, leukopenia, neutropenia, oculogyric episodes, psychosis, rash, slurred speech, urinary retention, visual disturbances, vomiting, weakness

Overdosage/Toxicology Symptoms include nausea, vomiting, slurred speech, blurred vision, lethargy, hallucinations, seizures, and myoclonic jerking. Following GI decontamination, treatment should be directed at reducing CNS stimulation and at maintaining cardiovascular function. Seizures can be treated with diazepam, while lidocaine infusion may be required for cardiac dysrhythmias.

Drug Interactions

Increased Effect/Toxicity: Anticholinergics (benztropine and trihexyphenidyl) may potentiate CNS side effects of amantadine. Hydrochlorothiazide, triamterene, and/or trimethoprim may increase toxicity of amantadine; monitor for altered response.

Ethanol/Nutrition/Herb Interactions Ethanol: Avoid ethanol (may increase CNS adverse effects).

Stability Protect from freezing

Mechanism of Action As an antiviral, blocks the uncoating of influenza A virus preventing penetration of virus into host; antiparkinsonian activity may be due to its blocking the reuptake of dopamine into presynaptic neurons or by increasing dopamine release from presynaptic fibers

Pharmacodynamics/Kinetics

Onset of action: Antidyskinetic: Within 48 hours

Absorption: Well absorbed

Distribution: V_d: Normal: 4.4 ± 0.2 L/kg; Renal failure: 5.1 ± 0.2 L/kg; in saliva, tear film, and nasal secretions; in animals, tissue (especially lung) concentrations higher than serum concentrations; crosses blood-brain barrier

Protein binding: Normal renal function: ~67%; Hemodialysis: ~59%

Metabolism: Not appreciable, small amounts of an acetyl metabolite identified

(Continued)

Amantadine *(Continued)*

Half-life elimination: 10-28 hours; Impaired renal function: 7-10 days

Time to peak: 1-4 hours

Excretion: Urine (80% to 90% as unchanged drug)

Usual Dosage Oral:

Children: Influenza A treatment:

1-9 years (<45 kg): 5-9 mg/kg/day in 1-2 divided doses to a maximum of 150 mg/day

10-12 years: 100-200 mg/day in 1-2 divided doses

Influenza prophylaxis: Administer for 10-21 days following exposure if the vaccine is concurrently given or for 90 days following exposure if the vaccine is unavailable or contraindicated and re-exposure is possible

Adults:

Drug-induced extrapyramidal symptoms: 100 mg twice daily; may increase to 300-400 mg/day, if needed

Parkinson's disease or Creutzfeldt-Jakob disease (unlabeled use): 100 mg twice daily as sole therapy; may increase to 400 mg/day if needed with close monitoring; initial dose: 100 mg/day if with other serious illness or with high doses of other anti-Parkinson drugs

Influenza A viral infection: 200 mg/day in 1-2 divided doses; initiate within 24-48 hours after onset of symptoms; discontinue as soon as possible based on clinical response (generally within 3-5 days or within 24-48 hours after symptoms disappear)

Influenza prophylaxis: 200 mg/day in 1-2 doses; minimum 10-day course of therapy following exposure if the vaccine is concurrently given or for 90 days following exposure if the vaccine is unavailable or contraindicated and re-exposure is possible

Elderly patients should take the drug in 2 daily doses rather than a single dose to avoid adverse neurologic reactions

Dosing interval in renal impairment:

Cl_{cr} 50-60 mL/minute: Administer 200 mg alternating with 100 mg/day

Cl_{cr} 30-50 mL/minute: Administer 100 mg/day

Cl_{cr} 20-30 mL/minute: Administer 200 mg twice weekly

Cl_{cr} 10-20 mL/minute: Administer 100 mg 3 times/week

Cl_{cr} <10 mL/minute: Administer 200 mg alternating with 100 mg every 7 days

Hemodialysis: Slightly hemodialyzable (5% to 20%); no supplemental dose is needed

Peritoneal dialysis: No supplemental dose is needed

Continuous arterio-venous or venous-venous hemofiltration: No supplemental dose is needed

Monitoring Parameters Renal function, Parkinson's symptoms, mental status, influenza symptoms, blood pressure

Patient Information Do not abruptly discontinue therapy, it may precipitate a parkinsonian crisis; may impair ability to perform activities requiring mental alertness or coordination; must take throughout flu season or for at least 10 days following vaccination for effective prophylaxis; take second dose of the day in early afternoon to decrease incidence of insomnia

Nursing Implications If insomnia occurs, the last daily dose should be given several hours before retiring; assess parkinsonian symptoms prior to and throughout course of therapy

Additional Information Patients with intolerable CNS side effects often do better with rimantadine.

Dosage Forms

Capsule, as hydrochloride: 100 mg

Syrup, as hydrochloride (Symmetrel®): 50 mg/5 mL (480 mL) [raspberry flavor]

Tablet, as hydrochloride (Symmetrel®): 100 mg

♦ **Amantadine Hydrochloride** *see* Amantadine *on page 65*

♦ **Amaphen®** *see* Butalbital Compound *on page 197*

♦ **Amaryl®** *see* Glimepiride *on page 631*

♦ **Amatine® (Can)** *see* Midodrine *on page 912*

♦ **Ambien®** *see* Zolpidem *on page 1445*

♦ **Ambi® Skin Tone [OTC]** *see* Hydroquinone *on page 686*

♦ **AmBisome®** *see* Amphotericin B (Liposomal) *on page 91*

Amcinonide *(am SIN oh nide)*

Related Information

Corticosteroids Comparison *on page 1495*

U.S. Brand Names Cyclocort®

Canadian Brand Names Cyclocort®

Therapeutic Category Anti-inflammatory Agent; Corticosteroid, Topical (High Potency)

Use Relief of the inflammatory and pruritic manifestations of corticosteroid-responsive dermatoses (high potency corticosteroid)

Pregnancy Risk Factor C

Contraindications Hypersensitivity to amcinonide or any component of the formulation; use on the face, groin, or axilla

Warnings/Precautions Adverse systemic effects may occur when used on large areas of the body, denuded areas, for prolonged periods of time, with an occlusive dressing, and/or in infants or small children; occlusive dressings should not be used in presence of infection or weeping lesions

Adverse Reactions Frequency not defined.

Dermatologic: Acne, hypopigmentation, allergic dermatitis, maceration of the skin, skin atrophy, striae, miliaria, telangiectasia

Endocrine & metabolic: HPA suppression, Cushing's syndrome, growth retardation

Local: Burning, itching, irritation, dryness, folliculitis, hypertrichosis

Systemic: Suppression of HPA axis, Cushing's syndrome, hyperglycemia; these reactions occur more frequently with occlusive dressings

Miscellaneous: Secondary infection

Overdosage/Toxicology Symptoms include cushingoid appearance (systemic), muscle weakness (systemic), and osteoporosis (systemic) all with long-term use only. When consumed in excessive quantities for prolonged periods, systemic hypercorticism and adrenal suppression may occur; in those cases, discontinuation and withdrawal of the corticosteroid should be done judiciously.

Mechanism of Action Stimulates the synthesis of enzymes needed to decrease inflammation, suppress mitotic activity, and cause vasoconstriction

Pharmacodynamics/Kinetics
Absorption: Adequate through intact skin; increases with skin inflammation or occlusion
Metabolism: Hepatic
Excretion: Urine and feces

Usual Dosage Adults: Topical: Apply in a thin film 2-3 times/day. Therapy should be discontinued when control is achieved; if no improvement is seen, reassessment of diagnosis may be necessary.

Patient Information Before applying, gently wash area to reduce risk of infection; apply a thin film to cleansed area and rub in gently and thoroughly until medication vanishes; avoid exposure to sunlight, severe sunburn may occur

Nursing Implications Assess for worsening of rash or fever

Dosage Forms
Cream, topical: 0.1% (15 g, 30 g, 60 g)
Lotion, topical: 0.1% (20 mL, 60 mL)
Ointment, topical: 0.1% (15 g, 30 g, 60 g)

Amifostine (am i FOS teen)

U.S. Brand Names Ethyol®
Canadian Brand Names Ethyol®
Synonyms Ethiofos; Gammaphos
Therapeutic Category Antidote, Cisplatin

Use Reduce the incidence of moderate to severe xerostomia in patients undergoing postoperative radiation treatment for head and neck cancer, where the radiation port includes a substantial portion of the parotid glands. Reduce the cumulative renal toxicity associated with repeated administration of cisplatin in patients with advanced ovarian cancer or nonsmall cell lung cancer. In these settings, the clinical data does not suggest that the effectiveness of cisplatin-based chemotherapy regimens is altered by amifostine.

Pregnancy Risk Factor C

Contraindications Hypersensitivity to aminothiol compounds or mannitol

Warnings/Precautions Limited data are currently available regarding the preservation of antitumor efficacy when amifostine is administered prior to cisplatin therapy in settings other than advanced ovarian cancer or nonsmall cell lung cancer. Amifostine should therefore not be used in patients receiving chemotherapy for other malignancies in which chemotherapy can produce a significant survival benefit or cure, except in the context of a clinical study.

Patients who are hypotensive or in a state of dehydration should not receive amifostine. Interrupt antihypertensive therapy for 24 hours before amifostine. Patients receiving antihypertensive therapy that cannot be stopped for 24 hours preceding amifostine treatment also should not receive amifostine. Patients should be adequately hydrated prior to amifostine infusion and kept in a supine position during the infusion. Blood pressure should be monitored every 5 minutes during the infusion. If hypotension requiring interruption of therapy occurs, patients should be placed in the Trendelenburg position and given an infusion of normal saline using a separate I.V. line.

It is recommended that antiemetic medication, including dexamethasone 20 mg I.V. and a serotonin 5-HT$_3$ receptor antagonist be administered prior to and in conjunction with amifostine. Rare hypersensitivity reactions, including anaphylaxis, have been reported. Discontinue if allergic reaction occurs; do not rechallenge.

Reports of clinically relevant hypocalcemia are rare, but serum calcium levels should be monitored in patients at risk of hypocalcemia, such as those with nephrotic syndrome.

Adverse Reactions
>10%:
Cardiovascular: Flushing; hypotension (62%) (see Additional Information)
Central nervous system: Chills, dizziness, somnolence
Gastrointestinal: Nausea/vomiting (may be severe)
Respiratory: Sneezing
Miscellaneous: Feeling of warmth/coldness, hiccups
<1% (Limited to important or life-threatening): Apnea, anaphylactoid reactions, anaphylaxis, arrhythmia, atrial fibrillation, erythema multiforme; hypersensitivity reactions (fever, rash, hypoxia, dyspnea, laryngeal edema); hypocalcemia, mild rashes, myocardial ischemia, rigors, seizure, Stevens-Johnson syndrome, toxic epidermal necrolysis

Overdosage/Toxicology Symptoms include increased nausea, vomiting, and hypotension. Treatment includes infusion of normal saline and other supportive measures, as clinically indicated.
(Continued)

Amifostine (Continued)

Drug Interactions

Increased Effect/Toxicity: Special consideration should be given to patients receiving antihypertensive medications or other drugs that could potentiate hypotension.

Stability

Store intact vials of lyophilized powder at room temperature (20°C to 25°C/68°F to 77°F)

Reconstitute with 9.7 mL of sterile 0.9% sodium chloride. The reconstituted solution (500 mg/10 mL) is chemically stable for up to 5 hours at room temperature (25°C) or up to 24 hours under refrigeration (2°C to 8°C).

Amifostine should be further diluted in 0.9% sodium chloride to a concentration of 5-40 mg/mL and is chemically stable for up to 5 hours at room temperature (25°C) or up to 24 hours under refrigeration (2°C to 8°C)

Mechanism of Action Prodrug that is dephosphorylated by alkaline phosphatase in tissues to a pharmacologically active free thiol metabolite that can reduce the toxic effects of cisplatin. The free thiol is available to bind to, and detoxify, reactive metabolites of cisplatin; and can also act as a scavenger of free radicals that may be generated in tissues exposed to cisplatin.

Pharmacodynamics/Kinetics

Distribution: V_d: 3.5 L

Metabolism: Hepatic dephosphorylation to two metabolites (active-free thiol and disulfide)

Half-life elimination: 9 minutes

Excretion: Urine

Clearance, plasma: 2.17 L/minute

Usual Dosage Adults: I.V. (refer to individual protocols): 910 mg/m^2 administered once daily as a 15-minute I.V. infusion, starting 30 minutes prior to chemotherapy

Reduction of xerostomia from head and neck radiation: 200 mg/m^2 I.V. (as a 3-minute infusion) once daily, starting 15-30 minutes before standard fraction radiation therapy

Note: 15-minute infusion is better tolerated than more extended infusions. Further reductions in infusion times have not been systematically investigated. The infusion of amifostine should be interrupted if the systolic blood pressure (mm Hg) decreases significantly from the following baseline values:

Decrease of 20 if baseline systolic blood pressure <100

Decrease of 25 if baseline systolic blood pressure 100-119

Decrease of 30 if baseline systolic blood pressure 120-139

Decrease of 40 if baseline systolic blood pressure 140-179

Decrease of 50 if baseline systolic blood pressure ≥180

Mean onset of hypotension is 14 minutes into the 15-minute infusion and the mean duration was 6 minutes. Hypotension should be treated with fluid infusion and postural management of the patient (supine or Trendelenburg position). If the blood pressure returns to normal within 5 minutes and the patient is asymptomatic, the infusion may be restarted so that the full dose of amifostine may be administered. If the full dose of amifostine cannot be administered, the dose of amifostine for subsequent cycles should be 740 mg/m^2.

Administration I.V.: Administer over 15 minutes; administration as a longer infusion is associated with a higher incidence of side effects

Monitoring Parameters Blood pressure should be monitored every 5 minutes during the infusion

Additional Information Mean onset of hypotension is 14 minutes into the 15-minute infusion and the mean duration was 6 minutes.

Dosage Forms Powder for injection: 500 mg

♦ **Amigesic**® see Salsalate on page 1220

Amikacin (am i KAY sin)

Related Information

Aminoglycoside Dosing and Monitoring on page 1470

Antimicrobial Drugs of Choice on page 1588

U.S. Brand Names Amikin®

Canadian Brand Names Amikin®

Synonyms Amikacin Sulfate

Therapeutic Category Antibiotic, Aminoglycoside

Use Treatment of serious infections due to organisms resistant to gentamicin and tobramycin including *Pseudomonas*, *Proteus*, *Serratia*, and other gram-positive bacilli (bone infections, respiratory tract infections, endocarditis, and septicemia); documented infection of mycobacterial organisms susceptible to amikacin

Pregnancy Risk Factor C

Contraindications Hypersensitivity to amikacin sulfate or any component of the formulation; cross-sensitivity may exist with other aminoglycosides

Warnings/Precautions Dose and/or frequency of administration must be monitored and modified in patients with renal impairment; drug should be discontinued if signs of ototoxicity, nephrotoxicity, or hypersensitivity occur; ototoxicity is proportional to the amount of drug given and the duration of treatment; tinnitus or vertigo may be indications of vestibular injury and impending bilateral irreversible damage; renal damage is usually reversible

Adverse Reactions

1% to 10%:

Central nervous system: Neurotoxicity

Otic: Ototoxicity (auditory), ototoxicity (vestibular)

Renal: Nephrotoxicity

<1% (Limited to important or life-threatening): Allergic reaction, dyspnea, eosinophilia

Overdosage/Toxicology Symptoms include ototoxicity, nephrotoxicity, and neuromuscular toxicity. Treatment of choice, following a single acute overdose, appears to be the maintenance of good urine output of at least 3 mL/kg/hour. Dialysis is of questionable value in the enhancement of aminoglycoside elimination. If required, hemodialysis is preferred over peritoneal dialysis in patients with normal renal function.

AMILORIDE

Drug Interactions

Increased Effect/Toxicity: Amikacin may increase or prolong the effect of neuromuscular blocking agents. Concurrent use of amphotericin (or other nephrotoxic drugs) may increase the risk of amikacin-induced nephrotoxicity. The risk of ototoxicity from amikacin may be increased with other ototoxic drugs.

Stability Stable for 24 hours at room temperature and 2 days at refrigeration when mixed in D_5W, $D_5^1/_4NS$, $D_5^1/_2NS$, NS, LR

Mechanism of Action Inhibits protein synthesis in susceptible bacteria by binding to 30S ribosomal subunits

Pharmacodynamics/Kinetics

Absorption: I.M.: May be delayed in the bedridden patient

Distribution: Primarily into extracellular fluid (highly hydrophilic); penetrates blood-brain barrier when meninges inflamed; crosses placenta

Relative diffusion of antimicrobial agents from blood into CSF: Good only with inflammation (exceeds usual MICs)

CSF:blood level ratio: Normal meninges: 10% to 20%; Inflamed meninges: 15% to 24%

Half-life elimination (dependent on renal function and age):

Infants: Low birthweight (1-3 days): 7-9 hours; Full-term >7 days: 4-5 hours

Children: 1.6-2.5 hours

Adults: Normal renal function: 1.4-2.3 hours; Anuria/end-stage renal disease: 28-86 hours

Time to peak, serum: I.M.: 45-120 minutes

Excretion: Urine (94% to 98%)

Usual Dosage Individualization is critical because of the low therapeutic index

Use of ideal body weight (IBW) for determining the mg/kg/dose appears to be more accurate than dosing on the basis of total body weight (TBW)

In morbid obesity, dosage requirement may best be estimated using a dosing weight of IBW + 0.4 (TBW - IBW)

Initial and periodic peak and trough plasma drug levels should be determined, particularly in critically ill patients with serious infections or in disease states known to significantly alter aminoglycoside pharmacokinetics (eg, cystic fibrosis, burns, or major surgery)

Infants, Children, and Adults: I.M., I.V.: 5-7.5 mg/kg/dose every 8 hours

Some clinicians suggest a daily dose of 15-20 mg/kg for all patients with normal renal function. This dose is at least as efficacious with similar, if not less, toxicity than conventional dosing.

Dosing interval in renal impairment: Some patients may require larger or more frequent doses if serum levels document the need (ie, cystic fibrosis or febrile granulocytopenic patients)

Cl_{cr} ≥60 mL/minute: Administer every 8 hours

Cl_{cr} 40-60 mL/minute: Administer every 12 hours

Cl_{cr} 20-40 mL/minute: Administer every 24 hours

Cl_{cr} <20 mL/minute: Loading dose, then monitor levels

Hemodialysis: Dialyzable (50% to 100%); administer dose postdialysis or administer $^2/_3$ normal dose as a supplemental dose postdialysis and follow levels

Peritoneal dialysis: Dose as Cl_{cr} <20 mL/minute: Follow levels

Continuous arteriovenous or venovenous hemodiafiltration effects: Dose as for Cl_{cr} 10-40 mL/minute and follow levels

Administration Administer I.M. injection in large muscle mass

Monitoring Parameters Urinalysis, BUN, serum creatinine, appropriately timed peak and trough concentrations, vital signs, temperature, weight, I & O, hearing parameters

Reference Range

Sample size: 0.5-2 mL blood (red top tube) or 0.1-1 mL serum (separated)

Therapeutic levels:

Peak:

Life-threatening infections: 25-30 µg/mL

Serious infections: 20-25 µg/mL

Urinary tract infections: 15-20 µg/mL

Trough:

Serious infections: 1-4 µg/mL

Life-threatening infections: 4-8 µg/mL

Toxic concentration: Peak: >35 µg/mL; Trough: >10 µg/mL

Timing of serum samples: Draw peak 30 minutes after completion of 30-minute infusion or at 1 hour following initiation of infusion or I.M. injection; draw trough within 30 minutes prior to next dose

Test Interactions Penicillin may decrease aminoglycoside serum concentrations *in vitro*

Patient Information Report loss of hearing, ringing or roaring in the ears, or feeling of fullness in head

Nursing Implications Aminoglycoside levels measured from blood taken from Silastic® central catheters can sometimes give falsely high readings (draw levels from alternate lumen or peripheral stick, if possible)

Additional Information Sodium content of 1 g: 29.9 mg (1.3 mEq)

Dosage Forms Injection, solution, as sulfate: 50 mg/mL (2 mL, 4 mL); 62.5 mg/mL (8 mL); 250 mg/mL (2 mL, 4 mL) [contains metabisulfite]

♦ **Amikacin Sulfate** *see* Amikacin *on page 68*

♦ **Amikin®** *see* Amikacin *on page 68*

Amiloride (a MIL oh ride)

Related Information

Heart Failure *on page 1663*

U.S. Brand Names Midamor®

Canadian Brand Names Midamor®

Synonyms Amiloride Hydrochloride

Therapeutic Category Diuretic, Potassium Sparing

(Continued)

69

Amiloride *(Continued)*

Use Counteracts potassium loss induced by other diuretics in the treatment of hypertension or edematous conditions including CHF, hepatic cirrhosis, and hypoaldosteronism; usually used in conjunction with more potent diuretics such as thiazides or loop diuretics

Unlabeled/Investigational Use Investigational: Cystic fibrosis; reduction of lithium-induced polyuria

Pregnancy Risk Factor B

Contraindications Hypersensitivity to amiloride or any component of the formulation; presence of elevated serum potassium levels (>5.5 mEq/L); if patient is receiving other potassium-conserving agents (eg, spironolactone, triamterene) or potassium supplementation (medicine, potassium-containing salt substitutes, potassium-rich diet); anuria; acute or chronic renal insufficiency; evidence of diabetic nephropathy. Patients with evidence of renal impairment or diabetes mellitus should not receive this medicine without close, frequent monitoring of serum electrolytes and renal function.

Warnings/Precautions Use cautiously in patients with severe hepatic insufficiency; may cause hyperkalemia (serum levels >5.5 mEq/L) which, if uncorrected, is potentially fatal; medication should be discontinued if potassium level are >6.5 mEq/L

Adverse Reactions

1% to 10%:

Central nervous system: Headache, fatigue, dizziness

Endocrine & metabolic: Hyperkalemia, hyperchloremic metabolic acidosis, dehydration, hyponatremia, gynecomastia

Gastrointestinal: Nausea, diarrhea, vomiting, abdominal pain, gas pain, appetite changes, constipation

Genitourinary: Impotence

Neuromuscular & skeletal: Muscle cramps, weakness

Respiratory: Cough, dyspnea

<1% (Limited to important or life-threatening): Alopecia, arrhythmias, bladder spasms, chest pain, dyspnea, dysuria, GI bleeding, increased intraocular pressure, jaundice, orthostatic hypotension, palpitations, polyuria

Overdosage/Toxicology Clinical signs are consistent with dehydration and electrolyte disturbance. Large amounts may result in life-threatening hyperkalemia (>6.5 mEq/L). This can be treated with I.V. glucose (dextrose 25% in water), with rapid-acting insulin, with concurrent I.V. sodium bicarbonate and, if needed, Kayexalate® oral or rectal solutions in sorbitol. Persistent hyperkalemia may require dialysis.

Drug Interactions

Increased Effect/Toxicity: Increased risk of amiloride-associated hyperkalemia with triamterene, spironolactone, angiotensin-converting enzyme (ACE) inhibitors, potassium preparations, cyclosporine, tacrolimus, and indomethacin. Amiloride may increase the toxicity of amantadine and lithium by reduction of renal excretion. Quinidine and amiloride together may increase risk of malignant arrhythmias.

Decreased Effect: Decreased effect of amiloride with use of nonsteroidal anti-inflammatory agents. Amoxicillin's absorption may be reduced with concurrent use.

Ethanol/Nutrition/Herb Interactions Food: Hyperkalemia may result if amiloride is taken with potassium-containing foods.

Mechanism of Action Interferes with potassium/sodium exchange (active transport) in the distal tubule, cortical collecting tubule and collecting duct by inhibiting sodium, potassium-ATPase; decreases calcium excretion; increases magnesium loss

Pharmacodynamics/Kinetics

Onset of action: 2 hours

Duration: 24 hours

Absorption: ~15% to 25%

Distribution: V_d: 350-380 L

Protein binding: 23%

Metabolism: No active metabolites

Half-life elimination: Normal renal function: 6-9 hours; End-stage renal disease: 8-144 hours

Time to peak, serum: 6-10 hours

Excretion: Urine and feces (equal amounts as unchanged drug)

Usual Dosage Oral:

Children: Although safety and efficacy have not been established by the FDA in children, a dosage of 0.625 mg/kg/day has been used in children weighing 6-20 kg.

Adults: 5-10 mg/day (up to 20 mg)

Elderly: Initial: 5 mg once daily or every other day

Dosing adjustment in renal impairment:

Cl_{cr} 10-50 mL/minute: Administer at 50% of normal dose.

Cl_{cr} <10 mL/minute: Avoid use.

Dietary Considerations Do not use salt substitutes or low salt milk without checking with your healthcare provider, too much potassium can be as harmful as too little.

Monitoring Parameters I & O, daily weights, blood pressure, serum electrolytes, renal function

Test Interactions ↑ potassium (S)

Patient Information Take with food or milk; avoid salt substitutes; because of high potassium content, avoid bananas and oranges; report any muscle cramps, weakness, nausea, or dizziness; use caution operating machinery or performing other tasks requiring alertness

Nursing Implications Assess fluid status via daily weights, I & O ratios, standing and supine blood pressures; observe for hyperkalemia; if ordered once daily, dose should be given in the morning

Additional Information Medication should be discontinued if potassium level exceeds 6.5 mEq/L. Combined with hydrochlorothiazide as Moduretic®. Amiloride is considered an alternative to triamterene or spironolactone.

Dosage Forms Tablet, as hydrochloride: 5 mg

Amiloride and Hydrochlorothiazide (a MIL oh ride & hye droe klor oh THYE a zide)

U.S. Brand Names Moduretic®

Canadian Brand Names Alti-Amiloride HCTZ; Apo®-Amilzide; Moduret®; Moduretic®; Novamilor; Nu-Amilzide

Synonyms Hydrochlorothiazide and Amiloride

Therapeutic Category Antihypertensive Agent, Combination

Use Potassium-sparing diuretic; antihypertensive

Pregnancy Risk Factor B

Usual Dosage Adults: Oral: Start with 1 tablet/day, then may be increased to 2 tablets/day if needed; usually given in a single dose

Additional Information Complete prescribing information for this medication should be consulted for additional detail.

Dosage Forms Tablet: Amiloride hydrochloride 5 mg and hydrochlorothiazide 50 mg

♦ **Amiloride Hydrochloride** *see Amiloride on page 69*

♦ **2-Amino-6-Mercaptopurine** *see Thioguanine on page 1318*

♦ **2-Amino-6-Trifluoromethoxy-benzothiazole** *see Riluzole on page 1196*

♦ **Aminobenzylpenicillin** *see Ampicillin on page 93*

Aminocaproic Acid (a mee noe ka PROE ik AS id)

U.S. Brand Names Amicar®

Canadian Brand Names Amicar®

Therapeutic Category Hemostatic Agent

Use Treatment of excessive bleeding from fibrinolysis

Pregnancy Risk Factor C

Contraindications Disseminated intravascular coagulation; evidence of an intravascular clotting process

Warnings/Precautions Rapid I.V. administration of the undiluted drug is not recommended. Aminocaproic acid may accumulate in patients with decreased renal function. Intrarenal obstruction may occur secondary to glomerular capillary thrombosis or clots in the renal pelvis and ureters. Do not use in hematuria of upper urinary tract origin unless possible benefits outweigh risks. Use with caution in patients with cardiac, renal, or hepatic disease. Do not administer without a definite diagnosis of laboratory findings indicative of hyperfibrinolysis. Inhibition of fibrinolysis may promote clotting or thrombosis. Subsequently, use with great caution in patients with or at risk for veno-occlusive disease of the liver. Benzyl alcohol is used as a preservative, therefore, these products should not be used in the neonate. Do not administer with factor IX complex concentrates or anti-inhibitor coagulant complexes.

Adverse Reactions

>10%: Gastrointestinal: Anorexia, nausea

1% to 10%:

Cardiovascular: Hypotension, bradycardia, arrhythmia

Central nervous system: Dizziness, headache, malaise, fatigue

Dermatologic: Rash (measles-like skin rash or itching on face and/or palms of hands); masculinization and hirsutism in females

Endocrine & metabolic: Adrenocortical insufficiency

Gastrointestinal: GI irritation, vomiting, cramps, diarrhea

Hematologic: Decreased platelet function, elevated serum enzymes, leukopenia, agranulocytosis, thrombocytopenia

Neuromuscular & skeletal: Myopathy, weakness

Otic: Tinnitus

Respiratory: Nasal congestion

<1% (Limited to important or life-threatening): Convulsions, renal failure, rhabdomyolysis

Overdosage/Toxicology Symptoms include nausea, diarrhea, delirium, hepatic necrosis, and thromboembolism.

Drug Interactions

Increased Effect/Toxicity: Increased risk of hypercoagulability with oral contraceptives, estrogens. Should not be administered with factor IX complex concentrated or anti-inhibitor complex concentrates due to an increased risk of thrombosis.

Mechanism of Action Competitively inhibits activation of plasminogen to plasmin, also, a lesser antiplasmin effect

Pharmacodynamics/Kinetics

Onset of action: ~1-72 hours

Distribution: Widely through intravascular and extravascular compartments

Metabolism: Minimal hepatic

Half-life elimination: 1-2 hours

Time to peak: Oral: Within 2 hours

Excretion: Urine (68% to 86% as unchanged drug)

Usual Dosage In the management of acute bleeding syndromes, oral dosage regimens are the same as the I.V. dosage regimens in adults and children

Chronic bleeding: Oral, I.V.: 5-30 g/day in divided doses at 3- to 6-hour intervals

Acute bleeding syndrome:

Children: Oral, I.V.: 100 mg/kg or 3 g/m^2 during the first hour, followed by continuous infusion at the rate of 33.3 mg/kg/hour or 1 g/m^2/hour; total dosage should not exceed 18 g/m^2/24 hours

Traumatic hyphema: Oral: 100 mg/kg/dose every 6-8 hours

Adults:

Oral: For elevated fibrinolytic activity, administer 5 g during first hour, followed by 1-1.25 g/hour for approximately 8 hours or until bleeding stops

I.V.: 4-5 g in 250 mL of diluent during first hour followed by continuous infusion at the rate of 1-1.25 g/hour in 50 mL of diluent, continue for 8 hours or until bleeding stops

Maximum daily dose: Oral, I.V.: 30 g

(Continued)

Aminocaproic Acid *(Continued)*

Dosing adjustment in renal impairment: Oliguria or ESRD: Reduce to 15% to 25% of usual dose

Administration Administration by infusion using appropriate I.V. solution (dextrose 5% or 0.9% sodium chloride); rapid I.V. injection (IVP) should be avoided since hypotension, bradycardia, and arrhythmia may result. Aminocaproic acid may accumulate in patients with decreased renal function.

Monitoring Parameters Fibrinogen, fibrin split products, creatine phosphokinase (with long-term therapy)

Reference Range Therapeutic concentration: >130 µg/mL (concentration necessary for inhibition of fibrinolysis)

Test Interactions ↑ potassium, creatine phosphokinase [CPK] (S)

Patient Information Report any signs of bleeding; change positions slowly to minimize dizziness

Nursing Implications Administration by infusion using appropriate I.V. solution (dextrose 5% or sodium chloride 0.9%); rapid I.V. injection (IVP) should be avoided since hypotension, bradycardia, and arrhythmia may result. Aminocaproic acid may accumulate in patients with decreased renal function.

Dosage Forms
Injection, solution: 250 mg/mL (20 mL) [contains benzyl alcohol]
Syrup: 1.25 g/5 mL (480 mL) [raspberry flavor]
Tablet: 500 mg

♦ **Amino-Cerv™ Vaginal Cream** *see Urea on page 1391*

Aminoglutethimide *(a mee noe gloo TETH i mide)*

U.S. Brand Names Cytadren®

Therapeutic Category Adrenal Steroid Inhibitor; Antiadrenal Agent; Antineoplastic Agent, Miscellaneous

Use In postmenopausal patients with breast cancer; third-line salvage agent for metastatic prostate cancer; suppression of adrenal function in selected patients with Cushing's syndrome

Pregnancy Risk Factor D

Usual Dosage Adults: Oral:
250 mg every 6 hours may be increased at 1- to 2-week intervals to a total of 2 g/day; administer in divided doses, 2-3 times/day to reduce incidence of nausea and vomiting. Follow adrenal cortical response by careful monitoring of plasma cortisol until the desired level of suppression is achieved.
Mineralocorticoid (fludrocortisone) replacement therapy may be necessary in up to 50% of patients. If glucocorticoid replacement therapy is necessary, 20-30 mg hydrocortisone orally in the morning will replace endogenous secretion.

Dosing adjustment in renal impairment: Dose reduction may be necessary

Additional Information Complete prescribing information for this medication should be consulted for additional detail.

Dosage Forms Tablet, scored: 250 mg

♦ **Aminoglycoside Dosing and Monitoring** *see page 1470*

Aminolevulinic Acid *(a MEE noh lev yoo lin ik AS id)*

U.S. Brand Names Levulan® Kerastick™

Canadian Brand Names Levulan®

Synonyms Aminolevulinic Acid Hydrochloride

Therapeutic Category Photosensitizing Agent, Topical; Porphyrin Agent, Topical

Use Treatment of nonhyperkeratotic actinic keratoses of the face or scalp; to be used in conjunction with blue light illumination

Pregnancy Risk Factor C

Pregnancy/Breast-Feeding Implications No adequate or well-controlled studies in pregnant women. Should be used during pregnancy only if clearly needed; excretion in breast milk is unknown; use caution in breast-feeding.

Contraindications Hypersensitivity to aminolevulinic acid or any component of the formulation; individuals with cutaneous photosensitivity at wavelengths of 400-450 nm; porphyria; allergy to porphyrins

Warnings/Precautions For external use only. Do not apply to eyes or mucous membranes. Treatment site will become photosensitive following application. Patients should be instructed to avoid exposure to sunlight, bright indoor lights, or tanning beds during the period prior to blue light treatment. Should be applied by a qualified health professional to avoid application to perilesional skin. Has not been tested in individuals with coagulation defects (acquired or inherited).

Adverse Reactions
Transient stinging, burning, itching, erythema, and edema result from the photosensitizing properties of this agent. Symptoms subside between 1 minute and 24 hours after turning off the blue light illuminator. Severe stinging or burning was reported in at least 50% of patients from at least one lesional site treatment.
>10%: Dermatologic: Severe stinging or burning (50%), scaling of the skin/crusted skin (64% to 71%), hyperpigmentation/hypopigmentation (22% to 36%), itching (14% to 25%), erosion (2% to 14%)
1% to 10%:
Central nervous system: Dysesthesia (0% to 2%)
Dermatologic: Skin ulceration (2% to 4%), vesiculation (4% to 5%), pustular drug eruption (0% to 4%), skin disorder (5% to 12%)
Hematologic: Bleeding/hemorrhage (2% to 4%)
Local: Wheal/flare (2% to 7%), local pain (1%), tenderness (1%), edema (1%), scabbing (0% to 2%)

Overdosage/Toxicology Monitoring and supportive care are recommended. Patients should be advised to avoid incidental exposure to intense light sources for at least 40 hours. Consequences of exceeding the recommended topical dosage are not known.

Drug Interactions
  Increased Effect/Toxicity: Photosensitizing agents such as griseofulvin, thiazide diuretics, sulfonamides, sulfonylureas, phenothiazines, and tetracyclines theoretically may increase the photosensitizing potential of aminolevulinic acid.

Stability Store at 25°C (77°F). Topical solution should be used immediately following solution preparation and must be completed within 2 hours of solution preparation.

Mechanism of Action Aminolevulinic acid is a metabolic precursor of protoporphyrin IX (PpIX), which is a photosensitizer. Photosensitization following application of aminolevulinic acid topical solution occurs through the metabolic conversion to PpIX. When exposed to light of appropriate wavelength and energy, accumulated PpIX produces a photodynamic reaction.

Pharmacodynamics/Kinetics
  PpIX:
    Peak fluorescence intensity: 11 hours ± 1 hour
    Half-life, mean clearance for lesions: 30 ± 10 hours

Usual Dosage Adults: Topical: Apply to actinic keratoses (**not** perilesional skin) followed 14-18 hours later by blue light illumination. Application/treatment may be repeated at a treatment site after 8 weeks.

Administration Actinic keratoses targeted for treatment should be clean and dry prior to application. Follow instructions for solution preparation and application. Solution is applied directly to the lesion, but not the perilesional skin, using the supplied applicator. Should not be applied to periorbital area or allowed to contact ocular or mucous membranes. Blue light exposure should follow between 14 and 18 hours after the application.

Patient Information Avoid exposure to sunlight, bright indoor lights, or tanning beds during the period prior to blue light treatment. Wear a wide-brimmed hat to protect from exposure. Sunscreens do not protect against photosensitization by this agent.

Additional Information Use in conjunction with the BLU-U™ Blue Light Photodynamic Therapy Illuminator.

Dosage Forms Solution, topical: 20% (with applicator)

♦ **Aminolevulinic Acid Hydrochloride** *see Aminolevulinic Acid on page 72*
♦ **Amino-Opti-E® [OTC]** *see Vitamin E on page 1423*
♦ **Aminophyllin™** *see Theophylline Salts on page 1310*
♦ **Aminophylline** *see Theophylline Salts on page 1310*

Aminosalicylate Sodium (a MEE noe sa LIS i late SOW dee um)

Canadian Brand Names Nemasol® Sodium

Synonyms Para-Aminosalicylate Sodium; PAS

Therapeutic Category Anti-inflammatory Agent; Antitubercular Agent; Nonsteroidal Anti-inflammatory Drug (NSAID), Oral

Use Adjunctive treatment of tuberculosis used in combination with other antitubercular agents; has also been used in Crohn's disease

Pregnancy Risk Factor C

Contraindications Hypersensitivity to aminosalicylate sodium or any component of the formulation

Warnings/Precautions Use with caution in patients with hepatic or renal dysfunction, patients with gastric ulcer, patients with CHF, and patients who are sodium restricted

Adverse Reactions
  1% to 10%: Gastrointestinal: Nausea, vomiting, diarrhea, abdominal pain
  <1% (Limited to important or life-threatening): Agranulocytosis, fever, hemolytic anemia, hepatitis jaundice, leukopenia, thrombocytopenia, vasculitis

Overdosage/Toxicology Acute overdose results in crystalluria and renal failure, nausea, and vomiting. Alkalinization of the urine with sodium bicarbonate and forced diuresis can prevent crystalluria and nephrotoxicity.

Drug Interactions
  Decreased Effect: Aminosalicylate sodium may decrease serum levels of digoxin and vitamin B_{12}.

Mechanism of Action Aminosalicylic acid (PAS) is a highly specific bacteriostatic agent active against *M. tuberculosis*. Structurally related to para-aminobenzoic acid (PABA) and its mechanism of action is thought to be similar to the sulfonamides, a competitive antagonism with PABA; disrupts plate biosynthesis in sensitive organisms.

Pharmacodynamics/Kinetics
  Absorption: Readily, >90%
  Metabolism: Hepatic acetylated, >50%
  Half-life elimination: Reduced with renal dysfunction
  Excretion: Urine (>80% as unchanged drug and metabolites)

Usual Dosage Oral:
  Children: 150 mg/kg/day in 3-4 equally divided doses
  Adults: 150 mg/kg/day in 2-3 equally divided doses (usually 12-14 g/day)
  Dosing adjustment in renal impairment:
    Cl_{cr} 10-50 mL/minute: Administer 50% to 75% of dose
    Cl_{cr} <10 mL/minute: Administer 50% of dose
    Administer after hemodialysis

Dietary Considerations May be taken with food.

Patient Information Notify physician if persistent sore throat, fever, unusual bleeding or bruising, persistent nausea, vomiting, or abdominal pain occurs; do not stop taking before consulting your physician; take with food or meals; do not use products that are brown or purple; store in a cool, dry place away from sunlight

Nursing Implications Do not administer if discolored

Dosage Forms Tablet: 500 mg

♦ **5-Aminosalicylic Acid** *see Mesalamine on page 866*

♦ **Aminoxin® [OTC]** *see Pyridoxine on page 1162*

Amiodarone (a MEE oh da rone)

Related Information
Antiarrhythmic Drugs Comparison *on page 1478*

U.S. Brand Names Cordarone®; Pacerone®

Canadian Brand Names Alti-Amiodarone; Cordarone®; Gen-Amiodarone; Novo-Amiodarone

Synonyms Amiodarone Hydrochloride

Therapeutic Category Antiarrhythmic Agent, Class III

Use
Oral: Management of life-threatening recurrent ventricular fibrillation (VF) or hemodynamically unstable ventricular tachycardia (VT)

I.V.: Initiation of treatment and prophylaxis of frequency recurring VF and unstable VT in patients refractory to other therapy. Also, used for patients when oral amiodarone is indicated, but who are unable to take oral medication.

Unlabeled/Investigational Use
Conversion of atrial fibrillation to normal sinus rhythm; maintenance of normal sinus rhythm
Prevention of postoperative atrial fibrillation during cardiothoracic surgery
Paroxysmal supraventricular tachycardia (SVT)
Control of rapid ventricular rate due to accessory pathway conduction in pre-excited atrial arrhythmias [ACLS guidelines]
After defibrillation and epinephrine in cardiac arrest with persistent ventricular tachycardia (VT) or ventricular fibrillation (VF) [ACLS guidelines]
Control of hemodynamically stable VT, polymorphic VT or wide-complex tachycardia of uncertain origin [ACLS guidelines]

Pregnancy Risk Factor D

Pregnancy/Breast-Feeding Implications May cause fetal harm when administered to a pregnant woman, leading to congenital goiter and hypo- or hyperthyroidism.

Contraindications Hypersensitivity to amiodarone or any component of the formulation; severe sinus-node dysfunction; second- and third-degree heart block (except in patients with a functioning artificial pacemaker); bradycardia causing syncope (except in patients with a functioning artificial pacemaker); cisapride, ritonavir, sparfloxacin, moxifloxacin, gatifloxacin; pregnancy; breast-feeding

Warnings/Precautions Not considered first-line antiarrhythmic due to high incidence of significant and potentially fatal toxicity (ie, hypersensitivity pneumonitis or interstitial/alveolar pneumonitis, hepatic failure, heart block, bradycardia or exacerbated arrhythmias), especially with large doses; reserve for use in arrhythmias refractory to other therapy; hospitalize patients while loading dose is administered; use cautiously in elderly due to predisposition to toxicity; use very cautiously and with close monitoring in patients with thyroid or liver disease. Due to an extensive tissue distribution and prolonged elimination period, the time at which a life-threatening arrhythmia will recur following discontinued therapy or an interaction with subsequent treatment may occur is unpredictable; patients must be observed carefully and extreme caution taken when other antiarrhythmic agents are substituted after discontinuation of amiodarone. Caution in surgical patients; may enhance hemodynamic effect of anesthetics. Corneal microdeposits occur in a majority of patients. Safety and efficacy in pediatric patients have not been established.

Adverse Reactions With large dosages (>400 mg/day), adverse reactions occur in ~75% of patients and require discontinuation in 5% to 20%.

>10%:
Cardiovascular: Hypotension (I.V., 16%)
Central nervous system: Between 20% and 40% of patients experience some form of neurologic adverse events (see Central Nervous System and Neuromuscular & Skeletal effects: 1% to 10% category)
Gastrointestinal: Nausea, vomiting

1% to 10%:
Cardiovascular: Congestive heart failure, arrhythmias (including atropine-resistant bradycardia, heart block, sinus arrest, ventricular tachycardia), myocardial depression, flushing, edema. Additional effects associated with I.V. administration include asystole, cardiac arrest, electromechanical dissociation, ventricular tachycardia and cardiogenic shock.
Central nervous system: Fever, fatigue, involuntary movements, incoordination, malaise, sleep disturbances, ataxia, dizziness, headache
Dermatologic: Photosensitivity (10%)
Endocrine & metabolic: Hypothyroidism or hyperthyroidism (less common), decreased libido
Gastrointestinal: Constipation, anorexia, abdominal pain, abnormal salivation, abnormal taste (oral form)
Genitourinary: noninfectious epididymitis (3% to 11%)
Hematologic: Coagulation abnormalities
Hepatic: Abnormal LFTs
Local: Phlebitis (I.V., with concentrations >3 mg/mL)
Neuromuscular & skeletal: Paresthesia, tremor, muscular weakness, peripheral neuropathy
Ocular: Visual disturbances, corneal microdeposits (occur in a majority of patients, and lead to visual disturbance in ~10%); other ocular symptoms are listed under the <1% category
Respiratory: Pulmonary toxicity has been estimated to occur at a frequency between 2% and 7% of patients (some reports indicate a frequency as high as 17%). Toxicity may present as hypersensitivity pneumonitis, pulmonary fibrosis (cough, fever, malaise), pulmonary inflammation, interstitial pneumonitis, or alveolar pneumonitis; other rare pulmonary toxicities are listed under the <1% category.
Miscellaneous: Abnormal smell (oral form)

<1% (Limited to important or life-threatening): Acute intracranial hypertension (I.V.), alopecia, anaphylactic shock, angioedema, aplastic anemia, ARDS (postoperative), atrial fibrillation, bone marrow granuloma, brain stem dysfunction, bronchiolitis obliterans organizing pneumonia (BOOP), cholestasis, cirrhosis, delirium, discoloration of skin (slate-blue), dyskinesias, encephalopathy, hypotension (with oral form), impotence, increased QT interval, leukocytoclastic vasculitis, neutropenia, nodal arrhythmia, optic neuritis, optic neuropathy, pancreatitis, pancytopenia, Parkinsonian symptoms, pleuritis, pseudotumor cerebri, pulmonary edema, rash, severe hepatotoxicity (potentially fatal hepatitis), Stevens-Johnson syndrome, thrombocytopenia, toxic epidermal necrolysis, vasculitis, ventricular fibrillation

Overdosage/Toxicology Symptoms include extensions of pharmacologic effect, sinus bradycardia and/or heart block, hypotension and QT prolongation. Patients should be monitored for several days following ingestion. Intoxication with amiodarone necessitates EKG monitoring. Bradycardia may be atropine resistant. Injectable isoproterenol or a temporary pacemaker may be required.

Drug Interactions

Cytochrome P450 Effect: CYP3A3/4 enzyme substrate; CYP2C9, 2D6, and 3A3/4 enzyme inhibitor

Increased Effect/Toxicity: Note: Due to the long half-life of amiodarone, drug interactions may take 1 or more weeks to develop. Use of amiodarone with diltiazem, verapamil, digoxin, beta-blockers, and other drugs which delay AV conduction may cause excessive AV block (amiodarone may also decrease the metabolism of some of these agents - see below). Amprenavir, cimetidine, nelfinavir, and ritonavir increase amiodarone levels. Amiodarone may increase the levels of digoxin (reduce dose by 50% on initiation), clonazepam, cyclosporine, flecainide (decrease dose up to 33%), metoprolol, phenothiazines, phenytoin, procainamide (reduce dose), propranolol, quinidine, tricyclic antidepressants, and warfarin. Concurrent use of fentanyl may lead to bradycardia, sinus arrest, and hypotension. The effect of drugs which prolong the QT interval, including amitriptyline, astemizole, bepridil, cisapride, disopyramide, erythromycin, gatifloxacin, haloperidol, imipramine, moxifloxacin, quinidine, pimozide, procainamide, sotalol, sparfloxacin, theophylline, and thioridazine may be increased. Cisapride, gatifloxacin, moxifloxacin, and sparfloxacin are contraindicated. Amiodarone may alter thyroid function and response to thyroid supplements. Amiodarone enhances the myocardial depressant and conduction defects of inhalation anesthetics (monitor).

Decreased Effect: Amiodarone blood levels may be decreased by phenytoin and rifampin. Amiodarone may alter thyroid function and response to thyroid supplements; monitor closely.

Ethanol/Nutrition/Herb Interactions

Food: Increases the rate and extent of absorption of amiodarone.

Herb/Nutraceutical: St John's wort may decrease amiodarone levels or enhance photosensitization. Avoid ephedra (may worsen arrhythmia). Avoid dong quai.

Stability I.V. infusions >2 hours must be administered in glass or polyolefin bottles; **incompatible** with aminophylline, cefamandole, cefazolin, heparin, and sodium bicarbonate; store at room temperature; protect from light

Mechanism of Action Class III antiarrhythmic agent which inhibits adrenergic stimulation, prolongs the action potential and refractory period in myocardial tissue; decreases AV conduction and sinus node function

Pharmacodynamics/Kinetics

Onset of action: Oral: 3 days to 3 weeks; I.V.: May be more rapid

Peak effect: 1 week to 5 months

Duration after discontinuing therapy: 7-50 days

Note: Mean onset of effect and duration after discontinuation may be shorter in children than adults

Distribution: V_d: 66 L/kg (range: 18-148 L/kg); crosses placenta; enters breast milk in concentrations higher than maternal plasma concentrations

Protein binding: 96%

Metabolism: Hepatic, major metabolite active; possible enterohepatic recirculation

Bioavailability: ~50%

Half-life elimination: 40-55 days (range: 26-107 days); shorter in children than adults

Excretion: Feces; urine (<1% as unchanged drug)

Usual Dosage

Oral:

Children (calculate doses for children <1 year on body surface area): Loading dose: 10-15 mg/kg/day or 600-800 mg/1.73 m^2/day for 4-14 days or until adequate control of arrhythmia or prominent adverse effects occur (this loading dose may be given in 1-2 divided doses/day). Dosage should then be reduced to 5 mg/kg/day or 200-400 mg/1.73 m^2/day given once daily for several weeks. If arrhythmia does not recur, reduce to lowest effective dosage possible. Usual daily minimal dose: 2.5 mg/kg/day; maintenance doses may be given for 5 of 7 days/week.

Adults: Ventricular arrhythmias: 800-1600 mg/day in 1-2 doses for 1-3 weeks, then when adequate arrhythmia control is achieved, decrease to 600-800 mg/day in 1-2 doses for 1 month; maintenance: 400 mg/day. Lower doses are recommended for supraventricular arrhythmias.

I.V.:

Children (safety and efficacy of amiodarone use in children has not been fully established): Ventricular arrhythmias: A multicenter study (Perry, 1996; n=40; mean age 5.4 years with 24 of 40 children <2 years of age) used an I.V. loading dose of 5 mg/kg that was divided into five 1 mg/kg aliquots, with each aliquot given over 5-10 minutes. Additional 1-5 mg/kg doses could be administered 30 minutes later in a similar fashion if needed. The mean loading dose was 6.3 mg/kg. A maintenance dose (continuous infusion of 10-15 mg/kg/day) was administered to 21 of the 40 patients. Further studies are needed.

Note: I.V. administration at low flow rates (potentially associated with use in pediatrics) may result in leaching of plasticizers (DEHP) from intravenous tubing. DEHP may

(Continued)

Amiodarone (Continued)

adversely affect male reproductive tract development. Alternative means of dosing and administration (1 mg/kg aliquots) may need to be considered.

Adults:

Stable VT or SVT (unlabeled uses): First 24 hours: 1000 mg according to following regimen

Step 1: 150 mg (100 mL) over first 10 minutes (mix 3 mL in 100 mL D_5W)

Step 2: 360 mg (200 mL) over next 6 hours (mix 18 mL in 500 mL D_5W): 1 mg/minute

Step 3: 540 mg (300 mL) over next 18 hours: 0.5 mg/minute

Note: After the first 24 hours: 0.5 mg/minute utilizing concentration of 1-6 mg/mL

Breakthrough VF or VT: 150 mg supplemental doses in 100 mL D_5W over 10 minutes

Pulseless VF or VT: I.V. push: Initial: 300 mg in 20-30 mL NS or D_5W; if VF or VT recurs, supplemental dose of 150 mg followed by infusion of 1 mg/minute for 6 hours, then 0.5 mg/minute (maximum daily dose: 2.2 g)

Note: When switching from I.V. to oral therapy, use the following as a guide:

<1-week I.V. infusion: 800-1600 mg/day

1- to 3-week I.V. infusion: 600-800 mg/day

>3-week I.V. infusion: 400 mg/day

Recommendations for conversion to intravenous amiodarone after oral administration: During long-term amiodarone therapy (ie, ≥4 months), the mean plasma-elimination half-life of the active metabolite of amiodarone is 61 days. Replacement therapy may not be necessary in such patients if oral therapy is discontinued for a period <2 weeks, since any changes in serum amiodarone concentrations during this period may **not** be clinically significant.

Dosing adjustment in hepatic impairment: Probably necessary in substantial hepatic impairment.

Hemodialysis: Not dialyzable (0% to 5%); supplemental dose is not necessary.

Peritoneal dialysis effects: Not dialyzable (0% to 5%); supplemental dose is not necessary.

Dietary Considerations Administer consistently with regard to meals.

Administration

Oral: Administer consistently with regard to meals. Take in divided doses with meals if high daily dose or if GI upset occurs. If GI intolerance occurs with single-dose therapy, use twice daily dosing.

I.V.: Give I.V. therapy using an infusion pump through a central line or a peripheral line at a concentration of <2 mg/mL. **Note:** I.V. administration at low flow rates (potentially associated with use in pediatrics) may result in leaching of plasticizers (DEHP) from intravenous tubing. DEHP may adversely affect male reproductive tract development. Alternative means of dosing and administration (1 mg/kg aliquots) may need to be considered.

Monitoring Parameters Monitor heart rate (EKG) and rhythm throughout therapy; assess patient for signs of thyroid dysfunction (thyroid function tests and liver enzymes), lethargy, edema of the hands, feet, weight loss, and pulmonary toxicity (baseline pulmonary function tests)

Reference Range Therapeutic: 0.5-2.5 mg/L (SI: 1-4 µmol/L) (parent); desethyl metabolite is active and is present in equal concentration to parent drug

Test Interactions Thyroid function tests: Amiodarone partially inhibits the peripheral conversion of thyroxine (T_4) to triiodothyronine (T_3); serum T_4 and reverse triiodothyronine (rT_3) concentrations may be increased and serum T_3 may be decreased; most patients remain clinically euthyroid, however, clinical hypothyroidism or hyperthyroidism may occur

Patient Information Take with food; use sunscreen or stay out of sun to prevent burns; skin discoloration is reversible; photophobia may make sunglasses necessary; do not discontinue abruptly; regular blood work for thyroid functions tests and ophthalmologic exams are necessary; notify physician if persistent dry cough or shortness of breath occurs

Nursing Implications Muscle weakness may present a great hazard for ambulation

Dosage Forms

Injection, solution, as hydrochloride: 50 mg/mL (3 mL) [contains benzyl alcohol and polysorbate (Tween®) 80]

Tablet, scored, as hydrochloride: 200 mg

Cordarone®: 200 mg

Pacerone®: 200 mg, 400 mg

Extemporaneous Preparations A 5 mg/mL oral suspension has been made from tablets and has an expected stability of 91 days under refrigeration; three 200 mg tablets are crushed in a mortar, 90 mL of methylcellulose 1%, and 10 mL of syrup (syrup NF (85% sucrose in water) or flavored syrup) are added in small amounts and triturated until uniform; purified water USP is used to make a quantity sufficient to 120 mL

Nahata MC and Hipple TF, *Pediatric Drug Formulations*, 2nd ed, Cincinnati, OH: Harvey Whitney Books Co, 1992.

♦ **Amiodarone Hydrochloride** *see* Amiodarone *on page 74*

♦ **Amitone® [OTC]** *see* Calcium Carbonate *on page 207*

Amitriptyline (a mee TRIP ti leen)

Related Information

Antidepressant Agents Comparison *on page 1482*

U.S. Brand Names Elavil®; Vanatrip®

Canadian Brand Names Apo®-Amitriptyline; Elavil®

Synonyms Amitriptyline Hydrochloride

Therapeutic Category Antidepressant, Tricyclic; Antimigraine Agent

Use Relief of symptoms of depression

Unlabeled/Investigational Use Analgesic for certain chronic and neuropathic pain; prophylaxis against migraine headaches; treatment of depressive disorders in children

Pregnancy Risk Factor D

Contraindications Hypersensitivity to amitriptyline or any component of the formulation (cross-sensitivity with other tricyclics may occur); use of MAO inhibitors within past 14 days; acute recovery phase following myocardial infarction; concurrent use of cisapride; pregnancy

Warnings/Precautions Often causes drowsiness/sedation, resulting in impaired performance of tasks requiring alertness (ie, operating machinery or driving). Sedative effects may be additive with other CNS depressants and/or ethanol. The degree of sedation is very high relative to other antidepressants. May worsen psychosis in some patients or precipitate a shift to mania or hypomania in patients with bipolar disease. May cause hyponatremia/SIADH. May increase the risks associated with electroconvulsive therapy. This agent should be discontinued, when possible, prior to elective surgery. Therapy should not be abruptly discontinued in patients receiving high doses for prolonged periods.

May cause orthostatic hypotension; the risk of this problem is very high relative to other antidepressants. Use with caution in patients at risk of hypotension or in patients where transient hypotensive episodes would be poorly tolerated (cardiovascular disease or cerebrovascular disease). The degree of anticholinergic blockade produced by this agent is very high relative to other cyclic antidepressants; use with caution in patients with urinary retention, benign prostatic hyperplasia, narrow-angle glaucoma, xerostomia, visual problems, constipation, or a history of bowel obstruction. May alter glucose control - use with caution in patients with diabetes.

Use caution in patients with depression, particularly if suicidal risk may be present. Use with caution in patients with a history of cardiovascular disease (including previous MI, stroke, tachycardia, or conduction abnormalities). The risk of conduction abnormalities with this agent is high relative to other antidepressants. May lower seizure threshold - use caution in patients with a previous seizure disorder or condition predisposing to seizures such as brain damage, alcoholism, or concurrent therapy with other drugs which lower the seizure threshold. Use with caution in hyperthyroid patients or those receiving thyroid supplementation. Use with caution in patients with hepatic or renal dysfunction and in elderly patients. Not recommended for use in patients <12 years of age.

Adverse Reactions Anticholinergic effects may be pronounced; moderate to marked sedation can occur (tolerance to these effects usually occurs).

Frequency not defined.
Cardiovascular: Orthostatic hypotension, tachycardia, nonspecific EKG changes, changes in AV conduction
Central nervous system: Restlessness, dizziness, insomnia, sedation, fatigue, anxiety, impaired cognitive function, seizures, extrapyramidal symptoms
Dermatologic: Allergic rash, urticaria, photosensitivity
Gastrointestinal: Weight gain, xerostomia, constipation
Genitourinary: Urinary retention
Ocular: Blurred vision, mydriasis
Miscellaneous: Diaphoresis

Overdosage/Toxicology Symptoms include agitation, confusion, hallucinations, urinary retention, hypothermia, hypotension, ventricular tachycardia, and seizures. Following initiation of essential overdose management, toxic symptoms should be treated. Sodium bicarbonate is indicated when the QRS interval is >0.10 seconds or the QT_c is >0.42 seconds. Ventricular arrhythmias often respond to phenytoin 15-20 mg/kg (adults) with concurrent systemic alkalinization (sodium bicarbonate 0.5-2 mEq/kg I.V.). Arrhythmias unresponsive to this therapy may respond to lidocaine 1 mg/kg I.V. followed by a titrated infusion. Physostigmine (1-2 mg slow I.V. for adults or 0.5 mg slow I.V. for children) may be indicated in reversing cardiac arrhythmias that are due to vagal blockade, or for anticholinergic effects, but should only be used as a last measure in life-threatening situations. Seizures usually respond to diazepam I.V. boluses (5-10 mg for adults up to 30 mg or 0.25-0.4 mg/kg/dose for children up to 10 mg/dose). If seizures are unresponsive or recur, phenytoin or phenobarbital may be required.

Drug Interactions
Cytochrome P450 Effect: CYP1A2, 2C9, 2C19, 2D6, and 3A3/4 enzyme substrate
Increased Effect/Toxicity: Amitriptyline increases the effects of amphetamines, anticholinergics, other CNS depressants (sedatives, hypnotics, or ethanol), carbamazepine, tolazamide, chlorpropamide, and warfarin. When used with MAO inhibitors, hyperpyrexia, hypertension, tachycardia, confusion, seizures, and **deaths have been reported** (serotonin syndrome). Serotonin syndrome has also been reported with ritonavir (rare). The SSRIs (to varying degrees), cimetidine, fenfluramine, grapefruit juice, indinavir, methylphenidate, ritonavir, quinidine, diltiazem, valproate, and verapamil inhibit the metabolism of TCAs and clinical toxicity may result. Use of lithium with a TCA may increase the risk for neurotoxicity. Phenothiazines may increase concentration of some TCAs and TCAs may increase the concentration of phenothiazines. Pressor response to I.V. epinephrine, norepinephrine, and phenylephrine may be enhanced in patients receiving TCAs (**Note:** Effect is unlikely with epinephrine or levonordefrin dosages typically administered as infiltration in combination with local anesthetics). Combined use of beta-agonists or drugs which prolong QT_c (including quinidine, procainamide, disopyramide, cisapride, sparfloxacin, gatifloxacin, moxifloxacin) with TCAs may predispose patients to cardiac arrhythmias.
Decreased Effect: Carbamazepine, phenobarbital, and rifampin may increase the metabolism of amitriptyline resulting in a decreased effect of amitriptyline. Amitriptyline inhibits the antihypertensive response to bethanidine, clonidine, debrisoquin, guanadrel, guanethidine, guanabenz, or guanfacine. Cholestyramine and colestipol may bind TCAs and reduce their absorption.

Ethanol/Nutrition/Herb Interactions
Ethanol: Avoid ethanol (may increase CNS depression).
Food: Grapefruit juice may inhibit the metabolism of some TCAs and clinical toxicity may result.
Herb/Nutraceutical: St John's wort may decrease amitriptyline levels. Avoid valerian, St John's wort, kava kava, gotu kola (may increase CNS depression).

Stability Protect injection and Elavil® 10 mg tablets from light
(Continued)

Amitriptyline *(Continued)*

Mechanism of Action Increases the synaptic concentration of serotonin and/or norepineph-rine in the central nervous system by inhibition of their reuptake by the presynaptic neuronal membrane

Pharmacodynamics/Kinetics

Onset of action: Migraine prophylaxis: 6 weeks, higher dosage may be required in heavy smokers because of increased metabolism; Depression: 3-4 weeks, reduce dosage to lowest effective level

Distribution: Crosses placenta; enters breast milk

Metabolism: Hepatic to nortriptyline (active), hydroxy and conjugated derivatives; may be impaired in the elderly

Half-life elimination: Adults: 9-25 hours (15-hour average)

Time to peak, serum: ~4 hours

Excretion: Urine; feces (small amounts)

Usual Dosage

Children:

Chronic pain management (unlabeled use): Oral: Initial: 0.1 mg/kg at bedtime, may advance as tolerated over 2-3 weeks to 0.5-2 mg/kg at bedtime

Depressive disorders (unlabeled use): Oral: Initial doses of 1 mg/kg/day given in 3 divided doses with increases to 1.5 mg/kg/day have been reported in a small number of children (n=9) 9-12 years of age; clinically, doses up to 3 mg/kg/day (5 mg/kg/day if monitored closely) have been proposed

Adolescents: Depressive disorders: Oral: Initial: 25-50 mg/day; may administer in divided doses; increase gradually to 100 mg/day in divided doses

Adults:

Depression:

Oral: 50-150 mg/day single dose at bedtime or in divided doses; dose may be gradually increased up to 300 mg/day

I.M.: 20-30 mg 4 times/day

Pain management (unlabeled use): Oral: Initial: 25 mg at bedtime; may increase as tolerated to 100 mg/day

Dosing interval in hepatic impairment: Use with caution and monitor plasma levels and patient response

Hemodialysis: Nondialyzable

Administration Not recommended for I.V.

Monitoring Parameters Monitor blood pressure and pulse rate prior to and during initial therapy; evaluate mental status; monitor weight; EKG in older adults and patients with cardiac disease

Reference Range Therapeutic: Amitriptyline and nortriptyline 100-250 ng/mL (SI: 360-900 nmol/L); nortriptyline 50-150 ng/mL (SI: 190-570 nmol/L); Toxic: >0.5 µg/mL; plasma levels do not always correlate with clinical effectiveness

Test Interactions May cause false positive reaction to EMIT immunoassay for imipramine

Patient Information Avoid alcohol; do not discontinue medication abruptly; may cause urine to turn blue-green; may cause drowsiness; full effect may not occur for 3-6 weeks; dry mouth may be helped by sips of water, sugarless gum, or hard candy

Nursing Implications May increase appetite and possibly a craving for sweets

Dosage Forms

Injection, as hydrochloride: 10 mg/mL (10 mL)

Tablet, as hydrochloride: 10 mg, 25 mg, 50 mg, 75 mg, 100 mg, 150 mg

Amitriptyline and Chlordiazepoxide

(a mee TRIP ti leen & klor dye az e POKS ide)

U.S. Brand Names Limbitrol®; Limbitrol® DS

Canadian Brand Names Limbitrol®

Synonyms Chlordiazepoxide and Amitriptyline

Therapeutic Category Antidepressant, Tricyclic

Use Treatment of moderate to severe anxiety and/or agitation and depression

Restrictions C-IV

Pregnancy Risk Factor D

Usual Dosage Initial: 3-4 tablets in divided doses; this may be increased to 6 tablets/day as required; some patients respond to smaller doses and can be maintained on 2 tablets

Additional Information Complete prescribing information for this medication should be consulted for additional detail.

Dosage Forms Tablet:

5-12.5 (Limbitrol®): Amitriptyline hydrochloride 12.5 mg and chlordiazepoxide 5 mg

10-25 (Limbitrol® DS): Amitriptyline hydrochloride 25 mg and chlordiazepoxide 10 mg

Amitriptyline and Perphenazine (a mee TRIP ti leen & per FEN a zeen)

U.S. Brand Names Etrafon®; Triavil®

Canadian Brand Names Etrafon®; Triavil®

Synonyms Perphenazine and Amitriptyline

Therapeutic Category Antidepressant/Phenothiazine

Use Treatment of patients with moderate to severe anxiety and depression

Unlabeled/Investigational Use Depression with psychotic features

Pregnancy Risk Factor D

Usual Dosage Oral: 1 tablet 2-4 times/day

Additional Information Complete prescribing information for this medication should be consulted for additional detail.

Dosage Forms Tablet:

2-10 (Etrafon®, Triavil®): Amitriptyline hydrochloride 10 mg and perphenazine 2 mg

2-25 (Etrafon®, Triavil®): Amitriptyline hydrochloride 25 mg and perphenazine 2 mg

4-10: Amitriptyline hydrochloride 10 mg and perphenazine 4 mg

4-25 (Etrafon®, Triavil®): Amitriptyline hydrochloride 25 mg and perphenazine 4 mg

4-50: Amitriptyline hydrochloride 50 mg and perphenazine 4 mg

♦ **Amitriptyline Hydrochloride** *see Amitriptyline on page 76*

Amlexanox (am LEKS an oks)

U.S. Brand Names Aphthasol™

Therapeutic Category Anti-inflammatory Agent

Use Treatment of aphthous ulcers (ie, canker sores)

Unlabeled/Investigational Use Allergic disorders

Pregnancy Risk Factor B

Usual Dosage Administer (0.5 cm - $^1/_4$") directly on ulcers 4 times/day following oral hygiene, after meals, and at bedtime

Additional Information Complete prescribing information for this medication should be consulted for additional detail.

Dosage Forms Paste: 5% (5 g)

Amlodipine (am LOE di peen)

Related Information

Calcium Channel Blockers Comparison *on page 1494*

U.S. Brand Names Norvasc®

Canadian Brand Names Norvasc®

Therapeutic Category Antihypertensive Agent; Calcium Channel Blocker

Use Treatment of hypertension and angina

Pregnancy Risk Factor C

Pregnancy/Breast-Feeding Implications Teratogenic and embryotoxic effects have been demonstrated in small animals. No well-controlled studies have been conducted in pregnant women. Use in pregnancy only when clearly needed and when the benefits outweigh the potential hazard to the fetus.

Clinical effects on the fetus: No data on crossing the placenta

Breast-feeding/lactation: No data on crossing into breast milk

Contraindications Hypersensitivity to amlodipine or any component of the formulation

Warnings/Precautions Use with caution and titrate dosages for patients with impaired renal or hepatic function; use caution when treating patients with congestive heart failure, sick-sinus syndrome, severe left ventricular dysfunction, hypertrophic cardiomyopathy (especially obstructive), concomitant therapy with beta-blockers or digoxin, edema, or increased intra-cranial pressure with cranial tumors; do not abruptly withdraw (may cause chest pain); elderly may experience hypotension and constipation more readily.

Adverse Reactions

>10%: Cardiovascular: Peripheral edema (1.8% to 14.6% dose-related)

1% to 10%:

Cardiovascular: Flushing (0.7% to 2.6%), palpitations (0.7% to 4.5%)

Central nervous system: Headache (7.3%; similar to placebo)

Dermatologic: Rash (1% to 2%), pruritus (1% to 2%)

Endocrine & metabolic: Male sexual dysfunction (1% to 2%)

Gastrointestinal: Nausea (2.9%), abdominal pain (1% to 2%), dyspepsia (1% to 2%), gingival hyperplasia

Neuromuscular & skeletal: Muscle cramps (1% to 2%), weakness (1% to 2%)

Respiratory: Dyspnea (1% to 2%), pulmonary edema (15% from PRAISE trial, CHF population)

<1% (Limited to important or life-threatening): Abnormal dreams, agitation alopecia, amnesia, anxiety, apathy, arrhythmias, ataxia, bradycardia, cardiac failure, depersonalization, depression, erythema multiforme, exfoliative dermatitis, extrapyramidal symptoms, gastritis, gynecomastia, hypotension, leukocytoclastic vasculitis, migraine, nonthrombocytopenic purpura, paresthesia, peripheral ischemia, photosensitivity, postural hypotension, purpura, rash, skin discoloration, Stevens-Johnson syndrome, syncope, thrombocytopenia, tinnitus, urticaria, vertigo, xerophthalmia

Overdosage/Toxicology

Primary cardiac symptoms of calcium blocker overdose include hypotension and brady-cardia. Hypotension is caused by peripheral vasodilation, myocardial depression, and bradycardia. Bradycardia results from sinus bradycardia, second- or third-degree atrioven-tricular block, or sinus arrest with junctional rhythm. Intraventricular conduction is usually not affected, so QRS duration is normal (verapamil prolongs the P-R interval and bepridil prolongs the QT interval and may cause ventricular arrhythmias, including torsade de pointes).

Noncardiac symptoms include confusion, stupor, nausea, vomiting, metabolic acidosis, and hyperglycemia. Following initial gastric decontamination, if possible, repeated calcium administration may promptly reverse depressed cardiac contractility (but not sinus node depression or peripheral vasodilation). Glucagon, epinephrine, and inamrinone (amrinone) may treat refractory hypotension. Glucagon and epinephrine also increase the heart rate (outside the U.S., 4-aminopyridine may be available as an antidote). Dialysis and hemoper-fusion are not effective in enhancing elimination, although repeat-dose activated charcoal may serve as an adjunct with sustained-release preparations.

In a few reported cases, overdose with calcium channel blockers has been associated with hypotension and bradycardia, initially refractory to atropine, but becoming more responsive to this agent when larger doses (approaching 1 g/hour for more than 24 hours) of calcium chloride were administered.

(Continued)

Amlodipine *(Continued)*

Drug Interactions
Cytochrome P450 Effect: CYP3A3/4 enzyme substrate
Increased Effect/Toxicity: Azole antifungals (itraconazole, ketoconazole, fluconazole), erythromycin, and other inhibitors of cytochrome P450 isoenzyme 3A4 may inhibit amlodipine's metabolism. Grapefruit juice may modestly increase amlodipine levels. Cyclosporine levels may be increased by amlodipine. Blood pressure-lowering effects of sildenafil are additive with amlodipine.
Decreased Effect: Rifampin (and potentially other enzyme inducers) increase the metabolism of amlodipine. Calcium may reduce the calcium channel blocker's hypotensive effects.
Ethanol/Nutrition/Herb Interactions Herb/Nutraceutical: St John's wort may decrease amlodipine levels. Avoid dong quai if using for hypertension (has estrogenic activity). Avoid ephedra, yohimbe, ginseng (may worsen hypertension). Avoid garlic (may have increased antihypertensive effects).
Stability Store at room temperature of 15°C to 30°C (59°F to 86°F).
Mechanism of Action Inhibits calcium ion from entering the "slow channels" or select voltage-sensitive areas of vascular smooth muscle and myocardium during depolarization, producing a relaxation of coronary vascular smooth muscle and coronary vasodilation; increases myocardial oxygen delivery in patients with vasospastic angina
Pharmacodynamics/Kinetics
Onset of action: 30-50 minutes
Peak effect: 6-12 hours
Duration: 24 hours
Absorption: Oral: Well absorbed
Protein binding: 93%
Metabolism: Hepatic, >90% to inactive metabolite
Bioavailability: 64% to 90%
Half-life elimination: 30-50 hours
Excretion: Urine
Usual Dosage Adults: Oral:
Hypertension: Initial dose: 2.5-5 mg once daily; usual dose: 5 mg once daily; maximum dose: 10 mg once daily. In general, titrate in 2.5 mg increments over 7-14 days.
Angina: Usual dose: 5-10 mg; use lower doses for elderly or those with hepatic insufficiency (eg, 2.5-5 mg).
Dialysis: Hemodialysis and peritoneal dialysis does not enhance elimination. Supplemental dose is not necessary.
Dosage adjustment in hepatic impairment: Administer 2.5 mg once daily.
Elderly: Dosing should start at the lower end of dosing range due to possible increased incidence of hepatic, renal, or cardiac impairment. Elderly patients also show decreased clearance of amlodipine.
Dietary Considerations May be taken without regard to meals.
Administration May be taken without regard to meals.
Patient Information Take as prescribed; do not stop abruptly without consulting prescriber. You may experience headache (if unrelieved, consult prescriber), nausea or vomiting (frequent small meals may help), or constipation (increased dietary bulk and fluids may help). May cause drowsiness; use caution when driving or engaging in tasks that require alertness until response to drug is known. Report unrelieved headache, vomiting, constipation, palpitations, peripheral or facial swelling, weight gain >5 lb/week, or respiratory changes.
Nursing Implications Do not discontinue abruptly; report any dizziness, shortness of breath, palpitations, or edema
Dosage Forms Tablet: 2.5 mg, 5 mg, 10 mg
Extemporaneous Preparations A 1 mg/mL suspension was stable for 91 days when refrigerated or 56 days when kept at room temperature when compounded as follows: Triturate fifty 5 mg tablets in a mortar, reduce to a fine powder. In a graduate, mix Ora-Sweet® 125 mL and Ora-Plus® 125 mL together. Add small amount of this mixture to the powder to make a paste. Add the remainder in small quantities while mixing. Shake well before using.

Nahata MC, Morosco RS, and Hipple TF, 4th ed, *Pediatric Drug Formulations*, Cincinnati, OH: Harvey Whitney Books Co, 2000.

Amlodipine and Benazepril (am LOE di peen & ben AY ze pril)

U.S. Brand Names Lotrel®
Canadian Brand Names Lotrel®
Synonyms Benazepril and Amlodipine
Therapeutic Category Angiotensin-Converting Enzyme (ACE) Inhibitor Combination; Antihypertensive Agent, Combination
Use Treatment of hypertension
Pregnancy Risk Factor C/D (2nd and 3rd trimesters)
Usual Dosage Adults: Oral: 1 capsule daily
Additional Information Complete prescribing information for this medication should be consulted for additional detail.
Dosage Forms
Capsule:
Amlodipine 2.5 mg and benazepril hydrochloride 10 mg
Amlodipine 5 mg and benazepril hydrochloride 10 mg
Amlodipine 5 mg and benazepril hydrochloride 20 mg

♦ **Ammonapse** *see* Sodium Phenylbutyrate *on page 1248*

Ammonium Chloride (a MOE nee um KLOR ide)

Therapeutic Category Diuretic, Miscellaneous; Metabolic Alkalosis Agent; Urinary Acidifying Agent
Use Diuretic or systemic and urinary acidifying agent; treatment of hypochloremic states
Pregnancy Risk Factor C

Contraindications Severe hepatic and renal dysfunction; patients with primary respiratory acidosis

Warnings/Precautions Safety and efficacy not established in children, use with caution in infants

Adverse Reactions Frequency not defined.
Central nervous system: Headache (with large doses), coma, mental confusion
Dermatologic: Rash
Endocrine & metabolic: Hypokalemia (with large doses), metabolic acidosis, potassium and sodium may be decreased, hyperchloremia,
Gastrointestinal: Vomiting, gastric irritation, nausea
Hepatic: Ammonia may be increased
Local: Pain at site of injection
Respiratory: Hyperventilation (with large doses)

Overdosage/Toxicology Symptoms include acidosis, headache, drowsiness, confusion, hyperventilation, and hypokalemia. Administer sodium bicarbonate or lactate to treat acidosis. Administer supplemental potassium for hypokalemia.

Stability Avoid excessive heat; protect from freezing (will precipitate crystals); if crystals form, warm at room temperature in water bath; compatible with normal saline

Mechanism of Action Increases acidity by increasing free hydrogen ion concentration

Pharmacodynamics/Kinetics
Absorption: Well absorbed; complete within 3-6 hours
Metabolism: Hepatic
Excretion: Urine

Usual Dosage Metabolic alkalosis: The following equations represent different methods of correction utilizing either the serum HCO_3^-, the serum chloride, or the base excess

Dosing of mEq NH_4Cl via the chloride-deficit method (hypochloremia):
Dose of mEq NH_4Cl = [0.2 L/kg x body weight (kg)] x [103 - observed serum chloride]; administer 100% of dose over 12 hours, then re-evaluate
Note: 0.2 L/kg is the estimated chloride space and 103 is the average normal serum chloride concentration

Dosing of mEq NH_4Cl via the bicarbonate-excess method (refractory hypochloremic metabolic alkalosis):
Dose of NH_4Cl = [0.5 L/kg x body weight (kg)] x (observed serum HCO_3^- - 24); administer 50% of dose over 12 hours, then re-evaluate
Note: 0.5 L/kg is the estimated bicarbonate space and 24 is the average normal serum bicarbonate concentration

Dosing of mEq NH_4Cl via the base-excess method:
Dose of NH_4Cl = [0.3 L/kg x body weight (kg)] x measured base excess (mEq/L); administer 50% of dose over 12 hours, then re-evaluate
Note: 0.3 L/kg is the estimated extracellular bicarbonate and base excess is measured by the chemistry lab and reported with arterial blood gases

These equations will yield different requirements of ammonium chloride
Equation #1 is inappropriate to use if the patient has severe metabolic alkalosis without hypochloremia or if the patient has uremia
Equation #3 is the most useful for the first estimation of ammonium chloride dosage
Children: Urinary acidifying agents: Oral, I.V.: 75 mg/kg/day in 4 divided doses; maximum daily dose: 6 g
Adults: Urinary acidifying agent/diuretic:
Oral: 1-2 g every 4-6 hours
I.V.: 1.5 g/dose every 6 hours

Administration Dilute to 0.2 mEq/mL and infuse I.V. over 3 hours; maximum concentration: 0.4 mEq/mL; maximum rate of infusion: 1 mEq/kg/hour

Patient Information Take oral dose after meals

Nursing Implications
Rapid I.V. injection may increase the likelihood of ammonia toxicity; dilute to 0.2 mEq/mL and infuse I.V. over 3 hours; maximum concentration: 0.4 mEq/mL; maximum rate of infusion: 1 mEq/kg/hour
Monitor serum electrolytes, serum ammonia

Dosage Forms
Injection: 26.75% [5 mEq/mL] (20 mL)
Tablet: 500 mg
Tablet, enteric coated: 486 mg

Amobarbital (am oh BAR bi tal)

U.S. Brand Names Amytal®
Canadian Brand Names Amytal®
Synonyms Amylobarbitone
Therapeutic Category Anticonvulsant; Barbiturate; Hypnotic; Sedative
Use
Oral: Hypnotic in short-term treatment of insomnia; reduce anxiety and provide sedation preoperatively
I.M., I.V.: Control status epilepticus or acute seizure episodes; control acute episodes of agitated behavior in psychosis and in "Amytal® Interviewing" for narcoanalysis
Restrictions C-II
Pregnancy Risk Factor D
Usual Dosage
Children: Oral:
Sedation: 6 mg/kg/day divided every 6-8 hours
Insomnia: 2 mg/kg or 70 mg/m^2/day in 4 equally divided doses
Hypnotic: 2-3 mg/kg
Adults:
Insomnia: Oral: 65-200 mg at bedtime
Sedation: Oral: 30-50 mg 2-3 times/day
Preanesthetic: Oral: 200 mg 1-2 hours before surgery
(Continued)

Amobarbital *(Continued)*

Hypnotic:
 Oral: 65-200 mg at bedtime
 I.M., I.V.: 65-500 mg, should not exceed 500 mg I.M. or 1000 mg I.V.
Acute episode of agitated behavior:
 Oral: 30-50 mg 2-3 times/day
 I.M., I.V.: 65-500 mg, should not exceed 500 mg I.M. or 1000 mg I.V.
Status epilepticus/acute seizure episode: I.M., I.V.: 65-500 mg, should not exceed 500 mg I.M. or 1000 mg I.V.
Amobarbital (Amytal®) interview: I.V.: 50 mg/minute for total dose up to 300 mg

Additional Information Complete prescribing information for this medication should be consulted for additional detail.

Dosage Forms
 Capsule, as sodium: 65 mg, 200 mg
 Injection, as sodium: 250 mg, 500 mg
 Tablet: 30 mg, 50 mg, 100 mg

Amobarbital and Secobarbital *(am oh BAR bi tal & see koe BAR bi tal)*

U.S. Brand Names Tuinal®
Synonyms Secobarbital and Amobarbital
Therapeutic Category Barbiturate
Use Short-term treatment of insomnia
Restrictions C-II
Pregnancy Risk Factor D
Usual Dosage Adults: Oral: 1-2 capsules at bedtime
Additional Information Complete prescribing information for this medication should be consulted for additional detail.
Dosage Forms Capsule: Amobarbital 50 mg and secobarbital 50 mg

♦ **AMO Vitrax**® *see* Sodium Hyaluronate *on page 1247*

Amoxapine *(a MOKS a peen)*

Related Information
 Antidepressant Agents Comparison *on page 1482*
U.S. Brand Names Asendin® [DSC]
Canadian Brand Names Asendin®
Therapeutic Category Antidepressant, Tricyclic
Use Treatment of depression, psychotic depression, depression accompanied by anxiety or agitation
Pregnancy Risk Factor C
Contraindications Hypersensitivity to amoxapine or any component of the formulation; use of MAO inhibitors within past 14 days; acute recovery phase following myocardial infarction
Warnings/Precautions May cause sedation, resulting in impaired performance of tasks requiring alertness (ie, operating machinery or driving). Sedative effects may be additive with other CNS depressants and/or ethanol. The degree of sedation is moderate relative to other antidepressants. May worsen psychosis in some patients or precipitate a shift to mania or hypomania in patients with bipolar disease. May increase the risks associated with electroconvulsive therapy. This agent should be discontinued, when possible, prior to elective surgery. Therapy should not be abruptly discontinued in patients receiving high doses for prolonged periods.

May cause extrapyramidal symptoms, including pseudoparkinsonism, acute dystonic reactions, akathisia, and tardive dyskinesia (risk of these reactions is low). May be associated with neuroleptic malignant syndrome.

May cause orthostatic hypotension (risk is moderate relative to other antidepressants) - use with caution in patients at risk of hypotension or in patients where transient hypotensive episodes would be poorly tolerated (cardiovascular disease or cerebrovascular disease). The degree of anticholinergic blockade produced by this agent is moderate relative to other cyclic antidepressants - use caution in patients with urinary retention, benign prostatic hyperplasia, narrow-angle glaucoma, xerostomia, visual problems, constipation, or history of bowel obstruction.

Use caution in patients with suicidal risk. Use with caution in patients with a history of cardiovascular disease (including previous MI, stroke, tachycardia, or conduction abnormalities). The risk of conduction abnormalities with this agent is moderate relative to other antidepressants. May lower seizure threshold - use caution in patients with a previous seizure disorder or condition predisposing to seizures such as brain damage, alcoholism, or concurrent therapy with other drugs which lower the seizure threshold. Use with caution in hyperthyroid patients or those receiving thyroid supplementation. Use with caution in patients with hepatic or renal dysfunction and in elderly patients. Tolerance develops in 1-3 months in some patients; close medical follow-up is essential.

Adverse Reactions
>10%:
 Central nervous system: Drowsiness
 Gastrointestinal: Xerostomia, constipation
1% to 10%:
 Central nervous system: Dizziness, headache, confusion, nervousness, restlessness, insomnia, ataxia, excitement, anxiety
 Dermatologic: Edema, skin rash
 Endocrine: Elevated prolactin levels
 Gastrointestinal: Nausea
 Neuromuscular & skeletal: Tremor, weakness
 Ocular: Blurred vision
 Miscellaneous: Diaphoresis

<1% (Limited to important or life-threatening): Agranulocytosis, allergic reactions, diarrhea, extrapyramidal symptoms, galactorrhea, hypertension, impotence, incoordination, increased intraocular pressure, leukopenia, menstrual irregularity, mydriasis, neuroleptic malignant syndrome, numbness, painful ejaculation, paresthesia, photosensitivity, seizures, SIADH, syncope, tardive dyskinesia, testicular edema, tinnitus, urinary retention, vomiting

Overdosage/Toxicology Symptoms include grand mal convulsions, acidosis, coma, and renal failure. Following initiation of essential overdose management, toxic symptoms should be treated. Sodium bicarbonate is indicated when the QRS interval is >0.10 seconds or the QT_c is >0.42 seconds. Ventricular arrhythmias often respond to phenytoin 15-20 mg/kg (adults) with concurrent systemic alkalinization (sodium bicarbonate 0.5-2 mEq/kg I.V.). Arrhythmias unresponsive to this therapy may respond to lidocaine 1 mg/kg I.V. followed by a titrated infusion. Physostigmine (1-2 mg slow I.V. for adults or 0.5 mg slow I.V. for children) may be indicated in reversing cardiac arrhythmias that are due to vagal blockade, or for anticholinergic effects, but should only be used as a last measure in life-threatening situations. Seizures usually respond to diazepam I.V. boluses (5-10 mg for adults up to 30 mg or 0.25-0.4 mg/kg/dose for children up to 10 mg/dose). If seizures are unresponsive or recur, phenytoin or phenobarbital may be required.

Drug Interactions

Cytochrome P450 Effect: CYP1A2, 2C9, 2C19, 2D6, and 3A3/4 enzyme substrate

Increased Effect/Toxicity: Amoxapine increases the effects of amphetamines, anticholinergics, other CNS depressants (sedatives, hypnotics, or ethanol), chlorpropamide, tolazamide, and warfarin. When used with MAO inhibitors, hyperpyrexia, hypertension, tachycardia, confusion, seizures, and **deaths have been reported** (serotonin syndrome). Serotonin syndrome has also been reported with ritonavir (rare). The SSRIs (to varying degrees), cimetidine, grapefruit juice, indinavir, methylphenidate, ritonavir, quinidine, diltiazem, and verapamil inhibit the metabolism of TCAs and clinical toxicity may result. Use of lithium with a TCA may increase the risk for neurotoxicity. Phenothiazines may increase concentration of some TCAs and TCAs may increase the concentration of phenothiazines. Pressor response to I.V. epinephrine, norepinephrine, and phenylephrine may be enhanced in patients receiving TCAs (**Note:** Effect is unlikely with epinephrine or levonordefrin dosages typically administered as infiltration in combination with local anesthetics). Combined use of beta-agonists or drugs which prolong QT_c (including quinidine, procainamide, disopyramide, cisapride, sparfloxacin, gatifloxacin, moxifloxacin) with TCAs may predispose patients to cardiac arrhythmias.

Decreased Effect: Carbamazepine, phenobarbital, and rifampin may increase the metabolism of amoxapine resulting in decreased effect of amoxapine. Amoxapine inhibits the antihypertensive effects of bethanidine, clonidine, debrisoquin, guanadrel, guanethidine, guanabenz, or guanfacine. Cholestyramine and colestipol may bind TCAs and reduce their absorption.

Ethanol/Nutrition/Herb Interactions

Ethanol: Avoid ethanol (may increase CNS depression).

Food: Grapefruit juice may inhibit the metabolism of some TCAs and clinical toxicity may result.

Herb/Nutraceutical: Avoid valerian, St John's wort, SAMe, kava kava.

Mechanism of Action Reduces the reuptake of serotonin and norepinephrine. The metabolite, 7-OH-amoxapine has significant dopamine receptor blocking activity similar to haloperidol.

Pharmacodynamics/Kinetics

Onset of action: Therapeutic: Usually 1-2 weeks

Absorption: Rapid and well absorbed

Distribution: V_d: 0.9-1.2 L/kg; enters breast milk

Protein binding: 80%

Metabolism: Primarily hepatic

Half-life elimination: Parent drug: 11-16 hours; Active metabolite (8-hydroxy): Adults: 30 hours

Time to peak, serum: 1-2 hours

Excretion: Urine (as unchanged drug and metabolites)

Usual Dosage Oral:

Children: Not established in children <16 years of age.

Adolescents: Initial: 25-50 mg/day; increase gradually to 100 mg/day; may administer as divided doses or as a single dose at bedtime

Adults: Initial: 25 mg 2-3 times/day, if tolerated, dosage may be increased to 100 mg 2-3 times/day; may be given in a single bedtime dose when dosage <300 mg/day

Elderly: Initial: 25 mg at bedtime increased by 25 mg weekly for outpatients and every 3 days for inpatients if tolerated; usual dose: 50-150 mg/day, but doses up to 300 mg may be necessary

Maximum daily dose:

Inpatient: 600 mg

Outpatient: 400 mg

Monitoring Parameters Monitor blood pressure and pulse rate prior to and during initial therapy evaluate mental status; monitor weight; EKG in older adults

Reference Range Therapeutic: Amoxapine: 20-100 ng/mL (SI: 64-319 nmol/L); 8-OH amoxapine: 150-400 ng/mL (SI: 478-1275 nmol/L); both: 200-500 ng/mL (SI: 637-1594 nmol/L)

Patient Information Dry mouth may be helped by sips of water, sugarless gum, or hard candy; avoid alcohol; very important to maintain established dosage regimen; photosensitivity to sunlight occur, do not discontinue abruptly; full effect may not occur for 3-4 weeks; full dosage may be taken at bedtime to avoid daytime sedation

Nursing Implications May increase appetite and possibly a craving for sweets; recognize signs of neuroleptic malignant syndrome and tardive dyskinesia

Additional Information Extrapyramidal reactions and tardive dyskinesia may occur.

Dosage Forms Tablet: 25 mg, 50 mg, 100 mg, 150 mg

Amoxicillin (a moks i SIL in)

Related Information
Animal and Human Bites Guidelines *on page 1584*
Antimicrobial Drugs of Choice *on page 1588*
Community-Acquired Pneumonia in Adults *on page 1603*
Helicobacter pylori Treatment *on page 1668*
Prevention of Bacterial Endocarditis *on page 1563*
Treatment of Sexually Transmitted Diseases *on page 1609*

U.S. Brand Names Amoxicot®; Amoxil®; Moxilin®; Trimox®; Wymox®

Canadian Brand Names Amoxil®; Apo®-Amoxi; Gen-Amoxicillin; Lin-Amox; Novamoxin®; Nu-Amoxi; Scheinpharm™ Amoxicillin

Synonyms Amoxicillin Trihydrate; Amoxycillin; *p*-Hydroxyampicillin

Therapeutic Category Antibiotic, Penicillin

Use Treatment of otitis media, sinusitis, and infections caused by susceptible organisms involving the respiratory tract, skin, and urinary tract; prophylaxis of bacterial endocarditis in patients undergoing surgical or dental procedures; as part of a multidrug regimen for *H. pylori* eradication

Unlabeled/Investigational Use Postexposure prophylaxis for anthrax exposure with documented susceptible organisms

Pregnancy Risk Factor B

Contraindications Hypersensitivity to amoxicillin, penicillin, or any component of the formulation

Warnings/Precautions In patients with renal impairment, doses and/or frequency of administration should be modified in response to the degree of renal impairment; a high percentage of patients with infectious mononucleosis have developed rash during therapy with amoxicillin; a low incidence of cross-allergy with other beta-lactams and cephalosporins exists

Adverse Reactions
Central nervous system: Hyperactivity, agitation, anxiety, insomnia, confusion, convulsions, behavioral changes, dizziness

Dermatologic: Erythematous maculopapular rashes, erythema multiforme, Stevens-Johnson syndrome, exfoliative dermatitis, toxic epidermal necrolysis, hypersensitivity vasculitis, urticaria

Gastrointestinal: Nausea, vomiting, diarrhea, hemorrhagic colitis, pseudomembranous colitis

Hematologic: Anemia, hemolytic anemia, thrombocytopenia, thrombocytopenia purpura, eosinophilia, leukopenia, agranulocytosis

Hepatic: Elevated AST (SGOT) and ALT (SGPT), cholestatic jaundice, hepatic cholestasis, acute cytolytic hepatitis

Overdosage/Toxicology Symptoms of penicillin overdose include neuromuscular hypersensitivity (agitation, hallucinations, asterixis, encephalopathy, confusion, and seizures) and electrolyte imbalance (with potassium or sodium salts), especially in renal failure. Hemodialysis may be helpful to aid in the removal of the drug from the blood, otherwise most treatment is supportive or symptom directed.

Drug Interactions
Increased Effect/Toxicity: Disulfiram and probenecid may increase amoxicillin levels. Amoxicillin may increase the effects of oral anticoagulants (warfarin). Theoretically, allopurinol taken with amoxicillin has an additive potential for amoxicillin rash.

Decreased Effect: Efficacy of oral contraceptives may be reduced by amoxicillin. Decreased effectiveness with tetracyclines and chloramphenicol.

Stability Oral suspension remains stable for 7 days at room temperature or 14 days if refrigerated; unit-dose antibiotic oral syringes are stable for 48 hours

Mechanism of Action Inhibits bacterial cell wall synthesis by binding to one or more of the penicillin binding proteins (PBPs); which in turn inhibits the final transpeptidation step of peptidoglycan synthesis in bacterial cell walls, thus inhibiting cell wall biosynthesis. Bacteria eventually lyse due to ongoing activity of cell wall autolytic enzymes (autolysins and murein hydrolases) while cell wall assembly is arrested.

Pharmacodynamics/Kinetics
Absorption: Oral: Rapid and nearly complete; food does not interfere

Distribution: Widely to most body fluids and bone; poor penetration into cells, eyes, and across normal meninges

Pleural fluids, lungs, and peritoneal fluid; high urine concentrations are attained; also into synovial fluid, liver, prostate, muscle, and gallbladder; penetrates into middle ear effusions, maxillary sinus secretions, tonsils, sputum, and bronchial secretions; crosses placenta; low concentrations enter breast milk

CSF:blood level ratio: Normal meninges: <1%; Inflamed meninges: 8% to 90%

Protein binding: 17% to 20%

Metabolism: Partial

Half-life elimination:
Neonates, full term: 3.7 hours
Infants and Children: 1-2 hours
Adults: Normal renal function: 0.7-1.4 hours
Cl$_{cr}$ <10 mL/minute: 7-21 hours

Time to peak: Capsule: 2 hours; Suspension: 1 hour

Excretion: Urine (80% as unchanged drug); lower in neonates

Usual Dosage Oral:
Children: 20-50 mg/kg/day in divided doses every 8 hours

Acute otitis media due to highly-resistant strains of *S. pneumoniae*: Doses as high as 80-90 mg/kg/day divided every 12 hours have been used

Subacute bacterial endocarditis prophylaxis: 50 mg/kg 1 hour before procedure

Anthrax exposure (unlabeled use): **Note:** Postexposure prophylaxis only with documented susceptible organisms:
<40 kg: 15 mg/kg every 8 hours
≥40 kg: 500 mg every 8 hours

Adults: 250-500 mg every 8 hours or 500-875 mg twice daily; maximum dose: 2-3 g/day

Endocarditis prophylaxis: 2 g 1 hour before procedure

Helicobacter pylori eradication: 1000 mg twice daily; requires combination therapy with at least one other antibiotic and an acid-suppressing agent (proton pump inhibitor or H_2 blocker)

Anthrax exposure (unlabeled use): **Note:** Postexposure prophylaxis only with documented susceptible organisms: 500 mg every 8 hours

Dosing interval in renal impairment:

Cl_{cr} 10-50 mL/minute: Administer every 12 hours

Cl_{cr} <10 mL/minute: Administer every 24 hours

Dialysis: Moderately dialyzable (20% to 50%) by hemo- or peritoneal dialysis; approximately 50 mg of amoxicillin per liter of filtrate is removed by continuous arteriovenous or venovenous hemofiltration; dose as per Cl_{cr} <10 mL/minute guidelines

Dietary Considerations May be taken with food.

Monitoring Parameters With prolonged therapy, monitor renal, hepatic, and hematologic function periodically; assess patient at beginning and throughout therapy for infection; monitor for signs of anaphylaxis during first dose

Test Interactions May interfere with urinary glucose tests using cupric sulfate (Benedict's solution, Clinitest®); may inactivate aminoglycosides *in vitro*

Patient Information Report diarrhea promptly; entire course of medication (10-14 days) should be taken to ensure eradication of organism; may interfere with oral contraceptives; females should report symptoms of vaginitis; pediatric drops may be placed on child's tongue or added to formula, milk, etc

Nursing Implications

Assess patient at beginning and throughout therapy for infection; observe for signs and symptoms of anaphylaxis; obtain specimens for C&S before the first dose; administer around-the-clock rather than 3 times/day, etc (ie, 8-4-12, not 9-1-5) to promote less variation in peak and trough serum levels

With prolonged therapy, monitor renal, hepatic, and hematologic function periodically

Dosage Forms

Capsule, as trihydrate: 250 mg, 500 mg

Amoxicot®, Amoxil®, Moxilin®, Trimox®: 250 mg, 500 mg

Wymox®: 250 mg

Powder for oral suspension, as trihydrate: 125 mg/5 mL (5 mL, 80 mL, 100 mL, 150 mL); 250 mg/5 mL (5 mL, 80 mL, 100 mL, 150 mL)

Amoxicot®: 125 mg/5 mL (100 mL, 150 mL); 250 mg/5 mL (100 mL, 150 mL)

Powder for oral suspension [drops], as trihydrate (Amoxil®): 50 mg/mL (15 mL, 30 mL) [strawberry flavor]

Tablet, chewable, as trihydrate: 125 mg, 200 mg, 250 mg, 400 mg

Amoxil® [cherry-banana-peppermint flavor]: 200 mg [contains phenylalanine 1.82 mg/tablet], 400 mg [contains phenylalanine 3.64 mg/tablet]

Tablet, film coated (Amoxil®): 500 mg, 875 mg

Amoxicillin and Clavulanate Potassium

(a moks i SIL in & klav yoo LAN ate poe TASS ee um)

Related Information

Animal and Human Bites Guidelines *on page 1584*

Antimicrobial Drugs of Choice *on page 1588*

U.S. Brand Names Augmentin®; Augmentin ES-600™

Canadian Brand Names Augmentin®; Clavulin®

Synonyms Amoxicillin and Clavulanic Acid

Therapeutic Category Antibiotic, Penicillin; Antibiotic, Penicillin & Beta-lactamase Inhibitor

Use Treatment of otitis media, sinusitis, and infections caused by susceptible organisms involving the lower respiratory tract, skin and skin structure, and urinary tract; spectrum same as amoxicillin with additional coverage of beta-lactamase producing *B. catarrhalis, H. influenzae, N. gonorrhoeae,* and *S. aureus* (not MRSA). The expanded coverage of this combination makes it a useful alternative when amoxicillin resistance is present and patients cannot tolerate alternative treatments.

Pregnancy Risk Factor B

Contraindications Hypersensitivity to amoxicillin, clavulanic acid, penicillin, or any component of the formulation; concomitant use of disulfiram; history of cholestatic jaundice or hepatic dysfunction with amoxicillin/clavulanate potassium therapy

Warnings/Precautions Prolonged use may result in superinfection. In patients with renal impairment, doses and/or frequency of administration should be modified in response to the degree of renal impairment; high percentage of patients with infectious mononucleosis have developed rash during therapy; a low incidence of cross-allergy with other beta-lactams and cephalosporins exists; incidence of diarrhea is higher than with amoxicillin alone. Due to differing content of clavulanic acid, not all formulations are interchangeable. Some products contain phenylalanine.

Adverse Reactions

>10%: Gastrointestinal: Diarrhea (3% to 34%; incidence varies upon dose and regimen used)

1% to 10%:

Dermatologic: Diaper rash, skin rash, urticaria

Gastrointestinal: Loose stools, nausea, vomiting

Genitourinary: Vaginitis

Miscellaneous: Moniliasis

<1% (Limited to important or life-threatening): Abdominal discomfort, cholestatic jaundice, flatulence, headache, hepatic dysfunction, prothrombin time increased, thrombocytosis

Additional adverse reactions seen with **ampicillin-class antibiotics:** Agitation, agranulocytosis, ALT elevated, anaphylaxis, anemia, angioedema, anxiety, AST elevated, behavioral changes, black "hairy" tongue, confusion, convulsions, dizziness, enterocolitis, eosinophilia, erythema multiforme, exanthematous pustulosis, exfoliative dermatitis, gastritis, glossitis, hematuria, hemolytic anemia, hemorrhagic colitis, indigestion, insomnia, hyperactivity, interstitial nephritis, leukopenia, mucocutaneous candidiasis, pruritus, pseudomembranous colitis, (Continued)

Amoxicillin and Clavulanate Potassium *(Continued)*

serum sickness-like reaction, Stevens-Johnson syndrome, stomatitis, thrombocytopenia, thrombocytopenic purpura, tooth discoloration, toxic epidermal necrolysis

Overdosage/Toxicology Symptoms of overdose may include abdominal pain, diarrhea, drowsiness, rash, hyperactivity, stomach pain, and vomiting. Electrolyte imbalance may occur, especially in renal failure. Hemodialysis may be helpful to aid in removal of the drug from blood, otherwise, treatment is supportive or symptom directed.

Drug Interactions

Increased Effect/Toxicity: Probenecid may increase amoxicillin levels. Increased effect of anticoagulants with amoxicillin. Allopurinol taken with Augmentin® has an additive potential for rash.

Decreased Effect: Efficacy of oral contraceptives may be reduced when taken with Augmentin®.

Stability Store dry powder at room temperature of 25°C (77°F). Reconstitute powder for oral suspension with appropriate amount of water as specified on the bottle. Shake vigorously until suspended. Reconstituted oral suspension should be kept in refrigerator. Discard unused suspension after 10 days. Unit-dose antibiotic oral syringes are stable for 48 hours.

Mechanism of Action Clavulanic acid binds and inhibits beta-lactamases that inactivate amoxicillin resulting in amoxicillin having an expanded spectrum of activity. Amoxicillin inhibits bacterial cell wall synthesis by binding to one or more of the penicillin binding proteins (PBPs); which in turn inhibits the final transpeptidation step of peptidoglycan synthesis in bacterial cell walls, thus inhibiting cell wall biosynthesis. Bacteria eventually lyse due to ongoing activity of cell wall autolytic enzymes (autolysins and murein hydrolases) while cell wall assembly is arrested.

Pharmacodynamics/Kinetics Amoxicillin pharmacokinetics are not affected by clavulanic acid.

Amoxicillin: See Amoxicillin monograph.

Clavulanic acid:

Metabolism: Hepatic

Excretion: Urine (30% to 40% as unchanged drug)

Usual Dosage Note: Dose is based on the amoxicillin component; see "Augmentin® Product-Specific Considerations table".

Infants <3 months: 30 mg/kg/day divided every 12 hours using the 125 mg/5 mL suspension

Children ≥3 months and <40 kg:

Otitis media: 90 mg/kg/day divided every 12 hours for 10 days

Lower respiratory tract infections, severe infections, sinusitis: 45 mg/kg/day divided every 12 hours **or** 40 mg/kg/day divided every 8 hours

Less severe infections: 25 mg/kg/day divided every 12 hours or 20 mg/kg/day divided every 8 hours

Children >40 kg and Adults: 250-500 mg every 8 hours or 875 mg every 12 hours

Dosing interval in renal impairment:

Cl_{cr} <30 mL/minute: Do not use 875 mg tablet

Cl_{cr} 10-30 mL/minute: 250-500 mg every 12 hours

Cl_{cr} <10 mL/minute: 250-500 every 24 hours

Hemodialysis: Moderately dializable (20% to 50%)

250-500 mg every 24 hours; administer dose during and after dialysis

Peritoneal dialysis: Moderately dializable (20% to 50%)

Amoxicillin: Administer 250 mg every 12 hours

Clavulanic acid: Dose for Cl_{cr} <10 mL/minute

Continuous arteriovenous or venovenous hemofiltration effects:

Amoxicillin: ~50 mg of amoxicillin/L of filtrate is removed

Clavulanic acid: Dose for Cl_{cr} <10 mL/minute

Augmentin® Product-Specific Considerations

Strength	Form	Consideration
125 mg	CT, S	q8h dosing
	S	For adults having difficulty swallowing tablets, 125 mg/5 mL suspension may be substituted for 500 mg tablet.
200 mg	CT, S	q12h dosing
	CT	Contains phenylalanine
	S	For adults having difficulty swallowing tablets, 200 mg/5 mL suspension may be substituted for 875 mg tablet.
250 mg	CT, S, T	q8h dosing
	CT	Contains phenylalanine
	T	Not for use in patients <40 kg
	CT, T	Tablet and chewable tablet are not interchangeable due to differences in clavulanic acid.
	S	For adults having difficulty swallowing tablets, 250 mg/5 mL suspension may be substituted for 500 mg tablet.
400 mg	CT, S	q12h dosing
	CT	Contains phenylalanine
	S	For adults having difficulty swallowing tablets, 400 mg/5 mL suspension may be substituted for 875 mg tablet.
500 mg	T	q8h or q12h dosing
600 mg	S	q12 h dosing
		Contains phenylalanine
		Not for use in adults or children ≥40 kg
		600 mg/5 mL suspension is not equivalent to or interchangeable with 200 mg/5 mL or 400 mg/5 mL due to differences in clavulanic acid.
875 mg	T	Not for use in Cl_{cr} <30 mL/minute

Legend: CT = chewable tablet, S = suspension, T = tablet

Dietary Considerations May be taken with meals or on an empty stomach; take with meals to increase absorption and decrease GI intolerance; may mix with milk, formula, or juice. Some products contain phenylalanine; avoid use in phenylketonurics. All dosage forms contain potassium.

Administration Administer around-the-clock to promote less variation in peak and trough serum levels. Administer with food to decrease stomach upset; shake suspension well before use.

Monitoring Parameters Assess patient at beginning and throughout therapy for infection; with prolonged therapy, monitor renal, hepatic, and hematologic function periodically; monitor for signs of anaphylaxis during first dose

Test Interactions May interfere with urinary glucose tests using cupric sulfate (Benedict's solution, Clinitest®, Fehling's solution); may inactivate aminoglycosides *in vitro*

Patient Information Report diarrhea promptly; entire course of medication (10-14 days) should be taken to ensure eradication of organism; females should report onset of symptoms of candidal vaginitis; may interfere with the effects of oral contraceptives

Nursing Implications Two 250 mg tablets are not equivalent to a 500 mg tablet (both tablet sizes contain equivalent clavulanate)

Dosage Forms
Powder for oral suspension:
125: Amoxicillin trihydrate 125 mg and clavulanate potassium 31.25 mg per 5 mL (75 mL, 100 mL, 150 mL) [banana flavor]
200: Amoxicillin 200 mg and clavulanate potassium 28.5 mg per 5 mL (50 mL, 75 mL, 100 mL) [contains phenylalanine 7 mg/5 mL; orange-raspberry flavor]
250: Amoxicillin trihydrate 250 mg and clavulanate potassium 62.5 mg per 5 mL (75 mL, 100 mL, 150 mL) [orange flavor]
400: Amoxicillin 400 mg and clavulanate potassium 57 mg per 5 mL (50 mL, 75 mL, 100 mL) [contains phenylalanine 7 mg/5 mL; orange-raspberry flavor]
600 (ES-600™): Amoxicillin 600 mg and clavulanic potassium 42.9 mg per 5 mL (50 mL, 75 mL, 100 mL, 150 mL) [contains phenylalanine 7 mg/5 mL; orange-raspberry flavor]
Tablet:
250: Amoxicillin trihydrate 250 mg and clavulanate potassium 125 mg
500: Amoxicillin trihydrate 500 mg and clavulanate potassium 125 mg
875: Amoxicillin trihydrate 875 mg and clavulanate potassium 125 mg
Tablet, chewable:
125: Amoxicillin trihydrate 125 mg and clavulanate potassium 31.25 mg [lemon-lime flavor]
200: Amoxicillin trihydrate 200 mg and clavulanate potassium 28.5 mg [contains phenylalanine 2.1 mg/tablet; cherry-banana flavor]
250: Amoxicillin trihydrate 250 mg and clavulanate potassium 62.5 mg [lemon-lime flavor]
400: Amoxicillin trihydrate 400 mg and clavulanate potassium 57 mg [contains phenylalanine 4.2 mg/tablet; cherry-banana flavor]

- ♦ **Amoxicillin and Clavulanic Acid** *see* Amoxicillin and Clavulanate Potassium *on page 85*
- ♦ **Amoxicillin, Lansoprazole, and Clarithromycin** *see* Lansoprazole, Amoxicillin, and Clarithromycin *on page 776*
- ♦ **Amoxicillin Trihydrate** *see* Amoxicillin *on page 84*
- ♦ **Amoxicot®** *see* Amoxicillin *on page 84*
- ♦ **Amoxil®** *see* Amoxicillin *on page 84*
- ♦ **Amoxycillin** *see* Amoxicillin *on page 84*
- ♦ **Amphetamine and Dextroamphetamine** *see* Dextroamphetamine and Amphetamine *on page 389*
- ♦ **Amphocin®** *see* Amphotericin B (Conventional) *on page 88*
- ♦ **Amphojel® [OTC]** *see* Aluminum Hydroxide *on page 63*
- ♦ **Amphotec®** *see* Amphotericin B Cholesteryl Sulfate Complex *on page 87*

Amphotericin B Cholesteryl Sulfate Complex
(am foe TER i sin bee kole LES te ril SUL fate KOM plecks)

U.S. Brand Names Amphotec®

Synonyms ABCD; Amphotericin B Colloidal Dispersion

Therapeutic Category Antifungal Agent, Systemic

Use Treatment of invasive aspergillosis in patients who have failed amphotericin B deoxycholate treatment, or who have renal impairment or experience unacceptable toxicity which precludes treatment with amphotericin B deoxycholate in effective doses.

Pregnancy Risk Factor B

Pregnancy/Breast-Feeding Implications Breast-feeding/lactation: Due to limited data, consider discontinuing nursing during therapy

Contraindications Hypersensitivity to amphotericin B or any component of the formulation

Warnings/Precautions Anaphylaxis has been reported with amphotericin B-containing drugs. If severe respiratory distress occurs, the infusion should be immediately discontinued. During the initial dosing, the drug should be administered under close clinical observation. Infusion reactions, sometimes, severe, usually subside with continued therapy - manage with decreased rate of infusion and pretreatment with antihistamines/corticosteroids.

Adverse Reactions
>10%: Central nervous system: Chills, fever
1% to 10%:
Cardiovascular: Hypotension, tachycardia
Central nervous system: Headache
Dermatologic: Rash
Endocrine & metabolic: Hypokalemia, hypomagnesemia
Gastrointestinal: Nausea, diarrhea, abdominal pain
Hematologic: Thrombocytopenia
Hepatic: LFT change
Neuromuscular & skeletal: Rigors
Renal: Elevated creatinine
(Continued)

Amphotericin B Cholesteryl Sulfate Complex *(Continued)*

Respiratory: Dyspnea

Note: Amphotericin B colloidal dispersion has an improved therapeutic index compared to conventional amphotericin B, and has been used safely in patients with amphotericin B-related nephrotoxicity; however, continued decline of renal function has occurred in some patients.

Overdosage/Toxicology Symptoms include renal dysfunction, anemia, thrombocytopenia, granulocytopenia, fever, nausea, and vomiting. Treatment is supportive.

Drug Interactions

Increased Effect/Toxicity: Toxic effect with other nephrotoxic drugs (eg, cyclosporine and aminoglycosides) may be additive. Corticosteroids may increase potassium depletion caused by amphotericin. Amphotericin B may predispose patients receiving digitalis glycosides or neuromuscular blocking agents to toxicity secondary to hypokalemia.

Decreased Effect: Pharmacologic antagonism may occur with azole antifungals (ketoconazole, miconazole, etc).

Stability

Store intact vials under refrigeration.

Reconstitute 50 mg and 100 mg vials with 10 mL and 20 mL of SWI, respectively. The reconstituted vials contain 5 mg/mL of amphotericin B. Shake the vial gently by hand until all solid particles have dissolved. After reconstitution, the solution should be refrigerated at 2°C to 8°C/36°F to 46°F and used within 24 hours.

Further dilute amphotericin B colloidal dispersion with dextrose 5% in water. Concentrations of 0.1-2 mg/mL in dextrose 5% in water are stable for 14 days at 4°C and 23°C if protected from light, however, due to the occasional formation of subvisual particles, solutions should be used within 48 hours.

Incompatible with sodium chloride solutions

Mechanism of Action Binds to ergosterol altering cell membrane permeability in susceptible fungi and causing leakage of cell components with subsequent cell death

Pharmacodynamics/Kinetics

Distribution: V_d: Total volume increases with higher doses, reflects increasing uptake by tissues (with 4 mg/kg/day = 4 L/kg); predominantly distributed in the liver; concentrations in kidneys and other tissues are lower than observed with conventional amphotericin B

Half-life elimination: 28-29 hours (increases with higher doses)

Usual Dosage Children and Adults: I.V.:

Premedication: For patients who experience chills, fever, hypotension, nausea, or other nonanaphylactic infusion-related immediate reactions, premedicate with the following drugs, 30-60 minutes prior to drug administration: a nonsteroidal (eg, ibuprofen, choline magnesium trisalicylate, etc) with or without diphenhydramine; or acetaminophen with diphenhydramine; or hydrocortisone 50-100 mg. If the patient experiences rigors during the infusion, meperidine may be administered.

Range: 3-4 mg/kg/day (infusion of 1 mg/kg/hour); maximum: 7.5 mg/kg/day

Monitoring Parameters Liver function tests, electrolytes, BUN, Cr, temperature, CBC, I/O, signs of hypokalemia (muscle weakness, cramping, drowsiness, EKG changes)

Nursing Implications May premedicate with acetaminophen and diphenhydramine 30 minutes prior to infusion; meperidine may help reduce rigors; avoid injection faster than 1 mg/kg/hour

Additional Information Controlled trials which compare the original formulation of amphotericin B to the newer liposomal formulations (ie, Amphotec®) are lacking. Thus, comparative data discussing differences among the formulations should be interpreted cautiously. Although the risk of nephrotoxicity and infusion-related adverse effects may be less with Amphotec®, the efficacy profiles of Amphotec® and the original amphotericin formulation are comparable. Consequently, Amphotec® should be restricted to those patients who cannot tolerate or fail a standard amphotericin B formulation.

Dosage Forms Suspension for injection: 50 mg (20 mL); 100 mg (50 mL)

♦ **Amphotericin B Colloidal Dispersion** *see* Amphotericin B Cholesteryl Sulfate Complex *on page 87*

Amphotericin B (Conventional) (am foe TER i sin bee con VEN sha nal)

Related Information

Antifungal Agents Comparison *on page 1484*

Desensitization Protocols *on page 1525*

USPHA/IDSA Guidelines for the Prevention of Opportunistic Infections in Persons With HIV *on page 1574*

U.S. Brand Names Amphocin®; Fungizone®

Canadian Brand Names Fungizone®

Synonyms Amphotericin B Desoxycholate

Therapeutic Category Antifungal Agent, Systemic; Antifungal Agent, Topical

Use Treatment of severe systemic and central nervous system infections caused by susceptible fungi such as *Candida* species, *Histoplasma capsulatum*, *Cryptococcus neoformans*, *Aspergillus* species, *Blastomyces dermatitidis*, *Torulopsis glabrata*, and *Coccidioides immitis*; fungal peritonitis; irrigant for bladder fungal infections; and topically for cutaneous and mucocutaneous candidal infections; used in fungal infection in patients with bone marrow transplantation, amebic meningoencephalitis, ocular aspergillosis (intraocular injection), candidal cystitis (bladder irrigation), chemoprophylaxis (low-dose I.V.), immunocompromised patients at risk of aspergillosis (intranasal/nebulized), refractory meningitis (intrathecal), coccidioidal arthritis (intra-articular/I.M.).

Low-dose amphotericin B 0.1-0.25 mg/kg/day has been administered after bone marrow transplantation to reduce the risk of invasive fungal disease. Alternative routes of administration and extemporaneous preparations have been used when standard antifungal therapy is not available (eg, inhalation, intraocular injection, subconjunctival application, intracavitary administration into various joints and the pleural space).

Pregnancy Risk Factor B

Contraindications Hypersensitivity to amphotericin or any component of the formulation

Warnings/Precautions Anaphylaxis has been reported with amphotericin B-containing drugs. During the initial dosing, the drug should be administered under close clinical observation. Avoid additive toxicity with other nephrotoxic drugs; drug-induced renal toxicity usually improves with interrupting therapy, decreasing dosage, or increasing dosing interval. I.V. amphotericin is used primarily for the treatment of patients with progressive and potentially fatal fungal infections; topical preparations may stain clothing. Infusion reactions are most common 1-3 hours after starting the infusion and diminish with continued therapy. Use amphotericin B with caution in patients with decreased renal function.

Adverse Reactions
Systemic:
>10%:
Cardiovascular: Hypotension, tachypnea
Central nervous system: Fever, chills, headache (less frequent with I.T.), malaise
Endocrine & metabolic: Hypokalemia, hypomagnesemia
Gastrointestinal: Anorexia, nausea (less frequent with I.T.), vomiting (less frequent with I.T.), diarrhea, heartburn, cramping epigastric pain
Hematologic: Normochromic-normocytic anemia
Neuromuscular & skeletal: Generalized pain, including muscle and joint pains (less frequent with I.T.)
Renal: Decreased renal function and renal function abnormalities including: azotemia, renal tubular acidosis, nephrocalcinosis
Local: Pain at injection site with or without phlebitis or thrombophlebitis (incidence may increase with peripheral infusion of admixtures >0.1 mg/mL)
1% to 10%:
Cardiovascular: Hypertension, flushing
Central nervous system: Delirium, arachnoiditis, pain along lumbar nerves (especially I.T. therapy)
Genitourinary: Urinary retention
Hematologic: Leukocytosis
Neuromuscular & skeletal: Paresthesia (especially with I.T. therapy)
<1% (Limited to important or life-threatening): Acute liver failure, agranulocytosis, anuria, bone marrow suppression, cardiac arrest, coagulation defects, convulsions, dyspnea, hearing loss, leukopenia, maculopapular rash, renal failure, renal tubular acidosis, thrombocytopenia, vision changes

Overdosage/Toxicology Symptoms include cardiac arrest, renal dysfunction, anemia, thrombocytopenia, granulocytopenia, fever, nausea, and vomiting. Treatment is supportive.

Drug Interactions
Increased Effect/Toxicity: Use of amphotericin with other nephrotoxic drugs (eg, cyclosporine and aminoglycosides) may result in additive toxicity. Amphotericin may increase the toxicity of flucytosine. Antineoplastic agents may increase the risk of amphotericin-induced nephrotoxicity, bronchospasms, and hypotension. Corticosteroids may increase potassium depletion caused by amphotericin. Amphotericin B may predispose patients receiving digitalis glycosides or neuromuscular-blocking agents to toxicity secondary to hypokalemia.

Decreased Effect: Pharmacologic antagonism may occur with azole antifungal agents (ketoconazole, miconazole).

Stability
Reconstitute only with sterile water without preservatives, not bacteriostatic water. **Benzyl alcohol, sodium chloride, or other electrolyte solutions may cause precipitation.**
Short-term exposure (<24 hours) to light during I.V. infusion does **not** appreciably affect potency
Reconstituted solutions with sterile water for injection and kept in the dark remain stable for 24 hours at room temperature and 1 week when refrigerated
Stability of parenteral admixture at room temperature (25°C): 24 hours; at refrigeration (4°C): 2 days
Standard diluent: Dose/250-500 mL D_5W

Mechanism of Action Binds to ergosterol altering cell membrane permeability in susceptible fungi and causing leakage of cell components with subsequent cell death

Pharmacodynamics/Kinetics
Distribution: Minimal amounts enter the aqueous humor, bile, CSF (inflamed or noninflamed meninges), amniotic fluid, pericardial fluid, pleural fluid, and synovial fluid
Protein binding, plasma: 90%
Half-life elimination: Biphasic: Initial: 15-48 hours; Terminal: 15 days
Time to peak: Within 1 hour following a 4- to 6-hour dose
Excretion: Urine (2% to 5% as biologically active form); ~40% eliminated over a 7-day period and may be detected in urine for at least 7 weeks after discontinued use

Usual Dosage
I.V.: Premedication: For patients who experience chills, fever, hypotension, nausea, or other nonanaphylactic infusion-related immediate reactions, premedicate with the following drugs, 30-60 minutes prior to drug administration: a nonsteroidal (eg, ibuprofen, choline magnesium trisalicylate, etc) with or without diphenhydramine; or acetaminophen with diphenhydramine; or hydrocortisone 50-100 mg. If the patient experiences rigors during the infusion, meperidine may be administered.
Infants and Children:
Test dose: I.V.: 0.1 mg/kg/dose to a maximum of 1 mg; infuse over 30-60 minutes. Many clinicians believe a test dose is unnecessary.
Maintenance dose: 0.25-1 mg/kg/day given once daily; infuse over 2-6 hours. Once therapy has been established, amphotericin B can be administered on an every-other-day basis at 1-1.5 mg/kg/dose; cumulative dose: 1.5-2 g over 6-10 week.
Adults:
Test dose: 1 mg infused over 20-30 minutes. Many clinicians believe a test dose is unnecessary.
(Continued)

Amphotericin B (Conventional) *(Continued)*

Maintenance dose: Usual: 0.25-1.5 mg/kg/day; 1-1.5 mg/kg over 4-6 hours every other day may be given once therapy is established; aspergillosis, mucormycosis, rhinocerebral phycomycosis often require 1-1.5 mg/kg/day; do not exceed 1.5 mg/kg/day

Duration of therapy varies with nature of infection: Usual duration is 4-12 weeks or cumulative dose of 1-4 g

I.T.: Meningitis, coccidioidal or cryptococcal:

Children.: 25-100 mcg every 48-72 hours; increase to 500 mcg as tolerated

Adults: Initial: 25-300 mcg every 48-72 hours; increase to 500 mcg to 1 mg as tolerated; maximum total dose: 15 mg has been suggested

Oral: 1 mL (100 mg) 4 times/day

Topical: Apply to affected areas 2-4 times/day for 1-4 weeks of therapy depending on nature and severity of infection

Bladder irrigation: Candidal cystitis: Irrigate with 50 mcg/mL solution instilled periodically or continuously for 5-10 days or until cultures are clear

Dosing adjustment in renal impairment: If renal dysfunction is due to the drug, the daily total can be decreased by 50% or the dose can be given every other day; I.V. therapy may take several months

Dialysis: Poorly dialyzed; no supplemental dosage necessary when using hemo- or peritoneal dialysis or continuous arteriovenous or venovenous hemodiafiltration effects

Administration in dialysate: Children and Adults: 1-2 mg/L of peritoneal dialysis fluid either with or without low-dose I.V. amphotericin B (a total dose of 2-10 mg/kg given over 7-14 days). Precipitate may form in ionic dialysate solutions.

Monitoring Parameters Renal function (monitor frequently during therapy), electrolytes (especially potassium and magnesium), liver function tests, temperature, PT/PTT, CBC; monitor input and output; monitor for signs of hypokalemia (muscle weakness, cramping, drowsiness, EKG changes, etc)

Reference Range Therapeutic: 1-2 μg/mL (SI: 1-2.2 μmol/L)

Patient Information Amphotericin cream may slightly discolor skin and stain clothing; good personal hygiene may reduce the spread and recurrence of lesions; avoid covering topical applications with occlusive bandages; most skin lesions require 1-3 weeks of therapy; report any cramping, muscle weakness, or pain at or near injection site

Nursing Implications May be infused over 2-6 hours

Additional Information Premedication with diphenhydramine and acetaminophen may reduce the severity of acute infusion-related reactions. Meperidine reduces the duration of amphotericin B-induced rigors and chilling. Hydrocortisone may be used in patients with severe or refractory infusion-related reactions. Bolus infusion of normal saline immediately preceding, or immediately preceding and following amphotericin B may reduce drug-induced nephrotoxicity. Risk of nephrotoxicity increases with amphotericin B doses >1 mg/kg/day. Infusion of admixtures more concentrated than 0.25 mg/mL should be limited to patients absolutely requiring volume contraction. Amphotericin B does not have a bacteriostatic constituent, subsequently admixture expiration is determined by sterility more than chemical stability.

Dosage Forms

Cream: 3% (20 g)

Lotion: 3% (30 mL)

Powder for injection, lyophilized, as desoxycholate: 50 mg

Suspension, oral: 100 mg/mL (24 mL with dropper)

♦ **Amphotericin B Desoxycholate** *see* Amphotericin B (Conventional) *on page 88*

Amphotericin B (Lipid Complex) (am foe TER i sin bee LIP id KOM pleks)

U.S. Brand Names Abelcet®

Canadian Brand Names Abelcet®

Synonyms ABLC

Therapeutic Category Antifungal Agent, Systemic

Use Treatment of aspergillosis or any type of progressive fungal infection in patients who are refractory to or intolerant of conventional amphotericin B therapy

Pregnancy Risk Factor B

Pregnancy/Breast-Feeding Implications Breast-feeding/lactation: Due to limited data, consider discontinuing nursing during therapy

Contraindications Hypersensitivity to amphotericin or any component of the formulation

Warnings/Precautions Anaphylaxis has been reported with amphotericin B-containing drugs. If severe respiratory distress occurs, the infusion should be immediately discontinued. During the initial dosing, the drug should be administered under close clinical observation. Acute reactions (including fever and chills) may occur 1-2 hours after starting an intravenous infusion. These reactions are usually more common with the first few doses and generally diminish with subsequent doses.

Adverse Reactions Nephrotoxicity and infusion-related hyperpyrexia, rigor, and chilling are reduced relative to amphotericin deoxycholate.

>10%:

Central nervous system: Chills, fever

Renal: Increased serum creatinine

Miscellaneous: Multiple organ failure

1% to 10%:

Cardiovascular: Hypotension, cardiac arrest

Central nervous system: Headache, pain

Dermatologic: Rash

Endocrine & metabolic: Bilirubinemia, hypokalemia, acidosis

Gastrointestinal: Nausea, vomiting, diarrhea, gastrointestinal hemorrhage, abdominal pain

Renal: Renal failure

Respiratory: Respiratory failure, dyspnea, pneumonia

Drug Interactions

Increased Effect/Toxicity: See Drug Interactions - Increased Effect/Toxicity in Amphotericin B monograph.

Decreased Effect: Pharmacologic antagonism may occur with azole antifungal agents (ketoconazole, miconazole).

Stability 100 mg vials in 20 mL of suspension in single-use vials (no preservative is present). Intact vials should be stored at 2°C to 8°C (35°F to 46°F) and protected from exposure to light; do not freeze intact vials. Shake the vial gently until there is no evidence of any yellow sediment at the bottom. Withdraw the appropriate dose and filter the contents (5 micron filter) prior to dilution. Dilute into D_5W to a final concentration of 1 mg/mL. For pediatric patients and patients with cardiovascular disease, the drug may be diluted with D_5W to a final concentration of 2 mg/mL.

Do not dilute with saline solutions or mix with other drugs or electrolytes - compatibility has not been established

Do not use an in-line filter <5 microns

Diluted solution is stable for up to 15 hours at 2°C to 8°C (38°F to 46°F) and an additional 6 hours at room temperature

Mechanism of Action Binds to ergosterol altering cell membrane permeability in susceptible fungi and causing leakage of cell components with subsequent cell death

Pharmacodynamics/Kinetics

Distribution: V_d: Increases with higher doses; reflects increased uptake by tissues (131 L/kg with 5 mg/kg/day)

Half-life elimination: ~24 hours

Excretion: Clearance: Increases with higher doses (5 mg/kg/day): 400 mL/hour/kg

Usual Dosage Children and Adults: I.V.:

Premedication: For patients who experience chills, fever, hypotension, nausea, or other nonanaphylactic infusion-related immediate reactions, premedicate with the following drugs, 30-60 minutes prior to drug administration: a nonsteroidal (eg, ibuprofen, choline magnesium trisalicylate, etc) with or without diphenhydramine; or acetaminophen with diphenhydramine; or hydrocortisone 50-100 mg. If the patient experiences rigors during the infusion, meperidine may be administered.

Range: 2.5-5 mg/kg/day as a single infusion

Dosing adjustment in renal impairment: None necessary; effects of renal impairment are not currently known

Hemodialysis: No supplemental dosage necessary

Peritoneal dialysis: No supplemental dosage necessary

Continuous arteriovenous or venovenous hemofiltration: No supplemental dosage necessary

Monitoring Parameters Renal function (monitor frequently during therapy), electrolytes (especially potassium and magnesium), liver function tests, temperature, PT/PTT, CBC; monitor input and output; monitor for signs of hypokalemia (muscle weakness, cramping, drowsiness, EKG changes, etc)

Nursing Implications I.V. therapy may take several months; personal hygiene is very important to help reduce the spread and recurrence of lesions; most skin lesions require 1-3 weeks of therapy; report any hearing loss

Additional Information As a modification of dimyristoyl phosphatidylcholine:dimyristoyl phosphatidylglycerol 7:3 (DMPC:DMPG) liposome, amphotericin B lipid-complex has a higher drug to lipid ratio and the concentration of amphotericin B is 33 M. ABLC is a ribbon-like structure, not a liposome.

Controlled trials which compare the original formulation of amphotericin B to the newer liposomal formulations (ie, Abelcet®) are lacking. Thus, comparative data discussing differences among the formulations should be interpreted cautiously. Although the risk of nephrotoxicity and infusion-related adverse effects may be less with Abelcet®, the efficacy profiles of Abelcet® and the original amphotericin formulation are comparable. Consequently, Abelcet® should be restricted to those patients who cannot tolerate or fail a standard amphotericin B formulation.

Dosage Forms Injection, suspension: 5 mg/mL (10 mL, 20 mL)

Amphotericin B (Liposomal) (am foe TER i sin bee lye po SO mal)

U.S. Brand Names AmBisome®

Canadian Brand Names AmBisome®

Synonyms L-AmB

Therapeutic Category Antifungal Agent, Systemic

Use Empirical therapy for presumed fungal infection in febrile, neutropenic patients. Treatment of patients with *Aspergillus* species, *Candida* species and/or *Cryptococcus* species infections refractory to amphotericin B desoxycholate, or in patients where renal impairment or unacceptable toxicity precludes the use of amphotericin B desoxycholate. Treatment of cryptococcal meningitis in HIV-infected patients. Treatment of visceral leishmaniasis; in immunocompromised patients with visceral leishmaniasis treated with amphotericin B (liposomal), relapse rates were high following initial clearance of parasites.

Pregnancy Risk Factor B

Contraindications Hypersensitivity to amphotericin B or any component of the formulation unless, in the opinion of the treating physician, the benefit of therapy outweighs the risk

Warnings/Precautions Anaphylaxis has been reported with amphotericin B desoxycholate and amphotericin B-containing drugs. During the initial dosing period, patients should be under close clinical observation. If severe respiratory distress occurs, the infusion should be immediately discontinued and the patient should not receive further infusions. Acute reactions (including fever and chills) may occur 1-2 hours after starting an intravenous infusion. These reactions are usually more common with the first few doses and generally diminish with subsequent doses.

Adverse Reactions Percentage of adverse reactions is dependent upon population studied and may vary with respect to premedications and underlying illness.

(Continued)

Amphotericin B (Liposomal) *(Continued)*

>10%:

Cardiovascular: Peripheral edema (15%), edema (12% to 14%), tachycardia (9% to 18%), hypotension (7% to 14%), hypertension (8% to 20%), chest pain (8% to 12%), hypervolemia (8% to 12%)

Central nervous system: Chills (29% to 48%), insomnia (17% to 22%), headache (9% to 20%), anxiety (7% to 14%), pain (14%), confusion (9% to 13%)

Dermatologic: Rash (5% to 25%), pruritus (11%)

Endocrine & metabolic: Hypokalemia (31% to 51%), hypomagnesemia (15% to 50%), hyperglycemia (8% to 23%), hypocalcemia (5% to 18%), hyponatremia (8% to 12%)

Gastrointestinal: Nausea (16% to 40%), vomiting (10% to 32%), diarrhea (11% to 30%), abdominal pain (7% to 20%), constipation (15%), anorexia (10% to 14%),

Hematologic: Anemia (27% to 48%), blood transfusion reaction (9% to 18%), leukopenia (15% to 17%), thrombocytopenia (6% to 13%)

Hepatic: Increased alkaline phosphatase (7% to 22%), increased BUN (7% to 21%), bilirubinemia (9% to 18%), increased ALT (15%), increased AST (13%), abnormal liver function tests (not specified) (4% to 13%)

Local: Phlebitis (9% to 11%)

Neuromuscular & skeletal: Weakness (6% to 13%), back pain (12%)

Renal: Increased creatinine (18% to 40%), hematuria (14%)

Respiratory: Dyspnea (18% to 23%), lung disorder (14% to 18%), increased cough (2% to 18%), epistaxis (8% to 15%), pleural effusion (12%), rhinitis (11%)

Miscellaneous: Sepsis (7% to 14%), infection (11% to 12%)

2% to 10% (Limited to important or life-threatening):

Cardiovascular: Arrhythmia, atrial fibrillation, bradycardia, cardiac arrest, cardiomegaly, postural hypotension,

Central nervous system: Agitation, coma, convulsion, depression, dizziness (7% to 8%), hallucinations, malaise, somnolence

Dermatologic: Alopecia, rash, petechia, purpura, skin discoloration, urticaria

Endocrine & metabolic: Acidosis, hypernatremia (4%), hyperchloremia, hyperkalemia, hypermagnesemia, hyperphosphatemia, hypophosphatemia

Gastrointestinal: Gastrointestinal hemorrhage (10%), hematemesis, gum/oral hemorrhage, ileus, ulcerative stomatitis

Genitourinary: Vaginal hemorrhage

Hematologic: Coagulation disorder, hemorrhage, decreased prothrombin, thrombocytopenia

Hepatic: Hepatocellular damage, veno-occlusive liver disease

Local: Injection site inflammation

Neuromuscular & skeletal: Arthralgia, bone pain, dystonia, paresthesia, rigors, tremor

Ocular: Conjunctivitis, eye hemorrhage

Renal: Acute kidney failure, toxic nephropathy

Respiratory: Asthma, atelectasis, hemoptysis, pulmonary edema, respiratory alkalosis, respiratory failure, hypoxia (6% to 8%)

Miscellaneous: Allergic reaction, cell-mediated immunological reaction, flu-like syndrome, procedural complication (8% to 10%), diaphoresis (7%)

<1% (Limited to important or life-threatening): Agranulocytosis, angioedema, cyanosis/hypoventilation, erythema, hemorrhagic cystitis, pulmonary edema, urticaria

Overdosage/Toxicology Toxicity due to overdose has not been defined. Repeated daily doses up to 7.5 mg/kg have been administered in clinical trials with no reported dose-related toxicity. If overdosage should occur, cease administration immediately. Symptomatic supportive measures should be instituted. Particular attention should be given to monitoring renal function.

Drug Interactions

Increased Effect/Toxicity: Drug interactions have not been studied in a controlled manner; however, drugs that interact with conventional amphotericin B may also interact with amphotericin B liposome for injection. The following drug interactions have been described for conventional amphotericin B. See Drug Interactions - Increased Effect/Toxicity in Amphotericin B monograph.

Stability Must be reconstituted using sterile water for injection, USP (without a bacteriostatic agent). Follow package insert instructions carefully for preparation. Do not reconstitute with saline or add saline to the reconstituted concentration, or mix with other drugs. The use of any solution other than those recommended, or the presence of a bacteriostatic agent in the solution, may cause precipitation.

Must be diluted with 5% dextrose injection to a final concentration of 1-2 mg/mL prior to administration. Lower concentrations (0.2-0.5 mg/mL) may be appropriate for infants and small children to provide sufficient volume for infusion.

Injection should commence within 6 hours of dilution with 5% dextrose injection.

An in-line membrane filter may be used for the intravenous infusion; provided, THE MEAN PORE DIAMETER OF THE FILTER SHOULD NOT BE LESS THAN 1 (one) MICRON.

Mechanism of Action Binds to ergosterol altering cell membrane permeability in susceptible fungi and causing leakage of cell components with subsequent cell death

Pharmacodynamics/Kinetics

Distribution: V_d: 131 L/kg

Half-life elimination: Terminal: 174 hours

Usual Dosage Children and Adults: I.V.:

Note: Premedication: For patients who experience chills, fever, hypotension, nausea, or other nonanaphylactic infusion-related immediate reactions, premedicate with the following drugs, 30-60 minutes prior to drug administration: a nonsteroidal (eg, ibuprofen, choline magnesium trisalicylate, etc) with or without diphenhydramine; or acetaminophen with diphenhydramine; or hydrocortisone 50-100 mg. If the patient experiences rigors during the infusion, meperidine may be administered.

Empiric therapy: Recommended initial dose: 3 mg/kg/day

Systemic fungal infections (*Aspergillus, Candida, Cryptococcus*): Recommended initial dose of 3-5 mg/kg/day

Cryptococcal meningitis in HIV-infected patients: 6 mg/kg/day
Treatment of visceral leishmaniasis:
Immunocompetent patients: 3 mg/kg/day on days 1-5, and 3 mg/kg/day on days 14 and 21; a repeat course may be given in patients who do not achieve parasitic clearance
Immunocompromised patients: 4 mg/kg/day on days 1-5, and 4 mg/kg/day on days 10, 17, 24, 31, and 38
Dosing adjustment in renal impairment: None necessary; effects of renal impairment are not currently known
Hemodialysis: No supplemental dosage necessary
Peritoneal dialysis effects: No supplemental dosage necessary
Continuous arteriovenous or venovenous hemofiltration: No supplemental dosage necessary
Administration Should be administered by intravenous infusion, using a controlled infusion device, over a period of approximately 2 hours. Infusion time may be reduced to approximately 1 hour in patients in whom the treatment is well-tolerated. If the patient experiences discomfort during infusion, the duration of infusion may be increased. Administer at a rate of 2.5 mg/kg/hour; infusion bag or syringe should be shaken before start of infusion. If infusion time exceeds 2 hours, the contents of the infusion bag should be mixed every 2 hours by shaking.
Monitoring Parameters Renal function (monitor frequently during therapy), electrolytes (especially potassium and magnesium), liver function tests, temperature, PT/PTT, CBC; monitor input and output; monitor for signs of hypokalemia (muscle weakness, cramping, drowsiness, EKG changes, etc)
Additional Information Amphotericin B, liposomal is a true single bilayer liposomal drug delivery system. Liposomes are closed, spherical vesicles created by mixing specific proportions of amphophilic substances such as phospholipids and cholesterol so that they arrange themselves into multiple concentric bilayer membranes when hydrated in aqueous solutions. Single bilayer liposomes are then formed by microemulsification of multilamellar vesicles using a homogenizer. Amphotericin B, liposomal consists of these unilamellar bilayer liposomes with amphotericin B intercalated within the membrane. Due to the nature and quantity of amphophilic substances used, and the lipophilic moiety in the amphotericin B molecule, the drug is an integral part of the overall structure of the amphotericin B liposomal liposomes. Amphotericin B, liposomal contains true liposomes that are <100 nm in diameter.
Dosage Forms Injection, powder for reconstitution: 50 mg

Ampicillin (am pi SIL in)
Related Information
Animal and Human Bites Guidelines *on page 1584*
Antibiotic Treatment of Adults With Infective Endocarditis *on page 1585*
Antimicrobial Drugs of Choice *on page 1588*
Community-Acquired Pneumonia in Adults *on page 1603*
Desensitization Protocols *on page 1525*
Prevention of Bacterial Endocarditis *on page 1563*
U.S. Brand Names Marcillin®; Principen®
Canadian Brand Names Apo®-Ampi; Novo-Ampicillin; Nu-Ampi
Synonyms Aminobenzylpenicillin; Ampicillin Sodium; Ampicillin Trihydrate
Therapeutic Category Antibiotic, Penicillin
Use Treatment of susceptible bacterial infections (nonbeta-lactamase-producing organisms); susceptible bacterial infections caused by streptococci, pneumococci, nonpenicillinase-producing staphylococci, *Listeria*, meningococci; some strains of *H. influenzae*, *Salmonella*, *Shigella*, *E. coli*, *Enterobacter*, and *Klebsiella*
Pregnancy Risk Factor B
Contraindications Hypersensitivity to ampicillin, any component of the formulation, or other penicillins
Warnings/Precautions Dosage adjustment may be necessary in patients with renal impairment; a low incidence of cross-allergy with other beta-lactams exists; high percentage of patients with infectious mononucleosis have developed rash during therapy with ampicillin. Appearance of a rash should be carefully evaluated to differentiate a nonallergic ampicillin rash from a hypersensitivity reaction. Ampicillin rash occurs in 5% to 10% of children receiving ampicillin and is a generalized dull red, maculopapular rash, generally appearing 3-14 days after the start of therapy. It normally begins on the trunk and spreads over most of the body. It may be most intense at pressure areas, elbows, and knees.
Adverse Reactions
>10%: Local: Pain at injection site
1% to 10%:
Dermatologic: Rash (appearance of a rash should be carefully evaluated to differentiate, if possible; nonallergic ampicillin rash from hypersensitivity reaction; incidence is higher in patients with viral infections, *Salmonella* infections, lymphocytic leukemia, or patients that have hyperuricemia)
Gastrointestinal: Diarrhea, vomiting, oral candidiasis, abdominal cramps
Miscellaneous: Allergic reaction (includes serum sickness, urticaria, angioedema, bronchospasm, hypotension, etc)
<1% (Limited to important or life-threatening): Decreased lymphocytes, eosinophilia, granulocytopenia, hemolytic anemia, interstitial nephritis (rare), leukopenia, penicillin encephalopathy, seizures (with large I.V. doses or patients with renal dysfunction), thrombocytopenia, thrombocytopenic purpura
Overdosage/Toxicology Symptoms of penicillin overdose include neuromuscular hypersensitivity (agitation, hallucinations, asterixis, encephalopathy, confusion, and seizures) and electrolyte imbalance (with potassium or sodium salts), especially in renal failure. Hemodialysis may be helpful to aid in the removal of the drug from the blood, otherwise most treatment is supportive or symptom directed.
Drug Interactions
Increased Effect/Toxicity: Ampicillin increases the effect of disulfiram and anticoagulants. Probenecid may increase penicillin levels. Theoretically, allopurinol taken with ampicillin has an additive potential for rash.
(Continued)

Ampicillin (Continued)

Decreased Effect: Efficacy of oral contraceptives may be reduced with ampicillin.

Ethanol/Nutrition/Herb Interactions Food: Food decreases ampicillin absorption rate; may decrease ampicillin serum concentration.

Stability Oral suspension is stable for 7 days at room temperature or for 14 days under refrigeration; solutions for I.M. or direct I.V. should be used within 1 hour; solutions for I.V. infusion will be inactivated by dextrose at room temperature; if dextrose-containing solutions are to be used, the resultant solution will only be stable for 2 hours versus 8 hours in the 0.9% sodium chloride injection. D_5W has limited stability.

Minimum volume: Concentration should not exceed 30 mg/mL due to concentration-dependent stability restrictions. Manufacturer may supply as either the anhydrous or the trihydrate form.

Stability of parenteral admixture in NS at room temperature (25°C): 8 hours

Stability of parenteral admixture in NS at refrigeration temperature (4°C): 2 days

Standard diluent: 500 mg/50 mL NS; 1 g/50 mL NS; 2 g/100 mL NS

Mechanism of Action Inhibits bacterial cell wall synthesis by binding to one or more of the penicillin binding proteins (PBPs); which in turn inhibits the final transpeptidation step of peptidoglycan synthesis in bacterial cell walls, thus inhibiting cell wall biosynthesis. Bacteria eventually lyse due to ongoing activity of cell wall autolytic enzymes (autolysins and murein hydrolases) while cell wall assembly is arrested.

Pharmacodynamics/Kinetics

Absorption: Oral: 50%

Distribution: Bile, blister, and tissue fluids; penetration into CSF occurs with inflamed meninges only, good only with inflammation (exceeds usual MICs)

Normal meninges: Nil; Inflamed meninges: 5% to 10%

Protein binding: 15% to 25%

Half-life elimination:

Neonates: 2-7 days: 4 hours; 8-14 days: 2.8 hours; 15-30 days: 1.7 hours

Children and Adults: 1-1.8 hours

Anuria/end-stage renal disease: 7-20 hours

Time to peak: Oral: Within 1-2 hours

Excretion: Urine (~90% as unchanged drug) within 24 hours

Usual Dosage

Neonates: I.M., I.V.:

Postnatal age ≤7 days:

≤2000 g: Meningitis: 50 mg/kg/dose every 12 hours; other infections: 25 mg/kg/dose every 12 hours

>2000 g: Meningitis: 50 mg/kg/dose every 8 hours; other infections: 25 mg/kg/dose every 8 hours

Postnatal age >7 days:

<1200 g: Meningitis: 50 mg/kg/dose every 12 hours; other infections: 25 mg/kg/dose every 12 hours

1200-2000 g: Meningitis: 50 mg/kg/dose every 8 hours; other infections: 25 mg/kg/dose every 8 hours

>2000 g: Meningitis: 50 mg/kg/dose every 6 hours; other infections: 25 mg/kg/dose every 6 hours

Infants and Children: I.M., I.V.: 100-400 mg/kg/day in doses divided every 4-6 hours

Meningitis: 200 mg/kg/day in doses divided every 4-6 hours; maximum dose: 12 g/day

Children: Oral: 50-100 mg/kg/day in doses divided every 6 hours; maximum dose: 2-3 g/day

Adults:

Oral: 250-500 mg every 6 hours

I.M.: 500 mg to 1.5 g every 4-6 hours

I.V.: 500 mg to 3 g every 4-6 hours; maximum dose: 12 g/day

Sepsis/meningitis: 150-250 mg/kg/24 hours divided every 3-4 hours

Dosing interval in renal impairment:

Cl_{cr} 30-50 mL/minute: Administer every 6-8 hours

Cl_{cr} 10-30 mL/minute: Administer every 8-12 hours

Cl_{cr} <10 mL/minute: Administer every 12 hours

Hemodialysis: Moderately dialyzable (20% to 50%); administer dose after dialysis

Peritoneal dialysis: Moderately dialyzable (20% to 50%)

Administer 250 mg every 12 hours

Continuous arteriovenous or venovenous hemofiltration effects: Dose as for Cl_{cr} 10-50 mL/minute; ~50 mg of ampicillin per liter of filtrate is removed

Dietary Considerations Take on an empty stomach 1 hour before or 2 hours after meals.

Administration Administer orally on an empty stomach (ie, 1 hour prior to, or 2 hours after meals) to increase total absorption

Monitoring Parameters With prolonged therapy monitor renal, hepatic, and hematologic function periodically; observe signs and symptoms of anaphylaxis during first dose

Test Interactions May interfere with urinary glucose tests using cupric sulfate (Benedict's solution, Clinitest®); may inactivate aminoglycosides *in vitro*

Patient Information Food decreases rate and extent of absorption; take oral on an empty stomach, if possible (ie, 1 hour prior to, or 2 hours after meals); report diarrhea promptly; entire course of medication should be taken to ensure eradication of organism; females should report onset of symptoms of candidal vaginitis; may interfere with the effects of oral contraceptives

Nursing Implications Ampicillin and gentamicin should not be mixed in the same I.V. tubing or administered concurrently

Additional Information

Sodium content of 5 mL suspension (250 mg/5 mL): 10 mg (0.4 mEq)

Sodium content of 1 g: 66.7 mg (3 mEq)

Dosage Forms

Capsule: 250 mg, 500 mg

Marcillin®: 500 mg

Principen®: 250 mg, 500 mg
Injection, powder for reconstitution, as sodium: 125 mg, 250 mg, 500 mg, 1 g, 2 g, 10 g
Powder for oral suspension (Principen®): 125 mg/5 mL (100 mL, 200 mL); 250 mg/5 mL (100 mL, 200 mL)

Ampicillin and Sulbactam (am pi SIL in & SUL bak tam)

Related Information
Antimicrobial Drugs of Choice *on page 1588*
Community-Acquired Pneumonia in Adults *on page 1603*
Treatment of Sexually Transmitted Diseases *on page 1609*

U.S. Brand Names Unasyn®

Canadian Brand Names Unasyn®

Synonyms Sulbactam and Ampicillin

Therapeutic Category Antibiotic, Anaerobic; Antibiotic, Penicillin; Antibiotic, Penicillin & Beta-lactamase Inhibitor

Use Treatment of susceptible bacterial infections involved with skin and skin structure, intra-abdominal infections, gynecological infections; spectrum is that of ampicillin plus organisms producing beta-lactamases such as *S. aureus, H. influenzae, E. coli, Klebsiella, Acineto-bacter, Enterobacter,* and anaerobes

Pregnancy Risk Factor B

Contraindications Hypersensitivity to ampicillin, sulbactam, penicillins, or any component of the formulations

Warnings/Precautions Dosage adjustment may be necessary in patients with renal impairment; a low incidence of cross-allergy with other beta-lactams exists; high percentage of patients with infectious mononucleosis have developed rash during therapy with ampicillin. Appearance of a rash should be carefully evaluated to differentiate a nonallergic ampicillin rash from a hypersensitivity reaction.

Adverse Reactions
>10%: Local: Pain at injection site (I.M.)
1% to 10%:
  Dermatologic: Rash
  Gastrointestinal: Diarrhea
  Local: Pain at injection site (I.V.)
  Miscellaneous: Allergic reaction (may include serum sickness, urticaria, bronchospasm, hypotension, etc)
<1% (Limited to important or life-threatening): Interstitial nephritis (rare), leukopenia, neutropenia, penicillin encephalopathy, pseudomembranous colitis, seizures (with large I.V. doses or patients with renal dysfunction), thrombocytopenia, thrombophlebitis

Overdosage/Toxicology Symptoms of penicillin overdose include neuromuscular hypersensitivity (agitation, hallucinations, asterixis, encephalopathy, confusion, and seizures) and electrolyte imbalance (with potassium or sodium salts), especially in renal failure. Hemodialysis may be helpful to aid in the removal of the drug from the blood, otherwise most treatment is supportive or symptom directed.

Drug Interactions
Increased Effect/Toxicity: Disulfiram or probenecid can increase ampicillin levels. Theoretically, allopurinol taken with ampicillin has an additive potential for rash.
Decreased Effect: Efficacy of oral contraceptives may be reduced with ampicillin and sulbactam.

Stability I.M. and direct I.V. administration: Use within 1 hour after preparation; reconstitute with sterile water for injection or 0.5% or 2% lidocaine hydrochloride injection (I.M.); sodium chloride 0.9% (NS) is the diluent of choice for I.V. piggyback use, solutions made in NS are stable up to 72 hours when refrigerated whereas dextrose solutions (same concentration) are stable for only 4 hours

Mechanism of Action The addition of sulbactam, a beta-lactamase inhibitor, to ampicillin extends the spectrum of ampicillin to include some beta-lactamase producing organisms; inhibits bacterial cell wall synthesis by binding to one or more of the penicillin binding proteins (PBPs); which in turn inhibits the final transpeptidation step of peptidoglycan synthesis in bacterial cell walls, thus inhibiting cell wall biosynthesis. Bacteria eventually lyse due to ongoing activity of cell wall autolytic enzymes (autolysins and murein hydrolases) while cell wall assembly is arrested.

Pharmacodynamics/Kinetics
Ampicillin: See Ampicillin monograph.
Sulbactam:
  Distribution: Bile, blister, and tissue fluids
  Protein binding: 38%
  Half-life elimination: Normal renal function: 1-1.3 hours
  Excretion: Urine (~75% to 85% as unchanged drug) within 8 hours

Usual Dosage Unasyn® (ampicillin/sulbactam) is a combination product. Each 3 g vial contains 2 g of ampicillin and 1 g of sulbactam. Sulbactam has very little antibacterial activity by itself, but effectively extends the spectrum of ampicillin to include beta-lactamase producing strains that are resistant to ampicillin alone. Therefore, dosage recommendations for Unasyn® are based on the ampicillin component.
I.M., I.V.:
  Children (3 months to 12 years): 100-200 mg ampicillin/kg/day (150-300 mg Unasyn®) divided every 6 hours; maximum dose: 8 g ampicillin/day (12 g Unasyn®)
  Adults: 1-2 g ampicillin (1.5-3 g Unasyn®) every 6-8 hours; maximum dose: 8 g ampicillin/day (12 g Unasyn®)
Dosing interval in renal impairment:
  Cl_{cr} 15-29 mL/minute: Administer every 12 hours
  Cl_{cr} 5-14 mL/minute: Administer every 24 hours

Monitoring Parameters With prolonged therapy, monitor hematologic, renal, and hepatic function; monitor for signs of anaphylaxis during first dose

Test Interactions May interfere with urinary glucose tests using cupric sulfate (Benedict's solution, Clinitest®); may inactivate aminoglycosides *in vitro*
(Continued)

Ampicillin and Sulbactam *(Continued)*

Nursing Implications Ampicillin and gentamicin should not be mixed in the same I.V. tubing or administered concurrently

Additional Information Sodium content of 1.5 g injection: 115 mg (5 mEq)

Dosage Forms

Powder for injection:

1.5 g [ampicillin sodium 1 g and sulbactam sodium 0.5 g]

3 g [ampicillin sodium 2 g and sulbactam sodium 1 g]

15 g [ampicillin sodium 10 g and sulbactam sodium 5 g] [bulk package]

♦ **Ampicillin Sodium** *see* Ampicillin *on page 93*

♦ **Ampicillin Trihydrate** *see* Ampicillin *on page 93*

Amprenavir *(am PREN a veer)*

Related Information

Antiretroviral Agents Comparison *on page 1488*

Antiretroviral Therapy for HIV Infection *on page 1595*

Management of Healthcare Worker Exposures to HIV, HBV, HCV *on page 1555*

U.S. Brand Names Agenerase®

Canadian Brand Names Agenerase®

Therapeutic Category Antiretroviral Agent, Protease Inhibitor; Protease Inhibitor

Use Treatment of HIV infections in combination with at least two other antiretroviral agents; oral solution should only be used when capsules or other protease inhibitors are not therapeutic options

Pregnancy Risk Factor C

Pregnancy/Breast-Feeding Implications It is not known if amprenavir crosses the human placenta and there are no clinical studies currently underway to evaluate its use in pregnant women. Pregnancy and protease inhibitors are both associated with an increased risk of hyperglycemia. Glucose levels should be closely monitored. Health professionals are encouraged to contact the antiretroviral pregnancy registry to monitor outcomes of pregnant women exposed to antiretroviral medications (1-800-258-4263).

Contraindications Hypersensitivity to amprenavir or any component of the formulation; concurrent therapy with rifampin, astemizole, bepridil, cisapride, dihydroergotamine, ergotamine, midazolam, pimozide, triazolam, lovastatin, and simvastatin; severe previous allergic reaction to sulfonamides; oral solution is contraindicated in infants or children <4 years of age, pregnant women, patients with renal or hepatic failure, and patients receiving concurrent metronidazole or disulfiram

Warnings/Precautions Because of hepatic metabolism and effect on cytochrome P450 enzymes, amprenavir should be used with caution in combination with other agents metabolized by this system (see Contraindications and Drug Interactions). Avoid concurrent use of St John's wort (may lead to loss of virologic response and/or resistance). Use with caution in patients with diabetes mellitus, sulfonamide allergy, hepatic impairment, or hemophilia. Additional vitamin E supplements should be avoided. Concurrent use of sildenafil should be avoided. Certain ethnic populations (Asians, Eskimos, Native Americans) may be at increased risk of propylene glycol-associated adverse effects; therefore, use of the oral solution of amprenavir should be avoided. Use oral solution only when capsules or other protease inhibitors are not options.

Adverse Reactions Protease inhibitors cause dyslipidemia which includes elevated cholesterol and triglycerides and a redistribution of body fat centrally to cause "protease paunch," buffalo hump, facial atrophy, and breast enlargement. These agents also cause hyperglycemia.

>10%:

Dermatologic: Rash (28%)

Endocrine & metabolic: Hyperglycemia (37% to 41%), hypertriglyceridemia (36% to 47%)

Gastrointestinal: Nausea (38% to 73%), vomiting (20% to 29%), diarrhea (33% to 56%)

Miscellaneous: Perioral tingling/numbness

1% to 10%:

Central nervous system: Depression (4% to 15%), headache, paresthesia, fatigue

Dermatologic: Stevens-Johnson syndrome (1% of total, 4% of patients who develop a rash)

Endocrine & metabolic: Hypercholesterolemia (4% to 9%)

Gastrointestinal: Taste disorders (1% to 10%)

Overdosage/Toxicology Monitor for signs and symptoms of propylene glycol toxicity (seizures, stupor, tachycardia, hyperosmolality, lactic acidosis, renal toxicity, hemolysis) if the oral solution is administered.

Drug Interactions

Cytochrome P450 Effect: CYP3A3/4 enzyme substrate; CYP3A3/4 enzyme inhibitor

Increased Effect/Toxicity: Concurrent use of cisapride, pimozide, quinidine, and rifampin is contraindicated. Serum concentrations/effect of many benzodiazepines may be increased; concurrent use of midazolam or triazolam is contraindicated. Concurrent use of ergot alkaloids (dihydroergotamine, ergotamine, ergonovine, methylergonovine) with amprenavir is also contraindicated (may cause vasospasm and peripheral ischemia).

Concurrent use of oral solution with disulfiram or metronidazole is contraindicated (risk of propylene glycol toxicity). Serum concentrations of amiodarone, lidocaine, quinidine and other antiarrhythmics may be increased, potentially leading to toxicity. HMG-CoA reductase inhibitors serum concentrations may be increased by amprenavir, increasing the risk of myopathy/rhabdomyolysis; lovastatin and simvastatin are contraindicated; fluvastatin and pravastatin may be safer alternatives. Serum concentrations/effect of benzodiazepines, calcium channel blockers, cyclosporine, itraconazole, ketoconazole, rifabutin, tacrolimus, tricyclic antidepressants may be increased. May increase warfarin's effects, monitor INR.

Sildenafil serum concentrations may be increased by amprenavir; when used concurrently, do not exceed a maximum sildenafil dose of 25 mg in a 48-hour period. Concurrent therapy with ritonavir may result in increased serum concentrations: dosage adjustment is recommended. Clarithromycin, indinavir, nelfinavir may increase serum concentrations of amprenavir.

Decreased Effect: Enzyme-inducing agents (rifampin, phenobarbital, phenytoin) may decrease serum concentrations/effect of amprenavir; rifampin is contraindicated. The administration of didanosine (buffered formulation) should be separated from amprenavir by 1 hour to limit interaction between formulations. Serum concentrations of estrogen may be decreased, use alternative (nonhormonal) forms of contraception. Dexamethasone may decrease the therapeutic effect of amprenavir. Efavirenz and nevirapine may decrease serum concentrations of amprenavir (dosing for combinations not established). Avoid St John's wort (may lead to subtherapeutic concentrations of amprenavir).

Ethanol/Nutrition/Herb Interactions
Ethanol: Avoid ethanol with amprenavir oral solution.
Food: Levels increased sixfold with high-fat meals.
Herb/Nutraceutical: Amprenavir serum concentration may be decreased by St John's wort; avoid concurrent use. Formulations contain vitamin E; avoid additional supplements.

Mechanism of Action Binds to the protease activity site and inhibits the activity of the enzyme. HIV protease is required for the cleavage of viral polyprotein precursors into individual functional proteins found in infectious HIV. Inhibition prevents cleavage of these polyproteins, resulting in the formation of immature, noninfectious viral particles.

Pharmacodynamics/Kinetics
Absorption: 63%
Distribution: 430 L
Protein binding: 90%
Metabolism: Hepatic via CYP450 isoenzymes (primarily CYP3A4)
Bioavailability: Not established (increased sixfold with high-fat meal)
Half-life elimination: 7.1-10.6 hours
Time to peak: 1-2 hours
Excretion: Feces (75%); urine (14% as metabolites)

Usual Dosage Oral: **Note:** Capsule and oral solution are **not** interchangeable on a mg-per-mg basis.
Capsule:
Children 4-12 years and older (<50 kg): 20 mg/kg twice daily or 15 mg/kg 3 times daily; maximum: 2400 mg/day
Children >13 years (>50 kg) and Adults: 1200 mg twice daily
Note: Dosage adjustments for amprenavir when administered in combination therapy:
Efavirenz: Adjustments necessary for both agents:
Amprenavir 1200 mg 3 times/day (single protease inhibitor) **or**
Amprenavir 1200 mg twice daily plus ritonavir 200 mg twice daily
Ritonavir: Adjustments necessary for both agents:
Amprenavir 1200 mg plus ritonavir 200 mg once daily **or**
Amprenavir 600 mg plus ritonavir 100 mg twice daily
Solution:
Children 4-12 years or older (up to 16 years weighing <50 kg): 22.5 mg/kg twice daily or 17 mg/kg 3 times daily; maximum: 2800 mg/day
Children 13-16 years (weighing at least 50 kg) or >16 years and Adults: 1400 mg twice daily

Dosage adjustment in renal impairment: Oral solution is contraindicated in renal failure.
Dosage adjustment in hepatic impairment:
Child-Pugh score between 5-8:
Capsule: 450 mg twice daily
Solution: 513 mg twice daily; contraindicated in hepatic failure
Child-Pugh score between 9-12:
Capsule: 300 mg twice daily
Solution: 342 mg twice daily; contraindicated in hepatic failure

Dietary Considerations May be taken with or without food; do not take with high-fat meal.

Patient Information Advise prescriber of any previous reactions to sulfonamides. Do not take this medication with antacids or high-fat meals. Do not take additional vitamin E supplements. Do not take any prescription medications, over-the-counter products or herbal products, especially St John's wort, without consulting prescriber. For women using oral contraceptives, an alternative method of contraception should be used.

Additional Information Capsules contain 109 int. units of vitamin E per capsule; oral solution contains 46 int. units of vitamin E per mL. Propylene glycol is included in the oral solution; a dose of 22.5 mg/kg twice daily corresponds to an intake of 1650 mg/kg of propylene glycol. Capsule and oral solution are not interchangeable on a mg-per-mg basis.

Dosage Forms
Capsule: 50 mg, 150 mg
Solution, oral [use only when there are no other options]: 15 mg/mL (240 mL) [contains propylene glycol 550 mg/mL and vitamin E 46 int. units/mL; grape-bubblegum-peppermint flavor]

♦ **AMPT** see Metyrosine on page 906
♦ **Amrinone Lactate** see Inamrinone on page 714
♦ **Amvisc®** see Sodium Hyaluronate on page 1247
♦ **Amvisc® Plus** see Sodium Hyaluronate on page 1247

Amyl Nitrite (AM il NYE trite)
Synonyms Isoamyl Nitrite
Therapeutic Category Antidote, Cyanide; Vasodilator, Coronary
Use Coronary vasodilator in angina pectoris; adjunct in treatment of cyanide poisoning; produce changes in the intensity of heart murmurs
Pregnancy Risk Factor X
(Continued)

Amyl Nitrite *(Continued)*

Usual Dosage Nasal inhalation:
Cyanide poisoning: Children and Adults: Inhale the vapor from a 0.3 mL crushed ampul every minute for 15-30 seconds until I.V. sodium nitrite infusion is available
Angina: Adults: 1-6 inhalations from 1 crushed ampul; may repeat in 3-5 minutes

Additional Information Complete prescribing information for this medication should be consulted for additional detail.

Dosage Forms Vapor for inhalation [crushable glass perles]: 0.3 mL

♦ **Amylobarbitone** *see Amobarbital on page 81*

♦ **Amytal®** *see Amobarbital on page 81*

♦ **Anacin PM Aspirin Free [OTC]** *See Acetaminophen and Diphenhydramine on page 25*

♦ **Anadrol®** *see Oxymetholone on page 1027*

♦ **Anafranil®** *see ClomiPRAMINE on page 315*

Anagrelide *(an AG gre lide)*

U.S. Brand Names Agrylin®
Canadian Brand Names Agrylin®
Synonyms Anagrelide Hydrochloride
Therapeutic Category Platelet Reducing Agent
Use Treatment of thrombocythemia (ET), secondary to myeloproliferative disorders, to reduce the elevated platelet count and the risk of thrombosis, and to ameliorate associated symptoms (including thrombohemorrhagic events)
Pregnancy Risk Factor C
Usual Dosage Adults: Oral: 0.5 mg 4 times/day or 1 mg twice daily
Maintain for ≥1 week, then adjust to the lowest effective dose to reduce and maintain platelet count <600,000/µL ideally to the normal range; the dose must not be increased by >0.5 mg/day in any 1 week; maximum dose: 10 mg/day or 2.5 mg/dose
Elderly: There are no special requirements for dosing in the elderly
Additional Information Complete prescribing information for this medication should be consulted for additional detail.
Dosage Forms Capsule: 0.5 mg, 1 mg

♦ **Anagrelide Hydrochloride** *see Anagrelide on page 98*

Anakinra *(an a KIN ra)*

U.S. Brand Names Kineret™
Synonyms IL-1Ra; Interleukin-1 Receptor antagonist
Therapeutic Category Antirheumatic, Disease Modifying; Interleukin-1 Receptor Antagonist
Use Reduction of signs and symptoms of moderately- to severely-active rheumatoid arthritis in adult patients who have failed one or more disease-modifying antirheumatic drugs (DMARDs); may be used alone or in combination with DMARDs (other than tumor necrosis factor-blocking agents)
Pregnancy Risk Factor B
Pregnancy/Breast-Feeding Implications No evidence of impaired fertility or harm to fetus in animal models; however, there are no controlled trials in pregnant women.
Contraindications Hypersensitivity to *E.coli*-derived proteins, anakinra, or any component of the formulation; patients with active infections (including chronic or local infection)
Warnings/Precautions Anakinra may affect defenses against infections and malignancies. Safety and efficacy in patients with immunosuppression or chronic infections have not been evaluated. Discontinue administration if patient develops a serious infection. Do not start drug administration in patients with an active infection. Patients with asthma may be at an increased risk of serious infections. Should not be used in combination with tumor necrosis factor antagonists, unless no satisfactory alternatives exist, and then only with extreme caution. Impact on the development and course of malignancies is not fully defined.

Use caution in patients with a history of significant hematologic abnormalities; has been associated with uncommon, but significant decreases in hematologic parameters (particularly neutrophil counts). Patients must be advised to seek medical attention if they develop signs and symptoms suggestive of blood dyscrasias. Discontinue if significant hematologic abnormalities are confirmed.

Patients should be brought up to date with all immunizations before initiating therapy. Live vaccines should not be given concurrently. Patients with a significant exposure to varicella virus should temporarily discontinue anakinra. Hypersensitivity reactions may occur. Impact on the development and course of malignancies is not fully defined. The safety of anakinra has not been studied in children <18 years of age.

Adverse Reactions
>10%
Central nervous system; headache (12%)
Local: Injection site reaction (majority mild, typically lasting 14-28 days, characterized by erythema, ecchymosis, inflammation and pain; up to 71%)
Miscellaneous: Infection (40% versus 35% in placebo; serious infections in 2% to 7%)
1% to 10%
Gastrointestinal: Nausea (8%), diarrhea (7%), abdominal pain (5%)
Hematologic: Decreased WBCs (8%)
Respiratory: Sinusitis (7%)
Miscellaneous: Flu-like symptoms (6%)
<1% (Limited to important or life-threatening): Neutropenia (0.3%)
Overdosage/Toxicology No serious toxicities have been reported following administration of high doses of anakinra (up to 35 times the typical dosage for rheumatoid arthritis).
Drug Interactions
Increased Effect/Toxicity: Concurrent use of anakinra and etanercept has been associated with an increased risk of serious infection. Use caution with other drugs known to

block or decrease the activity of tumor necrosis factor (TNF); includes infliximab and thalidomide.

Stability Store in refrigerator at 2°C to 8°C (36°F to 46°F). Protect from light. Do not freeze.

Mechanism of Action Binds to the interleukin-1 (IL-1) receptor. IL-1 is induced by inflammatory stimuli and mediates a variety of immunological responses, including degradation of cartilage (loss of proteoglycans) and stimulation of bone resorption.

Pharmacodynamics/Kinetics
Bioavailability: S.C.: 95%
Half-life elimination: Terminal: 4-6 hours
Time to peak: S.C.: 3-7 hours

Usual Dosage Adults: S.C.: Rheumatoid arthritis: 100 mg once daily (administer at approximately the same time each day)

Dosage adjustment in renal impairment: No specific guidelines for adjustment (clearance decreased by 70% to 75% in patients with Cl_{cr} <30 mL/minute)

Administration Rotate injection sites (thigh, abdomen, upper arm); injection should be given at least 1 inch away from previous injection site. Do not shake. Provided in single-use, preservative free syringes with 27 gauge needles; discard any unused portion.

Monitoring Parameters Neutrophil counts should be assessed prior to initiation of treatment, and repeated every month for the first 3 months of treatment, then quarterly up to 1 year.

Patient Information If self-injecting, follow instructions for injection and disposal of needles exactly. If redness, swelling, or irritation appears at the injection site, contact prescriber. Do not have any vaccinations while using this medication without consulting prescriber first. Immediately report skin rash, unusual muscle or bone weakness, or signs of respiratory flu or other infection (eg, chills, fever, sore throat, easy bruising or bleeding, mouth sores, unhealed sores).

Additional Information Anakinra is produced by recombinant DNA/*E. coli* technology.

Dosage Forms Injection, prefilled glass syringe [preservative free]: 100 mg/0.67 mL (1 mL)

♦ **Analpram-HC®** *see* Pramoxine and Hydrocortisone *on page 1117*
♦ **Anamine® [OTC]** *see* Chlorpheniramine and Pseudoephedrine *on page 279*
♦ **Anandron® (Can)** *see* Nilutamide *on page 983*
♦ **Anaplex® [OTC]** *see* Chlorpheniramine and Pseudoephedrine *on page 279*
♦ **Anaprox®** *see* Naproxen *on page 958*
♦ **Anaprox® DS (Can)** *see* Naproxen *on page 958*
♦ **Anaspaz®** *see* Hyoscyamine *on page 692*

Anastrozole (an AS troe zole)

U.S. Brand Names Arimidex®
Canadian Brand Names Arimidex®
Therapeutic Category Antineoplastic Agent, Hormone (Antiestrogen); Aromatase Inhibitor
Use Treatment of locally-advanced or metastatic breast cancer (ER-positive or hormone receptor unknown) in postmenopausal women; treatment of advanced breast cancer in postmenopausal women with disease progression following tamoxifen therapy; patients with ER-negative disease and patients who did not respond to tamoxifen therapy rarely responded to anastrozole

Pregnancy Risk Factor D

Pregnancy/Breast-Feeding Implications Clinical effects on the fetus: Anastrozole can cause fetal harm when administered to a pregnant woman. It is not known if anastrozole is excreted in human breast milk, use caution if administered to a nursing woman.

Contraindications Hypersensitivity to anastrozole or any component of the formulation; pregnancy

Warnings/Precautions Use with caution in patients with hyperlipidemias; mean serum total cholesterol and LDL cholesterol occurs in patients receiving anastrozole; exclude pregnancy before initiating therapy. Safety and efficacy in pediatric patients have not been established.

Adverse Reactions
>5%:
Central nervous system: Headache, dizziness, depression
Cardiovascular: Flushing, peripheral edema, chest pain
Dermatologic: Rash
Gastrointestinal: Little to mild nausea (10%), vomiting, diarrhea, abdominal pain, anorexia, dry mouth
Genitourinary: Pelvic pain
Neuromuscular & skeletal: Increased bone and tumor pain, muscle weakness, paresthesia
Respiratory: Dyspnea, cough, pharyngitis
2% to 5%:
Cardiovascular: Hypertension, thrombophlebitis
Central nervous system: Somnolence, confusion, insomnia, anxiety, nervousness, fever, malaise, accidental injury
Dermatologic: Hair thinning, pruritus
Endocrine & metabolic: Breast pain
Gastrointestinal: Weight loss
Genitourinary: Urinary tract infection
Hematologic: Anemia, leukopenia
Neuromuscular & skeletal: Myalgia, arthralgia, pathological fracture, neck pain
Respiratory: Sinusitis, bronchitis, rhinitis
Miscellaneous: Flu-like syndrome, infection

Overdosage/Toxicology Symptoms include severe irritation to the stomach (necrosis, gastritis, ulceration and hemorrhage). There is no specific antidote. Treatment must be symptomatic. Vomiting may be induced if the patient is alert. Dialysis may be helpful because anastrozole is not highly protein bound. Treatment consists of general supportive care, including frequent monitoring of all vital signs and close observation.

(Continued)

Anastrozole *(Continued)*

Drug Interactions

Cytochrome P450 Effect: CYP3A3/4 enzyme substrate; CYP1A2, 2C8, 2C9, and 3A3/4 enzyme inhibitor (only at high concentrations)

Increased Effect/Toxicity: At therapeutic concentrations, it is unlikely that coadministration of anastrozole with other drugs will result in clinically significant inhibition of cytochrome P450-mediated drug metabolism. Inhibitors of CYP3A4 may increase anastrozole concentrations.

Ethanol/Nutrition/Herb Interactions Herb/Nutraceutical: St John's wort may decrease anastrozole levels.

Mechanism of Action Potent and selective nonsteroidal aromatase inhibitor. It significantly lowers serum estradiol concentrations and has no detectable effect on formation of adrenal corticosteroids or aldosterone. In postmenopausal women, the principal source of circulating estrogen is conversion of adrenally generated androstenedione to estrone by aromatase in peripheral tissues.

Pharmacodynamics/Kinetics

Absorption: Well absorbed; not affected by food

Protein binding, plasma: 40%

Metabolism: Extensively hepatic (85%)

Half-life elimination: 50 hours

Excretion: Urine (11%)

Usual Dosage Breast cancer: Adults: Oral (refer to individual protocols): 1 mg once daily

Dosage adjustment in renal impairment: Because only about 10% is excreted unchanged in the urine, dosage adjustment in patients with renal insufficiency is not necessary

Dosage adjustment in hepatic impairment: Plasma concentrations in subjects with hepatic cirrhosis were within the range concentrations in normal subjects across all clinical trials; therefore, no dosage adjustment is needed

Test Interactions Lab test abnormalities: GGT, AST, ALT, alkaline phosphatase, total cholesterol and LDL increased; threefold elevations of mean serum GGT levels have been observed among patients with liver metastases. These changes were likely related to the progression of liver metastases in these patients, although other contributing factors could not be ruled out. Mean serum total cholesterol levels increased by 0.5 mmol/L among patients.

Nursing Implications Use with caution in patients with hyperlipidemias; mean serum total cholesterol and LDL cholesterol occurs in patients receiving anastrozole

Dosage Forms Tablet: 1 mg

- ◆ **Anatuss® DM [OTC]** *see* Guaifenesin, Pseudoephedrine, and Dextromethorphan *on page 648*
- ◆ **Anbesol® [OTC]** *see* Benzocaine *on page 154*
- ◆ **Anbesol® Baby [OTC]** *see* Benzocaine *on page 154*
- ◆ **Anbesol® Maximum Strength [OTC]** *see* Benzocaine *on page 154*
- ◆ **Ancef®** *see* Cefazolin *on page 240*
- ◆ **Ancobon®** *see* Flucytosine *on page 567*
- ◆ **Andehist NR Syrup** *see* Brompheniramine and Pseudoephedrine *on page 185*
- ◆ **Andriol® (Can)** *see* Testosterone *on page 1302*
- ◆ **Androderm®** *see* Testosterone *on page 1302*
- ◆ **AndroGel®** *see* Testosterone *on page 1302*
- ◆ **Android®** *see* MethylTESTOSTERone *on page 898*
- ◆ **Andropository (Can)** *see* Testosterone *on page 1302*
- ◆ **Anectine® Chloride** *see* Succinylcholine *on page 1264*
- ◆ **Anectine® Flo-Pack®** *see* Succinylcholine *on page 1264*
- ◆ **Anergan®** *see* Promethazine *on page 1139*
- ◆ **Anestacon®** *see* Lidocaine *on page 801*
- ◆ **Aneurine Hydrochloride** *see* Thiamine *on page 1316*
- ◆ **Anexate® (Can)** *see* Flumazenil *on page 570*
- ◆ **Anexsia®** *see* Hydrocodone and Acetaminophen *on page 676*
- ◆ **Angiomax®** *see* Bivalirudin *on page 174*
- ◆ **Angiotensin Agents Comparison** *see page 1473*
- ◆ **Animal and Human Bites Guidelines** *see page 1584*
- ◆ **Anodynos-DHC®** *see* Hydrocodone and Acetaminophen *on page 676*
- ◆ **Anoquan®** *see* Butalbital Compound *on page 197*
- ◆ **Ansaid® (Can)** *see* Flurbiprofen *on page 585*
- ◆ **Ansaid® Oral** *see* Flurbiprofen *on page 585*
- ◆ **Ansamycin** *see* Rifabutin *on page 1192*
- ◆ **Antabuse®** *see* Disulfiram *on page 426*
- ◆ **Antacid Drug Interactions** *see page 1477*
- ◆ **Antagon®** *see* Ganirelix *on page 620*
- ◆ **Antazoline and Naphazoline** *see* Naphazoline and Antazoline *on page 958*
- ◆ **Anthra-Derm®** *see* Anthralin *on page 100*
- ◆ **Anthraforte® (Can)** *see* Anthralin *on page 100*

Anthralin *(AN thra lin)*

U.S. Brand Names Anthra-Derm®; Drithocreme®; Drithocreme® HP 1%; Dritho-Scalp®; Micanol®

Canadian Brand Names Anthraforte®; Anthranol®; Anthrascalp®; Micanol®

Synonyms Dithranol

Therapeutic Category Antipsoriatic Agent, Topical; Keratolytic Agent

Use Treatment of psoriasis (quiescent or chronic psoriasis)

Pregnancy Risk Factor C

Usual Dosage Adults: Topical: Generally, apply once a day or as directed. The irritant potential of anthralin is directly related to the strength being used and each patient's individual tolerance. Always commence treatment for at least one week using the lowest strength possible.

Skin application: Apply sparingly only to psoriatic lesions and rub gently and carefully into the skin until absorbed. Avoid applying an excessive quantity which may cause unnecessary soiling and staining of the clothing or bed linen.

Scalp application: Comb hair to remove scalar debris and, after suitably parting, rub cream well into the lesions, taking care to prevent the cream from spreading onto the forehead

Remove by washing or showering; optimal period of contact will vary according to the strength used and the patient's response to treatment. Continue treatment until the skin is entirely clear (ie, when there is nothing to feel with the fingers and the texture is normal)

Additional Information Complete prescribing information for this medication should be consulted for additional detail.

Dosage Forms

Cream: 0.1% (50 g); 0.25% (50 g); 0.5% (50 g); 1% (50 g)

Ointment, topical: 0.1% (42.5 g); 0.25% (42.5 g); 0.5% (42.5 g); 1% (42.5 g)

♦ **Anthranol® (Can)** *see* Anthralin *on page 100*

♦ **Anthrascalp® (Can)** *see* Anthralin *on page 100*

Anthrax Vaccine Adsorbed *Not Commercially Available*

(AN thraks vak SEEN ad SORBED)

U.S. Brand Names BioThrax™

Synonyms AVA

Therapeutic Category Vaccine

Use Immunization against *Bacillus anthracis*. Recommended for individuals who may come in contact with animal products which come from anthrax endemic areas and may be contaminated with *Bacillus anthracis* spores; recommended for high-risk persons such as veterinarians and other handling potentially infected animals. Routine immunization for the general population is not recommended.

The Department of Defense is implementing an anthrax vaccination program against the biological warfare agent anthrax, which will be administered to all active duty and reserve personnel.

Unlabeled/Investigational Use Postexposure prophylaxis in combination with antibiotics

Restrictions Presently, all anthrax vaccine lots are owned by the U.S. Department of Defense. The Centers for Disease Control (CDC) does not currently recommend routine vaccination of the general public.

Pregnancy Risk Factor D

Pregnancy/Breast-Feeding Implications Reproduction studies have not been conducted. Use during pregnancy only if clearly needed. Unpublished data from the Department of Defense suggest the vaccine may be linked with an increased number of birth defects when given during pregnancy. Excretion in breast milk is unknown; use caution in breast-feeding women.

Contraindications Hypersensitivity to anthrax vaccine or any component of the formulation; severe anaphylactic reaction to a previous dose of anthrax vaccine; history of anthrax; history of Guillain-Barré syndrome

Warnings/Precautions Immediate treatment for anaphylactic/anaphylactoid reaction should be available during vaccine use. Patients with a history of Guillain-Barré syndrome should not be given the vaccine unless there is a clear benefit that outweighs the potential risk of recurrence. Defer dosing during acute respiratory disease or other active infection; defer dosing during short-term corticosteroid therapy, chemotherapy or radiation; additional dose required in patients on long-term corticosteroid therapy; discontinue immunization in patients with chills or fever associated with administration; use caution with latex allergy; immune response may be decreased with immunodeficiency; safety and efficacy in children <18 years of age or adults >65 years of age have not been established

Adverse Reactions (Includes pre- and post-licensure data; systemic reactions reported more often in women than in men)

>10%:

Central nervous system: Malaise (4% to 11%)

Local: Tenderness (58% to 71%), erythema (12% to 43%), subcutaneous nodule (4% to 39%), induration (8% to 21%), warmth (11% to 19%), local pruritus (7% to 19%)

Neuromuscular & skeletal: Arm motion limitation (7% to 12%)

1% to 10%:

Central nervous system: Headache (4% to 7%), fever (<1% to 7%)

Gastrointestinal: Anorexia (4%), vomiting (4%), nausea (<1% to 4%)

Local: Mild local reactions (edema/induration <30mm) (9%), edema (8%)

Neuromuscular & skeletal: Myalgia (4% to 7%)

Respiratory: Respiratory difficulty (4%)

<1% (Limited to important or life-threatening): Anaphylaxis, arthralgia, cardiomyopathy, cellulitis, chills, body aches, delayed hypersensitivity reaction (started approximately day 17), dizziness, encephalitis, facial palsy, fatigue, Guillain-Barré syndrome, idiopathic thrombocytopenia purpura, inflammatory arthritis, injection site pain/tenderness, moderate local reactions (edema/induration >30 mm and <120 mm), peripheral swelling, seizure, severe local reactions (edema/induration >120 mm in diameter or accompanied by marked limitation of arm motion or marked axillary node tenderness), sudden cardiac arrest, systemic lupus erythematosus

Drug Interactions

Decreased Effect: Effect of vaccine may be decreased with chemotherapy, corticosteroids (high doses, ≥14 days), immunosuppressant agents and radiation therapy; consider waiting at least 3 months between discontinuing therapy and administering vaccine.

Stability Store under refrigeration at 2°C to 8°C (36°F to 46°F); do not freeze

(Continued)

Anthrax Vaccine Adsorbed *Not Commercially Available* (Continued)

Mechanism of Action Active immunization against *Bacillus anthracis*. The vaccine is prepared from a cell-free filtrate of *B. anthracis*, but no dead or live bacteria.

Pharmacodynamics/Kinetics Duration: Unknown; may be 1-2 years following two inoculations based on animal data

Usual Dosage S.C.:

Children <18 years: Safety and efficacy have not been established

Children ≥18 years and Adults:

Primary immunization: Three injections of 0.5 mL each given 2 weeks apart, followed by three additional injections given at 6-, 12-, and 18 months; it is not necessary to restart the series if a dose is not given on time; resume as soon as practical

Subsequent booster injections: 0.5 mL at 1-year intervals are recommended for immunity to be maintained

Elderly: Safety and efficacy have not been established for patients >65 years of age

Administration Administer S.C.; shake well before use. Do not use if discolored or contains particulate matter. Do not use the same site for more than one injection. Do not mix with other injections. After administration, massage injection site to disperse the vaccine. Federal law requires that the date of administration, the vaccine manufacturer, lot number of vaccine, and the administering person's name, title and address be entered into the patient's permanent medical record.

Monitoring Parameters Monitor for local reactions, chills, fever, anaphylaxis

Patient Information The anthrax vaccine is used to protect against anthrax disease. Anthrax disease can be a skin disease, caused by contact with infected animals or animal products. It can also be caused by inhalation of anthrax spores. Immunization using the vaccine consists of a series of 6 injections. The vaccine should be used by people who may be exposed to the anthrax bacteria, such as laboratory workers, veterinarians, and military personnel. You should not use the vaccine if you have already had anthrax disease. Most people receiving the vaccine will experience soreness, redness, or itching at the injection site, which should clear up within 48 hours. Contact your prescriber immediately if you experience a fever, difficulty breathing, hoarseness, wheezing, fast heart beat, hives, dizziness, paleness, or swelling of the throat. Consult with your prescriber if you are pregnant or breast-feeding.

Nursing Implications Epinephrine 1:1000 should be available in case of anaphylactic reaction. Do not use the same site for more than one injection.

Additional Information Local reactions increase in severity by the fifth dose. Moderate local reactions (>5 cm) may be pruritic and may occur if given to a patient with a previous history of anthrax infection. Federal law requires that the date of administration, the vaccine manufacturer, lot number of vaccine, and the administering person's name, title and address be entered into the patient's permanent medical record.

Dosage Forms Injection, suspension: 5 mL [vial stopper contains dry natural rubber]

♦ **Antiarrhythmic Drugs Comparison** *see page 1478*

♦ **AntibiOtic® Otic** *see Neomycin, Polymyxin B, and Hydrocortisone on page 969*

♦ **Antibiotic Treatment of Adults With Infective Endocarditis** *see page 1585*

♦ **Anticonvulsants by Seizure Type** *see page 1481*

♦ **Antidepressant Agents Comparison** *see page 1482*

♦ **Antidigoxin Fab Fragments, Ovine** *see Digoxin Immune Fab on page 405*

♦ **Antidiuretic Hormone** *see Vasopressin on page 1408*

♦ **Antifungal Agents Comparison** *see page 1484*

Antihemophilic Factor (Human) (an tee hee moe FIL ik FAK tor HYU man)

U.S. Brand Names Alphanate®; Hemofil® M; Humate-P®; Koāte®-DVI; Monarc® M; Monoclate-P®

Canadian Brand Names Hemofil® M; Humate-P®

Synonyms AHF (Human); Factor VIII (Human)

Therapeutic Category Antihemophilic Agent; Blood Product Derivative

Use Management of hemophilia A for patients in whom a deficiency in factor VIII has been demonstrated; can be of significant therapeutic value in patients with acquired factor VIII inhibitors not exceeding 10 Bethesda units/mL

Humate-P®: In addition, indicated as treatment of spontaneous bleeding in patients with severe von Willebrand disease and in mild and moderate von Willebrand disease where desmopressin is known or suspected to be inadequate

Orphan status: Alphanate®: Management of von Willebrand disease

Pregnancy Risk Factor C

Pregnancy/Breast-Feeding Implications Safety and efficacy in pregnant women have not been established. Use during pregnancy only if clearly needed. Parvovirus B19, which may be present in the solution, may seriously affect a pregnant woman.

Contraindications Hypersensitivity to any component of the formulation or to mouse protein (Monoclate-P®, Hemofil® M)

Warnings/Precautions Risk of viral transmission is not totally eradicated. Because antihemophilic factor is prepared from pooled plasma, it may contain the causative agent of viral hepatitis and other viral diseases. Hepatitis B vaccination is recommended for all patients. Hepatitis A vaccination is also recommended for seronegative patients. Antihemophilic factor contains trace amounts of blood groups A and B isohemagglutinins and when large or frequently repeated doses are given to individuals with blood groups A, B, and AB, the patient should be monitored for signs of progressive anemia and the possibility of intravascular hemolysis should be considered. Natural rubber latex is a component of Hemofil® M packaging. Products vary by preparation method; final formulations contain human albumin.

Adverse Reactions <1% (Limited to important or life-threatening): Acute hemolytic anemia, allergic reactions (rare), anaphylaxis (rare), anemia, blurred vision, chest tightness, chills, edema, fever, headache, hyperfibrinogenemia, increased bleeding tendency, itching, jittery feeling, lethargy, nausea, paresthesias, pruritus, somnolence, stinging at the infusion site, stomach discomfort, tachycardia, tingling, vasomotor reactions with rapid infusion, vomiting

Overdosage/Toxicology Massive doses have been reported to cause acute hemolytic anemia, increased bleeding tendency, or hyperfibrinogenemia. Occurrence is rare.

Stability Store under refrigeration, 2°C to 8°C (36°F to 46°F); avoid freezing. Use within 3 hours of reconstitution; gently agitate or rotate vial after adding diluent, do not shake vigorously. Do not refrigerate after reconstitution, precipitation may occur.

Alphanate®: May be stored at room temperature for ≤2 months

Hemofil® M: May be stored at room temperature for ≤12 months

Humate-P®, Koāte®-DVI; Monoclate-P®: May also be stored at room temperature for ≤6 months

If refrigerated, the dried concentrate and diluent should be warmed to room temperature before reconstitution.

Mechanism of Action Protein (factor VIII) in normal plasma which is necessary for clot formation and maintenance of hemostasis; activates factor X in conjunction with activated factor IX; activated factor X converts prothrombin to thrombin, which converts fibrinogen to fibrin, and with factor XIII forms a stable clot

Pharmacodynamics/Kinetics Half-life elimination: Mean: 12-17 hours with hemophilia A; consult specific product labeling

Usual Dosage Children and Adults: I.V.: Individualize dosage based on coagulation studies performed prior to treatment and at regular intervals during treatment; 1 AHF unit is the activity present in 1 mL of normal pooled human plasma; dosage should be adjusted to actual vial size currently stocked in the pharmacy. (General guidelines presented; consult individual product labeling for specific dosing recommendations.)

Dosage based on desired factor VIII increase (%):
To calculate dosage needed based on desired factor VIII increase (%):
Body weight (kg) x 0.5 int. units/kg x desired factor VIII increase (%) = int. units factor VIII required
For example:
50 kg x 0.5 int. units/kg x 30 (% increase) = 750 int. units factor VIII

Dosage based on expected factor VIII increase (%):
It is also possible to calculate the **expected** % factor VIII increase:
(# int. units administered x 2%/int. units/kg) divided by body weight (kg) = expected % factor VIII increase
For example:
(1400 int. units x 2%/int. units/kg) divided by 70 kg = 40%

General guidelines:
Minor Hemorrhage: Required peak postinfusion AHF level: 20% to 40% (10-20 int. units/kg), repeat dose every 12-24 hours for 1-3 days until bleeding is resolved or healing achieved; mild superficial or early hemorrhages may respond to a single dose

Moderate hemorrhage: Required peak postinfusion AHF level: 30% to 60% (15-30 int. units/kg): Infuse every 12-24 hours for ≥3 days until pain and disability are resolved
Alternatively, a loading dose to achieve 50% (25 int. units/kg) may be given, followed by 10-15 int. units/kg dose given every 8-12 hours; may be needed for >7 days

Severe/life-threatening hemorrhage: Required peak postinfusion AHF level: 60% to 100% (30-50 int. units/kg): Infuse every 8-24 hours until threat is resolved
Alternatively, a loading dose to achieve 80% to 100% (40-50 int. units/kg) may be given, followed by 20-25 int. units/kg dose given every 8-12 hours for ≥14 days

Minor surgery: Required peak postinfusion AHF level: 30% to 80% (15-40 int. units/kg): Highly dependent upon procedure and specific product recommendations; for some procedures, may be administered as a single infusion plus oral antifibrinolytic therapy within 1 hour; in other procedures, may repeat dose every 12-24 hours as needed

Major surgery: Required peak pre- and postsurgery AHF level: 80% to 100% (40-50 int. units/kg): Administer every 6-24 hours until healing is complete (10-14 days)

Prophylaxis: May also be given on a regular schedule to prevent bleeding

If bleeding is not controlled with adequate dose, test for presence of inhibitor. It may not be possible or practical to control bleeding if inhibitor titers >10 Bethesda units/mL; antihemophilic factor (porcine) may be considered as an alternative

von Willebrand disease:
Treatment of hemorrhage in von Willebrand disease (Humate-P®): 1 int. units of factor VIII per kg of body weight would be expected to raise circulating vWR:RCof approximately 3.5-4 int. units/dL

Type 1, mild (if desmopressin is not appropriate): Major hemorrhage:
Loading dose: 40-60 int. units/kg
Maintenance dose: 40-50 int. units/kg every 8-12 hours for 3 days, keeping vWF:RCof nadir >50%; follow with 40-50 int. units/kg daily for up to 7 days

Type 1, moderate or severe:
Minor hemorrhage: 40-50 int. units/kg for 1-2 doses
Major hemorrhage:
Loading dose: 50-75 int. units/kg
Maintenance dose: 40-60 int. units/kg daily for up to 7 days

Types 2 and 3:
Minor hemorrhage: 40-50 int. units/kg for 1-2 doses
Major hemorrhage:
Loading dose: 60-80 int. units/kg
Maintenance dose: 40-60 int. units/kg every 8-12 hours for 3 days, keeping vWF:RCof nadir >50%; follow with 40-60 int. units/kg daily for up to 7 days

Elderly: Response in the elderly is not expected to differ from that of younger patients; dosage should be individualized

Administration Total dose may be administered over 5-10 minutes (maximum: 10 mL/minute); infuse Monoclate-P® at 2 mL/minute; adapt based on patient response

Monitoring Parameters Heart rate and blood pressure (before and during I.V. administration); AHF levels prior to and during treatment; in patients with circulating inhibitors, the
(Continued)

Antihemophilic Factor (Human) *(Continued)*

inhibitor level should be monitored; hematocrit; monitor for signs and symptoms of intravascular hemolysis; bleeding

Reference Range Average normal antihemophilic factor plasma activity ranges: 50% to 150%
Level to prevent spontaneous hemorrhage: 5%
Required peak postinfusion AHF activity in blood (as % of normal or units/dL plasma):
Early hemarthrosis, muscle bleed, or oral bleed: 20% to 40%
More extensive hemarthrosis, muscle bleed, or hematoma: 30% to 60%
Life-threatening bleeds (such as head injury, throat bleed, severe abdominal pain): 80% to 100%
Minor surgery, including tooth extraction: 60% to 80%
Major surgery: 80% to 100% (pre- and postoperative)

Patient Information This medication can only be given intravenously. Report sudden-onset headache, rash, chest or back pain, wheezing, or respiratory difficulties, hives, itching, low grade fever, nausea, vomiting, tiredness, decreased appetite to prescriber. Wear identification indicating that you have a hemophilic condition.

Nursing Implications Reduce rate of administration, or temporarily discontinue, if patient experiences any adverse reactions; possibility of hypersensitivity reactions (hives, chest tightness, itching, wheezing, hypotension)

Dosage Forms Injection, human [single-dose vial]: Labeling on cartons and vials indicates number of int. units

Antihemophilic Factor (Porcine) (an tee hee moe FIL ik FAK ter POR seen)

U.S. Brand Names Hyate:C®

Synonyms AHF (Porcine); Factor VIII (Porcine)

Therapeutic Category Antihemophilic Agent; Blood Product Derivative

Use Management of hemophilia A in patients with antibodies to human factor VIII (consider use of human factor VIII in patients with antibody titer of <5 Bethesda units/mL); management of previously nonhemophilic patients with spontaneously-acquired inhibitors to human factor VIII, regardless of initial antihuman inhibitor titer

Pregnancy Risk Factor C

Pregnancy/Breast-Feeding Implications Safety and efficacy in pregnant women have not been established. Use during pregnancy only if clearly needed.

Contraindications Hypersensitivity to porcine or any component of the formulation

Warnings/Precautions Rarely administration has been associated with anaphylaxis; epinephrine, hydrocortisone, and facilities for cardiopulmonary resuscitation should be available in case such a reaction occurs; infusion may be followed by a rise in plasma levels of antibody to both human and porcine factor VIII; inhibitor levels should be monitored both pre- and post-treatment

Adverse Reactions Reactions tend to lessen in frequency and severity as further infusions are given; hydrocortisone and/or antihistamines may help to prevent or alleviate side effects and may be prescribed as precautionary measures

1% to 10%:
Central nervous system: Fever, headache, chills
Dermatologic: Rashes
Gastrointestinal: Nausea, vomiting
<1% (Limited to important or life-threatening): Anaphylaxis, thrombocytopenia

Overdosage/Toxicology Massive doses of antihemophilic factor (human) have been reported to cause acute hemolytic anemia, increased bleeding tendency, or hyperfibrinogenemia. Occurrence is rare.

Stability Store at -15°C to -20°C (5°F to -4°F); warm to 20°C to 37°C (68°F to 98.6°F) prior to reconstitution; use within 3 hours of mixing

Mechanism of Action Factor VIII is the coagulation portion of the factor VIII complex in plasma. Factor VIII acts as a cofactor for factor IX to activate factor X in the intrinsic pathway of blood coagulation.

Pharmacodynamics/Kinetics Half-life elimination: 10-11 hours (patients without detectable inhibitors)

Usual Dosage Clinical response should be used to assess efficacy

Initial dose:
Antibody level to human factor VIII <50 Bethesda units/mL: 100-150 porcine units/kg (body weight) is recommended
Antibody level to human factor VIII >50 Bethesda units/mL: Activity of the antibody to antihemophilic (porcine) should be determined; **an antiporcine antibody level** >20 Bethesda units/mL indicates that the patient is unlikely to benefit from treatment; for lower titers, a dose of 100-150 porcine units/kg is recommended
The initial dose may also be calculated using the following method:
1. Determine patient's antibody titer against porcine factor VIII
2. Calculate average plasma volume:
(body weight kg) (average blood volume) (1 - hematocrit) = plasma volume
(body weight kg) (80 mL/kg) (1 - hematocrit) = plasma volume
Note: A hematocrit of 50% = 0.5 for the equation
3. Neutralizing dose:
(plasma volume mL) (antibody titer Bethesda units/mL) = neutralizing dose units
This is the predicted dose required to neutralize the circulating antibodies. An incremental dose must be added to the neutralizing dose in order to increase the plasma factor VIII to the desired level.
4. Incremental dose:
(desired plasma factor VIII level) (body weight) divided by 1.5 = incremental dose units
5. Total dose = neutralizing dose + incremental dose = total dose units
If a patient has previously been treated with Hyate:C®, this may provide a guide to his likely response and, therefore, assist in estimation of the preliminary dose

Subsequent doses: Following administration of the initial dose, if the recovery of factor VIII in the patient's plasma is not sufficient, another larger dose should be administered; if recovery after the second dose is still insufficient, a third and larger dose may prove effective. Once appropriate factor VIII levels are achieved, dosing can be repeated every 6-8 hours.

Administration Administer by I.V. route only; infuse slowly, 2-5 mL/minute

Monitoring Parameters Factor VIII levels pre- and postinfusion; inhibitor levels to human and/or porcine factor VIII pre- and postinfusion; heart rate and blood pressure (before and during I.V. administration); bleeding

Antibody levels to human factor VIII >50 Bethesda units/mL: Activity of the antibody to antihemophilic factor (porcine) should be determined

Antiporcine antibody level >20 Bethesda units/mL: Patient may not benefit from treatment

Reference Range

Average normal antihemophilic factor plasma activity range: 50% to 150%

Level to prevent spontaneous hemorrhage: 5%

Patient Information This medication can only be given intravenously. Report sudden-onset headache, rash, chest or back pain, or respiratory difficulties to prescriber. Wear identification indicating that you have a hemophilic condition.

Nursing Implications The assayed amount of activity is stated on the label, but may vary depending on the type of assay and hemophilic substrate plasma used. Product must be used within 3 hours of reconstitution. Infuse slowly; infusion rate should be 2-5 mL/minute. Hydrocortisone and/or antihistamines may help to prevent or alleviate side effects, and may be prescribed as precautionary measures. Monitor factor VIII levels pre- and postinfusion.

Additional Information Sodium ion concentration is not more than 200 mmol/L. The assayed amount of activity is stated on the label, but may vary depending on the type of assay and hemophilic substrate plasma used.

Dosage Forms Powder for injection, lyophilized: 400-700 porcine units to be reconstituted with 20 mL SWFI

Antihemophilic Factor (Recombinant)
(an tee hee moe FIL ik FAK tor ree KOM be nant)

U.S. Brand Names Helixate® FS; Kogenate® FS; Recombinate™; ReFacto®

Canadian Brand Names Kogenate®; Recombinate™

Synonyms AHF (Recombinant); Factor VIII (Recombinant); rAHF

Therapeutic Category Antihemophilic Agent

Use Management of hemophilia A for patients in whom a deficiency in factor VIII has been demonstrated; can be of significant therapeutic value in patients with acquired factor VIII inhibitors not exceeding 10 Bethesda units/mL

Orphan drug: ReFacto®: Control and prevention of hemorrhagic episodes; surgical prophylaxis for hemophilia A (congenital factor VIII deficiency or classic hemophilia)

Pregnancy Risk Factor C

Pregnancy/Breast-Feeding Implications Safety and efficacy in pregnant women has not been established. Use during pregnancy only if clearly needed.

Contraindications Hypersensitivity to mouse or hamster protein (Helixate® FS, Kogenate® FS); hypersensitivity to mouse, hamster, or bovine protein (Recombinate™, ReFacto®); hypersensitivity to any component of the formulation

Warnings/Precautions Monitor for signs of formation of antibodies to factor VIII; may occur at anytime but more common in young children with severe hemophilia. Monitor for allergic hypersensitivity reactions. Products vary by preparation method. Recombinate™ is stabilized using human albumin. Helixate® FS and Kogenate® FS are stabilized with sucrose.

Adverse Reactions <1% (Limited to important or life-threatening): Allergic reactions, anaphylaxis, angina pectoris, depersonalization, dyspnea, epistaxis, fever, headache, injection site reactions (burning, pruritus, erythema), nausea, rash, somnolence, urticaria, vasodilation, venous catheter access complications, vomiting

Overdosage/Toxicology Massive doses of antihemophilic factor (human) have been reported to cause acute hemolytic anemia, increased bleeding tendency, or hyperfibrinogenemia. Occurrence is rare.

Stability Store under refrigeration, 2°C to 8°C (36°F to 46°F); avoid freezing. Use within 3 hours of reconstitution; gently agitate or rotate vial after adding diluent, do not shake vigorously. Do not refrigerate after reconstitution, a precipitation may occur.

Kogenate® FS: Avoid prolonged exposure to light during storage.

Recombinate™, ReFacto®: May also be stored at room temperature for up to 3 months; avoid prolonged exposure to light during storage

If refrigerated, the dried concentrate and diluent should be warmed to room temperature before reconstitution.

Mechanism of Action Protein (factor VIII) in normal plasma which is necessary for clot formation and maintenance of hemostasis; activates factor X in conjunction with activated factor IX; activated factor X converts prothrombin to thrombin, which converts fibrinogen to fibrin, and with factor XIII forms a stable clot

Pharmacodynamics/Kinetics Half-life elimination: Mean: 14-16 hours

Usual Dosage Children and Adults: I.V.: Individualize dosage based on coagulation studies performed prior to treatment and at regular intervals during treatment; 1 AHF unit is the activity present in 1 mL of normal pooled human plasma; dosage should be adjusted to actual vial size currently stocked in the pharmacy. (General guidelines presented; consult individual product labeling for specific dosing recommendations.)

Dosage based on desired factor VIII increase (%):

To calculate dosage needed based on desired factor VIII increase (%):

Body weight (kg) x 0.5 int. units/kg x desired factor VIII increase (%) = int. units factor VIII required

For example:

50 kg x 0.5 int. units/kg x 30 (% increase) = 750 int. units factor VIII

(Continued)

Antihemophilic Factor (Recombinant) *(Continued)*

Dosage based on expected factor VIII increase (%):
It is also possible to calculate the **expected** % factor VIII increase:
(# int. units administered x 2%/int. units/kg) divided by body weight (kg) = expected % factor VIII increase
For example:
(1400 int. units x 2%/int. units/kg) divided by 70 kg = 40%

General guidelines:
Minor hemorrhage: Required peak postinfusion AHF level: 20% to 40% (10-20 int. units/kg); mild superficial or early hemorrhages may respond to a single dose; may repeat dose every 12-24 hours for 1-3 days until bleeding is resolved or healing achieved
Moderate hemorrhage/minor surgery: Required peak postinfusion AHF level: 30% to 60% (15-30 int. units/kg); repeat dose at 12-24 hours if needed; some products suggest continuing for ≥3 days until pain and disability are resolved
Severe/life-threatening hemorrhage: Required peak postinfusion AHF level: Initial dose: 80% to 100% (40-50 int. units/kg); maintenance dose: 40% to 50% (20-25 int. units/kg) every 8-12 hours until threat is resolved
Major surgery: Required peak pre- and postsurgery AHF level: ~100% (50 int. units/kg) give first dose prior to surgery and repeat every 6-12 hours until healing complete (10-14 days)
Prophylaxis: May also be given on a regular schedule to prevent bleeding
If bleeding is not controlled with adequate dose, test for presence of inhibitor. It may not be possible or practical to control bleeding if inhibitor titers >10 Bethesda units/mL; antihemophilic factor (porcine) may be considered as an alternative

Elderly: Response in the elderly is not expected to differ from that of younger patients; dosage should be individualized
Administration Total dose may be administered over 5-10 minutes (maximum: 10 mL/minute); adapt based on patient response
Monitoring Parameters Heart rate and blood pressure (before and during I.V. administration); AHF levels prior to and during treatment; in patients with circulating inhibitors, the inhibitor level should be monitored; bleeding
Reference Range Average normal antihemophilic factor plasma activity ranges: 50% to 150%
Level to prevent spontaneous hemorrhage: 5%
Required peak postinfusion AHF activity in blood (as % of normal or units/dL plasma):
Early hemarthrosis, muscle bleed, or oral bleed: 20% to 40%
More extensive hemarthrosis, muscle bleed, or hematoma: 30% to 60%
Life-threatening bleeds (such as head injury, throat bleed, severe abdominal pain): 80% to 100%
Minor surgery, including tooth extraction: 60% to 80%
Major surgery: 80% to 100% (pre- and postoperative)
Patient Information This medication can only be given intravenously. Report hives, itching, wheezing, sudden-onset headache, rash, chest or back pain, or other respiratory difficulties to prescriber. Wear identification indicating that you have a hemophilic condition.
Nursing Implications Reduce rate of administration, or temporarily discontinue, if patient experiences any adverse reactions; possibility of hypersensitivity reactions (hives, chest tightness, itching, wheezing, hypotension)
Dosage Forms
Powder for injection, recombinant [preservative free]:
Helixate® FS, Kogenate® FS: 250 int. units/vial, 500 int. units/vial, 1000 int. units/vial [contains sucrose 28 mg/vial]
Recombinate™: 250 int. units/vial, 500 int. units/vial, 1000 int. units/vial [contains human albumin 12.5 mg/mL]
ReFacto®: 250 int. units/vial, 500 units/vial, 1000 int. units/vial

♦ **Antihist-1® [OTC]** *see Clemastine on page 308*

Anti-inhibitor Coagulant Complex
(an tee-in HI bi tor coe AG yoo lant KOM pleks)
U.S. Brand Names Autoplex® T; Feiba VH Immuno®
Canadian Brand Names Feiba® VH Immuno
Synonyms Coagulant Complex Inhibitor
Therapeutic Category Antihemophilic Agent; Blood Product Derivative
Use Patients with factor VIII inhibitors who are to undergo surgery or those who are bleeding
Pregnancy Risk Factor C
Contraindications Disseminated intravascular coagulation; patients with normal coagulation mechanism
Warnings/Precautions Products are prepared from pooled human plasma; such plasma may contain the causative agents of viral diseases. Tests used to control efficacy such as APTT, WBCT, and TEG do not correlate with clinical efficacy. Dosing to normalize these values may result in DIC. Identification of the clotting deficiency as caused by factor VIII inhibitors is essential prior to starting therapy. Use with extreme caution in patients with impaired hepatic function.
Adverse Reactions <1% (Limited to important or life-threatening): Chills, disseminated intravascular coagulation, fever, headache, hypotension, rash, urticaria
Overdosage/Toxicology Rapid infusion may cause hypotension. Excessive administration can cause DIC.
Stability Store at 2°C to 8°C (36°F to 46°F); use within 1-3 hours after reconstitution
Usual Dosage Dosage range: 25-100 factor VIII correctional units per kg depending on the severity of hemorrhage
Test Interactions ↑ ↓ PT, ↑ ↓ PTT, ↓ WBCT, ↓ fibrin, ↓ platelets, ↑ fibrin split products
Nursing Implications Monitor for hypotension, may reinitiate infusion at a slower rate; have epinephrine ready to treat hypersensitivity reactions

Dosage Forms
Injection:
Autoplex® T: Each bottle is labeled with correctional units of factor VIII [with heparin 2 units]
Feiba VH Immuno®: Each bottle is labeled with correctional units of factor VIII [heparin free]

♦ **Antilirium®** *see* Physostigmine *on page 1081*
♦ **Antimicrobial Drugs of Choice** *see page 1588*
♦ **Antimigraine Drugs Comparison** *see page 1485*
♦ **Antiminth® [OTC]** *see* Pyrantel Pamoate *on page 1159*
♦ **Antipsychotic Agents Comparison** *see page 1486*

Antipyrine and Benzocaine (an tee PYE reen & BEN zoe kane)
U.S. Brand Names Allergen®; Auralgan®; Auroto®
Canadian Brand Names Auralgan®
Synonyms Benzocaine and Antipyrine
Therapeutic Category Otic Agent, Analgesic; Otic Agent, Cerumenolytic
Use Temporary relief of pain and reduction of swelling associated with acute congestive and serous otitis media, swimmer's ear, otitis externa; facilitates ear wax removal
Pregnancy Risk Factor C
Usual Dosage Otic: Fill ear canal; moisten cotton pledget, place in external ear, repeat every 1-2 hours until pain and congestion is relieved; for ear wax removal instill drops 3-4 times/day for 2-3 days
Additional Information Complete prescribing information for this medication should be consulted for additional detail.
Dosage Forms
Solution, otic: Antipyrine 5.4% and benzocaine 1.4% (10 mL, 15 mL)
Allergen®, Auroto®: Antipyrine 5.4% and benzocaine 1.4% (15 mL)
Auralgan®: Antipyrine 5.4% and benzocaine 1.4% (10 mL)

♦ **Antiretroviral Agents Comparison** *see page 1488*
♦ **Antiretroviral Therapy for HIV Infection** *see page 1595*
♦ **Antispas®** *see* Dicyclomine *on page 397*

Antithrombin III (an tee THROM bin three)
U.S. Brand Names Thrombate III™
Canadian Brand Names Thrombate III®
Synonyms AT III; Heparin Cofactor I
Therapeutic Category Blood Product Derivative
Use Agent for hereditary antithrombin III deficiency; has been used effectively for acquired antithrombin III deficiencies related to disseminated intravascular coagulation (DIC); may be useful during acute management of hepatic veno-occlusive disease
Orphan drug:
ATnativ®: Treatment of hereditary antithrombin III deficiency in connection with surgical or obstetrical procedures; treatment of thromboembolism
Thrombate III™: Replacement therapy in congenital deficiency of antithrombin III for prevention and treatment of thrombosis and pulmonary emboli
Pregnancy Risk Factor C
Contraindications Hypersensitivity to antithrombin III or any component of the formulation
Warnings/Precautions Test methods and treatment methods may not totally eradicate HBAg and HIV from pooled plasma used in processing of this product
Adverse Reactions
1% to 10%: Central nervous system: Dizziness (2%)
<1% (Limited to important or life-threatening): Abdominal cramps, bowel fullness, chest pain, chest tightness, cramps, diuretic effects, dyspnea, edema, fever, film over eye, fluid overload, foul taste in mouth, hematoma formation, hives, lightheadedness, nausea, thrombocytopenia, urticaria, vasodilatory effects
Overdosage/Toxicology Levels of 150% to 200% have been documented in patients with no signs or symptoms of complications.
Drug Interactions
Increased Effect/Toxicity: Heparin's anticoagulant effects are potentiated by antithrombin III. Risk of hemorrhage with antithrombin III may be increased by thrombolytic agents, oral anticoagulants (warfarin), and drugs which affect platelet function (eg, aspirin, NSAIDs, dipyridamole, ticlopidine, clopidogrel, and IIb/IIIa antagonists).
Stability Store under refrigeration at 2°C to 8°C (36°F to 46°F); reconstitute with diluent (SWFI) provided (10 mL/500 int. units, 20 mL/1000 int. units); bring to room temperature prior to administration; **do not shake**; use within 3 hours of reconstitution
Mechanism of Action Antithrombin III is the primary physiologic inhibitor of *in vivo* coagulation. It is an alpha₂-globulin. Its principal actions are the inactivation of thrombin, plasmin, and other active serine proteases of coagulation, including factors IXa, Xa, XIa, XIIa, and VIIa. The inactivation of proteases is a major step in the normal clotting process. The strong activation of clotting enzymes at the site of every bleeding injury facilitates fibrin formation and maintains normal hemostasis. Thrombosis in the circulation would be caused by active serine proteases if they were not inhibited by antithrombin III after the localized clotting process. Patients with congenital deficiency are in a prethrombotic state, even if asymptomatic, as evidenced by elevated plasma levels of prothrombin activation fragment, which are normalized following infusions of antithrombin III concentrate.
Usual Dosage Adults: After first dose of antithrombin III, level should increase to 120% of normal; thereafter maintain at levels >80%. Generally, achieved by administration of maintenance doses once every 24 hours. Initially and until patient is stabilized, measure antithrombin III level at least twice daily, thereafter once daily and always immediately before next infusion. 1 unit = quantity of antithrombin III in 1 mL of normal pooled human plasma; administration of 1 unit/1 kg raises AT-III level by 1% to 2%; assume plasma volume of 40 mL/kg.
(Continued)

Antithrombin III *(Continued)*

Initial dosage (units) = [desired AT-III level % - baseline AT-III level %] x body weight (kg) divided by 1%/units/kg (eg, if a 70 kg adult patient had a baseline AT-III level of 57%, the initial dose would be (120% - 57%) x 70/1%/units/kg = 4410 units).

Measure antithrombin III preceding and 30 minutes after dose to calculate *in vivo* recovery rate; maintain level within normal range for 2-8 days depending on type of surgery or procedure.

Administration Infuse over 5-10 minutes; rate of infusion is 50 units/minute (1 mL/minute) not to exceed 100 units/minute (2 mL/minute)

Monitoring Parameters Monitor antithrombin III levels during treatment period

Reference Range Maintain antithrombin III level in plasma >80%

Nursing Implications Infuse over 5-10 minutes; rate of infusion: 50 units/minute (1 mL/minute) not to exceed 100 units/minute (2 mL/minute)

Dosage Forms Injection, powder for reconstitution [with diluent]: 500 int. units, 1000 int. units

♦ **Antithymocyte Globulin (Equine)** *see Lymphocyte Immune Globulin on page 829*

Antithymocyte Globulin (Rabbit) *(an te THY moe site GLOB yu lin (RAB bit)*

U.S. Brand Names Thymoglobulin®

Synonyms Antithymocyte Immunoglobulin; ATG

Therapeutic Category Immunosuppressant Agent

Use Treatment of renal transplant acute rejection in conjunction with concomitant immunosuppression

Contraindications Patients with history of allergy or anaphylaxis to rabbit proteins, or who have an acute viral illness

Warnings/Precautions Infusion may produce fever and chills. To minimize, the first dose should be infused over a minimum of 6 hours into a high-flow vein. Also, premedication with corticosteroids, acetaminophen, and/or an antihistamine and/or slowing the infusion rate may reduce reaction incidence and intensity.

Prolonged use or overdosage of Thymoglobulin® in association with other immunosuppressive agents may cause over-immunosuppression resulting in severe infections and may increase the incidence of lymphoma or post-transplant lymphoproliferative disease (PTLD) or other malignancies. Appropriate antiviral, antibacterial, antiprotozoal, and/or antifungal prophylaxis is recommended.

Thymoglobulin® should only be used by physicians experienced in immunosuppressive therapy for the treatment of renal transplant patients. Medical surveillance is required during the infusion. In rare circumstances, anaphylaxis has been reported with use. In such cases, the infusion should be terminated immediately. Medical personnel should be available to treat patients who experience anaphylaxis. Emergency treatment such as 0.3-0.5 mL aqueous epinephrine (1:1000 dilution) subcutaneously and other resuscitative measures including oxygen, intravenous fluids, antihistamines, corticosteroids, pressor amines, and airway management, as clinically indicated, should be provided. Thymoglobulin® or other rabbit immunoglobulins should not be administered again for such patients. Thrombocytopenia or neutropenia may result from cross-reactive antibodies and is reversible following dose adjustments.

Adverse Reactions

>10%:

Central nervous system: Fever, chills, headache

Dermatologic: Rash

Endocrine & metabolic: Hyperkalemia

Gastrointestinal: Abdominal pain, diarrhea

Hematologic: Leukopenia, thrombocytopenia

Neuromuscular & skeletal: Weakness

Respiratory: Dyspnea

Miscellaneous: Systemic infection, pain

1% to 10%:

Gastrointestinal: Gastritis

Respiratory: Pneumonia

Miscellaneous: Sensitivity reactions: Anaphylaxis may be indicated by hypotension, respiratory distress, serum sickness, viral infection

Stability

Store intact vials under refrigeration (2°C to 8°C/36°F to 46°F); protect from light and do not freeze

Reconstitute 25 mg vial with diluent provided by manufacturer (SWFI >5 mL). Roll vial gently to dissolve powder. Use contents of vial within 4 hours of reconstitution. Dilute dosage to a final concentration of 0.5 mg/mL in 0.9% sodium chloride injection or 5% dextrose injection. Gently invert admixture 1-2 times to mix solution. Use admixture immediately.

Mechanism of Action May involve elimination of antigen-reactive T-lymphocytes (killer cells) in peripheral blood or alteration of T-cell function

Pharmacodynamics/Kinetics Half-life elimination, plasma: 2-3 days

Usual Dosage I.V.: 1.5 mg/kg/day for 7-14 days

Administration For I.V. use only; administer via central line; use of high flow veins will minimize the occurrence of phlebitis and thrombosis; administer by slow I.V. infusion through an in-line filter with pore size of 0.2 micrometer over a minimum of 6 hours for the first infusion and over at least 4 hours on subsequent days of therapy.

Monitoring Parameters Lymphocyte profile, CBC with differential and platelet count, vital signs during administration

Nursing Implications For I.V. use only; mild itching and erythema can be treated with antihistamines; infuse first dose over at least 6 hours; any severe systemic reaction to the skin test such as generalized rash, tachycardia, dyspnea, hypotension, or anaphylaxis should preclude further therapy. **Epinephrine and resuscitative equipment should be nearby.** Patient may need to be pretreated with an antipyretic, antihistamine, and/or corticosteroid.

Dosage Forms Injection [with diluent]: 25 mg vials

- **Antithymocyte Immunoglobulin** *see* Antithymocyte Globulin (Rabbit) *on page 108*
- **Antithymocyte Immunoglobulin** *see* Lymphocyte Immune Globulin *on page 829*
- **Anti-Tuss® Expectorant [OTC]** *see* Guaifenesin *on page 645*
- **Antivert®** *see* Meclizine *on page 846*
- **Antizol®** *see* Fomepizole *on page 599*
- **Antrizine®** *see* Meclizine *on page 846*
- **Anturane®** *see* Sulfinpyrazone *on page 1276*
- **Anucort-HC® Suppository** *see* Hydrocortisone *on page 682*
- **Anusol® HC 1 [OTC]** *see* Hydrocortisone *on page 682*
- **Anusol® HC 2.5% [OTC]** *see* Hydrocortisone *on page 682*
- **Anusol-HC® Suppository** *see* Hydrocortisone *on page 682*
- **ANX®** *see* HydrOXYzine *on page 691*
- **Anzemet®** *see* Dolasetron *on page 433*
- **APAP** *see* Acetaminophen *on page 22*
- **APAP and Tramadol** *see* Acetaminophen and Tramadol *on page 26*
- **Aphedrid™ [OTC]** *see* Triprolidine and Pseudoephedrine *on page 1380*
- **Aphthasol™** *see* Amlexanox *on page 79*
- **Aplisol®** *see* Tuberculin Tests *on page 1386*
- **Aplonidine** *see* Apraclonidine *on page 111*
- **Apo-Acebutolol (Can)** *see* Acebutolol *on page 21*
- **Apo®-Acetaminophen (Can)** *see* Acetaminophen *on page 22*
- **Apo®-Acetazolamide (Can)** *see* AcetaZOLAMIDE *on page 29*
- **Apo®-Acyclovir (Can)** *see* Acyclovir *on page 34*
- **Apo®-Allopurinol (Can)** *see* Allopurinol *on page 52*
- **Apo®-Alpraz (Can)** *see* Alprazolam *on page 55*
- **Apo®-Amilzide (Can)** *see* Amiloride and Hydrochlorothiazide *on page 71*
- **Apo®-Amitriptyline (Can)** *see* Amitriptyline *on page 76*
- **Apo®-Amoxi (Can)** *see* Amoxicillin *on page 84*
- **Apo®-Ampi (Can)** *see* Ampicillin *on page 93*
- **Apo®-ASA (Can)** *see* Aspirin *on page 120*
- **Apo®-Atenol (Can)** *see* Atenolol *on page 125*
- **Apo®-Baclofen (Can)** *see* Baclofen *on page 144*
- **Apo®-Beclomethasone (Can)** *see* Beclomethasone *on page 149*
- **Apo®-Benztropine (Can)** *see* Benztropine *on page 157*
- **Apo® Bromocriptine (Can)** *see* Bromocriptine *on page 184*
- **Apo®-Buspirone (Can)** *see* BusPIRone *on page 194*
- **Apo®-C (Can)** *see* Ascorbic Acid *on page 116*
- **Apo®-Cal (Can)** *see* Calcium Carbonate *on page 207*
- **Apo®-Capto (Can)** *see* Captopril *on page 218*
- **Apo®-Carbamazepine (Can)** *see* Carbamazepine *on page 221*
- **Apo®-Cefaclor (Can)** *see* Cefaclor *on page 237*
- **Apo®-Cefadroxil (Can)** *see* Cefadroxil *on page 238*
- **Apo®-Cephalex (Can)** *see* Cephalexin *on page 261*
- **Apo®-Cetirizine (Can)** *see* Cetirizine *on page 265*
- **Apo®-Chlorax (Can)** *see* Clidinium and Chlordiazepoxide *on page 309*
- **Apo®-Chlordiazepoxide (Can)** *see* Chlordiazepoxide *on page 274*
- **Apo®-Chlorpropamide (Can)** *see* ChlorproPAMIDE *on page 284*
- **Apo®-Chlorthalidone (Can)** *see* Chlorthalidone *on page 284*
- **Apo®-Cimetidine (Can)** *see* Cimetidine *on page 293*
- **Apo®-Clomipramine (Can)** *see* ClomiPRAMINE *on page 315*
- **Apo®-Clonazepam (Can)** *see* Clonazepam *on page 316*
- **Apo®-Clonidine (Can)** *see* Clonidine *on page 318*
- **Apo®-Clorazepate (Can)** *see* Clorazepate *on page 322*
- **Apo®-Cloxi (Can)** *see* Cloxacillin *on page 324*
- **Apo®-Cromolyn (Can)** *see* Cromolyn Sodium *on page 337*
- **Apo®-Cyclobenzaprine (Can)** *see* Cyclobenzaprine *on page 340*
- **Apo®-Desipramine (Can)** *see* Desipramine *on page 376*
- **Apo®-Diazepam (Can)** *see* Diazepam *on page 390*
- **Apo®-Diclo (Can)** *see* Diclofenac *on page 393*
- **Apo®-Diclo SR (Can)** *see* Diclofenac *on page 393*
- **Apo®-Diflunisal (Can)** *see* Diflunisal *on page 401*
- **Apo®-Diltiaz (Can)** *see* Diltiazem *on page 409*
- **Apo®-Diltiaz CD (Can)** *see* Diltiazem *on page 409*
- **Apo®-Diltiaz SR (Can)** *see* Diltiazem *on page 409*
- **Apo®-Dipyridamole FC (Can)** *see* Dipyridamole *on page 422*
- **Apo®-Divalproex (Can)** *see* Valproic Acid and Derivatives *on page 1398*
- **Apo®-Doxazosin (Can)** *see* Doxazosin *on page 439*
- **Apo®-Doxepin (Can)** *see* Doxepin *on page 440*
- **Apo®-Doxy (Can)** *see* Doxycycline *on page 448*
- **Apo®-Doxy Tabs (Can)** *see* Doxycycline *on page 448*
- **Apo®-Erythro Base (Can)** *see* Erythromycin (Systemic) *on page 486*
- **Apo®-Erythro E-C (Can)** *see* Erythromycin (Systemic) *on page 486*
- **Apo®-Erythro-ES (Can)** *see* Erythromycin (Systemic) *on page 486*

- Apo®-Erythro-S (Can) *see* Erythromycin (Systemic) *on page 486*
- Apo®-Etodolac (Can) *see* Etodolac *on page 532*
- Apo®-Famotidine (Can) *see* Famotidine *on page 543*
- Apo®-Fenofibrate (Can) *see* Fenofibrate *on page 548*
- Apo®-Feno-Micro (Can) *see* Fenofibrate *on page 548*
- Apo®-Ferrous Gluconate (Can) *see* Ferrous Gluconate *on page 556*
- Apo®-Ferrous Sulfate (Can) *see* Ferrous Sulfate *on page 557*
- Apo®-Fluconazole (Can) *see* Fluconazole *on page 565*
- Apo®-Flunisolide (Can) *see* Flunisolide *on page 572*
- Apo®-Fluoxetine (Can) *see* Fluoxetine *on page 578*
- Apo®-Fluphenazine (Can) *see* Fluphenazine *on page 581*
- Apo®-Flurazepam (Can) *see* Flurazepam *on page 584*
- Apo®-Flurbiprofen (Can) *see* Flurbiprofen *on page 585*
- Apo-Flutamide (Can) *see* Flutamide *on page 586*
- Apo®-Fluvoxamine (Can) *see* Fluvoxamine *on page 593*
- Apo®-Folic (Can) *see* Folic Acid *on page 595*
- Apo®-Furosemide (Can) *see* Furosemide *on page 612*
- Apo®-Gain (Can) *see* Minoxidil *on page 919*
- Apo®-Gemfibrozil (Can) *see* Gemfibrozil *on page 624*
- Apo®-Glyburide (Can) *see* GlyBURIDE *on page 635*
- Apo®-Haloperidol (Can) *see* Haloperidol *on page 654*
- Apo®-Hydralazine (Can) *see* HydrALAZINE *on page 671*
- Apo®-Hydro (Can) *see* Hydrochlorothiazide *on page 674*
- Apo®-Hydroxyzine (Can) *see* HydrOXYzine *on page 691*
- Apo®-Ibuprofen (Can) *see* Ibuprofen *on page 697*
- Apo®-Imipramine (Can) *see* Imipramine *on page 708*
- Apo®-Indapamide (Can) *see* Indapamide *on page 715*
- Apo®-Indomethacin (Can) *see* Indomethacin *on page 717*
- Apo®-Ipravent (Can) *see* Ipratropium *on page 740*
- Apo®-ISDN (Can) *see* Isosorbide Dinitrate *on page 750*
- Apo®-K (Can) *see* Potassium Chloride *on page 1108*
- Apo®-Keto (Can) *see* Ketoprofen *on page 763*
- Apo®-Ketoconazole (Can) *see* Ketoconazole *on page 762*
- Apo®-Keto-E (Can) *see* Ketoprofen *on page 763*
- Apo®-Ketorolac (Can) *see* Ketorolac *on page 764*
- Apo®-Keto SR (Can) *see* Ketoprofen *on page 763*
- Apo®-Ketotifen (Can) *see* Ketotifen *on page 767*
- Apo®-Levocarb (Can) *see* Levodopa and Carbidopa *on page 791*
- Apo®-Lisinopril (Can) *see* Lisinopril *on page 809*
- Apo®-Loperamide (Can) *see* Loperamide *on page 816*
- Apo®-Lorazepam (Can) *see* Lorazepam *on page 821*
- Apo®-Lovastatin (Can) *see* Lovastatin *on page 825*
- Apo®-Loxapine (Can) *see* Loxapine *on page 826*
- Apo®-Mefenamic (Can) *see* Mefenamic Acid *on page 850*
- Apo®-Megestrol (Can) *see* Megestrol *on page 852*
- Apo®-Meprobamate (Can) *see* Meprobamate *on page 861*
- Apo®-Metformin (Can) *see* Metformin *on page 875*
- Apo®-Methazide (Can) *see* Methyldopa and Hydrochlorothiazide *on page 892*
- Apo®-Methyldopa (Can) *see* Methyldopa *on page 891*
- Apo®-Metoclop (Can) *see* Metoclopramide *on page 900*
- Apo®-Metoprolol (Can) *see* Metoprolol *on page 902*
- Apo®-Metronidazole (Can) *see* Metronidazole *on page 904*
- Apo®-Minocycline (Can) *see* Minocycline *on page 918*
- Apo®-Nabumetone (Can) *see* Nabumetone *on page 947*
- Apo®-Nadol (Can) *see* Nadolol *on page 948*
- Apo®-Napro-Na (Can) *see* Naproxen *on page 958*
- Apo®-Napro-Na DS (Can) *see* Naproxen *on page 958*
- Apo®-Naproxen (Can) *see* Naproxen *on page 958*
- Apo®-Naproxen SR (Can) *see* Naproxen *on page 958*
- Apo®-Nifed (Can) *see* NIFEdipine *on page 981*
- Apo®-Nifed PA (Can) *see* NIFEdipine *on page 981*
- Apo®-Nitrofurantoin (Can) *see* Nitrofurantoin *on page 987*
- Apo®-Nizatidine (Can) *see* Nizatidine *on page 992*
- Apo®-Norflox (Can) *see* Norfloxacin *on page 994*
- Apo®-Nortriptyline (Can) *see* Nortriptyline *on page 996*
- Apo®-Oflox (Can) *see* Ofloxacin *on page 1004*
- Apo®-Oxazepam (Can) *see* Oxazepam *on page 1020*
- Apo®-Pentoxifylline SR Nu-Pentoxifylline SR (Can) *see* Pentoxifylline *on page 1061*
- Apo®-Pen VK (Can) *see* Penicillin V Potassium *on page 1055*
- Apo®-Perphenazine (Can) *see* Perphenazine *on page 1066*
- Apo®-Pindol (Can) *see* Pindolol *on page 1086*
- Apo®-Piroxicam (Can) *see* Piroxicam *on page 1093*
- Apo®-Prazo (Can) *see* Prazosin *on page 1120*
- Apo®-Prednisone (Can) *see* PredniSONE *on page 1124*

- Apo®-Primidone (Can) *see* Primidone *on page 1127*
- Apo®-Procainamide (Can) *see* Procainamide *on page 1130*
- Apo®-Propranolol (Can) *see* Propranolol *on page 1149*
- Apo®-Quinidine (Can) *see* Quinidine *on page 1168*
- Apo®-Ranitidine (Can) *see* Ranitidine *on page 1178*
- Apo®-Salvent (Can) *see* Albuterol *on page 41*
- Apo®-Selegiline (Can) *see* Selegiline *on page 1228*
- Apo®-Sertraline (Can) *see* Sertraline *on page 1231*
- Apo®-Sotalol (Can) *see* Sotalol *on page 1252*
- Apo®-Sucralate (Can) *see* Sucralfate *on page 1266*
- Apo®-Sulfatrim (Can) *see* Sulfamethoxazole and Trimethoprim *on page 1273*
- Apo®-Sulfinpyrazone (Can) *see* Sulfinpyrazone *on page 1276*
- Apo®-Sulin (Can) *see* Sulindac *on page 1278*
- Apo®-Tamox (Can) *see* Tamoxifen *on page 1286*
- Apo®-Temazepam (Can) *see* Temazepam *on page 1292*
- Apo®-Terazosin (Can) *see* Terazosin *on page 1298*
- Apo®-Tetra (Can) *see* Tetracycline *on page 1306*
- Apo®-Thioridazine (Can) *see* Thioridazine *on page 1321*
- Apo®-Ticlopidine (Can) *see* Ticlopidine *on page 1331*
- Apo®-Timol (Can) *see* Timolol *on page 1334*
- Apo®-Timop (Can) *see* Timolol *on page 1334*
- Apo®-Tolbutamide (Can) *see* TOLBUTamide *on page 1344*
- Apo®-Trazodone D (Can) *see* Trazodone *on page 1362*
- Apo®-Triazide (Can) *see* Hydrochlorothiazide and Triamterene *on page 675*
- Apo®-Triazo (Can) *see* Triazolam *on page 1370*
- Apo®-Trifluoperazine (Can) *see* Trifluoperazine *on page 1372*
- Apo®-Trihex (Can) *see* Trihexyphenidyl *on page 1374*
- Apo®-Trimip (Can) *see* Trimipramine *on page 1378*
- Apo®-Verap (Can) *see* Verapamil *on page 1412*
- Apo®-Zidovudine (Can) *see* Zidovudine *on page 1435*
- APPG *see* Penicillin G Procaine *on page 1054*

Apraclonidine (a pra KLOE ni deen)
U.S. Brand Names Iopidine®
Canadian Brand Names Iopidine®
Synonyms Aplonidine; Apraclonidine Hydrochloride; p-Aminoclonidine
Therapeutic Category Alpha₂-Adrenergic Agonist Agent, Ophthalmic; Sympathomimetic Agent, Ophthalmic
Use Prevention and treatment of postsurgical intraocular pressure elevation
Pregnancy Risk Factor C
Usual Dosage Adults: Ophthalmic:
  0.5%: Instill 1-2 drops in the affected eye(s) 3 times/day; since apraclonidine 0.5% will be used with other ocular glaucoma therapies, use an approximate 5-minute interval between instillation of each medication to prevent washout of the previous dose
  1%: Instill 1 drop in operative eye 1 hour prior to anterior segment laser surgery, second drop in eye immediately upon completion of procedure
  Dosing adjustment in renal impairment: Although the topical use of apraclonidine has not been studied in renal failure patients, structurally related clonidine undergoes a significant increase in half-life in patients with severe renal impairment; close monitoring of cardiovascular parameters in patients with impaired renal function is advised if they are candidates for topical apraclonidine therapy
  Dosing adjustment in hepatic impairment: Close monitoring of cardiovascular parameters in patients with impaired liver function is advised because the systemic dosage form of clonidine is partially metabolized in the liver
  Additional Information Complete prescribing information for this medication should be consulted for additional detail.
Dosage Forms Solution, ophthalmic, as hydrochloride: 0.5% (5 mL, 10 mL); 1% (0.1 mL)

- Apraclonidine Hydrochloride *see* Apraclonidine *on page 111*
- Apresazide® [DSC] *see* Hydralazine and Hydrochlorothiazide *on page 673*
- Apresoline® [DSC] *see* HydrALAZINE *on page 671*
- Apri® *see* Ethinyl Estradiol and Desogestrel *on page 510*
- Aprodine® [OTC] *see* Triprolidine and Pseudoephedrine *on page 1380*
- Aprodine® w/C *see* Triprolidine, Pseudoephedrine, and Codeine *on page 1381*

Aprotinin (a proe TYE nin)
U.S. Brand Names Trasylol®
Canadian Brand Names Trasylol®
Therapeutic Category Blood Product Derivative; Hemostatic Agent
Use Reduction or prevention of blood loss in patients undergoing coronary artery bypass surgery when a high risk of excessive bleeding exists, including open heart reoperation, pre-existing coagulopathies, operations on the great vessels, and when a patient's beliefs prohibit blood transfusions
Pregnancy Risk Factor B
Contraindications Hypersensitivity to aprotinin or any component of the formulation
Warnings/Precautions Anaphylactic reactions are possible. Hypersensitivity reactions are more common with repeated use especially when re-exposure is within 6 months. All patients should receive a test dose at least 10 minutes before loading dose. Patients with a history of allergic reactions to drugs or other agents may be more likely to develop a reaction. (Continued)

Aprotinin *(Continued)*

Adverse Reactions

1% to 10%:

Cardiovascular: Atrial fibrillation, myocardial infarction, heart failure, atrial flutter, ventricular tachycardia, hypotension, supraventricular tachycardia

Central nervous system: Fever, mental confusion

Local: Phlebitis

Renal: Increased potential for postoperative renal dysfunction

Respiratory: Dyspnea, bronchoconstriction

<1% (Limited to important or life-threatening): Cerebral embolism, cerebrovascular events, convulsions, hemolysis, liver damage, pulmonary edema

Overdosage/Toxicology The maximum amount of aprotinin that can safely be given has not yet been determined. One case report of aprotinin overdose was associated with the development of hepatic and renal failure and eventually death. Autopsy demonstrated severe hepatic necrosis and extensive renal tubular and glomerular necrosis. The relationship with these findings and aprotinin remains unclear.

Drug Interactions

Increased Effect/Toxicity: Heparin and aprotinin prolong ACT; the ACT becomes a poor measure of adequate anticoagulation with the concurrent use of these drugs. Use with succinylcholine or tubocurarine may produce prolonged or recurring apnea.

Decreased Effect: Aprotinin blocks the fibrinolytic activity of thrombolytic agents (alteplase, streptokinase). The antihypertensive effects of captopril (and other ACE inhibitors) may be blocked; avoid concurrent use.

Stability Vials should be stored between 2°C and 25°C and protected from freezing; it is **incompatible** with corticosteroids, heparin, tetracyclines, amino acid solutions, and fat emulsion

Mechanism of Action Serine protease inhibitor; inhibits plasmin, kallikrein, and platelet activation producing antifibrinolytic effects; a weak inhibitor of plasma pseudocholinesterase. It also inhibits the contact phase activation of coagulation and preserves adhesive platelet glycoproteins making them resistant to damage from increased circulating plasmin or mechanical injury occurring during bypass

Pharmacodynamics/Kinetics

Half-life elimination: 2.5 hours

Excretion: Urine

Usual Dosage

Test dose: **All** patients should receive a 1 mL I.V. test dose at least 10 minutes prior to the loading dose to assess the potential for allergic reactions. **Note:** To avoid physical incompatibility with heparin when adding to pump-prime solution, each agent should be added during recirculation to assure adequate dilution.

Regimen A (standard dose):

2 million units (280 mg) loading dose I.V. over 20-30 minutes

2 million units (280 mg) into pump prime volume

500,000 units/hour (70 mg/hour) I.V. during operation

Regimen B (low dose):

1 million units (140 mg) loading dose I.V. over 20-30 minutes

1 million units (140 mg) into pump prime volume

250,000 units/hour (35 mg/hour) I.V. during operation

Administration All intravenous doses should be administered through a central line

Monitoring Parameters Bleeding times, prothrombin time, activated clotting time, platelet count, red blood cell counts, hematocrit, hemoglobin and fibrinogen degradation products; for toxicity also include renal function tests and blood pressure

Reference Range Antiplasmin effects occur when plasma aprotinin concentrations are 125 KIU/mL and antikallikrein effects occur when plasma levels are 250-500 KIU/mL; it remains unknown if these plasma concentrations are required for clinical benefits to occur during cardiopulmonary bypass; **Note:** KIU = Kallikrein inhibitor unit

Test Interactions Aprotinin prolongs whole blood clotting time of heparinized blood as determined by the Hemochrom® method or similar surface activation methods. Patients may require additional heparin even in the presence of activated clotting time levels that appear to represent adequate anticoagulation.

Nursing Implications All intravenous doses should be administered through a central line

Dosage Forms Injection: 1.4 mg/mL [10,000 KIU/mL] (100 mL, 200 mL)

- ♦ **Aquacare® [OTC]** *see* Urea *on page 1391*
- ♦ **Aquachloral® Supprettes®** *see* Chloral Hydrate *on page 270*
- ♦ **Aquacort® (Can)** *see* Hydrocortisone *on page 682*
- ♦ **AquaMEPHYTON®** *see* Phytonadione *on page 1082*
- ♦ **Aquaphyllin®** *see* Theophylline Salts *on page 1310*
- ♦ **Aquasol A®** *see* Vitamin A *on page 1421*
- ♦ **Aquasol E® [OTC]** *see* Vitamin E *on page 1423*
- ♦ **Aquatensen®** *see* Methyclothiazide *on page 890*
- ♦ **Aquazide®** *see* Hydrochlorothiazide *on page 674*
- ♦ **Aqueous Procaine Penicillin G** *see* Penicillin G Procaine *on page 1054*
- ♦ **Aqueous Testosterone** *see* Testosterone *on page 1302*
- ♦ **Ara-A** *see* Vidarabine *on page 1414*
- ♦ **Arabinofuranosyladenine** *see* Vidarabine *on page 1414*
- ♦ **Arabinosylcytosine** *see* Cytarabine *on page 350*
- ♦ **Ara-C** *see* Cytarabine *on page 350*
- ♦ **Aralen® (Can)** *see* Chloroquine *on page 277*
- ♦ **Aralen® Phosphate** *see* Chloroquine *on page 277*
- ♦ **Aramine®** *see* Metaraminol *on page 874*
- ♦ **Aranesp™** *see* Darbepoetin Alfa *on page 365*

♦ **Arava™** *see* Leflunomide *on page 777*
♦ **Arduan®** *see* Pipecuronium *on page 1089*
♦ **Aredia®** *see* Pamidronate *on page 1032*

Argatroban (ar GA troh ban)

Therapeutic Category Anticoagulant, Thrombin Inhibitor

Use Prophylaxis or treatment of thrombosis in adults with heparin-induced thrombocytopenia

Pregnancy Risk Factor B

Pregnancy/Breast-Feeding Implications No adequate and well-controlled studies have been done in pregnant women. Argatroban should be used in pregnant women only if clearly needed. It is not known if argatroban is excreted in human milk. Because of the serious potential of adverse effects to the nursing infant, a decision to discontinue nursing or discontinue argatroban should be considered.

Contraindications Hypersensitivity to argatroban or any component of the formulation; overt major bleeding

Warnings/Precautions Hemorrhage can occur at any site in the body. Extreme caution should be used when there is an increased danger of hemorrhage, such as severe hypertension, immediately following lumbar puncture, spinal anesthesia, major surgery (including brain, spinal cord, or eye surgery), congenital or acquired bleeding disorders, and gastrointestinal ulcers. Use caution with hepatic dysfunction. Concomitant use with warfarin will cause increased prolongation of the PT and INR greater than that of warfarin alone; alternative guidelines for monitoring therapy should be followed. Safety and efficacy for use with other thrombolytic agents has not been established. Discontinue all parenteral anticoagulants prior to starting therapy. Allow reversal of heparin's effects before initiation. Patients with hepatic dysfunction may require >4 hours to achieve full reversal of argatroban's anticoagulant effect following treatment. For adult use; safety and efficacy in children <18 years of age have not been established.

Adverse Reactions As with all anticoagulants, bleeding is the major adverse effect of argatroban. Hemorrhage may occur at virtually any site. Risk is dependent on multiple variables, including the intensity of anticoagulation and patient susceptibility.

>10%:
  Gastrointestinal: Gastrointestinal bleed (minor, 14%)
  Genitourinary: Genitourinary bleed and hematuria (minor, 12%)
1% to 10%:
  Cardiovascular: Hypotension (7%), cardiac arrest (6%), ventricular tachycardia (5%), atrial fibrillation (3%), cerebrovascular disorder (3%)
  Central nervous system: Fever (7%), pain (5%), intracranial bleeding (1%, only observed in patients also receiving streptokinase or tissue plasminogen activator)
  Gastrointestinal: Diarrhea (6%), nausea (5%), vomiting (4%), abdominal pain (3%), bleeding (major, 2%)
  Genitourinary: Urinary tract infection (5%)
  Hematologic: Decreased hemoglobin <2 g/dL and hematocrit (minor, 10%)
  Local: Bleeding at the injection site (minor, 2% to 5%)
  Renal: Abnormal renal function (3%)
  Respiratory: Dyspnea (8%), coughing (3%), hemoptysis (minor, 3%), pneumonia (3%)
  Miscellaneous: Sepsis (6%), infection (4%)
<1% (Limited to important or life-threatening): Allergic reactions including cough, dyspnea, rash, bullous eruption, and vasodilation (increased to 14% in patients also receiving thrombolytic therapy and/or contrast media); decreased hemoglobin and hematocrit (major, 0.7%); genitourinary bleeding and hematuria (major, 0.9%); limb and below-the-knee stump bleed; multisystem hemorrhage and DIC

Overdosage/Toxicology No specific antidote is available. Treatment should be symptomatic and supportive. Discontinue or decrease infusion to control excessive anticoagulation with or without bleeding. Reversal of anticoagulant effects may be longer than 4 hours in patients with hepatic impairment.

Drug Interactions

Cytochrome P450 Effect: CYP3A4/5 enzyme substrate (minor pathway)

Increased Effect/Toxicity: Drugs which affect platelet function (eg, aspirin, NSAIDs, dipyridamole, ticlopidine, clopidogrel), anticoagulants, or thrombolytics may potentiate the risk of hemorrhage. Sufficient time must pass after heparin therapy is discontinued; allow heparin's effect on the aPTT to decrease
  Concomitant use of argatroban with warfarin increases PT and INR greater than that of warfarin alone. Argatroban is commonly continued during the initiation of warfarin therapy to assure anticoagulation and to protect against possible transient hypercoagulability.

Stability Store at 25°C (77°F). Protect from light. Once mixed, final concentration should be 1 mg/mL. The prepared solution is stable for 24 hours at 25°C (77°F) in ambient indoor light. Do not expose to direct sunlight. Prepared solutions are stable for 48 hours at 2°C to 8°C when stored in the dark.

Mechanism of Action A direct, highly selective thrombin inhibitor. Reversibly binds to the active thrombin site of free and clot-associated thrombin. Inhibits fibrin formation; activation of coagulation factors V, VIII, and XIII; protein C; and platelet aggregation.

Pharmacodynamics/Kinetics

Onset of action: Immediate
Distribution: 174 mL/kg
Protein binding: Albumin: 20%; α_1-acid glycoprotein: 35%
Metabolism: Hepatic via hydroxylation and aromatization. Metabolism via CYP3A4/5 to four known metabolites plays a minor role. Unchanged argatroban is the major plasma component. Plasma concentration of metabolite M1 is 0% to 20% of the parent drug and is 3- to 5-fold weaker.
Half-life elimination: 39-51 minutes; ≤181 minutes with hepatic dysfunction
Time to peak: Steady-state: 1-3 hours
Excretion: Feces (65%); urine (22%); low quantities of metabolites M2-4 in urine
(Continued)

113

Argatroban *(Continued)*

Usual Dosage I.V.: Adults:

Initial dose: 2 mcg/kg/minute

Maintenance dose: Measure aPTT after 2 hours, adjust dose until the steady-state aPTT is 1.5-3.0 times the initial baseline value, not exceeding 100 seconds; dosage should not exceed 10 mcg/kg/minute

Conversion to oral anticoagulant: Because there may be a combined effect on the INR when argatroban is combined with warfarin, loading doses of warfarin should not be used. Warfarin therapy should be started at the expected daily dose.

Patients receiving ≤2 mcg/kg/minute of argatroban: Argatroban therapy can be stopped when the combined INR on warfarin and argatroban is >4; repeat INR measurement in 4-6 hours; if INR is below therapeutic level, argatroban therapy may be restarted. Repeat procedure daily until desired INR on warfarin alone is obtained.

Patients receiving >2 mcg/kg/minute of argatroban: Reduce dose of argatroban to 2 mcg/kg/minute; measure INR for argatroban and warfarin 4-6 hours after dose reduction; argatroban therapy can be stopped when the combined INR on warfarin and argatroban is >4. Repeat INR measurement in 4-6 hours; if INR is below therapeutic level, argatroban therapy may be restarted. Repeat procedure daily until desired INR on warfarin alone is obtained.

Dosage adjustment in renal impairment: No adjustment is necessary

Dosage adjustment in hepatic impairment: Decreased clearance and increased elimination half-life are seen with hepatic impairment; dose should be reduced. Initial dose for moderate hepatic impairment is 0.5 mcg/kg/minute.

Elderly: No adjustment is necessary for patients with normal liver function

Administration Solution **must be diluted to 1 mg/mL** prior to administration. May be mixed with 0.9% sodium chloride injection, 5% dextrose injection, or lactated Ringer's injection. To prepare solution for I.V. administration, dilute each 250 mg vial with 250 mL of diluent (500 mg with 500 mL of diluent). Mix by repeated inversion for one minute. A slight but brief haziness may occur prior to mixing. Do not mix with other medications. The prepared solution is stable for 24 hours at 25°C (77°F) in ambient indoor light. Do not expose to direct sunlight. Prepared solutions are stable for 48 hours at 2°C to 8°C when stored in the dark.

Monitoring Parameters Obtain baseline aPTT prior to start of therapy. Check aPTT 2 hours after start of therapy to adjust dose, keeping the steady-state aPTT 1.5-3 times the initial baseline value (not exceeding 100 seconds). Monitor hemoglobin, hematocrit, signs and symptoms of bleeding.

Test Interactions Argatroban produces dose-dependent effects on PT, INR, ACT, and TT, however, therapeutic ranges are not established.

Patient Information This drug can only be administered by injection. You may have a tendency to bleed easily while taking this drug; brush teeth with soft brush, floss with waxed floss, use electric razor, avoid scissors or sharp knives, and potentially harmful activities. Report fever, confusion, persistent nausea or GI upset, unusual bleeding (including bleeding gums, nosebleed, blood in urine, dark stool), bruising, pain in joints or back, swelling or pain at injection site.

Nursing Implications Solution **must be diluted to 1 mg/mL** prior to administration. May be mixed with 0.9% sodium chloride injection, 5% dextrose injection, or lactated Ringer's injection. Do not mix with other medications. Do not expose diluted solution to direct sunlight, however, light-resistant containers are not necessary with exposure to ambient light. Obtain baseline aPTT prior to start of therapy. Check aPTT 2 hours after start of therapy to adjust dose, keeping the steady-state aPTT 1.5-3 times the initial baseline value (not exceeding 100 seconds). Patients should be monitored for bleeding.

Additional Information Platelet counts recovered by day 3 in 53% of patients with heparin-induced thrombocytopenia and in 58% of patients with heparin-induced thrombocytopenia with thrombosis syndrome.

Dosage Forms Injection: 100 mg/mL (2.5 mL)

♦ **Argesic®-SA** *see* Salsalate *on page 1220*

Arginine *(AR ji neen)*

U.S. Brand Names R-Gene®

Synonyms Arginine Hydrochloride

Therapeutic Category Diagnostic Agent, Pituitary Function; Metabolic Alkalosis Agent

Use Pituitary function test (growth hormone); management of severe, uncompensated, metabolic alkalosis (pH ≥7.55) **after** optimizing therapy with sodium and potassium supplements

Unlabeled/Investigational Use Treatment of metabolic acidosis

Pregnancy Risk Factor C

Usual Dosage I.V.:

Pituitary function test:

Children: 500 mg kg/dose administered over 30 minutes

Adults: 30 g (300 mL) administered over 30 minutes

Inborn errors of urea synthesis: Initial: 0.8 g/kg, then 0.2-0.8 g/kg/day as a continuous infusion

Metabolic alkalosis: Children and Adults: *Arginine hydrochloride is a fourth-line treatment for uncompensated metabolic alkalosis after sodium chloride, potassium chloride, and ammonium chloride supplementation has been optimized.*

Arginine dose (G) = weight (kg) x 0.1 x (HCO$_3^-$ - 24) where HCO$_3^-$ = the patient's serum bicarbonate concentration in mEq/L

Give ½ to ⅓ dose calculated then re-evaluate

Note: Arginine hydrochloride should never be used as an alternative to chloride supplementation but used in the patient who is unresponsive to sodium chloride or potassium chloride supplementation

Hypochloremia: Children and Adults: Arginine dose (mL) = 0.4 x weight (kg) x (103-Cl⁻) where Cl⁻ = the patient's serum chloride concentration in mEq/L

Give ½ to ⅓ dose calculated then re-evaluate

Additional Information Complete prescribing information for this medication should be consulted for additional detail.

Dosage Forms Injection, solution, as hydrochloride: 10% [100 mg/mL = 950 mOsm/L] (300 mL) [contains chloride 0.475 mEq/mL]

- ♦ **Arginine Hydrochloride** *see* Arginine *on page 114*
- ♦ **8-Arginine Vasopressin** *see* Vasopressin *on page 1408*
- ♦ **Aricept®** *see* Donepezil *on page 434*
- ♦ **Arimidex®** *see* Anastrozole *on page 99*
- ♦ **Aristocort®** *see* Triamcinolone *on page 1366*
- ♦ **Aristocort® A** *see* Triamcinolone *on page 1366*
- ♦ **Aristocort® Forte** *see* Triamcinolone *on page 1366*
- ♦ **Aristocort® Intralesional** *see* Triamcinolone *on page 1366*
- ♦ **Aristospan® (Can)** *see* Triamcinolone *on page 1366*
- ♦ **Aristospan® Intra-Articular** *see* Triamcinolone *on page 1366*
- ♦ **Aristospan® Intralesional** *see* Triamcinolone *on page 1366*
- ♦ **Arixtra®** *see* Fondaparinux *on page 602*
- ♦ **Arm-a-Med® Isoetharine** *see* Isoetharine *on page 747*
- ♦ **Armour® Thyroid** *see* Thyroid *on page 1326*
- ♦ **Aromasin®** *see* Exemestane *on page 537*

Arsenic Trioxide (AR se nik tri OKS id)

U.S. Brand Names Trisenox™

Therapeutic Category Antineoplastic Agent, Miscellaneous

Use Induction of remission and consolidation in patients with acute promyelocytic leukemia (APL) which is specifically characterized by t(15;17) translocation or PML/RAR-alpha gene expression. Should be used only in those patients who have relapsed or are refractory to retinoid and anthracycline chemotherapy.

Orphan drug: Treatment of myelodysplastic syndrome; multiple myeloma; chronic myeloid leukemia (CML); acute myelocytic leukemia (AML)

Pregnancy Risk Factor D

Pregnancy/Breast-Feeding Implications There are no adequate and well-controlled studies in pregnant women. May cause harm to the fetus. Pregnancy should be avoided. Excreted in human breast milk, do not breast-feed.

Contraindications Hypersensitivity to arsenic or any component of the formulation; pregnancy

Warnings/Precautions The U.S. Food and Drug Administration (FDA) currently recommends that procedures for proper handling and disposal of antineoplastic agents be considered. For use only by physicians experienced with the treatment of acute leukemia. A baseline 12-lead EKG, serum electrolytes (potassium, calcium, magnesium), and creatinine should be obtained. Correct electrolyte abnormalities prior to treatment and monitor potassium and magnesium levels during therapy (potassium should stay >4 mEq/dL and magnesium >1.8 mg/dL). Correct QT_c >500 msec prior to treatment. Discontinue therapy and hospitalize patient if QT_c >500 msec, syncope or irregular heartbeats develop during therapy. May prolong the QT interval. May lead to torsade de pointes or complete AV block. Risk factors for torsade de pointes include congestive heart failure, a history of torsade de pointes, pre-existing QT interval prolongation, patients taking potassium-wasting diuretics, and conditions which cause hypokalemia or hypomagnesemia. If possible, discontinue all medications known to prolong the QT interval. May cause retinoic-acid-acute promyelocytic leukemia (RA-APL) syndrome or APL differentiation syndrome. High-dose steroids have been used for treatment. May lead to the development of hyperleukocytosis. Use with caution in renal impairment. Safety and efficacy in children <5 years of age have not been established (limited experience with children 5-16 years of age).

Adverse Reactions

>10%:

Cardiovascular: Tachycardia (55%), edema (40%), QT interval >500 msec (38%), chest pain (25%), hypotension (25%)

Central nervous system: Fatigue (63%), fever (63%), headache (60%), insomnia (43%), anxiety (30%), dizziness (23%), depression (20%), pain (15%)

Dermatologic: Dermatitis (43%), pruritus (33%), bruising (20%)

Endocrine & metabolic: Hypokalemia (50%), hyperglycemia (45%), hypomagnesemia (45%), hyperkalemia (18%)

Gastrointestinal: Nausea (75%), abdominal pain (58%), vomiting (58%), diarrhea (53%), sore throat (40%), constipation (28%), anorexia (23%)

Genitourinary: Vaginal hemorrhage (13%)

Hematologic: Leukocytosis (50%), APL differentiation syndrome (23%), thrombocytopenia (19%), anemia (14%), febrile neutropenia (13%)

Hepatic: Elevated ALT (20%), elevated AST (13%)

Local: Injection site: Pain (20%), erythema (13%)

Neuromuscular & skeletal: Rigors (38%), arthralgia (33%), paresthesia (33%), myalgia (25%), bone pain (23%), back pain (18%), tremor (13%)

Respiratory: Cough (65%), dyspnea (53%), epistaxis (25%), hypoxia (23%), pleural effusion (20%), wheezing (13%)

1% to 10% (Limited to important or life-threatening):

Cardiovascular: Hypotension (10%), abnormal EKG (not QT prolongation) (7%)

Central nervous system: Convulsion (8%), somnolence (8%), agitation (5%), coma (5%), confusion (5%)

Dermatologic: Hyperpigmentation (8%), urticaria (8%), local exfoliation (5%)

Endocrine & metabolic: Hypocalcemia (10%), hypoglycemia (8%), acidosis (5%)

Gastrointestinal: Gastrointestinal hemorrhage (8%), hemorrhagic diarrhea (8%), oral blistering (8%)

Genitourinary: Intermenstrual bleeding (8%), incontinence (5%)

Hematologic: Neutropenia (10%), DIC (8%), hemorrhage (8%)

(Continued)

Arsenic Trioxide *(Continued)*

Otic: Tinnitus (5%)
Renal: Renal failure (8%), renal impairment (8%)
Respiratory: Hemoptysis (8%)
Miscellaneous: Hypersensitivity (5%), sepsis (5%)

Overdosage/Toxicology Symptoms of arsenic toxicity include convulsions, muscle weakness, and confusion. Discontinue treatment and begin chelation therapy. One suggested adult protocol is dimercaprol 3 mg/kg I.M. every 4 hours. Continue until life-threatening toxicity has subsided. Follow with penicillamine 250 mg orally up to 4 times/day (total daily dose ≤1 g).

Drug Interactions

Increased Effect/Toxicity: Use caution with medications causing hypokalemia or hypomagnesemia (ampho B, aminoglycosides, diuretics, cyclosporin). Use caution with medications that prolong the QT interval, avoid concurrent use if possible; includes type Ia and type III antiarrhythmic agents, selected quinolones (sparfloxacin, gatifloxacin, moxifloxacin, grepafloxacin), cisapride, thioridazine, and other agents.

Ethanol/Nutrition/Herb Interactions

Food: Avoid seafood (due to presence of arsenic as arsenobetaine and arsenocholine).
Herb/Nutraceutical: Avoid homeopathic products (arsenic is present in some homeopathic medications).

Stability Store at room temperature, 25°C (77°F); do not freeze. Following dilution, stable for 24 hours at room temperature or 48 hours when refrigerated.

Mechanism of Action Not fully understood; causes *in vitro* morphological changes and DNA fragmentation to NB4 human promyelocytic leukemia cells; also damages or degrades the fusion protein PML-RAR alpha

Pharmacodynamics/Kinetics

Metabolism: Hepatic; pentavalent arsenic is reduced to trivalent arsenic (active) by arsenate reductase; trivalent arsenic is methylated to monomethylarsinic acid, which is then converted to dimethylarsinic acid via methyltransferases
Excretion: Urine (as methylated metabolite); disposition not yet studied

Usual Dosage I.V.: Children >5 years and Adults:

Induction: 0.15 mg/kg/day; administer daily until bone marrow remission; maximum induction: 60 doses
Consolidation: 0.15 mg/kg/day starting 3-6 weeks after completion of induction therapy; maximum consolidation: 25 doses over 5 weeks

Dosage adjustment in renal impairment: Safety and efficacy have not been established; use with caution due to renal elimination
Dosage adjustment in hepatic impairment: Safety and efficacy have not been established
Elderly: Safety and efficacy have not been established; clinical trials included patients ≤72 years of age; use with caution due to the increased risk of renal impairment in the elderly

Administration Dilute in 100-250 mL D$_5$W or 0.9% sodium chloride. Does not contain a preservative; properly discard unused portion. Do not mix with other medications. Infuse over 1-2 hours. If acute vasomotor reactions occur, may infuse over a maximum of 4 hours. Does not require administration via a central venous catheter.

Monitoring Parameters Baseline then weekly 12-lead EKG, baseline then twice weekly serum electrolytes, hematologic and coagulation profiles at least twice weekly; more frequent monitoring may be necessary in unstable patients

Patient Information Check other medications with prescriber. Some medications may not mix well. Avoid homeopathic, herbal, or over-the-counter medications during treatment without approval of prescriber. You may not be alert. Avoid driving, doing other tasks or hobbies until until response to drug is known. May cause fatigue, fever, nausea, vomiting, diarrhea, cough, or headache. Contact prescriber immediately for unexplained fever, shortness of breath, lightheadedness, passing out, rapid heartbeats, or weight gain. EKG and blood tests will be performed regularly during treatment.

Nursing Implications Do not mix with other medications. Infuse over 1-2 hours. If acute vasomotor reactions occur, may infuse up to 4 hours. Monitor potassium and magnesium levels during treatment (potassium should stay >4 mEq/dL and magnesium >1.8 mg/dL). Monitor QT interval; QT$_c$ >500 msec should be corrected.

Additional Information Arsenic is stored in liver, kidney, heart, lung, hair, and nails. Arsenic trioxide is a human carcinogen.

Dosage Forms Injection: 1 mg/mL (10 mL)

♦ **Artane®** *see* Trihexyphenidyl *on page 1374*
♦ **Arthropan® [OTC]** *see* Choline Salicylate *on page 288*
♦ **Arthrotec®** *see* Diclofenac and Misoprostol *on page 395*
♦ **ASA** *see* Aspirin *on page 120*
♦ **5-ASA** *see* Mesalamine *on page 866*
♦ **Asacol®** *see* Mesalamine *on page 866*
♦ **Asaphen (Can)** *see* Aspirin *on page 120*
♦ **Asaphen E.C. (Can)** *see* Aspirin *on page 120*

Ascorbic Acid *(a SKOR bik AS id)*

U.S. Brand Names C-500-GR™ [OTC]; Cecon® [OTC]; Cevi-Bid® [OTC]; C-Gram [OTC]; Dull-C® [OTC]; Vita-C® [OTC]

Canadian Brand Names Apo®-C; Proflavanol C™; Revitalose C-1000®

Synonyms Vitamin C

Therapeutic Category Urinary Acidifying Agent; Vitamin, Water Soluble

Use Prevention and treatment of scurvy and to acidify the urine

Unlabeled/Investigational Use Investigational: In large doses to decrease the severity of "colds"; dietary supplementation; a 20-year study was recently completed involving 730 individuals which indicates a possible decreased risk of death by stroke when ascorbic acid at doses ≥45 mg/day was administered

Pregnancy Risk Factor A/C (dose exceeding RDA recommendation)

Warnings/Precautions Diabetics and patients prone to recurrent renal calculi (eg, dialysis patients) should not take excessive doses for extended periods of time (some studies point to as little as 100 mg/day)

Adverse Reactions

1% to 10%: Renal: Hyperoxaluria (incidence dose-related)

<1% (Limited to important or life-threatening): Dizziness, faintness, fatigue, flank pain, headache

Overdosage/Toxicology Symptoms include renal calculi, nausea, gastritis, and diarrhea. Diuresis with forced fluids may be useful following massive ingestion.

Drug Interactions

Increased Effect/Toxicity: Ascorbic acid enhances iron absorption from the GI tract. Concomitant ascorbic acid taken with oral contraceptives may increase contraceptive effect.

Decreased Effect: Ascorbic acid and fluphenazine may decrease fluphenazine levels. Ascorbic acid and warfarin may decrease anticoagulant effect. Changes in dose of ascorbic acid when taken with oral contraceptives may reduce the contraceptive effect.

Stability Injectable form should be stored under refrigeration (2°C to 8°C); protect oral dosage forms from light; is rapidly oxidized when in solution in air and alkaline media

Mechanism of Action Not fully understood; necessary for collagen formation and tissue repair; involved in some oxidation-reduction reactions as well as other metabolic pathways, such as synthesis of carnitine, steroids, and catecholamines and conversion of folic acid to folinic acid

Pharmacodynamics/Kinetics

Absorption: Oral: Readily absorbed; an active process thought to be dose dependent

Distribution: Large

Metabolism: Hepatic via oxidation and sulfation

Excretion: Urine (when high blood levels)

Usual Dosage Oral, I.M., I.V., S.C.:

Recommended daily allowance (RDA):

<6 months: 30 mg

6 months to 1 year: 35 mg

1-3 years: 15 mg; upper limit of intake should not exceed 400 mg/day

4-8 years: 25 mg; upper limit of intake should not exceed 650 mg/day

9-13 years: 45 mg; upper limit of intake should not exceed 1200 mg/day

14-18 years: Upper limit of intake should not exceed 1800 mg/day

Male: 75 mg

Female: 65 mg

Adults: Upper limit of intake should not exceed 2000 mg/day

Male: 90 mg

Female: 75 mg;

Pregnant female:

≤18 years: 80 mg; upper limit of intake should not exceed 1800 mg/day

19-50 years: 85 mg; upper limit of intake should not exceed 2000 mg/day

Lactating female:

≤18 years: 15 mg; upper limit of intake should not exceed 1800 mg/day

19-50 years: 20 mg; upper limit of intake should not exceed 2000 mg/day

Adult smoker: Add an additional 35 mg/day

Children:

Scurvy: 100-300 mg/day in divided doses for at least 2 weeks

Urinary acidification: 500 mg every 6-8 hours

Dietary supplement: 35-100 mg/day

Adults:

Scurvy: 100-250 mg 1-2 times/day for at least 2 weeks

Urinary acidification: 4-12 g/day in 3-4 divided doses

Prevention and treatment of colds: 1-3 g/day

Dietary supplement: 50-200 mg/day

Administration Avoid rapid I.V. injection

Monitoring Parameters Monitor pH of urine when using as an acidifying agent

Test Interactions False-positive urinary glucose with cupric sulfate reagent, false-negative urinary glucose with glucose oxidase method; false-negative stool occult blood 48-72 hours after ascorbic acid ingestion

Nursing Implications Avoid rapid I.V. injection

Additional Information Sodium content of 1 g: ~5 mEq

Dosage Forms

Capsule: 500 mg, 1000 mg

C-500-GR™: 500 mg

Capsule, timed release: 500 mg

Crystal (Vita-C®): 4 g/teaspoonful (100 g)

Injection, solution: 250 mg/mL (2 mL, 30 mL); 500 mg/mL (50 mL)

Cenolate®: 500 mg/mL (1 mL, 2 mL) [contains sodium hydrosulfite]

Powder, solution (Dull-C®): 4 g/teaspoonful (100 g, 500 g)

Solution, oral (Cecon®): 90 mg/mL (50 mL)

Tablet: 100 mg, 250 mg, 500 mg, 1000 mg

C-Gram: 1000 mg

Tablet, chewable: 100 mg, 250 mg, 500 mg [some products may contain aspartame]

Tablet, timed release: 500 mg, 1000 mg, 1500 mg

Cevi-Bid®: 500 mg

♦ **Asendin® [DSC]** *see* Amoxapine *on page 82*

♦ **Asmalix®** *see* Theophylline Salts *on page 1310*

Asparaginase (a SPEAR a ji nase)

U.S. Brand Names Elspar®

Canadian Brand Names Elspar®; Kidrolase®

Synonyms *E. coli* Asparaginase; *Erwinia* Asparaginase; L-asparaginase; NSC-106977 (*Erwinia*); NSC-109229 (*E. coli*)

Therapeutic Category Antineoplastic Agent, Protein Synthesis Inhibitor

Use Treatment of acute lymphocytic leukemia, lymphoma; induction therapy

Pregnancy Risk Factor C

Pregnancy/Breast-Feeding Implications Clinical effects on the fetus: Based on limited reports in humans, the use of asparaginase does not seem to pose a major risk to the fetus when used in the 2nd and 3rd trimesters, or when exposure occurs prior to conception in either females or males. Because of the teratogenicity observed in animals and the lack of human data after 1st trimester exposure, asparaginase should be used cautiously, if at all, during this period.

Contraindications Hypersensitivity to asparaginase or any component of the formulation; history of anaphylaxis to asparaginase; if a reaction occurs to Elspar®, obtain **Erwinia L-asparaginase** and use with caution; pancreatitis (active or any history of)

Warnings/Precautions The U.S. Food and Drug Administration (FDA) currently recommends that procedures for proper handling and disposal of antineoplastic agents be considered. Monitor for severe allergic reactions. May alter hepatic function. Use cautiously in patients with an underlying coagulopathy.

Risk factors for allergic reactions:
Route of administration: I.V. administration is more likely to cause a reaction than I.M. or S.C.
Prolonged therapy dose: Doses >6000-12,000 units/m^2 increase the risk of a reaction.
Previous therapy: Patients who have received previous cycles of asparaginase have an increased risk.
Intermittent therapy: Intervals of even a few days between doses increase the risk.

Up to 33% of patients who have an allergic reaction to *E. coli* asparaginase will also react to the *Erwinia* form or pegaspargase.

A test dose is often recommended prior to the first dose of asparaginase, or prior to restarting therapy after a hiatus of several days. Most commonly, 0.1-0.2 mL of a 20-250 units/mL (2-50 units) is injected intradermally, and the patient observed for 15-30 minutes. **False-negative rates of up to 80% to test doses of 2-50 units are reported.** Desensitization should be performed in patients found to be hypersensitive by the intradermal test dose or who have received previous courses of therapy with the drug.

Adverse Reactions Note: Immediate effects: Fever, chills, nausea, and vomiting occur in 50% to 60% of patients.

>10%:
Central nervous system: Fatigue, somnolence, depression, hallucinations, agitation, disorientation or convulsions (10% to 60%), stupor, confusion, coma (25%)
Endocrine & metabolic: Fever, chills (50% to 60%), hyperglycemia (10%)
Gastrointestinal: Nausea, vomiting (50% to 60%), anorexia, abdominal cramps (70%), acute pancreatitis (15%, may be severe in some patients)
Hematologic: Hypofibrinogenemia and depression of clotting factors V and VIII, variable decreased in factors VII and IX, severe protein C deficiency and decrease in antithrombin III (may be dose-limiting or fatal)
Hepatic: Transient elevations of transaminases, bilirubin, and alkaline phosphatase
Hypersensitivity: Acute allergic reactions (fever, rash, urticaria, arthralgia, hypotension, angioedema, bronchospasm, anaphylaxis (15% to 35%); may be dose-limiting in some patients, may be fatal)
Renal: Azotemia (66%)
1% to 10%:
Endocrine & metabolic: Hyperuricemia
Gastrointestinal: Stomatitis
<1% (Limited to important or life-threatening): Acute renal failure, coma (may be due to elevated NH$_4$ levels), diabetes mellitus (transient), fever, hallucinations, ketoacidosis, laryngeal spasm, Parkinsonism symptoms (tremor), seizures
Inhibition of protein synthesis will cause a decrease in production of albumin, insulin (resulting in hyperglycemia), serum lipoprotein, antithrombin III, and clotting factors II, V, VII, VIII, IX, and X. The loss of the later two proteins may result in either thrombotic or hemorrhagic events. These protein losses occur in 100% of patients.
Myelosuppressive: Myelosuppression is uncommon and usually mild; Onset (days): 7; Nadir (days): 14; Recovery (days): 21

Overdosage/Toxicology Symptoms include nausea and diarrhea.

Drug Interactions

Increased Effect/Toxicity: Increased toxicity has been noticed when asparaginase is administered with vincristine (neuropathy) and prednisone (hyperglycemia). Decreased metabolism when used with cyclophosphamide. Increased hepatotoxicity when used with mercaptopurine.

Decreased Effect: Asparaginase terminates methotrexate action.

Stability Intact vials of powder should be refrigerated (<8°C); lyophilized powder should be reconstituted with 1-5 mL sterile water for I.V. administration or NS for I.M. use, reconstituted solutions are stable 1 week at room temperature; shake well but not too vigorously; use of a 5 micron in-line filter is recommended to remove fiber-like particles in the solution (not 0.2 micron filter - has been associated with some loss of potency).

Standard I.M. dilution: 5000 international units/mL: 2 mL/syringe
Usually no >2 mL/injection site, however, contact RN first to clarify administration route.
Standard I.V. dilution: Dose/50-250 mL NS or D$_5$W
Stable for 8 hours at room temperature or refrigeration

Mechanism of Action Some malignant cells (ie, lymphoblastic leukemia cells and those of lymphocyte derivation) must acquire the amino acid asparagine from surrounding fluid such as blood, whereas normal cells can synthesize their own asparagine. Asparaginase is an enzyme that deaminates asparagine to aspartic acid and ammonia in the plasma and extracellular fluid and therefore deprives tumor cells of the amino acid for protein synthesis.

There are two purified preparations of the enzyme: one from *Escherichia coli* and one from *Erwinia carotovora*. These two preparations vary slightly in the gene sequencing and have slight differences in enzyme characteristics. Both are highly specific for asparagine and have less than 10% activity for the D-isomer. The preparation from *E. coli* has had the most use in clinical and research practice.

Pharmacodynamics/Kinetics
Absorption: I.M.: Produces peak blood levels 50% lower than those from I.V. administration
Distribution: V_d: 4-5 L/kg; 70% to 80% of plasma volume; does not penetrate CSF
Metabolism: Systemically degraded
Half-life elimination: 8-30 hours
Excretion: Urine (trace amounts)
   Clearance: Unaffected by age, renal function, or hepatic function

Usual Dosage Refer to individual protocols; dose must be individualized based upon clinical response and tolerance of the patient
Children:
   I.V.:
      Infusion for induction in combination with vincristine and prednisone: 1000 units/kg/day for 10 days
      Consolidation: 6000-10,000 units/m²/day for 14 days
   I.M.: In combination with vincristine and prednisone: 6000 units/m² on days 4, 7, 10, 13, 16, 19, 22, 25, 28
Adults:
   I.V. infusion single agent for induction:
      200 units/kg/day for 28 days **or**
      5000-10,000 units/m²/day for 7 days every 3 weeks **or**
      10,000-40,000 units every 2-3 weeks
   I.M. as single agent: 6000-12,000 units/m²; reconstitution to 10,000 units/mL may be necessary. (See pediatric dosage for combination therapy.)

Some institutions recommended the following precautions for asparaginase administration: Have parenteral epinephrine, diphenhydramine, and hydrocortisone available at the bedside. Have a freely running I.V. in place. Have a physician readily accessible. Monitor the patient closely for 30-60 minutes. Avoid administering the drug at night.

Some practitioners recommend a desensitization regimen for patients who react to a test dose, or are being retreated following a break in therapy. Doses are doubled and given every 10 minutes until the total daily dose for that day has been administered. See table.

Asparaginase Desensitization

Injection No.	Elspar Dose (IU)	Accumulated Total Dose
1	1	1
2	2	3
3	4	7
4	8	15
5	16	31
6	32	63
7	64	127
8	128	255
9	256	511
10	512	1023
11	1024	2047
12	2048	4095
13	4096	8191
14	8192	16,383
15	16,384	32,767
16	32,768	65,535
17	65,536	131,071
18	131,072	262,143

For example, if a patient was to receive a total dose of 4000 units, he/she would receive injections 1 through 12 during the desensitization

Administration Must only be given as a deep intramuscular injection into a large muscle; use two injection sites for I.M. doses >2 mL

May be administered I.V. infusion in 50 mL of D_5W or NS over more than 30 minutes; a small test dose (0.1 mL of a dilute 20 unit/mL solution) should be given first

Occasionally, gelatinous fiber-like particles may develop on standing; filtration through a 5-micron filter during administration will remove the particles with no loss of potency; some loss of potency has been observed with the use of a 0.2 micron filter

Monitoring Parameters Vital signs during administration, CBC, urinalysis, amylase, liver enzymes, prothrombin time, renal function tests, urine dipstick for glucose, blood glucose, uric acid

Test Interactions ↓ thyroxine and thyroxine-binding globulin

Patient Information This medication can only be given I.M. or I.V. It is vital to maintain good hydration (2-3 L/day of fluids unless instructed to restrict fluid intake) and good nutritional (Continued)

Asparaginase *(Continued)*

status (small frequent meals may help). You may experience acute gastric disturbances (eg, nausea or vomiting); frequent mouth care or lozenges may help or antiemetic may be prescribed. Report any respiratory difficulty, skin rash, or acute anxiety immediately. Report unusual fever or chills, confusion, agitation, depression, yellowing of skin or eyes, unusual bleeding or bruising, unhealed sores, or vaginal discharge. Contraceptive measures are recommended during therapy.

Nursing Implications Appropriate agents for maintenance of an adequate airway and treatment of a hypersensitivity reaction (antihistamine, epinephrine, oxygen, I.V. corticosteroids) should be readily available. Be prepared to treat anaphylaxis at each administration; monitor for onset of abdominal pain and mental status changes.

Additional Information The *E. coli* and the *Erwinia* strains of asparaginase differ slightly in their gene sequencing, and have slight differences in their enzyme characteristics. Both are highly specific for asparagine and have <10% activity for the D-isomer. The *E. coli* form is more commonly used, with the *Erwinia* variety usually being used only in patients who demonstrate allergic reactions to the other form.

Dosage Forms
Injection:
10,000 units/10 mL
10,000 units/vial (*Erwinia*)

♦ **A-Spas® S/L** *see Hyoscyamine on page 692*

♦ **Aspercin [OTC]** *see Aspirin on page 120*

♦ **Aspercin Extra [OTC]** *see Aspirin on page 120*

♦ **Aspergum® [OTC]** *see Aspirin on page 120*

Aspirin *(AS pir in)*

Related Information
Antacid Drug Interactions *on page 1477*
Salicylates *on page 1692*

U.S. Brand Names Ascriptin® [OTC]; Ascriptin® Arthritis Pain [OTC]; Ascriptin® Enteric [OTC]; Ascriptin® Extra Strength [OTC]; Aspercin [OTC]; Aspercin Extra [OTC]; Aspergum® [OTC]; Bayer® Aspirin [OTC]; Bayer® Aspirin Extra Strength [OTC]; Bayer® Aspirin Regimen Adult Low Strength [OTC]; Bayer® Aspirin Regimen Adult Low Strength with Calcium [OTC]; Bayer® Aspirin Regimen Children's [OTC]; Bayer® Aspirin Regimen Regular Strength [OTC]; Bayer® Plus Extra Strength [OTC]; Bufferin® [OTC]; Bufferin® Arthritis Strength [OTC]; Bufferin® Extra Strength [OTC]; Easprin®; Ecotrin® [OTC]; Ecotrin® Low Adult Strength [OTC]; Ecotrin® Maximum Strength [OTC]; Halfprin® [OTC]; St. Joseph® Pain Reliever [OTC]; Sureprin 81™ [OTC]; ZORprin®

Canadian Brand Names Apo®-ASA; Asaphen; Asaphen E.C.; Entrophen®; Novasen

Synonyms Acetylsalicylic Acid; ASA

Therapeutic Category Analgesic, Salicylate; Anti-inflammatory Agent; Antiplatelet Agent; Antipyretic; Nonsteroidal Anti-inflammatory Drug (NSAID), Oral; Platelet Aggregation Inhibitor; Salicylate

Use Treatment of mild to moderate pain, inflammation, and fever; may be used as prophylaxis of myocardial infarction; prophylaxis of stroke and/or transient ischemic episodes; management of rheumatoid arthritis, rheumatic fever, osteoarthritis, and gout (high dose); adjunctive therapy in revascularization procedures (coronary artery bypass graft [CABG], percutaneous transluminal coronary angioplasty [PTCA], carotid endarterectomy)

Unlabeled/Investigational Use Low doses have been used in the prevention of pre-eclampsia, recurrent spontaneous abortions, prematurity, fetal growth retardation (including complications associated with autoimmune disorders such as lupus or antiphospholipid syndrome)

Pregnancy Risk Factor C/D (full-dose aspirin in 3rd trimester - expert analysis)

Contraindications Hypersensitivity to salicylates, other NSAIDs, or any component of the formulation; asthma; rhinitis; nasal polyps; inherited or acquired bleeding disorders (including factor VII and factor IX deficiency); do not use in children (<16 years of age) for viral infections (chickenpox or flu symptoms), with or without fever, due to a potential association with Reye's syndrome; pregnancy (3rd trimester especially)

Warnings/Precautions Use with caution in patients with platelet and bleeding disorders, renal dysfunction, dehydration, erosive gastritis, or peptic ulcer disease. Heavy ethanol use (>3 drinks/day) can increase bleeding risks. Avoid use in severe renal failure or in severe hepatic failure. Discontinue use if tinnitus or impaired hearing occurs. Caution in mild-moderate renal failure (only at high dosages). Patients with sensitivity to tartrazine dyes, nasal polyps and asthma may have an increased risk of salicylate sensitivity. Surgical patients should avoid ASA if possible, for 1-2 weeks prior to surgery, to reduce the risk of excessive bleeding.

Adverse Reactions As with all drugs which may affect hemostasis, bleeding is associated with aspirin. Hemorrhage may occur at virtually any site. Risk is dependent on multiple variables including dosage, concurrent use of multiple agents which alter hemostasis, and patient susceptibility. Many adverse effects of aspirin are dose-related, and are extremely rare at low dosages. Other serious reactions are idiosyncratic, related to allergy or individual sensitivity. Accurate estimation of frequencies is not possible.

Central nervous system: Fatigue, insomnia, nervousness, agitation, confusion, dizziness, headache, lethargy, cerebral edema, hyperthermia, coma

Cardiovascular: Hypotension, tachycardia, dysrhythmias, edema

Dermatologic: Rash, angioedema, urticaria

Endocrine & metabolic: Acidosis, hyperkalemia, dehydration, hypoglycemia (children), hyperglycemia, hypernatremia (buffered forms)

Gastrointestinal: Nausea, vomiting, dyspepsia, epigastric discomfort, heartburn, stomach pains, gastrointestinal ulceration (6% to 31%), gastric erosions, gastric erythema, duodenal ulcers

Hematologic: Anemia, disseminated intravascular coagulation, prolongation of prothrombin times, coagulopathy, thrombocytopenia, hemolytic anemia, bleeding, iron-deficiency anemia

Hepatic: Hepatotoxicity, increased transaminases, hepatitis (reversible)

Neuromuscular & skeletal: Rhabdomyolysis, weakness, acetabular bone destruction (OA)

Otic: Hearing loss, tinnitus

Renal: Interstitial nephritis, papillary necrosis, proteinuria, renal failure (including cases caused by rhabdomyolysis), increased BUN, increased serum creatinine

Respiratory: Asthma, bronchospasm, dyspnea, laryngeal edema, hyperpnea, tachypnea, respiratory alkalosis, noncardiogenic pulmonary edema

Miscellaneous: Anaphylaxis, prolonged pregnancy and labor, stillbirths, low birth weight, peripartum bleeding, Reye's syndrome

Case reports: Colonic ulceration, esophageal stricture, esophagitis with esophageal ulcer, esophageal hematoma, oral mucosal ulcers (aspirin-containing chewing gum), coronary artery spasm, conduction defect and atrial fibrillation (toxicity), delirium, ischemic brain infarction, colitis, rectal stenosis (suppository), cholestatic jaundice, periorbital edema, rhinosinusitis

Overdosage/Toxicology Refer to the nomogram in "Toxicology Information" *on page 1693* in the Appendix. Symptoms include tinnitus, headache, dizziness, confusion, metabolic acidosis, hyperpyrexia, hypoglycemia, and coma. Treatment should also be based upon symptomatology. See "Salicylates" *on page 1692* in the Appendix.

Drug Interactions

Increased Effect/Toxicity: Aspirin may increase methotrexate serum levels/toxicity and may displace valproic acid from binding sites which can result in toxicity. NSAIDs and aspirin increase GI adverse effects (ulceration). Aspirin with oral anticoagulants (warfarin), thrombolytic agents, heparin, low molecular weight heparins, and antiplatelet agents (ticlopidine, clopidogrel, dipyridamole, NSAIDs, and IIb/IIIa antagonists) may increase risk of bleeding. Bleeding times may be additionally prolonged with verapamil. The effects of older sulfonylurea agents (tolazamide, tolbutamide) may be potentiated due to displacement from plasma proteins. This effect does not appear to be clinically significant for newer sulfonylurea agents (glyburide, glipizide, glimepiride).

Decreased Effect: The effects of ACE inhibitors may be blunted by aspirin administration (may be significant only at higher aspirin dosages). Aspirin may decrease the effects of beta-blockers, loop diuretics (furosemide), thiazide diuretics, and probenecid. Aspirin may cause a decrease in NSAIDs serum concentration and decrease the effects of probenecid. Increased serum salicylate levels when taken with with urine acidifiers (ammonium chloride, methionine).

Ethanol/Nutrition/Herb Interactions

Ethanol: Avoid ethanol (may enhance gastric mucosal damage).

Food: Food may decrease the rate but not the extent of oral absorption.

Folic acid: Hyperexcretion of folate; folic acid deficiency may result, leading to macrocytic anemia.

Iron: With chronic aspirin use and at doses of 3-4 g/day, iron-deficiency anemia may result.

Sodium: Hypernatremia resulting from buffered aspirin solutions or sodium salicylate containing high sodium content. Avoid or use with caution in CHF or any condition where hypernatremia would be detrimental.

Benedictine liqueur, prunes, raisins, tea, and gherkins: Potential salicylate accumulation.

Fresh fruits containing vitamin C: Displace drug from binding sites, resulting in increased urinary excretion of aspirin.

Herb/Nutraceutical: Avoid cat's claw, dong quai, evening primrose, feverfew, garlic, ginger, ginkgo, red clover, horse chestnut, green tea, ginseng (all have additional antiplatelet activity). Limit curry powder, paprika, licorice; may cause salicylate accumulation. These foods contain 6 mg salicylate/100 g. An ordinarily American diet contains 10-200 mg/day of salicylate.

Stability Keep suppositories in refrigerator, do not freeze; hydrolysis of aspirin occurs upon exposure to water or moist air, resulting in salicylate and acetate, which possess a vinegar-like odor; do not use if a strong odor is present

Mechanism of Action Inhibits prostaglandin synthesis, acts on the hypothalamus heat-regulating center to reduce fever, blocks prostaglandin synthetase action which prevents formation of the platelet-aggregating substance thromboxane A_2

Pharmacodynamics/Kinetics

Duration: 4-6 hours

Absorption: Rapid

Distribution: V_d: 10 L; readily into most body fluids and tissues

Metabolism: Hydrolyzed to salicylate (active) by esterases in GI mucosa, red blood cells, synovial fluid, and blood; metabolism of salicylate occurs primarily by hepatic conjugation; metabolic pathways are saturable

Bioavailability: 50% to 75% reaches systemic circulation

Half-life elimination: Parent drug: 15-20 minutes; Salicylates (dose dependent): 3 hours at lower doses (300-600 mg), 5-6 hours (after 1 g), 10 hours with higher doses

Time to peak, serum: ~1-2 hours

Excretion: Urine (10% as salicylic acid, 75% as salicyluric acid)

Usual Dosage

Children:

Analgesic and antipyretic: Oral, rectal: 10-15 mg/kg/dose every 4-6 hours, up to a total of 4 g/day

Anti-inflammatory: Oral: Initial: 60-90 mg/kg/day in divided doses; usual maintenance: 80-100 mg/kg/day divided every 6-8 hours; monitor serum concentrations

Antiplatelet effects: Adequate pediatric studies have not been performed; pediatric dosage is derived from adult studies and clinical experience and is not well established; suggested doses have ranged from 3-5 mg/kg/day to 5-10 mg/kg/day given as a single daily dose. Doses are rounded to a convenient amount (eg, 1/2 of 80 mg tablet).

Mechanical prosthetic heart valves: 6-20 mg/kg/day given as a single daily dose (used in combination with an oral anticoagulant in children who have systemic embolism

(Continued)

Aspirin *(Continued)*

despite adequate oral anticoagulation therapy (INR 2.5-3.5) and used in combination with low-dose anticoagulation (INR 2-3) and dipyridamole when full-dose oral anticoagulation is contraindicated)

Blalock-Taussig shunts: 3-5 mg/kg/day given as a single daily dose

Kawasaki disease: Oral: 80-100 mg/kg/day divided every 6 hours; monitor serum concentrations; after fever resolves: 3-5 mg/kg/day once daily; in patients without coronary artery abnormalities, give lower dose for at least 6-8 weeks or until ESR and platelet count are normal; in patients with coronary artery abnormalities, low-dose aspirin should be continued indefinitely

Antirheumatic: Oral: 60-100 mg/kg/day in divided doses every 4 hours

Adults:

Analgesic and antipyretic: Oral, rectal: 325-650 mg every 4-6 hours up to 4 g/day

Anti-inflammatory: Oral: Initial: 2.4-3.6 g/day in divided doses; usual maintenance: 3.6-5.4 g/day; monitor serum concentrations

Myocardial infarction prophylaxis: 75-325 mg/day; use of a lower aspirin dosage has been recommended in patients receiving ACE inhibitors

Acute myocardial infarction: 160-325 mg/day

CABG: 325 mg/day starting 6 hours following procedure

PTCA: Initial: 80-325 mg/day starting 2 hours before procedure; longer pretreatment durations (up to 24 hours) should be considered if lower dosages (80-100 mg) are used

Carotid endarterectomy: 81-325 mg/day preoperatively and daily thereafter

Acute stroke : 160-325 mg/day, initiated within 48 hours (in patients who are not candidates for thrombolytics and not receiving systemic anticoagulation)

Stroke prevention/TIA: 30-325 mg/day (dosages up to 1300 mg/day in 2-4 divided doses have been used in clinical trials)

Pre-eclampsia prevention (unlabeled use): 60-80 mg/day during gestational weeks 13-26 (patient selection criteria not established)

Dosing adjustment in renal impairment: Cl_{cr} <10 mL/minute: Avoid use.

Hemodialysis: Dialyzable (50% to 100%)

Dosing adjustment in hepatic disease: Avoid use in severe liver disease.

Dietary Considerations Take with food or large volume of water or milk to minimize GI upset.

Administration Do not crush sustained release or enteric coated tablet. Administer with food or a full glass of water to minimize GI distress

Reference Range Timing of serum samples: Peak levels usually occur 2 hours after ingestion. Salicylate serum concentrations correlate with the pharmacological actions and adverse effects observed. The serum salicylate concentration (mcg/mL) and the corresponding clinical correlations are as follows: See table.

Serum Salicylate: Clinical Correlations

Serum Salicylate Concentration (mcg/mL)	Desired Effects	Adverse Effects/Intoxication
~100	Antiplatelet Antipyresis Analgesia	GI intolerance and bleeding, hypersensitivity, hemostatic defects
150-300	Anti-inflammatory	Mild salicylism
250-400	Treatment of rheumatic fever	Nausea/vomiting, hyperventilation, salicylism, flushing, sweating, thirst, headache, diarrhea, and tachycardia
>400-500		Respiratory alkalosis, hemorrhage, excitement, confusion, asterixis, pulmonary edema, convulsions, tetany, metabolic acidosis, fever, coma, cardiovascular collapse, renal and respiratory failure

Test Interactions False-negative results for glucose oxidase urinary glucose tests (Clinistix®); false-positives using the cupric sulfate method (Clinitest®); also, interferes with Gerhardt test, VMA determination; 5-HIAA, xylose tolerance test and T_3 and T_4

Patient Information Watch for bleeding gums or any signs of GI bleeding; take with food or milk to minimize GI distress, notify physician if ringing in ears or persistent GI pain occurs; avoid other concurrent aspirin or salicylate-containing products

Nursing Implications Do not crush sustained release or enteric coated tablet

Dosage Forms

Caplet, buffered:

Ascriptin® Arthritis Pain: 325 mg [contains aluminum hydroxide, calcium carbonate, and magnesium hydroxide]

Ascriptin® Extra Strength: 500 mg [contains aluminum hydroxide, calcium carbonate, and magnesium hydroxide]

Gelcap:

Bayer® Aspirin: 325 mg

Bayer® Aspirin Extra Strength: 500 mg

Gum (Aspergum®): 227 mg

Suppository, rectal: 60 mg, 120 mg, 125 mg, 200 mg, 300 mg, 325 mg, 600 mg, 650 mg

Tablet: 325 mg, 500 mg

Aspercin: 325 mg

Aspercin Extra, Bayer® Aspirin Extra Strength: 500 mg

Bayer® Aspirin: 325 mg [film coated]

Tablet, buffered:

Ascriptin®: 325 mg [contains aluminum hydroxide, calcium carbonate, and magnesium hydroxide]

Bayer® Plus Extra Strength: 500 mg [contains calcium carbonate]

Bufferin®: 325 mg [contains citric acid]
Bufferin® Arthritis Strength, Bufferin® Extra Strength: 500 mg [contains citric acid]
Tablet, chewable: 81 mg
  Bayer® Aspirin Regimen Children's Chewable, St. Joseph® Pain Reliever: 81 mg
Tablet, controlled release (ZORprin®): 800 mg
Tablet, enteric coated: 81 mg, 162 mg, 325 mg, 500 mg, 650 mg, 975 mg
  Ascriptin® Enteric, Bayer® Aspirin Regimen Adult Low Strength, Ecotrin® Adult Low Strength, St. Joseph Pain Reliever: 81 mg
  Bayer® Aspirin Regimen Adult Low Strength with Calcium: 81 mg [contains calcium carbonate 250 mg]
  Bayer® Aspirin Regimen Regular Strength, Ecotrin®: 325 mg
  Easprin®: 975 mg
  Ecotrin® Maximum Strength: 500 mg
  Halfprin®: 81 mg, 162 mg
  Surexin 81™: 81 mg

♦ **Aspirin, Acetaminophen, and Caffeine** see Acetaminophen, Aspirin, and Caffeine on page 26
♦ **Aspirin and Carisoprodol** see Carisoprodol and Aspirin on page 229

Aspirin and Codeine (AS pir in & KOE deen)
Canadian Brand Names Coryphen® Codeine
Synonyms Codeine and Aspirin
Therapeutic Category Analgesic, Narcotic
Use Relief of mild to moderate pain
Restrictions C-III
Pregnancy Risk Factor D
Usual Dosage Oral:
  Children:
    Aspirin: 10 mg/kg/dose every 4 hours
    Codeine: 0.5-1 mg/kg/dose every 4 hours
  Adults: 1-2 tablets every 4-6 hours as needed for pain
  Dosing adjustment in renal impairment:
    Cl$_{cr}$ 10-50 mL/minute: Administer 75% of dose
    Cl$_{cr}$ <10 mL/minute: Avoid use
  Dosing interval in hepatic disease: Avoid use in severe liver disease
Additional Information Complete prescribing information for this medication should be consulted for additional detail.
Dosage Forms Tablet:
  #3: Aspirin 325 mg and codeine phosphate 30 mg
  #4: Aspirin 325 mg and codeine phosphate 60 mg

Aspirin and Extended-Release Dipyridamole
(AS pir in & ek STEN did ri LEES dye peer ID a mole)
U.S. Brand Names Aggrenox™
Canadian Brand Names Aggrenox®
Synonyms Aspirin and Extended-Release Dipyridamole; Dipyridamole and Aspirin
Therapeutic Category Antiplatelet Agent
Use Reduction in the risk of stroke in patients who have had transient ischemia of the brain or completed ischemic stroke due to thrombosis
Pregnancy Risk Factor B (dipyridamole); D (aspirin)
Pregnancy/Breast-Feeding Implications Aggrenox™ should be used in pregnancy only if the benefit justifies the potential risk to the fetus. It should not be used in the 3rd trimester of pregnancy.
Contraindications Hypersensitivity to dipyridamole, aspirin, or any component of the formulation; allergy to NSAIDs; patients with asthma, rhinitis, and nasal polyps; bleeding disorders (factor VII or IX deficiencies); children <16 years of age with viral infections; pregnancy (especially 3rd trimester)
Warnings/Precautions Patients who consume ≥3 alcoholic drinks per day are at risk of bleeding. Cautious use in patients with inherited or acquired bleeding disorders including those of liver disease or vitamin K deficiency. Watch for signs and symptoms of GI ulcers and bleeding. Avoid use in patients with active peptic ulcer disease. Discontinue use if dizziness, tinnitus, or impaired hearing occurs. Stop 1-2 weeks before elective surgical procedures to avoid bleeding. Use caution in the elderly who are at high risk for adverse events. Cautious use in patients with hypotension, patients with unstable angina, recent MI, and hepatic dysfunction. Avoid in patients with severe renal failure. Safety and efficacy in children have not been established.
Adverse Reactions
  >10%:
    Central nervous system: Headache (38%)
    Gastrointestinal: Dyspepsia, abdominal pain (18%), nausea (16%), diarrhea (13%)
  1% to 10%:
    Cardiovascular: Cardiac failure (2%)
    Central nervous system: Pain (6%), seizures (2%), fatigue (6%), malaise (2%), syncope (1%), amnesia (2%), confusion (1%), somnolence (1%)
    Dermatologic: Purpura (1%)
    Gastrointestinal: Vomiting (8%), bleeding (4%), rectal bleeding (2%), hemorrhoids (1%), hemorrhage (1%), anorexia (1%)
    Hematologic: Anemia (2%)
    Neuromuscular & skeletal: Back pain (5%), weakness (2%), arthralgia (6%), arthritis (2%), arthrosis (1%), myalgia (1%)
    Respiratory: Cough (2%), upper respiratory tract infections (1%), epistaxis (2%)
(Continued)

Aspirin and Extended-Release Dipyridamole *(Continued)*

<1% (Limited to important or life-threatening): Intracranial hemorrhage (0.6%), allergic reaction, coma, paresthesia, cerebral hemorrhage, subarachnoid hemorrhage, ulceration, deafness, arrhythmia, cholelithiasis, jaundice, uterine hemorrhage, bronchospasm, hemoptysis, pulmonary edema, pruritus, urticaria, renal failure, angina pectoris, cerebral edema, pancreatitis, Reye's syndrome, hematemesis, anaphylaxis, hepatitis, hepatic failure, rhabdomyolysis, prolonged PT time, disseminated intravascular coagulation, thrombocytopenia, stillbirths, lower weight infants, antepartum and postpartum bleeding, tachypnea, dyspnea, rash, alopecia, angioedema, Stevens-Johnson syndrome, interstitial nephritis, papillary necrosis, allergic vasculitis, anemia (aplastic), pancytopenia

Overdosage/Toxicology Symptoms of dipyridamole overdose might predominate because of the ratio of dipyridamole to aspirin. Symptoms may include hypotension and peripheral vasodilation. Treatment would include I.V. fluids and possibly vasopressors. Careful medical management is necessary.

Drug Interactions
Increased Effect/Toxicity: Refer to individual agents.
Decreased Effect: Refer to individual agents.

Ethanol/Nutrition/Herb Interactions Ethanol: Avoid ethanol (due to GI irritation).

Stability Store at 25°C (77°F); excursions permitted to 15°C to 30°C (59°F to 86°F); protect from excessive moisture

Mechanism of Action The antithrombotic action results from additive antiplatelet effects. Dipyridamole inhibits the uptake of adenosine into platelets, endothelial cells, and erythrocytes. Aspirin inhibits platelet aggregation by irreversible inhibition of platelet cyclooxygenase and thus inhibits the generation of thromboxane A2.

Pharmacodynamics/Kinetics
Aggrenox™:
Half-life elimination: Salicylic acid: 1.71 hours
Time to peak: 0.63 hours
Aspirin: See Aspirin monograph.
Dipyridamole:
Distribution: V_d: 92 L
Protein binding: 99%
Metabolism: Hepatic via conjugation with glucuronic acid
Half-life elimination: 13.6 hours
Time to peak: 2 hours
Excretion: Feces (95% as glucuronide metabolite); urine (5%)

Usual Dosage Adults: Oral: 1 capsule (dipyridamole 200 mg, aspirin 25 mg) twice daily.
Dosage adjustment in renal impairment: Avoid use in patients with severe renal dysfunction (Cl_{cr} <10 mL/minute). Studies have not been done in patients with renal impairment.
Dosage adjustment in hepatic impairment: Avoid use in patients with severe hepatic impairment; studies have not been done in patients with varying degrees of hepatic impairment
Elderly: Plasma concentrations were 40% higher, but specific dosage adjustments have not been recommended

Dietary Considerations May be taken with or without food.

Administration Capsule should be swallowed whole; do not crush or chew. May be given with or without food.

Monitoring Parameters Hemoglobin, hematocrit, signs or symptoms of bleeding, signs or symptoms of stroke or transient ischemic attack

Patient Information Swallow capsule whole without chewing or crushing; monitor for signs and symptoms of bleeding or another stroke or transient ischemic attack

Nursing Implications Monitor for signs and symptoms of bleeding or another stroke or transient ischemic attack

Dosage Forms Capsule: Dipyridamole (extended release) 200 mg and aspirin 25 mg

♦ **Aspirin and Hydrocodone** *see* Hydrocodone and Aspirin *on page 677*

Aspirin and Meprobamate *(AS pir in & me proe BA mate)*
U.S. Brand Names Equagesic®
Canadian Brand Names 292 MEP®
Synonyms Meprobamate and Aspirin
Therapeutic Category Skeletal Muscle Relaxant
Use Adjunct to treatment of skeletal muscular disease in patients exhibiting tension and/or anxiety
Restrictions C-IV
Pregnancy Risk Factor D
Usual Dosage Oral: 1 tablet 3-4 times/day
Additional Information Complete prescribing information for this medication should be consulted for additional detail.
Dosage Forms Tablet: Aspirin 325 mg and meprobamate 200 mg

♦ **Aspirin and Methocarbamol** *see* Methocarbamol and Aspirin *on page 884*

♦ **Aspirin and Oxycodone** *see* Oxycodone and Aspirin *on page 1026*

♦ **Aspirin® Backache (Can)** *see* Methocarbamol and Aspirin *on page 884*

♦ **Aspirin, Caffeine and Acetaminophen** *see* Acetaminophen, Aspirin, and Caffeine *on page 26*

♦ **Aspirin, Carisoprodol, and Codeine** *see* Carisoprodol, Aspirin, and Codeine *on page 230*

♦ **Aspirin Free Anacin® Maximum Strength [OTC]** *see* Acetaminophen *on page 22*

♦ **Aspirin, Orphenadrine, and Caffeine** *see* Orphenadrine, Aspirin, and Caffeine *on page 1015*

♦ **Assessment of Liver Function** *see page 1464*

♦ **Assessment of Renal Function** *see page 1465*

- **Astelin®** *see Azelastine on page 137*
- **Asthma** *see page 1645*
- **AsthmaHaler®** *see Epinephrine on page 470*
- **Astramorph™ PF** *see Morphine Sulfate on page 936*
- **Atacand®** *see Candesartan on page 214*
- **Atacand HCT™** *see Candesartan and Hydrochlorothiazide on page 215*
- **Atapryl®** *see Selegiline on page 1228*
- **Atarax®** *see HydrOXYzine on page 691*
- **Atasol® (Can)** *see Acetaminophen on page 22*

Atenolol (a TEN oh lole)

Related Information
Beta-Blockers Comparison *on page 1491*
Hypertension *on page 1675*

U.S. Brand Names Tenormin®

Canadian Brand Names Apo®-Atenol; Gen-Atenolol; Novo-Atenol; Nu-Atenol; PMS-Atenolol; Rhoxal-atenolol; Scheinpharm Atenolol; Tenolin; Tenormin®

Therapeutic Category Antianginal Agent; Antihypertensive Agent; Beta-Adrenergic Blocker

Use Treatment of hypertension, alone or in combination with other agents; management of angina pectoris, postmyocardial infarction patients

Unlabeled/Investigational Use Acute ethanol withdrawal, supraventricular and ventricular arrhythmias, and migraine headache prophylaxis

Pregnancy Risk Factor D

Pregnancy/Breast-Feeding Implications
Clinical effects on the fetus: Crosses the placenta; persistent beta-blockade, bradycardia, IUGR; IUGR probably related to maternal hypertension.
Breast-feeding/lactation: Crosses into breast milk.
Clinical effects on the infant: Symptoms have been reported of beta-blockade including cyanosis, hypothermia, bradycardia.

Contraindications Hypersensitivity to atenolol or any component of the formulation; sinus bradycardia; sinus node dysfunction; heart block greater than first-degree (except in patients with a functioning artificial pacemaker); cardiogenic shock; uncompensated cardiac failure; pulmonary edema; pregnancy

Warnings/Precautions Safety and efficacy in children have not been established. Administer cautiously in compensated heart failure and monitor for a worsening of the condition (efficacy of atenolol in heart failure has not been established). Avoid abrupt discontinuation in patients with a history of CAD; slowly wean while monitoring for signs and symptoms of ischemia. Use caution with concurrent use of beta-blockers and either verapamil or diltiazem; bradycardia or heart block can occur. Avoid concurrent I.V. use of both agents. Beta-blockers should be avoided in patients with bronchospastic disease (asthma) and peripheral vascular disease (may aggravate arterial insufficiency). Atenolol, with B1 selectivity, has been used cautiously in bronchospastic disease with close monitoring. Use cautiously in diabetics - may mask hypoglycemic symptoms. May mask signs of thyrotoxicosis. May cause fetal harm when administered in pregnancy. Use cautiously in the renally impaired (dosage adjustment required). Use care with anesthetic agents which decrease myocardial function. Caution in myasthenia gravis.

Adverse Reactions
1% to 10%:
Cardiovascular: Persistent bradycardia, hypotension, chest pain, edema, heart failure, second- or third-degree AV block, Raynaud's phenomenon
Central nervous system: Dizziness, fatigue, insomnia, lethargy, confusion, mental impairment, depression, headache, nightmares
Gastrointestinal: Constipation, diarrhea, nausea
Genitourinary: Impotence
Miscellaneous: Cold extremities
<1% (Limited to important or life-threatening): Alopecia, dyspnea (especially with large doses), elevated liver enzymes, hallucinations, impotence, lupus syndrome, Peyronie's disease, positive ANA, psoriaform rash, psychosis, thrombocytopenia, wheezing

Overdosage/Toxicology Symptoms include cardiac disturbances, CNS toxicity, bronchospasm, hypoglycemia and hyperkalemia. The most common cardiac symptoms include hypotension and bradycardia. Atrioventricular block, intraventricular conduction disturbances, cardiogenic shock, and asystole may occur with severe overdose, especially with membrane-depressant drugs (eg, propranolol). CNS effects include convulsions, coma, and respiratory arrest (commonly seen with propranolol and other membrane-depressant and lipid-soluble drugs). Treatment is symptomatic for seizures, hypotension, hyperkalemia, and hypoglycemia. Bradycardia and hypotension resistant to atropine, isoproterenol, or pacing may respond to glucagon. Wide QRS defects caused the membrane-depressant poisoning may respond to hypertonic sodium bicarbonate. Repeat-dose charcoal, hemoperfusion, or hemodialysis may be helpful in removal of only those beta-blockers with a small V_d, long half-life, or low intrinsic clearance (acebutolol, atenolol, nadolol, sotalol).

Drug Interactions
Increased Effect/Toxicity: Atenolol may increase the effects of other drugs which slow AV conduction (digoxin, verapamil, diltiazem), alpha-blockers (prazosin, terazosin), and alpha-adrenergic stimulants (epinephrine, phenylephrine). Atenolol may mask the tachycardia from hypoglycemia caused by insulin and oral hypoglycemics. In patients receiving concurrent therapy, the risk of hypertensive crisis is increased when either clonidine or the beta-blocker is withdrawn. Reserpine has been shown to enhance the effect of atenolol. Beta-blockers may increase the action or levels of ethanol, disopyramide, nondepolarizing muscle relaxants, and theophylline although the effects are difficult to predict.

Decreased Effect: Decreased effect of atenolol with aluminum salts, barbiturates, calcium salts, cholestyramine, colestipol, NSAIDs, penicillins (ampicillin), rifampin, salicylates, and sulfinpyrazone due to decreased bioavailability and plasma levels. Beta-blockers may decrease the effect of sulfonylureas.

(Continued)

Atenolol *(Continued)*

Ethanol/Nutrition/Herb Interactions
Food: Atenolol serum concentrations may be decreased if taken with food.

Herb/Nutraceutical: Avoid dong quai if using for hypertension (has estrogenic activity). Avoid ephedra, yohimbe, ginseng (may worsen hypertension). Avoid garlic (may have increased antihypertensive effect).

Stability Protect from light

Mechanism of Action
Competitively blocks response to beta-adrenergic stimulation, selectively blocks beta$_1$-receptors with little or no effect on beta$_2$-receptors except at high doses

Pharmacodynamics/Kinetics
Onset of action: Peak effect: Oral: 2-4 hours

Duration: Normal renal function: 12-24 hours

Absorption: Incomplete

Distribution: Low lipophilicity; does not cross blood-brain barrier

Protein binding: 3% to 15%

Metabolism: Limited hepatic

Half-life elimination: Beta:

    Neonates: ≤35 hours; Mean: 16 hours

    Children: 4.6 hours; children >10 years may have longer half-life (>5 hours) compared to children 5-10 years (<5 hours)

    Adults: Normal renal function: 6-9 hours, longer with renal impairment; End-stage renal disease: 15-35 hours

Excretion: Feces (50%); urine (40% as unchanged drug)

Usual Dosage
Oral:

    Children: 0.8-1 mg/kg/dose given daily; range of 0.8-1.5 mg/kg/day; maximum dose: 2 mg/kg/day

    Adults:

        Hypertension: 50 mg once daily, may increase to 100 mg/day. Doses >100 mg are unlikely to produce any further benefit.

        Angina pectoris: 50 mg once daily, may increase to 100 mg/day. Some patients may require 200 mg/day.

        Postmyocardial infarction: Follow I.V. dose with 100 mg/day or 50 mg twice daily for 6-9 days postmyocardial infarction.

I.V.:

    Hypertension: Dosages of 1.25-5 mg every 6-12 hours have been used in short-term management of patients unable to take oral enteral beta-blockers

    Postmyocardial infarction: Early treatment: 5 mg slow I.V. over 5 minutes; may repeat in 10 minutes. If both doses are tolerated, may start oral atenolol 50 mg every 12 hours or 100 mg/day for 6-9 days postmyocardial infarction.

Dosing interval for oral atenolol in renal impairment:

    Cl$_{cr}$ 15-35 mL/minute: Administer 50 mg/day maximum.

    Cl$_{cr}$ <15 mL/minute: Administer 50 mg every other day maximum.

Hemodialysis: Moderately dialyzable (20% to 50%) via hemodialysis; administer dose postdialysis or administer 25-50 mg supplemental dose.

Peritoneal dialysis: Elimination is not enhanced; supplemental dose is not necessary.

Dietary Considerations May be taken without regard to meals.

Administration
Administer I.V. at 1 mg/minute; intravenous administration requires a cardiac monitor and blood pressure monitor

Monitoring Parameters
Monitor blood pressure, apical and radial pulses, fluid I & O, daily weight, respirations, and circulation in extremities before and during therapy

Test Interactions ↑ glucose; ↓ HDL

Patient Information
Adhere to dosage regimen; watch for postural hypotension; **abrupt withdrawal of the drug should be avoided**; take at the same time each day; may mask diabetes symptoms; notify physician if any adverse effects occur; use with caution while driving or performing tasks requiring alertness; may be taken without regard to meals

Nursing Implications
Modify dosage in patients with renal insufficiency; administer by slow I.V. injection at a rate not to exceed 1 mg/minute; the injection can be administered undiluted or diluted with a compatible I.V. solution

Monitor blood pressure, heart rate, fluid I & O, daily weight, respiratory rate

Dosage Forms
Injection, solution: 0.5 mg/mL (10 mL)

Tablet: 25 mg, 50 mg, 100 mg

Extemporaneous Preparations
A 2 mg/mL atenolol oral liquid compounded from tablets and a commercially available oral diluent was found to be stable for up to 40 days when stored at 5°C or 25°C.

Garner SS, Wiest DB, and Reynolds ER, "Stability of Atenolol in an Extemporaneously Compounded Oral Liquid," *Am J Hosp Pharm*, 1994, 51(4):508-11.

Atenolol and Chlorthalidone *(a TEN oh lole & klor THAL i done)*

U.S. Brand Names Tenoretic®

Canadian Brand Names Tenoretic®

Synonyms Chlorthalidone and Atenolol

Therapeutic Category Antihypertensive Agent, Combination

Use Treatment of hypertension with a cardioselective beta-blocker and a diuretic

Pregnancy Risk Factor D

Usual Dosage Adults: Oral: Initial (based on atenolol component): 50 mg once daily, then individualize dose until optimal dose is achieved

Additional Information Complete prescribing information for this medication should be consulted for additional detail.

Dosage Forms
Tablet:
  50: Atenolol 50 mg and chlorthalidone 25 mg
  100: Atenolol 100 mg and chlorthalidone 25 mg

♦ **ATG** *see* Antithymocyte Globulin (Rabbit) *on page 108*
♦ **ATG** *see* Lymphocyte Immune Globulin *on page 829*
♦ **Atgam**® *see* Lymphocyte Immune Globulin *on page 829*
♦ **AT III** *see* Antithrombin III *on page 107*
♦ **Ativan**® *see* Lorazepam *on page 821*
♦ **Atolone**® *see* Triamcinolone *on page 1366*

Atorvastatin (a TORE va sta tin)
Related Information
Antacid Drug Interactions *on page 1477*
Hyperlipidemia Management *on page 1670*
Lipid-Lowering Agents *on page 1505*
U.S. Brand Names Lipitor®
Canadian Brand Names Lipitor™
Therapeutic Category Antilipemic Agent, HMG-CoA Reductase Inhibitor; HMG-CoA Reductase Inhibitor
Use Adjunct to diet for the reduction of elevated total and LDL cholesterol, apolipoprotein B, and triglyceride levels in patients with hypercholesterolemia (types IIA, IIB, and IIC); adjunctive therapy to diet for treatment of elevated serum triglyceride levels (type IV); treatment of primary dysbetalipoproteinemia (type III) in patients who do not respond adequately to diet; to increase HDL cholesterol in patients with primary hypercholesterolemia (heterozygous familial and nonfamilial) and mixed dyslipidemia (Fredrickson types IIa and IIb). Also may be used in hypercholesterolemic patients without clinically evident heart disease to reduce the risk of myocardial infarction, to reduce the risk for revascularization, and reduce the risk of death due to cardiovascular causes
Pregnancy Risk Factor X
Contraindications Hypersensitivity to atorvastatin or any component of the formulation; active liver disease; unexplained persistent elevations of serum transaminases; pregnancy
Warnings/Precautions Liver function must be monitored by periodic laboratory assessment. Rhabdomyolysis with acute renal failure has occurred. Risk is increased with concurrent use of clarithromycin, danazol, diltiazem, fluvoxamine, indinavir, nefazodone, nelfinavir, ritonavir, verapamil, troleandomycin, cyclosporine, fibric acid derivatives, erythromycin, niacin, or azole antifungals. Weigh the risk versus benefit when combining any of these drugs with atorvastatin. Discontinue in any patient experiencing an acute or serious condition predisposing to renal failure secondary to rhabdomyolysis.
Adverse Reactions
>10%: Central nervous system: Headache (3% to 17%)
2% to 10%:
  Cardiovascular: Chest pain, peripheral edema
  Central nervous system: Weakness (0% to 4%), insomnia, dizziness
  Dermatologic: Rash (1% to 4%)
  Gastrointestinal: Abdominal pain (0% to 4%), constipation (0% to 3%), diarrhea (0% to 4%), dyspepsia (1% to 3%), flatulence (1% to 3%), nausea
  Genitourinary: Urinary tract infection
  Neuromuscular & skeletal: Arthralgia (0% to 5%), myalgia (0% to 6%), back pain (0% to 4%), arthritis
  Respiratory: Sinusitis (0% to 6%), pharyngitis (0% to 3%), bronchitis, rhinitis
  Miscellaneous: Infection (2% to 10%), flu-like syndrome (0% to 3%), allergic reaction (0% to 3%)
<2% (Limited to important or life-threatening): Alopecia, anaphylaxis, angina, angioneurotic edema, arrhythmia, bullous rashes, cholestatic jaundice, deafness, dyspnea, erythema multiforme, esophagitis, facial paralysis, glaucoma gout, hepatitis, hyperkinesias, impotence, migraine, myasthenia, myopathy, myositis, nephritis, pancreatitis, paresthesia, peripheral neuropathy, petechiae, photosensitivity, postural hypotension, pruritus, rectal hemorrhage, rhabdomyolysis, somnolence, Stevens-Johnson syndrome, syncope, tendinous contracture, thrombocytopenia, tinnitus, torticollis, toxic epidermal necrolysis, urticaria, vaginal hemorrhage, vomiting
Overdosage/Toxicology Few symptoms of overdose anticipated. Treatment is supportive.
Drug Interactions
Cytochrome P450 Effect: CYP3A3/4 enzyme substrate
Increased Effect/Toxicity: Inhibitors of CYP3A3/4 (amprenavir, clarithromycin, cyclosporine, diltiazem, fluvoxamine, erythromycin, fluconazole, indinavir, itraconazole, ketoconazole, miconazole, nefazodone, nelfinavir, ritonavir, troleandomycin, and verapamil) may increase atorvastatin blood levels and may increase the risk of atorvastatin-induced myopathy and rhabdomyolysis. The risk of myopathy and rhabdomyolysis due to concurrent use of a CYP3A3/4 inhibitor with atorvastatin is probably less than lovastatin or simvastatin. Cyclosporine, clofibrate, fenofibrate, gemfibrozil, and niacin also may increase the risk of myopathy and rhabdomyolysis. The effect/toxicity of levothyroxine may be increased by atorvastatin. Levels of digoxin and ethinyl estradiol may be increased by atorvastatin.
Decreased Effect: Colestipol, antacids decreased plasma concentrations but effect on LDL cholesterol was not altered. Cholestyramine may decrease absorption of atorvastatin when administered concurrently.
Ethanol/Nutrition/Herb Interactions
Food: Atorvastatin serum concentrations may be increased by grapefruit juice; avoid concurrent use.
Herb/Nutraceutical: St John's wort may decrease atorvastatin levels.
Mechanism of Action Inhibitor of 3-hydroxy-3-methylglutaryl coenzyme A (HMG-CoA) reductase, the rate limiting enzyme in cholesterol synthesis (reduces the production of mevalonic
(Continued)

Atorvastatin (Continued)

acid from HMG-CoA); this then results in a compensatory increase in the expression of LDL receptors on hepatocyte membranes and a stimulation of LDL catabolism

Pharmacodynamics/Kinetics
Onset of action: Initial changes: 3-5 days; Maximal reduction in plasma cholesterol and triglycerides: 2 weeks
Absorption: Rapid
Protein binding: 98%
Metabolism: Undergoes enterohepatic recycling; not a prodrug; metabolized to active ortho- and parahydroxylated derivates and an inactive beta-oxidation product
Half-life elimination: Parent drug: 14 hours
Time to peak, serum: 1-2 hours
Excretion: Urine (2% as unchanged drug)

Usual Dosage Adults: Oral: Initial: 10 mg once daily, titrate up to 80 mg/day if needed
Dosing adjustment in renal impairment: No dosage adjustment is necessary.
Dosing adjustment in hepatic impairment: Do not use in active liver disease.

Dietary Considerations Before initiation of therapy, patients should be placed on a standard cholesterol-lowering diet for 3-6 months and the diet should be continued during drug therapy.

Monitoring Parameters Lipid levels after 2-4 weeks; LFTs, CPK

It is recommended that liver function tests (LFTs) be performed prior to and at 12 weeks following both the initiation of therapy and any elevation in dose, and periodically (eg, semiannually) thereafter

Patient Information May take with food if desired; may take without regard to time of day
Dosage Forms Tablet: 10 mg, 20 mg, 40 mg, 80 mg

Atovaquone (a TOE va kwone)

Related Information
Malaria Treatment on page 1607
U.S. Brand Names Mepron™
Canadian Brand Names Mepron®
Therapeutic Category Antiprotozoal
Use Acute oral treatment of mild to moderate *Pneumocystis carinii* pneumonia (PCP) in patients who are intolerant to co-trimoxazole; prophylaxis of PCP in patients intolerant to co-trimoxazole; treatment/suppression of *Toxoplasma gondii* encephalitis, primary prophylaxis of HIV-infected persons at high risk for developing *Toxoplasma gondii* encephalitis
Pregnancy Risk Factor C
Contraindications Life-threatening allergic reaction to the drug or formulation
Warnings/Precautions Has only been indicated in mild to moderate PCP; use with caution in elderly patients due to potentially impaired renal, hepatic, and cardiac function
Adverse Reactions
>10%:
Central nervous system: Headache, fever, insomnia, anxiety
Dermatologic: Rash
Gastrointestinal: Nausea, diarrhea, vomiting
Respiratory: Cough
1% to 10%:
Central nervous system: Dizziness
Dermatologic: Pruritus
Endocrine & metabolic: Hypoglycemia, hyponatremia
Gastrointestinal: Abdominal pain, constipation, anorexia, heartburn
Hematologic: Anemia, neutropenia, leukopenia
Hepatic: Elevated amylase and liver enzymes
Neuromuscular & skeletal: Weakness
Renal: Elevated BUN/creatinine
Respiratory: Cough
Miscellaneous: Oral *Monilia*

Drug Interactions
Increased Effect/Toxicity: Possible increased toxicity with other highly protein-bound drugs.
Decreased Effect: Rifamycins (rifampin) used concurrently decrease the steady-state plasma concentrations of atovaquone.

Ethanol/Nutrition/Herb Interactions Food: Ingestion with a fatty meals increases absorption.
Stability Do not freeze
Mechanism of Action Has not been fully elucidated; may inhibit electron transport in mitochondria inhibiting metabolic enzymes

Pharmacodynamics/Kinetics
Absorption: Significantly increased with a high-fat meal
Distribution: 3.5 L/kg
Protein binding: >99%
Metabolism: Enterohepatic cycling
Bioavailability: Tablet: 23%; Suspension: 47%
Half-life elimination: 2-3 days
Excretion: Feces (94% as unchanged drug)

Usual Dosage Oral: Adolescents 13-16 years and Adults:
Prevention of PCP: 1500 mg once daily with food
Treatment of mild to moderate PCP: 750 mg twice daily with food for 21 days

Patient Information Take only prescribed dose; take each dose with a meal, preferably one with high fat content
Nursing Implications Notify physician if patient is unable to eat significant amounts of food on an ongoing basis
Dosage Forms Suspension, oral: 750 mg/5 mL (5 mL, 210 mL) [citrus flavor]

Atovaquone and Proguanil (a TOE va kwone & pro GWA nil)

U.S. Brand Names Malarone™

Canadian Brand Names Malarone™

Synonyms Proguanil and Atovaquone

Therapeutic Category Antimalarial Agent

Use Prevention or treatment of acute, uncomplicated *P. falciparum* malaria

Pregnancy Risk Factor C

Pregnancy/Breast-Feeding Implications Use in pregnant women only if the potential benefit outweighs the possible risk to the fetus. Because falciparum malaria can cause maternal death and fetal loss, pregnant women traveling to malaria-endemic areas must use personal protection against mosquito bites. It is unknown if atovaquone is excreted in human milk, proguanil is excreted in small quantities; use with caution in nursing women.

Contraindications Hypersensitivity to atovaquone, proguanil, or any component of the formulation

Warnings/Precautions Not indicated for severe or complicated malaria. Absorption of atovaquone may be decreased in patients who have diarrhea or vomiting; monitor closely and consider use of an antiemetic. If severe, consider use of an alternative antimalarial. Administer with caution to patients with pre-existing renal disease. Not for use in patients <11 kg. Delayed cases of *P. falciparum* malaria may occur after stopping prophylaxis. Recrudescent infections or infections following prophylaxis with this agent should be treated with an alternative agent(s).

Adverse Reactions The following adverse reactions were reported in ≥5% of adults taking atovaquone/proguanil in treatment doses.

>10%: Gastrointestinal: Abdominal pain (17%), nausea (12%), vomiting (12% adults, 10% to 13% children)

1% to 10%:
Central nervous system: Headache (10%), dizziness (5%)
Dermatologic: Pruritus (6% children)
Gastrointestinal: Diarrhea (8%), anorexia (5%)
Neuromuscular & skeletal: Weakness (8%)

Adverse reactions reported in placebo-controlled clinical trials when used for prophylaxis. In general, reactions were similar to those seen with placebo:

>10%:
Central nervous system: Headache (22% adults, 19% children)
Gastrointestinal: Abdominal pain (33% children)
Neuromuscular & skeletal: Myalgia (12% adults)

1% to 10%:
Central nervous system: Fever (5% adults, 6% children)
Gastrointestinal: Abdominal pain (9% adults), diarrhea (6% adults, 2% children), dyspepsia (3% adults), gastritis (3% adults), vomiting (1% adults, 7% children)
Neuromuscular & skeletal: Back pain (8% adults)
Respiratory: Upper respiratory tract infection (8% adults), cough (6% adults, 9% children)
Miscellaneous: Flu-like syndrome (2% adults, 9% children)

In addition, 54% of adults in the placebo-controlled trials reported any adverse event (65% for placebo) and 60% of children reported adverse events (62% for placebo).

Case report: Anaphylaxis

Overdosage/Toxicology

Atovaquone: Overdoses of up to 31,500 mg have been reported. Rash has been reported as well as methemoglobinemia in one patient also taking dapsone. There is no known antidote and it is unknown if it is dialyzable.

Proguanil: Single doses of 1500 mg and 700 mg twice daily for two weeks have been reported without toxicity. Reversible hair loss, scaling of skin, reversible aphthous ulceration, and hematologic side effects have occurred. Epigastric discomfort and vomiting would also be expected. There have been no reported overdoses with the atovaquone/proguanil combination.

Drug Interactions

Cytochrome P450 Effect: Proguanil: CYP2C19 enzyme substrate

Decreased Effect: Metoclopramide decreases bioavailability of atovaquone. Rifampin decreases atovaquone levels by 50%. Tetracycline decreases plasma concentrations of atovaquone by 40%.

Ethanol/Nutrition/Herb Interactions Food: Atovaquone taken with dietary fat increases the rate and extent of absorption.

Stability Store tablets at 25°C (77°F)

Mechanism of Action

Atovaquone: Selectively inhibits parasite mitochondrial electron transport.

Proguanil: The metabolite cycloguanil inhibits dihydrofolate reductase, disrupting deoxythymidylate synthesis. Together, atovaquone/cycloguanil affect the erythrocytic and exoerythrocytic stages of development.

Pharmacodynamics/Kinetics

Atovaquone: See Atovaquone monograph.

Proguanil:
Absorption: Extensive
Distribution: 42 L/kg
Protein binding: 75%
Metabolism: Hepatic to active metabolite, cycloguanil (via CYP2C19) and 4-chlorophenylbiguanide
Half-life elimination: 12-21 hours
Excretion: Urine (40% to 60%)

(Continued)

Atovaquone and Proguanil *(Continued)*

Usual Dosage Oral (doses given in mg of atovaquone and proguanil):
  Children (dosage based on body weight):
    Prevention of malaria: Start 1-2 days prior to entering a malaria-endemic area, continue throughout the stay and for 7 days after returning. Take as a single dose, once daily.
      11-20 kg: Atovaquone/proguanil 62.5 mg/25 mg
      21-30 kg: Atovaquone/proguanil 125 mg/50 mg
      31-40 kg: Atovaquone/proguanil 187.5 mg/75 mg
      >40 kg: Atovaquone/proguanil 250 mg/100 mg
    Treatment of acute malaria: Take as a single dose, once daily for 3 consecutive days.
      11-20 kg: Atovaquone/proguanil 250 mg/100 mg
      21-30 kg: Atovaquone/proguanil 500 mg/200 mg
      31-40 kg: Atovaquone/proguanil 750 mg/300 mg
      >40 kg: Atovaquone/proguanil 1 g/400 mg
  Adults:
    Prevention of malaria: Atovaquone/proguanil 250 mg/100 mg once daily; start 1-2 days prior to entering a malaria-endemic area, continue throughout the stay and for 7 days after returning
    Treatment of acute malaria: Atovaquone/proguanil 1 g/400 mg as a single dose, once daily for 3 consecutive days
  Dosage adjustment in renal impairment: No information available, use with caution.
  Dosage adjustment in hepatic impairment: No information available
  Elderly: Use with caution due to possible decrease in renal and hepatic function, as well as possible decreases in cardiac function, concomitant diseases, or other drug therapy.
Dietary Considerations Must be taken with food or a milky drink.
Administration Dose should be given at the same time each day with food or a milky drink. If vomiting occurs within 1 hour of administration, repeat the dose.
Patient Information This medication is used to prevent or to treat malaria. It should be taken at the same time each day with food or a milky drink. If vomiting occurs within 1 hour of taking your dose, you may repeat the dose. Wear protective clothing and use insect repellents and bednets to help prevent malaria exposure. Notify your prescriber if you develop a fever after returning from or while visiting a malaria-endemic area.
Nursing Implications Give with food or a milky drink. If patient vomits within 1 hour of administration, repeat the dose.
Dosage Forms
  Tablet: Atovaquone 250 mg and proguanil hydrochloride 100 mg
  Tablet, pediatric: Atovaquone 62.5 mg and proguanil hydrochloride 25 mg

Atracurium *(a tra KYOO ree um)*

Related Information
  Neuromuscular Blocking Agents Comparison *on page 1508*
U.S. Brand Names Tracrium®
Synonyms Atracurium Besylate
Therapeutic Category Neuromuscular Blocker Agent, Nondepolarizing; Skeletal Muscle Relaxant
Use Adjunct to general anesthesia to facilitate endotracheal intubation and to relax skeletal muscles during surgery; to facilitate mechanical ventilation in ICU patients; does not relieve pain or produce sedation
Pregnancy Risk Factor C
Contraindications Hypersensitivity to atracurium besylate or any component of the formulation
Warnings/Precautions Reduce initial dosage and inject slowly (over 1-2 minutes) in patients in whom substantial histamine release would be potentially hazardous (eg, patients with clinically important cardiovascular disease); maintenance of an adequate airway and respiratory support is critical; certain clinical conditions may result in potentiation or antagonism of neuromuscular blockade:
    Potentiation: Electrolyte abnormalities, severe hyponatremia, severe hypocalcemia, severe hypokalemia, hypermagnesemia, neuromuscular diseases, acidosis, acute intermittent porphyria, renal failure, hepatic failure
    Antagonism: Alkalosis, hypercalcemia, demyelinating lesions, peripheral neuropathies, diabetes mellitus

  Increased sensitivity in patients with myasthenia gravis, Eaton-Lambert syndrome; resistance in burn patients (>30% of body) for period of 5-70 days postinjury; resistance in patients with muscle trauma, denervation, immobilization, infection, chronic treatment with atracurium. Bradycardia may be more common with atracurium than with other neuromuscular blocking agents since it has no clinically significant effects on heart rate to counteract the bradycardia produced by anesthetics.
Adverse Reactions Mild, rare, and generally suggestive of histamine release
  1% to 10%: Cardiovascular: Bradycardia, flushing, hypotension, tachycardia
  <1%: Bronchial secretions, erythema, itching, urticaria, wheezing
  In the ICU setting, reports of prolonged paralysis and generalized myopathy following discontinuation of agent (may be minimized by appropriately monitoring degree of blockade)

  Causes of prolonged neuromuscular blockade:
    Excessive drug administration
    Cumulative drug effect, decreased metabolism/excretion (hepatic and/or renal impairment)
    Accumulation of active metabolites
    Electrolyte imbalance (hypokalemia, hypocalcemia, hypermagnesemia, hypernatremia)
    Hypothermia
Overdosage/Toxicology Symptoms include respiratory depression and cardiovascular collapse. Neostigmine 1-3 mg slow I.V. push in adults (0.5 mg in children) antagonizes the neuromuscular blockade, and should be administered with or immediately after atropine 1-1.5 mg I.V. push (adults). This may be especially useful in the presence of bradycardia.

Drug Interactions

Increased Effect/Toxicity: Increased effects are possible with aminoglycosides, beta-blockers, clindamycin, calcium channel blockers, halogenated anesthetics, imipenem, ketamine, lidocaine, loop diuretics (furosemide), macrolides (case reports), magnesium sulfate, procainamide, quinidine, quinolones, tetracyclines, and vancomycin. May increase risk of myopathy when used with high- dose corticosteroids for extended periods.

Decreased Effect: Effect of nondepolarizing neuromuscular blockers may be reduced by carbamazepine (chronic use), corticosteroids (also associated with myopathy - see increased effect), phenytoin (chronic use), sympathomimetics, and theophylline.

Stability Refrigerate; unstable in alkaline solutions; **compatible** with D_5W, D_5NS, and NS; do not dilute in LR

Mechanism of Action Blocks neural transmission at the myoneural junction by binding with cholinergic receptor sites

Pharmacodynamics/Kinetics

Onset of action: 2-3 minutes (dose dependent)

Duration: Recovery begins in 20-35 minutes following initial dose of 0.4-0.5 mg/kg under balanced anesthesia; recovery to 95% of control takes 60-70 minutes

Metabolism: Undergoes ester hydrolysis and Hofmann elimination (nonbiologic process independent of renal, hepatic, or enzymatic function); metabolites have no neuromuscular blocking properties; laudanosine, a product of Hofmann elimination, is a CNS stimulant and can accumulate (via prolonged use in ICU patients (no documented evidence of CNS excitation in patients with prolonged administration)

Half-life elimination: Biphasic: Adults: Initial (distribution): 2 minutes; Terminal: 20 minutes

Usual Dosage I.V. (not to be used I.M.): Dose to effect; doses will vary due to interpatient variability; use ideal body weight for obese patients

Children 1 month to 2 years: Initial: 0.3-0.5 mg/kg followed by 0.25 mg/kg maintenance doses as needed to maintain neuromuscular blockade

Children >2 years to Adults: 0.4-0.5 mg/kg, then 0.08-0.1 mg/kg 20-45 minutes after initial dose to maintain neuromuscular block, followed by repeat doses of 0.08-0.1 mg/kg at 15- to 25-minute intervals

Initial dose after succinylcholine for intubation (balanced anesthesia): Adults: 0.2-0.4 mg/kg

Pretreatment/priming: 10% of intubating dose given 3-5 minutes before initial dose

Continuous infusion:

Surgery: Initial: 9-10 mcg/kg/minute at initial signs of recovery from bolus dose; block usually maintained by a rate of 5-9 mcg/kg/minute under balanced anesthesia

ICU: Block usually maintained by rate of 11-13 mcg/kg/minute (rates for pediatric patients may be higher)

See table.

Atracurium Besylate Infusion Chart

Drug Delivery Rate (mcg/kg/min)	Infusion Rate (mL/kg/min) 0.2 mg/mL (20 mg/100 mL)	Infusion Rate (mL/kg/min) 0.5 mg/mL (50 mg/100 mL)
5	0.025	0.01
6	0.03	0.012
7	0.035	0.014
8	0.04	0.016
9	0.045	0.018
10	0.05	0.02

Dosage adjustment for hepatic or renal impairment is not necessary

Administration May be given undiluted as a bolus injection; not for I.M. injection due to tissue irritation; administration via infusion requires the use of an infusion pump; use infusion solutions within 24 hours of preparation

Monitoring Parameters Vital signs (heart rate, blood pressure, respiratory rate); degree of muscle relaxation (via peripheral nerve stimulator and presence of spontaneous movement); renal function (serum creatinine, BUN) and liver function when in ICU

Patient Information May be difficult to talk because of head and neck muscle blockade

Nursing Implications Not for I.M. injection due to tissue irritation

Additional Information Atracurium is classified as an intermediate-duration neuromuscular-blocking agent. It does not appear to have a cumulative effect on the duration of blockade. It does not relieve pain or produce sedation.

Dosage Forms

Injection, as besylate: 10 mg/mL (5 mL, 10 mL)

Injection, as besylate [preservative free]: 10 mg/mL (5 mL)

♦ **Atracurium Besylate** see Atracurium on page 130

♦ **Atromid-S®** see Clofibrate on page 313

Atropine (A troe peen)

Related Information

Adult ACLS Algorithms on page 1632

Cycloplegic Mydriatics Comparison on page 1498

Pediatric ALS Algorithms on page 1628

U.S. Brand Names Atropine-Care®; Atropisol®; Isopto® Atropine; Sal-Tropine™

Canadian Brand Names Atropisol®; Isopto® Atropine

Synonyms Atropine Sulfate

Therapeutic Category Anticholinergic Agent; Anticholinergic Agent, Ophthalmic; Antidote, Organophosphate Poisoning; Antispasmodic Agent, Gastrointestinal; Bronchodilator; Ophthalmic Agent, Mydriatic

(Continued)

ATROPINE

Atropine *(Continued)*

Use Preoperative medication to inhibit salivation and secretions; treatment of symptomatic sinus bradycardia; antidote for organophosphate pesticide poisoning; to produce mydriasis and cycloplegia for examination of the retina and optic disc and accurate measurement of refractive errors; uveitis; AV block (nodal level); ventricular asystole; treatment of GI disorders (eg, peptic ulcer disease, irritable bowel syndrome, hypermotility of colon)

Pregnancy Risk Factor C

Contraindications Hypersensitivity to atropine or any component of the formulation; narrow-angle glaucoma; adhesions between the iris and lens; tachycardia; unstable cardiovascular status in acute hemorrhage; obstructive GI disease; paralytic ileus; intestinal atony of the elderly or debilitated patient; severe ulcerative colitis; toxic megacolon complicating ulcerative colitis; hepatic disease; obstructive uropathy; renal disease; myasthenia gravis; asthma; thyrotoxicosis; Mobitz type II block

Warnings/Precautions Use with caution in children with spastic paralysis; use with caution in elderly patients. Low doses cause a paradoxical decrease in heart rates. Some commercial products contain sodium metabisulfite, which can cause allergic-type reactions. May accumulate with multiple inhalational administration, particularly in the elderly. Heat prostration may occur in hot weather. Use with caution in patients with autonomic neuropathy, prostatic hyperplasia, hyperthyroidism, congestive heart failure, cardiac arrhythmias, chronic lung disease, biliary tract disease; anticholinergic agents are generally not well tolerated in the elderly and their use should be avoided when possible; atropine is rarely used except as a preoperative agent or in the acute treatment of bradyarrhythmias.

Adverse Reactions
>10%:
  Dermatologic: Dry, hot skin
  Gastrointestinal: Impaired GI motility, constipation, dry throat, dry mouth
  Local: Irritation at injection site
  Respiratory: Dry nose
  Miscellaneous: Diaphoresis (decreased)
1% to 10%:
  Dermatologic: Increased sensitivity to light
  Endocrine & metabolic: Decreased flow of breast milk
  Gastrointestinal: Dysphagia
<1% (Limited to important or life-threatening): Ataxia, blurred vision, bradycardia (doses <0.5 mg), confusion, delirium, drowsiness, elderly may be at increased risk for confusion and hallucinations, fatigue, headache, increased intraocular pain, loss of memory, mydriasis, orthostatic hypotension, palpitations, restlessness, tachycardia, ventricular fibrillation, ventricular tachycardia

Overdosage/Toxicology Symptoms include dilated, unreactive pupils; blurred vision; hot, dry flushed skin; dryness of mucous membranes; difficulty in swallowing, foul breath, diminished or absent bowel sounds, urinary retention, tachycardia, hyperthermia, and hypertension, increased respiratory rate. Anticholinergic toxicity is caused by strong binding of the drug to cholinergic receptors. Anticholinesterase inhibitors reduce acetylcholinesterase, the enzyme that breaks down acetylcholine and thereby allows acetylcholine to accumulate and compete for receptor binding with the offending anticholinergic. For anticholinergic overdose with severe life-threatening symptoms, physostigmine 1-2 mg (0.5 mg or 0.02 mg/kg for children) S.C. or slow I.V. may be given to reverse these effects.

Drug Interactions
Increased Effect/Toxicity: Amantadine, antihistamines, phenothiazines, and TCAs may increase anticholinergic effects of atropine when used concurrently. Sympathomimetic amines may cause tachyarrhythmias; avoid concurrent use.
Decreased Effect: Effect of some phenothiazines may be antagonized. Levodopa effects may be decreased (limited clinical validation). Drugs with cholinergic mechanisms (metoclopramide, cisapride, bethanechol) decrease anticholinergic effects of atropine.

Stability Store injection at <40°C; avoid freezing.

Mechanism of Action Blocks the action of acetylcholine at parasympathetic sites in smooth muscle, secretory glands and the CNS; increases cardiac output, dries secretions, antagonizes histamine and serotonin

Pharmacodynamics/Kinetics
Onset of action: I.V.: Rapid
Absorption: Complete
Distribution: Widely throughout the body; crosses placenta; trace amounts enter breast milk; crosses blood-brain barrier
Metabolism: Hepatic
Half-life elimination: 2-3 hours
Excretion: Urine (30% to 50% as unchanged drug and metabolites)

Usual Dosage
Neonates, Infants, and Children: Doses <0.1 mg have been associated with paradoxical bradycardia.
  Preanesthetic: Oral, I.M., I.V., S.C.:
    <5 kg: 0.02 mg/kg/dose 30-60 minutes preop then every 4-6 hours as needed. Use of a minimum dosage of 0.1 mg in neonates <5 kg will result in dosages >0.02 mg/kg. There is no documented minimum dosage in this age group.
    >5 kg: 0.01-0.02 mg/kg/dose to a maximum 0.4 mg/dose 30-60 minutes preop; minimum dose: 0.1 mg
  Bradycardia: I.V., intratracheal: 0.02 mg/kg, minimum dose 0.1 mg, maximum single dose: 0.5 mg in children and 1 mg in adolescents; may repeat in 5-minute intervals to a maximum total dose of 1 mg in children or 2 mg in adolescents. (**Note:** For intratracheal administration, the dosage must be diluted with normal saline to a total volume of 1-2 mL). When treating bradycardia in neonates, reserve use for those patients unresponsive to improved oxygenation and epinephrine.

Children:
  Mydriasis, cycloplegia (preprocedure): Ophthalmic: 0.5% solution: Instill 1-2 drops twice daily for 1-3 days before the procedure
  Uveitis: Ophthalmic: 0.5% solution: Instill 1-2 drops up to 3 times/day
Adults (doses <0.5 mg have been associated with paradoxical bradycardia):
  Asystole or pulseless electrical activity: I.V.: 1 mg; repeat in 3-5 minutes if asystole persists; total dose of 0.04 mg/kg; may give intratracheally in 10 mL NS (intratracheal dose should be 2-2.5 times the I.V. dose)
  Preanesthetic: I.M., I.V., S.C.: 0.4-0.6 mg 30-60 minutes preop and repeat every 4-6 hours as needed
  Bradycardia: I.V.: 0.5-1 mg every 5 minutes, not to exceed a total of 3 mg or 0.04 mg/kg; may give intratracheally in 10 mL NS (intratracheal dose should be 2-2.5 times the I.V. dose)
  Neuromuscular blockade reversal: I.V.: 25-30 mcg/kg 60 seconds before neostigmine or 7-10 mcg/kg in combination with edrophonium
  Organophosphate or carbamate poisoning: I.V.: 1-2 mg/dose every 10-20 minutes until atropine effect (dry flushed skin, tachycardia, mydriasis, fever) is observed, then every 1-4 hours for at least 24 hours; up to 50 mg in first 24 hours and 2 g over several days may be given in cases of severe intoxication
  GI disorders: Oral: 0.4-0.6 mg every 4-6 hours
  Ophthalmic:
    Solution: 1%:
      Mydriasis, cycloplegia (preprocedure): Instill 1-2 drops 1 hour before the procedure.
      Uveitis: Instill 1-2 drops 4 times/day.
    Ointment: Uveitis: Apply a small amount in the conjunctival sac up to 3 times/day. Compress the lacrimal sac by digital pressure for 1-3 minutes after instillation.
Administration I.V.: Administer undiluted by rapid I.V. injection; slow injection may result in paradoxical bradycardia
Monitoring Parameters Heart rate, blood pressure, pulse, mental status; intravenous administration requires a cardiac monitor
Patient Information Maintain good oral hygiene habits because lack of saliva may increase chance of cavities. Observe caution while driving or performing other tasks requiring alertness, as drug may cause drowsiness, dizziness, or blurred vision. Notify physician if rash, flushing, or eye pain occurs, or if difficulty in urinating, constipation, or sensitivity to light becomes severe or persists. Do not allow dropper bottle or tube to touch eye during administration.
Nursing Implications Observe for tachycardia if patient has cardiac problems
Additional Information May give intratracheal in 1 mg/10 mL dilution only.
Dosage Forms
  Injection, solution, as sulfate: 0.1 mg/mL (5 mL, 10 mL); 0.4 mg/mL (1 mL, 20 mL); 0.5 mg/mL (1 mL); 1 mg/mL (1 mL)
  Ointment, ophthalmic, as sulfate: 1% (3.5 g)
  Solution, ophthalmic, as sulfate: 1% (5 mL, 15 mL)
    Atropine-Care®: 1% (2 mL)
    Atropisol®: 1% (1 mL)
    Isopto® Atropine: 1% (5 mL, 15 mL)
  Tablet, as sulfate (Sal-Tropine™): 0.4 mg

Auranofin (au RANE oh fin)

U.S. Brand Names Ridaura®
Canadian Brand Names Ridaura®
Therapeutic Category Gold Compound
Use Management of active stage of classic or definite rheumatoid arthritis in patients that do not respond to or tolerate other agents; psoriatic arthritis; adjunctive or alternative therapy for pemphigus
Pregnancy Risk Factor C
Contraindications Renal disease, history of blood dyscrasias, congestive heart failure, exfoliative dermatitis, necrotizing enterocolitis, history of anaphylactic reactions
Warnings/Precautions NSAIDs and corticosteroids may be discontinued after starting gold therapy; therapy should be discontinued if platelet count falls to <100,000/mm³; WBC <4000, granulocytes <1500/mm³, explain possibility of adverse effects and their manifestations; use with caution in patients with renal or hepatic impairment
Adverse Reactions
  >10%:
    Dermatologic: Itching, rash
    Gastrointestinal: Stomatitis
    Ocular: Conjunctivitis
    Renal: Proteinuria
  1% to 10%:
    Dermatologic: Urticaria, alopecia
(Continued)

Auranofin *(Continued)*

Gastrointestinal: Glossitis

Hematologic: Eosinophilia, leukopenia, thrombocytopenia

Renal: Hematuria

<1%: Agranulocytosis, anemia, angioedema, aplastic anemia, dysphagia, GI hemorrhage, gingivitis, hepatotoxicity, interstitial pneumonitis, metallic taste, peripheral neuropathy, ulcerative enterocolitis

Overdosage/Toxicology Symptoms include hematuria, proteinuria, fever, nausea, vomiting, and diarrhea. Signs of gold toxicity include decrease in hemoglobin, leukopenia, granulocytes and platelets, proteinuria, hematuria, pruritus, or persistent diarrhea. Advise patients to report any symptoms of toxicity. Metallic taste may indicate stomatitis. For mild gold poisoning, dimercaprol 2.5 mg/kg 4 times/day for 2 days, or for more severe forms of gold intoxication, dimercaprol 3 mg/kg every 4 hours for 2 days, should be initiated. After 2 days the initial dose should be repeated twice daily on the third day and once daily thereafter for 10 days. Other chelating agents have been used with some success.

Drug Interactions

Increased Effect/Toxicity: Toxicity of penicillamine, antimalarials, hydroxychloroquine, cytotoxic agents, and immunosuppressants may be increased.

Stability Store in tight, light-resistant containers at 15°C to 30°C

Mechanism of Action The exact mechanism of action of gold is unknown; gold is taken up by macrophages which results in inhibition of phagocytosis and lysosomal membrane stabilization; other actions observed are decreased serum rheumatoid factor and alterations in immunoglobulins. Additionally, complement activation is decreased, prostaglandin synthesis is inhibited, and lysosomal enzyme activity is decreased.

Pharmacodynamics/Kinetics

Onset of action: Delayed; therapeutic response may require as long as 3-4 months

Duration: Prolonged

Absorption: Oral: ~20% gold in dose is absorbed

Protein binding: 60%

Half-life elimination: 21-31 days (dependent upon single or multiple dosing)

Time to peak, serum: ~2 hours

Excretion: Urine (60% of absorbed gold); remainder in feces

Usual Dosage Oral:

Children: Initial: 0.1 mg/kg/day divided daily; usual maintenance: 0.15 mg/kg/day in 1-2 divided doses; maximum: 0.2 mg/kg/day in 1-2 divided doses

Adults: 6 mg/day in 1-2 divided doses; after 3 months may be increased to 9 mg/day in 3 divided doses; if still no response after 3 months at 9 mg/day, discontinue drug

Dosing adjustment in renal impairment:

Cl_{cr} 50-80 mL/minute: Reduce dose to 50%

Cl_{cr} <50 mL/minute: Avoid use

Monitoring Parameters Monitor urine for protein; CBC and platelets; monitor for mouth ulcers and skin reactions; may monitor auranofin serum levels

Reference Range Gold: Normal: 0-0.1 µg/mL (SI: 0-0.0064 µmol/L); Therapeutic: 1-3 µg/mL (SI: 0.06-0.18 µmol/L); Urine: <0.1 µg/24 hours

Test Interactions May enhance the response to a tuberculin skin test

Patient Information Minimize exposure to sunlight; benefits from drug therapy may take as long as 3 months to appear; notify physician of pruritus, rash, sore mouth; metallic taste may occur; take shortly after a meal or light snack, can be given as bedtime dose if drowsiness occurs; optimum effect may take 2-4 weeks to be achieved; avoid alcohol; be aware of possible photosensitivity reaction; may cause painful erections; avoid sudden changes in position

Nursing Implications Discontinue therapy if platelet count falls <100,000/mm³

Dosage Forms Capsule: 3 mg [29% gold]

◆ **Auro® Ear Drops [OTC]** *see* Carbamide Peroxide *on page 224*

◆ **Aurolate®** *see* Gold Sodium Thiomalate *on page 639*

Aurothioglucose *(aur oh thye oh GLOO kose)*

U.S. Brand Names Solganal®

Canadian Brand Names Solganal®

Therapeutic Category Gold Compound

Use Adjunctive treatment in adult and juvenile active rheumatoid arthritis; alternative or adjunct in treatment of pemphigus; psoriatic patients who do not respond to NSAIDs

Pregnancy Risk Factor C

Contraindications Renal disease, history of blood dyscrasias, congestive heart failure, exfoliative dermatitis, hepatic disease, SLE, history of hypersensitivity

Warnings/Precautions Use with caution in patients with impaired renal or hepatic function; NSAIDs and corticosteroids may be discontinued over time after initiating gold therapy; explain the possibility of adverse reactions before initiating therapy; pregnancy should be ruled out before therapy is started; therapy should be discontinued if platelet counts fall to <100,000/mm³, WBC <4000/mm³, granulocytes <1500/mm³

Adverse Reactions

>10%:

Dermatologic: Itching, rash, exfoliative dermatitis, reddened skin

Gastrointestinal: Gingivitis, glossitis, metallic taste, stomatitis

1% to 10%: Renal: Proteinuria

<1% (Limited to important or life-threatening): agranulocytosis, allergic reaction (severe), anaphylactic shock, aplastic anemia, corneal ulcers, EEG abnormalities, encephalitis, eosinophilia, hepatotoxicity, interstitial pneumonitis, leukopenia, nephrotic syndrome, peripheral neuropathy, pulmonary fibrosis, thrombocytopenia, ulcerative enterocolitis

Overdosage/Toxicology Symptoms include hematuria, proteinuria, fever, nausea, vomiting, and diarrhea. Signs of gold toxicity include decrease in hemoglobin, leukopenia, granulocytes and platelets, proteinuria, hematuria, pruritus, stomatitis, persistent diarrhea, rash, or metallic taste. Advise patients to report any symptoms of toxicity. For mild gold poisoning, dimercaprol 2.5 mg/kg 4 times/day for 2 days, or for more severe forms of gold intoxication, dimercaprol 3-5 mg/kg every 4 hours for 2 days, should be initiated. Then after 2 days the initial dose should be repeated twice daily on the third day, and once daily thereafter for 10 days. Other chelating agents have been used with some success.

Drug Interactions
Increased Effect/Toxicity: Toxicity of penicillamine, antimalarials, hydroxychloroquine, cytotoxic agents, and immunosuppressants may be increased.

Stability Protect from light and store at 15°C to 30°C

Mechanism of Action Unknown, may decrease prostaglandin synthesis or may alter cellular mechanisms by inhibiting sulfhydryl systems

Pharmacodynamics/Kinetics
Absorption: I.M.: Erratic and slow
Distribution: Crosses placenta; enters breast milk
Protein binding: 95% to 99%
Half-life elimination: 3-27 days (dependent upon single or multiple dosing)
Time to peak, serum: 4-6 hours
Excretion: Urine (70%); feces (30%)

Usual Dosage I.M.: Doses should initially be given at weekly intervals
Children 6-12 years: Initial: 0.25 mg/kg/dose first week; increment at 0.25 mg/kg/dose increasing with each weekly dose; maintenance: 0.75-1 mg/kg/dose weekly not to exceed 25 mg/dose to a total of 20 doses, then every 2-4 weeks
Adults: 10 mg first week; 25 mg second and third week; then 50 mg/week until 800 mg to 1 g cumulative dose has been given; if improvement occurs without adverse reactions, administer 25-50 mg every 2-3 weeks, then every 3-4 weeks

Administration Administer by deep I.M. injection into the upper outer quadrant of the gluteal region

Monitoring Parameters CBC with differential, platelet count, urinalysis, baseline renal and liver function tests

Reference Range Gold: Normal: 0-0.1 µg/mL (SI: 0-0.0064 µmol/L); Therapeutic: 1-3 µg/mL (SI: 0.06-0.18 µmol/L); Urine: <0.1 µg/24 hours

Patient Information Minimize exposure to sunlight; benefits from drug therapy may take as long as 3 months to appear; notify physician of pruritus, rash, sore mouth; metallic taste may occur

Nursing Implications Therapy should be discontinued if platelet count falls <100,000/mm³; vial should be thoroughly shaken before withdrawing a dose; explain the possibility of adverse reactions before initiating therapy; advise patients to report any symptoms of toxicity

Dosage Forms Injection, suspension [gold 50%]: 50 mg/mL (10 mL)

Azatadine (a ZA ta deen)

U.S. Brand Names Optimine®
Canadian Brand Names Optimine®
Synonyms Azatadine Maleate
Therapeutic Category Antihistamine, H₁ Blocker
Use Treatment of perennial and seasonal allergic rhinitis and chronic urticaria
Pregnancy Risk Factor B
Contraindications Hypersensitivity to azatadine, any component of the formulation, or to other related antihistamines including cyproheptadine; patients taking MAO inhibitors should not use azatadine
Warnings/Precautions Sedation and somnolence are the most commonly reported adverse effects. Use with caution in patients with narrow-angle glaucoma, stenosing peptic ulcer, urinary bladder obstruction, prostatic hyperplasia, asthmatic attacks.
Adverse Reactions
>10%:
Central nervous system: Slight to moderate drowsiness
Respiratory: Thickening of bronchial secretions
(Continued)

Azatadine *(Continued)*

1% to 10%:
Central nervous system: Headache, fatigue, nervousness, dizziness
Gastrointestinal: Appetite increase, weight gain, nausea, diarrhea, abdominal pain, dry mouth
Neuromuscular & skeletal: Arthralgia
Respiratory: Pharyngitis
<1% (Limited to important or life-threatening): Hepatitis, bronchospasm, epistaxis
Overdosage/Toxicology Symptoms include CNS depression or stimulation, dry mouth, flushed skin, fixed and dilated pupils, apnea. There is no specific treatment for antihistamine overdose, however, clinical toxicity is mostly due to anticholinergic effects. Anticholinesterase inhibitors may be useful by reducing acetylcholinesterase. Anticholinesterase inhibitors include physostigmine, neostigmine, pyridostigmine, and edrophonium. For anticholinergic overdose with severe life-threatening symptoms, physostigmine 1-2 mg (0.5 mg or 0.02 mg/kg for children) slow I.V. may be given to reverse these effects.
Drug Interactions
Increased Effect/Toxicity: Potential for increased side effects when used with procarbazine, CNS depressants, tricyclic antidepressants, and alcohol.
Ethanol/Nutrition/Herb Interactions Ethanol: Avoid ethanol (may increase CNS depression).
Mechanism of Action Azatadine is a piperidine-derivative antihistamine; has both anticholinergic and antiserotonin activity; has been demonstrated to inhibit mediator release from human mast cells *in vitro*; mechanism of this action is suggested to prevent calcium entry into the mast cell through voltage-dependent calcium channels
Pharmacodynamics/Kinetics
Onset of action: 1-2 hours
Absorption: Rapid and extensive
Metabolism: Hepatic
Half-life elimination: ~8.7 hours
Time to peak: 4 hours
Excretion: Urine (~20% as unchanged drug) within 48 hours
Usual Dosage Children >12 years and Adults: Oral: 1-2 mg twice daily
Patient Information May cause drowsiness; avoid alcohol; can impair coordination and judgment
Nursing Implications Assist with ambulation
Dosage Forms Tablet, as maleate: 1 mg

Azatadine and Pseudoephedrine *(a ZA ta deen & soo doe e FED rin)*

U.S. Brand Names Rynatan® Tablet; Trinalin®
Canadian Brand Names Trinalin®
Synonyms Pseudoephedrine and Azatadine
Therapeutic Category Antihistamine/Decongestant Combination
Use Perennial and seasonal allergic rhinitis and other allergic symptoms including urticaria
Pregnancy Risk Factor C
Usual Dosage Adults: 1 tablet twice daily
Additional Information Complete prescribing information for this medication should be consulted for additional detail.
Dosage Forms Tablet: Azatadine maleate 1 mg and pseudoephedrine sulfate 120 mg

♦ **Azatadine Maleate** *see Azatadine on page 135*

Azathioprine *(ay za THYE oh preen)*

U.S. Brand Names Imuran®
Canadian Brand Names Alti-Azathioprine; Gen-Azathioprine; Imuran®
Synonyms Azathioprine Sodium
Therapeutic Category Antineoplastic Agent, Miscellaneous; Immunosuppressant Agent
Use Adjunct with other agents in prevention of rejection of solid organ transplants; also used in severe active rheumatoid arthritis unresponsive to other agents; other autoimmune diseases (ITP, SLE, MS, Crohn's disease)
Pregnancy Risk Factor D
Contraindications Hypersensitivity to azathioprine or any component of the formulation; pregnancy
Warnings/Precautions Chronic immunosuppression increases the risk of neoplasia; has mutagenic potential to both men and women and with possible hematologic toxicities; use with caution in patients with liver disease, renal impairment; monitor hematologic function closely
Adverse Reactions Dose reduction or temporary withdrawal allows reversal
>10%:
Central nervous system: Fever, chills
Gastrointestinal: Nausea, vomiting, anorexia, diarrhea
Hematologic: Thrombocytopenia, leukopenia, anemia
Miscellaneous: Secondary infection
1% to 10%:
Dermatologic: Rash
Hematologic: Pancytopenia
Hepatic: Hepatotoxicity
<1% (Limited to important or life-threatening): Hypotension, alopecia, veno-occlusive disease (potentially fatal), pneumonitis retinopathy, dyspnea, rare hypersensitivity reactions
Overdosage/Toxicology Symptoms include nausea, vomiting, diarrhea, and hematologic toxicity. Following initiation of essential overdose management, symptomatic and supportive treatment should be instituted. Dialysis has been reported to remove significant amounts of the drug and its metabolites, and should be considered as a treatment option in those patients who deteriorate despite established forms of therapy.

Drug Interactions

Increased Effect/Toxicity: Allopurinol may increase serum levels of azathioprine's active metabolite (6-MP). Decrease azathioprine dose to $1/3$ to $1/4$ of normal dose. Azathioprine and ACE inhibitors may induce severe leukopenia. Azathioprine and methotrexate may result in elevated levels of the metabolite 6-MP.

Decreased Effect: Azathioprine and cyclosporine may result in a decrease in cyclosporine levels. Azathioprine and nondepolarizing neuromuscular blockers may cause the action of the neuromuscular blocker to be decreased or reversed. Azathioprine and anticoagulants may result in decreased action of the anticoagulant.

Ethanol/Nutrition/Herb Interactions Herb/Nutraceutical: Avoid cat's claw, echinacea (have immunostimulant properties).

Stability

Stability of parenteral admixture at room temperature (25°C): 24 hours
Stability of parenteral admixture at refrigeration temperature (4°C): 16 days
Stable in neutral or acid solutions, but is hydrolyzed to mercaptopurine in alkaline solutions

Mechanism of Action Azathioprine is an imidazolyl derivative of 6-mercaptopurine; antagonizes purine metabolism and may inhibit synthesis of DNA, RNA, and proteins; may also interfere with cellular metabolism and inhibit mitosis

Pharmacodynamics/Kinetics

Distribution: Crosses placenta
Protein binding: ~30%
Metabolism: Extensively by hepatic xanthine oxidase to 6-mercaptopurine (active)
Half-life elimination: Parent drug: 12 minutes; 6-mercaptopurine: 0.7-3 hours; End-stage renal disease: Slightly prolonged
Excretion: Urine (primarily as metabolites)

Usual Dosage I.V. dose is equivalent to oral dose (dosing should be based on ideal body weight):

Children and Adults: Solid organ transplantation: Oral, I.V.: 2-5 mg/kg/day to start, then 1-2 mg/kg/day maintenance
Adults: Rheumatoid arthritis: Oral: 1 mg/kg/day for 6-8 weeks; increase by 0.5 mg/kg every 4 weeks until response or up to 2.5 mg/kg/day

Dosing adjustment in renal impairment:
Cl_{cr} 10-50 mL/minute: Administer 75% of normal dose daily
Cl_{cr} <10 mL/minute: Administer 50% of normal dose daily
Hemodialysis: Slightly dialyzable (5% to 20%)
Administer dose posthemodialysis: CAPD effects: Unknown; CAVH effects: Unknown

Dietary Considerations May be taken with food.

Administration Azathioprine can be administered IVP over 5 minutes at a concentration not to exceed 10 mg/mL **or** azathioprine can be further diluted with normal saline or D_5W and administered by intermittent infusion over 15-60 minutes

Monitoring Parameters CBC, platelet counts, total bilirubin, alkaline phosphatase

Patient Information Response in rheumatoid arthritis may not occur for up to 3 months; do not stop taking without the physician's approval, do not have any vaccinations before checking with your physician; check with your physician if you have a persistent sore throat, unusual bleeding or bruising, or fatigue. Contraceptive measures are recommended during therapy.

Nursing Implications Can be administered IVP over 5 minutes at a concentration not to exceed 10 mg/mL; or azathioprine can be further diluted with normal saline or D_5W and administered by intermittent infusion over 15-60 minutes

Dosage Forms

Injection, powder for reconstitution, as sodium: 100 mg
Tablet, scored: 50 mg

Extemporaneous Preparations A 50 mg/mL suspension compounded from twenty 50 mg tablets, distilled water, Cologel® 5 mL, and then adding 2:1 simple syrup/cherry syrup mixture to a total volume of 20 mL, was stable for 8 weeks when stored in the refrigerator

Handbook on Extemporaneous Formulations, Bethesda, MD: American Society of Hospital Pharmacists, 1987.

♦ **Azathioprine Sodium** *see* Azathioprine *on page 136*

Azelaic Acid (a zeh LAY ik AS id)

U.S. Brand Names Azelex®; Finevin™
Therapeutic Category Acne Products; Topical Skin Product, Acne
Use Topical treatment of mild to moderate inflammatory acne vulgaris
Pregnancy Risk Factor B
Usual Dosage Topical: Adolescents >12 years and Adults: Acne vulgaris: After skin is thoroughly washed and patted dry, gently but thoroughly massage a thin film of azelaic acid cream into the affected areas twice daily, in the morning and evening. The duration of use can vary and depends on the severity of the acne. In the majority of patients with inflammatory lesions, improvement of the condition occurs within 4 weeks.
Additional Information Complete prescribing information for this medication should be consulted for additional detail.
Dosage Forms
Cream, topical:
Azelex®: 20% (30 g, 50 g)
Finevin™: 20% (30 g)

Azelastine (a ZEL as teen)

U.S. Brand Names Astelin®; Optivar™
Canadian Brand Names Astelin®
Synonyms Azelastine Hydrochloride
Therapeutic Category Antihistamine; Antihistamine, Nasal; Antihistamine, Ophthalmic
(Continued)

Azelastine *(Continued)*

Use
Nasal spray: Treatment of the symptoms of seasonal allergic rhinitis such as rhinorrhea, sneezing, and nasal pruritus in children ≥5 years of age and adults; treatment of the symptoms of vasomotor rhinitis in children ≥12 years of age and adults

Ophthalmic: Treatment of itching of the eye associated with seasonal allergic conjunctivitis in children ≥3 years of age and adults

Pregnancy Risk Factor C

Pregnancy/Breast-Feeding Implications
There are no adequate and well-controlled studies in pregnant women. Animal reproduction studies have shown toxic effects to the fetus. Use during pregnancy only if the potential benefit to the mother outweighs the possible risk to the fetus. Excretion in breast milk is unknown; use caution.

Contraindications
Hypersensitivity to azelastine or any component of the formulation

Warnings/Precautions
Nasal spray: May cause drowsiness in some patients; instruct patient to use caution when driving or operating machinery. Effects may be additive with CNS depressants and/or ethanol.

Ophthalmic: Solution contains benzalkonium chloride; wait at least 10 minutes after instilling solution before inserting soft contact lenses. Do not use contact lenses if eyes are red.

Adverse Reactions

Nasal spray:
>10%:
Central nervous system: Headache (15%), somnolence (12%)
Gastrointestinal: Bitter taste (20%)

2% to 10%:
Central nervous system: Dizziness (2%), fatigue (2%)
Gastrointestinal: Nausea (3%), weight gain (2%), dry mouth (3%)
Respiratory: Nasal burning (4%), pharyngitis (4%), paroxysmal sneezing (3%), rhinitis (2%), epistaxis (2%)

<2% (Limited to important or life-threatening): Depression, anxiety, depersonalization, sleep disorder, ulcerative stomatitis, vomiting, bronchospasm, allergic reactions, anaphylactoid reaction, chest pain, dyspnea, involuntary muscle contractions, paresthesia, pruritus, rash, urinary retention

Ophthalmic:
>10%:
Central nervous system: Headache (15%)
Ocular: Transient burning/stinging (30%)

1% to 10%:
Central nervous system: Fatigue
Genitourinary: Bitter taste (10%)
Ocular: Conjunctivitis, eye pain, blurred vision (temporary)
Respiratory: Asthma, dyspnea, pharyngitis
Miscellaneous: Flu-like syndrome

Overdosage/Toxicology
There have been no reported overdoses with azelastine. Increased somnolence is likely to occur. Supportive measures should be employed.

Drug Interactions
Increased Effect/Toxicity: May cause additive sedation when concomitantly administered with other CNS depressant medications. Cimetidine can increase the AUC and C_{max} of azelastine by as much as 65%.

Ethanol/Nutrition/Herb Interactions
Ethanol: Avoid ethanol (may cause increased somnolence or fatigue).

Stability
Nasal spray: Store upright at controlled room temperature of 20°C to 25°C (68°F to 77°F); stable for 3 months after opening

Ophthalmic solution: Store upright between 2°C to 25°C (36°F to 77°F)

Mechanism of Action
Competes with histamine at H_1-receptor sites on effector cells and inhibits the release of histamine and other mediators involved in the allergic response. When used intranasally, reduces hyper-reactivity of the airways; increases the motility of bronchial epithelial cilia, improving mucociliary transport

Pharmacodynamics/Kinetics
Onset of action: Peak effect: Nasal spray: 3 hours; Ophthalmic solution: 3 minutes
Duration: Nasal spray: 12 hours; Ophthalmic solution: 8 hours
Protein binding: 88%
Metabolism: Hepatic via CYP450 enzyme system; active metabolite, desmethylazelastine
Bioavailability: Intranasal: 40%
Half-life elimination: 22 hours
Time to peak, serum: 2-3 hours

Usual Dosage
Children ≥5-11 years: Seasonal allergic rhinitis: Intranasal: 1 spray each nostril twice daily
Children ≥12 years and Adults: Seasonal allergic rhinitis or vasomotor rhinitis: Intranasal: 2 sprays (137 mcg/spray) each nostril twice daily
Children ≥3 years and Adults: Itching eyes due to seasonal allergic conjunctivitis: Ophthalmic: Instill 1 drop into affected eye(s) twice daily

Administration
Intranasal: Before initial use of the nasal spray, the delivery system should be primed with 4 sprays or until a fine mist appears. If 3 or more days have elapsed since last use, the delivery system should be reprimed.

Patient Information
Causes drowsiness and may impair ability to perform hazardous activities requiring mental alertness or physical coordination; avoid spraying in eyes

Dosage Forms
Solution, intranasal spray (Astelin®): 1 mg/mL [137 mcg/spray] (17 mL) [contains benzalkonium chloride]

Solution, ophthalmic (Optivar™): 0.05% (6 mL) [contains benzalkonium chloride]

♦ **Azelastine Hydrochloride** *see Azelastine on page 137*

♦ **Azelex®** *see Azelaic Acid on page 137*

♦ **Azidothymidine** *see Zidovudine on page 1435*

♦ **Azidothymidine, Abacavir, and Lamivudine** *see Abacavir, Lamivudine, and Zidovudine on page 17*

Azithromycin *(az ith roe MYE sin)*

Related Information
Antimicrobial Drugs of Choice *on page 1588*
Community-Acquired Pneumonia in Adults *on page 1603*
Prevention of Bacterial Endocarditis *on page 1563*
Treatment of Sexually Transmitted Diseases *on page 1609*
USPHA/IDSA Guidelines for the Prevention of Opportunistic Infections in Persons With HIV *on page 1574*

U.S. Brand Names Zithromax®; Zithromax® Z-PAK®

Canadian Brand Names Zithromax®; Zithromax® Z-PAK®

Synonyms Azithromycin Dihydrate

Therapeutic Category Antibiotic, Macrolide

Use
Children: Treatment of acute otitis media due to *H. influenzae*, *M. catarrhalis*, or *S. pneumoniae*; pharyngitis/tonsillitis due to *S. pyogenes*
Adults:
   Treatment of mild to moderate upper and lower respiratory tract infections, infections of the skin and skin structure, and sexually transmitted diseases due to susceptible strains of *C. trachomatis*, *M. catarrhalis*, *H. influenzae*, *S. aureus*, *S. pneumoniae*, *Mycoplasma pneumoniae*, and *C. psittaci*; community-acquired pneumonia, pelvic inflammatory disease (PID)
   Prevention of (or to delay onset of) infection with *Mycobacterium avium* complex (MAC)
   Prevention or (or to delay onset of) or treatment of MAC in patients with advanced HIV infection
   Prophylaxis of bacterial endocarditis in patients who are allergic to penicillin and undergoing surgical or dental procedures

Pregnancy Risk Factor B

Contraindications Hypersensitivity to azithromycin, other macrolide antibiotics, or any component of the formulation; hepatic impairment; use with pimozide

Warnings/Precautions Use with caution in patients with hepatic dysfunction; may mask or delay symptoms of incubating gonorrhea or syphilis, so appropriate culture and susceptibility tests should be performed prior to initiating azithromycin; pseudomembranous colitis has been reported with use of macrolide antibiotics; safety and efficacy have not been established in children <6 months of age with acute otitis media and in children <2 years of age with pharyngitis/tonsillitis

Adverse Reactions
1% to 10%: Gastrointestinal: Diarrhea, nausea, abdominal pain, cramping, vomiting (especially with high single-dose regimens)
<1% (Limited to important or life-threatening): Allergic reactions angioedema, cholestatic jaundice, eosinophilia, hypertrophic pyloric stenosis, nephritis, ototoxicity, rash, thrombophlebitis, ventricular arrhythmias

Overdosage/Toxicology Symptoms include nausea, vomiting, diarrhea, and prostration. Treatment is supportive and symptomatic.

Drug Interactions
Increased Effect/Toxicity: Concurrent use of pimozide is contraindicated due to potential cardiotoxicity. The manufacturer warns that azithromycin potentially may increase levels of tacrolimus, phenytoin, ergot alkaloids, alfentanil, astemizole, terfenadine, bromocriptine, carbamazepine, cyclosporine, digoxin, disopyramide, and triazolam. However, azithromycin did not affect the response/levels of carbamazepine, terfenadine, theophylline, or warfarin in specific interaction studies; caution is advised when administered together.
Decreased Effect: Decreased azithromycin peak serum concentrations with aluminum- and magnesium-containing antacids (by 24%), however, total absorption is unaffected.

Ethanol/Nutrition/Herb Interactions Food: Rate and extent of GI absorption may be altered depending upon the formulation. Azithromycin suspension, not tablet form, has significantly increased absorption (46%) with food; absorption may be decreased with capsule formulation.

Stability Store intact vials of injection at room temperature. Reconstitute the 500 mg vial with 4.8 mL of sterile water for injection and shake until all of the drug is dissolved. Each mL contains 100 mg azithromycin. Reconstituted solution is stable for 24 hours when stored below 30°C/86°F.
The initial solution should be further diluted to a concentration of 1 mg/mL (500 mL) to 2 mg/mL (250 mL) in 0.9% sodium chloride, 5% dextrose in water, and lactated Ringer's. The diluted solution is stable for 24 hours at or below room temperature (30°C or 86°F) and for 7 days if stored under refrigeration (5°C or 41°F).
Other medications should not be infused simultaneously through the same I.V. line.

Mechanism of Action Inhibits RNA-dependent protein synthesis at the chain elongation step; binds to the 50S ribosomal subunit resulting in blockage of transpeptidation

Pharmacodynamics/Kinetics
Absorption: Rapid
Distribution: Extensive tissue; distributes well into skin, lungs, sputum, tonsils, and cervix; penetration into CSF is poor
Protein binding (concentration dependent): 7% to 50%
Metabolism: Hepatic
Bioavailability: 37%; variable effect (increased with oral suspension, decreased with capsule, unchanged with tablet)
Half-life elimination: Terminal: 68 hours
Time to peak, serum: 2.3-4 hours
(Continued)

Azithromycin *(Continued)*

Excretion: Feces (50% as unchanged drug); urine (~5% to 12%)

Usual Dosage

Oral:

Children ≥6 months:

Community-acquired pneumonia: 10 mg/kg on day 1 (maximum: 500 mg/day) followed by 5 mg/kg/day once daily on days 2-5 (maximum: 250 mg/day)

Otitis media:

1-day regimen: 30 mg/kg as a single dose

3-day regimen: 10 mg/kg once daily for 3 days

5-day regimen: 10 mg/kg on day 1 (maximum: 250 mg/day) followed by 5 mg/kg/day once daily on days 2-5 (maximum: 250 mg/day)

Children ≥2 years: Pharyngitis, tonsillitis: 12 mg/kg/day once daily for 5 days (maximum: 500 mg/day)

Children:

M. avium-infected patients with acquired immunodeficiency syndrome: Not currently FDA approved for use; 10-20 mg/kg/day once daily (maximum: 40 mg/kg/day) has been used in clinical trials; prophylaxis for first episode of MAC: 5-12 mg/kg/day once daily (maximum: 500 mg/day)

Prophylaxis for bacterial endocarditis: 15 mg/kg 1 hour before procedure

Adolescents ≥16 years and Adults:

Respiratory tract, skin and soft tissue infections: 500 mg on day 1 followed by 250 mg/day on days 2-5 (maximum: 500 mg/day)

Nongonococcal urethritis/cervicitis (due to *C. trachomatis*): 1 g as a single dose

Prophylaxis of disseminated *M. avium* complex disease in patient with advanced HIV infection: 1200 mg once weekly (may be combined with rifabutin)

Treatment of disseminated *M. avium* complex disease in patient with advanced HIV infection: 600 mg daily (in combination with ethambutol 15 mg/kg)

Prophylaxis for bacterial endocarditis: 500 mg 1 hour prior to the procedure

I.V.: Adults:

Community-acquired pneumonia: 500 mg as a single dose for at least 2 days, follow I.V. therapy by the oral route with a single daily dose of 500 mg to complete a 7-10 day course of therapy

Pelvic inflammatory disease (PID): 500 mg as a single dose for 1-2 days, follow I.V. therapy by the oral route with a single daily dose of 250 mg to complete a 7-day course of therapy

Dietary Considerations Capsule should be administered 1 hour before or 2 hours following meals. Oral suspension may be administered with or without food. Tablet may be administered with food to decrease GI effects.

Administration

I.V.: Other medications should not be infused simultaneously through the same I.V. line.

Oral: Suspension and tablet may be taken without regard to food.

Monitoring Parameters Liver function tests, CBC with differential

Patient Information Take as directed. Take all of prescribed medication. Do not discontinue until prescription is completed. Take capsule form 1 hour before or 2 hours after meals; suspension may be taken with or without food; tablet form may be taken with meals to decrease GI effects. Do not take with aluminum- or magnesium-containing antacids.

Nursing Implications

Do not administer concurrently with aluminum or magnesium antacids

Monitor liver function tests; tolerance to medication; respiratory, cardiac, and fluid status of nursing home patients being treated for pneumonia

Parenteral: Infusate concentration and rate of infusion for azithromycin for injection should be either 1 mg/mL over 3 hours or 2 mg/mL over 1 hour

Additional Information Capsules are no longer being produced in the United States.

Dosage Forms

Injection, powder for reconstitution, as dihydrate: 500 mg

Powder for oral suspension, as dihydrate: 100 mg/5 mL (15 mL); 200 mg/5 mL (15 mL, 22.5 mL, 30 mL); 1 g [single-dose packet]

Tablet, as dihydrate: 250 mg, 600 mg

Zithromax® Z-PAK® [unit-dose pack]: 250 mg (6s)

◆ **Azithromycin Dihydrate** *see Azithromycin on page 139*

◆ **Azmacort®** *see Triamcinolone on page 1366*

◆ **Azo-Dine® [OTC]** *see Phenazopyridine on page 1068*

◆ **Azo-Gesic® [OTC]** *see Phenazopyridine on page 1068*

◆ **Azopt®** *see Brinzolamide on page 184*

◆ **Azo-Standard®** *see Phenazopyridine on page 1068*

◆ **AZT** *see Zidovudine on page 1435*

◆ **AZT + 3TC** *see Zidovudine and Lamivudine on page 1437*

◆ **AZT, Abacavir, and Lamivudine** *see Abacavir, Lamivudine, and Zidovudine on page 17*

◆ **Azthreonam** *see Aztreonam on page 140*

Aztreonam *(AZ tree oh nam)*

Related Information

Antimicrobial Drugs of Choice *on page 1588*

Community-Acquired Pneumonia in Adults *on page 1603*

U.S. Brand Names Azactam®

Canadian Brand Names Azactam®

Synonyms Azthreonam

Therapeutic Category Antibiotic, Miscellaneous

Use Treatment of patients with urinary tract infections, lower respiratory tract infections, septicemia, skin/skin structure infections, intra-abdominal infections, and gynecological infections caused by susceptible gram-negative bacilli; often useful in patients with allergies to penicillins or cephalosporins

Pregnancy Risk Factor B

Contraindications Hypersensitivity to aztreonam or any component of the formulation

Warnings/Precautions Rare cross-allergenicity to penicillins and cephalosporins; requires dosing adjustment in renal impairment

Adverse Reactions
1% to 10%:
  Dermatologic: Rash
  Gastrointestinal: Diarrhea, nausea, vomiting
  Local: Thrombophlebitis, pain at injection site
<1% (Limited to important or life-threatening): Anaphylaxis, bronchospasm, *C. difficile*-associated diarrhea, erythema multiforme, exfoliative dermatitis, hepatitis, hypotension, jaundice, leukocytosis, neutropenia, pancytopenia, pruritus, pseudomembranous colitis, purpura, seizures, thrombocytopenia, toxic epidermal necrolysis, urticaria, vaginal candidiasis, vertigo

Overdosage/Toxicology Symptoms include seizures. If necessary, dialysis can reduce the drug concentration in the blood.

Drug Interactions
  Decreased Effect: Avoid antibiotics that induce beta-lactamase production (cefoxitin, imipenem).

Stability Reconstituted solutions are colorless to light yellow straw and may turn pink upon standing without affecting potency; use reconstituted solutions and I.V. solutions (in NS and D_5W) within 48 hours if kept at room temperature (25°C) or 7 days under refrigeration (4°C)

Mechanism of Action Inhibits bacterial cell wall synthesis by binding to one or more of the penicillin binding proteins (PBPs); which in turn inhibits the final transpeptidation step of peptidoglycan synthesis in bacterial cell walls, thus inhibiting cell wall biosynthesis. Bacteria eventually lyse due to ongoing activity of cell wall autolytic enzymes (autolysins and murein hydrolases) while cell wall assembly is arrested. Monobactam structure makes cross-allergenicity with beta-lactams unlikely.

Pharmacodynamics/Kinetics
Absorption: I.M.: Well absorbed; I.M. and I.V. doses produce comparable serum concentrations
Distribution: Widely to most body fluids and tissues; crosses placenta; enters breast milk
  V_d: Neonates: 0.26-0.36 L/kg; Children: 0.2-0.29 L/kg; Adults: 0.2 L/kg
  Relative diffusion of antimicrobial agents from blood into CSF: Good only with inflammation (exceeds usual MICs)
  CSF:blood level ratio: Meninges: Inflamed: 8% to 40%; Normal: ~1%
Protein binding: 56%
Metabolism: Hepatic (minor %)
Half-life elimination:
  Neonates: <7 days, ≤2.5 kg: 5.5-9.9 hours; <7 days, >2.5 kg: 2.6 hours; 1 week to 1 month: 2.4 hours
  Children 2 months to 12 years: 1.7 hours
  Adults: Normal renal function: 1.7-2.9 hours
  End-stage renal disease: 6-8 hours
Time to peak: I.M., I.V. push: Within 60 minutes; I.V. infusion: 1.5 hours
Excretion: Urine (60% to 70% as unchanged drug); feces (~13% to 15%)

Usual Dosage
Neonates: I.M., I.V.:
  Postnatal age ≤7 days:
    <2000 g: 30 mg/kg/dose every 12 hours
    >2000 g: 30 mg/kg/dose every 8 hours
  Postnatal age >7 days:
    <1200 g: 30 mg/kg/dose every 12 hours
    1200-2000 g: 30 mg/kg/dose every 8 hours
    >2000 g: 30 mg/kg/dose every 6 hours
Children >1 month: I.M., I.V.: 90-120 mg/kg/day divided every 6-8 hours
  Cystic fibrosis: 50 mg/kg/dose every 6-8 hours (ie, up to 200 mg/kg/day); maximum: 6-8 g/day
Adults:
  Urinary tract infection: I.M., I.V.: 500 mg to 1 g every 8-12 hours
  Moderately severe systemic infections: 1 g I.V. or I.M. or 2 g I.V. every 8-12 hours
  Severe systemic or life-threatening infections (especially caused by *Pseudomonas aeruginosa*): I.V.: 2 g every 6-8 hours; maximum: 8 g/day
  Dosing adjustment in renal impairment: Adults:
    Cl_{cr} >50 mL/minute: 500 mg to 1 g every 6-8 hours
    Cl_{cr} 10-50 mL/minute: 50% to 75% of usual dose given at the usual interval
    Cl_{cr} <10 mL/minute: 25% of usual dosage given at the usual interval
  Hemodialysis: Moderately dialyzable (20% to 50%); administer dose postdialysis or supplemental dose of 500 mg after dialysis
  Peritoneal dialysis: Administer as for Cl_{cr} <10 mL/minute
  Continuous arteriovenous or venovenous hemofiltration: Dose as for Cl_{cr} 10-50 mL/minute

Administration Administer by IVP over 3-5 minutes or by intermittent infusion over 20-60 minutes at a final concentration not to exceed 20 mg/mL

Monitoring Parameters Periodic liver function test; monitor for signs of anaphylaxis during first dose

Test Interactions May interfere with urine glucose tests containing cupric sulfate (Benedict's solution, Clinitest®)

Nursing Implications Administer by IVP over 3-5 minutes at a maximum concentration of 66 mg/mL or by intermittent infusion over 20-60 minutes at a final concentration not to exceed 20 mg/mL

Additional Information Although marketed as an agent similar to aminoglycosides, aztreonam is a monobactam antimicrobial with almost pure gram-negative aerobic activity. It
(Continued)

Aztreonam *(Continued)*

cannot be used for gram-positive infections. Aminoglycosides are often used for synergy in gram-positive infections.

Dosage Forms
Powder for injection: 500 mg, 1 g, 2 g
Infusion [premixed]: 1 g (50 mL); 2 g (50 mL)

♦ **Azulfidine®** *see Sulfasalazine on page 1275*
♦ **Azulfidine® EN-tabs®** *see Sulfasalazine on page 1275*
♦ **Babee® Teething® [OTC]** *see Benzocaine on page 154*
♦ **B-A-C®** *see Butalbital Compound on page 197*
♦ **Bacid® [OTC]** *see Lactobacillus on page 770*
♦ **Baciguent® [OTC]** *see Bacitracin on page 142*
♦ **Baci-IM®** *see Bacitracin on page 142*
♦ **Bacillus Calmette-Guérin (BCG) Live** *see BCG Vaccine on page 148*

Bacitracin *(bas i TRAY sin)*

U.S. Brand Names AK-Tracin®; Baciguent® [OTC]; Baci-IM®
Canadian Brand Names Baciguent®
Therapeutic Category Antibiotic, Ophthalmic; Antibiotic, Topical; Antibiotic, Miscellaneous
Use Treatment of susceptible bacterial infections mainly has activity against gram-positive bacilli; due to toxicity risks, systemic and irrigant uses of bacitracin should be limited to situations where less toxic alternatives would not be effective; oral administration has been successful in antibiotic-associated colitis and has been used for enteric eradication of vancomycin-resistant enterococci (VRE)
Pregnancy Risk Factor C
Contraindications Hypersensitivity to bacitracin or any component of the formulation; I.M. use is contraindicated in patients with renal impairment
Warnings/Precautions Prolonged use may result in overgrowth of nonsusceptible organisms; I.M. use may cause renal failure due to tubular and glomerular necrosis; **do not administer intravenously** because severe thrombophlebitis occurs
Adverse Reactions 1% to 10%:
Cardiovascular: Hypotension, edema of the face/lips, tightness of chest
Central nervous system: Pain
Dermatologic: Rash, itching
Gastrointestinal: Anorexia, nausea, vomiting, diarrhea, rectal itching
Hematologic: Blood dyscrasias
Miscellaneous: Diaphoresis
Overdosage/Toxicology Symptoms include nephrotoxicity (parenteral), nausea, and vomiting (oral).
Drug Interactions
Increased Effect/Toxicity: Nephrotoxic drugs, neuromuscular blocking agents, and anesthetics (increased neuromuscular blockade).
Stability For I.M. use; bacitracin sterile powder should be dissolved in 0.9% sodium chloride injection containing 2% procaine hydrochloride; once reconstituted, bacitracin is stable for 1 week under refrigeration (2°C to 8°C); sterile powder should be stored in the refrigerator; do not use diluents containing parabens
Mechanism of Action Inhibits bacterial cell wall synthesis by preventing transfer of mucopeptides into the growing cell wall
Pharmacodynamics/Kinetics
Duration: 6-8 hours
Absorption: Poor from mucous membranes and intact or denuded skin; rapidly following I.M. administration; not absorbed by bladder irrigation, but absorption can occur from peritoneal or mediastinal lavage
Distribution: CSF: Nil even with inflammation
Protein binding, plasma: Minimal
Time to peak, serum: I.M.: 1-2 hours
Excretion: Urine (10% to 40%) within 24 hours
Usual Dosage Do not administer I.V.:
Infants: I.M.:
≤2.5 kg: 900 units/kg/day in 2-3 divided doses
>2.5 kg: 1000 units/kg/day in 2-3 divided doses
Children: I.M.: 800-1200 units/kg/day divided every 8 hours
Adults: Antibiotic-associated colitis: Oral: 25,000 units 4 times/day for 7-10 days
Children and Adults:
Topical: Apply 1-5 times/day
Ophthalmic, ointment: Instill ¼" to ½" ribbon every 3-4 hours into conjunctival sac for acute infections, or 2-3 times/day for mild to moderate infections for 7-10 days
Irrigation, solution: 50-100 units/mL in normal saline, lactated Ringer's, or sterile water for irrigation; soak sponges in solution for topical compresses 1-5 times/day or as needed during surgical procedures
Administration For I.M. administration, confirm any orders for parenteral use; pH of urine should be kept >6 by using sodium bicarbonate; bacitracin sterile powder should be dissolved in 0.9% sodium chloride injection containing 2% procaine hydrochloride; do not use diluents containing parabens
Monitoring Parameters I.M.: Urinalysis, renal function tests
Patient Information Ophthalmic ointment may cause blurred vision; do not share eye medications with others

Ophthalmic administration: Tilt head back, place medication in conjunctival sac and close eyes; apply light finger pressure on lacrimal sac for 1 minute following instillation
Topical bacitracin should not be used for longer than 1 week unless directed by a physician

Nursing Implications For I.M. administration, pH of urine should be kept above 6 by using sodium bicarbonate

Additional Information 1 unit is equivalent to 0.026 mg

Dosage Forms
Injection, powder for reconstitution (Baci-IM®): 50,000 units
Ointment, ophthalmic (AK-Tracin®): 500 units/g (3.5 g)
Ointment, topical: 500 units/g (0.9 g, 15 g, 30 g, 120 g, 454 g)
Baciguent®: 500 units/g (15 g, 30 g)

Bacitracin and Polymyxin B (bas i TRAY sin & pol i MIKS in bee)

U.S. Brand Names AK-Poly-Bac®; Betadine® First Aid Antibiotics + Moisturizer [OTC]; Polysporin® Ophthalmic; Polysporin® Topical [OTC]

Canadian Brand Names LID-Pack®; Optimyxin®; Optimyxin Plus®; Polycidin® Ophthalmic Ointment

Synonyms Polymyxin B and Bacitracin

Therapeutic Category Antibiotic, Ophthalmic; Antibiotic, Topical

Use Treatment of superficial infections caused by susceptible organisms

Pregnancy Risk Factor C

Usual Dosage Children and Adults:
Ophthalmic ointment: Instill ½" ribbon in the affected eye(s) every 3-4 hours for acute infections or 2-3 times/day for mild to moderate infections for 7-10 days
Topical ointment/powder: Apply to affected area 1-4 times/day; may cover with sterile bandage if needed

Additional Information Complete prescribing information for this medication should be consulted for additional detail.

Dosage Forms
Ointment, ophthalmic (AK-Poly-Bac®, Polysporin®): Bacitracin 500 units and polymyxin B sulfate 10,000 units per g (3.5 g)
Ointment, topical [OTC]: Bacitracin 500 units and polymyxin B sulfate 10,000 units per g in white petrolatum (15 g, 30 g)
Betadine® First Aid Antibiotics + Moisturizer: Bacitracin 500 units and polymyxin B sulfate 10,000 units per g (14 g)
Polysporin®: Bacitracin 500 units and polymyxin B sulfate 10,000 units per g (15g, 30 g)
Powder, topical (Polysporin®): Bacitracin 500 units and polymyxin B sulfate 10,000 units per g (10 g)

Bacitracin, Neomycin, and Polymyxin B
(bas i TRAY sin, nee oh MYE sin & pol i MIKS in bee)

U.S. Brand Names Mycitracin® [OTC]; Neosporin® Ophthalmic Ointment; Neosporin® Topical [OTC]; Triple Antibiotic®

Canadian Brand Names Neosporin® Ophthalmic Ointment; Neotopic®

Synonyms Neomycin, Bacitracin, and Polymyxin B; Polymyxin B, Bacitracin, and Neomycin

Therapeutic Category Antibiotic, Ophthalmic; Antibiotic, Topical

Use Helps prevent infection in minor cuts, scrapes and burns; short-term treatment of superficial external ocular infections caused by susceptible organisms

Pregnancy Risk Factor C

Usual Dosage Children and Adults:
Ophthalmic: Ointment: Instill ½" into the conjunctival sac every 3-4 hours for 7-10 days for acute infections; apply ½" 2-3 times/day for mild to moderate infections for 7-10 days
Topical: Apply 1-4 times/day to infected area and cover with sterile bandage as needed

Additional Information Complete prescribing information for this medication should be consulted for additional detail.

Dosage Forms
Ointment, ophthalmic (Neosporin®): Bacitracin 400 units, neomycin sulfate 3.5 mg, and polymyxin B sulfate 10,000 units per g (3.5 g)
Ointment, topical (Triple Antibiotic®): Bacitracin 400 units, neomycin sulfate 3.5 mg, and polymyxin B sulfate 5000 units per g (0.9 g, 15 g, 30 g, 454 g)
Mycitracin®: Bacitracin 400 units, neomycin sulfate 3.5 mg, and polymyxin B sulfate 5000 units per g (14 g)
Neosporin®: Bacitracin 400 units, neomycin sulfate 3.5 mg, and polymyxin B sulfate 5000 units per g (0.9 g, 15 g, 30 g)

Bacitracin, Neomycin, Polymyxin B, and Hydrocortisone
(bas i TRAY sin, nee oh MYE sin, pol i MIKS in bee & hye droe KOR ti sone)

U.S. Brand Names AK-Spore® H.C.; Cortisporin® Ointment

Canadian Brand Names Cortisporin®

Synonyms Hydrocortisone, Bacitracin, Neomycin, and Polymyxin B; Neomycin, Bacitracin, Polymyxin B, and Hydrocortisone; Polymyxin B, Bacitracin, Neomycin, and Hydrocortisone

Therapeutic Category Antibiotic, Ophthalmic; Antibiotic, Otic; Antibiotic, Topical; Anti-inflammatory Agent; Corticosteroid, Ophthalmic; Corticosteroid, Otic; Corticosteroid, Topical (Low Potency)

Use Prevention and treatment of susceptible superficial topical infections

Pregnancy Risk Factor C

Usual Dosage Children and Adults:
Ophthalmic: Ointment: Instill ½" ribbon to inside of lower lid every 3-4 hours until improvement occurs
Topical: Apply sparingly 2-4 times/day. Therapy should be discontinued when control is achieved; if no improvement is seen, reassessment of diagnosis may be necessary.

Additional Information Complete prescribing information for this medication should be consulted for additional detail.

Dosage Forms
Ointment, ophthalmic (AK-Spore® H.C., Cortisporin®): Bacitracin 400 units, neomycin sulfate 3.5 mg, polymyxin B sulfate 10,000 units, and hydrocortisone 10 mg per g (3.5 g)
(Continued)

Bacitracin, Neomycin, Polymyxin B, and Hydrocortisone
(Continued)

Ointment, topical (Cortisporin®): Bacitracin 400 units, neomycin sulfate 3.5 mg, polymyxin B sulfate 10,000 units, and hydrocortisone 10 mg per g (15 g)

Bacitracin, Neomycin, Polymyxin B, and Lidocaine
(bas i TRAY sin, nee oh MYE sin, pol i MIKS in bee & LYE doe kane)

U.S. Brand Names Spectrocin Plus® [OTC]

Therapeutic Category Antibiotic, Topical

Use Prevention and treatment of susceptible superficial topical infections

Usual Dosage Adults: Topical: Apply 1-4 times/day to infected areas; cover with sterile bandage if needed

Additional Information Complete prescribing information for this medication should be consulted for additional detail.

Dosage Forms Ointment, topical: Bacitracin 500 units, neomycin base 3.5 mg, polymyxin B sulfate 5000 units, and lidocaine 40 mg per g (15 g, 30 g)

Baclofen (BAK loe fen)
U.S. Brand Names Lioresal®

Canadian Brand Names Apo®-Baclofen; Gen-Baclofen; Lioresal®; Liotec; Novo-Baclofen; Nu-Baclo; PMS-Baclofen

Therapeutic Category Skeletal Muscle Relaxant

Use Treatment of reversible spasticity associated with multiple sclerosis or spinal cord lesions
Orphan drug: Intrathecal: Treatment of intractable spasticity caused by spinal cord injury, multiple sclerosis, and other spinal disease (spinal ischemia or tumor, transverse myelitis, cervical spondylosis, degenerative myelopathy)

Unlabeled/Investigational Use Intractable hiccups, intractable pain relief, bladder spasticity, trigeminal neuralgia, cerebral palsy, Huntington's chorea

Pregnancy Risk Factor C

Contraindications Hypersensitivity to baclofen or any component of the formulation

Warnings/Precautions Use with caution in patients with seizure disorder, impaired renal function; avoid abrupt withdrawal of the drug; elderly are more sensitive to the effects of baclofen and are more likely to experience adverse CNS effects at higher doses.

Adverse Reactions
>10%:
Central nervous system: Drowsiness, vertigo, dizziness, psychiatric disturbances, insomnia, slurred speech, ataxia, hypotonia
Neuromuscular & skeletal: Weakness
1% to 10%:
Cardiovascular: Hypotension
Central nervous system: Fatigue, confusion, headache, insomnia
Dermatologic: Rash
Gastrointestinal: Nausea, constipation
Genitourinary: Polyuria
<1% (Limited to important or life-threatening): Chest pain, dyspnea, dysuria, enuresis, hematuria, impotence, inability to ejaculate, nocturia, palpitations, syncope, urinary retention

Overdosage/Toxicology Symptoms include vomiting, muscle hypotonia, salivation, drowsiness, coma, seizures, and respiratory depression. Atropine has been used to improve ventilation, heart rate, blood pressure, and core body temperature. Following initiation of essential overdose management, symptomatic and supportive treatment should be instituted.

Drug Interactions
Increased Effect/Toxicity: Baclofen may decrease the clearance of ibuprofen or other NSAIDs and increase the potential for renal toxicity. Effects may be additive with CNS depressants.

Ethanol/Nutrition/Herb Interactions
Ethanol: Avoid ethanol (may increase CNS depression).
Herb/Nutraceutical: Avoid valerian, St John's wort, kava kava, gotu kola.

Mechanism of Action Inhibits the transmission of both monosynaptic and polysynaptic reflexes at the spinal cord level, possibly by hyperpolarization of primary afferent fiber terminals, with resultant relief of muscle spasticity

Pharmacodynamics/Kinetics
Onset of action: 3-4 days
Peak effect: 5-10 days
Absorption: Oral: Rapid; dose dependent
Protein binding: 30%
Metabolism: Hepatic (15% of dose)
Half-life elimination: 3.5 hours
Time to peak, serum: Oral: Within 2-3 hours
Excretion: Urine and feces (85% as unchanged drug)

Usual Dosage
Oral (avoid abrupt withdrawal of drug):
Children:
2-7 years: Initial: 10-15 mg/24 hours divided every 8 hours; titrate dose every 3 days in increments of 5-15 mg/day to a maximum of 40 mg/day
≥8 years: Maximum: 60 mg/day in 3 divided doses
Adults: 5 mg 3 times/day, may increase 5 mg/dose every 3 days to a maximum of 80 mg/day
Hiccups: Adults: Usual effective dose: 10-20 mg 2-3 times/day
Intrathecal:
Test dose: 50-100 mcg, doses >50 mcg should be given in 25 mcg increments, separated by 24 hours

Maintenance: After positive response to test dose, a maintenance intrathecal infusion can be administered via an implanted intrathecal pump. Initial dose via pump: Infusion at a 24-hour rate dosed at twice the test dose.

Dosing adjustment in renal impairment: It is necessary to reduce dosage in renal impairment but there are no specific guidelines available

Hemodialysis: Poor water solubility allows for accumulation during chronic hemodialysis. Low-dose therapy is recommended. There have been several case reports of accumulation of baclofen resulting in toxicity symptoms (organic brain syndrome, myoclonia, deceleration and steep potentials in EEG) in patients with renal failure who have received normal doses of baclofen.

Administration For screening dosages, dilute with preservative-free sodium chloride to a final concentration of 50 mcg/mL for bolus injection into the subarachnoid space; for maintenance infusions, concentrations of 500-2000 mcg/mL may be used

Test Interactions ↑ alkaline phosphatase, AST, glucose, ammonia (B); ↓ bilirubin (S)

Patient Information Take with food or milk; abrupt withdrawal after prolonged use may cause anxiety, hallucinations, tachycardia or spasticity; may cause drowsiness and impair coordination and judgment

Nursing Implications Epileptic patients should be closely monitored; supervise ambulation; avoid abrupt withdrawal of the drug

Dosage Forms

Injection, solution, intrathecal [preservative free]: 50 mcg/mL (1 mL); 500 mcg/mL (20 mL); 2000 mcg/mL (5 mL)

Tablet: 10 mg, 20 mg

Extemporaneous Preparations Make a 5 mg/mL suspension by crushing fifteen 20 mg tablets; wet with glycerin, gradually add 45 mL simple syrup in 3 x 5 mL aliquots to make a total volume of 60 mL; refrigerate; stable 35 days

Johnson CE and Hart SM, "Stability of an Extemporaneously Compounded Baclofen Oral Liquid," *Am J Hosp Pharm*, 1993, 50:2353-5.

- ♦ **Bactocill**® *see* Oxacillin *on page 1016*
- ♦ **BactoShield**® [OTC] *see* Chlorhexidine Gluconate *on page 275*
- ♦ **Bactrim**™ *see* Sulfamethoxazole and Trimethoprim *on page 1273*
- ♦ **Bactrim**™ **DS** *see* Sulfamethoxazole and Trimethoprim *on page 1273*
- ♦ **Bactroban**® *see* Mupirocin *on page 941*
- ♦ **Bactroban**® **Nasal** *see* Mupirocin *on page 941*
- ♦ **Baking Soda** *see* Sodium Bicarbonate *on page 1243*
- ♦ **BAL** *see* Dimercaprol *on page 412*
- ♦ **Baldex**® *see* Dexamethasone *on page 380*
- ♦ **BAL in Oil**® *see* Dimercaprol *on page 412*
- ♦ **Balminil**® **Decongestant (Can)** *see* Pseudoephedrine *on page 1155*
- ♦ **Balminil DM D (Can)** *see* Pseudoephedrine and Dextromethorphan *on page 1157*
- ♦ **Balminil DM + Decongestant + Expectorant (Can)** *see* Guaifenesin, Pseudoephedrine, and Dextromethorphan *on page 648*
- ♦ **Balminil DM E (Can)** *see* Guaifenesin and Dextromethorphan *on page 646*
- ♦ **Balminil Expectorant (Can)** *see* Guaifenesin *on page 645*

Balsalazide (bal SAL a zide)

U.S. Brand Names Colazal™

Synonyms Balsalazide Disodium

Therapeutic Category 5-Aminosalicylic Acid Derivative; Anti-inflammatory Agent

Use Treatment of mild to moderate active ulcerative colitis

Pregnancy Risk Factor B

Pregnancy/Breast-Feeding Implications No adequate and well-controlled studies have been done in pregnant women. Balsalazide should be used in pregnant women only if clearly needed. It is not known if balsalazide is excreted in human milk. Caution should be used in administering balsalazide to a nursing woman.

Contraindications Hypersensitivity to salicylates, components of the formulation, or metabolites of balsalazide

Warnings/Precautions Pyloric stenosis may prolong gastric retention of balsalazide capsules. Renal toxicity has been observed with other mesalamine (5-aminosalicylic acid) products, use with caution in patients with known renal disease. May exacerbate symptoms of colitis. Safety and efficacy of use beyond 12 weeks has not been established. For adult use; safety and efficacy in children has not been established.

Adverse Reactions 1% to 10%:

Central nervous system: Headache (8%), insomnia (2%), fatigue (2%), fever (2%), pain (2%), dizziness (1%)

Gastrointestinal: Abdominal pain (6%), diarrhea (5%), nausea (5%), vomiting (4%), anorexia (2%), dyspepsia (2%), flatulence (2%), rectal bleeding (2%), cramps (1%), constipation (1%), dry mouth (1%), frequent stools (1%)

Genitourinary: Urinary tract infection (1%)

Neuromuscular & skeletal: Arthralgia (4%), back pain (2%), myalgia (1%)

Respiratory: Respiratory infection (4%), cough (2%), pharyngitis (2%), rhinitis (2%), sinusitis (1%)

Miscellaneous: Flu-like syndrome (1%)

Additional adverse reactions reported **with mesalamine products** (limited to important or life-threatening): Acute intolerance syndrome (cramping, abdominal pain, bloody diarrhea, fever, headache, pruritus, rash), alopecia, cholestatic jaundice, cirrhosis, elevated liver function tests, eosinophilic pneumonitis, hepatocellular damage, hepatotoxicity, jaundice, Kawasaki-like syndrome, liver failure, liver necrosis, nephrotic syndrome, pancreatitis, pericarditis, renal dysfunction

(Continued)

Balsalazide *(Continued)*

Overdosage/Toxicology Treatment is supportive and should include correction of any electrolyte abnormalities.

Drug Interactions

Decreased Effect: No studies have been conducted. Oral antibiotics may potentially interfere with 5-aminosalicylic acid release in the colon.

Ethanol/Nutrition/Herb Interactions Food: The effect of food on absorption has not been studied.

Stability Store at room temperature (25°C/77°F)

Mechanism of Action Balsalazide is a prodrug, converted by bacterial azoreduction to 5-aminosalicylic acid (active), 4-aminobenzoyl-β-alanine (inert), and their metabolites. 5-aminosalicylic acid may decrease inflammation by blocking the production of arachidonic acid metabolites topically in the colon mucosa.

Pharmacodynamics/Kinetics

Onset of action: Delayed; may require several days to weeks

Absorption: Very low and variable

Protein binding: ≥99%

Metabolism: Azoreduced in the colon to 5-aminosalicylic acid (active), 4-aminobenzoyl-β-alanine (inert), and N-acetylated metabolites

Half-life elimination: Primary effect is topical (colonic mucosa), systemic half-life not determined

Time to peak: 1-2 hours

Excretion: Feces (65% as 5-aminosalicylic acid, 4-aminobenzoyl-β-alanine, and N-acetylated metabolites); urine (25% as N-acetylated metabolites); Parent drug: Urine or feces (<1%)

Usual Dosage Oral:

Adults: 2.25 g (three 750 mg capsules) 3 times/day for 8-12 weeks

Elderly: No specific dosage adjustment available

Dosage adjustment in renal impairment: No information available with balsalazide; renal toxicity has been observed with other 5-aminosalicylic acid products, use with caution

Dosage adjustment in hepatic impairment: No specific dosage adjustment available

Dietary Considerations Each capsule contains ~86 mg of sodium.

Patient Information Take as directed; do not chew or open capsules. Report abdominal pain, unresolved diarrhea, severe headache, or chest pain to prescriber.

Dosage Forms Capsule: 750 mg

♦ **Balsalazide Disodium** *see Balsalazide on page 145*

♦ **Bancap®** *see Butalbital Compound on page 197*

♦ **Bancap HC®** *see Hydrocodone and Acetaminophen on page 676*

♦ **Banophen® [OTC]** *see DiphenhydrAMINE on page 414*

♦ **Banophen® Decongestant [OTC]** *see Diphenhydramine and Pseudoephedrine on page 415*

♦ **Barbidonna®** *see Hyoscyamine, Atropine, Scopolamine, and Phenobarbital on page 694*

♦ **Baridium®** *see Phenazopyridine on page 1068*

♦ **Basaljel® (Can)** *see Aluminum Hydroxide on page 63*

Basiliximab *(ba si LIK si mab)*

U.S. Brand Names Simulect®

Canadian Brand Names Simulect®

Therapeutic Category Immunosuppressant Agent; Monoclonal Antibody

Use Prophylaxis of acute organ rejection in renal transplantation

Pregnancy Risk Factor B (manufacturer)

Pregnancy/Breast-Feeding Implications IL-2 receptors play an important role in the development of the immune system. Use in pregnant women only when benefit exceeds potential risk to the fetus. Women of childbearing potential should use effective contraceptive measures before beginning treatment and for 2 months after completion of therapy with this agent.

It is not known whether basiliximab is excreted in human milk. Because many immunoglobulins are secreted in milk and the potential for serious adverse reactions exists, a decision should be made whether to discontinue nursing or discontinue the drug, taking into account the importance of the drug to the mother.

Contraindications Hypersensitivity basiliximab, murine proteins, or any component of the formulation

Warnings/Precautions To be used as a component of immunosuppressive regimen which includes cyclosporine and corticosteroids. Only physicians experienced in transplantation and immunosuppression should prescribe, and patients should receive the drug in a facility with adequate equipment and staff capable of providing the laboratory and medical support required for transplantation.

The incidence of lymphoproliferative disorders and/or opportunistic infections may be increased by immunosuppressive therapy. Severe hypersensitivity reactions, occurring within 24 hours, have been reported. Reactions, including anaphylaxis, have occurred both with the initial exposure and/or following re-exposure after several months. Use caution during re-exposure to a subsequent course of therapy in a patient who has previously received basiliximab. Discontinue the drug permanently if a reaction occurs. Medications for the treatment of hypersensitivity reactions should be available for immediate use. Treatment may result in the development of human antimurine antibodies (HAMA); however, limited evidence suggesting the use of muromonab-CD3 or other murine products is not precluded.

Adverse Reactions Administration of basiliximab did not appear to increase the incidence or severity of adverse effects in clinical trials. Adverse events were reported in 96% of both the placebo and basiliximab groups.

>10%:

Cardiovascular: Peripheral edema, hypertension, atrial fibrillation

Central nervous system: Fever, headache, insomnia, pain

Dermatologic: Wound complications, acne
Endocrine & metabolic: Hypokalemia, hyperkalemia, hyperglycemia, hyperuricemia, hypo-phosphatemia, hypercholesterolemia
Gastrointestinal: Constipation, nausea, diarrhea, abdominal pain, vomiting, dyspepsia
Genitourinary: Urinary tract infection
Hematologic: Anemia
Neuromuscular & skeletal: Tremor
Respiratory: Dyspnea, infection (upper respiratory)
Miscellaneous: Viral infection

3% to 10% (Limited to important or life-threatening):
Cardiovascular: Chest pain, cardiac failure, hypotension, arrhythmia, tachycardia, edema, angina pectoris
Central nervous system: Hypoesthesia, neuropathy, agitation, anxiety, depression
Dermatologic: Cyst, hypertrichosis, pruritus, rash
Endocrine & metabolic: Dehydration, diabetes mellitus, fluid overload, hypercalcemia, hyperlipidemia, hypoglycemia, hypomagnesemia, acidosis, hypertriglyceridemia, hypo-calcemia, hyponatremia
Gastrointestinal: GI hemorrhage, gingival hyperplasia, melena, esophagitis, ulcerative stomatitis
Genitourinary: Impotence, genital edema, albuminuria, hematuria, renal tubular necrosis, urinary retention
Hematologic: Hematoma, hemorrhage, thrombocytopenia, thrombosis, polycythemia, leukopenia
Neuromuscular & skeletal: Arthralgia, arthropathy, paresthesia
Ocular: Cataract, conjunctivitis, abnormal vision
Respiratory: Bronchospasm, pulmonary edema
Miscellaneous: Sepsis, infection, increased glucocorticoids

Postmarketing and/or case reports: Severe hypersensitivity reactions, including anaphylaxis, have been reported. Symptoms may include hypotension, tachycardia, cardiac failure, dyspnea, bronchospasm, pulmonary edema, urticaria, rash, pruritus, sneezing, capillary leak syndrome, and respiratory failure.

Overdosage/Toxicology There have been no reports of overdose.

Drug Interactions
Increased Effect/Toxicity: Basiliximab is an immunoglobulin; specific drug interactions have not been evaluated, but are not anticipated.
Decreased Effect: Basiliximab is an immunoglobulin; specific drug interactions have not been evaluated, but are not anticipated. It is not known if the immune response to vaccines will be impaired during or following basiliximab therapy.

Stability Store intact vials under refrigeration 2°C to 8°C (36°F to 46°F). Reconstitute 20 mg vials with 5 mL of sterile water for injection, USP. Shake the vial gently to dissolve. It is recommended that after reconstitution, the solution should be used immediately. If not used immediately, it can be stored at 2°C to 8°C for up to 24 hours or at room temperature for up to 4 hours. Discard the reconstituted solution within 24 hours. Further dilute reconstituted solution to a volume of 50 mL with 0.9% sodium chloride or dextrose 5% in water. When mixing the solution, gently invert the bag to avoid foaming. Do not shake.

Mechanism of Action Chimeric (murine/human) monoclonal antibody which blocks the alpha-chain of the interleukin-2 (IL-2) receptor complex; this receptor is expressed on acti-vated T lymphocytes and is a critical pathway for activating cell-mediated allograft rejection

Pharmacodynamics/Kinetics
Duration: Mean: 36 days (determined by IL-2R alpha saturation)
Distribution: Mean: V_d: Children: 5.2 ± 2.8 L; Adults: 8.6 L
Half-life elimination: Children: 9.4 days; Adults: Mean: 7.2 days
Excretion: Clearance: Children: 20 mL/hour; Adults: Mean: 41 mL/hour

Usual Dosage Note: Patients previously administered basiliximab should only be re-exposed to a subsequent course of therapy with extreme caution.
I.V.:
Children <35 kg: Renal transplantation: 10 mg within 2 hours prior to transplant surgery, followed by a second 10 mg dose 4 days after transplantation; the second dose should be withheld if complications occur (including severe hypersensitivity reactions or graft loss)
Children ≥35 kg and Adults: Renal transplantation: 20 mg within 2 hours prior to transplant surgery, followed by a second 20 mg dose 4 days after transplantation; the second dose should be withheld if complications occur (including severe hypersensitivity reactions or graft loss)
Dosing adjustment/comments in renal or hepatic impairment: No specific dosing adjust-ment recommended

Administration Intravenous infusion over 20-30 minutes via central or peripheral intravenous line

Monitoring Parameters Signs and symptoms of acute rejection

Dosage Forms Injection, powder for reconstitution: 20 mg

♦ **Baycol**® see Cerivastatin *Withdrawn From U.S. Market* on page 264
♦ **Bayer**® **Aspirin [OTC]** see Aspirin on page 120
♦ **Bayer**® **Aspirin Extra Strength [OTC]** see Aspirin on page 120
♦ **Bayer**® **Aspirin Regimen Adult Low Strength [OTC]** see Aspirin on page 120
♦ **Bayer**® **Aspirin Regimen Adult Low Strength with Calcium [OTC]** see Aspirin on page 120
♦ **Bayer**® **Aspirin Regimen Children's [OTC]** see Aspirin on page 120
♦ **Bayer**® **Aspirin Regimen Regular Strength [OTC]** see Aspirin on page 120
♦ **Bayer**® **Plus Extra Strength [OTC]** see Aspirin on page 120
♦ **BayGam**® see Immune Globulin (Intramuscular) on page 710
♦ **BayHep B**™ see Hepatitis B Immune Globulin on page 661
♦ **BayRab**® see Rabies Immune Globulin (Human) on page 1174

- **BayRho-D®** *see* Rh₀(D) Immune Globulin (Intramuscular) *on page 1187*
- **BayRho-D® Mini-Dose** *see* Rh₀(D) Immune Globulin (Intramuscular) *on page 1187*
- **BayTet™** *see* Tetanus Immune Globulin (Human) *on page 1304*
- **Baza® Antifungal [OTC]** *see* Miconazole *on page 908*
- **B-Caro-T™** *see* Beta-Carotene *on page 161*
- **BCG, Live** *see* BCG Vaccine *on page 148*

BCG Vaccine (bee see jee vak SEEN)

U.S. Brand Names TheraCys®; TICE® BCG
Canadian Brand Names ImmuCyst®; Oncotice™; Pacis™
Synonyms Bacillus Calmette-Guérin (BCG) Live; BCG, Live
Therapeutic Category Biological Response Modulator; Vaccine, Live Bacteria
Use Immunization against tuberculosis and immunotherapy for cancer; treatment of bladder cancer

BCG vaccine is not routinely recommended for use in the U.S. for prevention of tuberculosis
BCG vaccine is strongly recommended for infants and children with negative tuberculin skin tests who:

> are at high risk of intimate and prolonged exposure to persistently untreated or ineffectively treated patients with infectious pulmonary tuberculosis, and
> cannot be removed from the source of exposure, and
> cannot be placed on long-term preventive therapy
> are continuously exposed with tuberculosis who have bacilli resistant to isoniazid and rifampin

BCG is also recommended for tuberculin-negative infants and children in groups in which the rate of new infections exceeds 1% per year and for whom the usual surveillance and treatment programs have been attempted but are not operationally feasible

BCG should be administered with caution to persons in groups at high risk for HIV infection or persons known to be severely immunocompromised. Although limited data suggest that the vaccine may be safe for use in asymptomatic children infected with HIV, BCG vaccination is not recommended for HIV infected adults or for persons with symptomatic disease. Until further research can clearly define the risks and benefits of BCG vaccination for this population, vaccination should be restricted to persons at exceptionally high risk for tuberculosis infection. HIV infected persons thought to be infected with *Mycobacterium tuberculosis* should be strongly recommended for tuberculosis preventive therapy.

Pregnancy Risk Factor C
Usual Dosage Children >1 month and Adults:

Immunization against tuberculosis (TICE® BCG): 0.2-0.3 mL percutaneous; initial lesion usually appears after 10-14 days consisting of small red papule at injection site and reaches maximum diameter of 3 mm in 4-6 weeks; conduct postvaccinal tuberculin test (ie, 5 TU of PPD) in 2-3 months; if test is negative, repeat vaccination

Immunotherapy for bladder cancer:

Intravesical treatment: Instill into bladder for 2 hours

TheraCys®: One dose diluted in 50 mL NS (preservative free) instilled into bladder once weekly for 6 weeks followed by one treatment at 3, 6, 12, 18, and 24 months after initial treatment

TICE® BCG: One dose diluted in 50 mL NS (preservative free) instilled into the bladder once weekly for 6 weeks followed by once monthly for 6-12 months

Additional Information Complete prescribing information for this medication should be consulted for additional detail.
Dosage Forms Injection, powder for reconstitution, intravesical:

TheraCys®: 81 mg [supplied with diluent]
TICE® BCG: 50 mg

- **BCNU** *see* Carmustine *on page 230*
- **B Complex** *see* Vitamins (Multiple) *on page 1424*
- **B Complex With C** *see* Vitamins (Multiple) *on page 1424*

Becaplermin (be KAP ler min)

U.S. Brand Names Regranex®
Canadian Brand Names Regranex®
Synonyms Recombinant Human Platelet-Derived Growth Factor B; rPDGF-BB
Therapeutic Category Growth Factor, Platelet-derived; Topical Skin Product
Use Debridement adjunct for the treatment of diabetic ulcers that occur on the lower limbs and feet
Pregnancy Risk Factor C
Contraindications Hypersensitivity to becaplermin or any component of the formulation; known neoplasm(s) at the site(s) of application; active infection at ulcer site
Warnings/Precautions Concurrent use of corticosteroids, cancer chemotherapy, or other immunosuppressive agents; ulcer wounds related to arterial or venous insufficiency. Thermal, electrical, or radiation burns at wound site. Malignancy (potential for tumor proliferation, although unproven; topical absorption is minimal). Should not be used in wounds that close by primary intention. For external use only.
Adverse Reactions <1%: Erythema with purulent discharge, exuberant granulation tissue, local pain, skin ulceration, tunneling of ulcer, ulcer infection
Stability Refrigerate at 2°C to 8°C (36°F to 46°F); do not freeze
Mechanism of Action Recombinant B-isoform homodimer of human platelet-derived growth factor (rPDGF-BB) which enhances formation of new granulation tissue, induces fibroblast proliferation, and differentiation to promote wound healing
Pharmacodynamics/Kinetics
Onset of action: Complete healing: 15% of patients within 8 weeks, 25% at 10 weeks
Absorption: Minimal
Distribution: Binds to PGDF-beta receptors in normal skin and granulation tissue

Usual Dosage Adults: Topical:

Diabetic ulcers: Apply appropriate amount of gel once daily with a cotton swab or similar tool, as a coating over the ulcer

The amount of becaplermin to be applied will vary depending on the size of the ulcer area. To calculate the length of gel applied to the ulcer, measure the greatest length of the ulcer by the greatest width of the ulcer in inches. Tube size will determine the formula used in the calculation. For a 15 or 7.5 g tube, multiply length x width x 0.6. For a 2 g tube, multiply length x width x 1.3.

Note: If the ulcer does not decrease in size by ~30% after 10 weeks of treatment or complete healing has not occurred in 20 weeks, continued treatment with becaplermin gel should be reassessed.

Monitoring Parameters Ulcer volume (pressure ulcers); wound area; evidence of closure; drainage (diabetic ulcers); signs/symptoms of toxicity (erythema, local infections)

Patient Information

Hands should be washed thoroughly before applying. The tip of the tube should not come into contact with the ulcer or any other surface; the tube should be recapped tightly after each use. A cotton swab, tongue depressor, or other application aid should be used to apply gel.

Step-by-step instructions for application:

Squeeze the calculated length of gel on to a clean, firm, nonabsorbable surface (wax paper)

With a clean cotton swab, tongue depressor, or similar application aid, spread the measured gel over the ulcer area to obtain an even layer

Cover with a saline-moistened gauze dressing. After ~12 hours, the ulcer should be gently rinsed with saline or water to remove residual gel and covered with a saline-moistened gauze dressing (**without** gel).

Dosage Forms Gel, topical: 0.01% (15 g)

Beclomethasone (be kloe METH a sone)

Related Information

Asthma *on page 1645*

Estimated Clinical Comparability of Doses for Inhaled Corticosteroids *on page 1652*

U.S. Brand Names Beclovent® [DSC]; Beconase®; Beconase® AQ; QVAR™; Vancenase® AQ 84 mcg; Vancenase® Pockethaler®; Vanceril®

Canadian Brand Names Alti-Beclomethasone; Apo®-Beclomethasone; Gen-Beclo; Nu-Beclomethasone; Propaderm®; QVAR™; Rivanase AQ; Vancenase®; Vanceril®

Synonyms Beclomethasone Dipropionate

Therapeutic Category Anti-inflammatory Agent, Inhalant; Corticosteroid, Inhalant; Corticosteroid, Intranasal

Use

Oral inhalation: Maintenance and prophylactic treatment of asthma; includes those who require corticosteroids and those who may benefit from a dose reduction/elimination of systemically administered corticosteroids. Not for relief of acute bronchospasm

Nasal aerosol: Symptomatic treatment of seasonal or perennial rhinitis and to prevent recurrence of nasal polyps following surgery

Pregnancy Risk Factor C

Pregnancy/Breast-Feeding Implications Data does not support an association between drug and congenital defects in humans

Clinical effects on fetus: No data on crossing the placenta or effects on the fetus

Breast-feeding/lactation: No data on crossing into breast milk or effects on the infant

Contraindications Hypersensitivity to beclomethasone or any component of the formulation; status asthmaticus

Warnings/Precautions Not to be used in status asthmaticus or for the relief of acute bronchospasm; safety and efficacy in children <6 years of age have not been established. May cause suppression of hypothalamic-pituitary-adrenal (HPA) axis, particularly in younger children or in patients receiving high doses for prolonged periods. Particular care is required when patients are transferred from systemic corticosteroids to inhaled products due to possible adrenal insufficiency or withdrawal from steroids, including an increase in allergic symptoms. Patients receiving 20 mg per day of prednisone (or equivalent) may be most susceptible. Fatalities have occurred due to adrenal insufficiency in asthmatic patients during and after transfer from systemic corticosteroids to aerosol steroids; aerosol steroids do **not** provide the systemic steroid needed to treat patients having trauma, surgery, or infections. Withdrawal and discontinuation of the corticosteroid should be done slowly and carefully.

Controlled clinical studies have shown that orally-inhaled and intranasal corticosteroids may cause a reduction in growth velocity in pediatric patients. (In studies of orally-inhaled corticosteroids, the mean reduction in growth velocity was approximately 1 centimeter per year [range 0.3-1.8 cm per year] and appears to be related to dose and duration of exposure.) The growth of pediatric patients receiving inhaled corticosteroids, should be monitored routinely (eg, via stadiometry). To minimize the systemic effects of orally-inhaled and intranasal corticosteroids, each patient should be titrated to the lowest effective dose.

May suppress the immune system, patients may be more susceptible to infection. Use with caution in patients with systemic infections or ocular herpes simplex. Avoid exposure to chickenpox and measles. Corticosteroids should be used with caution in patients with diabetes, hypertension, osteoporosis, peptic ulcer, glaucoma, cataracts, or tuberculosis. Use caution in hepatic impairment. Beclovent® Oral Inhaler, Beconase® Nasal Inhaler, and Vanceril® Oral Inhaler contain chlorofluorocarbons (CFCs).

Adverse Reactions Frequency not defined.

Central nervous system: Agitation, depression, dizziness, dysphonia, headache, lightheadedness, mental disturbances

Dermatologic: Acneiform lesions, angioedema, atrophy, bruising, pruritus, purpura, striae, rash, urticaria

Endocrine & metabolic: Cushingoid features, growth velocity reduction in children and adolescents, HPA function suppression

(Continued)

Beclomethasone *(Continued)*

Gastrointestinal: Dry/irritated nose, throat and mouth, hoarseness, localized *Candida* or *Aspergillus* infections, loss of smell, loss of taste, nausea, unpleasant smell, unpleasant taste, vomiting, weight gain

Local: Nasal spray: Burning, epistaxis, localized *Candida* infections, nasal septum perforation (rare), nasal stuffiness, nosebleeds, rhinorrhea, sneezing, transient irritation, ulceration of nasal mucosa (rare)

Ocular: Cataracts, glaucoma, increased intraocular pressure

Respiratory: Cough, paradoxical bronchospasm, pharyngitis, sinusitis, wheezing

Miscellaneous: Anaphylactic/anaphylactoid reactions, death (due to adrenal insufficiency, reported during and after transfer from systemic corticosteroids to aerosol in asthmatic patients), immediate and delayed hypersensitivity reactions

Overdosage/Toxicology Symptoms include irritation and burning of the nasal mucosa, sneezing, intranasal and pharyngeal *Candida* infections, nasal ulceration, epistaxis, rhinorrhea, nasal stuffiness, and headache. When consumed in excessive quantities, systemic hypercorticism and adrenal suppression may occur; in those cases, discontinuation and withdrawal of the corticosteroid should be done judiciously.

Drug Interactions

Increased Effect/Toxicity: The addition of salmeterol has been demonstrated to improve response to inhaled corticosteroids (as compared to increasing steroid dosage).

Stability Do not store near heat or open flame. Do not puncture canisters. Store at room temperature. Rest QVAR™ on concave end of canister with actuator on top.

Mechanism of Action Controls the rate of protein synthesis, depresses the migration of polymorphonuclear leukocytes, fibroblasts, reverses capillary permeability, and lysosomal stabilization at the cellular level to prevent or control inflammation

Pharmacodynamics/Kinetics

Onset of action: Therapeutic effect: 1-4 weeks

Absorption: Readily absorbed; quickly hydrolyzed by pulmonary esterases prior to absorption

Distribution: Beclomethasone: 20 L; active metabolite: 424 L

Protein binding: 87%

Metabolism: Hepatic via CYP3A4 to active metabolites

Bioavailability: Of active metabolite, 44% following nasal inhalation (43% from swallowed portion)

Half-life elimination: Initial: 3 hours

Excretion: Feces (60%); urine (12%)

Usual Dosage Nasal inhalation and oral inhalation dosage forms are not to be used interchangeably

Aqueous inhalation, nasal:

Vancenase® AQ, Beconase® AQ: Children ≥6 years and Adults: 1-2 inhalations each nostril twice daily; total dose 168-336 mcg/day

Vancenase® AQ 84 mcg: Children ≥6 years and Adults: 1-2 inhalations in each nostril once daily; total dose 168-336 mcg/day

Intranasal (Vancenase®, Beconase®):

Children 6-12 years: 1 inhalation in each nostril 3 times/day; total dose 252 mcg/day

Children ≥12 years and Adults: 1 inhalation in each nostril 2-4 times/day or 2 inhalations each nostril twice daily (total dose 168-336 mcg/day); usual maximum maintenance: 1 inhalation in each nostril 3 times/day (252 mcg/day)

Oral inhalation (doses should be titrated to the lowest effective dose once asthma is controlled):

Beclovent®, Vanceril®:

Children 6-12 years: 1-2 inhalations 3-4 times/day (alternatively: 2-4 inhalations twice daily); maximum dose: 10 inhalations/day (420 mcg)

Children ≥12 years and Adults: 2 inhalations 3-4 times/day (alternatively: 4 inhalations twice daily); maximum dose: 20 inhalations/day (840 mcg/day); patients with severe asthma: Initial: 12-16 inhalations/day (divided 3-4 times/day); dose should be adjusted downward according to patient's response

Vanceril® 84 mcg double strength:

Children 6-12 years: 2 inhalations twice daily; maximum dose: 5 inhalations/day (420 mcg)

Children ≥12 years and Adults: 2 inhalations twice daily; maximum dose: 10 inhalations/day (840 mcg); patients with severe asthma: Initial: 6-8 inhalations/day (divided twice daily); dose should be adjusted downward according to patient's response

QVAR™:

Children ≥ 12 years and Adults:

Patients previously on bronchodilators only: Initial dose 40-80 mcg twice daily; maximum dose 320 mcg twice day

Patients previously on inhaled corticosteroids: Initial dose 40-160 mcg twice daily; maximum dose 320 mcg twice daily

NIH Guidelines (NIH, 1997) (give in divided doses):

Children:

"Low" dose: 84-336 mcg/day (42 mcg/puff: 2-8 puffs/day or 84 mcg/puff: 1-4 puffs/day)

"Medium" dose: 336-672 mcg/day (42 mcg/puff: 8-16 puffs/day or 84 mcg/puff: 4-8 puffs/day)

"High" dose: >672 mcg/day (42 mcg/puff: >16 puffs/day or 84 mcg/puff >8 puffs/day)

Adults:

"Low" dose: 168-504 mcg/day (42 mcg/puff: 4-12 puffs/day or 84 mcg/puff: 2-6 puffs/day)

"Medium" dose: 504-840 mcg/day (42 mcg/puff: 12-20 puffs/day or 84 mcg/puff: 6-10 puffs/day)

"High" dose: >840 mcg/day (42 mcg/puff: >20 puffs/day or 84 mcg/puff: >10 puffs/day)

Administration

Aerosol inhalation: Shake container thoroughly before using

Aerosol inhalation, oral: Consider use of a spacer device for children <8 years of age requiring a metered dose inhaler (MDI)

Patient Information Rinse mouth and throat after use to prevent *Candida* infection, report sore throat or mouth lesions to physician. Inhaled beclomethasone makes many asthmatics cough, to reduce chance, inhale drug slowly or use prescribed inhaled bronchodilator 5 minutes before beclomethasone is used; keep inhaler clean and unobstructed, wash in warm water and dry thoroughly; shake thoroughly before using.

Nursing Implications Take drug history of patients with perennial rhinitis, may be drug related; check mucous membranes for signs of fungal infection

Additional Information Effects of inhaled/intranasal steroids on growth have been observed in the absence of laboratory evidence of HPA axis suppression, suggesting that growth velocity is a more sensitive indicator of systemic corticosteroid exposure in pediatric patients than some commonly used tests of HPA axis function. The long-term effects of this reduction in growth velocity associated with orally-inhaled and intranasal corticosteroids, including the impact on final adult height, are unknown. The potential for "catch up" growth following discontinuation of treatment with inhaled corticosteroids has not been adequately studied.

Dosage Forms

Aerosol for oral inhalation, as dipropionate:

Beclovent® [DSC], Vanceril®: 42 mcg/inhalation [200 metered doses] (16.8 g)

QVAR™: 40 mcg/inhalation [100 metered doses] (7.3 g); 80 mcg/inhalation [100 metered doses] (7.3 g)

Vanceril® Double Strength: 84 mcg/inhalation [40 metered doses] (5.4 g), 84 mcg/inhalation [120 metered doses] (12.2 g)

Aerosol, intranasal, as dipropionate (Beconase®, Vancenase®): 42 mcg/inhalation: [80 metered doses] (6.7 g); [200 metered doses] (16.8 g)

Suspension, intranasal, aqueous, as dipropionate [spray]:

Beconase® AQ, Vancenase® AQ 0.042%: 42 mcg/inhalation [≥200 metered doses] (25 g)

Vancenase® AQ Double Strength: 84 mcg per inhalation [120 actuations] (19 g)

♦ **Beclomethasone Dipropionate** *see Beclomethasone on page 149*

♦ **Beclovent® [DSC]** *see Beclomethasone on page 149*

♦ **Beconase®** *see Beclomethasone on page 149*

♦ **Beconase® AQ** *see Beclomethasone on page 149*

♦ **Becotin® Pulvules®** *see Vitamins (Multiple) on page 1424*

♦ **Bedoz (Can)** *see Cyanocobalamin on page 339*

♦ **Behenyl Alcohol** *see Docosanol on page 430*

Belladonna and Opium (bel a DON a & OH pee um)

U.S. Brand Names B&O Supprettes®

Synonyms Opium and Belladonna

Therapeutic Category Analgesic, Narcotic; Antispasmodic Agent, Urinary

Use Relief of moderate to severe pain associated with rectal or bladder tenesmus that may occur in postoperative states and neoplastic situations; pain associated with ureteral spasms not responsive to non-narcotic analgesics and to space intervals between injections of opiates

Restrictions C-II

Pregnancy Risk Factor C

Contraindications Glaucoma; severe renal or hepatic disease; bronchial asthma; respiratory depression; convulsive disorders; acute alcoholism; premature labor

Warnings/Precautions Usual precautions of opiate agonist therapy should be observed; infants <3 months of age are more susceptible to respiratory depression, use with caution and generally in reduced doses in this age group

Adverse Reactions

>10%:

Dermatologic: Dry skin

Gastrointestinal: Constipation, dry throat, dry mouth

Local: Irritation at injection site

Respiratory: Dry nose

Miscellaneous: Diaphoresis (decreased)

1% to 10%:

Dermatologic: Increased sensitivity to light

Endocrine & metabolic: Decreased flow of breast milk

Gastrointestinal: Dysphagia

<1% (Limited to important or life-threatening): Ataxia, CNS depression, increased intraocular pain, loss of memory, orthostatic hypotension, respiratory depression, tachycardia, ventricular fibrillation

Overdosage/Toxicology Primary attention should be directed to ensuring adequate respiratory exchange. Opiate agonist-induced respiratory depression may be reversed with parenteral naloxone hydrochloride. Anticholinergic toxicity may be caused by strong binding of a belladonna alkaloid to cholinergic receptors. Anticholinesterase inhibitors reduce acetylcholinesterase, the enzyme that breaks down acetylcholine and thereby allows acetylcholine to accumulate and compete for receptor binding with the offending anticholinergic. For an overdose with severe life-threatening symptoms, physostigmine 1-2 mg (0.5 mg or 0.02 mg/kg for children) S.C. or slow I.V., may be given to reverse these effects.

Drug Interactions

Increased Effect/Toxicity: Additive effects with CNS depressants. May increase effects of digoxin and atenolol. Coadministration with other anticholinergic agents (phenothiazines, tricyclic antidepressants, amantadine, and antihistamines) may increase effects such as dry mouth, constipation, and urinary retention.

Decreased Effect: May decrease effects of drugs with cholinergic mechanisms. Antipsychotic efficacy of phenothiazines may be decreased.

Ethanol/Nutrition/Herb Interactions Ethanol: Avoid ethanol (may increase sedation).

Stability Store at 15°C to 30°C (avoid freezing)

Mechanism of Action Anticholinergic alkaloids act primarily by competitive inhibition of the muscarinic actions of acetylcholine on structures innervated by postganglionic cholinergic (Continued)

Belladonna and Opium (Continued)

neurons and on smooth muscle; resulting effects include antisecretory activity on exocrine glands and intestinal mucosa and smooth muscle relaxation. Contains many narcotic alkaloids including morphine; its mechanism for gastric motility inhibition is primarily due to this morphine content; it results in a decrease in digestive secretions, an increase in GI muscle tone, and therefore a reduction in GI propulsion.

Pharmacodynamics/Kinetics
    Belladonna: See Belladonna monograph.
    Opium:
        Onset of action: Within 30 minutes
        Metabolism: Hepatic, with formation of glucuronide metabolites

Usual Dosage Adults: Rectal: 1 suppository 1-2 times/day, up to 4 doses/day

Test Interactions ↑ aminotransferase [ALT (SGPT)/AST (SGOT)] (S)

Patient Information May cause drowsiness and blurred vision

Nursing Implications Prior to rectal insertion, the finger and suppository should be moistened; assist with ambulation, monitor for CNS depression

Dosage Forms Suppository:
    #15 A: Belladonna extract 16.2 mg and opium 30 mg
    #16 A: Belladonna extract 16.2 mg and opium 60 mg

Belladonna, Phenobarbital, and Ergotamine Tartrate

(bel a DON a, fee noe BAR bi tal, & er GOT a meen TAR trate)

U.S. Brand Names Bellamine S; Bel-Phen-Ergot S®; Bel-Tabs

Canadian Brand Names Bellergal® Spacetabs®

Synonyms Belladonna, Phenobarbital, and Ergotamine Tartrate; Ergotamine Tartrate, Belladonna, and Phenobarbital; Phenobarbital, Belladonna, and Ergotamine Tartrate

Therapeutic Category Ergot Alkaloid and Derivative

Use Management and treatment of menopausal disorders, GI disorders, and recurrent throbbing headache

Pregnancy Risk Factor X

Usual Dosage Oral: 1 tablet each morning and evening

Additional Information Complete prescribing information for this medication should be consulted for additional detail.

Dosage Forms Tablet: Belladonna alkaloids 0.2 mg, phenobarbital 40 mg, and ergotamine tartrate 0.6 mg

♦ **Bellamine S** see Belladonna, Phenobarbital, and Ergotamine Tartrate on page 152

♦ **Bellatal®** see Hyoscyamine, Atropine, Scopolamine, and Phenobarbital on page 694

♦ **Bellergal® Spacetabs® (Can)** see Belladonna, Phenobarbital, and Ergotamine Tartrate on page 152

♦ **Bel-Phen-Ergot S®** see Belladonna, Phenobarbital, and Ergotamine Tartrate on page 152

♦ **Bel-Tabs** see Belladonna, Phenobarbital, and Ergotamine Tartrate on page 152

♦ **Benadryl® [OTC]** see DiphenhydrAMINE on page 414

♦ **Benadryl® Decongestant Allergy [OTC]** see Diphenhydramine and Pseudoephedrine on page 415

Benazepril (ben AY ze pril)

Related Information
    Angiotensin Agents Comparison on page 1473

U.S. Brand Names Lotensin®

Canadian Brand Names Lotensin®

Synonyms Benazepril Hydrochloride

Therapeutic Category Angiotensin-Converting Enzyme (ACE) Inhibitor; Antihypertensive Agent

Use Treatment of hypertension, either alone or in combination with other antihypertensive agents; treatment of left ventricular dysfunction after myocardial infarction

Pregnancy Risk Factor C/D (2nd and 3rd trimesters)

Pregnancy/Breast-Feeding Implications

Clinical effects on the fetus: No data available on crossing the placenta. Cranial defects, hypocalvaria/acalvaria, oligohydramnios, persistent anuria following delivery, hypotension, renal defects, renal dysgenesis/dysplasia, renal failure, pulmonary hypoplasia, limb contractures secondary to oligohydramnios and stillbirth reported. ACE inhibitors should be avoided during pregnancy.

Breast-feeding/lactation: Crosses into breast milk. AAP considers **compatible** with breast-feeding.

Contraindications Hypersensitivity to benazepril or any component of the formulation; angioedema or serious hypersensitivity related to previous treatment with an ACE inhibitor; bilateral renal artery stenosis; primary hyperaldosteronism; patients with idiopathic or hereditary angioedema; pregnancy (2nd and 3rd trimesters)

Warnings/Precautions Anaphylactic reactions can occur. Angioedema can occur at any time during treatment (especially following first dose). Careful blood pressure monitoring with first dose (hypotension can occur especially in volume depleted patients). Dosage adjustment needed in renal impairment. Use with caution in hypovolemia; collagen vascular diseases; valvular stenosis (particularly aortic stenosis); hyperkalemia; or before, during, or immediately after anesthesia. Avoid rapid dosage escalation which may lead to renal insufficiency. Hypersensitivity reactions may be seen during hemodialysis with high-flux dialysis membranes (eg, AN69). Deterioration in renal function can occur with initiation. Use with caution in unilateral renal artery stenosis and pre-existing renal insufficiency.

Adverse Reactions
    1% to 10%:
        Cardiovascular: Postural dizziness (1.5%)

Central nervous system: Headache (6.2%), dizziness (3.6%), fatigue (2.4%), somnolence (1.6%)

Endocrine & metabolic: Hyperkalemia (1%), increased uric acid

Gastrointestinal: Nausea (1.3%)

Renal: Increased serum creatinine (2%), worsening of renal function may occur in patients with bilateral renal artery stenosis or hypovolemia

Respiratory: Cough (1.2% to 10%)

<1% (Limited to important or life-threatening): Alopecia, angina, angioedema, asthma, dermatitis, dyspnea, hemolytic anemia, hypersensitivity, hypotension, impotence, insomnia, pancreatitis, paresthesia, photosensitivity, postural hypotension (0.3%), rash, shock, Stevens-Johnson syndrome, syncope, thrombocytopenia, vomiting

Eosinophilic pneumonitis, neutropenia, anaphylaxis, renal insufficiency and renal failure have been reported with other ACE inhibitors. In addition, a syndrome including fever, myalgia, arthralgia, interstitial nephritis, vasculitis, rash, eosinophilia, and elevated ESR has been reported to be associated with ACE inhibitors.

Overdosage/Toxicology Mild hypotension has been the only toxic effect seen with acute overdose; bradycardia may also occur. Hyperkalemia occurs even with therapeutic doses, especially in patients with renal insufficiency and those taking NSAIDs. Following initiation of essential overdose management, toxic symptom treatment and supportive treatment should be initiated. Hypotension usually responds to I.V. fluids or Trendelenburg positioning.

Drug Interactions

Increased Effect/Toxicity: Potassium supplements, co-trimoxazole (high dose), angiotensin II receptor antagonists (candesartan, losartan, irbesartan, etc), or potassium-sparing diuretics (amiloride, spironolactone, triamterene) may result in elevated serum potassium levels when combined with benazepril. ACE inhibitor effects may be increased by phenothiazines or probenecid (increases levels of captopril). ACE inhibitors may increase serum concentrations/effects of digoxin, lithium, and sulfonlyureas. Diuretics have additive hypotensive effects with ACE inhibitors, and hypovolemia increases the potential for adverse renal effects of ACE inhibitors. In patients with compromised renal function, coadministration with nonsteroidal anti-inflammatory drugs may result in further deterioration of renal function. Allopurinol and ACE inhibitors may cause a higher risk of hypersensitivity reaction when taken concurrently.

Decreased Effect: Aspirin (high dose) may reduce the therapeutic effects of ACE inhibitors; at low dosages this does not appear to be significant. Rifampin may decrease the effect of ACE inhibitors. Antacids may decrease the bioavailability of ACE inhibitors (may be more likely to occur with captopril); separate administration times by 1-2 hours. NSAIDs, specifically indomethacin, may reduce the hypotensive effects of ACE inhibitors.

Ethanol/Nutrition/Herb Interactions Herb/Nutraceutical: Avoid dong quai if using for hypertension (has estrogenic activity). Avoid ephedra, yohimbe, ginseng (may worsen hypertension). Avoid garlic (may have increased antihypertensive effect).

Mechanism of Action Competitive inhibition of angiotensin I being converted to angiotensin II, a potent vasoconstrictor, through the angiotensin I-converting enzyme (ACE) activity, with resultant lower levels of angiotensin II which causes an increase in plasma renin activity and a reduction in aldosterone secretion

Pharmacodynamics/Kinetics

Reduction in plasma angiotensin-converting enzyme activity:
Peak effect: 1-2 hours after 2-20 mg dose
Duration: >90% inhibition for 24 hours after 5-20 mg dose

Reduction in blood pressure:
Peak effect: 2-4 hours after single dose; 2 weeks with continuous therapy

Absorption: Rapid (37%); food does not alter significantly; metabolite (benazeprilat) itself unsuitable for oral administration due to poor absorption

Distribution: V_d: ~8.7 L

Metabolism: Rapidly and extensively hepatic to its active metabolite, benazeprilat, via enzymatic hydrolysis; extensive first-pass effect; completely eliminated from plasma in 4 hours

Half-life elimination: Effective: 10-11 hours; Benazeprilat: Terminal: 22 hours

Time to peak: Parent drug: 1-1.5 hours

Excretion: Clearance: Nonrenal clearance (ie, biliary, metabolic) appears to contribute to the elimination of benazepril (11% to 12%), particularly patients with severe renal impairment; hepatic clearance is the main elimination route of unchanged benazepril

Dialysis: ~6% of metabolite removed in 4 hours of dialysis following 10 mg of benazepril administered 2 hours prior to procedure; parent compound was not found in the dialysate

Usual Dosage Adults: Oral: Initial: 10 mg/day in patients not receiving a diuretic; 20-40 mg/day as a single dose or 2 divided doses; base dosage adjustments on peak (2-6 hours after dosing) and trough responses.

Dosing interval in renal impairment: Cl_{cr} <30 mL/minute: Administer 5 mg/day initially; maximum daily dose: 40 mg.

Hemodialysis: Moderately dialyzable (20% to 50%); administer dose postdialysis or administer 25% to 35% supplemental dose.

Peritoneal dialysis: Supplemental dose is not necessary.

Administration Discontinue diuretics 2-3 days prior to benazepril initiation; if the diuretics cannot be discontinued, begin benazepril at 5 mg

Patient Information May be taken in disregard of meals; notify physician of persistent cough or other side effects; do not stop therapy except under prescriber advice; may cause dizziness, fainting, and lightheadedness, especially in first week of therapy; sit and stand up slowly; may cause changes in taste or rash; do not add a salt substitute (potassium) without advice of physician

Nursing Implications Watch for hypotensive effect within 1-3 hours of first dose or new higher dose; discontinue therapy immediately if angioedema of the face, extremities, lips, tongue, or glottis occurs

Dosage Forms Tablet, as hydrochloride: 5 mg, 10 mg, 20 mg, 40 mg

♦ **Benazepril and Amlodipine** *see* Amlodipine and Benazepril *on page 80*

Benazepril and Hydrochlorothiazide
(ben AY ze pril & hye droe klor oh THYE a zide)

U.S. Brand Names Lotensin® HCT

Canadian Brand Names Lotrel®

Synonyms Hydrochlorothiazide and Benazepril

Therapeutic Category Angiotensin-Converting Enzyme (ACE) Inhibitor Combination; Antihypertensive Agent, Combination

Use Treatment of hypertension

Pregnancy Risk Factor C/D (2nd and 3rd trimesters)

Usual Dosage Dose is individualized

Additional Information Complete prescribing information for this medication should be consulted for additional detail.

Dosage Forms Tablet:
  Benazepril 5 mg and hydrochlorothiazide 6.25 mg
  Benazepril 10 mg and hydrochlorothiazide 12.5 mg
  Benazepril 20 mg and hydrochlorothiazide 12.5 mg
  Benazepril 20 mg and hydrochlorothiazide 25 mg

♦ **Benazepril Hydrochloride** *see Benazepril on page 152*

♦ **BeneFix™** *see Factor IX Complex (Human) on page 539*

♦ **Benemid® [DSC]** *see Probenecid on page 1129*

Bentoquatam (BEN toe kwa tam)
U.S. Brand Names IvyBlock® [OTC]

Synonyms Quaternium-18 Bentonite

Therapeutic Category Topical Skin Product

Use Skin protectant for the prevention of allergic contact dermatitis to poison oak, ivy, and sumac

Contraindications Hypersensitivity to bentoquatam or any component of the formulation

Warnings/Precautions Use with caution in patients with history of allergic-type responses to medications (especially topical formulations); open wounds, psoriatic lesions, or other cutaneous conditions. Use with caution in patients who are postexposure to poison oak, ivy, or sumac (lack of efficacy).

Adverse Reactions <1% (Limited to important or life-threatening): Erythema

Mechanism of Action An organoclay substance which is capable of absorbing or binding to urushiol, the active principle in poison oak, ivy, and sumac. Bentoquatam serves as a barrier, blocking urushiol skin contact/absorption.

Pharmacodynamics/Kinetics Absorption: Has not been studied

Usual Dosage Children >6 years and Adults: Topical: Apply to skin 15 minutes prior to potential exposure to poison ivy, poison oak, or poison sumac, and reapply every 4 hours

Monitoring Parameters Signs and symptoms of exposure to poison oak, ivy, or sumac (rash, swelling, blisters)

Patient Information Do not use this medication if you have had an allergic reaction to bentoquatam. Do not use this medication on children <6 years of age, unless ordered by your child's physician. Do not use this medication to treat a rash caused by poison ivy, oak, or sumac.

Use this medication on your skin only. Read and follow the instructions on the medicine label. The medication must be used at least 15 minutes **before** you are exposed to poison ivy, poison oak, or poison sumac. Shake the bottle well before each use. Rub a thin layer of the lotion on your skin to form a smooth moist layer. When the lotion dries, you will see a clay-like coating on the protected parts of your skin. You will need to apply more lotion on your skin at least every 4 hours or sooner if the medication rubs off. Do not use the medication in or near your eyes. If you do get the medication in your eyes, rinse them well with cool water for at least 20 minutes. Tell your physician if you have eye redness or eye pain that does not go away.

Dosage Forms Lotion: 5% (120 mL)

♦ **Bentyl®** *see Dicyclomine on page 397*

♦ **Bentylol® (Can)** *see Dicyclomine on page 397*

♦ **Benuryl™ (Can)** *see Probenecid on page 1129*

♦ **Benylin® 3.3 mg-D-E (Can)** *see Guaifenesin, Pseudoephedrine, and Codeine on page 648*

♦ **Benylin® DM-D (Can)** *see Pseudoephedrine and Dextromethorphan on page 1157*

♦ **Benylin® DM-D-E (Can)** *see Guaifenesin, Pseudoephedrine, and Dextromethorphan on page 648*

♦ **Benylin® DM-E (Can)** *see Guaifenesin and Dextromethorphan on page 646*

♦ **Benylin® E Extra Strength (Can)** *see Guaifenesin on page 645*

♦ **Benylin® Expectorant [OTC]** *see Guaifenesin and Dextromethorphan on page 646*

♦ **Benzacot®** *see Trimethobenzamide on page 1375*

♦ **Benzamycin®** *see Erythromycin and Benzoyl Peroxide on page 485*

♦ **Benzathine Benzylpenicillin** *see Penicillin G Benzathine on page 1051*

♦ **Benzathine Penicillin G** *see Penicillin G Benzathine on page 1051*

♦ **Benzazoline Hydrochloride** *see Tolazoline on page 1344*

♦ **Benzene Hexachloride** *see Lindane on page 806*

♦ **Benzhexol Hydrochloride** *see Trihexyphenidyl on page 1374*

♦ **Benzmethyzin** *see Procarbazine on page 1133*

Benzocaine (BEN zoe kane)
U.S. Brand Names Americaine® [OTC]; Americaine® Anesthetic Lubricant; Anbesol® [OTC]; Anbesol® Baby [OTC]; Anbesol® Maximum Strength [OTC]; Babee® Teething® [OTC]; Benzodent® [OTC]; Chiggerex® [OTC]; Chiggertox® [OTC]; Cylex® [OTC]; Detane® [OTC]; Foille® [OTC]; Foille® Medicated First Aid [OTC]; Foille® Plus [OTC]; HDA® Toothache [OTC];

Hurricaine®; Lanacane® [OTC]; Mycinettes® [OTC]; Orabase®-B [OTC]; Orajel® [OTC]; Orajel® Baby [OTC]; Orajel® Baby Nighttime [OTC]; Orajel® Maximum Strength [OTC]; Orasol® [OTC]; Solarcaine® [OTC]; Trocaine® [OTC]; Zilactin®-B [OTC]; Zilactin® Baby [OTC]

Canadian Brand Names Anbesol® Baby; Zilactin-B®; Zilactin Baby®

Synonyms Ethyl Aminobenzoate

Therapeutic Category Local Anesthetic, Ester Derivative; Local Anesthetic, Oral; Local Anesthetic, Otic; Local Anesthetic, Topical

Use Temporary relief of pain associated with local anesthetic for pruritic dermatosis, pruritus, minor burns, acute congestive and serous otitis media, swimmer's ear, otitis externa, toothache, minor sore throat pain, canker sores, hemorrhoids, rectal fissures, anesthetic lubricant for passage of catheters and endoscopic tubes; nonprescription diet aid

Pregnancy Risk Factor C

Contraindications Hypersensitivity to benzocaine, other ester-type local anesthetics, or any component of the formulation; secondary bacterial infection of area; ophthalmic use; see package labeling for specific contraindications

Warnings/Precautions Not intended for use when infections are present

Adverse Reactions Dose-related and may result in high plasma levels

1% to 10%:
    Dermatologic: Angioedema, contact dermatitis
    Local: Burning, stinging

<1% (Limited to important or life-threatening): Edema, methemoglobinemia in infants, urethritis, urticaria

Overdosage/Toxicology Methemoglobinemia has been reported with benzocaine in oral overdose. Treatment is primarily symptomatic and supportive. Termination of anesthesia by pneumatic tourniquet inflation should be attempted when the agent is administered by infiltration or regional injection. Methemoglobinemia may be treated with methylene blue, 1-2 mg/kg I.V. infused over several minutes. Seizures commonly respond to diazepam, while hypotension responds to I.V. fluids and Trendelenburg positioning. Bradyarrhythmias (when the heart rate is <60) can be treated with I.V., I.M., or S.C. atropine 15 mcg/kg. With the development of metabolic acidosis, I.V. sodium bicarbonate 0.5-2 mEq/kg and ventilatory assistance should be instituted.

Drug Interactions
    Decreased Effect: May antagonize actions of sulfonamides.

Mechanism of Action Ester local anesthetic blocks both the initiation and conduction of nerve impulses by decreasing the neuronal membrane's permeability to sodium ions, which results in inhibition of depolarization with resultant blockade of conduction

Pharmacodynamics/Kinetics
    Absorption: Topical: Poor to intact skin; well absorbed from mucous membranes and traumatized skin
    Metabolism: Hydrolyzed in plasma and liver (to a lesser extent) by cholinesterase
    Excretion: Urine (as metabolites)

Usual Dosage
    Children and Adults:
        Mucous membranes: Dosage varies depending on area to be anesthetized and vascularity of tissues
        Oral mouth/throat preparations: Refer to specific package labeling or as directed by physician
        Topical: Apply to affected area as needed

Dietary Considerations When used as a nonprescription diet aid, take just prior to food consumption.

Patient Information Do not eat for 1 hour after application to oral mucosa; chemical burns should be neutralized before application of benzocaine; avoid application to large areas of broken skin, especially in children

Nursing Implications Patient should not eat within 1 hour after application to oral mucosa

Dosage Forms
    Aerosol, oral spray (Hurricaine®): 20% (60 mL) [cherry flavor]
    Aerosol, topical spray:
        Americaine®: 20% (20 mL, 120 mL)
        Foille®: 5% (97.5 mL) [contains chloroxylenol 0.63%]
        Foille® Plus: 5% (105 mL) [contains chloroxylenol 0.63% and alcohol 57.33%]
        Solarcaine®: 20% (90 mL, 120 mL, 135 mL) [contains triclosan, alcohol 0.13%]
    Cream, topical: 5% (30 g, 454 g)
        Lanacane®: 20% (30g)
    Gel, oral:
        Anbesol® 6.3% (7.5 g)
        Anbesol® Baby, Detane®, Orajel® Baby: 7.5% (7.5 g, 10 g, 15 g)
        Anbesol® Maximum Strength, Orajel® Maximum Strength: 20% (6 g, 7.5 g, 10 g)
        HDA® Toothache: 6.5% (15 mL) [contains benzyl alcohol]
        Hurricaine®: 20% (5 g, 30 g) [mint, pina colada, watermelon, and wild cherry flavors]
        Orabase-B®: 20% (7 g)
        Orajel®, Orajel® Baby Nighttime, Zilactin®-B, Zilactin® Baby: 10% (6 g, 7.5 g, 10 g)
    Gel, topical (Americaine® Anesthetic Lubricant): 20% (2.5 g, 28 g) [contains 0.1% benzethonium chloride
    Liquid, oral:
        Anbesol®, Orasol®: 6.3% (9 mL, 15 mL, 30 mL)
        Anbesol® Maximum Strength: 20% (9 mL, 14 mL)
        Hurricaine®: 20% (30 mL) [pina colada and wild cherry flavors]
        Orajel®: 10% (13 mL) [contains tartrazine]
        Orajel® Baby: 7.5% (13 mL)
    Liquid, topical (Chiggertox®): 2% (30 mL)
    Lotion, oral (Babee® Teething): 2.5% (15 mL)
    Lozenge:
        Cylex®, Mycinettes®: 15 mg [Cylex® contains cetylpyridinium chloride 5 mg]
        Trocaine®: 10 mg

(Continued)

Benzocaine *(Continued)*

Ointment, oral (Benzodent®): 20% (30 g)
Ointment, topical:
Chiggerex®: 2% (52 g)
Foille® Medicated First Aid: 5% (3.5 g, 28 g) [contains chloroxylenol 0.1%, benzyl alcohol; corn oil base]
Paste, oral (Orabase®-B): 20% (7 g)

♦ **Benzocaine and Antipyrine** *see Antipyrine and Benzocaine on page 107*
♦ **Benzocaine and Cetylpyridinium Chloride** *see Cetylpyridinium and Benzocaine on page 267*

Benzocaine, Butyl Aminobenzoate, Tetracaine, and Benzalkonium Chloride

(BEN zoe kane, BYOO til a meen oh BENZ oh ate, TET ra kane, & benz al KOE nee um KLOR ide)
U.S. Brand Names Cetacaine®
Synonyms Tetracaine Hydrochloride, Benzocaine Butyl Aminobenzoate, and Benzalkonium Chloride
Therapeutic Category Local Anesthetic
Use Topical anesthetic to control pain or gagging
Pregnancy Risk Factor C
Usual Dosage Apply to affected area for approximately 1 second or less
Additional Information Complete prescribing information for this medication should be consulted for additional detail.
Dosage Forms
Aerosol, topical: Benzocaine 14%, butyl aminobenzoate 2%, tetracaine 2%, and benzalkonium chloride 0.5% (56 g)
Gel, topical: Benzocaine 14%, butyl aminobenzoate 2%, tetracaine 2%, and benzalkonium chloride 0.5% (29 g)
Liquid, topical: Benzocaine 14%, butyl aminobenzoate 2%, tetracaine 2%, and benzalkonium chloride 0.5% (56 mL)

Benzocaine, Gelatin, Pectin, and Sodium Carboxymethylcellulose

(BEN zoe kane, JEL a tin, PEK tin, & SOW dee um kar box ee meth il SEL yoo lose)
U.S. Brand Names Orabase® With Benzocaine [OTC]
Therapeutic Category Local Anesthetic
Use Topical anesthetic and emollient for oral lesions
Pregnancy Risk Factor C
Usual Dosage Apply 2-4 times/day
Additional Information Complete prescribing information for this medication should be consulted for additional detail.
Dosage Forms Paste: Benzocaine 20%, gelatin, pectin, and sodium carboxymethylcellulose (5 g, 15 g)

♦ **Benzodent® [OTC]** *see Benzocaine on page 154*
♦ **Benzodiazepines Comparison** *see page 1490*

Benzonatate *(ben ZOE na tate)*

U.S. Brand Names Tessalon®
Canadian Brand Names Tessalon®
Therapeutic Category Antitussive; Cough Preparation; Local Anesthetic, Oral
Use Symptomatic relief of nonproductive cough
Pregnancy Risk Factor C
Contraindications Hypersensitivity to benzonatate, related compounds (such as tetracaine), or any component of the formulation
Adverse Reactions 1% to 10%:
Central nervous system: Sedation, headache, dizziness, mental confusion, visual hallucinations, vague "chilly" sensation
Dermatologic: Rash
Gastrointestinal: Constipation, nausea, vomiting, GI upset
Neuromuscular & skeletal: Numbness in chest
Ocular: Burning sensation in eyes
Respiratory: Nasal congestion
Overdosage/Toxicology Symptoms include restlessness, tremor, and CNS stimulation. The drug's local anesthetic activity can reduce the patient's gag reflex and, therefore, may contradict the use of ipecac following ingestion, this is especially true when the capsules are chewed. Gastric lavage may be indicated if initiated early on following an acute ingestion or in comatose patients. The remaining treatment is supportive and symptomatic.
Mechanism of Action Tetracaine congener with antitussive properties; suppresses cough by topical anesthetic action on the respiratory stretch receptors
Pharmacodynamics/Kinetics
Onset of action: Therapeutic: 15-20 minutes
Duration: 3-8 hours
Usual Dosage Children >10 years and Adults: Oral: 100 mg 3 times/day or every 4 hours up to 600 mg/day
Monitoring Parameters Monitor patient's chest sounds and respiratory pattern
Patient Information Swallow capsule whole (do not break or chew capsule); use of hard candy may increase saliva flow to aid in protecting pharyngeal mucosa
Nursing Implications Change patient position every 2 hours to prevent pooling of secretions in lung; capsules are not to be crushed
Dosage Forms Capsule: 100 mg, 200 mg

♦ **Benzoyl Peroxide and Erythromycin** *see* Erythromycin and Benzoyl Peroxide *on page 485*

Benzoyl Peroxide and Hydrocortisone
(BEN zoe il peer OKS ide & hye droe KOR ti sone)
U.S. Brand Names Vanoxide-HC®
Canadian Brand Names Vanoxide-HC
Synonyms Hydrocortisone and Benzoyl Peroxide
Therapeutic Category Acne Products
Use Treatment of acne vulgaris and oily skin
Pregnancy Risk Factor C
Usual Dosage Shake well; apply thin film 1-3 times/day, gently massage into skin
Additional Information Complete prescribing information for this medication should be consulted for additional detail.
Dosage Forms Lotion: Benzoyl peroxide 5% and hydrocortisone acetate 0.5% (25 mL)

Benztropine (BENZ troe peen)
Related Information
Parkinson's Agents *on page 1513*
U.S. Brand Names Cogentin®
Canadian Brand Names Apo®-Benztropine; Cogentin®
Synonyms Benztropine Mesylate
Therapeutic Category Anticholinergic Agent; Anti-Parkinson's Agent, Anticholinergic
Use Adjunctive treatment of Parkinson's disease; treatment of drug-induced extrapyramidal symptoms (except tardive dyskinesia)
Pregnancy Risk Factor C
Contraindications Hypersensitivity to benztropine or any component of the formulation; pyloric or duodenal obstruction, stenosing peptic ulcers; bladder neck obstructions; achalasia; myasthenia gravis; children <3 years of age
Warnings/Precautions Use with caution in older children (dose has not been established). Use with caution in hot weather or during exercise. May cause anhidrosis and hyperthermia, which may be severe. The risk is increased in hot environments, particularly in the elderly, alcoholics, patients with CNS disease, and those with prolonged outdoor exposure.

Elderly patients frequently develop increased sensitivity and require strict dosage regulation - side effects may be more severe in elderly patients with atherosclerotic changes. Use with caution in patients with tachycardia, cardiac arrhythmias, hypertension, hypotension, prostatic hyperplasia, (especially in the elderly), any tendency toward urinary retention, liver or kidney disorders, and obstructive disease of the GI or GU tract. When given in large doses or to susceptible patients, may cause weakness and inability to move particular muscle groups.

May be associated with confusion or hallucinations (generally at higher dosages). Intensification of symptoms or toxic psychosis may occur in patients with mental disorders.
Adverse Reactions Frequency not defined.
Cardiovascular: Tachycardia
Central nervous system: Confusion, disorientation, memory impairment, toxic psychosis, visual hallucinations
Dermatologic: Rash
Endocrine & metabolic: Heat stroke, hyperthermia
Gastrointestinal: Xerostomia, nausea, vomiting, constipation, ileus
Genitourinary: Urinary retention, dysuria
Ocular: Blurred vision, mydriasis
Miscellaneous: Fever
Overdosage/Toxicology Symptoms include CNS depression, confusion, nervousness, hallucinations, dizziness, blurred vision, nausea, vomiting, and hyperthermia. For anticholinergic overdose with severe life-threatening symptoms, physostigmine 1-2 mg (0.5 mg or 0.02 mg/kg for children) S.C. or slow I.V., may be given to reverse these effects. Anticholinergic toxicity is caused by strong binding of the drug to cholinergic receptors. Anticholinesterase inhibitors reduce acetylcholinesterase, the enzyme that breaks down acetylcholine and thereby allows acetylcholine to accumulate and compete for receptor binding with the offending anticholinergic.
Drug Interactions
Increased Effect/Toxicity: Central and/or peripheral anticholinergic syndrome can occur when benztropine is administered with amantadine, rimantadine, narcotic analgesics, phenothiazines and other antipsychotics (especially with high anticholinergic activity), tricyclic antidepressants, quinidine and some other antiarrhythmics, and antihistamines. Benztropine may increase the absorption of digoxin.
Decreased Effect: May increase gastric degradation of levodopa and decrease the amount of levodopa absorbed by delaying gastric emptying. Therapeutic effects of cholinergic agents (tacrine, donepezil) and neuroleptics may be antagonized.
Ethanol/Nutrition/Herb Interactions Ethanol: Avoid ethanol (may increase CNS depression).
Mechanism of Action Possesses both anticholinergic and antihistaminic effects. *In vitro* anticholinergic activity approximates that of atropine; *in vivo* it is only about half as active as atropine. Animal data suggest its antihistaminic activity and duration of action approach that of pyrilamine maleate. May also inhibit the reuptake and storage of dopamine and thereby, prolong the action of dopamine.
Pharmacodynamics/Kinetics
Onset of action: Oral: Within 1 hour; Parenteral: Within 15 minutes
Duration: 6-48 hours
Metabolism: Hepatic
Excretion: Urine
(Continued)

157

Benztropine *(Continued)*

Usual Dosage Use in children ≤3 years of age should be reserved for life-threatening emergencies

Drug-induced extrapyramidal symptom: Oral, I.M., I.V.:

Children >3 years: 0.02-0.05 mg/kg/dose 1-2 times/day
Adults: 1-4 mg/dose 1-2 times/day

Acute dystonia: Adults: I.M., I.V.: 1-2 mg

Parkinsonism: Oral:

Adults: 0.5-6 mg/day in 1-2 divided doses; if one dose is greater, administer at bedtime; titrate dose in 0.5 mg increments at 5- to 6-day intervals

Elderly: Initial: 0.5 mg once or twice daily; increase by 0.5 mg as needed at 5-6 days; maximum: 4 mg/day

Monitoring Parameters Symptoms of EPS or Parkinson's, pulse, anticholinergic effects

Patient Information Take after meals or with food if GI upset occurs; do not discontinue drug abruptly; notify physician if adverse GI effects, rapid or pounding heartbeat, confusion, eye pain, rash, fever, or heat intolerance occurs. Observe caution when performing hazardous tasks or those that require alertness such as driving, as may cause drowsiness. Avoid alcohol and other CNS depressants. May cause dry mouth - adequate fluid intake or hard sugar-free candy may relieve. Difficult urination or constipation may occur - notify physician if effects persist; may increase susceptibility to heat stroke.

Nursing Implications No significant difference in onset of I.M. or I.V. injection, therefore, there is usually no need to use the I.V. route. Improvement is sometimes noticeable a few minutes after injection.

Dosage Forms

Injection, solution, as mesylate: 1 mg/mL (2 mL)
Tablet, as mesylate: 0.5 mg, 1 mg, 2 mg

♦ **Benztropine Mesylate** *see* Benztropine *on page 157*
♦ **Benzylpenicillin Benzathine** *see* Penicillin G Benzathine *on page 1051*
♦ **Benzylpenicillin Potassium** *see* Penicillin G (Parenteral/Aqueous) *on page 1053*
♦ **Benzylpenicillin Sodium** *see* Penicillin G (Parenteral/Aqueous) *on page 1053*

Benzylpenicilloyl-polylysine *(BEN zil pen i SIL oyl pol i LIE seen)*

Related Information

Skin Tests *on page 1533*

U.S. Brand Names Pre-Pen®

Synonyms Penicilloyl-polylysine; PPL

Therapeutic Category Diagnostic Agent, Penicillin Allergy Skin Test

Use Adjunct in assessing the risk of administering penicillin (penicillin or benzylpenicillin) in adults with a history of clinical penicillin hypersensitivity

Pregnancy Risk Factor C

Pregnancy/Breast-Feeding Implications Safety for use during pregnancy has not been established

Contraindications Known hypersensitivity to penicillin or any component of the formulation

Adverse Reactions Frequency not defined.

Cardiovascular: Hypotension
Dermatologic: Angioneurotic edema, pruritus, erythema, urticaria
Local: Intense local inflammatory response at skin test site, wheal (locally)
Respiratory: Dyspnea
Miscellaneous: Systemic allergic reactions occur rarely

Drug Interactions

Decreased Effect: Corticosteroids and other immunosuppressive agents may inhibit the immune response to the skin test.

Stability Refrigerate; discard if left at room temperature for longer than one day

Mechanism of Action Elicits IgE antibodies which produce type I accelerate urticarial reactions to penicillins

Usual Dosage PPL is administered by a scratch technique or by intradermal injection. For initial testing, PPL should always be applied via the scratch technique. **Do not administer intradermally to patients who have positive reactions to a scratch test.** PPL test alone does not identify those patients who react to a minor antigenic determinant and does not appear to reliably predict the occurrence of late reactions.

Scratch test: Use scratch technique with a 20-gauge needle to make 3-5 mm nonbleeding scratch on epidermis, apply a small drop of solution to scratch, rub in gently with applicator or toothpick. A positive reaction consists of a pale wheal surrounding the scratch site which develops within 10 minutes and ranges from 5-15 mm or more in diameter.

Intradermal test: Use intradermal test with a tuberculin syringe with a 26- to 30-gauge short bevel needle; a dose of 0.01-0.02 mL is injected intradermally. A control of 0.9% sodium chloride should be injected at least 1.5" from the PPL test site. Most skin responses to the intradermal test will develop within 5-15 minutes.

Interpretation:

(-) Negative: No reaction
(±) Ambiguous: Wheal only slightly larger than original bleb with or without erythematous flare and larger than control site
(+) Positive: Itching and marked increase in size of original bleb
Control site should be reactionless

Administration PPL is administered by a scratch technique or by intradermal injection. For initial testing, PPL should always be applied via the scratch technique. Do not give intradermally to patients who have positive reactions to a scratch test. Have epinephrine 1:1000 immediately available.

Nursing Implications Always use scratch test for initial testing; have epinephrine 1:1000 immediately available

Dosage Forms Injection, solution: 0.25 mL

Bepridil (BE pri dil)

Related Information
Calcium Channel Blockers Comparison *on page 1494*

U.S. Brand Names Vascor®

Canadian Brand Names Vascor®

Synonyms Bepridil Hydrochloride

Therapeutic Category Antianginal Agent; Calcium Channel Blocker

Use Treatment of chronic stable angina; due to side effect profile, reserve for patients who have been intolerant of other antianginal therapy; bepridil may be used alone or in combination with nitrates or beta-blockers

Pregnancy Risk Factor C

Contraindications Hypersensitivity to bepridil or any component of the formulation, calcium channel blockers, or adenosine; history of serious ventricular or atrial arrhythmias (especially tachycardia or those associated with accessory conduction pathways), uncompensated cardiac insufficiency, congenital QT interval prolongation, patients taking other drugs that prolong the QT interval; concurrent administration with ritonavir, amprenavir, or sparfloxacin

Warnings/Precautions Use with great caution in patients with history of IHSS, second or third degree AV block, cardiogenic shock; reserve for patients in whom other antianginals have failed. Carefully titrate dosages for patients with impaired renal or hepatic function; use caution when treating patients with congestive heart failure, significant hypotension, severe left ventricular dysfunction, hypertrophic cardiomyopathy (especially obstructive), concomitant therapy with beta-blockers or digoxin, edema, or increased intracranial pressure with cranial tumors; do not abruptly withdraw (may cause chest pain); elderly may experience hypotension and constipation more readily.

If dosage reduction does not maintain the QT within a safe range (not to exceed 0.52 seconds during therapy), discontinue the medication; has class I antiarrhythmic properties and can induce new arrhythmias, including VT/VF; it can also cause torsade de pointes type ventricular tachycardia due to its ability to prolong the QT interval; avoid use in patients in the immediate period postinfarction.

Adverse Reactions
>10%:
 Central nervous system: Dizziness
 Gastrointestinal: Nausea, dyspepsia

1% to 10%:
 Cardiovascular: Bradycardia, edema, palpitations, QT prolongation (dose-related; up to 5% with prolongation of ≥25%), congestive heart failure (1%)
 Central nervous system: Nervousness, headache (7% to 13%), drowsiness, psychiatric disturbances (<2%), insomnia (2% to 3%)
 Dermatologic: Rash (≤2%)
 Endocrine & metabolic: Sexual dysfunction
 Gastrointestinal: Diarrhea, anorexia, xerostomia, constipation, abdominal pain, dyspepsia, flatulence
 Neuromuscular & skeletal: Weakness (7% to 14%), tremor (<9%), paresthesia (3%)
 Ocular: Blurred vision
 Otic: Tinnitus
 Respiratory: Rhinitis, dyspnea (≤9%), cough (≤2%)
 Miscellaneous (≤2%): Flu syndrome, diaphoresis

<1% (Limited to important or life-threatening): Akathisia, arrhythmia, leukopenia, neutropenia, ventricular torsade de pointes (0.01% to 1%)

Overdosage/Toxicology
Primary cardiac symptoms of calcium blocker overdose include hypotension and bradycardia. Hypotension is caused by peripheral vasodilation, myocardial depression, and bradycardia. Bradycardia results from sinus bradycardia, second- or third-degree atrioventricular block, or sinus arrest with junctional rhythm. Intraventricular conduction is usually not affected so QRS duration is normal (verapamil prolongs the P-R interval and bepridil prolongs the QT and may cause ventricular arrhythmias, including torsade de pointes).

Noncardiac symptoms include confusion, stupor, nausea, vomiting, metabolic acidosis, and hyperglycemia. Following initial gastric decontamination, if possible, repeated calcium administration may promptly reverse depressed cardiac contractility (but not sinus node depression or peripheral vasodilation). Glucagon, epinephrine, and inamrinone (amrinone) may treat refractory hypotension. Glucagon and epinephrine also increase the heart rate (outside the U.S., 4-aminopyridine may be available as an antidote). Dialysis and hemoperfusion are not effective in enhancing elimination, although repeat-dose activated charcoal may serve as an adjunct with sustained-release preparations.

In a few reported cases, overdose with calcium channel blockers has been associated with hypotension and bradycardia, initially refractory to atropine, but becoming more responsive to this agent when larger doses (approaching 1 g/hour for more than 24 hours) of calcium chloride were administered.

Drug Interactions
Cytochrome P450 Effect: CYP3A3/4 enzyme substrate

Increased Effect/Toxicity: Use with H_2 blockers may increase bioavailability of bepridil. Use of bepridil with beta-blockers may increase cardiac depressant effects on AV conduction. Bepridil may increase serum levels/effects of carbamazepine, cyclosporine, digitalis, quinidine, and theophylline. Concurrent use of fentanyl with bepridil may increase hypotension. Use with amprenavir, ritonavir, sparfloxacin (possibly also gatifloxacin and moxifloxacin) may increase risk of bepridil toxicity, especially its cardiotoxicity. Use with cisapride may increase the risk of malignant arrhythmias, concurrent use is contraindicated.

Ethanol/Nutrition/Herb Interactions Herb/Nutraceutical: St John's wort may decrease bepridil levels. Avoid dong quai if using for hypertension (has estrogenic activity). Avoid ephedra, yohimbe, ginseng (may worsen hypertension). Avoid garlic (may have increased antihypertensive effect).

Mechanism of Action Bepridil, a type 4 calcium antagonist, possesses characteristics of the traditional calcium antagonists, inhibiting calcium ion from entering the "slow channels" or

(Continued)

Bepridil (Continued)

select voltage-sensitive areas of vascular smooth muscle and myocardium during depolarization and producing a relaxation of coronary vascular smooth muscle and coronary vasodilation. However, bepridil may also inhibit fast sodium channels (inward), which may account for some of its side effects (eg, arrhythmias); a direct bradycardia effect of bepridil has been postulated via direct action on the S-A node.

Pharmacodynamics/Kinetics
Onset of action: 1 hour
Absorption: 100%
Protein binding: >99%
Metabolism: Hepatic
Bioavailability: 60%
Half-life elimination: 24 hours
Time to peak: 2-3 hours
Excretion: Urine (as metabolites)

Usual Dosage Adults: Oral: Initial: 200 mg/day, then adjust dose at 10-day intervals until optimal response is achieved; usual dose: 300 mg/day; maximum daily dose: 400 mg

Dosage adjustment in renal impairment: Risk of toxic reactions is greater in patients with renal impairment; dose selection should be cautious, usually starting at the low end of the dosage range

Elderly: Peak concentrations and half-life are markedly increased in the elderly (>74 years); dose selection should be cautious, usually starting at the low end of the dosage range

Monitoring Parameters EKG and serum electrolytes, blood pressure, signs and symptoms of congestive heart failure; elderly may need very close monitoring due to underlying cardiac and organ system defects

Reference Range 1-2 ng/mL

Test Interactions ↑ aminotransferases, ↑ CPK, LDH

Patient Information May cause cardiac arrhythmias if potassium is low; can be taken with food or meals, maintain potassium supplementation as directed, routine EKGs will be necessary during start of therapy or dosage changes; notify physician if the following occur: irregular heartbeat, shortness of breath, pronounced dizziness, constipation, or hypotension

Nursing Implications EKG required; patient should be hospitalized during initiation or escalation of therapy

Dosage Forms Tablet, as hydrochloride: 200 mg, 300 mg

♦ **Bepridil Hydrochloride** see Bepridil on page 159

Beractant (ber AKT ant)

U.S. Brand Names Survanta®

Canadian Brand Names Survanta®

Synonyms Bovine Lung Surfactant; Natural Lung Surfactant

Therapeutic Category Lung Surfactant

Use Prevention and treatment of respiratory distress syndrome (RDS) in premature infants

Prophylactic therapy: Body weight <1250 g in infants at risk for developing or with evidence of surfactant deficiency (administer within 15 minutes of birth)

Rescue therapy: Treatment of infants with RDS confirmed by x-ray and requiring mechanical ventilation (administer as soon as possible - within 8 hours of age)

Warnings/Precautions Rapidly affects oxygenation and lung compliance and should be restricted to a highly supervised use in a clinical setting with immediate availability of clinicians experienced with intubation and ventilatory management of premature infants. If transient episodes of bradycardia and decreased oxygen saturation occur, discontinue the dosing procedure and initiate measures to alleviate the condition; produces rapid improvements in lung oxygenation and compliance that may require immediate reductions in ventilator settings and FiO_2.

Adverse Reactions During the dosing procedure:
>10%: Cardiovascular: Transient bradycardia
1% to 10%: Respiratory: Oxygen desaturation
<1% (Limited to important or life-threatening): Apnea, endotracheal tube blockage, hypercarbia, hypertension, hypotension, increased probability of post-treatment nosocomial sepsis, pulmonary air leaks, pulmonary interstitial emphysema, vasoconstriction

Stability Refrigerate; protect from light, prior to administration warm by standing at room temperature for 20 minutes or held in hand for 8 minutes; **artificial warming methods should not be used**; unused, unopened vials warmed to room temperature may be returned to the refrigerator within 8 hours of warming only once

Mechanism of Action Replaces deficient or ineffective endogenous lung surfactant in neonates with respiratory distress syndrome (RDS) or in neonates at risk of developing RDS. Surfactant prevents the alveoli from collapsing during expiration by lowering surface tension between air and alveolar surfaces.

Pharmacodynamics/Kinetics Alveolar clearance is rapid

Usual Dosage
Prophylactic treatment: Administer 100 mg phospholipids (4 mL/kg) intratracheal as soon as possible; as many as 4 doses may be administered during the first 48 hours of life, no more frequently than 6 hours apart. The need for additional doses is determined by evidence of continuing respiratory distress; if the infant is still intubated and requiring at least 30% inspired oxygen to maintain a PaO_2 ≤80 torr.

Rescue treatment: Administer 100 mg phospholipids (4 mL/kg) as soon as the diagnosis of RDS is made; may repeat if needed, no more frequently than every 6 hours to a maximum of 4 doses

Administration
For intratracheal administration only
Suction infant prior to administration; inspect solution to verify complete mixing of the suspension

Administer intratracheally by instillation through a 5-French end-hole catheter inserted into the infant's endotracheal tube

Administer the dose in four 1 mL/kg aliquots. Each quarter-dose is instilled over 2-3 seconds; each quarter-dose is administered with the infant in a different position; slightly downward inclination with head turned to the right, then repeat with head turned to the left; then slightly upward inclination with head turned to the right, then repeat with head turned to the left.

Monitoring Parameters Continuous EKG and transcutaneous O_2 saturation should be monitored during administration; frequent arterial blood gases are necessary to prevent postdosing hyperoxia and hypocarbia

Nursing Implications Do not shake; if settling occurs during storage, swirl gently

Additional Information Each mL contains 25 mg phospholipids suspended in 0.9% sodium chloride solution. Contents of 1 mL: 0.5-1.75 mg triglycerides, 1.4-3.5 mg free fatty acids, and <1 mg protein.

Dosage Forms Suspension for inhalation: 25 mg/mL (4 mL, 8 mL)

♦ **Berocca®** *see* Vitamin B Complex With Vitamin C and Folic Acid *on page 1422*

♦ **Beta-2®** *see* Isoetharine *on page 747*

♦ **Beta-Blockers Comparison** *see page 1491*

Beta-Carotene (BAY ta KARE oh teen)

U.S. Brand Names A-Caro-25®; B-Caro-T™; Lumitene™

Therapeutic Category Vitamin, Fat Soluble

Unlabeled/Investigational Use Prophylaxis and treatment of polymorphous light eruption; prophylaxis against photosensitivity reactions in erythropoietic protoporphyria

Pregnancy Risk Factor C

Usual Dosage Oral:

Children <14 years: 30-150 mg/day

Adults: 30-300 mg/day

Additional Information Complete prescribing information for this medication should be consulted for additional detail.

Dosage Forms

Capsule: 10,000 int. units (6 mg); 25,000 int. units (15 mg)

A-Caro-25®, B-Caro-T™: 25,000 int. units (15 mg)

Lumitene™: 50,000 int. units (30 mg)

Tablet: 10,000 int. units

♦ **Betaderm (Can)** *see* Betamethasone *on page 161*

♦ **Betadine® [OTC]** *see* Povidone-Iodine *on page 1114*

♦ **Betadine® 5% Sterile Ophthalmic Prep Solution** *see* Povidone-Iodine *on page 1114*

♦ **Betadine® First Aid Antibiotics + Moisturizer [OTC]** *see* Bacitracin and Polymyxin B *on page 143*

♦ **9-Beta-D-ribofuranosyladenine** *see* Adenosine *on page 37*

♦ **Betagan® (Can)** *see* Levobunolol *on page 788*

♦ **Betagan® [OTC]** *see* Povidone-Iodine *on page 1114*

♦ **Betagan® Liquifilm®** *see* Levobunolol *on page 788*

Betaine Anhydrous (BAY ta een an HY drus)

U.S. Brand Names Cystadane®

Canadian Brand Names Cystadane™

Therapeutic Category Homocystinuria Agent

Use Orphan drug: Treatment of homocystinuria to decrease elevated homocysteine blood levels; included within the category of homocystinuria are deficiencies or defects in cystathionine beta-synthase (CBS), 5,10-methylenetetrahydrofolate reductase (MTHFR), and cobalamin cofactor metabolism (CBL).

Pregnancy Risk Factor C

Usual Dosage

Children <3 years: Dosage may be started at 100 mg/kg/day and then increased weekly by 100 mg/kg increments

Children ≥3 years and Adults: Oral: 6 g/day administered in divided doses of 3 g twice daily. Dosages of up to 20 g/day have been necessary to control homocysteine levels in some patients.

Dosage in all patients can be gradually increased until plasma homocysteine is undetectable or present only in small amounts

Additional Information Complete prescribing information for this medication should be consulted for additional detail.

Dosage Forms Powder for oral solution: 1 g/scoop (180 g) [1 scoop = 1.7 mL]

♦ **Betaject™ (Can)** *see* Betamethasone *on page 161*

♦ **Betaloc® (Can)** *see* Metoprolol *on page 902*

♦ **Betaloc® Durules® (Can)** *see* Metoprolol *on page 902*

Betamethasone (bay ta METH a sone)

Related Information

Corticosteroids Comparison *on page 1495*

U.S. Brand Names Alphatrex®; Betatrex®; Beta-Val®; Celestone®; Celestone® Phosphate; Celestone® Soluspan®; Diprolene®; Diprolene® AF; Diprosone®; Luxiq™; Maxivate®; Valisone® [DSC]

Canadian Brand Names Betaderm; Betaject™; Betnesol®; Betnovate®; Celestoderm®-EV/2; Celestoderm®-V; Celestone® Soluspan®; Diprolene® Glycol; Diprosone®; Ectosone; Prevex® B; Taro-Sone®; Topilene®; Topisone®; Valisone® Scalp Lotion

Synonyms Betamethasone Dipropionate; Betamethasone Dipropionate, Augmented; Betamethasone Sodium Phosphate; Betamethasone Valerate; Flubenisolone

(Continued)

Betamethasone *(Continued)*

Therapeutic Category Anti-inflammatory Agent; Corticosteroid, Systemic; Corticosteroid, Topical (Low Potency); Corticosteroid, Topical (Medium Potency); Corticosteroid, Topical (High Potency); Glucocorticoid

Use Inflammatory dermatoses such as seborrheic or atopic dermatitis, neurodermatitis, anogenital pruritus, psoriasis, inflammatory phase of xerosis

Pregnancy Risk Factor C

Pregnancy/Breast-Feeding Implications Clinical effects on the fetus: There are no reports linking the use of betamethasone with congenital defects in the literature; betamethasone is often used in patients with premature labor [26-34 weeks gestation] to stimulate fetal lung maturation

Contraindications Hypersensitivity to betamethasone or any component of the formulation; systemic fungal infections

Warnings/Precautions Not to be used in status asthmaticus or for the relief of acute bronchospasm; topical use in patients ≤12 years of age is not recommended. May cause suppression of hypothalamic-pituitary-adrenal (HPA) axis, particularly in younger children or in patients receiving high doses for prolonged periods. Particular care is required when patients are transferred from systemic corticosteroids to inhaled products due to possible adrenal insufficiency or withdrawal from steroids, including an increase in allergic symptoms. Patients receiving 20 mg per day of prednisone (or equivalent) may be most susceptible. Fatalities have occurred due to adrenal insufficiency in asthmatic patients during and after transfer from systemic corticosteroids to aerosol steroids; aerosol steroids do **not** provide the systemic steroid needed to treat patients having trauma, surgery, or infections. Withdrawal and discontinuation of the corticosteroid should be done slowly and carefully

Controlled clinical studies have shown that orally-inhaled and intranasal corticosteroids may cause a reduction in growth velocity in pediatric patients. (In studies of orally-inhaled corticosteroids, the mean reduction in growth velocity was approximately 1 centimeter per year [range 0.3-1.8 cm per year] and appears to be related to dose and duration of exposure.) The growth of pediatric patients receiving inhaled corticosteroids, should be monitored routinely (eg, via stadiometry). To minimize the systemic effects of orally-inhaled and intranasal corticosteroids, each patient should be titrated to the lowest effective dose.

May suppress the immune system, patients may be more susceptible to infection. Use with caution in patients with systemic infections or ocular herpes simplex. Avoid exposure to chickenpox and measles.

Use with caution in patients with hypothyroidism, cirrhosis, ulcerative colitis; do not use occlusive dressings on weeping or exudative lesions and general caution with occlusive dressings should be observed; discontinue if skin irritation or contact dermatitis should occur; do not use in patients with decreased skin circulation

Adverse Reactions

Systemic:

>10%:

Central nervous system: Insomnia, nervousness

Gastrointestinal: Increased appetite, indigestion

1% to 10%:

Central nervous system: Dizziness or lightheadedness, headache

Dermatologic: Hirsutism, hypopigmentation

Endocrine & metabolic: Diabetes mellitus

Neuromuscular & skeletal: Arthralgia

Ocular: Cataracts, glaucoma

Respiratory: Epistaxis

Miscellaneous: Diaphoresis

<1% (Limited to important or life-threatening): Alkalosis, amenorrhea, Cushing's syndrome, delirium, euphoria, glucose intolerance, growth suppression, hallucinations, hyperglycemia, hypokalemia, pituitary-adrenal (HPA) axis suppression, pseudotumor cerebri, psychoses, seizures, sodium and water retention, vertigo

Topical:

1% to 10%:

Dermatologic: Itching, allergic contact dermatitis, erythema, dryness papular rashes, folliculitis, furunculosis, pustules, pyoderma, vesiculation, hyperesthesia, skin infection (secondary)

Local: Burning, irritation

<1% (Limited to important or life-threatening): Cataracts (posterior subcapsular), Cushing's syndrome, glaucoma, hypokalemic syndrome

Overdosage/Toxicology When consumed in excessive quantities for prolonged periods, systemic hypercorticism and adrenal suppression may occur; in those cases, discontinuation and withdrawal of the corticosteroid should be done judiciously.

Drug Interactions

Cytochrome P450 Effect: CYP3A3/4 enzyme substrate

Increased Effect/Toxicity: Inhibitors of CYP3A4 (including erythromycin, diltiazem, itraconazole, ketoconazole, quinidine, and verapamil) may decrease metabolism of betamethasone.

Decreased Effect: May induce cytochrome P450 enzymes, which may lead to decreased effect of any drug metabolized by P450 (ie, barbiturates, phenytoin, rifampin). Decreased effectiveness of salicylates when taken with betamethasone.

Ethanol/Nutrition/Herb Interactions

Ethanol: Avoid ethanol (may enhance gastric mucosal irritation).

Food: Betamethasone interferes with calcium absorption.

Herb/Nutraceutical: Avoid cat's claw, echinacea (have immunostimulant properties).

Mechanism of Action Controls the rate of protein synthesis, depresses the migration of polymorphonuclear leukocytes, fibroblasts, reverses capillary permeability, and lysosomal stabilization at the cellular level to prevent or control inflammation

Pharmacodynamics/Kinetics

Protein binding: 64%

Metabolism: Hepatic

Half-life elimination: 6.5 hours

Time to peak, serum: I.V.: 10-36 minutes

Excretion: Urine (<5% as unchanged drug)

Usual Dosage Base dosage on severity of disease and patient response

Children: Use lowest dose listed as initial dose for adrenocortical insufficiency (physiologic replacement)

I.M.: 0.0175-0.125 mg base/kg/day divided every 6-12 hours **or** 0.5-7.5 mg base/m²/day divided every 6-12 hours

Oral: 0.0175-0.25 mg/kg/day divided every 6-8 hours **or** 0.5-7.5 mg/m²/day divided every 6-8 hours

Topical:

≤12 years: Use is not recommended.

>12 years: Apply a thin film twice daily; use minimal amount for shortest period of time to avoid HPA axis suppression

Adolescents and Adults:

Oral: 2.4-4.8 mg/day in 2-4 doses; range: 0.6-7.2 mg/day

I.M.: Betamethasone sodium phosphate and betamethasone acetate: 0.6-9 mg/day (generally, ⅓ to ½ of oral dose) divided every 12-24 hours

Foam: Apply twice daily, once in the morning and once at night to scalp

Dosing adjustment in hepatic impairment: Adjustments may be necessary in patients with liver failure because betamethasone is extensively metabolized in the liver

Adults:

Intrabursal, intra-articular, intradermal: 0.25-2 mL

Intralesional: Rheumatoid arthritis/osteoarthritis:

Very large joints: 1-2 mL

Large joints: 1 mL

Medium joints: 0.5-1 mL

Small joints: 0.25-0.5 mL

Topical: Apply thin film 2-4 times/day. Therapy should be discontinued when control is achieved; if no improvement is seen, reassessment of diagnosis may be necessary.

Dietary Considerations May be taken with food to decrease GI distress.

Administration

Oral: Not for alternate day therapy; once daily doses should be given in the morning.

I.M.: Do **not** give injectable sodium phosphate/acetate suspension I.V.

Topical: Apply topical sparingly to areas. Not for use on broken skin or in areas of infection. Do not apply to wet skin unless directed. Do not apply to face or inguinal area. Do not cover with occlusive dressing.

Patient Information Take oral with food or milk; apply topical sparingly to areas and gently rub in until it disappears, not for use on broken skin or in areas of infection; do not apply to face or inguinal areas

Nursing Implications Apply topical sparingly to areas; not for use on broken skin or in areas of infection; do not apply to wet skin unless directed; do not apply to face or inguinal area. Not for alternate day therapy; once daily doses should be given in the morning; do not administer injectable sodium phosphate/acetate suspension I.V.

Dosage Forms

Cream, topical, as dipropionate: 0.05% (15 g, 45 g, 60 g)

Alphatrex®, Diprosone®: 0.05% (15 g, 45 g)

Maxivate®: 0.05% (45 g)

Cream, topical, as dipropionate augmented (Diprolene® AF): 0.05% (15 g, 50 g)

Cream, topical, as valerate: 0.1% (15 g, 45 g)

Betatrex®, Valisone® [DSC]: 0.1% (15 g, 45 g)

Beta-Val®: 0.1% (15 g, 45 g)

Foam, topical, as valerate (Luxiq™): 0.12% (50 g, 100 g) [contains alcohol 60.4%]

Gel, topical, as dipropionate augmented (Diprolene®): 0.05% (15 g, 50 g)

Injection, solution, as sodium phosphate (Celestone® Phosphate): 4 mg/mL (5 mL) [equivalent to 3 mg betamethasone/mL]

Injection, suspension (Celestone® Soluspan®): Betamethasone sodium phosphate 3 mg/mL and betamethasone acetate 3 mg/mL [6 mg/mL] (5 mL)

Lotion, topical, as dipropionate: 0.05% (20 mL, 60 mL)

Alphatrex®, Maxivate®: 0.05% (60 mL)

Diprosone®: 0.05% (20 mL, 60 mL)

Lotion, topical, as dipropionate augmented (Diprolene®): 0.05% (30 mL, 60 mL)

Lotion, topical, as valerate (Beta-Val®, Betatrex®, Valisone® [DSC]): 0.1% (60 mL)

Ointment, topical, as dipropionate: 0.05% (15 g, 45 g)

Alphatrex®, Maxivate®: 0.05% (45 g)

Diprosone®: 0.05% (15 g, 45 g)

Ointment, topical, as dipropionate augmented: 0.05% (15 g, 45 g, 50 g)

Diprolene®: 0.05% (15 g, 50 g)

Ointment, topical, as valerate (Betatrex®, Valisone® [DSC]): 0.1% (15 g, 45 g)

Syrup, as base (Celestone®): 0.6 mg/5 mL (118 mL)

Tablet, as base (Celestone®): 0.6 mg

Betamethasone and Clotrimazole (bay ta METH a sone & kloe TRIM a zole)

U.S. Brand Names Lotrisone®

Canadian Brand Names Lotriderm®

Synonyms Clotrimazole and Betamethasone

Therapeutic Category Antifungal/Corticosteroid; Corticosteroid, Topical

Use Topical treatment of various dermal fungal infections (including tinea pedis, cruris, and corpora in patients ≥17 years of age)

Pregnancy Risk Factor C

(Continued)

Betamethasone and Clotrimazole *(Continued)*

Usual Dosage

Children <17 years: Do not use

Children ≥17 years and Adults:

Tinea corporis, tinea cruris: Topical: Massage into affected area twice daily, morning and evening; do not use for longer than 2 weeks; re-evaluate after 1 week if no clinical improvement; do not exceed 45 g cream/week or 45 mL lotion/week

Tinea pedis: Topical: Massage into affected area twice daily, morning and evening; do not use for longer than 4 weeks; re-evaluate after 2 weeks if no clinical improvement; do not exceed 45 g cream/week or 45 mL lotion/week

Elderly: Use with caution; skin atrophy and skin ulceration (rare) have been reported in patients with thinning skin; do not use for diaper dermatitis or under occlusive dressings

Additional Information Complete prescribing information for this medication should be consulted for additional detail.

Dosage Forms

Cream: Betamethasone dipropionate 0.05% and clotrimazole 1% (15 g, 45 g)

Lotion: Betamethasone dipropionate 0.05% and clotrimazole 1% (30 mL)

- ◆ **Betamethasone Dipropionate** *see* Betamethasone *on page 161*
- ◆ **Betamethasone Dipropionate, Augmented** *see* Betamethasone *on page 161*
- ◆ **Betamethasone Sodium Phosphate** *see* Betamethasone *on page 161*
- ◆ **Betamethasone Valerate** *see* Betamethasone *on page 161*
- ◆ **Betapace®** *see* Sotalol *on page 1252*
- ◆ **Betapace AF™** *see* Sotalol *on page 1252*
- ◆ **Betasept® [OTC]** *see* Chlorhexidine Gluconate *on page 275*
- ◆ **Betaseron®** *see* Interferon Beta-1b *on page 736*
- ◆ **Betatrex®** *see* Betamethasone *on page 161*
- ◆ **Beta-Val®** *see* Betamethasone *on page 161*
- ◆ **Betaxin® (Can)** *see* Thiamine *on page 1316*

Betaxolol *(be TAKS oh lol)*

Related Information

Beta-Blockers Comparison *on page 1491*

Glaucoma Drug Therapy Comparison *on page 1499*

U.S. Brand Names Betoptic® S; Kerlone®

Canadian Brand Names Betoptic® S

Synonyms Betaxolol Hydrochloride

Therapeutic Category Antihypertensive Agent; Beta-Adrenergic Blocker; Beta-Adrenergic Blocker, Ophthalmic

Use Treatment of chronic open-angle glaucoma and ocular hypertension; management of hypertension

Pregnancy Risk Factor C (manufacturer); D (2nd and 3rd trimesters - expert analysis)

Contraindications Hypersensitivity to betaxolol or any component of the formulation; sinus bradycardia; heart block greater than first-degree (except in patients with a functioning artificial pacemaker); cardiogenic shock; uncompensated cardiac failure; pulmonary edema; pregnancy (2nd and 3rd trimester)

Warnings/Precautions Administer cautiously in compensated heart failure and monitor for a worsening of the condition. Avoid abrupt discontinuation in patients with a history of CAD; slowly wean while monitoring for signs and symptoms of ischemia. Use caution with concurrent use of beta-blockers and either verapamil or diltiazem; bradycardia or heart block can occur. Use caution in patients with PVD (can aggravate arterial insufficiency). In general, beta-blockers should be avoided in patients with bronchospastic disease. Betaxolol, with B1 selectivity, should be used cautiously in bronchospastic disease with close monitoring. Use cautiously in diabetics because it can mask prominent hypoglycemic symptoms. Can mask signs of thyrotoxicosis. Can cause fetal harm when administered in pregnancy. Dosage adjustment required in severe renal impairment and those on dialysis. Use care with anesthetic agents which decrease myocardial function.

Adverse Reactions

Ophthalmic:

>10%: Ocular: Conjunctival hyperemia

1% to 10%:

Ocular: Anisocoria, corneal punctate keratitis, keratitis, corneal staining, decreased corneal sensitivity, eye pain, vision disturbances

Systemic:

>10%:

Central nervous system: Drowsiness, insomnia

Endocrine & metabolic: Decreased sexual ability

1% to 10%:

Cardiovascular: Bradycardia, palpitations, edema, congestive heart failure, reduced peripheral circulation

Central nervous system: Mental depression

Gastrointestinal: Diarrhea or constipation, nausea, vomiting, stomach discomfort

Respiratory: Bronchospasm

Miscellaneous: Cold extremities

<1% (Limited to important or life-threatening): Chest pain, thrombocytopenia

Overdosage/Toxicology Symptoms of intoxication include cardiac disturbances, CNS toxicity, bronchospasm, hypoglycemia and hyperkalemia. The most common cardiac symptoms include hypotension and bradycardia. Atrioventricular block, intraventricular conduction disturbances, cardiogenic shock, and asystole may occur with severe overdose, especially with membrane-depressant drugs (eg, propranolol). CNS effects include convulsions, coma, and respiratory arrest (commonly seen with propranolol and other membrane-depressant and lipid-soluble drugs). Treatment is symptomatic for seizures, hypotension, hyperkalemia, and hypoglycemia. Bradycardia and hypotension resistant to atropine, isoproterenol, or pacing may respond to glucagon. Wide QRS defects caused by membrane-depressant poisoning may respond to hypertonic sodium bicarbonate. Repeat-dose charcoal, hemoperfusion, or hemodialysis may be helpful in removal of only those beta-blockers with a small V_d, long half-life, or low intrinsic clearance (acebutolol, atenolol, nadolol, sotalol).

Drug Interactions
  Cytochrome P450 Effect: CYP1A2 and 2D6 enzyme substrate
  Increased Effect/Toxicity: The heart rate lowering effects of betaxolol are additive with other drugs which slow AV conduction (digoxin, verapamil, diltiazem). Reserpine increases the effects of betaxolol. Concurrent use of betaxolol may increase the effects of alpha-blockers (prazosin, terazosin), alpha-adrenergic stimulants (epinephrine, phenylephrine), and the vasoconstrictive effects of ergot alkaloids. Betaxolol may mask the tachycardia from hypoglycemia caused by insulin and oral hypoglycemics. In patients receiving concurrent therapy, the risk of hypertensive crisis is increased when either clonidine or the beta-blocker is withdrawn. Beta-blockers may increase the action or levels of ethanol, disopyramide, nondepolarizing muscle relaxants, and theophylline although the effects are difficult to predict.
  Decreased Effect: Decreased effect of betaxolol with aluminum salts, barbiturates, calcium salts, cholestyramine, colestipol, NSAIDs, penicillins (ampicillin), rifampin, salicylates, and sulfinpyrazone due to decreased bioavailability and plasma levels. Beta-blockers may decrease the effect of sulfonylureas.

Ethanol/Nutrition/Herb Interactions Herb/Nutraceutical: Avoid dong quai if using for hypertension (has estrogenic activity). Avoid ephedra, yohimbe, ginseng (may worsen hypertension). Avoid garlic (may have increased antihypertensive effect).

Stability Avoid freezing

Mechanism of Action Competitively blocks beta$_1$-receptors, with little or no effect on beta$_2$-receptors; ophthalmic reduces intraocular pressure by reducing the production of aqueous humor

Pharmacodynamics/Kinetics
  Onset of action: Ophthalmic: 30 minutes; Oral: 1-1.5 hours
  Duration: Ophthalmic: ≥12 hours
  Absorption: Ophthalmic: Some systemic; Oral: ~100%
  Metabolism: Multiple metabolites: Hepatic
  Half-life elimination: Oral: 12-22 hours
  Time to peak: Ophthalmic: ~2 hours; Oral: 1.5-6 hours
  Excretion: Urine

Usual Dosage Adults:
  Ophthalmic: Instill 1 drop twice daily.
  Oral: 10 mg/day; may increase dose to 20 mg/day after 7-14 days if desired response is not achieved. Initial dose in elderly: 5 mg/day.
  Dosage adjustment in renal impairment: Administer 5 mg/day. Can increase every 2 weeks up to a maximum of 20 mg/day.
  Cl_{cr} <10 mL/minute: Administer 50% of usual dose.

Administration Ophthalmic: Shake well before using. Tilt head back and instill in eye. Keep eye open and do not blink for 30 seconds. Apply gentle pressure to lacrimal sac for 1 minute. Wipe away excess from skin. Do not touch applicator to eye and do not contaminate tip of applicator.

Monitoring Parameters Ophthalmic: Intraocular pressure. Systemic: Blood pressure, pulse

Patient Information Intended for twice daily dosing; keep eye open and do not blink for 30 seconds after instillation; wear sunglasses to avoid photophobic discomfort; apply gentle pressure to lacrimal sac during and immediately following instillation (1 minute)

Nursing Implications Monitor for systemic effect of beta-blockade

Dosage Forms
  Solution, ophthalmic, as hydrochloride: 0.5% (5 mL, 10 mL, 15 mL) [contains benzalkonium chloride]
  Suspension, ophthalmic, as hydrochloride (Betoptic® S): 0.25% (2.5 mL, 10 mL, 15 mL) [contains benzalkonium chloride]
  Tablet, as hydrochloride (Kerlone®): 10 mg, 20 mg

♦ **Betaxolol Hydrochloride** *see* Betaxolol *on page 164*

♦ **Betaxon®** *see* Levobetaxolol *on page 788*

Bethanechol (be THAN e kole)

U.S. Brand Names Urecholine®

Canadian Brand Names Duvoid®; Myotonachol®; Urecholine®

Synonyms Bethanechol Chloride

Therapeutic Category Cholinergic Agent

Use Nonobstructive urinary retention and retention due to neurogenic bladder; treatment and prevention of bladder dysfunction caused by phenothiazines; diagnosis of flaccid or atonic neurogenic bladder; gastroesophageal reflux

Pregnancy Risk Factor C

Contraindications Hypersensitivity to bethanechol or any component of the formulation; mechanical obstruction of the GI or GU tract or when the strength or integrity of the GI or bladder wall is in question; hyperthyroidism, peptic ulcer disease, epilepsy, obstructive pulmonary disease, bradycardia, vasomotor instability, atrioventricular conduction defects, hypotension, or parkinsonism; **contraindicated for I.M. or I.V. use due to a likely severe cholinergic reaction**

Warnings/Precautions Potential for reflux infection if the sphincter fails to relax as bethanechol contracts the bladder; use with caution when administering to nursing women, as it is unknown if the drug is excreted in breast milk; safety and efficacy in children <5 years of age have not been established; syringe containing atropine should be readily available for treatment of serious side effects; for S.C. injection only; do not administer I.M. or I.V.
(Continued)

Bethanechol (Continued)

Adverse Reactions

Oral: <1% (Limited to important or life-threatening): Blurred vision, borborygmi, diaphoresis, dyspnea, excessive salivation, hypotension with reflex tachycardia, urinary frequency, miosis, vasomotor response

Subcutaneous:

1% to 10%:

Cardiovascular: Hypotension with reflex tachycardia, flushed skin

Central nervous system: Malaise, headache

Gastrointestinal: Belching, abdominal cramps, nausea, diarrhea, excessive salivation, borborygmi

Genitourinary: Urinary frequency

Ocular: Blurred vision, miosis

Respiratory: Dyspnea, wheezing

Miscellaneous: Diaphoresis, vasomotor response

Overdosage/Toxicology Symptoms include nausea, vomiting, abdominal cramps, diarrhea, involuntary defecation, flushed skin, hypotension, and bronchospasm. Atropine is the treatment of choice for intoxications manifesting with significant muscarinic symptoms. Atropine I.V. 0.6 mg every 3-60 minutes (or 0.01 mg/kg I.V. every 2 hours if needed for children) should be repeated to control symptoms and then continued as needed for 1-2 days following the acute ingestion. Epinephrine 0.1-1 mg S.C. may be useful in reversing severe cardiovascular or pulmonary sequelae.

Drug Interactions

Increased Effect/Toxicity: Bethanechol and ganglionic blockers may cause a critical fall in blood pressure. Cholinergic drugs or anticholinesterase agents may have additive effects with bethanechol.

Decreased Effect: Procainamide, quinidine may decrease the effects of bethanechol. Anticholinergic agents (atropine, antihistamines, TCAs, phenothiazines) may decrease effects.

Mechanism of Action Stimulates cholinergic receptors in the smooth muscle of the urinary bladder and gastrointestinal tract resulting in increased peristalsis, increased GI and pancreatic secretions, bladder muscle contraction, and increased ureteral peristaltic waves

Pharmacodynamics/Kinetics

Onset of action: Oral: 30-90 minutes; S.C.: 5-15 minutes

Duration: Oral: Up to 6 hours; S.C.: 2 hours

Absorption: Oral: Variable

Usual Dosage

Children:

Oral:

Abdominal distention or urinary retention: 0.6 mg/kg/day divided 3-4 times/day

Gastroesophageal reflux: 0.1-0.2 mg/kg/dose given 30 minutes to 1 hour before each meal to a maximum of 4 times/day

S.C.: 0.15-0.2 mg/kg/day divided 3-4 times/day

Adults:

Oral: 10-50 mg 2-4 times/day

S.C.: 2.5-5 mg 3-4 times/day, up to 7.5-10 mg every 4 hours for neurogenic bladder

Dietary Considerations Should be taken 1 hour before meals or 2 hours after meals.

Administration Do **not** administer I.V. or I.M., a severe cholinergic reaction may occur

Monitoring Parameters Observe closely for side effects

Test Interactions ↑ lipase, AST, amylase (S), bilirubin, aminotransferase [ALT (SGPT)/AST (SGOT)] (S)

Patient Information Oral should be taken 1 hour before meals or 2 hours after meals to avoid nausea or vomiting; may cause abdominal discomfort, salivation, diaphoresis, or flushing; notify physician if these symptoms become pronounced; rise slowly from sitting/lying down

Nursing Implications Have bedpan readily available, if administered for urinary retention

Dosage Forms Tablet, as chloride: 5 mg, 10 mg, 25 mg, 50 mg

♦ **Bethanechol Chloride** *see Bethanechol on page 165*

♦ **Betimol®** *see Timolol on page 1334*

♦ **Betnesol® (Can)** *see Betamethasone on page 161*

♦ **Betnovate® (Can)** *see Betamethasone on page 161*

♦ **Betoptic® S** *see Betaxolol on page 164*

Bexarotene (beks AIR oh teen)

U.S. Brand Names Targretin®

Canadian Brand Names Targretin®

Therapeutic Category Retinoic Acid Derivative; Vitamin A Derivative

Use

Oral: Treatment of cutaneous manifestations of cutaneous T-cell lymphoma in patients who are refractory to at least one prior systemic therapy

Topical: Treatment of cutaneous lesions in patients with cutaneous T-cell lymphoma (stage 1A and 1B) who have refractory or persistent disease after other therapies or who have not tolerated other therapies

Pregnancy Risk Factor X

Pregnancy/Breast-Feeding Implications Bexarotene caused birth defects when administered orally to pregnant rats. It must not be given to a pregnant woman or a woman who intends to become pregnant. If a woman becomes pregnant while taking the drug, it must be stopped immediately and appropriate counseling be given. It is not known whether bexarotene is excreted in human milk. Contraindicated in breast-feeding.

Contraindications Hypersensitivity to bexarotene or any component of the formulation; pregnancy

Warnings/Precautions Pregnancy test needed 1 week before initiation and every month thereafter. Effective contraception must be in place one month before initiation, during therapy, and for at least 1 month after discontinuation. Male patients with sexual partners who are pregnant, possibly pregnant, or who could become pregnant, must use condoms during sexual intercourse during treatment and for 1 month after last dose. In a majority of patients, it induces major lipid abnormalities in triglyceride, total cholesterol, and HDL, and is reversible on discontinuation. Use extreme caution in patients with underlying hypertriglyceridemia. Pancreatitis secondary to hypertriglyceridemia has been reported. Monitor for liver function test abnormalities and discontinue drug if tests are three times the upper limit of normal values for AST (SGOT), ALT (SGPT) or bilirubin. Hypothyroidism occurs in about a third of patients. Monitor for signs and symptoms of infection about 4-8 weeks after initiation (leukopenia may occur). Any new visual abnormalities experienced by the patient should be evaluated by an ophthalmologist (cataracts can form, or worsen, especially in the geriatric population). May cause photosensitization. Safety and efficacy are not established in the pediatric population. Avoid use in hepatically impaired patients. Limit additional vitamin A intake to <15,000 int. units/day. Use caution with diabetic patients: monitor for hypoglycemia.

Adverse Reactions First percentage is at a dose of 300 mg/m^2/day; the second percentage is at a dose >300 mg/m^2/day. Grade 3 and grade 4 events that occurred more frequently in patients at both doses were hyperlipidemia, hypertriglyceridemia, pruritus, headache, peripheral edema, leukopenia, rash, and hypercholesterolemia. Frequency of events was dose-related.

>10%:
  Cardiovascular: Peripheral edema (13% to 11%)
  Central nervous system: Headache (30% to 42%), chills (10% to 13%)
  Dermatologic: Rash (17% to 23%), exfoliative dermatitis (10% to 28%)
  Endocrine & metabolic: Hyperlipidemia (about 79% in both dosing ranges), hypercholesterolemia (32% to 62%), hypothyroidism (29% to 53%)
  Hematologic: Leukopenia (17% to 47%)
  Neuromuscular & skeletal: Weakness (20% to 45%)
  Miscellaneous: Infection (13% to 23%)

<10% (Limited to important or life-threatening):
  Cardiovascular: Hemorrhage, hypertension, angina pectoris, right heart failure, tachycardia, cerebrovascular accident
  Central nervous system: Fever (5% to 17%), insomnia (5% to 11%), subdural hematoma, syncope, depression, agitation, ataxia
  Dermatologic: Dry skin (about 10% for both dosing ranges), alopecia (4% to 11%), skin ulceration, maculopapular rash, vesicular bullous rash, cheilitis
  Endocrine & metabolic: Hypoproteinemia, hyperglycemia
  Gastrointestinal: Abdominal pain (11% to 4%), nausea (16% to 8%), diarrhea (7% to 42%), vomiting (4% to 13%), anorexia (2% to 23%), colitis, gastroenteritis, gingivitis, melena, pancreatitis
  Genitourinary: Albuminuria, hematuria, dysuria
  Hematologic: Hypochromic anemia (4% to 13%), anemia (6% to 25%), eosinophilia, thrombocythemia, coagulation time increased, lymphocytosis, thrombocytopenia
  Hepatic: LDH increase (7% to 13%), hepatic failure
  Neuromuscular & skeletal: Back pain (2% to 11%), arthralgia, myalgia, myasthenia, neuropathy
  Ocular: Conjunctivitis, blepharitis, corneal lesion, visual field defects, keratitis
  Otic: Ear pain, otitis externa
  Renal: Renal dysfunction
  Respiratory: Pharyngitis, rhinitis, dyspnea, pleural effusion, bronchitis, increased cough, lung edema, hemoptysis, hypoxia
  Miscellaneous: Flu-like syndrome (4% to 13%), infection (1% to 13%)

Topical:
  Cardiovascular: Edema (10%)
  Central nervous system: Headache (14%), weakness (6%), pain (30%)
  Dermatologic: Rash (14% to 72%), pruritus (6% to 40%), contact dermatitis (14%), exfoliative dermatitis (6%)
  Hematologic: Leukopenia (6%), lymphadenopathy (6%)
  Neuromuscular & skeletal: Paresthesia (6%)
  Respiratory: Cough (6%), pharyngitis (6%)
  Miscellaneous: Diaphoresis (6%), infection (18%)

Overdosage/Toxicology Doses up to 1000 mg/m^2/day have been used in humans without acute toxic effects. Any overdose should be treated with supportive care focused on the symptoms exhibited.

Drug Interactions
  Cytochrome P450 Effect: CYP3A3/4 enzyme substrate
  Increased Effect/Toxicity: Bexarotene plasma concentrations may be increased by azole antifungals, clarithromycin, erythromycin, fluvoxamine, nefazodone, quinine, ritonavir, gemfibrozil, or grapefruit juice.
  Decreased Effect: Bexarotene plasma levels may be decreased by rifampin, phenytoin, phenobarbital, or nafcillin.

Ethanol/Nutrition/Herb Interactions
  Food: Take with a fat-containing meal. Bexarotene serum levels may be increased by grapefruit juice; avoid concurrent use.
  Herb/Nutraceutical: Avoid dong quai, St John's wort (may also cause photosensitization). Additional vitamin A supplements may lead to vitamin A toxicity (dry skin, irritation, arthralgias, myalgias, abdominal pain, hepatic changes). St John's wort may decrease bexarotene levels.

Stability Store at 2°C to 25°C (36°F to 77°F); protect from light

Mechanism of Action The exact mechanism in the treatment of cutaneous T-cell lymphoma is unknown. Binds and activates retinoid X receptor subtypes. Retinoid receptor subtypes can form heterodimers with various receptor partners such as retinoic acid receptors, vitamin D receptor, thyroid receptor, and peroxisome proliferator activator receptors. Once activated, these receptors function as transcription factors that regulate the expression of genes which (Continued)

Bexarotene (Continued)

control cellular differentiation and proliferation. Bexarotene inhibits the growth *in vitro* of some tumor cell lines of hematopoietic and squamous cell origin.

Pharmacodynamics/Kinetics
Absorption: Significantly improved by a fat-containing meal

Protein binding: >99%

Metabolism: CYP3A3/4 enzyme system is involved; four metabolites identified; oxidative metabolites are further metabolized by glucuronidation

Half-life elimination: 7 hours

Time to peak: 2 hours

Excretion: Primarily feces; urine (<1% as unchanged drug and metabolites)

Usual Dosage
Adults: Oral: 300 mg/m²/day taken as a single daily dose. If there is no tumor response after 8 weeks and the initial dose was well tolerated, then an increase to 400 mg/m²/day can be made with careful monitoring. Maintain as long as the patient is deriving benefit.

If the initial dose is not tolerated, then it may be adjusted to 200 mg/m²/day, then to 100 mg/m²/day or temporarily suspended if necessary to manage toxicity

Dosing adjustment in renal impairment: No studies have been conducted; however, renal insufficiency may result in significant protein binding changes and alter pharmacokinetics of bexarotene

Dosing adjustment in hepatic impairment: No studies have been conducted; however, hepatic impairment would be expected to result in decreased clearance of bexarotene due to the extensive hepatic contribution to elimination

Gel: Apply once every other day for first week, then increase on a weekly basis to once daily, 2 times/day, 3 times/day, and finally 4 times/day, according to tolerance

Monitoring Parameters If female, pregnancy test 1 week before initiation then monthly while on bexarotene; lipid panel before initiation, then weekly until lipid response established and then at 8-week intervals thereafter; baseline LFTs, repeat at 1, 2, and 4 weeks after initiation then at 8-week intervals thereafter if stable; baseline and periodic thyroid function tests; baseline CBC with periodic monitoring

Patient Information
Oral: Take with a fat-containing meal. Get pregnancy test before starting therapy and then every month thereafter while on the medicine. Do not get pregnant while taking this medicine. Use 2 forms of birth control 1 month before, during, and for at least a month after completion of therapy. For male patients, protect your partner against pregnancy by wearing a condom. Continue using protection for 1 month after last dose. Take at a similar time daily. Call your prescriber if you have a fever, chills, or any signs of infection. You are at risk of infections: stay away from crowds and people with viruses. Wash your hands frequently. Check vitamin A intake with your prescriber. You should avoid large amounts of vitamin A.

Topical gel: Allow gel to dry before covering. Avoid applying to normal skin or mucous membranes. Do not use occlusive dressings.

Nursing Implications Educate patient about medicine and frequency of laboratory monitoring

Dosage Forms
Capsule: 75 mg

Gel: 1% (60 g)

♦ **Bextra**® *see* Valdecoxib *on page 1395*

♦ **Biavax**®ₗₗ *see* Rubella and Mumps Vaccines (Combined) *on page 1216*

♦ **Biaxin**® *see* Clarithromycin *on page 306*

♦ **Biaxin**® XL *see* Clarithromycin *on page 306*

Bicalutamide (bye ka LOO ta mide)

U.S. Brand Names Casodex®

Canadian Brand Names Casodex®

Therapeutic Category Antiandrogen; Antineoplastic Agent, Miscellaneous

Use In combination therapy with LHRH agonist analogues in treatment of advanced prostatic carcinoma

Pregnancy Risk Factor X

Contraindications Hypersensitivity to bicalutamide or any component of the formulation; not for use in women, particularly in nonserious or nonlife-threatening conditions; pregnancy

Warnings/Precautions Rare cases of death or hospitalization due to hepatitis have been reported postmarketing. Use with caution in moderate to severe hepatic dysfunction. Hepatotoxicity generally occurs within the first 3-4 months of use. Baseline liver function tests should be obtained and repeated regularly during the first 4 months of treatment, and periodically thereafter. Additionally, patients should be monitored for signs and symptoms of liver dysfunction. Bicalutamide should be discontinued if patients have jaundice or ALT is two times the upper limit of normal. May cause gynecomastia in a high percentage of patients.

Adverse Reactions
10%:

Cardiovascular: Flushing (hot flashes), chest pain

Gastrointestinal: Abdominal pain, constipation, nausea

Neuromuscular & skeletal: Weakness

Miscellaneous: Pain (general)

1% to 10%:

Cardiovascular: Hypertension, chest pain pectoris, congestive heart failure, edema, peripheral edema

Central nervous system: Anxiety, headache, dizziness, depression, confusion, somnolence, nervousness, fever, chills, insomnia

Dermatologic: Dry skin, pruritus, alopecia, rash

Endocrine & metabolic: Breast pain, diabetes mellitus (hyperglycemia), decreased libido, dehydration, gout, impotency

inal: Diarrhea, vomiting, anorexia, heartburn, rectal hemorrhage, dry mouth,
eight gain/loss

y: Polyuria, urinary impairment, dysuria, urinary retention, urinary urgency
: Anemia

line phosphatase increased

ar & skeletal: Muscle weakness, arthritis, myalgia, leg cramps, pathological
ck pain, hypertonia, neuropathy

nine increased

Cough increased, dyspnea, pharyngitis, bronchitis, pneumonia, rhinitis, lung

: Sepsis, neoplasma

icology Symptoms include hypoactivity, ataxia, anorexia, vomiting, slow
lacrimation. Treatment is supportive with no benefit of dialysis. Induce

ct/Toxicity: Bicalutamide may displace warfarin from protein binding sites
may result in an increased anticoagulant effect, especially when bicalutamide
therapy is started after the patient is already on warfarin.

Stability Store at room temperature

Mechanism of Action Pure nonsteroidal antiandrogen that binds to androgen receptors; specifically a competitive inhibitor for the binding of dihydrotestosterone and testosterone; prevents testosterone stimulation of cell growth in prostate cancer

Pharmacodynamics/Kinetics

Absorption: Rapid and complete

Protein binding: 96%

Metabolism: Extensive; stereospecific metabolism

Half-life elimination: Up to 10 days; active enantiomer 5.8 days

Usual Dosage Adults: Oral: 1 tablet once daily (morning or evening), with or without food. It is recommended that bicalutamide be taken at the same time each day; start treatment with bicalutamide at the same time as treatment with an LHRH analog.

Dosage adjustment in renal impairment: None necessary as renal impairment has no significant effect on elimination

Dosage adjustment in liver impairment: Limited data in subjects with severe hepatic impairment suggest that excretion of bicalutamide may be delayed and could lead to further accumulation. Use with caution in patients with moderate to severe hepatic impairment.

Dietary Considerations May be taken with or without food.

Administration Dose should be taken at the same time each day with or without food; start treatment at the same time as treatment with an LHRH analog

Monitoring Parameters Serum prostate-specific antigen, alkaline phosphatase, acid phosphatase, or prostatic acid phosphatase; prostate gland dimensions; skeletal survey; liver scans; chest x-rays; physical exam every 3 months; bone scan every 3-6 months; CBC, EKG, echocardiograms, and serum testosterone and luteinizing hormone (periodically). Liver function tests should be obtained at baseline and repeated regularly during the first 4 months of treatment, and periodically thereafter; monitor for signs and symptoms of liver dysfunction. (discontinue if jaundice is noted or ALT is two or more times the upper limit of normal).

Patient Information Take as directed and do not alter dose or discontinue without consulting prescriber. Take at the same time each day with or without food; void before taking medication. Diabetics should monitor serum glucose closely and notify prescriber of changes; this medication can alter hypoglycemic requirements. You may lose your hair and experience impotency. May cause dizziness, confusion, or drowsiness (use caution when driving or engaging in tasks that require alertness until response to drug is known); nausea or vomiting (small frequent meals, frequent mouth care, sucking lozenges, or chewing gum may help); or constipation (increased dietary fiber, fruit, or fluid and increased exercise may help). Report easy bruising or bleeding; yellowing of skin or eyes; change in color of urine or stool; unresolved CNS changes (nervousness, chills, insomnia, somnolence); skin rash, redness, or irritation; chest pain or palpitations; difficulty breathing; urinary retention or inability to void; muscle weakness, tremors, or pain; persistent nausea, vomiting, diarrhea, or constipation; or other unusual signs or adverse reactions.

Nursing Implications Administer at the same time as treatment with LHRH analog

Dosage Forms Tablet: 50 mg

♦ **Bicillin® C-R** *see* Penicillin G Benzathine and Procaine Combined *on page 1052*

♦ **Bicillin® C-R 900/300** *see* Penicillin G Benzathine and Procaine Combined *on page 1052*

♦ **Bicillin® L-A** *see* Penicillin G Benzathine *on page 1051*

♦ **Bicitra®** *see* Sodium Citrate and Citric Acid *on page 1246*

♦ **BiCNU®** *see* Carmustine *on page 230*

♦ **Biltricide®** *see* Praziquantel *on page 1120*

Bimatoprost (bi MAT oh prost)

Related Information

Glaucoma Drug Therapy Comparison *on page 1499*

U.S. Brand Names Lumigan™

Therapeutic Category Prostaglandin, Ophthalmic

Use Reduction of intraocular pressure (IOP) in patients with open-angle glaucoma or ocular hypertension; should be used in patients who are intolerant of other IOP-lowering medications or failed treatment with another IOP-lowering medication

Pregnancy Risk Factor C

Pregnancy/Breast-Feeding Implications Excretion in breast milk unknown; use caution

Contraindications Hypersensitivity to bimatoprost or any component of the formulation

Warnings/Precautions May cause permanent changes in eye color (increases the amount of brown pigment in the iris), the eyelid skin, and eyelashes. In addition, may increase the length
(Continued)

Bimatoprost *(Continued)*

and/or number of eyelashes (may vary between eyes). Use caution in patients with intraocular inflammation, aphakic patients, pseudophakic patients with a torn posterior lens capsule, or patients with risk factors for macular edema. Contains benzalkonium chloride (may be adsorbed by contact lenses) Safety and efficacy have not been determined for use in patients with renal or hepatic impairment, angle closure, inflammatory or neovascular glaucoma. Safety and efficacy in pediatric patients not established.

Adverse Reactions

>10%: Ocular (15% to 45%): Conjunctival hyperemia, growth of eyelashes, ocular pruritus
1% to 10%:
Central nervous system: Headache (1% to 5%)
Dermatologic: Hirsutism (1% to 5%)
Hepatic: Abnormal liver function tests (1% to 5%)
Neuromuscular & skeletal: Weakness (1% to 5%)
Ocular:
3% to 10%: Blepharitis, burning, cataract, dryness, eyelid redness, eyelash darkening, foreign body sensation, irritation, pain, pigmentation of periocular skin, superficial punctate keratitis, visual disturbance
1% to 3%: Allergic conjunctivitis, asthenopia, conjunctival edema, discharge, increased iris pigmentation, photophobia, tearing
Respiratory: Upper respiratory tract infection (10%)
<1% (Limited to important or life-threatening): Bacterial keratitis (caused by inadvertent contamination of multiple-dose ophthalmic solutions), iritis

Overdosage/Toxicology No information available. Treatment is symptom directed and supportive.

Stability Store between 15°C to 25°C (59°F to 77°F)

Mechanism of Action As a synthetic analog of prostaglandin with ocular hypotensive activity, bimatoprost decreases intraocular pressure by increasing the outflow of aqueous humor.

Pharmacodynamics/Kinetics

Onset of action: Reduction of IOP: ~4 hours
Peak effect: Maximum reduction of IOP: ~8-12 hours
Distribution: 0.67 L/kg
Protein binding: ~88%
Metabolism: Undergoes oxidation, N-demethylation, and glucuronidation after reaching systemic circulation; forms metabolites
Half-life elimination: I.V.: 45 minutes
Time to peak: 10 minutes
Excretion: Urine (67%); feces (25%)

Usual Dosage Ophthalmic: Adult: Open-angle glaucoma or ocular hypertension: Instill 1 drop into affected eye(s) once daily in the evening; do not exceed once-daily dosing (may decrease IOP-lowering effect). If used with other topical ophthalmic agents, separate administration by at least 5 minutes.

Administration May be used with other eye drops to lower intraocular pressure. If using more than one ophthalmic product, wait at least 5 minutes in between application of each medication. Remove contact lenses prior to administration and wait 15 minutes before reinserting.

Patient Information Wash hands before instilling. Sit or lie down to instill. Open eye, look at ceiling, and instill prescribed amount of solution. Apply gentle pressure to inner corner of eye. Do not let tip of applicator touch eye; do not contaminate tip of applicator (contamination may cause eye infection leading to possible eye damage or vision loss). Contact prescriber concerning continued use of drops if eye infection develops, trauma occurs to the eye, and prior to eye surgery. This product contains benzalkonium chloride which may be adsorbed by contact lenses; remove contacts prior to administration and wait 15 minutes before reinserting. May cause permanent changes in eye color (increases the amount of brown pigment in the iris), eyelid, and eyelashes. May also increase the length and/or number of eyelashes. Changes may occur slowly (months to years). May be used with other eye drops to lower intraocular pressure. If using more than one eye drop medicine, wait at least 5 minutes in between application of each medication. Notify prescriber if conjunctivitis or eyelid reactions occur with use of this product.

Nursing Implications May be used with other eye drops to lower intraocular pressure. If using more than one ophthalmic product, wait at least 5 minutes in between application of each medication.

Additional Information The IOP-lowering effect was shown to be 7-8 mm Hg in clinical studies.

Dosage Forms Solution, ophthalmic: 0.03% (2.5 mL, 5 mL) [contains benzalkonium chloride]

- **Biocef** *see* Cephalexin *on page 261*
- **Biodine [OTC]** *see* Povidone-Iodine *on page 1114*
- **Biofed-PE® [OTC]** *see* Triprolidine and Pseudoephedrine *on page 1380*
- **Biohist® LA** *see* Carbinoxamine and Pseudoephedrine *on page 225*
- **Biolon™ (Can)** *see* Sodium Hyaluronate *on page 1247*
- **Bio-Statin®** *see* Nystatin *on page 1001*
- **BioThrax™** *see* Anthrax Vaccine Adsorbed *Not Commercially Available on page 101*
- **Bismatrol® [OTC]** *see* Bismuth *on page 170*

Bismuth *(BIZ muth)*

Related Information

Antimicrobial Drugs of Choice *on page 1588*
Helicobacter pylori Treatment *on page 1668*

U.S. Brand Names Bismatrol® [OTC]; Colo-Fresh™ [OTC]; Diotame® [OTC]; Pepto-Bismol® [OTC]; Pepto-Bismol® Maximum Strength [OTC]

Synonyms Bismuth Subgallate; Bismuth Subsalicylate; Pink Bismuth

Therapeutic Category Antidiarrheal

Use Symptomatic treatment of mild, nonspecific diarrhea; indigestion, nausea, control of traveler's diarrhea (enterotoxigenic *Escherichia coli*); as part of a multidrug regimen for *H. pylori* eradication to reduce the risk of duodenal ulcer recurrence; subgallate formulation to control fecal odors in colostomy, ileostomy, or fecal incontinence

Pregnancy Risk Factor C/D (3rd trimester)

Contraindications Do not use subsalicylate in patients with influenza or chickenpox because of risk of Reye's syndrome; hypersensitivity to salicylates or any component of the formulation; history of severe GI bleeding; history of coagulopathy; pregnancy (3rd trimester)

Warnings/Precautions Subsalicylate should be used with caution if patient is taking aspirin; use with caution in children, especially those <3 years of age and those with viral illness; may be neurotoxic with very large doses

Adverse Reactions

>10%: Gastrointestinal: Discoloration of the tongue (darkening), grayish black stools

<1% (Limited to important or life-threatening): Anxiety, confusion, headache, hearing loss, impaction may occur in infants and debilitated patients, mental depression, muscle spasms, slurred speech, tinnitus, weakness

Overdosage/Toxicology

Symptoms of toxicity: **Subsalicylate:** Hyperpnea, nausea, vomiting, tinnitus, hyperpyrexia, metabolic acidoses/respiratory alkalosis, tachycardia, and confusion; seizures in severe overdose, pulmonary or cerebral edema, respiratory failure, cardiovascular collapse, coma, and death. **Note:** Each 262.4 mg tablet of bismuth subsalicylate contains an equivalent of 130 mg aspirin; 150 mg/kg of aspirin is considered to be toxic. Serious life-threatening toxicity occurs with >300 mg/kg.

Treatment: Gastrointestinal decontamination (activated charcoal for immediate release formulations (10 x dose of ASA in g), whole bowel irrigation for enteric coated tablets or when serially increasing ASA plasma levels indicate the presence of an intestinal bezoar), supportive and symptomatic treatment with emphasis on correcting fluid, electrolyte, blood glucose and acid-base disturbances; elimination is enhanced with urinary alkalinization (sodium bicarbonate infusion with potassium), multiple-dose activated charcoal, and hemodialysis.

Symptoms of toxicity: **Bismuth:** Rare with short-term administrations of bismuth salts; encephalopathy, methemoglobinemia, seizures

Treatment: Gastrointestinal decontamination; chelation with dimercaprol in doses of 3 mg/kg or penicillamine 100 mg/kg/day for 5 days can hasten recovery from bismuth-induced encephalopathy; methylene blue 1-2 mg/kg in a 1% sterile aqueous solution I.V. push over 4-6 minutes for methemoglobinemia. This may be repeated within 60 minutes if necessary, up to a total dose of 7 mg/kg. Seizures usually respond to I.V. diazepam.

Drug Interactions

Increased Effect/Toxicity: Toxicity of aspirin, warfarin, and/or hypoglycemics may be increased.

Decreased Effect: The effects of tetracyclines and uricosurics may be decreased.

Mechanism of Action Bismuth subsalicylate exhibits both antisecretory and antimicrobial action. This agent may provide some anti-inflammatory action as well. The salicylate moiety provides antisecretory effect and the bismuth exhibits antimicrobial directly against bacterial and viral gastrointestinal pathogens. Bismuth has some antacid properties.

Pharmacodynamics/Kinetics

Absorption: Minimal (<1%) across GI tract, salt (eg, salicylate) may be readily absorbed (80%); bismuth subsalicylate is rapidly cleaved to bismuth and salicylic acid in the stomach

Distribution: Salicylate: V_d: 170 mL/kg

Protein binding, plasma: Bismuth and salicylate: >90%

Metabolism: Bismuth: Oral: Salts undergo chemical dissociation; Salicylate: Extensively hepatic

Half-life elimination: Terminal: Bismuth: 21-72 days; Salicylate: 2-5 hours

Excretion: Bismuth: Urine and feces; Salicylate: 10% (as unchanged drug)

Clearance: Bismuth: 50 mL/minute

Usual Dosage Oral:

Nonspecific diarrhea: Subsalicylate:

Children: Up to 8 doses/24 hours:

3-6 years: $1/3$ tablet or 5 mL (regular strength) every 30 minutes to 1 hour as needed

6-9 years: $2/3$ tablet or 10 mL (regular strength) every 30 minutes to 1 hour as needed

9-12 years: 1 tablet or 15 mL (regular strength) every 30 minutes to 1 hour as needed

Adults: 2 tablets or 30 mL every 30 minutes to 1 hour as needed up to 8 doses/24 hours

Prevention of traveler's diarrhea: 2.1 g/day or 2 tablets 4 times/day before meals and at bedtime

Helicobacter pylori eradication: 524 mg 4 times/day with meals and at bedtime; requires combination therapy

Control of fecal odor in ileostomy or colostomy: Subgallate: 1-2 tablets 3 times/day with meals (maximum: 5 tablets/day)

Dosing adjustment in renal impairment: Should probably be avoided in patients with renal failure

Test Interactions Increased uric acid, increased AST; bismuth absorbs x-rays and may interfere with diagnostic procedures of GI tract

Patient Information Chew tablet well or shake suspension well before using; may darken stools; if diarrhea persists for more than 2 days, consult a physician; can turn tongue black; tinnitus may indicate toxicity and use should be discontinued

Nursing Implications Seek causes for diarrhea; monitor for tinnitus; may aggravate or cause gout attack; may enhance bleeding if used with anticoagulants

Dosage Forms

Liquid, as subsalicylate: 262 mg/15 mL (240 mL, 360 mL, 480 mL); 525 mg/15 mL (240 mL, 360 mL)

Bismatrol®: 262 mg/15 mL (240 mL)

Diotame®: 262 mg/15 mL (30 mL)

Pepto-Bismol®: 262 mg/15 mL (120 mL, 240 mL, 360 mL, 480 mL) [wintergreen flavor]

(Continued)

Bismuth *(Continued)*

Pepto-Bismol® Maximum Strength: 525 mg/15 mL (120 mL, 240 mL, 360 mL) [wintergreen flavor]

Tablet, as subgallate (Colo-Fresh™): 324 mg

Tablet, chewable, as subsalicylate (Diaotame®, Bismatrol®, Pepto-Bismol®): 262 mg

♦ **Bismuth Subgallate** *see Bismuth on page 170*

♦ **Bismuth Subsalicylate** *see Bismuth on page 170*

Bismuth Subsalicylate, Metronidazole, and Tetracycline

(BIZ muth sub sa LIS i late, me troe NI da zole, & tet ra SYE kleen)

U.S. Brand Names Helidac®

Synonyms Bismuth Subsalicylate, Tetracycline, and Metronidazole; Metronidazole, Bismuth Subsalicylate, and Tetracycline; Metronidazole, Tetracycline, and Bismuth Subsalicylate; Tetracycline, Bismuth Subsalicylate, and Metronidazole; Tetracycline, Metronidazole, and Bismuth Subsalicylate

Therapeutic Category Antidiarrheal

Use In combination with an H_2 antagonist, as part of a multidrug regimen for *H. pylori* eradication to reduce the risk of duodenal ulcer recurrence

Pregnancy Risk Factor D (tetracycline); B (metronidazole)

Usual Dosage Adults: Chew 2 bismuth subsalicylate 262.4 mg tablets, swallow 1 metronidazole 250 mg tablet, and swallow 1 tetracycline 500 mg capsule 4 times/day at meals and bedtime, plus an H_2 antagonist (at the appropriate dose) for 14 days; follow with 8 oz of water; the H_2 antagonist should be continued for a total of 28 days

Additional Information Complete prescribing information for this medication should be consulted for additional detail.

Dosage Forms Each package contains 14 blister cards (2-week supply); each card contains the following:

Capsule: Tetracycline hydrochloride: 500 mg (4)

Tablet:

Bismuth subsalicylate [chewable]: 262.4 mg (8)

Metronidazole: 250 mg (4)

♦ **Bismuth Subsalicylate, Tetracycline, and Metronidazole** *see Bismuth Subsalicylate, Metronidazole, and Tetracycline on page 172*

Bisoprolol *(bis OH proe lol)*

Related Information

Beta-Blockers Comparison *on page 1491*

Heart Failure *on page 1663*

U.S. Brand Names Zebeta®

Canadian Brand Names Monocor®; Zebeta®

Synonyms Bisoprolol Fumarate

Therapeutic Category Antihypertensive Agent; Beta-Adrenergic Blocker

Use Treatment of hypertension, alone or in combination with other agents

Unlabeled/Investigational Use Angina pectoris, supraventricular arrhythmias, PVCs

Pregnancy Risk Factor C (manufacturer); D (2nd and 3rd trimesters - expert analysis)

Contraindications Hypersensitivity to bisoprolol or any component of the formulation; sinus bradycardia; heart block greater than first-degree (except in patients with a functioning artificial pacemaker); cardiogenic shock; uncompensated cardiac failure; pulmonary edema; pregnancy (2nd and 3rd trimesters)

Warnings/Precautions Use with caution in patients with inadequate myocardial function, bronchospastic disease, hyperthyroidism, undergoing anesthesia; and in those with impaired hepatic function. Acute withdrawal may exacerbate symptoms (gradually taper over a 2-week period). Use caution in patients with PVD (can aggravate arterial insufficiency). Use caution with concurrent use with verapamil or diltiazem; bradycardia or heart block can occur. Bisoprolol should be used cautiously in bronchospastic disease with close monitoring. Use cautiously in diabetics because it can mask prominent hypoglycemic symptoms. Can mask signs of thyrotoxicosis. Can cause fetal harm when administered in pregnancy. Use care with anesthetic agents which decrease myocardial function.

Adverse Reactions

>10%

Central nervous system: Drowsiness, insomnia

Endocrine & metabolic: Decreased sexual ability

1% to 10%:

Cardiovascular: Bradycardia, palpitations, edema, congestive heart failure, reduced peripheral circulation

Central nervous system: Mental depression

Gastrointestinal: Diarrhea or constipation, nausea, vomiting, stomach discomfort

Ocular: Mild ocular stinging and discomfort, tearing, photophobia, decreased corneal sensitivity, keratitis

Respiratory: Bronchospasm

Miscellaneous: Cold extremities

<1% (Limited to important or life-threatening): Arrhythmias, confusion (especially in the elderly), depression, dyspnea, hallucinations, leukopenia, orthostatic hypotension, psoriasiform eruption, thrombocytopenia

Overdosage/Toxicology Symptoms include cardiac disturbances, CNS toxicity, bronchospasm, hypoglycemia and hyperkalemia. The most common cardiac symptoms include hypotension and bradycardia. Atrioventricular block, intraventricular conduction disturbances, cardiogenic shock, and asystole may occur with severe overdose, especially with membrane-depressant drugs (eg, propranolol). CNS effects include convulsions, coma, and respiratory arrest (commonly seen with propranolol and other membrane-depressant and lipid-soluble drugs). Treatment is symptomatic for seizures, hypotension, hyperkalemia, and hypoglycemia. Bradycardia and hypotension resistant to atropine, isoproterenol, or pacing may respond to glucagon. Wide QRS defects caused by membrane-depressant poisoning may respond to hypertonic sodium bicarbonate. Repeat-dose charcoal, hemoperfusion, or hemodialysis may be helpful in removal of only those beta-blockers with a small V_d, long half-life, or low intrinsic clearance (acebutolol, atenolol, nadolol, sotalol).

Drug Interactions
  Cytochrome P450 Effect: CYP2D6 enzyme substrate
  Increased Effect/Toxicity: Bisoprolol may increase the effects of other drugs which slow AV conduction (digoxin, verapamil, diltiazem), alpha-blockers (prazosin, terazosin), and alpha-adrenergic stimulants (epinephrine, phenylephrine). Bisoprolol may mask the tachycardia from hypoglycemia caused by insulin and oral hypoglycemics. In patients receiving concurrent therapy, the risk of hypertensive crisis is increased when either clonidine or the beta-blocker is withdrawn. Reserpine has been shown to enhance the effect of beta-blockers. Beta-blockers may increase the action or levels of ethanol, disopyramide, nondepolarizing muscle relaxants, and theophylline although the effects are difficult to predict.
  Decreased Effect: Decreased effect of bisoprolol with aluminum salts, barbiturates, calcium salts, cholestyramine, colestipol, NSAIDs, penicillins (ampicillin), rifampin, and salicylates due to decreased bioavailability and plasma levels. The effect of sulfonylureas may be decreased by beta-blockers.

Ethanol/Nutrition/Herb Interactions Herb/Nutraceutical: Avoid dong quai if using for hypertension (has estrogenic activity). Avoid ephedra, yohimbe, ginseng (may worsen hypertension). Avoid garlic (may have increased antihypertensive effect).

Mechanism of Action Selective inhibitor of beta$_1$-adrenergic receptors; competitively blocks beta$_1$-receptors, with little or no effect on beta$_2$-receptors at doses <10 mg

Pharmacodynamics/Kinetics
  Onset of action: 1-2 hours
  Absorption: Rapid and almost complete
  Distribution: Widely; highest concentrations in heart, liver, lungs, and saliva; crosses blood-brain barrier; enters breast milk
  Protein binding: 26% to 33%
  Metabolism: Extensively hepatic; significant first-pass effect
  Half-life elimination: 9-12 hours
  Time to peak: 1.7-3 hours
  Excretion: Urine (3% to 10% as unchanged drug); feces (<2%)

Usual Dosage Oral:
  Adults: 5 mg once daily, may be increased to 10 mg, and then up to 20 mg once daily, if necessary
  Elderly: Initial dose: 2.5 mg/day; may be increased by 2.5-5 mg/day; maximum recommended dose: 20 mg/day
  Dosing adjustment in renal/hepatic impairment: Cl_{cr} <40 mL/minute: Initial: 2.5 mg/day; increase cautiously.
  Hemodialysis: Not dialyzable

Dietary Considerations May be taken without regard to meals.

Monitoring Parameters Blood pressure, EKG, neurologic status

Test Interactions ↑ thyroxine (S), cholesterol (S), glucose; ↑ triglycerides, uric acid; ↓ HDL

Patient Information Do not discontinue abruptly (angina may be precipitated); notify physician if CHF symptoms become worse or side effects occur; take at the same time each day; may mask diabetes symptoms; consult pharmacist or physician before taking with other adrenergic drugs (eg, cold medications); use with caution while driving or performing tasks requiring alertness; may be taken without regard to meals

Nursing Implications
  Modify dosage in patients with renal insufficiency
  Patient's therapeutic response may be evaluated by monitoring of blood pressure, apical and radial pulses, fluid I & O, daily weight, respirations, and circulation in extremities before and during therapy; monitor for CNS side effects

Dosage Forms Tablet, as fumarate: 5 mg, 10 mg

Bisoprolol and Hydrochlorothiazide
(bis OH proe lol & hye droe klor oh THYE a zide)

U.S. Brand Names Ziac®
Canadian Brand Names Ziac™
Synonyms Hydrochlorothiazide and Bisoprolol
Therapeutic Category Antihypertensive Agent, Combination
Use Treatment of hypertension
Pregnancy Risk Factor C/D (2nd and 3rd trimesters)
Usual Dosage Adults: Oral: Dose is individualized, given once daily
Additional Information Complete prescribing information for this medication should be consulted for additional detail.
Dosage Forms Tablet:
  Bisoprolol fumarate 2.5 mg and hydrochlorothiazide 6.25 mg
  Bisoprolol fumarate 5 mg and hydrochlorothiazide 6.25 mg
  Bisoprolol fumarate 10 mg and hydrochlorothiazide 6.25 mg

♦ **Bisoprolol Fumarate** *see* Bisoprolol *on page 172*
♦ **Bistropamide** *see* Tropicamide *on page 1384*

Bitolterol (bye TOLE ter ole)
Related Information
  Bronchodilators, Comparison of Inhaled Sympathomimetics *on page 1493*
U.S. Brand Names Tornalate® [DSC]
Canadian Brand Names Tornalate®
Synonyms Bitolterol Mesylate
Therapeutic Category Beta$_2$-Adrenergic Agonist Agent; Bronchodilator
Use Prevention and treatment of bronchial asthma and bronchospasm
(Continued)

Bitolterol *(Continued)*

Pregnancy Risk Factor C

Contraindications Hypersensitivity to bitolterol or any component of the formulation

Warnings/Precautions Use with caution in patients with unstable vasomotor symptoms, diabetes, hyperthyroidism, prostatic hyperplasia or a history of seizures; also use caution in the elderly and those patients with cardiovascular disorders such as coronary artery disease, arrhythmias, and hypertension; excessive use may result in cardiac arrest and death; do not use concurrently with other sympathomimetic bronchodilators. Safety and efficacy have not been established in children ≤12 years of age.

Adverse Reactions

>10%: Neuromuscular & skeletal: Trembling

1% to 10%:
Cardiovascular: Flushing of face, hypertension, pounding heartbeat
Central nervous system: Dizziness, lightheadedness, nervousness, headache
Gastrointestinal: Dry mouth, nausea
Respiratory: Bronchial irritation, coughing

<1% (Limited to important or life-threatening): Arrhythmias, chest pain, paradoxical broncho-spasm, tachycardia

Overdosage/Toxicology Symptoms include tremor, dizziness, nervousness, headache, nausea, and coughing. Treatment is symptomatic and supportive. In cases of severe over-dose, supportive therapy should be instituted, and prudent use of a cardioselective beta-adrenergic blocker (eg, atenolol or metoprolol) should be considered, keeping in mind the potential for induction of bronchoconstriction in an asthmatic individual. Dialysis has not been shown to be of value in the treatment of an overdose with this agent.

Drug Interactions

Increased Effect/Toxicity: Increased toxicity with MAO inhibitors, tricyclic antidepressants, sympathomimetic agents (eg, amphetamine, dopamine, dobutamine), inhaled anesthetics (eg, enflurane). Increased toxicity (cardiotoxicity) with aminophylline, theophylline, or oxtriphylline.

Decreased Effect: Decreased effect with beta-adrenergic blockers (eg, propranolol).

Mechanism of Action Selectively stimulates beta$_2$-adrenergic receptors in the lungs producing bronchial smooth muscle relaxation; minor beta$_1$ activity

Pharmacodynamics/Kinetics

Onset of action: Rapid
Duration: 4-8 hours
Metabolism: Inhalation: Bitolterol prodrug is hydrolyzed to colterol (active)
Half-life elimination: 3 hours
Time to peak, serum (colterol): Inhalation: ~1 hour
Excretion: Urine and feces

Usual Dosage Children >12 years and Adults:

Bronchospasm: 2 inhalations at an interval of at least 1-3 minutes, followed by a third inhalation if needed

Prevention of bronchospasm: 2 inhalations every 8 hours; do not exceed 3 inhalations every 6 hours or 2 inhalations every 4 hours

Administration Administer around-the-clock rather than 3 times/day, to promote less variation in peak and trough serum levels

Monitoring Parameters Assess lung sounds, pulse, and blood pressure before administration and during peak of medication; observe patient for wheezing after administration

Patient Information Do not exceed recommended dosage, excessive use may lead to adverse effects or loss of effectiveness; shake canister well before use; administer pressurized inhalation during the second half of inspiration, as the airways are open, water and the aerosol distribution is more extensive. If more than one inhalation per dose is necessary, wait at least 1 full minute between inhalations - second inhalation is best delivered after 10 minutes. May cause nervousness, restlessness, and insomnia; if these effects continue after dosage reduction, notify physician. Also notify physician if palpitations, tachycardia, chest pain, muscle tremors, dizziness, headache, flushing, or if breathing difficulty persists.

Nursing Implications Before using, the inhaler must be shaken well

Dosage Forms

Aerosol for oral inhalation, as mesylate: 0.8% [370 mcg/metered spray; 300 inhalations] (15 mL)

Solution for oral inhalation, as mesylate: 0.2% (10 mL, 30 mL, 60 mL)

♦ **Bitolterol Mesylate** *see* Bitolterol *on page 173*

Bivalirudin *(bye VAL i roo din)*

U.S. Brand Names Angiomax®

Synonyms Hirulog

Therapeutic Category Anticoagulant

Use Anticoagulant used in conjunction with aspirin for patients with unstable angina undergoing percutaneous transluminal coronary angioplasty (PTCA)

Pregnancy Risk Factor B

Pregnancy/Breast-Feeding Implications Although animal studies have not shown harm to the fetus, safety and efficacy for use in pregnant women have not been established. Bivalirudin is used in conjunction with aspirin, which may lead to maternal or fetal adverse effects, especially during the third trimester. Use during pregnancy only if clearly needed. It is not known if bivalirudin is excreted in human milk; use with caution if given to a breast-feeding woman.

Contraindications Hypersensitivity to bivalirudin or any component of the formulation; active major bleeding

Warnings/Precautions Safety and efficacy have not been established when used with platelet inhibitors other than aspirin, in patients with unstable angina not undergoing PTCA, in patients with other coronary syndromes, or in pediatric patients. As with all anticoagulants, bleeding may occur at any site and should be considered following an unexplained fall in blood pressure or hematocrit, or any unexplained symptom. Use with caution in patients with disease states associated with increased risk of bleeding.

Adverse Reactions As with all anticoagulants, bleeding is the major adverse effect of bivalirudin. Hemorrhage may occur at virtually any site. Risk is dependent on multiple variables, including the intensity of anticoagulation and patient susceptibility. Additional adverse effects are often related to idiosyncratic reactions, and the frequency is difficult to estimate. Adverse reactions reported were generally less than those seen with heparin.

>10%:
    Cardiovascular: Hypotension (12% bivalirudin vs 17% heparin)
    Central nervous system: Pain (15%), headache (12%)
    Gastrointestinal: Nausea (15%)
    Neuromuscular & skeletal: Back pain (42% vs 44% heparin)

1% to 10%:
    Cardiovascular: Hypertension (6%), bradycardia (5%)
    Central nervous system: Insomnia (7%), anxiety (6%), fever (5%), nervousness (5%)
    Gastrointestinal: Vomiting (6%), dyspepsia (5%), abdominal pain (5%)
    Genitourinary: Urinary retention (4%)
    Hematologic: Major hemorrhage (4% bivalirudin vs 9% heparin), transfusion required (2% bivalirudin vs 6% heparin)
    Local: Injection site pain (8%)
    Neuromuscular & skeletal: Pelvic pain (6%)

<1% (Limited to important or life-threatening): Cerebral ischemia, confusion, facial paralysis, intracranial bleeding, kidney failure, pulmonary edema, retroperitoneal bleeding, syncope, ventricular fibrillation

Overdosage/Toxicology There are no reports of overdose. Discontinue bivalirudin and monitor patients for signs of bleeding. Bivalirudin is hemodialyzable (~25% removed).

Drug Interactions
    Increased Effect/Toxicity: Aspirin may increase anticoagulant effect of bivalirudin (Note: All clinical trials included coadministration of aspirin). Limited drug interaction studies have not yet shown pharmacodynamic interactions between bivalirudin and ticlopidine, abciximab, or low molecular weight heparin (low molecular weight heparin was discontinued at least 8 hours prior to bivalirudin administration).

Stability Prior to and following reconstitution, bivalirudin vials should be stored at 2°C to 8°C. Final dilutions of 0.5 mg/mL or 5 mg/mL are stable at room temperature for up to 24 hours.

Mechanism of Action Bivalirudin acts as a specific and reversible direct thrombin inhibitor, binding to circulating and clot-bound thrombin. Shows linear dose- and concentration-dependent prolongation of ACT, aPTT, PT and TT.

Pharmacodynamics/Kinetics
    Onset of action: Immediate
    Duration: Coagulation times return to baseline ~1 hour following discontinuation of infusion
    Distribution: 0.2 L/kg
    Protein binding, plasma: Does not bind other than thrombin
    Half-life elimination: Normal renal function: 25 minutes; Cl_{cr} 10-29 mL/minute: 57 minutes
    Excretion: Urine, proteolytic cleavage

Usual Dosage Adults: Anticoagulant in patients with unstable angina undergoing PTCA (treatment should be started just prior to PTCA): I.V.: Initial: Bolus: 1 mg/kg, followed by continuous infusion: 2.5 mg/kg/hour over 4 hours; if needed, infusion may be continued at 0.2 mg/kg/hour for up to 20 hours; patients should also receive aspirin 300-325 mg/day
    Dosage adjustment in renal impairment: Infusion dose should be reduced based on degree of renal impairment; initial bolus dose remains unchanged; monitor activated coagulation time (ACT)
        Cl_{cr} ≥60 mL/minute: No adjustment required
        Cl_{cr} 30-59 mL/minute: Decrease infusion dose by 20%
        Cl_{cr} 10-29 mL/minute: Decrease infusion dose by 60%
        Dialysis-dependent patients (off dialysis): Decrease infusion dose by 90%
        Clearance of bivalirudin remains 1.8-fold greater than the glomerular filtration rate, regardless of the degree in renal impairment.
    Dosage adjustment in hepatic impairment: No dosage adjustment is needed
    Elderly: No dosage adjustment is needed in elderly patients with normal renal function. Puncture site hemorrhage and catheterization site hemorrhage were seen in more patients ≥65 years of age than in patients <65 years of age

Administration For I.V. administration only. To prepare infusion, reconstitute each 250 mg vial with 5 mL sterile water for injection; further dilute with 5% dextrose in water or 0.9% sodium chloride for injection; final concentration should be 5 mg/mL for the initial continuous infusion (50 mL/250 mg vial). If needed, a lower concentration bag should be prepared for the low rate infusion; final concentration should be 0.5 mg/mL. Do not mix with other medications.

Monitoring Parameters Manufacturer recommends monitoring of ACT in patients with renal impairment. Although the ACT was checked after 5 minutes and 45 minutes in clinical trials, the bivalirudin dose was not titrated to the ACT.

Patient Information This drug can only be administered by injection. You may have a tendency to bleed easily while taking this drug; brush teeth with soft brush, floss with waxed floss, use electric razor, avoid scissors or sharp knives, and potentially harmful activities. Report chest pain; unusual bleeding or bruising (bleeding gums, nosebleed, blood in urine, dark stool); pain in joints or back; or numbness, tingling, swelling, or pain at injection site. Notify prescriber if pregnant. Consult prescriber if breast-feeding.

Nursing Implications To be administered via I.V. line only. Do not mix with other medications.

Additional Information There is limited clinical experience using bivalirudin in patients undergoing PTCA with heparin-induced thrombocytopenia/heparin-induced thrombocytopenia-thrombosis syndrome. Open-label use has shown adequate anticoagulation in these patients.

Dosage Forms Injection, powder for reconstitution: 250 mg

◆ **Blenoxane**® *see Bleomycin on page 176*

♦ **Bleo** *see* Bleomycin *on page 176*

Bleomycin (blee oh MYE sin)

U.S. Brand Names Blenoxane®

Canadian Brand Names Blenoxane®

Synonyms Bleo; Bleomycin Sulfate; BLM; NSC-125066

Therapeutic Category Antineoplastic Agent, Antibiotic

Use Treatment of squamous cell carcinomas, melanomas, sarcomas, testicular carcinoma, Hodgkin's lymphoma, and non-Hodgkin's lymphoma

Orphan drug: Sclerosing agent for malignant pleural effusion

Pregnancy Risk Factor D

Contraindications Hypersensitivity to bleomycin sulfate or any component of the formulation; severe pulmonary disease; pregnancy

Warnings/Precautions The U.S. Food and Drug Administration (FDA) currently recommends that procedures for proper handling and disposal of antineoplastic agents be considered. Occurrence of pulmonary fibrosis is higher in elderly patients and in those receiving >400 units total and in smokers and patients with prior radiation therapy. A severe idiosyncratic reaction consisting of hypotension, mental confusion, fever, chills and wheezing (similar to anaphylaxis) has been reported in 1% of lymphoma patients treated with bleomycin. Since these reactions usually occur after the first or second dose, careful monitoring is essential after these doses. Check lungs prior to each treatment for fine rales (1st sign). Follow manufacturer recommendations for administering O_2 during surgery to patients who have received bleomycin.

Adverse Reactions

>10%:

Cardiovascular: Raynaud's phenomenon

Central nervous system: Mild febrile reaction, fever, chills, patients may become febrile after intracavitary administration

Dermatologic: Pruritic erythema

Integument: ~50% of patients will develop erythema, induration, and hyperkeratosis and peeling of the skin; hyperpigmentation, alopecia, nailbed changes may occur; this appears to be dose-related and is reversible after cessation of therapy

Gastrointestinal: Mucocutaneous toxicity, stomatitis, nausea, vomiting, anorexia

Emetic potential: Moderately low (10% to 30%)

Local: Phlebitis, pain at tumor site

Irritant chemotherapy

Respiratory: Pneumonitis

1% to 10%:

Dermatologic: Alopecia

Gastrointestinal: Weight loss

Respiratory: Pulmonary fibrosis and death

Respiratory effects are dose-related when total dose is >400 units or with single doses >30 units; manifested as an acute or chronic interstitial pneumonitis with interstitial fibrosis, hypoxia, and death; symptoms include cough, dyspnea, and bilateral pulmonary infiltrates noted on CXR; it is controversial whether steroids improve symptoms of bleomycin pulmonary toxicity

Miscellaneous: Idiosyncratic: Similar to anaphylaxis and occurs in 1% of lymphoma patients; may include hypotension, confusion, fever, chills, and wheezing. May be immediate or delayed for several hours; symptomatic treatment includes volume expansion, vasopressor agents, antihistamines, and steroids

<1% (Limited to important or life-threatening): Hepatotoxicity, myocardial infarction, myelosuppression (rare), renal toxicity, scleroderma-like skin changes, stroke

Overdosage/Toxicology Symptoms include chills, fever, pulmonary fibrosis, and hyperpigmentation.

Drug Interactions

Increased Effect/Toxicity: Bleomycin with digoxin may result in elevated serum digoxin levels due to decreased renal clearance. CCNU (lomustine) increases severity of leukopenia. Results in delayed bleomycin elimination due to a decrease in creatinine clearance secondary to cisplatin.

Decreased Effect: Bleomycin and digitalis glycosides may decrease plasma levels of digoxin. Concomitant therapy with phenytoin results in decreased phenytoin levels, possibly due to decreased oral absorption.

Stability

Refrigerate intact vials of powder; intact vials are stable for up to one month at 45°C

Reconstitute powder with 1-5 mL SWI or NS which is stable at room temperature for 28 days or in refrigerator for 14 days; may use bacteriostatic agent if prolonged storage is necessary

Incompatible with amino acid solutions, aminophylline, ascorbic acid, cefazolin, cisplatin, cytarabine, furosemide, diazepam, hydrocortisone sodium succinate, methotrexate, mitomycin, nafcillin, penicillin G

Compatible with amikacin, cyclophosphamide, dexamethasone, diphenhydramine, doxorubicin, fluorouracil, gentamicin, heparin, hydrocortisone mesna, phenytoin, sodium phosphate, streptomycin, tobramycin, vinblastine, vincristine

Standard I.V. dilution: Dose/50-1000 mL NS or D_5W

Stable for 96 hours at room temperature and 14 days under refrigeration

Mechanism of Action Inhibits synthesis of DNA; binds to DNA leading to single- and double-strand breaks; isolated from *Streptomyces verticillus*

Pharmacodynamics/Kinetics

Absorption: I.M. and intrapleural administration: 30% serum concentrations I.V. administration; intraperitoneal and S.C. routes produce serum concentrations equal to those of I.V.

Distribution: V_d: 22 L/m²; highest concentrations in skin, kidney, lung, heart tissues; lowest in testes and GI tract; does not cross blood-brain barrier

Protein binding: 1%

Metabolism: By several tissues including liver, GI tract, skin, lungs, kidney, and serum
Half-life elimination: Biphasic: Dependent upon renal function:
  Normal renal function: Initial: 1.3 hours; Terminal: 9 hours
  End-stage renal disease: Initial: 2 hours; Terminal: 30 hours
Time to peak, serum: I.M.: Within 30 minutes
Excretion: Urine (50% to 70% as active drug)

Usual Dosage Refer to individual protocols; 1 unit = 1 mg
May be administered I.M., I.V., S.C., or intracavitary
Children and Adults:
  Test dose for lymphoma patients: I.M., I.V., S.C.: Because of the possibility of an anaphylactoid reaction, ≤2 units of bleomycin for the first 2 doses; monitor vital signs every 15 minutes; wait a minimum of 1 hour before administering remainder of dose; if no acute reaction occurs, then the regular dosage schedule may be followed
  Single-agent therapy:
    I.M./I.V./S.C.: Squamous cell carcinoma, lymphoma, testicular carcinoma: 0.25-0.5 units/kg (10-20 units/m^2) 1-2 times/week
    CIV: 15 units/m^2 over 24 hours daily for 4 days
  Combination-agent therapy:
    I.M./I.V.: 3-4 units/m^2
    I.V.: ABVD: 10 units/m^2 on days 1 and 15
    Maximum cumulative lifetime dose: 400 units
  Pleural sclerosing: 60-240 units as a single infusion. Dose may be repeated at intervals of several days if fluid continues to accumulate (mix in 50-100 mL of D_5W, NS, or SWFI); may add lidocaine 100-200 mg to reduce local discomfort.
  Dosing adjustment in renal impairment:
    Cl_{cr} 10-50 mL/minute: Administer 75% of normal dose
    Cl_{cr} <10 mL/minute: Administer 50% of normal dose
  Hemodialysis: None
  CAPD effects: None
  CAVH effects: None
  Adults: Intracavitary injection for malignant pleural effusion: 60 international units (range of 15-120 units; dose generally does not exceed 1 unit/kg) in 50-100 mL SWI

Administration I.V. doses should be administered slowly (≤1 unit/minute); I.M. or S.C. may cause pain at injection site

Monitoring Parameters Pulmonary function tests (total lung volume, forced vital capacity, carbon monoxide diffusion), renal function, chest x-ray, temperature initially, CBC with differential and platelet count

Patient Information You may experience loss of appetite, nausea, vomiting, mouth sores; small frequent meals, frequent mouth care with soft swab, frequent mouth rinses, sucking lozenges, or chewing gum may help; if unresolved, notify prescriber. You may experience fever or chills (will usually resolve); redness, peeling, or increased color of skin, or loss of hair (reversible after cessation of therapy). Report any change in respiratory status; difficulty breathing; wheezing; air hunger; increased secretions; difficulty expectorating secretions; confusion; unresolved fever or chills; sores in mouth; vaginal itching, burning, or discharge; sudden onset of dizziness; or acute headache. Contraceptive measures are recommended during therapy.

Nursing Implications Patients should be closely monitored for signs of pulmonary toxicity; check body weight at regular intervals

Dosage Forms Injection, powder for reconstitution, as sulfate: 15 units, 30 units [1 unit = 1 mg]

- ♦ **Bleomycin Sulfate** *see* Bleomycin *on page 176*
- ♦ **Bleph®-10** *see* Sulfacetamide *on page 1268*
- ♦ **Blephamide®** *see* Sulfacetamide and Prednisolone *on page 1269*
- ♦ **Blis-To-Sol® [OTC]** *see* Tolnaftate *on page 1347*
- ♦ **BLM** *see* Bleomycin *on page 176*
- ♦ **Blocadren®** *see* Timolol *on page 1334*
- ♦ **Bluboro® [OTC]** *see* Aluminum Sulfate and Calcium Acetate *on page 64*
- ♦ **Bonamine™ (Can)** *see* Meclizine *on page 846*
- ♦ **Bonine® [OTC]** *see* Meclizine *on page 846*

Bosentan (boe SEN tan)

U.S. Brand Names Tracleer™

Therapeutic Category Endothelin Antagonist

Use Treatment of pulmonary artery hypertension (PAH) in patients with World Health Organization (WHO) Class III or IV symptoms to improve exercise capacity and decrease the rate of clinical deterioration

Unlabeled/Investigational Use Investigational: Congestive heart failure

Restrictions Bosentan (Tracleer™) is available only through a limited distribution program directly from the manufacturer (Actelion Pharmaceuticals 1-866-228-3546). It will not be available through wholesalers or individual pharmacies.

Pregnancy Risk Factor X

Pregnancy/Breast-Feeding Implications Based on animal studies, bosentan is likely to produce major birth defects if used by pregnant women. Pregnancy must be excluded prior to initiation of therapy, and effective contraception must be maintained throughout treatment. Hormonal contraception is not recommended as the sole contraceptive therapy due to a potential lack of efficacy in patients receiving bosentan. Breast-feeding is not recommended.

Contraindications Hypersensitivity to bosentan or any component of the formulation; concurrent use of cyclosporine or glyburide; pregnancy

Warnings/Precautions Avoid use in moderate to severe hepatic impairment. Avoid use in patients with elevated serum transaminases (>3 times upper limit of normal) at baseline; dosage adjustment recommended if elevations occur during therapy. Monitor hepatic function closely (at least monthly). Treatment should be stopped in patients who develop elevated (Continued)

177

Bosentan (Continued)

transaminases (ALT or AST) in combination with symptoms of hepatic injury (unusual fatigue, jaundice, nausea, vomiting, abdominal pain, and/or fever) or elevated serum bilirubin ≥2 times upper limit of normal.

Use in pregnancy is contraindicated; exclude pregnancy prior to initiation of therapy; patients must be instructed to use effective, nonhormonal contraception throughout treatment. May cause dose-related decreases in hemoglobin and hematocrit (monitoring of hemoglobin is recommended). Safety and efficacy in pediatric patients have not been established.

Adverse Reactions
>10% :

Central nervous system: Headache (16% to 22%)

Gastrointestinal: Dyspepsia (4%)

Hematologic: Decreased hemoglobin (≥1 g/dL in up to 57%; typically in first 6 weeks of therapy)

Hepatic: Increased serum transaminases (>3 times upper limit of normal; up to 11%)

Respiratory: Nasopharyngitis (11%)

1% to 10%:

Cardiovascular: Flushing (7% to 9%), edema (lower limb, 8%; generalized 4%), hypotension (7%), palpitations (5%)

Central nervous system: Fatigue (4%)

Dermatologic: Pruritus (4%)

Hematologic: Anemia (3%)

Hepatic: Abnormal hepatic function (6% to 8%)

Overdosage/Toxicology
No specific experience in overdose. Symptoms may include headache, nausea, vomiting, and hypotension. Treatment is supportive.

Drug Interactions
Cytochrome P450 Effect: CYP2C9 and CYP3A3/4 enzyme substrate; CYP2C9 and CYP3A3/4 enzyme inducer

Increased Effect/Toxicity: Increased effect/toxicity: An increased risk of serum transaminase elevations was observed during concurrent therapy with glyburide; concurrent use is contraindicated. Cyclosporine increases serum concentrations of bosentan (approximately 3-4 times baseline). Concurrent use of cyclosporine is contraindicated. Ketoconazole may increase the serum concentrations of bosentan; concentrations are increased approximately two-fold; monitor for increased effects.

Many interactions have not been specifically evaluated, but may be extrapolated from similar interactions with inducers/inhibitors of CYP3A3/4 and CYP2C9 isoenzymes. Inhibitors of CYP2C9 or CYP3A3/4 may increase the serum concentrations of bosentan; inhibitors include amiodarone, cimetidine, clarithromycin, erythromycin, delavirdine, diltiazem, dirithromycin, disulfiram, fluoxetine, fluvoxamine, grapefruit juice, indinavir, itraconazole, ketoconazole, nefazodone, nevirapine, propoxyphene, quinupristin-dalfopristin, ritonavir, saquinavir, sulfonamides, verapamil, zafirlukast, zileuton

Decreased Effect: Decreased effect: Bosentan may enhance the metabolism of cyclosporine, decreasing its serum concentrations by ~50%; effect on sirolimus and/or tacrolimus has not been specifically evaluated, but may be similar. Concurrent use of cyclosporine is contraindicated. Bosentan may increase the metabolism of selected anticonvulsants (ethosuximide, phenytoin, tiagabine, and zonisamide), antipsychotics, atorvastatin, calcium channel blockers, corticosteroids, doxycycline, estrogens, hormonal contraceptives, lovastatin, protease inhibitors, simvastatin, and warfarin. Bosentan may enhance the metabolism of methadone resulting in methadone withdrawal.

Ethanol/Nutrition/Herb Interactions
Food: Does not affect bioavailability of bosentan.

Herb/Nutraceutical: Avoid St John's wort (may decrease serum concentrations of bosentan).

Stability
Store at 20°C to 25°C (68°F to 77°F).

Mechanism of Action
Blocks endothelin receptors on vascular endothelium and smooth muscle. Stimulation of these receptors is associated with vasoconstriction. Although bosentan blocks both ET_A and ET_B receptors, the affinity is higher for the A subtype. Improvement in symptoms of pulmonary artery hypertension and a decrease in the rate of clinical deterioration have been demonstrated in clinical trials.

Pharmacodynamics/Kinetics
Distribution: V_d: 18 L

Protein binding, plasma: >98% to albumin

Metabolism: Hepatic via CYP2C9 and 3A3/4; to three primary metabolites (one having pharmacologic activity)

Bioavailability: 50%

Half-life elimination: 5 hours (increased in heart failure, possibly in PAH)

Excretion: Feces (as metabolites); urine (<3% as unchanged drug)

Usual Dosage
Oral: Adults: Initial: 62.5 mg twice daily for 4 weeks; increase to maintenance dose of 125 mg twice daily; adults <40 kg should be maintained at 62.5 mg twice daily

Note: When discontinuing treatment, consider a reduction in dosage to 62.5 mg twice daily for 3-7 days (to avoid clinical deterioration).

Dosage adjustment in renal impairment: No dosage adjustment required.

Dosage adjustment in hepatic impairment: Avoid use in patients with **pretreatment** moderate to severe hepatic insufficiency.

Modification based on transaminase elevation:

If any elevation, regardless of degree, is accompanied by clinical symptoms of hepatic injury (unusual fatigue, nausea, vomiting, abdominal pain, fever, or jaundice) or a serum bilirubin ≥2 times the upper limit of normal, treatment should be stopped.

AST/ALT >3 times but ≤5 times upper limit of normal: Confirm with additional test; if confirmed, reduce dose or interrupt treatment. Monitor transaminase levels at least every 2 weeks. May continue or reintroduce treatment, as appropriate, following return to pretreatment values. Begin with initial dose (above) and recheck transaminases within 3 days

AST/ALT >5 times but ≤8 times upper limit of normal: Confirm with additional test; if confirmed, stop treatment. Monitor transaminase levels at least every 2 weeks. May reintroduce treatment, as appropriate, following return to pretreatment values.

AST/ALT >8 times upper limit of normal: Stop treatment.

Dietary Considerations May be taken with or without food.

Administration May be administered with or without food, once in the morning and once in the evening.

Monitoring Parameters Serum transaminase (AST and ALT) should be determined prior to the initiation of therapy and at monthly intervals thereafter. A woman of childbearing potential must have a negative pregnancy test prior to the initiation of therapy and monthly thereafter. Hemoglobin and hematocrit should be measured at baseline, at 1 month and 3 months of treatment, and every 3 months thereafter. Monitor for clinical signs and symptoms of liver injury.

Patient Information May be taken with or without food. Report unusual fatigue, nausea, vomiting, abdominal pain, and/or yellowing of the skin/eyes to prescriber immediately. Do not get pregnant while taking this medication. A woman of childbearing potential must use an effective nonhormonal method of contraception during treatment with this medication.

Dosage Forms Tablet: 62.5 mg, 125 mg

♦ **B&O Supprettes**® *see* Belladonna and Opium *on page 151*

♦ **Botox**® *see* Botulinum Toxin Type A *on page 179*

Botulinum Toxin Type A (BOT yoo lin num TOKS in type aye)

U.S. Brand Names Botox®

Canadian Brand Names Botox®

Therapeutic Category Neuromuscular Blocker Agent, Toxin; Ophthalmic Agent, Toxin

Use Treatment of strabismus and blepharospasm associated with dystonia (including benign essential blepharospasm or VII nerve disorders in patients ≥12 years of age); cervical dystonia (spasmodic torticollis) in patients ≥16 years of age

Orphan drug: Treatment of dynamic muscle contracture in pediatric cerebral palsy patients

Unlabeled/Investigational Use Treatment of oromandibular dystonia, spasmodic dysphonia (laryngeal dystonia) and other dystonias (ie, writer's cramp, focal task-specific dystonias); migraine treatment and prophylaxis; cosmetic use to decrease lines and wrinkles of the face and neck; chronic anal fissure

Pregnancy Risk Factor C (manufacturer)

Pregnancy/Breast-Feeding Implications Human reproduction studies have not been conducted. Avoid use in pregnancy.

Contraindications Hypersensitivity to albumin, botulinum toxin, or any component of the formulation; infection at the proposed injection site(s); pregnancy. Relative contraindications include diseases of neuromuscular transmission; coagulopathy including therapeutic anticoagulation; uncooperative patient

Warnings/Precautions Higher doses or more frequent administration may result in neutralizing antibody formation and loss of efficacy. Product contains albumin and may carry a remote risk of virus transmission. Use caution if there is inflammation, excessive weakness, or atrophy at the proposed injection site(s). Have appropriate support in case of anaphylactic reaction. Use with caution in patients taking aminoglycosides or other drugs that interfere which neuromuscular transmission. Ensure adequate contraception in women of childbearing years. Long-term effects of chronic therapy unknown.

Cervical dystonia: Dysphagia is common. It may be severe requiring alternative feeding methods. Risk factors include smaller neck muscle mass, bilateral injections into the sternocleidomastoid muscle or injections into the levator scapulae. Dysphasia may be associated with increased risk of upper respiratory infection.

Blepharospasm: Reduced blinking from injection of the orbicularis muscle can lead to corneal exposure and ulceration.

Strabismus: Retrobulbar hemorrhages may occur from needle penetration into orbit. Spatial disorientation, double vision, or past pointing may occur if one or more extraocular muscles are paralyzed. Covering the affected eye may help. Careful testing of corneal sensation, avoidance of lower lid injections, and treatment of epithelial defects necessary.

Adverse Reactions Adverse effects usually occur in 1 week and may last up to several months

>10% :

Central nervous system: Headache (cervical dystonia: up to 11%; can occur with other uses)

Gastrointestinal: Dysphagia (cervical dystonia: 19%)

Neuromuscular & skeletal: Neck pain (cervical dystonia: 11%)

Ocular: Ptosis (blepharospasm: 10% to 40%; strabismus: 1% to 38%), vertical deviation (strabismus: 17%)

Respiratory: Upper respiratory infection (cervical dystonia: 12%),

2% to 10%:

Central nervous system: Dizziness (cervical dystonia), speech disorder (cervical dystonia), fever (cervical dystonia), drowsiness (cervical dystonia)

Gastrointestinal: Xerostomia (cervical dystonia), nausea (cervical dystonia)

Local: Injection site reaction

Neuromuscular & skeletal: Back pain (cervical dystonia), hypertonia (cervical dystonia), weakness (cervical dystonia)

Ocular: Dry eyes (blepharospasm: 6%), superficial punctate keratitis (blepharospasm: 6%)

Respiratory: Cough (cervical dystonia), rhinitis (cervical dystonia)

Miscellaneous: Flu syndrome (cervical dystonia)

<2% (Limited to important or life-threatening): Acute angle-closure glaucoma (blepharospasm), allergic reactions, anterior segment eye ischemia (strabismus) arrhythmia, brachial plexopathy (cervical dystonia), ciliary ganglion damage (strabismus), corneal perforation (blepharospasm), diplopia (cervical dystonia, blepharospasm), dysphonia (cervical dystonia), dyspnea (cervical dystonia), ectropion (blepharospasm), entropion (Continued)

Botulinum Toxin Type A *(Continued)*

(blepharospasm), exacerbation of myasthenia gravis (blepharospasm), lagophthalmos (blepharospasm), myocardial infarction, ptosis (cervical dystonia), reduced blinking leading to corneal ulceration (blepharospasm), retrobulbar hemorrhage (strabismus), syncope (blepharospasm), vitreous hemorrhage (strabismus)

Overdosage/Toxicology Systemic weakness or muscle paralysis could occur for up to several weeks after overdose. Signs and symptoms of overdose are not apparent immediately. An antitoxin is available if there is immediate knowledge of an overdose or misinjection. Contact Allergan for additional information at (800) 433-8871 or (714) 246-5954. The antitoxin will not reverse toxin-induced muscle weakness already present.

Drug Interactions

Increased Effect/Toxicity: Aminoglycosides, neuromuscular-blocking agents

Stability Store undiluted vials in a freezer at or below -5°C (23°F). Administer within 4 hours after the vial is removed from the freezer and reconstituted. Reconstitute with sterile normal saline without a preservative. Reconstitute vials with 1 mL of diluent to get 10 units per 0.1 mL; 2 mL of diluent to get 5 units per 0.1 mL; 4 mL of diluent to get 2.5 units per 0.1 mL; 8 mL of diluent to get 1.25 units per 0.1 mL. Mix gently. After reconstitution, store in refrigerator (2°C to 8°C) and use within 4 hours (does not contain preservative). Do not freeze.

Mechanism of Action Botulinum A toxin is a neurotoxin produced by *Clostridium botulinum*, spore-forming anaerobic bacillus, which appears to affect only the presynaptic membrane of the neuromuscular junction in humans, where it prevents calcium-dependent release of acetylcholine and produces a state of denervation. Muscle inactivation persists until new fibrils grow from the nerve and form junction plates on new areas of the muscle-cell walls.

Pharmacodynamics/Kinetics

Onset of action (improvement):
Blepharospasm: ~3 days
Cervical dystonia: ~2 weeks
Strabismus: ~1-2 days

Duration:
Blepharospasm: ~3 months
Cervical dystonia: <3 months
Strabismus: ~2-6 weeks

Absorption: Not expected to be present in peripheral blood at recommended doses

Time to peak:
Blepharospasm: 1-2 weeks
Cervical dystonia: ~6 weeks
Strabismus: Within first week

Usual Dosage I.M.:

Children ≥16 years and Adults: Cervical dystonia: For dosing guidance, the mean dose is 236 units (25th to 75th percentile range 198-300 units) divided among the affected muscles in patients previously treated with botulinum toxin. Initial dose in previously untreated patients should be lower. Sequential dosing should be based on the patient's head and neck position, localization of pain, muscle hypertrophy, patient response, and previous adverse reactions. The total dose injected into the sternocleidomastoid muscles should be ≤100 units to decrease the occurrence of dysphagia.

Children ≥12 years and Adults:

Blepharospasm: Initial dose: 1.25-2.5 units injected into the medial and lateral pretarsal orbicularis oculi of the upper and lower lid; dose may be increased up to twice the previous dose if the response from the initial dose lasted ≤2 months; maximum dose per site: 5 units; cumulative dose in a 30-day period: ≤200 units. Tolerance may occur if treatments are given more often than every 3 months, but the effect is not usually permanent.

Strabismus:

Initial dose:

Vertical muscles and for horizontal strabismus <20 prism diopters: 1.25-2.5 units in any one muscle

Horizontal strabismus of 20-50 prism diopters: 2.5-5 units in any one muscle

Persistent VI nerve palsy >1 month: 1.5-2.5 units in the medial rectus muscle

Re-examine patients 7-14 days after each injection to assess the effect of that dose. Subsequent doses for patients experiencing incomplete paralysis of the target may be increased up to twice the previous administered dose. The maximum recommended dose as a single injection for any one muscle is 25 units. Do not administer subsequent injections until the effects of the previous dose are gone.

Elderly: No specific adjustment recommended

Dosage adjustment in renal impairment: No specific adjustment recommended

Dosage adjustment in hepatic impairment: No specific adjustment recommended

Administration

Cervical dystonia: Use 25-, 27-, or 30-gauge needle for superficial muscles and a longer 22-gauge needle for deeper musculature; electromyography may help localize the involved muscles

Blepharospasm: Use a 27- or 30-gauge needle without electromyography guidance. Avoid injecting near the levator palpebrae superioris (may decrease ptosis); avoid medial lower lid injections (may decrease diplopia). Apply pressure at the injection site to prevent ecchymosis in the soft eyelid tissues.

Strabismus injections: Must use surgical exposure or electromyographic guidance; use the electrical activity recorded from the tip of the injections needle as a guide to placement within the target muscle. Local anesthetic and ocular decongestant should be given before injection. The volume of injection should be 0.05-0.15 mL per muscle. Many patients will require additional doses because of inadequate response to initial dose.

Patient Information This medicine is given in a clinic or hospital setting by a prescriber. It is given as an injection. It is not a cure, but may be given on a periodic basis to help with spasms. Tell your prescriber if you have any nerve diseases or any infections where the shot might be given. Patients with blepharospasm may not have been very active. Start activity slowly and increase as you see how you feel. Call prescriber as soon as possible if you have trouble swallowing, speaking, or breathing. May have double vision or other problems where covering the eye with a patch may help.

Nursing Implications To alleviate spatial disorientation or double vision in strabismic patients, cover the affected eye; have epinephrine ready for hypersensitivity reactions

Additional Information Units of biological activity of Botox® cannot be compared with units of any other botulinum toxin.

Dosage Forms Injection, powder for reconstitution: 100 units *Clostridium botulinum* toxin type A

Botulinum Toxin Type B (BOT yoo lin num TOKS in type bee)

U.S. Brand Names Myobloc®

Therapeutic Category Neuromuscular Blocker Agent, Toxin

Use Treatment of cervical dystonia (spasmodic torticollis)

Unlabeled/Investigational Use Treatment of cervical dystonia in patients who have developed resistance to botulinum toxin type A

Pregnancy Risk Factor C (manufacturer)

Pregnancy/Breast-Feeding Implications Neither animal or human reproduction studies have been conducted. Avoid use in pregnancy. Excretion into breast milk unknown/not recommended.

Contraindications Hypersensitivity to albumin, botulinum toxin, or any component of the formulation; infection at the injection site(s); pregnancy; coadministration of agents known to potentiate neuromuscular blockade. Relative contraindications include diseases of neuromuscular transmission; coagulopathy, including therapeutic anticoagulation; inability of patient to cooperate.

Warnings/Precautions Higher doses or more frequent administration may result in neutralizing antibody formation and loss of efficacy. Product contains albumin and may carry a remote risk of virus transmission. Use caution if there is inflammation, excessive weakness, or atrophy at the proposed injection site(s). Concurrent use of botulinum toxin type A or within <4 months of type B is not recommended. Have appropriate support in case of anaphylactic reaction. Use with caution in patients taking aminoglycosides or other drugs that interfere with neuromuscular transmission. Ensure adequate contraception in women of childbearing years. Long-term effects of chronic therapy unknown. Increased risk of dysphagia and respiratory complications. Safety and efficacy in children have not been established.

Adverse Reactions

>10%:
  Central nervous system: Headache (10% to 16%), pain (6% to 13%; placebo 10%)
  Gastrointestinal: Dysphagia (10% to 25%), xerostomia (3% to 34%)
  Local: Injection site pain (12% to 16%)
  Neuromuscular & skeletal: Neck pain (up to 17%; placebo: 16%)
  Miscellaneous: Infection (13% to 19%; placebo: 15%)

1% to 10%:
  Cardiovascular: Chest pain, vasodilation, peripheral edema
  Central nervous system: Dizziness (3% to 6%), fever, malaise, migraine, anxiety, tremor, hyperesthesia, somnolence, confusion, vertigo
  Dermatologic: Pruritus, bruising
  Gastrointestinal: Nausea (3% to 10%; placebo: 5%), dyspepsia (up to 10%; placebo: 5%), vomiting, stomatitis, taste perversion
  Genitourinary: Urinary tract infection, cystitis, vaginal moniliasis
  Hematologic: Serum neutralizing activity
  Neuromuscular & skeletal: Torticollis (up to 8%; placebo: 7%), arthralgia (up to 7%; placebo: 5%), back pain (up to 7%; placebo: 3%), myasthenia (3% to 6%; placebo: 3%), weakness (up to 6%; placebo: 4%), arthritis
  Ocular: Amblyopia, abnormal vision
  Otic: Otitis media, tinnitus
  Respiratory: Cough (3% to 7%; placebo: 3%), rhinitis (1% to 5%; placebo: 6%), dyspnea, pneumonia
  Miscellaneous: Flu-syndrome (6% to 9%), allergic reaction, viral infection, abscess, cyst

Overdosage/Toxicology Systemic weakness or muscle paralysis could occur for up to several weeks after overdose. Signs and symptoms of overdose are not apparent immediately. An antitoxin is available if there is immediate knowledge of an overdose or misinjection. Contact Elan Pharmaceuticals for additional information at (888) 638-7605 and your State Health Department to process a request for antitoxin through the CDC. The antitoxin will not reverse toxin-induced muscle weakness already present.

Drug Interactions

Increased Effect/Toxicity: Aminoglycosides, neuromuscular-blocking agents, botulinum toxin type A, other agents which may block neuromuscular transmission

Stability Store vials under refrigeration at 2°C to 8°C (36°F to 46°F) for up to 21 months. May be diluted with normal saline; once diluted, use within 4 hours. Does not contain preservative. Single-use vial. Do not shake; do not freeze. Do not mix with any other medicines.

Mechanism of Action Botulinum B toxin is a neurotoxin produced by *Clostridium botulinum*, spore-forming anaerobic bacillus. It cleaves synaptic Vesicle Association Membrane Protein (VAMP; synaptobrevin) which is a component of the protein complex responsible for docking and fusion of the synaptic vesicle to the presynaptic membrane. By blocking neurotransmitter release, botulinum B toxin paralyzes the muscle.

Pharmacodynamics/Kinetics

Duration: 12-16 weeks
Absorption: Not expected to be present in peripheral blood at recommended doses

Usual Dosage

Children: Not established in pediatric patients
Adults: Cervical dystonia: I.M.: Initial: 2500-5000 units divided among the affected muscles in patients **previously treated** with botulinum toxin; initial dose in **previously untreated** patients should be lower. Subsequent dosing should be optimized according to patient's response.

(Continued)

Botulinum Toxin Type B *(Continued)*

Elderly: No dosage adjustments required, but limited experience in patients ≥75 years old

Dosage adjustment in renal impairment: No specific adjustment recommended

Dosage adjustment in hepatic impairment: No specific adjustment recommended

Patient Information This medicine is given in a clinic or hospital setting by a prescriber. It is given as an injection. It is not a cure, but may be given on a periodic basis to help with spasms. Tell your prescriber if you have any nerve diseases or any infections where the injection might be given. Call your prescriber as soon as possible if you have trouble swallowing, speaking, breathing, or any muscle weakness.

Additional Information Units of biological activity of Myobloc® cannot be compared with units of any other botulinum toxin.

Dosage Forms Injection, solution [single-dose vial]: 5000 units/mL (0.5 mL, 1 mL, 2 mL) [contains albumin 0.05%]

Botulinum Toxoid, Pentavalent Vaccine (Against Types A, B, C, D, and E Strains of *C. botulinum*)

(BOT yoo lin num pen ta VAY lent [aye, bee, cee, dee, ee] TOKS oyd)

Synonyms Botulinum Toxoid, Pentavalent Vaccine (Against Types A / B / C / D / E Strains of *C. botulinum*)

Therapeutic Category Toxoid

Unlabeled/Investigational Use Investigational: Prophylaxis of botulism in personnel working with *C. botulinum* cultures

Additional Information Complete prescribing information for this medication should be consulted for additional detail.

♦ **Botulinum Toxoid, Pentavalent Vaccine (Against Types A / B / C / D / E Strains of *C. botulinum*)** *see* Botulinum Toxoid, Pentavalent Vaccine (Against Types A, B, C, D, and E Strains of *C. botulinum*) *on page 182*

♦ **Bovine Lung Surfactant** *see* Beractant *on page 160*

♦ **Breast-Feeding and Drugs** *see page 1709*

♦ **Breathe Free® [OTC]** *see* Sodium Chloride *on page 1245*

♦ **Breathe Right® Saline [OTC]** *see* Sodium Chloride *on page 1245*

♦ **Breonesin® [OTC]** *see* Guaifenesin *on page 645*

♦ **Brethaire® [DSC]** *see* Terbutaline *on page 1300*

♦ **Brethine®** *see* Terbutaline *on page 1300*

Bretylium (bre TIL ee um)

Related Information

Adult ACLS Algorithms *on page 1632*

Antiarrhythmic Drugs Comparison *on page 1478*

Pediatric ALS Algorithms *on page 1628*

Synonyms Bretylium Tosylate

Therapeutic Category Antiarrhythmic Agent, Class III

Use Treatment of ventricular tachycardia and fibrillation; treatment of other serious ventricular arrhythmias resistant to lidocaine

Pregnancy Risk Factor C

Contraindications Hypersensitivity to bretylium or any component of the formulation; severe aortic stenosis; severe pulmonary hypertension

Warnings/Precautions Hypotension occurs frequently. Keep patients supine until tolerance develops. Patients with fixed cardiac output (severe pulmonary hypertension or aortic stenosis) may experience severe hypotension due to decrease in peripheral resistance without ability to increase cardiac output. Reduce dose in renal failure patients. May have prolonged half-life in the elderly. Transient hypertension and increased frequency of arrhythmias may occur initially. Rapid I.V. injection may result in transient blood pressure changes, nausea, and vomiting. Use only in areas where there is equipment and staff familiar with management of life-threatening arrhythmias. Use continuous cardiac and blood pressure monitoring. Keep patients supine (postural hypotension common). Adjust dose in patients with impaired renal function. Give to a pregnant woman only if clearly needed.

Adverse Reactions

>10%: Cardiovascular: Hypotension (both postural and supine)

1% to 10%: Gastrointestinal: Nausea, vomiting

<1% (Limited to important or life-threatening): Bradycardia, chest pain, dyspnea, flushing, increase in premature ventricular contractions (PVCs), nasal congestion, postural hypotension, renal impairment, respiratory depression, syncope, transient initial hypertension

Overdosage/Toxicology Symptoms include significant hypertension followed by severe hypotension due to inhibition of catecholamine release. After GI decontamination, supportive treatment is required. **Note:** Quinidine and other type Ia should not be used to treat cardiotoxicity caused by bretylium. Continuously monitor vital signs and EKG for a minimum of 6 hours after exposure and admit the patient for 24 hours of intensive monitoring if there is evidence of toxicity. Dialysis and hemoperfusion are unlikely to assist.

Drug Interactions

Increased Effect/Toxicity: Other antiarrhythmic agents may potentiate or antagonize cardiac effects of bretylium. Toxic effects may be additive. The vasopressor effects of catecholamines may be enhanced by bretylium. Toxicity of agents which may prolong QT interval (including cisapride, tricyclic antidepressants, antipsychotics, erythromycin, Class Ia and Class III antiarrhythmics) and specific quinolones (sparfloxacin, gatifloxacin, moxifloxacin) may be increased. Digoxin toxicity may be aggravated by bretylium.

Stability Standard diluent: 2 g/250 mL D₅W; the premix infusion should be stored at room temperature and protected from freezing

Mechanism of Action Class III antiarrhythmic; after an initial release of norepinephrine at the peripheral adrenergic nerve terminals, inhibits further release by postganglionic nerve endings in response to sympathetic nerve stimulation

Pharmacodynamics/Kinetics
Onset of action: I.M.: May require 2 hours; I.V.: 6-20 minutes
Peak effect: 6-9 hours
Duration: 6-24 hours
Protein binding: 1% to 6%
Metabolism: None
Half-life elimination: 7-11 hours; Mean: 4-17 hours; End-stage renal disease: 16-32 hours
Excretion: Urine (70% to 80% as unchanged drug) within 24 hours

Usual Dosage Note: Patients should undergo defibrillation/cardioversion before and after bretylium doses as necessary.
Children (**Note:** Not well established, although the following dosing has been suggested):
I.M.: 2-5 mg/kg as a single dose
I.V.: Acute ventricular fibrillation: Initial: 5 mg/kg, then attempt electrical defibrillation; repeat with 10 mg/kg if ventricular fibrillation persists at 15- to 30-minute intervals to maximum total of 30 mg/kg.
Maintenance dose: I.M., I.V.: 5 mg/kg every 6 hours
Adults:
Immediate life-threatening ventricular arrhythmias (ventricular fibrillation, unstable ventricular tachycardia): Initial dose: I.V.: 5 mg/kg (undiluted) over 1 minute; if arrhythmia persists, administer 10 mg/kg (undiluted) over 1 minute and repeat as necessary (usually at 15- to 30-minute intervals) up to a total dose of 30-35 mg/kg.
Other life-threatening ventricular arrhythmias:
Initial dose: I.M., I.V.: 5-10 mg/kg, may repeat every 1-2 hours if arrhythmia persists; administer I.V. dose (diluted) over 8-10 minutes.
Maintenance dose: I.M.: 5-10 mg/kg every 6-8 hours; I.V. (diluted): 5-10 mg/kg every 6 hours; I.V. infusion (diluted): 1-2 mg/minute (little experience with doses >40 mg/kg/day)
Example dilution: 2 g/250 mL D_5W (infusion pump should be used for I.V. infusion administration)
Rate of I.V. infusion: 1-4 mg/minute
1 mg/minute = 7 mL/hour
2 mg/minute = 15 mL/hour
3 mg/minute = 22 mL/hour
4 mg/minute = 30 mL/hour

Dosing adjustment in renal impairment:
Cl_{cr} 10-50 mL/minute: Administer 25% to 50% of dose.
Cl_{cr} <10 mL/minute: Administer 25% of dose.
Dialysis: Not dialyzable (0% to 5%) via hemo- or peritoneal dialysis; supplemental doses are not needed.

Administration I.M. injection in adults should not exceed 5 mL volume in any one site
Monitoring Parameters EKG, heart rate, blood pressure; requires a cardiac monitor
Patient Information Anticipate vomiting
Nursing Implications Monitor EKG and blood pressure throughout therapy; onset of action may be delayed 15-30 minutes; rapid infusion may result in nausea and vomiting
Dosage Forms
Injection, solution, as tosylate: 50 mg/mL (10 mL)
Injection, solution, as tosylate [premixed in D_5W]: 2 mg/mL (250 mL); 4 mg/mL (250 mL)

♦ **Bretylium Tosylate** see Bretylium on page 182
♦ **Brevibloc®** see Esmolol on page 488
♦ **Brevicon®** see Ethinyl Estradiol and Norethindrone on page 522
♦ **Brevicon® 0.5/35 (Can)** see Ethinyl Estradiol and Norethindrone on page 522
♦ **Brevicon® 1/35 (Can)** see Ethinyl Estradiol and Norethindrone on page 522
♦ **Brevital® (Can)** see Methohexital on page 884
♦ **Brevital® Sodium** see Methohexital on page 884
♦ **Bricanyl® [DSC]** see Terbutaline on page 1300
♦ **Brietal Sodium® (Can)** see Methohexital on page 884

Brimonidine (bri MOE ni deen)

Related Information
Antacid Drug Interactions on page 1477
Glaucoma Drug Therapy Comparison on page 1499
U.S. Brand Names Alphagan®; Alphagan® P
Canadian Brand Names Alphagan™
Synonyms Brimonidine Tartrate
Therapeutic Category Alpha$_2$-Adrenergic Agonist Agent, Ophthalmic; Sympathomimetic
Use Lowering of intraocular pressure (IOP) in patients with open-angle glaucoma or ocular hypertension
Pregnancy Risk Factor B
Usual Dosage Ophthalmic: Children ≥2 years of age and Adults: Glaucoma (Alphagan®, Alphagan® P): Instill 1 drop in affected eye(s) 3 times/day (approximately every 8 hours)
Additional Information Complete prescribing information for this medication should be consulted for additional detail.
Dosage Forms Solution, ophthalmic, as tartrate:
Alphagan®: 0.2% (5 mL, 10 mL, 15 mL) [contains benzalkonium chloride]
Alphagan® P: 0.15% (5 mL, 10 mL, 15 mL) [contains Purite® 0.005% as preservative]

♦ **Brimonidine Tartrate** see Brimonidine on page 183

Brinzolamide (brin ZOH la mide)
Related Information
  Glaucoma Drug Therapy Comparison *on page 1499*
U.S. Brand Names Azopt®
Canadian Brand Names Azopt™
Therapeutic Category Carbonic Anhydrase Inhibitor
Use Lowers intraocular pressure to treat glaucoma in patients with ocular hypertension or open-angle glaucoma
Pregnancy Risk Factor C
Usual Dosage Adults: Ophthalmic: Instill 1 drop in affected eye(s) 3 times/day
Additional Information Complete prescribing information for this medication should be consulted for additional detail.
Dosage Forms Suspension, ophthalmic: 1% (5 mL, 10 mL, 15 mL) [contains benzalkonium chloride]

◆ **British Anti-Lewisite** *see* Dimercaprol *on page 412*
◆ **Brodspec®** *see* Tetracycline *on page 1306*
◆ **Brofed® [OTC]** *see* Brompheniramine and Pseudoephedrine *on page 185*
◆ **Bromanate® [OTC]** *see* Brompheniramine and Pseudoephedrine *on page 185*
◆ **Bromfed® [OTC]** *see* Brompheniramine and Pseudoephedrine *on page 185*
◆ **Bromfed-PD® [OTC]** *see* Brompheniramine and Pseudoephedrine *on page 185*
◆ **Bromfenex®** *see* Brompheniramine and Pseudoephedrine *on page 185*
◆ **Bromfenex® PD** *see* Brompheniramine and Pseudoephedrine *on page 185*

Bromocriptine (broe moe KRIP teen)
Related Information
  Parkinson's Agents *on page 1513*
U.S. Brand Names Parlodel®
Canadian Brand Names Apo® Bromocriptine; Parlodel®; PMS-Bromocriptine
Synonyms Bromocriptine Mesylate
Therapeutic Category Anti-Parkinson's Agent, Dopamine Agonist; Dopaminergic Agent (Antiparkinson's); Ergot Alkaloid and Derivative
Use
  Amenorrhea with or without galactorrhea; infertility or hypogonadism; prolactin-secreting adenomas; acromegaly; Parkinson's disease
  A previous indication for prevention of postpartum lactation was withdrawn voluntarily by Sandoz Pharmaceuticals Corporation
Unlabeled/Investigational Use Neuroleptic malignant syndrome
Pregnancy Risk Factor B
Contraindications Hypersensitivity to bromocriptine, ergot alkaloids, or any component of the formulation; uncontrolled hypertension; severe ischemic heart disease or peripheral vascular disorders; pregnancy (risk to benefit evaluation must be performed in women who become pregnant during treatment for acromegaly, prolactinoma, or Parkinson's disease - hypertension during treatment should generally result in efforts to withdraw)
Warnings/Precautions Use with caution in patients with impaired renal or hepatic function, a history of psychosis, or cardiovascular disease (myocardial infarction, arrhythmia). Patients who receive bromocriptine during and immediately following pregnancy as a continuation of previous therapy (ie, acromegaly) should be closely monitored for cardiovascular effects. Discontinuation of bromocriptine in patients with macroadenomas has been associated with rapid regrowth of tumor and increased prolactin serum levels. Use with caution in patients with a history of peptic ulcer disease, dementia, or concurrent antihypertensive therapy. Safety and effectiveness in patients <15 years of age have not been established.
Adverse Reactions
  >10%:
    Central nervous system: Headache, dizziness
    Gastrointestinal: Nausea
  1% to 10%:
    Cardiovascular: Orthostatic hypotension
    Central nervous system: Fatigue, lightheadedness, drowsiness
    Gastrointestinal: Anorexia, vomiting, abdominal cramps, constipation
    Respiratory: Nasal congestion
  <1% (Limited to important or life-threatening): Arrhythmias, hair loss, insomnia, paranoia, visual hallucinations
Overdosage/Toxicology Symptoms include nausea, vomiting, and hypotension. Hypotension, when unresponsive to I.V. fluids or Trendelenburg positioning, often responds to norepinephrine infusions started at 0.1-0.2 mcg/kg/minute followed by a titrated infusion.
Drug Interactions
  Cytochrome P450 Effect: CYP3A3/4 enzyme substrate
  Increased Effect/Toxicity: Isometheptene and phenylpropanolamine (and other sympathomimetics) should be avoided in patients receiving bromocriptine - may increase risk of hypertension and seizure. Erythromycin, fluvoxamine, and nefazodone may increase bromocriptine concentrations.
  Decreased Effect: Antipsychotics may inhibit bromocriptine's ability to lower prolactin.
Ethanol/Nutrition/Herb Interactions
  Ethanol: Avoid ethanol (may increase GI side effects or ethanol intolerance).
  Herb/Nutraceutical: St John's wort may decrease bromocriptine levels.
Mechanism of Action Semisynthetic ergot alkaloid derivative and a dopamine receptor agonist which activates postsynaptic dopamine receptors in the tuberoinfundibular and nigrostriatal pathways
Pharmacodynamics/Kinetics
  Protein binding: 90% to 96%
  Metabolism: Majority hepatic

Half-life elimination: Biphasic: Initial: 6-8 hours; Terminal: 50 hours

Time to peak, serum: 1-2 hours

Excretion: Feces; urine (2% to 6% as unchanged drug)

Usual Dosage Adults: Oral:

Parkinsonism: 1.25 mg 2 times/day, increased by 2.5 mg/day in 2- to 4-week intervals (usual dose range is 30-90 mg/day in 3 divided doses), though elderly patients can usually be managed on lower doses

Neuroleptic malignant syndrome: 2.5-5 mg 3 times/day

Hyperprolactinemia: 2.5 mg 2-3 times/day

Acromegaly: Initial: 1.25-2.5 mg increasing as necessary every 3-7 days; usual dose: 20-30 mg/day

Prolactin-secreting adenomas: Initial: 1.25-2.5 mg/day; daily range 2.5-10 mg.

Dosing adjustment in hepatic impairment: No guidelines are available, however, may be necessary

Dietary Considerations May be taken with food to decrease GI distress.

Monitoring Parameters Monitor blood pressure closely as well as hepatic, hematopoietic, and cardiovascular function

Patient Information Take with food or milk; drowsiness commonly occurs upon initiation of therapy; limit use of alcohol; avoid exposure to cold; incidence of side effects is high (68%) with nausea the most common; hypotension occurs commonly with initiation of therapy, usually upon rising after prolonged sitting or lying

Discontinue immediately if pregnant; may restore fertility; women desiring not to become pregnant should use mechanical contraceptive means

Nursing Implications Raise bed rails and institute safety measures; aid patient with ambulation; may cause postural hypotension and drowsiness

Additional Information Usually used with levodopa or levodopa/carbidopa to treat Parkinson's disease. When adding bromocriptine, the dose of levodopa/carbidopa can usually be decreased.

Dosage Forms

Capsule, as mesylate: 5 mg

Tablet, as mesylate: 2.5 mg

♦ **Bromocriptine Mesylate** *see* Bromocriptine *on page 184*

Brompheniramine and Pseudoephedrine

(brome fen IR a meen & soo doe e FED rin)

U.S. Brand Names Andehist NR Syrup; Brofed® [OTC]; Bromanate® [OTC]; Bromfed® [OTC]; Bromfed-PD® [OTC]; Bromfenex®; Bromfenex® PD; Children's Dimetapp® Elixir Cold & Allergy [OTC]; Iofed®; Iofed® PD

Synonyms Pseudoephedrine and Brompheniramine

Therapeutic Category Antihistamine/Decongestant Combination

Use Temporary relief of symptoms of seasonal and perennial allergic rhinitis, and vasomotor rhinitis, including nasal obstruction

Pregnancy Risk Factor C

Usual Dosage Oral:

Capsule, sustained release:

Based on 60 mg pseudoephedrine:

Children 6-12 years: 1 capsule every 12 hours

Children ≥12 years and Adults: 1-2 capsules every 12 hours

Based on 120 mg pseudoephedrine: Children ≥12 years and Adults: 1 capsule every 12 hours

Elixir: Children >12 years and Adults:

Brompheniramine 2 mg/pseudoephedrine 30 mg per 5 mL: 10 mL every 4-6 hours, up to 40 mL/day

Brompheniramine 4 mg/pseudoephedrine 30 mg per 5 mL: 10 mL 3 times/day

Tablet: Based on 60 mg pseudoephedrine: Children >12 years and Adults: 1 tablet every 4 hours

Additional Information Complete prescribing information for this medication should be consulted for additional detail.

Dosage Forms

Capsule, extended release:

Bromfed®, Bromfenex®, Iofed®: Brompheniramine maleate 12 mg and pseudoephedrine hydrochloride 120 mg

Bromfed-PD®, Bromfenex® PD, Iofed® PD: Brompheniramine maleate 6 mg and pseudoephedrine hydrochloride 60 mg

Elixir:

Brofed®: Brompheniramine maleate 4 mg and pseudoephedrine hydrochloride 30 mg per 5 mL (480 mL)

Bromanate®: Brompheniramine maleate 1 mg and pseudoephedrine sulfate 15 mg per 5 mL (120 mL, 240 mL, 480 mL) [alcohol free; grape flavor]

Children's Dimetapp® Elixir Cold & Allergy: Brompheniramine maleate 1 mg and pseudoephedrine hydrochloride 15 mg per 5 mL (240 mL) [alcohol free; sugar free; grape flavor]

Syrup (Andehist NR): Brompheniramine maleate 4 mg and pseudoephedrine sulfate 45 mg per 5 mL (473 mL) [raspberry flavor]

Tablet (Bromfed®): Brompheniramine maleate 4 mg and pseudoephedrine hydrochloride 60 mg

♦ **Brompheril® [OTC]** *see* Dexbrompheniramine and Pseudoephedrine *on page 383*

♦ **Bronchial®** *see* Theophylline and Guaifenesin *on page 1310*

♦ **Bronchodilators, Comparison of Inhaled Sympathomimetics** *see page 1493*

♦ **Broncho Saline®** *see* Sodium Chloride *on page 1245*

♦ **Bronitin®** *see* Epinephrine *on page 470*

♦ **Bronkodyl®** *see* Theophylline Salts *on page 1310*

♦ **Bronkometer®** *see* Isoetharine *on page 747*

- **Bronkosol®** *see Isoetharine on page 747*
- **Brontex® Liquid** *see Guaifenesin and Codeine on page 646*
- **Brontex® Tablet** *see Guaifenesin and Codeine on page 646*
- **B-type Natriuretic Peptide (Human)** *see Nesiritide on page 971*

Budesonide (byoo DES oh nide)

Related Information
Asthma *on page 1645*
Estimated Clinical Comparability of Doses for Inhaled Corticosteroids *on page 1652*

U.S. Brand Names Entocort™ EC; Pulmicort Respules®; Pulmicort Turbuhaler®; Rhinocort®; Rhinocort® Aqua™

Canadian Brand Names Entocort®; Gen-Budesonide AQ; Pulmicort®; Rhinocort® Turbuhaler®

Therapeutic Category Corticosteroid, Inhalant; Corticosteroid, Intranasal; Corticosteroid, Topical (Medium Potency)

Use
Intranasal: Children ≥6 years of age and Adults: Management of symptoms of seasonal or perennial rhinitis

Nebulization: Children 12 months to 8 years: Maintenance and prophylactic treatment of asthma

Oral capsule: Treatment of active Crohn's disease (mild to moderate) involving the ileum and/or ascending colon

Oral inhalation: Maintenance and prophylactic treatment of asthma; includes patients who require corticosteroids and those who may benefit from systemic dose reduction/elimination

Pregnancy Risk Factor C/B (Pulmicort Turbuhaler®)

Pregnancy/Breast-Feeding Implications No adequate or well-controlled studies in pregnant women; use only if potential benefit to the mother outweighs the possible risk to the fetus. Hypoadrenalism has been reported in infants.

Contraindications Hypersensitivity to budesonide or any component of the formulation
Inhalation: Contraindicated in primary treatment of status asthmaticus, acute episodes of asthma; not for relief of acute bronchospasm

Warnings/Precautions May cause hypercorticism and/or suppression of hypothalamic-pituitary-adrenal (HPA) axis, particularly in younger children or in patients receiving high doses for prolonged periods. Particular care is required when patients are transferred from systemic corticosteroids to products with lower systemic bioavailability (ie, inhalation). May lead to possible adrenal insufficiency or withdrawal from steroids, including an increase in allergic symptoms. Patients receiving prolonged therapy of ≥20 mg per day of prednisone (or equivalent) may be most susceptible. Aerosol steroids do **not** provide the systemic steroid needed to treat patients having trauma, surgery, or infections.

Controlled clinical studies have shown that orally-inhaled and intranasal corticosteroids may cause a reduction in growth velocity in pediatric patients. (In studies of orally-inhaled corticosteroids, the mean reduction in growth velocity was approximately 1 centimeter per year [range 0.3-1.8 cm per year] and appears to be related to dose and duration of exposure.) To minimize the systemic effects of orally-inhaled and intranasal corticosteroids, each patient should be titrated to the lowest effective dose. Growth should be routinely monitored in pediatric patients.

May suppress the immune system, patients may be more susceptible to infection. Use with caution in patients with systemic infections or ocular herpes simplex. Avoid exposure to chickenpox and measles. Corticosteroids should be used with caution in patients with diabetes, hypertension, osteoporosis, peptic ulcer, glaucoma, cataracts, or tuberculosis. Use caution in hepatic impairment. Enteric-coated capsules should not be crushed or chewed.

Adverse Reactions Reaction severity varies by dose and duration; not all adverse reactions have been reported with each dosage form.

>10%:
  Central nervous system: Oral capsule: Headache (up to 21%)
  Gastrointestinal: Oral capsule: Nausea (up to 11%)
  Respiratory: Respiratory infection, rhinitis
  Miscellaneous: Symptoms of HPA axis suppression and/or hypercorticism (acne, easy bruising, fat redistribution, striae, edema) may occur in >10% of patients following administration of dosage forms which result in higher systemic exposure (ie, oral, inhalation), but may be less frequent than rates observed with comparator drugs (prednisolone). These symptoms may be rare (<1%) following administration via methods which result in lower exposures (topical).

1% to 10%:
  Cardiovascular: Syncope, edema, hypertension
  Central nervous system: Chest pain, dysphonia, emotional lability, fatigue, fever, insomnia, migraine, nervousness, pain, dizziness, vertigo
  Dermatologic: Bruising, contact dermatitis, eczema, pruritus, pustular rash, rash
  Endocrine & metabolic: Hypokalemia, adrenal insufficiency
  Gastrointestinal: Abdominal pain, anorexia, diarrhea, dry mouth, dyspepsia, gastroenteritis, oral candidiasis, taste perversion, vomiting, weight gain, flatulence
  Hematologic: Cervical lymphadenopathy, purpura, leukocytosis
  Neuromuscular & skeletal: Arthralgia, fracture, hyperkinesis, hypertonia, myalgia, neck pain, weakness, paresthesia, back pain
  Ocular: Conjunctivitis, eye infection
  Otic: Earache, ear infection, external ear infection
  Respiratory: Bronchitis, bronchospasm, cough, epistaxis, nasal irritation, pharyngitis, sinusitis, stridor
  Miscellaneous: Allergic reaction, flu-like syndrome, herpes simplex, infection, moniliasis, viral infection, voice alteration

<1% (Limited to important or life-threatening): Aggressive reactions, alopecia, angioedema, avascular necrosis of the femoral head, benign intracranial hypertension, depression, dyspnea, growth suppression, hoarseness, hypersensitivity reactions (immediate and delayed; include rash, contact dermatitis, angioedema, bronchospasm), intermenstrual bleeding, irritability, nasal septum perforation, osteoporosis, psychosis, somnolence

Overdosage/Toxicology Symptoms of overdose with inhaled formulations include irritation and burning of the nasal mucosa, sneezing, intranasal and pharyngeal *Candida* infections, nasal ulceration, epistaxis, rhinorrhea, nasal stuffiness, and headache. When consumed in excessive quantities, systemic hypercorticism and adrenal suppression may occur; in those cases, discontinuation and withdrawal of the corticosteroid should be done judiciously. Treatment should be symptomatic and supportive.

Drug Interactions
Cytochrome P450 Effect: CYP3A3/4 enzyme substrate
Increased Effect/Toxicity: Cimetidine may decrease the clearance and increase the bioavailability of budesonide, increasing its serum concentrations. In addition, CYP3A3/4 inhibitors may increase the serum level and/or toxicity of budesonide this effect was shown with ketoconazole, but not erythromycin. Other potential inhibitors include amiodarone, cimetidine, clarithromycin, delavirdine, diltiazem, dirithromycin, disulfiram, fluoxetine, fluvoxamine, grapefruit juice, indinavir, itraconazole, ketoconazole, nefazodone, nevirapine, propoxyphene, quinupristin-dalfopristin, ritonavir, saquinavir, verapamil, zafirlukast, zileuton. The addition of salmeterol has been demonstrated to improve response to inhaled corticosteroids (as compared to increasing steroid dosage).

Decreased Effect: CYP3A3/4 inducers (including carbamazepine, phenytoin, phenobarbital, rifampin) may decrease budesonide levels and/or effects. Theoretically, proton pump inhibitors (omeprazole, pantoprazole) alter gastric pH may affect the rate of dissolution of enteric-coated capsules. Administration with omeprazole did not alter kinetics of budesonide capsules.

Ethanol/Nutrition/Herb Interactions
Food: Grapefruit juice may double systemic exposure of orally-administered budesonide. Administration of capsules with a high-fat meal delays peak concentration, but does not alter the extent of absorption.

Herb/Nutraceutical: St John's wort may decrease budesonide levels.

Stability
Nebulizer: Store upright at 20°C to 25°C (68°F to 77°F) and protect from light. Do not refrigerate or freeze. Once aluminum package is opened, solution should be used within 2 weeks. Continue to protect from light.

Nasal inhaler: Store with valve up at 15°C to 30°C (59°F to 86°F). Use within 6 months after opening aluminum pouch. Protect from high humidity.

Nasal spray: Store with valve up at 20°C to 25°C (68°F to 77°F) and protect from light. Do not freeze.

Mechanism of Action Controls the rate of protein synthesis, depresses the migration of polymorphonuclear leukocytes, fibroblasts, reverses capillary permeability, and lysosomal stabilization at the cellular level to prevent or control inflammation

Pharmacodynamics/Kinetics
Onset of action: Respules™: 2-8 days; Rhinocort® Aqua™: ~10 hours; Turbuhaler®: 24 hours
Peak effect: Respules™: 4-6 weeks; Rhinocort® Aqua™: ~2 weeks; Turbuhaler®: 1-2 weeks

Absorption: Capsule: Rapid and complete

Distribution: 2.2-3.9 L/kg

Protein binding: 85% to 90%

Metabolism: Hepatic via CYP3A3/4 to two metabolites (16 alpha-hydroxyprednisolone and 6 beta-hydroxybudesonide; minor activity)

Bioavailability: Limited by high first-pass effect; Capsule: 9% to 21%; Respules™: 6%; Turbuhaler®: 6% to 13%; Nasal: 34%

Half-life elimination: 2-3.6 hours

Time to peak: Capsule: 30-600 minutes (variable in Crohn's disease); Respules™: 10-30 minutes; Turbuhaler®: 1-2 hours; Nasal: 1 hour

Excretion: Urine (60%) and feces as metabolites

Usual Dosage
Nasal inhalation: Children ≥6 years and Adults:
Rhinocort®: Initial: 8 sprays (4 sprays/nostril) per day (256 mcg/day), given as either 2 sprays in each nostril in the morning and evening or as 4 sprays in each nostril in the morning; after symptoms decrease (usually by 3-7 days), reduce dose slowly every 2-4 weeks to the smallest amount needed to control symptoms

Rhinocort® Aqua™: 64 mcg/day as a single 32 mcg spray in each nostril. Some patients who do not achieve adequate control may benefit from increased dosage. A reduced dosage may be effective after initial control is achieved.

Maximum dose: Children <12 years: 128 mcg/day; Adults: 256 mcg/day

Nebulization: Children 12 months to 8 years: Pulmicort Respules™: Titrate to lowest effective dose once patient is stable; start at 0.25 mg/day or use as follows:
Previous therapy of bronchodilators alone: 0.5 mg/day administered as a single dose or divided twice daily (maximum daily dose: 0.5 mg)
Previous therapy of inhaled corticosteroids: 0.5 mg/day administered as a single dose or divided twice daily (maximum daily dose: 1 mg)
Previous therapy of oral corticosteroids: 1 mg/day administered as a single dose or divided twice daily (maximum daily dose: 1 mg)

Oral inhalation:
Children ≥6 years:
Previous therapy of bronchodilators alone: 200 mcg twice initially which may be increased up to 400 mcg twice daily
Previous therapy of inhaled corticosteroids: 200 mcg twice initially which may be increased up to 400 mcg twice daily

(Continued)

Budesonide *(Continued)*

Previous therapy of oral corticosteroids: The highest recommended dose in children is 400 mcg twice daily

Adults:

Previous therapy of bronchodilators alone: 200-400 mcg twice initially which may be increased up to 400 mcg twice daily

Previous therapy of inhaled corticosteroids: 200-400 mcg twice initially which may be increased up to 800 mcg twice daily

Previous therapy of oral corticosteroids: 400-800 mcg twice daily which may be increased up to 800 mcg twice daily

NIH Guidelines (NIH, 1997) (give in divided doses twice daily):

Children:

"Low" dose: 100-200 mcg/day

"Medium" dose: 200-400 mcg/day (1-2 inhalations/day)

"High" dose: >400 mcg/day (>2 inhalation/day)

Adults:

"Low" dose: 200-400 mcg/day (1-2 inhalations/day)

"Medium" dose: 400-600 mcg/day (2-3 inhalations/day)

"High" dose: >600 mcg/day (>3 inhalation/day)

Oral: Adults: Crohn's disease: 9 mg once daily in the morning; safety and efficacy have not been established for therapy duration >8 weeks; recurring episodes may be treated with a repeat 8-week course of treatment

Note: Treatment may be tapered to 6 mg once daily for 2 weeks prior to complete cessation. Patients receiving CYP3A3/4 inhibitors should be monitored closely for signs and symptoms of hypercorticism; dosage reduction may be required.

Dosage adjustment in hepatic impairment: Monitor closely for signs and symptoms of hypercorticism; dosage reduction may be required.

Dietary Considerations Avoid grapefruit juice when using oral capsules.

Administration

Inhalation: Inhaler should be shaken well immediately prior to use; while activating inhaler, deep breathe for 3-5 seconds, hold breath for ~10 seconds and allow ≥1 minute between inhalations. Rinse mouth with water after use to reduce aftertaste and incidence of candidiasis.

Nebulization: Shake well before using. Use Pulmicort Respules™ with jet nebulizer connected to an air compressor; administer with mouthpiece or facemask. Do not use ultrasonic nebulizer. Do not mix with other medications in nebulizer. Rinse mouth following treatments to decrease risk of oral candidiasis (wash face if using face mask).

Oral capsule: Capsule should be swallowed whole; do not crush or chew.

Monitoring Parameters Monitor growth in pediatric patients.

Patient Information Use as directed; do not increase dosage or discontinue abruptly without consulting prescriber. Report acute nervousness or inability to sleep; severe sneezing or nosebleed; difficulty breathing, sore throat, hoarseness, or bronchitis; respiratory difficulty or bronchospasms; disturbed menstrual pattern; vision changes; loss of taste or smell perception; or worsening of condition or lack of improvement. May be more susceptible to infection; avoid exposure to chickenpox and measles unless immunity has been established

Inhalation/nebulization: This is not a bronchodilator and will not relieve acute asthma attacks. It may take several days for you to realize full effects of treatment. If you are also using an inhaled bronchodilator, wait 10 minutes before using this steroid aerosol. You may experience dizziness, anxiety, or blurred vision (rise slowly from sitting or lying position and use caution when driving or engaging in tasks requiring alertness until response to drug is known); or taste disturbance or aftertaste (frequent mouth care and mouth rinses may help). Rinse mouth with water following oral treatments to decrease risk of oral candidiasis (wash face if using face mask).

Oral capsule: Swallow whole; do not crush or chew capsule.

Additional Information Effects of inhaled/intranasal steroids on growth have been observed in the absence of laboratory evidence of HPA axis suppression, suggesting that growth velocity is a more sensitive indicator of systemic corticosteroid exposure in pediatric patients than some commonly used tests of HPA axis function. The long-term effects of this reduction in growth velocity associated with orally-inhaled and intranasal corticosteroids, including the impact on final adult height, are unknown. The potential for "catch up" growth following discontinuation of treatment with inhaled corticosteroids has not been adequately studied.

Dosage Forms

Capsule, enteric coated (Entocort™ EC): 3 mg

Powder for oral inhalation (Pulmicort Turbuhaler®): 200 mcg/inhalation (104 g) [delivers ~160 mcg/inhalation; 200 metered doses]

Suspension for nasal inhalation (Rhinocort®): 50 mcg/inhalation (7 g) [delivers ~32 mcg/inhalation; 200 metered doses]

Suspension, nasal [spray] (Rhinocort® Aqua™): 32 mcg/inhalation (8.6 g) [120 metered doses]

Suspension for oral inhalation (Pulmicort Respules®): 0.25 mg/2 mL (30s), 0.5 mg/2 mL (30s)

♦ **Bufferin® [OTC]** *see* Aspirin *on page 120*

♦ **Bufferin® Arthritis Strength [OTC]** *see* Aspirin *on page 120*

♦ **Bufferin® Extra Strength [OTC]** *see* Aspirin *on page 120*

Bumetanide *(byoo MET a nide)*

Related Information

Heart Failure *on page 1663*

Sulfonamide Derivatives *on page 1515*

U.S. Brand Names Bumex®

Canadian Brand Names Bumex®; Burinex®

Therapeutic Category Antihypertensive Agent; Diuretic, Loop

Use Management of edema secondary to congestive heart failure or hepatic or renal disease including nephrotic syndrome; may be used alone or in combination with antihypertensives in the treatment of hypertension; can be used in furosemide-allergic patients

Pregnancy Risk Factor C (manufacturer); D (expert analysis)

Contraindications Hypersensitivity to bumetanide, any component of the formulation, or sulfonylureas; anuria; patients with hepatic coma or in states of severe electrolyte depletion until the condition improves or is corrected; pregnancy (based on expert analysis)

Warnings/Precautions Profound diuresis with fluid and electrolyte loss is possible; close medical supervision and dose evaluation is required; use caution when dosing in patients with hepatic failure; use caution in patients with known hypersensitivity to sulfonamides or thiazides (due to possible cross-sensitivity; avoid in history of severe reactions)

Chemical similarities are present among sulfonamides, sulfonylureas, carbonic anhydrase inhibitors, thiazides, and loop diuretics (except ethacrynic acid). Use in patients with sulfonylurea allergy is specifically contraindicated in product labeling, however a risk of cross-reaction exists in patients with allergy to any of these compounds; avoid use when previous reaction has been severe.

Excessive amounts can lead to profound diuresis with fluid and electrolyte loss; close medical supervision and dose evaluation is required; *in vitro* studies using pooled sera from critically ill neonates have shown bumetanide to be a potent displacer of bilirubin; avoid use in neonates at risk for kernicterus.

Adverse Reactions

>10%:
    Endocrine & metabolic: Hyperuricemia (18%), hypochloremia (15%), hypokalemia (15%)
    Renal: Azotemia (11%)

1% to 10%:
    Central nervous system: Dizziness (1%)
    Endocrine & metabolic: Hyponatremia (9%), hyperglycemia (7%), variations in phosphorus (5%), CO_2 content (4%), bicarbonate (3%), and calcium (2%)
    Neuromuscular & skeletal: Muscle cramps (1%)
    Otic: Ototoxicity (1%)
    Renal: Increased serum creatinine (7%)

<1% (Limited to important or life-threatening): Asterixis, dehydration, encephalopathy, hypernatremia, hypotension, impaired hearing, orthostatic hypotension, pruritus, rash, renal failure, vertigo, vomiting

Overdosage/Toxicology Symptoms include electrolyte depletion, and volume depletion. Treatment is primarily symptomatic and supportive.

Drug Interactions

Increased Effect/Toxicity: Bumetanide-induced hypokalemia may predispose to digoxin toxicity and may increase the risk of arrhythmia with drugs which may prolong QT interval, including type Ia and type III antiarrhythmic agents, cisapride, terfenadine, and some quinolones (sparfloxacin, gatifloxacin, and moxifloxacin). The risk of toxicity from lithium and salicylates (high dose) may be increased by loop diuretics. Hypotensive effects and/or adverse renal effects of ACE inhibitors and NSAIDs are potentiated by bumetanide-induced hypovolemia. The effects of peripheral adrenergic-blocking drugs or ganglionic blockers may be increased by bumetanide.

Bumetanide may increase the risk of ototoxicity with other ototoxic agents (aminoglycosides, cis-platinum), especially in patients with renal dysfunction. Synergistic diuretic effects occur with thiazide-type diuretics. Diuretics tend to be synergistic with other antihypertensive agents, and hypotension may occur.

Decreased Effect: Glucose tolerance may be decreased by loop diuretics, requiring adjustment of hypoglycemic agents. Cholestyramine or colestipol may reduce bioavailability of bumetanide. Indomethacin (and other NSAIDs) may reduce natriuretic and hypotensive effects of diuretics. Hypokalemia may reduce the efficacy of some antiarrhythmics.

Ethanol/Nutrition/Herb Interactions Herb/Nutraceutical: Avoid ephedra, yohimbe, ginseng (may worsen hypertension). Avoid dong quai if using for hypertension (has estrogenic activity). Avoid garlic (may have increased antihypertensive effect).

Stability I.V. infusion solutions should be used within 24 hours after preparation; light sensitive, discoloration may occur when exposed to light

Mechanism of Action Inhibits reabsorption of sodium and chloride in the ascending loop of Henle and proximal renal tubule, interfering with the chloride-binding cotransport system, thus causing increased excretion of water, sodium, chloride, magnesium, phosphate and calcium; it does not appear to act on the distal tubule

Pharmacodynamics/Kinetics

Onset of action: Oral, I.M.: 0.5-1 hour; I.V.: 2-3 minutes
Duration: 6 hours
Distribution: V_d: 13-25 L/kg
Protein binding: 95%
Metabolism: Partial, hepatic
Half-life elimination: Infants <6 months: Possibly 2.5 hours; Children and Adults: 1-1.5 hours
Excretion: Primarily urine (as unchanged drug and metabolites)

Usual Dosage

Oral, I.M., I.V.:
    Neonates (see Warnings/Precautions): 0.01-0.05 mg/kg/dose every 24-48 hours
    Infants and Children: 0.015-0.1 mg/kg/dose every 6-24 hours (maximum dose: 10 mg/day)
Adults:
    Edema:
        Oral: 0.5-2 mg/dose (maximum dose: 10 mg/day) 1-2 times/day
        I.M., I.V.: 0.5-1 mg/dose; may repeat in 2-3 hours for up to 2 doses if needed (maximum dose: 10 mg/day)
        Continuous I.V. infusion: 0.9-1 mg/hour
    Hypertension: Oral: 0.5 mg daily (range: 1-4 mg/day, maximum dose: 5 mg/day); for larger doses, divide into 2-3 doses daily

Dietary Considerations May require increased intake of potassium-rich foods.

(Continued)

Bumetanide *(Continued)*

Administration Administer I.V. slowly, over 1-2 minutes; an alternate-day schedule or a 3-4 daily dosing regimen with rest periods of 1-2 days in between may be the most tolerable and effective regimen for the continued control of edema; reserve I.V. administration for those unable to take oral medications

Monitoring Parameters Blood pressure, serum electrolytes, renal function

Patient Information May be taken with food or milk; rise slowly from a lying or sitting position to minimize dizziness, lightheadedness or fainting; also use extra care when exercising, standing for long periods of time, and during hot weather; take last dose of day early in the evening to prevent nocturia

Nursing Implications Be alert to complaints about hearing difficulty

Dosage Forms
Injection, solution: 0.25 mg/mL (2 mL, 4 mL, 10 mL)
Tablet: 0.5 mg, 1 mg, 2 mg
Bumex®: 0.5 mg, 1 mg, 2 mg

♦ **Bumex®** *see* Bumetanide *on page 188*
♦ **Buminate®** *see* Albumin *on page 40*
♦ **Buphenyl®** *see* Sodium Phenylbutyrate *on page 1248*

Bupivacaine *(byoo PIV a kane)*

U.S. Brand Names Marcaine®; Marcaine® Spinal; Sensorcaine®; Sensorcaine®-MPF
Canadian Brand Names Marcaine®; Sensorcaine®
Synonyms Bupivacaine Hydrochloride
Therapeutic Category Local Anesthetic, Injectable
Use Local anesthetic (injectable) for peripheral nerve block, infiltration, sympathetic block, caudal or epidural block, retrobulbar block
Pregnancy Risk Factor C
Contraindications Hypersensitivity to bupivacaine hydrochloride, amide-type local anesthetics (etidocaine, lidocaine, mepivacaine, prilocaine, ropivacaine) or any component of the formulation (para-aminobenzoic acid or parabens in specific formulations); not to be used for obstetrical paracervical block anesthesia
Warnings/Precautions Use with caution in patients with hepatic impairment. Some commercially available formulations contain sodium metabisulfite, which may cause allergic-type reactions; not recommended for use in children <12 years of age. The solution for spinal anesthesia should not be used in children <18 years of age. **Do not use solutions containing preservatives for caudal or epidural block.** Local anesthetics have been associated with rare occurrences of sudden respiratory arrest; convulsions due to systemic toxicity leading to cardiac arrest have also been reported, presumably following unintentional intravascular injection. The 0.75% is **not** recommended for obstetrical anesthesia. A test dose is recommended prior to epidural administration (prior to initial dose) and all reinforcing doses with continuous catheter technique.
Adverse Reactions 1% to 10%:
Cardiovascular: Cardiac arrest, hypotension, bradycardia, palpitations
Central nervous system: Seizures, restlessness, anxiety, dizziness
Gastrointestinal: Nausea, vomiting
Neuromuscular & skeletal: Weakness
Ocular: Blurred vision
Otic: Tinnitus
Respiratory: Apnea
Overdosage/Toxicology Treatment is primarily symptomatic and supportive. Termination of anesthesia by pneumatic tourniquet inflation should be attempted when the agent is administered by infiltration or regional injection. Seizures commonly respond to diazepam, while hypotension responds to I.V. fluids and Trendelenburg positioning. Bradyarrhythmias (when the heart rate is <60) can be treated with I.V., or S.C. atropine 15 mcg/kg. With the development of metabolic acidosis, I.V. sodium bicarbonate 0.5-2 mEq/kg and ventilatory assistance should be instituted. Methemoglobinemia should be treated with methylene blue 1-2 mg/kg in a 1% sterile aqueous solution I.V. push over 4-6 minutes, repeated up to a total dose of 7 mg/kg.
Drug Interactions
Increased Effect/Toxicity: Increased effect if used with hyaluronidase. Bupivacaine used in conjunction with epinephrine in patients on beta-blockers, ergot-type oxytocics, MAO inhibitors, tricyclic antidepressants, phenothiazines, vasopressors, or isoproterenol may result in prolonged hypotension or hypertension.
Stability Solutions with epinephrine should be protected from light
Mechanism of Action Blocks both the initiation and conduction of nerve impulses by decreasing the neuronal membrane's permeability to sodium ions, which results in inhibition of depolarization with resultant blockade of conduction
Pharmacodynamics/Kinetics
Onset of action: Anesthesia (route dependent): 4-10 minutes
Duration: 1.5-8.5 hours
Metabolism: Hepatic
Half-life elimination (age dependent): Neonates: 8.1 hours; Adults: 1.5-5.5 hours
Excretion: Urine (~6%)
Usual Dosage Dose varies with procedure, depth of anesthesia, vascularity of tissues, duration of anesthesia and condition of patient. Some formulations contain metabisulfites (in epinephrine-containing injection); do not use solutions containing preservatives for caudal or epidural block.
Local anesthesia: Infiltration: 0.25% infiltrated locally; maximum: 175 mg
Caudal block (with or without epinephrine, preservative free):
Children: 1-3.7 mg/kg
Adults: 15-30 mL of 0.25% or 0.5%

Epidural block (other than caudal block - with or without epinephrine, preservative free):
Administer in 3-5 mL increments, allowing sufficient time to detect toxic manifestations of inadvertent I.V. or I.T. administration:
Children: 1.25 mg/kg/dose
Adults: 10-20 mL of 0.25% or 0.5%
Surgical procedures requiring a high degree of muscle relaxation and prolonged effects **only**: 10-20 mL of 0.75% (**Note:** Not to be used in obstetrical cases)
Maxillary and mandibular infiltration and nerve block: 9 mg (1.8 mL) of 0.5% (with epinephrine) per injection site; a second dose may be administered if necessary to produce adequate anesthesia after allowing up to 10 minutes for onset, up to a maximum of 90 mg per dental appointment
Obstetrical anesthesia: Incremental dose: 3-5 mL of 0.5% (not exceeding 50-100 mg in any dosing interval); allow sufficient time to detect toxic manifestations or inadvertent I.V. or I.T. injection
Peripheral nerve block: 5 mL of 0.25 or 0.5%; maximum: 400 mg/day
Sympathetic nerve block: 20-50 mL of 0.25%
Retrobulbar anesthesia: 2-4 mL of 0.75%
Spinal anesthesia: Solution of 0.75% bupivacaine in 8.25% dextrose is used:
Lower extremity and perineal procedures: 1 mL
Lower abdominal procedures: 1.6 mL
Obstetrical:
Normal vaginal delivery: 0.8 mL (higher doses may be required in some patients)
Cesarean section: 1-1.4 mL

Administration Solutions containing preservatives should not be used for epidural or caudal blocks

Monitoring Parameters Monitor fetal heart rate during paracervical anesthesia

Patient Information Do not chew food in anesthetized region to prevent traumatizing tongue, lip, or buccal mucosa; single dose is usually sufficient in most applications

Dosage Forms
Injection, solution, as hydrochloride [preservative free]: 0.25% [2.5 mg/mL] (20 mL, 30 mL, 50 mL); 0.5% [5 mg/mL] (20 mL, 30 mL); 0.75% [7.5 mg/mL] (20 mL, 30 mL)
Marcaine®: 0.25% [2.5 mg/mL] (10 mL, 30 mL, 50 mL); 0.5% [5 mg/mL] (10 mL, 30 mL); 0.75% [7.5 mg/mL] (10 mL, 30 mL)
Marcaine® Spinal: 0.75% [7.5 mg/mL] (2 mL) [in dextrose 8.25%]
Sensorcaine®-MPF: 0.25% [2.5 mg/mL] (10 mL, 30 mL); 0.5% [5 mg/mL] (10 mL, 30 mL); 0.75% [7.5 mg/mL] (10 mL, 30 mL)
Injection, solution, as hydrochloride [with preservative]: 0.25% [2.5 mg/mL] (10 mL, 30 mL, 50 mL); 0.5% [5 mg/mL] (10 mL, 30 mL, 50 mL); 0.75% [7.5 mg/mL] (10 mL, 30 mL)
Marcaine®, Sensorcaine®: 0.25% [2.5 mg/mL] (50 mL); 0.5% [5 mg/mL] (50 mL) [contains methylparaben]
Injection, solution, with epinephrine 1:200,000, as hydrochloride [preservative free]:
Marcaine®: 0.25% [2.5 mg/mL] (10 mL, 30 mL, 50 mL); 0.5% [5 mg/mL] (3 mL, 10 mL, 30 mL); 0.75% [7.5 mg/mL] (30 mL) [contains sodium metabisulfite]
Sensorcaine®-MPF: 0.25% [2.5 mg/mL] (10 mL, 30 mL); 0.5% [5 mg/mL] (5 mL, 10 mL, 30 mL) [contains sodium metabisulfite]
Injection, solution, with epinephrine 1:200,000, as hydrochloride [with preservative] (Marcaine®, Sensorcaine®): 0.25% [2.5 mg/mL] (50 mL); 0.5% [5 mg/mL] (50 mL) [contains methylparaben and sodium metabisulfite]

♦ **Bupivacaine Hydrochloride** *see* Bupivacaine *on page 190*
♦ **Buprenex®** *see* Buprenorphine *on page 191*

Buprenorphine (byoo pre NOR feen)

Related Information
Narcotic Agonists Comparison *on page 1506*
U.S. Brand Names Buprenex®
Canadian Brand Names Buprenex®
Synonyms Buprenorphine Hydrochloride
Therapeutic Category Analgesic, Narcotic
Use Management of moderate to severe pain
Unlabeled/Investigational Use Heroin and opioid withdrawal
Restrictions C-V
Pregnancy Risk Factor C
Pregnancy/Breast-Feeding Implications Excreted in breast milk; breast-feeding is not recommended.
Contraindications Hypersensitivity to buprenorphine or any component of the formulation
Warnings/Precautions Use with caution in patients with hepatic dysfunction or possible neurologic injury; may precipitate abstinence syndrome in narcotic-dependent patients; tolerance or drug dependence may result from extended use
Adverse Reactions
>10%: Central nervous system: Sedation
1% to 10%:
Cardiovascular: Hypotension
Central nervous system: Respiratory depression, dizziness, headache
Gastrointestinal: Vomiting, nausea
Ocular: Miosis
Miscellaneous: Diaphoresis
<1% (Limited to important or life-threatening): Blurred vision, bradycardia, confusion, constipation, cyanosis, depression, diplopia, dyspnea, euphoria, hypertension, nervousness, paresthesia, pruritus, slurred speech, tachycardia, urinary retention, xerostomia
Overdosage/Toxicology Symptoms include CNS depression, pinpoint pupils, hypotension, and bradycardia. Treatment includes airway support, establishment of an I.V. line, and administration of naloxone 2 mg I.V. (0.01 mg/kg for children), with repeat administration as necessary, up to a total of 10 mg.
(Continued)

Buprenorphine *(Continued)*

Drug Interactions

Cytochrome P450 Effect: CYP3A3/4 enzyme substrate

Increased Effect/Toxicity: Barbiturate anesthetics and other CNS depressants may produce additive respiratory and CNS depression. Respiratory and CV collapse was reported in a patient who received diazepam and buprenorphine. Effects may be additive with other CNS depressants. CYP3A3/4 inhibitors may increase serum levels/toxicty of buprenorphine (inhibitors include amiodarone, cimetidine, clarithromycin, erythromycin, delavirdine, diltiazem, dirithromycin, disulfiram, fluoxetine, fluvoxamine, grapefruit juice, indinavir, itraconazole, ketoconazole, nefazodone, nevirapine, propoxyphene, quinupristin-dalfopristin, ritonavir, saquinavir, verapamil, zafirlukast, and zileuton); monitor for altered effects; a decrease in buprenorphine dosage may be required.

Decreased Effect: Enzyme inducers may reduce serum concentrations of buprenorphine, resulting in loss of efficacy (includes barbiturates, carbamazepine, phenytoin rifabutin, and rifampin). Naltrexone may antagonize the effect of narcotic analgesics; concurrent use or use within 7-10 days is contraindicated.

Ethanol/Nutrition/Herb Interactions

Ethanol: Avoid ethanol (may increase CNS depression).

Herb/Nutraceutical: Avoid valerian, St John's wort, kava kava, gotu kola (may increase CNS depression).

Stability Protect from excessive heat >40°C (104°F) and light

Compatible with 0.9% sodium chloride, lactated Ringer's solution, 5% dextrose in water, scopolamine, haloperidol, glycopyrrolate, droperidol, and hydroxyzine

Incompatible with diazepam, lorazepam

Mechanism of Action Buprenorphine exerts its analgesic effect via high affinity binding to μ opiate receptors in the CNS; displays both agonist and antagonist activity

Pharmacodynamics/Kinetics

Onset of action: Analgesic: 10-30 minutes

Duration: 6-8 hours

Absorption: I.M., S.C.: 30% to 40%

Distribution: V_d: 97-187 L/kg

Protein binding: High

Metabolism: Mainly hepatic; extensive first-pass effect

Half-life elimination: 2.2-3 hours

Excretion: Feces (70%); urine (20% as unchanged drug)

Usual Dosage Long-term use is not recommended

I.M., slow I.V.:

Children ≥13 years and Adults:

Moderate to severe pain: 0.3-0.6 mg every 6 hours as needed

Heroin or opiate withdrawal (unlabeled use): Variable; 0.1-0.4 mg every 6 hours

Elderly: Moderate to severe pain: 0.15 mg every 6 hours; elderly patients are more likely to suffer from confusion and drowsiness compared to younger patients

Administration Administer I.V. dose slowly.

Monitoring Parameters Pain relief, respiratory and mental status, CNS depression, blood pressure

Patient Information May cause drowsiness

Nursing Implications Gradual withdrawal of drug is necessary to avoid withdrawal symptoms

Additional Information 0.3 mg = 10 mg morphine or 75 mg meperidine, has longer duration of action than either agent

Dosage Forms Injection, solution, as hydrochloride: 0.3 mg/mL (1 mL)

♦ **Buprenorphine Hydrochloride** *see Buprenorphine on page 191*

BuPROPion *(byoo PROE pee on)*

Related Information

Antidepressant Agents Comparison *on page 1482*

U.S. Brand Names Wellbutrin®; Wellbutrin SR®; Zyban®

Canadian Brand Names Wellbutrin®; Zyban™

Therapeutic Category Antidepressant, Miscellaneous

Use Treatment of depression; adjunct in smoking cessation

Unlabeled/Investigational Use Attention-deficit/hyperactivity disorder (ADHD)

Pregnancy Risk Factor B

Contraindications Hypersensitivity to bupropion or any component of the formulation; seizure disorder; anorexia/bulimia; use of MAO inhibitors within 14 days

Warnings/Precautions Seizure risk is increased at total daily dosage >450 mg, individual dosages >150 mg, or by sudden, large increments in dose. The risk of seizures is increased in patients with a history of seizures, head trauma, CNS tumor, abrupt discontinuation of sedative-hypnotics or ethanol, medications which lower seizure threshold, stimulants, or hypoglycemic agents. May cause CNS stimulation (restlessness, anxiety, insomnia) or anorexia. Use with caution in patients where weight loss is not desirable. The incidence of sexual dysfunction with bupropion is generally lower than with SSRIs.

Use caution in patients with cardiovascular disease, history of hypertension, or coronary artery disease; treatment-emergent hypertension (including some severe cases) has been reported, both with bupropion alone and in combination with nicotine transdermal systems.

Use with caution in patients with hepatic or renal dysfunction and in elderly patients. Elderly patients may be at greater risk of accumulation during chronic dosing. May cause motor or cognitive impairment in some patients, use with caution if tasks requiring alertness such as operating machinery or driving are undertaken. May worsen psychosis in some patients or precipitate a shift to mania or hypomania in patients with bipolar disease. Use caution in patients with suicidal risk.

Arthralgia, myalgia, and fever with rash and other symptoms suggestive of delayed hypersensitivity resembling serum sickness reported

Adverse Reactions
>10%:
Cardiovascular: Tachycardia
Central nervous system: Agitation, insomnia, headache, dizziness, sedation
Gastrointestinal: Nausea, vomiting, xerostomia, constipation
Neuromuscular & skeletal: Tremor
Ocular: Blurred vision
Respiratory: Rhinitis
Miscellaneous: Diaphoresis
1% to 10%:
Cardiovascular: Hypertension (2.5% alone, up to 6.1% in combination with nicotine patch), palpitations
Central nervous system: Anxiety, nervousness, confusion, hostility, abnormal dreams
Dermatologic: Rash, acne, dry skin
Endocrine & metabolic: Hyper- or hypoglycemia
Gastrointestinal: Anorexia, diarrhea, dyspepsia
Neuromuscular & skeletal: Arthralgia, myalgia
Otic: Tinnitus
Postintroduction adverse reactions: Extrasystoles, myocardial infarction, orthostatic hypotension, phlebitis, pulmonary embolism, and third degree heart block. Arthralgia, myalgia, and fever with rash and other symptoms suggestive of delayed hypersensitivity resembling serum sickness reported. Hypertension (in some cases severe) requiring acute treatment has been reported in patients receiving bupropion alone and in combination with nicotine replacement therapy.

Overdosage/Toxicology
Symptoms include labored breathing, salivation, arched back, ataxia, convulsions, sedation, coma, and respiratory depression, especially with coingestion of ethanol. Bupropion may cause sinus tachycardia and seizures. Treatment is supportive following initial decontamination with activated charcoal (lavage with massive and recent doses). Treat seizures with I.V. benzodiazepines and supportive therapies. Dialysis may be of limited value after drug absorption because of slow tissue-to-plasma diffusion.

Drug Interactions
Cytochrome P450 Effect: CYP2B6 enzyme substrate; CYP3A3/4 enzyme substrate (minor)
Increased Effect/Toxicity: Treatment-emergent hypertension may occur in patients treated with bupropion and nicotine patch. Cimetidine may inhibit the metabolism (increase clinical/adverse effects) of bupropion. Toxicity of bupropion is enhanced by levodopa and phenelzine (MAO inhibitors). Risk of seizures may be increased with agents that may lower seizure threshold (antipsychotics, antidepressants, theophylline, abrupt discontinuation of benzodiazepines, systemic steroids).
Decreased Effect: Carbamazepine, phenobarbital, and phenytoin may increase the metabolism (decrease clinical effect) of bupropion.

Ethanol/Nutrition/Herb Interactions
Ethanol: Ethanol (may increase CNS depression).
Herb/Nutraceutical : Avoid valerian, St John's wort, SAMe, gotu kola, kava kava (may increase CNS depression).

Mechanism of Action
Antidepressant structurally different from all other previously marketed antidepressants; like other antidepressants the mechanism of bupropion's activity is not fully understood; weak inhibitor of the neuronal uptake of serotonin, norepinephrine, and dopamine

Pharmacodynamics/Kinetics
Onset of therapeutic effect: >2 weeks
Absorption: Rapid
Distribution: V_d: 19-21 L/kg
Protein binding: 82% to 88%
Metabolism: Extensively hepatic to multiple metabolites
Half-life elimination: 14 hours
Time to peak, serum: ~3 hours

Usual Dosage
Oral:
Children and Adolescents: ADHD (unlabeled use): 1.4-6 mg/kg/day
Adults:
Depression:
Immediate release: 100 mg 3 times/day; begin at 100 mg twice daily; may increase to a maximum dose of 450 mg/day
Sustained release: Initial: 150 mg/day in the morning; may increase to 150 mg twice daily by day 4 if tolerated; target dose: 300 mg/day given as 150 mg twice daily; maximum dose: 400 mg/day given as 200 mg twice daily
Smoking cessation: Initiate with 150 mg once daily for 3 days; increase to 150 mg twice daily; treatment should continue for 7-12 weeks
Elderly: Depression: 50-100 mg/day, increase by 50-100 mg every 3-4 days as tolerated; there is evidence that the elderly respond at 150 mg/day in divided doses, but some may require a higher dose
Dosing adjustment/comments in renal or hepatic impairment: Patients with renal or hepatic failure should receive a reduced dosage initially and be closely monitored

Monitoring Parameters
Body weight

Reference Range
Therapeutic levels (trough, 12 hours after last dose): 50-100 ng/mL

Patient Information
Take in equally divided doses 3-4 times/day to minimize the risk of seizures; avoid alcohol; do not take more than recommended dose or more than 150 mg in a single dose; do not discontinue abruptly, it may take 3-4 weeks for full effect; may impair driving or other motor or cognitive skills and judgment

As part of a smoking cessation program, bupropion can provide beneficial effects, but must be taken on a regular basis. Bupropion is only part of the total remedy for smoking cessation and must be combined with behavior and lifestyle modifications.

Nursing Implications
Be aware that drug may cause seizures
(Continued)

BuPROPion *(Continued)*

Dosage Forms
Tablet (Wellbutrin®): 75 mg, 100 mg
Tablet, sustained release:
Wellbutrin® SR: 100 mg, 150 mg
Zyban®: 150 mg

- ◆ **Burinex® (Can)** *see Bumetanide on page 188*
- ◆ **Burow's Otic** *see Aluminum Acetate and Acetic Acid on page 62*
- ◆ **BuSpar®** *see BusPIRone on page 194*
- ◆ **Buspirex (Can)** *see BusPIRone on page 194*

BusPIRone *(byoo SPYE rone)*

U.S. Brand Names BuSpar®
Canadian Brand Names Apo®-Buspirone; BuSpar®; Buspirex; Bustab®; Gen-Buspirone; Lin-Buspirone; Novo-Buspirone; Nu-Buspirone; PMS-Buspirone
Synonyms Buspirone Hydrochloride
Therapeutic Category Antianxiety Agent
Use Management of generalized anxiety disorder (GAD)
Unlabeled/Investigational Use Management of aggression in mental retardation and secondary mental disorders; major depression; potential augmenting agent for antidepressants; premenstrual syndrome
Pregnancy Risk Factor B
Contraindications Hypersensitivity to buspirone or any component of the formulation
Warnings/Precautions Safety and efficacy not established in children <18 years of age; use in hepatic or renal impairment is not recommended; does not prevent or treat withdrawal from benzodiazepines. Low potential for cognitive or motor impairment. Use with MAO inhibitors may result in hypertensive reactions.
Adverse Reactions
>10%: Central nervous system: Dizziness
1% to 10%:
Central nervous system: Drowsiness, EPS, serotonin syndrome, confusion, nervousness, lightheadedness, excitement, anger, hostility, headache
Dermatologic: Rash
Gastrointestinal: Diarrhea, nausea
Neuromuscular & skeletal: Muscle weakness, numbness, paresthesia, incoordination, tremor
Ocular: Blurred vision, tunnel vision
Miscellaneous: Diaphoresis, allergic reactions
Overdosage/Toxicology Symptoms include dizziness, drowsiness, pinpoint pupils, nausea, and vomiting. There is no known antidote for buspirone. Treatment is supportive.
Drug Interactions
Cytochrome P450 Effect: CYP3A3/4 enzyme substrate
Increased Effect/Toxicity: Concurrent use of buspirone with SSRIs or trazodone may cause serotonin syndrome. Erythromycin, clarithromycin, diltiazem, itraconazole, ketoconazole, verapamil, and grapefruit juice may result in increases in buspirone concentrations. Buspirone should not be used concurrently with an MAO inhibitor due to reports of increased blood pressure; theoretically, a selective MAO type B inhibitors (selegiline) has a lower risk of this reaction. Concurrent use of buspirone with nefazodone may increase risk of CNS adverse events; limit buspirone initial dose (eg, 2.5 mg/day).
Decreased Effect: Enzyme inducers (phenobarbital, carbamazepine, phenytoin, rifampin) may reduce serum concentrations of buspirone resulting in loss of efficacy.
Ethanol/Nutrition/Herb Interactions
Ethanol: Ethanol (may increase CNS depression).
Food: Food may decrease the absorption of buspirone, but it may also decrease the first-pass metabolism, thereby increasing the bioavailability of buspirone. Grapefruit juice may cause increased buspirone concentrations; avoid concurrent use.
Herb/Nutraceutical: St John's wort may decrease buspirone levels or increase CNS depression. Avoid valerian, gotu kola, kava kava (may increase CNS depression).
Mechanism of Action The mechanism of action of buspirone is unknown. Buspirone has a high affinity for serotonin 5-HT$_{1A}$ and 5-HT$_2$ receptors, without affecting benzodiazepine-GABA receptors; buspirone has moderate affinity for dopamine D$_2$ receptors
Pharmacodynamics/Kinetics
Protein binding: 86%
Metabolism: Hepatic via oxidation; extensive first-pass effect
Half-life elimination: 2-3 hours
Time to peak, serum: ~1 hour
Usual Dosage Oral:
Generalized anxiety disorder:
Children and Adolescents: Initial: 5 mg daily; increase in increments of 5 mg/day at weekly intervals as needed, to a maximum dose of 60 mg/day divided into 2-3 doses
Adults: Oral: 15 mg/day (7.5 mg twice daily); may increase in increments of 5 mg/day every 2-4 days to a maximum of 60 mg/day; target dose for most people is 30 mg/day (15 mg twice daily)
Dosing adjustment in renal or hepatic impairment: Buspirone is metabolized by the liver and excreted by the kidneys. Patients with impaired hepatic or renal function demonstrated increased plasma levels and a prolonged half-life of buspirone. Therefore, use in patients with severe hepatic or renal impairment cannot be recommended.
Monitoring Parameters Mental status, symptoms of anxiety
Patient Information Report any change in senses (ie, smelling, hearing, vision); cautious use with alcohol is recommended; cannot be substituted for benzodiazepines unless directed by a physician; takes 2-3 weeks to see the full effect of this medication; if you miss a dose, do **not** double your next dose

Nursing Implications Monitor mental status

Additional Information Has shown little potential for abuse; needs continuous use. Because of slow onset, not appropriate for "as needed" (prn) use or for brief, situational anxiety. Ineffective for treatment of benzodiazepine or ethanol withdrawal.

Dosage Forms Tablet, as hydrochloride: 5 mg, 7.5 mg, 10 mg, 15 mg, 30 mg

BuSpar®: 5 mg, 10 mg, 15 mg, 30 mg

♦ **Buspirone Hydrochloride** *see BusPIRone on page 194*

♦ **Bustab® (Can)** *see BusPIRone on page 194*

Busulfan (byoo SUL fan)

U.S. Brand Names Busulfex®; Myleran®

Canadian Brand Names Busulfex®; Myleran®

Therapeutic Category Antineoplastic Agent, Alkylating Agent

Use

Oral: Chronic myelogenous leukemia and bone marrow disorders, such as polycythemia vera and myeloid metaplasia, conditioning regimens for bone marrow transplantation

I.V.: Combination therapy with cyclophosphamide as a conditioning regimen prior to allogeneic hematopoietic progenitor cell transplantation for chronic myelogenous leukemia

Pregnancy Risk Factor D

Contraindications Hypersensitivity to busulfan or any component of the formulation; failure to respond to previous courses; pregnancy

Warnings/Precautions The U.S. Food and Drug Administration (FDA) currently recommends that procedures for proper handling and disposal of antineoplastic agents be considered. May induce severe bone marrow hypoplasia; reduce or discontinue dosage at first sign, as reflected by an abnormal decrease in any of the formed elements of the blood; use with caution in patients recently given other myelosuppressive drugs or radiation treatment. If white blood count is high, hydration and allopurinol should be employed to prevent hyperuricemia. Use caution in patients predisposed to seizures. Discontinue if lung toxicity develops. Busulfan has been causally related to the development of secondary malignancies (tumors and acute leukemias). Busulfan has been associated with ovarian failure (including failure to achieve puberty) in females.

Adverse Reactions

>10%:

Dermatologic: Skin hyperpigmentation (busulfan tan), urticaria, erythema, alopecia

Endocrine & metabolic: Ovarian suppression, amenorrhea, sterility

Genitourinary: Azoospermia, testicular atrophy; malignant tumors have been reported in patients on busulfan therapy

Hematologic: Severe pancytopenia, leukopenia, thrombocytopenia, anemia, and bone marrow suppression are common and patients should be monitored closely while on therapy; since this is a delayed effect (busulfan affects the stem cells), the drug should be discontinued temporarily at the first sign of a large or rapid fall in any blood element; some patients may develop bone marrow fibrosis or chronic aplasia which is probably due to the busulfan toxicity; in large doses, busulfan is myeloablative and is used for this reason in BMT

Myelosuppressive:

WBC: Moderate

Platelets: Moderate

Onset (days): 7-10

Nadir (days): 14-21

Recovery (days): 28

1% to 10%:

Cardiovascular: Hypotension

Central nervous system: Confusion,

Dermatologic: Hyperpigmentation

Endocrine & metabolic: Amenorrhea, hyperuricemia

Gastrointestinal: Nausea, stomatitis, anorexia, vomiting, diarrhea; drug has little effect on the GI mucosal lining

Emetic potential: Low (<10%)

Hepatic: Elevated LFTs

Neuromuscular & skeletal: Weakness

Ocular: Cataracts

Respiratory: Bronchopulmonary dysplasia

<1% (Limited to important or life-threatening): Adrenal suppression, gynecomastia, isolated cases of hemorrhagic cystitis have been reported, hepatic dysfunction; after long-term or high-dose therapy, a syndrome known as busulfan lung may occur; this syndrome is manifested by a diffuse interstitial pulmonary fibrosis and persistent cough, fever, rales, and dyspnea. May be relieved by corticosteroids.

BMT:

Central nervous system: Generalized or myoclonic seizures and loss of consciousness, abnormal electroencephalographic findings

Gastrointestinal: Mucositis, anorexia, moderately emetogenic

Hepatic: Veno-occlusive disease (VOD), hyperbilirubinemia

Miscellaneous: Transient pain at tumor sites, transient autoimmune disorders

Overdosage/Toxicology Symptoms include leukopenia and thrombocytopenia. Induction of vomiting or gastric lavage with charcoal is indicated for recent ingestions. The effects of dialysis are unknown.

Drug Interactions

Cytochrome P450 Effect: CYP3A3/4 enzyme substrate

Increased Effect/Toxicity: Itraconazole or other cytotoxic agents may increase risk of pulmonary toxicity.

Ethanol/Nutrition/Herb Interactions

Ethanol: Avoid ethanol due to GI irritation.

Food: No clear or firm data on the effect of food on busulfan bioavailability.

(Continued)

Busulfan *(Continued)*

Herb/Nutraceutical: St John's wort may decrease busulfan levels.

Stability Store unopened ampuls under refrigeration at 2°C to 8°C (36°F to 46°F).

Dilute busulfan injection in 0.9% sodium chloride injection or dextrose 5% in water. The dilution volume should be ten times the volume of busulfan injection, ensuring that the final concentration of busulfan is ≥0.5 mg/mL. This solution is stable for up to 8 hours at room temperature (25°C) but the infusion must also be completed within that 8-hour time frame. Dilution of busulfan injection in 0.9% sodium chloride is stable for up to 12 hours at refrigeration (2°C to 8°C) but the infusion must also be completed within that 12-hour time frame.

Mechanism of Action Reacts with N-7 position of guanosine and interferes with DNA replication and transcription of RNA. Busulfan has a more marked effect on myeloid cells (and is, therefore, useful in the treatment of CML) than on lymphoid cells. The drug is also very toxic to hematopoietic stem cells (thus its usefulness in high doses in BMT preparative regimens). Busulfan exhibits little immunosuppressive activity. Interferes with the normal function of DNA by alkylation and cross-linking the strands of DNA.

Pharmacodynamics/Kinetics

Duration: 28 days

Absorption: Rapid and complete

Distribution: V_d: ~1 L/kg; into CSF and saliva with levels similar to plasma

Protein binding: ~14%

Metabolism: Extensively hepatic (may increase with multiple dosing)

Half-life elimination: After first dose: 3.4 hours; After last dose: 2.3 hours

Time to peak, serum: Oral: Within 4 hours; I.V.: Within 5 minutes

Excretion: Urine (10% to 50% as metabolites) within 24 hours, (<2% as unchanged drug)

Usual Dosage Busulfan should be based on adjusted ideal body weight because actual body weight, ideal body weight, or other factors can produce significant differences in busulfan clearance among lean, normal, and obese patients; refer to individual protocols

Children:

For remission induction of CML: Oral: 0.06-0.12 mg/kg/day **OR** 1.8-4.6 mg/m²/day; titrate dosage to maintain leukocyte count above 40,000/mm³; reduce dosage by 50% if the leukocyte count reaches 30,000-40,000/mm³; discontinue drug if counts fall to ≤20,000/mm³

BMT marrow-ablative conditioning regimen: Oral: 1 mg/kg/dose (ideal body weight) every 6 hours for 16 doses

Adults:

For remission induction of CML: Oral: 4-8 mg/day (may be as high as 12 mg/day); Maintenance doses: Controversial, range from 1-4 mg/day to 2 mg/week; treatment is continued until WBC reaches 10,000-20,000 cells/mm³ at which time drug is discontinued; when WBC reaches 50,000/mm³, maintenance dose is resumed

BMT marrow-ablative conditioning regimen:

Oral: 1 mg/kg/dose (ideal body weight) every 6 hours for 16 doses

I.V.: 0.8 mg/kg (ideal body weight or actual body weight, whichever is lower) every 6 hours for 4 days (a total of 16 doses)

I.V. dosing in morbidly obese patients: Dosing should be based on adjusted ideal body weight (AIBW) which should be calculated as ideal body weight (IBW) + 0.25 times (actual weight minus ideal body weight)

AIBW = IBW + 0.25 x (AW - IBW)

Cyclophosphamide, in combination with busulfan, is given on each of two days as a 1-hour infusion at a dose of 160 mg/m² beginning on day 3, 6 hours following the 16th dose of busulfan

Unapproved use:

Polycythemia vera: 2-6 mg/day

Thrombocytosis: 4-6 mg/day

Administration Intravenous busulfan should be administered via a CENTRAL venous catheter as a 2-hour infusion - every 6 hours for 4 consecutive days for a total of 16 doses

Monitoring Parameters CBC with differential and platelet count, hemoglobin, liver function tests

Patient Information Take oral medication as directed with chilled liquids. Maintain adequate hydration (2-3 L/day of fluids unless instructed to restrict fluid intake) to help prevent kidney complications. Avoid alcohol, acidic or spicy foods, aspirin, or OTC medications unless approved by prescriber. Brush teeth with soft toothbrush or cotton swab. You may lose head hair or experience darkening of skin color (reversible when medication is discontinued), amenorrhea, sterility, or skin rash. You may experience nausea, vomiting, anorexia, or constipation (small frequent meals, increased exercise, and increased dietary fruit or fiber may help). You will be more susceptible to infection (avoid crowds or contagious persons, and do not receive any vaccinations unless approved by prescriber). Report palpitations or chest pain, excessive dizziness, confusion, respiratory difficulty, numbness or tingling of extremities, unusual bruising or bleeding, pain or changes in urination, or other adverse effects. Contraceptive measures are recommended during therapy.

Nursing Implications

Avoid I.M. injection if platelet count falls <100,000/mm³

Monitor CBC with differential and platelet count, hemoglobin, liver function tests

Dosage Forms

Injection, solution (Busulfex®): 6 mg/mL (10 mL)

Tablet (Myleran®): 2 mg

♦ **Busulfex®** *see* Busulfan *on page 195*

Butabarbital *(byoo ta BAR bi tal)*

U.S. Brand Names Butisol Sodium®

Therapeutic Category Barbiturate; Hypnotic; Sedative

Use Sedative; hypnotic

Restrictions C-III

Pregnancy Risk Factor D

Contraindications Hypersensitivity to barbiturates or any component of the formulation; porphyria; pregnancy

Warnings/Precautions May cause CNS depression, which may impair physical or mental abilities. Patients must be cautioned about performing tasks which require mental alertness (ie, operating machinery or driving). Effects with other sedative drugs or ethanol may be potentiated. May cause respiratory depression or hypotension. Use with caution in hemodynamically unstable patients or patients with respiratory disease. Potential for drug dependency exists; abrupt cessation may precipitate withdrawal, including status epilepticus in epileptic patients. Use caution in elderly, debilitated, renally impaired, hepatic impairment, or pediatric patients. May cause paradoxical responses, including agitation and hyperactivity, particularly in acute pain and pediatric patients. Use with caution in patients with depression or suicidal tendencies, or in patients with a history of drug abuse. Tolerance, psychological and physical dependence may occur with prolonged use.

Adverse Reactions
>10%: Central nervous system: Dizziness, lightheadedness, drowsiness, "hangover" effect
1% to 10%:
Central nervous system: Confusion, mental depression, unusual excitement, nervousness, faint feeling, headache, insomnia, nightmares
Gastrointestinal: Constipation, nausea, vomiting
<1% (Limited to important or life-threatening): Agranulocytosis, angioedema, dependence, exfoliative dermatitis, hallucinations, hypotension, megaloblastic anemia, rash, respiratory depression, Stevens-Johnson syndrome, thrombocytopenia, thrombophlebitis

Overdosage/Toxicology Symptoms include slurred speech, confusion, nystagmus, tachycardia, and hypotension. If hypotension occurs, administer I.V. fluids and place the patient in the Trendelenburg position. If unresponsive, an I.V. vasopressor (eg, dopamine, epinephrine) may be required. Forced alkaline diuresis is of no value in the treatment of intoxications with short-acting barbiturates. Charcoal hemoperfusion or hemodialysis may be useful in harder-to-treat intoxications, especially in the presence of very high serum barbiturate levels.

Drug Interactions
Cytochrome P450 Effect: Note: Barbiturates are cytochrome P450 enzyme inducers. Patients should be monitored when these drugs are started or stopped for a decreased or increased therapeutic effect respectively.
Increased Effect/Toxicity: When butabarbital is combined with other CNS depressants, ethanol, narcotic analgesics, antidepressants, or benzodiazepines, additive respiratory and CNS depression may occur. Barbiturates may enhance the hepatotoxic potential of acetaminophen overdoses. Chloramphenicol, MAO inhibitors, valproic acid, and felbamate may inhibit barbiturate metabolism. Barbiturates may impair the absorption of griseofulvin, and may enhance the nephrotoxic effects of methoxyflurane.
Decreased Effect: Barbiturates such as butabarbital are hepatic enzyme inducers, and may increase the metabolism of antipsychotics, some beta-blockers (unlikely with atenolol and nadolol), calcium channel blockers, chloramphenicol, cimetidine, corticosteroids, cyclosporine, disopyramide, doxycycline, ethosuximide, felbamate, furosemide, griseofulvin, lamotrigine, phenytoin, propafenone, quinidine, tacrolimus, TCAs, and theophylline. Barbiturates may increase the metabolism of estrogens and reduce the efficacy of oral contraceptives; an alternative method of contraception should be considered. Barbiturates inhibit the hypoprothrombinemic effects of oral anticoagulants via increased metabolism. Barbiturates may enhance the metabolism of methadone resulting in methadone withdrawal.

Ethanol/Nutrition/Herb Interactions
Ethanol: Avoid ethanol (may increase CNS depression).
Herb/Nutraceutical: Avoid valerian, St John's wort, kava kava, gotu kola (may increase CNS depression).

Mechanism of Action Interferes with transmission of impulses from the thalamus to the cortex of the brain resulting in an imbalance in central inhibitory and facilitatory mechanisms

Pharmacodynamics/Kinetics
Distribution: V_d: 0.8 L/kg
Protein binding: 26%
Metabolism: Hepatic
Half-life elimination: 1.6 days to 5.8 days
Time to peak, serum: 40-60 minutes
Excretion: Urine (as metabolites)

Usual Dosage Oral:
Children: Preoperative sedation: 2-6 mg/kg/dose (maximum: 100 mg)
Adults:
Sedative: 15-30 mg 3-4 times/day
Hypnotic: 50-100 mg
Preop: 50-100 mg 1-1$^{1}/_{2}$ hours before surgery

Reference Range Therapeutic: Not established; Toxic: 28-73 µg/mL

Patient Information May cause drowsiness, avoid alcohol or other CNS depressants, may impair judgment and coordination; may cause physical and psychological dependence with prolonged use; do not exceed recommended dose

Nursing Implications Raise bed rails; initiate safety measures; aid with ambulation; monitor for CNS depression

Dosage Forms
Elixir, as sodium: 30 mg/5 mL (480 mL) [contains alcohol 7%]
Tablet, as sodium: 30 mg, 50 mg

Butalbital Compound (byoo TAL bi tal KOM pound)

U.S. Brand Names Amaphen®; Anoquan®; Axotal®; B-A-C®; Bancap®; Endolor®; Esgic®; Femcet®; Fiorgen PF®; Fioricet®; Fiorinal®; G-1®; Isollyl® Improved; Lanorinal®; Margesic®; Marnal®; Medigesic®; Phrenilin®; Phrenilin® Forte; Repan®; Sedapap-10®; Triad®; Triapin®; Two-Dyne®
(Continued)

Butalbital Compound *(Continued)*

Canadian Brand Names Tecnal®

Therapeutic Category Barbiturate

Use Relief of symptomatic complex of tension or muscle contraction headache

Restrictions C-III (Fiorinal®)

Pregnancy Risk Factor D

Contraindications Patients with porphyria, known hypersensitivity to butalbital or any component

Warnings/Precautions Children and teenagers should not use for chickenpox or flu symptoms before a physician is consulted about Reye's syndrome (Fiorinal®).

Adverse Reactions

>10%:

Central nervous system: Dizziness, lightheadedness, drowsiness, "hangover" effect

Gastrointestinal: Nausea, heartburn, stomach pains, dyspepsia, epigastric discomfort

1% to 10%:

Central nervous system: Confusion, mental depression, unusual excitement, nervousness, faint feeling, headache, insomnia, nightmares, fatigue

Dermatologic: Rash

Gastrointestinal: Constipation, vomiting, gastrointestinal ulceration

Hematologic: Hemolytic anemia

Neuromuscular & skeletal: Weakness

Respiratory: Dyspnea

Miscellaneous: Anaphylactic shock

<1%: Agranulocytosis, bronchospasm, exfoliative dermatitis, hallucinations, hepatotoxicity, hypotension, impaired renal function, iron deficiency anemia, jitters, leukopenia, megaloblastic anemia, occult bleeding, prolongation of bleeding time, respiratory depression, Stevens-Johnson syndrome, thrombocytopenia, thrombophlebitis

Drug Interactions

Increased Effect/Toxicity: Propoxyphene, benzodiazepines, CNS depressants, valproic acid, methylphenidate, chloramphenicol

Decreased Effect: Phenothiazines, haloperidol, quinidine, cyclosporine, TCAs, corticosteroids, theophylline, ethosuximide, warfarin, oral contraceptives, chloramphenicol, griseofulvin, doxycycline, beta-blockers

Mechanism of Action Butalbital, like other barbiturates, has a generalized depressant effect on the central nervous system (CNS). Barbiturates have little effect on peripheral nerves or muscle at usual therapeutic doses. However, at toxic doses serious effects on the cardiovascular system and other peripheral systems may be observed. These effects may result in hypotension or skeletal muscle weakness. While all areas of the central nervous system are acted on by barbiturates, the mesencephalic reticular activating system is extremely sensitive to their effects. Barbiturates act at synapses where gamma-aminobenzoic acid is a neurotransmitter, but they have an effect in other areas as well.

Usual Dosage Adults: Oral: 1-2 tablets or capsules every 4 hours; not to exceed 6/day

Dosing interval in renal or hepatic impairment: Should be reduced

Dietary Considerations Alcohol: Additive CNS effects, avoid use

Patient Information Children and teenagers should not use this product; may cause drowsiness, avoid alcohol or other CNS depressants, may impair judgment and coordination; may cause physical and psychological dependence with prolonged use; do not exceed recommended dose

Nursing Implications Raise bed rails; initiate safety measures; aid with ambulation; monitor for CNS depression

Dosage Forms

Capsule, with acetaminophen:

Amaphen®, Anoquan®, Butace®, Endolor®, Esgic®, Femcet®, G-1®, Margesic®, Medigesic®, Repan®, Triad®, Two-Dyne®: Butalbital 50 mg, caffeine 40 mg, and acetaminophen 325 mg

Bancap®, Triapin®: Butalbital 50 mg and acetaminophen 325 mg

Phrenilin® Forte: Butalbital 50 mg and acetaminophen 650 mg

Capsule, with aspirin: (Fiorgen PF®, Fiorinal®, Isollyl® Improved, Lanorinal®, Marnal®): Butalbital 50 mg, caffeine 40 mg, and aspirin 325 mg

Tablet, with acetaminophen:

Esgic®, Fioricet®, Repan®: Butalbital 50 mg, caffeine 40 mg, and acetaminophen 325 mg

Phrenilin®: Butalbital 50 mg and acetaminophen 325 mg

Sedapap-10®: Butalbital 50 mg and acetaminophen 650 mg

Tablet, with aspirin:

Axotal®: Butalbital 50 mg and aspirin 650 mg

B-A-C®: Butalbital 50 mg, caffeine 40 mg, and aspirin 650 mg

Fiorinal®, Isollyl® Improved, Lanorinal®, Marnal®: Butalbital 50 mg, caffeine 40 mg, and aspirin 325 mg

Butenafine *(byoo TEN a feen)*

U.S. Brand Names Mentax®

Synonyms Butenafine Hydrochloride

Therapeutic Category Antifungal Agent, Topical

Use Topical treatment of tinea pedis (athlete's foot), tinea cruris (jock itch), tinea corporis (ringworm), and tinea versicolor

Pregnancy Risk Factor B

Contraindications Hypersensitivity to butenafine or any component of the formulation

Warnings/Precautions Only for topical use (not ophthalmic, vaginal, or internal routes); patients sensitive to other allylamine antifungals may cross-react with butenafine; has not been studied in immunocompromised patients

Adverse Reactions

>1%: Dermatologic: Burning, stinging, irritation, erythema, pruritus (2%)

<1% (Limited to important or life-threatening): Contact dermatitis

Mechanism of Action Butenafine exerts antifungal activity by blocking squalene epoxidation, resulting in inhibition of ergosterol synthesis (antidermatophyte and *Sporothrix schenckii* activity). In higher concentrations, the drug disrupts fungal cell membranes (anticandidal activity).

Pharmacodynamics/Kinetics
Absorption: Minimally systemic
Metabolism: Hepatic; principle metabolite via hydroxylation
Half-life elimination: 35 hours
Time to peak, serum: 6 hours

Usual Dosage Children >12 years and Adults: Topical:
Tinea corporis, tinea cruris, or tinea versicolor: Apply once daily for 2 weeks to affected area and surrounding skin
Tinea pedis: Apply once daily for 4 weeks or twice daily for 7 days to affected area and surrounding skin (7-day regimen may have lower efficacy)

Monitoring Parameters Culture and KOH exam, clinical signs of tinea pedis

Patient Information Report any signs of rash or allergy to your physician immediately; do not apply other topical medications on the same area as butenafine unless directed by your physician

Dosage Forms Cream, as hydrochloride: 1% (15 g, 30 g)

♦ **Butenafine Hydrochloride** *see* Butenafine *on page 198*

♦ **Butisol Sodium**® *see* Butabarbital *on page 196*

Butoconazole (byoo toe KOE na zole)

Related Information
Treatment of Sexually Transmitted Diseases *on page 1609*
U.S. Brand Names Gynazole-1™; Mycelex®-3 [OTC]
Canadian Brand Names Femstat® One
Synonyms Butoconazole Nitrate
Therapeutic Category Antifungal Agent, Imidazole Derivative; Antifungal Agent, Vaginal
Use Local treatment of vulvovaginal candidiasis
Pregnancy Risk Factor C (use only in 2nd or 3rd trimester)
Pregnancy/Breast-Feeding Implications No adequate and well-controlled studies have been conducted in pregnant women. However, butoconazole has been used during pregnancy. Use should be limited to the 2nd and 3rd trimesters only. It is not known if butoconazole is excreted in human breast milk, use with caution if administered to a nursing woman.
Contraindications Hypersensitivity to butoconazole or any component of the formulation
Warnings/Precautions If irritation or sensitization occurs, discontinue use. Contains mineral oil which may weaken latex or rubber products (condoms, vaginal contraceptive diaphragms); do not use these products within 72 hours of treatment. HIV infection should be considered in sexually-active women with difficult to eradicate recurrent vaginal yeast infections. OTC product is not for use in women with a first-time vaginal yeast infection. Safety and efficacy in females <12 years have not been established.
Adverse Reactions
Gastrointestinal: Abdominal pain or cramping
Genitourinary: Pelvic pain; vulvar/vaginal burning, itching, soreness, and swelling
Stability Store at 15°C to 30°C (59°F to 86°F)
Mechanism of Action Increases cell membrane permeability in susceptible fungi (*Candida*)
Pharmacodynamics/Kinetics
Absorption: 2%
Metabolism: Not reported
Time to peak: 12-24 hours
Usual Dosage Adults:
Femstat®-3 [OTC]: Insert 1 applicatorful (~5 g) intravaginally at bedtime for 3 consecutive days
Gynazole-1™: Insert 1 applicatorful (~5 g) intravaginally as a single dose; treatment may need to be extended for up to 6 days in pregnant women (use in pregnancy during 2nd or 3rd trimester only)
Patient Information May cause burning or stinging on application; dispose of applicator after use. If symptoms of vaginitis persist, contact prescriber. Do not use OTC product if you have abdominal pain, fever, or foul-smelling discharge. Contact prescriber if infection does not clear within 3 days. Do not use tampons while using this medication. This medication contains mineral oil, which may cause damage to condoms or diaphragms; use another method of birth control during treatment.
Nursing Implications May cause burning or stinging on application; if symptoms of vaginitis persist, contact physician
Additional Information Gynazole-1™: This product is delivered in a base allowing the active ingredient to remain vaginally for 4 days. It is associated with less leakage and can therefore be applied at anytime during the day or night (per product information, Gynazole-1™).
Dosage Forms
Cream, vaginal, as nitrate:
Mycelex®-3: 2% (20 g) [with disposable applicator]
Gynazole-1™ [prefilled applicator]: 2% (5 g)

♦ **Butoconazole Nitrate** *see* Butoconazole *on page 199*

Butorphanol (byoo TOR fa nole)

Related Information
Narcotic Agonists Comparison *on page 1506*
U.S. Brand Names Stadol®; Stadol® NS
Canadian Brand Names Stadol NS™
Synonyms Butorphanol Tartrate
Therapeutic Category Analgesic, Narcotic
(Continued)

Butorphanol *(Continued)*

Use

Parenteral: Management of moderate to severe pain; preoperative medication; supplement to balanced anesthesia; management of pain during labor

Nasal spray: Management of moderate to severe pain, including migraine headache pain

Restrictions C-IV

Pregnancy Risk Factor C/D (prolonged use or high doses at term)

Contraindications Hypersensitivity to butorphanol or any component of the formulation; avoid use in opiate-dependent patients who have not been detoxified, may precipitate opiate withdrawal; pregnancy (prolonged use or high doses at term)

Warnings/Precautions May cause CNS depression; use with caution in patients with hepatic/renal dysfunction, may elevate CSF pressure, may increase cardiac workload; tolerance of drug dependence may result from extended use. Concurrent use of sumatriptan nasal spray and butorphanol nasal spray may increase risk of transient high blood pressure.

Adverse Reactions

>10%:

Central nervous system: Drowsiness (43%), dizziness (19%), insomnia (Stadol® NS)

Gastrointestinal: Nausea/vomiting (13%)

Respiratory: Nasal congestion (Stadol® NS)

1% to 10%:

Cardiovascular: Vasodilation, palpitations

Central nervous system: Lightheadedness, headache, lethargy, anxiety, confusion, euphoria, somnolence

Dermatologic: Pruritus

Gastrointestinal: Anorexia, constipation, xerostomia, stomach pain, unpleasant aftertaste

Neuromuscular & skeletal: Tremor, paresthesia, weakness

Ocular: Blurred vision

Otic: Ear pain, tinnitus

Respiratory: Bronchitis, cough, dyspnea, epistaxis, nasal irritation, pharyngitis, rhinitis, sinus congestion, sinusitis, upper respiratory infection

Miscellaneous: Diaphoresis (increased)

<1% (Limited to important or life-threatening): Dependence (with prolonged use), depression, difficulty speaking (transient), dyspnea, hallucinations, hypertension, nightmares, paradoxical CNS stimulation, rash, respiratory depression, syncope, tinnitus, vertigo, withdrawal symptoms

Stadol® NS: Apnea, chest pain, convulsions, delusions, depressions, edema, hypertension, shallow breathing, tachycardia

Overdosage/Toxicology Symptoms include respiratory depression, cardiac and CNS depression. Treatment includes airway support, establishment of an I.V. line and administration of naloxone 2 mg I.V. (0.01 mg/kg for children), with repeat administration as necessary, up to a total of 10 mg.

Drug Interactions

Increased Effect/Toxicity: Increased toxicity with CNS depressants, phenothiazines, barbiturates, skeletal muscle relaxants, alfentanil, guanabenz, and MAO inhibitors.

Ethanol/Nutrition/Herb Interactions

Ethanol: Avoid or limit ethanol (may increase CNS depression). Watch for sedation.

Herb/Nutraceutical: Avoid valerian, St John's wort, kava kava, gotu kola (may increase CNS depression).

Stability Store at room temperature, protect from freezing; **incompatible** when mixed in the same syringe with diazepam, dimenhydrinate, methohexital, pentobarbital, secobarbital, thiopental

Mechanism of Action Mixed narcotic agonist-antagonist with central analgesic actions; binds to opiate receptors in the CNS, causing inhibition of ascending pain pathways, altering the perception of and response to pain; produces generalized CNS depression

Pharmacodynamics/Kinetics

Onset of action: I.M.: 5-10 minutes; I.V.: <10 minutes; Nasal: Within 15 minutes

Peak effect: I.M.: 0.5-1 hour; I.V.: 4-5 minutes

Duration: I.M., I.V.: 3-4 hours; Nasal: 4-5 hours

Absorption: Rapid and well

Protein binding: 80%

Metabolism: Hepatic

Half-life elimination: 2.5-4 hours

Excretion: Primarily urine

Usual Dosage Adults:

Parenteral:

Moderate to severe pain:

I.M. Initial: 2 mg, may repeat every 3-4 hours as needed

I.V.: Initial: 1 mg, may repeat every 3-4 hours as needed

Preoperative medication: I.M.: 2 mg 60-90 minutes before surgery

Supplement to balanced anesthesia: I.V.: 2 mg shortly before induction and/or an incremental dose of 0.5-1 mg (up to 0.06 mg/kg), depending on previously administered sedative, analgesic, and hypnotic medications

Pain during labor (fetus >37 weeks gestation and no signs of fetal distress):

I.M., I.V.: 1-2 mg; may repeat in 4 hours

Note: Alternative analgesia should be used for pain associated with delivery or if delivery is anticipated within 4 hours

Nasal spray:

Moderate to severe pain (including migraine headache pain): Initial: 1 spray (~1 mg per spray) in 1 nostril; if adequate pain relief is not achieved within 60-90 minutes, an additional 1 spray in 1 nostril may be given; may repeat initial dose sequence in 3-4 hours after the last dose as needed

Alternatively, an initial dose of 2 mg (1 spray in each nostril) may be used in patients who will be able to remain recumbent (in the event drowsiness or dizziness occurs); additional 2 mg doses should not be given for 3-4 hours

Note: In some clinical trials, an initial dose of 2 mg (as 2 doses 1 hour apart or 2 mg initially - 1 spray in each nostril) has been used, followed by 1 mg in 1 hour; side effects were greater at these dosages

Dosage adjustment in renal impairment:
I.M., I.V.: Initial dosage should generally be $1/2$ of the recommended dose; repeated dosing must be based on initial response rather than fixed intervals, but generally should be at least 6 hours apart

Nasal spray: Initial dose should not exceed 1 mg; a second dose may be given after 90-120 minutes

Dosage adjustment in hepatic impairment:
I.M., I.V.: Initial dosage should generally be $1/2$ of the recommended dose; repeated dosing must be based on initial response rather than fixed intervals, but generally should be at least 6 hours apart

Nasal spray: Initial dose should not exceed 1 mg; a second dose may be given after 90-120 minutes

Elderly:
I.M., I.V.: Initial dosage should generally be $1/2$ of the recommended dose; repeated dosing must be based on initial response rather than fixed intervals, but generally should be at least 6 hours apart

Nasal Spray: Initial dose should not exceed 1 mg; a second dose may be given after 90-120 minutes

Administration Intranasal: Consider avoiding simultaneous intranasal migraine sprays; may want to separate by at least 30 minutes

Monitoring Parameters Pain relief, respiratory and mental status, blood pressure

Reference Range 0.7-1.5 ng/mL

Patient Information May cause drowsiness; avoid alcohol

Nursing Implications Observe for excessive sedation or confusion, respiratory depression; raise bed rails; aid with ambulation; consider avoiding simultaneous intranasal migraine sprays (may want to separate by at least 30 minutes)

Dosage Forms
Injection, solution, as tartrate [preservative free] (Stadol®): 1 mg/mL (1 mL); 2 mg/mL (1 mL, 2 mL)
Injection, solution, as tartrate [with preservative] (Stadol®): 2 mg/mL (10 mL)
Solution, intranasal spray, as tartrate (Stadol® NS): 10 mg/mL (2.5 mL) [14-15 doses]

♦ **Butorphanol Tartrate** *see Butorphanol on page 199*

♦ **BW-430C** *see Lamotrigine on page 773*

♦ **Byclomine®** *see Dicyclomine on page 397*

♦ **Bydramine® Cough Syrup [OTC]** *see DiphenhydrAMINE on page 414*

♦ **C2B8** *see Rituximab on page 1204*

♦ **C7E3** *see Abciximab on page 17*

♦ **311C90** *see Zolmitriptan on page 1443*

♦ **C-500-GR™ [OTC]** *see Ascorbic Acid on page 116*

Cabergoline (ca BER goe leen)

Related Information
Parkinson's Agents *on page 1513*

U.S. Brand Names Dostinex®

Therapeutic Category Ergot Alkaloid and Derivative

Use Treatment of hyperprolactinemic disorders, either idiopathic or due to pituitary adenomas

Unlabeled/Investigational Use Adjunct for the treatment of Parkinson's disease

Pregnancy Risk Factor B

Contraindications Hypersensitivity to cabergoline, any component of the formulation, or ergot derivatives; patients with uncontrolled hypertension

Warnings/Precautions Initial doses >1 mg may cause orthostatic hypotension. Use caution when patients are receiving other medications which may reduce blood pressure. Not indicated for the inhibition or suppression of physiologic lactation since it has been associated with cases of hypertension, stroke, and seizures. Because cabergoline is extensively metabolized by the liver, careful monitoring in patients with hepatic impairment is warranted. Female patients should instruct the physician if they are pregnant, become pregnant, or intend to become pregnant. Should not be used in patients with pregnancy-induced hypertension unless benefit outweighs potential risk. Do not give to postpartum women who are breast-feeding or planning to breast-feed. In all patients, prolactin concentrations should be monitored monthly until normalized.

Adverse Reactions
>10%:
Central nervous system: Headache (26%), dizziness (17%)
Gastrointestinal: Nausea (29%)
1% to 10%:
Body as whole: Asthenia (6%), fatigue (5%), syncope (1%), influenza-like symptoms (1%), malaise (1%), periorbital edema (1%), peripheral edema (1%)
Cardiovascular: Hot flashes (3%), hypotension (1%), dependent edema (1%), palpitations (1%)
Central nervous system: Vertigo (4%), depression (3%), somnolence (2%), anxiety (1%), insomnia (1%), impaired concentration (1%), nervousness (1%)
Dermatologic: Acne (1%), pruritus (1%)
Endocrine: Breast pain (2%), dysmenorrhea (1%)
Gastrointestinal: Constipation (7%), abdominal pain (5%), dyspepsia (5%), vomiting (4%), xerostomia (2%), diarrhea (2%), flatulence (2%), throat irritation (1%), toothache (1%), anorexia (1%)
(Continued)

201

Cabergoline *(Continued)*

Neuromuscular & skeletal: Pain (2%), arthralgia (1%), paresthesias (2%)
Ocular: Abnormal vision (1%)
Respiratory: Rhinitis (1%)

Overdosage/Toxicology An overdose may produce nasal congestion, syncope, hallucinations, or hypotension. Measures to support blood pressure should be taken if necessary.

Drug Interactions

Increased Effect/Toxicity: Additive hypotensive effects may occur when cabergoline is administered with antihypertensive medications; dosage adjustment of the antihypertensive medication may be required.

Decreased Effect: Dopamine antagonists (eg, phenothiazines, butyrophenones, thioxanthenes, or metoclopramide) may reduce the therapeutic effects of cabergoline and should not be used concomitantly.

Mechanism of Action Cabergoline is a long-acting dopamine receptor agonist with a high affinity for D_2 receptors; prolactin secretion by the anterior pituitary is predominantly under hypothalamic inhibitory control exerted through the release of dopamine

Pharmacodynamics/Kinetics

Distribution: Extensive, particularly to the pituitary
Protein binding: 40% to 42%
Metabolism: Extensively hepatic; minimal CYP450 metabolism
Half-life elimination: 63-69 hours
Time to peak: 2-3 hours

Usual Dosage Initial dose: Oral: 0.25 mg twice weekly; the dose may be increased by 0.25 mg twice weekly up to a maximum of 1 mg twice weekly according to the patient's serum prolactin level. Dosage increases should not occur more rapidly than every 4 weeks. Once a normal serum prolactin level is maintained for 6 months, the dose may be discontinued and prolactin levels monitored to determine if cabergoline is still required. The durability of efficacy beyond 24 months of therapy has not been established.

Elderly: No dosage recommendations suggested, but start at the low end of the dosage range

Patient Information Patient should be instructed to notify physician if she suspects she is pregnant, becomes pregnant, or intends to become pregnant during therapy with cabergoline. A pregnancy test should be done if there is any suspicion of pregnancy and continuation of treatment should be discussed with physician.

Additional Information Bromocriptine and cabergoline are the only drugs indicated for the treatment of hyperprolactinemia. In the largest comparative clinical trial, prolactin levels normalized in 77% of patients treated with cabergoline compared to 59% of patients treated with bromocriptine. In that trial, 3% of patients discontinued treatment due to adverse effects in the cabergoline group versus 12% of patients in the bromocriptine group. In addition to the improved safety and efficacy profile, cabergoline (administered twice weekly) is more convenient than bromocriptine (administered 1-3 times/day) for patients to take.

If the drug is used to prevent lactation, a single 1 mg dose is recommended on the first day after delivery. The drug is not approved for the inhibition of established lactation and should only be used to prevent lactation when there are medical reasons whereby which the potential benefits of therapy outweigh the risks, since it has been associated with cases of hypertension, stroke, and seizures.

Dosage Forms Tablet: 0.5 mg

♦ **Caelyx® (Can)** *see* DOXOrubicin *on page 443*

♦ **Cafatine®** *see* Ergotamine *on page 483*

♦ **Cafergor® (Can)** *see* Ergotamine *on page 483*

♦ **Cafergot®** *see* Ergotamine *on page 483*

♦ **Caffeine, Acetaminophen, and Aspirin** *see* Acetaminophen, Aspirin, and Caffeine *on page 26*

Caffeine and Sodium Benzoate *(KAF een & SOW dee um BEN zoe ate)*

Synonyms Sodium Benzoate and Caffeine

Therapeutic Category Diuretic, Miscellaneous

Use Emergency stimulant in acute circulatory failure, diuretic, relief of spinal puncture headache

Pregnancy Risk Factor C

Usual Dosage

Adults:
Stimulant/diuretic: I.M., I.V.: 500 mg, maximum single dose: 1 g
Spinal puncture headaches:
I.V.: 500 mg in 1000 mL NS infused over 1 hour, followed by 1000 mL NS infused over 1 hour; a second course of caffeine can be given for unrelieved headache pain in 4 hours.
Oral: 300 mg
Children: Stimulant: I.M., I.V., S.C.: 8 mg/kg every 4 hours as needed

Additional Information Complete prescribing information for this medication should be consulted for additional detail.

Dosage Forms Injection: Caffeine 125 mg and sodium benzoate 125 mg per mL (2 mL)

♦ **Caffeine, Aspirin, and Acetaminophen** *see* Acetaminophen, Aspirin, and Caffeine *on page 26*

♦ **Caffeine, Hydrocodone, Chlorpheniramine, Phenylephrine, and Acetaminophen** *see* Hydrocodone, Chlorpheniramine, Phenylephrine, Acetaminophen, and Caffeine *on page 682*

♦ **Caffeine, Orphenadrine, and Aspirin** *see* Orphenadrine, Aspirin, and Caffeine *on page 1015*

♦ **Calan®** *see* Verapamil *on page 1412*

♦ **Calan® SR** *see* Verapamil *on page 1412*

♦ **Cal Carb-HD® [OTC]** *see* Calcium Carbonate *on page 207*

- **Calci-Chew™ [OTC]** *see* Calcium Carbonate *on page 207*
- **Calciday-667® [OTC]** *see* Calcium Carbonate *on page 207*

Calcifediol (kal si fe DYE ole)

U.S. Brand Names Calderol®

Canadian Brand Names Calderol®

Synonyms 25-HCC; 25-Hydroxycholecalciferol; 25-Hydroxyvitamin D_3

Therapeutic Category Vitamin, Fat Soluble

Use Treatment and management of metabolic bone disease associated with chronic renal failure or hypocalcemia in patients on chronic renal dialysis

Pregnancy Risk Factor C (manufacturer); A/D (dose exceeding RDA recommendation) (expert analysis)

Contraindications Hypersensitivity to calcifediol or any component of the formulation; malabsorption syndrome; hypervitaminosis D; significantly decreased renal function; hypercalcemia; pregnancy (dose exceeding RDA)

Warnings/Precautions Adequate (supplemental) dietary calcium is necessary for clinical response to vitamin D; calcium-phosphate product (serum calcium times phosphorus) must not exceed 70; avoid hypercalcemia

Adverse Reactions Frequency not defined.

Cardiovascular: Hypotension, cardiac arrhythmias, hypertension
Central nervous system: Irritability, headache, somnolence, seizures (rare)
Dermatologic: Pruritus,
Endocrine & metabolic: Hypercalcemia, polydipsia, hypermagnesemia
Gastrointestinal: Nausea, vomiting, constipation, anorexia, pancreatitis, metallic taste, xerostomia
Hepatic: Elevated LFTs
Neuromuscular & skeletal: Myalgia, bone pain,
Ocular: Conjunctivitis, photophobia
Renal: Polyuria

Overdosage/Toxicology Toxicity rarely occurs from acute overdose. Symptoms of chronic overdose include hypercalcemia, hypercalciuria with weakness, altered mental status, GI upset, renal tubular injury, and occasionally cardiac arrhythmias. Following withdrawal of the drug, treatment consists of bed rest, liberal fluid intake, reduced calcium intake, and cathartic administration. Severe hypercalcemia requires I.V. hydration and forced diuresis. I.V. saline may increase excretion of calcium. Calcitonin, cholestyramine, prednisone, sodium EDTA, biphosphonates, and mithramycin have all been used successfully to treat the more resistant cases of vitamin D-induced hypercalcemia.

Drug Interactions

Increased Effect/Toxicity: The effect of calcifediol is increased with thiazide diuretics. Additive effect with antacids (magnesium).

Decreased Effect: The effect of calcifediol is decreased when taken with cholestyramine or colestipol.

Stability Store in light-resistant container

Mechanism of Action Vitamin D analog that (along with calcitonin and parathyroid hormone) regulates serum calcium homeostasis by promoting absorption of calcium and phosphorus in the small intestine; promotes renal tubule resorption of phosphate; increases rate of accretion and resorption in bone minerals

Pharmacodynamics/Kinetics

Absorption: Rapid from small intestines
Distribution: Activated in kidneys; stored in liver and fat depots
Half-life elimination: 12-22 days
Time to peak: Within 4 hours
Excretion: Feces

Usual Dosage Oral: Hepatic osteodystrophy:

Infants: 5-7 mcg/kg/day
Children and Adults: Usual dose: 20-100 mcg/day or 20-200 mcg every other day; titrate to obtain normal serum calcium/phosphate levels; increase dose at 4-week intervals; initial dose: 300-350 mcg/week, administered daily or on alternate days

Test Interactions ↑ calcium (S), cholesterol (S), magnesium, BUN, AST, ALT; ↓ alk phos

Patient Information Compliance with dose, diet, and calcium supplementation is essential; avoid taking magnesium supplements or magnesium-containing antacids; notify physician if weakness, lethargy, headache, and decreased appetite occur

Nursing Implications Monitor calcium and phosphate levels closely; monitor symptoms of hypercalcemia

Dosage Forms Capsule: 20 mcg, 50 mcg

- **Calciferol™** *see* Ergocalciferol *on page 481*
- **Calcijex™** *see* Calcitriol *on page 204*
- **Calcimar®** *see* Calcitonin *on page 204*
- **Calci-Mix™ [OTC]** *see* Calcium Carbonate *on page 207*

Calcipotriene (kal si POE try een)

U.S. Brand Names Dovonex®

Therapeutic Category Topical Skin Product; Vitamin, Fat Soluble

Use Treatment of moderate plaque psoriasis

Pregnancy Risk Factor C

Usual Dosage Adults: Topical: Apply in a thin film to the affected skin twice daily and rub in gently and completely

Additional Information Complete prescribing information for this medication should be consulted for additional detail.

Dosage Forms

Cream, topical: 0.005% (30 g, 60 g, 100 g)
Ointment, topical: 0.005% (30 g, 60 g, 100 g)
Solution, topical: 0.005% (60 mL)

♦ **Calcite-500 (Can)** *see* Calcium Carbonate *on page 207*

Calcitonin (kal si TOE nin)

U.S. Brand Names Calcimar®; Miacalcin®

Canadian Brand Names Calcimar®; Caltine®; Miacalcin® NS

Synonyms Calcitonin (Salmon)

Therapeutic Category Antidote, Hypercalcemia

Use Calcitonin (salmon): Treatment of Paget's disease of bone (osteitis deformans); adjunctive therapy for hypercalcemia; used in postmenopausal osteoporosis and osteogenesis imperfecta

Pregnancy Risk Factor C

Contraindications Hypersensitivity to salmon protein or gelatin diluent

Warnings/Precautions A skin test should be performed prior to initiating therapy of calcitonin salmon; have epinephrine immediately available for a possible hypersensitivity reaction

Adverse Reactions
>10%:
　　Cardiovascular: Facial flushing
　　Gastrointestinal: Nausea, diarrhea, anorexia
　　Local: Edema at injection site
1% to 10%:
　　Genitourinary: Polyuria
　　Neuromuscular & skeletal: Back/joint pain
　　Respiratory: Nasal bleeding/crusting (following intranasal administration)
<1% (Limited to important or life-threatening): Dyspnea

Overdosage/Toxicology Symptoms include nausea, vomiting, hypocalcemia, and tetany.

Drug Interactions
Decreased Effect: Calcitonin may be antagonized by calcium and vitamin D in treating hypercalcemia.

Stability
Salmon calcitonin: Injection: Store under refrigeration at 2°C to 6°C/36°F to 43°F; stable for up to 2 weeks at room temperature; NS has been recommended for the dilution to prepare a skin test
Salmon calcitonin: Nasal: Store unopened bottle under refrigeration at 2°C to 8°C; once the pump has been activated, store at room temperature

Mechanism of Action Structurally similar to human calcitonin; it directly inhibits osteoclastic bone resorption; promotes the renal excretion of calcium, phosphate, sodium, magnesium and potassium by decreasing tubular reabsorption; increases the jejunal secretion of water, sodium, potassium, and chloride

Pharmacodynamics/Kinetics
Hypercalcemia:
　　Onset of action: ~2 hours
　　Duration: 6-8 hours
Distribution: Does not cross placenta
Half-life elimination: S.C.: 1.2 hours
Excretion: Urine (as inactive metabolites)

Usual Dosage Salmon calcitonin:
Children: Dosage not established
Adults:
　　Paget's disease: I.M., S.C.: Initial: 100 units/day; maintenance: 50 units/day or 50-100 units every 1-3 days
　　Hypercalcemia: Initial: I.M., S.C.: 4 units/kg every 12 hours; may increase up to 8 units/kg every 12 hours to a maximum of every 6 hours
　　Osteogenesis imperfecta: I.M., S.C.: 2 units/kg 3 times/week
　　Postmenopausal osteoporosis:
　　　　I.M., S.C.: 100 units/day
　　　　Intranasal: 200 units (1 spray)/day

Dietary Considerations Adequate vitamin D and calcium intake is essential for osteoporosis. Patients with Paget's disease and hypercalcemia should follow a low calcium diet as prescribed.

Monitoring Parameters Serum electrolytes and calcium; alkaline phosphatase and 24-hour urine collection for hydroxyproline excretion (Paget's disease); serum calcium

Reference Range Therapeutic: <19 pg/mL (SI: 19 ng/L) basal, depending on the assay

Patient Information Nasal spray: Notify physician if you develop significant nasal irritation. To activate the pump, hold the bottle upright and depress the two white side arms toward the bottle six times until a faint spray is emitted. The pump is activated once this first faint spray has been emitted; at this point, firmly place the nozzle into the bottle. It is not necessary to reactivate the pump before each daily use. Alternate nostrils with the spray formulation.

Nursing Implications Skin test should be performed prior to administration of salmon calcitonin; refrigerate; I.M. administration is preferred if the volume to injection exceeds 2 mL

Dosage Forms
Injection, salmon calcitonin (Calcimar®): 200 units/mL (2 mL)
Solution, intranasal, salmon calcitonin [spray] (Miacalcin®): 200 units/activation (0.09 mL/dose) (2 mL glass bottle with pump)

♦ **Calcitonin (Salmon)** *see* Calcitonin *on page 204*

Calcitriol (kal si TRYE ole)

Related Information
Antacid Drug Interactions *on page 1477*
U.S. Brand Names Calcijex™; Rocaltrol®
Canadian Brand Names Rocaltrol®

Synonyms 1,25 Dihydroxycholecalciferol

Therapeutic Category Vitamin, Fat Soluble

Use Management of hypocalcemia in patients on chronic renal dialysis; reduce elevated parathyroid hormone levels

Unlabeled/Investigational Use Decrease severity of psoriatic lesions in psoriatic vulgaris; vitamin D resistant rickets

Pregnancy Risk Factor C (manufacturer); A/D (dose exceeding RDA recommendation) (expert analysis)

Contraindications Hypercalcemia; vitamin D toxicity; abnormal sensitivity to the effects of vitamin D; malabsorption syndrome; pregnancy (dose exceeding RDA)

Warnings/Precautions Adequate dietary (supplemental) calcium is necessary for clinical response to vitamin D; maintain adequate fluid intake; calcium-phosphate product (serum calcium times phosphorus) must not exceed 70; avoid hypercalcemia or use with renal function impairment and secondary hyperparathyroidism

Adverse Reactions
>10%: Endocrine & metabolic: Hypercalcemia (33%)
Frequency not defined:
Cardiovascular: Cardiac arrhythmias, hypertension, hypotension
Central nervous system: Headache, irritability, seizures (rare), somnolence
Dermatologic: Pruritus
Endocrine & metabolic: Hypermagnesemia, polydipsia
Gastrointestinal: Anorexia, constipation, metallic taste, nausea, pancreatitis, vomiting, xerostomia
Hepatic: Elevated LFTs
Neuromuscular & skeletal: Bone pain, myalgia
Ocular: Conjunctivitis, photophobia
Renal: Polyuria

Overdosage/Toxicology Toxicity rarely occurs from acute overdose. Symptoms of chronic overdose include hypercalcemia, hypercalciuria with weakness, altered mental status, GI upset, renal tubular injury, and occasionally cardiac arrhythmias. Following withdrawal of the drug, treatment consists of bed rest, liberal fluid intake, reduced calcium intake, and cathartic administration. Severe hypercalcemia requires I.V. hydration and forced diuresis. I.V. saline may increase excretion of calcium. Calcitonin, cholestyramine, prednisone, sodium EDTA, biphosphonates, and mithramycin have all been used successfully to treat the more resistant cases of vitamin D-induced hypercalcemia.

Drug Interactions
Increased Effect/Toxicity: Risk of hypercalcemia with thiazide diuretics. Risk of hyper-magnesemia with magnesium-containing antacids.
Decreased Effect: Cholestyramine and colestipol decrease absorption/effect of calcitriol.

Stability Store in tight, light-resistant container; calcitriol degrades upon prolonged exposure to light

Mechanism of Action Promotes absorption of calcium in the intestines and retention at the kidneys thereby increasing calcium levels in the serum; decreases excessive serum phosphatase levels, parathyroid hormone levels, and decreases bone resorption; increases renal tubule phosphate resorption

Pharmacodynamics/Kinetics
Onset of action: ~2-6 hours
Duration: 3-5 days
Absorption: Oral: Rapid
Metabolism: Primarily to 1,24,25-trihydroxycholecalciferol and 1,24,25-trihydroxy ergocalciferol
Half-life elimination: 3-8 hours
Excretion: Primarily feces; urine (4% to 6%)

Usual Dosage Individualize dosage to maintain calcium levels of 9-10 mg/dL
Renal failure:
Children:
Oral: 0.25-2 mcg/day have been used (with hemodialysis); 0.014-0.041 mcg/kg/day (not receiving hemodialysis); increases should be made at 4- to 8-week intervals
I.V.: 0.01-0.05 mcg/kg 3 times/week if undergoing hemodialysis
Adults:
Oral: 0.25 mcg/day or every other day (may require 0.5-1 mcg/day); increases should be made at 4- to 8-week intervals
I.V.: 0.5 mcg/day 3 times/week (may require from 0.5-3 mcg/day given 3 times/week) if undergoing hemodialysis
Hypoparathyroidism/pseudohypoparathyroidism: Oral (evaluate dosage at 2- to 4-week intervals):
Children:
<1 year: 0.04-0.08 mcg/kg once daily
1-5 years: 0.25-0.75 mcg once daily
Children >6 years and Adults: 0.5-2 mcg once daily
Vitamin D-dependent rickets: Children and Adults: Oral: 1 mcg once daily
Vitamin D-resistant rickets (familial hypophosphatemia): Children and Adults: Oral: Initial: 0.015-0.02 mcg/kg once daily; maintenance: 0.03-0.06 mcg/kg once daily; maximum dose: 2 mcg once daily
Hypocalcemia in premature infants: Oral: 1 mcg once daily for 5 days
Hypocalcemic tetany in premature infants: I.V.: 0.05 mcg/kg once daily for 5-12 days
Elderly: No dosage recommendations, but start at the lower end of the dosage range

Monitoring Parameters Monitor symptoms of hypercalcemia (weakness, fatigue, somnolence, headache, anorexia, dry mouth, metallic taste, nausea, vomiting, cramps, diarrhea, muscle pain, bone pain and irritability)

Reference Range Calcium (serum) 9-10 mg/dL (4.5-5 mEq/L) but do not include the I.V. dosages; phosphate: 2.5-5 mg/dL

Test Interactions ↑ calcium, cholesterol, magnesium, BUN, AST, ALT, calcium (S), cholesterol (S); ↓ alkaline phosphatase
(Continued)

Calcitriol *(Continued)*

Patient Information Compliance with dose, diet, and calcium supplementation is essential; notify physician if weakness, lethargy, headache, and decreased appetite occur; avoid taking magnesium supplements or magnesium-containing antacids

Nursing Implications
May be administered as a bolus dose I.V. through the catheter at the end of hemodialysis
Monitor serum calcium and phosphate levels during therapy

Dosage Forms
Capsule: 0.25 mcg, 0.5 mcg
Injection: 1 mcg/mL (1 mL); 2 mcg/mL (1 mL)
Solution, oral: 1 mcg/mL

Calcium Acetate *(KAL see um AS e tate)*

U.S. Brand Names PhosLo®

Therapeutic Category Antidote, Hyperphosphatemia; Calcium Salt; Electrolyte Supplement, Oral; Electrolyte Supplement, Parenteral

Use
Oral: Control of hyperphosphatemia in end-stage renal failure; does not promote aluminum absorption
I.V.: Calcium supplementation in parenteral nutrition therapy

Pregnancy Risk Factor C

Contraindications Hypersensitivity to any component of the formulation; hypercalcemia, renal calculi

Warnings/Precautions Calcium absorption is impaired in achlorhydria (common in elderly - try alternate salt, administer with food); administration is followed by increased gastric acid secretion within 2 hours of administration; while hypercalcemia and hypercalciuria may result when therapeutic replacement amounts are given for prolonged periods, they are most likely to occur in hypoparathyroid patients receiving high doses of vitamin D

Adverse Reactions
Mild hypercalcemia (calcium: >10.5 mg/dL to ≤12 mg/dL) may be asymptomatic or manifest itself as constipation, anorexia, nausea, and vomiting
More severe hypercalcemia (calcium: >12 mg/dL) is associated with confusion, delirium, stupor, and coma
Postmarketing and/or case reports: Pruritus, allergic reaction

Overdosage/Toxicology Acute single ingestions of calcium salts may produce mild gastrointestinal distress, but hypercalcemia or other toxic manifestations are extremely unlikely. Treatment is supportive.

Drug Interactions
Increased Effect/Toxicity: High doses of calcium with thiazide diuretics may result in milk-alkali syndrome and hypercalcemia; monitor response. Calcium salts may decrease T_4 absorption; separate dose from levothyroxine by at least 4 hours. Calcium acetate may potentiate digoxin toxicity.
Decreased Effect: Absorption of tetracycline, atenolol (and potentially other beta-blockers), iron, quinolone antibiotics, alendronate, sodium fluoride, and zinc absorption may be significantly decreased; space administration times. Effects of calcium channel blockers (eg, verapamil) effects may be diminished. Polystyrene sulfonate's potassium-binding ability may be reduced; avoid concurrent administration.

Stability Admixture incompatibilities: Carbonates, phosphates, sulfates, tartrates

Mechanism of Action Combines with dietary phosphate to form insoluble calcium phosphate which is excreted in feces

Pharmacodynamics/Kinetics
Absorption: Requires vitamin D; minimal unless chronic, high doses are given; calcium is absorbed in soluble, ionized form; solubility of calcium is increased in an acid environment
Distribution: Crosses placenta; enters breast milk
Excretion: Primarily feces (as unabsorbed calcium); urine (20%)

Usual Dosage
Dietary Reference Intake:
0-6 months: 210 mg/day
7-12 months: 270 mg/day
1-3 years: 500 mg/day
4-8 years: 800 mg/day
Adults, Male/Female:
9-18 years: 1300 mg/day
19-50 years: 1000 mg/day
≥51 years: 1200 mg/day
Female: Pregnancy: Same as for Adults, Male/Female
Female: Lactating: Same as for Adults, Male/Female

Oral: Adults, on dialysis: Initial: 1334 mg with each meal, can be increased gradually to bring the serum calcium value <6 mg/dL as long as hypercalcemia does not develop (usual dose: 2001-2868 mg calcium acetate with each meal); do not give additional calcium supplements
I.V.: Dose is dependent on the requirements of the individual patient; in central venous total parental nutrition (TPN), calcium is administered at a concentration of 5 mEq (10 mL)/L of TPN solution; the additive maintenance dose in neonatal TPN is 0.5 mEq calcium/kg/day (1.0 mL/kg/day)
Neonates: 70-200 mg/kg/day
Infants and Children: 70-150 mg/kg/day
Adolescents: 18-35 mg/kg/day

Dietary Considerations Oral dosage forms must be administered with meals to be effective.

Administration Administer with meals.

Monitoring Parameters Serum calcium, serum phosphate; for control of hypophosphatemia, serum calcium times phosphate should not exceed 66

Reference Range

Serum calcium: 8.4-10.2 mg/dL

Due to a poor correlation between the serum ionized calcium (free) and total serum calcium, particularly in states of low albumin or acid/base imbalances, direct measurement of ionized calcium is recommended

In low albumin states, the corrected **total** serum calcium may be estimated by this equation (assuming a normal albumin of 4 g/dL)

Corrected total calcium = total serum calcium + 0.8 (4.0 - measured serum albumin)

or

Corrected calcium = measured calcium - measured albumin + 4.0

Patient Information Can take with food; do not take calcium supplements within 1-2 hours of taking other medicine by mouth or eating large amounts of fiber-rich foods; do not use nonprescription antacids or drink large amounts of alcohol, caffeine-containing beverages, or use tobacco

Additional Information Calcium acetate binds to phosphorus in the GI tract better than other calcium salts due to its lower solubility and subsequent reduced absorption and increased formation of calcium phosphate.

12.7 mEq calcium/g; 250 mg/g elemental calcium (25% elemental calcium)

Dosage Forms Elemental calcium listed in brackets

Capsule (PhosLo®): 333.5 mg [84.5 mg]; 667 mg [169 mg]

Gelcap (PhosLo®): 667 mg [169 mg]

Injection: 0.5 mEq calcium/mL [calcium acetate/mL 39.55 mg] (10 mL, 50 mL, 100 mL)

♦ **Calcium Acetate and Aluminum Sulfate** *see* Aluminum Sulfate and Calcium Acetate *on page 64*

Calcium Carbonate (KAL see um KAR bun ate)

U.S. Brand Names Alka-Mints® [OTC]; Amitone® [OTC]; Cal Carb-HD® [OTC]; Calci-Chew™ [OTC]; Calciday-667® [OTC]; Calci-Mix™ [OTC]; Cal-Plus® [OTC]; Caltrate® 600 [OTC]; Caltrate, Jr.® [OTC]; Chooz® [OTC]; Dicarbosil® [OTC]; Equilet® [OTC]; Florical® [OTC]; Gencalc® 600 [OTC]; Mallamint® [OTC]; Nephro-Calci® [OTC]; Os-Cal® 500 [OTC]; Oyst-Cal 500 [OTC]; Oystercal® 500; Rolaids® Calcium Rich [OTC]; Tums® [OTC]; Tums® E-X Extra Strength Tablet [OTC]; Tums® Ultra [OTC]

Canadian Brand Names Apo®-Cal; Calcite-500; Caltrate®; Os-Cal®

Therapeutic Category Antacid; Antidote, Hyperphosphatemia; Calcium Salt; Electrolyte Supplement, Oral

Use As an antacid, and treatment and prevention of calcium deficiency or hyperphosphatemia (eg, osteoporosis, osteomalacia, mild/moderate renal insufficiency, hypoparathyroidism, postmenopausal osteoporosis, rickets); has been used to bind phosphate

Pregnancy Risk Factor C

Pregnancy/Breast-Feeding Implications Available evidence suggests safe use during pregnancy and breast-feeding

Contraindications Hypercalcemia, renal calculi, hypophosphatemia

Warnings/Precautions Calcium carbonate absorption is impaired in achlorhydria (common in elderly - use alternate salt, administer with food); administration is followed by increased gastric acid secretion within 2 hours of administration; while hypercalcemia and hypercalciuria may result when therapeutic replacement amounts are given for prolonged periods, they are most likely to occur in hypoparathyroid patients receiving high doses of vitamin D

Adverse Reactions Well tolerated

1% to 10%:

Central nervous system: Headache

Endocrine & metabolic: Hypophosphatemia, hypercalcemia

Gastrointestinal: Constipation, laxative effect, acid rebound, nausea, vomiting, anorexia, abdominal pain, xerostomia, flatulence

Miscellaneous: Milk-alkali syndrome with very high, chronic dosing and/or renal failure (headache, nausea, irritability, and weakness or alkalosis, hypercalcemia, renal impairment)

Overdosage/Toxicology Acute single ingestions of calcium salts may produce mild gastrointestinal distress, but hypercalcemia or other toxic manifestations are extremely unlikely. Treatment is supportive.

Drug Interactions

Increased Effect/Toxicity: High doses of calcium with thiazide diuretics may result in milk-alkali syndrome and hypercalcemia; monitor response. Calcium salts may decrease T_4 absorption; separate dose from levothyroxine by at least 4 hours. Calcium acetate may potentiate digoxin toxicity.

Decreased Effect: Absorption of tetracycline, atenolol (and potentially other beta-blockers), iron, quinolone antibiotics, alendronate, sodium fluoride, and zinc absorption may be significantly decreased; space administration times. Effects of calcium channel blockers (eg, verapamil) effects may be diminished. Polystyrene sulfonate's potassium-binding ability may be reduced; avoid concurrent administration.

Ethanol/Nutrition/Herb Interactions Food: Food may increase calcium absorption. Calcium may decrease iron absorption. Bran, foods high in oxalates, or whole grain cereals may decrease calcium absorption.

Stability Admixture **incompatibilities** include carbonates, phosphates, sulfates, tartrates

Mechanism of Action As dietary supplement, used to prevent or treat negative calcium balance; in osteoporosis, it helps to prevent or decrease the rate of bone loss. The calcium in calcium salts moderates nerve and muscle performance and allows normal cardiac function. Also used to treat hyperphosphatemia in patients with advanced renal insufficiency by combining with dietary phosphate to form insoluble calcium phosphate, which is excreted in feces. Calcium salts as antacids neutralize gastric acidity resulting in increased gastric an duodenal bulb pH; they additionally inhibit proteolytic activity of peptic if the pH is increased >4 and increase lower esophageal sphincter tone.

(Continued)

CALCIUM CARBONATE AND MAGNESIUM HYDROXIDE

Calcium Carbonate *(Continued)*

Pharmacodynamics/Kinetics

Absorption: Requires vitamin D; minimal unless chronic, high doses are given; calcium is absorbed in soluble, ionized form; solubility of calcium is increased in an acid environment

Distribution: Crosses placenta; enters breast milk

Excretion: Primarily feces (as unabsorbed calcium); urine (20%)

Usual Dosage Oral (dosage is in terms of elemental calcium):

Dietary Reference Intake:

0-6 months: 210 mg/day

7-12 months: 270 mg/day

1-3 years: 500 mg/day

4-8 years: 800 mg/day

Adults, Male/Female:

9-18 years: 1300 mg/day

19-50 years: 1000 mg/day

≥51 years: 1200 mg/day

Female: Pregnancy: Same as for Adults, Male/Female

Female: Lactating: Same as for Adults, Male/Female

Hypocalcemia (dose depends on clinical condition and serum calcium level): Dose expressed in mg of **elemental calcium**

Neonates: 50-150 mg/kg/day in 4-6 divided doses; not to exceed 1 g/day

Children: 45-65 mg/kg/day in 4 divided doses

Adults: 1-2 g or more/day in 3-4 divided doses

Adults:

Dietary supplementation: 500 mg to 2 g divided 2-4 times/day

Antacid: Dosage based on acid-neutralizing capacity of specific product; generally, 1-2 tablets or 5-10 mL every 2 hours; maximum: 7000 mg calcium carbonate per 24 hours; specific product labeling should be consulted

Adults >51 years: Osteoporosis: 1200 mg/day

Dosing adjustment in renal impairment: Cl_{cr} <25 mL/minute: Dosage adjustments may be necessary depending on the serum calcium levels

Dietary Considerations As a dietary supplement, should be given with meals to increase absorption. May decrease iron absorption, so should be administered 1-2 hours before or after iron supplementation; limit intake of with bran, foods high in oxalates or whole grain cereals which may decrease calcium absorption.

Reference Range

Serum calcium: 8.4-10.2 mg/dL: Monitor plasma calcium levels if using calcium salts as electrolyte supplements for deficiency

Due to a poor correlation between the serum ionized calcium (free) and total serum calcium, particularly in states of low albumin or acid/base imbalances, direct measurement of ionized calcium is recommended

In low albumin states, the corrected **total** serum calcium may be estimated by: Corrected total calcium = total serum calcium + 0.8 (4.0 - measured serum albumin)

Test Interactions ↑ calcium (S); ↓ magnesium

Patient Information Shake suspension well; chew tablets thoroughly; take with large quantities of water or juice; do not take calcium supplements within 1-2 hours of taking other medicine by mouth or eating large amounts of fiber-rich foods; do not take other antacids or calcium supplements or drink large amounts of alcohol or caffeine-containing beverages; if the maximum dosage of antacids is required for >2 weeks, consult your physician

Nursing Implications Monitor serum calcium levels

Additional Information 20 mEq calcium/g; 400 mg elemental calcium/g calcium carbonate (40% elemental calcium)

Dosage Forms Elemental calcium listed in brackets

Capsule: 1500 mg [600 mg]

Calci-Mix™: 1250 mg [500 mg]

Florical®: 364 mg [145.6 mg] with sodium fluoride 8.3 mg

Powder (Cal Carb-HD®): 6.5 g/packet [2.6 g]

Suspension, oral: 1250 mg/5 mL [500 mg]

Tablet: 650 mg [260 mg], 1500 mg [600 mg]

Calciday-667®: 667 mg [267 mg]

Cal-Plus®, Caltrate® 600, Gencalc® 600, Nephro-Calci®: 1500 mg [600 mg]

Florical®: 364 mg [145.6 mg] with sodium fluoride 8.3 mg

Os-Cal® 500, Oyst-Cal 500, Oystercal® 500: 1250 mg [500 mg]

Tablet, chewable:

Alka-Mints®: 850 mg [340 mg]

Amitone®: 350 mg [140 mg]

Calci-Chew™, Os-Cal® 500: 1.25 g [500 mg]

Caltrate, Jr.®: 750 mg [300 mg]

Chooz®, Dicarbosil®, Equilet®, Tums®: 500 mg [200 mg]

Mallamint®: 420 mg [168 mg]

Rolaids® Calcium Rich: 550 mg [220 mg]

Tums® E-X Extra Strength: 750 mg [300 mg]

Tums® Ultra®: 1000 mg [400 mg]

Calcium Carbonate and Magnesium Hydroxide

(KAL see um KAR bun ate & mag NEE zhum hye DROKS ide)

U.S. Brand Names Mylanta® Gelcaps® [OTC]; Mylanta® Tablets [OTC]; Mylanta® Ultra Tablet [OTC]; Rolaids® [OTC]

Synonyms Magnesium Hydroxide and Calcium Carbonate

Therapeutic Category Antacid

Use Hyperacidity

Usual Dosage Adults: Oral: 2-4 tablets between meals, at bedtime, or as directed by healthcare provider

Additional Information Complete prescribing information for this medication should be consulted for additional detail.

Dosage Forms
Gelcap: Calcium carbonate 550 mg and magnesium hydroxide 125 mg
Tablet, chewable:
Mylanta®: Calcium carbonate 350 mg and magnesium hydroxide 150 mg
Mylanta® Ultra: Calcium carbonate 700 mg and magnesium hydroxide 300 mg
Rolaids®: Calcium carbonate 550 mg and magnesium hydroxide 110 mg

♦ **Calcium Carbonate, Magnesium Hydroxide, and Famotidine** *see* Famotidine, Calcium Carbonate, and Magnesium Hydroxide *on page 544*
♦ **Calcium Channel Blockers Comparison** *see page 1494*

Calcium Chloride (KAL see um KLOR ide)

Therapeutic Category Calcium Salt; Electrolyte Supplement, Parenteral

Use Cardiac resuscitation when epinephrine fails to improve myocardial contractions, cardiac disturbances of hyperkalemia, hypocalcemia, or calcium channel blocking agent toxicity; emergent treatment of hypocalcemic tetany, treatment of hypermagnesemia

Pregnancy Risk Factor C

Contraindications In ventricular fibrillation during cardiac resuscitation, hypercalcemia, and in patients with risk of digitalis toxicity, renal or cardiac disease; not recommended in treatment of asystole and electromechanical dissociation

Warnings/Precautions Avoid too rapid I.V. administration (<1 mL/minute) and extravasation; use with caution in digitalized patients, respiratory failure, or acidosis; hypercalcemia may occur in patients with renal failure, and frequent determination of serum calcium is necessary; avoid metabolic acidosis (ie, administer only 2-3 days then change to another calcium salt)

Adverse Reactions <1% (Limited to important or life-threatening): Bradycardia, cardiac arrhythmias, coma, decreased serum magnesium, elevated serum amylase, erythema, hypercalcemia, hypercalciuria, hypotension, lethargy, mania, muscle weakness, syncope, tissue necrosis, vasodilation, ventricular fibrillation

Overdosage/Toxicology Symptoms include lethargy, nausea, vomiting, and coma. Following withdrawal of the drug, treatment consists of bed rest, liberal fluid intake, reduced calcium intake, and cathartic administration. Severe hypercalcemia requires I.V. hydration and forced diuresis. Urine output should be monitored and maintained at >3 mL/kg/hour. I.V. saline and natriuretic agents (eg, furosemide) can quickly and significantly increase excretion of calcium.

Drug Interactions
Increased Effect/Toxicity: High doses of calcium with thiazide diuretics may result in milk-alkali syndrome and hypercalcemia; monitor response. Calcium may potentiate digoxin toxicity.
Decreased Effect: Effects of calcium channel blockers (eg, verapamil) effects may be diminished.

Stability
Do not refrigerate solutions; IVPB solutions/I.V. infusion solutions are stable for 24 hours at room temperature
Maximum concentration in parenteral nutrition solutions: 15 mEq/L of calcium and 30 mmol/L of phosphate
Incompatible with sodium bicarbonate, carbonates, phosphates, sulfates, and tartrates

Mechanism of Action Moderates nerve and muscle performance via action potential excitation threshold regulation

Pharmacodynamics/Kinetics
Distribution: Crosses placenta; enters breast milk
Excretion: Primarily feces (as unabsorbed calcium); urine (20%)

Usual Dosage Note: Calcium chloride is 3 times as potent as calcium gluconate
Cardiac arrest in the presence of hyperkalemia or hypocalcemia, magnesium toxicity, or calcium antagonist toxicity: I.V.:
Infants and Children: 20 mg/kg; may repeat in 10 minutes if necessary
Adults: 2-4 mg/kg (10% solution), repeated every 10 minutes if necessary
Hypocalcemia: I.V.:
Children (manufacturer's recommendation): 2.7-5 mg/kg/dose every 4-6 hours
Alternative pediatric dosing: Infants and Children: 10-20 mg/kg/dose (infants <1 mEq; children 1-7 mEq), repeat every 4-6 hours if needed
Adults: 500 mg to 1 g (7-14 mEq)/dose repeated every 4-6 hours if needed
Hypocalcemic tetany: I.V.:
Infants and Children: 10 mg/kg (0.5-0.7 mEq/kg) over 5-10 minutes; may repeat after 6-8 hours or follow with an infusion with a maximum dose of 200 mg/kg/day
Adults: 1 g over 10-30 minutes; may repeat after 6 hours
Hypocalcemia secondary to citrated blood transfusion: I.V.:
Neonates, Infants, and Children: Give 0.45 mEq **elemental** calcium for each 100 mL citrated blood infused
Adults: 1.35 mEq calcium with each 100 mL of citrated blood infused
Dosing adjustment in renal impairment: Cl_{cr} <25 mL/minute: Dosage adjustments may be necessary depending on the serum calcium levels

Administration Rapid I.V. injection at a maximum rate of 50 mg/minute; for I.V. infusion, dilute to a maximum concentration of 20 mg/mL and infuse over 1 hour or no greater than 45-90 mg/kg/hour (0.6-1.2 mEq/kg/hour); administration via a central or deep vein is preferred

Reference Range
Serum calcium: 8.4-10.2 mg/dL
Due to a poor correlation between the serum ionized calcium (free) and total serum calcium, particularly in states of low albumin or acid/base imbalances, direct measurement of ionized calcium is recommended
In low albumin states, the corrected **total** serum calcium may be estimated by this equation (assuming a normal albumin of 4 g/dL)

(Continued)

Calcium Chloride *(Continued)*

Corrected total calcium = total serum calcium + 0.8 (4.0 - measured serum albumin)
or
Corrected calcium = measured calcium - measured albumin + 4.0
Serum/plasma chloride: 95-108 mEq/L

Test Interactions ↑ calcium (S); ↓ magnesium

Nursing Implications Do not inject calcium chloride I.M. or administer S.C. or use scalp, small hand or foot veins for I.V. administration since severe necrosis and sloughing may occur. Monitor EKG if calcium is infused faster than 2.5 mEq/minute; usual: 0.7-1.5 mEq/minute (0.5-1 mL/minute); **stop the infusion if the patient complains of pain or discomfort.** Warm to body temperature; administer slowly, do not exceed 1 mL/minute (inject into ventricular cavity - not myocardium); **do not infuse calcium chloride in the same I.V. line as phosphate-containing solutions**.

Extravasation treatment (example):
Hyaluronidase: Add 1 mL NS to 150 unit vial to make 150 units/mL of concentration; mix 0.1 mL of above with 0.9 mL NS in 1 mL syringe to make final concentration = 15 units/mL

Additional Information 14 mEq calcium/g (10 mL); 270 mg elemental calcium/g calcium chloride (27% elemental calcium)

Dosage Forms Elemental calcium listed in brackets
Injection: 10% = 100 mg/mL [27.2 mg/mL, 1.36 mEq/mL] (10 mL)

♦ **Calcium Disodium Edetate** *see* Edetate Calcium Disodium *on page 456*
♦ **Calcium Disodium Versenate®** *see* Edetate Calcium Disodium *on page 456*
♦ **Calcium EDTA** *see* Edetate Calcium Disodium *on page 456*

Calcium Glubionate *(KAL see um gloo BYE oh nate)*

U.S. Brand Names Neo-Calglucon® [OTC]

Therapeutic Category Calcium Salt

Use Adjunct in treatment and prevention of postmenopausal osteoporosis; treatment and prevention of calcium depletion or hyperphosphatemia (eg, osteoporosis, osteomalacia, mild/moderate renal insufficiency, hypoparathyroidism, rickets)

Pregnancy Risk Factor C

Contraindications Hypercalcemia, renal calculi, ventricular fibrillation

Warnings/Precautions Calcium absorption is impaired in achlorhydria (common in elderly - try alternate salt, administer with food); administration is followed by increased gastric acid secretion within 2 hours of administration; while hypercalcemia and hypercalciuria may result when therapeutic replacement amounts are given for prolonged periods, they are most likely to occur in hypoparathyroid patients receiving high doses of vitamin D

Adverse Reactions
Mild hypercalcemia (calcium: >10.5 mg/dL) may be asymptomatic or manifest itself as constipation, anorexia, nausea, and vomiting
More severe hypercalcemia (calcium: >12 mg/dL) is associated with confusion, delirium, stupor, and coma

<1% (Limited to important or life-threatening): Abdominal pain, anorexia, constipation, headache, hypercalcemia, hypophosphatemia, nausea, thirst, vomiting

Overdosage/Toxicology Acute single ingestions of calcium salts may produce mild gastrointestinal distress, but hypercalcemia or other toxic manifestations are extremely unlikely. Treatment is supportive.

Drug Interactions
Increased Effect/Toxicity: High doses of calcium with thiazide diuretics may result in milk-alkali syndrome and hypercalcemia; monitor response. Calcium salts may decrease T_4 absorption; separate dose from levothyroxine by at least 4 hours. Calcium acetate may potentiate digoxin toxicity.
Decreased Effect: Absorption of tetracycline, atenolol (and potentially other beta-blockers), iron, quinolone antibiotics, alendronate, sodium fluoride, and zinc absorption may be significantly decreased; space administration times. Effects of calcium channel blockers (eg, verapamil) effects may be diminished. Polystyrene sulfonate's potassium-binding ability may be reduced; avoid concurrent administration.

Ethanol/Nutrition/Herb Interactions Food: Food may increase calcium absorption. Calcium may decrease iron absorption. Bran, foods high in oxalates, or whole grain cereals may decrease calcium absorption.

Mechanism of Action As dietary supplement, used to prevent or treat negative calcium balance; in osteoporosis, it helps to prevent or decrease the rate of bone loss. The calcium in calcium salts moderates nerve and muscle performance and allows normal cardiac function.

Pharmacodynamics/Kinetics
Absorption: Requires vitamin D; minimal unless chronic, high doses are given; calcium is absorbed in soluble, ionized form; solubility of calcium is increased in an acid environment
Distribution: Crosses placenta; enters breast milk
Excretion: Primarily feces (as unabsorbed calcium); urine (20%)

Usual Dosage Dosage is in terms of **elemental** calcium
Dietary Reference Intake:
0-6 months: 210 mg/day
7-12 months: 270 mg/day
1-3 years: 500 mg/day
4-8 years: 800 mg/day
Adults, Male/Female:
9-18 years: 1300 mg/day
19-50 years: 1000 mg/day
≥51 years: 1200 mg/day
Female: Pregnancy: Same as for Adults, Male/Female
Female: Lactating: Same as for Adults, Male/Female

Syrup is a hyperosmolar solution; dosage is in terms of calcium glubionate, elemental calcium is in parentheses

Neonatal hypocalcemia: 1200 mg (77 mg Ca^{++})/kg/day in 4-6 divided doses

Maintenance: Infants and Children: 600-2000 mg (38-128 mg Ca^{++})/kg/day in 4 divided doses up to a maximum of 9 g (575 mg Ca^{++})/day

Adults: 6-18 g (~0.5-1 g Ca^{++})/day in divided doses

Dosing adjustment in renal impairment: Cl$_{cr}$ <25 mL/minute: Dosage adjustments may be necessary depending on the serum calcium levels

Dietary Considerations Should be taken 1-3 hours after meals; may decrease iron absorption so should be administered 1-2 hours before or after iron supplementation; limit intake of bran, foods high in oxalates or whole grain cereals which may decrease calcium absorption.

Reference Range

Serum calcium: 8.4-10.2 mg/dL: Monitor plasma calcium levels if using calcium salts as electrolyte supplements for deficiency

Due to a poor correlation between the serum ionized calcium (free) and total serum calcium, particularly in states of low albumin or acid/base imbalances, direct measurement of ionized calcium is recommended

In low albumin states, the corrected **total** serum calcium may be estimated by: Corrected total calcium = total serum calcium + 0.8 (4.0 - measured serum albumin)

Test Interactions ↑ calcium (S); ↓ magnesium

Patient Information Do not take calcium supplements within 1-2 hours of taking other medicine by mouth or eating large amounts of fiber-rich foods; do not take other calcium-containing products or antacids, drink large amounts of alcohol or caffeine-containing beverages

Nursing Implications Monitor serum calcium, magnesium, phosphate

Additional Information 3.3 mEq calcium/g; 64 mg elemental calcium/g calcium glubionate (6% elemental calcium)

Dosage Forms Elemental calcium listed in brackets

Syrup: 1.8 g/5 mL [115 mg/5 mL] (480 mL)

Calcium Gluceptate (KAL see um gloo SEP tate)

Therapeutic Category Calcium Salt; Electrolyte Supplement, Parenteral

Use Treatment of cardiac disturbances of hyperkalemia, hypocalcemia, or calcium channel blocker toxicity; cardiac resuscitation when epinephrine fails to improve myocardial contractions; treatment of hypermagnesemia and hypocalcemia

Pregnancy Risk Factor C

Usual Dosage Dose expressed in mg of calcium gluceptate (elemental calcium is in parentheses)

Cardiac resuscitation in the presence of hypocalcemia, hyperkalemia, magnesium toxicity, or calcium channel blocker toxicity: I.V.:

Children: 110 mg (9 mg Ca^{++})/kg/dose

Adults: 1.1-1.5 g (90-123 mg Ca^{++})

Hypocalcemia:

I.M.:

Children: 200-500 mg (16.4-41 mg Ca^{++})/kg/day divided every 6 hours

Adults: 500 mg to 1.1 g/dose as needed

I.V.: Adults: 1.1-4.4 g (90-360 mg Ca^{++}) administered slowly as needed (≤2 mL/minute)

After citrated blood administration: Children and Adults: I.V.: 0.45 mEq Ca^{++}/100 mL blood infused

Dosing adjustment in renal impairment: Cl$_{cr}$ <25 mL/minute: Dosage adjustments may be necessary depending on the serum calcium levels

Additional Information Complete prescribing information for this medication should be consulted for additional detail.

Dosage Forms Elemental calcium listed in brackets

Injection: 220 mg/mL [18 mg/mL, 0.9 mEq/mL] (5 mL)

Calcium Gluconate (KAL see um GLOO koe nate)

Therapeutic Category Calcium Salt; Electrolyte Supplement, Oral; Electrolyte Supplement, Parenteral

Use Treatment and prevention of hypocalcemia; treatment of tetany, cardiac disturbances of hyperkalemia, cardiac resuscitation when epinephrine fails to improve myocardial contractions, hypocalcemia, or calcium channel blocker toxicity; calcium supplementation

Pregnancy Risk Factor C

Contraindications In ventricular fibrillation during cardiac resuscitation; patients with risk of digitalis toxicity, renal or cardiac disease, hypercalcemia, renal calculi, hypophosphatemia

Warnings/Precautions Avoid too rapid I.V. administration and avoid extravasation. Use with caution in digitalized patients, severe hyperphosphatemia, respiratory failure or acidosis. May produce cardiac arrest. Hypercalcemia may occur in patients with renal failure, frequent determination of serum calcium is necessary.

Adverse Reactions <1% (Limited to important or life-threatening): Abdominal pain, bradycardia, cardiac arrhythmias, coma, constipation, decreased serum magnesium, elevated serum amylase, erythema, hypercalcemia, hypercalciuria, hypotension, lethargy, mania, muscle weakness, nausea, syncope, tissue necrosis, vasodilation, ventricular fibrillation, vomiting

Overdosage/Toxicology Acute single oral ingestions of calcium salts may produce mild gastrointestinal distress, but hypercalcemia or other toxic manifestations are extremely unlikely. Symptoms of hypercalcemia include lethargy, nausea, vomiting, and coma. Treatment is supportive. Severe hypercalcemia following parenteral overdose requires I.V. hydration. Urine output should be monitored and maintained at >3 mL/kg/hour. I.V. saline and natriuretic agents (eg, furosemide) can quickly and significantly increase excretion of calcium into urine.

(Continued)

Calcium Gluconate (Continued)

Drug Interactions

Increased Effect/Toxicity: High doses of calcium with thiazide diuretics may result in milk-alkali syndrome and hypercalcemia; monitor response. Oral administration of calcium salts may decrease T_4 absorption; separate dose from levothyroxine by at least 4 hours. Calcium acetate may potentiate digoxin toxicity.

Decreased Effect: Absorption of tetracycline, atenolol (and potentially other beta-blockers), iron, quinolone antibiotics, alendronate, sodium fluoride, and zinc absorption may be significantly decreased by oral calcium administration; space administration times. Effects of calcium channel blockers (eg, verapamil) effects may be diminished. Polystyrene sulfonate's potassium-binding ability may be reduced; avoid concurrent oral administration.

Stability

Do not refrigerate solutions; IVPB solutions/I.V. infusion solutions are stable for 24 hours at room temperature

Standard diluent: 1 g/100 mL D_5W or NS; 2 g/100 mL D_5W or NS

Maximum concentration in parenteral nutrition solutions is 15 mEq/L of calcium and 30 mmol/L of phosphate

Incompatible with sodium bicarbonate, carbonates, phosphates, sulfates, and tartrates

Mechanism of Action As dietary supplement, used to prevent or treat negative calcium balance; in osteoporosis, it helps to prevent or decrease the rate of bone loss. The calcium in calcium salts moderates nerve and muscle performance and allows normal cardiac function.

Pharmacodynamics/Kinetics

Absorption: Requires vitamin D; minimal unless chronic, high doses are given; calcium is absorbed in soluble, ionized form; solubility of calcium is increased in an acid environment

Distribution: Crosses placenta; enters breast milk

Excretion: Primarily feces (as unabsorbed calcium); urine (20%)

Usual Dosage Dosage is in terms of **elemental** calcium

Dietary Reference Intake:

0-6 months: 210 mg/day

7-12 months: 270 mg/day

1-3 years: 500 mg/day

4-8 years: 800 mg/day

Adults, Male/Female:

9-18 years: 1300 mg/day

19-50 years: 1000 mg/day

≥51 years: 1200 mg/day

Female: Pregnancy: Same as for Adults, Male/Female

Female: Lactating: Same as for Adults, Male/Female

Dosage expressed in terms of **calcium gluconate**

Hypocalcemia: I.V.:

Neonates: 200-800 mg/kg/day as a continuous infusion or in 4 divided doses

Infants and Children: 200-500 mg/kg/day as a continuous infusion or in 4 divided doses

Adults: 2-15 g/24 hours as a continuous infusion or in divided doses

Hypocalcemia: Oral:

Children: 200-500 mg/kg/day divided every 6 hours

Adults: 500 mg to 2 g 2-4 times/day

Osteoporosis/bone loss: Oral: 1000-1500 mg in divided doses/day

Hypocalcemia secondary to citrated blood infusion: I.V.: Give 0.45 mEq **elemental** calcium for each 100 mL citrated blood infused

Hypocalcemic tetany: I.V.:

Neonates: 100-200 mg/kg/dose, may follow with 500 mg/kg/day in 3-4 divided doses or as an infusion

Infants and Children: 100-200 mg/kg/dose (0.5-0.7 mEq/kg/dose) over 5-10 minutes; may repeat every 6-8 hours **or** follow with an infusion of 500 mg/kg/day

Adults: 1-3 g (4.5-16 mEq) may be administered until therapeutic response occurs

Calcium antagonist toxicity, magnesium intoxication, or cardiac arrest in the presence of hyperkalemia or hypocalcemia: Calcium chloride is recommended calcium salt: I.V.:

Infants and Children: 60-100 mg/kg/dose (maximum: 3 g/dose)

Adults: 500-800 mg; maximum: 3 g/dose

Maintenance electrolyte requirements for total parenteral nutrition: I.V.: Daily requirements:

Adults: 8-16 mEq/1000 kcal/24 hours

Dosing adjustment in renal impairment: Cl_{cr} <25 mL/minute: Dosage adjustments may be necessary depending on the serum calcium levels

Administration Rapid I.V. injection at a maximum rate of 50 mg/minute; for I.V. infusion, dilute to a maximum concentration of 50 mg/mL and infuse over 1 hour or no greater than 120-240 mg/hour (0.6-1.2 mEq calcium/kg/hour)

Reference Range

Serum calcium: 8.4-10.2 mg/dL: Monitor plasma calcium levels if using calcium salts as electrolyte supplements for deficiency

Due to a poor correlation between the serum ionized calcium (free) and total serum calcium, particularly in states of low albumin or acid/base imbalances, direct measurement of ionized calcium is recommended

In low albumin states, the corrected **total** serum calcium may be estimated by: Corrected total calcium = total serum calcium + 0.8 (4.0 - measured serum albumin)

Test Interactions ↑ calcium (S); ↓ magnesium

Patient Information Do not take calcium supplements within 1-2 hours of taking other medicine by mouth or eating large amounts of fiber-rich foods; do not drink large amounts of alcohol or caffeine-containing beverages; take with food

Nursing Implications

Extravasation treatment (example):

Hyaluronidase: Add 1 mL NS to 150 unit vial to make 150 units/mL of concentration; mix 0.1 mL of above with 0.9 mL NS in 1 mL syringe to make final concentration = 15 units/mL

Do not infuse calcium gluconate solutions in the same I.V. line as phosphate-containing solutions (eg, TPN)

Additional Information 4.5 mEq calcium/g; 90 mg elemental calcium/g calcium gluconate (9% elemental calcium)

Dosage Forms Elemental calcium listed in brackets
Injection: 10% = 100 mg/mL [9 mg/mL] (10 mL, 50 mL, 100 mL, 200 mL)
Tablet: 500 mg [45 mg], 650 mg [58.5 mg], 975 mg [87.75 mg], 1 g [90 mg]

♦ **Calcium Leucovorin** *see Leucovorin on page 782*
♦ **Calderol®** *see Calcifediol on page 203*

Calfactant (kaf AKT ant)

U.S. Brand Names Infasurf®

Therapeutic Category Lung Surfactant

Use Prevention of respiratory distress syndrome (RDS) in premature infants at high risk for RDS and for the treatment ("rescue") of premature infants who develop RDS

Prophylaxis: Therapy at birth with calfactant is indicated for premature infants <29 weeks of gestational age at significant risk for RDS. Should be administered as soon as possible, preferably within 30 minutes after birth.

Treatment: For infants ≤72 hours of age with RDS (confirmed by clinical and radiologic findings) and requiring endotracheal intubation.

Warnings/Precautions Rapidly affects oxygenation and lung compliance and should be restricted to highly supervised use in a clinical setting with immediate availability of clinicians experienced with intubation and ventilatory management of premature infants; if transient episodes of bradycardia and decreased oxygen saturation occur, discontinue the dosing procedure and initiate measures to alleviate the condition; produces rapid improvement in lung oxygenation and compliance that may require immediate reductions in ventilator settings and FiO₂; for intratracheal administration only

Adverse Reactions
Cardiovascular: Bradycardia (34%), cyanosis (65%)
Respiratory: Airway obstruction (39%), reflux (21%), requirement for manual ventilation (16%), reintubation (1% to 10%)

Overdosage/Toxicology There have been no known reports of overdosage. While there are no known adverse effects of excess lung surfactant, overdoses would result in overloading the lungs with an isotonic solution. Ventilation should be supported until clearance of the liquid is accomplished.

Stability Gentle swirling or agitation of the vial of suspension is often necessary for redispersion. **Do not shake.** Visible flecks of the suspension and foaming under the surface are normal. Calfactant should be stored at refrigeration (2°C to 8°C/36°F to 46°F). Warming before administration is not necessary. Unopened and unused vials of calfactant that have been warmed to room temperature can be returned to the refrigeration storage within 24 hours for future use. Repeated warming to room temperature should be avoided. Each single-use vial should be entered only once and the vial with any unused material should be discarded after the initial entry.

Mechanism of Action Endogenous lung surfactant is essential for effective ventilation because it modifies alveolar surface tension, thereby stabilizing the alveoli. Lung surfactant deficiency is the cause of respiratory distress syndrome (RDS) in premature infants and lung surfactant restores surface activity to the lungs of these infants.

Pharmacodynamics/Kinetics No human studies of absorption, biotransformation, or excretion of calfactant have been performed

Usual Dosage Intratracheal administration **only**: Each dose is 3 mL/kg body weight at birth; should be administered every 12 hours for a total of up to 3 doses

Administration Gentle swirling or agitation of the vial is often necessary for redispersion as injection suspension settles during storage; do **not** shake; visible flecks in the suspension and foaming at the surface are normal; does not require reconstitution; do not dilute or sonicate

Should be administered intratracheally through an endotracheal tube. Dose is drawn into a syringe from the single-use vial using a 20-gauge or larger needle with care taken to avoid excessive foaming. Should be administered in 2 aliquots of 1.5 mL/kg each. After each aliquot is instilled, the infant should be positioned with either the right or the left side dependent. Administration is made while ventilation is continued over 20-30 breaths for each aliquot, with small bursts timed only during the inspiratory cycles. A pause followed by evaluation of the respiratory status and repositioning should separate the two aliquots.

Monitoring Parameters Following administration, patients should be carefully monitored so that oxygen therapy and ventilatory support can be modified in response to changes in respiratory status

Additional Information Each mL = 35 mg total phospholipids (including 26 mg phosphatidylcholine, of which 16 mg is desaturated phosphatidylcholine) and 0.65 protein (including 0.26 mg SP-B)

Dosage Forms Suspension, intratracheal: 6 mL (35 mg/mL)

♦ **Calmylin with Codeine (Can)** *see Guaifenesin, Pseudoephedrine, and Codeine on page 648*
♦ **Cal-Plus® [OTC]** *see Calcium Carbonate on page 207*
♦ **Caltine® (Can)** *see Calcitonin on page 204*
♦ **Caltrate® (Can)** *see Calcium Carbonate on page 207*
♦ **Caltrate® 600 [OTC]** *see Calcium Carbonate on page 207*
♦ **Caltrate, Jr.® [OTC]** *see Calcium Carbonate on page 207*
♦ **Campath®** *see Alemtuzumab on page 46*
♦ **Campath-1H** *see Alemtuzumab on page 46*
♦ **Camphorated Tincture of Opium** *see Paregoric on page 1039*
♦ **Camptosar®** *see Irinotecan on page 742*
♦ **Camptothecin-11** *see Irinotecan on page 742*

- Canasa™ *see* Mesalamine *on page 866*
- Cancidas® *see* Caspofungin *on page 236*

Candesartan (kan de SAR tan)

Related Information
Angiotensin Agents Comparison *on page 1473*

U.S. Brand Names Atacand®

Canadian Brand Names Atacand®

Synonyms Candesartan Cilexetil

Therapeutic Category Angiotensin II Receptor Antagonist (ARB); Antihypertensive Agent

Use Alone or in combination with other antihypertensive agents in treating essential hypertension; may have an advantage over losartan due to minimal metabolism requirements and consequent use in mild to moderate hepatic impairment

Pregnancy Risk Factor C/D (2nd and 3rd trimesters)

Pregnancy/Breast-Feeding Implications Avoid use in the nursing mother, if possible, since candesartan may be excreted in breast milk. The drug should be discontinued as soon as possible when pregnancy is detected. Drugs which act directly on renin-angiotensin can cause fetal and neonatal morbidity and death.

Contraindications Hypersensitivity to candesartan or any component of the formulation; hypersensitivity to other A-II receptor antagonists; primary hyperaldosteronism; bilateral renal artery stenosis; pregnancy (2nd and 3rd trimesters)

Warnings/Precautions Avoid use or use smaller dose in volume-depleted patients. Drugs which alter renin-angiotensin system have been associated with deterioration in renal function, including oliguria, acute renal failure and progressive azotemia. Use with caution in patients with renal artery stenosis (unilateral or bilateral) to avoid decrease in renal function; use caution in patients with pre-existing renal insufficiency (may decrease renal perfusion).

Adverse Reactions May be associated with worsening of renal function in patients dependent on renin-angiotensin-aldosterone system.

Cardiovascular: Flushing, chest pain, peripheral edema, tachycardia, palpitations, angina, myocardial infarction,

Central nervous system: Dizziness, lightheadedness, drowsiness, fatigue, headache, vertigo, anxiety, depression, somnolence, fever

Dermatologic: Angioedema, rash (>0.5%)

Endocrine & metabolic: Hyperglycemia, hypertriglyceridemia

Gastrointestinal: Nausea, diarrhea, vomiting, dyspepsia, gastroenteritis

Genitourinary: Hyperuricemia, hematuria

Neuromuscular & skeletal: Back pain, arthralgia, paresthesias, increased CPK, myalgia, weakness

Respiratory: Upper respiratory tract infection, pharyngitis, rhinitis, bronchitis, cough, sinusitis, epistaxis, dyspnea

Miscellaneous: Diaphoresis (increased)

<1% (Limited to important or life-threatening): Agranulocytosis, dyspnea, hepatitis, leukopenia, neutropenia, paresthesias, vomiting

Overdosage/Toxicology Symptoms include hypotension and tachycardia. Treatment is supportive.

Drug Interactions
Cytochrome P450 Effect: Not metabolized by cytochrome P450

Increased Effect/Toxicity: The risk of lithium toxicity may be increased by candesartan; monitor lithium levels. Concurrent use with potassium-sparing diuretics (amiloride, spironolactone, triamterene), potassium supplements, or trimethoprim (high-dose) may increase the risk of hyperkalemia.

Ethanol/Nutrition/Herb Interactions
Food: Food reduces the time to maximal concentration and increases the C_{max}.

Herb/Nutraceutical: Avoid dong quai if using for hypertension (has estrogenic activity). Avoid ephedra, yohimbe, ginseng (may worsen hypertension). Avoid garlic (may have increased antihypertensive effect).

Mechanism of Action Candesartan is an angiotensin receptor antagonist. Angiotensin II acts as a vasoconstrictor. In addition to causing direct vasoconstriction, angiotensin II also stimulates the release of aldosterone. Once aldosterone is released, sodium as well as water are reabsorbed. The end result is an elevation in blood pressure. Candesartan binds to the AT1 angiotensin II receptor. This binding prevents angiotensin II from binding to the receptor thereby blocking the vasoconstriction and the aldosterone secreting effects of angiotensin II.

Pharmacodynamics/Kinetics
Onset of action: 2-3 hours
Peak effect: 6-8 hours
Duration: >24 hours
Distribution: V_d: 0.13 L/kg
Protein binding: 99%
Metabolism: To candesartan by the intestinal wall cells
Bioavailability: 15%
Half-life elimination (dose dependent): 5-9 hours
Time to peak: 3-4 hours
Excretion: Urine (26%)
Clearance: Total body: 0.37 mL/kg/minute; Renal: 0.19 mL/kg/minute

Usual Dosage Adults: Oral: Usual dose is 4-32 mg once daily; dosage must be individualized. Blood pressure response is dose-related over the range of 2-32 mg. The usual recommended starting dose of 16 mg once daily when it is used as monotherapy in patients who are not volume depleted. It can be administered once or twice daily with total daily doses ranging from 8-32 mg. Larger doses do not appear to have a greater effect and there is relatively little experience with such doses.

No initial dosage adjustment is necessary for elderly patients (although higher concentrations (C_{max}) and AUC were observed in these populations), for patients with mildly impaired renal function, or for patients with mildly impaired hepatic function.

Monitoring Parameters Supine blood pressure, electrolytes, serum creatinine, BUN, urinalysis, symptomatic hypotension, and tachycardia

Patient Information Patients of childbearing age should be informed about the consequences of 2nd- and 3rd-trimester exposure to drugs that act on the renin-angiotensin system, and that these consequences do not appear to have resulted from intrauterine drug exposure that has been limited to the 1st trimester. Patients should report pregnancy to their physician as soon as possible.

Dosage Forms Tablet, as cilexetil: 4 mg, 8 mg, 16 mg, 32 mg

Candesartan and Hydrochlorothiazide
(kan de SAR tan & hye droe klor oh THYE a zide)

U.S. Brand Names Atacand HCT™

Synonyms Candesartan Cilexetil and Hydrochlorothiazide

Therapeutic Category Angiotensin II Antagonist Combination

Use Treatment of hypertension; combination product should not be used for initial therapy

Pregnancy Risk Factor C/D (2nd and 3rd trimesters)

Usual Dosage Adults: Oral: Replacement therapy: Combination product can be substituted for individual agents; maximum therapeutic effect would be expected within 4 weeks

Usual dosage range:

Candesartan: 8-32 mg/day, given once daily or twice daily in divided doses

Hydrochlorothiazide: 12.5-50 mg once daily

Dosage adjustment in renal impairment: Serum levels of candesartan are increased and the half-life of hydrochlorothiazide is prolonged in patients with renal impairment. Do not use if Cl_{cr} <30 mL/minute

Dosage adjustment in hepatic impairment: Use with caution

Elderly: No initial dosage adjustment is recommended in patients with normal renal and hepatic function; some patients may have increased sensitivity

Additional Information Complete prescribing information for this medication should be consulted for additional detail.

Dosage Forms

Tablet:

Atacand HCT™ 16-12.5: Candesartan 16 mg and hydrochlorothiazide 12.5 mg

Atacand HCT™ 32-12.5: Candesartan 32 mg and hydrochlorothiazide 12.5 mg

♦ **Candesartan Cilexetil** see Candesartan on page 214

♦ **Candesartan Cilexetil and Hydrochlorothiazide** see Candesartan and Hydrochlorothiazide on page 215

♦ **Candistatin® (Can)** see Nystatin on page 1001

♦ **Canesten® Topical, Canesten® Vaginal (Can)** see Clotrimazole on page 323

♦ **Capastat® Sulfate** see Capreomycin on page 218

Capecitabine (ka pe SITE a been)

U.S. Brand Names Xeloda®

Canadian Brand Names Xeloda®

Therapeutic Category Antineoplastic Agent, Antimetabolite

Use

Treatment of metastatic colorectal cancer.

Treatment of metastatic breast cancer in combination with docetaxel after failure of prior anthracycline therapy.

Monotherapy treatment of metastatic breast cancer resistant to both paclitaxel and an anthracycline-containing chemotherapy regimen or resistant to paclitaxel and for whom further anthracycline therapy is not indicated (eg, patients who have received cumulative doses of 400 mg/m² of doxorubicin or doxorubicin equivalents). Resistance is defined as progressive disease while on treatment, with or without an initial response, or relapse within 6 months of completing treatment with an anthracycline-containing adjuvant regimen.

Pregnancy Risk Factor D

Pregnancy/Breast-Feeding Implications There are no adequate and well-controlled studies using capecitabine in pregnant women; however, fetal harm may occur. Women of childbearing potential should avoid pregnancy. It is not known if the drug is excreted in breast milk. Because of the potential for serious adverse reactions in nursing infants, it is recommended that nursing be discontinued when receiving capecitabine therapy.

Contraindications Hypersensitivity to capecitabine, fluorouracil, or any component of the formulation; severe renal impairment (Cl_{cr} <30 mL/minute); pregnancy

Warnings/Precautions The U.S. Food and Drug Administration (FDA) currently recommends that procedures for proper handling and disposal of antineoplastic agents be considered. Use with caution in patients with bone marrow suppression, poor nutritional status, on warfarin therapy, ≥80 years of age, or renal or hepatic dysfunction. Dosing adjustment required in moderate renal impairment (Cl_{cr} 30-50 mL/minute). The drug should be discontinued if intractable diarrhea, stomatitis, bone marrow suppression, or myocardial ischemia develop. Use with caution in patients who have received extensive pelvic radiation or alkylating therapy. Use cautiously with warfarin; altered coagulation parameters and bleeding have been reported.

Capecitabine can cause severe diarrhea; median time to first occurrence is 31 days; subsequent doses should be reduced after grade 3 or 4 diarrhea

Hand-and-foot syndrome (palmar-plantar erythrodysesthesia or chemotherapy-induced acral erythema) is characterized by numbness, dysesthesia/paresthesia, tingling, painless or painful swelling, erythema, desquamation, blistering, and severe pain. If grade 2 or 3 hand-and-foot syndrome occurs, interrupt administration of capecitabine until the event resolves or (Continued)

215

Capecitabine *(Continued)*

decreases in intensity to grade 1. Following grade 3 hand-and-foot syndrome, decrease subsequent doses of capecitabine.

There has been cardiotoxicity associated with fluorinated pyrimidine therapy, including myocardial infarction, angina, dysrhythmias, cardiogenic shock, sudden death, and EKG changes. These adverse events may be more common in patients with a history of coronary artery disease.

Adverse Reactions Frequency listed derived from monotherapy trials.

>10%:

Cardiovascular: Edema (9% to 15%)

Central nervous system: Fatigue (~40%), fever (12% to 18%), pain (colorectal cancer: 12%)

Dermatologic: Palmar-plantar erythrodysesthesia (hand-and-foot syndrome) (~55%, may be dose limiting), dermatitis (27% to 37%)

Gastrointestinal: Diarrhea (~55%, may be dose limiting), mild to moderate nausea (43% to 53%), vomiting (27% to 37%), stomatitis (~25%), decreased appetite (colorectal cancer: 26%), anorexia (23%), abdominal pain (20% to 35%), constipation (~15%)

Hematologic: Lymphopenia (94%), anemia (72% to 80%; Grade 3/4: <1% to 3%), neutropenia (13% to 26%; Grade 3/4: 1% to 2%), thrombocytopenia (24%; Grade 3/4: 1% to 3%)

Hepatic: Increased bilirubin (22% to 48%)

Neuromuscular & skeletal: Paresthesia (21%)

Ocular: Eye irritation (~15%)

Respiratory: Dyspnea (colorectal cancer: 14%)

5% to 10%:

Cardiovascular: Venous thrombosis (colorectal cancer: 8%), chest pain (colorectal cancer: 6%)

Central nervous system: Headache (~10%), dizziness (~8%), insomnia (8%), mood alteration (colorectal cancer: 5%), depression (colorectal cancer: 5%)

Dermatologic: Nail disorders (7%), skin discoloration (colorectal cancer: 7%), alopecia (colorectal cancer: 6%)

Endocrine & metabolic: Dehydration (7%)

Gastrointestinal: Motility disorder (colorectal cancer: 10%), oral discomfort (colorectal cancer: 10%), dyspepsia (8%), upper GI inflammatory disorders (colorectal cancer: 8%), hemorrhage (colorectal cancer: 6%), ileus (colorectal cancer: 6%), taste disturbance (colorectal cancer: 6%)

Neuromuscular & skeletal: Back pain (colorectal cancer: 10%), myalgia (9%), neuropathy (colorectal cancer: 10%), arthralgia (colorectal cancer: 8%), limb pain (colorectal cancer: 6%)

Respiratory: Cough (7%), sore throat (2%), epistaxis (3%)

Ocular: Abnormal vision (colorectal cancer: 5%)

Miscellaneous: Viral infection (colorectal cancer: 5%)

<5% (Limited to important or life-threatening): Angina, asthma, cardiac arrest, cardiac failure, cardiomyopathy, cerebral vascular accident, dysrhythmia, encephalopathy, gastric ulcer, GI hemorrhage, hepatitis, hepatic failure, hepatic fibrosis, hypersensitivity, idiopathic thrombocytopenia purpura, ileus, infections, intestinal obstruction (~1%), myocardial infarction, myocardial ischemia, myocarditis, necrotizing enterocolitis, pericardial effusion, thrombocytopenic purpura, pancytopenia, photosensitivity, pneumonia, pulmonary embolism, radiation recall syndrome, sepsis, toxic dilation of intestine, vertigo

Overdosage/Toxicology Symptoms include myelosuppression, nausea, vomiting, diarrhea, and alopecia. No specific antidote exists. Monitor hematologically for at least 4 weeks. Treatment is supportive.

Drug Interactions

Increased Effect/Toxicity: Taking capecitabine immediately before an aluminum hydroxide/magnesium hydroxide antacid or a meal increases the absorption of capecitabine. The concentration of capecitabine's active metabolite (5-fluorouracil) is increased and its toxicity may be enhanced by leucovorin. Deaths from severe enterocolitis, diarrhea, and dehydration have been reported in elderly patients receiving weekly leucovorin and fluorouracil. Response to warfarin may be increased by capecitabine; changes may occur days to months after starting or stopping capecitabine therapy. Capecitabine may increase serum levels/effects of drugs metabolized by CYP2C9.

Ethanol/Nutrition/Herb Interactions Food: Food reduced the rate and extent of absorption of capecitabine.

Stability Tablets are stored at room temperature of 25°C (77°F).

Mechanism of Action Capecitabine is a prodrug of fluorouracil. It undergoes hydrolysis in the liver and tissues to form fluorouracil which is the active moiety. Fluorouracil is a fluorinated pyrimidine antimetabolite that inhibits thymidylate synthetase, blocking the methylation of deoxyuridylic acid to thymidylic acid, interfering with DNA, and to a lesser degree, RNA synthesis. Fluorouracil appears to be phase specific for the G_1 and S phases of the cell cycle.

Pharmacodynamics/Kinetics

Absorption: Rapid and extensive

Protein binding: <60%; 35% to albumin

Metabolism: Hepatic: Inactive metabolites: 5'-deoxy-5-fluorocytidine, 5'-deoxy-5-fluorouridine; Tissue: Active metabolite: 5-fluorouracil

Half-life elimination: 0.5-1 hour

Time to peak: 1.5 hours; peak fluorouracil level: 2 hours

Excretion: Urine (96%, 50% as α-fluoro-β-alanine)

Usual Dosage Oral:

Adults: 2500 mg/m²/day in 2 divided doses (~12 hours apart) at the end of a meal for 2 weeks followed by a 1-week rest period given as 3-week cycles

Capecitabine dose calculation according to BSA table: The following can be used to determine the total daily dose (mg) based on a dosing level of 2500 mg/m²/day. (The number of tablets per dose, given morning and evening, are also listed): See table.

Capecitabine Dose Calculation According to BSA Table

Dose Level 2500 mg/m²/day		# of tablets per dose (morning and evening)	
Surface Area (m²)	Total Daily Dose (mg)	150 mg	500 mg
≤1.25	3000	0	3
1.26-1.37	3300	1	3
1.38-1.51	3600	2	3
1.52-1.65	4000	0	4
1.66-1.77	4300	1	4
1.78-1.91	4600	2	4
1.92-2.05	5000	0	5
2.06-2.17	5300	1	5
≥2.18	5600	2	5

Dosing adjustment in renal impairment: Baseline calculation of creatinine clearance is required (Cockroft-Gault per manufacturer)

Note: In any patient with renal insufficiency, carefully monitor and interrupt therapy if grade 2-, 3-, or 4 toxicity develops.

Cl_{cr} 50-80 mL/minute: No adjustment of initial dose

Cl_{cr} 30-50 mL/minute: Reduce initial dose to 1900 mg/m²/day (25% reduction in dose)

Cl_{cr} <30 mL/minute: Do not use

Dosing adjustment in hepatic impairment:

Mild to moderate impairment: No starting dose adjustment is necessary; however, carefully monitor patients

Severe hepatic impairment: Patients have not been studied

Dosing adjustment in elderly patients: The elderly may be pharmacodynamically more sensitive to the toxic effects of 5-fluorouracil. Use with caution in monitoring the effects of capecitabine. Insufficient data are available to provide dosage modifications.

Dosage modification guidelines: Carefully monitor patients for toxicity. Toxicity caused by capecitabine administration may be managed by symptomatic treatment, dose interruptions, and adjustment of dose. Once the dose has been reduced, it should not be increased at a later time.

Dosage reduction for toxicity: The starting dose may be reduced by 25% in patients experiencing significant adverse effects at the full starting dose if symptoms persist, a further reduction (to 50% of the starting dose) may be considered. These recommendations were based on clinical studies reported at the 36th Annual Meeting of the American Society of Clinical Oncology (ASCO). See table.

Recommended Dose Modifications

Toxicity NCI Grades	During a Course of Therapy	Dose Adjustment for Next Cycle (% of starting dose)
Grade 1	Maintain dose level	Maintain dose level
Grade 2		
1st appearance	Interrupt until resolved to grade 0-1	100%
2nd appearance	Interrupt until resolved to grade 0-1	75%
3rd appearance	Interrupt until resolved to grade 0-1	50%
4th appearance	Discontinue treatment permanently	
Grade 3		
1st appearance	Interrupt until resolved to grade 0-1	75%
2nd appearance	Interrupt until resolved to grade 0-1	50%
3rd appearance	Discontinue treatment permanently	
Grade 4		
1st appearance	Discontinue permanently OR If physician deems it to be in the patient's best interest to continue, interrupt until resolved to grade 0-1	50%

Dietary Considerations Because current safety and efficacy data are based upon administration with food, it is recommended that capecitabine be administered with food. In all clinical trials, patients were instructed to administer capecitabine within 30 minutes after a meal.

Administration Capecitabine is administered orally, usually in two divided doses taken 12 hours apart. Doses should be taken after meals with water.

Monitoring Parameters Renal function should be estimated at baseline to determine initial dose; during therapy, CBC with differential, hepatic function, and renal function should be monitored

Patient Information Take with food or within 30 minutes after meal. Avoid use of antacids within 2 hours of taking capecitabine. Do not crush, chew, or dissolve tablets. You will need frequent blood tests while taking this medication. Maintain adequate hydration (2-3 L/day of fluids unless instructed to restrict fluid intake). You may experience lethargy, dizziness, visual changes, confusion, anxiety (avoid driving or engaging in tasks requiring alertness until response to drug is known). For nausea, vomiting, loss of appetite, or dry mouth, small, frequent meals, chewing gum, or sucking lozenges may help. You may experience loss of hair (will grow back when treatment is discontinued). You may experience photosensitivity (use sunscreen, wear protective clothing and eyewear, and avoid direct sunlight). You may (Continued)

Capecitabine *(Continued)*

experience dry, itchy, skin, and dry or irritated eyes (avoid contact lenses). You will be more susceptible to infection; avoid crowds or infected persons. Report chills or fever, confusion, persistent or violent vomiting or stomach pain, persistent diarrhea, respiratory difficulty, chest pain or palpitations, unusual bleeding or bruising, bone pain, muscle spasms/tremors, or vision changes immediately.

Dosage Forms Tablet: 150 mg, 500 mg

♦ **Capex™** *see Fluocinolone on page 572*

♦ **Capital® and Codeine** *see Acetaminophen and Codeine on page 24*

♦ **Capoten®** *see Captopril on page 218*

♦ **Capozide®** *see Captopril and Hydrochlorothiazide on page 221*

Capreomycin *(kap ree oh MYE sin)*

Related Information
Antimicrobial Drugs of Choice *on page 1588*
Tuberculosis Treatment Guidelines *on page 1612*

U.S. Brand Names Capastat® Sulfate

Synonyms Capreomycin Sulfate

Therapeutic Category Antibiotic, Miscellaneous; Antitubercular Agent

Use Treatment of tuberculosis in conjunction with at least one other antituberculosis agent

Pregnancy Risk Factor C

Contraindications Hypersensitivity to capreomycin sulfate or any component of the formulation

Warnings/Precautions Use in patients with renal insufficiency or pre-existing auditory impairment must be undertaken with great caution, and the risk of additional eighth nerve impairment or renal injury should be weighed against the benefits to be derived from therapy. Since other parenteral antituberculous agents (eg, streptomycin) also have similar and sometimes irreversible toxic effects, particularly on eighth cranial nerve and renal function, simultaneous administration of these agents with capreomycin is not recommended. Use with nonantituberculous drugs (ie, aminoglycoside antibiotics) having ototoxic or nephrotoxic potential should be undertaken only with great caution.

Adverse Reactions
>10%:
Otic: Ototoxicity [subclinical hearing loss (11%), clinical loss (3%)], tinnitus
Renal: Nephrotoxicity (36%, increased BUN)
1% to 10%: Hematologic: Eosinophilia (dose-related, mild)
<1% (Limited to important or life-threatening): Hypersensitivity (urticaria, rash, fever); hypokalemia, leukocytosis; pain, induration, and bleeding at injection site; thrombocytopenia (rare); vertigo

Overdosage/Toxicology Symptoms include renal failure, ototoxicity, and thrombocytopenia. Treatment is supportive.

Drug Interactions
Increased Effect/Toxicity: May increase effect/duration of nondepolarizing neuromuscular blocking agents. Additive toxicity (nephrotoxicity and ototoxicity), respiratory paralysis may occur with aminoglycosides (eg, streptomycin).
Decreased Effect:
Increased effect/duration of nondepolarizing neuromuscular blocking agents
Additive toxicity (nephrotoxicity and ototoxicity, respiratory paralysis): Aminoglycosides (eg, streptomycin)

Mechanism of Action Capreomycin is a cyclic polypeptide antimicrobial. It is administered as a mixture of capreomycin IA and capreomycin IB. The mechanism of action of capreomycin is not well understood. Mycobacterial species that have become resistant to other agents are usually still sensitive to the action of capreomycin. However, significant cross-resistance with viomycin, kanamycin, and neomycin occurs.

Pharmacodynamics/Kinetics
Half-life elimination: Normal renal function: 4-6 hours
Time to peak, serum: I.M.: ~1 hour
Excretion: Urine (as unchanged drug)

Usual Dosage I.M.:
Infants and Children: 15 mg/kg/day, up to 1 g/day maximum
Adults: 15-20 mg/kg/day up to 1 g/day for 60-120 days, followed by 1 g 2-3 times/week
Dosing interval in renal impairment: Adults:
Cl$_{cr}$ >100 mL/minute: Administer 13-15 mg/kg every 24 hours
Cl$_{cr}$ 80-100 mL/minute: Administer 10-13 mg/kg every 24 hours
Cl$_{cr}$ 60-80 mL/minute: Administer 7-10 mg/kg every 24 hours
Cl$_{cr}$ 40-60 mL/minute: Administer 11-14 mg/kg every 48 hours
Cl$_{cr}$ 20-40 mL/minute: Administer 10-14 mg/kg every 72 hours
Cl$_{cr}$ <20 mL/minute: Administer 4-7 mg/kg every 72 hours

Reference Range 10 μg/mL

Patient Information Report any hearing loss to physician immediately; do not discontinue without notifying physician

Nursing Implications The solution for injection may acquire a pale straw color and darken with time; this is not associated with a loss of potency or development of toxicity

Dosage Forms Injection, as sulfate: 100 mg/mL (10 mL)

♦ **Capreomycin Sulfate** *see Capreomycin on page 218*

Captopril *(KAP toe pril)*

Related Information
Angiotensin Agents Comparison *on page 1473*
Antacid Drug Interactions *on page 1477*
Heart Failure *on page 1663*

Hypertension *on page 1675*
U.S. Brand Names Capoten®
Canadian Brand Names Alti-Captopril; Apo®-Capto; Capoten™; Gen-Captopril; Novo-Captopril®; Nu-Capto®; PMS-Captopril®
Synonyms ACE
Therapeutic Category Angiotensin-Converting Enzyme (ACE) Inhibitor; Antihypertensive Agent
Use Management of hypertension; treatment of congestive heart failure, left ventricular dysfunction after myocardial infarction, diabetic nephropathy
Unlabeled/Investigational Use Treatment of hypertensive crisis, rheumatoid arthritis; diagnosis of anatomic renal artery stenosis, hypertension secondary to scleroderma renal crisis; diagnosis of aldosteronism, idiopathic edema, Bartter's syndrome, postmyocardial infarction for prevention of ventricular failure; increase circulation in Raynaud's phenomenon, hypertension secondary to Takayasu's disease
Pregnancy Risk Factor C/D (2nd and 3rd trimesters)
Pregnancy/Breast-Feeding Implications
Clinical effects on the fetus: No data available on crossing the placenta. Cranial defects, hypocalvaria/acalvaria, oligohydramnios, persistent anuria following delivery, hypotension, renal defects, renal dysgenesis/dysplasia, renal failure, pulmonary hypoplasia, limb contractures secondary to oligohydramnios and stillbirth reported. ACE inhibitors should be avoided during pregnancy.

Breast-feeding/lactation: Crosses into breast milk. AAP considers **compatible** with breast-feeding.
Contraindications Hypersensitivity to captopril or any component of the formulation; angioedema related to previous treatment with an ACE inhibitor; primary hyperaldosteronism; idiopathic or hereditary angioedema; bilateral renal artery `stenosis; pregnancy (2nd or 3rd trimester)
Warnings/Precautions Anaphylactic reactions can occur. Angioedema can occur at any time during treatment (especially following first dose). Careful blood pressure monitoring with first dose (hypotension can occur especially in volume depleted patients. Use with caution in collagen vascular diseases; valvular stenosis (particularly aortic stenosis); hyperkalemia; or before, during, or immediately after anesthesia. Avoid rapid dosage escalation which may lead to renal insufficiency. Neutropenia/agranulocytosis with myeloid hyperplasia can rarely occur. If patient has renal impairment then a baseline WBC with differential and serum creatinine should be evaluated and monitored closely during the first 3 months of therapy. Hypersensitivity reactions may be seen during hemodialysis with high-flux dialysis membranes (eg, AN69). Deterioration in renal function can occur with initiation.

Use with caution and decrease dosage in patients with renal impairment (especially renal artery stenosis), severe congestive heart failure, or with coadministered diuretic therapy; experience in children is limited. Severe hypotension may occur in patients who are sodium and/or volume depleted, initiate lower doses and monitor closely when starting therapy in these patients; ACE inhibitors may be preferred agents in elderly patients with congestive heart failure and diabetes mellitus (diabetic proteinuria is reduced, minimal CNS effects, and enhanced insulin sensitivity); however due to decreased renal function, tolerance must be carefully monitored.

Adverse Reactions
1% to 10%:
Cardiovascular: Hypotension (1% to 2.5%), tachycardia (1%), chest pain (1%), palpitation (1%)

Dermatologic: Rash (maculopapular or urticarial) (4% to 7%), pruritus (2%); in patients with rash, a positive ANA and/or eosinophilia has been noted in 7% to 10%.

Endocrine & metabolic: Hyperkalemia (1% to 11%)

Renal: Proteinuria (1%), increased serum creatinine, worsening of renal function (may occur in patients with bilateral renal artery stenosis or hypovolemia)

Respiratory: Cough (0.5% to 2%)

Miscellaneous: Hypersensitivity reactions (rash, pruritus, fever, arthralgia, and eosinophilia) have occurred in 4% to 7% of patients (depending on dose and renal function); dysgeusia - loss of taste or diminished perception (2% to 4%)

Neutropenia may occur in up to 3.7% of patients with renal insufficiency or collagen-vascular disease.

Frequency not defined:
Cardiovascular: Angioedema, cardiac arrest, cerebrovascular insufficiency, rhythm disturbances, orthostatic hypotension, syncope, flushing, pallor, angina, myocardial infarction, Raynaud's syndrome, congestive heart failure

Central nervous system: Ataxia, confusion, depression, nervousness, somnolence

Dermatologic: Bullous pemphigus, erythema multiforme, Stevens-Johnson syndrome, exfoliative dermatitis

Endocrine & metabolic: Increased serum transaminases, increased serum bilirubin, increased alkaline phosphatase, gynecomastia

Gastrointestinal: Pancreatitis, glossitis, dyspepsia

Genitourinary: Urinary frequency, impotence

Hematologic: Anemia, thrombocytopenia, pancytopenia, agranulocytosis, anemia

Hepatic: Jaundice, hepatitis, hepatic necrosis (rare), cholestasis, hyponatremia (symptomatic)

Neuromuscular & skeletal: Asthenia, myalgia, myasthenia

Ocular: Burred vision

Renal: Renal insufficiency, renal failure, nephrotic syndrome, polyuria, oliguria

Respiratory: Bronchospasm, eosinophilic pneumonitis, rhinitis

Miscellaneous: Anaphylactoid reactions

Postmarketing and/or case reports: Alopecia, aplastic anemia, exacerbations of Huntington's disease, Guillain-Barré syndrome, hemolytic anemia, Kaposi's sarcoma, pericarditis, seizures (in premature infants), systemic lupus erythematosus. A syndrome which may include fever, myalgia, arthralgia, interstitial nephritis, vasculitis, rash, eosinophilia, and elevated ESR has been reported for captopril and other ACE inhibitors.

(Continued)

Captopril *(Continued)*

Overdosage/Toxicology Mild hypotension has been the only toxic effect seen with acute overdose; bradycardia may also occur. Hyperkalemia occurs even with therapeutic doses, especially in patients with renal insufficiency and those taking NSAIDs. Following initiation of essential overdose management, toxic symptom treatment and supportive treatment should be initiated. Hypotension usually responds to I.V. fluids or Trendelenburg positioning.

Drug Interactions

Cytochrome P450 Effect: CYP2D6 enzyme substrate

Increased Effect/Toxicity: Potassium supplements, co-trimoxazole (high dose), angiotensin II receptor antagonists (candesartan, losartan, irbesartan, etc), or potassium-sparing diuretics (amiloride, spironolactone, triamterene) may result in elevated serum potassium levels when combined with captopril. ACE inhibitor effects may be increased by phenothiazines or probenecid (increases levels of captopril). ACE inhibitors may increase serum concentrations/effects of digoxin, lithium, and sulfonlyureas.

Diuretics have additive hypotensive effects with ACE inhibitors, and hypovolemia increases the potential for adverse renal effects of ACE inhibitors. In patients with compromised renal function, coadministration with nonsteroidal anti-inflammatory drugs may result in further deterioration of renal function. Allopurinol and ACE inhibitors may cause a higher risk of hypersensitivity reaction when taken concurrently.

Decreased Effect: Aspirin (high dose) may reduce the therapeutic effects of ACE inhibitors; at low dosages this does not appear to be significant. Rifampin may decrease the effect of ACE inhibitors. Antacids may decrease the bioavailability of ACE inhibitors (may be more likely to occur with captopril); separate administration times by 1-2 hours. NSAIDs, specifically indomethacin, may reduce the hypotensive effects of ACE inhibitors. More likely to occur in low renin or volume dependent hypertensive patients.

Ethanol/Nutrition/Herb Interactions

Food: Captopril serum concentrations may be decreased if taken with food. Long-term use of captopril may result in a zinc deficiency which can result in a decrease in taste perception.

Herb/Nutraceutical: Avoid dong quai if using for hypertension (has estrogenic activity). Avoid ephedra, yohimbe, ginseng (may worsen hypertension). Avoid garlic (may have increased antihypertensive effect).

Stability Unstable in aqueous solutions; to prepare solution for oral administration, mix prior to administration and use within 10 minutes

Mechanism of Action Competitive inhibitor of angiotensin-converting enzyme (ACE); prevents conversion of angiotensin I to angiotensin II, a potent vasoconstrictor; results in lower levels of angiotensin II which causes an increase in plasma renin activity and a reduction in aldosterone secretion

Pharmacodynamics/Kinetics

Onset of action: Peak effect: Blood pressure reduction: 1-1.5 hours after dose

Duration: Dose related, may require several weeks of therapy before full hypotensive effect

Absorption: 60% to 75%; food decreases absorption by 30% to 40%

Protein binding: 25% to 30%

Metabolism: 50%

Half-life elimination (dependent upon renal and cardiac function):
Adults, normal: 1.9 hours; Congestive heart failure: 2.06 hours; Anuria: 20-40 hours

Excretion: Urine (95%) within 24 hours

Usual Dosage Note: Dosage must be titrated according to patient's response; use lowest effective dose. Oral:

Infants: Initial: 0.15-0.3 mg/kg/dose; titrate dose upward to maximum of 6 mg/kg/day in 1-4 divided doses; usual required dose: 2.5-6 mg/kg/day

Children: Initial: 0.5 mg/kg/dose; titrate upward to maximum of 6 mg/kg/day in 2-4 divided doses

Older Children: Initial: 6.25-12.5 mg/dose every 12-24 hours; titrate upward to maximum of 6 mg/kg/day

Adolescents: Initial: 12.5-25 mg/dose given every 8-12 hours; increase by 25 mg/dose to maximum of 450 mg/day

Adults:

Acute hypertension (urgency/emergency): 12.5-25 mg, may repeat as needed (may be given sublingually, but no therapeutic advantage demonstrated)

Hypertension:
Initial dose: 12.5-25 mg 2-3 times/day; may increase by 12.5-25 mg/dose at 1- to 2-week intervals up to 50 mg 3 times/day; add diuretic before further dosage increases
Maximum dose: 150 mg 3 times/day

Congestive heart failure:
Initial dose: 6.25-12.5 mg 3 times/day in conjunction with cardiac glycoside and diuretic therapy; initial dose depends upon patient's fluid/electrolyte status
Target dose: 50 mg 3 times/day
Maximum dose: 150 mg 3 times/day

LVD after MI: Initial dose: 6.25 mg followed by 12.5 mg 3 times/day; then increase to 25 mg 3 times/day during next several days and then over next several weeks to target dose of 50 mg 3 times/day

Diabetic nephropathy: 25 mg 3 times/day; other antihypertensives often given concurrently

Dosing adjustment in renal impairment:

Cl_{cr} 10-50 mL/minute: Administer at 75% of normal dose.

Cl_{cr} <10 mL/minute: Administer at 50% of normal dose.

Note: Smaller dosages given every 8-12 hours are indicated in patients with renal dysfunction; renal function and leukocyte count should be carefully monitored during therapy.

Hemodialysis: Moderately dialyzable (20% to 50%); administer dose postdialysis or administer 25% to 35% supplemental dose.

Peritoneal dialysis: Supplemental dose is not necessary.

Dietary Considerations Should be taken at least 1 hour before or 2 hours after eating.

Monitoring Parameters BUN, serum creatinine, urine dipstick for protein, complete leukocyte count, and blood pressure

Test Interactions ↑ BUN, creatinine, potassium, positive Coombs' [direct]; ↓ cholesterol (S); may cause false-positive results in urine acetone determinations using sodium nitroprusside reagent

Patient Information Take 1 hour before meals; do not stop therapy except under prescriber advice; notify physician if you develop sore throat, fever, swelling, rash, difficult breathing, irregular heartbeats, chest pains, or cough. May cause dizziness, fainting, and lightheadedness, especially in first week of therapy; sit and stand up slowly; do not add a salt substitute (potassium) without advice of physician.

Nursing Implications Watch for hypotensive effect within 1-3 hours of first dose or new higher dose

Dosage Forms Tablet: 12.5 mg, 25 mg, 50 mg, 100 mg

Extemporaneous Preparations Captopril has limited stability in aqueous preparations. The addition of an antioxidant (sodium ascorbate) has been shown to increase the stability of captopril in solution; captopril (1 mg/mL) in syrup with methylcellulose is stable for 7 days stored either at 4°C or 22°C; captopril (1 mg/mL) in distilled water (no additives) is stable for 14 days if stored at 4°C and 7 days if stored at 22°C; captopril (1 mg/mL) with sodium ascorbate (5 mg/mL) in distilled water is stable for 56 days at 4°C and 14 days at 22°C. Captopril 0.75 mg/mL was found stable for up to 60 days at 5°C and 25°C in a 1:1 mixture of Ora-Sweet® and Ora-Plus®, in Ora-Sweet® SF and Ora-Plus®, and in cherry syrup.

Powder papers can also be made; powder papers are stable for 12 weeks when stored at room temperature

Allen LV and Erickson III MA, "Stability of Baclofen, Captopril, Diltiazem Hydrochloride, Dipyridamole, and Flecainide Acetate in Extemporaneously Compounded Oral Liquids," *Am J Health Syst Pharm*, 1996, 53:2179-84.

Nahata MC, Morosco RS, and Hipple TF, "Stability of Captopril in Three Liquid Dosage Forms," *Am J Hosp Pharm*, 1994, 51(1):95-96.

Taketomo CK, Chu SA, Cheng MH, et al, "Stability of Captopril in Powder Papers Under Three Storage Conditions," *Am J Hosp Pharm*, 1990;47(8):1799-1801.

Captopril and Hydrochlorothiazide
(KAP toe pril & hye droe klor oh THYE a zide)

U.S. Brand Names Capozide®

Canadian Brand Names Capozide®

Synonyms Hydrochlorothiazide and Captopril

Therapeutic Category Angiotensin-Converting Enzyme (ACE) Inhibitor Combination; Antihypertensive Agent, Combination

Use Management of hypertension and treatment of congestive heart failure

Pregnancy Risk Factor C/D (2nd and 3rd trimesters)

Usual Dosage Adults: Oral: Hypertension: Initial: Single tablet (captopril 25 mg/hydrochlorothiazide 15 mg) taken once daily; daily dose of captopril should not exceed 150 mg; daily dose of hydrochlorothiazide should not exceed 50 mg

Additional Information Complete prescribing information for this medication should be consulted for additional detail.

Dosage Forms
Tablet:
25/15: Captopril 25 mg and hydrochlorothiazide 15 mg
25/25: Captopril 25 mg and hydrochlorothiazide 25 mg
50/15: Captopril 50 mg and hydrochlorothiazide 15 mg
50/25: Captopril 50 mg and hydrochlorothiazide 25 mg

♦ **Carac™** see Fluorouracil on page 576
♦ **Carafate®** see Sucralfate on page 1266
♦ **Carapres® (Can)** see Clonidine on page 318

Carbachol (KAR ba kole)

Related Information
Glaucoma Drug Therapy Comparison on page 1499

U.S. Brand Names Carbastat®; Carboptic®; Isopto® Carbachol; Miostat® Intraocular

Canadian Brand Names Carbastat®; Isopto® Carbachol; Miostat®

Synonyms Carbacholine; Carbamylcholine Chloride

Therapeutic Category Cholinergic Agent, Ophthalmic; Ophthalmic Agent, Miotic

Use Lowers intraocular pressure in the treatment of glaucoma; cause miosis during surgery

Pregnancy Risk Factor C

Usual Dosage Adults:
Ophthalmic: Instill 1-2 drops up to 3 times/day
Intraocular: 0.5 mL instilled into anterior chamber before or after securing sutures

Additional Information Complete prescribing information for this medication should be consulted for additional detail.

Dosage Forms
Solution, intraocular (Carbastat®, Miostat®): 0.01% (1.5 mL)
Solution, ophthalmic, topical:
Carboptic®: 3% (15 mL)
Isopto® Carbachol: 0.75% (15 mL, 30 mL); 1.5% (15 mL, 30 mL); 2.25% (15 mL); 3% (15 mL, 30 mL)

♦ **Carbacholine** see Carbachol on page 221

Carbamazepine (kar ba MAZ e peen)

Related Information
Anticonvulsants by Seizure Type on page 1481
Depression on page 1655
Epilepsy & Seizure Treatment on page 1659

U.S. Brand Names Carbatrol®; Epitol®; Tegretol®; Tegretol®-XR

(Continued)

Carbamazepine *(Continued)*

Canadian Brand Names Apo®-Carbamazepine; Gen-Carbamazepine CR; Novo-Carbamaz®; Nu-Carbamazepine®; PMS-Carbamazepine; Taro-Carbamazepin; Tegretol®

Synonyms CBZ

Therapeutic Category Anticonvulsant

Use Partial seizures with complex symptomatology (psychomotor, temporal lobe), generalized tonic-clonic seizures (grand mal), mixed seizure patterns; pain relief of trigeminal or glosso-pharyngeal neuralgia

Unlabeled/Investigational Use Treatment of bipolar disorders and other affective disorders, resistant schizophrenia, ethanol withdrawal, restless leg syndrome, psychotic behavior associated with dementia, post-traumatic stress disorders

Pregnancy Risk Factor D

Pregnancy/Breast-Feeding Implications
Clinical effects on the fetus: Crosses the placenta. Dysmorphic facial features, cranial defects, cardiac defects, spina bifida, IUGR, and multiple other malformations reported. Epilepsy itself, number of medications, genetic factors, or a combination of these probably influence the teratogenicity of anticonvulsant therapy. Benefit:risk ratio usually favors continued use during pregnancy and breast-feeding.
Breast-feeding/lactation: Crosses into breast milk. AAP considers **compatible** with breast-feeding.

Contraindications Hypersensitivity to carbamazepine or any component of the formulation; may have cross-sensitivity with tricyclic antidepressants; marrow depression; MAO inhibitor use; pregnancy (may harm fetus)

Warnings/Precautions MAO inhibitors should be discontinued for a minimum of 14 days before carbamazepine is begun; administer with caution to patients with history of cardiac damage or hepatic disease; potentially fatal blood cell abnormalities have been reported following treatment; early detection of hematologic change is important; advise patients of early signs and symptoms including fever, sore throat, mouth ulcers, infections, easy bruising, petechial or purpuric hemorrhage; carbamazepine is not effective in absence, myoclonic or akinetic seizures; exacerbation of certain seizure types have been seen after initiation of carbamazepine therapy in children with mixed seizure disorders. Elderly may have increased risk of SIADH-like syndrome.

Adverse Reactions Frequency not defined.
Cardiovascular: Edema, congestive heart failure, syncope, bradycardia, hypertension or hypotension, AV block, arrhythmias, thrombophlebitis, thromboembolism, lymphadenopathy
Central nervous system: Sedation, dizziness, fatigue, ataxia, confusion, headache, slurred speech, aseptic meningitis (case report)
Dermatologic: Rash, urticaria, toxic epidermal necrolysis, Stevens-Johnson syndrome, photosensitivity reaction, alterations in skin pigmentation, exfoliative dermatitis, erythema multiforme, purpura, alopecia
Endocrine & metabolic: Hyponatremia, SIADH, fever, chills
Gastrointestinal: Nausea, vomiting, gastric distress, abdominal pain, diarrhea, constipation, anorexia, pancreatitis
Genitourinary: Urinary retention, urinary frequency, azotemia, renal failure, impotence
Hematologic: Aplastic anemia, agranulocytosis, eosinophilia, leukopenia, pancytopenia, thrombocytopenia, bone marrow suppression, acute intermittent porphyria, leukocytosis
Hepatic: Hepatitis, abnormal liver function tests, jaundice, hepatic failure
Neuromuscular & skeletal: Peripheral neuritis
Ocular: Blurred vision, nystagmus, lens opacities, conjunctivitis
Otic: Tinnitus, hyperacusis
Miscellaneous: Hypersensitivity (including multiorgan reactions, may include vasculitis, disorders mimicking lymphoma, eosinophilia, hepatosplenomegaly), diaphoresis

Overdosage/Toxicology Symptoms include dizziness ataxia, drowsiness, nausea, vomiting, tremor, agitation, nystagmus, urinary retention, dysrhythmias, coma, seizures, twitches, respiratory depression, and neuromuscular disturbances. Provide general supportive care. Activated charcoal is effective at binding certain chemicals and this is especially true for carbamazepine. Other treatment is supportive/symptomatic. Treatment consists of inducing emesis or gastric lavage. EKG should also be monitored to detect cardiac dysfunction. Monitor blood pressure, body temperature, pupillary reflexes, bladder function for several days following ingestion.

Drug Interactions
Cytochrome P450 Effect: CYP2C8 and 3A3/4 enzyme substrate; CYP1A2, 2C, and 3A3/4 inducer
Note: Carbamazepine (CBZ) is a heteroinducer. It induces its own metabolism as well as the metabolism of other drugs. If CBZ is added to a drug regimen, serum concentrations may decrease. Conversely, if CBZ is part of an ongoing regimen and it is discontinued, elevated concentrations of the other drugs may result.
Increased Effect/Toxicity: Carbamazepine levels/toxicity may be increased by amprenavir (and possibly other protease inhibitors), cimetidine, clarithromycin, danazol, diltiazem, erythromycin, felbamate, fluoxetine, fluvoxamine, isoniazid, lamotrigine, metronidazole, propoxyphene, verapamil, fluconazole, itraconazole, and ketoconazole. Carbamazepine may enhance the hepatotoxic potential of acetaminophen. Neurotoxicity may result in patients receiving lithium and carbamazepine concurrently.
Decreased Effect: Carbamazepine may decrease the effect of benzodiazepines, citalopram, clozapine, corticosteroids, cyclosporine, doxycycline, ethosuximide, felbamate, felodipine, haloperidol, mebendazole, methadone, oral contraceptives, phenytoin, tacrolimus, theophylline, thyroid hormones, tricyclic antidepressants, valproic acid, and warfarin. Carbamazepine suspension is incompatible with chlorpromazine solution and thioridazine liquid. Schedule carbamazepine suspension at least 1-2 hours apart from other liquid medicinals.

Ethanol/Nutrition/Herb Interactions
Ethanol: Avoid ethanol (may increase CNS depression).

Food: Carbamazepine serum levels may be increased if taken with food. Carbamazepine serum concentration may be increased if taken with grapefruit juice; avoid concurrent use.

Herb/Nutraceutical: Avoid evening primrose (seizure threshold decreased). Avoid valerian, St John's wort, kava kava, gotu kola (may increase CNS depression).

Mechanism of Action In addition to anticonvulsant effects, carbamazepine has anticholinergic, antineuralgic, antidiuretic, muscle relaxant and antiarrhythmic properties; may depress activity in the nucleus ventralis of the thalamus or decrease synaptic transmission or decrease summation of temporal stimulation leading to neural discharge by limiting influx of sodium ions across cell membrane or other unknown mechanisms; stimulates the release of ADH and potentiates its action in promoting reabsorption of water; chemically related to tricyclic antidepressants

Pharmacodynamics/Kinetics

Onset of action: Several days to reach steady-state concentrations

Absorption: Slow

Distribution: V_d: Neonates: 1.5 L/kg; Children: 1.9 L/kg; Adults: 0.59-2 L/kg

Protein binding: 75% to 90%; may be decreased in newborns

Metabolism: Hepatic to active epoxide metabolite; induces liver enzymes to increase metabolism.

Bioavailability: 85%

Half-life elimination: Initial: 18-55 hours; Multiple dosing: Children: 8-14 hours; Adults: 12-17 hours

Time to peak, serum: Unpredictable, 4-8 hours

Excretion: Urine (1% to 3% as unchanged drug)

Usual Dosage Oral (dosage must be adjusted according to patient's response and serum concentrations):

Children:

<6 years: Initial: 5 mg/kg/day; dosage may be increased every 5-7 days to 10 mg/kg/day; then up to 20 mg/kg/day if necessary; administer in 2-4 divided doses

6-12 years: Initial: 100 mg twice daily or 10 mg/kg/day in 2 divided doses; increase by 100 mg/day at weekly intervals depending upon response; usual maintenance: 20-30 mg/kg/day in 2-4 divided doses (maximum dose: 1000 mg/day)

Children >12 years and Adults: 200 mg twice daily to start, increase by 200 mg/day at weekly intervals until therapeutic levels achieved; usual dose: 400-1200 mg/day in 2-4 divided doses; maximum dose: 12-15 years: 1000 mg/day, >15 years: 1200 mg/day; some patients have required up to 1.6-2.4 g/day

Trigeminal or glossopharyngeal neuralgia: Initial: 100 mg twice daily with food, gradually increasing in increments of 100 mg twice daily as needed; usual maintenance: 400-800 mg daily in 2 divided doses; maximum dose: 1200 mg/day

Elderly: 100 mg 1-2 times daily, increase in increments of 100 mg/day at weekly intervals until therapeutic level is achieved; usual dose: 400-1000 mg/day

Dosing adjustment in renal impairment: Cl_{cr} <10 mL/minute: Administer 75% of dose

Dietary Considerations Drug may cause GI upset, take with large amount of water or food to decrease GI upset. May need to split doses to avoid GI upset.

Administration

Suspension dosage form must be given on a 3-4 times/day schedule versus tablets which can be given 2-4 times/day. When carbamazepine suspension has been combined with chlorpromazine or thioridazine solutions a precipitate forms which may result in loss of effect. Therefore, it is recommended that the carbamazepine suspension dosage form not be administered at the same time with other liquid medicinal agents or diluents. Since a given dose of suspension will produce higher peak levels than the same dose given as the tablet form, patients given the suspension should be started on lower doses and increased slowly to avoid unwanted side effects.

Extended release tablets should be inspected for damage. Damaged extended release tablets (without release portal) should not be administered.

Monitoring Parameters CBC with platelet count, reticulocytes, serum iron, liver function tests, urinalysis, BUN, serum carbamazepine levels, thyroid function tests, serum sodium; observe patient for excessive sedation, especially when instituting or increasing therapy

Reference Range

Timing of serum samples: Absorption is slow, peak levels occur 6-8 hours after ingestion of the first dose; the half-life ranges from 8-60 hours, therefore, steady-state is achieved in 2-5 days

Therapeutic levels: 4-12 µg/mL (SI: 25-51 µmol/L)

Toxic concentration: >15 µg/mL; patients who require higher levels of 8-12 µg/mL (SI: 34-51 µmol/L) should be watched closely. Side effects including CNS effects occur commonly at higher dosage levels. If other anticonvulsants are given therapeutic range is 4-8 µg/mL.

Patient Information Take with food, may cause drowsiness, periodic blood test monitoring required; notify physician if you observe bleeding, bruising, jaundice, abdominal pain, pale stools, mental disturbances, fever, chills, sore throat, or mouth ulcers

Nursing Implications Observe patient for excessive sedation; suspension dosage form must be given on a 3-4 times/day schedule versus tablets which can be given 2-4 times/day

Additional Information Investigationally, loading doses of the suspension (10 mg/kg for children <12 years of age and 8 mg/kg for children >12 years of age) were given (via NG or ND tubes followed by 5-10 mL of water to flush through tube) to PICU patients with frequent seizures/status. Five of 6 patients attained mean Cp of 4.3 mcg/mL and 7.3 mcg/mL at 1 and 2 hours postload. Concurrent enteral feeding or ileus may delay absorption.

Dosage Forms

Capsule, extended release: 200 mg, 300 mg

Suspension, oral: 100 mg/5 mL (450 mL) [citrus-vanilla flavor]

Tablet: 200 mg

Tablet, chewable: 100 mg

Tablet, extended release: 100 mg, 200 mg, 400 mg

♦ **Carbamide** see Urea on page 1391

Carbamide Peroxide (KAR ba mide per OKS ide)

U.S. Brand Names Auro® Ear Drops [OTC]; Debrox® Otic [OTC]; E•R•O Ear [OTC]; Gly-Oxide® Oral [OTC]; Mollifene® Ear Wax Removing Formula [OTC]; Murine® Ear Drops [OTC]; Orajel® Perioseptic® [OTC]; Proxigel® Oral [OTC]

Synonyms Urea Peroxide

Therapeutic Category Anti-infective Agent, Oral; Otic Agent, Cerumenolytic

Use Relief of minor inflammation of gums, oral mucosal surfaces and lips including canker sores and dental irritation; emulsify and disperse ear wax

Pregnancy Risk Factor C

Usual Dosage Children and Adults:

Gel: Gently massage on affected area 4 times/day; do not drink or rinse mouth for 5 minutes after use

Oral solution (should not be used for >7 days): Oral preparation should not be used in children <3 years of age; apply several drops undiluted on affected area 4 times/day after meals and at bedtime; expectorate after 2-3 minutes **or** place 10 drops onto tongue, mix with saliva, swish for several minutes, expectorate

Otic:

Children <12 years: Tilt head sideways and individualize the dose according to patient size; 3 drops (range: 1-5 drops) twice daily for up to 4 days, tip of applicator should not enter ear canal; keep drops in ear for several minutes by keeping head tilted and placing cotton in ear

Children ≥12 years and Adults: Tilt head sideways and instill 5-10 drops twice daily up to 4 days, tip of applicator should not enter ear canal; keep drops in ear for several minutes by keeping head tilted and placing cotton in ear

Additional Information Complete prescribing information for this medication should be consulted for additional detail.

Dosage Forms

Gel, oral (Proxigel®): 10% (34 g)

Solution, oral:

Gly-Oxide®: 10% in glycerin (15 mL, 60 mL)

Orajel® Perioseptic®: 15% in glycerin (13.3 mL)

Solution, otic (Auro® Ear Drops, Debrox®, E•R•O Ear, Mollifene® Ear Wax Removing, Murine® Ear Drops): 6.5% in glycerin (15 mL, 30 mL)

- ♦ **Carbamylcholine Chloride** *see* Carbachol *on page 221*
- ♦ **Carbastat®** *see* Carbachol *on page 221*
- ♦ **Carbatrol®** *see* Carbamazepine *on page 221*

Carbenicillin (kar ben i SIL in)

U.S. Brand Names Geocillin®

Synonyms Carbenicillin Indanyl Sodium; Carindacillin

Therapeutic Category Antibiotic, Penicillin

Use Treatment of serious urinary tract infections and prostatitis caused by susceptible gram-negative aerobic bacilli

Pregnancy Risk Factor B

Contraindications Hypersensitivity to carbenicillin, penicillins, or any component of the formulation

Warnings/Precautions Do not use in patients with severe renal impairment (Cl_{cr} <10 mL/minute); dosage modification required in patients with impaired renal and/or hepatic function. Use with caution in patients with history of hypersensitivity to cephalosporins.

Adverse Reactions

>10%: Gastrointestinal: Diarrhea

1% to 10%: Gastrointestinal: Nausea, bad taste, vomiting, flatulence, glossitis

<1% (Limited to important or life-threatening): Anemia, elevated LFTs, eosinophilia, epigastric distress, furry tongue, headache, hematuria, hypersensitivity reactions, hyperthermia, hypokalemia, leukopenia, neutropenia, rash, thrombocytopenia, urticaria

Overdosage/Toxicology Symptoms include neuromuscular hypersensitivity and convulsions. Many beta-lactam containing antibiotics have the potential to cause neuromuscular hyperirritability or convulsive seizures. Hemodialysis may be helpful to aid in the removal of the drug from the blood, otherwise, most treatment is supportive or symptom directed.

Drug Interactions

Increased Effect/Toxicity: Increased bleeding effects if taken with high doses of heparin or oral anticoagulants. Aminoglycosides may be synergistic against selected organisms. Probenecid and disulfiram may increase levels of penicillins (carbenicillin).

Decreased Effect: Decreased efficacy of oral contraceptives is possible with carbenicillin. Decreased effectiveness with tetracyclines.

Mechanism of Action Inhibits bacterial cell wall synthesis by binding to one or more of the penicillin binding proteins (PBPs); which in turn inhibits the final transpeptidation step of peptidoglycan synthesis in bacterial cell walls, thus inhibiting cell wall biosynthesis. Bacteria eventually lyse due to ongoing activity of cell wall autolytic enzymes (autolysins and murein hydrolases) while cell wall assembly is arrested.

Pharmacodynamics/Kinetics

Absorption: 30% to 40%

Distribution: Crosses placenta; small amounts enter breast milk; distributes into bile; low concentrations attained in CSF

Half-life elimination: Children: 0.8-1.8 hours; Adults: 1-1.5 hours, prolonged to 10-20 hours with renal insufficiency

Time to peak, serum: Normal renal function: 0.5-2 hours; concentrations are inadequate for treatment of systemic infections

Excretion: Urine (~80% to 99% as unchanged drug)

Usual Dosage Oral:

Children: 30-50 mg/kg/day divided every 6 hours; maximum dose: 2-3 g/day

Adults: 1-2 tablets every 6 hours for urinary tract infections or 2 tablets every 6 hours for prostatitis

Dosing interval in renal impairment: Adults:

Cl$_{cr}$ 10-50 mL/minute: Administer 382-764 mg every 12-24 hours

Cl$_{cr}$ <10 mL/minute: Administer 382-764 mg every 24-48 hours

Moderately dialyzable (20% to 50%)

Dietary Considerations Should be taken with water on empty stomach.

Monitoring Parameters Renal, hepatic, and hematologic function tests

Reference Range Therapeutic: Not established; Toxic: >250 µg/mL (SI: >660 µmol/L)

Test Interactions May interfere with urinary glucose tests using cupric sulfate (Benedict's solution, Clinitest®); may inactivate aminoglycosides *in vitro*; false-positive urine or serum proteins

Patient Information Tablets have a bitter taste; take with a full glass of water; take all medication for 7-14 days, do not skip doses; may interfere with oral contraceptives

Nursing Implications

Administer around-the-clock to promote less variation in peak and trough serum levels

Watch for increased edema, rales, or signs of congestion, bruising, or bleeding; monitor renal, hepatic, and hematologic function tests

Additional Information Sodium content of 382 mg tablet: 23 mg (1 mEq)

Dosage Forms Tablet, film coated: 382 mg

♦ **Carbenicillin Indanyl Sodium** *see* Carbenicillin *on page 224*

Carbidopa (kar bi DOE pa)

U.S. Brand Names Lodosyn®

Therapeutic Category Anti-Parkinson's Agent, Dopamine Agonist; Dopaminergic Agent (Antiparkinson's)

Use Given with levodopa in the treatment of parkinsonism to enable a lower dosage of levodopa to be used and a more rapid response to be obtained and to decrease side-effects; for details of administration and dosage, see Levodopa; has no effect without levodopa

Pregnancy Risk Factor C

Usual Dosage Adults: Oral: 70-100 mg/day; maximum daily dose: 200 mg

Additional Information Complete prescribing information for this medication should be consulted for additional detail.

Dosage Forms Tablet: 25 mg

♦ **Carbidopa and Levodopa** *see* Levodopa and Carbidopa *on page 791*

Carbinoxamine and Pseudoephedrine

(kar bi NOKS a meen & soo doe e FED rin)

U.S. Brand Names Biohist® LA; Carbiset®; Carbiset-TR®; Carbodec®; Carbodec® TR Tablet; Cardec-S® Syrup; Rondec® Drops; Rondec® Filmtab®; Rondec-TR®

Synonyms Pseudoephedrine and Carbinoxamine

Therapeutic Category Adrenergic Agonist Agent; Antihistamine, H$_1$ Blocker; Decongestant

Use Temporary relief of nasal congestion, running nose, sneezing, itching of nose or throat, and itchy, watery eyes due to the common cold, hay fever, or other respiratory allergies

Pregnancy Risk Factor C

Usual Dosage Oral:

Children:

Drops:

1-3 months: 0.25 mL 4 times/day

3-6 months: 0.5 mL 4 times/day

6-9 months: 0.75 mL 4 times/day

9-18 months: 1 mL 4 times/day

Syrup:

18 months to 6 years: 2.5 mL 3-4 times/day

>6 years: 5 mL 2-4 times/day

Adults:

Liquid: 5 mL 4 times/day

Tablets: 1 tablet 4 times/day

Tablets, sustained release: 1 tablet every 12 hours

Additional Information Complete prescribing information for this medication should be consulted for additional detail.

Dosage Forms

Solution, oral [drops]: Carbinoxamine maleate 2 mg and pseudoephedrine hydrochloride 25 mg per mL (30 mL with dropper)

Syrup: Carbinoxamine maleate 4 mg and pseudoephedrine hydrochloride 60 mg per 5 mL (120 mL, 480 mL)

Tablet, film coated: Carbinoxamine maleate 4 mg and pseudoephedrine hydrochloride 60 mg

Tablet, sustained release: Carbinoxamine maleate 8 mg and pseudoephedrine hydrochloride 120 mg

♦ **Carbinoxamine, Dextromethorphan, and Pseudoephedrine** *see* Carbinoxamine, Pseudoephedrine, and Dextromethorphan *on page 225*

Carbinoxamine, Pseudoephedrine, and Dextromethorphan

(kar bi NOKS a meen, soo doe e FED rin, & deks troe meth OR fan)

U.S. Brand Names Carbodec DM®; Cardec DM®; Pseudo-Car® DM; Rondamine-DM® Drops; Rondec®-DM; Tussafed® Drops

Synonyms Carbinoxamine, Dextromethorphan, and Pseudoephedrine; Dextromethorphan, Carbinoxamine, and Pseudoephedrine; Dextromethorphan, Pseudoephedrine, and Carbinoxamine; Pseudoephedrine, Carbinoxamine, and Dextromethorphan; Pseudoephedrine, Dextromethorphan, and Carbinoxamine

Therapeutic Category Antihistamine/Decongestant/Antitussive

(Continued)

Carbinoxamine, Pseudoephedrine, and Dextromethorphan
(Continued)

Use Relief of coughs and upper respiratory symptoms, including nasal congestion, associated with allergy or the common cold

Pregnancy Risk Factor C

Usual Dosage

Infants: Drops:
1-3 months: $1/4$ mL 4 times/day
3-6 months: $1/2$ mL 4 times/day
6-9 months: $3/4$ mL 4 times/day
9-18 months: 1 mL 4 times/day
Children $1^{1}/_{2}$ to 6 years: Syrup: 2.5 mL 4 times/day
Children >6 years and Adults: Syrup: 5 mL 4 times/day

Additional Information Complete prescribing information for this medication should be consulted for additional detail.

Dosage Forms

Solution, oral [drops]: Carbinoxamine maleate 2 mg, pseudoephedrine hydrochloride 25 mg, and dextromethorphan hydrobromide 4 mg per mL (30 mL)

Syrup: Carbinoxamine maleate 4 mg, pseudoephedrine hydrochloride 60 mg, and dextromethorphan hydrobromide 15 mg per 5 mL (120 mL, 480 mL, 4000 mL)

- ♦ **Carbiset**® *see* Carbinoxamine and Pseudoephedrine *on page 225*
- ♦ **Carbiset-TR**® *see* Carbinoxamine and Pseudoephedrine *on page 225*
- ♦ **Carbocaine**® *see* Mepivacaine *on page 861*
- ♦ **Carbodec**® *see* Carbinoxamine and Pseudoephedrine *on page 225*
- ♦ **Carbodec DM**® *see* Carbinoxamine, Pseudoephedrine, and Dextromethorphan *on page 225*
- ♦ **Carbodec**® **TR Tablet** *see* Carbinoxamine and Pseudoephedrine *on page 225*
- ♦ **Carbolith**™ **(Can)** *see* Lithium *on page 811*

Carboplatin (KAR boe pla tin)
U.S. Brand Names Paraplatin®
Canadian Brand Names Paraplatin-AQ
Synonyms CBDCA
Therapeutic Category Antineoplastic Agent, Alkylating Agent; Antineoplastic Agent, Irritant
Use Initial treatment of ovarian cancer; secondary treatment of advanced ovarian cancer
Unlabeled/Investigational Use Lung cancer, head and neck cancer, endometrial cancer, esophageal cancer, bladder cancer, breast cancer, cervical cancer, CNS tumors, germ cell tumors, osteogenic sarcoma, and high-dose therapy with stem cell/bone marrow support
Pregnancy Risk Factor D
Contraindications History of severe allergic reaction to cisplatin, carboplatin, other platinum-containing formulations, mannitol, or any component of the formulation; pregnancy
Warnings/Precautions The U.S. Food and Drug Administration (FDA) currently recommends that procedures for proper handling and disposal of antineoplastic agents be considered. High doses have resulted in severe abnormalities of liver function tests. Bone marrow suppression, which may be severe, and vomiting are dose related; reduce dosage in patients with bone marrow suppression and impaired renal function. Clinically significant hearing loss has been reported to occur in pediatric patients when carboplatin was administered at higher than recommended doses in combination with other ototoxic agents. Increased risk of allergic reactions in patients previously exposed to platinum therapy. When administered as sequential infusions, taxane derivatives (docetaxel, paclitaxel) should be administered before platinum derivatives (carboplatin, cisplatin) to limit myelosuppression and to enhance efficacy.

Adverse Reactions

>10%:
Endocrine & metabolic: Electrolyte abnormalities such as hypocalcemia and hypomagnesemia, hyponatremia, hypokalemia
Gastrointestinal: Nausea, vomiting, stomatitis
Emetic potential: Moderate
Time course for nausea and vomiting: Onset: 2-6 hours; Duration: 1-48 hours
Hematologic: Neutropenia, leukopenia, thrombocytopenia, anemia
Myelosuppressive: Dose-limiting toxicity
WBC: Severe (dose-dependent)
Platelets: Severe
Nadir: 21-24 days
Recovery: 28-35 days
Hepatic: Abnormal liver function tests
Local: Pain at injection site
Neuromuscular & skeletal: Weakness
Otic: Hearing loss at high tones (above speech ranges) has been reported in up to 19% in one series; clinically important ototoxicity is not usually seen; routine audiometric testing is not recommended
1% to 10%:
Dermatologic: Alopecia
Gastrointestinal: Diarrhea, anorexia
Hematologic: Hemorrhagic complications
Neuromuscular & skeletal: Peripheral neuropathy (4% to 6%; up to 10% in older and/or previously-treated patients)
Otic: Ototoxicity
<1% (Limited to important or life-threatening): Neurotoxicity has only been noted in patients previously treated with cisplatin; anaphylaxis, hypertension, malaise, nephrotoxicity (uncommon), rash, secondary malignancies, urticaria
BMT:
Dermatologic: Alopecia
Endocrine & metabolic: Hypokalemia, hypomagnesemia

Gastrointestinal: Nausea, vomiting, mucositis
Hepatic: Elevated liver function tests
Renal: Nephrotoxicity

Overdosage/Toxicology Symptoms include bone marrow suppression and hepatic toxicity.

Drug Interactions

Increased Effect/Toxicity: Nephrotoxic drugs; aminoglycosides increase risk of ototoxicity. When administered as sequential infusions, observational studies indicate a potential for increased toxicity when platinum derivatives (carboplatin, cisplatin) are administered before taxane derivatives (docetaxel, paclitaxel).

Ethanol/Nutrition/Herb Interactions Herb/Nutraceutical: Avoid black cohosh, dong quai in estrogen-dependent tumors.

Stability

Store intact vials at room temperature (15°C to 30°C/59°F to 86°F) and protect from light

Reconstitute powder to yield a final concentration of 10 mg/mL which is stable for 5 days at room temperature (25°C)

Aluminum needles should not be used for administration due to binding with the platinum ion

Compatible with etoposide

Standard I.V. dilution: Dose/250-1000 mL D_5W

Further dilution to a concentration as low as 0.5 mg/mL is stable at room temperature (25°C) or under refrigeration for 8 days in D_5W

Mechanism of Action Analogue of cisplatin which covalently binds to DNA; possible cross-linking and interference with the function of DNA

Pharmacodynamics/Kinetics

Distribution: V_d: 16 L/kg; Into liver, kidney, skin, and tumor tissue

Protein binding: 0%; platinum is 30% irreversibly bound

Metabolism: Minimally to aquated and hydroxylated compounds

Half-life elimination: Terminal: 22-40 hours; Cl_{cr} >60 mL/minute: 2.5-5.9 hours

Excretion: Urine (~60% to 90%) within 24 hours

Usual Dosage IVPB, I.V. infusion, intraperitoneal (refer to individual protocols):

Children:

Solid tumor: 300-600 mg/m^2 once every 4 weeks

Brain tumor: 175 mg/m^2 once weekly for 4 weeks with a 2-week recovery period between courses; dose is then adjusted on platelet count and neutrophil count values

Adults:

Ovarian cancer: Usual doses range from 360 mg/m^2 I.V. every 3 weeks single agent therapy to 300 mg/m^2 every 4 weeks as combination therapy

In general, however, single intermittent courses of carboplatin should not be repeated until the neutrophil count is at least 2000 and the platelet count is at least 100,000

The following dose adjustments are modified from a controlled trial in previously treated patients with ovarian carcinoma. Blood counts were done weekly, and the recommendations are based on the lowest post-treatment platelet or neutrophil value.

Carboplatin dosage adjustment based on pretreatment platelet counts

- Platelets >100,000 cells/mm^3 and neutrophils >2000 cells/mm^3: Adjust dose 125% from prior course
- Platelets 50-100,000 cells/mm^3 and neutrophils 500-2000 cells/mm^3: No dose adjustment
- Platelets <50,000 cells/mm^3 and neutrophils <500 cells/mm^3: Adjust dose 75% from prior course

Carboplatin dosage adjustment based on the Egorin formula (based on platelet counts):

Previously untreated patients:

$$\text{dosage (mg/m}^2) = (0.091) \frac{(Cl_{cr})}{(BSA)} \frac{(\text{Pretreat Plt count - Plt nadir count desired} \times 100)}{(\text{Pretreatment Plt count})} + 86$$

Previously treated patients with heavily myelosuppressive agents:

$$\text{dosage (mg/m}^2) = (0.091) \frac{(Cl_{cr})}{(BSA)} \frac{[(\text{Pretreat Plt count - Plt nadir count desired} \times 100) - 17]}{(\text{Pretreatment Plt count})} + 86$$

Autologous BMT: I.V.: 1600 mg/m^2 (total dose) divided over 4 days **requires BMT (ie, FATAL without BMT)**

Dosing adjustment in hepatic impairment: There are no published studies available on the dosing of carboplatin in patients with impaired liver function. Human data regarding the biliary elimination of carboplatin are not available; however, pharmacokinetic studies in rabbits and rats reflect a biliary excretion of 0.4% to 0.7% of the dose (ie, 0.05 mL/minute/kg biliary clearance).

Dosing adjustment in renal impairment: These dosing recommendations apply to the initial course of treatment. Subsequent dosages should be adjusted according to the patient's tolerance based on the degree of bone marrow suppression.

Cl_{cr} <60 mL/minute: Increased risk of severe bone marrow suppression. In renally impaired patients who received single agent carboplatin therapy, the incidence of severe leukopenia, neutropenia, or thrombocytopenia has been about 25% when the following dosage modifications have been used:

Cl_{cr} 41-59 mL/minute: Recommended dose on day 1 is 250 mg/m^2

Cl_{cr} 16-40 mL/minute: Recommended dose on day 1 is 200 mg/m^2

Cl_{cr} <15 mL/minute: The data available for patients with severely impaired kidney function are too limited to permit a recommendation for treatment

or

Dosing adjustment in renal impairment: CALVERT FORMULA

Total dose (mg) = Target AUC (mg/mL/minute) x (GFR [mL/minute] + 25)

Note: The dose of carboplatin calculated is TOTAL mg DOSE not mg/m^2. AUC is the area under the concentration versus time curve.

(Continued)

Carboplatin *(Continued)*

Target AUC value will vary depending upon:
Number of agents in the regimen
Treatment status (ie, previously untreated or treated)
For single agent carboplatin/no prior chemotherapy: Total dose (mg): 6-8 (GFR + 25)
For single agent carboplatin/prior chemotherapy: Total dose (mg): 4-6 (GFR + 25)
For combination chemotherapy/no prior chemotherapy: Total dose (mg): 4.5-6 (GFR + 25)
For combination chemotherapy/prior chemotherapy: A reasonable approach for these patients would be to use a target AUC value <5 for the initial cycle

Note: The Jelliffe formula (below) substantially underestimates the creatinine clearance in patients with a serum creatinine <1.5 mg/dL. However, the Jelliffe formula is more accurate in estimating creatinine clearance in patients with significant renal impairment than the Cockroft and Gault formula.

Cl_{cr} (mL/minute/1.73 m^2) for males = 98 - [(0.8) (Age - 20)]/S_{cr}

Cl_{cr} (mL/minute/1.73 m^2) for females = 98 - [(0.8) (Age - 20)]/S_{cr} multiplied by 90%

Intraperitoneal: 200-650 mg/m^2 in 2 L of dialysis fluid have been administered into the peritoneum of ovarian cancer patients

Administration
Do not use needles or I.V. administration sets containing aluminum parts that may come in contact with carboplatin (aluminum can react causing precipitate formation and loss of potency)
Administer as IVPB over 15 minutes up to a continuous intravenous infusion over 24 hours; may also be administered intraperitoneally

Monitoring Parameters CBC (with differential and platelet count), serum electrolytes, urinalysis, creatinine clearance, liver function tests

Patient Information Maintain adequate nutrition (frequent small meals may help) and adequate hydration (2-3 L/day of fluids unless instructed to restrict fluid intake). Nausea and vomiting may be severe; request antiemetic. You will be susceptible to infection; avoid crowds or exposure to infection. Report sore throat, fever, chills, unusual fatigue or unusual bruising/bleeding, difficulty breathing, muscle cramps or twitching, or change in hearing acuity. Contraceptive measures are recommended during therapy.

Nursing Implications Needle or intravenous administration sets containing aluminum parts should not be used in the administration or preparation of carboplatin (aluminum can interact with carboplatin resulting in precipitate formation and loss of potency); administer by I.V. intermittent infusion over 15 minutes to 1 hour, or by continuous infusion (continuous infusion regimens may be less toxic than the bolus route); reconstituted carboplatin 10 mg/mL should be further diluted to a final concentration of 0.5-2 mg/mL with D$_5$W or NS for administration

Dosage Forms Powder for injection, lyophilized: 50 mg, 150 mg, 450 mg

♦ **Carboprost** *see Carboprost Tromethamine on page 228*

Carboprost Tromethamine *(KAR boe prost tro METH a meen)*

U.S. Brand Names Hemabate™
Canadian Brand Names Hemabate™
Synonyms Carboprost
Therapeutic Category Abortifacient; Prostaglandin
Use Termination of pregnancy and refractory postpartum uterine bleeding
Unlabeled/Investigational Use Investigational: Hemorrhagic cystitis
Pregnancy Risk Factor X
Contraindications Hypersensitivity to carboprost tromethamine or any component of the formulation; acute pelvic inflammatory disease; pregnancy
Warnings/Precautions Use with caution in patients with history of asthma, hypotension or hypertension, cardiovascular, adrenal, renal or hepatic disease, anemia, jaundice, diabetes, epilepsy or compromised uteri
Adverse Reactions
>10%: Gastrointestinal: Diarrhea, vomiting, nausea
1% to 10%:
Cardiovascular: Flushing
Central nervous system: Dizziness, headache
Gastrointestinal: Stomach cramps
<1% (Limited to important or life-threatening): Abnormal taste, asthma, bladder spasms, blurred vision, bradycardia or tachycardia, breast tenderness, coughing, drowsiness, dry mouth, dystonia, fever, hiccups, hematemesis, hypertension, hypotension, myalgia, nervousness, respiratory distress, septic shock, vasovagal syndrome, vertigo
Drug Interactions
Increased Effect/Toxicity: Toxicity may be increased by oxytocic agents.
Stability Refrigerate ampuls
Bladder irrigation: Dilute immediately prior to administration in NS; stability unknown
Mechanism of Action Carboprost tromethamine is a prostaglandin similar to prostaglandin F$_2$ alpha (dinoprost) except for the addition of a methyl group at the C-15 position. This substitution produces longer duration of activity than dinoprost; carboprost stimulates uterine contractility which usually results in expulsion of the products of conception and is used to induce abortion between 13-20 weeks of pregnancy. Hemostasis at the placentation site is achieved through the myometrial contractions produced by carboprost.
Usual Dosage Adults: I.M.:
Abortion: Initial: 250 mcg, then 250 mcg at 1½-hour to 3½-hour intervals depending on uterine response; a 500 mcg dose may be given if uterine response is not adequate after several 250 mcg doses; do not exceed 12 mg total dose or continuous administration for >2 days
Refractory postpartum uterine bleeding: Initial: 250 mcg; may repeat at 15- to 90-minute intervals to a total dose of 2 mg
Bladder irrigation for hemorrhagic cystitis (refer to individual protocols): [0.4-1.0 mg/dL as solution] 50 mL instilled into bladder 4 times/day for 1 hour

Administration Do not inject I.V.; may result in bronchospasm, hypertension, vomiting, and anaphylaxis

Nursing Implications Do not inject I.V. (may result in bronchospasm, hypertension, vomiting and anaphylaxis)

Dosage Forms Injection: Carboprost 250 mcg and tromethamine 83 mcg per mL (1 mL)

Carisoprodol (kar eye soe PROE dole)

U.S. Brand Names Soma®

Canadian Brand Names Soma®

Synonyms Carisoprodate; Isobamate

Therapeutic Category Skeletal Muscle Relaxant

Use Skeletal muscle relaxant

Pregnancy Risk Factor C

Contraindications Hypersensitivity to carisoprodol, meprobamate or any component of the formulation; acute intermittent porphyria

Warnings/Precautions May cause CNS depression, which may impair physical or mental abilities. Effects with other sedative drugs or ethanol may be potentiated. Use with caution in patients with hepatic/renal dysfunction. Tolerance or drug dependence may result from extended use.

Adverse Reactions

>10%: Central nervous system: Drowsiness

1% to 10%:

Cardiovascular: Tachycardia, tightness in chest, flushing of face, syncope

Central nervous system: Mental depression, allergic fever, dizziness, lightheadedness, headache, paradoxical CNS stimulation

Dermatologic: Angioedema, dermatitis (allergic)

Gastrointestinal: Nausea, vomiting, stomach cramps

Neuromuscular & skeletal: Trembling

Ocular: Burning eyes

Respiratory: Dyspnea

Miscellaneous: Hiccups

<1% (Limited to important or life-threatening): Aplastic anemia, clumsiness, eosinophilia, erythema multiforme, leukopenia, rash, urticaria

Overdosage/Toxicology Symptoms include CNS depression, stupor, coma, shock, and respiratory depression. Treatment is supportive following attempts to enhance drug elimination. Hypotension should be treated with I.V. fluids and/or Trendelenburg positioning.

Drug Interactions

Cytochrome P450 Effect: CYP2C19 enzyme substrate

Increased Effect/Toxicity: Ethanol, CNS depressants, psychotropic drugs, and phenothiazines may increase toxicity.

Ethanol/Nutrition/Herb Interactions Ethanol: Avoid ethanol (may increase CNS depression).

Mechanism of Action Precise mechanism is not yet clear, but many effects have been ascribed to its central depressant actions

Pharmacodynamics/Kinetics

Onset of action: ~30 minutes

Duration: 4-6 hours

Distribution: Crosses placenta; high concentrations enter breast milk

Metabolism: Hepatic

Half-life elimination: 8 hours

Excretion: Urine

Usual Dosage Adults: Oral: 350 mg 3-4 times/day; take last dose at bedtime; compound: 1-2 tablets 4 times/day

Monitoring Parameters Look for relief of pain and/or muscle spasm and avoid excessive drowsiness

Patient Information May cause drowsiness or dizziness; avoid alcohol and other CNS depressants

Nursing Implications Raise bed rails; institute safety measures; assist with ambulation

Dosage Forms Tablet: 350 mg

Carisoprodol and Aspirin (kar eye soe PROE dole & AS pir in)

U.S. Brand Names Soma® Compound

Synonyms Aspirin and Carisoprodol

Therapeutic Category Skeletal Muscle Relaxant

(Continued)

Carisoprodol and Aspirin *(Continued)*

Use Skeletal muscle relaxant

Pregnancy Risk Factor C/D (full-dose aspirin in 3rd trimester)

Usual Dosage Adults: Oral: 1-2 tablets 4 times/day

Additional Information Complete prescribing information for this medication should be consulted for additional detail.

Dosage Forms Tablet: Carisoprodol 200 mg and aspirin 325 mg

Carisoprodol, Aspirin, and Codeine
(kar eye soe PROE dole, AS pir in, and KOE deen)

U.S. Brand Names Soma® Compound w/Codeine

Synonyms Aspirin, Carisoprodol, and Codeine; Codeine, Aspirin, and Carisoprodol

Therapeutic Category Skeletal Muscle Relaxant

Use Skeletal muscle relaxant

Restrictions C-III

Pregnancy Risk Factor C/D (full-dose aspirin in 3rd trimester)

Usual Dosage Adults: Oral: 1 or 2 tablets 4 times/day

Additional Information Complete prescribing information for this medication should be consulted for additional detail.

Dosage Forms Tablet: Carisoprodol 200 mg, aspirin 325 mg, and codeine phosphate 16 mg

♦ **Carmol® [OTC]** *see* Urea *on page 1391*

♦ **Carmol-HC®** *see* Urea and Hydrocortisone *on page 1391*

♦ **Carmol® Scalp** *see* Sulfacetamide *on page 1268*

Carmustine (kar MUS teen)

U.S. Brand Names BiCNU®; Gliadel®

Canadian Brand Names BiCNU®

Synonyms BCNU

Therapeutic Category Antineoplastic Agent, Alkylating Agent (Nitrosourea); Antineoplastic Agent, Vesicant; Vesicant

Use Treatment of brain tumors (glioblastoma, brainstem glioma, medulloblastoma, astrocytoma, ependymoma, and metastatic brain tumors), multiple myeloma, Hodgkin's disease, non-Hodgkin's lymphomas, melanoma, lung cancer, colon cancer

Gliadel®: Adjunct to surgery in patients with recurrent glioblastoma multiforme

Pregnancy Risk Factor D

Pregnancy/Breast-Feeding Implications Carmustine can cause fetal harm if administered to a pregnant woman. It is not known if carmustine is excreted in human breast milk. Due to potential harm to infant, breast-feeding is not recommended.

Contraindications Hypersensitivity to carmustine or any component of the formulation; myelosuppression (from previous chemotherapy or other causes); pregnancy

Warnings/Precautions The U.S. Food and Drug Administration (FDA) currently recommends that procedures for proper handling and disposal of antineoplastic agents be considered. Administer with caution to patients with depressed platelet, leukocyte or erythrocyte counts, renal or hepatic impairment. Bone marrow depression, notably thrombocytopenia and leukopenia, may lead to bleeding and overwhelming infections in an already compromised patient; will last for at least 6 weeks after a dose, **do not give courses more frequently than every 6 weeks because the toxicity is cumulative.**

Baseline pulmonary function tests are recommended. Delayed onset pulmonary fibrosis occurring up to 17 years after treatment has been reported in children (1-16 years) who received carmustine in cumulative doses ranging from 770-1800 mg/m^2 combined with cranial radiotherapy for intracranial tumors.

Adverse Reactions

>10%:

Cardiovascular: Hypotension is associated with **high-dose** administration secondary to the high content of the diluent

Central nervous system: Dizziness, ataxia; Wafers: Seizures (54%) postoperatively

Dermatologic: Hyperpigmentation of skin

Gastrointestinal: Nausea and vomiting occur within 2-4 hours after drug injection; dose-related

Emetic potential:

<200 mg: Moderately high (60% to 90%)

≥200 mg: High (>90%)

Time course of nausea/vomiting: Onset: 2-6 hours; Duration: 4-6 hours

Hematologic: Myelosuppressive: Delayed, occurs 4-6 weeks after administration and is dose-related; usually persists for 1-2 weeks; thrombocytopenia is usually more severe than leukopenia. Myelofibrosis and preleukemic syndromes have been reported.

WBC: Moderate

Platelets: Severe

Onset (days): 14

Nadir (days): 21-35

Recovery (days): 42-50

Local: Burning at injection site

Irritant chemotherapy: Pain at injection site

Ocular: Ocular toxicity, and retinal hemorrhages

1% to 10%:

Dermatologic: Facial flushing is probably due to the alcohol used in reconstitution, alopecia

Gastrointestinal: Stomatitis, diarrhea, anorexia

Hematologic: Anemia

<1% (Limited to important or life-threatening): Reversible toxicity; increased LFTs in 20%; fibrosis occurs mostly in patients treated with prolonged total doses >1400 mg/m^2 or with

bone marrow transplantation doses; risk factors include a history of lung disease, concomitant bleomycin, or radiation therapy; PFTs should be conducted prior to therapy and monitored; patients with predicted FVC or DLCO <70% are at a higher risk; azotemia; decrease in kidney size; renal failure

BMT:
Cardiovascular: Hypotension (infusion-related), arrhythmias (infusion-related)
Central nervous system: Encephalopathy, ethanol intoxication, seizures, fever
Endocrine & metabolic: Hyperprolactinemia and hypothyroidism in patients with brain tumors treated with radiation
Gastrointestinal: Severe nausea and vomiting
Hepatic Hepatitis, hepatic veno-occlusive disease
Pulmonary: Dyspnea

Overdosage/Toxicology Symptoms include nausea, vomiting, thrombocytopenia, and leukopenia. There are no known antidotes and treatment is primarily symptomatic and supportive.

Drug Interactions
Increased Effect/Toxicity: Carmustine given in combination with cimetidine is reported to cause bone marrow depression. Carmustine given in combination with etoposide is reported to cause severe hepatic dysfunction with hyperbilirubinemia, ascites, and thrombocytopenia.

Ethanol/Nutrition/Herb Interactions Ethanol: Avoid ethanol (due to GI irritation).

Stability
Store intact vials under refrigeration; vials are stable for 36 days at room temperature
Initially dilute with 3 mL of absolute alcohol diluent. Further dilute with 27 mL SWI to result in a concentration of 3.3 mg/mL with 10% alcohol. Initial solutions are stable for 8 hours at room temperature (25°C) and 24 hours at refrigeration (2°C to 8°C) and protected from light.
Further dilution in D_5W or NS is stable for 8 hours at room temperature (25°C) and 48 hours at refrigeration (4°C) in glass or Excel® protected from light
Incompatible with sodium bicarbonate; **compatible** with cisplatin

Standard I.V. dilution: Dose/150-500 mL D_5W or NS
Must use glass or Excel® containers for administration
Protect from light
Stable for 8 hours at room temperature (25°C) and 48 hours under refrigeration (4°C)

Mechanism of Action Interferes with the normal function of DNA by alkylation and crosslinking the strands of DNA, and by possible protein modification

Pharmacodynamics/Kinetics
Distribution: Readily crosses blood-brain barrier producing CSF levels equal to 15% to 70% of blood plasma levels; enters breast milk; highly lipid soluble
Metabolism: Rapid
Half-life elimination: Biphasic: Initial: 1.4 minutes; Secondary: 20 minutes (active metabolites: plasma half-life of 67 hours)
Excretion: Urine (~60% to 70%) within 96 hours; lungs (6% to 10% as CO_2)

Usual Dosage I.V. (refer to individual protocols):
Children: 200-250 mg/m² every 4-6 weeks as a single dose
Adults: Usual dosage (per manufacturer labeling): 150-200 mg/m² every 6-8 weeks as a single dose or divided into daily injections on 2 successive days
Next dose is to be determined based on hematologic response to the previous dose. Repeat dose should not be administered until circulating blood elements have returned to acceptable levels (leukocytes >4000, platelets >100,000), usually 6 weeks
Listed are the suggested carmustine doses, based upon the nadir after the prior dose.
• Leukocytes >4000 mm³ and platelets >100,000 mm³: Give 100% of prior dose
• Leukocytes 3000-3999 mm³ and platelets 75,000-99,999 mm³: Give 100% of prior dose
• Leukocytes 2000-2999 mm³ and platelets 25,000-74,999 mm³: Give 70% of prior dose
• Leukocytes <2000 mm³ and platelets <25,000 mm³: Give 50% of prior dose
Primary brain cancer:
150-200 mg/m² every 6-8 weeks as a single dose or divided into daily injections on 2 successive days
20-65 mg/m² every 4-6 weeks
0.5-1 mg/kg every 4-6 weeks
40-80 mg/m²/day for 3 days every 6-8 weeks
Autologous BMT: ALL OF THE FOLLOWING DOSES ARE FATAL WITHOUT BMT
Combination therapy: Up to 300-900 mg/m²
Single-agent therapy: Up to 1200 mg/m² (fatal necrosis is associated with doses >2 g/m²)
Adjunct to surgery in patients with recurrent glioblastoma multiforme (Gliadel®): Implantation: Up to 8 wafers may be placed in the resection cavity (total dose 62.6 mg); should the size and shape not accommodate 8 wafers, the maximum number of wafers allowed should be placed
Hemodialysis: Supplemental dosing is not required
Dosing adjustment in hepatic impairment: Dosage adjustment may be necessary; however, no specific guidelines are available

Administration
Significant absorption to PVC containers - should be administered in either glass or Excel® container
Infuse I.V. infusion over ≥15-45 minutes is recommended to minimize severe burning/vein irritation; longer infusion times (1-2 hours) can alleviate venous pain/irritation
High-dose carmustine: Maximum rate of infusion of ≤3 mg/m²/minute to avoid excessive flushing, agitation, and hypotension; infusions should run over at least 2 hours; some investigational protocols dictate shorter infusions.
Wafers should only be handled by persons wearing surgical gloves (double gloves recommended). Dispose of outer gloves in biohazard waste container after use. A surgical instrument dedicated to the handling of wafers should be used. In the event of removal, wafers should be handled as a potentially cytotoxic agent.

(Continued)

Carmustine *(Continued)*

Monitoring Parameters CBC with differential and platelet count, pulmonary function, liver function, and renal function tests; monitor blood pressure during administration

Patient Information This drug can only be administered by infusion. Limit oral intake for 4-6 hours before therapy. Do not use alcohol, aspirin-containing products, and OTC medications without consulting prescriber. It is important to maintain adequate nutrition and hydration during therapy (2-3 L/day of fluids unless instructed to restrict fluid intake); frequent small meals may help. Take 2-3 L/day of fluids. You may experience nausea or vomiting (frequent small meals, frequent mouth care, sucking lozenges, or chewing gum may help). If this is ineffective, consult prescriber for antiemetic medication. You may experience loss of hair (reversible). You will be more susceptible to infection (avoid crowds and exposure to infection as much as possible). You will be more sensitive to sunlight; use sunblock, wear protective clothing and dark glasses, or avoid direct exposure to sunlight. Frequent mouth care with soft toothbrush or cotton swabs and frequent mouth rinses may help relieve mouth sores. Report fever, chills, unusual bruising or bleeding, signs of infection, excessive fatigue, yellowing of eyes or skin, or change in color of urine or stool. Contraceptive measures are recommended during therapy.

Nursing Implications Must administer in glass containers; accidental skin contact may cause transient burning and brown discoloration of the skin

Additional Information Baseline pulmonary function tests are recommended. Delayed onset pulmonary fibrosis occurring up to 17 years after treatment has been reported in children (1-16 years) who received carmustine in cumulative doses ranging from 770-1800 mg/m^2 combined with cranial radiotherapy for intracranial tumors.

Dosage Forms
Powder for injection [with 3 mL absolute alcohol as diluent]: 100 mg/vial
Wafer (Gliadel®): 7.7 mg carmustine

♦ **Carnitor®** *see Levocarnitine on page 789*
♦ **Carrington Antifungal [OTC]** *see Miconazole on page 908*

Carteolol *(KAR tee oh lole)*

Related Information
Beta-Blockers Comparison *on page 1491*
Glaucoma Drug Therapy Comparison *on page 1499*

U.S. Brand Names Cartrol® Oral; Ocupress® Ophthalmic
Canadian Brand Names Cartrol® Oral; Ocupress® Ophthalmic
Synonyms Carteolol Hydrochloride
Therapeutic Category Antihypertensive Agent; Beta-Adrenergic Blocker; Beta-Adrenergic Blocker, Ophthalmic
Use Management of hypertension; treatment of chronic open-angle glaucoma and intraocular hypertension
Pregnancy Risk Factor C (manufacturer); D (2nd and 3rd trimesters - expert analysis)
Contraindications Hypersensitivity to carteolol or any component of the formulation; sinus bradycardia; heart block greater than first-degree (except in patients with a functioning artificial pacemaker); cardiogenic shock; bronchial asthma, bronchospasm, or COPD; uncompensated cardiac failure; pulmonary edema; pregnancy (2nd and 3rd trimesters)
Warnings/Precautions Avoid abrupt discontinuation in patients with a history of CAD; slowly wean while monitoring for signs and symptoms of ischemia. Use caution in patients with PVD (can aggravate arterial insufficiency). Use caution with concurrent use of beta-blockers and either verapamil or diltiazem; bradycardia or heart block can occur. Patients with bronchospastic disease should not receive beta-blockers. Use cautiously in diabetics because it can mask prominent hypoglycemic symptoms. Can mask signs of thyrotoxicosis. Can cause fetal harm when administered in pregnancy. Dosage adjustment is required in patients with renal dysfunction. Use care with anesthetic agents that decrease myocardial function. Beta-blockers with intrinsic sympathomimetic activity have not been demonstrated to be of value in congestive heart failure. Some products contain sulfites which can cause allergic reactions. Response diminished over time.

Adverse Reactions
Ophthalmic:
>10%: Ocular: Conjunctival hyperemia
1% to 10%: Ocular: Anisocoria, corneal punctate keratitis, corneal staining, decreased corneal sensitivity, eye pain, vision disturbances
Systemic:
>10%:
Central nervous system: Drowsiness, insomnia
Endocrine & metabolic: Decreased sexual ability
1% to 10%:
Cardiovascular: Bradycardia, palpitations, edema, congestive heart failure, reduced peripheral circulation
Central nervous system: Mental depression
Gastrointestinal: Diarrhea or constipation, nausea, vomiting, stomach discomfort
Respiratory: Bronchospasm
Miscellaneous: Cold extremities
<1% (Limited to important or life-threatening): Arrhythmias, chest pain, confusion (especially in the elderly), depression, dyspnea, hallucinations, headache, leukopenia, nervousness, orthostatic hypotension, polyuria, psoriasiform eruption, thrombocytopenia

Overdosage/Toxicology Symptoms include cardiac disturbances, CNS toxicity, bronchospasm, hypoglycemia, and hyperkalemia. The most common cardiac symptoms include hypotension and bradycardia. Atrioventricular block, intraventricular conduction disturbances, cardiogenic shock, and asystole may occur with severe overdose, especially with membrane-depressant drugs (eg, propranolol). CNS effects include convulsions, coma, and respiratory arrest (commonly seen with propranolol and other membrane-depressant and lipid-soluble drugs). Treatment is symptomatic for seizures, hypotension, hyperkalemia, and hypoglycemia. Bradycardia and hypotension resistant to atropine, isoproterenol, or pacing may respond to glucagon. Wide QRS defects caused by membrane-depressant poisoning may respond to hypertonic sodium bicarbonate. Repeat-dose charcoal, hemoperfusion, or hemodialysis may be helpful in removal of only those beta-blockers with a small V_d, long half-life, or low intrinsic clearance (acebutolol, atenolol, nadolol, sotalol).

Drug Interactions

Increased Effect/Toxicity: Carteolol may increase the effects of other drugs which slow AV conduction (digoxin, verapamil, diltiazem), alpha-blockers (prazosin, terazosin), and alpha-adrenergic stimulants (epinephrine, phenylephrine). Carteolol may mask the tachycardia from hypoglycemia caused by insulin and oral hypoglycemics. In patients receiving concurrent therapy, the risk of hypertensive crisis is increased when either clonidine or the beta-blocker is withdrawn. Reserpine has been shown to enhance the effect of beta-blockers. Beta-blockers may increase the action or levels of ethanol, disopyramide, nondepolarizing muscle relaxants, and theophylline although the effects are difficult to predict.

Decreased Effect: Decreased effect of beta-blockers with aluminum salts, barbiturates, calcium salts, cholestyramine, colestipol, NSAIDs, penicillins (ampicillin), rifampin, salicylates, and sulfinpyrazone due to decreased bioavailability and plasma levels. Beta-blockers may decrease the effect of sulfonylureas (possibly hyperglycemia). Nonselective beta-blockers blunt the effect of beta-2 adrenergic agonists (albuterol).

Ethanol/Nutrition/Herb Interactions Herb/Nutraceutical: Avoid dong quai if using for hypertension (has estrogenic activity). Avoid ephedra, yohimbe, ginseng (may worsen hypertension). Avoid garlic (may have increased antihypertensive effect).

Mechanism of Action Blocks both beta$_1$- and beta$_2$-receptors and has mild intrinsic sympathomimetic activity; has negative inotropic and chronotropic effects and can significantly slow AV nodal conduction

Pharmacodynamics/Kinetics

Onset of action: Oral: 1-1.5 hours
Peak effect: 2 hours
Duration: 12 hours
Absorption: Oral: 80%
Protein binding: 23% to 30%
Metabolism: 30% to 50%
Half-life elimination: 6 hours
Excretion: Urine (as metabolites)

Usual Dosage Adults:

Oral: 2.5 mg as a single daily dose, with a maintenance dose normally 2.5-5 mg once daily; doses >10 mg do not increase response and may in fact decrease effect.
Ophthalmic: Instill 1 drop in affected eye(s) twice daily.
Dosing interval in renal impairment: Oral:
Cl_{cr} >60 mL/minute/1.73 m^2: Administer every 24 hours.
Cl_{cr} 20-60 mL/minute/1.73 m^2: Administer every 48 hours.
Cl_{cr} <20 mL/minute/1.73 m^2: Administer every 72 hours.

Monitoring Parameters Ophthalmic: Intraocular pressure; Systemic: Blood pressure, pulse, CNS status

Patient Information Intended for twice daily dosing; keep eye open and do not blink for 30 seconds after instillation; wear sunglasses to avoid photophobic discomfort; apply gentle pressure to lacrimal sac during and immediately following instillation (1 minute); do not discontinue medication abruptly, sudden stopping of medication may precipitate or cause angina; consult pharmacist or physician before taking with other adrenergic drugs (eg, cold medications); notify physician if any systemic side effects occur; use with caution while driving or performing tasks requiring alertness; may mask signs of hypoglycemia in diabetics; may be taken without regard to meals

Nursing Implications Advise against abrupt withdrawal; monitor orthostatic blood pressures, apical and peripheral pulse, and mental status changes (ie, confusion, depression)

Dosage Forms

Solution, ophthalmic, as hydrochloride (Ocupress®): 1% (5 mL, 10 mL)
Tablet, as hydrochloride (Cartrol®): 2.5 mg, 5 mg

♦ **Carteolol Hydrochloride** *see* Carteolol *on page 232*

♦ **Cartia® XT** *see* Diltiazem *on page 409*

♦ **Cartrol® Oral** *see* Carteolol *on page 232*

Carvedilol (KAR ve dil ole)

Related Information

Beta-Blockers Comparison *on page 1491*
Heart Failure *on page 1663*

U.S. Brand Names Coreg®
Canadian Brand Names Coreg™
Therapeutic Category Alpha-/Beta- Adrenergic Blocker; Antihypertensive Agent; Beta-Adrenergic Blocker

Use Management of hypertension; can be used alone or in combination with other agents, especially thiazide-type diuretics; mild to severe heart failure of ischemic or cardiomyopathic origin usually in addition to standardized therapy.

Unlabeled/Investigational Use Angina pectoris

Pregnancy Risk Factor C (manufacturer); D (2nd and 3rd trimesters - expert analysis)

Pregnancy/Breast-Feeding Implications Use during pregnancy only if the potential benefit justifies the risk.

Contraindications Hypersensitivity to carvedilol or any component of the formulation; patients with decompensated cardiac failure requiring intravenous inotropic therapy; bronchial asthma or related bronchospastic conditions; second- or third-degree AV block, sick sinus syndrome, and severe bradycardia (except in patients with a functioning artificial pacemaker); cardiogenic shock; severe hepatic impairment; pregnancy (2nd and 3rd trimesters)

Warnings/Precautions Use with caution in patients with congestive heart failure treated with digitalis, diuretic, or ACE inhibitor since AV conduction may be slowed; discontinue therapy if (Continued)

Carvedilol *(Continued)*

any evidence of liver injury occurs; use caution in patients with peripheral vascular disease, those undergoing anesthesia, in hyperthyroidism and diabetes mellitus. If no other antihypertensive is tolerated, very small doses may be cautiously used in patients with bronchospastic disease. Abrupt withdrawal of the drug should be avoided, drug should be discontinued over 1-2 weeks; do not use in pregnant or nursing women; may potentiate hypoglycemia in a diabetic patient and mask signs and symptoms; safety and efficacy in children have not been established.

Adverse Reactions Note: Frequency ranges include data from hypertension and heart failure trials. Higher rates of adverse reactions have generally been noted in patients with congestive heart failure. However, the frequency of adverse effects associated with placebo is also increased in this population. Events occurring at a frequency > placebo in clinical trials.

>10%:
Central nervous system: Dizziness (6% to 32%), fatigue (4% to 24%)
Endocrine & metabolic: Hyperglycemia (5% to 12%), weight gain (10% to 12%)
Gastrointestinal: Diarrhea (2% to 12%)
Neuromuscular & skeletal: Weakness (11%)
Respiratory: Upper respiratory tract infection (14% to 18%)

1% to 10%:
Cardiovascular: Bradycardia (2% to 10%), hypotension (9% to 14%), hypertension (3%), AV block (3%), angina (2% to 6%), postural hypotension (2%), syncope (3% to 8%), dependent edema (4%), palpitations, peripheral edema (1% to 7%), generalized edema (5% to 6%)
Central nervous system: Pain (9%), headache (5% to 8%), fever (3%), paresthesia (2%), somnolence (2%), insomnia (2%), malaise, hypesthesia, vertigo
Endocrine & metabolic: Gout (6%), hypercholesterolemia (4%), dehydration (2%), hyperkalemia (3%), hypervolemia (2%), hypertriglyceridemia (1%), hyperuricemia, hypoglycemia, hyponatremia
Gastrointestinal: Nausea (4% to 9%), vomiting (6%), melena, periodontitis
Genitourinary: Urinary tract infection (2% to 3%), hematuria (3%), impotence
Hematologic: Thrombocytopenia (1% to 2%), decreased prothrombin, purpura
Hepatic: Increased transaminases, increased alkaline phosphatase
Neuromuscular & skeletal: Back pain (2% to 7%), arthralgia (6%), myalgia (3%), muscle cramps
Ocular: Blurred vision (3% to 5%)
Renal: Increased BUN (6%), abnormal renal function, albuminuria, glycosuria, increased creatinine (3%), kidney failure
Respiratory: Sinusitis (5%), bronchitis (5%), pharyngitis (2% to 3%), rhinitis (2%), increased cough (5%)
Miscellaneous: Infection (2%), injury (3% to 6%), increased diaphoresis (3%), viral infection (2%), allergy, sudden death

<1% (Limited to important or life-threatening): Aggravated depression, anaphylactoid reaction, anemia, aplastic anemia (rare, all events occurred in patients receiving other medications capable of causing this effect); asthma, AV block (complete), bronchospasm, bundle branch block, convulsion, diabetes mellitus, exfoliative dermatitis, GI hemorrhage, leukopenia, migraine, myocardial ischemia, neuralgia, pancytopenia, peripheral ischemia, pulmonary edema, Stevens-Johnson syndrome

Additional events from clinical trials in heart failure patients occurring at a frequency >2% but equal to or less than the frequency reported in patients receiving placebo: Anemia, arthritis, asthenia, cardiac failure, chest pain, coughing, depression, dyspepsia, flatulence, headache, hyperkalemia, leg cramps, nausea, pain, palpitation, rash, sinusitis, upper respiratory infection

Overdosage/Toxicology Symptoms include cardiac disturbances, CNS toxicity, bronchospasm, hypoglycemia, and hyperkalemia. The most common cardiac symptoms include hypotension and bradycardia. Atrioventricular block, intraventricular conduction disturbances, cardiogenic shock, and asystole may occur with severe overdose, especially with membrane-depressant drugs (eg, propranolol). CNS effects include convulsions, coma, and respiratory arrest, commonly seen with propranolol and other membrane-depressant and lipid-soluble drugs. Treatment is symptomatic for seizures, hypotension, hyperkalemia, and hypoglycemia. Bradycardia and hypotension resistant to atropine, isoproterenol, or pacing may respond to glucagon. Wide QRS defects caused by membrane-depressant poisoning may respond to hypertonic sodium bicarbonate. Repeat-dose charcoal, hemoperfusion, or hemodialysis may be helpful in removal of only those beta-blockers with a small V_d, long half-life, or low intrinsic clearance (acebutolol, atenolol, nadolol, sotalol).

Drug Interactions

Cytochrome P450 Effect: CYP1A2, 2E1, 2C9 (major), 2C19, 2D6 (major), 3A3/4 enzyme substrate

Increased Effect/Toxicity: Clonidine and cimetidine increase the serum levels and effects of carvedilol. Carvedilol may increase the levels of cyclosporine. Carvedilol may increase the effects of other drugs which slow AV conduction (digoxin, verapamil, diltiazem), alpha-blockers (prazosin, terazosin), and alpha-adrenergic stimulants (epinephrine, phenylephrine). Carvedilol may mask the tachycardia from hypoglycemia caused by insulin and oral hypoglycemics. In patients receiving concurrent therapy, the risk of hypertensive crisis is increased when either clonidine or the beta-blocker is withdrawn. Reserpine has been shown to enhance the effect of beta-blockers. Beta-blockers may increase the action or levels of disopyramide, and theophylline although the effects are difficult to predict.

Decreased Effect: Rifampin may reduce the plasma concentration of carvedilol by up to 70%. Decreased effect of beta-blockers has also occurred with antacids, barbiturates, calcium channel blockers, cholestyramine, colestipol, NSAIDs, penicillins (ampicillin), and salicylates due to decreased bioavailability and plasma levels. Beta-blockers may decrease the effect of sulfonylureas. Nonselective beta-blockers blunt the effect of beta-2 adrenergic agonists (albuterol).

Ethanol/Nutrition/Herb Interactions Herb/Nutraceutical: Avoid dong quai if using for hypertension (has estrogenic activity). Avoid ephedra, yohimbe, ginseng (may worsen hypertension). Avoid garlic (may have increased antihypertensive effect).

Stability Store at 30°C (86°F).

Mechanism of Action As a racemic mixture, carvedilol has nonselective beta-adrenoreceptor and alpha-adrenergic blocking activity. No intrinsic sympathomimetic activity has been documented. Associated effects in hypertensive patients include reduction of cardiac output, exercise- or beta agonist-induced tachycardia, reduction of reflex orthostatic tachycardia, vasodilation, decreased peripheral vascular resistance (especially in standing position), decreased renal vascular resistance, reduced plasma renin activity, and increased levels of atrial natriuretic peptide. In CHF, associated effects include decreased pulmonary capillary wedge pressure, decreased pulmonary artery pressure, decreased heart rate, decreased systemic vascular resistance, increased stroke volume index, and decreased right arterial pressure (RAP).

Pharmacodynamics/Kinetics
Onset of action: 1-2 hours
 Peak antihypertensive effect: ~1-2 hours
Absorption: Rapid; food decreases the rate but not extent of absorption; administration with food minimizes risks of orthostatic hypotension
Distribution: V_d: 115 L
Protein binding: <98%, primarily to albumin
Metabolism: Extensively hepatic, primarily by aromatic ring oxidation and glucuronidation (2% excreted unchanged); three active metabolites (4-hydroxyphenyl metabolite is 13 times more potent than parent drug for beta-blockade); first-pass effect; plasma concentrations in the elderly and those with cirrhotic liver disease are 50% and 4-7 times higher, respectively
Bioavailability: 25% to 35%
Half-life elimination: 7-10 hours
Excretion: Primarily feces

Usual Dosage Oral: Adults: Reduce dosage if heart rate drops to <55 beats/minute.
Hypertension: 6.25 mg twice daily; if tolerated, dose should be maintained for 1-2 weeks, then increased to 12.5 mg twice daily. Dosage may be increased to a maximum of 25 mg twice daily after 1-2 weeks. Maximum dose: 50 mg/day
Congestive heart failure: 3.125 mg twice daily for 2 weeks; if this dose is tolerated, may increase to 6.25 mg twice daily. Double the dose every 2 weeks to the highest dose tolerated by patient. (Prior to initiating therapy, other heart failure medications should be stabilized and fluid retention minimized.)
Maximum recommended dose:
 Mild to moderate heart failure:
  <85 kg: 25 mg twice daily
  >85 kg: 50 mg twice daily
 Severe heart failure: 25 mg twice daily
Angina pectoris (unlabeled use): 25-50 mg twice daily
 Dosing adjustment in renal impairment: None necessary
 Dosing adjustment in hepatic impairment: Use is contraindicated in liver dysfunction.

Dietary Considerations Should be taken with food to minimize the risk of orthostatic hypotension.

Administration Administer with food.

Monitoring Parameters Heart rate, blood pressure (base need for dosage increase on trough blood pressure measurements and for tolerance on standing systolic pressure 1 hour after dosing); renal studies, BUN, liver function

Test Interactions Increased hepatic enzymes, BUN, NPN, alkaline phosphatase; decreased HDL

Patient Information Take with food to minimize the risk of hypotension; do not interrupt or discontinue using carvedilol without a physician's advice; use care to avoid standing abruptly or standing still for long periods; lie down if dizziness or faintness occurs and consult a physician for a reduced dosage; contact lens wearers may experience dry eyes

Nursing Implications Minimize risk of bradycardia with initiation of treatment with a low dose, slow upward titration, and administration with food; decrease dose if pulse rate drops <55 beats per minute

Additional Information Fluid retention during therapy should be treated with an increase in diuretic dosage.

Dosage Forms Tablet: 3.125 mg, 6.25 mg, 12.5 mg, 25 mg

Cascara Sagrada (kas KAR a sah GRAH dah)

Related Information
 Laxatives, Classification and Properties *on page 1504*

Synonyms Cascara Sagrada

Therapeutic Category Laxative, Stimulant

Use Temporary relief of constipation; sometimes used with milk of magnesia ("black and white" mixture)

Pregnancy Risk Factor C

Contraindications Nausea; vomiting; abdominal pain; fecal impaction; intestinal obstruction; GI bleeding; appendicitis; congestive heart failure

Warnings/Precautions Excessive use can lead to electrolyte imbalance, fluid imbalance, vitamin deficiency, steatorrhea, osteomalacia, cathartic colon, and dependence; should be avoided during nursing because it may have a laxative effect on the infant

Adverse Reactions 1% to 10%:
Central nervous system: Faintness
Endocrine & metabolic: Electrolyte and fluid imbalance
Gastrointestinal: Abdominal cramps, nausea, diarrhea
Genitourinary: Discoloration of urine (reddish pink or brown)
(Continued)

235

Cascara Sagrada *(Continued)*

Drug Interactions
Decreased Effect: Decreased effect of oral anticoagulants.

Stability Protect from light and heat

Mechanism of Action Direct chemical irritation of the intestinal mucosa resulting in an increased rate of colonic motility and change in fluid and electrolyte secretion

Pharmacodynamics/Kinetics
Onset of action: 6-10 hours
Absorption: Oral: Poorly from small intestine
Metabolism: Hepatic

Usual Dosage Note: Cascara sagrada fluid extract is 5 times more potent than cascara sagrada aromatic fluid extract
Oral (aromatic fluid extract):
Infants: 1.25 mL/day (range: 0.5-1.5 mL) as needed
Children 2-11 years: 2.5 mL/day (range: 1-3 mL) as needed
Children ≥12 years and Adults: 5 mL/day (range: 2-6 mL) as needed at bedtime (1 tablet as needed at bedtime)

Dietary Considerations Administer on empty stomach for rapid effect.

Test Interactions ↓ calcium (S), ↓ potassium (S)

Patient Information Should not be used regularly for more than 1 week

Nursing Implications Cascara sagrada fluid extract is 5 times more potent than cascara sagrada aromatic fluid extract

Dosage Forms
Aromatic fluid extract: 120 mL, 473 mL
Tablet: 325 mg

♦ **Casodex®** *see* Bicalutamide *on page 168*

Caspofungin *(kas poe FUN jin)*

Related Information
Antifungal Agents Comparison *on page 1484*

U.S. Brand Names Cancidas®

Synonyms Caspofungin Acetate

Therapeutic Category Antifungal Agent, Systemic

Use Treatment of invasive *Aspergillus* infection in patients who do not tolerate or do not respond to other antifungal therapies (including amphotericin B, lipid formulations of amphotericin B, or itraconazole); has not been studied as initial therapy for aspergillosis

Pregnancy Risk Factor C

Pregnancy/Breast-Feeding Implications No adequate and well-controlled studies in pregnant women. Should be used during pregnancy only if potential benefit justifies the potential risk to the fetus. Embryotoxicity has been demonstrated in animal studies. Excretion in breast milk unknown.

Contraindications Hypersensitivity to caspofungin or any component of the formulation

Warnings/Precautions Has not been studied as initial therapy for *Aspergillus* infection. Avoid concurrent use of cyclosporine. Limited data are available concerning treatment regimens involving higher daily dosages (>50 mg/day) or treatment durations longer than 2 weeks.

Adverse Reactions Note: Listing includes some reactions/frequencies noted during investigational use for indications other than *Aspergillus*.

>10%:
Central nervous system: Headache (up to 11%), fever (3% to 26%)
Hepatic: Increased serum alkaline phosphatase (3% to 11%), increased transaminases (up to 13%)
Local: Infusion site reactions (2% to 12%), phlebitis (up to 16%)
1% to 10%:
Cardiovascular: Flushing (3%), edema (up to 3%)
Central nervous system: Fever (3%), headache, chills (up to 3%), pain (1% to 5%), paresthesia (1% to 3%)
Dermatologic: Rash (<1% to 4%), pruritus (2% to 3%), erythema (1% to 2%)
Endocrine & metabolic: Decreased serum potassium (3%)
Gastrointestinal: Nausea (3% to 6%), vomiting (1% to 3%), abdominal pain, diarrhea (1% to 4%)
Hematologic: Increased eosinophils (3%), decreased hemoglobin (3% to 12%), decreased neutrophils (2% to 3%), increased WBC (5% to 6%), anemia (up to 4%)
Hepatic: Increased serum alkaline phosphatase (3%)
Local: Infusion site reactions (3%), induration (up to 3%)
Neuromuscular & skeletal: Myalgia (up to 3%)
Renal: Proteinuria (5%), hematuria (2%), increased serum creatinine (<1% to 2%), increased urinary WBCs (up to 8%)
Miscellaneous: Flu-like syndrome (3%)
<1% (Limited to important or life-threatening): Adult respiratory distress syndrome (ARDS), anaphylaxis, dyspnea, dystonia, facial swelling, pruritus, pulmonary edema, rash, stridor

Overdosage/Toxicology No experience with overdosage has been reported. Caspofungin is not dialyzable. Treatment is symptomatic and supportive.

Drug Interactions
Increased Effect/Toxicity: Concurrent administration of cyclosporine may increase caspofungin concentrations. In limited experience, a high frequency of elevated hepatic serum transaminases was observed.
Decreased Effect: Caspofungin may decrease blood concentrations of tacrolimus. In limited experience, some enzyme inducers decreased the serum concentrations of caspofungin.

Stability Store vials at 2°C to 8°C (36°F to 46°F). Reconstituted solution may be stored at less than 25°C (77°F) for 1 hour prior to preparation of infusion solution. Infusion solutions may be stored at less than 25°C (77°F) and should be used within 24 hours. Do not mix with dextrose-containing solutions. Do not coadminister with other medications.

Mechanism of Action Inhibits synthesis of β(1,3)-D-glucan, an essential component of the cell wall of susceptible fungi. Highest activity in regions of active cell growth. Mammalian cells do not require β(1,3)-D-glucan, limiting potential toxicity.

Pharmacodynamics/Kinetics
Protein binding: 97% to albumin
Metabolism: Slowly, via hydrolysis and *N*-acetylation as well as by spontaneous degradation, with subsequent metabolism to component amino acids
Half-life elimination: Beta (distribution): 9-11 hours; Terminal: 40-50 hours
Excretion: Urine (41%) and feces (35%) as unchanged drug and metabolites

Usual Dosage I.V.:
Children: Safety and efficacy in pediatric patients have not been established
Adults: *Aspergillus* infection (invasive):
Initial dose: 70 mg infused slowly (over 1 hour)
Subsequent dosing: 50 mg/day (infused over 1 hour)
Duration of treatment should be determined by patient status and clinical response (limited experience beyond 2 weeks of therapy); efficacy of 70 mg/day dose (in patients not responding to 50 mg/day) has not been adequately studied, although this dose appears to be well tolerated
Patients receiving carbamazepine, dexamethasone, efavirenz, nelfinavir, nevirapine, phenytoin, and rifampin (and possibly other enzyme inducers) may require an increased daily dose of caspofungin (70 mg/day) if response to 50 mg/day is inadequate.
Elderly: The number of patients >65 years of age in clinical studies was not sufficient to establish whether a difference in response may be anticipated.

Dosage adjustment in renal impairment: No specific dosage adjustment is required; supplemental dose is not required following dialysis

Dosage adjustment in hepatic impairment:
Patients with mild hepatic impairment (Child-Pugh score 5 to 6): No adjustment necessary
Patients with moderate hepatic insufficiency (Child-Pugh score 7 to 9): Reduce daily dose to 35 mg (after initial 70 mg dose)

Administration Infuse slowly, over 1 hour; monitor during infusion; isolated cases of possible histamine-related reactions have occurred during clinical trials (rash, flushing, pruritus, facial edema)

Patient Information This drug can only be administered I.V., and therapy may take several days to weeks. During infusion, report immediately any chills, chest pain, difficulty breathing, tightness in throat, or other adverse reaction. You may experience nausea or vomiting (small frequent meals, frequent mouth care, sucking lozenges, or chewing gum may help). Report any skin rash, changes in color of urine or stool, persistent GI distress, alteration in voiding or bowel patterns, pain at injection site, or other adverse reactions.

Nursing Implications Infuse slowly over 1 hour; do not mix with dextrose-containing solutions; do not coadminister with other medications. Dosage adjustment may be needed in patients with hepatic impairment. Possible histamine-related reactions have occurred during clinical trials (rash, flushing, pruritus, facial edema).

Dosage Forms Powder for injection, as acetate: 50 mg, 70 mg

- **Caspofungin Acetate** see Caspofungin on page 236
- **Cataflam®** see Diclofenac on page 393
- **Catapres®** see Clonidine on page 318
- **Catapres-TTS®-1** see Clonidine on page 318
- **Catapres-TTS®-2** see Clonidine on page 318
- **Catapres-TTS®-3** see Clonidine on page 318
- **Cathflo™ Activase®** see Alteplase on page 59
- **Caverject®** see Alprostadil on page 57
- **CBDCA** see Carboplatin on page 226
- **CBZ** see Carbamazepine on page 221
- **CCNU** see Lomustine on page 814
- **2-CdA** see Cladribine on page 305
- **CDDP** see Cisplatin on page 301
- **Ceclor®** see Cefaclor on page 237
- **Ceclor® CD** see Cefaclor on page 237
- **Cecon® [OTC]** see Ascorbic Acid on page 116
- **Cedax®** see Ceftibuten on page 254
- **Cedocard®-SR (Can)** see Isosorbide Dinitrate on page 750
- **CeeNU®** see Lomustine on page 814

Cefaclor (SEF a klor)
Related Information
Antimicrobial Drugs of Choice on page 1588
U.S. Brand Names Ceclor®; Ceclor® CD
Canadian Brand Names Apo®-Cefaclor; Ceclor®; Novo-Cefaclor; Nu-Cefaclor; PMS-Cefaclor; Scheinpharm Cefaclor
Therapeutic Category Antibiotic, Cephalosporin (Second Generation)
Use Infections caused by susceptible organisms including *Staphylococcus aureus* and *H. influenzae*; treatment of otitis media, sinusitis, and infections involving the respiratory tract, skin and skin structure, bone and joint, and urinary tract
Pregnancy Risk Factor B
Contraindications Hypersensitivity to cefaclor, any component of the formulation, or other cephalosporins
Warnings/Precautions Modify dosage in patients with severe renal impairment; prolonged use may result in superinfection; a low incidence of cross-hypersensitivity to penicillins exists
(Continued)

Cefaclor (Continued)

Adverse Reactions
1% to 10%:
Gastrointestinal: Diarrhea (1.5%)
Hematologic: Eosinophilia (2%)
Hepatic: Elevated transaminases (2.5%)
Dermatologic: Rash (maculopapular, erythematous, or morbilliform) (1% to 1.5%)
<1% (Limited to important or life-threatening): Agitation, anaphylaxis, angioedema, arthralgia, cholestatic jaundice, CNS irritability, confusion, dizziness, hallucinations, hemolytic anemia, hepatitis, hyperactivity, insomnia, interstitial nephritis, nausea, nervousness, neutropenia, prolonged PT, pruritus, pseudomembranous colitis, seizures, serum-sickness, somnolence, Stevens-Johnson syndrome, urticaria, vaginitis, vomiting

Reactions reported with other cephalosporins include abdominal pain, cholestasis, fever, hemorrhage, renal dysfunction, superinfection, toxic nephropathy

Overdosage/Toxicology
After acute overdose, most agents cause only nausea, vomiting, and diarrhea, although neuromuscular hypersensitivity and seizures are possible, especially in patients with renal insufficiency. Many beta-lactam antibiotics have the potential to cause neuromuscular hyperirritability or seizures. Hemodialysis may be helpful to aid in removal of the drug from the blood, but is not usually indicated; otherwise, most treatment is supportive or symptom directed, following GI decontamination.

Drug Interactions
Increased Effect/Toxicity: Probenecid may decrease cephalosporin elimination. Furosemide, aminoglycosides when taken with cefaclor may result in additive nephrotoxicity. Bleeding may occur when administered with anticoagulants.

Ethanol/Nutrition/Herb Interactions
Food: Cefaclor serum levels may be decreased slightly if taken with food.

Stability
Refrigerate suspension after reconstitution; discard after 14 days; do not freeze

Mechanism of Action
Inhibits bacterial cell wall synthesis by binding to one or more of the penicillin-binding proteins (PBPs) which in turn inhibits the final transpeptidation step of peptidoglycan synthesis in bacterial cell walls, thus inhibiting cell wall biosynthesis. Bacteria eventually lyse due to ongoing activity of cell wall autolytic enzymes (autolysins and murein hydrolases) while cell wall assembly is arrested.

Pharmacodynamics/Kinetics
Absorption: Well absorbed, acid stable
Distribution: Widely throughout the body and reaches therapeutic concentration in most tissues and body fluids, including synovial, pericardial, pleural, peritoneal fluids; bile, sputum, and urine; bone, myocardium, gallbladder, skin and soft tissue; crosses placenta; enters breast milk
Protein binding: 25%
Metabolism: Partially
Half-life elimination: 0.5-1 hour; prolonged with renal impairment
Time to peak: Capsule: 60 minutes; Suspension: 45 minutes
Excretion: Urine (80% as unchanged drug)

Usual Dosage
Oral:
Children >1 month: 20-40 mg/kg/day divided every 8-12 hours; maximum dose: 2 g/day (total daily dose may be divided into two doses for treatment of otitis media or pharyngitis)
Adults: 250-500 mg every 8 hours
Extended release tablets: 500 mg every 12 hours for 7 days for acute bacterial exacerbations of or secondary infections with chronic bronchitis or 375 mg every 12 hour for 10 days for pharyngitis or tonsillitis or for uncomplicated skin and skin structure infections
Dosing adjustment in renal impairment: Cl_{cr} <50 mL/minute: Administer 50% of dose
Hemodialysis: Moderately dialyzable (20% to 50%)

Dietary Considerations
May be taken with or without food.

Monitoring Parameters
Assess patient at beginning and throughout therapy for infection; monitor for signs of anaphylaxis during first dose

Test Interactions
Positive direct Coombs', false-positive urinary glucose test using cupric sulfate (Benedict's solution, Clinitest®, Fehling's solution), false-positive serum or urine creatinine with Jaffé reaction

Patient Information
Chilling of the oral suspension improves flavor (do not freeze); report persistent diarrhea; entire course of medication (10-14 days) should be taken to ensure eradication of organism; may interfere with oral contraceptives; females should report symptoms of vaginitis

Nursing Implications
With prolonged therapy, monitor CBC and stool frequency periodically

Dosage Forms
Capsule: 250 mg, 500 mg
Powder for oral suspension: 125 mg/5 mL (75 mL, 150 mL); 187 mg/5 mL (50 mL, 100 mL); 250 mg/5 mL (75 mL, 150 mL); 375 mg/5 mL (50 mL, 100 mL) [strawberry flavor]
Tablet, extended release: 375 mg, 500 mg

Cefadroxil (sef a DROKS il)

Related Information
Prevention of Bacterial Endocarditis on page 1563

U.S. Brand Names
Duricef®

Canadian Brand Names
Apo®-Cefadroxil; Duricef™; Novo-Cefadroxil

Synonyms
Cefadroxil Monohydrate

Therapeutic Category
Antibiotic, Cephalosporin (First Generation)

Use
Treatment of susceptible bacterial infections, including those caused by group A beta-hemolytic Streptococcus; prophylaxis against bacterial endocarditis in patients who are allergic to penicillin and undergoing surgical or dental procedures

Pregnancy Risk Factor
B

Contraindications
Hypersensitivity to cefadroxil, other cephalosporins, or any component of the formulation

Warnings/Precautions Modify dosage in patients with severe renal impairment; prolonged use may result in superinfection; use with caution in patients with a history of penicillin allergy especially IgE-mediated reactions (eg, anaphylaxis, urticaria); may cause antibiotic-associated colitis or colitis secondary to *C. difficile*

Adverse Reactions

1% to 10%: Gastrointestinal: Diarrhea

<1% (Limited to important or life-threatening): Abdominal pain, agranulocytosis, anaphylaxis, angioedema, arthralgia, cholestasis, dyspepsia, erythema multiforme, fever, nausea, neutropenia, pruritus, pseudomembranous colitis, rash (maculopapular and erythematous), serum sickness, Stevens-Johnson syndrome, thrombocytopenia, transaminases increased, urticaria, vaginitis, vomiting

Reactions reported with other cephalosporins include abdominal pain, aplastic anemia, BUN increased, creatinine increased, eosinophilia, hemolytic anemia, hemorrhage, pancytopenia, prolonged prothrombin time, renal dysfunction, seizures, superinfection, toxic epidermal necrolysis, toxic nephropathy

Overdosage/Toxicology After acute overdose, most agents cause only nausea, vomiting, and diarrhea, although neuromuscular hypersensitivity and seizures are possible, especially in patients with renal insufficiency. Many beta-lactam antibiotics have the potential to cause neuromuscular hyperirritability or seizures. Hemodialysis may be helpful to aid in removal of the drug from the blood, but is not usually indicated; otherwise, most treatment is supportive or symptom directed, following GI decontamination.

Drug Interactions

Increased Effect/Toxicity: Bleeding may occur when administered with anticoagulants. Probenecid may decrease cephalosporin elimination.

Ethanol/Nutrition/Herb Interactions Food: Concomitant administration with food, infant formula, or cow's milk does **not** significantly affect absorption.

Stability Refrigerate suspension after reconstitution; discard after 14 days

Mechanism of Action Inhibits bacterial cell wall synthesis by binding to one or more of the penicillin-binding proteins (PBPs) which in turn inhibits the final transpeptidation step of peptidoglycan synthesis in bacterial cell walls, thus inhibiting cell wall biosynthesis. Bacteria eventually lyse due to ongoing activity of cell wall autolytic enzymes (autolysins and murein hydrolases) while cell wall assembly is arrested.

Pharmacodynamics/Kinetics

Absorption: Rapid and well absorbed

Distribution: Widely throughout the body and reaches therapeutic concentrations in most tissues and body fluids, including synovial, pericardial, pleural, and peritoneal fluids; bile, sputum, and urine; bone, myocardium, gallbladder, skin and soft tissue; crosses placenta; enters breast milk

Protein binding: 20%

Half-life elimination: 1-2 hours; 20-24 hours in renal failure

Time to peak, serum: 70-90 minutes

Excretion: Urine (>90% as unchanged drug)

Usual Dosage Oral:

Children: 30 mg/kg/day divided twice daily up to a maximum of 2 g/day

Adults: 1-2 g/day in 2 divided doses

Prophylaxis against bacterial endocarditis:

Children: 50 mg/kg 1 hour prior to the procedure

Adults: 2 g 1 hour prior to the procedure

Dosing interval in renal impairment:

Cl_{cr} 10-25 mL/minute: Administer every 24 hours

Cl_{cr} <10 mL/minute: Administer every 36 hours

Monitoring Parameters Observe for signs and symptoms of anaphylaxis during first dose

Test Interactions Positive direct Coombs', false-positive urinary glucose test using cupric sulfate (Benedict's solution, Clinitest®, Fehling's solution), false-positive serum or urine creatinine with Jaffé reaction

Patient Information Report persistent diarrhea; entire course of medication (10-14 days) should be taken to ensure eradication of organism; may interfere with oral contraceptives; females should report symptoms of vaginitis

Nursing Implications Administer around-the-clock to promote less variation in peak and trough serum levels

Dosage Forms

Capsule, as monohydrate: 500 mg

Suspension, oral, as monohydrate: 125 mg/5 mL, 250 mg/5 mL, 500 mg/5 mL (50 mL, 100 mL)

Tablet, as monohydrate: 1 g

♦ **Cefadroxil Monohydrate** *see* Cefadroxil *on page 238*

♦ **Cefadyl**® *see* Cephapirin *on page 262*

Cefamandole (sef a MAN dole)

U.S. Brand Names Mandol®

Synonyms Cefamandole Nafate

Therapeutic Category Antibiotic, Cephalosporin (Second Generation)

Use Treatment of susceptible bacterial infection; mainly respiratory tract, skin and skin structure, bone and joint, urinary tract and gynecologic, septicemia; surgical prophylaxis. Active against methicillin-sensitive staphylococci, many streptococci, and various gram-negative bacilli including *E. coli*, some *Klebsiella*, *P. mirabilis*, *H. influenzae*, and *Moraxella*.

Pregnancy Risk Factor B

Contraindications Hypersensitivity to cefamandole, any component of the formulation, or other cephalosporins

Warnings/Precautions Modify dosage in patients with severe renal impairment; prolonged use may result in superinfection; although rare, cefamandole may interfere with hemostasis via destruction of vitamin K producing intestinal bacteria, prevention of activation of prothrombin by the attachment of a methyltetrazolethiol side chain, and by an immune-

(Continued)

Cefamandole (Continued)

mediated thrombocytopenia. Use with caution in patients with a history of penicillin allergy especially IgE-mediated reactions (eg, anaphylaxis, urticaria); may cause antibiotic-associated colitis or colitis secondary to *C. difficile*.

Adverse Reactions Contains MTT side chain which may lead to increased risk of hypoprothrombinemia and bleeding.

1% to 10%:
  Gastrointestinal: Diarrhea
  Local: Thrombophlebitis
<1% (Limited to important or life-threatening): Anaphylaxis, BUN increased, cholestasis, creatinine increased, eosinophilia, fever, nausea, neutropenia, prolonged PT, pseudomembranous colitis, rash (maculopapular and erythematous), thrombocytopenia, transaminases increased, urticaria, vomiting

Reactions reported with other cephalosporins include abdominal pain, aplastic anemia, hemolytic anemia, hemorrhage, pancytopenia, renal dysfunction, seizures, Stevens-Johnson syndrome, superinfection, toxic epidermal necrolysis, nephropathy, vaginitis

Overdosage/Toxicology Symptoms include neuromuscular hypersensitivity and convulsions, especially in patients with renal insufficiency. Many beta-lactam antibiotics have the potential to cause neuromuscular hyperirritability or seizures. Hemodialysis may be helpful to aid in removal of the drug from the blood; otherwise, most treatment is supportive or symptom directed.

Drug Interactions

Increased Effect/Toxicity: Disulfiram-like reaction has been reported when taken within 72 hours of ethanol consumption. Increased cefamandole plasma levels when taken with probenecid. Aminoglycosides, furosemide when taken with cefamandole may increase nephrotoxicity. Increase in hypoprothrombinemic effect with warfarin or heparin and cefamandole.

Ethanol/Nutrition/Herb Interactions Ethanol: Avoid ethanol (possible disulfiram reaction).

Stability After reconstitution, CO_2 gas is liberated which allows solution to be withdrawn without injecting air; solution is stable for 24 hours at room temperature and 96 hours when refrigerated; for I.V., infusion in NS and D_5W is stable for 24 hours at room temperature, 1 week when refrigerated, or 26 weeks when frozen

Mechanism of Action Inhibits bacterial cell wall synthesis by binding to one or more of the penicillin-binding proteins (PBPs) which in turn inhibits the final transpeptidation step of peptidoglycan synthesis in bacterial cell walls, thus inhibiting cell wall biosynthesis. Bacteria eventually lyse due to ongoing activity of cell wall autolytic enzymes (autolysins and murein hydrolases) while cell wall assembly is arrested.

Pharmacodynamics/Kinetics

Distribution: Well throughout the body, except CSF; poor penetration even with inflamed meninges
Protein binding: 56% to 78%
Metabolism: Extensive enterohepatic circulation
Half-life elimination: 30-60 minutes
Time to peak, serum: I.M.: 1-2 hours
Excretion: Primarily urine (as unchanged drug); feces (high concentrations)

Usual Dosage I.M., I.V.:
Children: 50-150 mg/kg/day in divided doses every 4-8 hours
Adults: Usual dose: 500-1000 mg every 4-8 hours; in life-threatening infections: 2 g every 4 hours may be needed

Dosing interval in renal impairment:
  Cl_{cr} 25-50 mL/minute: 1-2 g every 8 hours
  Cl_{cr} 10-25 mL/minute: 1 g every 8 hours
  Cl_{cr} <10 mL/minute: 1 g every 12 hours
  Hemodialysis: Moderately dialyzable (20% to 50%)

Monitoring Parameters Monitor for signs of bruising or bleeding; observe for signs and symptoms of anaphylaxis during first dose

Test Interactions Positive direct Coombs', false-positive urinary glucose test using cupric sulfate (Benedict's solution, Clinitest®, Fehling's solution), false-positive serum or urine creatinine with Jaffé reaction

Nursing Implications Do not admix with aminoglycosides in same bottle/bag; observe for signs and symptoms of anaphylaxis during first dose

Dosage Forms Powder for injection, as nafate: 1 g (10 mL, 100 mL); 2 g (20 mL, 100 mL); 10 g (100 mL)

♦ **Cefamandole Nafate** *see* Cefamandole *on page 239*

Cefazolin (sef A zoe lin)

Related Information
  Animal and Human Bites Guidelines *on page 1584*
  Antibiotic Treatment of Adults With Infective Endocarditis *on page 1585*
  Community-Acquired Pneumonia in Adults *on page 1603*
  Prevention of Bacterial Endocarditis *on page 1563*
  Prevention of Wound Infection & Sepsis in Surgical Patients *on page 1569*

U.S. Brand Names Ancef®; Kefzol®

Canadian Brand Names Ancef®; Kefzol®

Synonyms Cefazolin Sodium

Therapeutic Category Antibiotic, Cephalosporin (First Generation)

Use Treatment of gram-positive bacilli and cocci (except enterococcus); some gram-negative bacilli including *E. coli*, *Proteus*, and *Klebsiella* may be susceptible

Pregnancy Risk Factor B

Contraindications Hypersensitivity to cefazolin sodium, any component of the formulation, or other cephalosporins

Warnings/Precautions Modify dosage in patients with severe renal impairment; prolonged use may result in superinfection; use with caution in patients with a history of penicillin allergy especially IgE-mediated reactions (eg, anaphylaxis, urticaria); may cause antibiotic-associated colitis or colitis secondary to *C. difficile*

Adverse Reactions

1% to 10%:

Gastrointestinal: Diarrhea

Local: Pain at injection site

<1% (Limited to important or life-threatening): Abdominal cramps, anaphylaxis, anorexia, eosinophilia, fever, leukopenia, nausea, neutropenia, oral candidiasis, phlebitis, pruritus, pseudomembranous colitis, rash, seizures, Stevens-Johnson syndrome, thrombocytopenia, thrombocytosis, transaminases increased, vaginitis, vomiting

Reactions reported with other cephalosporins include abdominal pain, aplastic anemia, cholestasis, hemolytic anemia, hemorrhage, pancytopenia, prolonged prothrombin time, renal dysfunction, superinfection, toxic epidermal necrolysis, toxic nephropathy

Overdosage/Toxicology Symptoms include neuromuscular hypersensitivity and convulsions especially with renal insufficiency. Many beta-lactam antibiotics have the potential to cause neuromuscular hyperirritability or seizures. Hemodialysis may be helpful to aid in removal of the drug from the blood; otherwise, most treatment is supportive or symptom directed.

Drug Interactions

Increased Effect/Toxicity: High-dose probenecid decreases clearance and increases effect of cefazolin. Aminoglycosides increase nephrotoxic potential when taken with cefazolin.

Stability

Store intact vials at room temperature and protect from temperatures exceeding 40°C

DUPLEX™ container: Store at 20°C to 25°C (68°F to 77°F); excursions permitted to 15°C to 30°C (59°F to 86°F) prior to activation

Reconstituted solutions of cefazolin are light yellow to yellow

Protection from light is recommended for the powder and for the reconstituted solutions

Reconstituted solutions are stable for 24 hours at room temperature and for 10 days under refrigeration

DUPLEX™: Following activation, stable for 24 hours at room temperature and for 7 days under refrigeration

Stability of parenteral admixture at room temperature (25°C): 48 hours

Stability of parenteral admixture at refrigeration temperature (4°C): 14 days

Standard diluent: 1 g/50 mL D_5W; 2 g/50 mL D_5W

Mechanism of Action Inhibits bacterial cell wall synthesis by binding to one or more of the penicillin-binding proteins (PBPs) which in turn inhibits the final transpeptidation step of peptidoglycan synthesis in bacterial cell walls, thus inhibiting cell wall biosynthesis. Bacteria eventually lyse due to ongoing activity of cell wall autolytic enzymes (autolysins and murein hydrolases) while cell wall assembly is arrested.

Pharmacodynamics/Kinetics

Distribution: Widely into most body tissues and fluids including gallbladder, liver, kidneys, bone, sputum, bile, pleural, and synovial; CSF penetration is poor; crosses placenta; enters breast milk

Protein binding: 74% to 86%

Metabolism: Minimally hepatic

Half-life elimination: 90-150 minutes; prolonged with renal impairment

Time to peak, serum: I.M.: 0.5-2 hours

Excretion: Urine (80% to 100% as unchanged drug)

Usual Dosage I.M., I.V.:

Children >1 month: 25-100 mg/kg/day divided every 6-8 hours; maximum: 6 g/day

Adults: 250 mg to 2 g every 6-12 (usually 8) hours, depending on severity of infection; maximum dose: 12 g/day

Prophylaxis against bacterial endocarditis:

Infants and Children: 25 mg/kg 30 minutes before procedure; maximum dose: 1 g

Adults: 1 g 30 minutes before procedure

Dosing adjustment in renal impairment:

Cl_{cr} 10-30 mL/minute: Administer every 12 hours

Cl_{cr} <10 mL/minute: Administer every 24 hours

Hemodialysis: Moderately dialyzable (20% to 50%); administer dose postdialysis or administer supplemental dose of 0.5-1 g after dialysis

Peritoneal dialysis: Administer 0.5 g every 12 hours

Continuous arteriovenous or venovenous hemofiltration: Dose as for Cl_{cr} 10-30 mL/minute; removes 30 mg of cefazolin per liter of filtrate per day

Monitoring Parameters Renal function periodically when used in combination with other nephrotoxic drugs, hepatic function tests, CBC; monitor for signs of anaphylaxis during first dose

Test Interactions Positive direct Coombs', false-positive urinary glucose test using cupric sulfate (Benedict's solution, Clinitest®, Fehling's solution), false-positive serum or urine creatinine with Jaffé reaction

Nursing Implications Do not admix with aminoglycosides in same bottle/bag; observe for signs and symptoms of anaphylaxis during first dose

Additional Information Sodium content of 1 g: 47 mg (2 mEq)

Dosage Forms

Infusion, as sodium [premixed in D_5W, frozen] (Ancef®): 500 mg (50 mL); 1 g (50 mL)

Powder for injection, as sodium [with 50 mL D_5W in DUPLEX™ container]: 500 mg, 1 g

Powder for injection, as sodium (Ancef®, Kefzol®): 500 mg, 1 g, 10 g, 20 g

♦ **Cefazolin Sodium** *see Cefazolin on page 240*

Cefdinir (SEF di ner)

U.S. Brand Names Omnicef®

Canadian Brand Names Omnicef®

(Continued)

Cefdinir (Continued)

Synonyms CFDN

Therapeutic Category Antibiotic, Cephalosporin (Third Generation)

Use Treatment of community-acquired pneumonia, acute exacerbations of chronic bronchitis, acute bacterial otitis media, acute maxillary sinusitis, pharyngitis/tonsillitis, and uncomplicated skin and skin structure infections.

Pregnancy Risk Factor B

Contraindications Hypersensitivity to cefdinir, other cephalosporins, any component of the formulation, or related antibiotics

Warnings/Precautions Administer cautiously to penicillin-sensitive patients. There is evidence of partial cross-allergenicity and cephalosporins cannot be assumed to be an absolutely safe alternative to penicillin in the penicillin-allergic patient. Serum sickness-like reactions have been reported. Signs and symptoms occur after a few days of therapy and resolve a few days after drug discontinuation with no serious sequelae. Pseudomembranous colitis occurs.

Adverse Reactions

1% to 10%

Dermatologic: Cutaneous moniliasis (1%)

Gastrointestinal: Diarrhea (8%), rash (3%), vomiting (1%), increased GGT (1%)

<1% (Limited to important or life-threatening): Acute renal failure, anaphylaxis, asthma exacerbation, cardiac failure, chest pain, cholestasis, coagulopathy, DIC, edema, enterocolitis, eosinophilic pneumonia, erythema multiforme, erythema nodosum, exfoliative dermatitis, fever, granulocytopenia, hemolytic anemia, hemorrhagic colitis, hepatic failure, hepatitis, hypertension, idiopathic interstitial pneumonia, ileus, involuntary movements, ITP, jaundice, laryngeal edema, leukopenia, loss of consciousness, myocardial infarction, nausea, nephropathy, pancytopenia, peptic ulcer, pseudomembranous colitis, rash, respiratory failure, rhabdomyolysis, shock, Stevens-Johnson syndrome, thrombocytopenia, toxic epidermal necrolysis, upper gastrointestinal bleeding, vaginal moniliasis, vasculitis

Reactions reported with other cephalosporins include angioedema, aplastic anemia, asterixis, dizziness, encephalopathy, fever, headache, hemorrhage, interstitial nephritis, neuromuscular excitability, prolonged PT, seizures, serum-sickness reactions, superinfection, toxic nephropathy

Overdosage/Toxicology After acute overdose, most agents cause only nausea, vomiting, and diarrhea, although neuromuscular hypersensitivity and seizures are possible, especially in patients with renal insufficiency. Hemodialysis may be helpful to aid in the removal of the drug from the blood but not usually indicated, otherwise, most treatment is supportive or symptom directed following GI decontamination.

Drug Interactions

Increased Effect/Toxicity: Probenecid increases the effects of cephalosporins by decreasing the renal elimination in those which are secreted by tubular secretion. Anticoagulant effects may be increased when administered with cephalosporins.

Stability Oral suspension should be mixed with 39 mL water for the 60 mL bottle and 65 mL of water for the 120 mL bottle. After mixing, the suspension can be stored at room temperature (25°C/77°F). The suspension may be used for 10 days. The suspension should be shaken well before each administration.

Mechanism of Action Inhibits bacterial cell wall synthesis by binding to one or more of the penicillin-binding proteins (PBPs) which in turn inhibits the final transpeptidation step of peptidoglycan synthesis in bacterial cell walls, thus inhibiting cell wall biosynthesis. Bacteria eventually lyse due to ongoing activity of cell wall autolytic enzymes (autolysins and murein hydrolases) while cell wall assembly is arrested.

Pharmacodynamics/Kinetics

Protein binding: 60% to 70%

Metabolism: Minimal

Bioavailability: Capsule: 16% to 21%; suspension 25%

Half-life elimination: 100 minutes

Excretion: Primarily urine

Usual Dosage Oral:

Children: 7 mg/kg/dose twice daily for 5-10 days or 14 mg/kg/dose once daily for 10 days (maximum: 600 mg/day)

Adolescents and Adults: 300 mg twice daily or 600 mg once daily for 10 days

Dosing adjustment in renal impairment: Cl_{cr} <30 mL/minute: 300 mg once daily

Hemodialysis removes cefdinir; recommended initial dose: 300 mg (or 7 mg/kg/dose) every other day. At the conclusion of each hemodialysis session, 300 mg (or 7 mg/kg/dose) should be given. Subsequent doses (300 mg or 7 mg/kg/dose) should be administered every other day.

Monitoring Parameters Observe for signs and symptoms of anaphylaxis during first dose

Dosage Forms

Capsule: 300 mg

Suspension, oral: 125 mg/5 mL (60 mL, 100 mL)

Cefditoren (sef de TOR en)

U.S. Brand Names Spectracef™

Synonyms Cefditoren Pivoxil

Therapeutic Category Antibiotic, Cephalosporin; Antibiotic, Cephalosporin (Third Generation)

Use Treatment of acute bacterial exacerbation of chronic bronchitis (due to susceptible organisms including *Haemophilus influenzae*, *Haemophilus parainfluenzae*, *Streptococcus pneumoniae*-penicillin susceptible only, *Moraxella catarrhalis*); pharyngitis or tonsillitis (*Streptococcus pyogenes*); and uncomplicated skin and skin-structure infections (*Staphylococcus aureus*-not MRSA, *Streptococcus pyogenes*)

Pregnancy Risk Factor B

Pregnancy/Breast-Feeding Implications There are no adequate and well-controlled studies in pregnant women; use only if clearly needed. Excretion in breast milk is unknown; use caution.

Contraindications Hypersensitivity to cefditoren, other cephalosporins, milk protein, or any component of the formulation; carnitine deficiency

Warnings/Precautions Use with caution in patients with a history of penicillin allergy, especially IgE-mediated reactions (eg, anaphylaxis, urticaria); may cause antibiotic-associated colitis or colitis secondary to *C. difficile*. Use caution in patients with renal or hepatic impairment. Cefditoren causes renal excretion of carnitine, do not use in patients with carnitine deficiency; not for long-term therapy due to the possible development of carnitine deficiency over time. Cefditoren tablets contain sodium caseinate, which may cause hypersensitivity reactions in patients with milk protein hypersensitivity; this does not affect patients with lactose intolerance. Safety and efficacy have not been established in children <12 years of age.

Adverse Reactions
>10%: Gastrointestinal: Diarrhea (11% to 14%)
1% to 10%:
Central nervous system: Headache (2%)
Endocrine & metabolic: Glucose increased (1%)
Gastrointestinal: Nausea (4% to 6%), abdominal pain (2%), dyspepsia (1% to 2%), vomiting (1%)
Genitourinary: Vaginal moniliasis (3% to 6%)
Hematologic: Hematocrit decreased (2%)
Renal: Hematuria (3%), urinary white blood cells increased (2%)
<1% (Limited to important or life-threatening): Allergic reaction, BUN increased, coagulation time increased, positive direct Coombs' test, pseudomembranous colitis, rash, thrombocytopenia
Additional adverse effects seen with cephalosporin antibiotics: Anaphylaxis, aplastic anemia, cholestasis, erythema multiforme, hemorrhage, hemolytic anemia, renal dysfunction, reversible hyperactivity, serum sickness-like reaction, Stevens-Johnson syndrome, toxic epidermal necrolysis, toxic nephropathy

Drug Interactions
Increased Effect/Toxicity: Increased levels of cefditoren with probenecid.
Decreased Effect: Antacids and H_2 receptor antagonists decrease cefditoren levels.
Ethanol/Nutrition/Herb Interactions Food: Moderate- to high-fat meals increase bioavailability and maximum plasma concentration.

Stability Store at controlled room temperature of 25°C (77°F). Protect from light and moisture.

Mechanism of Action Inhibits bacterial cell wall synthesis by binding to one or more of the penicillin binding proteins (PBPs); which in turn inhibits the final transpeptidation step of peptidoglycan synthesis in bacterial cell walls, thus inhibiting cell wall biosynthesis. Bacteria eventually lyse due to ongoing activity of cell wall autolytic enzymes (autolysins and murein hydrolases) while cell wall assembly is arrested.

Pharmacodynamics/Kinetics
Distribution: 9.3 ± 1.6 L
Protein binding: 88% (*in vitro*), primarily to albumin
Metabolism: Cefditoren pivoxil is hydrolyzed to cefditoren (active) and pivalate
Bioavailability: ~14% to 16%, increased by moderate to high-fat meal
Half-life elimination: 1.6 ± 0.4 hours
Time to peak: 1.5-3 hours
Excretion: Urine (as cefditoren and pivaloylcarnitine)

Usual Dosage Oral: Children ≥12 years and Adults:
Acute bacterial exacerbation of chronic bronchitis: 400 mg twice daily for 10 days
Pharyngitis, tonsillitis, uncomplicated skin and skin structure infections: 200 mg twice daily for 10 days
Elderly: Refer to adult dosing
Dosage adjustment in renal impairment:
Cl_{cr} 30-49 mL/minute: Maximum dose: 200 mg twice daily
Cl_{cr} <30 mL/minute: Maximum dose: 200 mg once daily
End-stage renal disease: Appropriate dosing not established
Dosage adjustment in hepatic impairment:
Mild or moderate impairment: Adjustment not required
Severe impairment (Child-Pugh class C): Specific guidelines not available

Dietary Considerations Cefditoren should be taken with meals. Plasma carnitine levels are decreased during therapy (39% with 200 mg dosing; 63% with 400 mg dosing); normal concentrations return within 7-10 days after treatment is discontinued.

Administration Should be administered with meals.

Monitoring Parameters Assess patient at beginning and throughout therapy for infection; monitor for signs of anaphylaxis during first dose.

Test Interactions May cause a false-negative ferricyanide test; false-positive urine glucose test when using Clinitest®

Patient Information Complete full course of medication to ensure eradication of organism. Report persistent diarrhea. Females should report symptoms of vaginitis; may interfere with oral contraceptives.

Dosage Forms Tablet, as pivoxil: 200 mg [equivalent to cefditoren] [contains sodium caseinate]

♦ **Cefditoren Pivoxil** *see* Cefditoren *on page 242*

Cefepime (SEF e pim)
Related Information
Antimicrobial Drugs of Choice *on page 1588*
Community-Acquired Pneumonia in Adults *on page 1603*
U.S. Brand Names Maxipime®
Canadian Brand Names Maxipime®
(Continued)

Cefepime *(Continued)*

Synonyms Cefepime Hydrochloride

Therapeutic Category Antibiotic, Cephalosporin (Fourth Generation)

Use Treatment of uncomplicated and complicated urinary tract infections, including pyelone-phritis caused by typical urinary tract pathogens; monotherapy for febrile neutropenia; uncomplicated skin and skin structure infections caused by *Streptococcus pyogenes*; moderate to severe pneumonia caused by pneumococcus, *Pseudomonas aeruginosa*, and other gram-negative organisms; complicated intra-abdominal infections (in combination with metronidazole). Also active against methicillin-susceptible staphylococci, *Enterobacter* sp, and many other gram-negative bacilli.

Children 2 months to 16 years: Empiric therapy of febrile neutropenia patients, uncomplicated skin/soft tissue infections, pneumonia, and uncomplicated/complicated urinary tract infections.

Pregnancy Risk Factor B

Contraindications Hypersensitivity to cefepime, any component of the formulation, or other cephalosporins

Warnings/Precautions Modify dosage in patients with severe renal impairment; prolonged use may result in superinfection; use with caution in patients with a history of penicillin or cephalosporin allergy, especially IgE-mediated reactions (eg, anaphylaxis, urticaria); may cause antibiotic-associated colitis or colitis secondary to *C. difficile*

Adverse Reactions

>10%: Hematologic: Positive Coombs' test without hemolysis

1% to 10%:

Dermatologic: Rash, pruritus

Gastrointestinal: : Diarrhea, nausea, vomiting

Central nervous system: Fever (1%), headache (1%)

Local: Pain, erythema at injection site

<1% (Limited to important or life-threatening): Agranulocytosis, anaphylactic shock, anaphylaxis, encephalopathy, leukopenia, myoclonus, neuromuscular excitability, neutropenia, seizures, thrombocytopenia

Other reactions with cephalosporins include aplastic anemia, erythema multiforme, hemolytic anemia, hemorrhage, pancytopenia, prolonged PT, renal dysfunction, Stevens-Johnson syndrome, superinfection, toxic epidermal necrolysis, toxic nephropathy, vaginitis

Overdosage/Toxicology Symptoms include neuromuscular hypersensitivity and convulsions. Many beta-lactam antibiotics have the potential to cause neuromuscular hyperirritability or seizures. Hemodialysis may be helpful to aid in the removal of the drug from the blood, however, most often treatment is supportive and symptom directed.

Drug Interactions

Increased Effect/Toxicity: High-dose probenecid decreases clearance and increases effect of cefepime. Aminoglycosides increase nephrotoxic potential when taken with cefepime.

Stability Cefepime is **compatible** and stable with normal saline, D_5W, and a variety of other solutions for 24 hours at room temperature and 7 days refrigerated

Mechanism of Action Inhibits bacterial cell wall synthesis by binding to one or more of the penicillin-binding proteins (PBPs) which in turn inhibits the final transpeptidation step of peptidoglycan synthesis in bacterial cell walls, thus inhibiting cell wall biosynthesis. Bacteria eventually lyse due to ongoing activity of cell wall autolytic enzymes (autolysis and murein hydrolases) while cell wall assembly is arrested.

Pharmacodynamics/Kinetics

Absorption: I.M.: Rapid and complete

Distribution: V_d: Adults: 14-20 L; penetrates into inflammatory fluid at concentrations ~80% of serum levels and into bronchial mucosa at levels ~60% of those reached in the plasma; crosses blood-brain barrier

Protein binding, plasma: 16% to 19%

Metabolism: Minimal

Half-life elimination: 2 hours

Time to peak: 0.5-1.5 hours

Excretion: Urine (85% as unchanged drug)

Usual Dosage I.V.:

Children:

Febrile neutropenia: 50 mg/kg every 8 hours for 7-10 days

Uncomplicated skin/soft tissue infections, pneumonia, and complicated/uncomplicated UTI: 50 mg/kg twice daily

Adults:

Most infections: 1-2 g every 12 hours for 5-10 days; higher doses or more frequent administration may be required in pseudomonal infections

Urinary tract infections, uncomplicated: 500 mg every 12 hours

Cefepime Hydrochloride

Creatinine Clearance (mL/minute)	Recommended Maintenance Schedule			
>60 Normal recommended dosing schedule	500 mg every 12 hours	1 g every 12 hours	2 g every 12 hours	2 g every 8 hours
30-60	500 mg every 24 hours	1 g every 24 hours	2 g every 24 hours	2 g every 12 hours
11-29	500 mg every 24 hours	500 mg every 24 hours	1 g every 24 hours	2 g every 24 hours
<11	250 mg every 24 hours	250 mg every 24 hours	500 mg every 24 hours	1 g every 24 hours

Monotherapy for febrile neutropenic patients: 2 g every 8 hours for 7 days or until the neutropenia resolves

Dosing adjustment in renal impairment: Adults: Recommended maintenance schedule based on creatinine clearance (mL/minute), compared to normal dosing schedule: See table on previous page.

Hemodialysis: Removed by dialysis; administer supplemental dose of 250 mg after each dialysis session

Peritoneal dialysis: Removed to a lesser extent than hemodialysis; administer 250 mg every 48 hours

Continuous arteriovenous or venovenous hemofiltration: Dose as normal Cl_{cr} (eg, >30 mL/minute)

Administration May be administered either I.M. or I.V.

Monitoring Parameters Obtain specimen for culture and sensitivity prior to the first dose; monitor for signs of anaphylaxis during first dose

Test Interactions Positive direct Coombs', false-positive urinary glucose test using cupric sulfate (Benedict's solution, Clinitest®, Fehling's solution), false-positive serum or urine creatinine with Jaffé reaction, false-positive urinary proteins and steroids

Patient Information Report side effects such as diarrhea, dyspepsia, headache, blurred vision, and lightheadedness to your physician

Nursing Implications Do not admix with aminoglycosides in the same bottle/bag; observe for signs and symptoms of bacterial infection, including defervescence; observe for anaphylaxis during first dose

Dosage Forms
Infusion, as hydrochloride (ADD-Vantage®): 1 g, 2 g
Infusion, piggyback, as hydrochloride: 1 g (100 mL); 2 g (100 mL)
Powder for injection, as hydrochloride: 500 mg, 1 g, 2 g

♦ Cefepime Hydrochloride see Cefepime on page 243

Cefixime (sef IKS eem)

Related Information
Antimicrobial Drugs of Choice on page 1588
Treatment of Sexually Transmitted Diseases on page 1609

U.S. Brand Names Suprax®

Canadian Brand Names Suprax®

Therapeutic Category Antibiotic, Cephalosporin (Third Generation)

Use Treatment of urinary tract infections, otitis media, respiratory infections due to susceptible organisms including *S. pneumoniae* and *S. pyogenes*, *H. influenzae* and many Enterobacteriaceae; documented poor compliance with other oral antimicrobials; outpatient therapy of serious soft tissue or skeletal infections due to susceptible organisms; single-dose oral treatment of uncomplicated cervical/urethral gonorrhea due to *N. gonorrhoeae*

Pregnancy Risk Factor B

Contraindications Hypersensitivity to cefixime, any component of the formulation, or other cephalosporins

Warnings/Precautions Prolonged use may result in superinfection; modify dosage in patients with renal impairment; use with caution in patients with a history of penicillin allergy especially IgE-mediated reactions (eg, anaphylaxis, urticaria); may cause antibiotic-associated colitis or colitis secondary to *C. difficile*

Adverse Reactions
>10%: Gastrointestinal: Diarrhea (16%)
1% to 10%: Gastrointestinal: Abdominal pain, nausea, dyspepsia, flatulence
<1% (Limited to important or life-threatening): BUN increased, candidiasis, creatinine increased, dizziness, eosinophilia, erythema multiforme, fever, headache, leukopenia, prolonged PT, pruritus, pseudomembranous colitis, rash, serum sickness-like reaction, Stevens-Johnson syndrome, thrombocytopenia, transaminases increased, urticaria, vaginitis, vomiting
Other reactions with cephalosporins include agranulocytosis, anaphylaxis, aplastic anemia, cholestasis, colitis, hemolytic anemia, hemorrhage, interstitial nephritis, neutropenia, pancytopenia, renal dysfunction, seizures, superinfection, toxic epidermal necrolysis, toxic nephropathy

Overdosage/Toxicology After acute overdose, most agents cause only nausea, vomiting, and diarrhea, although neuromuscular hypersensitivity and seizures are possible, especially in patients with renal insufficiency. Many beta-lactam antibiotics have the potential to cause neuromuscular hyperirritability or seizures. Hemodialysis may be helpful to aid in removal of the drug from the blood but is not usually indicated; otherwise, most treatment is supportive or symptom directed, following GI decontamination.

Drug Interactions
Increased Effect/Toxicity: Probenecid increases cefixime concentration. Cefixime may increase carbamazepine.

Ethanol/Nutrition/Herb Interactions Food: Delays cefixime absorption.

Stability After reconstitution, suspension may be stored for 14 days at room temperature

Mechanism of Action Inhibits bacterial cell wall synthesis by binding to one or more of the penicillin binding proteins (PBPs); which in turn inhibits the final transpeptidation step of peptidoglycan synthesis in bacterial cell walls, thus inhibiting cell wall biosynthesis. Bacteria eventually lyse due to ongoing activity of cell wall autolytic enzymes (autolysins and murein hydrolases) while cell wall assembly is arrested.

Pharmacodynamics/Kinetics
Absorption: 40% to 50%
Distribution: Widely throughout the body and reaches therapeutic concentration in most tissues and body fluids, including synovial, pericardial, pleural, peritoneal; bile, sputum, and urine; bone, myocardium, gallbladder, and skin and soft tissue
Protein binding: 65%
Half-life elimination: Normal renal function: 3-4 hours; Renal failure: Up to 11.5 hours
(Continued)

Cefixime *(Continued)*

Time to peak, serum: 2-6 hours; peak serum concentrations are 15% to 50% higher for oral suspension versus tablets; presence of food delays the time to reach peak concentrations

Excretion: Primarily urine (50% of absorbed dose as active drug); feces (10%)

Usual Dosage Oral:

Children: 8 mg/kg/day divided every 12-24 hours

Adolescents and Adults: 400 mg/day divided every 12-24 hours

Uncomplicated cervical/urethral gonorrhea due to *N. gonorrhoeae*: 400 mg as a single dose

For *S. pyogenes* infections, treat for 10 days; use suspension for otitis media due to increased peak serum levels as compared to tablet form

Dosing adjustment in renal impairment:

Cl_{cr} 21-60 mL/minute or with renal hemodialysis: Administer 75% of the standard dose

Cl_{cr} <20 mL/minute or with CAPD: Administer 50% of the standard dose

Moderately dialyzable (10%)

Dietary Considerations May be taken with food.

Administration Oral: May be administered with or without food; administer with food to decrease GI distress

Monitoring Parameters With prolonged therapy, monitor renal and hepatic function periodically; observe for signs and symptoms of anaphylaxis during first dose

Test Interactions Positive direct Coombs', false-positive urinary glucose test using cupric sulfate (Benedict's solution, Clinitest®, Fehling's solution), false-positive serum or urine creatinine with Jaffé reaction

Patient Information Report diarrhea promptly; entire course of medication (10-14 days) should be taken to ensure eradication of organism; may interfere with oral contraceptives, females should report symptoms of vaginitis

Nursing Implications Modify dosage in patients with renal impairment

Additional Information Otitis media should be treated with the suspension since it results in higher peak blood levels than the tablet.

Dosage Forms

Powder for oral suspension: 100 mg/5 mL (50 mL, 100 mL) [strawberry flavor]

Tablet, film coated: 200 mg, 400 mg

- **Cefizox®** *see* Ceftizoxime *on page 255*
- **Cefobid®** *see* Cefoperazone *on page 246*
- **Cefol® Filmtab®** *see* Vitamins (Multiple) *on page 1424*

Cefoperazone *(sef oh PER a zone)*

U.S. Brand Names Cefobid®

Canadian Brand Names Cefobid®

Synonyms Cefoperazone Sodium

Therapeutic Category Antibiotic, Cephalosporin (Third Generation)

Use Treatment of susceptible bacterial infection; mainly respiratory tract, skin and skin structure, bone and joint, urinary tract and gynecologic as well as septicemia. Active against a variety of gram-negative bacilli, some gram-positive cocci, and has some activity against *Pseudomonas aeruginosa*.

Pregnancy Risk Factor B

Contraindications Hypersensitivity to cefoperazone, any component of the formulation, or other cephalosporins

Warnings/Precautions Modify dosage in patients with severe renal or hepatic impairment; prolonged use may result in superinfection; although rare, cefoperazone may interfere with hemostasis via destruction of vitamin K-producing intestinal bacteria, prevention of activation of prothrombin by the attachment of a methyltetrazolethiol side chain, and by an immune-mediated thrombocytopenia; use with caution in patients with a history of penicillin allergy especially IgE-mediated reactions (eg, anaphylaxis, urticaria); may cause antibiotic-associated colitis or colitis secondary to *C. difficile*

Adverse Reactions Contains MTT side chain which may lead to increased risk of hypoprothrombinemia and bleeding.

1% to 10%:

Dermatologic: Rash (maculopapular or erythematous) (2%)

Gastrointestinal: Diarrhea (3%)

Hematologic: Decreased neutrophils (2%), decreased hemoglobin or hematocrit (5%), eosinophilia (10%)

Hepatic: Increased transaminases (5% to 10%)

<1% (Limited to important or life-threatening): Bleeding, BUN increased, creatinine increased, drug fever, hypoprothrombinemia, induration at injection site, nausea, pain at injection site, phlebitis, pseudomembranous colitis, vomiting

Other reactions with cephalosporins include agranulocytosis, anaphylaxis, aplastic anemia, cholestasis, colitis, hemolytic anemia, pancytopenia, renal dysfunction, seizures, Stevens-Johnson syndrome, superinfection, toxic epidermal necrolysis, toxic nephropathy

Overdosage/Toxicology Symptoms include neuromuscular hypersensitivity and convulsions, especially with renal insufficiency. Many beta-lactam antibiotics have the potential to cause neuromuscular hyperirritability or seizures. Hemodialysis may be helpful to aid in removal of the drug from the blood; otherwise, most treatment is supportive or symptom directed.

Drug Interactions

Increased Effect/Toxicity: Probenecid may decrease cephalosporin elimination resulting in increased levels. Furosemide, aminoglycosides in combination with cefoperazone may result in additive nephrotoxicity.

Ethanol/Nutrition/Herb Interactions

Ethanol: Avoid ethanol (may cause a disulfiram-like reaction).

Food: Cefoperazone may decrease vitamin K synthesis by suppressing GI flora; vitamin K deficiency may occur and result in an increased risk of hemorrhage; patients at risk include those with malabsorption states (eg, cystic fibrosis) or poor nutritional status.

Stability Reconstituted solution and I.V. infusion in NS or D_5W solution are stable for 24 hours at room temperature, 5 days when refrigerated or 3 weeks, when frozen; after freezing, thawed solution is stable for 48 hours at room temperature or 10 days when refrigerated

Mechanism of Action Inhibits bacterial cell wall synthesis by binding to one or more of the penicillin-binding proteins (PBPs) which in turn inhibits the final transpeptidation step of peptidoglycan synthesis in bacterial cell walls, thus inhibiting cell wall biosynthesis. Bacteria eventually lyse due to ongoing activity of cell wall autolytic enzymes (autolysins and murein hydrolases) while cell wall assembly is arrested.

Pharmacodynamics/Kinetics

Distribution: Widely in most body tissues and fluids; highest concentrations in bile; low penetration in CSF; variable when meninges are inflamed; crosses placenta; small amounts enter breast milk

Half-life elimination: 2 hours; higher with hepatic disease or biliary obstruction

Time to peak, serum: I.M.: 1-2 hours

Excretion: Primarily feces via the biliary tract (70% to 75%); urine (20% to 30% as unchanged drug)

Usual Dosage I.M., I.V.:

Children: 100-150 mg/kg/day divided every 8-12 hours; up to 12 g/day

Adults: 2-4 g/day in divided doses every 12 hours; up to 12 g/day

Dosing adjustment in hepatic impairment: Reduce dose 50% in patients with advanced liver cirrhosis; maximum daily dose: 4 g

Dietary Considerations May block activity of vitamin K. Monitor prothrombin time and administer vitamin K as needed.

Monitoring Parameters Monitor for coagulation abnormalities and diarrhea; observe for signs and symptoms of anaphylaxis during first dose

Test Interactions Positive direct Coombs', false-positive urinary glucose test using cupric sulfate (Benedict's solution, Clinitest®, Fehling's solution), false-positive serum or urine creatinine with Jaffé reaction

Nursing Implications Do not admix with aminoglycosides in same bottle/bag

Additional Information Sodium content of 1 g: 34.5 mg (1.5 mEq); contains the *N*-methylthiotetrazole (NMTT) side chain

Dosage Forms

Injection, as sodium [premixed, frozen]: 1 g (50 mL); 2 g (50 mL)

Powder for injection, as sodium: 1 g, 2 g

♦ **Cefoperazone Sodium** *see* Cefoperazone *on page 246*

♦ **Cefotan®** *see* Cefotetan *on page 248*

Cefotaxime (sef oh TAKS eem)

Related Information

Antibiotic Treatment of Adults With Infective Endocarditis *on page 1585*

Antimicrobial Drugs of Choice *on page 1588*

Community-Acquired Pneumonia in Adults *on page 1603*

Treatment of Sexually Transmitted Diseases *on page 1609*

U.S. Brand Names Claforan®

Canadian Brand Names Claforan®

Synonyms Cefotaxime Sodium

Therapeutic Category Antibiotic, Cephalosporin (Third Generation)

Use Treatment of susceptible infection in respiratory tract, skin and skin structure, bone and joint, urinary tract, gynecologic as well as septicemia, and documented or suspected meningitis. Active against most gram-negative bacilli (not *Pseudomonas*) and gram-positive cocci (not enterococcus). Active against many penicillin-resistant pneumococci.

Pregnancy Risk Factor B

Contraindications Hypersensitivity to cefotaxime, any component of the formulation, or other cephalosporins

Warnings/Precautions Modify dosage in patients with severe renal impairment; prolonged use may result in superinfection; a potentially life-threatening arrhythmia has been reported in patients who received a rapid bolus injection via central line. Use caution in patients with colitis; minimize tissue inflammation by changing infusion sites when needed. Use with caution in patients with a history of penicillin allergy especially IgE-mediated reactions (eg, anaphylaxis, urticaria); may cause antibiotic-associated colitis or colitis secondary to *C. difficile*.

Adverse Reactions

1% to 10%:

Dermatologic: Rash, pruritus

Gastrointestinal: Diarrhea, nausea, vomiting, colitis

Local: Pain at injection site

<1% (Limited to important or life-threatening): Anaphylaxis, arrhythmias (after rapid I.V. injection via central catheter), BUN increased, candidiasis, creatinine increased, eosinophilia, erythema multiforme, fever, headache, interstitial nephritis, neutropenia, phlebitis, pseudomembranous colitis, Stevens-Johnson syndrome, thrombocytopenia, transaminases increased, toxic epidermal necrolysis, urticaria, vaginitis

Reactions reported with other cephalosporins include agranulocytosis, aplastic anemia, cholestasis, hemolytic anemia, hemorrhage, pancytopenia, renal dysfunction, seizures, superinfection, toxic nephropathy.

Overdosage/Toxicology Usually well tolerated even in overdose; convulsions are possible. Many beta-lactam antibiotics have the potential to cause neuromuscular hyperirritability or seizures. Hemodialysis may be helpful to aid in removal of the drug from the blood; otherwise, most treatment is supportive or symptom directed.

(Continued)

Cefotaxime (Continued)

Drug Interactions

Increased Effect/Toxicity: Probenecid may decrease cephalosporin elimination resulting in increased levels. Furosemide, aminoglycosides in combination with cefotaxime may result in additive nephrotoxicity.

Stability Reconstituted solution is stable for 12-24 hours at room temperature and 7-10 days when refrigerated and for 13 weeks when frozen; for I.V. infusion in NS or D_5W, solution is stable for 24 hours at room temperature, 5 days when refrigerated, or 13 weeks when frozen in Viaflex® plastic containers; thawed solutions previously of frozen premixed bags are stable for 24 hours at room temperature or 10 days when refrigerated

Mechanism of Action Inhibits bacterial cell wall synthesis by binding to one or more of the penicillin-binding proteins (PBPs) which in turn inhibits the final transpeptidation step of peptidoglycan synthesis in bacterial cell walls, thus inhibiting cell wall biosynthesis. Bacteria eventually lyse due to ongoing activity of cell wall autolytic enzymes (autolysins and murein hydrolases) while cell wall assembly is arrested.

Pharmacodynamics/Kinetics

Distribution: Widely to body tissues and fluids including aqueous humor, ascitic and prostatic fluids, bone; penetrates CSF best when meninges are inflamed; crosses placenta; enters breast milk

Metabolism: Partially hepatic to active metabolite, desacetylcefotaxime

Half-life elimination:

Cefotaxime: Premature neonates <1 week: 5-6 hours; Full-term neonates <1 week: 2-3.4 hours; Adults: 1-1.5 hours; prolonged with renal and/or hepatic impairment

Desacetylcefotaxime: 1.5-1.9 hours (prolonged with renal impairment)

Time to peak, serum: I.M.: Within 30 minutes

Excretion: Urine (as unchanged drug and metabolites)

Usual Dosage

Infants and Children 1 month to 12 years: I.M., I.V.: <50 kg: 50-180 mg/kg/day in divided doses every 4-6 hours

Meningitis: 200 mg/kg/day in divided doses every 6 hours

Children >12 years and Adults:

Uncomplicated infections: I.M., I.V.: 1 g every 12 hours

Moderate/severe infections: I.M., I.V.: 1-2 g every 8 hours

Infections commonly needing higher doses (eg, septicemia): I.V.: 2 g every 6-8 hours

Life-threatening infections: I.V.: 2 g every 4 hours

Preop: I.M., I.V.: 1 g 30-90 minutes before surgery

C-section: 1 g as soon as the umbilical cord is clamped, then 1 g I.M., I.V. at 6- and 12-hour intervals

Dosing interval in renal impairment:

Cl_{cr} 10-50 mL/minute: Administer every 8-12 hours

Cl_{cr} <10 mL/minute: Administer every 24 hours

Hemodialysis: Moderately dialyzable

Dosing adjustment in hepatic impairment: Moderate dosage reduction is recommended in severe liver disease

Continuous arteriovenous or venovenous hemodiafiltration effects: Administer 1 g every 12 hour

Administration Can be administered IVP over 3-5 minutes or I.V. intermittent infusion over 15-30 minutes

Monitoring Parameters Observe for signs and symptoms of anaphylaxis during first dose; CBC with differential (especially with long courses)

Test Interactions Positive direct Coombs', false-positive urinary glucose test using cupric sulfate (Benedict's solution, Clinitest®, Fehling's solution), false-positive serum or urine creatinine with Jaffé reaction

Nursing Implications Cefotaxime can be administered IVP over 3-5 minutes or I.V. intermittent infusion over 15-30 minutes; do not admix with aminoglycosides in same bottle/bag; observe for signs and symptoms of anaphylaxis during first dose

Additional Information Sodium content of 1 g: 50.6 mg (2.2 mEq)

Dosage Forms

Infusion, as sodium [premixed in D_5W, frozen]: 1 g (50 mL); 2 g (50 mL)

Powder for injection, as sodium: 500 mg, 1 g, 2 g, 10 g

♦ **Cefotaxime Sodium** see Cefotaxime on page 247

Cefotetan (SEF oh tee tan)

Related Information

Animal and Human Bites Guidelines on page 1584

Antimicrobial Drugs of Choice on page 1588

Prevention of Wound Infection & Sepsis in Surgical Patients on page 1569

Treatment of Sexually Transmitted Diseases on page 1609

U.S. Brand Names Cefotan®

Canadian Brand Names Cefotan®

Synonyms Cefotetan Disodium

Therapeutic Category Antibiotic, Anaerobic; Antibiotic, Cephalosporin (Second Generation)

Use Less active against staphylococci and streptococci than first generation cephalosporins, but active against anaerobes including *Bacteroides fragilis*; active against gram-negative enteric bacilli including *E. coli*, *Klebsiella*, and *Proteus*; used predominantly for respiratory tract, skin and skin structure, bone and joint, urinary tract and gynecologic as well as septicemia; surgical prophylaxis; intra-abdominal infections and other mixed infections

Pregnancy Risk Factor B

Contraindications Hypersensitivity to cefotetan, any component of the formulation, or other cephalosporins

Warnings/Precautions Modify dosage in patients with severe renal impairment; prolonged use may result in superinfection; although cefotetan contains the methyltetrazolethiol side chain, bleeding has not been a significant problem; use with caution in patients with a history of penicillin allergy especially IgE-mediated reactions (eg, anaphylaxis, urticaria); may cause antibiotic-associated colitis or colitis secondary to *C. difficile*

Adverse Reactions Contains MTT side chain which may lead to increased risk of hypoprothrombinemia and bleeding.

1% to 10%:
 Gastrointestinal: Diarrhea (1.3%)
 Hepatic: Increased transaminases (1.2%)
 Miscellaneous: Hypersensitivity reactions (1.2%)
<1% (Limited to important or life-threatening): Agranulocytosis, anaphylaxis, bleeding, BUN increased, creatinine increased, eosinophilia, fever, hemolytic anemia, leukopenia, nausea, nephrotoxicity, phlebitis, prolonged PT, pruritus, pseudomembranous colitis, rash, thrombocytopenia, thrombocytosis, urticaria, vomiting
Other reactions with cephalosporins include agranulocytosis, aplastic anemia, cholestasis, colitis, hemolytic anemia, hemorrhage, pancytopenia, renal dysfunction, seizures, Stevens-Johnson syndrome, superinfection, toxic epidermal necrolysis, toxic nephropathy

Overdosage/Toxicology Symptoms include neuromuscular hypersensitivity and convulsions especially with renal insufficiency. Many beta-lactam antibiotics have the potential to cause neuromuscular hyperirritability or seizures. Hemodialysis may be helpful to aid in removal of the drug from the blood; otherwise, most treatment is supportive or symptom directed.

Drug Interactions
 Increased Effect/Toxicity: Probenecid may decrease cephalosporin elimination. Furosemide, aminoglycosides in combination with cefotetan may result in additive nephrotoxicity. May cause disulfiram-like reaction with concomitant ethanol use. Effects of warfarin may be enhanced by cefotetan (due to effects on gastrointestinal flora).

Ethanol/Nutrition/Herb Interactions Ethanol: Avoid ethanol (may cause a disulfiram-like reaction).

Stability Reconstituted solution is stable for 24 hours at room temperature and 96 hours when refrigerated; for I.V. infusion in NS or D$_5$W solution and after freezing, thawed solution is stable for 24 hours at room temperature or 96 hours when refrigerated; frozen solution is stable for 12 weeks

Mechanism of Action Inhibits bacterial cell wall synthesis by binding to one or more of the penicillin-binding proteins (PBPs) which in turn inhibits the final transpeptidation step of peptidoglycan synthesis in bacterial cell walls, thus inhibiting cell wall biosynthesis. Bacteria eventually lyse due to ongoing activity of cell wall autolytic enzymes (autolysins and murein hydrolases) while cell wall assembly is arrested.

Pharmacodynamics/Kinetics
 Distribution: Widely to body tissues and fluids including bile, sputum, prostatic, peritoneal; low concentrations enter CSF; crosses placenta; enters breast milk
 Protein binding: 76% to 90%
 Half-life elimination: 3-5 hours
 Time to peak, serum: I.M.: 1.5-3 hours
 Excretion: Primarily urine (as unchanged drug); feces (20%)

Usual Dosage I.M., I.V.:
 Children: 20-40 mg/kg/dose every 12 hours
 Adults: 1-6 g/day in divided doses every 12 hours; usual dose: 1-2 g every 12 hours for 5-10 days; 1-2 g may be given every 24 hours for urinary tract infection
 Dosing interval in renal impairment:
  Cl$_{cr}$ 10-30 mL/minute: Administer every 24 hours
  Cl$_{cr}$ <10 mL/minute: Administer every 48 hours
 Hemodialysis: Slightly dialyzable (5% to 20%); administer ¼ the usual dose every 24 hours on days between dialysis; administer ½ the usual dose on the day of dialysis.
 Continuous arteriovenous or venovenous hemodiafiltration effects: Administer 750 mg every 12 hours

Dietary Considerations Sodium content of 1 g: 34.5 mg (1.5 mEq)

Administration
 I.M.: Inject deep I.M. into large muscle mass.
 I.V.: Inject direct I.V. over 3-5 minutes. Infuse intermittent infusion over 30 minutes

Monitoring Parameters Observe for signs and symptoms of anaphylaxis during first dose

Test Interactions Positive direct Coombs', false-positive urinary glucose test using cupric sulfate (Benedict's solution, Clinitest®, Fehling's solution), false-positive serum or urine creatinine with Jaffé reaction

Nursing Implications Do not admix with aminoglycosides in same bottle/bag

Dosage Forms
 Infusion, as disodium [premixed, frozen]: 1 g (50 mL); 2 g (50 mL)
 Powder for injection, as disodium: 1 g, 2 g, 10 g

♦ **Cefotetan Disodium** *see* Cefotetan *on page 248*

Cefoxitin (se FOKS i tin)

Related Information
 Antimicrobial Drugs of Choice *on page 1588*
 Prevention of Wound Infection & Sepsis in Surgical Patients *on page 1569*
 Treatment of Sexually Transmitted Diseases *on page 1609*

U.S. Brand Names Mefoxin®

Canadian Brand Names Mefoxin®

Synonyms Cefoxitin Sodium

Therapeutic Category Antibiotic, Anaerobic; Antibiotic, Cephalosporin (Second Generation)

Use Less active against staphylococci and streptococci than first generation cephalosporins, but active against anaerobes including *Bacteroides fragilis*; active against gram-negative enteric bacilli including *E. coli*, *Klebsiella*, and *Proteus*; used predominantly for respiratory tract, skin and skin structure, bone and joint, urinary tract and gynecologic as well as septicemia; surgical prophylaxis; intra-abdominal infections and other mixed infections; indicated for bacterial *Eikenella corrodens* infections

(Continued)

Cefoxitin *(Continued)*

Pregnancy Risk Factor B

Contraindications Hypersensitivity to cefoxitin, any component of the formulation, or other cephalosporins

Warnings/Precautions Use with caution in patients with history of colitis; cefoxitin may increase resistance of organisms by inducing beta-lactamase; modify dosage in patients with severe renal impairment; prolonged use may result in superinfection; use with caution in patients with a history of penicillin allergy especially IgE-mediated reactions (eg, anaphylaxis, urticaria); may cause antibiotic-associated colitis or colitis secondary to *C. difficile*

Adverse Reactions

1% to 10%: Gastrointestinal: Diarrhea

<1% (Limited to important or life-threatening): Anaphylaxis, angioedema, bone marrow suppression, BUN increased, creatinine increased, dyspnea, eosinophilia, exacerbation of myasthenia gravis, exfoliative dermatitis, fever, hemolytic anemia, hypotension, interstitial nephritis, jaundice, leukopenia, nausea, nephrotoxicity (with aminoglycosides), phlebitis, prolonged PT, pruritus, pseudomembranous colitis, rash, thrombocytopenia, thrombophlebitis, toxic epidermal necrolysis, transaminases increased, vomiting

Other reactions with cephalosporins include agranulocytosis, aplastic anemia, cholestasis, colitis, erythema multiforme, hemolytic anemia, hemorrhage, pancytopenia, renal dysfunction, seizures, serum-sickness reactions, Stevens-Johnson syndrome, superinfection, toxic epidermal necrolysis, toxic nephropathy, urticaria, vaginitis

Overdosage/Toxicology Symptoms include neuromuscular hypersensitivity and convulsions especially with renal insufficiency. Many beta-lactam antibiotics have the potential to cause neuromuscular hyperirritability or seizures. Hemodialysis may be helpful to aid in removal of the drug from the blood; otherwise, most treatment is supportive or symptom directed.

Drug Interactions

Increased Effect/Toxicity: Probenecid may decrease cephalosporin elimination. Furosemide, aminoglycosides in combination with cefoxitin may result in additive nephrotoxicity.

Stability Reconstituted solution is stable for 24 hours at room temperature and 48 hours when refrigerated; I.V. infusion in NS or D_5W solution is stable for 24 hours at room temperature, 1 week when refrigerated, or 26 weeks when frozen; after freezing, thawed solution is stable for 24 hours at room temperature or 5 days when refrigerated

Mechanism of Action Inhibits bacterial cell wall synthesis by binding to one or more of the penicillin-binding proteins (PBPs) which in turn inhibits the final transpeptidation step of peptidoglycan synthesis in bacterial cell walls, thus inhibiting cell wall biosynthesis. Bacteria eventually lyse due to ongoing activity of cell wall autolytic enzymes (autolysins and murein hydrolases) while cell wall assembly is arrested.

Pharmacodynamics/Kinetics

Distribution: Widely to body tissues and fluids including pleural, synovial, ascitic, bile; poorly penetrates into CSF even with inflammation of the meninges; crosses placenta; small amounts enter breast milk

Protein binding: 65% to 79%

Half-life elimination: 45-60 minutes; increases significantly with renal insufficiency

Time to peak, serum: I.M. 20-30 minutes

Excretion: Urine (85% as unchanged drug)

Usual Dosage

Infants >3 months and Children: I.M., I.V.:

Mild to moderate infection: 80-100 mg/kg/day in divided doses every 4-6 hours

Severe infection: 100-160 mg/kg/day in divided doses every 4-6 hours; maximum dose: 12 g/day

Perioperative prophylaxis: 30-40 mg/kg 30-60 minutes prior to surgery followed by 30-40 mg/kg/dose every 6 hours for no more than 24 hours after surgery depending on the procedure

Adolescents and Adults: I.M., I.V.: Perioperative prophylaxis: 1-2 g 30-60 minutes prior to surgery followed by 1-2 g every 6-8 hours for no more than 24 hours after surgery depending on the procedure

Adults: I.M., I.V.: 1-2 g every 6-8 hours (I.M. injection is painful); up to 12 g/day

Pelvic inflammatory disease:

Inpatients: I.V.: 2 g every 6 hours **plus** doxycycline 100 mg I.V. or 100 mg orally every 12 hours until improved, followed by doxycycline 100 mg orally twice daily to complete 14 days

Outpatients: I.M.: 2 g **plus** probenecid 1 g orally as a single dose, followed by doxycycline 100 mg orally twice daily for 14 days

Dosing interval in renal impairment:

Cl_{cr} 30-50 mL/minute: Administer 1-2 g every 8-12 hours

Cl_{cr} 10-29 mL/minute: Administer 1-2 g every 12-24 hours

Cl_{cr} 5-9 mL/minute: Administer 0.5-1 g every 12-24 hours

Cl_{cr} <5 mL/minute: Administer 0.5-1 g every 24-48 hours

Hemodialysis: Moderately dialyzable (20% to 50%); administer a loading dose of 1-2 g after each hemodialysis; maintenance dose as noted above based on Cl_{cr}

Continuous arteriovenous or venovenous hemodiafiltration effects: Dose as for Cl_{cr} 10-50 mL/minute

Administration

I.M.: Inject deep I.M. into large muscle mass.

I.V.: Inject direct I.V. over 3-5 minutes. Infuse intermittent infusion over 30 minutes.

Monitoring Parameters Monitor renal function periodically when used in combination with other nephrotoxic drugs; observe for signs and symptoms of anaphylaxis during first dose

Test Interactions Positive direct Coombs', false-positive urinary glucose test using cupric sulfate (Benedict's solution, Clinitest®, Fehling's solution), false-positive serum or urine creatinine with Jaffé reaction

Nursing Implications Administer around-the-clock rather than 4 times/day, 3 times/day, etc (ie, 12-6-12-6, not 9-1-5-9) to promote less variation in peak and trough serum levels; modify dosage in patients with renal insufficiency; can be administered IVP over 3-5 minutes at a maximum concentration of 100 mg/mL or I.V. intermittent infusion over 10-60 minutes at a final concentration for I.V. administration not to exceed 40 mg/mL

Additional Information Sodium content of 1 g: 53 mg (2.3 mEq)

Dosage Forms
Infusion, as sodium [premixed in D₅W, frozen]: 1 g (50 mL); 2 g (50 mL)
Powder for injection, as sodium: 1 g, 2 g, 10 g

♦ **Cefoxitin Sodium** *see* Cefoxitin *on page 249*

Cefpodoxime (sef pode OKS eem)

Related Information
Antimicrobial Drugs of Choice *on page 1588*
Community-Acquired Pneumonia in Adults *on page 1603*

U.S. Brand Names Vantin®

Canadian Brand Names Vantin®

Synonyms Cefpodoxime Proxetil

Therapeutic Category Antibiotic, Cephalosporin (Third Generation)

Use Treatment of susceptible acute, community-acquired pneumonia caused by *S. pneumoniae* or nonbeta-lactamase producing *H. influenzae*; acute uncomplicated gonorrhea caused by *N. gonorrhoeae*; uncomplicated skin and skin structure infections caused by *S. aureus* or *S. pyogenes*; acute otitis media caused by *S. pneumoniae*, *H. influenzae*, or *M. catarrhalis*; pharyngitis or tonsillitis; and uncomplicated urinary tract infections caused by *E. coli*, *Klebsiella*, and *Proteus*

Pregnancy Risk Factor B

Contraindications Hypersensitivity to cefpodoxime, any component of the formulation, or other cephalosporins

Warnings/Precautions Modify dosage in patients with severe renal impairment; prolonged use may result in superinfection; a low incidence of cross-hypersensitivity to penicillins exists

Adverse Reactions
>10%:
Dermatologic: Diaper rash (12.1%)
Gastrointestinal: Diarrhea in infants and toddlers (15.4%)
1% to 10%:
Central nervous system: Headache (1.1%)
Dermatologic: Rash (1.4%)
Gastrointestinal: Diarrhea (7.2%), nausea (3.8%), abdominal pain (1.6%), vomiting (1.1% to 2.1%)
Genitourinary: Vaginal infections (3.1%)
<1% (Limited to important or life-threatening): Anaphylaxis, anxiety, appetite decreased, chest pain, cough, dizziness, epistaxis, eye itching, fatigue, fever, flatulence, flushing, fungal skin infection, hypotension, insomnia, malaise, nightmares, pruritus, pseudomembranous colitis, purpuric nephritis, salivation decreased, taste alteration, tinnitus, vaginal candidiasis, weakness
Other reactions with cephalosporins include agranulocytosis, aplastic anemia, cholestasis, colitis, erythema multiforme, hemolytic anemia, hemorrhage, interstitial nephritis, toxic nephropathy, pancytopenia, renal dysfunction, seizures, serum-sickness reactions, Stevens-Johnson syndrome, superinfection, toxic epidermal necrolysis, urticaria, vaginitis

Overdosage/Toxicology After acute overdose, most agents cause only nausea, vomiting, and diarrhea, although neuromuscular hypersensitivity and seizures are possible, especially in patients with renal insufficiency. Many beta-lactam antibiotics have the potential to cause neuromuscular hyperirritability or seizures. Hemodialysis may be helpful to aid in removal of the drug from the blood but not usually indicated; otherwise, most treatment is supportive or symptom directed, following GI decontamination.

Drug Interactions
Increased Effect/Toxicity: Probenecid may decrease cephalosporin elimination. Furosemide, aminoglycosides in combination with cefpodoxime may result in additive nephrotoxicity.
Decreased Effect: Antacids and H₂-receptor antagonists reduce absorption and serum concentration of cefpodoxime.

Ethanol/Nutrition/Herb Interactions Food: Food delays absorption; cefpodoxime serum levels may be increased if taken with food.

Stability After mixing, keep suspension in refrigerator, shake well before using; discard unused portion after 14 days

Mechanism of Action Inhibits bacterial cell wall synthesis by binding to one or more of the penicillin-binding proteins (PBPs) which in turn inhibits the final transpeptidation step of peptidoglycan synthesis in bacterial cell walls, thus inhibiting cell wall biosynthesis. Bacteria eventually lyse due to ongoing activity of cell wall autolytic enzymes (autolysins and murein hydrolases) while cell wall assembly is arrested.

Pharmacodynamics/Kinetics
Absorption: Rapid and well (50%), acid stable; enhanced in the presence of food or low gastric pH
Distribution: Good tissue penetration, including lung and tonsils; penetrates into pleural fluid
Protein binding: 18% to 23%
Metabolism: De-esterified in GI tract to active metabolite, cefpodoxime
Half-life elimination: 2.2 hours; prolonged with renal impairment
Time to peak: Within 1 hour
Excretion: Urine (80% as unchanged drug) in 24 hours

Usual Dosage Oral:
Children 2 months to 12 years:
Acute otitis media: 10 mg/kg/day divided every 12 hours (400 mg/day) for 5 days (maximum: 200 mg/dose)
Acute maxillary sinusitis: 10 mg/kg/day divided every 12 hours for 10 days (maximum: 200 mg/dose)
(Continued)

Cefpodoxime *(Continued)*

Pharyngitis/tonsillitis: 10 mg/kg/day in 2 divided doses for 5-10 days (maximum: 100 mg/dose)

Children ≥12 years and Adults:

Acute community-acquired pneumonia and bacterial exacerbations of chronic bronchitis: 200 mg every 12 hours for 14 days and 10 days, respectively

Acute maxillary sinusitis: 200 mg every 12 hours for 10 days

Skin and skin structure: 400 mg every 12 hours for 7-14 days

Uncomplicated gonorrhea (male and female) and rectal gonococcal infections (female): 200 mg as a single dose

Pharyngitis/tonsillitis: 100 mg every 12 hours for 5-10 days

Uncomplicated urinary tract infection: 100 mg every 12 hours for 7 days

Dosing adjustment in renal impairment: Cl_{cr} <30 mL/minute: Administer every 24 hours

Hemodialysis: Administer dose 3 times/week following hemodialysis

Dietary Considerations May be taken with food.

Monitoring Parameters Observe for signs and symptoms of anaphylaxis during first dose

Test Interactions Positive direct Coombs', false-positive urinary glucose test using cupric sulfate (Benedict's solution, Clinitest®, Fehling's solution), false-positive serum or urine creatinine with Jaffé reaction

Patient Information Take with food; chilling improves flavor (do not freeze); report persistent diarrhea; entire course of medication (10-14 days) should be taken to ensure eradication of organism; may interfere with oral contraceptives; females should report symptoms of vaginitis

Nursing Implications Assess patient at beginning and throughout therapy for infection; administer around-the-clock to promote less variation in peak and trough serum levels

Dosage Forms

Granules for oral suspension, as proxetil: 50 mg/5 mL (100 mL); 100 mg/5 mL (100 mL) [lemon creme flavor]

Tablet, film coated, as proxetil: 100 mg, 200 mg

♦ **Cefpodoxime Proxetil** *see* Cefpodoxime *on page 251*

Cefprozil *(sef PROE zil)*

Related Information

Community-Acquired Pneumonia in Adults *on page 1603*

U.S. Brand Names Cefzil®

Canadian Brand Names Cefzil™

Therapeutic Category Antibiotic, Cephalosporin (Second Generation)

Use Treatment of otitis media and infections involving the respiratory tract and skin and skin structure; active against methicillin-sensitive staphylococci, many streptococci, and various gram-negative bacilli including *E. coli*, some *Klebsiella*, *P. mirabilis*, *H. influenzae*, and *Moraxella*.

Pregnancy Risk Factor B

Contraindications Hypersensitivity to cefprozil, any component of the formulation, or other cephalosporins

Warnings/Precautions Modify dosage in patients with severe renal impairment; prolonged use may result in superinfection; use with caution in patients with a history of penicillin allergy especially IgE-mediated reactions (eg, anaphylaxis, urticaria); may cause antibiotic-associated colitis or colitis secondary to *C. difficile*

Adverse Reactions

1% to 10%:

Central nervous system: Dizziness (1%)

Dermatologic: Diaper rash (1.5%)

Gastrointestinal: Diarrhea (2.9%), nausea (3.5%), vomiting (1%), abdominal pain (1%)

Genitourinary: Vaginitis, genital pruritus (1.6%)

Hepatic: Increased transaminases (2%)

Miscellaneous: Superinfection

<1% (Limited to important or life-threatening): Anaphylaxis, angioedema, arthralgia, BUN increased, cholestatic jaundice, confusion, creatinine increased, eosinophilia, erythema multiforme, fever, headache, hyperactivity, insomnia, leukopenia, pseudomembranous colitis, rash, serum sickness, somnolence, Stevens-Johnson syndrome, thrombocytopenia, urticaria

Other reactions with cephalosporins include agranulocytosis, aplastic anemia, colitis, hemolytic anemia, hemorrhage, interstitial nephritis, pancytopenia, renal dysfunction, seizures, superinfection, toxic epidermal necrolysis, toxic nephropathy, vaginitis

Overdosage/Toxicology After acute overdose, most agents cause only nausea, vomiting, and diarrhea, although neuromuscular hypersensitivity and seizures are possible, especially in patients with renal insufficiency. Many beta-lactam antibiotics have the potential to cause neuromuscular hyperirritability or seizures. Hemodialysis may be helpful to aid in removal of the drug from the blood but not usually indicated; otherwise, most treatment is supportive or symptom directed, following GI decontamination.

Drug Interactions

Increased Effect/Toxicity: Probenecid may decrease cephalosporin elimination. Furosemide, aminoglycosides in combination with cefprozil may result in additive nephrotoxicity.

Ethanol/Nutrition/Herb Interactions Food: Food delays cefprozil absorption.

Mechanism of Action Inhibits bacterial cell wall synthesis by binding to one or more of the penicillin-binding proteins (PBPs) which in turn inhibits the final transpeptidation step of peptidoglycan synthesis in bacterial cell walls, thus inhibiting cell wall biosynthesis. Bacteria eventually lyse due to ongoing activity of cell wall autolytic enzymes (autolysins and murein hydrolases) while cell wall assembly is arrested.

Pharmacodynamics/Kinetics

Absorption: Well absorbed (94%)

Distribution: Low amounts enter breast milk

Protein binding: 35% to 45%

Half-life elimination: Normal renal function: 1.3 hours
Peak serum levels: Fasting: 1.5 hours
Excretion: Urine (61% as unchanged drug)

Usual Dosage Oral:
Infants and Children >6 months to 12 years: Otitis media: 15 mg/kg every 12 hours for 10 days
Pharyngitis/tonsillitis:
Children 2-12 years: 7.5 -15 mg/kg/day divided every 12 hours for 10 days (administer for >10 days if due to *S. pyogenes*); maximum: 1 g/day
Children >13 years and Adults: 500 mg every 24 hours for 10 days
Uncomplicated skin and skin structure infections:
Children 2-12 years: 20 mg/kg every 24 hours for 10 days; maximum: 1 g/day
Children >13 years and Adults: 250 mg every 12 hours, or 500 mg every 12-24 hours for 10 days
Secondary bacterial infection of acute bronchitis or acute bacterial exacerbation of chronic bronchitis: 500 mg every 12 hours for 10 days
Dosing adjustment in renal impairment: Cl$_{cr}$ <30 mL/minute: Reduce dose by 50%
Hemodialysis: Reduced by hemodialysis; administer dose after the completion of hemodialysis

Dietary Considerations May be taken with food.
Administration Administer around-the-clock to promote less variation in peak and trough serum levels. Chilling the reconstituted oral suspension improves flavor (do not freeze).
Monitoring Parameters Assess patient at beginning and throughout therapy for infection; monitor for signs of anaphylaxis during first dose
Test Interactions Positive direct Coombs', false-positive urinary glucose test using cupric sulfate (Benedict's solution, Clinitest®, Fehling's solution), false-positive serum or urine creatinine with Jaffé reaction
Patient Information Chilling improves flavor (do not freeze); report persistent diarrhea; entire course of medication (10-14 days) should be taken to ensure eradication of organism; may interfere with oral contraceptives; females should report symptoms of vaginitis
Nursing Implications
Administer around-the-clock to promote less variation in peak and trough serum levels
Assess patient at beginning and throughout therapy for infection
Dosage Forms
Powder for oral suspension, as anhydrous: 125 mg/5 mL (50 mL, 75 mL, 100 mL); 250 mg/5 mL (50 mL, 75 mL, 100 mL)
Tablet, as anhydrous: 250 mg, 500 mg

Ceftazidime (SEF tay zi deem)
Related Information
Antimicrobial Drugs of Choice *on page 1588*
U.S. Brand Names Ceptaz™; Fortaz®; Tazicef®; Tazidime®
Canadian Brand Names Ceptaz®; Fortaz®; Tazidime®
Therapeutic Category Antibiotic, Cephalosporin (Third Generation)
Use Treatment of documented susceptible *Pseudomonas aeruginosa* infection and infections due to other susceptible aerobic gram-negative organisms; empiric therapy of a febrile, granulocytopenic patient
Pregnancy Risk Factor B
Contraindications Hypersensitivity to ceftazidime, any component of the formulation, or other cephalosporins
Warnings/Precautions Modify dosage in patients with severe renal impairment; prolonged use may result in superinfection; use with caution in patients with a history of penicillin allergy especially IgE-mediated reactions (eg, anaphylaxis, urticaria); may cause antibiotic-associated colitis or colitis secondary to *C. difficile*
Adverse Reactions
1% to 10%:
Gastrointestinal: Diarrhea (1.3%)
Local: Pain at injection site (1.4%)
Miscellaneous: Hypersensitivity reactions (2%)
<1% (Limited to important or life-threatening): Anaphylaxis, angioedema, asterixis, BUN increased, candidiasis, creatinine increased, dizziness, encephalopathy, eosinophilia, erythema multiforme, fever, headache, hemolytic anemia, leukopenia, nausea, neuromuscular excitability, paresthesia, phlebitis, pruritus, pseudomembranous colitis, rash, Stevens-Johnson syndrome, thrombocytosis, toxic epidermal necrolysis, transaminases increased, vaginitis, vomiting
Other reactions with cephalosporins include agranulocytosis, aplastic anemia, BUN increased, cholestasis, colitis, creatinine increased, hemolytic anemia, hemorrhage, interstitial nephritis, pancytopenia, prolonged PT, renal dysfunction, seizures, serum-sickness reactions, superinfection, toxic nephropathy, urticaria
Overdosage/Toxicology Symptoms include neuromuscular hypersensitivity and convulsions, especially with renal insufficiency. Many beta-lactam antibiotics have the potential to cause neuromuscular hyperirritability or seizures. Hemodialysis may be helpful to aid in removal of the drug from the blood, otherwise, most treatment is supportive or symptom directed.
Drug Interactions
Increased Effect/Toxicity: Probenecid may decrease cephalosporin elimination. Aminoglycosides: *in vitro* studies indicate additive or synergistic effect against some strains of Enterobacteriaceae and *Pseudomonas aeruginosa*. Furosemide, aminoglycosides in combination with ceftazidime may result in additive nephrotoxicity.
Stability Reconstituted solution and I.V. infusion in NS or D$_5$W solution are stable for 24 hours at room temperature, 10 days when refrigerated, or 12 weeks when frozen; after freezing, thawed solution is stable for 24 hours at room temperature or 4 days when refrigerated; 96 hours under refrigeration, after mixing
(Continued)

Ceftazidime (Continued)

Mechanism of Action Inhibits bacterial cell wall synthesis by binding to one or more of the penicillin-binding proteins (PBPs) which in turn inhibits the final transpeptidation step of peptidoglycan synthesis in bacterial cell walls, thus inhibiting cell wall biosynthesis. Bacteria eventually lyse due to ongoing activity of cell wall autolytic enzymes (autolysins and murein hydrolases) while cell wall assembly is arrested.

Pharmacodynamics/Kinetics

Distribution: Widely throughout the body including bone, bile, skin, CSF (higher concentrations achieved when meninges are inflamed), endometrium, heart, pleural and lymphatic fluids

Protein binding: 17%

Half-life elimination: 1-2 hours, prolonged with renal impairment; Neonates <23 days: 2.2-4.7 hours

Time to peak, serum: I.M.: ~1 hour

Excretion: Urine (80% to 90% as unchanged drug)

Usual Dosage

Neonates 0-4 weeks: I.V.: 30 mg/kg every 12 hours

Infants and Children 1 month to 12 years: I.V.: 30-50 mg/kg/dose every 8 hours; maximum dose: 6 g/day

Adults: I.M., I.V.: 500 mg to 2 g every 8-12 hours

Urinary tract infections: 250-500 mg every 12 hours

Dosing interval in renal impairment:

Cl_{cr} 30-50 mL/minute: Administer every 12 hours

Cl_{cr} 10-30 mL/minute: Administer every 24 hours

Cl_{cr} <10 mL/minute: Administer every 48-72 hours

Hemodialysis: Dialyzable (50% to 100%)

Continuous arteriovenous or venovenous hemodiafiltration effects: Dose as for Cl_{cr} 30-50 mL/minute

Administration Any carbon dioxide bubbles that may be present in the withdrawn solution should be expelled prior to injection; administer around-the-clock to promote less variation in peak and trough serum levels; ceftazidime can be administered IVP over 3-5 minutes or I.V. intermittent infusion over 15-30 minutes; do not admix with aminoglycosides in same bottle/bag; final concentration for I.V. administration should not exceed 100 mg/mL

Monitoring Parameters Observe for signs and symptoms of anaphylaxis during first dose

Test Interactions Positive direct Coombs', false-positive urinary glucose test using cupric sulfate (Benedict's solution, Clinitest®, Fehling's solution), false-positive serum or urine creatinine with Jaffé reaction

Nursing Implications

Parenteral: Any carbon dioxide bubbles that may be present in the withdrawn solution should be expelled prior to injection; ceftazidime can be administered IVP over 3-5 minutes at a maximum concentration of 100 mg/mL or I.V. intermittent infusion over 15-30 minutes at a final concentration of ≤40 mg/mL

Monitor serum creatinine with concurrent use of an aminoglycoside; a change in renal function necessitates a change in dose

Additional Information Sodium content of 1 g: 2.3 mEq. With some organisms, resistance may develop during treatment (including *Enterobacter* spp and *Serratia* spp); consider combination therapy or periodic susceptibility testing for organisms with inducible resistance (see Warnings/Precautions).

Dosage Forms

Infusion [premixed, frozen] (Fortaz®): 1 g (50 mL); 2 g (50 mL)

Powder for injection: 500 mg, 1 g, 2 g, 6 g, 10 g

Ceftibuten (sef TYE byoo ten)

U.S. Brand Names Cedax®

Therapeutic Category Antibiotic, Cephalosporin (Third Generation)

Use Oral cephalosporin for treatment of bronchitis, otitis media, and pharyngitis/tonsillitis due to *H. influenzae* and *M. catarrhalis*, both beta-lactamase-producing and nonproducing strains, as well as *S. pneumoniae* (weak) and *S. pyogenes*

Pregnancy Risk Factor B

Contraindications Hypersensitivity to ceftibuten, any component of the formulation, or other cephalosporins

Warnings/Precautions Modify dosage in patients with severe renal impairment, prolonged use may result in superinfection; use with caution in patients with a history of penicillin allergy, especially IgE-mediated reactions (eg, anaphylaxis, urticaria); may cause antibiotic-associated colitis or colitis secondary to *C. difficile*

Adverse Reactions

1% to 10%:

Central nervous system: Headache (3%), dizziness (1%)

Gastrointestinal: Nausea (4%), diarrhea (3%), dyspepsia (2%), vomiting (1%), abdominal pain (1%)

Hematologic: Increased eosinophils (3%), decreased hemoglobin (2%), thrombocytosis

Hepatic: Increased ALT (1%), increased bilirubin (1%)

Renal: Increased BUN (4%)

<1% (Limited to important or life-threatening): Agitation, anorexia, candidiasis, constipation, creatinine increased, diaper rash, dry mouth, dyspnea, dysuria, fatigue, insomnia, irritability, leukopenia, nasal congestion, paresthesia, rash, rigors, transaminases increased, urticaria

Other reactions with cephalosporins include agranulocytosis, anaphylaxis, angioedema, aplastic anemia, asterixis, candidiasis, cholestasis, colitis, encephalopathy, erythema multiforme, fever, hemolytic anemia, hemorrhage, interstitial nephritis, neuromuscular excitability, pancytopenia, paresthesia, prolonged PT, pruritus, pseudomembranous colitis, renal dysfunction, seizures, serum-sickness reactions, Stevens-Johnson syndrome, superinfection, toxic epidermal necrolysis, toxic nephropathy, vaginitis

Overdosage/Toxicology After acute overdose, most agents cause only nausea, vomiting, and diarrhea, although neuromuscular hypersensitivity and seizures are possible, especially in patients with renal insufficiency. Many beta-lactam antibiotics have the potential to cause neuromuscular hyperirritability or seizures. Hemodialysis may be helpful to aid in removal of the drug from the blood but not usually indicated; otherwise, most treatment is supportive or symptom directed, following GI decontamination.

Drug Interactions

Increased Effect/Toxicity: High-dose probenecid decreases clearance. Aminoglycosides in combination with ceftibuten may increase nephrotoxic potential.

Stability Reconstituted suspension is stable for 14 days in the refrigerator

Mechanism of Action Inhibits bacterial cell wall synthesis by binding to one or more of the penicillin-binding proteins (PBPs) which in turn inhibits the final transpeptidation step of peptidoglycan synthesis in bacterial cell walls, thus inhibiting cell wall biosynthesis. Bacteria eventually lyse due to ongoing activity of cell wall autolytic enzymes (autolysins and murein hydrolases) while cell wall assembly is arrested.

Pharmacodynamics/Kinetics

Absorption: Rapid; food decreases peak concentrations, delays T_{max}, and lowers AUC

Distribution: V_d: Children: 0.5 L/kg; Adults: 0.21 L/kg

Half-life elimination: 2 hours

Time to peak: 2-3 hours

Excretion: Urine

Usual Dosage Oral:

Children <12 years: 9 mg/kg/day for 10 days; maximum daily dose: 400 mg

Children ≥12 years and Adults: 400 mg once daily for 10 days; maximum: 400 mg

Dosage adjustment in renal impairment:

Cl_{cr} 30-49 mL/minute: Administer 4.5 mg/kg or 200 mg every 24 hours

Cl_{cr} <29 mL/minute: Administer 2.25 mg/kg or 100 mg every 24 hours

Dietary Considerations

Capsule: Take without regard to food.

Suspension: Take 2 hours before or 1 hour after meals.

Monitoring Parameters Observe for signs and symptoms of anaphylaxis during first dose; with prolonged therapy, monitor renal, hepatic, and hematologic function periodically

Test Interactions Positive direct Coombs', false-positive urinary glucose test using cupric sulfate (Benedict's solution, Clinitest®, Fehling's solution), false-positive serum or urine creatinine with Jaffé reaction

Patient Information Must be administered at least 2 hours before meals or 1 hour after a meal; shake suspension well before use; suspension may be kept for 14 days if stored in refrigerator; discard any unused portion after 14 days; report prolonged diarrhea; entire course of medication should be taken to ensure eradication of organism; take at the same time each day to maintain adequate blood levels; may interfere with oral contraceptive; females should report symptoms of vaginitis

Nursing Implications After mixing suspension, may be kept for 14 days if stored in refrigerator; discard any unused portion after 14 days; must be administered at least 2 hours before meals or 1 hour after a meal; shake suspension well before use

Additional Information Oral suspension contains 1 g of sucrose per 5 mL

Dosage Forms

Capsule: 400 mg

Powder for oral suspension: 90 mg/5 mL (30 mL, 60 mL, 120 mL); 180 mg/5 mL (30 mL, 60 mL, 120 mL) [cherry flavor]

◆ **Ceftin**® see Cefuroxime on page 258

Ceftizoxime (sef ti ZOKS eem)

Related Information

Antimicrobial Drugs of Choice on page 1588

Treatment of Sexually Transmitted Diseases on page 1609

U.S. Brand Names Cefizox®

Canadian Brand Names Cefizox®

Synonyms Ceftizoxime Sodium

Therapeutic Category Antibiotic, Cephalosporin (Third Generation)

Use Treatment of susceptible bacterial infection, mainly respiratory tract, skin and skin structure, bone and joint, urinary tract and gynecologic, as well as septicemia; active against many gram-negative bacilli (not *Pseudomonas*), some gram-positive cocci (not *Enterococcus*), and some anaerobes

Pregnancy Risk Factor B

Contraindications Hypersensitivity to ceftizoxime, any component of the formulation, or other cephalosporins

Warnings/Precautions Modify dosage in patients with severe renal impairment, prolonged use may result in superinfection; use with caution in patients with a history of penicillin allergy, especially IgE-mediated reactions (eg, anaphylaxis, urticaria); may cause antibiotic-associated colitis or colitis secondary to *C. difficile*

Adverse Reactions

1% to 10%:

Central nervous system: Fever

Dermatologic: Rash, pruritus

Hematologic: Eosinophilia, thrombocytosis

Hepatic: Elevated transaminases, alkaline phosphatase

Local: Pain, burning at injection site

<1% (Limited to important or life-threatening): Anaphylaxis, anemia, bilirubin increased, BUN increased, creatinine increased, diarrhea, injection site reactions, leukopenia, nausea, neutropenia, numbness, paresthesia, phlebitis, thrombocytopenia, vaginitis, vomiting

Other reactions reported with cephalosporins include agranulocytosis, angioedema, aplastic anemia, asterixis, candidiasis, cholestasis, colitis, encephalopathy, erythema multiforme, (Continued)

Ceftizoxime *(Continued)*

hemolytic anemia, hemorrhage, interstitial nephritis, neuromuscular excitability, pancytopenia, prolonged PT, pseudomembranous colitis, renal dysfunction, seizures, serum-sickness reactions, Stevens-Johnson syndrome, superinfection, toxic epidermal necrolysis,
toxic nephropathy

Overdosage/Toxicology Symptoms include neuromuscular hypersensitivity and convulsions
especially with renal insufficiency. Many beta-lactam antibiotics have the potential to cause
neuromuscular hyperirritability or seizures. Hemodialysis may be helpful to aid in removal of
the drug from the blood; otherwise, most treatment is supportive or symptom directed.

Drug Interactions

Increased Effect/Toxicity: Probenecid may decrease cephalosporin elimination. Furosemide, aminoglycosides in combination with ceftizoxime may result in additive nephrotoxicity.

Stability Reconstituted solution is stable for 24 hours at room temperature and 96 hours when
refrigerated; for I.V. infusion in NS or D_5W solution is stable for 24 hours at room temperature,
96 hours when refrigerated or 12 weeks when frozen; after freezing, thawed solution is stable
for 24 hours at room temperature or 10 days when refrigerated

Mechanism of Action Inhibits bacterial cell wall synthesis by binding to one or more of the
penicillin-binding proteins (PBPs) which in turn inhibits the final transpeptidation step of
peptidoglycan synthesis in bacterial cell walls, thus inhibiting cell wall biosynthesis. Bacteria
eventually lyse due to ongoing activity of cell wall autolytic enzymes (autolysins and murein
hydrolases) while cell wall assembly is arrested.

Pharmacodynamics/Kinetics

Distribution: V_d: 0.35-0.5 L/kg; widely into most body tissues and fluids including gallbladder,
liver, kidneys, bone, sputum, bile, pleural and synovial fluids; has good CSF penetration;
crosses placenta; small amounts enter breast milk

Protein binding: 30%

Half-life elimination: 1.6 hours; Cl_{cr} <10 mL/minute: 25 hours

Time to peak, serum: I.M.: 0.5-1 hour

Excretion: Urine (as unchanged drug)

Usual Dosage I.M., I.V.:

Children ≥6 months: 150-200 mg/kg/day divided every 6-8 hours (maximum of 12 g/24 hours)

Adults: 1-2 g every 8-12 hours, up to 2 g every 4 hours or 4 g every 8 hours for life-
threatening infections

Dosing adjustment in renal impairment: Adults:

Cl_{cr} 10-30 mL/minute: Administer 1 g every 12 hours

Cl_{cr} <10 mL/minute: Administer 1 g every 24 hours

Moderately dialyzable (20% to 50%)

Continuous arteriovenous or venovenous hemodiafiltration effects: Dose as for Cl_{cr} 10-50 mL/
minute

Monitoring Parameters Observe for signs and symptoms of anaphylaxis during first dose

Test Interactions Positive direct Coombs', false-positive urinary glucose test using cupric
sulfate (Benedict's solution, Clinitest®, Fehling's solution), false-positive serum or urine creatinine with Jaffé reaction

Nursing Implications Do not admix with aminoglycosides in same bottle/bag

Additional Information Sodium content of 1 g: 60 mg (2.6 mEq)

Dosage Forms

Injection, as sodium [in D_5W, frozen]: 1 g (50 mL); 2 g (50 mL)

Powder for injection, as sodium: 500 mg, 1 g, 2 g, 10 g

♦ **Ceftizoxime Sodium** *see Ceftizoxime on page 255*

Ceftriaxone *(sef trye AKS one)*

Related Information

Animal and Human Bites Guidelines *on page 1584*

Antibiotic Treatment of Adults With Infective Endocarditis *on page 1585*

Antimicrobial Drugs of Choice *on page 1588*

Community-Acquired Pneumonia in Adults *on page 1603*

Treatment of Sexually Transmitted Diseases *on page 1609*

U.S. Brand Names Rocephin®

Canadian Brand Names Rocephin®

Synonyms Ceftriaxone Sodium

Therapeutic Category Antibiotic, Cephalosporin (Third Generation)

Use Treatment of lower respiratory tract infections, skin and skin structure infections, bone and
joint infections, intra-abdominal and urinary tract infections, sepsis and meningitis due to
susceptible organisms; documented or suspected infection due to susceptible organisms in
home care patients and patients without I.V. line access; treatment of documented or
suspected gonococcal infection or chancroid; emergency room management of patients at
high risk for bacteremia, periorbital or buccal cellulitis, salmonellosis or shigellosis, and
pneumonia of unestablished etiology (<5 years of age); treatment of Lyme disease, depends
on the stage of the disease (used in Stage II and Stage III, but not stage I; doxycycline is the
drug of choice for Stage I)

Pregnancy Risk Factor B

Contraindications Hypersensitivity to ceftriaxone sodium, any component of the formulation,
or other cephalosporins; **do not use in hyperbilirubinemic neonates**, particularly those
who are premature since ceftriaxone is reported to displace bilirubin from albumin binding
sites

Warnings/Precautions Modify dosage in patients with severe renal impairment, prolonged
use may result in superinfection; use with caution in patients with a history of penicillin
allergy, especially IgE-mediated reactions (eg, anaphylaxis, urticaria); may cause antibiotic-
associated colitis or colitis secondary to *C. difficile*

Adverse Reactions

1% to 10%:
Dermatologic: Rash (2%)
Gastrointestinal: Diarrhea (3%)
Hematologic: Eosinophilia (6%), thrombocytosis (5%), leukopenia (2%)
Hepatic: Elevated transaminases (3.1% to 3.3%)
Local: Pain, induration at injection site (I.V. 1%); warmth, tightness, induration (5% to 17%) following I.M. injection
Renal: Increased BUN (1%)

<1% (Limited to important or life-threatening): Agranulocytosis, anaphylaxis, anemia, basophilia, bronchospasm, candidiasis, chills, diaphoresis, dizziness, dysgeusia, flushing, gallstones, glycosuria, headache, hematuria, hemolytic anemia, jaundice, leukocytosis, lymphocytosis, lymphopenia, monocytosis, nausea, nephrolithiasis, neutropenia, phlebitis, prolonged or decreased PT, pruritus, renal precipitations, renal stones, serum sickness, thrombocytopenia, urinary casts, vaginitis, vomiting; increased alkaline phosphatase, bilirubin, and creatinine

Reactions reported with other cephalosporins include angioedema, aplastic anemia, asterixis, cholestasis, colitis, encephalopathy, erythema multiforme, hemorrhage, interstitial nephritis, neuromuscular excitability, pancytopenia, paresthesia, pseudomembranous colitis, renal dysfunction, seizures, superinfection, Stevens-Johnson syndrome, toxic epidermal necrolysis, toxic nephropathy

Overdosage/Toxicology Symptoms include neuromuscular hypersensitivity and convulsions especially with renal insufficiency. Many beta-lactam antibiotics have the potential to cause neuromuscular hyperirritability or seizures. Hemodialysis may be helpful to aid in removal of the drug from the blood; otherwise, most treatment is supportive or symptom directed.

Drug Interactions

Increased Effect/Toxicity: Aminoglycosides may result in synergistic antibacterial activity. High-dose probenecid decreases clearance. Aminoglycosides increase nephrotoxic potential.

Stability Reconstituted solution (100 mg/mL) is stable for 3 days at room temperature and 3 days when refrigerated; for I.V. infusion in NS or D_5W solution is stable for 3 days at room temperature, 10 days when refrigerated, or 26 weeks when frozen; after freezing, thawed solution is stable for 3 days at room temperature or 10 days when refrigerated

Mechanism of Action Inhibits bacterial cell wall synthesis by binding to one or more of the penicillin-binding proteins (PBPs) which in turn inhibits the final transpeptidation step of peptidoglycan synthesis in bacterial cell walls, thus inhibiting cell wall biosynthesis. Bacteria eventually lyse due to ongoing activity of cell wall autolytic enzymes (autolysins and murein hydrolases) while cell wall assembly is arrested.

Pharmacodynamics/Kinetics

Absorption: I.M.: Well absorbed
Distribution: Widely throughout the body including gallbladder, lungs, bone, bile, CSF (higher concentrations achieved when meninges are inflamed); crosses placenta; enters amniotic fluid and breast milk
Protein binding: 85% to 95%
Half-life elimination: Normal renal and hepatic function: 5-9 hours
Neonates: Postnatal (1-4 days old): 16 hours; 9-30 days old: 9 hours
Time to peak, serum: I.M.: 1-2 hours
Excretion: Urine (33% to 65% as unchanged drug); feces

Usual Dosage I.M., I.V.:

Neonates:
Postnatal age ≤7 days: 50 mg/kg/day given every 24 hours
Postnatal age >7 days:
≤2000 g: 50 mg/kg/day given every 24 hours
>2000 g: 50-75 mg/kg/day given every 24 hours
Gonococcal prophylaxis: 25-50 mg/kg as a single dose (dose not to exceed 125 mg)
Gonococcal infection: 25-50 mg/kg/day (maximum dose: 125 mg) given every 24 hours for 10-14 days
Infants and Children: 50-75 mg/kg/day in 1-2 divided doses every 12-24 hours; maximum: 2 g/24 hours
Meningitis: 100 mg/kg/day divided every 12-24 hours, up to a maximum of 4 g/24 hours; loading dose of 75 mg/kg/dose may be given at start of therapy
Otitis media: I.M.: 50 mg/kg as a single dose (maximum: 1 g)
Uncomplicated gonococcal infections, sexual assault, and STD prophylaxis: I.M.: 125 mg as a single dose plus doxycycline
Complicated gonococcal infections:
Infants: I.M., I.V.: 25-50 mg/kg/day in a single dose (maximum: 125 mg/dose); treat for 7 days for disseminated infection and 7-14 days for documented meningitis
<45 kg: 50 mg/kg/day once daily; maximum: 1 g/day; for ophthalmia, peritonitis, arthritis, or bacteremia: 50-100 mg/kg/day divided every 12-24 hours; maximum: 2 g/day for meningitis or endocarditis
>45 kg: 1 g/day once daily for disseminated gonococcal infections; 1-2 g dose every 12 hours for meningitis or endocarditis
Acute epididymitis: I.M.: 250 mg in a single dose
Adults: 1-2 g every 12-24 hours (depending on the type and severity of infection); maximum dose: 2 g every 12 hours for treatment of meningitis
Uncomplicated gonorrhea: I.M.: 250 mg as a single dose
Surgical prophylaxis: 1 g 30 minutes to 2 hours before surgery

Dosing adjustment in renal or hepatic impairment: No change necessary
Hemodialysis: Not dialyzable (0% to 5%); administer dose postdialysis
Peritoneal dialysis: Administer 750 mg every 12 hours
Continuous arteriovenous or venovenous hemofiltration: Removes 10 mg of ceftriaxone per liter of filtrate per day

Monitoring Parameters Observe for signs and symptoms of anaphylaxis
(Continued)

Ceftriaxone *(Continued)*

Test Interactions Positive direct Coombs', false-positive urinary glucose test using cupric sulfate (Benedict's solution, Clinitest®, Fehling's solution), false-positive serum or urine creatinine with Jaffé reaction

Nursing Implications For I.M. injection, the maximum concentration is 250 mg/mL; ceftriaxone can be diluted with 1:1 water and 1% lidocaine for I.M. administration. Do not admix with aminoglycosides in same bottle/bag.

Additional Information Sodium content of 1 g: 60 mg (2.6 mEq)

Dosage Forms
Infusion, as sodium [premixed, frozen]: 1 g [in $D_{3.8}W$] (50 mL); 2 g [in $D_{2.4}W$] (50 mL)
Powder for injection, as sodium: 250 mg, 500 mg, 1 g, 2 g, 10 g

♦ **Ceftriaxone Sodium** *see* Ceftriaxone *on page 256*

Cefuroxime *(se fyoor OKS eem)*

Related Information
Antimicrobial Drugs of Choice *on page 1588*
Community-Acquired Pneumonia in Adults *on page 1603*
Prevention of Wound Infection & Sepsis in Surgical Patients *on page 1569*

U.S. Brand Names Ceftin®; Kefurox®; Zinacef®

Canadian Brand Names Ceftin®; Kefurox®; Zinacef®

Synonyms Cefuroxime Axetil; Cefuroxime Sodium

Therapeutic Category Antibiotic, Cephalosporin (Second Generation)

Use Treatment of infections caused by staphylococci, group B streptococci, *H. influenzae* (type A and B), *E. coli*, *Enterobacter*, *Salmonella*, and *Klebsiella*; treatment of susceptible infections of the lower respiratory tract, otitis media, urinary tract, skin and soft tissue, bone and joint, sepsis and gonorrhea

Pregnancy Risk Factor B

Contraindications Hypersensitivity to cefuroxime, any component of the formulation, or other cephalosporins

Warnings/Precautions Modify dosage in patients with severe renal impairment, prolonged use may result in superinfection; use with caution in patients with a history of penicillin allergy, especially IgE-mediated reactions (eg, anaphylaxis, urticaria); may cause antibiotic-associated colitis or colitis secondary to *C. difficile*; tablets and oral suspension are not bioequivalent (do not substitute on a mg-per-mg basis)

Adverse Reactions
1% to 10%:
Hematologic: Eosinophilia (7%), decreased hemoglobin and hematocrit (10%)
Hepatic: Increased transaminases (4%), increased alkaline phosphatase (2%)
Local: Thrombophlebitis (1.7%)
<1% (Limited to important or life-threatening): Anaphylaxis, angioedema, BUN increased, cholestasis, colitis, creatinine increased, diarrhea, dizziness, erythema multiforme, fever, GI bleeding, hemolytic anemia, headache, hepatitis, interstitial nephritis, jaundice, leukopenia, nausea, neutropenia, pain at injection site, pancytopenia, prolonged PT/INR, pseudomembranous colitis, rash, seizures, Stevens-Johnson syndrome, stomach cramps, thrombocytopenia, toxic epidermal necrolysis, vaginitis, vomiting
Other reactions with cephalosporins include agranulocytosis, aplastic anemia, asterixis, colitis, encephalopathy, hemorrhage, neuromuscular excitability, serum-sickness reactions, superinfection, toxic nephropathy

Overdosage/Toxicology After acute overdose, most agents cause only nausea, vomiting, and diarrhea, although neuromuscular hypersensitivity and seizures are possible, especially in patients with renal insufficiency. Many beta-lactam antibiotics have the potential to cause neuromuscular hyperirritability or seizures. Hemodialysis may be helpful to aid in removal of the drug from the blood but not usually indicated; otherwise, most treatment is supportive and symptom directed, following GI decontamination.

Drug Interactions
Increased Effect/Toxicity: High-dose probenecid decreases clearance. Aminoglycosides in combination with cefuroxime may result in additive nephrotoxicity.

Ethanol/Nutrition/Herb Interactions Food: Bioavailability is increased with food; cefuroxime serum levels may be increased if taken with food or dairy products.

Stability Reconstituted solution is stable for 24 hours at room temperature and 48 hours when refrigerated; I.V. infusion in NS or D_5W solution is stable for 24 hours at room temperature, 7 days when refrigerated, or 26 weeks when frozen; after freezing, thawed solution is stable for 24 hours at room temperature or 21 days when refrigerated

Mechanism of Action Inhibits bacterial cell wall synthesis by binding to one or more of the penicillin-binding proteins (PBPs) which in turn inhibits the final transpeptidation step of peptidoglycan synthesis in bacterial cell walls, thus inhibiting cell wall biosynthesis. Bacteria eventually lyse due to ongoing activity of cell wall autolytic enzymes (autolysins and murein hydrolases) while cell wall assembly is arrested.

Pharmacodynamics/Kinetics
Absorption: Oral (cefuroxime axetil): Increases with food
Distribution: Widely to body tissues and fluids; crosses blood-brain barrier; therapeutic concentrations achieved in CSF even when meninges are not inflamed; crosses placenta; enters breast milk
Protein binding: 33% to 50%
Bioavailability, axetil: Oral: Tablet: 37% (empty stomach) to 52% (after meal)
Half-life elimination:
Neonates: ≤3 days old : 5.1-5.8 hours; 6-14 days old: 2-4.2 hours; 3-4 weeks old: 1-1.5 hours
Adults: 1-2 hours; prolonged in renal impairment
Time to peak, serum: I.M.: ~15-60 minutes; I.V.: 2-3 minutes
Excretion: Urine (66% to 100% as unchanged drug)

Usual Dosage Note: Cefuroxime axetil film-coated tablets and oral suspension are not bioequivalent and are not substitutable on a mg/mg basis

Children ≥3 months to 12 years:
Pharyngitis, tonsillitis: Oral:
Suspension: 20 mg/kg/day (maximum: 500 mg/day) in 2 divided doses for 10 days
Tablet: 125 mg every 12 hours for 10 days
Acute otitis media, impetigo: Oral:
Suspension: 30 mg/kg/day (maximum: 1 g/day) in 2 divided doses for 10 days
Tablet: 250 mg twice daily for 10 days
I.M., I.V.: 75-150 mg/kg/day divided every 8 hours; maximum dose: 6 g/day
Meningitis: Not recommended (doses of 200-240 mg/kg/day divided every 6-8 hours have been used); maximum dose: 9 g/day
Acute bacterial maxillary sinusitis:
Suspension: 30 mg/kg/day in 2 divided doses for 10 days; maximum dose: 1 g/day
Tablet: 250 mg twice daily for 10 days

Children ≥13 years and Adults:
Oral: 250-500 mg twice daily for 10 days (5 days in selected patients with acute bronchitis)
Uncomplicated urinary tract infection: 125-250 mg every 12 hours for 7-10 days
Uncomplicated gonorrhea: 1 g as a single dose
Early Lyme disease: 500 mg twice daily for 20 days
I.M., I.V.: 750 mg to 1.5 g/dose every 8 hours or 100-150 mg/kg/day in divided doses every 6-8 hours; maximum: 6 g/24 hours

Dosing adjustment in renal impairment:
Cl_{cr} 10-20 mL/minute: Administer every 12 hours
Cl_{cr} <10 mL/minute: Administer every 24 hours
Hemodialysis: Dialyzable (25%)
Continuous arteriovenous or venovenous hemodiafiltration effects: Dose as for Cl_{cr} 10-20 mL/minute

Dietary Considerations May be taken with food.

Administration
Oral: Administer around-the-clock to promote less variation in peak and trough serum levels.
Oral suspension: Administer with food. Shake well before use.
I.M.: Inject deep I.M. into large muscle mass.
I.V.: Inject direct I.V. over 3-5 minutes. Infuse intermittent infusion over 15-30 minutes.

Monitoring Parameters Observe for signs and symptoms of anaphylaxis during first dose; with prolonged therapy, monitor renal, hepatic, and hematologic function periodically; monitor prothrombin time in patients at risk of prolongation during cephalosporin therapy (nutritionally-deficient, prolonged treatment, renal or hepatic disease)

Test Interactions Positive direct Coombs', false-positive urinary glucose test using cupric sulfate (Benedict's solution, Clinitest®, Fehling's solution), false-positive serum or urine creatinine with Jaffé reaction

Patient Information Report prolonged diarrhea; entire course of medication (10-14 days) should be taken to ensure eradication of organism; may interfere with oral contraceptives; females should report symptoms of vaginitis

Nursing Implications Do not admix with aminoglycosides in same bottle/bag; obtain specimens for culture and sensitivity prior to the first dose

Additional Information Sodium content of 1 g: 54.2 mg (2.4 mEq)

Dosage Forms
Infusion, as sodium [premixed, frozen] (Zinacef®): 750 mg (50 mL); 1.5 g (50 mL)
Powder for injection, as sodium: 750 mg, 1.5 g, 7.5 g
Kefurox®, Zinacef®: 750 mg, 1.5 g, 7.5 g
Powder for oral suspension, as axetil (Ceftin®): 125 mg/5 mL (50 mL, 100 mL, 200 mL); 250 mg/5 mL (50 mL, 100 mL) [tutti-frutti flavor]
Tablet, as axetil (Ceftin®): 125 mg, 250 mg, 500 mg

♦ **Cefuroxime Axetil** *see Cefuroxime on page 258*

♦ **Cefuroxime Sodium** *see Cefuroxime on page 258*

♦ **Cefzil®** *see Cefprozil on page 252*

♦ **Celebrex®** *see Celecoxib on page 259*

Celecoxib (se le KOKS ib)

Related Information
Nonsteroidal Anti-Inflammatory Agents Comparison *on page 1512*

U.S. Brand Names Celebrex®

Canadian Brand Names Celebrex™

Therapeutic Category Analgesic, COX-2 Inhibitor; Nonsteroidal Anti-inflammatory Drug (NSAID), COX-2 Selective

Use Relief of the signs and symptoms of osteoarthritis; relief of the signs and symptoms of rheumatoid arthritis in adults; decreasing intestinal polyps in familial adenomatous polyposis (FAP); management of acute pain; treatment of primary dysmenorrhea

Pregnancy Risk Factor C/D (3rd trimester)

Pregnancy/Breast-Feeding Implications In late pregnancy may cause premature closure of the ductus arteriosus. In animal studies, celecoxib has been found to be excreted in milk; it is not known whether celecoxib is excreted in human milk. Because many drugs are excreted in milk, and the potential for serious adverse reactions exists, a decision should be made whether to discontinue nursing or discontinue the drug, taking into account the importance of the drug to the mother.

Contraindications Hypersensitivity to celecoxib, any component of the formulation, sulfonamides, aspirin, or other nonsteroidal anti-inflammatory drugs (NSAIDs); pregnancy (3rd trimester)

Warnings/Precautions Gastrointestinal irritation, ulceration, bleeding, and perforation may occur with NSAIDs (it is unclear whether celecoxib is associated with rates of these events which are similar to nonselective NSAIDs). Use with caution in patients with a history of GI disease (bleeding or ulcers), decreased renal function, hepatic disease, congestive heart (Continued)

Celecoxib (Continued)

failure, hypertension, or asthma. Anaphylactoid reactions may occur, even with no prior exposure to celecoxib. Use caution in patients with known or suspected deficiency of CYP2C9 isoenzyme. Safety and efficacy have not been established in patients <18 years of age.

Adverse Reactions
>10%: Central nervous system: Headache (15.8%)

2% to 10%:
   Cardiovascular: Peripheral edema (2.1%)
   Central nervous system: Insomnia (2.3%), dizziness (2%)
   Dermatologic : Skin rash (2.2%)
   Gastrointestinal: Dyspepsia (8.8%), diarrhea (5.6%), abdominal pain (4.1%), nausea (3.5%), flatulence (2.2%)
   Neuromuscular & skeletal: Back pain (2.8%)
   Respiratory: Upper respiratory tract infection (8.1%), sinusitis (5%), pharyngitis (2.3%), rhinitis (2%)
   Miscellaneous: Accidental injury (2.9%)

<2% (Limited to important or life-threatening): Acute renal failure, albuminuria, allergic reactions, alopecia, arthralgia, ataxia, bronchospasm, cerebrovascular accident, colitis, congestive heart failure, cystitis, diabetes mellitus, dyspnea, dysuria, ecchymosis, esophageal perforation, esophagitis, flu-like syndrome, gangrene, gastroenteritis, gastroesophageal reflux, gastrointestinal bleeding, glaucoma, conjunctivitis, deafness, hematuria, hypertension, hypokalemia, intestinal perforation, melena, migraine, myalgia, myocardial infarction, neuralgia, neuropathy, pancreatitis, paresthesia, photosensitivity, prostate disorder, pulmonary embolism, rash, renal calculi, sepsis, stomatitis, sudden death, syncope, thrombocytopenia, thrombophlebitis, tinnitus, urticaria, vaginal bleeding, vaginitis, ventricular fibrillation, vertigo, vomiting

Overdosage/Toxicology
Symptoms may include epigastric pain, drowsiness, lethargy, nausea, and vomiting. Gastrointestinal bleeding may occur. Rare manifestations include hypertension, respiratory depression, coma, and acute renal failure. Treatment is symptomatic and supportive. Forced diuresis, hemodialysis and/or urinary alkalinization may not be useful.

Drug Interactions
Cytochrome P450 Effect: CYP2C9 enzyme substrate, CYP2D6 enzyme inhibitor

Increased Effect/Toxicity: Fluconazole increases celecoxib concentrations twofold. Other inhibitors of cytochrome P450 isoenzyme 2C9 (ie, amiodarone, fluoxetine, sulfonamides, ritonavir, zafirlukast) theoretically may result in significant increases in celecoxib concentrations. Lithium concentrations may be increased by celecoxib. Celecoxib may be used with low-dose aspirin, however rates of gastrointestinal bleeding may be increased with coadministration. Celecoxib has been associated with increased prothrombin times and some bleeding episodes (predominantly in elderly patients) during warfarin therapy.

Decreased Effect: Efficacy of thiazide diuretics, loop diuretics (furosemide), or ACE-inhibitors may be diminished by celecoxib.

Ethanol/Nutrition/Herb Interactions
Ethanol: Avoid ethanol (increased GI irritation).
Food: Peak concentrations are delayed and AUC is increased by 10% to 20% when taken with a high-fat meal.

Stability Store at controlled room temperature of 25°C (77°F).

Mechanism of Action Inhibits prostaglandin synthesis by decreasing the activity of the enzyme, cyclooxygenase-2 (COX-2), which results in decreased formation of prostaglandin precursors. Celecoxib does not inhibit cyclooxygenase-1 (COX-1) at therapeutic concentrations.

Pharmacodynamics/Kinetics
Distribution: V_d (apparent): 400 L
Protein binding: 97% to albumin
Metabolism: Hepatic via CYP2C9; forms inactive metabolites
Bioavailability, absolute: Has not been determined
Half-life elimination: 11 hours
Time to peak: 3 hours
Excretion: Urine (as metabolites, <3% as unchanged drug)

Usual Dosage
Adults: Oral:
   Acute pain or primary dysmenorrhea: Initial dose: 400 mg, followed by an additional 200 mg if needed on day 1; maintenance dose: 200 mg twice daily as needed
   Familial adenomatous polyposis (FAP): 400 mg twice daily
   Osteoarthritis: 200 mg/day as a single dose or in divided dose twice daily
   Rheumatoid arthritis: 100-200 mg twice daily
   Elderly: No specific adjustment is recommended. However, the AUC in elderly patients may be increased by 50% as compared to younger subjects. Use the lowest recommended dose in patients weighing <50 kg.
   Dosing adjustment in renal impairment: No specific dosage adjustment is recommended; not recommended in patients with advanced renal disease
   Dosing adjustment in hepatic impairment: Reduced dosage is recommended (AUC may be increased by 40% to 180%); decrease dose by 50% in patients with moderate hepatic impairment (Child-Pugh class II)

Dietary Considerations Lower doses (200 mg twice daily) may be taken without regard to meals. Larger doses should be taken with food to improve absorption.

Monitoring Parameters Periodic LFTs; in patients treated for FAP, continue routine endoscopic exams

Patient Information Patients should be informed of the signs and symptoms of gastrointestinal bleeding. Gastrointestinal bleeding may occur as well as ulceration and perforation; pain may or may not be present. If gastric upset occurs, take with food, milk, or antacid; if gastric upset persists, contact physician.

Dosage Forms Capsule: 100 mg, 200 mg

- **Celestoderm®-EV/2 (Can)** see Betamethasone on page 161
- **Celestoderm®-V (Can)** see Betamethasone on page 161
- **Celestone®** see Betamethasone on page 161
- **Celestone® Phosphate** see Betamethasone on page 161
- **Celestone® Soluspan®** see Betamethasone on page 161
- **Celexa™** see Citalopram on page 304
- **CellCept®** see Mycophenolate on page 943
- **Celontin®** see Methsuximide on page 890
- **Cenafed® [OTC]** see Pseudoephedrine on page 1155
- **Cenafed® Plus Tablet [OTC]** see Triprolidine and Pseudoephedrine on page 1380
- **Cena-K®** see Potassium Chloride on page 1108
- **Cenestin™** see Estrogens (Conjugated A/Synthetic) on page 497
- **Cenestin (Can)** see Estrogens (Conjugated/Equine) on page 498
- **Cenolate®** see Sodium Ascorbate on page 1243
- **Cēpacol® Anesthetic Troches [OTC]** see Cetylpyridinium and Benzocaine on page 267

Cephalexin (sef a LEKS in)

Related Information
Animal and Human Bites Guidelines on page 1584
Prevention of Bacterial Endocarditis on page 1563

U.S. Brand Names Biocef; Keflex®; Keftab®

Canadian Brand Names Apo®-Cephalex; Keftab®; Novo-Lexin®; Nu-Cephalex®; PMS-Cephalexin

Synonyms Cephalexin Hydrochloride; Cephalexin Monohydrate

Therapeutic Category Antibiotic, Cephalosporin (First Generation)

Use Treatment of susceptible bacterial infections, including those caused by group A beta-hemolytic *Streptococcus, Staphylococcus, Klebsiella pneumoniae, E. coli, Proteus mirabilis,* and *Shigella;* predominantly used for lower respiratory tract, urinary tract, skin and soft tissue, and bone and joint; prophylaxis against bacterial endocarditis in high-risk patients undergoing surgical or dental procedures who are allergic to penicillin

Pregnancy Risk Factor B

Contraindications Hypersensitivity to cephalexin, any component of the formulation, or other cephalosporins

Warnings/Precautions Modify dosage in patients with severe renal impairment, prolonged use may result in superinfection; use with caution in patients with a history of penicillin allergy, especially IgE-mediated reactions (eg, anaphylaxis, urticaria); may cause antibiotic-associated colitis or colitis secondary to *C. difficile*

Adverse Reactions
1% to 10%: Gastrointestinal: Diarrhea

<1% (Limited to important or life-threatening): Abdominal pain, agitation, anaphylaxis, anemia, angioedema, arthralgia, cholestasis, confusion, dizziness, dyspepsia, eosinophilia, erythema multiforme, fatigue, gastritis, hallucinations, headache, hepatitis, interstitial nephritis, nausea, neutropenia, pseudomembranous colitis, rash, serum-sickness reaction, Stevens-Johnson syndrome, thrombocytopenia, toxic epidermal necrolysis, transaminases increased, urticaria, vomiting

Other reactions with cephalosporins include agranulocytosis, anaphylaxis, aplastic anemia, asterixis, colitis, encephalopathy, hemolytic anemia, hemorrhage, neuromuscular excitability, pancytopenia, prolonged PT, seizures, superinfection, vomiting

Overdosage/Toxicology After acute overdose, most agents cause only nausea, vomiting, and diarrhea, although neuromuscular hypersensitivity and seizures are possible, especially in patients with renal insufficiency. Many beta-lactam antibiotics have the potential to cause neuromuscular hyperirritability or seizures. Hemodialysis may be helpful to aid in removal of the drug from the blood but not usually indicated; otherwise, most treatment is supportive or symptom directed, following GI decontamination.

Drug Interactions
Increased Effect/Toxicity: High-dose probenecid may decrease clearance of cephalexin. Aminoglycosides in combination with cephalexin may result in additive nephrotoxicity.

Ethanol/Nutrition/Herb Interactions Food: Peak antibiotic serum concentration is lowered and delayed, but total drug absorbed is not affected. Cephalexin serum levels may be decreased if taken with food.

Stability Refrigerate suspension after reconstitution; discard after 14 days

Mechanism of Action Inhibits bacterial cell wall synthesis by binding to one or more of the penicillin-binding proteins (PBPs) which in turn inhibits the final transpeptidation step of peptidoglycan synthesis in bacterial cell walls, thus inhibiting cell wall biosynthesis. Bacteria eventually lyse due to ongoing activity of cell wall autolytic enzymes (autolysins and murein hydrolases) while cell wall assembly is arrested.

Pharmacodynamics/Kinetics
Absorption: Delayed in young children; may be decreased up to 50% in neonates

Distribution: Widely into most body tissues and fluids, including gallbladder, liver, kidneys, bone, sputum, bile, and pleural and synovial fluids; CSF penetration is poor; crosses placenta; enters breast milk

Protein binding: 6% to 15%

Half-life elimination: Neonates: 5 hours old; Children 3-12 months: 2.5 hours; Adults: 0.5-1.2 hours; prolonged with renal impairment

Time to peak, serum: ~1 hour

Excretion: Urine (80% to 100% as unchanged drug) within 8 hours

Usual Dosage Oral:
Children: 25-50 mg/kg/day every 6 hours; severe infections: 50-100 mg/kg/day in divided doses every 6 hours; maximum: 3 g/24 hours

Adults: 250-1000 mg every 6 hours; maximum: 4 g/day

(Continued)

Cephalexin *(Continued)*

Prophylaxis of bacterial endocarditis (dental, oral, respiratory tract, or esophageal procedures):
Children: 50 mg/kg 1 hour prior to procedure
Adults: 2 g 1 hour prior to procedure

Dosing adjustment in renal impairment: Adults:
Cl_{cr} 10-40 mL/minute: 250-500 mg every 8-12 hours
Cl_{cr} <10 mL/minute: 250 mg every 12-24 hours
Hemodialysis: Moderately dialyzable (20% to 50%)

Dietary Considerations Take without regard to food. If GI distress, take with food.

Administration Administer on an empty stomach (ie, 1 hour prior to, or 2 hours after meals) to increase total absorption

Monitoring Parameters With prolonged therapy monitor renal, hepatic, and hematologic function periodically; monitor for signs of anaphylaxis during first dose

Test Interactions Positive direct Coombs', false-positive urinary glucose test using cupric sulfate (Benedict's solution, Clinitest®, Fehling's solution), false-positive serum or urine creatinine with Jaffé reaction, false-positive urinary proteins and steroids

Patient Information Report prolonged diarrhea; entire course of medication (10-14 days) should be taken to ensure eradication of organism; may interfere with oral contraceptives; females should report symptoms of vaginitis

Nursing Implications Administer around-the-clock rather than 4 times/day to promote less variation in peak and trough serum levels

Dosage Forms
Capsule, as monohydrate: 250 mg, 500 mg
Tablet, as hydrochloride: 500 mg
Tablet, as monohydrate: 250 mg, 500 mg, 1 g
Powder for oral suspension, as monohydrate: 125 mg/5 mL (5 mL unit dose, 60 mL, 100 mL, 200 mL); 250 mg/5 mL (5 mL unit dose, 100 mL, 200 mL)

♦ **Cephalexin Hydrochloride** *see Cephalexin on page 261*
♦ **Cephalexin Monohydrate** *see Cephalexin on page 261*

Cephalothin *(sef A loe thin)*
Canadian Brand Names Ceporacin®
Synonyms Cephalothin Sodium
Therapeutic Category Antibiotic, Cephalosporin (First Generation)
Use Treatment of infections when caused by susceptible strains in respiratory, genitourinary, gastrointestinal, skin and soft tissue, bone and joint infections; septicemia; treatment of susceptible gram-positive bacilli and cocci (never enterococcus); some gram-negative bacilli including *E. coli*, *Proteus*, and *Klebsiella* may be susceptible
Pregnancy Risk Factor B
Usual Dosage I.M., I.V.:
Neonates:
Postnatal age <7 days:
<2000 g: 20 mg every 12 hours
>2000 g: 20 mg every 8 hours
Postnatal age >7 days:
<2000 g: 20 mg every 8 hours
>2000 g: 20 mg every 6 hours
Children: 75-125 mg/kg/day divided every 4-6 hours; maximum dose: 10 g in a 24-hour period
Adults: 500 mg to 2 g every 4-6 hours
Dosing interval in renal impairment:
Cl_{cr} 10-50 mL/minute: Administer every 6-8 hours
Cl_{cr} <10 mL/minute: Administer every 12 hours
Continuous arteriovenous or venovenous hemodiafiltration effects: Administer 1 g every 8 hours
Additional Information Complete prescribing information for this medication should be consulted for additional detail.
Dosage Forms Powder for injection, as sodium: 1 g, 2 g (50 mL)

♦ **Cephalothin Sodium** *see Cephalothin on page 262*

Cephapirin *(sef a PYE rin)*
U.S. Brand Names Cefadyl®
Canadian Brand Names Cefadyl®
Synonyms Cephapirin Sodium
Therapeutic Category Antibiotic, Cephalosporin (First Generation)
Use Treatment of infections when caused by susceptible strains in respiratory, genitourinary, gastrointestinal, skin and soft tissue, bone and joint infections, septicemia; treatment of susceptible gram-positive bacilli and cocci (never enterococcus); some gram-negative bacilli including *E. coli*, *Proteus*, and *Klebsiella* may be susceptible
Pregnancy Risk Factor B
Contraindications Hypersensitivity to cephapirin sodium, any component of the formulation, or other cephalosporins
Warnings/Precautions Modify dosage in patients with severe renal impairment, prolonged use may result in superinfection; use with caution in patients with a history of penicillin allergy, especially IgE-mediated reactions (eg, anaphylaxis, urticaria); may cause antibiotic-associated colitis or colitis secondary to *C. difficile*
Adverse Reactions
1% to 10%: Gastrointestinal: Diarrhea
<1% (Limited to important or life-threatening): CNS irritation, fever, leukopenia, rash, seizures, thrombocytopenia, transaminases increased, urticaria

Other reactions with cephalosporins include agranulocytosis, anaphylaxis, angioedema, aplastic anemia, asterixis, cholestasis, dizziness, encephalopathy, erythema multiforme, fever, headache, hemoglobin decreased, hemolytic anemia, hemorrhage, interstitial nephritis, nausea, neuromuscular excitability, pain at injection site, pancytopenia, prolonged PT, pseudomembranous colitis, seizures, serum-sickness reactions, Stevens-Johnson syndrome, superinfection, toxic epidermal necrolysis, toxic nephropathy, vaginitis, vomiting

Overdosage/Toxicology Symptoms include neuromuscular hypersensitivity and convulsions especially with renal insufficiency. Many beta-lactam antibiotics have the potential to cause neuromuscular hyperirritability or seizures. Hemodialysis may be helpful to aid in removal of the drug from the blood; otherwise, most treatment is supportive or symptom directed.

Drug Interactions

Increased Effect/Toxicity: High-dose probenecid decreases clearance of cephapirin. Aminoglycosides in combination with cephapirin may result in additive nephrotoxicity.

Stability Reconstituted solution is stable for 24 hours at room temperature and 10 days when refrigerated; for I.V. infusion in NS or D_5W solution is stable for 24 hours at room temperature, 10 days when refrigerated or 14 days when frozen; after freezing, thawed solution is stable for 12 hours at room temperature or 10 days when refrigerated

Mechanism of Action Inhibits bacterial cell wall synthesis by binding to one or more of the penicillin-binding proteins (PBPs) which in turn inhibits the final transpeptidation step of peptidoglycan synthesis in bacterial cell walls, thus inhibiting cell wall biosynthesis. Bacteria eventually lyse due to ongoing activity of cell wall autolytic enzymes (autolysins and murein hydrolases) while cell wall assembly is arrested.

Pharmacodynamics/Kinetics

Distribution: Widely into most body tissues and fluids including gallbladder, liver, kidneys, bone, sputum, bile, and pleural and synovial fluids; CSF penetration is poor; crosses placenta; small amounts enter breast milk

Protein binding: 22% to 25%

Metabolism: Partially hepatic, renal, and in plasma to metabolites (50% active)

Half-life elimination: 36-60 minutes

Time to peak, serum: I.M.: ~30 minutes; I.V.: ~5 minutes

Excretion: Urine (60% to 85% as unchanged drug)

Usual Dosage I.M., I.V.:

Children: 10-20 mg/kg/dose every 6 hours up to 4 g/24 hours

Adults: 500 mg to 1 g every 6 hours up to 12 g/day

Perioperative prophylaxis: 1-2 g 30 minutes to 1 hour prior to surgery and every 6 hours as needed for 24 hours following

Dosing interval in renal impairment:

Cl_{cr} 10-50 mL/minute: Administer every 6-8 hours

Cl_{cr} <10 mL/minute: Administer every 12 hours

Continuous arteriovenous or venovenous hemodiafiltration effects: Administer 1 g every 8 hours

Monitoring Parameters Observe for signs and symptoms of anaphylaxis during first dose

Test Interactions Positive direct Coombs', false-positive urinary glucose test using cupric sulfate (Benedict's solution, Clinitest®, Fehling's solution), false-positive serum or urine creatinine with Jaffé reaction, false-positive urinary proteins and steroids

Nursing Implications Do not admix with aminoglycosides in same bottle/bag; obtain specimens for culture and sensitivity prior to administration of first dose

Additional Information Sodium content of 1 g: 55.2 mg (2.4 mEq)

Dosage Forms Powder for injection, as sodium: 500 mg, 1 g, 2 g, 4 g

♦ **Cephapirin Sodium** see Cephapirin on page 262

Cephradine (SEF ra deen)

U.S. Brand Names Velosef®

Therapeutic Category Antibiotic, Cephalosporin (First Generation)

Use Treatment of infections when caused by susceptible strains in respiratory, genitourinary, gastrointestinal, skin and soft tissue, bone and joint infections; treatment of susceptible gram-positive bacilli and cocci (never enterococcus); some gram-negative bacilli including *E. coli*, *Proteus*, and *Klebsiella* may be susceptible

Pregnancy Risk Factor B

Contraindications Hypersensitivity to cephradine, any component of the formulation, or cephalosporins

Warnings/Precautions Modify dosage in patients with severe renal impairment, prolonged use may result in superinfection; use with caution in patients with a history of penicillin allergy, especially IgE-mediated reactions (eg, anaphylaxis, urticaria); may cause antibiotic-associated colitis or colitis secondary to *C. difficile*

Adverse Reactions

1% to 10%: Gastrointestinal: Diarrhea

<1% (Limited to important or life-threatening): BUN increased, creatinine increased, nausea, pseudomembranous colitis, rash, vomiting

Other reactions with cephalosporins include agranulocytosis, anaphylaxis, angioedema, aplastic anemia, asterixis, cholestasis, dizziness, encephalopathy, erythema multiforme, fever, headache, hemolytic anemia, hemorrhage, interstitial nephritis, leukopenia, neuromuscular excitability, neutropenia, pancytopenia, prolonged PT, seizures, serum-sickness reactions, Stevens-Johnson syndrome, superinfection, toxic epidermal necrolysis, toxic nephropathy, vaginitis

Overdosage/Toxicology Symptoms include neuromuscular hypersensitivity and convulsions especially with renal insufficiency. Many beta-lactam antibiotics have the potential to cause neuromuscular hyperirritability or seizures. Hemodialysis may be helpful to aid in removal of the drug from the blood; otherwise, most treatment is supportive or symptom directed.

Drug Interactions

Increased Effect/Toxicity: High-dose probenecid decreases clearance of cephradine. Aminoglycosides in combination with cephradine may result in additive nephrotoxicity.

(Continued)

Cephradine *(Continued)*

Ethanol/Nutrition/Herb Interactions Food: Food delays cephradine absorption but does not decrease extent.

Mechanism of Action Inhibits bacterial cell wall synthesis by binding to one or more of the penicillin-binding proteins (PBPs) which in turn inhibits the final transpeptidation step of peptidoglycan synthesis in bacterial cell walls, thus inhibiting cell wall biosynthesis. Bacteria eventually lyse due to ongoing activity of cell wall autolytic enzymes (autolysins and murein hydrolases) while cell wall assembly is arrested.

Pharmacodynamics/Kinetics

Absorption: Well absorbed

Distribution: Widely into most body tissues and fluids including gallbladder, liver, kidneys, bone, sputum, bile, and pleural and synovial fluids; CSF penetration is poor; crosses placenta; enters breast milk

Protein binding: 18% to 20%

Half-life elimination: 1-2 hours (prolonged in renal impairment)

Time to peak, serum: 1-2 hours

Excretion: Urine (~80% to 90% as unchanged drug) within 6 hours

Usual Dosage Oral:

Children ≥9 months: 25-50 mg/kg/day in divided doses every 6 hours

Adults: 250-500 mg every 6-12 hours

Dosing adjustment in renal impairment: Adults:

Cl_{cr} 10-50 mL/minute: 250 mg every 6 hours

Cl_{cr} <10 mL/minute: 125 mg every 6 hours

Dietary Considerations May administer with food to decrease GI distress.

Monitoring Parameters Observe for signs and symptoms of anaphylaxis during first dose

Test Interactions Positive direct Coombs', false-positive urinary glucose test using cupric sulfate (Benedict's solution, Clinitest®, Fehling's solution), false-positive serum or urine creatinine with Jaffé reaction, false-positive urinary proteins and steroids

Patient Information Take until gone, do not miss doses; report diarrhea promptly; entire course of medication (10-14 days) should be taken to ensure eradication of organism; may interfere with oral contraceptives; females should report symptoms of vaginitis

Nursing Implications Administer around-the-clock to promote less variation in peak and trough serum levels

Dosage Forms

Capsule: 250 mg, 500 mg

Powder for oral suspension: 125 mg/5 mL (5 mL, 100 mL, 200 mL); 250 mg/5 mL (5 mL, 100 mL, 200 mL)

♦ **Ceporacin®** (Can) *see* Cephalothin *on page 262*

♦ **Ceptaz™** *see* Ceftazidime *on page 253*

♦ **Cerebyx®** *see* Fosphenytoin *on page 609*

♦ **Ceredase®** *see* Alglucerase *on page 51*

♦ **Cerezyme®** *see* Imiglucerase *on page 705*

♦ **Cerivastatin Sodium** *see* Cerivastatin *Withdrawn From U.S. Market on page 264*

Cerivastatin *Withdrawn From U.S. Market* (se RIV a stat in)

U.S. Brand Names Baycol®

Canadian Brand Names Baycol®

Synonyms Cerivastatin Sodium

Therapeutic Category Antilipemic Agent, HMG-CoA Reductase Inhibitor; HMG-CoA Reductase Inhibitor

Use In conjunction with diet, reduces total and LDL serum cholesterol, apolipoprotein B, and triglycerides, and increases HDL-C concentrations in patients with primary hypercholesterolemia and mixed dyslipidemia (Fredrickson types IIa and IIb)

Pregnancy Risk Factor X

Pregnancy/Breast-Feeding Implications Breast-feeding is not recommended by manufacturer.

Contraindications Hypersensitivity to cerivastatin or any component of the formulation; active liver disease; unexplained persistent elevations of serum transaminases; concurrent use of gemfibrozil; pregnancy; breast-feeding

Warnings/Precautions Liver function must be monitored by periodic laboratory assessment. Rhabdomyolysis with acute renal failure has occurred. Risk is increased in patients receiving an initial dose >0.4 mg/day or with concurrent use of clarithromycin, cyclosporine, danazol, diltiazem, fibric acid derivatives, fluvoxamine, indinavir, nefazodone, nelfinavir, ritonavir, verapamil, troleandomycin, erythromycin, niacin, or azole antifungals. Weigh the risk versus benefit when combining any of these drugs with cerivastatin. Use with caution in patients who have a history of liver disease and/or consume substantial quantities of ethanol. Temporarily discontinue in any patient experiencing an acute or serious condition predisposing to renal failure secondary to rhabdomyolysis. Has not been evaluated in homozygous familial hypercholesterolemia.

Adverse Reactions

1% to 10%:

Cardiovascular: Chest pain (2%), peripheral edema (2%)

Central nervous system: Weakness (3%), insomnia (2%), headache (0.4% to 6%)

Gastrointestinal: Abdominal pain (1% to 3%), diarrhea (2% to 4%)

Neuromuscular & skeletal: Arthralgia (4%), myalgia (2%)

Respiratory: Cough (2%)

<1% (Limited to important or life-threatening): **Note:** Includes class-related events not necessarily reported with cerivastatin therapy and postmarketing case reports: Alopecia, anaphylaxis, angioedema, anxiety, arthritis, cataracts, cholestatic jaundice, cirrhosis, decreased libido, depression, dermatomyositis, dyspnea, eosinophilia, erythema multiforme, facial paresis, fatty liver, fever, fulminant hepatic necrosis, gynecomastia, hemolytic anemia, hepatitis, hepatoma, hypersensitivity reaction, impotence, increased CPK (>10x normal),

increased ESR, leukopenia, muscle cramps, myopathy, ophthalmoplegia, pancreatitis, paresthesia, peripheral nerve palsy, peripheral neuropathy, photosensitivity, polymyalgia rheumatica, positive ANA, psychic disturbance, purpura, rash, renal failure (secondary to rhabdomyolysis), rhabdomyolysis, skin discoloration, Stevens-Johnson syndrome, systemic lupus erythematosus-like syndrome, thrombocytopenia, thyroid dysfunction, toxic epidermal necrolysis, tremor, urticaria, vasculitis, vertigo, vomiting

Drug Interactions

Cytochrome P450 Effect: CYP2C8 and 3A3/4 enzyme substrate

Increased Effect/Toxicity: Inhibitors of CYP3A3/4 (amprenavir, clarithromycin, cyclosporine, diltiazem, fluvoxamine, erythromycin, fluconazole, indinavir, itraconazole, ketoconazole, miconazole, nefazodone, nelfinavir, ritonavir, troleandomycin, and verapamil) increase cerivastatin blood levels and may increase the risk of myopathy and rhabdomyolysis. Cyclosporine, clofibrate, fenofibrate, gemfibrozil, and niacin also may increase the risk of myopathy and rhabdomyolysis. The effect/toxicity of levothyroxine may be increased by cerivastatin. Digoxin, norethindrone, and ethinyl estradiol levels may be increased. Effects are additive with other lipid-lowering therapies.

Decreased Effect: When cerivastatin is taken within 1 before or up to 2 hours after cholestyramine, a decrease in absorption of cerivastatin can occur.

Ethanol/Nutrition/Herb Interactions

Food: Cerivastatin serum concentration may be increased by grapefruit juice; avoid concurrent use.

Herb/Nutraceutical: St John's wort may decrease cerivastatin levels.

Stability Store at 25°C (77°F).

Mechanism of Action As an HMG-CoA reductase inhibitor, cerivastatin competitively inhibits 3-hydroxyl-3-methylglutaryl-coenzyme A (HMG-CoA) reductase, the enzyme that catalyzes the rate-limiting step in cholesterol biosynthesis

Pharmacodynamics/Kinetics

Peak effect: ~2 weeks

Distribution: V_d: 0.3 L/kg

Protein binding, plasma: >99%; 80% to albumin

Metabolism: Hepatic; active metabolite, demethylation and hydroxylation

Bioavailability: 60%

Half-life elimination: 2-3 hours

Time to peak: 1-3 hours

Excretion: Feces (70%); urine (26% as metabolites)

Usual Dosage Note: Beginning therapy at a starting dose >0.4 mg increases the risk of myopathy and rhabdomyolysis

Adults: Oral: 0.4 mg once daily in the evening; may be taken with or without food; maximum effect of a given dose will be seen in 4 weeks; monitor lipid levels and adjust dose at that time; dosing range: 0.2-0.8 mg/day

Dosing adjustment with renal impairment: Moderate to severe impairment (<60 mL/minute): Starting dose: 0.2-0.3 mg

Dosing adjustment in hepatic impairment: Avoidance suggested; no guidelines for dosage reduction available.

Dietary Considerations May be taken without regard to meals.

Administration Administer with or without food.

Monitoring Parameters Serum total cholesterol, LDL, HDL, triglycerides, apolipoprotein B, diet, weight, LFTs (test liver function prior to initiation, at 6 and 12 weeks after initiation or first dose, and periodically thereafter)

Patient Information Call physician if you experience unexplained fever, rash, muscle pain, GI upset, or headache

Dosage Forms Tablet, as sodium: 0.2 mg, 0.3 mg, 0.4 mg, 0.8 mg

♦ **Cerose-DM**® **[OTC]** see Chlorpheniramine, Phenylephrine, and Dextromethorphan on page 280

♦ **Cerubidine**® see DAUNOrubicin Hydrochloride on page 368

♦ **Cerumenex**® see Triethanolamine Polypeptide Oleate-Condensate on page 1372

♦ **Cervidil**™ **(Can)** see Dinoprostone on page 412

♦ **Cervidil**® **Vaginal Insert** see Dinoprostone on page 412

♦ **C.E.S.** see Estrogens (Conjugated/Equine) on page 498

♦ **Cetacaine**® see Benzocaine, Butyl Aminobenzoate, Tetracaine, and Benzalkonium Chloride on page 156

♦ **Cetacort**® see Hydrocortisone on page 682

♦ **Cetafen**® **[OTC]** see Acetaminophen on page 22

♦ **Cetafen Extra**® **[OTC]** see Acetaminophen on page 22

♦ **Cetamide**® see Sulfacetamide on page 1268

♦ **Cetapred**® see Sulfacetamide and Prednisolone on page 1269

Cetirizine (se TI ra zeen)

U.S. Brand Names Zyrtec®

Canadian Brand Names Apo®-Cetirizine; Reactine™

Synonyms Cetirizine Hydrochloride; P-071; UCB-P071

Therapeutic Category Antihistamine, H_1 Blocker

Use Perennial and seasonal allergic rhinitis and other allergic symptoms including urticaria; chronic idiopathic urticaria

Pregnancy Risk Factor B

Contraindications Hypersensitivity to cetirizine, hydroxyzine, or any component of the formulation

Warnings/Precautions Cetirizine should be used cautiously in patients with hepatic or renal dysfunction, the elderly and in nursing mothers. Doses >10 mg/day may cause significant drowsiness

(Continued)

Cetirizine *(Continued)*

Adverse Reactions
>10%: Central nervous system: Headache has been reported to occur in 10% to 12% of patients, drowsiness has been reported in as much as 26% of patients on high doses
1% to 10%:
Central nervous system: Somnolence, fatigue, dizziness
Gastrointestinal: Dry mouth

Overdosage/Toxicology Symptoms include seizures, sedation, and hypotension. There is no specific treatment for antihistamine overdose, however, clinical toxicity is mostly due to anticholinergic effects. Anticholinesterase inhibitors may be useful by reducing acetylcholinesterase. For anticholinergic overdose with severe life-threatening symptoms, physostigmine 1-2 mg (0.5 mg or 0.02 mg/kg for children) slow I.V. may be given to reverse these effects.

Drug Interactions
Increased Effect/Toxicity: Increased toxicity with CNS depressants and anticholinergics.
Ethanol/Nutrition/Herb Interactions Ethanol: Avoid ethanol (may increase CNS depression).

Mechanism of Action Competes with histamine for H_1-receptor sites on effector cells in the gastrointestinal tract, blood vessels, and respiratory tract

Pharmacodynamics/Kinetics
Onset of action: 15-30 minutes
Absorption: Rapid
Metabolism: Limited hepatic metabolism
Half-life elimination: 8-11 hours
Time to peak, serum: 30-60 minutes

Usual Dosage
Children 2-5 years: Initial dose: 2.5 mg, may be increased to 2.5 mg every 12 hours or up to 5 mg/day
Children ≥6 years and Adults: Oral: 5-10 mg once daily, depending upon symptom severity
Dosing interval in renal/hepatic impairment: Cl_{cr} ≤31 mL/minute: Administer 5 mg once daily

Monitoring Parameters Relief of symptoms, sedation and anticholinergic effects

Dosage Forms
Syrup, as hydrochloride: 5 mg/5 mL (120 mL)
Tablet, as hydrochloride: 5 mg, 10 mg

♦ **Cetirizine Hydrochloride** *see Cetirizine on page 265*

Cetrorelix *(set roe REL iks)*
U.S. Brand Names Cetrotide™
Synonyms Cetrorelix Acetate
Therapeutic Category Antigonadotropic Agent
Use Inhibits premature luteinizing hormone (LH) surges in women undergoing controlled ovarian stimulation
Pregnancy Risk Factor X
Pregnancy/Breast-Feeding Implications Animal studies have shown fetal resorption and implantation losses following administration. Resorption resulting in fetal loss would be expected if used in a pregnant woman. It is unknown if cetrorelix is excreted in human milk, do not use in breast-feeding women.
Contraindications Hypersensitivity to cetrorelix or any component of the formulation; extrinsic peptide hormones, mannitol, gonadotropin releasing hormone (GnRH) or GnRH analogs; pregnancy
Warnings/Precautions Should only be prescribed by fertility specialists. Pregnancy should be excluded before treatment is begun.

Adverse Reactions
1% to 10%:
Central nervous system: Headache (1%)
Endocrine & metabolic: Ovarian hyperstimulation syndrome, WHO grade II or III (3%)
Gastrointestinal: Nausea (1%)
Hepatic: Increased ALT, AST, GGT, and alkaline phosphatase (1% to 2%)
Postmarketing and/or case reports: Severe anaphylactic reaction (cough, rash, hypotension) occurred in one patient following several months of treatment in a study not related to fertility. Congenital abnormalities and stillbirths have been reported, however the relationship to cetrorelix treatment has not been established. Local injection site reactions (bruising, erythema, itching, pruritus, redness, swelling) have also been reported.

Overdosage/Toxicology No cases of overdose have been reported. In nonfertility studies, single doses of up to 120 mg have been well tolerated.

Drug Interactions
Increased Effect/Toxicity: No formal studies have been performed.
Decreased Effect: No formal studies have been performed.

Stability Store in outer carton. Once mixed, solution should be used immediately.
0.25 mg vials: Store under refrigeration at 2°C to 8°C (36°F to 46°F)
3 mg vials: Store at controlled room temperature at 25°C (77°F)

Mechanism of Action Competes with naturally occurring GnRH for binding on receptors of the pituitary. This delays luteinizing hormone surge, preventing ovulation until the follicles are of adequate size.

Pharmacodynamics/Kinetics
Onset of action: 0.25 mg dose: 2 hours; 3 mg dose: 1 hour
Metabolism: Transformed by peptidases; cetrorelix and peptides (1-9), (1-7), (1-6), and (1-4) are found in the bile; peptide (1-4) is the predominant metabolite
Bioavailability: 85%
Half-life elimination: 0.25 mg dose: 5 hours; 0.25 mg multiple dose: 20.6 hours; 3 mg dose: 62.8 hours
Time to peak: 0.25 mg dose: 1 hour; 3 mg dose: 1.5 hours

Excretion: Feces (5% to 10% as unchanged drug and metabolites); urine (2% to 4% as unchanged drug); occurs within 24 hours

Usual Dosage S.C.: Adults: Female: Used in conjunction with controlled ovarian stimulation therapy using gonadotropins (FSH, HMG):

Single-dose regimen: 3 mg given when serum estradiol levels show appropriate stimulation response, usually stimulation day 7 (range days 5-9). If hCG is not administered within 4 days, continue cetrorelix at 0.25 mg/day until hCG is administered

Multiple-dose regimen: 0.25 mg morning or evening of stimulation day 5, or morning of stimulation day 6; continue until hCG is administered.

Dosing adjustment in renal impairment: No specific guidelines are available.

Dosing adjustment in hepatic impairment: No specific guidelines are available.

Elderly: Not intended for use in women ≥65 years of age (Phase 2 and Phase 3 studies included women 19-40 years of age)

Administration Cetrorelix is administered by S.C. injection following proper aseptic technique procedures. Injections should be to the lower abdomen, preferably around the navel. The injection site should be rotated daily. The needle should be inserted completely into the skin at a 45-degree angle.

Monitoring Parameters Ultrasound to assess follicle size

Patient Information An instructional leaflet will be provided if you will be administering this medication to yourself. Instructions will be given on how to administer S.C. injections and proper disposal of syringes and needles. Give at a similar time each day as instructed by prescriber. Do not skip doses. Keep all ultrasound appointments. Report any sudden weight gain, abdominal discomfort, or shortness of breath to prescriber. Do not take if pregnant.

Nursing Implications Teach patient/spouse to give S.C. injections. When mixing solution, gently agitate, avoid forming bubbles. Discuss ultrasound schedule and timing of other medications used.

Dosage Forms

Injection, prefilled glass syringe [single-dose vial]:
0.25 mg with 1 mL SWFI
3 mg with 3 mL SWFI

♦ **Cetrorelix Acetate** see Cetrorelix on page 266

♦ **Cetrotide**™ see Cetrorelix on page 266

Cetylpyridinium and Benzocaine (SEE til peer i DI nee um & BEN zoe kane)

U.S. Brand Names Cēpacol® Anesthetic Troches [OTC]

Synonyms Benzocaine and Cetylpyridinium Chloride; Cetylpyridinium Chloride and Benzocaine

Therapeutic Category Local Anesthetic

Use Symptomatic relief of sore throat

Pregnancy Risk Factor C

Usual Dosage Antiseptic/anesthetic: Oral: Dissolve in mouth as needed for sore throat

Additional Information Complete prescribing information for this medication should be consulted for additional detail.

Dosage Forms Troche: Cetylpyridinium chloride 1:1500 and benzocaine 10 mg per troche (18s)

♦ **Cetylpyridinium Chloride and Benzocaine** see Cetylpyridinium and Benzocaine on page 267

♦ **Cevi-Bid**® [OTC] see Ascorbic Acid on page 116

Cevimeline (se vi ME leen)

U.S. Brand Names Evoxac™

Canadian Brand Names Evoxac™

Synonyms Cevimeline Hydrochloride

Therapeutic Category Cholinergic Agent

Use Treatment of symptoms of dry mouth in patients with Sjögren's syndrome

Pregnancy Risk Factor C

Pregnancy/Breast-Feeding Implications There are no adequate or well-controlled studies in pregnant women. Use only if potential benefit justifies potential risk to the fetus. Excretion in breast milk is unknown/not recommended.

Contraindications Hypersensitivity to cevimeline or any component of the formulation; uncontrolled asthma; narrow-angle glaucoma; acute iritis; other conditions where miosis is undesirable

Warnings/Precautions May alter cardiac conduction and/or heart rate; use caution in patients with significant cardiovascular disease, including angina, myocardial infarction, or conduction disturbances. Cevimeline has the potential to increase bronchial smooth muscle tone, airway resistance, and bronchial secretions; use with caution in patients with controlled asthma, COPD, or chronic bronchitis. May cause decreased visual acuity (particularly at night and in patients with central lens changes) and impaired depth perception. Patients should be cautioned about driving at night or performing hazardous activities in reduced lighting. May cause a variety of parasympathomimetic effects, which may be particularly dangerous in elderly patients; excessive sweating may lead to dehydration in some patients.

Use with caution in patients with a history of biliary stones or nephrolithiasis; cevimeline may induce smooth muscle spasms, precipitating cholangitis, cholecystitis, biliary obstruction, renal colic, or ureteral reflux in susceptible patients. Patients with a known or suspected deficiency of CYP2D6 may be at higher risk of adverse effects. Safety and efficacy has not been established in pediatric patients.

Adverse Reactions

>10%:
Central nervous system: Headache (14%; placebo 20%)
Gastrointestinal: Nausea (14%), diarrhea (10%)
Respiratory: Rhinitis (11%), sinusitis (12%), upper respiratory infection (11%)
Miscellaneous: Increased diaphoresis (19%)

(Continued)

Cevimeline *(Continued)*

1% to 10%:

Cardiovascular: Peripheral edema, chest pain, edema, palpitation

Central nervous system: Dizziness (4%), fatigue (3%), pain (3%), insomnia (2%), anxiety (1%), fever, depression, migraine, vertigo

Dermatologic: Rash (4%; placebo 6%), pruritus, skin disorder, erythematous rash

Endocrine & metabolic: Hot flashes (2%)

Gastrointestinal: Dyspepsia (8%; placebo 9%), abdominal pain (8%), vomiting (5%), excessive salivation (2%), constipation, salivary gland pain, dry mouth, sialoadenitis, ulcerative stomatitis

Genitourinary: Urinary tract infection (6%), vaginitis, cystitis

Hematologic: Anemia

Local: Abscess

Neuromuscular & skeletal: back pain (5%), arthralgia (4%), skeletal pain (3%), rigors (1%), hypertonia, tremor, myalgia

Ocular: Conjunctivitis (4%), abnormal vision, eye pain, eye abnormality, xerophthalmia

Otic: Earache, otitis media

Respiratory: Coughing (6%), bronchitis (4%), pneumonia, epistaxis

Miscellaneous: Flu-like syndrome, infection, fungal infection, allergy, hiccups

<1% (Limited to important or life-threatening): Aggravated multiple sclerosis, aggressive behavior, alopecia, angina, anterior chamber hemorrhage, aphasia, apnea, arrhythmia, arthropathy, avascular necrosis (femoral head), bronchospasm, bullous eruption, bundle branch block, cholelithiasis, coma, deafness, delirium, depersonalization, dyskinesia, eosinophilia, esophageal stricture, esophagitis, fall, gastric ulcer, gastrointestinal hemorrhage, gingival hyperplasia, glaucoma, granulocytopenia, hallucination, hematuria, hypothyroidism, ileus, impotence, intestinal obstruction, leukopenia, lymphocytosis, manic reaction, myocardial infarction, neuropathy, paralysis, paranoia, paresthesia, peptic ulcer, pericarditis, peripheral ischemia, photosensitivity reaction, pleural effusion, pulmonary embolism, pulmonary fibrosis, renal calculus, seizure, sepsis, somnolence, syncope, systemic lupus erythematosus, tenosynovitis, thrombocytopenia, thrombocytopenic purpura, thrombophlebitis, T-wave inversion, urinary retention, vasculitis

Overdosage/Toxicology Symptoms may include headache, visual disturbances, lacrimation, sweating, gastrointestinal spasm, nausea, vomiting, diarrhea, A-V block, mental confusion, tremor, cardiac depression, bradycardia, tachycardia, or bronchospasm. Atropine may be of value as an antidote, and epinephrine may be required for bronchoconstriction. Additional treatment is supportive. The effect of hemodialysis is unknown.

Drug Interactions

Cytochrome P450 Effect: CYP2D6 and 3A3/4 substrate

Increased Effect/Toxicity: Drugs which inhibit CYP2D6 (including amiodarone, fluoxetine, paroxetine, quinidine, ritonavir) or CYP3A3/4 (including diltiazem, erythromycin, itraconazole, ketoconazole, verapamil) may increase levels of cevimeline. The effects of other cholinergic agents may be increased during concurrent administration with cevimeline. Concurrent use of cevimeline and beta-blockers may increase the potential for conduction disturbances.

Decreased Effect: Anticholinergic agents (atropine, TCAs, phenothiazines) may antagonize the effects of cevimeline.

Stability Store at 25°C (77°F)

Mechanism of Action Binds to muscarinic (cholinergic) receptors, causing an increase in secretion of exocrine glands (including salivary glands)

Pharmacodynamics/Kinetics

Distribution: V_d: 6 L/kg

Protein binding: <20%

Metabolism: Hepatic via CYP2D6 and CYP3A3/4

Half-life elimination: 5 hours

Time to peak: 1.5-2 hours

Excretion: Urine (as metabolites and unchanged drug)

Usual Dosage Adults: Oral: 30 mg 3 times/day

Dosage adjustment in renal/hepatic impairment: Not studied; no specific dosage adjustment is recommended

Elderly: No specific dosage adjustment is recommended; however, use caution when initiating due to potential for increased sensitivity

Dietary Considerations Take with or without food.

Patient Information May be taken with or without food; take with food if medicine causes upset stomach. May cause decreased visual acuity (particularly at night and in patients with central lens changes) and impaired depth perception; patients should be cautioned about driving at night or performing hazardous activities in reduced lighting.

Dosage Forms Capsule: 30 mg

- ◆ **Cevimeline Hydrochloride** *see* Cevimeline *on page 267*
- ◆ **CFDN** *see* Cefdinir *on page 241*
- ◆ **CGP-42446** *see* Zoledronic Acid *on page 1442*
- ◆ **CGP 57148B** *see* Imatinib *on page 703*
- ◆ **C-Gram [OTC]** *see* Ascorbic Acid *on page 116*
- ◆ **Charcadole® (Can)** *see* Charcoal *on page 268*
- ◆ **Charcadole®, Aqueous (Can)** *see* Charcoal *on page 268*
- ◆ **Charcadole® TFS (Can)** *see* Charcoal *on page 268*
- ◆ **CharcoAid® [OTC]** *see* Charcoal *on page 268*

Charcoal *(CHAR kole)*

Related Information

Toxicology Information *on page 1693*

U.S. Brand Names Actidose® [OTC]; Actidose-Aqua® [OTC]; CharcoAid® [OTC]; Charcocaps® [OTC]; Liqui-Char® [OTC]

Canadian Brand Names Charcadole®; Charcadole®, Aqueous; Charcadole® TFS
Synonyms Activated Carbon; Activated Charcoal; Adsorbent Charcoal; Liquid Antidote; Medicinal Carbon; Medicinal Charcoal
Therapeutic Category Antidiarrheal; Antidote, Adsorbent; Antiflatulent
Use Emergency treatment in poisoning by drugs and chemicals; repetitive doses for gastric dialysis in uremia to adsorb various waste products, and repetitive doses have proven useful to enhance the elimination of certain drugs (eg, theophylline, phenobarbital, and aspirin)
Pregnancy Risk Factor C
Contraindications Not effective for cyanide, mineral acids, caustic alkalis, organic solvents, iron, ethanol, methanol poisoning, lithium; do not use charcoal with sorbitol in patients with fructose intolerance; charcoal with sorbitol is not recommended in children <1 year.
Warnings/Precautions When using charcoal, induce vomiting with ipecac before administering activated charcoal since charcoal adsorbs ipecac syrup; charcoal may cause vomiting which is hazardous in petroleum distillate and caustic ingestions; if charcoal in sorbitol is administered, doses should be limited to prevent excessive fluid and electrolyte losses; do not mix charcoal with milk, ice cream, or sherbet
Adverse Reactions >10%:
Gastrointestinal: Vomiting, diarrhea with sorbitol, constipation
Miscellaneous: Stools will turn black
Drug Interactions
Decreased Effect: Charcoal decreases the effect of ipecac syrup. Charcoal effect is reduced when taken with milk, ice cream, or sherbet.
Ethanol/Nutrition/Herb Interactions Food: Milk, ice cream, sherbet, or marmalade may reduce charcoal's effectiveness.
Stability Adsorbs gases from air, store in closed container
Mechanism of Action Adsorbs toxic substances or irritants, thus inhibiting GI absorption; adsorbs intestinal gas; the addition of sorbitol results in hyperosmotic laxative action causing catharsis
Pharmacodynamics/Kinetics Excretion: Feces (as charcoal)
Usual Dosage Oral:
Acute poisoning:
Charcoal with sorbitol: Single-dose:
Children 1-12 years: 1-2 g/kg/dose or 15-30 g or approximately 5-10 times the weight of the ingested poison; 1 g adsorbs 100-1000 mg of poison; the use of repeat oral charcoal with sorbitol doses is not recommended. In young children, sorbitol should be repeated no more than 1-2 times/day.
Adults: 30-100 g
Charcoal in water:
Single-dose:
Infants <1 year: 1 g/kg
Children 1-12 years: 15-30 g or 1-2 g/kg
Adults: 30-100 g or 1-2 g/kg
Multiple-dose:
Infants <1 year: 0.5 g/kg every 4-6 hours
Children 1-12 years: 20-60 g or 0.5-1 g/kg every 2-6 hours until clinical observations, serum drug concentration have returned to a subtherapeutic range, or charcoal stool apparent
Adults: 20-60 g or 0.5-1 g/kg every 2-6 hours
Gastric dialysis: Adults: 20-50 g every 6 hours for 1-2 days
Intestinal gas, diarrhea, GI distress: Adults: 520-975 mg after meals or at first sign of discomfort; repeat as needed to a maximum dose of 4.16 g/day
Administration Flavoring agents (eg, chocolate) and sorbitol can enhance charcoal's palatability; marmalade, milk, ice cream, and sherbet should be avoided since they can reduce charcoal's effectiveness
Patient Information Charcoal causes the stools to turn black; should not be used prior to calling a poison control center or a physician
Nursing Implications Charcoal slurries that are too concentrated may clog airways, if aspirated; often given with a laxative or cathartic; check for presence of bowel sounds before administration
Dosage Forms
Capsule (Charcocaps®): 260 mg
Granules, activated (CharcoAid®-G): 15 g (120 mL)
Liquid, activated:
Actidose-Aqua®: 15 g (72 mL); 25 g (120 mL); 50 g (240 mL)
CharcoAid® 2000: 15 g (72 mL); 50 g (240 mL)
Liqui-Char®: 15 g (75 mL); 25 g (120 mL); 30 g (120 mL)
Liquid, activated, with propylene glycol: 12.5 g (60 mL); 25 g (120 mL)
Liquid, activated, with sorbitol:
Actidose®: 25 g (120 mL); 50 g (240 mL)
CharcoAid® 2000: 15 g (72 mL); 50 g (240 mL)
Liqui-Char®: 25 g (120 mL); 50 g (240 mL)
Powder for suspension, activated: 15 g, 30 g, 40 g, 120 g, 240 g

- **Children's Advil®** [OTC] *see* Ibuprofen *on page 697*
- **Children's Dimetapp® Elixir Cold & Allergy** [OTC] *see* Brompheniramine and Pseudoephedrine *on page 185*
- **Children's Motrin®** [OTC] *see* Ibuprofen *on page 697*
- **Children's Nostril®** *see* Phenylephrine *on page 1075*
- **Children's Silfedrine®** [OTC] *see* Pseudoephedrine *on page 1155*
- **Children's Sudafed® Cough & Cold** *see* Pseudoephedrine and Dextromethorphan *on page 1157*
- **Children's Sudafed® Nasal Decongestant** [OTC] *see* Pseudoephedrine *on page 1155*
- **Children's Tylenol® Cold** [OTC] *see* Acetaminophen, Chlorpheniramine, and Pseudoephedrine *on page 27*
- **Children's Tylenol® Sinus** [OTC] *see* Acetaminophen and Pseudoephedrine *on page 25*
- **Children's Vitamins** *see* Vitamins (Multiple) *on page 1424*
- **Chirocaine®** *see* Levobupivacaine *on page 788*
- **Chlorafed®** [OTC] *see* Chlorpheniramine and Pseudoephedrine *on page 279*
- **Chloral** *see* Chloral Hydrate *on page 270*

Chloral Hydrate (KLOR al HYE drate)
Related Information
Depression *on page 1655*
U.S. Brand Names Aquachloral® Supprettes®
Canadian Brand Names PMS-Chloral Hydrate
Synonyms Chloral; Hydrated Chloral; Trichloroacetaldehyde Monohydrate
Therapeutic Category Hypnotic; Sedative
Use Short-term sedative and hypnotic (<2 weeks), sedative/hypnotic for diagnostic procedures; sedative prior to EEG evaluations
Restrictions C-IV
Pregnancy Risk Factor C
Contraindications Hypersensitivity to chloral hydrate or any component of the formulation; hepatic or renal impairment; gastritis or ulcers; severe cardiac disease
Warnings/Precautions Use with caution in patients with porphyria; use with caution in neonates, drug may accumulate with repeated use, prolonged use in neonates associated with hyperbilirubinemia; tolerance to hypnotic effect develops, therefore, not recommended for use >2 weeks; taper dosage to avoid withdrawal with prolonged use; trichloroethanol (TCE), a metabolite of chloral hydrate, is a carcinogen in mice; there is no data in humans. Chloral hydrate is considered a second line hypnotic agent in the elderly. Recent interpretive guidelines from the Health Care Financing Administration (HCFA) discourage the use of chloral hydrate in residents of long-term care facilities.
Adverse Reactions Frequency not defined.
Central nervous system: Ataxia, disorientation, sedation, excitement (paradoxical), dizziness, fever, headache, confusion, lightheadedness, nightmares, hallucinations, drowsiness, "hangover" effect
Dermatologic: Rash, urticaria
Gastrointestinal: Gastric irritation, nausea, vomiting, diarrhea, flatulence
Hematologic: Leukopenia, eosinophilia, acute intermittent porphyria
Miscellaneous: Physical and psychological dependence may occur with prolonged use of large doses
Overdosage/Toxicology Symptoms include hypotension, respiratory depression, coma, hypothermia, cardiac arrhythmias. Treatment is supportive and symptomatic. Lidocaine or propranolol may be used for ventricular dysrhythmias, while isoproterenol or atropine may be required for torsade de pointes. Activated charcoal may prevent drug absorption.
Drug Interactions
Cytochrome P450 Effect: CYP2E1 enzyme substrate
Increased Effect/Toxicity: Chloral hydrate and ethanol (and other CNS depressants) have additive CNS depressant effects; monitor for CNS depression. Chloral hydrate's metabolite may displace warfarin from its protein binding sites resulting in an increase in the hypoprothrombinemic response to warfarin; warfarin dosages may need to be adjusted. Diaphoresis, flushing, and hypertension have occurred in patients who received I.V. furosemide within 24 hours after administration of chloral hydrate; consider using a benzodiazepine.
Ethanol/Nutrition/Herb Interactions
Ethanol: Avoid ethanol (may increase CNS depression).
Herb/Nutraceutical: Avoid valerian, St John's wort, kava kava, gotu kola (may increase CNS depression).
Stability Sensitive to light; exposure to air causes volatilization; store in light-resistant, airtight container
Mechanism of Action Central nervous system depressant effects are due to its active metabolite trichloroethanol, mechanism unknown
Pharmacodynamics/Kinetics
Onset of action: Peak effect: 0.5-1 hour
Duration: 4-8 hours
Absorption: Oral, rectal: Well absorbed
Distribution: Crosses placenta; negligible amounts enter breast milk
Metabolism: Rapidly to trichloroethanol (active metabolite); variable amounts hepatically and renally to trichloroacetic acid (inactive)
Half-life elimination: Active metabolite: 8-11 hours
Excretion: Urine (as metabolites); feces (small amounts)
Usual Dosage
Children:
Sedation or anxiety: Oral, rectal: 5-15 mg/kg/dose every 8 hours (maximum: 500 mg/dose)
Prior to EEG: Oral, rectal: 20-25 mg/kg/dose, 30-60 minutes prior to EEG; may repeat in 30 minutes to maximum of 100 mg/kg or 2 g total

Hypnotic: Oral, rectal: 20-40 mg/kg/dose up to a maximum of 50 mg/kg/24 hours or 1 g/dose or 2 g/24 hours

Sedation during nonpainful procedure: Oral: 50-75 mg/kg/dose 30-60 minutes prior to procedure; may repeat 30 minutes after initial dose if needed, to a total maximum dose of 120 mg/kg or 1 g total

Adults: Oral, rectal:

Sedation, anxiety: 250 mg 3 times/day

Hypnotic: 500-1000 mg at bedtime or 30 minutes prior to procedure, not to exceed 2 g/24 hours

Dosing adjustment/comments in renal impairment: Cl_{cr} <50 mL/minute: Avoid use
Hemodialysis: Dialyzable (50% to 100%); supplemental dose is not necessary

Dosing adjustment/comments in hepatic impairment: Avoid use in patients with severe hepatic impairment

Administration Do not crush capsule, contains drug in liquid form

Monitoring Parameters Vital signs, O_2 saturation and blood pressure with doses used for conscious sedation

Test Interactions False-positive urine glucose using Clinitest® method; may interfere with fluorometric urine catecholamine and urinary 17-hydroxycorticosteroid tests

Patient Information Take a capsule with a full glass of water or fruit juice; swallow capsules whole, do not chew; avoid alcohol and other CNS depressants; avoid activities needing good psychomotor coordination until CNS effects are known; drug may cause physical or psychological dependence; avoid abrupt discontinuation after prolonged use; if taking at home prior to a diagnostic procedure, have someone else transport

Nursing Implications Gastric irritation may be minimized by diluting dose in water or other oral liquid

Additional Information Not an analgesic

Dosage Forms

Capsule: 500 mg

Suppository, rectal: 324 mg, 500 mg, 648 mg

Syrup: 500 mg/5 mL (5 mL, 10 mL, 480 mL)

Chlorambucil (klor AM byoo sil)

U.S. Brand Names Leukeran®

Canadian Brand Names Leukeran®

Therapeutic Category Antineoplastic Agent, Alkylating Agent

Use Management of chronic lymphocytic leukemia, Hodgkin's and non-Hodgkin's lymphoma; breast and ovarian carcinoma; Waldenström's macroglobulinemia, testicular carcinoma, thrombocythemia, choriocarcinoma

Pregnancy Risk Factor D

Pregnancy/Breast-Feeding Implications Clinical effects on the fetus: Carcinogenic and mutagenic in humans

Contraindications Hypersensitivity to chlorambucil or any component of the formulation; pregnancy

Warnings/Precautions The U.S. Food and Drug Administration (FDA) currently recommends that procedures for proper handling and disposal of antineoplastic agents be considered. Use with caution in patients with seizure disorder and bone marrow suppression; reduce initial dosage if patient has received radiation therapy, myelosuppressive drugs or has a depressed baseline leukocyte or platelet count within the previous 4 weeks. Can severely suppress bone marrow function; affects human fertility; carcinogenic in humans and probably mutagenic and teratogenic as well; chromosomal damage has been documented; secondary AML may be associated with chronic therapy.

Adverse Reactions

>10%:

Hematologic: Myelosuppressive: Use with caution when receiving radiation; bone marrow suppression frequently occurs and occasionally bone marrow failure has occurred; blood counts should be monitored closely while undergoing treatment; leukopenia, thrombocytopenia, anemia

WBC: Moderate

Platelets: Moderate

Onset (days): 7

Nadir (days): 10-14

Recovery (days): 28

1% to 10%:

Dermatologic: Skin rashes

Endocrine & metabolic: Hyperuricemia, menstrual changes

Gastrointestinal: Nausea, vomiting, diarrhea, oral ulceration are all infrequent

Emetic potential: Low (<10%)

<1% (Limited to important or life-threatening): Agitation, angioneurotic edema, ataxia, confusion, drug fever, epidermal necrolysis, erythema multiforme, fertility impairment (has caused chromosomal damage in men, both reversible and permanent sterility have occurred in both sexes; can produce amenorrhea in females), generalized or focal seizures (rarely), hallucination, hepatic necrosis, hepatotoxicity, increased incidence of AML, muscular twitching, myoclonia, oral ulceration, peripheral neuropathy, pulmonary fibrosis, secondary malignancies, skin hypersensitivity, Stevens-Johnson syndrome, tremors, urticaria, weakness

Overdosage/Toxicology Symptoms include vomiting, ataxia, coma, seizures, and pancytopenia. There are no known antidotes for chlorambucil intoxication. Treatment is mainly supportive, directed at decontaminating the GI tract and controlling symptoms. Blood products may be used to treat hematologic toxicity.

Drug Interactions

Decreased Effect: Patients may experience impaired immune response to vaccines; possible infection after administration of live vaccines in patients receiving immunosuppressants.

(Continued)

Chlorambucil *(Continued)*

Ethanol/Nutrition/Herb Interactions
Ethanol: Avoid ethanol (may increase GI irritation).
Food: Avoid acidic foods and hot foods. Avoid spices.

Stability Store at room temperature; protect from light.

Mechanism of Action Interferes with DNA replication and RNA transcription by alkylation and cross-linking the strands of DNA

Pharmacodynamics/Kinetics
Absorption: 70% to 80% (with meals)
Distribution: V_d: 0.14-0.24 L/kg
Protein binding: ~99%
Metabolism: Hepatic; active metabolite: Phenylacetic acid mustard
Bioavailability: Decreases by 10% to 20% with food
Half-life elimination: 1.5 hours; phenylacetic acid mustard: 2.5 hours
Excretion: Urine (60% primarily as metabolites, <1% as unchanged drug)

Usual Dosage Oral (refer to individual protocols):
Children:
General short courses: 0.1-0.2 mg/kg/day **OR** 4.5 mg/m²/day for 3-6 weeks for remission induction (usual: 4-10 mg/day); maintenance therapy: 0.03-0.1 mg/kg/day (usual: 2-4 mg/day)
Nephrotic syndrome: 0.1-0.2 mg/kg/day every day for 5-15 weeks with low-dose prednisone
Chronic lymphocytic leukemia (CLL):
Biweekly regimen: Initial: 0.4 mg/kg/dose every 2 weeks; increase dose by 0.1 mg/kg every 2 weeks until a response occurs and/or myelosuppression occurs
Monthly regimen: Initial: 0.4 mg/kg, increase dose by 0.2 mg/kg every 4 weeks until a response occurs and/or myelosuppression occurs
Malignant lymphomas:
Non-Hodgkin's lymphoma: 0.1 mg/kg/day
Hodgkin's lymphoma: 0.2 mg/kg/day
Adults: 0.1-0.2 mg/kg/day **OR** 3-6 mg/m²/day for 3-6 weeks, then adjust dose on basis of blood counts. Pulse dosing has been used in CLL as intermittent, biweekly, or monthly doses of 0.4 mg/kg and increased by 0.1 mg/kg until the disease is under control or toxicity ensues. An alternate regimen is 14 mg/m²/day for 5 days, repeated every 21-28 days.
Hemodialysis: Supplemental dosing is not necessary
Peritoneal dialysis: Supplemental dosing is not necessary

Administration May divide single daily dose if nausea and vomiting occur. Take 1 hour before or 2 hours after meals.

Monitoring Parameters Liver function tests, CBC, leukocyte counts, platelets, serum uric acid

Patient Information Take exactly as directed. Maintain adequate hydration (2-3 L/day of fluids unless instructed to restrict fluid intake). Avoid alcohol, acidic, spicy, or hot foods, aspirin, or OTC medications unless approved by prescriber. Hair may be lost during treatment (reversible). You may experience menstrual irregularities and/or sterility. You will be more susceptible to infection; avoid crowds and exposure to infection. Frequent mouth care with a soft toothbrush or cotton swab may reduce occurrence of mouth sores. Report easy bruising or bleeding; fever or chills; numbness, pain, or tingling of extremities; muscle cramping or weakness; unusual swelling of extremities; menstrual irregularities; or any difficulty breathing. Contraceptive measures are recommended during therapy.

Nursing Implications Stability: Protect from light

Dosage Forms Tablet: 2 mg [sugar coated]

Extemporaneous Preparations A 2 mg/mL suspension was stable for 7 days when refrigerated and compounded as follows: Pulverize sixty 2 mg tablets; levigate with a small amount of glycerin; add 20 mL Cologel® and levigate until a uniform mixture is obtained; add a 2:1 simple syrup/cherry syrup mixture to make a total volume of 60 mL

Handbook on Extemporaneous Formulations, Bethesda, MD: American Society of Hospital Pharmacists, 1987.

Chloramphenicol *(klor am FEN i kole)*

Related Information
Antimicrobial Drugs of Choice *on page 1588*
Community-Acquired Pneumonia in Adults *on page 1603*

U.S. Brand Names Chloromycetin®; Chloroptic®; Ocu-Chlor®

Canadian Brand Names Chloromycetin®; Diochloram®; Pentamycetin®

Therapeutic Category Antibiotic, Anaerobic; Antibiotic, Ophthalmic; Antibiotic, Otic; Antibiotic, Miscellaneous

Use Treatment of serious infections due to organisms resistant to other less toxic antibiotics or when its penetrability into the site of infection is clinically superior to other antibiotics to which the organism is sensitive; useful in infections caused by *Bacteroides, H. influenzae, Neisseria meningitidis, Salmonella,* and *Rickettsia;* active against many vancomycin-resistant enterococci

Pregnancy Risk Factor C

Pregnancy/Breast-Feeding Implications Embryotoxic and teratogenic in animals, but no adequate, well-controlled trials in pregnant women. Has been shown to cross placental barrier. Excreted in breast milk (even with topical application); breast-feeding is not recommended.

Contraindications Hypersensitivity to chloramphenicol or any component of the formulation

Warnings/Precautions Use with caution in patients with impaired renal or hepatic function and in neonates; reduce dose with impaired liver function; use with care in patients with glucose 6-phosphate dehydrogenase deficiency. Serious and fatal blood dyscrasias have occurred after both short-term and prolonged therapy, including reports associated with topical treatment; should not be used when less potentially toxic agents are effective; prolonged use may result in superinfection.

Adverse Reactions

Ophthalmic:

1% to 10%:

Local: Burning or stinging

Ocular: Blurred vision

Miscellaneous: Hypersensitivity reactions

<1% (Limited to important or life-threatening): Blood dyscrasias

Systemic:

1% to 10%:

Gastrointestinal: Diarrhea, nausea, vomiting

Hematologic: Blood dyscrasias

<1% (Limited to important or life-threatening): Aplastic anemia, bone marrow suppression, enterocolitis, gray baby syndrome, headache, nightmares, optic neuritis, peripheral neuropathy, stomatitis

Three major toxicities associated with chloramphenicol include:

Aplastic anemia (idiosyncratic reaction, any route of administration; usually occurs 3 weeks to 12 months after initial exposure to chloramphenicol)

Bone marrow suppression (dose-related; serum concentrations >25 µg/mL)

Gray baby syndrome (circulatory collapse, cyanosis, acidosis, abdominal distention, myocardial depression, coma, and death). Appears to be associated with serum levels ≥50 µg/mL; may result from drug accumulation in patients with impaired hepatic or renal function.

Topical:

>10%: Miscellaneous: Hypersensitivity reactions

<1% (Limited to important or life-threatening): Blood dyscrasias

Overdosage/Toxicology Symptoms include anemia, metabolic acidosis, hypotension, and hypothermia. Treatment is supportive following GI decontamination.

Drug Interactions

Cytochrome P450 Effect: CYP2C9 enzyme inhibitor

Increased Effect/Toxicity: Chloramphenicol increases serum concentrations of chlorpropamide, phenytoin, and oral anticoagulants.

Decreased Effect: Phenobarbital and rifampin may decrease serum concentrations of chloramphenicol.

Ethanol/Nutrition/Herb Interactions Food: May decrease intestinal absorption of vitamin B_{12} may have increased dietary need for riboflavin, pyridoxine, and vitamin B_{12}.

Stability Refrigerate ophthalmic solution; parenteral reconstituted solutions remain stable for 30 days; use only clear solutions; frozen solutions remain stable for 6 months

Mechanism of Action Reversibly binds to 50S ribosomal subunits of susceptible organisms preventing amino acids from being transferred to growing peptide chains thus inhibiting protein synthesis

Pharmacodynamics/Kinetics

Distribution: To most tissues and body fluids; readily crosses placenta; enters breast milk

CSF:blood level ratio: Normal meninges: 66%; Inflamed meninges: >66%

Protein binding: 60%

Metabolism: Extensively hepatic (90%) to inactive metabolites, principally by glucuronidation, chloramphenicol palmitate is hydrolyzed by lipases in the GI tract to the active base; chloramphenicol sodium succinate is hydrolyzed by esterases to active base

Half-life elimination

Normal renal function: 1.6-3.3 hours

End-stage renal disease: 3-7 hours

Cirrhosis: 10-12 hours

Neonates: Postnatal: 1-2 days old: 24 hours; 10-16 days old: 10 hours

Time to peak: Oral: Within 0.5-3 hours

Excretion: Urine (5% to 15%); Neonates: Urine (6% to 80% as unchanged drug), feces (4%)

Usual Dosage

Meningitis: I.V.: Infants >30 days and Children: 50-100 mg/kg/day divided every 6 hours

Other infections: I.V.:

Infants >30 days and Children: 50-75 mg/kg/day divided every 6 hours; maximum daily dose: 4 g/day

Adults: 50-100 mg/kg/day in divided doses every 6 hours; maximum daily dose: 4 g/day

Ophthalmic: Children and Adults: Instill 1-2 drops 4-6 times/day or 1.25 cm ($^1/_2$" of ointment every 3-4 hours); increase interval between applications after 72 hours to 2-3 times/day; treatment should continue for ~7 days

Otic solution: Instill 2-3 drops into ear 3 times/day

Topical: Gently rub into the affected area 1-4 times/day

Dosing adjustment/comments in hepatic impairment: Avoid use in severe liver impairment as increased toxicity may occur

Hemodialysis: Slightly dialyzable (5% to 20%) via hemo- and peritoneal dialysis; no supplemental doses needed in dialysis or continuous arteriovenous or veno-venous hemofiltration

Dietary Considerations May have increased dietary need for riboflavin, pyridoxine, and vitamin B_{12}.

Administration Do not administer I.M.

Monitoring Parameters CBC with reticulocyte and platelet counts, periodic liver and renal function tests, serum drug concentration

Reference Range

Therapeutic levels:

Meningitis:

Peak: 15-25 µg/mL; toxic concentration: >40 µg/mL

Trough: 5-15 µg/mL

Other infections:

Peak: 10-20 µg/mL

Trough: 5-10 µg/mL

(Continued)

Chloramphenicol *(Continued)*

Timing of serum samples: Draw levels 1.5 hours and 3 hours after completion of I.V. or oral dose; trough levels may be preferred; should be drawn ≤1 hour prior to dose

Nursing Implications Draw peak level 2 hours post oral dose or draw peak levels 90 minutes after the end of a 30-minute infusion; trough levels should be drawn just prior to the next dose; can be administered IVP over 5 minutes at a maximum concentration of 100 mg/mL, or I.V. intermittent infusion over 15-30 minutes at a final concentration for administration of ≤20 mg/mL

Additional Information Sodium content of 1 g injection: 51.8 mg (2.25 mEq)

Dosage Forms
Capsule: 250 mg
Ointment, ophthalmic: 1% [10 mg/g] (3.5 g)
Chloromycetin®, Chloroptic® S.O.P., Ocu-Chlor®: 1% [10 mg/g] (3.5 g)
Powder for injection, as sodium succinate: 1 g
Powder for ophthalmic solution (Chloromycetin®): 25 mg/vial (15 mL)
Solution: 0.5% [5 mg/mL] (7.5 mL, 15 mL)
Solution, ophthalmic (Chloroptic®, Ocu-Chlor®): 0.5% [5 mg/mL] (2.5 mL, 7.5 mL, 15 mL)
Solution, otic (Chloromycetin®): 0.5% (15 mL)

Chlordiazepoxide *(klor dye az e POKS ide)*

Related Information
Antacid Drug Interactions *on page 1477*
Benzodiazepines Comparison *on page 1490*
U.S. Brand Names Librium®
Canadian Brand Names Apo®-Chlordiazepoxide; Novo-Poxide®
Synonyms Methaminodiazepoxide Hydrochloride
Therapeutic Category Benzodiazepine; Hypnotic; Sedative
Use Management of anxiety disorder or for the short-term relief of symptoms of anxiety; withdrawal symptoms of acute alcoholism; preoperative apprehension and anxiety
Restrictions C-IV
Pregnancy Risk Factor D
Contraindications Hypersensitivity to chlordiazepoxide or any component of the formulation (cross-sensitivity with other benzodiazepines may exist); narrow-angle glaucoma (not in product labeling: however, benzodiazepines are contraindicated); pregnancy
Warnings/Precautions Active metabolites with extended half-lives may lead to delayed accumulation and adverse effects. Use with caution in elderly or debilitated patients, pediatric patients, patients with hepatic disease (including alcoholics) or renal impairment, patients with respiratory disease or impaired gag reflex, patients with porphyria.

Parenteral administration should be avoided in comatose patients or shock. Adequate resuscitative equipment/personnel should be available, and appropriate monitoring should be conducted at the time of injection and for several hours following administration. The parenteral formulation should be diluted for I.M. administration with the supplied diluent only. This diluent should not be used when preparing the drug for intravenous administration.

Causes CNS depression (dose-related) resulting in sedation, dizziness, confusion, or ataxia which may impair physical and mental capabilities. Patients must be cautioned about performing tasks which require mental alertness (ie, operating machinery or driving). Use with caution in patients receiving other CNS depressants or psychoactive agents (lithium, phenothiazines). Effects with other sedative drugs or ethanol may be potentiated. Benzodiazepines have been associated with falls and traumatic injury and should be used with extreme caution in patients who are at risk of these events (especially the elderly).

Use caution in patients with depression, particularly if suicidal risk may be present. Use with caution in patients with a history of drug dependence. Benzodiazepines have been associated with dependence and acute withdrawal symptoms on discontinuation or reduction in dose. Acute withdrawal, including seizures, may be precipitated in patients after administration of flumazenil to patients receiving long-term benzodiazepine therapy.

Benzodiazepines have been associated with anterograde amnesia. Paradoxical reactions, including hyperactive or aggressive behavior have been reported with benzodiazepines, particularly in adolescent/pediatric or psychiatric patients. Does not have analgesic, antidepressant, or antipsychotic properties.

Adverse Reactions
>10%:
Central nervous system: Drowsiness, fatigue, ataxia, lightheadedness, memory impairment, dysarthria, irritability
Dermatologic: Rash
Endocrine & metabolic: Decreased libido, menstrual disorders
Gastrointestinal: Xerostomia, decreased salivation, increased or decreased appetite, weight gain/loss
Genitourinary: Micturition difficulties
1% to 10%:
Cardiovascular: Hypotension
Central nervous system: Confusion, dizziness, disinhibition, akathisia, increased libido
Dermatologic: Dermatitis
Gastrointestinal: Increased salivation
Genitourinary: Sexual dysfunction, incontinence
Neuromuscular & skeletal: Rigidity, tremor, muscle cramps
Otic: Tinnitus
Respiratory: Nasal congestion
Overdosage/Toxicology Symptoms include hypotension, respiratory depression, coma, hypothermia, and cardiac arrhythmias. Treatment for benzodiazepine overdose is supportive. Flumazenil has been shown to selectively block the binding of benzodiazepines to CNS

receptors, resulting in a reversal of benzodiazepine-induced CNS depression. Respiratory depression may not be reversed.

Drug Interactions
Cytochrome P450 Effect: CYP3A3/4 enzyme substrate
Increased Effect/Toxicity: Chlordiazepoxide potentiates the CNS depressant effects of narcotic analgesics, barbiturates, phenothiazines, ethanol, antihistamines, MAO inhibitors, sedative-hypnotics, and cyclic antidepressants. Serum concentrations/effects of chlordiazepoxide may be increased by inhibitors of CYP3A3/4, including cimetidine, ciprofloxacin, clarithromycin, clozapine, diltiazem, disulfiram, digoxin, erythromycin, ethanol, fluconazole, fluoxetine, fluvoxamine, grapefruit juice, isoniazid, itraconazole, ketoconazole, labetalol, levodopa, loxapine, metoprolol, metronidazole, miconazole, nefazodone, omeprazole, phenytoin, rifabutin, rifampin, troleandomycin, valproic acid, and verapamil.
Decreased Effect: Carbamazepine, rifampin, rifabutin may enhance the metabolism of chlordiazepoxide and decrease its therapeutic effect.

Ethanol/Nutrition/Herb Interactions
Ethanol: Avoid ethanol (may increase CNS depression).
Food: Serum concentrations/effects may be increased with grapefruit juice, but unlikely because of high oral bioavailability of chlordiazepoxide.
Herb/Nutraceutical: Avoid valerian, St John's wort, kava kava, gotu kola (may increase CNS depression).

Stability Refrigerate injection; protect from light; **incompatible** when mixed with Ringer's solution, normal saline, ascorbic acid, benzquinamide, heparin, phenytoin, promethazine, secobarbital

Mechanism of Action Binds to stereospecific benzodiazepine receptors on the postsynaptic GABA neuron at several sites within the central nervous system, including the limbic system, reticular formation. Enhancement of the inhibitory effect of GABA on neuronal excitability results in increased neuronal membrane permeability to chloride ions. This shift in chloride ions results in hyperpolarization (a less excitable state) and stabilization.

Pharmacodynamics/Kinetics
Duration: 2-7 days
Absorption: I.M.: Results in lower peak plasma levels than oral
Distribution: V_d: 3.3 L/kg; crosses placenta; enters breast milk
Protein binding: 90% to 98%
Metabolism: Extensively hepatic to desmethyldiazepam (active and long-acting)
Half-life elimination: 6.6-25 hours; End-stage renal disease: 5-30 hours; Cirrhosis: 30-63 hours
Time to peak, serum: Oral: Within 2 hours
Excretion: Urine (minimal as unchanged drug)

Usual Dosage
Children:
<6 years: Not recommended
>6 years: Anxiety: Oral, I.M.: 0.5 mg/kg/24 hours divided every 6-8 hours
Adults:
Anxiety:
Oral: 15-100 mg divided 3-4 times/day
I.M., I.V.: Initial: 50-100 mg followed by 25-50 mg 3-4 times/day as needed
Preoperative anxiety: I.M.: 50-100 mg prior to surgery
Ethanol withdrawal symptoms: Oral, I.V.: 50-100 mg to start, dose may be repeated in 2-4 hours as necessary to a maximum of 300 mg/24 hours
Dosing adjustment in renal impairment: Cl_{cr} <10 mL/minute: Administer 50% of dose
Hemodialysis: Not dialyzable (0% to 5%)
Dosing adjustment/comments in hepatic impairment: Avoid use

Administration Up to 300 mg may be given I.M. or I.V. during a 6-hour period, but not more than this in any 24-hour period; do not use diluent provided with parenteral form for I.V. administration; dissolve with normal saline instead; I.V. form is a powder and should be reconstituted with 5 mL of sterile water or saline prior to administration

Monitoring Parameters Respiratory and cardiovascular status, mental status, check for orthostasis

Reference Range Therapeutic: 0.1-3 µg/mL (SI: 0-10 µmol/L); Toxic: >23 µg/mL (SI: >77 µmol/L)

Patient Information Avoid alcohol and other CNS depressants; avoid activities needing good psychomotor coordination until CNS effects are known; drug may cause physical or psychological dependence; avoid abrupt discontinuation after prolonged use, may cause drowsiness, poor balance

Nursing Implications Raise bed rails; initiate safety measures; aid with ambulation

Additional Information Abrupt discontinuation after sustained use (generally >10 days) may cause withdrawal symptoms.

Dosage Forms
Capsule, as hydrochloride: 5 mg, 10 mg, 25 mg
Powder for injection, as hydrochloride: 100 mg

◆ **Chlordiazepoxide and Amitriptyline** see Amitriptyline and Chlordiazepoxide on page 78
◆ **Chlordiazepoxide and Clidinium** see Clidinium and Chlordiazepoxide on page 309

Chlorhexidine Gluconate (klor HEKS i deen GLOO koe nate)

U.S. Brand Names BactoShield® [OTC]; Betasept® [OTC]; Dyna-Hex® [OTC]; Exidine® Scrub [OTC]; Hibiclens® [OTC]; Hibistat® [OTC]; Peridex® Oral Rinse; PerioChip®; PerioGard®
Therapeutic Category Antibacterial, Oral Rinse; Mouthwash
Use Skin cleanser for surgical scrub, cleanser for skin wounds, germicidal hand rinse, and as antibacterial dental rinse. Chlorhexidine is active against gram-positive and gram-negative organisms, facultative anaerobes, aerobes, and yeast.
Orphan drug: Peridex®: Oral mucositis with cytoreductive therapy when used for patients undergoing bone marrow transplant
Pregnancy Risk Factor B
(Continued)

Chlorhexidine Gluconate *(Continued)*

Contraindications Hypersensitivity to chlorhexidine gluconate or any component of the formulation

Warnings/Precautions Staining of oral surfaces, tooth restorations, and dorsum of tongue may occur; keep out of eyes and ears; for topical use only; there have been case reports of anaphylaxis following chlorhexidine disinfection

Adverse Reactions

>10%: Oral: Increase of tartar on teeth, changes in taste. Staining of oral surfaces (mucosa, teeth, dorsum of tongue) may be visible as soon as 1 week after therapy begins and is more pronounced when there is a heavy accumulation of unremoved plaque and when teeth fillings have rough surfaces. Stain does not have a clinically adverse effect but because removal may not be possible, patient with frontal restoration should be advised of the potential permanency of the stain.

1% to 10%: Gastrointestinal: Tongue irritation, oral irritation

<1% (Limited to important or life-threatening): Dyspnea, facial edema, nasal congestion

Overdosage/Toxicology Symptoms of oral overdose include gastric distress, nausea, or signs of ethanol intoxication.

Stability Store at room temperature

Mechanism of Action The bactericidal effect of chlorhexidine is a result of the binding of this cationic molecule to negatively charged bacterial cell walls and extramicrobial complexes. At low concentrations, this causes an alteration of bacterial cell osmotic equilibrium and leakage of potassium and phosphorous resulting in a bacteriostatic effect. At high concentrations of chlorhexidine, the cytoplasmic contents of the bacterial cell precipitate and result in cell death.

Pharmacodynamics/Kinetics

Absorption: ~30% retained in oral cavity following rinsing and slowly released into oral fluids; GI tract: poor

Time to peak, plasma: Detectable levels are not present after 12 hours

Excretion: Primarily feces (~90%); urine (<1%)

Usual Dosage Adults:

Oral rinse (Peridex®):

Precede use of solution by flossing and brushing teeth; completely rinse toothpaste from mouth. Swish 15 mL undiluted oral rinse around in mouth for 30 seconds, then expectorate. Caution patient not to swallow the medicine. Avoid eating for 2-3 hours after treatment. (The cap on bottle of oral rinse is a measure for 15 mL.)

When used as a treatment of gingivitis, the regimen begins with oral prophylaxis. Patient treats mouth with 15 mL chlorhexidine, swishes for 30 seconds, then expectorates. This is repeated twice daily (morning and evening). Patient should have a re-evaluation followed by a dental prophylaxis every 6 months.

Cleanser:

Surgical scrub: Scrub 3 minutes and rinse thoroughly, wash for an additional 3 minutes

Hand wash: Wash for 15 seconds and rinse

Hand rinse: Rub 15 seconds and rinse

Periodontal chip: Adults: One chip is inserted into a periodontal pocket with a probing pocket depth ≥5 mm. Up to 8 chips may be inserted in a single visit. Treatment is recommended every 3 months in pockets with a remaining depth ≥5 mm. If dislodgment occurs 7 days or more after placement, the subject is considered to have had the full course of treatment. If dislodgment occurs within 48 hours, a new chip should be inserted.

Administration Insertion of periodontal chip: Pocket should be isolated and surrounding area dried prior to chip insertion. The chip should be grasped using forceps with the rounded edges away from the forceps. The chip should be inserted into the periodontal pocket to its maximum depth. It may be maneuvered into position using the tips of the forceps or a flat instrument. The chip biodegrades completely and does not need to be removed. Patients should avoid dental floss at the site of PerioChip® insertion for 10 days after placement because flossing might dislodge the chip.

Patient Information

Oral rinse: Do not swallow, do not rinse after use; may cause reduced taste perception which is reversible; may cause discoloration of teeth

Topical administration is for external use only

Nursing Implications Inform patient that reduced taste perception during treatment is reversible with discontinuation of chlorhexidine

Dosage Forms

Chip, for periodontal pocket insertion (PerioChip®): 2.5 mg

Foam, topical, with isopropyl alcohol 4% (BactoShield®): 4% (180 mL)

Liquid, topical, with isopropyl alcohol 2%:

BactoShield® 2: 2% (960 mL)

Dyna-Hex® Skin Cleanser: 2% (120 mL, 240 mL, 480 mL, 960 mL, 4000 mL)

Liquid, topical, with isopropyl alcohol 4%:

BactoShield®, Betasept®, Exidine® Skin Cleanser, Hibiclens® Skin Cleanser: 4% (15 mL, 120 mL, 240 mL, 480 mL, 960 mL, 4000 mL)

Dyna-Hex® Skin Cleanser: 4% (120 mL, 240 mL, 480 mL, 4000 mL)

Rinse, oral (Peridex®, PerioGard®): 0.12% with alcohol 11.6% (480 mL) [mint flavor]

Rinse, topical (Hibistat® Hand Rinse): 0.5% with isopropyl alcohol 70% (120 mL, 240 mL)

Sponge/Brush (Hibiclens®): 4% with isopropyl alcohol 4% (22 mL)

Wipes (Hibistat®): 0.5% with isopropyl alcohol 70% (50s)

◆ **2-Chlorodeoxyadenosine** *see* Cladribine *on page 305*

◆ **Chloromycetin®** *see* Chloramphenicol *on page 272*

Chloroprocaine *(klor oh PROE kane)*

U.S. Brand Names Nesacaine®; Nesacaine®-MPF

Canadian Brand Names Nesacaine®-CE

Synonyms Chloroprocaine Hydrochloride

Therapeutic Category Local Anesthetic, Injectable

Use Infiltration anesthesia and peripheral and epidural anesthesia

Pregnancy Risk Factor C

Contraindications Hypersensitivity to chloroprocaine, other ester type anesthetics, or any component of the formulation; myasthenia gravis; concurrent use of bupivacaine; do not use for subarachnoid administration

Warnings/Precautions Use with caution in patients with cardiac disease, renal disease, and hyperthyroidism; convulsions and cardiac arrest have been reported presumably due to intravascular injection

Adverse Reactions <1% (Limited to important or life-threatening): Anaphylactoid reactions, anxiety, bradycardia, cardiovascular collapse, chills, confusion, disorientation, drowsiness, edema, hypotension, myocardial depression, nausea, respiratory arrest, restlessness, seizures, shivering, tinnitus, tremor, unconsciousness, vomiting

Overdosage/Toxicology Treatment is primarily symptomatic and supportive. Termination of anesthesia by pneumatic tourniquet inflation should be attempted when the agent is administered by infiltration or regional injection. Hypotension responds to I.V. fluids and Trendelenburg positioning. Other symptoms (seizures, bradyarrhythmias, metabolic acidosis, methemoglobinemia) respond to conventional treatments.

Drug Interactions

Increased Effect/Toxicity: Avoid concurrent use of bupivacaine due to safety and efficacy concerns.

Decreased Effect: The para-aminobenzoic acid metabolite of chloroprocaine may decrease the efficacy of sulfonamide antibiotics.

Mechanism of Action Chloroprocaine HCl is benzoic acid, 4-amino-2-chloro-2-(diethylamino) ethyl ester monohydrochloride. Chloroprocaine is an ester-type local anesthetic, which stabilizes the neuronal membranes and prevents initiation and transmission of nerve impulses thereby affecting local anesthetic actions. Local anesthetics including chloroprocaine, reversibly prevent generation and conduction of electrical impulses in neurons by decreasing the transient increase in permeability to sodium. The differential sensitivity generally depends on the size of the fiber; small fibers are more sensitive than larger fibers and require a longer period for recovery. Sensory pain fibers are usually blocked first, followed by fibers that transmit sensations of temperature, touch, and deep pressure. High concentrations block sympathetic somatic sensory and somatic motor fibers. The spread of anesthesia depends upon the distribution of the solution. This is primarily dependent on the volume of drug injected.

Pharmacodynamics/Kinetics

Onset of action: 6-12 minutes

Duration: 30-60 minutes

Usual Dosage Dosage varies with anesthetic procedure, the area to be anesthetized, the vascularity of the tissues, depth of anesthesia required, degree of muscle relaxation required, and duration of anesthesia; range: 1.5-25 mL of 2% to 3% solution; single adult dose should not exceed 800 mg

Infiltration and peripheral nerve block: 1% to 2%

Infiltration, peripheral and central nerve block, including caudal and epidural block: 2% to 3%, without preservatives

Administration Before injecting, withdraw syringe plunger to ensure injection is not into vein or artery

Nursing Implications Must have resuscitative equipment available

Dosage Forms

Injection, as hydrochloride (Nesacaine®) [with preservative]: 1% (30 mL); 2% (30 mL)

Injection, as hydrochloride (Nesacaine®-MPF) [preservative free]: 2% (20 mL); 3% (20 mL)

♦ **Chloroprocaine Hydrochloride** see Chloroprocaine on page 276

♦ **Chloroptic®** see Chloramphenicol on page 272

Chloroquine (KLOR oh kwin)

Related Information

Malaria Treatment on page 1607

Prevention of Malaria on page 1552

U.S. Brand Names Aralen® Phosphate

Canadian Brand Names Aralen®

Synonyms Chloroquine Phosphate

Therapeutic Category Amebicide; Antimalarial Agent

Use Suppression or chemoprophylaxis of malaria; treatment of uncomplicated or mild to moderate malaria; extraintestinal amebiasis

Unlabeled/Investigational Use Rheumatoid arthritis; discoid lupus erythematosus, scleroderma, pemphigus

Pregnancy Risk Factor C

Contraindications Hypersensitivity to chloroquine or any component of the formulation; retinal or visual field changes; patients with psoriasis

Warnings/Precautions Use with caution in patients with liver disease, G6PD deficiency, alcoholism or in conjunction with hepatotoxic drugs, psoriasis, porphyria may be exacerbated; retinopathy (irreversible) has occurred with long or high-dose therapy; discontinue drug if any abnormality in the visual field or if muscular weakness develops during treatment

Adverse Reactions Frequency not defined.

Cardiovascular: Hypotension (rare), EKG changes (rare)

Central nervous system: Fatigue, personality changes, headache

Dermatologic: Pruritus, hair bleaching, pleomorphic skin eruptions, alopecia, lichen planus eruptions, alopecia, mucosal pigmentary changes (blue-black)

Gastrointestinal: Nausea, diarrhea, vomiting, anorexia, stomatitis

Hematologic: Blood dyscrasias

Ocular: Retinopathy (including irreversible changes in some patients long-term or high dose), blurred vision

Otic: Nerve deafness, tinnitus

(Continued)

Chloroquine (Continued)

Overdosage/Toxicology Symptoms include headache, visual changes, cardiovascular collapse, seizures, abdominal cramps, vomiting, cyanosis, methemoglobinemia, leukopenia, respiratory and cardiac arrest. Following initial measures (immediate GI decontamination), treatment is supportive and symptomatic.

Drug Interactions

Increased Effect/Toxicity: Chloroquine serum concentrations may be elevated with concomitant cimetidine use.

Decreased Effect: Decreased absorption if administered concomitantly with kaolin and magnesium trisilicate.

Ethanol/Nutrition/Herb Interactions Ethanol: Avoid ethanol (may increase GI irritation).

Mechanism of Action Binds to and inhibits DNA and RNA polymerase; interferes with metabolism and hemoglobin utilization by parasites; inhibits prostaglandin effects; chloroquine concentrates within parasite acid vesicles and raises internal pH resulting in inhibition of parasite growth; may involve aggregates of ferriprotoporphyrin IX acting as chloroquine receptors causing membrane damage; may also interfere with nucleoprotein synthesis

Pharmacodynamics/Kinetics

Duration: Small amounts may be present in urine months following discontinuation of therapy

Absorption: Oral: Rapid (~89%)

Distribution: Widely in body tissues (eg, eyes, heart, kidneys, liver, lungs) where retention prolonged; crosses placenta; enters breast milk

Metabolism: Partially hepatic

Half-life elimination: 3-5 days

Time to peak, serum: 1-2 hours

Excretion: Urine (~70% as unchanged drug); acidification of urine increases elimination

Usual Dosage Oral **(dosage expressed in terms of mg of base):**

Suppression or prophylaxis of malaria:

Children: Administer 5 mg base/kg/week on the same day each week (not to exceed 300 mg base/dose); begin 1-2 weeks prior to exposure; continue for 4-6 weeks after leaving endemic area; if suppressive therapy is not begun prior to exposure, double the initial loading dose to 10 mg base/kg and administer in 2 divided doses 6 hours apart, followed by the usual dosage regimen

Adults: 300 mg/week (base) on the same day each week; begin 1-2 weeks prior to exposure; continue for 4-6 weeks after leaving endemic area; if suppressive therapy is not begun prior to exposure, double the initial loading dose to 600 mg base and administer in 2 divided doses 6 hours apart, followed by the usual dosage regimen

Acute attack:

Oral:

Children: 10 mg/kg on day 1, followed by 5 mg/kg 6 hours later and 5 mg/kg on days 2 and 3

Adults: 600 mg on day 1, followed by 300 mg 6 hours later, followed by 300 mg on days 2 and 3

I.M. (as hydrochloride):

Children: 5 mg/kg, repeat in 6 hours

Adults: Initial: 160-200 mg, repeat in 6 hours if needed; maximum: 800 mg first 24 hours; begin oral dosage as soon as possible and continue for 3 days until 1.5 g has been given

Extraintestinal amebiasis:

Children: Oral: 10 mg/kg once daily for 2-3 weeks (up to 300 mg base/day)

Adults:

Oral: 600 mg base/day for 2 days followed by 300 mg base/day for at least 2-3 weeks

I.M., as hydrochloride: 160-200 mg/day for 10 days; resume oral therapy as soon as possible

Dosing adjustment in renal impairment: Cl_{cr} <10 mL/minute: Administer 50% of dose

Hemodialysis: Minimally removed by hemodialysis

Dietary Considerations May be taken with meals to decrease GI upset.

Monitoring Parameters Periodic CBC, examination for muscular weakness, and ophthalmologic examination in patients receiving prolonged therapy

Patient Information Take with meals; report any visual disturbances or difficulty in hearing or ringing in the ears; tablets are bitter tasting; may cause diarrhea, loss of appetite, nausea, stomach pain; notify physician if these become severe

Nursing Implications

Chloroquine phosphate tablets have also been mixed with chocolate syrup or enclosed in gelatin capsules to mask the bitter taste

Monitor periodic CBC, examination for muscular weakness and ophthalmologic examination in patients receiving prolonged therapy

Dosage Forms

Injection, as hydrochloride: 50 mg/mL [equivalent to 40 mg base/mL] (5 mL)

Tablet, as phosphate: 250 mg [equivalent to 150 mg base]; 500 mg [equivalent to 300 mg base]

Extemporaneous Preparations A 10 mg chloroquine base/mL suspension is made by pulverizing two Aralen® 500 mg phosphate = 300 mg base/tablet, levigating with sterile water, and adding by geometric proportion, a significant amount of the cherry syrup and levigating until a uniform mixture is obtained; qs ad to 60 mL with cherry syrup, stable for up to 4 weeks when stored in the refrigerator or at a temperature of 29°C

Mirochnick M, Barnett E, Clarke DF, et al, "Stability of Chloroquine in an Extemporaneously Prepared Suspension Stored at Three Temperatures," *Pediatr Infect Dis J*, 1994, 13(9):827-8.

♦ **Chloroquine Phosphate** *see* Chloroquine *on page 277*

Chlorothiazide (klor oh THYE a zide)

Related Information
Sulfonamide Derivatives *on page 1515*
U.S. Brand Names Diuril®
Canadian Brand Names Diuril®
Therapeutic Category Antihypertensive Agent; Diuretic, Thiazide
Use Management of mild to moderate hypertension, or edema associated with congestive heart failure or nephrotic syndrome in patients unable to take oral hydrochlorothiazide; when a thiazide is the diuretic of choice
Pregnancy Risk Factor C (manufacturer); D (expert analysis)
Usual Dosage Note: The manufacturer states that I.V. and oral dosing are equivalent. Some clinicians may use lower I.V. doses, however, because of chlorothiazide's poor oral absorption.
Infants <6 months:
Oral: 20-40 mg/kg/day in 2 divided doses
I.V.: 2-8 mg/kg/day in 2 divided doses
Infants >6 months and Children:
Oral: 20 mg/kg/day in 2 divided doses
I.V.: 4 mg/kg/day
Adults:
Oral: 500 mg to 2 g/day divided in 1-2 doses
I.V.: 100-500 mg/day (for edema only)
Elderly: Oral: 500 mg once daily **or** 1 g 3 times/week
Additional Information Complete prescribing information for this medication should be consulted for additional detail.
Dosage Forms
Powder for injection, lyophilized, as sodium: 500 mg
Suspension, oral: 250 mg/5 mL (237 mL)
Tablet: 250 mg, 500 mg

♦ **Chlorpheniramine, Acetaminophen, and Pseudoephedrine** *see* Acetaminophen, Chlorpheniramine, and Pseudoephedrine *on page 27*

Chlorpheniramine and Acetaminophen
(klor fen IR a meen & a seet a MIN oh fen)
U.S. Brand Names Coricidin® [OTC]
Synonyms Acetaminophen and Chlorpheniramine
Therapeutic Category Antihistamine/Analgesic
Use Symptomatic relief of congestion, headache, aches and pains of colds and flu
Usual Dosage Adults: Oral: 2 tablets every 4 hours
Additional Information Complete prescribing information for this medication should be consulted for additional detail.
Dosage Forms Tablet: Chlorpheniramine maleate 2 mg and acetaminophen 325 mg

♦ **Chlorpheniramine and Hydrocodone** *see* Hydrocodone and Chlorpheniramine *on page 679*

Chlorpheniramine and Phenylephrine (klor fen IR a meen & fen il EF rin)
U.S. Brand Names Dallergy-D®; Ed A-Hist®; Histatab® Plus [OTC]; Histor-D®; Rolatuss® Plain; Ru-Tuss®
Synonyms Phenylephrine and Chlorpheniramine
Therapeutic Category Antihistamine/Decongestant Combination
Use Temporary relief of nasal congestion and eustachian tube congestion as well as runny nose, sneezing, itching of nose or throat, itchy and watery eyes
Pregnancy Risk Factor C
Usual Dosage Oral:
Children:
2-5 years: 2.5 mL every 4 hours
6-12 years: 5 mL every 4 hours
Adults: 10 mL every 4 hours
Additional Information Complete prescribing information for this medication should be consulted for additional detail.
Dosage Forms
Liquid:
Dallergy-D®, Histor-D®, Rolatuss® Plain, Ru-Tuss®: Chlorpheniramine maleate 2 mg and phenylephrine hydrochloride 5 mg per 5 mL
Ed A-Hist® Liquid: Chlorpheniramine maleate 4 mg and phenylephrine hydrochloride 10 mg per 5 mL
Tablet (Histatab® Plus): Chlorpheniramine maleate 2 mg and phenylephrine hydrochloride 5 mg

Chlorpheniramine and Pseudoephedrine
(klor fen IR a meen & soo doe e FED rin)
U.S. Brand Names Allerest® Maximum Strength [OTC]; Anamine® [OTC]; Anaplex® [OTC]; Chlorafed® [OTC]; Chlor-Trimeton® Allergy/Decongestant [OTC]; Codimal-LA® [OTC]; Codimal-LA® Half [OTC]; Co-Pyronil® 2 Pulvules® [OTC]; Deconamine® [OTC]; Deconamine® SR [OTC]; Fedahist® [OTC]; Hayfebrol® [OTC]; Histalet® [OTC]; Klerist-D® [OTC]; Pseudo-Gest Plus® [OTC]; Rhinosyn® [OTC]; Rhinosyn-PD® [OTC]; Ryna® [OTC]; Sudafed® Cold & Allergy [OTC]
Synonyms Pseudoephedrine and Chlorpheniramine
Therapeutic Category Antihistamine/Decongestant Combination
Use Relief of nasal congestion associated with the common cold, hay fever, and other allergies, sinusitis, eustachian tube blockage, and vasomotor and allergic rhinitis
Pregnancy Risk Factor C
(Continued)

Chlorpheniramine and Pseudoephedrine *(Continued)*

Usual Dosage Oral:
Capsule: One every 12 hours
Tablet: One 3-4 times/day

Additional Information Complete prescribing information for this medication should be consulted for additional detail.

Dosage Forms
Capsule (Co-Pyronil® 2 Pulvules®): Chlorpheniramine maleate 4 mg and pseudoephedrine hydrochloride 60 mg

Capsule, sustained release:
Codimal-LA® Half: Chlorpheniramine maleate 4 mg and pseudoephedrine hydrochloride 60 mg

Deconamine® SR: Chlorpheniramine maleate 8 mg and pseudoephedrine hydrochloride 120 mg

Liquid:
Anamine®, Anaplex®, Chlorafed®, Deconamine®, Hayfebrol®, Rhinosyn-PD®, Ryna®: Chlorpheniramine maleate 2 mg and pseudoephedrine sulfate 30 mg per 5 mL
Histalet®: Chlorpheniramine maleate 3 mg and pseudoephedrine sulfate 45 mg per 5 mL
Rhinosyn®: Chlorpheniramine maleate 2 mg and pseudoephedrine sulfate 60 mg per 5 mL

Tablet:
Allerest® Maximum Strength: Chlorpheniramine maleate 2 mg and pseudoephedrine hydrochloride 30 mg
Chlor-Trimeton® 4-Hour, Deconamine®, Fedahist®, Klerist-D®, Pseudo-Gest Plus®, Sudafed® Cold & Allergy: Chlorpheniramine maleate 4 mg and pseudoephedrine hydrochloride 60 mg
Chlor-Trimeton® 12-Hour: Chlorpheniramine maleate 8 mg and pseudoephedrine hydrochloride 120 mg

Chlorpheniramine, Ephedrine, Phenylephrine, and Carbetapentane

(klor fen IR a meen, e FED rin, fen il EF rin, & kar bay ta PEN tane)

U.S. Brand Names Rentamine® [OTC]; Rynatuss® [OTC]; Rynatuss® Pediatric Suspension [OTC]; Tri-Tannate Plus® [OTC]

Therapeutic Category Antihistamine/Decongestant/Antitussive

Use Symptomatic relief of cough with a decongestant and an antihistamine

Pregnancy Risk Factor C

Usual Dosage Oral:
Children:
<2 years: Titrate dose individually
2-6 years: 2.5-5 mL every 12 hours
>6 years: 5-10 mL every 12 hours
Adults: 1-2 tablets every 12 hours

Additional Information Complete prescribing information for this medication should be consulted for additional detail.

Dosage Forms
Liquid: Carbetapentane tannate 30 mg, ephedrine tannate 5 mg, phenylephrine tannate 5 mg, and chlorpheniramine tannate 4 mg per 5 mL
Tablet: Carbetapentane tannate 60 mg, ephedrine tannate 10 mg, phenylephrine tannate 10 mg, and chlorpheniramine tannate 5 mg per 5 mL

♦ **Chlorpheniramine, Hydrocodone, Phenylephrine, Acetaminophen, and Caffeine** *see* Hydrocodone, Chlorpheniramine, Phenylephrine, Acetaminophen, and Caffeine *on page 682*

Chlorpheniramine, Phenylephrine, and Codeine With Potassium Iodide

(klor fen IR a meen, fen il EF rin, & KOE deen with poe TASS ee um EYE oh dide)

U.S. Brand Names Pediacof®; Pedituss®

Therapeutic Category Antihistamine/Decongestant/Antitussive

Use Symptomatic relief of rhinitis, nasal congestion and cough due to colds or allergy

Restrictions C-V

Usual Dosage Children 6 months to 12 years: 1.25-10 mL every 4-6 hours

Additional Information Complete prescribing information for this medication should be consulted for additional detail.

Dosage Forms
Liquid:
Pediacof®: Chlorpheniramine maleate 0.75 mg, phenylephrine hydrochloride 2.5 mg, and codeine phosphate 5 mg with potassium iodide 75 mg per 5 mL with alcohol 5%
Pedituss®: Chlorpheniramine maleate 0.75 mg, phenylephrine hydrochloride 2.5 mg, and codeine phosphate 5 mg with potassium iodide 75 mg per 5 mL

Chlorpheniramine, Phenylephrine, and Dextromethorphan

(klor fen IR a meen, fen il EF rin, & deks troe meth OR fan)

U.S. Brand Names Cerose-DM® [OTC]

Therapeutic Category Antihistamine/Decongestant/Antitussive

Use Temporary relief of cough due to minor throat and bronchial irritation; relieves nasal congestion, runny nose and sneezing

Usual Dosage Oral:
Children 6-12 years: ½ teaspoonful every 4 hour as needed; maximum: 6 doses/24 hours
Children >12 years and Adults: 1 teaspoonful every 4 hours as needed; maximum: 6 doses/24 hours

Additional Information Complete prescribing information for this medication should be consulted for additional detail.

Dosage Forms Liquid: Chlorpheniramine maleate 4 mg, phenylephrine hydrochloride 10 mg, and dextromethorphan hydrobromide 15 mg per 5 mL

Chlorpheniramine, Phenylephrine, and Methscopolamine
(klor fen IR a meen, fen il EF rin, & meth skoe POL a meen)
U.S. Brand Names D.A.II™; Dallergy®; Dura-Vent®/DA; Extendryl; Extendryl JR; Extendryl SR
Therapeutic Category Antihistamine/Decongestant/Anticholinergic
Use Treatment of upper respiratory symptoms such as respiratory congestion, allergic rhinitis, vasomotor rhinitis, sinusitis, and allergic skin reactions of urticaria and angioedema
Pregnancy Risk Factor C
Usual Dosage
Children 6-11 years: Relief of respiratory symptoms: Oral:
D.A.II™: One tablet every 12 hours
D.A. Chewable®, Extendryl chewable tablet: One tablet every 4 hours; do not exceed 4 doses in 24 hours
Dallergy®: One-half caplet every 12 hours
Dura-Vent®/DA: One-half tablet every 12 hours
Extendryl JR: One capsule every 12 hours
Extendryl syrup: 2.5-5 mL, may repeat up to every 4 hours depending on age and body weight
Children ≥12 years and Adults: Relief of respiratory symptoms: Oral: **Note:** If disturbances in urination occur in patients without renal impairment, medication should be discontinued for 1-2 days and should then be restarted at a lower dose
D.A.II™: Two tablets every 12 hours
Dallergy®, Extendryl SR: 1 capsule every 12 hours
Dura-Vent®/DA: One tablet every 12 hours
D.A. Chewable®, Extendryl: 1-2 chewable tablets every 4 hours
Extendryl syrup: 5-10 mL every 3-4 hours (4 times/day)
Elderly: Use with caution, may have increased adverse reactions
Dosage adjustment in renal impairment: Use is not recommended
Additional Information Complete prescribing information for this medication should be consulted for additional detail.
Dosage Forms
Caplet, sustained release (Dallergy®): Chlorpheniramine maleate 8 mg, phenylephrine hydrochloride 20 mg, and methscopolamine nitrate 2.5 mg
Capsule:
Extendryl JR: Chlorpheniramine maleate 4 mg, phenylephrine hydrochloride 10 mg, and methscopolamine nitrate 1.25 mg
Extendryl SR: Chlorpheniramine maleate 8 mg, phenylephrine hydrochloride 20 mg, and methscopolamine nitrate 2.5 mg
Syrup (Extendryl): Chlorpheniramine maleate 2 mg, phenylephrine hydrochloride 10 mg, and methscopolamine nitrate 1.25 mg per 5 mL [root beer flavor]
Tablet:
D.A.II™: Chlorpheniramine maleate 4 mg, phenylephrine hydrochloride 10 mg, and methscopolamine nitrate 1.25 mg
Dura-Vent®/DA: Chlorpheniramine maleate 8 mg, phenylephrine hydrochloride 20 mg, and methscopolamine nitrate 2.5 mg
Tablet, chewable:
D.A. Chewable®: Chlorpheniramine maleate 2 mg, phenylephrine hydrochloride 10 mg, and methscopolamine nitrate 1.25 mg [orange flavor, phenylalanine 7.5 mg/tablet]
Extendryl: Chlorpheniramine maleate 2 mg, phenylephrine hydrochloride 10 mg, and methscopolamine nitrate 1.25 mg [root beer flavor]

Chlorpheniramine, Phenylephrine, and Phenyltoloxamine
(klor fen IR a meen, fen il EF rin, & fen il tole LOKS a meen)
U.S. Brand Names Comhist®; Comhist® LA
Therapeutic Category Antihistamine/Decongestant Combination
Use Symptomatic relief of rhinitis and nasal congestion due to colds or allergy
Pregnancy Risk Factor C
Usual Dosage Oral: 1 capsule every 8-12 hours or 1-2 tablets 3 times/day
Additional Information Complete prescribing information for this medication should be consulted for additional detail.
Dosage Forms
Capsule, sustained release (Comhist® LA): Chlorpheniramine maleate 4 mg, phenylephrine hydrochloride 20 mg, and phenyltoloxamine citrate 50 mg
Tablet (Comhist®): Chlorpheniramine maleate 2 mg, phenylephrine hydrochloride 10 mg, and phenyltoloxamine citrate 25 mg

♦ **Chlorpheniramine, Pseudoephedrine, and Acetaminophen** see Acetaminophen, Chlorpheniramine, and Pseudoephedrine on page 27

Chlorpheniramine, Pseudoephedrine, and Codeine
(klor fen IR a meen, soo doe e FED rin, & KOE deen)
U.S. Brand Names Codehist® DH; Decohistine® DH; Dihistine® DH; Ryna-C®
Therapeutic Category Antihistamine/Decongestant/Antitussive
Use Temporary relief of cough associated with minor throat or bronchial irritation or nasal congestion due to common cold, allergic rhinitis, or sinusitis
Restrictions C-V
Pregnancy Risk Factor C
Usual Dosage Oral:
Children:
25-50 lb: 1.25-2.50 mL every 4-6 hours, up to 4 doses in 24-hour period
50-90 lb: 2.5-5 mL every 4-6 hours, up to 4 doses in 24-hour period
Adults: 10 mL every 4-6 hours, up to 4 doses in 24-hour period
(Continued)

Chlorpheniramine, Pseudoephedrine, and Codeine *(Continued)*

Additional Information Complete prescribing information for this medication should be consulted for additional detail.

Dosage Forms Liquid: Chlorpheniramine maleate 2 mg, pseudoephedrine hydrochloride 30 mg, and codeine phosphate 10 mg (120 mL, 480 mL)

Chlorpheniramine, Pyrilamine, and Phenylephrine

(klor fen IR a meen, pye RIL a meen, & fen il EF rin)

U.S. Brand Names Rhinatate®; R-Tannamine®; R-Tannate®; Rynatan® Pediatric Suspension; Tanoral®; Triotann®; Tri-Tannate®

Therapeutic Category Antihistamine/Decongestant Combination

Use Symptomatic relief of nasal congestion associated with upper respiratory tract condition

Pregnancy Risk Factor C

Usual Dosage
Children:
2-6 years: 2.5-5 mL (pediatric suspension) every 12 hours
>6 years: 5-10 mL (pediatric suspension) every 12 hours
Adults: 1-2 tablets every 12 hours

Additional Information Complete prescribing information for this medication should be consulted for additional detail.

Dosage Forms
Suspension, pediatric: Chlorpheniramine tannate 2 mg, pyrilamine tannate 12.5 mg, and phenylephrine tannate 5 mg per 5 mL
Tablet: Chlorpheniramine tannate 8 mg, pyrilamine maleate 25 mg, and phenylephrine tannate 25 mg

♦ **Chlorpromanyl® (Can)** *see* ChlorproMAZINE *on page 282*

ChlorproMAZINE (klor PROE ma zeen)

Related Information
Antacid Drug Interactions *on page 1477*
Antipsychotic Agents Comparison *on page 1486*

U.S. Brand Names Thorazine®

Canadian Brand Names Chlorpromanyl®; Largactil®

Synonyms Chlorpromazine Hydrochloride; CPZ

Therapeutic Category Antiemetic; Antipsychotic Agent, Phenothiazine; Phenothiazine Derivative

Use Control of mania; treatment of schizophrenia; control of nausea and vomiting; relief of restlessness and apprehension before surgery; acute intermittent porphyria; adjunct in the treatment of tetanus; intractable hiccups; combativeness and/or explosive hyperexcitable behavior in children 1-12 years of age and in short-term treatment of hyperactive children

Unlabeled/Investigational Use Management of psychotic disorders

Pregnancy Risk Factor C

Contraindications Hypersensitivity to chlorpromazine or any component of the formulation (cross-reactivity between phenothiazines may occur); severe CNS depression; coma

Warnings/Precautions Safety in children <6 months of age has not been established; use with caution in patients with seizures, bone marrow suppression, or severe liver disease
Significant hypotension may occur, especially when the drug is administered parenterally; injection contains benzyl alcohol; injection also contains sulfites which may cause allergic reaction
Tardive dyskinesia: Prevalence rate may be 40% in elderly; development of the syndrome and the irreversible nature are proportional to duration and total cumulative dose over time. May be reversible if diagnosed early in therapy.
Extrapyramidal reactions are more common in elderly with up to 50% developing these reactions after 60 years of age. Drug-induced **Parkinson's syndrome** occurs often. **Akathisia** is the most common extrapyramidal symptom in elderly.
Increased confusion, memory loss, psychotic behavior, and agitation frequently occur as a consequence of anticholinergic effects
Orthostatic hypotension is due to alpha-receptor blockade, the elderly are at greater risk for orthostatic hypotension
Antipsychotic associated sedation in nonpsychotic patients is extremely unpleasant due to feelings of depersonalization, derealization, and dysphoria
Life-threatening arrhythmias have occurred at therapeutic doses of antipsychotics

Adverse Reactions Frequency not defined.
Cardiovascular: Postural hypotension, tachycardia, dizziness, nonspecific QT changes
Central nervous system: Drowsiness, dystonias, akathisia, pseudoparkinsonism, tardive dyskinesia, neuroleptic malignant syndrome, seizures
Dermatologic: Photosensitivity, dermatitis, skin pigmentation (slate gray)
Endocrine & metabolic: Lactation, breast engorgement, false-positive pregnancy test, amenorrhea, gynecomastia, hyper- or hypoglycemia
Gastrointestinal: Xerostomia, constipation, nausea
Genitourinary: Urinary retention, ejaculatory disorder, impotence
Hematologic: Agranulocytosis, eosinophilia, leukopenia, hemolytic anemia, aplastic anemia, thrombocytopenic purpura
Hepatic: Jaundice
Ocular: Blurred vision, corneal and lenticular changes, epithelial keratopathy, pigmentary retinopathy

Overdosage/Toxicology Symptoms include deep sleep, coma, extrapyramidal symptoms, abnormal involuntary muscle movements, and hypotension. Following initiation of essential overdose management, toxic symptom treatment and supportive treatment should be initiated. Hypotension usually responds to I.V. fluids or Trendelenburg positioning. If unresponsive to these measures, the use of a parenteral inotrope may be required. Seizures commonly respond to diazepam (I.V. 5-10 mg bolus in adults every 15 minutes if needed up to a total of 30 mg; I.V. 0.25-0.4 mg/kg/dose up to a total of 10 mg in children) or to phenytoin or phenobarbital; critical cardiac arrhythmias often respond to I.V. phenytoin (15 mg/kg up to 1 g), while other antiarrhythmics can be used. Neuroleptics often cause extrapyramidal symptoms (eg, dystonic reactions) requiring management with anticholinergic agents such as benztropine mesylate I.V. 1-2 mg (adults) may be effective. These agents are generally effective within 2-5 minutes.

Drug Interactions

Cytochrome P450 Effect: CYP1A2, 2D6, and 3A3/4 enzyme substrate; CYP2D6 enzyme inhibitor

Increased Effect/Toxicity: Effects on CNS depression may be additive when chlorpromazine is combined with CNS depressants (narcotic analgesics, ethanol, barbiturates, cyclic antidepressants, antihistamines, or sedative-hypnotics). Chlorpromazine may increase the effects/toxicity of anticholinergics, antihypertensives, lithium (rare neurotoxicity), trazodone, or valproic acid. Concurrent use with TCA may produce increased toxicity or altered therapeutic response. Chloroquine and propranolol may increase chlorpromazine concentrations. Hypotension may occur when chlorpromazine is combined with epinephrine. May increase the risk of arrhythmia when combined with antiarrhythmics, cisapride, pimozide, sparfloxacin, or other drugs which prolong QT interval.

Decreased Effect: Phenothiazines inhibit the ability of bromocriptine to lower serum prolactin concentrations. Benztropine (and other anticholinergics) may inhibit the therapeutic response to chlorpromazine and excess anticholinergic effects may occur. Cigarette smoking and barbiturates may enhance the hepatic metabolism of chlorpromazine. Antihypertensive effects of guanethidine and guanadrel may be inhibited by chlorpromazine. Chlorpromazine may inhibit the antiparkinsonian effect of levodopa. Chlorpromazine and possibly other low potency antipsychotics may reverse the pressor effects of epinephrine.

Ethanol/Nutrition/Herb Interactions

Ethanol: Avoid ethanol (may increase CNS depression).

Herb/Nutraceutical: Avoid St John's wort (may decrease chlorpromazine levels, increase photosensitization, or enhance sedative effect). Avoid dong quai (may enhance photosensitization). Avoid kava kava, gotu kola, valerian (may increase CNS depression).

Stability Protect from light; a slightly yellowed solution does not indicate potency loss, but a markedly discolored solution should be discarded; diluted injection (1 mg/mL) with NS and stored in 5 mL vials remains stable for 30 days

Mechanism of Action Blocks postsynaptic mesolimbic dopaminergic receptors in the brain; exhibits a strong alpha-adrenergic blocking effect and depresses the release of hypothalamic and hypophyseal hormones; believed to depress the reticular activating system, thus affecting basal metabolism, body temperature, wakefulness, vasomotor tone, and emesis

Pharmacodynamics/Kinetics

Distribution: Crosses placenta; enters breast milk

Metabolism: Extensively hepatic to active and inactive metabolites

Half-life elimination: Biphasic: Initial: 2 hours; Terminal: 30 hours

Time to peak, serum: Oral: 1-2 hours

Excretion: Urine (<1% as unchanged drug) within 24 hours

Usual Dosage

Children ≥6 months:

Schizophrenia/psychoses:

Oral: 0.5-1 mg/kg/dose every 4-6 hours; older children may require 200 mg/day or higher

I.M., I.V.: 0.5-1 mg/kg/dose every 6-8 hours

<5 years (22.7 kg): Maximum: 40 mg/day

5-12 years (22.7-45.5 kg): Maximum: 75 mg/day

Nausea and vomiting:

Oral: 0.5-1 mg/kg/dose every 4-6 hours as needed

I.M., I.V.: 0.5-1 mg/kg/dose every 6-8 hours

<5 years (22.7 kg): Maximum: 40 mg/day

5-12 years (22.7-45.5 kg): Maximum: 75 mg/day

Rectal: 1 mg/kg/dose every 6-8 hours as needed

Adults:

Schizophrenia/psychoses:

Oral: Range: 30-2000 mg/day in 1-4 divided doses, initiate at lower doses and titrate as needed; usual dose: 400-600 mg/day; some patients may require 1-2 g/day

I.M., I.V.: Initial: 25 mg, may repeat (25-50 mg) in 1-4 hours, gradually increase to a maximum of 400 mg/dose every 4-6 hours until patient is controlled; usual dose: 300-800 mg/day

Intractable hiccups: Oral, I.M.: 25-50 mg 3-4 times/day

Nausea and vomiting:

Oral: 10-25 mg every 4-6 hours

I.M., I.V.: 25-50 mg every 4-6 hours

Rectal: 50-100 mg every 6-8 hours

Elderly: Behavioral symptoms associated with dementia: Initial: 10-25 mg 1-2 times/day; increase at 4- to 7-day intervals by 10-25 mg/day. Increase dose intervals (bid, tid, etc) as necessary to control behavior response or side effects; maximum daily dose: 800 mg; gradual increases (titration) may prevent some side effects or decrease their severity.

Dosing adjustment/comments in hepatic impairment: Avoid use in severe hepatic dysfunction

Administration

Oral: Dilute oral concentrate solution in juice before administration. Chlorpromazine concentrate is not compatible with carbamazepine suspension; schedule dosing at least 1-2 hours apart from each other. **Note:** Avoid skin contact with oral suspension or solution; may cause contact dermatitis.

I.V.: Direct of intermittent infusion: Infuse 1 mg or portion thereof over 1 minute.

Monitoring Parameters Orthostatic blood pressures; tremors; gait changes, abnormal movement in trunk, neck, buccal area, or extremities; monitor target behaviors for which the agent is given; watch for hypotension when administering I.M. or I.V.

(Continued)

ChlorproMAZINE (Continued)

Reference Range
Therapeutic: 50-300 ng/mL (SI: 157-942 nmol/L)
Toxic: >750 ng/mL (SI: >2355 nmol/L); serum concentrations poorly correlate with expected response

Test Interactions
False-positives for phenylketonuria, amylase, uroporphyrins, urobilinogen. May cause false-positive pregnancy test.

Patient Information
Do not stop taking unless informed by your physician; oral concentrate must be diluted in 2-4 oz of liquid (water, fruit juice, carbonated drinks, milk, or pudding); do not take antacid within 1 hour of taking drug; avoid alcohol; avoid excess sun exposure (use sun block); may cause drowsiness, rise slowly from recumbent position; use of supportive stockings may help prevent orthostatic hypotension

Nursing Implications
Avoid contact of oral solution or injection with skin (contact dermatitis)

Additional Information
Avoid rectal administration in immunocompromised patients.

Dosage Forms
Capsule, sustained action, as hydrochloride: 30 mg, 75 mg, 150 mg, 200 mg, 300 mg
Injection, as hydrochloride: 25 mg/mL (1 mL, 2 mL, 10 mL)
Solution, oral concentrate, as hydrochloride: 30 mg/mL (120 mL); 100 mg/mL (60 mL, 240 mL)
Suppository, rectal, as base: 25 mg, 100 mg
Syrup, as hydrochloride: 10 mg/5 mL (120 mL)
Tablet, as hydrochloride: 10 mg, 25 mg, 50 mg, 100 mg, 200 mg

♦ Chlorpromazine Hydrochloride see ChlorproMAZINE on page 282

ChlorproPAMIDE (klor PROE pa mide)

Related Information
Antacid Drug Interactions on page 1477
Hypoglycemic Drugs & Thiazolidinedione Information on page 1502
Sulfonamide Derivatives on page 1515

U.S. Brand Names
Diabinese®

Canadian Brand Names
Apo®-Chlorpropamide; Diabinese™

Therapeutic Category
Antidiabetic Agent, Sulfonylurea; Hypoglycemic Agent, Oral; Sulfonylurea Agent

Use
Management of blood sugar in type 2 diabetes mellitus (noninsulin dependent, NIDDM)

Unlabeled/Investigational Use
Neurogenic diabetes insipidus

Pregnancy Risk Factor
C

Usual Dosage
Oral: The dosage of chlorpropamide is variable and should be individualized based upon the patient's response
Initial dose:
Adults: 250 mg/day in mild to moderate diabetes in middle-aged, stable diabetic
Elderly: 100-125 mg/day in older patients
Subsequent dosages may be increased or decreased by 50-125 mg/day at 3- to 5-day intervals
Maintenance dose: 100-250 mg/day; severe diabetics may require 500 mg/day; avoid doses >750 mg/day

Dosing adjustment/comments in renal impairment: Cl_{cr} <50 mL/minute: Avoid use
Hemodialysis: Removed with hemoperfusion
Peritoneal dialysis: Supplemental dose is not necessary

Dosing adjustment in hepatic impairment: Dosage reduction is recommended. Conservative initial and maintenance doses are recommended in patients with liver impairment because chlorpropamide undergoes extensive hepatic metabolism.

Additional Information
Complete prescribing information for this medication should be consulted for additional detail.

Dosage Forms
Tablet: 100 mg, 250 mg

Chlorthalidone (klor THAL i done)

Related Information
Heart Failure on page 1663
Sulfonamide Derivatives on page 1515

U.S. Brand Names
Hygroton® [DSC]; Thalitone®

Canadian Brand Names
Apo®-Chlorthalidone

Therapeutic Category
Antihypertensive Agent; Diuretic, Miscellaneous

Use
Management of mild to moderate hypertension when used alone or in combination with other agents; treatment of edema associated with congestive heart failure or nephrotic syndrome. Recent studies have found chlorthalidone effective in the treatment of isolated systolic hypertension in the elderly.

Pregnancy Risk Factor
B (manufacturer); D (expert analysis)

Usual Dosage
Oral:
Children (nonapproved): 2 mg/kg/dose 3 times/week or 1-2 mg/kg/day
Adults: 25-100 mg/day or 100 mg 3 times/week
Elderly: Initial: 12.5-25 mg/day or every other day; there is little advantage to using doses >25 mg/day

Dosing adjustment in renal impairment: Cl_{cr} <10 mL/minute: Administer every 48 hours

Additional Information
Complete prescribing information for this medication should be consulted for additional detail.

Dosage Forms
Tablet: 25 mg, 50 mg, 100 mg
Thalitone®: 15 mg

♦ Chlorthalidone and Atenolol see Atenolol and Chlorthalidone on page 126
♦ Chlorthalidone and Clonidine see Clonidine and Chlorthalidone on page 320

♦ **Chlor-Trimeton® Allergy/Decongestant [OTC]** *see* Chlorpheniramine and Pseudoephedrine *on page 279*

♦ **Chlor-Tripolon ND® (Can)** *see* Loratadine and Pseudoephedrine *on page 820*

Chlorzoxazone (klor ZOKS a zone)

U.S. Brand Names Parafon Forte® DSC

Canadian Brand Names Parafon Forte®; Strifon Forte®

Therapeutic Category Centrally Acting Muscle Relaxant; Skeletal Muscle Relaxant

Use Symptomatic treatment of muscle spasm and pain associated with acute musculoskeletal conditions

Pregnancy Risk Factor C

Contraindications Hypersensitivity to chlorzoxazone or any component of the formulation; impaired liver function

Adverse Reactions Frequency not defined.

Central nervous system: Dizziness, drowsiness lightheadedness, paradoxical stimulation, malaise

Dermatologic: Rash, petechiae, ecchymoses (rare), angioneurotic edema

Gastrointestinal: Nausea, vomiting, stomach cramps

Genitourinary: Urine discoloration

Hepatic: Liver dysfunction

Miscellaneous: Anaphylaxis (very rare)

Overdosage/Toxicology Symptoms include nausea, vomiting, diarrhea, drowsiness, dizziness, headache, absent tendon reflexes, and hypotension. Treatment is supportive following attempts to enhance drug elimination. Hypotension should be treated with I.V. fluids and/or Trendelenburg positioning. Dialysis and hemoperfusion and osmotic diuresis have all been useful in reducing serum drug concentrations. Patients should be observed for possible relapses due to incomplete gastric emptying.

Drug Interactions

Cytochrome P450 Effect: CYP2E1 enzyme substrate

Increased Effect/Toxicity: Increased effect/toxicity when taken with ethanol or CNS depressants.

Ethanol/Nutrition/Herb Interactions Ethanol: Avoid ethanol (may increase CNS depression).

Mechanism of Action Acts on the spinal cord and subcortical levels by depressing polysynaptic reflexes

Pharmacodynamics/Kinetics

Onset of action: ~1 hour

Duration: 6-12 hours

Absorption: Readily absorbed

Metabolism: Extensively hepatic via glucuronidation

Excretion: Urine (as conjugates)

Usual Dosage Oral:

Children: 20 mg/kg/day or 600 mg/m^2/day in 3-4 divided doses

Adults: 250-500 mg 3-4 times/day up to 750 mg 3-4 times/day

Monitoring Parameters Periodic liver functions tests

Patient Information May cause drowsiness or dizziness; avoid alcohol and other CNS depressants

Nursing Implications Raise bed rails; institute safety measures; assist with ambulation

Dosage Forms

Caplet (Parafon Forte® DSC): 500 mg

Tablet: 250 mg

♦ **Cholac®** *see* Lactulose *on page 770*

♦ **Choledyl®** *see* Theophylline Salts *on page 1310*

Cholera Vaccine (KOL er a vak SEEN)

Canadian Brand Names Mutacol Berna®

Therapeutic Category Vaccine, Inactivated Bacteria

Use The World Health Organization no longer recommends cholera vaccination for travel to or from cholera-endemic areas. Some countries may still require evidence of a complete primary series or a booster dose given within 6 months of arrival. Vaccination should not be considered as an alternative to continued careful selection of foods and water. Ideally, cholera and yellow fever vaccines should be administered at least 3 weeks apart.

Pregnancy Risk Factor C

Contraindications Presence of any acute illness, history of severe systemic reaction, or allergic response following a prior dose of cholera vaccine

Warnings/Precautions There is no data on the safety of cholera vaccination during pregnancy. Use in pregnancy should reflect actual increased risk. Persons who have had severe local or systemic reactions to a previous dose should not be revaccinated. Have epinephrine (1:1000) available for immediate use.

Adverse Reactions All serious adverse reactions must be reported to the U.S. Department of Health and Human Services (DHHS) Vaccine Adverse Event Reporting System (VAERS) 1-800-822-7967.

>10%:

Central nervous system: Malaise, fever, headache

Local: Pain, edema, tenderness, erythema, and induration at injection site

Stability Refrigerate, avoid freezing

Mechanism of Action Inactivated vaccine producing active immunization

Usual Dosage

Children:

6 months to 4 years: Two 0.2 mL doses I.M./S.C. 1 week to 1 month apart; booster doses (0.2 mL I.M./S.C.) every 6 months

(Continued)

Cholera Vaccine (Continued)

5-10 years: Two 0.3 mL doses I.M./S.C. or two 0.2 mL intradermal doses 1 week to 1 month apart; booster doses (0.3 mL I.M./S.C. or 0.2 mL I.D.) every 6 months

Children ≥10 years and Adults: Two 0.5 mL doses given I.M./S.C. or two 0.2 mL doses I.D. 1 week to 1 month apart; booster doses (0.5 mL I.M. or S.C. or 0.2 mL I.D.) every 6 months

Administration For patients at risk of hemorrhage following intramuscular injection, the ACIP recommends "it should be administered intramuscularly if, in the opinion of the physician familiar with the patients bleeding risk, the vaccine can be administered with reasonable safety by this route. If the patient receives antihemophilia or other similar therapy, intramuscular vaccination can be scheduled shortly after such therapy is administered. A fine needle (23 gauge or smaller) can be used for the vaccination and firm pressure applied to the site (without rubbing) for at least 2 minutes. The patient should be instructed concerning the risk of hematoma from the injection."

Patient Information Local reactions can occur up to 7 days after injection

Nursing Implications Defer immunization in individuals with moderate or severe febrile illness

Additional Information Inactivated bacteria vaccine. Federal law requires that the date of administration, the vaccine manufacturer, lot number of vaccine, and the administering person's name, title and address be entered into the patient's permanent medical record.

Dosage Forms Injection: Suspension of killed *Vibrio cholerae* (Inaba and Ogawa types) 8 units of each serotype per mL (1.5 mL, 20 mL)

Cholestyramine Resin (koe LES teer a meen REZ in)

Related Information

Hyperlipidemia Management *on page 1670*

Lipid-Lowering Agents *on page 1505*

U.S. Brand Names LoCHOLEST®; LoCHOLEST® Light; Prevalite®; Questran®; Questran® Light

Canadian Brand Names Novo-Cholamine; Novo-Cholamine Light; PMS-Cholestyramine; Questran®; Questran® Light Sugar Free

Therapeutic Category Antilipemic Agent, Bile Acid Sequestrant

Use Adjunct in the management of primary hypercholesterolemia; pruritus associated with elevated levels of bile acids; diarrhea associated with excess fecal bile acids; binding toxicologic agents; pseudomembranous colitis

Pregnancy Risk Factor C

Contraindications Hypersensitivity of bile acid sequestering resins or any component of the formulation; complete biliary obstruction; bowel obstruction

Warnings/Precautions Use with caution in patients with constipation (GI dysfunction) and patients with phenylketonuria (Questran® Light contains aspartame). Overdose may result in GI obstruction. Not to be taken simultaneously with many other medicines (decreased absorption). Treat any diseases contributing to hypercholesterolemia first. May interfere with fat-soluble vitamins (A, D, E, K) and folic acid. Chronic use may be associated with bleeding problems (especially in high doses).

Adverse Reactions

>10%: Gastrointestinal: Constipation, heartburn, nausea, vomiting, stomach pain

1% to 10%:

Central nervous system: Headache

Gastrointestinal: Belching, bloating, diarrhea

<1% (Limited to important or life-threatening): Gallstones or pancreatitis, GI bleeding, hyperchloremic acidosis, hypoprothrombinemia (secondary to vitamin K deficiency), peptic ulcer, steatorrhea or malabsorption syndrome

Overdosage/Toxicology Symptoms include GI obstruction. Treatment is supportive.

Drug Interactions

Decreased Effect: Cholestyramine resin may cause decreased absorption of digitalis glycosides (oral), warfarin, thyroid hormones, thiazide diuretics, propranolol, phenobarbital, amiodarone, methotrexate, NSAIDs, and other drugs.

Ethanol/Nutrition/Herb Interactions

Food: Cholestyramine (especially high doses or long-term therapy) may decrease the absorption of folic acid, calcium, and iron.

Herb/Nutraceutical: Cholestyramine (especially high doses or long-term therapy) may decrease the absorption of fat-soluble vitamins (vitamins A, D, E, and K).

Stability Suspension may be used for up to 48 hours after refrigeration.

Mechanism of Action Forms a nonabsorbable complex with bile acids in the intestine, releasing chloride ions in the process; inhibits enterohepatic reuptake of intestinal bile salts and thereby increases the fecal loss of bile salt-bound low density lipoprotein cholesterol

Pharmacodynamics/Kinetics

Onset of action: Peak effect: 21 days

Absorption: None

Excretion: Feces (as insoluble complex with bile acids)

Usual Dosage Oral (dosages are expressed in terms of anhydrous resin):

Powder:

Children: 240 mg/kg/day in 3 divided doses; need to titrate dose depending on indication

Adults: 4 g 1-2 times/day to a maximum of 24 g/day and 6 doses/day

Dialysis: Not removed by hemo- or peritoneal dialysis; supplemental doses not necessary with dialysis or continuous arteriovenous or venovenous hemofiltration

Dietary Considerations Supplementation of vitamins A, D, E, and K, folic acid, and iron may be required with high-dose, long-term therapy.

Test Interactions ↑ prothrombin time; ↓ cholesterol (S), iron (B)

Patient Information Do not administer the powder in its dry form, mix with fluid or with applesauce; chew bars thoroughly; drink plenty of fluids; take other medications 1 hour before or 4-6 hours after binding resin; GI adverse reactions may decrease over time with continued use; adhere to prescribed diet

Nursing Implications Administer warfarin and other drugs at least 1 hour prior to or 4-6 hours after cholestyramine because cholestyramine may bind to them, decreasing their total absorption. (**Note:** Cholestyramine itself may cause hypoprothrombinemia in patients with impaired enterohepatic circulation.)

Dosage Forms

Powder: 4 g of resin/9 g of powder (9 g, 378 g)

Powder for oral suspension:

With aspartame: 4 g of resin/5 g of powder (5 g, 210 g)

With phenylalanine: 4 g of resin/5.5 g of powder (60s)

Choline Magnesium Trisalicylate (KOE leen mag NEE zhum trye sa LIS i late)

Related Information

Antacid Drug Interactions *on page 1477*

Salicylates *on page 1692*

U.S. Brand Names Tricosal®; Trilisate®

Canadian Brand Names Trilisate®

Therapeutic Category Analgesic, Salicylate; Anti-inflammatory Agent; Nonsteroidal Anti-inflammatory Drug (NSAID), Oral; Salicylate

Use Management of osteoarthritis, rheumatoid arthritis, and other arthritis; salicylate salts may not inhibit platelet aggregation and, therefore, should not be substituted for aspirin in the prophylaxis of thrombosis; acute painful shoulder

Pregnancy Risk Factor C/D (3rd trimester)

Pregnancy/Breast-Feeding Implications Excreted in breast milk; peak levels occur 9-12 hours after dose; use caution if used during breast-feeding

Contraindications Hypersensitivity to salicylates, other nonacetylated salicylates, other NSAIDs, or any component of the formulation; tartrazine dye hypersensitivity; bleeding disorders; pregnancy (3rd trimester)

Warnings/Precautions Use with caution in patients with impaired renal function, dehydration, erosive gastritis, or peptic ulcer; avoid use in patients with suspected varicella or influenza (salicylates have been associated with Reye's syndrome in children <16 years of age when used to treat symptoms of chickenpox or the flu). Discontinue use 1 week prior to surgical procedures.

Elderly are a high-risk population for adverse effects from nonsteroidal anti-inflammatory agents. As many as 60% of elderly can develop peptic ulceration and/or hemorrhage asymptomatically. Use lowest effective dose for shortest period possible. Tinnitus or impaired hearing may indicate toxicity. Tinnitus may be a difficult and unreliable indication of toxicity due to age-related hearing loss or eighth cranial nerve damage. CNS adverse effects may be observed in the elderly at lower doses than younger adults.

Adverse Reactions

<20%:

Gastrointestinal: Nausea, vomiting, diarrhea, heartburn, dyspepsia, epigastric pain, constipation

Ocular: Tinnitus

<2%:

Central nervous system: Headache, lightheadedness, dizziness, drowsiness, lethargy

Ocular: Hearing impairment

<1% (Limited to important or life-threatening): Anorexia, BUN increased, creatinine increased, dysgeusia, edema, epistaxis, gastric ulceration, occult bleeding, pruritus, rash, weight gain

Overdosage/Toxicology Symptoms include tinnitus, vomiting, acute renal failure, hyperthermia, irritability, seizures, coma, and metabolic acidosis. For acute ingestions, determine serum salicylate levels 6 hours after ingestion. The "Done" nomogram may be helpful for estimating the severity of aspirin poisoning and directing treatment using serum salicylate levels. Treatment can also be based upon symptomatology. See "Salicylates" *on page 1692* in the Appendix.

Drug Interactions

Increased Effect/Toxicity: Choline magnesium trisalicylate may increase the hypoprothrombinemic effect of warfarin.

Decreased Effect: Antacids may decrease choline magnesium trisalicylate absorption/salicylate concentrations.

Ethanol/Nutrition/Herb Interactions

Ethanol: Avoid ethanol (may enhance gastric mucosal irritation).

Food: May decrease the rate but not the extent of oral absorption.

Herb/Nutraceutical: Avoid cat's claw, dong quai, evening primrose, feverfew, garlic, ginger, ginkgo, red clover, horse chestnut, green tea, ginseng (all have additional antiplatelet activity). Limit curry powder, paprika, licorice, Benedictine liqueur, prunes, raisins, tea, and gherkins; may cause salicylate accumulation. These foods contain 6 mg salicylate/100 g.

Mechanism of Action Inhibits prostaglandin synthesis; acts on the hypothalamus heat-regulating center to reduce fever; blocks the generation of pain impulses

Pharmacodynamics/Kinetics

Onset of action: Peak effect: ~2 hours

Absorption: Stomach and small intestines

Distribution: Readily into most body fluids and tissues; crosses placenta; enters breast milk

Half-life elimination (dose dependent): Low dose: 2-3 hours; High dose: 30 hours

Time to peak, serum: ~2 hours

Usual Dosage Oral (based on total salicylate content):

Children <37 kg: 50 mg/kg/day given in 2 divided doses

Adults: 500 mg to 1.5 g 2-3 times/day; usual maintenance dose: 1-4.5 g/day

Dosing adjustment/comments in renal impairment: Avoid use in severe renal impairment

Dietary Considerations Take with food or large volume of water or milk to minimize GI upset. Liquid may be mixed with fruit juice just before drinking.

Magnesium: Hypermagnesemia resulting from magnesium salicylate; avoid or use with caution in renal insufficiency.

(Continued)

Choline Magnesium Trisalicylate *(Continued)*

Administration Liquid may be mixed with fruit juice just before drinking. Do not administer with antacids. Take with a full glass of water and remain in an upright position for 15-30 minutes after administration.

Monitoring Parameters Serum magnesium with high dose therapy or in patients with impaired renal function; serum salicylate levels, renal function, hearing changes or tinnitus, abnormal bruising, weight gain and response (ie, pain)

Reference Range Salicylate blood levels for anti-inflammatory effect: 150-300 µg/mL; analgesia and antipyretic effect: 30-50 µg/mL

Test Interactions False-negative results for glucose oxidase urinary glucose tests (Clinistix®); false-positives using the cupric sulfate method (Clinitest®); also, interferes with Gerhardt test (urinary ketone analysis), VMA determination; 5-HIAA, xylose tolerance test, and T_3 and T_4; increased PBI

Patient Information Take with food; do not take with antacids; watch for bleeding gums or any signs of GI bleeding; take with food or milk to minimize GI distress, notify physician if ringing in ears or persistent GI pain occurs

Nursing Implications Liquid may be mixed with fruit juice just before drinking; do not administer with antacids

Additional Information Contains choline salicylate 293 mg and magnesium salicylate 362 mg per tablet or 5 mL of liquid. Salicylate salts do not inhibit platelet aggregation and, therefore, should not be substituted for aspirin in the prophylaxis of thrombosis.

Dosage Forms
Liquid: 500 mg/5 mL total salicylate (293 mg/5 mL choline salicylate and 362 mg/5 mL magnesium salicylate)
Tablet:
500 mg total salicylate (293 mg choline salicylate and 362 mg magnesium salicylate)
750 mg total salicylate (440 mg choline salicylate and 544 mg magnesium salicylate)
1000 mg total salicylate (587 mg choline salicylate and 725 mg magnesium salicylate)

Choline Salicylate (KOE leen sa LIS i late)

Related Information
Antacid Drug Interactions *on page 1477*
Salicylates *on page 1692*
U.S. Brand Names Arthropan® [OTC]
Canadian Brand Names Teejel®
Therapeutic Category Analgesic, Salicylate; Anti-inflammatory Agent; Nonsteroidal Anti-inflammatory Drug (NSAID), Oral; Salicylate
Use Temporary relief of pain of rheumatoid arthritis, rheumatic fever, osteoarthritis, and other conditions for which oral salicylates are recommended; useful in patients in which there is difficulty in administering doses in a tablet or capsule dosage form, because of the liquid dosage form
Pregnancy Risk Factor C/D (3rd trimester)
Contraindications Hypersensitivity to salicylates or any component or other nonacetylated salicylates; pregnancy (3rd trimester)
Warnings/Precautions Use with caution in patients with impaired renal function, dehydration, erosive gastritis, or peptic ulcer; avoid use in patients with suspected varicella or influenza (salicylates have been associated with Reye's syndrome in children <16 years of age when used to treat symptoms of chickenpox or the flu); tinnitus or impaired hearing may indicate toxicity

Adverse Reactions
>10%: Gastrointestinal: Dyspepsia, epigastric discomfort, heartburn, nausea, stomach pains
1% to 10%:
Central nervous system: Fatigue
Dermatologic: Skin rash
Gastrointestinal: Gastrointestinal ulceration
Hematologic: Hemolytic anemia
Neuromuscular & skeletal: Weakness
Respiratory: Dyspnea
Miscellaneous: Anaphylactic shock
<1% (Limited to important or life-threatening): Bronchospasm, hepatotoxicity, impaired renal function, leukopenia, prolongation of bleeding time, thrombocytopenia

Overdosage/Toxicology Symptoms include tinnitus, vomiting, acute renal failure, hyperthermia, irritability, seizures, coma, and metabolic acidosis. For acute ingestions, determine serum salicylate levels 6 hours after ingestion. The "Done" nomogram may be helpful for estimating the severity of aspirin poisoning and directing treatment using serum salicylate levels. Treatment can also be based upon symptomatology. See "Salicylates" *on page 1692* in the Appendix.

Drug Interactions
Increased Effect/Toxicity: Effect of warfarin may be increased.
Decreased Effect: Decreased effect of salicylates with antacids. Effect of ACE-inhibitors and diuretics may be decreased by concurrent therapy with NSAIDs.
Mechanism of Action Inhibits prostaglandin synthesis; acts on the hypothalamus heat-regulating center to reduce fever; blocks the generation of pain impulses
Pharmacodynamics/Kinetics
Absorption: Stomach and small intestines in ~2 hours
Distribution: Readily into most body fluids and tissues; crosses placenta; enters breast milk
Protein binding: 75% to 90%
Metabolism: Hepatically hydrolyzed to salicylate
Half-life elimination (dose dependent): Low dose: 2-3 hours; High dose: 30 hours
Time to peak, serum: 1-2 hours
Excretion: Urine

Usual Dosage
Children >12 years and Adults: Oral: 5 mL (870 mg) every 3-4 hours, if necessary, but not more than 6 doses in 24 hours
Rheumatoid arthritis: 870-1740 mg (5-10 mL) up to 4 times/day
Dosing adjustment/comments in renal impairment: Avoid use in severe renal impairment
Dietary Considerations May be taken with food.
Test Interactions False-negative results for Clinistix® urine test; false-positive results with Clinitest®
Patient Information Take with food; do not take with antacids; watch for bleeding gums or any signs of GI bleeding; take with food or milk to minimize GI distress, notify physician if ringing in ears or persistent GI pain occurs
Nursing Implications Liquid may be mixed with fruit juice just before drinking; do not administer with antacids
Dosage Forms Liquid: 870 mg/5 mL (240 mL, 480 mL) [mint flavor]

♦ **Choline Theophyllinate** see Theophylline Salts on page 1310

Chondroitin Sulfate-Sodium Hyaluronate
(kon DROY tin SUL fate-SOW de um hye al yoor ON ate)
U.S. Brand Names Viscoat®
Synonyms Sodium Hyaluronate-Chrondroitin Sulfate
Therapeutic Category Ophthalmic Agent, Viscoelastic
Use Surgical aid in anterior segment procedures, protects corneal endothelium and coats intraocular lens thus protecting it
Pregnancy Risk Factor C
Contraindications Hypersensitivity to hyaluronate
Warnings/Precautions Product is extracted from avian tissues and contains minute amounts of protein, potential risks of hypersensitivity may exist. Intraocular pressure may be elevated as a result of pre-existing glaucoma, compromised outflow and by operative procedures and sequelae, including coma, compromised outflow and by operative procedures and sequelae, including enzymatic zonulysis, absence of an iridectomy, trauma to filtration structures and by blood and lenticular remnants in the anterior chamber. Monitor IOP, especially during the immediate postoperative period.
Adverse Reactions 1% to 10%: Ocular: Increased intraocular pressure
Stability Store at 2°C to 8°C (36°F to 46°F); do not freeze.
Mechanism of Action Functions as a tissue lubricant and is thought to play an important role in modulating the interactions between adjacent tissues
Pharmacodynamics/Kinetics
Absorption: Intravitreous injection: diffusion occurs slowly
Excretion: By Canal of Schlemm
Usual Dosage Carefully introduce (using a 27-gauge needle or cannula) into anterior chamber after thoroughly cleaning the chamber with a balanced salt solution
Administration May inject prior to or following delivery of the crystalline lens. Instillation prior to lens delivery provides additional protection to corneal endothelium, protecting it from possible damage arising from surgical instrumentation. May also be used to coat intraocular lens and tips of surgical instruments prior to implantation surgery. May inject additional solution during anterior segment surgery to fully maintain the solution lost during surgery. At the end of surgery, remove solution by thoroughly irrigating with a balanced salt solution.
Test Interactions False-negative results for Clinistix® urine test; false-positive results with Clinitest®
Dosage Forms Solution, ophthalmic: Sodium chondroitin 40 mg and sodium hyaluronate 30 mg (0.25 mL, 0.5 mL)

♦ **Chooz® [OTC]** see Calcium Carbonate on page 207
♦ **Choriogonadotropin Alfa** see Chorionic Gonadotropin (Recombinant) on page 289

Chorionic Gonadotropin (Human)
Therapeutic Category Gonadotropin; Ovulation Stimulator

Chorionic Gonadotropin (Recombinant)
(kor ee ON ik goe NAD oh troe pin ree KOM be nant)
U.S. Brand Names Ovidrel®
Synonyms Choriogonadotropin Alfa; r-hCG
Therapeutic Category Gonadotropin; Ovulation Stimulator
Use As part of an assisted reproductive technology (ART) program, induces ovulation in infertile females who have been pretreated with follicle stimulating hormones (FSH); induces ovulation and pregnancy in infertile females when the cause of infertility is functional
Pregnancy Risk Factor X
Pregnancy/Breast-Feeding Implications Ectopic pregnancy, premature labor, postpartum fever, and spontaneous abortion have been reported in clinical trials. Congenital abnormalities have also been observed, however the incidence is similar during natural conception. It is unknown if hCG is excreted in human milk, use caution if administered to a nursing woman.
Contraindications Hypersensitivity to hCG preparations or any component of the formulation; primary ovarian failure; uncontrolled thyroid or adrenal dysfunction; uncontrolled organic intracranial lesion (ie, pituitary tumor); abnormal uterine bleeding, ovarian cyst or enlargement of undetermined origin; sex hormone dependent tumors; pregnancy
Warnings/Precautions For use by infertility specialists; may cause ovarian hyperstimulation syndrome (OHSS); if severe, treatment should be discontinued and patient should be hospitalized. OHSS results in a rapid (<24 hours to 7 days) accumulation of fluid in the peritoneal cavity, thorax, and possibly the pericardium, which may become more severe if pregnancy occurs; monitor for ovarian enlargement; use may lead to multiple births; risk of arterial thromboembolism with hCG products; safety and efficacy in pediatric and geriatric patients have not been established.
(Continued)

Chorionic Gonadotropin (Recombinant) *(Continued)*

Adverse Reactions

2% to 10%:

Endocrine & metabolic: Ovarian cyst (3%), ovarian hyperstimulation (<2% to 3%)

Gastrointestinal: Abdominal pain (3% to 4%), nausea (3%), vomiting (3%)

Local: Injection site: Pain (8%), bruising (3% to 5%), reaction (<2% to 3%), inflammation (<2% to 2%)

Miscellaneous: Postoperative pain (5%)

<2% (Limited to important or life-threatening): Abdominal enlargement, albuminuria, back pain, breast pain, cardiac arrhythmia, cervical carcinoma, cervical lesion, cough, diarrhea, dizziness, dysuria, ectopic pregnancy, emotional lability, fever, flatulence, genital herpes, genital moniliasis, headache, heart murmur, hiccups, hot flashes, hyperglycemia, insomnia, intermenstrual bleeding, leukocytosis, leukorrhea, malaise, paresthesias, pharyngitis, pruritus, rash, upper respiratory tract infection, urinary incontinence, urinary tract infection, vaginal hemorrhage, vaginitis

In addition, the following have been reported with menotropin therapy: Adnexal torsion, hemoperitoneum, mild to moderate ovarian enlargement, pulmonary and vascular complications. Ovarian neoplasms have also been reported (rare) with multiple drug regimens used for ovarian induction (relationship not established).

Overdosage/Toxicology Information not reported

Drug Interactions

Increased Effect/Toxicity: Specific drug interaction studies have not been conducted.

Stability Store in original package under refrigeration or at room temperature, 2°C to 25°C (36°F to 77°F). Protect from light.

Mechanism of Action Luteinizing hormone analogue produced by recombinant DNA techniques; stimulates rupture of the ovarian follicle once follicular development has occurred.

Pharmacodynamics/Kinetics

Distribution: V_d: 5.9 ± 1 L

Bioavailability: 40%

Half-life elimination: Initial: 4 hours; Terminal: 29 hours

Time to peak: 12-24 hours

Excretion: Urine ($1/10^{th}$ of dose)

Usual Dosage S.C.:

Adults: Female:

Assisted reproductive technologies (ART) and ovulation induction: 250 mcg given 1 day following the last dose of follicle stimulating agent. Use only after adequate follicular development has been determined. Hold treatment when there is an excessive ovarian response.

Elderly: Safety and efficacy have not been established

Dosage adjustment in renal impairment: Safety and efficacy have not been established

Dosage adjustment in hepatic impairment: Safety and efficacy have not been established

Administration Prior to administration, mix vial with 1 mL sterile water for injection. Gently mix by rotating vial to dissolve powder; do not shake. Use only if solution is clear and colorless. For S.C. use only; inject into stomach area. Use immediately following reconstitution.

Monitoring Parameters Ultrasound and/or estradiol levels to assess follicle development; ultrasound to assess number and size of follicles; ovulation (basal body temperature, serum progestin level, menstruation, sonography)

Test Interactions May interfere with interpretation of pregnancy tests; may cross-react with radioimmunoassay of luteinizing hormone and other gonadotropins

Patient Information Instructions will be given on how to administer S.C. injections and proper disposal of syringes and needles. Use exactly as instructed by prescriber. Keep all ultrasound appointments. Report sudden weight gain, severe pelvic pain, nausea, vomiting, or shortness of breath to prescriber. Do not take if pregnant. As with other hCG products, there is a risk of multiple births associated with treatment. Avoid strenuous exercise, especially those with pelvic involvement.

Nursing Implications Should be administered by S.C. injection only. Patients should be taught how to reconstitute, administer r-hCG, and dispose of needles and syringes properly.

Additional Information Clinical studies have shown r-hCG to be clinically and statistically equivalent to urinary-derived hCG products.

Dosage Forms Injection [single-dose vial]: 285 mcg r-hCG per vial with 1 mL SWFI [delivers 250 mcg r-hCG following reconstitution]

♦ **Chronovera® (Can)** *see* Verapamil *on page 1412*

♦ **Chronulac®** *see* Lactulose *on page 770*

Ciclopirox *(sye kloe PEER oks)*

U.S. Brand Names Loprox®; Penlac™

Canadian Brand Names Loprox®; Penlac™

Synonyms Ciclopirox Olamine

Therapeutic Category Antifungal Agent, Topical

Use

Cream/lotion: Treatment of tinea pedis (athlete's foot), tinea cruris (jock itch), tinea corporis (ringworm), cutaneous candidiasis, and tinea versicolor (pityriasis)

Lacquer: Topical treatment of mild to moderate onychomycosis of the fingernails and toenails due to *Trichophyton rubrum*

Pregnancy Risk Factor B

Contraindications Hypersensitivity to ciclopirox or any component of the formulation; avoid occlusive wrappings or dressings

Warnings/Precautions For external use only; avoid contact with eyes; nail lacquer is for topical use only and has not been studied in conjunction with systemic therapy

Adverse Reactions 1% to 10%:

Dermatologic: Pruritus

Local: Irritation, redness, burning, or pain

Mechanism of Action Inhibiting transport of essential elements in the fungal cell causing problems in synthesis of DNA, RNA, and protein

Pharmacodynamics/Kinetics

Absorption: <2% through intact skin

Distribution: To epidermis, corium (dermis), including hair, hair follicles, and sebaceous glands

Protein binding: 94% to 98%

Half-life elimination: 1.7 hours

Excretion: Urine and feces (small amounts)

Usual Dosage Children >10 years and Adults:

Cream/lotion: Apply twice daily, gently massage into affected areas; if no improvement after 4 weeks of treatment, re-evaluate the diagnosis

Lacquer: Apply to affected nails daily (as a part of a comprehensive management program for onychomycosis)

Patient Information Avoid contact with eyes; if sensitivity or irritation occurs, discontinue use

Nursing Implications Avoid contact with eyes; if sensitivity or irritation occurs, discontinue use

Dosage Forms

Cream, topical, as olamine: 1% (15 g, 30 g, 90 g)

Lotion, topical, as olamine: 1% (30 mL, 60 mL)

Solution, nail lacquer, topical: 8% (3.3 mL)

♦ **Ciclopirox Olamine** see Ciclopirox on page 290

Cidofovir (si DOF o veer)

U.S. Brand Names Vistide®

Therapeutic Category Antiviral Agent, Nonantiretroviral; Antiviral Agent, Parenteral

Use Treatment of cytomegalovirus (CMV) retinitis in patients with acquired immunodeficiency syndrome (AIDS). **Note:** Should be administered with probenecid.

Pregnancy Risk Factor C

Pregnancy/Breast-Feeding Implications

Clinical effect on the fetus: Although studies are inconclusive, adenocarcinomas have occurred in animal studies with cidofovir; use during pregnancy only if the potential benefit justifies the potential risk to the fetus

Breast-feeding/lactation: Excretion of cidofovir into breast milk is unknown

Contraindications Patients with hypersensitivity to cidofovir and in patients with a history of clinically severe hypersensitivity to probenecid or other sulfa-containing medications

Warnings/Precautions Dose-dependent nephrotoxicity requires dose adjustment or discontinuation if changes in renal function occur during therapy (eg, proteinuria, glycosuria, decreased serum phosphate, uric acid or bicarbonate, and elevated creatinine); avoid use in patients with creatinine >1.5 mg/dL; Cl$_{cr}$ <55 mL/minute; use great caution with elderly patients; neutropenia and ocular hypotony have also occurred; safety and efficacy have not been established in children; administration must be accompanied by oral probenecid and intravenous saline prehydration; prepare admixtures in a class two laminar flow hood, wearing protective gear; dispose of cidofovir as directed

Adverse Reactions

>10%:

Central nervous system: Infection, chills, fever, headache, amnesia, anxiety, confusion, seizures, insomnia

Dermatologic: Alopecia, rash, acne, skin discoloration

Gastrointestinal: Nausea, vomiting, diarrhea, anorexia, abdominal pain, constipation, heartburn, gastritis

Hematologic: Thrombocytopenia, neutropenia, anemia

Neuromuscular & skeletal: Weakness, paresthesia

Ocular: Amblyopia, conjunctivitis, ocular hypotony

Renal: Tubular damage, proteinuria, Cr elevations

Respiratory: Asthma, bronchitis, coughing, dyspnea, pharyngitis

1% to 10%:

Cardiovascular: Hypotension, pallor, syncope, tachycardia

Central nervous system: Dizziness, hallucinations, depression, somnolence, malaise

Dermatologic: Pruritus, urticaria

Endocrine & metabolic: Hyperglycemia, hyperlipidemia, hypocalcemia, hypokalemia, dehydration

Gastrointestinal: Abnormal taste, stomatitis

Genitourinary: Glycosuria, urinary incontinence, urinary tract infections

Neuromuscular & skeletal: Skeletal pain

Ocular: Retinal detachment, iritis, uveitis, decreased intraocular pressure, abnormal vision

Renal: Hematuria

Respiratory: Pneumonia, rhinitis, sinusitis

Miscellaneous: Diaphoresis, allergic reactions

<1% (Limited to important or life-threatening): Fanconi syndrome, hepatic failure, increased bicarbonate excretion, iritis, metabolic acidosis, pancreatitis, uveitis

Overdosage/Toxicology Acute toxicity has not been reported, however, hemodialysis and hydration may reduce drug plasma concentrations. Probenecid may assist in decreasing active tubular secretion.

Drug Interactions

Increased Effect/Toxicity: Drugs with nephrotoxic potential (eg, amphotericin B, aminoglycosides, foscarnet, and I.V. pentamidine) should be avoided during cidofovir therapy.

Stability Store at controlled room temperature 20°C to 25°C (68°F to 77°F). Cidofovir infusion admixture should be administered within 24 hours of preparation at room temperature or refrigerated. Admixtures should be allowed to equilibrate to room temperature prior to use.

(Continued)

Cidofovir *(Continued)*

Mechanism of Action Cidofovir is converted to cidofovir diphosphate which is the active intracellular metabolite; cidofovir diphosphate suppresses CMV replication by selective inhibition of viral DNA synthesis. Incorporation of cidofovir into growing viral DNA chain results in reductions in the rate of viral DNA synthesis.

Pharmacodynamics/Kinetics The following pharmacokinetic data is based on a combination of cidofovir administered with probenecid:
Distribution: V_d: 0.54 L/kg; does not cross significantly into CSF
Protein binding: <6%
Metabolism: Minimal; phosphorylation occurs intracellularly
Half-life elimination, plasma: ~2.6 hours
Excretion: Urine

Usual Dosage
Induction: 5 mg/kg I.V. over 1 hour once weekly for 2 consecutive weeks
Maintenance: 5 mg/kg over 1 hour once every other week
Administer with probenecid - 2 g orally 3 hours prior to each cidofovir dose and 1 g at 2 and 8 hours after completion of the infusion (total: 4 g)
Hydrate with 1 L of 0.9% NS I.V. prior to cidofovir infusion; a second liter may be administered over a 1- to 3-hour period immediately following infusion, if tolerated
Dosing adjustment in renal impairment:
Cl_{cr} 41-55 mL/minute: 2 mg/kg
Cl_{cr} 30-40 mL/minute: 1.5 mg/kg
Cl_{cr} 20-29 mL/minute: 1 mg/kg
Cl_{cr} <19 mL/minute: 0.5 mg/kg
If the creatinine increases by 0.3-0.4 mg/dL, reduce the cidofovir dose to 3 mg/kg; discontinue therapy for increases ≥0.5 mg/dL or development of ≥3+ proteinuria

Monitoring Parameters Renal function (Cr, BUN, UAs), LFTs, WBCs, intraocular pressure and visual acuity

Patient Information Cidofovir is not a cure for CMV retinitis; regular follow-up ophthalmologic exams and careful monitoring of renal function are necessary; probenecid must be administered concurrently with cidofovir; report rash immediately to your physician; avoid use during pregnancy; use contraception during and for 3 months following treatment

Nursing Implications Administration of probenecid with a meal may decrease associated nausea; acetaminophen and antihistamines may ameliorate hypersensitivity reactions; dilute in 100 mL 0.9% saline; administer probenecid and I.V. saline before each infusion; allow the admixture to come to room temperature before administration

Dosage Forms Injection: 75 mg/mL (5 mL)

Cilostazol *(sil OH sta zol)*

U.S. Brand Names Pletal®
Canadian Brand Names Pletal®
Synonyms OPC13013
Therapeutic Category Phosphodiesterase Enzyme Inhibitor; Platelet Aggregation Inhibitor
Use Symptomatic management of peripheral vascular disease, primarily intermittent claudication; currently being investigated for the treatment of acute coronary syndromes and for graft patency improvement in percutaneous coronary interventions with or without stenting
Unlabeled/Investigational Use Investigational: Treatment of acute coronary syndromes and for graft patency improvement in percutaneous coronary interventions with or without stenting
Pregnancy Risk Factor C
Pregnancy/Breast-Feeding Implications In animal studies, abnormalities of the skeletal, renal and cardiovascular system were increased. In addition, the incidence of stillbirth and decreased birth weights were increased. It is not known whether cilostazol is excreted in human milk. Because of the potential risk to nursing infants, a decision to discontinue nursing the drug or discontinue nursing should be made.
Contraindications Hypersensitivity to cilostazol or any component of the formulation; heart failure (of any severity)
Warnings/Precautions Use with caution in patients receiving platelet aggregation inhibitors (effects are unknown), hepatic impairment (not studied). Use with caution in patients receiving inhibitors of CYP3A4 (such as ketoconazole or erythromycin) or inhibitors of CYP2C19 (such as omeprazole); use with caution in severe underlying heart disease; use is not recommended in nursing mothers
Adverse Reactions
>10%:
Central nervous system: Headache (27% to 34%)
Gastrointestinal: Abnormal stools (12% to 15%), diarrhea (12% to 19%)
Miscellaneous: Infection (10% to 14%)
2% to 10%:
Cardiovascular: Peripheral edema (7% to 9%), palpitation (5% to 10%), tachycardia (4%)
Central nervous system: Dizziness (9% to 10%)
Gastrointestinal: Dyspepsia (6%), nausea (6% to 7%), abdominal pain (4% to 5%), flatulence (2% to 3%)
Neuromuscular & skeletal: Back pain (6% to 7%), myalgia (2% to 3%)
Respiratory: Rhinitis (7% to 12%), pharyngitis (7% to 10%), cough (3% to 4%)
<2% (Limited to important or life-threatening): Arrhythmia, blindness, cardiac arrest, hemorrhage, cerebral infarction/ischemia, cholelithiasis, colitis, congestive heart failure, duodenal ulcer, esophageal hemorrhage, esophagitis, gout, hematemesis, hemorrhage, hypotension, melena, myocardial infarction/ischemia, neuralgia, peptic ulcer, postural hypotension, purpura, retinal hemorrhage, retroperitoneal hemorrhage, syncope, urticaria, vaginal hemorrhage
Overdosage/Toxicology Experience with overdosage in humans is limited. Headache, diarrhea, hypotension, tachycardia and/or cardiac arrhythmias may occur. Treatment is symptomatic and supportive. Hemodialysis is unlikely to be of value. In some animal models, high-dose or long-term administration was associated with a variety of cardiovascular lesions,

including endocardial hemorrhage, hemosiderin deposition and left ventricular fibrosis, coronary arteritis, and periarteritis.

Drug Interactions
 Cytochrome P450 Effect: CYP2C19 (minor) and 3A4 (major) enzyme substrate
 Increased Effect/Toxicity: Cilostazol serum concentrations may be increased by erythromycin, diltiazem, and omeprazole. Increased concentrations of cilostazol may be anticipated during concurrent therapy with other inhibitors of CYP3A4 (ie, clarithromycin, ketoconazole, itraconazole, fluconazole, miconazole, fluvoxamine, fluoxetine, nefazodone, and sertraline) or inhibitors of CYP2C19. Aspirin-induced inhibition of platelet aggregation is potentiated by concurrent cilostazol. The effect on platelet aggregation with other antiplatelet drugs is unknown.

Ethanol/Nutrition/Herb Interactions Food: Taking cilostazol with a high-fat meal may increase peak concentration by 90%. Avoid concurrent ingestion of grapefruit juice due to the potential to inhibit CYP3A4.

Mechanism of Action Cilostazol and its metabolites are inhibitors of phosphodiesterase III. As a result cyclic AMP is increased leading to inhibition of platelet aggregation and vasodilation. Other effects of phosphodiesterase III inhibition include increased cardiac contractility, accelerated AV nodal conduction, increased ventricular automaticity, heart rate, and coronary blood flow.

Pharmacodynamics/Kinetics
 Onset of action: 2-4 weeks; may require up to 12 weeks
 Protein binding: 97% to 98%
 Metabolism: Hepatic via CYP3A4 and 2C19; at least one metabolite has significant activity
 Half-life elimination: 11-13 hours
 Excretion: Urine (74%) and feces (20%) as metabolites

Usual Dosage Adults: Oral: 100 mg twice daily taken at least one-half hour before or 2 hours after breakfast and dinner; dosage should be reduced to 50 mg twice daily during concurrent therapy with inhibitors of CYP3A4 or CYP2C19 (see Drug Interactions)

Dietary Considerations It is best to take cilostazol 30 minutes before or 2 hours after meals.

Dosage Forms Tablet: 50 mg, 100 mg

♦ **Ciloxan**™ *see* Ciprofloxacin *on page 295*

Cimetidine (sye MET i deen)
Related Information
 Antacid Drug Interactions *on page 1477*
 Depression *on page 1655*
U.S. Brand Names Tagamet®; Tagamet® HB [OTC]
Canadian Brand Names Apo®-Cimetidine; Gen-Cimetidine; Novo-Cimetidine®; Nu-Cimet®; PMS-Cimetidine; Tagamet®; Tagamet® HB
Therapeutic Category Antihistamine, H₂ Blocker; Histamine H₂ Antagonist
Use Short-term treatment of active duodenal ulcers and benign gastric ulcers; long-term prophylaxis of duodenal ulcer; gastric hypersecretory states; gastroesophageal reflux; prevention of upper GI bleeding in critically ill patients
Unlabeled/Investigational Use Part of a multidrug regimen for *H. pylori* eradication to reduce the risk of duodenal ulcer recurrence
Pregnancy Risk Factor B
Contraindications Hypersensitivity to cimetidine, any component of the formulation, or other H₂ antagonists
Warnings/Precautions Adjust dosages in renal/hepatic impairment or patients receiving drugs metabolized through the P450 system
Adverse Reactions
 1% to 10%:
  Central nervous system: Headache, dizziness, agitation, drowsiness
  Gastrointestinal: Diarrhea, nausea, vomiting
 <1% (Limited to important or life-threatening): Agranulocytosis, AST and ALT increased, bradycardia, creatinine increased, hypotension, neutropenia, tachycardia, thrombocytopenia
Overdosage/Toxicology Treatment is primarily symptomatic and supportive. There is no experience with intentional overdose. Reported ingestions of 20 g have resulted in transient side effects. with recommended doses. Animal data have shown respiratory failure, tachycardia, muscle tremors, vomiting, restlessness, hypotension, salivation, emesis, and diarrhea.
Drug Interactions
 Cytochrome P450 Effect: CYP3A3/4 enzyme substrate; CYP1A2, 2C9, 2C18, 2C19, 2D6, and 3A3/4 enzyme inhibitor
 Increased Effect/Toxicity: Cimetidine increases warfarin's effect in a dose-related manner. Cimetidine may increase serum concentrations of alfentanil, amiodarone, benzodiazepines (except lorazepam, oxazepam, temazepam), beta-blockers (except atenolol, betaxolol, bisoprolol, nadolol, penbutolol), calcium channel blockers, carbamazepine, cisapride (avoid concurrent use), citalopram, flecainide, lidocaine, melphalan, meperidine, metronidazole, moricizine, paroxetine, phenytoin, procainamide, propafenone, quinidine, quinolone antibiotics, tacrine, TCAs, theophylline, and triamterene. Cimetidine increases carmustine's myelotoxicity; avoid concurrent use.
 Decreased Effect: Ketoconazole, fluconazole, itraconazole (especially capsule) decrease serum concentration; avoid concurrent use with H₂ antagonists. Delavirdine's absorption is decreased; avoid concurrent use with H₂ antagonists.
Ethanol/Nutrition/Herb Interactions
 Ethanol: Avoid ethanol (may enhance gastric mucosal irritation).
 Food: Cimetidine may increase serum caffeine levels if taken with caffeine. Cimetidine peak serum levels may be decreased if taken with food.
 Herb/Nutraceutical: St John's wort may decrease cimetidine levels.
 (Continued)

Cimetidine *(Continued)*

Stability
Intact vials of cimetidine should be stored at room temperature and protected from light; cimetidine may precipitate from solution upon exposure to cold but can be redissolved by warming without degradation

Stability at room temperature:
Prepared bags: 7 days
Premixed bags: Manufacturer expiration dating and out of overwrap stability: 15 days
Stable in parenteral nutrition solutions for up to 7 days when protected from light

Physically incompatible with barbiturates, amphotericin B, and cephalosporins

Mechanism of Action Competitive inhibition of histamine at H_2-receptors of the gastric parietal cells resulting in reduced gastric acid secretion, gastric volume and hydrogen ion concentration reduced

Pharmacodynamics/Kinetics
Onset of action: 1 hour
Duration: 6 hours
Distribution: Crosses placenta; enters breast milk
Protein binding: 20%
Bioavailability: 60% to 70%
Half-life elimination: Neonates: 3.6 hours; Children: 1.4 hours; Adults: Normal renal function: 2 hours
Time to peak, serum: Oral: 1-2 hours
Excretion: Primarily urine (as unchanged drug); feces (some)

Usual Dosage
Children: Oral, I.M., I.V.: 20-40 mg/kg/day in divided doses every 6 hours
Adults:
Short-term treatment of active ulcers:
Oral: 300 mg 4 times/day or 800 mg at bedtime or 400 mg twice daily for up to 8 weeks
I.M., I.V.: 300 mg every 6 hours or 37.5 mg/hour by continuous infusion; I.V. dosage should be adjusted to maintain an intragastric pH ≥5
Patients with an active bleed: Administer cimetidine as a continuous infusion (see above)
Duodenal ulcer prophylaxis: Oral: 400-800 mg at bedtime
Gastric hypersecretory conditions: Oral, I.M., I.V.: 300-600 mg every 6 hours; dosage not to exceed 2.4 g/day
Helicobacter pylori eradication (unlabeled use): 400 mg twice daily; requires combination therapy with antibiotics

Dosing adjustment/interval in renal impairment: Children and Adults:
Cl_{cr} 20-40 mL/minute: Administer every 8 hours or 75% of normal dose
Cl_{cr} 0-20 mL/minute: Administer every 12 hours or 50% of normal dose
Hemodialysis: Slightly dialyzable (5% to 20%)

Dosing adjustment/comments in hepatic impairment: Usual dose is safe in mild liver disease but use with caution and in reduced dosage in severe liver disease; increased risk of CNS toxicity in cirrhosis suggested by enhanced penetration of CNS

Administration Administer with meals so that the drug's peak effect occurs at the proper time (peak inhibition of gastric acid secretion occurs at 1 and 3 hours after dosing in fasting subjects and approximately 2 hours in nonfasting subjects; this correlates well with the time food is no longer in the stomach offering a buffering effect)

Monitoring Parameters CBC, gastric pH, occult blood with GI bleeding; monitor renal function to correct dose.

Test Interactions Increased creatinine, AST, ALT

Patient Information Take with or immediately after meals; take 1 hour before or 2 hours after antacids; may cause drowsiness, impaired judgment, or coordination; avoid excessive alcohol

Nursing Implications
Modify dosage in patients with renal impairment; can be administered as a slow I.V. push over a minimum of 15 minutes at a concentration not to exceed 15 mg/mL; or preferably as an I.V. intermittent or I.V. continuous infusion. Intermittent infusions are administered over 15-30 minutes at a final concentration not to exceed 6 mg/mL; for patients with an active bleed, preferred method of administration is continuous infusion
Monitor blood pressure with I.V. push administration; CBC

Dosage Forms
Infusion, as hydrochloride, in NS: 300 mg (50 mL)
Injection, as hydrochloride: 150 mg/mL (2 mL, 8 mL)
Liquid, oral, as hydrochloride: 200 mg/20 mL; 300 mg/5 mL with alcohol 2.8% (5 mL, 240 mL) [mint-peach flavor]
Tablet: 100 mg, 200 mg, 300 mg, 400 mg, 800 mg

♦ Cinobac® **(Can)** *see* Cinoxacin *on page 294*
♦ Cinobac® **Pulvules®** *see* Cinoxacin *on page 294*

Cinoxacin *(sin OKS a sin)*
Related Information
Antacid Drug Interactions *on page 1477*
U.S. Brand Names Cinobac® Pulvules®
Canadian Brand Names Cinobac®
Therapeutic Category Antibiotic, Quinolone
Use Treatment of urinary tract infections
Pregnancy Risk Factor B
Contraindications Hypersensitivity to cinoxacin, any component of the formulation, or other quinolones; history of convulsive disorders
Warnings/Precautions CNS stimulation may occur (tremor, restlessness, confusion, and very rarely hallucinations or seizures). Use with caution in patients with known or suspected

CNS disorders or renal impairment. Not recommended in children <18 years of age, ciprofloxacin (a related compound), has caused a transient arthropathy in children; prolonged use may result in superinfection; modify dosage in patients with renal impairment. Tendon inflammation and/or rupture have been reported with other quinolone antibiotics. Discontinue at first sign of tendon inflammation or pain. Quinolones may exacerbate myasthenia gravis.

Severe hypersensitivity reactions, including anaphylaxis, have occurred with quinolone therapy. If an allergic reaction occurs (itching, urticaria, dyspnea, facial edema, loss of consciousness, tingling, cardiovascular collapse), discontinue drug immediately. Prolonged use may result in superinfection; pseudomembranous colitis may occur and should be considered in all patients who present with diarrhea.

Adverse Reactions Generally well tolerated

Central nervous system: Confusion, dizziness, headache, insomnia, seizures (rare)

Gastrointestinal: Abdominal pain, anorexia, belching, diarrhea, flatulence, GI bleeding, heartburn, nausea

Hematologic: Thrombocytopenia (rare)

Ocular: Photophobia

Otic: Tinnitus

Overdosage/Toxicology Symptoms include acute renal failure and seizures. Treatment includes GI decontamination and supportive care. Not removed by peritoneal or hemodialysis.

Drug Interactions

Increased Effect/Toxicity: Quinolones may cause increased levels of azlocillin, cyclosporine, and caffeine/theophylline. Azlocillin, cimetidine, loop diuretics (furosemide, torsemide), and probenecid increase quinolone levels (decreased renal secretion). An increased incidence of seizures may occur with foscarnet or NSAIDs. The hypoprothrombinemic effect of warfarin is enhanced by some quinolone antibiotics.

Decreased Effect: Metal cations (magnesium, aluminum, iron, and zinc) bind quinolones in the gastrointestinal tract and inhibit absorption (by up to 98%). Due to electrolyte content, antacids, electrolyte supplements, sucralfate, quinapril, and some didanosine formulations should be avoided. Levofloxacin should be administered 4 hours before or 8 hours (a minimum of 2 hours before and 2 hours after) after these agents. Antineoplastic agents may decrease the absorption of quinolones.

Mechanism of Action Inhibits microbial synthesis of DNA with resultant inhibition of protein synthesis

Pharmacodynamics/Kinetics

Absorption: Oral: Rapid and complete; food decreases peak levels by 30% but not total amount absorbed

Distribution: Crosses placenta; concentrates in prostate tissue

Protein binding: 60% to 80%

Half-life elimination: 1.5 hours; prolonged in renal impairment

Time to peak, serum: 2-3 hours

Excretion: Urine (~60% as unchanged drug)

Usual Dosage Children >12 years and Adults: Oral: 1 g/day in 2-4 doses for 7-14 days

Dosing interval in renal impairment:

Cl_{cr} 20-50 mL/minute: 250 mg twice daily

Cl_{cr} <20 mL/minute: 250 mg/day

Patient Information May be taken with food to minimize upset stomach; avoid antacid use; drink fluid liberally; may cause dizziness; use caution when driving or performing other tasks requiring alertness

Nursing Implications Hold antacids for 3-4 hours after giving

Dosage Forms Capsule: 250 mg, 500 mg

♦ **Cipro**® see Ciprofloxacin on page 295

Ciprofloxacin (sip roe FLOKS a sin)

Related Information

Antacid Drug Interactions on page 1477

Antimicrobial Drugs of Choice on page 1588

Desensitization Protocols on page 1525

Treatment of Sexually Transmitted Diseases on page 1609

Tuberculosis Treatment Guidelines on page 1612

USPHA/IDSA Guidelines for the Prevention of Opportunistic Infections in Persons With HIV on page 1574

U.S. Brand Names Ciloxan™; Cipro®

Canadian Brand Names Ciloxan®; Cipro®

Synonyms Ciprofloxacin Hydrochloride

Therapeutic Category Antibiotic, Ophthalmic; Antibiotic, Quinolone

Use Treatment of documented or suspected infections of the lower respiratory tract, sinuses, skin and skin structure, bone/joints, and urinary tract (including prostatitis) due to susceptible bacterial strains; especially indicated for pseudomonal infections and those due to multidrug-resistant gram-negative organisms, chronic bacterial prostatitis, infectious diarrhea, complicated gram-negative and anaerobic intra-abdominal infections (with metronidazole) due to E. coli (enteropathic strains), B. fragilis, P. mirabilis, K. pneumoniae, P. aeruginosa, Campylobacter jejuni or Shigella; approved for acute sinusitis caused by H. influenzae or M. catarrhalis; also used in treatment of typhoid fever due to Salmonella typhi (although eradication of the chronic typhoid carrier state has not been proven), osteomyelitis when parenteral therapy is not feasible, acute uncomplicated cystitis in females, to reduce incidence or progression of disease following exposure to aerolized Bacillus anthracis, febrile neutropenia (with piperacillin), and sexually-transmitted diseases such as uncomplicated cervical and urethral gonorrhea due to Neisseria gonorrhoeae; used ophthalmologically for superficial ocular infections (corneal ulcers, conjunctivitis) due to susceptible strains

Pregnancy Risk Factor C

Pregnancy/Breast-Feeding Implications Reports of arthropathy (observed in immature animals and reported rarely in humans) has limited the use of fluoroquinolones in pregnancy. (Continued)

Ciprofloxacin (Continued)

According to the FDA, the Teratogen Information System concluded that therapeutic doses during pregnancy are unlikely to produce substantial teratogenic risk, but data are insufficient to say that there is no risk. In general, reports of exposure have been limited to short durations of therapy in the first trimester. When considering treatment for life-threatening infection and/or prolonged duration of therapy (such as in anthrax), the potential risk to the fetus must be balanced against the severity of the potential illness.

Contraindications Hypersensitivity to ciprofloxacin, any component of the formulation, or other quinolones

Warnings/Precautions Not recommended in children <18 years of age (exception - postexposure treatment of inhalational anthrax); has caused transient arthropathy in children; CNS stimulation may occur (tremor, restlessness, confusion, and very rarely hallucinations or seizures); use with caution in patients with known or suspected CNS disorder; green discoloration of teeth in newborns has been reported; prolonged use may result in superinfection. Tendon inflammation and/or rupture have been reported with ciprofloxacin and other quinolone antibiotics. Discontinue at first sign of tendon inflammation or pain. Quinolones may exacerbate myasthenia gravis.

Severe hypersensitivity reactions, including anaphylaxis, have occurred with quinolone therapy. If an allergic reaction occurs (itching, urticaria, dyspnea, facial edema, loss of consciousness, tingling, cardiovascular collapse), discontinue drug immediately.

Adverse Reactions

1% to 10%:
Central nervous system: Headache (1%), restlessness (1%)
Dermatologic: Rash (1%)
Gastrointestinal: Nausea (5%), diarrhea (2%), vomiting (2%), abdominal pain (2%)
Hepatic: Elevated ALT/AST (2%)
Renal: Elevated serum creatinine (1%)

<1% (Limited to important or life-threatening): Acute renal failure, agranulocytosis, allergic reactions, angina pectoris, arthralgia, cardiopulmonary arrest, cholestatic jaundice, confusion, dyspnea, erythema multiforme, gastrointestinal bleeding, hallucinations, joint pain, myocardial infarction, nightmares, photosensitivity, prolongation of PT, pseudomembranous colitis, ruptured tendons, seizures, Stevens-Johnson syndrome, syncope, toxic epidermal necrolysis

Overdosage/Toxicology Symptoms include acute renal failure and seizures. Treatment includes GI decontamination and supportive care. Not removed by peritoneal or hemodialysis.

Drug Interactions

Cytochrome P450 Effect: CYP1A2 enzyme inhibitor

Increased Effect/Toxicity: Ciprofloxacin increases the levels/effect of cyclosporine, caffeine, theophylline, and warfarin. The CNS-stimulating effect of some quinolones may be enhanced by NSAIDs, and foscarnet has been associated with an increased risk of seizures with some quinolones. Serum levels of some quinolones are increased by loop diuretics, probenecid, and cimetidine (and possibly other H_2-blockers) due to altered renal elimination. This effect may be more important for quinolones with high percentage of renal elimination than with ciprofloxacin.

Decreased Effect: Enteral feedings may decrease plasma concentrations of ciprofloxacin probably by >30% inhibition of absorption. Aluminum/magnesium products, didanosine, quinapril, and sucralfate may decrease absorption of ciprofloxacin by ≥90% if administered concurrently. (Administer ciprofloxacin at least 4 hours and preferably 6 hours after the dose of these agents.) Calcium, iron, zinc, and multivitamins with minerals products may decrease absorption of ciprofloxacin significantly if administered concurrently. (Administer ciprofloxacin 2 hours before dose or at least 2 hours after the dose of these agents). Antineoplastic agents may decrease quinolone absorption. Intravenous ciprofloxacin may decrease serum phenytoin concentrations.

Ethanol/Nutrition/Herb Interactions

Food: Food decreases rate, but not extent, of absorption. Ciprofloxacin serum levels may be decreased if taken with dairy products. Ciprofloxacin may increase serum caffeine levels if taken with caffeine.

Herb/Nutraceutical: Avoid dong quai, St John's wort (may also cause photosensitization).

Stability Refrigeration and room temperature: Prepared bags: 14 days; Premixed bags: Manufacturer expiration dating

Mechanism of Action Inhibits DNA-gyrase in susceptible organisms; inhibits relaxation of supercoiled DNA and promotes breakage of double-stranded DNA

Pharmacodynamics/Kinetics

Absorption: Oral: Rapid (~50% to 85%)

Distribution: Widely throughout body; tissue concentrations often exceed serum concentrations especially in kidneys, gallbladder, liver, lungs, gynecological tissue, and prostatic tissue; CSF concentrations: 10% (noninflamed meninges), 14% to 37% (inflamed meninges); crosses placenta; enters breast milk

Protein binding: 16% to 43%

Metabolism: Partially hepatic

Half-life elimination: Children: 2.5 hours; Adults: Normal renal function: 3-5 hours

Time to peak: Oral: 0.5-2 hours

Excretion: Urine (30% to 50% as unchanged drug); feces (20% to 40%)

Usual Dosage

Children (see Warnings/Precautions):
Oral: 20-30 mg/kg/day in 2 divided doses; maximum: 1.5 g/day
Cystic fibrosis: 20-40 mg/kg/day divided every 12 hours
Anthrax:
Inhalational (postexposure prophylaxis): 10-15 mg/kg/dose every 12 hours for 60 days; maximum: 500 mg/dose
Cutaneous (treatment): 10-15 mg/kg every 12 hours for 60 days; amoxicillin 80 mg/kg/day divided every 8 hours is an option for completion of treatment after clinical

improvement. **Note:** In the presence of systemic involvement, extensive edema, lesions on head/neck, refer to I.V. dosing for treatment of inhalational/gastrointestinal/oropharyngeal anthrax

I.V.: 15-20 mg/kg/day divided every 12 hours

Cystic fibrosis: 15-30 mg/kg/day divided every 8-12 hours

Anthrax:

Inhalational (postexposure prophylaxis): 10 mg/kg/dose every 12 hours; do **not** exceed 400 mg/dose (800 mg/day)

Inhalational/gastrointestinal/oropharyngeal (treatment): Initial: 10-15 mg/kg every 12 hours for 60 days (maximum: 500 mg/dose); switch to oral therapy when clinically appropriate; refer to Adults dosing for notes on combined therapy and duration

Adults: Oral:

Urinary tract infection: 250-500 mg every 12 hours for 7-10 days, depending on severity of infection and susceptibility

Cystitis, uncomplicated (in females): 100 mg or 250 mg every 12 hours for 3 days

Lower respiratory tract, skin/skin structure infections: 500-750 mg twice daily for 7-14 days depending on severity and susceptibility

Bone/joint infections: 500-750 mg twice daily for 4-6 weeks, depending on severity and susceptibility

Infectious diarrhea: 500 mg every 12 hours for 5-7 days

Typhoid fever: 500 mg every 12 hours for 10 days

Urethral/cervical gonococcal infections: 500 mg as a single dose (CDC recommends concomitant doxycycline or azithromycin due to developing resistance; avoid use in Asian or Western Pacific travelers)

Disseminated gonococcal infection: 500 mg twice daily to complete 7 days of therapy (initial treatment with ceftriaxone 1 g I.M./I.V. daily for 24-48 hours after improvement begins)

Chancroid: 500 mg twice daily for 3 days

Mild to moderate sinusitis: 500 mg every 12 hours for 10 days

Chronic bacterial prostatitis: 500 mg every 12 hours for 28 days

Anthrax:

Inhalational (postexposure prophylaxis): 500 mg every 12 hours for 60 days

Cutaneous (treatment): 500 mg every 12 hours for 60 days. **Note:** In the presence of systemic involvement, extensive edema, lesions on head/neck, refer to I.V. dosing for treatment of inhalational/gastrointestinal/oropharyngeal anthrax

Adults: I.V.:

Lower respiratory tract, skin/skin structure infection, or bone/ joint infections:

Mild to moderate: 400 mg every 12 hours for 7-14 days

Severe or complicated: 400 mg every 8 hours for 7-14 days

Nosocomial pneumonia (mild to moderate to severe): 400 mg every 8 hours

Prostatitis (chronic, bacterial): 400 mg every 12 hours

Sinusitis (acute): 400 mg every 12 hours

Urinary tract infection:

Mild to moderate: 200 mg every 12 hours for 7-10 days

Severe or complicated: 400 mg every 12 hours for 7-10 days

Febrile neutropenia (with piperacillin): 400 mg every 8 hours for 7-14 days

Intra-abdominal infection (with metronidazole): 400 mg every 12 hours

Anthrax:

Inhalational (postexposure prophylaxis): 400 mg every 12 hours

Inhalational/gastrointestinal/oropharyngeal (treatment): 400 mg every 12 hours. **Note:** Initial treatment should include two or more agents predicted to be effective (per CDC recommendations). Agents suggested for use in conjunction with ciprofloxacin or doxycycline include rifampin, vancomycin, imipenem, penicillin, ampicillin, chloramphenicol, clindamycin, and clarithromycin. May switch to oral antimicrobial therapy when clinically appropriate. Continue combined therapy for 60 days.

Elderly: No adjustment needed in patients with normal renal function

Ophthalmic:

Solution: Children >1 year and Adults: Instill 1-2 drops in eye(s) every 2 hours while awake for 2 days and 1-2 drops every 4 hours while awake for the next 5 days

Ointment: Children >2 years and Adults: Apply a ½" ribbon into the conjunctival sac 3 times/day for the first 2 days, followed by a ½" ribbon applied twice daily for the next 5 days

Dosing adjustment in renal impairment:

Cl_{cr} 30-50 mL/minute: Oral: 250-500 mg every 12 hours

Cl_{cr} 5-29 mL/minute:

Oral: 250-500 mg every 18 hours

I.V.: 200-400 mg every 18-24 hours

Dialysis: Only small amounts of ciprofloxacin are removed by hemo- or peritoneal dialysis (<10%); usual dose: 250-500 mg every 24 hours following dialysis

Continuous arteriovenous or venovenous hemodiafiltration effects: Administer 200-400 mg I.V. every 12 hours

Dietary Considerations

Food: Drug may cause GI upset; take without regard to meals (manufacturer prefers that drug is taken 2 hours after meals).

Dairy products, oral multivitamins, and mineral supplements: Absorption of ciprofloxacin is decreased by divalent and trivalent cations. The manufacturer states that the usual dietary intake of calcium has not been shown to interfere with ciprofloxacin absorption. Products may be taken 6 hours before or 2 hours following a dose of ciprofloxacin.

Caffeine: Patients consuming regular large quantities of caffeinated beverages may need to restrict caffeine intake if excessive cardiac or CNS stimulation occurs.

Administration

Oral: May administer with food to minimize GI upset; avoid antacid use; maintain proper hydration and urine output. Oral suspension should not be administered through feeding (Continued)

Ciprofloxacin *(Continued)*

tubes (due to its physical characteristics). Patients should avoid chewing on the microcapsules if the suspension is administered orally. Separate oral administration from drugs which may impair absorption (see Drug Interactions).

Parenteral: Administer by slow I.V. infusion over 60 minutes to reduce the risk of venous irritation (burning, pain, erythema, and swelling); final concentration for administration should not exceed 2 mg/mL

Monitoring Parameters Patients receiving concurrent ciprofloxacin, theophylline, or cyclosporine should have serum levels monitored

Reference Range Therapeutic: 2.6-3 µg/mL; Toxic: >5 µg/mL

Patient Information Take as directed, preferably on an empty stomach, 2 hours after meals. Swallow oral suspension, do not chew microcapsules. Take entire prescription even if feeling better. Maintain adequate hydration (2-3 L/day of fluids unless instructed to restrict fluid intake) to avoid concentrated urine and crystal formation. You may experience nausea, vomiting, or anorexia (small frequent meals, frequent mouth care, sucking lozenges, or chewing gum may help). You may experience increased sensitivity to sunlight; use sunblock, wear protective clothing and dark glasses, or avoid direct exposure to sunlight. Report immediately any signs of skin rash, joint or back pain, or difficulty breathing. Report unusual fever or chills; vaginal itching or foul-smelling vaginal discharge; easy bruising or bleeding. Report immediately any pain, inflammation, or rupture of tendon.

Dosage Forms
Infusion, as hydrochloride [in D$_5$W]: 400 mg (200 mL)
Infusion, as hydrochloride [in NS or D$_5$W]: 200 mg (100 mL)
Injection, as hydrochloride: 200 mg (20 mL); 400 mg (40 mL)
Ointment, ophthalmic, as hydrochloride: 3.33 mg/g [0.3% base] (3.5 g)
Solution, ophthalmic, as hydrochloride: 3.33 mg/g [0.3% base] (2.5 mL, 5 mL. 10 mL)
Suspension, oral: 250 mg/5 mL (100 mL); 500 mg/5 mL (100 mL)
Tablet, as hydrochloride: 100 mg, 250 mg, 500 mg, 750 mg

Ciprofloxacin and Hydrocortisone

(sip roe FLOKS a sin & hye droe KOR ti sone)

U.S. Brand Names Cipro® HC Otic

Canadian Brand Names Cipro® HC

Synonyms Hydrocortisone and Ciprofloxacin

Therapeutic Category Antibiotic/Corticosteroid, Otic

Use Treatment of acute otitis externa, sometimes known as "swimmer's ear"

Usual Dosage Children >1 year of age and Adults: Otic: The recommended dosage for all patients is three drops of the suspension in the affected ear twice daily for seven day; twice-daily dosing schedule is more convenient for patients than that of existing treatments with hydrocortisone, which are typically administered three or four times a day; a twice-daily dosage schedule may be especially helpful for parents and caregivers of young children

Additional Information Complete prescribing information for this medication should be consulted for additional detail.

Dosage Forms Suspension, otic: Ciprofloxacin hydrochloride 0.2% and hydrocortisone 1%

♦ **Ciprofloxacin Hydrochloride** *see* Ciprofloxacin *on page 295*

♦ **Cipro® HC (Can)** *see* Ciprofloxacin and Hydrocortisone *on page 298*

♦ **Cipro® HC Otic** *see* Ciprofloxacin and Hydrocortisone *on page 298*

Cisapride *U.S. - Available Via Limited-Access Protocol Only*

(SIS a pride)

U.S. Brand Names Propulsid®

Therapeutic Category Cholinergic Agent; Gastroprokinetic Agent

Use Treatment of nocturnal symptoms of gastroesophageal reflux disease (GERD); has demonstrated effectiveness for gastroparesis, refractory constipation, and nonulcer dyspepsia

Pregnancy Risk Factor C

Contraindications

Hypersensitivity to cisapride or any component of the formulations; GI hemorrhage, mechanical obstruction, GI perforation, or other situations when GI motility stimulation is dangerous

Serious cardiac arrhythmias including ventricular tachycardia, ventricular fibrillation, torsade de pointes, and QT prolongation have been reported in patients taking cisapride with other drugs that inhibit CYP3A4. Some of these events have been fatal. Concomitant oral or intravenous administration of the following drugs with cisapride may lead to elevated cisapride blood levels and is contraindicated:

Antibiotics: Oral or I.V. erythromycin, clarithromycin, troleandomycin
Antidepressants: Nefazodone
Antifungals: Oral or I.V. fluconazole, itraconazole, miconazole, oral ketoconazole
Protease inhibitors: Indinavir, ritonavir, amprenavir

Cisapride is also contraindicated for patients with a prolonged electrocardiographic QT intervals (QT$_c$ >450 msec), a history of QT$_c$ prolongation, or known family history of congenital long QT syndrome; clinically significant bradycardia, renal failure, history of ventricular arrhythmias, ischemic heart disease, and congestive heart failure; uncorrected electrolyte disorders (hypokalemia, hypomagnesemia); respiratory failure; and concomitant medications known to prolong the QT interval and increase the risk of arrhythmia, such as certain antiarrhythmics, certain antipsychotics, certain antidepressants, astemizole, bepridil, sparfloxacin, and terodiline. The preceding lists of drugs are not comprehensive. Cisapride should not be used in patients with uncorrected hypokalemia or hypomagnesemia or who might experience rapid reduction of plasma potassium such as those administered potassium-wasting diuretics and/or insulin in acute settings.

Warnings/Precautions Safety and effectiveness in children have not been established.

On March 24, 2000 the FDA announced that the manufacturer of cisapride would voluntarily withdraw its product from the U.S. market on July 14, 2000. This decision

was based on 341 reports of heart rhythm abnormalities including 80 reports of deaths. The company will continue to make the drug available to patients who meet specific clinical eligibility criteria for a limited-access protocol (contact 1-800-JANSSEN). Serious cardiac arrhythmias including ventricular tachycardia, ventricular fibrillation, torsade de pointes, and QT prolongation have been reported in patients taking this drug. Many of these patients also took drugs expected to increase cisapride blood levels by inhibiting the cytochrome P450 3A4 enzymes that metabolize cisapride. These drugs include clarithromycin, erythromycin, troleandomycin, nefazodone, fluconazole, itraconazole, ketoconazole, indinavir and ritonavir. Some of these events have been fatal. Cisapride is contraindicated in patients taking any of these drugs. **QT prolongation, torsade de pointes (sometimes with syncope), cardiac arrest and sudden death have been reported in patients taking cisapride without the above-mentioned contraindicated drugs.** Most patients had disorders that may have predisposed them to arrhythmias with cisapride. Cisapride is contraindicated for those patients with: history of prolonged electrocardiographic QT intervals; renal failure; history of ventricular arrhythmias, ischemic heart disease, and congestive heart failure; uncorrected electrolyte disorders (hypokalemia, hypomagnesemia); respiratory failure; and concomitant medications known to prolong the QT interval and increase the risk of arrhythmia, such as certain antiarrhythmics, including those of Class 1A (such as quinidine and procainamide) and Class III (such as sotalol); tricyclic antidepressants (such as amitriptyline); certain tetracyclic antidepressants (such as maprotiline); certain antipsychotic medications (such as certain phenothiazines and sertindole); protease inhibitors, astemizole, bepridil, sparfloxacin and terodiline. (The preceding lists of drugs are not comprehensive.) Recommended doses of cisapride should not be exceeded.

Patients should have a baseline ECG and an electrolyte panel (magnesium, calcium, potassium) prior to initiating cisapride (see Contraindications). Potential benefits should be weighed against risks prior administration of cisapride to patients who have or may develop prolongation of cardiac conduction intervals, particularly QT_c. These include patients with conditions that could predispose them to the development of serious arrhythmias, such as multiple organ failure, COPD, apnea and advanced cancer. Cisapride should not be used in patients with uncorrected hypokalemia or hypomagnesemia, such as those with severe dehydration, vomiting or malnutrition, or those taking potassium-wasting diuretics. Cisapride should not be used in patients who might experience rapid reduction of plasma potassium, such as those administered potassium-wasting diuretics and/or insulin in acute settings.

Adverse Reactions
>10%:
Central nervous system: Headache
Gastrointestinal: Diarrhea (dose dependent)
1% to 10%:
Cardiovascular: Tachycardia
Central nervous system: Extrapyramidal effects, somnolence, fatigue, insomnia, anxiety
Dermatologic: Rash
Gastrointestinal: Abdominal cramping, constipation, nausea
Respiratory: Sinusitis, rhinitis, coughing, upper respiratory tract infection, increased incidence of viral infection
<1% (Limited to important or life-threatening): Apnea, bronchospasm, gynecomastia, hyperprolactinemia, methemoglobinemia, photosensitivity, psychiatric disturbances, seizures (have been reported only in patients with a history of seizures)

Drug Interactions
Cytochrome P450 Effect: CYP3A3/4 enzyme substrate
Increased Effect/Toxicity: Cisapride may increase blood levels of warfarin, diazepam, cimetidine, ranitidine, and CNS depressants. The risk of cisapride-induced malignant arrhythmias may be increased by azole antifungals (fluconazole, itraconazole, ketoconazole, miconazole), antiarrhythmics (Class Ia; quinidine, procainamide, and Class III; amiodarone, sotalol), bepridil, cimetidine, maprotiline, macrolide antibiotics (erythromycin, clarithromycin, troleandomycin), molindone, nefazodone, protease inhibitors (amprenavir, indinavir, nelfinavir, ritonavir), phenothiazines (eg, prochlorperazine, promethazine), sertindole, tricyclic antidepressants (eg amitriptyline), and some quinolone antibiotics (sparfloxacin, gatifloxacin, moxifloxacin). Cardiovascular disease or electrolyte imbalances (potentially due to diuretic therapy) increase the risk of malignant arrhythmias.
Decreased Effect: Cisapride may decrease the effect of atropine and digoxin.

Ethanol/Nutrition/Herb Interactions
Ethanol: Avoid ethanol (may increase CNS depression).
Food: Coadministration of grapefruit juice with cisapride increases the bioavailability of cisapride and concomitant use should be avoided.
Herb/Nutraceutical: St John's wort may decrease cisapride levels.

Mechanism of Action Enhances the release of acetylcholine at the myenteric plexus. *In vitro* studies have shown cisapride to have serotonin-4 receptor agonistic properties which may increase gastrointestinal motility and cardiac rate; increases lower esophageal sphincter pressure and lower esophageal peristalsis; accelerates gastric emptying of both liquids and solids.

Pharmacodynamics/Kinetics
Onset of action: 0.5-1 hour
Protein binding: 97.5% to 98%
Metabolism: Extensively to norcisapride
Bioavailability: 35% to 40%
Half-life elimination: 6-12 hours
Excretion: Urine and feces (<10%)

Usual Dosage Oral:
Children: 0.15-0.3 mg/kg/dose 3-4 times/day; maximum: 10 mg/dose
Adults: Initial: 10 mg 4 times/day at least 15 minutes before meals and at bedtime; in some patients the dosage will need to be increased to 20 mg to obtain a satisfactory result

Nursing Implications Safety and effectiveness in children have not been established. Although cisapride does not affect psychomotor function nor induce sedation or drowsiness
(Continued)

Cisapride *U.S. - Available Via Limited-Access Protocol Only* (Continued)

when used alone, advise patients that the sedative effects of benzodiazepines and of ethanol may be accelerated.

Additional Information IMPORTANT NOTE: On March 24, 2000, the FDA announced that the manufacturer of cisapride would voluntarily withdraw its product from the U.S. market on July 14, 2000. This decision was based on 341 reports of heart rhythm abnormalities including 80 reports of deaths. The company will continue to make the drug available to patients who meet specific clinical eligibility criteria for a limited-access protocol (contact 1-800-JANSSEN).

Dosage Forms
Suspension, oral: 1 mg/mL (450 mL) [cherry cream flavor]
Tablet, scored: 10 mg, 20 mg

Cisatracurium (sis a tra KYOO ree um)

Related Information
Neuromuscular Blocking Agents Comparison *on page 1508*
U.S. Brand Names Nimbex®
Canadian Brand Names Nimbex®
Synonyms Cisatracurium Besylate
Therapeutic Category Neuromuscular Blocker Agent, Nondepolarizing; Skeletal Muscle Relaxant
Use Adjunct to general anesthesia to facilitate endotracheal intubation and to relax skeletal muscles during surgery; to facilitate mechanical ventilation in ICU patients; does not relieve pain or produce sedation
Pregnancy Risk Factor C
Contraindications Hypersensitivity to cisatracurium besylate or any component of the formulation
Warnings/Precautions Certain clinical conditions may result in potentiation or antagonism of neuromuscular blockade:
Potentiation: Electrolyte abnormalities, severe hyponatremia, severe hypocalcemia, severe hypokalemia, hypermagnesemia, neuromuscular diseases, acidosis, acute intermittent porphyria, renal failure, hepatic failure
Antagonism: Alkalosis, hypercalcemia, demyelinating lesions, peripheral neuropathies, diabetes mellitus

Increased sensitivity in patients with myasthenia gravis, Eaton-Lambert syndrome; resistance in burn patients (>30% of body) for period of 5-70 days postinjury; resistance in patients with muscle trauma, denervation, immobilization, infection
Adverse Reactions <1%: Effects are minimal and transient, bradycardia and hypotension, flushing, rash, bronchospasm
Overdosage/Toxicology Symptoms include respiratory depression and cardiovascular collapse. Neostigmine 1-3 mg slow I.V. push in adults (0.5 mg in children) antagonizes the neuromuscular blockade, and should be administered with or immediately after atropine 1-1.5 mg I.V. push (adults). This may be especially useful in the presence of bradycardia.
Drug Interactions
Increased Effect/Toxicity: Increased effects are possible with aminoglycosides, beta-blockers, clindamycin, calcium channel blockers, halogenated anesthetics, imipenem, ketamine, lidocaine, loop diuretics (furosemide), macrolides (case reports), magnesium sulfate, procainamide, quinidine, quinolones, tetracyclines, and vancomycin. May increase risk of myopathy when used with high-dose corticosteroids for extended periods.
Decreased Effect: Effect of nondepolarizing neuromuscular blockers may be reduced by carbamazepine (chronic use), corticosteroids (also associated with myopathy - see increased effect), phenytoin (chronic use), sympathomimetics, and theophylline.
Stability Refrigerate intact vials at 2°C to 8°C/36°F to 46°F; use vials within 21 days upon removal from the refrigerator to room temperature (25°C to 77°F). Dilutions of 0.1-0.2 mg/mL in 0.9% sodium chloride or dextrose 5% in water are stable for up to 24 hours at room temperature. **Incompatible** with sodium bicarbonate, ketorolac, propofol; **compatible** with alfentanil, droperidol, fentanyl, midazolam, and sufentanil.
Mechanism of Action Blocks neural transmission at the myoneural junction by binding with cholinergic receptor sites
Pharmacodynamics/Kinetics
Onset of action: I.V.: 2-3 minutes
Peak effect: 3-5 minutes
Duration: Recovery begins in 20-35 minutes when anesthesia is balanced; recovery is attained in 90% of patients in 25-93 minutes
Metabolism: Undergoes rapid nonenzymatic degradation in the bloodstream, additional metabolism occurs via ester hydrolysis; some active metabolites
Half-life elimination: 22 minutes
Usual Dosage I.V. (not to be used I.M.):
Operating room administration:
Children 2-12 years: Intubating doses: 0.1 mg over 5-15 seconds during either halothane or opioid anesthesia. (**Note:** When given during stable opioid/nitrous oxide/oxygen anesthesia, 0.1 mg/kg produces maximum neuromuscular block in an average of 2.8 minutes and clinically effective block for 28 minutes.)
Adults: Intubating doses: 0.15-0.2 mg/kg as component of propofol/nitrous oxide/oxygen induction-intubation technique. (**Note:** May produce generally good or excellent conditions for tracheal intubation in 1.5-2 minutes with clinically effective duration of action during propofol anesthesia of 55-61 minutes.); initial dose after succinylcholine for intubation: 0.1 mg/kg; maintenance dose: 0.03 mg/kg 40-60 minutes after initial dose, then at ~20-minute intervals based on clinical criteria
Children ≥2 years and Adults: Continuous infusion: After an initial bolus, a diluted solution can be given by continuous infusion for maintenance of neuromuscular blockade during

extended surgery; adjust the rate of administration according to the patient's response as determined by peripheral nerve stimulation. An initial infusion rate of 3 mcg/kg/minute may be required to rapidly counteract the spontaneous recovery of neuromuscular function; thereafter, a rate of 1-2 mcg/kg/minute should be adequate to maintain continuous neuromuscular block in the 89% to 99% range in most pediatric and adult patients. Consider reduction of the infusion rate by 30% to 40% when administering during stable isoflurane, enflurane, sevoflurane, or desflurane anesthesia. Spontaneous recovery from neuromuscular blockade following discontinuation of infusion of cisatracurium may be expected to proceed at a rate comparable to that following single bolus administration.

Intensive care unit administration: Follow the principles for infusion in the operating room. At initial signs of recovery from bolus dose, begin the infusion at a dose of 3 mcg/kg/minute and adjust rates accordingly; dosage ranges of 0.5-10 mcg/kg/minute have been reported. If patient is allowed to recover from neuromuscular blockade, readministration of a bolus dose may be necessary to quickly re-establish neuromuscular block prior to reinstituting the infusion. See table.

Cisatracurium Besylate Infusion Chart

Drug Delivery Rate (mcg/kg/min)	Infusion Rate (mL/kg/min) 0.1 mg/mL (10 mg/100 mL)	Infusion Rate (mL/kg/min) 0.4 mg/mL (40 mg/100 mL)
1	0.01	0.0025
1.5	0.015	0.00375
2	0.02	0.005
3	0.03	0.0075
5	0.05	0.0125

Dosing adjustment in renal impairment: Because slower times to onset of complete neuromuscular block were observed in renal dysfunction patients, extending the interval between the administration of cisatracurium and intubation attempt may be required to achieve adequate intubation conditions.

Administration Administer I.V. only; the use of a peripheral nerve stimulator will permit the most advantageous use of cisatracurium, minimize the possibility of overdosage or underdosage and assist in the evaluation of recovery

Give undiluted as a bolus injection; not for I.M. injection, too much tissue irritation; continuous administration requires the use of an infusion pump

Monitoring Parameters Vital signs (heart rate, blood pressure, respiratory rate)

Patient Information May be difficult to talk because of head and neck muscle blockade

Nursing Implications Neuromuscular blocking potency is 3 times that of atracurium; maximum block is up to 2 minutes longer than for equipotent doses of atracurium

Additional Information Cisatracurium is classified as an intermediate-duration neuromuscular-blocking agent. It does not appear to have a cumulative effect on the duration of blockade. Neuromuscular-blocking potency is 3 times that of atracurium; maximum block is up to 2 minutes longer than for equipotent doses of atracurium.

Dosage Forms Injection, as besylate: 2 mg/mL (5 mL, 10 mL); 10 mg/mL (20 mL)

♦ **Cisatracurium Besylate** see Cisatracurium on page 300

Cisplatin (SIS pla tin)

U.S. Brand Names Platinol®; Platinol®-AQ

Canadian Brand Names Platinol®-AQ

Synonyms CDDP

Therapeutic Category Antineoplastic Agent, Alkylating Agent; Antineoplastic Agent, Vesicant; Vesicant

Use Treatment of head and neck, breast, testicular, and ovarian cancer; Hodgkin's and non-Hodgkin's lymphoma; neuroblastoma; sarcomas; bladder, gastric, lung, esophageal, cervical, and prostate cancer; myeloma, melanoma, mesothelioma, small cell lung cancer, and osteosarcoma

Pregnancy Risk Factor D

Contraindications Hypersensitivity to cisplatin, other platinum-containing compounds, or any component of the formulation (anaphylactic-like reactions have been reported); pre-existing renal insufficiency; myelosuppression; hearing impairment; pregnancy

Warnings/Precautions The U.S. Food and Drug Administration (FDA) currently recommends that procedures for proper handling and disposal of antineoplastic agents be considered. All patients should receive adequate hydration prior to and for 24 hours after cisplatin administration, with or without mannitol and/or furosemide, to ensure good urine output and decrease the chance of nephrotoxicity; reduce dosage in renal impairment. Cumulative renal toxicity may be severe; dose-related toxicities include myelosuppression, nausea, and vomiting; cumulative ototoxicity, especially pronounced in children, is manifested by tinnitus or loss of high frequency hearing and occasionally, deafness. **Serum magnesium, as well as other electrolytes, should be monitored both before and within 48 hours after cisplatin therapy.** Patients who are magnesium depleted should receive replacement therapy before the cisplatin is administered. When administered as sequential infusions, taxane derivatives (docetaxel, paclitaxel) should be administered before platinum derivatives (carboplatin, cisplatin) to limit myelosuppression and to enhance efficacy.

Adverse Reactions

>10%:

Endocrine & metabolic: Hyperuricemia

Gastrointestinal: Nausea and vomiting (76% to 100%, dose related, may last up to 1 week)

Emetic potential:

<75 mg: Moderately high (60% to 90%)

≥75 mg: High (>90%)

(Continued)

Cisplatin *(Continued)*

Time course of nausea/vomiting: Onset: 1-4 hours; Duration: 12-96 hours

Hematologic: Myelosuppressive: Mild with moderate doses, mild to moderate with high-dose therapy

WBC: Mild

Platelets: Mild

Onset (days): 10

Nadir (days): 14-23

Recovery (days): 21-39

Neuromuscular & skeletal: Peripheral neuropathy (dose-related), ototoxicity (10% to 30%)

Otic: Ototoxicity (especially pronounced in children)

Renal: Nephrotoxicity: acute renal failure and chronic renal insufficiency

Miscellaneous: Anaphylactic reaction

1% to 10%:

Gastrointestinal: Anorexia

Local: **Irritant chemotherapy**

<1% (Limited to important or life-threatening): Arrhythmias, blurred vision, bradycardia, cerebral blindness, hemolytic anemia, liver enzymes increased, mild alopecia, mouth sores, optic neuritis, papilledema

BMT:

Central nervous system: Peripheral and autonomic neuropathy, ototoxicity

Endocrine & metabolic: Hypokalemia, hypomagnesemia

Gastrointestinal: Highly emetogenic

Hematologic: Myelosuppression

Renal: Acute renal failure, increased serum creatinine, azotemia

Miscellaneous: Transient pain at tumor, transient autoimmune disorders

Overdosage/Toxicology Symptoms include severe myelosuppression, intractable nausea and vomiting, kidney and liver failure, deafness, ocular toxicity, and neuritis. There is no known antidote. Hemodialysis appears to have little effect. Treatment is supportive therapy.

Drug Interactions

Increased Effect/Toxicity: Cisplatin and ethacrynic acid have resulted in severe ototoxicity in animals. Delayed bleomycin elimination with decreased glomerular filtration rate. When administered as sequential infusions, observational studies indicate a potential for increased toxicity when platinum derivatives (carboplatin, cisplatin) are administered before taxane derivatives (docetaxel, paclitaxel).

Decreased Effect: Sodium thiosulfate theoretically inactivates drug systemically; has been used clinically to reduce systemic toxicity with intraperitoneal administration of cisplatin.

Ethanol/Nutrition/Herb Interactions Herb/Nutraceutical: Avoid black cohosh, dong quai in estrogen-dependent tumors.

Stability

Store intact vials at room temperature (15°C to 25°C/59°F to 77°F); protect from light

Do not refrigerate solution - a precipitate may form. If inadvertently refrigerated, the precipitate will slowly dissolve within hours to days, when placed at room temperature. The precipitate may be dissolved without loss of potency by warming solution to 37°C/98.6°F.

Multidose (preservative-free) vials: After initial entry into the vial, solution is stable for 28 days protected from light or for at least 7 days under fluorescent room light at room temperature

Further dilution **stability is dependent on the chloride ion concentration** and should be mixed in solutions of NS (at least 0.3% NaCl). Further dilution in NS, D_5/0.45% NaCl or D_5/NS to a concentration of 0.05-2 mg/mL are stable for 72 hours at 4°C to 25°C in combination with mannitol; may administer 12.5-50 g mannitol/L

Do **NOT** administer with D_5W and other chloride-lacking solutions because nephrotoxicity increases in solutions which do not contain a chloride ion.

Aluminum-containing I.V. infusion sets and needles should NOT be used due to binding with the platinum

Incompatible with sodium bicarbonate

Standard I.V. dilution: Dose/250-1000 mL NS, D_5/NS or D_5/0.45% NaCl

Stable for 72 hours at 4°C to 25°C (in combination with mannitol)

Mechanism of Action Inhibits DNA synthesis by the formation of DNA cross-links; denatures the double helix; covalently binds to DNA bases and disrupts DNA function; may also bind to proteins; the *cis*-isomer is 14 times more cytotoxic than the *trans*-isomer; both forms cross-link DNA but cis-platinum is less easily recognized by cell enzymes and, therefore, not repaired. Cisplatin can also bind two adjacent guanines on the same strand of DNA producing intrastrand cross-linking and breakage.

Pharmacodynamics/Kinetics

Distribution: I.V.: Rapidly into tissue; high concentrations in kidneys, liver, ovaries, uterus, and lungs

Protein binding: >90%

Metabolism: Nonenzymatic; inactivated (in both cell and bloodstream) by sulfhydryl groups; covalently binds to glutathione and thiosulfate

Half-life elimination: Initial: 20-30 minutes; Beta: 60 minutes; Terminal: ~24 hours; Secondary half-life: 44-73 hours

Excretion: Urine (>90%); feces (10%)

Usual Dosage I.V. (refer to individual protocols):

An estimated Cl_{cr} should be on all cisplatin chemotherapy orders along with other patient parameters (ie, patient's height, weight, and body surface area). Pharmacy and nursing staff should check the Cl_{cr} on the order and determine the appropriateness of cisplatin dosing.

The manufacturer recommends that subsequent cycles should only be given when serum creatinine <1.5 mg/dL, WBC ≥4,000/mm³, platelets ≥ 100,000/mm³, and BUN <25.

It is recommended that a 24-hour urine creatinine clearance be checked prior to a patient's first dose of cisplatin and periodically thereafter (ie, after every 2-3 cycles of cisplatin)

Pretreatment hydration with 1-2 L of chloride-containing fluid is recommended prior to cisplatin administration; adequate hydration and urinary output (>100 mL/hour) should be maintained for 24 hours after administration

If the dose prescribed is a reduced dose, then this should be indicated on the chemo-therapy order

Children: Various dosage schedules range from 30-100 mg/m^2 once every 2-3 weeks; may also dose similar to adult dosing

Recurrent brain tumors: 60 mg/m^2 once daily for 2 consecutive days every 3-4 weeks

Adults:

Advanced bladder cancer: 50-70 mg/m^2 every 3-4 weeks

Head and neck cancer: 100-120 mg/m^2 every 3-4 weeks

Testicular cancer: 10-20 mg/m^2/day for 5 days repeated every 3-4 weeks

Metastatic ovarian cancer: 75-100 mg/m^2 every 3 weeks

Intraperitoneal: cisplatin has been administered intraperitoneal with systemic sodium thio-sulfate for ovarian cancer; doses up to 90-270 mg/m^2 have been administered and retained for 4 hours before draining

Dosing adjustment in renal impairment:

Cl$_{cr}$ 10-50 mL/minute: Administer 50% of normal dose

Cl$_{cr}$ <10 mL/minute: Do not administer

Hemodialysis: Partially cleared by hemodialysis; administer dose posthemodialysis

CAPD effects: Unknown

CAVH effects: Unknown

Administration

I.V.: Rate of administration has varied from a 15- to 120-minute infusion, 1 mg/minute infusion, 6- to 8-hour infusion, 24-hour infusion, or per protocol

Maximum rate of infusion of 1 mg/minute in patients with CHF

Pretreatment hydration with 1-2 L of fluid is recommended prior to cisplatin administration; adequate hydration and urinary output (>100 mL/hour) should be maintained for 24 hours after administration

Needles, syringes, catheters, or I.V. administration sets that contain aluminum parts should not be used for administration of drug

Monitoring Parameters Renal function tests (serum creatinine, BUN, Cl$_{cr}$), electrolytes (particularly magnesium, calcium, potassium); hearing test, neurologic exam (with high dose), liver function tests periodically, CBC with differential and platelet count; urine output, urinalysis

Patient Information This drug can only be given I.V. and numerous adverse side effects can occur. Maintaining adequate hydration is extremely important to help avoid kidney damage (2-3 L/day of fluids unless instructed to restrict fluid intake). Nausea and vomiting can be severe and can be delayed for up to 48 hours after infusion and last for 1 week; consult prescriber immediately for appropriate antiemetic medication. May cause hair loss (revers-ible). You will be susceptible to infection; avoid crowds or infectious situations (do not have any vaccinations without consulting prescriber). Report all unusual symptoms promptly to prescriber. Contraceptive measures are recommended during therapy.

Nursing Implications Perform pretreatment hydration (see Usual Dosage); monitor for possible anaphylactoid reaction; monitor renal, hematologic, otic, and neurologic function frequently

Management of extravasation:

Large extravasations (>20 mL) of concentrated solutions (>0.5 mg/mL) produce tissue necrosis. **Treatment is not recommended unless a large amount of highly concentrated solution is extravasated.**

Mix 4 mL of 10% sodium thiosulfate with 6 mL sterile water for injection: Inject 1-4 mL through existing I.V. line cannula. Administer 1 mL for each mL extravasated; inject S.C. if needle is removed.

Additional Information

Sodium content: 9 mg/mL (equivalent to 0.9% sodium chloride solution)

Osmolality of Platinol®-AQ = 285-286 mOsm

Comments on specific toxicities:

Gastrointestinal: Cisplatin is one of the most emetogenic agents used in cancer chemo-therapy; nausea and vomiting occur in 76% to 100% of patients and is dose-related. Prophylactic antiemetics should always be prescribed; nausea and vomiting may last up to 1 week after therapy.

Nephrotoxicity: Related to elimination, protein binding, and uptake of cisplatin. Two types of nephrotoxicity: Acute renal failure and chronic renal insufficiency.

Acute renal failure and azotemia is a dose-dependent process and can be minimized with proper administration and prophylaxis. Damage to the proximal tubules by unbound cisplatin is suspected to cause the toxicity. It is manifested as increased BUN/creatinine, oliguria, protein wasting, and potassium, calcium, and magnesium wasting.

Chronic renal dysfunction can develop in patients receiving multiple courses of cisplatin. Slow release of tissue-bound cisplatin may contribute to chronic nephrotoxicity. Mani-festations of this toxicity are varied, and can include sodium and water wasting, nephropathy, hyperuricemia, decreased Cl$_{cr}$, and magnesium wasting.

Recommendations for minimizing nephrotoxicity include:

Prepare cisplatin in saline-containing vehicles

Infuse dose over 24 hours

Vigorous hydration (125-150 mL/hour) before, during, and after cisplatin administration

Simultaneous administration of either mannitol or furosemide

Pretreatment with amifostine

Avoid other nephrotoxic agents (aminoglycosides, amphotericin, etc)

Neurotoxicity: Peripheral neuropathy is dose- and duration-dependent. The mechanism is through axonal degeneration with subsequent damage to the long sensory nerves. Toxicity can first be noted at cumulative doses of 200 mg/m^2, with measurable toxicity at cumulative doses >350 mg/m^2. This process is irreversible and progressive with continued therapy.

Ototoxicity: Ototoxicity occurs in 10% to 30%, and is manifested as high frequency hearing loss. Baseline audiography should be performed. Ototoxicity is especially pronounced in children.

(Continued)

Cisplatin *(Continued)*

Anaphylactic reaction occurs within minutes after intravenous or intraperitoneal administration and can be controlled with epinephrine, antihistamines, and steroids.

Dosage Forms

Injection, aqueous: 1 mg/mL (50 mL, 100 mL, 200 mL)

Powder for injection: 10 mg, 50 mg

♦ **13-*cis*-Retinoic Acid** *see* Isotretinoin *on page 753*

Citalopram *(sye TAL oh pram)*

Related Information

Antidepressant Agents Comparison *on page 1482*

Selective Serotonin Reuptake Inhibitor (SSRIs) Pharmacokinetics *on page 1514*

U.S. Brand Names Celexa™

Canadian Brand Names Celexa®

Synonyms Citalopram Hydrobromide; Nitalapram

Therapeutic Category Antidepressant, Serotonin Reuptake Inhibitor

Use Treatment of depression

Unlabeled/Investigational Use Investigational: Treatment of dementia, smoking cessation, ethanol abuse, obsessive-compulsive disorder (OCD) in children, diabetic neuropathy

Pregnancy Risk Factor C

Pregnancy/Breast-Feeding Implications Animal reproductive studies have revealed adverse effects on fetal and postnatal development (at doses higher than human therapeutic doses). Should be used in pregnancy only if potential benefit justifies potential risk. Citalopram is excreted in human milk; a decision should be made whether to continue or discontinue nursing or discontinue the drug.

Contraindications Hypersensitivity to citalopram or any component of the formulation; hypersensitivity or other adverse sequelae during therapy with other SSRIs; concomitant use with MAO inhibitors or within 2 weeks of discontinuing MAO inhibitors.

Warnings/Precautions As with all antidepressants, use with caution in patients with a history of mania (may activate hypomania/mania). Use with caution in patients with a history of seizures and patients at high risk of suicide. Has potential to impair cognitive/motor performance - should use caution operating hazardous machinery. Elderly and patients with hepatic insufficiency should receive lower dosages. Use with caution in renal insufficiency and other concomitant illness (due to limited drug experience). May cause hyponatremia/SIADH.

Adverse Reactions

>10%:

Central nervous system: Somnolence, insomnia

Gastrointestinal: Nausea, xerostomia

Miscellaneous: Diaphoresis

<10%:

Central nervous system: Anxiety, anorexia, agitation, yawning

Dermatologic: Rash, pruritus

Endocrine & metabolic: Sexual dysfunction

Gastrointestinal: Diarrhea, dyspepsia, vomiting, abdominal pain, weight gain

Neuromuscular & skeletal: Tremor, arthralgia, myalgia

Respiratory: Cough, rhinitis, sinusitis

Overdosage/Toxicology Symptoms include dizziness, nausea, vomiting, sweating, tremor, somnolence, and sinus tachycardia. Rare symptoms have included amnesia, confusion, coma, seizures, hyperventilation, and EKG changes (including QT_c prolongation, ventricular arrhythmia, and torsade de pointes). Management is supportive.

Drug Interactions

Cytochrome P450 Effect: CYP2C19 and 3A3/4 enzyme substrate; CYP2D6, 1A2, and 2C19 enzyme inhibitor (weak)

Increased Effect/Toxicity:

MAO inhibitors: Citalopram should not be used with nonselective MAO inhibitors (phenelzine, isocarboxazid) or other drugs with MAO inhibition (linezolid); fatal reactions have been reported. Wait 5 weeks after stopping citalopram before starting a nonselective MAO inhibitor and 2 weeks after stopping an MAO inhibitor before starting citalopram. Concurrent selegiline has been associated with mania, hypertension, or serotonin syndrome (risk may be reduced relative to nonselective MAO inhibitors).

Combined used of SSRIs and amphetamines, buspirone, meperidine, nefazodone, serotonin agonists (such as sumatriptan), sibutramine, other SSRIs, sympathomimetics, ritonavir, tramadol, and venlafaxine may increase the risk of serotonin syndrome. Risk of hyponatremia may increase with concurrent use of loop diuretics (bumetanide, furosemide, torsemide). Citalopram may increase the hypoprothrombinemic response to warfarin. Inhibitors of CYP3A3/4 or CYP2C19 may increase serum levels/effects of citalopram.

Combined use of sumatriptan (and other serotonin agonists) may result in toxicity; weakness, hyper-reflexia, and incoordination have been observed with sumatriptan and SSRIs. In addition, concurrent use may theoretically increase the risk of serotonin syndrome; includes sumatriptan, naratriptan, rizatriptan, and zolmitriptan.

Decreased Effect: Cyproheptadine may inhibit the effects of serotonin reuptake inhibitors.

Ethanol/Nutrition/Herb Interactions

Ethanol: Avoid ethanol (may increase CNS depression).

Herb/Nutraceutical: Avoid valerian, St John's wort, SAMe, kava kava, and gotu kola (may increase CNS depression).

Stability Store below 25°C.

Mechanism of Action A bicyclic phthalane derivative, citalopram selectively inhibits serotonin reuptake in the presynaptic neurons

Pharmacodynamics/Kinetics

Onset of action: Usually >2 weeks

Distribution: V_d: 12 L/kg

Protein binding, plasma: ~80%

Metabolism: Extensively hepatic, including CYP450 oxidase system, to N-demethylated, N-oxide, and deaminated metabolites

Bioavailability: 80%

Half-life elimination: 24-48 hours; average 35 hours (doubled with hepatic impairment)

Time to peak, serum: 1-6 hours, average within 4 hours

Excretion: Urine (10% as unchanged drug)

Clearance: Systemic: 330 mL/minute

Mild to moderate renal impairment may reduce clearance

Usual Dosage Oral:

Children and Adolescents: OCD (unlabeled use): 10-40 mg/day

Adults: Depression: Initial: 20 mg/day, generally with an increase to 40 mg/day; doses of more than 40 mg are not usually necessary. Should a dose increase be necessary, it should occur in 20 mg increments at intervals of no less than 1 week. Maximum dose: 60 mg/day; reduce dosage in elderly or those with hepatic impairment.

Dietary Considerations May be taken without regard to food.

Monitoring Parameters Monitor patient periodically for symptom resolution, heart rate, blood pressure, liver function tests, and CBC with continued therapy

Patient Information Citalopram does not impair psychomotor performance, nevertheless, patients receiving treatment may have an impaired ability to drive or operate machinery; they should be warned of this possibility and advised to avoid these tasks if so affected

Dosage Forms

Solution, oral: 10 mg/5 mL [peppermint flavor] [sugar free, alcohol free]

Tablet, as hydrobromide: 20 mg, 40 mg

♦ **Citalopram Hydrobromide** *see Citalopram on page 304*
♦ **Citrate of Magnesia** *see Magnesium Citrate on page 832*
♦ **Citric Acid and Potassium Citrate** *see Potassium Citrate and Citric Acid on page 1110*
♦ **Citro-Mag® (Can)** *see Magnesium Citrate on page 832*
♦ **Citrovorum Factor** *see Leucovorin on page 782*
♦ **CI-719** *see Gemfibrozil on page 624*
♦ **CL184116** *see Porfimer on page 1104*
♦ **Cla** *see Clarithromycin on page 306*

Cladribine *(KLA dri been)*

U.S. Brand Names Leustatin™

Canadian Brand Names Leustatin®

Synonyms 2-CdA; 2-Chlorodeoxyadenosine

Therapeutic Category Antineoplastic Agent, Antimetabolite (Purine)

Use Treatment of hairy cell leukemia, chronic lymphocytic leukemia, non-Hodgkin's lymphomas, progressive multiple sclerosis

Pregnancy Risk Factor D

Contraindications Hypersensitivity to cladribine or any component of the formulation; pregnancy

Warnings/Precautions The U.S. Food and Drug Administration (FDA) currently recommends that procedures for proper handling and disposal of antineoplastic agents be considered. Because of its myelosuppressive properties, cladribine should be used with caution in patients with pre-existing hematologic or immunologic abnormalities; prophylactic administration of allopurinol should be considered in patients receiving cladribine because of the potential for hyperuricemia secondary to tumor lysis; appropriate antibiotic therapy should be administered promptly in patients exhibiting signs and symptoms of neutropenia and infection.

Adverse Reactions

>10%:

Central nervous system: Fatigue, headache, fever (temperature ≥101°F has been associated with the use of cladribine in approximately 66% of patients in the first month of therapy. Although 69% of patients developed fevers, <33% of febrile events were associated with documented infection)

Dermatologic: Rash

Gastrointestinal: Nausea and vomiting

Emetic potential: Mild (10% to 30%)

Hematologic: Anemia (severe); thrombocytopenia; neutropenia; bone marrow suppression

Nadir: 5-10 days

Recovery 4-8 weeks

Note: CD4 counts nadir at 4-6 months after treatments. Patients should be considered immunosuppressed for up to 1 year after cladribine therapy.

1% to 10%:

Cardiovascular: Edema, tachycardia, phlebitis

Central nervous system: Dizziness, insomnia, pain, chills, malaise

Dermatologic: Pruritus, erythema

Gastrointestinal: Constipation, diarrhea, abdominal pain

Local: Injection site reactions

Neuromuscular & skeletal: Myalgia, arthralgia, weakness

Respiratory: Coughing, dyspnea

Miscellaneous: Diaphoresis, trunk pain

Ethanol/Nutrition/Herb Interactions Ethanol: Avoid ethanol (due to GI irritation).

Stability Store intact vials under refrigeration (2°C to 8°C/36°F to 46°F). Dilutions in 500 mL NS are stable for 72 hours. Stable in PVC containers for 24 hours at room temperature (15°C to 30°C/59°F to 86°F) and 7 days in Pharmacia Deltec® cassettes. Solutions for 7-day infusion should be prepared in bacteriostatic NS.

Incompatible with D₅W

Reconstitution: **7-day infusion:** Prepare with bacteriostatic 0.9% sodium chloride. Both cladribine and diluent should be passed through a sterile 0.22 micron hydrophilic filter as it is

(Continued)

305

Cladribine *(Continued)*

being introduced into the infusion reservoir. The calculated dose of cladribine should first be added to the infusion reservoir through a filter then the bacteriostatic 0.9% sodium chloride should be added to the reservoir to obtain a total volume of 100 mL.

Mechanism of Action A purine nucleoside analogue; prodrug which is activated via phosphorylation by deoxycytidine kinase to a 5'-triphosphate derivative. This active form incorporates into susceptible cells and into DNA to result in the breakage of DNA strand and shutdown of DNA synthesis. This also results in a depletion of nicotinamide adenine dinucleotide and adenosine triphosphate (ATP). The induction of strand breaks results in a drop in the cofactor nicotinamide adenine dinucleotide and disruption of cell metabolism. ATP is depleted to deprive cells of an important source of energy. Cladribine effectively kills resting as well as dividing cells.

Pharmacodynamics/Kinetics
Distribution: V_d: 4.52 ± 2.82 L/kg
Protein binding, plasma: 20%
Half-life elimination: Biphasic: Alpha: 25 minutes; Beta: 6.7 hours; Terminal, mean: Normal renal function: 5.4 hours
Excretion: Urine
Clearance: Estimated systemic: 640 mL/hour/kg

Usual Dosage I.V.: Refer to individual protocols.
Pediatrics: Acute leukemias: Optimum dose not determined; 6.2-7.5 mg/m²/day continuous infusion for days 1-5; maximum tolerated dose was 8.9 mg/m²/day.
Adults:
Hairy cell leukemia: Continuous infusion:
0.09-0.1 mg/kg/day days 1-7; may be repeated every 28-35 days **or**
3.4 mg/m²/day S.C. days 1-7
Chronic lymphocytic leukemia: Continuous infusion:
0.1 mg/kg/day days 1-7 **or**
0.028-0.14 mg/kg/day as a 2-hour infusion days 1-5
Chronic myelogenous leukemia: 15 mg/m²/day as a 1-hour infusion days 1-5; if no response increase second course to 20 mg/m²/day.

Administration Single daily infusion: Administer diluted in an infusion bag containing 500 mL of 0.9% sodium chloride and repeated for a total of 7 consecutive days

7-day infusion: Prepare with bacteriostatic 0.9% sodium chloride. Both cladribine and diluent should be passed through a sterile 0.22 micron hydrophilic filter as it is being introduced into the infusion reservoir. The calculated dose of cladribine (7 days x 0.09 mg/kg) should first be added to the infusion reservoir through a filter then the bacteriostatic 0.9% sodium chloride should be added to the reservoir to obtain a total volume of 100 mL.

Nursing Implications Monitor periodic assessment of peripheral blood counts, particularly during the first 4-8 weeks post-treatment, is recommended to detect the development of anemia, neutropenia, and thrombocytopenia and for early detection of any potential sequelae (ie, infection or bleeding)

Dosage Forms Injection [preservative free]: 1 mg/mL (10 mL)

♦ **Claforan**® *see* Cefotaxime *on page 247*

♦ **Clarinex**® *see* Desloratadine *on page 377*

Clarithromycin *(kla RITH roe mye sin)*

Related Information
Antimicrobial Drugs of Choice *on page 1588*
Community-Acquired Pneumonia in Adults *on page 1603*
Helicobacter pylori Treatment *on page 1668*
Prevention of Bacterial Endocarditis *on page 1563*
USPHA/IDSA Guidelines for the Prevention of Opportunistic Infections in Persons With HIV *on page 1574*

U.S. Brand Names Biaxin®; Biaxin® XL
Canadian Brand Names Biaxin®
Synonyms Cla
Therapeutic Category Antibiotic, Macrolide
Use
Adults:
Pharyngitis/tonsillitis due to susceptible *S. pyogenes*
Acute maxillary sinusitis and acute exacerbation of chronic bronchitis due to susceptible *H. influenzae, M. catarrhalis*, or *S. pneumoniae*
Pneumonia due to susceptible *H. influenzae, Mycoplasma pneumoniae, S. pneumoniae*, or *Chlamydia pneumoniae* (TWAR);
Uncomplicated skin/skin structure infections due to susceptible *S. aureus, S. pyogenes*
Disseminated mycobacterial infections due to *M. avium* or *M. intracellulare*
Prevention of disseminated mycobacterial infections due to *M. avium* complex (MAC) disease (eg, patients with advanced HIV infection)
Duodenal ulcer disease due to *H. pylori* in regimens with other drugs including amoxicillin and lansoprazole or omeprazole, ranitidine bismuth citrate, bismuth subsalicylate, tetracycline, and/or an H_2 antagonist
Alternate antibiotic for prophylaxis of bacterial endocarditis in patients who are allergic to penicillin and undergoing surgical or dental procedures
Children:
Pharyngitis/tonsillitis, acute maxillary sinusitis, uncomplicated skin/skin structure infections, and mycobacterial infections due to the above organisms
Acute otitis media (*H. influenzae, M. catarrhalis*, or *S. pneumoniae*)
Prevention of disseminated mycobacterial infections due to MAC disease in patients with advanced HIV infection
Pregnancy Risk Factor C

Pregnancy/Breast-Feeding Implications There are no adequate and well-controlled studies in pregnant women. Due to adverse fetal effects reported in animal studies, the manufacturer recommends that clarithromycin not be used in a pregnant woman unless there are no alternatives to therapy. It is not known if clarithromycin is excreted in human milk, although other antibiotics in this class are; use with caution in a nursing woman.

Contraindications Hypersensitivity to clarithromycin, erythromycin, or any macrolide antibiotic; use with pimozide, astemizole, cisapride, terfenadine; combination with ranitidine bismuth citrate should not be used in patients with history of acute porphyria or Cl_{cr} <25 mL/minute

Warnings/Precautions Dosage adjustment required with severe renal impairment, decreased dosage or prolonged dosing interval may be appropriate; antibiotic-associated colitis has been reported with use of clarithromycin. Macrolides (including clarithromycin) have been associated with rare QT prolongation and ventricular arrhythmias, including torsade de pointes. Safety and efficacy in children <6 months of age have not been established.

Adverse Reactions

1% to 10%:
Central nervous system: Headache (adults and children 2%)
Dermatologic: Rash (children 3%)
Gastrointestinal: Diarrhea (adults 6%, children 6%); vomiting (children 6%); nausea (adults 3%); abnormal taste (adults 7%); heartburn (adults 2%); abdominal pain (adults 2%, children 3%)
Hepatic: Elevated prothrombin time (1%)
Renal: Elevated BUN (4%)

<1% (Limited to important or life-threatening): Anaphylaxis, *Clostridium difficile* colitis, dyspnea, hallucinations, hepatitis, hypoglycemia, jaundice, leukopenia, manic behavior, neuromuscular blockade (case reports), neutropenia, psychosis, QT prolongation, Stevens-Johnson syndrome, thrombocytopenia, torsade de pointes, toxic epidermal necrolysis, tremor, ventricular tachycardia, vertigo

Overdosage/Toxicology Symptoms include nausea, vomiting, diarrhea, prostration, reversible pancreatitis, hearing loss with or without tinnitus, or vertigo. Treatment includes symptomatic and supportive care.

Drug Interactions

Cytochrome P450 Effect: CYP3A3/4 enzyme substrate; CYP1A2 and 3A3/4 enzyme inhibitor

Increased Effect/Toxicity: Serum levels of astemizole, cisapride, pimozide, and terfenadine may be increased, potentially resulting in QT prolongation, or torsade de pointes (malignant ventricular arrhythmias). In addition, risk of malignant arrhythmias may be increased with some quinolone antibiotics (sparfloxacin, gatifloxacin, or moxifloxacin), and concurrent use is contraindicated. Digoxin serum levels may be increased by clarithromycin; digoxin toxicity and potentially fatal arrhythmias have been reported; monitor digoxin levels.

Due to inhibition of CYP3A4, serum levels on many drugs may be increased, including alfentanil (and possibly other narcotic analgesics), benzodiazepines (particularly those metabolized by CYP3A4, including alprazolam and triazolam), bromocriptine, buspirone, calcium channel blockers (felodipine, verapamil, and potentially others metabolized by CYP3A4), carbamazepine, cilostazol, clozapine, cyclosporine, delavirdine, disopyramide, indinavir, loratadine, oral contraceptives, phenytoin (inconsistently - some patients may have decreased levels), rifabutin, sildenafil, tacrolimus, theophylline, valproic acid, and warfarin, and zidovudine (peak levels but not AUC).

The effect of neuromuscular blocking agents may be potentiated by clarithromycin (case reports). Fluconazole and ritonavir increase clarithromycin serum concentrations. Concurrent use or ergot alkaloids may lead to acute ergot toxicity (severe peripheral vasospasm and dysesthesia).

Decreased Effect: Although phenytoin and zidovudine serum levels may be increased by clarithromycin, other evidence suggested levels may be decreased in some patients.

Ethanol/Nutrition/Herb Interactions
Food: Delays absorption; total absorption remains unchanged.
Herb/Nutraceutical: St John's wort may decrease clarithromycin levels.

Stability Store tablets and granules for oral suspension at controlled room temperature. Reconstituted oral suspension should not be refrigerated because it might gel; microencapsulated particles of clarithromycin in suspension is stable for 14 days when stored at room temperature

Mechanism of Action Exerts its antibacterial action by binding to 50S ribosomal subunit resulting in inhibition of protein synthesis. The 14-OH metabolite of clarithromycin is twice as active as the parent compound against certain organisms.

Pharmacodynamics/Kinetics
Absorption: Highly stable in presence of gastric acid (unlike erythromycin); food delays but does not affect extent of absorption
Distribution: Widely into most body tissues except CNS
Metabolism: Partially converted to 14-OH clarithromycin (active metabolite)
Bioavailability: 50%
Half-life elimination: 5-7 hours
Time to peak: 2-4 hours
Excretion: Primarily urine
Clearance: Approximates normal GFR

Usual Dosage Oral:
Children ≥6 months: 15 mg/kg/day divided every 12 hours for 10 days
Mycobacterial infection (prevention and treatment): 7.5 mg/kg twice daily, up to 500 mg twice daily
Prophylaxis of bacterial endocarditis: 15 mg/kg 1 hour before procedure (maximum dose: 500 mg)
(Continued)

Clarithromycin *(Continued)*

Adults:

Usual dose: 250-500 mg every 12 hours **or** 1000 mg (two 500 mg extended release tablets) once daily for 7-14 days

Upper respiratory tract: 250-500 mg every 12 hours for 10-14 days

Pharyngitis/tonsillitis: 250 mg every 12 hours for 10 days

Acute maxillary sinusitis: 500 mg every 12 hours **or** 1000 mg (two 500 mg extended release tablets) once daily for 14 days

Lower respiratory tract: 250-500 mg every 12 hours for 7-14 days

Acute exacerbation of chronic bronchitis due to:

M. catarrhalis and *S. pneumoniae*: 250 mg every 12 hours **or** 1000 mg (two 500 mg extended release tablets) once daily for 7-14 days

H. influenzae: 500 mg every 12 hours for 7-14 days

Pneumonia due to:

C. pneumoniae, M. pneumoniae, and *S. pneumoniae*: 250 mg every 12 hours for 7-14 days **or** 1000 mg (two 500 mg extended release tablets) once daily for 7 days

H. influenzae: 250 mg every 12 hours for 7 days **or** 1000 mg (two 500 mg extended release tablets) once daily for 7 days

Mycobacterial infection (prevention and treatment): 500 mg twice daily (use with other antimycobacterial drugs, eg, ethambutol, clofazimine, or rifampin)

Prophylaxis of bacterial endocarditis: 500 mg 1 hour prior to procedure

Uncomplicated skin and skin structure: 250 mg every 12 hours for 7-14 days

Helicobacter pylori: Combination regimen with bismuth subsalicylate, tetracycline, clarithromycin, and an H_2-receptor antagonist; or combination of omeprazole and clarithromycin; 250 mg twice daily to 500 mg 3 times/day

Dosing adjustment in renal impairment:

Cl_{cr} <30 mL/minute: Half the normal dose or double the dosing interval

In combination with ranitidine bismuth citrate: If Cl_{cr} <25 mL/minute, clarithromycin use is contraindicated

In combination with ritonavir:

Cl_{cr} 30-60 mL/minute: Decrease clarithromycin dose by 50%

Cl_{cr} <30 mL/minute: Decrease clarithromycin dose by 75%

Dosing adjustment in hepatic impairment: No dosing adjustment is needed as long as renal function is normal

Elderly: Pharmacokinetics are similar to those in younger adults; may have age-related reductions in renal function; monitor and adjust dose if necessary

Dietary Considerations May be taken with or without meals; may be taken with milk. Biaxin® XL should be taken with food.

Administration Clarithromycin may be given with or without meals. Give every 12 hours rather than twice daily to avoid peak and trough variation.

Biaxin® XL: Should be given with food. Do not crush or chew extended release tablet.

Patient Information May be taken with meals; finish all medication; do not skip doses; do not refrigerate oral suspension, more palatable when taken at room temperature; do not crush or chew extended-release tablets

Nursing Implications Monitor patients receiving clarithromycin and drugs known to interact with erythromycin

Dosage Forms

Granules for oral suspension: 125 mg/5 mL (50 mL, 100 mL); 187.5 mg/5 mL (100 mL); 250 mg/5 mL (50 mL, 100 mL)

Tablet, film coated: 250 mg, 500 mg

Tablet, film coated, extended release: 500 mg

♦ **Clarithromycin, Lansoprazole, and Amoxicillin** *see* Lansoprazole, Amoxicillin, and Clarithromycin *on page 776*

♦ **Claritin®** *see* Loratadine *on page 819*

♦ **Claritin-D® 12-Hour** *see* Loratadine and Pseudoephedrine *on page 820*

♦ **Claritin-D® 24-Hour** *see* Loratadine and Pseudoephedrine *on page 820*

♦ **Claritin® Extra (Can)** *see* Loratadine and Pseudoephedrine *on page 820*

♦ **Claritin® RediTabs®** *see* Loratadine *on page 819*

♦ **Clavulin® (Can)** *see* Amoxicillin and Clavulanate Potassium *on page 85*

♦ **Clear Eyes® [OTC]** *see* Naphazoline *on page 957*

♦ **Clear Eyes® ACR [OTC]** *see* Naphazoline *on page 957*

♦ **Clear Tussin® 30** *see* Guaifenesin and Dextromethorphan *on page 646*

Clemastine *(KLEM as teen)*

U.S. Brand Names Antihist-1® [OTC]; Tavist®; Tavist®-1 [OTC]

Synonyms Clemastine Fumarate

Therapeutic Category Antihistamine, H_1 Blocker

Use Perennial and seasonal allergic rhinitis and other allergic symptoms including urticaria

Pregnancy Risk Factor B

Contraindications Hypersensitivity to clemastine or any component of the formulation; narrow-angle glaucoma

Warnings/Precautions Safety and efficacy have not been established in children <6 years of age; bladder neck obstruction, symptomatic prostate hypertrophy, asthmatic attacks, and stenosing peptic ulcer

Adverse Reactions

>10%:

Central nervous system: Dyscoordination, sedation, slight to moderate somnolence

Gastrointestinal: Epigastric distress

Respiratory: Thickening of bronchial secretions

1% to 10%:

Central nervous system: Fatigue, headache, increased dizziness, nervousness

Gastrointestinal: Appetite increase, diarrhea, nausea, weight gain, xerostomia

Neuromuscular & skeletal: Arthralgia
Respiratory: Pharyngitis
<1% (Limited to important or life-threatening): Angioedema, bronchospasm, depression, edema, epistaxis, hepatitis, myalgia, palpitations, paresthesia, photosensitivity, rash

Overdosage/Toxicology Symptoms include anemia, metabolic acidosis, hypotension, and hypothermia. There is no specific treatment for an antihistamine overdose, however, clinical toxicity is mostly due to anticholinergic effects. For anticholinergic overdose with severe life-threatening symptoms, physostigmine 1-2 mg (0.5 mg or 0.02 mg/kg for children) slow I.V. may be given to reverse these effects.

Drug Interactions
Increased Effect/Toxicity: CNS depressants may increase the degree of sedation and respiratory depression with antihistamines. May increase the absorption of digoxin. Central and/or peripheral anticholinergic syndrome can occur when administered with amantadine, rimantadine, narcotic analgesics, phenothiazines and other antipsychotics (especially with high anticholinergic activity), tricyclic antidepressants, quinidine, disopyramide, procainamide, and antihistamines.

Decreased Effect: May increase gastric degradation of levodopa and decrease the amount of levodopa absorbed by delaying gastric emptying. Therapeutic effects of cholinergic agents (tacrine, donepezil) and neuroleptics may be antagonized.

Ethanol/Nutrition/Herb Interactions Ethanol: Avoid ethanol (may increase CNS depression).

Mechanism of Action Competes with histamine for H_1-receptor sites on effector cells in the gastrointestinal tract, blood vessels, and respiratory tract

Pharmacodynamics/Kinetics
Onset of action: Peak effect: Therapeutic: 5-7 hours
Duration: 8-16 hours
Absorption: Almost complete
Metabolism: Hepatic
Excretion: Urine

Usual Dosage Oral:
Infants and Children <6 years: 0.05 mg/kg/day as **clemastine base** or 0.335-0.67 mg/day clemastine fumarate (0.25-0.5 mg base/day) divided into 2 or 3 doses; maximum daily dosage: 1.34 mg (1 mg base)
Children 6-12 years: 0.67-1.34 mg clemastine fumarate (0.5-1 mg base) twice daily; do not exceed 4.02 mg/day (3 mg/day base)
Children ≥12 years and Adults: 1.34 mg clemastine fumarate (1 mg base) twice daily to 2.68 mg (2 mg base) 3 times/day; do not exceed 8.04 mg/day (6 mg base)
Elderly: Lower doses should be considered in patients >60 years

Monitoring Parameters Look for a reduction of rhinitis, urticaria, eczema, pruritus, or other allergic symptoms

Patient Information Avoid alcohol; may cause drowsiness, may impair coordination or judgment

Nursing Implications Raise bed rails, institute safety measures, assist with ambulation

Dosage Forms
Syrup, as fumarate: 0.67 mg/5 mL with alcohol 5.5% (120 mL) [citrus flavor]
Tablet, as fumarate: 1.34 mg, 2.68 mg

♦ **Clemastine Fumarate** *see* Clemastine *on page 308*
♦ **Cleocin®** *see* Clindamycin *on page 309*
♦ **Cleocin 3®** *see* Clindamycin *on page 309*
♦ **Cleocin HCl®** *see* Clindamycin *on page 309*
♦ **Cleocin T®** *see* Clindamycin *on page 309*

Clidinium and Chlordiazepoxide (kli DI nee um & klor dye az e POKS ide)
U.S. Brand Names Librax®
Canadian Brand Names Apo®-Chlorax; Librax®
Synonyms Chlordiazepoxide and Clidinium
Therapeutic Category Anticholinergic Agent
Use Adjunct treatment of peptic ulcer; treatment of irritable bowel syndrome
Pregnancy Risk Factor D
Usual Dosage Oral: 1-2 capsules 3-4 times/day, before meals or food and at bedtime
Additional Information Complete prescribing information for this medication should be consulted for additional detail.
Dosage Forms Capsule: Clidinium bromide 2.5 mg and chlordiazepoxide hydrochloride 5 mg

♦ **Climacteron® (Can)** *see* Estradiol and Testosterone *on page 495*
♦ **Climara®** *see* Estradiol *on page 491*
♦ **Clinda-Derm®** *see* Clindamycin *on page 309*

Clindamycin (klin da MYE sin)
Related Information
Animal and Human Bites Guidelines *on page 1584*
Antimicrobial Drugs of Choice *on page 1588*
Community-Acquired Pneumonia in Adults *on page 1603*
Prevention of Bacterial Endocarditis *on page 1563*
Prevention of Wound Infection & Sepsis in Surgical Patients *on page 1569*
Treatment of Sexually Transmitted Diseases *on page 1609*
USPHA/IDSA Guidelines for the Prevention of Opportunistic Infections in Persons With HIV *on page 1574*
U.S. Brand Names Cleocin®; Cleocin 3®; Cleocin HCl®; Cleocin T®; Clinda-Derm®; Clindets® Pledgets; C/T/S®
Canadian Brand Names Alti-Clindamycin; Dalacin® C
Synonyms Clindamycin Hydrochloride; Clindamycin Phosphate
(Continued)

Clindamycin *(Continued)*

Therapeutic Category Acne Products; Antibiotic, Anaerobic; Antibiotic, Topical; Antibiotic, Miscellaneous

Use Treatment against aerobic and anaerobic streptococci (except enterococci), most staphylococci, *Bacteroides* sp and *Actinomyces*; used topically in treatment of severe acne, vaginally for *Gardnerella vaginalis* or bacterial vaginosis; alternate treatment for toxoplasmosis; prophylaxis in the prevention of bacterial endocarditis in high-risk patients undergoing surgical or dental procedures in patients allergic to penicillin; may be useful in PCP

Pregnancy Risk Factor B

Contraindications Hypersensitivity to clindamycin or any component of the formulation; previous pseudomembranous colitis; hepatic impairment

Warnings/Precautions Dosage adjustment may be necessary in patients with severe hepatic dysfunction; can cause severe and possibly fatal colitis; use with caution in patients with a history of pseudomembranous colitis; discontinue drug if significant diarrhea, abdominal cramps, or passage of blood and mucus occurs

Adverse Reactions

Systemic:

>10%: Gastrointestinal: Diarrhea, abdominal pain

1% to 10%:

Cardiovascular: Hypotension

Dermatologic: Urticaria, rashes, Stevens-Johnson syndrome

Gastrointestinal: Pseudomembranous colitis, nausea, vomiting

Local: Thrombophlebitis, sterile abscess at I.M. injection site

Miscellaneous: Fungal overgrowth, hypersensitivity

<1% (Limited to important or life-threatening): Granulocytopenia, neutropenia, polyarthritis, renal dysfunction (rare), thrombocytopenia

Topical:

>10%: Dermatologic: Dryness, scaliness, or peeling of skin (lotion)

1% to 10%:

Dermatologic: Contact dermatitis, irritation

Gastrointestinal: Diarrhea (mild), abdominal pain

Miscellaneous: Hypersensitivity

<1% (Limited to important or life-threatening): Diarrhea (severe), nausea, pseudomembranous colitis, vomiting

Vaginal:

>10%: Genitourinary: Vaginitis or vulvovaginal pruritus (from *Candida albicans*), painful intercourse

1% to 10%:

Central nervous system: Dizziness, headache

Gastrointestinal: Diarrhea, nausea, vomiting, stomach cramps

Overdosage/Toxicology Following GI decontamination, symptoms of overdose include diarrhea, nausea, and vomiting. Treatment is supportive.

Drug Interactions

Cytochrome P450 Effect: CYP3A3/4 enzyme substrate

Increased Effect/Toxicity: Increased duration of neuromuscular blockade when given in conjunction with tubocurarine and pancuronium.

Ethanol/Nutrition/Herb Interactions

Food: Peak concentrations may be delayed with food.

Herb/Nutraceutical: St John's wort may decrease clindamycin levels.

Stability Do **not** refrigerate reconstituted oral solution because it will thicken; oral solution is stable for 2 weeks at room temperature following reconstitution; I.V. infusion solution in NS or D₅W solution is stable for 16 days at room temperature

Mechanism of Action Reversibly binds to 50S ribosomal subunits preventing peptide bond formation thus inhibiting bacterial protein synthesis; bacteriostatic or bactericidal depending on drug concentration, infection site, and organism

Pharmacodynamics/Kinetics

Absorption: Topical: ~10%; Oral: Rapid (90%)

Distribution: High concentrations in bone and urine; no significant levels in CSF, even with inflamed meninges; crosses placenta; enters breast milk

Metabolism: Hepatic

Bioavailability: Topical: <1%

Half-life elimination: Neonates: Premature: 8.7 hours; Full-term: 3.6 hours; Adults: 1.6-5.3 hours, average: 2-3 hours

Time to peak, serum: Oral: Within 60 minutes; I.M.: 1-3 hours

Excretion: Urine (10%) and feces (~4%) as active drug and metabolites

Usual Dosage Avoid in neonates (contains benzyl alcohol)

Infants and Children:

Oral: 8-20 mg/kg/day as hydrochloride; 8-25 mg/kg/day as palmitate in 3-4 divided doses; minimum dose of palmitate: 37.5 mg 3 times/day

I.M., I.V.:

<1 month: 15-20 mg/kg/day

>1 month: 20-40 mg/kg/day in 3-4 divided doses

Children: Prevention of bacterial endocarditis: Oral: 20 mg/kg 1 hour before procedure with no follow-up dose needed; for patients allergic to penicillin and unable to take oral medications: 20 mg/kg I.V. within 30 minutes before procedure

Children and Adults: Topical: Apply a thin film twice daily

Adults:

Oral: 150-450 mg/dose every 6-8 hours; maximum dose: 1.8 g/day

Prevention of bacterial endocarditis in patients unable to take amoxicillin: Oral: 600 mg 1 hour before procedure with no follow-up dose needed; for patients allergic to penicillin and unable to take oral medications: 600 mg I.V. within 30 minutes before procedure

I.M., I.V.: 1.2-1.8 g/day in 2-4 divided doses; maximum dose: 4.8 g/day

Pelvic inflammatory disease: I.V.: 900 mg every 8 hours with gentamicin 2 mg/kg, then 1.5 mg/kg every 8 hours; continue after discharge with doxycycline 100 mg twice daily to complete 14 days of total therapy

Pneumocystis carinii pneumonia:
Oral: 300-450 mg 4 times/day with primaquine
I.M., I.V.: 1200-2400 mg/day with pyrimethamine
I.V.: 600 mg 4 times/day with primaquine

Bacterial vaginosis:
Oral: 300 mg twice daily for 7 days
Intravaginal:
Suppositories: Insert one ovule (100 mg clindamycin) daily into vagina at bedtime for 3 days
Cream: One full applicator inserted intravaginally once daily before bedtime for 3 or 7 consecutive days

Dosing adjustment in hepatic impairment: Adjustment recommended in patients with severe hepatic disease

Dietary Considerations May be taken with food.

Administration Administer oral dosage form with a full glass of water to minimize esophageal ulceration

Monitoring Parameters Observe for changes in bowel frequency, monitor for colitis and resolution of symptoms; during prolonged therapy monitor CBC, liver and renal function tests periodically

Patient Information Report any severe diarrhea immediately and do not take antidiarrheal medication; take each oral dose with a full glass of water; finish all medication; do not skip doses; should not engage in sexual intercourse during treatment with vaginal product; avoid contact of topical gel/solution with eyes, abraded skin, or mucous membranes

Nursing Implications
Administer by I.V. intermittent infusion over at least 10-60 minutes, at a rate **not** to exceed 30 mg/minute; final concentration for administration should not exceed 12 mg/mL
Observe for changes in bowel frequency; during prolonged therapy monitor CBC, liver and renal function tests periodically

Dosage Forms
Capsule, as hydrochloride: 75 mg, 150 mg, 300 mg
Cream, vaginal: 2% (40 g)
Gel, topical, as phosphate: 1% [10 mg/g] (7.5 g, 30 g)
Granules for oral solution, as palmitate: 75 mg/5 mL (100 mL)
Infusion, as phosphate [in D_5W]: 300 mg (50 mL); 600 mg (50 mL)
Injection, as phosphate: 150 mg/mL (2 mL, 4 mL, 6 mL, 50 mL, 60 mL)
Lotion: 1% [10 mg/mL] (60 mL)
Pledgets: 1%
Solution, topical, as phosphate: 1% [10 mg/mL] (30 mL, 60 mL, 480 mL)
Suppository, vaginal: 2.5 g (clindamycin 100 mg)

♦ **Clindamycin Hydrochloride** *see* Clindamycin *on page 309*
♦ **Clindamycin Phosphate** *see* Clindamycin *on page 309*
♦ **Clindets® Pledgets** *see* Clindamycin *on page 309*
♦ **Clinoril®** *see* Sulindac *on page 1278*

Clioquinol (klye oh KWIN ole)

U.S. Brand Names Vioform® [OTC]
Synonyms Iodochlorhydroxyquin
Therapeutic Category Antifungal Agent, Topical
Use Topically in the treatment of tinea pedis, tinea cruris, and skin infections caused by dermatophytic fungi (ringworm)
Pregnancy Risk Factor C
Usual Dosage Children and Adults: Topical: Apply 2-3 times/day; do not use for longer than 7 days
Additional Information Complete prescribing information for this medication should be consulted for additional detail.
Dosage Forms
Cream, topical: 3% (30 g)
Ointment, topical: 3% (30 g)

Clobetasol (kloe BAY ta sol)

Related Information
Corticosteroids Comparison *on page 1495*
U.S. Brand Names Cormax®; Olux™; Temovate®
Canadian Brand Names Alti-Clobetasol; Dermovate®; Gen-Clobetasol; Novo-Clobetasol®
Synonyms Clobetasol Propionate
Therapeutic Category Anti-inflammatory Agent; Corticosteroid, Topical (Very High Potency)
Use Short-term relief of inflammation of moderate to severe corticosteroid-responsive dermatoses (very high potency topical corticosteroid)
Pregnancy Risk Factor C
Usual Dosage
Children: Use in children <12 years of age is **not** recommended
Adults: Topical:
Apply twice daily for up to 2 weeks with no more than 50 g/week. Therapy should be discontinued when control is achieved; if no improvement is seen, reassessment of diagnosis may be necessary.
Foam: Scalp: Apply to affected scalp twice daily for up to 2 weeks (≤50 g/week)
Additional Information Complete prescribing information for this medication should be consulted for additional detail.
(Continued)

Clobetasol (Continued)

Dosage Forms
Cream, topical, as propionate: 0.05% (15 g, 30 g, 45 g)
Cream, topical, as propionate, in emollient base: 0.05% (15 g, 30 g, 60 g)
Foam for scalp application, topical, as propionate (Olux™): 0.05% (100 g)
Gel, topical, as propionate: 0.05% (15 g, 30 g, 45 g)
Ointment, topical, as propionate: 0.05% (15 g, 30 g, 45 g)
Solution topical, as propionate [scalp application]: 0.05% (25 mL, 50 mL)

♦ **Clobetasol Propionate** *see Clobetasol on page 311*
♦ **Clocort® Maximum Strength** *see Hydrocortisone on page 682*

Clocortolone (kloe KOR toe lone)

Related Information
Corticosteroids Comparison *on page 1495*
U.S. Brand Names Cloderm®
Canadian Brand Names Cloderm®
Synonyms Clocortolone Pivalate
Therapeutic Category Corticosteroid, Topical (Medium Potency)
Use Inflammation of corticosteroid-responsive dermatoses (intermediate-potency topical corticosteroid)
Pregnancy Risk Factor C
Contraindications Hypersensitivity to clocortolone or any component of the formulation; viral, fungal, or tubercular skin lesions
Warnings/Precautions Adrenal suppression can occur if used for >14 days
Adverse Reactions
1% to 10%:
  Dermatologic: Itching, erythema
  Local: Burning, dryness, irritation, papular rashes
<1% (Limited to important or life-threatening): Acneiform eruptions, hypertrichosis, hypopigmentation, maceration of skin, miliaria, perioral dermatitis, skin atrophy, striae
Mechanism of Action Stimulates the synthesis of enzymes needed to decrease inflammation, suppress mitotic activity, and cause vasoconstriction
Pharmacodynamics/Kinetics
Absorption: Percutaneous absorption is variable and dependent upon many factors including vehicle used, integrity of epidermis, dose, and use of occlusive dressings; small amounts enter circulatory system via skin
Metabolism: Hepatic
Excretion: Urine and feces
Usual Dosage Adults: Apply sparingly and gently; rub into affected area from 1-4 times/day. Therapy should be discontinued when control is achieved; if no improvement is seen, reassessment of diagnosis may be necessary.
Patient Information A thin film of cream or ointment is effective; do not overuse; do not use tight-fitting diapers or plastic pants on children being treated in the diaper area; use only as prescribed, and for no longer than the period prescribed; apply sparingly in light film; rub in lightly; avoid contact with eyes; notify physician if condition being treated persists or worsens
Nursing Implications For external use only; do not use on open wounds; apply sparingly to occlusive dressings; should not be used in the presence of open or weeping lesions
Dosage Forms Cream, topical, as pivalate: 0.1% (15 g, 45 g)

♦ **Clocortolone Pivalate** *see Clocortolone on page 312*
♦ **Cloderm®** *see Clocortolone on page 312*

Clofazimine (kloe FA zi meen)

Related Information
Antimicrobial Drugs of Choice *on page 1588*
Tuberculosis Treatment Guidelines *on page 1612*
U.S. Brand Names Lamprene®
Canadian Brand Names Lamprene®
Synonyms Clofazimine Palmitate
Therapeutic Category Antibiotic, Miscellaneous; Leprostatic Agent
Use Orphan drug: Treatment of dapsone-resistant leprosy; multibacillary dapsone-sensitive leprosy; erythema nodosum leprosum; *Mycobacterium avium-intracellulare* (MAI) infections
Pregnancy Risk Factor C
Contraindications Hypersensitivity to clofazimine or any component of the formulation
Warnings/Precautions Use with caution in patients with GI problems; dosages >100 mg/day should be used for as short a duration as possible; skin discoloration may lead to depression
Adverse Reactions
>10%:
  Dermatologic: Dry skin
  Gastrointestinal: Abdominal pain, nausea, vomiting, diarrhea
  Miscellaneous: Pink to brownish-black discoloration of the skin and conjunctiva
1% to 10%:
  Dermatologic: Rash, pruritus
  Endocrine & metabolic: Elevated blood sugar
  Gastrointestinal: Fecal discoloration
  Genitourinary: Discoloration of urine
  Ocular: Irritation of the eyes
  Miscellaneous: Discoloration of sputum, sweat
<1% (Limited to important or life-threatening): Acneiform eruptions, bowel obstruction, diminished vision, eosinophilia, eosinophilic enteritis, erythroderma, GI bleeding, giddiness, hepatitis, hypokalemia, jaundice, monilial cheilosis, neuralgia, phototoxicity
Overdosage/Toxicology Following GI decontamination, treatment is supportive.

Drug Interactions
  Decreased Effect: Combined use may decrease effect with dapsone (unconfirmed).
Ethanol/Nutrition/Herb Interactions
  Food: The presence of food increases the extent of absorption.
Stability Protect from moisture
Mechanism of Action Binds preferentially to mycobacterial DNA to inhibit mycobacterial growth; also has some anti-inflammatory activity through an unknown mechanism
Pharmacodynamics/Kinetics
  Absorption: Slowly (45% to 70%)
  Distribution: Highly lipophilic; deposited primarily in fatty tissue and cells of the reticuloendo-thelial system; taken up by macrophages throughout the body; distributed to breast milk, mesenteric lymph nodes, adrenal glands, subcutaneous fat, liver, bile, gallbladder, spleen, small intestine, muscles, bones, and skin; does not appear to cross blood-brain barrier; remains in tissues for prolonged periods
  Metabolism: Partially hepatic to two metabolites
  Half-life elimination: Terminal: 8 days; Tissue: 70 days
  Time to peak, serum: 1-6 hours (chronic therapy)
  Excretion: Primarily feces; urine (negligible amounts as unchanged drug); sputum, saliva, and sweat (small amounts)
Usual Dosage Oral:
  Children: Leprosy: 1 mg/kg/day every 24 hours in combination with dapsone and rifampin
  Adults:
    Dapsone-resistant leprosy: 100 mg/day in combination with one or more antileprosy drugs for 3 years; then alone 100 mg/day
    Dapsone-sensitive multibacillary leprosy: 100 mg/day in combination with two or more antileprosy drugs for at least 2 years and continue until negative skin smears are obtained, then institute single drug therapy with appropriate agent
    Erythema nodosum leprosum: 100-200 mg/day for up to 3 months or longer then taper dose to 100 mg/day when possible
    Pyoderma gangrenosum: 300-400 mg/day for up to 12 months
  Dosing adjustment in hepatic impairment: Should be considered in severe hepatic dysfunction
Dietary Considerations May be taken with meals.
Patient Information Drug may cause a pink to brownish-black discoloration of the skin, conjunctiva, tears, sweat, urine, feces, and nasal secretions; although reversible, may take months to years to disappear after therapy is complete; take with meals
Nursing Implications Monitor for GI complaints
Dosage Forms Capsule, as palmitate: 50 mg

♦ **Clofazimine Palmitate** see Clofazimine on page 312

Clofibrate (kloe FYE brate)
  Related Information
    Lipid-Lowering Agents on page 1505
  U.S. Brand Names Atromid-S®
  Therapeutic Category Antilipemic Agent, Fibric Acid
  Use Adjunct to dietary therapy in the management of hyperlipidemias associated with high triglyceride levels (types III, IV, V); primarily lowers triglycerides and very low density lipoprotein
  Pregnancy Risk Factor C
  Contraindications Hypersensitivity to clofibrate or any component of the formulation; significant hepatic or renal dysfunction; primary biliary cirrhosis
  Warnings/Precautions Clofibrate has been shown to be tumorigenic in animal studies; increased risk of cholelithiasis, cholecystitis; discontinue if lipid response is not obtained; no evidence substantiates a beneficial effect on cardiovascular mortality; anemia and leukopenia have been reported; elevations in serum transaminases can be seen; use with caution in peptic ulcer disease; flu-like symptoms may occur. Be careful in patient selection; this is not a first- or second-line choice; other agents may be more suitable.
  Adverse Reactions Frequency not defined.
    Common: Gastrointestinal: Nausea, diarrhea
    Less common:
      Central nervous system: Headache, dizziness, fatigue
      Gastrointestinal: Vomiting, loose stools, heartburn, flatulence, abdominal distress, epigastric pain
      Neuromuscular & skeletal: Muscle cramping, aching, weakness, myalgia
    Frequency not defined:
      Central nervous system: Fever
      Cardiovascular: Chest pain, cardiac arrhythmias
      Dermatologic: Rash, urticaria, pruritus, alopecia, dry,brittle hair, toxic epidermal necrolysis, erythema multiforme, Stevens-Johnson syndrome
      Endocrine & metabolic: Polyphagia, gynecomastia, hyperkalemia
      Gastrointestinal: Stomatitis, gallstones, pancreatitis, gastritis, peptic ulcer, weight gain
      Genitourinary: Impotence, decreased libido
      Hematologic: Leukopenia, anemia, eosinophilia, agranulocytosis, thrombocytopenic purpura
      Hepatic: Increased liver function test, hepatomegaly, jaundice
      Local: Thrombophlebitis
      Neuromuscular & skeletal: Myalgia, myopathy, myositis, arthralgia, rhabdomyolysis, increased creatinine phosphokinase (CPK), rheumatoid arthritis, tremor
      Ocular: Photophobic
      Renal: Dysuria, hematuria, proteinuria, renal toxicity (allergic), rhabdomyolysis-induced renal failure
      Miscellaneous: Flu-like syndrome, increased diaphoresis, systemic lupus erythematosus
(Continued)

Clofibrate *(Continued)*

Overdosage/Toxicology Symptoms include nausea, vomiting, diarrhea, GI distress. Following GI decontamination, treatment is supportive.

Drug Interactions

Cytochrome P450 Effect: CYP3A3/4 enzyme substrate

Increased Effect/Toxicity: Clofibrate may increase effects of warfarin, insulin, and sulfonylureas. Clofibrate's levels may be increased with probenecid. HMG-CoA reductase inhibitors (atorvastatin, cerivastatin, fluvastatin, lovastatin, pravastatin, simvastatin) may increase the risk of myopathy and rhabdomyolysis. The manufacturer warns against the concomitant use. However, combination therapy with statins has been used in some patients with resistant hyperlipidemias (with great caution).

Decreased Effect: Rifampin (and potentially other inducers of CYP3A4) may reduce blood levels of clofibrate.

Mechanism of Action Mechanism is unclear but thought to reduce cholesterol synthesis and triglyceride hepatic-vascular transference

Pharmacodynamics/Kinetics

Absorption: Complete

Distribution: V_d: 5.5 L/kg; crosses placenta

Protein binding: 95%

Metabolism: Intestinal transformation required to activate drug; hepatic to an inactive glucuronide ester

Half-life elimination: 6-24 hours, increases significantly with reduced renal function; Anuria: 110 hours

Time to peak, serum: 3-6 hours

Excretion: Urine (40% to 70%)

Usual Dosage Adults: Oral: 500 mg 4 times/day; some patients may respond to lower doses

Dosing interval in renal impairment:

Cl_{cr} >50 mL/minute: Administer every 6-12 hours

Cl_{cr} 10-50 mL/minute: Administer every 12-18 hours

Cl_{cr} <10 mL/minute: Avoid use

Hemodialysis: Elimination is not enhanced via hemodialysis; supplemental dose is not necessary

Monitoring Parameters Serum lipids, cholesterol and triglycerides, LFTs, CBC

Test Interactions ↑ creatine phosphokinase [CPK] (S); ↓ alkaline phosphatase (S), cholesterol (S), glucose, uric acid (S)

Patient Information If GI upset occurs, may be taken with food; notify physician of chest pain, shortness of breath, irregular heartbeat, severe stomach pain with nausea and vomiting, persistent fever, sore throat, or unusual bleeding or bruising; adhere to prescribed diet

Nursing Implications Monitor serum lipids, LFTs, CBC

Dosage Forms Capsule: 500 mg

♦ Clomid® *see* ClomiPHENE *on page 314*

ClomiPHENE *(KLOE mi feen)*

U.S. Brand Names Clomid®; Milophene®; Serophene®

Canadian Brand Names Clomid®; Milophene®; Serophene®

Synonyms Clomiphene Citrate

Therapeutic Category Ovulation Stimulator

Use Treatment of ovulatory failure in patients desiring pregnancy

Unlabeled/Investigational Use Male infertility

Pregnancy Risk Factor X

Contraindications Hypersensitivity to clomiphene citrate or any of its components; liver disease; abnormal uterine bleeding; enlargement or development of ovarian cyst; uncontrolled thyroid or adrenal dysfunction in the presence of an organic intracranial lesion such as pituitary tumor; pregnancy

Warnings/Precautions Patients unusually sensitive to pituitary gonadotropins (eg, polycystic ovary disease); multiple pregnancies, blurring or other visual symptoms can occur, ovarian hyperstimulation syndrome, and abdominal pain

Adverse Reactions

>10%: Endocrine & metabolic: Hot flashes, ovarian enlargement

1% to 10%:

Cardiovascular: Thromboembolism

Central nervous system: Mental depression, headache

Endocrine & metabolic: Breast enlargement (males), breast discomfort (females), abnormal menstrual flow, ovarian cyst formation, ovarian enlargement, premenstrual syndrome, uterine fibroid enlargement

Gastrointestinal: Distention, bloating, nausea, vomiting

Hepatic: Hepatotoxicity

Ocular: Blurring of vision, diplopia, floaters, after-images, phosphenes, photophobia, scotoma

<1% (Limited to important or life-threatening): Alopecia (reversible), polyuria

Drug Interactions

Decreased Effect: Decreased response when used with danazol. Decreased estradiol response when used with clomiphene.

Stability Protect from light

Mechanism of Action Induces ovulation by stimulating the release of pituitary gonadotropins

Pharmacodynamics/Kinetics

Metabolism: Enterohepatically circulated

Half-life elimination: 5-7 days

Excretion: Primarily feces; urine (small amounts)

Usual Dosage Adults: Oral:

Male (infertility): 25 mg/day for 25 days with 5 days rest, or 100 mg every Monday, Wednesday, Friday

Female (ovulatory failure): 50 mg/day for 5 days (first course); start the regimen on or about the fifth day of cycle. The dose should be increased only in those patients who do not ovulate in response to cyclic 50 mg Clomid®. A low dosage or duration of treatment course is particularly recommended if unusual sensitivity to pituitary gonadotropin is suspected, such as in patients with polycystic ovary syndrome.

If ovulation does not appear to occur after the first course of therapy, a second course of 100 mg/day (two 50 mg tablets given as a single daily dose) for 5 days should be given. This course may be started as early as 30 days after the previous one after precautions are taken to exclude the presence of pregnancy. Increasing the dosage or duration of therapy beyond 100 mg/day for 5 days is not recommended. The majority of patients who are going to ovulate will do so after the first course of therapy. If ovulation does not occur after 3 courses of therapy, further treatment is not recommended and the patient should be re-evaluated. If 3 ovulatory responses occur, but pregnancy has not been achieved, further treatment is not recommended. If menses does not occur after an ovulatory response, the patient should be re-evaluated. Long-term cyclic therapy is not recommended beyond a total of about 6 cycles.

Reference Range FSH and LH are expected to peak 5-9 days after completing clomiphene; ovulation assessed by basal body temperature or serum progesterone 2 weeks after last clomiphene dose

Test Interactions Clomiphene may increase levels of serum thyroxine and thyroxine-binding globulin (TBG)

Patient Information May cause visual disturbances, dizziness, lightheadedness; if possibility of pregnancy, stop the drug and consult your physician

Nursing Implications May cause visual disturbances, dizziness, lightheadedness; if possibility of pregnancy, stop the drug and consult your physician

Dosage Forms Tablet, as citrate: 50 mg

♦ **Clomiphene Citrate** see ClomiPHENE on page 314

ClomiPRAMINE (kloe MI pra meen)

Related Information
Antidepressant Agents Comparison on page 1482

U.S. Brand Names Anafranil®

Canadian Brand Names Anafranil®; Apo®-Clomipramine; Gen-Clomipramine; Novo-Clopramine

Synonyms Clomipramine Hydrochloride

Therapeutic Category Antidepressant, Tricyclic

Use Treatment of obsessive-compulsive disorder (OCD)

Unlabeled/Investigational Use Depression, panic attacks, chronic pain

Pregnancy Risk Factor C

Pregnancy/Breast-Feeding Implications There are no adequate studies in pregnant women. Withdrawal symptoms (including dizziness, nausea, vomiting, headache, malaise, sleep disturbance, hyperthermia, and/or irritability) have been observed in neonates whose mothers took clomipramine up to delivery. Use in pregnancy only if the benefits to the mother outweigh the potential risks to the fetus.

Contraindications Hypersensitivity to clomipramine, other tricyclic agents, or any component of the formulation; use of MAO inhibitors within 14 days; use in a patient during the acute recovery phase of MI

Warnings/Precautions Seizures are likely and are dose-related; can be additive when coadministered with other drugs that can lower the seizure threshold. Use with caution in patients with asthma, bladder outlet destruction, narrow-angle glaucoma. Has been associated with a high incidence of sexual dysfunction. Weight gain may occur. May cause sedation, resulting in impaired performance of tasks requiring alertness (ie, operating machinery or driving). Sedative effects may be additive with other CNS depressants and/or ethanol. The degree of sedation is very high relative to other antidepressants. May worsen psychosis in some patients or precipitate a shift to mania or hypomania in patients with bipolar disease. May increase the risks associated with electroconvulsive therapy. This agent should be discontinued, when possible, prior to elective surgery. Therapy should not be abruptly discontinued in patients receiving high doses for prolonged periods.

May cause orthostatic hypotension (risk is moderate-high relative to other antidepressants) - use with caution in patients at risk of hypotension or in patients where transient hypotensive episodes would be poorly tolerated (cardiovascular disease or cerebrovascular disease). The degree of anticholinergic blockade produced by this agent is very high relative to other cyclic antidepressants - use caution in patients with urinary retention, benign prostatic hyperplasia, narrow-angle glaucoma, xerostomia, visual problems, constipation, or history of bowel obstruction.

Use caution in patients with suicidal risk. Use with caution in patients with a history of cardiovascular disease (including previous MI, stroke, tachycardia, or conduction abnormalities). The risk conduction abnormalities with this agent is high relative to other antidepressants. Use with caution in hyperthyroid patients or those receiving thyroid supplementation. Use with caution in patients with hepatic or renal dysfunction and in elderly patients. Safety and efficacy in pediatric patients <10 years of age have not been established.

Adverse Reactions
>10%:
Central nervous system: Dizziness, drowsiness, headache, insomnia, nervousness
Endocrine & metabolic: Libido changes
Gastrointestinal: Xerostomia, constipation, increased appetite, nausea, weight gain, dyspepsia, anorexia, abdominal pain
Neuromuscular & skeletal: Fatigue, tremor, myoclonus
Miscellaneous: Increased diaphoresis
1% to 10%:
Cardiovascular: Hypotension, palpitations, tachycardia
(Continued)

ClomiPRAMINE *(Continued)*

Central nervous system: Confusion, hypertonia, sleep disorder, yawning, speech disorder, abnormal dreaming, paresthesia, memory impairment, anxiety, twitching, impaired coordination, agitation, migraine, depersonalization, emotional lability, flushing, fever

Dermatologic: Rash, pruritus, dermatitis

Gastrointestinal: Diarrhea, vomiting

Genitourinary: Difficult urination

Ocular: Blurred vision, eye pain

<1% (Limited to important or life-threatening): Alopecia, galactorrhea, hyperacusis, marrow depression, photosensitivity, reflux, seizures, SIADH

Overdosage/Toxicology Symptoms include agitation, confusion, hallucinations, urinary retention, hypothermia, hypotension, tachycardia, ventricular tachycardia, seizures, and coma. Following initiation of essential overdose management, toxic symptoms should be treated. Sodium bicarbonate is indicated when the QRS interval is >0.10 seconds or the QT_c is >0.42 seconds. Ventricular arrhythmias and EKG abnormalities (eg, QRS widening) often respond to systemic alkalinization (sodium bicarbonate 0.5-2 mEq/kg I.V.) and/or phenytoin 15-20 mg/kg (adults). Arrhythmias unresponsive to this therapy may respond to lidocaine 1 mg/kg I.V. followed by a titrated infusion. Physostigmine (1-2 mg slow I.V. for adults or 0.5 mg slow I.V. for children) may be indicated in reversing life-threatening cardiac arrhythmias. Seizures usually respond to diazepam I.V. boluses (5-10 mg for adults up to 30 mg or 0.25-0.4 mg/kg/dose for children up to 10 mg/dose). If seizures are unresponsive or recur, phenytoin or phenobarbital may be required.

Drug Interactions

Cytochrome P450 Effect: CYP1A2, 2C19, 2D6, and 3A3/4 enzyme substrate; CYP2D6 enzyme inhibitor

Increased Effect/Toxicity: Clomipramine increases the effects of amphetamines, anticholinergics, lithium, other CNS depressants (sedatives, hypnotics, ethanol), chlorpropamide, tolazamide, phenothiazines, and warfarin. When used with MAO inhibitors or other serotonergic drugs, serotonin syndrome may occur. Serotonin syndrome has also been reported with ritonavir (rare). Clomipramine serum concentrations/toxicity may be increased by SSRIs (to varying degrees), cimetidine, grapefruit juice, indinavir, methylphenidate, ritonavir, quinidine, diltiazem, phenothiazines, and verapamil. Pressor response to I.V. epinephrine, norepinephrine, and phenylephrine may be enhanced in patients receiving TCAs (**Note:** Effect is unlikely with epinephrine or levonordefrin dosages typically administered as infiltration in combination with local anesthetics). Combined use of beta-agonists or drugs which prolong QT_c (including quinidine, procainamide, disopyramide, cisapride, sparfloxacin, gatifloxacin, moxifloxacin) with TCAs may predispose patients to cardiac arrhythmias.

Decreased Effect: Clomipramine serum concentrations/effect may be decreased by carbamazepine, cholestyramine, colestipol, phenobarbital, and rifampin. Clomipramine inhibits the antihypertensive response to bethanidine, clonidine, debrisoquin, guanadrel, guanethidine, guanabenz, and guanfacine.

Ethanol/Nutrition/Herb Interactions

Ethanol: Avoid ethanol (may increase CNS depression).

Food: Serum concentrations/toxicity may be increased by grapefruit juice.

Herb/Nutraceutical: Avoid valerian, St John's wort, SAMe, kava kava.

Mechanism of Action Clomipramine appears to affect serotonin uptake while its active metabolite, desmethylclomipramine, affects norepinephrine uptake

Pharmacodynamics/Kinetics

Onset of action: Usually >2 weeks to therapeutic effect

Absorption: Rapid

Metabolism: Hepatic to desmethylclomipramine (active); extensive first-pass effect

Half-life elimination: 20-30 hours

Usual Dosage Oral: Initial:

Children:

<10 years: Safety and efficacy have not been established.

≥10 years: OCD: 25 mg/day; gradually increase, as tolerated, to a maximum of 3 mg/kg/day or 200 mg/day (whichever is smaller)

Adults: OCD: 25 mg/day and gradually increase, as tolerated, to 100 mg/day the first 2 weeks, may then be increased to a total of 250 mg/day maximum

Monitoring Parameters Pulse rate and blood pressure prior to and during therapy; EKG/cardiac status in older adults and patients with cardiac disease

Patient Information May cause seizures; caution should be used in activities that require alertness like driving, operating machinery, or swimming; effect of drug may take several weeks to appear

Nursing Implications Monitor pulse rate and blood pressure prior to and during therapy, evaluate mental status

Dosage Forms Capsule, as hydrochloride: 25 mg, 50 mg, 75 mg

♦ **Clomipramine Hydrochloride** *see ClomiPRAMINE on page 315*

♦ **Clonapam (Can)** *see Clonazepam on page 316*

Clonazepam *(kloe NA ze pam)*

Related Information

Anticonvulsants by Seizure Type *on page 1481*

Benzodiazepines Comparison *on page 1490*

Epilepsy & Seizure Treatment *on page 1659*

U.S. Brand Names Klonopin™

Canadian Brand Names Alti-Clonazepam; Apo®-Clonazepam; Clonapam; Gen-Clonazepam; Klonopin™; Novo-Clonazepam; Nu-Clonazepam; PMS-Clonazepam; Rho-Clonazepam; Rivotril®

Therapeutic Category Anticonvulsant; Benzodiazepine

Use Alone or as an adjunct in the treatment of petit mal variant (Lennox-Gastaut), akinetic, and myoclonic seizures; petit mal (absence) seizures unresponsive to succimides; panic disorder with or without agoraphobia

Unlabeled/Investigational Use Restless legs syndrome; neuralgia; multifocal tic disorder; parkinsonian dysarthria; bipolar disorder; adjunct therapy for schizophrenia

Restrictions C-IV

Pregnancy Risk Factor D

Pregnancy/Breast-Feeding Implications

Clinical effects on the fetus: Two reports of cardiac defects; respiratory depression, lethargy, hypotonia may be observed in newborns exposed near time of delivery. Epilepsy itself, number of medications, genetic factors, or a combination of these probably influence the teratogenicity of anticonvulsant therapy. Benefit:risk ratio usually favors continued use during pregnancy and breast-feeding.

Breast-feeding/lactation: Crosses into breast milk

Clinical effects on the infant: CNS depression, respiratory depression reported. No recommendation from the AAP.

Contraindications Hypersensitivity to clonazepam or any component of the formulation (cross-sensitivity with other benzodiazepines may exist); significant liver disease; narrow-angle glaucoma; pregnancy

Warnings/Precautions Use with caution in elderly or debilitated patients, patients with hepatic disease (including alcoholics), or renal impairment. Use with caution in patients with respiratory disease or impaired gag reflex or ability to protect the airway from secretions (salivation may be increased). Worsening of seizures may occur when added to patients with multiple seizure types. Concurrent use with valproic acid may result in absence status. Monitoring of CBC and liver function tests has been recommended during prolonged therapy.

Causes CNS depression (dose-related) resulting in sedation, dizziness, confusion, or ataxia which may impair physical and mental capabilities. Patients must be cautioned about performing tasks which require mental alertness (ie, operating machinery or driving). Use with caution in patients receiving other CNS depressants or psychoactive agents. Effects with other sedative drugs or ethanol may be potentiated. Benzodiazepines have been associated with falls and traumatic injury and should be used with extreme caution in patients who are at risk of these events (especially the elderly).

Use caution in patients with depression, particularly if suicidal risk may be present. Use with caution in patients with a history of drug dependence. Benzodiazepines have been associated with dependence and acute withdrawal symptoms, including seizures, on discontinuation or reduction in dose. Acute withdrawal, including seizures, may be precipitated in patients after administration of flumazenil to patients receiving long-term benzodiazepine therapy.

Benzodiazepines have been associated with anterograde amnesia. Paradoxical reactions, including hyperactive or aggressive behavior, have been reported with benzodiazepines, particularly in adolescent/pediatric or psychiatric patients. Does not have analgesic, antidepressant, or antipsychotic properties.

Adverse Reactions

>10%: Central nervous system: Drowsiness

1% to 10%:

Central nervous system: Dizziness, abnormal coordination, ataxia, dysarthria, depression, memory disturbance, fatigue

Dermatologic: Dermatitis, allergic reactions

Endocrine & metabolic: Decreased libido

Gastrointestinal: Anorexia, constipation, diarrhea, xerostomia

Respiratory: Upper respiratory tract infection, sinusitis, rhinitis, coughing

<1% (Limited to important or life-threatening): Blood dyscrasias, menstrual irregularities

Overdosage/Toxicology May produce somnolence, confusion, ataxia, diminished reflexes, or coma. Treatment for benzodiazepine overdose is supportive. Flumazenil has been shown to selectively block the binding of benzodiazepines to CNS receptors, resulting in a reversal of benzodiazepine-induced CNS depression, but not respiratory depression.

Drug Interactions

Cytochrome P450 Effect: CYP3A4 enzyme substrate

Increased Effect/Toxicity: Combined use of clonazepam and valproic acid has been associated with absence seizures. Clonazepam potentiates the CNS depressant effects of narcotic analgesics, barbiturates, phenothiazines, ethanol, antihistamines, MAO inhibitors, sedative-hypnotics, and cyclic antidepressants. Serum levels and/or toxicity of clonazepam may be increased by inhibitors of CYP3A3/4, including cimetidine, ciprofloxacin, clarithromycin, clozapine, delavirdine, diltiazem, disulfiram, digoxin, erythromycin, ethanol, fluconazole, fluoxetine, fluvoxamine, grapefruit juice, indinavir, isoniazid, itraconazole, ketoconazole, loxapine, metoprolol, metronidazole, miconazole, nefazodone, nevirapine, quinupristin/dalfopristin, omeprazole, phenytoin, rifabutin, rifampin, ritonavir, saquinavir, troleandomycin, verapamil, zafirlukast, and zileuton.

Decreased Effect: The combined use of clonazepam and valproic acid has been associated with absence seizures. Carbamazepine, rifampin, rifabutin may enhance the metabolism of clonazepam and decrease its therapeutic effect.

Ethanol/Nutrition/Herb Interactions

Ethanol: Avoid ethanol (may increase CNS depression).

Food: Clonazepam serum concentration is unlikely to be increased by grapefruit juice because of clonazepam's high oral bioavailability.

Herb/Nutraceutical: St John's wort may decrease clonazepam levels. Avoid valerian, St John's wort, kava kava, gotu kola (may increase CNS depression).

Mechanism of Action The exact mechanism is unknown, but believed to be related to its ability to enhance the activity of GABA; suppresses the spike-and-wave discharge in absence seizures by depressing nerve transmission in the motor cortex

Pharmacodynamics/Kinetics

Onset of action: 20-60 minutes

Duration: Infants and young children: 6-8 hours; Adults: ≤12 hours

(Continued)

Clonazepam *(Continued)*

Absorption: Well absorbed

Distribution: Adults: V_d: 1.5-4.4 L/kg

Protein binding: 85%

Metabolism: Extensively hepatic; glucuronide and sulfate conjugation

Half-life elimination: Children: 22-33 hours; Adults: 19-50 hours

Time to peak, serum: 1-3 hours; Steady-state: 5-7 days

Excretion: Urine (<2% as unchanged drug); metabolites excreted as glucuronide or sulfate conjugates

Usual Dosage Oral:

Children <10 years or 30 kg: Seizure disorders:

Initial daily dose: 0.01-0.03 mg/kg/day (maximum: 0.05 mg/kg/day) given in 2-3 divided doses; increase by no more than 0.5 mg every third day until seizures are controlled or adverse effects seen

Usual maintenance dose: 0.1-0.2 mg/kg/day divided 3 times/day, not to exceed 0.2 mg/kg/day

Adults:

Seizure disorders:

Initial daily dose not to exceed 1.5 mg given in 3 divided doses; may increase by 0.5-1 mg every third day until seizures are controlled or adverse effects seen (maximum: 20 mg/day)

Usual maintenance dose: 0.05-0.2 mg/kg; do not exceed 20 mg/day

Panic disorder: 0.25 mg twice daily; increase in increments of 0.125-0.25 mg twice daily every 3 days; target dose: 1 mg/day (maximum: 4 mg/day)

Elderly: Initiate with low doses and observe closely

Hemodialysis: Supplemental dose is not necessary

Monitoring Parameters CBC, liver function tests

Reference Range Relationship between serum concentration and seizure control is not well established

Timing of serum samples: Peak serum levels occur 1-3 hours after oral ingestion; the half-life is 20-40 hours; therefore, steady-state occurs in 5-7 days

Therapeutic levels: 20-80 ng/mL; Toxic concentration: >80 ng/mL

Patient Information Avoid alcohol and other CNS depressants; avoid activities needing good psychomotor coordination until CNS effects are known; drug may cause physical or psychological dependence; avoid abrupt discontinuation after prolonged use

Nursing Implications Observe patient for excess sedation, respiratory depression; raise bed rails, initiate safety measures, assist with ambulation

Additional Information Ethosuximide or valproic acid may be preferred for treatment of absence (petit mal) seizures. Clonazepam-induced behavioral disturbances may be more frequent in mentally handicapped patients. Abrupt discontinuation after sustained use (generally >10 days) may cause withdrawal symptoms. Flumazenil, a competitive benzodiazepine antagonist at the CNS receptor site, reverses benzodiazepine-induced CNS depression.

Dosage Forms Tablet: 0.5 mg, 1 mg, 2 mg

Extemporaneous Preparations A 0.1 mg/mL oral suspension has been made using five 2 mg tablets, purified water USP (10 mL) and methylcellulose 1% (qs ad 100 mL); the expected stability of this preparation is 2 weeks if stored under refrigeration; shake well before use

Nahata MC and Hipple TF, *Pediatric Drug Formulations*, 2nd ed, Cincinnati, OH: Harvey Whitney Books Co, 1992.

Clonidine *(KLON i deen)*

Related Information

Depression *on page 1655*

Hypertension *on page 1675*

U.S. Brand Names Catapres®; Catapres-TTS®-1; Catapres-TTS®-2; Catapres-TTS®-3; Duraclon™

Canadian Brand Names Apo®-Clonidine; Carapres®; Dixarit®; Novo-Clonidine®; Nu-Clonidine®

Synonyms Clonidine Hydrochloride

Therapeutic Category Alpha$_2$-Adrenergic Agonist Agent; Antihypertensive Agent; Antimigraine Agent

Use Management of mild to moderate hypertension; either used alone or in combination with other antihypertensives

Orphan drug: Duraclon™: For continuous epidural administration as adjunctive therapy with intraspinal opiates for treatment of cancer pain in patients tolerant to or unresponsive to intraspinal opiates

Unlabeled/Investigational Use Heroin or nicotine withdrawal; severe pain; dysmenorrhea; vasomotor symptoms associated with menopause; ethanol dependence; prophylaxis of migraines; glaucoma; diabetes-associated diarrhea; impulse control disorder, attention-deficit/hyperactivity disorder (ADHD), clozapine-induced sialorrhea

Pregnancy Risk Factor C

Pregnancy/Breast-Feeding Implications

Clinical effects on the fetus: Crosses the placenta. Caution should be used with this drug due to the potential of rebound hypertension with abrupt discontinuation.

Breast-feeding/lactation: Crosses into breast milk. AAP has NO RECOMMENDATION.

Contraindications Hypersensitivity to clonidine hydrochloride or any component of the formulation

Warnings/Precautions Gradual withdrawal is needed (over 1 week for oral, 2-4 days with epidural) if drug needs to be stopped. Patients should be instructed about abrupt discontinuation (causes rapid increase in BP and symptoms of sympathetic overactivity). In patients on both a beta-blocker and clonidine where withdrawal of clonidine is necessary, withdraw the beta-blocker first and several days before clonidine. Then slowly decrease clonidine.

Use with caution in patients with severe coronary insufficiency; conduction disturbances; recent MI, CVA, or chronic renal insufficiency. Caution in sinus node dysfunction. Discontinue within 4 hours of surgery then restart as soon as possible after. Clonidine injection should be administered via a continuous epidural infusion device. Epidural clonidine is not recommended for perioperative, obstetrical, or postpartum pain. It is not recommended for use in patients with severe cardiovascular disease or hemodynamic instability. In all cases, the epidural may lead to cardiovascular instability (hypotension, bradycardia). May cause significant CNS depression and xerostomia. Caution in patients with pre-existing CNS disease or depression. Elderly may be at greater risk for CNS depressive effects, favoring other agents in this population.

Adverse Reactions Incidence of adverse events is not always reported.

>10%:

Central nervous system: Drowsiness (35% oral, 12% transdermal), dizziness (16% oral, 2% transdermal)

Dermatologic: Transient localized skin reactions characterized by pruritus, and erythema (15% to 50% transdermal)

Gastrointestinal: Dry mouth (40% oral, 25% transdermal)

1% to 10%:

Cardiovascular: Orthostatic hypotension (3% oral)

Central nervous system: Headache (1% oral, 5% transdermal), sedation (3% transdermal), fatigue (6% transdermal), lethargy (3% transdermal), insomnia (2% transdermal), nervousness (3% oral, 1% transdermal), mental depression (1% oral)

Dermatologic: Rash (1% oral), allergic contact sensitivity (5% transdermal), localized vesiculation (7%), hyperpigmentation (5% at application site), edema (3%), excoriation (3%), burning (3%), throbbing, blanching (1%), papules (1%), and generalized macular rash (1%) has occurred in patients receiving transdermal clonidine.

Endocrine & metabolic: Sodium and water retention, sexual dysfunction (3% oral, 2% transdermal), impotence (3% oral, 2% transdermal), weakness (10% transdermal)

Gastrointestinal: Nausea (5% oral, 1% transdermal), vomiting (5% oral), anorexia and malaise (1% oral), constipation (10% oral, 1% transdermal), dry throat (2% transdermal), taste disturbance (1% transdermal), weight gain (1% oral)

Genitourinary: Nocturia (1% oral)

Hepatic: Liver function test (mild abnormalities, 1% oral)

Miscellaneous: Withdrawal syndrome (1% oral)

<1% (Limited to important or life-threatening): Abdominal pain, agitation, alopecia, angioedema, AV block, behavioral changes, blurred vision, bradycardia, chest pain, congestive heart failure, contact dermatitis (transdermal), CVA, delirium, depression, dryness of the eyes, EKG abnormalities, gynecomastia, hallucinations, hepatitis, increased sensitivity to ethanol, localized hypo- or hyperpigmentation (transdermal), nightmares, orthostatic symptoms, pseudo-obstruction rash, Raynaud's phenomenon, syncope, tachycardia, thrombocytopenia, urinary retention, urticaria, vomiting, withdrawal syndrome

Overdosage/Toxicology Symptoms include bradycardia, CNS depression, hypothermia, diarrhea, respiratory depression, and apnea. Treatment is primarily supportive and symptomatic. Hypotension usually responds to I.V. fluids and Trendelenburg positioning. Naloxone may be utilized in treating CNS depression and/or apnea and should be given I.V. 0.4-2 mg, with repeated doses as needed, or as an infusion.

Drug Interactions

Increased Effect/Toxicity: Concurrent use with antipsychotics (especially low potency), narcotic analgesics, or nitroprusside may produce additive hypotensive effects. Clonidine may decrease the symptoms of hypoglycemia with oral hypoglycemic agents or insulin. Alcohol, barbiturates, and other CNS depressants may have additive CNS effects when combined with clonidine. Epidural clonidine may prolong the sensory and motor blockade of local anesthetics. Clonidine may increase cyclosporine (and perhaps tacrolimus) serum concentrations. Beta-blockers may potentiate bradycardia in patients receiving clonidine and may increase the rebound hypertension of withdrawal. Tricyclic antidepressants may also enhance the hypertensive response associated with abrupt clonidine withdrawal.

Decreased Effect: Tricyclic antidepressants (TCAs) antagonize the hypotensive effects of clonidine.

Ethanol/Nutrition/Herb Interactions

Ethanol: Avoid ethanol (may increase CNS depression).

Herb/Nutraceutical: Avoid dong quai if using for hypertension (has estrogenic activity). Avoid ephedra, yohimbe, ginseng (may worsen hypertension). Avoid valerian, St John's wort, kava kava, gotu kola (may increase CNS depression).

Mechanism of Action Stimulates alpha$_2$-adrenoceptors in the brain stem, thus activating an inhibitory neuron, resulting in reduced sympathetic outflow from the CNS, producing a decrease in peripheral resistance, renal vascular resistance, heart rate, and blood pressure; epidural clonidine may produce pain relief at spinal presynaptic and postjunctional alpha$_2$-adrenoceptors by preventing pain signal transmission; pain relief occurs only for the body regions innervated by the spinal segments where analgesic concentrations of clonidine exist

Pharmacodynamics/Kinetics

Onset of action: Oral: 0.5-1 hour

Duration: 6-10 hours

Distribution: V$_d$: Adults: 2.1 L/kg; highly lipid soluble; distributes readily into extravascular sites

Protein binding: 20% to 40%

Metabolism: Hepatic (enterohepatic recirculation); extensively metabolized to inactive metabolites

Bioavailability: 75% to 95%

Half-life elimination: Adults: Normal renal function: 6-20 hours; Renal impairment: 18-41 hours

Time to peak: 2-4 hours

Excretion: Urine (65%, 32% as unchanged drug); feces (22%)

(Continued)

Clonidine *(Continued)*

Usual Dosage

Children:

Oral:

Hypertension: Initial: 5-10 mcg/kg/day in divided doses every 8-12 hours; increase gradually at 5- to 7-day intervals to 25 mcg/kg/day in divided doses every 6 hours; maximum: 0.9 mg/day

Clonidine tolerance test (test of growth hormone release from pituitary): 0.15 mg/m^2 or 4 mcg/kg as single dose

ADHD (unlabeled use): Initial: 0.05 mg/day; increase every 3-7 days by 0.05 mg/day to 3-5 mcg/kg/day given in divided doses 3-4 times/day (maximum dose: 0.3-0.4 mg/day)

Epidural infusion: Pain management: Reserved for patients with severe intractable pain, unresponsive to other analgesics or epidural or spinal opiates: Initial: 0.5 mcg/kg/hour; adjust with caution, based on clinical effect

Adults:

Oral:

Acute hypertension (urgency): Initial 0.1-0.2 mg; may be followed by additional doses of 0.1 mg every hour, if necessary, to a maximum total dose of 0.6 mg

Hypertension: Initial dose: 0.1 mg twice daily, usual maintenance dose: 0.2-1.2 mg/day in 2-4 divided doses; maximum recommended dose: 2.4 mg/day

Nicotine withdrawal symptoms: 0.1 mg twice daily to maximum of 0.4 mg/day for 3-4 weeks

Transdermal: Hypertension: Apply once every 7 days; for initial therapy start with 0.1 mg and increase by 0.1 mg at 1- to 2-week intervals; dosages >0.6 mg do not improve efficacy

Epidural infusion: Pain management: Starting dose: 30 mcg/hour; titrate as required for relief of pain or presence of side effects; minimal experience with doses >40 mcg/hour; should be considered an adjunct to intraspinal opiate therapy

Elderly: Initial: 0.1 mg once daily at bedtime, increase gradually as needed

Dosing adjustment in renal impairment: Cl$_{cr}$ <10 mL/minute: Administer 50% to 75% of normal dose initially

Dialysis: Not dialyzable (0% to 5%) via hemo- or peritoneal dialysis; supplemental dose not necessary

Dietary Considerations Hypertensive patients may need to decrease sodium and calories in diet.

Administration

Oral: Do not discontinue clonidine abruptly. if needed, gradually reduce dose over 2-4 days to avoid rebound hypertension

Transdermal patch: Patches should be applied weekly at bedtime to a clean, hairless area of the upper outer arm or chest. Rotate patch sites weekly. Redness under patch may be reduced if a topical corticosteroid spray is applied to the area before placement of the patch.

Monitoring Parameters Blood pressure, standing and sitting/supine, mental status, heart rate

Reference Range Therapeutic: 1-2 ng/mL (SI: 4.4-8.7 nmol/L)

Patient Information Do not discontinue drug except on instruction of physician; check daily to be sure patch is present; may cause drowsiness, impaired coordination, and judgment; use extreme caution while driving or operating machines

Nursing Implications Patches should be applied weekly at bedtime to a clean, hairless area of the upper outer arm or chest; rotate patch sites weekly; redness under patch may be reduced if a topical corticosteroid spray is applied to the area before placement of the patch; if needed, gradually reduce dose over 2-4 days to avoid rebound hypertension; during epidural administration, monitor cardiovascular and respiratory status carefully

Additional Information Transdermal clonidine should only be used in patients unable to take oral medication. The transdermal product is much more expensive than oral clonidine and produces no better therapeutic effects.

Dosage Forms

Injection, as hydrochloride [preservative free]: 100 mcg/mL (10 mL); 500 mcg/mL (10 mL)

Patch, transdermal, as hydrochloride [7-day duration]:

Catapres-TTS®-1: 0.1 mg/day (4s)

Catapres-TTS®-2: 0.2 mg/day (4s)

Catapres-TTS®-3: 0.3 mg/day (4s)

Tablet, as hydrochloride: 0.1 mg, 0.2 mg, 0.3 mg

Clonidine and Chlorthalidone *(KLON i deen & klor THAL i done)*

U.S. Brand Names Combipres®

Synonyms Chlorthalidone and Clonidine

Therapeutic Category Antihypertensive Agent, Combination

Use Management of mild to moderate hypertension

Pregnancy Risk Factor C

Usual Dosage Oral: 1 tablet 1-2 times/day; maximum: 0.6 mg clonidine and 30 mg chlorthalidone

Additional Information Complete prescribing information for this medication should be consulted for additional detail.

Dosage Forms

Tablet:

0.1: Clonidine 0.1 mg and chlorthalidone 15 mg

0.2: Clonidine 0.2 mg and chlorthalidone 15 mg

0.3: Clonidine 0.3 mg and chlorthalidone 15 mg

♦ **Clonidine Hydrochloride** *see* Clonidine *on page 318*

Clopidogrel (kloh PID oh grel)

U.S. Brand Names Plavix®

Canadian Brand Names Plavix™

Synonyms Clopidogrel Bisulfate

Therapeutic Category Antiplatelet Agent; Platelet Aggregation Inhibitor

Use Reduce atherosclerotic events (myocardial infarction, stroke, vascular deaths) in patients with atherosclerosis documented by recent myocardial infarction (MI), recent stroke, or established peripheral arterial disease; prevention of thrombotic complications after coronary stenting; acute coronary syndrome (unstable angina or non-Q-wave MI)

Unlabeled/Investigational Use In aspirin-allergic patients, prevention of coronary artery bypass graft closure (saphenous vein)

Pregnancy Risk Factor B

Contraindications Hypersensitivity to clopidogrel or any component of the formulation; active pathological bleeding such as PUD or intracranial hemorrhage; coagulation disorders

Warnings/Precautions Cases of thrombotic thrombocytopenic purpura (TTP) have been reported, usually within the first 2 weeks of therapy. Patients receiving anticoagulants or other antiplatelet drugs concurrently, liver disease, patients having a previous hypersensitivity or other untoward effects related to ticlopidine, hypertension, renal impairment, history of bleeding or hemostatic disorders or drug-related hematologic disorders, and in patients scheduled for major surgery consider discontinuing 5 days prior to that surgery

Adverse Reactions As with all drugs which may affect hemostasis, bleeding is associated with clopidogrel. Hemorrhage may occur at virtually any site. Risk is dependent on multiple variables, including the concurrent use of multiple agents which alter hemostasis and patient susceptibility.

>10%: Gastrointestinal: The overall incidence of gastrointestinal events (including abdominal pain, vomiting, dyspepsia, gastritis and constipation) has been documented to be 27% compared to 30% in patients receiving aspirin.

3% to 10%:
Cardiovascular: Chest pain (8%), edema (4%), hypertension (4%)
Central nervous system: Headache (3% to 8%), dizziness (2% to 6%), depression (4%), fatigue (3%), general pain (6%)
Dermatologic: Rash (4%), pruritus (3%)
Endocrine & metabolic: Hypercholesterolemia (4%)
Gastrointestinal: Abdominal pain (2% to 6%), dyspepsia (2% to 5%), diarrhea (2% to 5%), nausea (3%)
Genitourinary: Urinary tract infection (3%)
Hematologic: Purpura (5%), epistaxis (3%)
Hepatic: Liver function test abnormalities (<3%; discontinued in 0.11%)
Neuromuscular & skeletal: Arthralgia (6%), back pain (6%)
Respiratory: Dyspnea (5%), rhinitis (4%), bronchitis (4%), coughing (3%), upper respiratory infections (9%)
Miscellaneous: Flu-like syndrome (8%)
<1% (Limited to important or life-threatening): Agranulocytosis, allergic reaction, anaphylactoid reaction, angioedema, aplastic anemia, bilirubinemia, bronchospasm, bullous eruption, fatty liver, fever, granulocytopenia, hematuria, hemoptysis, hemothorax, hepatitis, hypochromic anemia, intracranial hemorrhage (0.4%), ischemic necrosis, leukopenia, maculopapular rash, menorrhagia, neutropenia (0.05%), ocular hemorrhage, pulmonary hemorrhage, purpura, retroperitoneal bleeding, thrombocytopenia, thrombotic thrombocytopenic purpura, urticaria

Overdosage/Toxicology Symptoms of acute toxicity include vomiting, prostration, difficulty breathing, and gastrointestinal hemorrhage. Only one case of overdose with clopidogrel has been reported to date; no symptoms were reported with this case and no specific treatments were required. Based on its pharmacology, platelet transfusions may be an appropriate treatment when attempting to reverse the effects of clopidogrel. After decontamination, treatment is symptomatic and supportive.

Drug Interactions

Cytochrome P450 Effect: CYP2C9 enzyme inhibitor (high concentrations - *in vitro*)

Increased Effect/Toxicity: At high concentrations, clopidogrel may interfere with the metabolism of amiodarone, cisapride, cyclosporine, diltiazem, fluvastatin, irbesartan, losartan, oral hypoglycemics, paclitaxel, phenytoin, quinidine, sildenafil, tamoxifen, torsemide, verapamil, and some NSAIDs which may result in toxicity. Clopidogrel and naproxen resulted in an increase of GI occult blood loss. Anticoagulants (warfarin, thrombolytics, drotrecogin alfa) or other antiplatelet agents may increase the risk of bleeding.

Ethanol/Nutrition/Herb Interactions Herb/Nutraceutical: Avoid cat's claw, dong quai, evening primrose, feverfew, garlic, ginger, ginkgo, red clover, horse chestnut, green tea, ginseng (all have additional antiplatelet activity).

Stability Store at 25°C (77°F); excursions permitted to 15°C to 3°C (59°F to 86°F).

Mechanism of Action Blocks the ADP receptors, which prevent fibrinogen binding at that site and thereby reduce the possibility of platelet adhesion and aggregation

Pharmacodynamics/Kinetics

Onset of action: Inhibition of platelet aggregation detected: 2 hours after 300 mg administered; after second day of treatment with 50-100 mg/day
Peak effect: 50-100 mg/day: Bleeding time: 5-6 days; Platelet function: 3-7 days
Metabolism: Extensively hepatic via hydrolysis; biotransformation to carboxyl acid derivative (active metabolite that inhibits platelet aggregation)
Half-life elimination: ~8 hours
Time to peak, serum: ~1 hour
Excretion: Urine

Usual Dosage Oral: Adults:

Recent MI, recent stroke, or established arterial disease: 75 mg once daily
Acute coronary syndrome: Initial: 300 mg loading dose, followed by 75 mg once daily (in combination with aspirin 75-325 mg once daily)

(Continued)

Clopidogrel *(Continued)*

Prevention of coronary artery bypass graft closure (saphenous vein): Aspirin-allergic patients (unlabeled use): Loading dose: 300 mg 6 hours following procedure; maintenance: 50-100 mg/day

Dosing adjustment in renal impairment and elderly: None necessary

Dietary Considerations May be taken without regard to meals.

Monitoring Parameters Signs of bleeding; hemoglobin and hematocrit periodically

Patient Information Report any unusual or prolonged bleeding or fever; inform your physician before starting any new medications, changing your diet, or undergoing any procedures that may be associated with a risk of bleeding

Dosage Forms Tablet, as bisulfate: 75 mg

♦ **Clopidogrel Bisulfate** *see Clopidogrel on page 321*

Clorazepate *(klor AZ e pate)*

Related Information

Antacid Drug Interactions *on page 1477*
Benzodiazepines Comparison *on page 1490*
Epilepsy & Seizure Treatment *on page 1659*

U.S. Brand Names Tranxene®

Canadian Brand Names Apo®-Clorazepate; Novo-Clopate®; Tranxene®

Synonyms Clorazepate Dipotassium

Therapeutic Category Anticonvulsant; Benzodiazepine; Sedative

Use Treatment of generalized anxiety disorder; management of ethanol withdrawal; adjunct anticonvulsant in management of partial seizures

Restrictions C-IV

Pregnancy Risk Factor D

Contraindications Hypersensitivity to clorazepate or any component of the formulation (cross-sensitivity with other benzodiazepines may exist); narrow-angle glaucoma; pregnancy

Warnings/Precautions Not recommended for use in patients <9 years of age or patients with depressive or psychotic disorders. Use with caution in elderly or debilitated patients, patients with hepatic disease (including alcoholics), or renal impairment. Active metabolites with extended half-lives may lead to delayed accumulation and adverse effects. Use with caution in patients with respiratory disease or impaired gag reflex. Use is not recommended in patients with depressive disorders or psychoses. Avoid use in patients with sleep apnea.

Causes CNS depression (dose-related) resulting in sedation, dizziness, confusion, or ataxia which may impair physical and mental capabilities. Patients must be cautioned about performing tasks which require mental alertness (ie, operating machinery or driving). Use with caution in patients receiving other CNS depressants or psychoactive agents. Effects with other sedative drugs or ethanol may be potentiated. Benzodiazepines have been associated with falls and traumatic injury and should be used with extreme caution in patients who are at risk of these events (especially the elderly).

Use caution in patients with depression, particularly if suicidal risk may be present. Use with caution in patients with a history of drug dependence. Benzodiazepines have been associated with dependence and acute withdrawal symptoms on discontinuation or reduction in dose. Acute withdrawal, including seizures, may be precipitated in patients after administration of flumazenil to patients receiving long-term benzodiazepine therapy.

Benzodiazepines have been associated with anterograde amnesia. Paradoxical reactions, including hyperactive or aggressive behavior, have been reported with benzodiazepines, particularly in adolescent/pediatric or psychiatric patients. Does not have analgesic, antidepressant, or antipsychotic properties.

Adverse Reactions Frequency not defined.

Cardiovascular: Hypotension

Central nervous system: Drowsiness, fatigue, ataxia, lightheadedness, memory impairment, insomnia, anxiety, headache, depression, slurred speech, confusion, nervousness, dizziness, irritability

Dermatologic: Rash

Endocrine & metabolic: Decreased libido

Gastrointestinal: Xerostomia, constipation, diarrhea, decreased salivation, nausea, vomiting, increased or decreased appetite

Neuromuscular & skeletal: Dysarthria, tremor

Ocular: Blurred vision, diplopia

Overdosage/Toxicology May produce somnolence, confusion, ataxia, diminished reflexes, and coma. Treatment for benzodiazepine overdose is supportive. Mechanical ventilation is rarely required. Flumazenil has been shown to selectively block the binding of benzodiazepines to CNS receptors, resulting in a reversal of benzodiazepine-induced CNS depression, but not respiratory depression.

Drug Interactions

Cytochrome P450 Effect: CYP3A3/4 enzyme substrate

Increased Effect/Toxicity: Clorazepate potentiates the CNS depressant effects of narcotic analgesics, barbiturates, phenothiazines, ethanol, antihistamines, MAO inhibitors, sedative-hypnotics, and cyclic antidepressants. Serum concentrations/toxicity of clorazepate may be increased by inhibitors of CYP3A3/4, including amprenavir, cimetidine, ciprofloxacin, clarithromycin, clozapine, diltiazem, disulfiram, digoxin, erythromycin, ethanol, fluconazole, fluoxetine, fluvoxamine, grapefruit juice, isoniazid, itraconazole, ketoconazole, labetalol, levodopa, loxapine, metoprolol, metronidazole, miconazole, nefazodone, nelfinavir, omeprazole, phenytoin, rifabutin, rifampin, ritonavir, troleandomycin, valproic acid, and verapamil.

Decreased Effect: Carbamazepine, rifampin, rifabutin may enhance the metabolism of clorazepate and decrease its therapeutic effect.

Ethanol/Nutrition/Herb Interactions

Ethanol: Avoid ethanol (may increase CNS depression).

Food: Serum concentrations/toxicity may be increased by grapefruit juice.

Herb/Nutraceutical: Avoid valerian, St John's wort, kava kava, gotu kola (may increase CNS depression).

Mechanism of Action Binds to stereospecific benzodiazepine receptors on the postsynaptic GABA neuron at several sites within the central nervous system, including the limbic system, reticular formation. Enhancement of the inhibitory effect of GABA on neuronal excitability results in increased neuronal membrane permeability to chloride ions. This shift in chloride ions results in hyperpolarization (a less excitable state) and stabilization.

Pharmacodynamics/Kinetics

Onset of action: ~1 hour

Duration: Variable, 8-24 hours

Distribution: Crosses placenta; appears in urine

Metabolism: Rapidly decarboxylated to desmethyldiazepam (active) in acidic stomach prior to absorption; hepatically to oxazepam (active)

Half-life elimination: Adults: Desmethyldiazepam: 48-96 hours; Oxazepam: 6-8 hours

Time to peak, serum: ~1 hour

Excretion: Primarily urine

Usual Dosage Oral:

Children 9-12 years: Anticonvulsant: Initial: 3.75-7.5 mg/dose twice daily; increase dose by 3.75 mg at weekly intervals, not to exceed 60 mg/day in 2-3 divided doses

Children >12 years and Adults: Anticonvulsant: Initial: Up to 7.5 mg/dose 2-3 times/day; increase dose by 7.5 mg at weekly intervals, not to exceed 90 mg/day

Adults:

Anxiety:

Regular release tablets (Tranxene® T-Tab®): 7.5-15 mg 2-4 times/day

Sustained release (Tranxene®-SD): 11.25 or 22.5 mg once daily at bedtime

Ethanol withdrawal: Initial: 30 mg, then 15 mg 2-4 times/day on first day; maximum daily dose: 90 mg; gradually decrease dose over subsequent days

Monitoring Parameters Respiratory and cardiovascular status, excess CNS depression

Reference Range Therapeutic: 0.12-1 µg/mL (SI: 0.36-3.01 µmol/L)

Patient Information Avoid alcohol and other CNS depressants; avoid activities needing good psychomotor coordination until CNS effects are known; drug may cause physical or psychological dependence; avoid abrupt discontinuation after prolonged use

Nursing Implications Observe patient for excess sedation, respiratory depression; raise bed rails, initiate safety measures, assist with ambulation

Additional Information Abrupt discontinuation after sustained use (generally >10 days) may cause withdrawal symptoms.

Dosage Forms

Tablet, as dipotassium:

Tranxene®-SD™: 22.5 mg [once daily]

Tranxene®-SD™ Half Strength: 11.25 mg [once daily]

Tranxene® T-Tab®: 3.75 mg, 7.5 mg, 15 mg

♦ **Clorazepate Dipotassium** see Clorazepate on page 322

♦ **Clotrimaderm (Can)** see Clotrimazole on page 323

Clotrimazole (kloe TRIM a zole)

Related Information

Treatment of Sexually Transmitted Diseases on page 1609

USPHA/IDSA Guidelines for the Prevention of Opportunistic Infections in Persons With HIV on page 1574

U.S. Brand Names Cruex® [OTC]; Gyne-Lotrimin® [OTC]; Gyne-Lotrimin® 3 [OTC]; Gynix® [OTC]; Lotrimin®; Lotrimin® AF [OTC]; Mycelex®; Mycelex®-3; Mycelex®-7 [OTC]; Mycelex® Twin Pack [OTC]; Trivagizole 3™

Canadian Brand Names Canesten® Topical, Canesten® Vaginal; Clotrimaderm; Scheinpharm™ Clotrimazole; Trivagizole-3®

Therapeutic Category Antifungal Agent, Oral Nonabsorbed; Antifungal Agent, Topical; Antifungal Agent, Vaginal

Use Treatment of susceptible fungal infections, including oropharyngeal candidiasis, dermatophytoses, superficial mycoses, and cutaneous candidiasis, as well as vulvovaginal candidiasis; limited data suggest that clotrimazole troches may be effective for prophylaxis against oropharyngeal candidiasis in neutropenic patients

Pregnancy Risk Factor B (topical); C (troches)

Contraindications Hypersensitivity to clotrimazole or any component of the formulation

Warnings/Precautions Clotrimazole should not be used for treatment of systemic fungal infection; safety and effectiveness of clotrimazole lozenges (troches) in children <3 years of age have not been established; when using topical formulation, avoid contact with eyes

Adverse Reactions

Oral:

>10%: Hepatic: Abnormal liver function tests

1% to 10%:

Gastrointestinal: Nausea and vomiting may occur in patients on clotrimazole troches

Local: Mild burning, irritation, stinging to skin or vaginal area

Vaginal:

1% to 10%: Genitourinary: Vulvar/vaginal burning

<1% (Limited to important or life-threatening): Burning or itching of penis of sexual partner; polyuria; vulvar itching, soreness, edema, or discharge

Drug Interactions

Cytochrome P450 Effect: CYP3A3/4 and 3A5-7 enzyme inhibitor

Mechanism of Action Binds to phospholipids in the fungal cell membrane altering cell wall permeability resulting in loss of essential intracellular elements

Pharmacodynamics/Kinetics

Absorption: Topical: Negligible through intact skin

(Continued)

Clotrimazole *(Continued)*

Time to peak, serum:
Oral topical: Salivary levels occur within 3 hours following 30 minutes of dissolution time
Vaginal cream: High vaginal levels: 8-24 hours
Vaginal tablet: High vaginal levels: 1-2 days
Excretion: Feces (as metabolites)

Usual Dosage
Children >3 years and Adults:
Oral:
Prophylaxis: 10 mg troche dissolved 3 times/day for the duration of chemotherapy or until steroids are reduced to maintenance levels
Treatment: 10 mg troche dissolved slowly 5 times/day for 14 consecutive days
Topical (cream, lotion, solution): Apply twice daily; if no improvement occurs after 4 weeks of therapy, re-evaluate diagnosis
Children >12 years and Adults:
Vaginal:
Cream:
1%: Insert 1 applicatorful vaginal cream daily (preferably at bedtime) for 7 consecutive days
2%: Insert 1 applicatorful vaginal cream daily (preferably at bedtime) for 3 consecutive days
Tablet: Insert 100 mg/day for 7 days or 500 mg single dose
Topical (cream, lotion, solution): Apply to affected area twice daily (morning and evening) for 7 consecutive days

Administration
Oral: Allow to dissolve slowly over 15-30 minutes.
Topical: Avoid contact with eyes. For external use only. Apply sparingly. Protect hands with latex gloves. Do not use occlusive dressings.

Monitoring Parameters Periodic liver function tests during oral therapy with clotrimazole lozenges

Patient Information Oral: Do not swallow oral medication whole; allow to dissolve slowly in mouth. You may experience nausea or vomiting (small frequent meals, frequent mouth care, chewing gum, or sucking lozenges may help). Report signs of opportunistic infection (eg, white plaques in mouth, fever, chills, perianal itching or vaginal discharge, fatigue, unhealed wounds or sores).

Topical: Wash hands before applying or wear gloves. Apply thin film of gel, lotion, or solution to affected area. May apply porous dressing. Report persistent burning, swelling, itching, worsening of condition, or lack of response to therapy.

Vaginal: Wash hands before using. Insert full applicator into vagina gently and expel cream, or insert tablet into vagina, at bedtime. Wash applicator with soap and water following use. Remain lying down for 30 minutes following administration. Avoid intercourse during therapy (sexual partner may experience penile burning or itching). Report adverse reactions (eg, vulvar itching, frequent urination), worsening of condition, or lack of response to therapy. Contact prescriber if symptoms do not improve within 3 days or you do not feel well within 7 days. Do not use tampons until therapy is complete. Contact prescriber immediately if you experience abdominal pain, fever, or foul-smelling discharge.

Nursing Implications
Administer around-the-clock rather than 4 times/day, 3 times/day, etc (ie, 12-6-12-6, not 9-1-5-9) to promote less variation in peak and trough serum levels
Monitor periodic liver function tests during oral therapy with clotrimazole lozenges

Dosage Forms
Combination pack:
Gyne-Lotrimin®, Mycelex®-7: Vaginal tablet 100 mg (7s) and vaginal cream 1% (7 g)
Gyne-Lotrimin® 3: Vaginal tablet 200 mg and vaginal cream 1% (7 g)
Mycelex® Twin Pack: Vaginal tablet 500 mg (1s) and vaginal cream 1% (7 g)
Cream, topical (Lotrimin®, Lotrimin® AF, Mycelex®, Mycelex® OTC): 1% (15 g, 30 g, 45 g, 90 g)
Cream, vaginal:
Gyne-Lotrimin®, Mycelex®-7: 1% (45 g, 90 g)
Gyne-Lotrimin® 3, Mycelex®-3, Trivagizole 3™: 2% (25 g)
Lotion (Lotrimin®): 1% (30 mL)
Solution, topical (Lotrimin®, Lotrimin® AF, Mycelex®, Mycelex® OTC): 1% (10 mL, 30 mL)
Tablet, vaginal:
Gyne-Lotrimin®, Mycelex®-7: 100 mg (7s)
Mycelex®-G: 500 mg (1s)
Troche (Mycelex®): 10 mg

♦ **Clotrimazole and Betamethasone** *see* Betamethasone and Clotrimazole *on page 163*

Cloxacillin *(kloks a SIL in)*

U.S. Brand Names Cloxapen®
Canadian Brand Names Apo®-Cloxi; Novo-Cloxin®; Nu-Cloxi®
Synonyms Cloxacillin Sodium
Therapeutic Category Antibiotic, Penicillin
Use Treatment of susceptible bacterial infections, notably penicillinase-producing staphylococci causing respiratory tract, skin and skin structure, bone and joint, urinary tract infections
Pregnancy Risk Factor B
Contraindications Hypersensitivity to cloxacillin, any component of the formulation, or penicillins
Warnings/Precautions Monitor PT if patient concurrently on warfarin, elimination of drug is slow in renally impaired; use with caution in patients allergic to cephalosporins due to a low incidence of cross-hypersensitivity

Adverse Reactions

1% to 10%: Gastrointestinal: Nausea, diarrhea, abdominal pain

<1% (Limited to important or life-threatening): Agranulocytosis, anemia, BUN increased, creatinine increased, eosinophilia, fever, hematuria, hemolytic anemia, hepatotoxicity, hypersensitivity, interstitial nephritis, leukopenia, neutropenia, prolonged PT, pseudomembranous colitis, rash (maculopapular to exfoliative), seizures with extremely high doses and/or renal failure, serum sickness-like reactions, thrombocytopenia, transient elevated LFTs, vaginitis, vomiting

Overdosage/Toxicology Symptoms of penicillin overdose include neuromuscular hypersensitivity (agitation, hallucinations, asterixis, encephalopathy, confusion, and seizures) and electrolyte imbalance (with potassium or sodium salts), especially in renal failure. Hemodialysis may be helpful to aid in the removal of the drug from the blood, otherwise, most treatment is supportive or symptom directed.

Drug Interactions

Increased Effect/Toxicity: Probenecid and disulfiram may increase levels of penicillins (cloxacillin). The hypoprothrombinemic effects of warfarin may be increased.

Decreased Effect: The efficacy of oral contraceptives may be reduced.

Stability Refrigerate oral solution after reconstitution; discard after 14 days; stable for 3 days at room temperature

Mechanism of Action Inhibits bacterial cell wall synthesis by binding to one or more of the penicillin-binding proteins (PBPs) which in turn inhibits the final transpeptidation step of peptidoglycan synthesis in bacterial cell walls, thus inhibiting cell wall biosynthesis. Bacteria eventually lyse due to ongoing activity of cell wall autolytic enzymes (autolysins and murein hydrolases) while cell wall assembly is arrested.

Pharmacodynamics/Kinetics

Absorption: Oral: ~50%

Distribution: Widely to most body fluids and bone; penetration into cells, into eye, and across normal meninges is poor; crosses placenta; enters breast milk; inflammation increases amount that crosses blood-brain barrier

Protein binding: 90% to 98%

Metabolism: Significantly hepatic to active and inactive metabolites

Half-life elimination: 0.5-1.5 hours; prolonged with renal impairment and in neonates

Time to peak, serum: 0.5-2 hours

Excretion: Urine and feces

Usual Dosage Oral:

Children >1 month (<20 kg): 50-100 mg/kg/day in divided doses every 6 hours; up to a maximum of 4 g/day

Children (>20 kg) and Adults: 250-500 mg every 6 hours

Hemodialysis: Not dialyzable (0% to 5%)

Dietary Considerations Should be taken 1 hour before or 2 hours after meals with water.

Monitoring Parameters Observe for signs and symptoms of anaphylaxis during first dose

Test Interactions May interfere with urinary glucose tests using cupric sulfate (Benedict's solution, Clinitest®); may inactivate aminoglycosides *in vitro*; false-positive urine and serum proteins; false-positive in uric acid, urinary steroids

Patient Information Take 1 hour before or 2 hours after meals; finish all medication; do not skip doses

Nursing Implications Monitor CBC with differential, urinalysis, BUN, serum creatinine, and liver enzymes

Additional Information

Sodium content of 250 mg capsule: 13.8 mg (0.6 mEq)

Sodium content of suspension 5 mL of 125 mg/5 mL: 11 mg (0.48 mEq)

Dosage Forms

Capsule, as sodium: 250 mg, 500 mg

Powder for oral suspension, as sodium: 125 mg/5 mL (100 mL, 200 mL)

♦ **Cloxacillin Sodium** see Cloxacillin on page 324

♦ **Cloxapen**® see Cloxacillin on page 324

Clozapine (KLOE za peen)

Related Information

Antipsychotic Agents Comparison on page 1486

U.S. Brand Names Clozaril®

Canadian Brand Names Clozaril®

Therapeutic Category Antipsychotic Agent, Atypical

Use Treatment of refractory schizophrenia

Unlabeled/Investigational Use Schizoaffective disorder, bipolar disorder, childhood psychosis

Pregnancy Risk Factor B

Contraindications Hypersensitivity to clozapine or any component of the formulation; history of agranulocytosis or granulocytopenia with clozapine; uncontrolled epilepsy; severe central nervous system depression or comatose state; myeloproliferative disorders or use with other agents which have a well-known risk of agranulocytosis or bone marrow suppression

In patients with WBC ≤3500 cells/mm³ before therapy; if WBC falls to <3000 cells/mm³ during therapy the drug should be withheld until signs and symptoms of infection disappear and WBC rises to >3000 cells/mm³

Warnings/Precautions Medication should not be stopped abruptly; taper off over 1-2 weeks. If conditions warrant abrupt discontinuation (leukopenia), monitor patient for psychosis and cholinergic rebound (headache, nausea, vomiting, diarrhea). WBC testing should occur weekly for the first 6 months of therapy; thereafter, if acceptable, WBC counts are maintained (WBC ≥3000/mm³, ANC ≥1500/mm³) then WBC counts can be monitored every other week. WBCs must be monitored weekly for the first 4 weeks after therapy discontinuation. Significant risk of agranulocytosis, potentially life-threatening. Use with caution in patients receiving other marrow suppressive agents.

(Continued)

Clozapine *(Continued)*

Cognitive and/or motor impairment (sedation) is common with clozapine, resulting in impaired performance of tasks requiring alertness (ie, operating machinery or driving).

May cause orthostatic hypotension and tachycardia; use with caution in patients at risk of hypotension or in patients where transient hypotensive episodes would be poorly tolerated (cardiovascular disease or cerebrovascular disease). Concurrent use of psychotropics and benzodiazepines may increase the risk of severe cardiopulmonary reactions. Use with caution in patients at risk of seizures, including those with a history of seizures, head trauma, brain damage, alcoholism, or concurrent therapy with medications which may lower seizure threshold.

Clozapine's potential for extrapyramidal symptoms appears to be extremely low. May cause anticholinergic effects; use with caution in patients with urinary retention, benign prostatic hyperplasia, narrow-angle glaucoma, xerostomia, visual problems, constipation, or history of bowel obstruction.

Rare cases of thromboembolism, including pulmonary embolism and stroke resulting in fatalities, have been associated with clozapine. Myocarditis, pericarditis, pericardial effusion, and congestive heart failure have also been associated with clozapine. Fatalities due to myocarditis have been reported; highest risk in the first month of therapy, however, later cases also reported. Myocarditis should be considered in patients who present with signs/symptoms of heart failure (dyspnea, tachypnea, unexplained fatigue), chest pain, palpitations, new electrocardiographic abnormalities (arrhythmias, ST-T wave abnormalities), or unexplained fever. Patients with tachycardia during the first month of therapy should be closely monitored for other signs of myocarditis. Discontinue clozapine if myocarditis is suspected; do not rechallenge in patients with clozapine-related myocarditis.

Adverse Reactions

>10%:

Cardiovascular: Tachycardia, orthostasis (up to 25%)

Central nervous system: Drowsiness, dizziness

Gastrointestinal: Constipation, weight gain, diarrhea, sialorrhea

Genitourinary: Urinary incontinence

1% to 10%:

Cardiovascular: EKG changes, hypertension, hypotension, syncope

Central nervous system: Akathisia, seizures, headache, nightmares, akinesia, confusion, insomnia, fatigue, myoclonic jerks

Dermatologic: Rash

Gastrointestinal: Abdominal discomfort, heartburn, xerostomia, nausea, vomiting

Hematologic: Eosinophilia, leukopenia

Neuromuscular & skeletal: Tremor

Miscellaneous: Diaphoresis (increased), fever

<1% (Limited to important or life-threatening): Agranulocytosis, arrhythmias, congestive heart failure, diabetes mellitus, granulocytopenia, hyperglycemia, impotence, myocardial infarction, myocarditis, narrow-angle glaucoma, neuroleptic malignant syndrome, pericardial effusion, pericarditis, pulmonary embolism, rigidity, stroke, tardive dyskinesia, thrombocytopenia, thromboembolism

Overdosage/Toxicology
Symptoms include altered states of consciousness, tachycardia, hypotension, hypersalivation, and respiratory depression. Following initiation of essential overdose management, toxic symptom treatment and supportive treatment should be initiated. Hypotension usually responds to I.V. fluids or Trendelenburg positioning. If unresponsive to these measures, the use of a parenteral inotrope may be required. Seizures commonly respond to diazepam (I.V. 5-10 mg bolus in adults every 15 minutes, if needed, up to a total of 30 mg; I.V. 0.25-0.4 mg/kg/dose up to a total of 10 mg in children), or to phenytoin or phenobarbital. Critical cardiac arrhythmias often respond to I.V. phenytoin (15 mg/kg up to 1 g), while other antiarrhythmics can be used. Neuroleptics often cause extrapyramidal symptoms (eg, dystonic reactions) requiring management with anticholinergic agents such as benztropine mesylate I.V. 1-2 mg (adults) may be effective. These agents are generally effective within 2-5 minutes.

Drug Interactions

Cytochrome P450 Effect: CYP1A2, 2C (minor), 2D6 (minor), 2E1, 3A3/4 enzyme substrate

Increased Effect/Toxicity: May potentiate anticholinergic and hypotensive effects of other drugs. Benzodiazepines in combination with clozapine may produce respiratory depression and hypotension, especially during the first few weeks of therapy. May potentiate effect/toxicity of risperidone. Clozapine serum concentrations may be increased by inhibitors of CYP1A2, CYP2D6, and CYP3A3/4. The list of inhibitors is extensive, but includes amiodarone, cimetidine, ciprofloxacin, clarithromycin, delavirdine, diltiazem, erythromycin, fluoxetine, fluvoxamine, indinavir, isoniazid, itraconazole, ketoconazole, nefazodone, paroxetine, quinidine, ritonavir, saquinavir, sertraline, verapamil, zafirlukast, and zileuton.

Decreased Effect: Carbamazepine, phenytoin, primidone, and valproic acid may increase the hepatic metabolism (decrease serum levels) of clozapine. Cigarette smoking (nicotine) may enhance the metabolism of clozapine. Clozapine may reverse the pressor effect of epinephrine (avoid in treatment of drug-induced hypotension).

Ethanol/Nutrition/Herb Interactions

Ethanol: Avoid ethanol (may increase CNS depression).

Herb/Nutraceutical: St John's wort may decrease clozapine levels. Avoid kava kava, gotu kola, valerian, St John's wort (may increase CNS depression).

Stability
Dispensed in "clozapine patient system" packaging.

Mechanism of Action
Clozapine is a weak dopamine$_1$ and dopamine$_2$ receptor blocker, but blocks D$_1$-D$_5$ receptors; in addition, it blocks the serotonin$_2$, alpha-adrenergic, histamine H$_1$, and cholinergic receptors

Pharmacodynamics/Kinetics

Protein binding, serum: 97%

Metabolism: Extensively hepatic

Half-life elimination: 12 hours (range: 4-66 hours)

Time to peak: 2.5 hours

Excretion: Urine (~50%) and feces (30%) with trace amounts of unchanged drug

Usual Dosage Oral: If dosing is interrupted for >48 hours, therapy must be re-initiated at 12.5-25 mg/day; may be increased more rapidly than with initial titration.

Children and Adolescents: Childhood psychosis (unlabeled use): Initial: 25 mg/day; increase to a target dose of 25-400 mg/day

Adults: Schizophrenia: Initial: 25 mg once or twice daily; increased, as tolerated to a target dose of 300-450 mg/day after 2-4 weeks, but may require doses as high as 600-900 mg/day

Elderly: Schizophrenia: Dose selection and titration should be cautious

Note: In the event of planned termination of clozapine, gradual reduction in dose over a 1- to 2-week period is recommended. If conditions warrant abrupt discontinuation (leukopenia), monitor patient for psychosis and cholinergic rebound (headache, nausea, vomiting, diarrhea).

Dietary Considerations May be taken without regard to food.

Monitoring Parameters Complete blood count weekly for 6 months then every other week thereafter, if clozapine is discontinued, continue monitoring for 1 month. WBC testing should occur weekly for the first 6 months of therapy; thereafter, if acceptable, WBC counts are maintained (WBC ≥3000/mm^3, ANC ≥1500/mm^3) then WBC counts can be monitored every other week. WBCs must be monitored weekly for the first 4 weeks after therapy discontinuation. EKG, liver function tests should also be monitored.

Patient Information Report any lethargy, fever, sore throat, flu-like symptoms, or any other signs or symptoms of infection; may cause drowsiness; frequent blood samples must be taken; do not stop taking even if you think it is not working

Nursing Implications Benign, self-limiting temperature elevations sometimes occur during the first 3 weeks of treatment, weekly CBC mandatory for first 6 months

Dosage Forms Tablet: 25 mg, 100 mg

♦ **Clozaril**® *see Clozapine on page 325*

♦ **CMV-IGIV** *see Cytomegalovirus Immune Globulin (Intravenous-Human) on page 353*

♦ **CoActifed**® **(Can)** *see Triprolidine, Pseudoephedrine, and Codeine on page 1381*

♦ **Coagulant Complex Inhibitor** *see Anti-inhibitor Coagulant Complex on page 106*

♦ **Coagulation Factor VIIa** *see Factor VIIa (Recombinant) on page 538*

Cocaine (koe KANE)

Synonyms Cocaine Hydrochloride

Therapeutic Category Local Anesthetic, Ester Derivative; Local Anesthetic, Topical

Use Topical anesthesia for mucous membranes

Restrictions C-II

Pregnancy Risk Factor C/X (nonmedicinal use)

Pregnancy/Breast-Feeding Implications Excreted in breast milk; cocaine intoxication of infants who are receiving breast milk from their mothers abusing cocaine has been reported

Contraindications Hypersensitivity to cocaine or any component of the topical solution; ophthalmologic anesthesia (causing sloughing of the corneal epithelium); pregnancy (nonmedicinal use)

Warnings/Precautions For topical use only. Limit to office and surgical procedures only. Resuscitative equipment and drugs should be immediately available when any local anesthetic is used. Debilitated, elderly patients, acutely ill patients, and children should be given reduced doses consistent with their age and physical status. Use caution in patients with severely traumatized mucosa and sepsis in the region of the proposed application. Use with caution in patients with cardiovascular disease or a history of cocaine abuse. In patients being treated for cardiovascular complication of cocaine abuse, avoid beta-blockers for treatment.

Adverse Reactions

>10%:

Central nervous system: CNS stimulation

Gastrointestinal: Loss of taste perception

Respiratory: Rhinitis, nasal congestion

Miscellaneous: Loss of smell

1% to 10%:

Cardiovascular: Heart rate (decreased) with low doses, tachycardia with moderate doses, hypertension, cardiomyopathy, cardiac arrhythmias, myocarditis, QRS prolongation, Raynaud's phenomenon, cerebral vasculitis, thrombosis, fibrillation (atrial), flutter (atrial), sinus bradycardia, congestive heart failure, pulmonary hypertension, sinus tachycardia, tachycardia (supraventricular), arrhythmias (ventricular), vasoconstriction

Central nervous system: Fever, nervousness, restlessness, euphoria, excitation, headache, psychosis, hallucinations, agitation, seizures, slurred speech, hyperthermia, dystonic reactions, cerebral vascular accident, vasculitis, clonic-tonic reactions, paranoia, sympathetic storm

Dermatologic: Skin infarction, pruritus, madarosis

Gastrointestinal: Nausea, anorexia, colonic ischemia, spontaneous bowel perforation

Genitourinary: Priapism, uterine rupture

Hematologic: Thrombocytopenia

Neuromuscular & skeletal: Chorea (extrapyramidal), paresthesia, tremors, fasciculations

Ocular: Mydriasis (peak effect at 45 minutes; may last up to 12 hours), sloughing of the corneal epithelium, ulceration of the cornea, iritis, mydriasis, chemosis

Renal: Myoglobinuria, necrotizing vasculitis

Respiratory: Tachypnea, nasal mucosa damage (when snorting), hyposmia, bronchiolitis obliterans organizing pneumonia

Miscellaneous: "Washed-out" syndrome

Overdosage/Toxicology Symptoms include anxiety, excitement, confusion, nausea, vomiting, headache, rapid pulse, irregular respiration, delirium, fever, seizures, respiratory

(Continued)

Cocaine *(Continued)*

arrest, hallucinations, dilated pupils, muscle spasms, sensory aberrations, and cardiac arrhythmias. Fatal dose: Oral: 500 mg to 1.2 g; severe toxic effects have occurred with doses as low as 20 mg. Since no specific antidote for cocaine exists, serious toxic effects are treated symptomatically. Maintain airway and respiration. Attempt delay of absorption (if ingested) with activated charcoal, gastric lavage or emesis. Seizures are treated with diazepam while propranolol or labetalol may be useful for life-threatening arrhythmias, agitation, and/or hypertension.

Drug Interactions

Cytochrome P450 Effect: CYP3A3/4 enzyme substrate

Increased Effect/Toxicity: Increased toxicity with MAO inhibitors. Use with epinephrine may cause extreme hypertension and/or cardiac arrhythmias.

Stability Store in well closed, light-resistant containers

Mechanism of Action Ester local anesthetic blocks both the initiation and conduction of nerve impulses by decreasing the neuronal membrane's permeability to sodium ions, which results in inhibition of depolarization with resultant blockade of conduction; interferes with the uptake of norepinephrine by adrenergic nerve terminals producing vasoconstriction

Pharmacodynamics/Kinetics Following topical administration to mucosa:

Onset of action: ~1 minute

Peak effect: ~5 minutes

Duration: ≥30 minutes, dose dependent; cocaine metabolites may appear in urine of neonates up to 5 days after birth due to maternal cocaine use shortly before birth

Absorption: Well absorbed through mucous membranes; limited by drug-induced vasoconstriction; enhanced by inflammation

Distribution: Enters breast milk

Metabolism: Hepatic; major metabolites are ecgonine methyl ester and benzoyl ecgonine

Half-life elimination: 75 minutes

Excretion: Primarily urine (<10% as unchanged drug and metabolites)

Usual Dosage Dosage depends on the area to be anesthetized, tissue vascularity, technique of anesthesia, and individual patient tolerance; use the lowest dose necessary to produce adequate anesthesia should be used, not to exceed 1 mg/kg. Use reduced dosages for children, elderly, or debilitated patients.

Topical application (ear, nose, throat, bronchoscopy): Concentrations of 1% to 4% are used. Concentrations >4% are not recommended because of potential for increased incidence and severity of systemic toxic reactions.

Monitoring Parameters Vital signs

Reference Range Therapeutic: 100-500 ng/mL (SI: 330 nmol/L); Toxic: >1000 ng/mL (SI: >3300 nmol/L)

Nursing Implications Use only on mucous membranes of the oral, laryngeal, and nasal cavities, do not use on extensive areas of broken skin

Additional Information Cocaine intoxication of infants who are receiving breast milk from their mothers abusing cocaine has been reported.

Dosage Forms

Powder, as hydrochloride: 5 g, 25 g

Solution, topical, as hydrochloride: 4% [40 mg/mL] (4 mL, 10 mL); 10% [100 mg/mL] (4 mL, 10 mL)

Solution, viscous, topical, as hydrochloride: 4% [40 mg/mL] (4 mL, 10 mL); 10% [100 mg/mL] (4 mL, 10 mL)

◆ **Cocaine Hydrochloride** *see Cocaine on page 327*

◆ **Codafed® Expectorant** *see Guaifenesin, Pseudoephedrine, and Codeine on page 648*

◆ **Codehist® DH** *see Chlorpheniramine, Pseudoephedrine, and Codeine on page 281*

Codeine *(KOE deen)*

Related Information

Narcotic Agonists Comparison *on page 1506*

Synonyms Codeine Phosphate; Codeine Sulfate; Methylmorphine

Therapeutic Category Analgesic, Narcotic; Antitussive

Use Treatment of mild to moderate pain; antitussive in lower doses; dextromethorphan has equivalent antitussive activity but has much lower toxicity in accidental overdose

Restrictions C-II

Pregnancy Risk Factor C/D (prolonged use or high doses at term)

Contraindications Hypersensitivity to codeine or any component of the formulation; pregnancy (prolonged use or high doses at term)

Warnings/Precautions Use with caution in patients with hypersensitivity reactions to other phenanthrene derivative opioid agonists (morphine, hydrocodone, hydromorphone, levorphanol, oxycodone, oxymorphone); respiratory diseases including asthma, emphysema, COPD, or severe liver or renal insufficiency; some preparations contain sulfites which may cause allergic reactions; tolerance or drug dependence may result from extended use

Not recommended for use for cough control in patients with a productive cough; not recommended as an antitussive for children <2 years of age; the elderly may be particularly susceptible to the CNS depressant and confusion as well as constipating effects of narcotics

Not approved for I.V. administration (although this route has been used clinically). If given intravenously, must be given slowly and the patient should be lying down. Rapid intravenous administration of narcotics may increase the incidence of serious adverse effects, in part due to limited opportunity to assess response prior to administration of the full dose. Access to respiratory support should be immediately available.

Adverse Reactions

>10%:

Central nervous system: Drowsiness

Gastrointestinal: Constipation

1% to 10%:
> Cardiovascular: Tachycardia or bradycardia, hypotension
> Central nervous system: Dizziness, lightheadedness, false feeling of well being, malaise, headache, restlessness, paradoxical CNS stimulation, confusion
> Dermatologic: Rash, urticaria
> Gastrointestinal: Dry mouth, anorexia, nausea, vomiting
> Hepatic: Increased transaminases
> Genitourinary: Decreased urination, ureteral spasm
> Local: Burning at injection site
> Neuromuscular & skeletal: Weakness
> Ocular: Blurred vision
> Respiratory: Dyspnea
> Miscellaneous: Physical and psychological dependence, histamine release

<1% (Limited to important or life-threatening): Convulsions, hallucinations, insomnia, mental depression, nightmares

Overdosage/Toxicology Symptoms include CNS and respiratory depression, gastrointestinal cramping, and constipation. Treatment includes naloxone 2 mg I.V. (0.01 mg/kg for children), with repeat administration as necessary, up to a total of 10 mg.

Drug Interactions
> **Cytochrome P450 Effect:** CYP2D6 and 3A3/4 enzyme substrate; CYP2D6 enzyme inhibitor
> **Increased Effect/Toxicity:** May cause severely increased toxicity of codeine when taken with CNS depressants, phenothiazines, tricyclic antidepressants, other narcotic analgesics, guanabenz, MAO inhibitors, and neuromuscular blockers.
> **Decreased Effect:** Decreased effect with cigarette smoking.

Ethanol/Nutrition/Herb Interactions
> Ethanol: Avoid or limit ethanol (may increase CNS depression). Watch for sedation.
> Herb/Nutraceutical: St John's wort may decrease codeine levels. Avoid valerian, St John's wort, kava kava, gotu kola (may increase CNS depression).

Stability Store injection between 15°C to 30°C, avoid freezing; do not use if injection is discolored or contains a precipitate; protect injection from light

Mechanism of Action Binds to opiate receptors in the CNS, causing inhibition of ascending pain pathways, altering the perception of and response to pain; causes cough supression by direct central action in the medulla; produces generalized CNS depression

Pharmacodynamics/Kinetics
> Onset of action: Oral: 0.5-1 hour; I.M.: 10-30 minutes
> Peak effect: Oral: 1-1.5 hours; I.M.: 0.5-1 hour
> Duration: 4-6 hours
> Absorption: Oral: Adequate
> Distribution: Crosses placenta; enters breast milk
> Protein binding: 7%
> Metabolism: Hepatic to morphine (active)
> Half-life elimination: 2.5-3.5 hours
> Excretion: Urine (3% to 16% as unchanged drug, norcodeine, and free and conjugated morphine)

Usual Dosage
> Analgesic: **Note:** Doses should be titrated to appropriate analgesic effect and side effects; when changing routes of administration, note that oral dose is 2/3 as effective as parenteral dose
>> Children: Oral, I.M., S.C.: 0.5-1 mg/kg/dose every 4-6 hours as needed; maximum: 60 mg/dose
>> Adults: Oral, I.M., I.V., S.C.: 30 mg/dose; range: 15-60 mg every 4-6 hours as needed
> Antitussive: Oral (for nonproductive cough):
>> Children: 1-1.5 mg/kg/day in divided doses every 4-6 hours as needed: Alternative dose according to age:
>>> 2-6 years: 2.5-5 mg every 4-6 hours as needed; maximum: 30 mg/day
>>> 6-12 years: 5-10 mg every 4-6 hours as needed; maximum: 60 mg/day
>> Adults: 10-20 mg/dose every 4-6 hours as needed; maximum: 120 mg/day

Dosing adjustment in renal impairment:
> Cl_{cr} 10-50 mL/minute: Administer 75% of dose
> Cl_{cr} <10 mL/minute: Administer 50% of dose

Dosing adjustment in hepatic impairment: Probably necessary in hepatic insufficiency

Administration Not approved for I.V. administration (although this route has been used clinically). If given intravenously, must be given slowly and the patient should be lying down. Rapid intravenous administration of narcotics may increase the incidence of serious adverse effects, in part due to limited opportunity to assess response prior to administration of the full dose. Access to respiratory support should be immediately available.

Monitoring Parameters Pain relief, respiratory and mental status, blood pressure, heart rate

Reference Range Therapeutic: Not established; Toxic: >1.1 µg/mL

Patient Information Avoid alcohol; may cause drowsiness, impaired judgment, or coordination; may cause physical and psychological dependence with prolonged use

Nursing Implications Observe patient for excessive sedation, respiratory depression, implement safety measures, assist with ambulation

Dosage Forms
> Injection, as phosphate: 30 mg (1 mL, 2 mL); 60 mg (1 mL, 2 mL)
> Solution, oral, as phosphate: 15 mg/5 mL
> Tablet, as sulfate: 15 mg, 30 mg, 60 mg
> Tablet, soluble, as phosphate: 30 mg, 60 mg
> Tablet, soluble, as sulfate: 15 mg, 30 mg, 60 mg

♦ **Codeine and Acetaminophen** see Acetaminophen and Codeine on page 24
♦ **Codeine and Aspirin** see Aspirin and Codeine on page 123
♦ **Codeine and Guaifenesin** see Guaifenesin and Codeine on page 646
♦ **Codeine and Promethazine** see Promethazine and Codeine on page 1141

- **Codeine, Aspirin, and Carisoprodol** see Carisoprodol, Aspirin, and Codeine *on page 230*
- **Codeine, Guaifenesin, and Pseudoephedrine** see Guaifenesin, Pseudoephedrine, and Codeine *on page 648*
- **Codeine Phosphate** see Codeine *on page 328*
- **Codeine, Promethazine, and Phenylephrine** see Promethazine, Phenylephrine, and Codeine *on page 1142*
- **Codeine, Pseudoephedrine, and Triprolidine** see Triprolidine, Pseudoephedrine, and Codeine *on page 1381*
- **Codeine Sulfate** see Codeine *on page 328*
- **Codiclear® DH** see Hydrocodone and Guaifenesin *on page 679*
- **Codimal-LA® [OTC]** see Chlorpheniramine and Pseudoephedrine *on page 279*
- **Codimal-LA® Half [OTC]** see Chlorpheniramine and Pseudoephedrine *on page 279*
- **Cod Liver Oil** see Vitamin A and Vitamin D *on page 1422*
- **Cogentin®** see Benztropine *on page 157*
- **Co-Gesic®** see Hydrocodone and Acetaminophen *on page 676*
- **Cognex®** see Tacrine *on page 1282*
- **Colace® [OTC]** see Docusate *on page 430*
- **Colax-C® (Can)** see Docusate *on page 430*
- **Colazal™** see Balsalazide *on page 145*

Colchicine (KOL chi seen)

Therapeutic Category Anti-inflammatory Agent

Use Treatment of acute gouty arthritis attacks and prevention of recurrences of such attacks; management of familial Mediterranean fever

Unlabeled/Investigational Use Primary biliary cirrhosis

Pregnancy Risk Factor C (oral); D (parenteral)

Contraindications Hypersensitivity to colchicine or any component of the formulation; serious renal, gastrointestinal, hepatic, or cardiac disorders; blood dyscrasias; pregnancy (parenteral)

Warnings/Precautions Severe local irritation can occur following S.C. or I.M. administration; use with caution in debilitated patients or elderly patients or patients with severe GI, renal, or liver disease

Adverse Reactions

>10%: Gastrointestinal: Nausea, vomiting, diarrhea, abdominal pain

1% to 10%:
  Dermatologic: Alopecia
  Gastrointestinal: Anorexia

<1% (Limited to important or life-threatening): Agranulocytosis, aplastic anemia, arrhythmias (with intravenous administration), bone marrow suppression, hepatotoxicity

Overdosage/Toxicology Symptoms include nausea, vomiting, abdominal pain, shock, kidney damage, muscle weakness, burning in throat, watery to bloody diarrhea, hypotension, anuria, cardiovascular collapse, delirium, and convulsions. Treatment includes gastric lavage and measures to prevent shock, hemodialysis or peritoneal dialysis. Atropine and morphine may relieve abdominal pain.

Drug Interactions

Increased Effect/Toxicity: Increased toxicity may be seen when taken with sympathomimetic agents or CNS depressant (effects are enhanced). Alkalizing agents potentiate effects of colchicine.

Decreased Effect: Vitamin B_{12} absorption may be decreased with colchicine. Acidifying agents inhibit action of colchicine.

Ethanol/Nutrition/Herb Interactions

Ethanol: Avoid ethanol.

Food: Cyanocobalamin (vitamin B_{12}): Malabsorption of the substrate. May result in macrocytic anemia or neurologic dysfunction.

Stability Protect tablets from light; I.V. colchicine is **incompatible** with I.V. solutions with preservatives; **incompatible** with dextrose

Mechanism of Action Decreases leukocyte motility, decreases phagocytosis in joints and lactic acid production, thereby reducing the deposition of urate crystals that perpetuates the inflammatory response

Pharmacodynamics/Kinetics

Onset of action: Oral: Pain relief: ~12 hours if adequately dosed

Distribution: Concentrates in leukocytes, kidney, spleen, and liver; does not distribute in heart, skeletal muscle, and brain

Protein binding: 10% to 31%

Metabolism: Partially deacetylated hepatically

Half-life elimination: 12-30 minutes; End-stage renal disease: 45 minutes

Time to peak, serum: Oral: 0.5-2 hours, declining for the next 2 hours before increasing again due to enterohepatic recycling

Excretion: Primarily feces; urine (10% to 20%)

Usual Dosage

Familial Mediterranean fever: Prophylaxis: Oral:
  Children:
    ≤5 years: 0.5 mg/day
    >5 years: 1-1.5 mg/day in 2-3 divided doses
  Adults: 1-2 mg daily in divided doses (occasionally reduced to 0.6 mg/day in patients with GI intolerance)

Gouty arthritis, acute attacks: Adults:
  Oral: Initial: 0.5-1.2 mg, then 0.5-0.6 mg every 1-2 hours or 1-1.2 mg every 2 hours until relief or GI side effects (nausea, vomiting, or diarrhea) occur to a maximum total dose of 8 mg; wait 3 days before initiating another course of therapy
  I.V.: Initial: 1-3 mg, then 0.5 mg every 6 hours until response, not to exceed 4 mg/day; if pain recurs, it may be necessary to administer a daily dose of 1-2 mg for several days,

however, do not administer more colchicine by any route for at least 7 days after a full course of I.V. therapy (4 mg), transfer to oral colchicine in a dose similar to that being given I.V.

Gouty arthritis, prophylaxis of recurrent attacks: Adults: Oral: 0.5-0.6 mg/day or every other day; patients who are to undergo surgical procedures may receive 0.5-0.6 mg 3 times/day for 3 days before and 3 days after surgery

Dosing adjustment in renal impairment:

Cl_{cr} <50 mL/minute: Avoid chronic use or administration

Cl_{cr} <10 mL/minute: Decrease dose by 75% for treatment of acute attacks

Hemodialysis: Not dialyzable (0% to 5%); supplemental dose is not necessary

Peritoneal dialysis: Supplemental dose is not necessary

Dietary Considerations May need to supplement with vitamin B_{12}.

Administration Injection should be made over 2-5 minutes into tubing of free-flowing I.V. with compatible fluid; do not administer I.M. or S.C.

Monitoring Parameters CBC and renal function test

Test Interactions May cause false-positive results in urine tests for erythrocytes or hemoglobin

Patient Information Avoid alcohol; discontinue if nausea or vomiting occurs; if taking for acute attack, discontinue as soon as pain resolves or if nausea, vomiting, or diarrhea occurs

Nursing Implications Severe local irritation can occur following S.C. or I.M. administration; extravasation can cause tissue irritation; administer I.V. over 2-5 minutes into tubing of free-flowing I.V. with compatible fluid; administer orally with water and maintain adequate fluid intake

Dosage Forms
Injection: 0.5 mg/mL (2 mL)
Tablet: 0.5 mg, 0.6 mg

Colchicine and Probenecid (KOL chi seen & proe BEN e sid)

Synonyms Probenecid and Colchicine

Therapeutic Category Antigout Agent

Use Treatment of chronic gouty arthritis when complicated by frequent, recurrent acute attacks of gout

Pregnancy Risk Factor C

Usual Dosage Adults: Oral: 1 tablet daily for 1 week, then 1 tablet twice daily thereafter

Additional Information Complete prescribing information for this medication should be consulted for additional detail.

Dosage Forms Tablet: Colchicine 0.5 mg and probenecid 0.5 g

Colesevelam (koh le SEV a lam)

Related Information
Hyperlipidemia Management on page 1670
Lipid-Lowering Agents on page 1505

U.S. Brand Names WelChol™

Canadian Brand Names WelChol™

Therapeutic Category Antilipemic Agent, Bile Acid Sequestrant

Use Adjunctive therapy to diet and exercise in the management of elevated LDL in primary hypercholesterolemia (Fredrickson type IIa) when used alone or in combination with an HMG-CoA reductase inhibitor

Pregnancy Risk Factor B

Pregnancy/Breast-Feeding Implications Use only in pregnancy if clearly needed. No breast-feeding recommendations.

Contraindications Hypersensitivity to colesevelam or any component of the formulation; bowel obstruction

Warnings/Precautions Use caution in treating patients with serum triglyceride levels >300 mg/dL (excluded from trials). Safety and efficacy has not been established in pediatric patients. Use caution in dysphagia, swallowing disorders, severe GI motility disorders, major GI tract surgery, pregnancy, nursing mothers, and in patients susceptible to fat-soluble vitamin deficiencies (vitamins A,D,E and K). Minimal effects are seen on HDL-C and triglyceride levels. Secondary causes of hypercholesterolemia should be excluded before initiation.

Adverse Reactions
>10%: Gastrointestinal: Constipation (11%)
2% to 10%:
Gastrointestinal: Dyspepsia (8%)
Neuromuscular & skeletal: Weakness (4%), myalgia (2%)
Respiratory: Pharyngitis (3%)

Overdosage/Toxicology Systemic toxicity is low since the drug is not absorbed.

Drug Interactions
Increased Effect/Toxicity: Refer to Decreased Effect.
Decreased Effect: Sustained-release verapamil AUC and C_{max} were reduced. Clinical significance unknown.
Digoxin, lovastatin, metoprolol, quinidine, valproic acid, or warfarin absorption was not significantly affected with concurrent administration.
Clinical effects of atorvastatin, lovastatin, and simvastatin were not changed by concurrent administration.

Stability Store at room temperature. Protect from moisture.

Mechanism of Action Colesevelam binds bile acids including glycocholic acid in the intestine, impeding their reabsorption. Increases the fecal loss of bile salt-bound LDL-C

Pharmacodynamics/Kinetics
Peak effect: Therapeutic: ~2 weeks
Absorption: Insignificant
Excretion: Urine (0.05%) after 1 month of chronic dosing
(Continued)

Colesevelam (Continued)

Usual Dosage Adult: Oral:

Monotherapy: 3 tablets twice daily with meals or 6 tablets once daily with a meal; maximum dose: 7 tablets/day

Combination therapy with an HMG-CoA reductase inhibitor: 4-6 tablets daily; maximum dose: 6 tablets/day

Dosage adjustment in renal impairment: No recommendations made

Dosage adjustment in hepatic impairment: No recommendations made

Elderly: No recommendations made

Dietary Considerations Take with meal(s). Follow dietary guidelines.

Monitoring Parameters Serum cholesterol, LDL, and triglyceride levels should be obtained before initiating treatment and periodically thereafter (in accordance with NCEP guidelines)

Patient Information Take once or twice daily with meals. Follow diet and exercise plan as recommended by prescriber. Tell prescriber if you are pregnant, plan on getting pregnant, or are breast-feeding.

Nursing Implications Give with meal(s). Make sure patient understands dietary guidelines.

Dosage Forms Tablet: 625 mg

♦ **Colestid®** see Colestipol on page 332

Colestipol (koe LES ti pole)

Related Information

Hyperlipidemia Management on page 1670

Lipid-Lowering Agents on page 1505

U.S. Brand Names Colestid®

Canadian Brand Names Colestid®

Synonyms Colestipol Hydrochloride

Therapeutic Category Antilipemic Agent, Bile Acid Sequestrant

Use Adjunct in management of primary hypercholesterolemia; regression of arteriolosclerosis; relief of pruritus associated with elevated levels of bile acids; possibly used to decrease plasma half-life of digoxin in toxicity

Pregnancy Risk Factor C

Contraindications Hypersensitivity to bile acid sequestering resins or any component of the formulation; bowel obstruction

Warnings/Precautions Not to be taken simultaneously with many other medicines (decreased absorption). Avoid in patients with high triglycerides, GI dysfunction (constipation); fecal impaction may occur; hemorrhoids may be worsened. May be associated with increased bleeding tendency as a result of hypothrombinemia secondary to vitamin K deficiency; may cause depletion of vitamins A, D, and E, and folic acid.

Adverse Reactions

>10%: Gastrointestinal: Constipation

1% to 10%:

Central nervous system: Headache, dizziness, anxiety, vertigo, drowsiness, fatigue

Gastrointestinal: Abdominal pain and distention, belching, flatulence, nausea, vomiting, diarrhea

<1% (Limited to important or life-threatening): Cholecystitis, cholelithiasis, dyspnea breath, gallstones, GI bleeding, malabsorption syndrome, peptic ulceration

Overdosage/Toxicology Symptoms include GI obstruction, nausea, and GI distress. Treatment is supportive.

Drug Interactions

Decreased Effect: Colestipol can reduce the absorption of numerous medications when used concurrently. Give other medications 1 hour before or 4 hours after giving colestipol. Medications which may be affected include HMG-CoA reductase inhibitors, thiazide diuretics, propranolol (and potentially other beta-blockers), corticosteroids, thyroid hormones, digoxin, valproic acid, NSAIDs, loop diuretics, sulfonylureas, troglitazone (and potentially other agents in this class - pioglitazone and rosiglitazone).

Warfarin and other oral anticoagulants: Absorption is reduced by cholestyramine and may also be reduced by colestipol. Separate administration times (as detailed above).

Mechanism of Action Binds with bile acids to form an insoluble complex that is eliminated in feces; it thereby increases the fecal loss of bile acid-bound low density lipoprotein cholesterol

Pharmacodynamics/Kinetics Absorption: None

Usual Dosage Adults: Oral:

Granules: 5-30 g/day given once or in divided doses 2-4 times/day; initial dose: 5 g 1-2 times/day; increase by 5 g at 1- to 2-month intervals

Tablets: 2-16 g/day; initial dose: 2 g 1-2 times/day; increase by 2 g at 1- to 2-month intervals

Administration Dry powder should be added to at least 90 mL of liquid and stirred until completely mixed; other drugs should be administered at least 1 hour before or 4 hours after colestipol

Test Interactions ↑ prothrombin time; ↓ cholesterol (S)

Patient Information Take granules in water or fruit juice (~90 mL) or sprinkled on food, swallow tablets whole with plenty of fluids; other drugs should not be taken at least 1 hour before or 4 hours after colestipol; rinse glass with small amount of liquid to ensure full dose is taken

Nursing Implications Dry powder should be added to at least 90 mL of liquid and stirred until completely mixed; other drugs should be administered at least 1 hour before or 4 hours after colestipol

Dosage Forms

Granules, as hydrochloride: 5 g packet, 300 g, 500 g

Tablet, as hydrochloride: 1 g

♦ **Colestipol Hydrochloride** see Colestipol on page 332

Colfosceril Palmitate (kole FOS er il PALM i tate)

U.S. Brand Names Exosurf Neonatal®

Canadian Brand Names Exosurf® Neonatal

Synonyms Dipalmitoylphosphatidylcholine; DPPC; Synthetic Lung Surfactant

Therapeutic Category Lung Surfactant

Use Neonatal respiratory distress syndrome:

Prophylactic therapy: Body weight <1350 g in infants at risk for developing RDS; body weight >1350 g in infants with evidence of pulmonary immaturity

Rescue therapy: Treatment of infants with RDS based on respiratory distress not attributable to any other causes and chest radiographic findings consistent with RDS

Contraindications Hypersensitivity to colfosceril palmitate or any component of the formulation

Warnings/Precautions Pulmonary hemorrhaging may occur especially in infants <700 g. Mucous plugs may have formed in the endotracheal tube in those infants whose ventilation was markedly impaired during or shortly after dosing. If chest expansion improves substantially, the ventilator PIP setting should be reduced immediately. Hyperoxia and hypocarbia (hypocarbia can decrease blood flow to the brain) may occur requiring appropriate ventilator adjustments.

Adverse Reactions 1% to 10%: Respiratory: Pulmonary hemorrhage, apnea, mucous plugging, decrease in transcutaneous O_2 of >20%

Stability Reconstituted suspension should be used immediately and unused portion discarded; store at room temperature of 15°C to 30°C (59°F to 86°F); do not refrigerate.

Mechanism of Action Replaces deficient or ineffective endogenous lung surfactant in neonates with respiratory distress syndrome (RDS) or in neonates at risk of developing RDS; reduces surface tension and stabilizes the alveoli from collapsing

Pharmacodynamics/Kinetics

Absorption: Intratracheal: Absorbed from alveolus

Metabolism: Catabolized and reutilized for further synthesis and secretion in lung tissue

Usual Dosage For intratracheal use only. Neonates:

Prophylactic treatment: Administer 5 mL/kg (as two 2.5 mL/kg half-doses) as soon as possible; the second and third doses should be administered at 12 and 24 hours later to those infants remaining on ventilators

Rescue treatment: Administer 5 mL/kg (as two 2.5 mL/kg half-doses) as soon as the diagnosis of RDS is made; the second 5 mL/kg (as two 2.5 mL/kg half-doses) dose should be administered 12 hours later

Administration Reconstitute with 8 mL preservative-free sterile water for injection; each mL contains 13.5 mg colfosceril; if the suspension appears to separate, gently swirl vial to resuspend contents; do not use if persistent large flakes or particulates appear

Intratracheal: For intratracheal administration only. Suction infant prior to administration; inspect solution to verify complete mixing of the suspension. Administer via sideport on the special endotracheal tube adapter without interrupting mechanical ventilation. Administer the dose in two 2.5 mL/kg aliquots. Each half-dose is instilled slowly over 1-2 minutes in small bursts with each inspiration. After the first 2.5 mL/kg dose, turn the infants head and torso 45° to the right for 30 seconds, then return to the midline position and administer the second dose as above. Following the second dose, turn the infant's head and torso 45° to the left for 30 seconds and return the infant to the midline position.

Monitoring Parameters Continuous EKG and transcutaneous O_2 saturation should be monitored during administration; frequent ABG sampling is necessary to prevent postdosing hyperoxia and hypocarbia

Dosage Forms Powder for injection, lyophilized: 108 mg (10 mL)

Colistimethate (koe lis ti METH ate)

U.S. Brand Names Coly-Mycin® M

Canadian Brand Names Coly-Mycin® M

Synonyms Colistimethate Sodium

Therapeutic Category Antibiotic, Miscellaneous

Use Treatment of infections due to sensitive strains of certain gram-negative bacilli which are resistant to other antibacterials or in patients allergic to other antibacterials

Not FDA approved: Used as inhalation in the prevention of *Pseudomonas aeruginosa* respiratory tract infections in immunocompromised patients, and used as inhalation adjunct agent for the treatment of *P. aeruginosa* infections in patients with cystic fibrosis and other seriously ill or chronically ill patients

Pregnancy Risk Factor B

Contraindications Hypersensitivity to colistimethate or any component of the formulation

Warnings/Precautions Use with caution in patients with pre-existing renal disease

Adverse Reactions 1% to 10%: Respiratory arrest, nephrotoxicity, GI upset, vertigo, slurring of speech, urticaria

Drug Interactions

Increased Effect/Toxicity: Other nephrotoxic drugs, neuromuscular blocking agents.

Stability Freshly prepare any infusion and use for no longer than 24 hours.

Mechanism of Action Hydrolyzed to colistin, which acts as a cationic detergent which damages the bacterial cytoplasmic membrane causing leaking of intracellular substances and cell death

Pharmacodynamics/Kinetics

Distribution: Widely, except for CNS, synovial, pleural, and pericardial fluids

Half-life elimination: 1.5-8 hours; Anuria: ≤2-3 days

Time to peak: ~2 hours

Excretion: Primarily urine (as unchanged drug)

Usual Dosage Children and Adults:

I.M., I.V.: 2.5-5 mg/kg/day in 2-4 divided doses

Inhalation: 75 mg in 3 mL NS (4 mL total) via nebulizer twice daily

(Continued)

Colistimethate *(Continued)*

Dosing interval in renal impairment: Adults:
S_{cr} 0.7-1.2 mg/dL: 100-125 mg 2-4 times/day
S_{cr} 1.3-1.5 mg/dL: 75-115 mg twice daily
S_{cr} 1.6-2.5 mg/dL: 66-150 mg once or twice daily
S_{cr} 2.6-4 mg/dL: 100-150 mg every 36 hours

Nursing Implications Freshly prepare and use within 24 hours

Dosage Forms Powder for injection, lyophilized: 150 mg

♦ **Colistimethate Sodium** *see Colistimethate on page 333*

Colistin, Neomycin, and Hydrocortisone

(koe LIS tin, nee oh MYE sin & hye droe KOR ti sone)

U.S. Brand Names Coly-Mycin® S Otic; Cortisporin®-TC Otic

Synonyms Hydrocortisone, Colistin, and Neomycin; Neomycin, Colistin, and Hydrocortisone

Therapeutic Category Antibiotic/Corticosteroid, Otic

Use Treatment of superficial and susceptible bacterial infections of the external auditory canal; for treatment of susceptible bacterial infections of mastoidectomy and fenestration cavities

Pregnancy Risk Factor C

Usual Dosage
Children: 3 drops in affected ear 3-4 times/day
Adults: 4 drops in affected ear 3-4 times/day

Additional Information Complete prescribing information for this medication should be consulted for additional detail.

Dosage Forms
Suspension, otic:
Coly-Mycin® S Otic Drops: Colistin sulfate 0.3%, neomycin sulfate 0.47%, and hydrocortisone acetate 1% (5 mL, 10 mL)
Cortisporin®-TC: Colistin sulfate 0.3%, neomycin sulfate 0.33%, and hydrocortisone acetate 1% (5 mL, 10 mL)

♦ **Collagen** *see Microfibrillar Collagen Hemostat on page 909*

Collagenase (KOL la je nase)

U.S. Brand Names Plaquase®; Santyl®

Canadian Brand Names Santyl®

Therapeutic Category Enzyme, Topical Debridement

Use Promotes debridement of necrotic tissue in dermal ulcers and severe burns
Orphan drug: Injection: Treatment of Peyronie's disease; treatment of Dupytren's disease

Pregnancy Risk Factor C

Usual Dosage Topical: Apply once daily (or more frequently if the dressing becomes soiled)

Additional Information Complete prescribing information for this medication should be consulted for additional detail.

Dosage Forms
Ointment, topical (Santyl®): 250 units/g (15 g, 30 g)
Powder for injection (Plaquase®): 10,000 units/vial

♦ **Colo-Fresh™ [OTC]** *see Bismuth on page 170*
♦ **Coly-Mycin® M** *see Colistimethate on page 333*
♦ **Coly-Mycin® S Otic** *see Colistin, Neomycin, and Hydrocortisone on page 334*
♦ **Colyte®** *see Polyethylene Glycol-Electrolyte Solution on page 1101*
♦ **Combantrin™ (Can)** *see Pyrantel Pamoate on page 1159*
♦ **CombiPatch™** *see Estradiol and Norethindrone on page 494*
♦ **Combipres®** *see Clonidine and Chlorthalidone on page 320*
♦ **Combivent®** *see Ipratropium and Albuterol on page 741*
♦ **Combivir®** *see Zidovudine and Lamivudine on page 1437*
♦ **Comhist®** *see Chlorpheniramine, Phenylephrine, and Phenyltoloxamine on page 281*
♦ **Comhist® LA** *see Chlorpheniramine, Phenylephrine, and Phenyltoloxamine on page 281*
♦ **Community-Acquired Pneumonia in Adults** *see page 1603*
♦ **Compazine®** *see Prochlorperazine on page 1134*
♦ **Compound E** *see Cortisone Acetate on page 335*
♦ **Compound F** *see Hydrocortisone on page 682*
♦ **Compound S** *see Zidovudine on page 1435*
♦ **Compound S, Abacavir, and Lamivudine** *see Abacavir, Lamivudine, and Zidovudine on page 17*
♦ **Compoz® Gel Caps [OTC]** *see DiphenhydrAMINE on page 414*
♦ **Compoz® Nighttime Sleep Aid [OTC]** *see DiphenhydrAMINE on page 414*
♦ **Compro™** *see Prochlorperazine on page 1134*
♦ **Comtan®** *see Entacapone on page 468*
♦ **Comtrex® Allergy-Sinus [OTC]** *see Acetaminophen, Chlorpheniramine, and Pseudoephedrine on page 27*
♦ **Comtrex® Non-Drowsy Cough and Cold [OTC]** *see Acetaminophen, Dextromethorphan, and Pseudoephedrine on page 27*
♦ **Comvax®** *see Haemophilus b Conjugate and Hepatitis B Vaccine on page 650*
♦ **Concerta™** *see Methylphenidate on page 894*
♦ **Congess® Jr** *see Guaifenesin and Pseudoephedrine on page 647*
♦ **Congess® Sr** *see Guaifenesin and Pseudoephedrine on page 647*
♦ **Congest (Can)** *see Estrogens (Conjugated/Equine) on page 498*
♦ **Congestac®** *see Guaifenesin and Pseudoephedrine on page 647*
♦ **Conjugated Estrogen and Methyltestosterone** *see Estrogens and Methyltestosterone on page 496*

- **Constant-T**® *see* Theophylline Salts *on page 1310*
- **Constilac**® *see* Lactulose *on page 770*
- **Constulose**® *see* Lactulose *on page 770*
- **Contac**® Cold 12 Hour Relief Non Drowsy **(Can)** *see* Pseudoephedrine *on page 1155*
- **Contac**® Cough, Cold and Flu Day & Night™ **(Can)** *see* Acetaminophen, Dextromethorphan, and Pseudoephedrine *on page 27*
- **Contac**® Severe Cold and Flu/Non-Drowsy **[OTC]** *see* Acetaminophen, Dextromethorphan, and Pseudoephedrine *on page 27*
- **Contrast Media Reactions, Premedication for Prophylaxis** *see page 1653*
- **Convulsive Status Epilepticus** *see page 1661*
- **Copaxone**® *see* Glatiramer Acetate *on page 630*
- **Copolymer-1** *see* Glatiramer Acetate *on page 630*
- **Co-Pyronil**® 2 Pulvules® **[OTC]** *see* Chlorpheniramine and Pseudoephedrine *on page 279*
- **Cordarone**® *see* Amiodarone *on page 74*
- **Cordran**® *see* Flurandrenolide *on page 583*
- **Cordran**® SP *see* Flurandrenolide *on page 583*
- **Coreg**® *see* Carvedilol *on page 233*
- **Corgard**® *see* Nadolol *on page 948*
- **Coricidin**® **[OTC]** *see* Chlorpheniramine and Acetaminophen *on page 279*
- **Corlopam**® *see* Fenoldopam *on page 550*
- **Cormax**® *see* Clobetasol *on page 311*
- **Cortaid**® Maximum Strength **[OTC]** *see* Hydrocortisone *on page 682*
- **Cortaid**® With Aloe **[OTC]** *see* Hydrocortisone *on page 682*
- **Cortamed**® **(Can)** *see* Hydrocortisone *on page 682*
- **Cortate**® **(Can)** *see* Hydrocortisone *on page 682*
- **Cortatrigen**® Otic *see* Neomycin, Polymyxin B, and Hydrocortisone *on page 969*
- **Cort-Dome**® *see* Hydrocortisone *on page 682*
- **Cortef**® *see* Hydrocortisone *on page 682*
- **Cortef**® Feminine Itch *see* Hydrocortisone *on page 682*
- **Cortenema**® *see* Hydrocortisone *on page 682*
- **Corticaine**® *see* Hydrocortisone *on page 682*
- **Corticosteroids Comparison** *see page 1495*
- **Cortifoam**® *see* Hydrocortisone *on page 682*
- **Cortimyxin**® **(Can)** *see* Neomycin and Polymyxin B *on page 968*
- **Cortimyxin**® **(Can)** *see* Neomycin, Polymyxin B, and Hydrocortisone *on page 969*
- **Cortisol** *see* Hydrocortisone *on page 682*

Cortisone Acetate (KOR ti sone AS e tate)

Related Information
Corticosteroids Comparison *on page 1495*
Canadian Brand Names Cortone®
Synonyms Compound E
Therapeutic Category Anti-inflammatory Agent; Corticosteroid, Adrenal; Corticosteroid, Systemic; Diagnostic Agent, Adrenocortical Insufficiency; Glucocorticoid; Mineralocorticoid
Use Management of adrenocortical insufficiency
Pregnancy Risk Factor D
Contraindications Hypersensitivity to cortisone acetate or any component of the formulation; serious infections, except septic shock or tuberculous meningitis; administration of live virus vaccines
Warnings/Precautions Use with caution in patients with hypothyroidism, cirrhosis, hypertension, congestive heart failure, ulcerative colitis, thromboembolic disorders, osteoporosis, convulsive disorders, peptic ulcer, diabetes mellitus, myasthenia gravis; prolonged therapy (>5 days) of pharmacologic doses of corticosteroids may lead to hypothalamic-pituitary-adrenal suppression, the degree of adrenal suppression varies with the degree and duration of glucocorticoid therapy; this must be taken into consideration when taking patients off steroids
Adverse Reactions
>10%:
  Central nervous system: Insomnia, nervousness
  Gastrointestinal: Increased appetite, indigestion
1% to 10%:
  Dermatologic: Hirsutism
  Endocrine & metabolic: Diabetes mellitus
  Neuromuscular & skeletal: Arthralgia
  Ocular: Cataracts, glaucoma
  Respiratory: Epistaxis
<1% (Limited to important or life-threatening): Alkalosis, Cushing's syndrome, delirium, edema, euphoria, fractures, hallucinations, hypersensitivity reactions, hypertension, hypokalemia, muscle wasting, myalgia, osteoporosis, pancreatitis, peptic ulcer, pituitary-adrenal axis suppression, pseudotumor cerebri, psychoses, seizures, skin atrophy, ulcerative esophagitis
Overdosage/Toxicology When consumed in excessive quantities for prolonged periods, systemic hypercorticism and adrenal suppression may occur; in these cases, discontinuation and withdrawal of the corticosteroid should be done judiciously. Cushingoid changes from continued administration of large doses results in moon face, central obesity, striae, hirsutism, acne, ecchymoses, hypertension, osteoporosis, myopathy, sexual dysfunction, diabetes, hyperlipidemia, peptic ulcer, increased susceptibility to infection, and electrolyte and fluid imbalance.
(Continued)

Cortisone Acetate (Continued)

Drug Interactions

Cytochrome P450 Effect: CYP3A3/4 enzyme substrate

Increased Effect/Toxicity: Estrogens may increase cortisone effects. Cortisone may increase ulcerogenic potential of NSAIDs, and may increase potassium deletion due to diuretics.

Decreased Effect: Enzyme inducers (barbiturates, phenytoin, rifampin) may decrease cortisone effects. Effect of live virus vaccines may be decreased. Anticholinesterase agents may decrease effect of cortisone.

Cortisone may decrease effects of warfarin and salicylates.

Ethanol/Nutrition/Herb Interactions Food: Limit caffeine intake.

Mechanism of Action Decreases inflammation by suppression of migration of polymorphonuclear leukocytes and reversal of increased capillary permeability

Pharmacodynamics/Kinetics

Onset of action: Peak effect: Oral: ~2 hours; I.M.: 20-48 hours

Duration: 30-36 hours

Absorption: Slow

Distribution: Muscles, liver, skin, intestines, and kidneys; crosses placenta; enters breast milk

Metabolism: Hepatic to inactive metabolites

Half-life elimination: 0.5-2 hours; End-stage renal disease: 3.5 hours

Excretion: Urine and feces

Usual Dosage If possible, administer glucocorticoids before 9 AM to minimize adrenocortical suppression; dosing depends upon the condition being treated and the response of the patient; **Note:** Supplemental doses may be warranted during times of stress in the course of withdrawing therapy

Children:

Anti-inflammatory or immunosuppressive: Oral: 2.5-10 mg/kg/day **or** 20-300 mg/m^2/day in divided doses every 6-8 hours

Physiologic replacement: Oral: 0.5-0.75 mg/kg/day **or** 20-25 mg/m^2/day in divided doses every 8 hours

Adults:

Anti-inflammatory or immunosuppressive: Oral: 25-300 mg/day in divided doses every 12-24 hours

Physiologic replacement: Oral: 25-35 mg/day

Hemodialysis: Supplemental dose is not necessary

Peritoneal dialysis: Supplemental dose is not necessary

Dietary Considerations May need diet with increased potassium, pyridoxine, vitamin C, vitamin D, folate, calcium, and phosphorus and decreased sodium; may be taken with food to decrease GI distress.

Administration Insoluble in water.

Patient Information Take with meals or take with food or milk; do not discontinue drug without notifying physician

Nursing Implications Withdraw gradually following long-term therapy

Dosage Forms Tablet: 5 mg, 10 mg, 25 mg

- ◆ **Cortisporin® (Can)** *see* Bacitracin, Neomycin, Polymyxin B, and Hydrocortisone *on page 143*
- ◆ **Cortisporin®** *see* Neomycin, Polymyxin B, and Hydrocortisone *on page 969*
- ◆ **Cortisporin® Ointment** *see* Bacitracin, Neomycin, Polymyxin B, and Hydrocortisone *on page 143*
- ◆ **Cortisporin® Ophthalmic Suspension** *see* Neomycin, Polymyxin B, and Hydrocortisone *on page 969*
- ◆ **Cortisporin®-TC Otic** *see* Colistin, Neomycin, and Hydrocortisone *on page 334*
- ◆ **Cortizone®-5 [OTC]** *see* Hydrocortisone *on page 682*
- ◆ **Cortizone®-10 [OTC]** *see* Hydrocortisone *on page 682*
- ◆ **Cortoderm (Can)** *see* Hydrocortisone *on page 682*
- ◆ **Cortone® (Can)** *see* Cortisone Acetate *on page 335*
- ◆ **Cortrosyn®** *see* Cosyntropin *on page 336*
- ◆ **Corvert®** *see* Ibutilide *on page 699*
- ◆ **Coryphen® Codeine (Can)** *see* Aspirin and Codeine *on page 123*
- ◆ **Cosmegen®** *see* Dactinomycin *on page 356*
- ◆ **Cosopt®** *see* Dorzolamide and Timolol *on page 438*

Cosyntropin (koe sin TROE pin)

U.S. Brand Names Cortrosyn®

Canadian Brand Names Cortrosyn®

Synonyms Synacthen; Tetracosactide

Therapeutic Category Diagnostic Agent, Adrenocortical Insufficiency

Use Diagnostic test to differentiate primary adrenal from secondary (pituitary) adrenocortical insufficiency

Pregnancy Risk Factor C

Contraindications Hypersensitivity to cosyntropin or any component of the formulation

Warnings/Precautions Use with caution in patients with pre-existing allergic disease or a history of allergic reactions to corticotropin

Adverse Reactions

1% to 10%:

Cardiovascular: Flushing

Central nervous system: Mild fever

Dermatologic: Pruritus

Gastrointestinal: Chronic pancreatitis

<1% (Limited to important or life-threatening): Hypersensitivity reactions

Stability Reconstitute with NS

Stability of parenteral admixture at room temperature (25°C): 24 hours
Stability of parenteral admixture at refrigeration temperature (4°C): 21 days
I.V. infusion in NS or D$_5$W is stable 12 hours at room temperature

Mechanism of Action Stimulates the adrenal cortex to secrete adrenal steroids (including hydrocortisone, cortisone), androgenic substances, and a small amount of aldosterone

Pharmacodynamics/Kinetics
Distribution: Crosses placenta
Time to peak, serum: I.M., IVP: ~1 hour; plasma cortisol levels rise in healthy individuals within 5 minutes

Usual Dosage
Adrenocortical insufficiency: I.M., I.V. (over 2 minutes): Peak plasma cortisol concentrations usually occur 45-60 minutes after cosyntropin administration
Neonates: 0.015 mg/kg/dose
Children <2 years: 0.125 mg
Children >2 years and Adults: 0.25-0.75 mg
When greater cortisol stimulation is needed, an I.V. infusion may be used:
Children >2 years and Adults: 0.25 mg administered at 0.04 mg/hour over 6 hours
Congenital adrenal hyperplasia evaluation: 1 mg/m^2/dose up to a maximum of 1 mg

Administration Administer I.V. doses over 2 minutes

Reference Range Normal baseline cortisol; increase in serum cortisol after cosyntropin injection of >7 μg/dL or peak response >18 μg/dL; plasma cortisol concentrations should be measured immediately before and exactly 30 minutes after a dose

Test Interactions Decreased effect: Spironolactone, hydrocortisone, cortisone

Nursing Implications Patient should not receive corticosteroids or spironolactone the day prior and the day of the test

Additional Information Each 0.25 mg of cosyntropin is equivalent to 25 units of corticotropin

Dosage Forms Powder for injection: 0.25 mg

Cromolyn Sodium (KROE moe lin SOW dee um)

Related Information
Asthma on page 1645

U.S. Brand Names Crolom®; Gastrocrom®; Intal®; Nasalcrom® [OTC]; Opticrom®

Canadian Brand Names Apo®-Cromolyn; Intal®; Nalcrom®; Nu-Cromolyn; Opticrom®

Synonyms Cromoglycic Acid; Disodium Cromoglycate; DSCG

Therapeutic Category Antiallergic, Inhalation; Antiallergic, Ophthalmic

Use Adjunct in the prophylaxis of allergic disorders, including rhinitis, giant papillary conjunctivitis, and asthma; inhalation product may be used for prevention of exercise-induced bronchospasm; oral product is used for systemic mastocytosis, food allergy, and treatment of inflammatory bowel disease; **cromolyn is a prophylactic drug with no benefit for acute situations**

Pregnancy Risk Factor B

Pregnancy/Breast-Feeding Implications
Clinical effects on the fetus: No data on whether cromolyn crosses the placenta or clinical effects on the fetus. Available evidence suggests safe use during pregnancy.
Breast-feeding/lactation: No data on whether cromolyn crosses into breast milk or clinical effects on the infant

Contraindications Hypersensitivity to cromolyn or any component of the formulation; acute asthma attacks

Warnings/Precautions Severe anaphylactic reactions may occur rarely; cromolyn is a prophylactic drug with no benefit for acute situations; do not use in patients with severe renal or hepatic impairment; caution should be used when withdrawing the drug or tapering the dose as symptoms may reoccur; use with caution in patients with a history of cardiac arrhythmias

Adverse Reactions
>10%:
Gastrointestinal: Unpleasant taste (inhalation aerosol)
Respiratory: Hoarseness, coughing
1% to 10%:
Dermatologic: Angioedema
Gastrointestinal: Xerostomia
(Continued)

Cromolyn Sodium *(Continued)*

Genitourinary: Dysuria

Respiratory: Sneezing, nasal congestion

<1% (Limited to important or life-threatening): Anaphylactic reactions, arthralgia, diarrhea, dizziness, eosinophilic pneumonia, headache, lacrimation, nasal burning, nausea, ocular stinging, pulmonary infiltrates, rash, throat irritation, urticaria, vomiting, wheezing

Overdosage/Toxicology Symptoms include bronchospasm, laryngeal edema, and dysuria.

Stability Nebulizer solution is **compatible** with metaproterenol sulfate, isoproterenol hydrochloride, 0.25% isoetharine hydrochloride, epinephrine hydrochloride, terbutaline sulfate, and 20% acetylcysteine solution for at least 1 hour after their admixture; store nebulizer solution protected from direct light

Mechanism of Action Prevents the mast cell release of histamine, leukotrienes and slow-reacting substance of anaphylaxis by inhibiting degranulation after contact with antigens

Pharmacodynamics/Kinetics

Absorption:

Inhalation: ~8% reaches lungs upon inhalation; well absorbed

Oral: 0.5% to 2%

Half-life elimination: 80-90 minutes

Time to peak, serum: Inhalation: ~15 minutes

Excretion: Urine and feces (equal amounts as unchanged drug); exhaled gases (small amounts)

Usual Dosage

Oral:

Systemic mastocytosis:

Neonates and preterm Infants: Not recommended

Infants and Children <2 years: 20 mg/kg/day in 4 divided doses; may increase in patients 6 months to 2 years of age if benefits not seen after 2-3 weeks; do not exceed 30 mg/kg/day

Children 2-12 years: 100 mg 4 times/day; not to exceed 40 mg/kg/day

Children >12 years and Adults: 200 mg 4 times/day

Food allergy and inflammatory bowel disease:

Children <2 years: Not recommended

Children 2-12 years: Initial dose: 100 mg 4 times/day; may double the dose if effect is not satisfactory within 2-3 weeks; not to exceed 40 mg/kg/day

Children >12 years and Adults: Initial dose: 200 mg 4 times/day; may double the dose if effect is not satisfactory within 2-3 weeks; up to 400 mg 4 times/day

Once desired effect is achieved, dose may be tapered to lowest effective dose

Inhalation:

For chronic control of asthma, taper frequency to the lowest effective dose (ie, 4 times/day to 3 times/day to twice daily):

Nebulization solution: Children >2 years and Adults: Initial: 20 mg 4 times/day; usual dose: 20 mg 3-4 times/day

Metered spray:

Children 5-12 years: Initial: 2 inhalations 4 times/day; usual dose: 1-2 inhalations 3-4 times/day

Children ≥12 years and Adults: Initial: 2 inhalations 4 times/day; usual dose: 2-4 inhalations 3-4 times/day

Prevention of allergen- or exercise-induced bronchospasm: Administer 10-15 minutes prior to exercise or allergen exposure but no longer than 1 hour before:

Nebulization solution: Children >2 years and Adults: Single dose of 20 mg

Metered spray: Children >5 years and Adults: Single dose of 2 inhalations

Ophthalmic: Children >4 years and Adults: 1-2 drops in each eye 4-6 times/day

Nasal: Allergic rhinitis (treatment and prophylaxis): Children ≥2 years and Adults: 1 spray into each nostril 3-4 times/day; may be increased to 6 times/day (symptomatic relief may require 2-4 weeks)

Dietary Considerations Should be taken at least 30 minutes before meals.

Administration

Oral concentrate: Open ampul and squeeze contents into glass of water; stir well; administer at least 30 minutes before meals and at bedtime; do not mix with juice, milk, or food.

Oral inhalation: Shake canister gently before use; do not immerse canister in water.

Nasal inhalation: Clear nasal passages by blowing nose prior to use.

Monitoring Parameters Periodic pulmonary function tests

Patient Information Do not discontinue abruptly; not effective for acute relief of symptoms; must be taken on a regularly scheduled basis; do not mix oral capsule with fruit juice, milk, or foods

Nursing Implications Advise patient to clear as much mucus as possible before inhalation treatments

Dosage Forms

Solution for oral inhalation [spray] (Intal®): 800 mcg/spray (8.1 g)

Solution for nebulization: 10 mg/mL (2 mL)

Intal®: 10 mg/mL (2 mL)

Solution, intranasal [spray] (Nasalcrom® [OTC]): 40 mg/mL (13 mL)

Solution, ophthalmic (Crolom®, Opticrom®): 4% (2.5 mL, 10 mL)

Solution, oral, as sodium (Gastrocrom®): 100 mg/5 mL

Crotamiton *(kroe TAM i tonn)*

U.S. Brand Names Eurax® Topical

Therapeutic Category Scabicidal Agent

Use Treatment of scabies (*Sarcoptes scabiei*) and symptomatic treatment of pruritus

Pregnancy Risk Factor C

Contraindications Hypersensitivity to crotamiton or any component of the formulation; patients who manifest a primary irritation response to topical medications

Warnings/Precautions Avoid contact with face, eyes, mucous membranes, and urethral meatus; do not apply to acutely inflamed or raw skin; for external use only

Adverse Reactions <1% (Limited to important or life-threatening): Contact dermatitis, irritation, pruritus, warm sensation

Overdosage/Toxicology Symptoms of ingestion include burning sensation in mouth; irritation of the buccal, esophageal and gastric mucosa, nausea, vomiting, and abdominal pain. There is no specific antidote. General measures to eliminate the drug and reduce its absorption, combined with symptomatic treatment, are recommended.

Mechanism of Action Crotamiton has scabicidal activity against *Sarcoptes scabiei*; mechanism of action unknown

Usual Dosage Topical:

Scabicide: Children and Adults: Wash thoroughly and scrub away loose scales, then towel dry; apply a thin layer and massage drug onto skin of the entire body from the neck to the toes (with special attention to skin folds, creases, and interdigital spaces). Repeat application in 24 hours. Take a cleansing bath 48 hours after the final application. Treatment may be repeated after 7-10 days if live mites are still present.

Pruritus: Massage into affected areas until medication is completely absorbed; repeat as necessary

Patient Information For topical use only; all contaminated clothing and bed linen should be washed to avoid reinfestation

Nursing Implications Lotion: Shake well before using; avoid contact with face, eyes, mucous membranes, and urethral meatus

Dosage Forms

Cream: 10% (60 g)

Lotion: 10% (60 mL, 454 mL)

♦ **Cruex®** [OTC] *see* Clotrimazole *on page 323*

♦ **Cryselle™** *see* Ethinyl Estradiol and Norgestrel *on page 528*

♦ **Crystalline Penicillin** *see* Penicillin G (Parenteral/Aqueous) *on page 1053*

♦ **Crystal Violet** *see* Gentian Violet *on page 630*

♦ **Crystamine®** *see* Cyanocobalamin *on page 339*

♦ **Crysti 1000®** *see* Cyanocobalamin *on page 339*

♦ **Crystodigin®** [DSC] *see* Digitoxin **Not Available in U.S.** *on page 402*

♦ **CSA** *see* CycloSPORINE *on page 345*

♦ **C/T/S®** *see* Clindamycin *on page 309*

♦ **CTX** *see* Cyclophosphamide *on page 342*

♦ **Cuprimine®** *see* Penicillamine *on page 1050*

♦ **Cutivate™** *see* Fluticasone *on page 587*

♦ **CyA** *see* CycloSPORINE *on page 345*

Cyanocobalamin (sye an oh koe BAL a min)

U.S. Brand Names Crystamine®; Crysti 1000®; Cyanoject®; Cyomin®; Ener-B®; Nascobal®

Canadian Brand Names Bedoz; Scheinpharm B12

Synonyms Vitamin B_{12}

Therapeutic Category Vitamin, Water Soluble

Use Treatment of pernicious anemia; vitamin B_{12} deficiency; increased B_{12} requirements due to pregnancy, thyrotoxicosis, hemorrhage, malignancy, liver or kidney disease

Pregnancy Risk Factor A/C (dose exceeding RDA recommendation); C (nasal gel)

Contraindications Hypersensitivity to cyanocobalamin or any component of the formulation, cobalt; patients with hereditary optic nerve atrophy, Leber's disease

Warnings/Precautions I.M. route used to treat pernicious anemia; vitamin B_{12} deficiency for >3 months results in irreversible degenerative CNS lesions; treatment of vitamin B_{12} megaloblastic anemia may result in severe hypokalemia, sometimes, fatal, when anemia corrects due to cellular potassium requirements. B_{12} deficiency masks signs of polycythemia vera; vegetarian diets may result in B_{12} deficiency; pernicious anemia occurs more often in gastric carcinoma than in general population. Patients with Leber's disease may suffer rapid optic atrophy when treated with vitamin B_{12}.

Adverse Reactions

1% to 10%:

Central nervous system: Headache (2% to 11%), anxiety, dizziness, pain, nervousness, hypoesthesia

Dermatologic: Itching

Gastrointestinal: Sore throat, nausea and vomiting, dyspepsia, diarrhea

Neuromuscular & skeletal: Weakness (1% to 4%), back pain, arthritis, myalgia, paresthesia, abnormal gait

Respiratory: Dyspnea, rhinitis

<1% (Limited to important or life-threatening): Anaphylaxis, congestive heart failure, peripheral vascular thrombosis, pulmonary edema, urticaria

Drug Interactions

Decreased Effect: Ethanol decreases B_{12} absorption. Chloramphenicol, cholestyramine, cimetidine, colchicine, neomycin, PAS, and potassium may reduce absorption and/or effect of cyanocobalamin.

Stability Clear pink to red solutions are stable at room temperature; protect from light; **incompatible** with chlorpromazine, phytonadione, prochlorperazine, warfarin, ascorbic acid, dextrose, heavy metals, oxidizing or reducing agents

Mechanism of Action Coenzyme for various metabolic functions, including fat and carbohydrate metabolism and protein synthesis, used in cell replication and hematopoiesis

Pharmacodynamics/Kinetics

Absorption: From the terminal ileum in presence of calcium; gastric "intrinsic factor" must be present to transfer the compound across the intestinal mucosa

Distribution: Principally stored in the liver, also stored in the kidneys and adrenals

Protein binding: To transcobalamin II

(Continued)

Cyanocobalamin *(Continued)*

Metabolism: Converted in tissues to active coenzymes methylcobalamin and deoxyadenosyl-cobalamin

Usual Dosage

Recommended daily allowance (RDA):
Children: 0.3-2 mcg
Adults: 2 mcg

Nutritional deficiency:
Intranasal gel: 500 mcg once weekly
Oral: 25-250 mcg/day

Anemias: I.M. or deep S.C. (oral is not generally recommended due to poor absorption and I.V. is not recommended due to more rapid elimination):

Pernicious anemia, congenital (if evidence of neurologic involvement): 1000 mcg/day for at least 2 weeks; maintenance: 50-100 mcg/month or 100 mcg for 6-7 days; if there is clinical improvement, give 100 mcg every other day for 7 doses, then every 3-4 days for 2-3 weeks; follow with 100 mcg/month for life. Administer with folic acid if needed.

Children: 30-50 mcg/day for 2 or more weeks (to a total dose of 1000-5000 mcg), then follow with 100 mcg/month as maintenance dosage

Adults: 100 mcg/day for 6-7 days; if improvement, administer same dose on alternate days for 7 doses; then every 3-4 days for 2-3 weeks; once hematologic values have returned to normal, maintenance dosage: 100 mcg/month. **Note:** Use only parenteral therapy as oral therapy is not dependable.

Hematologic remission (without evidence of nervous system involvement): Intranasal gel: 500 mcg once weekly

Vitamin B$_{12}$ deficiency:
Children:
Neurologic signs: 100 mcg/day for 10-15 days (total dose of 1-1.5 mg), then once or twice weekly for several months; may taper to 60 mcg every month
Hematologic signs: 10-50 mcg/day for 5-10 days, followed by 100-250 mcg/dose every 2-4 weeks
Adults: Initial: 30 mcg/day for 5-10 days; maintenance: 100-200 mcg/month

Schilling test: I.M.: 1000 mcg

Administration I.M. or deep S.C. are preferred routes of administration

Monitoring Parameters Serum potassium, erythrocyte and reticulocyte count, hemoglobin, hematocrit

Reference Range Normal range of serum B$_{12}$ is 150-750 pg/mL; this represents 0.1% of total body content. Metabolic requirements are 2-5 µg/day; years of deficiency required before hematologic and neurologic signs and symptoms are seen. Occasional patients with significant neuropsychiatric abnormalities may have no hematologic abnormalities and normal serum cobalamin levels, 200 pg/mL (SI: >150 pmol/L), or more commonly between 100-200 pg/mL (SI: 75-150 pmol/L). There exists evidence that people, particularly elderly whose serum cobalamin concentrations <300 pg/mL, should receive replacement parenteral therapy; this recommendation is based upon neuropsychiatric disorders and cardiovascular disorders associated with lower sodium cobalamin concentrations.

Test Interactions Methotrexate, pyrimethamine, and most antibiotics invalidate folic acid and vitamin B$_{12}$ diagnostic microbiological blood assays

Patient Information Pernicious anemia will require monthly injections for life

Nursing Implications Oral therapy is markedly inferior to parenteral therapy; monitor potassium concentrations during early therapy

Dosage Forms

Gel, intranasal (Nascobal®): 500 mcg/0.1 mL (5 mL)
Injection: 100 mcg/mL (1 mL, 10 mL, 30 mL); 1000 mcg/mL (1 mL, 10 mL, 30 mL)
Tablet [OTC]: 50 mcg, 100 mcg, 250 mcg, 500 mcg, 1000 mcg

♦ **Cyanocobalamin, Folic Acid, and Pyridoxine** *see Folic Acid, Cyanocobalamin, and Pyridoxine on page 596*

♦ **Cyanoject®** *see Cyanocobalamin on page 339*

♦ **Cyclen® (Can)** *see Ethinyl Estradiol and Norgestimate on page 525*

♦ **Cyclessa®** *see Ethinyl Estradiol and Desogestrel on page 510*

Cyclobenzaprine *(sye kloe BEN za preen)*

U.S. Brand Names Flexeril®

Canadian Brand Names Apo®-Cyclobenzaprine; Flexeril®; Flexitec; Gen-Cyclobenzaprine; Novo-Cycloprine®; Nu-Cyclobenzaprine

Synonyms Cyclobenzaprine Hydrochloride

Therapeutic Category Skeletal Muscle Relaxant

Use Treatment of muscle spasm associated with acute painful musculoskeletal conditions; supportive therapy in tetanus

Pregnancy Risk Factor B

Contraindications Hypersensitivity to cyclobenzaprine or any component of the formulation; do not use concomitantly or within 14 days of MAO inhibitors; hyperthyroidism; congestive heart failure; arrhythmias

Warnings/Precautions Cyclobenzaprine shares the toxic potentials of the tricyclic antidepressants and the usual precautions of tricyclic antidepressant therapy should be observed; use with caution in patients with urinary hesitancy or angle-closure glaucoma

Adverse Reactions

>10%:
Central nervous system: Drowsiness, dizziness, lightheadedness
Gastrointestinal: Dry mouth

1% to 10%:
Cardiovascular: Edema of the face/lips, syncope
Gastrointestinal: Bloated feeling
Genitourinary: Problems in urinating, polyuria

Neuromuscular & skeletal: Problems in speaking, muscle weakness

Ocular: Blurred vision

Otic: Tinnitus

<1% (Limited to important or life-threatening): Angioedema, dermatitis, dysuria, hepatitis, rash, syncope

Overdosage/Toxicology Symptoms include difficulty breathing, drowsiness, syncope, seizures, tachycardia, hallucinations, and vomiting. Following initiation of essential overdose management, toxic symptoms should be treated. Ventricular arrhythmias often respond to systemic alkalinization (sodium bicarbonate 0.5-2 mEq/kg I.V.) and/or phenytoin 15-20 mg/kg (adults). Arrhythmias unresponsive to this therapy may respond to lidocaine 1 mg/kg I.V. followed by a titrated infusion. Physostigmine (1-2 mg I.V. slowly for adults or 0.5 mg I.V. slowly for children) may be indicated in reversing life-threatening cardiac arrhythmias. Seizures usually respond to diazepam I.V. boluses (5-10 mg for adults up to 30 mg, or 0.25-0.4 mg/kg/dose for children up to 10 mg/dose). If seizures are unresponsive or recur, phenytoin or phenobarbital may be required.

Drug Interactions

Cytochrome P450 Effect: CYP1A2, 2D6, and 3A3/4 enzyme substrate

Increased Effect/Toxicity: Because of cyclobenzaprine's similarities to the tricyclic antidepressants, there may be additive toxicities and side effects similar to tricyclic antidepressants. Cyclobenzaprine's toxicity may also be additive with other agents with anticholinergic properties. Cyclobenzaprine may enhance effects of alcohol, barbiturates, and other CNS depressants. See Warnings/Precautions for MAO inhibitor precautions.

Decreased Effect: Cyclobenzaprine may block effect of guanethidine.

Ethanol/Nutrition/Herb Interactions

Ethanol: Avoid ethanol (may increase CNS depression).

Herb/Nutraceutical: St John's wort may decrease cyclobenzaprine levels. Avoid valerian, St John's wort, kava kava, gotu kola (may increase CNS depression).

Mechanism of Action Centrally acting skeletal muscle relaxant pharmacologically related to tricyclic antidepressants; reduces tonic somatic motor activity influencing both alpha and gamma motor neurons

Pharmacodynamics/Kinetics

Onset of action: ~1 hour

Duration: 8 to >24 hours

Absorption: Completely

Metabolism: Hepatic; may undergo enterohepatic recycling

Time to peak, serum: 3-8 hours

Excretion: Urine (as inactive metabolites); feces (as unchanged drug)

Usual Dosage Oral: **Note:** Do not use longer than 2-3 weeks

Children: Dosage has not been established

Adults: 20-40 mg/day in 2-4 divided doses; maximum dose: 60 mg/day

Patient Information Drug may impair ability to perform hazardous activities requiring mental alertness or physical coordination, such as operating machinery or driving a motor vehicle

Nursing Implications Raise bed rails, institute safety measures, assist with ambulation

Dosage Forms Tablet, as hydrochloride: 10 mg

♦ **Cyclobenzaprine Hydrochloride** *see Cyclobenzaprine on page 340*

♦ **Cyclocort®** *see Amcinonide on page 66*

♦ **Cyclogyl®** *see Cyclopentolate on page 341*

♦ **Cyclomen® (Can)** *see Danazol on page 362*

♦ **Cyclomydril®** *see Cyclopentolate and Phenylephrine on page 341*

Cyclopentolate (sye kloe PEN toe late)

Related Information

Cycloplegic Mydriatics Comparison *on page 1498*

U.S. Brand Names AK-Pentolate®; Cyclogyl®; I-Pentolate®

Canadian Brand Names Cyclogyl®; Diopentolate®

Synonyms Cyclopentolate Hydrochloride

Therapeutic Category Anticholinergic Agent, Ophthalmic; Ophthalmic Agent, Mydriatic

Use Diagnostic procedures requiring mydriasis and cycloplegia

Pregnancy Risk Factor C

Usual Dosage Ophthalmic:

Neonates and Infants: **Note:** Cyclopentolate and phenylephrine combination formulation is the preferred agent for use in neonates and infants due to lower cyclopentolate concentration and reduced risk for systemic reactions

Children: Instill 1 drop of 0.5%, 1%, or 2% in eye followed by 1 drop of 0.5% or 1% in 5 minutes, if necessary

Adults: Instill 1 drop of 1% followed by another drop in 5 minutes; 2% solution in heavily pigmented iris

Additional Information Complete prescribing information for this medication should be consulted for additional detail.

Dosage Forms Solution, ophthalmic, as hydrochloride: 0.5% (2 mL, 5 mL, 15 mL); 1% (2 mL, 5 mL, 15 mL); 2% (2 mL, 5 mL, 15 mL)

Cyclopentolate and Phenylephrine (sye kloe PEN toe late & fen il EF rin)

U.S. Brand Names Cyclomydril®

Synonyms Phenylephrine and Cyclopentolate

Therapeutic Category Anticholinergic/Adrenergic Agonist

Use Induce mydriasis greater than that produced with cyclopentolate HCl alone

Pregnancy Risk Factor C

Usual Dosage Ophthalmic: Neonates, Infants, Children, and Adults: Instill 1 drop into the eye every 5-10 minutes, for up to 3 doses, approximately 40-50 minutes before the examination

Additional Information Complete prescribing information for this medication should be consulted for additional detail.

(Continued)

Cyclopentolate and Phenylephrine *(Continued)*

Dosage Forms Solution, ophthalmic: Cyclopentolate hydrochloride 0.2% and phenylephrine hydrochloride 1% (2 mL, 5 mL)

♦ **Cyclopentolate Hydrochloride** *see Cyclopentolate on page 341*

Cyclophosphamide *(sye kloe FOS fa mide)*

U.S. Brand Names Cytoxan®; Neosar®
Canadian Brand Names Cytoxan®; Procytox®
Synonyms CPM; CTX; CYT; NSC-26271
Therapeutic Category Antineoplastic Agent, Alkylating Agent
Use

Oncologic: Treatment of Hodgkin's and non-Hodgkin's lymphoma, Burkitt's lymphoma, chronic lymphocytic leukemia (CLL), chronic myelocytic leukemia (CML), acute myelocytic leukemia (AML), acute lymphocytic leukemia (ALL), mycosis fungoides, multiple myeloma, neuroblastoma, retinoblastoma, rhabdomyosarcoma, Ewing's sarcoma; breast, testicular, endometrial, ovarian, and lung cancers, and in conditioning regimens for bone marrow transplantation

Nononcologic: Prophylaxis of rejection for kidney, heart, liver, and bone marrow transplants, severe rheumatoid disorders, nephrotic syndrome, Wegener's granulomatosis, idiopathic pulmonary hemosideroses, myasthenia gravis, multiple sclerosis, systemic lupus erythematosus, lupus nephritis, autoimmune hemolytic anemia, idiopathic thrombocytic purpura (ITP), macroglobulinemia, and antibody-induced pure red cell aplasia

Pregnancy Risk Factor D

Contraindications Hypersensitivity to cyclophosphamide or any component of the formulation; pregnancy

Warnings/Precautions The U.S. Food and Drug Administration (FDA) currently recommends that procedures for proper handling and disposal of antineoplastic agents be considered. Possible dosage adjustment needed for renal or hepatic failure; use with caution in patients with bone marrow suppression.

Adverse Reactions

>10%:

Dermatologic: Alopecia (40% to 60%) but hair will usually regrow although it may be a different color and/or texture. Hair loss usually begins 3-6 weeks after the start of therapy.

Endocrine & metabolic: Fertility: May cause sterility; interferes with oogenesis and spermatogenesis; may be irreversible in some patients; gonadal suppression (amenorrhea)

Gastrointestinal: Nausea and vomiting occur more frequently with larger doses, usually beginning 6-10 hours after administration; anorexia, diarrhea, mucositis, and stomatitis are also seen

Genitourinary: Severe, potentially fatal acute hemorrhagic cystitis, believed to be a result of chemical irritation of the bladder by acrolein, a cyclophosphamide metabolite, occurs in 7% to 12% of patients and has been reported in up to 40% of patients in some series. Patients should be encouraged to drink plenty of fluids (3-4 L/day) during therapy, void frequently, and avoid taking the drug at night. With large I.V. doses, I.V. hydration is usually recommended. The use of mesna and/or continuous bladder irrigation is rarely needed for doses <2 g/m^2.

Hematologic: Thrombocytopenia and anemia are less common than leukopenia
Onset: 7 days
Nadir: 10-14 days
Recovery: 21 days

1% to 10%:

Central nervous system: Headache

Dermatologic: Skin rash, facial flushing

Renal: SIADH may occur, usually with doses >50 mg/kg (or 1 g/m^2); renal tubular necrosis, which usually resolves with discontinuation of the drug, is also reported

Respiratory: Nasal congestion occurs when I.V. doses are administered too rapidly (large doses via 30-60 minute infusion); patients experience runny eyes, rhinorrhea, sinus congestion, and sneezing during or immediately after the infusion. If needed, a decongestant or decongestant/antihistamine (eg, pseudoephedrine or pseudoephedrine/triprolidine) can be used to prevent or relieve these symptoms.

<1% (Limited to important or life-threatening): High-dose therapy may cause cardiac dysfunction manifested as congestive heart failure; cardiac necrosis or hemorrhagic myocarditis has occurred rarely, but may be fatal. Cyclophosphamide may also potentiate the cardiac toxicity of anthracyclines. Other adverse reactions include anaphylactic reactions, darkening of skin/fingernails, dizziness, hemorrhagic colitis, hemorrhagic ureteritis, hepatotoxicity, hyperglycemia, hyperuricemia, hypokalemia, jaundice, renal tubular necrosis, secondary malignancy, Stevens-Johnson syndrome, toxic epidermal necrolysis; interstitial pneumonitis and pulmonary fibrosis are occasionally seen with high doses

BMT:

Cardiovascular: Heart failure, cardiac necrosis, pericardial tamponade

Endocrine & metabolic: Hyponatremia

Gastrointestinal: Severe nausea and vomiting

Miscellaneous: Hemorrhagic cystitis, secondary malignancy

Overdosage/Toxicology Symptoms include myelosuppression, alopecia, nausea, and vomiting. Treatment is supportive. Cyclophosphamide is moderately dialyzable (20% to 50%).

Drug Interactions

Cytochrome P450 Effect: CYP2B6, 2D6, and 3A3/4 enzyme substrate

Increased Effect/Toxicity: Allopurinol may cause an increase in bone marrow depression and may result in significant elevations of cyclophosphamide cytotoxic metabolites.

Anesthetic agents: Cyclophosphamide reduces serum pseudocholinesterase concentrations and may prolong the neuromuscular blocking activity of succinylcholine. Use with caution with halothane, nitrous oxide, and succinylcholine.

Chloramphenicol causes prolonged cyclophosphamide half-life and increased toxicity.

Cimetidine inhibits hepatic metabolism of drugs and may decrease the activation of cyclophosphamide.

Doxorubicin: Cyclophosphamide may enhance cardiac toxicity of anthracyclines.

Phenobarbital and phenytoin induce hepatic enzymes and cause a more rapid production of cyclophosphamide metabolites with a concurrent decrease in the serum half-life of the parent compound.

Tetrahydrocannabinol results in enhanced immunosuppression in animal studies.

Thiazide diuretics: Leukopenia may be prolonged.

Decreased Effect: Cyclophosphamide may decrease digoxin serum levels.

Ethanol/Nutrition/Herb Interactions Herb/Nutraceutical: St John's wort may decrease cyclobenzaprine levels. Avoid black cohosh, dong quai in estrogen-dependent tumors.

Stability Store intact vials of powder at room temperature (15°C to 30°C/59°F to 86°F). Reconstituted solutions are stable for 24 hours at room temperature and 6 days at refrigeration (2°C to 8°C/36°F to 46°F). Further dilutions in D$_5$W or NS are stable for 24 hours at room temperature and 6 days at refrigeration.

Reconstitute vials with sterile water, normal saline, or 5% dextrose to a concentration of 20 mg/mL.

Mechanism of Action Cyclophosphamide is an alkylating agent that prevents cell division by cross-linking DNA strands and decreasing DNA synthesis. It is a cell cycle phase nonspecific agent. Cyclophosphamide also possesses potent immunosuppressive activity. Cyclophosphamide is a prodrug that must be metabolized to active metabolites in the liver.

Pharmacodynamics/Kinetics
Absorption: Oral: Well absorbed
Distribution: Well; V$_d$: 0.48-0.71 L/kg; crosses placenta; crosses into CSF (not high enough to treat meningeal leukemia)
Protein binding: 10% to 56%
Metabolism: Hepatic into its active components: acrolein, 4-aldophosphamide, 4-hydroperoxycyclophosphamide, and nor-nitrogen mustard
Bioavailability: >75%
Half-life elimination: 4-8 hours
Time to peak, serum: Oral: ~1 hour
Excretion: Urine (<30% as unchanged drug, 85% to 90% as metabolites)

Usual Dosage Refer to individual protocols
Patients with compromised bone marrow function may require a 33% to 50% reduction in initial loading dose
Children:
SLE: I.V.: 500-750 mg/m^2 every month; maximum dose: 1 g/m^2
JRA/vasculitis: I.V.: 10 mg/kg every 2 weeks
Children and Adults:
Oral: 50-100 mg/m^2/day as continuous therapy or 400-1000 mg/m^2 in divided doses over 4-5 days as intermittent therapy
I.V.:
Single Doses: 400-1800 mg/m^2 (30-50 mg/kg) per treatment course (1-5 days) which can be repeated at 2-4 week intervals
MAXIMUM SINGLE DOSE WITHOUT BMT is 7 g/m^2 (190 mg/kg) SINGLE AGENT THERAPY
Continuous daily doses: 60-120 mg/m^2 (1-2.5 mg/kg) per day
Autologous BMT: IVPB: 50 mg/kg/dose x 4 days or 60 mg/kg/dose for 2 days; total dose is usually divided over 2-4 days
Nephrotic syndrome: Oral: 2-3 mg/kg/day every day for up to 12 weeks when corticosteroids are unsuccessful
Dosing adjustment in renal impairment: A large fraction of cyclophosphamide is eliminated by hepatic metabolism
Some authors recommend no dose adjustment unless severe renal insufficiency (Cl$_{cr}$ <20 mL/minute)
Cl$_{cr}$ >10 mL/minute: Administer 100% of normal dose
Cl$_{cr}$ <10 mL/minute: Administer 75% of normal dose
Hemodialysis: Moderately dialyzable (20% to 50%); administer dose posthemodialysis or administer supplemental 50% dose
CAPD effects: Unknown
CAVH effects: Unknown
Dosing adjustment in hepatic impairment: Some authors recommend dosage reductions (of up to 30%); however, the pharmacokinetics of cyclophosphamide are not significantly altered in the presence of hepatic insufficiency. Cyclophosphamide undergoes hepatic transformation in the liver to its 4-hydroxycyclophosphamide, which breaks down to its active form, phosphoramide mustard.

Dietary Considerations Tablets should be administered during or after meals.

Administration
May be administered I.M., I.P., intrapleurally, IVPB, or continuous I.V. infusion
I.V. infusions may be administered over 1-2 hours
Doses >500 mg to approximately 1 g may be administered over 20-30 minutes
May also be administered slow IVP in lower doses
Force fluids up to 2 L/day to minimize bladder toxicity; high-dose regimens should be accompanied by vigorous hydration ± MESNA therapy
Tablets are not scored and should not be cut or crushed

Monitoring Parameters CBC with differential and platelet count, BUN, UA, serum electrolytes, serum creatinine
(Continued)

Cyclophosphamide *(Continued)*

Patient Information Tablets may be taken during or after meals to reduce GI effects. Maintain adequate fluid balance (2-3 L/day of fluids unless instructed to restrict fluid intake). Void frequently and report any difficulty or pain with urination. May cause hair loss (reversible after treatment), sterility, or amenorrhea (sometimes reversible). If you are diabetic, you will need to monitor serum glucose closely to avoid hypoglycemia. You may be more susceptible to infection; avoid crowds and unnecessary exposure to infection. Report unusual bleeding or bruising; persistent fever or sore throat; blood in urine, stool (black stool), or vomitus; delayed healing of any wounds; skin rash; yellowing of skin or eyes; or changes in color of urine or stool. Contraceptive measures are recommended during therapy.

Nursing Implications Encourage adequate hydration and frequent voiding to help prevent hemorrhagic cystitis

Additional Information May be used in combination with mesna to prevent hemorrhagic cystitis. Rarely required for doses <1.5-2 g/m^2.

Dosage Forms
Powder for injection, lyophilized: 100 mg, 200 mg, 500 mg, 1 g, 2 g
Tablet: 25 mg, 50 mg

Extemporaneous Preparations A 2 mg/mL oral elixir was stable for 14 days when refrigerated when made as follows: Reconstitute a 200 mg vial with aromatic elixir, withdraw the solution, and add sufficient aromatic elixir to make a final volume of 100 mL (store in amber glass container).

Brook D, Davis RE, and Bequette RJ, "Chemical Stability of Cyclophosphamide in Aromatic Elixir U.S.P.," *Am J Health Syst Pharm*, 1973, 30:618-20.

♦ **Cycloplegic Mydriatics Comparison** see page 1498

CycloSERINE *(sye kloe SER een)*

Related Information
Antimicrobial Drugs of Choice on page 1588
Depression on page 1655
Tuberculosis Treatment Guidelines on page 1612
U.S. Brand Names Seromycin® Pulvules®
Therapeutic Category Antibiotic, Miscellaneous; Antitubercular Agent
Use Adjunctive treatment in pulmonary or extrapulmonary tuberculosis; has been studied for use in Gaucher's disease
Pregnancy Risk Factor C
Contraindications Hypersensitivity to cycloserine or any component of the formulation
Warnings/Precautions Epilepsy, depression, severe anxiety, psychosis, severe renal insufficiency, chronic alcoholism
Adverse Reactions Frequency not defined.
Cardiovascular: Cardiac arrhythmias
Central nervous system: Drowsiness, headache, dizziness, vertigo, seizures, confusion, psychosis, paresis, coma
Dermatologic: Rash
Endocrine & metabolic: Vitamin B$_{12}$ deficiency
Hematologic: Folate deficiency
Hepatic: Liver enzymes increased
Neuromuscular & skeletal: Tremor
Overdosage/Toxicology Symptoms include confusion, agitation, CNS depression, psychosis, coma, and seizures. Decontaminate with activated charcoal. Can be hemodialyzed. Management is supportive. Administer pyridoxine 100-300 mg/day to reduce neurotoxic effects. Acute toxicity can occur with ingestions >1 g, chronic toxicity can occur with ingestions >500 mg/day.
Drug Interactions
Increased Effect/Toxicity: Alcohol, isoniazid, and ethionamide increase toxicity of cycloserine. Cycloserine inhibits the hepatic metabolism of phenytoin and may increase risk of epileptic seizures.
Ethanol/Nutrition/Herb Interactions
Ethanol: Avoid ethanol (may increase CNS depression).
Food: May increase vitamin B$_{12}$ and folic acid dietary requirements.
Mechanism of Action Inhibits bacterial cell wall synthesis by competing with amino acid (D-alanine) for incorporation into the bacterial cell wall; bacteriostatic or bactericidal
Pharmacodynamics/Kinetics
Absorption: ~70% to 90%
Distribution: Widely to most body fluids and tissues including CSF, breast milk, bile, sputum, lymph tissue, lungs, and ascitic, pleural, and synovial fluids; crosses placenta
Half-life elimination: Normal renal function: 10 hours
Metabolism: Hepatic
Time to peak, serum: 3-4 hours
Excretion: Urine (60% to 70% as unchanged drug) within 72 hours; feces (small amounts); remainder metabolized
Usual Dosage Some of the neurotoxic effects may be relieved or prevented by the concomitant administration of pyridoxine
Tuberculosis: Oral:
Children: 10-20 mg/kg/day in 2 divided doses up to 1000 mg/day for 18-24 months
Adults: Initial: 250 mg every 12 hours for 14 days, then administer 500 mg to 1 g/day in 2 divided doses for 18-24 months (maximum daily dose: 1 g)
Dosing interval in renal impairment:
Cl$_{cr}$ 10-50 mL/minute: Administer every 24 hours
Cl$_{cr}$ <10 mL/minute: Administer every 36-48 hours
Dietary Considerations May be taken with food; may increase vitamin B$_{12}$ and folic acid dietary requirements.

Monitoring Parameters Periodic renal, hepatic, hematological tests, and plasma cycloserine concentrations

Reference Range Toxicity is greatly increased at levels >30 µg/mL

Patient Information May cause drowsiness; notify physician if skin rash, mental confusion, dizziness, headache, or tremors occur; do not skip doses; do not drink excessive amounts of alcoholic beverages

Nursing Implications

Some of the neurotoxic effects may be relieved or prevented by the concomitant administration of pyridoxine

Monitor periodic renal, hepatic, hematological tests, and plasma cycloserine concentrations

Dosage Forms Capsule: 250 mg

♦ **Cyclosporin A** see CycloSPORINE on page 345

CycloSPORINE (SYE kloe spor een)

U.S. Brand Names Gengraf™; Neoral®; Sandimmune®; Sandimmune® Oral

Canadian Brand Names Neoral®; Sandimmune® I.V.

Synonyms CSA; CyA; Cyclosporin A

Therapeutic Category Immunosuppressant Agent

Use Prophylaxis of organ rejection in kidney, liver, and heart transplants, has been used with azathioprine and/or corticosteroids; severe, active rheumatoid arthritis (RA) not responsive to methotrexate alone; severe, recalcitrant plaque psoriasis in nonimmunocompromised adults unresponsive to or unable to tolerate other systemic therapy

Unlabeled/Investigational Use Short-term, high-dose cyclosporine as a modulator of multidrug resistance in cancer treatment; allogenic bone marrow transplants for prevention and treatment of graft-versus-host disease; also used in some cases of severe autoimmune disease (ie, SLE, myasthenia gravis) that are resistant to corticosteroids and other therapy; focal segmental glomerulosclerosis

Pregnancy Risk Factor C

Pregnancy/Breast-Feeding Implications Cyclosporine crosses the placenta. Based on clinical use, premature births and low birth weight were consistently observed. Use only if the benefit to the mother outweighs the possible risks to the fetus. Enters breast milk, use is contraindicated. The AAP considers cyclosporine to be "contraindicated" during breast-feeding.

Contraindications Hypersensitivity to cyclosporine or any component of the formulation. Rheumatoid arthritis and psoriasis: Abnormal renal function, uncontrolled hypertension, malignancies. Concomitant treatment with PUVA or UVB therapy, methotrexate, other immunosuppressive agents, coal tar, or radiation therapy are also contraindications for use in patients with psoriasis.

Warnings/Precautions Dose-related risk of nephrotoxicity and hepatotoxicity; monitor. Use caution with other potentially nephrotoxic drugs. Increased risk of lymphomas and other malignancies. Increased risk of infection. May cause hypertension. Use caution when changing dosage forms. Monitor cyclosporine concentrations closely following the addition, modification, or deletion of other medications; live, attenuated vaccines may be less effective; use should be avoided.

Transplant patients: May cause significant hyperkalemia and hyperuricemia, seizures (particularly if used with high dose corticosteroids), and encephalopathy. To avoid toxicity or possible organ rejection, make dose adjustments based on cyclosporine blood concentrations. Anaphylaxis has been reported with I.V. use; reserve for patients who cannot take oral form.

Psoriasis: Patients should avoid excessive sun exposure; safety and efficacy in children <18 have not been established

Rheumatoid arthritis: Safety and efficacy for use in juvenile rheumatoid arthritis have not been established

Products may contain corn oil, castor oil, ethanol, or propylene glycol; injection also contains Cremophor® EL (polyoxyethylated castor oil).

Adverse Reactions Note: Adverse reactions reported generally reflect dosages used in transplantation, range is approximate/may overlap. [Reactions reported for rheumatoid arthritis (RA) are based on cyclosporine (modified) 2.5 mg/kg/day versus placebo.]

>10%:
  Cardiovascular: Hypertension (13% to 53%; RA 8%; psoriasis 25% to 27%)
  Central nervous system: Headache (2% to 15%; RA 17%, psoriasis 14% to 16%)
  Dermatologic: Hirsutism (21% to 45%), hypertrichosis (5% to 19%)
  Endocrine & metabolic: Increased triglycerides (psoriasis 15%), female reproductive disorder (psoriasis 8% to 11%)
  Gastrointestinal: Nausea (RA 23%), diarrhea (RA 12%), gum hyperplasia (4% to 16%), abdominal discomfort (RA 15%), dyspepsia (RA 12%)
  Neuromuscular & skeletal: Tremor (12% to 55%)
  Renal: Renal dysfunction/nephropathy (25% to 38%; RA 10%, psoriasis 21%), creatinine elevation ≥50% (RA 24%), increased creatinine (psoriasis 16% to 20%)
  Respiratory: Upper respiratory infection (psoriasis 8% to 11%)
  Miscellaneous: Infection (psoriasis 24% to 25%)

1% to 10% (All indications, frequency range approximate):
  Cardiovascular: Hypertension, edema, chest pain, arrhythmia, cardiac failure, myocardial infarction
  Central nervous system: Dizziness, seizures (up to 5%), psychiatric events (up to 5%), pain, insomnia, depression, migraine, anxiety, vertigo
  Dermatologic: Purpura, pruritus, acne, skin disorder, urticaria
  Endocrine & metabolic: Menstrual disorder, diabetes mellitus, goiter, hyperkalemia, hyperuricemia, hypoglycemia, hyperglycemia, gynecomastia
  Gastrointestinal: Vomiting, nausea, diarrhea, flatulence, gingivitis, gum hyperplasia, constipation, dry mouth, gastritis, gingival bleeding, taste perversion,

(Continued)

CycloSPORINE *(Continued)*

Genitourinary: Leukorrhea, urinary incontinence
Hematologic: Anemia, leukopenia, thrombocytopenia
Hepatic: Bilirubinemia, hepatotoxicity (<1% to 7%)
Neuromuscular & skeletal: Paresthesia, tremor, leg cramps/muscle contractions
Renal: Increased BUN, hematuria, renal abscess
Respiratory: Cough, dyspnea, bronchospasm, sinusitis
Miscellaneous: Infection, allergy, lymphoma, flu-like syndrome

<1% (Limited to important or life-threatening): Allergic reaction, bleeding disorder, deafness, death (due to renal deterioration), encephalopathy, gout, hyperbilirubinemia, hyperkalemia, impaired consciousness, increased cholesterol, increased uric acid, mild hypomagnesemia, neurotoxicity, upper GI bleeding, vestibular disorder

Overdosage/Toxicology Symptoms include hepatotoxicity, nephrotoxicity, nausea, vomiting, and tremor. CNS secondary to direct action of the drug may not be reflected in serum concentrations, may be more predictable by renal magnesium loss.

Drug Interactions

Cytochrome P450 Effect: CYP3A3/4 enzyme substrate; CYP3A3/4 enzyme inhibitor

Increased Effect/Toxicity: Increased toxicity:

Drugs that increase cyclosporine concentrations: Allopurinol, metoclopramide, nicardipine, octreotide

CYP3A3/4 inhibitors: Serum level and/or toxicity of cyclosporine may be increased. Inhibitors include amiodarone, bromocriptine, cimetidine, clarithromycin, danazol, erythromycin, delavirdine, diltiazem, disulfiram, fluconazole, fluoxetine, fluvoxamine, grapefruit juice, indinavir, itraconazole, ketoconazole, nefazodone, nevirapine, propoxyphene, quinupristin-dalfopristin, ritonavir, saquinavir, verapamil, zafirlukast, zileuton.

Drugs that enhance nephrotoxicity of cyclosporine: Aminoglycosides, amphotericin B, acyclovir, cimetidine, ketoconazole, lovastatin, melphalan, NSAIDs, ranitidine, trimethoprim and sulfamethoxazole, tacrolimus

Cyclosporine increases toxicity of: Digoxin, diuretics, methotrexate, nifedipine

Decreased Effect:

Drugs that decrease cyclosporine concentrations: Carbamazepine, nafcillin, phenobarbital, phenytoin, rifampin, isoniazid, ticlopidine

Cyclosporine decreases effect of: Live vaccines

Ethanol/Nutrition/Herb Interactions

Food: Grapefruit juice increases absorption; unsupervised use should be avoided.

Herb/Nutraceutical: Avoid St John's wort; as an enzyme inducer, it may increase the metabolism of and decrease plasma levels of cyclosporine. Avoid cat's claw, echinacea (have immunostimulant properties).

Stability

Capsule: Store at controlled room temperature

Injection: Store at controlled room temperature; do not refrigerate. Ampuls should be protected from light.

Oral solution: Store at controlled room temperature; do not refrigerate. Use within 2 months after opening; should be mixed in glass containers

Reconstitution:

Sandimmune® injection: Injection should be further diluted [1 mL (50 mg) of concentrate in 20-100 mL of D_5W or NS] for administration by intravenous infusion. Light protection is not required for intravenous admixtures of cyclosporine.

Stability of injection of parenteral admixture at room temperature (25°C) is 6 hours in PVC; 24 hours in Excel®, PAB® containers, or glass.

Polyoxyethylated castor oil (Cremophor® EL) surfactant in cyclosporine injection may leach phthalate from PVC containers such as bags and tubing. The actual amount of diethylhexyl phthalate (DEHP) plasticizer leached from PVC containers and administration sets may vary in clinical situations, depending on surfactant concentration, bag size, and contact time.

Compatibility:

Neoral® oral solution: Orange juice, apple juice; avoid changing diluents frequently; mix thoroughly and drink at once

Sandimmune® oral solution: Milk, chocolate milk, orange juice; avoid changing diluents frequently; mix thoroughly and drink at once

Mechanism of Action Inhibition of production and release of interleukin II and inhibits interleukin II-induced activation of resting T-lymphocytes

Pharmacodynamics/Kinetics

Absorption: Oral:

Cyclosporine (non-modified): Erratically and incompletely absorbed; dependent on presence of food, bile acids, and GI motility; larger oral doses are needed in pediatrics due to shorter bowel length and limited intestinal absorption

Cyclosporine (modified): Erratically and incompletely absorbed; increased absorption, up to 30% when compared to cyclosporine (non-modified); absorption less dependent on food, bile acids, or GI motility when compared to cyclosporine (non-modified)

Distribution: Widely in tissues and body fluids including the liver, pancreas, and lungs; crosses placenta; enters breast milk

V_{dss}: 4-6 L/kg in renal, liver, and marrow transplant recipients (slightly lower values in cardiac transplant patients; children <10 years have higher values)

Protein binding: 90% to 98% to lipoproteins

Metabolism: Extensively hepatic via CYP450 system; forms at least 25 metabolites; extensive first-pass effect following oral administration

Bioavailability: Oral:

Cyclosporine (non-modified): Dependent on patient population and transplant type (<10% in adult liver transplant patients and as high as 89% in renal transplant patients); bioavailability of Sandimmune® capsules and oral solution are equivalent; bioavailability of oral solution is ~30% of the I.V. solution

Children: 28% (range: 17% to 42%); gut dysfunction common in BMT patients and oral bioavailability is further reduced

Cyclosporine (modified): Bioavailability of Neoral® capsules and oral solution are equivalent:

Children: 43% (range: 30% to 68%)

Adults: 23% greater than with cyclosporine (non-modified) in renal transplant patients; 50% greater in liver transplant patients

Half-life elimination: Oral: May be prolonged in patients with hepatic dysfunction and lower in pediatric patients due to the higher metabolism rate

Cyclosporine (non-modified): Biphasic: Alpha: 1.4 hours; Terminal: 19 hours (range: 10-27 hours)

Cyclosporine (modified): Biphasic: Terminal: 8.4 hours (range: 5-18 hours)

Time to peak, serum: Oral:

Cyclosporine (non-modified): 2-6 hours; some patients have a second peak at 5-6 hours

Cyclosporine (modified): Renal transplant: 1.5-2 hours

Excretion: Primarily feces; urine (6%, 0.1% as unchanged drug and metabolites)

Usual Dosage Note: Neoral® and Sandimmune® are not bioequivalent and cannot be used interchangeably

Children: Transplant: Refer to adult dosing; children may require, and are able to tolerate, larger doses than adults.

Adults:

Newly-transplanted patients: Adjunct therapy with corticosteroids is recommended. Initial dose should be given 4-12 hours prior to transplant or may be given postoperatively; adjust initial dose to achieve desired plasma concentration

Oral: Dose is dependent upon type of transplant and formulation:

Cyclosporine (modified):

Renal: 9 ±3 mg/kg/day, divided twice daily

Liver: 8 ±4 mg/kg/day, divided twice daily

Heart: 7 ±3 mg/kg/day, divided twice daily

Cyclosporine (non-modified): Initial dose: 15 mg/kg/day as a single dose (range 14-18 mg/kg); lower doses of 10-14 mg/kg/day have been used for renal transplants. Continue initial dose daily for 1-2 weeks; taper by 5% per week to a maintenance dose of 5-10 mg/kg/day; some renal transplant patients may be dosed as low as 3 mg/kg/day

When using the non-modified formulation, cyclosporine levels may increase in liver transplant patients when the T-tube is closed; dose may need decreased

I.V.: Cyclosporine (non-modified): Initial dose: 5-6 mg/kg/day as a single dose (⅓ the oral dose), infused over 2-6 hours; use should be limited to patients unable to take capsules or oral solution; patients should be switched to an oral dosage form as soon as possible

Conversion to cyclosporine (modified) from cyclosporine (non-modified): Start with daily dose previously used and adjust to obtain preconversion cyclosporine trough concentration. Plasma concentrations should be monitored every 4-7 days and dose adjusted as necessary, until desired trough level is obtained. When transferring patients with previously poor absorption of cyclosporine (non-modified), monitor trough levels at least twice weekly (especially if initial dose exceeds 10 mg/kg/day); high plasma levels are likely to occur.

Rheumatoid arthritis: Oral: Cyclosporine (modified): Initial dose: 2.5 mg/kg/day, divided twice daily; salicylates, NSAIDs, and oral glucocorticoids may be continued (refer to Drug Interactions); dose may be increased by 0.5-0.75 mg/kg/day if insufficient response is seen after 8 weeks of treatment; additional dosage increases may be made again at 12 weeks (maximum dose: 4 mg/kg/day). Discontinue if no benefit is seen by 16 weeks of therapy.

Note: Increase the frequency of blood pressure monitoring after each alteration in dosage of cyclosporine. Cyclosporine dosage should be decreased by 25% to 50% in patients with no history of hypertension who develop sustained hypertension during therapy and, if hypertension persists, treatment with cyclosporine should be discontinued.

Psoriasis: Oral: Cyclosporine (modified): Initial dose: 2.5 mg/kg/day, divided twice daily; dose may be increased by 0.5 mg/kg/day if insufficient response is seen after 4 weeks of treatment. Additional dosage increases may be made every 2 weeks if needed; (maximum dose: 4 mg/kg/day). Discontinue if no benefit is seen by 6 weeks of therapy. Once patients are adequately controlled, the dose should be decreased to the lowest effective dose. Doses lower than 2.5 mg/kg/day may be effective. Treatment longer than 1 year is not recommended.

Note: Increase the frequency of blood pressure monitoring after each alteration in dosage of cyclosporine. Cyclosporine dosage should be decreased by 25% to 50% in patients with no history of hypertension who develop sustained hypertension during therapy and, if hypertension persists, treatment with cyclosporine should be discontinued.

Focal segmental glomerulosclerosis: Initial: 3 mg/kg/day divided every 12 hours

Autoimmune diseases: 1-3 mg/kg/day

Dosage adjustment in renal impairment: For severe psoriasis:

Serum creatinine levels ≥25% above pretreatment levels: Take another sample within 2 weeks; if the level remains ≥25% above pretreatment levels, decrease dosage of cyclosporine (modified) by 25% to 50%. If two dosage adjustments do not reverse the increase in serum creatinine levels, treatment should be discontinued.

Serum creatinine levels ≥50% above pretreatment levels: Decrease cyclosporine dosage by 25% to 50%. If two dosage adjustments do not reverse the increase in serum creatinine levels, treatment should be discontinued.

Hemodialysis: Supplemental dose is not necessary.

Peritoneal dialysis: Supplemental dose is not necessary.

Dosage adjustment in hepatic impairment: Probably necessary; monitor levels closely

Dietary Considerations Administer this medication consistently with relation to time of day and meals.

Administration

Oral solution: May dilute Neoral® oral solution with orange juice or apple juice. May dilute Sandimmune® oral solution with milk, chocolate milk, or orange juice. Avoid changing diluents frequently. Mix thoroughly and drink at once. Use syringe provided to measure

(Continued)

CycloSPORINE (Continued)

dose. Mix in a glass container and rinse container with more diluent to ensure total dose is taken. Do not rinse syringe before or after use (may cause dose variation).

I.V.: Following dilution, intravenous admixture should be administered over 2-6 hours. Discard solution after 24 hours. Anaphylaxis has been reported with I.V. use; reserve for patients who cannot take oral form. Patients should be under continuous observation for at least the first 30 minutes of the infusion, and should be monitored frequently thereafter. Maintain patent airway; other supportive measures and agents for treating anaphylaxis should be present when I.V. drug is given.

Monitoring Parameters Monitor blood pressure and serum creatinine after any cyclosporine dosage changes or addition, modification, or deletion of other medications. Monitor plasma concentrations periodically.

Transplant patients: Cyclosporine trough levels, serum electrolytes, renal function, hepatic function, blood pressure, lipid profile

Psoriasis therapy: Baseline blood pressure, serum creatinine (2 levels each), BUN, CBC, serum magnesium, potassium, uric acid, lipid profile. Biweekly monitoring of blood pressure, complete blood count, and levels of BUN, uric acid, potassium, lipids, and magnesium during the first 3 months of treatment for psoriasis. Monthly monitoring is recommended after this initial period. Also evaluate any atypical skin lesions prior to therapy. Increase the frequency of blood pressure monitoring after each alteration in dosage of cyclosporine. Cyclosporine dosage should be decreased by 25% to 50% in patients with no history of hypertension who develop sustained hypertension during therapy and, if hypertension persists, treatment with cyclosporine should be discontinued.

Rheumatoid arthritis: Baseline blood pressure, and serum creatinine (2 levels each); serum creatinine every 2 weeks for first 3 months, then monthly if patient is stable. Increase the frequency of blood pressure monitoring after each alteration in dosage of cyclosporine. Cyclosporine dosage should be decreased by 25% to 50% in patients with no history of hypertension who develop sustained hypertension during therapy and, if hypertension persists, treatment with cyclosporine should be discontinued.

Reference Range Reference ranges are method dependent and specimen dependent; use the same analytical method consistently

Method-dependent and specimen-dependent: Trough levels should be obtained:

Oral: 12-18 hours after dose (chronic usage)

I.V.: 12 hours after dose **or** immediately prior to next dose

Therapeutic range: Not absolutely defined, dependent on organ transplanted, time after transplant, organ function and CsA toxicity:

General range of 100-400 ng/mL

Toxic level: Not well defined, nephrotoxicity may occur at any level

Test Interactions Specific whole blood, HPLC assay for cyclosporine may be falsely elevated if sample is drawn from the same line through which dose was administered (even if flush has been administered and/or dose was given hours before).

Patient Information Use glass container for liquid solution (do not use plastic or styrofoam cup). Diluting oral solution improves flavor. May dilute Neoral® oral solution with orange juice or apple juice. May dilute Sandimmune® oral solution with milk, chocolate milk, or orange juice. Avoid changing what you mix with your cyclosporine. Mix thoroughly and drink at once. Use syringe provided to measure dose. Mix in a glass container and rinse container with more juice/milk to ensure total dose is taken. Do not rinse syringe before or after use (may cause dose variation). Take dose at the same time each day. You will be susceptible to infection; avoid crowds and exposure to any infectious diseases. Do not have any vaccinations without consulting prescriber. Practice good oral hygiene to reduce gum inflammation; see dentist regularly during treatment. Report severe headache; unusual hair growth or deepening of voice; mouth sores or swollen gums; persistent nausea, vomiting, or abdominal pain; muscle pain or cramping; unusual swelling of extremities, weight gain, or change in urination; or chest pain or rapid heartbeat. Increases in blood pressure or damage to the kidney are possible. Your prescriber will need to monitor closely. Do not change one brand of cyclosporine for another; any changes must be done by your prescriber. If you are taking this medication for psoriasis, your risk of cancer may be increased when taking additional medications.

Nursing Implications Anaphylaxis has been reported with I.V. use; reserve for patients who cannot take oral form. Patients should be under continuous observation for at least the first 30 minutes of the infusion, and should be monitored frequently thereafter. Maintain patent airway; other supportive measures and agents for treating anaphylaxis should be present when I.V. drug is given. Do not administer liquid from plastic or styrofoam cup. Diluting oral solution improves flavor. May dilute Neoral® oral solution with orange juice or apple juice. May dilute Sandimmune® oral solution with milk, chocolate milk, or orange juice. Stir well; do not allow to stand before drinking; rinse with more diluent to ensure that the total dose is taken; after use, dry outside of pipette; do not rinse with water or other cleaning agents; may cause inflamed gums

Additional Information Cyclosporine (modified): Refers to the capsule dosage formulation of cyclosporine in an aqueous dispersion (previously referred to as "microemulsion"). Cyclosporine (modified) has increased bioavailability as compared to cyclosporine (non-modified) and cannot be used interchangeably without close monitoring.

In July, 2000, SangCya® (cyclosporine, modified) was voluntarily recalled due to lack of bioequivalency with Neoral® oral solution when mixed in apple juice. The product was allowed to remain in pharmacies to provide a transition time for changing patients to another cyclosporine product. Patients who were previously stabilized on this product should be instructed not to change how they mix their medication until they can be switched to another product. (SangCya® was previously marketed as a generic Neoral® oral solution.)

Dosage Forms

Cyclosporine, modified:

Capsule, soft gel:

Gengraf™: 25 mg, 100 mg [contains ethanol, castor oil, propylene glycol]

Neoral®: 25 mg, 100 mg [contains dehydrated ethanol, corn oil, castor oil]

Solution, oral:
    Neoral®: 100 mg/mL (50 mL) [contains dehydrated ethanol, corn oil, castor oil, propylene glycol]
    SangCya®: 100 mg/mL (50 mL) [no longer available as of 7/00]
Cyclosporine, non-modified (Sandimmune®):
    Capsule, soft gel: 25 mg, 50 mg, 100 mg [contains dehydrated ethanol, corn oil]
    Injection: 50 mg/mL (5 mL) [contains Cremophor® EL (polyoxyethylated castor oil) and ethanol]
    Solution, oral: 100 mg/mL (50 mL) [contains olive oil and ethanol]

♦ **Cycofed® Pediatric** see Guaifenesin, Pseudoephedrine, and Codeine on page 648
♦ **Cyklokapron®** see Tranexamic Acid on page 1357
♦ **Cylert®** see Pemoline on page 1048
♦ **Cylex® [OTC]** see Benzocaine on page 154
♦ **Cyomin®** see Cyanocobalamin on page 339

Cyproheptadine (si proe HEP ta deen)

U.S. Brand Names Periactin®

Canadian Brand Names Periactin®

Synonyms Cyproheptadine Hydrochloride

Therapeutic Category Antihistamine, H₁ Blocker

Use Perennial and seasonal allergic rhinitis and other allergic symptoms including urticaria

Unlabeled/Investigational Use Appetite stimulation, blepharospasm, cluster headaches, migraine headaches, Nelson's syndrome, pruritus, schizophrenia, spinal cord damage associated spasticity, and tardive dyskinesia

Pregnancy Risk Factor B

Contraindications Hypersensitivity to cyproheptadine or any component of the formulation; narrow-angle glaucoma; bladder neck obstruction; acute asthmatic attack; stenosing peptic ulcer; GI tract obstruction; concurrent use of MAO inhibitors; avoid use in premature and term newborns due to potential association with SIDS

Warnings/Precautions Do not use in neonates, safety and efficacy have not been established in children <2 years of age; symptomatic prostate hypertrophy; antihistamines are more likely to cause dizziness, excessive sedation, syncope, toxic confusion states, and hypotension in the elderly. In case reports, cyproheptadine has promoted weight gain in anorexic adults, though it has not been specifically studied in the elderly. All cases of weight loss or decreased appetite should be adequately assessed.

Adverse Reactions

>10%:
    Central nervous system: Slight to moderate drowsiness
    Respiratory: Thickening of bronchial secretions

1% to 10%:
    Central nervous system: Headache, fatigue, nervousness, dizziness
    Gastrointestinal: Appetite stimulation, nausea, diarrhea, abdominal pain, dry mouth
    Neuromuscular & skeletal: Arthralgia
    Respiratory: Pharyngitis

<1% (Limited to important or life-threatening): Bronchospasm, CNS stimulation, depression, epistaxis, hemolytic anemia, hepatitis, leukopenia, sedation, seizures, thrombocytopenia

Overdosage/Toxicology Symptoms include CNS depression or stimulation, dry mouth, flushed skin, fixed and dilated pupils, and apnea. There is no specific treatment for an antihistamine overdose, however, clinical toxicity is mostly due to anticholinergic effects. Anticholinesterase inhibitors may be useful by reducing acetylcholinesterase. Anticholinesterase inhibitors include physostigmine, neostigmine, pyridostigmine, and edrophonium. For anticholinergic overdose with severe life-threatening symptoms, physostigmine 1-2 mg (0.5 mg or 0.02 mg/kg for children) slow I.V. may be given to reverse these effects.

Drug Interactions

Increased Effect/Toxicity: Cyproheptadine may potentiate the effect of CNS depressants. MAO inhibitors may cause hallucinations when taken with cyproheptadine.

Ethanol/Nutrition/Herb Interactions Ethanol: Avoid ethanol (may increase CNS sedation).

Mechanism of Action A potent antihistamine and serotonin antagonist, competes with histamine for H₁-receptor sites on effector cells in the gastrointestinal tract, blood vessels, and respiratory tract

Pharmacodynamics/Kinetics

Metabolism: Almost completely
Excretion: Urine (>50% primarily as metabolites); feces (~25%)

Usual Dosage Oral:

Children:
    Allergic conditions: 0.25 mg/kg/day or 8 mg/m²/day in 2-3 divided doses **or**
        2-6 years: 2 mg every 8-12 hours (not to exceed 12 mg/day)
        7-14 years: 4 mg every 8-12 hours (not to exceed 16 mg/day)
    Migraine headaches: 4 mg 2-3 times/day

Children ≥12 years and Adults: Spasticity associated with spinal cord damage: 4 mg at bedtime; increase by a 4 mg dose every 3-4 days; average daily dose: 16 mg in divided doses; not to exceed 36 mg/day

Children >13 years and Adults: Appetite stimulation (anorexia nervosa): 2 mg 4 times/day; may be increased gradually over a 3-week period to 8 mg 4 times/day

Adults:
    Allergic conditions: 4-20 mg/day divided every 8 hours (not to exceed 0.5)
    Cluster headaches: 4 mg 4 times/day
    Migraine headaches: 4-8 mg 3 times/day

Dosage adjustment in hepatic impairment: Reduce dosage in patients with significant hepatic dysfunction

Test Interactions Diagnostic antigen skin test results may be suppressed; false positive serum TCA screen

(Continued)

Cyproheptadine *(Continued)*

Patient Information May cause drowsiness; may stimulate appetite; avoid alcohol and other CNS depressants; may impair judgment and coordination

Nursing Implications Raise bed rails, institute safety measures, assist with ambulation

Additional Information May stimulate appetite; in case reports, cyproheptadine has promoted weight gain in anorexic adults.

Dosage Forms

Syrup, as hydrochloride: 2 mg/5 mL with alcohol 5% (473 mL)

Tablet, as hydrochloride: 4 mg

♦ **Cyproheptadine Hydrochloride** *see Cyproheptadine on page 349*

♦ **Cystadane®** *see Betaine Anhydrous on page 161*

♦ **Cystagon®** *see Cysteamine on page 350*

Cysteamine *(sis TEE a meen)*

U.S. Brand Names Cystagon®

Synonyms Cysteamine Bitartrate

Therapeutic Category Anticystine Agent; Urinary Tract Product

Use Orphan drug: Treatment of nephropathic cystinosis

Pregnancy Risk Factor C

Usual Dosage Initiate therapy with $^1/_4$ to $^1/_8$ of maintenance dose; titrate slowly upward over 4-6 weeks

Children <12 years: Oral: Maintenance: 1.3 g/m^2/day divided into 4 doses

Children >12 years and Adults (>110 lbs): 2 g/day in 4 divided doses; dosage may be increased to 1.95 g/m^2/day if cystine levels are <1 nmol/$^1/_2$ cystine/mg protein, although intolerance and incidence of adverse events may be increased

Additional Information Complete prescribing information for this medication should be consulted for additional detail.

Dosage Forms Capsule, as bitartrate: 50 mg, 150 mg

♦ **Cysteamine Bitartrate** *see Cysteamine on page 350*

♦ **Cystistat® (Can)** *see Sodium Hyaluronate on page 1247*

♦ **Cystospaz®** *see Hyoscyamine on page 692*

♦ **Cystospaz-M®** *see Hyoscyamine on page 692*

♦ **CYT** *see Cyclophosphamide on page 342*

♦ **Cytadren®** *see Aminoglutethimide on page 72*

Cytarabine *(sye TARE a been)*

U.S. Brand Names Cytosar-U®

Canadian Brand Names Cytosar®

Synonyms Arabinosylcytosine; Ara-C; Cytarabine Hydrochloride; Cytosine Arabinosine Hydrochloride

Therapeutic Category Antineoplastic Agent, Antimetabolite (Purine)

Use Ara-C is one of the most active agents in leukemia; also active against lymphoma, meningeal leukemia, and meningeal lymphoma; has little use in the treatment of solid tumors

Pregnancy Risk Factor D

Contraindications Hypersensitivity to cytarabine or any component of the formulation; pregnancy

Warnings/Precautions The U.S. Food and Drug Administration (FDA) currently recommends that procedures for proper handling and disposal of antineoplastic agents are considered. Use with caution in pregnant women or women of childbearing age and in infants; must monitor drug tolerance, protect and maintain a patient compromised by drug toxicity that includes bone marrow suppression with leukopenia, thrombocytopenia and anemia along with nausea, vomiting, diarrhea, abdominal pain, oral ulceration and hepatic impairment; marked bone marrow suppression necessitates dosage reduction by a decrease in the number of days of administration.

Adverse Reactions

>10%:

High-dose therapy toxicities: Cerebellar toxicity, conjunctivitis (make sure the patient is on steroid eye drops during therapy), corneal keratitis, hyperbilirubinemia, pulmonary edema, pericarditis, and tamponade

Central nervous system: Seizures (when given I.T.), cerebellar toxicity (ataxia, dysarthria, and dysdiadochokinesia; dose-related)

Dermatologic: Oral/anal ulceration, rash

Gastrointestinal: Nausea, vomiting, anorexia, stomatitis, mucositis

Emetic potential:

<500 mg: Moderately low (10% to 30%)

500 mg to 1500 mg: Moderately high (60% to 90%)

>1-1.5 g: High (>90%)

Time course of nausea/vomiting: Onset: 1-3 hours; Duration: 3-8 hours

Hematologic: Bleeding, leukopenia, thrombocytopenia

Myelosuppressive: Occurs within the first week of treatment and lasts for 10-14 days; primarily manifested as granulocytopenia, but anemia can also occur

WBC: Severe

Platelets: Severe

Onset (days): 4-7

Nadir (days): 14-18

Recovery (days): 21-28

Hepatic: Hepatic dysfunction, mild jaundice, increased transaminases

1% to 10%:

Cardiovascular: Cardiomegaly

Central nervous system: Dizziness, headache, somnolence, confusion, neuritis, malaise

Dermatologic: Skin freckling, itching, alopecia, cellulitis at injection site

Endocrine & metabolic: Hyperuricemia or uric acid nephropathy
Gastrointestinal: Esophagitis, diarrhea
Genitourinary: Urinary retention
Hematologic: Megaloblastic anemia
Hepatic: Hepatotoxicity
Local: Thrombophlebitis
Neuromuscular & skeletal: Myalgia, bone pain, peripheral neuropathy
Respiratory: Syndrome of sudden respiratory distress progressing to pulmonary edema, pneumonia
Miscellaneous: Sepsis
<1% (Limited to important or life-threatening): Pancreatitis

BMT:
Dermatologic: Rash, desquamation may occur following cytarabine and TBI
Gastrointestinal: Severe nausea and vomiting, mucositis, diarrhea
Neurologic:
Cerebellar toxicity: Nystagmus, dysarthria, dysdiadochokinesia, slurred speech
Cerebral toxicity: Somnolence, confusion
Ocular: Photophobia, excessive tearing, blurred vision, local discomfort, chemical conjunctivitis
Respiratory: Noncardiogenic pulmonary edema (onset 22-27 days following completion of therapy)

Overdosage/Toxicology Symptoms include myelosuppression, megaloblastosis, nausea, vomiting, respiratory distress, and pulmonary edema. A syndrome of sudden respiratory distress progressing to pulmonary edema and cardiomegaly has been reported following high doses.

Drug Interactions
Increased Effect/Toxicity: Alkylating agents and radiation, purine analogs, and methotrexate when coadminstered with cytarabine result in increased toxic effects.
Decreased Effect: Decreased effect of gentamicin, flucytosine. Decreased digoxin oral tablet absorption.

Stability Store intact vials of powder at room temperature 15°C to 30°C (59°F to 86°F)

WARNING: Bacteriostatic diluent should not be used for the preparation of either high doses or intrathecal doses of cytarabine
Reconstitute with SWI, D$_5$W or NS; dilute to a concentration of 100 mg/mL as follows; reconstituted solutions are stable for 48 hours at 15°C to 30°C
100 mg vial = 1 mL
500 mg vial = 5 mL
1 g vial = 10 mL
2 g vial = 20 mL
Further dilution in D$_5$W or NS is stable for 8 days at room temperature (25°C)

Standard I.V. dilution:
I.V. push: Dose/syringe (concentration: 100 mg/mL)
Maximum syringe size for IVP is 30 mL syringe and syringe should be ≤75% full
IVPB: Dose/100 mL D$_5$W or NS
CIV: Dose/250-1000 mL D$_5$W or NS
Compatible with calcium, idarubicin, magnesium, potassium chloride, and vincristine
Incompatible with 5-FU, gentamicin, heparin, insulin, methylprednisolone, nafcillin, oxacillin, penicillin G sodium

Intrathecal solutions in 3-20 mL lactated Ringer's are stable for 7 days at room temperature (30°C); however, should be used within 24 hours due to sterility concerns

Standard intrathecal dilutions: Dose/3-5 mL lactated Ringer's ± methotrexate (12 mg) ± hydrocortisone (15-50 mg)
Compatible with methotrexate and hydrocortisone in lactated Ringer's or NS for 24 hours at room temperature (25°C)

Mechanism of Action Inhibition of DNA synthesis. Cytosine gains entry into cells by a carrier process, and then must be converted to its active compound, aracytidine triphosphate. Cytosine is a purine analog and is incorporated into DNA; however, the primary action is inhibition of DNA polymerase resulting in decreased DNA synthesis and repair. The degree of cytotoxicity correlates linearly with incorporation into DNA; therefore, incorporation into the DNA is responsible for drug activity and toxicity. Cytarabine is specific for the S phase of the cell cycle.

Pharmacodynamics/Kinetics
Distribution: V$_d$: Total body water; widely and rapidly since it enters the cells readily; crosses blood-brain barrier with CSF levels of 40% to 50% of plasma level
Metabolism: Primarily hepatic; aracytidine triphosphate is the active moiety; about 86% to 96% of dose is metabolized to inactive uracil arabinoside
Half-life elimination: Initial: 7-20 minutes; Terminal: 0.5-2.6 hours
Excretion: Urine (~80% as metabolites) within 24-36 hours

Usual Dosage I.V. bolus, IVPB, and CIV doses of cytarabine are very different. Bolus doses are relatively well tolerated since the drug is rapidly metabolized; but are associated with greater neurotoxicity. Continuous infusion uniformly results in myelosuppression. Refer to individual protocols. Children and Adults:
Remission induction:
I.V.: 100-200 mg/m^2/day for 5-10 days; a second course, beginning 2-4 weeks after the initial therapy, may be required in some patients.
I.T.: 5-75 mg/m^2 every 2-7 days until CNS findings normalize; or age-based dosing:
<1 year: 20 mg
1-2 years: 30 mg
2-3 years: 50 mg
>3 years: 75 mg
Remission maintenance:
I.V.: 70-200 mg/m^2/day for 2-5 days at monthly intervals
I.M., S.C.: 1-1.5 mg/kg single dose for maintenance at 1- to 4-week intervals
(Continued)

Cytarabine *(Continued)*

High-dose therapies:

Doses as high as 1-3 g/m^2 have been used for refractory or secondary leukemias or refractory non-Hodgkin's lymphoma.

Doses of 3 g/m^2 every 12 hours for up to 12 doses have been used

Bone marrow transplant: 1.5 g/m^2 continuous infusion over 48 hours

Hemodialysis: Supplemental dose is not necessary.

Peritoneal dialysis: Supplemental dose is not necessary.

Dosage adjustment in hepatic impairment: Dose may need to be adjusted since cytarabine is partially detoxified in the liver.

Administration

Can be administered I.M., IVP, I.V. infusion, I.T., or S.C. at a concentration not to exceed 100 mg/mL.

I.V. may be administered either as a bolus, IVPB (high doses of >500 mg/m^2) or continuous intravenous infusion (doses of 100-200 mg/m^2)

I.V. doses of >200 mg/m^2 may produce conjunctivitis which can be ameliorated with prophylactic use of corticosteroid (0.1% dexamethasone) eye drops. Dexamethasone eye drops should be administered at 1-2 drops every 6 hours for 2-7 days after cytarabine is done.

Monitoring Parameters Liver function tests, CBC with differential and platelet count, serum creatinine, BUN, serum uric acid

Patient Information This drug can only be given by infusion or injection. During therapy, maintain adequate hydration (2-3 L/day of fluids unless instructed to restrict fluid intake). You will be more susceptible to infection; avoid crowds and exposure to infection. Do not have any vaccinations without consulting prescriber. Small frequent meals, frequent mouth care, sucking lozenges, or chewing gum may reduce incidence of nausea or vomiting or loss of appetite. If these measures are ineffective, consult prescriber for antiemetic medication. Report immediately any signs of CNS changes or change in gait, easy bruising or bleeding, yellowing of eyes or skin, change in color of urine or blackened stool, respiratory difficulty, or palpitations. Contraceptive measures are recommended during therapy.

Nursing Implications Administer corticosteroid eye drops around the clock prior to, during, and after high-dose Ara-C for prophylaxis of conjunctivitis; pyridoxine has been administered on days of high-dose Ara-C therapy for prophylaxis of CNS toxicity. Can be administered I.M., IVP, I.V. infusion, or S.C. at a concentration not to exceed 100 mg/mL; high-dose regimens are usually administered by I.V. infusion over 1-3 hours or as I.V. continuous infusion; for I.T. use, reconstitute with preservative free saline or preservative free lactated Ringer's solution.

Additional Information

Supplied with diluent containing benzyl alcohol, which should not be used when preparing either high-dose or I.T. doses.

Latex-free products: 100 mg, 500 mg, 1 g, 2 g vials (Cytosar-U®) by Pharmacia-Upjohn

Dosage Forms

Powder for injection, as hydrochloride: 100 mg, 500 mg, 1 g, 2 g

Cytosar-U®: 100 mg, 500 mg, 1 g, 2 g

♦ **Cytarabine Hydrochloride** *see* Cytarabine *on page 350*

Cytarabine (Liposomal) *(sye TARE a been lip po SOE mal)*

U.S. Brand Names DepoCyt™

Canadian Brand Names DepoCyt™

Therapeutic Category Antineoplastic Agent, Antimetabolite (Purine)

Use Treatment of neoplastic (lymphomatous) meningitis

Pregnancy Risk Factor D

Pregnancy/Breast-Feeding Implications Cytarabine may cause fetal harm if a pregnant woman is exposed systemically. Excretion in breast milk is unknown, however, breast-feeding is not recommended.

Contraindications Hypersensitivity to cytarabine or any component of the formulation; active meningeal infection; pregnancy

Warnings/Precautions The U.S. Food and Drug Administration (FDA) currently recommends that procedures for proper handling and disposal of antineoplastic agents are considered. The incidence and severity of chemical arachnoiditis is reduced by coadministration with dexamethasone. May cause neurotoxicity. Blockage to CSF flow may increase the risk of neurotoxicity. Safety and use in pediatric patients has not been established.

Adverse Reactions Chemical arachnoiditis is commonly observed, and may include neck pain, neck rigidity, headache, fever, nausea, vomiting, and back pain. It may occur in up to 100% of cycles without dexamethasone prophylaxis. The incidence is reduced to 33% when dexamethasone is used concurrently.

>10%:

Central nervous system: Headache (28%), confusion (14%), somnolence (12%), fever (11%), pain (11%)

Gastrointestinal: Vomiting (12%), nausea (11%)

1% to 10%:

Cardiovascular: Peripheral edema (7%)

Gastrointestinal: Constipation (7%)

Genitourinary: Incontinence (3%)

Hematologic: Neutropenia (9%), thrombocytopenia (8%), anemia (1%)

Neuromuscular & skeletal: Back pain (7%), weakness (19%), abnormal gait (4%)

<1% (Limited to important or life-threatening): Anaphylaxis, neck pain

Overdosage/Toxicology No overdosage with liposomal cytarabine has been reported. Symptoms of cytarabine overdose (when administered systemically) include myelosuppression, megaloblastosis, nausea, vomiting, respiratory distress, and pulmonary edema. A syndrome of sudden respiratory distress, progressing to pulmonary edema and cardiomegaly, has been reported following high doses. Exchange of CSF with isotonic saline, a procedure used in intrathecal cytarabine overdose, may be considered in the event of an overdose of the liposomal product.

Drug Interactions

Increased Effect/Toxicity: No formal studies of interactions with other medications have been conducted. The limited systemic exposure minimizes the potential for interaction between liposomal cytarabine and other medications.

Decreased Effect: No formal studies of interactions with other medications have been conducted. The limited systemic exposure minimizes the potential for interaction between liposomal cytarabine and other medications.

Stability Store under refrigeration (2°C to 8°C). Protect from freezing and avoid aggressive agitation. Solutions should be used within 4 hours of withdrawal from the vial. Particles may settle in diluent over time, and may be resuspended by gentle agitation or inversion of the vial.

Mechanism of Action This is a sustained-release formulation of the active ingredient cytarabine, which acts through inhibition of DNA synthesis; cell cycle-specific for the S phase of cell division; cytosine gains entry into cells by a carrier process, and then must be converted to its active compound; cytosine acts as an analog and is incorporated into DNA; however, the primary action is inhibition of DNA polymerase resulting in decreased DNA synthesis and repair; degree of its cytotoxicity correlates linearly with its incorporation into DNA; therefore, incorporation into the DNA is responsible for drug activity and toxicity

Pharmacodynamics/Kinetics

Absorption: Systemic exposure following intrathecal administration is negligible since transfer rate from CSF to plasma is slow

Metabolism: In plasma to ara-U (inactive)

Half-life elimination, CSF: 100-263 hours

Time to peak, CSF: Intrathecal: ~5 hours

Excretion: Primarily urine (as metabolites - ara-U)

Usual Dosage Adults:

Induction: 50 mg intrathecally every 14 days for a total of 2 doses (weeks 1 and 3)

Consolidation: 50 mg intrathecally every 14 days for 3 doses (weeks 5, 7, and 9), followed by an additional dose at week 13

Maintenance: 50 mg intrathecally every 28 days for 4 doses (weeks 17, 21, 25, and 29)

If drug-related neurotoxicity develops, the dose should be reduced to 25 mg. If toxicity persists, treatment with liposomal cytarabine should be discontinued.

Note: Patients should be started on dexamethasone 4 mg twice daily (oral or I.V.) for 5 days, beginning on the day of liposomal cytarabine injection

Administration For intrathecal use only. Dose should be removed from vial immediately before administration (must be administered within 4 hours of removal). An in-line filter should **not** be used. Vials are intended for a single use and contain no preservative. Administer directly into the CSF via an intraventricular reservoir or by direct injection into the lumbar sac. Injection should be made slowly (over 1-5 minutes). Patients should lie flat for 1 hour after lumbar puncture. Patients should be monitored closely for immediate toxic reactions.

Monitoring Parameters Monitor closely for signs of an immediate reaction

Test Interactions Since cytarabine liposomes are similar in appearance to WBCs, care must be taken in interpreting CSF examinations in patients receiving liposomal cytarabine

Patient Information Notify physician of any fever, sore throat, bleeding, or bruising; contraceptive measures are recommended during therapy

Dosage Forms Injection: 10 mg/mL (5 mL)

♦ **Cytochrome P-450 and Drug Metabolism** see page 1516
♦ **CytoGam®** see Cytomegalovirus Immune Globulin (Intravenous-Human) on page 353

Cytomegalovirus Immune Globulin (Intravenous-Human)

(sye toe meg a low VYE rus i MYUN GLOB yoo lin in tra VEE nus HYU man)

U.S. Brand Names CytoGam®

Synonyms CMV-IGIV

Therapeutic Category Immune Globulin

Use Prophylaxis of cytomegalovirus (CMV) disease associated with kidney, lung, liver, pancreas, and heart transplants; concomitant use with ganciclovir should be considered in organ transplants (other than kidney) from CMV seropositive donors to CMV seronegative recipients; has been used as adjunct therapy in the treatment of CMV disease in immunocompromised patients

Pregnancy Risk Factor C

Pregnancy/Breast-Feeding Implications Reproduction studies have not been conducted

Contraindications Hypersensitivity to CMV-IGIV, other immunoglobulins, or any component of the formulation; immunoglobulin A deficiency

Warnings/Precautions Monitor for anaphylactic reactions during infusion. May theoretically transmit blood-borne viruses. Use with caution in patients with renal insufficiency, diabetes mellitus, patients >65 years of age, volume depletion, sepsis, paraproteinemia, or patients on concomitant nephrotoxic drugs. Stabilized with sucrose and albumin, contains no preservative.

Adverse Reactions

<6%:

Cardiovascular: Flushing

Central nervous system: Fever, chills

Gastrointestinal: Nausea, vomiting

Neuromuscular & skeletal: Arthralgia, back pain, muscle cramps

Respiratory: Wheezing

<1%: Blood pressure decreased

Postmarketing and/or case reports: Acute renal failure, acute tubular necrosis, AMS, anaphylactic shock, angioneurotic edema, anuria, BUN increase, serum creatinine increase, oliguria, osmotic nephrosis, proximal tubular nephropathy

Overdosage/Toxicology Symptoms related to volume overload would be expected to occur with overdose. Treatment is symptom directed and supportive.

(Continued)

Cytomegalovirus Immune Globulin (Intravenous-Human)
(Continued)

Drug Interactions
Decreased Effect: Decreased effect of live vaccines may be seen if given within 3 months of IGIV administration. Defer vaccination or revaccinate.

Stability Store between 2°C and 8°C (35.6°F and 46.4°F). Use reconstituted product within 6 hours; do not admix with other medications; do not use if turbid. Do not shake vials. Dilution is not recommended. Infusion with other products is not recommended. If unavoidable, may be piggybacked into an I.V. line of sodium chloride, 2.5% dextrose in water, 5% dextrose in water, 10% dextrose in water, or 20% dextrose in water. Do not dilute more than 1:2.

Mechanism of Action CMV-IGIV is a preparation of immunoglobulin G derived from pooled healthy blood donors with a high titer of CMV antibodies; administration provides a passive source of antibodies against cytomegalovirus

Usual Dosage I.V.: Adults:
Kidney transplant:
  Initial dose (within 72 hours of transplant): 150 mg/kg/dose
  2-, 4-, 6-, and 8 weeks after transplant: 100 mg/kg/dose
  12 and 16 weeks after transplant: 50 mg/kg/dose
Liver, lung, pancreas, or heart transplant:
  Initial dose (within 72 hours of transplant): 150 mg/kg/dose
  2-, 4-, 6-, and 8 weeks after transplant: 150 mg/kg/dose
  12 and 16 weeks after transplant: 100 mg/kg/dose
Severe CMV pneumonia: Various regimens have been used, including 400 mg/kg CMV-IGIV in combination with ganciclovir on days 1, 2, 7, or 8, followed by 200 mg/kg CMV-IGIV on days 14 and 21
Elderly: Use with caution in patients >65 years of age, may be at increased risk of renal insufficiency

Dosage adjustment in renal impairment: Use with caution; specific dosing adjustments are not available. Infusion rate should be the minimum practical; do not exceed 180 mg/kg/hour

Administration Administer through an I.V. line containing an in-line filter (pore size 15 micron) using an infusion pump. Do not mix with other infusions; do not use if turbid. Begin infusion within 6 hours of entering vial, complete infusion within 12 hours.

Infuse at 15 mg/kg/hour. If no adverse reactions occur within 30 minutes, may increase rate to 30 mg/kg/hour. If no adverse reactions occur within the second 30 minutes, may increase rate to 60 mg/kg/hour; maximum rate of infusion: 75 mL/hour. When infusing subsequent doses, may decrease titration interval from 30 minutes to 15 minutes. If patient develops nausea, back pain, or flushing during infusion, slow the rate or temporarily stop the infusion. Discontinue if blood pressure drops or in case of anaphylactic reaction.

Monitoring Parameters Vital signs (throughout infusion), flushing, chills, muscle cramps, back pain, fever, nausea, vomiting, wheezing, decreased blood pressure, or anaphylaxis; renal function and urine output

Nursing Implications I.V. use only; administer as separate infusion; if administering via a pre-existing line, dilute no more than 1:2. Patients should not be volume depleted prior to infusion. Do not shake vials, do not use if turbid. If patient develops a minor side effect (flushing, back pain, nausea), slow the rate of or temporarily interrupt the infusion; can restart after symptoms resolve at tolerated dose. Stop infusion if blood pressure drops or anaphylaxis occurs. Have epinephrine and diphenhydramine available in case of anaphylactic reaction.

Dosage Forms Powder for injection, lyophilized, detergent treated: 2500 mg ±500 mg (50 mL); 1000 mg ±200 mg (20 mL)

- Cytomel® *see* Liothyronine *on page 808*
- Cytosar® **(Can)** *see* Cytarabine *on page 350*
- Cytosar-U® *see* Cytarabine *on page 350*
- Cytosine Arabinosine Hydrochloride *see* Cytarabine *on page 350*
- Cytotec® *see* Misoprostol *on page 921*
- Cytovene® *see* Ganciclovir *on page 618*
- Cytoxan® *see* Cyclophosphamide *on page 342*
- D-3-Mercaptovaline *see* Penicillamine *on page 1050*
- d4T *see* Stavudine *on page 1259*

Dacarbazine *(da KAR ba zeen)*
U.S. Brand Names DTIC-Dome®
Canadian Brand Names DTIC®
Synonyms DIC; Dimethyl Triazeno Imidazol Carboxamide; DTIC; Imidazole Carboxamide
Therapeutic Category Antineoplastic Agent, Vesicant; Antineoplastic Agent, Miscellaneous; Vesicant
Use Treatment of malignant melanoma, Hodgkin's disease, soft-tissue sarcomas, fibrosarcomas, rhabdomyosarcoma, islet cell carcinoma, medullary carcinoma of the thyroid, and neuroblastoma
Pregnancy Risk Factor C
Contraindications Hypersensitivity to dacarbazine or any component
Warnings/Precautions The U.S. Food and Drug Administration (FDA) currently recommends that procedures for proper handling and disposal of antineoplastic agents be considered. Use with caution in patients with bone marrow suppression; in patients with renal and/or hepatic impairment since dosage reduction may be necessary; avoid extravasation of the drug.
Adverse Reactions
>10%:
  Local: Pain and burning at infusion site
    Irritant chemotherapy
  Gastrointestinal: Anorexia; moderate to severe nausea and vomiting in 90% of patients and lasting up to 12 hours after administration; nausea and vomiting are dose-related and

occur more frequently when given as a one-time dose, as opposed to a less intensive 5-day course; diarrhea may also occur

Hematologic: Anemia, leukopenia, thrombocytopenia
  Emetic potential:
  <500 mg: Moderately high (60% to 90%)
  ≥500 mg: High (>90%)
  Time course of nausea/vomiting: Onset: 1-2 hours; Duration: 2-4 hours

1% to 10%:
  Cardiovascular: Facial flushing
  Central nervous system: Headache
  Dermatologic: Alopecia, rash
  Flu-like effects: Fever, malaise, headache, myalgia, and sinus congestion may last up to several days after administration
  Gastrointestinal: Anorexia, metallic taste
  Hematologic: Myelosuppressive: Mild to moderate is common and dose-related dose-limiting toxicity
    WBC: Mild (primarily leukocytes)
    Platelets: Mild
    Onset (days): 7
    Nadir (days): 21-25
    Recovery (days): 21-28
  Neuromuscular & skeletal: Paresthesias
  Respiratory: Sinus congestion

<1% (Limited to important or life-threatening): Alopecia, elevated LFTs, headache, hepatic vein thrombosis, hepatocellular necrosis, orthostatic hypotension, photosensitivity reactions, polyneuropathy, seizures

BMT:
  Cardiovascular: Hypotension (infusion-related)
  Gastrointestinal: Severe nausea and vomiting

Overdosage/Toxicology Symptoms include myelosuppression and diarrhea. There are no known antidotes and treatment is primarily symptomatic and supportive.

Drug Interactions
  Decreased Effect: Metabolism may be increased by drugs that induce hepatic enzymes (carbamazepine, phenytoin, phenobarbital, and rifampin), potentially leading to decreased efficacy. Patients may experience impaired immune response to vaccines; possible infection after administration of live vaccines in patients receiving immunosuppressants.

Ethanol/Nutrition/Herb Interactions
  Ethanol: Avoid ethanol (due to GI irritation).
  Herb/Nutraceutical: Avoid dong quai, St John's wort (may also cause photosensitization).

Stability
  Store intact vials under refrigeration (2°C to 8°C) and protect from light; vials are stable for 4 weeks at room temperature
  Reconstitute with a minimum of 2 mL (100 mg vial) or 4 mL (200 mg vial) of SWI, D_5W, or NS; dilute to a concentration of 10 mg/mL as follows; reconstituted solution is stable for 24 hours at room temperature (20°C) and 96 hours under refrigeration (4°C)
    100 mg vial = 9.9 mL
    200 mg vial = 19.7 mL
    500 mg vial = 49.5 mL
  Further dilution in 200-500 mL of D_5W or NS is stable for 24 hours at room temperature and protected from light
  Decomposed drug turns pink

  Standard I.V. dilution:
    Dose/250-500 mL D_5W or NS
    Stable for 24 hours at room temperature and refrigeration (4°C) when protected from light

Mechanism of Action Alkylating agent which forms methylcarbonium ions that attack nucleophilic groups in DNA; cross-links strands of DNA resulting in the inhibition of DNA, RNA, and protein synthesis, but the exact mechanism of action is still unclear; originally developed as a purine antimetabolite, but it does not interfere with purine synthesis; metabolism by the host is necessary for activation of dacarbazine, then the methylated species acts by alkylation of nucleic acids; dacarbazine is active in all phases of the cell cycle

Pharmacodynamics/Kinetics
  Onset of action: I.V.: 18-24 days
  Distribution: V_d: 0.6 L/kg, exceeding total body water; suggesting binding to some tissue (probably liver)
  Protein binding: 5%
  Metabolism: Extensively hepatic; hepatobiliary excretion is probably of some importance; metabolites may also have an antineoplastic effect
  Half-life elimination: Biphasic: Initial: 20-40 minutes; Terminal: 5 hours
  Excretion: Urine (~30% to 50% as unchanged drug)

Usual Dosage Refer to individual protocols. Some dosage regimens include:
  Intra-arterial: 50-400 mg/m² for 5-10 days
  I.V.:
    ABVD for Hodgkin's disease: 375 mg/m² days 1 and 15 every 4 weeks
    Metastatic melanoma (alone or in combination with other agents): 150-250 mg/m² days 1-5 every 3-4 weeks
    Metastatic melanoma: 850 mg/m² every 3 weeks
  High dose: Bone marrow/blood cell transplantation: I.V.: 1-3 g/m²; maximum dose as a single agent: 3.38 g/m²; generally combined with other high-dose chemotherapeutic drugs
  Dosage adjustment in renal/hepatic impairment: No guidelines exist for adjustment

Monitoring Parameters CBC (with differential, erythrocyte, and platelet count), liver function tests

Patient Information Limit oral intake for 4-6 hours before therapy. Do not use alcohol, aspirin-containing products, and/or OTC medications without consulting prescriber. It is important to maintain adequate nutrition and hydration (2-3 L/day of fluids unless instructed to restrict fluid

(Continued)

Dacarbazine *(Continued)*

intake) during therapy; frequent small meals may help. You may experience nausea or vomiting (frequent small meals, frequent mouth care, sucking lozenges, or chewing gum may help). If this is ineffective, consult prescriber for antiemetic medication. You may experience loss of hair (reversible); you will be more susceptible to infection (avoid crowds and exposure to infection as much as possible); you will be more sensitive to sunlight; use sunblock, wear protective clothing and dark glasses, or avoid direct exposure to sunlight. Flu-like symptoms (eg, malaise, fever, myalgia) may occur 1 week after infusion and persist for 1-3 weeks; consult prescriber for severe symptoms. Report fever, chills, unusual bruising or bleeding, signs of infection, excessive fatigue, yellowing of eyes or skin, or change in color of urine or stool. Contraceptive measures are recommended during therapy.

Nursing Implications

Extravasation management: Local pain, burning sensation, and irritation at the injection site may be relieved by local application of hot packs; if extravasation occurs, apply cold packs; protect exposed tissue from light following extravasation

Dosage Forms Injection: 100 mg (10 mL, 20 mL); 200 mg (20 mL, 30 mL); 500 mg (50 mL)

Daclizumab *(dac KLYE zue mab)*

U.S. Brand Names Zenapax®

Canadian Brand Names Zenapax®

Therapeutic Category Immunosuppressant Agent

Use In combination with other standard immunosuppressants (eg, cyclosporine and corticosteroids), daclizumab reduces the incidence of acute rejection in renal transplant recipients. Weekly daclizumab has not been ineffective in prevention of graft-versus-host disease.

Pregnancy Risk Factor C

Contraindications Hypersensitivity to daclizumab or any component of the formulation

Warnings/Precautions Only physicians experienced in immunosuppressive therapy and management of organ transplant patients should prescribe daclizumab. Manage patients receiving the drug in facilities equipped and staffed with adequate laboratory and supportive medical resources. Readministration of daclizumab after an initial course of therapy has not been studied in humans. The potential risks of such readministration, specifically those associated with immunosuppression or the occurrence of anaphylaxis/anaphylactoid reactions, are not known.

Adverse Reactions Although reported adverse events are frequent, when daclizumab is compared with placebo the incidence of adverse effects is similar between the two groups. Many of the adverse effects reported during clinical trial use of daclizumab may be related to the patient population, transplant procedure, and concurrent transplant medications.

≥2%:

Cardiovascular: Bleeding, hypertension, hypotension, tachycardia, thrombosis, edema
Central nervous system: Headache, tremor, dizziness, prickly sensation, fatigue, fever
Dermatologic: Acne, hirsutism, increased diaphoresis, pruritus
Endocrine & metabolic: Dehydration, diabetes mellitus
Gastrointestinal: Abdominal pain or distension, constipation, diarrhea, dyspepsia, epigastric pain, flatulence, gastritis, nausea, vomiting
Genitourinary: Dysuria, oliguria, hematuria, renal dysfunction
Neuromuscular & skeletal: Back pain, leg cramps, musculoskeletal pain
Ocular: Blurred vision
Respiratory: Atelectasis, coughing, dyspnea, hypoxia, pharyngitis, pleural effusion, rhinitis
Miscellaneous: Infectious complications

Overdosage/Toxicology Overdose has not been reported. A maximum tolerated dose has not been determined in patients. A dose of 1.5 mg/kg has been administered to bone marrow transplant recipients without any associated adverse events.

Stability Refrigerate vials at 2°C to 8°C/36°F to 46°F. Do not shake or freeze; protect undiluted solution against direct sunlight. Dose should be further diluted in 50 mL 0.9% sodium chloride solution. Diluted solution is stable for 24 hours at 4°C or for 4 hours at room temperature.

Mechanism of Action Daclizumab is a chimeric (90% human, 10% murine) monoclonal IgG antibody produced by recombinant DNA technology. Daclizumab inhibits immune reactions by binding and blocking the alpha-chain of the interleukin-2 receptor (CD25) located on the surface of activated lymphocytes.

Pharmacodynamics/Kinetics

Distribution: V_d: Central compartment: 2.5 L; Peripheral compartment: 3.4 L
Half-life elimination (estimated): Terminal: 20 days

Usual Dosage Daclizumab is used adjunctively with other immunosuppressants (eg, cyclosporine, corticosteroids, mycophenolate mofetil, and azathioprine): I.V.:

Children: Use same weight-based dose as adults

Adults:

Immunoprophylaxis against acute renal allograft rejection: 1 mg/kg infused over 15 minutes within 24 hours before transplantation (day 0), then every 14 days for 4 doses

Treatment of graft-versus-host disease (limited data): 0.5-1.5 mg/kg, repeat same dosage for transient response. Repeat doses have been administered 11-48 days following the initial dose.

Administration Daclizumab dose should be diluted in 50 mL NS solution. When mixing the solution, gently invert the bag to avoid foaming; do not shake. Daclizumab solution should be administered within 4 hours of preparation if stored at room temperature; infuse over a 15-minute period via a peripheral or central vein

Dosage Forms Injection: 5 mg/mL (5 mL)

Dactinomycin *(dak ti noe MYE sin)*

U.S. Brand Names Cosmegen®

Canadian Brand Names Cosmegen®

Synonyms ACT; Actinomycin D

Therapeutic Category Antineoplastic Agent, Antibiotic; Antineoplastic Agent, Vesicant; Vesicant

Use Treatment of testicular tumors, melanoma, choriocarcinoma, Wilms' tumor, neuroblastoma, retinoblastoma, rhabdomyosarcoma, uterine sarcomas, Ewing's sarcoma, Kaposi's sarcoma, sarcoma botryoides, and soft tissue sarcoma

Pregnancy Risk Factor C

Pregnancy/Breast-Feeding Implications Malformations reported in animal studies. No controlled studies in pregnant women. Use only when potential benefit justifies potential risk to the fetus. It is not known if dactinomycin is excreted in human breast milk. Due to the potential for serious reactions in the infant, breast-feeding is not recommended.

Contraindications Hypersensitivity to dactinomycin or any component of the formulation; patients with concurrent or recent chickenpox or herpes zoster; avoid in infants <6 months of age

Warnings/Precautions The U.S. Food and Drug Administration (FDA) currently recommends that procedures for proper handling and disposal of antineoplastic agents be considered. Drug is extremely irritating to tissues and must be administered I.V.; if extravasation occurs during I.V. use, severe damage to soft tissues will occur. Dosage is calculated in micrograms and must be calculated on the basis of body surface area (BSA) in obese or edematous patients. Use with caution in patients who have received radiation therapy (particularly within 2 months of irradiation for right-sided Wilms' tumor) or in the presence of hepatobiliary dysfunction; reduce dosage in patients who are receiving radiation therapy simultaneously. Increased incidence of second primary tumors following treatment; long-term monitoring of cancer survivors is needed.

Adverse Reactions

>10%:

Central nervous system: Unusual fatigue, malaise, fever

Dermatologic: Alopecia (reversible), skin eruptions, acne, increased pigmentation of previously irradiated skin

Extravasation: An irritant and should be administered through a rapidly running I.V. line; extravasation can lead to tissue necrosis, pain, and ulceration

Vesicant chemotherapy

Endocrine & metabolic: Hypocalcemia

Gastrointestinal: **Highly emetogenic**

Severe nausea and vomiting occurs in most patients and persists for up to 24 hours; stomatitis, anorexia, abdominal pain, esophagitis, diarrhea

Time course of nausea/vomiting: Onset: 2-5 hours; Duration: 4-24 hours

Hematologic: Myelosuppressive: Dose-limiting toxicity; anemia, aplastic anemia, agranulocytosis, pancytopenia

WBC: Moderate

Platelets: Moderate

Onset (days): 7

Nadir (days): 14-21

Recovery (days): 21-28

1% to 10%: Gastrointestinal: Diarrhea, mucositis

<1% (Limited to important or life-threatening): Anaphylactoid reaction, hepatitis, hyperuricemia, LFT abnormalities

Overdosage/Toxicology Symptoms include myelosuppression, nausea, vomiting, glossitis, and oral ulceration. There are no known antidotes and treatment is primarily symptomatic and supportive.

Drug Interactions

Increased Effect/Toxicity: Dactinomycin potentiates the effects of radiation therapy. Radiation may cause skin erythema which may become severe. Also associated with GI toxicity.

Ethanol/Nutrition/Herb Interactions Ethanol: Avoid ethanol (due to GI irritation).

Stability

Store intact vials at controlled room temperature 15°C to 30°C (59°F to 86°F) and protect from light, humidity, and heat;

Dilute with 1.1 mL of preservative-free SWI to yield a final concentration of 500 mcg/mL; do not use preservative diluent as precipitation may occur. Solution is chemically stable for 24 hours at room temperature (25°C). Significant binding of the drug occurs with micrometer nitrocellulose filter materials.

Compatible with D_5W or NS

Standard I.V. dilution:

I.V. push: Dose/syringe (500 mcg/mL)

IVPB: Dose/50 mL D_5W or NS

Stable for 24 hours at room temperature

Mechanism of Action Binds to the guanine portion of DNA intercalating between guanine and cytosine base pairs inhibiting DNA and RNA synthesis and protein synthesis; product of *Streptomyces parvullus* (a yeast species)

Pharmacodynamics/Kinetics

Distribution: High concentrations found in bone marrow and tumor cells, submaxillary gland, liver, and kidney; crosses placenta; poor CSF penetration

Metabolism: Minimal

Half-life elimination: 36 hours

Time to peak, serum: I.V.: 2-5 minutes

Excretion: Bile (50%); feces (14%); urine (~10% as unchanged drug)

Usual Dosage Refer to individual protocols: I.V.:

Dactinomycin doses are almost ALWAYS expressed in MICROGRAMS rather than milligrams. Some practitioners recommend calculation of the dosage for obese or edematous patients on the basis of body surface area in an effort to relate dosage to lean body mass.

Children >6 months: 15 mcg/kg/day for 5 days **or** 2.5 mg/m² given over 1-week period; a second course may be given after at least 3 weeks have elapsed, provided all signs of toxicity have disappeared

(Continued)

Dactinomycin (Continued)

Adults: Usual dose: 500 mcg daily for a maximum of 5 days; dosage should not exceed 15 mcg/kg/day or 400-600 mcg/m²/day for 5 days; a second course may be given after at least 3 weeks have elapsed, provided all signs of toxicity have disappeared

Children >6 months and Adults: Other regimens have included:

0.75-2 mg/m² as a single dose given at intervals of 1-4 weeks

400-600 mcg/m²/day for 5 days, repeated every 3-6 weeks

Dosing in renal impairment: No adjustment necessary

Administration

Administer slow I.V. push over 10-15 minutes

An in-line cellulose membrane filter should not be used during administration of dactinomycin solutions; do not administer I.M. or S.C.

Avoid extravasation: Extremely damaging to soft tissue and will cause a severe local reaction if extravasation occurs

Monitoring Parameters CBC with differential and platelet count, liver function tests, and renal function tests

Test Interactions May interfere with bioassays of antibacterial drug levels

Patient Information Limit oral intake for 4-6 hours before therapy. Do not use alcohol, aspirin-containing products, and/or OTC medications without consulting prescriber. It is important to maintain adequate nutrition and hydration (2-3 L/day of fluids unless instructed to restrict fluid intake) during therapy; frequent small meals may help. You may experience nausea or vomiting (frequent small meals, frequent mouth care, sucking lozenges, or chewing gum may help). If this is ineffective, consult prescriber for antiemetic medication. You may experience loss of hair (reversible); you will be more susceptible to infection (avoid crowds and exposure to infection as much as possible); you will be more sensitive to sunlight; use sunblock, wear protective clothing and dark glasses, or avoid direct exposure to sunlight. Flu-like symptoms (eg, malaise, fever, myalgia) may occur 1 week after infusion and persist for 1-3 weeks; consult prescriber for severe symptoms. Report fever, chills, unusual bruising or bleeding, signs of infection, excessive fatigue, yellowing of eyes or skin, or change in color of urine or stool. Contraceptive measures are recommended during therapy.

Nursing Implications Care should be taken to avoid extravasation of the drug; an in-line cellulose membrane filter should not be used during administration of dactinomycin solutions; do not administer I.M. or S.C.

Management of extravasation: Apply ice immediately for 30-60 minutes; then alternate off/on every 15 minutes for one day. Data is not currently available regarding potential antidotes for dactinomycin. If accidental skin contact should occur, irrigate affected area with water for at least 15 minutes

Dosage Forms Injection, powder for reconstitution: Dactinomycin 0.5 mg and mannitol 20 mg

- ◆ **D.A.II™** see Chlorpheniramine, Phenylephrine, and Methscopolamine on page 281
- ◆ **Dakin's Solution** see Sodium Hypochlorite Solution on page 1248
- ◆ **Dalacin® C (Can)** see Clindamycin on page 309
- ◆ **Dalalone®** see Dexamethasone on page 380
- ◆ **Dalalone D.P.®** see Dexamethasone on page 380
- ◆ **Dalalone L.A.®** see Dexamethasone on page 380
- ◆ **Dallergy®** see Chlorpheniramine, Phenylephrine, and Methscopolamine on page 281
- ◆ **Dallergy-D®** see Chlorpheniramine and Phenylephrine on page 279
- ◆ **Dalmane®** see Flurazepam on page 584
- ◆ **d-Alpha Tocopherol** see Vitamin E on page 1423

Dalteparin (dal TE pa rin)

Related Information

Heparin Comparison on page 1501

U.S. Brand Names Fragmin®

Canadian Brand Names Fragmin®

Therapeutic Category Low Molecular Weight Heparin

Use Prevention of deep vein thrombosis which may lead to pulmonary embolism, in patients requiring abdominal surgery who are at risk for thromboembolism complications (ie, patients >40 years of age, obesity, patients with malignancy, history of deep vein thrombosis or pulmonary embolism, and surgical procedures requiring general anesthesia and lasting longer than 30 minutes); prevention of DVT in patients undergoing hip surgery; acute treatment of unstable angina or non-Q-wave myocardial infarction; prevention of ischemic complications in patients on concurrent aspirin therapy

Unlabeled/Investigational Use Active treatment of deep vein thrombosis

Pregnancy Risk Factor B

Contraindications Hypersensitivity to dalteparin or any component of the formulation; thrombocytopenia associated with a positive in vitro test for antiplatelet antibodies in the presence of dalteparin; hypersensitivity to pork products; patient with active major bleeding; not for I.M. or I.V. use

Warnings/Precautions Use with caution in patients with pre-existing thrombocytopenia, recent childbirth, subacute bacterial endocarditis, peptic ulcer disease, pericarditis or pericardial effusion, liver or renal function impairment, recent lumbar puncture, vasculitis, concurrent use of aspirin (increased bleeding risk), previous hypersensitivity to heparin, heparin-associated thrombocytopenia. If thromboembolism develops despite dalteparin prophylaxis, dalteparin should be discontinued and appropriate treatment should be initiated.

Use with caution in patients with known hypersensitivity to methylparaben or propylparaben. Monitor patient closely for signs or symptoms of bleeding. Certain patients are at increased risk of bleeding. Risk factors include bacterial endocarditis; congenital or acquired bleeding disorders; active ulcerative or angiodysplastic GI diseases; severe uncontrolled hypertension; hemorrhagic stroke; or use shortly after brain, spinal, or ophthalmology surgery; in patient treated concomitantly with platelet inhibitors; recent GI bleeding; thrombocytopenia or platelet defects; severe liver disease; hypertensive or diabetic retinopathy; or in patients undergoing invasive procedures. Use with caution in patients with severe renal failure (has not been studied). Safety and efficacy in pediatric patients have not been established. Rare cases of thrombocytopenia with thrombosis have occurred. Multidose vials contain benzyl alcohol and should not be used in pregnant women. Heparin can cause hyperkalemia by affecting aldosterone. Similar reactions could occur with LMWHs. Monitor for hyperkalemia. Discontinue therapy if platelets are <100,000/mm^3.

Patients with recent or anticipated neuraxial anesthesia (epidural or spinal anesthesia) are at risk of spinal or epidural hematoma and subsequent paralysis. Consider risk versus benefit prior to neuraxial anesthesia. Risk is increased by concomitant agents which may alter hemostasis, as well as traumatic or repeated epidural or spinal puncture. Patient should be observed closely for bleeding if dalteparin is administered during or immediately following diagnostic lumbar puncture, epidural anesthesia, or spinal anesthesia.

Adverse Reactions
1% to 10%
> Hematologic: Bleeding (3% to 5 %), wound hematoma (0.1% to 3%)
> Local: Pain at injection site (up to 12%), injection site hematoma (0.2% to 7%)
<1% (Limited to important or life-threatening): Allergic reaction (fever, pruritus, rash, injection site reaction, bullous eruption), anaphylactoid reaction, gastrointestinal bleeding, injection site hematoma, operative site bleeding, skin necrosis, thrombocytopenia (including heparin-induced thrombocytopenia). Spinal or epidural hematomas can occur following neuraxial anesthesia or spinal puncture, resulting in paralysis. Risk is increased in patients with indwelling epidural catheters or concomitant use of other drugs affecting hemostasis, osteoporosis (3-6 month use).

Drug Interactions
Increased Effect/Toxicity: The risk of bleeding with dalteparin may be increased by drugs which affect platelet function (eg, aspirin, NSAIDs, dipyridamole, ticlopidine, clopidogrel), oral anticoagulants, and thrombolytic agents. Although the risk of bleeding may be increased during concurrent warfarin therapy, dalteparin is commonly continued during the initiation of warfarin therapy to assure anticoagulation and to protect against possible transient hypercoagulability.

Ethanol/Nutrition/Herb Interactions Herb/Nutraceutical: Avoid cat's claw, dong quai, evening primrose, garlic, ginseng (all have additional antiplatelet activity).

Stability Store at temperatures 20°C to 25°C (68°F to 77°F).

Mechanism of Action Low molecular weight heparin analog with a molecular weight of 4000-6000 daltons; the commercial product contains 3% to 15% heparin with a molecular weight <3000 daltons, 65% to 78% with a molecular weight of 3000-8000 daltons and 14% to 26% with a molecular weight >8000 daltons; while dalteparin has been shown to inhibit both factor Xa and factor IIa (thrombin), the antithrombotic effect of dalteparin is characterized by a higher ratio of antifactor Xa to antifactor IIa activity (ratio = 4)

Pharmacodynamics/Kinetics
Onset of action: 1-2 hours
Duration: >12 hours
Time to peak, serum: 4 hours
Half-life elimination (route dependent): 2-5 hours

Usual Dosage Adults: S.C.:
Low-moderate risk patients undergoing abdominal surgery: 2500 int. units 1-2 hours prior to surgery, then once daily for 5-10 days postoperatively
High-risk patients undergoing abdominal surgery: 5000 int. units 1-2 hours prior to surgery and then once daily for 5-10 days postoperatively
Patients undergoing total hip surgery: **Note:** Three treatment options are currently available. Dose is given for 5-10 days, although up to 14 days of treatment have been tolerated in clinical trials:
Postoperative start:
> Initial: 2500 int. units 4-8 hours* after surgery
> Maintenance: 5000 int. units once daily; start at least 6 hours after postsurgical dose
Preoperative (starting day of surgery):
> Initial: 2500 int. units within 2 hours before surgery
> Adjustment: 2500 int. units 4-8 hours* after surgery
> Maintenance: 5000 int. units once daily; start at least 6 hours after postsurgical dose
Preoperative (starting evening prior to surgery):
> Initial: 5000 int. units 10-14 hours before surgery
> Adjustment: 5000 int. units 4-8 hours* after surgery
> Maintenance: 5000 int. units once daily, allowing 24 hours between doses
*Dose may be delayed if hemostasis is not yet achieved.
Patients with unstable angina or non-Q-wave myocardial infarction: 120 int. units/kg body weight (maximum dose: 10,000 int. units) every 12 hours for 5-8 days with concurrent aspirin therapy. Discontinue dalteparin once patient is clinically stable.

Dosing adjustment in renal impairment: Half-life is increased in patients with chronic renal failure, use with caution, accumulation can be expected; specific dosage adjustments have not been recommended

Dosing adjustment in hepatic impairment: Use with caution in patients with hepatic insufficiency; specific dosage adjustments have not been recommended

Administration For deep S.C. injection only. May be injected in a U-shape to the area surrounding the navel, the upper outer side of the thigh, or the upper outer quadrangle of the buttock. Vary injection site daily. Use thumb and forefinger to lift a fold of skin when injecting dalteparin to the navel area or thigh. Insert needle at a 45- to 90-degree angle. The entire length of needle should be inserted.

Administration once daily beginning prior to surgery and continuing 5-10 days after surgery prevents deep vein thrombosis in patients at risk for thromboembolic complications. For unstable angina or non-Q-wave myocardial infarction, dalteparin is administered every 12 hours until the patient is stable (5-8 days).
(Continued)

Dalteparin *(Continued)*

Monitoring Parameters Periodic CBC including platelet count; stool occult blood tests; monitoring of PT and PTT is not necessary

Additional Information Multiple dose vial contains 14 mg/mL benzyl alcohol.

Dosage Forms

Injection [multidose vial]: 95,000 int. units (9.5 mL) [10,000 antifactor Xa int. units/mL]

Injection, prefilled syringe: Antifactor Xa 2500 int. units per 0.2 mL; antifactor Xa 5000 int. units per 0.2 mL

Danaparoid *(da NAP a roid)*

Related Information

Heparin Comparison *on page 1501*

U.S. Brand Names Orgaran®

Canadian Brand Names Orgaran®

Synonyms Danaparoid Sodium

Therapeutic Category Heparinoid

Use Prevention of postoperative deep vein thrombosis following elective hip replacement surgery

Unlabeled/Investigational Use Systemic anticoagulation for patients with heparin-induced thrombocytopenia: factor Xa inhibition is used to monitor degree of anticoagulation if necessary

Pregnancy Risk Factor B

Contraindications Hypersensitivity to danaparoid or thrombocytopenia associated with a positive *in vitro* test for antiplatelet antibodies in the presence of danaparoid; hypersensitivity to pork products or to sulfites (contains metabisulfite); patients with active major bleeding; severe hemorrhagic diathesis (hemophilia, idiopathic thrombocytopenic purpura); not for I.M. or I.V. use

Warnings/Precautions Do not administer intramuscularly. Danaparoid shows a low cross-sensitivity with antiplatelet antibodies in individuals with type II heparin-induced thrombocytopenia. This product contains sodium sulfite which may cause allergic-type reactions, including anaphylactic symptoms and life-threatening asthmatic episodes in susceptible people; this is seen more frequently in asthmatics.

Carefully monitor patients receiving low molecular weight heparins or heparinoids. These drugs, when used concurrently with spinal or epidural anesthesia or spinal puncture, may cause bleeding or hematomas within the spinal column. Increased pressure on the spinal cord may result in permanent paralysis if not detected and treated immediately.

Use with caution in patients with known hypersensitivity to methylparaben or propylparaben. Use with caution in patients with history of heparin-induced thrombocytopenia. Monitor patient closely for signs or symptoms of bleeding. Certain patients are at increased risk of bleeding. Risk factors include bacterial endocarditis; congenital or acquired bleeding disorders; active ulcerative or angioplastic GI diseases; severe uncontrolled hypertension; hemorrhagic stroke; use shortly after brain, spinal, or ophthalmology surgery; patient treated concomitantly with platelet inhibitors; recent GI bleeding; thrombocytopenia or platelet defects; severe liver disease; hypertensive or diabetic retinopathy; or patients undergoing invasive procedures. Use with caution in patients with severe renal failure (has not been studied). Safety and efficacy in pediatric patients have not been established. Heparin can cause hyperkalemia by affecting aldosterone. A similar reaction could occur with danaparoid. Monitor for hyperkalemia. Discontinue therapy if platelets are <100,000/mm^3.

Note: Danaparoid is **not** effectively antagonized by protamine sulfate. No other antidote is available, so extreme caution is needed in monitoring dose given and resulting Xa inhibition effect.

Adverse Reactions As with all anticoagulants, bleeding is the major adverse effect of danaparoid. Hemorrhage may occur at virtually any site. Risk is dependent on multiple variables.

>10%:

Central nervous system: Fever (22.2%)

Gastrointestinal: Nausea (4.1% to 14.3%), constipation (3.5% to 11.3%)

1% to 10%:

Cardiovascular: Peripheral edema (3.3%), edema (2.6%)

Central nervous system: Insomnia (3.1%), headache (2.6%), asthenia (2.3%), dizziness (2.3%), pain (8.7%)

Dermatologic: Rash (2.1% to 4.8%), pruritus (3.9%)

Gastrointestinal: Vomiting (2.9%)

Genitourinary: Urinary tract infection (2.6% to 4.0%), urinary retention (2.0%)

Hematologic: Anemia (2.2%)

Local: Injection site pain (7.6% to 13.7%), injection site hematoma (5%)

Neuromuscular & skeletal: Joint disorder (2.6%)

Miscellaneous: Infection (2.1%)

<1% (Limited to important or life-threatening): Spinal or epidural hematomas can occur following neuraxial anesthesia or spinal puncture, resulting in paralysis. Risk is increased in patients with indwelling epidural catheters or concomitant use of other drugs affecting hemostasis, thrombocytopenia, hyperkalemia, wound infection, skin rash, allergic reaction.

Overdosage/Toxicology Symptom include hemorrhage. Protamine zinc has been used to reverse effects.

Drug Interactions

Increased Effect/Toxicity: The risk of hemorrhage associated with danaparoid may be increased with thrombolytic agents, oral anticoagulants (warfarin) and drugs which affect platelet function (eg, aspirin, NSAIDs, dipyridamole, ticlopidine, clopidogrel).

Ethanol/Nutrition/Herb Interactions Herb/Nutraceutical: Avoid cat's claw, dong quai, evening primrose, feverfew, garlic, ginger, ginkgo, red clover, horse chestnut, green tea, and ginseng (all have additional antiplatelet activity).

Stability Store intact vials or ampuls under refrigeration

Mechanism of Action Prevents fibrin formation in coagulation pathway via thrombin generation inhibition by anti-Xa and anti-IIa effects.

Pharmacodynamics/Kinetics

Onset of action: Peak effect: S.C.: Maximum antifactor Xa and antithrombin (antifactor IIa) activities occur in 2-5 hours

Half-life elimination, plasma: Mean: Terminal: ~24 hours

Excretion: Primarily urine

Usual Dosage S.C.:

Children: Safety and effectiveness have not been established.

Adults:

Prevention of DVT following hip replacement: S.C.: 750 anti-Xa units twice daily; beginning 1-4 hours before surgery and then not sooner than 2 hours after surgery and every 12 hours until the risk of DVT has diminished. The average duration of therapy is 7-10 days.

Adults: Treatment: Based on diagnosis/indication: See table.

Adult Danaparoid Treatment Dosing Regimens

	Body Weight (kg)	I.V. Bolus aFXaU	Long–Term Infusion aFXaU	Level of aFXaU/mL	Monitoring
Deep Vein Thrombosis OR Acute Pulmonary Embolism	<55	1250	400 units/h over 4 h then	0.5-0.8	Days 1-3 daily, then every alternate day
	55-90	2500	300 units/h over 4 h, then		
	>90	3750	150-200 units/h maintenance dose		
Deep Vein Thrombosis OR Pulmonary Embolism >5 d old	<90	1250	S.C.: 3 x 750/d	<0.5	Not necessary
	>90	1250	S.C.: 3 x 1250/d		
Embolectomy	<90	2500 preoperatively	S.C.: 2 x 1250/d postoperatively	<0.4	Not necessary
	>90 and high risk	2500 preoperatively	150-200 units/hour I.V.; perioperative arterial irrigation, if necessary: 750 units/20 mL NaCl	0.5-0.8	Days 1-3 daily, then every alternate day
Peripheral Arterial Bypass		2500 preoperatively	150-200 units/h	0.5-0.8	Days 1-3 daily, then every alternate day
Cardiac Catheter	<90	2500 preoperatively			
	>90	3750 preoperatively			
Surgery (excluding vascular)			S.C.: 750, 1-4 h preoperatively S.C.: 750, 2-5 h postoperatively, then 2 x 750/d	<0.35	Not necessary

Dosing adjustment in elderly and severe renal impairment: Adjustment may be necessary. Patients with serum creatinine levels ≥2.0 mg/dL should be carefully monitored.

Hemodialysis: See table.

Hemodialysis With Danaparoid Sodium

Dialysis on alternate days	Dosage prior to dialysis in aFXaU (dosage for body wt <55 kg)	
First dialysis	3750 (<55 kg 2500)	
Second dialysis	3750 (<55 kg 2000)	
Further dialysis:		
aFXa level before dialysis (eg, day 5)	Bolus before next dialysis, aFXaU (eg, day 7)	aFXa level during dialysis
<0.3	3000 (<55 kg 2000)	0.5-0.8
0.3-0.35	2500 (<55 kg 2000)	
0.35-0.4	2000 (<55 kg 1500)	
>0.4	No bolus; if fibrin strands occur, 1500 aFXaU I.V.	
Monitoring: 30 minutes before dialysis and after 4 hours of dialysis		
Daily Dialysis		
First dialysis	3750 (<55 kg 2500)	
Second dialysis	2500 (<55 kg 2000)	
Further dialyses	See above	
As with "dialysis on alternate days", always take the aFXa activity preceding the previous dialysis as a basis for the current dosage.		

(Continued)

Danaparoid *(Continued)*

Monitoring Parameters Platelets, occult blood, and anti-Xa activity, if available; the monitoring of PT and/or PTT is not necessary

Additional Information A 750 anti-Xa unit dose of danaparoid is approximately equivalent to 55 mg of danaparoid.

Dosage Forms Injection, as sodium: 750 anti-Xa units/0.6 mL

♦ **Danaparoid Sodium** *see* Danaparoid *on page 360*

Danazol *(DA na zole)*

U.S. Brand Names Danocrine®

Canadian Brand Names Cyclomen®; Danocrine®

Therapeutic Category Androgen; Antigonadotropic Agent

Use Treatment of endometriosis, fibrocystic breast disease, and hereditary angioedema

Pregnancy Risk Factor X

Pregnancy/Breast-Feeding Implications Pregnancy should be ruled out prior to treatment using a sensitive test (beta subunit test, if available). Nonhormonal contraception should be used during therapy. May cause androgenic effects to the female fetus; clitoral hypertrophy, labial fusion, urogenital sinus defect, vaginal atresia, and ambiguous genitalia have been reported. Enters breast milk; breast-feeding is contraindicated.

Contraindications Hypersensitivity to danazol or any component of the formulation; undiagnosed genital bleeding; pregnancy; breast-feeding; porphyria; markedly impaired hepatic, renal, or cardiac function

Warnings/Precautions Use with caution in patients with seizure disorders, migraine, or conditions influenced by edema. Thromboembolism, thrombotic, and thrombophlebitic events have been reported (including life-threatening or fatal strokes). Peliosis hepatis and benign hepatic adenoma have been reported with long-term use. May cause benign intracranial hypertension. Breast cancer should be ruled out prior to treatment for fibrocystic breast disease. May increase risk of atherosclerosis and coronary artery disease. May cause nonreversible androgenic effects. Pregnancy must be ruled out prior to treatment. Safety and efficacy in pediatric patients have not been established.

Adverse Reactions Frequency not defined.

Cardiovascular: Benign intracranial hypertension (rare), edema, flushing, hypertension, diaphoresis

Central nervous system: Anxiety (rare), chills (rare), convulsions (rare), depression, dizziness, emotional lability, fainting, fever (rare), Guillain-Barré syndrome, headache, nervousness, sleep disorders, tremor

Dermatologic: Acne, hair loss, mild hirsutism, maculopapular rash, papular rash, petechial rash, pruritus, purpuric rash, seborrhea, Stevens-Johnson syndrome (rare), photosensitivity (rare), urticaria, vesicular rash

Endocrine & metabolic: Amenorrhea (which may continue post therapy), breast size reduction, clitoris hypertrophy, glucose intolerance, HDL decreased, LDL increased, libido changes, nipple discharge, menstrual disturbances (spotting, altered timing of cycle), semen abnormalities (changes in volume, viscosity, sperm count/motility), spermatogenesis reduction

Gastrointestinal: Appetite changes (rare), bleeding gums (rare), constipation, gastroenteritis, nausea, pancreatitis (rare), vomiting, weight gain

Genitourinary: Vaginal dryness, vaginal irritation, pelvic pain

Hematologic: Eosinophilia, erythrocytosis (reversible), leukocytosis, leukopenia, platelet count increased, polycythemia, RBC increased, thrombocytopenia

Hepatic: Cholestatic jaundice, hepatic adenoma, jaundice, liver enzymes (elevated), malignant tumors (after prolonged use), peliosis hepatis

Neuromuscular & skeletal: Back pain, carpal tunnel syndrome (rare), CPK abnormalities, extremity pain, joint lockup, joint pain, joint swelling, muscle cramps, neck pain, paresthesias, spasms, weakness

Ocular: Cataracts (rare), visual disturbances

Renal: Hematuria

Respiratory: Nasal congestion (rare)

Miscellaneous: Voice change (hoarseness, sore throat, instability, deepening of pitch)

Drug Interactions

Cytochrome P450 Effect: CYP3A3/4 enzyme inhibitor

Increased Effect/Toxicity: Danazol may increase serum levels of carbamazepine, cyclosporine, tacrolimus, and warfarin leading to toxicity; dosage adjustment may be needed; monitor. Concomitant use of danazol and HMG-CoA reductase inhibitors may lead to severe myopathy or rhabdomyolysis. Danazol may enhance the glucose-lowering effect of hypoglycemic agents.

Decreased Effect: Danazol may decrease effectiveness of hormonal contraceptives. Nonhormonal birth control methods are recommended.

Ethanol/Nutrition/Herb Interactions Food: Delays time to peak; high-fat meal increases plasma concentration

Stability Store at controlled room temperature of 15°C to 30°C (59°F to 86°F).

Mechanism of Action Suppresses pituitary output of follicle-stimulating hormone and luteinizing hormone that causes regression and atrophy of normal and ectopic endometrial tissue; decreases rate of growth of abnormal breast tissue; reduces attacks associated with hereditary angioedema by increasing levels of C4 component of complement

Pharmacodynamics/Kinetics

Onset of action: Therapeutic: ~4 weeks

Metabolism: Extensively hepatic, primarily to 2-hydroxymethylethisterone

Half-life elimination: 4.5 hours (variable)

Time to peak, serum: Within 2 hours

Excretion: Urine

Usual Dosage Adults: Oral:

Female: Endometriosis: Initial: 200-400 mg/day in 2 divided doses for mild disease; individualize dosage. Usual maintenance dose: 800 mg/day in 2 divided doses to achieve amenorrhea and rapid response to painful symptoms. Continue therapy uninterrupted for 3-6 months (up to 9 months).

Female: Fibrocystic breast disease: Range: 100-400 mg/day in 2 divided doses

Male/Female: Hereditary angioedema: Initial: 200 mg 2-3 times/day; after favorable response, decrease the dosage by 50% or less at intervals of 1-3 months or longer if the frequency of attacks dictates. If an attack occurs, increase the dosage by up to 200 mg/day.

Monitoring Parameters Signs and symptoms of intracranial hypertension (papilledema, headache, nausea, vomiting), lipoproteins, androgenic changes, hepatic function

Test Interactions Testosterone, androstenedione, dehydroepiandrosterone

Patient Information Notify physician if masculinity effects occur; virilization may occur in female patients; report menstrual irregularities; male patients report persistent penile erections; all patients should report persistent GI distress, diarrhea, or jaundice

Nursing Implications Notify physician if masculinity effects occur

Dosage Forms Capsule: 50 mg, 100 mg, 200 mg

♦ **Danocrine**® *see Danazol on page 362*

♦ **Dantrium**® *see Dantrolene on page 363*

Dantrolene (DAN troe leen)

U.S. Brand Names Dantrium®

Canadian Brand Names Dantrium®

Synonyms Dantrolene Sodium

Therapeutic Category Antidote, Malignant Hyperthermia; Hyperthermia, Treatment; Skeletal Muscle Relaxant

Use Treatment of spasticity associated with spinal cord injury, stroke, cerebral palsy, or multiple sclerosis; treatment of malignant hyperthermia

Unlabeled/Investigational Use Neuroleptic malignant syndrome (NMS)

Pregnancy Risk Factor C

Contraindications Active hepatic disease; should not be used where spasticity is used to maintain posture or balance

Warnings/Precautions Use with caution in patients with impaired cardiac function or impaired pulmonary function; has potential for hepatotoxicity; overt hepatitis has been most frequently observed between the third and twelfth month of therapy; hepatic injury appears to be greater in females and in patients >35 years of age

Adverse Reactions

>10%:

Central nervous system: Drowsiness, dizziness, lightheadedness, fatigue

Dermatologic: Rash

Gastrointestinal: Diarrhea (mild), vomiting

Neuromuscular & skeletal: Muscle weakness

1% to 10%:

Cardiovascular: Pleural effusion with pericarditis

Central nervous system: Chills, fever, headache, insomnia, nervousness, mental depression

Gastrointestinal: Diarrhea (severe), constipation, anorexia, stomach cramps

Ocular: Blurred vision

Respiratory: Respiratory depression

<1% (Limited to important or life-threatening): Confusion, hepatic necrosis, hepatitis, seizures

Overdosage/Toxicology Symptoms include CNS depression, hypotension, nausea, and vomiting. For decontamination, lavage/activated charcoal with cathartic; do not use ipecac. Hypotension can be treated with isotonic I.V. fluids with the patient placed in the Trendelenburg position. Dopamine or norepinephrine can be given if hypotension is refractory to the above therapy.

Drug Interactions

Increased Effect/Toxicity: Increased toxicity with estrogens (hepatotoxicity), CNS depressants (sedation), MAO inhibitors, phenothiazines, clindamycin (increased neuromuscular blockade), verapamil (hyperkalemia and cardiac depression), warfarin, clofibrate, and tolbutamide.

Ethanol/Nutrition/Herb Interactions

Ethanol: Avoid ethanol (may increase CNS depression).

Herb/Nutraceutical: Avoid valerian, St John's wort, kava kava, gotu kola (may increase CNS depression).

Stability Reconstitute vial by adding 60 mL of sterile water for injection USP (**not bacteriostatic water for injection**); protect from light; use within 6 hours; avoid glass bottles for I.V. infusion

Mechanism of Action Acts directly on skeletal muscle by interfering with release of calcium ion from the sarcoplasmic reticulum; prevents or reduces the increase in myoplasmic calcium ion concentration that activates the acute catabolic processes associated with malignant hyperthermia

Pharmacodynamics/Kinetics

Absorption: Oral: Slow and incomplete

Metabolism: Hepatic

Half-life elimination: 8.7 hours

Excretion: Urine (25% as unchanged drug and metabolites); feces (45% to 50%)

Usual Dosage

Spasticity: Oral:

Children: Initial: 0.5 mg/kg/dose twice daily, increase frequency to 3-4 times/day at 4- to 7-day intervals, then increase dose by 0.5 mg/kg to a maximum of 3 mg/kg/dose 2-4 times/day up to 400 mg/day

Adults: 25 mg/day to start, increase frequency to 2-4 times/day, then increase dose by 25 mg every 4-7 days to a maximum of 100 mg 2-4 times/day or 400 mg/day

(Continued)

Dantrolene *(Continued)*

Malignant hyperthermia: Children and Adults:
  Preoperative prophylaxis:
    Oral: 4-8 mg/kg/day in 4 divided doses, begin 1-2 days prior to surgery with last dose 3-4 hours prior to surgery
    I.V.: 2.5 mg/kg ~1¼ hours prior to anesthesia and infused over 1 hour with additional doses as needed and individualized
  Crisis: I.V.: 2.5 mg/kg; may repeat dose up to cumulative dose of 10 mg/kg; if physiologic and metabolic abnormalities reappear, repeat regimen
  Postcrisis follow-up: Oral: 4-8 mg/kg/day in 4 divided doses for 1-3 days; I.V. dantrolene may be used when oral therapy is not practical; individualize dosage beginning with 1 mg/kg or more as the clinical situation dictates
Neuroleptic malignant syndrome (unlabeled use): I.V.: 1 mg/kg; may repeat dose up to maximum cumulative dose of 10 mg/kg, then switch to oral dosage

Administration I.V.: Therapeutic or emergency dose can be administered with rapid continuous I.V. push. Follow-up doses should be administered over 2-3 minutes.

Monitoring Parameters Motor performance should be monitored for therapeutic outcomes; nausea, vomiting, and liver function tests should be monitored for potential hepatotoxicity; intravenous administration requires cardiac monitor and blood pressure monitor

Patient Information Avoid unnecessary exposure to sunlight (or use sunscreen, protective clothing); avoid alcohol and other CNS depressants; patients should use caution while driving or performing other tasks requiring alertness

Nursing Implications Exercise caution at meals on the day of administration because difficulty swallowing and choking has been reported; avoid extravasation as is a tissue irritant

Dosage Forms
Capsule, as sodium: 25 mg, 50 mg, 100 mg
Powder for injection, as sodium: 20 mg

Extemporaneous Preparations A 5 mg/mL suspension may be made by adding five 100 mg capsules to a citric acid solution (150 mg citric acid powder in 10 mL water) and then adding syrup to a total volume of 100 mL; stable 2 days in refrigerator

Nahata MC and Hipple TF, *Pediatric Drug Formulations*, 1st ed, Cincinnati, OH: Harvey Whitney Books Co, 1990.

♦ **Dantrolene Sodium** *see Dantrolene on page 363*

Dapiprazole *(DA pi pray zole)*

U.S. Brand Names Rêv-Eyes™
Synonyms Dapiprazole Hydrochloride
Therapeutic Category Alpha-Adrenergic Blocking Agent, Ophthalmic
Use Reverse dilation due to drugs (adrenergic or parasympathomimetic) after eye exams
Pregnancy Risk Factor B
Usual Dosage Adults: Ophthalmic: Instill 2 drops followed 5 minutes later by an additional 2 drops into the conjunctiva of each eye; should not be used more frequently than once a week in the same patient
Additional Information Complete prescribing information for this medication should be consulted for additional detail.
Dosage Forms Powder, ophthalmic, lyophilized, as hydrochloride: 25 mg [0.5% solution when mixed with supplied diluent]

♦ **Dapiprazole Hydrochloride** *see Dapiprazole on page 364*

Dapsone *(DAP sone)*

Related Information
Antimicrobial Drugs of Choice *on page 1588*
USPHA/IDSA Guidelines for the Prevention of Opportunistic Infections in Persons With HIV *on page 1574*
Canadian Brand Names Avlosulfon®
Synonyms Diaminodiphenylsulfone
Therapeutic Category Antibiotic, Sulfone; Leprostatic Agent
Use Treatment of leprosy and dermatitis herpetiformis (infections caused by *Mycobacterium leprae*); prophylaxis of toxoplasmosis in severely immunocompromised patients; alternative agent for *Pneumocystis carinii* pneumonia prophylaxis (given alone) and treatment (given with trimethoprim); may be useful in relapsing polychondritis, prophylaxis of malaria, inflammatory bowel disorders, leishmaniasis, rheumatic/connective tissue disorders, brown recluse spider bites
Pregnancy Risk Factor C
Contraindications Hypersensitivity to dapsone or any component of the formulation
Warnings/Precautions Use with caution in patients with severe anemia, G6PD, methemoglobin reductase or hemoglobin M deficiency; hypersensitivity to other sulfonamides; aplastic anemia, agranulocytosis and other severe blood dyscrasias have resulted in death; monitor carefully; serious dermatologic reactions (including toxic epidermal necrolysis) are rare but potential occurrences; sulfone reactions may also occur as potentially fatal hypersensitivity reactions; these, but not leprosy reactional states, require drug discontinuation
Adverse Reactions
>10%:
  Hematologic: Hemolytic anemia, methemoglobinemia with cyanosis
  Dermatologic: Skin rash
1% to 10%:
  Central nervous system: Reactional states
  Hematologic: Dose-related hemolysis,
<1% (Limited to important or life-threatening): Agranulocytosis, cholestatic jaundice, exfoliative dermatitis, hepatitis, leukopenia, peripheral neuropathy

Overdosage/Toxicology Symptoms include nausea, vomiting, confusion, hyperexcitability, seizures, cyanosis, hemolysis, methemoglobinemia, sulfhemoglobinemia, metabolic acidosis, hallucinations, and hepatitis. Following decontamination, methylene blue 1-2 mg/kg I.V. is the treatment of choice if MHb level is >15%; may repeat every 6-8 hours for 2-3 days if needed. If hemolysis is present, give I.V. fluids and alkalinize urine to prevent acute tubular necrosis.

Drug Interactions

Cytochrome P450 Effect: CYP2C9, 2E1, and 3A3/4 enzyme substrate

Increased Effect/Toxicity: Folic acid antagonists (methotrexate) may increase the risk of hematologic reactions of dapsone; probenecid decreases dapsone excretion; trimethoprim with dapsone may increase toxic effects of both drugs Dapsone levels may be increased by protease inhibitors (amprenavir, nelfinavir, ritonavir).

Decreased Effect: Para-aminobenzoic acid and rifampin levels are decreased when given with dapsone.

Ethanol/Nutrition/Herb Interactions Herb/Nutraceutical: St John's wort may decrease dapsone levels.

Stability Protect from light

Mechanism of Action Competitive antagonist of para-aminobenzoic acid (PABA) and prevents normal bacterial utilization of PABA for the synthesis of folic acid

Pharmacodynamics/Kinetics

Absorption: Well absorbed

Distribution: V_d: 1.5 L/kg; throughout total body water and present in all tissues, especially liver and kidney

Metabolism: Hepatic

Half-life elimination: 30 hours (range: 10-50 hours)

Excretion: Urine

Usual Dosage Oral:

Leprosy:

Children: 1-2 mg/kg/24 hours, up to a maximum of 100 mg/day

Adults: 50-100 mg/day for 3-10 years

Dermatitis herpetiformis: Adults: Start at 50 mg/day, increase to 300 mg/day, or higher to achieve full control, reduce dosage to minimum level as soon as possible

Pneumocystis carinii pneumonia:

Prophylaxis:

Children >1 month: 2 mg/kg/day once daily (maximum dose: 100 mg/day) or 4 mg/kg/dose once weekly (maximum dose: 200 mg)

Adults: 100 mg/day

Treatment: Adults: 100 mg/day in combination with trimethoprim (15-20 mg/kg/day) for 21 days

Dosing in renal impairment: No specific guidelines are available

Dietary Considerations Do not administer with antacids, alkaline foods, or drugs.

Monitoring Parameters Monitor patient for signs of jaundice and hemolysis; CBC weekly for first month, monthly for 6 months, and semiannually thereafter

Patient Information Frequent blood tests are required during early therapy; discontinue if rash develops and contact physician if persistent sore throat, fever, malaise, or fatigue occurs; may cause photosensitivity

Dosage Forms Tablet: 25 mg, 100 mg

Extemporaneous Preparations One report indicated that dapsone may not be well absorbed when administered to children as suspensions made from pulverized tablets

Mirochnick M, Clarke D, Brenn A, et al, "Low Serum Dapsone Concentrations in Children Receiving an Extemporaneously Prepared Oral Formulation," [Abstract Th B 365], APS-SPR, Baltimore, MD: 1992.

Jacobus Pharmaceutical Company (609) 921-7447 makes a 2 mg/mL proprietary liquid formulation available under an IND for the prophylaxis of *Pneumocystis carinii* pneumonia

♦ **Daraprim**® *see* Pyrimethamine *on page 1163*

Darbepoetin Alfa (dar be POE e tin AL fa)

U.S. Brand Names Aranesp™

Synonyms Erythropoiesis Stimulating Protein

Therapeutic Category Colony-Stimulating Factor; Growth Factor; Recombinant Human Erythropoietin

Use Treatment of anemia associated with chronic renal failure, including patients on dialysis (end-stage renal disease) and patients not on dialysis

Unlabeled/Investigational Use Treatment of anemia associated with chronic cancer

Pregnancy Risk Factor C

Pregnancy/Breast-Feeding Implications There are no adequate and well-controlled studies in pregnant women. Darbepoetin alfa should be used in a pregnant woman only if potential benefit justifies the potential risk to the fetus.

Contraindications Hypersensitivity to darbepoetin or any component of the formulation (including polysorbate 80 and/or albumin); uncontrolled hypertension

Warnings/Precautions Erythropoietic therapies may be associated with an increased risk of cardiovascular and/or neurologic events in chronic renal failure. Hemoglobin should be managed carefully; avoid increases >1 g/dL in any 2-week period, and do not exceed a target hemoglobin of 12 g/dL. It is recommended that the dose be decreased if the hemoglobin increase exceeds 1 g/dL in any 2-week period. Prior to and during therapy, iron stores must be evaluated. Supplemental iron is recommended in any patient with a serum ferritin <100 mcg/mL or serum transferrin saturation <20%.

Use with caution in patients with hypertension or with a history of seizures. Blood pressure and neurologic status should be carefully monitored during therapy. **Not** recommended for acute correction of severe anemia or as a substitute for transfusion. Consider discontinuing in patients who receive a renal transplant.

(Continued)

Darbepoetin Alfa *(Continued)*

Prior to treatment, correct or exclude deficiencies of vitamin B_{12} and/or folate, as well as other factors which may impair erythropoiesis (aluminum toxicity, inflammatory conditions, infections). Poor response should prompt evaluation of these potential factors, as well as possible malignant processes, occult blood loss, hemolysis, and/or bone marrow fibrosis.

Safety and efficacy in patients with underlying hematologic diseases have not been established, including porphyria, thalassemia, hemolytic anemia, and sickle cell disease. Safety and efficacy in pediatric patients have not been established.

Adverse Reactions Note: Frequency of adverse events cited may be, in part, a reflection of population in which the drug is used and/or associated with dialysis procedures.

>10%:

Cardiovascular: Hypertension (23%), hypotension (22%), peripheral edema (11%), arrhythmia (10%)

Central nervous system: Headache (16%)

Gastrointestinal: Diarrhea (16%), vomiting (15%), nausea (14%), abdominal pain (12%)

Neuromuscular & skeletal: Myalgia (21%), arthralgia (11%), limb pain (10%)

Respiratory: Upper respiratory infection (14%), dyspnea (12%), cough (10%)

Miscellaneous: Infection (27%)

1% to 10%:

Cardiovascular: Angina/chest pain (6% to 8%), fluid overload (6%), congestive heart failure (6%), myocardial infarction (2%)

Central nervous system: Fatigue (9%), fever (9%), dizziness (8%), seizure (1%), stroke (1%), transient ischemic attack (1%)

Dermatologic: Pruritus (8%)

Gastrointestinal: Constipation (5%)

Local: Injection site pain (7%)

Neuromuscular & skeletal: Back pain (8%), weakness (5%)

Respiratory: Bronchitis (6%)

Miscellaneous: Vascular access thrombosis (8%, annualized rate 0.22 events per patient year), vascular access infection (6%), influenza-like symptoms (6%), vascular access hemorrhage (6%)

Overdosage/Toxicology The maximum amount of darbepoetin has not been determined. However, cardiovascular and neurologic adverse events have been correlated to excessive and/or rapid rise in hemoglobin. Phlebotomy may be performed if clinically indicated.

Ethanol/Nutrition/Herb Interactions Ethanol: Should be avoided due to adverse effects on erythropoiesis.

Stability Store at 2°C to 8°C (36°F to 46°F). Do not freeze or shake. Protect from light. Do not dilute or administer with other solutions.

Mechanism of Action Induces erythropoiesis by stimulating the division and differentiation of committed erythroid progenitor cells; induces the release of reticulocytes from the bone marrow into the bloodstream, where they mature to erythrocytes. There is a dose response relationship with this effect. This results in an increase in reticulocyte counts followed by a rise in hematocrit and hemoglobin levels. When administered S.C. or I.V., darbepoetin's half-life is ~3 times that of epoetin alfa concentrations.

Pharmacodynamics/Kinetics

Onset of action: Increased hemoglobin levels not generally observed until 2-6 weeks after initiating treatment

Absorption: S.C.: Slow

Distribution: V_d: 0.06 L/kg

Bioavailability: S.C.: ~37% (range: 30% to 50%)

Half-life elimination: Terminal: I.V.: 21 hours, S.C.: 49 hours; **Note:** Half-life is ~3 times as long as epoetin alfa

Time to peak: S.C.: 34 hours (range: 24-72 hours)

Usual Dosage I.V., S.C.:

Correction of anemia:

Initial: 0.45 mcg/kg once weekly; dosage should be titrated to limit increases in hemoglobin to <1 g/dL over any 2-week interval, with a target concentration of <12 g/dL.

Maintenance: Titrated to hematologic response. Some patients may require doses <0.45 mcg/kg once weekly. Selected patients may be managed by administering S.C. doses every 2 weeks.

Conversion from epoetin alfa to darbepoetin alfa: Initial: Estimate dosage based on weekly epoetin alfa dosage; see table:

Conversion From Epoetin Alfa to Darbepoetin Alfa

Previous Dosage of Epoetin Alfa (units/week)	Darbopoetin Alfa Dosage (mcg/week)
<2500	6.25
2500-4999	12.5
5000-10,999	25
11,000-17,999	40
18,000-33,999	60
34,000-89,999	100
≥90,000	200

Note: In patients receiving epoetin alfa 2-3 times per week, darbepoetin alfa is administered once weekly. In patients receiving epoetin alfa once weekly, darbepoetin alfa is administered once every 2 weeks.

Dosage adjustment: It is recommended that the dosage of darbepoetin should be decreased if the hemoglobin increases >1 g/dL in any 2-week period. If the increase in hemoglobin is <1 g/dL over 4 weeks and iron stores are adequate, increase by ~25% of the previous dose. Further increases may be made at 4-week intervals. If the hemoglobin is increasing and approaches the target value of 12 g/dL, decrease weekly dosage by ~25%. If hemoglobin exceeds the target value, hold dose until hemoglobin is <12 g/dL and reduce dose by 25%.

Dosage adjustment in renal impairment: Dosage requirements for patients with chronic renal failure who do not require dialysis may be lower than in dialysis patients. Monitor patients closely during the time period in which a dialysis regimen is initiated, dosage requirement may increase.

Dietary Considerations Supplemental iron intake may be required in patients with low iron stores.

Administration May be administered by S.C. or I.V. injection. Do not shake. Do not dilute or administer in conjunction with other drug solutions. Discard any unused portion of the vial. Discontinue immediately if signs/symptoms of anaphylaxis occur.

Monitoring Parameters Hemoglobin (weekly); prior to and during therapy, iron stores must be evaluated (supplemental iron is recommended in any patient with a serum ferritin <100 mcg/mL or serum transferrin saturation <20%)

Patient Information You will require frequent blood tests to determine appropriate dosage. Do not take other medications, vitamin or iron supplements, or make significant changes in your diet without consulting prescriber. Report signs or symptoms of edema (eg, swollen extremities, difficulty breathing, rapid weight gain), onset of severe headache, acute back pain, chest pain, or muscular tremors or seizure activity. Be careful to check blood pressure regularly. Inform prescriber if you are or intend to be pregnant. Consult prescriber if breastfeeding.

Additional Information Due to the delayed onset of erythropoiesis, darbepoetin is of no value in the acute treatment of anemia. Emergency/stat orders for darbepoetin are inappropriate.

Dosage Forms
Injection, with polysorbate 80 0.05 mg/mL [preservative free, single-dose vial]: 25 mcg/mL (1 mL); 40 mcg/mL (1 mL); 60 mcg/mL (1 mL); 100 mcg/mL (1 mL); 200 mcg/mL (1 mL)
Injection, with human albumin 2.5 mg/mL [preservative free, single-dose vial]: 25 mcg/mL (1 mL); 40 mcg/mL (1 mL); 60 mcg/mL (1 mL); 100 mcg/mL (1 mL); 200 mcg/mL (1 mL)

♦ **Darvocet-N® 50** *see* Propoxyphene and Acetaminophen *on page 1148*
♦ **Darvocet-N® 100** *see* Propoxyphene and Acetaminophen *on page 1148*
♦ **Darvon®** *see* Propoxyphene *on page 1147*
♦ **Darvon® Compound-65 Pulvules®** *see* Propoxyphene and Aspirin *on page 1148*
♦ **Darvon-N®** *see* Propoxyphene *on page 1147*
♦ **Daunomycin** *see* DAUNOrubicin Hydrochloride *on page 368*

DAUNOrubicin Citrate (Liposomal)
(daw noe ROO bi sin SI trate lip po SOE mal)

U.S. Brand Names DaunoXome®

Therapeutic Category Antineoplastic Agent, Anthracycline; Antineoplastic Agent, Antibiotic

Use First-line cytotoxic therapy for advanced HIV-associated Kaposi's sarcoma

Pregnancy Risk Factor D

Contraindications Hypersensitivity to daunorubicin or any component of the formulation; pregnancy

Warnings/Precautions The U.S. Food and Drug Administration (FDA) currently recommends that procedures for proper handling and disposal of antineoplastic agents be considered.

The primary toxicity is myelosuppression, especially off the granulocytic series, which may be severe, with much less marked effects on platelets and erythroid series. Potential cardiac toxicity, particularly in patients who have received prior anthracyclines or who have pre-existing cardiac disease, may occur. Refer to Daunorubicin monograph.

Although grade 3-4 injection site inflammation has been reported in patients treated with the liposomal daunorubicin, no instances of local tissue necrosis were observed with extravasation. However, refer to daunorubicin monograph and avoid extravasation.

Reduce dosage in patients with impaired hepatic function. Hyperuricemia can be induced secondary to rapid lysis of leukemic cells. As a precaution, administer allopurinol prior to initiating antileukemic therapy.

Adverse Reactions
>10%:
Dermatologic: Alopecia (reversible)
Gastrointestinal: Mild nausea or vomiting occurs in 50% of patients within the first 24 hours; esophagitis or stomatitis may occur 3-7 days after administration, but is not as severe as that caused by doxorubicin
Time course for nausea/vomiting: Onset: 1-3 hours; Duration: 4-24 hours
Genitourinary: Discoloration of urine (red)
1% to 10%:
Cardiovascular: Congestive heart failure; maximum lifetime dose: Refer to Warnings/Precautions
Dermatologic: Darkening or redness of skin
Endocrine & metabolic: Hyperuricemia
Gastrointestinal: GI ulceration, diarrhea
Hematologic: Myelosuppressive: Dose-limiting toxicity; occurs in all patients; leukopenia is more significant than thrombocytopenia
WBC: Severe
Platelets: Severe
Onset (days): 7
Nadir (days): 14
Recovery (days): 21-28
Local: **Vesicant chemotherapy**
<1% (Limited to important or life-threatening): Elevation in serum bilirubin, AST, and alkaline phosphatase; myocarditis; pericarditis
(Continued)

DAUNOrubicin Citrate (Liposomal) *(Continued)*

Overdosage/Toxicology Symptoms of acute overdose are increased severity of the observed dose-limiting toxicities of therapeutic doses, such as myelosuppression (especially granulocytopenia), fatigue, nausea, and vomiting. Treatment is symptomatic.

Drug Interactions

Decreased Effect: Patients may experience impaired immune response to vaccines; possible infection after administration of live vaccines in patients receiving immunosuppressants.

Ethanol/Nutrition/Herb Interactions Ethanol: Avoid ethanol (due to GI irritation).

Stability Store intact vials under refrigeration (2°C to 8°C/36°F to 46°F). Reconstitute liposomal daunorubicin 1:1 with 5% dextrose injection before administration. Store reconstituted solution for a maximum of 6 hours. Do not freeze and protect from light. Do not use an in-line filter for intravenous infusion.

Mechanism of Action Liposomes have been shown to penetrate solid tumors more effectively, possibly because of their small size and longer circulation time. Once in tissues, daunorubicin is released. Daunorubicin inhibits DNA and RNA synthesis by intercalation between DNA base pairs and by steric obstruction; and intercalates at points of local uncoiling of the double helix. Although the exact mechanism is unclear, it appears that direct binding to DNA (intercalation) and inhibition of DNA repair (topoisomerase II inhibition) result in blockade of DNA and RNA synthesis and fragmentation of DNA.

Pharmacodynamics/Kinetics

Distribution: V_d: 3-6.4 L

Metabolism: Similar to daunorubicin, but metabolite plasma levels are low

Half-life elimination: Distribution: 4.4 hours; Terminal: 3-5 hours

Excretion: Primarily feces; some urine

Clearance, plasma: 17.3 mL/minute

Usual Dosage Refer to individual protocols. Adults: I.V.:

20-40 mg/m^2 every 2 weeks

100 mg/m^2 every 3 weeks

Dosing adjustment in renal impairment: Serum creatinine >3 mg/dL: Administer 50% of normal dose

Dosing adjustment in hepatic impairment:

Bilirubin 1.2-3 mg/dL: Administer 75% of normal dose

Bilirubin >3 mg/dL: Administer 50% of normal dose

Administration Infuse over 1 hour; do not mix with other drugs. **Extravasation management:** Infiltration can cause severe inflammation, tissue necrosis, and ulceration. If the drug is infiltrated, consult institutional policy, apply ice to the area, and elevate the limb.

Monitoring Parameters Observe patient closely and monitor chemical and laboratory tests extensively. Evaluate cardiac, renal, and hepatic function prior to each course of treatment. Repeat blood counts prior to each dose and withhold if the absolute granulocyte count is <750 cells/mm^3. Monitor serum uric acid levels.

Dosage Forms Injection: 2 mg/mL (equivalent to 50 mg daunorubicin base) (1 mL, 4 mL, 10 mL unit packs)

DAUNOrubicin Hydrochloride (daw noe ROO bi sin hye droe KLOR ide)

U.S. Brand Names Cerubidine®

Canadian Brand Names Cerubidine®

Synonyms Daunomycin; DNR; Rubidomycin Hydrochloride

Therapeutic Category Antineoplastic Agent, Anthracycline; Antineoplastic Agent, Antibiotic; Antineoplastic Agent, Vesicant; Vesicant

Use Treatment of acute lymphocytic (ALL) and nonlymphocytic (ANLL) leukemias

Pregnancy Risk Factor D

Pregnancy/Breast-Feeding Implications May cause fetal harm when administered to a pregnant woman. Animal studies have shown an increased incidence of fetal abnormalities. Excretion in breast milk is unknown; breast-feeding is not recommended.

Contraindications Hypersensitivity to daunorubicin or any component of the formulation; congestive heart failure or arrhythmias; previous therapy with high cumulative doses of daunorubicin and/or doxorubicin; pre-existing bone marrow suppression; pregnancy

Warnings/Precautions The U.S. Food and Drug Administration (FDA) currently recommends that procedures for proper handling and disposal of antineoplastic agents be considered. I.V. use only, severe local tissue necrosis will result if extravasation occurs; reduce dose in patients with impaired hepatic, renal, or biliary function; severe myelosuppression is possible when used in therapeutic doses. Total cumulative dose should take into account previous or concomitant treatment with cardiotoxic agents or irradiation of chest.

Irreversible myocardial toxicity may occur as total dosage approaches:

550 mg/m^2 in adults

400 mg/m^2 in patients receiving chest radiation

300 mg/m^2 in children >2 years of age or

10 mg/kg in children <2 years; this may occur during therapy or several months after therapy

Adverse Reactions

>10%:

Dermatologic: Alopecia (reversible)

Gastrointestinal: Mild nausea or vomiting occurs in 50% of patients within the first 24 hours; esophagitis or stomatitis may occur 3-7 days after administration, but is not as severe as that caused by doxorubicin

Time course for nausea/vomiting: Onset: 1-3 hours; Duration: 4-24 hours

Genitourinary: Discoloration of urine (red)

1% to 10%:

Cardiovascular: Congestive heart failure; maximum lifetime dose: Refer to Warnings/Precautions

Dermatologic: Darkening or redness of skin

Endocrine & metabolic: Hyperuricemia

Gastrointestinal: GI ulceration, diarrhea

Hematologic: Myelosuppressive: Dose-limiting toxicity; occurs in all patients; leukopenia is more significant than thrombocytopenia

  WBC: Severe

  Platelets: Severe

  Onset (days): 7

  Nadir (days): 14

  Recovery (days): 21-28

Local: **Vesicant chemotherapy**

<1% (Limited to important or life-threatening): Elevation in serum bilirubin, AST, and alkaline phosphatase; myocarditis; pericarditis

Overdosage/Toxicology Symptoms include myelosuppression, nausea, vomiting, and stomatitis. There are no known antidotes. Treatment is primarily symptomatic and supportive.

Drug Interactions

Decreased Effect: Patients may experience impaired immune response to vaccines; possible infection after administration of live vaccines in patients receiving immunosuppressants.

Ethanol/Nutrition/Herb Interactions Ethanol: Avoid ethanol (due to GI irritation).

Stability

Store intact vials at room temperature and protect from light

Dilute vials with 4 mL SWI for a final concentration of 5 mg/mL; reconstituted solution is stable for 4 days at 15°C to 25°C

  Protect from fluorescent light to decrease photo-inactivation after storage in solution for several days; protect from direct sunlight

  Decomposed drug turns purple

  For I.V. push administration, desired dose is withdrawn into a syringe containing 10-15 mL NS

  Further dilution in D$_5$W, LR, or NS is stable for 24 hours at room temperature (25°C) and up to 4 weeks if protected from light

  Incompatible with dexamethasone, heparin, sodium bicarbonate, 5-FU

Standard I.V. dilution:

  I.V. push: Dose/syringe (initial concentration is 5 mg/mL; however, qs to 10-15 mL with NS) . Maximum syringe size for IVP is a 30 mL syringe and syringe should be <75% full

  IVPB: Dose/50-100 mL NS or D$_5$W

  Stable for 24 hours at room temperature (25°C)

Mechanism of Action Inhibition of DNA and RNA synthesis, by intercalating between DNA base pairs and by steric obstruction; is not cell cycle-specific for the S phase of cell division; daunomycin is preferred over doxorubicin for the treatment of ANLL because of its dose-limiting toxicity (myelosuppression) is not of concern in the therapy of this disease; has less mucositis associated with its use

Pharmacodynamics/Kinetics

Distribution: Many body tissues, particularly the liver, kidneys, lung, spleen, and heart; not into CNS; crosses placenta; V$_d$: 40 L/kg

Metabolism: Primarily hepatic to daunorubicinol (active)

Half-life elimination: Distribution: 2 minutes; Elimination: 14-20 hours; Terminal: 18.5 hours; Daunorubicinol plasma half-life: 24-48 hours

Excretion: Feces (40%); urine (~25% as unchanged drug and metabolites)

Usual Dosage I.V. (refer to individual protocols):

Children:

  ALL combination therapy: Remission induction: 25-45 mg/m^2 on day 1 every week for 4 cycles **or** 30-45 mg/m^2/day for 3 days

  AML combination therapy: Induction: I.V. continuous infusion: 30-60 mg/m^2/day on days 1-3 of cycle

  Note: In children <2 years or <0.5 m^2, daunorubicin should be based on weight - mg/kg: 1 mg/kg per protocol with frequency dependent on regimen employed

  Cumulative dose should not exceed 300 mg/m^2 in children >2 years or 10 mg/kg in children <2 years

Adults:

  Range: 30-60 mg/m^2/day for 3-5 days, repeat dose in 3-4 weeks

  AML: Single agent induction: 60 mg/m^2/day for 3 days; repeat every 3-4 weeks

  AML: Combination therapy induction: 45 mg/m^2/day for 3 days of the first course of induction therapy; subsequent courses: Every day for 2 days

  ALL combination therapy: 45 mg/m^2/day for 3 days

  Cumulative dose should not exceed 400-600 mg/m^2

Dosing adjustment in renal impairment:

Cl$_{cr}$ <10 mL/minute: Administer 75% of normal dose

S$_{cr}$ >3 mg/dL: Administer 50% of normal dose

Dosing adjustment in hepatic impairment:

Serum bilirubin 1.2-3 mg/dL or AST 60-180 int. units: Reduce dose to 75%

Serum bilirubin 3.1-5 mg/dL or AST >180 int. units: Reduce dose to 50%

Serum bilirubin >5 mg/dL: Omit use

Administration Administer IVP over 1-5 minutes into the tubing of a rapidly infusing I.V. solution of D$_5$W or NS; daunorubicin has also been diluted in 100 mL of D$_5$W or NS and infused over 15-30 minutes

Avoid extravasation, can cause severe tissue damage; flush with 5-10 mL of I.V. solution before and after drug administration

Monitoring Parameters CBC with differential and platelet count, liver function test, EKG, ventricular ejection fraction, renal function test

Patient Information This medication can only be administered I.V. During therapy, do not use alcohol, aspirin-containing products, and/or OTC medications without consulting prescriber. It is important to maintain adequate nutrition and hydration (2-3 L/day of fluids unless instructed to restrict fluid intake) during therapy; frequent small meals may help. You may experience nausea or vomiting (frequent small meals, frequent mouth care, sucking lozenges, or chewing gum may help). You may experience loss of hair (reversible); you will be more (Continued)

DAUNOrubicin Hydrochloride (Continued)

susceptible to infection (avoid crowds and exposure to infection as much as possible). Urine may turn red (normal). Yogurt or buttermilk may help reduce diarrhea (if unresolved, contact prescriber for medication relief). Report fever, chills, unusual bruising or bleeding, signs of infection, abdominal pain or blood in stools, excessive fatigue, yellowing of eyes or skin, swelling of extremities, difficulty breathing, or unresolved diarrhea. Contraceptive measures are recommended during therapy.

Nursing Implications Daunorubicin is a vesicant and should never be administered I.M. or S.C.

Extravasation management:

Apply ice immediately for 30-60 minutes; then alternate off/on every 15 minutes for one day Topical cooling may be achieved using ice packs or cooling pad with circulating ice water; cooling of site for 24 hours as tolerated by the patient. Elevate and rest extremity 24-48 hours, then resume normal activity as tolerated. Application of cold inhibits vesicant's cytotoxicity.

Application of heat or sodium bicarbonate can be harmful and is contraindicated

If pain, erythema, and/or swelling persist beyond 48 hours, refer patient immediately to plastic surgeon for consultation and possible debridement

Dosage Forms Powder for injection, lyophilized: 5 mg/mL (4 mL, 10 mL)

* **DaunoXome®** see DAUNOrubicin Citrate (Liposomal) on page 367
* **1-Day™ [OTC]** see Tioconazole on page 1337
* **Daypro™** see Oxaprozin on page 1019
* **DC 240® Softgels® [OTC]** see Docusate on page 430
* **DCF** see Pentostatin on page 1061
* **DDAVP®** see Desmopressin on page 378
* **ddC** see Zalcitabine on page 1431
* **ddI** see Didanosine on page 397
* **1-Deamino-8-D-Arginine Vasopressin** see Desmopressin on page 378
* **Debrisan® [OTC]** see Dextranomer on page 387
* **Debrox® Otic [OTC]** see Carbamide Peroxide on page 224
* **Decadron®** see Dexamethasone on page 380
* **Decadron®-LA** see Dexamethasone on page 380
* **Decadron® Phosphate** see Dexamethasone on page 380
* **Deca-Durabolin®** see Nandrolone on page 956
* **Decaject®** see Dexamethasone on page 380
* **Decaject-LA®** see Dexamethasone on page 380
* **Decaspray®** see Dexamethasone on page 380
* **Declomycin®** see Demeclocycline on page 373
* **Decofed® [OTC]** see Pseudoephedrine on page 1155
* **Decohistine® DH** see Chlorpheniramine, Pseudoephedrine, and Codeine on page 281
* **Decohistine® Expectorant** see Guaifenesin, Pseudoephedrine, and Codeine on page 648
* **Deconamine® [OTC]** see Chlorpheniramine and Pseudoephedrine on page 279
* **Deconamine® SR [OTC]** see Chlorpheniramine and Pseudoephedrine on page 279
* **Deconsal® II** see Guaifenesin and Pseudoephedrine on page 647
* **Deconsal® Sprinkle®** see Guaifenesin and Phenylephrine on page 647
* **Defen-LA®** see Guaifenesin and Pseudoephedrine on page 647

Deferoxamine (de fer OKS a meen)

U.S. Brand Names Desferal®

Canadian Brand Names Desferal®

Synonyms Deferoxamine Mesylate

Therapeutic Category Antidote, Aluminum Toxicity; Antidote, Iron Toxicity

Use Acute iron intoxication when serum iron is >450-500 µg/dL or when clinical signs of significant iron toxicity exist; chronic iron overload secondary to multiple transfusions; diagnostic test for iron overload; iron overload secondary to congenital anemias; hemochromatosis; removal of corneal rust rings following surgical removal of foreign bodies

Unlabeled/Investigational Use Investigational: Treatment of aluminum accumulation in renal failure; treatment of aluminum-induced bone disease

Pregnancy Risk Factor C

Contraindications Hypersensitivity to deferoxamine or any component of the formulation; patients with anuria, primary hemochromatosis

Warnings/Precautions Use with caution in patients with severe renal disease, pyelonephritis; may increase susceptibility to Yersinia enterocolitica. Ocular and auditory disturbances, as well as growth retardation (children only), have been reported following prolonged administration. Has been associated with adult respiratory distress syndrome (ARDS) following excessively high-dose treatment of acute intoxication.

Adverse Reactions Frequency not defined.

Cardiovascular: Flushing, hypotension, tachycardia, shock, edema

Central nervous system: Convulsions, fever, dizziness, neuropathy, paresthesia, seizures, exacerbation of aluminum-related encephalopathy (dialysis), coma, aphasia, agitation

Dermatologic: Erythema, urticaria, pruritus, rash, cutaneous wheal formation

Endocrine & metabolic: Hypocalcemia

Gastrointestinal: Abdominal discomfort, diarrhea

Genitourinary: Dysuria

Hematologic: Thrombocytopenia, leukopenia

Local: Pain and induration at injection site

Neuromuscular & skeletal: Leg cramps

Ocular: Blurred vision, visual loss, scotoma, visual field defects, impaired vision, optic neuritis, cataracts, retinal pigmentary abnormalities

Otic: Hearing loss, tinnitus
Renal: Renal impairment, acute renal failure
Respiratory: Acute respiratory distress syndrome (with dyspnea, cyanosis)
Miscellaneous: Anaphylaxis

Overdosage/Toxicology Symptoms include hypotension, blurring of vision, diarrhea, leg cramps, and tachycardia. Treatment is symptomatic and supportive.

Drug Interactions
Increased Effect/Toxicity: May cause loss of consciousness when administered with prochlorperazine. Concomitant treatment with vitamin C (>500 mg/day) has been associated with cardiac impairment.

Stability Protect from light; reconstituted solutions (sterile water) may be stored at room temperature for 7 days

Mechanism of Action Complexes with trivalent ions (ferric ions) to form ferrioxamine, which are removed by the kidneys

Pharmacodynamics/Kinetics
Absorption: Oral: <15%
Metabolism: Hepatic to ferrioxamine
Half-life elimination: Parent drug: 6.1 hours; Ferrioxamine: 5.8 hours
Excretion: Urine (as unchanged drug and metabolites)

Usual Dosage
Children and Adults:
Acute iron toxicity: I.V. route is used when severe toxicity is evidenced by systemic symptoms (coma, shock, metabolic acidosis, or severe gastrointestinal bleeding) or potentially severe intoxications (serum iron level >500 µg/dL). When severe symptoms are not present, the I.M. route may be preferred; however, the use of deferoxamine in situations where the serum iron concentration is <500 µg/dL or when severe toxicity is not evident is a subject of some clinical debate.
Dose: For the first 1000 mg, infuse at 15 mg/kg/hour (although rates up to 40-50 mg/kg/hour have been given in patients with massive iron intoxication); may be followed by 500 mg every 4 hours for up to 2 doses; subsequent doses of 500 mg have been administered every 4-12 hours
Maximum recommended dose: 6 g/day (however, doses as high as 16-37 g have been administered)
Children:
Chronic iron overload: S.C.: 20-40 mg/kg/day over 8-12 hours (via a portable, controlled infusion device)
Aluminum-induced bone disease: 20-40 mg/kg every hemodialysis treatment, frequency dependent on clinical status of the patient
Adults: Chronic iron overload:
I.M.: 500-1000 mg/day; in addition, 2000 mg should be given with each unit of blood transfused (administer separately from blood)
I.V.: 2 g after each unit of blood infusion at 15 mg/kg/hour
S.C.: 1-2 g every day over 8-24 hours
Dosing adjustment in renal impairment: Cl_{cr} <10 mL/minute: Administer 50% of dose
Has been used investigationally as a single 40 mg/kg I.V. dose over 2 hours, to promote mobilization of aluminum from tissue stores as an aid in the diagnosis of aluminum-associated osteodystrophy

Administration Administer I.M., slow S.C., or I.V. infusion
I.M.: I.M. administration is preferred in patients not in shock. Add 2 mL sterile water to 500 mg vial. For I.M. or S.C. administration, no further dilution is required.
I.V.: The manufacturer states that the I.M. route is preferred; however, the I.V. route is generally preferred in patients with severe toxicity (ie, patients in shock). Urticaria, hypotension, and shock have occurred following rapid I.V. administration; maximum I.V. rate: 15 mg/kg/hour for first 1000 mg; subsequent dosing, if needed, should not exceed 125 mg/hour

Monitoring Parameters Serum iron, total iron-binding capacity; ophthalmologic exam (fundoscopy, slit-lamp exam) and audiometry with chronic therapy

Patient Information May turn urine pink; blood and urine tests are necessary to follow therapy

Nursing Implications Iron chelate colors urine salmon pink

Dosage Forms Powder for injection, as mesylate: 500 mg, 2 g

♦ **Deferoxamine Mesylate** *see Deferoxamine on page 370*
♦ **Dehydral® (Can)** *see Methenamine on page 881*
♦ **Delatestryl®** *see Testosterone on page 1302*

Delavirdine (de la VIR deen)
Related Information
Antiretroviral Agents Comparison *on page 1488*
Antiretroviral Therapy for HIV Infection *on page 1595*
Management of Healthcare Worker Exposures to HIV, HBV, HCV *on page 1555*
U.S. Brand Names Rescriptor®
Canadian Brand Names Rescriptor®
Synonyms U-90152S
Therapeutic Category Antiretroviral Agent, Non-nucleoside Reverse Transcriptase Inhibitor (NNRTI)
Use Treatment of HIV-1 infection in combination with at least two additional antiretroviral agents
Pregnancy Risk Factor C
Pregnancy/Breast-Feeding Implications It is not known if delavirdine crosses the human placenta. Health professionals are encouraged to contact the antiretroviral pregnancy registry to monitor outcomes of pregnant women exposed to antiretroviral medications (1-800-258-4263).
(Continued)

Delavirdine (Continued)

Contraindications Hypersensitivity to delavirdine or any component of the formulation; concurrent use of alprazolam, astemizole, cisapride, ergot alkaloids, midazolam, pimozide, or triazolam

Warnings/Precautions Avoid use with benzodiazepines, cisapride, clarithromycin, dapsone, enzyme-inducing anticonvulsants (carbamazepine, phenytoin, phenobarbital, rifampin, rifabutin, St John's wort, or terfenadine); may lead to loss of efficacy or development of resistance. Concurrent use of lovastatin or simvastatin should be avoided (use caution with other statins). Use with amphetamines, antacids, antiarrhythmics, benzodiazepines (alprazolam, midazolam, and triazolam are contraindicated), clarithromycin, dihydropyridine, calcium channel blockers, dapsone, immunosuppressants, methadone, oral contraceptives, or sildenafil.

Use with caution in patients with hepatic or renal dysfunction; due to rapid emergence of resistance, delavirdine should not be used as monotherapy; cross-resistance may be conferred to other non-nucleoside reverse transcriptase inhibitors. Long-term effects of delavirdine are not known. Safety and efficacy have not been established in children. Rash, which occurs frequently, may require discontinuation of therapy; usually occurs within 1-3 weeks and lasts <2 weeks. Most patients may resume therapy following a treatment interruption.

Adverse Reactions

>10%: Dermatologic: Rash (3.2% required discontinuation)

1% to 10%:

Central nervous system: Headache, fatigue

Dermatologic: Pruritus

Gastrointestinal: Nausea, diarrhea, vomiting

Metabolic: Increased ALT (SGPT), increased AST (SGOT)

<1% (Limited to important or life-threatening): Acute renal failure, allergic reaction, alopecia, angioedema, ataxia, chest pain, confusion, dermal leukocytoblastic vasculitis, desquamation, dyspnea, eosinophilia, epistaxis, erythema multiforme, ethanol intolerance, granulocytosis, hallucination, hematuria, hemolytic anemia, hepatic failure, hepatitis (nonspecific), neuropathy, neutropenia, nystagmus, pancytopenia, paralysis, paranoid symptoms, postural hypotension, proteinuria, renal calculi, rhabdomyolysis, Stevens-Johnson syndrome, syncope, thrombocytopenia, vertigo, vesiculobullous rash

Overdosage/Toxicology Human reports of overdose with delavirdine are not available. GI decontamination and supportive measures are recommended, dialysis is unlikely to be of benefit in removing the drug since it is extensively metabolized by the liver and is highly protein bound.

Drug Interactions

Cytochrome P450 Effect: CYP2D6 and 3A3/4 enzyme substrate; CYP2D6 and 3A3/4 enzyme inhibitor

Increased Effect/Toxicity: Delavirdine concentrations may be increased by clarithromycin, ketoconazole, and fluoxetine. Delavirdine increases plasma concentrations of alprazolam, amiodarone, amphetamines, amprenavir, astemizole, bepridil, calcium channel blockers (dihydropyridine-type), cisapride, clarithromycin, dapsone, dexamethasone, ergot alkaloids, flecainide, HMG-CoA reductase inhibitors, indinavir, methadone, midazolam, pimozide, propafenone, quinidine, rifabutin, saquinavir, sildenafil, terfenadine, triazolam, and warfarin.

Decreased Effect: Decreased plasma concentrations of delavirdine with carbamazepine, dexamethasone, phenobarbital, phenytoin, rifabutin, rifampin, didanosine, and saquinavir. Decreased absorption of delavirdine with antacids, histamine-2 receptor antagonists, proton pump inhibitors (omeprazole, lansoprazole), and didanosine. Delavirdine decreases plasma concentrations of didanosine.

Ethanol/Nutrition/Herb Interactions Herb/Nutraceutical: Delavirdine serum concentration may be decreased by St John's wort; avoid concurrent use.

Mechanism of Action Delavirdine binds directly to reverse transcriptase, blocking RNA-dependent and DNA-dependent DNA polymerase activities

Pharmacodynamics/Kinetics

Absorption: Rapid

Distribution: Low concentration in saliva and semen; CSF 0.4% concurrent plasma concentration

Protein binding: ~98%, primarily albumin

Metabolism: Hepatic via CYP3A3/4 and 2D6 (**Note:** May reduce CYP3A activity and inhibit its own metabolism.)

Bioavailability: 85%

Half-life elimination: 2-11 hours

Time to peak, plasma: 1 hour

Excretion: Urine (51%, <5% as unchanged drug); feces (44%); nonlinear kinetics exhibited

Usual Dosage Adults: Oral: 400 mg 3 times/day

Dietary Considerations May be taken without regard to food.

Administration Patients with achlorhydria should take the drug with an acidic beverage; antacids and delavirdine should be separated by 1 hour

Monitoring Parameters Liver function tests if administered with saquinavir

Patient Information Stay under the care of a physician when using delavirdine; notify your physician if a rash occurs or symptoms of rash with fever, blistering, oral lesions, conjunctivitis, swelling, or muscle/joint pain. Consult pharmacist or physician prior to taking any other medications (including over-the-counter medications and herbal products) due to the potential for drug interactions.

Additional Information Potential compliance problems, frequency of administration, and adverse effects should be discussed with patients before initiating therapy to help prevent the emergence of resistance.

Dosage Forms Tablet: 100 mg, 200 mg

Extemporaneous Preparations A dispersion of delavirdine may be prepared by adding 4 tablets to at least 3 oz of water; allow to stand for a few minutes and stir until uniform dispersion; drink immediately; rinse glass and mouth following ingestion to ensure total dose administered

- **Delcort**® *see* Hydrocortisone *on page 682*
- **Delestrogen**® *see* Estradiol *on page 491*
- **Delta-Cortef**® *see* PrednisoLONE *on page 1122*
- **Deltacortisone** *see* PredniSONE *on page 1124*
- **Deltadehydrocortisone** *see* PredniSONE *on page 1124*
- **Deltahydrocortisone** *see* PrednisoLONE *on page 1122*
- **Deltasone**® *see* PredniSONE *on page 1124*
- **Delta-Tritex**® *see* Triamcinolone *on page 1366*
- **Demadex**® *see* Torsemide *on page 1352*

Demecarium (dem e KARE ee um)

Related Information
Glaucoma Drug Therapy Comparison *on page 1499*
U.S. Brand Names Humorsol®
Canadian Brand Names Humorsol®
Synonyms Demecarium Bromide
Therapeutic Category Cholinergic Agent, Ophthalmic; Ophthalmic Agent, Miotic
Use Management of chronic simple glaucoma, chronic and acute angle-closure glaucoma; strabismus
Pregnancy Risk Factor C
Usual Dosage Children/Adults: Ophthalmic:
Glaucoma: Instill 1 drop into eyes twice weekly to a maximum dosage of 1 or 2 drops twice daily for up to 4 months
Strabismus:
Diagnosis: Instill 1 drop daily for 2 weeks, then 1 drop every 2 days for 2-3 weeks. If eyes become straighter, an accommodative factor is demonstrated.
Therapy: Instill not more than 1 drop at a time in both eyes every day for 2-3 weeks. Then reduce dosage to 1 drop every other day for 3-4 weeks and re-evaluate. Continue at 1 drop every 2 days to 1 drop twice a week and evaluate the patient's condition every 4-12 weeks. If improvement continues, reduce dose to 1 drop once a week and eventually off of medication. Discontinue therapy after 4 months if control of the condition still requires 1 drop every 2 days.
Additional Information Complete prescribing information for this medication should be consulted for additional detail.
Dosage Forms Solution, ophthalmic, as bromide: 0.125% (5 mL); 0.25% (5 mL)

- **Demecarium Bromide** *see* Demecarium *on page 373*

Demeclocycline (dem e kloe SYE kleen)

U.S. Brand Names Declomycin®
Canadian Brand Names Declomycin®
Synonyms Demeclocycline Hydrochloride; Demethylchlortetracycline
Therapeutic Category Antibiotic, Tetracycline Derivative
Use Treatment of susceptible bacterial infections (acne, gonorrhea, pertussis and urinary tract infections) caused by both gram-negative and gram-positive organisms; used when penicillin is contraindicated (other agents are preferred)
Unlabeled/Investigational Use Treatment of chronic syndrome of inappropriate secretion of antidiuretic hormone (SIADH)
Pregnancy Risk Factor D
Contraindications Hypersensitivity to demeclocycline, tetracyclines, or any component of the formulation; pregnancy
Warnings/Precautions Do not administer to children <8 years of age; photosensitivity reactions occur frequently with this drug, avoid prolonged exposure to sunlight, do not use tanning equipment
Adverse Reactions
1% to 10%:
Dermatologic: Photosensitivity
Gastrointestinal: Nausea, diarrhea
<1%: Pericarditis, increased intracranial pressure, bulging fontanels in infants, dermatologic effects, pruritus, exfoliative dermatitis, diabetes insipidus syndrome, vomiting, esophagitis, anorexia, abdominal cramps, paresthesia, acute renal failure, azotemia, superinfections, anaphylaxis, pigmentation of nails
Overdosage/Toxicology Symptoms include diabetes insipidus, nausea, anorexia, and diarrhea. Following GI decontamination, treatment is supportive.
Drug Interactions
Increased Effect/Toxicity: Increased effect of warfarin, digoxin when taken with demeclocycline.
Decreased Effect: Decreased effect with antacids (aluminum, calcium, zinc, or magnesium), bismuth salts, sodium bicarbonate, barbiturates, carbamazepine, and hydantoins. Decreased effect of oral contraceptives, penicillins.
Ethanol/Nutrition/Herb Interactions
Food: Demeclocycline serum levels may be decreased if taken with food.
Herb/Nutraceutical: Avoid dong quai, St John's wort (may also cause photosensitization).
Stability Tetracyclines form toxic products when outdated or when exposed to light, heat, or humidity (Fanconi-like syndrome)
Mechanism of Action Inhibits protein synthesis by binding with the 30S and possibly the 50S ribosomal subunit(s) of susceptible bacteria; may also cause alterations in the cytoplasmic membrane; inhibits the action of ADH in patients with chronic SIADH
Pharmacodynamics/Kinetics
Onset of action: SIADH: Several days
(Continued)

Demeclocycline *(Continued)*

Absorption: ~50% to 80%; food and dairy products reduce absorption
Protein binding: 41% to 50%
Metabolism: Hepatic (small amounts) to inactive metabolites; enterohepatically recycled
Half-life elimination: Reduced renal function: 10-17 hours
Time to peak, serum: 3-6 hours
Excretion: Urine (42% to 50% as unchanged drug)

Usual Dosage Oral:
Children ≥8 years: 8-12 mg/kg/day divided every 6-12 hours
Adults: 150 mg 4 times/day or 300 mg twice daily
Uncomplicated gonorrhea (penicillin sensitive): 600 mg stat, 300 mg every 12 hours for 4 days (3 g total)
SIADH: 900-1200 mg/day or 13-15 mg/kg/day divided every 6-8 hours initially, then decrease to 600-900 mg/day

Dosing adjustment/comments in renal/hepatic impairment: Should be avoided in patients with renal/hepatic dysfunction
Dietary Considerations Should be taken 1 hour before or 2 hours after food or milk with plenty of fluid.
Administration Administer 1 hour before or 2 hours after food or milk with plenty of fluid
Monitoring Parameters CBC, renal and hepatic function
Test Interactions May interfere with tests for urinary glucose (false-negative urine glucose using Clinistix®, Tes-Tape®)
Patient Information Avoid prolonged exposure to sunlight or sunlamps; avoid taking antacids before tetracyclines
Dosage Forms Tablet, as hydrochloride: 150 mg, 300 mg

Denileukin Diftitox *(de ni LOO kin DIF ti toks)*

U.S. Brand Names ONTAK®
Therapeutic Category Antineoplastic Agent, Miscellaneous
Use Treatment of patients with persistent or recurrent cutaneous T-cell lymphoma whose malignant cells express the CD25 component of the IL-2 receptor
Pregnancy Risk Factor C
Pregnancy/Breast-Feeding Implications Animal reproduction studies have not been conducted. Should be given to a pregnant mother only if clearly needed. The excretion of denileukin diftitox in breast milk is unknown, however, it is recommended that a breast-feeding woman who is treated with denileukin diftitox should discontinue nursing.
Contraindications Hypersensitivity to denileukin diftitox, diphtheria toxin, interleukin-2, or any component of the formulation
Warnings/Precautions Acute hypersensitivity reactions, including anaphylaxis, may occur; most events occur during or within 24 hours of the first dose of a treatment cycle. Has been associated with a delayed-onset vascular leak syndrome, which may be severe. The onset of symptoms of vascular leak syndrome usually occurred within the first 2 weeks of infusion and may persist or worsen after cessation of denileukin diftitox. Pre-existing low serum albumin levels may predict or predispose to vascular leak syndrome. Denileukin diftitox may impair immune function. Use with caution in patients with pre-existing cardiovascular disease and in patients >65 years of age.
Adverse Reactions The occurrence of adverse events diminishes after the first two treatment courses. Infusion-related hypersensitivity reactions have been reported in 69% of patients.

Has been associated with vascular leak syndrome (27%), characterized by hypotension, edema, or hypoalbuminemia, usually developing within the first 2 weeks of infusion. Six percent of patients who developed this syndrome required hospitalization. The symptoms may persist or even worsen despite cessation of denileukin diftitox.

>10%:
Cardiovascular: Edema (47%), hypotension (36%), chest pain (24%), vasodilation (22%), tachycardia (12%)
Central nervous system: Fever/chills (81%), headache (26%), pain (48%), dizziness (22%), nervousness (11%)
Dermatologic: Rash (34%), pruritus (20%)
Endocrine & metabolic: Hypoalbuminemia (83%), hypocalcemia (17%)
Gastrointestinal: Nausea/vomiting (64%), anorexia (36%), diarrhea (29%), weight loss (14%)
Hematologic: Decreased lymphocyte count (34%), anemia (18%)
Hepatic: Increased transaminases (61%)
Neuromuscular & skeletal: Asthenia (66%), myalgia (17%)
Respiratory: Dyspnea (29%), increased cough (26%), pharyngitis (17%), rhinitis (13%)
Miscellaneous: Hypersensitivity (69%), infection (48%), vascular leak syndrome (27%), increased diaphoresis (10%), paresthesia (13%)

1% to 10%:
Cardiovascular: Hypertension (6%), arrhythmias (6%), myocardial infarction (1%)
Central nervous system: Insomnia (9%), confusion (8%)
Endocrine & metabolic: Dehydration (9%), hypokalemia (6%), hyperthyroidism (<5%), hypothyroidism (<5%)
Gastrointestinal: Constipation (9%), dyspepsia (7%), dysphagia (6%), pancreatitis (<5%)

Genitourinary: Hematuria (10%), albuminuria (10%), pyuria (10%)
Hematologic: Thrombotic events (7%), thrombocytopenia (8%), leukopenia (6%)
Local: Injection site reaction (8%)
Miscellaneous: Anaphylaxis (1%)
Neuromuscular & skeletal: Arthralgia (8%)
Renal: Increased creatinine (7%), acute renal insufficiency (<5%)

Overdosage/Toxicology Although there is no human experience in overdose, dose-limiting toxicities include nausea, vomiting, fever, chills and persistent asthenia. Treatment is supportive and symptom directed. Fluid balance and hepatic and renal function should be closely monitored.

Stability
Storage: Store frozen at or below -10°C; cannot be refrozen
Reconstitution: Must be brought to room temperature (25°C or 77°F) before preparing the dose. DO NOT HEAT vials. Thaw in refrigerator for not >24 hours or at room temperature for 1-2 hours. Avoid vigorous agitation. Solution may be mixed by gentle swirling.
Compatibility: DO NOT use glass syringes or containers

Mechanism of Action Denileukin diftitox is a fusion protein (a combination of amino acid sequences from diphtheria toxin and interleukin-2) which selectively delivers the cytotoxic activity of diphtheria toxin to targeted cells. It interacts with the high-affinity IL-2 receptor on the surface of malignant cells to inhibit intracellular protein synthesis, rapidly leading to cell death.

Pharmacodynamics/Kinetics
Distribution: V_d = 0.06-0.08 L/kg
Metabolism: Hepatic via proteolytic degradation (animal studies)
Half-life elimination: Distribution: 2-5 minutes; Terminal: 70-80 minutes

Usual Dosage Adults: I.V.: A treatment cycle consists of 9 or 18 mcg/kg/day for 5 consecutive days administered every 21 days. The optimal duration of therapy has not been determined. Only 2% of patients who failed to demonstrate a response (at least a 25% decrease in tumor burden) prior to the fourth cycle responded to subsequent treatment.

Administration For I.V. use only. Should be infused over at least 15 minutes. Should not be given as an I.V. bolus. Patients should be closely observed during the infusion for symptoms of hypersensitivity. If a patient experiences a reaction, the severity of the reaction should be evaluated, and a decision should be made to either reduce the rate or discontinue the infusion. Resuscitation equipment must be readily available. Delay therapy if serum albumin is <3 g/dL.

Monitoring Parameters Prior to administration, malignant cells should be tested for expression of CD25. The patient should have a CBC, blood chemistry panel, renal and hepatic function tests as well as a serum albumin level. These tests should be repeated at weekly intervals during therapy. During the infusion, the patient should be monitored for symptoms of an acute hypersensitivity reaction. After infusion, the patient should be monitored for the development of a delayed vascular leak syndrome (usually in the first 2 weeks), including careful monitoring of weight, blood pressure, and serum albumin.

Nursing Implications Patients should be closely observed during the infusion for symptoms of hypersensitivity or capillary leak syndrome.

Additional Information Formulation includes EDTA and polysorbate 20, and has a pH of 6.9-7.2.

Dosage Forms Injection: 150 mcg/mL (2 mL)

- **Dermovate® (Can)** *see* Clobetasol *on page 311*
- **Dermtex® HC With Aloe** *see* Hydrocortisone *on page 682*
- **DES** *see* Diethylstilbestrol *on page 400*
- **Desensitization Protocols** *see page 1525*
- **Deserpidine and Methyclothiazide** *see* Methyclothiazide and Deserpidine *on page 891*
- **Desferal®** *see* Deferoxamine *on page 370*
- **Desiccated Thyroid** *see* Thyroid *on page 1326*

Desipramine (des IP ra meen)

Related Information
Antidepressant Agents Comparison *on page 1482*

U.S. Brand Names Norpramin®

Canadian Brand Names Alti-Desipramine; Apo®-Desipramine; Norpramin®; Novo-Desipramine; Nu-Desipramine; PMS-Desipramine

Synonyms Desipramine Hydrochloride; Desmethylimipramine Hydrochloride

Therapeutic Category Antidepressant, Tricyclic

Use Treatment of depression

Unlabeled/Investigational Use Analgesic adjunct in chronic pain; peripheral neuropathies; substance-related disorders; attention-deficit/hyperactivity disorder (ADHD)

Pregnancy Risk Factor C

Contraindications Hypersensitivity to desipramine, drugs of similar chemical class, or any component of the formulation; use of MAO inhibitors within 14 days; use in a patient during the acute recovery phase of MI

Warnings/Precautions May cause sedation, resulting in impaired performance of tasks requiring alertness (ie, operating machinery or driving). Sedative effects may be additive with other CNS depressants and/or ethanol. The degree of sedation is low-moderate relative to other antidepressants. May worsen psychosis in some patients or precipitate a shift to mania or hypomania in patients with bipolar disease. May cause hyponatremia/SIADH. May increase the risks associated with electroconvulsive therapy. This agent should be discontinued, when possible, prior to elective surgery. Therapy should not be abruptly discontinued in patients receiving high doses for prolonged periods.

May cause orthostatic hypotension (risk is moderate relative to other antidepressants) - use with caution in patients at risk of hypotension or in patients where transient hypotensive episodes would be poorly tolerated (cardiovascular disease or cerebrovascular disease). The degree of anticholinergic blockade produced by this agent is low relative to other cyclic antidepressants - however, caution should be used in patients with urinary retention, benign prostatic hyperplasia, narrow-angle glaucoma, xerostomia, visual problems, constipation, or a history of bowel obstruction.

Use caution in patients with suicidal risk. Use with caution in patients with a history of cardiovascular disease (including previous MI, stroke, tachycardia, or conduction abnormalities). The risk conduction abnormalities with this agent is moderate relative to other antidepressants. Use caution in patients with a previous seizure disorder or condition predisposing to seizures such as brain damage, alcoholism, or concurrent therapy with other drugs which lower the seizure threshold. Use with caution in hyperthyroid patients or those receiving thyroid supplementation. Use with caution in patients with hepatic or renal dysfunction and in elderly patients.

Adverse Reactions Frequency not defined.

Cardiovascular: Arrhythmias, hypotension, hypertension, palpitations, heart block, tachycardia

Central nervous system: Dizziness, drowsiness, headache, confusion, delirium, hallucinations, nervousness, restlessness, parkinsonian syndrome, insomnia, disorientation, anxiety, agitation, hypomania, exacerbation of psychosis, incoordination, seizures, extrapyramidal symptoms

Dermatologic: Alopecia, photosensitivity, skin rash, urticaria

Endocrine & metabolic: Breast enlargement, galactorrhea, SIADH

Gastrointestinal: Xerostomia, decreased lower esophageal sphincter tone may cause GE reflux, constipation, nausea, unpleasant taste, weight gain/loss, anorexia, abdominal cramps, diarrhea, heartburn

Genitourinary: Difficult urination, sexual dysfunction, testicular edema

Hematologic: Agranulocytosis, eosinophilia, purpura, thrombocytopenia

Hepatic: Cholestatic jaundice, increased liver enzyme

Neuromuscular & skeletal: Fine muscle tremors, weakness, numbness, tingling, paresthesia of extremities, ataxia

Ocular: Blurred vision, disturbances of accommodation, mydriasis, increased intraocular pressure

Miscellaneous: Diaphoresis (excessive), allergic reactions

Overdosage/Toxicology Symptoms include severe hypotension, agitation, confusion, hyperthermia, urinary retention, CNS depression (including coma), cyanosis, dry mucous membranes, cardiac arrhythmias, seizures, changes in EKG (particularly in QRS axis and width), transient visual hallucinations, stupor, and muscle rigidity. Following GI decontamination, treatment is supportive. Sodium bicarbonate is indicated when the QRS interval is ≥0.10 seconds or the QT_c is >0.42 seconds. Ventricular arrhythmias and EKG changes (eg, QRS widening) often respond with concurrent systemic alkalinization (sodium bicarbonate 0.5-2 mEq/kg I.V.). Arrhythmias unresponsive to phenytoin 15-20 mg/kg (adults) may respond to lidocaine 1 mg/kg I.V. followed by a titrated infusion. Physostigmine (1-2 mg slow I.V. for adults or 0.5 mg slow I.V. for children) may be indicated in reversing life-threatening cardiac arrhythmias. Seizures usually respond to diazepam I.V. boluses (5-10 mg for adults up to 30 mg or 0.25-0.4 mg/kg/dose for children up to 10 mg/dose). If seizures are unresponsive or recur, phenytoin or phenobarbital may be required.

Drug Interactions
Cytochrome P450 Effect: CYP1A2 and 2D6 enzyme substrate; CYP2D6 inhibitor

Increased Effect/Toxicity: Desipramine increases the effects of amphetamines, anticholinergics, other CNS depressants (sedatives, hypnotics, or ethanol), chlorpropamide, tolazamide, and warfarin. When used with MAO inhibitors, serotonin syndrome may occur. Serotonin syndrome has also been reported with ritonavir (rare). The SSRIs (to varying degrees), cimetidine, grapefruit juice, indinavir, methylphenidate, ritonavir (and other protease inhibitors), quinidine, diltiazem, and verapamil inhibit the metabolism of TCAs and clinical toxicity may result. Use of lithium with a TCA may increase the risk for neurotoxicity. Phenothiazines may increase concentration of some TCAs and TCAs may increase concentration of phenothiazines. Pressor response to I.V. epinephrine, norepinephrine, and phenylephrine may be enhanced in patients receiving TCAs (**Note:** Effect is unlikely with epinephrine or levonordefrin dosages typically administered as infiltration in combination with local anesthetics). Combined use of beta-agonists or drugs which prolong QT_c (including quinidine, procainamide, disopyramide, cisapride, sparfloxacin, gatifloxacin, moxifloxacin) with TCAs may predispose patients to cardiac arrhythmias.

Decreased Effect: Desipramine's serum levels/effect may be decreased by carbamazepine, cholestyramine, colestipol, phenobarbital, and rifampin. Desipramine inhibits the antihypertensive effect of to bethanidine, clonidine, debrisoquin, guanadrel, guanethidine, guanabenz, or guanfacine.

Ethanol/Nutrition/Herb Interactions
Ethanol: Avoid ethanol (may increase CNS depression).

Food: Grapefruit juice may inhibit the metabolism of some TCAs and clinical toxicity may result.

Herb/Nutraceutical: Avoid valerian, St John's wort, SAMe, kava kava (may increase risk of serotonin syndrome and/or excessive sedation).

Mechanism of Action
Traditionally believed to increase the synaptic concentration of norepinephrine (and to a lesser extent, serotonin) in the central nervous system by inhibition of its reuptake by the presynaptic neuronal membrane. However, additional receptor effects have been found including desensitization of adenyl cyclase, down regulation of beta-adrenergic receptors, and down regulation of serotonin receptors.

Pharmacodynamics/Kinetics
Onset of action: 1-3 weeks; Maximum antidepressant effect: >2 weeks

Absorption: Well absorbed

Metabolism: Hepatic

Half-life elimination: Adults: 7-60 hours

Time to peak, plasma: 4-6 hours

Excretion: Urine (70%)

Usual Dosage
Oral (dose is generally administered at bedtime):

Children 6-12 years: Depression: 10-30 mg/day or 1-3 mg/kg/day in divided doses; do not exceed 5 mg/kg/day

Adolescents: Depression: Initial: 25-50 mg/day; gradually increase to 100 mg/day in single or divided doses (maximum: 150 mg/day)

Adults: Depression: Initial: 75 mg/day in divided doses; increase gradually to 150-200 mg/day in divided or single dose (maximum: 300 mg/day)

Elderly: Depression: Initial dose: 10-25 mg/day; increase by 10-25 mg every 3 days for inpatients and every week for outpatients if tolerated; usual maintenance dose: 75-100 mg/day, but doses up to 150 mg/day may be necessary

Hemodialysis/peritoneal dialysis: Supplemental dose is not necessary

Monitoring Parameters
Monitor blood pressure and pulse rate prior to and during initial therapy evaluate mental status; monitor weight; EKG in older adults and those patients with cardiac disease; blood levels are useful for therapeutic monitoring

Reference Range
Plasma levels do not always correlate with clinical effectiveness

Timing of serum samples: Draw trough just before next dose

Therapeutic: 50-300 ng/mL

In elderly patients the response rate is greatest with steady-state plasma concentrations >115 ng/mL

Possible toxicity: >300 ng/mL

Toxic: >1000 ng/mL

Patient Information
Avoid alcohol; do not discontinue medication abruptly; may cause urine to turn blue-green; may cause drowsiness; avoid unnecessary exposure to sunlight; sugarless hard candy or gum can help with dry mouth; full effect may not occur for 3-4 weeks

Nursing Implications
May increase appetite

Monitor blood pressure and pulse rate prior to and during initial therapy; evaluate mental status; monitor weight

Additional Information
Less sedation and anticholinergic effects than with amitriptyline or imipramine

Dosage Forms Tablet, as hydrochloride: 10 mg, 25 mg, 50 mg, 75 mg, 100 mg, 150 mg

- **Desipramine Hydrochloride** *see Desipramine on page 376*
- **Desitin® [OTC]** *see Zinc Oxide, Cod Liver Oil, and Talc on page 1439*

Desloratadine (des lor AT a deen)
U.S. Brand Names Clarinex®

Therapeutic Category Antihistamine, H_1 Blocker

Use Relief of nasal and non-nasal symptoms of seasonal allergic rhinitis (SAR) and perennial allergic rhinitis (PAR); treatment of chronic idiopathic urticaria (CIU)

Pregnancy Risk Factor C

Pregnancy/Breast-Feeding Implications There are no adequate and well-controlled studies in pregnant women. Use during pregnancy only if clearly needed. Enters in breast milk; breast-feeding not recommended.

(Continued)

Desloratadine *(Continued)*

Contraindications Hypersensitivity to desloratadine, loratadine, or any component of the formulation

Warnings/Precautions Dose should be adjusted in patients with liver or renal impairment. Use with caution in patients known to be slow metabolizers of desloratadine (incidence of side effects may be increased). Safety and efficacy have not been established for children <12 years of age.

Adverse Reactions
>10%: Central nervous system: Headache (14%)
1% to 10%:
Central nervous system: Fatigue (2% to 5%), somnolence (2%), dizziness (4%)
Endocrine & metabolic: Dysmenorrhea (2%)
Gastrointestinal: Dry mouth (3%), nausea (5%), dyspepsia (3%)
Neuromuscular & skeletal: Myalgia (3%)
Respiratory: Pharyngitis (3% to 4%)
Postmarketing and/or case reports: Anaphylaxis, bilirubin elevated, dyspnea, edema, hypersensitivity reactions, liver enzymes elevated, pruritus, rash, tachycardia, urticaria

Overdosage/Toxicology Information is limited to doses studied during clinical trials (up to 45 mg/day). Symptoms included somnolence, and small increases in heart rate and QT_c interval (not clinically significant). In the event of an overdose, treatment should be symptom-directed and supportive. Desloratadine and its metabolite are not removed by hemodialysis.

Drug Interactions
Increased Effect/Toxicity: With concurrent use of desloratadine and erythromycin or ketoconazole, the C_{max} and AUC of desloratadine and its metabolite are increased; however, no clinically-significant changes in the safety profile of desloratadine were observed in clinical studies.

Ethanol/Nutrition/Herb Interactions Food: Does not affect bioavailability.

Stability Store between 2°C to 25°C (36°F to 77°F); protect from moisture and excessive heat (temperatures ≥30°C/86°F)

Mechanism of Action Desloratadine, a major metabolite of loratadine, is a long-acting tricyclic antihistamine with selective peripheral histamine H_1 receptor antagonistic activity and additional anti-inflammatory properties.

Pharmacodynamics/Kinetics
Protein binding: Desloratadine: 82% to 87%; 3-hydroxydesloratadine: 85% to 89%
Metabolism: Hepatic to an active metabolite, 3-hydroxydesloratadine (specific enzymes not identified); undergoes glucuronidation. Metabolism may be decreased in slow metabolizers of desloratadine. Not expected to affect or be affected by medications metabolized by CYP isoenzymes with normal doses.
Half-life elimination: 27 hours
Time to peak: 3 hours
Excretion: Urine and feces (as metabolites)

Usual Dosage Oral: Adults and Children ≥12 years: 5 mg once daily
Dosage adjustment in renal/hepatic impairment: 5 mg every other day ·

Dietary Considerations May be taken with or without food.

Administration May be taken with or without food.

Patient Information May be taken with or without food. Do not increase dose or take more often than recommended by prescriber. Drowsiness, tiredness, headache, or dry mouth may occur. Notify prescriber for increased heart beat, rash, itching or shortness of breath. Notify prescriber if pregnant; breast-feeding is not recommended.

Dosage Forms Tablet: 5 mg

♦ **Desmethylimipramine Hydrochloride** *see Desipramine on page 376*

Desmopressin *(des moe PRES in)*

U.S. Brand Names DDAVP®; Stimate™
Canadian Brand Names DDAVP®; Octostim®
Synonyms 1-Deamino-8-D-Arginine Vasopressin; Desmopressin Acetate
Therapeutic Category Antihemophilic Agent; Hemostatic Agent; Vasopressin Analog, Synthetic
Use Treatment of diabetes insipidus and controlling bleeding in mild hemophilia, von Willebrand disease, and thrombocytopenia (eg, uremia); primary nocturnal enuresis
Pregnancy Risk Factor B
Contraindications Hypersensitivity to desmopressin or any component of the formulation; avoid using in patients with type IIB or platelet-type von Willebrand disease, or patients with <5% factor VIII activity level
Warnings/Precautions Avoid overhydration especially when drug is used for its hemostatic effect

Adverse Reactions
1% to 10%:
Cardiovascular: Facial flushing
Central nervous system: Headache, dizziness
Gastrointestinal: Nausea, abdominal cramps
Genitourinary: Vulval pain
Local: Pain at the injection site
Respiratory: Nasal congestion (intranasal use)
<1% (Limited to important or life-threatening): Increase in blood pressure

Overdosage/Toxicology Symptoms include drowsiness, headache, confusion, anuria, and water intoxication.

Drug Interactions
Increased Effect/Toxicity: Chlorpropamide, fludrocortisone may increase ADH response.
Decreased Effect: Demeclocycline and lithium may decrease ADH response.
Ethanol/Nutrition/Herb Interactions Ethanol: Avoid ethanol (may decrease antidiuretic effect).

Stability Keep in refrigerator, avoid freezing; discard discolored solutions; nasal solution stable for 3 weeks at room temperature; injection stable for 2 weeks at room temperature

Mechanism of Action Enhances reabsorption of water in the kidneys by increasing cellular permeability of the collecting ducts; possibly causes smooth muscle constriction with resultant vasoconstriction; raises plasma levels of von Willebrand factor and factor VIII

Pharmacodynamics/Kinetics
Intranasal administration:
Onset of action: ADH: ~1 hour
Peak effect: 1-5 hours
Duration: 5-21 hours
I.V. infusion:
Onset of increased factor VIII activity: 15-30 minutes
Peak effect: 1.5-3 hours
Absorption: Nasal: Slow; 10% to 20%
Metabolism: Unknown
Half-life elimination: Terminal: 75 minutes

Usual Dosage
Children:
Diabetes insipidus: 3 months to 12 years: Intranasal (using 100 mcg/mL nasal solution): Initial: 5 mcg/day (0.05 mL/day) divided 1-2 times/day; range: 5-30 mcg/day (0.05-0.3 mL/day) divided 1-2 times/day; adjust morning and evening doses separately for an adequate diurnal rhythm of water turnover
Hemophilia: >3 months: I.V. 0.3 mcg/kg; may repeat dose if needed; begin 30 minutes before procedure; dilute I.V. dose in 50 mL 0.9% sodium chloride and infuse over 15-30 minutes
Nocturnal enuresis: ≥6 years: Intranasal (using 100 mcg/mL nasal solution): Initial: 20 mcg (0.2 mL) at bedtime; range: 10-40 mcg; it is recommended that $^1/_2$ of the dose be given in each nostril
Children ≥12 years and Adults:
Diabetes insipidus:
I.V., S.C.: 2-4 mcg/day in 2 divided doses or $^1/_{10}$ of the maintenance intranasal dose; dilute I.V. dose in 50 mL 0.9% sodium chloride and infuse over 15-30 minutes
Intranasal (using 100 mcg/mL nasal solution): 5-40 mcg/day (0.05-0.4 mL) divided 1-3 times/day; adjust morning and evening doses separately for an adequate diurnal rhythm of water turnover. **Note:** The nasal spray pump can only deliver doses of 10 mcg (0.1 mL) or multiples of 10 mcg (0.1 mL), if doses other than this are needed, the rhinal tube delivery system is preferred.
Mild hemophilia A, mild to moderate von Willebrand disease:
I.V.: 0.3-0.4 mcg/kg by slow infusion, begin 30 minutes before procedure; dilute I.V. dose in 50 mL 0.9% sodium chloride and infuse over 15-30 minutes
Nasal spray: Using high concentration spray: 2-4 mcg/kg/dose; <50 kg: 150 mcg (1 spray); >50 kg: 300 mcg (1 spray each nostril); repeat use is determined by the patient's clinical condition and laboratory work; if using preoperatively, administer 2 hours before surgery
Oral: Begin therapy 12 hours after the last intranasal dose for patients previously on intra-nasal therapy
Children: Initial: 0.05 mg; fluid restrictions are required in children to prevent hyponatremia and water intoxication
Adults: 0.05 mg twice daily; adjust individually to optimal therapeutic dose. Total daily dose should be increased or decreased (range: 0.1-1.2 mg divided 2-3 times/day) as needed to obtain adequate antidiuresis.

Administration For I.V. administration, dilute in 10-50 mL 0.9% sodium chloride and infuse over 15-30 minutes

Monitoring Parameters Blood pressure and pulse should be monitored during I.V. infusion
Diabetes insipidus: Fluid intake, urine volume, specific gravity, plasma and urine osmolality, serum electrolytes
Hemophilia: Factor VIII antigen levels, aPTT, bleeding time (for von Willebrand disease and thrombocytopathies)

Patient Information Avoid overhydration; notify physician if headache, shortness of breath, heartburn, nausea, abdominal cramps, or vulval pain occur

Nursing Implications Parenteral: Dilute to a maximum concentration of 0.5 mcg/mL in normal saline and infuse over 15-30 minutes

Dosage Forms
Injection, as acetate (DDAVP®): 4 mcg/mL (1 mL, 10 mL)
Solution, intranasal, as acetate [spray]:
DDAVP®: 100 mcg/mL (2.5 mL, 5 mL)
Stimate™: 1.5 mg/mL (2.5 mL)
Tablet, as acetate (DDAVP®): 0.1 mg, 0.2 mg

♦ **Desmopressin Acetate** *see* Desmopressin *on page 378*
♦ **Desocort®** (Can) *see* Desonide *on page 379*
♦ **Desogen®** *see* Ethinyl Estradiol and Desogestrel *on page 510*
♦ **Desogestrel and Ethinyl Estradiol** *see* Ethinyl Estradiol and Desogestrel *on page 510*

Desonide (DES oh nide)

U.S. Brand Names DesOwen®; Tridesilon®
Canadian Brand Names Desocort®; Scheinpharm Desonide
Therapeutic Category Anti-inflammatory Agent; Corticosteroid, Topical (Low Potency); Corticosteroid, Topical (Medium Potency)
Use Adjunctive therapy for inflammation in acute and chronic corticosteroid responsive derma-tosis (low potency corticosteroid)
Pregnancy Risk Factor C
(Continued)

Desonide *(Continued)*

Usual Dosage Corticosteroid responsive dermatoses: Topical: Apply 2-4 times/day sparingly. Therapy should be discontinued when control is achieved; if no improvement is seen, reassessment of diagnosis may be necessary.

Additional Information Complete prescribing information for this medication should be consulted for additional detail.

Dosage Forms
Cream, topical: 0.05% (15 g, 60 g)
Lotion, topical: 0.05% (60 mL, 120 mL)
Ointment, topical: 0.05% (15 g, 60 g)

♦ **DesOwen®** *see* Desonide *on page 379*

Desoximetasone *(des oks i MET a sone)*

Related Information
Corticosteroids Comparison *on page 1495*

U.S. Brand Names Topicort®; Topicort®-LP

Canadian Brand Names Taro-Desoximetasone; Topicort®

Therapeutic Category Corticosteroid, Topical (Medium Potency); Corticosteroid, Topical (High Potency)

Use Relieves inflammation and pruritic symptoms of corticosteroid-responsive dermatosis (intermediate- to high-potency topical corticosteroid)

Pregnancy Risk Factor C

Usual Dosage Desoximetasone is a potent fluorinated topical corticosteroid. Therapy should be discontinued when control is achieved; if no improvement is seen, reassessment of diagnosis may be necessary.

Children: Apply sparingly in a very thin film to affected area 1-2 times/day
Adults: Apply sparingly to affected area in a thin film twice daily

Additional Information Complete prescribing information for this medication should be consulted for additional detail.

Dosage Forms
Cream, topical:
Topicort®: 0.25% (15 g, 60 g, 120 g)
Topicort®-LP: 0.05% (15 g, 60 g)
Gel, topical (Topicort®): 0.05% (15 g, 60 g)
Ointment, topical (Topicort®): 0.25% (15 g, 60 g)

♦ **Desoxyephedrine Hydrochloride** *see* Methamphetamine *on page 879*

♦ **Desoxyn®** *see* Methamphetamine *on page 879*

♦ **Desoxyn® Gradumet®** *see* Methamphetamine *on page 879*

♦ **Desoxyphenobarbital** *see* Primidone *on page 1127*

♦ **Desoxyribonuclease and Fibrinolysin** *see* Fibrinolysin and Desoxyribonuclease *on page 560*

♦ **Desyrel®** *see* Trazodone *on page 1362*

♦ **Detane® [OTC]** *see* Benzocaine *on page 154*

♦ **Detrol™** *see* Tolterodine *on page 1347*

♦ **Detrol® LA** *see* Tolterodine *on page 1347*

♦ **Dettussin® Liquid** *see* Hydrocodone and Pseudoephedrine *on page 681*

♦ **Dexacidin®** *see* Neomycin, Polymyxin B, and Dexamethasone *on page 969*

♦ **Dexacort® Phosphate Turbinaire®** *see* Dexamethasone *on page 380*

Dexamethasone *(deks a METH a sone)*

Related Information
Corticosteroids Comparison *on page 1495*

U.S. Brand Names AK-Dex®; Baldex®; Dalalone®; Dalalone D.P.®; Dalalone L.A.®; Decadron®; Decadron®-LA; Decadron® Phosphate; Decaject®; Decaject-LA®; Decaspray®; Dexacort® Phosphate Turbinaire®; Dexasone®; Dexasone® L.A.; Dexone®; Dexone® LA; Hexadrol®; Hexadrol® Phosphate; Maxidex®; Solurex®; Solurex L.A.®

Canadian Brand Names Decadron®; Dexasone®; Diodex®; Hexadrol® Phosphate; Maxidex®; PMS-Dexamethasone

Synonyms Dexamethasone Acetate; Dexamethasone Sodium Phosphate

Therapeutic Category Antiemetic; Anti-inflammatory Agent; Anti-inflammatory Agent, Inhalant; Anti-inflammatory Agent, Ophthalmic; Corticosteroid, Inhalant; Corticosteroid, Ophthalmic; Corticosteroid, Systemic; Corticosteroid, Topical (Low Potency); Glucocorticoid

Use Systemically and locally for chronic swelling; allergic, hematologic, neoplastic, and autoimmune diseases; may be used in management of cerebral edema, septic shock, as a diagnostic agent, antiemetic

Unlabeled/Investigational Use General indicator consistent with depression; diagnosis of Cushing's syndrome

Pregnancy Risk Factor C

Pregnancy/Breast-Feeding Implications Dexamethasone has been used in patients with premature labor (26-34 weeks gestation) to stimulate fetal lung maturation

Clinical effects on the fetus: Crosses the placenta; transient leukocytosis reported. Available evidence suggests safe use during pregnancy
Breast-feeding/lactation: No data on crossing into breast milk or effects on the infant

Contraindications Hypersensitivity to dexamethasone or any component of the formulation; active untreated infections; ophthalmic use in viral, fungal, or tuberculosis diseases of the eye

Warnings/Precautions Use with caution in patients with hypothyroidism, cirrhosis, hypertension, congestive heart failure, ulcerative colitis, thromboembolic disorders. Corticosteroids should be used with caution in patients with diabetes, osteoporosis, peptic ulcer, glaucoma, cataracts, or tuberculosis. Use caution in hepatic impairment. Because of the risk of adverse effects, systemic corticosteroids should be used cautiously in the elderly in the smallest possible dose and for the shortest possible time.

May cause suppression of hypothalamic-pituitary-adrenal (HPA) axis, particularly in younger children or in patients receiving high doses for prolonged periods. Particular care is required when patients are transferred from systemic corticosteroids to inhaled products due to possible adrenal insufficiency or withdrawal from steroids, including an increase in allergic symptoms. Patients receiving 20 mg per day of prednisone (or equivalent) may be most susceptible. Fatalities have occurred due to adrenal insufficiency in asthmatic patients during and after transfer from systemic corticosteroids to aerosol steroids; aerosol steroids do **not** provide the systemic steroid needed to treat patients having trauma, surgery, or infections

Controlled clinical studies have shown that orally-inhaled and intranasal corticosteroids may cause a reduction in growth velocity in pediatric patients. (In studies of orally-inhaled corticosteroids, the mean reduction in growth velocity was approximately 1 centimeter per year [range 0.3-1.8 cm per year] and appears to be related to dose and duration of exposure.) The growth of pediatric patients receiving inhaled corticosteroids, should be monitored routinely (eg, via stadiometry). To minimize the systemic effects of orally-inhaled and intranasal corticosteroids, each patient should be titrated to the lowest effective dose.

May suppress the immune system, patients may be more susceptible to infection. Use with caution in patients with systemic infections or ocular herpes simplex. Avoid exposure to chickenpox and measles.

Adverse Reactions
Systemic:
>10%:
   Central nervous system: Insomnia, nervousness
   Gastrointestinal: Increased appetite, indigestion
1% to 10%:
   Dermatologic: Hirsutism
   Endocrine & metabolic: Diabetes mellitus
   Neuromuscular & skeletal: Arthralgia
   Ocular: Cataracts
   Respiratory: Epistaxis
<1% (Limited to important or life-threatening): Abdominal distention, acne, amenorrhea, bone growth suppression, bruising, Cushing's syndrome, delirium, euphoria, hallucinations, headache, hyperglycemia, hyperpigmentation, hypersensitivity reactions, mood swings, muscle wasting, pancreatitis, seizures, skin atrophy, sodium and water retention, ulcerative esophagitis
Topical: <1% (Limited to important or life-threatening): Acneiform eruptions, allergic contact dermatitis, burning, dryness, folliculitis, hypertrichosis, hypopigmentation, irritation, itching, miliaria, perioral dermatitis, secondary infection, skin atrophy, skin maceration, striae
Overdosage/Toxicology Symptoms include moon face, central obesity, hypertension, psychosis, hallucinations, diabetes, hyperlipidemia, peptic ulcer, increased susceptibility to infection, electrolyte and fluid imbalance. When consumed in excessive quantities, systemic hypercorticism and adrenal suppression may occur; in those cases, discontinuation and withdrawal of the corticosteroid should be done judiciously.

Drug Interactions
Cytochrome P450 Effect: CYP3A3/4 enzyme substrate; CYP3A3/4 enzyme inducer; CYP3A3/4 enzyme inhibitor
Decreased Effect: Barbiturates, phenytoin, and rifampin may cause decreased dexamethasone effects. Dexamethasone decreases effect of salicylates, vaccines, and toxoids.

Ethanol/Nutrition/Herb Interactions
Ethanol: Avoid ethanol (may enhance gastric mucosal irritation).
Food: Dexamethasone interferes with calcium absorption. Limit caffeine.
Herb/Nutraceutical: Avoid cat's claw, echinacea (have immunostimulant properties).

Stability
Dexamethasone 4 mg/mL injection solution is clear and colorless and dexamethasone 24 mg/mL injection solution is clear and colorless to light yellow. Injection solution should be protected from light and freezing.
Stability of injection of parenteral admixture at room temperature (25°C): 24 hours
Stability of injection of parenteral admixture at refrigeration temperature (4°C): 2 days; protect from light and freezing
Standard diluent: 4 mg/50 mL D_5W; 10 mg/50 mL D_5W
Minimum volume: 50 mL D_5W

Mechanism of Action Decreases inflammation by suppression of migration of polymorphonuclear leukocytes and reversal of increased capillary permeability; suppresses normal immune response

Pharmacodynamics/Kinetics
Onset of action: Acetate: Prompt
Duration of metabolic effect: 72 hours; acetate is a long-acting repository preparation
Metabolism: Hepatic
Half-life elimination: Normal renal function: 1.8-3.5 hours; Biological half-life: 36-54 hours
Time to peak, serum: Oral: 1-2 hours; I.M.: ~8 hours
Excretion: Urine and feces

Usual Dosage
Children:
   Antiemetic (prior to chemotherapy): I.V. (should be given as sodium phosphate): 10 mg/m²/dose (maximum: 20 mg) for first dose then 5 mg/m²/dose every 6 hours as needed
   Anti-inflammatory immunosuppressant: Oral, I.M., I.V. (injections should be given as sodium phosphate): 0.08-0.3 mg/kg/day **or** 2.5-10 mg/m²/day in divided doses every 6-12 hours
   Extubation or airway edema: Oral, I.M., I.V. (injections should be given as sodium phosphate): 0.5-2 mg/kg/day in divided doses every 6 hours beginning 24 hours prior to extubation and continuing for 4-6 doses afterwards
(Continued)

Dexamethasone *(Continued)*

Cerebral edema: I.V. (should be given as sodium phosphate): Loading dose: 1-2 mg/kg/ dose as a single dose; maintenance: 1-1.5 mg/kg/day (maximum: 16 mg/day) in divided doses every 4-6 hours for 5 days then taper for 5 days, then discontinue

Bacterial meningitis in infants and children >2 months: I.V. (should be given as sodium phosphate): 0.6 mg/kg/day in 4 divided doses every 6 hours for the first 4 days of antibiotic treatment; start dexamethasone at the time of the first dose of antibiotic

Physiologic replacement: Oral, I.M., I.V.: 0.03-0.15 mg/kg/day or 0.6-0.75 mg/m^2/day in divided doses every 6-12 hours

Adults:

Antiemetic:

Prophylaxis: Oral, I.V.: 10-20 mg 15-30 minutes before treatment on each treatment day

Continuous infusion regimen: Oral or I.V.: 10 mg every 12 hours on each treatment day

Mildly emetogenic therapy: Oral, I.M., I.V.: 4 mg every 4-6 hours

Delayed nausea/vomiting: Oral:

8 mg every 12 hours for 2 days; then

4 mg every 12 hours for 2 days **or**

20 mg 1 hour before chemotherapy; then

10 mg 12 hours after chemotherapy; then

8 mg every 12 hours for 4 doses; then

4 mg every 12 hours for 4 doses

Anti-inflammatory:

Oral, I.M., I.V. (injections should be given as sodium phosphate): 0.75-9 mg/day in divided doses every 6-12 hours

I.M. (as acetate): 8-16 mg; may repeat in 1-3 weeks

Intralesional (as acetate): 0.8-1.6 mg

Intra-articular/soft tissue (as acetate): 4-16 mg; may repeat in 1-3 weeks

Intra-articular, intralesional, or soft tissue (as sodium phosphate): 0.4-6 mg/day

Ophthalmic:

Ointment: Apply thin coating into conjunctival sac 3-4 times/day; gradually taper dose to discontinue

Suspension: Instill 2 drops into conjunctival sac every hour during the day and every other hour during the night; gradually reduce dose to every 3-4 hours, then to 3-4 times/day

Topical: Apply 1-4 times/day. Therapy should be discontinued when control is achieved; if no improvement is seen, reassessment of diagnosis may be necessary.

Chemotherapy: Oral, I.V.: 40 mg every day for 4 days, repeated every 4 weeks (VAD regimen)

Cerebral edema: I.V. 10 mg stat, 4 mg I.M./I.V. (should be given as sodium phosphate) every 6 hours until response is maximized, then switch to oral regimen, then taper off if appropriate; dosage may be reduced after 24 days and gradually discontinued over 5-7 days

Dexamethasone suppression test (depression indicator) or diagnosis for Cushing's syndrome (unlabeled uses): Oral: 1 mg at 11 PM, draw blood at 8 AM the following day for plasma cortisol determination

Physiological replacement: Oral, I.M., I.V. (should be given as sodium phosphate): 0.03-0.15 mg/kg/day **OR** 0.6-0.75 mg/m^2/day in divided doses every 6-12 hours

Treatment of shock:

Addisonian crisis/shock (ie, adrenal insufficiency/responsive to steroid therapy): I.V. (given as sodium phosphate): 4-10 mg as a single dose, which may be repeated if necessary

Unresponsive shock (ie, unresponsive to steroid therapy): I.V. (given as sodium phosphate): 1-6 mg/kg as a single I.V. dose or up to 40 mg initially followed by repeat doses every 2-6 hours while shock persists

Hemodialysis: Supplemental dose is not necessary

Peritoneal dialysis: Supplemental dose is not necessary

Dietary Considerations May be taken with meals to decrease GI upset. May need diet with increased potassium, pyridoxine, vitamin C, vitamin D, folate, calcium, and phosphorus.

Administration

Oral: Administer with meals to decrease GI upset.

I.M.: Acetate injection is **not** for I.V. use.

Topical: For external use. Do not use on open wounds. Apply sparingly to occlusive dressings. Should not be used in the presence of open or weeping lesions.

Monitoring Parameters Hemoglobin, occult blood loss, serum potassium, and glucose

Reference Range Dexamethasone suppression test, overnight: 8 AM cortisol <6 µg/100 mL (dexamethasone 1 mg); plasma cortisol determination should be made on the day after giving dose

Patient Information Notify physician of any signs of infection or injuries during therapy; inform physician or dentist before surgery if you are taking a corticosteroid; may cause GI upset, take with food; do not overuse; use only as prescribed and for no longer than the period prescribed; notify physician if condition being treated persists or worsens

Topical: Thin film of cream or ointment is effective, do not overuse; do not use tight-fitting diapers or plastic pants on children being treated in the diaper area; use only as prescribed, and for no longer than the period prescribed; rub in lightly; avoid contact with eyes; notify physician if condition being treated persists or worsens

Nursing Implications Topical formation is for external use, do not use on open wounds; apply sparingly to occlusive dressings; should not be used in the presence of open or weeping lesions; **acetate injection is not for I.V. use**

Additional Information Not suitable for every-other-day dosing due to long duration of effect. Effects of inhaled/intranasal steroids on growth have been observed in the absence of laboratory evidence of HPA axis suppression, suggesting that growth velocity is a more sensitive indicator of systemic corticosteroid exposure in pediatric patients than some commonly used tests of HPA axis function. The long-term effects of this reduction in growth velocity associated with orally-inhaled and intranasal corticosteroids, including the impact on final adult height, are unknown. The potential for "catch up" growth following discontinuation of treatment with inhaled corticosteroids has not been adequately studied.

Dosage Forms
Aerosol, topical: 0.04% (25 g)
Cream, as sodium phosphate: 0.1% (15 g, 30 g)
Elixir: 0.5 mg/5 mL (5 mL, 20 mL, 100 mL, 120 mL, 237 mL, 240 mL, 500 mL)
Injection, as acetate suspension: 8 mg/mL (1 mL, 5 mL); 16 mg/mL (1 mL, 5 mL)
Injection, as sodium phosphate: 4 mg/mL (1 mL, 5 mL, 10 mL, 25 mL, 30 mL); 10 mg/mL (1 mL, 10 mL); 20 mg/mL (5 mL); 24 mg/mL (5 mL, 10 mL)
Ointment, ophthalmic, as sodium phosphate: 0.05% (3.5 g)
Solution, oral: 0.5 mg/5 mL (5 mL, 20 mL, 500 mL)
Solution, oral concentrate: 0.5 mg/0.5 mL (30 mL) (30% alcohol)
Suspension, ophthalmic, as sodium phosphate: 0.1% with methylcellulose 0.5% (5 mL, 15 mL)
Tablet: 0.25 mg, 0.5 mg, 0.75 mg, 1 mg, 1.5 mg, 2 mg, 4 mg, 6 mg
Tablet, therapeutic pack: 6 x 1.5 mg; 8 x 0.75 mg

♦ **Dexamethasone Acetate** *see Dexamethasone on page 380*
♦ **Dexamethasone and Neomycin** *see Neomycin and Dexamethasone on page 968*
♦ **Dexamethasone and Tobramycin** *see Tobramycin and Dexamethasone on page 1342*
♦ **Dexamethasone, Neomycin, and Polymyxin B** *see Neomycin, Polymyxin B, and Dexamethasone on page 969*
♦ **Dexamethasone Sodium Phosphate** *see Dexamethasone on page 380*
♦ **Dexasone®** *see Dexamethasone on page 380*
♦ **Dexasone® L.A.** *see Dexamethasone on page 380*
♦ **Dexasporin®** *see Neomycin, Polymyxin B, and Dexamethasone on page 969*

Dexbrompheniramine and Pseudoephedrine
(deks brom fen EER a meen & soo doe e FED rin)
U.S. Brand Names Brompheril® [OTC]; Disobrom® [OTC]; Disophrol® Chronotabs® [OTC]; Drixomed®; Drixoral® Cold & Allergy [OTC]; Histrodrix®; Resporal®
Canadian Brand Names Drixoral®
Synonyms Pseudoephedrine and Dexbrompheniramine
Therapeutic Category Antihistamine/Decongestant Combination
Use Relief of symptoms of upper respiratory mucosal congestion in seasonal and perennial nasal allergies, acute rhinitis, rhinosinusitis and eustachian tube blockage
Pregnancy Risk Factor B
Usual Dosage Children >12 years and Adults: Oral: 1 timed release tablet every 12 hours, may require 1 tablet every 8 hours
Additional Information Complete prescribing information for this medication should be consulted for additional detail.
Dosage Forms Tablet, timed release (Disobrom®, Drixomed®, Drixoral® Cold & Allergy, Histrodrix®, Resporal®): Dexbrompheniramine maleate 6 mg and pseudoephedrine sulfate 120 mg

Dexchlorpheniramine (deks klor fen EER a meen)
U.S. Brand Names Polaramine®
Canadian Brand Names Polaramine®
Synonyms Dexchlorpheniramine Maleate
Therapeutic Category Antihistamine, H_1 Blocker
Use Perennial and seasonal allergic rhinitis and other allergic symptoms including urticaria
Pregnancy Risk Factor B
Usual Dosage Oral:
Children:
2-5 years: 0.5 mg every 4-6 hours (do not use timed release)
6-11 years: 1 mg every 4-6 hours or 4 mg timed release at bedtime
Adults: 2 mg every 4-6 hours or 4-6 mg timed release at bedtime or every 8-10 hours
Additional Information Complete prescribing information for this medication should be consulted for additional detail.
Dosage Forms
Syrup, as maleate: 2 mg/5 mL with alcohol 6% (480 mL) [orange flavor]
Tablet, as maleate: 2 mg
Tablet, sustained action, as maleate: 4 mg, 6 mg

♦ **Dexchlorpheniramine Maleate** *see Dexchlorpheniramine on page 383*
♦ **Dexedrine®** *see Dextroamphetamine on page 388*
♦ **Dexferrum®** *see Iron Dextran Complex on page 745*
♦ **Dexiron™ (Can)** *see Iron Dextran Complex on page 745*

Dexmedetomidine (deks MED e toe mi deen)
U.S. Brand Names Precedex™
Canadian Brand Names Precedex™
Synonyms Dexmedetomidine Hydrochloride
Therapeutic Category Alpha-Adrenergic Agonist - Central-Acting (Alpha$_2$-Agonists); Sedative
Use Sedation of initially intubated and mechanically ventilated patients during treatment in an intensive care setting; duration of infusion should not exceed 24 hours
Unlabeled/Investigational Use Unlabeled uses include premedication prior to anesthesia induction with thiopental; relief of pain and reduction of opioid dose following laparoscopic tubal ligation; as an adjunct anesthetic in ophthalmic surgery; treatment of shivering; premedication to attenuate the cardiostimulatory and postanesthetic delirium of ketamine
Pregnancy Risk Factor C
(Continued)

Dexmedetomidine *(Continued)*

Pregnancy/Breast-Feeding Implications Caution should be exercised when administered to a nursing woman

Contraindications Hypersensitivity to dexmedetomidine or any component of the formulation; use outside of an intensive care setting

Warnings/Precautions Should be administered only by persons skilled in management of patients in intensive care setting. Patients should be continuously monitored. Episodes of bradycardia, hypotension, and sinus arrest have been associated with dexmedetomidine. Use caution in patients with heart block, severe ventricular dysfunction, hypovolemia, diabetes, chronic hypertension, and elderly. Use with caution in patients receiving vasodilators or drugs which decrease heart rate. If medical intervention is required, treatment may include stopping or decreasing the infusion; increasing the rate of I.V. fluid administration, use of pressor agents, and elevation of the lower extremities. Transient hypertension has been primarily observed during the dose in association with the initial peripheral vasoconstrictive effects of dexmedetomidine. Treatment of this is not generally necessary; however, reduction of infusion rate may be desirable.

Adverse Reactions
>10%:
  Cardiovascular: Hypotension (30%)
  Gastrointestinal: Nausea (11%)
1% to 10%:
  Cardiovascular: Bradycardia (8%), atrial fibrillation (7%)
  Central nervous system: Pain (3%)
  Hematologic: Anemia (3%), leukocytosis (2%)
  Renal: Oliguria (2%)
  Respiratory: Hypoxia (6%), pulmonary edema (2%), pleural effusion (3%)
  Miscellaneous: Infection (2%), thirst (2%)

Overdosage/Toxicology In reports of overdosages where the blood concentration was 13 times the upper boundary of the therapeutic range, first degree A-V block and second degree heart block occurred. No hemodynamic compromise was noted with A-V block and heart block resolved spontaneously within one minute. Two patients who received a 2 mcg/kg loading dose over 10 minutes experienced bradycardia and/or hypotension. One patient who received a loading dose of undiluted dexmedetomidine (19.4 mcg/kg) had cardiac arrest and was successfully resuscitated.

Drug Interactions
Cytochrome P450 Effect: CYP2A6 enzyme substrate
Increased Effect/Toxicity:
  Possible enhanced effects and pharmacodynamic interaction with sedatives, hypnotics, opioids, and anesthetics; monitor and decrease the dose as necessary of each agent and/or dexmedetomidine. Enhanced effects may occur with sevoflurane, isoflurane, propofol, alfentanil, and midazolam.
  Hypotension and/or bradycardia may be increased by vasodilators and heart rate-lowering agents.

Stability Compatible with lactated Ringer's, 5% dextrose in water, 0.9% sodium chloride in water, 20% mannitol, thiopental, etomidate, vecuronium, pancuronium, succinylcholine, atracurium, mivacurium, glycopyrrolate, phenylephrine, atropine, midazolam, morphine, fentanyl, and a plasma substitute

May adsorb to certain types of natural rubber; use components made with synthetic or coated natural rubber gaskets whenever possible

Mechanism of Action Selective alpha$_2$-adrenoceptor agonist with sedative properties; alpha$_1$ activity was observed at high doses or after rapid infusions

Pharmacodynamics/Kinetics
Onset of action: Rapid
Distribution: V$_{ss}$: Approximately 118 L; rapid
Protein binding: 94%
Metabolism: Undergoes complete biotransformation involving both direct glucuronidation and CYP2A6
Half-life elimination: 6 minutes; Terminal: 2 hours
Excretion: Urine (95%); feces (4%)

Usual Dosage Individualized and titrated to desired clinical effect
Adults: I.V.: Solution must be diluted prior to administration. Initial: Loading infusion of 1 mcg/kg over 10 minutes, followed by a maintenance infusion of 0.2-0.7 mcg/kg/hour; not indicated for infusions lasting >24 hours
Elderly (>65 years of age): Dosage reduction may need to be considered. No specific guidelines available. Dose selections should be cautious, at the low end of dosage range; titration should be slower, allowing adequate time to evaluate response.

Dosage adjustment in hepatic impairment: Dosage reduction may need to be considered. No specific guidelines available.

Administration Administer using a controlled infusion device. Must be diluted in 0.9% sodium chloride solution to achieve the required concentration prior to administration. Advisable to use administration components made with synthetic or coated natural rubber gaskets. Parenteral products should be inspected visually for particulate matter and discoloration prior to administration.

Monitoring Parameters Level of sedation, heart rate, respiration, rhythm

Nursing Implications Must be diluted in 0.9% sodium chloride solution to achieve the required concentration prior to administration. Advisable to use administration components made with synthetic or coated natural rubber gaskets. Parenteral products should be inspected visually for particulate matter and discoloration prior to administration.

Dosage Forms Injection: 100 mcg/mL (2 mL vial, 2 mL ampul)

♦ **Dexmedetomidine Hydrochloride** *see* Dexmedetomidine *on page 383*

Dexmethylphenidate (dex meth il FEN i date)
U.S. Brand Names Focalin™
Synonyms Dexmethylphenidate Hydrochloride
Therapeutic Category Central Nervous System Stimulant
Use Treatment of attention-deficit/hyperactivity disorder (ADHD)
Restrictions C-II
Pregnancy Risk Factor C
Usual Dosage Oral: Children ≥6 years and Adults: Treatment of ADHD: Initial: 2.5 mg twice daily in patients not currently taking methylphenidate; dosage may be adjusted in 2.5-5 mg increments at weekly intervals (maximum dose: 20 mg/day); doses should be taken at least 4 hours apart

When switching from methylphenidate to dexmethylphenidate, the starting dose of dexmethylphenidate should be half that of methylphenidate (maximum dose: 20 mg/day)

Safety and efficacy for long-term use of dexmethylphenidate have not yet been established. Patients should be re-evaluated at appropriate intervals to assess continued need of the medication.

Dose reductions and discontinuation: Reduce dose or discontinue in patients with paradoxical aggravation. Discontinue if no improvement is seen after one month of treatment.
Additional Information Complete prescribing information for this medication should be consulted for additional detail.
Dosage Forms Tablet, as hydrochloride: 2.5 mg, 5 mg, 10 mg

♦ **Dexmethylphenidate Hydrochloride** see Dexmethylphenidate on page 385
♦ **Dexone®** see Dexamethasone on page 380
♦ **Dexone® LA** see Dexamethasone on page 380

Dexpanthenol (deks PAN the nole)
U.S. Brand Names Ilopan®; Panthoderm® Cream [OTC]
Synonyms Pantothenyl Alcohol
Therapeutic Category Gastrointestinal Agent, Stimulant
Use Prophylactic use to minimize paralytic ileus, treatment of postoperative distention; topical to relieve itching and to aid healing
Pregnancy Risk Factor C
Usual Dosage
Children and Adults: Relief of itching and aid in skin healing: Topical: Apply to affected area 1-2 times/day
Adults:
Relief of gas retention: Oral: 2-3 tablets 3 times/day
Prevention of postoperative ileus: I.M.: 250-500 mg stat, repeat in 2 hours, followed by doses every 6 hours until danger passes
Paralyzed ileus: I.M.: 500 mg stat, repeat in 2 hours, followed by doses every 6 hours, if needed
Additional Information Complete prescribing information for this medication should be consulted for additional detail.
Dosage Forms
Cream (Panthoderm®): 2% (30 g, 60 g)
Injection (Ilopan®): 250 mg/mL (2 mL, 10 mL, 30 mL)
Tablet: 50 mg with choline bitartrate 25 mg

Dexrazoxane (deks ray ZOKS ane)
U.S. Brand Names Zinecard®
Canadian Brand Names Zinecard®
Synonyms ICRF-187
Therapeutic Category Cardioprotective Agent
Use Reduction of the incidence and severity of cardiomyopathy associated with doxorubicin administration in women with metastatic breast cancer who have received a cumulative doxorubicin dose of 300 mg/m^2 and who would benefit from continuing therapy with doxorubicin. It is not recommended for use with the initiation of doxorubicin therapy.
Pregnancy Risk Factor C
Pregnancy/Breast-Feeding Implications
Clinical effects on the fetus: Avoid use in pregnant women unless the potential benefit justifies the potential risk to the fetus
Breast-feeding/lactation: Discontinue nursing during dexrazoxane therapy
Contraindications Do not use with chemotherapy regimens that do not contain an anthracycline
Warnings/Precautions Dexrazoxane may add to the myelosuppression caused by chemotherapeutic agents. There is some evidence that the use of dexrazoxane concurrently with the initiation of fluorouracil, doxorubicin, and cyclophosphamide (FAC) therapy interferes with the antitumor efficacy of the regimen, and this use is not recommended. Dexrazoxane should only be used in those patients who have received a cumulative doxorubicin dose of 300 mg/m^2 and are continuing with doxorubicin therapy. Dexrazoxane does not eliminate the potential for anthracycline-induced cardiac toxicity. Carefully monitor cardiac function.
Adverse Reactions Adverse experiences are likely attributable to the FAC regimen, with the exception of pain on injection that was observed mainly with dexrazoxane. Patients receiving FAC with dexrazoxane experienced more severe leukopenia, granulocytopenia, and thrombocytopenia at nadir than patients receiving FAC without dexrazoxane; but recovery counts were similar for the two groups.

1% to 10%: Dermatologic: Urticaria, recall skin reaction, extravasation
Overdose/Toxicology Management includes supportive care until resolution of myelosuppression and related conditions is complete. Management of overdose should include treatment of infections, fluid regulation, and management of nutritional requirements. Retention of
(Continued)

Dexrazoxane *(Continued)*

a significant dose fraction of the unchanged drug in the plasma pool, minimal tissue partitioning or binding, and availability of >90% of systemic drug levels in the unbound form, suggest that dexrazoxane could be removed using conventional peritoneal or hemodialysis.

Drug Interactions
Decreased Effect: The use of dexrazoxane concurrently with the initiation of FAC therapy may interfere with the antitumor efficacy of the regimen, and this use is not recommended.

Stability
Store intact vials at controlled room temperature (15°C to 30°C/59°F to 86°F). Reconstituted and diluted solutions are stable for 6 hours at controlled room temperature or under refrigeration (2°C to 8°C/36°F to 46°F).

Must be reconstituted with 0.167 Molar (M/6) sodium lactate injection to a concentration of 10 mg dexrazoxane/mL sodium lactate. Reconstituted dexrazoxane solution may be diluted with either 0.9% sodium chloride injection or 5% dextrose injection to a concentration of 1.3-5 mg/mL in intravenous infusion bags.

Caution should be exercised in the handling and preparation of the reconstituted solution; the use of gloves is recommended. If dexrazoxane powder or solutions contact the skin or mucosae, immediately wash with soap and water.

Mechanism of Action Derivative of EDTA and potent intracellular chelating agent. The mechanism of cardioprotectant activity is not fully understood. Appears to be converted intracellularly to a ring-opened chelating agent that interferes with iron-mediated free radical generation thought to be responsible, in part, for anthracycline-induced cardiomyopathy.

Pharmacodynamics/Kinetics
Distribution: V_d: 22-22.4 L/m^2
Protein binding: None
Half-life elimination: 2.1-2.5 hours
Excretion: Urine (42%)
Clearance, renal: 3.35 L/hour/m^2; Plasma: 6.25-7.88 L/hour/m^2

Usual Dosage Adults: I.V.: The recommended dosage ratio of dexrazoxane:doxorubicin is 10:1 (eg, 500 mg/m^2 dexrazoxane:50 mg/m^2 doxorubicin). Administer the reconstituted solution by slow I.V. push or rapid I.V. infusion from a bag. After completing the infusion, and prior to a total elapsed time of 30 minutes (from the beginning of the dexrazoxane infusion), administer the I.V. injection of doxorubicin.

Administration Doxorubicin should not be administered prior to the I.V. injection of dexrazoxane. Administer dexrazoxane by slow I.V. push or rapid drip I.V. infusion from a bag. Administer doxorubicin within 30 minutes after beginning the infusion with dexrazoxane.

Monitoring Parameters Since dexrazoxane will always be used with cytotoxic drugs, and since it may add to the myelosuppressive effects of cytotoxic drugs, frequent complete blood counts are recommended

Nursing Implications Observe for signs and symptoms of cardiac toxicity, infection, and anemia

Additional Information Reimbursement Guarantee Program: 1-800-808-9111

Dosage Forms Powder for injection, lyophilized: 250 mg, 500 mg (10 mg/mL when reconstituted)

Dextran *(DEKS tran)*

U.S. Brand Names Gentran®; LMD®; Macrodex®; Rheomacrodex®
Canadian Brand Names Gentran®
Synonyms Dextran 40; Dextran 70; Dextran, High Molecular Weight; Dextran, Low Molecular Weight
Therapeutic Category Plasma Volume Expander, Colloid
Use Blood volume expander used in treatment of shock or impending shock when blood or blood products are not available; dextran 40 is also used as a priming fluid in cardiopulmonary bypass and for prophylaxis of venous thrombosis and pulmonary embolism in surgical procedures associated with a high risk of thromboembolic complications
Pregnancy Risk Factor C
Contraindications Hypersensitivity to dextran or any component of the formulation; marked hemostatic defects (thrombocytopenia, hypofibrinogenemia) of all types including those caused by drugs; marked cardiac decompensation; renal disease with severe oliguria or anuria
Warnings/Precautions Hypersensitivity reactions have been reported (dextran 40 rarely causes a reaction), usually early in the infusion. Monitor closely during infusion initiation for signs or symptoms of a hypersensitivity reaction. Dextran 1 is indicated for prophylaxis of serious anaphylactic reactions to dextran infusions. Administration can cause fluid or solute overload. Use caution in patients with fluid overload. Use with caution in patients with active hemorrhage. Use caution in patients receiving corticosteroids. Renal failure has been reported. Fluid status including urine output should be monitored closely. Exercise care to prevent a depression of hematocrit <30% (can cause hemodilution). Observe for signs of bleeding.
Adverse Reactions <1% (Limited to important or life-threatening): Mild hypotension, tightness of chest, wheezing
Overdosage/Toxicology Symptoms include fluid overload, pulmonary edema, increased bleeding time, and decreased platelet function. Treatment is supportive; blood products containing clotting factors may be necessary.
Stability Store at room temperature; discard partially used containers
Mechanism of Action Produces plasma volume expansion by virtue of its highly colloidal starch structure, similar to albumin
Pharmacodynamics/Kinetics
Onset of action: Minutes to 1 hour (depending upon the molecular weight polysaccharide administered)
Excretion: Urine (~75%) within 24 hours

Usual Dosage I.V. (requires an infusion pump): Dose and infusion rate are dependent upon the patient's fluid status and must be individualized:

Volume expansion/shock:
Children: Total dose should not exceed 20 mL/kg during first 24 hours

Adults: 500-1000 mL at a rate of 20-40 mL/minute; maximum daily dose: 20 mL/kg for first 24 hours; 10 mL/kg/day thereafter; therapy should not be continued beyond 5 days

Pump prime (Dextran 40): Varies with the volume of the pump oxygenator; generally, the 10% solution is added in a dose of 1-2 g/kg

Prophylaxis of venous thrombosis/pulmonary embolism (Dextran 40): Begin during surgical procedure and give 50-100 g on the day of surgery; an additional 50 g (500 mL) should be administered every 2-3 days during the period of risk (up to 2 weeks postoperatively); usual maximum infusion rate for nonemergency use: 4 mL/minute

Dosing in renal and/or hepatic impairment: Use with extreme caution

Administration For I.V. infusion only (use an infusion pump). Infuse initial 500 mL at a rate of 20-40 mL/minute if hypervolemic. Reduce rate for additional infusion to 4 mL/minute. **Observe patients closely for anaphylactic reaction.**

Monitoring Parameters Observe patient for signs of circulatory overload and/or monitor central venous pressure; observe patients closely during the first minute of infusion and have other means of maintaining circulation should dextran therapy result in an anaphylactoid reaction; monitor hemoglobin and hematocrit, electrolytes, serum protein

Nursing Implications Patients should be well hydrated at the start of therapy; discontinue dextran if urine specific gravity is low, and/or if oliguria or anuria occurs, or if there is a precipitous rise in central venous pressure or sign of circulatory overloading

Additional Information Dextran 40 is known as low molecular weight dextran (LMD®) and has an average molecular weight of 40,000; dextran 75 has an average molecular weight of 75,000. Dextran 70 has an average molecular weight of 70,000; sodium content of 500 mL is 77 mEq, with pH ranging from 3.0-7.0.

Dosage Forms
Injection, high molecular weight:
Dextran: 6% dextran 75 in sodium chloride 0.9% (500 mL)
Gentran®, Macrodex: 6% dextran 70 in sodium chloride 0.9% (500 mL)
Macrodex®: 6% dextran 70 in dextrose 5% (500 mL)
Macrodex®: 6% dextran 75 in dextrose 5% (500 mL)
Injection, low molecular weight (Gentran®, LMD®, Rheomacrodex®):
10% dextran 40 in dextrose 5% (500 mL)
10% dextran 40 in sodium chloride 0.9% (500 mL)

Dextran 1 (DEKS tran won)

U.S. Brand Names Promit®

Therapeutic Category Dextran Adjunct; Plasma Volume Expander, Colloid

Use Prophylaxis of serious anaphylactic reactions to I.V. infusion of dextran

Pregnancy Risk Factor C

Contraindications Hypersensitivity to dextrans or any component of the formulation; **dextran** contraindicated

Warnings/Precautions Severe hypotension and bradycardia can occur. If any reaction occurs, do not administer dextran. Mild dextran-induced anaphylactic reactions are not prevented.

Adverse Reactions <1% (Limited to important or life-threatening): Mild hypotension, tightness of chest, wheezing

Stability Protect from freezing

Mechanism of Action Binds to dextran-reactive immunoglobulin without bridge formation and no formation of large immune complexes

Usual Dosage I.V. (time between dextran 1 and dextran solution should not exceed 15 minutes):

Children: 0.3 mL/kg 1-2 minutes before I.V. infusion of dextran
Adults: 20 mL 1-2 minutes before I.V. infusion of dextran

Nursing Implications Do not dilute or admix with dextrans

Dosage Forms Injection: 150 mg/mL (20 mL)

♦ **Dextran 40** see Dextran on page 386
♦ **Dextran 70** see Dextran on page 386
♦ **Dextran, High Molecular Weight** see Dextran on page 386
♦ **Dextran, Low Molecular Weight** see Dextran on page 386

Dextranomer (deks TRAN oh mer)

U.S. Brand Names Debrisan® [OTC]

Therapeutic Category Topical Skin Product

Use Clean exudative ulcers and wounds such as venous stasis ulcers, decubitus ulcers, and infected traumatic and surgical wounds; no controlled studies have found dextranomer to be more effective than conventional therapy

Pregnancy Risk Factor C

Contraindications Hypersensitivity to dextranomer or any component of the formulation; deep fistulas or sinus tracts

Warnings/Precautions Do not use in deep fistulas or any area where complete removal is not assured; do not use on dry wounds (ineffective); avoid contact with eyes

Adverse Reactions 1% to 10%:
Local: Transitory pain, blistering
Dermatologic: Maceration may occur, erythema
Hematologic: Bleeding

Mechanism of Action Dextranomer is a network of dextran-sucrose beads possessing a great many exposed hydroxy groups; when this network is applied to an exudative wound surface, the exudate is drawn by capillary forces generated by the swelling of the beads, with vacuum forces producing an upward flow of exudate into the network

(Continued)

Dextranomer *(Continued)*

Usual Dosage Debride and clean wound prior to application; apply to affected area once or twice daily in a ¼" layer; apply a dressing and seal on all four sides; removal should be done by irrigation

Patient Information For external use only; avoid contact with eyes; contact physician if condition worsens or persists beyond 14-21 days

Nursing Implications Sprinkle beads into ulcer (or apply paste) to ¼" thickness; change dressings 1-4 times/day depending on drainage; change dressing before it is completely dry to facilitate removal

Dosage Forms
Beads, topical: 4 g, 25 g, 60 g, 120 g
Paste, topical: 10 g foil packets

Dextroamphetamine *(deks troe am FET a meen)*

Related Information
Antacid Drug Interactions *on page 1477*

U.S. Brand Names Dexedrine®

Canadian Brand Names Dexedrine®

Synonyms Dextroamphetamine Sulfate

Therapeutic Category Amphetamine; Anorexiant; Central Nervous System Stimulant, Amphetamine

Use Narcolepsy; attention-deficit/hyperactivity disorder (ADHD)

Unlabeled/Investigational Use Exogenous obesity; depression; abnormal behavioral syndrome in children (minimal brain dysfunction)

Restrictions C-II

Pregnancy Risk Factor C

Contraindications Hypersensitivity or idiosyncrasy to dextroamphetamine or other sympathomimetic amines. Patients with advanced arteriosclerosis, symptomatic cardiovascular disease, moderate to severe hypertension (stage II or III), hyperthyroidism, glaucoma, diabetes mellitus, agitated states, patients with a history of drug abuse, and during or within 14 days following MAO inhibitor therapy. Stimulant medications are contraindicated for use in children with attention-deficit/hyperactivity disorders and concomitant Tourette's syndrome or tics.

Warnings/Precautions Use with caution in patients with psychopathic personalities, cardiovascular disease, HTN, angina, and glaucoma. Use with caution in patients with bipolar disorder, cardiovascular disease, seizure disorder, insomnia, porphyria, mild hypertension (stage I), or history of substance abuse. May exacerbate symptoms of behavior and thought disorder in psychotic patients. Stimulants may unmask tics in individuals with coexisting Tourette's syndrome. Potential for drug dependency exists - avoid abrupt discontinuation in patients who have received for prolonged periods. Use in weight reduction programs only when alternative therapy has been ineffective. Products may contain tartrazine - use with caution in potentially sensitive individuals. Stimulant use in children has been associated with growth suppression.

Adverse Reactions Frequency not defined.
Cardiovascular: Palpitations, tachycardia, hypertension, cardiomyopathy
Central nervous system: Overstimulation, euphoria, dyskinesia, dysphoria, exacerbation of motor and phonic tics, restlessness, insomnia, dizziness, headache, psychosis, Tourette's syndrome
Dermatologic: Rash, urticaria
Endocrine & metabolic: Changes in libido
Gastrointestinal: Diarrhea, constipation, anorexia, weight loss, xerostomia, unpleasant taste
Genitourinary: Impotence
Neuromuscular & skeletal: Tremor

Overdosage/Toxicology Symptoms include restlessness, tremor, confusion, hallucinations, panic, dysrhythmias, nausea, and vomiting. There is no specific antidote for dextroamphetamine intoxication and the bulk of treatment is supportive. Hyperactivity and agitation usually respond to reduced sensory input; however, with extreme agitation, haloperidol (2-5 mg I.M. for adults) may be required. Hyperthermia is best treated with external cooling measures; when severe or unresponsive, muscle paralysis with pancuronium may be needed. Hypertension is usually transient and generally does not require treatment unless severe. For diastolic blood pressures >110 mm Hg, a nitroprusside infusion should be initiated. Seizures usually respond to diazepam I.V. and/or phenytoin maintenance regimens.

Drug Interactions
Increased Effect/Toxicity: Dextroamphetamine may precipitate hypertensive crisis or serotonin syndrome in patients receiving MAO inhibitors (selegiline >10 mg/day, isocarboxazid, phenelzine, tranylcypromine, furazolidone). Serotonin syndrome has also been associated with combinations of amphetamines and SSRIs; these combinations should be avoided. TCAs may enhance the effects of amphetamines. Large doses of antacids or urinary alkalinizers increase the half-life and duration of action of amphetamines. May precipitate arrhythmias in patients receiving general anesthetics.

Decreased Effect: Amphetamines inhibit the antihypertensive response to guanethidine and guanadrel. Urinary acidifiers decrease the half-life and duration of action of amphetamines.

Ethanol/Nutrition/Herb Interactions
Ethanol: Avoid ethanol (may increase CNS depression).
Food: Dextroamphetamine serum levels may be altered if taken with acidic food, juices, or vitamin C.
Herb/Nutraceutical: Avoid ephedra (may cause hypertension or arrhythmias).

Stability Protect from light

Mechanism of Action Blocks reuptake of dopamine and norepinephrine from the synapse, thus increases the amount of circulating dopamine and norepinephrine in cerebral cortex to reticular activating system; inhibits the action of monoamine oxidase and causes catecholamines to be released. Peripheral actions include elevated blood pressure, weak bronchodilator, and respiratory stimulant action.

Pharmacodynamics/Kinetics

Onset of action: 1-1.5 hours

Distribution: V_d: Adults: 3.5-4.6 L/kg; distributes into CNS; mean CSF concentrations are 80% of plasma; enters breast milk

Metabolism: Hepatic via CYP450 monooxygenase and glucuronidation

Half-life elimination: Adults: 10-13 hours

Time to peak, serum: Immediate release tablet: ~3 hours

Excretion: Urine (as unchanged drug and inactive metabolites)

Usual Dosage Oral:

Children:

Narcolepsy: 6-12 years: Initial: 5 mg/day; may increase at 5 mg increments in weekly intervals until side effects appear (maximum dose: 60 mg/day)

ADHD:

3-5 years: Initial: 2.5 mg/day given every morning; increase by 2.5 mg/day in weekly intervals until optimal response is obtained; usual range: 0.1-0.5 mg/kg/dose every morning with maximum of 40 mg/day

≥6 years: 5 mg once or twice daily; increase in increments of 5 mg/day at weekly intervals until optimal response is obtained; usual range: 0.1-0.5 mg/kg/dose every morning (5-20 mg/day) with maximum of 40 mg/day

Children >12 years and Adults:

Narcolepsy: Initial: 10 mg/day, may increase at 10 mg increments in weekly intervals until side effects appear; maximum: 60 mg/day

Exogenous obesity (unlabeled use): 5-30 mg/day in divided doses of 5-10 mg 30-60 minutes before meals

Dietary Considerations Should be taken 30 minutes before meals and at least 6 hours before bedtime.

Administration Administer as single dose in morning or as divided doses with breakfast and lunch

Monitoring Parameters Growth in children and CNS activity in all

Patient Information Take during day to avoid insomnia; do not discontinue abruptly, may cause physical and psychological dependence with prolonged use

Nursing Implications Last daily dose should be given 6 hours before retiring; do not crush sustained release drug product

Dosage Forms

Capsule, sustained release, as sulfate: 5 mg, 10 mg, 15 mg

Tablet, as sulfate: 5 mg, 10 mg (5 mg tablets contain tartrazine)

Dextroamphetamine and Amphetamine

(deks troe am FET a meen & am FET a meen)

U.S. Brand Names Adderall®; Adderall XR™

Synonyms Amphetamine and Dextroamphetamine

Therapeutic Category Amphetamine; Central Nervous System Stimulant, Amphetamine

Use Attention-deficit/hyperactivity disorder (ADHD); narcolepsy

Restrictions C-II

Pregnancy Risk Factor C

Usual Dosage Oral: **Note:** Use lowest effective individualized dose; administer first dose as soon as awake

ADHD:

Children: <3 years: Not recommended

Children: 3-5 years (Adderall®): Initial 2.5 mg/day given every morning; increase daily dose in 2.5 mg increments at weekly intervals until optimal response is obtained (maximum dose: 40 mg/day given in 1-3 divided doses); use intervals of 4-6 hours between additional doses

Children: ≥6 years:

Adderall®: Initial: 5 mg 1-2 times/day; increase daily dose in 5 mg increments at weekly intervals until optimal response is obtained (usual maximum: 40 mg/day given in 1-3 divided doses); use intervals of 4-6 hours between additional doses

Adderall XR™: 10 mg once daily in the morning; if needed, may increase daily dose in 10 mg increments at weekly intervals (maximum dose: 30 mg/day)

Narcolepsy: Adderall®

Children: 6-12 years: Initial: 5 mg/day; increase daily dose in 5 mg at weekly intervals until optimal response is obtained (maximum dose: 60 mg/day given in 1-3 divided doses)

Children >12 years and Adults: Initial: 10 mg/day; increase daily dose in 10 mg increments at weekly intervals until optimal response is obtained (maximum dose: 60 mg/day given in 1-3 divided doses)

Additional Information Complete prescribing information for this medication should be consulted for additional detail.

Dosage Forms

Capsule (Adderall XR™):

10 mg [dextroamphetamine sulfate 2.5 mg, dextroamphetamine saccharate 2.5 mg and amphetamine aspartate monohydrate 2.5 mg, amphetamine sulfate 2.5 mg] (equivalent to amphetamine base 6.3 mg)

20 mg [dextroamphetamine sulfate 5 mg, dextroamphetamine saccharate 5 mg and amphetamine aspartate monohydrate 5 mg, amphetamine sulfate 5 mg] (equivalent to amphetamine base 12.5 mg)

30 mg [dextroamphetamine sulfate 7.5 mg, dextroamphetamine saccharate 7.5 mg and amphetamine aspartate monohydrate 7.5 mg, amphetamine sulfate 7.5 mg] (equivalent to amphetamine base 18.8 mg)

(Continued)

Dextroamphetamine and Amphetamine *(Continued)*

Tablet (Adderall®):

5 mg [dextroamphetamine sulfate 1.25 mg, dextroamphetamine saccharate 1.25 mg and amphetamine aspartate 1.25 mg, amphetamine sulfate 1.25 mg] (equivalent to amphetamine base 3.13 mg)

7.5 mg [dextroamphetamine 1.875 mg, dextroamphetamine saccharate 1.875 mg and amphetamine aspartate 1.875 mg, amphetamine sulfate 1.875 mg] (equivalent to amphetamine base 4.7 mg)

10 mg [dextroamphetamine sulfate 2.5 mg, dextroamphetamine saccharate 2.5 mg and amphetamine aspartate 2.5 mg, amphetamine sulfate 2.5 mg] (equivalent to amphetamine base 6.3 mg)

12.5 mg [dextroamphetamine sulfate 3.125 mg, dextroamphetamine saccharate 3.125 mg and amphetamine aspartate 3.125 mg, amphetamine sulfate 3.125 mg] (equivalent to amphetamine base 7.8 mg)

15 mg [dextroamphetamine sulfate 3.75 mg, dextroamphetamine saccharate 3.75 mg and amphetamine aspartate 3.75 mg, amphetamine sulfate 3.75 mg] (equivalent to amphetamine base 9.4 mg)

20 mg [dextroamphetamine sulfate 5 mg, dextroamphetamine saccharate 5 mg and amphetamine aspartate 5 mg, amphetamine sulfate 5 mg] (equivalent to amphetamine base 12.6 mg)

30 mg [dextroamphetamine sulfate 7.5 mg, dextroamphetamine saccharate 7.5 mg and amphetamine aspartate 7.5 mg, amphetamine sulfate 7.5 mg] (equivalent to amphetamine base 18.8 mg)

- ♦ **Dextroamphetamine Sulfate** *see* Dextroamphetamine *on page 388*
- ♦ **Dextromethorphan, Acetaminophen, and Pseudoephedrine** *see* Acetaminophen, Dextromethorphan, and Pseudoephedrine *on page 27*
- ♦ **Dextromethorphan and Guaifenesin** *see* Guaifenesin and Dextromethorphan *on page 646*
- ♦ **Dextromethorphan and Promethazine** *see* Promethazine and Dextromethorphan *on page 1141*
- ♦ **Dextromethorphan and Pseudoephedrine** *see* Pseudoephedrine and Dextromethorphan *on page 1157*
- ♦ **Dextromethorphan, Carbinoxamine, and Pseudoephedrine** *see* Carbinoxamine, Pseudoephedrine, and Dextromethorphan *on page 225*
- ♦ **Dextromethorphan, Guaifenesin, and Pseudoephedrine** *see* Guaifenesin, Pseudoephedrine, and Dextromethorphan *on page 648*
- ♦ **Dextromethorphan, Pseudoephedrine, and Carbinoxamine** *see* Carbinoxamine, Pseudoephedrine, and Dextromethorphan *on page 225*
- ♦ **Dextropropoxyphene** *see* Propoxyphene *on page 1147*
- ♦ **Dey-Lute® Isoetharine** *see* Isoetharine *on page 747*
- ♦ **DFMO** *see* Eflornithine *on page 461*
- ♦ **DFP** *see* Isoflurophate *on page 747*
- ♦ **DHAD** *see* Mitoxantrone *on page 925*
- ♦ **DHC®** *see* Hydrocodone and Acetaminophen *on page 676*
- ♦ **DHC Plus®** *see* Dihydrocodeine Compound *on page 407*
- ♦ **DHE** *see* Dihydroergotamine *on page 407*
- ♦ **D.H.E. 45®** *see* Dihydroergotamine *on page 407*
- ♦ **DHPG Sodium** *see* Ganciclovir *on page 618*
- ♦ **DHT™** *see* Dihydrotachysterol *on page 409*
- ♦ **Diaβeta®** *see* GlyBURIDE *on page 635*
- ♦ **Diabetes Mellitus Treatment** *see page 1657*
- ♦ **Diabetic Tussin® DM [OTC]** *see* Guaifenesin and Dextromethorphan *on page 646*
- ♦ **Diabetic Tussin® EX [OTC]** *see* Guaifenesin and Dextromethorphan *on page 645*
- ♦ **Diabinese®** *see* ChlorproPAMIDE *on page 284*
- ♦ **Dialume® [OTC]** *see* Aluminum Hydroxide *on page 63*
- ♦ **Diaminodiphenylsulfone** *see* Dapsone *on page 364*
- ♦ **Diamox®** *see* AcetaZOLAMIDE *on page 29*
- ♦ **Diamox Sequels®** *see* AcetaZOLAMIDE *on page 29*
- ♦ **Diar-Aid® [OTC]** *see* Loperamide *on page 816*
- ♦ **Diarr-Eze (Can)** *see* Loperamide *on page 816*
- ♦ **Diastat® (Can)** *see* Diazepam *on page 390*
- ♦ **Diastat® Rectal Delivery System** *see* Diazepam *on page 390*
- ♦ **Diazemuls® (Can)** *see* Diazepam *on page 390*

Diazepam *(dye AZ e pam)*

Related Information

Adult ACLS Algorithms *on page 1632*
Antacid Drug Interactions *on page 1477*
Benzodiazepines Comparison *on page 1490*
Convulsive Status Epilepticus *on page 1661*
Febrile Seizures *on page 1660*

U.S. Brand Names Diastat® Rectal Delivery System; Diazepam Intensol®; Valium®

Canadian Brand Names Apo®-Diazepam; Diastat®; Diazemuls®; Valium®; Vivol®

Therapeutic Category Antianxiety Agent; Anticonvulsant; Benzodiazepine; Sedative

Use Management of anxiety disorders, ethanol withdrawal symptoms; skeletal muscle relaxant; treatment of convulsive disorders

Orphan drug: Viscous solution for rectal administration: Management of selected, refractory epilepsy patients on stable regimens of antiepileptic drugs (AEDs) requiring intermittent use of diazepam to control episodes of increased seizure activity

Unlabeled/Investigational Use Panic disorders; preoperative sedation, light anesthesia, amnesia

Restrictions C-IV

Pregnancy Risk Factor D

Pregnancy/Breast-Feeding Implications

Clinical effects on the fetus: Crosses the placenta. Oral clefts reported, however, more recent data does not support an association between drug and oral clefts; inguinal hernia, cardiac defects, spina bifida, dysmorphic facial features, skeletal defects, multiple other malformations reported; hypotonia and withdrawal symptoms reported following use near time of delivery

Breast-feeding/lactation: Crosses into breast milk

Clinical effects on the infant: Sedation; AAP reports that USE MAY BE OF CONCERN.

Contraindications Hypersensitivity to diazepam or any component of the formulation (cross-sensitivity with other benzodiazepines may exist); narrow-angle glaucoma; not for use in children <6 months of age (oral) or <30 days of age (parenteral); pregnancy

Warnings/Precautions Diazepam has been associated with increasing the frequency of grand mal seizures. Withdrawal has also been associated with an increase in the seizure frequency. Use with caution in drugs which may decrease diazepam metabolism. Use with caution in elderly or debilitated patients, patients with hepatic disease (including alcoholics), or renal impairment. Active metabolites with extended half-lives may lead to delayed accumulation and adverse effects. Use with caution in patients with respiratory disease or impaired gag reflex.

Acute hypotension, muscle weakness, apnea, and cardiac arrest have occurred with parenteral administration. Acute effects may be more prevalent in patients receiving concurrent barbiturates, narcotics, or ethanol. Appropriate resuscitative equipment and qualified personnel should be available during administration and monitoring. Avoid use of the injection in patients with shock, coma, or acute ethanol intoxication. Intra-arterial injection or extravasation of the parenteral formulation should be avoided. Parenteral formulation contains propylene glycol, which has been associated with toxicity when administered in high dosages.

Causes CNS depression (dose-related) resulting in sedation, dizziness, confusion, or ataxia which may impair physical and mental capabilities. Patients must be cautioned about performing tasks which require mental alertness (ie, operating machinery or driving). Use with caution in patients receiving other CNS depressants or psychoactive agents. Effects with other sedative drugs or ethanol may be potentiated. The dosage of narcotics should be reduced by approximately 1/3 when diazepam is added. Benzodiazepines have been associated with falls and traumatic injury and should be used with extreme caution in patients who are at risk of these events (especially the elderly).

Use caution in patients with depression, particularly if suicidal risk may be present. Use with caution in patients with a history of drug dependence. Benzodiazepines have been associated with dependence and acute withdrawal symptoms on discontinuation or reduction in dose. Acute withdrawal, including seizures, may be precipitated in patients after administration of flumazenil to patients receiving long-term benzodiazepine therapy.

Diazepam has been associated with anterograde amnesia. Paradoxical reactions, including hyperactive or aggressive behavior, have been reported with benzodiazepines, particularly in adolescent/pediatric or psychiatric patients. Does not have analgesic, antidepressant, or antipsychotic properties.

Adverse Reactions Frequency not defined.

Cardiovascular: Hypotension

Central nervous system: Drowsiness, ataxia, amnesia, slurred speech, paradoxical excitement or rage, fatigue, insomnia, memory impairment, headache, anxiety, depression, vertigo, confusion

Dermatologic: Rash

Endocrine & metabolic: Changes in libido

Gastrointestinal: Changes in salivation, constipation, nausea

Genitourinary: Incontinence, urinary retention

Hepatic: Jaundice

Local: Phlebitis, pain with injection

Neuromuscular & skeletal: Dysarthria, tremor

Ocular: Blurred vision, diplopia

Respiratory: Decrease in respiratory rate, apnea

Overdosage/Toxicology Symptoms include somnolence, confusion, coma, hypoactive reflexes, dyspnea, hypotension, slurred speech, and impaired coordination. Treatment for benzodiazepine overdose is supportive. Rarely is mechanical ventilation required. Flumazenil has been shown to selectively block the binding of benzodiazepines to CNS receptors, resulting in a reversal of benzodiazepine-induced CNS depression, but not respiratory depression.

Drug Interactions

Cytochrome P450 Effect: CYP2B6, 2C8/9, 2C19, 3A3/4, 3A5-7 enzyme substrate; CYP2C19 and 3A3/4 enzyme inhibitor

Increased Effect/Toxicity: Diazepam potentiates the CNS depressant effects of narcotic analgesics, barbiturates, phenothiazines, ethanol, antihistamines, MAO inhibitors, sedative-hypnotics, and cyclic antidepressants. Diazepam effect/toxicity may be increased by inhibitors of CYP3A3/4, including amprenavir, cimetidine, ciprofloxacin, clarithromycin, clozapine, diltiazem, disulfiram, digoxin, erythromycin, ethanol, fluconazole, fluoxetine, fluvoxamine, grapefruit juice, isoniazid, itraconazole, ketoconazole, labetalol, levodopa, loxapine, metoprolol, metronidazole, miconazole, nefazodone, nelfinavir, omeprazole, phenytoin, rifabutin, rifampin, ritonavir, troleandomycin, valproic acid, and verapamil.

Decreased Effect: Carbamazepine, rifampin, and rifabutin may enhance the metabolism of diazepam and decrease its therapeutic effect.

Ethanol/Nutrition/Herb Interactions

Ethanol: Avoid ethanol (may increase CNS depression).

(Continued)

Diazepam (Continued)

Food: Diazepam serum levels may be increased if taken with food. Diazepam effect/toxicity may be increased by grapefruit juice; avoid concurrent use.

Herb/Nutraceutical: St John's wort may decrease diazepam levels. Avoid valerian, St John's wort, kava kava, gotu kola (may increase CNS depression).

Stability

Protect parenteral dosage form from light; potency is retained for up to 3 months when kept at room temperature; most stable at pH 4-8, hydrolysis occurs at pH <3; do not mix I.V. product with other medications

Rectal gel: Store at 25°C (77°F); excursion permitted to 15°C to 30°C (59°F to 86°F).

Mechanism of Action Binds to stereospecific benzodiazepine receptors on the postsynaptic GABA neuron at several sites within the central nervous system, including the limbic system, reticular formation. Enhancement of the inhibitory effect of GABA on neuronal excitability results by increased neuronal membrane permeability to chloride ions. This shift in chloride ions results in hyperpolarization (a less excitable state) and stabilization.

Pharmacodynamics/Kinetics

I.V.: Status epilepticus:
Onset of action: Almost immediate
Duration: 20-30 minutes
Absorption: Oral: 85% to 100%, more reliable than I.M.
Protein binding: 98%
Metabolism: Hepatic
Half-life elimination: Parent drug: Adults: 20-50 hours; increased half-life in neonates, elderly, and those with severe hepatic disorders; Active major metabolite (desmethyldiazepam): 50-100 hours; may be prolonged in neonates

Usual Dosage Oral absorption is more reliable than I.M.

Children:
Conscious sedation for procedures: Oral: 0.2-0.3 mg/kg (maximum: 10 mg) 45-60 minutes prior to procedure
Sedation/muscle relaxant/anxiety:
Oral: 0.12-0.8 mg/kg/day in divided doses every 6-8 hours
I.M., I.V.: 0.04-0.3 mg/kg/dose every 2-4 hours to a maximum of 0.6 mg/kg within an 8-hour period if needed
Status epilepticus:
Infants 30 days to 5 years: I.V.: 0.05-0.3 mg/kg/dose given over 2-3 minutes, every 15-30 minutes to a maximum total dose of 5 mg; repeat in 2-4 hours as needed **or** 0.2-0.5 mg/kg/dose every 2-5 minutes to a maximum total dose of 5 mg
>5 years: I.V.: 0.05-0.3 mg/kg/dose given over 2-3 minutes every 15-30 minutes to a maximum total dose of 10 mg; repeat in 2-4 hours as needed **or** 1 mg/dose given over 2-3 minutes, every 2-5 minutes to a maximum total dose of 10 mg
Rectal: 0.5 mg/kg, then 0.25 mg/kg in 10 minutes if needed
Anticonvulsant (acute treatment): Rectal gel formulation:
Infants <6 months: Not recommended
Children <2 years: Safety and efficacy have not been studied
Children 2-5 years: 0.5 mg/kg
Children 6-11 years: 0.3 mg/kg
Children ≥12 years and Adults: 0.2 mg/kg
Note: Dosage should be rounded upward to the next available dose, 2.5, 5, 10, 15, and 20 mg/dose; dose may be repeated in 4-12 hours if needed; do not use more than 5 times per month or more than once every 5 days
Adolescents: Conscious sedation for procedures:
Oral: 10 mg
I.V.: 5 mg, may repeat with ½ dose if needed
Adults:
Anxiety/sedation/skeletal muscle relaxant:
Oral: 2-10 mg 2-4 times/day
I.M., I.V.: 2-10 mg, may repeat in 3-4 hours if needed
Status epilepticus: I.V.: 5-10 mg every 10-20 minutes, up to 30 mg in an 8-hour period; may repeat in 2-4 hours if necessary
Rapid tranquilization of agitated patient (administer every 30-60 minutes): Oral: 5-10 mg; average total dose for tranquilization: 20-60 mg
Elderly: Oral: Initial:
Anxiety: 1-2 mg 1-2 times/day; increase gradually as needed, rarely need to use >10 mg/day (watch for hypotension and excessive sedation)
Skeletal muscle relaxant: 2-5 mg 2-4 times/day
Hemodialysis: Not dialyzable (0% to 5%); supplemental dose is not necessary
Dosing adjustment in hepatic impairment: Reduce dose by 50% in cirrhosis and avoid in severe/acute liver disease

Administration Intensol® should be diluted before use; diazepam does not have any analgesic effects

In children, do not exceed 1-2 mg/minute IVP; adults 5 mg/minute

Monitoring Parameters Respiratory, cardiovascular, and mental status; check for orthostasis

Reference Range Therapeutic: Diazepam: 0.2-1.5 µg/mL (SI: 0.7-5.3 µmol/L); N-desmethyldiazepam (nordiazepam): 0.1-0.5 µg/mL (SI: 0.35-1.8 µmol/L)

Test Interactions False-negative urinary glucose determinations when using Clinistix® or Diastix®

Patient Information Avoid alcohol and other CNS depressants; avoid activities needing good psychomotor coordination until CNS effects are known; drug may cause physical or psychological dependence; avoid abrupt discontinuation after prolonged use

Nursing Implications Provide safety measures (ie, side rails, night light, and call button); supervise ambulation

Additional Information Intensol® should be diluted before use; diazepam does not have any analgesic effects.

Dosage Forms
 Gel, rectal delivery system (Diastat®):
  Adult rectal tip (6 cm): 5 mg/mL (10 mg, 15 mg, 20 mg) [twin packs]
  Pediatric rectal tip (4.4 cm): 5 mg/mL (2.5 mg, 5 mg, 10 mg) [twin packs]
 Injection: 5 mg/mL (1 mL, 2 mL, 5 mL, 10 mL)
 Solution, oral: 5 mg/5 mL (5 mL, 10 mL, 500 mL) [wintergreen-spice flavor]
 Solution, oral concentrate (Diazepam Intensol®): 5 mg/mL (30 mL)
 Tablet: 2 mg, 5 mg, 10 mg

♦ **Diazepam Intensol®** *see* Diazepam *on page 390*

Diazoxide (dye az OKS ide)
Related Information
 Hypertension *on page 1675*
U.S. Brand Names Hyperstat® I.V.; Proglycem®
Canadian Brand Names Hyperstat® I.V.; Proglycem®
Therapeutic Category Antihypertensive Agent; Antihypoglycemic Agent
Use
 Oral: Hypoglycemia related to islet cell adenoma, carcinoma, hyperplasia, or adenomatosis, nesidioblastosis, leucine sensitivity, or extrapancreatic malignancy
 I.V.: Severe hypertension
Pregnancy Risk Factor C
Usual Dosage
 Hypertension: Children and Adults: I.V.: 1-3 mg/kg up to a maximum of 150 mg in a single injection; repeat dose in 5-15 minutes until blood pressure adequately reduced; repeat administration at intervals of 4-24 hours; monitor the blood pressure closely; do not use longer than 10 days
 Hyperinsulinemic hypoglycemia: Oral: **Note:** Use lower dose listed as initial dose
  Newborns and Infants: 8-15 mg/kg/day in divided doses every 8-12 hours
  Children and Adults: 3-8 mg/kg/day in divided doses every 8-12 hours
  Dosing adjustment in renal impairment: None
  Dialysis: Elimination is not enhanced via hemo- or peritoneal dialysis; supplemental dose is not necessary
Additional Information Complete prescribing information for this medication should be consulted for additional detail.
Dosage Forms
 Capsule (Proglycem®): 50 mg
 Injection (Hyperstat®): 15 mg/mL (1 mL, 20 mL)
 Suspension, oral (Proglycem®): 50 mg/mL (30 mL) [chocolate-mint flavor]

♦ **Dibent®** *see* Dicyclomine *on page 397*
♦ **Dibenzyline®** *see* Phenoxybenzamine *on page 1072*
♦ **DIC** *see* Dacarbazine *on page 354*
♦ **Dicarbosil® [OTC]** *see* Calcium Carbonate *on page 207*
♦ **Dichloralphenazone, Acetaminophen, and Isometheptene** *see* Acetaminophen, Isometheptene, and Dichloralphenazone *on page 28*
♦ **Dichloralphenazone, Isometheptene, and Acetaminophen** *see* Acetaminophen, Isometheptene, and Dichloralphenazone *on page 28*

Dichlorodifluoromethane and Trichloromonofluoromethane
(dye klor oh dye flor oh METH ane & tri klor oh mon oh flor oh METH ane)
U.S. Brand Names Fluori-Methane®
Synonyms Trichloromonofluoromethane and Dichlorodifluoromethane
Therapeutic Category Analgesic, Topical
Use Management of pain associated with injections
Usual Dosage Invert bottle over treatment area approximately 12" away from site of application; open dispenseal spring valve completely, allowing liquid to flow in a stream from the bottle. The rate of spraying is approximately 10 cm/second and should be continued until entire muscle has been covered.
Additional Information Complete prescribing information for this medication should be consulted for additional detail.
Dosage Forms Aerosol, topical: Dichlorodifluoromethane 15% and trichloromonofluoromethane 85% (103 mL)

♦ **Dichysterol** *see* Dihydrotachysterol *on page 409*

Diclofenac (dye KLOE fen ak)
Related Information
 Nonsteroidal Anti-Inflammatory Agents Comparison *on page 1512*
U.S. Brand Names Cataflam®; Solaraze™; Voltaren®; Voltaren®-XR
Canadian Brand Names Apo®-Diclo; Apo®-Diclo SR; Cataflam®; Diclotec; Novo-Difenac®; Novo-Difenac K; Novo-Difenac-SR®; Nu-Diclo; Nu-Diclo-SR; PMS-Diclofenac; PMS-Diclofenac SR; Riva-Diclofenac; Riva-Diclofenac-K; Voltaren®; Voltaren Ophtha®; Voltaren Rapide®
Synonyms Diclofenac Potassium; Diclofenac Sodium
Therapeutic Category Nonsteroidal Anti-inflammatory Drug (NSAID), Oral
Use
 Immediate-release tablets: Acute treatment of mild to moderate pain; ankylosing spondylitis; primary dysmenorrhea; acute and chronic treatment of rheumatoid arthritis, osteoarthritis
 Delayed-release tablets: Acute and chronic treatment of rheumatoid arthritis, osteoarthritis, ankylosing spondylitis
 Extended-release tablets: Chronic treatment of osteoarthritis, rheumatoid arthritis
 Ophthalmic solution: Postoperative inflammation following cataract extraction; temporary relief of pain and photophobia in patients undergoing corneal refractive surgery
(Continued)

Diclofenac *(Continued)*

Topical gel: Actinic keratosis (AK) in conjunction with sun avoidance

Unlabeled/Investigational Use Juvenile rheumatoid arthritis

Pregnancy Risk Factor B/D (3rd trimester)

Pregnancy/Breast-Feeding Implications Safety and efficacy in pregnant women have not been established. Exposure late in pregnancy may lead to premature closure of the ductus arteriosus and may inhibit uterine contractions. Diclofenac may be excreted in human milk; use with caution in breast-feeding women.

Contraindications Hypersensitivity to diclofenac, any component of the formulation, aspirin or other nonsteroidal anti-inflammatory drugs (NSAIDs), including patients who experience bronchospasm, asthma, rhinitis, or urticaria following NSAID or aspirin; porphyria; pregnancy (3rd trimester)

Warnings/Precautions Use with caution in patients with congestive heart failure, dehydration, hypertension, decreased renal or hepatic function, history of GI disease, active gastrointestinal ulceration or bleeding, or those receiving anticoagulants. Anaphylactoid reactions have been reported with NSAID use, even without prior exposure; may be more common in patients with the aspirin triad. Use with caution in patients with pre-existing asthma. Rare cases of severe hepatic reactions (including necrosis, jaundice, fulminant hepatitis) have been reported. Vision changes (including changes in color) have been rarely reported with oral diclofenac. Topical gel should not be applied to the eyes, open wounds, infected areas, or to exfoliative dermatitis. Monitor patients for 1 year following application of ophthalmic drops for corneal refractive procedures. Patients using ophthalmic drops should not wear soft contact lenses. Ophthalmic drops may slow/delay healing or prolong bleeding time following surgery. Elderly are at a high risk for adverse effects from nonsteroidal anti-inflammatory agents. As many as 60% of elderly can develop peptic ulceration and/or hemorrhage asymptomatically.

Use lowest effective dose for shortest period possible. Use of NSAIDs can compromise existing renal function especially when Cl_{cr} is <30 mL/minute. CNS adverse effects such as confusion, agitation, and hallucination are generally seen in overdose or high-dose situations; however, elderly may demonstrate these adverse effects at lower doses than younger adults. Withhold for at least 4-6 half-lives prior to surgical or dental procedures.

Adverse Reactions

>10%:
Local: Application site reactions (gel): Pruritus (31% to 52%), rash (35% to 46%), contact dermatitis (19% to 33%), dry skin (25% to 27%), pain (15% to 26%), exfoliation (6% to 24%), paresthesia (8% to 20%)
Ocular: Ophthalmic drops (incidence may be dependent upon indication): Lacrimation (30%), keratitis (28%), elevated IOP (15%), transient burning/stinging (15%)

1% to 10%:
Central nervous system: Headache (7%), dizziness (3%)
Dermatologic: Pruritus (1% to 3%), rash (1% to 3%)
Endocrine & metabolic: Fluid retention (1% to 3%)
Gastrointestinal: Abdominal cramps (3% to 9%), abdominal pain (3% to 9%), constipation (3% to 9%), diarrhea (3% to 9%), flatulence (3% to 9%), indigestion (3% to 9%), nausea (3% to 9%), abdominal distention (1% to 3%), peptic ulcer/GI bleed (0.6% to 2%)
Hepatic: Increased ALT/AST (2%)
Local: Application site reactions (gel): Edema (4%)
Ocular: Ophthalmic drops: Abnormal vision, acute elevated IOP, blurred vision, conjunctivitis, corneal deposits, corneal edema, corneal opacity, corneal lesions, discharge, eyelid swelling, injection, iritis, irritation, itching, lacrimation disorder, ocular allergy
Otic: Tinnitus (1% to 3%)

<1% (Limited to important or life-threatening): Oral dosage forms: Acute renal failure, agranulocytosis, allergic purpura, alopecia, anaphylactoid reactions, anaphylaxis, angioedema, aplastic anemia, aseptic meningitis, asthma, bullous eruption, cirrhosis, congestive heart failure, eosinophilia, erythema multiforme major, GI hemorrhage, hearing loss, hemolytic anemia, hepatic necrosis, hepatitis, hepatorenal syndrome, interstitial nephritis, jaundice, laryngeal edema, leukopenia, nephrotic syndrome, pancreatitis, papillary necrosis, photosensitivity, purpura, Stevens-Johnson syndrome, swelling of lips and tongue, thrombocytopenia, urticaria, visual changes, vomiting

Overdosage/Toxicology Symptoms include acute renal failure, vomiting, drowsiness, and leukocytosis. Management of nonsteroidal anti-inflammatory drug (NSAID) intoxication is primarily supportive and symptomatic. Fluid therapy is commonly effective in managing hypotension that may occur following an acute NSAID overdose, except when due to acute blood loss.

Drug Interactions

Cytochrome P450 Effect: CYP2C8 and 2C9 enzyme substrate; CYP2C9 enzyme inhibitor
Increased Effect/Toxicity: Increased toxicity of digoxin, methotrexate, cyclosporine, lithium, insulin, sulfonylureas, potassium-sparing diuretics, warfarin, and aspirin.
Decreased Effect: Decreased effect of diclofenac with aspirin. Decreased effect of thiazides, furosemide.

Ethanol/Nutrition/Herb Interactions

Ethanol: Avoid ethanol (may enhance gastric mucosal irritation).
Herb/Nutraceutical: Avoid cat's claw, dong quai, evening primrose, feverfew, garlic, ginger, ginkgo, red clover, horse chestnut, green tea, ginseng (all have additional antiplatelet activity).

Stability Store above 30°C (86°F); protect from moisture, store in tight container.

Mechanism of Action Inhibits prostaglandin synthesis by decreasing the activity of the enzyme, cyclo-oxygenase, which results in decreased formation of prostaglandin precursors. Mechanism of action for the treatment of AK has not been established.

Pharmacodynamics/Kinetics

Onset of action: Cataflam® has a more rapid onset of action than does the sodium salt (Voltaren®), because it dissolves in the stomach instead of the duodenum
Absorption: Topical gel: 10%

Protein binding: 99% to albumin

Metabolism: Hepatic to several metabolites

Half-life elimination: 2 hours

Time to peak, serum: Cataflam®: ~1 hour; Voltaren®: ~2 hours

Excretion: Primarily urine (65%); feces (35%)

Usual Dosage Adults:

Oral:

Analgesia/primary dysmenorrhea: Starting dose: 50 mg 3 times/day; maximum dose: 150 mg/day

Rheumatoid arthritis: 150-200 mg/day in 2-4 divided doses (100 mg/day of sustained release product)

Osteoarthritis: 100-150 mg/day in 2-3 divided doses (100-200 mg/day of sustained release product)

Ankylosing spondylitis: 100-125 mg/day in 4-5 divided doses

Ophthalmic:

Cataract surgery: Instill 1 drop into affected eye 4 times/day beginning 24 hours after cataract surgery and continuing for 2 weeks

Corneal refractive surgery: Instill 1-2 drops into affected eye within the hour prior to surgery, within 15 minutes following surgery, and then continue for 4 times/day, up to 3 days

Topical: Apply gel to lesion area twice daily for 60-90 days

Dosage adjustment in renal impairment: Monitor closely in patients with significant renal impairment

Dosage adjustment in hepatic impairment: No specific dosing recommendations

Elderly: No specific dosing recommendations; elderly may demonstrate adverse effects at lower doses than younger adults, and >60% may develop asymptomatic peptic ulceration with or without hemorrhage; monitor renal function

Dietary Considerations May be taken with food to decrease GI distress.

Monitoring Parameters Monitor CBC, liver enzymes; monitor urine output and BUN/serum creatinine; occult blood loss, hemoglobin, hematocrit

Patient Information Oral: Serious gastrointestinal bleeding can occur as well as ulceration and perforation. Pain may or may not be present. Avoid aspirin and aspirin-containing products while taking this medication. If gastric upset occurs, take with food, milk, or antacid. If gastric adverse effects persist, contact physician. May cause drowsiness, dizziness, blurred vision, and confusion. Use caution when performing tasks that require alertness (eg, driving). Do not take for more than 3 days for fever or 10 days for pain without physician's advice.

Ophthalmic: Apply gentle pressure to inner corner of eye for 30 seconds. Do not use any other eye preparation for at least 10 minutes. May cause sensitivity to bright light. Do not wear soft contact lenses.

Topical gel: Avoid sun during therapy. Cover lesion with gel and smooth into skin gently. You may not notice complete healing until 30 days after therapy is completed. Do not cover lesion with occlusive dressings or apply sunscreens, cosmetics, or other medications to affected area.

Nursing Implications Do not crush tablets. Topical gel: Cover lesion with gel and smooth into skin gently. Do not cover lesion with occlusive dressings or apply sunscreens, cosmetics, or other medications to affected area.

Additional Information Diclofenac potassium = Cataflam®; potassium content: 5.8 mg (0.15 mEq) per 50 mg tablet

Dosage Forms

Gel, as sodium (Solaraze™): 30 mg/g (25 g, 50 g)

Solution, ophthalmic, as sodium (Voltaren®): 0.1% (2.5 mL, 5 mL)

Tablet, as potassium (Cataflam®): 50 mg

Tablet, delayed release: 25 mg, 50 mg, 75 mg

Tablet, enteric coated, as sodium: 25 mg, 50 mg, 75 mg

Voltaren®: 25 mg, 50 mg, 75 mg

Tablet, extended release, as sodium (Voltaren®-XR): 100 mg

Diclofenac and Misoprostol (dye KLOE fen ak & mye soe PROST ole)

U.S. Brand Names Arthrotec®

Canadian Brand Names Arthrotec®

Synonyms Misoprostol and Diclofenac

Therapeutic Category Analgesic, Nonsteroidal Anti-inflammatory Drug; Prostaglandin

Use The diclofenac component is indicated for the treatment of osteoarthritis and rheumatoid arthritis; the misoprostol component is indicated for the prophylaxis of NSAID-induced gastric and duodenal ulceration

Pregnancy Risk Factor X

Usual Dosage Oral:

Adults:

Arthrotec® 50:

Osteoarthritis: 1 tablet 2-3 times/day

Rheumatoid arthritis: 1 tablet 3-4 times/day

For both regimens, if not tolerated by patient, the dose may be reduced to 1 tablet twice daily

Arthrotec® 75:

Patients who cannot tolerate full daily Arthrotec® 50 regimens: 1 tablet twice daily

Note: The use of these tablets may not be as effective at preventing GI ulceration

Elderly: No specific dosage adjustment is recommended; may require reduced dosage due to lower body weight; monitor renal function

Additional Information Complete prescribing information for this medication should be consulted for additional detail.

Dosage Forms Tablet: Diclofenac 50 mg and misoprostol 200 mcg; diclofenac 75 mg and misoprostol 200 mcg

- **Diclofenac Potassium** *see Diclofenac on page 393*
- **Diclofenac Sodium** *see Diclofenac on page 393*
- **Diclotec (Can)** *see Diclofenac on page 393*

Dicloxacillin (dye kloks a SIL in)

U.S. Brand Names Dycill®; Pathocil®
Canadian Brand Names Dycill®; Pathocil®
Synonyms Dicloxacillin Sodium
Therapeutic Category Antibiotic, Penicillin
Use Treatment of systemic infections such as pneumonia, skin and soft tissue infections, and osteomyelitis caused by penicillinase-producing staphylococci
Pregnancy Risk Factor B
Contraindications Hypersensitivity to dicloxacillin, penicillin, or any component of the formulation
Warnings/Precautions Monitor PT if patient concurrently on warfarin; elimination of drug is slow in neonates; use with caution in patients allergic to cephalosporins; bad taste of suspension may make compliance difficult
Adverse Reactions
1% to 10%: Gastrointestinal: Nausea, diarrhea, abdominal pain
<1% (Limited to important or life-threatening): Agranulocytosis, eosinophilia, hemolytic anemia, hepatotoxicity, hypersensitivity, interstitial nephritis, leukopenia, neutropenia, prolonged PT, pseudomembranous colitis, rash (maculopapular to exfoliative), seizures with extremely high doses and/or renal failure, serum sickness-like reactions, thrombocytopenia, vaginitis, vomiting
Overdosage/Toxicology Symptoms of penicillin overdose include neuromuscular hypersensitivity (agitation, hallucinations, asterixis, encephalopathy, confusion, seizures) and electrolyte imbalance (with potassium or sodium salts), especially in renal failure. Hemodialysis may be helpful to aid in removal of the drug from the blood, otherwise, most treatment is supportive or symptom directed.
Drug Interactions
Increased Effect/Toxicity: Disulfiram, probenecid may increase penicillin levels. Increased effect of (warfarin) anticoagulants.
Decreased Effect: Efficacy of oral contraceptives may be reduced when taken with dicloxacillin.
Ethanol/Nutrition/Herb Interactions Food: Decreases drug absorption rate; decreases drug serum concentration.
Stability Refrigerate suspension after reconstitution; discard after 14 days if refrigerated or 7 days if kept at room temperature; unit dose antibiotic oral syringes are stable for 48 hours
Mechanism of Action Inhibits bacterial cell wall synthesis by binding to one or more of the penicillin binding proteins (PBPs); which in turn inhibits the final transpeptidation step of peptidoglycan synthesis in bacterial cell walls, thus inhibiting cell wall biosynthesis. Bacteria eventually lyse due to ongoing activity of cell wall autolytic enzymes (autolysins and murein hydrolases) while cell wall assembly is arrested.
Pharmacodynamics/Kinetics
Absorption: 35% to 76%; food decreases rate and extent of absorption
Distribution: Throughout body with highest concentrations in kidney and liver; CSF penetration is low; crosses placenta; enters breast milk
Protein binding: 96%
Half-life elimination: 0.6-0.8 hours; slightly prolonged with renal impairment
Time to peak, serum: 0.5-2 hours
Excretion: Feces; urine (56% to 70% as unchanged drug); prolonged in neonates
Usual Dosage Oral:
Use in newborns not recommended
Children <40 kg: 12.5-25 mg/kg/day divided every 6 hours; doses of 50-100 mg/kg/day in divided doses every 6 hours have been used for therapy of osteomyelitis
Children >40 kg and Adults: 125-250 mg every 6 hours
Dosage adjustment in renal impairment: Not necessary
Hemodialysis: Not dialyzable (0% to 5%); supplemental dosage not necessary
Peritoneal dialysis: Supplemental dosage not necessary
Continuous arteriovenous or venovenous hemofiltration: Supplemental dosage not necessary
Dietary Considerations Administer on an empty stomach 1 hour before or 2 hours after meals.
Monitoring Parameters Monitor prothrombin time if patient concurrently on warfarin; monitor for signs of anaphylaxis during first dose
Test Interactions False-positive urine and serum proteins; false-positive in uric acid, urinary steroids; may interfere with urinary glucose tests using cupric sulfate (Benedict's solution, Clinitest®); may inactivate aminoglycosides *in vitro*
Patient Information Take until all medication used; take 1 hour before or 2 hours after meals, do not skip doses
Nursing Implications
Administer around-the-clock rather than 4 times/day, 3 times/day, etc (ie, 12-6-12-6, not 9-1-5-9) to promote less variation in peak and trough serum levels
Monitor periodic monitoring of CBC, urinalysis, BUN, serum creatinine, and liver enzymes during prolonged therapy
Additional Information
Sodium content of 250 mg capsule: 13 mg (0.6 mEq)
Sodium content of suspension 65 mg/5 mL: 27 mg (1.2 mEq)
Dosage Forms
Capsule, as sodium: 125 mg, 250 mg, 500 mg
Powder for oral suspension, as sodium: 62.5 mg/5 mL (80 mL, 100 mL, 200 mL)

- **Dicloxacillin Sodium** *see Dicloxacillin on page 396*

Dicyclomine (dye SYE kloe meen)

U.S. Brand Names Antispas®; Bentyl®; Byclomine®; Dibent®; Di-Spaz®; Or-Tyl®
Canadian Brand Names Bentylol®; Formulex®; Lomine
Synonyms Dicyclomine Hydrochloride; Dicycloverine Hydrochloride
Therapeutic Category Antispasmodic Agent, Gastrointestinal
Use Treatment of functional disturbances of GI motility such as irritable bowel syndrome
    Other reported use: Urinary incontinence
Pregnancy Risk Factor B
Usual Dosage
  Oral:
    Infants >6 months: 5 mg/dose 3-4 times/day
    Children: 10 mg/dose 3-4 times/day
    Adults: Begin with 80 mg/day in 4 equally divided doses, then increase up to 160 mg/day
  I.M. **(should not be used I.V.):** Adults: 80 mg/day in 4 divided doses (20 mg/dose)
Additional Information Complete prescribing information for this medication should be consulted for additional detail.
Dosage Forms
  Capsule, as hydrochloride: 10 mg
  Injection, as hydrochloride: 10 mg/mL (2 mL, 10 mL)
  Syrup, as hydrochloride: 10 mg/5 mL (118 mL, 473 mL, 946 mL)
  Tablet, as hydrochloride: 20 mg

♦ **Dicyclomine Hydrochloride** *see* Dicyclomine *on page 397*
♦ **Dicycloverine Hydrochloride** *see* Dicyclomine *on page 397*

Didanosine (dye DAN oh seen)

Related Information
  Antiretroviral Agents Comparison *on page 1488*
  Antiretroviral Therapy for HIV Infection *on page 1595*
  Management of Healthcare Worker Exposures to HIV, HBV, HCV *on page 1555*
U.S. Brand Names Videx®; Videx® EC
Canadian Brand Names Videx™
Synonyms ddl; Dideoxyinosine
Therapeutic Category Antiretroviral Agent, Nucleoside Reverse Transcriptase Inhibitor (NRTI) [Adenosine Analog]
Use Treatment of HIV infection; always to be used in combination with at least two other antiretroviral agents
Pregnancy Risk Factor B
Pregnancy/Breast-Feeding Implications Cases of fatal and nonfatal lactic acidosis, with or without pancreatitis, have been reported in pregnant women. It is not known if pregnancy itself potentiates this known side effect; however, pregnant women may be at increased risk of lactic acidosis and liver damage. Hepatic enzymes and electrolytes should be monitored frequently during the 3rd trimester of pregnancy. Use during pregnancy only if the potential benefit to the mother outweighs the potential risk of this complication.
  Clinical effects on the fetus: Phase I/II studies have shown limited placental transfer. Health professionals are encouraged to contact the antiretroviral pregnancy registry to monitor outcomes of pregnant women exposed to antiretroviral medications (1-800-258-4263).
Contraindications Hypersensitivity to didanosine or any component of the formulation
Warnings/Precautions Pancreatitis (sometimes fatal) has been reported, incidence is dose related. Risk factors for developing pancreatitis include a previous history of the condition, concurrent cytomegalovirus or *Mycobacterium avium-intracellulare* infection, and concomitant use of stavudine, pentamidine, or co-trimoxazole. Discontinue didanosine if clinical signs of pancreatitis occur. Lactic acidosis and severe hepatomegaly with steatosis (sometimes fatal) have occurred with antiretroviral nucleoside analogues, including didanosine. Pregnant women may be at increased risk of lactic acidosis and liver damage.

Peripheral neuropathy occurs in ~20% of patients receiving the drug. Retinal changes (including retinal depigmentation) and optic neuritis have been reported in adults and children using didanosine. Patients should undergo retinal examination every 6-12 months. Use with caution in patients with decreased renal or hepatic function, phenylketonuria, sodium-restricted diets, or with edema, congestive heart failure, or hyperuricemia. Twice-daily dosing is the preferred dosing frequency for didanosine tablets. Didanosine sustained release capsules are indicated for once-daily use.
Adverse Reactions As reported in monotherapy studies; risk of toxicity may increase when combined with other agent.

>10%:
  Gastrointestinal: Increased amylase (15% to 17%), abdominal pain (7% to 13%), diarrhea (19% to 28%)
  Neuromuscular & skeletal: Peripheral neuropathy (17% to 20%)
1% to 10%:
  Dermatologic: Rash, pruritus
  Endocrine & metabolic: Increased uric acid
  Gastrointestinal: Pancreatitis; patients >65 years of age had a higher frequency of pancreatitis than younger patients
  Hepatic: Increased SGOT, increased SGPT, increased alkaline phosphatase
Postmarketing and/or case reports: Alopecia, anaphylactoid reaction, anemia, anorexia, arthralgia, diabetes mellitus, granulocytopenia, hepatitis, hypersensitivity, lactic acidosis/hepatomegaly, leukopenia, liver failure, myalgia, myopathy, neuritis, optic renal impairment, pain, retinal depigmentation, rhabdomyolysis, seizures, thrombocytopenia, weakness
Overdosage/Toxicology Chronic overdose may cause pancreatitis, peripheral neuropathy, diarrhea, hyperuricemia, and hepatic impairment. There is no known antidote for didanosine overdose. Treatment is symptomatic.
(Continued)

Didanosine *(Continued)*

Drug Interactions

Increased Effect/Toxicity: Concomitant administration of other drugs which have the potential to cause peripheral neuropathy or pancreatitis may increase the risk of these toxicities Allopurinol may increase didanosine concentration; avoid concurrent use. Concomitant use of antacids with buffered tablet or pediatric didanosine solution may potentiate adverse effects of aluminum- or magnesium-containing antacids. Ganciclovir may increase didanosine concentration; monitor. Hydroxyurea may precipitate didanosine-induced pancreatitis if added to therapy; concomitant use is not recommended.

Decreased Effect: Didanosine buffered tablets and buffered pediatric solution may decrease absorption of quinolones or tetracyclines (administer 2 hours prior to didanosine buffered formulations). Didanosine should be held during PCP treatment with pentamidine. Didanosine may decrease levels of indinavir. Drugs whose absorption depends on the level of acidity in the stomach such as ketoconazole, itraconazole, and dapsone should be administered at least 2 hours prior to the buffered formulations of didanosine (not affected by sustained release capsules). Methadone may decrease didanosine concentrations.

Ethanol/Nutrition/Herb Interactions

Ethanol: Avoid ethanol (increases risk of pancreatitis).

Food: Decreases AUC and C_{max}. Didanosine serum levels may be decreased by 55% if taken with food.

Stability Tablets and sustained release capsules should be stored in tightly closed bottles at 15°C to 30°C; tablets undergo rapid degradation when exposed to an acidic environment; tablets dispersed in water are stable for 1 hour at room temperature; reconstituted buffered solution is stable for 4 hours at room temperature; pediatric solution, when reconstituted with antacid as directed, is stable for 30 days if refrigerated

Mechanism of Action Didanosine, a purine nucleoside analogue and the deamination product of dideoxyadenosine (ddA), inhibits HIV replication *in vitro* in both T cells and monocytes. Didanosine is converted within the cell to the mono-, di-, and triphosphates of ddA. These ddA triphosphates act as substrate and inhibitor of HIV reverse transcriptase substrate and inhibitor of HIV reverse transcriptase thereby blocking viral DNA synthesis and suppressing HIV replication.

Pharmacodynamics/Kinetics

Absorption: Subject to degradation by acidic pH of stomach; some formulations are buffered to resist acidic pH; ≤50% reduction in peak plasma concentration is observed in presence of food. Sustained release capsules contain enteric-coated beadlets which dissolve in the small intestine.

Distribution: V_d: Children: 35.6 L/m²; Adults: 1.08 L/kg

Protein binding: <5%

Metabolism: Has not been evaluated in humans; studies conducted in dogs, show extensive metabolism with allantoin, hypoxanthine, xanthine, and uric acid being the major metabolites found in urine

Bioavailability: 42%

Half-life elimination:

Children and Adolescents: 0.8 hour

Adults: Normal renal function: 1.5 hours; however, its active metabolite ddATP has an intracellular half-life >12 hours *in vitro*; Impaired renal function: 2.5-5 hours

Time to peak: Buffered tablets: 0.67 hours; sustained release capsules: 2 hours

Excretion: Urine (~55% as unchanged drug)

Clearance: Total body: Averages 800 mL/minute

Usual Dosage Treatment of HIV infection: Oral (administer on an empty stomach):

Children: 180 mg/m²/day divided every 12 hours **or** dosing is based on body surface area (m²) as follows:

BSA ≤0.4 m²: 25 mg twice daily (tablets)

BSA 0.5-0.7 m²: 50 mg twice daily (tablets)

BSA 0.8-1.0 m²: 75 mg twice daily (tablets)

BSA 1.1-1.4 m²: 100 mg twice daily (tablets)

Children <1 year should receive 1 tablet per dose and children >1 year should receive 2-4 tablets per dose for adequate buffering and absorption; tablets should be chewed or dispersed

Adults: Dosing based on patient weight:

Note: Preferred dosing frequency is twice daily for didanosine tablets

Tablets:

<60 kg: 125 mg twice daily or 250 mg once daily

≥60 kg: 200 mg twice daily or 400 mg once daily

Recommended Dose (mg) of Didanosine by Body Weight

Creatinine Clearance (mL/min)	≥60 kg			<60 kg		
	Tablet* (mg)	Buffered Powder† (mg)	Sustained Release Capsule (mg)	Tablet* (mg)	Buffered Powder† (mg)	Sustained Release Capsule (mg)
≥60	400 qd or 200 bid	250 bid	400 qd	250 qd or 125 bid	167 bid	250 qd
30-59	200 qd or 100 bid	100 bid	200 qd	150 qd or 75 bid	100 bid	125 qd
10-29	150 qd	167 qd	125 qd	100 qd	100 bid	125 qd
<10	100 qd	100 qd	125 qd	75 qd	100 qd	‡

*Chewable/dispersible buffered tablet; 2 tablets must be taken with each dose; different strengths of tablets may be combined to yield the recommended dose.

†Buffered powder for oral solution

‡Not suitable for use in patients <60 kg with Cl_cr <10 mL/minute; use alternate formulation

Note: Adults should receive 2-4 tablets per dose for adequate buffering and absorption; tablets should be chewed or dispersed; didanosine has also been used as 300 mg once daily

Buffered Powder:
  <60 kg: 167 mg twice daily
  ≥60 kg: 250 mg twice daily
Sustained release capsule:
  <60 kg: 250 mg once daily
  ≥60 kg: 400 mg once daily

Dosage adjustment in renal impairment: Dosing based on patient weight, creatinine clearance, and dosage form: See table.

Hemodialysis: Removed by hemodialysis (40% to 60%)

Dosage adjustment in hepatic impairment: Should be considered; monitor for toxicity

Elderly patients have a higher frequency of pancreatitis (10% versus 5% in younger patients); monitor renal function and dose accordingly

Dietary Considerations Do not mix with fruit juice or other acid-containing liquid; administer at least 1 hour before or 2 hours after eating. Each chewable tablet contains 36.5 mg phenylalanine and 8.6 mEq magnesium. Each single-dose powder packet (for oral solution) contains 1380 mg sodium.

Administration
Chewable/dispersible buffered tablets: At least 2 tablets, but no more than 4 tablets, should be taken together to allow adequate buffering. Tablets may be chewed or dispersed prior to consumption. To disperse, dissolve in 1 oz water, stir until uniform dispersion is formed, and drink immediately. May also add 1 oz of clear apple juice to initial dispersion if additional flavor is needed. The apple juice dilution is stable for 1 hour at room temperature.

Buffered powder for oral solution: Pour contents of packet into 4 ounces of water. Mix until dissolved and drink immediately. Do not mix with fruit juice.

Pediatric powder for oral solution: Prior to dispensing, the powder should be mixed with purified water USP to an initial concentration of 20 mg/mL and then further diluted with an appropriate antacid suspension to a final mixture of 10 mg/mL. Shake well prior to use.

Monitoring Parameters Serum potassium, uric acid, creatinine; hemoglobin, CBC with neutrophil and platelet count, CD4 cells; viral load; liver function tests, amylase; weight gain; perform dilated retinal exam every 6 months

Patient Information Take as directed, 1 hour before or 2 hours after eating. You will be susceptible to infection; avoid crowds. Report numbness or tingling of fingers, toes, or feet; abdominal pain; or persistent nausea or vomiting. Should have a retinal exam every 6-12 months. Notify prescriber if you are pregnant or plan to be pregnant. Do not breast-feed. HIV-infected mothers are discouraged from breast-feeding to decrease potential transmission of HIV.

Chewable/dispersible tablets: Chew tablets thoroughly and/or dissolve in water

Single-dose buffered powder for oral solution: Pour powder into 4 oz of liquid, stir, and drink immediately; do not mix with fruit juice or other acid-containing liquids

Sustained release capsules should be swallowed whole; do not chew, crush or open the capsule

Pediatric oral solution: Shake well before use; store in refrigerator; discard after 30 days

Nursing Implications Administer liquified powder immediately after dissolving; avoid creating dust if powder spilled, use wet mop or damp sponge

Additional Information Sodium content of buffered tablets: 264.5 mg (11.5 mEq)

Dosage Forms
Capsule, sustained release: 125 mg, 200 mg, 250 mg, 400 mg
Powder for oral solution, buffered [single-dose packet]: 100 mg, 167 mg, 250 mg
  Powder for oral solution, reconstituted, pediatric: 2 g, 4 g
Tablet, buffered, chewable/dispersible: 25 mg, 50 mg, 100 mg, 150 mg, 200 mg [mint flavor]

♦ **Dideoxycytidine** *see* Zalcitabine *on page 1431*
♦ **Dideoxyinosine** *see* Didanosine *on page 397*
♦ **Didronel®** *see* Etidronate Disodium *on page 531*

Diethylpropion (dye eth il PROE pee on)

Related Information
Antacid Drug Interactions *on page 1477*
Obesity Treatment Guidelines for Adults *on page 1685*

U.S. Brand Names Tenuate®; Tenuate® Dospan®

Canadian Brand Names Tenuate®; Tenuate® Dospan®

Synonyms Amfepramone; Diethylpropion Hydrochloride

Therapeutic Category Anorexiant

Use Short-term adjunct in a regimen of weight reduction based on exercise, behavioral modification, and caloric reduction in the management of exogenous obesity for patients with an initial body mass index ≥30 kg/m² or ≥27 kg/m² in the presence of other risk factors (diabetes, hypertension)

Unlabeled/Investigational Use Migraine

Restrictions C-IV

Pregnancy Risk Factor B

Usual Dosage Adults: Oral:
Tablet: 25 mg 3 times/day before meals or food
Tablet, controlled release: 75 mg at midmorning

Additional Information Complete prescribing information for this medication should be consulted for additional detail.

Dosage Forms
Tablet, as hydrochloride: 25 mg
Tablet, controlled release, as hydrochloride: 75 mg

♦ **Diethylpropion Hydrochloride** *see Diethylpropion on page 399*

Diethylstilbestrol (dye eth il stil BES trole)
U.S. Brand Names Stilphostrol®
Canadian Brand Names Honvol®; Stilbestrol
Synonyms DES; Diethylstilbestrol Diphosphate Sodium; Stilbestrol
Therapeutic Category Estrogen Derivative; Estrogen Derivative, Oral; Estrogen Derivative, Parenteral
Use Palliative treatment of inoperable metastatic prostatic carcinoma and postmenopausal inoperable, progressing breast cancer
Pregnancy Risk Factor X
Contraindications Undiagnosed vaginal bleeding; breast cancer except in select patients with metastatic disease; pregnancy
Warnings/Precautions Use with caution in patients with a history of thromboembolism, stroke, myocardial infarction (especially >40 years of age who smoke), liver tumor, hypertension, cardiac, renal or hepatic insufficiency; estrogens have been reported to increase the risk of endometrial carcinoma; do not use estrogens during pregnancy
Adverse Reactions
>10%:
Cardiovascular: Peripheral edema
Endocrine & metabolic: Enlargement of breasts (female and male), breast tenderness
Gastrointestinal: Nausea, anorexia, bloating
1% to 10%:
Central nervous system: Headache, migraine headache
Endocrine & metabolic: Increased libido (female), decreased libido (male)
Gastrointestinal: Vomiting, diarrhea
<1% (Limited to important or life-threatening): Alterations in frequency and flow of menses, amenorrhea, anxiety, breast tumors, decreased glucose tolerance, depression, dizziness, edema, gallbladder obstruction, GI distress, hepatitis, hypertension, increased susceptibility to *Candida* infection, increased triglycerides and LDL, intolerance to contact lenses, myocardial infarction, nausea, stroke, thromboembolism
Overdosage/Toxicology Symptoms include nausea.
Drug Interactions
Decreased Effect: Barbiturates, phenytoin, and rifampin may decrease steroids.
Stability Intravenous solution should be stored at room temperature and away from direct light; solution is stable for 3 days as long as cloudiness or precipitation has not occurred
Mechanism of Action Competes with estrogenic and androgenic compounds for binding onto tumor cells and thereby inhibits their effects on tumor growth
Pharmacodynamics/Kinetics
Metabolism: Hepatic
Excretion: Urine and feces
Usual Dosage Adults:
Male:
Prostate carcinoma (inoperable, progressing):
Oral: Diphosphate 50 mg 3 times/day; increase up to 200 mg or more 3 times/day; maximum daily dose: 1 g
I.V.: Administer 0.5 g, dissolved in 250 mL of saline or D_5W, administer slowly the first 10-15 minutes then adjust rate so that the entire amount is given in 1 hour; repeat for ≥5 days depending on patient response, then repeat 0.25-0.5 g 1-2 times for one week or change to oral therapy
Female: Postmenopausal (inoperable, progressing) breast carcinoma: Oral: 15 mg/day
Dietary Considerations Should be taken with food to decrease GI distress.
Administration I.V. infusion: Dilute 0.5-1 g in 250-500 mL D_5W or NS; give 1-2 mL/minute for 10-15 minutes, then infuse remaining solution over 1 hour
Test Interactions
Increased prothrombin and factors VII, VIII, IX, X
Decreased antithrombin III
Increased platelet aggregability
Increased thyroid-binding globulin
Increased total thyroid hormone (T_4)
Decreased serum folate concentration
Increased serum triglycerides/phospholipids
Patient Information Patients should inform their physicians if signs or symptoms of thromboembolic or thrombotic disorders including sudden severe headache or vomiting, disturbance of vision or speech, loss of vision, numbness or weakness in an extremity, sharp or crushing chest pain, calf pain, shortness of breath, severe abdominal pain or mass, mental depression or unusual bleeding.
Nursing Implications Administer 0.5 g I.V., dissolved in 250 mL of saline or D_5W, administer slowly the first 10-15 minutes then adjust rate so that the entire amount is administered in 1 hour
Dosage Forms
Injection, as diphosphate sodium: 0.25 g (5 mL)
Tablet: 50 mg

♦ **Diethylstilbestrol Diphosphate Sodium** *see Diethylstilbestrol on page 400*

Difenoxin and Atropine (dye fen OKS in & A troe peen)
U.S. Brand Names Motofen®
Synonyms Atropine and Difenoxin
Therapeutic Category Antidiarrheal
Use Treatment of diarrhea
Restrictions C-IV
Pregnancy Risk Factor C

Usual Dosage Adults: Oral: Initial: 2 tablets, then 1 tablet after each loose stool; 1 tablet every 3-4 hours, up to 8 tablets in a 24-hour period; if no improvement after 48 hours, continued administration is not indicated

Additional Information Complete prescribing information for this medication should be consulted for additional detail.

Dosage Forms Tablet: Difenoxin hydrochloride 1 mg and atropine sulfate 0.025 mg

♦ **Differin®** *see* Adapalene *on page 36*

Diflorasone (dye FLOR a sone)

Related Information

Corticosteroids Comparison *on page 1495*

U.S. Brand Names Maxiflor®; Psorcon™; Psorcon™ E

Canadian Brand Names Florone®; Psorcon™

Synonyms Diflorasone Diacetate

Therapeutic Category Corticosteroid, Topical (High Potency); Corticosteroid, Topical (Very High Potency)

Use Relieves inflammation and pruritic symptoms of corticosteroid-responsive dermatosis (high to very high potency topical corticosteroid)

Maxiflor®: High potency topical corticosteroid
Psorcon™: Very high potency topical corticosteroid

Pregnancy Risk Factor C

Contraindications Hypersensitivity to diflorasone

Warnings/Precautions Use with caution in patients with impaired circulation; skin infections

Adverse Reactions <1% (Limited to important or life-threatening): Arthralgia, burning, dryness, folliculitis, itching, maceration, muscle atrophy, secondary infection

Overdosage/Toxicology Symptoms include moon face, central obesity, hypertension, diabetes, hyperlipidemia, peptic ulcer, increased susceptibility to infection, electrolyte and fluid imbalance, psychosis, and hallucinations. When consumed in excessive quantities, systemic hypercorticism and adrenal suppression may occur; in those cases, discontinuation and withdrawal of the corticosteroid should be done judiciously.

Mechanism of Action Decreases inflammation by suppression of migration of polymorphonuclear leukocytes and reversal of increased capillary permeability

Pharmacodynamics/Kinetics

Absorption: Negligible, around 1% reaches dermal layers or systemic circulation; occlusive dressings increase absorption percutaneously

Metabolism: Primarily hepatic

Usual Dosage Topical: Apply ointment sparingly 1-3 times/day; apply cream sparingly 2-4 times/day. Therapy should be discontinued when control is achieved; if no improvement is seen, reassessment of diagnosis may be necessary.

Patient Information A thin film of cream or ointment is effective; do not overuse; do not use tight-fitting diapers or plastic pants on children being treated in the diaper area; use only as prescribed, and for no longer than the period prescribed; apply sparingly in light film; rub in lightly; avoid contact with eyes; notify physician if condition being treated persists or worsens

Nursing Implications For external use only; do not use on open wounds; apply sparingly to occlusive dressings; should not be used in the presence of open or weeping lesions

Dosage Forms

Cream, topical, as diacetate: 0.05% (15 g, 30 g, 60 g)
Ointment, topical, as diacetate: 0.05% (15 g, 30 g, 60 g)

♦ **Diflorasone Diacetate** *see* Diflorasone *on page 401*

♦ **Diflucan®** *see* Fluconazole *on page 565*

Diflunisal (dye FLOO ni sal)

Related Information

Nonsteroidal Anti-Inflammatory Agents Comparison *on page 1512*

U.S. Brand Names Dolobid®

Canadian Brand Names Apo®-Diflunisal; Novo-Diflunisal; Nu-Diflunisal

Therapeutic Category Analgesic, Nonsteroidal Anti-inflammatory Drug; Anti-inflammatory Agent; Nonsteroidal Anti-inflammatory Drug (NSAID), Oral

Use Management of inflammatory disorders usually including rheumatoid arthritis and osteoarthritis; can be used as an analgesic for treatment of mild to moderate pain

Pregnancy Risk Factor C (1st and 2nd trimesters); D (3rd trimester)

Contraindications Hypersensitivity to diflunisal or any component of the formulation; may be a cross-sensitivity with other nonsteroidal anti-inflammatory agents including aspirin; should not be used in patients with active GI bleeding; pregnancy (3rd trimester)

Warnings/Precautions Peptic ulceration and GI bleeding have been reported; platelet function and bleeding time are inhibited; ophthalmologic effects; impaired renal function, use lower dosage; dehydration; peripheral edema; possibility of Reye's syndrome; elevation in liver tests. Withhold for at least 4-6 half-lives prior to surgical or dental procedures.

Adverse Reactions

1% to 10%:

Cardiovascular: Chest pain, arrhythmias

Central nervous system: Dizziness, headache

Dermatologic: Rash

Endocrine & metabolic: Fluid retention

Gastrointestinal: Abdominal cramps, bloated feeling, constipation, diarrhea, indigestion, nausea, vomiting, mouth soreness

Genitourinary: Vaginal bleeding

Otic: Tinnitus

<1% (Limited to important or life-threatening): Agranulocytosis, angioedema, chest pain, dyspnea, edema, erythema multiforme, exfoliative dermatitis, hallucinations, hearing loss, hemolytic anemia, hepatitis, interstitial nephritis, itching, mental depression, nephrotic

(Continued)

Diflunisal *(Continued)*

syndrome, renal impairment, seizures, Stevens-Johnson syndrome, thrombocytopenia, toxic epidermal necrolysis, urticaria, vasculitis, wheezing

Overdosage/Toxicology Symptoms include drowsiness, nausea, vomiting, hyperventilation, tachycardia, tinnitus, stupor, coma, renal failure, and leukocytosis. Management of nonsteroidal anti-inflammatory drug (NSAID) intoxication is primarily supportive and symptomatic. Fluid therapy is commonly effective in managing hypotension that may occur following an acute NSAID overdose, except when due to acute blood loss.

Drug Interactions

Increased Effect/Toxicity: May cause increased toxicity of cyclosporine, digoxin, methotrexate, anticoagulants, phenytoin, sulfonylureas, sulfonamides, lithium, indomethacin, hydrochlorothiazide, and acetaminophen (levels) when coadministered with diflunisal.

Decreased Effect: Decreased effect with antacids, aspirin.

Ethanol/Nutrition/Herb Interactions

Ethanol: Avoid ethanol (may enhance gastric mucosal irritation).

Herb/Nutraceutical: Avoid cat's claw, dong quai, evening primrose, feverfew, garlic, ginger, ginkgo, red clover, horse chestnut, green tea, ginseng (all have additional antiplatelet activity).

Mechanism of Action Inhibits prostaglandin synthesis by decreasing the activity of the enzyme, cyclo-oxygenase, which results in decreased formation of prostaglandin precursors

Pharmacodynamics/Kinetics

Onset of action: Analgesic: ~1 hour

Duration: 8-12 hours

Absorption: Well absorbed

Distribution: Enters breast milk

Metabolism: Extensively hepatic

Half-life elimination: 8-12 hours; prolonged with renal impairment

Time to peak, serum: 2-3 hours

Excretion: Urine (~3% as unchanged drug, 90% as glucuronide conjugates) within 72-96 hours

Usual Dosage Adults: Oral:

Pain: Initial: 500-1000 mg followed by 250-500 mg every 8-12 hours; maximum daily dose: 1.5 g

Inflammatory condition: 500-1000 mg/day in 2 divided doses; maximum daily dose: 1.5 g

Dosing adjustment in renal impairment: Cl_{cr} <50 mL/minute: Administer 50% of normal dose

Dietary Considerations Should be taken with food to decrease GI distress.

Test Interactions Decrease in uric acid (S), increase in salicylate levels (S), increase in bleeding time

Patient Information May cause GI upset, take with water, milk, or meals; do not take aspirin with diflunisal, swallow tablets whole, do not crush or chew

Nursing Implications Do not crush tablet

Additional Information Diflunisal is a salicylic acid derivative which is chemically different than aspirin and is not metabolized to salicylic acid. It is not considered a salicylate. Diflunisal 500 mg is equal in analgesic efficacy to aspirin 650 mg, acetaminophen 650 mg, and acetaminophen 650 mg/propoxyphene napsylate 100 mg, but has a longer duration of effect (8-12 hours). Not recommended as an antipyretic. Not found to be clinically useful to treat fever; at doses ≥2 g/day, platelets are reversibly inhibited in function. Diflunisal is uricosuric at 500-750 mg/day; causes less GI and renal toxicity than aspirin and other NSAIDs; fecal blood loss is $^1/_2$ that of aspirin at 2.6 g/day.

Dosage Forms Tablet: 250 mg, 500 mg

♦ **Digibind**® *see Digoxin Immune Fab on page 405*

♦ **DigiFab**™ *see Digoxin Immune Fab on page 405*

Digitoxin *Not Available in U.S.* (di ji TOKS in)

U.S. Brand Names Crystodigin® [DSC]

Therapeutic Category Antiarrhythmic Agent, Miscellaneous; Cardiac Glycoside

Use Treatment of congestive heart failure, atrial fibrillation, atrial flutter, paroxysmal atrial tachycardia, and cardiogenic shock

Pregnancy Risk Factor C

Usual Dosage Oral:

Children: Doses are very individualized; **when recommended**, digitalizing dose is as follows:

<1 year: 0.045 mg/kg

1-2 years: 0.04 mg/kg

>2 years: 0.03 mg/kg which is equivalent to 0.75 mg/m^2

Maintenance: Approximately $^1/_{10}$ of the digitalizing dose

Adults: Oral:

Rapid loading dose: Initial: 0.6 mg followed by 0.4 mg and then 0.2 mg at intervals of 4-6 hours

Slow loading dose: 0.2 mg twice daily for a period of 4 days followed by a maintenance dose

Maintenance: 0.05-0.3 mg/day

Most common dose: 0.15 mg/day

Dosing adjustment in renal impairment: Cl_{cr} <10 mL/minute: Administer 50% to 75% of normal dose.

Hemodialysis: Not dialyzable (0% to 5%)

Dosing adjustment in hepatic impairment: Dosage reduction is necessary in severe liver disease.

Additional Information Complete prescribing information for this medication should be consulted for additional detail.

Dosage Forms Tablet: 0.1 mg, 0.2 mg

Digoxin (di JOKS in)

Related Information
Adult ACLS Algorithms *on page 1632*
Antacid Drug Interactions *on page 1477*
Antiarrhythmic Drugs Comparison *on page 1478*
Heart Failure *on page 1663*

U.S. Brand Names Lanoxicaps®; Lanoxin®

Canadian Brand Names Lanoxicaps®; Lanoxin®

Therapeutic Category Antiarrhythmic Agent, Miscellaneous; Cardiac Glycoside

Use Treatment of congestive heart failure and to slow the ventricular rate in tachyarrhythmias such as atrial fibrillation, atrial flutter, and supraventricular tachycardia (paroxysmal atrial tachycardia); cardiogenic shock

Pregnancy Risk Factor C

Contraindications Hypersensitivity to digoxin or any component of the formulation; hypersensitivity to cardiac glycosides (another may be tried); history of toxicity; ventricular tachycardia or fibrillation; idiopathic hypertrophic subaortic stenosis; constrictive pericarditis; amyloid disease; second- or third-degree heart block (except in patients with a functioning artificial pacemaker); Wolff-Parkinson-White syndrome and atrial fibrillation concurrently

Warnings/Precautions Use with caution in patients with hypoxia, myxedema, hypothyroidism, acute myocarditis; patients with incomplete AV block (Stokes-Adams attack) may progress to complete block with digitalis drug administration; use with caution in patients with acute myocardial infarction, severe pulmonary disease, advanced heart failure, idiopathic hypertrophic subaortic stenosis, Wolff-Parkinson-White syndrome, sick-sinus syndrome (bradyarrhythmias), amyloid heart disease, and constrictive cardiomyopathies; adjust dose with renal impairment and when verapamil, quinidine or amiodarone are added to a patient on digoxin; elderly and neonates may develop exaggerated serum/tissue concentrations due to age-related alterations in clearance and pharmacodynamic differences; exercise will reduce serum concentrations of digoxin due to increased skeletal muscle uptake; recent studies indicate photopsia, chromatopsia and decreased visual acuity may occur even with therapeutic serum drug levels; reduce or hold dose 1-2 days before elective electrical cardioversion

Adverse Reactions Incidence of reactions are not always reported.

Cardiovascular: Heart block; first-, second- (Wenckebach), or third-degree heart block; asystole; atrial tachycardia with block; AV dissociation; accelerated junctional rhythm; ventricular tachycardia or ventricular fibrillation; PR prolongation; ST segment depression

Central nervous system: Visual disturbances (blurred or yellow vision), headache (3.2%), weakness, dizziness (4.9%), apathy, confusion, mental disturbances (4.1%), anxiety, depression, hallucinations, fever

Dermatologic: Maculopapular rash (1.6%), erythematous, scarlatiniform, papular, vesicular or bullous rashes, urticaria, pruritus, facial, angioneurotic or laryngeal edema, shedding of fingernails or toenails, alopecia

Gastrointestinal: Nausea (3.2%), vomiting (1.6%), diarrhea (3.2%), abdominal pain

<1% (Limited to important or life-threatening): Abdominal pain, anorexia, eosinophilia, gynecomastia, hemorrhagic necrosis of the intestines, increased plasma estrogen and decreased serum luteinizing hormone in men and postmenopausal women and decreased plasma testosterone in men, intestinal ischemia, palpitations, sexual dysfunction, thrombocytopenia, unifocal or multiform ventricular premature contractions (especially bigeminy or trigeminy), vaginal cornification

Any arrhythmia in a child on digoxin should be considered as digoxin toxicity. The gastrointestinal and central nervous system symptoms are not frequently seen in children.

Overdosage/Toxicology Symptoms of acute overdose include vomiting, hyperkalemia, sinus bradycardia, S-A arrest and A-V block are common, ventricular tachycardia, and fibrillation. Symptoms of chronic intoxication include visual disturbances, weakness, sinus bradycardia, atrial fibrillation with slowed ventricular response, and ventricular arrhythmias. After GI decontamination, treat hyperkalemia if >5.5 mEq/L with sodium bicarbonate and glucose with insulin or Kayexalate®. Treat bradycardia or heart block with atropine or pacemaker and other arrhythmias with conventional antiarrhythmics. Use Digibind® for severe hyperkalemia, symptomatic arrhythmias unresponsive to other drugs, and for prophylactic treatment in massive overdose.

Drug Interactions

Increased Effect/Toxicity: Beta-blocking agents (propranolol), verapamil, and diltiazem may have additive effects on heart rate. Carvedilol has additive effects on heart rate and inhibits the metabolism of digoxin. Digoxin levels may be increased by amiodarone (reduce digoxin dose 50%), bepridil, cyclosporine, diltiazem, indomethacin, itraconazole, some macrolides (erythromycin, clarithromycin), methimazole, nitrendipine, propafenone, propylthiouracil, quinidine (reduce digoxin dose 33% to 50% on initiation), tetracyclines, and verapamil. Moricizine may increase the toxicity of digoxin (mechanism undefined). Spironolactone may interfere with some digoxin assays, but may also increase blood levels directly. Succinylcholine administration to patients on digoxin has been associated with an increased risk of arrhythmias. Rare cases of acute digoxin toxicity have been associated with parenteral calcium (bolus) administration. The following medications have been associated with increased digoxin blood levels which appear to be of limited clinical significance: Famciclovir, flecainide, ibuprofen, fluoxetine, nefazodone, cimetidine, famotidine, ranitidine, omeprazole, trimethoprim.

Decreased Effect: Amiloride and spironolactone may reduce the inotropic response to digoxin. Cholestyramine, colestipol, kaolin-pectin, and metoclopramide may reduce digoxin absorption. Levothyroxine (and other thyroid supplements) may decrease digoxin blood levels. Penicillamine has been associated with reductions in digoxin blood levels The following reported interactions appear to be of limited clinical significance: Aminoglutethimide, aminosalicylic acid, aluminum-containing antacids, sucralfate, sulfasalazine, neomycin, ticlopidine.

(Continued)

Digoxin (Continued)

Ethanol/Nutrition/Herb Interactions

Food: Digoxin peak serum levels may be decreased if taken with food. Meals containing increased fiber (bran) or foods high in pectin may decrease oral absorption of digoxin.

Herb/Nutraceutical: Avoid ephedra (risk of cardiac stimulation). Avoid natural licorice (causes sodium and water retention and increases potassium loss).

Stability Protect elixir and injection from light; solution **compatibility**: D_5W, $D_{10}W$, NS, sterile water for injection (when diluted fourfold or greater)

Mechanism of Action

Congestive heart failure: Inhibition of the sodium/potassium ATPase pump which acts to increase the intracellular sodium-calcium exchange to increase intracellular calcium leading to increased contractility

Supraventricular arrhythmias: Direct suppression of the AV node conduction to increase effective refractory period and decrease conduction velocity - positive inotropic effect, enhanced vagal tone, and decreased ventricular rate to fast atrial arrhythmias. Atrial fibrillation may decrease sensitivity and increase tolerance to higher serum digoxin concentrations.

Pharmacodynamics/Kinetics

Onset of action: Oral: 1-2 hours; I.V.: 5-30 minutes

Peak effect: Oral: 2-8 hours; I.V.: 1-4 hours

Duration: Adults: 3-4 days both forms

Absorption: By passive nonsaturable diffusion in the upper small intestine; food may delay, but does not affect extent of absorption

Distribution:

Normal renal function: 6-7 L/kg

V_d: Extensive to peripheral tissues, with a distinct distribution phase which lasts 6-8 hours; concentrates in heart, liver, kidney, skeletal muscle, and intestines. Heart/serum concentration is 70:1. Pharmacologic effects are delayed and do not correlate well with serum concentrations during distribution phase.

Hyperthyroidism: Increased V_d

Hyperkalemia, hyponatremia: Decreased digoxin distribution to heart and muscle

Hypokalemia: Increased digoxin distribution to heart and muscles

Concomitant quinidine therapy: Decreased V_d

Chronic renal failure: 4-6 L/kg

Decreased sodium/potassium ATPase activity - decreased tissue binding

Neonates, full term: 7.5-10 L/kg

Children: 16 L/kg

Adults: 7 L/kg, decreased with renal disease

Protein binding: 30% (in uremic patients, digoxin is displaced from plasma protein binding sites)

Metabolism: By sequential sugar hydrolysis in the stomach or by reduction of lactone ring by intestinal bacteria (in ~10% of population, gut bacteria may metabolize up to 40% of digoxin dose); metabolites may contribute to therapeutic and toxic effects of digoxin; metabolism is reduced with CHF

Bioavailability: Oral (formulation dependent): Elixir: 75% to 85%; Tablets: 70% to 80%

Half-life elimination (age, renal and cardiac function dependent):

Neonates: Premature: 61-170 hours; Full-term: 35-45 hours

Infants: 18-25 hours

Children: 35 hours

Adults: 38-48 hours

Adults, anephric: 4-6 days

Half-life elimination: Parent drug: 38 hours; Metabolites: Digoxigenin: 4 hours; Monodigitoxoside: 3-12 hours

Time to peak, serum: Oral: ~1 hour

Excretion: Urine (50% to 70% as unchanged drug)

Usual Dosage When changing from oral (tablets or liquid) or I.M. to I.V. therapy, dosage should be reduced by 20% to 25%. Refer to the following: See table.

Dosage Recommendations for Digoxin

Age	Total Digitalizing Dose† (mcg/kg*)		Daily Maintenance Dose‡ (mcg/kg*)	
	P.O.	I.V. or I.M.	P.O.	I.V. or I.M.
Preterm infant*	20-30	15-25	5-7.5	4-6
Full-term infant*	25-35	20-30	6-10	5-8
1 mo - 2 y*	35-60	30-50	10-15	7.5-12
2-5 y*	30-40	25-35	7.5-10	6-9
5-10 y*	20-35	15-30	5-10	4-8
>10 y*	10-15	8-12	2.5-5	2-3
Adults	0.75-1.5 mg	0.5-1 mg	0.125-0.5 mg	0.1-0.4 mg

*Based on lean body weight and normal renal function for age. Decrease dose in patients with ↓ renal function; digitalizing dose often not recommended in infants and children.

†Give one-half of the total digitalizing dose (TDD) in the initial dose, then give one-quarter of the TDD in each of two subsequent doses at 8- to 12-hour intervals. Obtain EKG 6 hours after each dose to assess potential toxicity.

‡Divided every 12 hours in infants and children <10 years of age. Given once daily to children >10 years of age and adults.

Dosing adjustment/interval in renal impairment:

Cl_{cr} 10-50 mL/minute: Administer 25% to 75% of dose or every 36 hours

Cl_{cr} <10 mL/minute: Administer 10% to 25% of dose or every 48 hours

Reduce loading dose by 50% in ESRD

Hemodialysis: Not dialyzable (0% to 5%)

Dietary Considerations Maintain adequate amounts of potassium in diet to decrease risk of hypokalemia (hypokalemia may increase risk of digoxin toxicity).

Monitoring Parameters
When to draw serum digoxin concentrations: Digoxin serum concentrations are monitored because digoxin possesses a narrow therapeutic serum range; the therapeutic endpoint is difficult to quantify and digoxin toxicity may be life-threatening. Digoxin serum levels should be drawn **at least 4 hours after an intravenous dose** and **at least 6 hours after an oral dose (optimally 12-24 hours after a dose).**

Initiation of therapy:
If a loading dose is given: Digoxin serum concentration may be drawn within 12-24 hours after the initial loading dose administration. Levels drawn this early may confirm the relationship of digoxin plasma levels and response but are of little value in determining maintenance doses.

If a loading dose is not given: Digoxin serum concentration should be obtained after 3-5 days of therapy

Maintenance therapy:
Trough concentrations should be followed just prior to the next dose or at a minimum of 4 hours after an I.V. dose and at least 6 hours after an oral dose

Digoxin serum concentrations should be obtained within 5-7 days (approximate time to steady-state) after any dosage changes. Continue to obtain digoxin serum concentrations 7-14 days after any change in maintenance dose. **Note:** In patients with end-stage renal disease, it may take 15-20 days to reach steady-state.

Additionally, patients who are receiving potassium-depleting medications such as diuretics, should be monitored for potassium, magnesium, and calcium levels

Digoxin serum concentrations should be obtained whenever any of the following conditions occur:
Questionable patient compliance or to evaluate clinical deterioration following an initial good response
Changing renal function
Suspected digoxin toxicity
Initiation or discontinuation of therapy with drugs (amiodarone, quinidine, verapamil) which potentially interact with digoxin; if quinidine therapy is started; digoxin levels should be drawn within the first 24 hours after starting quinidine therapy, then 7-14 days later or empirically skip one day's digoxin dose and decrease the daily dose by 50%
Any disease changes (hypothyroidism)
Heart rate and rhythm should be monitored along with periodic EKGs to assess both desired effects and signs of toxicity
Follow closely (especially in patients receiving diuretics or amphotericin) for decreased serum potassium and magnesium or increased calcium, all of which predispose to digoxin toxicity
Assess renal function
Be aware of drug interactions

Reference Range
Digoxin therapeutic serum concentrations:
Congestive heart failure: 0.8-2 ng/mL
Arrhythmias: 1.5-2.5 ng/mL
Adults: <0.5 ng/mL; probably indicates underdigitalization unless there are special circumstances
Toxic: >2.5 ng/mL; tachyarrhythmias commonly require levels >2 ng/mL
Digoxin-like immunoreactive substance (DLIS) may cross-react with digoxin immunoassay. DLIS has been found in patients with renal and liver disease, congestive heart failure, neonates, and pregnant women (3rd trimester).

Patient Information Do not discontinue medication without checking with physician; notify physician if loss of appetite or visual changes occur

Nursing Implications Observe patients for noncardiac signs of toxicity, ie, anorexia, vision changes (blurred), confusion, and depression

Dosage Forms
Capsule: 50 mcg, 100 mcg, 200 mcg
Elixir, pediatric: 50 mcg/mL with alcohol 10% (60 mL) [lime flavor]
Injection: 250 mcg/mL (1 mL, 2 mL)
Injection, pediatric: 100 mcg/mL (1 mL)
Tablet: 125 mcg, 250 mcg, 500 mcg

Digoxin Immune Fab (di JOKS in i MYUN fab)

U.S. Brand Names Digibind®; DigiFab™
Canadian Brand Names Digibind®
Synonyms Antidigoxin Fab Fragments, Ovine
Therapeutic Category Antidote, Digoxin
Use Treatment of life-threatening or potentially life-threatening digoxin intoxication, including:
• acute digoxin ingestion (ie, >10 mg in adults or >4 mg in children)
• chronic ingestions leading to steady-state digoxin concentrations > 6 ng/mL in adults or >4 ng/mL in children
• manifestations of digoxin toxicity due to overdose (life-threatening ventricular arrhythmias, progressive bradycardia, second- or third-degree heart block not responsive to atropine, serum potassium >5 mEq/L in adults or >6 mEq/L in children)

Pregnancy Risk Factor C
Pregnancy/Breast-Feeding Implications Animal reproduction studies have not been conducted. Safety and efficacy in pregnant women have not been established. Use during pregnancy only if clearly needed.
Contraindications Hypersensitivity to sheep products or any component of the formulation
Warnings/Precautions Use with caution in renal or cardiac failure; allergic reactions possible (sheep product)-skin testing not routinely recommended; epinephrine should be immediately available, Fab fragments may be eliminated more slowly in patients with renal failure, heart
(Continued)

Digoxin Immune Fab *(Continued)*

failure may be exacerbated as digoxin level is reduced; total serum digoxin concentration may rise precipitously following administration of Digibind®, but this will be almost entirely bound to the Fab fragment and not able to react with receptors in the body; Digibind® will interfere with digitalis immunoassay measurements - this will result in clinically misleading serum digoxin concentrations until the Fab fragment is eliminated from the body (several days to >1 week after Digibind® administration). Hypokalemia has been reported to occur following reversal of digitalis intoxication as has exacerbation of underlying heart failure. Serum digoxin levels drawn prior to therapy may be difficult to evaluate if 6-8 hours have not elapsed after the last dose of digoxin (time to equilibration between serum and tissue); redigitalization should not be initiated until Fab fragments have been eliminated from the body, which may occur over several days or greater than a week in patients with impaired renal function.

Adverse Reactions Frequency not defined.

Cardiovascular: Effects (due to withdrawal of digitalis) include exacerbation of low cardiac output states and congestive heart failure, rapid ventricular response in patients with atrial fibrillation; postural hypotension

Endocrine & metabolic: Hypokalemia

Local: Phlebitis

Miscellaneous: Allergic reactions, serum sickness

Overdosage/Toxicology Symptoms include delayed serum sickness. Treatment of serum sickness includes acetaminophen, histamine$_1$ and possibly histamine$_2$ blockers and cortico-steroids.

Drug Interactions

Increased Effect/Toxicity: Digoxin: Following administration of digoxin immune Fab, serum digoxin levels are markedly increased due to bound complexes (may be clinically misleading, since bound complex cannot interact with receptors).

Stability Should be refrigerated (2°C to 8°C). Reconstitute by adding 4 mL sterile water, resulting in 10 mg/mL for I.V. infusion. The reconstituted solution may be further diluted with NS to a convenient volume (eg, 1 mg/mL). Reconstituted solutions should be used within 4 hours if refrigerated. For very small doses, vial can be reconstituted by adding an additional 36 mL of sterile isotonic saline, to achieve a final concentration of 1 mg/mL.

Mechanism of Action Digoxin immune antigen-binding fragments (Fab) are specific antibodies for the treatment of digitalis intoxication in carefully selected patients; binds with molecules of digoxin or digitoxin and then is excreted by the kidneys and removed from the body

Pharmacodynamics/Kinetics

Onset of action: I.V.: Improvement in 2-30 minutes for toxicity

Half-life elimination: 15-20 hours; prolonged with renal impairment

Excretion: Urine; level declines to undetectable amounts in 5-7 days

Usual Dosage Each vial of Digibind® 38 mg or DigiFab™ 40 mg will bind ~0.5 mg of digoxin or digitoxin.

Estimation of the dose is based on the body burden of digitalis. This may be calculated if the amount ingested is known or the postdistribution serum drug level is known (round dose to the nearest whole vial). See table.

Digoxin Immune Fab

Tablets Ingested (0.25 mg)	Fab Dose (vials)
5	2
10	4
25	10
50	20
75	30
100	40
150	60
200	80

Fab dose based on serum drug level postdistribution:

Digoxin: No. of vials = level (ng/mL) x body weight (kg) divided by 100

Digitoxin: No. of vials = digitoxin (ng/mL) x body weight (kg) divided by 1000

If neither amount ingested nor drug level are known, dose empirically as follows:

For acute toxicity: 20 vials, administered in 2 divided doses to decrease the possibility of a febrile reaction, and to avoid fluid overload in small children.

For chronic toxicity: 6 vials; for infants and small children (≤20kg), a single vial may be sufficient

Administration Continuous I.V. infusion over ≥30 minutes is preferred. May give by bolus injection if cardiac arrest is imminent. Small doses (infants/small children) may be administered using tuberculin syringe. Stopping the infusion and restarting at a slower rate may help if infusion-related reactions occur.

Monitoring Parameters Serum potassium, serum digoxin concentration prior to first dose of digoxin immune Fab; **digoxin levels will greatly increase with digoxin immune Fab use and are not an accurate determination of body stores**; standard digoxin concentration measurements may be misleading until Fab fragments are eliminated from the body.

Patients with renal failure should be monitored for a prolonged period for re-intoxication with digoxin following the re-release of bound digoxin into the blood.

Test Interactions Digoxin immune Fab interferes with digitalis immunoassay test leading to misleading digoxin serum concentrations until the Fab fragments are eliminated from the body. If possible, take digoxin serum levels prior to the administration of digoxin immune Fab; keeping in mind the time the last dose of digoxin was taken.

Dosage Forms Powder for injection, lyophilized:
Digibind®: 38 mg
DigiFab™: 40 mg

♦ **Dihematoporphyrin Ether** see Porfimer on page 1104

♦ **Dihistine® DH** see Chlorpheniramine, Pseudoephedrine, and Codeine on page 281

♦ **Dihistine® Expectorant** see Guaifenesin, Pseudoephedrine, and Codeine on page 648

♦ **Dihydrex®** see DiphenhydrAMINE on page 414

Dihydrocodeine Compound (dye hye droe KOE deen KOM pound)
U.S. Brand Names DHC Plus®; Synalgos®-DC
Therapeutic Category Analgesic, Narcotic
Use Management of mild to moderate pain that requires relaxation
Restrictions C-III
Pregnancy Risk Factor B/D (prolonged use or high doses at term)
Contraindications Hypersensitivity to dihydrocodeine or any component of the formulation; pregnancy (prolonged use or high doses at term)
Warnings/Precautions Use with caution in patients with hypersensitivity reactions to other phenanthrene derivative opioid agonists (morphine, hydrocodone, hydromorphone, levorphanol, oxycodone, oxymorphone); respiratory diseases including asthma, emphysema, COPD, or severe liver or renal insufficiency; some preparations contain sulfites which may cause allergic reactions; dextromethorphan has equivalent antitussive activity but has much lower toxicity in accidental overdose; tolerance of drug dependence may result from extended use

Adverse Reactions
>10%:
Central nervous system: Lightheadedness, dizziness, drowsiness, sedation
Dermatologic: Pruritus, skin reactions
Gastrointestinal: Nausea, vomiting, constipation
1% to 10%:
Cardiovascular: Hypotension, palpitations, bradycardia, peripheral vasodilation
Central nervous system: Increased intracranial pressure
Endocrine & metabolic: Antidiuretic hormone release
Gastrointestinal: Biliary tract spasm
Genitourinary: Urinary tract spasm
Ocular: Miosis
Respiratory: Respiratory depression
Miscellaneous: Histamine release, physical and psychological dependence with prolonged use

Overdosage/Toxicology Treatment includes naloxone 2 mg I.V. (0.01 mg/kg for children), with repeat administration as necessary, up to a total of 10 mg.

Drug Interactions
Cytochrome P450 Effect: CYP2D6 enzyme substrate
Increased Effect/Toxicity: MAO inhibitors may increase adverse symptoms.
Ethanol/Nutrition/Herb Interactions Ethanol: Avoid ethanol (may increase CNS depression).
Mechanism of Action Binds to opiate receptors in the CNS, causing inhibition of ascending pain pathways, altering the perception of and response to pain; causes cough suppression by direct central action in the medulla; produces generalized CNS depression
Pharmacodynamics/Kinetics
Onset of action: 10-30 minutes
Duration: 4-6 hours
Half-life elimination, serum: 3.8 hours
Time to peak, serum: 30-60 minutes
Usual Dosage
Adults: Oral: 1-2 capsules every 4-6 hours as needed for pain
Elderly: Initial dosing should be cautious (low end of adult dosing range)
Patient Information Avoid alcohol; may cause drowsiness, impaired judgment or coordination; may cause physical and psychological dependence with prolonged use
Nursing Implications Observe patient for excessive sedation, respiratory depression; implement safety measures, assist with ambulation
Dosage Forms
Capsule:
DHC Plus®: Dihydrocodeine bitartrate 16 mg, acetaminophen 356.4 mg, and caffeine 30 mg
Synalgos®-DC: Dihydrocodeine bitartrate 16 mg, aspirin 356.4 mg, and caffeine 30 mg

Dihydroergotamine (dye hye droe er GOT a meen)
U.S. Brand Names D.H.E. 45®; Migranal® Nasal Spray
Canadian Brand Names Migranal®
Synonyms DHE; Dihydroergotamine Mesylate
Therapeutic Category Ergot Alkaloid and Derivative
Use Treatment of migraine headache with or without aura; injection also indicated for treatment of cluster headaches
Unlabeled/Investigational Use Adjunct for DVT prophylaxis for hip surgery, for orthostatic hypotension, xerostomia secondary to antidepressant use, and pelvic congestion with pain
Pregnancy Risk Factor X
Pregnancy/Breast-Feeding Implications Dihydroergotamine is oxytocic and should not be used during pregnancy. Ergot derivatives inhibit prolactin and it is known that ergotamine is excreted in breast milk (vomiting, diarrhea, weak pulse, and unstable blood pressure have been reported in nursing infants). It is not known if dihydroergotamine would also cause these (Continued)

Dihydroergotamine *(Continued)*

effects, however, it is likely that it is excreted in human breast milk. Do not use in nursing women.

Contraindications Hypersensitivity to dihydroergotamine or any component of the formulation; high-dose aspirin therapy; uncontrolled hypertension, ischemic heart disease, angina pectoris, history of MI, silent ischemia, or coronary artery vasospasm including Prinzmetal's angina; hemiplegic or basilar migraine; peripheral vascular disease; sepsis; severe hepatic or renal dysfunction; following vascular surgery; avoid use within 24 hours of sumatriptan, zolmitriptan, other serotonin agonists, or ergot-like agents; avoid during or within 2 weeks of discontinuing MAO inhibitors; concurrent use with ritonavir, nelfinavir, and amprenavir; pregnancy

Warnings/Precautions Do not give to patients with risk factors for CAD until a cardiovascular evaluation has been performed; if evaluation is satisfactory, the healthcare provider should administer the first dose and cardiovascular status should be periodically evaluated. May cause vasospastic reactions; persistent vasospasm may lead to gangrene or death in patients with compromised circulation. Discontinue if signs of vasoconstriction develop. Rare reports of increased blood pressure in patients without history of hypertension. Rare reports of adverse cardiac events (acute MI, life-threatening arrhythmias, death) have been reported following use of the injection. Cerebral hemorrhage, subarachnoid hemorrhage, and stroke have also occurred following use of the injection. Not for prolonged use. Safety and efficacy in pediatric patients have not been established.

Adverse Reactions

>10%: Nasal spray: Respiratory: Rhinitis (26%)

1% to 10%: Nasal spray:
Central nervous system: Dizziness (4%), somnolence (3%)
Endocrine & metabolic: Hot flashes (1%)
Gastrointestinal: Nausea (10%), taste disturbance (8%), vomiting (4%), diarrhea (2%)
Local: Application site reaction (6%)
Neuromuscular & skeletal: Weakness (1%), stiffness (1%)
Respiratory: Pharyngitis (3%)

<1% (Limited to important or life-threatening): Injection and nasal spray: Cerebral hemorrhage, coronary artery vasospasm, hypertension, myocardial infarction, paresthesia, peripheral cyanosis, peripheral ischemia, rash, stroke, subarachnoid hemorrhage, ventricular fibrillation, ventricular tachycardia. Pleural and retroperitoneal fibrosis have been reported following prolonged use of the injection.

Overdosage/Toxicology Symptoms include peripheral ischemia, paresthesia, headache, nausea, and vomiting. Activated charcoal is effective at binding certain chemicals; this is especially true for ergot alkaloids.

Drug Interactions

Cytochrome P450 Effect: CYP3A enzyme inhibitor

Increased Effect/Toxicity: Concurrent use of protease inhibitors (amprenavir, nelfinavir, and ritonavir) may increase toxicity of dihydroergotamine (use is contraindicated). Increased effect of heparin. Increased toxicity with erythromycin, clarithromycin, nitroglycerin, propranolol, and troleandomycin. Potential for serotonin syndrome if combined with other serotonergic drugs.

Stability

Injection: Store below 25°C (77°F), do not refrigerate or freeze; protect from heat and light

Nasal spray: Prior to use, store below 25°C (77°F), do not refrigerate or freeze; once spray applicator has been prepared, use within 8 hours; discard any unused solution

Mechanism of Action Ergot alkaloid alpha-adrenergic blocker directly stimulates vascular smooth muscle to vasoconstrict peripheral and cerebral vessels; also has effects on serotonin receptors

Pharmacodynamics/Kinetics

Onset of action: 15-30 minutes
Duration: 3-4 hours
Distribution: V_d: 14.5 L/kg
Protein binding: 90%
Metabolism: Extensively hepatic
Half-life elimination: 1.3-3.9 hours
Time to peak, serum: I.M.: 15-30 minutes
Excretion: Primarily feces; urine (10% mostly as metabolites)

Usual Dosage Adults:

I.M., S.C.: 1 mg at first sign of headache; repeat hourly to a maximum dose of 3 mg total; maximum dose: 6 mg/week

I.V.: 1 mg at first sign of headache; repeat hourly up to a maximum dose of 2 mg total; maximum dose: 6 mg/week

Intranasal: 1 spray (0.5 mg) of nasal spray should be administered into each nostril; repeat as needed within 15 minutes, up to a total of 4 sprays in any 24-hour period and no more than 8 sprays in a week

Dosing adjustment in renal impairment: Contraindicated in severe renal impairment

Dosing adjustment in hepatic impairment: Dosage reductions are probably necessary but specific guidelines are not available; contraindicated in severe hepatic dysfunction

Elderly: Patients >65 years of age were not included in controlled clinical studies

Administration Prior to administration of nasal spray the nasal spray applicator must be primed (pumped 4 times); in order to let the drug be absorbed through the skin in the nose, patients should not inhale deeply through the nose while spraying or immediately after spraying; for best results, treatment should be initiated at the first symptom or sign of an attack; however, nasal spray can be used at any stage of a migraine attack

Reference Range Minimum concentration for vasoconstriction is reportedly 0.06 ng/mL

Patient Information Rare feelings of numbness or tingling of fingers, toes, or face may occur. Avoid using this medication if you are pregnant, have heart disease, hypertension, liver disease, infection, itching.

Nasal spray: Do not assemble sprayer until you are ready to use it; prime as instructed. Do not tilt head back or inhale through nose while spraying.

Additional Information Nasal spray contains caffeine.

Dosage Forms

Injection, as mesylate: 1 mg/mL (1 mL)
Solution, intranasal, as mesylate [spray]: 4 mg/mL [0.5 mg/spray] (1 mL)

◆ **Dihydroergotamine Mesylate** *see Dihydroergotamine on page 407*

◆ **Dihydroergotoxine** *see Ergoloid Mesylates on page 482*

◆ **Dihydrogenated Ergot Alkaloids** *see Ergoloid Mesylates on page 482*

◆ **Dihydrohydroxycodeinone** *see Oxycodone on page 1024*

◆ **Dihydromorphinone** *see Hydromorphone on page 685*

Dihydrotachysterol (dye hye droe tak ISS ter ole)

U.S. Brand Names DHT™; Hytakerol®

Canadian Brand Names Hytakerol®

Synonyms Dichysterol

Therapeutic Category Vitamin, Fat Soluble

Use Treatment of hypocalcemia associated with hypoparathyroidism; prophylaxis of hypocalcemic tetany following thyroid surgery

Pregnancy Risk Factor A/D (dose exceeding RDA recommendation)

Usual Dosage Oral:

Hypoparathyroidism:
Infants and young Children: Initial: 1-5 mg/day for 4 days, then 0.1-0.5 mg/day
Older Children and Adults: Initial: 0.8-2.4 mg/day for several days followed by maintenance doses of 0.2-1 mg/day
Nutritional rickets: 0.5 mg as a single dose or 13-50 mcg/day until healing occurs
Renal osteodystrophy: Maintenance: 0.25-0.6 mg/24 hours adjusted as necessary to achieve normal serum calcium levels and promote bone healing

Additional Information Complete prescribing information for this medication should be consulted for additional detail.

Dosage Forms

Capsule (Hytakerol®): 0.125 mg
Solution, oral concentrate (DHT™): 0.2 mg/mL (30 mL)
Tablet (DHT™): 0.125 mg, 0.2 mg, 0.4 mg

◆ **1,25 Dihydroxycholecalciferol** *see Calcitriol on page 204*

◆ **Diiodohydroxyquin** *see Iodoquinol on page 738*

◆ **Diisopropyl Fluorophosphate** *see Isoflurophate on page 747*

◆ **Dilacor® XR** *see Diltiazem on page 409*

◆ **Dilantin®** *see Phenytoin on page 1077*

◆ **Dilatrate®-SR** *see Isosorbide Dinitrate on page 750*

◆ **Dilaudid®** *see Hydromorphone on page 685*

◆ **Dilaudid-5®** *see Hydromorphone on page 685*

◆ **Dilaudid-HP®** *see Hydromorphone on page 685*

◆ **Dilaudid-HP-Plus® (Can)** *see Hydromorphone on page 685*

◆ **Dilaudid® Sterile Powder (Can)** *see Hydromorphone on page 685*

◆ **Dilaudid-XP® (Can)** *see Hydromorphone on page 685*

Diloxanide Furoate (dye LOKS ah nide FYOOR oh ate)

U.S. Brand Names Furamide®

Therapeutic Category Amebicide

Use Treatment of amebiasis (asymptomatic cyst passers)

Additional Information Complete prescribing information for this medication should be consulted for additional detail.

◆ **Diltia® XT** *see Diltiazem on page 409*

Diltiazem (dil TYE a zem)

Related Information

Adult ACLS Algorithms *on page 1632*
Antiarrhythmic Drugs Comparison *on page 1478*
Calcium Channel Blockers Comparison *on page 1494*
Hypertension *on page 1675*

U.S. Brand Names Cardizem®; Cardizem® CD; Cardizem® SR; Cartia® XT; Dilacor® XR; Diltia® XT; Tiamate®; Tiazac®

Canadian Brand Names Alti-Diltiazem; Alti-Diltiazem CD; Apo®-Diltiaz; Apo®-Diltiaz CD; Apo®-Diltiaz SR; Cardizem®; Cardizem® CD; Cardizem® SR; Gen-Diltiazem; Gen-Diltiazem SR; Novo-Diltiazem; Novo-Diltiazem SR; Nu-Diltiaz; Nu-Diltiaz-CD; Rhoxal-diltiazem SR; Syn-Diltiazem®; Tiazac®

Synonyms Diltiazem Hydrochloride

Therapeutic Category Antianginal Agent; Antiarrhythmic Agent, Class IV; Antihypertensive Agent; Calcium Channel Blocker

Use

Capsule: Essential hypertension (sustained release only, alone or in combination); chronic stable angina or angina from coronary artery spasm
Injection: Atrial fibrillation or atrial flutter; paroxysmal supraventricular tachycardia (PSVT)

Unlabeled/Investigational Use Investigational: Therapy of Duchenne muscular dystrophy

Pregnancy Risk Factor C

Pregnancy/Breast-Feeding Implications

Clinical effects on the fetus: Teratogenic and embryotoxic effects have been demonstrated in small animals given doses 5-10 times the adult dose (mg/kg)

(Continued)

Diltiazem *(Continued)*

Breast-feeding/lactation: Freely diffuses into breast milk; however, the AAP considers diltiazem to be **compatible** with breast-feeding. Available evidence suggest safe use during breast-feeding.

Contraindications Hypersensitivity to diltiazem or any component of the formulation; sick sinus syndrome; second- or third-degree AV block (except in patients with a functioning artificial pacemaker); hypotension (systolic <90 mm Hg); acute MI and pulmonary congestion by x-ray

Warnings/Precautions Use with caution and titrate dosages for patients with hypotension or patients taking antihypertensives, impaired renal or hepatic function, or when treating patients with congestive heart failure. Use caution with concomitant therapy with beta-blockers or digoxin. Monitor LFTs during therapy since these enzymes may rarely be increased and symptoms of hepatic injury may occur; usually reverses with drug discontinuation; avoid abrupt withdrawal of calcium blockers since rebound angina is theoretically possible.

Adverse Reactions

>10%: Gastrointestinal: Gingival hyperplasia (21%)

1% to 10%:

Cardiovascular: Sinus bradycardia (2% to 6%), first-degree AV block (2% to 8%), EKG abnormality (4%), peripheral edema (dose-related 5% to 8%), flushing (2% to 3%), hypotension (1%), palpitations (1%)

Central nervous system: Dizziness (3% to 7%), headache (5% to 12%), somnolence (1%), insomnia (1%)

Gastrointestinal: Nausea (1% to 2%), constipation (2%), dyspepsia (1%)

Neuromuscular & skeletal: Weakness (3% to 5%)

Dermatological: Rash (1% to 2%)

Renal: Polyuria (1%)

<1% (Limited to important or life-threatening): Agranulocytosis, akathisia, amnesia, angina, arrhythmia, AV block, bundle branch block, congestive heart failure, depression, dysgeusia, dyspnea, erythema multiforme, exfoliative dermatitis, gait abnormalities, hallucinations, hyperglycemia, impotence, leukocytopenia (overdose), mania, myoclonus, nocturia, osteoarticular pain, paresthesia, Parkinsonian-like syndrome, personality change, photosensitivity, pruritus, psychosis, sexual dysfunction, Stevens-Johnson syndrome, syncope, thrombocytopenia, tinnitus, toxic epidermal necrolysis (TEN), tremor, urticaria, vomiting

Overdosage/Toxicology

Primary cardiac symptoms of calcium blocker overdose include hypotension and bradycardia. Hypotension is caused by peripheral vasodilation, myocardial depression, and bradycardia. Bradycardia results from sinus bradycardia, second- or third-degree atrioventricular block, or sinus arrest with junctional rhythm. Intraventricular conduction is usually not affected, so QRS duration is normal (verapamil prolongs the P-R interval and bepridil prolongs the QT interval and may cause ventricular arrhythmias, including torsade de pointes).

Noncardiac symptoms include confusion, stupor, nausea, vomiting, metabolic acidosis, and hyperglycemia. Following initial gastric decontamination, if possible, repeated calcium administration may promptly reverse depressed cardiac contractility (but not sinus node depression or peripheral vasodilation). Glucagon, epinephrine, and inamrinone (amrinone) may treat refractory hypotension. Glucagon and epinephrine also increase the heart rate (outside the U.S., 4-aminopyridine may be available as an antidote). Dialysis and hemoperfusion are not effective in enhancing elimination, although repeat-dose activated charcoal may serve as an adjunct with sustained-release preparations.

In a few reported cases, overdose with calcium channel blockers has been associated with hypotension and bradycardia, initially refractory to atropine, but becoming more responsive to this agent when larger doses (approaching 1 g/hour for more than 24 hours) of calcium chloride were administered.

Drug Interactions

Cytochrome P450 Effect: CYP3A3/4 enzyme substrate; CYP1A2, 2D6, and 3A3/4 enzyme inhibitor

Increased Effect/Toxicity: Diltiazem effects may be additive with amiodarone, beta-blockers, or digoxin, which may lead to bradycardia, other conduction delays, and decreased cardiac output. Serum concentrations/toxicity of diltiazem may be increased by inhibitors of CYP3A3/4, including amprenavir, cimetidine, ciprofloxacin, clarithromycin, clozapine, diltiazem, disulfiram, digoxin, erythromycin, ethanol, fluconazole, fluoxetine, fluvoxamine, isoniazid, itraconazole, ketoconazole, labetalol, levodopa, loxapine, metoprolol, metronidazole, miconazole, nefazodone, nelfinavir, omeprazole, phenytoin, rifabutin, rifampin, ritonavir, troleandomycin, valproic acid, and verapamil. Diltiazem may increase serum levels/toxicity of alfentanil (possibly fentanyl and sufentanil), some benzodiazepines (specifically midazolam and triazolam), carbamazepine, cisapride (QT prolongation, arrhythmia), cyclosporine, digoxin, HMG-CoA reductase inhibitors (atorvastatin, lovastatin, simvastatin), lithium (neurotoxicity), midazolam, moricizine, and tacrolimus.

Decreased Effect: Rifampin markedly reduces diltiazem serum levels resulting in decreased diltiazem effect. Coadministration with other cytochrome P450 enzyme inducers should be avoided (includes phenytoin, barbiturates, and carbamazepine).

Ethanol/Nutrition/Herb Interactions

Ethanol: Avoid ethanol (may increase risk of hypotension or vasodilation).

Food: Diltiazem serum levels may be elevated if taken with food. Serum concentrations were not altered by grapefruit juice in small clinical trials.

Herb/Nutraceutical: St John's wort may decrease diltiazem levels. Avoid dong quai if using for hypertension (has estrogenic activity). Avoid ephedra (may worsen arrhythmia or hypertension). Avoid yohimbe, ginseng (may worsen hypertension). Avoid garlic (may have increased antihypertensive effect).

Stability Store injections in refrigerator at 2°C to 8°C (36°F to 46°F); stable for 24 hours

Mechanism of Action Inhibits calcium ion from entering the "slow channels" or select voltage-sensitive areas of vascular smooth muscle and myocardium during depolarization, producing a relaxation of coronary vascular smooth muscle and coronary vasodilation; increases myocardial oxygen delivery in patients with vasospastic angina

Pharmacodynamics/Kinetics
Onset of action: Oral: Short-acting tablets: 30-60 minutes
Absorption: 80% to 90%
Distribution: V_d: 3-13 L/kg; enters breast milk
Protein binding: 77% to 85%
Metabolism: Hepatic; extensive first-pass effect; following single I.V. injection, plasma concentrations of N-monodesmethyldiltiazem and desacetyldiltiazem are typically undetectable; however, these metabolites accumulate to detectable concentrations following 24-hour constant rate infusion. N-monodesmethyldiltiazem appears to have 20% of the potency of diltiazem; desacetyldiltiazem is about 50% as potent as the parent compound.
Bioavailability: ~40% to 60%
Half-life elimination: 4-6 hours, may increase with renal impairment; 5-7 hours with sustained release
Time to peak, serum: Short-acting tablets: 2-3 hours; Sustained release: 6-11 hours
Excretion: Urine and feces (primarily as metabolites)

Usual Dosage Adults:
Angina: Oral: Usual starting dose: 30 mg 4 times/day; sustained release: 120-180 mg once daily; dosage should be increased gradually at 1- to 2-day intervals until optimum response is obtained. Doses up to 360 mg/day have been effectively used. Hypertension is controllable with single daily doses of sustained release products, or divided daily doses of regular release products, in the range of 240-360 mg/day.
Sustained-release capsules:
Cardizem® SR: Initial: 60-120 mg twice daily; adjust to maximum antihypertensive effect (usually within 14 days); usual range: 240-360 mg/day
Cardizem® CD, Tiazac®: Hypertension: Total daily dose of short-acting administered once daily or initially 180 or 240 mg once daily; adjust to maximum effect (usually within 14 days); maximum: 480 mg/day; usual range: 240-360 mg/day
Cardizem® CD: Angina: Initial: 120-180 mg once daily; maximum: 480 mg once/day
Dilacor® XR:
Hypertension: 180-240 mg once daily; maximum: 540 mg/day; usual range: 180-480 mg/day; use lower dose in elderly
Angina: Initial: 120 mg/day; titrate slowly over 7-14 days up to 480 mg/day, as needed
I.V. (requires an infusion pump):
• Initial bolus dose: 0.25 mg/kg actual body weight over 2 minutes (average adult dose: 20 mg)
• Repeat bolus dose (may be administered after 15 minutes if the response is inadequate.): 0.35 mg/kg actual body weight over 2 minutes (average adult dose: 25 mg)
• Continuous infusion (infusions >24 hours or infusion rates >15 mg/hour are not recommended.): Initial infusion rate of 10 mg/hour; rate may be increased in 5 mg/hour increments up to 15 mg/hour as needed; some patients may respond to an initial rate of 5 mg/hour.

If Cardizem® injectable is administered by continuous infusion for >24 hours, the possibility of decreased diltiazem clearance, prolonged elimination half-life, and increased diltiazem and/or diltiazem metabolite plasma concentrations should be considered.

Conversion from I.V. diltiazem to oral diltiazem: Start oral approximately 3 hours after bolus dose.
Oral dose (mg/day) is approximately equal to [rate (mg/hour) x 3 + 3] x 10.
3 mg/hour = 120 mg/day
5 mg/hour = 180 mg/day
7 mg/hour = 240 mg/day
11 mg/hour = 360 mg/day

Dosing comments in renal/hepatic impairment: Use with caution as extensively metabolized by the liver and excreted in the kidneys and bile.
Dialysis: Not removed by hemo- or peritoneal dialysis; supplemental dose is not necessary.

Administration
Oral: Do not crush sustained release capsules; they may be opened and sprinkled on a spoonful of applesauce. Applesauce should be swallowed without chewing, followed by drinking a glass of water.
I.V.: Bolus doses given over 2 minutes with continuous EKG and blood pressure monitoring. Continuous infusion should be via infusion pump.

Monitoring Parameters Liver function tests, blood pressure, EKG

Patient Information Sustained release products should be taken in the morning; do not crush or chew; limit caffeine intake; notify physician if angina pain is not reduced when taking this drug, irregular heartbeat, shortness of breath, swelling, dizziness, constipation, nausea, or hypotension occurs; do not stop therapy without advice of physician

Nursing Implications Do not crush sustained release capsules

Dosage Forms
Capsule, sustained release, as hydrochloride: 60 mg, 90 mg, 120 mg, 180 mg, 240 mg, 300 mg
Cardizem® CD, Cartia® XT: 120 mg, 180 mg, 240 mg, 300 mg
Cardizem® SR: 60 mg, 90 mg, 120 mg
Dilacor® XR: 180 mg, 240 mg
Diltia XT®: 120 mg, 180 mg, 240 mg
Tiazac®: 120 mg, 180 mg, 240 mg, 300 mg, 360 mg, 420 mg
Injection, as hydrochloride: 5 mg/mL (5 mL, 10 mL)
Cardizem®: 5 mg/mL (5 mL, 10 mL)
Cardizem® Lyo-Ject®: 5 mg/mL (5 mL)
Injection for infusion, as hydrochloride (Cardizem® Monovial®): 100 mg
Tablet, as hydrochloride (Cardizem®): 30 mg, 60 mg, 90 mg, 120 mg
Tablet, extended release, as hydrochloride (Tiamate®): 120 mg, 180 mg, 240 mg
(Continued)

Diltiazem *(Continued)*

Extemporaneous Preparations A 12 mg/mL oral liquid preparation made from tablets (regular, not sustained release) and 3 different vehicles (cherry syrup, a 1:1 mixture of Ora-Sweet® and Ora-Plus®, or a 1:1 mixture of Ora-Sweet® SF and Ora-Plus®) was stable for 60 days when stored in amber plastic prescription bottles in the dark at room temperature (25°C) or under refrigeration (5°C); grind sixteen 90 mg tablets in a mortar into a fine powder; add 10 mL of the vehicle and mix well to form a uniform paste; mix while adding the vehicle in geometric proportions to **almost** 120 mL; transfer to a calibrated bottle and qs ad with vehicle to 120 mL; label "shake well" and "protect from light".

Allen LV and Erickson MA, "Stability of Baclofen, Captopril, Diltiazem Hydrochloride, Dipyridamole, and Flecainide Acetate in Extemporaneously Compounded Oral Liquids," *Am J Health Sys Pharm*, 1996, 53(18):2179-84.

♦ **Diltiazem Hydrochloride** *see* Diltiazem *on page 409*

♦ **Dimacol® Caplets [OTC]** *see* Guaifenesin, Pseudoephedrine, and Dextromethorphan *on page 648*

Dimercaprol *(dye mer KAP role)*

U.S. Brand Names BAL in Oil®

Synonyms BAL; British Anti-Lewisite; Dithioglycerol

Therapeutic Category Antidote, Arsenic Toxicity; Antidote, Gold Toxicity; Antidote, Lead Toxicity; Antidote, Mercury Toxicity

Use Antidote to gold, arsenic (except arsine), and mercury poisoning (except nonalkyl mercury); adjunct to edetate calcium disodium in lead poisoning; possibly effective for antimony, bismuth, chromium, copper, nickel, tungsten, or zinc

Pregnancy Risk Factor C

Contraindications Hepatic insufficiency (unless due to arsenic poisoning); do not use on iron, cadmium, or selenium poisoning

Warnings/Precautions Potentially a nephrotoxic drug, use with caution in patients with oliguria or glucose 6-phosphate dehydrogenase deficiency; keep urine alkaline to protect kidneys; administer all injections deep I.M. at different sites

Adverse Reactions

>10%:
  Cardiovascular: Hypertension, tachycardia (dose-related)
  Central nervous system: Headache

1% to 10%: Gastrointestinal: Nausea, vomiting

<1% (Limited to important or life-threatening): Abscess formation, blepharospasm, burning eyes; burning sensation of the lips, mouth, throat, and penis; convulsions, dysuria, fever, increased PT, myalgia, nephrotoxicity, nervousness, pain at the injection site, paresthesia, salivation, thrombocytopenia, transient neutropenia

Drug Interactions

Increased Effect/Toxicity: Toxic complexes with iron, cadmium, selenium, or uranium.

Stability Do not mix in the same syringe with edetate calcium disodium

Mechanism of Action Sulfhydryl group combines with ions of various heavy metals to form relatively stable, nontoxic, soluble chelates which are excreted in urine

Pharmacodynamics/Kinetics

Distribution: To all tissues including the brain
Metabolism: Rapidly to inactive products
Time to peak, serum: 0.5-1 hour
Excretion: Urine

Usual Dosage Children and Adults: Deep I.M.:

Arsenic, mercury, and gold poisoning: 3 mg/kg every 4-6 hours for 2 days, then every 12 hours for 7-10 days or until recovery (initial dose may be up to 5 mg if severe poisoning)
Lead poisoning (in conjunction with calcium EDTA): For symptomatic acute encephalopathy or blood level >100 mcg/dL: 4-5 mg/kg every 4 hours for 3-5 days

Administration Administer deep I.M. only; keep urine alkaline to protect renal function

Test Interactions Iodine ^{131}I thyroidal uptake values may be decreased

Patient Information Frequent blood and urine tests may be required

Nursing Implications Urine should be kept alkaline because chelate dissociates in acid media

Dosage Forms Injection: 100 mg/mL (3 mL)

♦ **Dimetapp® Decongestant Liqui-Gels® [OTC]** *see* Pseudoephedrine *on page 1155*

♦ **β,β-Dimethylcysteine** *see* Penicillamine *on page 1050*

♦ **Dimethyl Triazeno Imidazol Carboxamide** *see* Dacarbazine *on page 354*

Dinoprostone *(dye noe PROST one)*

U.S. Brand Names Cervidil® Vaginal Insert; Prepidil® Vaginal Gel; Prostin E₂® Vaginal Suppository

Canadian Brand Names Cervidil™; Prepidil®; Prostin® E2

Synonyms PGE₂; Prostaglandin E₂

Therapeutic Category Abortifacient; Prostaglandin

Use

Gel: Promote cervical ripening prior to labor induction; usage for gel include any patient undergoing induction of labor with an unripe cervix, most commonly for pre-eclampsia, eclampsia, postdates, diabetes, intrauterine growth retardation, and chronic hypertension
Suppositories: Terminate pregnancy from 12th through 28th week of gestation; evacuate uterus in cases of missed abortion or intrauterine fetal death; manage benign hydatidiform mole
Vaginal insert: Initiation and/or cervical ripening in patients at or near term in whom there is a medical or obstetrical indication for the induction of labor

Pregnancy Risk Factor C

Contraindications

Vaginal insert: Hypersensitivity to prostaglandins; fetal distress (suspicion or clinical evidence unless delivery is imminent); unexplained vaginal bleeding during this pregnancy; strong suspicion of marked cephalopelvic disproportion; patients in whom oxytoxic drugs are contraindicated or when prolonged contraction of the uterus may be detrimental to fetal safety or uterine integrity (including previous cesarean section or major uterine surgery); greater than 6 previous term pregnancies; patients already receiving oxytoxic drugs

Gel: Hypersensitivity to prostaglandins or any constituents of the cervical gel, history of asthma, contracted pelvis, malpresentation of the fetus

Gel: The following are "relative" contraindications and should only be considered by the physician under these circumstances: Patients in whom vaginal delivery is not indicated (ie, herpes genitalia with a lesion at the time of delivery); prior uterine surgery, breech presentation, multiple gestation, polyhydramnios, premature rupture of membranes

Suppository: Hypersensitivity to dinoprostone, acute pelvic inflammatory disease, uterine fibroids, cervical stenosis

Warnings/Precautions Dinoprostone should be used only by medically trained personnel in a hospital; caution in patients with cervicitis, infected endocervical lesions, acute vaginitis, compromised (scarred) uterus or history of asthma, hypertension or hypotension, epilepsy, diabetes mellitus, anemia, jaundice, or cardiovascular, renal, or hepatic disease. Oxytocin should not be used simultaneously with Prepidil® (>6 hours of the last dose of Prepidil®).

Adverse Reactions

>10%:
Central nervous system: Headache
Gastrointestinal: Vomiting, diarrhea, nausea

1% to 10%:
Cardiovascular: Bradycardia
Central nervous system: Fever
Neuromuscular & skeletal: Back pain

<1% (Limited to important or life-threatening): Bronchospasm, cardiac arrhythmias, chills, coughing, dizziness, dyspnea, flushing, hot flashes, hypotension, pain, shivering, syncope, tightness of the chest, vasomotor and vasovagal reactions, wheezing

Overdosage/Toxicology Symptoms include vomiting, bronchospasm, hypotension, chest pain, abdominal cramps, and uterine contractions. Treatment is symptomatic.

Drug Interactions

Increased Effect/Toxicity: Increased effect of oxytocics.

Stability Suppositories must be kept frozen, store in freezer not above -20°F (-4°C); bring to room temperature just prior to use; cervical gel should be stored under refrigeration 2°C to 8°C (36°F to 46°F)

Mechanism of Action A synthetic prostaglandin E_2 abortifacient that stimulates uterine contractions similar to those seen during natural labor

Pharmacodynamics/Kinetics

Onset of action (uterine contractions): Within 10 minutes
Duration: Up to 2-3 hours
Absorption: Vaginal: Slow
Metabolism: In many tissues including the kidney, lungs, and spleen
Excretion: Primarily urine; feces (small amounts)

Usual Dosage

Abortifacient: Insert 1 suppository high in vagina, repeat at 3- to 5-hour intervals until abortion occurs up to 240 mg (maximum dose); continued administration for longer than 2 days is not advisable

Cervical ripening:
Gel:
Intracervical: 0.25-1 mg
Intravaginal: 2.5 mg
Suppositories: Intracervical: 2-3 mg
Vaginal Insert (Cervidil®): 10 mg (to be removed at the onset of active labor or after 12 hours)

Administration

Vaginal insert: One vaginal insert in placed transversely in the posterior fornix of the vaginal immediately after removal from its foil package. Patients should remain in the recumbent position for 2 hours after insertion, but thereafter may be ambulatory

Endocervical gel: Intracervically: For cervical ripening, patient should be supine in the dorsal position

Nursing Implications Bring suppository to room temperature just prior to use; patient should remain recumbent for 2 hours following insertion; commercially available suppositories should not be used for extemporaneous preparation of any other dosage form of drug

Dosage Forms

Gel, endocervical: 0.5 mg in 3 g syringes [each package contains a 10 mm and 20 mm shielded catheter]
Insert, vaginal (Cervidil®): 10 mg
Suppository, vaginal: 20 mg

- **Dionephrine® (Can)** *see* Phenylephrine *on page 1075*
- **Diopentolate® (Can)** *see* Cyclopentolate *on page 341*
- **Diopred® (Can)** *see* PrednisoLONE *on page 1122*
- **Dioptimyd® (Can)** *see* Sulfacetamide and Prednisolone *on page 1269*
- **Dioptrol® (Can)** *see* Neomycin, Polymyxin B, and Dexamethasone *on page 969*
- **Diosulf™ (Can)** *see* Sulfacetamide *on page 1268*
- **Diotame® [OTC]** *see* Bismuth *on page 170*
- **Diotrope® (Can)** *see* Tropicamide *on page 1384*
- **Diovan®** *see* Valsartan *on page 1402*
- **Diovan HCT®** *see* Valsartan and Hydrochlorothiazide *on page 1403*
- **Diovol® (Can)** *see* Aluminum Hydroxide and Magnesium Hydroxide *on page 64*
- **Diovol® Ex (Can)** *see* Aluminum Hydroxide and Magnesium Hydroxide *on page 64*
- **Diovol Plus® (Can)** *see* Aluminum Hydroxide, Magnesium Hydroxide, and Simethicone *on page 64*
- **Dipalmitoylphosphatidylcholine** *see* Colfosceril Palmitate *on page 333*
- **Dipentum®** *see* Olsalazine *on page 1007*
- **Diphenacen-50®** *see* DiphenhydrAMINE *on page 414*
- **Diphenatol®** *see* Diphenoxylate and Atropine *on page 416*
- **Diphen® Cough [OTC]** *see* DiphenhydrAMINE *on page 414*
- **Diphenhist [OTC]** *see* DiphenhydrAMINE *on page 414*

DiphenhydrAMINE (dye fen HYE dra meen)

Related Information
Contrast Media Reactions, Premedication for Prophylaxis *on page 1653*

U.S. Brand Names AllerMax® [OTC]; Banophen® [OTC]; Benadryl® [OTC]; Bydramine® Cough Syrup [OTC]; Compoz® Gel Caps [OTC]; Compoz® Nighttime Sleep Aid [OTC]; Dihydrex®; Diphenacen-50®; Diphen® Cough [OTC]; Diphenhist [OTC]; Dormin® [OTC]; Genahist®; Hyrexin-50®; Maximum Strength Nytol® [OTC]; Miles Nervine® [OTC]; Nordryl®; Nytol® [OTC]; Siladryl® [OTC]; Silphen® Cough [OTC]; Sleep-eze 3® Oral [OTC]; Sleepinal® [OTC]; Sleepwell 2-nite® [OTC]; Sominex® [OTC]; Tusstat®; Twilite® [OTC]; Uni-Bent® Cough Syrup; 40 Winks® [OTC]

Canadian Brand Names Allerdryl®; Allernix®; Benadryl®; Nytol™; Nytol™ Extra Strength; PMS-Diphenhydramine

Synonyms Diphenhydramine Hydrochloride

Therapeutic Category Antidote, Hypersensitivity Reactions; Antihistamine, H₁ Blocker; Sedative

Use Symptomatic relief of allergic symptoms caused by histamine release which include nasal allergies and allergic dermatosis; can be used for mild nighttime sedation; prevention of motion sickness and as an antitussive; has antinausea and topical anesthetic properties; treatment of antipsychotic-induced extrapyramidal symptoms

Pregnancy Risk Factor B

Contraindications Hypersensitivity to diphenhydramine or any component of the formulation; acute asthma; not for use in neonates

Warnings/Precautions Causes sedation, caution must be used in performing tasks which require alertness (ie, operating machinery or driving). Sedative effects of CNS depressants or ethanol are potentiated. Use with caution in patients with angle-closure glaucoma, pyloroduodenal obstruction (including stenotic peptic ulcer), urinary tract obstruction (including bladder neck obstruction and symptomatic prostatic hypertrophy), hyperthyroidism, increased intraocular pressure, and cardiovascular disease (including hypertension and tachycardia). Diphenhydramine has high sedative and anticholinergic properties, so it may not be considered the antihistamine of choice for prolonged use in the elderly. May cause paradoxical excitation in pediatric patients, and can result in hallucinations, coma, and death in overdose. Some preparations contain sodium bisulfite; syrup formulations may contain alcohol.

Adverse Reactions Frequency not defined.
Cardiovascular: Hypotension, palpitations, tachycardia
Central nervous system: Sedation, sleepiness, dizziness, disturbed coordination, headache, fatigue, nervousness, paradoxical excitement, insomnia, euphoria, confusion
Dermatologic: Photosensitivity, rash, angioedema, urticaria
Gastrointestinal: Nausea, vomiting, diarrhea, abdominal pain, xerostomia, appetite increase, weight gain, dry mucous membranes, anorexia
Genitourinary: Urinary retention, urinary frequency, difficult urination
Hematologic: Hemolytic anemia, thrombocytopenia, agranulocytosis
Neuromuscular & skeletal: Tremor, paresthesia
Ocular: blurred vision
Respiratory: Thickening of bronchial secretions

Overdosage/Toxicology Symptoms include CNS stimulation or depression. Overdose may result in death in infants and children. There is no specific treatment for antihistamine overdose, however, clinical toxicity is mostly due to anticholinergic effects. Anticholinesterase inhibitors (eg, physostigmine, neostigmine, pyridostigmine, or edrophonium) may be useful by reducing acetylcholinesterase. For anticholinergic overdose with severe life-threatening symptoms, physostigmine 1-2 mg (0.5 mg or 0.02 mg/kg for children) slow I.V. may be given to reverse these effects.

Drug Interactions
Cytochrome P450 Effect: CYP2D6 enzyme substrate
Increased Effect/Toxicity: CNS depressants may increase the degree of sedation and respiratory depression with diphenhydramine. May increase the absorption of digoxin. Central and/or peripheral anticholinergic syndrome can occur when administered with amantadine, rimantadine, narcotic analgesics, phenothiazines and other antipsychotics (especially with high anticholinergic activity), tricyclic antidepressants, quinidine, disopyramide, procainamide, and antihistamines. Syrup should not be given to patients taking

drugs that can cause disulfiram reactions (ie, metronidazole, chlorpropamide) due to high alcohol content.

Decreased Effect: May increase gastric degradation of levodopa and decrease the amount of levodopa absorbed by delaying gastric emptying. Therapeutic effects of cholinergic agents (tacrine, donepezil) and neuroleptics may be antagonized.

Ethanol/Nutrition/Herb Interactions
Ethanol: Avoid ethanol (may increase CNS depression).
Herb/Nutraceutical: Avoid valerian, St John's wort, kava kava, gotu kola (may increase CNS depression).

Stability Protect from light; the following drugs are **incompatible** with diphenhydramine when mixed in the same syringe: Amobarbital, amphotericin B, cephalothin, diatrizoate, foscarnet, heparin, hydrocortisone, hydroxyzine, pentobarbital, phenobarbital, phenytoin, prochlorperazine, promazine, promethazine, tetracycline, thiopental

Mechanism of Action Competes with histamine for H_1-receptor sites on effector cells in the gastrointestinal tract, blood vessels, and respiratory tract; anticholinergic and sedative effects are also seen

Pharmacodynamics/Kinetics
Onset of action: Maximum sedative effect: 1-3 hours; I.V.: More rapid
Duration: 4-7 hours
Bioavailability: Oral: 40% to 60%
Protein binding: 78%
Metabolism: Extensively hepatic; smaller degrees in pulmonary and renal systems; significant first-pass effect
Half-life elimination: 2-8 hours; Elderly: 13.5 hours
Time to peak, serum: 2-4 hours

Usual Dosage
Children:
Oral, I.M., I.V.:
Treatment of moderate to severe allergic reactions: 5 mg/kg/day or 150 mg/m²/day in divided doses every 6-8 hours, not to exceed 300 mg/day
Minor allergic rhinitis or motion sickness:
2 to <6 years: 6.25 mg every 4-6 hours; maximum: 37.5 mg/day
6 to <12 years: 12.5-25 mg every 4-6 hours; maximum: 150 mg/day
≥12 years: 25-50 mg every 4-6 hours; maximum: 300 mg/day
Night-time sleep aid: 30 minutes before bedtime:
2 to <12 years: 1 mg/kg/dose; maximum: 50 mg/dose
≥12 years: 50 mg
Oral: Antitussive:
2 to <6 years: 6.25 mg every 4 hours; maximum 37.5 mg/day
6 to <12 years: 12.5 mg every 4 hours; maximum 75 mg/day
≥12 years: 25 mg every 4 hours; maximum 150 mg/day
I.M., I.V.: Treatment of dystonic reactions: 0.5-1 mg/kg/dose
Adults:
Oral: 25-50 mg every 6-8 hours
Minor allergic rhinitis or motion sickness: 25-50 mg every 4-6 hours; maximum: 300 mg/day
Moderate to severe allergic reactions: 25-50 mg every 4 hours, not to exceed 400 mg/day
Nighttime sleep aid: 50 mg at bedtime
I.M., I.V.: 10-50 mg in a single dose every 2-4 hours, not to exceed 400 mg/day
Dystonic reaction: 50 mg in a single dose; may repeat in 20-30 minutes if necessary
Topical: For external application, not longer than 7 days

Monitoring Parameters Relief of symptoms, mental alertness

Reference Range
Antihistamine effects at levels >25 ng/mL
Drowsiness at levels 30-40 ng/mL
Mental impairment at levels >60 ng/mL
Therapeutic: Not established
Toxic: >0.1 µg/mL

Test Interactions May suppress the wheal and flare reactions to skin test antigens

Patient Information May cause drowsiness; swallow whole, do not crush or chew sustained release product; avoid alcohol, may impair coordination and judgment

Nursing Implications Raise bed rails, institute safety measures, assist with ambulation

Additional Information Its use as a sleep aid is discouraged due to its anticholinergic effects.

Dosage Forms
Capsule, as hydrochloride: 25 mg, 50 mg
Cream, as hydrochloride: 1%, 2%
Elixir, as hydrochloride: 12.5 mg/5 mL (5 mL, 10 mL, 20 mL, 120 mL, 480 mL, 3780 mL)
Injection, as hydrochloride: 10 mg/mL (10 mL, 30 mL); 50 mg/mL (1 mL, 10 mL)
Liquid, as hydrochloride: 6.25/5 mL
Lotion, as hydrochloride: 1% (75 mL)
Solution, topical, as hydrochloride [spray]: 1% (60 mL), 2%
Syrup, as hydrochloride: 12.5 mg/5 mL (5 mL, 120 mL, 240 mL, 480 mL, 3780 mL)
Tablet, as hydrochloride: 25 mg, 50 mg
Tablet, chewable, as hydrochloride: 12.5 mg

♦ **Diphenhydramine and Acetaminophen** see Acetaminophen and Diphenhydramine on page 25

Diphenhydramine and Pseudoephedrine
(dye fen HYE dra meen & soo doe e FED rin)

U.S. Brand Names Actifed® Allergy (Night) [OTC]; Banophen® Decongestant [OTC]; Benadryl® Decongestant Allergy [OTC]

Synonyms Pseudoephedrine and Diphenhydramine
(Continued)

Diphenhydramine and Pseudoephedrine *(Continued)*

Therapeutic Category Antihistamine/Decongestant Combination

Use Relief of symptoms of upper respiratory mucosal congestion in seasonal and perennial nasal allergies, acute rhinitis, rhinosinusitis, and eustachian tube blockage

Usual Dosage Based on **pseudoephedrine** component:
Adults: Oral: 60 mg every 4-6 hours, maximum: 240 mg/day

Additional Information Complete prescribing information for this medication should be consulted for additional detail.

Dosage Forms

Capsule (Banophen®): Diphenhydramine hydrochloride 25 mg and pseudoephedrine hydrochloride 60 mg

Tablet:

Actifed® Allergy (Night): Diphenhydramine hydrochloride 25 mg and pseudoephedrine hydrochloride 30 mg

Benadryl® Decongestant Allergy: Diphenhydramine hydrochloride 25 mg and pseudoephedrine hydrochloride 60 mg

♦ **Diphenhydramine Hydrochloride** *see* DiphenhydrAMINE *on page 414*

Diphenoxylate and Atropine *(dye fen OKS i late & A troe peen)*

U.S. Brand Names Diphenatol®; Lomocot®; Lomotil®; Lonox®

Canadian Brand Names Lomotil®

Synonyms Atropine and Diphenoxylate

Therapeutic Category Antidiarrheal

Use Treatment of diarrhea

Restrictions C-V

Pregnancy Risk Factor C

Contraindications Hypersensitivity to diphenoxylate, atropine, or any component of the formulation; severe liver disease; jaundice; dehydration; narrow-angle glaucoma; not for use in children <2 years of age

Warnings/Precautions High doses may cause physical and psychological dependence with prolonged use; use with caution in patients with ulcerative colitis, dehydration, and hepatic dysfunction; reduction of intestinal motility may be deleterious in diarrhea resulting from *Shigella*, *Salmonella*, toxigenic strains of *E. coli*, and from pseudomembranous enterocolitis associated with broad spectrum antibiotics; children may develop signs of atropinism (dryness of skin and mucous membranes, thirst, hyperthermia, tachycardia, urinary retention, flushing) even at the recommended dosages; if there is no response with 48 hours, the drug is unlikely to be effective and should be discontinued; if chronic diarrhea is not improved symptomatically within 10 days at maximum dosage of 20 mg/day, control is unlikely with further use.

Adverse Reactions

1% to 10%:

Central nervous system: Nervousness, restlessness, dizziness, drowsiness, headache, mental depression

Gastrointestinal: Paralytic ileus, dry mouth, megacolon

Genitourinary: Urinary retention and difficult urination

Ocular: Blurred vision

Respiratory: Respiratory depression

<1% (Limited to important or life-threatening): Abdominal discomfort, nausea, pancreatitis, stomach cramps, tachycardia, vomiting

Overdosage/Toxicology Symptoms include drowsiness, hypotension, blurred vision, flushing, dry mouth, and miosis. Treatment includes administration of activated charcoal to reduce bioavailability of diphenoxylate. Treatment includes naloxone 2 mg I.V. (0.01 mg/kg for children), with repeat administration as necessary, up to a total of 10 mg. For anticholinergic overdose with severe life-threatening symptoms, physostigmine 1-2 mg (0.5 mg or 0.02 mg/kg for children) S.C. or slow I.V. may be given to reverse these effects.

Drug Interactions

Increased Effect/Toxicity: MAO inhibitors (hypertensive crisis), CNS depressants when taken with diphenoxylate may result in increased adverse effects, antimuscarinics (paralytic ileus). May prolong half-life of drugs metabolized in liver.

Ethanol/Nutrition/Herb Interactions Ethanol: Avoid ethanol (may increase CNS depression).

Stability Protect from light

Mechanism of Action Diphenoxylate inhibits excessive GI motility and GI propulsion; commercial preparations contain a subtherapeutic amount of atropine to discourage abuse

Pharmacodynamics/Kinetics

Atropine: See Atropine monograph.

Diphenoxylate:

Onset of action: Antidiarrheal: 45-60 minutes

Peak effect: Antidiarrheal: ~2 hours

Duration: Antidiarrheal: 3-4 hours

Absorption: Well absorbed

Metabolism: Extensively hepatic to diphenoxylic acid (active)

Half-life elimination: Diphenoxylate: 2.5 hours

Time to peak, serum: 2 hours

Excretion: Primarily feces (as metabolites); urine (~14% with <1% as unchanged drug)

Usual Dosage Oral:

Children (use with caution in young children due to variable responses): Liquid: 0.3-0.4 mg of diphenoxylate/kg/day in 2-4 divided doses **or**

<2 years: Not recommended

2-5 years: 2 mg of diphenoxylate 3 times/day

5-8 years: 2 mg of diphenoxylate 4 times/day

8-12 years: 2 mg of diphenoxylate 5 times/day

Adults: 15-20 mg/day of diphenoxylate in 3-4 divided doses; maintenance: 5-15 mg/day in 2-3 divided doses

Monitoring Parameters Watch for signs of atropinism (dryness of skin and mucous membranes, tachycardia, thirst, flushing); monitor number and consistency of stools; observe for signs of toxicity, fluid and electrolyte loss, hypotension, and respiratory depression

Patient Information Drowsiness, dizziness, dry mouth; use caution while driving or performing hazardous tasks; avoid alcohol or other CNS depressants; do not exceed prescribed dose; report persistent diarrhea, fever, or palpitations to physician

Nursing Implications Raise bed rails, institute safety measures

Dosage Forms

Solution, oral: Diphenoxylate hydrochloride 2.5 mg and atropine sulfate 0.025 mg per 5 mL (4 mL, 10 mL, 60 mL)

Tablet: Diphenoxylate hydrochloride 2.5 mg and atropine sulfate 0.025 mg

♦ **Diphenylhydantoin** *see Phenytoin on page 1077*

Diphtheria and Tetanus Toxoid (dif THEER ee a & TET a nus TOKS oyd)

Related Information

Adverse Events and Vaccination *on page 1553*
Immunization Recommendations *on page 1538*
Recommendations of the Advisory Committee on Immunization Practices (ACIP) *on page 1540*
Skin Tests *on page 1533*

Synonyms DT; Td; Tetanus and Diphtheria Toxoid

Therapeutic Category Toxoid

Use Active immunity against diphtheria and tetanus when pertussis vaccine is contraindicated; tetanus prophylaxis in wound management

DT: Infants and children through 6 years of age
Td: Children and adults ≥7 years of age

Pregnancy Risk Factor C

Pregnancy/Breast-Feeding Implications Clinical effects on the fetus: Td and tetanus vaccines are not known to cause special problems for pregnant women or their unborn babies. While physicians do not usually recommend giving any drugs or vaccines to pregnant women, Advisory Committee on Immunization Practices (ACIP) recommends unvaccinated pregnant women (without previous immunization) receive Td, two doses 4-8 weeks apart during the 2nd and 3rd trimesters, if delivery will be under nonhygenic circumstances.

Contraindications Patients receiving immunosuppressive agents, prior anaphylactic, allergic, or systemic reactions; hypersensitivity to diphtheria and tetanus toxoid or any component of the formulation; acute respiratory infection or other active infection

Warnings/Precautions History of a neurologic reaction or immediate hypersensitivity reaction following a previous dose. History of severe local reaction (Arthus-type) following previous dose (such individuals should not be given further routine or emergency doses of tetanus and diphtheria toxoids for 10 years). Do not confuse pediatric DT with adult diphtheria and tetanus toxoid (Td), absorbed (Td) is used in patients >7 years of age; primary immunization should be postponed until the second year of life due to possibility of CNS damage or convulsion; have epinephrine 1:1000 available.

Adverse Reactions All serious adverse reactions must be reported to the U.S. Department of Health and Human Services (DDHS) Vaccine Adverse Event Reporting System (VAERS) 1-800-822-7967.

>10%: Central nervous system: Fretfulness, drowsiness

1% to 10%:
Central nervous system: Persistent crying
Gastrointestinal: Anorexia, vomiting

<1% (Limited to important or life-threatening): Arthus-type hypersensitivity reactions, convulsions (rarely), edema, hypotension, pain, pruritus, redness, tachycardia, tenderness, transient fever, urticaria

Stability Refrigerate

Usual Dosage I.M.:

Infants and Children (DT):

6 weeks to 1 year: Three 0.5 mL doses at least 4 weeks apart; administer a reinforcing dose 6-12 months after the third injection

1-6 years: Two 0.5 mL doses at least 4 weeks apart; reinforcing dose 6-12 months after second injection; if final dose is given after seventh birthday, use adult preparation

4-6 years (booster immunization): 0.5 mL; not necessary if all 4 doses were given after fourth birthday - routinely administer booster doses at 10-year intervals with the adult preparation

Tetanus Prophylaxis in Wound Management

Number of Prior Tetanus Toxoid Doses	Clean, Minor Wounds		All Other Wounds	
	Td*	TIG†	Td*	TIG†
Unknown or <3	Yes	No	Yes	Yes
≥3‡	No#	No	No¶	No

*Adult tetanus and diphtheria toxoids; use pediatric preparations (DT or DTP) if the patient is <7 years old.

†Tetanus immune globulin.

‡If only three doses of fluid tetanus toxoid have been received, a fourth dose of toxoid, preferably an adsorbed toxoid, should be given.

#Yes, if >10 years since last dose.

¶Yes, if >5 years since last dose.

Adapted from Report of the Committee on Infectious Diseases, American Academy of Pediatrics, Elk Grove Village, IL: American Academy of Pediatrics, 1986.

(Continued)

Diphtheria and Tetanus Toxoid *(Continued)*

Children >7 years and Adults: Should receive Td; 2 primary doses of 0.5 mL each, given at an interval of 4-6 weeks; third (reinforcing) dose of 0.5 mL 6-12 months later; boosters every 10 years.

Tetanus prophylaxis in wound management (Use of tetanus toxoid (Td*) and/or tetanus immune globulin (TIG) depends upon the number of prior tetanus toxoid doses and type of wound): See table on previous page.

Administration For patients at risk of hemorrhage following intramuscular injection, the ACIP recommends "it should be administered intramuscularly if, in the opinion of the physician familiar with the patients bleeding risk, the vaccine can be administered with reasonable safety by this route. If the patient receives antihemophilia or other similar therapy, intramuscular vaccination can be scheduled shortly after such therapy is administered. A fine needle (23 gauge or smaller) can be used for the vaccination and firm pressure applied to the site (without rubbing) for at least 2 minutes. The patient should be instructed concerning the risk of hematoma from the injection."

Patient Information DT, Td and T vaccines cause few problems (mild fever or soreness, swelling, and redness/knot at the injection site); these problems usually last 1-2 days, but this does not nearly as often as with DTP vaccine

Nursing Implications Shake well before giving

Additional Information Pediatric dosage form should only be used in patients ≤6 years of age. Federal law requires that the date of administration, the vaccine manufacturer, lot number of vaccine, and the administering person's name, title, and address be entered into the patient's permanent medical record.

Since protective tetanus and diphtheria antibodies decline with age, only 28% of persons >70 years of age in the U.S. are believed to be immune to tetanus, and most of the tetanus-induced deaths occur in people >60 years of age, it is advisable to offer Td especially to the elderly concurrent with their influenza and other immunization programs if history of vaccination is unclear; boosters should be given at 10-year intervals; earlier for wounds

DT contains higher proportions of diphtheria toxoid than Td.

Dosage Forms
Injection, adult:
Diphtheria 2 Lf units and tetanus 2 Lf units per 0.5 mL (5 mL) [Massachusetts Biological Laboratories]
Diphtheria 2 Lf units and tetanus 5 Lf units per 0.5 mL (0.5 mL, 5 mL) [Wyeth]
Diphtheria 2 Lf units and tetanus 5 Lf units per 0.5 mL (5 mL) [Lederle, Aventis/Pasteur]
Injection, pediatric:
Diphtheria 6.7 Lf units and tetanus 5 Lf units per 0.5 mL (5 mL) [Aventis/Pasteur]
Diphtheria 7.5 Lf units and tetanus 7.5 Lf units per 0.5 mL (5 mL) [Massachusetts Biological Laboratories]
Diphtheria 10 Lf units and tetanus 5 Lf units per 0.5 mL (0.5 mL, 5 mL) [Wyeth-Ayerst]
Diphtheria 12.5 Lf units and tetanus 5 Lf units per 0.5 mL (5 mL) [Lederle]

♦ **Diphtheria CRM$_{197}$ Protein** *see* Pneumococcal Conjugate Vaccine (7-Valent) *on page 1097*

♦ **Diphtheria CRM$_{197}$ Protein Conjugate** *see* Haemophilus b Conjugate Vaccine *on page 651*

Diphtheria, Tetanus Toxoids, and Acellular Pertussis Vaccine
(dif THEER ee a, TET a nus TOKS oyds & ay CEL yoo lar per TUS sis vak SEEN)

Related Information
Adverse Events and Vaccination *on page 1553*
Immunization Recommendations *on page 1538*
Recommendations of the Advisory Committee on Immunization Practices (ACIP) *on page 1540*
Recommended Childhood Immunization Schedule - US - 2002 *on page 1539*
Recommended Immunization Schedule for HIV-Infected Children *on page 1543*
USPHA/IDSA Guidelines for the Prevention of Opportunistic Infections in Persons With HIV *on page 1574*

U.S. Brand Names Infanrix®; Tripedia®

Canadian Brand Names Adacel®

Synonyms DTaP

Therapeutic Category Toxoid; Vaccine

Use Active immunization against diphtheria, tetanus, and pertussis from age 6 weeks through seventh birthday

Pregnancy Risk Factor C

Pregnancy/Breast-Feeding Implications Clinical effects on the fetus: Animal reproduction studies have not been conducted. It is not known whether the vaccine can cause fetal harm when administered to a pregnant woman or can affect reproductive capacity; **not** recommended for use in a pregnant woman or any patient ≥7 years of age

Contraindications Hypersensitivity to diphtheria and tetanus toxoids, pertussis, or any component of the formulation; children ≥7 years of age; moderate or severe febrile illness (postpone vaccine); immediate anaphylactic reaction following previous dose; history of any of the following effects from previous administration of pertussis vaccine - anaphylactic reaction, convulsions, focal neurologic signs, or encephalopathy

Warnings/Precautions Carefully consider use in patients with history of any of the following effects from previous administration of pertussis vaccine: >105°F fever (40.5°C) within 48 hours of unknown cause, convulsions with or without fever occurring within 3 days, screaming episodes lasting ≥3 hours and occurring within 48 hours, shock or collapse within 48 hours; use with caution in children with coagulation disorders (including thrombocytopenia) where intramuscular injections should not be used; patients who are immunocompromised may have reduced response; may be used in patients with HIV infection; defer immunization during outbreaks of poliomyelitis. Use caution in patients with history of seizure disorder, progressive neurologic disease, or conditions predisposing to seizures; ACIP and APP guidelines recommend deferring immunization until health status can be assessed and condition stabilized. Products may contain thimerosal; packaging may contain natural latex rubber; safety and efficacy in children <6 weeks of age have not been established

Adverse Reactions All serious adverse reactions must be reported to the U.S. Department of Health and Human Services (DDHS) Vaccine Adverse Event Reporting System (VAERS) 1-800-822-7967.

Incidence of erythema, swelling and fever increase with successive doses

>10%:
 Central nervous system: Drowsiness, irritability
 Gastrointestinal: Decreased appetite
 Local: Redness, swelling

1% to 10%:
 Central nervous system: Fever
 Gastrointestinal: Vomiting
 Local: Pain, redness ≥3 cm, swelling ≥3 cm, tenderness
 Miscellaneous: High-pitched/unusual crying

<1% (Limited to important or life-threatening): Hypotonic-hyporesponsive episode, persistent crying ≥3 hours

Drug Interactions
 Increased Effect/Toxicity: Increased bleeding/bruising with anticoagulants.
 Decreased Effect: Vaccine effect may be decreased with corticosteroids and immunosuppressant agents. Consider deferring vaccine for 1 month after agent is discontinued.

Stability Refrigerate at 2°C to 8°C (35°F to 46°F); do not freeze

Mechanism of Action Promotes active immunity to diphtheria, tetanus, and pertussis by inducing production of specific antibodies and antitoxins.

Usual Dosage
 Children 6 weeks to <7 years: I.M.: 0.5 mL
  Primary series: Three doses, usually given at 2-, 4-, and 6 months of age; may be given as early as 6 weeks of age and repeated every 4-8 weeks; use same product for all 3 doses
  Booster series:
   Fourth dose: Given at ~15-20 months of age, but at least 6 months after third dose
   Fifth dose: Given at 5-6 years of age, prior to starting school or kindergarten; if the fourth dose is given at ≥4 years of age, the fifth dose may be omitted

 Children ≥7 years and Adults: Tetanus and diphtheria toxoids for adult use (Td) preparation is the preferred agent

Administration Administer only I.M. in anterolateral aspect of thigh or deltoid muscle of upper arm

For patients at risk of hemorrhage following intramuscular injection, the ACIP recommends "it should be administered intramuscularly if, in the opinion of the physician familiar with the patients bleeding risk, the vaccine can be administered with reasonable safety by this route. If the patient receives antihemophilia or other similar therapy, intramuscular vaccination can be scheduled shortly after such therapy is administered. A fine needle (23 gauge or smaller) can be used for the vaccination and firm pressure applied to the site (without rubbing) for at least 2 minutes. The patient should be instructed concerning the risk of hematoma from the injection."

Patient Information A nodule may be palpable at the injection site for a few weeks. Reactions to the vaccine, if seen, usually occur within 3 days. Mild reactions include sore arm or leg, fever, fussiness, decreased appetite, tiredness, or vomiting. Contact prescriber for any of the following less common reactions: Nonstop crying for 3 hours or more, fever of 105°F or higher, seizures, or if your child becomes limp, pale, or less alert. Reactions to the DTaP vaccine are less likely to occur then those previously seen with the DTP vaccine. It is important that each child receive all the recommended doses in the series in order to be fully immunized. This vaccine is not used in adults or children >7 years of age.

Nursing Implications Acetaminophen or ibuprofen may reduce or prevent fever; shake well before administering; the child's medical record should document that the small risk of postvaccination seizure and the benefits of the pertussis vaccination were discussed with the patient; parents or guardians should be questioned prior to administration of vaccine as to any adverse reactions from previous dose. Provide Vaccine Information Materials, as required by National Childhood Vaccine Injury Act of 1986, prior to immunization. Epinephrine 1:1000 and other appropriate agents should be available to control immediate allergic reactions.

Additional Information DTaP may be given for the fourth and fifth doses in children who started immunization with DTP vaccine. In patients who cannot be given pertussis vaccine, DT for pediatric use should be given to complete the series.

TriHIBit® is Tripedia® vaccine used to reconstitute ActHIB® (Haemophilus b conjugate) vaccine. The combination can be used for the DTaP dose given at 15-18 months when Tripedia® was used for the initial doses and a primary series of HIB vaccine has been given.

Federal law requires that the date of administration, the vaccine manufacturer, lot number of vaccine, and the administering person's name, title and address be entered into the patient's permanent medical record.

Dosage Forms
 Injection:
  Infanrix®: Diphtheria 25 Lf units, tetanus 10 Lf units, and acellular pertussis vaccine 25 mcg per 0.5 mL (0.5 mL)
  Tripedia®: Diphtheria 6.7 Lf units, tetanus 5 Lf units, and acellular pertussis vaccine 46.8 mcg per 0.5 mL (7.5 mL) [contains thimerosal]
  Note: Tripedia® vaccine is also used to reconstitute ActHIB® to prepare TriHIBit® vaccine (diphtheria, tetanus toxoids, and acellular pertussis vaccine and Haemophilus influenzae b conjugate vaccine combination)

Diphtheria, Tetanus Toxoids, and Acellular Pertussis Vaccine and *Haemophilus influenzae* b Conjugate Vaccine

(dif THEER ee a, TET a nus TOKS oyds & ay CEL yoo lar per TUS sis vak SEEN & hem OF fi lus in floo EN za bee KON joo gate vak SEEN)

U.S. Brand Names TriHIBit®

Therapeutic Category Toxoid; Vaccine, Inactivated Bacteria

Use Active immunization of children 15-18 months of age for prevention of diphtheria, tetanus, pertussis, and invasive disease caused by *H. influenzae* type b.

Contraindications Any contraindication of the component vaccines (see individual monographs); contraindicated in children <15 months of age

Usual Dosage Children >15 months of age: I.M.: 0.5 mL (as part of a general vaccination schedule; see individual vaccines). Vaccine should be used within 30 minutes of reconstitution.

Administration For patients at risk of hemorrhage following intramuscular injection, the ACIP recommends "it should be administered intramuscularly if, in the opinion of the physician familiar with the patients bleeding risk, the vaccine can be administered with reasonable safety by this route. If the patient receives antihemophilia or other similar therapy, intramuscular vaccination can be scheduled shortly after such therapy is administered. A fine needle (23 gauge or smaller) can be used for the vaccination and firm pressure applied to the site (without rubbing) for at least 2 minutes. The patient should be instructed concerning the risk of hematoma from the injection."

Additional Information TriHIBit® is Tripedia® vaccine used to reconstitute ActHIB® (*Haemophilus* b conjugate) vaccine. The combination can be used for the DTaP dose given at 15-18 months when Tripedia® was used for the initial doses and a primary series of HIB vaccine has been given. Federal law requires that the date of administration, the vaccine manufacturer, lot number of vaccine, and the administering person's name, title and address be entered into the patient's permanent medical record.

Dosage Forms Injection: 5 Lf units tetanus toxoid, 6.7 Lf units diphtheria toxoid, 46.8 mcg pertussis antigens, and 10 mcg *H. influenzae* type b purified capsular polysaccharide [Tripedia® vaccine is used to reconstitute ActHIB®] (0.5 mL)

Diphtheria, Tetanus Toxoids, and Whole-Cell Pertussis Vaccine

(dif THEER ee a & TET a nus TOKS oyds & hole-sel per TUS sis vak SEEN)

Related Information

Recommended Immunization Schedule for HIV-Infected Children *on page 1543*

U.S. Brand Names Tri-Immunol® [DSC]

Canadian Brand Names Pentacel™

Synonyms DPT; DTP; DTwP

Therapeutic Category Toxoid and Vaccine

Use Active immunization of infants and children through 6 years of age (between 2 months and the seventh birthday) against diphtheria, tetanus, and pertussis; recommended for primary immunization; start immunization if whooping cough or diphtheria is present in the community. **ACIP recommends exclusive use of acellular pertussis vaccine for all doses of the pertussis vaccine series.**

For children who are severely immunocompromised or who are infected with HIV, DTP vaccine is indicated in the same schedule and dose as for immunocompetent children, including the use of acellular pertussis-containing vaccines (DTaP) as a booster. Although no specific studies with pertussis vaccine are available, if immunosuppressive therapy is to be discontinued shortly, it would be reasonable to defer immunization until at least 3 months after the patient last received therapy; otherwise, the patient should be vaccinated while still receiving therapy.

Pregnancy Risk Factor C

Contraindications

Hypersensitivity to diphtheria and tetanus toxoids or pertussis vaccine, thimerosal, or any component of the formulation; thrombocytopenia

Children >7 years of age history of any of the following effects from previous administration of pertussis vaccine precludes further use

Temperature of 105°F or higher **within 2 days** after getting DTP

Shock-collapse (becoming blue or pale, limp, and not responsive) **within 2 days** after getting DTP

Convulsion **within 3 days** after getting DTP

Crying that cannot be stopped which lasts for more than 3 hours at a time **within 2 days** after getting DTP

Warnings/Precautions Do not use DTP for treatment of actual tetanus, diphtheria, or whooping cough infections. The child's medical record should document that the small risk of past vaccination seizure and the benefits of the pertussis vaccination were discussed with the patient. If adverse reactions occurred with previous doses, immunization should be completed with diphtheria and tetanus toxoid absorbed (pediatric); have epinephrine 1:1000 available.

Adverse Reactions All serious adverse reactions must be reported to the U.S. Department of Health and Human Services (DHHS) Vaccine Adverse Event Reporting System (VAERS). Reporting forms and information about reporting requirements or completion of the form can be obtained from VAERS through a toll-free number 1-800-822-7967.

<1% (Limited to important or life-threatening): Arthralgia, chills, collapse, convulsions, erythema, focal neurological signs, induration, local tenderness, malaise, mild to moderate fever, rash, screaming episodes, shock, sleepiness, swelling, urticaria

Stability Refrigerate

Mechanism of Action Promotes active immunity to diphtheria, tetanus, and pertussis by inducing production of specific antibodies and antitoxins.

Usual Dosage For pediatric use only. Do not give to patients >7 years of age; primary immunization for children 2-6 years of age, ideally beginning at the age of 2-3 months

Primary immunization: Administer 0.5 mL I.M. on three occasions at 8-week intervals with a re-enforcing dose administered at 15-18 months of age

The booster doses are given when children are 4-6 years of age, 0.5 mL I.M.

For booster doses thereafter, use the recommended dose of diphtheria and tetanus toxoids, adsorbed (adults) every 10 years; for patients not receiving immunization at usual times, consult authoritative source

Administration Administer I.M. only

Patient Information Most children have little or no problem from the DTP shot; many children will have fever or soreness, swelling, and redness where the shot was given. Usually these problems are mild and last 1-2 days. Some children will be cranky, drowsy, or not want to eat during this time.

Nursing Implications Acetaminophen 10-15 mg/kg before and every 4 hours to 12-24 hours may reduce fever; give vaccine only I.M.

The child's medical record should document that the small risk of past vaccination seizure and the benefits of the pertussis vaccination were discussed with the patient

Additional Information Inactivated/killed bacterial vaccine. Federal law requires that the date of administration, the vaccine manufacturer, lot number of vaccine, and the administering person's name, title, and address be entered into the patient's permanent medical record. DTaP may be given for the fourth and fifth doses in children who started immunization with DTP vaccine.

Dosage Forms Injection: 0.5 mL

Diphtheria, Tetanus Toxoids, Whole-Cell Pertussis, and *Haemophilus influenzae* Type b Conjugate Vaccines

(dif THEER ee a, TET a nus TOKS oyds, hole-sel per TUS sis, & hem OF fil us in floo EN za type bee CON ju gate vak SEENS)

U.S. Brand Names Tetramune® [DSC]

Synonyms DTwP-HIB

Therapeutic Category Toxoid

Use Active immunization of infants and children through 5 years of age (between 2 months and the sixth birthday) against diphtheria, tetanus, and pertussis and *Haemophilus* b disease when indications for immunization with DTP vaccine and HIB vaccine coincide

Pregnancy Risk Factor B

Contraindications Hypersensitivity to *Haemophilus* b polysaccharide vaccine (thimerosal) or any component of the formulation; children with any febrile illness or active infection; children who are immunosuppressed or receiving immunosuppressive therapy; patients >7 years of age, patients with cancer, immunodeficiencies, an acute respiratory infection, or any other active infection; children with a history of neurologic disorders should not receive the pertussis any component of the formulation; history of any of the following effects from previous administration of pertussis vaccine precludes further use: fever >103°F (39.4°C), convulsions, focal neurologic signs, screaming episodes, shock, collapse, sleepiness or encephalopathy; hypersensitivity to diphtheria and tetanus toxoids or pertussis vaccine; do not use DTP for treatment of actual tetanus, diphtheria or whooping cough infections

Warnings/Precautions If adverse reactions occurred with previous doses, immunization should be completed with diphtheria and tetanus toxoid absorbed (pediatric); any febrile illness or active infection is reason for delaying use of *Haemophilus* b conjugate vaccine

Adverse Reactions

>10%:

Central nervous system: Fever, chills, irritability, restlessness, drowsiness

Local: Erythema, edema, induration, pain and warmth at injection site

1% to 10%:

Dermatologic: Rash

Gastrointestinal: Vomiting, diarrhea, loss of appetite

<1% (Limited to important or life-threatening): Arthralgia, chills, collapse, convulsions, focal neurological signs, increased risk of *Haemophilus* b infections in the week after vaccination, local tenderness, malaise, rarely allergic or anaphylactic reactions, screaming episodes, shock, sleepiness, urticaria

Stability Keep in refrigerator, may be frozen (not diluent) without affecting potency; unopened vials are stable for up to 24 hours at <70°C

Mechanism of Action Promotes active immunity to diphtheria, tetanus, pertussis, and *H. influenzae* by inducing production of specific antibodies and antitoxins.

Usual Dosage The primary immunization for children 2 months to 5 years of age, ideally beginning at the age of 2-3 months or at 6-week check-up. Administer 0.5 mL I.M. on 3 occasions at ~2-month intervals, followed by a fourth 0.5 mL dose at ~15 months of age.

Administration Administer I.M. only

Patient Information A nodule may be palpable at the injection site for a few weeks

Nursing Implications

Acetaminophen 10-15 mg/kg before and every 4 hours to 12-24 hours may reduce or prevent fever

Shake well before administering

The child's medical record should document that the small risk of past vaccination seizure and the benefits of the pertussis vaccination were discussed with the patient

Additional Information Inactivated bacterial vaccine. Federal law requires that the date of administration, the vaccine manufacturer, lot number of vaccine, and the administering person's name, title, and address be entered into the patient's permanent medical record. (**Note:** Diphtheria and Tetanus Toxoids, and Acellular Pertussis and *Haemophilus influenzae* Type B Conjugate Vaccine is Tripedia®/ActHIB®.)

Dosage Forms Injection: Diphtheria toxoid 12.5 Lf units, tetanus toxoid 5 Lf units, and whole-cell pertussis vaccine 4 units, and *Haemophilus influenzae* type b oligosaccharide 10 mcg per 0.5 mL (5 mL)

♦ **Diphtheria Toxoid Conjugate** *see Haemophilus b Conjugate Vaccine on page 651*
♦ **Dipivalyl Epinephrine** *see Dipivefrin on page 422*

Dipivefrin (dye PI ve frin)
Related Information
Glaucoma Drug Therapy Comparison *on page 1499*
U.S. Brand Names AKPro®; Propine®
Canadian Brand Names Ophtho-Dipivefrin™; PMS-Dipivefrin; Propine®
Synonyms Dipivalyl Epinephrine; Dipivefrin Hydrochloride; DPE
Therapeutic Category Adrenergic Agonist Agent, Ophthalmic; Ophthalmic Agent, Vasoconstrictor
Use Reduces elevated intraocular pressure in chronic open-angle glaucoma; also used to treat ocular hypertension, low tension, and secondary glaucomas
Pregnancy Risk Factor B
Usual Dosage Adults: Ophthalmic: Instill 1 drop every 12 hours into the eyes
Additional Information Complete prescribing information for this medication should be consulted for additional detail.
Dosage Forms Solution, ophthalmic, as hydrochloride: 0.1% (5 mL, 10 mL, 15 mL)

♦ **Dipivefrin Hydrochloride** *see Dipivefrin on page 422*
♦ **Diprivan®** *see Propofol on page 1145*
♦ **Diprolene®** *see Betamethasone on page 161*
♦ **Diprolene® AF** *see Betamethasone on page 161*
♦ **Diprolene® Glycol (Can)** *see Betamethasone on page 161*
♦ **Dipropylacetic Acid** *see Valproic Acid and Derivatives on page 1398*
♦ **Diprosone®** *see Betamethasone on page 161*

Dipyridamole (dye peer ID a mole)
U.S. Brand Names Persantine®
Canadian Brand Names Apo®-Dipyridamole FC; Novo-Dipiradol; Persantine®
Therapeutic Category Antiplatelet Agent; Platelet Aggregation Inhibitor; Vasodilator, Coronary
Use Maintains patency after surgical grafting procedures including coronary artery bypass; used with warfarin to decrease thrombosis in patients after artificial heart valve replacement; used with aspirin to prevent coronary artery thrombosis; in combination with aspirin or warfarin to prevent other thromboembolic disorders. Dipyridamole may also be given 2 days prior to open heart surgery to prevent platelet activation by extracorporeal bypass pump and as a diagnostic agent in CAD.
Unlabeled/Investigational Use Treatment of proteinuria in pediatric renal disease
Pregnancy Risk Factor B
Contraindications Hypersensitivity to dipyridamole or any component of the formulation
Warnings/Precautions Use caution in patients with hypotension. Use caution in patients on other antiplatelet agents or anticoagulation. Severe adverse reactions have occurred rarely with I.V. administration. Use the I.V. form with caution in patients with bronchospastic disease or unstable angina. Have aminophylline ready in case of urgency or emergency with I.V. use.
Adverse Reactions
>10%:
  Cardiovascular: Exacerbation of angina pectoris (19.7% - I.V.)
  Central nervous system: Dizziness (13.6% - P.O.), headache (12.2% - I.V.)
1% to 10%:
  Cardiovascular: Hypotension (4.6%), hypertension (1.5%), blood pressure lability (1.6%), EKG abnormalities (ST-T changes, extrasystoles), chest pain, tachycardia (3.2% - I.V.)
  Central nervous system: Headache (2.3% - I.V.), flushing (3.4% - I.V.), fatigue (1.2% - I.V.)
  Dermatologic: Rash (2.3% - P.O.)
  Gastrointestinal: Abdominal distress (6.1% - P.O.), nausea (4.6% - I.V.)
  Neuromuscular & skeletal: Paresthesia (1.3% - I.V.)
  Respiratory: Dyspnea (2.6% - I.V.)
<1% (Limited to important or life-threatening):
  I.V.: Arrhythmias (ventricular tachycardia, bradycardia, AV block, SVT, atrial fibrillation, asystole), bronchospasm, depersonalization, intermittent claudication, myocardial infarction, orthostatic hypotension, syncope, vertigo
  P.O.: Angina pectoris, liver dysfunction.
  Case reports: Epistaxis, esophageal hematoma, gallstones, pharyngeal bleeding, rapidly progressive glomerulonephritis, respiratory arrest (I.V.), thrombotic thrombocytopenic purpura
Overdosage/Toxicology Symptoms include hypotension and peripheral vasodilation. Dialysis is not effective. Treatment includes fluids and vasopressors although hypotension is often transient.
Drug Interactions
  Increased Effect/Toxicity: Dipyridamole enhances the risk of bleeding with aspirin (and other antiplatelet agents), heparin, low-molecular weight heparins, and warfarin. Adenosine blood levels and pharmacologic effects are increased with dipyridamole; consider reduced doses of adenosine.
  Decreased Effect: Decreased vasodilation from I.V. dipyridamole when given to patients taking theophylline. Theophylline may reduce the pharmacologic effects of dipyridamole (hold theophylline preparations for 36-48 hours before dipyridamole facilitated stress test).
Ethanol/Nutrition/Herb Interactions Herb/Nutraceutical: Avoid cat's claw, dong quai, evening primrose, feverfew, garlic, ginger, ginkgo, red clover, horse chestnut, green tea, ginseng (all have additional antiplatelet activity).
Stability Do not freeze, protect I.V. preparation from light
Mechanism of Action Inhibits the activity of adenosine deaminase and phosphodiesterase, which causes an accumulation of adenosine, adenine nucleotides, and cyclic AMP; these

mediators then inhibit platelet aggregation and may cause vasodilation; may also stimulate release of prostacyclin or PGD_2; causes coronary vasodilation

Pharmacodynamics/Kinetics
  Absorption: Readily, but variable
  Distribution: Adults: V_d: 2-3 L/kg
  Protein binding: 91% to 99%
  Metabolism: Hepatic
  Half-life elimination: Terminal: 10-12 hours
  Time to peak, serum: 2-2.5 hours
  Excretion: Feces (as glucuronide conjugates and unchanged drug)

Usual Dosage
  Children: Oral: 3-6 mg/kg/day in 3 divided doses
    Doses of 4-10 mg/kg/day have been used investigationally to treat proteinuria in pediatric renal disease
    Mechanical prosthetic heart valves: Oral: 2-5 mg/kg/day (used in combination with an oral anticoagulant in children who have systemic embolism despite adequate oral anticoagulant therapy, and used in combination with low-dose oral anticoagulation (INR 2-3) plus aspirin in children in whom full-dose oral anticoagulation is contraindicated)
  Adults:
    Oral: 75-400 mg/day in 3-4 divided doses
    Evaluation of coronary artery disease: I.V.: 0.14 mg/kg/minute for 4 minutes; maximum dose: 60 mg
  Hemodialysis: Significant drug removal is unlikely based on physiochemical characteristics

Dietary Considerations Should be taken with water 1 hour before meals.

Administration I.V.: Dilute in at least a 1:2 ratio with normal saline, $^1/_2$NS, or D_5W; infusion of undiluted dipyridamole may cause local irritation

Patient Information Notify physician or pharmacist if taking other medications that affect bleeding, such as NSAIDs or warfarin

Nursing Implications Monitor blood pressure, heart rate, EKG (stress test)

Dosage Forms
  Injection: 5 mg/mL (2 mL, 10 mL)
  Tablet: 25 mg, 50 mg, 75 mg

Extemporaneous Preparations A 10 mg/mL oral suspension has been made using four 25 mg tablets and purified water USP qs ad to 10 mL; expected stability is 3 days. Dipyridamole 10 mg/mL was stable for up to 60 days at 5°C and 25°C in 1:1 mixtures of Ora-Sweet® and Ora-Plus®, Ora-Sweet® SF and Ora-Plus® and in cherry syrup

Allen LV and Erickson III MA, "Stability of Baclofen, Captopril, Diltiazem, Hydrochloride, Dipyridamole, and Flecainide Acetate in Extemporaneously Compounded Oral Liquids," *Am J Health Syst Pharm*, 1996, 53:2179-84.

Nahata MC and Hipple TF, *Pediatric Drug Formulations*, 2nd ed, Cincinnati, OH: Harvey Whitney Books Co, 1992.

♦ **Dipyridamole and Aspirin** see Aspirin and Extended-Release Dipyridamole on page 123

Dirithromycin (dye RITH roe mye sin)

U.S. Brand Names Dynabac®
Therapeutic Category Antibiotic, Macrolide
Use Treatment of mild to moderate upper and lower respiratory tract infections due to *Moraxella catarrhalis*, *Streptococcus pneumoniae*, *Legionella pneumophila*, *H. influenzae*, or *S. pyogenes*, ie, acute exacerbation of chronic bronchitis, secondary bacterial infection of acute bronchitis, community-acquired pneumonia, pharyngitis/tonsillitis, and uncomplicated infections of the skin and skin structure due to *Staphylococcus aureus*

Pregnancy Risk Factor C
Pregnancy/Breast-Feeding Implications
  Clinical effects on the fetus: Animal studies indicate the use of dirithromycin during pregnancy should be avoided if possible
  Breast-feeding/lactation: Use caution when administering to nursing women

Contraindications Hypersensitivity to any macrolide or component of dirithromycin; use with pimozide

Warnings/Precautions Contrary to potential serious consequences with other macrolides (eg, cardiac arrhythmias), the combination of terfenadine and dirithromycin has not shown alteration of terfenadine metabolism; however, caution should be taken during coadministration of dirithromycin and terfenadine; pseudomembranous colitis has been reported and should be considered in patients presenting with diarrhea subsequent to therapy with dirithromycin

Adverse Reactions
  1% to 10%:
    Central nervous system: Headache, dizziness, vertigo, insomnia
    Dermatologic: Rash, pruritus, urticaria
    Endocrine & metabolic: Hyperkalemia
    Gastrointestinal: Abdominal pain, nausea, diarrhea, vomiting, dyspepsia, flatulence
    Hematologic: Thrombocytosis, eosinophilia, segmented neutrophils
    Neuromuscular & skeletal: Weakness, pain, increased CPK
    Respiratory: Increased cough, dyspnea
  <1% (Limited to important or life-threatening): Depression, flu-like syndrome, hemoptysis, leukocytosis, monocytosis, neutropenia, paresthesia, somnolence, syncope, tinnitus, thrombocytopenia

Overdosage/Toxicology Symptoms include nausea, vomiting, abdominal pain, and diarrhea. Treatment is supportive. Dialysis has not been found to be effective.

Drug Interactions
  Cytochrome P450 Effect: CYP3A3/4 enzyme inhibitor
  Increased Effect/Toxicity: Absorption of dirithromycin is slightly enhanced with concomitant antacids and H_2 antagonists. Dirithromycin may, like erythromycin, increase the effect

(Continued)

Dirithromycin *(Continued)*

of alfentanil, anticoagulants, bromocriptine, carbamazepine, cyclosporine, digoxin, disopyramide, ergots, methylprednisolone, cisapride, astemizole, and triazolam.

Note: Interactions with nonsedating antihistamines (eg, astemizole and terfenadine) or theophylline are not known to occur; however, caution is advised with coadministration.

Mechanism of Action After being converted during intestinal absorption to its active form, erythromycylamine, dirithromycin inhibits protein synthesis by binding to the 50S ribosomal subunits of susceptible microorganisms

Pharmacodynamics/Kinetics
Absorption: Rapidly absorbed
Distribution: V_d: 800 L; rapidly and widely (higher levels in tissues than plasma)
Protein binding: 14% to 30%
Metabolism: Hydrolyzed to erythromycylamine
Bioavailability: 10%
Half-life elimination: 8 hours (range: 2-36 hours)
Time to peak: 4 hours
Excretion: Feces (81% to 97%)

Usual Dosage Adults: Oral: 500 mg once daily for 5-14 days (14 days required for treatment of community-acquired pneumonia due to *Legionella, Mycoplasma,* or *S. pneumoniae;* 10 days is recommended for treatment of *S. pyogenes* pharyngitis/tonsillitis)

Dosing adjustment in renal impairment: None necessary
Dosing adjustment in hepatic impairment: None needed in mild dysfunction; not studied in moderate to severe dysfunction

Dietary Considerations Administer with food or within 1 hour of eating.
Administration Administer with food or within an hour following a meal
Monitoring Parameters Temperature, CBC
Patient Information Take with food or within an hour following a meal; do not cut, chew, or crush tablets; entire course of medication should be taken to ensure eradication of organism
Nursing Implications Do not crush tablets
Dosage Forms Tablet, enteric coated: 250 mg

♦ **Disalcid®** *see Salsalate on page 1220*

♦ **Disalicylic Acid** *see Salsalate on page 1220*

♦ **Disobrom® [OTC]** *see Dexbrompheniramine and Pseudoephedrine on page 383*

♦ **Disodium Cromoglycate** *see Cromolyn Sodium on page 337*

♦ **d-Isoephedrine Hydrochloride** *see Pseudoephedrine on page 1155*

♦ **Disophrol® Chronotabs® [OTC]** *see Dexbrompheniramine and Pseudoephedrine on page 383*

Disopyramide *(dye soe PEER a mide)*

Related Information
Antiarrhythmic Drugs Comparison *on page 1478*
U.S. Brand Names Norpace®; Norpace® CR
Canadian Brand Names Norpace®; Rythmodan®; Rythmodan®-LA
Synonyms Disopyramide Phosphate
Therapeutic Category Antiarrhythmic Agent, Class I-A
Use Suppression and prevention of unifocal and multifocal atrial and premature, ventricular premature complexes, coupled ventricular tachycardia; effective in the conversion of atrial fibrillation, atrial flutter, and paroxysmal atrial tachycardia to normal sinus rhythm and prevention of the recurrence of these arrhythmias after conversion by other methods
Pregnancy Risk Factor C
Contraindications Hypersensitivity to disopyramide or any component of the formulation; cardiogenic shock; pre-existing second- or third-degree heart block (except in patients with a functioning artificial pacemaker); congenital QT syndrome; sick sinus syndrome
Warnings/Precautions Monitor closely for hypotension during the initiation of therapy. Avoid concurrent use with other medications with prolong QT interval or decrease myocardial contractility. Pre-existing urinary retention, family history, or existing angle-closure glaucoma, myasthenia gravis, congestive heart failure unless caused by an arrhythmias, widening of QRS complex during therapy or QT interval (>25% to 50% of baseline QRS complex or QT interval), sick-sinus syndrome or WPW may require decrease in dosage; disopyramide ineffective in hypokalemia and potentially toxic with hyperkalemia. Due to changes in total clearance (decreased) in elderly, monitor closely; the anticholinergic action may be intolerable and require discontinuation. May precipitate or exacerbate CHF. Due to significant anticholinergic effects, do not use in patients with urinary retention, BPH, glaucoma, or myasthenia gravis. Reduce dosage in renal or hepatic impairment. The extended release form is not recommended for Cl_{cr} <40 mL/minute. In patients with atrial fibrillation or flutter, block the AV node before initiating. Use caution in Wolff-Parkinson-White syndrome or bundle branch block.
Adverse Reactions The most common adverse effects are related to cholinergic blockade. The most serious adverse effects of disopyramide are hypotension and congestive heart failure.

>10%:
Gastrointestinal: Xerostomia (32%), constipation (11%)
Genitourinary: Urinary hesitancy (14% to 23%)
1% to 10%:
Cardiovascular: Congestive heart failure, hypotension, cardiac conduction disturbance, edema, syncope, chest pain
Central nervous system: Fatigue, headache, malaise, dizziness, nervousness
Dermatologic: Rash, generalized dermatoses, pruritus
Endocrine & metabolic: Hypokalemia, elevated cholesterol, elevated triglycerides

Gastrointestinal: Dry throat, nausea, abdominal distension, flatulence, abdominal bloating, anorexia, diarrhea, vomiting, weight gain

Genitourinary: Urinary retention, urinary frequency, urinary urgency, impotence (1% to 3%)

Neuromuscular & skeletal: Muscle weakness, muscular pain

Ocular: Blurred vision, dry eyes

Respiratory: Dyspnea

<1% (Limited to important or life-threatening): Agranulocytosis, AV block, cholestatic jaundice, depression, dysuria, creatinine increased, gynecomastia, hepatotoxicity, hypoglycemia, BUN increased, insomnia, new or worsened arrhythmias (proarrhythmic effect), paresthesia, psychotic reaction, respiratory distress, thrombocytopenia, transaminases increased. Rare cases of lupus have been reported (generally in patients previously receiving procainamide), peripheral neuropathy, psychosis, toxic cutaneous blisters

Overdosage/Toxicology

Has a low toxic therapeutic ratio and may easily produce fatal intoxication (acute toxic dose: 1 g in adults). Symptoms include sinus bradycardia, sinus node arrest or asystole; PR, QRS, or QT interval prolongation; torsade de pointes (polymorphous ventricular tachycardia) and depressed myocardial contractility; depressed myocardium, along with alpha-adrenergic or ganglionic blockade, may result in hypotension and pulmonary edema. Other effects are anticholinergic (dry mouth, dilated pupils, and delirium) as well as seizures, coma and respiratory arrest.

Treatment is primarily symptomatic and effects usually respond to conventional therapies (fluids, positioning, vasopressors, anticonvulsants, antiarrhythmics). **Note:** Do not use other type Ia or Ic antiarrhythmic agents to treat ventricular tachycardia. Sodium bicarbonate may treat wide QRS intervals or hypotension. Markedly impaired conduction or high degree A-V block, unresponsive to bicarbonate, indicates consideration of a pacemaker.

Drug Interactions

Cytochrome P450 Effect: CYP3A3/4 enzyme substrate

Increased Effect/Toxicity: Disopyramide may increase the effects/toxicity of anticholinergics, beta-blockers, flecainide, procainamide, quinidine, or propafenone. Digoxin and quinidine serum concentrations may be increased by disopyramide. Erythromycin and clarithromycin may increase disopyramide serum concentrations, increasing toxicity (widening QT interval).

Disopyramide effect/toxicity may be additive with drugs which may prolong the QT interval - amiodarone, amitriptyline, astemizole, bepridil, cisapride (use is contraindicated), disopyramide, erythromycin, haloperidol, imipramine, pimozide, quinidine, sotalol, and thioridazine. In addition concurrent use with sparfloxacin, gatifloxacin, and moxifloxacin may result in additional prolongation of the QT interval; concurrent use is contraindicated.

Decreased Effect: Hepatic microsomal enzyme inducing agents (eg, phenytoin, phenobarbital, rifampin) may increase metabolism of disopyramide leading to a decreased effect. Anticoagulants may have decreased prothrombin times after discontinuation of disopyramide.

Ethanol/Nutrition/Herb Interactions

Ethanol: Avoid ethanol (may increase CNS depression).

Herb/Nutraceutical: St John's wort may decrease disopyramide levels. Avoid ephedra (may worsen arrhythmia).

Stability Extemporaneously prepared suspension is stable for 4 weeks refrigerated

Mechanism of Action Class Ia antiarrhythmic: Decreases myocardial excitability and conduction velocity; reduces disparity in refractory between normal and infarcted myocardium; possesses anticholinergic, peripheral vasoconstrictive, and negative inotropic effects

Pharmacodynamics/Kinetics

Onset of action: 0.5-3.5 hours

Duration: 1.5-8.5 hours

Absorption: 60% to 83%

Protein binding: 20% to 60% (concentration dependent)

Metabolism: Hepatic to inactive metabolites

Half-life elimination: Adults: 4-10 hours, increased with hepatic or renal disease

Excretion: Urine (40% to 60% as unchanged drug); feces (10% to 15%)

Usual Dosage Oral:

Children:

<1 year: 10-30 mg/kg/24 hours in 4 divided doses

1-4 years: 10-20 mg/kg/24 hours in 4 divided doses

4-12 years: 10-15 mg/kg/24 hours in 4 divided doses

12-18 years: 6-15 mg/kg/24 hours in 4 divided doses

Adults:

<50 kg: 100 mg every 6 hours or 200 mg every 12 hours (controlled release)

>50 kg: 150 mg every 6 hours or 300 mg every 12 hours (controlled release); if no response, increase to 200 mg every 6 hours. Maximum dose required for patients with severe refractory ventricular tachycardia is 400 mg every 6 hours.

Elderly: Dose with caution, starting at the lower end of dosing range

Dosing adjustment in renal impairment: 100 mg (nonsustained release) given at the following intervals, based on creatinine clearance (mL/minute):

Cl_{cr} 30-40 mL/minute: Administer every 8 hours

Cl_{cr} 15-30 mL/minute: Administer every 12 hours

Cl_{cr} <15 mL/minute: Administer every 24 hours

or alter the dose as follows:

Cl_{cr} 30-<40 mL/minute: Reduce dose 50%

Cl_{cr} 15-30 mL/minute: Reduce dose 75%

Dialysis: Not dialyzable (0% to 5%) by hemo- or peritoneal methods; supplemental dose is not necessary.

Dosing interval in hepatic impairment: 100 mg every 6 hours or 200 mg every 12 hours (controlled release)

Dietary Considerations Should be taken on an empty stomach.

Administration Administer around-the-clock rather than 4 times/day (ie, 12-6-12-6, not 9-1-5-9) to promote less variation in peak and trough serum levels

(Continued)

Disopyramide (Continued)

Monitoring Parameters EKG, blood pressure, urinary retention, CNS anticholinergic effects (confusion, agitation, hallucinations, etc)

Reference Range
Therapeutic concentration:
Atrial arrhythmias: 2.8-3.2 µg/mL
Ventricular arrhythmias 3.3-7.5 µg/mL
Toxic concentration: >7 µg/mL

Patient Information Notify physician if urinary retention or worsening CHF; do not break or chew sustained release capsules

Nursing Implications Do not crush controlled release capsules

Dosage Forms
Capsule, as phosphate: 100 mg, 150 mg
Capsule, sustained action, as phosphate: 100 mg, 150 mg

Extemporaneous Preparations Extemporaneous suspensions in cherry syrup (1 mg/mL and 10 mg/mL) are stable for 4 weeks in amber glass bottles stored at 5°C, 30°C, or at room temperature; shake well before use; do not use extended release capsules for this suspension

Mathur LK, Lai PK, and Shively CD, "Stability of Disopyramide Phosphate in Cherry Syrup," *J Hosp Pharm*, 1982, 39(2):309-10.

♦ **Disopyramide Phosphate** *see Disopyramide on page 424*

♦ **Disotate®** *see Edetate Disodium on page 457*

♦ **Di-Spaz®** *see Dicyclomine on page 397*

Disulfiram (dye SUL fi ram)

Related Information
Depression *on page 1655*

U.S. Brand Names Antabuse®

Canadian Brand Names Antabuse®

Therapeutic Category Aldehyde Dehydrogenase Inhibitor Agent; Antialcoholic Agent

Use Management of chronic alcoholism

Pregnancy Risk Factor C

Contraindications Hypersensitivity to disulfiram and related compounds or any component of the formulation; patients receiving or using ethanol, metronidazole, paraldehyde, or ethanol-containing preparations like cough syrup or tonics; psychosis; severe myocardial disease and coronary occlusion

Warnings/Precautions Use with caution in patients with diabetes, hypothyroidism, seizure disorders, nephritis (acute or chronic); hepatic cirrhosis or insufficiency; should never be administered to a patient when he/she is in a state of alcohol intoxication, or without his/her knowledge. Patient must receive appropriate counseling, including information on "disguised" forms of alcohol (tonics, mouthwashes, etc) and the duration of the drug's activity (up to 14 days). Severe (sometimes fatal) hepatitis and/or hepatic failure have been associated with disulfiram. May occur in patients with or without prior history of abnormal hepatic function.

Adverse Reactions Frequency not defined.
Central nervous system: Drowsiness, headache, fatigue, psychosis
Dermatologic: Rash, acneiform eruptions, allergic dermatitis
Gastrointestinal: Metallic or garlic-like aftertaste
Genitourinary: Impotence
Hepatic: Hepatitis
Neuromuscular & skeletal: Peripheral neuritis, polyneuritis, peripheral neuropathy
Ocular: Optic neuritis

Overdosage/Toxicology Management of disulfiram reaction: Institute support measures to restore blood pressure (pressors and fluids); monitor for hypokalemia.

Drug Interactions
Cytochrome P450 Effect: CYP2C9 and 2E1 enzyme inhibitor, both disulfiram and diethyldithiocarbamate (disulfiram metabolite) are CYP3A3/4 inhibitors
Increased Effect/Toxicity: Disulfiram may increase serum concentrations of benzodiazepines that undergo oxidative metabolism (all but oxazepam, lorazepam, temazepam). Disulfiram increases phenytoin and theophylline serum concentrations; toxicity may occur. Disulfiram inhibits the metabolism of warfarin resulting in an increased hypoprothrombinemic response. Disulfiram results in severe ethanol intolerance (disulfiram reaction) secondary to disulfiram's ability to inhibit aldehyde dehydrogenase; this combination should be avoided. Combined use with isoniazid, metronidazole, or MAO inhibitors may result in adverse CNS effects; this combination should be avoided. Some pharmaceutic dosage forms include ethanol, including elixirs and intravenous trimethoprim-sulfamethoxazole (contains 10% ethanol as a solubilizing agent); these may inadvertently provoke a disulfiram reaction.

Ethanol/Nutrition/Herb Interactions Ethanol: Disulfiram inhibits ethanol's usual metabolism. Avoid all ethanol. Patients can have a disulfiram reaction (headache, nausea, vomiting, chest, or abdominal pain) if they drink ethanol concurrently. Avoid cough syrups and elixirs containing ethanol. Avoid vinegars, cider, extracts, and foods containing ethanol.

Mechanism of Action Disulfiram is a thiuram derivative which interferes with aldehyde dehydrogenase. When taken concomitantly with alcohol, there is an increase in serum acetaldehyde levels. High acetaldehyde causes uncomfortable symptoms including flushing, nausea, thirst, palpitations, chest pain, vertigo, and hypotension. This reaction is the basis for disulfiram use in postwithdrawal long-term care of alcoholism.

Pharmacodynamics/Kinetics
Onset of action: Full effect: 12 hours
Duration: ~1-2 weeks after last dose
Absorption: Rapid
Metabolism: To diethylthiocarbamate

Usual Dosage Adults: Oral: Do not administer until the patient has abstained from ethanol for at least 12 hours

Initial: 500 mg/day as a single dose for 1-2 weeks; maximum daily dose is 500 mg
Average maintenance dose: 250 mg/day; range: 125-500 mg; duration of therapy is to continue until the patient is fully recovered socially and a basis for permanent self control has been established; maintenance therapy may be required for months or even years

Monitoring Parameters Hypokalemia; liver function tests at baseline and after 10-14 days of treatment; CBC, serum chemistries, liver function tests should be monitored during therapy

Patient Information Notify prescriber of any respiratory difficulty, weakness, nausea, vomiting, decreased appetite, yellowing of skin or eyes, or dark-colored urine. Avoid alcohol, including products containing ethanol (cough and cold syrups), or use ethanol-containing skin products for at least 3 days and preferably 14 days after stopping this medication or while taking this medication; not for treatment of alcohol intoxication; may cause drowsiness; tablets can be crushed or mixed with water

Nursing Implications Administration of any medications containing ethanol including topicals is contraindicated

Dosage Forms Tablet: 250 mg, 500 mg

DOBUTamine (doe BYOO ta meen)

Related Information
Adrenergic Agonists, Cardiovascular Comparison *on page 1469*
Adult ACLS Algorithms *on page 1632*
Antacid Drug Interactions *on page 1477*

U.S. Brand Names Dobutrex®
Canadian Brand Names Dobutrex®
Synonyms Dobutamine Hydrochloride
Therapeutic Category Adrenergic Agonist Agent; Sympathomimetic
Use Short-term management of patients with cardiac decompensation
Unlabeled/Investigational Use Positve inotropic agent for use in myocardial dysfunction of sepsis

Pregnancy Risk Factor B
Contraindications Hypersensitivity to dobutamine or sulfites (some contain sodium metabisulfate), or any component of the formulation; idiopathic hypertrophic subaortic stenosis (IHSS)

Warnings/Precautions Can see an increase in heart rate. Patients with atrial fibrillation may experience an increase in ventricular response. An increase in blood pressure is more common, but occasionally a patient may become hypotensive. May exacerbate ventricular ectopy. If needed, correct hypovolemia first to optimize hemodynamics. Ineffective in the presence of mechanical obstruction such as severe aortic stenosis. Use caution post-MI (can increase myocardial oxygen demand). Use cautiously in the elderly starting at lower end of the dosage range.

Adverse Reactions Incidence of adverse events is not always reported.
Cardiovascular: Increased heart rate, increased blood pressure, increased ventricular ectopic activity, hypotension, premature ventricular beats (5%, dose-related), anginal pain (1% to 3%), nonspecific chest pain (1% to 3%), palpitations (1% to 3%)
Central nervous system: Fever (1% to 3%), headache (1% to 3%), paresthesia
Endocrine & metabolic: Slight decrease in serum potassium
Gastrointestinal: Nausea (1% to 3%)
Hematologic: Thrombocytopenia (isolated cases)
Local: Phlebitis, local inflammatory changes and pain from infiltration, cutaneous necrosis (isolated cases)
Neuromuscular & skeletal: Mild leg cramps
Respiratory: Dyspnea (1% to 3%)

Overdosage/Toxicology Symptoms include fatigue, nervousness, tachycardia, hypertension, and arrhythmias. Reduce rate of administration or discontinue infusion until condition stabilizes.

Drug Interactions
Increased Effect/Toxicity: General anesthetics (eg, halothane or cyclopropane) and usual doses of dobutamine have resulted in ventricular arrhythmias in animals. Bretylium and may potentiate dobutamine's effects. Beta-blockers (nonselective ones) may increase hypertensive effect; avoid concurrent use. Cocaine may cause malignant arrhythmias. Guanethidine, MAO inhibitors, methyldopa, reserpine, and tricyclic antidepressants can increase the pressor response to sympathomimetics.

Decreased Effect: Beta-adrenergic blockers may decrease effect of dobutamine and increase risk of severe hypotension.

(Continued)

DOBUTamine *(Continued)*

Stability Remix solution every 24 hours; store reconstituted solution under refrigeration for 48 hours or 6 hours at room temperature; pink discoloration of solution indicates slight oxidation but **no** significant loss of potency.

Stability of parenteral admixture at room temperature (25°C): 48 hours; at refrigeration (4°C): 7 days

Standard adult diluent: 250 mg/500 mL D_5W; 500 mg/500 mL D_5W

Incompatible with heparin, cefazolin, penicillin, and sodium bicarbonate; **incompatible** in alkaline solutions (sodium bicarbonate)

Compatible with dopamine, epinephrine, isoproterenol, lidocaine

Mechanism of Action Stimulates beta$_1$-adrenergic receptors, causing increased contractility and heart rate, with little effect on beta$_2$- or alpha-receptors

Pharmacodynamics/Kinetics

Onset of action: I.V.: 1-10 minutes

Peak effect: 10-20 minutes

Metabolism: In tissues and hepatically to inactive metabolites

Half-life elimination: 2 minutes

Excretion: Urine (as metabolites)

Usual Dosage Administration requires the use of an infusion pump; I.V. infusion:

Neonates: 2-15 mcg/kg/minute, titrate to desired response

Children and Adults: 2.5-20 mcg/kg/minute; maximum: 40 mcg/kg/minute, titrate to desired response. See table.

Infusion Rates of Various Dilutions of Dobutamine

Desired Delivery Rate (mcg/kg/min)	Infusion Rate (mL/kg/min)	
	500 mcg/mL*	1000 mcg/mL†
2.5	0.005	0.0025
5.0	0.01	0.005
7.5	0.015	0.0075
10.0	0.02	0.01
12.5	0.025	0.0125
15.0	0.03	0.015

* 500 mg per liter or 250 mg per 500 mL of diluent.

†1000 mg per liter or 250 mg per 250 mL of diluent.

Administration Use infusion device to control rate of flow; administer into large vein. Do not administer through same I.V. line as heparin, hydrocortisone sodium succinate, cefazolin, or penicillin.

To prepare for infusion:

$$\frac{6 \times \text{weight (kg)} \times \text{desired dose (mcg/kg/min)}}{\text{I.V. infusion rate (mL/h)}} = \text{mg of drug to be added to 100 mL of I.V. fluid}$$

Monitoring Parameters Blood pressure, EKG, heart rate, CVP, RAP, MAP, urine output; if pulmonary artery catheter is in place, monitor CI, PCWP, and SVR; also monitor serum potassium

Nursing Implications Management of extravasation: Phentolamine: Mix 5 mg with 9 mL of NS; inject a small amount of this dilution into extravasation area; blanching should reverse immediately. Monitor site; if blanching should recur, additional injections of phentolamine may be needed.

Additional Information Dobutamine lowers central venous pressure and wedge pressure but has little effect on pulmonary vascular resistance.

Dobutamine therapy should be avoided in patients with stable heart failure due to an increase in mortality. In patients with intractable heart failure, dobutamine may be used as a short-term infusion to provide symptomatic benefit. It is not known whether short-term dobutamine therapy in end-stage heart failure has any outcome benefit.

Dobutamine infusion during echocardiography is used as a cardiovascular stress. Wall motion abnormalities developing with increasing doses of dobutamine may help to identify ischemic and/or hibernating myocardium.

Dosage Forms Infusion, as hydrochloride: 12.5 mg/mL (20 mL)

♦ **Dobutamine Hydrochloride** *see* DOBUTamine *on page 427*

♦ **Dobutrex**® *see* DOBUTamine *on page 427*

Docetaxel *(doe se TAKS el)*

U.S. Brand Names Taxotere®

Canadian Brand Names Taxotere®

Therapeutic Category Antineoplastic Agent, Antimicrotubular

Use Treatment of patients with locally advanced or metastatic breast cancer who have progressed during anthracycline-based therapy or have relapsed during anthracycline-based adjuvant therapy; treatment of patients with locally advanced or metastatic nonsmall cell lung cancer after failure of prior platinum-based chemotherapy

Unlabeled/Investigational Use Investigational: Treatment of gastric, pancreatic, head and neck, ovarian, soft tissue sarcoma, and melanoma

Pregnancy Risk Factor D

Contraindications Hypersensitivity to docetaxel, Polysorbate 80®, or any component of the formulation; pre-existing bone marrow suppression; pregnancy

Warnings/Precautions Early studies reported severe hypersensitivity reactions characterized by hypotension, bronchospasms, or minor reactions characterized by generalized rash/erythema. The overall incidence was 25% in patients who did not receive premedication.

Fluid retention syndrome characterized by pleural effusions, ascites, edema, and weight gain (2-15 kg) has also been reported. It has not been associated with cardiac, pulmonary, renal, hepatic, or endocrine dysfunction. The incidence and severity of the syndrome increase sharply at cumulative doses ≥400 mg/m².

Premedication to reduce fluid retention and hypersensitivity reactions: Oral dexametha-sone 8 mg twice daily for 5 days starting one day prior to docetaxel exposure. There is also data to support that a 3-day corticosteroid regimen (oral dexamethasone 8 mg twice daily for 3 days starting one day prior to docetaxel exposure) was as effective as the standard 5-day regimen in reducing the incidence and severity of fluid retention. In addition, the 3-day regimen had a more favorable safety profile.

Neutropenia was the dose-limiting toxicity; however this rarely resulted in treatment delays and prophylactic colony stimulating factors have not been routinely used. Patients with increased liver function tests experienced more episodes of neutropenia with a greater number of severe infections. Patients with an absolute neutrophil count <1500 cells/mm³ should not receive docetaxel.

Docetaxel preparation should be performed in a Class II laminar flow biologic safety cabinet. Personnel should be wearing surgical gloves and a closed front surgical gown with knit cuffs. Appropriate safety equipment is recommended for preparation, administration, and disposal of antineoplastics. If docetaxel contacts the skin, wash and flush thoroughly with water.

When administered as sequential infusions, taxane derivatives (docetaxel, paclitaxel) should be administered before platinum derivatives (carboplatin, cisplatin) to limit myelosuppression and to enhance efficacy.

Adverse Reactions
>10%:
Allergic: Angioedema, rash, flushing, fever, hypotension (30%); patients should be premedicated with dexamethasone starting the day before docetaxel administration
Dermatologic: Alopecia (80%); nail banding, onycholysis (28%); hypo- or hyperpigmenta-tion (28%)
Endocrine & metabolic: Fluid retention, including peripheral edema, pleural effusions, and ascites (17% to 70%), may be more common at cumulative doses ≥400 mg/m²
Gastrointestinal: Mucositis (45%), may be dose-limiting; mild to moderate nausea and vomiting (40% to 80%), diarrhea (25%)
Hematologic: Myelosuppression, neutropenia, thrombocytopenia, anemia
Onset: 4-7 days
Nadir: 5-9 days
Recovery: 21 days
Hepatic: Increased transaminase levels (18%)
Neuromuscular & skeletal: Peripheral neuropathies (13%)
1% to 10%:
Cardiovascular: Myocardial infarction
Dermatologic: Rash and skin eruptions (6%)
Gastrointestinal: GI perforation, neutropenic enterocolitis
Hepatic: Increased bilirubin (9%)
Neuromuscular & skeletal: Paresthesia, dysesthesia, pain/burning sensation (7%), may be related to prior cisplatin therapy and/or high (500-700 mg/m²) cumulative doses of docetaxel

Drug Interactions
Cytochrome P450 Effect: CYP3A3/4 enzyme substrate
Increased Effect/Toxicity: Increased toxicity with cytochrome P450 substrate agents. Possibility of an inhibition of metabolism of docetaxel in patients treated with ketoconazole, erythromycin, terfenadine, astemizole, or cyclosporine. When administered as sequential infusions, observational studies indicate a potential for increased toxicity when platinum derivatives (carboplatin, cisplatin) are administered before taxane derivatives (docetaxel, paclitaxel).

Ethanol/Nutrition/Herb Interactions
Ethanol: Avoid ethanol (due to GI irritation).
Herb/Nutraceutical: St John's wort (may docetaxel decrease levels).

Stability Store intact vials at refrigeration (2°C to 8°C/36°F to 47°F) and protect from light. Intact vials of solution should be further diluted with 13% (w/w) ethanol/water to a final concentration of 10 mg/mL.

Docetaxel dose should be further diluted with 0.9% sodium chloride or 5% dextrose in water to a final concentration of 0.3-0.9 mg/mL and must be prepared in a glass bottle, polypro-pylene, or polyolefin plastic bag to prevent leaching of plasticizers.

Non-PVC tubing **must** be used. Diluted solutions are stable for up to 4 weeks at room temperature (15°C to 25°C/59°F to 77°F) in polyolefin containers. (Thiesen J and Kramer I, *Pharm World Sci*, 1999, 21(3):137-41.)

Although the stability of some antineoplastic agents may be long, it is probably considered good pharmaceutical practice to allow a maximum expiration dating of 24 hours due to possible sterility concerns.

Mechanism of Action Semisynthetic agent prepared from a noncytotoxic precursor which is extracted from the needles of the European Yew *Taxus baccata*. Docetaxel differs structur-ally from the prototype taxoid, paclitaxel, by substitutions at the C-10 and C-5 positions. It is an antimicrotubule agent, but exhibits a unique mechanism of action. Unlike other antimicrotubule agents that induce microtubule disassembly (eg, vinca alkaloids and colchi-cine), docetaxel promotes the assembly of microtubules from tubulin dimers, and inhibits the depolymerization of tubulin which leads to bundles of microtubules in the cell.

Pharmacodynamics/Kinetics Administered by I.V. infusion and exhibits linear pharmacoki-netics at the recommended dosage range

Distribution: Extensive extravascular distribution and/or tissue binding; V_{dss}: 113 L (mean steady state)
Protein binding: 94%, mainly to alpha₁-acid glycoprotein, albumin, and lipoproteins
Metabolism: Hepatic; oxidation; CYP3A3/4
(Continued)

Docetaxel *(Continued)*

Half-life elimination: Alpha, beta, gamma: 4 minutes, 36 minutes, and 11.1 hours, respectively

Excretion: Feces (75%); urine (6%); ~80% within 48 hours
Clearance: Total body: Mean: 21 L/hour/m^2

Usual Dosage Corticosteroids (oral dexamethasone 8 mg twice daily for 3 days or 5 days starting 1 day prior to docetaxel administration) are necessary to reduce the potential for hypersensitivity and severe fluid retention

Adults: I.V. infusion: Refer to individual protocols:
Locally advanced or metastatic carcinoma of the breast: 60-100 mg/m^2 over 1 hour every 3 weeks

Nonsmall-cell lung cancer: I.V.: 75 mg/m^2 over 1 hour every 3 weeks

Dosage adjustment in patients who are initially started at 100 mg/m^2 (>1 week), cumulative cutaneous reactions, or severe peripheral neuropathy: 75 mg/m^2

Note: If the patient continues to experience these adverse reactions, the dosage should be reduced to 55 mg/m^2 or therapy should be discontinued

Dosing adjustment in hepatic impairment:
Total bilirubin ≥ the upper limit of normal (ULN), or AST/ALT >1.5 times the ULN concomitant with alkaline phosphatase >2.5 times the ULN: Docetaxel **should not be administered** secondary to increased incidence of treatment-related mortality

Administration
Anaphylactoid-like reactions have been reported: Premedication with dexamethasone (8 mg orally twice daily for 5 days starting one day prior to administration of docetaxel)
Administer I.V. infusion over 1-hour

Monitoring Parameters Monitor for hypersensitivity reactions and fluid retention

Patient Information This medication can only be administered I.V. During therapy, do not use alcohol, aspirin-containing products, and/or OTC medications without consulting prescriber. It is important to maintain adequate nutrition and hydration (2-3 L/day of fluids unless instructed to restrict fluid intake) during therapy; frequent small meals may help. You may experience nausea or vomiting (frequent small meals, frequent mouth care, sucking lozenges, or chewing gum may help); you may experience loss of hair (reversible); you will be more susceptible to infection (avoid crowds and exposure to infection as much as possible). Urine may turn red-brown (normal). Yogurt or buttermilk may help reduce diarrhea (if unresolved, contact prescriber for medication relief). Report swelling of extremities, difficulty breathing, unusual weight gain, abdominal distention, fever, chills, unusual bruising or bleeding, signs of infection, excessive fatigue, or unresolved diarrhea. Contraceptive measures are recommended during therapy.

Dosage Forms Injection: 20 mg/0.5 mL (0.5 mL); 80 mg/2 mL (2 mL)

Docosanol *(doe KOE san ole)*
U.S. Brand Names Abreva™ [OTC]
Synonyms Behenyl Alcohol; *n*-Docosanol
Therapeutic Category Antiviral Agent, Nonantiretroviral; Antiviral Agent, Topical
Use Treatment of herpes simplex of the face or lips
Contraindications Hypersensitivity to docosanol or any component of the formulation
Warnings/Precautions For external use only. Do not apply to inside of mouth or around eyes. Not for use in children <12 years of age.
Adverse Reactions Limited information; headache reported (frequency similar to placebo)
Stability Store at 20°C to 25°C (68°F to 77°F); do not freeze.
Mechanism of Action Prevents viral entry and replication at the cellular level
Usual Dosage Children ≥12 years and Adults: Topical: Apply 5 times/day to affected area of face or lips. Start at first sign of cold sore or fever blister and continue until healed.
Patient Information Wash hands before and after applying cream. Begin treatment at first tingle of cold sore or fever blister. Rub into area gently, but completely. Do not apply directly to inside of mouth or around eyes. Contact prescriber if sore gets worse or does not heal within 10 days. Do not share this product with others, may spread infection. Notify healthcare professional if pregnant or breast-feeding.
Dosage Forms Cream, topical: 10% (2 g)

Docusate *(DOK yoo sate)*
Related Information
Laxatives, Classification and Properties *on page 1504*
U.S. Brand Names Colace® [OTC]; DC 240® Softgels® [OTC]; Diocto® [OTC]; DOS® Softgel® [OTC]; D-S-S® [OTC]; Ex-Lax® Stool Softener [OTC]; Modane® Soft [OTC]; Regulax SS® [OTC]; Surfak® [OTC]
Canadian Brand Names Albert® Docusate; Colace®; Colax-C®; PMS-Docusate Calcium; PMS-Docusate Sodium; Regulex®; Selax®; Soflax™
Synonyms Dioctyl Calcium Sulfosuccinate; Dioctyl Sodium Sulfosuccinate; Docusate Calcium; Docusate Potassium; Docusate Sodium; DOSS; DSS
Therapeutic Category Laxative, Surfactant; Stool Softener
Use Stool softener in patients who should avoid straining during defecation and constipation associated with hard, dry stools; prophylaxis for straining (Valsalva) following myocardial infarction. A safe agent to be used in elderly; some evidence that doses <200 mg are ineffective; stool softeners are unnecessary if stool is well hydrated or "mushy" and soft; shown to be ineffective used long-term.
Unlabeled/Investigational Use Ceruminolytic
Pregnancy Risk Factor C
Contraindications Hypersensitivity to docusate or any component of the formulation; concomitant use of mineral oil; intestinal obstruction, acute abdominal pain, nausea, or vomiting
Warnings/Precautions Prolonged, frequent or excessive use may result in dependence or electrolyte imbalance

Adverse Reactions 1% to 10%:
Gastrointestinal: Intestinal obstruction, diarrhea, abdominal cramping
Miscellaneous: Throat irritation

Overdosage/Toxicology Symptoms include abdominal cramps, diarrhea, fluid loss, and hypokalemia. Treatment is symptomatic.

Drug Interactions
Increased Effect/Toxicity: Increased toxicity with mineral oil, phenolphthalein.
Decreased Effect: Decreased effect of warfarin with high doses of docusate.

Mechanism of Action Reduces surface tension of the oil-water interface of the stool resulting in enhanced incorporation of water and fat allowing for stool softening

Pharmacodynamics/Kinetics Onset of action: 12-72 hours

Usual Dosage Docusate salts are interchangeable; the amount of sodium or calcium per dosage unit is clinically insignificant

Infants and Children <3 years: Oral: 10-40 mg/day in 1-4 divided doses
Children: Oral:
3-6 years: 20-60 mg/day in 1-4 divided doses
6-12 years: 40-150 mg/day in 1-4 divided doses
Adolescents and Adults: Oral: 50-500 mg/day in 1-4 divided doses
Older Children and Adults: Rectal: Add 50-100 mL of docusate liquid to enema fluid (saline or water); administer as retention or flushing enema

Ceruminolytic (unlabeled use): Intra-aural: Administer 1 mL of docusate sodium in 2 mL syringes; if no clearance in 15 minutes, irrigate with 50-100 mL normal saline (this method is 80% effective)

Dietary Considerations Should be taken with a full glass of water, milk, or fruit juice.

Test Interactions ↓ potassium (S), ↓ chloride (S)

Patient Information Adults: Docusate should be taken with a full glass of water; do not use if abdominal pain, nausea, or vomiting are present; laxative use should be used for a short period of time (<1 week); prolonged use may result in abuse, dependence, as well as fluid and electrolyte loss; notify physician if bleeding occurs or if constipation is not relieved

Nursing Implications Docusate liquid should be given with milk, fruit juice, or infant formula to mask the bitter taste

Dosage Forms
Capsule, as calcium (Surfak® Liquigel): 240 mg
Capsule, as sodium:
Colace®: 50 mg, 100 mg
DOS® Softgel®: 100 mg, 250 mg
D-S-S®: 100 mg
Modane® Soft: 100 mg
Regulax SS®: 100 mg
Liquid, as sodium (Colace®, Diocto®): 150 mg/15 mL (480 mL)
Syrup, as sodium: 50 mg/15 mL (15 mL, 30 mL)
Colace®, Diocto®: 60 mg/15 mL (480 mL)
Tablet, as sodium (Ex-Lax® Stool Softener): 100 mg

♦ **Docusate Calcium** see Docusate on page 430
♦ **Docusate Potassium** see Docusate on page 430
♦ **Docusate Sodium** see Docusate on page 430

Dofetilide (doe FET il ide)

Related Information
Antiarrhythmic Drugs Comparison on page 1478

U.S. Brand Names Tikosyn™

Canadian Brand Names Tikosyn™

Therapeutic Category Antiarrhythmic Agent, Class III

Use Maintenance of normal sinus rhythm in patients with chronic atrial fibrillation/atrial flutter of longer than 1-week duration who have been converted to normal sinus rhythm; conversion of atrial fibrillation and atrial flutter to normal sinus rhythm

Pregnancy Risk Factor C

Pregnancy/Breast-Feeding Implications Dofetilide has been shown to adversely affect *in utero* growth, organogenesis, and survival of rats and mice. There are no adequate and well controlled studies in pregnant women. Dofetilide should be used with extreme caution in pregnant women and in women of childbearing age only when the benefit to the patient unequivocally justifies the potential risk to the fetus.

Contraindications Hypersensitivity to dofetilide or any component of the formulation; patients with paroxysmal atrial fibrillation; patients with congenital or acquired long QT syndromes; do not use if a baseline QT interval or QT_c is >440 msec (500 msec in patients with ventricular conduction abnormalities); severe renal impairment (estimated Cl_{cr} <20 mL/minute); concurrent use with verapamil, cimetidine, trimethoprim (alone or in combination with sulfamethoxazole), ketoconazole, prochlorperazine, or megestrol; baseline heart rate <50 beats/minute; other drugs that prolong QT intervals (phenothiazines, cisapride, bepridil, tricyclic antidepressants, certain oral macrolides: sparfloxacin, gatifloxacin, moxifloxacin); hypokalemia or hypomagnesemia; concurrent amiodarone

Warnings/Precautions Note: Must be initiated (or reinitiated) in a setting with continuous monitoring and staff familiar with the recognition and treatment of life-threatening arrhythmias. Patients must be monitored with continuous EKG for a minimum of 3 days, or for a minimum of 12 hours after electrical or pharmacological cardioversion to normal sinus rhythm, whichever is greater. Patients should be readmitted for continuous monitoring if dosage is later increased.

Reserve for patients who are highly symptomatic with atrial fibrillation/atrial flutter; torsade de pointes significantly increases with doses >500 mcg twice daily; hold Class Ia or Class II antiarrhythmics for at least three half-lives prior to starting dofetilide; use in patients on amiodarone therapy only if serum amiodarone level is <0.3 mg/L or if amiodarone was (Continued)

Dofetilide *(Continued)*

stopped for >3 months previously; correct hypokalemia or hypomagnesemia before initiating dofetilide and maintain within normal limits during treatment.

Patients with sick sinus syndrome or with second or third-degree heart block should not receive dofetilide unless a functional pacemaker is in place. Defibrillation threshold is reduced in patients with ventricular tachycardia or ventricular fibrillation undergoing implantation of a cardioverter-defibrillator device. Safety and efficacy in children (<18 years old) have not been established. Use with caution in renal impairment; not recommended in patients receiving drugs which may compete for renal secretion via cationic transport. Use with caution in patients with severe hepatic impairment.

Adverse Reactions

Supraventricular arrhythmia patients (incidence > placebo)

>10%: Central nervous system: Headache (11%)

2% to 10%:

Central nervous system: Dizziness (8%), insomnia (4%)

Cardiovascular: Ventricular tachycardia (2.6% to 3.7%), chest pain (10%), torsade de pointes (3.3% in CHF patients and 0.9% in patients with a recent MI; up to 10.5% in patients receiving doses in excess of those recommended). Torsade de pointes occurs most frequently within the first 3 days of therapy.

Dermatologic: Rash (3%)

Gastrointestinal: Nausea (5%), diarrhea (3%), abdominal pain (3%)

Neuromuscular & skeletal: Back pain (3%)

Respiratory: Dyspnea (6%), respiratory tract infection (7%)

Miscellaneous: Flu syndrome (4%)

<2% (Limited to important or life-threatening): Angioedema, AV block (0.4% to 1.5%), bundle branch block, cardiac arrest, facial paralysis, flaccid paralysis, heart block, hepatotoxicity, myocardial infarction, paralysis, paresthesia, stroke, syncope, ventricular fibrillation (0% to 0.4%)

Overdosage/Toxicology The major dose-related toxicity is torsade de pointes. Treatment should be symptomatic and supportive. Watch for excessive prolongation of the QT interval in overdose situations. Continuous cardiac monitoring is necessary. A charcoal slurry is helpful when given early (15 minutes) after the overdose. Isoproterenol infusion into anesthetized dogs with cardiac pacing has been shown to correct atrial and ventricular effective refractory periods caused by dofetilide. General treatment measures, override pacing, and magnesium therapy appear to be effective in the management of dofetilide-induced torsade de pointes.

Drug Interactions

Cytochrome P450 Effect: CYP3A3/4 enzyme substrate (minor)

Increased Effect/Toxicity: Dofetilide concentrations are increased by cimetidine, verapamil, ketoconazole, and trimethoprim (concurrent use of these agents is contraindicated). Dofetilide levels may also be increased by renal cationic transport inhibitors (including triamterene, metformin, amiloride, and megestrol) or inhibitors of cytochrome P450 isoenzyme 3A3/4 (including amiodarone, azole antifungal agents, clarithromycin, cannabinoids, diltiazem, erythromycin, nefazodone, norfloxacin, protease inhibitors, quinidine, serotonin reuptake inhibitors. verapamil, and zafirlukast). Diuretics and other drugs which may deplete potassium and/or magnesium (aminoglycoside antibiotics, amphotericin, cyclosporine) may increase dofetilide's toxicity (torsade de pointes).

Ethanol/Nutrition/Herb Interactions Herb/Nutraceutical: St John's wort may decrease dofetilide levels. Avoid ephedra (may worsen arrhythmia).

Mechanism of Action Vaughan Williams Class III antiarrhythmic activity. Blockade of the cardiac ion channel carrying the rapid component of the delayed rectifier potassium current. Dofetilide has no effect on sodium channels, adrenergic alpha-receptors, or adrenergic beta-receptors. It increases the monophasic action potential duration due to delayed repolarization. The increase in the QT interval is a function of prolongation of both effective and functional refractory periods in the His-Purkinje system and the ventricles. Changes in cardiac conduction velocity and sinus node function have not been observed in patients with or without structural heart disease. PR and QRS width remain the same in patients with pre-existing heart block and or sick sinus syndrome.

Pharmacodynamics/Kinetics

Absorption: >90%

Distribution: V_d: 3 L/kg

Protein binding: 60% to 70%

Metabolism: Hepatically by CYP3A3/4, but low affinity for it; metabolites formed by N-dealkylation and N-oxidation

Bioavailability: >90%

Half-life elimination: 10 hours

Time to peak: Fasting: 2-3 hours

Excretion: Urine (80%, 80% as unchanged drug and 20% as inactive or minimally active metabolites); renal elimination consists of glomerular filtration and active tubular secretion via cationic transport system

Usual Dosage Adults: Oral:

Note: QT or QT_c must be determined prior to first dose. If QT_c >440 msec (>500 msec in patients with ventricular conduction abnormalities), dofetilide is contraindicated (see Contraindications and Warnings/Precautions).

Initial: 500 mcg orally twice daily. Initial dosage must be adjusted in patients with estimated Cl_{cr} <60 mL/minute (see Dosage Adjustment in Renal Impairment). Dofetilide may be initiated at lower doses than recommended based on physician discretion.

Modification of dosage in response to initial dose:

QT_c interval should be measured 2-3 hours after the initial dose. If the QT_c >15% of baseline, or if the QT_c is >500 msec (550 msec in patients with ventricular conduction abnormalities) dofetilide should be adjusted. If the starting dose is 500 mcg twice daily, then adjust to 250 mcg twice daily. If the starting dose was 250 mcg twice daily, then adjust to 125 mcg twice daily. If the starting dose was 125 mcg twice daily then adjust to 125 mcg every day.

Continued monitoring for doses 2-5:
QT$_c$ interval must be determined 2-3 hours after each subsequent dose of dofetilide for in-hospital doses 2-5. If the measured QT$_c$ is >500 msec (550 msec in patients with ventricular conduction abnormalities) at any time, dofetilide should be discontinued.
Chronic therapy (following the 5th dose):
QT or QT$_c$ and creatinine clearance should be evaluated every 3 months. If QT$_c$ >500 msec (>550 msec in patients with ventricular conduction abnormalities), dofetilide should be discontinued.

Dosage adjustment in renal impairment:
Cl$_{cr}$ >60 mL/minute: Administer 500 mcg twice daily.
Cl$_{cr}$ 40-60 mL/minute: Administer 250 mcg twice daily.
Cl$_{cr}$ 20-39 mL/minute: Administer 125 mcg twice daily.
Cl$_{cr}$ <20 mL/minute: Contraindicated in this group.

Dosage adjustment in hepatic impairment: No dosage adjustments required in Child-Pugh Class A and B. Patients with severe hepatic impairment were not studied.

Elderly: No specific dosage adjustments are recommended based on age, however careful assessment of renal function is particularly important in this population.

Monitoring Parameters EKG monitoring with attention to QT$_c$ and occurrence of ventricular arrhythmias, baseline serum creatinine and changes in serum creatinine. Check serum potassium and magnesium levels if on medications where these electrolyte disturbances can occur, or if patient has a history of hypokalemia or hypomagnesemia. QT or QT$_c$ must be monitored at specific times prior to the first dose and during the first 3 days of therapy. Thereafter, QT or QT$_c$ and creatinine clearance must be evaluated at 3-month intervals.

Patient Information Take with or without food; take exactly the way it was prescribed; do not stop this medicine without talking with your physician; never take an extra dose; if you miss a dose just take your normal amount at the next scheduled time. If you take more medicine than you should call your physician now. If you cannot reach your physician, go to the nearest emergency room (take your medicine with you). Tell your physician about any new medicines before taking them; not all medicines mix well with this one. Call your physician now if you faint, become dizzy, have fast heartbeats, severe diarrhea, unusual sweating, vomiting, no appetite, or more thirst than normal. You may feel tired, weak, or have numbness, tingling, muscle cramps, constipation, vomiting, or rapid heartbeats if you have a low potassium level.

Nursing Implications Patient must be carefully instructed concerning how to take this medicine, what to do if a dose is missed, which over-the-counter medications to avoid (eg, cimetidine), and the recognition of serious adverse events. Patients should be cautioned not to stop taking this medication without talking with their prescriber. Measure QT$_c$ as outlined in dosing information and discuss results with physician, monitor EKG for any tachyarrhythmias, and monitor for changes in renal function and signs/symptoms of electrolyte imbalance. A patient resource kit is available.

Dosage Forms Capsule: 125 mcg, 250 mcg, 500 mcg

♦ **Dolacet®** see Hydrocodone and Acetaminophen on page 676

Dolasetron (dol A se tron)

U.S. Brand Names Anzemet®
Canadian Brand Names Anzemet™
Synonyms Dolasetron Mesylate
Therapeutic Category Antiemetic, Serotonin Antagonist; 5-HT$_3$ Receptor Antagonist; Serotonin Antagonist
Use Prevention of nausea and vomiting associated with emetogenic cancer chemotherapy, including initial and repeat courses; prevention of postoperative nausea and vomiting and treatment of postoperative nausea and vomiting (injectable form only)
Pregnancy Risk Factor B
Contraindications Hypersensitivity to dolasetron or any component of the formulation
Warnings/Precautions Dolasetron should be administered with caution in patients who have or may develop prolongation of cardiac conduction intervals, particularly QT$_c$ intervals. These include patients with hypokalemia or hypomagnesemia, patients taking diuretics with potential for inducing electrolyte abnormalities, patients with congenital QT syndrome, patients taking antiarrhythmic drugs or other drugs which lead to QT prolongation, and cumulative high-dose anthracycline therapy.
Adverse Reactions Dolasetron may cause EKG changes which are directly related to the concentration of hydrodolasetron, its active metabolite. Other adverse effects include:

Cancer patients:
>10%
Central nervous system: Headache (24%)
Gastrointestinal: Diarrhea (15%)
1% to 10% (occurring >2% and > placebo):
Central nervous system: Fever (4.3%), fatigue (3.6%), pain (2.4%), dizziness (2.2%), chills (2.0%)
Gastrointestinal: Increased transaminase levels (3.6%), abdominal pain (3.2%)
Cardiovascular: Hypertension (2.9%)
Postoperative patients:
1% to 10% (occurring >2% and > placebo):
Central nervous system: Headache (9.4%), dizziness (5.5%), drowsiness (2.4%), pain (2.4%)
Genitourinary: Urinary retention (2.4%)
<1% (Limited to important or life-threatening):
Patients in clinical trials involving either cancer patients or surgery: Anaphylaxis, arrhythmias, bronchospasm, hypotension

Overdosage/Toxicology In animal toxicity studies, doses 6.3-12.6 times the recommended human dose (based upon surface area) were lethal. Symptoms of acute poisoning included tremors, depression, and convulsions. There is no known specific antidote for dolasetron. Patients with suspected overdose should be managed with supportive therapy.
(Continued)

433

Dolasetron *(Continued)*

Drug Interactions

Cytochrome P450 Effect: CYP2D6 and 3A3/4 enzyme substrate

Increased Effect/Toxicity: Increased blood levels of active metabolite may occur during concurrent administration of cimetidine and atenolol. Inhibitors of this isoenzyme may increase blood levels of active metabolite. Due to the potential to potentiate QT_c prolongation, drugs which may prolong QT interval directly (eg, antiarrhythmics) or by causing alterations in electrolytes (eg, diuretics) should be used with caution.

Decreased Effect: Blood levels of active metabolite are decreased during coadministration of rifampin.

Ethanol/Nutrition/Herb Interactions Herb/Nutraceutical: St John's wort may decrease dolasetron levels.

Stability After dilution, I.V. dolasetron is stable under normal lighting conditions at room temperature for 24 hours or under refrigeration for 48 hours with the following **compatible** intravenous fluids: 0.9% sodium chloride injection, 5% dextrose injection, 5% dextrose and 0.45% sodium chloride injection, 5% dextrose and lactated Ringer's injection, lactated Ringer's injection, and 10% mannitol injection

Mechanism of Action Selective serotonin receptor (5-HT$_3$) antagonist, blocking serotonin both peripherally (primary site of action) and centrally at the chemoreceptor trigger zone

Pharmacodynamics/Kinetics

Metabolism: Hepatic to a reduced alcohol (active metabolite MDL 74,156)

Half-life elimination: Dolasetron: 10 minutes; MDL 74,156: 8 hours

Usual Dosage

Children <2 years: Not recommended for use

Nausea and vomiting associated with chemotherapy (including initial and repeat courses):

Children 2-16 years:

Oral: 1.8 mg/kg within 1 hour before chemotherapy; maximum: 100 mg/dose

I.V.: 1.8 mg/kg ~30 minutes before chemotherapy; maximum: 100 mg/dose

Adults:

Oral: 200 mg single dose

I.V.:

0.6-5 mg/kg as a single dose

50 mg 1-2 minute bolus

2.4-3 mg/kg 20-minute infusion

Prevention of postoperative nausea and vomiting:

Children 2-16 years:

Oral: 1.2 mg/kg within 2 hours before surgery; maximum: 100 mg/dose

I.V.: 0.35 mg/kg (maximum: 12.5 mg) ~15 minutes before stopping anesthesia

Adults:

Oral: 100 mg within 2 hours before surgery

I.V.: 12.5 mg ~15 minutes before stopping anesthesia

Treatment of postoperative nausea and vomiting: I.V. (only):

Children: 0.35 mg/kg (maximum: 12.5 mg) as soon as needed

Adults: 12.5 mg as soon as needed

Dosing adjustment for elderly, renal/hepatic impairment: No dosage adjustment is recommended

Administration I.V. injection may be given either undiluted IVP over 30 seconds or diluted to 50 mL and infused as an IVPB over 15 minutes. Dolasetron injection may be diluted in apple or apple-grape juice and taken orally (**Note:** Timing and doses are different with oral and I.V. routes of administration)

Monitoring Parameters Liver function tests, blood pressure and pulse, and EKG in patients with cardiovascular disease

Nursing Implications Dolasetron injection may be diluted in apple or apple-grape juice and taken orally

Additional Information Efficacy of dolasetron, for chemotherapy treatment, is enhanced with concomitant administration of dexamethasone 20 mg (increases complete response from 50% to 76%). Oral administration of the intravenous solution is equivalent to tablets. A single I.V. dose of dolasetron mesylate (1.8 or 2.4 mg/kg) has comparable safety and efficacy to a single 32 mg I.V. dose of ondansetron in patients receiving cisplatin chemotherapy.

Dosage Forms

Injection, as mesylate: 20 mg/mL (0.625 mL, 5 mL)

Tablet, as mesylate: 50 mg, 100 mg

- **Dolasetron Mesylate** *see Dolasetron on page 433*
- **Dolobid®** *see Diflunisal on page 401*
- **Dolophine®** *see Methadone on page 877*
- **Domeboro® [OTC]** *see Aluminum Sulfate and Calcium Acetate on page 64*
- **Dome Paste Bandage** *see Zinc Gelatin on page 1438*

Donepezil *(doh NEP e zil)*

U.S. Brand Names Aricept®

Canadian Brand Names Aricept®

Synonyms E2020

Therapeutic Category Acetylcholinesterase Inhibitor; Cholinergic Agent

Use Treatment of mild to moderate dementia of the Alzheimer's type

Unlabeled/Investigational Use Attention-deficit/hyperactivity disorder (ADHD)

Pregnancy Risk Factor C

Contraindications Hypersensitivity to donepezil, piperidine derivatives, or any component of the formulation

Warnings/Precautions Cholinesterase inhibitors may have vagotonic effects. May cause bradycardia and/or heart block; syncopal episodes have been associated with donepezil. Use with caution in patients with sick sinus syndrome or other supraventricular cardiac conduction abnormalities, in patients with seizures, COPD, or asthma; avoid use in nursing mothers. Use with caution in patients at risk of ulcer disease (ie, previous history or NSAID use), or in patients with bladder outlet obstruction. May cause diarrhea, nausea, and/or vomiting, which may be dose-related.

Adverse Reactions

>10%:

Central nervous system: Headache

Gastrointestinal: Nausea, diarrhea

1% to 10%:

Cardiovascular: Syncope, chest pain, hypertension, atrial fibrillation, hypotension, hot flashes

Central nervous system: Fatigue, insomnia, dizziness, depression, abnormal dreams, somnolence

Dermatologic: Bruising

Gastrointestinal: Anorexia, vomiting, weight loss, fecal incontinence, GI bleeding, bloating, epigastric pain

Genitourinary: Frequent urination

Neuromuscular & skeletal: Muscle cramps, arthritis, body pain

<1% (Limited to significant or life-threatening): Cholecystitis, congestive heart failure, delusions, dysarthria, dysphasia, dyspnea, eosinophilia, hallucinations, heart block, hemolytic anemia, hyponatremia, intracranial hemorrhage, neuroleptic malignant syndrome, pancreatitis, paresthesia, rash, seizures, thrombocytopenia

Overdosage/Toxicology Donepezil can cause cholinergic crisis characterized by severe nausea, vomiting, salivation, sweating, bradycardia, hypotension, cardiovascular collapse, and convulsions. Increased muscle weakness is a possibility and may result in death if respiratory muscles are involved.

Tertiary anticholinergics, such as atropine, may be used as an antidote. I.V. atropine sulfate titrated to effect is recommended, with an initial dose of 1-2 mg I.V., and with subsequent doses based on clinical response. Atypical blood pressure and heart rate increases have been reported with other cholinomimetics when coadministered with quaternary anticholinergics (eg, glycopyrrolate). Implement general supportive measures.

Drug Interactions

Cytochrome P450 Effect: CYP2D6 and 3A3/4 enzyme substrate

Increased Effect/Toxicity: Ketoconazole and quinidine inhibit donepezil's metabolism *in vitro* and may increase toxicity. A synergistic effect may be seen with concurrent administration of succinylcholine or cholinergic agonists (bethanechol).

Decreased Effect: Donepezil levels may be decreased by enzyme inducers (phenytoin, carbamazepine, dexamethasone, rifampin, and phenobarbital). Anticholinergic agents (benztropine) may inhibit the effects of donepezil.

Ethanol/Nutrition/Herb Interactions Herb/Nutraceutical: St John's wort may decrease donepezil levels.

Mechanism of Action Alzheimer's disease is characterized by cholinergic deficiency in the cortex and basal forebrain, which contributes to cognitive deficits. Donepezil reversibly and noncompetitively inhibits centrally-active acetylcholinesterase, the enzyme responsible for hydrolysis of acetylcholine. This appears to result in increased concentrations of acetylcholine available for synaptic transmission in the central nervous system.

Pharmacodynamics/Kinetics

Duration: May be prolonged, particularly in elderly

Absorption: Well absorbed

Half-life elimination: 70 hours

Time to peak, plasma: 3-4 hours

Usual Dosage Oral:

Children: ADHD (unlabeled use): 5 mg/day

Adults: Dementia of Alzheimer's type: Initial: 5 mg/day at bedtime; may increase to 10 mg/day at bedtime after 4-6 weeks

Monitoring Parameters Behavior, mood, bowel function

Additional Information Donepezil does not significantly elevate liver enzymes.

Dosage Forms Tablet: 5 mg, 10 mg

♦ **Donnatal®** *see* Hyoscyamine, Atropine, Scopolamine, and Phenobarbital *on page 694*

DOPamine (DOE pa meen)

Related Information

Adrenergic Agonists, Cardiovascular Comparison *on page 1469*

Adult ACLS Algorithms *on page 1632*

Antacid Drug Interactions *on page 1477*

U.S. Brand Names Intropin®

Canadian Brand Names Intropin®

Synonyms Dopamine Hydrochloride

Therapeutic Category Adrenergic Agonist Agent; Sympathomimetic; Vesicant

Use Adjunct in the treatment of shock (eg, MI, open heart surgery, renal failure, cardiac decompensation, etc) which persists after adequate fluid volume replacement

Unlabeled/Investigational Use Symptomatic bradycardia or heart block unresponsive to atropine or pacing

Pregnancy Risk Factor C

Contraindications Hypersensitivity to sulfites (commercial preparation contains sodium bisulfite); pheochromocytoma; ventricular fibrillation

Warnings/Precautions Use with caution in patients with cardiovascular disease or cardiac arrhythmias or patients with occlusive vascular disease. Correct hypovolemia and electrolytes when used in hemodynamic support. May cause increases in HR and arrhythmia. Avoid infiltration - may cause severe tissue necrosis. Use with caution in post-MI patients.

Adverse Reactions Frequency not defined.

Most frequent:

Cardiovascular: Ectopic beats, tachycardia, anginal pain, palpitations, hypotension, vasoconstriction

(Continued)

DOPamine (Continued)

Central nervous system: Headache
Gastrointestinal: Nausea and vomiting
Respiratory: Dyspnea

Infrequent:

Cardiovascular: Aberrant conduction, bradycardia, widened QRS complex, ventricular arrhythmias (high dose), gangrene (high dose), hypertension

Central nervous system: Anxiety

Endocrine & metabolic: Piloerection, serum glucose increased (usually not above normal limits)

Local: Extravasation of dopamine can cause tissue necrosis and sloughing of surrounding tissues

Ocular: Intraocular pressure increased, dilated pupils

Renal: Azotemia, polyuria

Overdosage/Toxicology Symptoms include severe hypertension, cardiac arrhythmias, and acute renal failure. **Important:** Antidote for peripheral ischemia: To prevent sloughing and necrosis in ischemic areas, the area should be infiltrated as soon as possible with 10-15 mL of saline solution containing 5-10 mg of Regitine® (brand of phentolamine), an adrenergic blocking agent. A syringe with a fine hypodermic needle should be used, and the solution liberally infiltrated throughout the ischemic area. Sympathetic blockade with phentolamine causes immediate and conspicuous local hyperemic changes if the area is infiltrated within 12 hours. Therefore, phentolamine should be given as soon as possible after the extravasation is noted.

Drug Interactions

Increased Effect/Toxicity: Dopamine's effects are prolonged and intensified by MAO inhibitors, alpha- and beta-adrenergic blockers, cocaine, general anesthetics, methyldopa, phenytoin, reserpine, and TCAs.

Decreased Effect: Tricyclic antidepressants may have a decreased effect when coadministered with dopamine. Guanethidine's hypotensive effects may only be partially reversed; may need to use a direct-acting sympathomimetic.

Stability Protect from light; solutions that are darker than slightly yellow should not be used; **incompatible** with alkaline solutions or iron salts; **compatible** when coadministered with dobutamine, epinephrine, isoproterenol, and lidocaine

Mechanism of Action Stimulates both adrenergic and dopaminergic receptors, lower doses are mainly dopaminergic stimulating and produce renal and mesenteric vasodilation, higher doses also are both dopaminergic and beta$_1$-adrenergic stimulating and produce cardiac stimulation and renal vasodilation; large doses stimulate alpha-adrenergic receptors

Pharmacodynamics/Kinetics

Children: Dopamine has exhibited nonlinear kinetics in children; with medication changes, may not achieve steady-state for ~1 hour rather than 20 minutes

Onset of action: Adults: 5 minutes

Duration: Adults: <10 minutes

Metabolism: Renal, hepatic, plasma; 75% to inactive metabolites by monoamine oxidase and 25% to norepinephrine

Half-life elimination: 2 minutes

Excretion: Urine (as metabolites)

Clearance: Neonates: Varies and appears to be age related; clearance is more prolonged with combined hepatic and renal dysfunction

Usual Dosage I.V. infusion (administration requires the use of an infusion pump):

Neonates: 1-20 mcg/kg/minute continuous infusion, titrate to desired response.

Children: 1-20 mcg/kg/minute, maximum: 50 mcg/kg/minute continuous infusion, titrate to desired response.

Adults: 1-5 mcg/kg/minute up to 20 mcg/kg/minute, titrate to desired response. Infusion may be increased by 1-4 mcg/kg/minute at 10- to 30-minute intervals until optimal response is obtained.

If dosages >20-30 mcg/kg/minute are needed, a more direct-acting pressor may be more beneficial (ie, epinephrine, norepinephrine).

The hemodynamic effects of dopamine are dose-dependent:

Low-dose: 1-3 mcg/kg/minute, increased renal blood flow and urine output

Intermediate-dose: 3-10 mcg/kg/minute, increased renal blood flow, heart rate, cardiac contractility, and cardiac output

High-dose: >10 mcg/kg/minute, alpha-adrenergic effects begin to predominate, vasoconstriction, increased blood pressure

Administration Administer into large vein to prevent the possibility of extravasation (central line administration); monitor continuously for free flow; use infusion device to control rate of flow; administration into an umbilical arterial catheter is not recommended; when discontinuing the infusion, gradually decrease the dose of dopamine (sudden discontinuation may cause hypotension).

To prepare for infusion:

$$\frac{6 \times \text{weight (kg)} \times \text{desired dose (mcg/kg/min)}}{\text{I.V. infusion rate (mL/h)}} = \begin{array}{l} \text{mg of drug to be added to} \\ \text{100 mL of I.V. fluid} \end{array}$$

Monitoring Parameters Blood pressure, EKG, heart rate, CVP, RAP, MAP, urine output; if pulmonary artery catheter is in place, monitor CI, PCWP, SVR, and PVR

Nursing Implications Extravasation: Due to short half-life, withdrawal of drug is often only necessary treatment. Use phentolamine as antidote; mix 5 mg with 9 mL of NS; inject a small amount of this dilution into extravasated area; blanching should reverse immediately. Monitor site; if blanching should recur, additional injections of phentolamine may be needed.

Additional Information Dopamine is most frequently used for treatment of hypotension because of its peripheral vasoconstrictor action. In this regard, dopamine is often used together with dobutamine and minimizes hypotension secondary to dobutamine-induced vasodilation. Thus, pressure is maintained by increased cardiac output (from dobutamine) and vasoconstriction (by dopamine). It is critical neither dopamine nor dobutamine be used in patients in the absence of correcting any hypovolemia as a cause of hypotension.

Low-dose dopamine is often used in the intensive care setting for presumed beneficial effects on renal function. However, there is no clear evidence that low-dose dopamine confers any renal or other benefit. Indeed, dopamine may act on dopamine receptors in the carotid bodies causing chemoreflex suppression. In patients with heart failure, dopamine may inhibit breathing and cause pulmonary shunting. Both these mechanisms would act to decrease minute ventilation and oxygen saturation. This could potentially be deleterious in patients with respiratory compromise and patients being weaned from ventilators.

Dosage Forms
Infusion, as hydrochloride [in D$_5$W]: 0.8 mg/mL (250 mL, 500 mL); 1.6 mg/mL (250 mL, 500 mL); 3.2 mg/mL (250 mL, 500 mL)
Injection, as hydrochloride: 40 mg/mL (5 mL, 10 mL, 20 mL); 80 mg/mL (5 mL, 20 mL); 160 mg/mL (5 mL)

♦ **Dopamine Hydrochloride** see DOPamine on page 435
♦ **Dopar**® see Levodopa on page 790
♦ **Dopram**® see Doxapram on page 439
♦ **Doral**® see Quazepam on page 1164
♦ **Dormin**® [OTC] see DiphenhydrAMINE on page 414

Dornase Alfa (DOOR nase AL fa)
U.S. Brand Names Pulmozyme®
Canadian Brand Names Pulmozyme™
Synonyms DNase; Recombinant Human Deoxyribonuclease
Therapeutic Category Enzyme
Use Management of cystic fibrosis patients to reduce the frequency of respiratory infections that require parenteral antibiotics, and to improve pulmonary function
Unlabeled/Investigational Use Treatment of chronic bronchitis
Pregnancy Risk Factor B
Contraindications Hypersensitivity to dornase alfa, Chinese hamster ovary cell products (eg, epoetin alfa), or any component of the formulation
Warnings/Precautions No clinical trials have been conducted to demonstrate safety and effectiveness of dornase in children <5 years of age, in patients with pulmonary function <40% of normal, or in patients for longer treatment periods >12 months; no data exists regarding safety during lactation
Adverse Reactions
>10%:
Cardiovascular: Chest pain
Respiratory: Pharyngitis
Miscellaneous: Voice alteration
1% to 10%:
Dermatologic: Rash
Ocular: Conjunctivitis
Respiratory: Laryngitis, cough, dyspnea, hemoptysis, rhinitis, hoarse throat, wheezing
Stability Must be stored in the refrigerator at 2°C to 8°C (36°F to 46°F) and protected from strong light; should not be exposed to room temperature for a total of 24 hours
Mechanism of Action The hallmark of cystic fibrosis lung disease is the presence of abundant, purulent airway secretions composed primarily of highly polymerized DNA. The principal source of this DNA is the nuclei of degenerating neutrophils, which is present in large concentrations in infected lung secretions. The presence of this DNA produces a viscous mucous that may contribute to the decreased mucociliary transport and persistent infections that are commonly seen in this population. Dornase alfa is a deoxyribonuclease (DNA) enzyme produced by recombinant gene technology. Dornase selectively cleaves DNA, thus reducing mucous viscosity and as a result, airflow in the lung is improved and the risk of bacterial infection may be decreased.
Pharmacodynamics/Kinetics
Onset of action: Nebulization: Enzyme levels are measured in sputum in ~15 minutes
Duration: Rapidly declines
Usual Dosage Inhalation:
Children >3 months to Adults: 2.5 mg once daily through selected nebulizers; experience in children <5 years is limited
Patients unable to inhale or exhale orally throughout the entire treatment period may use Pari-Baby™ nebulizer. Some patients may benefit from twice daily administration.
Administration Nebulization: Should not be diluted or mixed with any other drugs in the nebulizer, this may inactivate the drug
Nursing Implications Should not be diluted or mixed with any other drugs in the nebulizer, this may inactivate the drug
Dosage Forms Solution for nebulization: 1 mg/mL (2.5 mL)

♦ **Doryx**® see Doxycycline on page 448

Dorzolamide (dor ZOLE a mide)
Related Information
Glaucoma Drug Therapy Comparison on page 1499
U.S. Brand Names Trusopt®
Canadian Brand Names Trusopt®
Synonyms Dorzolamide Hydrochloride
Therapeutic Category Carbonic Anhydrase Inhibitor
Use Lowers intraocular pressure to treat glaucoma in patients with ocular hypertension or open-angle glaucoma
Pregnancy Risk Factor C
Usual Dosage Adults: Glaucoma: Instill 1 drop in the affected eye(s) 3 times/day
(Continued)

Dorzolamide *(Continued)*

Additional Information Complete prescribing information for this medication should be consulted for additional detail.

Dosage Forms Solution, ophthalmic, as hydrochloride: 2%

Dorzolamide and Timolol *(dor ZOLE a mide & TYE moe lole)*

U.S. Brand Names Cosopt®

Canadian Brand Names Cosopt®

Synonyms Timolol and Dorzolamide

Therapeutic Category Beta-Adrenergic Blocker; Carbonic Anhydrase Inhibitor

Use Lowers intraocular pressure to treat glaucoma in patients with ocular hypertension or open-angle glaucoma

Usual Dosage Adults: ophthalmic: One drop in eye(s) twice daily

Additional Information Complete prescribing information for this medication should be consulted for additional detail.

Dosage Forms Solution, ophthalmic: Dorzolamide 2% and timolol 0.5% (5 mL, 10 mL)

♦ **Dorzolamide Hydrochloride** *see* Dorzolamide *on page 437*

♦ **DOSS** *see* Docusate *on page 430*

♦ **DOS® Softgel® [OTC]** *see* Docusate *on page 430*

♦ **Dostinex®** *see* Cabergoline *on page 201*

♦ **Dovonex®** *see* Calcipotriene *on page 203*

Doxacurium *(doks a KYOO ri um)*

Related Information
Neuromuscular Blocking Agents Comparison *on page 1508*

U.S. Brand Names Nuromax®

Canadian Brand Names Nuromax™

Synonyms Doxacurium Chloride

Therapeutic Category Neuromuscular Blocker Agent, Nondepolarizing; Skeletal Muscle Relaxant

Use Adjunct to general anesthesia to facilitate endotracheal intubation and to relax skeletal muscles during surgery; to facilitate mechanical ventilation in ICU patients; does not relieve pain or produce sedation; the characteristics of this agent make it especially useful in procedures requiring careful maintenance of hemodynamic stability for prolonged periods

Pregnancy Risk Factor C

Contraindications Hypersensitivity to doxacurium or any component of the formulation

Warnings/Precautions Use with caution in the elderly, effects and duration are more variable; product contains benzyl alcohol, use with caution in newborns; use with caution in patients with renal or hepatic impairment; certain clinical conditions may result in potentiation or antagonism of neuromuscular blockade:

Potentiation: Electrolyte abnormalities, severe hyponatremia, severe hypocalcemia, severe hypokalemia, hypermagnesemia, neuromuscular diseases, acidosis, acute intermittent porphyria, renal failure, hepatic failure

Antagonism: Alkalosis, hypercalcemia, demyelinating lesions, peripheral neuropathies, diabetes mellitus

Increased sensitivity in patients with myasthenia gravis, Eaton-Lambert syndrome; resistance in burn patients (>30% of body) for period of 5-70 days postinjury; resistance in patients with muscle trauma, denervation, immobilization, infection; does not counteract bradycardia produced by anesthetics/vagal stimulation.

Adverse Reactions <1% (Limited to important or life-threatening): Diplopia, fever, hypotension, **produces little, if any, histamine release**, respiratory insufficiency and apnea, skeletal muscle weakness, urticaria, wheezing

In the ICU setting, reports of prolonged paralysis and generalized myopathy following discontinuation of agent (may be minimized by appropriately monitoring degree of blockade)

Overdosage/Toxicology Overdosage is manifested by prolonged neuromuscular blockage. Treatment is supportive. Reverse blockade with neostigmine, pyridostigmine, or edrophonium.

Drug Interactions

Increased Effect/Toxicity: Increased effects are possible with aminoglycosides, betablockers, clindamycin, calcium channel blockers, halogenated anesthetics, imipenem, ketamine, lidocaine, loop diuretics (furosemide), macrolides (case reports), magnesium sulfate, procainamide, quinidine, quinolones, tetracyclines, and vancomycin. May increase risk of myopathy when used with high- dose corticosteroids for extended periods.

Decreased Effect: Effect of nondepolarizing neuromuscular blockers may be reduced by carbamazepine (chronic use), corticosteroids (also associated with myopathy - see increased effect), phenytoin (chronic use), sympathomimetics, and theophylline.

Stability Stable for 24 hours at room temperature when diluted, up to 0.1 mg/mL in dextrose 5% or normal saline; compatible with sufentanil, alfentanil, and fentanyl

Mechanism of Action Prevents depolarization of muscle membrane and subsequent muscle contraction by acting as a competitive antagonist to acetylcholine at the alpha subunits of the nicotinic cholinergic receptors on the motor endplates in skeletal muscle, also interferes with the mobilization of acetylcholine presynaptically; the neuromuscular blockade can be pharmacologically reversed with an anticholinesterase agent (neostigmine, edrophonium, pyridostigmine)

Pharmacodynamics/Kinetics
Onset of action: 5-11 minutes
Duration: 30 minutes (range: 12-54 minutes)
Protein binding: 30%
Excretion: Primarily urine and feces (as unchanged drug); recovery time is longer in elderly

Usual Dosage Administer I.V.; dose to effect; doses will vary due to interpatient variability; use ideal body weight for obese patients

Surgery:
  Children >2 years: Initial: 0.03-0.05 mg/kg followed by maintenance doses of 0.005-0.01 mg/kg after 30-45 minutes
  Adults: 0.05-0.08 mg/kg with thiopental/narcotic or 0.025 mg/kg after initial dose of succinylcholine for intubation; initial maintenance dose of 0.005-0.01 mg/kg after 100-160 minutes followed by repeat doses every 30-45 minutes
Pretreatment/priming: 10% of intubating dose given 3-5 minutes before initial dose
ICU: 0.05 mg/kg bolus followed by 0.025 mg/kg every 2-3 hours or 0.25-0.75 mcg/kg/minute once initial recovery from bolus dose observed

Dosing adjustment in renal impairment: Reduce initial dose and titrate carefully as duration may be prolonged

Administration May be given rapid I.V. injection undiluted or via a continuous infusion using an infusion pump; use infusion solutions within 24 hours of preparation

Monitoring Parameters Blockade is monitored with a peripheral nerve stimulator, should also evaluate EKG, blood pressure, and heart rate

Nursing Implications Blockade is monitored with a peripheral nerve stimulator, should also evaluate EKG, blood pressure, and heart rate

Additional Information Doxacurium is a long-acting nondepolarizing neuromuscular blocker with virtually no cardiovascular side effects. Characteristics of this agent make it especially useful in procedures requiring careful maintenance of hemodynamic stability for prolonged periods; reduce dosage in renal or hepatic impairment. It does not relieve pain or produce sedation. It does not appear to have a cumulative effect on duration of blockade.

Dosage Forms Injection, as chloride: 1 mg/mL (5 mL)

♦ **Doxacurium Chloride** *see* Doxacurium *on page 438*

Doxapram (DOKS a pram)
U.S. Brand Names Dopram®
Canadian Brand Names Dopram®
Synonyms Doxapram Hydrochloride
Therapeutic Category Central Nervous System Stimulant, Nonamphetamine; Respiratory Stimulant
Use Respiratory and CNS stimulant for respiratory depression secondary to anesthesia, drug-induced CNS depression; acute hypercapnia secondary to COPD
Pregnancy Risk Factor B
Usual Dosage Contains a significant amount of benzyl alcohol (0.9%); I.V.: Adults:
Respiratory depression following anesthesia:
  Intermittent injection: Initial: 0.5-1 mg/kg; may repeat at 5-minute intervals (only in patients who demonstrate initial response); maximum total dose: 2 mg/kg
  I.V. infusion: Initial: 5 mg/minute until adequate response or adverse effects seen; decrease to 1-3 mg/minute; maximum total dose: 4 mg/kg
Drug-induced CNS depression:
  Intermittent injection: Initial: 1-2 mg/kg, repeat after 5 minutes; may repeat at 1-2 hour intervals (until sustained consciousness); maximum 3 g/day
  I.V. infusion: Initial: Bolus dose of 2 mg/kg, repeat after 5 minutes. If no response, wait 1-2 hours and repeat. If some stimulation is noted, initiate infusion at 1-3 mg/minute (depending on size of patient/depth of CNS depression); suspend infusion if patient begins to awaken. Infusion should not be continued for >2 hours. May reinstitute infusion as described above, including bolus, after rest interval of 30 minutes to 2 hours; maximum: 3 g/day
Acute hypercapnia secondary to COPD: I.V. infusion: Initial: Initiate infusion at 1-2 mg/minute (depending on size of patient/depth of CNS depression); may increase to maximum rate of 3 mg/minute; infusion should not be continued for >2 hours. Monitor arterial blood gases prior to initiation of infusion and at 30-minute intervals during the infusion (to identify possible development of acidosis/CO_2 retention). Additional infusions are not recommended (per manufacturer).
Hemodialysis: Not dialyzable

Additional Information Complete prescribing information for this medication should be consulted for additional detail.

Dosage Forms Injection, as hydrochloride: 20 mg/mL (20 mL)

♦ **Doxapram Hydrochloride** *see* Doxapram *on page 439*

Doxazosin (doks AY zoe sin)
U.S. Brand Names Cardura®
Canadian Brand Names Apo®-Doxazosin; Cardura-1™; Cardura-2™; Cardura-4™; Gen-Doxazosin; Novo-Doxazosin
Therapeutic Category Alpha-Adrenergic Blocking Agent, Oral; Antihypertensive Agent
Use Treatment of hypertension alone or in conjunction with diuretics, cardiac glycosides, ACE inhibitors, or calcium antagonists (particularly appropriate for those with hypertension and other cardiovascular risk factors such as hypercholesterolemia and diabetes mellitus); treatment of urinary outflow obstruction and/or obstructive and irritative symptoms associated with benign prostatic hyperplasia (BPH), particularly useful in patients with troublesome symptoms who are unable or unwilling to undergo invasive procedures, but who require rapid symptomatic relief
Pregnancy Risk Factor C
Contraindications Hypersensitivity to quinazolines (prazosin, terazosin), doxazosin, or any component of the formulation
Warnings/Precautions Use with caution in patients with renal impairment. Can cause marked hypotension and syncope with sudden loss of consciousness with the first dose. Prostate cancer should be ruled out before starting for BPH. Anticipate a similar effect if

(Continued)

Doxazosin (Continued)

therapy is interrupted for a few days, if dosage is increased rapidly, or if another antihypertensive drug is introduced.

Adverse Reactions

>10%: Central nervous system: Dizziness (16% to 19%), headache (10% to 14%)

1% to 10%:

Cardiovascular: Orthostatic hypotension (dose-related; 0.3% up to 10%), edema (3% to 4%), hypotension (2%), palpitation (1% to 2%), chest pain (1% to 2%), arrhythmia (1%), syncope (2%), flushing (1%)

Central nervous system: Fatigue (8% to 12%), somnolence (3% to 5%), nervousness (2%), pain (2%), vertigo (2%), insomnia (1%), anxiety (1%), paresthesia (1%), movement disorder (1%), ataxia (1%), hypertonia (1%), depression (1%), weakness (1%)

Dermatologic: Rash (1%), pruritus (1%)

Endocrine & metabolic: Sexual dysfunction (2%)

Gastrointestinal: Abdominal pain (2%), diarrhea (2%), dyspepsia (1% to 2%), nausea (2% to 3%), xerostomia (1% to 2%), constipation (1%), flatulence (1%)

Genitourinary: Urinary tract infection (1%), impotence (1%), polyuria (2%), incontinence (1%)

Neuromuscular & skeletal: Back pain (2%), arthritis (1%), muscle weakness (1%), myalgia (1%), muscle cramps (1%)

Ocular: Abnormal vision (1% to 2%), conjunctivitis (1%)

Otic: Tinnitus (1%)

Respiratory: Rhinitis (3%), dyspnea (1% to 3%), respiratory disorder (1%), epistaxis (1%)

Miscellaneous: Flu-like syndrome (1%), increased diaphoresis (1%)

<1% (Limited to important or life-threatening): Agitation, alopecia, amnesia, angina, bronchospasm, cataplexy, depersonalization, eczema, emotional lability, enuresis, fecal incontinence, fever, gout, hot flashes, impaired concentration, infection, leukopenia, myocardial infarction, paranoia, paresis, peripheral ischemia, photophobia, purpura, renal calculus, rigors, stroke, syncope, systemic lupus erythematosus, urticaria

Overdosage/Toxicology Symptoms include severe hypotension, drowsiness, and tachycardia. Hypotension usually responds to I.V. fluids, Trendelenburg positioning, or a parenteral vasoconstrictor. Treatment is primarily supportive and symptomatic.

Drug Interactions

Increased Effect/Toxicity: Increased hypotensive effect with beta-blockers, diuretics, ACE inhibitors, calcium channel blockers, and other antihypertensive medications.

Decreased Effect: Decreased hypotensive effect with NSAIDs.

Ethanol/Nutrition/Herb Interactions Herb/Nutraceutical: Avoid dong quai if using for hypertension (has estrogenic activity). Avoid ephedra, yohimbe, ginseng (may worsen hypertension). Avoid saw palmetto when used for BPH (due to limited experience with this combination). Avoid garlic (may have increased antihypertensive effect).

Mechanism of Action Competitively inhibits postsynaptic alpha-adrenergic receptors which results in vasodilation of veins and arterioles and a decrease in total peripheral resistance and blood pressure; approximately 50% as potent on a weight by weight basis as prazosin

Pharmacodynamics/Kinetics Not significantly affected by increased age

Duration: >24 hours

Half-life elimination: 22 hours

Time to peak, serum: 2-3 hours

Usual Dosage Oral:

Adults: 1 mg once daily in morning or evening; may be increased to 2 mg once daily. Thereafter titrate upwards, if needed, over several weeks, balancing therapeutic benefit with doxazosin-induced postural hypotension

Hypertension: Maximum dose: 16 mg/day

BPH: Maximum dose: 8 mg/day

Elderly: Initial: 0.5 mg once daily

Administration Syncope may occur usually within 90 minutes of the initial dose.

Monitoring Parameters Blood pressure, standing and sitting/supine

Test Interactions Increased urinary VMA 17%, norepinephrine metabolite 42%

Patient Information Rise from sitting/lying position carefully; may cause dizziness; report to physician if painful persistent erection occurs; take the first dose at bedtime

Nursing Implications Syncope may occur usually within 90 minutes of the initial dose

Additional Information First-dose hypotension occurs less frequently with doxazosin as compared to prazosin; this may be due to its slower onset of action.

Dosage Forms Tablet: 1 mg, 2 mg, 4 mg, 8 mg

Doxepin (DOKS e pin)

Related Information

Antidepressant Agents Comparison on page 1482

U.S. Brand Names Sinequan®; Zonalon® Cream

Canadian Brand Names Alti-Doxepin; Apo®-Doxepin; Novo-Doxepin; Sinequan™; Zonalon

Synonyms Doxepin Hydrochloride

Therapeutic Category Antianxiety Agent; Antidepressant, Tricyclic

Use

Oral: Depression

Topical: Short-term (<8 days) management of moderate pruritus in adults with atopic dermatitis or lichen simplex chronicus

Unlabeled/Investigational Use Analgesic for certain chronic and neuropathic pain; anxiety

Pregnancy Risk Factor C

Contraindications Hypersensitivity to doxepin, drugs from similar chemical class, or any component of the formulation; narrow-angle glaucoma; urinary retention; use of MAO inhibitors within 14 days; use in a patient during acute recovery phase of MI

Warnings/Precautions Often causes sedation, which may result in impaired performance of tasks requiring alertness (ie, operating machinery or driving). Sedative effects may be additive with other CNS depressants and/or ethanol. The degree of sedation is very high relative to other antidepressants. May worsen psychosis in some patients or precipitate a shift to mania or hypomania in patients with bipolar disease. May increase the risks associated with electroconvulsive therapy. This agent should be discontinued, when possible, prior to elective surgery. Therapy should not be abruptly discontinued in patients receiving high doses for prolonged periods.

May cause orthostatic hypotension (risk is moderate relative to other antidepressants) - use with caution in patients at risk of hypotension or in patients where transient hypotensive episodes would be poorly tolerated (cardiovascular disease or cerebrovascular disease). The degree of anticholinergic blockade produced by this agent is high relative to other cyclic antidepressants - use caution in patients with benign prostatic hypertrophy, xerostomia, visual problems, constipation, or history of bowel obstruction.

Use caution in patients with suicidal risk. Use with caution in patients with a history of cardiovascular disease (including previous MI, stroke, tachycardia, or conduction abnormalities). The risk conduction abnormalities with this agent is moderate relative to other antidepressants. Use caution in patients with a previous seizure disorder or condition predisposing to seizures such as brain damage, alcoholism, or concurrent therapy with other drugs which lower the seizure threshold. Use with caution in hyperthyroid patients or those receiving thyroid supplementation. Use with caution in patients with hepatic or renal dysfunction and in elderly patients. Use in children <12 years of age has not been established.

Adverse Reactions Frequency not defined.
  Cardiovascular: Hypotension, hypertension, tachycardia
  Central nervous system: Drowsiness, dizziness, headache, disorientation, ataxia, confusion, seizure
  Dermatologic: Alopecia, photosensitivity, rash, pruritus
  Endocrine & metabolic: Breast enlargement, galactorrhea, SIADH, increase or decrease in blood sugar, increased or decreased libido
  Gastrointestinal: Xerostomia, constipation, vomiting, indigestion, anorexia, aphthous stomatitis, nausea, unpleasant taste, weight gain, diarrhea, trouble with gums, decreased lower esophageal sphincter tone may cause GE reflux
  Genitourinary: Urinary retention, testicular edema
  Hematologic: Agranulocytosis, leukopenia, eosinophilia, thrombocytopenia, purpura
  Neuromuscular & skeletal: Weakness, tremors, numbness, paresthesia, extrapyramidal symptoms, tardive dyskinesia
  Ocular: Blurred vision
  Otic: Tinnitus
  Miscellaneous: Diaphoresis (excessive), allergic reactions

Overdosage/Toxicology Symptoms include confusion, hallucinations, seizures, urinary retention, hypothermia, hypotension, tachycardia, and cyanosis. Following initiation of essential overdose management, toxic symptoms should be treated. Sodium bicarbonate is indicated when the QRS interval is >0.10 seconds or the QT_c interval is >0.42 seconds. Ventricular arrhythmias often respond to systemic alkalinization with or without phenytoin 15-20 mg/kg (adults) (sodium bicarbonate 0.5-2 mEq/kg I.V.). Arrhythmias unresponsive to this therapy may respond to lidocaine 1 mg/kg I.V. followed by a titrated infusion. Physostigmine (1-2 mg slow I.V. for adults or 0.5 mg slow I.V. for children) may be indicated in reversing life-threatening cardiac arrhythmias. Seizures usually respond to diazepam I.V. boluses (5-10 mg for adults up to 30 mg or 0.25-0.4 mg/kg/dose for children up to 10 mg/dose). If seizures are unresponsive or recur, phenytoin or phenobarbital may be required.

Drug Interactions
  Cytochrome P450 Effect: CYP2D6 enzyme substrate
  Increased Effect/Toxicity: Doxepin increases the effects of amphetamines, anticholinergics, other CNS depressants (sedatives, hypnotics, or ethanol), chlorpropamide, tolazamide, and warfarin. When used with MAO inhibitors, hyperpyrexia, hypertension, tachycardia, confusion, seizures, and **deaths have been reported** (serotonin syndrome). Serotonin syndrome has also been reported with ritonavir (rare). The SSRIs (to varying degrees), cimetidine, grapefruit juice, indinavir, methylphenidate, ritonavir, quinidine, diltiazem, and verapamil inhibit the metabolism of TCAs and clinical toxicity may result. Use of lithium with a TCA may increase the risk for neurotoxicity. Phenothiazines may increase concentration of some TCAs and TCAs may increase concentration of phenothiazines. Pressor response to I.V. epinephrine, norepinephrine, and phenylephrine may be enhanced in patients receiving TCAs (**Note:** Effect is unlikely with epinephrine or levonordefrin dosages typically administered as infiltration in combination with local anesthetics). Combined use of beta-agonists or drugs which prolong QT_c (including quinidine, procainamide, disopyramide, cisapride, sparfloxacin, gatifloxacin, moxifloxacin) with TCAs may predispose patients to cardiac arrhythmias.
  Decreased Effect: Carbamazepine, phenobarbital, and rifampin may increase the metabolism of doxepin resulting in decreased effect of doxepin. Doxepin inhibits the antihypertensive response to bethanidine, clonidine, debrisoquin, guanadrel, guanethidine, guanabenz, and guanfacine. Cholestyramine and colestipol may bind TCAs and reduce their absorption.

Ethanol/Nutrition/Herb Interactions
  Ethanol: Avoid ethanol (may increase CNS depression).
  Food: Grapefruit juice may inhibit the metabolism of some TCAs and clinical toxicity may result.
  Herb/Nutraceutical: Avoid valerian, St John's wort, SAMe, kava kava (may increase risk of serotonin syndrome and/or excessive sedation).

Stability Protect from light
Mechanism of Action Increases the synaptic concentration of serotonin and norepinephrine in the central nervous system by inhibition of their reuptake by the presynaptic neuronal membrane
(Continued)

441

Doxepin *(Continued)*

Pharmacodynamics/Kinetics

Peak effect: Antidepressant: Usually >2 weeks; Anxiolytic: may occur sooner
Distribution: Crosses placenta; enters breast milk
Protein binding: 80% to 85%
Metabolism: Hepatic; metabolites include desmethyldoxepin (active)
Half-life elimination: Adults: 6-8 hours
Excretion: Urine

Usual Dosage Oral (entire daily dose may be given at bedtime):

Depression or anxiety (unlabeled use):
Children: 1-3 mg/kg/day in single or divided doses
Adolescents: Initial: 25-50 mg/day in single or divided doses; gradually increase to 100 mg/day
Adults: Initial: 30-150 mg/day at bedtime or in 2-3 divided doses; may gradually increase up to 300 mg/day; single dose should not exceed 150 mg; select patients may respond to 25-50 mg/day
Elderly: Use a lower dose and adjust gradually
Dosing adjustment in hepatic impairment: Use a lower dose and adjust gradually

Topical: Adults: Apply a thin film 4 times/day with at least 3- to 4-hour interval between applications. **Note:** Low-dose (25-50 mg) oral administration has also been used to treat pruritus, but systemic effects are increased.

Monitoring Parameters Monitor blood pressure and pulse rate prior to and during initial therapy; monitor mental status, weight; EKG in older adults

Reference Range Therapeutic: 30-150 ng/mL; Toxic: >500 ng/mL; utility of serum level monitoring is controversial

Test Interactions ↑ glucose

Patient Information Avoid unnecessary exposure to sunlight; avoid alcohol; do not discontinue medication abruptly; may cause urine to turn blue-green; may cause drowsiness; can use sugarless gum or hard candy for dry mouth; full effect may not occur for 4-6 weeks

Nursing Implications May increase appetite; may cause drowsiness, raise bed rails, institute safety precautions

Dosage Forms

Capsule, as hydrochloride (Sinequan®): 10 mg, 25 mg, 50 mg, 75 mg, 100 mg, 150 mg
Cream (Zonalon®): 5% (30 g, 45 g)
Solution, oral concentrate, as hydrochloride (Sinequan®): 10 mg/mL (120 mL)

♦ **Doxepin Hydrochloride** *see Doxepin on page 440*

Doxercalciferol *(doks er kal sif e FEER ole)*

U.S. Brand Names Hectorol®
Canadian Brand Names Hectorol®
Therapeutic Category Vitamin D Analog
Use Reduction of elevated intact parathyroid hormone (iPTH) in the management of secondary hyperparathyroidism in patients on chronic hemodialysis
Pregnancy Risk Factor B
Pregnancy/Breast-Feeding Implications Reproduction in animals (usual and high dose) do not reveal teratogenic or fetotoxic effects. Studies in humans are lacking. Excretion in breast milk is unknown. Other vitamin D derivatives are excreted in breast milk; there is a potential for adverse effects. Therefore, breast-feeding should be discontinued or doxercalciferol discontinued, depending upon importance of the drug to the mother.
Contraindications History of hypercalcemia or evidence of vitamin D toxicity; hyperphosphatemia should be corrected before initiating therapy
Warnings/Precautions Other forms of vitamin D should be discontinued when doxercalciferol is started. Overdose from vitamin D is dangerous and needs to be avoided. Careful dosage titration and monitoring can minimize risk. Hyperphosphatemia exacerbates secondary hyperparathyroidism, diminishing the effect of doxercalciferol. Hyperphosphatemia needs to be corrected for best results. Use with caution in patients with hepatic impairment. Safety and efficacy have not been established in pediatrics.

Adverse Reactions

>10%:
Cardiovascular: Edema (34.4%)
Central nervous system: Headache (28%), malaise (28%), dizziness (11.5%)
Gastrointestinal: Nausea/vomiting (34%)
Respiratory: Dyspnea (11.5%)
1% to 10%:
Cardiovascular: Bradycardia (6.6%)
Central nervous system: Sleep disorder (3.3%)
Dermatologic: Pruritus (8.2%)
Gastrointestinal: Anorexia (4.9%), constipation (3.3%), dyspepsia (4.9%)
Neuromuscular & skeletal: Arthralgia (4.9%)
Miscellaneous: Abscess (3.3%)

Overdosage/Toxicology Doxercalciferol, in excess, can cause hypercalcemia, hypercalciuria, hyperphosphatemia, and oversuppression of PTH secretion. Some signs and symptoms of hypercalcemia include anorexia, nausea, vomiting, constipation, polyuria, weakness, fatigue, confusion, stupor, and coma. Following withdrawal of the drug and calcium supplements, hypercalcemia treatment consists of a low calcium diet and monitoring. Adjustments of calcium in the dialysis bath can also be made if necessary. When calcium levels normalize, doxercalciferol can be restarted. Reduce each dose by at least 2.5 mcg. Monitor serum calcium levels closely.

Drug Interactions

Increased Effect/Toxicity: Doxercalciferol toxicity may be increased by concurrent use of other vitamin D supplements or magnesium-containing antacids and supplements.

Decreased Effect: Absorption of doxercalciferol is reduced with mineral oil and cholestyramine.

Stability Store at controlled room temperature (15°C to 30°C/59°F to 86°F); protect injection from light

Mechanism of Action Doxercalciferol is metabolized to the active form of vitamin D. The active form of vitamin D controls the intestinal absorption of dietary calcium, the tubular reabsorption of calcium by the kidneys, and in conjunction with PTH, the mobilization of calcium from the skeleton.

Pharmacodynamics/Kinetics
Metabolism: Hepatically via CYP27
Half-life elimination: Active metabolite: 32-37 hours; up to 96 hours

Usual Dosage
Oral:
If the iPTH >400 pg/mL, then the initial dose is 10 mcg 3 times/week at dialysis. The dose is adjusted at 8-week intervals based upon the iPTH levels.
If the iPTH level is decreased by 50% and >300 pg/mL, then the dose can be increased to 12.5 mcg 3 times/week for 8 more weeks. This titration process can continue at 8-week intervals up to a maximum dose of 20 mcg 3 times/week. Each increase should be by 2.5 mcg/dose.
If the iPTH is between 150-300 pg/mL, maintain the current dose.
If the iPTH is <100 pg/mL, then suspend the drug for 1 week; resume doxercalciferol at a reduced dose. Decrease each dose (not weekly dose) by at least 2.5 mcg.
I.V.:
If the iPTH >400 pg/mL, then the initial dose is 4 mcg 3 times/week after dialysis, administered as a bolus dose
If the iPTH level is decreased by 50% and >300 pg/mL, then the dose can be increased by 1-2 mcg at 8-week intervals as necessary
If the iPTH is between 150-300 pg/mL, maintain the current dose.
If the iPTH is <100 pg/mL, then suspend the drug for 1 week; resume doxercalciferol at a reduced dose (at least 1 mcg lower)

Monitoring Parameters Before initiating, check iPTH, serum calcium and phosphorus. Check weekly thereafter until stable. Serum iPTH, calcium, phosphorus, and alkaline phosphatase should be monitored.

Reference Range Serum calcium times phosphorus product should be less than 70

Patient Information Be clear on dose and directions for taking. Stop other vitamin D products. Do not miss doses. Avoid magnesium-containing antacids and supplements. Report headache, dizziness, weakness, sleepiness, severe nausea, vomiting, and difficulty thinking or concentrating to your prescriber. Do not take over-the-counter medicines or supplements without first consulting your prescriber. Follow diet and calcium supplements as directed by your prescriber.

Dosage Forms
Capsule: 2.5 mcg
Injection: 2 mcg/mL

♦ Doxil® see DOXOrubicin (Liposomal) on page 445

DOXOrubicin (doks oh ROO bi sin)

U.S. Brand Names Adriamycin PFS®; Adriamycin RDF®; Rubex®
Canadian Brand Names Adriamycin®; Caelyx®
Synonyms ADR; Doxorubicin Hydrochloride; Hydroxydaunomycin Hydrochloride
Therapeutic Category Antineoplastic Agent, Anthracycline; Antineoplastic Agent, Antibiotic; Vesicant
Use Treatment of leukemias, lymphomas, multiple myeloma, osseous and nonosseous sarcomas, mesotheliomas, germ cell tumors of the ovary or testis, and carcinomas of the head and neck, thyroid, lung, breast, stomach, pancreas, liver, ovary, bladder, prostate, uterus, and neuroblastoma
Pregnancy Risk Factor D
Contraindications Hypersensitivity to doxorubicin or any component of the formulation; congestive heart failure or arrhythmias; previous therapy with high cumulative doses of doxorubicin and/or daunorubicin; pre-existing bone marrow suppression; pregnancy
Warnings/Precautions The U.S. Food and Drug Administration (FDA) currently recommends that procedures for proper handling and disposal of antineoplastic agents be considered. Total dose should not exceed 550 mg/m² or 400 mg/m² in patients with previous or concomitant treatment (with daunorubicin, cyclophosphamide, or irradiation of the cardiac region); irreversible myocardial toxicity may occur as total dosage approaches 550 mg/m². A baseline cardiac evaluation (EKG, LVEF, +/- ECHO) is recommended, especially in patients with risk factors for increased cardiac toxicity. I.V. use only, severe local tissue necrosis will result if extravasation occurs; reduce dose in patients with impaired hepatic function; severe myelosuppression is also possible.

Adverse Reactions
>10%:
Dermatologic: Alopecia
Gastrointestinal: Acute nausea and vomiting may be seen in 21% to 55% of patients; mucositis, ulceration, and necrosis of the colon, anorexia, and diarrhea, stomatitis, esophagitis
Emetic potential:
≤20 mg: Moderately low (10% to 30%)
>20 mg or <60 mg: Moderate (30% to 60%)
≥60 mg: Moderately high (60% to 90%)
Time course for nausea/vomiting: Onset: 1-3 hours; Duration 4-24 hours
Genitourinary: Discoloration of urine (red)
Hematologic: Myelosuppressive: 60% to 80% of patients will have leukopenia; dose-limiting toxicity
WBC: Moderate
(Continued)

DOXOrubicin *(Continued)*

Platelets: Moderate
Onset (days): 7
Nadir (days): 10-14
Recovery (days): 21-28

Local: **Vesicant chemotherapy**

1% to 10%:

Cardiovascular: Acute: Arrhythmias, heart block, pericarditis-myocarditis, facial flushing; Delayed: Congestive heart failure (related to cumulative dose; usually a maximum total lifetime dose of 450-550 mg/m^2; possibly higher if given by continuous infusion in breast cancer),

Dermatologic: Hyperpigmentation of nail beds, erythematous streaking along the vein if administered rapidly

Endocrine & metabolic: Hyperuricemia

<1% (Limited to important or life-threatening):

Pediatric patients may be at increased risk of later neoplastic disease, particularly acute myeloid leukemia (pediatric patients). Prepubertal growth failure may result from intensive chemotherapy regimens.

Radiation recall: Noticed in patients who have had prior irradiation; reactions include redness, warmth, erythema, and dermatitis in the radiation port. Can progress to severe desquamation and ulceration. Occurs 5-7 days after doxorubicin administration; local therapy with topical corticosteroids and cooling have given the best relief.

Overdosage/Toxicology Symptoms include myelosuppression, nausea, vomiting, and myocardial toxicity.

Drug Interactions

Cytochrome P450 Effect: CYP3A3/4 enzyme substrate; CYP2D6 enzyme inhibitor

Increased Effect/Toxicity: Allopurinol may enhance the antitumor activity of doxorubicin (animal data only). Cyclosporine may increase doxorubicin levels, enhancing hematologic toxicity or may induce coma or seizures. Cyclophosphamide enhances the cardiac toxicity of doxorubicin by producing additional myocardial cell damage. Mercaptopurine increases doxorubicin toxicities. Streptozocin greatly enhances leukopenia and thrombocytopenia. Verapamil alters the cellular distribution of doxorubicin and may result in increased cell toxicity by inhibition of the P-glycoprotein pump. Paclitaxel reduces doxorubicin clearance and increases toxicity if administered prior to doxorubicin. High doses of progesterone enhance toxicity (neutropenia and thrombocytopenia). Based on mouse studies, cardiotoxicity may be enhanced by verapamil. Concurrent therapy with actinomycin-D may result in recall pneumonitis following radiation.

Decreased Effect: Doxorubicin may decrease plasma levels and effectiveness of digoxin and phenytoin. Phenobarbital increases elimination (decreases effect) of doxorubicin.

Ethanol/Nutrition/Herb Interactions

Ethanol: Avoid ethanol (due to GI irritation).

Herb/Nutraceutical: St John's wort may decrease doxorubicin levels. Avoid black cohosh, dong quai in estrogen-dependent tumors.

Stability

Store intact vials of solution under refrigeration (2°C to 8°C) and protect from light; store intact vials of lyophilized powder at room temperature (15°C to 30°C). Gensia formulation of generic doxorubicin is stable for up to 30 days at room temperature.

Reconstitute lyophilized powder with SWI or NS to a final concentration of 2 mg/mL as follows. Reconstituted solution is stable for 7 days at room temperature (25°C) and 15 days under refrigeration (5°C) when protected from light.

10 mg vial = 5 mL
20 mg vial = 10 mL
50 mg vial = 25 mL

Further dilution in D$_5$W or NS is stable for 48 hours at room temperature (25°C) when protected from light

Unstable in solutions with a pH <3 or >7; avoid aluminum needles and bacteriostatic diluents as precipitation occurs; decomposing drug turns purple; protect from direct sunlight

Incompatible with aminophylline, cephalothin, dexamethasone, diazepam, fluorouracil, furosemide, heparin, hydrocortisone, sodium bicarbonate

Y-site compatible with bleomycin, cyclophosphamide, dacarbazine, vinblastine, vincristine

Standard I.V. dilution:

I.V. push: Dose/syringe (concentration: 2 mg/mL)

Maximum syringe size for IVP is a 30 mL syringe and syringe should be ≤75% full

Syringes are stable for 7 days at room temperature (25°C) and 15 days under refrigeration (5°C) when protected from light

IVPB: Dose/50-100 mL D$_5$W or NS

IVPB solutions are stable for 48 hours at room temperature (25°C) when protected from light

Mechanism of Action Inhibition of DNA and RNA synthesis by intercalation between DNA base pairs and by steric obstruction. Doxorubicin intercalates at points of local uncoiling of the double helix. Although the exact mechanism is unclear, it appears that direct binding to DNA (intercalation) and inhibition of DNA repair (topoisomerase II inhibition) result in blockade of DNA and RNA synthesis and fragmentation of DNA. Doxorubicin is also a powerful iron chelator; the iron-doxorubicin complex can bind DNA and cell membranes and produce free radicals that immediately cleave the DNA and cell membranes.

Pharmacodynamics/Kinetics

Absorption: Oral: Poor (<50%)

Distribution: V$_d$: 25 L/kg; to many body tissues, particularly liver, spleen, kidney, lung, heart; does not distribute into the CNS; crosses placenta

Protein binding, plasma: 70%

Metabolism: Primarily hepatic to doxorubicinol (active), then to inactive aglycones, conjugated sulfates, and glucuronides

Half-life elimination:
　Distribution: 10 minutes
　Elimination: Doxorubicin: 1-3 hours; Metabolites: 3-3.5 hours
　Terminal: 17-30 hours
　Male: 54 hours; female: 35 hours
Excretion: Feces (~40% to 50% as unchanged drug); urine (~3% to 10% as metabolites, 1% doxorubicinol, <1% adrimycine aglycones, and unchanged drug)
　Clearance: Male: 113 L/hour; female: 44 L/hour
Usual Dosage Refer to individual protocols. I.V.:
Children:
　35-75 mg/m² as a single dose, repeat every 21 days **or**
　20-30 mg/m² once weekly **or**
　60-90 mg/m² given as a continuous infusion over 96 hours every 3-4 weeks
Adults:
　Usual or typical dose: 60-75 mg/m² as a single dose, repeat every 21 days **or** other dosage regimens like 20-30 mg/m²/day for 2-3 days, repeat in 4 weeks **or** 20 mg/m² once weekly
　　The lower dose regimen should be given to patients with decreased bone marrow reserve, prior therapy or marrow infiltration with malignant cells
Currently the maximum cumulative dose is 550 mg/m² or 450 mg/m² in patients who have received RT to the mediastinal areas; a baseline MUGA should be performed prior to initiating treatment. If the LVEF is <30% to 40%, therapy should not be instituted; LVEF should be monitored during therapy.
Doxorubicin has also been administered intraperitoneal (phase I in refractory ovarian cancer patients) and intra-arterially.
Dosing adjustment in renal impairment:
　Mild to moderate renal failure: Adjustment is not required
　Cl_cr <10 mL/minute: Administer 75% of normal dose
Hemodialysis: Supplemental dose is not necessary
Dosing adjustment in hepatic impairment:
　Bilirubin 1.2-3 mg/dL: Administer 50% of dose
　Bilirubin 3.1-5 mg/dL: Administer 25% of dose
　Bilirubin >5 mg/dL: Do not administer drug
Administration
　Administer I.V. push over 1-2 minutes or IVPB; may be further diluted in either NS of D₅W for I.V. administration. Continuous infusions must be administered via central line.
　Avoid extravasation, associated with severe ulceration and soft tissue necrosis; flush with 5-10 mL of I.V. solution before and after drug administration
Monitoring Parameters CBC with differential and platelet count, echocardiogram, liver function tests
Patient Information This medication can only be administered I.V. During therapy, do not use alcohol, aspirin-containing products, and/or OTC medications without consulting prescriber. It is important to maintain adequate nutrition and hydration (2-3 L/day of fluids unless instructed to restrict fluid intake) during therapy; frequent small meals may help. You may experience nausea or vomiting (frequent small meals, frequent mouth care, sucking lozenges, or chewing gum may help). You may experience loss of hair (reversible); you will be more susceptible to infection (avoid crowds and exposure to infection as much as possible). Urine may turn red-brown (normal). Yogurt or buttermilk may help reduce diarrhea (if unresolved, contact prescriber for medication relief). Frequent mouth care and use of a soft toothbrush or cotton swabs may reduce mouth sores. May discolor urine (red/pink). Report fever, chills, unusual bruising or bleeding, signs of infection, abdominal pain or blood in stools, excessive fatigue, yellowing of eyes or skin, swelling of extremities, difficulty breathing, or unresolved diarrhea. Contraceptive measures are recommended during therapy.
Nursing Implications
　Local erythematous streaking along the vein and/or facial flushing may indicate too rapid a rate of administration
　Extravasation management:
　　Apply ice immediately for 30-60 minutes; then alternate off/on every 15 minutes for one day
　　Topical cooling may be achieved using ice packs or cooling pad with circulating ice water. Cooling of site for 24 hours as tolerated by the patient. Elevate and rest extremity 24-48 hours, then resume normal activity as tolerated. Application of cold inhibits vesicant's cytotoxicity.
　　Application of heat or sodium bicarbonate can be harmful and is contraindicated
　　If pain, erythema, and/or swelling persist beyond 48 hours, refer patient immediately to plastic surgeon for consultation and possible debridement
Dosage Forms
　Injection, as hydrochloride [preservative free]: 2 mg/mL (5 mL, 10 mL, 25 mL, 37.5 mL)
　Injection, aqueous, as hydrochloride, with NS: 2 mg/mL (5 mL, 10 mL, 25 mL, 100 mL)
　Powder for injection, lyophilized, as hydrochloride: 10 mg, 20 mg, 50 mg, 100 mg
　Powder for injection, lyophilized, rapid dissolution formula, as hydrochloride: 10 mg, 20 mg, 50 mg, 150 mg

♦ **Doxorubicin Hydrochloride** *see DOXOrubicin on page 443*
♦ **Doxorubicin Hydrochloride (Liposomal)** *see DOXOrubicin (Liposomal) on page 445*

DOXOrubicin (Liposomal) (doks oh ROO bi sin lip pah SOW mal)

U.S. Brand Names Doxil®
Canadian Brand Names Doxil®
Synonyms Doxorubicin Hydrochloride (Liposomal)
Therapeutic Category Antineoplastic Agent, Anthracycline; Antineoplastic Agent, Antibiotic
Use Treatment of AIDS-related Kaposi's sarcoma, breast cancer, ovarian cancer, solid tumors
Pregnancy Risk Factor D
Pregnancy/Breast-Feeding Implications Advise patients to avoid becoming pregnant (females) and to avoid causing pregnancy (males).
(Continued)

DOXOrubicin (Liposomal) *(Continued)*

Contraindications Hypersensitivity to doxorubicin, other anthracyclines, or any component of the formulation; pre-existing bone marrow suppression; pregnancy

Warnings/Precautions The U.S. Food and Drug Administration (FDA) currently recommends that procedures for proper handling and disposal of antineoplastic agents be considered. Total dose should not exceed 550 mg/m^2 or 400 mg/m^2 in patients with previous or concomitant treatment (with daunorubicin, cyclophosphamide, or irradiation of the cardiac region); irreversible myocardial toxicity may occur as total dosage approaches 550 mg/m^2. I.V. use only, severe local tissue necrosis will result if extravasation occurs; reduce dose in patients with impaired hepatic function; severe myelosuppression is also possible.

Adverse Reactions Information on adverse events is based on the experience reported in 753 patients with AIDS-related Kaposi's sarcoma enrolled in four studies.

>10%:
  Gastrointestinal: Nausea; emetic potential:
    ≤20 mg: Moderately low (10% to 30%)
    >20 mg or <75 mg: Moderate (30% to 60%)
    ≥75 mg: Moderately high (49%)
  Hematologic: Myelosuppressive: 60% to 80% of patients will have leukopenia; dose-limiting toxicity
    WBC: Moderate
    Platelets: Moderate
    Onset (days): 7
    Nadir (days): 10-14
    Recovery (days): 21-28
  Local: **Irritant chemotherapy**
1% to 10%:
  Cardiovascular: Cardiac toxicity (9.7%): Cardiomyopathy, congestive heart failure, arrhythmia, pericardial effusion, tachycardia, facial flushing
  Dermatologic: Hyperpigmentation of nail beds, erythematous streaking along the vein if administered rapidly
  Endocrine & metabolic: Hyperuricemia

Overdosage/Toxicology Symptoms include increased mucositis, leukopenia, and thrombocytopenia. In acute overdose, the severely myelosuppressed patient should be hospitalized and treated with antibiotics, platelet and granulocyte transfusions. Mucositis should be treated symptomatically.

Drug Interactions

Cytochrome P450 Effect: CYP3A3/4 enzyme substrate; CYP2D6 enzyme inhibitor

Increased Effect/Toxicity: No formal drug interaction studies have been conducted with doxorubicin hydrochloride liposome injection; however, it may interact with drugs known to interact with the conventional formulation of doxorubicin hydrochloride. Allopurinol may enhance the antitumor activity of doxorubicin (animal data only). Cyclosporine may induce coma or seizures. Cyclophosphamide enhances the cardiac toxicity of doxorubicin by producing additional myocardial cell damage. Mercaptopurine increases toxicities. Streptozocin greatly enhances leukopenia and thrombocytopenia. Verapamil alters the cellular distribution of doxorubicin and may result in increased cell toxicity by inhibition of the P-glycoprotein pump.

Decreased Effect: No formal drug interaction studies have been conducted with doxorubicin hydrochloride liposome injection; however, it may interact with drugs known to interact with the conventional formulation of doxorubicin hydrochloride. Doxorubicin may decrease plasma levels and effectiveness of digoxin and phenytoin. Phenobarbital increases elimination (decreases effect) of doxorubicin.

Ethanol/Nutrition/Herb Interactions

Ethanol: Avoid ethanol (due to GI irritation).

Herb/Nutraceutical: St John's wort may decrease doxorubicin levels. Avoid black cohosh, dong quai in estrogen-dependent tumors.

Stability Store intact vials of solution under refrigeration (2°C to 8°C) and avoid freezing. Prolonged freezing may adversely affect liposomal drug products, however, short-term freezing (<1 month) does not appear to have a deleterious effect.

The appropriate dose (up to a maximum of 90 mg) must be diluted in 250 mL of dextrose 5% in water prior to administration. Diluted doxorubicin hydrochloride liposome injection should be refrigerated at 2°C to 8°C and administered within 24 hours. **Do not use with in-line filters.**

Mechanism of Action Doxil® is doxorubicin hydrochloride encapsulated in long-circulating STEALTH® liposomes. Liposomes are microscopic vesicles composed of a phospholipid bilayer that are capable of encapsulating active drugs. Doxorubicin works through inhibition of topoisomerase-II at the point of DNA cleavage. A second mechanism of action is the production of free radicals (the hydroxy radical OH) by doxorubicin, which in turn can destroy DNA and cancerous cells. Doxorubicin is also a very powerful iron chelator, equal to deferoxamine. The iron-doxorubicin complex can bind DNA and cell membranes rapidly and produce free radicals that immediately cleave the DNA and cell membranes. Inhibits DNA and RNA synthesis by intercalating between DNA base pairs and by steric obstruction; active throughout entire cell cycle.

Pharmacodynamics/Kinetics

Distribution: V$_{dss}$: Confined mostly to the vascular fluid volume

Protein binding, plasma: Doxorubicin: 70%

Metabolism: Hepatic and in plasma to both active and inactive metabolites

Excretion: Urine (5% as doxorubicin or doxorubicinol)

Clearance: Mean: 0.041 L/hour/m^2

Usual Dosage Refer to individual protocols

I.V. (patient's ideal weight should be used to calculate body surface area): 20 mg/m^2 over 30 minutes, once every 3 weeks, for as long as patients respond satisfactorily and tolerate treatment.

AIDS-KS patients: I.V.: 20 mg/m²/dose over 30 minutes once every 3 weeks for as long as patients respond satisfactorily and tolerate treatment

Breast cancer: I.V.: 20-80 mg/m²/dose has been studied in a limited number of phase I/II trials

Ovarian cancer: I.V.: 50 mg/m²/dose repeated every 4 weeks (minimum of 4 courses is recommended)

Solid tumors: I.V.: 50-60 mg/m²/dose repeated every 3-4 weeks has been studied in a limited number of phase I/II trials

See table.

Recommended Dose Modification Guidelines

Toxicity Grade	Dose Adjustment
PALMAR-PLANTAR ERYTHRODYSESTHESIA	
1 (Mild erythema, swelling, or desquamation not interfering with daily activities)	Redose unless patient has experienced previous Grade 3 or 4 toxicity. If so, delay up to 2 weeks and decrease dose by 25%; return to original dosing interval.
2 (Erythema, desquamation, or swelling interfering with, but not precluding, normal physical activities; small blisters or ulcerations <2 cm in diameter)	Delay dosing up to 2 weeks or until resolved to Grade 0-1. If after 2 weeks there is no resolution, liposomal doxorubicin should be discontinued.
3 (Blistering, ulceration, or swelling interfering with walking or normal daily activities; cannot wear regular clothing)	Delay dosing up to 2 weeks or until resolved to Grade 0-1. Decrease dose by 25% and return to original dosing interval; if after 2 weeks there is no resolution, liposomal doxorubicin should be discontinued.
4 (Diffuse or local process causing infectious complications, or a bed-ridden state or hospitalization)	Delay dosing up to 2 weeks or until resolved to Grade 0-1. Decrease dose by 25% and return to original dosing interval. If after 2 weeks there is no resolution, liposomal doxorubicin should be discontinued.
STOMATITIS	
1 (Painless ulcers, erythema, or mild soreness)	Redose unless patient has experienced previous Grade 3 or 4 toxicity. If so, delay up to 2 weeks and decrease by 25%. Return to original dosing interval.
2 (Painful erythema, edema, or ulcers, but can eat)	Delay dosing up to 2 weeks or until resolved to Grade 0-1. If after 2 weeks there is no resolution, liposomal doxorubicin should be discontinued.
3 (Painful erythema, edema, or ulcers, but cannot eat)	Delay dosing up to 2 weeks or until resolved to Grade 0-1. Decrease dose by 25% and return to original dosing interval. If after 2 weeks there is no resolution, liposomal doxorubicin should be discontinued.
4 (Requires parenteral or enteral support)	Delay dosing up to 2 weeks or until resolved to Grade 0-1. Decrease dose by 25% and return to original dosing interval. If after 2 weeks there is no resolution, liposomal doxorubicin should be discontinued.

Dosing adjustment in hepatic impairment:
Bilirubin 1.2-3 mg/dL or AST 60-180 units/L: Administer 50% of dose
Bilirubin >3 mg/dL: Administer 25% of dose

See table.

Hematological Toxicity

Grade	ANC	Platelets	Modification
1	1500 - 1900	75,000 - 150,000	Resume treatment with no dose reduction
2	1000 - <1500	50,000 - <75,000	Wait until ANC ≥1500 and platelets ≥75,000; redose with no dose reduction
3	500 - 999	25,000 - <50,000	Wait until ANC ≥1500 and platelets ≥75,000; redose with no dose reduction
4	<500	<25,000	Wait until ANC ≥1500 and platelets ≥75,000; redose at 25% dose reduction or continue full dose with cytokine support

Administration
Administer IVPB over 30 minutes; administer at initial rate of 1 mg/minute to minimize risk of infusion reactions; further dilute in D₅W; do not administer as a bolus injection or undiluted solution

Do not administer intramuscular or subcutaneous

Avoid extravasation, associated with severe ulceration and soft tissue necrosis; flush with 5-10 mL of D₅W solution before and after drug administration

Monitoring Parameters CBC with differential and platelet count, echocardiogram, liver function tests

Patient Information This medication can only be administered I.V. During therapy, do not use alcohol, aspirin-containing products, and/or OTC medications without consulting prescriber. It is important to maintain adequate nutrition and hydration (2-3 L/day of fluids unless instructed to restrict fluid intake) during therapy; frequent small meals may help. You may experience nausea or vomiting (frequent small meals, frequent mouth care, sucking lozenges, or chewing gum may help). You may experience loss of hair (reversible); you will be more susceptible to infection (avoid crowds and exposure to infection as much as possible). Urine (Continued)

DOXOrubicin (Liposomal) *(Continued)*

may turn red-brown (normal). Yogurt or buttermilk may help reduce diarrhea (if unresolved, contact prescriber for medication relief). Frequent mouth care and use of a soft toothbrush or cotton swabs may reduce mouth sores. Report fever, chills, unusual bruising or bleeding, signs of infection, abdominal pain or blood in stools, excessive fatigue, yellowing of eyes or skin, darkening in color of urine or pale colored stools, swelling of extremities, difficulty breathing, or unresolved diarrhea. Contraceptive measures are recommended during therapy

Nursing Implications
Local erythematous streaking along the vein and/or facial flushing may indicate too rapid a rate of administration

Extravasation management:

Apply ice immediately for 30-60 minutes; then alternate off/on every 15 minutes for one day

Topical cooling may be achieved using ice packs or cooling pad with circulating ice water. Cooling of site for 24 hours as tolerated by the patient. Elevate and rest extremity 24-48 hours, then resume normal activity as tolerated. Application of cold inhibits vesicant's cytotoxicity.

Application of heat or sodium bicarbonate can be harmful and is contraindicated

If pain, erythema, and/or swelling persist beyond 48 hours, refer patient immediately to plastic surgeon for consultation and possible debridement

Dosage Forms Injection, as hydrochloride: 2 mg/mL (10 mL)

♦ **Doxy-100™** *see Doxycycline on page 448*

♦ **Doxycin (Can)** *see Doxycycline on page 448*

Doxycycline *(doks i SYE kleen)*

Related Information
Animal and Human Bites Guidelines *on page 1584*
Antimicrobial Drugs of Choice *on page 1588*
Community-Acquired Pneumonia in Adults *on page 1603*
Prevention of Malaria *on page 1552*
Prevention of Wound Infection & Sepsis in Surgical Patients *on page 1569*
Treatment of Sexually Transmitted Diseases *on page 1609*

U.S. Brand Names Adoxa™; Doryx®; Doxy-100™; Monodox®; Periostat®; Vibramycin®; Vibra-Tabs®

Canadian Brand Names Apo®-Doxy; Apo®-Doxy Tabs; Doxycin; Doxytec; Novo-Doxylin; Nu-Doxycycline; Vibra-Tabs™

Synonyms Doxycycline Calcium; Doxycycline Hyclate; Doxycycline Monohydrate

Therapeutic Category Antibiotic, Tetracycline Derivative

Use Principally in the treatment of infections caused by susceptible *Rickettsia*, *Chlamydia*, and *Mycoplasma* along with uncommon susceptible gram-negative and gram-positive organisms; alternative to mefloquine for malaria prophylaxis; treatment for syphilis in penicillin-allergic patients; often active against vancomycin-resistant enterococci; used for community-acquired pneumonia and other common infections due to susceptible organisms; anthrax due to *Bacillus anthracis*, including inhalational anthrax (postexposure), to reduce the incidence or progression of disease following exposure to aerolized *Bacillus anthracis*

Unlabeled/Investigational Use Sclerosing agent for pleural effusion injection

Pregnancy Risk Factor D

Pregnancy/Breast-Feeding Implications Exposure during the last half or pregnancy causes permanent yellow-gray-brown discoloration of the teeth. Tetracyclines also form a complex in bone-forming tissue, leading to a decreased fibula growth rate when given to premature infants.

According to the FDA, the Teratogen Information System concluded that therapeutic doses during pregnancy are unlikely to produce substantial teratogenic risk, but data are insufficient to say that there is no risk. In general, reports of exposure have been limited to short durations of therapy in the first trimester. When considering treatment for life-threatening infection and/or prolonged duration of therapy (such as in anthrax), the potential risk to the fetus must be balanced against the severity of the potential illness.

Contraindications Hypersensitivity to doxycycline, tetracycline or any component of the formulation; children <8 years of age, except in treatment of anthrax (including inhalational anthrax postexposure prophylaxis); severe hepatic dysfunction; pregnancy

Warnings/Precautions Do not use during pregnancy - use of tetracyclines during tooth development may cause permanent discoloration of the teeth and enamel hypoplasia; prolonged use may result in superinfection, including oral or vaginal candidiasis; photosensitivity reaction may occur with this drug; avoid prolonged exposure to sunlight or tanning equipment. Avoid in children ≤8 years of age.

Additional specific warnings for Periostat®: Effectiveness has not been established in patients with coexistent oral candidiasis; use with caution in patients with a history or predisposition to oral candidiasis

Adverse Reactions Frequency not defined.

Cardiovascular: Intracranial hypertension, pericarditis

Dermatologic: Angioneurotic edema, exfoliative dermatitis (rare), photosensitivity, rash, urticaria

Endocrine & metabolic: Brown/black discoloration of thyroid gland (no dysfunction reported)

Gastrointestinal: Anorexia, diarrhea, dysphagia, enterocolitis, esophagitis (rare), esophageal ulcerations (rare), glossitis, inflammatory lesions in anogenital region, tooth discoloration (children)

Hematologic: Eosinophilia, hemolytic anemia, neutropenia, thrombocytopenia

Renal: Increased BUN

Miscellaneous: Anaphylactoid purpura, anaphylaxis, bulging fontanels (infants), SLE exacerbation

Adverse effects in clinical trials with Periostat® occurring at a frequency greater than placebo included acid indigestion, bronchitis, common cold, diarrhea, dyspepsia, joint pain, menstrual cramp, nausea, pain, rash .

Overdosage/Toxicology Symptoms include nausea, anorexia, and diarrhea. Following GI decontamination, care is supportive only. Fluid support may be required for hypotension.

Drug Interactions
Cytochrome P450 Effect: CYP3A3/4 inhibitor

Increased Effect/Toxicity: Increased digoxin toxicity when taken with digoxin. Increased prothrombin time with warfarin.

Decreased Effect: Decreased levels of doxycycline may occur when taken with antacids containing aluminum, calcium, or magnesium. Decreased levels when taken with iron, bismuth subsalicylate, barbiturates, phenytoin, sucralfate, didanosine, quinapril, and carbamazepine. Tetracyclines decrease the contraceptive effect of oral contraceptives. Concurrent use of tetracycline and Penthrane® has been reported to result in fatal renal toxicity.

Ethanol/Nutrition/Herb Interactions
Ethanol: Chronic ethanol ingestion may reduce the serum concentration of doxycycline.
Food: Doxycycline serum levels may be slightly decreased if taken with food or milk. Administration with iron or calcium may decrease doxycycline absorption. May decrease absorption of calcium, iron, magnesium, zinc, and amino acids.
Herb/Nutraceutical: St John's wort may decrease doxycycline levels. Avoid dong quai, St John's wort (may also cause photosensitization).

Stability
Capsules/tablets: Store at controlled room temperature; protect from light
I.V. infusion: Following reconstitution with sterile water for injection, dilute to a final concentration of 0.1-1 mg/mL using a compatible solution. Solutions for I.V. infusion may be prepared using 0.9% sodium chloride, D_5W, Ringer's injection, lactated Ringer's, D_5LR. Protect from light. Stability varies based on solution.

Mechanism of Action Inhibits protein synthesis by binding with the 30S and possibly the 50S ribosomal subunit(s) of susceptible bacteria; may also cause alterations in the cytoplasmic membrane

Periostat® capsules (proposed mechanism): Has been shown to inhibit collagenase activity *in vitro*. Also has been noted to reduce elevated collagenase activity in the gingival crevicular fluid of patients with periodontal disease. Systemic levels do not reach inhibitory concentrations against bacteria.

Pharmacodynamics/Kinetics
Absorption: Oral: Almost completely; reduced by food or milk by 20%
Distribution: Widely into body tissues and fluids including synovial, pleural, prostatic, seminal fluids, and bronchial secretions; saliva, aqueous humor, and CSF penetration is poor; readily crosses placenta; enters breast milk
Protein binding: 90%
Metabolism: Not hepatic, instead, partially inactivated in GI tract by chelate formation
Half-life elimination: 12-15 hours (usually increases to 22-24 hours with multiple dosing); End-stage renal disease: 18-25 hours
Time to peak, serum: 1.5-4 hours
Excretion: Feces (30%); urine (23%)

Usual Dosage
Children:
Anthrax: Doxycycline should be used in children if antibiotic susceptibility testing, exhaustion of drug supplies, or allergic reaction preclude use of penicillin or ciprofloxacin. For treatment, the consensus recommendation does not include a loading dose for doxycycline.
Inhalational (postexposure prophylaxis) (*MMWR*, 2001, 50:889-893): Oral, I.V. (use oral route when possible):
≤8 years: 2.2 mg/kg every 12 hours for 60 days
>8 years and ≤45 kg: 2.2 mg/kg every 12 hours for 60 days
>8 years and >45 kg: 100 mg every 12 hours for 60 days
Cutaneous (treatment): Oral: See dosing for "Inhalational (postexposure prophylaxis)"
Note: In the presence of systemic involvement, extensive edema, and/or lesions on head/neck, doxycycline should initially be administered I.V.
Inhalational/gastrointestinal/oropharyngeal (treatment): I.V.: Refer to dosing for inhalational anthrax (postexposure prophylaxis); switch to oral therapy when clinically appropriate; refer to Adults dosing for "Note" on combined therapy and duration
Children ≥8 years (<45 kg): Oral, I.V.: 2-5 mg/kg/day in 1-2 divided doses, not to exceed 200 mg/day
Children ≥8 years (>45 kg) and Adults: Oral, I.V.: 100-200 mg/day in 1-2 divided doses
Acute gonococcal infection (PID) in combination with another antibiotic: 100 mg every 12 hours until improved, followed by 100 mg orally twice daily to complete 14 days
Community-acquired pneumonia: 100 mg twice daily
Lyme disease: Oral: 100 mg twice daily for 14-21 days
Early syphilis: 200 mg/day in divided doses for 14 days
Late syphilis: 200 mg/day in divided doses for 28 days
Uncomplicated chlamydial infections: 100 mg twice daily for ≥7 days
Endometritis, salpingitis, parametritis, or peritonitis: 100 mg I.V. twice daily with cefoxitin 2 g every 6 hours for 4 days and for ≥48 hours after patient improves; then continue with oral therapy 100 mg twice daily to complete a 10- to 14-day course of therapy
Sclerosing agent for pleural effusion injection (unlabeled use): 500 mg as a single dose in 30-50 mL of NS or SWI
Periodontitis: Oral (Periostat®): 20 mg twice daily as an adjunct following scaling and root planing; may be administered for up to 9 months. Safety beyond 12 months of treatment and efficacy beyond 9 months of treatment have not been established.
(Continued)

449

Doxycycline *(Continued)*

Adults:
Anthrax:
Inhalational (postexposure prophylaxis): Oral, I.V. (use oral route when possible): 100 mg every 12 hours for 60 days (*MMWR*, 2001, 50:889-93); **Note:** Preliminary recommendation, FDA review and update is anticipated.

Cutaneous (treatment): Oral: 100 mg every 12 hours for 60 days. **Note:** In the presence of systemic involvement, extensive edema, lesions on head/neck, refer to I.V. dosing for treatment of inhalational/gastrointestinal/oropharyngeal anthrax

Inhalational/gastrointestinal/oropharyngeal (treatment): I.V.: Initial: 100 mg every 12 hours; switch to oral therapy when clinically appropriate; some recommend initial loading dose of 200 mg, followed by 100 mg every 8-12 hours (*JAMA*, 1997, 278:399-411). **Note:** Initial treatment should include two or more agents predicted to be effective (per CDC recommendations). Agents suggested for use in conjunction with doxycycline or ciprofloxacin include rifampin, vancomycin, imipenem, penicillin, ampicillin, chloramphenicol, clindamycin, and clarithromycin. May switch to oral antimicrobial therapy when clinically appropriate. Continue combined therapy for 60 days

Dosing adjustment in renal impairment: Cl_{cr} <10 mL/minute: 100 mg every 24 hours

Dialysis: Not dialyzable; 0% to 5% by hemo- and peritoneal methods or by continuous arteriovenous or venovenous hemofiltration: No supplemental dosage necessary

Dietary Considerations Take with food if gastric irritation occurs. While administration with food may decrease GI absorption of doxycycline by up to 20%, administration on an empty stomach is not recommended due to GI intolerance. Of currently available tetracyclines, doxycycline has the least affinity for calcium.

Administration

Oral: Administer with adequate fluid to reduce risk of esophageal irritation and ulceration; may administer with meals to decrease GI upset

I.V.: Infuse I.V. doxycycline over 1-4 hours

Test Interactions False elevations of urine catecholamine levels; false-negative urine glucose using Clinistix®, Tes-Tape®

Patient Information Avoid unnecessary exposure to sunlight; finish all medication; do not skip doses. Consult prescriber if you are pregnant.

Nursing Implications Avoid extravasation

Dosage Forms

Capsule, as hyclate (Vibramycin®): 50 mg, 100 mg

Capsule, as monohydrate (Monodox®): 50 mg, 100 mg

Capsule, coated pellets, as hyclate (Doryx®): 100 mg

Powder for injection, as hyclate (Doxy-100™): 100 mg

Powder for oral suspension, as monohydrate (Vibramycin®): 25 mg/5 mL (60 mL) [raspberry flavor]

Syrup, as calcium (Vibramycin®): 50 mg/5 mL (480 mL) [raspberry-apple flavor]

Tablet, as hyclate:

Periostat®: 20 mg

Vibra-Tabs®: 100 mg

Tablet, as monohydrate (Adoxa™): 50 mg, 100 mg

Dronabinol *(droe NAB i nol)*

U.S. Brand Names Marinol®

Canadian Brand Names Marinol®

Synonyms Tetrahydrocannabinol; THC

Therapeutic Category Antiemetic

Use When conventional antiemetics fail to relieve the nausea and vomiting associated with cancer chemotherapy, AIDS-related anorexia

Restrictions C-III

Pregnancy Risk Factor C

Contraindications Hypersensitivity to dronabinol or any component of the formulation, or marijuana; should be avoided in patients with a history of schizophrenia

Warnings/Precautions Use with caution in patients with heart disease, hepatic disease, or seizure disorders. Reduce dosage in patients with severe hepatic impairment. May have potential for abuse; drug is psychoactive substance in marijuana. Monitor for possible psychotic reaction with first dose.

Adverse Reactions

>10%:

Central nervous system: Drowsiness (48%), sedation (53%), confusion (30%), dizziness (21%), detachment, anxiety, difficulty concentrating, mood change

Gastrointestinal: Increased appetite (may be troublesome when used as an antiemetic), xerostomia (38% to 50%)

1% to 10%:

Cardiovascular: Orthostatic hypotension, tachycardia

Central nervous system: Ataxia (4%), depression (7%), headache, vertigo, hallucinations (5%), memory lapse (4%)

Neuromuscular & skeletal: Paresthesia, weakness

<1% (Limited to important or life-threatening): Diaphoresis, diarrhea, myalgia, nightmares, syncope, tinnitus

Overdosage/Toxicology Symptoms include tachycardia, hypertension, and hypotension.

Drug Interactions

Cytochrome P450 Effect: CYP2C18 and 3A3/4 enzyme substrate

Increased Effect/Toxicity: Increased toxicity (drowsiness) with alcohol, barbiturates, and benzodiazepines.

Ethanol/Nutrition/Herb Interactions

Ethanol: Avoid ethanol (may increase CNS depression).

Herb/Nutraceutical: St John's wort may decrease dronabinol levels.

Stability Store in a cool place

Mechanism of Action Not well defined, probably inhibits the vomiting center in the medulla oblongata

Pharmacodynamics/Kinetics

Absorption: Oral: 90% to 95%; ~10% to 20% of dose gets into systemic circulation

Distribution: V_d: 2.5-6.4 L; tetrahydrocannabinol is highly lipophilic and distributes to adipose tissue

Protein binding: 97% to 99%

Metabolism: Hepatically to at least 50 metabolites, some of which are active; 11-hydroxyte-trahydrocannabinol (11-OH-THC) is the major metabolite; extensive first-pass effect

Half-life elimination: THC: 19-24 hours; THC metabolites: 49-53 hours

Time to peak, serum: 2-3 hours

Excretion: Feces (35% as unconjugated metabolites); urine (10% to 15% as acid metabolites and conjugates)

Usual Dosage Refer to individual protocols. Oral:

Antiemetic:

Children: 5 mg/m² starting 6-8 hours before chemotherapy and every 4-6 hours after to be continued for 12 hours after chemotherapy is discontinued

Adults: 5 mg/m² 1-3 hours before chemotherapy, then 5 mg/m²/dose every 2-4 hours after chemotherapy for a total of 4-6 doses/day; increase doses in increments of 2.5 mg/m² to a maximum of 15 mg/m²/dose.

Appetite stimulant: Initial: 2.5 mg twice daily (before lunch and dinner); titrate up to a maximum of 20 mg/day.

Monitoring Parameters CNS effects, heart rate, blood pressure

Reference Range Antinauseant effects: 5-10 ng/mL

Test Interactions ↓ FSH, ↓ LH, ↓ growth hormone, ↓ testosterone

Patient Information Avoid activities such as driving which require motor coordination, avoid alcohol and other CNS depressants; may impair coordination and judgment

Nursing Implications Raise bed rails, institute safety measures, assist with ambulation

Dosage Forms Capsule: 2.5 mg, 5 mg, 10 mg

Droperidol (droe PER i dole)

U.S. Brand Names Inapsine®

Therapeutic Category Antiemetic; Antipsychotic Agent, Miscellaneous

Use Antiemetic in surgical and diagnostic procedures; preoperative medication in patients when other treatments are ineffective or inappropriate

Pregnancy Risk Factor C

Pregnancy/Breast-Feeding Implications

Clinical effects on the fetus: Crosses the placenta

Breast-feeding/lactation: No data available

Contraindications Hypersensitivity to droperidol or any component of the formulation; known or suspected QT prolongation, including congenital long QT syndrome (prolonged QT_c is defined as >440 msec in males or >450 msec in females)

Warnings/Precautions Droperidol should be reserved for patients who fail to respond or do not tolerate other treatments. May alter cardiac conduction. Cases of QT prolongation and torsade de pointes have been reported, including some fatal cases, in patients treated within or even below normal dosage range. A 12-lead EKG is recommended prior to initiation; continued monitoring is recommended for 2-3 hours. Use extreme caution in patients with bradycardia (<50 bpm), cardiac disease, concurrent MAOI therapy, Class I and Class III antiarrhythmics or other drugs known to prolong QT interval, and electrolyte disturbances (hypokalemia or hypomagnesemia), including concomitant drugs which may alter electrolytes (diuretics).

Use with caution in patients with seizures, bone marrow suppression, or severe liver disease. May be sedating, use with caution in disorders where CNS depression is a feature. Caution in patients with hemodynamic instability, predisposition to seizures, subcortical brain damage, renal or respiratory disease. Esophageal dysmotility and aspiration have been associated (Continued)

Droperidol *(Continued)*

with antipsychotic use - use with caution in patients at risk of pneumonia (ie, Alzheimer's disease). Caution in breast cancer or other prolactin-dependent tumors (may elevate prolactin levels). May alter temperature regulation or mask toxicity of other drugs due to antiemetic effects. May cause orthostatic hypotension - use with caution in patients at risk of this effect or those who would tolerate transient hypotensive episodes (cerebrovascular disease, cardiovascular disease, or other medications which may predispose). Significant hypotension may occur; injection contains benzyl alcohol; injection also contains sulfites which may cause allergic reaction.

May cause anticholinergic effects (confusion, agitation, constipation, dry mouth, blurred vision, urinary retention). Therefore, they should be used with caution in patients with decreased gastrointestinal motility, urinary retention, BPH, xerostomia, or visual problems. Conditions which also may be exacerbated by cholinergic blockade include narrow-angle glaucoma (screening is recommended) and worsening of myasthenia gravis. Relative to other neuroleptics, droperidol has a low potency of cholinergic blockade.

May cause extrapyramidal symptoms, including pseudoparkinsonism, acute dystonic reactions, akathisia, and tardive dyskinesia (risk of these reactions is high relative to other neuroleptics). May be associated with neuroleptic malignant syndrome (NMS) or pigmentary retinopathy. Safety in children <6 months of age has not been established.

Adverse Reactions EKG changes, retinal pigmentation are more common than with chlorpromazine. Relative to other neuroleptics, droperidol has a low potency of cholinergic blockade.

>10%:
 Cardiovascular: QT_c prolongation (dose-dependent)
 Central nervous system: Restlessness, anxiety, extrapyramidal reactions, dystonic reactions, pseudoparkinsonian signs and symptoms, tardive dyskinesia, neuroleptic malignant syndrome (NMS), seizures, altered central temperature regulation, akathisia
 Endocrine & metabolic: Swelling of breasts
 Gastrointestinal: Weight gain, constipation
1% to 10%:
 Cardiovascular: Hypotension (especially orthostatic), tachycardia, abnormal T waves with prolonged ventricular repolarization
 Central nervous system: Hallucinations, sedation, drowsiness, persistent tardive dyskinesia
 Gastrointestinal: Nausea, vomiting
 Genitourinary: Dysuria
<1% (Limited to important or life-threatening): Adynamic ileus, agranulocytosis, alopecia, arrhythmia, cholestatic jaundice, decreased visual acuity (may be irreversible), heat stroke, hyperpigmentation, laryngospasm, leukopenia, neuroleptic malignant syndrome (NMS), obstructive jaundice, photosensitivity (rare), priapism, rash, respiratory depression, retinal pigmentation, tardive dystonia, torsade de pointes, urinary retention, ventricular tachycardia

Overdosage/Toxicology Symptoms include hypotension, tachycardia, hallucinations, and extrapyramidal symptoms. Prolonged QT interval, seizures, and arrhythmias have been reported. Following initiation of essential overdose management, toxic symptom and supportive treatment should be initiated. Hypotension usually responds to I.V. fluids or Trendelenburg positioning. If unresponsive to these measures, the use of a parenteral inotrope may be required (eg, norepinephrine 0.1-0.2 mcg/kg/minute titrated to response). Seizures commonly respond to diazepam (I.V. 5-10 mg bolus in adults every 15 minutes, if needed, up to a total of 30 mg; I.V. 0.25-0.4 mg/kg/dose up to a total of 10 mg in children) or to phenytoin or phenobarbital. Arrhythmia management is per ACLS protocols (**Note:** Potential for QT prolongation and/or torsade de pointes). Neuroleptics often cause extrapyramidal symptoms (eg, dystonic reactions) requiring management with diphenhydramine 1-2 mg/kg (adults), up to a maximum of 50 mg I.M. or slow I.V. push, followed by a maintenance dose for 48-72 hours. When these reactions are unresponsive to diphenhydramine, anticholinergic agents such as benztropine mesylate I.V. 1-2 mg (adults) may be effective. These agents are generally effective within 2-5 minutes.

Drug Interactions
 Increased Effect/Toxicity: Droperidol in combination with certain forms of conduction anesthesia may produce peripheral vasodilitation and hypotension. Droperidol and CNS depressants will likely have additive CNS effects. Droperidol and cyclobenzaprine may have an additive effect on prolonging the QT interval. Use caution with other agents known to prolong QT interval (Class I or Class III antiarrhythmics, some quinolone antibiotics, cisapride, some phenothiazines, pimozide, tricyclic antidepressants). Potassium- or magnesium-depleting agents (diuretics, aminoglycosides, amphotericin B, cyclosporine) may increase risk of arrhythmias.

Stability
 Droperidol ampuls/vials should be stored at room temperature and protected from light
 Stability of parenteral admixture at room temperature (25°C): 7 days
 Standard diluent: 2.5 mg/50 mL D_5W
 Incompatible with barbiturates

Mechanism of Action Butyrophenone derivative that produces tranquilization, sedation, and an antiemetic effect; other effects include alpha-adrenergic blockade, peripheral vascular dilation, and reduction of the pressor effect of epinephrine resulting in hypotension and decreased peripheral vascular resistance; may also reduce pulmonary artery pressure

Pharmacodynamics/Kinetics
 Onset of action: Peak effect: Parenteral: ~30 minutes
 Duration: Parenteral: 2-4 hours, may extend to 12 hours
 Metabolism: Hepatic
 Half-life elimination: Adults: 2.3 hours
 Excretion: Urine (75%); feces (22%)

Usual Dosage Titrate carefully to desired effect

Children 2-12 years: Nausea and vomiting: I.M., I.V.: 0.05-0.06 mg/kg (maximum initial dose: 0.1 mg/kg); additional doses may be repeated to achieve effect; administer additional doses with caution

Adults: Nausea and vomiting: I.M., I.V.: Initial: 2.5 mg; additional doses of 1.25 mg may be administered to achieve desired effect; administer additional doses with caution

Administration Administer I.M. or I.V.; I.V. should be administered slow IVP (over 2-5 minutes) or IVPB; EKG monitoring for 2-3 hours after administration is recommended

Monitoring Parameters To identify QT prolongation, a 12-lead EKG prior to use is recommended (use is contraindicated); continued EKG monitoring for 2-3 hours following administration is recommended. Blood pressure, heart rate, respiratory rate; observe for dystonias, extrapyramidal side effects, and temperature changes; serum potassium and magnesium levels

Nursing Implications
Parenteral: I.V. over 2-5 minutes
Monitor blood pressure, heart rate, respiratory rate

Additional Information Does not possess analgesic effects; has little or no amnesic properties.

Dosage Forms Solution for injection: 2.5 mg/mL (1 mL, 2 mL)

♦ **Drospirenone and Ethinyl Estradiol** see Ethinyl Estradiol and Drospirenone on page 511

Drotrecogin Alfa (dro TRE coe jin AL fa)

U.S. Brand Names Xigris™

Synonyms Activated Protein C, Human, Recombinant; Drotrecogin Alfa, Activated; Protein C (Activated), Human, Recombinant

Therapeutic Category Protein C (Activated)

Use Reduction of mortality from severe sepsis (associated with organ dysfunction) in adults at high risk of death (eg, APACHE II score ≥25)

Pregnancy Risk Factor C

Contraindications Hypersensitivity to drotrecogin alfa or any component of the formulation; active internal bleeding; recent hemorrhagic stroke (within 3 months); severe head trauma (within 2 months); recent intracranial or intraspinal surgery (within 2 months); intracranial neoplasm or mass lesion; evidence of cerebral herniation; presence of an epidural catheter; trauma with an increased risk of life-threatening bleeding

Warnings/Precautions Increases risk of bleeding; careful evaluation of risks and benefit is required prior to initiation (see Contraindications). Bleeding risk is increased in patients receiving concurrent therapeutic heparin, oral anticoagulants, glycoprotein IIb/IIIa antagonists, platelet aggregation inhibitors, or aspirin at a dosage of >650 mg/day (within 7 days). In addition, an increased bleeding risk is associated with prolonged INR (>3.0), gastrointestinal bleeding (within 6 weeks), decreased platelet count (<30,000/mm³), chronic dialysis patients (within 3 days), recent ischemic stroke (within 3 months), intracranial AV malformation or aneurysm, known bleeding diathesis, severe hepatic disease (chronic), or other condition where bleeding is a significant hazard or difficult to manage due to its location. Discontinue if significant bleeding occurs (may consider continued use after stabilization). Treatment interruption required for invasive procedures. APTT cannot be used to assess coagulopathy during treatment (PT/INR not affected).

Efficacy not established in adult patients at a low risk of death. Patients with pre-existing nonsepsis-related medical conditions with a poor prognosis (anticipated survival <28 days), HIV-infected patients with a CD4 count ≤50 cells/mm³, chronic dialysis patients, pre-existing hypercoagulable conditions, and patients who had received bone marrow, liver, lung, pancreas, or small bowel transplants were excluded from the clinical trial which established benefit. In addition, patients with a high body weight (>135 kg) were not evaluated. Safety and efficacy have not been established in pediatric patients.

Adverse Reactions As with all drugs which may affect hemostasis, bleeding is the major adverse effect associated with drotrecogin alfa. Hemorrhage may occur at virtually any site. Risk is dependent on multiple variables, including the dosage administered, concurrent use of multiple agents which alter hemostasis, and patient predisposition.

>10%
Dermatologic: Bruising
Gastrointestinal: Gastrointestinal bleeding

1% to 10%: Hematologic: Bleeding (serious 2.4% during infusion vs 3.5% during 28-day study period; individual events listed as <1%)

<1% (Limited to important or life-threatening): Gastrointestinal hemorrhage, genitourinary bleeding, immune reaction (antibody production), intracranial hemorrhage (0.2%; frequencies up to 2% noted in a previous trial without placebo control), intrathoracic hemorrhage, retroperitoneal bleeding, skin/soft tissue bleeding

Overdosage/Toxicology There has been no reported experience with overdose. Hemorrhagic complications are likely consequences of overdose. Treatment is supportive including immediate interruption of the infusion and monitoring for hemorrhagic complications. There is no known antidote.

Drug Interactions
Increased Effect/Toxicity: Concurrent use of antiplatelet agents, including aspirin (>650 mg/day, recent use within 7 days), cilostazol, clopidogrel, dipyridamole, ticlopidine, NSAIDs, or glycoprotein IIb/IIIa antagonists (recent use within 7 days) may increase risk of bleeding. Concurrent use of low molecular weight heparins or heparin at therapeutic rates of infusion may increase the risk of bleeding. However, the use of low-dose prophylactic heparin does not appear to affect safety. Recent use of thrombolytic agents (within 3 days) may increase the risk of bleeding. Recent use of warfarin (within 7 days or elevation of INR ≥3) may increase the risk of bleeding. Other drugs which interfere with coagulation may increase risk of bleeding (including antithrombin III, danaparoid, direct thrombin inhibitors).

Ethanol/Nutrition/Herb Interactions Herb/Nutraceutical: Recent use/intake of herbs with anticoagulant or antiplatelet activity (including cat's claw, feverfew, garlic, ginkgo, ginseng, and horse chestnut seed) may increase the risk of bleeding.

(Continued)

Drotrecogin Alfa *(Continued)*

Stability Store vials under refrigeration at 2°C to 8°C (36°F to 46°F). Protect from light. Do not freeze. Reconstitute 5 mg vials with 2.5 mL and 20 mg vials with 10 mL sterile water for injection (resultant concentration ~2 mg/mL). Must be further diluted (within 3 hours of reconstitution) in 0.9% sodium chloride, typically to a concentration between 100 mcg/mL and 200 mcg/mL when using infusion pump and between 100 mcg/mL and 1000 mcg/mL when infused via syringe pump. Although product information states administration must be completed within 12 hours of preparation, additional studies (data on file, Lilly Research Laboratories) show that the final solution is stable for 14 hours at 15°C to 30°C (59°F to 86°F). If not used immediately, a prepared solution may be stored in the refrigerator for up to 12 hours. The total expiration time (refrigeration and administration) should be ≤24 hours from time of preparation.

Mechanism of Action Inhibits factors Va and VIIIa, limiting thrombotic effects. Additional *in vitro* data suggest inhibition of plasminogen activator inhibitor-1 (PAF-1) resulting in profibrinolytic activity, inhibition of macrophage production of tumor necrosis factor, blocking of leukocyte adhesion, and limitation of thrombin-induced inflammatory responses. Relative contribution of effects on the reduction of mortality from sepsis is not completely understood.

Pharmacodynamics/Kinetics

Duration: Plasma nondetectable within 2 hours of discontinuation

Metabolism: Inactivated by endogenous plasma protease inhibitors; mean clearance: 40 L/hour; increased with severe sepsis (~50%)

Half-life elimination: 1.6 hours

Usual Dosage I.V.: Adults: 24 mcg/kg/hour for a total of 96 hours; stop infusion **immediately** if clinically-important bleeding is identified

Dosage adjustment in renal impairment: No specific adjustment recommended.

Administration Infuse separately from all other medications. Only dextrose, normal saline, dextrose/saline combinations, and lactated Ringer's solution may be infused through the same line. May administer via infusion pump or syringe pump. Administration of prepared solution must be completed within 12 hours of preparation. Suspend administration for 2 hours prior to invasive procedures or other procedure with significant bleeding risk; may continue treatment immediately following uncomplicated, minimally-invasive procedures, but delay for 12 hours after major invasive procedures/surgery.

Monitoring Parameters Monitor for signs and symptoms of bleeding, hemoglobin/hematocrit, PT/INR, platelet count

Test Interactions May interfere with one-stage coagulation assays based on the aPTT (such as factor VIII, IX, and XI assays).

Additional Information Prepared by recombinant DNA technology in human cell line

Dosage Forms Powder for injection [preservative free]: 5 mg, 20 mg

Dyclonine (DYE kloe neen)

U.S. Brand Names Dyclone®; Sucrets® [OTC]
Synonyms Dyclonine Hydrochloride
Therapeutic Category Local Anesthetic, Mucous Membrane; Local Anesthetic, Oral
Use Local anesthetic prior to laryngoscopy, bronchoscopy, or endotracheal intubation; use topically for temporary relief of pain associated with oral mucosa or anogenital lesions
Pregnancy Risk Factor C
Usual Dosage Use the lowest dose needed to provide effective anesthesia
Children and Adults:
Topical solution:
Mouth sores: 5-10 mL of 0.5% or 1% to oral mucosa (swab or swish and then spit) 3-4 times/day as needed; maximum single dose: 200 mg (40 mL of 0.5% solution or 20 mL of 1% solution)
Bronchoscopy: Use 2 mL of the 1% solution or 4 mL of the 0.5% solution sprayed onto the larynx and trachea every 5 minutes until the reflex has been abolished
Children >2 years and Adults: Lozenge: Slowly dissolve 1 lozenge in mouth every 2 hours as needed
Additional Information Complete prescribing information for this medication should be consulted for additional detail.
Dosage Forms
Lozenge, as hydrochloride: 1.2 mg, 2 mg, 3 mg
Solution, topical, as hydrochloride: 0.5% (30 mL); 1% (30 mL)

- ◆ **Dyclonine Hydrochloride** see Dyclonine on page 455
- ◆ **Dyflos** see Isoflurophate on page 747
- ◆ **Dymelor® [DSC]** see AcetoHEXAMIDE on page 31
- ◆ **Dynabac®** see Dirithromycin on page 423
- ◆ **Dynacin®** see Minocycline on page 918
- ◆ **DynaCirc®** see Isradipine on page 755
- ◆ **DynaCirc® CR** see Isradipine on page 755
- ◆ **Dyna-Hex® [OTC]** see Chlorhexidine Gluconate on page 275
- ◆ **Dyrenium®** see Triamterene on page 1369
- ◆ **E₂C and MPA** see Estradiol Cypionate and Medroxyprogesterone Acetate on page 495
- ◆ **7E3** see Abciximab on page 17
- ◆ **E2020** see Donepezil on page 434
- ◆ **Easprin®** see Aspirin on page 120

Echothiophate Iodide (ek oh THYE oh fate EYE oh dide)

Related Information
Glaucoma Drug Therapy Comparison on page 1499
U.S. Brand Names Phospholine Iodide®
Canadian Brand Names Phospholine Iodide®
Synonyms Ecostigmine Iodide
Therapeutic Category Ophthalmic Agent, Miotic
Use Used as miotic in treatment of open-angle glaucoma; may be useful in specific case of narrow-angle glaucoma; accommodative esotropia
Pregnancy Risk Factor C
Usual Dosage Adults:
Ophthalmic: Glaucoma: Instill 1 drop twice daily into eyes with 1 dose just prior to bedtime; some patients have been treated with 1 dose daily or every other day
Accommodative esotropia:
Diagnosis: Instill 1 drop of 0.125% once daily into both eyes at bedtime for 2-3 weeks
Treatment: Use lowest concentration and frequency which gives satisfactory response, with a maximum dose of 0.125% once daily, although more intensive therapy may be used for short periods of time
Additional Information Complete prescribing information for this medication should be consulted for additional detail.
Dosage Forms Powder for reconstitution, ophthalmic: 1.5 mg [0.03%] (5 mL); 3 mg [0.06%] (5 mL); 6.25 mg [0.125%] (5 mL); 12.5 mg [0.25%] (5 mL)

- ◆ **EC-Naprosyn®** see Naproxen on page 958
- ◆ **E. coli Asparaginase** see Asparaginase on page 118
- ◆ **E-Complex-600® [OTC]** see Vitamin E on page 1423

Econazole (e KONE a zole)

U.S. Brand Names Spectazole™
Canadian Brand Names Ecostatin®; Spectazole™
Synonyms Econazole Nitrate
Therapeutic Category Antifungal Agent, Topical
Use Topical treatment of tinea pedis (athlete's foot), tinea cruris (jock itch), tinea corporis (ringworm), tinea versicolor, and cutaneous candidiasis
Pregnancy Risk Factor C
Pregnancy/Breast-Feeding Implications Clinical effect on the fetus: Do not use during the 1st trimester of pregnancy, unless essential to a patient's welfare; use during the second and third trimesters only if clearly needed
Contraindications Hypersensitivity to econazole or any component of the formulation
Warnings/Precautions Discontinue drug if sensitivity or chemical irritation occurs; not for ophthalmic or intravaginal use
Adverse Reactions
1% to 10%: Genitourinary: Vulvar/vaginal burning
<1% (Limited to important or life-threatening): Burning or itching of penis of sexual partner; polyuria; vulvar itching, soreness, edema, or discharge
(Continued)

Econazole *(Continued)*

Mechanism of Action Alters fungal cell wall membrane permeability; may interfere with RNA and protein synthesis, and lipid metabolism

Pharmacodynamics/Kinetics
Absorption: <10%
Metabolism: Hepatic to more than 20 metabolites
Excretion: Urine; feces (<1%)

Usual Dosage Children and Adults: Topical:
Tinea pedis, tinea cruris, tinea corporis, tinea versicolor: Apply sufficient amount to cover affected areas once daily
Cutaneous candidiasis: Apply sufficient quantity twice daily (morning and evening)
Duration of treatment: Candidal infections and tinea cruris, versicolor, and corporis should be treated for 2 weeks and tinea pedis for 1 month; occasionally, longer treatment periods may be required

Patient Information For external use only; avoid eye contact; if condition worsens or persists, or irritation occurs, notify physician

Nursing Implications Candidal infections and tinea cruris, versicolor, and corporis should be treated for 2 weeks and tinea pedis for 1 month; occasionally, longer treatment periods may be required

Dosage Forms Cream, topical, as nitrate: 1% (15 g, 30 g, 85 g)

Edetate Calcium Disodium (ED e tate KAL see um dye SOW dee um)

U.S. Brand Names Calcium Disodium Versenate®

Synonyms Calcium Disodium Edetate; Calcium EDTA

Therapeutic Category Antidote, Lead Toxicity

Use Treatment of symptomatic acute and chronic lead poisoning or for symptomatic patients with high blood lead levels; used as an aid in the diagnosis of lead poisoning; possibly useful in poisoning by zinc, manganese, and certain heavy radioisotopes

Pregnancy Risk Factor B

Contraindications Severe renal disease, anuria

Warnings/Precautions Potentially nephrotoxic; renal tubular acidosis and fatal nephrosis may occur, especially with high doses; EKG changes may occur during therapy; do not exceed recommended daily dose; avoid rapid I.V. infusion in the management of lead encephalopathy, may increase intracranial pressure to lethal levels. If anuria, increasing proteinuria, or hematuria occurs during therapy, discontinue calcium EDTA. Minimize nephrotoxicity by adequate hydration, establishment of good urine output, avoidance of excessive doses, and limitation of continuous administration to ≤5 days.

Adverse Reactions Frequency not defined.
Cardiovascular: Arrhythmias, EKG changes, hypotension
Central nervous system: Chills, fever, headache
Dermatologic: Cheilosis, skin lesions
Endocrine & metabolic: Hypercalcemia
Gastrointestinal: Anorexia, GI upset, nausea, vomiting
Hematologic: Anemia, bone marrow suppression (transient)
Hepatic: Liver function test increased (mild)
Local: Thrombophlebitis following I.V. infusion (when concentration >5 mg/mL), pain at injection site following I.M. injection
Neuromuscular & skeletal: Arthralgia, numbness, tremor, paresthesia
Ocular: Lacrimation
Renal: Renal tubular necrosis, microscopic hematuria, proteinuria
Respiratory: Nasal congestion, sneezing
Miscellaneous: Zinc deficiency

Drug Interactions
Decreased Effect: Do not use simultaneously with zinc insulin preparations; do not mix in the same syringe with dimercaprol.

Stability Dilute with 0.9% sodium chloride or D_5W; physically **incompatible** with $D_{10}W$, LR, Ringer's injection

Mechanism of Action Calcium is displaced by divalent and trivalent heavy metals, forming a nonionizing soluble complex that is excreted in urine

Pharmacodynamics/Kinetics
Onset of action: Chelation of lead: I.V.: 1 hour
Absorption: I.M., S.C.: Well absorbed
Distribution: Into extracellular fluid; minimal CSF penetration
Half-life elimination, plasma: I.M.: 1.5 hours; I.V.: 20 minutes
Excretion: Urine (as metal chelates or unchanged drug); decreased GFR decreases elimination

Usual Dosage Several regimens have been recommended:

Diagnosis of lead poisoning: Mobilization test (not recommended by AAP guidelines): I.M., I.V.:

Children: 500 mg/m^2/dose (maximum dose: 1 g) as a single dose or divided into 2 doses

Adults: 500 mg/m^2/dose

Note: Urine is collected for 24 hours after first EDTA dose and analyzed for lead content; if the ratio of mcg of lead in urine to mg calcium EDTA given is >1, then test is considered positive; for convenience, an 8-hour urine collection may be done after a single 50 mg/kg I.M. (maximum dose: 1 g) or 500 mg/m^2 I.V. dose; a positive test occurs if the ratio of lead excretion to mg calcium EDTA >0.5-0.6.

Treatment of lead poisoning: Children and Adults (each regimen is specific for route):

Symptoms of lead encephalopathy and/or blood lead level >70 mcg/dL: Treat 5 days; give in conjunction with dimercaprol; wait a minimum of 2 days with no treatment before considering a repeat course:

I.M.: 250 mg/m^2/dose every 4 hours

I.V.: 50 mg/kg/day as 24-hour continuous I.V. infusion **or** 1-1.5 g/m^2 I.V. as either an 8- to 24-hour infusion or divided into 2 doses every 12 hours

Symptomatic lead poisoning **without** encephalopathy **or** asymptomatic with blood lead level >70 mcg/dL: Treat 3-5 days; treatment with dimercaprol is recommended until the blood lead level concentration <50 mcg/dL:

I.M.: 167 mg/m^2 every 4 hours

I.V.: 1 g/m^2 as an 8- to 24-hour infusion or divided every 12 hours

Asymptomatic **children** with blood lead level 45-69 mcg/dL: I.V.: 25 mg/kg/day for 5 days as an 8- to 24-hour infusion or divided into 2 doses every 12 hours

Depending upon the blood lead level, additional courses may be necessary; repeat at least 2-4 days and preferably 2-4 weeks apart

Adults with lead nephropathy: An alternative dosing regimen reflecting the reduction in renal clearance is based upon the serum creatinine. Refer to the following:

Dose of Ca EDTA based on serum creatinine:

S_{cr} ≤2 mg/dL: 1 g/m^2/day for 5 days*

S_{cr} 2-3 mg/dL: 500 mg/m^2/day for 5 days*

S_{cr} 3-4 mg/dL: 500 mg/m^2/dose every 48 hours for 3 doses*

S_{cr} >4 mg/dL: 500 mg/m^2/week*

*Repeat these regimens monthly until lead excretion is reduced toward normal.

Administration For intermittent I.V. infusion, administer the dose I.V. over at least 1 hour in asymptomatic patients, 2 hours in symptomatic patients; for I.V. continuous infusion, dilute to 2-4 mg/mL in D$_5$W or NS and infuse over at least 8 hours, usually over 12-24 hours; for I.M. injection, 1 mL of 1% procaine hydrochloride may be added to each mL of EDTA calcium to minimize pain at injection site

Monitoring Parameters BUN, creatinine, urinalysis, I & O, and EKG during therapy; intravenous administration requires a cardiac monitor, blood and urine lead concentrations

Test Interactions If calcium EDTA is given as a continuous I.V. infusion, stop the infusion for at least 1 hour before blood is drawn for lead concentration to avoid a falsely elevated value

Dosage Forms Injection: 200 mg/mL (5 mL)

Edetate Disodium (ED e tate dye SOW dee um)

U.S. Brand Names Chealamide®; Disotate®; Endrate®

Synonyms Edathamil Disodium; EDTA; Sodium Edetate

Therapeutic Category Antidote, Hypercalcemia; Chelating Agent, Parenteral

Use Emergency treatment of hypercalcemia; control digitalis-induced cardiac dysrhythmias (ventricular arrhythmias)

Pregnancy Risk Factor C

Contraindications Severe renal failure or anuria

Warnings/Precautions Use of this drug is recommended only when the severity of the clinical condition justifies the aggressive measures associated with this type of therapy; use with caution in patients with renal dysfunction, intracranial lesions, seizure disorders, coronary or peripheral vascular disease

Adverse Reactions Rapid I.V. administration or excessive doses may cause a sudden drop in serum calcium concentration which may lead to hypocalcemic tetany, seizures, arrhythmias, and death from respiratory arrest. Do **not** exceed recommended dosage and rate of administration.

1% to 10%: Gastrointestinal: Nausea, vomiting, abdominal cramps, diarrhea

<1% (Limited to important or life-threatening): Acute tubular necrosis, anemia, arrhythmias, back pain, chills, death from respiratory arrest, dermatologic lesions, eruptions, fever, headache, hypokalemia, hypomagnesemia, muscle cramps, nephrotoxicity, pain at the site of injection, paresthesia may occur, seizures, tetany, thrombophlebitis, transient hypotension

Overdosage/Toxicology Symptoms include hypotension, dysrhythmias, tetany, and seizures. Treatment includes immediate I.V. calcium salts for hypocalcemia-related adverse reactions. Replace calcium cautiously in patients on digitalis.

Drug Interactions

Increased Effect/Toxicity: Increased effect of insulin (edetate disodium may decrease blood glucose concentrations and reduce insulin requirements in diabetic patients treated with insulin).

Mechanism of Action Chelates with divalent or trivalent metals to form a soluble complex that is then eliminated in urine

Pharmacodynamics/Kinetics

Metabolism: None

Half-life elimination: 20-60 minutes

Time to peak: I.V.: 24-48 hours

Excretion: Following chelation: Urine (95%); chelates within 24-48 hours

(Continued)

Edetate Disodium *(Continued)*

Usual Dosage Hypercalcemia: I.V.:

Children: 40-70 mg/kg/day slow infusion over 3-4 hours or more to a maximum of 3 g/24 hours; administer for 5 days and allow 5 days between courses of therapy

Adults: 50 mg/kg/day over 3 or more hours to a maximum of 3 g/24 hours; a suggested regimen of 5 days followed by 2 days without drug and repeated courses up to 15 total doses

Digitalis-induced arrhythmias: Children and Adults: 15 mg/kg/hour (maximum dose: 60 mg/kg/day) as continuous infusion

Administration Parenteral: I.V.: Must be diluted before I.V. use in D_5W or NS to a maximum concentration of 30 mg/mL (3%) and infused over at least 3 hours; avoid extravasation; not for I.M. use

Monitoring Parameters Cardiac function (EKG monitoring); blood pressure during infusion; renal function should be assessed before and during therapy; monitor calcium, magnesium, and potassium levels; cardiac monitor required

Nursing Implications Avoid extravasation; patient should remain supine for a short period after infusion; infuse over 3-4 hours

Additional Information Sodium content of 1 g: 5.4 mEq

Dosage Forms Injection: 150 mg/mL (20 mL)

♦ **Edex®** *see* Alprostadil *on page 57*

Edrophonium *(ed roe FOE nee um)*

U.S. Brand Names Enlon®; Reversol®; Tensilon®

Canadian Brand Names Enlon®

Synonyms Edrophonium Chloride

Therapeutic Category Antidote, Neuromuscular Blocking Agent; Cholinergic Agent; Diagnostic Agent, Myasthenia Gravis

Use Diagnosis of myasthenia gravis; differentiation of cholinergic crises from myasthenia crises; reversal of nondepolarizing neuromuscular blockers; adjunct treatment of respiratory depression caused by curare overdose

Pregnancy Risk Factor C

Contraindications Hypersensitivity to edrophonium, sulfites, or any component of the formulation; GI or GU obstruction

Warnings/Precautions Use with caution in patients with bronchial asthma and those receiving a cardiac glycoside; atropine sulfate should always be readily available as an antagonist. Overdosage can cause cholinergic crisis which may be fatal. I.V. atropine should be readily available for treatment of cholinergic reactions.

Adverse Reactions Frequency not defined.

Cardiovascular: Arrhythmias (especially bradycardia), hypotension, decreased carbon monoxide, tachycardia, AV block, nodal rhythm, nonspecific EKG changes, cardiac arrest, syncope, flushing

Central nervous system: Convulsions, dysarthria, dysphonia, dizziness, loss of consciousness, drowsiness, headache

Dermatologic: Skin rash, thrombophlebitis (I.V.), urticaria

Gastrointestinal: Hyperperistalsis, nausea, vomiting, salivation, diarrhea, stomach cramps, dysphagia, flatulence

Genitourinary: Urinary urgency

Neuromuscular & skeletal: Weakness, fasciculations, muscle cramps, spasms, arthralgias

Ocular: Small pupils, lacrimation

Respiratory: Increased bronchial secretions, laryngospasm, bronchiolar constriction, respiratory muscle paralysis, dyspnea, respiratory depression, respiratory arrest, bronchospasm

Miscellaneous: Diaphoresis (increased), anaphylaxis, allergic reactions

Overdosage/Toxicology Symptoms include muscle weakness, nausea, vomiting, miosis, bronchospasm, and respiratory paralysis. Maintain an adequate airway. For muscarinic symptoms, the antidote is atropine. Pralidoxime (2-PAM) may also be needed to reverse severe muscle weakness or paralysis. Skeletal muscle effects of edrophonium are not alleviated by atropine.

Drug Interactions

Increased Effect/Toxicity: Digoxin may enhance bradycardia potential of edrophonium. Effects of succinylcholine, decamethonium, nondepolarizing muscle relaxants (eg, pancuronium, vecuronium) are prolonged by edrophonium. I.V. acetazolamide, neostigmine, physostigmine, and acute muscle weakness may increase the effects of edrophonium.

Decreased Effect: Atropine, nondepolarizing muscle relaxants, procainamide, and quinidine may antagonize the effects of edrophonium.

Mechanism of Action Inhibits destruction of acetylcholine by acetylcholinesterase. This facilitates transmission of impulses across myoneural junction and results in increased cholinergic responses such as miosis, increased tonus of intestinal and skeletal muscles, bronchial and ureteral constriction, bradycardia, and increased salivary and sweat gland secretions.

Pharmacodynamics/Kinetics

Onset of action: I.M.: 2-10 minutes; I.V.: 30-60 seconds

Duration: I.M.: 5-30 minutes: I.V.: 10 minutes

Distribution: V_d: 1.1 L/kg

Half-life elimination: 1.8 hours

Usual Dosage Usually administered I.V., however, if not possible, I.M. or S.C. may be used:

Infants:

I.M.: 0.5-1 mg

I.V.: Initial: 0.1 mg, followed by 0.4 mg if no response; total dose = 0.5 mg

Children:

Diagnosis: Initial: 0.04 mg/kg over 1 minute followed by 0.16 mg/kg if no response, to a maximum total dose of 5 mg for children <34 kg, or 10 mg for children >34 kg

I.M.:

<34 kg: 1 mg

>34 kg: 5 mg

Titration of oral anticholinesterase therapy: 0.04 mg/kg once given 1 hour after oral intake of the drug being used in treatment; if strength improves, an increase in neostigmine or pyridostigmine dose is indicated

Adults:

Diagnosis:

I.V.: 2 mg test dose administered over 15-30 seconds; 8 mg given 45 seconds later if no response is seen; test dose may be repeated after 30 minutes

I.M.: Initial: 10 mg; if no cholinergic reaction occurs, administer 2 mg 30 minutes later to rule out false-negative reaction

Titration of oral anticholinesterase therapy: 1-2 mg given 1 hour after oral dose of anticholinesterase; if strength improves, an increase in neostigmine or pyridostigmine dose is indicated

Reversal of nondepolarizing neuromuscular blocking agents (neostigmine with atropine usually preferred): I.V.: 10 mg over 30-45 seconds; may repeat every 5-10 minutes up to 40 mg

Termination of paroxysmal atrial tachycardia: I.V. rapid injection: 5-10 mg

Differentiation of cholinergic from myasthenic crisis: I.V.: 1 mg; may repeat after 1 minute. **Note:** Intubation and controlled ventilation may be required if patient has cholinergic crisis

Dosing adjustment in renal impairment: Dose may need to be reduced in patients with chronic renal failure

Administration Edrophonium is administered by direct I.V. injection; see Usual Dosage

Test Interactions ↑ aminotransferase [ALT (SGPT)/AST (SGOT)] (S), amylase (S)

Nursing Implications

Parenteral: Edrophonium is administered by direct I.V. injection

Monitor pre- and postinjection strength (cranial musculature is most useful); heart rate, respiratory rate, blood pressure

Additional Information Atropine should be administered along with edrophonium when reversing the effects of nondepolarizing agents to antagonize the cholinergic effects at the muscarinic receptors, especially bradycardia. It is important to recognize the difference in dose for diagnosis of myasthenia gravis versus reversal of muscle relaxant, a much larger dose is needed for desired effect of reversal of muscle paralysis.

Dosage Forms Injection, as chloride: 10 mg/mL (1 mL, 10 mL, 15 mL)

♦ **Edrophonium Chloride** see Edrophonium on page 458
♦ **ED-SPAZ**® see Hyoscyamine on page 692
♦ **EDTA** see Edetate Disodium on page 457
♦ **E.E.S.**® see Erythromycin (Systemic) on page 486

Efavirenz (e FAV e renz)

Related Information

Antiretroviral Agents Comparison on page 1488
Antiretroviral Therapy for HIV Infection on page 1595
Management of Healthcare Worker Exposures to HIV, HBV, HCV on page 1555

U.S. Brand Names Sustiva®

Canadian Brand Names Sustiva®

Therapeutic Category Antiretroviral Agent, Non-nucleoside Reverse Transcriptase Inhibitor (NNRTI)

Use Treatment of HIV-1 infections in combination with at least two other antiretroviral agents. Also has some activity against hepatitis B virus and herpes viruses.

Pregnancy Risk Factor C

Pregnancy/Breast-Feeding Implications Teratogenic effects have been observed in Primates receiving efavirenz; no studies in pregnant humans are currently planned. Pregnancy should be avoided. Women of childbearing potential should undergo pregnancy testing prior to initiation of efavirenz. Barrier contraception should be used in combination with other (hormonal) methods of contraception. Health professionals are encouraged to contact the antiretroviral pregnancy registry to monitor outcomes of pregnant women exposed to antiretroviral medications (1-800-258-4263).

Contraindications Clinically significant hypersensitivity efavirenz or any component of the formulation

Warnings/Precautions Do not use as single-agent therapy; avoid pregnancy; women of childbearing potential should undergo pregnancy testing prior to initiation of therapy; do not administer with other agents metabolized by CYP3A4 isoenzyme including cisapride, midazolam, triazolam or ergot alkaloids (potential for life-threatening adverse effects); history of mental illness/drug abuse (predisposition to psychological reactions); serious psychiatric side effects have been associated with efavirenz, including severe depression, suicide, paranoia, and mania; discontinue if severe rash (involving blistering, desquamation, mucosal involvement or fever) develops. Caution in patients with known or suspected hepatitis B or C infection (monitoring of liver function is recommended); hepatic impairment. Children are more susceptible to development of rash - prophylactic antihistamines may be used. Concomitant use with St John's wort is not recommended.

Adverse Reactions

>10%:

Central nervous system: Dizziness* (2% to 28%), depression (1% to 16%), insomnia (6% to 16%), anxiety (1% to 11%), pain* (1% to 13%)

Dermatologic: Rash* (NCI grade 1: 9% to 11%; NCI grade 2: 15% to 32%)

Endocrine & metabolic: HDL increased (25% to 35%), total cholesterol increased (20% to 40%)

Gastrointestinal: Diarrhea* (3% to 14%), nausea* (2% to 12%)

1% to 10%:

Central nervous system: Impaired concentration (2% to 8%), headache* (2% to 7%), somnolence (2% to 7%), fatigue (2% to 7%), abnormal dreams (1% to 6%), nervousness (2% to 6%), severe depression (2%), hallucinations (1%)

(Continued)

Efavirenz *(Continued)*

Dermatologic: Pruritus (1% to 9%), diaphoresis increased (1% to 2%)

Gastrointestinal: Vomiting* (6% to 7%), dyspepsia (3%), abdominal pain (1% to 3%), anorexia (1% to 2%)

*Adverse effect reported in ≥10% of patients 3-16 years of age

<1% (Limited to important or life-threatening): Aggressive reaction, agitation, allergic reaction, body fat accumulation/redistribution, convulsions, liver failure, manic reaction, neuropathy, paranoid reaction, Stevens-Johnson syndrome, suicide, visual abnormality

Overdosage/Toxicology Increased central nervous system symptoms and involuntary muscle contractions have been reported in accidental overdose. Treatment is supportive. Activated charcoal may enhance elimination. Dialysis is unlikely to remove the drug.

Drug Interactions

Cytochrome P450 Effect: CYP2C9, 2C19, and CYP3A3/4 enzyme inhibitor; CYP3A4 enzyme inducer

Increased Effect/Toxicity: Coadministration with medications metabolized by these enzymes may lead to increased concentration-related effects. Cisapride, midazolam, triazolam, and ergot alkaloids may result in life-threatening toxicities; concurrent use is contraindicated. The AUC of nelfinavir is increased (20%); AUC of both ritonavir and efavirenz are increased by 20% during concurrent therapy. The AUC of ethinyl estradiol is increased 37% by efavirenz (clinical significance unknown). May increase (or decrease) effect of warfarin.

Decreased Effect: Other inducers of this enzyme (including phenobarbital, rifampin, rifabutin, and St John's wort) may decrease serum concentrations of efavirenz. Concentrations of indinavir may be reduced; dosage increase to 1000 mg 3 times/day is recommended. Concentrations of saquinavir may be decreased (use as sole protease inhibitor is not recommended). The AUC of amprenavir may be decreased (36%). Plasma concentrations of clarithromycin are decreased (clinical significance unknown). Serum concentrations of methadone are decreased; monitor for withdrawal. May decrease (or increase) effect of warfarin.

Ethanol/Nutrition/Herb Interactions

Ethanol: Avoid ethanol (hepatic and CNS adverse effects).

Food: Avoid high-fat meals (increase the absorption of efavirenz).

Herb/Nutraceutical: St John's wort may decrease efavirenz serum levels. Avoid concurrent use.

Stability Store below 25°C (77°F).

Mechanism of Action As a non-nucleoside reverse transcriptase inhibitor, efavirenz has activity against HIV-1 by binding to reverse transcriptase. It consequently blocks the RNA-dependent and DNA-dependent DNA polymerase activities including HIV-1 replication. It does not require intracellular phosphorylation for antiviral activity.

Pharmacodynamics/Kinetics

Absorption: Increased 50% by fatty meals

Distribution: CSF concentrations exceed free fraction in serum

Protein binding: >99%, primarily to albumin

Metabolism: Hepatic

Half-life elimination: Single dose: 52-76 hours; after multiple doses: 40-55 hours

Time to peak: 3-8 hours

Excretion: Urine (14% to 34% as metabolites); feces (16% to 41% primarily as unchanged drug)

Usual Dosage Oral: Dosing at bedtime is recommended to limit central nervous system effects; should not be used as single-agent therapy

Children: Dosage is based on body weight

10 kg to <15 kg: 200 mg once daily

15 kg to <20 kg: 250 mg once daily

20 kg to <25 kg: 300 mg once daily

25 kg to <32.5 kg: 350 mg once daily

32.5 kg to <40 kg: 400 mg once daily

≥40 kg: 600 mg once daily

Adults: 600 mg once daily

Dosing adjustment in renal impairment: None recommended

Dosing comments in hepatic impairment: Limited clinical experience, use with caution

Dietary Considerations Should be taken on an empty stomach.

Administration Administer on an empty stomach.

Monitoring Parameters Serum transaminases (discontinuation of treatment should be considered for persistent elevations greater than five times the upper limit of normal), cholesterol, triglycerides, signs and symptoms of infection

Test Interactions False positive test for cannabinoids have been reported when the CEDIA DAU Multilevel THC assay is used. False positive results with other assays for cannabinoids have not been observed.

Patient Information Take efavirenz exactly as prescribed; report all side effects to your physician; do not alter dose or discontinue without consulting physician; many medications (OTC, herbals/supplements, prescription products) cannot be taken with efavirenz; may cause dizziness, drowsiness, impaired concentration, delusions or depression; taking at bedtime may minimize these effects; caution in performing potentially hazardous tasks such as operating machinery or driving; do not get pregnant; avoid high-fat meals

Dosage Forms

Capsule: 50 mg, 100 mg, 200 mg

Tablet: 600 mg

♦ **Effer-K™** *see* Potassium Bicarbonate and Potassium Citrate (Effervescent) *on page 1108*

♦ **Effexor®** *see* Venlafaxine *on page 1410*

♦ **Effexor® XR** *see* Venlafaxine *on page 1410*

♦ **Efidac/24® [OTC]** *see* Pseudoephedrine *on page 1155*

Eflornithine (ee FLOR ni theen)

U.S. Brand Names Vaniqa™

Synonyms DFMO; Eflornithine Hydrochloride

Therapeutic Category Antiprotozoal; Topical Skin Product

Use Cream: Females ≥12 years: Reduce unwanted hair from face and adjacent areas under the chin

Orphan status: Injection: Treatment of meningoencephalitic stage of *Trypanosoma brucei gambiense* infection (sleeping sickness)

Pregnancy Risk Factor C

Pregnancy/Breast-Feeding Implications There are no adequate and well-controlled studies of topical eflornithine cream in pregnant women. The potential benefits to the mother versus the possible risks to the fetus should be considered prior to use. It is not known if eflornithine hydrochloride is excreted in breast milk, use caution if administered to a nursing woman.

Contraindications Hypersensitivity to eflornithine or any component of the formulation

Warnings/Precautions

Injection: Must be diluted before use; frequent monitoring for myelosuppression should be done; use with caution in patients with a history of seizures and in patients with renal impairment; serial audiograms should be obtained; due to the potential for relapse, patients should be followed up for at least 24 months

Cream: For topical use by females only; discontinue if hypersensitivity occurs; safety and efficacy in children <12 years has not been studied

Adverse Reactions

Injection:

>10%: Hematologic (reversible): Anemia (55%), leukopenia (37%), thrombocytopenia (14%)

1% to 10%:

Central nervous system: Seizures (may be due to the disease) (8%), dizziness

Dermatologic: Alopecia

Gastrointestinal: Vomiting, diarrhea

Hematologic: Eosinophilia

Otic: Hearing impairment

<1% (Limited to important or life-threatening): Abdominal pain, anorexia, facial edema, headache, weakness

Topical:

>10%: Dermatologic: Acne (11% to 21%), pseudofolliculitis barbae (5% to 15%)

1% to 10%:

Central nervous system: Headache (4% to 5%), dizziness (1%), vertigo (0.3% to 1%)

Dermatologic: Pruritus (3% to 4%), burning skin (2% to 4%), tingling skin (1% to 4%), dry skin (2% to 3%), rash (1% to 3%), facial edema (0.3% to 3%), alopecia (1% to 2%), skin irritation (1% to 2%), erythema (up to 2%), ingrown hair (0.3% to 2%), folliculitis (up to 1%)

Gastrointestinal: Dyspepsia (2%), anorexia (0.7% to 2%)

<1% (Limited to important or life-threatening): Bleeding skin, cheilitis, contact dermatitis, herpes simplex, lip swelling, nausea, numbness, rosacea, weakness

Overdosage/Toxicology There is no known antidote. Treatment is supportive. In mice and rats CNS depression, seizures, and death have occurred. Overdose with the topical product is not expected due to low percutaneous penetration.

Drug Interactions

Increased Effect/Toxicity: Cream: Possible interactions with other topical products have not been studied.

Decreased Effect: Cream: Possible interactions with other topical products have not been studied.

Stability

Injection: Must be diluted before use and used within 24 hours of preparation

Cream: Store at controlled room temperature 25°C (77°F); do not freeze

Mechanism of Action Eflornithine exerts antitumor and antiprotozoal effects through specific, irreversible ("suicide") inhibition of the enzyme ornithine decarboxylase (ODC). ODC is the rate-limiting enzyme in the biosynthesis of putrescine, spermine, and spermidine, the major polyamines in nucleated cells. Polyamines are necessary for the synthesis of DNA, RNA, and proteins and are, therefore, necessary for cell growth and differentiation. Although many microorganisms and higher plants are able to produce polyamines from alternate biochemical pathways, all mammalian cells depend on ornithine decarboxylase to produce polyamines. Eflornithine inhibits ODC and rapidly depletes animal cells of putrescine and spermidine; the concentration of spermine remains the same or may even increase. Rapidly dividing cells appear to be most susceptible to the effects of eflornithine. Topically, the inhibition of ODC in the skin leads to a decreased rate of hair growth.

Pharmacodynamics/Kinetics

Absorption: Topical: <1%

Half-life elimination: I.V.: 3-3.5 hours; Topical: 8 hours

Excretion: Primarily urine (as unchanged drug)

Usual Dosage

Children ≥12 years and Adults: Females: Topical: Apply thin layer of cream to affected areas of face and adjacent chin twice daily, at least 8 hours apart

Adults: I.V. infusion: 100 mg/kg/dose given every 6 hours (over at least 45 minutes) for 14 days

Dosing adjustment in renal impairment: Injection: Dose should be adjusted although no specific guidelines are available

Administration Cream: Apply thin layer of eflornithine cream to affected areas of face and adjacent chin area twice daily, at least 8 hours apart. Rub in thoroughly. Hair removal techniques must still be continued; wait at least 5 minutes after removing hair to apply cream. Do not wash affected area for at least 8 hours following application.

Monitoring Parameters CBC with platelet counts

(Continued)

Eflornithine *(Continued)*

Patient Information

Injection: Report any persistent or unusual fever, sore throat, fatigue, bleeding, or bruising; frequent blood tests are needed during therapy.

Cream: For topical use only. This product will not prevent hair growth, but will decrease the rate of growth. You will still need to use hair removal techniques, such as shaving and plucking, while using eflornithine cream. Wait at least 5 minutes after removing hair to apply cream. Improvement can be seen within 4-8 weeks of use. Following discontinuation of use, pretreatment hair growth will be seen in about 8 weeks. Contact prescriber if skin irritation or intolerance develop. Do not wash affected area for at least 8 hours following application. You may apply cosmetics or make-up over the affected area once the cream has dried.

Nursing Implications Cream: Apply thin layer of cream to affected areas of face and adjacent chin area twice daily, at least 8 hours apart. Rub in thoroughly. Hair removal techniques must still be continued; wait at least 5 minutes after removing hair to apply cream. Do not wash affected area for at least 8 hours following application.

Dosage Forms

Cream, topical, as hydrochloride: 13.9% (30 g)

Injection, as hydrochloride: 200 mg/mL (100 mL) [orphan drug status]

- **Eflornithine Hydrochloride** *see* Eflornithine *on page 461*
- **Efudex®** *see* Fluorouracil *on page 576*
- **EHDP** *see* Etidronate Disodium *on page 531*
- **ELA-Max® [OTC]** *see* Lidocaine *on page 801*
- **Elase®** *see* Fibrinolysin and Desoxyribonuclease *on page 560*
- **Elase-Chloromycetin®** *see* Fibrinolysin and Desoxyribonuclease *on page 560*
- **Elavil®** *see* Amitriptyline *on page 76*
- **Eldecort®** *see* Hydrocortisone *on page 682*
- **Eldepryl®** *see* Selegiline *on page 1228*
- **Eldercaps® [OTC]** *see* Vitamins (Multiple) *on page 1424*
- **Eldopaque® [OTC]** *see* Hydroquinone *on page 686*
- **Eldopaque Forte®** *see* Hydroquinone *on page 686*
- **Eldoquin® [OTC]** *see* Hydroquinone *on page 686*
- **Eldoquin® Forte®** *see* Hydroquinone *on page 686*
- **Electrolyte Lavage Solution** *see* Polyethylene Glycol-Electrolyte Solution *on page 1101*
- **Eligard™** *see* Leuprolide *on page 783*
- **Elimite™** *see* Permethrin *on page 1065*
- **Elixophyllin®** *see* Theophylline Salts *on page 1310*
- **Ellence™** *see* Epirubicin *on page 472*
- **Elmiron®** *see* Pentosan Polysulfate Sodium *on page 1060*
- **Elocom® (Can)** *see* Mometasone Furoate *on page 932*
- **Elocon®** *see* Mometasone Furoate *on page 932*
- **Elspar®** *see* Asparaginase *on page 118*
- **Eltor® (Can)** *see* Pseudoephedrine *on page 1155*
- **Eltroxin® (Can)** *see* Levothyroxine *on page 799*
- **Emcyt®** *see* Estramustine *on page 495*
- **EMLA®** *see* Lidocaine and Prilocaine *on page 804*
- **Emo-Cort® (Can)** *see* Hydrocortisone *on page 682*
- **Empracet®-30 (Can)** *see* Acetaminophen and Codeine *on page 24*
- **Empracet®-60 (Can)** *see* Acetaminophen and Codeine *on page 24*
- **Emtec-30 (Can)** *see* Acetaminophen and Codeine *on page 24*
- **EmTet®** *see* Tetracycline *on page 1306*
- **E-Mycin®** *see* Erythromycin (Systemic) *on page 486*
- **ENA 713** *see* Rivastigmine *on page 1206*

Enalapril *(e NAL a pril)*

Related Information

Angiotensin Agents Comparison *on page 1473*

Heart Failure *on page 1663*

U.S. Brand Names Vasotec®; Vasotec® I.V.

Canadian Brand Names Vasotec®; Vasotec® I.V.

Synonyms Enalaprilat; Enalapril Maleate

Therapeutic Category Angiotensin-Converting Enzyme (ACE) Inhibitor; Antihypertensive Agent

Use Management of mild to severe hypertension; treatment of congestive heart failure, left ventricular dysfunction after myocardial infarction

Unlabeled/Investigational Use

Unlabeled: Hypertensive crisis, diabetic nephropathy, rheumatoid arthritis, diagnosis of anatomic renal artery stenosis, hypertension secondary to scleroderma renal crisis, diagnosis of aldosteronism, idiopathic edema, Bartter's syndrome, postmyocardial infarction for prevention of ventricular failure

Investigational: Severe congestive heart failure in infants, neonatal hypertension, acute pulmonary edema

Pregnancy Risk Factor C/D (2nd and 3rd trimesters)

Pregnancy/Breast-Feeding Implications

Clinical effects on the fetus: No data available on crossing the placenta. Cranial defects, hypocalvaria/acalvaria, oligohydramnios, persistent anuria following delivery, hypotension, renal defects, renal dysgenesis/dysplasia, renal failure, pulmonary hypoplasia, limb contractures secondary to oligohydramnios and stillbirth reported. ACE inhibitors should be avoided during pregnancy.

Breast-feeding/lactation: Crosses into breast milk. Detectable levels but appears clinically insignificant. AAP considers **compatible** with breast-feeding.

Contraindications Hypersensitivity to enalapril or enalaprilat; angioedema related to previous treatment with an ACE inhibitor; patients with idiopathic or hereditary angioedema; bilateral renal artery stenosis; primary hyperaldosteronism; pregnancy (2nd and 3rd trimesters)

Warnings/Precautions Anaphylactic reactions can occur. Angioedema can occur at any time during treatment (especially following first dose). Careful blood pressure monitoring with first dose (hypotension can occur especially in volume depleted patients). Dosage adjustment needed in renal impairment. Use with caution in hypovolemia; collagen vascular diseases; valvular stenosis (particularly aortic stenosis); hyperkalemia; or before, during, or immediately after anesthesia. Avoid rapid dosage escalation which may lead to renal insufficiency. Hypersensitivity reactions may be seen during hemodialysis with high-flux dialysis membranes (eg, AN69). Hyperkalemia may rarely occur. Neutropenia/agranulocytosis with myeloid hyperplasia can rarely occur. If patient has renal impairment then a baseline WBC with differential and serum creatinine should be evaluated and monitored closely during the first 3 months of therapy. Use with caution in unilateral renal artery stenosis and pre-existing renal insufficiency. Experience in children is limited.

Adverse Reactions Note: Frequency ranges include data from hypertension and heart failure trials. Higher rates of adverse reactions have generally been noted in patients with congestive heart failure. However, the frequency of adverse effects associated with placebo is also increased in this population.

1% to 10%:

Cardiovascular: Hypotension (0.9% to 6.7%), chest pain (2%), syncope (0.5% to 2%), orthostasis (2%), orthostatic hypotension (2%)

Central nervous system: Headache (2% to 5%), dizziness (4% to 8%), fatigue (2% to 3%), weakness (2%)

Dermatologic: Rash (1.5%) Gastrointestinal: Abnormal taste, abdominal pain, vomiting, nausea, diarrhea, anorexia, constipation

Neuromuscular & skeletal: Weakness

Renal: Increased serum creatinine (0.2% to 20%), worsening of renal function (in patients with bilateral renal artery stenosis or hypovolemia)

Respiratory (1% to 2%): Bronchitis, cough, dyspnea

<1% (Limited to important or life-threatening): Agranulocytosis, alopecia, angina pectoris, angioedema, ataxia, bronchospasm, cardiac arrest, cerebral vascular accident, depression, erythema multiforme, exfoliative dermatitis, giant cell arteritis, gynecomastia, hallucinations, hemolysis with G6PD, Henoch-Schönlein purpura, hepatitis, ileus, impotence, jaundice, lichen-form reaction, myocardial infarction, neutropenia, ototoxicity, pancreatitis, paresthesia, pemphigus, pemphigus foliaceus, photosensitivity, psychosis, pulmonary edema, sicca syndrome, Stevens-Johnson syndrome, systemic lupus erythematosus, toxic epidermal necrolysis, toxic pustuloderma, vertigo. Worsening of renal function may occur in patients with bilateral renal artery stenosis or in hypovolemic patients. A syndrome which may include fever, myalgia, arthralgia, interstitial nephritis, vasculitis, rash, eosinophilia and positive ANA, and elevated ESR has been reported for enalapril and other ACE inhibitors.

Overdosage/Toxicology Mild hypotension has been the only toxic effect seen with acute overdose. Bradycardia may also occur. Hyperkalemia occurs even with therapeutic doses, especially in patients with renal insufficiency, and those taking NSAIDs. Following initiation of essential overdose management, toxic symptom and supportive treatment should be initiated. Hypotension usually responds to I.V. fluids or Trendelenburg positioning.

Drug Interactions

Cytochrome P450 Effect: CYP3A3/4 enzyme substrate

Increased Effect/Toxicity: Potassium supplements, co-trimoxazole (high dose), angiotensin II receptor antagonists (candesartan, losartan, irbesartan, etc), or potassium-sparing diuretics (amiloride, spironolactone, triamterene) may result in elevated serum potassium levels when combined with enalapril. ACE inhibitor effects may be increased by phenothiazines or probenecid (increases levels of captopril). ACE inhibitors may increase serum concentrations/effects of digoxin, lithium, and sulfonlyureas.

Diuretics have additive hypotensive effects with ACE inhibitors, and hypovolemia increases the potential for adverse renal effects of ACE inhibitors. In patients with compromised renal function, coadministration with nonsteroidal anti-inflammatory drugs may result in further deterioration of renal function. Allopurinol and ACE inhibitors may cause a higher risk of hypersensitivity reaction when taken concurrently.

Decreased Effect: Aspirin (high dose) may reduce the therapeutic effects of ACE inhibitors; at low dosages this does not appear to be significant. Rifampin may decrease the effect of ACE inhibitors. Antacids may decrease the bioavailability of ACE inhibitors (may be more likely to occur with captopril); separate administration times by 1-2 hours. NSAIDs may reduce the hypotensive effects of ACE inhibitors. More likely to occur in low renin or volume dependent hypertensive patients.

Ethanol/Nutrition/Herb Interactions Herb/Nutraceutical: St John's wort may decrease enalapril levels. Avoid dong quai if using for hypertension (has estrogenic activity). Avoid ephedra, yohimbe, ginseng (may worsen hypertension). Avoid natural licorice (causes sodium and water retention and increases potassium loss). Avoid garlic (may have increased antihypertensive effect).

Stability Enalaprilat: Clear, colorless solution which should be stored at <30°C; I.V. is 24 hours at room temperature in D₅W or NS

Mechanism of Action Competitive inhibitor of angiotensin-converting enzyme (ACE); prevents conversion of angiotensin I to angiotensin II, a potent vasoconstrictor; results in lower levels of angiotensin II which causes an increase in plasma renin activity and a reduction in aldosterone secretion

Pharmacodynamics/Kinetics

Onset of action: Oral: ~1 hour

(Continued)

Enalapril *(Continued)*

Duration: Oral: 12-24 hours

Absorption: Oral: 55% to 75%

Protein binding: 50% to 60%

Metabolism: Enalapril is a prodrug which undergoes hepatic biotransformation to enalaprilat

Half-life elimination:

Enalapril: Adults: Healthy: 2 hours; With congestive heart failure: 3.4-5.8 hours

Enalaprilat: Infants 6 weeks to 8 months old: 6-10 hours; Adults: 35-38 hours

Time to peak, serum: Oral: Enalapril: 0.5-1.5 hours; Enalaprilat (active): 3-4.5 hours

Excretion: Primarily urine (60% to 80%); some feces

Usual Dosage Use lower listed initial dose in patients with hyponatremia, hypovolemia, severe congestive heart failure, decreased renal function, or in those receiving diuretics.

Oral: **Enalapril**: Children 1 month to 16 years: Hypertension: Initial: 0.08 mg/kg (up to 5 mg) once daily; adjust dosage based on patient response; doses >0.58 mg/kg (40 mg) have not been evaluated in pediatric patients

Investigational: Congestive heart failure: Initial oral doses of **enalapril**: 0.1 mg/kg/day increasing as needed over 2 weeks to 0.5 mg/kg/day have been used in infants

Investigational: Neonatal hypertension: I.V. doses of **enalaprilat**: 5-10 mcg/kg/dose administered every 8-24 hours have been used; monitor patients carefully; select patients may require higher doses

Adults:

Oral: **Enalapril**

Hypertension: 2.5-5 mg/day then increase as required, usual therapeutic dose for hypertension: 10-40 mg/day in 1-2 divided doses. **Note:** Initiate with 2.5 mg if patient is taking a diuretic which cannot be discontinued. May add a diuretic if blood pressure cannot be controlled with enalapril alone.

Heart failure: As standard therapy alone or with diuretics, beta-blockers, and digoxin, initiate with 2.5 mg once or twice daily (usual range: 5-20 mg/day in 2 divided doses; target: 40 mg)

Asymptomatic left ventricular dysfunction: 2.5 mg twice daily, titrated as tolerated to 20 mg/day

I.V.: **Enalaprilat**

Hypertension: 1.25 mg/dose, given over 5 minutes every 6 hours; doses as high as 5 mg/dose every 6 hours have been tolerated for up to 36 hours. **Note:** If patients are concomitantly receiving diuretic therapy, begin with 0.625 mg I.V. over 5 minutes; if the effect is not adequate after 1 hour, repeat the dose and administer 1.25 mg at 6-hour intervals thereafter; if adequate, administer 0.625 mg I.V. every 6 hours.

Heart failure: Avoid I.V. administration in patients with unstable heart failure or those suffering acute myocardial infarction.

Conversion from I.V. to oral therapy if not concurrently on diuretics: 5 mg once daily; subsequent titration as needed; if concurrently receiving diuretics and responding to 0.625 mg I.V. every 6 hours, initiate with 2.5 mg/day.

Dosing adjustment in renal impairment:

Oral: Enalapril:

Cl$_{cr}$ 30-80 mL/minute: Administer 5 mg/day titrated upwards to maximum of 40 mg.

Cl$_{cr}$ <30 mL/minute: Administer 2.5 mg day; titrated upward until blood pressure is controlled.

For heart failure patients with sodium <130 mEq/L or serum creatinine >1.6 mg/dL, initiate dosage with 2.5 mg/day, increasing to twice daily as needed. Increase further in increments of 2.5 mg/dose at >4-day intervals to a maximum daily dose of 40 mg.

I.V.: Enalaprilat:

Cl$_{cr}$ >30 mL/minute: Initiate with 1.25 mg every 6 hours and increase dose based on response.

Cl$_{cr}$ <30 mL/minute: Initiate with 0.625 mg every 6 hours and increase dose based on response.

Hemodialysis: Moderately dialyzable (20% to 50%); administer dose postdialysis (eg, 0.625 mg I.V. every 6 hours) or administer 20% to 25% supplemental dose following dialysis; Clearance: 62 mL/minute.

Peritoneal dialysis: Supplemental dose is not necessary, although some removal of drug occurs.

Dosing adjustment in hepatic impairment: Hydrolysis of enalapril to enalaprilat may be delayed and/or impaired in patients with severe hepatic impairment, but the pharmacodynamic effects of the drug do not appear to be significantly altered; no dosage adjustment.

Dietary Considerations Limit salt substitutes or potassium-rich diet.

Administration Administer direct IVP over at least 5 minutes or dilute up to 50 mL and infuse; discontinue diuretic, if possible, for 2-3 days before beginning enalapril therapy

Monitoring Parameters Blood pressure, renal function, WBC, serum potassium; blood pressure monitor required during intravenous administration

Test Interactions Positive Coombs' [direct]; may cause false-positive results in urine acetone determinations using sodium nitroprusside reagent

Patient Information Notify physician if vomiting, diarrhea, excessive perspiration, or dehydration should occur; also if swelling of face, lips, tongue, or difficulty in breathing occurs or if persistent cough develops

Nursing Implications May cause depression in some patients; discontinue if angioedema of the face, extremities, lips, tongue, or glottis occurs; watch for hypotensive effects within 1-3 hours of first dose or new higher dose

Dosage Forms

Injection, as enalaprilat: 1.25 mg/mL (1 mL, 2 mL)

Tablet, as maleate: 2.5 mg, 5 mg, 10 mg, 20 mg

Extemporaneous Preparations

An enalapril oral suspension (0.2 mg/mL) has been made using one 2.5 mg tablet and 12.5 mL sterile water; stability unknown; suspension should be used immediately and the remaining amount discarded

Young TE and Mangum OB, "Neofax®, '95: A Manual of Drugs Used in Neonatal Care," 8th ed, Columbus, OH: Ross Products Division, Abbott Laboratories, 1995, 85.

An enalapril oral suspension (1 mg/mL) has been made using 20 mg tablets and mL Bicitra®. Add 50 mL Bicitra® to a polyethylene terephthalate (PET) bottle containing ten 20 mg tablets and shake for at least 2 minutes. Let concentrate stand for 60 minutes. Following the 60-minute hold time, shake the concentration for an additional minute. Add 150 mL Bicitra® to the concentrate and shake the suspension to disperse the ingredients. The suspension should refrigerated at 2°C to 8°C (36°F to 46°F); it can be stored for up to 30 days. Shake suspension well before use.
Package labeling, Merck & Co, Inc, issued October 2000.

Enalapril and Felodipine (e NAL a pril & fe LOE di peen)
U.S. Brand Names Lexxel™
Canadian Brand Names Lexxel™
Synonyms Felodipine and Enalapril
Therapeutic Category Angiotensin-Converting Enzyme (ACE) Inhibitor Combination; Antihypertensive Agent, Combination
Use Treatment of hypertension, however, not indicated for initial treatment of hypertension; replacement therapy in patients receiving separate dosage forms (for patient convenience); when monotherapy with one component fails to achieve desired antihypertensive effect, or when dose-limiting adverse effects limit upward titration of monotherapy
Pregnancy Risk Factor C/D (2nd and 3rd trimesters)
Usual Dosage Adults: Oral: 1 tablet daily
Additional Information Complete prescribing information for this medication should be consulted for additional detail.
Dosage Forms
Tablet, extended release:
Enalapril maleate 5 mg and felodipine 2.5 mg
Enalapril maleate 5 mg and felodipine 5 mg

Enalapril and Hydrochlorothiazide
(e NAL a pril & hye droe klor oh THYE a zide)
U.S. Brand Names Vaseretic® 5-12.5; Vaseretic® 10-25
Canadian Brand Names Vaseretic®
Synonyms Hydrochlorothiazide and Enalapril
Therapeutic Category Angiotensin-Converting Enzyme (ACE) Inhibitor Combination; Antihypertensive Agent, Combination
Use Treatment of hypertension
Pregnancy Risk Factor C/D (2nd and 3rd trimesters)
Usual Dosage Oral: Dose is individualized
Additional Information Complete prescribing information for this medication should be consulted for additional detail.
Dosage Forms
Tablet:
Enalapril maleate 5 mg and hydrochlorothiazide 12.5 mg
Enalapril maleate 10 mg and hydrochlorothiazide 25 mg

- **Enalaprilat** see Enalapril on page 462
- **Enalapril Maleate** see Enalapril on page 462
- **Enbrel®** see Etanercept on page 504
- **Endal®** see Guaifenesin and Phenylephrine on page 647
- **Endantadine® (Can)** see Amantadine on page 65
- **End Lice® [OTC]** see Pyrethrins and Piperonyl Butoxide on page 1160
- **Endocet®** see Oxycodone and Acetaminophen on page 1026
- **Endocodone™** see Oxycodone on page 1024
- **Endodan®** see Oxycodone and Aspirin on page 1026
- **Endo®-Levodopa/Carbidopa (Can)** see Levodopa and Carbidopa on page 791
- **Endolor®** see Butalbital Compound on page 197
- **Endrate®** see Edetate Disodium on page 457
- **Enduron®** see Methyclothiazide on page 890
- **Enduronyl®** see Methyclothiazide and Deserpidine on page 891
- **Enduronyl® Forte** see Methyclothiazide and Deserpidine on page 891
- **Ener-B®** see Cyanocobalamin on page 339
- **Engerix-B®** see Hepatitis B Vaccine on page 662
- **Engerix-B® and Havrix®** see Hepatitis A Inactivated and Hepatitis B (Recombinant) Vaccine on page 660
- **Enhanced-potency Inactivated Poliovirus Vaccine** see Poliovirus Vaccine (Inactivated) on page 1100
- **Enlon®** see Edrophonium on page 458

Enoxaparin (ee noks a PA rin)
Related Information
Heparin Comparison on page 1501
U.S. Brand Names Lovenox®
Canadian Brand Names Lovenox®
Synonyms Enoxaparin Sodium
Therapeutic Category Low Molecular Weight Heparin
Use
Prevention of deep vein thrombosis following hip or knee replacement surgery or abdominal surgery in patients at risk for thromboembolic complications (high-risk patients include those with one or more of the following risk factors: >40 years of age, obese, general (Continued)

Enoxaparin *(Continued)*

anesthesia lasting >30 minutes, malignancy, history of deep vein thrombosis or pulmonary embolism)

Prevention of deep vein thrombosis in medical patients at risk for thromboembolic complications due to severely restricted mobility during acute illness

Inpatient treatment of acute deep vein thrombosis with and without pulmonary embolism when administered in conjunction with warfarin sodium

Outpatient treatment of acute deep vein thrombosis without pulmonary embolism when administered in conjunction with warfarin sodium

Prevention of ischemic complications of unstable angina and non-Q wave myocardial infarction (when administered with aspirin)

Pregnancy Risk Factor B

Pregnancy/Breast-Feeding Implications There are no adequate and well-controlled studies using enoxaparin in pregnant women. Animal studies have not shown teratogenic or fetotoxic effects. Postmarketing reports include congenital abnormalities (cause and effect not established) and also fetal death when used in pregnant women. In addition, prosthetic valve thrombosis, including fatal cases, has been reported in pregnant women receiving enoxaparin as thromboprophylaxis. It is not known if enoxaparin is excreted in breast milk; use caution if administered to a nursing woman.

Contraindications Hypersensitivity to enoxaparin or any component of the formulation; thrombocytopenia associated with a positive *in vitro* test for antiplatelet antibodies in the presence of enoxaparin; hypersensitivity to pork products; active major bleeding; not for I.M. or I.V. use

Warnings/Precautions Do not administer intramuscularly. **Patients with recent or anticipated neuraxial anesthesia (epidural or spinal anesthesia) are at risk of spinal or epidural hematoma and subsequent paralysis.** Consider risk versus benefit prior to neuraxial anesthesia; risk is increased by concomitant agents which may alter hemostasis, as well as traumatic or repeated epidural or spinal puncture. Patient should be observed closely for bleeding if enoxaparin is administered during or immediately following diagnostic lumbar puncture, epidural anesthesia, or spinal anesthesia.

Not recommended for thromboprophylaxis in patients with prosthetic heart valves (especially pregnant women). Not to be used interchangeably (unit for unit) with heparin or any other low molecular weight heparins. Cautious use in patient with history of heparin-induced thrombocytopenia. Monitor patient closely for signs or symptoms of bleeding. Certain patients are at increased risk of bleeding. Risk factors include bacterial endocarditis; congenital or acquired bleeding disorders; active ulcerative or angiodysplastic GI diseases; severe uncontrolled hypertension; hemorrhagic stroke; use shortly after brain, spinal, or ophthalmology surgery; patients treated concomitantly with platelet inhibitors; recent GI bleeding; thrombocytopenia or platelet defects; severe liver disease; hypertensive or diabetic retinopathy; or in patients undergoing invasive procedures. Cautious use in patients with severe renal failure (has not been studied). Safety and efficacy in pediatric patients have not been established. Use with caution in the elderly (delayed elimination may occur). Heparin can cause hyperkalemia by affecting aldosterone. Similar reactions could occur with LMWHs. Monitor for hyperkalemia. Discontinue therapy if platelets are <100,000/mm^3.

Adverse Reactions As with all anticoagulants, bleeding is the major adverse effect of enoxaparin. Hemorrhage may occur at virtually any site. Risk is dependent on multiple variables. At the recommended doses, single injections of enoxaparin do not significantly influence platelet aggregation or affect global clotting time (ie, PT or APTT).

1% to 10%:

Central nervous system: Fever (5% to 8%), confusion, pain

Dermatologic: Erythema, bruising

Gastrointestinal: Nausea (3%), diarrhea

Hematologic: Hemorrhage (5% to 13%), thrombocytopenia (2%), hypochromic anemia (2%)

Hepatic: Increased ALT/AST

Local: Injection site hematoma (9%), local reactions (irritation, pain, ecchymosis, erythema)

<1% (Limited to important or life-threatening): Allergic reaction, anaphylactoid reaction, eczematous plaques, hyperlipidemia, hypertriglyceridemia, itchy erythematous patches, pruritus, purpura, skin necrosis, thrombocytosis, urticaria, vesicobullous rash. Retroperitoneal or intracranial bleed (some fatal). Spinal or epidural hematomas can occur following neuraxial anesthesia or spinal puncture, resulting in paralysis. Risk is increased in patients with indwelling epidural catheters or concomitant use of other drugs affecting hemostasis. Cases of heparin-induced thrombocytopenia with thrombosis (some complicated by organ infarction, limb ischemia, or death) have been reported. Prosthetic valve thrombosis, including fatal cases, has been reported in pregnant women receiving enoxaparin as thromboprophylaxis.

Overdosage/Toxicology Symptoms include hemorrhage. Protamine sulfate has been used to reverse effects.

Drug Interactions

Increased Effect/Toxicity: Risk of bleeding with enoxaparin may be increased with thrombolytic agents, oral anticoagulants (warfarin), drugs which affect platelet function (eg, aspirin, NSAIDs, dipyridamole, ticlopidine, clopidogrel, and IIb/IIIa antagonists). Although the risk of bleeding may be increased during concurrent therapy with warfarin, enoxaparin is commonly continued during the initiation of warfarin therapy to assure anticoagulation and to protect against possible transient hypercoagulability. Some cephalosporins and penicillins may block platelet aggregation, theoretically increasing the risk of bleeding.

Ethanol/Nutrition/Herb Interactions Herb/Nutraceutical: Avoid cat's claw, dong quai, evening primrose, feverfew, garlic, ginger, ginkgo, red clover, horse chestnut, green tea, ginseng (all have additional antiplatelet activity).

Stability Store at 15°C to 25°C (59°F to 77°F); do not freeze; do not mix with other injections or infusions

Mechanism of Action Standard heparin consists of components with molecular weights ranging from 4000-30,000 daltons with a mean of 16,000 daltons. Heparin acts as an anticoagulant by enhancing the inhibition rate of clotting proteases by antithrombin III impairing normal hemostasis and inhibition of factor Xa. Low molecular weight heparins have a small effect on the activated partial thromboplastin time and strongly inhibit factor Xa. Enoxaparin is derived from porcine heparin that undergoes benzylation followed by alkaline depolymerization. The average molecular weight of enoxaparin is 4500 daltons which is distributed as (≤20%) 2000 daltons (≥68%) 2000-8000 daltons, and (≤15%) >8000 daltons. Enoxaparin has a higher ratio of antifactor Xa to antifactor IIa activity than unfractionated heparin.

Pharmacodynamics/Kinetics

Peak effect: S.C.: Antifactor Xa and antithrombin (antifactor IIa): 3-5 hours

Duration: 40 mg dose: Antifactor Xa activity: ~12 hours

Protein binding: Does not bind to heparin binding proteins

Half-life elimination, plasma: 2-4 times longer than standard heparin, independent of dose

Usual Dosage S.C.:

Children: Prophylaxis of DVT following abdominal, hip replacement or knee replacement surgery: Safety and effectiveness have not been established. Few studies have been conducted; the Fifth American College of Chest Physicians Consensus Conference on Antithrombotic Therapy (Michelson, 1998) recommends low molecular weight heparin as an alternative to heparin therapy in children ≥2 months with DVT or pulmonary embolism; the following initial doses and titration schedule, based on therapeutic antifactor Xa levels of 0.5-1 unit/mL, are recommended. **Note:** For treatment of DVT or pulmonary embolism in children ≥2 months of age, enoxaparin should be continued for 5-10 days and oral anticoagulation should be overlapped for 4-5 days (Michelson, 1998)

Infants >2 months and Children ≤18 years: Prophylaxis: Initial: 0.5 mg/kg every 12 hours; treatment: Initial: 1 mg/kg every 12 hours

Dosage titration:

Antifactor Xa <0.35 units/mL: Increase dose by 25%; repeat antifactor Xa level 4 hour after next dose

Antifactor Xa 0.35-0.49 units/mL: Increase dose by 10%; repeat antifactor Xa level 4 hour after next dose

Antifactor Xa 0.5-1 unit/mL: Keep same dosage; repeat antifactor Xa level next day, then 1 week later (4 hour after dose)

Antifactor Xa 1.1-1.5 units/mL: Decrease dose by 20%; repeat antifactor Xa level before next dose

Antifactor Xa 1.6-2 units/mL: Hold dose for 3 hour and decrease dose by 30%; repeat antifactor Xa level before next dose, then 4 hour after next dose

Antifactor Xa >2 units/mL: Hold all doses until antifactor Xa is 0.5 units/mL, then decrease dose by 40%; repeat antifactor Xa level before next dose and every 12 hour until antifactor Xa <0.5 units/mL

Adults:

DVT prophylaxis in hip replacement:

30 mg twice daily: First dose within 12-24 hours after surgery and every 12 hours until risk of deep vein thrombosis has diminished or the patient is adequately anticoagulated on warfarin. Average duration of therapy: 7-10 days.

40 mg once daily: First dose within 9-15 hours before surgery and daily until risk of deep vein thrombosis has diminished or the patient is adequately anticoagulated on warfarin. Average duration of therapy: 7-10 days unless warfarin is not given concurrently, then 40 mg S.C. once daily should be continued for 3 more weeks (4 weeks total).

DVT prophylaxis in knee replacement: 30 mg twice daily: First dose within 12-24 hours after surgery and every 12 hours until risk of deep vein thrombosis has diminished. Average duration of therapy: 7-10 days; maximum course: 14 days.

DVT prophylaxis in high-risk patients undergoing abdominal surgery: 40 mg once daily, with initial dose given 2 hours prior to surgery; usual duration: 7-10 days and up to 12 days has been tolerated in clinical trials.

DVT prophylaxis in medical patients with severely restricted mobility during acute illness: 40 mg once daily; usual duration: 6-11 days; up to 14 days was used in clinical trial

Treatment of acute proximal DVT: Start warfarin within 72 hours and continue enoxaparin until INR is between 2.0 and 3.0 (usually 7 days).

Inpatient treatment of DVT with or without pulmonary embolism: 1 mg/kg/dose every 12 hours or 1.5 mg/kg once daily.

Outpatient treatment of DVT without pulmonary embolism: 1 mg/kg/dose every 12 hours.

Prevention of ischemic complications with unstable angina or non-Q-wave myocardial infarction: 1 mg/kg twice daily in conjunction with oral aspirin therapy (100-325 mg once daily); treatment should be continued for a minimum of 2 days and continued until clinical stabilization (usually 2-8 days).

Elderly: Increased incidence of bleeding with doses of 1.5 mg/kg/day or 1 mg/kg every 12 hours; injection-associated bleeding and serious adverse reactions are also increased in the elderly. Careful attention should be paid to elderly patients <45 kg.

Dosing adjustment in renal impairment: Total clearance is lower and elimination is delayed in patients with renal failure; adjustment may be necessary in elderly and patients with severe renal impairment.

Hemodialysis: Supplemental dose is not necessary.

Peritoneal dialysis: Significant drug removal is unlikely based on physiochemical characteristics.

Administration Should be administered by deep S.C. injection to the left or right anterolateral and left or right posterolateral abdominal wall. To avoid loss of drug from the 30 mg and 40 mg syringes, do not expel the air bubble from the syringe prior to injection. In order to minimize bruising, do not rub injection site. An automatic injector (Lovenox EasyInjector™) is available with the 30 mg and 40 mg syringes to aid the patient with self-injections. **Note:** Enoxaparin is available in 100 mg/mL and 150 mg/mL concentrations.

(Continued)

Enoxaparin *(Continued)*

Monitoring Parameters Platelets, occult blood, and anti-Xa activity, if available; the monitoring of PT and/or PTT is not necessary

Nursing Implications Administer S.C. only; do not administer I.M. injection. When using the 30 and 40 mg prefilled syringes, do not expel air bubble from syringe before injection.

Dosage Forms

Injection, ampul, as sodium [preservative free]: 30 mg/0.3 mL

Injection, graduated prefilled syringe, as sodium [preservative free]: 60 mg/0.6 mL, 80 mg/0.8 mL, 90 mg/0.6 mL, 100 mg/mL, 120 mg/0.8 mL, 150 mg/mL

Injection, prefilled syringe, as sodium [preservative free]: 30 mg/0.3 mL, 40 mg/0.4 mL

♦ **Enoxaparin Sodium** *see* Enoxaparin *on page 465*

Entacapone *(en TA ka pone)*

Related Information

Parkinson's Agents *on page 1513*

U.S. Brand Names Comtan®

Canadian Brand Names Comtan®

Therapeutic Category Anti-Parkinson's Agent, COMT Inhibitor; Reverse COMT Inhibitor

Use Adjunct to levodopa/carbidopa therapy in patients with idiopathic Parkinson's disease who experience "wearing-off" symptoms at the end of a dosing interval

Pregnancy Risk Factor C

Pregnancy/Breast-Feeding Implications Not recommended

Contraindications Hypersensitivity to entacapone or any of component of the formulation

Warnings/Precautions Patient should not be treated concomitantly with entacapone and a nonselective MAO inhibitor. Orthostatic hypotension may be increased in patients on dopaminergic therapy in Parkinson's disease.

Adverse Reactions

>10%:

Gastrointestinal: Nausea (14%)

Neuromuscular & skeletal: Dyskinesia (25%), placebo (15%)

1% to 10%:

Cardiovascular: Orthostatic hypotension (4.3%), syncope (1.2%)

Central nervous system: Dizziness (8%), fatigue (6%), hallucinations (4%), anxiety (2%), somnolence (2%), agitation (1%)

Dermatologic: Purpura (2%)

Gastrointestinal: Diarrhea (10%), abdominal pain (8%), constipation (6%), vomiting (4%), dry mouth (3%), dyspepsia (2%), flatulence (2%), gastritis (1%), taste perversion (1%)

Genitourinary: Brown-orange urine discoloration (10%)

Neuromuscular & skeletal: Hyperkinesia (10%), hypokinesia (9%), back pain (4%), weakness (2%)

Respiratory: Dyspnea (3%)

Miscellaneous: Increased diaphoresis (2%), bacterial infection (1%)

<1% (Limited to important or life-threatening): Hyperpyrexia and confusion (resembling neuroleptic malignant syndrome), pulmonary fibrosis, retroperitoneal fibrosis, rhabdomyolysis

Overdosage/Toxicology There have been no reported cases of intentional or accidental overdose with this drug. COMT inhibition by entacapone treatment is dose-dependent.

Drug Interactions

Cytochrome P450 Effect: CYP1A2, 2A6, 2C9, 2C19, 2D6, 2E1, 3A3/4 enzyme inhibitor; these effects are seen only at concentrations higher than those achieved at recommended dosing.

Increased Effect/Toxicity: Cardiac effects with drugs metabolized by COMT (eg, epinephrine, isoproterenol, dopamine, apomorphine, bitolterol, dobutamine, methyldopa) increased other CNS depressants; nonselective MAO inhibitors are not recommended; chelates iron. Caution with drugs that interfere with glucuronidation, intestinal, biliary excretion, intestinal beta-glucuronidase (eg, probenecid, cholestyramine, erythromycin, chloramphenicol, rifampicin, ampicillin).

Decreased Effect: Entacapone is an iron chelator and an iron supplement should not be administered concurrently with this medicine.

Ethanol/Nutrition/Herb Interactions Ethanol: Avoid ethanol (may increase CNS adverse effects).

Mechanism of Action Entacapone is a reversible and selective inhibitor of catechol-O-methyltransferase (COMT). When entacapone is taken with levodopa, the pharmacokinetics are altered, resulting in more sustained levodopa serum levels compared to levodopa taken alone. The resulting levels of levodopa provide for increased concentrations available for absorption across the blood-brain barrier, thereby providing for increased CNS levels of dopamine, the active metabolite of levodopa.

Pharmacodynamics/Kinetics

Onset of action: Rapid

Peak effect: 1 hour

Absorption: Rapid

Distribution: I.V.: V_{dss}: 20 L

Protein binding: 98%, mainly to albumin

Metabolism: Isomerization to the *cis*-isomer, followed by direct glucuronidation of the parent and *cis*-isomer

Bioavailability: 35%

Half-life elimination: B phase: 0.4-0.7 hours; Y phase: 2.4 hours

Time to peak, serum: 1 hour

Excretion: Feces (90%); urine (10%)

Usual Dosage
Adults: Oral: 200 mg dose, up to a maximum of 8 times/day; maximum daily dose: 1600 mg/day. Always administer with levodopa/carbidopa. To optimize therapy, the levodopa/carbidopa dosage must be reduced, usually by 25%. This reduction is usually necessary when the patient is taking more than 800 mg of levodopa daily.

Dosage adjustment in hepatic impairment: Treat with caution and monitor carefully; AUC and C_{max} can be possibly doubled

Dietary Considerations Can take with or without food.

Administration Always administer in association with levodopa/carbidopa; can be combined with both the immediate and sustained release formulations of levodopa/carbidopa. Can be taken with or without food. Should not be abruptly withdrawn from patient's therapy due to significant worsening of symptoms.

Monitoring Parameters Signs and symptoms of Parkinson's disease; liver function tests, blood pressure, patient's mental status

Patient Information Take only as prescribed; can be taken with or without food. Possible nausea, hallucinations, and change in color of urine (not clinically relevant) may occur. Do not drive a car or operate other complex machinery until there is sufficient experience with entacapone. Do not withdraw medication unless advised by healthcare professional.

Dosage Forms Tablet: 200 mg

- ◆ **Entex® PSE** *see* Guaifenesin and Pseudoephedrine *on page 647*
- ◆ **Entocort® (Can)** *see* Budesonide *on page 186*
- ◆ **Entocort™ EC** *see* Budesonide *on page 186*
- ◆ **Entrophen® (Can)** *see* Aspirin *on page 120*
- ◆ **Entsol® [OTC]** *see* Sodium Chloride *on page 1245*
- ◆ **Enulose®** *see* Lactulose *on page 770*
- ◆ **Enzone®** *see* Pramoxine and Hydrocortisone *on page 1117*
- ◆ **Epaxal Berna® (Can)** *see* Hepatitis A Vaccine *on page 660*

Ephedrine (e FED rin)

Related Information
Antacid Drug Interactions *on page 1477*
Contrast Media Reactions, Premedication for Prophylaxis *on page 1653*

U.S. Brand Names Kondon's Nasal® [OTC]; Pretz-D® [OTC]

Synonyms Ephedrine Sulfate

Therapeutic Category Adrenergic Agonist Agent; Bronchodilator; Sympathomimetic

Use Treatment of bronchial asthma, nasal congestion, acute bronchospasm, idiopathic orthostatic hypotension

Pregnancy Risk Factor C

Contraindications Hypersensitivity to ephedrine or any component of the formulation; cardiac arrhythmias; angle-closure glaucoma; concurrent use of other sympathomimetic agents

Warnings/Precautions Blood volume depletion should be corrected before ephedrine therapy is instituted; use caution in patients with unstable vasomotor symptoms, diabetes, hyperthyroidism, prostatic hyperplasia, a history of seizures or those on other sympathomimetic agents; also use caution in the elderly and those patients with cardiovascular disorders such as coronary artery disease, arrhythmias, and hypertension. Ephedrine may cause hypertension resulting in intracranial hemorrhage. Long-term use may cause anxiety and symptoms of paranoid schizophrenia. Avoid as a bronchodilator; generally not used as a bronchodilator since new beta₂ agents are less toxic. Use with caution in the elderly, since it crosses the blood-brain barrier and may cause confusion.

Adverse Reactions Frequency not defined.
Cardiovascular: Hypertension, tachycardia, palpitations, elevation or depression of blood pressure, unusual pallor, chest pain, arrhythmias
Central nervous system: CNS stimulating effects, nervousness, anxiety, apprehension, fear, tension, agitation, excitation, restlessness, irritability, insomnia, hyperactivity, dizziness, headache
Gastrointestinal: Xerostomia, nausea, anorexia, GI upset, vomiting
Genitourinary: Painful urination
Neuromuscular & skeletal: Trembling, tremor (more common in the elderly), weakness
Respiratory: Dyspnea
Miscellaneous: Diaphoresis (increased)

Overdosage/Toxicology Symptoms include dysrhythmias, CNS excitation, respiratory depression, vomiting, and convulsions. There is no specific antidote for ephedrine intoxication and the bulk of the treatment is supportive. Hyperactivity and agitation usually respond to reduced sensory input; however, with extreme agitation, haloperidol (2-5 mg I.M. for adults) may be required. Hyperthermia is best treated with external cooling measures; or when severe or unresponsive, muscle paralysis with pancuronium may be needed. Hypertension is usually transient and generally does not require treatment unless severe. For diastolic blood pressures >110 mm Hg, a nitroprusside infusion should be initiated. Seizures usually respond to diazepam I.V. and/or phenytoin maintenance regimens.

Drug Interactions
Increased Effect/Toxicity: Increased (toxic) cardiac stimulation with other sympathomimetic agents, theophylline, cardiac glycosides, or general anesthetics. Increased blood pressure with atropine or MAO inhibitors.
Decreased Effect: Alpha- and beta-adrenergic blocking agents decrease ephedrine vasopressor effects.

Ethanol/Nutrition/Herb Interactions Herb/Nutraceutical: Avoid ephedra, yohimbe (may cause CNS stimulation).

Stability Protect all dosage forms from light

Mechanism of Action Releases tissue stores of epinephrine and thereby produces an alpha- and beta-adrenergic stimulation; longer-acting and less potent than epinephrine

Pharmacodynamics/Kinetics
Onset of action: Oral: Bronchodilation: 0.25-1 hour
(Continued)

Ephedrine *(Continued)*

Duration: Oral: 3-6 hours
Distribution: Crosses placenta; enters breast milk
Metabolism: Minimal hepatic
Half-life elimination: 2.5-3.6 hours
Excretion: Urine (60% to 77% as unchanged drug) within 24 hours

Usual Dosage

Children:
Oral, S.C.: 3 mg/kg/day or 25-100 mg/m^2/day in 4-6 divided doses every 4-6 hours
I.M., slow I.V. push: 0.2-0.3 mg/kg/dose every 4-6 hours

Adults:
Oral: 25-50 mg every 3-4 hours as needed
I.M., S.C.: 25-50 mg, parenteral adult dose should not exceed 150 mg in 24 hours
I.V.: 5-25 mg/dose slow I.V. push repeated after 5-10 minutes as needed, then every 3-4
hours not to exceed 150 mg/24 hours

Nasal spray:
Children 6-12 years: 1-2 sprays into each nostril, not more frequently than every 4 hours
Children ≥12 years and Adults: 2-3 sprays into each nostril, not more frequently than every
4 hours

Monitoring Parameters Blood pressure, pulse, urinary output, mental status; cardiac monitor
and blood pressure monitor required

Test Interactions Can cause a false-positive amphetamine EMIT assay

Patient Information May cause wakefulness or nervousness; take last dose 4-6 hours before
bedtime

Nursing Implications Do not administer unless solution is clear

Additional Information For I.V. administration, give the undiluted injection slowly. Additional
I.V. doses may be given 5-10 minutes if needed. Do not exceed adult parenteral dose of 150
mg/24 hours. Do not exceed pediatric dose of 3 mg/kg/24 hours; use the smallest effective
dose.

Dosage Forms

Capsule, as sulfate: 25 mg, 50 mg
Injection, as sulfate: 50 mg/mL (1 mL)
Jelly, as sulfate (Kondon's Nasal®): 1% (20 g)
Solution, as sulfate [spray] (Pretz-D®): 0.25% (50 mL)

♦ **Ephedrine Sulfate** *see Ephedrine on page 469*

♦ **Ephedrine, Theophylline and Phenobarbital** *see Theophylline, Ephedrine, and Phenobarbital on page 1310*

♦ **Epidermal Thymocyte Activating Factor** *see Aldesleukin on page 43*

♦ **Epifoam®** *see Pramoxine and Hydrocortisone on page 1117*

♦ **Epifrin®** *see Epinephrine on page 470*

♦ **Epilepsy & Seizure Treatment** *see page 1659*

♦ **E-Pilo® (Can)** *see Pilocarpine and Epinephrine on page 1084*

♦ **E-Pilo-x®** *see Pilocarpine and Epinephrine on page 1084*

Epinephrine *(ep i NEF rin)*

Related Information

Adrenergic Agonists, Cardiovascular Comparison *on page 1469*
Adult ACLS Algorithms *on page 1632*
Antacid Drug Interactions *on page 1477*
Bronchodilators, Comparison of Inhaled Sympathomimetics *on page 1493*
Glaucoma Drug Therapy Comparison *on page 1499*
Pediatric ALS Algorithms *on page 1628*

U.S. Brand Names Adrenalin®; AsthmaHaler®; Bronitin®; Epifrin®; EpiPen® Auto-Injector;
EpiPen® Jr Auto-Injector; Glaucon®; Primatene® Mist [OTC]; Sus-Phrine®

Canadian Brand Names Adrenalin®; Epipen®; Epipen® Jr.; Vaponefrin®

Synonyms Adrenaline; Epinephrine Bitartrate; Epinephrine Hydrochloride

Therapeutic Category Adrenergic Agonist Agent; Antidote, Hypersensitivity Reactions;
Bronchodilator; Sympathomimetic

Use Treatment of bronchospasms, anaphylactic reactions, cardiac arrest, management of
open-angle (chronic simple) glaucoma; added to local anesthetics to decrease systemic
absorption, increase duration of action, and decrease toxicity of the local anesthetic

Unlabeled/Investigational Use ACLS guidelines: Ventricular fibrillation (VF) or pulseless
ventricular tachycardia (VT) unresponsive to initial defibrillatory shocks; pulseless electrical
activity, asystole, hypotension unresponsive to volume resuscitation; symptomatic bradycardia or heart block unresponsive to atropine or pacing

Pregnancy Risk Factor C

Pregnancy/Breast-Feeding Implications

Clinical effects on the fetus: Crosses the placenta. Reported association with malformations
in 1 study; may be secondary to severe maternal disease.
Breast-feeding/lactation: No data on crossing into breast milk or clinical effects on the infant

Contraindications Hypersensitivity to epinephrine or any component of the formulation;
cardiac arrhythmias; angle-closure glaucoma

Warnings/Precautions Use with caution in elderly patients, patients with diabetes mellitus,
cardiovascular diseases (angina, tachycardia, myocardial infarction), thyroid disease, or
cerebral arteriosclerosis, Parkinson's; some products contain sulfites as preservatives. Rapid
I.V. infusion may cause death from cerebrovascular hemorrhage or cardiac arrhythmias. Oral
inhalation of epinephrine is **not** the preferred route of administration.

Adverse Reactions Frequency not defined.

Cardiovascular: Tachycardia (parenteral), pounding heartbeat, flushing, hypertension, pallor,
chest pain, increased myocardial oxygen consumption, cardiac arrhythmias, sudden death,
angina, vasoconstriction

Central nervous system: Nervousness, anxiety, restlessness, headache, dizziness, light-headedness, insomnia

Gastrointestinal: Nausea, vomiting, xerostomia,dry throat

Genitourinary: Acute urinary retention in patients with bladder outflow obstruction

Neuromuscular & skeletal: Weakness, trembling

Ocular: Precipitation or or exacerbation of narrow-angle glaucoma, transient stinging, burning, eye pain, allergic lid reaction, ocular irritation

Renal: Decreased renal and splanchnic blood flow

Respiratory: Wheezing, dyspnea

Miscellaneous: Diaphoresis (increased)

Overdosage/Toxicology Symptoms of overdose include arrhythmias, unusually large pupils, pulmonary edema, renal failure, metabolic acidosis; and hypertension, which may result in subarachnoid hemorrhage and hemiplegia. There is no specific antidote for epinephrine intoxication and the bulk of treatment is supportive. Hyperactivity and agitation usually respond to reduced sensory input; however, with extreme agitation, haloperidol (2-5 mg I.M. for adults) may be required. Hyperthermia is best treated with external cooling measures; or when severe or unresponsive, muscle paralysis with pancuronium may be needed. Hypertension is usually transient and generally does not require treatment unless severe. For diastolic blood pressures >110 mm Hg, a nitroprusside infusion should be initiated. Seizures usually respond to diazepam I.V. and/or phenytoin maintenance regimens.

Drug Interactions

Increased Effect/Toxicity: Increased cardiac irritability if administered concurrently with halogenated inhalation anesthetics, beta-blocking agents, or alpha-blocking agents.

Decreased Effect: Decreased bronchodilation with β-blockers. Decreases antihypertensive effects of methyldopa or guanethidine.

Ethanol/Nutrition/Herb Interactions Herb/Nutraceutical: Avoid ephedra, yohimbe (may cause CNS stimulation).

Stability

Epinephrine is sensitive to light and air; protection from light is recommended

Oxidation turns drug pink, then a brown color; **solutions should not be used if they are discolored or contain a precipitate**

Stability of injection of parenteral admixture at room temperature (25°C) or refrigeration (4°C): 24 hours

Standard diluent: 1 mg/250 mL NS

Compatible with dopamine, dobutamine, diltiazem

Incompatible with aminophylline, sodium bicarbonate or other alkaline solutions

Mechanism of Action Stimulates alpha-, beta$_1$-, and beta$_2$-adrenergic receptors resulting in relaxation of smooth muscle of the bronchial tree, cardiac stimulation, and dilation of skeletal muscle vasculature; small doses can cause vasodilation via beta$_2$-vascular receptors; large doses may produce constriction of skeletal and vascular smooth muscle; decreases production of aqueous humor and increases aqueous outflow; dilates the pupil by contracting the dilator muscle

Pharmacodynamics/Kinetics

Onset of action: Bronchodilation: S.C.: ~5-10 minutes; Inhalation: ~1 minute; Conjunctival instillation: IOP declines ~1 hour

Peak effect: Conjunctival instillation: 4-8 hours

Duration: Conjunctival instillation: Ocular effect: 12-24 hours

Distribution: Crosses placenta; enters breast milk

Metabolism: Taken up into the adrenergic neuron and metabolized by monoamine oxidase and catechol-o-methyltransferase; circulating drug hepatically metabolized

Excretion: Urine (as inactive metabolites metanephrine and the sulfate and hydroxy derivatives of mandelic acid, small amounts unchanged drug)

Usual Dosage

Neonates: Cardiac arrest: I.V.: Intratracheal: 0.01-0.03 mg/kg (0.1-0.3 mL/kg of **1:10,000** solution) every 3-5 minutes as needed; dilute intratracheal doses to 1-2 mL with normal saline

Infants and Children:

Bronchodilator: S.C.: 10 mcg/kg (0.01 mL/kg of **1:1000**) (single doses not to exceed 0.5 mg) **or** suspension (1:200): 0.005 mL/kg/dose (0.025 mg/kg/dose) to a maximum of 0.15 mL (0.75 mg for single dose) every 8-12 hours

Bradycardia:

I.V.: 0.01 mg/kg (0.1 mL/kg of **1:10,000** solution) every 3-5 minutes as needed (maximum: 1 mg/10 mL)

Intratracheal: 0.1 mg/kg (0.1 mL/kg of **1:1000** solution every 3-5 minutes); doses as high as 0.2 mg/kg may be effective

Asystole or pulseless arrest:

I.V. or intraosseous: **First dose:** 0.01 mg/kg (0.1 mL/kg of a **1:10,000** solution); **subsequent doses:** 0.1 mg/kg (0.1 mL/kg of a **1:1000** solution); doses as high as 0.2 mg/kg may be effective; repeat every 3-5 minutes

Intratracheal: 0.1 mg/kg (0.1 mL/kg of a **1:1000** solution); doses as high as 0.2 mg/kg may be effective

Hypersensitivity reaction: S.C.: 0.01 mg/kg every 15 minutes for 2 doses then every 4 hours as needed (single doses not to exceed 0.5 mg)

Refractory hypotension (refractory to dopamine/dobutamine): Continuous I.V. infusions of 0.1-1 mcg/kg/minute; titrate dosage to desired effect

Nebulization: 0.25-0.5 mL of 2.25% **racemic epinephrine** solution diluted in 3 mL normal saline, or L-epinephrine at an equivalent dose; racemic epinephrine 10 mg = 5 mg L-epinephrine; use lower end of dosing range for younger infants

Intranasal: Children ≥6 years and Adults: Apply locally as drops or spray or with sterile swab

Adults:

Asystole:

I.V.: 1 mg every 3-5 minutes; if this approach fails, alternative regimens include:

Intermediate: 2-5 mg every 3-5 minutes

Escalating: 1 mg, 3 mg, 5 mg at 3-minute intervals

(Continued)

Epinephrine (Continued)

High: 0.1 mg/kg every 3-5 minutes

Intratracheal: 1 mg (although optimal dose is unknown, doses of 2-2.5 times the I.V. dose may be needed)

Bronchodilator: I.M., S.C. (**1:1000**): 0.1-0.5 mg every 10-15 minutes to 4 hours

Hypersensitivity reaction: I.M., S.C.: 0.3-0.5 mg every 15-20 minutes if condition requires; if hypotension is present: 0.1 mg I.V. slowly over 5-10 minutes followed by continuous infusion 1-10 mcg/minute

Symptomatic bradycardia or heart block (not responsive to atropine or pacing): I.V. infusion: 1-10 mcg/minute; titrate to desired effect

Refractory hypotension (refractory to dopamine/dobutamine): Continuous I.V. infusion 1 mcg/minute (range: 1-10 mcg/minute); titrate dosage to desired effect; severe cardiac dysfunction may require doses >10 mcg/minute (up to 0.1 mcg/kg/minute)

Nebulization: Instill 8-15 drops into nebulizer reservoirs; administer 1-3 inhalations 4-6 times/day

Ophthalmic: Instill 1-2 drops in eye(s) once or twice daily; when treating open-angle glaucoma, the concentration and dosage must be adjusted to the response of the patient

Administration Central line administration only; intravenous infusions require an infusion pump

Endotracheal: Doses (2-2.5 times the I.V. dose) should be diluted to 10 mL with NS or distilled water prior to administration

Epinephrine can be administered S.C., I.M., I.V., or intracardiac injection

I.M. administration into the buttocks should be avoided

Desired pediatric intravenous infusion solution preparation: "RULE OF 6"

Simplified equation: 0.6 x weight (kg) = amount (mg) of drug to be added to 100 mL of I.V. fluid

When infused at 1 mL/hour, then it will deliver the drug at a rate of 0.1 mcg/kg/minute

Complex equation: 6 x desired dose (mcg/kg/minute) x body weight (kg) divided by desired rate (mL/hour) is the amount (mg) added to make 100 mL of solution

Preparation of adult I.V. infusion: Dilute 1 mg in 250 mL of D_5W or NS (4 mcg/mL); administer at an initial rate of 1 mcg/minute and increase to desired effects; at 20 mcg/minute pure alpha effects occur

1 mcg/minute: 15 mL/hour

2 mcg/minute: 30 mL/hour

3 mcg/minute: 45 mL/hour, etc

Monitoring Parameters Pulmonary function, heart rate, blood pressure, site of infusion for blanching, extravasation; cardiac monitor and blood pressure monitor required

Reference Range Therapeutic: 31-95 pg/mL (SI: 170-520 pmol/L)

Test Interactions ↑ bilirubin (S), catecholamines (U), glucose, uric acid (S)

Nursing Implications Patients should be cautioned to avoid the use of over-the-counter epinephrine inhalation products; beta$_2$-adrenergic agents for inhalation are preferred

Management of extravasation: Use phentolamine as antidote; mix 5 mg with 9 mL of NS; inject a small amount of this dilution into extravasated area; blanching should reverse immediately. Monitor site; if blanching should recur, additional injections of phentolamine may be needed.

Dosage Forms

Aerosol for oral inhalation (Primatene®): 0.2 mg/spray (15 mL, 22.5 mL)

Aerosol for oral inhalation, as bitartrate (AsthmaHaler®, Bronitin®, Primatene® Suspension): 0.3 mg/spray [epinephrine base 0.16 mg/spray] (10 mL, 15 mL, 22.5 mL)

Auto-injector:

EpiPen®: Delivers 0.3 mg I.M. of epinephrine 1:1000 (2 mL)

EpiPen® Jr.: Delivers 0.15 mg I.M. of epinephrine 1:2000 (2 mL)

Injection (Adrenalin®): 1 mg/mL [1:1000] (2 mL)

Injection for solution: 0.1 mg/mL [1:10,000] (10 mL)

Injection for solution, pediatric: 0.1 mg/mL [1:10,000] (5 mL)

Injection for suspension (Sus-Phrine®): 5 mg/mL [1:200] (0.3 mL, 5 mL)

Solution for oral inhalation:

Adrenalin®: 1% [10 mg/mL, 1:100] (7.5 mL)

AsthmaNefrin®, microNefrin®: Racepinephrine 2% [epinephrine base 1.125%] (7.5 mL, 15 mL, 30 mL)

Solution, intranasal [spray]: 0.1% [1 mg/mL, 1:1000] (30 mL)

Solution, ophthalmic, as borate (Epinal®): 0.5% (7.5 mL); 1% (7.5 mL)

Solution, ophthalmic, as hydrochloride (Epifrin®, Glaucon®): 0.1% (1 mL); 0.5% (15 mL); 1% (10 mL, 15 mL); 2% (10 mL, 15 mL)

♦ **Epinephrine and Lidocaine** see Lidocaine and Epinephrine on page 804

♦ **Epinephrine and Pilocarpine** see Pilocarpine and Epinephrine on page 1084

♦ **Epinephrine Bitartrate** see Epinephrine on page 470

♦ **Epinephrine Hydrochloride** see Epinephrine on page 470

♦ **Epipen® (Can)** see Epinephrine on page 470

♦ **EpiPen® Auto-Injector** see Epinephrine on page 470

♦ **Epipen® Jr. (Can)** see Epinephrine on page 470

♦ **EpiPen® Jr Auto-Injector** see Epinephrine on page 470

♦ **Epipodophyllotoxin** see Etoposide on page 533

Epirubicin (ep i ROO bi sin)

U.S. Brand Names Ellence™

Canadian Brand Names Ellence™; Pharmorubicin®

Therapeutic Category Antineoplastic Agent, Anthracycline; Antineoplastic Agent, Antibiotic

Use As a component of adjuvant therapy following primary resection of primary breast cancer in patients with evidence of axillary node tumor involvement

Pregnancy Risk Factor D

Pregnancy/Breast-Feeding Implications Epirubicin is mutagenic and carcinogenic. If a pregnant woman is treated with epirubicin, or if a woman becomes pregnant while receiving this drug, she should be informed of the potential hazard to the fetus. Women of childbearing potential should be advised to avoid becoming pregnant. Excretion in human breast milk is unknown, however other anthracyclines are excreted. Breast-feeding is contraindicated.

Contraindications Hypersensitivity to epirubicin, other anthracyclines, or anthracenediones; baseline neutrophil count <1500 cells/mm³; severe myocardial insufficiency; recent myocardial infarction; previous treatment with anthracyclines up to the maximum cumulative dose; severe hepatic dysfunction; pregnancy

Warnings/Precautions Should be administered only under the supervision of a physician experienced in the use of chemotherapy. The U.S. Food and Drug Administration (FDA) currently recommends that procedures for proper handling and disposal of antineoplastic agents be considered. The primary toxicity is myelosuppression, especially of the granulocytic series, with less marked effects on platelets and erythroid series.

Potential cardiotoxicity, particularly in patients who have received prior anthracyclines or who have pre-existing cardiac disease, may occur. Acute toxicity (primarily arrhythmias) and delayed toxicity (CHF) have been described. Delayed toxicity usually develops late in the course of therapy or within 2-3 months after completion, however, events with an onset of several months to years after termination of treatment have been described. The risk of delayed cardiotoxicity has been correlated to cumulative dose; 0.9% at 550 mg/m², 1.6% at 700 mg/m², 3.3% at 900 mg/m². The risk increases more steeply at dosages above 900 mg/m², and this dose should be exceeded only with extreme caution. Toxicity may be additive with other anthracyclines or anthracenediones.

Reduce dosage and use with caution in mild to moderate hepatic impairment or in severe renal dysfunction (serum creatinine >5 mg/dL). May cause tumor lysis syndrome or radiation recall. Treatment with anthracyclines may increase the risk of secondary leukemias. May cause premature menopause in premenopausal women. For I.V. administration only, severe local tissue necrosis will result if extravasation occurs. Epirubicin is emetogenic.

Adverse Reactions
>10%:
Central nervous system: Lethargy (1% to 46%)
Dermatologic: Alopecia (69% to 95%)
Endocrine & metabolic: Amenorrhea (69% to 72%), hot flashes (5% to 39%)
Gastrointestinal: Nausea, vomiting (83% to 92%), mucositis (9% to 59%), diarrhea (7% to 25%)
Hematologic: Leukopenia (49% to 80%), neutropenia (54% to 80%), anemia (13% to 72%), thrombocytopenia (5% to 49%)
Local: Injection site reactions (3% to 20%)
Vesicant chemotherapy.
Ocular: Conjunctivitis (1% to 15%)
Miscellaneous: Infection (15% to 21%)
1% to 10%:
Cardiovascular: Congestive heart failure (0.4% to 1.5%), decreased LVEF (asymptomatic) (1.4% to 1.8%)
Central nervous system: Fever (1% to 5%)
Dermatologic: Rash (1% to 9%), skin changes (0.7% to 5%)
Gastrointestinal: Anorexia (2% to 3%)
Other reactions (percentage not specified): Acute lymphoid leukemia, acute myelogenous leukemia (0.2% at 3 years), anaphylaxis, hypersensitivity, increased transaminases, photosensitivity reaction, premature menopause, radiation recall, skin and nail hyperpigmentation, urticaria

Overdosage/Toxicology Symptoms of overdose are generally extensions of known cytotoxic effects, including myelosuppression, mucositis, gastrointestinal bleeding, lactic acidosis, multiple organ failure, and death. Delayed development of congestive heart failure may also occur. Treatment is supportive.

Drug Interactions
Cytochrome P450 Effect: No systematic evaluation of the potential for interaction with inhibitors or inducers of cytochrome P450 isoenzymes has been performed.
Increased Effect/Toxicity: Cimetidine increased the blood levels of epirubicin (AUC increased by 50%).

Ethanol/Nutrition/Herb Interactions
Ethanol: Avoid ethanol (due to GI irritation).
Herb/Nutraceutical: St John's wort may decrease doxorubicin levels. Avoid black cohosh, dong quai in estrogen-dependent tumors.

Stability Store refrigerated (2°C to 8°C/36°F to 46°F). Protect from light. Solution should be used within 24 hours of penetrating the rubber stopper. Incompatible with heparin, fluorouracil, or any solution of alkaline pH.

Mechanism of Action Epirubicin is an anthracycline cytotoxic agent. The precise mechanism of its cytotoxic and antiproliferative effect has not been elucidated. Epirubicin is known to inhibit DNA and RNA synthesis by steric obstruction after intercalating between DNA base pairs; active throughout entire cell cycle. Intercalation triggers DNA cleavage by topoisomerase II, resulting in cytocidal activity. Epirubicin also inhibits DNA helicase, and generates cytotoxic free radicals.

Pharmacodynamics/Kinetics
Distribution: V_{ss} 21-27 L/kg
Protein binding: 77% to albumin
Metabolism: Extensive, via hepatic and extrahepatic (including RBCs) routes
Half-life elimination: Triphasic; Mean terminal: 33 hours
Excretion: Feces; urine (lesser extent)

Usual Dosage
Adults: I.V.:
Recommended starting dose: 100-120 mg/m². Epirubicin is given in repeated 3- to 4-week cycles with the total dose given on day 1 of each cycle or divided equally and given on
(Continued)

Epirubicin (Continued)

days 1 and 8 of each cycle. Patients receiving the 120 mg/m^2 regimen should also receive prophylactic antibiotics with TMP-SMX or a fluoroquinolone.

As a component of adjuvant therapy in patients with axillary-node positive breast cancer:
CEF-120: 60 mg/m^2 on days 1 and 8 of cycle (in combination with cyclophosphamide and 5-fluorouracil); cycle is repeated every 28 days for 6 cycles

FEC-100: 100 mg/m^2 on day 1 of cycle (in combination with 5-fluorouracil and cyclophosphamide); cycle is repeated every 21 days for 6 cycles

Dosage adjustment in bone marrow dysfunction:
Patients with heavy pretreatment, pre-existing bone marrow depression, or the presence of neoplastic bone marrow infiltration: Consider lower starting doses of 75-90 mg/m^2

Dosage modifications after the first treatment cycle: Nadir platelet counts <50,000/mm^3, ANC <250/mm^3, neutropenic fever, or grades 3/4 nonhematologic toxicity: Reduce day 1 dose in subsequent cycles to 75% of the current cycle. Day 1 chemotherapy in subsequent courses of treatment should be delayed until platelet counts are ≥100,000/mm^3, ANC ≥1500/mm^3, and nonhematologic toxicities have recovered to ≤ grade 1.

In addition, for patients receiving divided dose (day 1 and day 8) regimen:
Day 8 platelet counts 75,000-100,000/mm^3 and ANC 1000-1499/mm^3: Day 8 dose should be 75% of the day 1 dose

Day 8 platelet counts <75,000/mm^3, ANC <1000/mm^3, or grade 3 or 4 nonhematologic toxicity: Omit day 8 dose

Dosage adjustment in renal impairment: Severe renal impairment (serum creatinine >5 mg/dL): Lower doses should be considered

Dosage adjustment in hepatic impairment:
Bilirubin 1.2-3 mg/dL or AST 2-4 times the upper limit of normal: 50% of recommended starting dose
Bilirubin >3 mg/dL or AST >4 times the upper limit of normal: 25% of recommended starting dose

Elderly: Plasma clearance of epirubicin in elderly female patients was noted to be reduced by 35%. Although no initial dosage reduction is specifically recommended, particular care should be exercised in monitoring toxicity and adjusting subsequent dosage in elderly patients (particularly females >70 years).

Administration Administer I.V. into the tubing of a freely flowing intravenous infusion (0.9% sodium chloride or 5% glucose solution) over 3-5 minutes. Avoid extravasation, associated with severe ulceration and soft tissue necrosis; flush with 5-10 mL of I.V. solution before and after drug administration. Should not be mixed with other drugs in the same syringe. Incompatible with heparin, fluorouracil, or any solution of alkaline pH.

Monitoring Parameters Monitor injection site during infusion for possible extravasation or local reactions; CBC with differential and platelet count, liver function tests, renal function, EKG, and left ventricular ejection fraction

Patient Information Report any stinging or change in sensation during the infusion. This medication can only be administered I.V. During therapy, do not use alcohol, aspirin-containing products, and OTC medications without consulting prescriber. It is important to maintain adequate nutrition and hydration (2-3 L/day of fluids unless instructed to restrict fluid intake) during therapy; frequent small meals may help. You may experience nausea or vomiting (frequent small meals, frequent mouth care, sucking lozenges, or chewing gum may help). You may experience loss of hair (reversible); you will be more susceptible to infection (avoid crowds and exposure to infection as much as possible). Yogurt or buttermilk may help reduce diarrhea (if unresolved, contact prescriber for medication relief). Frequent mouth care and use of a soft toothbrush or cotton swabs may reduce mouth sores. May discolor urine (red/pink). Report fever, chills, unusual bruising or bleeding, signs of infection, abdominal pain or blood in stools, excessive fatigue, yellowing of eyes or skin, swelling of extremities, difficulty breathing, or unresolved diarrhea. Barrier contraceptive measures are recommended for both males and females while receiving this drug and for at least one month following administration. Risks of treatment include irreversible heart damage, treatment-related leukemia, and premature menopause in women.

Dosage Forms Injection: 2 mg/mL (25 mL, 100 mL)

♦ **Epitol**® see Carbamazepine on page 221
♦ **Epival**® **I.V. (Can)** see Valproic Acid and Derivatives on page 1398
♦ **Epivir**® see Lamivudine on page 771
♦ **Epivir-HBV**® see Lamivudine on page 771
♦ **EPO** see Epoetin Alfa on page 474

Epoetin Alfa (e POE e tin AL fa)

U.S. Brand Names Epogen®; Procrit®
Canadian Brand Names Eprex®
Synonyms EPO; Erythropoietin; rHuEPO-α
Therapeutic Category Colony-Stimulating Factor; Growth Factor; Recombinant Human Erythropoietin

Use
Treatment of anemia related to zidovudine therapy in HIV-infected patients; in patients when the endogenous erythropoietin level is ≤500 mU/mL and the dose of zidovudine is ≤4200 mg/week

Treatment of anemia in cancer patients on chemotherapy; in patients with nonmyeloid malignancies where anemia is caused by the effect of the concomitantly administered chemotherapy; to decrease the need for transfusions in patients who will be receiving chemotherapy for a minimum of 2 months

Reduction of allogeneic block transfusion in surgery patients scheduled to undergo elective, noncardiac, nonvascular surgery

Orphan drug: Epogen®: Treatment of anemia associated with end-stage renal disease; treatment of anemia associated with HIV infection or HIV treatment

Unlabeled/Investigational Use Anemia associated with rheumatic disease; hypogenerative anemia of Rh hemolytic disease; sickle cell anemia; acute renal failure; Gaucher's disease; Castleman's disease; paroxysmal nocturnal hemoglobinuria

Pregnancy Risk Factor C

Pregnancy/Breast-Feeding Implications Clinical effect on the fetus: Epoetin alfa has been shown to have adverse effects in rats when given in doses 5X the human dose. There are no adequate and well-controlled studies in pregnant women. Epoetin alfa should be used only if potential benefit justifies the potential risk to the fetus.

Contraindications Hypersensitivity to albumin (human) or mammalian cell-derived products; uncontrolled hypertension

Warnings/Precautions Use with caution in patients with porphyria, hypertension, or a history of seizures; prior to and during therapy, iron stores must be evaluated. It is recommended that the epoetin dose be decreased if the hematocrit increase exceeds 4 points in any 2-week period.

Pretherapy parameters:
Serum ferritin >100 ng/dL
Transferrin saturation (serum iron/iron binding capacity x 100) of 20% to 30%
Iron supplementation (usual oral dosing of 325 mg 2-3 times/day) should be given during therapy to provide for increased requirements during expansion of the red cell mass secondary to marrow stimulation by EPO unless iron stores are already in excess
For patients with endogenous serum EPO levels which are inappropriately low for hemoglobin level, documentation of the serum EPO level will help indicate which patients may benefit from EPO therapy. Serum EPO levels can be ordered routinely from Clinical Chemistry (red top serum separator tube). Refer to "Reference Range" for information on interpretation of EPO levels.

See table:

Factors Limiting Response to Epoetin Alfa

Factor	Mechanism
Iron deficiency	Limits hemoglobin synthesis
Blood loss/hemolysis	Counteracts epoetin alfa-stimulated erythropoiesis
Infection/inflammation	Inhibits iron transfer from storage to bone marrow
	Suppresses erythropoiesis through activated macrophages
Aluminum overload	Inhibits iron incorporation into heme protein
Bone marrow replacement Hyperparathyroidsm Metastatic, neoplastic	Limits bone marrow volume
Folic acid/vitamin B_{12} deficiency	Limits hemoglobin synthesis
Patient compliance	Self-administered epoetin alfa or iron therapy

Increased mortality has occurred when aggressive dosing is used in CHF or anginal patients undergoing hemodialysis. An Amgen-funded study determined that when patients were targeted for a hematocrit of 42% versus a less aggressive 30%, mortality was higher (35% versus 29%).

Adverse Reactions
>10%:
Cardiovascular: Hypertension
Central nervous system: Fatigue, headache, fever
1% to 10%:
Cardiovascular: Edema, chest pain, polycythemia
Central nervous system: Dizziness, seizures
Gastrointestinal: Nausea, vomiting, diarrhea
Hematologic: Clotted access
Neuromuscular & skeletal: Arthralgia, weakness
<1% (Limited to important or life-threatening): CVA/TIA, myocardial infarction

Overdosage/Toxicology Symptoms include erythrocytosis. Adequate airway and other supportive measures and agents for treating anaphylaxis should be present when I.V. drug is given.

Stability
Vials should be stored at 2°C to 8°C (36°F to 46°F); **do not freeze or shake**; single-use vials are stable 2 weeks at room temperature and multidose vials are stable for 1 week at room temperature
Single-dose 1 mL vial contains no preservative: Use one dose per vial; do not re-enter vial; discard unused portions
Multidose 2 mL vial contains preservative; store at 2°C to 8°C after initial entry and between doses; discard 21 days after initial entry
For minimal dilution: Mix with bacteriostatic 0.9% sodium chloride, containing 20 mL of 0.9% sodium chloride and benzyl alcohol as the bacteriostatic agent; dilutions of 1:10 and 1:20 (1 part to epoetin:19 parts sodium chloride) are stable for 18 hours at room temperature; results showed no loss of epoetin alfa after a 1:20 dilution; 250 mcg/mL albumin remaining after a 1:10 dilution of formulated epoetin alfa should be sufficient to prevent it from binding to commonly encountered containers

Mechanism of Action Induces erythropoiesis by stimulating the division and differentiation of committed erythroid progenitor cells; induces the release of reticulocytes from the bone marrow into the bloodstream, where they mature to erythrocytes. There is a dose response relationship with this effect. This results in an increase in reticulocyte counts followed by a rise in hematocrit and hemoglobin levels.

Pharmacodynamics/Kinetics
Onset of action: Several days
Peak effect: 2-3 weeks
(Continued)

Epoetin Alfa *(Continued)*

Distribution: V_d: 9 L; rapid in the plasma compartment; concentrated in liver, kidneys, and bone marrow

Metabolism: Some degradation does occur

Bioavailability: S.C.: ~21% to 31%; intraperitoneal epoetin: 3% (a few patients)

Half-life elimination: Circulating: Chronic renal failure: 4-13 hours; Normal volunteers: 20% shorter

Time to peak, serum: S.C.: 2-8 hours

Excretion: Feces (majority); urine (small amounts, 10% unchanged in normal volunteers)

Usual Dosage

Chronic renal failure patients: I.V., S.C.:

Initial dose: 50-100 units/kg 3 times/week

Reduce dose by 25 units/kg when
1) hematocrit approaches 36% **or**
2) when hematocrit increases >4 points in any 2-week period

Increase dose if hematocrit does not increase by 5-6 points after 8 weeks of therapy and hematocrit is below suggested target range

Suggested target hematocrit range: 30% to 36%

Maintenance dose: Individualize to target range

Dialysis patients: Median dose: 75 units/kg 3 times/week

Nondialysis patients: Doses of 75-150 units/kg

Zidovudine-treated, HIV-infected patients: Patients with erythropoietin levels >500 mU/mL are **unlikely** to respond

Initial dose: I.V., S.C.: 100 units/kg 3 times/week for 8 weeks

Increase dose by 50-100 units/kg 3 times/week if response is not satisfactory in terms of reducing transfusion requirements or increasing hematocrit after 8 weeks of therapy

Evaluate response every 4-8 weeks thereafter and adjust the dose accordingly by 50-100 units/kg increments 3 times/week

If patients have not responded satisfactorily to a 300 unit/kg dose 3 times/week, it is unlikely that they will respond to higher doses

Stop dose if hematocrit exceeds 40% and resume treatment at a 25% dose reduction when hematocrit drops to 36%

Cancer patients on chemotherapy: Treatment of patients with erythropoietin levels >200 mU/mL is **not recommended**

Initial dose: S.C.: 150 units/kg 3 times/week

Dose adjustment: If response is not satisfactory in terms of reducing transfusion requirement or increasing hematocrit after 8 weeks of therapy, the dose may be increased up to 300 units/kg 3 times/week. If patients do not respond, it is unlikely that they will respond to higher doses.

If hematocrit exceeds 40%, hold the dose until it falls to 36% and reduce the dose by 25% when treatment is resumed

Surgery patients: Prior to initiating treatment, obtain a hemoglobin to establish that is >10 mg/dL or ≤13 mg/dL

Initial dose: S.C.: 300 units/kg/day for 10 days before surgery, on the day of surgery, and for 4 days after surgery

Alternative dose: S.C.: 600 units/kg in once weekly doses (21, 14, and 7 days before surgery) plus a fourth dose on the day of surgery

Administration Dilute with an equal volume of normal saline and infuse over 1-3 minutes; it may be administered into the venous line at the end of the dialysis procedure

Monitoring Parameters

Careful monitoring of blood pressure is indicated; problems with hypertension have been noted especially in renal failure patients treated with rHuEPO. Other patients are less likely to develop this complication.

Suggested tests to be monitored and their frequency: See table.

Test	Initial Phase Frequency	Maintenance Phase Frequency
Hematocrit/hemoglobin*	2 x/week	2-4 x/month
Blood pressure	3 x/week	3 x/week
Serum ferritin	Monthly	Quarterly
Transferrin saturation	Monthly	Quarterly
Serum chemistries including CBC with differential, creatinine, blood urea nitrogen, potassium, phosphorous	Regularly per routine	Regularly per routine

*Hematocrit should be determined twice weekly until stabilization within the target range (30% to 36%), and twice weekly for at least 2-6 weeks after a dose increase.

Reference Range Guidelines should be based on the following figure or published literature

Guidelines for estimating appropriateness of endogenous EPO levels for varying levels of anemia via the EIA assay method: See figure. The reference range for erythropoietin in serum, for subjects with normal hemoglobin and hematocrit, is 4.1-22.2 mU/mL by the EIA method. Erythropoietin levels are typically inversely related to hemoglobin (and hematocrit) levels in anemias not attributed to impaired erythropoietin production.

Zidovudine-treated HIV patients: Available evidence indicates patients with endogenous serum erythropoietin levels >500 mU/mL are unlikely to respond

Cancer chemotherapy patients: Treatment of patients with endogenous serum erythropoietin levels >200 mU/mL is not recommended

Patient Information You will require frequent blood tests to determine appropriate dosage. Do not take other medications, vitamin or iron supplements, or make significant changes in your diet without consulting prescriber. Report signs or symptoms of edema (eg, swollen extremities, difficulty breathing, rapid weight gain), onset of severe headache, acute back pain, chest pain, muscular tremors, or seizure activity.

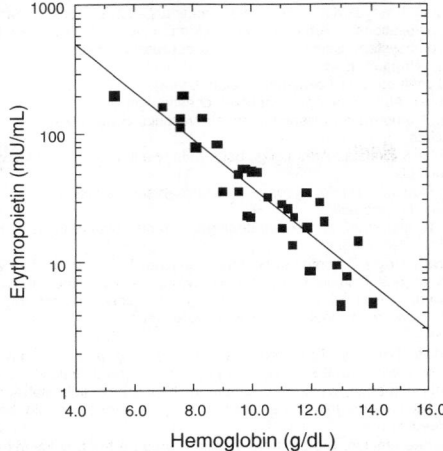

Hemoglobin (g/dL)

Nursing Implications Dilute with an equal volume of normal saline and infuse over 1-3 minutes; may be administered into the venous line at the end of the dialysis procedure

Additional Information Due to the delayed onset of erythropoiesis (7-10 days to ↑ reticulocyte count; 2-6 weeks to ↑ hemoglobin), erythropoietin is of no value in the acute treatment of anemia. Emergency/stat orders for erythropoietin are inappropriate.

Professional Services:
Amgen (Epogen®): 1-800-772-6436
Ortho Biotech (Procrit®): 1-800-325-7504
Reimbursement Assistance:
Amgen: 1-800-272-9376
Ortho Biotech: 1-800-553-3851

Dosage Forms
Solution, 1 mL [multidose vial] [with preservative]: 20,000 units/mL
Solution, 1 mL [single-dose vial] [preservative free]:
2000 units/mL
3000 units/mL
4000 units/mL
10,000 units/mL
40,000 units/mL
Solution, 2 mL [multidose vial] [with preservative]: 10,000 units/mL

♦ **Epogen®** see Epoetin Alfa on page 474

Epoprostenol (e poe PROST en ole)
U.S. Brand Names Flolan®
Canadian Brand Names Flolan®
Synonyms Epoprostenol Sodium; PGI₂; PGX; Prostacyclin
Therapeutic Category Prostaglandin
Use Orphan drug: Treatment of primary pulmonary hypertension; treatment of secondary pulmonary hypertension due to intrinsic precapillary pulmonary vascular disease
Unlabeled/Investigational Use Other potential uses include pulmonary hypertension associated with ARDS, SLE, or CHF; neonatal pulmonary hypertension; cardiopulmonary bypass surgery; hemodialysis; atherosclerosis; peripheral vascular disorders; and neonatal purpura fulminans
Pregnancy Risk Factor B
Contraindications Hypersensitivity to epoprostenol or to structurally-related compounds; chronic use in patients with CHF due to severe left ventricular systolic dysfunction
Warnings/Precautions Abrupt interruptions or large sudden reductions in dosage may result in rebound pulmonary hypertension; some patients with primary pulmonary hypertension have developed pulmonary edema during dose ranging, which may be associated with pulmonary veno-occlusive disease; during chronic use, unless contraindicated, anticoagulants should be coadministered to reduce the risk of thromboembolism. Clinical studies of epoprostenol in pulmonary hypertension did not include sufficient numbers of patients ≥65 years of age to substantiate its safety and efficacy in the geriatric population. As a result, in general, dose selection for an elderly patient should be cautious usually starting at the low end of the dosing range.
Adverse Reactions
>10%:
Cardiovascular: Flushing, tachycardia, shock, syncope, heart failure
Central nervous system: Fever, chills, anxiety, nervousness, dizziness, headache, hyperesthesia, pain
Gastrointestinal: Diarrhea, nausea, vomiting
Neuromuscular & skeletal: Jaw pain, myalgia, tremor, paresthesia
Respiratory: Hypoxia
Miscellaneous: Sepsis, flu-like symptoms
(Continued)

Epoprostenol *(Continued)*

1% to 10%:
  Cardiovascular: Bradycardia, hypotension, angina pectoris, edema, arrhythmias, pallor, cyanosis, palpitations, cerebrovascular accident, myocardial ischemia, chest pain
  Central nervous system: Seizures, confusion, depression, insomnia
  Dermatologic: Pruritus, rash
  Endocrine & metabolic: Hypokalemia, weight change
  Gastrointestinal: Abdominal pain, anorexia, constipation
  Hematologic: Hemorrhage, disseminated intravascular coagulation
  Hepatic: Ascites
  Neuromuscular & skeletal: Arthralgias, bone pain, weakness
  Ocular: Amblyopia
  Respiratory: Cough increase, dyspnea, epistaxis, pleural effusion
  Miscellaneous: Diaphoresis
<1% (Limited to important or life-threatening): Anemia, hypersplenism, hyperthyroidism, pancytopenia, splenomegaly

Overdosage/Toxicology Symptoms include headache, hypotension, tachycardia, nausea, vomiting, diarrhea, and flushing. If any of these symptoms occur, the infusion rate should be reduced until symptoms subside. If symptoms do not subside, consider drug discontinuation. No fatal events have been reported following overdosage.

Drug Interactions
  Increased Effect/Toxicity: The hypotensive effects of epoprostenol may be exacerbated by other vasodilators, diuretics, or by using acetate in dialysis fluids. Patients treated with anticoagulants (heparins, warfarin, thrombin inhibitors) or antiplatelet agents (ticlopidine, clopidogrel, IIb/IIIa antagonists, aspirin) and epoprostenol should be monitored for increased bleeding risk.

Stability Refrigerate ampuls; protect from freezing; prepare fresh solutions every 24 hours; stable only when reconstituted with the diluent solution packaged with the medication. See table.

Preparation of Epoprostenol Infusion

To make 100 mL of solution with concentration:	Directions
3000 ng/mL	Dissolve one 0.5 mg vial with 5 mL supplied diluent, withdraw 3 mL, and add to sufficient diluent to make a total of 100 mL.
5000 ng/mL	Dissolve one 0.5 mg vial with 5 mL supplied diluent, withdraw entire vial contents, and add a sufficient volume of diluent to make a total of 100 mL.
10,000 ng/mL	Dissolve two 0.5 mg vials each with 5 mL supplied diluent, withdraw entire vial contents, and add a sufficient volume of diluent to make a total of 100 mL.
15,000 ng/mL	Dissolve one 1.5 mg vial with 5 mL supplied diluent, withdraw entire vial contents, and add a sufficient volume of diluent to make a total of 100 mL.

Mechanism of Action Epoprostenol is also known as prostacyclin and PGI_2. It is a strong vasodilator of all vascular beds. In addition, it is a potent endogenous inhibitor of platelet aggregation. The reduction in platelet aggregation results from epoprostenol's activation of intracellular adenylate cyclase and the resultant increase in cyclic adenosine monophosphate concentrations within the platelets. Additionally, it is capable of decreasing thrombogenesis and platelet clumping in the lungs by inhibiting platelet aggregation.

Pharmacodynamics/Kinetics
  Metabolism: Rapidly hydrolyzed at neutral pH in blood and subject to some enzymatic degradation to one active metabolite, and 13 inactive metabolites
  Half-life elimination: 2.7-6 minutes; Continuous infusion: ~15 minutes
  Excretion: Urine (12% as unchanged drug)

Usual Dosage I.V.: The drug is administered by continuous intravenous infusion via a central venous catheter using an ambulatory infusion pump; during dose ranging it may be administered peripherally

  Acute dose ranging: The initial infusion rate should be 2 ng/kg/minute by continuous I.V. and increased in increments of 2 ng/kg/minute every 15 minutes or longer until dose-limiting effects are elicited (such as chest pain, anxiety, dizziness, changes in heart rate, dyspnea, nausea, vomiting, headache, hypotension and/or flushing)
  Continuous chronic infusion: Initial: 4 ng/kg/minute **less** than the maximum-tolerated infusion rate determined during acute dose ranging
    If maximum-tolerated infusion rate is <5 ng/kg/minute, the chronic infusion rate should be $^1/_2$ the maximum-tolerated acute infusion rate
  Dosage adjustments: Dose adjustments in the chronic infusion rate should be based on persistence, recurrence, or worsening of patient symptoms of pulmonary hypertension
    If symptoms persist or recur after improving, the infusion rate should be increased by 1-2 ng/kg/minute increments, every 15 minutes or greater; following establishment of a new chronic infusion rate, the patient should be observed and vital signs monitored.

Administration
  Using an ambulatory infusion pump, administer a chronic continuous infusion of epoprostenol through a central venous catheter. A peripheral intravenous catheter may be used during acute dose-ranging until central access is established. Consider a multilumen catheter if other intravenous therapies are routinely administered. During extended use at ambient temperatures exceeding 25°C (77°F), cold pouches with frozen gel packs were used during clinical trials.
  The ambulatory infusion pump should be small and lightweight, be able to adjust infusion rates in 2 ng/kg/minute increments, have occlusion, end of infusion, and low battery

alarms, have ±6% accuracy of the programmed rate, and have positive continuous or pulsatile pressure with intervals ≤3 minutes between pulses. The reservoir should be made of polyvinyl chloride, polypropylene, or glass. The infusion pumps used in clinical trials were CADD-1 HFX 5100 (Pharmacia Deltec), Walk-Med 410 C (Medfusion, Inc) and the Auto Syringe AS2F (Baxter HealthCare).

Monitoring Parameters Monitor for improvements in pulmonary function, decreased exertional dyspnea, fatigue, syncope and chest pain, pulmonary vascular resistance, pulmonary arterial pressure and quality of life. In addition, the pump device and catheters should be monitored frequently to avoid "system" related failure.

Patient Information Therapy with epoprostenol requires commitment to drug reconstitution, administration, and care of the permanent central venous catheter. The decision to receive epoprostenol should be based upon the understanding that there is a high likelihood that therapy will be needed for prolonged periods, possibly for life, and that the care of the catheter and infusion pump will be required and should be carefully considered. Promptly report any adverse drug reactions with epoprostenol, this may require dosage adjustments.

Nursing Implications Monitor arterial pressure; assess all vital functions; hypoxia, flushing, and tachycardia may indicate overdose. Epoprostenol must be reconstituted with manufacturer-supplied sterile diluent only and when given on an ongoing basis, it must be infused through a permanent indwelling central venous catheter via a portable infusion pump. Instruct patient to report ADRs since dosage adjustments may be necessary.

Additional Information All orders for epoprostenol are distributed only by Olsten Health Services. To order the drug or to request reimbursement assistance, call 1-800-935-6526.

Dosage Forms Injection, as sodium [with 50 mL sterile diluent]: 0.5 mg/vial, 1.5 mg/vial

♦ **Epoprostenol Sodium** *see* Epoprostenol *on page 477*

♦ **Eprex® (Can)** *see* Epoetin Alfa *on page 474*

Eprosartan (ep roe SAR tan)

Related Information
Angiotensin Agents Comparison *on page 1473*

U.S. Brand Names Teveten®

Therapeutic Category Angiotensin II Receptor Antagonist (ARB); Antihypertensive Agent

Use Treatment of hypertension; may be used alone or in combination with other antihypertensives

Pregnancy Risk Factor C (1st trimester); D (2nd and 3rd trimesters)

Contraindications Hypersensitivity to eprosartan or any component of the formulation; sensitivity to other A-II receptor antagonists; bilateral renal artery stenosis; primary hyperaldosteronism; pregnancy (2nd and 3rd trimesters)

Warnings/Precautions Avoid use or use a smaller dose in patients who are volume depleted; correct depletion first. Deterioration in renal function can occur with initiation. Use with caution in unilateral renal artery stenosis and pre-existing renal insufficiency; significant aortic/mitral stenosis. Safety and efficacy not established in pediatric patients.

Adverse Reactions
1% to 10%:
   Central nervous system: Fatigue (2%), depression (1%)
   Endocrine & metabolic: Hypertriglyceridemia (1%)
   Gastrointestinal: Abdominal pain (2%)
   Genitourinary: Urinary tract infection (1%)
   Respiratory: Upper respiratory tract infection (8%), rhinitis (4%), pharyngitis (4%), cough (4%)
   Miscellaneous: Viral infection (2%), injury (2%)
<1% (Limited to important or life-threatening): Angina, arthritis, asthma, ataxia, BUN increased, creatinine increased, eczema, edema, esophagitis, ethanol intolerance, gingivitis, gout, influenza-like symptoms, leg cramps, leukopenia, maculopapular rash, migraine, neuritis, neutropenia, paresthesia, peripheral ischemia, purpura, renal calculus, somnolence, tendonitis, thrombocytopenia, tinnitus, tremor, urinary incontinence, vertigo

Overdosage/Toxicology The most likely manifestations of overdose would be hypotension and tachycardia. Initiate supportive care for symptomatic hypotension.

Drug Interactions
   Increased Effect/Toxicity: Eprosartan may increase risk of lithium toxicity. May increase risk of hyperkalemia with potassium-sparing diuretics (eg, amiloride, potassium, spironolactone, triamterene), potassium supplements, or high doses of trimethoprim.

Ethanol/Nutrition/Herb Interactions Herb/Nutraceutical: Avoid dong quai if using for hypertension (has estrogenic activity). Avoid ephedra, yohimbe, ginseng (may worsen hypertension). Avoid garlic (may have increased antihypertensive effect).

Mechanism of Action Angiotensin II is formed from angiotensin I in a reaction catalyzed by angiotensin-converting enzyme (ACE, kininase II). Angiotensin II is the principal pressor agent of the renin-angiotensin system, with effects that include vasoconstriction, stimulation of synthesis and release of aldosterone, cardiac stimulation, and renal reabsorption of sodium. Eprosartan blocks the vasoconstrictor and aldosterone-secreting effects of angiotensin II by selectively blocking the binding of angiotensin II to the AT1 receptor in many tissues, such as vascular smooth muscle and the adrenal gland. Its action is therefore independent of the pathways for angiotensin II synthesis. Blockade of the renin-angiotensin system with ACE inhibitors, which inhibit the biosynthesis of angiotensin II from angiotensin I, is widely used in the treatment of hypertension. ACE inhibitors also inhibit the degradation of bradykinin, a reaction also catalyzed by ACE. Because eprosartan does not inhibit ACE (kininase II), it does not affect the response to bradykinin. Whether this difference has clinical relevance is not yet known. Eprosartan does not bind to or block other hormone receptors or ion channels known to be important in cardiovascular regulation.

Pharmacodynamics/Kinetics
   Half-life elimination: Terminal: 5-9 hours
   Time to peak, serum: Fasting: 1-2 hours
   Excretion: Clearance: 7.9 L/hour
   (Continued)

Eprosartan *(Continued)*

Usual Dosage Adults: Oral: Dosage must be individualized; can administer once or twice daily with total daily doses of 400-800 mg. Usual starting dose is 600 mg once daily as monotherapy in patients who are euvolemic. Limited clinical experience with doses >800 mg.
Dosage adjustment in renal impairment: No starting dosage adjustment is necessary; however, carefully monitor the patient
Dosage adjustment in hepatic impairment: No starting dosage adjustment is necessary; however, carefully monitor the patient

Elderly: No starting dosage adjustment is necessary; however, carefully monitor the patient
Patient Information May be taken with or without food; female patients should be counseled regarding appropriate birth control methods and to report any signs and symptoms of pregnancy. Monitor blood pressure regularly. Do not stop taking this medication without advising your healthcare professional. Take each dose at the same time each day. Take a missed dose as soon as possible, but do not double-up doses.
Dosage Forms
Tablet: 600 mg
Tablet, scored: 400 mg

♦ **Epsom Salts** *see* Magnesium Sulfate *on page 836*
♦ **EPT** *see* Teniposide *on page 1296*

Eptifibatide *(ep TIF i ba tide)*
Related Information
Glycoprotein Antagonists *on page 1500*
U.S. Brand Names Integrilin®
Canadian Brand Names Integrilin™
Synonyms Intrifiban
Therapeutic Category Antiplatelet Agent; Glycoprotein IIb/IIIa Inhibitor; Platelet Aggregation Inhibitor
Use Treatment of patients with acute coronary syndrome (UA/NQMI), including patients who are to be managed medically and those undergoing percutaneous coronary intervention (PCI including PTCA; intracoronary stenting)
Pregnancy Risk Factor B
Contraindications Hypersensitivity to eptifibatide or any component of the product; active abnormal bleeding or a history of bleeding diathesis within the previous 30 days; history of CVA within 30 days or a history of hemorrhagic stroke; severe hypertension (systolic blood pressure >200 mm Hg or diastolic blood pressure >110 mm Hg) not adequately controlled on antihypertensive therapy; major surgery within the preceding 6 weeks; current or planned administration of another parenteral GP IIb/IIIa inhibitor; thrombocytopenia; serum creatinine >4 mg/dL; dependency on renal dialysis
Warnings/Precautions Bleeding is the most common complication. Most major bleeding occurs at the arterial access site where the cardiac catheterization was done. When bleeding can not be controlled with pressure, discontinue infusion and heparin. Use caution in patients with platelet counts <100,000/mm^3, hemorrhagic retinopathy, or with other drugs that affect hemostasis. Concurrent use with thrombolytics has not been established as safe. Minimize other procedures including arterial and venous punctures, I.M. injections, nasogastric tubes, etc. Prior to sheath removal, the aPTT or ACT should be checked (do not remove unless aPTT is <45 seconds or the ACT <150 seconds).
Adverse Reactions Bleeding is the major drug-related adverse effect. Major bleeding was reported in 4.4% to 10.8%; minor bleeding was reported in 10.5% to 14.2%; requirement for transfusion was reported in 5.5% to 12.8%. Incidence of bleeding is also related to heparin intensity (aPTT goal 50-70 seconds). Patients weighing <70 kg may have an increased risk of major bleeding.

Cardiovascular: Hypotension
Local: Injection site reaction
Neuromuscular & skeletal: Back pain

1% to 10%: Hematologic: Thrombocytopenia (1.2% to 3.2%)
<1% (Limited to important or life-threatening): Anaphylaxis, GI hemorrhage, intracranial hemorrhage (0.5% to 0.7%), pulmonary hemorrhage
Overdosage/Toxicology Two cases of human overdosage have been reported. Neither case was eventful and were not associated with major bleeding. Symptoms of overdose in animal studies include loss of righting reflex, dyspnea, ptosis, decreased muscle tone, and petechial hemorrhages.
Drug Interactions
Increased Effect/Toxicity: Eptifibatide effect may be increased by other drugs which affect hemostasis include thrombolytics, oral anticoagulants, nonsteroidal anti-inflammatory agents, dipyridamole, heparin, low molecular weight heparins, ticlopidine, and clopidogrel. Avoid concomitant use of other IIb/IIIa inhibitors. Cephalosporins which contain the MTT side chain may theoretically increase the risk of hemorrhage. Use with aspirin and heparin may increase bleeding over aspirin and heparin alone. However, aspirin and heparin were used concurrently in the majority of patients in the major clinical studies of eptifibatide.
Stability Vials should be stored refrigerated at 2°C to 8°C (36°F to 46°F). Vials can be kept at room temperature for 2 months. Protect from light until administration. Do not use beyond the expiration date. Discard any unused portion left in the vial.

May be administered in same I.V. line as alteplase, atropine, dobutamine, heparin, lidocaine, meperidine, metoprolol, midazolam, morphine, nitroglycerin, verapamil, normal saline (infusion may contain up to 60 mEq/L KCl), or normal saline/D$_5$W (infusion may contain up to 60 mEq/L KCl).
Mechanism of Action Eptifibatide is a cyclic heptapeptide which blocks the platelet glycoprotein IIb/IIIa receptor, the binding site for fibrinogen, von Willebrand factor, and other ligands. Inhibition of binding at this final common receptor reversibly blocks platelet aggregation and prevents thrombosis.

Pharmacodynamics/Kinetics
Onset of action: Within 1 hour
Duration: Platelet function restored ~4 hours following discontinuation
Protein binding: ~25%
Half-life elimination: 2.5 hours
Excretion: Primarily urine (as eptifibatide and metabolites); significant renal impairment may alter disposition of this compound
Clearance: Total body: 55-58 mL/kg/hour; Renal: ~50% of total in healthy subjects

Usual Dosage I.V.: Adults:
Acute coronary syndrome: Bolus of 180 mcg/kg (maximum: 22.6 mg) over 1-2 minutes, begun as soon as possible following diagnosis, followed by a continuous infusion of 2 mcg/kg/minute (maximum: 15 mg/hour) until hospital discharge or initiation of CABG surgery, up to 72 hours. Concurrent aspirin (160-325 mg initially and daily thereafter) and heparin therapy (target aPTT 50-70 seconds) are recommended.
Percutaneous coronary intervention (PCI): Bolus of 180 mcg/kg (maximum: 22.6 mg) administered immediately before the initiation of PCI, followed by a continuous infusion of 2 mcg/kg/minute (maximum: 15 mg/hour). A second 180 mcg/kg bolus (maximum: 22.6 mg) should be administered 10 minutes after the first bolus. Infusion should be continued until hospital discharge or for up to 18-24 hours, whichever comes first; minimum of 12 hours of infusion is recommended. Concurrent aspirin (160-325 mg 1-24 hours before PCI and daily thereafter) and heparin therapy (ACT 200-300 seconds during PCI) are recommended. Heparin infusion after PCI is discouraged. In patients who undergo coronary artery bypass graft surgery, discontinue infusion prior to surgery.
Dosing adjustment in renal impairment:
Acute coronary syndrome: S_{cr} >2 mg/dL and <4 mg/dL: Use 180 mcg/kg bolus (maximum: 22.6 mg) and 1 mcg/kg/minute infusion (maximum: 7.5 mg/hour)
Percutaneous coronary intervention (PCI): Adults: S_{cr} >2 mg/dL and <4 mg/dL: Use 180 mcg/kg bolus (maximum: 22.6 mg) administered immediately before the initiation of PCI and followed by a continuous infusion of 1 mcg/kg/minute (maximum: 7.5 mg/hour). A second 180 mcg/kg (maximum: 22.6 mg) bolus should be administered 10 minutes after the first bolus.

Administration Visually inspect for discoloration or particulate matter prior to administration. The bolus dose should be withdrawn from the 10 mL vial into a syringe and administered by I.V. push over 1-2 minutes. Begin continuous infusion immediately following bolus administration, administered directly from the 100 mL vial. The 100 mL vial should be spiked with a vented infusion set.

Monitoring Parameters Coagulation parameters, signs/symptoms of excessive bleeding. Laboratory tests at baseline and monitoring during therapy: hematocrit and hemoglobin, platelet count, serum creatinine, PT/aPTT (maintain aPTT between 50-70 seconds unless PCI is to be performed), and ACT with PCI (maintain ACT between 200-300 seconds during PCI).

Nursing Implications Do not shake the vial; maintain bleeding precautions, avoid unnecessary arterial and venous punctures, use saline or heparin lock for blood drawing, assess sheath insertion site and distal pulses of affected leg every 15 minutes for the first hour and then every 1 hour for the next 6 hours. Arterial access site care is important to prevent bleeding. Care should be taken when attempting vascular access that only the anterior wall of the femoral artery is punctured, avoiding a Seldinger (through and through) technique for obtaining sheath access. Femoral vein sheath placement should be avoided unless needed. While the vascular sheath is in place, patients should be maintained on complete bed rest with the head of the bed at a 30° angle and the affected limb restrained in a straight position.

Observe patient for mental status changes, hemorrhage, assess nose and mouth mucous membranes, puncture sites for oozing, ecchymosis and hematoma formation, and examine urine, stool and emesis for presence of occult or frank blood; gentle care should be provided when removing dressings.

Dosage Forms Injection: 0.75 mg/mL (100 mL); 2 mg/mL (10 mL, 100 mL)

♦ **Equagesic®** see Aspirin and Meprobamate on page 124
♦ **Equanil®** see Meprobamate on page 861
♦ **Equilet® [OTC]** see Calcium Carbonate on page 207
♦ **Ercaf®** see Ergotamine on page 483
♦ **Ergamisol®** see Levamisole on page 786

Ergocalciferol (er goe kal SIF e role)
U.S. Brand Names Calciferol™; Drisdol®
Canadian Brand Names Drisdol®; Ostoforte®
Synonyms Activated Ergosterol; Viosterol; Vitamin D_2
Therapeutic Category Vitamin, Fat Soluble
Use Treatment of refractory rickets, hypophosphatemia, hypoparathyroidism
Pregnancy Risk Factor A/C (dose exceeding RDA recommendation)
Usual Dosage Oral dosing is preferred; I.M. therapy required with GI, liver, or biliary disease associated with malabsorption
Dietary supplementation (each mcg = 40 USP units):
Premature infants: 10-20 mcg/day (400-800 units), up to 750 mcg/day (30,000 units)
Infants and healthy Children: 10 mcg/day (400 units)
Adults: 10 mcg/day (400 units)
Renal failure:
Children: 100-1000 mcg/day (4000-40,000 units)
Adults: 500 mcg/day (20,000 units)
Hypoparathyroidism:
Children: 1.25-5 mg/day (50,000-200,000 units) and calcium supplements
Adults: 625 mcg to 5 mg/day (25,000-200,000 units) and calcium supplements
Vitamin D-dependent rickets:
Children: 75-125 mcg/day (3000-5000 units); maximum: 1500 mcg/day
Adults: 250 mcg to 1.5 mg/day (10,000-60,000 units)
(Continued)

Ergocalciferol *(Continued)*

Nutritional rickets and osteomalacia:
  Children and Adults (with normal absorption): 25-125 mcg/day (1000-5000 units)
  Children with malabsorption: 250-625 mcg/day (10,000-25,000 units)
  Adults with malabsorption: 250-7500 mcg (10,000-300,000 units)
Vitamin D-resistant rickets:
  Children: Initial: 1000-2000 mcg/day (40,000-80,000 units) with phosphate supplements;
    daily dosage is increased at 3- to 4-month intervals in 250-500 mcg (10,000-20,000
    units) increments
  Adults: 250-1500 mcg/day (10,000-60,000 units) with phosphate supplements
Familial hypophosphatemia: 10,000-80,000 units daily plus 1-2 g/day elemental phosphorus
Osteoporosis prophylaxis: Adults:
  51-70 years: 400 units/day
  >70 years: 600 units/day
  Maximum daily dose: 2000 units/day

Additional Information Complete prescribing information for this medication should be consulted for additional detail.

Dosage Forms
  Capsule (Drisdol®): 50,000 units [1.25 mg]
  Injection (Calciferol™): 500,000 units/mL [12.5 mg/mL] (1 mL)
  Liquid (Calciferol™, Drisdol®): 8000 units/mL [200 mcg/mL] (60 mL)

Ergoloid Mesylates *(ER goe loid MES i lates)*

U.S. Brand Names Germinal®; Hydergine®; Hydergine® LC
Canadian Brand Names Hydergine®
Synonyms Dihydroergotoxine; Dihydrogenated Ergot Alkaloids
Therapeutic Category Ergot Alkaloid and Derivative
Use Treatment of cerebrovascular insufficiency in primary progressive dementia, Alzheimer's dementia, and senile onset
Pregnancy Risk Factor C
Usual Dosage Adults: Oral: 1 mg 3 times/day up to 4.5-12 mg/day; up to 6 months of therapy may be necessary
Additional Information Complete prescribing information for this medication should be consulted for additional detail.
Dosage Forms
  Capsule, liquid (Hydergine® LC): 1 mg
  Liquid (Hydergine®): 1 mg/mL (100 mL)
  Tablet (Hydergine®): 1 mg
  Tablet, sublingual (Gerimal®, Hydergine®): 0.5 mg, 1 mg

♦ **Ergomar**® *see Ergotamine on page 483*
♦ **Ergometrine Maleate** *see Ergonovine on page 482*

Ergonovine *(er goe NOE veen)*

Synonyms Ergometrine Maleate; Ergonovine Maleate
Therapeutic Category Ergot Alkaloid and Derivative
Use Prevention and treatment of postpartum and postabortion hemorrhage caused by uterine atony or subinvolution
Unlabeled/Investigational Use Migraine headaches, diagnostically to identify Prinzmetal's angina

Pregnancy Risk Factor X
Pregnancy/Breast-Feeding Implications Prolonged constriction of the uterine vessels and/or increased myometrial tone may lead to reduced placental blood flow. This has contributed to fetal growth retardation in animals. Excreted in breast milk, breast-feeding is not recommended.
Contraindications Hypersensitivity to ergonovine or any component of the formulation; concurrent use with ritonavir, nelfinavir, or amprenavir; induction of labor, threatened spontaneous abortion, pregnancy
Warnings/Precautions Use with caution in patients with sepsis, heart disease, hypertension, or with hepatic or renal impairment; restore uterine responsiveness in calcium-deficient patients who do not respond to ergonovine by I.V. calcium administration; avoid prolonged use; discontinue if ergotism develops
Adverse Reactions
  1% to 10%: Gastrointestinal: Nausea, vomiting
  <1% (Limited to important or life-threatening): Bradycardia, cerebrovascular accidents, diaphoresis, dizziness, dyspnea, ergotism, headache, hypertension (sometimes extreme - treat with I.V. chlorpromazine), myocardial infarction, palpitations, seizures, shock, thrombophlebitis, tinnitus, transient chest pain
Overdosage/Toxicology Symptoms include gangrene (chronic), seizures (acute), chest pain, numbness in extremities, weak pulse, confusion, excitement, delirium, and hallucinations. Treatment is supportive following GI decontamination (for oral overdose). Administer I.V. or intra-arterial nitroprusside for arterial venospasm and nitroglycerin for coronary vasospasm.
Drug Interactions
  Increased Effect/Toxicity: Concomitant use with beta-adrenergic blockers may result in toxic peripheral ischemia, gangrene.
Stability Refrigerate injection, protect from light; store intact ampuls in refrigerator, stable for 60-90 days; do not use if discoloration occurs
Mechanism of Action Ergot alkaloid alpha-adrenergic agonist directly stimulates vascular smooth muscle to vasoconstrict peripheral and cerebral vessels; may also have antagonist effects on serotonin
Pharmacodynamics/Kinetics
  Onset of action: I.M.: ~2-5 minutes

Duration: I.M.: Uterine effect: 3 hours; I.V.: ~45 minutes

Metabolism: Hepatic

Excretion: Primarily feces; urine

Usual Dosage Adults: I.M., I.V. (I.V. should be reserved for emergency use only): 0.2 mg, repeat dose in 2-4 hours as needed

Administration I.V. doses should be administered over a period of not <1 minute; dilute in NS to 5 mL for I.V. administration

Patient Information May cause nausea, vomiting, dizziness, increased blood pressure, headache, ringing in the ears, chest pain, or shortness of breath

Nursing Implications I.V. use should be limited to patients with severe uterine bleeding or other life-threatening emergency situations

Dosage Forms Injection, as maleate: 0.2 mg/mL (1 mL)

♦ **Ergonovine Maleate** *see* Ergonovine *on page 482*

Ergotamine (er GOT a meen)

U.S. Brand Names Cafatine®; Cafergot®; Ercaf®; Ergomar®; Migranal®; Wigraine®

Canadian Brand Names Cafergot®; Ergomar®

Synonyms Ergotamine Tartrate; Ergotamine Tartrate and Caffeine

Therapeutic Category Adrenergic Blocking Agent; Antimigraine Agent, Prophylactic; Ergot Alkaloid and Derivative

Use Abort or prevent vascular headaches, such as migraine or cluster

Pregnancy Risk Factor X

Pregnancy/Breast-Feeding Implications Prolonged constriction of the uterine vessels and/or increased myometrial tone may lead to reduced placental blood flow. This has contributed to fetal growth retardation in animals. Excreted in breast milk, breast-feeding is not recommended.

Contraindications Hypersensitivity to ergotamine, caffeine, or any component of the formulation; peripheral vascular disease; hepatic or renal disease; coronary artery disease; hypertension; peptic ulcer disease; sepsis; concurrent use with ritonavir, nelfinavir, and amprenavir; pregnancy

Warnings/Precautions Avoid prolonged administration or excessive dosage because of the danger of ergotism (intense vasoconstriction) and gangrene; patients who take ergotamine for extended periods of time may become dependent on it. May be harmful due to reduction in cerebral blood flow; may precipitate angina, myocardial infarction, or aggravate intermittent claudication; therefore, not considered a drug of choice in the elderly.

Adverse Reactions

>10%:

Cardiovascular: Tachycardia, bradycardia, arterial spasm, claudication and vasoconstriction; rebound headache may occur with sudden withdrawal of the drug in patients on prolonged therapy; localized edema, peripheral vascular effects (numbness and tingling of fingers and toes)

Central nervous system: Drowsiness, dizziness

Gastrointestinal: Nausea, vomiting, diarrhea, dry mouth

Emetic potential: Moderate (10% to 60%)

1% to 10%:

Cardiovascular: Transient tachycardia or bradycardia, precordial distress and pain

Neuromuscular & skeletal: Weakness in the legs, abdominal or muscle pain, muscle pains in the extremities, paresthesia

Overdosage/Toxicology Symptoms include vasospastic effects, nausea, vomiting, lassitude, impaired mental function, hypotension, hypertension, unconsciousness, seizures, shock, and death. Treatment includes general supportive therapy, gastric lavage, or induction of emesis, and saline cathartic. Keep extremities warm. Activated charcoal is effective at binding certain chemicals, this is especially true for ergot alkaloids. Treatment is symptomatic, with heparin and vasodilators (nitroprusside). Use vasodilators with caution to avoid exaggerating any pre-existing hypotension.

Drug Interactions

Increased Effect/Toxicity:

Propranolol: One case of severe vasoconstriction with pain and cyanosis has been reported.

Erythromycin, troleandomycin, and other macrolide antibiotics: Monitor for signs of ergot toxicity.

Protease inhibitors (amprenavir, nelfinavir, and ritonavir): Toxicity of ergot alkaloids is increased (use is contraindicated)

Ethanol/Nutrition/Herb Interactions Food: Avoid tea, cola, and coffee (caffeine may increase GI absorption of ergotamine).

Mechanism of Action Has partial agonist and/or antagonist activity against tryptaminergic, dopaminergic and alpha-adrenergic receptors depending upon their site; is a highly active uterine stimulant; it causes constriction of peripheral and cranial blood vessels and produces depression of central vasomotor centers

Pharmacodynamics/Kinetics

Absorption: Oral, rectal: Erratic; enhanced by caffeine coadministration

Metabolism: Extensively hepatic

Bioavailability: <5%

Time to peak, serum: 0.5-3 hours following coadministration with caffeine

Excretion: Feces (90% as metabolites)

Usual Dosage

Oral:

Cafergot®: 2 tablets at onset of attack; then 1 tablet every 30 minutes as needed; maximum: 6 tablets per attack; do not exceed 10 tablets/week.

Ergostat®: 1 tablet under tongue at first sign, then 1 tablet every 30 minutes, 3 tablets/24 hours, 5 tablets/week

(Continued)

Ergotamine *(Continued)*

Rectal (Cafergot® suppositories, Wigraine® suppositories, Cafatine® suppositories): 1 at first sign of an attack; follow with second dose after 1 hour, if needed; maximum: 2 per attack; do not exceed 5/week.

Patient Information Any symptoms such as nausea, vomiting, numbness or tingling, and chest, muscle, or abdominal pain should be reported to the physician. Initiate therapy at first sign of attack. Do **not** exceed recommended dosage.

Nursing Implications Do not crush sublingual drug product

Dosage Forms

Solution, intranasal [spray] (Migranal®): 4 mg/mL (1 mL)

Suppository, rectal (Cafatine®, Cafergot®, Wigraine®): Ergotamine tartrate 2 mg and caffeine 100 mg (12s)

Tablet (Ercaf®, Wigraine®): Ergotamine tartrate 1 mg and caffeine 100 mg

Tablet, sublingual (Ergomar®): Ergotamine tartrate 2 mg

◆ **Ergotamine Tartrate** *see Ergotamine on page 483*

◆ **Ergotamine Tartrate and Caffeine** *see Ergotamine on page 483*

◆ **Ergotamine Tartrate, Belladonna, and Phenobarbital** *see Belladonna, Phenobarbital, and Ergotamine Tartrate on page 152*

◆ **E•R•O Ear [OTC]** *see Carbamide Peroxide on page 224*

Ertapenem *(er ta PEN em)*

U.S. Brand Names Invanz™

Synonyms Ertapenem Sodium; L-749,345; MK-0826

Therapeutic Category Antibiotic, Anaerobic; Antibiotic, Carbapenem

Use Treatment of moderate-severe, complicated intra-abdominal infections, skin and skin structure infections, pyelonephritis, acute pelvic infections, and community-acquired pneumonia. Antibacterial coverage includes aerobic gram-positive organisms, aerobic gram-negative organisms, anaerobic organisms.

Methicillin-resistant *Staphylococcus*, *Enterococcus* spp, penicillin-resistant strains of *Streptococcus pneumoniae*, beta-lactamase-positive strains of *Haemophilus influenzae* are **resistant** to ertapenem, as are most *Pseudomonas aeruginosa*.

Pregnancy Risk Factor B

Pregnancy/Breast-Feeding Implications No adequate and well-controlled studies in pregnant women. Use only if clearly needed.

Contraindications Hypersensitivity to ertapenem or any other component of the formulation; anaphylactic reactions to beta-lactam antibiotics. If using intramuscularly, known hypersensitivity to local anesthetics of the amide type (lidocaine is the diluent).

Warnings/Precautions Dosage adjustment required with impaired renal function; prolonged use may result in superinfection; use with caution in patients with CNS disorder (eg, brain lesions, history of seizures), compromised renal function, hypersensitivity to beta-lactams, the elderly; safety and efficacy in patients <18 years of age have not been established.

Adverse Reactions

1% to 10%:

Cardiovascular: Swelling/edema (3%), chest pain (1%), hypertension (0.7% to 2%), hypotension (1% to 2%), tachycardia (1% to 2%)

Central nervous system: Headache (6% to 7%), altered mental status (ie, agitation, confusion, disorientation, decreased mental acuity, changed mental status, somnolence, stupor) (3% to 5%), fever (2% to 5%), insomnia (3%), dizziness (2%), fatigue (1%), anxiety (0.8% to 1%)

Dermatologic: Rash (2% to 3%), pruritus (1% to 2%), erythema (1% to 2%)

Gastrointestinal: Diarrhea (9% to 10%), nausea (6% to 9%), abdominal pain (4%), vomiting (4%), constipation (3% to 4%), acid regurgitation (1% to 2%), dyspepsia (1%), oral candidiasis (0.1% to 1%)

Genitourinary: Vaginitis (1% to 3%)

Hematologic: Platelet count increased (4% to 7%), eosinophils increased (1% to 2%)

Hepatic: Hepatic enzyme elevations (7% to 9%), alkaline phosphatase increase (4% to 7%)

Local: Infused vein complications (5% to 7%), phlebitis/thrombophlebitis (1.5% to 2%), extravasation (0.7% to 2%)

Neuromuscular & skeletal: Leg pain (0.4% to 1%)

Respiratory: Dyspnea (1% to 3%), cough (1% to 2%), pharyngitis (0.7% to 1%), rales/rhonchi (0.5% to 1%), respiratory distress (0.2% to 1%)

<1% (Limited to important or life-threatening): Arrhythmia, asthma, asystole, atrial fibrillation, bradycardia, cardiac arrest, cholelithiasis, epistaxis, gastrointestinal hemorrhage, gout, heart failure, heart murmur, hypoxemia, ileus, pancreatitis, pseudomembranous colitis, pyloric stenosis, seizures (0.5%), subdural hemorrhage, syncope, urticaria, ventricular tachycardia, vertigo

Drug Interactions

Increased Effect/Toxicity: Probenecid decreases the renal clearance of ertapenem.

Stability Before reconstitution store at ≤25°C (77°F). Reconstituted I.V. solution may be stored at room temperature and used within 6 hours **or** refrigerated, stored for up to 24 hours and used within 4 hours after removal from refrigerator. Do not freeze.

I.M.: Reconstitute 1 g vial with 3.2 mL of 1% lidocaine HCl injection (without epinephrine). Shake well. Use within 1 hour after preparation.

I.V.: Reconstitute 1 g vial with 10 mL of water for injection, 0.9% sodium chloride injection, or bacteriostatic water for injection. Shake well. Transfer to 50 mL of 0.9% sodium chloride injection.

Do not mix with other medications. Do not use diluents containing dextrose.

Mechanism of Action Inhibits bacterial cell wall synthesis by binding to one or more of the penicillin binding proteins; which in turn inhibits the final transpeptidation step of peptidoglycan synthesis in bacterial cell walls, thus inhibiting cell wall biosynthesis. Bacteria eventually lyse due to ongoing activity of cell wall autolytic enzymes (autolysins and murein hydrolases) while cell wall assembly is arrested.

Pharmacodynamics/Kinetics
Absorption: I.M.: Almost complete
Distribution: V_{dss}: 8.2 L
Protein binding: Concentration-dependent; 85% at 300 mcg/mL, 95% at <100 mcg/mL
Metabolism: Hydrolysis to inactive metabolite
Bioavailability: I.M.: 90%
Half-life elimination: 4 hours
Time to peak: I.M.: 2.3 hours
Excretion: Urine (80% as unchanged drug and metabolite); feces (10%)

Usual Dosage Adults: I.V., I.M.: **Note:** I.V. therapy may be administered for up to 14 days; I.M. for up to 7 days
Intra-abdominal infection: 1 g/day for 5-14 days
Skin and skin structure infections: 1 g/day for 7-14 days
Community-acquired pneumonia: 1 g/day; duration of total antibiotic treatment: 10-14 days
Urinary tract infections/pyelonephritis: 1 g/day; duration of total antibiotic treatment: 10-14 days
Acute pelvic infections: 1 g/day for 3-10 days
Elderly: Refer to adult dosing.

Dosage adjustment in renal impairment: Cl_{cr} <30 mL/minute: 500 mg/day
Hemodialysis: When the daily dose is given within 6 hours prior to hemodialysis, a supplementary dose of 150 mg is required following hemodialysis.

Dosage adjustment in hepatic impairment: Adjustments cannot be recommended (lack of experience and research in this patient population).

Dietary Considerations Sodium content: 137 mg (~6 mEq) per gram of ertapenem

Administration
I.M.: Avoid injection into a blood vessel. Make sure patient does not have an allergy to lidocaine or another anesthetic of the amide type. Administer by deep I.M. injection into a large muscle mass (eg, gluteal muscle or lateral part of the thigh). Do not administer I.M. preparation or drug reconstituted for I.M. administration intravenously.
I.V.: Infuse over 30 minutes

Monitoring Parameters Periodic renal, hepatic, and hematopoietic assessment during prolonged therapy; neurological assessment

Patient Information Report warmth, swelling, irritation at infusion or injection site. Report unresolved nausea or vomiting (small, frequent meals may help). Report feelings of excessive dizziness, palpitations, visual disturbances, headache, diarrhea, and CNS changes. Report chills, or unusual discharge, or foul-smelling urine. Inform prescriber if you are or intend to be pregnant. Consult prescriber if breast-feeding

Nursing Implications
I.M.: Avoid injection into a blood vessel. Make sure patient does not have an allergy to lidocaine or another anesthetic of the amide type. Administer by deep I.M. injection into a large muscle mass (eg., gluteal muscle or lateral part of the thigh). Do not administer I.M. preparation or drug reconstituted for I.M. administration intravenously.
I.V.: Infuse over 30 minutes

Dosage Forms Powder for injection, as sodium: 1 g [ertapenem sodium 1.046 g = ertapenem 1 g]

♦ **Ertapenem Sodium** see Ertapenem on page 484
♦ **Erwinia Asparaginase** see Asparaginase on page 118
♦ **Erybid™ (Can)** see Erythromycin (Systemic) on page 486
♦ **Eryc®** see Erythromycin (Systemic) on page 486
♦ **EryPed®** see Erythromycin (Systemic) on page 486
♦ **Ery-Tab®** see Erythromycin (Systemic) on page 486
♦ **Erythrocin®** see Erythromycin (Systemic) on page 486
♦ **Erythrocin™ I.V. (Can)** see Erythromycin (Systemic) on page 486
♦ **Erythromid® (Can)** see Erythromycin (Systemic) on page 486

Erythromycin and Benzoyl Peroxide
(er ith roe MYE sin & BEN zoe il per OKS ide)

U.S. Brand Names Benzamycin®
Synonyms Benzoyl Peroxide and Erythromycin
Therapeutic Category Acne Products
Use Topical control of acne vulgaris
Pregnancy Risk Factor C
Usual Dosage Apply twice daily, morning and evening
Additional Information Complete prescribing information for this medication should be consulted for additional detail.
Dosage Forms Gel, topical: Erythromycin 30 mg and benzoyl peroxide 50 mg per g

Erythromycin and Sulfisoxazole (er ith roe MYE sin & sul fi SOKS a zole)

U.S. Brand Names Eryzole®; Pediazole®
Canadian Brand Names Pediazole®
Synonyms Sulfisoxazole and Erythromycin
Therapeutic Category Antibiotic, Macrolide Combination; Antibiotic, Sulfonamide Derivative
Use Treatment of susceptible bacterial infections of the upper and lower respiratory tract, otitis media in children caused by susceptible strains of *Haemophilus influenzae*, and many other infections in patients allergic to penicillin
Pregnancy Risk Factor C
(Continued)

Erythromycin and Sulfisoxazole *(Continued)*

Usual Dosage Oral (dosage recommendation is based on the product's erythromycin content):

Children ≥2 months: 50 mg/kg/day erythromycin and 150 mg/kg/day sulfisoxazole in divided doses every 6 hours; not to exceed 2 g erythromycin/day or 6 g sulfisoxazole/day for 10 days

Adults >45 kg: 400 mg erythromycin and 1200 mg sulfisoxazole every 6 hours

Dosing adjustment in renal impairment (sulfisoxazole must be adjusted in renal impairment):

Cl_{cr} 10-50 mL/minute: Administer every 8-12 hours

Cl_{cr} <10 mL/minute: Administer every 12-24 hours

Dosage Forms Suspension, oral: Erythromycin ethylsuccinate 200 mg and sulfisoxazole acetyl 600 mg per 5 mL (100 mL, 150 mL, 200 mL, 250 mL)

♦ **Erythromycin Base** *see* Erythromycin (Systemic) *on page 486*
♦ **Erythromycin Estolate** *see* Erythromycin (Systemic) *on page 486*
♦ **Erythromycin Ethylsuccinate** *see* Erythromycin (Systemic) *on page 486*
♦ **Erythromycin Gluceptate** *see* Erythromycin (Systemic) *on page 486*
♦ **Erythromycin Lactobionate** *see* Erythromycin (Systemic) *on page 486*
♦ **Erythromycin Stearate** *see* Erythromycin (Systemic) *on page 486*

Erythromycin (Systemic) *(er ith roe MYE sin sis TEM ik)*

Related Information

Antimicrobial Drugs of Choice *on page 1588*
Community-Acquired Pneumonia in Adults *on page 1603*
Prevention of Wound Infection & Sepsis in Surgical Patients *on page 1569*
Treatment of Sexually Transmitted Diseases *on page 1609*

U.S. Brand Names E.E.S.®; E-Mycin®; Eryc®; EryPed®; Ery-Tab®; Erythrocin®; PCE®

Canadian Brand Names Apo®-Erythro Base; Apo®-Erythro E-C; Apo®-Erythro-ES; Apo®-Erythro-S; Diomycin®; EES®; Erybid™; Eryc®; Erythrocin®; Erythrocin™ I.V.; Erythromid®; Ilosone®; Novo-Rythro Encap; Nu-Erythromycin-S; PCE®; PMS-Erythromycin

Synonyms Erythromycin Base; Erythromycin Estolate; Erythromycin Ethylsuccinate; Erythromycin Gluceptate; Erythromycin Lactobionate; Erythromycin Stearate

Therapeutic Category Antibiotic, Macrolide; Antibiotic, Ophthalmic

Use Treatment of susceptible bacterial infections including *S. pyogenes*, some *S. pneumoniae*, some *S. aureus*, *M. pneumoniae*, *Legionella pneumophila*, diphtheria, pertussis, chancroid, *Chlamydia*, erythrasma, *N. gonorrhoeae*, *E. histolytica*, syphilis and nongonococcal urethritis, and *Campylobacter* gastroenteritis; used in conjunction with neomycin for decontaminating the bowel

Unlabeled/Investigational Use Treatment of gastroparesis

Pregnancy Risk Factor B

Contraindications Hypersensitivity to erythromycin or any component of the formulation; pre-existing liver disease (erythromycin estolate); concomitant use with pimozide, terfenadine, astemizole, or cisapride; hepatic impairment

Warnings/Precautions Hepatic impairment with or without jaundice has occurred, it may be accompanied by malaise, nausea, vomiting, abdominal colic, and fever; discontinue use if these occur; avoid using erythromycin lactobionate in neonates since formulations may contain benzyl alcohol which is associated with toxicity in neonates; observe for superinfections. Macrolides have been associated with rare QT_c prolongation and ventricular arrhythmias, including torsade de pointes.

Adverse Reactions

Cardiovascular: Ventricular arrhythmias
Central nervous system: Headache (8%), pain (2%), fever,
Dermatitis: Rash (3%), pruritus (1%)
Gastrointestinal: Abdominal pain (8%), cramping, nausea (8%), oral candidiasis, vomiting (3%), diarrhea (7%), dyspepsia (2%), flatulence (2%), anorexia, pseudomembranous colitis, hypertrophic pyloric stenosis
Hematologic: Eosinophilia (1%)
Hepatic: Cholestatic jaundice (most common with estolate), increased liver function tests (2%)
Local: Phlebitis at the injection site, thrombophlebitis
Neuromuscular & skeletal: Weakness (2%)
Respiratory: Dyspnea (1%), cough (3%)
Miscellaneous: Hypersensitivity reactions, allergic reactions

Overdosage/Toxicology Symptoms include nausea, vomiting, and diarrhea. Treatment consists of general and supportive care only.

Drug Interactions

Cytochrome P450 Effect: CYP3A3/4 enzyme substrate; CYP1A2 and 3A3/4 enzyme inhibitor

Increased Effect/Toxicity: Erythromycin decreases clearance (increases effects) of alfentanil, bromocriptine, carbamazepine, cyclosporine, digoxin (10% of patients), disopyramide, ergot alkaloids, felodipine (and other dihydropyridine calcium channel blockers), methylprednisolone, protease inhibitors, tacrolimus, theophylline (as much as 60%), triazolam, valproate, and vinblastine. Erythromycin may increase concentrations of HMG-CoA reductase inhibitors (except fluvastatin, pravastatin), and increase risk of rhabdomyolysis. The effects of warfarin may be potentiated by erythromycin.

Cisapride, astemizole, and terfenadine should be avoided with use of erythromycin due to the risk of malignant arrhythmias. Sparfloxacin, gatifloxacin, or moxifloxacin with erythromycin may increase the risk of malignant arrhythmias; avoid concurrent use. Cardiotoxicity of pimozide may be enhanced by erythromycin, fatalities have occurred. Case reports of enhanced effects of neuromuscular blocking agents have been reported with erythromycin.

Erythromycin serum concentrations may be increased by amprenavir (and possibly other protease inhibitors).

Ethanol/Nutrition/Herb Interactions

Ethanol: Avoid ethanol (may decrease absorption of erythromycin or enhance ethanol effects).

Food: Increased drug absorption with meals; erythromycin serum levels may be altered if taken with food.

Herb/Nutraceutical: St John's wort may decrease erythromycin levels.

Stability

Erythromycin lactobionate should be reconstituted with sterile water for injection without preservatives to avoid gel formation; the reconstituted solution is stable for 2 weeks when refrigerated for 24 hours at room temperature

Erythromycin I.V. infusion solution is stable at pH 6-8. Stability of lactobionate is pH dependent; I.V. form has the longest stability in 0.9% sodium chloride (NS) and should be prepared in this base solution whenever possible. Do not use D_5W as a diluent unless sodium bicarbonate is added to solution. If I.V. must be prepared in D_5W, 0.5 mL of the 8.4% sodium bicarbonate solution should be added per each 100 mL of D_5W.

Stability of parenteral admixture at room temperature (25°C) and at refrigeration temperature (4°C): 24 hours

Standard diluent: 500 mg/250 mL D_5W/NS; 750 mg/250 mL D_5W/NS; 1 g/250 mL D_5W/NS

Refrigerate oral suspension

Mechanism of Action Inhibits RNA-dependent protein synthesis at the chain elongation step; binds to the 50S ribosomal subunit resulting in blockage of transpeptidation

Pharmacodynamics/Kinetics

Absorption: Oral: Variable but better with salt forms than with base form; 18% to 45%; ethylsuccinate may be better absorbed with food

Distribution: Crosses placenta; enters breast milk

Relative diffusion from blood into CSF: Minimal even with inflammation

CSF:blood level ratio: Normal meninges: 1% to 12%; Inflamed meninges: 7% to 25%

Protein binding: 75% to 90%

Metabolism: Hepatic via demethylation

Half-life elimination: Peak: 1.5-2 hours; End-stage renal disease: 5-6 hours

Time to peak, serum: Base: 4 hours; Ethylsuccinate: 0.5-2.5 hours; delayed in presence of food due to differences in absorption

Excretion: Primarily feces; urine (2% to 15% as unchanged drug)

Usual Dosage

Infants and Children (**Note:** 400 mg ethylsuccinate = 250 mg base, stearate, or estolate salts):

Oral: 30-50 mg/kg/day divided every 6-8 hours; may double doses in severe infections

Preop bowel preparation: 20 mg/kg erythromycin base at 1, 2, and 11 PM on the day before surgery combined with mechanical cleansing of the large intestine and oral neomycin

I.V.: Lactobionate: 20-40 mg/kg/day divided every 6 hours

Adults:

Oral:

Base: 250-500 mg every 6-12 hours

Ethylsuccinate: 400-800 mg every 6-12 hours

Preop bowel preparation: Oral: 1 g erythromycin base at 1, 2, and 11 PM on the day before surgery combined with mechanical cleansing of the large intestine and oral neomycin

I.V.: Lactobionate: 15-20 mg/kg/day divided every 6 hours or 500 mg to 1 g every 6 hours, or given as a continuous infusion over 24 hours (maximum: 4 g/24 hours)

Children and Adults: Ophthalmic: Instill ½" (1.25 cm) 2-8 times/day depending on the severity of the infection

Dialysis: Slightly dialyzable (5% to 20%); no supplemental dosage necessary in hemo or peritoneal dialysis or in continuous arteriovenous or venovenous hemofiltration

Erythromycin has been used as a prokinetic agent to improve gastric emptying time and intestinal motility. In adults, 200 mg was infused I.V. initially followed by 250 mg orally 3 times/day 30 minutes before meals. In children, erythromycin 3 mg/kg I.V. has been infused over 60 minutes initially followed by 20 mg/kg/day orally in 3-4 divided doses before meals or before meals and at bedtime

Dietary Considerations Drug may cause GI upset; may take with food.

Administration Can administer with food to decrease GI upset

Test Interactions False-positive urinary catecholamines

Patient Information Refrigerate after reconstitution, take until gone, do not skip doses; chewable tablets should not be swallowed whole; report to physician if persistent diarrhea occurs; discard any unused portion after 10 days; absorption of estolate, ethylsuccinate, and base in a delayed release form are unaffected by food; take stearate salt and nondelayed release tape preparations 2 hours before or after meals

Nursing Implications Some formulations may contain benzyl alcohol as a preservative; use with extreme care in neonates; do not crush enteric coated drug product; GI upset, including diarrhea, is common; I.V. infusion may be very irritating to the vein; if phlebitis/pain occurs with used dilution, consider diluting further (eg, 1:5) and administer over ≥20-60 minutes, if fluid status of the patient will tolerate, or consider administering in larger available vein

Additional Information Due to differences in absorption, 400 mg erythromycin ethylsuccinate produces the same serum levels as 250 mg erythromycin base, stearate, or estolate. Do not use D_5W as a diluent unless sodium bicarbonate is added to solution; infuse over 30 minutes.

Sodium content of oral suspension (ethylsuccinate) 200 mg/5 mL: 29 mg (1.3 mEq)

Sodium content of base Filmtab® 250 mg: 70 mg (3 mEq)

Dosage Forms

Capsule, as estolate: 250 mg

Capsule, delayed release, as base: 250 mg

Capsule, delayed release, enteric-coated pellets, as base (Eryc®): 250 mg

(Continued)

Erythromycin (Systemic) *(Continued)*

Granules for oral suspension, as ethylsuccinate (EryPed®): 200 mg/5 mL, 400 mg/5 mL (60 mL, 100 mL, 200 mL)

Injection, as gluceptate: 1000 mg (30 mL)

Ointment, ophthalmic, as base: 0.55 mg (3.5 g)

Powder for injection, as lactobionate: 500 mg, 1000 mg

Powder for oral suspension, as ethylsuccinate (E.E.S.®): 200 mg/5 mL (100 mL, 200 mL)

Suspension, oral, as estolate: 125 mg/5 mL (120 mL, 200 mL, 480 mL); 250 mg/5 mL (150 mL, 200 mL, 480 mL)

Suspension, oral, as ethylsuccinate (E.E.S.®, EryPed®): 200 mg/5 mL (5 mL, 100 mL, 200 mL, 480 mL); 400 mg/5 mL (5 mL, 60 mL, 100 mL, 200 mL, 480 mL)

Suspension, oral, as ethylsuccinate [drops] (EryPed®): 100 mg/2.5 mL (50 mL)

Tablet, as ethylsuccinate (E.E.S.®): 400 mg

Tablet, chewable, as ethylsuccinate (EryPed®): 200 mg

Tablet, delayed release, as base: 333 mg

Tablet, enteric coated, as base (E-Mycin®, Ery-Tab®): 250 mg, 333 mg, 500 mg

Tablet, film coated, as base: 250 mg, 500 mg

Tablet, film coated, as stearate (Erythrocin®): 250 mg, 500 mg

Tablet, polymer-coated particles, as base (PCE®): 333 mg, 500 mg

♦ **Erythropoiesis Stimulating Protein** *see* Darbepoetin Alfa *on page 365*

♦ **Erythropoietin** *see* Epoetin Alfa *on page 474*

♦ **Eryzole®** *see* Erythromycin and Sulfisoxazole *on page 485*

♦ **Esclim®** *see* Estradiol *on page 491*

♦ **Eserine® (Can)** *see* Physostigmine *on page 1081*

♦ **Eserine Salicylate** *see* Physostigmine *on page 1081*

♦ **Esgic®** *see* Butalbital Compound *on page 197*

♦ **Esidrix®** *see* Hydrochlorothiazide *on page 674*

♦ **Eskalith®** *see* Lithium *on page 811*

♦ **Eskalith CR®** *see* Lithium *on page 811*

Esmolol *(ES moe lol)*

Related Information

Antiarrhythmic Drugs Comparison *on page 1478*

Beta-Blockers Comparison *on page 1491*

Hypertension *on page 1675*

U.S. Brand Names Brevibloc®

Canadian Brand Names Brevibloc®

Synonyms Esmolol Hydrochloride

Therapeutic Category Antiarrhythmic Agent, Class II; Antihypertensive Agent; Beta-Adrenergic Blocker

Use Treatment of supraventricular tachycardia and atrial fibrillation/flutter (primarily to control ventricular rate); treatment of tachycardia and/or hypertension (especially intraoperative or postoperative)

Pregnancy Risk Factor C (manufacturer); D (2nd and 3rd trimesters - expert analysis)

Contraindications Hypersensitivity to esmolol or any component of the formulation; sinus bradycardia; heart block greater than first degree (except in patients with a functioning artificial pacemaker); cardiogenic shock; bronchial asthma; uncompensated cardiac failure; hypotension; pregnancy (2nd and 3rd trimesters)

Warnings/Precautions Hypotension is common; patients need close blood pressure monitoring. Administer cautiously in compensated heart failure and monitor for a worsening of the condition. Use caution in patients with PVD (can aggravate arterial insufficiency). Use caution with concurrent use of beta-blockers and either verapamil or diltiazem; bradycardia or heart block can occur. Avoid concurrent I.V. use of both agents. In general, beta-blockers should be avoided in patients with bronchospastic disease. Esmolol, a beta-1 selective beta-blocker, can be cautiously used in patients with bronchospastic disease. Monitor pulmonary status closely. Use cautiously in diabetics because it can mask prominent hypoglycemic symptoms. Can mask signs of thyrotoxicosis. Can cause fetal bradycardia when administered in the third trimester of pregnancy or at delivery. Use caution in patients with renal dysfunction (active metabolite retained). Do not use in the treatment of hypertension associated with vasoconstriction related to hypothermia. Concentrations >10 mcg/mL or infusion into small veins or through a butterfly catheter should be avoided (can cause thrombophlebitis). Extravasation can lead to skin necrosis and sloughing.

Adverse Reactions

>10%:

Cardiovascular: Asymptomatic hypotension (25%), symptomatic hypotension (12%)

Miscellaneous: Diaphoresis (10%)

1% to 10%:

Cardiovascular: Peripheral ischemia (1%)

Central nervous system: Dizziness (3%), somnolence (3%), confusion (2%), headache (2%), agitation (2%), fatigue (1%)

Gastrointestinal: Nausea (7%), vomiting (1%)

Local: Pain on injection (8%)

<1% (Limited to important or life-threatening): Alopecia, bronchospasm, chest pain, congestive heart failure, depression, dyspnea, edema, exfoliative dermatitis, heart block, infusion site reactions, paresthesia, pruritus, pulmonary edema, rigors, seizures, severe bradycardia/asystole (rare), skin necrosis (from extravasation), syncope, thrombophlebitis, urinary retention

Overdosage/Toxicology Symptoms include cardiac disturbances, CNS toxicity, bronchospasm, hypoglycemia and hyperkalemia. The most common cardiac symptoms include hypotension and bradycardia. Atrioventricular block, intraventricular conduction disturbances, cardiogenic shock, and asystole may occur with severe overdose, especially with membrane-depressant drugs (eg, propranolol). CNS effects include convulsions, coma, and respiratory arrest (commonly seen with propranolol and other membrane-depressant and lipid-soluble drugs). Treatment is symptomatic for seizures, hypotension, hyperkalemia, and hypoglycemia. Bradycardia and hypotension resistant to atropine, isoproterenol, or pacing may respond to glucagon. Wide QRS defects caused by membrane-depressant poisoning may respond to hypertonic sodium bicarbonate. Repeat-dose charcoal, hemoperfusion, or hemodialysis may be helpful in removal of only those beta-blockers with a small V_d, long half-life, or low intrinsic clearance (acebutolol, atenolol, nadolol, sotalol).

Drug Interactions

Increased Effect/Toxicity: Esmolol may increase the effect/toxicity of verapamil, and may increase potential for hypertensive crisis after or during withdrawal of either agent when combined with clonidine. Esmolol may extend the effect of neuromuscular blocking agents (succinylcholine). Esmolol may increase digoxin serum levels by 10% to 20% and may increase theophylline concentrations. Morphine may increase esmolol blood concentrations.

Decreased Effect: Decreased effect of beta-blockers with aluminum salts, barbiturates, calcium salts, cholestyramine, colestipol, NSAIDs, penicillins (ampicillin), rifampin, salicylates, and sulfinpyrazone due to decreased bioavailability and plasma levels. Beta-blockers may decrease the effect of sulfonylureas. Xanthines (eg, theophylline, caffeine) may decrease effects of esmolol.

Stability Clear, colorless to light yellow solution which should be stored at 25°C (77°F). Excursions permitted to 15°C to 30°C (59°F to 86°F).

Stability of parenteral admixture at room temperature (25°C) and at refrigeration temperature (4°C) is 24 hours (standard preparation: 5 g/500 mL or 2.5 g/250 mL NS or 5% dextrose). Premixed bags are stable until the expiration date assigned by the manufacturer, but should be used within 24 hours after withdrawal of the initial bolus, with any unused portion discarded.

Mechanism of Action Class II antiarrhythmic: Competitively blocks response to beta$_1$-adrenergic stimulation with little or no effect of beta$_2$-receptors except at high doses, no intrinsic sympathomimetic activity, no membrane stabilizing activity

Pharmacodynamics/Kinetics

Onset of action: Beta-blockade: I.V.: 2-10 minutes (quickest when loading doses are administered)

Duration: 10-30 minutes; prolonged following higher cumulative doses, extended duration of use

Protein binding: 55%

Metabolism: In blood by esterases

Half-life elimination: Adults: 9 minutes

Excretion: Urine (~69% as metabolites, 2% unchanged drug)

Usual Dosage I.V. infusion requires an infusion pump (must be adjusted to individual response and tolerance):

Children: A limited amount of information regarding esmolol use in pediatric patients is currently available. Some centers have utilized doses of 100-500 mcg/kg given over 1 minute for control of supraventricular tachycardias.

Loading doses of 500 mcg/kg/minute over 1 minute with maximal doses of 50-250 mcg/kg/minute (mean = 173) have been used in addition to nitroprusside to treat postoperative hypertension after coarctation of aorta repair.

Adults:

Intraoperative tachycardia and/or hypertension (immediate control): Initial bolus: 80 mg (~1 mg/kg) over 30 seconds, followed by a 150 mcg/kg/minute infusion, if necessary. Adjust infusion rate as needed to maintain desired heart rate and/or blood pressure, up to 300 mcg/kg/minute.

Supraventricular tachycardia or gradual control of postoperative tachycardia/hypertension: Loading dose: 500 mcg/kg over 1 minute; follow with a 50 mcg/kg/minute infusion for 4 minutes; response to this initial infusion rate may be a rough indication of the responsiveness of the ventricular rate.

Infusion may be continued at 50 mcg/kg/minute or, if the response is inadequate, titrated upward in 50 mcg/kg/minute increments (increased no more frequently than every 4 minutes) to a maximum of 200 mcg/kg/minute.

To achieve more rapid response, following the initial loading dose and 50 mcg/kg/minute infusion, rebolus with a second 500 mcg/kg loading dose over 1 minute, and increase the maintenance infusion to 100 mcg/kg/minute for 4 minutes. If necessary, a third (and final) 500 mcg/kg loading dose may be administered, prior to increasing to an infusion rate of 150 mcg/kg/minute. After 4 minutes of the 150 mcg/kg/minute infusion, the infusion rate may be increased to a maximum rate of 200 mcg/kg/minute (without a bolus dose).

Usual dosage range (SVT): 50-200 mcg/kg/minute with average dose of 100 mcg/kg/minute. For control of postoperative hypertension, as many as one-third of patients may require higher doses (250-300 mcg/kg/minute) to control blood pressure; the safety of doses >300 mcg/kg/minute has not been studied.

Esmolol: Hemodynamic effects of beta-blockade return to baseline within 20-30 minutes after discontinuing esmolol infusions.

Guidelines for withdrawal of therapy:

Transfer to alternative antiarrhythmic drug (propranolol, digoxin, verapamil).

Infusion should be reduced by 50% 30 minutes following the first dose of the alternative agent.

Following the second dose of the alternative drug, patient's response should be monitored and if control is adequate for the first hours, esmolol may be discontinued.

Dialysis: Not removed by hemo- or peritoneal dialysis; supplemental dose is not necessary.

Administration Infusions must be administered with an infusion pump. The concentrate (250 mg/mL ampul) is **not** for direct I.V. injection, but rather must first be diluted to a final concentration of 10 mg/mL (ie, 2.5 g in 250 mL or 5 g in 500 mL). Concentrations >10 mg/mL or infusion into small veins or through a butterfly catheter should be avoided (can cause thrombophlebitis). Decrease or discontinue infusion if hypotension or congestive heart failure (Continued)

Esmolol *(Continued)*

occur. Medication port of premixed bags should be used to withdraw only the initial bolus, if necessary (not to be used for withdrawal of additional bolus doses).

Monitoring Parameters Blood pressure, heart rate, MAP, EKG, respiratory rate, I.V. site; cardiac monitor and blood pressure monitor required

Test Interactions Increases cholesterol (S), glucose

Nursing Implications Decrease infusion or discontinue if hypotension, congestive heart failure, etc occur; The 250 mg/mL ampul is **not** for direct I.V. injection, but must first be diluted to a final concentration not to exceed 10 mg/mL (ie, 2.5 g in 250 mL or 5 g in 500 mL).

Dosage Forms Injection, as hydrochloride: 10 mg/mL (10 mL); 250 mg/mL (10 mL)

♦ **Esmolol Hydrochloride** *see* Esmolol *on page 488*

Esomeprazole *(es oh ME pray zol)*

Related Information

Helicobacter pylori Treatment *on page 1668*

U.S. Brand Names Nexium™

Synonyms Esomeprazole Magnesium

Therapeutic Category Gastric Acid Secretion Inhibitor; Proton Pump Inhibitor

Use Short-term (4-8 weeks) treatment of erosive esophagitis; maintaining symptom resolution and healing of erosive esophagitis; treatment of symptomatic gastroesophageal reflux disease; as part of a multidrug regimen for *Helicobacter pylori* eradication in patients with duodenal ulcer disease (active or history of within the past 5 years)

Pregnancy Risk Factor B

Pregnancy/Breast-Feeding Implications Animal studies in doses of ≤60 times the human dose show no harm to the fetus; excretion in breast milk unknown/contraindicated

Contraindications Hypersensitivity to esomeprazole, lansoprazole, omeprazole, rabeprazole, or any component of the formulation

Warnings/Precautions Relief of symptoms does not preclude the presence of a gastric malignancy. Atrophic gastritis (by biopsy) has been noted with long-term omeprazole therapy; this may also occur with esomeprazole. No reports of enterochromaffin-like (ECL) cell carcinoids, dysplasia, or neoplasia has occurred. Safety and efficacy in pediatric patients have not been established.

Adverse Reactions

1% to 10%:

Central nervous system: Headache (4% to 6%)

Gastrointestinal: Diarrhea (4%), nausea, flatulence, abdominal pain (4%), constipation, xerostomia

<1% (Limited to important or life-threatening): Allergic reactions, angina, angioedema, arthritis, asthma, confusion, depression, dyspnea, edema (facial, larynx, peripheral, tongue), goiter, hematuria, hypertension, hyponatremia, impotence, migraine, paresthesia, polymyalgia rheumatica, rash, thrombocytopenia, ulcerative stomatitis, urticaria, vertigo

Overdosage/Toxicology Treatment is symptom directed and supportive. Not dialyzable.

Drug Interactions

Cytochrome P450 Effect: CYP2C19 and 3A4 enzyme substrate

Increased Effect/Toxicity: Increased serum concentration of diazepam, digoxin, penicillins

Decreased Effect: Decreased absorption of dapsone, iron, itraconazole, ketoconazole and other drugs where an acidic stomach is required for absorption.

Ethanol/Nutrition/Herb Interactions Food: Absorption is decreased by 33% to 53% when taken with food.

Stability Store at 15°C to 30°C (59°F to 86°F). Keep container tightly closed. The contents of the capsule remain intact when exposed to tap water, orange juice, apple juice, and yogurt.

Mechanism of Action Proton pump inhibitor suppresses gastric acid secretion by inhibition of the H^+/K^+-ATPase in the gastric parietal cell

Pharmacodynamics/Kinetics

Distribution: V_{dss}: 16 L

Protein binding: 97%

Metabolism: Hepatic via CYP2C19 and 3A4 enzymes to hydroxy, desmethyl, and sulfone metabolites (all inactive)

Bioavailability: 90% with repeat dosing

Half-life elimination: 1-1.5 hours

Time to peak: 1.5 hours

Excretion: Urine (80%); feces (20%)

Usual Dosage Note: Delayed-release capsules should be swallowed whole and taken at least 1 hour before eating

Children: Safety and efficacy have not been established in pediatric patients

Adults: Oral:

Erosive esophagitis (healing): 20-40 mg once daily for 4-8 weeks; maintenance: 20 mg once daily

Symptomatic GERD: 20 mg once daily for 4 weeks

Helicobacter pylori eradication: 40 mg once daily; requires combination therapy

Elderly: No dosage adjustment needed

Dosage adjustment in renal impairment: No dosage adjustment needed

Dosage adjustment in hepatic impairment:

Mild to moderate liver impairment (Child-Pugh Class A or B): No dosage adjustment needed

Severe liver impairment (Child-Pugh Class C): Dose should not exceed 20 mg/day

Dietary Considerations Take at least 1 hour before meals.

Administration Capsule should be swallowed whole and taken at least 1 hour before eating. For patients with difficulty swallowing, open capsule and mix contents with 1 tablespoon of applesauce. Swallow immediately; mixture should not be chewed. The mixture should not be stored for future use.

Monitoring Parameters Susceptibility testing recommended in patients who fail *H. pylori* eradication regimen (esomeprazole, clarithromycin, and amoxicillin)

Patient Information Take on an empty stomach. Take 1 hour before meals. Swallow capsule whole. Do not chew, break, or crush. Take at a similar time everyday. For patients who have difficulty swallowing, put 1 tablespoon of applesauce in a bowl. Open esomeprazole capsule and sprinkle contents over applesauce. Mix and swallow now. The applesauce should not be hot and should be soft enough to swallow without chewing. Do not chew the mixture. It should not be stored for later use. Common side effects include headache, diarrhea, and abdominal pain. Notify prescriber if you have blood in the stool or toilet bowl, are vomiting blood, or have severe abdominal pain.

Nursing Implications Do not break or crush capsule. Instruct patient not to chew capsule.

Additional Information Esomeprazole is the S-isomer of omeprazole.

Dosage Forms Capsule, delayed release: 20 mg, 40 mg

- **Esomeprazole Magnesium** *see* Esomeprazole *on page 490*
- **Esoterica® Facial [OTC]** *see* Hydroquinone *on page 686*
- **Esoterica® Regular [OTC]** *see* Hydroquinone *on page 686*
- **Esoterica® Sensitive Skin Formula [OTC]** *see* Hydroquinone *on page 686*
- **Esoterica® Sunscreen [OTC]** *see* Hydroquinone *on page 686*

Estazolam (es TA zoe lam)

Related Information
Antacid Drug Interactions *on page 1477*
Benzodiazepines Comparison *on page 1490*

U.S. Brand Names ProSom™

Therapeutic Category Benzodiazepine; Hypnotic; Sedative

Use Short-term management of insomnia

Restrictions C-IV

Pregnancy Risk Factor X

Usual Dosage Adults: Oral: 1 mg at bedtime, some patients may require 2 mg; start at doses of 0.5 mg in debilitated or small elderly patients

Dosing adjustment in hepatic impairment: May be necessary

Additional Information Complete prescribing information for this medication should be consulted for additional detail.

Dosage Forms Tablet: 1 mg, 2 mg

- **Esterified Estrogen and Methyltestosterone** *see* Estrogens and Methyltestosterone *on page 496*
- **Esterified Estrogens** *see* Estrogens (Esterified) *on page 500*
- **Estimated Clinical Comparability of Doses for Inhaled Corticosteroids** *see page 1652*
- **Estinyl®** *see* Ethinyl Estradiol *on page 509*
- **Estrace®** *see* Estradiol *on page 491*
- **Estraderm®** *see* Estradiol *on page 491*

Estradiol (es tra DYE ole)

U.S. Brand Names Alora®; Climara®; Delestrogen®; Depo®-Estradiol; Esclim®; Estrace®; Estraderm®; Estring®; Gynodiol™; Vagifem®; Vivelle®; Vivelle-Dot™

Canadian Brand Names Climara®; Delestrogen®; Depo®-Estradiol; Estrace®; Estraderm®; Estring®; Estrogel®; Oesclim®; Vagifem®; Vivelle®

Synonyms Estradiol Cypionate; Estradiol Hemihydrate; Estradiol Transdermal; Estradiol Valerate

Therapeutic Category Contraceptive, Topical Patch; Contraceptive, Vaginal; Estrogen Derivative, Intramuscular; Estrogen Derivative, Oral; Estrogen Derivative, Topical; Estrogen Derivative, Vaginal

Use Treatment of moderate to severe vasomotor symptoms associated with menopause; treatment of vulvar and vaginal atrophy; hypoestrogenism (due to hypogonadism, castration, or primary ovarian failure); prostatic cancer (palliation), breast cancer (palliation), osteoporosis (prophylaxis); abnormal uterine bleeding due to hormonal imbalance; postmenopausal urogenital symptoms of the lower urinary tract (urinary urgency, dysuria)

Pregnancy Risk Factor X

Pregnancy/Breast-Feeding Implications Increased risk of fetal reproductive tract disorders and other birth defects; do not use during pregnancy. Excreted in human milk/use caution in breast-feeding women.

Contraindications Hypersensitivity to estradiol or any component of the formulation; undiagnosed abnormal vaginal bleeding; history of or current thrombophlebitis or thromboembolic disorders; carcinoma of the breast, except in appropriately selected patients being treated for metastatic disease; estrogen-dependent tumor; porphyria; pregnancy

Warnings/Precautions Unopposed estrogens may increase the risk of endometrial carcinoma in postmenopausal women. Use with caution in patients with diseases which may be exacerbated by fluid retention, including asthma, epilepsy, migraine, diabetes, cardiac or renal dysfunction. Use with caution in patients with a history of hypercalcemia, cardiovascular disease, and gallbladder disease. May increase blood pressure. Use with caution in patients with hepatic disease. May increase risk of venous thromboembolism. Estrogens may increase the risk of breast cancer (controversial/currently under study). Estrogen compounds are generally associated with lipid effects such as increased HDL-cholesterol and decreased LDL-cholesterol. Triglycerides may also be increased; use with caution in patients with familial defects of lipoprotein metabolism. Estrogens may cause premature closure of the epiphyses in young individuals. Safety and efficacy in pediatric patients have not been established. May increase size of pre-existing uterine leiomyomata. May increase the risk of benign hepatic adenoma, which may cause significant consequences in the event of rupture.
(Continued)

Estradiol *(Continued)*

Use vaginal tablets with caution in patients with severely atrophic vaginal mucosa or following gynecological surgery due to possible trauma from the applicator. Oral therapy may be more convenient for vaginal atrophy and stress incontinence.

Before prescribing estrogen therapy to postmenopausal women, the risks and benefits must be weighed for each patient. Women should be informed of these risks and benefits, as well as possible effects of progestin when added to estrogen therapy.

Adverse Reactions Frequency not defined.

Cardiovascular: Edema, hypertension, venous thromboembolism

Central nervous system: Dizziness, headache, mental depression, migraine

Dermatologic: Chloasma, erythema multiforme, erythema nodosum, hemorrhagic eruption, hirsutism, loss of scalp hair, melasma

Endocrine & metabolic: Breast enlargement, breast tenderness, changes in libido, increased thyroid-binding globulin, increased total thyroid hormone (T_4), increased serum triglycerides/phospholipids, increased HDL-cholesterol, decreased LDL-cholesterol, impaired glucose tolerance, hypercalcemia

Gastrointestinal: Abdominal cramps, bloating, cholecystitis, cholelithiasis, gallbladder disease, nausea, pancreatitis, vomiting, weight gain/loss

Genitourinary: Alterations in frequency and flow of menses, changes in cervical secretions, endometrial cancer, increased size of uterine leiomyomata, vaginal candidiasis

Vaginal: Trauma from applicator insertion may occur in women with severely atrophic vaginal mucosa

Hematologic: Aggravation of porphyria, decreased antithrombin III and antifactor Xa, increased levels of fibrinogen, increased platelet aggregability and platelet count; increased prothrombin and factors VII, VIII, IX, X

Hepatic: Cholestatic jaundice

Local: Transdermal patches: Burning, erythema, irritation, pruritus, rash

Neuromuscular & skeletal: Chorea

Ocular: Intolerance to contact lenses, steeping of corneal curvature

Respiratory: Pulmonary thromboembolism

Miscellaneous: Carbohydrate intolerance

Postmarketing events: Vivelle®; Anaphylaxis (isolated reports), elevated liver function tests (rare), leg pain

Overdosage/Toxicology Symptoms include fluid retention, jaundice, thrombophlebitis, nausea, and vomiting. Toxicity is unlikely following single exposures of excessive doses. Treatment following emesis and charcoal administration should be supportive and symptomatic.

Drug Interactions

Cytochrome P450 Effect: CYP1A2 and 3A3/4 enzyme substrate

Increased Effect/Toxicity: Estradiol with hydrocortisone increases corticosteroid toxic potential. Anticoagulants and estradiol increase the potential for thromboembolic events.

Decreased Effect: Rifampin, nelfinavir, and ritonavir decrease estradiol serum concentrations. Anticonvulsants which are enzyme inducers (barbiturates, carbamazepine, phenobarbital, phenytoin, primidone) may potentially decrease estrogen levels.

Ethanol/Nutrition/Herb Interactions

Ethanol: Avoid ethanol (routine use increases estrogen level and risk of breast cancer).

Food: Folic acid absorption may be decreased

Herb/Nutraceutical: St John's wort may decrease estradiol levels. Avoid black cohosh, dong quai (has estrogenic activity). Avoid red clover, saw palmetto, ginseng.

Mechanism of Action Estrogens are responsible for the development and maintenance of the female reproductive system and secondary sexual characteristics. Estradiol is the principle intracellular human estrogen and is more potent than estrone and estriol at the receptor level; it is the primary estrogen secreted prior to menopause. Following menopause, estrone and estrone sulfate are more highly produced. Estrogens modulate the pituitary secretion of gonadotropins, luteinizing hormone, and follicle-stimulating hormone through a negative feedback system; estrogen replacement reduces elevated levels of these hormones in postmenopausal women.

Pharmacodynamics/Kinetics

Absorption: Oral, topical: Well absorbed

Distribution: Crosses placenta; enters breast milk

Metabolism: Oral: Hepatic; oxidation and conjugation in GI tract; hydroxylated via CYP3A3/4 to metabolites; first-pass effect; enterohepatic recirculation

Protein binding: 37% to sex-hormone-binding globulin; 61% to albumin

Excretion: Primarily urine (as metabolites); feces (small amounts)

Usual Dosage All dosage needs to be adjusted based upon the patient's response

Oral:

Prostate cancer (androgen-dependent, inoperable, progressing): 10 mg 3 times/day for at least 3 months

Breast cancer (inoperable, progressing in appropriately selected patients): 10 mg 3 times/day for at least 3 months

Osteoporosis prophylaxis in postmenopausal females: 0.5 mg/day in a cyclic regimen (3 weeks on and 1 week off)

Female hypoestrogenism (due to hypogonadism, castration, or primary ovarian failure): 1-2 mg/day; titrate as necessary to control symptoms using minimal effective dose for maintenance therapy

Treatment of moderate to severe vasomotor symptoms associated with menopause: 1-2 mg/day, adjusted as necessary to limit symptoms; administration should be cyclic (3 weeks on, 1 week off). Patients should be re-evaluated at 3- to 6-month intervals to determine if treatment is still necessary.

I.M.

Prostate cancer: Valerate: ≥30 mg or more every 1-2 weeks

Moderate to severe vasomotor symptoms associated with menopause:
>> Cypionate: 1-5 mg every 3-4 weeks
>> Valerate: 10-20 mg every 4 weeks
> Female hypoestrogenism (due to hypogonadism):
>> Cypionate: 1.5-2 mg monthly
>> Valerate: 10-20 mg every 4 weeks

Transdermal: Indicated dose may be used continuously in patients without an intact uterus. May be given continuously or cyclically (3 weeks on, 1 week off) in patients with an intact uterus. When changing patients from oral to transdermal therapy, start transdermal patch 1 week after discontinuing oral hormone (may begin sooner if symptoms reappear within 1 week):

Once-weekly patch:
> Moderate to severe vasomotor symptoms associated with menopause (Climara®): Apply 0.025 mg/day patch once weekly. Adjust dose as necessary to control symptoms. Patients should be re-evaluated at 3- to 6-month intervals to determine if treatment is still necessary.
> Osteoporosis prophylaxis in postmenopausal women (Climara®): Apply patch once weekly; minimum effective dose 0.025 mg/day; adjust response to therapy by biochemical markers and bone mineral density

Twice-weekly patch:
> Moderate to severe vasomotor symptoms associated with menopause, vulvar/vaginal atrophy, female hypogonadism: Titrate to lowest dose possible to control symptoms, adjusting initial dose after the first month of therapy; re-evaluate therapy at 3- to 6-month intervals to taper or discontinue medication:
>> Alora®, Esclim®, Estraderm®, Vivelle-Dot™: Apply 0.05 mg patch twice weekly
>> Vivelle®: Apply 0.0375 mg patch twice weekly
> Prevention of osteoporosis in postmenopausal women:
>> Estraderm®: Apply 0.05 mg patch twice weekly
>> Vivelle®: Apply 0.025 mg patch twice weekly, adjust dose as necessary

Vaginal cream: Vulvar and vaginal atrophy: Insert 2-4 g/day intravaginally for 2 weeks, then gradually reduce to ½ the initial dose for 2 weeks, followed by a maintenance dose of 1 g 1-3 times/week

Vaginal ring: Postmenopausal vaginal atrophy, urogenital symptoms: Estring®: Following insertion, Estring® should remain in place for 90 days

Vaginal tablets: Atrophic vaginitis: Vagifem®: Initial: Insert 1 tablet once daily for 2 weeks; maintenance: Insert 1 tablet twice weekly; attempts to discontinue or taper medication should be made at 3- to 6-month intervals

Dosing adjustment in hepatic impairment:
> Mild to moderate liver impairment: Dosage reduction of estrogens is recommended
> Severe liver impairment: **Not recommended**

Dietary Considerations Ensure adequate calcium and vitamin D intake when used for the prevention of osteoporosis.

Administration
> Injection formulation: Intramuscular use only
> Transdermal patch: Aerosol topical corticosteroids applied under the patch may reduce allergic reactions. Do not apply transdermal system to breasts, but place on trunk of body (preferably abdomen). Rotate application sites.

Monitoring Parameters Yearly physical examination that includes blood pressure and Papanicolaou smear, breast exam, mammogram. Monitor for signs of endometrial cancer in female patients with uterus; rule out malignancy if unexplained vaginal bleeding occurs

Reference Range
> Children: <10 pg/mL (SI: <37 pmol/L)
> Male: 10-50 pg/mL (SI: 37-184 pmol/L)
> Female:
>> Premenopausal: 30-400 pg/mL (SI: 110-1468 pmol/L)
>> Postmenopausal: 0-30 pg/mL (SI: 0-110 pmol/L)

Test Interactions Pathologist should be advised of estrogen/progesterone therapy when specimens are submitted. Reduced response to metyrapone test.

Patient Information Patients should inform their physicians if signs or symptoms of any of the following occur: Thromboembolic or thrombotic disorders including sudden severe headache or vomiting, disturbance of vision or speech, loss of vision, numbness or weakness in an extremity, sharp or crushing chest pain, calf pain, shortness of breath, severe abdominal pain or mass, mental depression, or unusual bleeding.

Patients should discontinue taking the medication if they suspect they are pregnant or become pregnant. Notify physician if area under dermal patch becomes irritated or a rash develops. Patient package insert is available with product; insert vaginal product high into the vagina.

Nursing Implications Aerosol topical corticosteroids applied under the patch may reduce allergic reactions; do not apply transdermal system to breasts, but place on trunk of body (preferably abdomen); rotate application sites

Dosage Forms
> Cream, vaginal (Estrace®): 0.1 mg/g (42.5 g)
> Injection, as cypionate (Depo®-Estradiol): 5 mg/mL (5 mL) [chlorobutanol as preservative; in cottonseed oil]
> Injection, as valerate: 20 mg/mL (10 mL); 40 mg/mL (10 mL) [may contain benzyl alcohol; may be in castor oil]
>> Delestrogen®:
>>> 10 mg/mL (5 mL) [chlorobutanol as preservative; in sesame oil]
>>> 20 mg/mL (5 mL) [contains benzyl alcohol; in castor oil]
>>> 40 mg/mL (5 mL) [contains benzyl alcohol; in castor oil]
> Tablet, micronized, oral:
>> Estrace®: 0.5 mg, 1 mg, 2 mg
>> Gynodiol™: 0.5 mg, 1 mg, 1.5 mg, 2 mg

(Continued)

Estradiol *(Continued)*

Tablet, vaginal (Vagifem®): 25.8 mcg of estradiol hemihydrate [equivalent to 25 mcg estradiol]

Transdermal system:

Alora®:
0.05 mg/24 hours [18 cm²], total estradiol 1.5 mg
0.075 mg/24 hours [27 cm²], total estradiol 2.3 mg
0.1 mg/24 hours [36 cm²], total estradiol 3 mg

Climara®:
0.025 mg/24 hours [6.5 cm²], total estradiol 2.04 mg
0.05 mg/24 hours [12.5 cm²], total estradiol 3.9 mg
0.075 mg/24 hours [18.75 cm²], total estradiol 5.85 mg
0.1 mg/24 hours [25 cm²], total estradiol 7.8 mg

Esclim®, Vivelle®:
0.025 mg/day
0.0375 mg/day
0.05 mg/day
0.075 mg/day
0.1 mg/day

Estraderm®:
0.05 mg/24 hours [10 cm²], total estradiol 4 mg
0.1 mg/24 hours [20 cm²], total estradiol 8 mg

Vivelle-Dot™:
0.0375 mg/day
0.05 mg/day
0.075 mg/day
0.1 mg/day

Vaginal ring (Estring®): 2 mg gradually released over 90 days

Estradiol and Norethindrone (es tra DYE ole & nor eth IN drone)

U.S. Brand Names Activella™; CombiPatch™

Synonyms Norethindrone and Estradiol

Therapeutic Category Estrogen and Progestin Combination

Use Women with an intact uterus:

Tablet: Treatment of moderate to severe vasomotor symptoms associated with menopause; treatment of vulvar and vaginal atrophy; prophylaxis for postmenopausal osteoporosis

Transdermal patch: Treatment of moderate to severe vasomotor symptoms associated with menopause; treatment of vulvar and vaginal atrophy; treatment of hypoestrogenism due to hypogonadism, castration, or primary ovarian failure

Pregnancy Risk Factor X

Pregnancy/Breast-Feeding Implications Estrogens/progestins should not be used during pregnancy.

Contraindications Hypersensitivity to estrogens, progestins, or any components; carcinoma of the breast; estrogen-dependent tumor; undiagnosed abnormal vaginal bleeding; thrombophlebitis, thromboembolic disorders, or stroke; hysterectomy; pregnancy

Warnings/Precautions For use only in women with an intact uterus. Use with caution in patients with diseases that may be exacerbated by fluid retention, including asthma, epilepsy, migraine, diabetes, cardiac or renal dysfunction. Use with caution in patients with a history of hypercalcemia, cardiovascular disease, or gallbladder disease. May increase blood pressure. Use with caution in patients with liver dysfunction or disease. May increase risk of venous thromboembolism. Unopposed estrogens may increase the risk of endometrial carcinoma in postmenopausal women (incidence is less likely with the addition of progesterone). Estrogens may increase the risk of breast cancer; estrogen compounds are generally associated with lipid effects such as increased HDL-cholesterol, and decreased LDL-cholesterol; triglycerides may also be increased. Use with caution in patients with familial defects of lipoprotein metabolism. Safety and efficacy in children have not been established. May cause visual abnormalities. Discontinue if papilledema or renal vascular lesions develop.

Adverse Reactions Frequency not defined.

Cardiovascular: Altered blood pressure, cardiovascular accident, edema, venous thromboembolism

Central nervous system: Dizziness, fatigue, headache, insomnia, mental depression, migraine, nervousness

Dermatologic: Chloasma, erythema multiforme, erythema nodosum, hemorrhagic eruption, hirsutism, itching, loss of scalp hair, melasma, pruritus, skin rash

Endocrine & metabolic: Breast enlargement, breast tenderness, breast pain, changes in libido

Gastrointestinal: Abdominal pain, bloating, changes in appetite, flatulence, gallbladder disease, nausea, pancreatitis, vomiting, weight gain/loss

Genitourinary: Alterations in frequency and flow of menses, changes in cervical secretions, cystitis-like syndrome, increased size of uterine leiomyomata, premenstrual-like syndrome, vaginal candidiasis, vaginitis

Hematologic: Aggravation of porphyria

Hepatic: Cholestatic jaundice

Local: Application site reaction (transdermal patch)

Neuromuscular & skeletal: Arthralgia, back pain, chorea, myalgia, weakness

Ocular: Intolerance to contact lenses, steeping of corneal curvature

Respiratory: Pharyngitis, pulmonary thromboembolism, rhinitis

Miscellaneous: Allergic reactions, carbohydrate intolerance, flu-like syndrome

Pharmacodynamics/Kinetics

Activella:™
Bioavailability: Estradiol: 50%; Norethindrone: 100%
Half-life elimination: Estradiol: 12-14 hours; Norethindrone: 8-11 hours
Time to peak: Estradiol: 5-8 hours

See individual agents.

Usual Dosage Adults:
  Oral: 1 tablet daily
  Transdermal patch:
    Continuous combined regimen: Apply one patch twice weekly
    Continuous sequential regimen: Apply estradiol-only patch for first 14 days of cycle, followed by one CombiPatch™ applied twice weekly for the remaining 14 days of a 28-day cycle

Administration Transdermal patch: Apply to clean dry skin. Do not apply transdermal patch to breasts; apply to lower abdomen, avoiding waistline. Rotate application sites.

Dosage Forms
  Tablet (Activella™): Estradiol 1 mg and norethindrone acetate 0.5 mg (28s)
  Transdermal system (CombiPatch™):
    9 sq cm: Estradiol 0.05 mg and norethindrone acetate 0.14 mg per day
    16 sq cm: Estradiol 0.05 mg and norethindrone acetate 0.25 mg per day

Estradiol and Testosterone (es tra DYE ole & tes TOS ter one)
  U.S. Brand Names Depo-Testadiol®; Depotestogen®; Duo-Cyp®; Valertest No.1®
  Canadian Brand Names Climacteron®
  Synonyms Estradiol Cypionate and Testosterone Cypionate; Estradiol Valerate and Testosterone Enanthate; Testosterone and Estradiol
  Therapeutic Category Estrogen and Androgen Combination
  Use Vasomotor symptoms associated with menopause
  Pregnancy Risk Factor X
  Usual Dosage Adults: All dosage needs to be adjusted based upon the patient's response
  Additional Information Complete prescribing information for this medication should be consulted for additional detail.
  Dosage Forms
    Injection:
      Depo-Testadiol®, Depotestogen®, Duo-Cyp®: Estradiol cypionate 2 mg and testosterone cypionate 50 mg per mL in cottonseed oil (10 mL)
      Valertest No.1®: Estradiol valerate 4 mg and testosterone enanthate 90 mg per mL in sesame oil (10 mL)

♦ **Estradiol Cypionate** *see Estradiol on page 491*

Estradiol Cypionate and Medroxyprogesterone Acetate
  (es tra DYE ole sip pe OH nate & me DROKS ee proe JES te rone AS e tate)
  U.S. Brand Names Lunelle™
  Synonyms E$_2$C and MPA; Medroxyprogesterone Acetate and Estradiol Cypionate
  Therapeutic Category Contraceptive, Parenteral (Estrogen/Progestin)
  Use Prevention of pregnancy
  Pregnancy Risk Factor X
  Usual Dosage Adults: Female: I.M.: 0.5 mL
    First dose: Within first 5 days of menstrual period or within 5 days of a complete 1st trimester abortion; do not administer <4 weeks postpartum **if not breast-feeding** or <6 weeks postpartum **if breast-feeding**
    Maintenance dose: Monthly, every 28-30 days following previous injection; do not exceed 33 days; pregnancy must be ruled out if >33 days have past between injections; bleeding episodes cannot be used to guide injection schedule; shortening schedule may lead to menstrual pattern changes
    Switching from other forms of contraception: First injection should be given within 7 days of last active oral contraceptive pill; when switching from other methods, timing of injection should ensure continuous contraceptive coverage

    Elderly: Not for postmenopausal use

    Dosage adjustment in renal impairment: Studies have not been conducted; however, dosage adjustment is not anticipated due to hepatic metabolism
    Dosage adjustment in hepatic impairment: Contraindicated in hepatic dysfunction
  Additional Information Complete prescribing information for this medication should be consulted for additional detail.
  Dosage Forms Injection, suspension: Estradiol cypionate 5 mg and medroxyprogesterone acetate 25 mg per 0.5 mL

♦ **Estradiol Cypionate and Testosterone Cypionate** *see Estradiol and Testosterone on page 495*

♦ **Estradiol Hemihydrate** *see Estradiol on page 491*

♦ **Estradiol Transdermal** *see Estradiol on page 491*

♦ **Estradiol Valerate** *see Estradiol on page 491*

♦ **Estradiol Valerate and Testosterone Enanthate** *see Estradiol and Testosterone on page 495*

Estramustine (es tra MUS teen)
  U.S. Brand Names Emcyt®
  Canadian Brand Names Emcyt®
  Synonyms Estramustine Phosphate Sodium
  Therapeutic Category Antineoplastic Agent, Alkylating Agent; Antineoplastic Agent, Hormone; Antineoplastic Agent, Nitrogen Mustard
  Use Palliative treatment of prostatic carcinoma (progressive or metastatic)
  Pregnancy Risk Factor C
  Contraindications Hypersensitivity to estramustine or any component, estradiol or nitrogen mustard; active thrombophlebitis or thromboembolic disorders
  Warnings/Precautions The U.S. Food and Drug Administration (FDA) currently recommends that procedures for proper handling and disposal of antineoplastic agents be considered. Glucose tolerance may be decreased; elevated blood pressure may occur; exacerbation of
(Continued)

Estramustine *(Continued)*

peripheral edema or congestive heart disease may occur; use with caution in patients with impaired liver function, renal insufficiency, or metabolic bone diseases.

Adverse Reactions

>10%:

Cardiovascular: Edema

Endocrine & metabolic: Sodium retention, decreased libido, breast tenderness, breast enlargement

Gastrointestinal: Diarrhea, nausea

Hematologic: Thrombocytopenia

Respiratory: Dyspnea

1% to 10%:

Cardiovascular: Myocardial infarction

Central nervous system: Insomnia, lethargy

Gastrointestinal: Anorexia, flatulence, vomiting

Hematologic: Leukopenia

Local: Thrombophlebitis

Neuromuscular & skeletal: Leg cramps

Respiratory: Pulmonary embolism

<1% (Limited to important or life-threatening): Allergic reactions, anemia, angioedema, cardiac arrest, gynecomastia

Overdosage/Toxicology Symptoms include nausea, vomiting, and myelosuppression. There are no known antidotes. Treatment is primarily symptomatic and supportive.

Drug Interactions

Decreased Effect: Milk products and calcium-rich foods/drugs may impair the oral absorption of estramustine phosphate sodium.

Ethanol/Nutrition/Herb Interactions Food: Estramustine serum levels may be decreased if taken with dairy products.

Stability Refrigerate at 2°C to 8°C (36°F to 46°F); capsules may be stored outside of refrigerator for up to 24-48 hours without affecting potency

Mechanism of Action Mechanism is not completely clear, thought to act as an alkylating agent and as estrogen

Pharmacodynamics/Kinetics

Absorption: 75%

Metabolism:

GI tract: Initial dephosphorylation

Hepatic: Oxidation and hydrolysis; metabolites include estramustine, estrone, estradiol, nitrogen mustard

Half-life elimination: Terminal: 20-24 hours

Time to peak, serum: 2-3 hours

Excretion: Feces (2.9% to 4.8% as unchanged drug)

Usual Dosage Refer to individual protocols.

Oral: 10-16 mg/kg/day (14 mg/kg/day is most common) or 140 mg 4 times/day (some patients have been maintained for >3 years on therapy)

I.V.: 300 mg/day for 3-4 weeks, then 300-450 mg/week for 3-8 weeks (investigational)

Dietary Considerations Administer at least 1 hour before or 2 hours after eating.

Patient Information It may take several weeks to manifest effects of this medication. Store capsules in refrigerator. Do not take with milk or milk products. Preferable to take on empty stomach (1 hour before or 2 hours after meals). Small frequent meals and frequent mouth care may reduce incidence of nausea or vomiting. You may experience flatulence, diarrhea, decreased libido (reversible), breast tenderness or enlargement. Report sudden acute pain or cramping in legs or calves, chest pain, shortness of breath, weakness or numbness of arms or legs, difficulty breathing, or edema (increased weight, swelling of legs or feet); contraceptive measures are recommended during therapy.

Nursing Implications Administer on an empty stomach, particularly avoid taking with milk

Additional Information Although I.V. use is reported, no parenteral product is commercially available in the U.S.

Dosage Forms Capsule, as phosphate sodium: 140 mg

♦ **Estramustine Phosphate Sodium** *see* Estramustine *on page 495*

♦ **Estratab®** *see* Estrogens (Esterified) *on page 500*

♦ **Estratest®** *see* Estrogens and Methyltestosterone *on page 496*

♦ **Estratest® H.S.** *see* Estrogens and Methyltestosterone *on page 496*

♦ **Estring®** *see* Estradiol *on page 491*

♦ **Estrogel® (Can)** *see* Estradiol *on page 491*

♦ **Estrogenic Substance Aqueous** *see* Estrone *on page 502*

♦ **Estrogenic Substances, Conjugated** *see* Estrogens (Conjugated/Equine) *on page 498*

Estrogens and Methyltestosterone *(ES troe jenz & meth il tes TOS te rone)*

U.S. Brand Names Estratest®; Estratest® H.S.

Canadian Brand Names Estratest®

Synonyms Conjugated Estrogen and Methyltestosterone; Esterified Estrogen and Methyltestosterone

Therapeutic Category Estrogen and Androgen Combination

Use Vasomotor symptoms of menopause

Pregnancy Risk Factor X

Usual Dosage Adults: Female: Oral: Lowest dose that will control symptoms should be chosen, normally given 3 weeks on and 1 week off

Additional Information Complete prescribing information for this medication should be consulted for additional detail.

Dosage Forms
Tablet:
  Estratest®: Esterified estrogen 1.25 mg and methyltestosterone 2.5 mg
  Estratest® H.S.: Esterified estrogen 0.625 mg and methyltestosterone 1.25 mg

Estrogens (Conjugated) and Medroxyprogesterone
(ES troe jenz KON joo gate ed & me DROKS ee proe JES te rone)
U.S. Brand Names Premphase®; Prempro™
Canadian Brand Names Premphase®; Prempro™
Synonyms Medroxyprogesterone and Estrogens (Conjugated); MPA and Estrogens (Conjugated)
Therapeutic Category Estrogen and Progestin Combination
Use Women with an intact uterus: Treatment of moderate to severe vasomotor symptoms associated with menopause; treatment of atrophic vaginitis; osteoporosis (prophylaxis)
Pregnancy Risk Factor X
Usual Dosage Oral: Adults:
Treatment of moderate to severe vasomotor symptoms associated with menopause or treatment of atrophic vaginitis in females with an intact uterus:
  Premphase®: One maroon conjugated estrogen 0.625 mg tablet daily on days 1 through 14 and one light blue conjugated estrogen 0.625 mg/MPA 5 mg tablet daily on days 15 through 28; re-evaluate patients at 3- and 6-month intervals to determine if treatment is still necessary; monitor patients for signs of endometrial cancer; rule out malignancy if unexplained vaginal bleeding occurs
  Prempro™: One conjugated estrogen 0.625 mg/MPA 2.5 mg tablet daily; re-evaluate at 3- and 6-month intervals to determine if therapy is still needed; dose may be increased to one conjugated estrogen 0.625 mg/MPA 5 mg tablet daily in patients with bleeding or spotting, once malignancy has been ruled out
Osteoporosis prophylaxis in females with an intact uterus:
  Premphase®: One maroon conjugated estrogen 0.625 tablet daily on days 1 through 14 and one light blue conjugated estrogen 0.625 mg/MPA 5 mg tablet daily on days 15 through 28; monitor patients for signs of endometrial cancer; rule out malignancy if unexplained vaginal bleeding occurs
  Prempro™: One conjugated estrogen 0.625 mg/MPA 2.5 mg tablet daily; dose may be increased to one conjugated estrogen 0.625 mg/MPA 5 mg tablet daily; in patients with bleeding or spotting, once malignancy has been ruled out
Additional Information Complete prescribing information for this medication should be consulted for additional detail.
Dosage Forms
Tablet:
  Premphase®: Two separate tablets in therapy pack: Conjugated estrogens 0.625 mg (14s) and conjugated estrogen 0.625 mg/medroxyprogesterone acetate 5 mg (14s)
  Prempro™:
    Conjugated estrogens 0.625 mg and medroxyprogesterone acetate 2.5 mg (28s)
    Conjugated estrogens 0.625 mg and medroxyprogesterone acetate 5 mg (28s)

Estrogens (Conjugated A/Synthetic)
(ES troe jenz, KON joo gate ed, aye, sin THET ik)
U.S. Brand Names Cenestin™
Therapeutic Category Estrogen Derivative
Use Treatment of moderate to severe vasomotor symptoms of menopause
Pregnancy Risk Factor X
Contraindications Hypersensitivity to estrogens or any component of the formulation; undiagnosed vaginal bleeding; thrombophlebitis; thromboembolic disorders; liver disease; carcinoma of the breast; estrogen dependent tumor; pregnancy
Warnings/Precautions Use with caution in patients with a history of hypercalcemia, cardiac disease, and gallbladder disease. The addition of progestins may attenuate estrogen's effects on raising HDL and lowering LDL cholesterol. May increase blood pressure and serum triglycerides (in patients with familial dyslipidemias). Use caution in patients with hepatic disease or renal dysfunction; may increase risk of venous thromboembolism; estrogens have been reported to increase the risk of endometrial carcinoma and may increase the risk of breast cancer; safety and efficacy in children have not been established; do not use estrogens during pregnancy.
Adverse Reactions
 >10%:
  Cardiovascular: Palpitation (21%), peripheral edema (10%)
  Central nervous system; Headache (68%), insomnia (42%), paresthesia (33%), nervousness (28%), depression (28%), pain (11%), dizziness (11%)
  Endocrine & metabolic: Breast pain (29%), menorrhagia (14%)
  Gastrointestinal: Abdominal pain (28%), flatulence (29%), nausea (18%), dyspepsia (10%)
  Musculoskeletal: Myalgia (28%), arthralgia (25%), back pain (14%)
  Miscellaneous: Weakness (33%), infection (14%)
 1% to 10%:
  Central nervous system: Hypertonia (6%), fever (1%)
  Gastrointestinal: Vomiting (7%), constipation (6%), diarrhea (6%)
  Musculoskeletal: Leg cramps (10%)
  Respiratory: Pharyngitis (8%), rhinitis (8%), cough (6%)
  Additional adverse reactions associated with estrogen therapy: Aggravation of porphyria, alopecia, alterations in frequency and flow of menses, amenorrhea, anxiety, breast enlargement, breast tenderness, breast tumors, changes in cervical secretions, changes in corneal curvature, changes in libido, cholestatic jaundice, chorea chloasma, decreased glucose tolerance, erythema multiforme, erythema nodosum, GI distress, hirsutism, hypercalcemia, hypertension, increase in blood pressure, increased susceptibility to *Candida* infection, increased triglycerides and LDL, intolerance to contact lenses, melasma, myocardial infarction, pancreatitis, rash, stroke, thromboembolic disorder, weight gain/loss
(Continued)

497

Estrogens (Conjugated A/Synthetic) *(Continued)*

Overdosage/Toxicology Toxicity is unlikely following single exposures of excessive doses. Symptoms include fluid retention, jaundice, and thrombophlebitis. Treatment following emesis and charcoal administration should be supportive and symptomatic.

Drug Interactions

Increased Effect/Toxicity: Specific drug interactions have not been conducted for the synthetic preparation, however the following interactions have been noted for conjugated estrogens. Hydrocortisone increases corticosteroid toxic potential. Increased potential for thromboembolic events with anticoagulants.

Decreased Effect: Specific drug interactions have not been conducted for the synthetic preparation, however the following interactions have been noted for conjugated estrogens. Rifampin decreases estrogen serum concentrations (other enzyme inducers may share this effect).

Ethanol/Nutrition/Herb Interactions

Ethanol: Avoid ethanol (routine use increases estrogen level and risk of breast cancer).

Herb/Nutraceutical: St John's wort may decrease levels. Avoid black cohosh, dong quai (has estrogenic activity). Avoid red clover, saw palmetto, ginseng (due to potential hormonal effects).

Usual Dosage Adolescents and Adults: Moderate to severe vasomotor symptoms: Oral: 0.625 mg/day; may be titrated up to 1.25 mg/day. Attempts to discontinue medication should be made at 3- to 6-month intervals.

Patient Information

Patient package insert available with product

Women should inform their physicians if signs or symptoms of any of the following occur: Thromboembolic or thrombotic disorders including sudden severe headache or vomiting, disturbance of vision or speech, loss of vision, numbness or weakness in an extremity, sharp or crushing chest pain, calf pain, shortness of breath, severe abdominal pain or mass, mental depression, or unusual bleeding

Women should discontinue taking the medication if they suspect they are pregnant or become pregnant

Additional Information Not biologically equivalent to conjugated estrogens from equine source. Contains 9 unique estrogenic compounds (equine source contains at least 10 active estrogenic compounds).

Dosage Forms Tablet: 0.625 mg, 0.9 mg, 1.25 mg

Estrogens (Conjugated/Equine) (ES troe jenz KON joo gate ed, EE kwine)

Related Information

Depression *on page 1655*

U.S. Brand Names Premarin®

Canadian Brand Names Cenestin; C.E.S.®; Congest; PMS-Conjugated Estrogens; Premarin®

Synonyms C.E.S.; Estrogenic Substances, Conjugated

Therapeutic Category Estrogen Derivative; Estrogen Derivative, Intramuscular; Estrogen Derivative, Oral; Estrogen Derivative, Parenteral; Estrogen Derivative, Vaginal

Use Treatment of moderate to severe vasomotor symptoms associated with menopause; treatment of vulvar and vaginal atrophy; hypoestrogenism (due to hypogonadism, castration, or primary ovarian failure); prostatic cancer (palliation); breast cancer (palliation); osteoporosis (prophylaxis)

Unlabeled/Investigational Use Uremic bleeding; abnormal uterine bleeding

Pregnancy Risk Factor X

Pregnancy/Breast-Feeding Implications Increased risk of fetal reproductive tract disorders and other birth defects; do not use during pregnancy. Excreted in human milk; use caution in breast-feeding women.

Contraindications Hypersensitivity to estrogens or any component of the formulation; undiagnosed abnormal vaginal bleeding; history of or current thrombophlebitis or thromboembolic disorders; carcinoma of the breast (except in appropriately selected patients being treated for metastatic disease); estrogen-dependent tumor; pregnancy

Warnings/Precautions Unopposed estrogens may increase the risk of endometrial carcinoma in postmenopausal women. Use with caution in patients with diseases which may be exacerbated by fluid retention, including asthma, epilepsy, migraine, diabetes, cardiac or renal dysfunction. Use with caution in patients with a history of hypercalcemia, cardiovascular disease, and gallbladder disease. May increase blood pressure. Use with caution in patients with hepatic disease. May increase risk of venous thromboembolism. Estrogens may increase the risk of breast cancer (controversial/currently under study). Estrogen compounds are generally associated with lipid effects such as increased HDL-cholesterol and decreased LDL-cholesterol. Triglycerides may also be increased; use with caution in patients with familial defects of lipoprotein metabolism. Estrogens may cause premature closure of the epiphyses in young individuals. May increase size of pre-existing uterine leiomyomata. Before prescribing estrogen therapy to postmenopausal women, the risks and benefits must be weighed for each patient. Women should be informed of these risks and benefits, as well as possible effects of progestin when added to estrogen therapy. Safety and efficacy in pediatric patients have not been established.

Adverse Reactions Frequency not defined.

Cardiovascular: Edema, hypertension, venous thromboembolism

Central nervous system: Dizziness, headache, mental depression, migraine

Dermatologic: Chloasma, erythema multiforme, erythema nodosum, hemorrhagic eruption, hirsutism, loss of scalp hair, melasma

Endocrine & metabolic: Breast enlargement, breast tenderness, changes in libido, increased thyroid-binding globulin, increased total thyroid hormone (T_4), increased serum triglycerides/phospholipids, increased HDL-cholesterol, decreased LDL-cholesterol, impaired glucose tolerance, hypercalcemia

Gastrointestinal: Abdominal cramps, bloating, cholecystitis, cholelithiasis, gallbladder disease, nausea, pancreatitis, vomiting, weight gain/loss

Genitourinary: Alterations in frequency and flow of menses, changes in cervical secretions, endometrial cancer, increased size of uterine leiomyomata, vaginal candidiasis

Hematologic: Aggravation of porphyria, decreased antithrombin III and antifactor Xa, increased levels of fibrinogen, increased platelet aggregability and platelet count; increased prothrombin and factors VII, VIII, IX, X

Hepatic: Cholestatic jaundice

Neuromuscular & skeletal: Chorea

Miscellaneous: Carbohydrate intolerance

Ocular: Intolerance to contact lenses, steeping of corneal curvature

Respiratory: Pulmonary thromboembolism

Overdosage/Toxicology Toxicity is unlikely following single exposures of excessive doses. Effects noted after large doses include headache, nausea, and vomiting. Bleeding may occur in females. Treatment following emesis and charcoal administration should be supportive and symptomatic.

Drug Interactions

Cytochrome P450 Effect: May be a substrate for cytochrome isoenzymes (profile not defined)

Increased Effect/Toxicity: Hydrocortisone taken with estrogen may cause corticosteroid-induced toxicity. Increased potential for thromboembolic events with anticoagulants.

Decreased Effect: Rifampin, nelfinavir, and ritonavir decrease estradiol serum concentrations. Anticonvulsants which are enzyme inducers (barbiturates, carbamazepine, phenobarbital, phenytoin, primidone) may potentially decrease estrogen levels.

Ethanol/Nutrition/Herb Interactions

Ethanol: Avoid ethanol (routine use increases estrogen level and risk of breast cancer).

Food: Folic acid absorption may be decreased.

Herb/Nutraceutical: St John's wort may decrease levels. Avoid black cohosh, dong quai (has estrogenic activity). Avoid red clover, saw palmetto, ginseng (due to potential hormonal effects).

Stability

Injection: Refrigerate at 2°C to 8°C (36°F to 46°F) prior to reconstitution; following reconstitution, solution in stable for 60 days under refrigeration

Compatible with normal saline, dextrose, and inert sugar solutions

Incompatible with proteins, ascorbic acid, or solutions with acidic pH

Tablets, vaginal cream: Store at room temperature (25°C)

Mechanism of Action Conjugated estrogens contain a mixture of estrone sulfate, equilin sulfate, 17 alpha-dihydroequilin, 17 alpha-estradiol and 17 beta-dihydroequilin. Estrogens are responsible for the development and maintenance of the female reproductive system and secondary sexual characteristics. Estradiol is the principle intracellular human estrogen and is more potent than estrone and estriol at the receptor level; it is the primary estrogen secreted prior to menopause. Following menopause, estrone and estrone sulfate are more highly produced. Estrogens modulate the pituitary secretion of gonadotropins, luteinizing hormone, and follicle-stimulating hormone through a negative feedback system; estrogen replacement reduces elevated levels of these hormones in postmenopausal women.

Pharmacodynamics/Kinetics

Absorption: Well absorbed

Metabolism: Hepatic to inactive compounds

Excretion: Urine and feces

Usual Dosage Adults:

Male and Female:

Breast cancer palliation, metastatic disease in selected patients: Oral: 10 mg 3 times/day for at least 3 months

Uremic bleeding: I.V.: 0.6 mg/kg/day for 5 days

Androgen-dependent prostate cancer: Oral: 1.25-2.5 mg 3 times/day

Prevention of osteoporosis in postmenopausal women: Oral: 0.625 mg/day, cyclically* or daily, depending on medical assessment of patient

Moderate to severe vasomotor symptoms associated with menopause: Oral: 0.625 mg/day; lowest dose that will control symptoms should be used. Medication should be discontinued as soon as possible. May be given cyclically* or daily, depending on medical assessment of patient

Vulvar and vaginal atrophy:

Oral: 0.3-1.25 mg (or more) daily, depending on tissue response of the patient; lowest dose that will control symptoms should be used. Medication should be discontinued as soon as possible. May be given cyclically* or daily, depending on medical assessment of patient.

Vaginal cream: Intravaginal: ½ to 2 g/day given cyclically*

Female hypogonadism: Oral: 0.3-0.625 mg/day given cyclically*; adjust dose in response to symptoms and endometrium response; progestin treatment should be added to maintain bone mineral density

Female castration, primary ovarian failure: Oral: 1.25 mg/day given cyclically*; adjust according to severity of symptoms and patient response. For maintenance, adjust to the lowest effective dose.

Abnormal uterine bleeding:

Acute/heavy bleeding:

Oral: 1.25 mg, may repeat every 4 hours for 24 hours, followed by 1.25 mg once daily for 7-10 days

I.V.: 25 mg, may repeat every 4 hours up to 3 doses

Note: Oral/I.V.: Treatment should be followed by a low-dose oral contraceptive; medroxyprogesterone acetate along with or following estrogen therapy can also be given

Nonacute/lesser bleeding: Oral: 1.25 mg once daily for 7-10 days

*Cyclic administration: Either 3 weeks on, 1 week off **or** 25 days on, 5 days off

Dietary Considerations Ensure adequate calcium and vitamin D intake when used for the prevention of osteoporosis.

(Continued)

Estrogens (Conjugated/Equine) *(Continued)*

Administration May also be administered intramuscularly; when administered I.V., drug should be administered slowly to avoid the occurrence of a flushing reaction

Monitoring Parameters Yearly physical examination that includes blood pressure and Papanicolaou smear, breast exam, mammogram. Monitor for signs of endometrial cancer in female patients with uterus; rule out malignancy if unexplained vaginal bleeding occurs

Reference Range

Children: <10 µg/24 hours (SI: <35 µmol/day) (values at Mayo Medical Laboratories)

Adults:

Male: 15-40 µg/24 hours (SI: 52-139 µmol/day)

Female:

Menstruating: 15-80 µg/24 hours (SI: 52-277 µmol/day)

Postmenopausal: <20 µg/24 hours (SI: <69 µmol/day)

Test Interactions Pathologist should be advised of estrogen/progesterone therapy when specimens are submitted. Reduced response to metyrapone test.

Patient Information It is important to maintain schedule. Estrogens have been shown to increase the risk of endometrial cancer. Annual gynecologic and breast exams are important. You may experience nausea or vomiting (small frequent meals may help); abdominal pain; difficult/painful menstrual cycles; dizziness or mental depression; headaches; rash; breast pain; or increased/decreased libido. Report significant swelling of extremities, sudden acute pain in legs or calves, chest or abdomen; shortness of breath; severe headache or vomiting; weakness or numbness of arms or legs; or unusual vaginal bleeding. You may become intolerant to wearing contact lenses, notify prescriber if this occurs. If taking for prevention of osteoporosis, ask prescriber about calcium and vitamin D intake, and weight-bearing exercises.

Nursing Implications May also be administered intramuscularly; administer at bedtime to minimize occurrence of adverse effects; when administered I.V., drug should be administered slowly to avoid the occurrence of a flushing reaction. Monitor blood pressure.

Additional Information Contains 50% to 65% sodium estrone sulfate and 20% to 35% sodium equilin sulfate

Dosage Forms

Cream, vaginal: 0.625 mg/g (42.5 g)

Injection: 25 mg (5 mL)

Tablet: 0.3 mg, 0.625 mg, 0.9 mg, 1.25 mg, 2.5 mg

Estrogens (Esterified) *(ES troe jenz, es TER i fied)*

U.S. Brand Names Estratab®; Menest®

Canadian Brand Names Estratab®; Menest®

Synonyms Esterified Estrogens

Therapeutic Category Estrogen Derivative; Estrogen Derivative, Oral

Use Treatment of moderate to severe vasomotor symptoms associated with menopause; treatment of vulvar and vaginal atrophy; hypoestrogenism (due to hypogonadism, castration, or primary ovarian failure); prostatic cancer (palliation); breast cancer (palliation); osteoporosis (prophylaxis)

Pregnancy Risk Factor X

Pregnancy/Breast-Feeding Implications Increased risk of fetal reproductive tract disorders and other birth defects; do not use during pregnancy. Excreted in human milk; use caution in breast-feeding women

Contraindications Hypersensitivity to estrogens or any component of the formulation; undiagnosed abnormal vaginal bleeding; history of current thrombophlebitis or thromboembolic disorders; carcinoma of the breast, except in appropriately selected patients being treated for metastatic disease; estrogen-dependent tumor; pregnancy

Warnings/Precautions Unopposed estrogens may increase the risk of endometrial carcinoma in postmenopausal women. Use with caution in patients with diseases which may be exacerbated by fluid retention, including asthma, epilepsy, migraine, diabetes, cardiac or renal dysfunction. Use with caution in patients with a history of hypercalcemia, cardiovascular disease, and gallbladder disease. May increase blood pressure. Use with caution in patients with hepatic disease. May increase risk of venous thromboembolism. Estrogens may increase the risk of breast cancer (controversial/currently under study). Estrogen compounds are generally associated with lipid effects such as increased HDL-cholesterol, and decreased LDL-cholesterol. Triglycerides may also be increased; use with caution in patients with familial defects of lipoprotein metabolism. May increase size of pre-existing uterine leiomyomata. Before prescribing estrogen therapy to postmenopausal women, the risks and benefits must be weighed for each patient. Women should be informed of these risks and benefits, as well as possible effects of progestin when added to estrogen therapy. Estrogens may cause premature closure of the epiphyses in young individuals. Safety and efficacy in pediatric patients have not been established.

Adverse Reactions

Cardiovascular: Edema, hypertension, venous thromboembolism

Central nervous system: Dizziness, headache, mental depression, migraine

Dermatologic: Chloasma, erythema multiforme, erythema nodosum, hemorrhagic eruption, hirsutism, loss of scalp hair, melasma

Endocrine & metabolic: Breast enlargement, breast tenderness, changes in libido, increased thyroid-binding globulin, increased total thyroid hormone (T_4), increased serum triglycerides/phospholipids, increased HDL cholesterol, decreased LDL cholesterol, impaired glucose tolerance, hypercalcemia

Gastrointestinal: Abdominal cramps, bloating, cholecystitis, cholelithiasis, gallbladder disease, nausea, pancreatitis, vomiting, weight gain/loss

Genitourinary: Alterations in frequency and flow of menses, changes in cervical secretions, endometrial cancer, increased size of uterine leiomyomata, vaginal candidiasis

Hematologic: Aggravation of porphyria, decreased antithrombin III and antifactor Xa, increased levels of fibrinogen, increased platelet aggregability and platelet count; increased prothrombin and factors VII, VIII, IX, X

Hepatic: Cholestatic jaundice
Neuromuscular & skeletal: Chorea
Ocular: Intolerance to contact lenses, steeping of corneal curvature
Respiratory: Pulmonary thromboembolism
Miscellaneous: Carbohydrate intolerance

Overdosage/Toxicity Toxicity is unlikely following single exposures of excessive doses. Effects noted after large doses include headache, nausea, and vomiting. Bleeding may occur in females. Treatment following emesis and charcoal administration should be supportive and symptomatic.

Drug Interactions

Cytochrome P450 Effect: May induce and is a substrate for cytochrome isoenzymes (profile not defined); estradiol is a CYP1A2 enzyme inhibitor

Increased Effect/Toxicity: Hydrocortisone taken with estrogen may cause corticosteroid-induced toxicity. Increased potential for thromboembolic events with anticoagulants.

Decreased Effect: Rifampin, nelfinavir, and ritonavir decrease estradiol serum concentrations. Anticonvulsants which are enzyme inducers (barbiturates, carbamazepine, phenobarbital, phenytoin, primidone) may potentially decrease estrogen levels.

Ethanol/Nutrition/Herb Interactions

Ethanol: Avoid ethanol (routine use increases estrogen level and risk of breast cancer).
Food: Folic acid absorption may be decreased.
Herb/Nutraceutical: St John's wort may decrease levels. Avoid black cohosh, dong quai (has estrogenic activity). Avoid red clover, saw palmetto, ginseng (due to potential hormonal effects).

Stability Store below 30°C (86°F); protect from moisture

Mechanism of Action Esterified estrogens contain a mixture of estrogenic substances; the principle component is estrone. Preparations contain 75% to 85% sodium estrone sulfate and 6% to 15% sodium equilin sulfate such that the total is not <90%. Estrogens are responsible for the development and maintenance of the female reproductive system and secondary sexual characteristics. Estradiol is the principle intracellular human estrogen and is more potent than estrone and estriol at the receptor level; it is the primary estrogen secreted prior to menopause. In males and following menopause in females, estrone and estrone sulfate are more highly produced. Estrogens modulate the pituitary secretion of gonadotropins, luteinizing hormone, and follicle-stimulating hormone through a negative feedback system; estrogen replacement reduces elevated levels of these hormones.

Pharmacodynamics/Kinetics

Absorption: Readily
Metabolism: Rapidly hepatic to estrone sulfate, conjugated and unconjugated metabolites; first-pass effect
Excretion: Urine (as unchanged drug and as glucuronide and sulfate conjugates)

Usual Dosage Oral: Adults:

Prostate cancer (palliation): 1.25-2.5 mg 3 times/day

Female hypogonadism: 2.5-7.5 mg of estrogen daily for 20 days followed by a 10-day rest period. Administer cyclically (3 weeks on and 1 week off). If bleeding does not occur by the end of the 10-day period, repeat the same dosing schedule; the number of courses is dependent upon the responsiveness of the endometrium. If bleeding occurs before the end of the 10-day period, begin an estrogen-progestin cyclic regimen of 2.5-7.5 mg esterified estrogens daily for 20 days. During the last 5 days of estrogen therapy, give an oral progestin. If bleeding occurs before regimen is concluded, discontinue therapy and resume on the fifth day of bleeding.

Moderate to severe vasomotor symptoms associated with menopause: 1.25 mg/day administered cyclically (3 weeks on and 1 week off). If patient has not menstruated within the last 2 months or more, cyclic administration is started arbitrary. If the patient is menstruating, cyclical administration is started on day 5 of the bleeding. For short-term use only and should be discontinued as soon as possible. Re-evaluate at 3- to 6-month intervals for tapering or discontinuation of therapy.

Atopic vaginitis and kraurosis vulvae: 0.3 to ≥1.25 mg/day, depending on the tissue response of the individual patient. Administer cyclically. For short-term use only and should be discontinued as soon as possible. Re-evaluate at 3- to 6-month intervals for tapering or discontinuation of therapy.

Breast cancer (palliation): 10 mg 3 times/day for at least 3 months

Osteoporosis in postmenopausal women: Initial: 0.3 mg/day and increase to a maximum daily dose of 1.25 mg/day; initiate therapy as soon as possible after menopause; cyclically or daily, depending on medical assessment of patient. Monitor patients with an intact uterus for signs of endometrial cancer; rule out malignancy if unexplained vaginal bleeding occurs

Female castration and primary ovarian failure: 1.25 mg/day, cyclically. Adjust dosage upward or downward, according to the severity of symptoms and patient response. For maintenance, adjust dosage to lowest level that will provide effective control.

Dosing adjustment in hepatic impairment:

Mild to moderate liver impairment: Dosage reduction of estrogens is recommended
Severe liver impairment: **Not recommended**

Dietary Considerations Should be taken with food at same time each day. Ensure adequate calcium and vitamin D intake when used for the prevention of osteoporosis.

Monitoring Parameters Yearly physical examination that includes blood pressure, Papanicolaou smear, breast exam, and mammogram. Monitor for signs of endometrial cancer in female patients with uterus; rule out malignancy if unexplained vaginal bleeding occurs.

Test Interactions Pathologist should be advised of estrogen/progesterone therapy when specimens are submitted. Reduced response to metyrapone test.

Patient Information It is important to maintain schedule. Estrogens have been shown to increase the risk of endometrial cancer. Annual gynecologic and breast exams are important. You may experience nausea or vomiting (small frequent meals may help); abdominal pain; difficult/painful menstrual cycles; dizziness or mental depression; headaches; rash; breast pain; or increased/decreased libido. Report significant swelling of extremities, sudden acute (Continued)

Estrogens (Esterified) *(Continued)*

pain in legs or calves, chest or abdomen; shortness of breath; severe headache or vomiting; weakness or numbness of arms or legs; or unusual vaginal bleeding. You may become intolerant to wearing contact lenses, notify prescriber if this occurs. If taking for prevention of osteoporosis, ask prescriber about calcium and vitamin D intake, and weight-bearing exercises.

Dosage Forms Tablet: 0.3 mg, 0.625 mg, 1.25 mg, 2.5 mg

Estrone (ES trone)

U.S. Brand Names Kestrone®
Canadian Brand Names Oestrilin
Synonyms Estrogenic Substance Aqueous
Therapeutic Category Estrogen Derivative; Estrogen Derivative, Intramuscular
Use Hypogonadism; primary ovarian failure; vasomotor symptoms of menopause; prostatic carcinoma; inoperable breast cancer, kraurosis vulvae, abnormal uterine bleeding due to hormone imbalance
Pregnancy Risk Factor X
Contraindications Hypersensitivity to estrogens or any component of the formulation; thrombophlebitis; undiagnosed vaginal bleeding; pregnancy
Warnings/Precautions Use with caution in patients with asthma, epilepsy, migraine, diabetes, cardiac or renal dysfunction; estrogens may cause premature closure of the epiphyses in young individuals; safety and efficacy in children have not been established; estrogens have been reported to increase the risk of endometrial carcinoma, do not use estrogens during pregnancy

Adverse Reactions
Systemic:
>10%:
Cardiovascular: Peripheral edema
Endocrine & metabolic: Enlargement of breasts (female and male), breast tenderness
Gastrointestinal: Nausea, anorexia, bloating
1% to 10%:
Central nervous system: Headache, migraine headache
Endocrine & metabolic: Increased libido (female), decreased libido (male)
Gastrointestinal: Vomiting, diarrhea
<1% (Limited to important or life-threatening): Alterations in frequency and flow of menses, amenorrhea, anxiety, breast tumors, chloasma, decreased glucose tolerance, depression, dizziness, edema, gallbladder obstruction, GI distress, hepatitis, hypertension, increased susceptibility to *Candida* infection, increased triglycerides and LDL, intolerance to contact lenses, melasma, myocardial infarction, nausea, rash, stroke, thromboembolism
Vaginal:
1% to 10%:
Cardiovascular: Peripheral edema
Endocrine & metabolic: Breast tenderness, breast enlargement
Gastrointestinal: Anorexia, abdominal cramping
<1% (Limited to important or life-threatening): Alterations in frequency and flow of menses, anxiety, breast tenderness or enlargement, chloasma, cholestatic jaundice, decreased glucose tolerance, depression, dizziness, GI distress, headache, hypertension, increased susceptibility to *Candida* infection, increased triglycerides and LDL, melasma, migraine, myocardial infarction, nausea, rash, stroke, thromboembolism
Overdosage/Toxicology Toxicity is unlikely following single exposures of excessive doses. Symptoms include fluid retention, jaundice, and thrombophlebitis. Treatment should be supportive and symptomatic.

Drug Interactions
Increased Effect/Toxicity: Hydrocortisone taken with estrogen may cause corticosteroid-induced toxicity. Increased potential for thromboembolic events with anticoagulants. Estrone may increase the effect of carbamazepine, tricyclic antidepressants, and corticosteroids. Increased thromboembolic potential when estrone is taken with oral anticoagulants.
Decreased Effect: Rifampin decreases estrogen serum concentrations.
Mechanism of Action Estrone is a natural ovarian estrogenic hormone that is available as an aqueous mixture of water insoluble estrone and water soluble estrone potassium sulfate; all estrogens, including estrone, act in a similar manner; there is no evidence that there are biological differences among various estrogen preparations other than their ability to bind to cellular receptors inside the target cells
Pharmacodynamics/Kinetics Absorption: Readily
Usual Dosage Adults: I.M.:
Male: Prostatic carcinoma: 2-4 mg 2-3 times/week
Female:
Senile vaginitis and kraurosis vulvae: 0.1-0.5 mg 2-3 times/week; cyclical (3 weeks on and 1 week off)
Breast cancer (inoperable, progressing): 5 mg 3 or more times/week
Primary ovarian failure, hypogonadism: 0.1-1 mg/week, up to 2 mg/week in single or divided doses; cyclical (3 weeks on and 1 week off)
Abnormal uterine bleeding: Brief courses of intensive therapy: 2-5 mg/day for several days
Dosing adjustment in hepatic impairment:
Mild to moderate liver impairment: Dosage reduction of estrogens is recommended
Severe liver impairment: **Not recommended**
Administration Intramuscular injection only
Test Interactions
Decreased antithrombin III
Decreased serum folate concentration
Increased prothrombin and factors VII, VIII, IX, X
Increased platelet aggregability

Increased thyroid-binding globulin
Increased total thyroid hormone (T_4)
Increased serum triglycerides/phospholipids

Patient Information Patients should inform their physicians if signs or symptoms of any of the following occur: Thromboembolic or thrombotic disorders including sudden severe headache or vomiting, disturbance of vision or speech, loss of vision, numbness or weakness in an extremity, sharp or crushing chest pain, calf pain, shortness of breath, severe abdominal pain or mass, mental depression or unusual bleeding; patients should discontinue taking the medication if they suspect they are pregnant or become pregnant

Nursing Implications May also be administered intramuscularly; administer at bedtime to minimize occurrence of adverse effects; when administered I.V., drug should be administered slowly to avoid the occurrence of a flushing reaction

Dosage Forms Injection: 2 mg/mL (10 mL); 5 mg/mL (10 mL)

Estropipate (ES troe pih pate)

U.S. Brand Names Ogen®; Ortho-Est®

Canadian Brand Names Ogen®

Synonyms Piperazine Estrone Sulfate

Therapeutic Category Estrogen Derivative; Estrogen Derivative, Oral; Estrogen Derivative, Vaginal

Use Treatment of moderate to severe vasomotor symptoms associated with menopause; treatment of vulvar and vaginal atrophy; hypoestrogenism (due to hypogonadism, castration, or primary ovarian failure); osteoporosis (prophylaxis)

Pregnancy Risk Factor X

Pregnancy/Breast-Feeding Implications Increased risk of fetal reproductive tract disorders and other birth defects; do not use during pregnancy. Excreted in human milk/use caution in breast-feeding women.

Contraindications Hypersensitivity to estrogens or any component of the formulation; undiagnosed abnormal vaginal bleeding; history of or current thrombophlebitis or thrombo-embolic disorders; carcinoma of the breast, except in appropriately selected patients being treated for metastatic disease; estrogen-dependent tumor; pregnancy

Warnings/Precautions Unopposed estrogens may increase the risk of endometrial carci-noma in postmenopausal women. Use with caution in patients with diseases which may be exacerbated by fluid retention, including asthma, epilepsy, migraine, diabetes, cardiac or renal dysfunction. Use with caution in patients with a history of hypercalcemia, cardiovascular disease, and gallbladder disease. May increase blood pressure. Use with caution in patients with hepatic dysfunction. May increase risk of venous thromboembolism. Estrogens may increase the risk of breast cancer (controversial/currently under study). Estrogen compounds are generally associated with lipid effects such as increased HDL-cholesterol and decreased LDL-cholesterol. Triglycerides may also be increased; use with caution in patients with familial defects of lipoprotein metabolism. Estrogens may cause premature closure of the epiphyses in young individuals. May increase size of pre-existing uterine leiomyomata. Before prescribing estrogen therapy to postmenopausal women, the risks and benefits must be weighed for each patient. Women should be informed of these risks and benefits, as well as possible effects of progestin when added to estrogen therapy. Safety and efficacy in pediatric patients have not been established.

Adverse Reactions Frequency not defined.
Cardiovascular: Edema, hypertension, venous thromboembolism
Central nervous system: Dizziness, headache, mental depression, migraine
Dermatologic: Chloasma, erythema multiforme, erythema nodosum, hemorrhagic eruption, hirsutism, loss of scalp hair, melasma
Endocrine & metabolic: Breast enlargement, breast tenderness, changes in libido, increased thyroid-binding globulin, increased total thyroid hormone (T_4), increased serum triglycer-ides/phospholipids, increased HDL cholesterol, decreased LDL cholesterol, impaired glucose tolerance, hypercalcemia
Gastrointestinal: Abdominal cramps, bloating, cholecystitis, cholelithiasis, gallbladder disease, nausea, pancreatitis, vomiting, weight gain/loss
Genitourinary: Alterations in frequency and flow of menses, changes in cervical secretions, endometrial cancer, increased size of uterine leiomyomata, vaginal candidiasis
Hematologic: Aggravation of porphyria, decreased antithrombin III and antifactor Xa, increased levels of fibrinogen, increased platelet aggregability and platelet count; increased prothrombin and factors VII, VIII, IX, X
Hepatic: Cholestatic jaundice
Neuromuscular & skeletal: Chorea
Ocular: Intolerance to contact lenses, steeping of corneal curvature
Respiratory: Pulmonary thromboembolism
Miscellaneous: Carbohydrate intolerance

Overdosage/Toxicology Toxicity is unlikely following single exposures of excessive doses. Effects noted after large doses include headache, nausea, and vomiting. Bleeding may occur in females. Treatment following emesis and charcoal administration should be supportive and symptomatic.

Drug Interactions
Increased Effect/Toxicity: Hydrocortisone taken with estrogen may cause corticosteroid-induced toxicity. Increased potential for thromboembolic events with anticoagulants.
Decreased Effect: Rifampin, nelfinavir, and ritonavir decrease estradiol serum concentra-tions. Anticonvulsants which are enzyme inducers (barbiturates, carbamazepine, pheno-barbital, phenytoin, primidone) may potentially decrease estrogen levels.

Ethanol/Nutrition/Herb Interactions
Ethanol: Routine use increases estrogen level and risk of breast cancer; avoid ethanol.
Food: Folic acid absorption may be decreased.
Herb/Nutraceutical: St John's wort may decrease levels. Avoid black cohosh, dong quai (has estrogenic activity). Avoid red clover, saw palmetto, ginseng (due to potential hormonal effects).

(Continued)

503

Estropipate *(Continued)*

Stability
Tablet: Store below 25°C (77°F)
Vaginal cream: Store below 30°C (86°F)

Mechanism of Action Estrogens are responsible for the development and maintenance of the female reproductive system and secondary sexual characteristics. Estradiol is the principle intracellular human estrogen and is more potent than estrone and estriol at the receptor level; it is the primary estrogen secreted prior to menopause. In males and following menopause in females, estrone and estrone sulfate are more highly produced. Estrogens modulate the pituitary secretion of gonadotropins, luteinizing hormone, and follicle-stimulating hormone through a negative feedback system; estrogen replacement reduces elevated levels of these hormones. Estropipate is prepared from purified crystalline estrone that has been solubilized as the sulfate and stabilized with piperazine.

Pharmacodynamics/Kinetics
Absorption: Well absorbed
Metabolism: Hepatic and in target tissues; first-pass effect

Usual Dosage Adults:
Oral:
Moderate to severe vasomotor symptoms associated with menopause: Usual dosage range: 0.75-6 mg estropipate daily; use the lowest dose and regimen that will control symptoms, and discontinue as soon as possible. Attempt to discontinue or taper medication at 3- to 6-month intervals. If a patient with vasomotor symptoms has not menstruated within the last ≥2 months, start the cyclic administration arbitrarily. If the patient has menstruated, start cyclic administration on day 5 of bleeding.

Female hypogonadism: 1.5-9 mg estropipate daily for the first 3 weeks, followed by a rest period of 8-10 days; use the lowest dose and regimen that will control symptoms. Repeat if bleeding does not occur by the end of the rest period. The duration of therapy necessary to product the withdrawal bleeding will vary according to the responsiveness of the endometrium. If satisfactory withdrawal bleeding does not occur, give an oral progestin in addition to estrogen during the third week of the cycle.

Female castration or primary ovarian failure: 1.5-9 mg estropipate daily for the first 3 weeks of a theoretical cycle, followed by a rest period of 8-10 days; use the lowest dose and regimen that will control symptoms

Osteoporosis prophylaxis: 0.75 mg estropipate daily for 25 days of a 31-day cycle

Atrophic vaginitis or kraurosis vulvae: 0.75- 6 mg estropipate daily. Use the lowest dose and regimen that will control symptoms; administer cyclically

Intravaginal: Atrophic vaginitis or kraurosis vulvae: Instill 2-4 g/day intravaginally; use the lowest dose and regimen that will control symptoms; attempt to discontinue or taper medication at 3- to 6-month intervals

Dosing adjustment in hepatic impairment:
Mild to moderate liver impairment: Dosage reduction of estrogens is recommended
Severe liver impairment: **Not recommended**

Dietary Considerations Ensure adequate calcium and vitamin D intake when used for the prevention of osteoporosis.

Monitoring Parameters Yearly physical examination that includes blood pressure and Papanicolaou smear, breast exam, mammogram. Monitor for signs of endometrial cancer in female patients with uterus; rule out malignancy if unexplained vaginal bleeding occurs

Test Interactions Pathologist should be advised of estrogen/progesterone therapy when specimens are submitted. Reduced response to metyrapone test.

Patient Information It is important to maintain schedule. Estrogens have been shown to increase the risk of endometrial cancer. Annual gynecologic and breast exams are important. You may experience nausea or vomiting (small frequent meals may help); abdominal pain; difficult/painful menstrual cycles; dizziness or mental depression; headaches; rash; breast pain; or increased/decreased libido. Report significant swelling of extremities, sudden acute pain in legs or calves, chest or abdomen; shortness of breath; severe headache or vomiting; weakness or numbness of arms or legs; or unusual vaginal bleeding. You may become intolerant to wearing contact lenses, notify prescriber if this occurs. If taking for prevention of osteoporosis, ask prescriber about calcium and vitamin D intake, and weight-bearing exercises.

Intravaginal cream: Insert high in vagina; wash hands and applicator before and after application

Nursing Implications Patients should inform their physicians if signs or symptoms of any of the following occur: Thromboembolic or thrombotic disorders including sudden severe headache or vomiting, disturbance of vision or speech, loss of vision, numbness or weakness in an extremity, sharp or crushing chest pain, calf pain, shortness of breath, severe abdominal pain or mass, mental depression or unusual bleeding; patients should discontinue taking the medication if they suspect they are pregnant or become pregnant. Patient package insert is available; insert vaginal cream high into the vagina.

Dosage Forms
Cream, vaginal (Ogen®): 0.15% [estropipate 1.5 mg/g] (42.5 g tube)
Tablet (Ogen®, Ortho-Est®): 0.625 mg [estropipate 0.75 mg]; 1.25 mg [estropipate 1.5 mg]; 2.5 mg [estropipate 3 mg]

♦ **Estrostep® 21** *see* Ethinyl Estradiol and Norethindrone *on page 522*
♦ **Estrostep® Fe** *see* Ethinyl Estradiol and Norethindrone *on page 522*
♦ **ETAF** *see* Aldesleukin *on page 43*

Etanercept *(et a NER sept)*
U.S. Brand Names Enbrel®
Therapeutic Category Antirheumatic, Disease Modifying
Use Reduction in signs and symptoms of moderately to severely active rheumatoid arthritis, moderately to severely active polyarticular juvenile arthritis, or psoriatic arthritis in patients

who have had an inadequate response to one or more disease-modifying antirheumatic drugs (DMARDs)

Unlabeled/Investigational Use Crohn's disease

Pregnancy Risk Factor B

Pregnancy/Breast-Feeding Implications Developmental toxicity studies performed in animals have revealed no evidence of harm to the fetus. There are no studies in pregnant women; this drug should be used during pregnancy only if clearly needed.

It is not known whether etanercept is excreted in human milk or absorbed systemically after ingestion. Because many immunoglobulins are excreted in human milk, and because of the potential for serious adverse reactions in nursing infants from etanercept, a decision should be made whether to discontinue nursing or to discontinue the drug.

Contraindications Hypersensitivity to etanercept or any component of the formulation; patients with sepsis (mortality may be increased); active infections (including chronic or local infection)

Warnings/Precautions Etanercept may affect defenses against infections and malignancies. Safety and efficacy in patients with immunosuppression or chronic infections have not been evaluated. Discontinue administration if patient develops a serious infection. Do not start drug administration in patients with an active infection. Use caution in patients predisposed to infection, such as poorly-controlled diabetes.

Use caution in patients with pre-existing or recent-onset demyelinating CNS disorders. Use caution in patients with a history of significant hematologic abnormalities; has been associated with pancytopenia and aplastic anemia (rare). Discontinue if significant hematologic abnormalities are confirmed.

Treatment may result in the formation of autoimmune antibodies; cases of autoimmune disease have not been described.

Patients should be brought up to date with all immunizations before initiating therapy. Live vaccines should not be given concurrently. Patients with a significant exposure to varicella virus should temporarily discontinue etanercept. Treatment with varicella zoster immune globulin should be considered.

Adverse Reactions Events reported include those >3% with incidence higher than placebo.

>10%:
 Central nervous system: Headache (17%)
 Local: Injection site reaction (37%)
 Respiratory: Respiratory tract infection (38%), upper respiratory tract infection (29%), rhinitis (12%)
 Miscellaneous: Infection (35%), positive ANA (11%), positive antidouble-stranded DNA antibodies (15% by RIA, 3% by *Crithidia lucilae* assay)

≥3% to 10%:
 Central nervous system: Dizziness (7%)
 Dermatologic: Rash (5%)
 Gastrointestinal: Abdominal pain (5%), dyspepsia (4%), nausea (9%), vomiting (3%)
 Neuromuscular & skeletal: Weakness (5%)
 Respiratory: Pharyngitis (7%), respiratory disorder (5%), sinusitis (3%), cough (6%)

<3% (Limited to important or life-threatening): Alopecia, angioedema, aplastic anemia, cerebral ischemia, chest pain, cholecystitis, deep vein thrombosis, demyelinating CNS disorders, depression, dyspnea, flu syndrome, gastrointestinal hemorrhage, heart failure, infection (serious), malignancies, membranous glomerulopathy, myocardial infarction, myocardial ischemia, optic neuritis, pancreatitis, pancytopenia, paresthesia, polymyositis, pruritus, pulmonary disease, pulmonary embolism, seizures, stroke, thrombocytopenia, thrombophlebitis, tuberculosis, urticaria, vasculitis (cutaneous)

Pediatric patients (JRA): The percentages of patients reporting abdominal pain (17%) and vomiting (14.5%) was higher than in adult RA. Two patients developed varicella infection associated with aseptic meningitis which resolved without complications (see Warnings/Precautions).

Overdosage/Toxicology No dose-limiting toxicities have been observed during clinical trials. Single I.V. doses up to 60 mg/m² have been administered to healthy volunteers in an endotoxemia study, without evidence of dose-limiting toxicities.

Drug Interactions
 Increased Effect/Toxicity: Specific drug interaction studies have not been conducted with etanercept.
 Decreased Effect: Specific drug interaction studies have not been conducted with etanercept.

Stability The dose tray containing etanercept (sterile powder) must be refrigerated at 2°C to 8°C (36°F to 46°F). Do not freeze. Reconstituted solutions of etanercept should be administered as soon as possible after reconstitution. If not administered immediately after reconstitution, etanercept may be stored in the vial at 2°C to 8°C (36°F to 46°F) for up to 6 hours.

Mechanism of Action Etanercept is a recombinant DNA-derived protein composed of tumor necrosis factor receptor (TNFR) linked to the Fc portion of human IgG1. Etanercept binds tumor necrosis factor (TNF) and blocks its interaction with cell surface receptors. TNF plays an important role in the inflammatory processes of rheumatoid arthritis (RA) and the resulting joint pathology.

Pharmacodynamics/Kinetics
 Onset of action: ~2-3 weeks
 Half-life elimination: 115 hours (range: 98-300 hours)
 Time to peak: 72 hours (range: 48-96 hours)
 Excretion: Clearance: Children: 45.9 mL/hour/m²; Adults: 89 mL/hour (52 mL/hour/m²)

Usual Dosage
 Children 4-17 years: Juvenile rheumatoid arthritis: S.C.: 0.4 mg/kg (maximum: 25 mg dose) twice weekly; doses should be separated by 72-96 hours
 Adult: Rheumatoid arthritis, psoriatic arthritis: S.C.: 25 mg given twice weekly; doses should be separated by 72-96 hours; if the physician determines that it is appropriate, patients may self-inject after proper training in injection technique

(Continued)

Etanercept *(Continued)*

Elderly: Although greater sensitivity of some elderly patients cannot be ruled out, no overall differences in safety or effectiveness were observed

Administration Follow package instructions carefully for reconstitution. **Note:** The needle cover of the diluent syringe contains dry natural rubber (latex) which should not be handled by persons sensitive to this substance. Injection sites should be rotated. New injections should be given at least one inch from an old site and never into areas where the skin is tender, bruised, red, or hard.

Patient Information If self-injecting, follow instructions for injection and disposal of needles exactly. If redness, swelling, or irritation appears at the injection site, contact prescriber. Do not have any vaccinations while using this medication without consulting prescriber first. You may experience headache or dizziness (use caution when driving or engaging in tasks requiring alertness until response to drug is known). If stomach pain or cramping, unusual bleeding or bruising, persistent fever, paleness, blood in vomitus, stool, or urine occurs, stop taking medication and contact prescriber **immediately**. Also immediately report skin rash, unusual muscle or bone weakness, or signs of respiratory flu or other infection (eg, chills, fever, sore throat, easy bruising or bleeding, mouth sores, unhealed sores).

Nursing Implications Rotate injection sites (thigh, abdomen, upper arm); injection should be given at least 1 inch away from previous injection site

Dosage Forms Powder for injection: 25 mg

♦ **Ethacrynate Sodium** *see* Ethacrynic Acid *Not Currently Manufactured* on page 506

Ethacrynic Acid *Not Currently Manufactured* (eth a KRIN ik AS id)

U.S. Brand Names Edecrin® [DSC]

Canadian Brand Names Edecrin®

Synonyms Ethacrynate Sodium

Therapeutic Category Diuretic, Loop

Use Management of edema associated with congestive heart failure; hepatic cirrhosis or renal disease; short-term management of ascites due to malignancy, idiopathic edema, and lymphedema

Pregnancy Risk Factor B

Pregnancy/Breast-Feeding Implications

Clinical effects on the fetus: No data available. Generally, use of diuretics during pregnancy is avoided due to risk of decreased placental perfusion.

Breast-feeding/lactation: No data available

Contraindications Hypersensitivity to ethacrynic acid or any component of the formulation; anuria; history of severe watery diarrhea caused by this product; infants

Warnings/Precautions Use with caution in patients with advanced hepatic cirrhosis, diabetes mellitus, hypotension, dehydration, history of watery diarrhea from ethacrynic acid, hearing impairment; ototoxicity occurs more frequently than with other loop diuretics. Safety and efficacy in infants have not been established. Hypersensitivity reactions can rarely occur, however, ethacrynic acid has no cross-reactivity to sulfonamides or sulfonylureas. Monitor fluid status and renal function in an attempt to prevent oliguria, azotemia, and reversible increases in BUN and creatinine. Close medical supervision of aggressive diuresis required. Watch for and correct electrolyte disturbances. Coadministration of antihypertensives may increase the risk of hypotension. Increased risk of gastric hemorrhage associated with corticosteroid therapy.

Adverse Reactions Frequency not defined.

Central nervous system: Headache, fatigue, apprehension, confusion, fever, chills, encephalopathy (patients with pre-existing liver disease); vertigo

Dermatologic: Skin rash, Henoch-Schönlein purpura (in patient with rheumatic heart disease)

Endocrine & metabolic: Hyponatremia, hyperglycemia, variations in phosphorus, CO_2 content, bicarbonate, and calcium; reversible hyperuricemia, gout, hyperglycemia, hypoglycemia (occurred in two uremic patients who received doses above those recommended)

Gastrointestinal: Anorexia, malaise, abdominal discomfort or pain, dysphagia, nausea, vomiting, and diarrhea, gastrointestinal bleeding, acute pancreatitis (rare)

Genitourinary: Hematuria

Hepatic: Jaundice, abnormal liver function tests

Hematology: Agranulocytosis, severe neutropenia, thrombocytopenia

Local: Thrombophlebitis (with intravenous use), local irritation and pain,

Ocular: Blurred vision

Otic: Deafness, tinnitus, temporary or permanent deafness

Renal: Increased serum creatinine

Overdosage/Toxicology Symptoms include electrolyte depletion, volume depletion, dehydration, and circulatory collapse. Following GI decontamination, treatment is supportive. Hypotension responds to fluids and Trendelenburg positioning.

Drug Interactions

Increased Effect/Toxicity: Ethacrynic acid-induced hypokalemia may predispose to digoxin toxicity and may increase the risk of arrhythmia with drugs which may prolong QT interval, including type Ia and type III antiarrhythmic agents, cisapride, terfenadine, and some quinolones (sparfloxacin, gatifloxacin, and moxifloxacin). The risk of toxicity from lithium and salicylates (high dose) may be increased by loop diuretics. Hypotensive effects and/or adverse renal effects of ACE inhibitors and NSAIDs are potentiated by ethacrynic acid-induced hypovolemia. The effects of peripheral adrenergic-blocking drugs or ganglionic blockers may be increased by ethacrynic acid.

Ethacrynic acid may increase the risk of ototoxicity with other ototoxic agents (aminoglycosides, cis-platinum), especially in patients with renal dysfunction. Synergistic diuretic effects occur with thiazide-type diuretics. Diuretics tend to be synergistic with other antihypertensive agents, and hypotension may occur. Nephrotoxicity has been associated with concomitant use of cephaloridine or cephalexin.

Decreased Effect: Probenecid decreases diuretic effects of ethacrynic acid. Glucose tolerance may be decreased by loop diuretics, requiring adjustment of hypoglycemic agents.

Cholestyramine or colestipol may reduce bioavailability of ethacrynic acid. Indomethacin (and other NSAIDs) may reduce natriuretic and hypotensive effects of diuretics.

Mechanism of Action Inhibits reabsorption of sodium and chloride in the ascending loop of Henle and distal renal tubule, interfering with the chloride-binding cotransport system, thus causing increased excretion of water, sodium, chloride, magnesium, and calcium

Pharmacodynamics/Kinetics

Onset of action: Diuresis: Oral: ~30 minutes; I.V.: 5 minutes

Peak effect: Oral: 2 hours; I.V.: 30 minutes

Duration: Oral: 12 hours; I.V.: 2 hours

Absorption: Oral: Rapid

Metabolism: Hepatic (35% to 40%) to active cysteine conjugate

Protein binding: >90%

Half-life elimination: Normal renal function: 2-4 hours

Excretion: Feces and urine (30% to 60% as unchanged drug)

Usual Dosage I.V. formulation should be diluted in D_5W or NS (1 mg/mL) and infused over several minutes.

Children: Oral: 1 mg/kg/dose once daily; increase at intervals of 2-3 days as needed, to a maximum of 3 mg/kg/day.

Adults:

Oral: 50-200 mg/day in 1-2 divided doses; may increase in increments of 25-50 mg at intervals of several days; doses up to 200 mg twice daily may be required with severe, refractory edema.

I.V.: 0.5-1 mg/kg/dose (maximum: 100 mg/dose); repeat doses not routinely recommended; however, if indicated, repeat doses every 8-12 hours.

Dosing adjustment/comments in renal impairment: Cl_{cr} <10 mL/minute: Avoid use.

Dialysis: Not removed by hemo- or peritoneal dialysis; supplemental dose is not necessary.

Dietary Considerations This product may cause a potassium loss. Your healthcare provider may prescribe a potassium supplement, another medication to help prevent the potassium loss, or recommend that you eat foods high in potassium, especially citrus fruits. Do not change your diet on your own while taking this medication, especially if you are taking potassium supplements or medications to reduce potassium loss. Too much potassium can be as harmful as too little.

Administration Injection should **not** be given S.C. or I.M. due to local pain and irritation; single I.V. doses should not exceed 100 mg; if a second dose is needed, use a new injection site to avoid possible thrombophlebitis

Monitoring Parameters Blood pressure, renal function, serum electrolytes, and fluid status closely, including weight and I & O daily; hearing

Patient Information May be taken with food or milk; get up slowly from a lying or sitting position to minimize dizziness, lightheadedness, or fainting; also use extra care when exercising, standing for long periods of time, and during hot weather. Take in morning, take last dose of multiple doses before 6 PM unless instructed otherwise.

Nursing Implications

Tissue irritant; not to be administered I.M. or S.C.; dilute injection with 50 mL dextrose 5% or normal saline (1 mg/mL concentration resulting); may be injected without further dilution over a period of several minutes or infused over 20-30 minutes

Monitor blood pressure, serum electrolytes, renal function, hearing

Dosage Forms

Powder for injection, as ethacrynate sodium: 50 mg (50 mL)

Tablet: 25 mg, 50 mg

Extemporaneous Preparations To make a 1 mg/mL suspension: Dissolve 120 mg ethacrynic acid powder in a small amount of 10% alcohol. Add a small amount of 50% sorbitol solution and stir. Adjust pH to 7 with 0.1N sodium hydroxide solution. Add sufficient 50% sorbitol solution to make a final volume of 120 mL. (Methylparaben 6 mg and propylparaben 2.4 mg are added as preservatives.) Stable 220 days at room temperature.

Handbook on Extemporaneous Formulations, Bethesda, MD: American Society of Hospital Pharmacists, 1987.

Ethambutol (e THAM byoo tole)

Related Information

Antimicrobial Drugs of Choice *on page 1588*
Depression *on page 1655*
Desensitization Protocols *on page 1525*
Tuberculosis Prophylaxis *on page 1572*
Tuberculosis Treatment Guidelines *on page 1612*

U.S. Brand Names Myambutol®

Canadian Brand Names Etibi®; Myambutol®

Synonyms Ethambutol Hydrochloride

Therapeutic Category Antitubercular Agent

Use Treatment of tuberculosis and other mycobacterial diseases in conjunction with other antituberculosis agents

Pregnancy Risk Factor B

Contraindications Hypersensitivity to ethambutol or any component of the formulation; optic neuritis

Warnings/Precautions May cause optic neuritis, resulting in decreased visual acuity or other vision changes. Discontinue promptly in patients with changes in vision, color blindness, or visual defects (effects normally reversible, but reversal may require up to a year). Use only in children whose visual acuity can accurately be determined and monitored (not recommended for use in children <13 years of age unless the benefit outweighs the risk); dosage modification required in patients with renal insufficiency

Adverse Reactions Frequency not defined.

Central nervous system: Headache, confusion, disorientation, malaise, mental confusion, fever

Dermatologic: Rash, pruritus

(Continued)

Ethambutol *(Continued)*

Endocrine & metabolic: Acute gout or hyperuricemia
Gastrointestinal: Abdominal pain, anorexia, nausea, vomiting
Hepatic: Abnormal LFTs
Neuromuscular & skeletal: Peripheral neuritis
Ocular: Optic neuritis; symptoms may include decreased acuity, scotoma, color blindness, or visual defects (usually reversible with discontinuation, irreversible blindness has been described)
Miscellaneous: Anaphylaxis

Overdosage/Toxicology Symptoms include decreased visual acuity, anorexia, joint pain, and numbness of the extremities. Following GI decontamination, treatment is supportive.

Drug Interactions
  Decreased Effect: Ethambutol absorption is decreased when taken with aluminum salts.

Mechanism of Action Suppresses mycobacteria multiplication by interfering with RNA synthesis

Pharmacodynamics/Kinetics
Absorption: ~80%
Distribution: Widely throughout body; concentrated in kidneys, lungs, saliva, and red blood cells
  Relative diffusion from blood into CSF: Adequate with or without inflammation (exceeds usual MICs)
  CSF:blood level ratio: Normal meninges: 0%; Inflamed meninges: 25%
Protein binding: 20% to 30%
Metabolism: Hepatic, 20% to inactive metabolite
Half-life elimination: 2.5-3.6 hours; End-stage renal disease: 7-15 hours
Time to peak, serum: 2-4 hours
Excretion: Urine (~50%) and feces (20%) as unchanged drug

Usual Dosage Oral:
Ethambutol is generally not recommended in children whose visual acuity cannot be monitored. However, ethambutol should be considered for all children with organisms resistant to other drugs, when susceptibility to ethambutol has been demonstrated, or susceptibility is likely.
Note: A four-drug regimen (isoniazid, rifampin, pyrazinamide, and either streptomycin or ethambutol) is preferred for the initial, empiric treatment of TB. When the drug susceptibility results are available, the regimen should be altered as appropriate.
Children and Adults:
  Daily therapy: 15-25 mg/kg/day (maximum: 2.5 g/day)
  Directly observed therapy (DOT): Twice weekly: 50 mg/kg (maximum: 2.5 g)
  DOT: 3 times/week: 25-30 mg/kg (maximum: 2.5 g)
Adults: Treatment of disseminated *Mycobacterium avium* complex (MAC) in patients with advanced HIV infection: 15 mg/kg ethambutol in combination with azithromycin 600 mg daily
  Dosing interval in renal impairment:
  Cl_{cr} 10-50 mL/minute: Administer every 24-36 hours
  Cl_{cr} <10 mL/minute: Administer every 48 hours
  Hemodialysis: Slightly dialyzable (5% to 20%); Administer dose postdialysis
  Peritoneal dialysis: Dose for Cl_{cr} <10 mL/minute
  Continuous arteriovenous or venovenous hemofiltration: Administer every 24-36 hours

Dietary Considerations May be taken with food as absorption is not affected, may cause gastric irritation.
Monitoring Parameters Periodic visual testing in patients receiving >15 mg/kg/day; periodic renal, hepatic, and hematopoietic tests
Patient Information Report any visual changes or rash to physician; may cause stomach upset, take with food; do not take within 2 hours of aluminum-containing antacids
Nursing Implications
Reinforce compliance
Monitor visual testing periodically in patients receiving more than 15 mg/kg/day; periodic renal, hepatic, and hematopoietic tests
Dosage Forms Tablet, as hydrochloride: 100 mg, 400 mg

♦ **Ethambutol Hydrochloride** *see Ethambutol on page 507*
♦ **Ethamolin®** *see Ethanolamine Oleate on page 508*
♦ **Ethanoic Acid** *see Acetic Acid on page 31*

Ethanolamine Oleate *(ETH a nol a meen OH lee ate)*
U.S. Brand Names Ethamolin®
Synonyms Monoethanolamine
Therapeutic Category Sclerosing Agent
Use Orphan drug: Sclerosing agent used for bleeding esophageal varices
Pregnancy Risk Factor C
Contraindications Hypersensitivity to agent or oleic acid
Warnings/Precautions Fatal anaphylactic shock has been reported following administration; use with caution and decrease doses in patients with significant liver dysfunction (child class C), with concomitant cardiorespiratory disease, or in the elderly or critically ill
Adverse Reactions
1% to 10%:
  Central nervous system: Pyrexia (1.8%)
  Gastrointestinal: Esophageal ulcer (2%), esophageal stricture (1.3%)
  Respiratory: Pleural effusion (2%), pneumonia (1.2%)
  Miscellaneous: Retrosternal pain (1.6%)
<1% (Limited to important or life-threatening): Acute renal failure, anaphylaxis, esophagitis, injection necrosis, perforation

Overdosage/Toxicology Anaphylaxis and severe intramural necrosis can occur after administration of larger than normal volumes. Treatment is supportive with epinephrine, corticosteroids, fluids, and pressors.

Mechanism of Action Derived from oleic acid and similar in physical properties to sodium morrhuate; however, the exact mechanism of the hemostatic effect used in endoscopic injection sclerotherapy is not known. Intravenously injected ethanolamine oleate produces a sterile inflammatory response resulting in fibrosis and occlusion of the vein; a dose-related extravascular inflammatory reaction occurs when the drug diffuses through the venous wall. Autopsy results indicate that variceal obliteration occurs secondary to mural necrosis and fibrosis. Thrombosis appears to be a transient reaction.

Usual Dosage Adults: 1.5-5 mL per varix, up to 20 mL total or 0.4 mL/kg for a 50 kg patient; doses should be decreased in patients with severe hepatic dysfunction and should receive less than recommended maximum dose

Administration Use care to use acceptable technique to avoid necrosis

Nursing Implications Have epinephrine and resuscitative equipment nearby

Dosage Forms Injection: 5% [50 mg/mL] (2 mL)

Ethchlorvynol (eth klor VI nole)

U.S. Brand Names Placidyl®

Therapeutic Category Hypnotic; Sedative

Use Short-term management of insomnia

Restrictions C-IV

Pregnancy Risk Factor C

Usual Dosage Adults: Oral: 500-1000 mg at bedtime

Dosing adjustment in renal impairment: Cl_{cr} <50 mL/minute: Avoid use

Additional Information Complete prescribing information for this medication should be consulted for additional detail.

Dosage Forms Capsule: 200 mg, 500 mg, 750 mg

Ethinyl Estradiol (ETH in il es tra DYE ole)

U.S. Brand Names Estinyl®

Therapeutic Category Estrogen Derivative; Estrogen Derivative, Oral

Use Treatment of moderate to severe vasomotor symptoms associated with menopause; hypogonadism; prostatic cancer (palliation); breast cancer (palliation)

Pregnancy Risk Factor X

Pregnancy/Breast-Feeding Implications Increased risk of fetal reproductive tract disorders and other birth defects; do not use during pregnancy. Excreted in human milk; do not use in breast-feeding women (per manufacturer)

Contraindications Hypersensitivity to estrogens or any component of the formulation; undiagnosed abnormal vaginal bleeding; history of or current thrombophlebitis or thromboembolic disorders; carcinoma of the breast, except in appropriately selected patients being treated for metastatic disease; estrogen-dependent tumor; pregnancy

Warnings/Precautions Unopposed estrogens may increase the risk of endometrial carcinoma in postmenopausal women. Use with caution in patients with diseases which may be exacerbated by fluid retention, including asthma, epilepsy, migraine, diabetes, cardiac or renal dysfunction. Use with caution in patients with a history of hypercalcemia, cardiovascular disease, and gallbladder disease. May increase blood pressure. Use with caution in patients with hepatic disease. May increase risk of venous thromboembolism. Estrogens may increase the risk of breast cancer (controversial/currently under study). Estrogen compounds are generally associated with lipid effects such as increased HDL-cholesterol, and decreased LDL-cholesterol; triglycerides may also be increased. Use with caution in patients with familial defects of lipoprotein metabolism. May increase size of pre-existing uterine leiomyomata. Patients with a history of depression should be monitored, discontinue if depression recurs to a serious degree. Before prescribing estrogen therapy to postmenopausal women, the risks and benefits must be weighed for each patient. Women should be informed of these risks and benefits, as well as possible effects of progestin when added to estrogen therapy. Estrogens may cause premature closure of the epiphyses in young individuals. Safety and efficacy in pediatric patients have not been established. Some tablet formulations contain tartrazine.

Adverse Reactions Frequency not defined.

Cardiovascular: Edema, hypertension, venous thromboembolism

Central nervous system: Dizziness, headache, mental depression, migraine

Dermatologic: Chloasma, erythema multiforme, erythema nodosum, hemorrhagic eruption, hirsutism, loss of scalp hair, melasma

Endocrine & metabolic: Breast enlargement, breast tenderness, changes in libido, increased thyroid-binding globulin, increased total thyroid hormone (T_4), increased serum triglycerides/phospholipids, increased HDL-cholesterol, decreased LDL-cholesterol, impaired glucose tolerance, hypercalcemia

Gastrointestinal: Abdominal cramps, bloating, cholecystitis, cholelithiasis, gallbladder disease, nausea, pancreatitis, vomiting, weight gain/loss

Genitourinary: Alterations in frequency and flow of menses, changes in cervical secretions, endometrial cancer, increased size of uterine leiomyomata, vaginal candidiasis

Hematologic: Aggravation of porphyria, decreased antithrombin III and antifactor Xa, increased levels of fibrinogen, increased platelet aggregability and platelet count; increased prothrombin and factors VII, VIII, IX, X

Hepatic: Cholestatic jaundice

Neuromuscular & skeletal: Chorea

Ocular: Intolerance to contact lenses, steeping of corneal curvature

Respiratory: Pulmonary thromboembolism

Miscellaneous: Carbohydrate intolerance

(Continued)

Ethinyl Estradiol *(Continued)*

Overdosage/Toxicology Toxicity is unlikely following single exposures of excessive doses. Treatment following emesis and charcoal administration should be supportive and symptomatic. Effects noted after large doses include headache, nausea, and vomiting. Bleeding may occur in females.

Drug Interactions

Cytochrome P450 Effect: CYP3A3/4 enzyme substrate

Increased Effect/Toxicity: Hydrocortisone taken with estrogen may cause corticosteroid-induced toxicity. Increased potential for thromboembolic events with anticoagulants.

Decreased Effect: Rifampin, nelfinavir, and ritonavir decrease estradiol serum concentrations. Anticonvulsants which are enzyme inducers (barbiturates, carbamazepine, phenobarbital, phenytoin, primidone) may potentially decrease estrogen levels.

Ethanol/Nutrition/Herb Interactions

Ethanol: Routine use increases estrogen level and risk of breast cancer; avoid ethanol

Food: Folic acid absorption may be decreased

Herb/Nutraceutical: St John's wort may decrease levels. Avoid black cohosh, dong quai (has estrogenic activity). Avoid red clover, saw palmetto, ginseng (due to potential hormonal effects).

Stability Store between 2°C and 30°C (36°F and 86°F)

Mechanism of Action Estrogens are responsible for the development and maintenance of the female reproductive system and secondary sexual characteristics. Estradiol is the principle intracellular human estrogen and is more potent than estrone and estriol at the receptor level; it is the primary estrogen secreted prior to menopause. In males and following menopause in females, estrone and estrone sulfate are more highly produced. Estrogens modulate the pituitary secretion of gonadotropins, luteinizing hormone, and follicle-stimulating hormone through a negative feedback system; estrogen replacement reduces elevated levels of these hormones. Ethinyl estradiol is a synthetic derivative of estradiol. The addition of the ethinyl group prevents rapid degradation by the liver.

Pharmacodynamics/Kinetics

Absorption: Oral: Rapid and complete

Distribution: V_d: 2-4 L/kg

Protein binding: 50% to 97% primarily to albumin

Metabolism: Primarily hepatic via CYP3A3/4 isoenzyme; less first-pass effect than with estradiol; extensive enterohepatic recirculation; converted to estrone and estriol

Bioavailability: 38% to 55%

Half-life elimination: ~8-25 hours

Time to peak: Initial: 2-3 hours; Secondary: 12 hours

Excretion: Urine and feces (as metabolites)

Usual Dosage Oral: Adults:

Prostatic cancer (palliation): 0.15-2 mg/day

Female hypogonadism: 0.05 mg 1-3 times/day during the first 2 weeks of a theoretical menstrual cycle; follow with a progesterone during the last half of the arbitrary cycle; continue for 3-6 months. The patient should not be treated for the following 2 months to determine if additional therapy is needed.

Vasomotor symptoms associated with menopause: Usual dosage range: 0.02-0.05 mg/day; give cyclically for short-term use only and use the lowest dose that will control symptoms. Discontinue as soon as possible and administer cyclically (3 weeks on and 1 week off). Attempt to discontinue or taper medication at 3- to 6-month intervals. In severe cases (due to surgery or roentgenologic castration), doses of 0.05 mg 3 times/day may be needed initially; clinical improvement may be seen within a few weeks, decrease to lowest dose which will control symptoms

Breast cancer (palliation in appropriately selected postmenopausal women): 1 mg 3 times/day

Dosing adjustment in hepatic impairment:

Mild to moderate liver impairment: Dosage reduction of estrogens is recommended

Severe liver impairment: **Not recommended**

Dietary Considerations Ensure adequate calcium and vitamin D intake when used for the prevention of osteoporosis.

Monitoring Parameters Yearly physical examination that includes blood pressure, Papanicolaou smear, breast exam, and mammogram. Monitor for signs of endometrial cancer in female patients with uterus; rule out malignancy if unexplained vaginal bleeding occurs.

Test Interactions Pathologist should be advised of estrogen/progesterone therapy when specimens are submitted. Reduced response to metyrapone test.

Patient Information It is important to maintain schedule. Estrogens have been shown to increase the risk of endometrial cancer. Annual gynecologic and breast exams are important. You may experience nausea or vomiting (small frequent meals may help); abdominal pain; difficult/painful menstrual cycles; dizziness or mental depression; headaches; rash; breast pain; or increased/decreased libido. Report significant swelling of extremities, sudden acute pain in legs or calves, chest or abdomen; shortness of breath; severe headache or vomiting; weakness or numbness of arms or legs; or unusual vaginal bleeding. You may become intolerant to wearing contact lenses, notify prescriber if this occurs. If taking for prevention of osteoporosis, ask prescriber about calcium and vitamin D intake, and weight-bearing exercises.

Nursing Implications Monitor blood pressure

Dosage Forms Tablet: 0.02 mg [contains tartrazine], 0.05 mg

Ethinyl Estradiol and Desogestrel

(ETH in il es tra DYE ole & des oh JES trel)

U.S. Brand Names Apri®; Cyclessa®; Desogen®; Mircette®; Ortho-Cept®

Canadian Brand Names Marvelon®; Ortho-Cept®

Synonyms Desogestrel and Ethinyl Estradiol

Therapeutic Category Contraceptive, Oral

Use Prevention of pregnancy

Pregnancy Risk Factor X

Usual Dosage Oral: Adults: Female: Contraception:

Schedule 1 (Sunday starter): Dose begins on first Sunday after onset of menstruation; if the menstrual period starts on Sunday, take first tablet that very same day. **With a Sunday start, an additional method of contraception should be used until after the first 7 days of consecutive administration.**

For 21-tablet package: Dosage is 1 tablet daily for 21 consecutive days, followed by 7 days off of the medication; a new course begins on the 8th day after the last tablet is taken.

For 28-tablet package: Dosage is 1 tablet daily without interruption.

Schedule 2 (Day 1 starter): Dose starts on first day of menstrual cycle taking 1 tablet daily.

For 21-tablet package: Dosage is 1 tablet daily for 21 consecutive days, followed by 7 days off of the medication; a new course begins on the 8th day after the last tablet is taken.

For 28-tablet package: Dosage is 1 tablet daily without interruption.

If all doses have been taken on schedule and one menstrual period is missed, continue dosing cycle. If two consecutive menstrual periods are missed, pregnancy test is required before new dosing cycle is started.

Missed doses **monophasic formulations** (refer to package insert for complete information):

One dose missed: Take as soon as remembered or take 2 tablets next day

Two consecutive doses missed in the first 2 weeks: Take 2 tablets as soon as remembered or 2 tablets next 2 days. **An additional method of contraception should be used for 7 days after missed dose.**

Two consecutive doses missed in week 3 or three consecutive doses missed at any time:

Schedule 1 (Sunday starter): Continue to take 1 tablet daily until Sunday, then discard the rest of the pack, and a new pack is started that same day.

Schedule 2 (Day 1 starter): Current pack should be discarded, and a new pack started that same day. **An additional method of contraception should be used for 7 days after missed dose.**

Missed doses **biphasic/triphasic formulations** (refer to package insert for complete information):

One dose missed: Take as soon as remembered or take 2 tablets next day.

Two consecutive doses missed in week 1 or week 2 of the pack: Take 2 tablets as soon as remembered and 2 tablets the next day. Resume taking 1 tablet daily until the pack is empty. **An additional method of contraception should be used for 7 days after a missed dose.**

Two consecutive doses missed in week 3 of the pack; **an additional method of contraception must be used for 7 days after a missed dose:**

Schedule 1 (Sunday starter): Take 1 tablet every day until Sunday. Discard the remaining pack and start a new pack of pills on the same day.

Schedule 2 (Day 1 starter): Discard the remaining pack and start a new pack the same day.

Three or more consecutive doses missed; **an additional method of contraception must be used for 7 days after a missed dose:**

Schedule 1 (Sunday starter): Take 1 tablet every day until Sunday; on Sunday, discard the pack and start a new pack.

Schedule 2 (Day 1 starter): Discard the remaining pack and begin new pack of tablets starting on the same day.

Dosage adjustment in renal impairment: Specific guidelines not available; Use with caution

Dosage adjustment in hepatic impairment: Contraindicated in patients with hepatic impairment

Additional Information Complete prescribing information for this medication should be consulted for additional detail.

Dosage Forms Tablet:

Low-dose formulation: Mircette®:

Day 1-21: Ethinyl estradiol 0.02 mg and desogestrel 0.15 mg [21 white tablets]

Day 22-23: 2 inactive green tablets

Day 24-28: Ethinyl estradiol 0.01 mg [5 yellow tablets] (28s)

Monophasic formulations:

Apri® 28: Ethinyl estradiol 0.03 mg and desogestrel 0.15 mg [21 rose tablets] and 7 white inactive tablets (28s)

Desogen®: Ethinyl estradiol 0.03 mg and desogestrel 0.15 mg [21 white tablets] and 7 green inactive tablets (28s)

Ortho-Cept® 28: Ethinyl estradiol 0.03 mg and desogestrel 0.15 mg [21 orange tablets] and 7 green inactive tablets (28s)

Triphasic formulation: Cyclessa®:

Day 1-7:Ethinyl estradiol 0.025 mg and desogestrel 0.1 mg [7 light yellow tablets]

Day 8-14: Ethinyl estradiol 0.025 mg and desogestrel 0.125 mg [7 orange tablets]

Day 14-21: Ethinyl estradiol 0.025 mg and desogestrel 0.15 mg [7 red tablets]

Day 21-28: 7 green inactive tablets (28s)

Ethinyl Estradiol and Drospirenone

(ETH in il es tra DYE ole & droh SPYE re none)

U.S. Brand Names Yasmin®

Synonyms Drospirenone and Ethinyl Estradiol

Therapeutic Category Contraceptive, Oral

Use Prevention of pregnancy

Pregnancy Risk Factor X

Pregnancy/Breast-Feeding Implications In general, the use of oral contraceptives when inadvertently taken early in pregnancy have not been associated with teratogenic effects. Esophageal atresia was reported in one infant with a single-cycle exposure to ethinyl estradiol and drospirenone *in utero* (association not known). Pregnancy should be ruled out prior

(Continued)

Ethinyl Estradiol and Drospirenone (Continued)

to treatment and discontinued if pregnancy occurs. Due to increased risk of thromboembolism postpartum, do not start oral contraceptives earlier than 4-6 weeks following delivery. Enters breast milk; breast-feeding is not recommended.

Contraindications Hypersensitivity to ethinyl estradiol, drospirenone, or to any component of the formulation; thrombophlebitis or thromboembolic disorders (current or history of), cerebral vascular disease, coronary artery disease; known or suspected breast carcinoma, endometrial cancer, estrogen-dependent neoplasms, undiagnosed abnormal genital bleeding; renal insufficiency, hepatic dysfunction or tumor, adrenal insufficiency, cholestatic jaundice of pregnancy, jaundice with prior oral contraceptive use; heavy smoking (≥15 cigarettes/day) in patients >35 years of age; pregnancy

Warnings/Precautions Oral contraceptives do not protect against HIV infection or other sexually-transmitted diseases. The risk of cardiovascular side effects increases in women who smoke cigarettes, especially those who are >35 years of age; women who use oral contraceptives should be strongly advised not to smoke. Oral contraceptives may lead to increased risk of myocardial infarction, use with caution in patients with risk factors for coronary artery disease. May increase the risk of thromboembolism. Oral contraceptives may have a dose-related risk of vascular disease (decreases HDL), hypertension, and gallbladder disease; a preparation with the lowest effective estrogen/progesterone combination should be used. Women with high blood pressure should be encouraged to use another form of contraception. Oral contraceptives may cause glucose intolerance. Retinal thrombosis has been reported (rarely) with oral contraceptive use. Use with caution in patients with conditions that may be aggravated by fluid retention, depression, or patients with history of migraine. Not for use prior to menarche.

Drospirenone has antimineralocorticoid activity that may lead to hyperkalemia in patients with renal insufficiency, hepatic dysfunction, or adrenal insufficiency. Use caution with medications that may increase serum potassium.

Adverse Reactions

>1%:

Central nervous system: Depression, dizziness, emotional lability, headache, migraine, nervousness

Dermatologic: Acne, pruritus, rash

Endocrine & metabolic: Amenorrhea, dysmenorrhea, intermenstrual bleeding, menstrual irregularities

Gastrointestinal: Abdominal pain, diarrhea, gastroenteritis, nausea, vomiting

Genitourinary: Cystitis, leukorrhea, vaginal moniliasis, vaginitis

Neuromuscular & skeletal: Back pain, weakness

Respiratory: Bronchitis, pharyngitis, sinusitis, upper respiratory infection

Miscellaneous: Allergic reaction, flu-like syndrome, infection

Adverse reactions reported with other oral contraceptives: Appetite changes, antithrombin III decreased, arterial thromboembolism, benign liver tumors, breast changes, Budd-Chiari syndrome, carbohydrate intolerance, cataracts, cerebral hemorrhage, cerebral thrombosis, cervical changes, change in corneal curvature (steepening), cholestatic jaundice, colitis, contact lens intolerance, decreased lactation (postpartum), deep vein thrombosis, diplopia, edema, erythema multiforme, erythema nodosum; factors VII, VIII, IX, X increased; folate serum concentrations decreased, gallbladder disease, glucose intolerance, hemorrhagic eruption, hemolytic uremic syndrome, hepatic adenomas, hirsutism, hypercalcemia, hypertension, hyperglycemia, libido changes, melasma, mesenteric thrombosis, myocardial infarction, papilledema, platelet aggregability increased, porphyria, premenstrual syndrome, proptosis, prothrombin increased, pulmonary thromboembolism, renal function impairment, retinal thrombosis, sex hormone-binding globulin increased, thrombophlebitis, thyroid-binding globulin increased, total thyroid hormone (T_4) increased, triglycerides/phospholipids increased, vaginal candidiasis, weight changes

Overdosage/Toxicology May cause nausea; withdrawal bleeding may occur in females. Due to the antimineralocorticoid properties of drospirenone, monitor potassium and sodium serum concentrations and monitor for evidence of metabolic acidosis.

Drug Interactions

Cytochrome P450 Effect:

Ethinyl estradiol: CYP3A3/4 and 3A5-7 enzyme substrate; CYP1A2, 2C19, and 3A3/4 (weak) enzyme inhibitor

Drospirenone: CYP3A4 enzyme substrate; CYP1A1, CYP2C9, CYP2C19, and CYP3A4 enzyme inhibitor (weak)

Increased Effect/Toxicity: ACE inhibitors, aldosterone antagonists, angiotensin II receptor antagonists, heparin, NSAIDs (when taken daily, long term), and potassium-sparing diuretics increase risk of hyperkalemia with concomitant use. Acetaminophen, ascorbic acid, and atorvastatin may increase plasma concentrations of oral contraceptives. Ethinyl estradiol may increase plasma concentrations of cyclosporine, prednisolone, selegiline, and theophylline. Oral contraceptives may increase (or decrease) the effects of coumarin derivatives.

Decreased Effect: Oral contraceptives may decrease the plasma concentration of acetaminophen, clofibric acid, morphine, salicylic acid, and temazepam. Aminoglutethimide, anticonvulsants (carbamazepine, felbamate, phenobarbital, phenytoin, topiramate), phenylbutazone, rifampin, and ritonavir may increase metabolism leading to decreased effect of oral contraceptives. Oral contraceptives may decrease (or increase) the effects of coumarin derivatives.

Ethanol/Nutrition/Herb Interactions

Food: CNS effects of caffeine may be enhanced if oral contraceptives are used concurrently with caffeine. Grapefruit juice increases ethinyl estradiol concentrations; clinical implications are unclear.

Herb/Nutraceutical: St John's wort may decrease the effectiveness of oral contraceptives by inducing hepatic enzymes; may also result in breakthrough bleeding.

Stability Store at 25°C (77°F)

Mechanism of Action Combination oral contraceptives inhibit ovulation via a negative feedback mechanism on the hypothalamus, which alters the normal pattern of gonadotropin secretion of a follicle-stimulating hormone (FSH) and luteinizing hormone by the anterior pituitary. The follicular phase FSH and midcycle surge of gonadotropins are inhibited. In addition, oral contraceptives produce alterations in the genital tract, including changes in the cervical mucus, rendering it unfavorable for sperm penetration even if ovulation occurs. Changes in the endometrium may also occur, producing an unfavorable environment for nidation. Oral contraceptive drugs may alter the tubal transport of the ova through the fallopian tubes. Progestational agents may also alter sperm fertility. Drospirenone is a spironolactone analogue with antimineralocorticoid and antiandrogenic activity.

Pharmacodynamics/Kinetics

Ethinyl Estradiol: See Ethinyl Estradiol monograph.

Drospirenone:

Distribution: 4 L/kg

Protein binding: Serum proteins (excluding sex hormone-binding globulin and corticosteroid binding globulin): 97%

Metabolism: To inactive metabolites; minor metabolism in liver via CYP3A4

Bioavailability: 76%

Half-life elimination: 30 hours

Time to peak: 1-3 hours

Excretion: Urine and feces

Usual Dosage Oral: Adults: Female: Contraception: Dosage is 1 tablet daily for 28 consecutive days. Dose should be taken at the same time each day, either after the evening meal or at bedtime. Dosing may be started on the first day of menstrual period (Day 1 starter) or on the first Sunday after the onset of the menstrual period (Sunday starter).

Day 1 starter: Dose starts on first day of menstrual cycle taking 1 tablet daily.

Sunday starter: Dose begins on first Sunday after onset of menstruation; if the menstrual period starts on Sunday, take first tablet that very same day. **With a Sunday start, an additional method of contraception should be used until after the first 7 days of consecutive administration.**

If all doses have been taken on schedule and one menstrual period is missed, continue dosing cycle. If two consecutive menstrual periods are missed, pregnancy test is required before new dosing cycle is started.

If doses have been missed during the first 3 weeks and the menstrual period is missed, pregnancy should be ruled out prior to continuing treatment.

Missed doses (monophasic formulations) (refer to package insert for complete information):

One dose missed: Take as soon as remembered or take 2 tablets next day

Two consecutive doses missed in the first 2 weeks: Take 2 tablets as soon as remembered or 2 tablets next 2 days. **An additional method of contraception should be used for 7 days after missed dose.**

Two consecutive doses missed in week 3 or three consecutive doses missed at any time: **An additional method of contraception must be used for 7 days after a missed dose.**

Day 1 starter: Current pack should be discarded, and a new pack should be started that same day.

Sunday starter: Continue dose of 1 tablet daily until Sunday, then discard the rest of the pack, and a new pack should be started that same day.

Any number of doses missed in week 4: Continue taking one pill each day until pack is empty; no back-up method of contraception is needed

Dosage adjustment in renal impairment: Contraindicated in patients with renal dysfunction (Cl$_{cr}$ ≤50 mL/minute)

Dosage adjustment in hepatic impairment: Contraindicated in patients with hepatic dysfunction

Administration To be taken at the same time each day, either after the evening meal or at bedtime

Monitoring Parameters Blood pressure, pregnancy, serum potassium in high-risk patients and those on medications with potassium-retaining properties

Patient Information Take exactly as directed by prescriber (see package insert). An additional form of contraception should be used until after the first 7 consecutive days of administration. You are at risk of becoming pregnant if doses are missed. If you miss a dose, take as soon as possible or double the dose the next day. If two or more consecutive doses are missed, contact prescriber for restarting directions. Detailed and complete information on dosing and missed doses can be found in the package insert. If any number of doses are missed in week 4, continue taking one pill each day until pack is empty; no back-up method of contraception is needed. Be aware that some medications may reduce the effectiveness of oral contraceptives; an alternate form of contraception may be needed (see Drug Interactions).

It is important that you check your blood pressure monthly (on same day each month) and report any increased blood pressure to prescriber. Have an annual physical assessment, Pap smear, and vision exam while taking this medication.

Avoid smoking while taking this medication; smoking increases risk or adverse effects, including thromboembolic events and heart attacks. You may experience loss of appetite (small frequent meals will help); constipation (increased fluids, exercise, and dietary fiber, or stool softeners may help). If you are diabetic you should use accurate serum glucose testing to identify any changes in glucose tolerance; notify prescriber of significant changes so antidiabetic medication can be adjusted if necessary. Report immediately pain or muscle soreness; swelling, heat, or redness in calves; shortness of breath; sudden loss of vision; unresolved leg or foot swelling or weight gain (>5 lb); change in menstrual pattern (unusual bleeding, amenorrhea, breakthrough spotting); breast tenderness that does not go away; acute abdominal cramping; signs of vaginal infection (drainage, pain, itching); changes in CNS (blurred vision, confusion, acute anxiety, or unresolved depression); or other persistent (Continued)

Ethinyl Estradiol and Drospirenone *(Continued)*

adverse effects. precautions: This drug may cause severe fetal complication. If you suspect you may be pregnant, contact prescriber immediately. Breast-feeding is not recommended.

Dosage Forms Tablet: Ethinyl estradiol 0.03 mg and drospirenone 3 mg [21 yellow round active tablets and 7 white inert round tablets] (28s)

Ethinyl Estradiol and Ethynodiol Diacetate

(ETH in il es tra DYE ole & e thye noe DYE ole dye AS e tate)

U.S. Brand Names Demulen®; Zovia™

Canadian Brand Names Demulen® 30

Synonyms Ethynodiol Diacetate and Ethinyl Estradiol

Therapeutic Category Contraceptive, Oral (Intermediate Potency Estrogen, Intermediate Potency Progestin); Contraceptive, Oral (Low Potency Estrogen, Intermediate Potency Progestin); Contraceptive, Oral (Monophasic); Estrogen Derivative, Oral; Progestin

Use Prevention of pregnancy

Unlabeled/Investigational Use Treatment of hypermenorrhea, endometriosis, female hypogonadism

Pregnancy Risk Factor X

Pregnancy/Breast-Feeding Implications Breast-feeding: Not recommended; excreted in breast milk; combination oral contraceptives decrease the quality and quantity of breast milk.

Pregnancy should be ruled out prior to treatment and discontinued if pregnancy occurs. In general, the use of combination hormonal contraceptives when inadvertently taken early in pregnancy have not been associated with teratogenic effects. Due to increased risk of thromboembolism postpartum, combination hormonal contraceptives should not be started earlier than 4-6 weeks following delivery.

Contraindications Hypersensitivity to ethinyl estradiol, ethynodiol diacetate, or any component of the formulation; thrombophlebitis or thromboembolic disorders (current or history of), cerebral vascular disease, coronary artery disease, valvular heart disease with complications, severe hypertension; diabetes mellitus with vascular involvement; severe headache with focal neurological symptoms; known or suspected breast carcinoma, endometrial cancer, estrogen-dependent neoplasms, undiagnosed abnormal genital bleeding; hepatic dysfunction or tumor, cholestatic jaundice of pregnancy, jaundice with prior combination hormonal contraceptive use; major surgery with prolonged immobilization; heavy smoking (≥15 cigarettes/day) in patients >35 years of age; pregnancy

Warnings/Precautions Combination hormonal contraceptives do not protect against HIV infection or other sexually-transmitted diseases. The risk of cardiovascular side effects increases in women who smoke cigarettes, especially those who are >35 years of age; women who use combination hormonal contraceptives should be strongly advised not to smoke. Combination hormonal contraceptives may lead to increased risk of myocardial infarction, use with caution in patients with risk factors for coronary artery disease. May increase the risk of thromboembolism. Combination hormonal contraceptives may have a dose-related risk of vascular disease, hypertension, and gallbladder disease. Women with hypertension should be encouraged to use a nonhormonal form of contraception. The use of combination hormonal contraceptives has been associated with a slight increase in frequency of breast cancer, however, studies are not consistent. Combination hormonal contraceptives may cause glucose intolerance. Retinal thrombosis has been reported (rarely). Use with caution in patients with renal disease, conditions that may be aggravated by fluid retention, depression, or history of migraine. Not for use prior to menarche.

The minimum dosage combination of estrogen/progestin that will effectively treat the individual patient should be used. New patients should be started on products containing <50 mcg of estrogen per tablet.

Adverse Reactions Frequency not defined.

Cardiovascular: Arterial thromboembolism, cerebral hemorrhage, cerebral thrombosis, edema, hypertension, mesenteric thrombosis, myocardial infarction

Central nervous system: Depression, dizziness, headache, migraine, nervousness, premenstrual syndrome, stroke

Dermatologic: Acne, erythema multiforme, erythema nodosum, hirsutism, loss of scalp hair, melasma (may persist), rash (allergic)

Endocrine & metabolic: Amenorrhea, breakthrough bleeding, breast enlargement, breast secretion, breast tenderness, carbohydrate intolerance, lactation decreased (postpartum), glucose tolerance decreased, libido changes, menstrual flow changes, sex hormone-binding globulins (SHBG) increased, spotting, temporary infertility (following discontinuation), thyroid-binding globulin increased, triglycerides increased

Gastrointestinal: Abdominal cramps, appetite changes, bloating, cholestasis, colitis, gallbladder disease, jaundice, nausea, vomiting, weight gain/loss

Genitourinary: Cervical erosion changes, cervical secretion changes, cystitis-like syndrome, vaginal candidiasis, vaginitis

Hematologic: Antithrombin III decreased, folate levels decreased, hemolytic uremic syndrome, norepinephrine induced platelet aggregability increased, porphyria, prothrombin increased; factors VII, VIII, IX, and X increased

Hepatic: Benign liver tumors, Budd-Chiari syndrome, cholestatic jaundice, hepatic adenomas

Local: Thrombophlebitis

Ocular: Cataracts, change in corneal curvature (steepening), contact lens intolerance, optic neuritis, retinal thrombosis

Renal: Impaired renal function

Respiratory: Pulmonary thromboembolism

Miscellaneous: Hemorrhagic eruption

Overdosage/Toxicology Toxicity is unlikely following single exposures of excessive doses. Treatment following emesis and charcoal administration should be supportive and symptomatic.

Drug Interactions
    Cytochrome P450 Effect: Ethinyl estradiol: CYP3A3/4 enzyme substrate
    Increased Effect/Toxicity: Acetaminophen and ascorbic acid may increase plasma levels of estrogen component. Atorvastatin and indinavir increase plasma levels of combination hormonal contraceptives. Combination hormonal contraceptives increase the plasma levels of alprazolam, chlordiazepoxide, cyclosporine, diazepam, prednisolone, selegiline, theophylline, tricyclic antidepressants. Combination hormonal contraceptives may increase (or decrease) the effects of coumarin derivatives.
    Decreased Effect: Combination hormonal contraceptives may decrease plasma levels of acetaminophen, clofibric acid, lorazepam, morphine, oxazepam, salicylic acid, temazepam. Contraceptive effect decreased by acitretin, aminoglutethimide, amprenavir, anticonvulsants, griseofulvin, lopinavir, nelfinavir, nevirapine, penicillins (effect not consistent), rifampin, ritonavir, tetracyclines (effect not consistent). Combination hormonal contraceptives may decrease (or increase) the effects of coumarin derivatives.
Ethanol/Nutrition/Herb Interactions
    Food: CNS effects of caffeine may be enhanced if combination hormonal contraceptives are used concurrently with caffeine. Grapefruit juice increases ethinyl estradiol concentrations and would be expected to increase progesterone serum levels as well; clinical implications are unclear.
    Herb/Nutraceutical: St John's wort may decrease the effectiveness of combination hormonal contraceptives by inducing hepatic enzymes. Avoid dong quai and black cohosh (have estrogen activity). Avoid saw palmetto, red clover, ginseng.
Stability Store at controlled room temperature of 25°C (77°F).
Mechanism of Action Combination hormonal contraceptives inhibit ovulation via a negative feedback mechanism on the hypothalamus, which alters the normal pattern of gonadotropin secretion of a follicle-stimulating hormone (FSH) and luteinizing hormone by the anterior pituitary. The follicular phase FSH and midcycle surge of gonadotropins are inhibited. In addition, combination hormonal contraceptives produce alterations in the genital tract, including changes in the cervical mucus, rendering it unfavorable for sperm penetration even if ovulation occurs. Changes in the endometrium may also occur, producing an unfavorable environment for nidation. Combination hormonal contraceptive drugs may alter the tubal transport of the ova through the fallopian tubes. Progestational agents may also alter sperm fertility.
Pharmacodynamics/Kinetics
    Ethinyl Estradiol: See Ethinyl Estradiol monograph.
    Ethynodiol diacetate (converted to norethindrone)
        Metabolism: Hepatic conjugation
        Half-life elimination: Terminal: 5-14 hours
        See Norethindrone monograph.
Usual Dosage Oral: Adults: Female: Contraception:
    Schedule 1 (Sunday starter): Dose begins on first Sunday after onset of menstruation; if the menstrual period starts on Sunday, take first tablet that very same day. **With a Sunday start, an additional method of contraception should be used until after the first 7 days of consecutive administration.**
        For 21-tablet package: 1 tablet/day for 21 consecutive days, followed by 7 days off of the medication; a new course begins on the 8th day after the last tablet is taken.
        For 28-tablet package: 1 tablet/day without interruption.
    Schedule 2 (Day 1 starter): Dose starts on first day of menstrual cycle taking 1 tablet daily.
        For 21-tablet package: 1 tablet/day for 21 consecutive days, followed by 7 days off of the medication; a new course begins on the 8th day after the last tablet is taken.
        For 28-tablet package: 1 tablet/day without interruption.
    If all doses have been taken on schedule and one menstrual period is missed, continue dosing cycle. If two consecutive menstrual periods are missed, pregnancy test is required before new dosing cycle is started.
    Missed doses **monophasic formulations** (refer to package insert for complete information):
        One dose missed: Take as soon as remembered or take 2 tablets next day
        Two consecutive doses missed in the first 2 weeks: Take 2 tablets as soon as remembered or 2 tablets next 2 days. **An additional method of contraception should be used for 7 days after missed dose.**
        Two consecutive doses missed in week 3 or three consecutive doses missed at any time: **An additional method of contraception should be used for 7 days after missed dose:**
            Schedule 1 (Sunday starter): Continue dose of 1 tablet daily until Sunday, then discard the rest of the pack, and a new pack should be started that same day.
            Schedule 2 (Day 1 starter): Current package should be discarded, and a new pack should be started that same day.
    Dosage adjustment in renal impairment: Specific guidelines not available; use with caution
    Dosage adjustment in hepatic impairment: Contraindicated in patients with hepatic impairment
Dietary Considerations Should be taken with food at same time each day.
Administration Administer at the same time each day.
Monitoring Parameters Blood pressure, breast exam, Pap smear, and pregnancy; lipid profiles in patients being treated for hyperlipidemias
Patient Information
    Inform your physician if signs or symptoms of any of the following occur: Thromboembolic or thrombotic disorders including sudden severe headache or vomiting, disturbance of vision or speech, loss of vision, numbness or weakness in an extremity, sharp or crushing chest pain, calf pain, shortness of breath, severe abdominal pain or mass, mental depression or unusual bleeding.
    Discontinue taking the medication if you suspect you are pregnant or become pregnant
Nursing Implications Women should inform their physicians if signs or symptoms of any of the following occur: thromboembolic or thrombotic disorders including sudden severe headache or vomiting, disturbance of vision or speech, loss of vision, numbness or weakness in an extremity, sharp or crushing chest pain, calf pain, shortness of breath, severe abdominal
(Continued)

Ethinyl Estradiol and Ethynodiol Diacetate (Continued)

pain or mass, mental depression or unusual bleeding. Women should be advised to read package insert for missed-dose instructions. Women should discontinue taking the medication if they suspect they are pregnant or become pregnant.

Dosage Forms Tablet, monophasic formulations:

Demulin® 1/35-21: Ethinyl estradiol 0.035 mg and ethynodiol diacetate 1 mg [white tablets] (21s)

Demulin® 1/35-28: Ethinyl estradiol 0.035 mg and ethynodiol diacetate 1 mg [21 white tablets] and 7 blue inactive tablets (28s)

Demulin® 1/50-21: Ethinyl estradiol 0.05 mg and ethynodiol diacetate 1 mg [white tablets] (21s)

Demulin® 1/50-28: Ethinyl estradiol 0.05 mg and ethynodiol diacetate 1 mg [21 white tablets] and 7 pink inactive tablets (28s)

Zovia™ 1/35-21: Ethinyl estradiol 0.035 mg and ethynodiol diacetate 1 mg [light pink tablets] (21s)

Zovia™ 1/35-28: Ethinyl estradiol 0.035 mg and ethynodiol diacetate 1 mg [21 light pink tablets] and 7 white inactive tablets (28s)

Zovia™ 1/50-21: Ethinyl estradiol 0.05 mg and ethynodiol diacetate 1 mg [pink tablets] (21s)

Zovia™ 1/50-28: Ethinyl estradiol 0.05 mg and ethynodiol diacetate 1 mg [21 pink tablets] and 7 white inactive tablets (28s)

Ethinyl Estradiol and Etonogestrel

(ETH in il es tra DYE ole & et oh noe JES trel)

U.S. Brand Names NuvaRing®

Synonyms Etonogestrel and Ethinyl Estradiol

Therapeutic Category Contraceptive, Vaginal; Estrogen and Progestin Combination

Use Prevention of pregnancy

Restrictions Initially, this product will be available only through physicians' offices.

Pregnancy Risk Factor X

Pregnancy/Breast-Feeding Implications Pregnancy should be ruled out prior to treatment and discontinued if pregnancy occurs. In general, the use of combination hormonal contraceptives, when inadvertently used early in pregnancy, have not been associated with teratogenic effects. Due to increased risk of thromboembolism postpartum, do not start earlier than 4-6 weeks following delivery.

Contraindications Hypersensitivity to ethinyl estradiol, etonogestrel, or any component of the formulation; thrombophlebitis or thromboembolic disorders (current or history of), major surgery with prolonged immobilization, cerebral vascular disease, coronary artery disease, valvular heart disease with complications, severe hypertension; diabetes mellitus with vascular involvement; severe headache with focal neurological symptoms; known or suspected breast carcinoma, endometrial cancer, estrogen-dependent neoplasms, undiagnosed abnormal genital bleeding; hepatic dysfunction or tumor, cholestatic jaundice of pregnancy, jaundice with prior combination hormonal contraceptive use; heavy smoking (≥15 cigarettes/day) in patients >35 years of age; conditions which make the vagina susceptible to irritation or ulceration; pregnancy

Warnings/Precautions Combination hormonal contraceptive agents do not protect against HIV infection or other sexually-transmitted diseases. The risk of cardiovascular side effects increases in women who smoke cigarettes, especially those who are >35 years of age; women who use combination hormonal contraceptives should be strongly advised not to smoke. May lead to increased risk of myocardial infarction, use with caution in patients with risk factors for coronary artery disease. May increase the risk of thromboembolism. May have a dose-related risk of vascular disease, hypertension, and gallbladder disease. Women with hypertension should be encouraged to use another form of contraception. May cause glucose intolerance. Retinal thrombosis has been reported (rarely). Use with caution in patients with renal disease, conditions that may be aggravated by fluid retention, depression, or history of migraine. Not for use prior to menarche.

Vaginally-administered combination hormonal contraceptive agents may have a similar adverse effects associated with oral contraceptive products. In order to reduce some of the possible risks, the minimum dosage combination of estrogen/progestin that will effectively treat the individual patient should be used.

Adverse Reactions Adverse reactions associated with oral combination hormonal contraceptive agents are also likely to appear with vaginally-administered products (frequency difficult to anticipate). Refer to oral contraceptive monographs for additional information.

5% to 14%:

Central nervous system: Headache

Gastrointestinal: Nausea, weight gain

Genitourinary: Leukorrhea, vaginitis

Respiratory: Sinusitis, upper respiratory tract infection

Frequency not defined:

Central nervous system: Emotional lability

Genitourinary: Coital problems, device expulsion, foreign body sensation, vaginal discomfort

Overdosage/Toxicology Overdose with the vaginal ring is not likely. If broken, the ring will not release higher doses of hormonal agents. In the event of overdose, treatment should be symptom directed and supportive.

Drug Interactions

Cytochrome P450 Effect: Ethinyl estradiol and etonogestrel: CYP3A3/4 enzyme substrates

Increased Effect/Toxicity: Acetaminophen and ascorbic acid may increase plasma levels of estrogen component. Atorvastatin and indinavir increase plasma levels of combination hormonal contraceptives. Combination hormonal contraceptives increase the plasma levels of alprazolam, chlordiazepoxide, cyclosporine, diazepam, prednisolone, selegiline, theophylline, tricyclic antidepressants. Combination hormonal contraceptives may increase (or decrease) the effects of coumarin derivatives.

Decreased Effect: Combination hormonal contraceptives may decrease plasma levels of acetaminophen, clofibric acid, lorazepam, morphine, oxazepam, salicylic acid, temazepam. Contraceptive effect decreased by acitretin, aminoglutethimide, amprenavir, anticonvulsants, griseofulvin, lopinavir, nelfinavir, nevirapine, penicillins (effect not consistent), rifampin, ritonavir, tetracyclines (effect not consistent). Combination hormonal contraceptives may decrease (or increase) the effects of coumarin derivatives.

Ethanol/Nutrition/Herb Interactions

Food: CNS effects of caffeine may be enhanced if combination hormonal contraceptives are used concurrently with caffeine. Grapefruit juice increases ethinyl estradiol concentrations and would be expected to increase progesterone serum levels as well; clinical implications are unclear.

Herb/Nutraceutical: St John's wort may decrease the effectiveness of combination hormonal contraceptives by inducing hepatic enzymes. Avoid dong quai and black cohosh (have estrogen activity). Avoid saw palmetto, red clover, ginseng.

Stability Prior to dispensing, store under refrigeration, 2°C to 8°C (36°F to 46°F). After dispensing, may be stored at room temperature of 25°C (77°F) for up to 4 months. Avoid direct sunlight.

Mechanism of Action Combination hormonal contraceptives inhibit ovulation via a negative feedback mechanism on the hypothalamus, which alters the normal pattern of gonadotropin secretion of a follicle-stimulating hormone (FSH) and luteinizing hormone by the anterior pituitary. The follicular phase FSH and midcycle surge of gonadotropins are inhibited. In addition, combination hormonal contraceptives produce alterations in the genital tract, including changes in the cervical mucus, rendering it unfavorable for sperm penetration even if ovulation occurs. Changes in the endometrium may also occur, producing an unfavorable environment for nidation. Combination hormonal contraceptive drugs may alter the tubal transport of the ova through the fallopian tubes. Progestational agents may also alter sperm fertility.

Pharmacodynamics/Kinetics

NuvaRing®:

Duration: Serum levels (contraceptive effectiveness) decrease after 3 weeks of continuous use

Absorption: Rapid

Bioavailability: Ethinyl estradiol: ~56% Etonogestrel: 100%

Half-life: Ethinyl estradiol: 44.7 hours; Etonogestrel: 29.3 hours

Etonogestrel:

Absorption: Rapid

Protein binding: 32% to sex-hormone-binding globulin (SHBG) and 66% to albumin; SHBG capacity is affected by plasma ethinyl estradiol levels

Metabolism: Hepatic via CYP3A3/4; forms metabolites (activity not known)

Bioavailability: 100%

Half-life: 29.3 hours

Excretion: Urine, bile, and feces

Ethinyl Estradiol: See Ethinyl Estradiol monograph.

Usual Dosage Vaginal: Adults: Female: Contraception: One ring, inserted vaginally and left in place for 3 consecutive weeks, then removed for 1 week. A new ring is inserted 7 days after the last was removed (even if bleeding is not complete) and should be inserted at approximately the same time of day the ring was removed the previous week.

Initial treatment should begin as follows (pregnancy should always be ruled out first):

No hormonal contraceptive use in the past month: Using the first day of menstruation as "Day 1," insert the ring on or prior to "Day 5," even if bleeding is not complete. **An additional form of contraception should be used for the following 7 days.***

Switching from combination oral contraceptive: Ring should be inserted within 7 days after the last active tablet was taken and no later than the first day a new cycle of tablets would begin. Additional forms of contraception are not needed.

Switching from progestin-only contraceptive: **An additional form of contraception should be used for the following 7 days with any of the following.***

If previously using a progestin-only mini-pill, insert the ring on any day of the month; do not skip days between the last pill and insertion of the ring.

If previously using an implant, insert the ring on the same day of implant removal.

If previously using a progestin-containing IUD, insert the ring on day of IUD removal.

If previously using a progestin injection, insert the ring on the day the next injection would be given.

Following complete 1st trimester abortion: Insert ring within the first five days of abortion. If not inserted within five days, follow instructions for "No hormonal contraceptive use within the past month" and instruct patient to use a nonhormonal contraceptive in the interim.

Following delivery or 2nd trimester abortion: Insert ring 4 weeks postpartum (in women who are not breast-feeding) or following 2nd trimester abortion. **An additional form of contraception should be used for the following 7 days.***

If the ring is accidentally removed from the vagina at anytime during the 3-week period of use, it may be rinsed with cool or lukewarm water (not hot) and reinserted as soon as possible. If the ring is not reinserted within three hours, contraceptive effectiveness will be decreased. **An additional form of contraception should be used until the ring has been inserted for 7 continuous days.***

If the ring has been removed for longer than 1 week, pregnancy must be ruled out prior to restarting therapy. **An additional form of contraception should be used for the following 7 days.***

If the ring has been left in place for >3 weeks, a new ring should be inserted following a 1-week (ring-free) interval. Pregnancy must be ruled out prior to insertion and **an additional form of contraception should be used for the following 7 days.***

*Note: Diaphragms may interfere with proper ring placement, and therefore, are not recommended for use as an additional form of contraception.

Dosage adjustment in renal impairment: Specific guidelines not available; use with caution.

(Continued)

Ethinyl Estradiol and Etonogestrel *(Continued)*

Dosage adjustment in hepatic impairment: Contraindicated in patients with hepatic impairment

Administration Vaginal: Wash hands and remove ring from protective pouch (keep pouch for later ring disposal). Press sides of ring together between thumb and index finger and insert folded ring into vagina. Specific placement is not required for ring to be effective, but ring should be inserted far enough into the vagina as to be comfortable. To remove, hook index finger around rim and pull out. Vaginal ring **cannot** be disposed of in the toilet. New rings should be inserted at approximately the same time of day the ring was removed the previous week. If the ring accidentally falls out, it may be rinsed with cool or warm (not hot) water and replaced. However, it must be replaced within 3 hours. Refer to dosing if ring is out of place for >3 hours.

Monitoring Parameters Blood pressure, breast exam, Pap smear, and pregnancy; lipid profiles in patients being treated for hyperlipidemias

Patient Information Combination hormonal contraceptives do not protect against HIV or other sexually-transmitted diseases. Use exactly as directed by prescriber (also see package insert). You are at risk of becoming pregnant if schedule is not followed. Detailed and complete information can be found in the package insert. Be aware that some medications may reduce the effectiveness of combination hormonal contraceptives; an alternate form of contraception may be needed (diaphragms should not be used). Check all medicines (prescription and over-the-counter), herbal, and alternative products with prescriber. It is important that you check your blood pressure monthly (on same day each month) and that you have an annual physical assessment, Pap smear, and vision assessment while using this medication. Avoid smoking; smoking increases risk or adverse effects, including thromboembolic events and heart attacks. You may experience loss of appetite (small frequent meals will help); constipation (increased fluids, exercise, and dietary fiber, or stool softeners may help). Diabetics should use accurate serum glucose testing to identify any changes in glucose tolerance; notify prescriber of significant changes so antidiabetic medication can be adjusted if necessary. Report immediately pain or muscle soreness; swelling, heat, or redness in calves; shortness of breath; sudden loss of vision; unresolved leg or foot swelling; change in menstrual pattern (unusual bleeding, amenorrhea, breakthrough spotting); breast tenderness that does not go away; acute abdominal cramping; signs of vaginal infection (drainage, pain, itching); changes in CNS (blurred vision, confusion, acute anxiety, or unresolved depression); or significant weight gain (>5 lb/week). Notify prescriber for changes in contact lens tolerance. This medication should not be used during pregnancy. If you suspect you may be pregnant, contact prescriber immediately. Breast-feeding is not recommended.

Although rare, it is possible for the ring to slip out of the vagina. This may occur if not inserted properly, while removing a tampon, during bowel movements, straining or severe constipation, or in women with a prolapsed (dropped) uterus. If the ring accidentally falls out, it may be rinsed with cool or warm (not hot) water and replaced. However, it must be replaced within 3 hours. Refer to patient leaflet or contact prescriber for additional instructions if ring is out of place for >3 hours.

Dosage Forms Intravaginal ring [3-week duration]: Ethinyl estradiol 0.015 mg/day and etonogestrel 0.12 mg/day (1s, 3s)

Ethinyl Estradiol and Levonorgestrel

(ETH in il es tra DYE ole & LEE voe nor jes trel)

U.S. Brand Names Alesse®; Aviane™; Levlen®; Levlite™; Levora®; Nordette®; PREVEN™; Tri-Levlen®; Triphasil®; Trivora®

Canadian Brand Names Alesse®; Min-Ovral®; Preven™; Triphasil®; Triquilar®

Synonyms Levonorgestrel and Ethinyl Estradiol

Therapeutic Category Contraceptive, Emergency; Contraceptive, Oral (Intermediate Potency Estrogen, Low Potency Progestin); Contraceptive, Oral (Low Potency Estrogen, Low Potency Progestin); Contraceptive, Oral (Monophasic); Contraceptive, Oral (Triphasic); Emergency Contraception Estrogen Derivative, Oral Progestin

Use Prevention of pregnancy; postcoital contraception

Unlabeled/Investigational Use Treatment of hypermenorrhea, endometriosis, female hypogonadism

Pregnancy Risk Factor X

Pregnancy/Breast-Feeding Implications Breast-feeding is not recommended; excreted in breast milk; combination hormonal contraceptives decrease the quality and quantity of breast milk.

Pregnancy should be ruled out prior to treatment and discontinued if pregnancy occurs. In general, the use of combination hormonal contraceptives when inadvertently taken early in pregnancy have not been associated with teratogenic effects. Due to increased risk of thromboembolism postpartum, combination hormonal contraceptives should not be started earlier than 4-6 weeks following delivery.

Contraindications Hypersensitivity to ethinyl estradiol, levonorgestrel, or any component of the formulation; thrombophlebitis or thromboembolic disorders (current or history of); cerebral vascular disease, coronary artery disease, valvular heart disease with complications, severe hypertension; diabetes mellitus with vascular involvement; severe headache with focal neurological symptoms; known or suspected breast carcinoma, endometrial cancer, estrogen-dependent neoplasms, undiagnosed abnormal genital bleeding; hepatic dysfunction or tumor, cholestatic jaundice of pregnancy, jaundice with prior combination hormonal contraceptive use; major surgery with prolonged immobilization; heavy smoking (≥15 cigarettes/day) in patients >35 years of age; pregnancy

Warnings/Precautions Combination hormonal contraceptives do not protect against HIV infection or other sexually-transmitted diseases. The risk of cardiovascular side effects increases in women who smoke cigarettes, especially those who are >35 years of age; women who use combination hormonal contraceptives should be strongly advised not to smoke. Combination hormonal contraceptives may lead to increased risk of myocardial infarction, use with caution in patients with risk factors for coronary artery disease. May increase the risk of thromboembolism. Combination hormonal contraceptives may have a dose-related risk of vascular disease, hypertension, and gallbladder disease. Women with hypertension should be encouraged to use another form of contraception. The use of combination hormonal contraceptives has been associated with a slight increase in frequency of breast cancer, however, studies are not consistent. Combination hormonal contraceptives may cause glucose intolerance. Retinal thrombosis has been reported (rarely). Use with caution in patients with renal disease, conditions that may be aggravated by fluid retention, depression, or history of migraine. Not for use prior to menarche.

The minimum dosage combination of estrogen/progestin that will effectively treat the individual patient should be used. New patients should be started on products containing <50 mcg of estrogen per tablet.

Adverse Reactions Frequency not defined.

Cardiovascular: Arterial thromboembolism, cerebral hemorrhage, cerebral thrombosis, edema, hypertension, mesenteric thrombosis, myocardial infarction

Central nervous system: Depression, dizziness, headache, migraine, nervousness, premenstrual syndrome, stroke

Dermatologic: Acne, erythema multiforme, erythema nodosum, hirsutism, loss of scalp hair, melasma (may persist), rash (allergic)

Endocrine & metabolic: Amenorrhea, breakthrough bleeding, breast enlargement, breast secretion, breast tenderness, carbohydrate intolerance, lactation decreased (postpartum), glucose tolerance decreased, libido changes, menstrual flow changes, sex hormone-binding globulins (SHBG) increased, spotting, temporary infertility (following discontinuation), thyroid-binding globulin increased, triglycerides increased

Gastrointestinal: Abdominal cramps, appetite changes, bloating, cholestasis, colitis, gallbladder disease, jaundice, nausea, vomiting, weight gain/loss

Genitourinary: Cervical erosion changes, cervical secretion changes, cystitis-like syndrome, vaginal candidiasis, vaginitis

Hematologic: Antithrombin III decreased, folate levels decreased, hemolytic uremic syndrome, norepinephrine induced platelet aggregability increased, porphyria, prothrombin increased; factors VII, VIII, IX, and X increased

Hepatic: Benign liver tumors, Budd-Chiari syndrome, cholestatic jaundice, hepatic adenomas

Local: Thrombophlebitis

Ocular: Cataracts, change in corneal curvature (steepening), contact lens intolerance, optic neuritis, retinal thrombosis

Renal: Impaired renal function

Respiratory: Pulmonary thromboembolism

Miscellaneous: Hemorrhagic eruption

Overdosage/Toxicology Toxicity is unlikely following single exposures of excessive doses. Treatment following emesis and charcoal administration should be supportive and symptomatic.

Drug Interactions

Cytochrome P450 Effect: Ethinyl estradiol and levonorgestrel: CYP3A3/4 enzyme substrates

Increased Effect/Toxicity: Acetaminophen and ascorbic acid may increase plasma levels of estrogen component. Atorvastatin and indinavir increase plasma levels of combination hormonal contraceptives. Combination hormonal contraceptives increase the plasma levels of alprazolam, chlordiazepoxide, cyclosporine, diazepam, prednisolone, selegiline, theophylline, tricyclic antidepressants. Combination hormonal contraceptives may increase (or decrease) the effects of coumarin derivatives.

Decreased Effect: Combination hormonal contraceptives may decrease plasma levels of acetaminophen, clofibric acid, lorazepam, morphine, oxazepam, salicylic acid, temazepam. Contraceptive effect decreased by acitretin, aminoglutethimide, amprenavir, anticonvulsants, griseofulvin, lopinavir, nelfinavir, nevirapine, penicillins (effect not consistent), rifampin, ritonavir, tetracyclines (effect not consistent). Combination hormonal contraceptives may decrease (or increase) the effects of coumarin derivatives.

Ethanol/Nutrition/Herb Interactions

Food: CNS effects of caffeine may be enhanced if combination hormonal contraceptives are used concurrently with caffeine. Grapefruit juice increases ethinyl estradiol concentrations and would be expected to increase progesterone serum levels as well; clinical implications are unclear.

Herb/Nutraceutical: St John's wort may decrease the effectiveness of combination hormonal contraceptives by inducing hepatic enzymes. Avoid dong quai and black cohosh (have estrogen activity). Avoid saw palmetto, red clover, ginseng.

Stability Store at controlled room temperature of 25°C (77°F).

Mechanism of Action Combination hormonal contraceptives inhibit ovulation via a negative feedback mechanism on the hypothalamus, which alters the normal pattern of gonadotropin secretion of a follicle-stimulating hormone (FSH) and luteinizing hormone by the anterior pituitary. The follicular phase FSH and midcycle surge of gonadotropins are inhibited. In addition, combination hormonal contraceptives produce alterations in the genital tract, including changes in the cervical mucus, rendering it unfavorable for sperm penetration even if ovulation occurs. Changes in the endometrium may also occur, producing an unfavorable environment for nidation. Combination hormonal contraceptive drugs may alter the tubal transport of the ova through the fallopian tubes. Progestational agents may also alter sperm fertility.

Pharmacodynamics/Kinetics See individual agents.

Usual Dosage Oral: Adults: Female:

Contraception:

Schedule 1 (Sunday starter): Dose begins on first Sunday after onset of menstruation; if the menstrual period starts on Sunday, take first tablet that very same day. With a Sunday start, an additional method of contraception should be used until after the first 7 days of consecutive administration:

For 21-tablet package: 1 tablet/day for 21 consecutive days, followed by 7 days off of the medication; a new course begins on the 8th day after the last tablet is taken

For 28-tablet package: 1 tablet/day without interruption

(Continued)

Ethinyl Estradiol and Levonorgestrel *(Continued)*

Schedule 2 (Day 1 starter): Dose starts on first day of menstrual cycle taking 1 tablet/day:

For 21-tablet package: 1 tablet/day for 21 consecutive days, followed by 7 days off of the medication; a new course begins on the 8th day after the last tablet is taken

For 28-tablet package: 1 tablet/day without interruption

If all doses have been taken on schedule and one menstrual period is missed, continue dosing cycle. If two consecutive menstrual periods are missed, pregnancy test is required before new dosing cycle is started.

Missed doses **monophasic formulations** (refer to package insert for complete information):

One dose missed: Take as soon as remembered or take 2 tablets next day

Two consecutive doses missed in the first 2 weeks: Take 2 tablets as soon as remembered or 2 tablets next 2 days. An additional method of contraception should be used for 7 days after missed dose.

Two consecutive doses missed in week 3 or three consecutive doses missed at any time: An additional method of contraception must be used for 7 days after a missed dose:

Schedule 1 (Sunday starter): Continue dose of 1 tablet daily until Sunday, then discard the rest of the pack, and a new pack should be started that same day.

Schedule 2 (Day 1 starter): Current pack should be discarded, and a new pack should be started that same day.

Missed doses **biphasic/triphasic formulations** (refer to package insert for complete information):

One dose missed: Take as soon as remembered or take 2 tablets next day.

Two consecutive doses missed in week 1 or week 2 of the pack: Take 2 tablets as soon as remembered and 2 tablets the next day. Resume taking 1 tablet daily until the pack is empty. An additional method of contraception should be used for 7 days after a missed dose.

Two consecutive doses missed in week 3 of the pack: An additional method of contraception must be used for 7 days after a missed dose.

Schedule 1 (Sunday starter): Take 1 tablet every day until Sunday. Discard the remaining pack and start a new pack of pills on the same day.

Schedule 2 (Day 1 starter): Discard the remaining pack and start a new pack the same day.

Three or more consecutive doses missed: An additional method of contraception must be used for 7 days after a missed dose.

Schedule 1 (Sunday starter): Take 1 tablet every day until Sunday; on Sunday, discard the pack and start a new pack.

Schedule 2 (Day 1 starter): Discard the remaining pack and begin new pack of tablets starting on the same day.

Emergency contraception (PREVEN™): Initial: 2 tablets as soon as possible (but within 72 hours of unprotected intercourse), followed by a second dose of 2 tablets 12 hours later. Repeat dose or use antiemetic if vomiting occurs within 1 hour of dose.

Dosage adjustment in renal impairment: Specific guidelines not available; use with caution

Dosage adjustment in hepatic impairment: Contraindicated in patients with hepatic impairment

Dietary Considerations Should be taken at the same time each day.

Administration Administer at the same time each day.

Monitoring Parameters Blood pressure, breast exam, Pap smear, and pregnancy; lipid profiles in patients being treated for hyperlipidemias

Patient Information Inform your physician if signs or symptoms of any of the following occur: Thromboembolic or thrombotic disorders including sudden severe headache or vomiting, disturbance of vision or speech, loss of vision, numbness or weakness in an extremity, sharp or crushing chest pain, calf pain, shortness of breath, severe abdominal pain or mass, mental depression or unusual bleeding

If any doses are missed, alternative contraceptive methods should be used for the next 2 days or until 2 days into the new cycle

Discontinue taking the medication if you suspect you are pregnant or become pregnant

Emergency contraceptive kit (PREVEN™) is **not** recommended for ongoing pregnancy protection or as a routine form of contraception. PREVEN™ emergency contraceptive kit contains a pregnancy test. This test can be used to verify an existing pregnancy resulting from intercourse that occurred earlier in the concurrent menstrual cycle or the previous cycle. If a positive pregnancy result is obtained, the patient should **not** take the pills in the PREVEN™ kit. The patient should be instructed that if she vomits within 1 hour of taking either dose of the medication, she should contact her healthcare professional to discuss whether to repeat that dose or to take an antinausea medication.

Nursing Implications Women should inform their physicians if signs or symptoms of any of the following occur: thromboembolic or thrombotic disorders including sudden severe headache or vomiting, disturbance of vision or speech, loss of vision, numbness or weakness in an extremity, sharp or crushing chest pain, calf pain, shortness of breath, severe abdominal pain or mass, mental depression or unusual bleeding. Women should be advised to read package insert for missed-dose instructions. Women should discontinue taking the medication if they suspect they are pregnant or become pregnant.

Dosage Forms Tablet:

PREVEN™: Ethinyl estradiol 0.05 mg and levonorgestrel 0.25 mg (4s) [also available as a kit containing 4 tablets and a pregnancy test]

Low-dose formulations:

Alesse® 21: Ethinyl estradiol 0.02 mg and levonorgestrel 0.1 mg [pink tablets] (21s)

Alesse® 28: Ethinyl estradiol 0.02 mg and levonorgestrel 0.1 mg [21 pink tablets] and 7 light green inactive tablets (28s)

Aviane™ 28: Ethinyl estradiol 0.02 mg and levonorgestrel 0.1 mg [21 orange tablets] and 7 light green inactive tablets (28s)

Levlite™ 21:Ethinyl estradiol 0.02 mg and levonorgestrel 0.1 mg [pink tablets] (21s)

Levlite™ 28: Ethinyl estradiol 0.02 mg and levonorgestrel 0.1 mg [21 pink tablets] and 7 white inactive tablets (28s)

Monophasic formulations:

Levlen® 21: Ethinyl estradiol 0.03 mg and levonorgestrel 0.15 mg [light orange tablets] (21s)

Levlen® 28: Ethinyl estradiol 0.03 mg and levonorgestrel 0.15 mg [21 light orange tablets] and 7 pink inactive tablets (28s)

Levora® 21: Ethinyl estradiol 0.03 mg and levonorgestrel 0.15 mg [white tablets] (21s)

Levora® 28: Ethinyl estradiol 0.03 mg and levonorgestrel 0.15 mg [21 white tablets] and 7 peach inactive tablets (28s)

Nordette® 21:Ethinyl estradiol 0.03 mg and levonorgestrel 0.15 mg [light orange tablets] (21s)

Nordette® 28: Ethinyl estradiol 0.03 mg and levonorgestrel 0.15 mg [21 light orange tablets] and 7 pink inactive tablets (28s)

Triphasic formulations:

Tri-Levlen® 21, Triphasil® 21:

Day 1-6:Ethinyl estradiol 0.03 mg and levonorgestrel 0.05 mg [6 brown tablets]

Day 7-11: Ethinyl estradiol 0.04 mg and levonorgestrel 0.075 mg [5 white tablets]

Day 12-21:Ethinyl estradiol 0.03 mg and levonorgestrel 0.125 mg [10 light yellow tablets] (21s)

Trivora® 21:

Day 1-6: Ethinyl estradiol 0.03 mg and levonorgestrel 0.05 mg [6 blue tablets]

Day 7-11: Ethinyl estradiol 0.04 mg and levonorgestrel 0.075 mg [5 white tablets]

Day 12-21: Ethinyl estradiol 0.03 mg and levonorgestrel 0.125 mg [10 pink tablets] (21s)

Tri-Levlen® 28, Triphasil® 28:

Day 1-6:Ethinyl estradiol 0.03 mg and levonorgestrel 0.05 mg [6 brown tablets]

Day 7-11: Ethinyl estradiol 0.04 mg and levonorgestrel 0.075 mg [5 white tablets]

Day 12-21:Ethinyl estradiol 0.03 mg and levonorgestrel 0.125 mg [10 light yellow tablets]

Day 22-28: 7 light green inactive tablets (28s)

Trivora® 28:

Day 1-6: Ethinyl estradiol 0.03 mg and levonorgestrel 0.05 mg [6 blue tablets]

Day 7-11: Ethinyl estradiol 0.04 mg and levonorgestrel 0.075 mg [5 white tablets]

Day 12-21:Ethinyl estradiol 0.03 mg and levonorgestrel 0.125 mg [10 pink tablets]

Day 22-28: 7 peach inactive tablets (28s)

♦ **Ethinyl Estradiol and NGM** *see Ethinyl Estradiol and Norgestimate* *on page 525*

Ethinyl Estradiol and Norelgestromin

(ETH in il es tra DYE ole & nor el JES troe min)

U.S. Brand Names Ortho Evra™

Synonyms Norelgestromin and Ethinyl Estradiol

Therapeutic Category Contraceptive, Topical Patch; Estrogen and Progestin Combination

Use Prevention of pregnancy

Pregnancy Risk Factor X

Usual Dosage Topical: Adults: Female:

Contraception: Apply one patch each week for 3 weeks (21 total days); followed by one week that is patch-free. Each patch should be applied on the same day each week ("patch change day") and only one patch should be worn at a time. No more than 7 days should pass during the patch-free interval.

Schedule 1 (Sunday starter): Dose begins on first Sunday after onset of menstruation; if the menstrual period starts on Sunday, apply one patch that very same day. **With a Sunday start, an additional method of contraception (nonhormonal) should be used until after the first 7 days of consecutive administration.** Each patch change will then occur on Sunday.

Schedule 2 (Day 1 starter): Dose starts on first day of menstrual cycle, applying one patch during the first 24 hours of menstrual cycle. No back-up method of contraception is needed as long as the patch is applied on the first day of cycle. Each patch change will then occur on that same day of the week.

Additional dosing considerations:

No bleeding during patch-free week/missed menstrual period: If patch has been applied as directed, continue treatment on usual "patch change day". If used correctly, no bleeding during patch-free week does not necessarily indicate pregnancy. However, if no withdrawal bleeding occurs for 2 consecutive cycles, pregnancy should be ruled out. If patch has not been applied as directed, and one menstrual period is missed, pregnancy should be ruled out prior to continuing treatment.

If a patch becomes partially or completely detached for <24 hours: Try to reapply to same place, or replace with a new patch immediately. Do not reapply if patch is no longer sticky, if it is sticking to itself or another surface, or if it has material sticking to it.

If a patch becomes partially or completely detached for >24 hours (or time period is unknown): Apply a new patch and use this day of the week as the new "patch change day" from this point on. **An additional method of contraception (nonhormonal) should be used until after the first 7 days of consecutive administration.**

Switching from oral contraceptives: Apply first patch on the first day of withdrawal bleeding. If there is no bleeding within 5 days of taking the last active tablet, pregnancy must first be ruled out. If patch is applied later than the first day of bleeding, **an additional method of contraception (nonhormonal) should be used until after the first 7 days of consecutive administration**

Use after childbirth: Therapy should not be started <4 weeks after childbirth. Pregnancy should be ruled out prior to treatment if menstrual periods have not restarted. **An additional method of contraception (nonhormonal) should be used until after the first 7 days of consecutive administration.**

(Continued)

Ethinyl Estradiol and Norelgestromin *(Continued)*

Use after abortion or miscarriage: Therapy may be started immediately if abortion/miscarriage occur within the first trimester. If therapy is not started within 5 days, follow instructions for first time use. If abortion/miscarriage occur during the second trimester, therapy should not be started for at least 4 weeks. Follow directions for use after childbirth.

Dosage adjustment in renal impairment: Specific guidelines not available; use with caution
Dosage adjustment in hepatic impairment: Contraindicated in patients with hepatic impairment

Additional Information Complete prescribing information for this medication should be consulted for additional detail.

Dosage Forms Patch, topical: Ethinyl estradiol 0.75 mg and norelgestromin 6 mg [releases ethinyl estradiol 20 mcg and norelgestromin 150 mcg per day] (1s, 3s)

Ethinyl Estradiol and Norethindrone

(ETH in il es tra DYE ole & nor eth IN drone)

U.S. Brand Names Brevicon®; Estrostep® 21; Estrostep® Fe; femhrt®; Jenest™-28; Loestrin®; Loestrin® Fe; Microgestin™ Fe; Modicon®; Necon® 0.5/35; Necon® 1/35; Necon® 10/11; Norinyl® 1+35; Nortrel™; Ortho-Novum®; Ovcon®; Tri-Norinyl®

Canadian Brand Names Brevicon® 0.5/35; Brevicon® 1/35; FemHRT®; Loestrin™ 1.5.30; Minestrin™ 1/20; Ortho® 0.5/35; Ortho® 1/35; Ortho® 7/7/7; Select™ 1/35; Synphasic®

Synonyms Norethindrone Acetate and Ethinyl Estradiol

Therapeutic Category Contraceptive, Oral (Biphasic); Contraceptive, Oral (Intermediate Potency Estrogen, Intermediate Potency Progestin); Contraceptive, Oral (Intermediate Potency Estrogen, Low Potency Progestin); Contraceptive, Oral (Low Potency Estrogen, Low Potency Progestin); Contraceptive, Oral (Monophasic); Contraceptive, Oral (Triphasic); Estrogen Derivative, Oral; Progestin

Use Prevention of pregnancy; treatment of acne; moderate to severe vasomotor symptoms associated with menopause; prevention of osteoporosis

Unlabeled/Investigational Use Treatment of hypermenorrhea, endometriosis, female hypogonadism

Pregnancy Risk Factor X

Pregnancy/Breast-Feeding Implications Breast-feeding is not recommended; excreted in breast milk; combination oral contraceptives decrease the quality and quantity of breast milk.

Pregnancy should be ruled out prior to treatment and discontinued if pregnancy occurs. In general, the use of combination hormonal contraceptives when inadvertently taken early in pregnancy have not been associated with teratogenic effects. Due to increased risk of thromboembolism postpartum, combination hormonal contraceptives should not be started earlier than 4-6 weeks following delivery.

Contraindications Hypersensitivity to ethinyl estradiol, norethindrone, norethindrone acetate, or any component of the formulation; thrombophlebitis or thromboembolic disorders (current or history of), cerebral vascular disease, coronary artery disease, severe hypertension; diabetes mellitus with vascular involvement; severe headache with focal neurological symptoms; known or suspected breast carcinoma, endometrial cancer, estrogen-dependent neoplasms, undiagnosed abnormal genital bleeding; hepatic dysfunction or tumor, cholestatic jaundice of pregnancy, jaundice with prior combination hormonal contraceptive use; major surgery with prolonged immobilization; heavy smoking (≥15 cigarettes/day) in patients >35 years of age; pregnancy

Warnings/Precautions Combination hormonal contraceptives do not protect against HIV infection or other sexually-transmitted diseases. The risk of cardiovascular side effects increases in women who smoke cigarettes, especially those who are >35 years of age; women who use combination hormonal contraceptives should be strongly advised not to smoke. Combination hormonal contraceptives may lead to increased risk of myocardial infarction, use with caution in patients with risk factors for coronary artery disease. May increase the risk of thromboembolism. Combination hormonal contraceptives may have a dose-related risk of vascular disease, hypertension, and gallbladder disease. Women with hypertension should be encouraged to use another form of contraception. The use of combination hormonal contraceptives has been associated with a slight increase in frequency of breast cancer, however, studies are not consistent. Combination hormonal contraceptives may cause glucose intolerance. Retinal thrombosis has been reported (rarely). Use with caution in patients with renal disease, conditions that may be aggravated by fluid retention, depression, or history of migraine. Not for use prior to menarche.

The minimum dosage combination of estrogen/progestin that will effectively treat the individual patient should be used. New patients should be started on products containing <50 mcg of estrogen per tablet.

Acne: For use only in females ≥15 years, who also desire combination hormonal contraceptive therapy, are unresponsive to topical treatments, and have no contraindications to combination hormonal contraceptive use; treatment must continue for at least 6 months.

Vasomotor symptoms associated with menopause and prevention of osteoporosis: For use only in postmenopausal women with an intact uterus.

Adverse Reactions As reported with oral contraceptive agents. Frequency not defined.
Cardiovascular: Arterial thromboembolism, cerebral hemorrhage, cerebral thrombosis, edema, hypertension, mesenteric thrombosis, myocardial infarction
Central nervous system: Depression, dizziness, headache, migraine, nervousness, premenstrual syndrome, stroke
Dermatologic: Acne, erythema multiforme, erythema nodosum, hirsutism, loss of scalp hair, melasma (may persist), rash (allergic)
Endocrine & metabolic: Amenorrhea, breakthrough bleeding, breast enlargement, breast secretion, breast tenderness, carbohydrate intolerance, lactation decreased (postpartum), glucose tolerance decreased, libido changes, menstrual flow changes, sex hormone-binding globulins (SHBG) increased, spotting, temporary infertility (following discontinuation), thyroid-binding globulin increased, triglycerides increased

Gastrointestinal: Abdominal cramps, appetite changes, bloating, cholestasis, colitis, gall-bladder disease, jaundice, nausea, vomiting, weight gain/loss

Genitourinary: Cervical erosion changes, cervical secretion changes, cystitis-like syndrome, vaginal candidiasis, vaginitis

Hematologic: Antithrombin III decreased, folate levels decreased, hemolytic uremic syndrome, norepinephrine induced platelet aggregability increased, porphyria, prothrombin increased; factors VII, VIII, IX, and X

Hepatic: Benign liver tumors, Budd-Chiari syndrome, cholestatic jaundice, hepatic adenomas

Local: Thrombophlebitis

Ocular: Cataracts, change in corneal curvature (steepening), contact lens intolerance, optic neuritis, retinal thrombosis

Renal: Impaired renal function

Respiratory: Pulmonary thromboembolism

Miscellaneous: Hemorrhagic eruption

Drug Interactions

Cytochrome P450 Effect: Ethinyl estradiol: CYP3A3/4 enzyme substrate

Increased Effect/Toxicity: Acetaminophen and ascorbic acid may increase plasma levels of estrogen component. Atorvastatin and indinavir increase plasma levels of combination hormonal contraceptives. Combination hormonal contraceptives increase the plasma levels of alprazolam, chlordiazepoxide, cyclosporine, diazepam, prednisolone, selegiline, theophylline, tricyclic antidepressants. Combination hormonal contraceptives may increase (or decrease) the effects of coumarin derivatives.

Decreased Effect: Combination hormonal contraceptives may decrease plasma levels of acetaminophen, clofibric acid, lorazepam, morphine, oxazepam, salicylic acid, temazepam. Contraceptive effect decreased by acitretin, aminoglutethimide, amprenavir, anticonvulsants, griseofulvin, lopinavir, nelfinavir, nevirapine, penicillins (effect not consistent), rifampin, ritonavir, tetracyclines (effect not consistent), troglitazone. Oral contraceptives may decrease (or increase) the effects of coumarin derivatives.

Ethanol/Nutrition/Herb Interactions

Food: CNS effects of caffeine may be enhanced if combination hormonal contraceptives are used concurrently with caffeine. Grapefruit juice increases ethinyl estradiol concentrations and would be expected to increase progesterone serum levels as well; clinical implications are unclear. Norethindrone absorption is increased by 27% following administration with food.

Herb/Nutraceutical: St John's wort may decrease the effectiveness of combination hormonal contraceptives by inducing hepatic enzymes. Avoid dong quai and black cohosh (have estrogen activity). Avoid saw palmetto, red clover, ginseng.

Stability Store at controlled room temperature of 25°C (77°F).

Estrostep®: Protect from light.

Mechanism of Action Combination oral contraceptives inhibit ovulation via a negative feedback mechanism on the hypothalamus, which alters the normal pattern of gonadotropin secretion of a follicle-stimulating hormone (FSH) and luteinizing hormone by the anterior pituitary. The follicular phase FSH and midcycle surge of gonadotropins are inhibited. In addition, combination hormonal contraceptives produce alterations in the genital tract, including changes in the cervical mucus, rendering it unfavorable for sperm penetration even if ovulation occurs. Changes in the endometrium may also occur, producing an unfavorable environment for nidation. Combination hormonal contraceptive drugs may alter the tubal transport of the ova through the fallopian tubes. Progestational agents may also alter sperm fertility.

In postmenopausal women, exogenous estrogen is used to replace decreased endogenous production. The addition of progestin reduces the incidence of endometrial hyperplasia and risk of adenocarcinoma in women with an intact uterus.

Pharmacodynamics/Kinetics See individual agents.

Usual Dosage Oral:

Adolescents ≥15 years and Adults: Female: Acne: Estrostep®: Refer to dosing for contraception

Adults: Female:

Moderate to severe vasomotor symptoms associated with menopause: femhrt® 1/5: 1 tablet daily; patients should be re-evaluated at 3- to 6-month intervals to determine if treatment is still necessary

Prevention of osteoporosis: femhrt® 1/5: 1 tablet daily

Contraception:

Schedule 1 (Sunday starter): Dose begins on first Sunday after onset of menstruation; if the menstrual period starts on Sunday, take first tablet that very same day. With a Sunday start, an additional method of contraception should be used until after the first 7 days of consecutive administration.

For 21-tablet package: Dosage is 1 tablet daily for 21 consecutive days, followed by 7 days off of the medication; a new course begins on the 8th day after the last tablet is taken.

For 28-tablet package: Dosage is 1 tablet daily without interruption.

Schedule 2 (Day 1 starter): Dose starts on first day of menstrual cycle taking 1 tablet daily.

For 21-tablet package: Dosage is 1 tablet daily for 21 consecutive days, followed by 7 days off of the medication; a new course begins on the 8th day after the last tablet is taken.

For 28-tablet package: Dosage is 1 tablet daily without interruption.

If all doses have been taken on schedule and one menstrual period is missed, continue dosing cycle. If two consecutive menstrual periods are missed, pregnancy test is required before new dosing cycle is started.

Missed doses **monophasic formulations** (refer to package insert for complete information):

One dose missed: Take as soon as remembered or take 2 tablets next day Two consecutive doses missed in the first 2 weeks: Take 2 tablets as soon as remembered

(Continued)

Ethinyl Estradiol and Norethindrone *(Continued)*

or 2 tablets next 2 days. An additional method of contraception should be used for 7 days after missed dose.

Two consecutive doses missed in week 3 or three consecutive doses missed at any time: An additional method of contraception must be used for 7 days after a missed dose.

Schedule 1 (Sunday starter): Continue dose of 1 tablet daily until Sunday, then discard the rest of the pack, and a new pack should be started that same day.

Schedule 2 (Day 1 starter): Current pack should be discarded, and a new pack should be started that same day.

Missed doses **biphasic/triphasic formulations** (refer to package insert for complete information):

One dose missed: Take as soon as remembered or take 2 tablets next day.

Two consecutive doses missed in week 1 or week 2 of the pack: Take 2 tablets as soon as remembered and 2 tablets the next day. Resume taking 1 tablet daily until the pack is empty. An additional method of contraception should be used for 7 days after a missed dose.

Two consecutive doses missed in week 3 of the pack: An additional method of contraception must be used for 7 days after a missed dose.

Schedule 1 (Sunday Starter): Take 1 tablet every day until Sunday. Discard the remaining pack and start a new pack of pills on the same day.

Schedule 2 (Day 1 starter): Discard the remaining pack and start a new pack the same day.

Three or more consecutive doses missed: An additional method of contraception must be used for 7 days after a missed dose.

Schedule 1 (Sunday Starter): Take 1 tablet every day until Sunday; on Sunday, discard the pack and start a new pack.

Schedule 2 (Day 1 Starter): Discard the remaining pack and begin new pack of tablets starting on the same day.

Dosage adjustment in renal impairment: Specific guidelines not available; use with caution.

Dosage adjustment in hepatic impairment: Contraindicated in patients with hepatic impairment.

Dietary Considerations Should be taken at same time each day. May be taken with or without food.

Administration Administer at the same time each day.

Monitoring Parameters Blood pressure, breast exam, Pap smear, and pregnancy; lipid profiles in patients being treated for hyperlipidemias

Patient Information Take exactly as directed; use additional method of birth control during first week of administration of first cycle; photosensitivity may occur. Women should inform their physicians if signs or symptoms of any of the following occur thromboembolic or thrombotic disorders including sudden severe headache or vomiting, disturbance of vision or speech, loss of vision, numbness or weakness in an extremity, sharp or crushing chest pain, calf pain, shortness of breath, severe abdominal pain or mass, mental depression, or unusual bleeding.

When any doses are missed, alternative contraceptive methods should be used for the next 2 days or until 2 days into the new cycle

Women should discontinue taking the medication if they suspect they are pregnant or become pregnant

Nursing Implications Administer at bedtime to minimize occurrence of adverse effects.

Additional Information Norethindrone acetate 1 mg is equivalent to ethinyl estradiol 2.8 mcg.

Dosage Forms Tablet:

femhrt® 1/5: Ethinyl estradiol 0.005 mg and norethindrone acetate 1 mg [white tablets]

Monophasic formulations:

Brevicon®: Ethinyl estradiol 0.035 mg and norethindrone 0.5 mg [21 blue tablets] and 7 orange inactive tablets (28s)

Loestrin® 21 1/20: Ethinyl estradiol 0.02 mg and norethindrone acetate 1 mg [white tablets] (21s)

Loestrin® 21 1.5/30: Ethinyl estradiol 0.03 mg and norethindrone acetate 1.5 mg [green tablets] (21s)

Loestrin® Fe 1/20, Microgestin™ Fe 1/20: Ethinyl estradiol 0.02 mg and norethindrone acetate 1mg [21 white tablets] and ferrous fumarate 75 mg [7 brown tablets] (28s)

Loestrin® Fe 1.5/30, Microgestin™ Fe 1.5/30: Ethinyl estradiol 0.03 mg and norethindrone acetate 1.5 mg [21 green tablets] and ferrous fumarate 75 mg [7 brown tablets] (28s)

Modicon® 21: Ethinyl estradiol 0.035 mg and norethindrone 0.5 mg [white tablets] (21s)

Modicon® 28: Ethinyl estradiol 0.035 mg and norethindrone 0.5 mg [21 white tablets] and 7 green inactive tablets (28s)

Necon® 0.5/35-21: Ethinyl estradiol 0.035 mg and norethindrone 0.5 mg [light yellow tablets] (21s)

Necon® 0.5/35-28: Ethinyl estradiol 0.035 mg and norethindrone 0.5 mg [21 light yellow tablets] and 7 white inactive tablets (28s)

Necon® 1/35-21: Ethinyl estradiol 0.035 mg and norethindrone 1 mg [dark yellow tablets] (21s)

Necon® 1/35-28: Ethinyl estradiol 0.035 mg and norethindrone 1 mg [21 dark yellow tablets] and 7 white inactive tablets (28s)

Norinyl® 1+35: Ethinyl estradiol 0.035 mg and norethindrone 1 mg [21 yellow-green tablets] and 7 orange inactive tablets (28s)

Nortrel™ 0.5/35 mg:

Ethinyl estradiol 0.035 mg and norethindrone 0.5 mg [light yellow tablets] (21s)

Ethinyl estradiol 0.035 mg and norethindrone 0.5 mg [21 light yellow tablets] and 7 white inactive tablets (28s)

Nortrel™ 1/35 mg:
- Ethinyl estradiol 0.035 mg and norethindrone 1 mg [yellow tablets] (21s)
- Ethinyl estradiol 0.035 mg and norethindrone 1 mg [21 yellow tablets] and 7 white inactive tablets (28s)

Ortho-Novum® 1/35 21: Ethinyl estradiol 0.035 mg and norethindrone 1 mg [peach tablets] (21s)

Ortho-Novum® 1/35 28: Ethinyl estradiol 0.035 mg and norethindrone 1 mg [21 peach tablets] and 7 green inactive tablets (28s)

Ovcon® 35 21-day: Ethinyl estradiol 0.035 mg and norethindrone 0.4 mg [peach tablets] (21s)

Ovcon® 35 28-day: Ethinyl estradiol 0.035 mg and norethindrone 0.4 mg [21 peach tablets] and 7 green inactive tablets (28s)

Ovcon® 50: Ethinyl estradiol 0.05 mg and norethindrone 1 mg [21 yellow tablets] and 7 green inactive tablets (28s)

Biphasic formulations:

Jenest™-28:
- Day 1-7: Ethinyl estradiol 0.035 mg and norethindrone 0.5 mg [7 white tablets]
- Day 8-21: Ethinyl estradiol 0.035 mg and norethindrone 1 mg [14 peach tablets]
- Day 22-28: 7 green inactive tablets (28s)

Necon® 10/11-21:
- Day 1-10: Ethinyl estradiol 0.035 mg and norethindrone 0.5 mg [10 light yellow tablets]
- Day 11-21: Ethinyl estradiol 0.035 mg and norethindrone 1 mg [11 dark yellow tablets] (21s)

Necon® 10/11-28:
- Day 1-10: Ethinyl estradiol 0.035 mg and norethindrone 0.5 mg [10 light yellow tablets]
- Day 11-21: Ethinyl estradiol 0.035 mg and norethindrone 1 mg [11 dark yellow tablets]
- Day 22-28: 7 white inactive tablets (28s)

Ortho-Novum® 10/11-21:
- Day 1-10: Ethinyl estradiol 0.035 mg and norethindrone 0.5 mg [10 white tablets]
- Day 11-21: Ethinyl estradiol 0.035 mg and norethindrone 1 mg [11 peach tablet] (21s)

Ortho-Novum® 10/11-28:
- Day 1-10: Ethinyl estradiol 0.035 mg and norethindrone 0.5 mg [10 white tablets]
- Day 11-21: Ethinyl estradiol 0.035 mg and norethindrone 1 mg [11 peach tablet]
- Day 22-28: 7 green inactive tablets (28s)

Triphasic formulations:

Estrostep® 21:
- Day 1-5: Ethinyl estradiol 0.02 mg and norethindrone acetate 1mg [5 white triangular tablets]
- Day 6-12: Ethinyl estradiol 0.03 mg and norethindrone acetate 1 mg [7 white square tablets]
- Day 13-21: Ethinyl estradiol 0.035 mg and norethindrone acetate 1 mg [9 white round tablets] (21s)

Estrostep® Fe:
- Day 1-5: Ethinyl estradiol 0.02 mg and norethindrone acetate 1 mg [5 white triangular tablets]
- Day 6-12: Ethinyl estradiol 0.03 mg and norethindrone acetate 1 mg [7 white square tablets]
- Day 13-21: Ethinyl estradiol 0.035 mg and norethindrone acetate 1 mg [9 white round tablets]
- Day 22-28: Ferrous fumarate 75 mg [7 brown tablets] (28s)

Ortho-Novum® 7/7/7 21:
- Day 1-7: Ethinyl estradiol 0.035 mg and norethindrone 0.5 mg [7 white tablets]
- Day 8-14: Ethinyl estradiol 0.035 mg and norethindrone 0.75 mg [7 light peach tablets]
- Day 15-21: Ethinyl estradiol 0.035 mg and norethindrone 1 mg [7 peach tablet] (21s)

Ortho-Novum® 7/7/7 28:
- Day 1-7: Ethinyl estradiol 0.035 mg and norethindrone 0.5 mg [7 white tablets]
- Day 8-14: Ethinyl estradiol 0.035 mg and norethindrone 0.75 mg [7 light peach tablets]
- Day 15-21: Ethinyl estradiol 0.035 mg and norethindrone 1 mg [7 peach tablet]
- Day 22-28: 7 green inactive tablets (28s)

Tri-Norinyl® 28:
- Day 1-7: Ethinyl estradiol 0.035 mg and norethindrone 0.5 mg [7 blue tablets]
- Day 8-16: Ethinyl estradiol 0.035 mg and norethindrone 1 mg [9 yellow-green tablets]
- Day 17-21: Ethinyl estradiol 0.035 mg and norethindrone 0.5 mg [5 blue tablets]
- Day 22-28: 7 orange inactive tablets (28s)

Ethinyl Estradiol and Norgestimate

(ETH in il es tra DYE ole & nor JES ti mate)

U.S. Brand Names Ortho-Cyclen®; Ortho Tri-Cyclen®

Canadian Brand Names Cyclen®; Tri-Cyclen®

Synonyms Ethinyl Estradiol and NGM; Norgestimate and Ethinyl Estradiol

Therapeutic Category Contraceptive, Oral

Use Prevention of pregnancy; treatment of acne

Pregnancy Risk Factor X

Pregnancy/Breast-Feeding Implications Breast-feeding: Not recommended; excreted in breast milk; combination oral contraceptives decrease the quality and quantity of breast milk.

Pregnancy should be ruled out prior to treatment and discontinued if pregnancy occurs. In general, the use of combination hormonal contraceptives when inadvertently taken early in pregnancy have not been associated with teratogenic effects. Due to increased risk of thromboembolism postpartum, combination hormonal contraceptives should not be started earlier than 4-6 weeks following delivery.

Contraindications Hypersensitivity to ethinyl estradiol, norgestimate, or any component of the formulation; thrombophlebitis or thromboembolic disorders (current or history of), cerebral vascular disease, coronary artery disease, valvular heart disease with complications, severe (Continued)

Ethinyl Estradiol and Norgestimate *(Continued)*

hypertension; severe headache with focal neurological symptoms; known or suspected breast carcinoma, endometrial cancer, estrogen-dependent neoplasms, undiagnosed abnormal genital bleeding; hepatic dysfunction or tumor, cholestatic jaundice of pregnancy, jaundice with prior combination hormonal contraceptive use; heavy smoking (≥15 cigarettes/day) in patients >35 years of age; pregnancy

Warnings/Precautions Combination hormonal contraceptives do not protect against HIV infection or other sexually-transmitted diseases. The risk of cardiovascular side effects increases in women who smoke cigarettes, especially those who are >35 years of age; women who use combination hormonal contraceptives should be strongly advised not to smoke. Combination hormonal contraceptives may lead to increased risk of myocardial infarction, use with caution in patients with risk factors for coronary artery disease. May increase the risk of thromboembolism. Combination hormonal contraceptives may have a dose-related risk of vascular disease, hypertension, and gallbladder disease. Women with hypertension should be encouraged to use a nonhormonal form of contraception. The use of combination hormonal contraceptives has been associated with a slight increase in frequency of breast cancer, however, studies are not consistent. Combination hormonal contraceptives may cause glucose intolerance. Retinal thrombosis has been reported (rarely). Use with caution in patients with renal disease, conditions that may be aggravated by fluid retention, depression, or history of migraine. Not for use prior to menarche.

The minimum dosage combination of estrogen/progestin that will effectively treat the individual patient should be used. New patients should be started on products containing <50 mcg of estrogen per tablet.

Acne: For use only in females ≥15 years, who also desire combination hormonal contraceptive therapy, are unresponsive to topical treatments, and have no contraindications to combination hormonal contraceptive use; treatment must continue for at least 6 months.

Adverse Reactions Frequency not defined.

Cardiovascular: Arterial thromboembolism, cerebral hemorrhage, cerebral thrombosis, edema, hypertension, mesenteric thrombosis, myocardial infarction

Central nervous system: Depression, dizziness, headache, migraine, nervousness, premenstrual syndrome, stroke

Dermatologic: Acne, erythema multiforme, erythema nodosum, hirsutism, loss of scalp hair, melasma (may persist), rash (allergic)

Endocrine & metabolic: Amenorrhea, breakthrough bleeding, breast enlargement, breast secretion, breast tenderness, carbohydrate intolerance, lactation decreased (postpartum), glucose tolerance decreased, libido changes, menstrual flow changes, sex hormone-binding globulins (SHBG) increased, spotting, temporary infertility (following discontinuation), thyroid-binding globulin increased, triglycerides increased

Gastrointestinal: Abdominal cramps, appetite changes, bloating, cholestasis, colitis, gallbladder disease, jaundice, nausea, vomiting, weight gain/loss

Genitourinary: Cervical erosion changes, cervical secretion changes, cystitis-like syndrome, vaginal candidiasis, vaginitis

Hematologic: Antithrombin III decreased, folate levels decreased, hemolytic uremic syndrome, norepinephrine induced platelet aggregability increased, porphyria, prothrombin increased; factors VII, VIII, IX, and X increased

Hepatic: Benign liver tumors, Budd-Chiari syndrome, cholestatic jaundice, hepatic adenomas

Local: Thrombophlebitis

Ocular: Cataracts, change in corneal curvature (steepening), contact lens intolerance, optic neuritis, retinal thrombosis

Renal: Impaired renal function

Respiratory: Pulmonary thromboembolism

Miscellaneous: Hemorrhagic eruption

Overdosage/Toxicology Toxicity is unlikely following single exposures of excessive doses. May cause withdrawal bleeding in females. Treatment following emesis and charcoal administration should be supportive and symptomatic.

Drug Interactions

Cytochrome P450 Effect: Ethinyl estradiol: CYP3A3/4 enzyme substrate

Increased Effect/Toxicity: Acetaminophen and ascorbic acid may increase plasma levels of estrogen component. Atorvastatin and indinavir increase plasma levels of combination hormonal contraceptives. Combination hormonal contraceptives increase the plasma levels of alprazolam, chlordiazepoxide, cyclosporine, diazepam, prednisolone, selegiline, theophylline, tricyclic antidepressants. Combination hormonal contraceptives may increase (or decrease) the effects of coumarin derivatives.

Decreased Effect: Combination hormonal contraceptives may decrease plasma levels of acetaminophen, clofibric acid, lorazepam, morphine, oxazepam, salicylic acid, temazepam. Contraceptive effect decreased by acitretin, aminoglutethimide, amprenavir, anticonvulsants, griseofulvin, lopinavir, nelfinavir, nevirapine, penicillins (effect not consistent), rifampin, ritonavir, tetracyclines (effect not consistent). Combination hormonal contraceptives may decrease (or increase) the effects of coumarin derivatives.

Ethanol/Nutrition/Herb Interactions

Food: CNS effects of caffeine may be enhanced if combination hormonal contraceptives are used concurrently with caffeine. Grapefruit juice increases ethinyl estradiol concentrations and would be expected to increase progesterone serum levels as well; clinical implications are unclear.

Herb/Nutraceutical: St John's wort may decrease the effectiveness of combination hormonal contraceptives by inducing hepatic enzymes. Avoid dong quai and black cohosh (have estrogen activity). Avoid saw palmetto, red clover, ginseng.

Stability Store at controlled room temperature of 25°C (77°F).

Mechanism of Action Combination hormonal contraceptives inhibit ovulation via a negative feedback mechanism on the hypothalamus, which alters the normal pattern of gonadotropin secretion of a follicle-stimulating hormone (FSH) and luteinizing hormone by the anterior pituitary. The follicular phase FSH and midcycle surge of gonadotropins are inhibited. In addition, combination hormonal contraceptives produce alterations in the genital tract, including changes in the cervical mucus, rendering it unfavorable for sperm penetration even if ovulation occurs. Changes in the endometrium may also occur, producing an unfavorable environment for nidation. Combination hormonal contraceptive drugs may alter the tubal transport of the ova through the fallopian tubes. Progestational agents may also alter sperm fertility.

Pharmacodynamics/Kinetics

Ethinyl estradiol: See Ethinyl Estradiol monograph.

Norgestimate:

Absorption: Well absorbed

Protein binding: To albumin and sex-hormone-binding globulin (SHBG); SHBG capacity is affected by plasma ethinyl estradiol levels

Metabolism: Hepatic; forms 17-deacetylnorgestimate (major active metabolite) and other metabolites

Half-life elimination: 17-deacetylnorgestimate: 12-30 hours

Excretion: Urine and feces

Usual Dosage Oral:

Children ≥15 years and Adults: Female: Acne (Ortho Tri-Cyclen®): Refer to dosing for contraception

Adults: Female:

Contraception:

Schedule 1 (Sunday starter): Dose begins on first Sunday after onset of menstruation; if the menstrual period starts on Sunday, take first tablet that very same day. **With a Sunday start, an additional method of contraception should be used until after the first 7 days of consecutive administration.**

For 21-tablet package: Dosage is 1 tablet daily for 21 consecutive days, followed by 7 days off of the medication; a new course begins on the 8th day after the last tablet is taken.

For 28-tablet package: Dosage is 1 tablet daily without interruption.

Schedule 2 (Day 1 starter): Dose starts on first day of menstrual cycle taking 1 tablet daily.

For 21-tablet package: Dosage is 1 tablet daily for 21 consecutive days, followed by 7 days off of the medication; a new course begins on the 8th day after the last tablet is taken.

For 28-tablet package: Dosage is 1 tablet daily without interruption.

If all doses have been taken on schedule and one menstrual period is missed, continue dosing cycle. If two consecutive menstrual periods are missed, pregnancy test is required before new dosing cycle is started.

Missed doses **monophasic formulations** (refer to package insert for complete information):

One dose missed: Take as soon as remembered or take 2 tablets next day

Two consecutive doses missed in the first 2 weeks: Take 2 tablets as soon as remembered or 2 tablets next 2 days. **An additional method of contraception should be used for 7 days after missed dose.**

Two consecutive doses missed in week 3 or three consecutive doses missed at any time: **An additional method of contraception must be used for 7 days after a missed dose:**

Schedule 1 (Sunday starter): Continue dose of 1 tablet daily until Sunday, then discard the rest of the pack, and a new pack should be started that same day.

Schedule 2 (Day 1 starter): Current pack should be discarded, and a new pack should be started that same day.

Missed doses **biphasic/triphasic formulations** (refer to package insert for complete information):

One dose missed: Take as soon as remembered or take 2 tablets next day.

Two consecutive doses missed in week 1 or week 2 of the pack: Take 2 tablets as soon as remembered and 2 tablets the next day. Resume taking 1 tablet daily until the pack is empty. **An additional method of contraception must be used for 7 days after a missed dose.**

Two consecutive doses missed in week 3 of the pack. **An additional method of contraception must be used for 7 days after a missed dose.**

Schedule 1 (Sunday starter): Take 1 tablet every day until Sunday. Discard the remaining pack and start a new pack of pills on the same day.

Schedule 2 (Day 1 starter): Discard the remaining pack and start a new pack the same day.

Three or more consecutive doses missed. **An additional method of contraception must be used for 7 days after a missed dose.**

Schedule 1 (Sunday starter): Take 1 tablet every day until Sunday; on Sunday, discard the pack and start a new pack.

Schedule 2 (Day 1 starter): Discard the remaining pack and begin new pack of tablets starting on the same day.

Dosage adjustment in renal impairment: Specific guidelines not available; use with caution.

Dosage adjustment in hepatic impairment: Contraindicated in patients with hepatic impairment.

Dietary Considerations Should be taken at same time each day.

Administration Administer at the same time each day.

Monitoring Parameters Blood pressure, breast exam, Pap smear, and pregnancy; lipid profiles in patients being treated for hyperlipidemias

Patient Information Women should inform their physicians if signs or symptoms of any of the following occur: thromboembolic or thrombotic disorders including sudden severe headache or vomiting, disturbance of vision or speech, loss of vision, numbness or weakness in an extremity, sharp or crushing chest pain, calf pain, shortness of breath, severe abdominal pain or mass, mental depression or unusual bleeding. Women should be advised that when any doses are missed, alternative contraceptive methods should be used for the next 2 days or until 2 days into the new cycle; women should discontinue taking the medication if they suspect they are pregnant or become pregnant.

(Continued)

Ethinyl Estradiol and Norgestimate *(Continued)*

Nursing Implications Women should inform their physicians if signs or symptoms of any of the following occur: thromboembolic or thrombotic disorders including sudden severe headache or vomiting, disturbance of vision or speech, loss of vision, numbness or weakness in an extremity, sharp or crushing chest pain, calf pain, shortness of breath, severe abdominal pain or mass, mental depression or unusual bleeding. Women should be advised to read package insert for missed-dose instructions. Women should discontinue taking the medication if they suspect they are pregnant or become pregnant.

Dosage Forms Tablet:

Monophasic formulation (Ortho-Cyclen®): Ethinyl estradiol 0.035 mg and norgestimate 0.25 mg [21 blue tablets] and 7 green inactive tablets (28s)

Triphasic formulation (Ortho Tri-Cyclen®):

Day 1-7: Ethinyl estradiol 0.035 mg and norgestimate 0.18 mg [7 white tablets]

Day 8-14: Ethinyl estradiol 0.035 mg and norgestimate 0.215 mg [7 light blue tablets]

Day 15-21: Ethinyl estradiol 0.035 mg and norgestimate 0.25 mg [7 blue tablets]

Day 22-28: 7 green inactive tablets

Ethinyl Estradiol and Norgestrel (ETH in il es tra DYE ole & nor JES trel)

U.S. Brand Names Cryselle™; Lo/Ovral®; Low-Ogestrel®; Ogestrel®; Ovral®

Canadian Brand Names Ovral®

Synonyms Morning After Pill; Norgestrel and Ethinyl Estradiol

Therapeutic Category Contraceptive, Emergency; Contraceptive, Oral (Intermediate Potency Estrogen, High Potency Progestin); Contraceptive, Oral (Low Potency Estrogen, Intermediate Potency Progestin); Contraceptive, Oral (Monophasic); Estrogen Derivative, Oral; Progestin

Use Prevention of pregnancy; postcoital contraceptive or "morning after" pill

Unlabeled/Investigational Use Treatment of hypermenorrhea, endometriosis, female hypogonadism

Pregnancy Risk Factor X

Pregnancy/Breast-Feeding Implications Pregnancy should be ruled out prior to treatment and discontinued if pregnancy occurs. In general, the use of combination hormonal contraceptives when inadvertently taken early in pregnancy have not been associated with teratogenic effects. Due to increased risk of thromboembolism postpartum, combination hormonal contraceptives should not be started earlier than 4-6 weeks following delivery.

Contraindications Hypersensitivity to ethinyl estradiol, norgestrel, or any component of the formulation; thrombophlebitis or thromboembolic disorders (current or history of), cerebral vascular disease, coronary artery disease, valvular heart disease with complications, severe hypertension; diabetes mellitus with vascular involvement; severe headache with focal neurological symptoms; known or suspected breast carcinoma, endometrial cancer, estrogen-dependent neoplasms, undiagnosed abnormal genital bleeding; hepatic dysfunction or tumor, cholestatic jaundice of pregnancy, jaundice with prior combination hormonal contraceptive use; major surgery with prolonged immobilization; heavy smoking (≥15 cigarettes/day) in patients >35 years of age; pregnancy

Warnings/Precautions Combination hormonal contraceptives do not protect against HIV infection or other sexually-transmitted diseases. The risk of cardiovascular side effects increases in women who smoke cigarettes, especially those who are >35 years of age; women who use combination hormonal contraceptives should be strongly advised not to smoke. Combination hormonal contraceptives may lead to increased risk of myocardial infarction, use with caution in patients with risk factors for coronary artery disease. May increase the risk of thromboembolism. Combination hormonal contraceptives may have a dose-related risk of vascular disease, hypertension, and gallbladder disease. Women with hypertension should be encouraged to use another form of contraception. The use of combination hormonal contraceptives has been associated with a slight increase in frequency of breast cancer, however, studies are not consistent. Combination hormonal contraceptives may cause glucose intolerance. Retinal thrombosis has been reported (rarely). Use with caution in patients with renal disease, conditions that may be aggravated by fluid retention, depression, or history of migraine. Not for use prior to menarche.

The minimum dosage combination of estrogen/progestin that will effectively treat the individual patient should be used. New patients should be started on products containing <50 mcg of estrogen per tablet.

Adverse Reactions Frequency not defined.

Cardiovascular: Arterial thromboembolism, cerebral hemorrhage, cerebral thrombosis, edema, hypertension, mesenteric thrombosis, myocardial infarction

Central nervous system: Depression, dizziness, headache, migraine, nervousness, premenstrual syndrome, stroke

Dermatologic: Acne, erythema multiforme, erythema nodosum, hirsutism, loss of scalp hair, melasma (may persist), rash (allergic)

Endocrine & metabolic: Amenorrhea, breakthrough bleeding, breast enlargement, breast secretion, breast tenderness, carbohydrate intolerance, lactation decreased (postpartum), glucose tolerance decreased, libido changes, menstrual flow changes, sex hormone-binding globulins (SHBG) increased, spotting, temporary infertility (following discontinuation), thyroid-binding globulin increased, triglycerides increased

Gastrointestinal: Abdominal cramps, appetite changes, bloating, cholestasis, colitis, gallbladder disease, jaundice, nausea, vomiting, weight gain/loss

Genitourinary: Cervical erosion changes, cervical secretion changes, cystitis-like syndrome, vaginal candidiasis, vaginitis

Hematologic: Antithrombin III decreased, folate levels decreased, hemolytic uremic syndrome, norepinephrine induced platelet aggregability increased, porphyria, prothrombin increased; factors VII, VIII, IX, and X

Hepatic: Benign liver tumors, Budd-Chiari syndrome, cholestatic jaundice, hepatic adenomas

Local: Thrombophlebitis

Ocular: Cataracts, change in corneal curvature (steepening), contact lens intolerance, optic neuritis, retinal thrombosis

Renal: Impaired renal function

Respiratory: Pulmonary thromboembolism

Miscellaneous: Hemorrhagic eruption

Overdosage/Toxicology Toxicity is unlikely following single exposures of excessive doses. May cause withdrawal bleeding in females. Treatment following emesis and charcoal administration should be supportive and symptomatic.

Drug Interactions

Cytochrome P450 Effect: Ethinyl estradiol and norgestrel: CYP3A3/4 enzyme substrates

Increased Effect/Toxicity: Acetaminophen and ascorbic acid may increase plasma levels of estrogen component. Atorvastatin and indinavir increase plasma levels of combination hormonal contraceptives. Combination hormonal contraceptives increase the plasma levels of alprazolam, chlordiazepoxide, cyclosporine, diazepam, prednisolone, selegiline, theophylline, tricyclic antidepressants. Combination hormonal contraceptives may increase (or decrease) the effects of coumarin derivatives.

Decreased Effect: Combination hormonal contraceptives may decrease plasma levels of acetaminophen, clofibric acid, lorazepam, morphine, oxazepam, salicylic acid, temazepam. Contraceptive effect decreased by acitretin, aminoglutethimide, amprenavir, anticonvulsants, griseofulvin, lopinavir, nelfinavir, nevirapine, penicillins (effect not consistent), rifampin, ritonavir, tetracyclines (effect not consistent). Combination hormonal contraceptives may decrease (or increase) the effects of coumarin derivatives.

Ethanol/Nutrition/Herb Interactions

Food: CNS effects of caffeine may be enhanced if combination hormonal contraceptives are used concurrently with caffeine. Grapefruit juice increases ethinyl estradiol concentrations and would be expected to increase progesterone serum levels as well; clinical implications are unclear.

Herb/Nutraceutical: St John's wort may decrease the effectiveness of combination hormonal contraceptive by inducing hepatic enzymes. Avoid dong quai and black cohosh (have estrogen activity). Avoid saw palmetto, red clover, ginseng.

Stability Store at controlled room temperature of 25°C (77°F).

Mechanism of Action Combination hormonal contraceptives inhibit ovulation via a negative feedback mechanism on the hypothalamus, which alters the normal pattern of gonadotropin secretion of a follicle-stimulating hormone (FSH) and luteinizing hormone by the anterior pituitary. The follicular phase FSH and midcycle surge of gonadotropins are inhibited. In addition, combination hormonal contraceptives produce alterations in the genital tract, including changes in the cervical mucus, rendering it unfavorable for sperm penetration even if ovulation occurs. Changes in the endometrium may also occur, producing an unfavorable environment for nidation. Combination hormonal contraceptive drugs may alter the tubal transport of the ova through the fallopian tubes. Progestational agents may also alter sperm fertility.

Pharmacodynamics/Kinetics See individual agents.

Usual Dosage Oral: Adults: Female:

Contraception:

Schedule 1 (Sunday starter): Dose begins on first Sunday after onset of menstruation; if the menstrual period starts on Sunday, take first tablet that very same day. **With a Sunday start, an additional method of contraception should be used until after the first 7 days of consecutive administration.**

For 21-tablet package: Dosage is 1 tablet daily for 21 consecutive days, followed by 7 days off of the medication; a new course begins on the 8th day after the last tablet is taken.

For 28-tablet package: Dosage is 1 tablet daily without interruption.

Schedule 2 (Day 1 starter): Dose starts on first day of menstrual cycle taking 1 tablet daily.

For 21-tablet package: Dosage is 1 tablet daily for 21 consecutive days, followed by 7 days off of the medication; a new course begins on the 8th day after the last tablet is taken.

For 28-tablet package: Dosage is 1 tablet daily without interruption.

If all doses have been taken on schedule and one menstrual period is missed, continue dosing cycle. If two consecutive menstrual periods are missed, pregnancy test is required before new dosing cycle is started.

Missed doses **monophasic formulations** (refer to package insert for complete information):

One dose missed: Take as soon as remembered or take 2 tablets next day

Two consecutive doses missed in the first 2 weeks: Take 2 tablets as soon as remembered or 2 tablets next 2 days. **An additional method of contraception should be used for 7 days after missed dose.**

Two consecutive doses missed in week 3 or three consecutive doses missed at any time:

Schedule 1 (Sunday starter): Continue to take 1 tablet daily until Sunday, then discard the rest of the pack, and a new pack is started that same day.

Schedule 2 (Day 1 starter): Current pack should be discarded, and a new pack started that same day. **An additional method of contraception should be used for 7 days after missed dose.**

Postcoital contraception:

Ethinyl estradiol 0.03 mg and norgestrel 0.3 mg formulation: 4 tablets within 72 hours of unprotected intercourse and 4 tablets 12 hours after first dose

Ethinyl estradiol 0.05 mg and norgestrel 0.5 mg formulation: 2 tablets within 72 hours of unprotected intercourse and 2 tablets 12 hours after first dose

Dosage adjustment in renal impairment: Specific guidelines not available; use with caution.

Dosage adjustment in hepatic impairment: Contraindicated in patients with hepatic impairment.

Dietary Considerations Should be taken at same time each day.

Administration Administer at the same time each day.

Monitoring Parameters Blood pressure, breast exam, Pap smear, and pregnancy; lipid profiles in patients being treated for hyperlipidemias

Patient Information Take exactly as directed; use additional method of birth control during first week of administration of first cycle; photosensitivity may occur. Women should inform their physicians if signs or symptoms of any of the following occur: Thromboembolic or

(Continued)

Ethinyl Estradiol and Norgestrel *(Continued)*

thrombotic disorders including sudden severe headache or vomiting, disturbance of vision or speech, loss of vision, numbness or weakness in an extremity, sharp or crushing chest pain, calf pain, shortness of breath, severe abdominal pain or mass, mental depression or unusual bleeding. Women should be advised that when any doses are missed, alternative contraceptive methods should be used for the next 2 days or until 2 days into the new cycle Women should discontinue taking the medication if they suspect they are pregnant or become pregnant.

Nursing Implications Administer at bedtime to minimize occurrence of adverse effects

Dosage Forms Tablet, monophasic formulations:

Cryselle™: Ethinyl estradiol 0.03 mg and norgestrel 0.3 mg [21 white tablets] and 7 light green inactive tablets (28s)

Lo/Ovral®, Low-Ogestrel® 21: Ethinyl estradiol 0.03 mg and norgestrel 0.3 mg [white tablets] (21s)

Low-Ogestrel® 28: Ethinyl estradiol 0.03 mg and norgestrel 0.3 mg [21 white tablets] and 7 peach inactive tablets (28s)

Lo/Ovral® 28: Ethinyl estradiol 0.03 mg and norgestrel 0.3 mg [21 white tablets] and 7 pink inactive tablets (28s)

Ogestrel® 21, Ovral® 21: Ethinyl estradiol 0.05 mg and norgestrel 0.5 mg [white tablets] (21s)

Ogestrel® 28: Ethinyl estradiol 0.05 mg and norgestrel 0.5 mg [21 white tablets] and 7 peach inactive tablets (28s)

Ovral® 28: Ethinyl estradiol 0.05 mg and norgestrel 0.5 mg [21 white tablets] and 7 pink inactive tablets (28s)

♦ **Ethiofos** *see Amifostine on page 67*

Ethionamide *(e thye on AM ide)*

Related Information

Antimicrobial Drugs of Choice *on page 1588*

Tuberculosis Prophylaxis *on page 1572*

Tuberculosis Treatment Guidelines *on page 1612*

U.S. Brand Names Trecator®-SC

Canadian Brand Names Trecator®-SC

Therapeutic Category Antitubercular Agent

Use Treatment of tuberculosis and other mycobacterial diseases, in conjunction with other antituberculosis agents, when first-line agents have failed or resistance has been demonstrated

Pregnancy Risk Factor C

Contraindications Hypersensitivity to ethionamide or any component of the formulation; severe hepatic impairment

Warnings/Precautions Use with caution in patients receiving cycloserine or isoniazid, in diabetics

Adverse Reactions Frequency not defined.

Cardiovascular: Postural hypotension

Central nervous system: Psychiatric disturbances, drowsiness, dizziness, seizures, headache

Dermatologic: Rash, alopecia

Endocrine & metabolic: Hypothyroidism or goiter, hypoglycemia, gynecomastia

Gastrointestinal: Metallic taste, diarrhea, anorexia, nausea, vomiting, stomatitis, abdominal pain

Hematologic: Thrombocytopenia

Hepatic: Hepatitis (5%), jaundice

Neuromuscular & skeletal: Peripheral neuritis, weakness (common)

Ocular: Optic neuritis, blurred vision

Respiratory: Olfactory disturbances

Overdosage/Toxicology Symptoms include peripheral neuropathy, anorexia, and joint pain. Following GI decontamination, treatment is supportive. Pyridoxine may be given to prevent peripheral neuropathy.

Drug Interactions

Increased Effect/Toxicity: Cycloserine and isoniazid; increased hepatotoxicity with rifampin

Mechanism of Action Inhibits peptide synthesis

Pharmacodynamics/Kinetics

Absorption: Rapid

Distribution: Crosses placenta

Protein binding: 10%

Bioavailability: 80%

Half-life elimination: 2-3 hours

Time to peak, serum: ~3 hours

Excretion: Urine (as unchanged drug and active and inactive metabolites)

Usual Dosage Oral:

Children: 15-20 mg/kg/day in 2 divided doses, not to exceed 1 g/day

Adults: 500-1000 mg/day in 1-3 divided doses

Dosing adjustment in renal impairment: Cl_{cr} <50 mL/minute: Administer 50% of dose

Dietary Considerations Healthcare provider may recommend an increase in dietary intake of pyridoxine to prevent neurotoxic effects of ethionamide.

Monitoring Parameters Initial and periodic serum ALT and AST

Patient Information Take with meals; notify physician of persistent or severe stomach upset, loss of appetite, or metallic taste; frequent blood tests are needed for monitoring; increase dietary intake of pyridoxine

Nursing Implications

Neurotoxic effects may be relieved by the administration of pyridoxine

Monitor initial and periodic serum ALT and AST

Additional Information Neurotoxic effects may be relieved by the administration of pyridoxine.

Dosage Forms Tablet, sugar coated: 250 mg

◆ **Ethmozine**® *see Moricizine on page 934*

Ethosuximide (eth oh SUKS i mide)
Related Information
Anticonvulsants by Seizure Type *on page 1481*
Epilepsy & Seizure Treatment *on page 1659*
U.S. Brand Names Zarontin®
Canadian Brand Names Zarontin®
Therapeutic Category Anticonvulsant
Use Management of absence (petit mal) seizures
Pregnancy Risk Factor C
Usual Dosage Oral:
Children 3-6 years: Initial: 250 mg/day (or 15 mg/kg/day) in 2 divided doses; increase every 4-7 days; usual maintenance dose: 15-40 mg/kg/day in 2 divided doses
Children >6 years and Adults: Initial: 250 mg twice daily; increase by 250 mg as needed every 4-7 days, up to 1.5 g/day in 2 divided doses; usual maintenance dose: 20-40 mg/kg/day in 2 divided doses
Dosing comment in renal/hepatic dysfunction: Use with caution.
Additional Information Complete prescribing information for this medication should be consulted for additional detail.
Dosage Forms
Capsule: 250 mg
Syrup: 250 mg/5 mL (473 mL) [raspberry flavor]

◆ **Ethoxynaphthamido Penicillin Sodium** *see Nafcillin on page 950*
◆ **Ethyl Aminobenzoate** *see Benzocaine on page 154*
◆ **Ethylenediamine** *see Theophylline Salts on page 1310*
◆ **Ethynodiol Diacetate and Ethinyl Estradiol** *see Ethinyl Estradiol and Ethynodiol Diacetate on page 514*
◆ **Ethyol**® *see Amifostine on page 67*
◆ **Etibi**® **(Can)** *see Ethambutol on page 507*

Etidocaine (e TI doe kane)
U.S. Brand Names Duranest®
Canadian Brand Names Duranest®
Synonyms Etidocaine Hydrochloride
Therapeutic Category Local Anesthetic, Injectable
Use Infiltration anesthesia; peripheral nerve blocks; central neural blocks
Pregnancy Risk Factor B
Usual Dosage Varies with procedure; use 1% for peripheral nerve block, central nerve block, lumbar peridural caudal; use 1.5% for maxillary infiltration or inferior alveolar nerve block; use 1% or 1.5% for intra-abdominal or pelvic surgery, lower limb surgery, or caesarean section
Additional Information Complete prescribing information for this medication should be consulted for additional detail.
Dosage Forms
Injection, as hydrochloride: 1% [10 mg/mL] (30 mL)
Injection, with epinephrine 1:200,000, as hydrochloride: 1% [10 mg/mL] (30 mL); 1.5% [15 mg/mL] (20 mL)

◆ **Etidocaine Hydrochloride** *see Etidocaine on page 531*

Etidronate Disodium (e ti DROE nate dye SOW dee um)
U.S. Brand Names Didronel®
Canadian Brand Names Didronel®
Synonyms EHDP; Sodium Etidronate
Therapeutic Category Antidote, Hypercalcemia; Bisphosphonate Derivative
Use Symptomatic treatment of Paget's disease and heterotopic ossification due to spinal cord injury or after total hip replacement, hypercalcemia associated with malignancy
Pregnancy Risk Factor B (oral); C (parenteral)
Usual Dosage Adults: Oral formulation should be taken on an empty stomach 2 hours before any meal.
Paget's disease: Oral
Initial: 5-10 mg/kg/day (not to exceed 6 months) or 11-20 mg/kg/day (not to exceed 3 months). Doses >10 mg/kg/day are **not** recommended.
Retreatment: Initiate only after etidronate-free period ≥90 days. Monitor patients every 3-6 months. Retreatment regimens are the same as for initial treatment.
Heterotopic ossification: Oral:
Caused by spinal cord injury: 20 mg/kg/day for 2 weeks, then 10 mg/kg/day for 10 weeks; total treatment period: 12 weeks
Complicating total hip replacement: 20 mg/kg/day for 1 month preoperatively then 20 mg/kg/day for 3 months postoperatively; total treatment period is 4 months
Hypercalcemia associated with malignancy:
I.V. (dilute dose in at least 250 mL NS): 7.5 mg/kg/day for 3 days; there should be at least 7 days between courses of treatment
Oral: Start 20 mg/kg/day on the last day of infusion and continue for 30-90 days
Dosing adjustment in renal impairment:
S_{cr} 2.5-5 mg/dL: Use with caution
S_{cr} >5 mg/dL: **Not recommended**
Additional Information Complete prescribing information for this medication should be consulted for additional detail.
(Continued)

Etidronate Disodium (Continued)

Dosage Forms
Injection: 50 mg/mL (6 mL)
Tablet: 200 mg, 400 mg

♦ Etodine® [OTC] see Povidone-Iodine on page 1114

Etodolac (ee toe DOE lak)

Related Information
Nonsteroidal Anti-Inflammatory Agents Comparison on page 1512

U.S. Brand Names Lodine®; Lodine® XL

Canadian Brand Names Apo®-Etodolac; Gen-Etodolac; Lodine®; Utradol™

Synonyms Etodolic Acid

Therapeutic Category Analgesic, Nonsteroidal Anti-inflammatory Drug; Anti-inflammatory Agent; Nonsteroidal Anti-inflammatory Drug (NSAID), Oral

Use Acute and long-term use in the management of signs and symptoms of osteoarthritis and management of pain

Unlabeled/Investigational Use Rheumatoid arthritis

Pregnancy Risk Factor C/D (3rd trimester)

Contraindications Hypersensitivity to etodolac, aspirin, other NSAIDs, or any component of the formulation; active gastric/duodenal ulcer disease; pregnancy (3rd trimester)

Warnings/Precautions Use with caution in patients with congestive heart failure, hypertension, dehydration, decreased renal or hepatic function, history of GI disease (bleeding or ulcers), or those receiving anticoagulants. Elderly are at a high risk for adverse effects from nonsteroidal anti-inflammatory agents. As many as 60% of elderly can develop peptic ulceration and/or hemorrhage asymptomatically.

Use lowest effective dose for shortest period possible. Use of NSAIDs can compromise existing renal function especially when Cl_{cr} is <30 mL/minute. CNS adverse effects such as confusion, agitation, and hallucination are generally seen in overdose or high-dose situations; however, elderly may demonstrate these adverse effects at lower doses than younger adults. Withhold for at least 4-6 half-lives prior to surgical or dental procedures.

Adverse Reactions
1% to 10%:
Central nervous system: Headache, nervousness
Dermatologic: Itching, rash
Endocrine & metabolic: Fluid retention
Gastrointestinal: Abdominal cramps, heartburn, indigestion, nausea, vomiting, gastritis, GI hemorrhage, GI ulceration
Otic: Tinnitus
<1% (Limited to important or life-threatening): Acute renal failure, agranulocytosis, anemia, angioedema, arrhythmia, bone marrow suppression, congestive heart failure, dyspnea, erythema multiforme, exfoliative dermatitis, hemolytic anemia, hepatitis, hypertension, leukopenia, peripheral neuropathy, Stevens-Johnson syndrome, syncope, tachycardia, thrombocytopenia, toxic amblyopia, toxic epidermal necrolysis, urticaria

Overdosage/Toxicology Symptoms include acute renal failure, vomiting, drowsiness, and leukocytosis. Management of nonsteroidal anti-inflammatory drug (NSAID) intoxication is primarily supportive and symptomatic. Fluid therapy is commonly effective in managing hypotension that may occur following an acute NSAID overdose, except when due to acute blood loss.

Drug Interactions
Increased Effect/Toxicity: Etodolac may increase effect/toxicity of aspirin (GI irritation), lithium, methotrexate, digoxin, cyclosporine (nephrotoxicity), and warfarin (bleeding).
Decreased Effect: Decreased effect with aspirin. May reduce effect of some diuretics and antihypertensive effect of β-blockers.

Ethanol/Nutrition/Herb Interactions
Ethanol: Avoid ethanol (may enhance gastric mucosal irritation).
Food: Etodolac peak serum levels may be decreased if taken with food.
Herb/Nutraceutical: Avoid cat's claw, dong quai, evening primrose, feverfew, garlic, ginger, ginkgo, red clover, horse chestnut, green tea, ginseng (all have additional antiplatelet activity)

Stability Protect from moisture

Mechanism of Action Inhibits prostaglandin synthesis by decreasing the activity of the enzyme, cyclo-oxygenase, which results in decreased formation of prostaglandin precursors

Pharmacodynamics/Kinetics
Onset of action: Analgesic: 2-4 hours; Maximum anti-inflammatory effect: A few days
Absorption: Well absorbed
Distribution: V_d: 0.4 L/kg
Protein binding: High
Metabolism: Hepatic
Half-life elimination: 7 hours
Time to peak, serum: 1 hour
Excretion: Urine

Usual Dosage Single dose of 76-100 mg is comparable to the analgesic effect of aspirin 650 mg; in patients ≥65 years, no substantial differences in the pharmacokinetics or side-effects profile were seen compared with the general population

Adults: Oral:
Acute pain: 200-400 mg every 6-8 hours, as needed, not to exceed total daily doses of 1200 mg; for patients weighing <60 kg, total daily dose should not exceed 20 mg/kg/day
Osteoarthritis: Initial: 800-1200 mg/day given in divided doses: 400 mg 2 or 3 times/day; 300 mg 2, 3, or 4 times/day; 200 mg 3 or 4 times/day; total daily dose should not exceed 1200 mg; for patients weighing <60 kg, total daily dose should not exceed 20 mg/kg/day
Lodine® XL: 400-1000 mg once daily

Dietary Considerations May be taken with food to decrease GI distress.

Monitoring Parameters Monitor CBC, liver enzymes; in patients receiving diuretics, monitor urine output and BUN/serum creatinine

Test Interactions False-positive for urinary bilirubin and ketone ↑ bleeding time

Patient Information Do not crush tablets; take with food, milk, or water; report any signs of blood in stool

Dosage Forms

Capsule (Lodine®): 200 mg, 300 mg

Tablet (Lodine®): 400 mg, 500 mg

Tablet, extended release (Lodine® XL): 400 mg, 500 mg, 600 mg

♦ **Etodolic Acid** *see* Etodolac *on page 532*

Etomidate (e TOM i date)

Related Information

Adult ACLS Algorithms *on page 1632*

U.S. Brand Names Amidate®

Canadian Brand Names Amidate®

Therapeutic Category General Anesthetic

Use Induction and maintenance of general anesthesia

Unlabeled/Investigational Use Sedation for diagnosis of seizure foci

Pregnancy Risk Factor C

Contraindications Hypersensitivity to etomidate or any component of the formulation

Warnings/Precautions Consider exogenous corticosteroid replacement in patients undergoing severe stress

Adverse Reactions

>10%:

Gastrointestinal: Nausea, vomiting on emergence from anesthesia

Local: Pain at injection site (30% to 80%)

Neuromuscular & skeletal: Myoclonus (33%), transient skeletal movements, uncontrolled eye movements

1% to 10%: Hiccups

<1% (Limited to important or life-threatening): Apnea, arrhythmias, bradycardia, decreased cortisol synthesis, hypertension, hyperventilation, hypotension, hypoventilation, laryngospasm, tachycardia

Overdosage/Toxicology Symptoms include respiratory arrest and coma. Treatment is supportive.

Drug Interactions

Increased Effect/Toxicity: Fentanyl decreases etomidate elimination. Verapamil may increase the anesthetic and respiratory depressant effects of etomidate.

Stability Store at room temperature.

Mechanism of Action Ultrashort-acting nonbarbiturate hypnotic (benzylimidazole) used for the induction of anesthesia; chemically, it is a carboxylated imidazole which produces a rapid induction of anesthesia with minimal cardiovascular effects; produces EEG burst suppression at high doses

Pharmacodynamics/Kinetics

Onset of action: 30-60 seconds

Peak effect: 1 minute

Duration: 3-5 minutes; terminated by redistribution

Distribution: V_d: 2-4.5 L/kg

Protein binding: 76%;

Metabolism: Hepatic and plasma esterases

Half-life elimination: Terminal: 2.6 hours

Usual Dosage Children >10 years and Adults: I.V.: Initial: 0.2-0.6 mg/kg over 30-60 seconds for induction of anesthesia; maintenance: 5-20 mcg/kg/minute

Monitoring Parameters Cardiac monitoring and blood pressure required

Nursing Implications Store at room temperature.

Additional Information Etomidate decreases cerebral metabolism and cerebral blood flow while maintaining perfusion pressure. Premedication with opioids or benzodiazepines can decrease myoclonus. Etomidate can enhance somatosensory evoked potential recordings.

Dosage Forms Injection: 2 mg/mL (10 mL, 20 mL)

♦ **Etonogestrel and Ethinyl Estradiol** *see* Ethinyl Estradiol and Etonogestrel *on page 516*

♦ **Etopophos®** *see* Etoposide Phosphate *on page 535*

Etoposide (e toe POE side)

U.S. Brand Names Toposar®; VePesid®

Canadian Brand Names VePesid®

Synonyms Epipodophyllotoxin; VP-16; VP-16-213

Therapeutic Category Antineoplastic Agent, Podophyllotoxin Derivative

Use Treatment of lymphomas, ANLL, lung, testicular, bladder, and prostate carcinoma, hepatoma, rhabdomyosarcoma, uterine carcinoma, neuroblastoma, mycosis fungoides, Kaposi's sarcoma, histiocytosis, gestational trophoblastic disease, Ewing's sarcoma, Wilms' tumor, and brain tumors

Pregnancy Risk Factor D

Contraindications Hypersensitivity to etoposide or any component of the formulation; **intrathecal administration**; pregnancy

Warnings/Precautions The U.S. Food and Drug Administration (FDA) currently recommends that procedures for proper handling and disposal of antineoplastic agents be considered. Severe myelosuppression with resulting infection or bleeding may occur.

Dosage should be adjusted in patients with hepatic or renal impairment

(Continued)

Etoposide *(Continued)*

Adverse Reactions

>10%:

Dermatologic: Alopecia (reversible)

Gastrointestinal: Diarrhea, nausea, vomiting severe mucositis (with BMT doses), anorexia

Emetic potential: Moderately low (10% to 30%)

Hematologic: Anemia, leukopenia

WBC: Mild to severe

Platelets: Mild

Onset (days): 10

Nadir (days): granulocytes 7-14 days; platelets 9-16 days

Recovery (days): 21-28

1% to 10%:

Cardiovascular: Hypotension: Related to drug infusion time; may be related to vehicle used in the I.V. preparation (polysorbate 80 plus polyethylene glycol). Best to administer the drug over 1 hour.

Central nervous system: Unusual fatigue

Gastrointestinal: Stomatitis, diarrhea, abdominal pain, hepatic dysfunction

<1% (Limited to important or life-threatening): Tachycardia, neurotoxicity, peripheral neuropathy, toxic hepatitis (with high-dose therapy), flushing and bronchospasm (may be prevented by pretreatment with corticosteroids and antihistamines)

Irritant, thrombophlebitis has been reported

BMT:

Cardiovascular: Hypotension (infusion-related)

Dermatologic: Skin lesions resembling Stevens-Johnson syndrome, alopecia

Endocrine & metabolic: Metabolic acidosis

Gastrointestinal: Severe nausea and vomiting, mucositis

Hepatic: Hepatitis

Miscellaneous: Secondary malignancy, ethanol intoxication

Overdosage/Toxicology Symptoms include bone marrow depression, leukopenia, thrombocytopenia, nausea, and vomiting.

Drug Interactions

Cytochrome P450 Effect: CYP3A3/4 enzyme substrate

Increased Effect/Toxicity: The effects of etoposide may be increased by calcium antagonists (increased effects noted *in vitro*). Cyclosporine may increase the levels of etoposide. Etoposide may increase the effects/toxicity of methotrexate and warfarin. There have been reports of frequent hepatic dysfunction with hyperbilirubinemia, ascites, and thrombocytopenia when etoposide is combined with carmustine.

Ethanol/Nutrition/Herb Interactions

Ethanol: Avoid ethanol (may increase GI irritation).

Food: Administration of food does not affect GI absorption with doses ≤200 mg of injection.

Herb/Nutraceutical: St John's wort may decrease etoposide levels.

Stability

Store intact vials of injection at room temperature and protected from light; injection solution contains polyethylene glycol vehicle with absolute alcohol; store oral capsules under refrigeration

VP-16 should be further diluted in D_5W or NS for administration; diluted solutions have CONCENTRATION-DEPENDENT stability: More concentrated solutions have shorter stability times

At room temperature in D_5W or NS in polyvinyl chloride, the concentration is stable as follows:

0.2 mg/mL: 96 hours

0.4 mg/mL: 48 hours

0.6 mg/mL: 8 hours

1 mg/mL: 2 hours

2 mg/mL: 1 hour

20 mg/mL (undiluted): 24 hours

Y-site compatible with carboplatin, cytarabine, daunorubicin, mesna

Standard I.V. dilution:

Lower dose regimens (<1 g/dose):

Doses may be diluted in 100-1000 mL of D_5W or NS

If the concentration is less than or equal to 0.6 mg/mL, the bag should be mixed with the appropriate expiration dating

If the concentration is >0.6 mg/mL, the concentration is highly unstable and a syringe of UNDILUTED etoposide accompanied with the appropriate volume of diluent will be sent to the nursing unit to be mixed by the nursing staff just prior to administration

High dose regimens (>1g/dose):

Total dose should be drawn into an empty Viaflex® container and the appropriate amount of diluent (for a final concentration of 1 mg/mL) will be sent

Use the **2-Channel Pump Method**: Instill all of the etoposide dose into one viaflex container (concentration = 20 mg/mL). Infuse this into one channel (Baxter Flow-Guard 6300 Dual Channel Volumetric Infusion Pump - or any 2-channel infusion pump that does not require a "hard" plastic cassette). Infuse the indicated diluent (ie, D_5W or NS) at a rate of at least 20 times the infusion rate of the etoposide to simulate a 1 mg/mL concentration in the line. The etoposide should be Y-sited into the port most proximal to the patient. A 0.22 micron filter should be attached to the line after the Y-site and before entry into the patient.

Mechanism of Action Etoposide does not inhibit microtubular assembly. It has been shown to delay transit of cells through the S phase and arrest cells in late S or early G_2 phase. The drug may inhibit mitochondrial transport at the NADH dehydrogenase level or inhibit uptake of nucleosides into HeLa cells. Etoposide is a topoisomerase II inhibitor and appears to cause DNA strand breaks.

Pharmacodynamics/Kinetics

Absorption: Oral: 25% to 75%; significant inter- and intrapatient variation

Distribution: Average V_d: 3-36 L/m²; poor penetration across the blood-brain barrier; CSF concentrations <10% of plasma concentrations

Protein binding: 94% to 97%

Metabolism: Hepatic to hydroxy acid and cislactone metabolites

Half-life elimination: Terminal: 4-15 hours; Children: Normal renal/hepatic function: 6-8 hours

Time to peak, serum: Oral: 1-1.5 hours

Excretion: Adults: Urine (56%, 23% as unchanged drug) within 120 hours, feces (44%); Children: Urine (≤55% as unchanged drug)

Usual Dosage Refer to individual protocols:

Children: I.V.: 60-120 mg/m²/day for 3-5 days every 3-6 weeks

AML:

Remission induction: 150 mg/m²/day for 2-3 days for 2-3 cycles

Intensification or consolidation: 250 mg/m²/day for 3 days, courses 2-5

Brain tumor: 150 mg/m²/day on days 2 and 3 of treatment course

Neuroblastoma: 100 mg/m²/day over 1 hour on days 1-5 of cycle; repeat cycle every 4 weeks

BMT conditioning regimen used in patients with rhabdomyosarcoma or neuroblastoma: I.V. continuous infusion: 160 mg/m²/day for 4 days

Conditioning regimen for allogenic BMT: 60 mg/kg/dose as a single dose

Adults:

Small cell lung cancer:

Oral: Twice the I.V. dose rounded to the nearest 50 mg given once daily if total dose ≤400 mg or in divided doses if >400 mg

I.V.: 35 mg/m²/day for 4 days or 50 mg/m²/day for 5 days every 3-4 weeks total dose ≤400 mg/day or in divided doses if >400 mg/day

IVPB: 60-100 mg/m²/day for 3 days (with cisplatin)

CIV: 500 mg/m² over 24 hours every 3 weeks

Testicular cancer:

IVPB: 50-100 mg/m²/day for 5 days repeated every 3-4 weeks

I.V.: 100 mg/m² every other day for 3 doses repeated every 3-4 weeks

BMT/relapsed leukemia: I.V.: 2.4-3.5 g/m² or 25-70 mg/kg administered over 4-36 hours

Dosing adjustment in renal impairment:

Cl_{cr} 10-50 mL/minute: Administer 75% of normal dose

Cl_{cr} <10 mL/minute: Administer 50% of normal dose

Hemodialysis: Supplemental dose is not necessary

Peritoneal dialysis: Supplemental dose is not necessary

CAPD effects: Unknown

CAVH effects: Unknown

Dosing adjustment in hepatic impairment:

Bilirubin 1.5-3 mg/dL or AST 60-180 units: Reduce dose by 50%

Bilirubin 3-5 mg/dL or AST >180 units: Reduce by 75%

Bilirubin >5 mg/dL: Do not administer

Administration

Oral: Doses should be rounded to the nearest 50 mg; doses ≤400 mg/day should be given as a single daily dose; doses ≥400 mg/day should be given in 2-4 divided doses.

I.V.: As a bolus or 24-hour continuous infusion; bolus infusions are usually administered over at least 45-60 minutes. Infusion of doses in ≤30 minutes greatly increases the risk of hypotension.

Monitoring Parameters CBC with differential, platelet count, and hemoglobin, vital signs (blood pressure), bilirubin, and renal function tests

Patient Information During therapy, do not use alcohol, aspirin-containing products, and/or OTC medications without consulting prescriber. It is important to maintain adequate nutrition and hydration (2-3 L/day of fluids unless instructed to restrict fluid intake) during therapy; frequent small meals may help. You may experience mild nausea or vomiting (frequent small meals, frequent mouth care, sucking lozenges, or chewing gum may help). You may experience loss of hair (reversible); you will be more susceptible to infection (avoid crowds and exposure to infection as much as possible). Yogurt or buttermilk may help reduce diarrhea. Frequent mouth care and use of a soft toothbrush or cotton swabs may help prevent mouth sores. This drug may cause sterility or birth defects. Report extreme fatigue, pain or numbness in extremities, severe GI upset or diarrhea, bleeding or bruising, fever, chills, sore throat, vaginal discharge, difficulty breathing, yellowing of eyes or skin, and any changes in color of urine or stool. Contraceptive measures are recommended during therapy. The drug may be excreted in breast milk, therefore, an alternative form of feeding your baby should be used.

Nursing Implications

Extravasation treatment:

Inject 150-900 units of hyaluronidase S.C. clockwise into the infiltrated area using a 25-gauge needle; change the needle with each injection; apply heat immediately for 1 hour, repeat 4 times/day for 3-5 days

Application of cold or hydrocortisone is contraindicated.

If necessary, the injection may be used for oral administration; mix with orange juice, apple juice, or lemonade to a concentration of 0.4 mg/mL or less, and use within a 3-hour period

Dosage Forms

Capsule (VePesid®): 50 mg

Injection (Toposar®, VePesid®): 20 mg/mL (5 mL, 7.5 mL, 25 mL, 50 mL)

Etoposide Phosphate (e toe POE side FOS fate)

U.S. Brand Names Etopophos®

Therapeutic Category Antineoplastic Agent, Irritant; Antineoplastic Agent, Podophyllotoxin Derivative; Vesicant

Use Treatment of refractory testicular tumors and small cell lung cancer

Pregnancy Risk Factor D

(Continued)

Etoposide Phosphate *(Continued)*

Contraindications Hypersensitivity to etoposide, etoposide phosphate, or any component of the formulation; **intrathecal administration**; pregnancy

Warnings/Precautions The U.S. Food and Drug Administration (FDA) currently recommends that procedures for proper handling and disposal of antineoplastic agents be considered. Severe myelosuppression with resulting infection or bleeding may occur.

Dosage should be adjusted in patients with hepatic or renal impairment

Adverse Reactions Refer to Etoposide monograph *on page 533* for details

Overdosage/Toxicology Refer to Etoposide monograph *on page 533* for details

Drug Interactions

Increased Effect/Toxicity: Etoposide taken with warfarin may result in prolongation of bleeding times. Alteration of MTX transport has been found as a slow efflux of MTX and its polyglutamated form out of the cell, leading to intercellular accumulation of MTX. Calcium antagonists increase the rate of VP-16-induced DNA damage and cytotoxicity *in vitro*. Use with carmustine has shown reports of frequent hepatic dysfunction with hyperbilirubinemia, ascites, and thrombocytopenia. Cyclosporine may cause additive cytotoxic effects on tumor cells.

Ethanol/Nutrition/Herb Interactions

Ethanol: Avoid ethanol (may increase GI irritation).

Food: Administration of food does not affect GI absorption with doses ≤200 mg of injection.

Herb/Nutraceutical: St John's wort may decrease etoposide levels.

Stability

Store intact vials of injection under refrigeration 2°C to 8°C (36°F to 46°F); protect from light Reconstituted vials with 5 mL or 10 mL SWI, D_5W, NS, bacteriostatic SWI, or bacteriostatic NS to a concentration of 20 mg/mL or 10 mg/mL etoposide (22.7 mg/mL or 11.4 mg/mL etoposide phosphate), respectively. These solutions may be administered without further dilution or may be further diluted to a concentration as low as 0.1 mg/mL etoposide with either D_5W or NS. Solutions are stable in glass or plastic containers for at least 7 days at room temperature 20°C to 25°C (68°F to 77°F) or at least 31 days under refrigeration 2°C to 8°C (36°F to 47°F) for up to 24 hours.

Y-site **incompatible** with: Amphotericin B, cefepime hydrochloride, chlorpromazine hydrochloride, imipenem-cilastatin sodium, methylprednisolone sodium phosphate, mitomycin, prochlorperazine edisylate

Y-site **compatible** with: Bleomycin, carboplatin, carmustine, cisplatin, cyclophosphamide, cytarabine, dacarbazine, dactinomycin, daunorubicin, doxorubicin, floxuridine, fludarabine, fluorouracil, idarubicin, ifosfamide, methotrexate, mitoxantrone, paclitaxel, plicamycin, streptozocin, teniposide, thiotepa, vinblastine, vincristine, acyclovir, amikacin, ampicillin, ampicillin sodium-sulbactam sodium, aztreonam, cefazolin, cefoperazone, cefonicid, cefotaxime, cefotetan, cefoxitin, ceftazidime, ceftizoxime, ceftriaxone, cefuroxime, ciprofloxacin, clindamycin, doxycycline, fluconazole, ganciclovir, gentamicin, metronidazole, minocycline, netilmicin, ofloxacin, piperacillin, piperacillin sodium-tazobactam, ticarcillin, ticarcillin disodium-clavulanate potassium, tobramycin, trimethoprim-sulfamethoxazole, vancomycin, zidovudine, aminophylline, bumetanide, buprenorphine, butorphanol, calcium gluconate, cimetidine, dexamethasone, diphenhydramine, dobutamine, dopamine, droperidol, enalaprilat, famotidine, furosemide, gallium nitrate, granisetron, haloperidol, heparin, hydrocortisone sodium phosphate, hydrocortisone sodium succinate, hydroxyzine, leucovorin, lorazepam, magnesium sulfate, mannitol, meperidine, mesna, metoclopramide, morphine, nalbuphine, ondansetron, potassium chloride, promethazine, ranitidine, sodium bicarbonate

Mechanism of Action Etoposide phosphate is converted *in vivo* to the active moiety, etoposide, by dephosphorylation. Etoposide inhibits mitotic activity; inhibits cells from entering prophase; inhibits DNA synthesis. Initially thought to be mitotic inhibitors similar to podophyllotoxin, but actually have no effect on microtubule assembly. However, later shown to induce DNA strand breakage and inhibition of topoisomerase II (an enzyme which breaks and repairs DNA); etoposide acts in late S or early G2 phases.

Pharmacodynamics/Kinetics

Distribution: Average V_d: 3-36 L/m^2; poor penetration across blood-brain barrier; concentrations in CSF being <10% that of plasma

Protein binding: 94% to 97%

Metabolism: Hepatic (with a biphasic decay)

Half-life elimination: Terminal: 4-15 hours; Children: Normal renal/hepatic function: 6-8 hours

Excretion: Urine (as unchanged drug and metabolites, feces (2% to 16%); Children: I.V.: Urine (≤55% as unchanged drug)

Usual Dosage Refer to individual protocols. Adults:

Small cell lung cancer: I.V. (in combination with other approved chemotherapeutic drugs): **Equivalent doses of etoposide phosphate to an etoposide dosage** range of 35 mg/m^2/day for 4 days to 50 mg/m^2/day for 5 days. Courses are repeated at 3- to 4-week intervals after adequate recovery from any toxicity.

Testicular cancer: I.V. (in combination with other approved chemotherapeutic agents): **Equivalent dose of etoposide phosphate to etoposide dosage** range of 50-100 mg/m^2/day on days 1-5 to 100 mg/m^2/day on days 1, 3, and 5. Courses are repeated at 3- to 4-week intervals after adequate recovery from any toxicity.

Dosage adjustment in renal impairment:

Cl_{cr} 15-50 mL/minute: Administer 75% of normal dose

Cl_{cr} <15 mL minute: Data are not available and further dose reduction should be considered in these patients.

Hemodialysis: Supplemental dose is not necessary

Peritoneal dialysis: Supplemental dose is not necessary

CAPD effects: Unknown

CAVH effects: Unknown

Dosage adjustment in hepatic impairment:

Bilirubin 1.5-3 mg/dL or AST 60-180 units: Reduce dose by 50%

Bilirubin 3-5 mg/dL or AST >180 units: Reduce by 75%
Bilirubin >5 mg/dL: Do not administer

Administration I.V. infusion, usually over 5 minutes to 3 hours, infusions over 10-12 hours are reported. Unlike etoposide, etoposide phosphate may be administered rapidly without causing hypotension or anaphylactoid reactions.

Monitoring Parameters CBC with differential, platelet count, and hemoglobin, vital signs (blood pressure), bilirubin, and renal function tests

Patient Information This drug can only be administered by infusion. During therapy, do not use alcohol, aspirin-containing products, and/or OTC medications without consulting prescriber. It is important to maintain adequate nutrition and hydration (2-3 L/day of fluids unless instructed to restrict fluid intake) during therapy; frequent small meals may help. You may experience mild nausea or vomiting (frequent small meals, frequent mouth care, sucking lozenges, or chewing gum may help). You may experience loss of hair (reversible); you will be more susceptible to infection (avoid crowds and exposure to infection as much as possible). Yogurt or buttermilk may help reduce diarrhea. Frequent mouth care and use of a soft toothbrush or cotton swabs may help prevent mouth sores. This drug may cause sterility or birth defects. Report extreme fatigue, pain or numbness in extremities, severe GI upset or diarrhea, bleeding or bruising, fever, chills, sore throat, vaginal discharge, difficulty breathing, yellowing of eyes or skin, and any changes in color of urine or stool. Contraceptive measures should be used during therapy. The drug may cause permanent sterility and may cause birth defects. The drug may be excreted in breast milk, therefore, an alternative form of feeding your baby should be used.

Dosage Forms Powder for injection, lyophilized: 119.3 mg (100 mg base, 500 mg base)

Exemestane (ex e MES tane)

U.S. Brand Names Aromasin®
Canadian Brand Names Aromasin®
Therapeutic Category Antineoplastic Agent, Aromatase Inactivator
Use Treatment of advanced breast cancer in postmenopausal women whose disease has progressed following tamoxifen therapy
Pregnancy Risk Factor D
Pregnancy/Breast-Feeding Implications Exemestane can cause fetal harm when administered to a pregnant woman. It is not indicated for premenopausal women, but if exposure occurred during pregnancy, risk to the fetus and potential risk for loss of the pregnancy should be discussed.
Contraindications Hypersensitivity to exemestane or any component of the formulation; pregnancy
Warnings/Precautions Exemestane has been associated with prolonged gestation, abnormal or difficult labor, increased resorption, reduced number of live fetuses, decreased fetal weight, and retarded ossification in rats. Patients who are exposed to exemestane during pregnancy should be apprised of the possible hazard to the fetus and risk for loss of the pregnancy. Exemestane should not be administered concurrently with estrogen-containing drugs; and is not recommended for use in premenopausal women.

Adverse Reactions
>10%:
Central nervous system: Fatigue (22%), pain (13%), depression (13%), insomnia (11%), anxiety (10%)
Endocrine & metabolic: Hot flashes (13%)
Gastrointestinal: Nausea (18%)
1% to 10%:
Cardiovascular: Edema (7%), hypertension (5%), chest pain
Central nervous system: Dizziness (8%), headache (8%), fever (5%), hypoesthesia, confusion
Dermatologic: Rash, itching, alopecia
Gastrointestinal: Vomiting (7%), abdominal pain (6%), anorexia (6%), constipation (5%), diarrhea (4%), increased appetite (3%), dyspepsia
Genitourinary: Urinary tract infection
Neuromuscular & skeletal: Weakness, paresthesia, pathological fracture, arthralgia
Respiratory: Dyspnea (10%), cough (6%), bronchitis, sinusitis, pharyngitis, rhinitis
Miscellaneous: Influenza-like symptoms (6%), diaphoresis (6%), lymphedema, infection
<1% (Limited to important or life-threatening): GGT increased, transaminases increased,

A dose-dependent decrease in sex hormone-binding globulin has been observed with daily doses of 25 mg or more. Serum luteinizing hormone and follicle-stimulating hormone levels have increased with this medicine.

(Continued)

Exemestane *(Continued)*

Overdosage/Toxicology Daily doses as high as 800 mg have been used in healthy volunteers and 600 mg for 12 weeks in postmenopausal women with advanced breast cancer. If an overdose should occur, general supportive care would be indicated. Mice given 3200 mg/kg as a single dose died. This would be equivalent to 640 times the recommended human dose on a mg/m² basis. Rats and dogs died at higher single doses equivalent to 2000-4000 times the recommended human dose on a mg/m² basis.

Drug Interactions
Cytochrome P450 Effect: CYP3A3/4 enzyme substrate
Increased Effect/Toxicity: Although exemestane is a CYP3A4 substrate, ketoconazole, a CYP3A4 inhibitor, did not change the pharmacokinetics of exemestane. No other potential drug interactions have been evaluated.

Ethanol/Nutrition/Herb Interactions
Food: Plasma levels increased by 40% when exemestane was taken with a fatty meal.
Herb/Nutraceutical: St John's wort may decrease exemestane levels. Avoid black cohosh, dong quai in estrogen-dependent tumors.

Stability Store at 25°C (77°F)

Mechanism of Action Exemestane is an irreversible, steroidal aromatase inactivator. It prevents conversion of androgens to estrogens by tying up the enzyme aromatase. In breast cancers where growth is estrogen-dependent, this medicine will lower circulating estrogens.

Pharmacodynamics/Kinetics
Absorption: Rapid
Distribution: Extensive
Protein binding: 90%
Metabolism: Extensively hepatic; oxidation (CYP3A4) of methylene group, reduction of 17-keto group with formation of many secondary metabolites; metabolites are inactive or inhibit aromatase with decreased potency compared to parent drug
Half-life elimination: 24 hours
Time to peak: Women with breast cancer: 1.2 hours
Excretion: Urine (<1% as unchanged drug, 42% as metabolites); feces (42%)

Usual Dosage Adults: Oral: 25 mg once daily after a meal; treatment should continue until tumor progression is evident
Dosing adjustment in renal/hepatic impairment: Safety of chronic doses has not been studied

Patient Information Take after a meal; use caution if you have uncontrolled high blood pressure. Do not use in pregnancy or lactation. Avoid driving or doing other tasks or hobbies that require alertness until you know how this medicine affects you. Take at a similar time every day.

Nursing Implications Educate patient about getting blood pressure checked while on medicine, especially if there is a history of poor control. Encourage patient not to drive until she sees how the medicine affects her; it can cause fatigue and dizziness. Medication should be taken at a similar time every day and after a meal to decrease nausea and increase absorption.

Dosage Forms Tablet: 25 mg

Factor VIIa (Recombinant) *(FAK ter SEV en ree KOM be nant)*

U.S. Brand Names Novo-Seven®
Synonyms Coagulation Factor VIIa; rFVIIa
Therapeutic Category Antihemophilic Agent; Blood Product Derivative
Use Treatment of bleeding episodes in patients with hemophilia A or B when inhibitors to factor VIII or factor IX are present
Pregnancy Risk Factor C
Contraindications Hypersensitivity to Factor VII or any component of the formulation; hypersensitivity to mouse, hamster, or bovine proteins
Warnings/Precautions Patients should be monitored for signs and symptoms of activation of the coagulation system or thrombosis. Thrombotic events may be increased in patients with disseminated intravascular coagulation (DIC), advanced atherosclerotic disease, sepsis or crush injury. Decreased dosage or discontinuation is warranted in confirmed DIC. Efficacy with prolonged infusions and data evaluating this agent's long-term adverse effects are limited.
Adverse Reactions
1% to 10%:
Cardiovascular: Hypertension
Hematologic: Hemorrhage, decreased plasma fibrinogen
Musculoskeletal: Hemarthrosis
<1% (Limited to important or life-threatening): Abnormal renal function, allergic reactions, arthrosis, bradycardia, coagulation disorder, prothrombin decreased, disseminated intravascular coagulation (DIC), edema, headache, hypotension, increased fibrinolysis, injection-site reactions, pneumonia, pruritus, purpura, rash, vomiting

Overdosage/Toxicology Experience with human overdose is limited. An increased risk of thrombotic events may occur. Treatment is symptomatic and supportive.

Stability Store under refrigeration (2°C to 8°C/36°F to 46°F); reconstituted solutions may be stored at room temperature or under refrigeration, but must be infused within 3 hours of reconstitution

Mechanism of Action Recombinant factor VIIa, a vitamin K-dependent glycoprotein, promotes hemostasis by activating the extrinsic pathway of the coagulation cascade. It replaces deficient activated coagulation factor VII, which complexes with tissue factor and may activate coagulation factor X to Xa and factor IX to IXa. When complexed with other factors, coagulation factor Xa converts prothrombin to thrombin, a key step in the formation of a fibrin-platelet hemostatic plug.

Pharmacodynamics/Kinetics
Distribution: V_d: 103 mL/kg (78-139)
Half-life elimination: 2.3 hours (1.7-2.7)
Excretion: Clearance: 33 mL/kg/hour (27-49)

Usual Dosage Children and Adults: I.V. administration only: 90 mcg/kg every 2 hours until hemostasis is achieved or until the treatment is judged ineffective. The dose and interval may be adjusted based upon the severity of bleeding and the degree of hemostasis achieved. The duration of therapy following hemostasis has not been fully established; for patients experiencing severe bleeds, dosing should be continued at 3-6 hour intervals after hemostasis has been achieved and the duration of dosing should be minimized.

In clinical trials, dosages have ranged from 35-120 mcg/kg and a decision on the final therapeutic dosages was reached within 8 hours in the majority of patients

Administration I.V. administration only; reconstitute only with the specified volume of sterile water for injection, USP; administer within 3 hours after reconstitution

Monitoring Parameters Monitor for evidence of hemostasis; although the prothrombin time, aPTT, and factor VII clotting activity have no correlation with achieving hemostasis, these parameters may be useful as adjunct tests to evaluate efficacy and guide dose or interval adjustments

Dosage Forms Powder for injection: 1.2 mg, 4.8 mg

- ♦ **Factor VIII (Human)** *see* Antihemophilic Factor (Human) *on page 102*
- ♦ **Factor VIII (Porcine)** *see* Antihemophilic Factor (Porcine) *on page 104*
- ♦ **Factor VIII (Recombinant)** *see* Antihemophilic Factor (Recombinant) *on page 105*

Factor IX Complex (Human) (FAK ter nyne KOM pleks HYU man)

U.S. Brand Names AlphaNine® SD; BeneFix™; Hemonyne®; Konÿne® 80; Profilnine® SD; Proplex® T

Synonyms Prothrombin Complex Concentrate

Therapeutic Category Antihemophilic Agent

Use
Control bleeding in patients with factor IX deficiency (hemophilia B or Christmas disease)
Note: Factor IX concentrate containing **only** factor IX is also available and preferable for this indication.
Prevention/control of bleeding in hemophilia A patients with inhibitors to factor VIII
Prevention/control of bleeding in patients with factor VII deficiency
Emergency correction of the coagulopathy of warfarin excess in critical situations.

Pregnancy Risk Factor C

Contraindications Liver disease with signs of intravascular coagulation or fibrinolysis, not for use in factor VII deficiencies, patients undergoing elective surgery

Warnings/Precautions Use with caution in patients with liver dysfunction; prepared from pooled human plasma - the risk of viral transmission is not totally eradicated; monitor patients who receive repeated doses twice daily with PTT and prothrombin time and level of factor being replaced (eg, usually VII or IX); if PT is <10 seconds, this may indicate risk of hypercoagulable complication

Adverse Reactions
1% to 10%:
Central nervous system: Fever, headache, chills
Neuromuscular & skeletal: Tingling
Miscellaneous: Following rapid administration: Transient fever
<1% (Limited to important or life-threatening): Disseminated intravascular coagulation (DIC), flushing, nausea, somnolence, thrombosis following high dosages because of presence of activated clotting factors, tightness in chest, tightness in neck, urticaria, vomiting

Overdosage/Toxicology Symptoms include disseminated intravascular coagulation (DIC).

Drug Interactions
Increased Effect/Toxicity: Do not coadminister with aminocaproic acid; may increase risk for thrombosis.

Stability When stored at refrigerator temperature, 2°C to 8°C (36°F to 46°F), coagulation factor IX is stable for the period indicated by the expiration date on its label. Avoid freezing which may damage container for the diluent.
Stability of parenteral admixture at room temperature (25°C): 24 hours
Standard diluent: Dose in units/bag
Minimum volume: Use complete vial(s) for entire dose
Comments: Infusion rate should be 2 mL/minute

Mechanism of Action Replaces deficient clotting factor including factor X; hemophilia B, or Christmas disease, is an X-linked recessively inherited disorder of blood coagulation characterized by insufficient or abnormal synthesis of the clotting protein factor IX. Factor IX is a vitamin K-dependent coagulation factor which is synthesized in the liver. Factor IX is activated by factor XIa in the intrinsic coagulation pathway. Activated factor IX (IXa), in combination with factor VII:C activates factor X to Xa, resulting ultimately in the conversion of prothrombin to thrombin and the formation of a fibrin clot. The infusion of exogenous factor IX to replace the deficiency present in hemophilia B temporarily restores hemostasis.

(Continued)

Factor IX Complex (Human) *(Continued)*

Pharmacodynamics/Kinetics

Half-life elimination:
VII component: Initial: 4-6 hours; Terminal: 22.5 hours
IX component: 24 hours

Usual Dosage Children and Adults: Dosage is expressed in units of factor IX activity and must be individualized. I.V. only:

Formula for units required to raise blood level %:

Total blood volume (mL blood/kg) = 70 mL/kg (adults), 80 mL/kg (children)
Plasma volume = total blood volume (mL) x [1 - Hct (in decimals)]

For example, for a 70 kg adult with a Hct = 40%: Plasma volume = [70 kg x 70 mL/kg] x [1 - 0.4] = 2940 mL

To calculate number of units needed to increase level to desired range (highly individualized and dependent on patient's condition): Number of units = desired level increase [desired level - actual level] x plasma volume (in mL)

For example, for a 100% level in the above patient who has an actual level of 20%: Number of units needed = [1 (for a 100% level) - 0.2] x 2940 mL = 2352 units

As a general rule, the level of factor IX required for treatment of different conditions is listed below:

Minor Spontaneous Hemorrhage, Prophylaxis:
Desired levels of factor IX for hemostasis: 15% to 25%
Initial loading dose to achieve desired level: <20-30 units/kg
Frequency of dosing: Once; repeated in 24 hours if necessary
Duration of treatment: Once; repeated if necessary

Major Trauma or Surgery:
Desired levels of factor IX for hemostasis: 25% to 50%
Initial loading dose to achieve desired level: <75 units/kg
Frequency of dosing: Every 18-30 hours, depending on half-life and measured factor IX levels
Duration of treatment: Up to 10 days, depending upon nature of insult

Factor VIII inhibitor patients: 75 units/kg/dose; may be given every 6-12 hours
Anticoagulant overdosage: I.V.: 15 units/kg

Administration Solution should be infused at room temperature
I.V. administration only: Should be infused **slowly**: Start infusion at a rate of 2-3 mL/minute. If headache, flushing, changes in pulse rate or blood pressure appear, the infusion rate should be decreased. Initially, stop the infusion until the symptoms disappear, then resume the infusion at a slower rate. **Infuse at a rate not exceeding 3 mL/minute.**

Monitoring Parameters Levels of factors being replaced (eg, VII or IX), PT, PTT

Reference Range Average normal factor VII and factor IX levels are 50% to 150%; patients with severe hemophilia will have levels <1%, often undetectable. Moderate forms of the disease have levels of 1% to 10% while some mild cases may have 11% to 49% of normal factor IX.

Maintain factor IX plasma level at least 20% until hemostasis achieved after acute joint or muscle bleeding
In preparation for and following surgery:
Level to prevent spontaneous hemorrhage: 5%
Minimum level for hemostasis following trauma and surgery: 30% to 50%
Severe hemorrhage: >60%
Major surgery: >60% prior to procedure, 30% to 50% for several days after surgery, and >20% for 7-10 days thereafter

Patient Information Early signs of hypersensitivity reactions including hives, generalized urticaria, tightness of the chest, wheezing, hypotension, and anaphylaxis indicate discontinuation of use of the concentrate and physician should be contacted if these symptoms occur

Nursing Implications Early signs of hypersensitivity reactions including hives, generalized urticaria, tightness of the chest, wheezing, hypotension, and anaphylaxis indicate discontinuation of use of the concentrate and physician should be contacted if these symptoms occur

Dosage Forms
Injection:
AlphaNine® SD [single-dose vial]: Factors II, VII, IX, X
BeneFix™: 250 units, 500 units, 1000 units [purified factor IX recombinant]
Hemonyne®: 20 mL, 40 mL [factors II, VIII, IX, X]
Konÿne® 80: 20 mL, 40 mL [factors II, VII, I, X]
Profilnine® SD [single-dose vial]: Factors II, VII, IX, X
Proplex® T: 30 mL vial [factors II, VII, IX, X]

Factor IX (Purified/Human) *(FAK ter nyne, PURE eh fide HYU man)*

U.S. Brand Names Mononine®

Canadian Brand Names Immunine® VH

Therapeutic Category Antihemophilic Agent

Use Control bleeding in patients with factor IX deficiency (hemophilia B or Christmas disease) Mononine® contains **nondetectable levels of factors II, VII, and X** (<0.0025 units per factor IX unit using standard coagulation assays) and is, therefore, **NOT INDICATED** for replacement therapy of any of these clotting factors.

Mononine® is also **NOT INDICATED** in the treatment or reversal of coumarin-induced anticoagulation or in a hemorrhagic state caused by hepatitis-induced lack of production of liver dependent coagulation factors.

Pregnancy Risk Factor C

Contraindications Hypersensitivity to mouse protein or any component of the formulation

Warnings/Precautions Use with caution in patients with liver dysfunction; prepared from pooled human plasma - the risk of viral transmission is not totally eradicated; monitor patients who receive repeated doses twice daily with PTT and level of factor being replaced (eg, IX).

Observe closely for signs or symptoms of intravascular coagulation or thrombosis. Caution should be exercised when administering to patients with liver disease, postoperatively, neonates, or patients at risk of thromboembolic phenomena or disseminated intravascular coagulation because of the potential risk of thromboembolic complications.

Adverse Reactions
1% to 10%:
    Central nervous system: Fever, headache, chills
    Neuromuscular & skeletal: Tingling
    Miscellaneous: Following rapid administration: Transient fever
<1% (Limited to important or life-threatening): Disseminated intravascular coagulation (DIC), flushing, nausea, somnolence, thrombosis following high dosages because of presence of activated clotting factors, tightness in chest, tightness in neck, urticaria, vomiting

Overdosage/Toxicology Symptoms include disseminated intravascular coagulation (DIC).

Drug Interactions
    Increased Effect/Toxicity: Do not coadminister with aminocaproic acid; may increase risk for thrombosis.

Stability When stored at refrigerator temperature, 2°C to 8°C (36°F to 46°F), coagulation factor IX is stable for the period indicated by the expiration date on its label. Avoid freezing which may damage container for the diluent.
Stability of parenteral admixture at room temperature (25°C): 24 hours
Standard diluent: Dose in units/bag
Minimum volume: Use complete vial(s) for entire dose
Comments: Infusion rate should be up to 225 units/minute (2 mL/minute)

Mechanism of Action Replaces deficient clotting factor IX; concentrate of factor IX; hemophilia B, or Christmas disease, is an X-linked inherited disorder of blood coagulation characterized by insufficient or abnormal synthesis of the clotting protein factor IX. Factor IX is a vitamin K-dependent coagulation factor which is synthesized in the liver. Factor IX is activated by factor XIa in the intrinsic coagulation pathway. Activated factor IX (IXa), in combination with factor VII:C activates factor X to Xa, resulting ultimately in the conversion of prothrombin to thrombin and the formation of a fibrin clot. The infusion of exogenous factor IX to replace the deficiency present in hemophilia B temporarily restores hemostasis. Depending upon the patient's level of biologically active factor IX, clinical symptoms range from moderate skin bruising or excessive hemorrhage after trauma or surgery to spontaneous hemorrhage into joints, muscles, or internal organs including the brain. Severe or recurring hemorrhages can produce death, organ dysfunction, or orthopedic deformity.

Pharmacodynamics/Kinetics Half-life elimination: IX component: 23-31 hours

Usual Dosage Children and Adults: Dosage is expressed in units of factor IX activity and must be individualized. I.V. only:
    Formula for units required to raise blood level %:
      Number of Factor IX Units Required = body weight (in kg) x desired Factor IX level increase (% normal) x 1 unit/kg
      For example, for a 100% level a patient who has an actual level of 20%: Number of Factor IX Units needed = 70 kg x 80% x 1 Unit/kg = 5600 Units
As a general rule, the level of factor IX required for treatment of different conditions is listed below:

Minor Spontaneous Hemorrhage, Prophylaxis:
    Desired levels of factor IX for hemostasis: 15% to 25%
    Initial loading dose to achieve desired level: <20-30 units/kg
    Frequency of dosing: Once; repeated in 24 hours if necessary
    Duration of treatment: Once; repeated if necessary

Major Trauma or Surgery:
    Desired levels of factor IX for hemostasis: 25% to 50%
    Initial loading dose to achieve desired level: <75 units/kg
    Frequency of dosing: Every 18-30 hours, depending on half-life and measured factor IX levels
    Duration of treatment: Up to 10 days, depending upon nature of insult

Administration
Solution should be infused at room temperature
I.V. administration only:
    Should be infused **slowly**: The rate of administration should be determined by the response and comfort of the patient; intravenous dosage administration rates of up to 225 units/minute (~2 mL/minute) have been regularly tolerated without incident.
    Infuse at a rate not exceeding 2 mL/minute

Monitoring Parameters Levels of factors being replaced (eg, IX), PTT

Reference Range Average normal factor IX levels are 50% to 150%; patients with severe hemophilia will have levels <1%, often undetectable. Moderate forms of the disease have levels of 1% to 10% while some mild cases may have 11% to 49% of normal factor IX.

Maintain factor IX plasma level at least 20% until hemostasis achieved after acute joint or muscle bleeding
In preparation for and following surgery:
    Level to prevent spontaneous hemorrhage: 5%
    Minimum level for hemostasis following trauma and surgery: 30% to 50%
    Severe hemorrhage: >60%
    Major surgery: ≥50% prior to procedure, 30% to 50% for several days after surgery, and >20% for 10-14 days thereafter

Patient Information Early signs of hypersensitivity reactions including hives, generalized urticaria, tightness of the chest, wheezing, hypotension, and anaphylaxis indicate discontinuation of use of the concentrate and physician should be contacted if these symptoms occur

Nursing Implications Early signs of hypersensitivity reactions including hives, generalized urticaria, tightness of the chest, wheezing, hypotension, and anaphylaxis indicate discontinuation of use of the concentrate and physician should be contacted if these symptoms occur

Dosage Forms Factor IX units listed per vial and per lot to lot variation of factor IX
Injection: 250 units, 500 units, 1000 units

♦ **Factrel**® *see* Gonadorelin *on page 640*

Famciclovir (fam SYE kloe veer)

Related Information

Treatment of Sexually Transmitted Diseases *on page 1609*

U.S. Brand Names Famvir™

Canadian Brand Names Famvir®

Therapeutic Category Antiviral Agent, Oral

Use Management of acute herpes zoster (shingles) and recurrent episodes of genital herpes; treatment of recurrent herpes simplex in immunocompetent patients

Pregnancy Risk Factor B

Pregnancy/Breast-Feeding Implications

Clinical effects on the fetus: Use only if the benefit to the patient clearly exceeds the potential risk to the fetus

Breast-feeding/lactation: Due to potential for excretion of famciclovir in breast milk and for its associated tumorigenicity, discontinue nursing or discontinue the drug during lactation

Contraindications Hypersensitivity to famciclovir or any component of the formulation

Warnings/Precautions Has not been studied in immunocompromised patients or patients with ophthalmic or disseminated zoster; dosage adjustment is required in patients with renal insufficiency (Cl_{cr} <60 mL/minute) and in patients with noncompensated hepatic disease; safety and efficacy have not been established in children <18 years of age; animal studies indicated increases in incidence of carcinomas, mutagenic changes, and decreases in fertility with extremely large doses

Adverse Reactions

1% to 10%:

Central nervous system: Fatigue (4% to 6%), fever (1% to 3%), dizziness (3% to 5%), somnolence (1% to 2%), headache

Dermatologic: Pruritus (1% to 4%)

Gastrointestinal: Diarrhea (4% to 8%), vomiting (1% to 5%), constipation (1% to 5%), anorexia (1% to 3%), abdominal pain (1% to 4%), nausea

Neuromuscular & skeletal: Paresthesia (1% to 3%)

Respiratory: Sinusitis/pharyngitis (2%)

<1% (Limited to important or life-threatening): Arthralgia, rigors, upper respiratory infection

Overdosage/Toxicology Supportive and symptomatic care is recommended. Hemodialysis may enhance elimination.

Drug Interactions

Increased Effect/Toxicity:

Cimetidine: Penciclovir AUC may increase due to impaired metabolism.

Digoxin: C_{max} of digoxin increases by ~19%.

Probenecid: Penciclovir serum levels significantly increase.

Theophylline: Penciclovir AUC/C_{max} may increase and renal clearance decrease, although not clinically significant.

Ethanol/Nutrition/Herb Interactions Food: Rate of absorption and/or conversion to penciclovir and peak concentration are reduced with food, but bioavailability is not affected.

Mechanism of Action After undergoing rapid biotransformation to the active compound, penciclovir, famciclovir is phosphorylated by viral thymidine kinase in HSV-1, HSV-2, and VZV-infected cells to a monophosphate form; this is then converted to penciclovir triphosphate and competes with deoxyguanosine triphosphate to inhibit HSV-2 polymerase (ie, herpes viral DNA synthesis/replication is selectively inhibited)

Pharmacodynamics/Kinetics

Absorption: Food decreases maximum peak concentration and delays time to peak; AUC remains the same

Distribution: V_{dss}: 0.98-1.08 L/kg

Protein binding: 20%

Metabolism: Rapidly deacetylated and oxidized to penciclovir (not by CYP450)

Bioavailability: 77%

Half-life elimination: Penciclovir: 2-3 hours (10, 20, and 7 hours in HSV-1, HSV-2, and VZV-infected cells); increases with renal impairment

Time to peak: 0.9 hours; C_{max} and T_{max} are decreased and prolonged with noncompensated hepatic impairment

Excretion: Urine (>90% as unchanged drug)

Usual Dosage Initiate therapy as soon as herpes zoster is diagnosed: Adults: Oral:

Acute herpes zoster: 500 mg every 8 hours for 7 days

Recurrent herpes simplex in immunocompetent patients: 125 mg twice daily for 5 days

Genital herpes:

First episode: 250 mg 3 times/day for 7-10 days

Recurrent episodes: 125 mg twice daily for 5 days

Prophylaxis: 250 mg twice daily

Severe (hospitalized patients): 250 mg twice daily

Dosing interval in renal impairment:

Herpes zoster:

Cl_{cr} ≥60 mL/minute: Administer 500 mg every 8 hours

Cl_{cr} 40-59 mL/minute: Administer 500 mg every 12 hours

Cl_{cr} 20-39 mL/minute: Administer 500 mg every 24 hours

Cl_{cr} <20 mL/minute: Administer 250 mg every 24 hours

Recurrent genital herpes:

Cl_{cr} ≥40 mL/minute: Administer 125 mg every 12 hours

Cl_{cr} 20-39 mL/minute: Administer 125 mg every 24 hours

Cl_{cr} <20 mL/minute: Administer 125 mg every 48 hours

Suppression of recurrent genital herpes:

Cl_{cr} ≥40 mL/minute: Administer 250 mg every 12 hours

Cl_{cr} 20-39 mL/minute: Administer 125 mg every 12 hours

Cl_{cr} <20 mL/minute: Administer 125 mg every 24 hours

Recurrent orolabial or genital herpes in HIV-infected patients:
  Cl_{cr} ≥40 mL/minute: Administer 500 mg every 12 hours
  Cl_{cr} 20-39 mL/minute: Administer 500 mg every 24 hours
  Cl_{cr} <20 mL/minute: Administer 250 mg every 24 hours

Dietary Considerations May be taken with food or on an empty stomach.

Monitoring Parameters Periodic CBC during long-term therapy

Patient Information Initiate therapy as soon as herpes zoster is diagnosed; may take medication with food or on an empty stomach

Additional Information Most effective if therapy is initiated within 72 hours of initial lesion.

Dosage Forms Tablet: 125 mg, 250 mg, 500 mg

Famotidine (fa MOE ti deen)

U.S. Brand Names Mylanta AR® [DSC]; Pepcid®; Pepcid® AC [OTC]; Pepcid RPD™

Canadian Brand Names Alti-Famotidine; Apo®-Famotidine; Gen-Famotidine; Novo-Famotidine; Nu-Famotidine; Pepcid®; Pepcid AC®; Pepcid® I.V.; Rhoxal-famotidine; Ulcidine®

Therapeutic Category Antihistamine, H_2 Blocker; Histamine H_2 Antagonist

Use

Pepcid®: Therapy and treatment of duodenal ulcer, gastric ulcer, control gastric pH in critically ill patients, symptomatic relief in gastritis, gastroesophageal reflux, active benign ulcer, and pathological hypersecretory conditions

Pepcid® AC: Relief of heartburn, acid indigestion, and sour stomach

Unlabeled/Investigational Use Part of a multidrug regimen for *H. pylori* eradication to reduce the risk of duodenal ulcer recurrence

Pregnancy Risk Factor B

Pregnancy/Breast-Feeding Implications

Clinical effects on the fetus: Crosses the placenta. No data on effects on the fetus (insufficient data).

Breast-feeding/lactation: Crosses into breast milk. AAP has NO RECOMMENDATIONS.

Contraindications Hypersensitivity to famotidine, other H_2 antagonists, or any component of the formulation

Warnings/Precautions Modify dose in patients with renal impairment; orally-disintegrating and chewable tablets contain phenylalanine; multidose vials contain benzyl alcohol

Adverse Reactions

1% to 10%:
  Central nervous system: Headache, dizziness
  Gastrointestinal: Constipation, diarrhea

<1% (Limited to important or life-threatening): Agranulocytosis, bradycardia, bronchospasm, hypertension, AST/ALT increased or proteinuria, neutropenia, BUN/creatinine increased or proteinuria, neutropenia, palpitations, seizures, tachycardia, thrombocytopenia

Overdosage/Toxicology Symptoms include hypotension, tachycardia, vomiting, and drowsiness. Treatment is symptomatic and supportive.

Drug Interactions

Decreased Effect: Decreased serum levels of ketoconazole and itraconazole (reduced absorption).

Ethanol/Nutrition/Herb Interactions

Ethanol: Avoid ethanol (may cause gastric mucosal irritation).

Food: Famotidine bioavailability may be increased if taken with food.

Stability Reconstituted I.V. solution is stable for 48 hours at room temperature; I.V. infusion in NS or D_5W solution is stable for 7 days at room temperature; reconstituted oral solution is stable for 30 days at room temperature

Mechanism of Action Competitive inhibition of histamine at H_2 receptors of the gastric parietal cells, which inhibits gastric acid secretion

Pharmacodynamics/Kinetics

Onset of action: GI: Oral: Within 1 hour

Duration: 10-12 hours

Protein binding: 15% to 20%

Bioavailability: Oral: 40% to 50%

Half-life elimination: 2.5-3.5 hours (increases with renal impairment); Oliguria: 20 hours

Time to peak, serum: Oral: ~1-3 hours

Excretion: Urine (as unchanged drug)

Usual Dosage

Children: 1-16 years: Treatment duration and dose should be individualized

Peptic ulcer:
  Oral: 0.5 mg/kg/day at bedtime or divided twice daily (maximum dose: 40 mg/day); doses of up to 1 mg/kg/day have been used in clinical studies
  I.V.: 0.25 mg/kg every 12 hours (maximum dose: 40 mg/day); doses of up to 0.5 mg/kg have been used in clinical studies

GERD: Oral: 1 mg/kg/day divided twice daily (maximum dose: 40 mg twice daily); doses of up to 2 mg/kg/day have been used in clinical studies

Adults:
  Duodenal ulcer: Oral: Acute therapy: 40 mg/day at bedtime for 4-8 weeks; maintenance therapy: 20 mg/day at bedtime

  Helicobacter pylori eradication (unlabeled use): 40 mg once daily; requires combination therapy with antibiotics

  Gastric ulcer: Oral: Acute therapy: 40 mg/day at bedtime

  Hypersecretory conditions: Oral: Initial: 20 mg every 6 hours, may increase in increments up to 160 mg every 6 hours

  GERD: Oral: 20 mg twice daily for 6 weeks

  Esophagitis and accompanying symptoms due to GERD: Oral: 20 mg or 40 mg twice daily for up to 12 weeks

  Patients unable to take oral medication: I.V.: 20 mg every 12 hours

  Heartburn, indigestion, sour stomach: Pepcid® AC [OTC]: Oral: 10 mg every 12 hours; dose may be taken 15-60 minutes before eating foods known to cause heartburn

(Continued)

543

Famotidine *(Continued)*

Dosing adjustment in renal impairment:

Cl$_{cr}$ <50 mL/minute: Manufacturer recommendation: Administer 50% of dose **or** increase the dosing interval to every 36-48 hours (to limit potential CNS adverse effects).

Cl$_{cr}$ <10 mL/minute: Administer 50% of dose **or** increase dosing interval to every 36-48 hours.

Dietary Considerations Phenylalanine content:

Pepcid RPD™:

20 mg tablet contains 1.05 mg phenylalanine

40 mg tablet contains 2.1 mg phenylalanine

Pepcid® AC chewable: Each tablet contains 1.4 mg phenylalanine

Administration

I.V. infusion: Administer over 15-30 minutes

I.V. push: May be given undiluted (some centers dilute to a total volume of 5-10 mL); inject no faster that 10 mg/minute

Patient Information

Pepcid RPD™: Allow tablet to dissolve on tongue and swallow; no water is needed

Oral suspension: Shake well before use

Pepcid® AC: Do not use for more than 14 days unless recommended by prescriber

Nursing Implications

I.V. infusion: Administer over 15-30 minutes

I.V. push: May be given undiluted (some centers dilute to a total volume of 5-10 mL); inject no faster that 10 mg/minute

Dosage Forms

Gelcap (Pepcid® AC): 10 mg

Infusion [premixed in NS]: 20 mg (50 mL)

Injection [single-dose vial]: 10 mg/mL (2 mL, 4 mL)

Powder for oral suspension (Pepcid®): 40 mg/5 mL (50 mL) [cherry-banana-mint flavor]

Tablet (Pepcid® AC): 10 mg

Tablet, chewable (Pepcid® AC): 10 mg [contains 1.4 mg phenylalanine/tablet]

Tablet, film coated (Pepcid®): 20 mg, 40 mg

Tablet, orally disintegrating (Pepcid RPD™): 20 mg [contains 1.05 phenylalanine/tablet]; 40 mg [contains 2.1 mg phenylalanine/tablet]

Famotidine, Calcium Carbonate, and Magnesium Hydroxide

(fa MOE ti deen, KAL see um KAR bun ate, & mag NEE zhum hye DROKS ide)

U.S. Brand Names Pepcid® Complete [OTC]

Synonyms Calcium Carbonate, Magnesium Hydroxide, and Famotidine; Magnesium Hydroxide, Famotidine, and Calcium Carbonate

Therapeutic Category Antacid; Histamine H$_2$ Antagonist

Use Relief of heartburn due to acid indigestion

Contraindications Hypersensitivity to famotidine or other H$_2$ antagonists, calcium carbonate, magnesium hydroxide, or any component of the formulation. See individual agents for additional information.

Warnings/Precautions See individual agents

Adverse Reactions See individual agents

Drug Interactions

Increased Effect/Toxicity: Refer to individual agents.

Decreased Effect: Refer to individual agents.

Stability Store at 25°C to 30°C (77°F to 86°F); protect from moisture

Mechanism of Action

Famotidine: H$_2$ antagonist

Calcium carbonate: Antacid

Magnesium hydroxide: Antacid

Pharmacodynamics/Kinetics See individual agents.

Usual Dosage Children ≥12 years and Adults: Relief of heartburn due to acid indigestion: Oral: Pepcid® Complete: 1 tablet as needed; no more than 2 tablets in 24 hours; do **not** swallow whole, chew tablet completely before swallowing; do not use for longer than 14 days (see Additional Information for dosing ranges for individual ingredients)

Patient Information Do **not** swallow tablet whole; chew completely before swallowing. Contact prescriber if your symptoms last for more than 14 days. Should not be used in combination with other products for acid indigestion (prescription or over the counter). Certain foods are more likely to cause acid indigestion in some patients, including foods that are rich, spicy, fatty, or fried; chocolate; caffeine; alcohol; some fruits or vegetables. Avoid meals close to bedtime, eat slowly and avoid big meals to help decrease symptoms. Avoid smoking. Notify prescriber if you are pregnant or breast-feeding.

Additional Information Presented in dosage field is the specific OTC labeling for the indicated product. Dosing ranges of the individual ingredients include:

Adults:

Famotidine: Duodenal/gastric ulcer: 40 mg/day at bedtime

Calcium carbonate: Antacid: ≤3 g/day of elemental calcium

Magnesium hydroxide: Antacid: Approximately ≤5 g/day of magnesium hydroxide

Healthcare providers should also refer to the individual monographs for more specific information.

Dosage Forms Tablet, chewable (Pepcid® Complete): Famotidine 10 mg, calcium carbonate 800 mg, and magnesium hydroxide 165 mg

◆ **Famvir**™ *see* Famciclovir *on page 542*

◆ **Fansidar**® *see* Sulfadoxine and Pyrimethamine *on page 1271*

◆ **Fareston**® *see* Toremifene *on page 1351*

Fat Emulsion (fat e MUL shun)

U.S. Brand Names Intralipid®; Liposyn®; Nutrilipid®; Soyacal®

Canadian Brand Names Intralipid®

Synonyms Intravenous Fat Emulsion

Therapeutic Category Caloric Agent

Use Source of calories and essential fatty acids for patients requiring parenteral nutrition of extended duration

Pregnancy Risk Factor B/C

Contraindications Hypersensitivity to fat emulsion or any component of the formulation; severe egg or legume (soybean) allergies; pathologic hyperlipidemia, lipoid nephrosis pancreatitis with hyperlipemia

Warnings/Precautions Use caution in patients with severe liver damage, pulmonary disease, anemia, or blood coagulation disorder; use with caution in jaundiced, premature, and low birth weight children

Adverse Reactions Frequency not defined.

Cardiovascular: Cyanosis, flushing, chest pain

Central nervous system: Headache, dizziness

Endocrine & metabolic: Hyperlipemia

Gastrointestinal: Nausea, vomiting, diarrhea

Hematologic: Hypercoagulability, thrombocytopenia in neonates (rare)

Hepatic: Hepatomegaly

Local: Thrombophlebitis

Respiratory: Dyspnea

Miscellaneous: Sepsis, diaphoresis

Overdosage/Toxicology Too rapid administration results in fluid or fat overloading, causing dilution of serum electrolytes, overhydration, pulmonary edema, impaired pulmonary diffusion capacity, or metabolic acidosis. Treatment is supportive.

Stability May be stored at room temperature; do not store partly used bottles for later use; do not use if emulsion appears to be oiling out

Mechanism of Action Essential for normal structure and function of cell membranes

Pharmacodynamics/Kinetics

Metabolism: Undergoes lipolysis to free fatty acids which are utilized by reticuloendothelial cells

Half-life elimination: 0.5-1 hour

Usual Dosage Fat emulsion should not exceed 60% of the total daily calories

Premature Infants: Initial dose: 0.25-0.5 g/kg/day, increase by 0.25-0.5 g/kg/day to a maximum of 3 g/kg/day depending on needs/nutritional goals; limit to 1 g/kg/day if on phototherapy; maximum rate of infusion: 0.15 g/kg/hour (0.75 mL/kg/hour of 20% solution)

Infants and Children: Initial dose: 0.5-1 g/kg/day, increase by 0.5 g/kg/day to a maximum of 3 g/kg/day depending on needs/nutritional goals; maximum rate of infusion: 0.25 g/kg/hour (1.25 mL/kg/hour of 20% solution)

Adolescents and Adults: Initial dose: 1 g/kg/day, increase by 0.5-1 g/kg/day to a maximum of 2.5 g/kg/day of 10% and 3 g/kg/day of 20% depending on needs/nutritional goals; maximum rate of infusion: 0.25 g/kg/hour (1.25 mL/kg/hour of 20% solution); do not exceed 50 mL/hour (20%) or 100 mL/hour (10%)

Prevention of essential fatty acid deficiency (8% to 10% of total caloric intake): 0.5-1 g/kg/24 hours

Children: 5-10 mL/kg/day at 0.1 mL/minute then up to 100 mL/hour

Adults: 500 mL (10%) twice weekly at rate of 1 mL/minute for 30 minutes, then increase to 42 mL/hour (500 mL over 12 hours)

Note: At the onset of therapy, the patient should be observed for any immediate allergic reactions such as dyspnea, cyanosis, and fever; slower initial rates of infusion may be used for the first 10-15 minutes of the infusion (eg, 0.1 mL/minute of 10% or 0.05 mL/minute of 20% solution)

Administration May be simultaneously infused with amino acid dextrose mixtures by means of Y-connector located near infusion site. The 10% isotonic solution which has 1.1 cal/mL (10%) and may be administered peripherally; the 20% (2 cal/mL) is not recommended for use in low birth weight infants.

Monitoring Parameters Serum triglycerides; before initiation of therapy and at least weekly during therapy. Frequent (some advise daily) platelet counts should be performed in neonatal patients receiving parenteral lipids.

Nursing Implications May be simultaneously infused with amino acid dextrose mixtures by means of Y-connector located near infusion site

Dosage Forms Injection: 10% [100 mg/mL] (100 mL, 250 mL, 500 mL); 20% [200 mg/mL] (100 mL, 250 mL, 500 mL); 30% (500 mL)

♦ **5-FC** see Flucytosine on page 567

♦ **FC1157a** see Toremifene on page 1351

♦ **Febrile Seizures** see page 1660

♦ **Fedahist® [OTC]** see Chlorpheniramine and Pseudoephedrine on page 279

♦ **Fedahist® Expectorant [OTC]** see Guaifenesin and Pseudoephedrine on page 647

♦ **Feiba VH Immuno®** see Anti-inhibitor Coagulant Complex on page 106

Felbamate (FEL ba mate)

U.S. Brand Names Felbatol®

Therapeutic Category Anticonvulsant, Miscellaneous

Use Not as a first-line antiepileptic treatment; only in those patients who respond inadequately to alternative treatments and whose epilepsy is so severe that a substantial risk of aplastic anemia and/or liver failure is deemed acceptable in light of the benefits conferred by its use. Patient must be fully advised of risk and provide signed written informed consent. Felbamate can be used as either monotherapy or adjunctive therapy in the treatment of partial seizures (with and without generalization) and in adults with epilepsy.

(Continued)

Felbamate *(Continued)*

Orphan drug: Adjunctive therapy in the treatment of partial and generalized seizures associated with Lennox-Gastaut syndrome in children

Pregnancy Risk Factor C

Contraindications Hypersensitivity to felbamate or any component of the formulation; use with caution in those patients who have demonstrated hypersensitivity reactions to other carbamates

Adverse Reactions

>10%:

Central nervous system: Somnolence, headache, fatigue, dizziness

Gastrointestinal: Nausea, anorexia, vomiting, constipation

1% to 10%:

Cardiovascular: Chest pain, palpitations, tachycardia

Central nervous system: Depression or behavior changes, nervousness, anxiety, ataxia, stupor, malaise, agitation, psychological disturbances, aggressive reaction

Dermatologic: Skin rash, acne, pruritus

Gastrointestinal: Xerostomia, diarrhea, abdominal pain, weight gain, taste perversion

Neuromuscular & skeletal: Tremor, abnormal gait, paresthesia, myalgia

Ocular: Diplopia, abnormal vision

Respiratory: Sinusitis, pharyngitis

Miscellaneous: SGPT increase

<1% (Limited to important or life-threatening): Euphoria, hallucinations, leukocytosis, leukopenia, lymphadenopathy, migraine, suicide attempts, thrombocytopenia, urticaria

Overdosage/Toxicology Symptoms include sedation, gastrointestinal upset, and tachycardia. Provide general supportive care.

Drug Interactions

Cytochrome P450 Effect: CYP2C19 enzyme inhibitor

Increased Effect/Toxicity: Felbamate increases serum phenytoin, phenobarbital, and valproic acid concentrations which may result in toxicity; consider decreasing phenytoin or phenobarbital dosage by 25%. A decrease in valproic acid dosage may also be necessary.

Decreased Effect: Carbamazepine, phenytoin may decrease serum felbamate concentrations. Felbamate may decrease carbamazepine levels and increase levels of the active metabolite of carbamazepine (10,11-epoxide) resulting in carbamazepine toxicity; monitor for signs of carbamazepine toxicity (dizziness, ataxia, nystagmus, drowsiness).

Ethanol/Nutrition/Herb Interactions

Ethanol: Avoid ethanol (may increase CNS depression).

Food: Food does not affect absorption.

Herb/Nutraceutical: Avoid evening primrose (seizure threshold decreased).

Stability Store medication in tightly closed container at room temperature away from excessive heat.

Mechanism of Action Mechanism of action is unknown but has properties in common with other marketed anticonvulsants; has weak inhibitory effects on GABA-receptor binding, benzodiazepine receptor binding, and is devoid of activity at the MK-801 receptor binding site of the NMDA receptor-ionophore complex.

Pharmacodynamics/Kinetics

Absorption: Rapid and almost complete; food has no effect upon the tablet's absorption

Half-life elimination: 20-23 hours average

Time to peak, serum: ~3 hours

Excretion: Urine (40% to 50% as unchanged drug, 40% as inactive metabolites)

Usual Dosage Anticonvulsant:

Monotherapy: Children >14 years and Adults:

Initial: 1200 mg/day in divided doses 3 or 4 times/day; titrate previously untreated patients under close clinical supervision, increasing the dosage in 600 mg increments every 2 weeks to 2400 mg/day based on clinical response and thereafter to 3600 mg/day as clinically indicated

Conversion to monotherapy: Initiate at 1200 mg/day in divided doses 3 or 4 times/day, reduce the dosage of the concomitant anticonvulsant(s) by 20% to 33% at the initiation of felbamate therapy; at week 2, increase the felbamate dosage to 2400 mg/day while reducing the dosage of the other anticonvulsant(s) up to an additional 33% of their original dosage; at week 3, increase the felbamate dosage up to 3600 mg/day and continue to reduce the dosage of the other anticonvulsant(s) as clinically indicated

Adjunctive therapy: Children with Lennox-Gastaut and ages 2-14 years:

Week 1:

Felbamate: 15 mg/kg/day divided 3-4 times/day

Concomitant anticonvulsant(s): Reduce original dosage by 20% to 30%

Week 2:

Felbamate: 30 mg/kg/day divided 3-4 times/day

Concomitant anticonvulsant(s): Reduce original dosage up to an additional 33%

Week 3:

Felbamate: 45 mg/kg/day divided 3-4 times/day

Concomitant anticonvulsant(s): Reduce dosage as clinically indicated

Adjunctive therapy: Children >14 years and Adults:

Week 1:

Felbamate: 1200 mg/day initial dose

Concomitant anticonvulsant(s): Reduce original dosage by 20% to 33%

Week 2:

Felbamate: 2400 mg/day (therapeutic range)

Concomitant anticonvulsant(s): Reduce original dosage by up to an additional 33%

Week 3:

Felbamate: 3600 mg/day (therapeutic range)

Concomitant anticonvulsant(s): Reduce original dosage as clinically indicated

Dietary Considerations May be taken without regard to meals.

Administration Administer on an empty stomach for best absorption.

Monitoring Parameters Monitor serum levels of concomitant anticonvulsant therapy; monitor AST, ALT, and bilirubin weekly. Hematologic evaluations before therapy begins, frequently during therapy, and for a significant period after discontinuation.

Reference Range Not necessary to routinely monitor serum drug levels, since dose should be titrated to clinical response

Patient Information Take exactly as directed (do not increase dose or frequency or discontinue without consulting prescriber). While using this medication, do not use alcohol and other prescription or OTC medications (especially pain medications, sedatives, antihistamines, or hypnotics) without consulting prescriber. Maintain adequate hydration (2-3 L/day of fluids unless instructed to restrict fluid intake). You may experience drowsiness, dizziness, or blurred vision (use caution when driving or engaging in tasks requiring alertness until response to drug is known); nausea, vomiting, loss of appetite, or dry mouth (small frequent meals, frequent mouth care, chewing gum, or sucking lozenges may help). Wear identification of epileptic status and medications. Report CNS changes, mentation changes, or changes in cognition; muscle cramping, weakness, tremors, changes in gait; persistent GI symptoms (cramping, constipation, vomiting, anorexia); rash or skin irritations; unusual bruising or bleeding (mouth, urine, stool); cough, runny nose, sore throat, or difficulty breathing; worsening of seizure activity, or loss of seizure control. Inform prescriber if you are or intend to be pregnant. Breast-feeding is not recommended.

Nursing Implications Monitor serum levels of concomitant anticonvulsant therapy.

Additional Information Monotherapy has not been associated with gingival hyperplasia, impaired concentration, weight gain, or abnormal thinking. Because felbamate is the only drug shown effective in Lennox-Gastaut syndrome, it is considered an orphan drug for this indication.

Dosage Forms
Suspension, oral: 600 mg/5 mL (240 mL, 960 mL)
Tablet: 400 mg, 600 mg

◆ **Felbatol**® *see* Felbamate *on page 545*
◆ **Feldene**® *see* Piroxicam *on page 1093*

Felodipine (fe LOE di peen)

Related Information
Calcium Channel Blockers Comparison *on page 1494*
U.S. Brand Names Plendil®
Canadian Brand Names Plendil®; Renedil®
Therapeutic Category Antihypertensive Agent; Calcium Channel Blocker
Use Treatment of hypertension, congestive heart failure
Pregnancy Risk Factor C
Contraindications Hypersensitivity to felodipine, any component of the formulation, or other calcium channel blocker
Warnings/Precautions Use with caution and titrate dosages for patients with impaired renal or hepatic function; use caution when treating patients with congestive heart failure, sick-sinus syndrome, severe left ventricular dysfunction, hypertrophic cardiomyopathy (especially obstructive), concomitant therapy with beta-blockers or digoxin, edema, or increased intracranial pressure with cranial tumors; do not abruptly withdraw (may cause chest pain); elderly may experience hypotension and constipation more readily. Safety and efficacy in children have not been established. Dosage titration should occur after 14 days on a given dose.

Adverse Reactions
>10%: Central nervous system: Headache (11% to 15%)
2% to 10%: Cardiovascular: Peripheral edema (2% to 17%), tachycardia (0.4% to 2.5%), flushing (4% to 7%)
<1% (Limited to important or life-threatening): Angina, angioedema, anxiety, arrhythmia, CHF, CVA, libido decreased, depression, dizziness, gingival hyperplasia, dyspnea, dysuria, gynecomastia, hypotension, impotence, insomnia, irritability, leukocytoclastic vasculitis, myocardial infarction, nervousness, paresthesias, somnolence, syncope, urticaria, vomiting

Overdosage/Toxicology
Primary cardiac symptoms of calcium blocker overdose include hypotension and bradycardia. Hypotension is caused by peripheral vasodilation, myocardial depression, and bradycardia. Bradycardia results from sinus bradycardia, second- or third-degree atrioventricular block, or sinus arrest with junctional rhythm. Intraventricular conduction is usually not affected so QRS duration is normal (verapamil prolongs the P-R interval and bepridil prolongs the QT interval and may cause ventricular arrhythmias, including torsade de pointes).

Noncardiac symptoms include confusion, stupor, nausea, vomiting, metabolic acidosis and hyperglycemia. Following initial gastric decontamination, if possible, repeated calcium administration may promptly reverse depressed cardiac contractility (but not sinus node depression or peripheral vasodilation). Glucagon, epinephrine, and inamrinone (amrinone) may treat refractory hypotension. Glucagon and epinephrine also increase the heart rate (outside the U.S., 4-aminopyridine may be available as an antidote). Dialysis and hemoperfusion are not effective in enhancing elimination, although repeat-dose activated charcoal may serve as an adjunct with sustained-release preparations.

In a few reported cases, overdose with calcium channel blockers has been associated with hypotension and bradycardia, initially refractory to atropine, but becoming more responsive to this agent when larger doses (approaching 1 g/hour for more than 24 hours) of calcium chloride were administered.

Drug Interactions
Cytochrome P450 Effect: CYP3A3/4 enzyme substrate
Increased Effect/Toxicity: Inhibitors of CYP3A4, including azole antifungals (ketoconazole, itraconazole) and erythromycin, may inhibit calcium channel blocker metabolism, increasing the effects of felodipine. Beta-blockers may have increased pharmacokinetic or pharmacodynamic interactions with felodipine. Cyclosporine increases felodipine's serum
(Continued)

Felodipine *(Continued)*

concentration. Ethanol increases felodipine's absorption; watch for a greater hypotensive effect.

Decreased Effect: Felodipine may decrease pharmacologic actions of theophylline. Calcium may reduce the calcium channel blocker's effects, particularly hypotension. Carbamazepine significantly reduces felodipine's bioavailability; avoid this combination. Nafcillin decreases plasma concentration of felodipine; avoid this combination. Rifampin increases the metabolism of felodipine. Felodipine may decrease pharmacologic actions of theophylline.

Ethanol/Nutrition/Herb Interactions

Food: Increased therapeutic and vasodilator side effects, including severe hypotension and myocardial ischemia, may occur if felodipine is taken with grapefruit juice; avoid concurrent use. High-fat/carbohydrate meals will increase C_{max} by 60%; grapefruit juice will increase C_{max} by twofold.

Herb/Nutraceutical: St John's wort may decrease felodipine levels. Avoid dong quai if using for hypertension (has estrogenic activity). Avoid ephedra, yohimbe, ginseng (may worsen hypertension). Avoid garlic (may have increased antihypertensive effect).

Mechanism of Action Inhibits calcium ions from entering the "slow channels" or select voltage-sensitive areas of vascular smooth muscle and myocardium during depolarization, producing a relaxation of coronary vascular smooth muscle and coronary vasodilation; increases myocardial oxygen delivery in patients with vasospastic angina

Pharmacodynamics/Kinetics

Onset of action: 2-5 hours

Duration: 16-24 hours

Absorption: 100%; absolute: 20% due to first-pass effect

Protein binding: >99%

Metabolism: Hepatic; large first-pass effect

Half-life elimination: 11-16 hours

Excretion: Urine (as metabolites)

Usual Dosage

Adults: Oral: 2.5-10 mg once daily; usual initial dose: 5 mg; increase by 5 mg at 2-week intervals, as needed; maximum: 10 mg

Elderly: Begin with 2.5 mg/day

Dosing adjustment/comments in hepatic impairment: May require lower dosages (initial: 2.5 mg/day); monitor blood pressure

Dietary Considerations Should be taken without food.

Administration Do not crush or chew extended release tablets; swallow whole.

Patient Information Do not crush or chew tablets; do not discontinue abruptly; report any dizziness, shortness of breath, palpitations or edema occurs

Nursing Implications Do not crush extended release tablets

Additional Information Felodipine maintains renal and mesenteric blood flow during hemorrhagic shock in animals.

Dosage Forms Tablet, extended release: 2.5 mg, 5 mg, 10 mg

♦ **Felodipine and Enalapril** *see Enalapril and Felodipine on page 465*

♦ **Femara®** *see Letrozole on page 781*

♦ **Femcet®** *see Butalbital Compound on page 197*

♦ **femhrt®** *see Ethinyl Estradiol and Norethindrone on page 522*

♦ **Femiron® [OTC]** *see Ferrous Fumarate on page 555*

♦ **Femstat® One (Can)** *see Butoconazole on page 199*

♦ **Fenesin™** *see Guaifenesin on page 645*

♦ **Fenesin™ DM** *see Guaifenesin and Dextromethorphan on page 646*

Fenofibrate *(fen oh FYE brate)*

Related Information

Hyperlipidemia Management *on page 1670*

Lipid-Lowering Agents *on page 1505*

U.S. Brand Names TriCor®

Canadian Brand Names Apo®-Fenofibrate; Apo®-Feno-Micro; Gen-Fenofibrate Micro; Lipidil Micro®; Lipidil Supra®; Nu-Fenofibrate; PMS-Fenofibrate Micro; TriCor®

Synonyms Procetofene; Proctofene

Therapeutic Category Antilipemic Agent, Fibric Acid

Use Adjunct to dietary therapy for the treatment of adults with very high elevations of serum triglyceride levels (types IV and V hyperlipidemia) who are at risk of pancreatitis and who do not respond adequately to a determined dietary effort; safety and efficacy may be greater than that of clofibrate; adjunct to dietary therapy for the reduction of low density lipoprotein cholesterol (LDL-C), total cholesterol (total-C), triglycerides, and apolipoprotein B (apo B) in adult patients with primary hypercholesterolemia or mixed dyslipidemia (Fredrickson types IIa and IIb); its efficacy can be enhanced by combination with other hypolipidemic agents that have a different mechanism of action

Pregnancy Risk Factor C

Pregnancy/Breast-Feeding Implications Animal studies have shown embryocidal and teratogenic effect. There are no adequate and well-controlled studies in pregnant women. Use should be avoided, if possible, in pregnant women since the neonatal glucuronide conjugation pathways are immature.

Contraindications Hypersensitivity to fenofibrate or any component of the formulation; hepatic or severe renal dysfunction including primary biliary cirrhosis and unexplained persistent liver function abnormalities; pre-existing gallbladder disease

Warnings/Precautions Product reformulation has resulted in dosing changes; see Usual Dosage. The hypoprothrombinemic effect of anticoagulants is significantly increased with concomitant fenofibrate administration. Use with caution in patients with severe renal dysfunction. Hepatic transaminases can significantly elevate (dose-related). Regular monitoring of liver function tests is required. May cause cholelithiasis. Adjustments in warfarin therapy may be required with concurrent use. Use caution when combining fenofibrate with HMG-CoA reductase inhibitors (may lead to myopathy, rhabdomyolysis). The effect of CAD morbidity and mortality has not been established. Therapy should be withdrawn if an adequate response is not obtained after 2 months of therapy at the maximal daily dose (201 mg). Rare hypersensitivity reactions may occur. Dose adjustment is required for renal impairment and elderly patients. Safety and efficacy in children have not been established.

Adverse Reactions
1% to 10%:
Gastrointestinal: Abdominal pain (5%), constipation (2%)
Hepatic: Abnormal liver function test (7%), creatine phosphokinase increased (3%), ALT increased (3%), AST increased (3%)
Neuromuscular & skeletal: Back pain (3%)
Respiratory: Respiratory disorder (6%), rhinitis (2%)

Frequency not defined (limited to important or life-threatening): Allergic reaction, alopecia, angina pectoris, anxiety, arrhythmias, asthma, atrial fibrillation, cholecystitis, cholelithiasis, colitis, depression, diabetes mellitus, dyspnea, eosinophilia, esophagitis, gastritis, gout, gynecomastia, hypoglycemia, kidney function abnormality, leukopenia, lymphadenopathy, myasthenia, myocardial infarction, neuralgia, paresthesia, photosensitivity reaction, rash, thrombocytopenia, urolithiasis, urticaria, vertigo, vomiting

Overdosage/Toxicology Symptoms include nausea, vomiting, diarrhea, and GI distress. Treatment is supportive. Hemodialysis has no effect on removal of fenofibric acid from the plasma.

Drug Interactions
Increased Effect/Toxicity: The hypolipidemic effect of fenofibrate is increased when used with cholestyramine or colestipol. Fenofibrate may increase the effect of chlorpropamide and warfarin. Concurrent use of fenofibrate with HMG-CoA reductase inhibitors (atorvastatin, cerivastatin, fluvastatin, lovastatin, pravastatin, simvastatin) may increase the risk of myopathy and rhabdomyolysis. The manufacturer warns against concomitant use. However, combination therapy with statins has been used in some patients with resistant hyperlipidemias (with great caution).
Decreased Effect: Rifampin (and potentially other enzyme inducers) may decrease levels of fenofibrate.

Mechanism of Action Fenofibric acid is believed to increase VLDL catabolism by enhancing the synthesis of lipoprotein lipase; as a result of a decrease in VLDL levels, total plasma triglycerides are reduced by 30% to 60%; modest increase in HDL occurs in some hypertriglyceridemic patients

Pharmacodynamics/Kinetics
Absorption: 60% to 90% when given with meals
Distribution: Widely to most tissues except brain or eye; concentrates in liver, kidneys, and gut
Protein binding: >99%
Metabolism: Metabolized to its active form, fenofibric acid, by tissue and plasma esterases; undergoes inactivation by glucuronidation hepatically or renally
Half-life elimination: 21 hours; Elderly: 30 hours; Hepatic impairment: 44-54 hours
Time to peak: 4-6 hours
Excretion: Urine (60% to 93% as metabolites); feces (5% to 25%); hemodialysis has no effect on removal of fenofibric acid from plasma

Usual Dosage Oral: **Note:** As of September, 2001, a tablet formulation became available which will replace the capsules, as soon as existing supply is exhausted.
Adults:
Hypertriglyceridemia: Initial:
Capsule: 67 mg/day with meals, up to 200 mg/day
Tablet: 54 mg/day with meals, up to 160 mg/day
Hypercholesterolemia or mixed hyperlipidemia: Initial:
Capsule: 200 mg/day with meals
Tablet: 160 mg/day with meals
Elderly: Initial: 67 mg/day (capsule) or 54 mg/day (tablet)
Dosage adjustment in renal impairment: Decrease dose or increase dosing interval for patients with renal failure: Initial: 67 mg/day (capsule) or 54 mg/day (tablet)
Hemodialysis has no effect on removal of fenofibric acid from the plasma.

Dietary Considerations Take with food.

Administration 6-8 weeks of therapy is required to determine efficacy.

Monitoring Parameters Total serum cholesterol and triglyceride concentration and CLDL, LDL, and HDL levels should be measured periodically; if only marginal changes are noted in 6-8 weeks, the drug should be discontinued; serum transaminases should be measured every 3 months; if ALT values increase >100 units/L, therapy should be discontinued. Monitor LFTs prior to initiation, at 6 and 12 weeks after initiation of first dose, then periodically thereafter.

Patient Information Take with food. Do not change dosage or dosage form without consulting prescriber. Maintain diet and exercise program as prescribed. You may experience mild GI disturbances (eg, gas, diarrhea, constipation, nausea); inform prescriber if these are severe. Report skin rash or irritation, insomnia, unusual muscle pain or tremors, or persistent dizziness. Inform prescriber if you are or intend to be pregnant; consult prescriber if breastfeeding.

Additional Information In September, 2001, a tablet formulation of TriCor® was approved by the FDA. According to Abbott Laboratories, the tablet will replace the capsule formulation. It is important to note that the strengths of the tablet are not the same as the capsule. The tablet formulation has increased bioavailability, which produces equivalent plasma levels at lower doses. Patients previously taking the 200 mg capsule should be changed to the 160 mg tablet. Patients previously taking the 67 mg capsule should be changed to the 54 mg tablet. Tablets should be taken with food. Prescriptions for the capsules should be filled as written (Continued)

Fenofibrate *(Continued)*

until the supply of capsules is depleted; at that time a new prescription for tablets should be requested from the prescriber.

Dosage Forms
Capsule: 67 mg, 200 mg [Note: This dosage form to be discontinued.]
Tablet: 54 mg, 160 mg

Fenoldopam (fe NOL doe pam)

Related Information
Hypertension *on page 1675*

U.S. Brand Names Corlopam®

Canadian Brand Names Corlopam®

Synonyms Fenoldopam Mesylate

Therapeutic Category Antihypertensive Agent

Use Treatment of severe hypertension particularly I.V. and in patients with renal compromise; potential use for congestive heart failure

Contraindications Hypersensitivity of fenoldopam or any component of the formulation; hypersensitivity to sulfites (contains sodium metabisulfite)

Warnings/Precautions Use with caution in patients with cirrhosis, portal hypertension (due to possible increases in portal venous pressure), unstable angina, or glaucoma

Adverse Reactions Frequency not defined:
Cardiovascular: Angina, asymptomatic T wave flattening on EKG, chest pain, edema, facial flushing, fibrillation (atrial), flutter (atrial), hypotension, tachycardia
Central nervous system: Dizziness, headache
Gastrointestinal: Diarrhea, nausea, vomiting
Ocular: Intraocular pressure (increased)

Drug Interactions
Increased Effect/Toxicity: Concurrent acetaminophen may increase fenoldopam levels (30% to 70%). Beta-blockers increase the risk of hypotension.

Stability Store ampuls at room temperature; diluted solution is stable for ≤24 hours; discard any diluted solution that is not used after 24 hours

Mechanism of Action A selective postsynaptic dopamine agonist (D_1-receptors) which exerts hypotensive effects by decreasing peripheral vasculature resistance with increased renal blood flow, diuresis, and natriuresis; 6 times as potent as dopamine in producing renal vasodilitation; has minimal adrenergic effects

Pharmacodynamics/Kinetics
Onset of action: I.V.: 10 minutes
Duration: Oral: 2-4 hours; I.V.: 1 hour
Absorption: Oral: Good; peak serum levels at 1 hour
Distribution: V_d: 0.6 L/kg
Half-life elimination: I.V.: 9.8 minutes
Metabolism: Hepatic to multiple metabolites; the 8-sulfate metabolite may have some activity; extensive first-pass effect
Excretion: Urine (80%); feces (20%)

Usual Dosage I.V.: Severe hypertension: Initial: 0.1 mcg/kg/minute; may be increased in increments of 0.05-0.2 mcg/kg/minute until target blood pressure is achieved; average rate: 0.25-0.5 mcg/kg/minute; usual length of treatment is 1-6 hours with tapering of 12% every 15-30 minutes

Dosing adjustment in renal impairment: None required
Dosing adjustment in hepatic impairment: None published

Monitoring Parameters Blood pressure, heart rate, EKG, renal/hepatic function tests

Reference Range Mean plasma fenoldopam levels after a 2 hour infusion (at 0.5 μg/kg/minute) and a 100 mg dose is approximately 13 ng/mL and 50 ng/mL

Additional Information Suitable for use in patients whose condition is unstable or rapidly changing because the effects of the drug are predictable and easily reversible; it has been found to safely control blood pressure in patients with a variety of pre-existing conditions including kidney disease, liver disease, and heart failure. (Clinical benefit other than blood pressure reduction has not been established.) In none of these situations does the dose need to be adjusted, minimizing the risk of drug overdose in patients with these conditions. The drug is quickly metabolized into inactive substances before it is excreted; therefore, there are no toxic chemicals derived from the drug. Unlike the situation with some other intravenous antihypertensives, the patient does not need an arterial line for blood pressure monitoring; a blood pressure cuff is sufficient to monitor blood pressure lowering. Since the drug induces natriuresis, diuresis, and increased creatinine clearance, it may have an advantage over nitroprusside, especially in patients with severe renal insufficiency and in volume overloaded patients.

Dosage Forms Injection: 10 mg/mL (5 mL)

♦ **Fenoldopam Mesylate** *see Fenoldopam on page 550*

Fenoprofen (fen oh PROE fen)

Related Information
Nonsteroidal Anti-Inflammatory Agents Comparison *on page 1512*

U.S. Brand Names Nalfon®

Canadian Brand Names Nalfon®

Synonyms Fenoprofen Calcium

Therapeutic Category Analgesic, Nonsteroidal Anti-inflammatory Drug; Anti-inflammatory Agent; Nonsteroidal Anti-inflammatory Drug (NSAID), Oral

Use Symptomatic treatment of acute and chronic rheumatoid arthritis and osteoarthritis; relief of mild to moderate pain

Pregnancy Risk Factor B/D (3rd trimester)

Contraindications Hypersensitivity to fenoprofen, aspirin, or other NSAIDs; pregnancy (3rd trimester)

Warnings/Precautions Use with caution in patients with congestive heart failure, hypertension, dehydration, decreased renal or hepatic function, history of GI disease (bleeding or ulcers), or those receiving anticoagulants. Elderly are at a high risk for adverse effects from nonsteroidal anti-inflammatory agents. As many as 60% of elderly can develop peptic ulceration and/or hemorrhage asymptomatically.

Use lowest effective dose for shortest period possible. Use of NSAIDs can compromise existing renal function especially when Cl_{cr} is <30 mL/minute. CNS adverse effects such as confusion, agitation, and hallucination are generally seen in overdose or high-dose situations; however, elderly may demonstrate these adverse effects at lower doses than younger adults. Withhold for at least 4-6 half-lives prior to surgical or dental procedures.

Adverse Reactions
1% to 10%:
  Central nervous system: Headache, nervousness, dizziness
  Dermatologic: Itching, rash
  Endocrine & metabolic: Fluid retention
  Gastrointestinal: Abdominal cramps, heartburn, indigestion, nausea, vomiting
  Otic: Ringing in ears
  <1% (Limited to important or life-threatening): Congestive heart failure, hypertension, arrhythmias, tachycardia, erythema multiforme, toxic epidermal necrolysis, Stevens-Johnson syndrome, angioedema, GI ulceration, agranulocytosis, anemia, hemolytic anemia, bone marrow depression, leukopenia, thrombocytopenia, hepatitis, polyuria, acute renal failure, dyspnea

Overdosage/Toxicology Symptoms include acute renal failure, vomiting, drowsiness, and leukocytosis. Management of nonsteroidal anti-inflammatory drug (NSAID) intoxication is primarily supportive and symptomatic. Fluid therapy is commonly effective in managing hypotension that may occur following an acute NSAID overdose, except when due to acute blood loss.

Drug Interactions
  Increased Effect/Toxicity: Increased effect/toxicity of phenytoin, sulfonamides, sulfonylureas, salicylates, and oral anticoagulants.
  Decreased Effect: Decreased effect with phenobarbital.

Ethanol/Nutrition/Herb Interactions
  Ethanol: Avoid ethanol (may enhance gastric mucosal irritation).
  Food: Fenoprofen peak serum levels may be decreased if taken with food.
  Herb/Nutraceutical: Avoid cat's claw, dong quai, evening primrose, feverfew, garlic, ginger, ginkgo, red clover, horse chestnut, green tea, ginseng (all have additional antiplatelet activity).

Mechanism of Action Inhibits prostaglandin synthesis by decreasing the activity of the enzyme, cyclo-oxygenase, which results in decreased formation of prostaglandin precursors

Pharmacodynamics/Kinetics
  Onset of action: A few days
  Absorption: Rapid; 80%
  Distribution: Does not cross the placenta
  Protein binding: 99%
  Metabolism: Extensively hepatic
  Half-life elimination: 2.5-3 hours
  Time to peak, serum: ~2 hours
  Excretion: Urine (2% to 5% as unchanged drug); feces (small amounts)

Usual Dosage Adults: Oral:
  Rheumatoid arthritis: 300-600 mg 3-4 times/day up to 3.2 g/day
  Mild to moderate pain: 200 mg every 4-6 hours as needed

Dietary Considerations May be taken with food to decrease GI distress.

Monitoring Parameters Monitor CBC, liver enzymes; monitor urine output and BUN/serum creatinine in patients receiving diuretics

Reference Range Therapeutic: 20-65 µg/mL (SI: 82-268 µmol/L)

Test Interactions ↑ chloride (S), ↑ sodium (S)

Patient Information Do not crush tablets; take with food, milk, or water; report any signs of blood in stool

Nursing Implications Monitor CBC, liver enzymes; monitor urine output and BUN/serum creatinine in patients receiving diuretics

Dosage Forms
  Capsule, as calcium: 200 mg, 300 mg
  Tablet, as calcium: 600 mg

♦ **Fenoprofen Calcium** *see Fenoprofen on page 550*

Fentanyl (FEN ta nil)

Related Information
  Adult ACLS Algorithms *on page 1632*
  Narcotic Agonists Comparison *on page 1506*

U.S. Brand Names Actiq®; Duragesic®; Sublimaze®

Canadian Brand Names Actiq®; Duragesic®

Synonyms Fentanyl Citrate

Therapeutic Category Analgesic, Narcotic

Use Sedation, relief of pain, preoperative medication, adjunct to general or regional anesthesia, management of chronic pain (transdermal product)

Actiq® is indicated only for management of breakthrough cancer pain in patients who are tolerant to and currently receiving opioid therapy for persistent cancer pain.

Restrictions C-II

Pregnancy Risk Factor B/D (prolonged use or high doses at term)
(Continued)

Fentanyl (Continued)

Contraindications Hypersensitivity to fentanyl or any component of the formulation; increased intracranial pressure; severe respiratory depression; severe liver or renal insufficiency; pregnancy (prolonged use or high doses near term)

Actiq® must not be used in patients who are intolerant to opioids. Patients are considered opioid-tolerant if they are taking at least 60 mg morphine/day, 50 mcg transdermal fentanyl/hour, or an equivalent dose of another opioid for ≥1 week.

Warnings/Precautions Fentanyl shares the toxic potentials of opiate agonists, and precautions of opiate agonist therapy should be observed; use with caution in patients with bradycardia; rapid I.V. infusion may result in skeletal muscle and chest wall rigidity, impaired ventilation, respiratory distress, apnea, bronchoconstriction, laryngospasm; inject slowly over 3-5 minutes; nondepolarizing skeletal muscle relaxant may be required. Tolerance of drug dependence may result from extended use.

Actiq® should be used only for the care of cancer patients and is intended for use by specialists who are knowledgeable in treating cancer pain. Actiq® preparations contain an amount of medication that can be fatal to children. Keep all units out of the reach of children and discard any open units properly. Patients and caregivers should be counseled on the dangers to children including the risk of exposure to partially-consumed units. Safety and efficacy have not been established in children <16 years of age.

Topical patches: Serum fentanyl concentrations may increase approximately one-third for patients with a body temperature of 40°C secondary to a temperature-dependent increase in fentanyl release from the system and increased skin permeability. Patients who experience adverse reactions should be monitored for at least 12 hours after removal of the patch.

The elderly may be particularly susceptible to the CNS depressant and constipating effects of narcotics

Adverse Reactions

>10%:
Cardiovascular: Bradycardia, hypotension, peripheral vasodilation
Central nervous system: Drowsiness, sedation, increased intracranial pressure
Gastrointestinal: Nausea, vomiting
Endocrine & metabolic: Antidiuretic hormone release
Ocular: Miosis
Neuromuscular & skeletal: Chest wall rigidity

1% to 10%:
Cardiovascular: Cardiac arrhythmias, orthostatic hypotension
Central nervous system: Confusion, CNS depression
Gastrointestinal: Constipation
Ocular: Blurred vision
Respiratory: Apnea, postoperative respiratory depression

<1% (Limited to important or life-threatening): Bronchospasm, convulsions, hypercarbia, laryngospasm, respiratory depression

Overdosage/Toxicology Symptoms include CNS depression, respiratory depression, and miosis. Overdose treatment includes airway support, establishment of an I.V. line, and administration of naloxone 2 mg I.V. (0.01 mg/kg for children), with repeat administration as necessary, up to a total of 10 mg.

Drug Interactions

Cytochrome P450 Effect: CYP3A3/4 enzyme substrate

Increased Effect/Toxicity: Increased sedation with CNS depressants, phenothiazines. Tricyclic antidepressants may potentiate fentanyl's adverse effects. Potential for serotonin syndrome if combined with other serotonergic drugs. CYP3A3/4 inhibitors (including erythromycin, clarithromycin, ketoconazole, itraconazole, and protease inhibitors) may increase serum concentration of fentanyl.

Decreased Effect: CYP3A3/4 inducers (including carbamazepine, phenytoin, phenobarbital, rifampin) may decrease serum levels of fentanyl by increasing metabolism.

Ethanol/Nutrition/Herb Interactions

Ethanol: Avoid ethanol (may increase CNS depression).
Food: Glucose may cause hyperglycemia.
Herb/Nutraceutical: St John's wort may decrease fentanyl levels. Avoid valerian, St John's wort, kava kava, gotu kola (may increase CNS depression).

Stability

Injection formulation: Protect from light; **incompatible** when mixed in the same syringe with pentobarbital
Transmucosal: Store at controlled room temperature of 15°C to 30°C (59°F to 86°F)

Mechanism of Action Binds with stereospecific receptors at many sites within the CNS, increases pain threshold, alters pain reception, inhibits ascending pain pathways

Pharmacodynamics/Kinetics Respiratory depressant effect may last longer than analgesic effect

Onset of action: Analgesic: I.M.: 7-15 minutes; I.V.: Almost immediate; Transmucosal: 5-15 minutes
Peak effect: Transmucosal: Analgesic: 20-30 minutes
Duration: I.M.: 1-2 hours; I.V.: 0.5-1 hour; Transmucosal: Related to blood level
Absorption: Transmucosal: Rapid, ~25% from the buccal mucosa; 75% swallowed with saliva and slowly absorbed from gastrointestinal tract
Distribution: Highly lipophilic, redistributes into muscle and fat
Metabolism: Hepatic
Bioavailability: Transmucosal: ~50% (range: 36% to 71%)
Half-life elimination: 2-4 hours; Transmucosal: 6.6 hours (range: 5-15 hours)
Excretion: Urine (primarily as metabolites, 10% as unchanged drug)

Usual Dosage Doses should be titrated to appropriate effects; wide range of doses, dependent upon desired degree of analgesia/anesthesia

Children 1-12 years:

Sedation for minor procedures/analgesia: I.M., I.V.: 1-2 mcg/kg/dose; may repeat at 30- to 60-minute intervals. **Note:** Children 18-36 months of age may require 2-3 mcg/kg/dose

Continuous sedation/analgesia: Initial I.V. bolus: 1-2 mcg/kg then 1 mcg/kg/hour; titrate upward; usual: 1-3 mcg/kg/hour

Pain control: Transdermal: Not recommended

Children >12 years and Adults: Sedation for minor procedures/analgesia: I.M., I.V.: 0.5-1 mcg/kg/dose; higher doses are used for major procedures

Adults:

Preoperative sedation, adjunct to regional anesthesia, postoperative pain: I.M., I.V.: 50-100 mcg/dose

Continuous sedation/analgesia (including ICU settings): Initial I.V. bolus: 25-50 mcg; then 1 mcg/kg/hour; titrate upward; usual: 1-3 mcg/kg/hour

Adjunct to general anesthesia: I.M., I.V.: 2-50 mcg/kg

General anesthesia without additional anesthetic agents: I.V. 50-100 mcg/kg with O_2 and skeletal muscle relaxant

Breakthrough cancer pain: Adults: Transmucosal: Actiq® dosing should be individually titrated to provide adequate analgesia with minimal side effects. It is indicated only for management of breakthrough cancer pain in patients who are tolerant to and currently receiving opioid therapy for persistent cancer pain. An initial starting dose of 200 mcg should be used for the treatment of breakthrough cancer pain. Patients should be monitored closely in order to determine the proper dose. If redosing for the same episode is necessary, the second dose may be started 15 minutes after completion of the first dose. Dosing should be titrated so that the patient's pain can be treated with one single dose. Generally, 1-2 days is required to determine the proper dose of analgesia with limited side effects. Once the dose has been determined, consumption should be limited to 4 units/day or less. Patients needing more than 4 units/day should have the dose of their long-term opioid re-evaluated. If signs of excessive opioid effects occur before a dose is complete, the unit should be removed from the patients mouth immediately, and subsequent doses decreased.

Pain control: Adults: Transdermal: Initial: 25 mcg/hour system; if currently receiving opiates, convert to fentanyl equivalent and administer equianalgesic dosage titrated to minimize the adverse effects and provide analgesia. To convert patients from oral or parenteral opioids to Duragesic®, the previous 24-hour analgesic requirement should be calculated. This analgesic requirement should be converted to the equianalgesic oral morphine dose.

See tables.

Equianalgesic Doses of Opioid Agonists

Drug	Equianalgesic Dose (mg)	
	I.M.	P.O.
Codeine	130	200
Hydromorphone	1.5	7.5
Levorphanol	2	4
Meperidine	75	—
Methadone	10	20
Morphine	10	60
Oxycodone	15	30
Oxymorphone	1	10 (PR)

From *N Engl J Med*, 1985, 313:84-95.

Corresponding Doses of Oral/Intramuscular Morphine and Duragesic™

P.O. 24-Hour Morphine (mg/d)	I.M. 24-Hour Morphine (mg/d)	Duragesic™ Dose (mcg/h)
45-134	8-22	25
135-224	28-37	50
225-314	38-52	75
315-404	53-67	100
405-494	68-82	125
495-584	83-97	150
585-674	98-112	175
675-764	113-127	200
765-854	128-142	225
855-944	143-157	250
945-1034	158-172	275
1035-1124	173-187	300

Product information, Duragesic™ — Janssen Pharmaceutica, January, 1991.

The dosage should not be titrated more frequently than every 3 days after the initial dose or every 6 days thereafter. The majority of patients are controlled on every 72-hour administration, however, a small number of patients require every 48-hour administration.

Elderly >65 years: Transmucosal: Actiq®: Dose should be reduced to 2.5-5 mcg/kg; elderly have been found to be twice as sensitive as younger patients to the effects of fentanyl. Patients in this age group generally require smaller doses of Actiq® than younger patients

(Continued)

Fentanyl *(Continued)*

Dosing adjustment in renal impairment:
Cl$_{cr}$ 10-50 mL/minute: Administer at 75% of normal dose
Cl$_{cr}$ <10 mL/minute: Administer at 50% of normal dose

Dosing adjustment in renal/hepatic impairment: Actiq®: Although fentanyl kinetics may be altered in renal/hepatic disease, Actiq® can be used successfully in the management of breakthrough cancer pain. Doses should be titrated to reach clinical effect with careful monitoring of patients with severe renal/hepatic disease.

Dietary Considerations Glucose may cause hyperglycemia; monitor blood glucose concentrations.

Administration

I.V.: Muscular rigidity may occur with rapid I.V. administration. During prolonged administration, dosage requirements may decrease.

Transdermal: Patients with an elevated temperature may have increased fentanyl absorption transdermally. Observe for adverse effects; dosage adjustment may be needed. Pharmacologic and adverse effects can be seen after discontinuation of transdermal system. Observe patients for at least 12 hours after transdermal product is removed. Keep transdermal product (both used and unused) out of the reach of children. Do **not** use soap, alcohol, or other solvents to remove transdermal gel if it accidentally touches skin, as they may increase transdermal absorption; use copious amounts of water.

Transmucosal: Foil overwrap should be removed just prior to administration. Once removed, patient should place the unit in mouth and allow it to dissolve. Do **not** chew. Actiq® units may be occasionally moved from one side of the mouth to the other. The unit should be consumed over a period of 15 minutes. Unit should be removed after it is consumed or if patient has achieved an adequate response and/or shows signs of respiratory depression. For patients who have received transmucosal product within 6-12 hours, it is recommended that if other narcotics are required, they should be used at starting doses ¼ to ⅓ those usually recommended.

Monitoring Parameters Respiratory and cardiovascular status, blood pressure, heart rate

Patient Information Actiq® preparations contain an amount of medication that can be fatal to children. Keep all units out of the reach of children and discard any open units properly. Actiq® Welcome Kits are available which contain educational materials, safe storage and disposal instructions.

Nursing Implications

May cause rebound respiratory depression postoperatively

Patients with increased temperature may have increased fentanyl absorption transdermally, observe for adverse effects, dosage adjustment may be needed

Pharmacologic and adverse effects can be seen after discontinuation of transdermal system, observe patients for at least 12 hours after transdermal product removed; keep transdermal product (both used and unused) out of the reach of children

Do **not** use soap, alcohol, or other solvents to remove transdermal gel if it accidentally touches skin as they may increase transdermal absorption, use copious amounts of water

For patients who have received transmucosal product within 6-12 hours, it is recommended that if other narcotics are required, they should be used at starting doses ¼ to ⅓ those usually recommended.

Additional Information Disposal of Actiq® units: After consumption of a complete unit, the handle may be disposed of in a trash container that is out of the reach of children. For a partially-consumed unit, or a unit that still has any drug matrix remaining on the handle, the handle should be placed under hot running tap water until the drug matrix has dissolved. Special child-resistant containers are available to temporarily store partially consumed units that cannot be disposed of immediately.

Fentanyl is 50-100 times as potent as morphine; morphine 10 mg I.M. is equivalent to fentanyl 0.1-0.2 mg I.M.; fentanyl has less hypotensive effects than morphine or meperidine due to minimal or no histamine release. Keep transdermal product (both used and unused) out of the reach of children. Do **not** use soap, alcohol, or other solvents to remove transdermal gel if it accidentally touches skin as they may increase transdermal absorption, use copious amounts of water.

Dosage Forms

Injection, as citrate [preservative free]: 0.05 mg/mL (2 mL, 5 mL, 10 mL, 20 mL, 30 mL, 50 mL)

Lozenge, oral transmucosal, as citrate, mounted on a plastic radiopaque handle (Actiq®): 200 mcg, 400 mcg, 600 mcg, 800 mcg, 1200 mcg, 1600 mcg [raspberry flavor]

Transdermal system: 25 mcg/hour [10 cm²]; 50 mcg/hour [20 cm²]; 75 mcg/hour [30 cm²]; 100 mcg/hour [40 cm²] (all available in 5s)

Ferric Gluconate *(FER ik GLOO koe nate)*

U.S. Brand Names Ferrlecit®

Synonyms Sodium Ferric Gluconate

Therapeutic Category Iron Salt

Use Repletion of total body iron content in patients with iron-deficiency anemia who are undergoing hemodialysis in conjunction with erythropoietin therapy

Pregnancy Risk Factor B

Pregnancy/Breast-Feeding Implications There are no well-controlled studies available. Should be used in pregnancy only when the potential benefit to the mother clearly outweighs the potential risk to the fetus. It is not known if ferrous gluconate is excreted in human milk. Use caution if the drug is administered to women who are breast-feeding.

Contraindications Hypersensitivity to ferric gluconate or any component of the formulation; use in any anemia not caused by iron deficiency; heart failure (of any severity); iron overload

Warnings/Precautions Potentially serious hypersensitivity reactions may occur. Fatal immediate hypersensitivity reactions have occurred with other iron carbohydrate complexes. Avoid rapid administration. Flushing and transient hypotension may occur. May augment hemodialysis-induced hypotension. Use with caution in elderly patients. Safety and efficacy in pediatric patients have not been established. Contains benzyl alcohol; do not use in neonates. Administration rate should not exceed 2.1 mg/minute.

Adverse Reactions Major adverse reactions include hypotension and hypersensitivity reactions. Hypersensitivity reactions have included pruritus, chest pain, hypotension, nausea, abdominal pain, flank pain, fatigue and rash.

1% to 10%:

Cardiovascular: Hypotension (serious hypotension in 1%), chest pain, hypertension, syncope, tachycardia, angina, myocardial infarction, pulmonary edema, hypovolemia, peripheral edema

Central nervous system: Headache, fatigue, fever, malaise, dizziness, paresthesia, insomnia, agitation, somnolence, pain

Dermatologic: Pruritus, rash

Endocrine & metabolic: Hyperkalemia, hypoglycemia, hypokalemia

Gastrointestinal: Abdominal pain, nausea, vomiting, diarrhea, rectal disorder, dyspepsia, flatulence, melena

Genitourinary: Urinary tract infection

Hematologic: Anemia, abnormal erythrocytes, lymphadenopathy

Local: Injection site reactions, injection site pain

Neuromuscular & skeletal: Weakness, back pain, leg cramps, myalgia, arthralgia, paresthesia

Ocular: Blurred vision, conjunctivitis

Respiratory: Dyspnea, cough, rhinitis, upper respiratory infection, pneumonia

Miscellaneous: Hypersensitivity reactions, infection, rigors, chills, flu-like syndrome, sepsis, carcinoma, diaphoresis (increased)

<1% (Limited to important or life-threatening): Dry mouth, epigastric pain, groin pain, hemorrhage, hypertonia, nervousness

Overdosage/Toxicology Symptoms of iron overdose include CNS toxicity, acidosis, hepatic and renal impairment, hematemesis, and lethargy. Treatment is generally symptomatic and supportive, but severe overdoses may be treated with deferoxamine. Due to severe toxicity, serum iron ≥300 µg/mL requires treatment. Deferoxamine may be administered I.V. (80 mg/kg over 24 hours) or I.M. (40-90 mg/kg every 8 hours). The usual toxic dose of elemental iron is ≥35 mg/kg.

Drug Interactions

Decreased Effect: Chloramphenicol may decrease effect of ferric gluconate injection; ferric gluconate injection may decrease the absorption of oral iron

Stability Store at 20°C to 25°C (68°F to 77°F). For I.V. infusion, dilute 10 mL ferric gluconate in 100 mL 0.9% sodium chloride; use immediately after dilution. Do **not** mix with parenteral nutrition solutions or other medications.

Mechanism of Action Supplies a source to elemental iron necessary to the function of hemoglobin, myoglobin and specific enzyme systems; allows transport of oxygen via hemoglobin

Pharmacodynamics/Kinetics Half-life elimination: Bound: 1 hour

Usual Dosage Adults: A test dose of 2 mL diluted in 50 mL 0.9% sodium chloride over 60 minutes was previously recommended (not in current manufacturer labeling).

Repletion of iron in hemodialysis patients: I.V.: 125 mg elemental iron per 10 mL (either by I.V. infusion or slow I.V. injection). Most patients will require a cumulative dose of 1 g elemental iron over approximately 8 sequential dialysis treatments to achieve a favorable response.

Administration May be diluted prior to administration; avoid rapid administration. Infusion rate should not exceed 2.1 mg/minute. If administered undiluted, infuse slowly at a rate of up to 12.5 mg/minute. Monitor patient for hypotension or hypersensitivity reactions during infusion.

Monitoring Parameters Hemoglobin and hematocrit, serum ferritin, iron saturation; vital signs

Additional Information Contains benzyl alcohol 9 mg/mL

Dosage Forms Injection: 12.5 mg elemental iron/mL (5 mL) [contains benzyl alcohol 9 mg/mL]

♦ **Ferrlecit®** see Ferric Gluconate on page 554

♦ **Ferro-Sequels® [OTC]** see Ferrous Fumarate on page 555

Ferrous Fumarate (FER us FYOO ma rate)

U.S. Brand Names Femiron® [OTC]; Feostat® [OTC]; Ferro-Sequels® [OTC]; Hemocyte® [OTC]; Ircon® [OTC]; Nephro-Fer™ [OTC]; Span-FF®

Canadian Brand Names Palafer®

Therapeutic Category Iron Salt

Use Prevention and treatment of iron-deficiency anemias

Pregnancy Risk Factor A

Contraindications Hypersensitivity to iron salts or any component of the formulation; hemochromatosis, hemolytic anemia

Warnings/Precautions Avoid in patients with peptic ulcer, enteritis, or ulcerative colitis. Administration of iron for >6 months should be avoided except in patients with continuous bleeding or menorrhagia. Anemia in the elderly is often caused by "anemia of chronic disease" or associated with inflammation rather than blood loss. Iron stores are usually normal or increased, with a serum ferritin >50 ng/mL and a decreased total iron binding

(Continued)

Ferrous Fumarate (Continued)

capacity. Hence, the "anemia of chronic disease" is not secondary to iron deficiency but the inability of the reticuloendothelial system to reclaim available iron stores. Avoid in patients receiving frequent blood transfusions Avoid use in premature infants until the vitamin E stores, deficient at birth, are replenished.

Adverse Reactions

>10%: Gastrointestinal: Stomach cramping, constipation, nausea, vomiting, dark stools

1% to 10%:

Gastrointestinal: Heartburn, diarrhea, staining of teeth

Genitourinary: Discoloration of urine

<1% (Limited to important or life-threatening): Contact irritation

Overdosage/Toxicology Symptoms include acute GI irritation, erosion of GI mucosa, hepatic and renal impairment, coma, hematemesis, lethargy, and acidosis. Due to severe toxicity, serum iron ≥300 µg/mL requires treatment. Following treatment for fluid losses, metabolic acidosis, and shock, a severe iron overdose may be treated with deferoxamine. Deferoxamine may be administered I.V. (80 mg/kg over 24 hours) or I.M. (40-90 mg/kg every 8 hours). The usual toxic dose of elemental iron is ≥35 mg/kg.

Drug Interactions

Increased Effect/Toxicity: Concurrent administration of ≥200 mg vitamin C per 30 mg elemental iron increases absorption of oral iron.

Decreased Effect: Absorption of oral preparation of iron and tetracyclines are decreased when both of these drugs are given together. Absorption of fluoroquinolones, levodopa, methyldopa, and penicillamine may be decreased due to formation of a ferric ion-quinolone complex. Concurrent administration of antacids, H_2 blockers (cimetidine), or proton pump inhibitors may decrease iron absorption. Response to iron therapy may be delayed by chloramphenicol.

Ethanol/Nutrition/Herb Interactions Food: Cereals, dietary fiber, tea, coffee, eggs, and milk may decrease absorption.

Mechanism of Action Replaces iron found in hemoglobin, myoglobin, and enzymes; allows the transportation of oxygen via hemoglobin

Pharmacodynamics/Kinetics

Onset of action: Hematologic response: Oral, parenteral iron salts: ~3-10 days

Peak effect: Reticulocytosis: 5-10 days; hemoglobin values increase within 2-4 weeks

Absorption: Iron is absorbed in the duodenum and upper jejunum; in persons with normal iron stores 10% of an oral dose is absorbed, this is increased to 20% to 30% in persons with inadequate iron stores; food and achlorhydria will decrease absorption

Protein binding: To serum transferrin

Excretion: Urine, sweat, sloughing of intestinal mucosa, and menses

Usual Dosage Oral (dose expressed in terms of elemental iron):

Children:

Severe iron-deficiency anemia: 4-6 mg Fe/kg/day in 3 divided doses

Mild to moderate iron deficiency anemia: 3 mg Fe/kg/day in 1-2 divided doses

Prophylaxis: 1-2 mg Fe/kg/day

Adults:

Iron deficiency: 60-100 mg twice daily up to 60 mg 2 times/day

Prophylaxis: 60-100 mg/day

To avoid GI upset, start with a single daily dose and increase by 1 tablet/day each week or as tolerated until desired daily dose is achieved

Elderly: 200 mg 3-4 times/day

Dietary Considerations Should be taken with water or juice on an empty stomach; may be administered with food to prevent irritation; however, not with cereals, dietary fiber, tea, coffee, eggs, or milk.

Reference Range

Serum iron:

Male: 75-175 µg/dL (SI: 13.4-31.3 µmol/L)

Female: 65-165 µg/dL (SI: 11.6-29.5 µmol/L)

Total iron binding capacity: 230-430 µg/dL

Transferrin: 204-360 mg/dL

Percent transferrin saturation: 20% to 50%

Iron levels >300 µg/dL can be considered toxic, should be treated as an overdose

Patient Information May color stool black, take between meals for maximum absorption; may take with food if GI upset occurs, do not take with milk or antacids; keep out of reach of children

Nursing Implications Administer 2 hours prior to or 4 hours after antacids

Additional Information Elemental iron content of ferrous fumarate: 33%

Dosage Forms Elemental iron listed in brackets

Capsule, controlled release (Span-FF®): 325 mg [106 mg]

Solution, oral [drops] (Feostat®): 45 mg/0.6 mL [15 mg/0.6 mL] (60 mL)

Suspension, oral (Feostat®): 100 mg/5 mL [33 mg/5 mL] (240 mL)

Tablet: 325 mg [106 mg]

Femiron®: 63 mg [20 mg]

Hemocyte®: 324 mg [106 mg]

Nephro-Fer™: 350 mg [115 mg]

Tablet, chewable (Feostat®): 100 mg [33 mg] [chocolate flavor]

Tablet, timed release (Ferro-Sequels®): Ferrous fumarate 150 mg [50 mg]

Ferrous Gluconate (FER us GLOO koe nate)

U.S. Brand Names Fergon® [OTC]

Canadian Brand Names Apo®-Ferrous Gluconate

Therapeutic Category Iron Salt

Use Prevention and treatment of iron-deficiency anemias

Pregnancy Risk Factor A

Contraindications Hypersensitivity to iron salts or any component of the formulation; hemochromatosis, hemolytic anemia

Warnings/Precautions Administration of iron for >6 months should be avoided except in patients with continued bleeding, menorrhagia, or repeated pregnancies; avoid in patients with peptic ulcer, enteritis, or ulcerative colitis. Anemia in the elderly is often caused by "anemia of chronic disease" or associated with inflammation rather than blood loss. Iron stores are usually normal or increased, with a serum ferritin >50 ng/mL and a decreased total iron binding capacity. Hence, the "anemia of chronic disease" is not secondary to iron deficiency but the inability of the reticuloendothelial system to reclaim available iron stores.

Adverse Reactions
>10%: Gastrointestinal: Stomach cramping, constipation, nausea, vomiting, dark stools
1% to 10%:
Gastrointestinal: Heartburn, diarrhea, staining of teeth
Genitourinary: Discoloration of urine
<1% (Limited to important or life-threatening): Contact irritation

Overdosage/Toxicology Symptoms include acute GI irritation, erosion of GI mucosa, hepatic and renal impairment, coma, hematemesis, lethargy, and acidosis. Due to severe toxicity, serum iron ≥300 µg/mL requires treatment. Following treatment for fluid losses, metabolic acidosis, and shock, a severe iron overdose may be treated with deferoxamine. Deferoxamine may be administered I.V. (80 mg/kg over 24 hours) or I.M. (40-90 mg/kg every 8 hours). The usual toxic dose of elemental iron is ≥35 mg/kg.

Drug Interactions
Increased Effect/Toxicity: Concurrent administration of ≥200 mg vitamin C per 30 mg elemental iron increases absorption of oral iron.
Decreased Effect: Absorption of oral preparation of iron and tetracyclines are decreased when both of these drugs are given together. Absorption of fluoroquinolones, levodopa, methyldopa, and penicillamine may be decreased due to formation of a ferric ion-quinolone complex. Concurrent administration of antacids, H$_2$ blockers (cimetidine), or proton pump inhibitors may decrease iron absorption. Response to iron therapy may be delayed by chloramphenicol.

Ethanol/Nutrition/Herb Interactions Food: Cereals, dietary fiber, tea, coffee, eggs, and milk may decrease absorption.

Mechanism of Action Replaces iron found in hemoglobin, myoglobin, and enzymes; allows the transportation of oxygen via hemoglobin

Pharmacodynamics/Kinetics Onset of action: Hematologic response: Oral: 3-10 days; peak reticulocytosis occurs in 5-10 days, and hemoglobin values increase in ~2-4 weeks

Usual Dosage Oral (dose expressed in terms of elemental iron):
Children:
Severe iron-deficiency anemia: 4-6 mg Fe/kg/day in 3 divided doses
Mild to moderate iron deficiency anemia: 3 mg Fe/kg/day in 1-2 divided doses
Prophylaxis: 1-2 mg Fe/kg/day
Adults:
Iron deficiency: 60 mg twice daily up to 60 mg 4 times/day
Prophylaxis: 60 mg/day

Dietary Considerations Should be taken with water or juice on an empty stomach; may be administered with food to prevent irritation; however not with cereals, dietary fiber, tea, coffee, eggs, or milk.

Administration Administration of iron preparations to premature infants with vitamin E deficiency may cause increased red cell hemolysis and hemolytic anemia, therefore, vitamin E deficiency should be corrected if possible

Reference Range Therapeutic: Male: 75-175 µg/dL (SI: 13.4-31.3 µmol/L); Female: 65-165 µg/dL (SI: 11.6-29.5 µmol/L); serum iron level >300 µg/dL usually requires treatment of overdose due to severe toxicity

Test Interactions False-positive for blood in stool by the guaiac test

Patient Information May color stool black, take between meals for maximum absorption; may take with food if GI upset occurs, do not take with milk or antacids; keep out of reach of children

Nursing Implications
Administer 2 hours before or 4 hours after antacids
Monitor serum iron, total iron binding capacity, reticulocyte count, hemoglobin

Additional Information Elemental iron content of ferrous gluconate: 12%

Dosage Forms Elemental iron listed in brackets
Tablet: 300 mg [34 mg]; 325 mg [36 mg]
Fergon®: 240 mg [27 mg]

Ferrous Sulfate (FER us SUL fate)

U.S. Brand Names Feosol® [OTC]; Feratab® [OTC]; Fer-In-Sol® [OTC]; Fer-Iron® [OTC]; Slow FE® [OTC]

Canadian Brand Names Apo®-Ferrous Sulfate; Fer-In-Sol®; Ferodan™

Synonyms FeSO$_4$

Therapeutic Category Iron Salt

Use Prevention and treatment of iron-deficiency anemias

Pregnancy Risk Factor A

Contraindications Hypersensitivity to iron salts or any component of the formulation; hemochromatosis, hemolytic anemia

Warnings/Precautions Administration of iron for >6 months should be avoided except in patients with continued bleeding, menorrhagia, or repeated pregnancies; avoid in patients with peptic ulcer, enteritis, or ulcerative colitis. Anemia in the elderly is often caused by "anemia of chronic disease" or associated with inflammation rather than blood loss. Iron stores are usually normal or increased, with a serum ferritin >50 ng/mL and a decreased total iron binding capacity. Hence, the "anemia of chronic disease" is not secondary to iron deficiency but the inability of the reticuloendothelial system to reclaim available iron stores. (Continued)

Ferrous Sulfate *(Continued)*

Adverse Reactions
>10%: Gastrointestinal: GI irritation, epigastric pain, nausea, dark stool, vomiting, stomach cramping, constipation

1% to 10%:
Gastrointestinal: Heartburn, diarrhea
Genitourinary: Discoloration of urine
Miscellaneous: Liquid preparations may temporarily stain the teeth

<1% (Limited to important or life-threatening): Contact irritation

Overdosage/Toxicology
Symptoms include acute GI irritation, erosion of GI mucosa, hepatic and renal impairment, coma, hematemesis, lethargy, and acidosis. Due to severe toxicity, serum iron ≥300 μg/mL requires treatment. Following treatment for fluid losses, metabolic acidosis, and shock, a severe iron overdose may be treated with deferoxamine. Deferoxamine may be administered I.V. (80 mg/kg over 24 hours) or I.M. (40-90 mg/kg every 8 hours). The usual toxic dose of elemental iron is ≥35 mg/kg.

Drug Interactions
Increased Effect/Toxicity: Concurrent administration of ≥200 mg vitamin C per 30 mg elemental iron increases absorption of oral iron.

Decreased Effect: Absorption of oral preparation of iron and tetracyclines are decreased when both of these drugs are given together. Absorption of fluoroquinolones, levodopa, methyldopa, and penicillamine may be decreased due to formation of a ferric ion-quinolone complex. Concurrent administration of antacids, H_2 blockers (cimetidine), or proton pump inhibitors may decrease iron absorption. Response to iron therapy may be delayed by chloramphenicol.

Ethanol/Nutrition/Herb Interactions
Food: Cereals, dietary fiber, tea, coffee, eggs, and milk may decrease absorption.

Mechanism of Action
Replaces iron, found in hemoglobin, myoglobin, and other enzymes; allows the transportation of oxygen via hemoglobin

Pharmacodynamics/Kinetics
Onset of action: Hematologic response: Oral: ~3-10 days
Peak effect: Reticulocytosis: 5-10 days; hemoglobin increases within 2-4 weeks
Absorption: Iron is absorbed in the duodenum and upper jejunum; in persons with normal serum iron stores, 10% of an oral dose is absorbed; this is increased to 20% to 30% in persons with inadequate iron stores. Food and achlorhydria will decrease absorption
Protein binding: To transferrin
Excretion: Urine, sweat, sloughing of the intestinal mucosa, and menses

Usual Dosage
Oral:
Children **(dose expressed in terms of elemental iron)**:
Severe iron-deficiency anemia: 4-6 mg Fe/kg/day in 3 divided doses
Mild to moderate iron deficiency anemia: 3 mg Fe/kg/day in 1-2 divided doses
Prophylaxis: 1-2 mg Fe/kg/day up to a maximum of 15 mg/day
Adults **(dose expressed in terms of ferrous sulfate)**:
Iron deficiency: 300 mg twice daily up to 300 mg 4 times/day or 250 mg (extended release) 1-2 times/day
Prophylaxis: 300 mg/day

Dietary Considerations
Should be taken with water or juice on an empty stomach; may be administered with food to prevent irritation; however not with cereals, dietary fiber, tea, coffee, eggs, or milk.

Administration
Administer ferrous sulfate 2 hours prior to, or 4 hours after antacids

Reference Range
Serum iron:
Male: 75-175 μg/dL (SI: 13.4-31.3 μmol/L)
Female: 65-165 μg/dL (SI: 11.6-29.5 μmol/L)
Total iron binding capacity: 230-430 μg/dL
Transferrin: 204-360 mg/dL
Percent transferrin saturation: 20% to 50%

Test Interactions
False-positive for blood in stool by the guaiac test

Patient Information
May color stool black, take between meals for maximum absorption; may take with food if GI upset occurs, do not take with milk or antacids; keep out of reach of children

Nursing Implications
Administer 2 hours before or 4 hours after antacids
Monitor serum iron, total iron binding capacity, reticulocyte count, hemoglobin

Additional Information
Elemental iron content of iron salts in ferrous sulfate is 20% (ie, 300 mg ferrous sulfate is equivalent to 60 mg ferrous iron)

Dosage Forms
Elemental iron listed in brackets
Elixir (Feosol®): 220 mg/5 mL [44 mg/5 mL] with alcohol 5% (473 mL, 4000 mL)
Solution, oral [drops] (Fer-In-Sol®, Fer-Iron®): 75 mg/0.6 mL [15 mg/0.6 mL] (50 mL)
Syrup (Fer-In-Sol®): 90 mg/5 mL [18 mg/5 mL] with alcohol 5% (480 mL)
Tablet: 324 mg [65 mg]
Feratab®: 187 mg [60 mg]
Tablet, exsiccated (Feosol®) 200 mg [65 mg]
Tablet, exsiccated, timed release (Slow FE®): 160 mg [50 mg]

Ferrous Sulfate and Ascorbic Acid *(FER us SUL fate & a SKOR bik AS id)*

U.S. Brand Names Fero-Grad 500® [OTC]
Synonyms Ascorbic Acid and Ferrous Sulfate
Therapeutic Category Iron Salt; Vitamin
Use Treatment of iron deficiency in nonpregnant adults; treatment and prevention of iron deficiency in pregnant adults
Usual Dosage Adults: Oral: 1 tablet daily
Additional Information Complete prescribing information for this medication should be consulted for additional detail.

Dosage Forms Elemental iron listed in brackets
Tablet (Fero-Grad 500®): Ferrous sulfate 525 mg [105 mg] and ascorbic acid 500 mg

Ferrous Sulfate, Ascorbic Acid, and Vitamin B-Complex
(FER us SUL fate, a SKOR bik AS id, & VYE ta min bee KOM pleks)
U.S. Brand Names Iberet®-Liquid [OTC]; Iberet®-Liquid 500 [OTC]
Therapeutic Category Iron Salt; Vitamin
Use Conditions of iron deficiency with an increased needed for B-complex vitamins and vitamin C
Usual Dosage Oral:
Children 1-3 years: 5 mL twice daily after meals
Children >4 years and Adults: 10 mL 3 times/day after meals
Additional Information Complete prescribing information for this medication should be consulted for additional detail.
Dosage Forms
Liquid (components all per 15 mL):
Iberet®-Liquid:
Ascorbic acid: 112.5 mg
B_1: 4.5 mg
B_2: 4.5 mg
B_3: 22.5 mg
B_5: 7.5 mg
B_6: 3.75 mg
B_{12}: 18.75 mg
Ferrous sulfate: 78.75 mg
Iberet®-Liquid 500:
Ascorbic acid: 375 mg
B_1: 4.5 mg
B_2: 4.5 mg
B_3: 22.5 mg
B_5: 7.5 mg
B_6: 3.75 mg
B_{12}: 18.75 mg
Ferrous sulfate: 78.75 mg

Ferrous Sulfate, Ascorbic Acid, Vitamin B-Complex, and Folic Acid
(FER us SUL fate, a SKOR bik AS id, VYE ta min bee KOM pleks, & FOE lik AS id)
Therapeutic Category Vitamin
Use Treatment of iron deficiency and prevention of concomitant folic acid deficiency where there is an associated deficient intake or increased need for B-complex vitamins
Pregnancy Risk Factor A
Usual Dosage Adults: Oral: 1 tablet daily
Additional Information Complete prescribing information for this medication should be consulted for additional detail.
Dosage Forms
Tablet, controlled release:
Ascorbic acid: 500 mg
B_1: 6 mg
B_2: 6 mg
B_3: 30 mg
B_5: 10 mg
B_6: 5 mg
B_{12}: 25 mcg
Ferrous sulfate: 105 mg
Folic acid: 800 mcg

♦ **Fertinex®** see Follitropins on page 596
♦ **Fertinex®** see Urofollitropin on page 1391
♦ **Fertinorm® H.P. (Can)** see Urofollitropin on page 1391
♦ **FeSO₄** see Ferrous Sulfate on page 557
♦ **Feverall® [OTC]** see Acetaminophen on page 22

Fexofenadine (feks oh FEN a deen)
U.S. Brand Names Allegra®
Canadian Brand Names Allegra®
Synonyms Fexofenadine Hydrochloride
Therapeutic Category Antihistamine, H_1 Blocker
Use Nonsedating antihistamine indicated for the relief of seasonal allergic rhinitis and chronic idiopathic urticaria
Pregnancy Risk Factor C
Pregnancy/Breast-Feeding Implications There are no adequate and well-controlled studies in pregnant women; use during pregnancy only if potential benefit to mother outweighs possible risk to fetus. Excretion in breast milk is unknown; use caution in breast-feeding.
Contraindications Hypersensitivity to fexofenadine or any component of the formulation; breast-feeding
Warnings/Precautions Safety and efficacy in children <6 years of age have not been established.
Adverse Reactions
>10%: Central nervous system: Headache 11% (with once-daily dosing)
(Continued)

Fexofenadine *(Continued)*

1% to 10%:
Central nervous system: Fever (2%), dizziness (2%), pain (2%), drowsiness (1% to 2%), fatigue (1%)
Endocrine & metabolic: Dysmenorrhea (2%)
Gastrointestinal: Nausea (2%), dyspepsia (1%)
Neuromuscular & skeletal: Back pain (2% to 3%)
Otic: Otitis media (3%)
Respiratory: Cough (4%), upper respiratory tract infection (4%), sinusitis (2%)
Miscellaneous: Viral infection (3%)
<1% (Limited to important or life-threatening): Hypersensitivity reactions (anaphylaxis, angioedema, dyspnea, flushing, pruritus, rash, urticaria); insomnia, nervousness, sleep disorders, paroniria

Overdosage/Toxicology Limited overdose data describe dizziness, drowsiness, and dry mouth. Fexofenadine is not effectively removed by hemodialysis. Doses up to 690 mg twice daily were administered for 1 month without significant adverse effects. Treatment is supportive.

Drug Interactions
Cytochrome P450 Effect: CYP2D6 enzyme inhibitor (weak)
Increased Effect/Toxicity: Erythromycin and ketoconazole increased the levels of fexofenadine; however, no increase in adverse events or QT$_c$ intervals was noted. The effect of other macrolide agents or azoles has not been investigated.
Decreased Effect: Aluminum- and magnesium-containing antacids decrease plasma levels of fexofenadine; separate administration is recommended.

Ethanol/Nutrition/Herb Interactions
Ethanol: Avoid ethanol (although limited with fexofenadine, may increase risk of sedation).
Herb/Nutraceutical: St John's wort may decrease fexofenadine levels.

Stability Store capsules at controlled room temperature of 20°C to 25°C (68°F to 77°F). Protect from excessive moisture.

Mechanism of Action Fexofenadine is an active metabolite of terfenadine and like terfenadine it competes with histamine for H$_1$-receptor sites on effector cells in the gastrointestinal tract, blood vessels and respiratory tract; it appears that fexofenadine does not cross the blood brain barrier to any appreciable degree, resulting in a reduced potential for sedation

Pharmacodynamics/Kinetics
Onset of action: 60 minutes
Duration: Antihistaminic effect: ≥12 hours
Metabolism: ~5% mostly by gut flora; 0.5% to 1.5% by CYP450 enzymes
Half-life elimination: 14.4 hours
Time to peak, serum: ~2.6 hours
Excretion: Primarily feces (~80%) and urine (~11%) as unchanged drug

Usual Dosage Oral:
Children 6-11 years: 30 mg twice daily (once daily in children with impaired renal function)
Children ≥12 years and Adults:
Seasonal allergic rhinitis: 60 mg twice daily **or** 180 mg once daily
Chronic idiopathic urticaria: 60 mg twice daily
Dosing adjustment in renal impairment: Recommended initial doses of 60 mg once daily

Monitoring Parameters Relief of symptoms

Patient Information Although relatively uncommon (1.3%), fexofenadine may cause drowsiness; contact your physician or pharmacist if you experience drowsiness, upset stomach, increased pain or cramping during menstruation while taking this medication

Dosage Forms
Capsule, as hydrochloride: 60 mg
Tablet, as hydrochloride: 30 mg, 60 mg, 180 mg

Fexofenadine and Pseudoephedrine
(feks oh FEN a deen & soo doe e FED rin)

U.S. Brand Names Allegra-D®
Canadian Brand Names Allegra-D®
Synonyms Pseudoephedrine and Fexofenadine
Therapeutic Category Antihistamine/Decongestant Combination
Use Relief of symptoms associated with seasonal allergic rhinitis in adults and children 12 years of age and older. Symptoms treated effectively include sneezing, rhinorrhea, itchy nose/palate/ and/or throat, itchy/watery/red eyes, and nasal congestion.
Pregnancy Risk Factor C
Usual Dosage Oral: Adults: One tablet twice daily for adults and children 12 years of age and older. It is recommended that the administration with food should be avoided. A dose of one tablet once daily is recommended as the starting dose in patients with decreased renal function.
Additional Information Complete prescribing information for this medication should be consulted for additional detail.
Dosage Forms Tablet, extended release: Fexofenadine hydrochloride 60 mg and pseudoephedrine hydrochloride 120 mg

♦ **Fexofenadine Hydrochloride** *see* Fexofenadine *on page 559*
♦ **Fiberall® Powder [OTC]** *see* Psyllium *on page 1158*
♦ **Fiberall® Wafer [OTC]** *see* Psyllium *on page 1158*

Fibrinolysin and Desoxyribonuclease
(fye brin oh LYE sin & des oks i rye boe NOO klee ase)

U.S. Brand Names Elase®; Elase-Chloromycetin®
Synonyms Desoxyribonuclease and Fibrinolysin
Therapeutic Category Enzyme
Use Debriding agent; cervicitis; and irrigating agent in infected wounds

Pregnancy Risk Factor C
Usual Dosage
Ointment: 2-3 times/day
Wet dressing: 3-4 times/day
Additional Information Complete prescribing information for this medication should be consulted for additional detail.
Dosage Forms
Ointment, topical (Elase®): Fibrinolysin 1 unit and desoxyribonuclease 666.6 units per g (10 g, 30 g)
Ointment, topical (Elase-Chloromycetin®): Fibrinolysin 1 unit and desoxyribonuclease 666.6 units per g with chloramphenicol 10 mg per g (10 g, 30 g)

Filgrastim (fil GRA stim)
Related Information
Sargramostim *on page 1223*
U.S. Brand Names Neupogen®
Canadian Brand Names Neupogen®
Synonyms G-CSF; Granulocyte Colony Stimulating Factor
Therapeutic Category Colony-Stimulating Factor
Use Stimulation of granulocyte production in patients with malignancies, including myeloid malignancies; receiving myelosuppressive therapy associated with a significant risk of neutropenia; severe chronic neutropenia (SCN); receiving bone marrow transplantation (BMT); undergoing peripheral blood progenitor cell (PBPC) collection
Pregnancy Risk Factor C
Pregnancy/Breast-Feeding Implications Excretion in breast milk is unknown; use caution in breast-feeding.
Contraindications Hypersensitivity to filgrastim, *E. coli*-derived proteins, or any component of the formulation; concurrent myelosuppressive chemotherapy or radiation therapy
Warnings/Precautions Complete blood count and platelet count should be obtained prior to chemotherapy. Do not use G-CSF in the period 12-24 hours before to 24 hours after administration of cytotoxic chemotherapy because of the potential sensitivity of rapidly dividing myeloid cells to cytotoxic chemotherapy. Precaution should be exercised in the usage of G-CSF in any malignancy with myeloid characteristics. G-CSF can potentially act as a growth factor for any tumor type, particularly myeloid malignancies. Tumors of nonhematopoietic origin may have surface receptors for G-CSF.

Allergic-type reactions have occurred in patients receiving G-CSF with first or later doses. Reactions tended to occur more frequently with intravenous administration and within 30 minutes of infusion. Most cases resolved rapidly with antihistamines, steroids, bronchodilators, and/or epinephrine. Symptoms recurred in >50% of patients on rechallenge.
Adverse Reactions Effects are generally mild and dose related
>10%:
Central nervous system: Neutropenic fever, fever
Dermatologic: Alopecia
Gastrointestinal: Nausea, vomiting, diarrhea, mucositis, splenomegaly (more common in patients who prolonged (>14 days) treatment, usually subclinical)
Neuromuscular & skeletal: Medullary bone pain (24%):
1% to 10%:
Cardiovascular: Chest pain, fluid retention
Central nervous system: Headache
Dermatologic: Skin rash
Gastrointestinal: Anorexia, stomatitis, constipation
Hematologic: Leukocytosis
Local: Pain at injection site
Neuromuscular & skeletal: Weakness
Respiratory: Dyspnea, cough, sore throat
<1% (Limited to important or life-threatening): Pericarditis, thrombophlebitis, transient supraventricular arrhythmia
Overdosage/Toxicology No clinical adverse effects have been seen with high doses producing ANC >10,000/mm^3. After discontinuing in patients receiving myelosuppressive chemotherapy, there is a 50% decrease in circulating neutrophils within 1-2 days, and a return to pretreatment levels within 1-7 days.
Drug Interactions
Increased Effect/Toxicity: Drugs which may potentiate the release of neutrophils (eg, lithium) should be used with caution.

Comparative Effects — G-CSF vs. GM-CSF

Proliferation/Differentiation	G-CSF (Filgrastim)	GM-CSF (Sargramostim)
Neutrophils	Yes	Yes
Eosinophils	No	Yes
Macrophages	No	Yes
Neutrophil migration	Enhanced	Inhibited

Stability Intact vials should be kept refrigerated at 2°C to 8°C (36°F to 46°F); **do not freeze**. The drug is stable for 24 hours at room temperature of 15°C to 30°C (59°F to 86°F) in the vial or in a tuberculin syringe. Undiluted filgrastim in a tuberculin syringe is stable for up to 14 days under refrigeration.

Solutions for I.V. administration may be diluted in 5% dextrose in water to a concentration ≥15 mcg/mL. Diluted solutions are stable for up to 7 days at room temperature or under refrigeration.
(Continued)

Filgrastim *(Continued)*

Use of concentrations <15 mcg/mL is NOT recommended. Concentrations >5 mcg/mL and <15 mcg/mL require the addition of albumin (0.2% final albumin concentration) to prevent absorption by the container. Concentrations <5 mcg/mL are unstable and may precipitate.

Mechanism of Action Stimulates the production, maturation, and activation of neutrophils, G-CSF activates neutrophils to increase both their migration and cytotoxicity. See table on previous page.

Pharmacodynamics/Kinetics

Onset of action: ~24 hours; plateaus in 3-5 days

Duration: ANC decreases by 50% within 2 days after discontinuing G-CSF; white counts return to the normal range in 4-7 days; peak plasma levels can be maintained for up to 12 hours

Absorption: S.C.: 100%

Distribution: V_d: 150 mL/kg; no evidence of drug accumulation over a 11- to 20-day period

Metabolism: Systemic

Half-life elimination: 1.8-3.5 hours

Time to peak, serum: S.C.: 2-6 hours

Usual Dosage Refer to individual protocols.

Dosing, even in morbidly obese patients, should be based on actual body weight. Rounding doses to the nearest vial size often enhances patient convenience and reduces costs without compromising clinical response.

Myelosuppressive therapy: 5 mcg/kg/day - doses may be increased by 5 mcg/kg according to the duration and severity of the neutropenia.

Bone marrow transplantation: 5-10 mcg/kg/day - doses may be increased by 5 mcg/kg according to the duration and severity of neutropenia; recommended steps based on neutrophil response:

When ANC >1000/mm³ for 3 consecutive days: Reduce filgrastim dose to 5 mcg/kg/day

If ANC remains >1000/mm³ for 3 more consecutive days: Discontinue filgrastim

If ANC decreases to <1000/mm³: Resume at 5 mcg/kg/day

If ANC decreases <1000/mm³ during the 5 mcg/kg/day dose, increase filgrastim to 10 mcg/kg/day and follow the above steps

Peripheral blood progenitor cell (PBPC) collection: 10 mcg/kg/day **or** 5-8 mcg/kg twice daily in donors. The optimal timing and duration of growth factor stimulation has not been determined.

Severe chronic neutropenia:

Congenital: 6 mcg/kg twice daily

Idiopathic/cyclic: 5 mcg/kg/day

Not removed by hemodialysis

Administration May be administered undiluted by S.C. or by I.V. infusion over 15-60 minutes in D_5W; **incompatible** with sodium chloride solutions

Monitoring Parameters CBC and platelet count should be obtained twice weekly. Leukocytosis (white blood cell counts ≥100,000/mm³) has been observed in ~2% of patients receiving G-CSF at doses >5 mcg/kg/day. Monitor platelets and hematocrit regularly.

Reference Range No clinical benefit seen with ANC >10,000/mm³

Patient Information Follow directions for proper storage and administration of S.C. medication. Never reuse syringes or needles. You may experience bone pain (request analgesic); nausea or vomiting (small frequent meals may help); hair loss (reversible); or sore mouth (frequent mouth care with a soft toothbrush or cotton swab may help). Report unusual fever or chills; unhealed sores; severe bone pain; pain, redness, or swelling at injection site; unusual swelling of extremities or difficulty breathing; or chest pain and palpitations.

Nursing Implications Do not mix with sodium chloride solutions

Additional Information

Reimbursement Hotline: 1-800-272-9376

Professional Services [Amgen]: 1-800-77-AMGEN

Dosage Forms

Solution for injection [preservative free]: 300 mcg/mL (1 mL, 1.6 mL)

Neupogen® Singleject® [prefilled syringe]: 600 mcg/mL (0.5 mL, 0.8 mL)

Finasteride *(fi NAS teer ide)*

U.S. Brand Names Propecia®; Proscar®

Canadian Brand Names Propecia®; Proscar®

Therapeutic Category Antiandrogen; Antineoplastic Agent, Miscellaneous

Use

Propecia®: Treatment of male pattern hair loss in **men only**. Safety and efficacy were demonstrated in men between 18-41 years of age.

Proscar®: Treatment of symptomatic benign prostatic hyperplasia (BPH)

Unlabeled/Investigational Use Adjuvant monotherapy after radical prostatectomy in the treatment of prostatic cancer; female hirsutism

Pregnancy Risk Factor X

Contraindications Hypersensitivity to finasteride or any component of the formulation; pregnancy; not for use in children

Warnings/Precautions A minimum of 6 months of treatment may be necessary to determine whether an individual will respond to finasteride. Use with caution in those patients with liver function abnormalities. Carefully monitor patients with a large residual urinary volume or severely diminished urinary flow for obstructive uropathy. These patients may not be candidates for finasteride therapy.

Adverse Reactions

1% to 10%:

Endocrine & metabolic: Decreased libido

Genitourinary: <4% incidence of impotence, decreased volume of ejaculate

<1% (Limited to important or life-threatening): Hypersensitivity (pruritus, urticaria, swelling of face/lips), testicular pain

Drug Interactions

Cytochrome P450 Effect: CYP3A3/4 enzyme substrate

Ethanol/Nutrition/Herb Interactions

Food: Administration with food may delay the rate and reduce the extent of oral absorption.

Herb/Nutraceutical: St John's wort may decrease finasteride levels. Avoid saw palmetto (concurrent use has not been adequately studied).

Mechanism of Action Finasteride is a 4-azo analog of testosterone and is a competitive inhibitor of both tissue and hepatic 5-alpha reductase. This results in inhibition of the conversion of testosterone to dihydrotestosterone and markedly suppresses serum dihydrotestosterone levels; depending on dose and duration, serum testosterone concentrations may or may not increase. Testosterone-dependent processes such as fertility, muscle strength, potency, and libido are not affected by finasteride.

Pharmacodynamics/Kinetics

Onset of action: 3-6 months of ongoing therapy

Duration:

After a single oral dose as small as 0.5 mg: 65% depression of plasma dihydrotestosterone levels persists 5-7 days

After 6 months of treatment with 5 mg/day: Circulating dihydrotestosterone levels are reduced to castrate levels without significant effects on circulating testosterone; levels return to normal within 14 days of discontinuation of treatment

Absorption: May be reduced if administered with food

Protein binding: 90%

Metabolism: Hepatic; two active metabolites have been identified

Bioavailability: Mean: 63%

Half-life elimination, serum: Parent drug: ~5-17 hours (mean: 1.9 fasting, 4.2 with breakfast); Elderly: 8 hours; Adults: 6 hours (3-16); rate decreased in elderly, but no dosage adjustment needed

Time to peak, serum: 2-6 hours

Excretion: Urine (39%) and feces (57%) as metabolites

Usual Dosage Adults:

Male:

Benign prostatic hyperplasia (Proscar®): Oral: 5 mg/day as a single dose; clinical responses occur within 12 weeks to 6 months of initiation of therapy; long-term administration is recommended for maximal response

Male pattern baldness (Propecia®): Oral: 1 mg daily

Female: Hirsutism: Oral: 5 mg/day

Dosing adjustment in renal impairment: No dosage adjustment is necessary

Dosing adjustment in hepatic impairment: Use with caution in patients with liver function abnormalities because finasteride is metabolized extensively in the liver

Administration Administration with food may delay the rate and reduce the extent of oral absorption. Childbearing age women should not touch or handle this medication.

Monitoring Parameters Objective and subjective signs of relief of benign prostatic hyperplasia, including improvement in urinary flow, reduction in symptoms of urgency, and relief of difficulty in micturition

Nursing Implications Monitor objective and subjective signs of relief of benign prostatic hyperplasia, including improvement in urinary flow, reduction in symptoms of urgency, and relief of difficulty in micturition. Childbearing age women should not touch or handle this medication.

Dosage Forms

Tablet, film coated:

Propecia®: 1 mg

Proscar®: 5 mg

- **Finevin™** *see* Azelaic Acid *on page 137*
- **Fiorgen PF®** *see* Butalbital Compound *on page 197*
- **Fioricet®** *see* Butalbital Compound *on page 197*
- **Fiorinal®** *see* Butalbital Compound *on page 197*
- **Fisalamine** *see* Mesalamine *on page 866*
- **FK506** *see* Tacrolimus *on page 1283*
- **Flagyl®** *see* Metronidazole *on page 904*
- **Flagyl ER®** *see* Metronidazole *on page 904*
- **Flamazine® (Can)** *see* Silver Sulfadiazine *on page 1238*
- **Flarex®** *see* Fluorometholone *on page 575*

Flavoxate (fla VOKS ate)

U.S. Brand Names Urispas®

Canadian Brand Names Urispas®

Synonyms Flavoxate Hydrochloride

Therapeutic Category Antispasmodic Agent, Urinary

Use Antispasmodic to provide symptomatic relief of dysuria, nocturia, suprapubic pain, urgency, and incontinence due to detrusor instability and hyper-reflexia in elderly with cystitis, urethritis, urethrocystitis, urethrotrigonitis, and prostatitis

Pregnancy Risk Factor B

Usual Dosage Children >12 years and Adults: Oral: 100-200 mg 3-4 times/day; reduce the dose when symptoms improve

Additional Information Complete prescribing information for this medication should be consulted for additional detail.

Dosage Forms Tablet, film coated, as hydrochloride: 100 mg

- **Flavoxate Hydrochloride** *see* Flavoxate *on page 563*

Flecainide (fle KAY nide)

Related Information

Antacid Drug Interactions *on page 1477*
Antiarrhythmic Drugs Comparison *on page 1478*

U.S. Brand Names Tambocor™

Canadian Brand Names Tambocor™

Synonyms Flecainide Acetate

Therapeutic Category Antiarrhythmic Agent, Class I-C

Use Prevention and suppression of documented life-threatening ventricular arrhythmias (eg, sustained ventricular tachycardia); controlling symptomatic, disabling supraventricular tachycardias in patients without structural heart disease in whom other agents fail

Pregnancy Risk Factor C

Contraindications Hypersensitivity to flecainide or any component of the formulation; pre-existing second- or third-degree AV block or with right bundle branch block when associated with a left hemiblock (bifascicular block) (except in patients with a functioning artificial pacemaker); cardiogenic shock; coronary artery disease (based on CAST study results); concurrent use of ritonavir or amprenavir

Warnings/Precautions Pre-existing sinus node dysfunction, sick-sinus syndrome, history of congestive heart failure or myocardial dysfunction; increases in PR interval ≥300 MS, QRS ≥180 MS, QT_c interval increases, and/or new bundle-branch block; patients with pacemakers, renal impairment, and/or hepatic impairment. Not recommended for patients with chronic atrial fibrillation.

The manufacturer and FDA recommend that this drug be reserved for life-threatening ventricular arrhythmias unresponsive to conventional therapy. Its use for symptomatic nonsustained ventricular tachycardia, frequent premature ventricular complexes (PVCs), uniform and multiform PVCs and/or coupled PVCs is no longer recommended. Flecainide can worsen or cause arrhythmias with an associated risk of death. Proarrhythmic effects range from an increased number of PVCs to more severe ventricular tachycardias (eg, tachycardias that are more sustained or more resistant to conversion to sinus rhythm).

Adverse Reactions

>10%:
  Central nervous system: Dizziness (19% to 30%)
  Ocular: Visual disturbances (16%)
  Respiratory: Dyspnea (~10%)

1% to 10%:
  Cardiovascular: Palpitations (6%), chest pain (5%), edema (3.5%), tachycardia (1% to 3%), proarrhythmic (4% to 12%), sinus node dysfunction (1.2%)
  Central nervous system: Headache (4% to 10%), fatigue (8%), nervousness (5%) additional symptoms occurring at a frequency between 1% and 3%: fever, malaise, hypoesthesia, paresis, ataxia, vertigo, syncope, somnolence, tinnitus, anxiety, insomnia, depression
  Dermatologic: Rash (1% to 3%)
  Gastrointestinal: Nausea (9%), constipation (1%), abdominal pain (3%), anorexia (1% to 3%), diarrhea (0.7% to 3%)
  Neuromuscular & skeletal: Tremor (5%), weakness (5%), paresthesias (1%)
  Ocular: Diplopia (1% to 3%), blurred vision

<1% (Limited to important or life-threatening): Alopecia, alters pacing threshold, amnesia, angina, AV block, bradycardia, bronchospasm, congestive heart failure, corneal deposits, depersonalization, euphoria, exfoliative dermatitis, granulocytopenia, heart block, increased P-R, leukopenia, metallic taste, neuropathy, paradoxical increase in ventricular rate in atrial fibrillation/flutter, paresthesia, photophobia, pneumonitis, pruritus, QRS duration, swollen lips/tongue/mouth, tardive dyskinesia, thrombocytopenia, urinary retention, urticaria, ventricular arrhythmias

Overdosage/Toxicology Has a narrow therapeutic index; severe toxicity may occur slightly above the therapeutic range, especially if combined with other antiarrhythmic drugs. An acute single ingestion of twice the daily therapeutic dose is life-threatening. Symptoms include increased PR, QRS, and QT intervals; amplitude of the T wave, A-V block, bradycardia, hypotension, ventricular arrhythmias (monomorphic or polymorphic ventricular tachycardia), and asystole. Other symptoms include dizziness, blurred vision, headache, and GI upset. Treatment is supportive, using conventional treatment (fluids, positioning, anticonvulsants, antiarrhythmics). **Note:** Type Ia antiarrhythmic agents should not be used to treat cardiotoxicity caused by type Ic antiarrhythmics. Sodium bicarbonate may reverse QRS prolongation, bradycardia, and hypotension. Ventricular pacing may be needed. Hemodialysis is only of possible benefit for tocainide or flecainide overdose in patients with renal failure.

Drug Interactions

Cytochrome P450 Effect: CYP2D6 enzyme substrate

Increased Effect/Toxicity: Flecainide concentrations may be increased by amiodarone (reduce flecainide 25% to 33%), amprenavir, cimetidine, digoxin, propranolol, quinidine, and ritonavir. Beta-adrenergic blockers, disopyramide, verapamil may enhance flecainide's negative inotropic effects. Alkalinizing agents (ie, high-dose antacids, cimetidine, carbonic anhydrase inhibitors, sodium bicarbonate) may decrease flecainide clearance, potentially increasing toxicity. Propranolol blood levels are increased by flecainide.

Decreased Effect: Smoking and acid urine increase flecainide clearance.

Ethanol/Nutrition/Herb Interactions Food: Clearance may be decreased in patients following strict vegetarian diets due to urinary pH ≥8. Dairy products (milk, infant formula, yogurt) may interfere with the absorption of flecainide in infants; there is one case report of a neonate (GA 34 weeks PNA >6 days) who required extremely large doses of oral flecainide when administered every 8 hours with feedings ("milk feeds"); changing the feedings from "milk feeds" to 5% glucose feeds alone resulted in a doubling of the flecainide serum concentration and toxicity.

Mechanism of Action Class Ic antiarrhythmic; slows conduction in cardiac tissue by altering transport of ions across cell membranes; causes slight prolongation of refractory periods; decreases the rate of rise of the action potential without affecting its duration; increases electrical stimulation threshold of ventricle, His-Purkinje system; possesses local anesthetic and moderate negative inotropic effects

Pharmacodynamics/Kinetics
Absorption: Oral: Rapid
Distribution: Adults: V_d: 5-13.4 L/kg
Protein binding: 40% to 50% (alpha$_1$ glycoprotein)
Bioavailability: 85% to 90%
Metabolism: Hepatic
Half-life elimination: Infants: 11-12 hours; Children: 8 hours; Adults: 7-22 hours, increased with congestive heart failure or renal dysfunction; End-stage renal disease: 19-26 hours
Time to peak, serum: ~1.5-3 hours
Excretion: Urine (80% to 90%, 10% to 50% as unchanged drug and metabolites)

Usual Dosage Oral:
Children:
Initial: 3 mg/kg/day or 50-100 mg/m^2/day in 3 divided doses
Usual: 3-6 mg/kg/day or 100-150 mg/m^2/day in 3 divided doses; up to 11 mg/kg/day or 200 mg/m^2/day for uncontrolled patients with subtherapeutic levels
Adults:
Life-threatening ventricular arrhythmias:
Initial: 100 mg every 12 hours
Increase by 50-100 mg/day (given in 2 doses/day) every 4 days; maximum: 400 mg/day. Use of higher initial doses and more rapid dosage adjustments have resulted in an increased incidence of proarrhythmic events and congestive heart failure, particularly during the first few days. Do not use a loading dose. Use very cautiously in patients with history of congestive heart failure or myocardial infarction.
Prevention of paroxysmal supraventricular arrhythmias in patients with disabling symptoms but no structural heart disease:
Initial: 50 mg every 12 hours
Increase by 50 mg twice daily at 4-day intervals; maximum: 300 mg/day.
Dosing adjustment in severe renal impairment: Cl_{cr} <35 mL/minute: Decrease initial dose to 50 mg every 12 hours; increase doses at intervals >4 days monitoring EKG levels closely.
Dialysis: Not dialyzable (0% to 5%) via hemo- or peritoneal dialysis; no supplemental dose necessary.
Dosing adjustment/comments in hepatic impairment: Monitoring of plasma levels is recommended because of significantly increased half-life.
When transferring from another antiarrhythmic agent, allow for 2-4 half-lives of the agent to pass before initiating flecainide therapy.

Administration Administer around-the-clock to promote less variation in peak and trough serum levels

Monitoring Parameters EKG, blood pressure, pulse, periodic serum concentrations, especially in patients with renal or hepatic impairment

Reference Range Therapeutic: 0.2-1 µg/mL; pediatric patients may respond at the lower end of the recommended therapeutic range

Patient Information Notify physician if chest pain, faintness, or palpitations occurs; take only as prescribed

Nursing Implications Administer around-the-clock to promote less variation in peak and trough serum concentrations; monitor EKG

Dosage Forms Tablet, as acetate: 50 mg, 100 mg, 150 mg

Extemporaneous Preparations A 5 mg/mL suspension compounded from tablets and an oral flavored commercially available diluent (Roxane®) was stable for up to 45 days when stored at 5°C or 25°C in amber glass bottles. Flecainide 20 mg/mL was found stable for up to 60 days at 5°C and 25°C in a 1:1 preparation of Ora-Sweet® and Ora-Plus®, in Ora-Sweet® SF and Ora-Plus® and in cherry syrup

Allen LV and Erickson III MA, "Stability of Baclofen, Captopril, Diltiazem, Hydrochloride, Dipyridamole, and Flecainide Acetate in Extemporaneously Compounded Oral Liquids," *Am J Health Syst Pharm*, 53:2179-84.

Wiest DB, Garner SS, and Pagacz LR, "Stability of Flecainide Acetate in an Extemporaneously Compounded Oral Suspension," *Am J Hosp Pharm*, 1992, 49(6):1467-70.

Fluconazole (floo KOE na zole)

Related Information

U.S. Brand Names Diflucan®
(Continued)

Fluconazole *(Continued)*

Canadian Brand Names Apo®-Fluconazole; Diflucan™

Therapeutic Category Antifungal Agent, Systemic

Use Treatment of oral or vaginal candidiasis unresponsive to nystatin or clotrimazole; nonlife-threatening *Candida* infections (eg, cystitis, esophagitis); treatment of hepatosplenic candidiasis; treatment of other *Candida* infections in persons unable to tolerate amphotericin B; treatment of cryptococcal infections; secondary prophylaxis for cryptococcal meningitis in persons with AIDS; antifungal prophylaxis in allogeneic bone marrow transplant recipients

Oral fluconazole should be used in persons able to tolerate oral medications; parenteral fluconazole should be reserved for patients who are both unable to take oral medications and are unable to tolerate amphotericin B (eg, due to hypersensitivity or renal insufficiency)

Pregnancy Risk Factor C

Contraindications Hypersensitivity to fluconazole, other azoles, or any component of the formulation; concomitant administration with terfenadine, cisapride, or astemizole

Warnings/Precautions Should be used with caution in patients with renal and hepatic dysfunction or previous hepatotoxicity from other azole derivatives. Patients who develop abnormal liver function tests during fluconazole therapy should be monitored closely and discontinued if symptoms consistent with liver disease develop. **Should be used with caution in patients receiving cisapride.**

Adverse Reactions Frequency not always defined.

Cardiovascular: Pallor, angioedema

Central nervous system: Headache (2% to 13%), seizures, dizziness

Dermatologic: Rash (2%), alopecia, toxic epidermal necrolysis, Stevens-Johnson syndrome

Endocrine & metabolic: Hypertriglyceridemia, hypokalemia

Gastrointestinal: Nausea (4% to 7%), vomiting (2%), abdominal pain (2% to 6%), diarrhea (2% to 3%), taste perversion

Hematologic: Leukopenia, thrombocytopenia

Hepatic: Hepatic failure (rare), hepatitis, cholestasis, jaundice, increased ALT/AST, increased alkaline phosphatase

Respiratory: Dyspnea

Miscellaneous: Anaphylactic reactions (rare)

Overdosage/Toxicology Symptoms include decreased lacrimation, salivation, respiration, GI motility, urinary incontinence, and cyanosis. Treatment includes supportive measures. A 3-hour hemodialysis will remove 50% of the drug.

Drug Interactions

Cytochrome P450 Effect: CYP2C9 enzyme inducer; CYP2C9, 2C18, and 2C19 enzyme inhibitor and CYP3A3/4 enzyme inhibitor (weak)

Increased Effect/Toxicity: Fluconazole may increase serum concentrations/effects of cyclosporine, phenytoin, rifabutin, tacrolimus, theophylline, rifabutin, sulfonylureas, warfarin, and zidovudine. Fluconazole may also increase cisapride, terfenadine, or astemizole levels which has been associated with malignant arrhythmias. Hydrochlorothiazide may increase fluconazole levels.

Decreased Effect: Rifampin decreases concentrations of fluconazole.

Stability Parenteral admixture at room temperature (25°C): Manufacturer expiration dating; do not refrigerate

Standard diluent: 200 mg/100 mL NS (premixed); 400 mg/200 mL NS (premixed); 200 mg/100 mL D₅W (premixed); 400 mg/200 mL in D₅W (premixed)

Mechanism of Action Interferes with cytochrome P450 activity, decreasing ergosterol synthesis (principal sterol in fungal cell membrane) and inhibiting cell membrane formation

Pharmacodynamics/Kinetics

Distribution: Widely throughout body with good penetration into CSF, eye, peritoneal fluid, sputum, skin, and urine

Relative diffusion blood into CSF: Adequate with or without inflammation (exceeds usual MICs)

CSF:blood level ratio: Normal meninges: 70% to 80%; Inflamed meninges: >70% to 80%

Protein binding, plasma: 11% to 12%

Bioavailability: Oral: >90%

Half-life elimination: Normal renal function: 25-30 hours

Time to peak, serum: Oral: ~2-4 hours

Excretion: Urine (80% as unchanged drug)

Usual Dosage The daily dose of fluconazole is the same for oral and I.V. administration

Neonates: First 2 weeks of life, especially premature neonates: Same dose as older children every 72 hours

Children: Once-daily dosing by indication: See table.

Fluconazole — Once-Daily Dosing — Children

Indication	Day 1	Daily Therapy	Minimum Duration of Therapy
Oropharyngeal candidiasis	6 mg/kg	3 mg/kg	14 d
Esophageal candidiasis	6 mg/kg	3-12 mg/kg	21 d and for at least 2 wks following resolution of symptoms
Systemic candidiasis	—	6-12 mg/kg	28 d
Cryptococcal meningitis acute	12 mg/kg	6-12 mg/kg	10-12 wk after CSF culture becomes negative
relapse suppression	6 mg/kg	6 mg/kg	N/A

N/A = Not applicable

Adults: Oral, I.V.: Once-daily dosing by indication: See table on next page.

Fluconazole — Once-Daily Dosing — Adults

Indication	Day 1	Daily Therapy	Minimum Duration of Therapy
Oropharyngeal candidiasis	200 mg	100 mg	14 d
Esophageal candidiasis	200 mg	100 mg	21 d and for at least 14 d following resolution of symptoms
Prevention of candidiasis in bone marrow transplant	400 mg	400 mg	3 d before neutropenia, 7 d after neutrophils >1000 cells/mm^3
Candidiasis UTIs, peritonitis	50-200 mg	50-200 mg	N/A
Systemic candidiasis	400 mg	200 mg	28 d
Cryptococcal meningitis			10-12 wk after CSF culture becomes negative
acute	400 mg	200 mg	
relapse suppression	200 mg	200 mg	N/A
Vaginal candidiasis	150 mg	Single dose	N/A

N/A = Not applicable

Dosing adjustment/interval in renal impairment:
No adjustment for vaginal candidiasis single-dose therapy
For multiple dosing, administer usual load then adjust daily doses
Cl$_{cr}$ 11-50 mL/minute: Administer 50% of recommended dose or administer every 48 hours
Hemodialysis: One dose after each dialysis
Continuous arteriovenous or venovenous hemodiafiltration effects: Dose as for Cl$_{cr}$ 10-50 mL/minute

Dietary Considerations Take with or without regard to food.

Administration Parenteral fluconazole must be administered by I.V. infusion over approximately 1-2 hours; do not exceed 200 mg/hour when giving I.V. infusion; maximum rate of infusion: 200 mg/hour

Monitoring Parameters Periodic liver function tests (AST, ALT, alkaline phosphatase) and renal function tests, potassium

Patient Information May take with food; complete full course of therapy; contact physician or pharmacist if side effects develop; consider using an alternative method of contraception if taking concurrently with birth control pills

Nursing Implications Parenteral fluconazole must be administered by I.V. infusion over ~1-2 hours; do not exceed 200 mg/hour when administering I.V. infusion; final concentration for administration of 2 mg/mL; do not unwrap unit until ready for use; do not use if cloudy or precipitated

Dosage Forms
Injection: 2 mg/mL (100 mL, 200 mL)
Powder for oral suspension: 10 mg/mL (35 mL); 40 mg/mL (35 mL)
Tablet: 50 mg, 100 mg, 150 mg, 200 mg

Flucytosine (floo SYE toe seen)

Related Information
Antifungal Agents Comparison *on page 1484*

U.S. Brand Names Ancobon®

Canadian Brand Names Ancobon®

Synonyms 5-FC; 5-Flurocytosine

Therapeutic Category Antifungal Agent, Systemic

Use Adjunctive treatment of susceptible fungal infections (usually *Candida* or *Cryptococcus*); synergy with amphotericin B for certain fungal infections (*Cryptococcus* spp., *Candida* spp.)

Pregnancy Risk Factor C

Contraindications Hypersensitivity to flucytosine or any component

Warnings/Precautions Use with extreme caution in patients with renal impairment, bone marrow suppression, or in patients with AIDS; dosage modification required in patients with impaired renal function

Adverse Reactions Frequency not defined.
Central nervous system: Confusion, headache, hallucinations, dizziness, drowsiness, psychosis, parkinsonism, ataxia, sedation
Dermatologic: Rash, photosensitivity, pruritus, urticaria
Endocrine & metabolic: Temporary growth failure, hypoglycemia, hypokalemia
Gastrointestinal: Nausea, vomiting, diarrhea, abdominal pain, loss of appetite
Hematologic: Bone marrow suppression, anemia, leukopenia, thrombocytopenia
Hepatic: Elevated liver enzymes, hepatitis, jaundice, azotemia
Neuromuscular & skeletal: Peripheral neuropathy, paresthesia, weakness
Otic: Hearing loss
Renal: Elevated BUN and serum creatinine, renal failure
Respiratory: Respiratory arrest
Miscellaneous: Anaphylaxis

Overdosage/Toxicology Symptoms include nausea, vomiting, diarrhea, and bone marrow suppression. Treatment is supportive.

Drug Interactions
Increased Effect/Toxicity: Increased effect with amphotericin B. Amphotericin B-induced renal dysfunction may predispose patient to flucytosine accumulation and myelosuppression.

Ethanol/Nutrition/Herb Interactions Food: Food decreases the rate, but not the extent of absorption.

Stability Protect from light

Mechanism of Action Penetrates fungal cells and is converted to fluorouracil which competes with uracil interfering with fungal RNA and protein synthesis
(Continued)

Flucytosine (Continued)

Pharmacodynamics/Kinetics
Absorption: 75% to 90%

Distribution: Into CSF, aqueous humor, joints, peritoneal fluid, and bronchial secretions

Protein binding: 2% to 4%

Metabolism: Minimal

Half-life elimination: 3-8 hours; Anuria: As long as 200 hours; End-stage renal disease: 75-200 hours

Time to peak, serum: ~2-6 hours

Excretion: Urine (75% to 90% as unchanged drug)

Usual Dosage Children and Adults: Oral: 50-150 mg/kg/day in divided doses every 6 hours

Dosing interval in renal impairment: Use lower initial dose:

Cl_{cr} 20-40 mL/minute: Administer every 12 hours

Cl_{cr} 10-20 mL/minute: Administer every 24 hours

Cl_{cr} <10 mL/minute: Administer every 24-48 hours

Hemodialysis: Dialyzable (50% to 100%); administer dose posthemodialysis

Peritoneal dialysis: Adults: Administer 0.5-1 g every 24 hours

Continuous arteriovenous or venovenous hemodiafiltration effects: Dose as for Cl_{cr} 10-50 mL/minute

Monitoring Parameters Serum creatinine, BUN, alkaline phosphatase, AST, ALT, CBC; serum flucytosine concentrations

Reference Range
Therapeutic: 25-100 µg/mL (SI: 195-775 µmol/L); levels should not exceed 100-120 µg/mL to avoid toxic bone marrow depressive effects

Trough: Draw just prior to dose administration

Peak: Draw 2 hours after an oral dose administration

Test Interactions Flucytosine causes markedly false elevations in serum creatinine values when the Ektachem® analyzer is used

Patient Information Take capsules a few at a time with food over a 15-minute period to avoid nausea

Nursing Implications Administer around-the-clock rather than 4 times/day, 3 times/day, etc (ie, 12-6-12-6, not 9-1-5-9) to promote less variation in peak and trough serum levels; perform hematologic, renal and hepatic function tests

Dosage Forms Capsule: 250 mg, 500 mg

Extemporaneous Preparations Flucytosine oral liquid has been prepared by using the contents of ten 500 mg capsules triturated in a mortar and pestle with a small amount of distilled water; the mixture was transferred to a 500 mL volumetric flask; the mortar was rinsed several times with a small amount of distilled water and the fluid added to the flask; sufficient distilled water was added to make a total volume of 500 mL of a 10 mg/mL liquid; oral liquid was stable for 70 days when stored in glass or plastic prescription bottles at 4°C or for up to 14 days at room temperature.

Wintermeyer SM and Nahata MC, "Stability of Flucytosine in an Extemporaneously Compounded Oral Liquid," *Am J Health Syst Pharm*, 1996, 53:407-9.

♦ **Fludara**® *see Fludarabine on page 568*

Fludarabine (floo DARE a been)

U.S. Brand Names Fludara®

Canadian Brand Names Fludara®

Synonyms Fludarabine Phosphate

Therapeutic Category Antineoplastic Agent, Antimetabolite (Purine)

Use Salvage therapy of non-Hodgkin's lymphoma and acute leukemias

Orphan drug: Treatment of chronic lymphocytic leukemia (CLL), including refractory CLL

Pregnancy Risk Factor D

Contraindications Hypersensitivity of fludarabine or any component of the formulation; pregnancy

Warnings/Precautions The U.S. Food and Drug Administration (FDA) currently recommends that procedures for proper handling and disposal of antineoplastic agents be considered. Use with caution with renal insufficiency, patients with a fever, documented infection, or pre-existing hematological disorders (particularly granulocytopenia) or in patients with pre-existing central nervous system disorder (epilepsy), spasticity, or peripheral neuropathy. Use with caution in patients with pre-existing renal insufficiency. Life-threatening and sometimes fatal autoimmune hemolytic anemia have occurred.

Adverse Reactions
>10%:

Central nervous system: Fever, chills, fatigue, pain

Dermatologic: Rash

Gastrointestinal: Mild nausea, vomiting, diarrhea, stomatitis, GI bleeding

Genitourinary: Urinary infection

Hematologic: Anemia, thrombocytopenia, leukopenia; Myelosuppression: Dose-limiting toxicity; myelosuppression may not be related to cumulative dose

Granulocyte nadir: 13 days (3-25)

Platelet nadir: 16 days (2-32)

WBC nadir: 8 days

Recovery: 5-7 weeks

Neuromuscular & skeletal: Paresthesia, myalgia, weakness

Respiratory: Manifested as dyspnea and a nonproductive cough; lung biopsy has shown pneumonitis in some patients, pneumonia

Miscellaneous: Infection

1% to 10%:

Cardiovascular: Congestive heart failure, edema

Central nervous system: Malaise, headache

Dermatologic: Alopecia

Endocrine & metabolic: Hyperglycemia
Gastrointestinal: Anorexia
Emetic potential: Very low (<10%)
Ocular: Blurred vision
Otic: Hearing loss
<1% (Limited to important or life-threatening): Interstitial pneumonitis, life-threatening and sometimes fatal autoimmune hemolytic anemia (often recurs on rechallenge - steroid treatment may or may not be beneficial), metabolic acidosis, renal failure, reversible hepatotoxicity, severe neurotoxicity (reported with higher dose levels: most patients shown to have CNS demyelination; somnolence, blindness, coma, and death also occurred), tumor lysis syndrome

Overdosage/Toxicology There are clear, dose-dependent, toxic neurologic effects associated with fludarabine. Doses of 96 mg/m^2/day for 5-7 days are associated with a syndrome characterized by delayed blindness, coma, and death. Symptoms have appeared in 21-60 days following the last dose. Central nervous system toxicity has distinctive features of delayed onset and progressive encephalopathy, resulting in fatalities. It is reported at an incidence rate of 36% at high doses (≥96 mg/m^2/day for 5-7 days) and <0.2% for low doses (≤125 mg/m^2/course).

Drug Interactions
Increased Effect/Toxicity: Cytarabine when administered with or prior to a fludarabine dose competes for deoxycytidine kinase decreasing the metabolism of F-ara-A to the active F-ara-ATP (inhibits the antineoplastic effect of fludarabine); however, administering fludarabine prior to cytarabine may stimulate activation of cytarabine.

Ethanol/Nutrition/Herb Interactions Ethanol: Avoid ethanol (due to GI irritation).

Stability Store intact vials under refrigeration (2°C to 8°C/36°F to 46°F). Reconstituted vials are stable for 16 days at room temperature (15°C to 30°C/59°F to 86°F) or refrigerated. Solutions diluted in saline or dextrose are stable for 48 hours at room temperature or under refrigeration.
Reconstitute vials with 2 mL SWI to result in a concentration of 25 mg/mL.

Mechanism of Action Fludarabine is analogous to that of Ara-C and Ara-A. Following systemic administration, FAMP is rapidly dephosphorylated to 2-fluoro-Ara-A. 2-Fluoro-Ara-A enters the cell by a carrier-mediated transport process, then is phosphorylated intracellularly by deoxycytidine kinase to form the active metabolite 2-fluoro-Ara-ATP. 2-Fluoro-Ara-ATP inhibits DNA synthesis by inhibition of DNA polymerase and ribonucleotide reductase.

Pharmacodynamics/Kinetics
Distribution: V$_d$: 38-96 L/m^2; widely with extensive tissue binding
Metabolism: I.V.: Fludarabine phosphate is rapidly dephosphorylated to 2-fluoro-vidarabine, which subsequently enters tumor cells and is phosphorylated to the active triphosphate derivative; rapidly dephosphorylated in the serum
Bioavailability: 75%
Half-life elimination: 2-fluoro-vidarabine: 9 hours
Excretion: Urine (60%, 23% as 2-fluoro-vidarabine) within 24 hours

Usual Dosage I.V.:
Children:
Acute leukemia: 10 mg/m^2 bolus over 15 minutes followed by continuous infusion of 30.5 mg/m^2/day over 5 days **or**
10.5 mg/m^2 bolus over 15 minutes followed by 30.5 mg/m^2/day over 48 hours followed by cytarabine has been used in clinical trials
Solid tumors: 9 mg/m^2 bolus followed by 27 mg/m^2/day continuous infusion over 5 days
Adults:
Chronic lymphocytic leukemia: 25 mg/m^2/day over a 30-minute period for 5 days; 5-day courses are repeated every 28 days days
Non-Hodgkin's lymphoma: Loading dose: 20 mg/m^2 followed by 30 mg/m^2/day for 48 hours
Dosing in renal impairment:
Cl$_{cr}$ 30-70 mL/minute: Reduce dose by 20%
Cl$_{cr}$ <30 mL/minute: Not recommended

Administration Fludarabine is administered intravenously, usually as a 15- to 30-minute infusion; continuous infusions are occasionally used

Monitoring Parameters CBC with differential, platelet count, AST, ALT, creatinine, serum albumin, uric acid

Reference Range Peak plasma levels: 0.3-0.9 µg/mL following a short infusion of 25 mg/m^2

Nursing Implications Parenteral: Fludarabine phosphate has been administered by intermittent I.V. infusion over 15-30 minutes and by continuous infusion; in clinical trials the loading dose has been diluted in 20 mL D$_5$W and administered over 15 minutes and the continuous infusion diluted to 240 mL in D$_5$W and administered at a constant rate of 10 mL/hour; in other clinical studies fludarabine has been diluted to a concentration of 0.25 to 1 mg/mL in D$_5$W or sodium chloride 0.9%

Dosage Forms Powder for injection, lyophilized, as phosphate: 50 mg (6 mL)

♦ **Fludarabine Phosphate** *see* Fludarabine *on page 568*

Fludrocortisone (floo droe KOR ti sone)
Related Information
Corticosteroids Comparison *on page 1495*
U.S. Brand Names Florinef®
Canadian Brand Names Florinef®
Synonyms Fludrocortisone Acetate; Fluohydrisone Acetate; Fluohydrocortisone Acetate; 9α-Fluorohydrocortisone Acetate
Therapeutic Category Mineralocorticoid
Use Partial replacement therapy for primary and secondary adrenocortical insufficiency in Addison's disease; treatment of salt-losing adrenogenital syndrome
Pregnancy Risk Factor C
Contraindications Hypersensitivity to fludrocortisone or any component of the formulation; systemic fungal infections
(Continued)

Fludrocortisone *(Continued)*

Warnings/Precautions Taper dose gradually when therapy is discontinued; use with caution with Addison's disease, sodium retention and potassium loss

Adverse Reactions 1% to 10%:

Cardiovascular: Hypertension, edema, congestive heart failure

Central nervous system: Convulsions, headache, dizziness

Dermatologic: Acne, rash, bruising

Endocrine & metabolic: Hypokalemic alkalosis, suppression of growth, hyperglycemia, HPA suppression

Gastrointestinal: Peptic ulcer

Neuromuscular & skeletal: Muscle weakness

Ocular: Cataracts

Miscellaneous: Diaphoresis, anaphylaxis (generalized)

Overdosage/Toxicology Symptoms include hypertension, edema, hypokalemia, and excessive weight gain. When consumed in excessive quantities, systemic hypercorticism and adrenal suppression may occur; in those cases, discontinuation and withdrawal of the corticosteroid should be done judiciously.

Drug Interactions

Decreased Effect: Anticholinesterases effects are antagonized. Decreased corticosteroid effects by rifampin, barbiturates, and hydantoins. May decrease salicylate levels.

Mechanism of Action Promotes increased reabsorption of sodium and loss of potassium from renal distal tubules

Pharmacodynamics/Kinetics

Absorption: Rapid and complete

Protein binding: 42%

Metabolism: Hepatic

Half-life elimination, plasma: 30-35 minutes; Biological: 18-36 hours

Time to peak, serum: ~1.7 hours

Usual Dosage Oral:

Infants and Children: 0.05-0.1 mg/day

Adults: 0.1-0.2 mg/day with ranges of 0.1 mg 3 times/week to 0.2 mg/day

Addison's disease: Initial: 0.1 mg/day; if transient hypertension develops, reduce the dose to 0.05 mg/day. Preferred administration with cortisone (10-37.5 mg/day) or hydrocortisone (10-30 mg/day).

Salt-losing adrenogenital syndrome: 0.1-0.2 mg/day

Dietary Considerations Systemic use of mineralocorticoids/corticosteroids may require a diet with increased potassium, vitamins A, B_6, C, D, folate, calcium, zinc, and phosphorus, and decreased sodium. With fludrocortisone a decrease in dietary sodium is often not required as the increased retention of sodium is usually the desired therapeutic effect.

Administration Administration in conjunction with a glucocorticoid is preferable

Monitoring Parameters Monitor blood pressure and signs of edema when patient is on chronic therapy; very potent mineralocorticoid with high glucocorticoid activity; monitor serum electrolytes, serum renin activity, and blood pressure; monitor for evidence of infection

Patient Information Notify physician if dizziness, severe or continuing headaches, swelling of feet or lower legs or unusual weight gain occur

Nursing Implications Monitor blood pressure and signs of edema when patient is on chronic therapy; very potent mineralocorticoid with high glucocorticoid activity; monitor serum electrolytes, serum renin activity, and blood pressure; monitor evidence of infection; closely monitor patients with Addison's disease and stop treatment if a significant increase in weight or blood pressure, edema or cardiac enlargement occurs

Additional Information In patients with salt-losing forms of congenital adrenogenital syndrome, use along with cortisone or hydrocortisone. Fludrocortisone 0.1 mg has sodium retention activity equal to DOCA® 1 mg.

Dosage Forms Tablet, as acetate: 0.1 mg

♦ **Fludrocortisone Acetate** *see Fludrocortisone on page 569*

♦ **Flumadine®** *see Rimantadine on page 1197*

Flumazenil *(FLOO may ze nil)*

U.S. Brand Names Romazicon™

Canadian Brand Names Anexate®; Romazicon™

Therapeutic Category Antidote, Benzodiazepine

Use Benzodiazepine antagonist - reverses sedative effects of benzodiazepines used in general anesthesia; for management of benzodiazepine overdose; flumazenil does **not** antagonize the CNS effects of other GABA agonists (eg, ethanol, barbiturates, or general anesthetics), **does** not reverse narcotics

Pregnancy Risk Factor C

Contraindications Hypersensitivity to flumazenil, benzodiazepines, or any component of the formulation; patients given benzodiazepines for control of potentially life-threatening conditions (eg, control of intracranial pressure or status epilepticus); patients who are showing signs of serious cyclic-antidepressant overdosage

Warnings/Precautions

Risk of seizures = high-risk patients:

Patients on benzodiazepines for long-term sedation

Tricyclic antidepressant overdose patients

Concurrent major sedative-hypnotic drug withdrawal

Recent therapy with repeated doses of parenteral benzodiazepines

Myoclonic jerking or seizure activity prior to flumazenil administration

Hypoventilation: Does not reverse respiratory depression/hypoventilation or cardiac depression

Resedation: Occurs more frequently in patients where a large single dose or cumulative dose of a benzodiazepine is administered along with a neuromuscular blocking agent and multiple anesthetic agents

Flumazenil should be used with caution in the intensive care unit because of increased risk of unrecognized benzodiazepine dependence in such settings.

Does **not** antagonize the CNS effects of other GABA agonists (such as ethanol, barbiturates, or general anesthetics), nor does it reverse narcotics

Adverse Reactions
>10%: Gastrointestinal: Vomiting, nausea

1% to 10%:

Cardiovascular: Palpitations

Central nervous system: Headache, anxiety, nervousness, insomnia, abnormal crying, euphoria, depression, agitation, dizziness, emotional lability, ataxia, depersonalization, increased tears, dysphoria, paranoia

Endocrine & metabolic: Hot flashes

Gastrointestinal: Xerostomia

Local: Pain at injection site

Neuromuscular & skeletal: Tremor, weakness, paresthesia

Ocular: Abnormal vision, blurred vision

Respiratory: Dyspnea, hyperventilation

Miscellaneous: Diaphoresis

<1% (Limited to important or life-threatening): Bradycardia, chest pain, generalized convulsions, hypertension, tachycardia, ventricular extrasystoles, withdrawal syndrome

Drug Interactions
Increased Effect/Toxicity: Use with caution in overdosage involving mixed drug overdose. Toxic effects may emerge (especially with cyclic antidepressants) with the reversal of the benzodiazepine effect by flumazenil.

Stability For I.V. use only; **compatible** with D_5W, lactated Ringer's, or normal saline; once drawn up in the syringe or mixed with solution use within 24 hours; discard any unused solution after 24 hours

Mechanism of Action Competitively inhibits the activity at the benzodiazepine recognition site on the GABA/benzodiazepine receptor complex. Flumazenil does not antagonize the CNS effect of drugs affecting GABA-ergic neurons by means other than the benzodiazepine receptor (ethanol, barbiturates, general anesthetics) and does not reverse the effects of opioids

Flumazenil

Pediatric Dosage	
Further studies are needed	
Pediatric dosage for **reversal of conscious sedation:** Intravenously through a freely running intravenous infusion into a large vein to minimize pain at the injection site	
Initial dose	0.01 mg/kg over 15 seconds (maximum dose of 0.2 mg)
Repeat doses	0.005-0.01 mg/kg (maximum dose of 0.2 mg) repeated at 1-minute intervals
Maximum total cumulative dose	1 mg
Pediatric dosage for **management of benzodiazepine overdose:** Intravenously through a freely running intravenous infusion into a large vein to minimize pain at the injection site	
Initial dose	0.01 mg/kg (maximum dose: 0.2 mg)
Repeat doses	0.01 mg/kg (maximum dose of 0.2 mg) repeated at 1-minute intervals
Maximum total cumulative dose	1 mg
In place of repeat bolus doses, follow-up continuous infusions of 0.005-0.01 mg/kg/hour have been used; further studies are needed.	

Adult Dosage	
Adult dosage for **reversal of conscious sedation:** Intravenously through a freely running intravenous infusion into a large vein to minimize pain at the injection site	
Initial dose	0.2 mg intravenously over 15 seconds
Repeat doses	If desired level of consciousness is not obtained, 0.2 mg may be repeated at 1-minute intervals.
Maximum total cumulative dose	1 mg (usual dose 0.6-1 mg) **In the event of resedation:** Repeat doses may be given at 20-minute intervals with maximum of 1 mg/dose and 3 mg/hour
Adult dosage for **suspected benzodiazepine overdose:** Intravenously through a freely running intravenous infusion into a large vein to minimize pain at the injection site	
Initial dose	0.2 mg intravenously over 30 seconds
Repeat doses	0.5 mg over 30 seconds repeated at 1-minute intervals
Maximum total cumulative dose	3 mg (usual dose 1-3 mg) Patients with a partial response at 3 mg may require additional titration up to a total dose of 5 mg. If a patient has not responded 5 minutes after cumulative dose of 5 mg, the major cause of sedation is not likely due to benzodiazepines. **In the event of resedation:** May repeat doses at 20-minute intervals with maximum of 1 mg/dose and 3 mg/hour

Pharmacodynamics/Kinetics
Onset of action: 1-3 minutes; 80% response within 3 minutes

(Continued)

Flumazenil *(Continued)*

Peak effect: 6-10 minutes

Duration: Resedation: ~1 hour; duration related to dose given and benzodiazepine plasma concentrations; reversal effects of flumazenil may wear off before effects of benzodiazepine

Distribution: Initial V_d: 0.5 L/kg; V_{dss} 0.77-1.6 L/kg

Protein binding: 40% to 50%

Metabolism: Hepatic; dependent upon hepatic blood flow

Half-life elimination: Adults: Alpha: 7-15 minutes; Terminal: 41-79 minutes

Excretion: Feces; urine (0.2% as unchanged drug)

Usual Dosage

Children and Adults: I.V.: See table on previous page.

Resedation: Repeated doses may be given at 20-minute intervals as needed; repeat treatment doses of 1 mg (at a rate of 0.5 mg/minute) should be given at any time and no more than 3 mg should be given in any hour. After intoxication with high doses of benzodiazepines, the duration of a single dose of flumazenil is not expected to exceed 1 hour; if desired, the period of wakefulness may be prolonged with repeated low intravenous doses of flumazenil, or by an infusion of 0.1-0.4 mg/hour. Most patients with benzodiazepine overdose will respond to a cumulative dose of 1-3 mg and doses >3 mg do not reliably produce additional effects. Rarely, patients with a partial response at 3 mg may require additional titration up to a total dose of 5 mg. **If a patient has not responded 5 minutes after receiving a cumulative dose of 5 mg, the major cause of sedation is not likely to be due to benzodiazepines.**

Elderly: No differences in safety or efficacy have been reported. However, increased sensitivity may occur in some elderly patients.

Dosing in renal impairment: Not significantly affected by renal failure (Cl_{cr} <10 mL/minute) or hemodialysis beginning 1 hour after drug administration

Dosing in hepatic impairment: Initial dose of flumazenil used for initial reversal of benzodiazepine effects is not changed; however, subsequent doses in liver disease patients should be reduced in size or frequency

Monitoring Parameters Monitor patients for return of sedation or respiratory depression

Patient Information Flumazenil does not consistently reverse amnesia; do not engage in activities requiring alertness for 18-24 hours after discharge; resedation may occur in patients on long-acting benzodiazepines (such as diazepam)

Nursing Implications Parenteral: For I.V. use only; administer via freely running I.V. infusion into larger vein to decrease chance of pain, phlebitis

Dosage Forms Injection: 0.1 mg/mL (5 mL, 10 mL)

Flunisolide *(floo NISS oh lide)*

Related Information

Asthma *on page 1645*

Estimated Clinical Comparability of Doses for Inhaled Corticosteroids *on page 1652*

U.S. Brand Names AeroBid®; AeroBid®-M; Nasalide®; Nasarel®

Canadian Brand Names Alti-Flunisolide; Apo®-Flunisolide; Nasalide®; Rhinalar®

Therapeutic Category Anti-inflammatory Agent, Inhalant; Corticosteroid, Inhalant; Corticosteroid, Intranasal

Use Steroid-dependent asthma; nasal solution is used for seasonal or perennial rhinitis

Pregnancy Risk Factor C

Usual Dosage

Children >6 years:

Oral inhalation: 2 inhalations twice daily (morning and evening) up to 4 inhalations/day

Nasal: 1 spray each nostril twice daily (morning and evening), not to exceed 4 sprays/day each nostril

Adults:

Oral inhalation: 2 inhalations twice daily (morning and evening) up to 8 inhalations/day maximum

Nasal: 2 sprays each nostril twice daily (morning and evening); maximum dose: 8 sprays/day in each nostril

Additional Information Complete prescribing information for this medication should be consulted for additional detail.

Dosage Forms

Aerosol for oral inhalation:

AeroBid® Aerosol: 250 mcg/actuation [100 metered doses] (7 g)

AeroBid-M® Aerosol: 250 mcg/actuation [100 metered doses] (7 g) [menthol flavor]

Solution, intranasal [spray]:

Nasalide®: 25 mcg/actuation [200 sprays] (25 mL)

Nasarel®: 0.025% [200 actuations] (25 mL)

Fluocinolone *(floo oh SIN oh lone)*

Related Information

Corticosteroids Comparison *on page 1495*

U.S. Brand Names Capex™; Derma-Smoothe/FS®; FS Shampoo® [DSC]; Synalar®

Canadian Brand Names Capex®; Derma-Smoothe/FS®; Fluoderm; Synalar®

Synonyms Fluocinolone Acetonide

Therapeutic Category Anti-inflammatory Agent; Corticosteroid, Shampoo; Corticosteroid, Topical (Low Potency); Corticosteroid, Topical (Medium Potency); Corticosteroid, Topical (High Potency)

Use Relief of susceptible inflammatory dermatosis [low, medium, high potency topical corticosteroid]; psoriasis of the scalp; atopic dermatitis in children ≥2 years of age

Pregnancy Risk Factor C

Usual Dosage Topical:
  Children ≥2 years: Atopic dermatitis (Derma-Smoothe/FS®): Moisten skin; apply to affected area twice daily; do not use for longer than 4 weeks
  Children and Adults: Corticosteroid-responsive dermatoses: Cream, lotion, ointment, solution: Apply a thin layer to affected area 2-4 times/day; may use occlusive dressings to manage psoriasis or recalcitrant conditions
  Adults:
    Atopic dermatitis (Derma-Smoothe/FS®): Apply thin film to affected area 3 times/day
    Scalp psoriasis (Derma-Smoothe/FS®): Massage thoroughly into wet or dampened hair/scalp; cover with shower cap. Leave on overnight (or for at least 4 hours). Remove by washing hair with shampoo and rinsing thoroughly.
    Seborrheic dermatitis of the scalp (Capex™): Apply no more than 1 ounce to scalp once daily; work into lather and allow to remain on scalp for ~5 minutes. Remove from hair and scalp by rinsing thoroughly with water.
Additional Information Complete prescribing information for this medication should be consulted for additional detail.
Dosage Forms
  Cream, topical, as acetonide: 0.01% (15 g, 60 g); 0.025% (15 g, 60 g)
    Synalar®: 0.025% (15 g, 60 g)
  Oil, topical, as acetonide (Derma-Smoothe/FS®): 0.01% (120 mL) [contains peanut oil]
  Ointment, topical, as acetonide: 0.025% (15 g, 60 g)
    Synalar®: 0.025% (15 g, 30 g, 60 g)
  Shampoo, topical, as acetonide (Capex™): 0.01% (120 mL)
  Solution, topical, as acetonide: 0.01% (20 mL, 60 mL)
    Synalar®: 0.01% (20 mL, 60 mL)

♦ **Fluocinolone Acetonide** *see* Fluocinolone *on page 572*

Fluocinonide (floo oh SIN oh nide)
  Related Information
    Corticosteroids Comparison *on page 1495*
  U.S. Brand Names Lidex®; Lidex-E®
  Canadian Brand Names Lidemol®; Lidex®; Lyderm®; Lydonide; Tiamol®; Topsyn®
  Therapeutic Category Corticosteroid, Topical (High Potency)
  Use Anti-inflammatory, antipruritic, relief of inflammatory and pruritic manifestations [high potency topical corticosteroid]
  Pregnancy Risk Factor C
  Usual Dosage Children and Adults: Topical: Apply thin layer to affected area 2-4 times/day depending on the severity of the condition. Therapy should be discontinued when control is achieved; if no improvement is seen, reassessment of diagnosis may be necessary.
  Additional Information Complete prescribing information for this medication should be consulted for additional detail.
  Dosage Forms
    Cream: 0.05% (15 g, 30 g, 60 g, 120 g)
    Cream, anhydrous, emollient (Lidex®): 0.05% (15 g, 30 g, 60 g, 120 g)
    Cream, aqueous, emollient (Lidex-E®): 0.05% (15 g, 30 g, 60 g, 120 g)
    Gel, topical: 0.05% (15 g, 60 g)
      Lidex®: 0.05% (15 g, 30 g, 60 g, 120 g)
    Ointment, topical: 0.05% (15 g, 30 g, 60 g)
      Lidex®: 0.05% (15 g, 30 g, 60 g, 120 g)
    Solution, topical: 0.05% (20 mL, 60 mL)
      Lidex®: 0.05% (20 mL, 60 mL)

♦ **Fluoderm (Can)** *see* Fluocinolone *on page 572*
♦ **Fluogen®** *see* Influenza Virus Vaccine *on page 721*
♦ **Fluohydrisone Acetate** *see* Fludrocortisone *on page 569*
♦ **Fluohydrocortisone Acetate** *see* Fludrocortisone *on page 569*
♦ **Fluoracaine®** *see* Proparacaine and Fluorescein *on page 1144*
♦ **Fluor-A-Day® (Can)** *see* Fluoride *on page 574*

Fluorescein Sodium (FLURE e seen SOW dee um)
  U.S. Brand Names AK-Fluor; Fluorescite®; Fluorets® Ophthalmic Strips; Fluor-I-Strip®; Fluor-I-Strip-AT®; Fluress®; Ful-Glo® Ophthalmic Strips; Ophthifluor®
  Canadian Brand Names Diofluor™; Fluorescite®; Fluorets™
  Synonyms Soluble Fluorescein
  Therapeutic Category Diagnostic Agent, Ophthalmic Dye
  Use Demonstrates defects of corneal epithelium; diagnostic aid in ophthalmic angiography
  Pregnancy Risk Factor C (topical); X (parenteral)
  Usual Dosage
    Ophthalmic:
      Solution: Instill 1-2 drops of 2% solution and allow a few seconds for staining; wash out excess with sterile water or irrigating solution
      Strips: Moisten strip with sterile water. Place moistened strip at the fornix into the lower cul-de-sac close to the punctum. For best results, patient should close lid tightly over strip until desired amount of staining is obtained. Patient should blink several times after application.
      Removal of foreign bodies, sutures or tonometry (Fluress®): Instill 1 or 2 drops (single instillations) into each eye before operating
      Deep ophthalmic anesthesia (Fluress®): Instill 2 drops into each eye every 90 seconds up to 3 doses
    Injection: Prior to use, perform intradermal skin test; have epinephrine 1:1000, an antihistamine, and oxygen available
      Children: 3.5 mg/lb (7.5 mg/kg) injected rapidly into antecubital vein
      Adults: 500-750 mg injected rapidly into antecubital vein
  (Continued)

Fluorescein Sodium *(Continued)*

Additional Information Complete prescribing information for this medication should be consulted for additional detail.

Dosage Forms

Injection (AK-Fluor, Fluorescite®, Ophthifluor®): 10% [100 mg/mL] (5 mL); 25% [250 mg/mL] (2 mL, 3 mL)

Ophthalmic, solution: 2% [20 mg/mL] (1 mL, 2 mL, 15 mL)

Fluress®: 0.25% [2.5 mg/mL] with benoxinate 0.4% (5 mL)

Ophthalmic strip:

Fluorets®, Fluor-I-Strip-AT®: 1 mg

Fluor-I-Strip®: 9 mg

Ful-Glo®: 0.6 mg

♦ **Fluorescite®** *see Fluorescein Sodium on page 573*

♦ **Fluorets™ (Can)** *see Fluorescein Sodium on page 573*

♦ **Fluorets® Ophthalmic Strips** *see Fluorescein Sodium on page 573*

Fluoride *(FLOR ide)*

U.S. Brand Names ACT® [OTC]; Fluorigard® [OTC]; Fluorinse®; Fluoritab®; Flura-Drops®; Flura-Loz®; Gel-Kam®; Gel-Tin® [OTC]; Karidium®; Karigel®; Karigel®-N; Luride®; Luride® Lozi-Tab®; Luride®-SF Lozi-Tabs®; Minute-Gel®; Pediaflor®; Pharmaflur®; Phos-Flur®; Point-Two®; PreviDent®; PreviDent® 5000 Plus™; Stop® [OTC]; Thera-Flur®; Thera-Flur-N®

Canadian Brand Names Fluor-A-Day®; Fluotic®

Synonyms Acidulated Phosphate Fluoride; Sodium Fluoride; Stannous Fluoride

Therapeutic Category Mineral, Oral; Mineral, Oral Topical

Use Used exclusively in dental applications (prevention of dental caries)

Pregnancy Risk Factor C

Contraindications Hypersensitivity to fluoride, tartrazine, or any component of the formulation; when fluoride content of drinking water exceeds 0.7 ppm; low sodium or sodium-free diets; do not use 1 mg tablets in children <3 years of age or when drinking water fluoride content is ≥0.3 ppm; do not use 1 mg/5 mL rinse (as supplement) in children <6 years of age

Warnings/Precautions Prolonged ingestion with excessive doses may result in dental fluorosis and osseous changes; do **not** exceed recommended dosage; some products contain tartrazine

Adverse Reactions <1% (Limited to important or life-threatening): Discoloration of teeth, rash, nausea, vomiting

Overdosage/Toxicology Symptoms include hypersalivation, salty or soapy taste, epigastric pain, nausea, vomiting, diarrhea, rash, muscle weakness, tremor, seizures, cardiac failure, respiratory arrest, shock, and death. The fatal dose not known. Treatment consists of gastric lavage with $CaCl_2$ or $Ca(OH)_2$ solution. Administer a large quantity of milk at frequent intervals. $Al(OH)_3$ may also bind the fluoride ion.

Drug Interactions

Decreased Effect: Decreased effect/absorption with magnesium-, aluminum-, and calcium-containing products.

Stability Store in tight plastic containers (not glass)

Mechanism of Action Promotes remineralization of decalcified enamel; inhibits the cariogenic microbial process in dental plaque; increases tooth resistance to acid dissolution

Pharmacodynamics/Kinetics

Absorption: Oral: Rapid and complete; sodium fluoride; other soluble fluoride salts; calcium, iron, or magnesium may delay absorption

Distribution: 50% of fluoride is deposited in teeth and bone after ingestion; topical application works superficially on enamel and plaque; crosses placenta; enters breast milk

Excretion: Urine and feces

Usual Dosage Oral:

The recommended daily dose of oral fluoride supplement (mg), based on fluoride ion content (ppm) in drinking water (2.2 mg of sodium fluoride is equivalent to 1 mg of fluoride ion): See table.

Fluoride Ion

Fluoride Content of Drinking Water	Daily Dose, Oral (mg)
<0.3 ppm	
Birth - 6 mo	None
6 mo - 3 y	0.25
3-6 y	0.5
6-16 y	1
0.3-0.6 ppm	
Birth - 6 mo	None
6 mo - 3 y	None
3-6 y	0.25
6-16 y	0.5

Table from: Recommended dosage schedule of The American Dental Association, The American Academy of Pediatric Dentistry, and The American Academy of Pediatrics

Dental rinse or gel:

Children 6-12 years: 5-10 mL rinse or apply to teeth and spit daily after brushing

Adults: 10 mL rinse or apply to teeth and spit daily after brushing

PreviDent® rinse: Children >6 years and Adults: Once weekly, rinse 10 mL vigorously around and between teeth for 1 minute, then spit; this should be done preferably at bedtime, after thoroughly brushing teeth; for maximum benefit, do not eat, drink, or rinse mouth for at least 30 minutes after treatment; do not swallow

Fluorinse®: Children >6 years and Adults: Once weekly, vigorously swish 5-10 mL in mouth for 1 minute, then spit

Dietary Considerations Do not administer with milk; do **not** allow eating or drinking for 30 minutes after use.

Patient Information Take with food (but not milk) to eliminate GI upset; with dental rinse or dental gel do **not** swallow, do **not** eat or drink for 30 minutes after use

Nursing Implications Avoid giving with milk or dairy products

Dosage Forms Fluoride ion content listed in brackets

Cream, oral, as sodium (PreviDent® 5000 Plus™): 1.1% [2.5 mg per dose] (51 g)

Gel, topical, acidulated phosphate fluoride (Minute-Gel®): 1.23% (480 mL)

Gel, topical, sodium fluoride (Karigel®, Karigel®-N, PreviDent®): 1.1% [0.5%] (24 g, 30 g, 60 g, 120 g, 130 g, 250 g)

Gel, topical, stannous fluoride (Gel Kam®, Gel-Tin®, Stop®): 0.4% [0.1%] (60 g, 65 g, 105 g, 120 g)

Lozenge, as sodium (Flura-Loz®): 2.2 mg [1 mg] [raspberry flavor]

Solution, oral, as sodium (Phos-Flur®): 0.44 mg/mL [0.2 mg/mL] (250 mL, 500 mL, 3780 mL)

Solution, oral, as sodium [drops]:

Fluoritab®, Flura-Drops®: 0.55 mg/drop [0.25 mg/drop] (22.8 mL, 24 mL)

Karidium®: 0.275 mg/drop [0.125 mg/drop] (30 mL, 60 mL)

Luride®, Pediaflor®: 1.1 mg/mL [0.5 mg/mL] (50 mL)

Solution, topical, as sodium [rinse]:

ACT®, Fluorigard®: 0.05% [0.02%] (90 mL, 180 mL, 300 mL, 360 mL, 480 mL)

Fluorinse®, Point-Two®: 0.2% [0.09%] (240 mL, 480 mL, 3780 mL)

PreviDent®: 0.2% [9 mg per dose] (250 mL)

Tablet, as sodium (Flura®, Karidium®): 2.2 mg [1 mg]

Tablet, chewable:

Fluoritab®, Luride® Lozi-Tabs®, Pharmaflur®: 1.1 mg [0.5 mg]

Fluoritab®, Karidium®, Luride® Lozi-Tabs®, Luride®-SF Lozi-Tabs®, Pharmaflur®: 2.2 mg [1 mg]

♦ **Fluorigard®** [OTC] see Fluoride on page 574

♦ **Fluori-Methane®** see Dichlorodifluoromethane and Trichloromonofluoromethane on page 393

♦ **Fluorinse®** see Fluoride on page 574

♦ **Fluor-I-Strip®** see Fluorescein Sodium on page 573

♦ **Fluor-I-Strip-AT®** see Fluorescein Sodium on page 573

♦ **Fluoritab®** see Fluoride on page 574

♦ **9α-Fluorohydrocortisone Acetate** see Fludrocortisone on page 569

Fluorometholone (flure oh METH oh lone)

U.S. Brand Names Flarex®; Fluor-Op®; FML®; FML® Forte

Canadian Brand Names Flarex®; FML®; FML® Forte®

Therapeutic Category Anti-inflammatory Agent; Corticosteroid, Ophthalmic; Corticosteroid, Topical (Low Potency)

Use Treatment of steroid-responsive inflammatory conditions of the eye

Pregnancy Risk Factor C

Pregnancy/Breast-Feeding Implications The extent of systemic absorption is not known. Use with caution in pregnant or nursing women.

Contraindications Hypersensitivity to fluorometholone or any component of the formulation; viral diseases of the cornea and conjunctiva (including epithelial herpes simplex keratitis, vaccinia and varicella); mycobacterial or fungal infections of the eye; untreated eye infections which may be masked/enhanced by a steroid

Warnings/Precautions Not recommended in children <2 years of age; prolonged use may result in glaucoma, elevated intraocular pressure, or other ocular damage; may exacerbate severity of viral infections, use caution in patients with history of herpes simplex; re-evaluate after 2 days if symptoms have not improved; may delay healing following cataract surgery; some products contain sulfites

Adverse Reactions

Ocular: Anterior uveitis, burning upon application, cataract formation, conjunctival hyperemia, conjunctivitis, corneal ulcers, glaucoma with optic nerve damage, perforation of the globe, secondary ocular infection (bacterial, fungal, viral), intraocular pressure elevation, visual acuity and field defects, keratitis, mydriasis, stinging upon application, delayed wound healing

Miscellaneous: Systemic hypercorticoidism (rare) and taste perversion have also been reported

Overdosage/Toxicology When consumed in high doses over prolonged periods, systemic hypercorticism and adrenal suppression may occur; in those cases, discontinuation of the corticosteroid should be done judiciously.

Stability Store at room temperature

Mechanism of Action Decreases inflammation by suppression of migration of polymorpho-nuclear leukocytes and reversal of increased capillary permeability

Pharmacodynamics/Kinetics Absorption: Into aqueous humor with slight systemic absorption

Usual Dosage Children >2 years and Adults: Ophthalmic: Re-evaluate therapy if improvement is not seen within 2 days; use care not to discontinue prematurely; in chronic conditions, gradually decrease dosing frequency prior to discontinuing treatment

Ointment: Apply small amount (~1/2 inch ribbon) to conjunctival sac every 4 hours in severe cases; 1-3 times/day in mild to moderate cases

Solution: Instill 1-2 drops into conjunctival sac every hour during day, every 2 hours at night until favorable response is obtained, then use 1 drop every 4 hours; for mild to moderate inflammation, instill 1-2 drops into conjunctival sac 2-4 times/day

(Continued)

Fluorometholone *(Continued)*

Monitoring Parameters Intraocular pressure in patients with glaucoma or when used for ≥10 days; presence of secondary infections (including the development of fungal infections and exacerbation of viral infections)

Nursing Implications Use a separate container for each patient. Store suspension upright, shake well before using.

Dosage Forms

Ointment, ophthalmic (FML®): 0.1% (3.5 g)

Suspension, ophthalmic:

Flarex®: 0.1% (2.5 mL, 5 mL, 10 mL)

Fluor-Op®: 0.1% (5 mL, 10 mL, 15 mL)

FML®: 0.1% (1 mL, 5 mL, 10 mL, 15 mL)

FML® Forte: 0.25% (2 mL, 5 mL, 10 mL, 15 mL)

♦ **Fluorometholone and Sulfacetamide** *see* Sulfacetamide Sodium and Fluorometholone *on page 1269*

♦ **Fluor-Op®** *see* Fluorometholone *on page 575*

♦ **Fluoroplex®** *see* Fluorouracil *on page 576*

Fluorouracil *(flure oh YOOR a sil)*

U.S. Brand Names Adrucil®; Carac™; Efudex®; Fluoroplex®

Canadian Brand Names Adrucil®; Efudex®

Synonyms 5-Fluorouracil; 5-FU

Therapeutic Category Antineoplastic Agent, Antimetabolite (Pyrimidine)

Use Treatment of carcinomas of the breast, colon, head and neck, pancreas, rectum, or stomach; topically for the management of actinic or solar keratoses and superficial basal cell carcinomas

Pregnancy Risk Factor D (injection); X (topical)

Pregnancy/Breast-Feeding Implications There are no adequate and well-controlled studies in pregnant women, however, fetal defects and miscarriages have been reported following use of topical and intravenous products. Use is contraindicated during pregnancy. It is not known if fluorouracil is excreted in human milk, however, use during breast-feeding is not recommended.

Contraindications Hypersensitivity to fluorouracil or any component of the formulation; poor nutritional status; depressed bone marrow function; thrombocytopenia; potentially serious infections; major surgery within the previous month; dihydropyrimidine dehydrogenase (DPD) enzyme deficiency; pregnancy

Warnings/Precautions The U.S. Food and Drug Administration (FDA) currently recommends that procedures for proper handling and disposal of antineoplastic agents be considered. Use with caution in patients with impaired kidney or liver function. The drug should be discontinued if intractable vomiting or diarrhea, precipitous falls in leukocyte or platelet counts, stomatitis, hemorrhage, or myocardial ischemia occurs. Use with caution in patients who have had high-dose pelvic radiation or previous use of alkylating agents. Palmar-plantar erythrodysesthesia (hand-foot) syndrome has been associated with use. Patient should be hospitalized during initial course of therapy. Safety and efficacy have not been established in pediatric patients.

Adverse Reactions Toxicity depends on route and duration of infusion

>10%:

Dermatologic: Dermatitis, pruritic maculopapular rash, alopecia

Gastrointestinal (route and schedule dependent): Heartburn, nausea, vomiting, anorexia, stomatitis, esophagitis, anorexia, stomatitis, and diarrhea

Emetic potential:

<1000 mg: Moderately low (10% to 30%)

≥1000 mg: Moderate (30% to 60%)

Hematologic: Leukopenia; Myelosuppressive (tends to be more pronounced in patients receiving bolus dosing of 5-FU):

WBC: Moderate

Platelets: Mild to moderate

Onset (days): 7-10

Nadir (days): 14

Recovery (days): 21

Local: **Irritant chemotherapy**

1% to 10%:

Dermatologic: Dry skin

Gastrointestinal: GI ulceration

<1% (Limited to important or life-threatening): Cardiac enzyme abnormalities, chest pain, coagulopathy, dyspnea, EKG changes similar to ischemic changes, hepatotoxicity; hyperpigmentation of nailbeds, face, hands, and veins used in infusion; hypotension, palmarplantar syndrome (hand-foot syndrome), photosensitization

Cerebellar ataxia, headache, somnolence, ataxia are seen primarily in intracarotid arterial infusions for head and neck tumors.

Overdosage/Toxicology Symptoms include myelosuppression, nausea, vomiting, diarrhea, and alopecia. No specific antidote exists. Monitor hematologically for at least 4 weeks. Treatment is supportive.

Drug Interactions

Increased Effect/Toxicity: Leucovorin increases the folate pool and, in certain tumors, may promote TS inhibition and increase 5-FU activity. Leucovorin must be given before or with the 5-FU to prime the cells; it is not used as a rescue agent in this case. Allopurinol inhibits thymidine phosphorylase (an enzyme that activates 5-FU). The antitumor effect of 5-FU appears to be unaltered, but the toxicity is increased. Cimetidine results in increased plasma levels of 5-FU due to drug metabolism inhibition and reduction of liver blood flow induced by cimetidine.

Decreased Effect: Methotrexate: This interaction is schedule dependent; **5-FU should be given following MTX, not prior to.** If 5-FU is given first: 5-FU inhibits the TS binding and thus the reduced folate pool is not depleted, thereby negating the effect of MTX.

Ethanol/Nutrition/Herb Interactions
Ethanol: Avoid ethanol (due to GI irritation).
Herb/Nutraceutical: Avoid black cohosh, dong quai in estrogen-dependent tumors.

Stability
Injection: Store intact vials at room temperature and protect from light; slight discoloration does not usually denote decomposition
Topical: Store at controlled room temperature

Mechanism of Action A pyrimidine antimetabolite that interferes with DNA synthesis by blocking the methylation of deoxyuridylic acid; 5-FU rapidly enters the cell and is activated to the nucleotide level; there it inhibits thymidylate synthetase (TS), or is incorporated into RNA (most evident during the GI phase of the cell cycle). The reduced folate cofactor is required for tight binding to occur between the 5-FdUMP and TS.

Pharmacodynamics/Kinetics
Duration: ~3 weeks
Distribution: V_d: ~22% of total body water; penetrates extracellular fluid, CSF, and third space fluids (eg, pleural effusions and ascitic fluid)
Metabolism: Hepatic; 5-FU must be metabolized to be active. 90% metabolized; hepatically accomplished by a dehydrogenase enzyme; dose may need to be omitted in patients with liver failure (bilirubin >5 mg/dL)
Bioavailability: <75%, erratic and undependable
Half-life elimination: Biphasic: Initial: 6-20 minutes; doses of 400-600 mg/m^2 produce drug concentrations above the threshold for cytotoxicity for normal tissue and remain there for 6 hours; two metabolites, FdUMP and FUTP, have prolonged half-lives depending on the type of tissue; the clinical effect of these metabolites has not been determined
Excretion: Lung (large amounts as CO_2); urine (5% as unchanged drug) in 6 hours

Usual Dosage Adults:
Carcinoma of the breast, colon, pancreas, rectum, and stomach: Refer to individual protocols: All dosages are based on the patient's actual weight. However, the estimated lean body mass (dry weight) is used if the patient is obese or if there has been a spurious weight gain due to edema, ascites, or other forms of abnormal fluid retention.
I.V.: Manufacturers suggested dosing:
Initial sequence: 12 mg/kg once daily on days 1-4 (maximum daily dose: 800 mg); no treatment is given on day 5; if no toxicity is observed, administer 6 mg/kg on days 6, 8, 10, and 12; no treatment is given on days 7, 9, or 11
Poor risk patients/patients with poor nutritional status: 6 mg/kg once daily on days 1-3 (maximum dose: 400 mg); no therapy is given on day 4; if no toxicity is observed, administer 3 mg/kg on days 5, 7, and 9; no treatment is given on days 6 or 8
Maintenance: Repeat initial sequence every 30 days after last day of previous treatment **or** 10-15 mg/kg/week as a single dose (maximum 1 g/week, begin when toxic signs from initial course of treatment have subsided); further duration of treatment and dosage are dependent upon patient response; treatment has ranged from 9-45 courses over 12-60 months
Examples of other dosing regimens include:
Intermittent bolus dose in combination with other agents: 600 mg/m^2 every 3-4 weeks
Continuous infusion in combination with other agents: 1000 mg/m^2/day for 4-5 days every 3-4 weeks
Bolus dose in combination with leucovorin: 425 mg/m^2/day for 5 days every 4 weeks
Continuous protracted infusion: 200-300 mg/m^2/day

Actinic keratoses: Topical:
Carac™: Apply thin film to lesions once daily for up to 4 weeks, as tolerated
Efudex®: Apply cream or solution to lesions twice daily for 2-4 weeks; complete healing may not be evident for 1-2 months following treatment
Fluoroplex®: Apply to lesions twice daily for 2-6 weeks
Basal cell carcinoma: Topical: Efudex®: Apply 5% cream or solution to affected lesions twice daily for 3-6 weeks; treatment may be continued for up to 10-12 weeks

Dietary Considerations Increase dietary intake of thiamine.

Administration
I.V.: Preparation of fluorouracil should be performed in a Class II laminar flow biologic safety cabinet. Personnel should be wearing surgical gloves and a closed front surgical gown with knit cuffs. Appropriate safety equipment is recommended for preparation, administration, and disposal of antineoplastics. If fluorouracil comes in contact with skin, wash and flush thoroughly with water.
Topical: Apply 10 minutes after washing, rinsing, and drying the affected area. Apply using fingertip (wash hands immediately after application) or nonmetal applicator. Avoid eyes, nostrils, and mouth. Do not cover area with an occlusive dressing.

Monitoring Parameters CBC with differential and platelet count, renal function tests, liver function tests

Patient Information Avoid alcohol and all OTC drugs unless approved by your prescriber. Maintain adequate hydration (2-3 L/day of fluids unless instructed to restrict fluid intake) and nutrition (small frequent meals may help). You may experience sensitivity to sunlight (use sunblock, wear protective clothing, or avoid direct sunlight); susceptibility to infection (avoid crowds or infected persons or persons with contagious diseases); nausea, vomiting, diarrhea, or loss of appetite (frequent small meals may help - request medication); weakness, lethargy, dizziness, decreased vision (use caution when driving or engaging in tasks requiring alertness until response to drug is known); headache (request medication). Report signs and symptoms of infection (eg, fever, chills, sore throat, burning urination, vaginal itching or discharge, fatigue, mouth sores); bleeding (eg, black or tarry stools, easy bruising, unusual bleeding); vision changes; unremitting nausea, vomiting, or abdominal pain; CNS changes; respiratory difficulty; chest pain or palpitations; severe skin reactions to topical application; or any other adverse reactions. Contraceptive measures are recommended during therapy. The (Continued)

Fluorouracil *(Continued)*

drug may be excreted in breast milk, therefore, an alternative form of feeding your baby should be used.

Topical: Use as directed; do not overuse. Wash hands thoroughly before and after applying medication; avoid contact with eyes and mouth; avoid occlusive dressings; use a porous dressing. May cause local reaction (pain, burning, or swelling); if severe, contact prescriber.

Nursing Implications Cool to body temperature before using; after vial has been entered, any unused portion should be discarded within 1 hour; wash hands immediately after topical application of the 5% cream

Dosage Forms
Cream, topical:
Carac™: 0.5% (30 g)
Efudex®: 5% (25 g)
Fluoroplex®: 1% (30 g)
Injection (Adrucil®): 50 mg/mL (10 mL, 20 mL, 50 mL, 100 mL)
Solution, topical:
Efudex®: 2% (10 mL); 5% (10 mL)
Fluoroplex®: 1% (30 mL)

- ◆ **5-Fluorouracil** *see Fluorouracil on page 576*
- ◆ **Fluostigmin** *see Isoflurophate on page 747*
- ◆ **Fluotic® (Can)** *see Fluoride on page 574*

Fluoxetine *(floo OKS e teen)*

Related Information
Antidepressant Agents Comparison *on page 1482*
Selective Serotonin Reuptake Inhibitor (SSRIs) Pharmacokinetics *on page 1514*

U.S. Brand Names Prozac®; Prozac® Weekly™; Sarafem™

Canadian Brand Names Alti-Fluoxetine; Apo®-Fluoxetine; Gen-Fluoxetine; Novo-Fluoxetine; Nu-Fluoxetine; PMS-Fluoxetine; Prozac®; Rhoxal-fluoxetine; Scheinpharm™ Fluoxetine

Synonyms Fluoxetine Hydrochloride

Therapeutic Category Antidepressant, Serotonin Reuptake Inhibitor

Use Treatment of major depression; geriatric depression; treatment of binge-eating and vomiting in patients with moderate-to-severe bulimia nervosa; obsessive-compulsive disorder (OCD); premenstrual dysphoric disorder (PMDD)

Unlabeled/Investigational Use Selective mutism

Pregnancy Risk Factor C

Pregnancy/Breast-Feeding Implications Fluoxetine crosses the placenta

Contraindications Hypersensitivity to fluoxetine or any component of the formulation; patients receiving MAO inhibitors, thioridazine, or mesoridazine currently or within prior 14 days; an MAO inhibitor, thioridazine, or mesoridazine should not be initiated until 5 weeks after the discontinuation of fluoxetine

Warnings/Precautions Potential for severe reaction when used with MAO inhibitors - serotonin syndrome (hyperthermia, muscular rigidity, mental status changes/agitation, autonomic instability) may occur. Fluoxetine may elevate plasma levels of thioridazine and increase the risk of QT_c interval prolongation. This may lead to serious ventricular arrhythmias such as torsade de pointe-type arrhythmias and sudden death.

Fluoxetine use has been associated with occurrences of significant rash and allergic events, including vasculitis, lupus-like syndrome, laryngospasm, anaphylactoid reactions, and pulmonary inflammatory disease.

May precipitate a shift to mania or hypomania in patients with bipolar disease. May cause insomnia, anxiety, nervousness, or anorexia. Use with caution in patients where weight loss is undesirable. May impair cognitive or motor performance; caution operating hazardous machinery or driving. Use caution in patients with depression, particularly if suicidal risk may be present. Use caution in patients with a previous seizure disorder or condition predisposing to seizures such as brain damage, alcoholism, or concurrent therapy with other drugs which lower the seizure threshold. Use caution in patients with suicidal risk.

Use with caution in patients with hepatic or renal dysfunction and in elderly patients. May cause hyponatremia/SIADH. May increase the risks associated with electroconvulsive treatment. Use with caution in patients at risk of bleeding or receiving concurrent anticoagulant therapy; may cause impairment in platelet function. May alter glycemic control in patients with diabetes. Due to the long half-life of fluoxetine and its metabolites, the effects and interactions noted may persist for prolonged periods following discontinuation. May cause or exacerbate sexual dysfunction.

Adverse Reactions Predominant adverse effects are CNS and GI
>10%:
Central nervous system: Headache, nervousness (7% to 14%), insomnia (9% to 24%), anxiety, drowsiness
Gastrointestinal: Nausea, diarrhea, xerostomia, anorexia
Neuromuscular & skeletal: Weakness, tremor
1% to 10%:
Cardiovascular: Vasodilation, palpitation, hypertension
Central nervous system: Amnesia, confusion, emotional lability, sleep disorder, dizziness, agitation, yawning, pain, fever, abnormal dreams
Dermatologic: Rash, pruritus
Systemic events, possibly related to vasculitis (including lupus-like syndrome), have occurred rarely in patients with rash; may include lung, kidney, and/or hepatic involvement. Death has been reported.
Endocrine & metabolic: SIADH, hypoglycemia, hyponatremia (elderly or volume-depleted patients)
Gastrointestinal: Dyspepsia, increased appetite, constipation, vomiting, flatulence, weight gain/loss, abdominal pain, dyspepsia

Genitourinary: Sexual dysfunction, urinary frequency

Ocular: Abnormal vision

Respiratory: Pharyngitis

Miscellaneous: Diaphoresis, fever, flu syndrome, infection, abnormal thinking

<1% (Limited to important or life-threatening): Allergies, alopecia, anaphylactoid reactions, angina, arrhythmia, asthma, cataract, CHF, cholelithiasis, cholestatic jaundice, colitis, dyskinesia, dysphagia, eosinophilic pneumonia, erythema nodosum, esophagitis, euphoria, exfoliative dermatitis, extrapyramidal symptoms (rare), gout, hallucinations, heart arrest, hepatic failure/necrosis, hemorrhage, hyperprolactinemia, immune-related hemolytic anemia, laryngospasm, lupus-like syndrome, myocardial infarction, neuroleptic malignant syndrome (NMS), optic neuritis, pancreatitis, pancytopenia, photosensitivity reaction, postural hypotension, priapism, pulmonary embolism, pulmonary hypertension, QT prolongation, renal failure, serotonin syndrome, Stevens-Johnson syndrome, syncope, thrombocytopenia, thrombocytopenic purpura, vasculitis, ventricular tachycardia (including torsade de pointes), vomiting

Overdosage/Toxicology Symptoms include ataxia, sedation, coma, and EKG abnormalities (QT prolongation, torsade de pointes). Respiratory depression may occur, especially with coingestion of alcohol or other drugs. Seizures rarely occur. Treatment is supportive.

Drug Interactions

Cytochrome P450 Effect: CYP2D6 (minor) and CYP3A3/4 enzyme substrate; CYP2C9 enzyme inducer; CYP1A2 (high dose), 2C9, 2C19, 2D6, and 3A3/4 enzyme inhibitor

Increased Effect/Toxicity:

MAO inhibitors: Fluoxetine should not be used with nonselective MAO inhibitors (phenelzine, isocarboxazid) or other drugs with MAO inhibition (linezolid); fatal reactions have been reported. Wait 5 weeks after stopping fluoxetine before starting a nonselective MAO inhibitor and 2 weeks after stopping an MAO inhibitor before starting fluoxetine. Concurrent selegiline has been associated with mania, hypertension, or serotonin syndrome (risk may be reduced relative to nonselective MAO inhibitors).

Phenothiazines: Fluoxetine may inhibit the metabolism of thioridazine or mesoridazine, resulting in increased plasma levels and increasing the risk of QT_c interval prolongation. This may lead to serious ventricular arrhythmias, such as torsade de pointes-type arrhythmias and sudden death. Do not use together. Wait at least 5 weeks after discontinuing fluoxetine prior to starting thioridazine.

Combined used of SSRIs and amphetamines, buspirone, meperidine, nefazodone, serotonin agonists (such as sumatriptan), sibutramine, other SSRIs, sympathomimetics, ritonavir, tramadol, and venlafaxine may increase the risk of serotonin syndrome. Fluoxetine may increase serum levels/effects of benzodiazepines (alprazolam and diazepam), beta-blockers (except atenolol or nadolol), carbamazepine, carvedilol, clozapine, cyclosporine (and possibly tacrolimus), dextromethorphan, digoxin, haloperidol, HMG-CoA reductase inhibitors (lovastatin and simvastatin - increasing the risk of rhabdomyolysis), phenytoin, propafenone, trazodone, tricyclic antidepressants, and valproic acid. Concurrent lithium may increase risk of nephrotoxicity. Risk of hyponatremia may increase with concurrent use of loop diuretics (bumetanide, furosemide, torsemide). Fluoxetine may increase the hypoprothrombinemic response to warfarin.

Combined use of sumatriptan (and other serotonin agonists) may result in toxicity; weakness, hyper-reflexia, and incoordination have been observed with sumatriptan and SSRIs. In addition, concurrent use may theoretically increase the risk of serotonin syndrome; includes sumatriptan, naratriptan, rizatriptan, and zolmitriptan.

Decreased Effect: Cyproheptadine may inhibit the effects of serotonin reuptake inhibitors.

Ethanol/Nutrition/Herb Interactions

Ethanol: Avoid ethanol (may increase CNS depression). Depressed patients should avoid/limit intake.

Herb/Nutraceutical: Avoid valerian, St John's wort, kava kava, gotu kola (may increase CNS depression).

Stability All dosage forms should be stored at controlled room temperature of 15°C to 30°C (50°F to 86°F); oral liquid should be dispensed in a light-resistant container

Mechanism of Action Inhibits CNS neuron serotonin reuptake; minimal or no effect on reuptake of norepinephrine or dopamine; does not significantly bind to alpha-adrenergic, histamine, or cholinergic receptors

Pharmacodynamics/Kinetics

Absorption: Well absorbed; delayed 1-2 hours with weekly formulation

Protein binding: 95%

Metabolism: Hepatic, to norfluoxetine (active; equal to fluoxetine)

Half-life elimination: Parent drug: 2-3 days, Metabolite (norfluoxetine): 4-16 days; due to long half-life, resolution of adverse reactions after discontinuation may be slow

Time to peak: 4-8 hours

Excretion: Urine (2.5% to 5% as fluoxetine, 10% as norfluoxetine)

Note: Weekly formulation results in greater fluctuations between peak and trough concentrations of fluoxetine and norfluoxetine compared to once-daily dosing (24% daily/164% weekly; 17% daily/43% weekly, respectively). Trough concentrations are 76% lower for fluoxetine and 47% lower for norfluoxetine than the concentrations maintained by 20 mg once-daily dosing. Steady-state fluoxetine concentrations are ~50% lower following the once-weekly regimen compared to 20 mg once daily.

Usual Dosage Oral:

Children:

<5 years: No dosing information available

5-18 years: Initial: 5-10 mg/day; titrate upwards as needed (usual maximum dose: 60 mg/day)

Adults: 20 mg/day in the morning; may increase after several weeks by 20 mg/day increments; maximum: 80 mg/day; doses >20 mg should be divided into morning and noon doses. **Note:** Lower doses of 5-10 mg/day have been used for initial treatment.

Usual dosage range:

Bulimia nervosa: 60-80 mg/day

(Continued)

Fluoxetine *(Continued)*

Depression: 20-40 mg/day; patients maintained on Prozac® 20 mg/day may be changed to Prozac® Weekly™ 90 mg/week, starting dose 7 days after the last 20 mg/day dose
Obesity: 20-60 mg/day
OCD: 40-80 mg/day
PMDD (Sarafem™): 20 mg/day

Elderly: Depression: Some patients may require an initial dose of 10 mg/day with dosage increases of 10 and 20 mg every several weeks as tolerated; should not be taken at night unless patient experiences sedation

Dosing adjustment in renal impairment:
Single dose studies: Pharmacokinetics of fluoxetine and norfluoxetine were similar among subjects with all levels of impaired renal function, including anephric patients on chronic hemodialysis
Chronic administration: Additional accumulation of fluoxetine or norfluoxetine may occur in patients with severely impaired renal function
Hemodialysis: Not removed by hemodialysis

Dosing adjustment in hepatic impairment: Elimination half-life of fluoxetine is prolonged in patients with hepatic impairment; a lower or less frequent dose of fluoxetine should be used in these patients
Cirrhosis patients: Administer a lower dose or less frequent dosing interval
Compensated cirrhosis without ascites: Administer 50% of normal dose

Dietary Considerations May be taken with or without food.

Monitoring Parameters Signs and symptoms of depression, anxiety, sleep

Reference Range Therapeutic levels have not been well established
Therapeutic: Fluoxetine: 100-800 ng/mL (SI: 289-2314 nmol/L); Norfluoxetine: 100-600 ng/mL (SI: 289-1735 nmol/L)
Toxic: Fluoxetine plus norfluoxetine: >2000 ng/mL

Patient Information Avoid alcohol; take in morning to avoid insomnia; fluoxetine's potential stimulating and anorexic effects may be bothersome to some patients. Use sugarless hard candy for dry mouth; may cause drowsiness, improvement may take several weeks; rise slowly to prevent dizziness. If you miss a dose, take it as soon as you remember. However, if it is time for your next dose, skip the missed dose and take only your regularly scheduled dose. Do not take more than the daily amount that has been prescribed.

Nursing Implications Offer patient sugarless hard candy for dry mouth

Additional Information EKG may reveal S-T segment depression; not shown to be teratogenic in rodents; 15-60 mg/day, buspirone and cyproheptadine, may be useful in treatment of sexual dysfunction during treatment with a selective serotonin reuptake inhibitor.

Weekly capsules are a delayed release formulation containing enteric-coated pellets of fluoxetine hydrochloride, equivalent to 90 mg fluoxetine. Therapeutic equivalence of weekly formulation with daily formulation for delaying time to relapse has not been established.

Dosage Forms
Capsule, as hydrochloride:
Prozac®: 10 mg, 20 mg, 40 mg
Sarafem™: 10 mg, 20 mg
Capsule, sustained release, as hydrochloride (Prozac® Weekly™): 90 mg
Solution, oral, as hydrochloride (Prozac®): 20 mg/5 mL (120 mL) [contains 0.23% alcohol] [mint flavor]
Tablet, scored, as hydrochloride (Prozac®): 10 mg

Extemporaneous Preparations A 20 mg capsule may be mixed with 4 oz of water, apple juice, or Gatorade® to provide a solution that is stable for 14 days under refrigeration

♦ **Fluoxetine Hydrochloride** *see* Fluoxetine *on page 578*

Fluoxymesterone *(floo oks i MES te rone)*

U.S. Brand Names Halotestin®

Canadian Brand Names Halotestin®

Therapeutic Category Androgen

Use Replacement of endogenous testicular hormone; in females, used as palliative treatment of breast cancer

Unlabeled/Investigational Use Stimulation of erythropoiesis, angioneurotic edema

Restrictions C-III

Pregnancy Risk Factor X

Contraindications Hypersensitivity to fluoxymesterone or any component of the formulation; serious cardiac disease, liver or kidney disease; pregnancy

Warnings/Precautions May accelerate bone maturation without producing compensatory gain in linear growth in children; in prepubertal children perform radiographic examination of the hand and wrist every 6 months to determine the rate of bone maturation and to assess the effect of treatment on the epiphyseal centers

Adverse Reactions
>10%:
Male: Priapism
Female: Menstrual problems (amenorrhea), virilism, breast soreness
Cardiovascular: Edema
Dermatologic: Acne
1% to 10%:
Male: Prostatic carcinoma, hirsutism (increase in pubic hair growth), impotence, testicular atrophy
Cardiovascular: Edema
Gastrointestinal: GI irritation, nausea, vomiting
Genitourinary: Prostatic hyperplasia
Hepatic: Hepatic dysfunction
<1% (Limited to important or life-threatening): Cholestatic hepatitis, hepatic necrosis, leukopenia, polycythemia

Overdosage/Toxicology Symptoms include abnormal liver function tests and water retention.

Drug Interactions

Increased Effect/Toxicity: Fluoxymesterone may suppress clotting factors II, V, VII, and X; therefore, bleeding may occur in patients on anticoagulant therapy May elevate cyclosporine serum levels. May enhance hypoglycemic effect of insulin therapy; may decrease blood glucose concentrations and insulin requirements in patients with diabetes. Lithium may potentiate EPS and other CNS effect. May potentiate the effects of narcotics including respiratory depression

Decreased Effect: May decrease barbiturate levels and fluphenazine effectiveness.

Stability Protect from light

Mechanism of Action Synthetic androgenic anabolic hormone responsible for the normal growth and development of male sex hormones and development of male sex organs and maintenance of secondary sex characteristics; synthetic testosterone derivative with significant androgen activity; stimulates RNA polymerase activity resulting in an increase in protein production; increases bone development; halogenated derivative of testosterone with up to 5 times the activity of methyltestosterone

Pharmacodynamics/Kinetics

Absorption: Rapid

Protein binding: 98%

Metabolism: Hepatic; enterohepatic circulation

Half-life elimination: 10-100 minutes

Excretion: Urine (90%)

Usual Dosage Adults: Oral:

Male:

Hypogonadism: 5-20 mg/day

Delayed puberty: 2.5-20 mg/day for 4-6 months

Female: Inoperable breast carcinoma: 10-40 mg/day in divided doses for 1-3 months

Monitoring Parameters In prepubertal children, perform radiographic examination of the hand and wrist every 6 months

Test Interactions Decreased levels of thyroxine-binding globulin; decreased total T_4 serum levels; increased resin uptake of T_3 and T_4

Patient Information Take as directed; do not discontinue without consulting prescriber. Diabetics should monitor serum glucose closely and notify prescriber of changes; this medication can alter hypoglycemic requirements. You may experience acne, growth of body hair, loss of libido, impotence, or menstrual irregularity (usually reversible); nausea or vomiting (small frequent meals, frequent mouth care, sucking lozenges, or chewing gum may help). Report changes in menstrual pattern; deepening of voice or unusual growth of body hair; fluid retention (swelling of ankles, feet, or hands, difficulty breathing, or sudden weight gain); change in color of urine or stool; yellowing of eyes or skin; unusual bruising or bleeding; or other adverse reactions.

Nursing Implications In prepubertal children, perform radiographic examination of the hand and wrist every 6 months

Dosage Forms Tablet: 2 mg, 5 mg, 10 mg

Fluphenazine (floo FEN a zeen)

Related Information

Antacid Drug Interactions on page 1477

Antipsychotic Agents Comparison on page 1486

U.S. Brand Names Permitil®; Prolixin®; Prolixin Decanoate®; Prolixin Enanthate®

Canadian Brand Names Apo®-Fluphenazine; Modecate®; Moditen® Enanthate; Moditen® HCl; PMS-Fluphenazine Decanoate; Rho®-Fluphenazine Decanoate

Synonyms Fluphenazine Decanoate; Fluphenazine Enanthate; Fluphenazine Hydrochloride

Therapeutic Category Antipsychotic Agent, Phenothiazine; Phenothiazine Derivative

Use Management of manifestations of psychotic disorders and schizophrenia; depot formulation may offer improved outcome in individuals with psychosis who are nonadherent with oral antipsychotics

Unlabeled/Investigational Use Pervasive developmental disorder

Pregnancy Risk Factor C

Contraindications Hypersensitivity to fluphenazine or any component of the formulation (cross-reactivity between phenothiazines may occur); severe CNS depression; coma; subcortical brain damage; blood dyscrasias; hepatic disease

Warnings/Precautions Safety in children <6 months of age has not been established. May be sedating, use with caution in disorders where CNS depression is a feature. Use with caution in Parkinson's disease. Caution in patients with hemodynamic instability; bone marrow suppression; predisposition to seizures; severe cardiac, renal, or respiratory disease. Esophageal dysmotility and aspiration have been associated with antipsychotic use - use with caution in patients at risk of pneumonia (ie, Alzheimer's disease). Caution in breast cancer or other prolactin-dependent tumors (may elevate prolactin levels). May alter temperature regulation or mask toxicity of other drugs due to antiemetic effects. May alter cardiac conduction; life-threatening arrhythmias have occurred with therapeutic doses of phenothiazines. Hypotension may occur, particularly with I.M. administration. May cause orthostatic hypotension - use with caution in patients at risk of this effect or those who would tolerate transient hypotensive episodes (cerebrovascular disease, cardiovascular disease, or other medications which may predispose). Adverse effects of depot injections may be prolonged.

Phenothiazines may cause anticholinergic effects (confusion, agitation, constipation, dry mouth, blurred vision, urinary retention). Therefore, they should be used with caution in patients with decreased gastrointestinal motility, urinary retention, BPH, xerostomia, or visual problems. Conditions which also may be exacerbated by cholinergic blockade include narrow-angle glaucoma (screening is recommended) and worsening of myasthenia gravis. Relative to other antipsychotics, fluphenazine has a low potency of cholinergic blockade. (Continued)

Fluphenazine *(Continued)*

May cause extrapyramidal reactions, including pseudoparkinsonism, acute dystonic reactions, akathisia and tardive dyskinesia (risk of these reactions is high relative to other antipsychotics). May be associated with neuroleptic malignant syndrome (NMS) or pigmentary retinopathy.

Adverse Reactions Frequency not defined.

Cardiovascular: Hypotension, tachycardia, fluctuations in blood pressure, hypertension, arrhythmias, edema

Central nervous system: Parkinsonian symptoms, akathisia, dystonias, tardive dyskinesia, dizziness, hyper-reflexia, headache, cerebral edema, drowsiness, lethargy, restlessness, excitement, bizarre dreams, EEG changes, depression, seizures, NMS, altered central temperature regulation

Dermatologic: Increased sensitivity to sun, rash, skin pigmentation, itching, erythema, urticaria, seborrhea, eczema, dermatitis

Endocrine & metabolic: Changes in menstrual cycle, breast pain, amenorrhea, galactorrhea, gynecomastia, changes in libido, elevated prolactin, SIADH

Gastrointestinal: Weight gain, loss of appetite, salivation, xerostomia, constipation, paralytic ileus, laryngeal edema

Genitourinary: Ejaculatory disturbances, impotence, polyuria, bladder paralysis, enuresis

Hematologic: Agranulocytosis, leukopenia, thrombocytopenia, nonthrombocytopenic purpura, eosinophilia, pancytopenia

Hepatic: Cholestatic jaundice, hepatotoxicity

Neuromuscular & skeletal: Trembling of fingers, SLE, facial hemispasm

Ocular: Pigmentary retinopathy, cornea and lens changes, blurred vision, glaucoma

Respiratory: Nasal congestion, asthma

Overdosage/Toxicology Symptoms include deep sleep, hypotension, hypertension, dystonia, seizures, extrapyramidal symptoms, and respiratory failure. Following initiation of essential overdose management, toxic symptom and supportive treatment should be initiated. Hypotension usually responds to I.V. fluids or Trendelenburg positioning. If unresponsive to these measures, the use of a parenteral inotrope may be required. Seizures commonly respond to diazepam (I.V. 5-10 mg bolus in adults every 15 minutes, if needed, up to a total of 30 mg; I.V. 0.25-0.4 mg/kg/dose up to a total of 10 mg in children) or to phenytoin or phenobarbital. Cardiac arrhythmias often respond to I.V. lidocaine while other antiarrhythmics can be used. Neuroleptics often cause extrapyramidal symptoms (eg, dystonic reactions) requiring management with anticholinergic agents such as benztropine mesylate I.V. 1-2 mg (adults) may be effective. These agents are generally effective within 2-5 minutes.

Drug Interactions

Cytochrome P450 Effect: CYP2D6 enzyme substrate; CYP2D6 enzyme inhibitor

Increased Effect/Toxicity: Effects on CNS depression may be additive when fluphenazine is combined with CNS depressants (narcotic analgesics, ethanol, barbiturates, cyclic antidepressants, antihistamines, sedative-hypnotics). Fluphenazine may increase the effects/toxicity of anticholinergics, antihypertensives, lithium (rare neurotoxicity), trazodone, or valproic acid. Concurrent use with TCA may produce increased toxicity or altered therapeutic response. Chloroquine and propranolol may increase chlorpromazine concentrations. Hypotension may occur when fluphenazine is combined with epinephrine. May increase the risk of arrhythmia when combined with antiarrhythmics, cisapride, pimozide, sparfloxacin, or other drugs which prolong QT interval.

Decreased Effect: Phenothiazines inhibit the activity of guanethidine, guanadrel, levodopa, and bromocriptine. Barbiturates and cigarette smoking may enhance the hepatic metabolism of fluphenazine. Fluphenazine and possibly other low potency antipsychotics may reverse the pressor effects of epinephrine.

Ethanol/Nutrition/Herb Interactions

Ethanol: Avoid ethanol (may increase CNS depression).

Herb/Nutraceutical: Avoid dong quai, St John's wort (may also cause photosensitization). Avoid kava kava, gotu kola, valerian, St John's wort (may increase CNS depression).

Stability Avoid freezing; protect all dosage forms from light; clear or slightly yellow solutions may be used; should be dispensed in amber or opaque vials/bottles. Solutions may be diluted or mixed with fruit juices or other liquids but must be administered immediately after mixing; do not prepare bulk dilutions or store bulk dilutions.

Mechanism of Action Blocks postsynaptic mesolimbic dopaminergic D_1 and D_2 receptors in the brain; depresses the release of hypothalamic and hypophyseal hormones; believed to depress the reticular activating system thus affecting basal metabolism, body temperature, wakefulness, vasomotor tone, and emesis

Pharmacodynamics/Kinetics

Onset of action: I.M., S.C. (derivative dependent): Hydrochloride salt: ~1 hour

Peak effect: Neuroleptic: Decanoate: 48-96 hours

Duration: Hydrochloride salt: 6-8 hours; Decanoate (lasts the longest): 24-72 hours

Distribution: Crosses placenta; enters breast milk

Metabolism: Hepatic

Half-life elimination (derivative dependent): Enanthate: 84-96 hours; Hydrochloride: 33 hours; Decanoate: 163-232 hours

Usual Dosage

Children: Oral: Childhood-onset pervasive developmental disorder (unlabeled use): 0.04 mg/kg/day

Adults: Psychoses:

Oral: 0.5-10 mg/day in divided doses at 6- to 8-hour intervals; some patients may require up to 40 mg/day

I.M.: 2.5-10 mg/day in divided doses at 6- to 8-hour intervals (parenteral dose is ⅓ to ½ the oral dose for the hydrochloride salts)

I.M. (decanoate): 12.5 mg every 2 weeks

Conversion from hydrochloride to decanoate I.M. 0.5 mL (12.5 mg) decanoate every 3 weeks is approximately equivalent to 10 mg hydrochloride/day

I.M. (enanthate): 12.5-25 mg every 2 weeks

Hemodialysis: Not dialyzable (0% to 5%)

Administration Avoid contact of oral solution or injection with skin (contact dermatitis). Oral liquid should be diluted in the following **only**: water, saline, 7-UP®, homogenized milk, carbonated orange beverages, pineapple, apricot, prune, orange, V8® juice, tomato, and grapefruit juices. Do **not** dilute in beverages containing caffeine, tannics, or pectinate. Watch for hypotension when administering I.M.

Monitoring Parameters EKG monitoring for 48 hours

Reference Range Therapeutic: 5-20 ng/mL; correlation of serum concentrations and efficacy is controversial; most often dosed to best response

Patient Information Avoid alcohol; may cause drowsiness; do not discontinue without consulting physician

Nursing Implications Avoid contact of oral solution or injection with skin (contact dermatitis); watch for hypotension when administering I.M. or I.V.; oral liquid to be diluted in the following **only**: water, saline, 7-UP®, homogenized milk, carbonated orange beverages, pineapple, apricot, prune, orange, V8® juice, tomato, and grapefruit juices

Additional Information Less sedative and hypotensive effects than chlorpromazine

Dosage Forms

Elixir, as hydrochloride (Prolixin®): 2.5 mg/5 mL with alcohol 14% (60 mL, 473 mL)

Injection, as decanoate (Prolixin Decanoate®): 25 mg/mL (1 mL, 5 mL)

Injection, as enanthate (Prolixin Enanthate®): 25 mg/mL (5 mL)

Injection, as hydrochloride (Prolixin®): 2.5 mg/mL (10 mL)

Solution, oral concentrate, as hydrochloride:

Permitil®: 5 mg/mL with alcohol 1% (118 mL)

Prolixin®: 5 mg/mL with alcohol 14% (120 mL)

Tablet, as hydrochloride:

Permitil®: 2.5 mg, 5 mg, 10 mg

Prolixin®: 1 mg, 2.5 mg, 5 mg, 10 mg

- ♦ **Fluphenazine Decanoate** see Fluphenazine on page 581
- ♦ **Fluphenazine Enanthate** see Fluphenazine on page 581
- ♦ **Fluphenazine Hydrochloride** see Fluphenazine on page 581
- ♦ **Flura-Drops®** see Fluoride on page 574
- ♦ **Flura-Loz®** see Fluoride on page 574

Flurandrenolide (flure an DREN oh lide)

Related Information

Corticosteroids Comparison on page 1495

U.S. Brand Names Cordran®; Cordran® SP

Canadian Brand Names Cordran®

Synonyms Flurandrenolone

Therapeutic Category Anti-inflammatory Agent; Corticosteroid, Topical (Low Potency); Corticosteroid, Topical (Medium Potency)

Use Inflammation of corticosteroid-responsive dermatoses [medium potency topical corticosteroid]

Pregnancy Risk Factor C

Contraindications Hypersensitivity to flurandrenolide or any component of the formulation; viral, fungal, or tubercular skin lesions

Warnings/Precautions Adverse systemic effects may occur when used on large areas of the body, denuded areas, for prolonged periods of time, with an occlusive dressing, and/or in infants or small children

Adverse Reactions Frequency not defined.

Cardiovascular: Intracranial hypertension

Dermatologic: Itching, dry skin, folliculitis, hypertrichosis, acneiform eruptions, hyperpigmentation, perioral dermatitis, allergic contact dermatitis, skin atrophy, striae, miliaria, acne, maceration of the skin

Endocrine & metabolic: Cushing's syndrome, growth retardation, HPA suppression

Local: Burning, irritation

Miscellaneous: Secondary infection

Overdosage/Toxicology When consumed in excessive quantities, systemic hypercorticism and adrenal suppression may occur; in those cases, discontinuation and withdrawal of the corticosteroid should be done judiciously.

Mechanism of Action Decreases inflammation by suppression of migration of polymorphonuclear leukocytes and reversal of increased capillary permeability

Pharmacodynamics/Kinetics

Absorption: Adequate with intact skin; repeated applications lead to depot effects on skin, potentially resulting in enhanced percutaneous absorption

Metabolism: Hepatic

Excretion: Urine; feces (small amounts)

Usual Dosage Topical: Therapy should be discontinued when control is achieved; if no improvement is seen, reassessment of diagnosis may be necessary.

Children:

Ointment, cream: Apply sparingly 1-2 times/day

Tape: Apply once daily

Adults: Cream, lotion, ointment: Apply sparingly 2-3 times/day

Nursing Implications A thin film is effective; do not overuse; do not use tight-fitting diapers or plastic pants on children being treated in the diaper area; use only as prescribed, and for no longer than the period prescribed; apply sparingly in light film; rub in lightly; avoid contact with eyes; notify physician if condition being treated persists or worsens

Dosage Forms

Cream, emulsified, topical, as base (Cordran® SP): 0.025% (30 g, 60 g); 0.05% (15 g, 30 g, 60 g)

Lotion (Cordran®): 0.05% (15 mL, 60 mL)

Ointment, topical (Cordran®): 0.025% (30 g, 60 g); 0.05% (15 g, 30 g, 60 g)

Tape, topical (Cordran®): 4 mcg/cm^2 (7.5 cm x 60 cm, 7.5 cm x 200 cm rolls)

♦ **Flurandrenolone** *see Flurandrenolide on page 583*

Flurazepam (flure AZ e pam)

Related Information
Antacid Drug Interactions *on page 1477*
Benzodiazepines Comparison *on page 1490*

U.S. Brand Names Dalmane®

Canadian Brand Names Apo®-Flurazepam; Dalmane®; Somnol®

Synonyms Flurazepam Hydrochloride

Therapeutic Category Benzodiazepine; Hypnotic; Sedative

Use Short-term treatment of insomnia

Restrictions C-IV

Pregnancy Risk Factor X

Contraindications Hypersensitivity to flurazepam or any component of the formulation (cross-sensitivity with other benzodiazepines may exist); narrow-angle glaucoma; pregnancy

Warnings/Precautions Use with caution in patients receiving other CNS depressants, patients with low albumin, hepatic dysfunction, and in the elderly; do not use in pregnant women; may cause drug dependency; safety and efficacy have not been established in children <15 years of age

Adverse Reactions Frequency not defined.
Cardiovascular: Palpitations, chest pain
Central nervous system: Drowsiness, ataxia, lightheadedness, memory impairment, depression, headache, hangover effect, confusion, nervousness, dizziness, falling, apprehension, irritability, euphoria, slurred speech, restlessness, hallucinations, paradoxical reactions, talkativeness
Dermatologic: Rash, pruritus
Gastrointestinal: Xerostomia, constipation, increased/excessive salivation, heartburn, upset stomach, nausea, vomiting, diarrhea, increased or decreased appetite, bitter taste, weight gain/loss
Hematologic: Euphoria, granulocytopenia
Hepatic: Elevated SGOT/SGPT, total bilirubin, alkaline phosphatase; cholestatic jaundice
Neuromuscular & skeletal: Dysarthria, body/joint pain, reflex slowing, weakness
Ocular: Blurred vision, burning eyes, difficulty focusing
Otic: Tinnitus
Respiratory: Apnea, dyspnea
Miscellaneous: Diaphoresis, drug dependence

Overdosage/Toxicology Symptoms include respiratory depression, hypoactive reflexes, unsteady gait, and hypotension. Treatment for benzodiazepine overdose is supportive. Rarely is mechanical ventilation required. Flumazenil has been shown to selectively block the binding of benzodiazepines to CNS receptors, resulting in a reversal of benzodiazepine-induced CNS depression.

Drug Interactions
Cytochrome P450 Effect: CYP3A3/4 enzyme substrate
Increased Effect/Toxicity: Serum levels and response to flurazepam may be increased by amprenavir, cimetidine, ciprofloxacin, clarithromycin, clozapine, CNS depressants, diltiazem, disulfiram, digoxin, erythromycin, ethanol, fluconazole, fluoxetine, fluvoxamine, grapefruit juice, isoniazid, itraconazole, ketoconazole, labetalol, levodopa, loxapine, metoprolol, metronidazole, miconazole, nefazodone, nelfinavir, omeprazole, phenytoin, rifabutin, rifampin, ritonavir, troleandomycin, valproic acid, and verapamil.
Decreased Effect: Carbamazepine, rifampin, and rifabutin may enhance the metabolism of flurazepam and decrease its therapeutic effect; consider using an alternative sedative/hypnotic agent.

Ethanol/Nutrition/Herb Interactions
Ethanol: Avoid ethanol (may increase CNS depression).
Food: Serum levels and response to flurazepam may be increased by grapefruit juice, but unlikely because of flurazepam's high oral bioavailability.
Herb/Nutraceutical: Avoid valerian, St John's wort, kava kava, gotu kola (may increase CNS depression).

Stability Store in light-resistant containers

Mechanism of Action Binds to stereospecific benzodiazepine receptors on the postsynaptic GABA neuron at several sites within the central nervous system, including the limbic system, reticular formation. Enhancement of the inhibitory effect of GABA on neuronal excitability results by increased neuronal membrane permeability to chloride ions. This shift in chloride ions results in hyperpolarization (a less excitable state) and stabilization.

Pharmacodynamics/Kinetics
Onset of action: Hypnotic: 15-20 minutes
Peak effect: 3-6 hours
Duration: 7-8 hours
Metabolism: Hepatic to N-desalkylflurazepam (active)
Half-life elimination: Desalkylflurazepam:
Adults: Single dose: 74-90 hours; multiple dose: 111-113 hours
Elderly (61-85 years): Single dose: 120-160 hours; multiple dose: 126-158 hours

Usual Dosage Oral:
Children: Insomnia:
≤15 years: Dose not established
>15 years: 15 mg at bedtime
Adults: Insomnia: 15-30 mg at bedtime
Elderly: Insomnia: Oral: 15 mg at bedtime; avoid use if possible

Monitoring Parameters Respiratory and cardiovascular status

Reference Range Therapeutic: 0-4 ng/mL (SI: 0-9 nmol/L); Metabolite N-desalkylflurazepam: 20-110 ng/mL (SI: 43-240 nmol/L); Toxic: >0.12 µg/mL

Patient Information Avoid alcohol and other CNS depressants; avoid activities needing good psychomotor coordination until CNS effects are known; drug may cause physical or psychological dependence; avoid abrupt discontinuation after prolonged use

Nursing Implications Provide safety measures (ie, side rails, night light, and call button); remove smoking materials from area; supervise ambulation; avoid abrupt discontinuance in patients with prolonged therapy or seizure disorders

Dosage Forms Capsule, as hydrochloride: 15 mg, 30 mg

♦ **Flurazepam Hydrochloride** *see* Flurazepam *on page 584*

Flurbiprofen (flure BI proe fen)

Related Information
Nonsteroidal Anti-Inflammatory Agents Comparison *on page 1512*

U.S. Brand Names Ansaid® Oral; Ocufen® Ophthalmic

Canadian Brand Names Alti-Flurbiprofen; Ansaid®; Apo®-Flurbiprofen; Froben®; Froben-SR®; Novo-Flurprofen; Nu-Flurprofen; Ocufen™

Synonyms Flurbiprofen Sodium

Therapeutic Category Analgesic, Nonsteroidal Anti-inflammatory Drug; Anti-inflammatory Agent; Nonsteroidal Anti-inflammatory Drug (NSAID), Ophthalmic; Nonsteroidal Anti-inflammatory Drug (NSAID), Oral

Use
Oral: Acute or long-term treatment of signs and symptoms of rheumatoid arthritis and osteoarthritis
Ophthalmic: Inhibition of intraoperative miosis; prevention and management of postoperative ocular inflammation and postoperative cystoid macular edema remains to be determined

Pregnancy Risk Factor C/D (3rd trimester)

Contraindications Hypersensitivity to flurbiprofen or any component of the formulation; dendritic keratitis; pregnancy (3rd trimester)

Warnings/Precautions Use with caution in patients with congestive heart failure, hypertension, dehydration, decreased renal or hepatic function, history of GI disease (bleeding or ulcers), or those receiving anticoagulants. Elderly are at a high risk for adverse effects from nonsteroidal anti-inflammatory agents. As many as 60% of elderly can develop peptic ulceration and/or hemorrhage asymptomatically.

Use lowest effective dose for shortest period possible. Use of NSAIDs can compromise existing renal function especially when Cl_{cr} is <30 mL/minute. CNS adverse effects such as confusion, agitation, and hallucination are generally seen in overdose or high-dose situations; however, elderly may demonstrate these adverse effects at lower doses than younger adults. Withhold for at least 4-6 half-lives prior to surgical or dental procedures. Ophthalmic solution contains thimerosal.

Adverse Reactions
Ophthalmic:
>10%: Ocular: Slowing of corneal wound healing, mild ocular stinging, itching and burning eyes, ocular irritation
1% to 10%: Ocular: Eye redness
Systemic:
1% to 10%:
  Central nervous system: Headache, nervousness, dizziness
  Dermatologic: Itching, rash
  Endocrine & metabolic: Fluid retention
  Gastrointestinal: Abdominal cramps, heartburn, indigestion, nausea, vomiting
  Otic: Tinnitus
<1% (Limited to important or life-threatening): Acute renal failure, agranulocytosis, allergic reactions, angioedema, arrhythmias, aseptic meningitis, bone marrow suppression, CHF, dyspnea, erythema multiforme, GI ulceration, hallucinations, hemolytic anemia, hepatitis, hypertension, leukopenia, mental depression, peripheral neuropathy, Stevens-Johnson syndrome, thrombocytopenia, toxic amblyopia, toxic epidermal necrolysis, tachycardia, urticaria

Overdosage/Toxicology Symptoms include apnea, metabolic acidosis, coma, nystagmus, leukocytosis, and renal failure. Management of nonsteroidal anti-inflammatory drug (NSAID) intoxication is primarily supportive and symptomatic. Fluid therapy is commonly effective in managing hypotension that may occur following an acute NSAID overdose, except when due to acute blood loss. Seizures tend to be very short-lived and often do not require drug treatment, although recurrent seizures should be treated with I.V. diazepam. Since many of NSAIDs undergo enterohepatic cycling, multiple doses of charcoal may be needed to reduce the potential for delayed toxicities.

Drug Interactions
Cytochrome P450 Effect: CYP2C9 enzyme substrate; CYP2C9 enzyme inhibitor
Decreased Effect: Ophthalmic: When used with concurrent administration of flurbiprofen, acetylcholine chloride and carbachol have been shown to be ineffective. Reports of acetylcholine chloride and carbachol being ineffective when used with flurbiprofen.

Ethanol/Nutrition/Herb Interactions
Ethanol: Avoid ethanol (may enhance gastric mucosal irritation).
Food: Food may decrease the rate but not the extent of absorption.
Herb/Nutraceutical: Avoid cat's claw, dong quai, evening primrose, feverfew, garlic, ginger, ginkgo, red clover, horse chestnut, green tea, ginseng (all have additional antiplatelet activity).

Mechanism of Action Inhibits prostaglandin synthesis by decreasing the activity of the enzyme, cyclo-oxygenase, which results in decreased formation of prostaglandin precursors

Pharmacodynamics/Kinetics
Onset of action: ~1-2 hours
Metabolism: Hepatic biotransformation via CYP2C9
Half-life elimination: 5.7 hours
(Continued)

Flurbiprofen *(Continued)*

Time to peak: 1.5 hours
Excretion: Urine

Usual Dosage
Oral: Rheumatoid arthritis and osteoarthritis: 200-300 mg/day in 2-, 3-, or 4 divided doses
Ophthalmic: Instill 1 drop every 30 minutes, 2 hours prior to surgery (total of 4 drops to each affected eye)

Dietary Considerations Can be taken with food, milk, or antacid to decrease GI effects.

Patient Information Take the oral formulation with food to decrease any abdominal complaints. Eye drops may cause mild burning or stinging, notify physician if this becomes severe or persistent; do not touch dropper to eye, visual acuity may be decreased after administration.

Nursing Implications Care should be taken to avoid contamination of the solution container tip

Dosage Forms
Solution, ophthalmic, as sodium (Ocufen®): 0.03% (2.5 mL, 5 mL, 10 mL) [with thimerosal 0.005% as preservative]
Tablet, as sodium (Ansaid®): 50 mg, 100 mg

♦ **Flurbiprofen Sodium** *see Flurbiprofen on page 585*
♦ **Fluress®** *see Fluorescein Sodium on page 573*
♦ **5-Flurocytosine** *see Flucytosine on page 567*
♦ **FluShield®** *see Influenza Virus Vaccine on page 721*

Flutamide *(FLOO ta mide)*

U.S. Brand Names Eulexin®

Canadian Brand Names Apo-Flutamide; Euflex®; Eulexin®; Novo-Flutamide; PMS-Flutamide

Therapeutic Category Antiandrogen; Antineoplastic Agent, Miscellaneous

Use In combination therapy with LHRH agonist analogues in treatment of metastatic prostatic carcinoma. A study has shown that the addition of flutamide to leuprolide therapy in patients with advanced prostatic cancer increased median actuarial survival time to 34.9 months versus 27.9 months with leuprolide alone. To achieve benefit to combination therapy, both drugs need to be started simultaneously.

Unlabeled/Investigational Use Female hirsutism

Pregnancy Risk Factor D

Contraindications Hypersensitivity to flutamide or any component of the formulation; severe hepatic impairment; pregnancy

Warnings/Precautions The U.S. Food and Drug Administration (FDA) currently recommends that procedures for proper handling and disposal of antineoplastic agents be considered. Hospitalization and, rarely, death due to liver failure have been reported in patients taking flutamide. Elevated serum transaminase levels, jaundice, hepatic encephalopathy, and acute hepatic failure have been reported. Product labeling states flutamide is not for use in women, particularly for nonlife-threatening conditions. In some patients, the toxicity reverses after discontinuation of therapy. About 50% of the cases occur within the first 3 months of treatment. Serum transaminase levels should be measured prior to starting treatment, monthly for 4 months, and periodically thereafter. Liver function tests should be obtained at the first suggestion of liver dysfunction (nausea, vomiting, abdominal pain, fatigue, anorexia, "flu-like" symptoms, hyperbilirubinuria, jaundice, or right upper quadrant tenderness). Flutamide should be immediately discontinued any time a patient has jaundice, and/or an ALT level greater than twice the upper limit of normal. Flutamide should not be used in patients whose ALT values are greater than twice the upper limit of normal.

Patients who have taken flutamide, with glucose-6 phosphate dehydrogenase deficiency or hemoglobin M disease or smokers are at risk of toxicities associated aniline exposure, including methemoglobinemia, hemolytic anemia, and cholestatic jaundice. Monitor methemoglobin levels.

Adverse Reactions
>10%:
Endocrine & metabolic: Gynecomastia, hot flashes, breast tenderness, galactorrhea (9% to 42%); impotence; decreased libido; tumor flare
Gastrointestinal: Nausea, vomiting (11% to 12%)
Hepatic: Increased AST (SGOT) and LDH levels, transient, mild
1% to 10%:
Cardiovascular: Hypertension (1%), edema
Central nervous system: Drowsiness, confusion, depression, anxiety, nervousness, headache, dizziness, insomnia
Dermatologic: Pruritus, ecchymosis, photosensitivity, herpes zoster
Gastrointestinal: Anorexia, increased appetite, constipation, indigestion, upset stomach (4% to 6%); diarrhea
Hematologic: Anemia (6%), leukopenia (3%), thrombocytopenia (1%)
Neuromuscular & skeletal: Weakness (1%)
<1% (Limited to important or life-threatening): Hepatic failure, hepatitis, jaundice, malignant breast neoplasm (male), myocardial infarction, pulmonary embolism, sulfhemoglobinemia, thrombophlebitis, yellow discoloration of the urine

Overdosage/Toxicology Symptoms include hypoactivity, ataxia, anorexia, vomiting, slow respirations, and lacrimation. Induce vomiting. Management is supportive. There is no benefit from dialysis.

Drug Interactions
Cytochrome P450 Effect: CYP3A3/4 enzyme substrate
Increased Effect/Toxicity: Warfarin effects may be increased.

Ethanol/Nutrition/Herb Interactions
Food: No effect on bioavailability of flutamide.
Herb/Nutraceutical: St John's wort may decrease flutamide levels.

Stability Store at room temperature

Mechanism of Action Nonsteroidal antiandrogen that inhibits androgen uptake or inhibits binding of androgen in target tissues

Pharmacodynamics/Kinetics
Absorption: Rapid and complete
Metabolism: Extensively to more than 10 metabolites
Half-life elimination: 5-6 hours
Excretion: Primarily urine (as metabolites)

Usual Dosage Oral: Adults:
Prostatic carcinoma: 2 capsules every 8 hours for a total daily dose of 750 mg
Female hirsutism: 250 mg daily

Administration Contents of capsule may be opened and mixed with applesauce, pudding, or other soft foods; mixing with a beverage is not recommended

Monitoring Parameters Serum transaminase levels should be measured prior to starting treatment and should be repeated monthly for the first 4 months of therapy, and periodically thereafter. LFTs should be checked at the first sign or symptom of liver dysfunction (eg, nausea, vomiting, abdominal pain, fatigue, anorexia, flu-like symptoms, hyperbilirubinuria, jaundice, or right upper quadrant tenderness). Other parameters include tumor reduction, testosterone/estrogen, and phosphatase serum levels.

Patient Information Take as directed; do not discontinue without consulting prescriber. You may experience decreased libido, impotence, swelling of breasts, or decreased appetite (small frequent meals may help). Report chest pain or palpitation; acute abdominal pain; pain, tingling, or numbness of extremities; swelling of extremities or unusual weight gain; difficulty breathing; or other persistent adverse effects.

Dosage Forms Capsule: 125 mg

◆ **Flutex®** see Triamcinolone on page 1366

Fluticasone (floo TIK a sone)

Related Information
Asthma on page 1645
Corticosteroids Comparison on page 1495
Estimated Clinical Comparability of Doses for Inhaled Corticosteroids on page 1652

U.S. Brand Names Cutivate™; Flonase®; Flovent®; Flovent® Rotadisk®

Canadian Brand Names Cutivate™; Flonase®; Flovent®

Synonyms Fluticasone Propionate

Therapeutic Category Corticosteroid, Inhalant; Corticosteroid, Topical (Medium Potency)

Use
Inhalation: Maintenance treatment of asthma as prophylactic therapy. It is also indicated for patients requiring oral corticosteroid therapy for asthma to assist in total discontinuation or reduction of total oral dose. NOT indicated for the relief of acute bronchospasm.
Intranasal: Management of seasonal and perennial allergic rhinitis and nonallergic rhinitis in patients ≥4 years of age
Topical: Relief of inflammation and pruritus associated with corticosteroid-responsive dermatoses in patients ≥3 months of age

Pregnancy Risk Factor C

Pregnancy/Breast-Feeding Implications There are no adequate and well-controlled studies using inhaled fluticasone in pregnant women. Oral corticosteroid use has shown animals to be more prone to teratogenic effects than humans. Due to the natural increase in corticosteroid production during pregnancy, most women may require a lower steroid dose; use with caution. It is not known if fluticasone is excreted in human milk; use with caution in breast-feeding women.

Contraindications Hypersensitivity to fluticasone or any component of the formulation; primary treatment of status asthmaticus
Topical: Do not use if infection is present at treatment site, in the presence of skin atrophy, or for the treatment of rosacea or perioral dermatitis

Warnings/Precautions May cause suppression of hypothalamic-pituitary-adrenal (HPA) axis, particularly in younger children or in patients receiving high doses for prolonged periods. Fluticasone may cause less HPA axis suppression than therapeutically equivalent oral doses of prednisone. Particular care is required when patients are transferred from systemic corticosteroids to inhaled products due to possible adrenal insufficiency or withdrawal from steroids, including an increase in allergic symptoms. Patients receiving 20 mg per day of prednisone (or equivalent) may be most susceptible.

Controlled clinical studies have shown that orally-inhaled and intranasal corticosteroids may cause a reduction in growth velocity in pediatric patients. (In studies of orally-inhaled corticosteroids, the mean reduction in growth velocity was approximately 1 centimeter per year [range 0.3-1.8 cm per year] and appears to be related to dose and duration of exposure.) To minimize the systemic effects of orally-inhaled and intranasal corticosteroids, each patient should be titrated to the lowest effective dose.

May suppress the immune system, patients may be more susceptible to infection. Use with caution, if at all, in patients with systemic infections, active or quiescent tuberculosis infection, or ocular herpes simplex. Avoid exposure to chickenpox and measles.

Supplemental steroids (oral or parenteral) may be needed during stress or severe asthma attacks. Rare cases of vasculitis (Churg-Strauss syndrome) or other eosinophilic conditions can occur. Flovent® aerosol contains chlorofluorocarbons (CFCs).

Inhalation: Not to be used in status asthmaticus or for the relief of acute bronchospasm

Topical: May also cause suppression of HPA axis, especially when used on large areas of the body, denuded areas, for prolonged periods of time or with an occlusive dressing. Pediatric patients may be more susceptible to systemic toxicity. Safety and efficacy in pediatric patients <3 months of age have not been established.
(Continued)

Fluticasone *(Continued)*

Adverse Reactions

Oral or nasal inhalation: Frequency depends upon population studied and dosing used. Reactions reported are representative of multiple oral formulations.

>3%:

Central nervous system: Headache (2% to 22%), fever (1% to 7%)

Gastrointestinal: Nausea/vomiting (1% to 8%)

Neuromuscular & skeletal: Muscle injury (1% to 5%), musculoskeletal pain (1% to 5%), back problems (<1% to 4%)

Respiratory: Upper respiratory tract infection (14% to 22%), throat irritation (3% to 22%), nasal congestion (4% to 16%), pharyngitis (6% to 14%), oral candidiasis (<1% to 11%), sinusitis/sinus infection (3% to 10%), rhinitis (1% to 9%), dysphonia (<1% to 8%),

Miscellaneous: Viral infection (2% to 5%)

<3% (Limited to important or life-threatening): Aggression, agitation, cataracts, cholecystitis, Churg-Strauss syndrome, Cushingoid features, depression, dyspnea, eosinophilic conditions, fungal skin infection, gastroenteritis, glaucoma, goiter, growth velocity reduction (in children/adolescents), increased intraocular pressure, lower respiratory infections, migraine, mood disorders, nasopharyngitis, nervousness, nose/throat polyps, oral ulcerations, paradoxical bronchospasm, paralysis of cranial nerves, photodermatitis, pruritus, skin rash, throat constriction, urticaria, vasculitis

Overdosage/Toxicology When consumed in excessive quantities, systemic hypercorticism and adrenal suppression may occur; in those cases, discontinuation and withdrawal of the corticosteroid should be done judiciously.

Drug Interactions

Cytochrome P450 Effect: CYP3A3/4 enzyme substrate

Increased Effect/Toxicity:

CYP3A3/4 inhibitors: Serum level and/or toxicity of fluticasone may be increased; this effect was shown with ketoconazole, but not erythromycin. Other potential inhibitors include amiodarone, cimetidine, clarithromycin, delavirdine, diltiazem, dirithromycin, disulfiram, fluoxetine, fluvoxamine, grapefruit juice, indinavir, itraconazole, ketoconazole, nefazodone, nevirapine, propoxyphene, quinupristin-dalfopristin, ritonavir, saquinavir, verapamil, zafirlukast, zileuton.

Salmeterol: The addition of salmeterol has been demonstrated to improve response to inhaled corticosteroids (as compared to increasing steroid dosage).

Ethanol/Nutrition/Herb Interactions Herb/Nutraceutical: In theory, St John's wort may decrease serum levels of fluticasone by inducing CYP3A3/4 isoenzymes.

Stability

Aerosol, cream: Store between 2°C to 30°C (36°F to 86°F). Store aerosol with nozzle end down, protect from freezing and direct sunlight. Discard aerosol after labeled number of doses has been used.

Nasal spray: Store between 4°C to 30°C (39°F to 86°F). Discard after labeled number of doses has been used, even if bottle is not completely empty.

Powder for oral inhalation:

Flovent® Diskus®: Store at controlled room temperature, 20°C to 25°C (68°F to 77°F), in a dry place away from direct heat or sunlight. The 50 mcg strength should be discarded 6 weeks after opening protective wrap; the 100 mcg and 250 mcg strengths should be discarded 2 months after opening protective wrap (or when indicator reads "0", whichever comes first).

Flovent® Rotadisk®: Store at controlled room temperature, 20°C to 25°C (68°F to 77°F). Use blisters within 2 months of opening protective pouch.

Mechanism of Action Fluticasone belongs to a new group of corticosteroids which utilizes a fluorocarbothioate ester linkage at the 17 carbon position; extremely potent vasoconstrictive and anti-inflammatory activity; has a weak HPA inhibitory potency when applied topically, which gives the drug a high therapeutic index. The effectiveness of inhaled fluticasone is due to its direct local effect. The mechanism of action for all topical corticosteroids is believed to be a combination of three important properties: anti-inflammatory activity, immunosuppressive properties, and antiproliferative actions.

Pharmacodynamics/Kinetics

Absorption:

Cream: 5% (increased with inflammation)

Oral inhalation: Primarily via lungs, minimal GI absorption due to presystemic metabolism

Distribution: 4.2 L/kg

Protein binding: 91%

Metabolism: Hepatic via CYP3A4 to 17β-carboxylic acid (negligible activity)

Bioavailability: Oral inhalation: 14% to 30%

Excretion: Feces (as parent drug and metabolites); urine (<5% as metabolites)

Usual Dosage

Children:

Asthma: Inhalation, oral:

Flovent®: Children ≥12 years: Refer to adult dosing.

Flovent® Diskus® and Rotadisk®: **Note:** Titrate to the lowest effective dose once asthma stability is achieved; children previously maintained on Flovent® Rotadisk® may require dosage adjustments when transferred to Flovent® Diskus®

Children ≥4-11 years: Dosing based on previous therapy

Bronchodilator alone: Recommended starting dose: 50 mcg twice daily; highest recommended dose: 100 mcg twice daily

Inhaled corticosteroids: Recommended starting dose: 50 mcg twice daily; highest recommended dose: 100 mcg twice daily; a higher starting dose may be considered in patients previously requiring higher doses of inhaled corticosteroids

Children ≥11 years: Refer to adult dosing.

Inflammation/pruritus associated with corticosteroid-responsive dermatoses: Topical:

Children ≥3 months: Apply sparingly in a thin film twice daily; therapy should be discontinued when control is achieved. If no improvement is seen within 2 weeks, reassessment of diagnosis may be necessary. Safety and efficacy for use in pediatric patients <3 months have not been established.

Rhinitis: Intranasal: Children ≥4 years and Adolescents: Initial: 1 spray (50 mcg/spray) per nostril once daily; patients not adequately responding or patients with more severe symptoms may use 2 sprays (100 mcg) per nostril. Depending on response, dosage may be reduced to 100 mcg daily. Total daily dosage should not exceed 2 sprays in each nostril (200 mcg)/day. Dosing should be at regular intervals.

Adults:
  Asthma: Inhalation, oral: Note: Titrate to the lowest effective dose once asthma stability is achieved
  Flovent®: Dosing based on previous therapy
    Bronchodilator alone: Recommended starting dose: 88 mcg twice daily; highest recommended dose: 440 mcg twice daily
    Inhaled corticosteroids: Recommended starting dose: 88-220 mcg twice daily; highest recommended dose: 440 mcg twice daily; a higher starting dose may be considered in patients previously requiring higher doses of inhaled corticosteroids
    Oral corticosteroids: Recommended starting dose: 880 mcg twice daily; highest recommended dose: 880 mcg twice daily; starting dose is patient dependent. In patients on chronic oral corticosteroids therapy, reduce prednisone dose no faster than 2.5 mg/day on a weekly basis; begin taper after ≥1 week of fluticasone therapy
  Flovent® Diskus® and Rotadisk®: Dosing based on previous therapy
    Bronchodilator alone: Recommended starting dose 100 mcg twice daily; highest recommended dose: 500 mcg twice daily
    Inhaled corticosteroids: 100-250 mcg twice daily; highest recommended dose: 500 mcg twice daily; a higher starting dose may be considered in patients previously requiring higher doses of inhaled corticosteroids
    Oral corticosteroids: 500-1000 mcg twice daily; highest recommended dose: 1000 mcg twice daily; starting dose is patient dependent. In patients on chronic oral corticosteroids therapy, reduce prednisone dose no faster than 2.5 mg/day on a weekly basis; begin taper after ≥1 week of fluticasone therapy
  Inflammation/pruritus associated with corticosteroid-responsive dermatoses: Topical: Apply sparingly in a thin film twice daily; therapy should be discontinued when control is achieved. If no improvement is seen within 2 weeks, reassessment of diagnosis may be necessary.
  Rhinitis: Intranasal: Initial: 2 sprays (50 mcg/spray) per nostril once daily; may also be divided into 100 mcg twice a day. After the first few days, dosage may be reduced to 1 spray per nostril once daily for maintenance therapy. Dosing should be at regular intervals.

Dosage adjustment in hepatic impairment: Fluticasone is primarily cleared in the liver. Fluticasone plasma levels may be increased in patients with hepatic impairment, use with caution; monitor.

Elderly: No differences in safety have been observed in the elderly when compared to younger patients. Based on current data, no dosage adjustment is needed based on age.

Administration
  Aerosol inhalation: Shake container thoroughly before using. Take 3-5 deep breaths. Use inhaler on inspiration. Allow 1 full minute between inhalations. Rinse mouth with water after use to reduce aftertaste and incidence of candidiasis.
  Nasal spray: Shake bottle gently before using. Prime pump prior to first use (press 6 times until fine spray appears). Blow nose to clear nostrils. Insert applicator into nostril, keeping bottle upright, and close off the other nostril. Breathe in through nose. While inhaling, press pump to release spray. Nasal applicator may be removed and rinsed with warm water to clean.
  Powder for oral inhalation: Flovent® Diskus®: Do not use with a spacer device. Do not exhale into Diskus®. Do not wash or take apart. Use in horizontal position.
  Topical: Apply sparingly in a thin film of cream or ointment. Rub in lightly. Do not use for diaper dermatitis.

Monitoring Parameters Growth (adolescents and children); signs/symptoms of HPA axis suppression/adrenal insufficiency; possible eosinophilic conditions (including Churg-Strauss syndrome)

Patient Information Use as directed; do not overuse and use only for length of time prescribed.
  Inhalation: Rinse mouth after use; avoid spraying in eyes
    Powder for oral inhalation: Flovent® Diskus®: Do not attempt to take device apart. Do not use with a spacer device. Do not exhale into the Diskus®, use in a level horizontal position. Do not wash the mouthpiece. Use within 2 months of opening foil overwrap.
  Nasal spray: Shake gently before use. Use at regular intervals, no more frequently than directed. Report unusual cough or spasm; persistent nasal bleeding, burning, or irritation; or worsening of condition.
  Topical: For external use only. Apply thin film to affected area only; rub in lightly. Do not apply occlusive covering (including under diapers or plastic pants) unless advised by prescriber. Wash hand thoroughly after use; avoid contact with eyes. Notify prescriber if skin condition persists or worsens. Do not use for treatment of diaper dermatitis, or under diapers or plastic pants.

Nursing Implications Topical: A thin film of cream or ointment is effective; do not overuse; do not use tight-fitting diapers or plastic pants on children being treated in the diaper area; use only as prescribed, and for no longer than the period prescribed; apply sparingly in light film; rub in lightly; avoid contact with eyes; notify physician if condition being treated persists or worsens

Additional Information Effects of inhaled/intranasal steroids on growth have been observed in the absence of laboratory evidence of HPA axis suppression, suggesting that growth velocity is a more sensitive indicator of systemic corticosteroid exposure in pediatric patients than some commonly used tests of HPA axis function. The long-term effects of this reduction in growth velocity associated with orally-inhaled and intranasal corticosteroids, including the
(Continued)

Fluticasone *(Continued)*

impact on final adult height, are unknown. The potential for "catch up" growth following discontinuation of treatment with inhaled corticosteroids has not been adequately studied.

Dosage Forms
Aerosol for oral inhalation, as propionate (Flovent®):
44 mcg/inhalation (7.9 g) [60 metered doses], (13 g) [120 metered doses]
110 mcg/inhalation (7.9 g) [60 metered doses], (13 g) [120 metered doses]
220 mcg/inhalation (7.9 g) [60 metered doses], (13 g) [120 metered doses]
Cream, topical, as propionate (Cutivate™): 0.05% (15 g, 30 g, 60 g)
Ointment, topical, as propionate (Cutivate™): 0.005% (15 g, 30 g, 60 g)
Powder, for oral inhalation, as propionate:
50 mcg: 44 mcg/inhalation (60s)
100 mcg: 88 mcg/inhalation (60s)
250 mcg: 220 mcg/inhalation (60s)
Suspension, intranasal [spray] (Flonase®): 50 mcg/inhalation (16 g) [120 metered doses]

Fluticasone and Salmeterol (floo TIK a sone & sal ME te role)

U.S. Brand Names Advair™ Diskus®
Canadian Brand Names Advair™ Diskus®
Synonyms Salmeterol and Fluticasone
Therapeutic Category Beta$_2$-Adrenergic Agonist Agent; Corticosteroid, Inhalant
Use Maintenance treatment of asthma in adults and children ≥12 years; **not** for use for relief of acute bronchospasm

Pregnancy Risk Factor C
Pregnancy/Breast-Feeding Implications There are no adequate and well-controlled studies of fluticasone and/or salmeterol in pregnant women. Use only during pregnancy if the potential benefit to the mother outweighs the potential risk to the fetus. The use of fluticasone and/or salmeterol have not been studied in nursing women. It is not known if either are found in human breast milk. Use caution if administering to a nursing woman.

Contraindications Hypersensitivity to fluticasone, salmeterol, or any component of the formulation; status asthmaticus; acute episodes of asthma

Warnings/Precautions Do not use to transfer patients from oral corticosteroid therapy. Not for use in patients with rapidly deteriorating or life-threatening episodes of asthma. Fatalities have been reported. Not indicated for treatment of acute symptoms of asthma. Do not use in conjunction with other long-acting beta$_2$ agonist inhalers. Do not exceed recommended dosage; short acting beta$_2$ agonists should be used for acute symptoms and symptoms occurring between treatments. Monitor for increased use of short-acting beta$_2$ agonist inhalers; may be marker of a deteriorating asthma condition. Immediate hypersensitivity reactions (urticaria, angioedema, rash, bronchospasm) have been reported. Laryngeal spasm, irritation, swelling, stridor, and choking have also been reported. Rare cases of vasculitis (Churg-Strauss syndrome) have been reported with fluticasone use.

Corticosteroids may cause suppression of HPA axis, particularly in younger children or in patients receiving high doses for prolonged periods. Particular care is required when patients are transferred from systemic corticosteroids to inhaled products due to possible adrenal insufficiency or withdrawal from steroids, including an increase in allergic symptoms. Patients receiving ≥20 mg/day of prednisone (or equivalent) may be most susceptible. Controlled clinical studies have shown that inhaled and intranasal corticosteroids may cause a reduction in growth velocity in pediatric patients. Growth velocity provides a means of comparing the rate of growth among children of the same age.

May suppress the immune system; patients may be more susceptible to infection. Use with caution in patients with systemic infections or ocular herpes simplex. Avoid exposure to chickenpox and measles.

Beta agonists may cause elevation in blood pressure, heart rate, and result in excitement (CNS). Use with caution in patients with prostatic hyperplasia, diabetes, cardiovascular disorders, convulsive disorders, thyrotoxicosis, or patients who are sensitive to the effects of sympathomimetic amines. Paroxysmal bronchospasm (which can be fatal) has been reported with this and other inhaled agents. If this occurs, discontinue treatment. The elderly may be at greater risk of cardiovascular side effects; safety and efficacy have not been established in children <12 years of age.

Adverse Reactions
>10%:
Central nervous system: Headache (12% to 13%)
Respiratory: Pharyngitis (10% to 13%), upper respiratory tract infection (21% to 27%)
>3% to 10%:
Gastrointestinal: Diarrhea (2% to 4%), GI pain/discomfort (1% to 4%), oral candidiasis (1% to 4%), nausea/vomiting (4% to 6%)
Neuromuscular & skeletal: Musculoskeletal pain (2% to 4%)
Respiratory: Bronchitis (2% to 8%), cough (3% to 6%), hoarseness/dysphonia (2% to 5%), sinusitis (4% to 5%), upper respiratory tract inflammation (6% to 7%), viral respiratory tract infections (4%)
1% to 3%:
Cardiovascular: Chest symptoms, fluid retention, palpitations
Central nervous system: Compressed nerve syndromes, hypnagogic effects, pain, sleep disorders, tremors
Dermatologic: Hives, skin flakiness/ichthyosis, urticaria, viral skin infections
Gastrointestinal: Appendicitis, constipation, dental discomfort/pain, gastrointestinal disorder, gastrointestinal infections, gastrointestinal signs and symptoms (nonspecified), oral discomfort/pain, oral erythema/rash, oral ulcerations, unusual taste, viral GI infections (0% to 3%)
Hematologic: Contusions/hematomas, lymphatic signs and symptoms (nonspecified)
Hepatic: Abnormal liver function tests

Neuromuscular & skeletal: Arthralgia, articular rheumatism, bone/cartilage disorders, fractures, muscle injuries, muscle stiffness, tightness/rigidity

Ocular: Conjunctivitis, eye redness, keratitis

Otic: Ear signs and symptoms (nonspecified)

Respiratory: Blood in nasal mucosa, congestion, ear/nose/throat infections, lower respiratory tract infections, lower respiratory signs and symptoms (nonspecified), nasal irritation, nasal signs and symptoms (nonspecified), nasal sinus disorders, pneumonia, rhinitis, rhinorrhea/post nasal drip, sneezing, wheezing

Miscellaneous: Allergies/allergic reactions, bacterial infections, burns, candidiasis (0% to 3%), sweat/sebum disorders, sweating, viral infections, wounds and lacerations

<1% (Limited to important or life-threatening): Aphonia, arrhythmias, bronchospasm (paradoxical), Cushing syndrome, depression, dysmenorrhea, growth velocity reduction (in children/adolescents), hypercorticism, hyperglycemia, hypersensitivity reaction (immediate and delayed), influenza, laryngeal spasm/irritation, paradoxical tracheitis, paresthesia, photodermatitis, rare cases of vasculitis (Churg-Strauss syndrome), restlessness, stridor, ventricular tachycardia, vulvovaginitis, xerostomia

Overdosage/Toxicology
Fluticasone: When consumed in excessive quantities, systemic hypercorticism and adrenal suppression may occur; in those cases, discontinuation and withdrawal of the corticosteroid should be done judiciously.

Salmeterol: Signs and symptoms include excessive beta-adrenergic stimulation and exaggeration of adverse reactions; possible prolongation of the QT_c interval, leading to ventricular arrhythmias; hypokalemia, and hyperglycemia. Treatment includes prudent use of a cardioselective beta-adrenergic blocker (eg, atenolol or metoprolol); keeping in mind the potential for induction of bronchoconstriction in an asthmatic. Dialysis has not been shown to be of value.

Drug Interactions
Increased Effect/Toxicity: Diuretics (loop, thiazide): Hypokalemia from diuretics may be worsened by beta-agonists (dose related); use with caution. Ketoconazole and other CYP3A3/4 inhibitors may increase levels and/or effects of fluticasone. May cause increased cardiovascular toxicity with MAO inhibitors or tricyclic antidepressants; wait at least 2 weeks after discontinuing these agents to start fluticasone/salmeterol.

Decreased Effect: Beta-adrenergic blockers (eg, propranolol) may decreased the effect of salmeterol component and may cause bronchospasm in asthmatics; use with caution.

Stability Store at 20°C to 25°C (68°F to 77°F). Store in a dry place out of direct heat or sunlight. Keep out of reach of children. Diskus® device should be discarded 1 month after removal from foil pouch, or when dosing indicator reads "zero," whichever comes first. Device is not reusable.

Mechanism of Action Combination of fluticasone (corticosteroid) and salmeterol (long-acting beta₂ agonist) designed to improve pulmonary function and control over what is produced by either agent when used alone. Because fluticasone and salmeterol act locally in the lung, plasma levels do not predict therapeutic effect.

Fluticasone: The mechanism of action for all topical corticosteroids is believed to be a combination of three important properties: Anti-inflammatory activity, immunosuppressive properties, and antiproliferative actions. Fluticasone has extremely potent vasoconstrictive and anti-inflammatory actions.

Salmeterol: Relaxes bronchial smooth muscle by selective action on beta₂-receptors with little effect on heart rate

Pharmacodynamics/Kinetics
Advair™ Diskus®:
Onset of action: 30-60 minutes
Peak effect: ≥1 week for full effect
Duration: 12 hours
See individual agents.

Usual Dosage Do not use to transfer patients from systemic corticosteroid therapy
Children ≥12 and Adults: Oral inhalation: One inhalation twice daily, morning and evening, 12 hours apart

Advair™ Diskus® is available in 3 strengths, initial dose prescribed should be based upon previous asthma therapy. Dose should be increased after 2 weeks if adequate response is not achieved. Patients should be titrated to lowest effective dose once stable. (Because each strength contains salmeterol 50 mcg/inhalation, dose adjustments should be made by changing inhaler strength. No more than 1 inhalation of any strength should be taken more than twice a day). Maximum dose: Fluticasone 500 mcg/salmeterol 50 mcg, one inhalation twice daily.

Patients not currently on inhaled corticosteroids: Fluticasone 100 mcg/salmeterol 50 mcg
Patients currently using inhaled beclomethasone dipropionate:
≤420 mcg/day: Fluticasone 100 mcg/salmeterol 50 mcg
462-840 mcg/day: Fluticasone 250 mcg/salmeterol 50 mcg
Patients currently using inhaled budesonide:
≤400 mcg/day: Fluticasone 100 mcg/salmeterol 50 mcg
800-1200 mcg/day: Fluticasone 250 mcg/salmeterol 50 mcg
1600 mcg/day: Fluticasone 500 mcg/salmeterol 50 mcg
Patients currently using inhaled flunisolide:
≤1000 mcg/day: Fluticasone 100 mcg/salmeterol 50 mcg
1250-2000 mcg/day: Fluticasone 250 mcg/salmeterol 50 mcg
Patients currently using inhaled fluticasone propionate aerosol:
≤176 mcg/day: Fluticasone 100 mcg/salmeterol 50 mcg
440 mcg/day: Fluticasone 250 mcg/salmeterol 50 mcg
660-880 mcg/day: Fluticasone 500 mcg/salmeterol 50 mcg
Patients currently using inhaled fluticasone propionate powder:
≤200 mcg/day: Fluticasone 100 mcg/salmeterol 50 mcg
500 mcg/day: Fluticasone 250 mcg/salmeterol 50 mcg
1000 mcg/day: Fluticasone 500 mcg/salmeterol 50 mcg

(Continued)

Fluticasone and Salmeterol *(Continued)*

Patients currently using inhaled triamcinolone acetonide:
≤1000 mcg/day: Fluticasone 100 mcg/salmeterol 50 mcg
1100-1600 mcg/day: Fluticasone 250 mcg/salmeterol 50 mcg

Dosage adjustment in renal impairment: Specific guidelines are not available

Dosage adjustment in hepatic impairment: Fluticasone is cleared by hepatic metabolism. No dosing adjustment suggested. Use with caution in patients with impaired liver function.

Elderly: No differences in safety or effectiveness have been seen in studies of patients ≥65 years of age. However, increased sensitivity may be seen in the elderly. Use with caution in patients with concomitant cardiovascular disease.

Administration Not to be used with a spacer device. Do not wash the mouthpiece or other parts of the Diskus®; do not attempt to take device apart. Do not exhale into device.

Patient Information Use at regular intervals, as directed; do not overuse. Do not use for acute attacks. It may take ≥1 week to see full benefits from treatment. You may experience nervousness, dizziness, or fatigue (use caution when driving or engaging in tasks requiring alertness until response to drug is known); or dry mouth, stomach upset (frequent small meals, frequent mouth care, chewing gum, or sucking hard candy may help). Report unresolved GI upset; dizziness or fatigue; vision changes; chest pain, rapid heartbeat, or palpitations; insomnia; nervousness or hyperactivity; muscle cramping, tremors, or pain; unusual cough or spasm; or rash (hypersensitivity). Notify prescriber immediately if there is an increased need for short-acting beta$_2$ agonists, a decrease in peak flow, or general worsening of condition. May be more susceptible to infection; avoid exposure to chickenpox and measles unless immunity has been established.

Nursing Implications Not to be used for the relief of acute attacks. Patients should be instructed as to the correct use of the Diskus®.

Additional Information Effects of inhaled/intranasal steroids on growth have been observed in the absence of laboratory evidence of HPA axis suppression, suggesting that growth velocity is a more sensitive indicator of systemic corticosteroid exposure in pediatric patients than some commonly used tests of HPA axis function. The long-term effects of this reduction in growth velocity associated with orally-inhaled and intranasal corticosteroids, including the impact on final adult height, are unknown. The potential for "catch up" growth following discontinuation of treatment with inhaled corticosteroids has not been adequately studied.

Dosage Forms

Powder for oral inhalation (Advair™ Diskus®):
Fluticasone 100 mcg and salmeterol 50 mcg
Fluticasone 250 mcg and salmeterol 50 mcg
Fluticasone 500 mcg and salmeterol 50 mcg

♦ **Fluticasone Propionate** *see Fluticasone on page 587*

Fluvastatin *(FLOO va sta tin)*

Related Information
Hyperlipidemia Management *on page 1670*
Lipid-Lowering Agents *on page 1505*

U.S. Brand Names Lescol®; Lescol® XL

Canadian Brand Names Lescol®

Therapeutic Category Antilipemic Agent, HMG-CoA Reductase Inhibitor; HMG-CoA Reductase Inhibitor

Use To be used as a component of multiple risk factor intervention in patients at risk for atherosclerosis vascular disease due to hypercholesterolemia

Adjunct to dietary therapy to reduce elevated total cholesterol (total-C), LDL-C, triglyceride, and apolipoprotein B (apo-B) levels and to increase HDL-C in primary hypercholesterolemia and mixed dyslipidemia (Fredrickson types IIa and IIb); to slow the progression of coronary atherosclerosis in patients with coronary heart disease

Pregnancy Risk Factor X

Pregnancy/Breast-Feeding Implications Animal studies have shown delays in fetal skeletal development and fetal, neonatal, and maternal mortality. Congenital anomalies following use of other HMG-CoA reductase inhibitors in humans have been reported (rare). Use in women of childbearing potential only if they are highly unlikely to conceive; discontinue if pregnancy occurs. Fluvastatin is excreted in human breast milk (milk plasma ratio 2:1); do not use in breast-feeding women.

Contraindications Hypersensitivity to fluvastatin or any component of the formulation; active liver disease; unexplained persistent elevations of serum transaminases; pregnancy

Warnings/Precautions Secondary causes of hyperlipidemia should be ruled out prior to therapy. Liver function must be monitored by periodic laboratory assessment. Rhabdomyolysis with acute renal failure has occurred with fluvastatin and other HMG-CoA reductase inhibitors. Risk is increased with concurrent use of clarithromycin, danazol, diltiazem, fluvoxamine, indinavir, nefazodone, nelfinavir, ritonavir, verapamil, troleandomycin, cyclosporine, fibric acid derivatives, erythromycin, niacin, or azole antifungals. The risk of combining any of these drugs with fluvastatin is minimal. Temporarily discontinue in any patient experiencing an acute or serious condition predisposing to renal failure secondary to rhabdomyolysis. Use caution in patients with previous liver disease or heavy ethanol use. Treatment in patients <18 years of age is not recommended.

Adverse Reactions As reported with fluvastatin capsules; in general, adverse reactions reported with fluvastatin extended release tablet were similar, but the incidence was less.

1% to 10%:
Central nervous system: Headache (9%), fatigue (3%), insomnia (3%)
Gastrointestinal: Dyspepsia (8%), diarrhea (5%), abdominal pain (5%), nausea (3%)
Genitourinary: Urinary tract infection (2%)
Neuromuscular & skeletal: Myalgia (5%)
Respiratory: Sinusitis (3%), bronchitis (2%)

<1% (Limited to important or life-threatening) including additional class-related events (not necessarily reported with fluvastatin therapy): Alopecia, anaphylaxis, angioedema, arthralgia, arthritis, cataracts, cholestatic jaundice, cirrhosis, depression, dermatomyositis, dyspnea, elevated transaminases, eosinophilia, erectile dysfunction, erythema multiforme, facial paresis, fatty liver, fever, fulminant hepatic necrosis, gynecomastia, hemolytic anemia, hepatitis, hepatoma, hypersensitivity reaction, impotence, increased CPK (>10x normal), increased ESR, leukopenia, memory loss, muscle cramps, myopathy, nodules, ophthalmoplegia, pancreatitis, paresthesia, peripheral nerve palsy, peripheral neuropathy, photosensitivity, polymyalgia rheumatica, positive ANA, pruritus, psychic disturbance, purpura, rash, renal failure (secondary to rhabdomyolysis), rhabdomyolysis, skin discoloration, Stevens-Johnson syndrome, systemic lupus erythematosus-like syndrome, taste alteration, thrombocytopenia, thyroid dysfunction, toxic epidermal necrolysis, tremor, urticaria, vasculitis, vertigo

Overdosage/Toxicology GI complaints and elevated ALT (SGOT) and AST (SGPT) have been reported following large doses of the extended release tablets. In case of overdose, supportive measures should be instituted, as required. Dialyzability is not known.

Drug Interactions

Cytochrome P450 Effect: CYP2C9 enzyme substrate; CYP2C9, 2C18, and 2C19 enzyme inhibitor

Increased Effect/Toxicity: Cimetidine, omeprazole, ranitidine, and ritonavir may increase fluvastatin blood levels. Clofibrate, erythromycin, gemfibrozil, fenofibrate, and niacin may increase the risk of myopathy and rhabdomyolysis. Anticoagulant effect of warfarin may be increased by fluvastatin. Cholestyramine effect will be additive with fluvastatin if administration times are separated. Fluvastatin may increase C_{max} and decrease clearance of digoxin.

Decreased Effect: Administration of cholestyramine at the same time with fluvastatin reduces absorption and clinical effect of fluvastatin. Separate administration times by at least 4 hours. Rifampin and rifabutin may decrease fluvastatin blood levels.

Ethanol/Nutrition/Herb Interactions Food: Reduces rate but not the extent of absorption.

Stability Store at 25°C (77°F); protect from light

Mechanism of Action Acts by competitively inhibiting 3-hydroxyl-3-methylglutaryl-coenzyme A (HMG-CoA) reductase, the enzyme that catalyzes the reduction of HMG-CoA to mevalonate; this is an early rate-limiting step in cholesterol biosynthesis. HDL is increased while total, LDL and VLDL cholesterols, apolipoprotein B, and plasma triglycerides are decreased.

Pharmacodynamics/Kinetics

Protein binding: >98%

Metabolism: To inactive and active metabolites [oxidative metabolism via CYP2C9 (75%), 2C8 (~5%), and 3A4 (~20%) isoenzymes]; active forms do not circulate systemically; extensive first-pass hepatic extraction

Bioavailability: Absolute: Capsule: 24%; Extended release tablet: 29%

Half-life elimination: 1.2 hours

Excretion: Feces (90%): urine (5%)

Usual Dosage Adults: Oral:

Patients requiring ≥25% decrease in LDL-C: 40 mg capsule or 80 mg extended release tablet once daily in the evening; may also use 40 mg capsule twice daily

Patients requiring <25% decrease in LDL-C: 20 mg capsule once daily in the evening

Note: Dosing range: 20-80 mg/day; adjust dose based on response to therapy; maximum response occurs within 4-6 weeks

Dosage adjustment in renal impairment: Less than 6% excreted renally; no dosage adjustment needed with mild to moderate renal impairment; use with caution in severe impairment

Dosage adjustment in hepatic impairment: Levels may accumulate in patients with liver disease (increased AUC and C_{max}); use caution with severe hepatic impairment or heavy ethanol ingestion; contraindicated in active liver disease or unexplained transaminase elevations; decrease dose and monitor effects carefully in patients with hepatic insufficiency

Elderly: No dosage adjustment necessary based on age

Dietary Considerations Before initiation of therapy, patients should be placed on a standard cholesterol-lowering diet for 3-6 months and the diet should be continued during drug therapy. May be take without regard to meals.

Administration Patient should be placed on a standard cholesterol-lowering diet before and during treatment; fluvastatin may be taken without regard to meals; adjust dosage as needed in response to periodic lipid determinations during the first 4 weeks after a dosage change; lipid-lowering effects are additive when fluvastatin is combined with a bile-acid binding resin or niacin, however, it must be administered at least 2 hours following these drugs.

Monitoring Parameters Obtain baseline LFTs and total cholesterol profile; repeat tests at 12 weeks after initiation of therapy or elevation in dose, and periodically thereafter. Monitor LDL-C at intervals no less than 4 weeks.

Patient Information Avoid prolonged exposure to the sun and other ultraviolet light; report unexplained muscle pain or weakness, especially if accompanied by fever or malaise

Nursing Implications Monitor liver function tests and cholesterol profile. May be taken without regard to meals.

Dosage Forms

Capsule: 20 mg, 40 mg

Tablet, extended release: 80 mg

♦ **Fluviral S/F® (Can)** see Influenza Virus Vaccine on page 721

♦ **Fluvirin®** see Influenza Virus Vaccine on page 721

Fluvoxamine (floo VOKS a meen)

Related Information

Antidepressant Agents Comparison on page 1482

Selective Serotonin Reuptake Inhibitor (SSRIs) Pharmacokinetics on page 1514

(Continued)

Fluvoxamine *(Continued)*

U.S. Brand Names Luvox®

Canadian Brand Names Alti-Fluvoxamine; Apo®-Fluvoxamine; Gen-Fluvoxamine; Luvox®; Novo-Fluvoxamine; Nu-Fluvoxamine; PMS-Fluvoxamine

Therapeutic Category Antidepressant, Serotonin Reuptake Inhibitor

Use Treatment of obsessive-compulsive disorder (OCD) in children ≥8 years of age and adults

Unlabeled/Investigational Use Treatment of major depression; panic disorder; anxiety disorders in children

Pregnancy Risk Factor C

Contraindications Hypersensitivity to fluvoxamine or any component of the formulation; concurrent use with terfenadine, astemizole, pimozide, thioridazine, mesoridazine, or cisapride; use of MAO inhibitors within 14 days

Warnings/Precautions Potential for severe reaction when used with MAO inhibitors - serotonin syndrome (hyperthermia, muscular rigidity, mental status changes/agitation, autonomic instability) may occur. May precipitate a shift to mania or hypomania in patients with bipolar disease. Has a low potential to impair cognitive or motor performance - caution operating hazardous machinery or driving. Use caution in patients with suicidal risk. Use caution in patients with a previous seizure disorder or condition predisposing to seizures such as brain damage, alcoholism, or concurrent therapy with other drugs which lower the seizure threshold. Use with caution in patients with hepatic or renal dysfunction and in elderly patients. May cause hyponatremia/SIADH. Use with caution in patients with renal insufficiency or other concurrent illness (cardiovascular disease). Use with caution in patients at risk of bleeding or receiving concurrent anticoagulant therapy, although not consistently noted, fluvoxamine may cause impairment in platelet function. May cause or exacerbate sexual dysfunction.

Adverse Reactions

>10%:
Central nervous system: Headache, somnolence, insomnia, nervousness, dizziness
Gastrointestinal: Nausea, diarrhea, xerostomia
Neuromuscular & skeletal: Weakness

1% to 10%:
Cardiovascular: Palpitations
Central nervous system: Somnolence, headache, insomnia, dizziness, nervousness, mania, hypomania, vertigo, abnormal thinking, agitation, anxiety, malaise, amnesia, yawning, hypertonia, CNS stimulation, depression
Endocrine & metabolic: Decreased libido
Gastrointestinal: Abdominal pain, vomiting, dyspepsia, constipation, abnormal taste, anorexia, flatulence, weight gain
Genitourinary: Delayed ejaculation, impotence, anorgasmia, urinary frequency, urinary retention
Neuromuscular & skeletal: Tremors
Ocular: Blurred vision
Respiratory: Dyspnea
Miscellaneous: Diaphoresis

<1% (Limited to important or life-threatening): Acne, agranulocytosis, akinesia with fever, alopecia, anaphylaxis, anemia, angina, angioedema, aplastic anemia, ataxia, bradycardia, delayed menstruation, dermatitis, dry skin, dysuria, elevated liver transaminases, extrapyramidal reactions, Henoch-Schönlein purpura, hepatitis, lactation, leukocytosis, neuropathy, nocturia, pancreatitis, seizures, serotonin syndrome, SIADH, Stevens-Johnson syndrome, thrombocytopenia, torsade de pointes, toxic epidermal necrolysis, urticaria, vasculitis, ventricular tachycardia

Overdosage/Toxicology Symptoms include nausea, vomiting, somnolence, hypotension, hypokalemia, tachycardia, respiratory distress, and coma. Other symptoms reported in overdose (single- or multiple-drug ingestion) include bradycardia, EKG abnormalities, seizures, tremor, diarrhea, and increased reflexes. A specific antidote does not exist. Treatment is supportive. Although vomiting has not been extensive in overdose to date, patients should be monitored for fluid and electrolyte loss, and appropriate replacement therapy instituted when necessary.

Drug Interactions

Cytochrome P450 Effect: CYP1A2 enzyme substrate; CYP1A2, 2C9, 2C19, 2D6, and 3A3/4 enzyme inhibitor

Increased Effect/Toxicity:

MAO inhibitors: Fluvoxamine should not be used with nonselective MAO inhibitors (phenelzine, isocarboxazid) and drugs with MAO inhibitor properties (linezolid); fatal reactions have been reported. Wait 5 weeks after stopping fluvoxamine before starting a nonselective MAO inhibitor and 2 weeks after stopping an MAO inhibitor before starting fluvoxamine. Concurrent selegiline has been associated with mania, hypertension, or serotonin syndrome (risk may be reduced relative to nonselective MAO inhibitors).

Phenothiazines: Fluvoxamine may inhibit the metabolism of thioridazine or mesoridazine, resulting in increased plasma levels and increasing the risk of QT_c interval prolongation. This may lead to serious ventricular arrhythmias, such as torsade de pointes-type arrhythmias and sudden death. Do not use together. Wait at least 5 weeks after discontinuing fluvoxamine prior to starting thioridazine.

Combined used of SSRIs and amphetamines, buspirone, meperidine, nefazodone, serotonin agonists (such as sumatriptan), sibutramine, other SSRIs, sympathomimetics, ritonavir, tramadol, and venlafaxine may increase the risk of serotonin syndrome. Fluvoxamine may increase serum levels/effects of benzodiazepines (alprazolam and diazepam), beta-blockers (except atenolol or nadolol), carbamazepine, carvedilol, clozapine, cyclosporin (and possibly tacrolimus), dextromethorphan, digoxin, haloperidol, HMG-CoA reductase inhibitors (lovastatin and simvastatin - increasing the risk of rhabdomyolysis), mexiletine, phenytoin, propafenone, quinidine, tacrine, theophylline, trazodone, tricyclic antidepressants, and valproic acid. Concurrent lithium may increase risk of nephrotoxicity. Risk of hyponatremia may increase with concurrent use of loop diuretics (bumetanide, furosemide, torsemide). Fluvoxamine may increase the hypoprothrombinemic response to warfarin.

Combined use of sumatriptan (and other serotonin agonists) may result in toxicity; weakness, hyper-reflexia, and incoordination have been observed with sumatriptan and SSRIs. In addition, concurrent use may theoretically increase the risk of serotonin syndrome; includes sumatriptan, naratriptan, rizatriptan, and zolmitriptan.

Decreased Effect: Cyproheptadine, a serotonin antagonist, may inhibit the effects of serotonin reuptake inhibitors (fluvoxamine); monitor for altered antidepressant response.

Ethanol/Nutrition/Herb Interactions

Ethanol: Avoid ethanol. Depressed patients should avoid/limit intake.

Food: The bioavailability of melatonin has been reported to be increased by fluvoxamine.

Herb/Nutraceutical: Avoid valerian, St John's wort, SAMe, kava kava (may increase risk of serotonin syndrome and/or excessive sedation).

Stability Protect from high humidity and store at controlled room temperature 15°C to 30°C (59°F to 86°F); dispense in tight containers

Mechanism of Action Inhibits CNS neuron serotonin uptake; minimal or no effect on reuptake of norepinephrine or dopamine; does not significantly bind to alpha-adrenergic, histamine or cholinergic receptors

Pharmacodynamics/Kinetics

Onset of action: Therapeutic: >2 weeks

Absorption: Steady-state plasma concentrations have been noted to be 2-3 times higher in children than those in adolescents; female children demonstrated a significantly higher AUC than males

Half-life elimination: ~15 hours

Time to peak, plasma: 3-8 hours

Usual Dosage Oral: **Note:** When total daily dose exceeds 50 mg, the dose should be given in 2 divided doses:

Children 8-17 years: Initial: 25 mg at bedtime; adjust in 25 mg increments at 4- to 7-day intervals, as tolerated, to maximum therapeutic benefit: Range: 50-200 mg/day

Maximum: Children: 8-11 years: 200 mg/day; adolescents: 300 mg/day; lower doses may be effective in female versus male patients

Adults: Initial: 50 mg at bedtime; adjust in 50 mg increments at 4- to 7-day intervals; usual dose range: 100-300 mg/day; divide total daily dose into 2 doses; administer larger portion at bedtime

Elderly: Reduce dose, titrate slowly

Dosage adjustment in hepatic impairment: Reduce dose, titrate slowly

Monitoring Parameters Signs and symptoms of depression, anxiety, weight gain or loss, nutritional intake, sleep

Patient Information Its favorable side effect profile makes it a useful alternative to the traditional agents; use sugarless hard candy for dry mouth; avoid alcohol, may cause drowsiness; improvement may take several weeks; rise slowly to prevent dizziness. As with all psychoactive drugs, fluvoxamine may impair judgment, thinking, or motor skills, so use caution when operating hazardous machinery, including automobiles, especially early on into therapy. Inform your physician of any concurrent medications you may be taking.

Dosage Forms Tablet: 25 mg, 50 mg, 100 mg

♦ **Fluzone**® see Influenza Virus Vaccine on page 721
♦ **FML**® see Fluorometholone on page 575
♦ **FML**® **Forte** see Fluorometholone on page 575
♦ **FML-S**® see Sulfacetamide Sodium and Fluorometholone on page 1269
♦ **Focalin**™ see Dexmethylphenidate on page 385
♦ **Foille**® **[OTC]** see Benzocaine on page 154
♦ **Foille**® **Medicated First Aid [OTC]** see Benzocaine on page 154
♦ **Foille**® **Plus [OTC]** see Benzocaine on page 154
♦ **Folacin** see Folic Acid on page 595
♦ **Folacin, Vitamin B₁₂, and Vitamin B₆** see Folic Acid, Cyanocobalamin, and Pyridoxine on page 596
♦ **Folate** see Folic Acid on page 595

Folic Acid (FOE lik AS id)

U.S. Brand Names Folvite®

Canadian Brand Names Apo®-Folic

Synonyms Folacin; Folate; Pteroylglutamic Acid

Therapeutic Category Vitamin, Water Soluble

Use Treatment of megaloblastic and macrocytic anemias due to folate deficiency; dietary supplement to prevent neural tube defects

Pregnancy Risk Factor A/C (dose exceeding RDA recommendation)

Contraindications Pernicious, aplastic, or normocytic anemias

Warnings/Precautions Doses >0.1 mg/day may obscure pernicious anemia with continuing irreversible nerve damage progression. Resistance to treatment may occur with depressed hematopoiesis, alcoholism, deficiencies of other vitamins. Injection contains benzyl alcohol (1.5%) as preservative (use care in administration to neonates).

Adverse Reactions <1% (Limited to important or life-threatening): Bronchospasm

Drug Interactions

Decreased Effect: In folate-deficient patients, folic acid therapy may increase phenytoin metabolism which may lead to a decrease in the effect of phenytoin. Phenytoin, primidone, para-aminosalicylic acid, and sulfasalazine may decrease serum folate concentrations resulting in a folic acid deficiency. Concurrent administration of chloramphenicol and folic acid may result in antagonism of the hematopoietic response to folic acid.

(Continued)

Folic Acid *(Continued)*

Stability Incompatible with oxidizing and reducing agents and heavy metal ions

Mechanism of Action Folic acid is necessary for formation of a number of coenzymes in many metabolic systems, particularly for purine and pyrimidine synthesis; required for nucleoprotein synthesis and maintenance in erythropoiesis; stimulates WBC and platelet production in folate deficiency anemia

Pharmacodynamics/Kinetics
Onset of effect: Peak effect: Oral: 0.5-1 hour
Absorption: Proximal part of small intestine

Usual Dosage
Infants: 0.1 mg/day
Children <4 years: Up to 0.3 mg/day
Children >4 years and Adults: 0.4 mg/day
Pregnant and lactating women: 0.8 mg/day
RDA:
Adult male: 0.15-0.2 mg/day
Adult female: 0.15-0.18 mg/day

Administration Oral preferred, but may also be administered by deep I.M., S.C., or I.V. injection; a diluted solution for oral or for parenteral administration may be prepared by diluting 1 mL of folic acid injection (5 mg/mL), with 49 mL sterile water for injection; resulting solution is 0.1 mg folic acid per 1 mL

Reference Range Therapeutic: 0.005-0.015 µg/mL

Test Interactions Falsely low serum concentrations may occur with the *Lactobacillus casei* assay method in patients on anti-infectives (eg, tetracycline)

Patient Information Take folic acid replacement only under recommendation of physician

Nursing Implications
Oral, but may also be administered by deep I.M., S.C., or I.V. injection; a diluted solution for oral or for parenteral administration may be prepared by diluting 1 mL of folic acid injection (5 mg/mL), with 49 mL sterile water for injection; resulting solution is 0.1 mg folic acid per 1 mL
Monitor hemoglobin

Dosage Forms
Injection, as sodium folate: 5 mg/mL (10 mL)
Folvite®: 5 mg/mL (10 mL)
Tablet: 0.4 mg, 0.8 mg, 1 mg
Folvite®: 1 mg

Extemporaneous Preparations A 1 mg/mL folic acid solution may be prepared by crushing fifty 1 mg tablets. Dissolve in a small amount of distilled water, then add sufficient distilled water to make a final volume of 50 mL. Adjust the pH to 8 with sodium hydroxide. It is stable for 42 days at room temperature.

Nahata MC and Hipple TF, *Pediatric Drug Formulations*, Harvey Whitney Books Company, 1992.

Folic Acid, Cyanocobalamin, and Pyridoxine
(FOE lik AS id, sye an oh koe BAL a min, & peer i DOKS een)

U.S. Brand Names Foltx™

Synonyms Cyanocobalamin, Folic Acid, and Pyridoxine; Folacin, Vitamin B₁₂, and Vitamin B₆; Pyridoxine, Folic Acid, and Cyanocobalamin

Therapeutic Category Vitamin

Use Nutritional supplement in end-stage renal failure, dialysis, hyperhomocysteinemia, homocystinuria, malabsorption syndromes, dietary deficiencies

Usual Dosage Oral: Adults: 1 tablet daily

Additional Information Complete prescribing information for this medication should be consulted for additional detail.

Dosage Forms Tablet: Folic acid 2.5 mg, cyanocobalamin 1 mg, and pyridoxine 25 mg per tablet

♦ **Folinic Acid** *see Leucovorin on page 782*
♦ **Follistim®** *see Follitropins on page 596*
♦ **Follitropin Alfa** *see Follitropins on page 596*
♦ **Follitropin Alpha** *see Follitropins on page 596*
♦ **Follitropin Beta** *see Follitropins on page 596*

Follitropins (foe li TRO pins)

U.S. Brand Names Fertinex®; Follistim®; Gonal-F®

Canadian Brand Names Gonal-F®; Puregon™

Synonyms Follitropin Alfa; Follitropin Alpha; Follitropin Beta; Recombinant Human Follicle Stimulating Hormone; rFSH-alpha; rFSH-beta; rhFSH-alpha; rhFSH-beta; Urofollitropin

Therapeutic Category Ovulation Stimulator

Use
Urofollitropin (Fertinex®):
Polycystic ovary syndrome: Administered sequentially with hCG for the stimulation of follicular recruitment and development and the induction of ovulation in patients with polycystic ovary syndrome and infertility, who have failed to respond or conceive following adequate clomiphene citrate therapy
Follicle stimulation: Stimulation of the development of multiple follicles in ovulatory patients undergoing assisted reproductive technologies such as *in vitro* fertilization
Follitropin alfa (Gonal-F®) / follitropin beta (Follistim™):
Ovulation induction: Induction of ovulation and pregnancy in anovulatory infertile patients in whom the cause of infertility is functional and not caused by primary ovarian failure
Follicle stimulation: Stimulation of the development of multiple follicles in ovulatory patients undergoing assisted reproductive technologies such as *in vitro* fertilization

Spermatogenesis induction: Induction of spermatogenesis in adult males with primary and secondary hypogonadotropic hypogonadism in whom the cause of infertility is not due to primary testicular failure

Pregnancy Risk Factor X

Pregnancy/Breast-Feeding Implications Ectopic pregnancy, congenital abnormalities, and multiple births have been reported. The incidence of congenital abnormality is similar during natural conception. Excretion in breast milk unknown; breast-feeding is not recommended.

Contraindications Hypersensitivity to follitropins or any component of the formulation; high levels of FSH indicating primary gonadal failure (ovarian or testicular); uncontrolled thyroid or adrenal dysfunction; the presence of any cause of infertility other than anovulation; tumor of the ovary, breast, uterus, hypothalamus, testis, or pituitary gland; abnormal vaginal bleeding of undetermined origin; ovarian cysts or enlargement not due to polycystic ovary syndrome; pregnancy

Warnings/Precautions These medications should only be used by physicians who are thoroughly familiar with infertility problems and their management. To minimize risks, use only at the lowest effective dose. Monitor ovarian response with serum estradiol and vaginal ultrasound on a regular basis.

Ovarian enlargement which may be accompanied by abdominal distention or abdominal pain, occurs in ~20% of those treated with urofollitropin and hCG, and generally regresses without treatment within 2-3 weeks. Ovarian hyperstimulation syndrome, characterized by severe ovarian enlargement, abdominal pain/distention, nausea, vomiting, diarrhea, dyspnea, and oliguria, and may be accompanied by ascites, pleural effusion, hypovolemia, electrolyte imbalance, hemoperitoneum, and thromboembolic events is reported in about 6% of patients. If hyperstimulation occurs, stop treatment and hospitalize patient. This syndrome develops rapidly within 24 hours to several days and generally occurs during the 7-10 days immediately following treatment. Hemoconcentration associated with fluid loss into the abdominal cavity has occurred and should be assessed by fluid intake & output, weight, hematocrit, serum & urinary electrolytes, urine specific gravity, BUN and creatinine, and abdominal girth. Determinations should be performed daily or more often if the need arises. Treatment is primarily symptomatic and consists of bed rest, fluid and electrolyte replacement and analgesics. The ascitic, pleural and pericardial fluids should never be removed because of the potential danger of injury.

Serious pulmonary conditions (atelectasis, acute respiratory distress syndrome and exacerbation of asthma) have been reported. Thromboembolic events, both in association with and separate from ovarian hyperstimulation syndrome, have been reported.

Multiple pregnancies have been associated with these medications, including triplet and quintuplet gestations. Advise patient of the potential risk of multiple births before starting the treatment.

Adverse Reactions

2% to 10%:

Central nervous system: Headache, dizziness, fever

Dermatologic: Acne (male), dermoid cyst (male), dry skin, body rash, hair loss, hives

Endocrine & metabolic: Ovarian hyperstimulation syndrome, adnexal torsion, mild to moderate ovarian enlargement, abdominal pain, ovarian cysts, breast tenderness, gynecomastia (male)

Gastrointestinal: Nausea, vomiting, diarrhea, abdominal cramps, bloating, flatulence, dyspepsia

Genitourinary: Urinary tract infection, menstrual disorder, intermenstrual bleeding, dysmenorrhea, cervical lesion

Local: Pain, rash, swelling, or irritation at the site of injection

Neuromuscular & skeletal: Back pain, varicose veins (male)

Respiratory: Exacerbation of asthma, sinusitis, pharyngitis

Miscellaneous: Febrile reactions accompanied by chills, musculoskeletal, joint pains, malaise, headache, and fatigue; flu-like symptoms

<2% (Limited to important or life-threatening): Adnexal torsion, asthma, atelectasis, congenital abnormalities (incidence not greater than in general population), hemoperitoneum, hypotension, migraine, paresthesia, respiratory distress syndrome, somnolence, vaginal hemorrhage

Overdosage/Toxicology Aside from possible ovarian hyperstimulation and multiple gestations, little is known concerning the consequences of an acute overdose. Treatment is symptomatic.

Stability

Urofollitropin (Fertinex®): Lyophilized powder may be stored in the refrigerator or at room temperature (3°C to 25°C/37°F to 77°F). Protect from light; use immediately after reconstitution.

Urofollitropin (Fertinex®): Dissolve the contents of one or more ampuls of urofollitropin in 0.5-1 mL of sterile saline (concentration should not exceed 225 int. units/0.5 mL)

Follitropin alfa (Gonal-F®)/follitropin beta (Follistim®): Store powder refrigerated or at room temperature (2°C to 25°C/36°F to 77°F). Protect from light; use immediately after reconstitution.

Follitropin alfa (Gonal-F®):

Single-dose ampul: Dissolve the contents of one or more ampuls in 0.5-1 mL of sterile water for injection (concentration should not exceed 225 int. units/0.5 mL)

Multiple-dose vial: Dissolve the contents of the multidose vial with the contents of 1 prefilled syringe (bacteriostatic water for injection with 0.9% benzyl alcohol). **Do not shake.** Following reconstitution, store in refrigerator; protect from light; use within 28 days.

Follitropin beta (Follistim®): Inject 1 mL of 0.45% sodium chloride injection into vial of follitropin beta. **Do not shake,** but gently swirl until solution is clear; generally the follitropin beta dissolves immediately

Mechanism of Action Urofollitropin is a preparation of highly purified follicle-stimulating hormone (FSH) extracted from the urine of postmenopausal women. Follitropin alfa and follitropin beta are human FSH preparations of recombinant DNA origin. Follitropins stimulate (Continued)

Follitropins *(Continued)*

ovarian follicular growth in women who do not have primary ovarian failure, and stimulate spermatogenesis in men with hypogonadotrophic hypogonadism. FSH is required for normal follicular growth, maturation, gonadal steroid production, and spermatogenesis.

Pharmacodynamics/Kinetics

Onset of effect: Peak effect: Spermatogenesis, median: 165 days (range: 25-327 days); follicle development: Within cycle

Absorption: Rate limited: I.M., S.C.: Slower than elimination rate

Distribution: Mean V_d: Follitropin alfa: 10 L; Follitropin beta: 8 L

Bioavailability: Ranges from ~66% to 78% depending on agent

Half-life elimination:

Mean: S.C.: Follitropin alfa: 24-32 hours; Follitropin beta: ~30 hours

Mean terminal: Multiple dosing: I.M. follitropin alfa, S.C. Follitropin beta: ~30 hours

Time to peak:

Follitropin alfa: S.C.: 16 hours; I.M.: 25 hours

Follitropin beta: I.M.: 27 hours

Urofollitropin: S.C.: 15 hours; I.M.: 10 hours

Usual Dosage

Urofollitropin (Fertinex®): Adults: S.C.:

Polycystic ovary syndrome: Initial recommended dose of the first cycle: 75 int. units/day; consider dose adjustment after 5-7 days; additional dose adjustments may be considered based on individual patient response. The dose should not be increased more than twice in any cycle or by more than 75 int. units per adjustment. To complete follicular development and affect ovulation in the absence of an endogenous LH surge, give 5000 to 10,000 units hCG, 1 day after the last dose of urofollitropin. Withhold hCG if serum estradiol is >2000 pg/mL.

Individualize the initial dose administered in subsequent cycles for each patient based on her response in the preceding cycle. Doses of >300 int. units of FSH/day are not routinely recommended. As in the initial cycle, 5000-10,000 units of hCG must be given 1 day after the last dose of urofollitropin to complete follicular development and induce ovulation.

Give the lowest dose consistent with the expectation of good results. Over the course of treatment, doses may range between 75-300 int. units/day depending on individual patient response. Administer urofollitropin until adequate follicular development as indicated by serum estradiol and vaginal ultrasonography. A response is generally evident after 5-7 days.

Encourage the couple to have intercourse daily, beginning on the day prior to the administration of hCG until ovulation becomes apparent from the indices employed for determination of progestational activity. Take care to ensure insemination.

Follicle stimulation: For Assisted Reproductive Technologies, initiate therapy with urofollitropin in the early follicular phase (cycle day 2 or 3) at a dose of 150 int. units/day, until sufficient follicular development is attained. In most cases, therapy should not exceed 10 days.

Follitropin alfa (Gonal-F®): Adults: S.C.:

Ovulation induction: Female: Initial recommended dose of the first cycle: 75 int. units/day. Consider dose adjustment after 5-7 days; additional dose adjustments of up to 37.5 int. units may be considered after 14 days. Further dose increases of the same magnitude can be made, if necessary, every 7 days. To complete follicular development and affect ovulation in the absence of an endogenous LH surge, give 5000-10,000 units hCG, 1 day after the last dose of follitropin alfa. Withhold hCG if serum estradiol is >2000 pg/mL. Individualize the initial dose administered in subsequent cycles for each patient based on her response in the preceding cycle. Doses of >300 int. units of FSH/day are not routinely recommended. As in the initial cycle, 5000-10,000 units of hCG must be given 1 day after the last dose of urofollitropin to complete follicular development and induce ovulation.

Give the lowest dose consistent with the expectation of good results. Over the course of treatment, doses may range between 75-300 int. units/day depending on individual patient response. Administer urofollitropin until adequate follicular development as indicated by serum estradiol and vaginal ultrasonography. A response is generally evident after 5-7 days.

Encourage the couple to have intercourse daily, beginning on the day prior to the administration of hCG until ovulation becomes apparent from the indices employed for determination of progestational activity. Take care to ensure insemination.

Follicle stimulation: Female: Initiate therapy with follitropin alfa in the early follicular phase (cycle day 2 or 3) at a dose of 150 int. units/day, until sufficient follicular development is attained. In most cases, therapy should not exceed 10 days.

In patients undergoing Assisted Reproductive Technologies, whose endogenous gonadotropin levels are suppressed, initiate follitropin alfa at a dose of 225 int. units/day. Continue treatment until adequate follicular development is determined as determined by ultrasound in combination with measurement of serum estradiol levels. Consider adjustments to dose after 5 days based on the patient's response; adjust subsequent dosage every 3-5 days by ≤75-150 int. units additionally at each adjustment. Doses >450 int. units/day are not recommended. Once adequate follicular development is evident, administer hCG (5000-10,000 units) to induce final follicular maturation in preparation for oocyte.

Spermatogenesis induction: **Note:** Begin therapy with hCG pretreatment to normalize serum testosterone levels. Once normal levels are reached, follitropin beta therapy is initiated, and must be administered **concurrently** with hCG treatment.

Male: S.C.: 450 int. units/week given as 225 int. units twice weekly **or** 150 int. units 3 times/week with hCG; treatment response was noted at up to 12 months

Follitropin beta (Follistim®): Adults: S.C. or I.M.:

Ovulation induction: Stepwise approach: Initiate therapy with 75 int. units/day for up to 14 days. Increase by 37.5 int. units at weekly intervals until follicular growth or serum estradiol levels indicate an adequate response. The maximum, individualized, daily dose that has been safely used for ovulation induction in patients during clinical trials is 300 int. units. Treat the patient until ultrasonic visualizations or serum estradiol determinations indicate preovulatory conditions greater than or equal to normal values followed by 5000-10,000 units hCG.

During treatment and during a 2-week post-treatment period, examine patients at least every other day for signs of excessive ovarian stimulation. Discontinue follitropin beta administration if the ovaries become abnormally enlarged or abdominal pain occurs.

Encourage the couple to have intercourse daily, beginning on the day prior to the administration of hCG until ovulation becomes apparent from the indices employed for determination of progestational activity. Take care to ensure insemination.

Follicle stimulation: A starting dose of 150-225 int. units of follitropin beta is recommended for at least the first 4 days of treatment. The dose may be adjusted for the individual patient based upon their ovarian response. Daily maintenance doses ranging from 75-300 int. units for 6-12 days are usually sufficient, although longer treatment may be necessary. However, maintenance doses of up to 375-600 int. units may be necessary according to individual response. The maximum daily dose used in clinical studies is 600 int. units. When a sufficient number of follicles of adequate size are present, the final maturation of the follicles is induced by administering hCG at a dose of 5000-10,000 int. units. Oocyte retrieval is performed 34-36 hours later. Withhold hCG in cases where the ovaries are abnormally enlarged on the last day of follitropin beta therapy.

Administration
Urofollitropin (Fertinex®)/follitropin alpha (Gonal-F®): Administer S.C.
Follitropin beta (Follistim®): Administer S.C. or I.M. to female patients; administer S.C. only to males. The most convenient sites for S.C. injection are either in the abdomen around the navel or in the upper thigh. The best site for I.M. injection is the upper outer quadrant of the buttock muscle.

Monitoring Parameters Monitor sufficient follicular maturation. This may be directly estimated by sonographic visualization of the ovaries and endometrial lining or measuring serum estradiol levels. The combination of both ultrasonography and measurement of estradiol levels is useful for monitoring for the growth and development of follicles and timing hCG administration.

The clinical evaluation of estrogenic activity (changes in vaginal cytology and changes in appearance and volume of cervical mucus) provides an indirect estimate of the estrogenic effect upon the target organs and, therefore, it should only be used adjunctively with more direct estimates of follicular development (ultrasonography and serum estradiol determinations).

The clinical confirmation of ovulation is obtained by direct and indirect indices of progesterone production. The indices most generally used are: rise in basal body temperature, increase in serum progesterone, and menstruation following the shift in basal body temperature.

Spermatogenesis: Monitor serum testosterone levels, sperm count

Patient Information Discontinue immediately if possibility of pregnancy. Prior to therapy, inform patients of the following: Duration of treatment and monitoring required; possible adverse reactions; risk of multiple births.

Dosage Forms
Injection, powder for reconstitution [with diluent]:
    Follitropin alfa (Gonal-F®):
        37.5 int. units [1 mL ampul]
        75 int. units [1 mL ampul]
        150 int. units [1 mL ampul]
        1200 int. units (2 mL) [multidose vial]
    Follitropin beta (Follistim®): 75 int. units
    Urofollitropin (Fertinex®): 75 int. units, 150 int. units

♦ **Foltx**™ *see* Folic Acid, Cyanocobalamin, and Pyridoxine *on page 596*
♦ **Folvite®** *see* Folic Acid *on page 595*

Fomepizole (foe ME pi zole)

U.S. Brand Names Antizol®
Synonyms 4-Methylpyrazole; 4-MP
Therapeutic Category Antidote, Ethylene Glycol Toxicity; Antidote, Methanol Toxicity
Use Orphan drug: Treatment of methanol or ethylene glycol poisoning alone or in combination with hemodialysis
Unlabeled/Investigational Use Known or suspected propylene glycol toxicity
Pregnancy Risk Factor C
Pregnancy/Breast-Feeding Implications Clinical effects on the fetus: Reproduction studies have not been conducted; use in pregnant women only if the benefits clearly outweigh the risks
Contraindications Documented serious hypersensitivity reaction to fomepizole or other pyrazoles; hypersensitivity to any component of the formulation
Warnings/Precautions Should not be given undiluted or by bolus injection; fomepizole is metabolized in the liver and excreted in the urine, use caution with hepatic or renal impairment; hemodialysis should be used in patients with renal failure, significant or worsening metabolic acidosis, or ethylene glycol/methanol levels ≥50 mg/dL; monitor and manage adverse events of intoxication (respiratory distress syndrome, visual disturbances, hypocalcemia); safety and efficacy in pediatric patients have not been established
Adverse Reactions
>10%:
    Central nervous system: Headache (14%)
    Gastrointestinal: Nausea (11%)
1% to 10% (≤3% unless otherwise noted):
    Cardiovascular: Bradycardia, facial flush, hypotension, phlebosclerosis, shock, tachycardia
(Continued)

Fomepizole *(Continued)*

Central nervous system: Dizziness (6%), increased drowsiness (6%), agitation, anxiety, lightheadedness, seizure, vertigo

Dermatologic: Rash

Endocrine & metabolic: Increased liver function tests

Gastrointestinal: Bad/metallic taste (6%), abdominal pain, decreased appetite, diarrhea, heartburn, vomiting

Hematologic: Anemia, disseminated intravascular coagulation, eosinophilia, lymphangitis

Local: Application site reaction, inflammation at the injection site, pain during injection, phlebitis

Neuromuscular & skeletal: Backache

Ocular: Nystagmus, transient blurred vision, visual disturbances

Renal: Anuria

Respiratory: Abnormal smell, hiccups, pharyngitis

Miscellaneous: Multiorgan failure, speech disturbances

<1% (Limited to important or life-threatening): Mild allergic reactions (mild rash, eosinophilia)

Overdosage/Toxicology Nausea, dizziness, and vertigo were noted in healthy volunteers receiving 3-6 times the recommended dose. Dose-dependent CNS effects were short-lived in most subjects, but lasted up to 30 hours in one subject. Because fomepizole is dialyzable, dialysis may be useful in overdosage treatment.

Drug Interactions

Cytochrome P450 Effect: CYP450 mixed enzyme inducer

Ethanol/Nutrition/Herb Interactions Ethanol: Ethanol decreases the rate of fomepizole elimination by ~50%; conversely, fomepizole decreases the rate of elimination of ethanol by ~40%.

Stability Fomepizole diluted in 0.9% sodium chloride injection or dextrose 5% injection is stable for at least 24 hours when stored refrigerated or at room temperature; although, it is chemically and physically stable when diluted as recommended, sterile precautions should be observed because diluents generally do not contain preservatives.

After dilution, do not use beyond 24 hours. Fomepizole solidifies at temperatures <25°C (77°F). If the fomepizole solution has become solid in the vial, the solution should carefully be warmed by running the vial under warm water or by holding in the hand. Solidification does not affect the efficacy, safety, or stability of the drug.

Mechanism of Action Fomepizole competitively inhibits alcohol dehydrogenase, an enzyme which catalyzes the metabolism of ethanol, ethylene glycol, and methanol to their toxic metabolites. Ethylene glycol is metabolized to glycoaldehyde, then oxidized to glycolate, glyoxylate, and oxalate. Glycolate and oxalate are responsible for metabolic acidosis and renal damage. Methanol is metabolized to formaldehyde, then oxidized to formic acid. Formic acid is responsible for metabolic acidosis and visual disturbances.

Pharmacodynamics/Kinetics

Onset of effect: Peak effect: Maximum: 1.5-2 hours

Absorption: Oral: Readily absorbed

Distribution: V_d: 0.6-1.02 L/kg; rapidly into total body water

Protein binding: Negligible

Metabolism: Hepatic to 4-carboxypyrazole (80% to 85% of dose), 4-hydroxymethylpyrazole, and their N-glucuronide conjugates; following multiple doses, induces its own metabolism via CYP450 mixed-function oxidases after 30-40 hours

Half-life elimination: Has not been calculated; varies with dose

Excretion: Urine (1% to 3.5% as unchanged drug and metabolites)

Usual Dosage Adults: Ethylene glycol and methanol toxicity: I.V.: A loading dose of 15 mg/kg should be administered, followed by doses of 10 mg/kg every 12 hours for 4 doses, then 15 mg/kg every 12 hours thereafter until ethylene glycol levels have been reduced <20 mg/dL and patient is asymptomatic with normal pH

Dosage adjustment in renal impairment: Fomepizole and its metabolites are excreted in the urine; dialysis should be considered in addition to fomepizole in the case of renal failure, significant or worsening metabolic acidosis, or a measured ethylene glycol level of ≥50 mg/dL. Patients should be dialyzed to correct metabolic abnormalities and to lower the ethylene glycol level <50 mg/dL; fomepizole is dialyzable and the frequency of dosing should be increased to every 4 hours during hemodialysis

Fomepizole is dialyzable and the frequency of dosing should be increased to every 4 hours during hemodialysis

Dose at the beginning of hemodialysis:

If <6 hours since last fomepizole dose: Do not administer dose

If ≥6 hours since last fomepizole dose: Administer next scheduled dose

Dosing during hemodialysis: Dose every 4 hours

Dosing at the time hemodialysis is complete, based on time between last dose and the end of hemodialysis:

<1 hour: Do not administer dose at the end of hemodialysis

1-3 hours: Administer 1/2 of next scheduled dose

>3 hours: Administer next scheduled dose

Maintenance dose when off hemodialysis: Give next scheduled dose 12 hours from last dose administered.

Dosage adjustment in hepatic impairment: Fomepizole is metabolized in the liver; specific dosage adjustments have not been determined in patients with hepatic impairment

Administration The appropriate dose of fomepizole should be drawn from the vial with a syringe and injected into at least 100 mL of sterile 0.9% sodium chloride injection or dextrose 5% injection. All doses should be administered as a slow intravenous infusion (IVPB) over 30 minutes.

Monitoring Parameters Fomepizole plasma levels should be monitored; response to fomepizole; monitor plasma/urinary ethylene glycol or methanol levels, urinary oxalate (ethylene glycol), plasma/urinary osmolality, renal/hepatic function, serum electrolytes, arterial blood gases; anion and osmolar gaps, resolution of clinical signs and symptoms of ethylene glycol or methanol intoxication

Reference Range
Fomepizole: Concentrations 100-300 μmol/L (8.2-24.6 mg/L) should result in enzyme inhibition of alcohol dehydrogenase
Ethylene glycol: Lethal dose is ~1.4 mL/kg
Methanol: Lethal dose is ~1-2 mL/kg

Patient Information This medication is given to treat antifreeze or windshield wiper fluid ingestion. It can only be given by injection. If not treated, serious side effects will occur from ingesting these agents including kidney and/or eye damage, seizures, coma, and possibly death. The most common side effects from this medicine are headache and nausea. Notify prescriber if pregnant or breast-feeding.

Nursing Implications This agent is intended as an antidote for ethylene glycol poisoning, the main ingredient in antifreeze and coolants, which can cause severe CNS depression, severe metabolic acidosis, renal failure, coma, and possibly death. It is also used for the treatment of methanol poisoning, the main ingredient in windshield wiper fluid, which can also cause severe metabolic acidosis as well as visual disturbances. The most common reactions to be aware of with the use of this agent are minor allergic reactions, headache, nausea, and dizziness. It may be used alone or in combination with hemodialysis.

Additional Information Alternate therapies, including ethanol and hemodialysis, are difficult to use in children. Fomepizole's affinity for alcohol dehydrogenase is 8000 times greater than ethanol.

Dosage Forms Injection: 1 g/mL (1.5 mL)

Fomivirsen (foe MI vir sen)

U.S. Brand Names Vitravene™
Canadian Brand Names Vitravene™
Synonyms Fomivirsen Sodium
Therapeutic Category Antiviral Agent, Nonantiretroviral; Antiviral Agent, Ophthalmic
Use Local treatment of cytomegalovirus (CMV) retinitis in patients with acquired immunodeficiency syndrome who are intolerant or insufficiently responsive to other treatments for CMV retinitis or when other treatments for CMV retinitis are contraindicated

Pregnancy/Breast-Feeding Implications Studies have not been conducted in pregnant women. Should be used in pregnancy only when potential benefit to the mother outweighs the potential risk to the fetus. Excretion in human milk is unknown. Breast-feeding is contraindicated.

Contraindications Hypersensitivity to fomivirsen or any component

Warnings/Precautions For ophthalmic use via intravitreal injection only. Uveitis occurs frequently, particularly during induction dosing. Do not use in patients who have received intravenous or intravitreal cidofovir within 2-4 weeks (risk of exaggerated inflammation is increased). Patients should be monitored for CMV disease in the contralateral eye and/or extraocular disease. Commonly increases intraocular pressure - monitoring is recommended.

Adverse Reactions
5% to 10%:
Central nervous system: Fever, headache
Gastrointestinal: Abdominal pain, diarrhea, nausea, vomiting
Hematologic: Anemia
Neuromuscular & skeletal: Asthenia
Ocular: Uveitis, abnormal vision, anterior chamber inflammation, blurred vision, cataract, conjunctival hemorrhage, decreased visual acuity, loss of color vision, eye pain, increased intraocular pressure, photophobia, retinal detachment, retinal edema, retinal hemorrhage, retinal pigment changes, vitreitis
Respiratory: Pneumonia, sinusitis
Miscellaneous: Systemic CMV, sepsis, infection
2% to 5%:
Cardiovascular: Chest pain
Central nervous system: Confusion, depression, dizziness, neuropathy, pain
Endocrine & metabolic: Dehydration
Gastrointestinal: Abnormal LFTs, pancreatitis, anorexia, weight loss
Hematologic: Thrombocytopenia, lymphoma
Neuromuscular & skeletal: Back pain, cachexia
Ocular: Application site reaction, conjunctival hyperemia, conjunctivitis, corneal edema, decreased peripheral vision, eye irritation, keratic precipitates, optic neuritis, photopsia, retinal vascular disease, visual field defect, vitreous hemorrhage, vitreous opacity
Renal: Kidney failure
Respiratory: Bronchitis, dyspnea, cough
Miscellaneous: Allergic reaction, flu-like syndrome, diaphoresis (increased)

Stability Store between 2°C to 25°C (35°F to 77°F); protect from excessive heat or light

Mechanism of Action Inhibits synthesis of viral protein by binding to mRNA which blocks replication of cytomegalovirus through an antisense mechanism

Pharmacodynamics/Kinetics Pharmacokinetic studies have not been conducted in humans. In animal models, the drug is cleared from the eye after 7-10 days. It is metabolized by sequential nucleotide removal, with a small amount of the radioactivity from a dose appearing in the urine.

Usual Dosage Adults: Intravitreal injection: Induction: 330 mcg (0.05 mL) every other week for 2 doses, followed by maintenance dose of 330 mcg (0.05 mL) every 4 weeks
If progression occurs during maintenance, a repeat of the induction regimen may be attempted to establish resumed control. Unacceptable inflammation during therapy may be managed by temporary interruption, provided response has been established. Topical corticosteroids have been used to reduce inflammation.

Administration Administered by intravitreal injection following application of standard topical and/or local anesthetics and antibiotics.
(Continued)

Fomivirsen *(Continued)*

Monitoring Parameters Immediately after injection, light perception and optic nerve head perfusion should be monitored. Anterior chamber paracentesis may be necessary if perfusion is not complete within 7-10 minutes after injection. Subsequent patient evaluation should include monitoring for contralateral CMV infection or extraocular CMV disease, and intraocular pressure prior to each injection.

Additional Information Because the mechanism of action of fomivirsen is different than other antiviral agents active against CMV, fomivirsen may be active against isolates resistant to ganciclovir, foscarnet, or cidofovir. The converse may also be true.

Dosage Forms Injection, intravitreal: 6.6 mg/mL (0.25 mL)

♦ **Fomivirsen Sodium** *see Fomivirsen on page 601*

Fondaparinux *(fon da PARE i nuks)*

U.S. Brand Names Arixtra®

Synonyms Fondaparinux Sodium

Therapeutic Category Factor Xa Inhibitor

Use Prophylaxis of deep vein thrombosis (DVT) in patients undergoing surgery for hip fracture or hip or knee replacement

Unlabeled/Investigational Use Treatment of DVT

Pregnancy Risk Factor B

Pregnancy/Breast-Feeding Implications Reproductive animal studies have not shown any fetal harm. There are no adequate or well-controlled studies in pregnant women; use only if clearly needed. Excretion in breast milk is unknown; use caution in breast-feeding.

Contraindications Hypersensitivity to fondaparinux or any component of the formulation; severe renal impairment (Cl_{cr} <30 mL/minute); body weight <50 kg; active major bleeding; bacterial endocarditis; thrombocytopenia associated with a positive *in vitro* test for antiplatelet antibody in the presence of fondaparinux

Warnings/Precautions Patients with recent or anticipated neuraxial anesthesia (epidural or spinal anesthesia) are at risk of spinal or epidural hematoma and subsequent paralysis. Not to be used interchangeably (unit-for-unit) with heparin, low molecular weight heparins (LMWHs), or heparinoids. Use caution in patients with moderate renal dysfunction (Cl_{cr} 30-50 mL/minute). Discontinue if severe dysfunction or labile function develops.

Use caution in congenital or acquired bleeding disorders; active ulcerative or angiodysplastic gastrointestinal disease; hemorrhagic stroke; shortly after brain, spinal, or ophthalmologic surgery; or in patients taking platelet inhibitors. Discontinue agents that may enhance the risk of hemorrhage if possible. If thrombocytopenia occurs discontinue fondaparinux. Use caution in the elderly, patients with a history of heparin-induced thrombocytopenia, patients with a bleeding diathesis, uncontrolled hypertension, recent gastrointestinal ulceration, diabetic retinopathy, and hemorrhage. Safety and efficacy in pediatric patients have not been established.

Adverse Reactions As with all anticoagulants, bleeding is the major adverse effect. Hemorrhage may occur at any site. Risk appears increased by a number of factors including renal dysfunction, age (>75 years), and weight (<50 kg).

>10%:
  Central nervous system: Fever (14%)
  Gastrointestinal: Nausea (11%)
  Hematologic: Anemia (20%)

1% to 10%:
  Cardiovascular: Edema (9%), hypotension (4%), confusion (3%)
  Central nervous system: Insomnia (5%), dizziness (4%), headache (2%), pain (2%)
  Dermatologic: Rash (8%), purpura (4%), bullous eruption (3%)
  Endocrine & metabolic: Hypokalemia (4%)
  Gastrointestinal: Constipation (9%), vomiting (6%), diarrhea (3%), dyspepsia (2%)
  Genitourinary: Urinary tract infection (4%), urinary retention (3%)
  Hematologic: Moderate thrombocytopenia (50,000-100,000/mm^3: 3%), major bleeding (2% to 3%), minor bleeding (3% to 4%), hematoma (3%)
  Hepatic: SGOT increased (2%), SGPT increased (3%)
  Local: Injection site reaction (bleeding, rash, pruritus)
  Miscellaneous: Wound drainage increased (5%)

<1% (Limited to important or life-threatening): Severe thrombocytopenia (<50,000/mm^3)

Overdosage/Toxicology Treatment is symptom directed and supportive.

Drug Interactions

Increased Effect/Toxicity: Anticoagulants, antiplatelet agents, drotrecogin alfa, nonsteroidal anti-inflammatory agents, salicylates and thrombolytic agents may enhance the anticoagulant effect and/or increase the risk of bleeding.

Ethanol/Nutrition/Herb Interactions Herb/Nutraceutical: Avoid alfalfa, anise, bilberry, bladderwrack, bromelain, cat's claw, celery, coleus, cordyceps, dong quai, evening primrose oil, fenugreek, feverfew, garlic, ginger, ginkgo biloba, ginseng (American/Panax/Siberian), grape seed, green tea, guggul, horse chestnut seed, horseradish, licorice, prickly ash, red clover, reishi, sweet clover, turmeric, white willow (all possess anticoagulant or antiplatelet activity and as such, may enhance the anticoagulant effects of fondaparinux).

Stability Store at 15°C to 30°C (59°F to 86°F).

Mechanism of Action Fondaparinux is a synthetic pentasaccharide that causes an antithrombin III-mediated selective inhibition of factor Xa. Neutralization of factor Xa interrupts the blood coagulation cascade and inhibits thrombin formation and thrombus development.

Pharmacodynamics/Kinetics
  Absorption: Rapid and complete
  Distribution: V_d: 7-11 L; mainly in blood
  Protein binding: ≥94% (to antithrombin III)
  Bioavailability: 100%
  Half-life elimination: 17-21 hours; increases with worsening renal function
  Time to peak: 2-3 hours

Excretion: Urine (as unchanged drug)

Usual Dosage S.C.:

Adults: ≥50 kg: Usual dose: 2.5 mg once daily. **Note:** Initiate dose after hemostasis has been established, 6-8 hours postoperatively.

Elderly: Use caution, elimination may be prolonged; assess renal function before initiating therapy

Dosage adjustment in renal impairment:

Cl$_{cr}$ 30-50 mL/minute: Use caution

Cl$_{cr}$ <30 mL/minute: Contraindicated

Administration Do not administer I.M.; for S.C administration only. Do not mix with other injections or infusions.

Monitoring Parameters Periodic monitoring of CBC, serum creatinine, occult blood testing of stools recommended. Antifactor Xa activity of fondaparinux can be measured by the assay if fondaparinux is used as the calibrator. PT and aPTT are insensitive measures of fondaparinux activity.

Test Interactions International standards of heparin or LMWH are not the appropriate calibrators for antifactor Xa activity of fondaparinux.

Patient Information This drug can only be administered by injection. You may have a tendency to bleed easily while taking this drug; brush teeth with soft brush, floss with waxed floss, use electric razor, avoid scissors or sharp knives, and potentially harmful activities. Report unusual bleeding or bruising (bleeding gums, nosebleed, blood in urine, dark stool); any falls or accidents; new joint pain or swelling, dizziness, severe headache, shortness of breath, weakness, fainting or passing out. **Breast-feeding precaution:** Consult prescriber if breast-feeding.

Nursing Implications Administer only by S.C. injection. Monitor for bleeding problems.

Dosage Forms Injection, solution, as sodium [prefilled syringe]: 2.5 mg/0.5 mL

- **Fondaparinux Sodium** *see Fondaparinux on page 602*
- **Foradil® (Can)** *see Formoterol on page 603*
- **Foradil® Aerolizer™** *see Formoterol on page 603*

Formoterol (for MOH te rol)

U.S. Brand Names Foradil® Aerolizer™

Canadian Brand Names Foradil®; Oxeze® Turbuhaler®

Synonyms Formoterol Fumarate

Therapeutic Category Beta$_2$-Adrenergic Agonist Agent

Use Maintenance treatment of asthma and prevention of bronchospasm in patients ≥5 years of age with reversible obstructive airway disease, including patients with symptoms of nocturnal asthma, who require regular treatment with inhaled, short-acting beta$_2$ agonists; maintenance treatment of bronchoconstriction in patients with chronic obstructive pulmonary disease (COPD); prevention of exercise-induced bronchospasm in patients ≥12 years of age

Pregnancy Risk Factor C

Pregnancy/Breast-Feeding Implications When given orally to rats throughout organogenesis, formoterol caused delayed ossification and decreased fetal weight, but no malformations. There were no adverse events when given to pregnant rats in late pregnancy. Doses used were ≥70 times the recommended daily inhalation dose in humans. There are no adequate and well-controlled studies in pregnant women. Use only if benefit outweighs risk to the fetus. Beta agonists interfere with uterine contractility so use during labor only if benefit outweighs risk to the fetus. Unknown if excreted in breast milk; use caution during breast-feeding.

Contraindications Hypersensitivity to adrenergic amines, formoterol, or any component of the formulation; need for acute bronchodilation; within 2 weeks of MAO inhibitor use

Warnings/Precautions Formoterol is not meant to relieve acute asthmatic symptoms. Use short-acting beta$_2$ agonists for symptomatic relief of acute asthma symptoms only. Use with caution in patients with cardiovascular disorders, convulsive disorders, thyrotoxicosis, or others who are sensitive to the effects of sympathomimetic amines. Paroxysmal bronchospasm (which can be fatal) has been reported with this and other inhaled agents. If this occurs, discontinue treatment. Safety and efficacy have not been established in children <5 years of age.

Adverse Reactions Children are more likely to have infection, inflammation, abdominal pain, nausea, and dyspepsia.

>10%: Miscellaneous: Viral infection (17%)

1% to 10%:

Cardiovascular: Chest pain (2%)

Central nervous system: Tremor (2%), dizziness (2%), insomnia (2%), dysphonia (1%)

Dermatologic: Rash (1%)

Respiratory: Bronchitis (5%), infection (3%), dyspnea (2%), tonsillitis (1%)

<1% (Limited to important or life-threatening): Anaphylactic reactions (severe hypotension, angioedema), asthma exacerbation

Overdosage/Toxicology Signs and symptoms would be those associated with excessive beta-adrenergic stimulation. Treatment would include symptomatic and supportive care. Prudent use of a cardioselective beta-adrenergic blocker (eg, atenolol or metoprolol) may help reduce symptoms. Keep in mind the potential for induction of bronchoconstriction in an asthmatic.

Drug Interactions

Cytochrome P450 Effect: CYP2A6, CYP2C9, CYP2C19, CYP2D6 enzyme substrate

Increased Effect/Toxicity: Adrenergic agonists, antidepressants (tricyclic), beta-blockers, corticosteroids, diuretics, drugs that prolong QT$_c$ interval, MAO inhibitors, theophylline derivatives

Stability Prior to dispensing, store in refrigerator at 2°C to 8°C (36°F to 46°F); after dispensing, store at room temperature at 20°C to 25°C (68°F to 77°F). Protect from heat and moisture. Capsules should always be stored in the blister and only removed immediately before use. (Continued)

Formoterol *(Continued)*

Always check expiration date. Use within 4 months of purchase date or product expiration date, whichever comes first.

Mechanism of Action Relaxes bronchial smooth muscle by selective action on beta$_2$ receptors with little effect on heart rate. Formoterol has a long-acting effect.

Pharmacodynamics/Kinetics

Duration: Improvement in FEV$_1$ observed for 12 hours in most patients

Absorption: Rapidly into plasma

Protein binding: 61% to 64% *in vitro* at higher concentrations than achieved with usual dosing

Metabolism: By direct glucuronidation and O-demethylation; CYP2D6, CYP2C19, CYP2C9, CYP2A6 involved in O-demethylation

Half-life elimination: ~10-14 hours

Time to peak: Maximum improvement in FEV$_1$ in 1-3 hours

Excretion:

Children 5-12 years: Urine (6% as unchanged drug, 7% to 9% as direct glucuronide metabolites)

Adults: Urine (10% as unchanged drug, 15% to 18% as direct glucuronide metabolites)

Usual Dosage Inhalation:

Children ≥5 years and Adults: Asthma maintenance: 12 mcg capsule every 12 hours

Children ≥12 years and Adults: Exercise-induced bronchospasm: 12 mcg capsule at least 15 minutes before exercise on an "as needed" basis; additional doses should not be used for another 12 hours. **Note:** If already using for asthma maintenance then should not use additional doses for exercise-induced bronchospasm.

Adults: Maintenance treatment for COPD: 12 mcg capsule every 12 hours

Elderly: No specific dosing recommendations

Dosage adjustment in renal impairment: Not studied

Dosage adjustment in hepatic impairment: Not studied

Administration Remove capsule from foil blister **immediately** before use. Place capsule in the capsule-chamber in the base of the Aerolizer™ Inhaler. Must only use the Aerolizer™ Inhaler. Press both buttons **once only** and then release. Keep inhaler in a level, horizontal position. Do not exhale into inhaler. Tilt head slightly back and inhale (rapidly, steadily, and deeply). Hold breath as long as possible. If any powder remains in capsule, exhale and inhale again. Repeat until capsule is empty. Throw away empty capsule; do not leave in inhaler. Do not use a spacer with the Aerolizer™ Inhaler. Always keep capsules and inhaler dry.

Monitoring Parameters Peak flow meter

Patient Information Do not swallow this capsule. You will put the capsule in the Aerolizer™ Inhaler and inhale the contents of the capsule into your lungs. Only this inhaler can be used for this medicine. Do not use this inhaler to take any other medicines. Check inhaler use with prescriber at each visit. Using the inhaler the right way is very important. Do not use a space with this inhaler. Never wash inhaler; always keep it dry. Do not use more than 2 times per day. Separate doses by about 12 hours. Wear medical alert identification for asthma. To prevent exercise-induced wheezing, take at least 15 minutes before exercise. Do not take another dose for at least 12 hours. Common side effects include shakiness, fast heartbeats, headache, muscle cramps, pain, nervousness, and irritation of the mouth or throat. Notify prescriber if asthma is worsening, peak flow measurements decreasing, short-acting bronchodilator not working as well, chest pain or pressure, any rash, no improvement or feeling worse.

Dosage Forms Powder for oral inhalation, as fumarate [capsule]: 12 mcg [contains lactose 25 mg] (18s, 60s)

♦ **Formoterol Fumarate** *see* Formoterol *on page 603*

♦ **Formulex® (Can)** *see* Dicyclomine *on page 397*

♦ **5-Formyl Tetrahydrofolate** *see* Leucovorin *on page 782*

♦ **Fortaz®** *see* Ceftazidime *on page 253*

♦ **Fortovase®** *see* Saquinavir *on page 1221*

♦ **Fosamax®** *see* Alendronate *on page 48*

Foscarnet *(fos KAR net)*

Related Information

USPHA/IDSA Guidelines for the Prevention of Opportunistic Infections in Persons With HIV *on page 1574*

U.S. Brand Names Foscavir®

Canadian Brand Names Foscavir®

Synonyms PFA; Phosphonoformate; Phosphonoformic Acid

Therapeutic Category Antiviral Agent, Nonantiretroviral; Antiviral Agent, Parenteral

Use

Herpes virus infections suspected to be caused by acyclovir - (HSV, VZV) or ganciclovir - (CMV) resistant strains (this occurs almost exclusively in immunocompromised persons, eg, with advanced AIDS), who have received prolonged treatment for a herpes virus infection

CMV retinitis in persons with AIDS; other CMV infections in persons unable to tolerate ganciclovir; may be given in combination with ganciclovir in patients who relapse after monotherapy with either drug

Pregnancy Risk Factor C

Contraindications Hypersensitivity to foscarnet or any component of the formulation; Cl$_{cr}$ <0.4 mL/minute/kg during therapy

Warnings/Precautions Renal impairment occurs to some degree in the majority of patients treated with foscarnet; renal impairment may occur at any time and is usually reversible within 1 week following dose adjustment or discontinuation of therapy, however, several patients have died with renal failure within 4 weeks of stopping foscarnet; therefore, renal function should be closely monitored. Foscarnet is deposited in teeth and bone of young, growing animals; it has adversely affected tooth enamel development in rats; safety and effectiveness in children have not been studied. Imbalance of serum electrolytes or minerals occurs in 6% to 18% of patients (hypocalcemia, low ionized calcium, hypo- or hyperphosphatemia, hypomagnesemia or hypokalemia).

Patients with a low ionized calcium may experience perioral tingling, numbness, paresthesias, tetany, and seizures. Seizures have been experienced by up to 10% of AIDS patients. Risk factors for seizures include a low baseline absolute neutrophil count (ANC), impaired baseline renal function and low total serum calcium. Some patients who have experienced seizures have died, while others have been able to continue or resume foscarnet treatment after their mineral or electrolyte abnormality has been corrected, their underlying disease state treated, or their dose decreased. Foscarnet has been shown to be mutagenic *in vitro* and in mice at very high doses. Information on the use of foscarnet is lacking in the elderly; dose adjustments and proper monitoring must be performed because of the decreased renal function common in older patients.

Adverse Reactions
>10%:
  Central nervous system: Fever, headache, seizures
  Endocrine & metabolic: Electrolyte disorders (hyper- or hypocalcemia; hyper- or hypomagnesemia, hyper- or hypophosphatemia, or hypokalemia)
  Gastrointestinal: Nausea, diarrhea, vomiting
  Hematologic: Anemia
  Renal: Nephrotoxicity (abnormal renal function, decreased creatinine clearance)
1% to 10%:
  Central nervous system: Seizures (in up to 10% of HIV patients), fatigue, malaise, dizziness, hypoesthesia, depression, confusion, anxiety
  Dermatologic: Rash
  Gastrointestinal: Anorexia
  Hematologic: Granulocytopenia, leukopenia
  Local: Injection site pain
  Neuromuscular & skeletal: Paresthesia, involuntary muscle contractions, rigors, neuropathy (peripheral), weakness
  Ocular: Vision abnormalities
  Respiratory: Coughing, dyspnea
  Miscellaneous: Sepsis, diaphoresis (increased)
<1% (Limited to important or life-threatening): Arrhythmias, ascites, bradycardia, cardiac failure, cerebral edema, cholecystitis, cholelithiasis, hepatitis, hepatosplenomegaly, leg edema, peripheral edema, substernal chest pain, syncope, vocal cord paralysis

Overdosage/Toxicology Symptoms include seizures, renal dysfunction, perioral or limb paresthesias, and hypocalcemia. Treatment is supportive. Administer I.V. calcium salts for hypocalcemia.

Drug Interactions
Increased Effect/Toxicity: Concurrent use with ciprofloxacin (or other fluoroquinolone) increases seizure potential. Acute renal failure (reversible) has been reported with cyclosporine due most likely to a synergistic toxic effect. Nephrotoxic drugs (amphotericin B, I.V. pentamidine, aminoglycosides, etc) should be avoided, if possible, to minimize additive renal risk with foscarnet. Concurrent use of pentamidine also increases the potential for hypocalcemia. Protease inhibitors (ritonavir, saquinavir) have been associated with an increased risk of renal impairment during concurrent use of foscarnet

Stability
Foscarnet injection is a clear, colorless solution; it should be stored at room temperature and protected from temperatures >40°C and from freezing
Foscarnet should be diluted in D$_5$W or NS and transferred to PVC containers; stable for 24 hours at room temperature or refrigeration
For peripheral line administration, foscarnet **must** be diluted to 12 mg/mL with D$_5$W or NS
For central line administration, foscarnet may be administered undiluted
Incompatible with dextrose 30%, I.V. solutions containing calcium, magnesium, vancomycin, TPN

Mechanism of Action Pyrophosphate analogue which acts as a noncompetitive inhibitor of many viral RNA and DNA polymerases as well as HIV reverse transcriptase. Similar to ganciclovir, foscarnet is a virostatic agent. Foscarnet does not require activation by thymidine kinase.

Pharmacodynamics/Kinetics
Distribution: Up to 28% of cumulative I.V. dose may be deposited in bone
Metabolism: Biotransformation does not occur
Half-life elimination: ~3 hours
Excretion: Urine (≤28% as unchanged drug)

Usual Dosage
CMV retinitis: I.V.:
  Induction treatment: 60 mg/kg/dose every 8 hours **or** 100 mg/kg every 12 hours for 14-21 days
  Maintenance therapy: 90-120 mg/kg/day as a single infusion
Acyclovir-resistant HSV induction treatment: I.V.: 40 mg/kg/dose every 8-12 hours for 14-21 days
Dosage adjustment in renal impairment:
Induction and maintenance dosing schedules based on creatinine clearance (mL/minute/kg):
  See tables on next page.
  Hemodialysis:
  Foscarnet is highly removed by hemodialysis (30% in 4 hours HD)
  Doses of 50 mg/kg/dose posthemodialysis have been found to produce similar serum concentrations as doses of 90 mg/kg twice daily in patients with normal renal function
  Doses of 60-90 mg/kg/dose loading dose (posthemodialysis) followed by 45 mg/kg/dose posthemodialysis (3 times/week) with the monitoring of weekly plasma concentrations to maintain peak plasma concentrations in the range of 400-800 μMolar has been recommended by some clinicians

(Continued)

Foscarnet *(Continued)*

Continuous arteriovenous or venovenous hemodiafiltration effects: Dose as for Cl$_{cr}$ 10-50 mL/ minute

Induction Dosing of Foscarnet in Patients with Abnormal Renal Function

Cl$_{cr}$ (mL/min/kg)	HSV Equivalent to 40 mg/kg q12h	HSV Equivalent to 40 mg/kg q8h	CMV Equivalent to 60 mg/kg q8h	CMV Equivalent to 90 mg/kg q12h
<0.4	not recommended	not recommended	not recommended	not recommended
≥0.4-0.5	20 mg/kg every 24 hours	35 mg/kg every 24 hours	50 mg/kg every 24 hours	50 mg/kg every 24 hours
>0.5-0.6	25 mg/kg every 24 hours	40 mg/kg every 24 hours	60 mg/kg every 24 hours	60 mg/kg every 24 hours
>0.6-0.8	35 mg/kg every 24 hours	25 mg/kg every 12 hours	40 mg/kg every 12 hours	80 mg/kg every 24 hours
>0.8-1.0	20 mg/kg every 12 hours	35 mg/kg every 12 hours	50 mg/kg every 12 hours	50 mg/kg every 12 hours
>1.0-1.4	30 mg/kg every 12 hours	30 mg/kg every 8 hours	45 mg/kg every 8 hours	70 mg/kg every 12 hours
>1.4	40 mg/kg every 12 hours	40 mg/kg every 8 hours	60 mg/kg every 8 hours	90 mg/kg every 12 hours

Maintenance Dosing of Foscarnet in Patients with Abnormal Renal Function

Cl$_{cr}$ (mL/min/kg)	CMV Equivalent to 90 mg/kg q24h	CMV Equivalent to 120 mg/kg q24h
<0.4	not recommended	not recommended
≥0.4-0.5	50 mg/kg every 48 hours	65 mg/kg every 48 hours
>0.5-0.6	60 mg/kg every 48 hours	80 mg/kg every 48 hours
>0.6-0.8	80 mg/kg every 48 hours	105 mg/kg every 48 hours
>0.8-1.0	50 mg/kg every 24 hours	65 mg/kg every 24 hours
>1.0-1.4	70 mg/kg every 24 hours	90 mg/kg every 24 hours
>1.4	90 mg/kg every 24 hours	120 mg/kg every 24 hours

Administration
Foscarnet is administered by intravenous infusion, using an infusion pump, at a rate not exceeding 1 mg/kg/minute
Undiluted (24 mg/mL) solution can be administered without further dilution when using a central venous catheter for infusion
For peripheral vein administration, the solution **must** be diluted to a final concentration **not to exceed** 12 mg/mL
The recommended dosage, frequency, and rate of infusion should not be exceeded

Patient Information Close monitoring is important and any symptom of electrolyte abnormalities should be reported immediately; maintain adequate fluid intake and hydration; regular ophthalmic examinations are necessary. Foscarnet is not a cure; disease progression may occur during or following treatment. Report any numbness in the extremities, paresthesias, or perioral tingling.

Nursing Implications Do not administer by rapid or bolus injection; follow administration guidelines carefully

Additional Information Sodium loading with 500 mL of 0.9% sodium chloride solution before and after foscarnet infusion helps to minimize the risk of nephrotoxicity.

Dosage Forms Injection: 24 mg/mL (250 mL, 500 mL)

♦ Foscavir® *see Foscarnet on page 604*

Fosfomycin *(fos foe MYE sin)*

Related Information
Antimicrobial Drugs of Choice *on page 1588*

U.S. Brand Names Monurol™

Canadian Brand Names Monurol™

Synonyms Fosfomycin Tromethamine

Therapeutic Category Antibiotic, Miscellaneous

Use A single oral dose in the treatment of uncomplicated urinary tract infections in women due to susceptible strains of *E. coli* and *Enterococcus*; multiple doses have been investigated for complicated urinary tract infections in men; may have an advantage over other agents since it maintains high concentration in the urine for up to 48 hours

Pregnancy Risk Factor B

Pregnancy/Breast-Feeding Implications Breast-feeding/lactation: Milk concentration approximates 10% of plasma

Adverse Reactions
>1%:
Central nervous system: Headache
Dermatologic: Rash
Gastrointestinal: Diarrhea (2% to 8%), nausea, vomiting, epigastric discomfort, anorexia
<1% (Limited to important or life-threatening): Dizziness, drowsiness, fatigue, pruritus

Overdosage/Toxicology Symptomatic and supportive treatment is recommended in the event of an overdose.

Drug Interactions
Decreased Effect: Antacids or calcium salts may cause precipitate formation and decrease fosfomycin absorption. Increased gastrointestinal motility due to metoclopramide may

lower fosfomycin tromethamine serum concentrations and urinary excretion. This drug interaction possibly could be extrapolated to other medications which increase gastrointestinal motility.

Mechanism of Action As a phosphonic acid derivative, fosfomycin inhibits bacterial wall synthesis (bactericidal) by inactivating the enzyme, pyruvyl transferase, which is critical in the synthesis of cell walls by bacteria; the tromethamine salt is preferable to the calcium salt due to its superior absorption

Pharmacodynamics/Kinetics

Absorption: Well absorbed

Distribution: V_d: 2 L/kg; high concentrations in urine; well into other tissues; crosses maximally into CSF with inflamed meninges

Protein binding: Minimal (<3%)

Bioavailability: 34% to 58%

Half-life elimination: 4-8 hours; Cl_{cr} <10 mL/minute: 50 hours

Time to peak, serum: 2 hours

Excretion: Urine (as unchanged drug); high urinary levels (100 mcg/mL) persist for >48 hours

Usual Dosage Adults: Urinary tract infections: Oral:

Female: Single dose of 3 g in 4 oz of water

Male: 3 g once daily for 2-3 days for complicated urinary tract infections

Dosing adjustment in renal impairment: Decrease dose; 80% removed by dialysis, repeat dose after dialysis

Dosing adjustment in hepatic impairment: No dosage decrease needed

Administration Always mix with water before ingesting; do not administer in its dry form; pour contents of envelope into 90-120 mL of water (not hot), stir to dissolve and take immediately

Monitoring Parameters Signs and symptoms of urinary tract infection

Patient Information May be taken with or without food; avoid use of antacids or calcium salts within 4 hours before or 2 hours after taking fosfomycin; contact your physician if signs of allergy develop; if symptoms do not improve after 2-3 days, contact your prescriber

Additional Information Many gram-positive and gram-negative organisms such as staphylococci, pneumococci, *E. coli*, *Salmonella*, *Shigella*, *H. influenzae*, *Neisseria* spp, and some strains of *P. aeruginosa*, indole-negative *Proteus*, and *Providencia* are inhibited. *B. fragilis*, and anaerobic gram-negative cocci are resistant.

Dosage Forms Powder, as tromethamine: 3 g [mix in 4 oz water]

♦ **Fosfomycin Tromethamine** *see Fosfomycin on page 606*

Fosinopril (foe SIN oh pril)

Related Information

Angiotensin Agents Comparison *on page 1473*

Heart Failure *on page 1663*

U.S. Brand Names Monopril®

Canadian Brand Names Monopril™

Therapeutic Category Angiotensin-Converting Enzyme (ACE) Inhibitor; Antihypertensive Agent

Use Treatment of hypertension, either alone or in combination with other antihypertensive agents; treatment of congestive heart failure, left ventricular dysfunction after myocardial infarction

Pregnancy Risk Factor C/D (2nd and 3rd trimesters)

Contraindications Hypersensitivity to fosinopril or any component of the formulation; angioedema related to previous treatment with an ACE inhibitor; idiopathic or hereditary angioedema; bilateral renal artery stenosis; primary hyperaldosteronism; pregnancy (2nd and 3rd trimesters)

Warnings/Precautions Anaphylactic reactions can occur. Angioedema can occur at any time during treatment (especially following first dose). Careful blood pressure monitoring (hypotension can occur especially in volume depleted patients). Dosage adjustment needed in severe renal impairment (Cl_{cr} <10 mL/minute). Use with caution in hypovolemia; collagen vascular diseases; valvular stenosis (particularly aortic stenosis); hyperkalemia; or before, during, or immediately after anesthesia. Avoid rapid dosage escalation which may lead to renal insufficiency. Hypersensitivity reactions may be seen during hemodialysis with high-flux dialysis membranes (eg, AN69). Hyperkalemia may rarely occur. Neutropenia/agranulocytosis with myeloid hyperplasia can rarely occur. If patient has renal impairment, then a baseline WBC with differential and serum creatinine should be evaluated and monitored closely during initial therapy. Use with caution in unilateral renal artery stenosis and pre-existing renal insufficiency. Safety and efficacy in pediatric patients have not been established.

Adverse Reactions Note: Frequency ranges include data from hypertension and heart failure trials. Higher rates of adverse reactions have generally been noted in patients with congestive heart failure. However, the frequency of adverse effects associated with placebo is also increased in this population.

>10%: Central nervous system: Dizziness (1.6% to 11.9%)

1% to 10%:

Cardiovascular: Orthostatic hypotension (1.4% to 1.9%), palpitation (1.4%)

Central nervous system: Dizziness (1% to 2%; up to 12% in CHF patients), headache (3.2%), weakness (1.4%), fatigue (1% to 2%)

Endocrine & metabolic: Hyperkalemia (2.6%)

Gastrointestinal: Diarrhea (2.2%), nausea/vomiting (1.2% to 2.2%)

Hepatic: Increased transaminases

Neuromuscular & skeletal: Musculoskeletal pain (<1% to 3.3%), noncardiac chest pain (<1% to 2.2%)

Renal: Increased serum creatinine, worsening of renal function (in patients with bilateral renal artery stenosis or hypovolemia)

Respiratory: Cough (2.2% to 9.7%)

Miscellaneous: Upper respiratory infection (2.2%)

>1% but ≤ frequency in patients receiving placebo: Sexual dysfunction, fever, flu-like syndrome, dyspnea, rash, headache, insomnia

(Continued)

Fosinopril *(Continued)*

<1% (Limited to important or life-threatening): Anaphylactoid reaction, angina, angioedema, arthralgia, bronchospasm, cerebral infarction, cerebrovascular accident, eosinophilic vasculitis, gout, gynecomastia, hepatitis, hepatomegaly, myalgia, myocardial infarction, pancreatitis, paresthesia, photosensitivity, pleuritic chest pain, pruritus, rash, renal insufficiency, scleroderma, shock, sudden death, syncope, TIA, tinnitus, urticaria, vertigo. In a small number of patients, a symptom complex of cough, bronchospasm, and eosinophilia has been observed with fosinopril.

Other events reported with ACE inhibitors: Acute renal failure, agranulocytosis, anemia, aplastic anemia, bullous pemphigus, cardiac arrest, eosinophilic pneumonitis, exfoliative dermatitis, hemolytic anemia, hepatic failure, jaundice, neutropenia, pancytopenia, Stevens-Johnson syndrome, symptomatic hyponatremia, thrombocytopenia. In addition, a syndrome which may include fever, myalgia, arthralgia, interstitial nephritis, vasculitis, rash, eosinophilia and positive ANA, and elevated ESR has been reported for other ACE inhibitors.

Overdosage/Toxicology Mild hypotension has been the only toxic effect seen with acute overdose. Bradycardia may also occur; hyperkalemia occurs even with therapeutic doses, especially in patients with renal insufficiency and those taking NSAIDs. Following initiation of essential overdose management, toxic symptom and supportive treatment should be initiated. Hypotension usually responds to I.V. fluids or Trendelenburg positioning.

Drug Interactions

Increased Effect/Toxicity: Potassium supplements, co-trimoxazole (high dose), angiotensin II receptor antagonists (candesartan, losartan, irbesartan, etc), or potassium-sparing diuretics (amiloride, spironolactone, triamterene) may result in elevated serum potassium levels when combined with fosinopril. ACE inhibitor effects may be increased by phenothiazines or probenecid (increases levels of captopril). ACE inhibitors may increase serum concentrations/effects of digoxin, lithium, and sulfonlyureas.

Diuretics have additive hypotensive effects with ACE inhibitors, and hypovolemia increases the potential for adverse renal effects of ACE inhibitors. In patients with compromised renal function, coadministration with nonsteroidal anti-inflammatory drugs may result in further deterioration of renal function. Allopurinol and ACE inhibitors may cause a higher risk of hypersensitivity reaction when taken concurrently.

Decreased Effect: Aspirin (high dose) may reduce the therapeutic effects of ACE inhibitors; at low dosages this does not appear to be significant. Rifampin may decrease the effect of ACE inhibitors. Antacids may decrease the bioavailability of ACE inhibitors (may be more likely to occur with captopril); separate administration times by 1-2 hours. NSAIDs, specifically indomethacin, may reduce the hypotensive effects of ACE inhibitors. More likely to occur in low renin or volume dependent hypertensive patients.

Ethanol/Nutrition/Herb Interactions Herb/Nutraceutical: Avoid dong quai if using for hypertension (has estrogenic activity). Avoid ephedra, garlic, yohimbe, ginseng (may worsen hypertension).

Mechanism of Action Competitive inhibitor of angiotensin-converting enzyme (ACE); prevents conversion of angiotensin I to angiotensin II, a potent vasoconstrictor; results in lower levels of angiotensin II which causes an increase in plasma renin activity and a reduction in aldosterone secretion; a CNS mechanism may also be involved in hypotensive effect as angiotensin II increases adrenergic outflow from CNS; vasoactive kallikreins may be decreased in conversion to active hormones by ACE inhibitors, thus reducing blood pressure

Pharmacodynamics/Kinetics

Onset of action: 1 hour

Duration: 24 hours

Absorption: 36%

Protein binding: 95%

Metabolism: Fosinopril is a prodrug and is hydrolyzed to its active metabolite fosinoprilat by intestinal wall and hepatic esterases

Bioavailability: 36%

Half-life elimination, serum (fosinoprilat): 12 hours

Time to peak, serum: ~3 hours

Excretion: Urine and feces (as fosinoprilat and other metabolites in roughly equal proportions, 45% to 50%)

Usual Dosage Adults: Oral:

Hypertension: Initial: 10 mg/day; most patients are maintained on 20-40 mg/day. May need to divide the dose into two if trough effect is inadequate; discontinue the diuretic, if possible 2-3 days before initiation of therapy; resume diuretic therapy carefully, if needed.

Heart failure: Initial: 10 mg/day (5 mg if renal dysfunction present) and increase, as needed, to a maximum of 40 mg once daily over several weeks; usual dose: 20-40 mg/day. If hypotension, orthostasis, or azotemia occur during titration, consider decreasing concomitant diuretic dose, if any.

Dosing adjustment/comments in renal impairment: None needed since hepatobiliary elimination compensates adequately diminished renal elimination.

Hemodialysis: Moderately dialyzable (20% to 50%)

Monitoring Parameters Blood pressure (supervise for at least 2 hours after the initial dose or any increase for significant orthostasis); serum potassium, calcium, creatinine, BUN, WBC

Test Interactions Positive Coombs' [direct]; may cause false-positive results in urine acetone determinations using sodium nitroprusside reagent

Patient Information Notify physician if vomiting, diarrhea, excessive perspiration, or dehydration should occur; also if swelling of face, lips, tongue, or difficulty in breathing occurs or if persistent cough develops; may be taken with meals; do not stop therapy or add a potassium salt replacement without physician's advice

Nursing Implications May cause depression in some patients; discontinue if angioedema of the face, extremities, lips, tongue, or glottis occurs; watch for hypotensive effects within 1-3 hours of first dose or new higher dose

Dosage Forms Tablet: 10 mg, 20 mg, 40 mg

Fosphenytoin (FOS fen i toyn)

Related Information
Fosphenytoin and Phenytoin, Parenteral Comparison *on page 1498*

U.S. Brand Names Cerebyx®

Canadian Brand Names Cerebyx®

Synonyms Fosphenytoin Sodium

Therapeutic Category Anticonvulsant

Use Indicated for short-term parenteral administration when other means of phenytoin administration are unavailable, inappropriate or deemed less advantageous; the safety and effectiveness of fosphenytoin in this use has not been systematically evaluated for more than 5 days; may be used for the control of generalized convulsive status epilepticus and prevention and treatment of seizures occurring during neurosurgery

Pregnancy Risk Factor D

Pregnancy/Breast-Feeding Implications
Clinical effects on the fetus: Crosses placenta with fetal serum concentrations equal to those of mother; eye, cardiac, cleft palate, and skeletal malformations have been noted; fetal hydantoin syndrome associated with maternal ingestion of 100-800 mg/kg during 1st trimester

Breast-feeding/lactation: Distributes into breast milk

Contraindications Hypersensitivity to phenytoin, other hydantoins, or any component of the formulation; patients with sinus bradycardia, sinoatrial block, second- and third-degree AV block, or Adams-Stokes syndrome; occurrence of rash during treatment (should not be resumed if rash is exfoliative, purpuric, or bullous); not recommended for use in children <4 years of age; pregnancy

Warnings/Precautions Use with caution in patients with severe cardiovascular, hepatic, renal disease or diabetes mellitus; avoid abrupt discontinuation; dosing should be slowly reduced to avoid precipitation of seizures; increased toxicity with nephrotic syndrome patient; may increase frequency of petit mal seizures; use with caution in patients with porphyria, fever, or hypothyroidism

Adverse Reactions The more important adverse clinical events caused by the I.V. use of fosphenytoin or phenytoin are cardiovascular collapse and/or central nervous system depression. Hypotension can occur when either drug is administered rapidly by the I.V. route. Do not exceed a rate of 150 mg phenytoin equivalent/minute when administering fosphenytoin.

The adverse clinical events most commonly observed with the use of fosphenytoin in clinical trials were nystagmus, dizziness, pruritus, paresthesia, headache, somnolence, and ataxia. Paresthesia and pruritus were seen more often following fosphenytoin (versus phenytoin) administration and occurred more often with I.V. fosphenytoin than with I.M. administration. These events were dose- and rate-related (doses ≥15 mg/kg at a rate of 150 mg/minute). These sensations, generally described as itching, burning, or tingling are usually not at the infusion site. The location of the discomfort varied with the groin mentioned most frequently. The paresthesia and pruritus were transient events that occurred within several minutes of the start of infusion and generally resolved within 10 minutes after completion of infusion.

Transient pruritus, tinnitus, nystagmus, somnolence, and ataxia occurred 2-3 times more often at doses ≥15 mg/kg and rates ≥150 mg/minute.

I.V. administration (maximum dose/rate):
>10%:
Central nervous system: Nystagmus, dizziness, somnolence, ataxia
Dermatologic: Pruritus
1% to 10%:
Cardiovascular: Hypotension, vasodilation, tachycardia
Central nervous system: Stupor, incoordination, paresthesia, extrapyramidal syndrome, tremor, agitation, hypesthesia, dysarthria, vertigo, brain edema, headache
Gastrointestinal: Nausea, tongue disorder, dry mouth, vomiting
Ocular: Diplopia, amblyopia
Otic: Tinnitus, deafness
Neuromuscular & skeletal: Pelvic pain, muscle weakness, back pain
Miscellaneous: Taste perversion

I.M. administration (substitute for oral phenytoin):
1% to 10%:
Central nervous system: Nystagmus, tremor, ataxia, headache, incoordination, somnolence, dizziness, paresthesia, reflexes decreased
Dermatologic: Pruritus
Gastrointestinal: Nausea, vomiting
Hematologic/lymphatic: Ecchymosis
Neuromuscular & skeletal: Muscle weakness
<1% (Limited to important or life-threatening): Acidosis, acute hepatic failure, acute hepatotoxicity, alkalosis, anemia, atrial flutter, bundle branch block, cardiac arrest, cardiomegaly, cerebral hemorrhage, cerebral infarct, congestive heart failure, cyanosis, dehydration, hyperglycemia, hyperkalemia, hypertension, hypochromic anemia, hypokalemia, hypophosphatemia, ketosis, leukocytosis, leukopenia, lymphadenopathy, palpitations, postural hypotension, pulmonary embolus, QT interval prolongation, sinus bradycardia, syncope, thrombocytopenia, thrombophlebitis, ventricular extrasystoles

Overdosage/Toxicology Signs and symptoms include unsteady gait, tremors, hyperglycemia, chorea (extrapyramidal), gingival hyperplasia, gynecomastia, myoglobinuria, nephrotic syndrome, slurred speech, mydriasis, myoclonus, confusion, encephalopathy, hyperthermia, drowsiness, nausea, hypothermia, fever, hypotension, respiratory depression, hyper-reflexia, coma, systemic lupus erythematosus (SLE), ophthalmoplegia; as well as, leukopenia, neutropenia, agranulocytosis, and granulocytopenia. Treatment for hypotension is supportive. Treat with I.V. fluids and Trendelenburg positioning. Seizures may be controlled with lorazepam or diazepam 5-10 mg (0.25-0.4 mg/kg in children); intravenous albumin (25 g every 6 hours) has been used to increase the bound fraction of drug. Multiple (Continued)

Fosphenytoin (Continued)

dosing of activated charcoal may be effective. Peritoneal dialysis, diuresis, hemodialysis, hemoperfusion, and plasmapheresis are of little value.

Drug Interactions

Cytochrome P450 Effect: CYP2C9 and 2C19 enzyme substrate; CYP1A2, 2B6, 2C, 2C9, 2C18, 2C19, 2D6, 3A3/4, and 3A5-7 enzyme inducer

Increased Effect/Toxicity: Phenytoin may increase phenobarbital and primidone levels. Protein binding of phenytoin can be affected by valproic acid or salicylates. Serum phenytoin concentrations may be increased by cimetidine, felbamate, ethosuximide, methsuximide, chloramphenicol, disulfiram, fluconazole, omeprazole, isoniazid, trimethoprim, or sulfonamides.

Decreased Effect: No drugs are known to interfere with the conversion of fosphenytoin to phenytoin. Phenytoin may decrease the serum concentration or effectiveness of valproic acid, ethosuximide, felbamate, benzodiazepines, carbamazepine, lamotrigine, primidone, warfarin, oral contraceptives, corticosteroids, cyclosporine, theophylline, chloramphenicol, rifampin, doxycycline, quinidine, mexiletine, disopyramide, dopamine, or nondepolarizing skeletal muscle relaxants. Serum phenytoin concentrations may be decreased by rifampin, cisplatin, vinblastine, bleomycin, and folic acid.

Stability Refrigerated vials are stable for 2 years; at room temperature, stable for 3 months; I.V. solutions are stable for one day when refrigerated

Compatible with all diluents and does not require propylene glycol or ethanol for solubility

Mechanism of Action Diphosphate ester salt of phenytoin which acts as a water soluble prodrug of phenytoin; after administration, plasma esterases convert fosphenytoin to phosphate, formaldehyde and phenytoin as the active moiety; phenytoin works by stabilizing neuronal membranes and decreasing seizure activity by increasing efflux or decreasing influx of sodium ions across cell membranes in the motor cortex during generation of nerve impulses

Pharmacodynamics/Kinetics

Onset of action: May be more rapid due to more rapid infusion

Protein binding: 95% to 99% (albumin), can displace phenytoin and increase free fraction (up to 30% unbound) during the period required for conversion of fosphenytoin to phenytoin

Metabolism: Fosphenytoin is a prodrug of phenytoin and its anticonvulsant effects are attributable to phenytoin; converted via hydrolysis to phenytoin

Bioavailability: I.M.: 100%

Half-life: Variable (kinetics of phenytoin are saturable); mean: 12-29 hours

Conversion to phenytoin: Following I.V. administration conversion half-life elimination is 15 minutes; following I.M. administration, peak phenytoin levels are reached in 3 hours

Excretion: Urine, as metabolites (inactive)

See Phenytoin monograph for additional information.

Usual Dosage The dose, concentration in solutions, and infusion rates for fosphenytoin are expressed as phenytoin sodium equivalents; fosphenytoin should always be prescribed and dispensed in phenytoin sodium equivalents

Children 5-18 years: I.V.: A limited number of children have been studied. Seven children received a single I.V. loading dose of fosphenytoin 10-20 mg PE/kg for the treatment of acute generalized convulsive status epilepticus (Pellock, 1996). Some centers are using the phenytoin dosing guidelines in children and dosing fosphenytoin using PE doses equal to the phenytoin doses (ie, phenytoin 1 mg = fosphenytoin 1 mg PE). Further pediatric studies are needed.

Adults:

Status epilepticus: I.V.: Loading dose: Phenytoin equivalent: 15-20 mg/kg I.V. administered at 100-150 mg/minute

Nonemergent loading and maintenance dosing: I.V. or I.M.:

Loading dose: Phenytoin equivalent: 10-20 mg/kg I.V. or I.M. (maximum I.V. rate: 150 mg/minute)

Initial daily maintenance dose: Phenytoin equivalent: 4-6 mg/kg/day I.V. or I.M.

I.M. or I.V. substitution for oral phenytoin therapy: May be substituted for oral phenytoin sodium at the same total daily dose, however, Dilantin® capsules are ~90% bioavailable by the oral route; phenytoin, supplied as fosphenytoin, is 100% bioavailable by both the I.M. and I.V. routes; for this reason, plasma phenytoin concentrations may increase when I.M. or I.V. fosphenytoin is substituted for oral phenytoin sodium therapy; in clinical trials I.M. fosphenytoin was administered as a single daily dose utilizing either 1 or 2 injection sites; some patients may require more frequent dosing

Dosing adjustments in renal/hepatic impairment: Phenytoin clearance may be substantially reduced in cirrhosis and plasma level monitoring with dose adjustment advisable; free phenytoin levels should be monitored closely in patients with renal or hepatic disease or in those with hypoalbuminemia; furthermore, fosphenytoin clearance to phenytoin may be increased without a similar increase in phenytoin in these patients leading to increase frequency and severity of adverse events

Administration Since there is no precipitation problem with fosphenytoin, no I.V. filter is required; I.V. administration rate should not exceed 150 mg/minute

Monitoring Parameters Blood pressure, vital signs (with I.V. use), plasma level monitoring, CBC, liver function tests

Reference Range

Therapeutic: 10-20 µg/mL (SI: 40-79 µmol/L); toxicity is measured clinically, and some patients require levels outside the suggested therapeutic range

Toxic: 30-50 µg/mL (SI: 120-200 µmol/L)

Lethal: >100 µg/mL (SI: >400 µmol/L)

Manifestations of toxicity:

Nystagmus: 20 µg/mL (SI: 79 µmol/L)

Ataxia: 30 µg/mL (SI: 118.9 µmol/L)

Decreased mental status: 40 µg/mL (SI: 159 µmol/L)

Coma: 50 µg/mL (SI: 200 µmol/L)

Peak serum phenytoin level after a 375 mg I.M. fosphenytoin dose in healthy males: 5.7 µg/mL

Peak serum fosphenytoin levels and phenytoin levels after a 1.2 g infusion (I.V.) in healthy subjects over 30 minutes were 129 µg/mL and 17.2 µg/mL respectively

Test Interactions Increases glucose, alkaline phosphatase (S); decreases thyroxine (S), calcium (S); serum sodium increases in overdose setting

Nursing Implications I.V. injections should be followed by normal saline flushes through the same needle or I.V. catheter to avoid local irritation of the vein; must be diluted to concentrations <6 mg/mL, in normal saline, for I.V. infusion

Additional Information 1.5 mg fosphenytoin is approximately equivalent to 1 mg phenytoin. Equimolar fosphenytoin dose is 375 mg (75 mg/mL solution) to phenytoin 250 mg (50 mg/mL).

Dosage Forms Injection, as sodium: 75 mg/mL [equivalent to 50 mg/mL phenytoin sodium] (2 mL, 10 mL)

♦ **Fosphenytoin and Phenytoin, Parenteral Comparison** *see page 1498*
♦ **Fosphenytoin Sodium** *see Fosphenytoin on page 609*
♦ **Fragmin®** *see Dalteparin on page 358*
♦ **Froben® (Can)** *see Flurbiprofen on page 585*
♦ **Froben-SR® (Can)** *see Flurbiprofen on page 585*
♦ **Frova™** *see Frovatriptan on page 611*

Frovatriptan (froe va TRIP tan)

Related Information
Antimigraine Drugs Comparison *on page 1485*

U.S. Brand Names Frova™

Synonyms Frovatriptan Succinate

Therapeutic Category Antimigraine Agent, Serotonin 5-HT$_{1D}$ Agonist; Serotonin 5-HT$_{1B, 1D}$ Receptor Agonist

Use Acute treatment of migraine with or without aura in adults

Pregnancy Risk Factor C

Pregnancy/Breast-Feeding Implications There are no adequate and well-controlled studies using frovatriptan in pregnant women. Use only if potential benefit to the mother outweighs the potential risk to the fetus. It is unknown whether frovatriptan is excreted in human breast milk. Use caution if administered to a nursing woman.

Contraindications Hypersensitivity to frovatriptan or any component of the formulation; patients with ischemic heart disease or signs or symptoms of ischemic heart disease (including Prinzmetal's angina, angina pectoris, myocardial infarction, silent myocardial ischemia); cerebrovascular syndromes (including strokes, transient ischemic attacks); peripheral vascular syndromes (including ischemic bowel disease); uncontrolled hypertension; use within 24 hours of ergotamine derivatives; use within 24 hours of another 5-HT$_1$ agonist; management of hemiplegic or basilar migraine; prophylactic treatment of migraine; severe hepatic impairment

Warnings/Precautions Not intended for migraine prophylaxis, or treatment of cluster headaches, hemiplegic or basilar migraines. Cardiac events, cerebral/subarachnoid hemorrhage, and stroke have been reported with 5-HT$_1$ agonist administration. Do not give to patients with risk factors for CAD until a cardiovascular evaluation has been performed; if evaluation is satisfactory, the healthcare provider should administer the first dose and cardiovascular status should be periodically evaluated. Significant elevation in blood pressure, including hypertensive crisis, has also been reported on rare occasions in patients using other 5-HT$_{1D}$ agonists with and without a history of hypertension. Vasospasm-related reactions have been reported other than coronary artery vasospasm. Use with caution in patients with history of seizure disorder. Safety and efficacy in pediatric patients have not been established

Adverse Reactions
1% to 10%:
Cardiovascular: Chest pain (2%), flushing (4%), palpitation (1%)
Central nervous system: Dizziness (8%), fatigue (5%), headache (4%), hot or cold sensation (3%), anxiety (1%), dysesthesia (1%), hypoesthesia (1%), insomnia (1%), pain (1%)
Gastrointestinal: Hyposalivation (3%), dyspepsia (2%), abdominal pain (1%), diarrhea (1%), vomiting (1%)
Neuromuscular & skeletal: Paresthesia (4%), skeletal pain (3%)
Ocular: Visual abnormalities (1%)
Otic: Tinnitus (1%)
Respiratory: Rhinitis (1%), sinusitis (1%)
Miscellaneous: Diaphoresis (1%)
<1% (Limited to important or life-threatening): Abnormal dreaming, abnormal gait, abnormal lacrimation, abnormal reflexes, abnormal urine, agitation, amnesia, arthralgia, arthrosis, ataxia, back pain, bradycardia, bullous eruption, cheilitis, confusion, conjunctivitis, constipation, dehydration, depersonalization, depression, dysphagia, dyspnea, earache, EKG changes, emotional lability, epistaxis, eructation, esophagospasm, euphoria, eye pain, fever, gastroesophageal reflux, hiccup, hot flushes, hyperacusis, hyperesthesia, hypertonia, hyperventilation, hypocalcemia, hypoglycemia, hypotonia, impaired concentration, involuntary muscle contractions, laryngitis, leg cramps, malaise, micturition, muscle weakness, myalgia, nervousness, nocturia, peptic ulcer, personality disorder, polyuria, pruritus, purpura, renal pain, rigors, saliva increased, salivary gland pain, speech disorder, stomatitis, syncope, tachycardia, taste perversion, thirst, tongue paralysis, toothache, tremor, unspecified pain, urinary frequency, vertigo, weakness

Overdosage/Toxicology Single oral doses up to 100 mg have been reported without adverse effects. Treatment should be supportive and symptomatic. Monitor for at least 48 hours or until signs and symptoms subside. It is not known if hemodialysis or peritoneal dialysis is effective.
(Continued)

Frovatriptan *(Continued)*

Drug Interactions

Cytochrome P450 Effect: CYP1A2 enzyme substrate

Increased Effect/Toxicity: The effects of frovatriptan may be increased by CYP1A2 inhibitors (eg, cimetidine, ciprofloxacin, erythromycin), estrogen derivatives, propranolol. Ergot derivatives may increase the effects of frovatriptan (do not use within 24 hours of each other). SSRIs may exhibit additive toxicity with frovatriptan or other serotonin agonists (eg, antidepressants, dextromethorphan, tramadol) leading to serotonin syndrome.

Decreased Effect: The effects of frovatriptan may be decreased by CYP1A2 inducers (eg, carbamazepine, phenobarbital, phenytoin, ritonavir), ergotamine.

Ethanol/Nutrition/Herb Interactions Food: Food does not affect frovatriptan bioavailability.

Stability Store at room temperature of 25°C (77°F); protect from moisture and light.

Mechanism of Action Selective agonist for serotonin (5-HT$_{1B}$ and 5-HT$_{1D}$ receptor) in cranial arteries to cause vasoconstriction and reduces sterile inflammation associated with antidromic neuronal transmission correlating with relief of migraine.

Pharmacodynamics/Kinetics

Distribution: Male: 4.2 L/kg; Female: 3.0 L/kg

Protein binding: 15%

Metabolism: Primarily hepatic via CYP1A2 isoenzymes (forms metabolites)

Bioavailability: 20% to 30%

Half-life elimination: 26 hours

Time to peak: 2-4 hours

Excretion: Feces (62%); urine (32%)

Usual Dosage Oral: Adults: Migraine: 2.5 mg; if headache recurs, a second dose may be given if first dose provided some relief and at least 2 hours have elapsed since the first dose (maximum daily dose: 7.5 mg)

Dosage adjustment in renal impairment: No adjustment necessary

Dosage adjustment in hepatic impairment: No adjustment necessary in mild to moderate hepatic impairment; use with caution in severe impairment

Administration Take with fluids.

Patient Information Take at first sign of migraine attack. This drug is to be used to relieve your migraine, not to prevent or reduce number of attacks. If headache returns or is not fully resolved after first dose, the dose may be repeated after 2 hours. **Do not exceed 7.5 mg (3 tablets) in 24 hours.** Take tablet whole with fluids. **Do not take within 24 hours of any other migraine medication without first consulting prescriber.** You may experience some dizziness (use caution); hot flashes (cool room may help); nausea or vomiting (frequent small meals, frequent mouth care, sucking lozenges or chewing gum may help); or excess sweating (will resolve). Report chest tightness or pain; excessive drowsiness; acute abdominal pain; skin rash or burning sensation; muscle weakness, soreness, or numbness; or respiratory difficulty. Inform prescriber if you are or intend to become pregnant. Consult prescriber if breast-feeding.

Dosage Forms Tablet, as base: 2.5 mg

- ♦ **Frovatriptan Succinate** *see* Frovatriptan *on page 611*
- ♦ **Frusemide** *see* Furosemide *on page 612*
- ♦ **FS Shampoo® [DSC]** *see* Fluocinolone *on page 572*
- ♦ **5-FU** *see* Fluorouracil *on page 576*
- ♦ **Ful-Glo® Ophthalmic Strips** *see* Fluorescein Sodium *on page 573*
- ♦ **Fulvicin® P/G** *see* Griseofulvin *on page 644*
- ♦ **Fulvicin-U/F®** *see* Griseofulvin *on page 644*
- ♦ **Fungizone®** *see* Amphotericin B (Conventional) *on page 88*
- ♦ **Fungoid® Tincture [OTC]** *see* Miconazole *on page 908*
- ♦ **Furacin®** *see* Nitrofurazone *on page 988*
- ♦ **Furadantin®** *see* Nitrofurantoin *on page 987*
- ♦ **Furamide®** *see* Diloxanide Furoate *on page 409*

Furazolidone *(fyoor a ZOE li done)*

Related Information

Tyramine Content of Foods *on page 1737*

U.S. Brand Names Furoxone®

Canadian Brand Names Furoxone®

Therapeutic Category Antibiotic, Miscellaneous; Antidiarrheal; Antiprotozoal

Use Treatment of bacterial or protozoal diarrhea and enteritis caused by susceptible organisms *Giardia lamblia* and *Vibrio cholerae*

Pregnancy Risk Factor C

Usual Dosage Oral:

Children >1 month: 5-8 mg/kg/day in 4 divided doses for 7 days, not to exceed 400 mg/day or 8.8 mg/kg/day

Adults: 100 mg 4 times/day for 7 days

Additional Information Complete prescribing information for this medication should be consulted for additional detail.

Dosage Forms

Liquid: 50 mg/15 mL (60 mL, 473 mL)

Tablet: 100 mg

- ♦ **Furazosin** *see* Prazosin *on page 1120*

Furosemide *(fyoor OH se mide)*

Related Information

Adrenergic Agonists, Cardiovascular Comparison *on page 1469*

Adult ACLS Algorithms *on page 1632*

Heart Failure *on page 1663*

Sulfonamide Derivatives *on page 1515*
U.S. Brand Names Lasix®
Canadian Brand Names Apo®-Furosemide; Lasix®; Lasix® Special
Synonyms Frusemide
Therapeutic Category Antihypertensive Agent; Diuretic, Loop
Use Management of edema associated with congestive heart failure and hepatic or renal disease; alone or in combination with antihypertensives in treatment of hypertension
Pregnancy Risk Factor C
Pregnancy/Breast-Feeding Implications
Clinical effects on the fetus: Crosses the placenta. Increased fetal urine production, electrolyte disturbances reported. Generally, use of diuretics during pregnancy is avoided due to risk of decreased placental perfusion.
Breast-feeding/lactation: Crosses into breast milk; may suppress lactation. AAP has NO RECOMMENDATION.
Contraindications Hypersensitivity to furosemide, any component, or sulfonylureas; anuria; patients with hepatic coma or in states of severe electrolyte depletion until the condition improves or is corrected
Warnings/Precautions Loop diuretics are potent diuretics; close medical supervision and dose evaluation is required to prevent fluid and electrolyte imbalance; use caution with other nephrotoxic or ototoxic drugs; use caution in patients with known hypersensitivity to sulfonamides or thiazides (due to possible cross-sensitivity; avoid in history of severe reactions).

Chemical similarities are present among sulfonamides, sulfonylureas, carbonic anhydrase inhibitors, thiazides, and loop diuretics (except ethacrynic acid). Use in patients with sulfonylurea allergy is specifically contraindicated in product labeling, however a risk of cross-reaction exists in patients with allergy to any of these compounds; avoid use when previous reaction has been severe.
Adverse Reactions Frequency not defined.
Cardiovascular: Orthostatic hypotension, necrotizing angiitis, thrombophlebitis, chronic aortitis, acute hypotension, sudden death from cardiac arrest (with I.V. or I.M. administration)
Central nervous system: Paresthesias, vertigo, dizziness, lightheadedness, headache, blurred vision, xanthopsia, fever, restlessness
Dermatologic: Exfoliative dermatitis, erythema multiforme, purpura, photosensitivity, urticaria, rash, pruritus, cutaneous vasculitis
Endocrine & metabolic: Hyperglycemia, hyperuricemia, hypokalemia, hypochloremia, metabolic alkalosis, hypocalcemia, hypomagnesemia, gout, hypernatremia
Gastrointestinal: Nausea, vomiting, anorexia, oral and gastric irritation, cramping, diarrhea, constipation, pancreatitis, intrahepatic cholestatic jaundice, ischemia hepatitis
Genitourinary: Urinary bladder spasm, urinary frequency
Hematological: Aplastic anemia (rare), thrombocytopenia, agranulocytosis (rare), hemolytic anemia, leukopenia, anemia, purpura
Neuromuscular & skeletal: Muscle spasm, weakness
Otic: Hearing impairment (reversible or permanent with rapid I.V. or I.M. administration), tinnitus, reversible deafness (with rapid I.V. or I.M. administration)
Renal: Vasculitis, allergic interstitial nephritis, glycosuria, fall in glomerular filtration rate and renal blood flow (due to overdiuresis), transient rise in BUN
Miscellaneous: Anaphylaxis (rare), exacerbate or activate systemic lupus erythematosus
Overdosage/Toxicology Symptoms include electrolyte imbalance, volume depletion, hypotension, dehydration, hypokalemia and hypochloremic alkalosis. Following GI decontamination, treatment is supportive. Hypotension responds to fluids and Trendelenburg position.
Drug Interactions
Increased Effect/Toxicity: Furosemide-induced hypokalemia may predispose to digoxin toxicity and may increase the risk of arrhythmia with drugs which may prolong QT interval, including type Ia and type III antiarrhythmic agents, cisapride, terfenadine, and some quinolones (sparfloxacin, gatifloxacin, and moxifloxacin). The risk of toxicity from lithium and salicylates (high dose) may be increased by loop diuretics. Hypotensive effects and/or adverse renal effects of ACE inhibitors and NSAIDs are potentiated by furosemide-induced hypovolemia. The effects of peripheral adrenergic-blocking drugs or ganglionic blockers may be increased by furosemide.

Furosemide may increase the risk of ototoxicity with other ototoxic agents (aminoglycosides, cis-platinum), especially in patients with renal dysfunction. Synergistic diuretic effects occur with thiazide-type diuretics. Diuretics tend to be synergistic with other antihypertensive agents, and hypotension may occur.
Decreased Effect: Indomethacin, aspirin, phenobarbital, phenytoin, and NSAIDs may reduce natriuretic and hypotensive effects of furosemide. Colestipol, cholestyramine, and sucralfate may reduce the effect of furosemide; separate administration by 2 hours. Furosemide may antagonize the effect of skeletal muscle relaxants (tubocurarine). Glucose tolerance may be decreased by furosemide, requiring an adjustment in the dose of hypoglycemic agents. Metformin may decrease furosemide concentrations.
Ethanol/Nutrition/Herb Interactions
Food: Furosemide serum levels may be decreased if taken with food.
Herb/Nutraceutical: Avoid dong quai if using for hypertension (has estrogenic activity). Avoid ephedra, yohimbe, ginseng (may worsen hypertension). Limit intake of natural licorice. Avoid garlic (may have increased antihypertensive effect).
Stability
Furosemide injection should be stored at controlled room temperature and protected from light
Exposure to light may cause discoloration; do not use furosemide solutions if they have a yellow color
Refrigeration may result in precipitation or crystallization, however, resolubilization at room temperature or warming may be performed without affecting the drug's stability
Furosemide solutions are unstable in acidic media but very stable in basic media
I.V. infusion solution mixed in NS or D_5W solution is stable for 24 hours at room temperature
(Continued)

Furosemide *(Continued)*

Mechanism of Action Inhibits reabsorption of sodium and chloride in the ascending loop of Henle and distal renal tubule, interfering with the chloride-binding cotransport system, thus causing increased excretion of water, sodium, chloride, magnesium, and calcium

Pharmacodynamics/Kinetics

Onset of action: Diuresis: Oral: 30-60 minutes; I.M.: 30 minutes; I.V.: ~5 minutes
Peak effect: Oral: 1-2 hours
Duration: Oral: 6-8 hours; I.V.: 2 hours
Absorption: Oral: 60% to 67%
Protein binding: >98%
Metabolism: Minimally hepatic
Half-life elimination: Normal renal function: 0.5-1.1 hours; End-stage renal disease: 9 hours
Excretion: Urine (50% oral dose, 80% I.V. dose) within 24 hours; feces (as unchanged drug); nonrenal clearance increased in renal dysfunction

Usual Dosage

Infants and Children:

Oral: 1-2 mg/kg/dose increased in increments of 1 mg/kg/dose with each succeeding dose until a satisfactory effect is achieved to a maximum of 6 mg/kg/dose no more frequently than 6 hours.

I.M., I.V.: 1 mg/kg/dose, increasing by each succeeding dose at 1 mg/kg/dose at intervals of 6-12 hours until a satisfactory response up to 6 mg/kg/dose.

Adults:

Oral: 20-80 mg/dose initially increased in increments of 20-40 mg/dose at intervals of 6-8 hours; usual maintenance dose interval is twice daily or every day; may be titrated up to 600 mg/day with severe edematous states.

I.M., I.V.: 20-40 mg/dose, may be repeated in 1-2 hours as needed and increased by 20 mg/dose until the desired effect has been obtained. Usual dosing interval: 6-12 hours; for acute pulmonary edema, the usual dose is 40 mg I.V. over 1-2 minutes. If not adequate, may increase dose to 80 mg.

Continuous I.V. infusion: Initial I.V. bolus dose of 0.1 mg/kg followed by continuous I.V. infusion doses of 0.1 mg/kg/hour doubled every 2 hours to a maximum of 0.4 mg/kg/hour if urine output is <1 mL/kg/hour have been found to be effective and result in a lower daily requirement of furosemide than with intermittent dosing. Other studies have used a rate of ≤4 mg/minute as a continuous I.V. infusion.

Elderly: Oral, I.M., I.V.: Initial: 20 mg/day; increase slowly to desired response.

Refractory heart failure: Oral, I.V.: Doses up to 8 g/day have been used.

Dosing adjustment/comments in renal impairment: Acute renal failure: High doses (up to 1-3 g/day - oral/I.V.) have been used to initiate desired response; avoid use in oliguric states.

Dialysis: Not removed by hemo- or peritoneal dialysis; supplemental dose is not necessary.

Dosing adjustment/comments in hepatic disease: Diminished natriuretic effect with increased sensitivity to hypokalemia and volume depletion in cirrhosis; monitor effects, particularly with high doses.

Dietary Considerations This product may cause a potassium loss; your healthcare provider may prescribe a potassium supplement, another medication to help prevent the potassium loss, or recommend that you eat foods high in potassium, especially citrus fruits; do not change your diet on your own while taking this medication, especially if you are taking potassium supplements or medications to reduce potassium loss; too much potassium can be as harmful as too little; ideally, should be administered on an empty stomach; however, may be administered with food or milk if GI distress; do not mix with acidic solutions.

Administration I.V. injections should be given slowly over 1-2 minutes; maximum rate of administration for IVPB or infusion: 4 mg/minute; replace parenteral therapy with oral therapy as soon as possible

Monitoring Parameters Monitor weight and I & O daily; blood pressure, serum electrolytes, renal function; in high doses, monitor hearing

Patient Information May be taken with food or milk; rise slowly from a lying or sitting position to minimize dizziness, lightheadedness, or fainting; also use extra care when exercising, standing for long periods of time, and during hot weather; take last dose of day early in the evening to prevent nocturia

Nursing Implications I.V. injections should be administered slowly over 1-2 minutes; replace parenteral therapy with oral therapy as soon as possible; for continuous infusion furosemide in patients with severely impaired renal function, do not exceed 4 mg/minute; be alert to complaints about hearing difficulty; check the patient for orthostasis; may be administered undiluted direct I.V. at a maximum rate of 0.5 mg/kg/minute for doses <120 mg and 4 mg/minute for doses >120 mg; may also be diluted for infusion 1-2 mg/mL (maximum: 10 mg/mL) over 10-15 minutes (following maximum rate as above)

Additional Information Sodium content of 1 mL (injection): 0.162 mEq

Dosage Forms

Injection: 10 mg/mL (2 mL, 4 mL, 5 mL, 6 mL, 8 mL, 10 mL, 12 mL)
Solution, oral: 10 mg/mL (60 mL, 120 mL); 40 mg/5 mL (5 mL, 10 mL, 500 mL)
Tablet: 20 mg, 40 mg, 80 mg

♦ **Furoxone®** *see* Furazolidone *on page 612*

♦ **G-1®** *see* Butalbital Compound *on page 197*

Gabapentin *(GA ba pen tin)*

Related Information

Anticonvulsants by Seizure Type *on page 1481*
Epilepsy & Seizure Treatment *on page 1659*

U.S. Brand Names Neurontin®

Canadian Brand Names Neurontin™

Therapeutic Category Anticonvulsant

Use Adjunct for treatment of partial seizures with and without secondary generalized seizures in patients >12 years of age with epilepsy; adjunct for treatment of partial seizures in pediatric patients 3-12 years of age

Unlabeled/Investigational Use Bipolar disorder, chronic pain, social phobia

Pregnancy Risk Factor C

Pregnancy/Breast-Feeding Implications Clinical effects on the fetus: No data on crossing the placenta; there have been reports of normal pregnancy outcomes, as well as respiratory distress, pyloric stenosis, and inguinal hernia following 1st trimester exposure to gabapentin plus carbamazepine; epilepsy itself, number of medications, genetic factors, or a combination of these probably influence the teratogenicity of anticonvulsant therapy. Use during pregnancy only if the potential benefit to the mother outweighs the potential risk to the fetus. Gabapentin is excreted in human breast milk. A nursed infant could be exposed to ~1 mg/kg/day of gabapentin; the effect on the child is not known. Use in breast-feeding women only if the benefits to the mother outweigh the potential risk to the infant.

Contraindications Hypersensitivity to gabapentin or any component of the formulation

Warnings/Precautions Avoid abrupt withdrawal, may precipitate seizures; may be associated with a slight incidence (0.6%) of status epilepticus and sudden deaths (0.0038 deaths/patient year); use cautiously in patients with severe renal dysfunction; rat studies demonstrated an association with pancreatic adenocarcinoma in male rats; clinical implication unknown. May cause CNS depression, which may impair physical or mental abilities. Patients must be cautioned about performing tasks which require mental alertness (ie, operating machinery or driving). Effects with other sedative drugs or ethanol may be potentiated. Pediatric patients (3-12 years of age) have shown increased incidence of CNS-related adverse effects, including emotional lability, hostility, thought disorder, and hyperkinesia. Safety and efficacy in children <3 years of age have not been established.

Adverse Reactions As reported in patients >12 years of age, unless otherwise noted

>10%:
    Central nervous system: Somnolence (20%), dizziness (17%), ataxia (12%), fatigue (11% in adults)
    Miscellaneous: Viral infection (11% in children 3-12 years)

1% to 10%:
    Cardiovascular: Peripheral edema (2%)
    Central nervous system: Fever (10% in children 3-12 years), hostility (8% in children 3-12 years), somnolence (8% in children 3-12 years), emotional lability (4% to 6% in children 3-12 years), fatigue (3% in children 3-12 years), abnormal thinking (2% in children and adults), amnesia (2%), depression (2%), dizziness (2% in children 3-12 years), dysarthria (2%), nervousness (2%), abnormal coordination (1%), twitching (1%)
    Dermatologic: Pruritus (1%)
    Gastrointestinal: Nausea/vomiting (8% in children 3-12 years), weight gain (3% in adults and children), dyspepsia (2%), dry throat (2%), xerostomia (2%), appetite stimulation (1%), constipation (1%), dental abnormalities (1%)
    Genitourinary: Impotence (1%)
    Hematologic: Leukopenia (1%), decreased WBC (1%)
    Neuromuscular & skeletal: Tremor (7%), hyperkinesia (3% to 5% in children 3-12 years), back pain (2%), myalgia (2%)
    Ocular: Nystagmus (8%), diplopia (6%), blurred vision (4%)
    Respiratory: Rhinitis (4%), bronchitis (3% in children 3-12 years), pharyngitis (3%), coughing (2%), respiratory infection (2% in children 3-12 years)

<1% (Limited to important or life-threatening): Allergy, alopecia, angina pectoris, angioedema, erythema multiforme, ethanol intolerance, hepatitis, hyperlipidemia, hypertension, hyponatremia, intracranial hemorrhage, jaundice, new tumor formation/worsening of existing tumors, pancreatitis, peripheral vascular disorder, pneumonia, purpura, Stevens-Johnson syndrome, subdural hematoma, vertigo

Overdosage/Toxicology Acute oral overdoses up to 49 g have been reported; double vision, slurred speech, drowsiness, lethargy, and diarrhea were observed. Patients recovered with supportive care. Decontaminate using lavage/activated charcoal with cathartic. Multiple dosing of activated charcoal may be useful. Hemodialysis may be useful.

Drug Interactions

    Increased Effect/Toxicity: Cimetidine may increased gabapentin levels. Gabapentin may increase peak concentrations of norethindrone.

    Decreased Effect: Gabapentin does not modify plasma concentrations of standard anticonvulsant medications (eg, valproic acid, carbamazepine, phenytoin, or phenobarbital). Antacids reduce the bioavailability of gabapentin by 20%.

Ethanol/Nutrition/Herb Interactions

    Ethanol: Avoid ethanol (may increase CNS depression).
    Food: Does not change rate or extent of absorption.
    Herb/Nutraceutical: Avoid evening primrose (seizure threshold decreased). Avoid valerian, St John's wort, kava kava, gotu kola (may increase CNS depression).

Stability Store capsules and tablets at controlled room temperature. Oral solution should be stored under refrigeration, 2°C to 8°C (59°F to 86°F).

Mechanism of Action Exact mechanism of action is not known, but does have properties in common with other anticonvulsants; although structurally related to GABA, it does not interact with GABA receptors

Pharmacodynamics/Kinetics

    Absorption: 50% to 60%
    Distribution: V_d: 0.6-0.8 L/kg
    Protein binding: <3%
    Half-life elimination: 5-7 hours
    Excretion: Urine (56% to 80%)

Usual Dosage Oral:

    Children: Anticonvulsant:
        3-12 years: Initial: 10-15 mg/kg/day in 3 divided doses; titrate to effective dose over ~3 days; dosages of up to 50 mg/kg/day have been tolerated in clinical studies
        3-4 years: Effective dose: 40 mg/kg/day in 3 divided doses

(Continued)

Gabapentin *(Continued)*

≥5-12 years: Effective dose: 25-35 mg/kg/day in 3 divided doses
Note: If gabapentin is discontinued or if another anticonvulsant is added to therapy, it should be done slowly over a minimum of 1 week
Children >12 years and Adults:
Anticonvulsant: Initial: 300 mg 3 times/day; if necessary the dose may be increased using 300 mg or 400 mg capsules 3 times/day up to 1800 mg/day
Dosage range: 900-1800 mg administered in 3 divided doses at 8-hour intervals
Pain (unlabeled use): 300-1800 mg/day given in 3 divided doses has been the most common dosage range
Bipolar disorder (unlabeled use): 300-3000 mg/day given in 3 divided doses; **Note:** Does not appear to be effective as an adjunctive treatment for bipolar disorder (Pande AC, 2000)

Elderly: Studies in elderly patients have shown a decrease in clearance as age increases. This is most likely due to age-related decreases in renal function; dose reductions may be needed.

Dosing adjustment in renal impairment: Children ≥12 years and Adults:
Cl_{cr} >60 mL/minute: Administer 1200 mg/day (400 mg 3 times/day)
Cl_{cr} 30-60 mL/minute: Administer 600 mg/day (300 mg 2 times/day)
Cl_{cr} 15-30 mL/minute: Administer 300 mg/day (300 mg/day)
Cl_{cr} <15 mL/minute: Administer 150 mg/day (300 mg every other day)
Hemodialysis: 200-300 mg after each 4-hour dialysis following a loading dose of 300-400 mg
Dietary Considerations May take without regard to meals.
Administration Maximum time interval between multiple daily doses should not exceed 12 hours; administer first dose on first day at bedtime to avoid somnolence and dizziness
Monitoring Parameters Monitor serum levels of concomitant anticonvulsant therapy
Reference Range Minimum effective serum concentration may be 2 µg/mL
Test Interactions False positives have been reported with the Ames N-Multistix SG® dipstick test for urine protein
Patient Information Take only as prescribed; may cause dizziness, somnolence, and other symptoms and signs of CNS depression; do not operate machinery or drive a car until you have experience with the drug; may be administered without regard to meals. Do not stop making medication abruptly; may lead to an increased seizure activity.
Dosage Forms
Capsule: 100 mg, 300 mg, 400 mg
Solution, oral: 250 mg/5 mL
Tablet: 600 mg, 800 mg
Extemporaneous Preparations A 100 mg/mL suspension was stable for 91 days when refrigerated or 56 days when kept at room temperature when compounded as follows:
Triturate sixty-seven 300 mg tablets in a mortar, reduce to a fine powder, then add a small amount of one of the following vehicles to make a paste; then add the remaining vehicle in small quantities while mixing:
Vehicle 1. Methylcellulose 1% (100 mL) and Simple Syrup N.F. (100 mL) mixed together in a graduate, **or**
Vehicle 2. Ora-Sweet® (100 mL) and Ora-Plus® (100 mL) mixed together in a graduate
Shake well before using and keep in refrigerator

Nahata MC, Morosco RS, and Hipple TF, *Stability of Gabapentin in Extemporaneously Prepared Suspensions at Two Temperatures*, American Society of Health System Pharmacists Midyear Meeting, December 7-11, 1997.

♦ **Gabitril**® *see Tiagabine on page 1328*

Galantamine *(ga LAN ta meen)*
U.S. Brand Names Reminyl®
Synonyms Galantamine Hydrobromide
Therapeutic Category Acetylcholinesterase Inhibitor
Use Treatment of mild to moderate dementia of Alzheimer's disease
Pregnancy Risk Factor B
Pregnancy/Breast-Feeding Implications In animal studies, there was a slight increased in the incident of skeletal variations when given during organogenesis. Adequate, well-controlled studies in pregnant women do not exist. Should be used in pregnancy only if benefit outweighs potential risk to the fetus. Excretion in breast milk unknown/not recommended.
Contraindications Hypersensitivity to galantamine or any component of the formulation; severe liver dysfunction (Child-Pugh score 10-15); severe renal dysfunction (Cl_{cr} <9 mL/minute)
Warnings/Precautions Use caution in patients with supraventricular conduction delays (without a functional pacemaker in place) or patients taking medicines that slow conduction through SA or AV node. Use caution in peptic ulcer disease(or in patients at risk); seizure disorder; asthma; COPD; mild to moderate liver dysfunction; moderate renal dysfunction. May cause bladder outflow obstruction. May exaggerate neuromuscular blockade effects of succinylcholine and like agents. Safety and efficacy in children have not been established.
Adverse Reactions
>10%: Gastrointestinal: Nausea (6% to 24%), vomiting (4% to 13%), diarrhea (6% to 12%)
1% to 10%:
Cardiovascular: Bradycardia (2% to 3%), syncope (0.4% to 2.2%: dose-related), chest pain (≥1%)
Central nervous system: Dizziness (9%), headache (8%), depression (7%), fatigue (5%), insomnia (5%), somnolence (4%), tremor (3%)
Gastrointestinal: Anorexia (7% to 9%), weight loss (5% to 7%), abdominal pain (5%), dyspepsia (5%), flatulence (≥1%)
Genitourinary: Urinary tract infection (8%), hematuria (<1% to 3%), incontinence (≥1%)

Hematologic: Anemia (3%)

Respiratory: Rhinitis (4%)

<1% (Limited to important or life-threatening): Alkaline phosphatase increased, aphasia, apraxia, ataxia, atrial fibrillation, AV block, bundle branch block, convulsions, delirium, diverticulitis, dysphagia, epistaxis, esophageal perforation, heart failure, hypokinesia, hypotension, melena, palpitations, paranoid reaction, paresthesia, paroniria, postural hypotension, purpura, QT prolongation, rectal hemorrhage, renal calculi, supraventricular tachycardia, T-wave inversion, thrombocytopenia, ventricular tachycardia, vertigo

Overdosage/Toxicology Symptoms may include bradycardia, collapse, convulsions, defecation, gastrointestinal cramping, hypotension, lacrimation, muscle fasciculations, muscle weakness, respiratory depression, salivation, severe nausea, sweating, urination, and vomiting. Treatment is symptom directed and supportive. Atropine may be used as an antidote with an initial dose of 0.5-1 mg I.V., titrated to effect. An atypical response in blood pressure and heart rate has been reported. Effects of hemodialysis are unknown.

Drug Interactions

Cytochrome P450 Effect: CYP3A4, CYP2D6 enyzme substrates

Increased Effect/Toxicity: Succinylcholine: increased neuromuscular blockade. Amiodarone, beta-blockers without ISA activity, diltiazem, verapamil may increase bradycardia. NSAIDs increase risk of peptic ulcer. Cimetidine, ketoconazole, paroxetine, other CYP3A4 inhibitors, other CYP2D6 inhibitors increase levels of galantamine. Concurrent cholinergic agents may have synergistic effects. Digoxin may lead to AV block.

Decreased Effect: Anticholinergic agents are antagonized by galantamine. CYP inducers may decrease galantamine levels.

Ethanol/Nutrition/Herb Interactions

Ethanol: Avoid ethanol (may increase CNS adverse events).

Herb/Nutraceutical: St John's wort may decrease galantamine serum levels; avoid concurrent use.

Stability Store at 15°C to 30°C (59°F to 86°F). Do not freeze oral solution; protect from light.

Mechanism of Action Centrally-acting cholinesterase inhibitor (competitive and reversible). It elevates acetylcholine in cerebral cortex by slowing the degradation of acetylcholine. Modulates nicotinic acetylcholine receptor to increase acetylcholine from surviving presynaptic nerve terminals. May increase glutamate and serotonin levels.

Pharmacodynamics/Kinetics

Duration: Maximum inhibition of erythrocyte acetylcholinesterase ~40% at 1 hour post 10 mg oral dose; levels return to baseline at 30 hour

Absorption: Rapid and complete

Distribution: V_d 1.8-2.6 L/kg

Protein binding: 18%

Metabolism: Hepatic; linear, CYP2D6 and 3A4; metabolized to epigalanthaminone and galanthaminone both of which have acetylcholinesterase inhibitory activity 130 times less than galantamine

Bioavailability: 90%

Half-life elimination: 7 hours

Time to peak: 1 hour

Excretion: Urine (95%, 20% to 32% as unchanged drug and metabolites); feces (5%)

Usual Dosage Note: Take with breakfast and dinner. If therapy is interrupted for ≥3 days, restart at the lowest dose and increase to current dose.

Oral: Adults: Mild to moderate dementia of Alzheimer's: Initial: 4 mg twice a day for 4 weeks

If 8 mg per day tolerated, increase to 8 mg twice daily for ≥4 weeks

If 16 mg per day tolerated, increase to 12 mg twice daily

Range: 16-24 mg/day in 2 divided doses

Elderly: No dosage adjustment needed

Dosage adjustment in renal impairment:

Moderate renal impairment: Maximum dose: 16 mg/day.

Severe renal dysfunction (Cl_{cr} <9 mL/minute): Use is not recommended

Dosage adjustment in hepatic impairment:

Moderate liver dysfunction (Child-Pugh score 7-9): Maximum dose: 16 mg/day

Severe liver dysfunction (Child-Pugh score 10-15): Use is not recommended

Dietary Considerations Take with breakfast and dinner.

Administration Take with breakfast and dinner. If therapy is interrupted for ≥3 days, restart at the lowest dose and increase to current dose. If using oral solution, mix dose with 3-4 ounces of any nonalcoholic beverage; mix well and drink immediately.

Monitoring Parameters Mental status

Patient Information This medication will not cure Alzheimer's disease, but may help reduce symptoms. Use exactly as directed; do not increase dose or discontinue without consulting prescriber. Maintain adequate hydration (2-3 L/day) unless instructed to restrict fluids. May cause dizziness, sedation, hypotension, or tremor (use caution when driving or engaging in hazardous tasks, rise slowly from sitting or lying position, and use caution when climbing stairs until response to drug is known); diarrhea (boiled milk, yogurt, or buttermilk may help); or nausea or vomiting (frequent small meals, good mouth care, sucking lozenges, or chewing gum may help). Report persistent gastrointestinal disturbances; significantly increased salivation, sweating, or tearing; excessive fatigue, insomnia, dizziness, or depression; increased muscle, joint, or body pain or spasms; vision changes; respiratory changes, wheezing, or signs of dyspnea; chest pain or palpitations; or other adverse reactions.

Nursing Implications Have patient take with breakfast and dinner. If therapy is interrupted for ≥3 days, restart at the lowest dose and increase to current dose as per patient tolerance.

Dosage Forms

Solution, oral, as hydrobromide: 4 mg/mL (100 mL) [with calibrated pipette]

Tablet, as hydrobromide: 4 mg, 8 mg, 12 mg

◆ **Galantamine Hydrobromide** *see Galantamine on page 616*

Gallium Nitrate (GAL ee um NYE trate)

U.S. Brand Names Ganite™

Therapeutic Category Antidote, Hypercalcemia

Use Treatment of clearly symptomatic cancer-related hypercalcemia that has not responded to adequate hydration

Pregnancy Risk Factor C

Contraindications Hypersensitivity to any component of the formulation; serum creatinine >2.5 mg/dL

Warnings/Precautions Safety and efficacy in children have not been established. Concurrent use of gallium nitrate with other potentially nephrotoxic drugs may increase the risk for developing severe renal insufficiency in patients with cancer-related hypercalcemia; use with caution in patients with impaired renal function or dehydration

Adverse Reactions

>10%:

Endocrine & metabolic: Hypophosphatemia

Gastrointestinal: Nausea, vomiting, diarrhea, metallic taste

Renal: Renal toxicity

1% to 10%: Endocrine & metabolic: Hypocalcemia

<1% (Limited to important or life-threatening): Anemia, hearing impairment, optic neuritis

Overdosage/Toxicology Symptoms include nausea, vomiting, renal failure, hypocalcemia, and tetany. Treatment consists of supportive measures to ensure adequate hydration and use of calcium salts for hypocalcemia.

Drug Interactions

Increased Effect/Toxicity: Nephrotoxic drugs (eg, aminoglycosides, amphotericin B)

Stability Store at room temperature of 15°C to 30°C (59°F to 86°F); when diluted in NS or D_5W, stable for 48 hours at room temperature or 7 days under refrigeration at 2°C to 8°C (36°F to 46°F)

Mechanism of Action Primarily via inhibition of bone resorption with associated reduction in urinary calcium excretion. Gallium has increased the calcium content of newly mineralized bone following short-term treatment *in vitro*, and this effect combined with its ability to inhibit bone resorption has suggested the use of gallium for other disorders associated with increased bone loss.

Pharmacodynamics/Kinetics

Metabolism: None

Half-life elimination: Terminal: 25-111 hours

Excretion: Urine (≤70%)

Usual Dosage Adults:

I.V. infusion (over 24 hours): 200 mg/m² for 5 consecutive days in 1 L of NS or D_5W

Mild hypercalcemia/few symptoms: 100 mg/m²/day for 5 days in 1 L of NS or D_5W

Dosing adjustment/comments in renal impairment: Cl_{cr} <30 mL/minute: Avoid use

Monitoring Parameters Serum creatinine, BUN, and calcium

Reference Range Steady-state gallium serum levels: Generally obtained within 2 days following initiation of continuous I.V. infusions of gallium nitrate

Nursing Implications Patients should have adequate I.V. hydration, serum creatinine levels should be monitored during gallium nitrate therapy

Dosage Forms Injection: 25 mg/mL (20 mL)

♦ Gamimune® N *see* Immune Globulin (Intravenous) *on page 711*

♦ Gamma Benzene Hexachloride *see* Lindane *on page 806*

♦ Gammagard® *see* Immune Globulin (Intravenous) *on page 711*

♦ Gammagard® S/D *see* Immune Globulin (Intravenous) *on page 711*

♦ Gamma Globulin *see* Immune Globulin (Intramuscular) *on page 710*

♦ Gammaphos *see* Amifostine *on page 67*

♦ Gammar®-P I.V. *see* Immune Globulin (Intravenous) *on page 711*

Ganciclovir (gan SYE kloe veer)

Related Information

USPHA/IDSA Guidelines for the Prevention of Opportunistic Infections in Persons With HIV *on page 1574*

U.S. Brand Names Cytovene®; Vitrasert®

Canadian Brand Names Cytovene®; Vitrasert®

Synonyms DHPG Sodium; GCV Sodium; Nordeoxyguanosine

Therapeutic Category Antiviral Agent, Nonantiretroviral; Antiviral Agent, Parenteral

Use

Parenteral: Treatment of CMV retinitis in immunocompromised individuals, including patients with acquired immunodeficiency syndrome; prophylaxis of CMV infection in transplant patients; may be given in combination with foscarnet in patients who relapse after monotherapy with either drug

Oral: Alternative to the I.V. formulation for maintenance treatment of CMV retinitis in immunocompromised patients, including patients with AIDS, in whom retinitis is stable following appropriate induction therapy and for whom the risk of more rapid progression is balanced by the benefit associated with avoiding daily I.V. infusions.

Implant: Treatment of CMV retinitis

Pregnancy Risk Factor C

Contraindications Hypersensitivity to ganciclovir, acyclovir, or any component of the formulation; absolute neutrophil count <500/mm³; platelet count <25,000/mm³

Warnings/Precautions Dosage adjustment or interruption of ganciclovir therapy may be necessary in patients with neutropenia and/or thrombocytopenia and patients with impaired renal function. Use with extreme caution in children since long-term safety has not been determined and due to ganciclovir's potential for long-term carcinogenic and adverse reproductive effects; ganciclovir may adversely affect spermatogenesis and fertility; due to its mutagenic potential, contraceptive precautions for female and male patients need to be followed during and for at least 90 days after therapy with the drug; take care to administer only into veins with good blood flow.

Adverse Reactions

>10%:
  Central nervous system: Fever (38% to 48%)
  Dermatologic: Rash (15% oral, 10% I.V.)
  Gastrointestinal: Abdominal pain (17% to 19%), diarrhea (40%), nausea (25%), anorexia (15%), vomiting (13%)
  Hematologic: Anemia (20% to 25%), leukopenia (30% to 40%)

1% to 10%:
  Central nervous system: Confusion, neuropathy (8% to 9%), headache (4%)
  Dermatologic: Pruritus (5%)
  Hematologic: Thrombocytopenia (6%), neutropenia with ANC <500/mm^3 (5% oral, 14% I.V.)
  Neuromuscular & skeletal: Paresthesia (6% to 10%), weakness (6%)
  Ocular: Retinal detachment (8% oral, 11% I.V.; relationship to ganciclovir not established)
  Miscellaneous: Sepsis (4% oral, 15% I.V.)

<1% (Limited to important or life-threatening): Alopecia, arrhythmia, ataxia, bronchospasm, coma, dyspnea, encephalopathy, eosinophilia, exfoliative dermatitis, extrapyramidal symptoms, hemorrhage, nervousness, pancytopenia, psychosis, renal failure, seizures, SIADH, Stevens-Johnson syndrome, torsade de pointes, urticaria, visual loss

Overdosage/Toxicology Symptoms include neutropenia, vomiting, hypersalivation, bloody diarrhea, cytopenia, and testicular atrophy. Treatment is supportive. Hemodialysis removes 50% of drug. Hydration may be of some benefit.

Drug Interactions

Increased Effect/Toxicity: Immunosuppressive agents may increase hematologic toxicity of ganciclovir. Imipenem/cilastatin may increase seizure potential. Oral ganciclovir increases blood levels of zidovudine, although zidovudine decreases steady-state levels of ganciclovir. Since both drugs have the potential to cause neutropenia and anemia, some patients may not tolerate concomitant therapy with these drugs at full dosage. Didanosine levels are increased with concurrent ganciclovir. Other nephrotoxic drugs (eg, amphotericin and cyclosporine) may have additive nephrotoxicity with ganciclovir.

Decreased Effect: A decrease in blood levels of ganciclovir AUC may occur when used with didanosine.

Stability

Preparation should take place in a vertical laminar flow hood with the same precautions as antineoplastic agents

Intact vials should be stored at room temperature and protected from temperatures >40°C

Reconstitute powder with sterile water **not** bacteriostatic water because parabens may cause precipitation

Reconstituted solution is stable for 12 hours at room temperature, however, conflicting data indicates that reconstituted solution is stable for 60 days under refrigeration (4°C)

Drug product should be reconstituted immediately before use and any unused portion should be discarded

Stability of parenteral admixture at room temperature (25°C) and at refrigeration temperature (4°C): 5 days

Mechanism of Action Ganciclovir is phosphorylated to a substrate which competitively inhibits the binding of deoxyguanosine triphosphate to DNA polymerase resulting in inhibition of viral DNA synthesis

Pharmacodynamics/Kinetics

Bioavailability: Oral: Fasting: 5%; Following food: 6% to 9%; Following fatty meal: 28% to 31%

Distribution: V_d: 15.26 L/1.73 m^2; widely to all tissues including CSF and ocular tissue

Protein binding: 1% to 2%

Half-life elimination: 1.7-5.8 hours; increases with impaired renal function; End-stage renal disease: 5-28 hours

Excretion: Urine (80% to 99% as unchanged drug)

Usual Dosage

CMV retinitis: Slow I.V. infusion (dosing is based on total body weight):
  Children >3 months and Adults:
    Induction therapy: 5 mg/kg/dose every 12 hours for 14-21 days followed by maintenance therapy
    Maintenance therapy: 5 mg/kg/day as a single daily dose for 7 days/week or 6 mg/kg/day for 5 days/week

CMV retinitis: Oral: 1000 mg 3 times/day with food **or** 500 mg 6 times/day with food

Prevention of CMV disease in patients with advanced HIV infection and normal renal function: Oral: 1000 mg 3 times/day with food

Prevention of CMV disease in transplant patients: Same initial and maintenance dose as CMV retinitis except duration of initial course is 7-14 days, duration of maintenance therapy is dependent on clinical condition and degree of immunosuppression

Intravitreal implant: One implant for 5- to 8-month period; following depletion of ganciclovir, as evidenced by progression of retinitis, implant may be removed and replaced

Elderly: Refer to adult dosing; in general, dose selection should be cautious, reflecting greater frequency of organ impairment

Dosing adjustment in renal impairment:

I.V. (Induction):
  Cl_{cr} 50-69 mL/minute: Administer 2.5 mg/kg/dose every 12 hours
  Cl_{cr} 25-49 mL/minute: Administer 2.5 mg/kg/dose every 24 hours
  Cl_{cr} 10-24 mL/minute: Administer 1.25 mg/kg/dose every 24 hours
  Cl_{cr} <10 mL/minute: Administer 1.25 mg/kg/dose 3 times/week following hemodialysis

I.V. (Maintenance):
  Cl_{cr} 50-69 mL/minute: Administer 2.5 mg/kg/dose every 24 hours
  Cl_{cr} 25-49 mL/minute: Administer 1.25 mg/kg/dose every 24 hours
  Cl_{cr} 10-24 mL/minute: Administer 0.625 mg/kg/dose every 24 hours

(Continued)

Ganciclovir (Continued)

Cl_{cr} <10 mL/minute: Administer 0.625 mg/kg/dose 3 times/week following hemodialysis
Oral:
Cl_{cr} 50-69 mL/minute: Administer 1500 mg/day or 500 mg 3 times/day
Cl_{cr} 25-49 mL/minute: Administer 1000 mg/day or 500 mg twice daily
Cl_{cr} 10-24 mL/minute: Administer 500 mg/day
Cl_{cr} <10 mL/minute: Administer 500 mg 3 times/week following hemodialysis

Hemodialysis effects: Dialyzable (50%) following hemodialysis; administer dose postdialysis. During peritoneal dialysis, dose as for Cl_{cr} <10 mL/minute. During continuous arteriovenous or venovenous hemofiltration, administer 2.5 mg/kg/dose every 24 hours.

Dietary Considerations Sodium content of 500 mg vial: 46 mg

Administration The same precautions utilized with antineoplastic agents should be followed with ganciclovir administration. Ganciclovir should not be administered by I.M., S.C., or rapid IVP administration; administer by slow I.V. infusion over at least 1 hour at a final concentration for administration not to exceed 10 mg/mL. Oral ganciclovir should be administered with food.

Monitoring Parameters CBC with differential and platelet count, serum creatinine, ophthalmologic exams

Patient Information Ganciclovir is not a cure for CMV retinitis; regular ophthalmologic examinations should be done; close monitoring of blood counts should be done while on therapy and dosage adjustments may need to be made; take with food to increase absorption

Nursing Implications Must be prepared in vertical flow hood; use chemotherapy precautions during administration; discard appropriately

Dosage Forms
Capsule: 250 mg, 500 mg
Implant, intravitreal: 4.5 mg [released gradually over 5-8 months]
Powder for injection, lyophilized, as sodium: 500 mg (10 mL)

Ganirelix (ga ni REL ix)

U.S. Brand Names Antagon®
Canadian Brand Names Antagon®
Synonyms Ganirelix Acetate
Therapeutic Category Antigonadotropic Agent
Use Inhibits premature luteinizing hormone (LH) surges in women undergoing controlled ovarian hyperstimulation in fertility clinics.
Pregnancy Risk Factor X
Pregnancy/Breast-Feeding Implications Fetal resorption occurred in pregnant rats and rabbits. These effects are results of hormonal alterations and could result in fetal loss in humans. The drug should not be used in pregnant women. Breast-feeding is not recommended.
Contraindications Hypersensitivity of ganirelix or any component of the formulation; hypersensitivity to gonadotropin-releasing hormone or any other analog; known or suspected pregnancy
Warnings/Precautions Should only be prescribed by fertility specialists. The packaging contains natural rubber latex (may cause allergic reactions). Pregnancy must be excluded before starting medication.
Adverse Reactions
1% to 10%:
Central nervous system: Headache (3%)
Endocrine & metabolic: Ovarian hyperstimulation syndrome (2%)
Gastrointestinal: Abdominal pain (5%), nausea (1%), and abdominal pain (1%)
Genitourinary: Vaginal bleeding (2%)
Local: Injection site reaction (1%)
<1% (Limited to important or life-threatening): Congenital abnormalities
Overdosage/Toxicology No reports of human overdosage.
Drug Interactions
Increased Effect/Toxicity: No formal studies have been performed.
Decreased Effect: No formal studies have been performed.
Stability Store at controlled room temperature of 15°C to 30°C (59°F to 86°F)
Mechanism of Action Competitively blocks the gonadotropin-release hormone receptors on the pituitary gonadotroph and transduction pathway. This suppresses gonadotropin secretion and luteinizing hormone secretion preventing ovulation until the follicles are of adequate size.
Pharmacodynamics/Kinetics
Absorption: S.C.: Rapid
Distribution: Mean V_d: 43.7 L
Protein binding: 81.9%
Metabolism: Hepatic, to two primary metabolites (1-4 and 1-6 peptide)
Bioavailability: 91.1%
Half-life elimination: 16.2 hours
Time to peak: 1.1 hours
Excretion: Feces (75%) within 288 hours; urine (22%) within 24 hours
Usual Dosage Adult: S.C.: 250 mcg/day during the mid-to-late phase after initiating follicle-stimulating hormone on day 2 or 3 of cycle. Treatment should be continued daily until the day of chorionic gonadotropin administration.
Monitoring Parameters Ultrasound to assess the follicle's size
Patient Information Nurse to teach how to administer S.C. injections. Give at a similar time daily as instructed by fertility clinic. Do not skip doses. Keep all ultrasound appointments. Report any sudden weight gain, abdominal discomfort, or shortness of breath to clinic. Do not take if pregnant.
Nursing Implications Teach patient/spouse to give S.C. injections. Discuss ultrasound schedule and timing of other medications used.

Dosage Forms Injection [prefilled glass syringe]: 250 mcg/0.5 mL (with 27-gauge x ½ inch needle)

- ◆ **Ganirelix Acetate** *see* Ganirelix *on page 620*
- ◆ **Ganite™** *see* Gallium Nitrate *on page 618*
- ◆ **Gantanol®** *see* Sulfamethoxazole *on page 1272*
- ◆ **Gantrisin®** *see* SulfiSOXAZOLE *on page 1277*
- ◆ **Garamycin®** *see* Gentamicin *on page 627*
- ◆ **Garatec (Can)** *see* Gentamicin *on page 627*
- ◆ **Gastrocrom®** *see* Cromolyn Sodium *on page 337*

Gatifloxacin (gat i FLOKS a sin)

Related Information
Antacid Drug Interactions *on page 1477*
Antimicrobial Drugs of Choice *on page 1588*
Community-Acquired Pneumonia in Adults *on page 1603*

U.S. Brand Names Tequin®
Canadian Brand Names Tequin®
Therapeutic Category Antibiotic, Quinolone
Use Treatment of the following infections when caused by susceptible bacteria: Acute bacterial exacerbation of chronic bronchitis due to *S. pneumoniae, H. influenzae, H. parainfluenzae, M. catarrhalis,* or *S. aureus*; acute sinusitis due to *S. pneumoniae, H. influenzae*; community acquired pneumonia due to *S. pneumoniae, H. influenzae, H. parainfluenzae, M. catarrhalis, S. aureus, M. pneumoniae, C. pneumoniae,* or *L. pneumophilia*; uncomplicated urinary tract infections (cystitis) due to *E. coli, K. pneumoniae,* or *P. mirabilis*; complicated urinary tract infections due to *E. coli, K. pneumoniae,* or *P. mirabilis*; pyelonephritis due to *E. coli*; uncomplicated urethral and cervical gonorrhea; acute, uncomplicated rectal infections in women due to *N. gonorrhoeae*
Pregnancy Risk Factor C
Pregnancy/Breast-Feeding Implications No adequate or well-controlled studies in pregnant women. Should be used during pregnancy only when the potential benefit justifies the potential risk to the fetus.
Contraindications Hypersensitivity to gatifloxacin, other quinolone antibiotics, or any component of the formulation; known prolongation of QT interval, uncorrected hypokalemia, or concurrent administration of other medications known to prolong the QT interval (including Class Ia and Class III antiarrhythmics, cisapride, erythromycin, antipsychotics, and tricyclic antidepressants)
Warnings/Precautions Use with caution in patients with significant bradycardia or acute myocardial ischemia. May have potential to prolong QT interval; should avoid in patients with uncorrected hypokalemia, or concurrent administration of other medications known to prolong the QT interval (including class Ia and class III antiarrhythmics, cisapride, erythromycin, antipsychotics, and tricyclic antidepressants). Safety and effectiveness in pediatric patients (<18 years of age) have not been established. Experience in immature animals has resulted in permanent arthropathy. May cause increased CNS stimulation, increased intracranial pressure, convulsions, or psychosis. Use with caution in individuals at risk of seizures. Discontinue in patients who experience significant CNS adverse effects. Use caution in renal dysfunction (dosage adjustment required) and in severe hepatic insufficiency (no data available). Use caution in patients with diabetes - glucose regulation may be altered. Tendon inflammation and/or rupture has been reported with this and other quinolone antibiotics. Discontinue at first signs or symptoms of tendon or pain. Quinolones may exacerbate myasthenia gravis.

Severe hypersensitivity reactions, including anaphylaxis, have occurred with quinolone therapy. Prolonged use may result in superinfection; pseudomembranous colitis may occur and should be considered in all patients who present with diarrhea.

Adverse Reactions
3% to 10%:
Central nervous system: Headache (3%), dizziness (3%)
Gastrointestinal: Nausea (8%), diarrhea (4%)
Genitourinary: Vaginitis (6%)
Local: Injection site reactions (5%)
<3% (Limited to important or life-threatening): Allergic reaction, anaphylactic reaction, angioneurotic edema, ataxia, bradycardia, bronchospasm, chest pain, colitis, depersonalization, depression, dysphagia, dyspnea, ethanol intolerance, euphoria, gastrointestinal hemorrhage, hallucination, hepatitis, hyper-/hypoglycemia (severe), increased INR, increased prothrombin time, myasthenia, nonketotic hyperglycemia, palpitation, paresthesia, pseudomembranous colitis, psychosis, rash, seizures, tendon rupture, thrombocytopenia, tinnitus, torsade de pointes, vertigo, vomiting
Overdosage/Toxicology Potential symptoms of overdose include CNS excitation, seizures, QT prolongation, and arrhythmias (including torsade de pointes). Monitor by continuous EKG in the event of an overdose. Management is supportive and symptomatic. The drug is not removed by dialysis.
Drug Interactions
Increased Effect/Toxicity: Drugs which prolong QT interval (including Class Ia and Class III antiarrhythmics, erythromycin, cisapride, antipsychotics, and cyclic antidepressants) are contraindicated with gatifloxacin. Drugs which may induce bradycardia (eg, beta-blockers, amiodarone) should be avoided. Probenecid, loop diuretics, and cimetidine (possibly other H_2 antagonists) may increase the serum concentrations of gatifloxacin (based on experience with other quinolones). Digoxin levels may be increased in some patients by gatifloxacin. NSAIDs and foscarnet have been associated with an increased risk of seizures with some quinolones (not reported with gatifloxacin). The hypoprothrombinemic effect of warfarin is enhanced by some quinolone antibiotics. Monitoring of the INR during concurrent therapy is recommended by the manufacturer. Gatifloxacin may alter glucose control in patients receiving hypoglycemic agents with or without insulin.
(Continued)

Gatifloxacin *(Continued)*

Decreased Effect: Metal cations (magnesium, aluminum, iron, and zinc) inhibit intestinal absorption of gatifloxacin (by up to 98%). Antacids, electrolyte supplements, sucralfate, quinapril, and some didanosine formulations should be avoided. Gatifloxacin should be administered 4 hours before or 8 hours after these agents. Calcium carbonate was not found to alter the absorption of gatifloxacin. Antineoplastic agents, H_2 antagonists, and proton pump inhibitors may also decrease absorption of some quinolones. Gatifloxacin may alter glucose control in patients receiving hypoglycemic agents with or without insulin.

Ethanol/Nutrition/Herb Interactions Herb/Nutraceutical: Avoid dong quai, St John's wort (may also cause photosensitization).

Stability Store at 25°C (77°F). Do not freeze injection. Injection must be diluted to a concentration of 2 mg/mL prior to administration. Compatible with 5% dextrose in water, 0.9% sodium chloride, lactated Ringer's and 5% dextrose injection, 5% sodium bicarbonate injection, Plasma-Lyte® 56/5% dextrose injection. Compatible with 5% dextrose or 0.45% sodium chloride containing up to 20 mEq/L potassium chloride.

Mechanism of Action Gatifloxacin is a DNA gyrase inhibitor, and also inhibits topoisomerase IV. DNA gyrase (topoisomerase II) is an essential bacterial enzyme that maintains the superhelical structure of DNA. DNA gyrase is required for DNA replication and transcription, DNA repair, recombination, and transposition; inhibition is bactericidal.

Pharmacodynamics/Kinetics

Absorption: Oral: Well absorbed

Distribution: V_d: 1.5-2.0 L/kg; concentrates in alveolar macrophages and lung parenchyma

Protein binding: 20%

Metabolism: Only 1%; no interaction with hepatic microsomal enzymes

Bioavailability: 96%

Half-life elimination: 7.1-13.9 hours; ESRD/CAPD: 30-40 hours

Time to peak: Oral: 1 hour

Excretion: Urine (as unchanged drug); feces (5%)

Usual Dosage Adults: Oral, I.V.:

Acute bacterial exacerbation of chronic bronchitis: 400 mg every 24 hours for 5 days

Acute sinusitis: 400 mg every 24 hours for 10 days

Community-acquired pneumonia: 400 mg every 24 hours for 7-14 days

Uncomplicated urinary tract infections (cystitis): 400 mg single dose or 200 mg every 24 hours for 3 days

Complicated urinary tract infections: 400 mg every 24 hours for 7-10 days

Acute pyelonephritis: 400 mg every 24 hours for 7-10 days

Uncomplicated urethral gonorrhea in men, cervical or rectal gonorrhea in women: 400 mg single dose

Dosage adjustment in renal impairment: Creatinine clearance <40 mL/minute (or patients on hemodialysis/CAPD) should receive an initial dose of 400 mg, followed by a subsequent dose of 200 mg every 24 hours. Patients receiving single-dose or 3-day therapy for appropriate indications do not require dosage adjustment. Administer after hemodialysis.

Dosage adjustment in hepatic impairment: No dosage adjustment is required in mild-moderate hepatic disease. No data are available in severe hepatic impairment (Child-Pugh Class C).

Elderly: No dosage adjustment is required based on age, however, assessment of renal function is particularly important in this population.

Dietary Considerations May take with or without food, milk, or calcium supplements. Gatifloxacin should be taken 4 hours before supplements (including multivitamins) containing iron, zinc, or magnesium.

Administration Concentrated injection (10 mg/mL) must be diluted to 2 mg/mL prior to administration. No further dilution is required for premixed 100 mL and 200 mL solutions. Infuse over 60 minutes. Avoid rapid or bolus infusions.

Monitoring Parameters WBC, signs of infection

Patient Information May be taken with or without food. Drink plenty of fluids. Avoid exposure to direct sunlight during therapy and for several days following. Take gatifloxacin 4 hours before antacids or mineral supplements (iron, magnesium, or zinc). Contact your physician immediately if signs of allergy occur or if signs of tendon inflammation or pain occur. Do not discontinue therapy until your course has been completed. Take a missed dose as soon as possible, unless it is almost time for your next dose.

Dosage Forms

Injection: 10 mg/mL (20 mL, 40 mL)

Injection for infusion [premixed]: 2 mg/mL (100 mL, 200 mL)

Tablet: 200 mg, 400 mg

♦ **Gaviscon® Extra Strength [OTC]** *see* Aluminum Hydroxide and Magnesium Carbonate *on page 63*

♦ **Gaviscon® Liquid [OTC]** *see* Aluminum Hydroxide and Magnesium Carbonate *on page 63*

♦ **Gaviscon® Tablet [OTC]** *see* Aluminum Hydroxide and Magnesium Trisilicate *on page 64*

♦ **G-CSF** *see* Filgrastim *on page 561*

♦ **G-CSF (PEG Conjugate)** *see* Pegfilgrastim *on page 1045*

♦ **GCV Sodium** *see* Ganciclovir *on page 618*

♦ **Gee Gee® [OTC]** *see* Guaifenesin *on page 645*

Gelatin, Pectin, and Methylcellulose

(JEL a tin, PEK tin, & meth il SEL yoo lose)

U.S. Brand Names Orabase® Plain [OTC]

Therapeutic Category Topical Skin Product

Use Temporary relief from minor oral irritations

Usual Dosage Press small dabs into place until the involved area is coated with a thin film; do not try to spread onto area; may be used as often as needed

Additional Information Complete prescribing information for this medication should be consulted for additional detail.

Dosage Forms Paste, oral: 5 g

♦ **Gel-Kam**® *see* Fluoride *on page 574*
♦ **Gel-Tin**® **[OTC]** *see* Fluoride *on page 574*
♦ **Gelucast**® *see* Zinc Gelatin *on page 1438*
♦ **Gelusil**® **(Can)** *see* Aluminum Hydroxide and Magnesium Hydroxide *on page 64*
♦ **Gelusil**® **Extra Strength (Can)** *see* Aluminum Hydroxide and Magnesium Hydroxide *on page 64*

Gemcitabine (jem SITE a been)

U.S. Brand Names Gemzar®
Canadian Brand Names Gemzar®
Synonyms Gemcitabine Hydrochloride
Therapeutic Category Antineoplastic Agent, Antimetabolite
Use Adenocarcinoma of the pancreas; first-line therapy for patients with locally advanced (nonresectable stage II or stage III) or metastatic (stage IV) adenocarcinoma of the pancreas (indicated for patients previously treated with 5-FU); combination with cisplatin for the first-line treatment of patients with inoperable, locally advanced (stage IIIA or IIIB) or metastatic (stage IV) nonsmall-cell lung cancer
Pregnancy Risk Factor D
Contraindications Hypersensitivity to gemcitabine or any component of the formulation; pregnancy
Warnings/Precautions The U.S. Food & Drug Administration (FDA) recommends that procedures for proper handling and disposal of antineoplastic agents be considered. Prolongation of the infusion time >60 minutes and more frequent than weekly dosing have been shown to increase toxicity. Gemcitabine can suppress bone marrow function manifested by leukopenia, thrombocytopenia and anemia, and myelosuppression is usually the dose-limiting ototoxicity. The incidence of fever is 41% and gemcitabine may cause fever in the absence of clinical infection. Rash has been reported in 30% of patients - typically a macular or finely granular maculopapular pruritic eruption of mild to moderate severity involving the trunk and extremities. Gemcitabine should be used with caution in patients with pre-existing renal impairment (mild proteinuria and hematuria were commonly reported; hemolytic uremic syndrome has been reported) and hepatic impairment (associated with transient elevations of serum transaminases in $^2/_3$ of patients - but no evidence of increasing hepatic toxicity).

Adverse Reactions
>10%:
  Central nervous system: Fatigue, fever (40%), lethargy, pain (10% to 48%), somnolence (5% to 11%)
  Dermatologic: Alopecia (15%); mild to moderate rashes (5% to 32%)
  Endocrine & metabolic: Increased serum transaminase levels (~66%), mild, transient
  Gastrointestinal: Mild nausea, vomiting, anorexia (20% to 70%); stomatitis (10% to 14%)
  Hematologic: Myelosuppression (20% to 30%), primarily leukopenia, may be dose-limiting
  Neuromuscular & skeletal: Weakness (15% to 25%)
  Renal: Proteinuria, hematuria (45%), elevation of BUN
  Respiratory: Mild to moderate dyspnea (10% to 23%)
  Miscellaneous: Flu-like syndrome (myalgia, fever, chills, fatigue) (20% to 100%), may be dose-limiting
1% to 10%:
  Dermatologic: Pruritus (8%)
  Gastrointestinal: Mild diarrhea (7%), constipation (6%)
  Hematologic: Thrombocytopenia (~10%), anemia (6%)
  Hepatic: Elevated bilirubin (10%)
  Neuromuscular & skeletal: Paresthesia (2% to 10%), peripheral neuropathies (paresthesias, decreased tendon reflexes) (3.5%)
  Respiratory: Severe dyspnea (3%)
  Miscellaneous: Allergic reactions (4%), mild, usually edema, bronchospasm
<1% (Limited to important or life-threatening): Adult respiratory distress syndrome (ARDS), hemolytic-uremic syndrome, interstitial pneumonia, pulmonary edema

Overdosage/Toxicology Symptoms include myelosuppression, paresthesias, and severe rash. These were the principle effects seen when a single dose, as high as 5,700 mg/m², was administered by I.V. infusion over 30 minutes every 2 weeks. Monitor blood counts and administer supportive therapy as needed.

Drug Interactions
Decreased Effect: No confirmed interactions have been reported. No specific drug interaction studies have been conducted.

Ethanol/Nutrition/Herb Interactions Ethanol: Avoid ethanol (due to GI irritation).
Stability Store intact vials at room temperature (20°C to 25°C/68°F to 77°F). When reconstituted with preservative-free sodium chloride, the resulting solution has a concentration of 38 mg/mL **(NOT 40 mg/mL as indicated on earlier labeling).** Reconstituted vials and infusion solutions diluted in 0.9% sodium chloride are stable up to 24 hours.
Reconstitute with:
  200 mg vial with 5 mL 0.9% NaCl
  1000 mg vial with 25 mL 0.9% NaCl

Resulting solution is approximately 38 mg/mL, but is variable. A suggestion is to withdraw the entire solution into a syringe in order to determine the final concentration. The appropriate dose may be further diluted with 0.9% sodium chloride injection to concentrations as low as 0.1 mg/mL. Do not refrigerate.
Mechanism of Action Nucleoside analogue that primarily kills cells undergoing DNA synthesis (S-phase) and blocks the progression of cells through the G1/S-phase boundary
Pharmacodynamics/Kinetics
Distribution: V_d: Male: 15.6 mL mL/m²; Female: 11.3 L/m²
(Continued)

Gemcitabine *(Continued)*

Protein binding: Low

Metabolism: Hepatic, metabolites: di- and triphosphates (active); uridine derivative (inactive)

Half-life elimination: Infusion time: ≤1 hour: 32-94 minutes; Infusion time: 3-4 hours: 4-10.5 hours

Time to peak: 30 minutes

Excretion: Urine (99%, 92% to 98% as intact drug or inactive uridine metabolite); feces (<1%)

Usual Dosage Refer to individual protocols. I.V.:

Pancreatic cancer: 1000 mg/m^2 over 30 minutes weekly for 7 weeks followed by 1 week rest; repeat cycles 3 out of every 4 weeks.

Nonsmall cell lung cancer (in combination with cisplatin): 1000 mg/m^2 over 30 minutes on days 1, 8, 15; repeat every 28 days **or** 1250 mg/m^2 over 30 minutes on days 1, 8; repeat every 21 days.

Dosing reductions based on hematologic function: Patients who complete an entire 7-week initial cycle of gemcitabine therapy or a subsequent 3-week cycle at a dose of 1000 mg/m^2 may have the dose for subsequent cycles increased by 25% (1250 mg/m^2), provided that the absolute granulocyte count (AGC) and platelet nadirs exceed 1500 x 10^6/L and 100,000 x 10^6/L, respectively, and if nonhematologic toxicity has not been more than World Health Organization Grade 1

For patients who tolerate the subsequent course, at a dose of 1250 mg/m^2, the dose for the next cycle can be increased to 1500 mg/m^2, provided again that the AGC and platelet nadirs exceed 1500 x 10^6/L and 100,000 x 10^6/L, respectively, and again, if nonhematologic toxicity has not been greater than WHO Grade 1

Dosing adjustment in renal/hepatic impairment: Use with caution; gemcitabine has not been studied in patients with significant renal or hepatic dysfunction

Administration Gemcitabine is given intravenously, usually as a 30-minute bolus infusion. Infusions over several hours have been reported, but increase the risk of toxicity. Doses ≥2500 mg/m^2 should be diluted in a liter of fluid and infused over at least 4 hours.

Monitoring Parameters Patients should be monitored prior to each dose with a complete blood count (CBC), including differential and platelet count; suspension or modification of therapy should be considered when marrow suppression is detected. The diagnosis of hemolytic-uremic syndrome (HUS) should be considered if evidence of microangiopathic hemolysis is noted (elevation of bilirubin or LDH, reticulocytosis, severe thrombocytopenia, and/or renal failure).

Hepatic and renal function should be performed prior to initiation of therapy and periodically, thereafter

Dosage Forms Powder for injection, lyophilized, as hydrochloride: 20 mg/mL (10 mL, 50 mL)

♦ **Gemcitabine Hydrochloride** *see* Gemcitabine *on page 623*

Gemfibrozil *(jem FI broe zil)*

Related Information

Hyperlipidemia Management *on page 1670*

Lipid-Lowering Agents *on page 1505*

U.S. Brand Names Lopid®

Canadian Brand Names Apo®-Gemfibrozil; Gen-Gemfibrozil; Lopid®; Novo-Gemfibrozil; Nu-Gemfibrozil; PMS-Gemfibrozil

Synonyms CI-719

Therapeutic Category Antilipemic Agent, Fibric Acid

Use Treatment of hypertriglyceridemia in types IV and V hyperlipidemia for patients who are at greater risk for pancreatitis and who have not responded to dietary intervention

Pregnancy Risk Factor C

Contraindications Hypersensitivity to gemfibrozil or any component of the formulation; significant hepatic or renal dysfunction; primary biliary cirrhosis; pre-existing gallbladder disease

Warnings/Precautions Abnormal elevation of AST, ALT, LDH, bilirubin, and alkaline phosphatase has occurred; if no appreciable triglyceride or cholesterol lowering effect occurs after 3 months, the drug should be discontinued; not useful for type I hyperlipidemia; myositis may be more common in patients with poor renal function

Adverse Reactions

>10% Gastrointestinal: Dyspepsia (20%)

1% to 10%:

Central nervous system: Fatigue (4%), vertigo (2%), headache (1%)

Dermatologic: Eczema (2%), rash (2%)

Gastrointestinal: Abdominal pain (10%), diarrhea (7%), nausea/vomiting (3%), constipation (1%)

<1% (Limited to important or life-threatening): Alopecia, anaphylaxis, angioedema, bone marrow hypoplasia, cataracts, depression, dermatomyositis/polymyositis, drug-induced lupus-like syndrome, eosinophilia, exfoliative dermatitis, hypokalemia, impotence, intracranial hemorrhage, jaundice, laryngeal edema, leukopenia, myasthenia, myopathy, nephrotoxicity, pancreatitis, paresthesia, peripheral neuritis, photosensitivity, positive ANA, rash, Raynaud's phenomenon, retinal edema, rhabdomyolysis, seizures, syncope, thrombocytopenia, urticaria, vasculitis

Overdosage/Toxicology Symptoms include abdominal pain, diarrhea, nausea, and vomiting. Following GI decontamination, treatment is supportive.

Drug Interactions

Cytochrome P450 Effect: CYP3A3/4 enzyme substrate

Increased Effect/Toxicity: Gemfibrozil may potentiate the effects of bexarotene (avoid concurrent use), sulfonylureas (including glyburide, chlorpropamide), and warfarin. HMG-CoA reductase inhibitors (atorvastatin, fluvastatin, lovastatin, pravastatin, simvastatin) may increase the risk of myopathy and rhabdomyolysis. The manufacturer warns against the concurrent use of lovastatin. However, combination therapy with statins has been used in some patients with resistant hyperlipidemias (with great caution).

Decreased Effect: Cyclosporine's blood levels may be reduced during concurrent therapy. Rifampin may decreased gemfibrozil blood levels.

Ethanol/Nutrition/Herb Interactions Ethanol: Avoid ethanol to decrease triglycerides.

Mechanism of Action The exact mechanism of action of gemfibrozil is unknown, however, several theories exist regarding the VLDL effect; it can inhibit lipolysis and decrease subsequent hepatic fatty acid uptake as well as inhibit hepatic secretion of VLDL; together these actions decrease serum VLDL levels; increases HDL cholesterol; the mechanism behind HDL elevation is currently unknown

Pharmacodynamics/Kinetics

Onset of action: May require several days

Absorption: Well absorbed

Protein binding: 99%

Metabolism: Hepatic via oxidation to two inactive metabolites; undergoes enterohepatic recycling

Half-life elimination: 1.4 hours

Time to peak, serum: 1-2 hours

Excretion: Urine (70% primarily as unchanged drug)

Usual Dosage Adults: Oral: 1200 mg/day in 2 divided doses, 30 minutes before breakfast and dinner

Hemodialysis: Not removed by hemodialysis; supplemental dose is not necessary

Dietary Considerations Before initiation of therapy, patients should be placed on a standard cholesterol-lowering diet for 3-6 months and the diet should be continued during drug therapy.

Monitoring Parameters Serum cholesterol, LFTs

Patient Information May cause dizziness or blurred vision, abdominal or epigastric pain, diarrhea, nausea, or vomiting; notify physician if these become pronounced

Nursing Implications Monitor serum cholesterol; abnormal elevation of AST, ALT, LDH, bilirubin and alkaline phosphatase have occurred; if no appreciable triglyceride or cholesterol, lowering effect occurs after 3 months, the drug should be discontinued

Dosage Forms Tablet, film coated: 600 mg

Gemtuzumab Ozogamicin (gem TOO zoo mab oh zog a MY sin)

U.S. Brand Names Mylotarg™

Canadian Brand Names Mylotarg™

Therapeutic Category Antineoplastic Agent, Monoclonal Antibody

Use Treatment of acute myeloid leukemia (CD33 positive) in first relapse in patients who are ≥60 years of age and who are not considered candidates for cytotoxic chemotherapy.

Pregnancy Risk Factor D

Pregnancy/Breast-Feeding Implications May cause fetal harm when administered to a pregnant woman. Women of childbearing potential should avoid becoming pregnant while receiving treatment. If used in pregnancy, or if patient becomes pregnant during treatment, the patients should be apprised of potential hazard to the fetus. Excretion in breast milk unknown, breast feeding is not recommended.

Contraindications Hypersensitivity to gemtuzumab ozogamicin, calicheamicin derivatives, or any component of the formulation; patients with anti-CD33 antibody; pregnancy

Warnings/Precautions The U.S. Food and Drug Administration (FDA) currently recommends that procedures for proper handling and disposal of antineoplastic agents be considered. Safety and efficacy in patients with poor performance status and organ dysfunction have not been established.

Infusion-related events are common, generally reported to occur with the first dose at the end of the 2-hour intravenous infusion. These symptoms usually resolved after 2-4 hours with a supportive therapy of acetaminophen, diphenhydramine, and intravenous fluids. Fewer infusion-related events were observed after the second dose. Postinfusion reactions, which may include fever, chills, hypotension, or dyspnea, may occur during the first 24 hours after administration. **Infusion-related reactions may be severe (including anaphylaxis, pulmonary edema, or ARDS).** Symptomatic intrinsic lung disease or high peripheral blast counts may increase the risk of severe reactions. Consider discontinuation in patients who develop severe infusion-related reactions.

Severe myelosuppression occurs in all patients at recommended dosages. Use caution in patients with renal impairment (no clinical experience) and hepatic impairment (no clinical experience in patients with bilirubin >2 mg/dL). Tumor lysis syndrome may occur as a consequence of leukemia treatment, adequate hydration and prophylactic allopurinol must be instituted prior to use. Other methods to lower WBC <30,000 cells/mm³ may be considered (hydroxyurea or leukapheresis) to minimize the risk of tumor lysis syndrome, and/or severe infusion reactions. Has been associated with severe veno-occlusive disease or hepatotoxicity (risk may be increased by combination chemotherapy, previous hepatic disease, or hematopoietic stem cell transplant).

Adverse Reactions Percentages established in adults >60 years of age.

>10%:

Cardiovascular: Peripheral edema (21%), hypertension (20%), hypotension (16%)

Central nervous system: Chills (66%), fever (80%), headache (26%), pain (25%), dizziness (11%), insomnia (18%)

Dermatologic: Rash (23%), petechiae (21%), ecchymosis (15%)

Endocrine & metabolic: Hypokalemia (30%), hypokalemia

Gastrointestinal: Nausea (64%), vomiting (55%), diarrhea (38%), anorexia (31%), abdominal pain (29%), constipation (28%), stomatitis/mucositis (25%), abdominal distention (11%), dyspepsia (11%)

Hematologic: Neutropenia (98%; median recovery 40.5 days), thrombocytopenia (99%; median recovery 39 days); anemia (47%), bleeding (15%), lymphopenia

Hepatic: Hyperbilirubinemia (23%) increased LDH (18%), increased transaminases (9% to 17%)

Local: Local reaction (25%)

(Continued)

Gemtuzumab Ozogamicin *(Continued)*

Neuromuscular & skeletal: Weakness (45%), back pain (18%)
Respiratory: Dyspnea (36%), epistaxis (29%; severe 3%), cough (19%), pharyngitis (14%)
Miscellaneous: Infection (28%), sepsis (24%), neutropenic fever (20%)

1% to 10%:
Cardiovascular: Tachycardia (10%)
Central nervous system: Depression (10%), cerebral hemorrhage (2%), intracranial hemorrhage (2%)
Endocrine & metabolic: Hypomagnesemia (4%), hyperglycemia (2%)
Genitourinary: Hematuria (10%; severe 1%), vaginal hemorrhage (7%)
Hematologic: Hemorrhage (8%), disseminated intravascular coagulation (DIC) (2%)
Hepatic: Elevated PT
Neuromuscular & skeletal: Arthralgia (10%)
Respiratory: Rhinitis (10%), hypoxia (6%), pneumonia (10%), rhinitis (10%)

<1% (Limited to important or life-threatening): Acute respiratory distress syndrome, anaphylaxis, hepatic failure, hepatosplenomegaly, hypersensitivity reactions, jaundice, noncardiogenic pulmonary edema, renal failure, veno-occlusive disease

Overdosage/Toxicology Symptoms are unknown. General supportive measures should be instituted. Gemtuzumab ozogamicin is not dialyzable.

Drug Interactions
Increased Effect/Toxicity: No formal drug interaction studies have been conducted.
Decreased Effect: No formal drug interaction studies have been conducted.

Ethanol/Nutrition/Herb Interactions Ethanol: Avoid ethanol (due to GI irritation).

Stability
Storage: Light sensitive; protect from light. Store vials under refrigeration 2°C to 8°C (36°F to 46°F). Reconstituted vials may be stored under refrigeration for up to 8 hours.
Reconstitution: Prepare in biologic safety hood with the fluorescent light turned **off**. Allow to warm to room temperature prior to reconstitution. Reconstitute vial with 5 mL sterile water for injection, USP. Final concentration in vial is 1 mg/mL. Dilute desired dose in 100 mL of 0.9% sodium chloride injection. The resulting I.V. bag should be placed in a UV protectant bag and infused immediately.
Compatibility: No information (infuse via separate line)

Mechanism of Action Antibody to CD33 antigen, which is expressed on leukemic blasts in >80% of patients with acute myeloid leukemia (AML), as well as normal myeloid cells. Binding results in internalization of the antibody-antigen complex. Following internalization, the calicheamicin derivative is released inside the myeloid cell. The calicheamicin derivative binds to DNA resulting in double strand breaks and cell death. Pluripotent stem cells and nonhematopoietic cells are not affected.

Pharmacodynamics/Kinetics Half-life elimination: Calicheamicin: Total: Initial: 45 hours, Repeat dose: 60 hours; Unconjugated: 100 hours (no change noted in repeat dosing)

Usual Dosage I.V.: Adults ≥60 years: 9 mg/m², infused over 2 hours. The patient should receive diphenhydramine 50 mg orally and acetaminophen 650-1000 mg orally 1 hour prior to administration of each dose. Acetaminophen dosage should be repeated as needed every 4 hours for two additional doses. A full treatment course is a total of two doses administered with 14 days between doses. Full hematologic recovery is not necessary for administration of the second dose. There has been only limited experience with repeat courses of gemtuzumab ozogamicin.
Dosage adjustment in renal impairment: No recommendation (not studied)
Dosage adjustment in hepatic impairment: No recommendation (not studied)

Administration Administer as infusion only, over at least 2 hours. Do not administer I.V. push (bolus). Infuse through a separate line equipped with a low protein-binding 1.2 micron terminal filter. May be infused peripherally or through a central line. Premedication with acetaminophen and diphenhydramine should be administered prior to each infusion.

Monitoring Parameters Monitor vital signs during the infusion and for 4 hours following the infusion. Monitor for signs/symptoms of postinfusion reaction. Monitor electrolytes, LFTs, CBC with differential, and platelet counts frequently. Monitor for signs and symptoms of hepatitis reaction (weight gain, right upper quadrant abdominal pain, hepatomegaly, ascites).

Test Interactions None known

Patient Information This medication can only be administered I.V. During therapy do not use ethanol, aspirin-containing products, antiplatelet medications (ticlopidine, clopidogrel, or dipyridamole), OTC medications, or supplements/herbal products without consulting prescriber. It is important to maintain adequate nutrition and hydration. You may experience nausea and vomiting (small frequent meals, frequent mouth care, sucking lozenges or chewing gum may help). Frequent mouth care and use of a soft toothbrush or cotton swabs may reduce mouth sores. You will be susceptible to infection (avoid crowds and exposure to infection). Report fever, chills, unusual bruising or bleeding, signs of infection, dizziness, lightheadedness, difficulty breathing, or yellowing of the eyes or skin to prescriber. Keep all appointments and get required blood work done.

Nursing Implications Monitor vital signs during infusion and for 4 hours afterward. May be administered in an outpatient setting. Cover with UV protective bag during infusion. Premedicate with acetaminophen and diphenhydramine.

Dosage Forms Powder for injection: 5 mg

- ◆ **Genapap® Children [OTC]** *see* Acetaminophen *on page 22*
- ◆ **Genapap® Extra Strength [OTC]** *see* Acetaminophen *on page 22*
- ◆ **Genapap® Infant [OTC]** *see* Acetaminophen *on page 22*
- ◆ **Genaphed® [OTC]** *see* Pseudoephedrine *on page 1155*
- ◆ **Genaspor® [OTC]** *see* Tolnaftate *on page 1347*
- ◆ **Gen-Atenolol (Can)** *see* Atenolol *on page 125*
- ◆ **Genatuss® [OTC]** *see* Guaifenesin *on page 645*
- ◆ **Genatuss DM® [OTC]** *see* Guaifenesin and Dextromethorphan *on page 646*
- ◆ **Gen-Azathioprine (Can)** *see* Azathioprine *on page 136*
- ◆ **Gen-Baclofen (Can)** *see* Baclofen *on page 144*
- ◆ **Gen-Beclo (Can)** *see* Beclomethasone *on page 149*
- ◆ **Gen-Budesonide AQ (Can)** *see* Budesonide *on page 186*
- ◆ **Gen-Buspirone (Can)** *see* BusPIRone *on page 194*
- ◆ **Gencalc® 600 [OTC]** *see* Calcium Carbonate *on page 207*
- ◆ **Gen-Captopril (Can)** *see* Captopril *on page 218*
- ◆ **Gen-Carbamazepine CR (Can)** *see* Carbamazepine *on page 221*
- ◆ **Gen-Cimetidine (Can)** *see* Cimetidine *on page 293*
- ◆ **Gen-Clobetasol (Can)** *see* Clobetasol *on page 311*
- ◆ **Gen-Clomipramine (Can)** *see* ClomiPRAMINE *on page 315*
- ◆ **Gen-Clonazepam (Can)** *see* Clonazepam *on page 316*
- ◆ **Gen-Cyclobenzaprine (Can)** *see* Cyclobenzaprine *on page 340*
- ◆ **Gen-Diltiazem (Can)** *see* Diltiazem *on page 409*
- ◆ **Gen-Diltiazem SR (Can)** *see* Diltiazem *on page 409*
- ◆ **Gen-Divalproex (Can)** *see* Valproic Acid and Derivatives *on page 1398*
- ◆ **Gen-Doxazosin (Can)** *see* Doxazosin *on page 439*
- ◆ **Genebs® [OTC]** *see* Acetaminophen *on page 22*
- ◆ **Genebs® Extra Strength [OTC]** *see* Acetaminophen *on page 22*
- ◆ **Genesec® [OTC]** *see* Acetaminophen and Phenyltoloxamine *on page 25*
- ◆ **Gen-Etodolac (Can)** *see* Etodolac *on page 532*
- ◆ **Gen-Famotidine (Can)** *see* Famotidine *on page 543*
- ◆ **Gen-Fenofibrate Micro (Can)** *see* Fenofibrate *on page 548*
- ◆ **Gen-Fluoxetine (Can)** *see* Fluoxetine *on page 578*
- ◆ **Gen-Fluvoxamine (Can)** *see* Fluvoxamine *on page 593*
- ◆ **Gen-Gemfibrozil (Can)** *see* Gemfibrozil *on page 624*
- ◆ **Gen-Glybe (Can)** *see* GlyBURIDE *on page 635*
- ◆ **Gengraf™** *see* CycloSPORINE *on page 345*
- ◆ **Gen-Indapamide (Can)** *see* Indapamide *on page 715*
- ◆ **Gen-Ipratropium (Can)** *see* Ipratropium *on page 740*
- ◆ **Gen-K®** *see* Potassium Chloride *on page 1108*
- ◆ **Gen-Medroxy (Can)** *see* MedroxyPROGESTERone *on page 848*
- ◆ **Gen-Metformin (Can)** *see* Metformin *on page 875*
- ◆ **Gen-Metoprolol (Can)** *see* Metoprolol *on page 902*
- ◆ **Gen-Minocycline (Can)** *see* Minocycline *on page 918*
- ◆ **Gen-Naproxen EC (Can)** *see* Naproxen *on page 958*
- ◆ **Gen-Nortriptyline (Can)** *see* Nortriptyline *on page 996*
- ◆ **Genoptic®** *see* Gentamicin *on page 627*
- ◆ **Genoptic® S.O.P.** *see* Gentamicin *on page 627*
- ◆ **Genotropin®** *see* Human Growth Hormone *on page 667*
- ◆ **Genotropin Miniquick®** *see* Human Growth Hormone *on page 667*
- ◆ **Gen-Oxybutynin (Can)** *see* Oxybutynin *on page 1023*
- ◆ **Gen-Pindolol (Can)** *see* Pindolol *on page 1086*
- ◆ **Gen-Piroxicam (Can)** *see* Piroxicam *on page 1093*
- ◆ **Genpril® [OTC]** *see* Ibuprofen *on page 697*
- ◆ **Gen-Ranidine (Can)** *see* Ranitidine *on page 1178*
- ◆ **Gen-Selegiline (Can)** *see* Selegiline *on page 1228*
- ◆ **Gen-Sotalol (Can)** *see* Sotalol *on page 1252*
- ◆ **Gentacidin®** *see* Gentamicin *on page 627*
- ◆ **Gentak®** *see* Gentamicin *on page 627*

Gentamicin (jen ta MYE sin)

Related Information

Aminoglycoside Dosing and Monitoring *on page 1470*
Antibiotic Treatment of Adults With Infective Endocarditis *on page 1585*
Antimicrobial Drugs of Choice *on page 1588*
Community-Acquired Pneumonia in Adults *on page 1603*
Prevention of Bacterial Endocarditis *on page 1563*
Prevention of Wound Infection & Sepsis in Surgical Patients *on page 1569*
Treatment of Sexually Transmitted Diseases *on page 1609*

U.S. Brand Names Garamycin®; Genoptic®; Genoptic® S.O.P.; Gentacidin®; Gentak®; G-myticin®

Canadian Brand Names Alcomicin®; Diogent®; Garamycin®; Garatec; Scheinpharm Gentamicin

Synonyms Gentamicin Sulfate

Therapeutic Category Antibiotic, Aminoglycoside; Antibiotic, Ophthalmic; Antibiotic, Topical

(Continued)

Gentamicin *(Continued)*

Use Treatment of susceptible bacterial infections, normally gram-negative organisms including *Pseudomonas, Proteus, Serratia,* and gram-positive *Staphylococcus;* treatment of bone infections, respiratory tract infections, skin and soft tissue infections, as well as abdominal and urinary tract infections, endocarditis, and septicemia; used topically to treat superficial infections of the skin or ophthalmic infections caused by susceptible bacteria; prevention of bacterial endocarditis prior to dental or surgical procedures

Pregnancy Risk Factor C

Contraindications Hypersensitivity to gentamicin or other aminoglycosides

Warnings/Precautions Not intended for long-term therapy due to toxic hazards associated with extended administration; pre-existing renal insufficiency, vestibular or cochlear impairment, myasthenia gravis, hypocalcemia, conditions which depress neuromuscular transmission

Parenteral aminoglycosides have been associated with significant nephrotoxicity or ototoxicity; the ototoxicity may be directly proportional to the amount of drug given and the duration of treatment; tinnitus or vertigo are indications of vestibular injury and impending hearing loss; renal damage is usually reversible

Adverse Reactions

>10%:
    Central nervous system: Neurotoxicity (vertigo, ataxia)
    Neuromuscular & skeletal: Gait instability
    Otic: Ototoxicity (auditory), ototoxicity (vestibular)
    Renal: Nephrotoxicity, decreased creatinine clearance

1% to 10%:
    Cardiovascular: Edema
    Dermatologic: Skin itching, reddening of skin, rash

<1% (Limited to important or life-threatening): Agranulocytosis, allergic reaction, dyspnea, granulocytopenia, photosensitivity, pseudomotor cerebri, thrombocytopenia

Overdosage/Toxicology Symptoms include ototoxicity, nephrotoxicity, and neuromuscular toxicity. Serum level monitoring is recommended. The treatment of choice, following a single acute overdose, appears to be the maintenance of urine output of at least 3 mL/kg/hour. Dialysis is of questionable value in enhancing aminoglycoside elimination. If required, hemodialysis is preferred over peritoneal dialysis in patients with normal renal function. Careful hydration may be all that is required to promote diuresis and therefore enhance the drug's elimination. Chelation with penicillins is experimental.

Drug Interactions

Increased Effect/Toxicity: Penicillins, cephalosporins, amphotericin B, loop diuretics may increase nephrotoxic potential. Aminoglycosides may potentiate the effects of neuromuscular blocking agents.

Stability

Gentamicin is a colorless to slightly yellow solution which should be stored between 2°C to 30°C, but refrigeration is not recommended

I.V. infusion solutions mixed in NS or D_5W solution are stable for 24 hours at room temperature and refrigeration

Premixed bag: Manufacturer expiration date

Out of overwrap stability: 30 days

Mechanism of Action Interferes with bacterial protein synthesis by binding to 30S and 50S ribosomal subunits resulting in a defective bacterial cell membrane

Pharmacodynamics/Kinetics

Absorption: Oral: None

Distribution: Crosses placenta

V_d: Increased by edema, ascites, fluid overload; decreased with dehydration
    Neonates: 0.4-0.6 L/kg
    Children: 0.3-0.35 L/kg
    Adults: 0.2-0.3 L/kg

Relative diffusion from blood into CSF: Minimal even with inflammation

CSF:blood level ratio: Normal meninges: Nil; Inflamed meninges: 10% to 30%

Protein binding: <30%

Half-life elimination

Infants: <1 week old: 3-11.5 hours; 1 week to 6 months old: 3-3.5 hours

Adults: 1.5-3 hours; End-stage renal disease: 36-70 hours

Time to peak, serum: I.M.: 30-90 minutes; I.V.: 30 minutes after 30-minute infusion

Excretion: Urine (as unchanged drug)

Clearance: Directly related to renal function

Usual Dosage Individualization is critical because of the low therapeutic index; refer to "Aminoglycoside Dosing and Monitoring" *on page 1470* in the Appendix

Use of ideal body weight (IBW) for determining the mg/kg/dose appears to be more accurate than dosing on the basis of total body weight (TBW).

In morbid obesity, dosage requirement may best be estimated using a dosing weight of IBW + 0.4 (TBW - IBW)

Initial and periodic peak and trough plasma drug levels should be determined, particularly in critically ill patients with serious infections or in disease states known to significantly alter aminoglycoside pharmacokinetics (eg, cystic fibrosis, burns, or major surgery)

Newborns: Intrathecal: 1 mg every day

Infants >3 months: Intrathecal: 1-2 mg/day

Infants and Children <5 years: I.M., I.V.: 2.5 mg/kg/dose every 8 hours*

Cystic fibrosis: 2.5 mg/kg/dose every 6 hours

Children >5 years: I.M., I.V.: 1.5-2.5 mg/kg/dose every 8 hours*

Prevention of bacterial endocarditis: Dental, oral, upper respiratory procedures, GI/GU procedures: 2 mg/kg with ampicillin (50 mg/kg) 30 minutes prior to procedure

*Some patients may require larger or more frequent doses (eg, every 6 hours) if serum levels document the need (ie, cystic fibrosis or febrile granulocytopenic patients)

Adults: I.M., I.V.:
  Severe life-threatening infections: 2-2.5 mg/kg/dose
  Urinary tract infections: 1.5 mg/kg/dose
  Synergy (for gram-positive infections): 1 mg/kg/dose
  Prevention of bacterial endocarditis:
    Dental, oral, or upper respiratory procedures: 1.5 mg/kg not to exceed 80 mg with ampicillin (1-2 g) 30 minutes prior to procedure
    GI/GU surgery: 1.5 mg/kg not to exceed 80 mg with ampicillin 2 g 30 minutes prior to procedure
Some clinicians suggest a daily dose of 4-7 mg/kg for all patients with normal renal function. This dose is at least as efficacious with similar, if not less, toxicity than conventional dosing; see "Aminoglycoside Dosing and Monitoring" *on page 1470* in the Appendix
Children and Adults:
  Intrathecal: 4-8 mg/day
  Ophthalmic:
    Ointment: Instill $^1/_2$" (1.25 cm) 2-3 times/day to every 3-4 hours
    Solution: Instill 1-2 drops every 2-4 hours, up to 2 drops every hour for severe infections
  Topical: Apply 3-4 times/day to affected area
Dosing interval in renal impairment:
  Cl$_{cr}$ ≥60 mL/minute: Administer every 8 hours
  Cl$_{cr}$ 40-60 mL/minute: Administer every 12 hours
  Cl$_{cr}$ 20-40 mL/minute: Administer every 24 hours
  Cl$_{cr}$ <20 mL/minute: Loading dose, then monitor levels
  Hemodialysis: Dialyzable; removal by hemodialysis: 30% removal of aminoglycosides occurs during 4 hours of HD; administer dose after dialysis and follow levels
  Removal by continuous ambulatory peritoneal dialysis (CAPD):
    Administration via CAPD fluid:
      Gram-negative infection: 4-8 mg/L (4-8 mcg/mL) of CAPD fluid
      Gram-positive infection (ie, synergy): 3-4 mg/L (3-4 mcg/mL) of CAPD fluid
    Administration via I.V., I.M. route during CAPD: Dose as for Cl$_{cr}$ <10 mL/minute and follow levels
    Removal via continuous arteriovenous or venovenous hemofiltration: Dose as for Cl$_{cr}$ 10-40 mL/minute and follow levels
Dosing adjustment/comments in hepatic disease: Monitor plasma concentrations
Dietary Considerations Calcium, magnesium, potassium: Renal wasting may cause hypocalcemia, hypomagnesemia, and/or hypokalemia.
Monitoring Parameters Urinalysis, urine output, BUN, serum creatinine; hearing should be tested before, during, and after treatment; particularly in those at risk for ototoxicity or who will be receiving prolonged therapy (>2 weeks)
Reference Range
  Timing of serum samples: Draw peak 30 minutes after 30-minute infusion has been completed or 1 hour after I.M. injection; draw trough immediately before next dose
  Sample size: 0.5-2 mL blood (red top tube) or 0.1-1 mL serum (separated)
  Therapeutic levels:
    Peak:
      Serious infections: 6-8 µg/mL (12-17 µmol/L)
      Life-threatening infections: 8-10 µg/mL (17-21 µmol/L)
      Urinary tract infections: 4-6 µg/mL
      Synergy against gram-positive organisms: 3-5 µg/mL
    Trough:
      Serious infections: 0.5-1 µg/mL
      Life-threatening infections: 1-2 µg/mL
    Obtain drug levels after the third dose unless renal dysfunction/toxicity suspected
Test Interactions Penicillin may decrease aminoglycoside serum concentrations *in vitro*
Patient Information Report any dizziness or sensations of ringing or fullness in ears; do not touch ophthalmics to eye; use no other eye drops within 5-10 minutes of instilling ophthalmic
Nursing Implications Slower absorption and lower peak concentrations probably due to poor circulation in the atrophic muscle, may occur following I.M. injection in paralyzed patients (suggest I.V. route); aminoglycoside levels measured in blood taken from Silastic® central catheters can sometimes give falsely high readings (draw via separate lumen or peripheral site if possible, otherwise flush very well). Monitor serum creatinine and urine output; obtain drug levels after the third dose unless otherwise directed (eg, suspected toxicity or renal dysfunction). Peak levels are drawn 30 minutes after the end of a 30-minute infusion or 60 minutes following I.M. injection; trough levels are drawn within 30 minutes before the next dose. Separate administration of extended-spectrum penicillins (eg, carbenicillin, ticarcillin, piperacillin) from gentamicin in patients with severe renal impairment; gentamicin's efficacy may be reduced if given concurrently. Hearing should be tested before, during, and after treatment in patients at risk for ototoxicity.
Additional Information Gentamicin is the only aminoglycoside that is commercially available in a preservative-free solution for injection in a 2 mg/mL concentration and a 2 mL vial.
Dosage Forms
  Cream, topical, as sulfate (Garamycin®, G-myticin®): 0.1% (15 g)
  Infusion, as sulfate [in D$_5$W]: 60 mg, 80 mg, 100 mg
  Infusion, as sulfate [in NS]: 40 mg, 60 mg, 80 mg, 90 mg, 100 mg, 120 mg
  Injection, as sulfate: 40 mg/mL (1 mL, 1.5 mL, 2 mL, 20 mL)
  Injection, intrathecal, as sulfate [preservative free] (Garamycin®): 2 mg/mL (2 mL)
  Injection, pediatric, as sulfate: 10 mg/mL (2 mL)
  Ointment, ophthalmic, as sulfate: 0.3% [3 mg/g] (3.5 g)
    Garamycin®, Genoptic® S.O.P., Gentacidin®, Gentak®: 0.3% [3 mg/g] (3.5 g)
  Ointment, topical, as sulfate (Garamycin®, G-myticin®): 0.1% (15 g)
  Solution, ophthalmic, as sulfate: 0.3% (5 mL, 15 mL)
    Garamycin®, Genoptic®, Gentacidin®, Gentak®: 0.3% (1 mL, 5 mL, 15 mL)

◆ **Gentamicin and Prednisolone** *see* Prednisolone and Gentamicin *on page 1124*
◆ **Gentamicin Sulfate** *see* Gentamicin *on page 627*

- **Gen-Tamoxifen (Can)** *see* Tamoxifen *on page 1286*
- **Gen-Temazepam (Can)** *see* Temazepam *on page 1292*

Gentian Violet (JEN shun VYE oh let)

Synonyms Crystal Violet; Methylrosaniline Chloride

Therapeutic Category Antibacterial, Topical; Antifungal Agent, Topical

Use Treatment of cutaneous or mucocutaneous infections caused by *Candida albicans* and other superficial skin infections

Pregnancy Risk Factor C

Contraindications Hypersensitivity to gentian violet or any component of the formulation; ulcerated areas; porphyria

Warnings/Precautions Infants should be turned face down after application to minimize amount of drug swallowed; may result in tattooing of the skin when applied to granulation tissue; solution is for external use only; avoid contact with eyes

Adverse Reactions Frequency not defined.

Dermatologic: Vesicle formation

Gastrointestinal: Esophagitis, ulceration of mucous membranes,

Local: Burning, irritation

Respiratory: Laryngitis, laryngeal obstruction, tracheitis

Miscellaneous: Sensitivity reactions

Overdosage/Toxicology Signs and symptoms include laryngeal obstruction.

Mechanism of Action Topical antiseptic/germicide effective against some vegetative gram-positive bacteria, particularly *Staphylococcus* sp, and some yeast; it is much less effective against gram-negative bacteria and is ineffective against acid-fast bacteria

Usual Dosage Children and Adults: Topical: Apply 0.5% to 2% locally with cotton to lesion 2-3 times/day for 3 days, do not swallow and avoid contact with eyes

Patient Information Drug stains skin and clothing purple; do not apply to an ulcerative lesion; may result in "tattooing" of the skin; when used for the treatment of vaginal candidiasis, coitus should be avoided; insert vaginal product high into vagina. Use condoms or refrain from sexual intercourse to avoid reinfection.

Dosage Forms Solution, topical: 1% (30 mL); 2% (30 mL)

- **Gen-Ticlopidine (Can)** *see* Ticlopidine *on page 1331*
- **Gen-Timolol (Can)** *see* Timolol *on page 1334*
- **Gentran®** *see* Dextran *on page 386*
- **Gen-Trazodone (Can)** *see* Trazodone *on page 1362*
- **Gen-Triazolam (Can)** *see* Triazolam *on page 1370*
- **Gen-Verapamil (Can)** *see* Verapamil *on page 1412*
- **Gen-Verapamil SR (Can)** *see* Verapamil *on page 1412*
- **Geocillin®** *see* Carbenicillin *on page 224*
- **Geodon®** *see* Ziprasidone *on page 1440*
- **Geref®** *see* Sermorelin Acetate *on page 1230*
- **Geref® Diagnostic** *see* Sermorelin Acetate *on page 1230*
- **German Measles Vaccine** *see* Rubella Virus Vaccine (Live) *on page 1217*
- **Germinal®** *see* Ergoloid Mesylates *on page 482*
- **GG** *see* Guaifenesin *on page 645*
- **GI87084B** *see* Remifentanil *on page 1182*

Glatiramer Acetate (gla TIR a mer AS e tate)

U.S. Brand Names Copaxone®

Canadian Brand Names Copaxone®

Synonyms Copolymer-1

Therapeutic Category Biological, Miscellaneous

Use Treatment of relapsing-remitting type multiple sclerosis; studies indicate that it reduces the frequency of attacks and the severity of disability; appears to be most effective for patients with minimal disability

Pregnancy Risk Factor B

Pregnancy/Breast-Feeding Implications No adequate and well-controlled studies in pregnant women. Use in pregnancy only if clearly necessary. Excretion in breast milk is unknown; use caution in nursing women.

Contraindications Previous hypersensitivity to any component of the copolymer formulation, glatiramer acetate, or mannitol

Warnings/Precautions For S.C. use only, **not for I.V. administration**. Glatiramer acetate is antigenic, and may possibly lead to the induction of untoward host responses. Systemic postinjection reactions occur in a substantial percentage of patients (~10% in premarketing studies). Safety and efficacy have not been established in patients <18 years of age.

Adverse Reactions Reported in >2% of patients in placebo-controlled trials:

>10%:

Cardiovascular: Chest pain (21%)

Central nervous system: Pain (28%), vasodilation (27%), anxiety (23%), palpitations (17%)

Dermatologic: Pruritus (18%), rash (18%), diaphoresis (15%)

Gastrointestinal: Nausea (22%), diarrhea (12%)

Local: Injection site reactions: Pain (73%), erythema (66%), inflammation (49%), pruritus (40%), mass (27%), induration (13%), welt (11%)

Neuromuscular & skeletal: Weakness (41%), arthralgia (24%), hypertonia (22%), back pain (16%)

Respiratory: Dyspnea (19%), rhinitis (14%)

Miscellaneous: Infection (50%), flu-like syndrome (19%), lymphadenopathy (12%)

1% to 10%:

Cardiovascular: Peripheral edema (7%), facial edema (6%), edema (3%), tachycardia (5%), hypertension (1%)

Central nervous system: Fever (8%), vertigo (6%), migraine (5%), syncope (5%), agitation (4%), chills (4%), confusion (2%), nervousness (2%), speech disorder (2%), abnormal dreams (1%), emotional lability (1%), stupor (1%)

Dermatologic: Bruising (8%), erythema (4%), urticaria (4%), skin nodule (2%), eczema, herpes zoster, pustular rash, skin atrophy

Endocrine & metabolic: Dysmenorrhea (6%), amenorrhea (1%), menorrhagia (1%), vaginal hemorrhage (1%)

Gastrointestinal: Anorexia (8%), vomiting (6%), gastrointestinal disorder (5%), gastroenteritis (3%), weight gain (3%), oral moniliasis (1%), ulcerative stomatitis (1%), salivary gland enlargement

Genitourinary: Urinary urgency (10%), vaginal moniliasis (8%), hematuria (1%), impotence (1%)

Local: Injection site reactions: Hemorrhage (5%), urticaria (5%), edema (1%), atrophy (1%), abscess (1%), hypersensitivity (1%)

Neuromuscular & skeletal: Tremor (7%), foot drop (3%)

Ocular: Eye disorder (4%), nystagmus (2%), visual field defect (1%)

Otic: Ear pain (7%)

Respiratory: Bronchitis (9%), laryngismus (5%)

Miscellaneous: Neck pain (8%), bacterial infection (5%), herpes simplex (4%), cyst (2%)

<1% (Limited to important or life-threatening): Anaphylactoid reaction, angina, angioedema, aphasia, arrhythmia, blindness, carcinoma (breast, bladder, lung), cardiomyopathy, cholecystitis, cholelithiasis, cirrhosis, coma, congestive heart failure, corneal ulcer, esophageal ulcer, esophagitis, ethanol intolerance, gastrointestinal hemorrhage, GI carcinoma, glaucoma, gout, hallucinations, hematemesis, hepatitis, hepatomegaly, hypotension, leukopenia, lupus erythematosus, mania, meningitis, myocardial infarction, neuralgia, optic neuritis, pancreatitis, pancytopenia, paraplegia, pericardial effusion, photosensitivity, postural hypotension, priapism, pulmonary embolism, rash, renal failure, rheumatoid arthritis, seizures, sepsis, serum sickness, splenomegaly, stomatitis, stroke, suicide attempt, thrombocytopenia, thrombosis

Overdosage/Toxicology Well tolerated; no serious toxicities can be anticipated.

Stability Reconstituted product contains no preservative, use immediately; store unreconstituted product in refrigerator at 2°C to 8°C (36°F to 46°F); excursions to room temperature for up to 1 week do not have a negative impact on potency. Diluent may be stored at room temperature

Mechanism of Action Glatiramer is a mixture of random polymers of four amino acids; L-alanine, L-glutamic acid, L-lysine and L-tyrosine, the resulting mixture is antigenically similar to myelin basic protein, which is an important component of the myelin sheath of nerves; glatiramer is thought to suppress T-lymphocytes specific for a myelin antigen, it is also proposed that glatiramer interferes with the antigen-presenting function of certain immune cells opposing pathogenic T-cell function

Pharmacodynamics/Kinetics

Distribution: Small amounts of intact and partial hydrolyzed drug enter lymphatic circulation

Metabolism: S.C.: Large percentage hydrolyzed locally

Usual Dosage Adults: S.C.: 20 mg daily

Patient Information It is essential to provide the patient with proper handling and reconstitution instruction, since they will most likely have to self-administer the drug for an extended period

Dosage Forms Injection [single-dose vial] [with 1 mL vial diluent (SWFI)]: 20 mg of glatiramer and 40 mg mannitol [packaged in 2 mL vials]

♦ **Glaucoma Drug Therapy Comparison** *see page 1499*

♦ **Glaucon**® *see Epinephrine on page 470*

♦ **Gleevec**™ *see Imatinib on page 703*

♦ **Gliadel**® *see Carmustine on page 230*

♦ **Glibenclamide** *see GlyBURIDE on page 635*

Glimepiride (GLYE me pye ride)

Related Information

Antacid Drug Interactions *on page 1477*

Diabetes Mellitus Treatment *on page 1657*

Hypoglycemic Drugs & Thiazolidinedione Information *on page 1502*

U.S. Brand Names Amaryl®

Canadian Brand Names Amaryl®

Therapeutic Category Antidiabetic Agent, Sulfonylurea; Hypoglycemic Agent, Oral; Sulfonylurea Agent

Use Management of type 2 diabetes mellitus (noninsulin dependent, NIDDM) as an adjunct to diet and exercise to lower blood glucose or in combination with metformin; use in combination with insulin to lower blood glucose in patients whose hyperglycemia cannot be controlled by diet and exercise in conjunction with an oral hypoglycemic agent

Pregnancy Risk Factor C

Pregnancy/Breast-Feeding Implications Abnormal blood glucose levels are associated with a higher incidence of congenital abnormalities. Insulin is the drug of choice for the control of diabetes mellitus during pregnancy.

Contraindications Hypersensitivity to glimepiride, any component of the formulation, or sulfonamides; diabetic ketoacidosis (with or without coma)

Warnings/Precautions All sulfonylurea drugs are capable of producing severe hypoglycemia. Hypoglycemia is more likely to occur when caloric intake is deficient, after severe or prolonged exercise, when ethanol is ingested, or when more than one glucose-lowering drug is used.

Chemical similarities are present among sulfonamides, sulfonylureas, carbonic anhydrase inhibitors, thiazides, and loop diuretics (except ethacrynic acid). Use in patients with sulfonamide allergy is specifically contraindicated in product labeling, however a risk of cross-
(Continued)

Glimepiride *(Continued)*

reaction exists in patients with allergy to any of these compounds; avoid use when previous reaction has been severe.

Product labeling states oral hypoglycemic drugs may be associated with an increased cardio-vascular mortality as compared to treatment with diet alone or diet plus insulin. Data to support this association are limited, and several studies, including a large prospective trial (UKPDS) have not supported an association.

Adverse Reactions

1% to 10%:

Central nervous system: Headache, dizziness

Gastrointestinal: Nausea

<1% (Limited to important or life-threatening): Agranulocytosis, aplastic anemia, blood dyscrasias, bone marrow suppression, cholestatic jaundice, hemolytic anemia, hypogly-cemia, hyponatremia, thrombocytopenia

Overdosage/Toxicology Symptoms include low blood sugar, tingling of lips and tongue, nausea, yawning, confusion, agitation, tachycardia, sweating, convulsions, stupor, and coma. Intoxications with sulfonylureas can cause hypoglycemia and are best managed with glucose administration (orally for milder hypoglycemia or by injection in more severe forms). Patients should be monitored for a minimum of 24-48 hours after ingestion.

Drug Interactions

Cytochrome P450 Effect: CYP2C9 enzyme substrate

Increased Effect/Toxicity: Anticoagulants, androgens, fluconazole, miconazole, salicy-lates, gemfibrozil, sulfonamides, tricyclic antidepressants, probenecid, MAO inhibitors, beta-blockers, methyldopa, digitalis glycosides, urinary acidifiers may increase the hypo-glycemic effects of glimepiride.

Decreased Effect: There may be a decreased effect of glimepiride with corticosteroids, cholestyramine, estrogens, oral contraceptives, phenytoin, rifampin, thiazide and other diuretics, phenothiazines, NSAIDs, thyroid products, nicotinic acid, isoniazid, sympathomi-metics, urinary alkalinizers, and charcoal. **Note:** However, data from pooled data did **not** demonstrate drug interactions with calcium channel blockers, estrogens, NSAIDs, HMG-CoA reductase inhibitors, sulfonamides, or thyroid hormone.

Ethanol/Nutrition/Herb Interactions

Ethanol: Caution with ethanol (may cause hypoglycemia).

Herb/Nutraceutical: Caution with chromium, garlic, gymnema (may cause hypoglycemia).

Mechanism of Action Stimulates insulin release from the pancreatic beta cells; reduces glucose output from the liver; insulin sensitivity is increased at peripheral target sites

Pharmacodynamics/Kinetics

Onset of action: Peak effect: Blood glucose reductions: 2-3 hours

Duration: 24 hours

Protein binding: >99.5%

Absorption: 100%; delayed when given with food

Metabolism: Completely hepatic

Half-life elimination: 5-9 hours

Excretion: Urine and feces (as metabolites)

Usual Dosage Oral (allow several days between dose titrations):

Adults: Initial: 1-2 mg once daily, administered with breakfast or the first main meal; usual maintenance dose: 1-4 mg once daily; after a dose of 2 mg once daily, increase in increments of 2 mg at 1- to 2-week intervals based upon the patient's blood glucose response to a maximum of 8 mg once daily

Combination with insulin therapy (fasting glucose level for instituting combination therapy is in the range of >150 mg/dL in plasma or serum depending on the patient): initial recom-mended dose: 8 mg once daily with the first main meal

After starting with low-dose insulin, upward adjustments of insulin can be done approxi-mately weekly as guided by frequent measurements of fasting blood glucose. Once stable, combination-therapy patients should monitor their capillary blood glucose on an ongoing basis, preferably daily.

Dosing adjustment/comments in renal impairment: Cl_{cr} <22 mL/minute: Initial starting dose should be 1 mg and dosage increments should be based on fasting blood glucose levels

Dosing adjustment in hepatic impairment: No data available

Elderly: Initial: 1 mg/day; dose titration and maintenance dosing should be conservative to avoid hypoglycemia

Dietary Considerations Administer with breakfast or the first main meal of the day. Dietary modification based on ADA recommendations is a part of therapy. Decreases blood glucose concentration. Hypoglycemia may occur. Must be able to recognize symptoms of hypogly-cemia (palpitations, sweaty palms, lightheadedness).

Administration May be administered with a meal/food

Monitoring Parameters Urine for glucose and ketones; monitor for signs and symptoms of hypoglycemia (fatigue, excessive hunger, profuse sweating, numbness of extremities), fasting blood glucose, hemoglobin A_{1c}, fructosamine

Reference Range Target range: Adults:

Fasting blood glucose: <120 mg/dL

Glycosylated hemoglobin: <7%

Patient Information Patients must be counseled by someone experienced in diabetes educa-tion, signs and symptoms of hyper- and hypoglycemia, exercise and diet, blood glucose monitoring, and other related topics; eat regularly, do not skip meals; carry quick source of sugar; medical alert bracelet

Nursing Implications Patients who are NPO may need to have their dose held to avoid hypoglycemia

Dosage Forms Tablet: 1 mg, 2 mg, 4 mg

GlipiZIDE (GLIP i zide)

Related Information

Antacid Drug Interactions *on page 1477*
Hypoglycemic Drugs & Thiazolidinedione Information *on page 1502*
Sulfonamide Derivatives *on page 1515*

U.S. Brand Names Glucotrol®; Glucotrol® XL

Synonyms Glydiazinamide

Therapeutic Category Antidiabetic Agent, Sulfonylurea; Hypoglycemic Agent, Oral; Sulfonylurea Agent

Use Management of type 2 diabetes mellitus (noninsulin dependent, NIDDM)

Pregnancy Risk Factor C

Pregnancy/Breast-Feeding Implications

Clinical effects on the fetus: Crosses the placenta. Abnormal blood glucose levels are associated with a higher incidence of congenital abnormalities. Insulin is the drug of choice for the control of diabetes mellitus during pregnancy.

Breast-feeding/lactation: Due to risk of neonatal hypoglycemia, breast-feeding is contraindicated.

Contraindications Hypersensitivity to glipizide or any component of the formulation, other sulfonamides; type 1 diabetes mellitus (insulin dependent, IDDM)

Warnings/Precautions Use with caution in patients with severe hepatic disease; a useful agent since few drug to drug interactions and not dependent upon renal elimination of active drug

Chemical similarities are present among sulfonamides, sulfonylureas, carbonic anhydrase inhibitors, thiazides, and loop diuretics (except ethacrynic acid). Use in patients with sulfonamide allergy is specifically contraindicated in product labeling, however a risk of cross-reaction exists in patients with allergy to any of these compounds; avoid use when previous reaction has been severe.

Product labeling states oral hypoglycemic drugs may be associated with an increased cardiovascular mortality as compared to treatment with diet alone or diet plus insulin. Data to support this association are limited, and several studies, including a large prospective trial (UKPDS) have not supported an association.

At higher dosages, sulfonylureas may block the ATP-sensitive potassium channels, which have been suggested to increase the risk of cardiovascular events. In May, 2000, the National Diabetes Center (a patient advocacy group, not a government agency) issued a warning to avoid the use of sulfonylureas at higher dosages. The clinical data supporting an association is inconsistent, and there is no consensus within the medical community to support this assertion.

Adverse Reactions Frequency not defined.

Cardiovascular: Edema

Central nervous system: Headache

Dermatologic: Rash, urticaria, photosensitivity

Endocrine & metabolic: Hypoglycemia, hyponatremia, SIADH (rare)

Gastrointestinal: Anorexia, nausea, vomiting, diarrhea, epigastric fullness, constipation, heartburn

Hematologic: Blood dyscrasias, aplastic anemia, hemolytic anemia, bone marrow suppression, thrombocytopenia, agranulocytosis

Hepatic: Cholestatic jaundice, hepatic porphyria

Renal: Diuretic effect (minor)

Miscellaneous: Disulfiram-like reaction

Overdosage/Toxicology Symptoms include low blood sugar, tingling of lips and tongue, nausea, yawning, confusion, agitation, tachycardia, sweating, convulsions, stupor, and coma. Intoxications with sulfonylureas can cause hypoglycemia and are best managed with glucose administration (orally for milder hypoglycemia or by injection in more severe forms).

Drug Interactions

Increased Effect/Toxicity: Increased effects/hypoglycemic effects of glipizide with H_2 antagonists, anticoagulants, androgens, cimetidine, fluconazole, salicylates, gemfibrozil, sulfonamides, tricyclic antidepressants, probenecid, MAO inhibitors, methyldopa, digitalis glycosides, and urinary acidifiers.

Decreased Effect: Decreased effect of glipizide with beta-blockers, cholestyramine, hydantoins, rifampin, thiazide diuretics, urinary alkalinizers, and charcoal.

Ethanol/Nutrition/Herb Interactions

Ethanol: Caution with ethanol (may cause hypoglycemia or rare disulfiram reaction).

Food: A delayed release of insulin may occur if glipizide is taken with food. Should be administered 30 minutes before meals to avoid erratic absorption.

Herb/Nutraceutical: Caution with chromium, garlic, gymnema (may cause hypoglycemia).

Mechanism of Action Stimulates insulin release from the pancreatic beta cells; reduces glucose output from the liver; insulin sensitivity is increased at peripheral target sites

Pharmacodynamics/Kinetics

Onset of action: Peak effect: Blood glucose reductions: 1.5-2 hours

Duration: 12-24 hours

Absorption: Delayed when given with food

Protein binding: 92% to 99%

Metabolism: Hepatic with metabolites

Half-life elimination: 2-4 hours

Excretion: Urine (60% to 80%, 91% to 97% as metabolites); feces (11%)

Usual Dosage Oral (allow several days between dose titrations): Give ~30 minutes before a meal to obtain the greatest reduction in postprandial hyperglycemia

Adults: Initial: 5 mg/day; adjust dosage in 2.5-5 mg daily increments as determined by blood glucose response at intervals of several days. Maximum recommended once-daily dose: 15 mg; maximum recommended total daily dose: 40 mg; extended release (Glucotrol® XL) maximum recommended dose: 20 mg.

Elderly: Initial: 2.5 mg/day; increase by 2.5-5 mg/day at 1- to 2-week intervals

(Continued)

GlipiZIDE *(Continued)*

Dosing adjustment/comments in renal impairment: Cl_{cr} <10 mL/minute: Some investigators recommend not using

Dosing adjustment in hepatic impairment: Initial dosage should be 2.5 mg/day

Dietary Considerations Take glipizide before meals. Dietary modification based on ADA recommendations is a part of therapy. Decreases blood glucose concentration. Hypoglycemia may occur. Must be able to recognize symptoms of hypoglycemia (palpitations, sweaty palms, lightheadedness).

Administration Administer 30 minutes before a meal to achieve greatest reduction in postprandial hyperglycemia

Monitoring Parameters Urine for glucose and ketones; monitor for signs and symptoms of hypoglycemia (fatigue, excessive hunger, profuse sweating, numbness of extremities), fasting blood glucose, hemoglobin A_{1c}, fructosamine

Reference Range Target range: Adults:
Fasting blood glucose: <120 mg/dL
Glycosylated hemoglobin: <7%

Patient Information Patients must be counseled by someone experienced in diabetes education, signs and symptoms of hyper- and hypoglycemia, exercise and diet, blood glucose monitoring, and other related topics; eat regularly, do not skip meals; carry quick source of sugar; medical alert bracelet

Nursing Implications Patients who are NPO may need to have their dose held to avoid hypoglycemia

Dosage Forms
Tablet: 5 mg, 10 mg
Tablet, extended release: 2.5 mg, 5 mg, 10 mg

♦ **Glivec** *see* Imatinib *on page 703*

♦ **GlucaGen®** *see* Glucagon *on page 634*

Glucagon *(GLOO ka gon)*

U.S. Brand Names GlucaGen®

Therapeutic Category Antidote, Hypoglycemia; Diagnostic Agent, Gastrointestinal

Use Management of hypoglycemia; diagnostic aid in the radiologic examination of GI tract when a hypnotic state is needed

Unlabeled/Investigational Use Used with some success as a cardiac stimulant in management of severe cases of beta-adrenergic blocking agent overdosage

Pregnancy Risk Factor B

Contraindications Hypersensitivity to glucagon or any component of the formulation

Warnings/Precautions Use with caution in patients with a history of insulinoma and/or pheochromocytoma

Adverse Reactions
Gastrointestinal: Nausea, vomiting (high incidence with rapid administration of high doses)
Miscellaneous: Hypersensitivity reactions (hypotension, respiratory distress, urticaria)

Overdosage/Toxicology Symptoms include hypokalemia, nausea, and vomiting.

Drug Interactions
Increased Effect/Toxicity: Glucagon and warfarin - hypoprothrombinemic effects may be increased, possibly with bleeding.

Stability After reconstitution, use immediately; may be kept at 5°C for up to 48 hours if necessary

Mechanism of Action Stimulates adenylate cyclase to produce increased cyclic AMP, which promotes hepatic glycogenolysis and gluconeogenesis, causing a raise in blood glucose levels

Pharmacodynamics/Kinetics
Onset of action: Peak effect: Blood glucose levels: Parenteral: 5-20 minutes
Duration: 60-90 minutes
Metabolism: Hepatic; some inactivation occurring renally and in plasma
Half-life elimination, plasma: 3-10 minutes

Usual Dosage
Hypoglycemia or insulin shock therapy: I.M., I.V., S.C.:
Children: 0.025-0.1 mg/kg/dose, not to exceed 1 mg/dose, repeated in 20 minutes as needed
Adults: 0.5-1 mg, may repeat in 20 minutes as needed
If patient fails to respond to glucagon, I.V. dextrose must be given
Beta-blocker overdose (unlabeled use): I.V.: 3-10 mg **or** initially 0.5-5 mg bolus followed by continuous infusion 1-5 mg/hour
Diagnostic aid: Adults: I.M., I.V.: 0.25-2 mg 10 minutes prior to procedure

Administration Reconstitute powder for injection by adding 1 or 10 mL of sterile diluent to a vial containing 1 or 10 units of the drug, respectively, to provide solutions containing 1 mg of glucagon/mL; if dose to be administered is <2 mg of the drug → use only the diluent provided by the manufacturer; if >2 mg → use sterile water for injection; use immediately after reconstitution

Monitoring Parameters Blood pressure, blood glucose

Patient Information Instruct a close associate on how to prepare and administer as a treatment for insulin shock

Nursing Implications Parenteral: Dilute with manufacturer provided diluent resulting in 1 mg/mL; if doses exceeding 2 mg are used, dilute with sterile water instead of diluent; administer by direct I.V. injection

Additional Information 1 unit = 1 mg

Dosage Forms Powder for injection, lyophilized: 1 mg [1 unit]; 10 mg [10 units]

♦ **Glucocerebrosidase** *see* Alglucerase *on page 51*

♦ **GlucoNorm® (Can)** *see* Repaglinide *on page 1183*

♦ **Glucophage®** *see* Metformin *on page 875*

- **Glucophage® XR** *see Metformin on page 875*
- **Glucotrol®** *see GlipiZIDE on page 633*
- **Glucotrol® XL** *see GlipiZIDE on page 633*
- **Glucovance™** *see Glyburide and Metformin on page 636*
- **Glu-K® [OTC]** *see Potassium Gluconate on page 1110*
- **Glyate® [OTC]** *see Guaifenesin on page 645*
- **Glybenclamide** *see GlyBURIDE on page 635*
- **Glybenzcyclamide** *see GlyBURIDE on page 635*

GlyBURIDE (GLYE byoor ide)

Related Information
Antacid Drug Interactions *on page 1477*
Diabetes Mellitus Treatment *on page 1657*
Hypoglycemic Drugs & Thiazolidinedione Information *on page 1502*
Sulfonamide Derivatives *on page 1515*

U.S. Brand Names Diaβeta®; Glynase™ PresTab™; Micronase®

Canadian Brand Names Albert® Glyburide; Apo®-Glyburide; Diaβeta®; Euglucon®; Gen-Glybe; Novo-Glyburide; Nu-Glyburide; PMS-Glyburide

Synonyms Glibenclamide; Glybenclamide; Glybenzcyclamide

Therapeutic Category Antidiabetic Agent, Sulfonylurea; Hypoglycemic Agent, Oral; Sulfonylurea Agent

Use Management of type 2 diabetes mellitus (noninsulin dependent, NIDDM)

Unlabeled/Investigational Use Alternative to insulin in women for the treatment of gestational diabetes (11-33 weeks gestation)

Pregnancy Risk Factor C

Pregnancy/Breast-Feeding Implications
Clinical effects on the fetus: Crosses the placenta. Hypoglycemia; ear defects reported; other malformations reported but may have been secondary to poor maternal glucose control/diabetes. Insulin is the drug of choice for the control of diabetes mellitus during pregnancy.
Breast-feeding/lactation: No data available

Contraindications Hypersensitivity to glyburide, any component of the formulation, or other sulfonamides; type 1 diabetes mellitus (insulin dependent, IDDM), diabetic ketoacidosis with or without coma

Warnings/Precautions Elderly: Rapid and prolonged hypoglycemia (>12 hours) despite hypertonic glucose injections have been reported; age and hepatic and renal impairment are independent risk factors for hypoglycemia; dosage titration should be made at weekly intervals. Use with caution in patients with renal and hepatic impairment, malnourished or debilitated conditions, or adrenal or pituitary insufficiency.

Chemical similarities are present among sulfonamides, sulfonylureas, carbonic anhydrase inhibitors, thiazides, and loop diuretics (except ethacrynic acid). Use in patients with sulfonamide allergy is specifically contraindicated in product labeling, however a risk of cross-reaction exists in patients with allergy to any of these compounds; avoid use when previous reaction has been severe.

Product labeling states oral hypoglycemic drugs may be associated with an increased cardiovascular mortality as compared to treatment with diet alone or diet plus insulin. Data to support this association are limited, and several studies, including a large prospective trial (UKPDS) have not supported an association.

Adverse Reactions Frequency not defined.
Central nervous system: Headache, dizziness
Dermatologic: Pruritus, rash, urticaria, photosensitivity reaction
Gastrointestinal: Nausea, epigastric fullness, heartburn, constipation, diarrhea, anorexia
Endocrine & metabolic: Hypoglycemia, hyponatremia (SIADH reported with other sulfonylureas)
Genitourinary: Nocturia
Hematologic: Leukopenia, thrombocytopenia, hemolytic anemia, aplastic anemia, bone marrow suppression, agranulocytosis
Hepatic: Cholestatic jaundice, hepatitis
Neuromuscular & skeletal: Arthralgia, paresthesia
Ocular: Blurred vision
Renal: Diuretic effect (minor)

Overdosage/Toxicology Symptoms include severe hypoglycemia, seizures, cerebral damage, tingling of lips and tongue, nausea, yawning, confusion, agitation, tachycardia, sweating, convulsions, stupor, and coma. Intoxications with sulfonylureas can cause hypoglycemia and are best managed with glucose administration (orally for milder hypoglycemia or by injection in more severe forms).

Drug Interactions
Cytochrome P450 Effect: CYP3A3/4 enzyme substrate
Increased Effect/Toxicity: Increased hypoglycemic effects of glyburide may occur with oral anticoagulants (warfarin), phenytoin, other hydantoins, salicylates, NSAIDs, sulfonamides, and beta-blockers. Ethanol ingestion may cause disulfiram reactions.
Decreased Effect: Thiazides and other diuretics, corticosteroids may decrease effectiveness of glyburide.

Ethanol/Nutrition/Herb Interactions
Ethanol: Caution with ethanol (may cause hypoglycemia).
Herb/Nutraceutical: Caution with chromium, garlic, gymnema (may cause hypoglycemia).

Mechanism of Action Stimulates insulin release from the pancreatic beta cells; reduces glucose output from the liver; insulin sensitivity is increased at peripheral target sites

Pharmacodynamics/Kinetics
Onset of action: Serum insulin levels begin to increase 15-60 minutes after a single dose
Duration: ≤24 hours
Metabolism: To one moderately active and several inactive metabolites
Protein binding, plasma: >99%
(Continued)

GlyBURIDE (Continued)

Half-life elimination: 5-16 hours; may be prolonged with renal insufficiency or hepatic insufficiency

Time to peak, serum: Adults: 2-4 hours

Excretion: Feces (50%) and urine (50%) as metabolites

Usual Dosage Oral:

Adults:

Initial: 2.5-5 mg/day, administered with breakfast or the first main meal of the day. In patients who are more sensitive to hypoglycemic drugs, start at 1.25 mg/day.

Increase in increments of no more than 2.5 mg/day at weekly intervals based on the patient's blood glucose response

Maintenance: 1.25-20 mg/day given as single or divided doses; maximum: 20 mg/day

Elderly: Initial: 1.25-2.5 mg/day, increase by 1.25-2.5 mg/day every 1-3 weeks

Micronized tablets (Glynase™ PresTab™): Adults:

Initial: 1.5-3 mg/day, administered with breakfast or the first main meal of the day in patients who are more sensitive to hypoglycemic drugs, start at 0.75 mg/day. Increase in increments of no more than 1.5 mg/day in weekly intervals based on the patient's blood glucose response.

Maintenance: 0.75-12 mg/day given as a single dose or in divided doses. Some patients (especially those receiving >6 mg/day) may have a more satisfactory response with twice-daily dosing.

Dosing adjustment/comments in renal impairment: Cl$_{cr}$ <50 mL/minute: **Not recommended**

Dosing adjustment in hepatic impairment: Use conservative initial and maintenance doses and avoid use in severe disease

Dietary Considerations Should be taken with meals at the same time each day. Dietary modification based on ADA recommendations is a part of therapy. Decreases blood glucose concentration. Hypoglycemia may occur. Must be able to recognize symptoms of hypoglycemia (palpitations, sweaty palms, lightheadedness).

Administration Administer with meals at the same time each day.

Monitoring Parameters Signs and symptoms of hypoglycemia, fasting blood glucose, hemoglobin A$_{1c}$

Reference Range Target range: Adults:

Fasting blood glucose: <120 mg/dL

Glycosylated hemoglobin: <7%

Patient Information Patients must be counseled by someone experienced in diabetes education, signs and symptoms of hyper- and hypoglycemia, exercise and diet, blood glucose monitoring, and other related topics; eat regularly, do not skip meals; carry quick source of sugar; medical alert bracelet

Nursing Implications Patients who are anorexic or NPO, may need to have their dose held to avoid hypoglycemia

Dosage Forms

Tablet (Diaβeta®, Micronase®): 1.25 mg, 2.5 mg, 5 mg

Tablet, micronized (Glynase™ PresTab™): 1.5 mg, 3 mg, 4.5 mg, 6 mg

Glyburide and Metformin (GLYE byoor ide & met FOR min)

U.S. Brand Names Glucovance™

Synonyms Glyburide and Metformin Hydrochloride

Therapeutic Category Antidiabetic Agent, Sulfonylurea

Use Initial therapy for management of type 2 diabetes mellitus (noninsulin dependent, NIDDM) when hyperglycemia cannot be managed with diet and exercise alone. Second-line therapy for management of type 2 diabetes mellitus (noninsulin dependent, NIDDM) when hyperglycemia cannot be managed with a sulfonylurea or metformin along with diet and exercise.

Pregnancy Risk Factor B (manufacturer); C (expert analysis)

Pregnancy/Breast-Feeding Implications Abnormal blood glucose levels during pregnancy may be associated with an increased incidence of congenital abnormalities. Insulin is the drug of choice for the control of diabetes mellitus during pregnancy. Use glyburide/metformin during pregnancy only if clearly needed.

Glyburide: Crosses the placenta. Hypoglycemia, ear defects reported; other malformations reported but may have been secondary to poor maternal glucose control/diabetes.

Metformin: May partially cross the placenta.

Severe prolonged hypoglycemia has been reported in neonates whose mothers were taking sulfonylureas at the time of delivery. If the decision has been made to use glyburide/metformin during pregnancy, it should be discontinued at least 2 weeks prior to delivery.

Breast-feeding/lactation: No data available for glyburide, however, other sulfonylureas are excreted in breast milk. It is possible that hypoglycemia may occur in a nursing infant.

Contraindications Hypersensitivity to glyburide or other sulfonamides, metformin, or any component of the formulation; renal disease or renal dysfunction (serum creatinine ≥1.5 mg/dL in males or ≥1.4 mg/dL in females, or creatinine clearance <60 mL/minute) which may also result from conditions such as cardiovascular collapse, acute myocardial infarction, and septicemia; acute or chronic metabolic acidosis with or without coma (including diabetic ketoacidosis); discontinue at the time of or prior to the procedure in patients undergoing radiologic studies in which intravascular iodinated contrast materials are utilized, and withhold for 48 hours subsequent to the procedure; reinstitute only after renal function has been re-evaluated and found to be normal

Warnings/Precautions Age, hepatic and renal impairment are independent risk factors for hypoglycemia. Use with caution in patients with hepatic impairment, malnourished or debilitated conditions, or adrenal or pituitary insufficiency. Use caution in patients with renal impairment. Metformin is substantially excreted by the kidney. The risk of accumulation and lactic acidosis increases with the degree of impairment in renal function. Ethanol will potentiate this effect. Patients with renal function below the limit of normal for their age should not receive metformin. In elderly patients, renal function should be monitored regularly. Use of concomitant medications that may affect renal function (ie, affect tubular secretion) may affect metformin disposition. Suspend treatment for surgical procedures which restrict the intake of food and fluids; do not restart treatment until oral intake and renal function are normal.

Chemical similarities are present among sulfonamides, sulfonylureas, carbonic anhydrase inhibitors, thiazides, and loop diuretics (except ethacrynic acid). Use in patients with sulfonamide allergy is specifically contraindicated in product labeling, however a risk of cross-reaction exists in patients with allergy to any of these compounds; avoid use when previous reaction has been severe.

Product labeling states oral hypoglycemic drugs may be associated with an increased cardiovascular mortality as compared to treatment with diet alone or diet plus insulin. Data to support this association are limited, and several studies, including a large prospective trial (UKPDS) have not supported an association.

Adverse Reactions See individual agents

Overdosage/Toxicology
Glyburide: Symptoms include severe hypoglycemia, seizures, cerebral damage, tingling of lips and tongue, nausea, yawning, confusion, agitation, tachycardia, sweating, convulsions, stupor, and coma. Intoxications with sulfonylureas can cause hypoglycemia and are best managed with glucose administration (orally for milder hypoglycemia or by injection in more severe forms).
Metformin: Lactic acidosis may occur. Hemodialysis may be used in suspected cases of overdose.

Drug Interactions
Cytochrome P450 Effect: Glyburide: CYP3A3/4 enzyme substrate
Increased Effect/Toxicity: Refer to individual agents.
Decreased Effect: Refer to individual agents.

Ethanol/Nutrition/Herb Interactions
Ethanol: May cause hypoglycemia; incidence of lactic acidosis may be increased; a disulfiram-like reaction characterized by flushing, headache, nausea, vomiting, sweating, or tachycardia has been reported with sulfonylureas; avoid or limit use.
Food: Metformin decreases absorption of vitamin B_{12}. Metformin decreases absorption of folic acid.

Stability Store at 25°C (77°F)

Mechanism of Action The combination of glyburide and metformin is used to improve glycemic control in patients with type 2 diabetes mellitus by using two different, but complementary, mechanisms of action:
Glyburide: Stimulates insulin release from the pancreatic beta cells; reduces glucose output from the liver; insulin sensitivity is increased at peripheral target sites
Metformin: Decreases hepatic glucose production, decreasing intestinal absorption of glucose and improves insulin sensitivity (increases peripheral glucose uptake and utilization)

Pharmacodynamics/Kinetics
Glucovance™:
Bioavailability: 18% with 2.5 mg glyburide/500 mg metformin dose; 7% with 5 mg glyburide/500 mg metformin dose; bioavailability is greater than that of Micronase® brand of glyburide and therefore not bioequivalent
Time to peak: 2.75 hours when taken with food
Glyburide: See Glyburide monograph.
Metformin: This component of Glucovance™ is bioequivalent to metformin coadministration with glyburide.

Usual Dosage Adults: Oral: Dose should be individualized based on effectiveness and tolerance; titrate to minimum effective dose needed to achieve blood glucose control; **do not exceed maximum recommended doses**
Initial therapy: Glucovance™ 1.25 mg/250 mg once daily with a meal; patients with Hb A_{1c} >9% or fasting plasma glucose (FPG) >200 mg/dL may start with Glucovance™ 1.25 mg/250 mg twice daily with meals
Dosage increases may be made every 2 weeks, in increments of Glucovance™ 1.25 mg/250 mg, until a dose of glyburide 10 mg/metformin 2000 mg per day has been reached
Due to increased risk of hypoglycemia, do not start with Glucovance™ 5 mg/500 mg.
Second-line therapy: Patients previously treated with a sulfonylurea or metformin alone: Starting dose: Glucovance™ 2.5 mg/500 mg or Glucovance™ 5 mg/500 mg twice daily with the morning and evening meals; doses may be increased in increments no larger than glyburide 5 mg/metformin 500 mg, up to a maximum dose of glyburide 20 mg/metformin 2000 mg.
When switching patients previously on a sulfonylurea and metformin together, do not exceed the daily dose of glyburide (or glyburide equivalent) or metformin.

Dosage adjustment in renal impairment: Risk of lactic acidosis increases with degree of renal impairment; contraindicated in renal disease or renal dysfunction (see Contraindications)
Dosage adjustment in hepatic impairment: Use conservative initial and maintenance doses and avoid use in severe hepatic disease
Elderly: Conservative doses are recommended in the elderly due to potentially decreased renal function; **do not titrate to maximum dose**; should not be used in patients ≥80 years of age unless renal function is verified as normal

Dietary Considerations May cause GI upset; take with food to decrease GI upset. Dietary modification based on ADA recommendations is a part of therapy. Decreases blood glucose concentration. Hypoglycemia may occur. Must be able to recognize symptoms of hypoglycemia (palpitations, sweaty palms, lightheadedness). Monitor for signs and symptoms of vitamin B_{12} deficiency. Monitor for signs and symptoms of folic acid deficiency.

Administration Administer with a meal(s)

Monitoring Parameters Signs and symptoms of hypoglycemia, urine for glucose and ketones, FPG, Hb A_{1c}, and fructosamine. Initial and periodic monitoring of hematologic
(Continued)

Glyburide and Metformin *(Continued)*

parameters (eg, hemoglobin/hematocrit and red blood cell indices) and renal function should be performed. Monitor at least annually once patient is on maintenance therapy. While megaloblastic anemia has been rarely seen with metformin, if suspected, vitamin B_{12} deficiency should be excluded.

Reference Range Target range: Adults: Fasting blood glucose: <120 mg/dL; glycosylated hemoglobin: <7%

Patient Information This medication is used to control diabetes; it is not a cure. Other components of treatment plan are important: Follow prescribed diet, medication, and exercise regimen. Take exactly as directed. Do not change dose or discontinue without consulting prescriber. Avoid alcohol; could cause severe adverse reactions (hypoglycemia, lactic acidosis). Inform prescriber of all other prescription or OTC medications you are taking; do not introduce new medication without consulting prescriber. Do not take other medication within 2 hours of this medication unless so advised by prescriber. If you experience hypoglycemic reaction, contact prescriber immediately. Maintain regular dietary intake and exercise routine and always carry quick source of sugar with you. You may be more sensitive to sunlight (avoid direct sunlight, use sunscreen, and wear protective clothing and eyewear). You may experience side effects during first weeks of therapy (headache, nausea); consult prescriber if these persist. Nausea, vomiting and other gastrointestinal symptoms are common at the start of therapy and can be decreased by taking this medication with food. If these occur later in your therapy, notify prescriber. Report severe or persistent side effects, extended vomiting, or flu-like symptoms, skin rash, easy bruising or bleeding, or change in color of urine or stool. Discontinue medication and call your prescriber immediately if you have unexplained hyperventilation, myalgia, malaise, unusual tiredness, or other nonspecific symptoms.

Nursing Implications Patients who are anorexic or NPO may need to have their dose held to avoid hypoglycemia. Hypoglycemia may be masked in patients who are taking beta-blockers and in the elderly.

Dosage Forms
Tablet, film coated:
1.25 mg/250 mg: Glyburide 1.25 mg and metformin hydrochloride 250 mg
2.5 mg/500 mg: Glyburide 2.5 mg and metformin hydrochloride 500 mg
5 mg/500 mg: Glyburide 5 mg and metformin hydrochloride 500 mg

♦ **Glyburide and Metformin Hydrochloride** *see* Glyburide and Metformin *on page 636*

Glycerin, Lanolin, and Peanut Oil (GLIS er in, LAN oh lin, & PEE nut oyl)
U.S. Brand Names Massé® Breast Cream [OTC]
Therapeutic Category Topical Skin Product
Use Nipple care of pregnant and nursing women
Usual Dosage Apply as often as needed
Additional Information Complete prescribing information for this medication should be consulted for additional detail.
Dosage Forms Cream, topical: 2 oz

♦ **Glycerol Guaiacolate** *see* Guaifenesin *on page 645*

♦ **Glycerol-T®** *see* Theophylline and Guaifenesin *on page 1310*

♦ **Glyceryl Trinitrate** *see* Nitroglycerin *on page 989*

♦ **Glycofed®** *see* Guaifenesin and Pseudoephedrine *on page 647*

♦ **Glycon (Can)** *see* Metformin *on page 875*

♦ **Glycoprotein Antagonists** *see page 1500*

Glycopyrrolate (glye koe PYE roe late)
U.S. Brand Names Robinul®; Robinul® Forte
Synonyms Glycopyrronium Bromide
Therapeutic Category Anticholinergic Agent; Antispasmodic Agent, Gastrointestinal
Use Inhibit salivation and excessive secretions of the respiratory tract preoperatively; reversal of neuromuscular blockade; control of upper airway secretions; adjunct in treatment of peptic ulcer

Pregnancy Risk Factor B

Contraindications Hypersensitivity to glycopyrrolate or any component of the formulation; ulcerative colitis; narrow-angle glaucoma; acute hemorrhage; tachycardia; obstructive uropathy; paralytic ileus; obstructive disease of GI tract

Warnings/Precautions Not recommended in children <12 years of age for the management of peptic ulcer; infants, patients with Down syndrome, and children with spastic paralysis or brain damage may be hypersensitive to antimuscarine effects. Use caution in elderly, patients with autonomic neuropathy, hepatic or renal disease, ulcerative colitis may predispose megacolon, hyperthyroidism, CAD, CHF, arrhythmias, tachycardia, BPH, hiatal hernia, with reflux.

Adverse Reactions
>10%:
Dermatologic: Dry skin
Gastrointestinal: Constipation, dry throat, dry mouth
Local: Irritation at injection site
Respiratory: Dry nose
Miscellaneous: Diaphoresis (decreased)
1% to 10%:
Dermatologic: Increased sensitivity to light
Endocrine & metabolic: Decreased flow of breast milk
Gastrointestinal: Dysphagia
<1% (Limited to important or life-threatening): Increased intraocular pain, orthostatic hypotension, palpitations, tachycardia, ventricular fibrillation

Overdosage/Toxicology Symptoms include blurred vision, urinary retention, tachycardia, and absent bowel sounds. Anticholinergic toxicity is caused by strong binding of the drug to cholinergic receptors. For anticholinergic overdose with severe life-threatening symptoms, physostigmine 1-2 mg (0.5 mg or 0.02 mg/kg for children) S.C. or slow I.V. may be given to reverse these effects.

Drug Interactions

Increased Effect/Toxicity: Increased toxicity with amantadine and cyclopropane. Effects of other anticholinergic agents may be increased by glycopyrrolate.

Decreased Effect: Decreased effect of levodopa.

Stability Unstable at pH >6; **incompatible** with secobarbital (immediate precipitation), sodium bicarbonate (gas evolves), thiopental (immediate precipitation)

Mechanism of Action Blocks the action of acetylcholine at parasympathetic sites in smooth muscle, secretory glands, and the CNS

Pharmacodynamics/Kinetics

Onset of action: Oral: 50 minutes; I.M.: 20-40 minutes; I.V.: ~1 minute

Peak effect: Oral: ~1 hour

Duration: Vagal effect: 2-3 hours; Inhibition of salivation: Up to 7 hours; Anticholinergic: Oral: 8-12 hours

Absorption: Oral: Poor and erratic

Bioavailability: ~10%

Half-life: 20-40 minutes

Usual Dosage

Children:

Control of secretions:

Oral: 40-100 mcg/kg/dose 3-4 times/day

I.M., I.V.: 4-10 mcg/kg/dose every 3-4 hours; maximum: 0.2 mg/dose or 0.8 mg/24 hours

Intraoperative: I.V.: 4 mcg/kg not to exceed 0.1 mg; repeat at 2- to 3-minute intervals as needed

Preoperative: I.M.:

<2 years: 4.4-8.8 mcg/kg 30-60 minutes before procedure

>2 years: 4.4 mcg/kg 30-60 minutes before procedure

Children and Adults: Reverse neuromuscular blockade: I.V.: 0.2 mg for each 1 mg of neostigmine or 5 mg of pyridostigmine administered or 5-15 mcg/kg glycopyrrolate with 25-70 mcg/kg of neostigmine or 0.1-0.3 mg/kg of pyridostigmine (agents usually administered simultaneously, but glycopyrrolate may be administered first if bradycardia is present)

Adults:

Intraoperative: I.V.: 0.1 mg repeated as needed at 2- to 3-minute intervals

Preoperative: I.M.: 4.4 mcg/kg 30-60 minutes before procedure

Peptic ulcer:

Oral: 1-2 mg 2-3 times/day

I.M., I.V.: 0.1-0.2 mg 3-4 times/day

Administration For I.V. administration, glycopyrrolate may also be administered via the tubing of a running I.V. infusion of a compatible solution

Patient Information Maintain good oral hygiene habits, because lack of saliva may increase chance of cavities. Observe caution while driving or performing other tasks requiring alertness, as may cause drowsiness, dizziness, or blurred vision. Notify physician if skin rash, flushing or eye pain occurs; or if difficulty in urinating, constipation, or sensitivity to light becomes severe or persists.

Nursing Implications Monitor heart rate; anticholinergic effects

Dosage Forms

Injection, as bromide: 0.2 mg/mL (1 mL, 2 mL, 5 mL, 20 mL)

Robinul®: 0.2 mg/mL (1 mL, 2 mL, 5 mL, 20 mL)

Tablet, as bromide:

Robinul®: 1 mg

Robinul® Forte: 2 mg

Gold Sodium Thiomalate (gold SOW dee um thye oh MAL ate)

U.S. Brand Names Aurolate®

Canadian Brand Names Myochrysine®

Therapeutic Category Gold Compound

Use Treatment of progressive rheumatoid arthritis

Pregnancy Risk Factor C

Contraindications Hypersensitivity to gold compounds or any component of the formulation; systemic lupus erythematosus; history of blood dyscrasias; congestive heart failure, exfoliative dermatitis, colitis

Warnings/Precautions Frequent monitoring of patients for signs and symptoms of toxicity will prevent serious adverse reactions; nonsteroidal anti-inflammatory drugs (NSAIDs) and corticosteroids may be discontinued after initiating gold therapy; must not be injected I.V.

(Continued)

Gold Sodium Thiomalate (Continued)

Explain the possibility of adverse reactions before initiating therapy; signs of gold toxicity include decrease in hemoglobin, leukopenia, granulocytes and platelets; proteinuria, hematuria, pigmentation, pruritus, stomatitis or persistent diarrhea, rash, metallic taste; advise patient to report any symptoms of toxicity; use with caution in patients with liver or renal disease

Adverse Reactions

>10%:
  Dermatologic: Itching, rash
  Gastrointestinal: Stomatitis, gingivitis, glossitis
  Ocular: Conjunctivitis
1% to 10%:
  Dermatologic: Urticaria, alopecia
  Hematologic: Eosinophilia, leukopenia, thrombocytopenia
  Renal: Proteinuria, hematuria
<1% (Limited to important or life-threatening): Agranulocytosis, anemia, angioedema, aplastic anemia, dysphagia, GI hemorrhage, hepatotoxicity, interstitial pneumonitis, metallic taste, peripheral neuropathy, ulcerative enterocolitis

Overdosage/Toxicology Symptoms include hematuria, proteinuria, fever, nausea, vomiting, and diarrhea. For mild gold poisoning, dimercaprol 2.5 mg/kg 4 times/day for 2 days, or for more severe forms of gold intoxication, dimercaprol 3-5 mg/kg every 4 hours for 2 days should be initiated. Then after 2 days, the initial dose should be repeated twice daily on the third day, and once daily thereafter for 10 days. Other chelating agents have been used with some success.

Drug Interactions
  Decreased Effect: Penicillamine and acetylcysteine may decrease effect of gold sodium thiomalate.

Stability Should not be used if solution is darker than pale yellow.

Mechanism of Action Unknown, may decrease prostaglandin synthesis or may alter cellular mechanisms by inhibiting sulfhydryl systems

Pharmacodynamics/Kinetics
  Onset of action: Delayed; may require up to 3 months
  Half-life elimination: 5 days; may lengthen with multiple doses
  Time to peak, serum: 4-6 hours
  Excretion: Primarily urine (60% to 90%); feces (10% to 40%)

Usual Dosage I.M.:
  Children: Initial: Test dose of 10 mg is recommended, followed by 1 mg/kg/week for 20 weeks; maintenance: 1 mg/kg/dose at 2- to 4-week intervals thereafter for as long as therapy is clinically beneficial and toxicity does not develop. Administration for 2-4 months is usually required before clinical improvement is observed.
  Adults: 10 mg first week; 25 mg second week; then 25-50 mg/week until 1 g cumulative dose has been given; if improvement occurs without adverse reactions, administer 25-50 mg every 2-3 weeks for 2-20 weeks, then every 3-4 weeks indefinitely
  Dosing adjustment in renal impairment:
    Cl_{cr} 50-80 mL/minute: Administer 50% of normal dose
    Cl_{cr} <50 mL/minute: Avoid use

Administration Deep I.M. injection into the upper outer quadrant of the gluteal region addition of 0.1 mL of 1% lidocaine to each injection may reduce the discomfort associated with I.M. administration

Monitoring Parameters Signs and symptoms of gold toxicity, CBC with differential and platelet count, urinalysis

Reference Range Gold: Normal: 0-0.1 µg/mL (SI: 0-0.0064 µmol/L); Therapeutic: 1-3 µg/mL (SI: 0.06-0.18 µmol/L); Urine: <0.1 µg/24 hour

Patient Information Minimize exposure to sunlight; benefits from drug therapy may take as long as 3 months to appear; notify physician of pruritus, rash, sore mouth; metallic taste may occur

Nursing Implications Explain the possibility of adverse reactions before initiating therapy

Additional Information Approximately 50% gold

Dosage Forms Injection: 25 mg/mL (1 mL); 50 mg/mL (1 mL, 2 mL, 10 mL)

♦ GoLYTELY® *see Polyethylene Glycol-Electrolyte Solution on page 1101*

Gonadorelin (goe nad oh RELL in)

U.S. Brand Names Factrel®; Lutrepulse®

Canadian Brand Names Lutrepulse™

Synonyms GnRH; Gonadorelin Acetate; Gonadorelin Hydrochloride; Gonadotropin Releasing Hormone; LHRH; LRH; Luteinizing Hormone Releasing Hormone

Therapeutic Category Diagnostic Agent, Gonadotrophic Hormone; Gonadotropin

Use Evaluation of functional capacity and response of gonadotrophic hormones; evaluate abnormal gonadotropin regulation as in precocious puberty and delayed puberty.
  Orphan drug: Lutrepulse®: Induction of ovulation in females with hypothalamic amenorrhea

Pregnancy Risk Factor B

Contraindications Hypersensitivity to gonadorelin or any component of the formulation; women with any condition that could be exacerbated by pregnancy; patients who have ovarian cysts or causes of anovulation other than those of hypothalamic origin; any condition that may worsened by reproductive hormones

Warnings/Precautions Hypersensitivity and anaphylactic reactions have occurred following multiple-dose administration; multiple pregnancy is a possibility; use with caution in women in whom pregnancy could worsen pre-existing conditions (eg, pituitary prolactinemia). Multiple pregnancy is a possibility with Lutrepulse®.

Adverse Reactions 1% to 10%: Local: Pain at injection site

Overdosage/Toxicology Symptoms include abdominal discomfort, nausea, headache, and flushing. Treatment is symptomatic.

GOSERELIN

Drug Interactions
  Increased Effect/Toxicity: Increased levels/effect with androgens, estrogens, progestins, glucocorticoids, spironolactone, and levodopa.
  Decreased Effect: Decreased levels/effect with oral contraceptives, digoxin, phenothiazines, and dopamine antagonists.

Stability
  Factrel®: Prepare immediately prior to use; after reconstitution, store at room temperature and use within 1 day; discard unused portion
  Lutrepulse®: Store at room temperature; reconstitute with diluent immediately prior to use and transfer to plastic reservoir. The solution will supply 90 minute pulsatile doses for 7 consecutive days (Lutrepulse® pump).

Mechanism of Action Stimulates the release of luteinizing hormone (LH) from the anterior pituitary gland

Pharmacodynamics/Kinetics
  Onset of action: Peak effect: Maximal LH release: ~20 minutes
  Duration: 3-5 hours
  Half-life elimination: 4 minutes

Usual Dosage
  Diagnostic test: Children >12 years and Female Adults: I.V., S.C. hydrochloride salt: 100 mcg administered in women during early phase of menstrual cycle (day 1-7)
  Primary hypothalamic amenorrhea: Female Adults: Acetate: I.V.: 5 mcg every 90 minutes via Lutrepulse® pump kit at treatment intervals of 21 days (pump will pulsate every 90 minutes for 7 days)

Administration
  Factrel®: Dilute in 3 mL of normal saline; administer I.V. push over 30 seconds
  Lutrepulse®: A presterilized reservoir bag with the infusion catheter set supplied with the kit should be filled with the reconstituted solution and administered I.V. using the Lutrepulse® pump. Set the pump to deliver 25-50 mL of solution, based upon the dose, over a pulse period of 1 minute and at a pulse frequency of 90 minutes.

Monitoring Parameters LH, FSH

Nursing Implications Parenteral: Dilute in 3 mL of normal saline; administer I.V. push over 30 seconds

Dosage Forms
  Injection, as acetate (Lutrepulse®): 0.8 mg, 3.2 mg
  Injection, as hydrochloride (Factrel®): 100 mcg, 500 mcg

♦ **Gonadorelin Acetate** see Gonadorelin on page 640
♦ **Gonadorelin Hydrochloride** see Gonadorelin on page 640
♦ **Gonadotropin Releasing Hormone** see Gonadorelin on page 640
♦ **Gonal-F®** see Follitropins on page 596
♦ **Goody's® Extra Strength Headache Powder [OTC]** see Acetaminophen, Aspirin, and Caffeine on page 26
♦ **Goody's PM® Powder** see Acetaminophen and Diphenhydramine on page 25
♦ **Gormel® Creme [OTC]** see Urea on page 1391

Goserelin (GOE se rel in)

U.S. Brand Names Zoladex® Implant
Canadian Brand Names Zoladex®; Zoladex® LA
Synonyms Goserelin Acetate
Therapeutic Category Antineoplastic Agent, Miscellaneous; Gonadotropin Releasing Hormone Analog; Luteinizing Hormone-Releasing Hormone Analog

Use
  Prostate carcinoma: Palliative treatment of advanced carcinoma of the prostate. An alternative treatment of prostatic cancer when orchiectomy or estrogen administration are either not indicated or unacceptable to the patient. Combination with flutamide for the management of locally confined stage T2b-T4 (stage B2-C) carcinoma of the prostate.
  3.6 mg implant only:
    Endometriosis: Management of endometriosis, including pain relief and reduction of endometriotic lesions for the duration of therapy
    Advanced breast cancer: Palliative treatment of advanced breast cancer in pre- and perimenopausal women. Estrogen and progesterone receptor values may help to predict whether goserelin therapy is likely to be beneficial.
    Note: The 10.8 mg implant is not indicated in women as the data are insufficient to support reliable suppression of serum estradiol

Pregnancy Risk Factor X
Contraindications Hypersensitivity to goserelin or any component of the formulation; pregnancy (or potential to become pregnant)
Warnings/Precautions Initially, goserelin transiently increases serum levels of testosterone. Transient worsening of signs and symptoms, usually manifested by an increase in cancer-related pain which may be managed symptomatically, may develop during the first few weeks of treatment. Isolated cases of ureteral obstruction and spinal cord compression have been reported; patient's symptoms may initially worsen temporarily during first few weeks of therapy, cancer-related pain can usually be controlled by analgesics
Adverse Reactions Hormone replacement therapy may decrease vasomotor symptoms and loss of bone mineral density. Adverse reaction profile varies with gender and therapeutic use.

  >10%:
    Central nervous system: Headache (11%)
    Endocrine & metabolic: Hot flashes (53% to 62% of men, 100% of women), sexual dysfunction (15% to 21%), decreased libido, impotence, impaired erection (16% to 18%), tumor flare, bone pain (23% of women, 1% to 10% of men), vaginal dryness (10% to 14%)

(Continued)

Goserelin (Continued)

1% to 10%:

Cardiovascular: Anginal pain, arrhythmias, hypertension, thromboembolic events, congestive heart failure, myocardial infarction (1% to 5%), edema

Central nervous system: Lethargy (5% to 8%), anxiety, depression, dizziness, insomnia

Dermatologic: Urticaria, maculopapular rashes (10%)

Endocrine & metabolic: Gynecomastia, breast swelling (3% to 5%), bone loss, diaphoresis

Gastrointestinal: Abdominal pain, taste disturbances, diarrhea, nausea, vomiting (5%), anorexia

<1% (Limited to important or life-threatening): Spinal cord compression, ovarian cyst formation, pituitary apoplexy (following initiation in patients with functional pituitary adenoma)

Changes in blood pressure (usually transient) have been associated with goserelin use. Osteoporosis, decreased bone mineral density, and fracture have been reported rarely in men treated with goserelin.

Overdosage/Toxicology Treatment is symptomatic.

Stability Zoladex® should be stored at room temperature not to exceed 25°C or 77°F; protect from light; must be dispensed in an amber bag

Mechanism of Action LHRH synthetic analog of luteinizing hormone-releasing hormone also known as gonadotropin-releasing hormone (GnRH) incorporated into a biodegradable depot material which allows for continuous slow release over 28 days; mechanism of action is similar to leuprolide

Pharmacodynamics/Kinetics

Absorption: S.C.: Rapid and can be detected in serum in 10 minutes

Distribution: V_d: 13.7 L

Time to peak, serum: S.C.: 12-15 days

Half-life elimination: S.C. dose: 5 hours; Impaired renal function: 12 hours

Excretion: Urine within 4.2 hours

Usual Dosage

Adults: S.C.:

Monthly implant: 3.6 mg injected into upper abdomen every 28 days; while a delay of a few days is permissible, attempt to adhere to the 28-day schedule

3-month implant: 10.8 mg injected into the upper abdominal wall every 12 weeks; while a delay of a few days is permissible, attempt to adhere to the 12-week schedule

Prostate carcinoma: Intended for long-term administration

Endometriosis: Recommended duration: 6 months; retreatment is not recommended since safety data is not available. If symptoms recur after a course of therapy, and further treatment is contemplated, consider monitoring bone mineral density. Currently, there are no clinical data on the effect of treatment of benign gynecological conditions with goserelin for periods >6 months.

Dosing adjustment in renal/hepatic impairment: No adjustment is necessary

Administration

Do not remove the sterile syringe until immediately before use.

After cleaning with an alcohol swab, a local anesthetic may be used on an area of skin on the upper abdominal wall.

Stretch the patient's skin with one hand, and grip the needle with fingers around the barrel of the syringe. Insert the hypodermic needle into the SC fat. Do not try to aspirate with the goserelin syringe. If the needle is in a large vessel, blood will immediately appear in the syringe chamber.

Change the direction of the needle so it parallels the abdominal wall. Push the needle in until the barrel hub touches the patient's skin. Withdraw the needle 1 cm to create a space to discharge the drug; fully depress the plunger to discharge.

Withdraw needle and bandage the site. Confirm discharge by ensuring tip of the plunger is visible within the tip of the needle.

Test Interactions Serum alkaline phosphatase, serum acid phosphatase, serum testosterone, serum LH and FSH, serum estradiol

Patient Information This drug must be implanted into your stomach every 28 days; it is important to maintain appointment schedule. You may experience systemic hot flashes (cool clothes and temperatures may help), headache (analgesic may help), constipation (increased bulk and water in diet or stool softener may help), sexual dysfunction (decreased libido, decreased erection). Symptoms may worsen temporarily during first weeks of therapy. Report unusual nausea or vomiting, any chest pain, respiratory difficulty, unresolved dizziness, or constipation. Females must use reliable contraception during therapy.

Nursing Implications Do not try to aspirate with the goserelin syringe, if the needle is in a large vessel, blood will immediately appear in syringe chamber

Dosage Forms

Injection, 3-month implant [single-dose disposable syringe with 14-gauge hypodermic needle]: 10.8 mg

Injection, monthly implant [single-dose disposable syringe with 16-gauge hypodermic needle]: 3.6 mg

♦ **Goserelin Acetate** see Goserelin on page 641

♦ **GP 47680** see Oxcarbazepine on page 1021

♦ **GR1222311X** see Ranitidine Bismuth Citrate on page 1180

♦ **Gramicidin, Neomycin, and Polymyxin B** see Neomycin, Polymyxin B, and Gramicidin on page 969

Granisetron (gra NI se tron)

U.S. Brand Names Kytril®

Canadian Brand Names Kytril®

Therapeutic Category Antiemetic, Serotonin Antagonist; 5-HT₃ Receptor Antagonist; Serotonin Antagonist

Use Prophylaxis and treatment of chemotherapy-related emesis; may be prescribed for patients who are refractory to or have severe adverse reactions to standard antiemetic therapy. Prophylaxis of nausea and vomiting associated with radiation therapy, including total body irradiation and fractionated abdominal radiation. Granisetron may be prescribed for young patients (ie, <45 years of age who are more likely to develop extrapyramidal symptoms to high-dose metoclopramide) who are to receive highly emetogenic chemotherapeutic agents (see Additional Information); granisetron should not be prescribed for chemotherapeutic agents with a low emetogenic potential (eg, bleomycin, busulfan, cyclophosphamide <1000 mg, etoposide, 5-fluorouracil, vinblastine, vincristine)

Unlabeled/Investigational Use Prophylaxis and treatment of postoperative nausea and vomiting

Pregnancy Risk Factor B

Contraindications Previous hypersensitivity to granisetron, other 5-HT$_3$ receptor antagonists, or any component of the formulation

Warnings/Precautions Use with caution in patients with liver disease or in pregnant patients

Adverse Reactions
>10%:
Central nervous system: Headache (10% to 21%)
Gastrointestinal: Constipation (3% to 18%)
1% to 10%:
Cardiovascular: Hypertension (1%)
Central nervous system: Dizziness, insomnia, anxiety, somnolence, fever
Gastrointestinal: Abdominal pain, diarrhea (1% to 9%), dyspepsia
Hepatic: Elevated liver enzymes (5% to 6%)
Neuromuscular & skeletal: Weakness (5% to 18%)
<1% (Limited to important or life-threatening): Agitation, allergic reactions, anaphylaxis, angina, arrhythmias, atrial fibrillation, hot flashes, hypotension, syncope

Drug Interactions
Cytochrome P450 Effect: CYP3A3/4 enzyme substrate

Ethanol/Nutrition/Herb Interactions Herb/Nutraceutical: St John's wort may decrease granisetron levels.

Stability
I.V.: Stable when mixed in NS or D$_5$W for 24 hours at room temperature. Protect from light. Do not freeze vials.
Oral: Store tablet or oral solution at 15°C to 30°C (59°F to 86°F). Protect from light.

Mechanism of Action Selective 5-HT$_3$-receptor antagonist, blocking serotonin, both peripherally on vagal nerve terminals and centrally in the chemoreceptor trigger zone

Pharmacodynamics/Kinetics
Onset of action: Emesis: Controlled within 1-3 minutes
Duration: Generally up to 24 hours
Distribution: V$_d$: 2-3 L/kg; widely throughout body
Metabolism: Hepatic; some metabolites may have 5-HT$_3$ agonist activity
Half-life elimination: Cancer patients: 10-12 hours; Healthy volunteers: 3-4 hours
Excretion: Primarily nonrenal; urine (8% to 15% as unchanged drug)

Usual Dosage Refer to individual protocols or/and institutional guidelines. A number of different dosing schedules, for varying emetic potentials, have been reported.
Oral: 2 mg once daily or 1 mg every 12 hours on days of chemotherapy
Prophylaxis of radiation therapy-associated emesis: 2 mg once daily 1 hour before radiation therapy
Postoperative nausea and vomiting: 40 mcg/kg
I.V.:
Postoperative nausea and vomiting: 40 mcg/kg
Prophylaxis associated with cancer chemotherapy:
Within U.S.: 10 mcg/kg/dose (or 1 mg/dose): for some drugs (eg, carboplatin, cyclophosphamide) with a later onset of emetic action, 10 mcg/kg every 12 hours may be necessary.
Outside U.S.: 40 mcg/kg/dose (or 3 mg/dose); maximum: 9 mg/24 hours
Breakthrough: Repeat the dose 2-3 times within the first 24 hours as necessary (suggested by anecdotal information; **not** based on controlled trials, or generally recommended).
Note: Granisetron should only be given on the day(s) of chemotherapy
Dosing interval in renal impairment: No dosage adjustment required.
Dosing interval in hepatic impairment: Kinetic studies in patients with hepatic impairment showed that total clearance was approximately halved, however, standard doses were very well tolerated

Administration
Oral: Doses should be given up to 1 hour prior to initiation of chemotherapy/radiation
I.V.: Doses should be given at least 15 minutes prior to initiation of chemotherapy.

Nursing Implications Doses should be given at least 15 minutes prior to initiation of chemotherapy or 1 hour before radiation therapy

Additional Information
Agents with high emetogenic potential (>90%) (dose/m^2):
Amifostine
Azacitidine
Carmustine ≥200 mg/m^2
Cisplatin ≥50 mg/m^2
Cyclophosphamide ≥1 g/m^2
Cytarabine ≥1500 mg/m^2
Dacarbazine ≥500 mg/m^2
Dactinomycin
Doxorubicin ≥60 mg/m^2
Lomustine ≥60 mg/m^2
Mechlorethamine
Melphalan ≥100 mg/m^2
Streptozocin
Thiotepa ≥100 mg/m^2
(Continued)

Granisetron (Continued)

or two agents classified as having high or moderately high emetogenic potential as listed:

Agents with moderately high emetogenic potential (60% to 90%) (dose/m²):
Carboplatin 200-400 mg/m²
Carmustine <200 mg/m²
Cisplatin <50 mg/m²
Cyclophosphamide 600-999 mg/m²
Dacarbazine <500 mg/m²
Doxorubicin 21-59 mg/m²
Hexamethyl melamine
Ifosfamide ≥5000 mg/m²
Lomustine <60 mg/m²
Methotrexate ≥250 mg/m²
Pentostatin
Procarbazine

Dosage Forms
Injection [multidose vial]: 1 mg/mL (4 mL)
Injection [single dose]: 1 mg/mL (1 mL)
Solution, oral: 2 mg/10 mL (30 mL) [orange flavor]
Tablet: 1 mg

Extemporaneous Preparations A 0.2 mg/mL oral suspension may be prepared by crushing twelve (12) 1 mg tablets and mixing with 30 mL water and enough cherry syrup to provide a final volume of 60 mL; this preparation is stable for 14 days at room temperature or when refrigerated

♦ **Granulex** see Trypsin, Balsam Peru, and Castor Oil on page 1386
♦ **Granulocyte Colony Stimulating Factor** see Filgrastim on page 561
♦ **Granulocyte Colony Stimulating Factor (PEG Conjugate)** see Pegfilgrastim on page 1045
♦ **Granulocyte-Macrophage Colony Stimulating Factor** see Sargramostim on page 1223
♦ **Grifulvin® V** see Griseofulvin on page 644

Griseofulvin (gri see oh FUL vin)

Related Information
Antifungal Agents Comparison on page 1484
U.S. Brand Names Fulvicin® P/G; Fulvicin-U/F®; Grifulvin® V; Gris-PEG®
Canadian Brand Names Fulvicin® U/F
Synonyms Griseofulvin Microsize; Griseofulvin Ultramicrosize
Therapeutic Category Antifungal Agent, Systemic
Use Treatment of susceptible tinea infections of the skin, hair, and nails
Pregnancy Risk Factor C
Contraindications Hypersensitivity to griseofulvin or any component of the formulation; severe liver disease; porphyria (interferes with porphyrin metabolism)
Warnings/Precautions Safe use in children <2 years of age has not been established; during long-term therapy, periodic assessment of hepatic, renal, and hematopoietic functions should be performed; may cause fetal harm when administered to pregnant women; avoid exposure to intense sunlight to prevent photosensitivity reactions; hypersensitivity cross reaction between penicillins and griseofulvin is possible
Adverse Reactions
Central nervous system: Headache, fatigue, dizziness, insomnia, mental confusion
Dermatologic: Rash (most common), urticaria (most common), photosensitivity, angioneurotic edema (rare)
Gastrointestinal: Nausea, vomiting, epigastric distress, diarrhea, GI bleeding
Genitourinary: Menstrual irregularities (rare)
Hematologic: Leukopenia
Neuromuscular & skeletal: Paresthesia (rare)
Renal: Hepatotoxicity, proteinuria, nephrosis
Miscellaneous: Oral thrush, drug-induced lupus-like syndrome (rare)
Overdosage/Toxicology Symptoms include lethargy, vertigo, blurred vision, nausea, vomiting, and diarrhea. Following GI decontamination, treatment is supportive.
Drug Interactions
Cytochrome P450 Effect: CYP1A2 enzyme inducer
Increased Effect/Toxicity: Increased toxicity with ethanol, may cause tachycardia and flushing.
Decreased Effect: Barbiturates may decrease levels. Decreased warfarin activity. Decreased oral contraceptive effectiveness.
Ethanol/Nutrition/Herb Interactions
Ethanol: Avoid ethanol (may increase CNS depression). Ethanol will cause "disulfiram"-type reaction consisting of flushing, headache, nausea, and in some patients, vomiting and chest and/or abdominal pain.
Food: Griseofulvin concentrations may be increased if taken with food, especially with high-fat meals.
Mechanism of Action Inhibits fungal cell mitosis at metaphase; binds to human keratin making it resistant to fungal invasion
Pharmacodynamics/Kinetics
Absorption: Ultramicrosize griseofulvin absorption is almost complete; absorption of microsize griseofulvin is variable (25% to 70% of an oral dose); absorption enhanced by ingestion of a fatty meal (GI absorption of ultramicrosize is ~1.5 times that of microsize)
Distribution: Crosses placenta
Metabolism: Extensively hepatic
Half-life elimination: 9-22 hours
Excretion: Urine (<1% as unchanged drug); feces; perspiration

Usual Dosage Oral:
Children:
Microsize: 10-20 mg/kg/day in single or 2 divided doses
Ultramicrosize: >2 years: 5-10 mg/kg/day in single or 2 divided doses
Adults:
Microsize: 500-1000 mg/day in single or divided doses
Ultramicrosize: 330-375 mg/day in single or divided doses; doses up to 750 mg/day have been used for infections more difficult to eradicate such as tinea unguium
Duration of therapy depends on the site of infection:
Tinea corporis: 2-4 weeks
Tinea capitis: 4-6 weeks or longer
Tinea pedis: 4-8 weeks
Tinea unguium: 3-6 months or longer
Administration Oral: Administer with a fatty meal (peanuts or ice cream to increase absorption), or with food or milk to avoid GI upset
Monitoring Parameters Periodic renal, hepatic, and hematopoietic function tests
Test Interactions False-positive urinary VMA levels
Patient Information Avoid exposure to sunlight, take with fatty meal; if patient gets headache, it usually goes away with continued therapy; may cause dizziness, drowsiness, and impair judgment; do not take if pregnant; if you become pregnant, discontinue immediately
Nursing Implications Monitor periodic renal, hepatic, and hematopoietic function tests
Dosage Forms
Capsule, microsize: 250 mg
Suspension, oral, microsize (Grifulvin® V): 125 mg/5 mL with alcohol 0.2% (120 mL)
Tablet, microsize
Fulvicin-U/F®: 250 mg, 500 mg
Grifulvin® V: 125 mg, 250 mg
Tablet, ultramicrosize:
Fulvicin® P/G: 125 mg, 165 mg, 250 mg, 330 mg
Gris-PEG®: 125 mg, 250 mg

♦ **Griseofulvin Microsize** *see* Griseofulvin *on page 644*
♦ **Griseofulvin Ultramicrosize** *see* Griseofulvin *on page 644*
♦ **Gris-PEG®** *see* Griseofulvin *on page 644*
♦ **Growth Hormone** *see* Human Growth Hormone *on page 667*
♦ **Guaifed® [OTC]** *see* Guaifenesin and Pseudoephedrine *on page 647*
♦ **Guaifed-PD®** *see* Guaifenesin and Pseudoephedrine *on page 647*

Guaifenesin (gwye FEN e sin)
U.S. Brand Names Anti-Tuss® Expectorant [OTC]; Breonesin® [OTC]; Diabetic Tussin® EX [OTC]; Duratuss-G®; Fenesin™; Gee Gee® [OTC]; Genatuss® [OTC]; Glyate® [OTC]; Glycotuss® [OTC]; Glytuss® [OTC]; Guaifenex® LA; Guiatuss® [OTC]; Humibid® L.A.; Humibid® Sprinkle; Hytuss® [OTC]; Hytuss-2X® [OTC]; Liquibid®; Monafed®; Muco-Fen-LA®; Mytussin® [OTC]; Naldecon® Senior EX [OTC]; Organidin® NR; Pneumomist®; Respa-GF®; Robitussin® [OTC]; Scot-Tussin® [OTC]; Siltussin® [OTC]; Sinumist®-SR Capsulets®; Touro Ex®; Tusibron® [OTC]; Uni-tussin® [OTC]
Canadian Brand Names Balminil Expectorant; Benylin® E Extra Strength; Koffex Expectorant; Robitussin®
Synonyms GG; Glycerol Guaiacolate
Therapeutic Category Cough Preparation; Expectorant
Use Temporary control of cough due to minor throat and bronchial irritation
Pregnancy Risk Factor C
Contraindications Hypersensitivity to guaifenesin or any component of the formulation
Warnings/Precautions Not for persistent cough such as occurs with smoking, asthma, or emphysema or cough accompanied by excessive secretions
Adverse Reactions 1% to 10%:
Central nervous system: Drowsiness, headache
Dermatologic: Rash
Gastrointestinal: Nausea, vomiting, stomach pain
Overdosage/Toxicology Symptoms include vomiting, lethargy, coma, and respiratory depression. Treatment is supportive.
Drug Interactions
Increased Effect/Toxicity: May increase toxicity/effect of disulfiram, MAO inhibitors, metronidazole, and procarbazine.
Stability Protect from light
Mechanism of Action Thought to act as an expectorant by irritating the gastric mucosa and stimulating respiratory tract secretions, thereby increasing respiratory fluid volumes and decreasing phlegm viscosity
Pharmacodynamics/Kinetics
Absorption: Well absorbed
Metabolism: Hepatic, 60%
Half-life elimination: ~1 hour
Excretion: Urine (as unchanged drug and metabolites)
Usual Dosage Oral:
Children:
<2 years: 12 mg/kg/day in 6 divided doses
2-5 years: 50-100 mg every 4 hours, not to exceed 600 mg/day
6-11 years: 100-200 mg every 4 hours, not to exceed 1.2 g/day
Children >12 years and Adults: 200-400 mg every 4 hours to a maximum of 2.4 g/day
Test Interactions Possible color interference with determination of 5-HIAA and VMA
Patient Information Take with a large quantity of fluid to ensure proper action; if cough persists for more than 1 week or is accompanied by fever, rash, or persistent headache, physician should be consulted
(Continued)

Guaifenesin *(Continued)*

Nursing Implications Administer with large quantity of water to ensure proper action; some products contain alcohol

Additional Information Syrup contains 3.5% alcohol

Dosage Forms

Caplet, sustained release (Touro Ex®): 600 mg

Capsule (Breonesin®, Hytuss-2X®): 200 mg

Capsule, sustained release (Humibid® Sprinkle): 300 mg

Liquid:

Diabetic Tussin EX®, Organidin® NR, Tusibron®: 100 mg/5 mL (118 mL)

Naldecon® Senior EX: 200 mg/5 mL (118 mL, 480 mL)

Syrup (Anti-Tuss® Expectorant, Genatuss®, Glyate®, Guiatuss®, Mytussin®, Robitussin®, Scot-Tussin®, Siltussin®, Tusibron®, Uni-Tussin®): 100 mg/5 mL with alcohol 3.5% (30 mL, 120 mL, 240 mL, 473 mL, 946 mL)

Tablet:

Duratuss-G®: 1200 mg

Gee Gee®, Glytuss®, Organidin® NR: 200 mg

Hytuss®: 100 mg

Tablet, sustained release (Fenesin™, Guaifenex LA®, Humibid® L.A., Liquibid®, Monafed®, Muco-Fen-LA®, Pneumomist®, Respa-GF®, Sinumist®-SR Capsulets®): 600 mg

Guaifenesin and Codeine *(gwye FEN e sin & KOE deen)*

U.S. Brand Names Brontex® Liquid; Brontex® Tablet; Cheracol®; Guiatuss AC®; Guiatussin® With Codeine; Mytussin® AC; Robafen® AC; Robitussin® A-C; Tussi-Organidin® NR

Synonyms Codeine and Guaifenesin

Therapeutic Category Antitussive; Cough Preparation; Expectorant

Use Temporary control of cough due to minor throat and bronchial irritation

Restrictions C-V

Pregnancy Risk Factor C

Usual Dosage Oral:

Children:

2-6 years: 1-1.5 mg/kg codeine/day divided into 4 doses administered every 4-6 hours (maximum: 30 mg/24 hours)

6-12 years: 5 mL every 4 hours, not to exceed 30 mL/24 hours

Children >12 years and Adults: 5-10 mL every 6 hours not to exceed 60 mL/24 hours

Additional Information Complete prescribing information for this medication should be consulted for additional detail.

Dosage Forms

Liquid (Brontex®): Guaifenesin 75 mg and codeine phosphate 2.5 mg per 5 mL

Syrup (Cheracol®, Guaituss AC®, Guiatussin® with Codeine, Mytussin® AC, Robafen® AC, Robitussin® A-C, Tussi-Organidin® NR): Guaifenesin 100 mg and codeine phosphate 10 mg per 5 mL (60 mL, 120 mL, 480 mL)

Tablet (Brontex®): Guaifenesin 300 mg and codeine phosphate 10 mg

Guaifenesin and Dextromethorphan

(gwye FEN e sin & deks troe meth OR fan)

U.S. Brand Names Benylin® Expectorant [OTC]; Cheracol® D [OTC]; Clear Tussin® 30; Diabetic Tussin® DM [OTC]; Extra Action Cough Syrup [OTC]; Fenesin™ DM; Genatuss DM® [OTC]; Glycotuss-dM® [OTC]; Guaifenex® DM; GuiaCough® [OTC]; Guiatuss-DM® [OTC]; Halotussin® DM [OTC]; Humibid® DM [OTC]; Iobid DM®; Kolephrin® GG/DM [OTC]; Monafed® DM; Muco-Fen-DM®; Mytussin® DM [OTC]; Naldecon® Senior DX [OTC]; Phanatuss® Cough Syrup [OTC]; Phenadex® Senior [OTC]; Respa®-DM; Rhinosyn-DMX® [OTC]; Robafen DM® [OTC]; Robitussin®-DM [OTC]; Safe Tussin® 30 [OTC]; Scot-Tussin® Senior Clear [OTC]; Siltussin DM® [OTC]; Synacol® CF [OTC]; Syracol-CF® [OTC]; Tolu-Sed® DM [OTC]; Tusibron-DM® [OTC]; Tuss-DM® [OTC]; Tussi-Organidin® DM NR; Uni-tussin® DM [OTC]; Vicks® 44E [OTC]; Vicks® Pediatric Formula 44E [OTC]

Canadian Brand Names Balminil DM E; Benylin® DM-E; Koffex DM-Expectorant; Robi-tussin® DM

Synonyms Dextromethorphan and Guaifenesin

Therapeutic Category Antitussive; Cough Preparation; Expectorant

Use Temporary control of cough due to minor throat and bronchial irritation

Pregnancy Risk Factor C

Contraindications Hypersensitivity to guaifenesin, dextromethorphan, or any component of the formulation

Warnings/Precautions Should not be used for persistent or chronic cough such as that occurring with smoking, asthma, chronic bronchitis, or emphysema or for cough associated with excessive phlegm

Adverse Reactions See individual agents

Drug Interactions

Increased Effect/Toxicity: Refer to individual agents.

Decreased Effect: Refer to individual agents.

Stability Protect from light.

Mechanism of Action

Guaifenesin is thought to act as an expectorant by irritating the gastric mucosa and stimulating respiratory tract secretions, thereby increasing respiratory fluid volumes and decreasing phlegm viscosity

Dextromethorphan is a chemical relative of morphine lacking narcotic properties except in overdose; controls cough by depressing the medullary cough center

Pharmacodynamics/Kinetics

Onset of action: Oral: Antitussive: 15-30 minutes

See individual agents.

Usual Dosage Oral:

    Children: Dextromethorphan: 1-2 mg/kg/24 hours divided 3-4 times/day

    Children >12 years and Adults: 5 mL every 4 hours or 10 mL every 6-8 hours not to exceed 40 mL/24 hours

Patient Information Take with a large quantity of fluid to ensure proper action; if cough persists for more than one week, is recumbent, or is accompanied by fever, rash or persistent headache, physician should be consulted

Nursing Implications

    Administer with a large quantity of fluid

    The "NR" in Tussi-Organidin® DM NR means "Newly Reformulated"

Dosage Forms

    Capsule (Humibid® DM Sprinkles): Guaifenesin 300 mg and dextromethorphan hydrobromide 15 mg per 5 mL

    Syrup:

        Benylin® Expectorant: Guaifenesin 100 mg and dextromethorphan hydrobromide 5 mg per 5 mL (118 mL, 236 mL)

        Cheracol® D, Clear Tussin® 30, Diabetic Tussin® DM, Extra Action Cough Syrup, Genatuss® DM, Guiatuss DM®, Halotussin® DM, Mytussin® DM, Robitussin®-DM, Siltussin DM®, Tolu-Sed® DM, Tussin-DM®, Tussi-Organidin® DM NR, Uni-Tussin® DM: Guaifenesin 100 mg and dextromethorphan hydrobromide 10 mg per 5 mL (5 mL, 10 mL, 120 mL, 240 mL, 360 mL, 480 mL, 3780 mL)

        Clear Tussin® 30, GuiaCough®, Rhinosyn-DMX®, Safe Tussin® 30, Tusibron-DM®: Guaifenesin 100 mg and dextromethorphan hydrobromide 15 mg per 5 mL (120 mL, 240 mL, 480 mL)

        Kolephrin® GG/DM: Guaifenesin 150 mg and dextromethorphan hydrobromide 10 mg per 5 mL (120 mL)

        Naldecon® Senior DX: Guaifenesin 200 mg and dextromethorphan hydrobromide 10 mg per 5 mL (118 mL, 480 mL)

        Phanatuss®: Guaifenesin 85 mg and dextromethorphan hydrobromide 10 mg per 5 mL

        Scot Tussin® Sr: Guaifenesin 200 mg and dextromethorphan hydrobromide 15 mg per 5 mL

        Vicks® 44E: Guaifenesin 66.7 mg and dextromethorphan hydrobromide 6.7 mg per 5 mL

        Vicks® 44E Pediatric Formula: Guaifenesin 33.3 mg and dextromethorphan hydrobromide 3.3 mg per 5 mL

    Tablet, extended release:

        Fenesin™ DM, Guaifenex DM®, Humibid® DM, Iobid DM®, Monafed® DM, Muco-Fen DM®, Respa-DM®: Guaifenesin 600 mg and dextromethorphan hydrobromide 30 mg

        Glycotuss-dM®: Guaifenesin 100 mg and dextromethorphan hydrobromide 10 mg

        Synacol-CF®, Syracol-CF®: Guaifenesin 200 mg and dextromethorphan hydrobromide 15 mg

        Tuss-DM®: Guaifenesin 200 mg and dextromethorphan hydrobromide 10 mg

♦ **Guaifenesin and Hydrocodone** see Hydrocodone and Guaifenesin on page 679

Guaifenesin and Phenylephrine (gwye FEN e sin & fen il EF rin)

U.S. Brand Names Deconsal® Sprinkle®; Endal®; Sinupan®

Synonyms Phenylephrine and Guaifenesin

Therapeutic Category Decongestant

Use Symptomatic relief of those respiratory conditions where tenacious mucous plugs and congestion complicate the problem such as sinusitis, pharyngitis, bronchitis, asthma, and as an adjunctive therapy in serous otitis media

Usual Dosage Oral: Adults: 1 or 2 every 12 hours

    Product labeling: Adults: Endal®: 1-2 timed release tablets every 12 hours

Additional Information Complete prescribing information for this medication should be consulted for additional detail.

Dosage Forms

    Capsule, sustained release:

        Deconsal® Sprinkle®: Guaifenesin 300 mg and phenylephrine hydrochloride 10 mg

        Sinupan®: Guaifenesin 200 mg and phenylephrine hydrochloride 40 mg

    Tablet, timed release (Endal®): Guaifenesin 300 mg and phenylephrine hydrochloride 20 mg

Guaifenesin and Pseudoephedrine (gwye FEN e sin & soo doe e FED rin)

U.S. Brand Names Congess® Jr; Congess® Sr; Congestac®; Deconsal® II; Defen-LA®; Duratuss™; Entex® PSE; Eudal®-SR; Fedahist® Expectorant [OTC]; Glycofed®; Guaifed® [OTC]; Guaifed-PD®; Guaifenex® PSE; GuaiMAX-D®; Guaitab®; Guaivent®; Guai-Vent/PSE®; Histalet® X; Maxifed®; Maxifed-G®; Nasabid™; Respa-1st®; Respaire®-60 SR; Respaire®-120 SR; Robitussin-PE® [OTC]; Robitussin® Severe Congestion Liqui-Gels® [OTC]; Ru-Tuss® DE; Rymed®; Sinufed® Timecelles®; Touro LA®; Versacaps®; Zephrex®; Zephrex LA®

Canadian Brand Names Novahistex® Expectorant with Decongestant

Synonyms Pseudoephedrine and Guaifenesin

Therapeutic Category Decongestant; Expectorant

Use Enhance the output of respiratory tract fluid and reduce mucosal congestion and edema in the nasal passage

Pregnancy Risk Factor C

Usual Dosage Oral:

    Children:

        2-6 years: 2.5 mL every 4 hours not to exceed 15 mL/24 hours

        6-12 years: 5 mL every 4 hours not to exceed 30 mL/24 hours

    Children >12 years and Adults: 10 mL every 4 hours not to exceed 60 mL/24 hours

Additional Information Complete prescribing information for this medication should be consulted for additional detail.

(Continued)

Guaifenesin and Pseudoephedrine *(Continued)*

Dosage Forms
Capsule:
> Congess® Sr, Guai-Vent™: Guaifenesin 250 mg and pseudoephedrine hydrochloride 120 mg
>
> Robitussin® Severe Congestion Liqui-Gels®: Guaifenesin 200 mg and pseudoephedrine hydrochloride 30 mg
>
> Rymed®: Guaifenesin 250 mg and pseudoephedrine hydrochloride 30 mg

Capsule, extended release:
> Congess® Jr: Guaifenesin 125 mg and pseudoephedrine hydrochloride 60 mg
>
> Congess® Sr, Guaifed®, Respaire®-120 SR: Guaifenesin 250 mg and pseudoephedrine hydrochloride 120 mg
>
> Guaifed-PD®, Sinufed® Timecelles®, Versacaps®: Guaifenesin 300 mg and pseudoephedrine hydrochloride 60 mg
>
> Nasabid®: Guaifenesin 250 mg and pseudoephedrine hydrochloride 90 mg
>
> Respaire®-60 SR: Guaifenesin 200 mg and pseudoephedrine hydrochloride 60 mg

Syrup:
> Fedahist® Expectorant: Guaifenesin 200 mg and pseudoephedrine hydrochloride 20 mg per 5 mL
>
> Guaifed®: Guaifenesin 200 mg and pseudoephedrine hydrochloride 30 mg per 5 mL (120 mL, 240 mL)
>
> Guiatuss® PE, Robitussin-PE®, Rymed®: Guaifenesin 100 mg and pseudoephedrine hydrochloride 30 mg per 5 mL (120 mL, 240 mL, 480 mL)
>
> Histalet® X: Guaifenesin 200 mg and pseudoephedrine hydrochloride 45 mg per 5 mL (473 mL)

Tablet:
> Congestac®, Guiatab®, Zephrex®: Guaifenesin 400 mg and pseudoephedrine hydrochloride 60 mg
>
> Glycofed®: Guaifenesin 100 mg and pseudoephedrine hydrochloride 30 mg

Tablet, extended release:
> Deconsal® II, Defen-LA®, Guaifenex PSE® 60, Respa-1st®: Guaifenesin 600 mg and pseudoephedrine hydrochloride 60 mg
>
> Duratuss®, Entex® PSE, Guaifenex PSE® 120, GuaiMax-D®, Guai-Vent/PSE™, Ru-Tuss® DE, Sudex®, Zephrex LA®: Guaifenesin 600 mg and pseudoephedrine hydrochloride 120 mg
>
> Eudal®-SR, Histalet® X: Guaifenesin 400 mg and pseudoephedrine hydrochloride 120 mg
>
> Maxifed®: Guaifenesin 700 mg and pseudoephedrine hydrochloride 80 mg
>
> Maxifed-G®: Guaifenesin 550 mg and pseudoephedrine hydrochloride 60 mg
>
> Touro-LA®, Tuss-LA®, V-Dec-M®: Guaifenesin 500 mg and pseudoephedrine hydrochloride 120 mg

♦ **Guaifenesin and Theophylline** *see* Theophylline and Guaifenesin *on page 1310*

Guaifenesin, Pseudoephedrine, and Codeine
(gwye FEN e sin, soo doe e FED rin, & KOE deen)

U.S. Brand Names Codafed® Expectorant; Cycofed® Pediatric; Decohistine® Expectorant; Deproist® Expectorant With Codeine; Dihistine® Expectorant; Guaituss® DAC; Guiatussin® DAC; Halotussin® DAC; Isoclor® Expectorant; Mytussin® DAC; Nucofed®; Nucofed® Pediatric Expectorant; Nucotuss®; Phenhist® Expectorant; Robitussin®-DAC; Ryna-CX®; Tussar® SF Syrup

Canadian Brand Names Benylin® 3.3 mg-D-E; Calmylin with Codeine

Synonyms Codeine, Guaifenesin, and Pseudoephedrine; Pseudoephedrine, Guaifenesin, and Codeine

Therapeutic Category Antitussive/Decongestant/Expectorant

Use Temporarily relieves nasal congestion and controls cough due to minor throat and bronchial irritation; helps loosen phlegm and thin bronchial secretions to make coughs more productive

Restrictions C-III; C-V

Pregnancy Risk Factor C

Usual Dosage Oral:
> Children 6-12 years: 5 mL every 4 hours, not to exceed 40 mL/24 hours
>
> Children >12 years and Adults: 10 mL every 4 hours, not to exceed 40 mL/24 hours

Additional Information Complete prescribing information for this medication should be consulted for additional detail.

Dosage Forms
Liquid:
> Nucofed®, Nucotuss® (C-III): Guaifenesin 200 mg, pseudoephedrine hydrochloride 60 mg, and codeine phosphate 20 mg per 5 mL (480 mL)
>
> Codafed® Expectorant, Decohistine® Expectorant, Deproist® Expectorant with Codeine, Dihistine® Expectorant, Guiatuss DAC®, Guiatussin® DAC, Halotussin® DAC, Isoclor® Expectorant, Mytussin® DAC, Nucofed® Pediatric Expectorant, Phenhist® Expectorant, Robitussin®-DAC, Ryna-CX®, Tussar® SF (C-V): Guaifenesin 100 mg, pseudoephedrine hydrochloride 30 mg, and codeine phosphate 10 mg per 5 mL (120 mL, 480 mL, 4000 mL)

Guaifenesin, Pseudoephedrine, and Dextromethorphan
(gwye FEN e sin, soo doe e FED rin, & deks troe meth OR fan)

U.S. Brand Names Anatuss® DM [OTC]; Dimacol® Caplets [OTC]; Maxifed® DM; Rhinosyn-X® Liquid [OTC]; Ru-Tuss® Expectorant [OTC]; Sudafed® Cold & Cough Liquid Caps [OTC]

Canadian Brand Names Balminil DM + Decongestant + Expectorant; Benylin® DM-D-E; Koffex DM + Decongestant + Expectorant; Novahistex® DM Decongestant Expectorant; Novahistine® DM Decongestant Expectorant; Robitussin® Cough & Cold®

Synonyms Dextromethorphan, Guaifenesin, and Pseudoephedrine; Pseudoephedrine, Dextromethorphan, and Guaifenesin

Therapeutic Category Antitussive/Decongestant/Expectorant

Use Temporarily relieves nasal congestion and controls cough due to minor throat and bronchial irritation; helps loosen phlegm and thin bronchial secretions to make coughs more productive

Usual Dosage Adults: Oral: 2 capsules or 10 mL every 4 hours

Additional Information Complete prescribing information for this medication should be consulted for additional detail.

Dosage Forms

Capsule (Sudafed® Cold & Cough Liquid Caps): Guaifenesin 100 mg, pseudoephedrine hydrochloride 30 mg, and dextromethorphan hydrobromide 10 mg

Liquid (Rhinosyn-X® Liquid, Ru-Tuss® Expectorant): Guaifenesin 100 mg, pseudoephedrine hydrochloride 30 mg, and dextromethorphan hydrobromide 10 mg per 5 mL

Tablet, sustained release (Maxifed® DM): Guaifenesin 550 mg, pseudoephedrine hydrochloride 60 mg, and dextromethorphan hydrobromide 30 mg

- **Guaifenex® DM** see Guaifenesin and Dextromethorphan on page 646
- **Guaifenex® LA** see Guaifenesin on page 645
- **Guaifenex® PSE** see Guaifenesin and Pseudoephedrine on page 647
- **GuaiMAX-D®** see Guaifenesin and Pseudoephedrine on page 647
- **Guaitab®** see Guaifenesin and Pseudoephedrine on page 647
- **Guaituss AC®** see Guaifenesin and Codeine on page 646
- **Guaivent®** see Guaifenesin and Pseudoephedrine on page 647
- **Guai-Vent/PSE®** see Guaifenesin and Pseudoephedrine on page 647

Guanabenz (GWAHN a benz)

U.S. Brand Names Wytensin®

Canadian Brand Names Wytensin®

Synonyms Guanabenz Acetate

Therapeutic Category Alpha$_2$-Adrenergic Agonist Agent; Antihypertensive Agent

Use Management of hypertension

Pregnancy Risk Factor C

Usual Dosage Adults: Oral: Initial: 4 mg twice daily; increase in increments of 4-8 mg/day every 1-2 weeks to a maximum of 32 mg twice daily.

Dosing adjustment in hepatic impairment: Probably necessary

Additional Information Complete prescribing information for this medication should be consulted for additional detail.

Dosage Forms Tablet, as acetate: 4 mg, 8 mg

- **Guanabenz Acetate** see Guanabenz on page 649

Guanadrel (GWAHN a drel)

U.S. Brand Names Hylorel®

Canadian Brand Names Hylorel®

Synonyms Guanadrel Sulfate

Therapeutic Category Adrenergic Blocking Agent, Peripherally Acting; Antihypertensive Agent

Use Considered a second line agent in the treatment of hypertension, usually with a diuretic

Pregnancy Risk Factor B

Usual Dosage Oral:

Adults: Initial: 10 mg/day (5 mg twice daily); adjust dosage weekly or monthly until blood pressure is controlled, usual dosage: 20-75 mg/day, given twice daily. For larger dosage, 3-4 times/day dosing may be needed.

Elderly: Initial: 5 mg once daily

Dosing interval in renal impairment:

Cl$_{cr}$ 10-50 mL/minute: Administer every 12-24 hours.

Cl$_{cr}$ <10 mL/minute: Administer every 24-48 hours.

Additional Information Complete prescribing information for this medication should be consulted for additional detail.

Dosage Forms Tablet, as sulfate: 10 mg, 25 mg

- **Guanadrel Sulfate** see Guanadrel on page 649

Guanethidine (gwahn ETH i deen)

Related Information

Depression on page 1655

U.S. Brand Names Ismelin®

Synonyms Guanethidine Monosulfate

Therapeutic Category Alpha$_2$-Adrenergic Agonist Agent; Antihypertensive Agent

Use Treatment of moderate to severe hypertension

Pregnancy Risk Factor C

Usual Dosage Oral:

Children: Initial: 0.2 mg/kg/day; increase by 0.2 mg/kg/day at 7- to 10-day intervals to a maximum of 3 mg/kg/day.

Adults:

Ambulatory patients: Initial: 10 mg/day; increase at 5- to 7-day intervals to an average of 25-50 mg/day.

Hospitalized patients: Initial: 25-50 mg/day; increase by 25-50 mg/day or every other day to desired therapeutic response.

Elderly: Initial: 5 mg once daily

Dosing interval in renal impairment: Cl$_{cr}$ <10 mL/minute: Administer every 24-36 hours.

Additional Information Complete prescribing information for this medication should be consulted for additional detail.

Dosage Forms Tablet, as monosulfate: 10 mg, 25 mg

◆ **Guanethidine Monosulfate** *see Guanethidine on page 649*

Guanfacine (GWAHN fa seen)
U.S. Brand Names Tenex®
Canadian Brand Names Tenex®
Synonyms Guanfacine Hydrochloride
Therapeutic Category Alpha₂-Adrenergic Agonist Agent; Antihypertensive Agent
Use Management of hypertension
Pregnancy Risk Factor B
Usual Dosage Adults: Oral: Hypertension: 1 mg usually at bedtime, may increase if needed at 3- to 4-week intervals; 1 mg/day is most common dose
Additional Information Complete prescribing information for this medication should be consulted for additional detail.
Dosage Forms Tablet, as hydrochloride: 1 mg, 2 mg

◆ **Guanfacine Hydrochloride** *see Guanfacine on page 650*
◆ **GuiaCough® [OTC]** *see Guaifenesin and Dextromethorphan on page 646*
◆ **Guiatuss® [OTC]** *see Guaifenesin on page 645*
◆ **Guiatuss DAC®** *see Guaifenesin, Pseudoephedrine, and Codeine on page 648*
◆ **Guiatuss-DM® [OTC]** *see Guaifenesin and Dextromethorphan on page 646*
◆ **Guiatussin® DAC** *see Guaifenesin, Pseudoephedrine, and Codeine on page 648*
◆ **Guiatussin® With Codeine** *see Guaifenesin and Codeine on page 646*
◆ **G-well®** *see Lindane on page 806*
◆ **Gynazole-1™** *see Butoconazole on page 199*
◆ **Gynecort® [OTC]** *see Hydrocortisone on page 682*
◆ **GyneCure™ (Can)** *see Tioconazole on page 1337*
◆ **Gyne-Lotrimin® [OTC]** *see Clotrimazole on page 323*
◆ **Gyne-Lotrimin® 3 [OTC]** *see Clotrimazole on page 323*
◆ **Gynix® [OTC]** *see Clotrimazole on page 323*
◆ **Gynodiol™** *see Estradiol on page 491*
◆ **Habitrol® (Can)** *see Nicotine on page 979*
◆ **Habitrol™ Patch** *see Nicotine on page 979*

Haemophilus b Conjugate and Hepatitis B Vaccine
(he MOF i lus bee KON joo gate & hep a TYE tis bee vak SEEN)
U.S. Brand Names Comvax®
Synonyms *Haemophilus* b (meningococcal protein conjugate) Conjugate Vaccine; Hib
Therapeutic Category Vaccine
Use
Immunization against invasive disease caused by *H. influenzae* type b and against infection caused by all known subtypes of hepatitis B virus in infants 8 weeks to 15 months of age born of HB₅Ag-negative mothers
Infants born of HB₅Ag-positive mothers or mothers of unknown HB₅Ag status should receive hepatitis B immune globulin and hepatitis B vaccine (recombinant) at birth and should complete the hepatitis B vaccination series given according to a particular schedule
Pregnancy Risk Factor C
Contraindications Hypersensitivity to any component of the formulation
Warnings/Precautions If used in persons with malignancies or those receiving immunosuppressive therapy or who are otherwise immunocompromised, the expected immune response may not be obtained.

Patients who develop symptoms suggestive of hypersensitivity after an injection should not receive further injections of the vaccine.

The decision to administer or delay vaccination because of current or recent febrile illness depends on the severity of symptoms and the etiology of the disease. Immunization should be delayed during the course of an acute febrile illness.
Adverse Reactions When administered during the same visit that DTP, OPV, IPV, varicella virus vaccine, and M-M-R II vaccines are given, the rates of systemic reactions do not differ from those observed only when any of the vaccines are administered. **All serious adverse reactions must be reported to the U.S. Department of Health and Human Services (DHHS) Vaccine Adverse Event Reporting System (VAERS) 1-800-822-7967.**
>10%: Central nervous system: Acute febrile reactions
1% to 10%:
Central nervous system: Fever (up to 102.2°F), irritability, lethargy
Gastrointestinal: Anorexia, diarrhea
Local: Irritation at injection site
<1% (Limited to important or life-threatening): Allergic or anaphylactic reactions (difficulty in breathing, hives, itching, swelling of eyes, face, unusual tiredness or weakness), convulsions, fever (>102.2°F), vomiting
Stability Store at 2°C to 8°C (36°F to 48°F).
Mechanism of Action Hib conjugate vaccines use covalent binding of capsular polysaccharide of *Haemophilus influenzae* type b to OMPC carrier to produce an antigen which is postulated to convert a T-independent antigen into a T-dependent antigen to result in enhanced antibody response and on immunologic memory. Recombinant hepatitis B vaccine is a noninfectious subunit viral vaccine. The vaccine is derived from hepatitis B surface antigen (HB₅Ag) produced through recombinant DNA techniques from yeast cells. The portion of the hepatitis B gene which codes for HB₅Ag is cloned into yeast which is then cultured to produce hepatitis B vaccine.
Pharmacodynamics/Kinetics See individual agents.
Usual Dosage Infants (>8 weeks of age): I.M.: 0.5 mL at 2, 4, and 12-15 months of age (total of 3 doses)

If the recommended schedule cannot be followed, the interval between the first two doses should be at least 2 months and the interval between the second and third dose should be as close as possible to 8-11 months.

Modified Schedule: Children who receive one dose of hepatitis B vaccine at or shortly after birth may receive Comvax® on a schedule of 2,4, and 12-15 months of age

Administration Administer 0.5 mL I.M. into anterolateral thigh [data suggests that injections given in the buttocks frequently are given into fatty tissue instead of into muscle to result in lower seroconversion rates]; **do not administer intravenously, intradermally, or subcutaneously**

For patients at risk of hemorrhage following intramuscular injection, the ACIP recommends "it should be administered intramuscularly if, in the opinion of the physician familiar with the patients bleeding risk, the vaccine can be administered with reasonable safety by this route. If the patient receives antihemophilia or other similar therapy, intramuscular vaccination can be scheduled shortly after such therapy is administered. A fine needle (23 gauge or smaller) can be used for the vaccination and firm pressure applied to the site (without rubbing) for at least 2 minutes. The patient should be instructed concerning the risk of hematoma from the injection."

Patient Information May use acetaminophen for postdose fever

Nursing Implications Defer immunization if infection or febrile illness present

Additional Information Inactivated bacterial vaccine and inactivated viral vaccine. Federal law requires that the date of administration, the vaccine manufacturer, lot number of vaccine, and the administering person's name, title, and address be entered into the patient's permanent medical record.

Dosage Forms Injection: 7.5 mcg *Haemophilus* b PRP and 5 mcg HB$_s$Ag/0.5 mL

Haemophilus b Conjugate Vaccine
(he MOF fi lus bee KON joo gate vak SEEN)

Related Information

Haemophilus influenzae Vaccination *on page 1546*
Immunization Recommendations *on page 1538*
Recommendations of the Advisory Committee on Immunization Practices (ACIP) *on page 1540*
Recommended Immunization Schedule for HIV-Infected Children *on page 1543*
USPHA/IDSA Guidelines for the Prevention of Opportunistic Infections in Persons With HIV *on page 1574*

U.S. Brand Names ActHIB®; HibTITER®; PedvaxHIB®

Canadian Brand Names ActHIB®; PedvaxHIB®

Synonyms Diphtheria CRM$_{197}$ Protein Conjugate; Diphtheria Toxoid Conjugate; *Haemophilus* b Oligosaccharide Conjugate Vaccine; *Haemophilus* b Polysaccharide Vaccine; HbCV; Hib Polysaccharide Conjugate; PRP-D

Therapeutic Category Vaccine, Inactivated Bacteria

Use Routine immunization of children 2 months to 5 years of age against invasive disease caused by *H. influenzae*

Unimmunized children ≥5 years of age with a chronic illness known to be associated with increased risk of *Haemophilus influenzae* type b disease, specifically, persons with anatomic or functional asplenia or sickle cell anemia or those who have undergone splenectomy, should receive Hib vaccine.

Haemophilus b conjugate vaccines are not indicated for prevention of bronchitis or other infections due to *H. influenzae* in adults; adults with specific dysfunction or certain complement deficiencies who are at especially high risk of *H. influenzae* type b infection (HIV-infected adults); patients with Hodgkin's disease (vaccinated at least 2 weeks before the initiation of chemotherapy or 3 months after the end of chemotherapy)

Pregnancy Risk Factor C

Contraindications Children with any febrile illness or active infection, hypersensitivity to *Haemophilus* b polysaccharide vaccine (thimerosal), children who are immunosuppressed or receiving immunosuppressive therapy

Warnings/Precautions The carrier proteins used in HbOC (but not PRP-OMP) are chemically and immunologically related to toxoids contained in DTP vaccine. Earlier or simultaneous vaccination with diphtheria or tetanus toxoids may be required to elicit an optimal anti-PRP antibody response to HbOC. In contrast, the immunogenicity of PRP-OMP is not affected by vaccination with DTP. In infants in whom DTP or DT vaccination is deferred, PRP-OMP may be advantageous for *Haemophilus influenzae* type b vaccination.

Children with immunologic impairment: Children with chronic illness associated with increased risk of *Haemophilus influenzae* type b disease may have impaired anti-PRP antibody responses to conjugate vaccination. Examples include those with HIV infection, immunoglobulin deficiency, anatomic or functional asplenia, and sickle cell disease, as well as recipients of bone marrow transplants and recipients of chemotherapy for malignancy. Some children with immunologic impairment may benefit from more doses of conjugate vaccine than normally indicated.

Adverse Reactions When administered during the same visit that DTP vaccine is given, the rates of systemic reactions do not differ from those observed only when DTP vaccine is administered. **All serious adverse reactions must be reported to the U.S. Department of Health and Human Services (DHHS) Vaccine Adverse Event Reporting System (VAERS) 1-800-822-7967.**

25%:
Cardiovascular: Edema
Dermatologic: Local erythema
Local: Increased risk of *Haemophilus* b infections in the week after vaccination
Miscellaneous: Warmth
>10%: Acute febrile reactions
1% to 10%:
Central nervous system: Fever (up to 102.2°F), irritability, lethargy
(Continued)

Haemophilus b Conjugate Vaccine *(Continued)*

Gastrointestinal: Anorexia, diarrhea

Local: Irritation at injection site

<1% (Limited to important or life-threatening: Convulsions, dyspnea, edema of the eyes/face, fever (>102.2°F), itching, unusual fatigue, urticaria, vomiting, weakness

Stability Keep in refrigerator, may be frozen (not diluent) without affecting potency; reconstituted Hib-Imune® remains stable for only 8 hours, whereas HibVAX® remain stable for 30 days when refrigerated

Mechanism of Action Stimulates production of anticapsular antibodies and provides active immunity to *Haemophilus influenzae*

Pharmacodynamics/Kinetics Seroconversion following one dose of Hib vaccine for children 18 months or 24 months of age or older is 75% to 90% respectively.

Onset of action: Serum antibody response: 1-2 weeks

Duration: Immunity: 1.5 years

Usual Dosage Children: I.M.: 0.5 mL as a single dose should be administered according to one of the following "brand-specific" schedules; do not inject I.V. (see table)

Vaccination Schedule for *Haemophilus* b Conjugate Vaccines

Age at 1st Dose (mo)	HibTITER® Primary Series	HibTITER® Booster	PedvaxHIB® Primary Series	PedvaxHIB® Booster	ProHIBiT® Primary Series	ProHIBiT® Booster
2-6*	3 doses, 2 months apart	15 mo†	2 doses, 2 months apart	12 mo†		
7-11	2 doses, 2 months apart	15 mo†	2 doses, 2 months apart	15 mo†		
12-14	1 dose	15 mo†	1 dose	15 mo†		
15-60	1 dose	—	1 dose	—	1 dose	—

*It is not currently recommended that the various *Haemophilus* b conjugate vaccines be interchanged (ie, the same brand should be used throughout the entire vaccination series). If the health care provider does not know which vaccine was previously used, it is prudent that an infant, 2-6 months of age, be given a primary series of three doses.

†At least 2 months after previous dose.

Administration For patients at risk of hemorrhage following intramuscular injection, the ACIP recommends "it should be administered intramuscularly if, in the opinion of the physician familiar with the patients bleeding risk, the vaccine can be administered with reasonable safety by this route. If the patient receives antihemophilia or other similar therapy, intramuscular vaccination can be scheduled shortly after such therapy is administered. A fine needle (23 gauge or smaller) can be used for the vaccination and firm pressure applied to the site (without rubbing) for at least 2 minutes. The patient should be instructed concerning the risk of hematoma from the injection."

Test Interactions May interfere with interpretation of antigen detection tests

Patient Information May use acetaminophen for postdose fever

Nursing Implications Defer immunization if infection or febrile illness present. Do not administer I.V.

Additional Information Federal law requires that the date of administration, the vaccine manufacturer, lot number of vaccine, and the administering person's name, title, and address be entered into the patient's permanent medical record.

Dosage Forms

Injection:

ActHIB® [with 0.4% sodium chloride diluent]: Capsular polysaccharide 10 mcg and tetanus toxoid 24 mcg per 0.5 mL

HibTITER®: Capsular oligosaccharide 10 mcg and diphtheria CRM_{197} protein ~25 mcg per 0.5 mL (0.5 mL, 2.5 mL, 5 mL)

PedvaxHIB®: Purified capsular polysaccharide 15 mcg and *Neisseria meningitidis* OMPC 250 mcg per dose (0.5 mL)

♦ *Haemophilus* b (meningococcal protein conjugate) Conjugate Vaccine *see Haemophilus* b Conjugate and Hepatitis B Vaccine *on page 650*

♦ *Haemophilus* b Oligosaccharide Conjugate Vaccine *see Haemophilus* b Conjugate Vaccine *on page 651*

♦ *Haemophilus* b Polysaccharide Vaccine *see Haemophilus* b Conjugate Vaccine *on page 651*

♦ *Haemophilus influenzae* Vaccination *see page 1546*

Halazepam *(hal AZ e pam)*

Related Information

Antacid Drug Interactions *on page 1477*

Benzodiazepines Comparison *on page 1490*

U.S. Brand Names Paxipam®

Canadian Brand Names Paxipam®

Therapeutic Category Antianxiety Agent; Benzodiazepine

Use Management of anxiety disorders

Unlabeled/Investigational Use Hostility; ethanol withdrawal

Restrictions C-IV

Pregnancy Risk Factor D

Usual Dosage Oral:

Adults: 20-40 mg 3-4 times/day; optimal dosage usually ranges from 80-160 mg/day. If side effects occur with the starting dose, lower the dose.

Elderly ≥70 years or debilitated patients: 20 mg 1-2 times/day and adjust dose accordingly
Additional Information Complete prescribing information for this medication should be consulted for additional detail.
Dosage Forms Tablet: 20 mg, 40 mg

Halcinonide (hal SIN oh nide)
Related Information
Corticosteroids Comparison *on page 1495*
U.S. Brand Names Halog®; Halog®-E
Canadian Brand Names Halog®
Therapeutic Category Corticosteroid, Topical (Medium Potency); Corticosteroid, Topical (High Potency)
Use Inflammation of corticosteroid-responsive dermatoses [high potency topical corticosteroid]
Pregnancy Risk Factor C
Usual Dosage Children and Adults: Topical: Steroid-responsive dermatoses: Apply sparingly 1-3 times/day, occlusive dressing may be used for severe or resistant dermatoses; a thin film is effective; do not overuse. Therapy should be discontinued when control is achieved; if no improvement is seen, reassessment of diagnosis may be necessary.
Additional Information Complete prescribing information for this medication should be consulted for additional detail.
Dosage Forms
Cream, topical (Halog®): 0.1% (15 g, 30 g, 60 g, 240 g)
Cream, emollient base, topical (Halog®-E): 0.1% (30 g, 60 g)
Ointment, topical (Halog®): 0.1% (15 g, 30 g, 60 g, 240 g)
Solution, topical (Halog®): 0.1% (20 mL, 60 mL)

♦ **Halcion®** *see* Triazolam *on page 1370*
♦ **Haldol®** *see* Haloperidol *on page 654*
♦ **Haldol® Decanoate** *see* Haloperidol *on page 654*
♦ **Haley's M-O® [OTC]** *see* Magnesium Hydroxide and Mineral Oil Emulsion *on page 833*
♦ **Halfan®** *see* Halofantrine *on page 653*
♦ **Halfprin® [OTC]** *see* Aspirin *on page 120*

Halobetasol (hal oh BAY ta sol)
Related Information
Corticosteroids Comparison *on page 1495*
U.S. Brand Names Ultravate™
Canadian Brand Names Ultravate™
Synonyms Halobetasol Propionate
Therapeutic Category Corticosteroid, Topical (Very High Potency)
Use Relief of inflammatory and pruritic manifestations of corticosteroid-response dermatoses [very high potency topical corticosteroid]
Pregnancy Risk Factor C
Usual Dosage Children and Adults: Topical: Steroid-responsive dermatoses: Apply sparingly to skin twice daily, rub in gently and completely; treatment should not exceed 2 consecutive weeks and total dosage should not exceed 50 g/week. Therapy should be discontinued when control is achieved; if no improvement is seen, reassessment of diagnosis may be necessary.
Additional Information Complete prescribing information for this medication should be consulted for additional detail.
Dosage Forms
Cream, topical, as propionate: 0.05% (15 g, 45 g)
Ointment, topical, as propionate: 0.05% (15 g, 45 g)

♦ **Halobetasol Propionate** *see* Halobetasol *on page 653*

Halofantrine (ha loe FAN trin)
Related Information
Malaria Treatment *on page 1607*
U.S. Brand Names Halfan®
Synonyms Halofantrine Hydrochloride
Therapeutic Category Antimalarial Agent
Use Orphan drug: Treatment of mild to moderate acute malaria caused by susceptible strains of *Plasmodium falciparum* and *Plasmodium vivax*
Pregnancy Risk Factor X
Contraindications Family history of congenital QT_c prolongation; hypersensitivity to halofantrine or any component of the formulation; drugs or clinical conditions known to prolong QT_c intervals; previous treatment with mefloquine; known or suspected ventricular dysrhythmias; AV conduction abnormalities or unexplained syncope
Warnings/Precautions Monitor closely for decreased hematocrit and hemoglobin, patients with chronic liver disease
Adverse Reactions
1% to 10%:
Cardiovascular: Edema
Central nervous system: Malaise, headache (3%), dizziness (5%)
Dermatologic: Pruritus (3%)
Gastrointestinal: Nausea (3%), vomiting (4%), abdominal pain (9%), diarrhea (6%)
Hematologic: Leukocytosis
Hepatic: Elevated LFTs
Local: Tenderness
Neuromuscular & skeletal: Myalgia (1%), rigors (2%)
Respiratory: Cough
Miscellaneous: Lymphadenopathy
(Continued)

Halofantrine *(Continued)*

<1% (Limited to important or life-threatening): Anaphylactic shock, asthma, chest pain, confusion, depression, hypertensive crisis, hypotension, orthostasis, paresthesias, pulmonary edema, seizures, sterile abscesses, stroke, tetany, tinnitus, urticaria, ventricular arrhythmias

Drug Interactions

Cytochrome P450 Effect: CYP2D6 and 3A3/4 enzyme substrate

Increased Effect/Toxicity: Increased toxicity (QT_c interval prolongation) with other agents that cause QT_c interval prolongation, especially mefloquine

Mechanism of Action Similar to mefloquine; destruction of asexual blood forms, possible inhibition of proton pump

Pharmacodynamics/Kinetics

Absorption: Erratic and variable; serum levels are proportional to dose up to 1000 mg; smaller doses should be divided; may be increased 60% with high fat meals

Distribution: V_d: 570 L/kg; widely to most tissues

Metabolism: Hepatic to active metabolite

Half-life elimination: 23 hours; Metabolite: 82 hours; may be increased in active disease

Excretion: Urine (as unchanged drug)

Clearance: Parasite: Mean: 40-84 hours

Usual Dosage Oral:

Children <40 kg: 8 mg/kg every 6 hours for 3 doses; repeat in 1 week

Children ≥40 kg and Adults: 500 mg every 6 hours for 3 doses; repeat in 1 week

Monitoring Parameters CBC, LFTs, parasite counts

Test Interactions Increased serum transaminases, bilirubin

Patient Information Take on an empty stomach; avoid high fat meals; notify physician of persistent nausea, vomiting, abdominal pain, light stools, dark urine

Nursing Implications Monitor closely for jaundice, other signs of hepatotoxicity

Dosage Forms Tablet, as hydrochloride: 250 mg

♦ **Halofantrine Hydrochloride** *see Halofantrine on page 653*

♦ **Halog**® *see Halcinonide on page 653*

♦ **Halog**®**-E** *see Halcinonide on page 653*

Haloperidol *(ha loe PER i dole)*

Related Information

Antipsychotic Agents Comparison *on page 1486*

Depression *on page 1655*

U.S. Brand Names Haldol®; Haldol® Decanoate

Canadian Brand Names Apo®-Haloperidol; Haldol®; Novo-Peridol; Peridol; PMS-Haloperidol LA; Rho®-Haloperidol Decanoate

Synonyms Haloperidol Decanoate; Haloperidol Lactate

Therapeutic Category Antipsychotic Agent, Miscellaneous; Sedative

Use Treatment of psychoses; control of tics and vocal utterances of Tourette's disorder in children and adults; severe behavioral problems in children

Unlabeled/Investigational Use May be used for the emergency sedation of severely agitated or delirious patients; adjunctive treatment of ethanol dependence; antiemetic

Pregnancy Risk Factor C

Contraindications Hypersensitivity to haloperidol or any component of the formulation; Parkinson's disease; severe CNS depression; bone marrow suppression; severe cardiac or hepatic disease; coma

Warnings/Precautions Safety and efficacy have not been established in children <3 years of age. Use caution in patients with CNS depression and severe liver or cardiac disease. Hypotension may occur, particularly with parenteral administration. Decanoate form should never be administered I.V. Avoid in thyrotoxicosis. May be sedating, use with caution in disorders where CNS depression is a feature. Caution in patients with hemodynamic instability, predisposition to seizures, subcortical brain damage, renal or respiratory disease. Esophageal dysmotility and aspiration have been associated with antipsychotic use - use with caution in patients at risk of pneumonia (ie, Alzheimer's disease). Caution in breast cancer or other prolactin-dependent tumors (may elevate prolactin levels). May alter temperature regulation or mask toxicity of other drugs due to antiemetic effects. May alter cardiac conduction - life-threatening arrhythmias have occurred with therapeutic doses of antipsychotics. Adverse effects of decanoate may be prolonged. May cause orthostatic hypotension - use with caution in patients at risk of this effect or those who would tolerate transient hypotensive episodes (cerebrovascular disease, cardiovascular disease, or other medications which may predispose). Some tablets contain tartrazine.

May cause anticholinergic effects (confusion, agitation, constipation, dry mouth, blurred vision, urinary retention). Therefore, they should be used with caution in patients with decreased gastrointestinal motility, urinary retention, BPH, xerostomia, or visual problems. Conditions which also may be exacerbated by cholinergic blockade include narrow-angle glaucoma (screening is recommended) and worsening of myasthenia gravis. Relative to other neuroleptics, haloperidol has a low potency of cholinergic blockade.

May cause extrapyramidal reactions, including pseudoparkinsonism, acute dystonic reactions, akathisia, and tardive dyskinesia (risk of these reactions is high relative to other neuroleptics). May be associated with neuroleptic malignant syndrome (NMS) or pigmentary retinopathy.

Adverse Reactions Frequency not defined.

Cardiovascular: Hypotension, hypertension, tachycardia, arrhythmias, abnormal T waves with prolonged ventricular repolarization

Central nervous system: Restlessness, anxiety, extrapyramidal reactions, dystonic reactions, pseudoparkinsonian signs and symptoms, tardive dyskinesia, neuroleptic malignant syndrome (NMS), altered central temperature regulation, akathisia, tardive dystonia, insomnia, euphoria, agitation, drowsiness, depression, lethargy, headache, confusion, vertigo, seizures

Dermatologic: Hyperpigmentation, pruritus, rash, contact dermatitis, alopecia, photosensitivity (rare)

Endocrine & metabolic: Amenorrhea, galactorrhea, gynecomastia, sexual dysfunction, lactation, breast engorgement, mastalgia, menstrual irregularities, hyperglycemia, hypoglycemia, hyponatremia

Gastrointestinal: Nausea, vomiting, anorexia, constipation, diarrhea, hypersalivation, dyspepsia, xerostomia

Genitourinary: Urinary retention, priapism

Hematologic: Cholestatic jaundice, obstructive jaundice

Ocular: Blurred vision

Respiratory: Laryngospasm, bronchospasm

Miscellaneous: Heat stroke, diaphoresis

Overdosage/Toxicology Symptoms include deep sleep, dystonia, agitation, dysrhythmias, and extrapyramidal symptoms. Following initiation of essential overdose management, toxic symptom treatment and supportive treatment should be initiated. Critical cardiac arrhythmias often respond to I.V. lidocaine, while other antiarrhythmics can be used. Neuroleptics often cause extrapyramidal symptoms (eg, dystonic reactions) requiring management with anticholinergic agents such as benztropine mesylate I.V. 1-2 mg (adult). These agents are generally effective within 2-5 minutes.

Drug Interactions

Cytochrome P450 Effect: CYP1A2 (minor), CYP2D6 (minor), and 3A3/4 enzyme substrate; CYP2D6 enzyme inhibitor

Increased Effect/Toxicity: Haloperidol concentrations/effects may be increased by chloroquine, fluoxetine, paroxetine, propranolol, quinidine, and sulfadoxine-pyridoxine.

Haloperidol may increase the effects of antihypertensives, CNS depressants (ethanol, narcotics, sedative-hypnotics), lithium, trazodone, and TCAs. Haloperidol in combination with indomethacin may result in drowsiness, tiredness, and confusion.

Decreased Effect: Haloperidol may inhibit the ability of bromocriptine to lower serum prolactin concentrations. Benztropine (and other anticholinergics) may inhibit the therapeutic response to haloperidol and excess anticholinergic effects may occur. Barbiturates, carbamazepine, and cigarette smoking may enhance the hepatic metabolism of haloperidol. Haloperidol may inhibit the antiparkinsonian effect of levodopa; avoid this combination.

Ethanol/Nutrition/Herb Interactions

Ethanol: Avoid ethanol (may increase CNS depression).

Herb/Nutraceutical: Avoid valerian, St John's wort, kava kava, gotu kola (may increase CNS depression).

Stability

Protect oral dosage forms from light

Haloperidol lactate injection should be stored at controlled room temperature and protected from light, freezing and temperatures >40°C; exposure to light may cause discoloration and the development of a grayish-red precipitate over several weeks

Haloperidol lactate may be administered IVPB or I.V. infusion in D_5W solutions; NS solutions should not be used due to reports of decreased stability and incompatibility

Standardized dose: 0.5-100 mg/50-100 mL D_5W

Stability of standardized solutions is 38 days at room temperature (24°C)

Mechanism of Action Blocks postsynaptic mesolimbic dopaminergic D_1 and D_2 receptors in the brain; depresses the release of hypothalamic and hypophyseal hormones; believed to depress the reticular activating system thus affecting basal metabolism, body temperature, wakefulness, vasomotor tone, and emesis

Pharmacodynamics/Kinetics

Onset of action: Sedation: I.V.: ~1 hour

Duration: Decanoate: ~3 weeks

Distribution: Crosses placenta; enters breast milk

Protein binding: 90%

Metabolism: Hepatic to inactive compounds

Bioavailability: Oral: 60%

Half-life elimination: 20 hours

Time to peak, serum: 20 minutes

Excretion: Urine (33% to 40% as metabolites) within 5 days; feces (15%)

Usual Dosage

Children: 3-12 years (15-40 kg): Oral:

Initial: 0.05 mg/kg/day or 0.25-0.5 mg/day given in 2-3 divided doses; increase by 0.25-0.5 mg every 5-7 days; maximum: 0.15 mg/kg/day

Usual maintenance:

Agitation or hyperkinesia: 0.01-0.03 mg/kg/day once daily

Nonpsychotic disorders: 0.05-0.075 mg/kg/day in 2-3 divided doses

Psychotic disorders: 0.05-0.15 mg/kg/day in 2-3 divided doses

Children 6-12 years: Sedation/psychotic disorders: I.M. (as lactate): 1-3 mg/dose every 4-8 hours to a maximum of 0.15 mg/kg/day; change over to oral therapy as soon as able

Adults:

Psychosis:

Oral: 0.5-5 mg 2-3 times/day; usual maximum: 30 mg/day

I.M. (as lactate): 2-5 mg every 4-8 hours as needed

I.M. (as decanoate): Initial: 10-20 times the daily oral dose administered at 4-week intervals

Maintenance dose: 10-15 times initial oral dose; used to stabilize psychiatric symptoms

Sedation in the intensive care unit:

I.M., IVP, IVPB: May repeat bolus doses after 30 minutes until calm achieved then administer 50% of the maximum dose every 6 hours

Mild agitation: 0.5-2 mg

Moderate agitation: 2.5-5 mg

(Continued)

Haloperidol *(Continued)*

Severe agitation: 10-20 mg

Oral: Agitation: 5-10 mg

Continuous intravenous infusion (100 mg/100 mL D$_5$W): Rates of 1-40 mg/hour have been used

Rapid tranquilization of severely-agitated patient (unlabeled use): Administer every 30-60 minutes:

Oral: 5-10 mg

I.M.: 5 mg

Average total dose (oral or I.M.) for tranquilization: 10-20 mg

Elderly: Initial: Oral: 0.25-0.5 mg 1-2 times/day; increase dose at 4- to 7-day intervals by 0.25-0.5 mg/day; increase dosing intervals (twice daily, 3 times/day, etc) as necessary to control response or side effects

Hemodialysis/peritoneal dialysis: Supplemental dose is not necessary

Administration The decanoate injectable formulation should be administered I.M. only, **do not administer decanoate I.V.** Dilute the oral concentrate with water or juice before administration

Monitoring Parameters Monitor orthostatic blood pressures after initiation of therapy or a dose increase; observe for tremor and abnormal movement or posturing (extrapyramidal symptoms)

Reference Range

Therapeutic: 5-15 ng/mL (SI: 10-30 nmol/L) (psychotic disorders - less for Tourette's and mania)

Toxic: >42 ng/mL (SI: >84 nmol/L)

Patient Information May cause drowsiness, restlessness, avoid alcohol and other CNS depressants, rise slowly from recumbent position; use of supportive stockings may help prevent orthostatic hypotension; do not alter dosage or discontinue without consulting physician; oral concentrate must be diluted in 2-4 oz of liquid (water, fruit juice, carbonated drinks, milk, or pudding)

Nursing Implications Avoid skin contact with oral suspension or solution; may cause contact dermatitis

Dosage Forms

Injection, as decanoate: 50 mg/mL (1 mL, 5 mL); 100 mg/mL (1 mL, 5 mL)

Injection, as lactate: 5 mg/mL (1 mL, 2 mL, 2.5 mL, 10 mL)

Solution, oral concentrate, as lactate: 2 mg/mL (5 mL, 10 mL, 15 mL, 120 mL, 240 mL)

Tablet: 0.5 mg, 1 mg, 2 mg, 5 mg, 10 mg, 20 mg

- ◆ **Haloperidol Decanoate** *see Haloperidol on page 654*
- ◆ **Haloperidol Lactate** *see Haloperidol on page 654*

Haloprogin *Not Available in U.S.* (ha loe PROE jin)

Therapeutic Category Antifungal Agent, Topical

Use Topical treatment of tinea pedis (athlete's foot), tinea cruris (jock itch), tinea corporis (ringworm), tinea manuum caused by *Trichophyton rubrum*, *Trichophyton tonsurans*, *Trichophyton mentagrophytes*, *Microsporum canis*, or *Epidermophyton floccosum*; topical treatment of *Malassezia furfur*

Pregnancy Risk Factor B

Contraindications Hypersensitivity to haloprogin or any component of the formulation

Warnings/Precautions Safety and efficacy have not been established in children

Adverse Reactions Pruritus, folliculitis, vesicle formation, erythema, irritation, burning sensation

Mechanism of Action Interferes with fungal DNA replication to inhibit yeast cell respiration and disrupt its cell membrane

Pharmacodynamics/Kinetics

Absorption: Poorly through the skin (~11%)

Metabolism: To trichlorophenol

Excretion: Urine (75% as unchanged drug)

Usual Dosage Topical: Children and Adults: Apply liberally twice daily for 2-3 weeks; intertriginous areas may require up to 4 weeks of treatment

Patient Information Avoid contact with eyes; for external use only; improvement should occur within 4 weeks; discontinue use if sensitization or irritation occur

Nursing Implications Avoid contact with eyes; for external use only; improvement should occur within 4 weeks; discontinue use if sensitization or irritation occur

Dosage Forms

Cream, topical: 1% (15 g, 30 g)

Solution, topical: 1% with alcohol 75% (10 mL, 30 mL)

- ◆ **Halotestin®** *see Fluoxymesterone on page 580*
- ◆ **Halotussin® DAC** *see Guaifenesin, Pseudoephedrine, and Codeine on page 648*
- ◆ **Halotussin® DM [OTC]** *see Guaifenesin and Dextromethorphan on page 646*
- ◆ **Haltran® [OTC]** *see Ibuprofen on page 697*
- ◆ **Havrix®** *see Hepatitis A Vaccine on page 660*
- ◆ **Havrix® and Engerix-B®** *see Hepatitis A Inactivated and Hepatitis B (Recombinant) Vaccine on page 660*
- ◆ **Hayfebrol® [OTC]** *see Chlorpheniramine and Pseudoephedrine on page 279*
- ◆ **HbCV** *see Haemophilus b Conjugate Vaccine on page 651*
- ◆ **HBIG** *see Hepatitis B Immune Globulin on page 661*
- ◆ **hBNP** *see Nesiritide on page 971*
- ◆ **25-HCC** *see Calcifediol on page 203*
- ◆ **HCTZ** *see Hydrochlorothiazide on page 674*
- ◆ **HCTZ and Telmisartan** *see Telmisartan and Hydrochlorothiazide on page 1291*
- ◆ **HDA® Toothache [OTC]** *see Benzocaine on page 154*

- **HDCV** *see* Rabies Virus Vaccine *on page 1175*
- **Head & Shoulders® Intensive Treatment [OTC]** *see* Selenium Sulfide *on page 1229*
- **Healon®** *see* Sodium Hyaluronate *on page 1247*
- **Healon® GV** *see* Sodium Hyaluronate *on page 1247*
- **Heart Failure** *see page 1663*
- **Hectorol®** *see* Doxercalciferol *on page 442*
- *Helicobacter pylori* **Treatment** *see page 1668*
- **Helidac®** *see* Bismuth Subsalicylate, Metronidazole, and Tetracycline *on page 172*
- **Helistat®** *see* Microfibrillar Collagen Hemostat *on page 909*
- **Helixate® FS** *see* Antihemophilic Factor (Recombinant) *on page 105*
- **Hemabate™** *see* Carboprost Tromethamine *on page 228*
- **Hemocyte® [OTC]** *see* Ferrous Fumarate *on page 555*
- **Hemofil® M** *see* Antihemophilic Factor (Human) *on page 102*
- **Hemonyne®** *see* Factor IX Complex (Human) *on page 539*
- **Hemotene®** *see* Microfibrillar Collagen Hemostat *on page 909*
- **Hemril-HC® Uniserts®** *see* Hydrocortisone *on page 682*
- **Hepalean® (Can)** *see* Heparin *on page 657*
- **Hepalean® Leo (Can)** *see* Heparin *on page 657*
- **Hepalean®-LOK (Can)** *see* Heparin *on page 657*

Heparin (HEP a rin)

Related Information
Heparin Comparison *on page 1501*
U.S. Brand Names Hep-Lock®
Canadian Brand Names Hepalean®; Hepalean® Leo; Hepalean®-LOK
Synonyms Heparin Calcium; Heparin Lock Flush; Heparin Sodium
Therapeutic Category Anticoagulant
Use Prophylaxis and treatment of thromboembolic disorders
Pregnancy Risk Factor C
Contraindications Hypersensitivity to heparin or any component of the formulation; severe thrombocytopenia; uncontrolled active bleeding except when due to DIC; suspected intracranial hemorrhage; not for I.M. use; not for use when appropriate monitoring parameters cannot be obtained
Warnings/Precautions Use cautiously in patients with a documented hypersensitivity reaction and only in life-threatening situations. Hemorrhage is the most common complication. Monitor for signs and symptoms of bleeding. Certain patients are at increased risk of bleeding. Risk factors include bacterial endocarditis; congenital or acquired bleeding disorders; active ulcerative or angiodysplastic GI diseases; severe uncontrolled hypertension; hemorrhagic stroke; or use shortly after brain, spinal, or ophthalmology surgery; patient treated concomitantly with platelet inhibitors; conditions associated with increased bleeding tendencies (hemophilia, vascular purpura); recent GI bleeding; thrombocytopenia or platelet defects; severe liver disease; hypertensive or diabetic retinopathy; or in patients undergoing invasive procedures. A higher incidence of bleeding has been reported in patients >60 years of age, particularly women. They are also more sensitive to the dose.

Patients who develop thrombocytopenia on heparin may be at risk of developing a new thrombus ("White-clot syndrome"). Hypersensitivity reactions can occur. Osteoporosis can occur following long-term use (>6 months). Monitor for hyperkalemia. Discontinue therapy and consider alternatives if platelets are <100,000/mm³. Patients >60 years of age may require lower doses of heparin.

Some preparations contain benzyl alcohol as a preservative. In neonates, large amounts of benzyl alcohol (>100 mg/kg/day) have been associated with fatal toxicity (gasping syndrome). The use of preservative-free heparin is, therefore, recommended in neonates. Some preparations contain sulfite which may cause allergic reactions.

Heparin does not possess fibrinolytic activity and, therefore, cannot lyse established thrombi; discontinue heparin if hemorrhage occurs; severe hemorrhage or overdosage may require protamine

Adverse Reactions
Cardiovascular: Chest pain, vasospasm (possibly related to thrombosis), hemorrhagic shock
Central nervous system: Fever, headache, chills
Dermatologic: Unexplained bruising, urticaria, alopecia, dysesthesia pedis, purpura, eczema, cutaneous necrosis (following deep S.C. injection), erythematous plaques (case reports)
Endocrine & metabolic: Hyperkalemia (supression of aldosterone), rebound hyperlipidemia on discontinuation
Gastrointestinal: Nausea, vomiting, constipation, hematemesis
Genitourinary: Frequent or persistent erection
Hematologic: Hemorrhage, blood in urine, bleeding from gums, epistaxis, adrenal hemorrhage, ovarian hemorrhage, retroperitoneal hemorrhage, thrombocytopenia (see note)
Hepatic: Elevated liver enzymes (AST/ALT) Local: Irritation, ulceration, cutaneous necrosis have been rarely reported with deep S.C. injections, I.M. injection (not recommended) is associated with a high incidence of these effects
Neuromuscular & skeletal: Peripheral neuropathy, osteoporosis (chronic therapy effect)
Respiratory: Hemoptysis, pulmonary hemorrhage, asthma, rhinitis, bronchospasm (case reports)
Ocular: Conjunctivitis (allergic reaction)
Miscellaneous: Allergic reactions, anaphylactoid reactions

Note: Thrombocytopenia has been reported to occur at an incidence between 0% and 30%. It is often of no clinical significance. However, immunologically mediated heparin-induced thrombocytopenia has been estimated to occur in 1% to 2% of patients, and is marked by a progressive fall in platelet counts and, in some cases, thromboembolic complications (skin necrosis, pulmonary embolism, gangrene of the extremities, stroke or myocardial infarction); (Continued)

Heparin *(Continued)*

daily platelet counts for 5-7 days at initiation of therapy may help detect the onset of this complication.

Overdosage/Toxicology The primary symptom of overdose is bleeding. The antidote is protamine: 1 mg per 100 units of heparin. Discontinue all heparin if evidence of progressive immune thrombocytopenia occurs.

Drug Interactions
Increased Effect/Toxicity: The risk of hemorrhage associated with heparin may be increased by oral anticoagulants (warfarin), thrombolytics, dextran, and drugs which affect platelet function (eg, aspirin, NSAIDs, dipyridamole, ticlopidine, clopidogrel, IIb/IIIa antagonists). However, heparin is often used in conjunction with thrombolytic therapy or during the initiation of warfarin therapy to assure anticoagulation and to protect against possible transient hypercoagulability. Cephalosporins which contain the MTT side chain and parenteral penicillins (may inhibit platelet aggregation) may increase the risk of hemorrhage. Other drugs reported to increase heparin's anticoagulant effect include antihistamines, tetracycline, quinine, nicotine, and cardiac glycosides (digoxin).

Decreased Effect: Nitroglycerin (I.V.) may decrease heparin's anticoagulant effect. This interaction has not been validated in some studies, and may only occur at high nitroglycerin dosages.

Ethanol/Nutrition/Herb Interactions
Food: When taking for >6 months, may interfere with calcium absorption.

Herb/Nutraceutical: Avoid cat's claw, dong quai, evening primrose, feverfew, red clover, horse chestnut, garlic, green tea, ginseng, ginkgo (all have additional antiplatelet activity).

Stability
Heparin solutions are colorless to slightly yellow; minor color variations do not affect therapeutic efficacy

Heparin should be stored at controlled room temperature and protected from freezing and temperatures >40°C

Stability at room temperature and refrigeration:
Prepared bag: 24 hours
Premixed bag: After seal is broken 4 days
Out of overwrap stability: 30 days
Standard diluent: 25,000 units/500 mL D_5W (premixed)
Minimum volume: 250 mL D_5W

Mechanism of Action Potentiates the action of antithrombin III and thereby inactivates thrombin (as well as activated coagulation factors IX, X, XI, XII, and plasmin) and prevents the conversion of fibrinogen to fibrin; heparin also stimulates release of lipoprotein lipase (lipoprotein lipase hydrolyzes triglycerides to glycerol and free fatty acids)

Pharmacodynamics/Kinetics
Onset of action: Anticoagulation: I.V.: Immediate; S.C.: ~20-30 minutes
Absorption: Oral, rectal, I.M.: Erratic at best from all these routes of administration; S.C. absorption is also erratic, but considered acceptable for prophylactic use
Distribution: Does not cross placenta; does not enter breast milk
Metabolism: Hepatic; believed to be partially metabolized in the reticuloendothelial system
Half-life elimination: Mean: 1.5 hours; Range: 1-2 hours; affected by obesity, renal function, hepatic function, malignancy, presence of pulmonary embolism, and infections
Excretion: Urine (small amounts as unchanged drug)

Usual Dosage
Children:
Intermittent I.V.: Initial: 50-100 units/kg, then 50-100 units/kg every 4 hours
I.V. infusion: Initial: 50 units/kg, then 15-25 units/kg/hour; increase dose by 2-4 units/kg/hour every 6-8 hours as required
Adults:
Prophylaxis (low-dose heparin): S.C.: 5000 units every 8-12 hours
Intermittent I.V.: Initial: 10,000 units, then 50-70 units/kg (5000-10,000 units) every 4-6 hours
I.V. infusion (weight-based dosing per institutional nomogram recommended):
Acute coronary syndromes: MI: Fibrinolytic therapy:
Alteplase or reteplase with first or second bolus: Concurrent bolus of 60 units/kg (maximum: 4000 units), then 12 units/kg/hour (maximum: 1000 units/hour) as continuous infusion. Check aPTT every 4-6 hours; adjust to target of 1.5-2 times the upper limit of control (50-70 seconds in clinical trials); usual range 10-30 units/kg/hour. Duration of heparin therapy depends on concurrent therapy and the specific patient risks for systemic or venous thromboembolism.
Streptokinase: Heparin use optional depending on concurrent therapy and specific patient risks for systemic or venous thromboembolism (anterior MI, CHF, previous embolus, atrial fibrillation, LV thrombus): If heparin is administered, start when aPTT <2 times the upper limit of control; do not use a bolus, but initiate infusion adjusted to a target aPTT of 1.5-2 times the upper limit of control (50-70 seconds in clinical trials). If heparin is not administered by infusion, 7500-12,500 units S.C. every 12 hours (when aPTT <2 times the upper limit of control) is recommended.
Percutaneous coronary intervention: Heparin bolus and infusion may be administered to an activated clotting time (ACT) of 300-350 seconds if no concurrent GPIIb/IIIa receptor antagonist is administered or 200-250 seconds if a GPIIb/IIIa receptor antagonist is administered.
Treatment of unstable angina (high-risk and some intermediate-risk patients): Initial bolus of 60-70 units/kg (maximum: 5000 units), followed by an initial infusion of 12-15 units/kg/hour (maximum: 1000 units/hour). The American College of Chest Physicians consensus conference has recommended dosage adjustments to correspond to a therapeutic range equivalent to heparin levels of 0.3-0.7 units/mL by antifactor Xa determinations, which correlates with aPTT values between 60 and 80 seconds

Treatment of venous thromboembolism (DVT/PE): 80 units/kg I.V. push followed by continuous infusion of 18 units/kg/hour

Line flushing: When using daily flushes of heparin to maintain patency of single and double lumen central catheters, 10 units/mL is commonly used for younger infants (eg, <10 kg) while 100 units/mL is used for older infants, children, and adults. Capped PVC catheters and peripheral heparin locks require flushing more frequently (eg, every 6-8 hours). Volume of heparin flush is usually similar to volume of catheter (or slightly greater). Additional flushes should be given when stagnant blood is observed in catheter, after catheter is used for drug or blood administration, and after blood withdrawal from catheter.

Addition of heparin (0.5-1 unit/mL) to peripheral and central TPN has been shown to increase duration of line patency. The final concentration of heparin used for TPN solutions may need to be decreased to 0.5 units/mL in small infants receiving larger amounts of volume in order to avoid approaching therapeutic amounts. Arterial lines are heparinized with a final concentration of 1 unit/mL.

Using a standard heparin solution (25,000 units/500 mL D_5W), the following infusion rates can be used to achieve the listed doses.

For a dose of:

400 units/hour: Infuse at 8 mL/hour
500 units/hour: Infuse at 10 mL/hour
600 units/hour: Infuse at 12 mL/hour
700 units/hour: Infuse at 14 mL/hour
800 units/hour: Infuse at 16 mL/hour
900 units/hour: Infuse at 18 mL/hour
1000 units/hour: Infuse at 20 mL/hour
1100 units/hour: Infuse at 22 mL/hour
1200 units/hour: Infuse at 24 mL/hour
1300 units/hour: Infuse at 26 mL/hour
1400 units/hour: Infuse at 28 mL/hour
1500 units/hour: Infuse at 30 mL/hour
1600 units/hour: Infuse at 32 mL/hour
1700 units/hour: Infuse at 34 mL/hour
1800 units/hour: Infuse at 36 mL/hour
1900 units/hour: Infuse at 38 mL/hour
2000 units/hour: Infuse at 40 mL/hour

Dosing adjustments in the elderly: Patients >60 years of age may have higher serum levels and clinical response (longer aPTTs) as compared to younger patients receiving similar dosages; lower dosages may be required

Administration Do not administer I.M. due to pain, irritation, and hematoma formation; central venous catheters must be flushed with heparin solution when newly inserted, daily (at the time of tubing change), after blood withdrawal or transfusion, and after an intermittent infusion through an injectable cap. A volume of at least 10 mL of blood should be removed and discarded from a heparinized line before blood samples are sent for coagulation testing.

Monitoring Parameters Platelet counts, aPTT, hemoglobin, hematocrit, signs of bleeding

For intermittent I.V. injections, aPTT is measured 3.5-4 hours after I.V. injection

Note: Continuous I.V. infusion is preferred over I.V. intermittent injections. For full-dose heparin (ie, nonlow-dose), the dose should be titrated according to aPTT results. For anticoagulation, an aPTT 1.5-2.5 times normal is usually desired. Because of variation among hospitals in the control aPTT values, nomograms should be established at each institution, designed to achieve aPTT values in the target range (eg, for a control aPTT of 30 seconds, the target range [1.5-2.5 times control] would be 45-75 seconds). Measurements should be made prior to heparin therapy, 6 hours after initiation, and 6 hours after any dosage change, and should be used to adjust the heparin infusion until the aPTT exhibits a therapeutic level. When two consecutive aPTT values are therapeutic, the measurements may be made every 24 hours, and if necessary, dose adjustment carried out. In addition, a significant change in the patient's clinical condition (eg, recurrent ischemia, bleeding, hypotension) should prompt an immediate aPTT determination, followed by dose adjustment if necessary. Increase or decrease infusion by 2-4 units/kg/hour dependent upon aPTT.

Heparin infusion dose adjustment:
aPTT >3x control: Decrease infusion rate 50%
aPTT 2-3x control: Decrease infusion rate 25%
aPTT 1.5-2x control: No change
aPTT <1.5x control: Increase rate of infusion 25%; max 2500 units/hour

Reference Range Heparin: 0.3-0.5 unit/mL; aPTT: 1.5-2.5 times **the patient's baseline**

Test Interactions Increased thyroxine (S) (competitive protein binding methods); increased PT, increased aPTT, increased bleeding time

Nursing Implications Do not administer I.M. due to pain, irritation, and hematoma formation
Note: Heparin lock flush solution is intended only to maintain patency of I.V. devices and is **not** to be used for anticoagulant therapy

Dosage Forms
Infusion, porcine intestinal mucosa, as sodium:
D_5W: 40 units/mL (500 mL); 50 units/mL (250 mL, 500 mL); 100 units/mL (100 mL, 250 mL)
NaCl 0.45%: 2 units/mL (500 mL, 1000 mL); 50 units/mL (250 mL); 100 units/mL (250 mL)
NaCl 0.9%: 2 units/mL (500 mL, 1000 mL); 5 units/mL (1000 mL); 50 units/mL (250 mL, 500 mL, 1000 mL)
Injection, as sodium [lock flush] [**Note:** Heparin lock flush solution is intended only to maintain patency of I.V. devices and is **not** to be used for anticoagulant therapy]:
Beef lung source: 10 units/mL (1 mL, 2 mL, 2.5 mL, 3 mL, 5 mL, 10 mL, 30 mL); 100 units/mL (1 mL, 2 mL, 2.5 mL, 3 mL, 5 mL, 10 mL, 30 mL)
Porcine intestinal mucosa: 10 units/mL (1 mL, 2 mL, 10 mL, 30 mL); 100 units/mL (1 mL, 2 mL, 10 mL, 30 mL)
Porcine intestinal mucosa [preservative free]: 10 units/mL (1 mL); 100 units/mL (1 mL)
(Continued)

Heparin (Continued)

Injection, as sodium [multidose vial]:
Beef lung source [with preservative]: 1000 units/mL (5 mL, 10 mL, 30 mL); 5000 units/mL (10 mL); 10,000 units/mL (1 mL, 4 mL, 5 mL, 10 mL); 20,000 units/mL (2 mL, 5 mL); 40,000 units/mL (2 mL, 5 mL)
Porcine intestinal mucosa [with preservative]: 1000 units/mL (10 mL, 30 mL); 5000 units/mL (10 mL); 10,000 units/mL (4 mL); 20,000 units/mL (2 mL, 5 mL)
Injection, as sodium [single-dose vial]:
Beef lung: 1000 units/mL (1 mL); 5000 units/mL (1 mL); 10,000 units/mL (1 mL); 20,000 units/mL (1 mL); 40,000 units/mL (1 mL)
Porcine intestinal mucosa: 1000 units/mL (1 mL); 5000 units/mL (1 mL); 10,000 units/mL (1 mL); 20,000 units/mL (1 mL); 40,000 units/mL (1 mL)
Injection, porcine intestinal mucosa, as calcium [preservative free] [unit dose] (Calciparine®): 5000 units/dose (0.2 mL); 12,500 units/dose (0.5 mL); 20,000 units/dose (0.8 mL)
Injection, porcine intestinal mucosa, as sodium [with preservative] [unit dose]: 1000 units/dose (1 mL, 2 mL); 2500 units/dose (1 mL); 5000 units/dose (0.5 mL, 1 mL); 7500 units/dose (1 mL); 10,000 units/dose (1 mL); 15,000 units/dose (1 mL); 20,000 units/dose (1 mL)

♦ **Heparin Calcium** see Heparin on page 657
♦ **Heparin Cofactor I** see Antithrombin III on page 107
♦ **Heparin Comparison** see page 1501
♦ **Heparin Lock Flush** see Heparin on page 657
♦ **Heparin Sodium** see Heparin on page 657

Hepatitis A Inactivated and Hepatitis B (Recombinant) Vaccine
(hep a TYE tis aye in ak ti VAY ted & hep a TYE tis bee ree KOM be nant vak SEEN)
U.S. Brand Names Twinrix®
Canadian Brand Names Twinrix™
Synonyms Engerix-B® and Havrix®; Havrix® and Engerix-B®; Hepatitis B (Recombinant) and Hepatitis A Inactivated Vaccine
Therapeutic Category Vaccine
Use Active immunization against disease caused by hepatitis A virus and hepatitis B virus (all known subtypes) in populations desiring protection against or at high risk of exposure to these viruses.

Populations include travelers to areas of intermediate/high endemicity for **both** HAV and HBV; those at increased risk of HBV infection due to behavioral or occupational factors; patients with chronic liver disease; laboratory workers who handle live HAV and HBV; healthcare workers, police, and other personnel who render first-aid or medical assistance; workers who come in contact with sewage; employees of day care centers and correctional facilities; patients/staff of hemodialysis units; male homosexuals; patients frequently receiving blood products; military personnel; users of injectable illicit drugs; close household contacts of patients with hepatitis A and hepatitis B infection.
Pregnancy Risk Factor C
Usual Dosage I.M.: Adults: Primary immunization: Three doses (1 mL each) given on a 0-, 1-, and 6-month schedule
Additional Information Complete prescribing information for this medication should be consulted for additional detail.
Dosage Forms
Injection [single-dose vial]: Inactivated hepatitis A virus 720 ELISA units and hepatitis B surface antigen 20 mcg per mL (1 mL)
Injection, prefilled syringe [single-dose]: Inactivated hepatitis A virus 720 ELISA units and hepatitis B surface antigen 20 mcg per mL (1 mL)

Hepatitis A Vaccine (hep a TYE tis aye vak SEEN)
Related Information
Immunization Recommendations on page 1538
U.S. Brand Names Havrix®; VAQTA®
Canadian Brand Names Avaxim®; Epaxal Berna®; Havrix™; VAQTA®
Therapeutic Category Vaccine, Inactivated Virus
Use For populations desiring protection against hepatitis A or for populations at high risk of exposure to hepatitis A virus (travelers to developing countries, household and sexual contacts of persons infected with hepatitis A), child day care employees, patients with chronic liver disease, illicit drug users, male homosexuals, institutional workers (eg, institutions for the mentally and physically handicapped persons, prisons, etc), and healthcare workers who may be exposed to hepatitis A virus (eg, laboratory employees); protection lasts for approximately 15 years
Pregnancy Risk Factor C
Contraindications Hypersensitivity to hepatitis A vaccine or any component of the formulation
Warnings/Precautions Use caution in patients with serious active infection, cardiovascular disease, or pulmonary disorders; treatment for anaphylactic reactions should be immediately available
Adverse Reactions All serious adverse reactions must be reported to the U.S. Department of Health and Human Services (DHHS) Vaccine Adverse Event Reporting System (VAERS) 1-800-822-7967.
Percentage unknown: Fatigue, fever (rare), transient LFT abnormalities
>10%:
Central nervous system: Headache
Local: Pain, tenderness, and warmth
1% to 10%:
Endocrine & metabolic: Pharyngitis (1%)
Gastrointestinal: Abdominal pain (1%)

Local: Cutaneous reactions at the injection site (soreness, edema, and redness)

Mechanism of Action As an inactivated virus vaccine, hepatitis A vaccine offers active immunization against hepatitis A virus infection at an effective immune response rate in up to 99% of subjects

Pharmacodynamics/Kinetics
Onset of action (protection): 3 weeks after a single dose

Duration: Neutralizing antibodies have persisted for >3 years; unconfirmed evidence indicates that antibody levels may persist for 5-10 years

Usual Dosage I.M.:
Havrix®:

Children 2-18 years: 720 ELISA units (administered as 2 injections of 360 ELISA units [0.5 mL]) 15-30 days prior to travel with a booster 6-12 months following primary immunization; the deltoid muscle should be used for I.M. injection

Adults: 1440 ELISA units (1 mL) 15-30 days prior to travel with a booster 6-12 months following primary immunization; injection should be in the deltoid

VAQTA®:

Children 2-17 years: 25 units (0.5 mL) with 25 units (0.5 mL) booster to be given 6-18 months after primary immunization

Adults: 50 units (1 mL) with 50 units (1 mL) booster to be given 6 months after primary immunization

Administration For patients at risk of hemorrhage following intramuscular injection, the ACIP recommends "it should be administered intramuscularly if, in the opinion of the physician familiar with the patients bleeding risk, the vaccine can be administered with reasonable safety by this route. If the patient receives antihemophilia or other similar therapy, intramuscular vaccination can be scheduled shortly after such therapy is administered. A fine needle (23 gauge or smaller) can be used for the vaccination and firm pressure applied to the site (without rubbing) for at least 2 minutes. The patient should be instructed concerning the risk of hematoma from the injection."

Monitoring Parameters Liver function tests

Reference Range Seroconversion for Havrix®: Antibody >20 milli-international units/mL

Additional Information Some investigators suggest simultaneous or sequential administration of inactivated hepatitis A vaccine and immune globulin for postexposure protection, especially for travelers requiring rapid immunization, although a slight decrease in vaccine immunogenicity may be observed with this technique. Federal law requires that the date of administration, the vaccine manufacturer, lot number of vaccine, and the administering person's name, title and address be entered into the patient's permanent medical record.

Dosage Forms
Injection, adult, prefilled syringe [single-dose vial]:
Havrix®: 1440 ELISA units/mL
VAQTA®: 50 units/mL HAV protein
Injection, pediatric, prefilled syringe [single-dose vial] (Havrix®): 720 ELISA units/0.5 mL
Injection, pediatric/adolescent, prefilled syringe [single-dose vial] (VAQTA®): 25 units/0.5 mL HAV protein

Hepatitis B Immune Globulin (hep a TYE tis bee i MYUN GLOB yoo lin)

Related Information
Immunization Recommendations *on page 1538*
Postexposure Prophylaxis for Hepatitis B *on page 1549*

U.S. Brand Names BayHep B™; Nabi-HB®

Canadian Brand Names BayHep B™

Synonyms HBIG

Therapeutic Category Immune Globulin

Use Provide prophylactic passive immunity to hepatitis B infection to those individuals exposed; newborns of mothers known to be hepatitis B surface antigen positive; hepatitis B immune globulin is not indicated for treatment of active hepatitis B infections and is ineffective in the treatment of chronic active hepatitis B infection

Pregnancy Risk Factor C

Contraindications Hypersensitivity to hepatitis B immune globulin or any component of the formulation; allergies to gamma globulin or anti-immunoglobulin antibodies; allergies to thimerosal; IgA deficiency

Warnings/Precautions Have epinephrine 1:1000 available for anaphylactic reactions. As a product of human plasma, this product may potentially transmit disease; screening of donors, as well as testing and/or inactivation of certain viruses reduces this risk. Use caution in patients with thrombocytopenia or coagulation disorders (I.M. injections may be contraindicated), in patients with isolated IgA deficiency, or in patients with previous systemic hypersensitivity to human immunoglobulins. Not for intravenous administration.

Adverse Reactions
Central nervous system: Dizziness, malaise, fever, lethargy, chills
Dermatologic: Urticaria, angioedema, rash, erythema
Gastrointestinal: Vomiting, nausea
Genitourinary: Nephrotic syndrome
Local: Pain, tenderness, and muscular stiffness at injection site
Neuromuscular & skeletal: Arthralgia, myalgia
Miscellaneous: Anaphylaxis

Stability Refrigerate at 2°C to 8°C (36°F to 46°F); do not freeze

Mechanism of Action Hepatitis B immune globulin (HBIG) is a nonpyrogenic sterile solution containing 10% to 18% protein of which at least 80% is monomeric immunoglobulin G (IgG). HBIG differs from immune globulin in the amount of anti-HB_s. Immune globulin is prepared from plasma that is not preselected for anti-HB_s content. HBIG is prepared from plasma preselected for high titer anti-HB_s. In the U.S., HBIG has an anti-HB_s high titer >1:100,000 by IRA. There is no evidence that the causative agent of AIDS (HTLV-III/LAV) is transmitted by HBIG.

(Continued)

Hepatitis B Immune Globulin *(Continued)*

Pharmacodynamics/Kinetics
Absorption: Slow
Time to peak, serum: 1-6 days

Usual Dosage I.M.:
Newborns: Hepatitis B: 0.5 mL as soon after birth as possible (within 12 hours); may repeat at 3 months in order for a higher rate of prevention of the carrier state to be achieved; at this time an active vaccination program with the vaccine may begin

Adults: Postexposure prophylaxis: 0.06 mL/kg as soon as possible after exposure (ie, within 24 hours of needlestick, ocular, or mucosal exposure or within 14 days of sexual exposure); usual dose: 3-5 mL; repeat at 28-30 days after exposure

Note: HBIG may be administered at the same time (but at a different site) or up to 1 month preceding hepatitis B vaccination without impairing the active immune response

Administration I.M. injection only in gluteal or deltoid region; to prevent injury from injection, care should be taken when giving to patients with thrombocytopenia or bleeding disorders; has been administered intravenously in hepatitis B-positive liver transplant patients

Nursing Implications I.M. injection only; to prevent injury from injection care should be taken when administering to patients with thrombocytopenia or bleeding disorders; do not administer I.V.

Additional Information Has been administered intravenously in hepatitis B-positive liver transplant patients.

Dosage Forms
Injection [single-dose vial] (BayHep B™, Nabi-HB®): 1 mL, 5 mL
Injection, neonatal [single-dose vial] (BayHep B™): 0.5 mL

♦ **Hepatitis B Inactivated Virus Vaccine (plasma derived)** *see* Hepatitis B Vaccine *on page 662*

♦ **Hepatitis B Inactivated Virus Vaccine (recombinant DNA)** *see* Hepatitis B Vaccine *on page 662*

♦ **Hepatitis B (Recombinant) and Hepatitis A Inactivated Vaccine** *see* Hepatitis A Inactivated and Hepatitis B (Recombinant) Vaccine *on page 660*

Hepatitis B Vaccine (hep a TYE tis bee vak SEEN)

Related Information
Adverse Events and Vaccination *on page 1553*
Immunization Recommendations *on page 1538*
Postexposure Prophylaxis for Hepatitis B *on page 1549*
Recommendations of the Advisory Committee on Immunization Practices (ACIP) *on page 1540*
Recommended Childhood Immunization Schedule - US - 2002 *on page 1539*
Recommended Immunization Schedule for HIV-Infected Children *on page 1543*
USPHA/IDSA Guidelines for the Prevention of Opportunistic Infections in Persons With HIV *on page 1574*

U.S. Brand Names Engerix-B®; Recombivax HB®

Canadian Brand Names Engerix®-B; Recombivax HB®

Synonyms Hepatitis B Inactivated Virus Vaccine (plasma derived); Hepatitis B Inactivated Virus Vaccine (recombinant DNA)

Therapeutic Category Vaccine, Inactivated Virus

Use Immunization against infection caused by all known subtypes of hepatitis B virus, in individuals considered at high risk of potential exposure to hepatitis B virus or HB$_s$Ag-positive materials: See table.

Pre-exposure Prophylaxis for Hepatitis B
Health care workers[1]
Special patient groups (eg, adolescents, infants born to HB$_s$Ag–positive mothers, children born after 11/21/91, military personnel, etc)
Hemodialysis patients[2] (see dosing recommendations)
Recipients of certain blood products[3]
Lifestyle factors
Homosexual and bisexual men
Intravenous drug abusers
Heterosexually active persons with multiple sexual partners or recently acquired sexually transmitted diseases
Environmental factors
Household and sexual contacts of HBV carriers
Prison inmates
Clients and staff of institutions for the mentally handicapped
Residents, immigrants and refugees from areas with endemic HBV infection
International travelers at increased risk of acquiring HBV infection

[1]The risk of hepatitis B virus (HBV) infection for health care workers varies both between hospitals and within hospitals. Hepatitis B vaccination is recommended for all health care workers with blood exposure.

[2]Hemodialysis patients often respond poorly to hepatitis B vaccination; higher vaccine doses or increased number of doses are required. A special formulation of one vaccine is now available for such persons (Recombivax HB®, 40 mcg/mL). The anti-HB$_s$ (antibody to hepatitis B surface antigen) response of such persons should be tested after they are vaccinated, and those who have not responded should be revaccinated with 1-3 additional doses.

Patients with chronic renal disease should be vaccinated as early as possible, ideally before they require hemodialysis. In addition, their anti-HB$_s$ levels should be monitored at 6-12 month intervals to assess the need for revaccination.

[3]Patients with hemophilia should be immunized subcutaneously, not intramuscularly.

Pregnancy Risk Factor C

Pregnancy/Breast-Feeding Implications Reproduction studies have not been conducted. The ACIP suggests vaccination should be considered if otherwise indicated.

Contraindications Hypersensitivity to yeast, hepatitis B vaccine, or any component of the formulation

Warnings/Precautions Immediate treatment for anaphylactic/anaphylactoid reaction should be available during vaccine use; consider delaying vaccination during acute febrile illness; use caution with decreased cardiopulmonary function; unrecognized hepatitis B infection may be present, immunization may not prevent infection in these patients; patients >65 years may have lower response rates

Adverse Reactions All serious adverse reactions must be reported to the U.S. Department of Health and Human Services (DHHS) Vaccine Adverse Event Reporting System (VAERS) 1-800-822-7967.
Frequency not defined. The most common adverse effects reported with both products included injection site reactions (>10%).

Cardiovascular: Hypotension

Central nervous system: Agitation, chills, dizziness, fatigue, fever (≥37.5°C / 100°F), flushing, headache, insomnia, irritability, lightheadedness, malaise, vertigo

Dermatologic: Angioedema, petechiae, pruritus, rash, urticaria

Gastrointestinal: Abdominal pain, appetite decreased, cramps, diarrhea, dyspepsia, nausea, vomiting

Genitourinary: Dysuria

Local: Injection site reactions: Ecchymosis, erythema, induration, pain, nodule formation, soreness, swelling, tenderness, warmth

Neuromuscular & skeletal: Achiness, arthralgia, back pain, myalgia, neck pain, neck stiffness, paresthesia, shoulder pain, weakness

Otic: Earache

Respiratory: Cough, pharyngitis, rhinitis, upper respiratory tract infection

Miscellaneous: Lymphadenopathy, diaphoresis

Postmarketing and/or case reports: Alopecia, anaphylaxis, arthritis, Bell's palsy, bronchospasm, conjunctivitis, constipation, eczema, encephalitis, erythema nodosum, erythema multiforme, erythrocyte sedimentation rate increased, Guillain-Barré syndrome, herpes zoster, hypoesthesia, keratitis, liver enzyme elevation, migraine, multiple sclerosis, optic neuritis, palpitations, paresis, paresthesia, purpura, seizures, serum-sickness like syndrome (may be delayed days to weeks), Stevens-Johnson syndrome, syncope, tachycardia, thrombocytopenia, transverse myelitis, visual disturbances, vertigo

Drug Interactions
Decreased Effect: Decreased effect: Immunosuppressive agents

Stability Refrigerate at 2°C to 8°C (36°F to 46°F). Do not freeze.

Mechanism of Action Recombinant hepatitis B vaccine is a noninfectious subunit viral vaccine. The vaccine is derived from hepatitis B surface antigen (HB$_s$Ag) produced through recombinant DNA techniques from yeast cells. The portion of the hepatitis B gene which codes for HB$_s$Ag is cloned into yeast which is then cultured to produce hepatitis B vaccine.

Pharmacodynamics/Kinetics Duration of action: Following all 3 doses of hepatitis B vaccine, immunity will last ~5-7 years.

Usual Dosage I.M.:
Immunization regimen: Regimen consists of 3 doses (0, 1, and 6 months): First dose given on the elected date, second dose given 1 month later, third dose given 6 months after the first dose; see table.

Routine Immunization Regimen of Three I.M. Hepatitis B Vaccine Doses

Age	Initial		1 mo		6 mo	
	Recombivax HB® (mL)	Engerix-B® (mL)	Recombivax HB® (mL)	Engerix-B® (mL)	Recombivax HB® (mL)	Engerix-B® (mL)
Birth[1] - 19 y	0.5[2]	0.5[3]	0.5[2]	0.5[3]	0.5[2]	0.5[3]
≥20 y	1[4]	1[5]	1[4]	1[5]	1[4]	1[5]
Dialysis or immunocompromised patients[6]	1[7]	2[8]	1[7]	2[8]	1[7]	2[8]

[1]Infants born of HB$_s$ Ag **negative** mothers.
[2]5 mcg/0.5 mL pediatric/adolescent formulation
[3]10 mcg/0.5 mL formulation
[4]10 mcg/mL adult formulation
[5]20 mcg/mL formulation
[6]Revaccinate if anti-HB$_s$ <10 mIU/mL ≥1-2 months after third dose.
[7]40 mcg/mL dialysis formulation
[8]Two 1 mL doses given at different sites using the 40 mcg/2 mL dialysis formulation

Alternative dosing schedule for **Recombivax HB®:** Children 11-15 years (10 mcg/mL adult formulation): First dose of 1 mL given on the elected date, second dose given 4-6 months later

Alternative dosing schedules for **Engerix-B®:**
Children ≤10 years (10 mcg/0.5 mL formulation): High-risk children: 0.5 mL at 0, 1, 2, and 12 months; lower-risk children ages 5-10 who are candidates for an extended administration schedule may receive an alternative of 0.5 mL at 0, 12, and 24 months. If booster dose is needed, revaccinate with 0.5 mL.
Adolescents 11-19 years (20 mcg/mL formulation): 1 mL at 0, 1, and 6 months. High-risk adolescents: 1 mL at 0, 1, 2, and 12 months; lower-risk adolescents 11-16 years who are candidates for an extended administration schedule may receive an alternative regimen of 0.5 mL (using the 10 mcg/0.5 mL) formulation at 0, 12, and 24 months. If booster dose is needed, revaccinate with 20 mcg.
Adults ≥20 years: High-risk adults (20 mcg/mL formulation): 1 mL at 0, 1, 2, and 12 months. If booster dose is needed, revaccinate with 1 mL.

Postexposure prophylaxis: See table on next page.
(Continued)

Hepatitis B Vaccine *(Continued)*

Postexposure Prophylaxis
Recommended Dosage for Infants Born to
HB₅Ag-Positive Mothers

Treatment	Birth	Within 7 d	1 mo	6 mo
Engerix-B® (pediatric formulation 10 mcg/0.5 mL)[1]	Note[2]	0.5 mL[2]	0.5 mL	0.5 mL
Recombivax HB® (pediatric/adolescent formulation 5 mcg/0.5 mL)	Note[2]	0.5 mL[2]	0.5 mL	0.5 mL
Hepatitis B immune globulin	0.5 mL	—	—	—

[1]Note: An alternate regimen is administration of the vaccine at birth, within 7 days of birth, and 1, 2, and 12 months later.

[2]Note: The first dose may be given at birth at the same time as HBIG, but give in the opposite anterolateral thigh. This may better ensure vaccine absorption.

> **Administration** It is possible to interchange the vaccines for completion of a series or for booster doses; the antibody produced in response to each type of vaccine is comparable, however, the quantity of the vaccine will vary
>
> I.M. injection only; in adults, the deltoid muscle is the preferred site; the anterolateral thigh is the recommended site in infants and young children. Not for gluteal administration. Shake well prior to withdrawal and use.
>
> For patients at risk of hemorrhage following intramuscular injection, the ACIP recommends "it should be administered intramuscularly if, in the opinion of the physician familiar with the patients bleeding risk, the vaccine can be administered with reasonable safety by this route. If the patient receives antihemophilia or other similar therapy, intramuscular vaccination can be scheduled shortly after such therapy is administered. A fine needle (23 gauge or smaller) can be used for the vaccination and firm pressure applied to the site (without rubbing) for at least 2 minutes. The patient should be instructed concerning the risk of hematoma from the injection."
>
> Federal law requires that the date of administration, the vaccine manufacturer, lot number of vaccine, and the administering person's name, title, and address be entered into the patient's permanent medical record.
>
> **Patient Information** Must complete full course of injections for adequate immunization
> **Nursing Implications** Rare chance of anaphylactoid reaction; have epinephrine available
> **Additional Information** Inactivated virus vaccine. Federal law requires that the date of administration, the vaccine manufacturer, lot number of vaccine, and the administering person's name, title, and address be entered into the patient's permanent medical record.
> **Dosage Forms**
> Injection, suspension [recombinant DNA]:
>   Engerix-B®:
>   Adult: Hepatitis B surface antigen 20 mcg/mL (1 mL) [contains trace amounts of thimerosal]
>   Pediatric/adolescent: Hepatitis B surface antigen 10 mcg/0.5 mL (0.5 mL) [contains trace amounts of thimerosal]
>   Recombivax HB®:
>   Adult [with preservative]: Hepatitis B surface antigen 10 mcg/mL (1 mL, 3 mL)
>   Dialysis [with preservative]: Hepatitis B surface antigen 40 mcg/mL (1 mL)
>   Pediatric/adolescent [preservative free]: Hepatitis B surface antigen 5 mcg/0.5 mL (0.5 mL)
>   Pediatric/adolescent [with preservative]: Hepatitis B surface antigen 5 mcg/0.5 mL (0.5 mL)

- ◆ **Hep-Lock®** *see Heparin on page 657*
- ◆ **Heptovir® (Can)** *see Lamivudine on page 771*
- ◆ **Herb-Drug Interactions/Cautions** *see page 1723*
- ◆ **Herceptin®** *see Trastuzumab on page 1359*
- ◆ **HES** *see Hetastarch on page 664*
- ◆ **Hespan®** *see Hetastarch on page 664*

Hetastarch *(HET a starch)*

U.S. Brand Names Hespan®; Hextend®
Synonyms HES; Hydroxyethyl Starch
Therapeutic Category Plasma Volume Expander, Colloid
Use Blood volume expander used in treatment of shock or impending shock when blood or blood products are not available (does not have oxygen-carrying capacity and is not a substitute for blood or plasma)
Unlabeled/Investigational Use Has also been used as an adjunct in leukapheresis (Hextend® contraindicated for this use per manufacturer), as a priming fluid in pump oxygenators during cardiopulmonary bypass, and as a plasma volume expander during cardiopulmonary bypass.
Pregnancy Risk Factor C
Contraindications Severe bleeding disorders, renal failure with oliguria or anuria, or severe congestive heart failure; per the manufacturer, Hextend® is also contraindicated in the treatment of lactic acidosis and in leukapheresis
Warnings/Precautions Anaphylactoid reactions have occurred; use with caution in patients with thrombocytopenia (may interfere with platelet function); large volume may cause drops in hemoglobin concentrations; use with caution in patients at risk from overexpansion of blood volume, including the very young or aged patients, those with congestive heart failure or pulmonary edema; large volumes may interfere with platelet function and prolong PT and PTT times; use with caution in patients with history of liver disease; note electrolyte content of Hextend® including calcium, lactate, and potassium (see Additional Information); use caution

in situations where electrolyte and/or acid-base disturbances may be exacerbated (renal impairment, respiratory alkalosis). Safety and efficacy in pediatric patients have not been established.

Adverse Reactions Frequency not defined.
Cardiovascular: Circulatory overload, heart failure, peripheral edema
Central nervous system: Chills, fever, headache
Dermatologic: Itching, pruritus
Endocrine & metabolic: Increased amylase levels, parotid gland enlargement, elevated indirect bilirubin
Gastrointestinal: Vomiting
Hematologic: Bleeding, decreased factor VIII:C plasma levels, decreased plasma aggregation, decreased von Willebrand factor, dilutional coagulopathy; prolongation of PT, PTT, clotting time, and bleeding time; thrombocytopenia
Neuromuscular & skeletal: Myalgia
Miscellaneous: Anaphylactoid reactions, hypersensitivity

Overdosage/Toxicology Symptoms include heart failure, nausea, vomiting, circulatory overload, and bleeding. Treatment is supportive.

Stability Store at room temperature; do not freeze. Do not use if crystalline precipitate forms or is turbid deep brown. Change I.V. tubing or flush copiously with normal saline before adding blood.

Mechanism of Action Produces plasma volume expansion by virtue of its highly colloidal starch structure, similar to albumin

Pharmacodynamics/Kinetics
Onset of action: Volume expansion: I.V.: ~30 minutes
Duration: 24-36 hours
Metabolism: Molecules >50,000 daltons require enzymatic degradation by the reticuloendothelial system or amylases in the blood prior to urinary and fecal excretion
Excretion: Urine (~40%) within 24 hours; smaller molecular weight molecules readily excreted

Usual Dosage I.V. infusion (requires an infusion pump):
Children: Safety and efficacy have not been established
Shock:
Adults: 500-1000 mL (up to 1500 mL/day) or 20 mL/kg/day (up to 1500 mL/day); larger volumes (15,000 mL/24 hours) have been used safely in small numbers of patients
Leukapheresis: 250-700 mL hetastarch

Dosing adjustment in renal impairment: Cl_cr <10 mL/minute: Initial dose is the same but subsequent doses should be reduced by 20% to 50% of normal

Administration Administer I.V. only; infusion pump is required. May administer up to 1.2 g/kg/hour (20 mL/kg/hour). Change I.V. tubing or flush copiously with normal saline before adding blood. Anaphylactoid reactions can occur, have epinephrine and resuscitative equipment available. Do not use if crystalline precipitate forms or is turbid deep brown.

Monitoring Parameters Volume expansion: Blood pressure, heart rate, capillary refill time, CVP, RAP, MAP, urine output; if pulmonary artery catheter in place, monitor PCWP, SVR, and PVR; hemoglobin, hematocrit, cardiac index
Leukapheresis: CBC, total leukocyte and platelet counts, leukocyte differential count, hemoglobin, hematocrit, PT, PTT

Nursing Implications Anaphylactoid reactions can occur, have epinephrine and resuscitative equipment available

Additional Information Does not have oxygen-carrying capacity and is not a substitute for blood or plasma. Large volumes may interfere with platelet function and prolong PT and aPTT times. Hetastarch is a synthetic polymer derived from a waxy starch composed of amylopectin. Average molecular weight = 450,000; each 500 mL provides 77 mEq sodium chloride; each liter of Hextend® contains the following amounts of electrolytes: Sodium 143 mEq, chloride 124 mEq, lactate 28 mEq, calcium 5 mEq, magnesium 0.9 mEq, and potassium 0.3 mEq.

Dosage Forms
Infusion, in lactated electrolyte injection (Hextend®): 6% (500 mL, 1000 mL)
Infusion, in sodium chloride 0.9% (Hespan®): 6% (500 mL)

♦ **Hexachlorocyclohexane** *see* Lindane *on page 806*

Hexachlorophene (heks a KLOR oh feen)
U.S. Brand Names pHisoHex®
Canadian Brand Names pHisoHex®
Therapeutic Category Antibacterial, Topical; Soap
Use Surgical scrub and as a bacteriostatic skin cleanser; control an outbreak of gram-positive infection when other procedures have been unsuccessful
Pregnancy Risk Factor C
Usual Dosage Children and Adults: Topical: Apply 5 mL cleanser and water to area to be cleansed; lather and rinse thoroughly under running water
Additional Information Complete prescribing information for this medication should be consulted for additional detail.
Dosage Forms Liquid, topical (pHisoHex®): 3% (8 mL, 150 mL, 500 mL, 3840 mL)

♦ **Hexadrol®** *see* Dexamethasone *on page 380*
♦ **Hexadrol® Phosphate** *see* Dexamethasone *on page 380*
♦ **Hexalen®** *see* Altretamine *on page 62*
♦ **Hexamethylenetetramine** *see* Methenamine *on page 881*
♦ **Hexamethylmelamine** *see* Altretamine *on page 62*
♦ **Hexavitamin** *see* Vitamins (Multiple) *on page 1424*
♦ **Hexit™ (Can)** *see* Lindane *on page 806*
♦ **HEXM** *see* Altretamine *on page 62*
♦ **Hextend®** *see* Hetastarch *on page 664*

- **Hib** *see Haemophilus b Conjugate and Hepatitis B Vaccine on page 650*
- **Hiclens® [OTC]** *see Chlorhexidine Gluconate on page 275*
- **Hibistat® [OTC]** *see Chlorhexidine Gluconate on page 275*
- **Hib Polysaccharide Conjugate** *see Haemophilus b Conjugate Vaccine on page 651*
- **HibTITER®** *see Haemophilus b Conjugate Vaccine on page 651*
- **Hi-Cor® 1.0** *see Hydrocortisone on page 682*
- **Hi-Cor® 2.5** *see Hydrocortisone on page 682*
- **Hiprex®** *see Methenamine on page 881*
- **Hirulog** *see Bivalirudin on page 174*
- **Histafed® [OTC]** *see Triprolidine and Pseudoephedrine on page 1380*
- **Histalet® [OTC]** *see Chlorpheniramine and Pseudoephedrine on page 279*
- **Histalet® X** *see Guaifenesin and Pseudoephedrine on page 647*
- **Histatab® Plus [OTC]** *see Chlorpheniramine and Phenylephrine on page 279*
- **Hista-Tabs® [OTC]** *see Triprolidine and Pseudoephedrine on page 1380*
- **Histor-D®** *see Chlorpheniramine and Phenylephrine on page 279*

Histrelin (his TREL in)

U.S. Brand Names Supprelin™

Therapeutic Category Gonadotropin Releasing Hormone Analog; Luteinizing Hormone-Releasing Hormone Analog

Use Treatment of estrogen-associated gynecological disorders (eg, acute intermittent porphyria, endometriosis, leiomyomata uteri, premenstrual syndrome)

Orphan drug: Treatment of central precocious puberty

Pregnancy Risk Factor X

Usual Dosage

Central idiopathic precocious puberty: S.C.: Usual dose is 10 mcg/kg/day given as a single daily dose at the same time each day

Acute intermittent porphyria in women: S.C.: 5 mcg/day

Endometriosis: S.C.: 100 mcg/day

Leiomyomata uteri: S.C.: 20-50 mcg/day or 4 mcg/kg/day

Additional Information Complete prescribing information for this medication should be consulted for additional detail.

Dosage Forms Injection [single-use 7-day kit]: 120 mcg/0.6 mL; 300 mcg/0.6 mL; 600 mcg/0.6 mL

- **Histrodrix®** *see Dexbrompheniramine and Pseudoephedrine on page 383*
- **Histussin D® Liquid** *see Hydrocodone and Pseudoephedrine on page 681*
- **Hivid®** *see Zalcitabine on page 1431*
- **HMM** *see Altretamine on page 62*
- **HMS Liquifilm®** *see Medrysone on page 850*
- **HN₂** *see Mechlorethamine on page 845*

Homatropine (hoe MA troe peen)

Related Information

Cycloplegic Mydriatics Comparison *on page 1498*

U.S. Brand Names Isopto® Homatropine

Synonyms Homatropine Hydrobromide

Therapeutic Category Anticholinergic Agent, Ophthalmic; Ophthalmic Agent, Mydriatic

Use Producing cycloplegia and mydriasis for refraction; treatment of acute inflammatory conditions of the uveal tract

Pregnancy Risk Factor C

Contraindications Hypersensitivity to the drug or any component of the formulation; narrow-angle glaucoma, acute hemorrhage

Warnings/Precautions Use with caution in patients with hypertension, cardiac disease, or increased intraocular pressure; safety and efficacy not established in infants and young children, therefore, use with extreme caution due to susceptibility of systemic effects; use with caution in obstructive uropathy, paralytic ileus, ulcerative colitis, unstable cardiovascular status in acute hemorrhage

Adverse Reactions

>10%: Ocular: Blurred vision, photophobia

1% to 10%:

Local: Irritation

Ocular: Increased intraocular pressure

Respiratory: Congestion

<1% (Limited to important or life-threatening): Eczematoid dermatitis, edema, exudate, follicular conjunctivitis, somnolence, vascular congestion

Overdosage/Toxicology Symptoms include blurred vision, urinary retention, and tachycardia. Anticholinergic toxicity is caused by strong binding of the drug to cholinergic receptors. For anticholinergic overdose with severe life-threatening symptoms, physostigmine 1-2 mg (0.5 mg or 0.02 mg/kg for children) S.C. or slow I.V. may be given to reverse these effects.

Stability Protect from light

Mechanism of Action Blocks response of iris sphincter muscle and the accommodative muscle of the ciliary body to cholinergic stimulation resulting in dilation and loss of accommodation

Pharmacodynamics/Kinetics

Onset of action: Accommodation and pupil effect: Ophthalmic:

Maximum mydriatic effect: Within 10-30 minutes

Maximum cycloplegic effect: Within 30-90 minutes

Duration:

Mydriasis: 6 hours to 4 days

Cycloplegia: 10-48 hours

Usual Dosage

Children:

Mydriasis and cycloplegia for refraction: Instill 1 drop of 2% solution immediately before the procedure; repeat at 10-minute intervals as needed

Uveitis: Instill 1 drop of 2% solution 2-3 times/day

Adults:

Mydriasis and cycloplegia for refraction: Instill 1-2 drops of 2% solution or 1 drop of 5% solution before the procedure; repeat at 5- to 10-minute intervals as needed; maximum of 3 doses for refraction

Uveitis: Instill 1-2 drops of 2% or 5% 2-3 times/day up to every 3-4 hours as needed

Administration Ophthalmic instillation: Finger pressure should be applied to lacrimal sac for 1-2 minutes after instillation to decrease risk of absorption and systemic reactions

Dosage Forms

Solution, ophthalmic, as hydrobromide: 2% (1 mL, 5 mL); 5% (1 mL, 2 mL, 5 mL)

Isopto® Homatropine: 2% (5 mL, 15 mL); 5% (5 mL, 15 mL)

- ◆ **Homatropine and Hydrocodone** *see* Hydrocodone and Homatropine *on page 679*
- ◆ **Homatropine Hydrobromide** *see* Homatropine *on page 666*
- ◆ **Honvol® (Can)** *see* Diethylstilbestrol *on page 400*
- ◆ **Horse Antihuman Thymocyte Gamma Globulin** *see* Lymphocyte Immune Globulin *on page 829*
- ◆ **Hp-PAC® (Can)** *see* Lansoprazole, Amoxicillin, and Clarithromycin *on page 776*
- ◆ **Humalog®** *see* Insulin Preparations *on page 722*
- ◆ **Humalog® Mix25™ (Can)** *see* Insulin Preparations *on page 722*
- ◆ **Humalog® Mix 75/25™** *see* Insulin Preparations *on page 722*
- ◆ **Human Diploid Cell Cultures Rabies Vaccine** *see* Rabies Virus Vaccine *on page 1175*

Human Growth Hormone (HYU man grothe HOR mone)

U.S. Brand Names Genotropin®; Genotropin Miniquick®; Humatrope®; Norditropin®; Norditropin® Cartridges; Nutropin®; Nutropin AQ®; Nutropin Depot®; Protropin®; Saizen®; Serostim®

Canadian Brand Names Humatrope®; Nutropin® AQ; Nutropine®; Protropine®; Saizen®; Serostim®

Synonyms Growth Hormone; Somatrem; Somatropin

Therapeutic Category Growth Hormone

Use

Children:

Long-term treatment of growth failure due to lack of adequate endogenous growth hormone secretion (Genotropin®, Humatrope®, Norditropin®, Nutropin®, Nutropin AQ®, Nutropin® Depot™, Protropin®, Saizen®)

Long-term treatment of short stature associated with Turner syndrome (Humatrope®, Nutropin®, Nutropin AQ®)

Treatment of Prader-Willi syndrome (Genotropin®)

Treatment of growth failure associated with chronic renal insufficiency (CRI) up until the time of renal transplantation (Nutropin®, Nutropin AQ®)

Long-term treatment of growth failure in children born small for gestational age who fail to manifest catch-up growth by 2 years of age (Genotropin®)

Adults:

AIDS wasting or cachexia with concomitant antiviral therapy (Serostim®)

Replacement of endogenous growth hormone in patients with adult growth hormone deficiency who meet both of the following criteria (Genotropin®, Humatrope®, Nutropin®, Nutropin AQ®):

Biochemical diagnosis of adult growth hormone deficiency by means of a subnormal response to a standard growth hormone stimulation test (peak growth hormone ≤5 µg/L)

and

Adult-onset: Patients who have adult growth hormone deficiency whether alone or with multiple hormone deficiencies (hypopituitarism) as a result of pituitary disease, hypothalamic disease, surgery, radiation therapy, or trauma

or

Childhood-onset: Patients who were growth hormone deficient during childhood, confirmed as an adult before replacement therapy is initiated

Unlabeled/Investigational Use Investigational: Congestive heart failure

Pregnancy Risk Factor B/C (depending upon manufacturer)

Contraindications Hypersensitivity to growth hormone or any component of the formulation; growth promotion in pediatric patients with closed epiphyses; progression of any underlying intracranial lesion or actively growing intracranial tumor; acute critical illness due to complications following open heart or abdominal surgery; multiple accidental trauma or acute respiratory failure; evidence of active malignancy

Warnings/Precautions Use with caution in patients with diabetes or with risk factors for glucose intolerance; when administering to newborns, reconstitute with sterile water for injection; intracranial hypertension has been reported with growth hormone product, funduscopic examinations are recommended; progression of scoliosis may occur in children experiencing rapid growth; patients with growth hormone deficiency may develop slipped capital epiphyses more frequently, evaluate any child with new onset of a limp or with complaints of hip or knee pain; patients with Turner syndrome are at increased risk for otitis media and other ear/hearing disorders, cardiovascular disorders (including stroke, aortic aneurysm, hypertension), and thyroid disease, monitor carefully; products may contain benzyl alcohol, m-Cresol or glycerin, some products may be manufactured by recombinant DNA technology using *E. coli* as a precursor, consult specific product labeling. Not for I.V. injection.

(Continued)

Human Growth Hormone (Continued)

Adverse Reactions

Growth hormone deficiency: Antigrowth hormone antibodies, carpal tunnel syndrome (rare), fluid balance disturbances, glucosuria, gynocomastia (rare), headache, hematuria, hyperglycemia (mild), hypoglycemia, hypothyroidism, leukemia, lipoatrophy, muscle pain, increased growth of pre-existing nevi (rare), pain/ local reactions at the injection site, pancreatitis (rare), peripheral edema, exacerbation of psoriasis, seizures

Prader-Willi syndrome: Aggressiveness, arthralgia, edema, hair loss, headache, benign intracranial hypertension, myalgia

Turner syndrome: Humatrope®: Surgical procedures (45%), otitis media (43%), ear disorders (18%), hypothyroidism (13%), increased nevi (11%), peripheral edema (7%)

Adult growth hormone replacement: Increased ALT, increased AST, arthralgia, back pain, carpal tunnel syndrome, diabetes mellitus, fatigue, flu-like syndrome, generalized edema, gastritis, gynocomastia (rare), headache, hypoesthesia, joint disorder, myalgia, increased growth of pre-existing nevi, pain, pancreatitis (rare), paresthesia, peripheral edema, pharyngitis, rhinitis, stiffness in extremities, weakness

AIDS wasting or cachexia (limited): Serostim®: Musculoskeletal discomfort (54%), increased tissue turgor (27%), diarrhea (26%), neuropathy (26%), nausea (26%), fatigue (17%), albuminuria (15%), increased diaphoresis (14%), anorexia (12%), anemia (12%), increased AST (12%), insomnia (11%), tachycardia (11%), hyperglycemia (10%), increased ALT (10%)

Postmarketing and/or case reports: Diabetes, diabetic ketoacidosis, glucose intolerance

Small for gestational age: Mild, transient hyperglycemia; benign intracranial hypertension (rare); central precocious puberty; jaw prominence (rare); aggravation of pre-existing scoliosis (rare); injection site reactions; progression of pigmented nevi

Overdosage/Toxicology Symptoms of acute overdose may include initial hypoglycemia, hyperglycemia, fluid retention, headache, nausea, and vomiting. Long-term overdose may result in signs and symptoms of acromegaly.

Drug Interactions

Cytochrome P450 Effect: Limited data suggest somatropin may increase clearance of medications metabolized via CYP2B6, 2C, and 3A3/4.

Decreased Effect: Glucocorticoid therapy may inhibit growth-promoting effects. Growth hormone may induce insulin resistance in patients with diabetes mellitus; monitor glucose and adjust insulin dose as necessary.

Stability

Somatrem: Protropin®: Before and after reconstitution, store at 2°C to 8°C (36°F to 46°F), avoid freezing; when reconstituted with bacteriostatic water for injection; use within 14 days; when reconstituted with sterile water for injection, use immediately (only one dose per vial) and discard unused portion

Somatropin:

Genotropin®: Store at 2°C to 8°C (36°F to 46°F), do not freeze, protect from light

  1.5 mg cartridge: Following reconstitution, store under refrigeration and use within 24 hours; discard unused portion

  5.8 mg and 13.8 mg cartridge: Following reconstitution, store under refrigeration and use within 21 days

Miniquick®: Store in refrigerator prior to dispensing, but may be stored ≤25°C (77°F) for up to 3 months after dispensing; once reconstituted, solution must be refrigerated and used within 24 hours; discard unused portion

Humatrope®:

  Vial: Before and after reconstitution, store at 2°C to 8°C (36°F to 46°F), avoid freezing; when reconstituted with bacteriostatic water for injection, use within 14 days; when reconstituted with sterile water for injection, use within 24 hours and discard unused portion

  Cartridge: Before and after reconstitution, store at 2°C to 8°C (36°F to 46°F), avoid freezing; following reconstitution, stable for 14 days under refrigeration. Dilute with solution provided with cartridges **ONLY**; do not use diluent provided with vials

Norditropin®: Store at 2°C to 8°C (36°F to 46°F), do not freeze; avoid direct light

  Cartridge: Must be used within 4 weeks once inserted into pen

  Powder for injection: Must be used within 14 days of reconstitution

Nutropin®: Before and after reconstitution, store at 2°C to 8°C (36°F to 46°F), avoid freezing

  Vial: Reconstitute with bacteriostatic water for injection; use reconstituted vials within 14 days; when reconstituted with sterile water for injection, use immediately and discard unused portion

  AQ formulation: Use within 28 days following initial use

  Depot™: Before suspension, store at 2°C to 8°C (36°F to 46°F), avoid freezing; use suspended solution immediately; dilute only with diluent provided

Saizen®: Prior to reconstitution, store at room temperature 15°C to 30°C (59°F to 86°F); following reconstitution with bacteriostatic water for injection, reconstituted solution should be refrigerated and used within 14 days; when reconstituted with sterile water for injection, use immediately and discard unused portion

Serostim®: Prior to reconstitution, store at room temperature 15°C to 30°C (59°F to 86°F); reconstitute with sterile water for injection; store reconstituted solution under refrigeration and use within 24 hours, avoid freezing. Do not use if cloudy

Mechanism of Action Somatropin and somatrem are purified polypeptide hormones of recombinant DNA origin; somatropin contains the identical sequence of amino acids found in human growth hormone while somatrem's amino acid sequence is identical plus an additional amino acid, methionine; human growth hormone stimulates growth of linear bone, skeletal muscle, and organs; stimulates erythropoietin which increases red blood cell mass; exerts both insulin-like and diabetogenic effects

Pharmacodynamics/Kinetics Somatrem and somatropin have equivalent pharmacokinetic properties

Duration: Maintains supraphysiologic levels for 18-20 hours

Absorption: I.M., S.C.: Well absorbed

Metabolism: ~90% hepatic and renal

Half-life elimination: Dependent upon preparation and route of administration

Excretion: Urine

Usual Dosage

Children (individualize dose):

Growth hormone deficiency:

Somatrem: Protropin®: I.M., S.C.: Weekly dosage: 0.3 mg/kg divided into daily doses

Somatropin:

Genotropin®: S.C.: Weekly dosage: 0.16-0.24 mg/kg divided into 6-7 doses

Humatrope®: I.M., S.C.: Weekly dosage: 0.18 mg/kg; maximum replacement dose: 0.3 mg/kg/week; dosing should be divided into equal doses given 3 times/week on alternating days, 6 times/week, or daily

Norditropin®: S.C.: Weekly dosage: 0.024-0.034 mg/kg administered in the evening, divided into doses 6-7 times/week; cartridge and vial formulations are bioequivalent; cartridge formulation does not need to be reconstituted prior to use; cartridges must be administered using the corresponding color-coded NordiPen® injection pen

Nutropin® Depot™: S.C.:

Once-monthly injection: 1.5 mg/kg administered on the same day of each month; patients >15 kg will require more than 1 injection per dose

Twice-monthly injection: 0.75 mg/kg administered twice each month on the same days of each month (eg, days 1 and 15 of each month); patients >30 kg will require more than 1 injection per dose

Nutropin®, Nutropin® AQ: S.C.: Weekly dosage: 0.3 mg/kg divided into daily doses; pubertal patients: ≤0.7 mg/kg/week divided daily

Saizen®: I.M., S.C.: Weekly dosage: 0.06 mg/kg administered 3 times/week

Note: Therapy should be discontinued when patient has reached satisfactory adult height, when epiphyses have fused, or when the patient ceases to respond. Growth of 5 cm/year or more is expected, if growth rate does not exceed 2.5 cm in a 6-month period, double the dose for the next 6 months; if there is still no satisfactory response, discontinue therapy

Chronic renal insufficiency (CRI): Nutropin®, Nutropin® AQ: S.C.: Weekly dosage: 0.35 mg/kg divided into daily injections; continue until the time of renal transplantation

Dosage recommendations in patients treated for CRI who require dialysis:

Hemodialysis: Administer dose at night prior to bedtime or at least 3-4 hours after hemodialysis to prevent hematoma formation from heparin

CCPD: Administer dose in the morning following dialysis

CAPD: Administer dose in the evening at the time of overnight exchange

Turner syndrome: Humatrope®, Nutropin®, Nutropin® AQ: S.C.: Weekly dosage: ≤0.375 mg/kg divided into equal doses 3-7 times per week

Prader-Willi syndrome: Genotropin®: S.C.: Weekly dosage: 0.24 mg/kg divided in 6-7 doses

Small for gestational age: Genotropin®: S.C.: Weekly dosage: 0.48 mg/kg divided in 6-7 doses

Adults:

Growth hormone deficiency: To minimize adverse events in older or overweight patients, reduced dosages may be necessary. During therapy, dosage should be decreased if required by the occurrence of side effects or excessive IGF-I levels.

Somatropin:

Nutropin®, Nutropin® AQ: S.C.: ≤0.006 mg/kg/day; dose may be increased according to individual requirements, up to a maximum of 0.025 mg/kg/day in patients <35 years of age, or up to a maximum of 0.0125 mg/kg/day in patients ≥35 years of age

Humatrope®: S.C.: ≤0.006 mg/kg/day; dose may be increased according to individual requirements, up to a maximum of 0.0125 mg/kg/day

Genotropin®: S.C.: Weekly dosage: ≤0.04 mg/kg divided in 6-7 doses; dose may be increased at 4- to 8-week intervals according to individual requirements, to a maximum of 0.08 mg/kg/week

AIDS wasting or cachexia:

Serostim®: S.C.: Dose should be given once daily at bedtime; patients who continue to lose weight after 2 weeks should be re-evaluated for opportunistic infections or other clinical events; rotate injection sites to avoid lipodystrophy

Daily dose based on body weight:

<35 kg: 0.1 mg/kg

35-45 kg: 4 mg

45-55 kg: 5 mg

>55 kg: 6 mg

Dosage adjustment in renal impairment Reports indicate patients with chronic renal failure tend to have decreased clearance; specific dosing suggestions not available

Dosage adjustment in hepatic impairment: Clearance may be reduced in patients with severe hepatic dysfunction; specific dosing suggestions not available

Elderly: Patients ≥65 years of age may be more sensitive to the action of growth hormone and more prone to adverse effects; in general, dosing should be cautious, beginning at low end of dosing range

Administration Do not shake; administer S.C. or I.M.; refer to product labeling; when administering to newborns, reconstitute with sterile water for injection

Monitoring Parameters Growth curve, periodic thyroid function tests, bone age (annually), periodical urine testing for glucose, somatomedin C (IGF-I) levels; funduscopic examinations at initiation of therapy and periodically during treatment; serum phosphorus, alkaline phosphatase and parathyroid hormone. If growth deceleration is observed in children treated for growth hormone deficiency, and not due to other causes, evaluate for presence of antibody formation. Strict blood glucose monitoring in diabetic patients.

Somatrem (Protropin®): Consider changing to somatropin if antibody binding capacity is >2 mg/L

(Continued)

669

Human Growth Hormone *(Continued)*

Patient Information This medication can only be given by injection. You will be instructed how to prepare and administer the medication. Use a small enough syringe so that the prescribed dose can be drawn from the vial with reasonable accuracy; for I.M. injections, use a needle of sufficient length (≥1") to ensure that the injection reaches the muscle layer. Rotate injection sites. Dispose of needles and syringes properly. Follow storage instructions. Report the development of a severe headache, acute visual changes, a limp, or complaints of hip or knee pain to your prescriber. Contact prescriber if you become pregnant or are breast-feeding.

Nursing Implications Watch for glucose intolerance; instructions should be given to patients/caregivers who will be administering at home; ensure puncture-resistant container is provided for needle disposal

Dosage Forms
Powder for injection, lyophilized [rDNA origin]:
Somatrem: Protropin® [diluent contains benzyl alcohol]: 5 mg [~15 int. units]; 10 mg [~30 int. units]
Somatropin:
Genotropin® [preservative free]: 1.5 mg [4 int. units/mL] [delivers 1.3 mg/mL]
Genotropin® [with preservative]:
5.8 mg [15 int. units/mL] [delivers 5 mg/mL]
13.8 mg [36 int. units/mL] [delivers 12 mg/mL]
Genotropin Miniquick® [preservative free]: 0.2 mg, 0.4 mg, 0.6 mg, 0.8 mg, 1 mg, 1.2 mg, 1.4 mg, 1.6 mg, 1.8 mg, 2 mg [each strength delivers 0.25 mL]
Humatrope®: 5 mg [~15 int. units], 6 mg [18 int. units], 12 mg [36 int. units], 24 mg [72 int. units]
Norditropin® [diluent contains benzyl alcohol]: 4 mg [~12 int. units]; 8 mg [~24 int. units]
Nutropin® [diluent contains benzyl alcohol]: 5 mg [~15 int. units]; 10 mg [~30 int. units]
Nutropin Depot ® [preservative free]: 13.5 mg; 18 mg; 22.5 mg
Saizen® [diluent contains benzyl alcohol]: 5 mg [~15 int. units]
Serostim®: 4 mg [12 int. units]; 5 mg [15 int. units]; 6 mg [18 int. units]
Solution, for injection [rDNA origin]:
Somatropin:
Norditropin® Cartridges: 5 mg/1.5 mL (1.5 mL); 10 mg/1.5 mL (1.5 mL); 15 mg/1.5 mL (1.5 mL)
Nutropin AQ®: 5 mg/mL [~30 int. units/2 mL] (2 mL)

- **Humanized IgG1 Anti-CD52 Monoclonal Antibody** *see Alemtuzumab on page 46*
- **Human Thyroid Stimulating Hormone** *see Thyrotropin Alpha on page 1327*
- **Humate-P**® *see Antihemophilic Factor (Human) on page 102*
- **Humatin**® *see Paromomycin on page 1040*
- **Humatrope**® *see Human Growth Hormone on page 667*
- **Humegon**™ *see Menotropins on page 857*
- **Humibid**® **DM [OTC]** *see Guaifenesin and Dextromethorphan on page 646*
- **Humibid**® **L.A.** *see Guaifenesin on page 645*
- **Humibid**® **Sprinkle** *see Guaifenesin on page 645*
- **Humorsol**® *see Demecarium on page 373*
- **Humulin**® *see Insulin Preparations on page 722*
- **Humulin**® **50/50** *see Insulin Preparations on page 722*
- **Humulin**® **70/30** *see Insulin Preparations on page 722*
- **Humulin**® **L** *see Insulin Preparations on page 722*
- **Humulin**® **N** *see Insulin Preparations on page 722*
- **Humulin**® **R** *see Insulin Preparations on page 722*
- **Humulin**® **R (Concentrated) U-500** *see Insulin Preparations on page 722*
- **Hurricaine**® *see Benzocaine on page 154*
- **HXM** *see Altretamine on page 62*
- **Hyalgan**® *see Sodium Hyaluronate on page 1247*
- **Hyaluronic Acid** *see Sodium Hyaluronate on page 1247*

Hyaluronidase *(hye al yoor ON i dase)*

U.S. Brand Names Wydase®

Canadian Brand Names Wydase®

Therapeutic Category Antidote, Extravasation

Use Increases the dispersion and absorption of other drugs; increases rate of absorption of parenteral fluids given by hypodermoclysis; enhances diffusion of locally irritating or toxic drugs in the management of I.V. extravasation

Pregnancy Risk Factor C

Contraindications Hypersensitivity to hyaluronidase or any component of the formulation; do not inject in or around infected, inflamed, or cancerous areas

Warnings/Precautions Drug infiltrates in which hyaluronidase is contraindicated: Dopamine, alpha-adrenergic agonists; an intradermal skin test for sensitivity should be performed before actual administration using 0.02 mL of a 150 units/mL of hyaluronidase solution. Avoid overhydration in pediatric patients by controlling the rate and total volume.

Adverse Reactions Urticaria (rare), anaphylactic-like reactions (rare)
Case report: Cardiac fibrillation

Overdosage/Toxicology Symptoms include local edema, urticaria, erythema, chills, nausea, vomiting, and hypotension.

Drug Interactions
Decreased Effect: Salicylates, cortisone, ACTH, estrogens, antihistamines

Stability Reconstituted hyaluronidase solution remains stable for only 24 hours when stored in the refrigerator; do not use discolored solutions

Mechanism of Action Modifies the permeability of connective tissue through hydrolysis of hyaluronic acid, one of the chief ingredients of tissue cement which offers resistance to diffusion of liquids through tissues

Pharmacodynamics/Kinetics
Onset of action: S.C., I.D.: Immediate for treatment of extravasation
Duration: 24-48 hours

Usual Dosage
Infants and Children: Management of I.V. extravasation: S.C., intradermal: Reconstitute the 150 unit vial of lyophilized powder with 1 mL NS; take 0.1 mL of this solution and dilute with 0.9 mL NS to yield 15 units/mL; using a 25- or 26-gauge needle, five 0.2 mL injections are made subcutaneously or intradermally into the extravasation site at the leading edge, changing the needle after each injection; **Note:** Some sites utilize a 150 units/mL hyaluronidase solution and, without further dilution, administer 0.2 mL injections subcutaneously or intradermally into the extravasation site at the leading edge

Hypodermoclysis: S.C.: 15 units is added to each 100 mL of I.V. fluid to be administered
Premature Infants and Neonates: Volume of a single clysis should not exceed 25 mL/kg and the rate of administration should not exceed 2 mL/minute
Children <3 years: Volume of a single clysis should not exceed 200 mL
Children ≥3 years and Adults: Rate and volume of administration should not exceed those used for I.V. infusion

Adults:
Management of I.V. extravasation: Reconstitute the 150 unit vial of lyophilized powder with 1 mL normal saline; take 0.1 mL of this solution and dilute with 0.9 mL normal saline to yield 15 units/mL; using a 25- or 26-gauge needle, five 0.2 mL injections are made subcutaneously or intradermally into the extravasation site at the leading edge, changing the needle after each injection; **Note:** Some sites utilize a 150 units/mL hyaluronidase solution and, without further dilution, administer 0.2 mL injections subcutaneously or intradermally into the extravasation site at the leading edge
Absorption and dispersion of drugs: 150 units are added to the vehicle containing the drug
Hypodermoclysis: Refer to pediatric dosing

Administration Administer hyaluronidase within the first few minutes to 1 hour after the extravasation of a necrotizing agent is recognized; do not administer I.V.

Nursing Implications Appropriate drugs for the management of an acute hypersensitivity (epinephrine, corticosteroids, and antihistamines) should be readily available

Additional Information The USP hyaluronidase unit is equivalent to the turbidity-reducing (TR) unit and the International Unit. Each unit is defined as being the activity contained in 100 mcg of the International Standard Preparation.

Dosage Forms
Injection, stabilized solution: 150 units/mL (1 mL, 10 mL)
Powder for injection, lyophilized: 150 units, 1500 units

HydrALAZINE (hye DRAL a zeen)

Related Information
Depression on page 1655
Heart Failure on page 1663
Hypertension on page 1675

U.S. Brand Names Apresoline® [DSC]
Canadian Brand Names Apo®-Hydralazine; Apresoline®; Novo-Hylazin; Nu-Hydral
Synonyms Hydralazine Hydrochloride
Therapeutic Category Antihypertensive Agent; Vasodilator
Use Management of moderate to severe hypertension, congestive heart failure, hypertension secondary to pre-eclampsia/eclampsia; treatment of primary pulmonary hypertension
Pregnancy Risk Factor C
Pregnancy/Breast-Feeding Implications
Clinical effects on the fetus: Crosses the placenta. One report of fetal arrhythmia; transient neonatal thrombocytopenia and fetal distress reported following late 3rd trimester use. A large amount of clinical experience with the use of this drug for management of hypertension during pregnancy is available. Available evidence suggests safe use during pregnancy and breast-feeding.
Breast-feeding/lactation: Crosses into breast milk in extremely small amounts. AAP considers **compatible** with breast-feeding.
Contraindications Hypersensitivity to hydralazine or any component of the formulation; mitral valve rheumatic heart disease
Warnings/Precautions May cause a drug-induced lupus-like syndrome (more likely on larger doses, longer duration). Discontinue hydralazine in patients who develop SLE-like syndrome or positive ANA. Use with caution in patients with severe renal disease or cerebral vascular accidents or with known or suspected coronary artery disease; monitor blood pressure
(Continued)

HydrALAZINE *(Continued)*

closely with I.V. use; some formulations may contain tartrazines or sulfites. Slow acetylators, patients with decreased renal function, and patients receiving >200 mg/day (chronically) are at higher risk for SLE. Titrate dosage to patient's response. Usually administered with diuretic and a beta-blocker to counteract side effects of sodium and water retention and reflex tachycardia.

Adjust dose in severe renal dysfunction. Use with caution in CAD (increase in tachycardia may increase myocardial oxygen demand). Use with caution in pulmonary hypertension (may cause hypotension). Patients may be poorly compliant because of frequent dosing. Hydralazine-induced fluid and sodium retention may require addition or increased dosage of a diuretics.

Adverse Reactions Frequency not defined.

Cardiovascular: Tachycardia, angina pectoris, orthostatic hypotension (rare), dizziness (rare), paradoxical hypertension, peripheral edema, vascular collapse (rare), flushing

Central nervous system: Increased intracranial pressure (I.V., in patient with pre-existing increased intracranial pressure), fever (rare), chills (rare), anxiety*, disorientation*, depression*, coma*

Dermatologic: Rash (rare), urticaria (rash), pruritus (rash)

Gastrointestinal: Anorexia, nausea, vomiting, diarrhea, constipation, adynamic ileus

Genitourinary: Difficulty in micturition, impotence

Hematologic: Hemolytic anemia (rare), eosinophilia (rare), decreased hemoglobin concentration (rare), reduced erythrocyte count (rare), leukopenia (rare), agranulocytosis (rare), thrombocytopenia (rare)

Neuromuscular & skeletal: Rheumatoid arthritis, muscle cramps, weakness, tremors, peripheral neuritis (rare)

Ocular: Lacrimation, conjunctivitis

Respiratory: Nasal congestion, dyspnea

Miscellaneous: Drug-induced lupus-like syndrome (dose-related; fever, arthralgia, splenomegaly, lymphadenopathy, asthenia, myalgia, malaise, pleuritic chest pain, edema, positive ANA, positive LE cells, maculopapular facial rash, positive direct Coombs' test, pericarditis, pericardial tamponade), diaphoresis

*Seen in uremic patients and severe hypertension where rapidly escalating doses may have caused hypotension leading to these effects.

Overdosage/Toxicology Symptoms include hypotension, tachycardia, and shock. Hypotension usually responds to I.V. fluids, Trendelenburg positioning, or vasoconstrictors. Treatment is primarily supportive and symptomatic.

Drug Interactions

Increased Effect/Toxicity: Hydralazine may increase levels of beta-blockers (metoprolol, propranolol). Some beta-blockers (acebutolol, atenolol, and nadolol) are unlikely to be affected due to limited hepatic metabolism. Concurrent use of hydralazine with MAO inhibitors may cause a significant decrease in blood pressure. Propranolol may increase hydralazine serum concentrations.

Decreased Effect: NSAIDs (eg, indomethacin) may decrease the hemodynamic effects of hydralazine.

Ethanol/Nutrition/Herb Interactions

Ethanol: Avoid ethanol (may increase CNS depression).

Food: Food enhances bioavailability of hydralazine.

Herb/Nutraceutical: Avoid dong quai if using for hypertension (has estrogenic activity). Avoid ephedra, yohimbe, ginseng (may worsen hypertension). Avoid garlic (may have increased antihypertensive effect).

Stability Intact ampuls/vials of hydralazine should not be stored under refrigeration because of possible precipitation or crystallization. Hydralazine should be diluted in NS for IVPB administration due to decreased stability in D_5W. Stability of IVPB solution in NS is 4 days at room temperature.

Mechanism of Action Direct vasodilation of arterioles (with little effect on veins) with decreased systemic resistance

Pharmacodynamics/Kinetics

Onset of action: Oral: 20-30 minutes; I.V.: 5-20 minutes

Duration: Oral: 2-4 hours; I.V.: 2-6 hours

Distribution: Crosses placenta; enters breast milk

Metabolism: Hepatically acetylated; extensive first-pass effect (oral)

Protein binding: 85% to 90%

Bioavailability: 30% to 50%; enhanced by concurrent administration with food

Half-life elimination: Normal renal function: 2-8 hours; End-stage renal disease: 7-16 hours

Excretion: Urine (14% as unchanged drug)

Usual Dosage

Children:

Oral: Initial: 0.75-1 mg/kg/day in 2-4 divided doses; increase over 3-4 weeks to maximum of 7.5 mg/kg/day in 2-4 divided doses; maximum daily dose: 200 mg/day

I.M., I.V.: 0.1-0.2 mg/kg/dose (not to exceed 20 mg) every 4-6 hours as needed, up to 1.7-3.5 mg/kg/day in 4-6 divided doses

Adults:

Oral: Hypertension:

Initial dose: 10 mg 4 times/day for first 2-4 days; increase to 25 mg 4 times/day for the balance of the first week

Increase by 10-25 mg/dose gradually to 50 mg 4 times/day; 300 mg/day may be required for some patients

Oral: Congestive heart failure:

Initial dose: 10-25 mg 3-4 times/day

Adjustment: Dosage must be adjusted based on individual response

Target dose: 75 mg 4 times/day in combination with isosorbide dinitrate (40 mg 4 times/day)

Range: Typically 200-600 mg daily in 2-4 divided doses; dosages as high as 3 g/day have been used in some patients for symptomatic and hemodynamic improvement. Hydralazine 75 mg 4 times/day combined with isosorbide dinitrate 40 mg 4 times/day were shown in clinical trials to provide a mortality benefit in the treatment of CHF. Higher doses may be used for symptomatic and hemodynamic improvement following optimization of standard therapy.

I.M., I.V.:

Hypertension: Initial: 10-20 mg/dose every 4-6 hours as needed, may increase to 40 mg/dose; change to oral therapy as soon as possible.

Pre-eclampsia/eclampsia: 5 mg/dose then 5-10 mg every 20-30 minutes as needed.

Elderly: Oral: Initial: 10 mg 2-3 times/day; increase by 10-25 mg/day every 2-5 days.

Dosing interval in renal impairment:

Cl_{cr} 10-50 mL/minute: Administer every 8 hours.

Cl_{cr} <10 mL/minute: Administer every 8-16 hours in fast acetylators and every 12-24 hours in slow acetylators.

Hemodialysis: Supplemental dose is not necessary.

Peritoneal dialysis: Supplemental dose is not necessary.

Dietary Considerations Administer with meals.

Administration Inject over 1 minute. Hypotensive effect may be delayed and unpredictable in some patients.

Monitoring Parameters Blood pressure (monitor closely with I.V. use), standing and sitting/supine, heart rate, ANA titer

Patient Information Report flu-like symptoms, rise slowly from sitting/lying position; take with meals

Nursing Implications Aid with ambulation, rising may cause orthostasis

Dosage Forms

Injection, as hydrochloride: 20 mg/mL (1 mL)

Tablet, as hydrochloride: 10 mg, 25 mg, 50 mg, 100 mg

Extemporaneous Preparations An oral solution (20 mg/5 mL) has been made from 20 mL of the hydralazine injection (20 mg/mL), 8 mL of propylene glycol and purified water USP qs ad 100 mL; expected stability: 30 days if refrigerated

A flavored syrup (1.25 mg/mL) has been made using seventy-five hydralazine hydrochloride 50 mg tablets, dissolved in 250 mL of distilled water with 2250 g of Lycasin® (75% w/w maltitol syrup vehicle); edetate disodium 3 g and sodium saccharin 3 g dissolved in 50 mL distilled water was added; solution was preserved with 30 mL of a solution containing methylparaben 10% (w/v) and propylparaben 2% (w/v) in propylene glycol; flavored with 3 mL orange flavoring; qs ad to 3 L with distilled water and then pH adjusted to pH of 3.7 using glacial acetic acid; measured stability was 5 days at room temperature (25°C); less than 2% loss of hydralazine occurred at 2 weeks when syrup was stored at 5°C

Alexander KS, Pudipeddi M, and Parker GA, "Stability of Hydralazine Hydrochloride Syrup Compounded From Tablets," *Am J Hosp Pharm*, 1993, 50(4):683-6.

Nahata MC and Hipple TF, *Pediatric Drug Formulations*, 2nd ed, Cincinnati, OH: Harvey Whitney Books Co, 1992.

Hydralazine and Hydrochlorothiazide

(hye DRAL a zeen & hye droe klor oh THYE a zide)

U.S. Brand Names Apresazide® [DSC]

Synonyms Hydrochlorothiazide and Hydralazine

Therapeutic Category Antihypertensive Agent, Combination

Use Management of moderate to severe hypertension and treatment of congestive heart failure

Pregnancy Risk Factor C

Usual Dosage Adults: Oral: Take as directed; not to exceed 50 mg hydrochlorothiazide per day

Additional Information Complete prescribing information for this medication should be consulted for additional detail.

Dosage Forms

Capsule:

25/25: Hydralazine hydrochloride 25 mg and hydrochlorothiazide 25 mg

50/50: Hydralazine hydrochloride 50 mg and hydrochlorothiazide 50 mg

100/50: Hydralazine hydrochloride 100 mg and hydrochlorothiazide 50 mg

♦ **Hydralazine Hydrochloride** *see* HydrALAZINE *on page 671*

Hydralazine, Hydrochlorothiazide, and Reserpine

(hye DRAL a zeen, hye droe klor oh THYE a zide, & re SER peen)

U.S. Brand Names Hydrap-ES®; Ser-Ap-Es®

Synonyms Hydrochlorothiazide, Hydralazine, and Reserpine; Reserpine, Hydralazine, and Hydrochlorothiazide

Therapeutic Category Antihypertensive Agent, Combination

Use Treatment of hypertensive disorders

Pregnancy Risk Factor C

Usual Dosage Adults: Oral: 1-2 tablets 3 times/day

Additional Information Complete prescribing information for this medication should be consulted for additional detail.

Dosage Forms Tablet: Hydralazine 25 mg, hydrochlorothiazide 15 mg, and reserpine 0.1 mg

♦ **Hydrap-ES®** *see* Hydralazine, Hydrochlorothiazide, and Reserpine *on page 673*

♦ **Hydrated Chloral** *see* Chloral Hydrate *on page 270*

♦ **Hydrea®** *see* Hydroxyurea *on page 689*

♦ **Hydrocet®** *see* Hydrocodone and Acetaminophen *on page 676*

Hydrochlorothiazide (hye droe klor oh THYE a zide)

Related Information
Heart Failure *on page 1663*
Sulfonamide Derivatives *on page 1515*

U.S. Brand Names Aquazide®; Esidrix®; Ezide®; Hydrocot®; HydroDIURIL®; Microzide™; Oretic®

Canadian Brand Names Apo®-Hydro; HydroDIURIL®

Synonyms HCTZ

Therapeutic Category Antihypertensive Agent; Diuretic, Thiazide

Use Management of mild to moderate hypertension; treatment of edema in congestive heart failure and nephrotic syndrome

Unlabeled/Investigational Use Treatment of lithium-induced diabetes insipidus

Pregnancy Risk Factor B (manufacturer); D (expert analysis)

Contraindications Hypersensitivity to hydrochlorothiazide or any component of the formulation, thiazides, or sulfonamide-derived drugs; anuria; renal decompensation; pregnancy

Warnings/Precautions Avoid in severe renal disease (ineffective). Electrolyte disturbances (hypokalemia, hypochloremic alkalosis, hyponatremia) can occur. Use with caution in severe hepatic dysfunction; hepatic encephalopathy can be caused by electrolyte disturbances. Gout can be precipitate in certain patients with a history of gout, a familial predisposition to gout, or chronic renal failure. Cautious use in diabetics; may see a change in glucose control. Hypersensitivity reactions can occur. Can cause SLE exacerbation or activation. Use with caution in patients with moderate or high cholesterol concentrations. Photosensitization may occur. Correct hypokalemia before initiating therapy.

Chemical similarities are present among sulfonamides, sulfonylureas, carbonic anhydrase inhibitors, thiazides, and loop diuretics (except ethacrynic acid). Use in patients with sulfonamide allergy is specifically contraindicated in product labeling, however a risk of cross-reaction exists in patients with allergy to any of these compounds; avoid use when previous reaction has been severe.

Adverse Reactions
1% to 10%:
Cardiovascular: Orthostatic hypotension, hypotension
Dermatologic: Photosensitivity
Endocrine & metabolic: Hypokalemia
Gastrointestinal: Anorexia, epigastric distress
<1% (Limited to important or life-threatening): Agranulocytosis, allergic myocarditis, allergic reactions (possibly with life-threatening anaphylactic shock), alopecia, aplastic anemia, eosinophilic pneumonitis, erythema multiforme, exfoliative dermatitis, hemolytic anemia, hepatic function impairment, interstitial nephritis, leukopenia, renal failure, respiratory distress, Stevens-Johnson syndrome, thrombocytopenia, toxic epidermal necrolysis

Overdosage/Toxicology Symptoms include hypermotility, diuresis, lethargy, confusion, and muscle weakness. Following GI decontamination, therapy is supportive with I.V. fluids, electrolytes, and I.V. pressors if needed.

Drug Interactions
Increased Effect/Toxicity: Increased effect of hydrochlorothiazide with furosemide and other loop diuretics. Increased hypotension and/or renal adverse effects of ACE inhibitors may result in aggressively diuresed patients. Beta-blockers increase hyperglycemic effects of thiazides in type 2 diabetes mellitus. Cyclosporine and thiazides can increase the risk of gout or renal toxicity. Digoxin toxicity can be exacerbated if a thiazide induces hypokalemia or hypomagnesemia. Lithium toxicity can occur with thiazides due to reduced renal excretion of lithium. Thiazides may prolong the duration of action with neuromuscular blocking agents.

Decreased Effect: Effects of oral hypoglycemics may be decreased. Decreased absorption of hydrochlorothiazide with cholestyramine and colestipol. NSAIDs can decrease the efficacy of thiazides, reducing the diuretic and antihypertensive effects.

Ethanol/Nutrition/Herb Interactions
Food: Hydrochlorothiazide peak serum levels may be decreased if taken with food. This product may deplete potassium, sodium, and magnesium.
Herb/Nutraceutical: Avoid dong quai if using for hypertension (has estrogenic activity). Dong quai may also cause photosensitization. Avoid ephedra, ginseng, yohimbe (may worsen hypertension). Avoid garlic (may have increased antihypertensive effect).

Mechanism of Action Inhibits sodium reabsorption in the distal tubules causing increased excretion of sodium and water as well as potassium and hydrogen ions

Pharmacodynamics/Kinetics
Onset of action: Diuresis: ~2 hours
Peak effect: 4-6 hours
Duration: 6-12 hours
Absorption: ~50% to 80%
Distribution: 3.6-7.8 L/kg
Protein binding: 68%
Bioavailability: 50% to 80%
Half-life elimination: 5.6-14.8 hours
Time to peak: 1-2.5 hours
Excretion: Urine (as unchanged drug)

Usual Dosage Oral (effect of drug may be decreased when used every day):
Children (in pediatric patients, chlorothiazide may be preferred over hydrochlorothiazide as there are more dosage formulations [eg, suspension] available):
<6 months: 2-3 mg/kg/day in 2 divided doses
>6 months: 2 mg/kg/day in 2 divided doses
Adults:
Edema: 25-100 mg/day in 1-2 doses; maximum: 200 mg/day
Hypertension: 25-50 mg/day; minimal increase in response and more electrolyte disturbances are seen with doses >50 mg/day
Elderly: 12.5-25 mg once daily

Dosing adjustment/comments in renal impairment: Cl$_{cr}$ 25-50 mL/minute: Not effective

Monitoring Parameters Assess weight, I & O reports daily to determine fluid loss; blood pressure, serum electrolytes, BUN, creatinine

Test Interactions ↑ creatine phosphokinase [CPK] (S), ammonia (B), amylase (S), calcium (S), chloride (S), cholesterol (S), glucose, ↑ acid (S), ↓ chloride (S), magnesium, potassium (S), sodium (S); Tyramine and phentolamine tests, histamine tests for pheochromocytoma

Patient Information May be taken with food or milk; take early in day to avoid nocturia; take the last dose of multiple doses no later than 6 PM unless instructed otherwise. A few people who take this medication become more sensitive to sunlight and may experience skin rash, redness, itching, or severe sunburn, especially if sun block SPF ≥15 is not used on exposed skin areas. May increase blood glucose levels in diabetics.

Nursing Implications Take blood pressure with patient lying down and standing

Additional Information If given the morning of surgery it may render the patient volume depleted and blood pressure may be labile during general anesthesia. Effect of drug may be decreased when used every day.

Dosage Forms
Capsule: 12.5 mg
Solution, oral: 50 mg/5 mL (50 mL) [mint flavor]
Tablet: 25 mg, 50 mg, 100 mg

♦ **Hydrochlorothiazide and Amiloride** see Amiloride and Hydrochlorothiazide on page 71

♦ **Hydrochlorothiazide and Benazepril** see Benazepril and Hydrochlorothiazide on page 154

♦ **Hydrochlorothiazide and Bisoprolol** see Bisoprolol and Hydrochlorothiazide on page 173

♦ **Hydrochlorothiazide and Captopril** see Captopril and Hydrochlorothiazide on page 221

♦ **Hydrochlorothiazide and Enalapril** see Enalapril and Hydrochlorothiazide on page 465

♦ **Hydrochlorothiazide and Hydralazine** see Hydralazine and Hydrochlorothiazide on page 673

♦ **Hydrochlorothiazide and Irbesartan** see Irbesartan and Hydrochlorothiazide on page 742

♦ **Hydrochlorothiazide and Lisinopril** see Lisinopril and Hydrochlorothiazide on page 811

♦ **Hydrochlorothiazide and Losartan** see Losartan and Hydrochlorothiazide on page 824

♦ **Hydrochlorothiazide and Methyldopa** see Methyldopa and Hydrochlorothiazide on page 892

♦ **Hydrochlorothiazide and Moexipril** see Moexipril and Hydrochlorothiazide on page 931

♦ **Hydrochlorothiazide and Propranolol** see Propranolol and Hydrochlorothiazide on page 1151

♦ **Hydrochlorothiazide and Quinapril** see Quinapril and Hydrochlorothiazide on page 1168

Hydrochlorothiazide and Spironolactone
(hye droe klor oh THYE a zide & speer on oh LAK tone)

U.S. Brand Names Aldactazide®

Canadian Brand Names Aldactazide 25®; Aldactazide 50®; Novo-Spirozine

Synonyms Spironolactone and Hydrochlorothiazide

Therapeutic Category Antihypertensive Agent, Combination

Use Management of mild to moderate hypertension; treatment of edema in congestive heart failure and nephrotic syndrome, and cirrhosis of the liver accompanied by edema and/or ascites

Pregnancy Risk Factor C

Usual Dosage Oral:
Children: 1.66-3.3 mg/kg/day (of spironolactone) in 2-4 divided doses
Adults:
Hydrochlorothiazide 25 mg and spironolactone 25 mg: $^1/_2$-8 tablets daily
Hydrochlorothiazide 50 mg and spironolactone 50 mg: $^1/_2$-4 tablets daily in 1-2 doses

Additional Information Complete prescribing information for this medication should be consulted for additional detail.

Dosage Forms
Tablet:
25/25: Hydrochlorothiazide 25 mg and spironolactone 25 mg
50/50: Hydrochlorothiazide 50 mg and spironolactone 50 mg

♦ **Hydrochlorothiazide and Telmisartan** see Telmisartan and Hydrochlorothiazide on page 1291

Hydrochlorothiazide and Triamterene
(hye droe klor oh THYE a zide & trye AM ter een)

U.S. Brand Names Dyazide®; Maxzide®; Maxzide®-25

Canadian Brand Names Apo®-Triazide; Dyazide®; Novo-Triamzide; Nu-Triazide

Synonyms Triamterene and Hydrochlorothiazide

Therapeutic Category Antihypertensive Agent; Diuretic, Potassium Sparing; Diuretic, Thiazide

Use Management of mild to moderate hypertension; treatment of edema in congestive heart failure and nephrotic syndrome

Pregnancy Risk Factor C (per manufacturer)

Usual Dosage Adults: Oral:
Hydrochlorothiazide 25 mg and triamterene 37.5 mg: 1-2 tablets/capsules once daily
Hydrochlorothiazide 50 mg and triamterene 75 mg: $^1/_2$-1 tablet daily

Additional Information Complete prescribing information for this medication should be consulted for additional detail.

Dosage Forms
Capsule (Dyazide®): Hydrochlorothiazide 25 mg and triamterene 37.5 mg
Tablet:
Maxzide®: Hydrochlorothiazide 50 mg and triamterene 75 mg
Maxzide®-25: Hydrochlorothiazide 25 mg and triamterene 37.5 mg

- **Hydrochlorothiazide and Valsartan** *see* Valsartan and Hydrochlorothiazide *on page 1403*
- **Hydrochlorothiazide, Hydralazine, and Reserpine** *see* Hydralazine, Hydrochlorothiazide, and Reserpine *on page 673*
- **Hydrocil® [OTC]** *see* Psyllium *on page 1158*
- **Hydro Cobex®** *see* Hydroxocobalamin *on page 687*

Hydrocodone and Acetaminophen
(hye droe KOE done & a seet a MIN oh fen)

Related Information

Narcotic Agonists Comparison *on page 1506*

U.S. Brand Names Anexsia®; Anodynos-DHC®; Bancap HC®; Co-Gesic®; DHC®; Dolacet®; DuoCet™; Hydrocet®; Hydrogesic®; Hy-Phen®; Lorcet® 10/650; Lorcet®-HD; Lorcet® Plus; Lortab®; Margesic® H; Medipain 5®; Norco®; Stagesic®; T-Gesic®; Vicodin®; Vicodin® ES; Vicodin® HP; Zydone®

Synonyms Acetaminophen and Hydrocodone

Therapeutic Category Analgesic, Narcotic

Use Relief of moderate to severe pain; antitussive (hydrocodone)

Restrictions C-III

Pregnancy Risk Factor C

Contraindications Hypersensitivity to hydrocodone, acetaminophen, or any component of the formulation; CNS depression; severe respiratory depression

Warnings/Precautions Use with caution in patients with hypersensitivity reactions to other phenanthrene derivative opioid agonists (morphine, hydrocodone, hydromorphone, levorphanol, oxycodone, oxymorphone); tablets contain metabisulfite which may cause allergic reactions; tolerance or drug dependence may result from extended use

Adverse Reactions

Cardiovascular: Hypotension, bradycardia

Central nervous system: Lightheadedness, dizziness, sedation, drowsiness, fatigue, confusion

Gastrointestinal: Nausea, vomiting

Genitourinary: Decreased urination

Neuromuscular & skeletal: Weakness

Respiratory: Dyspnea

<1% (Limited to important or life-threatening): Biliary tract spasm, hallucinations, histamine release, physical and psychological dependence with prolonged use, urinary tract spasm

Overdosage/Toxicology Symptoms include hepatic necrosis, blood dyscrasias, and respiratory depression. Treatment consists of acetylcysteine 140 mg/kg orally (loading), followed by 70 mg/kg every 4 hours for 17 doses. Therapy should be initiated based upon laboratory analysis suggesting a high probability of hepatotoxic potential. Naloxone (2 mg I.V.) can also be used to reverse toxic effects of the opiate. Activated charcoal is effective at binding certain chemicals, and this is especially true for acetaminophen.

Drug Interactions

Increased Effect/Toxicity: Hydrocodone with other narcotic analgesics, CNS depressants, antianxiety agents, or antipsychotics may cause enhanced CNS depression. MAO inhibitors or tricyclic antidepressants with hydrocodone may increase the effect of either agent.

Decreased Effect: Decreased effect with phenothiazines

Ethanol/Nutrition/Herb Interactions

Ethanol: Avoid ethanol or limit to <3 drinks/day.

Food: Rate of absorption of acetaminophen may be decreased when administered with food high in carbohydrates.

Herb/Nutraceutical: Avoid valerian, St John's wort, SAMe, kava kava (may increase risk excessive sedation).

Pharmacodynamics/Kinetics

Acetaminophen: See Acetaminophen monograph.

Hydrocodone:

Onset of action: Narcotic analgesic: 10-20 minutes

Duration: 4-8 hours

Distribution: Crosses placenta

Metabolism: Hepatic; O-demethylation; N-demethylation and 6-ketosteroid reduction

Half-life elimination: 3.3-4.4 hours

Excretion: Urine

Usual Dosage Oral (doses should be titrated to appropriate analgesic effect); for children ≥12 years of age and adults, the dosage of acetaminophen should be limited to ≤4 g/day (and possibly less in patients with hepatic impairment or ethanol use)

Children:

Antitussive (hydrocodone): 0.6 mg/kg/day in 3-4 divided doses; even though dosing by hydrocodone, make sure to keep within age-specific acetaminophen doses as well

A single dose should not exceed 10 mg in children >12 years, 5 mg in children 2-12 years, and 1.25 mg in children <2 years of age

Analgesic (acetaminophen): Refer to Acetaminophen monograph

Adults: Analgesic: 1-2 tablets or capsules every 4-6 hours or 5-10 mL solution every 4-6 hours as needed for pain; do not exceed 4 g/day of acetaminophen

Hydrocodone 2.5-5 mg and acetaminophen 400-500 mg; maximum: 8 tablets/capsules per day

Hydrocodone 7.5 mg and acetaminophen: 400-650 mg; maximum: 6 tablets/capsules per day

Hydrocodone 2.5 mg and acetaminophen: 167 mg/5 mL (elixir/solution); maximum: 6 Tbsp/day

Hydrocodone 7.5 mg and acetaminophen 750 mg; maximum: 5 tablets/capsules per day

Hydrocodone 10 mg and acetaminophen: 350-660 mg; maximum: 6 tablets/day per product labeling

Do not exceed 4 g/day of acetaminophen

Monitoring Parameters Pain relief, respiratory and mental status, blood pressure

Patient Information May cause drowsiness; do not exceed recommended dose; do not take for more than 10 days without physician's advice

Nursing Implications Observe patient for excessive sedation, respiratory depression

Additional Information Acetaminophen dosing for pediatric patients: 10-15 mg/kg/dose **or alternatively,**

Up to 3 months: 40 mg
4-11 months: 80 mg
1-2 years: 120 mg
2-3 years: 160 mg
4-5 years: 240 mg
6-8 years: 320 mg
9-10 years: 400 mg
11 years: 480 mg

Dosage Forms

Capsule: Bancap HC®, Dolacet®, Hydrocet®, Hydrogesic®, Lorcet®-HD, Margesic® H, Medipain 5®, Norcet®, Stagesic®, T-Gesic®, Zydone®: Hydrocodone bitartrate 5 mg and acetaminophen 500 mg

Elixir (Lortab®): Hydrocodone bitartrate 2.5 mg and acetaminophen 167 mg per 5 mL with alcohol 7% (480 mL) [tropical fruit punch flavor]

Solution, oral (Lortab®): Hydrocodone bitartrate 2.5 mg and acetaminophen 167 mg per 5 mL with alcohol 7% (480 mL) [tropical fruit punch flavor]

Tablet:
Hydrocodone bitartrate 5 mg and acetaminophen 400 mg
Hydrocodone bitartrate 7.5 mg and acetaminophen 400 mg
Hydrocodone bitartrate 10 mg and acetaminophen 400 mg
Hydrocodone bitartrate 5 mg and acetaminophen 500 mg
Hydrocodone bitartrate 7.5 mg and acetaminophen 750 mg
Hydrocodone bitartrate 7.5 mg and acetaminophen 500 mg
Hydrocodone bitartrate 7.5 mg and acetaminophen 650 mg
Hydrocodone bitartrate 10 mg and acetaminophen 500 mg

Anexsia® 5/500, Anodynos-DHC®, Co-Gesic®, DuoCet™, DHC®; Hy-Phen®, Lorcet®-HD, Lortab® 5/500, Vicodin®: Hydrocodone bitartrate 5 mg and acetaminophen 500 mg
Anexsia® 7.5/650, Lorcet® Plus: Hydrocodone bitartrate 7.5 mg and acetaminophen 650 mg
Lorcet® 10/650: Hydrocodone bitartrate 10 mg and acetaminophen 650 mg
Lortab® 2.5/500: Hydrocodone bitartrate 2.5 mg and acetaminophen 500 mg
Lortab® 7.5/500: Hydrocodone bitartrate 7.5 mg and acetaminophen 500 mg
Lortab® 10/500: Hydrocodone bitartrate 10 mg and acetaminophen 500 mg
Norco®: Hydrocodone bitartrate 10 mg and acetaminophen 325 mg
Vicodin® ES: Hydrocodone bitartrate 7.5 mg and acetaminophen 750 mg
Vicodin® HP: Hydrocodone bitartrate 10 mg and acetaminophen 660 mg
Zydone®:
Hydrocodone bitartrate 5 mg and acetaminophen 400 mg
Hydrocodone bitartrate 7.5 mg and acetaminophen 400 mg
Hydrocodone bitartrate 10 mg and acetaminophen 400 mg

Hydrocodone and Aspirin (hye droe KOE done & AS pir in)

Related Information
Narcotic Agonists Comparison *on page 1506*

U.S. Brand Names Lortab® ASA

Synonyms Aspirin and Hydrocodone

Therapeutic Category Analgesic, Narcotic

Use Relief of moderate to moderately severe pain

Restrictions C-III

Pregnancy Risk Factor D

Contraindications
Based on **hydrocodone** component: Hypersensitivity to hydrocodone or any component of the formulation
Based on **aspirin** component: Hypersensitivity to salicylates, other NSAIDs, or any component of the formulation; asthma; rhinitis; nasal polyps; inherited or acquired bleeding disorders (including factor VII and factor IX deficiency); pregnancy (in 3rd trimester especially); do not use in children (<16 years) for viral infections (chickenpox or flu symptoms), with or without fever, due to a potential association with Reye's syndrome

Warnings/Precautions Use with caution in patients with impaired renal function, erosive gastritis, or peptic ulcer disease; children and teenagers should not use for chickenpox or flu symptoms before a physician is consulted about Reye's syndrome; tolerance or drug dependence may result from extended use

Based on **hydrocodone** component: Use with caution in patients with hypersensitivity reactions to other phenanthrene-derivative opioid agonists (morphine, codeine, hydromorphone, levorphanol, oxycodone, oxymorphone); should be used with caution in elderly or debilitated patients, and those with severe impairment of hepatic or renal function, prostatic hyperplasia, or urethral stricture.

Based on **aspirin** component: Use with caution in patients with platelet and bleeding disorders, renal dysfunction, dehydration, erosive gastritis, or peptic ulcer disease. Heavy ethanol use (>3 drinks/day) can increase bleeding risks. Avoid use in severe renal failure or in severe hepatic failure. Discontinue use if tinnitus or impaired hearing occurs. Caution in mild-moderate renal failure (only at high dosages). Patients with sensitivity to tartrazine dyes, nasal polyps and asthma may have an increased risk of salicylate sensitivity. Surgical patients should avoid ASA if possible, for 1-2 weeks prior to surgery, to reduce the risk of excessive bleeding.

Adverse Reactions
>10%:
Cardiovascular: Hypotension
(Continued)

Hydrocodone and Aspirin *(Continued)*

Central nervous system: Lightheadedness, dizziness, sedation, drowsiness, fatigue
Gastrointestinal: Nausea, heartburn, stomach pains, heartburn, epigastric discomfort
Neuromuscular & skeletal: Weakness

1% to 10%:
Cardiovascular: Bradycardia
Central nervous system: Confusion
Dermatologic: Rash
Gastrointestinal: Vomiting, gastrointestinal ulceration
Genitourinary: Decreased urination
Hematologic: Hemolytic anemia
Respiratory: Dyspnea
Miscellaneous: Anaphylactic shock

<1% (Limited to important or life-threatening): Biliary tract spasm, bronchospasm, hallucinations, hepatotoxicity, histamine release, leukopenia, occult bleeding, physical and psychological dependence with prolonged use, prolonged bleeding time, thrombocytopenia, urinary tract spasm

Overdosage/Toxicology The antidote for codeine is naloxone, 2 mg I.V. (0.01 mg/kg for children) with repeat administration, as necessary, up to a total of 10 mg. The "Done" nomogram is very helpful for estimating the severity of aspirin poisoning and directing treatment using serum salicylate levels. Treatment can also be based upon symptomatology. See Aspirin monograph.

Drug Interactions
Increased Effect/Toxicity:
Based on **hydrocodone** component: CNS depressants, MAO inhibitors, general anesthetics, and tricyclic antidepressants may potentiate the effects of opiate agonists; dextroamphetamine may enhance the analgesic effect of opiate agonists.

Based on **aspirin** component: May increase methotrexate serum levels/toxicity and may displace valproic acid from binding sites which can result in toxicity. NSAIDs and aspirin increase GI adverse effects (ulceration). Aspirin with oral anticoagulants (warfarin), thrombolytic agents, heparin, low molecular weight heparins, and antiplatelet agents (ticlopidine, clopidogrel, dipyridamole, NSAIDs, and IIb/IIIa antagonists) may increase risk of bleeding. Bleeding times may be additionally prolonged with verapamil. The effects of older sulfonylurea agents (tolazamide, tolbutamide) may be potentiated due to displacement from plasma proteins. This effect does not appear to be clinically significant for newer sulfonylurea agents (glyburide, glipizide, glimepiride).

Decreased Effect:
Based on **hydrocodone** component: Phenothiazines may antagonize the analgesic effect of opiate agonists

Based on **aspirin** component: The effects of ACE inhibitors may be blunted by aspirin administration (may be significant only at higher aspirin dosages). Aspirin may decrease the effects of beta-blockers, loop diuretics (furosemide), thiazide diuretics, and probenecid. Aspirin may cause a decrease in NSAIDs serum concentration and decrease the effects of probenecid. Increased serum salicylate levels when taken with with urine acidifiers (ammonium chloride, methionine).

Ethanol/Nutrition/Herb Interactions
Based on **hydrocodone** component: Ethanol: Avoid or limit ethanol (may increase CNS depression). Watch for sedation.

Based on **aspirin** component:
Ethanol: Avoid ethanol (may enhance gastric mucosal damage).
Food: Food may decrease the rate but not the extent of oral absorption. Take with food or large volume of water or milk to minimize GI upset.
Herb/Nutraceutical: Avoid cat's claw, dong quai, evening primrose, feverfew, garlic, ginger, ginkgo, red clover, horse chestnut, green tea, ginseng (all have additional antiplatelet activity).

Mechanism of Action
Based on **hydrocodone** component: Binds to opiate receptors in the CNS, altering the perception of and response to pain; suppresses cough in medullary center; produces generalized CNS depression

Based on **aspirin** component: Inhibits prostaglandin synthesis, acts on the hypothalamus heat-regulating center to reduce fever, blocks prostaglandin synthetase action which prevents formation of the platelet-aggregating substance thromboxane A_2

Pharmacodynamics/Kinetics
Aspirin: See Aspirin monograph.
Hydrocodone:
Onset of action: Narcotic analgesic: 10-20 minutes
Duration: 4-8 hours
Distribution: Crosses placenta
Metabolism: Hepatic; O-demethylation; N-demethylation and 6-ketosteroid reduction
Half-life elimination: 3.3-4.4 hours
Excretion: Urine

Usual Dosage Adults: Oral: 1-2 tablets every 4-6 hours as needed for pain

Administration Administer with food or a full glass of water to minimize GI distress

Monitoring Parameters Observe patient for excessive sedation, respiratory depression

Test Interactions Urine glucose, urinary 5-HIAA, serum uric acid

Patient Information May cause drowsiness; avoid alcohol; watch for bleeding gums or any signs of GI bleeding; take with food or milk to minimize GI distress, notify physician if ringing in ears or persistent GI pain occurs

Nursing Implications May cause drowsiness; avoid alcohol; watch for bleeding gums or any signs of GI bleeding; notify healthcare provider if ringing in ears or persistent GI pain occurs

Dosage Forms Tablet: Hydrocodone bitartrate 5 mg and aspirin 500 mg

Hydrocodone and Chlorpheniramine
(hye droe KOE done & klor fen IR a meen)

U.S. Brand Names Tussionex®

Synonyms Chlorpheniramine and Hydrocodone

Therapeutic Category Antihistamine/Antitussive

Use Symptomatic relief of cough and allergy

Restrictions C-III

Pregnancy Risk Factor C

Usual Dosage Oral:
Children 6-12 years: 2.5 mL every 12 hours; do not exceed 5 mL/24 hours
Adults: 5 mL every 12 hours; do not exceed 10 mL/24 hours

Additional Information Complete prescribing information for this medication should be consulted for additional detail.

Dosage Forms Syrup: Hydrocodone polistirex 10 mg and chlorpheniramine polistirex 8 mg per 5 mL (480 mL, 900 mL) [alcohol free]

Hydrocodone and Guaifenesin (hye droe KOE done & gwye FEN e sin)

U.S. Brand Names Codiclear® DH; HycoClear Tuss®; Hycotuss® Expectorant Liquid; Kwelcof®; Vicodin Tuss™

Synonyms Guaifenesin and Hydrocodone

Therapeutic Category Antitussive/Expectorant

Use Symptomatic relief of nonproductive coughs associated with upper and lower respiratory tract congestion

Restrictions C-III

Pregnancy Risk Factor C

Usual Dosage Oral:
Children:
<2 years: 0.3 mg/kg/day (hydrocodone) in 4 divided doses
2-12 years: 2.5 mL every 4 hours, after meals and at bedtime
>12 years: 5 mL every 4 hours, after meals and at bedtime
Adults: 5 mL every 4 hours, after meals and at bedtime, not >30 mL in a 24-hour period

Additional Information Complete prescribing information for this medication should be consulted for additional detail.

Dosage Forms Liquid: Hydrocodone bitartrate 5 mg and guaifenesin 100 mg per 5 mL (120 mL, 480 mL)

Hydrocodone and Homatropine (hye droe KOE done & hoe MA troe peen)

Related Information
Narcotic Agonists Comparison *on page 1506*

U.S. Brand Names Hycodan®; Hydromet®; Hydropane®; Hydrotropine®; Tussigon®

Synonyms Homatropine and Hydrocodone

Therapeutic Category Antitussive; Cough Preparation

Use Symptomatic relief of cough

Restrictions C-III

Pregnancy Risk Factor C

Contraindications Hypersensitivity to hydrocodone, homatropine, or any component of the formulation; increased intracranial pressure, narrow-angle glaucoma, depressed ventilation

Warnings/Precautions
Based on **hydrocodone** component: Use with caution in patients with hypersensitivity reactions to other phenanthrene derivative opioid agonists (morphine, codeine, hydromorphone, levorphanol, oxycodone, oxymorphone); should be used with caution in elderly or debilitated patients, and those with severe impairment of hepatic or renal function, prostatic hyperplasia, or urethral stricture. Also use caution in patients with head injury, increased intracranial pressure, acute abdomen, or impaired thyroid function. Hydrocodone suppresses the cough reflex; caution should be exercised when this agent is used postoperatively and in patients with pulmonary diseases (including asthma, emphysema, COPD); tolerance or drug dependence may result from extended use
Based on **homatropine** component: Use with caution in patients with hypertension, cardiac disease, or increased intraocular pressure; safety and efficacy not established in infants and young children, therefore, use with extreme caution due to susceptibility of systemic effects; use with caution in obstructive uropathy, paralytic ileus, ulcerative colitis, unstable cardiovascular status in acute hemorrhage; use with caution in children with spastic paralysis, in the elderly, and in patients with prostatic hyperplasia

Adverse Reactions
Cardiovascular: Bradycardia, tachycardia, hypotension, hypertension
Central nervous system: Lightheadedness, dizziness, sedation, drowsiness, fatigue, confusion, hallucinations
Gastrointestinal: Nausea, vomiting, xerostomia, anorexia, impaired GI motility
Genitourinary: Decreased urination, urinary tract spasm
Hepatic: Biliary tract spasm
Neuromuscular & skeletal: Weakness
Ocular: Diplopia, miosis, mydriasis, blurred vision
Respiratory: Dyspnea
Miscellaneous: Histamine release, physical and psychological dependence with prolonged use

Overdosage/Toxicology Symptoms include CNS and respiratory depression, gastrointestinal cramping, dilated, unreactive pupils; blurred vision; hot, dry, flushed skin; dry mucous membranes, difficulty swallowing, foul breath, diminished or absent bowel sounds, urinary retention, tachycardia, hyperthermia, hypertension, and increased respiratory rate. CNS depression is an extension of pharmacologic effect. Treatment is supportive. Administer naloxone 0.4 mg I.V. (0.01 mg/kg for children) with repeat administrations as necessary. Anticholinergic toxicity is caused by strong binding of the drug to cholinergic receptors. For (Continued)

Hydrocodone and Homatropine *(Continued)*

anticholinergic overdose with severe life-threatening symptoms, physostigmine 1-2 mg (0.5 or 0.02 mg/kg for children) S.C. or slow I.V. may be given to reverse these effects.

Drug Interactions
Increased Effect/Toxicity:
Based on **hydrocodone** component: Increased toxicity: CNS depressants, MAO inhibitors, general anesthetics, and tricyclic antidepressants may potentiate the effects of opiate agonists; dextroamphetamine may enhance the analgesic effect of opiate agonists
Based on **homatropine** component:
Phenothiazine and TCAs may increase anticholinergic effects when used concurrently. Sympathomimetic amines may cause tachyarrhythmias; avoid concurrent use
Decreased Effect: Based on **hydrocodone** component: Decreased effect: Phenothiazines may antagonize the analgesic effect of opiate agonists
Ethanol/Nutrition/Herb Interactions Ethanol: Avoid or limit ethanol (may increase CNS depression). Watch for sedation.

Mechanism of Action
Based on **hydrocodone** component: Binds to opiate receptors in the CNS, altering the perception of and response to pain; suppresses cough in medullary center; produces generalized CNS depression
Based on **homatropine** component: Blocks response of iris sphincter muscle and the accommodative muscle of the ciliary body to cholinergic stimulation resulting in dilation and loss of accommodation

Pharmacodynamics/Kinetics Duration: Hydrocodone: 4-6 hours

Usual Dosage Oral (based on hydrocodone component):
Children: 0.6 mg/kg/day in 3-4 divided doses; do not administer more frequently than every 4 hours
A single dose should not exceed 1.25 mg in children <2 years of age, 5 mg in children 2-12 years, and 10 mg in children >12 years
Adults: 10 mg every 4-6 hours, a single dose should not exceed 15 mg; do not administer more frequently than every 4 hours

Test Interactions ↑ ALT, AST (S)

Patient Information Avoid alcohol; may cause drowsiness and impair judgment or coordination; may cause physical and psychological dependence with prolonged use; lack of saliva may enhance cavities; maintain good oral hygiene; use caution while driving; may cause blurred vision; notify physician if difficulty in urinating or constipation becomes severe

Nursing Implications Dispense in light-resistant container; observe patient for excessive sedation, respiratory depression, implement safety measures, assist with ambulation

Dosage Forms
Syrup (Hycodan®, Hydromet®, Hydropane®, Hydrotropine®): Hydrocodone bitartrate 5 mg and homatropine methylbromide 1.5 mg per 5 mL (120 mL, 480 mL, 4000 mL)
Tablet (Hycodan®, Tussigon®): Hydrocodone bitartrate 5 mg and homatropine methylbromide 1.5 mg

Hydrocodone and Ibuprofen *(hye droe KOE done & eye byoo PROE fen)*

Related Information
Narcotic Agonists Comparison *on page 1506*
U.S. Brand Names Vicoprofen®
Canadian Brand Names Vicoprofen®
Synonyms Ibuprofen and Hydrocodone
Therapeutic Category Analgesic, Narcotic
Use Short-term (generally <10 days) management of moderate to severe acute pain; is not indicated for treatment of such conditions as osteoarthritis or rheumatoid arthritis
Restrictions C-III
Pregnancy Risk Factor C/D (3rd trimester)
Pregnancy/Breast-Feeding Implications Clinical effects on the fetus: As with other NSAID-containing products, this agent should be avoided in late pregnancy because it may cause premature closure of the ductus arteriosus
Contraindications Hypersensitivity to hydrocodone, ibuprofen, aspirin, other NSAIDs, or any component of the formulation; pregnancy (3rd trimester)
Warnings/Precautions As with any opioid analgesic agent, this agent should be used with caution in elderly or debilitated patients, and those with severe impairment of hepatic or renal function, hypothyroidism, Addison's disease, prostatic hyperplasia, or urethral stricture. The usual precautions should be observed and the possibility of respiratory depression should be kept in mind. Patients with head injury, increased intracranial pressure, acute abdomen, active peptic ulcer disease, history of upper GI disease, impaired thyroid function, asthma, hypertension, edema, heart failure, and any bleeding disorder should use this agent cautiously. Hydrocodone suppresses the cough reflex; as with opioids, caution should be exercised when this agent is used postoperatively and in patients with pulmonary disease.

Adverse Reactions
>10%:
Central nervous system: Headache (27%), dizziness (14%), sedation (22%)
Dermatologic: Rash, urticaria
Gastrointestinal: Constipation (22%), nausea (21%), dyspepsia (12%)
1% to 10%:
Cardiovascular: Bradycardia, palpitations (<3%), vasodilation (<3%), edema (3% to 9%)
Central nervous system: Headache, nervousness, confusion, fever (<3%), pain (3% to 9%), anxiety (3% to 9%), thought abnormalities
Dermatologic: Itching (3% to 9%)
Endocrine & metabolic: Fluid retention
Gastrointestinal: Vomiting (3% to 9%), anorexia, diarrhea (3% to 9%), xerostomia (3% to 9%), flatulence (3% to 9%), gastritis (<3%), melena (<3%), mouth ulcers (<3%)
Genitourinary: Polyuria (<3%)
Neuromuscular & skeletal: Weakness (3% to 9%)

Otic: Tinnitus
Respiratory: Dyspnea, hiccups, pharyngitis, rhinitis
Miscellaneous: Flu syndrome (<3%), infection (3% to 9%)
<1% (Limited to important or life-threatening): Acute renal failure, agranulocytosis, anemia, arrhythmias, aseptic meningitis, biliary tract spasm, bone marrow suppression, congestive heart failure, depression, diplopia, erythema multiforme, hallucinations, hemolytic anemia, hepatitis, histamine release, inhibition of platelet aggregation, leukopenia, neutropenia, peripheral neuropathy, physical and psychological dependence with prolonged use, Stevens-Johnson syndrome, thrombocytopenia, toxic amblyopia, toxic epidermal necrolysis, urinary tract spasm, urticaria

Overdosage/Toxicology Treat according to separate ingredient (hydrocodone and ibuprofen) toxicology.

Drug Interactions

Cytochrome P450 Effect: Ibuprofen: CYP2C8 and 2C9 enzyme substrate

Increased Effect/Toxicity: Anticholinergic agents taken with hydrocodone may cause paralytic ileus. Aspirin taken concomitantly may enhance adverse effects. Other CNS depressants (eg, antihistamines, alcohol, antipsychotics, etc) taken concomitantly may exhibit additive CNS toxicity. Warfarin taken with ibuprofen may result in additional risk of bleeding. Methotrexate taken with ibuprofen may enhance methotrexate toxicity. Furosemide taken with ibuprofen may reduce the effect of furosemide. Lithium taken with ibuprofen may elevate lithium serum levels.

Decreased Effect:

Based on **hydrocodone** component: Phenothiazines may antagonize the analgesic effect of opiate agonists opiate agonists

Based on **ibuprofen** component: Aspirin may decrease ibuprofen serum concentrations. Ibuprofen may decrease the effect of some antihypertensive agents (including ACE inhibitors and angiotensin antagonists) and diuretics.

Ethanol/Nutrition/Herb Interactions

Based on **hydrocodone** component: Ethanol: Avoid or limit ethanol (may increase CNS depression). Watch for sedation.

Based on **ibuprofen** component:

Ethanol: Avoid ethanol (may enhance gastric mucosal irritation).

Food: Ibuprofen peak serum levels may be decreased if taken with food.

Herb/Nutraceutical: Avoid cat's claw, dong quai, evening primrose, feverfew, garlic, ginger, ginkgo, red clover, horse chestnut, green tea, ginseng (all have additional antiplatelet activity).

Mechanism of Action

Based on **hydrocodone** component: Binds to opiate receptors in the CNS, altering the perception of and response to pain; suppresses cough in medullary center; produces generalized CNS depression

Based on **ibuprofen** component: Inhibits prostaglandin synthesis by decreasing the activity of the enzyme, cyclo-oxygenase, which results in decreased formation of prostaglandin precursors

Pharmacodynamics/Kinetics

Ibuprofen: See Ibuprofen monograph.

Hydrocodone:

Onset of action: Narcotic analgesic: 10-20 minutes

Duration: 4-8 hours

Distribution: Crosses placenta

Protein binding: Ibuprofen: 99%; Hydrocodone: 19% to 45%

Metabolism: Hepatic; O-demethylation; N-demethylation and 6-ketosteroid reduction

Half-life elimination: 3.3-4.4 hours

Time to peak: Ibuprofen: 1.8 hours; Hydrocodone: 1.7 hours

Excretion: Urine

Usual Dosage Adults: Oral: 1-2 tablets every 4-6 hours as needed for pain; maximum: 5 tablets/day

Patient Information Hydrocodone and ibuprofen, like other opioid-containing analgesics, may impair mental and/or physical abilities required for the performance of potentially hazardous tasks such as driving a car or operating machinery; patients should be cautioned accordingly. Alcohol and other CNS depressants may produce an additive CNS depression, when taken with this combination product, and should be avoided. This agent may be habit-forming. Patients should take the drug only for as long as it is prescribed, in the amounts prescribed, and no more frequently than prescribed.

Additional Information The antipyretic and anti-inflammatory activity of ibuprofen may reduce fever and inflammation, thus diminishing their utility as diagnostic signs in detecting complications of presumed noninfectious, noninflammatory painful conditions.

Dosage Forms Tablet: Hydrocodone bitartrate 7.5 mg and ibuprofen 200 mg

Hydrocodone and Pseudoephedrine

(hye droe KOE done & soo doe e FED rin)

U.S. Brand Names Detussin® Liquid; Histussin D® Liquid; Tyrodone® Liquid

Synonyms Pseudoephedrine and Hydrocodone

Therapeutic Category Cough and Cold Combination

Use Symptomatic relief of cough due to colds, nasal congestion, and cough

Restrictions C-III

Usual Dosage Oral: Adults: 5 mL 4 times/day

Additional Information Complete prescribing information for this medication should be consulted for additional detail.

Dosage Forms Liquid (Detussin®, Histussin D®, Tyrodone®): Hydrocodone bitartrate 5 mg and pseudoephedrine hydrochloride 60 mg per 5 mL

Hydrocodone, Chlorpheniramine, Phenylephrine, Acetaminophen, and Caffeine

(hye droe KOE done, klor fen IR a meen, fen il EF rin, a seet a MIN oh fen, & KAF een)

U.S. Brand Names Hycomine® Compound

Synonyms Acetaminophen, Caffeine, Hydrocodone, Chlorpheniramine, and Phenylephrine; Caffeine, Hydrocodone, Chlorpheniramine, Phenylephrine, and Acetaminophen; Chlorpheniramine, Hydrocodone, Phenylephrine, Acetaminophen, and Caffeine; Phenylephrine, Hydrocodone, Chlorpheniramine, Acetaminophen, and Caffeine

Therapeutic Category Antitussive

Use Symptomatic relief of cough and symptoms of upper respiratory infection

Restrictions C-III

Pregnancy Risk Factor C

Usual Dosage Adults: Oral: 1 tablet every 4 hours, up to 4 times/day

Additional Information Complete prescribing information for this medication should be consulted for additional detail.

Dosage Forms Tablet: Hydrocodone bitartrate 5 mg, chlorpheniramine maleate 2 mg, phenylephrine hydrochloride 10 mg, acetaminophen 250 mg, and caffeine 30 mg

♦ **Hydrocort**® *see* Hydrocortisone *on page 682*

Hydrocortisone (hye droe KOR ti sone)

Related Information

Corticosteroids Comparison *on page 1495*

U.S. Brand Names A-hydroCort®; Ala-Cort®; Ala-Scalp®; Anucort-HC® Suppository; Anusol® HC 1 [OTC]; Anusol® HC 2.5% [OTC]; Anusol-HC® Suppository; Cetacort®; Clocort® Maximum Strength; Cortaid® Maximum Strength [OTC]; Cortaid® With Aloe [OTC]; Cort-Dome®; Cortef®; Cortef® Feminine Itch; Cortenema®; Corticaine®; Cortifoam®; Cortizone®-5 [OTC]; Cortizone®-10 [OTC]; Delcort®; Dermacort®; DermiCort®; Dermolate® [OTC]; Dermtex® HC With Aloe; Eldecort®; Gynecort® [OTC]; Hemril-HC® Uniserts®; Hi-Cor® 1.0; Hi-Cor® 2.5; Hycort®; Hydrocort®; Hydrocortone® Acetate; Hydrocortone® Phosphate; HydroTex® [OTC]; Hytone®; LactiCare-HC®; Lanacort® [OTC]; Locoid®; Nutracort®; Orabase® HCA; Pandel®; Penecort®; Procort® [OTC]; Proctocort™; Scalpicin®; Solu-Cortef®; S-T Cort®; Synacort®; Tegrin®-HC [OTC]; Texacort®; Westcort®

Canadian Brand Names A-Hydrocort®; Aquacort®; Cortamed®; Cortate®; Cortef®; Cortenema®; Cortifoam™; Cortoderm; Emo-Cort®; Hycort™; Hyderm; Locoid®; Prevex® HC; Sarna® HC; Solu-Cortef®; Westcort®

Synonyms Compound F; Cortisol; Hydrocortisone Acetate; Hydrocortisone Buteprate; Hydrocortisone Butyrate; Hydrocortisone Cypionate; Hydrocortisone Sodium Phosphate; Hydrocortisone Sodium Succinate; Hydrocortisone Valerate

Therapeutic Category Anti-inflammatory Agent; Anti-inflammatory Agent, Rectal; Corticosteroid, Rectal; Corticosteroid, Systemic; Corticosteroid, Topical (Low Potency); Corticosteroid, Topical (Medium Potency); Glucocorticoid; Mineralocorticoid

Use Management of adrenocortical insufficiency; relief of inflammation of corticosteroid-responsive dermatoses (low and medium potency topical corticosteroid); adjunctive treatment of ulcerative colitis

Pregnancy Risk Factor C

Contraindications Hypersensitivity to hydrocortisone or any component of the formulation; serious infections, except septic shock or tuberculous meningitis; viral, fungal, or tubercular skin lesions

Warnings/Precautions

Use with caution in patients with hyperthyroidism, cirrhosis, nonspecific ulcerative colitis, hypertension, osteoporosis, thromboembolic tendencies, CHF, convulsive disorders, myasthenia gravis, thrombophlebitis, peptic ulcer, diabetes, glaucoma, cataracts, or tuberculosis. Use caution in hepatic impairment.

Acute adrenal insufficiency may occur with abrupt withdrawal after long-term therapy or with stress; young pediatric patients may be more susceptible to adrenal axis suppression from topical therapy

Because of the risk of adverse effects, systemic corticosteroids should be used cautiously in the elderly, in the smallest possible dose, and for the shortest possible time

Adverse Reactions

Systemic:

>10%:

Central nervous system: Insomnia, nervousness

Gastrointestinal: Increased appetite, indigestion

1% to 10%:

Central nervous system: Dizziness, lightheadedness, headache

Dermatologic: Hirsutism, hypopigmentation

Endocrine & metabolic: Diabetes mellitus

Neuromuscular & skeletal: Arthralgia

Ocular: Cataracts, glaucoma

Respiratory: Epistaxis

Miscellaneous: Diaphoresis

<1% (Limited to important or life-threatening): Alkalosis, amenorrhea, sodium and water retention, Cushing's syndrome, glucose intolerance, growth suppression, hyperglycemia, hypokalemia, pituitary-adrenal axis suppression, pseudotumor cerebri, seizures

Topical:

1% to 10%:

Dermatologic: Itching, allergic contact dermatitis, erythema, dryness papular rashes, folliculitis, furunculosis, pustules, pyoderma, vesiculation, hyperesthesia, skin infection (secondary)

Local: Burning, irritation

<1% (Limited to important or life-threatening): Cataracts (posterior subcapsular), Cushing's syndrome, glaucoma, hypokalemic syndrome

Overdosage/Toxicology Symptoms include cushingoid appearance (systemic), muscle weakness (systemic), and osteoporosis (systemic) - all with long-term use only. When consumed in excessive quantities for prolonged periods, systemic hypercorticism and adrenal suppression may occur. In those cases, discontinuation and withdrawal of the corticosteroid should be done judiciously.

Drug Interactions

Cytochrome P450 Effect: CYP2D6 and 3A3/4 enzyme substrate

Increased Effect/Toxicity: Hydrocortisone in combination with oral anticoagulants may increase prothrombin time. Potassium-depleting diuretics increase risk of hypokalemia. Cardiac glycosides increase risk of arrhythmias or digitalis toxicity secondary to hypokalemia.

Decreased Effect: Hydrocortisone may decrease the hypoglycemic effect of insulin. Phenytoin, phenobarbital, ephedrine, and rifampin increase metabolism of hydrocortisone resulting in a decreased steroid blood level.

Ethanol/Nutrition/Herb Interactions

Ethanol: Avoid ethanol (may enhance gastric mucosal irritation).

Food: Hydrocortisone interferes with calcium absorption.

Herb/Nutraceutical: St John's wort may decrease hydrocortisone levels. Avoid cat's claw, echinacea (have immunostimulant properties).

Stability

Hydrocortisone sodium phosphate and hydrocortisone sodium succinate are clear, light yellow solutions which are heat labile

After initial reconstitution, hydrocortisone sodium succinate solutions are stable for 3 days at room temperature and refrigeration if protected from light

Stability of parenteral admixture (Solu-Cortef®) at room temperature (25°C) and at refrigeration temperature (4°C) is concentration dependent

Minimum volume: Concentration should not exceed 1 mg/mL

Stability of concentration ≤1 mg/mL: 24 hours

Stability of concentration >1 mg/mL to <25 mg/mL: Unpredictable, 4-6 hours

Stability of concentration ≥25 mg/mL: 3 days

Standard diluent (Solu-Cortef®): 50 mg/50 mL D_5W; 100 mg/100 mL D_5W

Comments: Should be administered in a 0.1-1 mg/mL concentration due to stability problems

Mechanism of Action Decreases inflammation by suppression of migration of polymorphonuclear leukocytes and reversal of increased capillary permeability

Pharmacodynamics/Kinetics

Onset of action:

Hydrocortisone acetate: Slow

Hydrocortisone sodium phosphate (water soluble): Rapid

Hydrocortisone sodium succinate (water soluble): Rapid

Duration:

Hydrocortisone acetate: Long

Hydrocortisone sodium phosphate (water soluble): Short

Absorption: Rapid by all routes, except rectally

Metabolism: Hepatic

Half-life elimination: Biologic: 8-12 hours

Excretion: Urine (primarily as 17-hydroxysteroids and 17-ketosteroids)

Usual Dosage Dose should be based on severity of disease and patient response

Acute adrenal insufficiency: I.M., I.V.:

Infants and young Children: Succinate: 1-2 mg/kg/dose bolus, then 25-150 mg/day in divided doses every 6-8 hours

Older Children: Succinate: 1-2 mg/kg bolus then 150-250 mg/day in divided doses every 6-8 hours

Adults: Succinate: 100 mg I.V. bolus, then 300 mg/day in divided doses every 8 hours or as a continuous infusion for 48 hours; once patient is stable change to oral, 50 mg every 8 hours for 6 doses, then taper to 30-50 mg/day in divided doses

Chronic adrenal corticoid insufficiency: Adults: Oral: 20-30 mg/day

Anti-inflammatory or immunosuppressive:

Infants and Children:

Oral: 2.5-10 mg/kg/day **or** 75-300 mg/m²/day every 6-8 hours

I.M., I.V.: Succinate: 1-5 mg/kg/day **or** 30-150 mg/m²/day divided every 12-24 hours

Adolescents and Adults: Oral, I.M., I.V.: Succinate: 15-240 mg every 12 hours

Congenital adrenal hyperplasia: Oral: Initial: 10-20 mg/m²/day in 3 divided doses; a variety of dosing schedules have been used. **Note:** Inconsistencies have occurred with liquid formulations; tablets may provide more reliable levels. Doses must be individualized by monitoring growth, bone age, and hormonal levels. Mineralocorticoid and sodium supplementation may be required based upon electrolyte regulation and plasma renin activity.

Physiologic replacement: Children:

Oral: 0.5-0.75 mg/kg/day **or** 20-25 mg/m²/day every 8 hours

I.M.: Succinate: 0.25-0.35 mg/kg/day **or** 12-15 mg/m²/day once daily

Shock: I.M., I.V.: Succinate:

Children: Initial: 50 mg/kg, then repeated in 4 hours and/or every 24 hours as needed

Adolescents and Adults: 500 mg to 2 g every 2-6 hours

Status asthmaticus: Children and Adults: I.V.: Succinate: 1-2 mg/kg/dose every 6 hours for 24 hours, then maintenance of 0.5-1 mg/kg every 6 hours

Adults:

Rheumatic diseases:

Intralesional, intra-articular, soft tissue injection: Acetate:

Large joints: 25 mg (up to 37.5 mg)

Small joints: 10-25 mg

Tendon sheaths: 5-12.5 mg

Soft tissue infiltration: 25-50 mg (up to 75 mg)

Bursae: 25-37.5 mg

Ganglia: 12.5-25 mg

(Continued)

Hydrocortisone *(Continued)*

Stress dosing (surgery) in patients known to be adrenally-suppressed or on chronic systemic steroids: I.V.:

Minor stress (ie, inguinal herniorrhaphy): 25 mg/day for 1 day

Moderate stress (ie, joint replacement, cholecystectomy): 50-75 mg/day (25 mg every 8-12 hours) for 1-2 days

Major stress (pancreatoduodenectomy, esophagogastrectomy, cardiac surgery): 100-150 mg/day (50 mg every 8-12 hours) for 2-3 days

Dermatosis: Children >2 years and Adults: Topical: Apply to affected area 3-4 times/day (Buteprate: Apply once or twice daily). Therapy should be discontinued when control is achieved; if no improvement is seen, reassessment of diagnosis may be necessary.

Ulcerative colitis: Adults: Rectal: 10-100 mg 1-2 times/day for 2-3 weeks

Dietary Considerations Systemic use of corticosteroids may require a diet with increased potassium, vitamins A, B$_6$, C, D, folate, calcium, zinc, phosphorus, and decreased sodium.

Administration

Oral: Administer with food or milk to decrease GI upset

Parenteral: Hydrocortisone sodium succinate may be administered by I.M. or I.V. routes

I.V. bolus: Dilute to 50 mg/mL and administer over 30 seconds to several minutes (depending on the dose)

I.V. intermittent infusion: Dilute to 1 mg/mL and administer over 20-30 minutes

Topical: Apply a thin film to clean, dry skin and rub in gently

Monitoring Parameters Blood pressure, weight, serum glucose, and electrolytes

Reference Range Therapeutic: AM: 5-25 µg/dL (SI: 138-690 nmol/L), PM: 2-9 µg/dL (SI: 55-248 nmol/L) depending on test, assay

Patient Information Notify surgeon or dentist before surgical repair; oral formulation may cause GI upset, take with food; notify physician if any sign of infection occurs; avoid abrupt withdrawal when on long-term therapy. Before applying, gently wash area to reduce risk of infection; apply a thin film to cleansed area and rub in gently and thoroughly until medication vanishes; avoid exposure to sunlight, severe sunburn may occur.

Nursing Implications

Topical: Apply sparingly

I.V. bolus: Dilute to 50 mg/mL and administer over 3-5 minutes

I.V. intermittent infusion: Dilute to 1 mg/mL and administer over 20-30 minutes

Additional Information

Sodium content of 1 g (sodium succinate injection): 47.5 mg (2.07 mEq)

Hydrocortisone base topical cream, lotion, and ointments in concentrations of 0.25%, 0.5%, and 1% may be OTC or prescription depending on the product labeling

Dosage Forms

Aerosol, rectal, as acetate: 10% (20 g)

Aerosol, topical, as base: 0.5% (45 g, 58 g); 1% (45 mL)

Cream, as buteprate: 0.1%, 1% (15 g, 45 g)

Cream, as butyrate: 0.1% (15 g, 45 g)

Cream, rectal, as base: 1% (30 g); 2.5% (30 g)

Cream, topical, as acetate: 0.5% (15 g, 22.5 g, 30 g); 1% (15 g, 30 g, 120 g)

Cream, topical, as base: 0.2% (15 g, 30 g, 60 g, 120 g, 454 g); 0.5% (15 g, 30 g, 60 g, 120 g, 454 g); 1% (15 g, 20 g, 30 g, 60 g, 90 g, 120 g, 240 g, 454 g); 2.5% (15 g, 20 g, 30 g, 60 g, 120 g, 240 g, 454 g)

Cream, topical, as valerate: 0.2% (15 g, 45 g, 60 g)

Gel, topical, as base: 0.5% (15 g, 30 g); 1% (15 g, 30 g)

Injection, I.M./I.V., as sodium succinate: 100 mg, 250 mg, 500 mg, 1000 mg

Injection, I.M./I.V./S.C., as sodium phosphate: 50 mg/mL (2 mL, 10 mL)

Injection, suspension, as acetate: 25 mg/mL (5 mL, 10 mL); 50 mg/mL (5 mL, 10 mL)

Lotion, as acetate: 0.5%

Lotion, topical, as base: 0.25% (120 mL); 0.5% (30 mL, 60 mL, 120 mL); 1% (60 mL, 118 mL, 120 mL); 2% (30 mL); 2.5% (60 mL, 120 mL)

Ointment, ophthalmic, as acetate: 0.5%

Ointment, rectal, as base: 1% (30 g)

Ointment, topical, as acetate: 0.5% (15 g, 30 g); 1% (15 g, 21 g, 30 g)

Ointment, topical, as base: 0.2% (15 g, 30 g); 0.5% (30 g) ; 1% (15 g, 20 g, 28 g, 30 g, 60 g, 120 g, 240 g, 454 g); 2.5% (20 g, 30 g)

Ointment, topical, as butyrate: 0.1% (15 g, 45 g)

Ointment, topical, as valerate: 0.2% (15 g, 45 g, 60 g, 120 g)

Solution, topical, as base: 1% (45 mL, 75 mL, 120 mL)

Solution, topical, as butyrate: 0.1% (20 mL, 50 mL)

Suppositories, rectal, as acetate: 10 mg, 25 mg

Suspension, oral, as cypionate: 10 mg/5 mL (120 mL)

Suspension, rectal, as base: 100 mg/60 mL (7s)

Tablet, oral, as base: 5 mg, 10 mg, 20 mg

♦ **Hydrocortisone Acetate** *see* Hydrocortisone *on page 682*

♦ **Hydrocortisone, Acetic Acid, and Propylene Glycol Diacetate** *see* Acetic Acid, Propylene Glycol Diacetate, and Hydrocortisone *on page 31*

♦ **Hydrocortisone and Benzoyl Peroxide** *see* Benzoyl Peroxide and Hydrocortisone *on page 157*

♦ **Hydrocortisone and Ciprofloxacin** *see* Ciprofloxacin and Hydrocortisone *on page 298*

♦ **Hydrocortisone and Iodoquinol** *see* Iodoquinol and Hydrocortisone *on page 738*

♦ **Hydrocortisone and Neomycin** *see* Neomycin and Hydrocortisone *on page 968*

♦ **Hydrocortisone and Polymyxin B** *see* Polymyxin B and Hydrocortisone *on page 1103*

♦ **Hydrocortisone and Pramoxine** *see* Pramoxine and Hydrocortisone *on page 1117*

♦ **Hydrocortisone and Urea** *see* Urea and Hydrocortisone *on page 1391*

♦ **Hydrocortisone, Bacitracin, Neomycin, and Polymyxin B** *see* Bacitracin, Neomycin, Polymyxin B, and Hydrocortisone *on page 143*

♦ **Hydrocortisone Buteprate** *see* Hydrocortisone *on page 682*

- **Hydrocortisone Butyrate** *see Hydrocortisone on page 682*
- **Hydrocortisone, Colistin, and Neomycin** *see Colistin, Neomycin, and Hydrocortisone on page 334*
- **Hydrocortisone Cypionate** *see Hydrocortisone on page 682*
- **Hydrocortisone, Neomycin, and Polymyxin B** *see Neomycin, Polymyxin B, and Hydrocortisone on page 969*
- **Hydrocortisone, Propylene Glycol Diacetate, and Acetic Acid** *see Acetic Acid, Propylene Glycol Diacetate, and Hydrocortisone on page 31*
- **Hydrocortisone Sodium Phosphate** *see Hydrocortisone on page 682*
- **Hydrocortisone Sodium Succinate** *see Hydrocortisone on page 682*
- **Hydrocortisone Valerate** *see Hydrocortisone on page 682*
- **Hydrocortone® Acetate** *see Hydrocortisone on page 682*
- **Hydrocortone® Phosphate** *see Hydrocortisone on page 682*
- **Hydrocot®** *see Hydrochlorothiazide on page 674*
- **Hydro-Crysti-12®** *see Hydroxocobalamin on page 687*
- **HydroDIURIL®** *see Hydrochlorothiazide on page 674*

Hydroflumethiazide *Not Available in U.S.* (hye droe floo meth EYE a zide)
Related Information
  Sulfonamide Derivatives *on page 1515*
U.S. Brand Names Diucardin® [DSC]; Saluron® [DSC]
Canadian Brand Names Diucardin®; Saluron®
Therapeutic Category Antihypertensive Agent; Diuretic, Thiazide
Use Management of mild to moderate hypertension; treatment of edema in congestive heart failure and nephrotic syndrome
Pregnancy Risk Factor D
Usual Dosage Oral:
  Children (not approved): 1 mg/kg/24 hours
  Adults:
    Edema:
      Initial: 50 mg 1-2 times/day
      Maintenance: 25-200 mg/day (use divided doses when >100 mg/day)
    Hypertension:
      Initial: 50 mg twice daily
      Maintenance: 50-100 mg/day; maximum: 200 mg/day
Additional Information Complete prescribing information for this medication should be consulted for additional detail.
Dosage Forms Tablet: 50 mg

- **Hydrogesic®** *see Hydrocodone and Acetaminophen on page 676*
- **Hydromet®** *see Hydrocodone and Homatropine on page 679*
- **Hydromorph Contin® (Can)** *see Hydromorphone on page 685*

Hydromorphone (hye droe MOR fone)
Related Information
  Narcotic Agonists Comparison *on page 1506*
U.S. Brand Names Dilaudid®; Dilaudid-5®; Dilaudid-HP®
Canadian Brand Names Dilaudid®; Dilaudid-HP®; Dilaudid-HP-Plus®; Dilaudid® Sterile Powder; Dilaudid-XP®; Hydromorph Contin®; PMS-Hydromorphone
Synonyms Dihydromorphinone; Hydromorphone Hydrochloride
Therapeutic Category Analgesic, Narcotic; Antitussive
Use Management of moderate to severe pain; antitussive at lower doses
Restrictions C-II
Pregnancy Risk Factor B/D (prolonged use or high doses at term)
Contraindications Hypersensitivity to hydromorphone, any component of the formulation, or other phenanthrene derivative; pregnancy (prolonged use or high doses at term)
Warnings/Precautions Tablet and cough syrup contain tartrazine which may cause allergic reactions; hydromorphone shares toxic potential of opiate agonists, and precaution of opiate agonist therapy should be observed; extreme caution should be taken to avoid confusing the highly concentrated injection with the less concentrated injectable product, injection contains benzyl alcohol; use with caution in patients with hypersensitivity to other phenanthrene opiates, in patients with respiratory disease, or severe liver or renal failure; tolerance or drug dependence may result from extended use
Adverse Reactions
  Frequency not defined: Antidiuretic hormone release, biliary tract spasm, urinary tract spasm, miosis, histamine release, physical and psychological dependence; increased AST, ALT
  >10%:
    Cardiovascular: Palpitations, hypotension, peripheral vasodilation
    Central nervous system: Dizziness, lightheadedness, drowsiness
    Gastrointestinal: Anorexia
  1% to 10%:
    Cardiovascular: Tachycardia, bradycardia, flushing of face
    Central nervous system: CNS depression, increased intracranial pressure, fatigue, headache, nervousness, restlessness
    Gastrointestinal: Nausea, vomiting, constipation, stomach cramps, xerostomia
    Genitourinary: Decreased urination, ureteral spasm
    Hepatic: Increased LFTs
    Neuromuscular & skeletal: Trembling, weakness
    Respiratory: Respiratory depression, dyspnea
  <1% (Limited to important or life-threatening): Hallucinations, mental depression, myoclonus, paralytic ileus, pruritus, rash, seizures, urticaria
  (Continued)

Hydromorphone *(Continued)*

Overdosage/Toxicology Symptoms include CNS depression, respiratory depression, miosis, apnea, pulmonary edema, and convulsions. Treatment includes airway maintenance, I.V. line establishment, and administration of naloxone 2 mg I.V. (0.01 mg/kg for children), with repeat administration as necessary, up to a total of 10 mg.

Drug Interactions

Increased Effect/Toxicity: CNS depressants, phenothiazines, and tricyclic antidepressants may potentiate the adverse effects of hydromorphone.

Ethanol/Nutrition/Herb Interactions

Ethanol: Avoid ethanol (may increase CNS depression).

Herb/Nutraceutical: Avoid valerian, St John's wort, kava kava, gotu kola (may increase CNS depression).

Stability Store injection and oral dosage forms at 25°C (77°F). Protect tablets from light. A slightly yellowish discoloration has not been associated with a loss of potency; I.V. is **incompatible** when mixed with minocycline, prochlorperazine, sodium bicarbonate, tetracycline, thiopental.

Mechanism of Action Binds to opiate receptors in the CNS, causing inhibition of ascending pain pathways, altering the perception of and response to pain; causes cough supression by direct central action in the medulla; produces generalized CNS depression

Pharmacodynamics/Kinetics

Onset of action: Analgesic: 15-30 minutes

Peak effect: 0.5-1.5 hours

Duration: 4-5 hours

Metabolism: Hepatic; no active metabolites

Bioavailability: 62%

Half-life elimination: 1-3 hours

Excretion: Urine (primarily as glucuronide conjugates)

Usual Dosage

Doses should be titrated to appropriate analgesic effects; when changing routes of administration, note that oral doses are less than half as effective as parenteral doses (may be only one-fifth as effective)

Pain: Older Children and Adults:

Oral, I.M., I.V., S.C.: 1-4 mg/dose every 4-6 hours as needed; usual adult dose: 2 mg/dose

Rectal: 3 mg every 6-8 hours

Antitussive: Oral:

Children 6-12 years: 0.5 mg every 3-4 hours as needed

Children >12 years and Adults: 1 mg every 3-4 hours as needed

Dosing adjustment in hepatic impairment: Should be considered

Administration May be given S.C. or I.M.; for IVP, must be given slowly over 2-3 minutes (rapid IVP has been associated with an increase in side effects, especially respiratory depression and hypotension). Vial stopper contains latex.

Monitoring Parameters Pain relief, respiratory and mental status, blood pressure

Patient Information May cause drowsiness; avoid alcohol; take with food or milk to minimize GI distress

Nursing Implications Observe patient for oversedation, respiratory depression, implement safety measures

Additional Information Equianalgesic doses: Morphine 10 mg I.M. = hydromorphone 1.5 mg I.M.

Dosage Forms

Injection, as hydrochloride:

Dilaudid®: 1 mg/mL (1 mL); 2 mg/mL (1 mL, 20 mL); 4 mg/mL (1 mL)

Dilaudid-HP®: 10 mg/mL (1 mL, 2 mL, 5 mL)

Liquid, as hydrochloride (Dilaudid-5®): 1 mg/mL (1 mL, 4 mL, 8 mL, 120 mL, 250 mL, 480 mL, 500 mL)

Powder for injection, as hydrochloride (Dilaudid-HP®): 250 mg

Solution, oral, as hydrochloride: 5 mg/mL (120 mL, 250 mL, 500 mL) [raspberry flavor]

Suppository, rectal, as hydrochloride: 3 mg (6s)

Tablet, as hydrochloride: 2 mg, 4 mg, 8 mg

♦ **Hydromorphone Hydrochloride** *see* Hydromorphone *on page 685*

♦ **Hydromox®** *see* Quinethazone *on page 1168*

♦ **Hydropane®** *see* Hydrocodone and Homatropine *on page 679*

♦ **Hydroquinol** *see* Hydroquinone *on page 686*

Hydroquinone *(HYE droe kwin one)*

U.S. Brand Names Ambi® Skin Tone [OTC]; Eldopaque® [OTC]; Eldopaque Forte®; Eldoquin® [OTC]; Eldoquin® Forte®; Esoterica® Facial [OTC]; Esoterica® Regular [OTC]; Esoterica® Sensitive Skin Formula [OTC]; Esoterica® Sunscreen [OTC]; Melanex®; Melpaque HP®; Melquin HP® Melquin-3® [OTC]; Nuquin® Gel; Nuquin HP® Cream; Porcelana® [OTC]; Porcelana® Sunscreen [OTC]; Solaquin® [OTC]; Solaquin Forte®

Canadian Brand Names Eldopaque™; Eldoquin™; Neostrata® HQ; Solaquin™; Solaquin Forte™; Ultraquin™

Synonyms Hydroquinol; Quinol

Therapeutic Category Depigmenting Agent

Use Gradual bleaching of hyperpigmented skin conditions

Pregnancy Risk Factor C

Contraindications Hypersensitivity to hydroquinone or any component of the formulation; sunburn, depilatory usage

Warnings/Precautions Limit application to area no larger than face and neck or hands and arms

Adverse Reactions Frequency not defined.

Dermatologic: Dermatitis, dryness, erythema, stinging, inflammatory reaction, sensitization

Local: Irritation

Mechanism of Action Produces reversible depigmentation of the skin by suppression of melanocyte metabolic processes, in particular the inhibition of the enzymatic oxidation of tyrosine to DOPA (3,4-dihydroxyphenylalanine); sun exposure reverses this effect and will cause repigmentation.

Pharmacodynamics/Kinetics Onset and duration of depigmentation produced by hydroquinone varies among individuals

Usual Dosage Children >12 years and Adults: Topical: Apply thin layer and rub in twice daily

Patient Information Use sunscreens or clothing; do not use on irritated or denuded skin; stop using if rash or irritation develops; for external use only, avoid eye contact

Nursing Implications Use sunscreens or clothing; do not use on irritated or denuded skin; stop using if rash or irritation develops; for external use only, avoid contact with eyes

Dosage Forms
Cream, topical:
Eldopaque®, Eldoquin®, Esoterica® Facial, Esoterica® Regular, Porcelana® With Sunscreen: 2% (14.2 g, 28.4 g, 60 g, 85 g, 120 g)
Eldopaque Forte®, Eldoquin® Forte®, Melquin HP®: 4% (14.2 g, 28.4 g)
Esoterica® Sensitive Skin Formula: 1.5% (85 g)
Cream, topical, with sunscreen:
Esoterica® Sunscreen, Porcelana®, Solaquin®: 2% (28.4 g, 120 g)
Melpaque HP®, Nuquin HP®, Solaquin Forte®: 4% (14.2 g, 28.4 g)
Gel, topical, with sunscreen (Nuquin® Gel, Solaquin Forte® Gel): 4% (14.2 g, 28.4 g)
Solution, topical (Melanex®, Melquin-3®): 3% (30 mL)

♦ **HydroTex® [OTC]** *see Hydrocortisone on page 682*

♦ **Hydrotropine®** *see Hydrocodone and Homatropine on page 679*

Hydroxocobalamin (hye droks oh koe BAL a min)

U.S. Brand Names Hydro Cobex®; Hydro-Crysti-12®; LA-12®

Synonyms Vitamin B_{12}

Therapeutic Category Vitamin, Water Soluble

Use Treatment of pernicious anemia, vitamin B_{12} deficiency, increased B_{12} requirements due to pregnancy, thyrotoxicosis, hemorrhage, malignancy, liver or kidney disease

Unlabeled/Investigational Use Neuropathies, multiple sclerosis

Pregnancy Risk Factor A/C (dose exceeding RDA recommendation)

Contraindications Hypersensitivity to cyanocobalamin or any component of the formulation, cobalt; patients with hereditary optic nerve atrophy

Warnings/Precautions Some products contain benzoyl alcohol; avoid use in premature infants; an intradermal test dose should be performed for hypersensitivity; use only if oral supplementation not possible or when treating pernicious anemia

Adverse Reactions
1% to 10%:
Dermatologic: Itching
Gastrointestinal: Diarrhea
<1% (Limited to important or life-threatening): Peripheral vascular thrombosis

Stability Clear pink to red solutions are stable at room temperature; protect from light; incompatible with chlorpromazine, phytonadione, prochlorperazine, warfarin, ascorbic acid, dextrose, heavy metals, oxidizing or reducing agents; avoid freezing

Mechanism of Action Coenzyme for various metabolic functions, including fat and carbohydrate metabolism and protein synthesis, used in cell replication and hematopoiesis

Usual Dosage Vitamin B_{12} deficiency: I.M.:
Children: 1-5 mg given in single doses of 100 mcg over 2 or more weeks, followed by 30-50 mcg/month
Adults: 30 mcg/day for 5-10 days, followed by 100-200 mcg/month

Administration Administer I.M. only; may require coadministration of folic acid

Patient Information Therapy is required throughout life; do not take folic acid instead of B_{12} to prevent anemia

Nursing Implications Therapy is required throughout life; do not administer folic acid instead of B_{12} to prevent anemia

Dosage Forms Injection: 1000 mcg/mL (30 mL)

♦ **Hydroxycarbamide** *see Hydroxyurea on page 689*

Hydroxychloroquine (hye droks ee KLOR oh kwin)

U.S. Brand Names Plaquenil®

Canadian Brand Names Plaquenil®

Synonyms Hydroxychloroquine Sulfate

Therapeutic Category Antimalarial Agent

Use Suppression and treatment of acute attacks of malaria; treatment of systemic lupus erythematosus and rheumatoid arthritis

Unlabeled/Investigational Use Porphyria cutanea tarda, polymorphous light eruptions

Pregnancy Risk Factor C

Contraindications Hypersensitivity to hydroxychloroquine, 4-aminoquinoline derivatives, or any component of the formulation; retinal or visual field changes attributable to 4-aminoquinolines

Warnings/Precautions Use with caution in patients with hepatic disease, G6PD deficiency, psoriasis, and porphyria; long-term use in children is not recommended; perform baseline and periodic (6 months) ophthalmologic examinations; test periodically for muscle weakness

Adverse Reactions Frequency not defined.
Cardiovascular: Cardiomyopathy (rare, relationship to hydroxychloroquine unclear)
Central nervous system: Irritability, nervousness, emotional changes, nightmares, psychosis, headache, dizziness, vertigo, seizures, ataxia, lassitude
Dermatologic: Bleaching of hair, alopecia, pigmentation changes (skin and mucosal; black-blue color), rash (urticarial, morbilliform, lichenoid, maculopapular, purpuric, erythema
(Continued)

Hydroxychloroquine *(Continued)*

annulare centrifugum, Stevens-Johnson syndrome, acute generalized exanthematous pustulosis, and exfoliative dermatitis)

Endocrine & metabolic: Weight loss

Gastrointestinal: Anorexia, nausea, vomiting, diarrhea, abdominal cramping

Hematologic: Aplastic anemia, agranulocytosis, leukopenia, thrombocytopenia, hemolysis (in patients with glucose-6-phosphate deficiency)

Hepatic: Abnormal liver function/hepatic failure (isolated cases)

Neuromuscular & skeletal: Myopathy, palsy, or neuromyopathy leading to progressive weakness and atrophy of proximal muscle groups (may be associated with mild sensory changes, loss of deep tendon reflexes, and abnormal nerve conduction)

Ocular: Disturbance in accommodation, keratopathy, corneal changes/deposits (visual disturbances, blurred vision, photophobia - reversible on discontinuation), macular edema, atrophy, abnormal pigmentation, retinopathy (early changes reversible - may progress despite discontinuation if advanced), optic disc pallor/atrophy, attenuation of retinal arterioles, pigmentary retinopathy, scotoma, decreased visual acuity, nystagmus

Otic: Tinnitus, deafness

Miscellaneous: Exacerbation of porphyria and nonlight sensitive psoriasis

Overdosage/Toxicology Symptoms include headache, drowsiness, visual changes, cardiovascular collapse, and seizures, followed by respiratory and cardiac arrest. Treatment is symptomatic. Activated charcoal will bind the drug following GI decontamination. Urinary alkalinization will enhance renal elimination.

Drug Interactions

Increased Effect/Toxicity: Cimetidine increases levels of chloroquine and probably other 4-aminoquinolones.

Decreased Effect: Chloroquine and other 4-aminoquinolones absorption may be decreased due to GI binding with kaolin or magnesium trisilicate.

Ethanol/Nutrition/Herb Interactions Ethanol: Avoid ethanol (due to GI irritation).

Mechanism of Action Interferes with digestive vacuole function within sensitive malarial parasites by increasing the pH and interfering with lysosomal degradation of hemoglobin; inhibits locomotion of neutrophils and chemotaxis of eosinophils; impairs complement-dependent antigen-antibody reactions

Pharmacodynamics/Kinetics

Onset of action: Rheumatic disease: May require 4-6 weeks to respond

Absorption: Complete

Protein binding: 55%

Metabolism: Hepatic

Half-life elimination: 32-50 days

Time to peak: Rheumatic disease: Several months

Excretion: Urine (as metabolites and unchanged drug); may be enhanced by urinary acidification

Usual Dosage Note: Hydroxychloroquine sulfate 200 mg is equivalent to 155 mg hydroxychloroquine base and 250 mg chloroquine phosphate. Oral:

Children:

Chemoprophylaxis of malaria: 5 mg/kg (base) once weekly; should not exceed the recommended adult dose; begin 2 weeks before exposure; continue for 4-6 weeks after leaving endemic area; if suppressive therapy is not begun prior to the exposure, double the initial dose and give in 2 doses, 6 hours apart

Acute attack: 10 mg/kg (base) initial dose; followed by 5 mg/kg at 6, 24, and 48 hours

JRA or SLE: 3-5 mg/kg/day divided 1-2 times/day; avoid exceeding 7 mg/kg/day

Adults:

Chemoprophylaxis of malaria: 310 mg base weekly on same day each week; begin 2 weeks before exposure; continue for 4-6 weeks after leaving endemic area; if suppressive therapy is not begun prior to the exposure, double the initial dose and give in 2 doses, 6 hours apart

Acute attack: 620 mg first dose day 1; 310 mg in 6 hours day 1; 310 mg in 1 dose day 2; and 310 mg in 1 dose day 3

Rheumatoid arthritis: 310-465 mg/day to start taken with food or milk; increase dose until optimum response level is reached; usually after 4-12 weeks dose should be reduced by $\frac{1}{2}$ and a maintenance dose of 155-310 mg/day given

Lupus erythematosus: 310 mg every day or twice daily for several weeks depending on response; 155-310 mg/day for prolonged maintenance therapy

Dietary Considerations May be taken with food or milk.

Administration Administer with food or milk

Monitoring Parameters Ophthalmologic exam, CBC

Patient Information Take with food or milk; complete full course of therapy; wear sunglasses in bright sunlight; notify physician if blurring or other vision changes, ringing in the ears, or hearing loss occurs

Nursing Implications Periodic blood counts and eye examinations are recommended when patient is on chronic therapy

Dosage Forms Tablet, as sulfate: 200 mg [base 155 mg]

Extemporaneous Preparations A 25 mg/mL hydroxychloroquine sulfate suspension is made by removing the coating off of fifteen 200 mg hydroxychloroquine sulfate tablets with a towel moistened with alcohol; tablets are ground to a fine powder and levigated to a paste with 15 mL of Ora-Plus® suspending agent; add an additional 45 mL of suspending agent and levigate until a uniform mixture is obtained; qs ad to 120 mL with sterile water for irrigation; a 30 day expiration date is recommended, although stability testing has not been performed

Pesko LJ, "Compounding: Hydroxychloroquine," *Am Druggist*, 1993, 207:57.

Hydroxyprogesterone (hye droks ee proe JES te rone)

U.S. Brand Names Hylutin®; Prodrox®

Synonyms Hydroxyprogesterone Caproate

Therapeutic Category Progestin

Use Treatment of amenorrhea, abnormal uterine bleeding, endometriosis, uterine carcinoma

Pregnancy Risk Factor D

Contraindications Hypersensitivity to hydroxyprogesterone or any component of the formulation; thrombophlebitis; thromboembolic disorders; cerebral hemorrhage; liver impairment; carcinoma of the breast; undiagnosed vaginal bleeding; pregnancy

Warnings/Precautions Use with caution in patients with asthma, seizure disorders, migraine, cardiac or renal impairment, history of mental depression; use of any progestin during the first 4 months of pregnancy is not recommended; observe patients closely for signs and symptoms of thrombotic disorders

Adverse Reactions Frequency not defined.

Cardiovascular: Edema

Central nervous system: Mental depression, insomnia, fever, somnolence

Dermatologic: Melasma or chloasma, allergic rash with or without pruritus, acne, hirsutism

Endocrine & metabolic: Breakthrough bleeding, spotting, changes in menstrual flow, amenorrhea

Gastrointestinal: Anorexia, nausea, weight gain/loss

Genitourinary: Changes in cervical erosion and secretions, increased breast tenderness, galactorrhea

Hepatic: Cholestatic jaundice

Local: Pain at injection site

Neuromuscular & skeletal: Weakness

Overdosage/Toxicology Toxicity is unlikely following single exposures of excessive doses. Supportive treatment is adequate in most cases.

Drug Interactions

Decreased Effect: Rifampin may increase clearance of hydroxyprogesterone.

Stability Store at <40°C (15°C to 30°C); avoid freezing

Mechanism of Action Natural steroid hormone that induces secretory changes in the endometrium, promotes mammary gland development, relaxes uterine smooth muscle, blocks follicular maturation and ovulation and maintains pregnancy

Pharmacodynamics/Kinetics

Duration: Concentrations measurable for 3-4 weeks after injection

Metabolism: Hepatic

Time to peak, serum: I.M.: 3-7 days

Excretion: Urine

Usual Dosage Adults: Female: I.M.: *Long-acting progestin*

Amenorrhea: 375 mg; if no bleeding, begin cyclic treatment with estradiol valerate

Production of secretory endometrium and desquamation (Medical D and C): 125-250 mg administered on day 10 of cycle; repeat every 7 days until suppression is no longer desired.

Uterine carcinoma: 1 g one or more times/day (1-7 g/week) for up to 12 weeks

Administration Administer deep I.M. only

Test Interactions Thyroid function tests and liver function tests and endocrine function tests

Patient Information Take this medicine only as directed; do not exceed recommended dosage nor take it for a longer period of time; if you suspect you may have become pregnant, stop taking this medicine; take with food; patient package insert is available upon request; notify physician of pain in calves along with swelling and warmth, severe headache, visual disturbance

Nursing Implications Patients should receive a copy of the patient labeling for the drug

Dosage Forms Injection, as caproate (Hylutin®, Prodrox®): 250 mg/mL (5 mL)

♦ **Hydroxyprogesterone Caproate** *see* Hydroxyprogesterone *on page 689*

Hydroxyurea (hye droks ee yoor EE a)

U.S. Brand Names Droxia™; Hydrea®; Mylocel™

Canadian Brand Names Hydrea®

Synonyms Hydroxycarbamide

Therapeutic Category Antineoplastic Agent, Antimetabolite (Ribonucleotide Reductase Inhibitor)

Use CML in chronic phase; radiosensitizing agent in the treatment of primary brain tumors, head and neck tumors, uterine cervix and nonsmall cell lung cancer, and psoriasis; treatment of hematologic conditions such as essential thrombocythemia, polycythemia vera, hypereosinophilia, and hyperleukocytosis due to acute leukemia. Has shown activity against renal cell cancer, melanoma, ovarian cancer, head and neck cancer (excluding lip cancer), and prostate cancer.

Orphan drug: Droxia™: Sickle cell anemia: Specifically for patients >18 years of age who have had at least three "painful crises" in the previous year - to reduce frequency of these crises and the need for blood transfusions

Pregnancy Risk Factor D

Pregnancy/Breast-Feeding Implications Hydroxyurea is teratogenic and fetotoxic in animals; data on use during human pregnancy is limited. Effective contraception is recommended in women of childbearing potential.

Contraindications Hypersensitivity to hydroxyurea or any component of the formulation; severe anemia; severe bone marrow suppression; WBC <2500/mm³ or platelet count <100,000/mm³; pregnancy

Warnings/Precautions The U.S. Food and Drug Administration (FDA) currently recommends that procedures for proper handling and disposal of antineoplastic agents be considered. Use with caution in patients with renal impairment, in patients who have received prior irradiation therapy with exacerbation of postirradiation erythema, bone marrow suppression, erythrocytic (Continued)

Hydroxyurea (Continued)

abnormalities, mucositis, and in the elderly. May cause pancreatitis, neuropathy, or hepatotoxicity; risk is increased in HIV-infected patients receiving didanosine and/or stavudine. With long-term use (myeloproliferative disorders), secondary leukemias have been reported.

Adverse Reactions Frequency not defined.

Cardiovascular: Edema

Central nervous system: Drowsiness (with high doses), hallucinations, headache, dizziness, disorientation, seizures, fever, chills

Dermatologic: Erythema of the hands and face, maculopapular rash, pruritus, dry skin, dermatomyositis-like skin changes, hyperpigmentation, atrophy of skin and nails, scaling and violet papules (long-term use), nail banding, skin cancer

Endocrine & metabolic: Hyperuricemia

Gastrointestinal: Nausea, vomiting, stomatitis, anorexia, diarrhea, constipation, mucositis (potentiated in patients receiving radiation), pancreatitis, ulceration of buccal mucosa and GI epithelium (severe intoxication)

Emetic potential: Low (10% to 30%)

Genitourinary: Dysuria

Hematologic: Myelosuppression (primarily leukopenia); Dose-limiting toxicity, causes a rapid drop in leukocyte count (seen in 4-5 days in nonhematologic malignancy and more rapidly in leukemia); thrombocytopenia and anemia occur less often

Onset: 24-48 hours

Nadir: 10 days

Recovery: 7 days after stopping drug (reversal of WBC count occurs rapidly but the platelet count may take 7-10 days to recover)

Other hematologic effects include megaloblastic erythropoiesis, macrocytosis, hemolysis, decreased serum iron, persistent cytopenias, secondary leukemias (long-term use)

Hepatic: Elevation of hepatic enzymes, hepatotoxicity, hyperbilirubinemia (polycythemia vera)

Neuromuscular & skeletal: Weakness, peripheral neuropathy

Renal: Increased creatinine and BUN due to impairment of renal tubular function

Respiratory: Acute diffuse pulmonary infiltrates (rare), dyspnea, pulmonary fibrosis

Overdosage/Toxicology Symptoms include myelosuppression, facial swelling, hallucinations, and disorientation. Treatment is supportive.

Drug Interactions

Increased Effect/Toxicity: Zidovudine, zalcitabine, didanosine may increase synergy. The potential for neurotoxicity may increase with concomitant administration with fluorouracil. Hydroxyurea modulates the metabolism and cytotoxicity of cytarabine; dose reduction is recommended. Hydroxyurea may precipitate didanosine- or stavudine-induced pancreatitis, hepatotoxicity, or neuropathy; concomitant use is not recommended.

Stability Store capsules at room temperature; capsules may be opened and emptied into water (will not dissolve completely)

Mechanism of Action Thought to interfere (unsubstantiated hypothesis) with synthesis of DNA, during the S phase of cell division, without interfering with RNA synthesis; inhibits ribonucleoside diphosphate reductase, preventing conversion of ribonucleotides to deoxyribonucleotides; cell-cycle specific for the S phase and may hold other cells in the G_1 phase of the cell cycle.

Pharmacodynamics/Kinetics

Absorption: Readily (≥80%)

Distribution: Readily crosses blood-brain barrier; well into intestine, brain, lung, kidney tissues, effusions and ascites; enters breast milk

Metabolism: Hepatic; 50% degradation by enzymes of intestinal bacteria

Half-life elimination: 3-4 hours

Time to peak: ~2 hours

Excretion: Urine (80%, 50% as unchanged drug, 30% as urea); exhaled gases (as CO_2)

Usual Dosage Oral (refer to individual protocols): All dosage should be based on ideal or actual body weight, whichever is less:

Children:

No FDA-approved dosage regimens have been established; dosages of 1500-3000 mg/m² as a single dose in combination with other agents every 4-6 weeks have been used in the treatment of pediatric astrocytoma, medulloblastoma, and primitive neuroectodermal tumors

CML: Initial: 10-20 mg/kg/day once daily; adjust dose according to hematologic response

Adults: Dose should always be titrated to patient response and WBC counts; usual oral doses range from 10-30 mg/kg/day or 500-3000 mg/day; if WBC count falls to <2500 cells/mm³, or the platelet count to <100,000/mm³, therapy should be stopped for at least 3 days and resumed when values rise toward normal

Solid tumors:

Intermittent therapy: 80 mg/kg as a single dose every third day

Continuous therapy: 20-30 mg/kg/day given as a single dose/day

Concomitant therapy with irradiation: 80 mg/kg as a single dose every third day starting at least 7 days before initiation of irradiation

Resistant chronic myelocytic leukemia: Continuous therapy: 20-30 mg/kg as a single daily dose

HIV: 1000-1500 mg daily in a single dose or divided doses

Sickle cell anemia (moderate/severe disease): Initial: 15 mg/kg/day, increased by 5 mg/kg every 12 weeks if blood counts are in an acceptable range until the maximum tolerated dose of 35 mg/kg/day is achieved or the dose that does not produce toxic effects

Acceptable range:

Neutrophils ≥2500 cells/mm³

Platelets ≥95,000/mm³

Hemoglobin >5.3 g/dL, and

Reticulocytes ≥95,000/mm³ if the hemoglobin concentration is <9 g/dL

Toxic range:
Neutrophils <2000 cells/mm^3
Platelets <80,000/mm^3
Hemoglobin <4.5 g/dL
Reticulocytes <80,000/mm^3 if the hemoglobin concentration is <9 g/dL
Monitor for toxicity every 2 weeks; if toxicity occurs, stop treatment until the bone marrow recovers; restart at 2.5 mg/kg/day less than the dose at which toxicity occurs; if no toxicity occurs over the next 12 weeks, then the subsequent dose should be increased by 2.5 mg/kg/day; reduced dosage of hydroxyurea alternating with erythropoietin may decrease myelotoxicity and increase levels of fetal hemoglobin in patients who have not been helped by hydroxyurea alone

Dosing adjustment in renal impairment:
Cl$_{cr}$ 10-50 mL/minute: Administer 50% of normal dose
Cl$_{cr}$ <10 mL/minute: Administer 20% of normal dose
Hemodialysis: Supplemental dose is not necessary. Hydroxyurea is a low molecular weight compound with high aqueous solubility that may be freely dialyzable, however, clinical studies confirming this hypothesis have not been performed; peak serum concentrations are reached within 2 hours after oral administration and by 24 hours, the concentration in the serum is zero
CAPD effects: Unknown
CAVH effects: Dose for GFR 10-50 mL/minute

Administration Capsules may be opened and emptied into water (will not dissolve completely).

Monitoring Parameters CBC with differential, platelets, hemoglobin, renal function and liver function tests, serum uric acid

Patient Information Take capsules exactly on schedule directed by prescriber (dosage and timing will be specific to purpose of therapy). Contents of capsule may be emptied into a glass of water and taken immediately. You will require frequent monitoring and blood tests while taking this medication to assess effectiveness and monitor adverse reactions. You will be susceptible to infection; avoid crowds, infected persons, and persons with contagious diseases. You may experience nausea, vomiting, or loss of appetite (small frequent meals, frequent mouth care, sucking lozenges, or chewing gum may help); constipation (increased exercise, fluid, or dietary fiber may help); diarrhea (buttermilk, boiled milk, or yogurt may help); mouth sores (frequent mouth care will help). Report persistent vomiting, diarrhea, constipation, stomach pain, or mouth sores; skin rash, redness, irritation, or sores; painful or difficult urination; increased confusion, depression, hallucinations, lethargy, or seizures; persistent fever or chills, unusual fatigue, white plaques in mouth, vaginal discharge, or unhealed sores; unusual lassitude, weakness, or muscle tremors; easy bruising/bleeding; or blood in vomitus, stool, or urine. People not taking hydroxyurea should not be exposed to it; if powder from capsule is spilled, wipe up with damp, disposable towel immediately, and discard the towel in a closed container, such as a plastic bag; wash hands thoroughly. Contraceptive measures are recommended during therapy.

Additional Information Although I.V. use is reported, no parenteral product is commercially available in the U.S.

If WBC decreases to <2500/mm^3 or platelet count to <100,000/mm^3, interrupt therapy until values rise significantly toward normal. Treat anemia with whole blood replacement; do not interrupt therapy. Adequate trial period to determine effectiveness is 6 weeks. Almost all patients receiving hydroxyurea in clinical trials needed to have their medication stopped for a time to allow their low blood count to return to acceptable levels.

Dosage Forms
Capsule: 500 mg
Droxia™: 200 mg, 300 mg, 400 mg
Hydrea®: 500 mg
Tablet (Mylocel™): 1000 mg

♦ **25-Hydroxyvitamin D$_3$** *see* Calcifediol *on page 203*

HydrOXYzine (hye DROKS i zeen)

U.S. Brand Names ANX®; Atarax®; Hyzine-50®; Restall®; Vistacot®; Vistaril®
Canadian Brand Names Apo®-Hydroxyzine; Atarax™; Novo-Hydroxyzin; PMS-Hydroxyzine; Vistaril®
Synonyms Hydroxyzine Hydrochloride; Hydroxyzine Pamoate
Therapeutic Category Antianxiety Agent; Antiemetic; Antihistamine, H$_1$ Blocker; Sedative
Use Treatment of anxiety; preoperative sedative; antipruritic
Unlabeled/Investigational Use Antiemetic; ethanol withdrawal symptoms
Pregnancy Risk Factor C
Contraindications Hypersensitivity to hydroxyzine or any component of the formulation
Warnings/Precautions Causes sedation, caution must be used in performing tasks which require alertness (ie, operating machinery or driving). Sedative effects of CNS depressants or ethanol are potentiated. S.C., intra-arterial, and I.V. administration are not recommended since thrombosis and digital gangrene can occur; extravasation can result in sterile abscess and marked tissue induration; should be used with caution in patients with narrow-angle glaucoma, prostatic hypertrophy, and bladder neck obstruction; should also be used with caution in patients with asthma or COPD.

Anticholinergic effects are not well tolerated in the elderly. Hydroxyzine may be useful as a short-term antipruritic, but it is not recommended for use as a sedative or anxiolytic in the elderly.

Adverse Reactions Frequency not defined.
Central nervous system: Drowsiness, headache, fatigue, nervousness, dizziness
Gastrointestinal: Xerostomia
Neuromuscular & skeletal: Tremor, paresthesia, seizure
Ocular: Blurred vision
Respiratory: Thickening of bronchial secretions
(Continued)

HydrOXYzine (Continued)

Overdosage/Toxicology Symptoms include seizures, sedation, and hypotension. There is no specific treatment for antihistamine overdose, however, clinical toxicity is mostly due to anticholinergic effects. Anticholinesterase inhibitors may be useful by reducing acetylcholinesterase. For anticholinergic overdose with severe life-threatening symptoms, physostigmine 1-2 mg (0.5 mg or 0.02 mg/kg for children) slow I.V. may be given to reverse these effects.

Drug Interactions

Increased Effect/Toxicity: CNS depressants, anticholinergics, used in combination with hydroxyzine may result in additive effects.

Ethanol/Nutrition/Herb Interactions

Ethanol: Avoid ethanol (may increase CNS depression).

Herb/Nutraceutical: Avoid valerian, St John's wort, kava kava, gotu kola (may increase CNS depression).

Stability Protect from light; store at 15°C to 30°C and protected from freezing; I.V. is **incompatible** when mixed with aminophylline, amobarbital, chloramphenicol, dimenhydrinate, heparin, penicillin G, pentobarbital, phenobarbital, phenytoin, ranitidine, sulfisoxazole, vitamin B complex with C

Mechanism of Action Competes with histamine for H_1-receptor sites on effector cells in the gastrointestinal tract, blood vessels, and respiratory tract. Possesses skeletal muscle relaxing, bronchodilator, antihistamine, antiemetic, and analgesic properties.

Pharmacodynamics/Kinetics

Onset of action: 15-30 minutes

Duration: 4-6 hours

Absorption: Oral: Rapid

Metabolism: Exact fate is unknown

Half-life elimination: 3-7 hours

Time to peak: ~2 hours

Usual Dosage

Children:

I.M.: 0.5-1.1 mg/kg/dose every 4-6 hours as needed

Oral: 0.6 mg/kg/dose every 6 hours

Adults:

Antiemetic: I.M.: 25-100 mg/dose every 4-6 hours as needed

Anxiety: Oral: 25-100 mg 4 times/day; maximum dose: 600 mg/day

Preoperative sedation:

Oral: 50-100 mg

I.M.: 25-100 mg

Management of pruritus: Oral: 25 mg 3-4 times/day

Dosing interval in hepatic impairment: Change dosing interval to every 24 hours in patients with primary biliary cirrhosis

Administration For I.M. administration in children, injections should be made into the midlateral muscles of the thigh; S.C., intra-arterial, and I.V. administration **not** recommended since thrombosis and digital gangrene can occur

Monitoring Parameters Relief of symptoms, mental status, blood pressure

Patient Information Will cause drowsiness, avoid alcohol and other CNS depressants, avoid driving and other hazardous tasks until the CNS effects are known

Nursing Implications Extravasation can result in sterile abscess and marked tissue induration; provide safety measures (ie, side rails, night light, and call button); remove smoking materials from area; supervise ambulation

Additional Information Although not recommended in the product labeling due to the possibility of arterial and venous spasms, intravascular hemolysis, and orthostatic hypotension, hydroxyzine can be administered as a short (15- to 30-minute) I.V. infusion.

Hydroxyzine hydrochloride: Anxanil®, Atarax®, Hydroxacen®, Quiess®, Vistaril® injection, Vistazine®

Hydroxyzine pamoate: Hy-Pam®, Vistaril® capsule and suspension

Dosage Forms

Capsule, as pamoate: 25 mg, 50 mg, 100 mg

Injection, as hydrochloride: 25 mg/mL (1 mL, 2 mL, 10 mL); 50 mg/mL (1 mL, 2 mL, 10 mL)

Suspension, oral, as pamoate: 25 mg/5 mL (120 mL, 480 mL)

Syrup, as hydrochloride: 10 mg/5 mL (120 mL, 480 mL, 4000 mL)

Tablet, as hydrochloride: 10 mg, 25 mg, 50 mg, 100 mg

♦ **Hydroxyzine Hydrochloride** see HydrOXYzine on page 691
♦ **Hydroxyzine Pamoate** see HydrOXYzine on page 691
♦ **Hygroton® [DSC]** see Chlorthalidone on page 284
♦ **Hylorel®** see Guanadrel on page 649
♦ **Hylutin®** see Hydroxyprogesterone on page 689
♦ **Hyoscine** see Scopolamine on page 1225

Hyoscyamine (hye oh SYE a meen)

U.S. Brand Names Anaspaz®; A-Spas® S/L; Cystospaz®; Cystospaz-M®; ED-SPAZ®; Hyosine; Levbid®; Levsin®; Levsinex®; Levsin/SL®; NuLev™; Spacol; Spacol T/S; Symax SL; Symax SR

Canadian Brand Names Cystospaz®; Levsin®

Synonyms Hyoscyamine Sulfate; l-Hyoscyamine Sulfate

Therapeutic Category Anticholinergic Agent; Antispasmodic Agent, Gastrointestinal

Use

Oral: Adjunctive therapy for peptic ulcers, irritable bowel, neurogenic bladder/bowel; treatment of infant colic, GI tract disorders caused by spasm; to reduce rigidity, tremors, sialorrhea, and hyperhidrosis associated with parkinsonism; as a drying agent in acute rhinitis

Injection: Preoperative antimuscarinic to reduce secretions and block cardiac vagal inhibitory reflexes; to improve radiologic visibility of the kidneys; symptomatic relief of biliary and renal colic; reduce GI motility to facilitate diagnostic procedures (ie, endoscopy, hypotonic duodenography); reduce pain and hypersecretion in pancreatitis, certain cases of partial heart block associated with vagal activity; reversal of neuromuscular blockade

Pregnancy Risk Factor C

Pregnancy/Breast-Feeding Implications Crosses the placenta, effects to the fetus not known; use during pregnancy only if clearly needed. Excreted in breast milk; breast-feeding is not recommended.

Contraindications Hypersensitivity to belladonna alkaloids or any component of the formulation; glaucoma; obstructive uropathy; myasthenia gravis; obstructive GI tract disease, paralytic ileus, intestinal atony of elderly or debilitated patients, severe ulcerative colitis, toxic megacolon complicating ulcerative colitis; unstable cardiovascular status in acute hemorrhage, myocardial ischemia

Warnings/Precautions Heat prostration may occur in hot weather. Diarrhea may be a sign of incomplete intestinal obstruction, treatment should be discontinued if this occurs. May produce side effects as seen with other anticholinergic medications including drowsiness, dizziness, blurred vision, or psychosis. Children and the elderly may be more susceptible to these effects. Use with caution in children with spastic paralysis. Use with caution in patients with autonomic neuropathy, coronary heart disease, congestive heart failure, cardiac arrhythmias, prostatic hyperplasia, hyperthyroidism, hypertension, chronic lung disease, renal disease, and hiatal hernia associated with reflux esophagitis. Use with caution in the elderly, may precipitate undiagnosed glaucoma and/or severely impair memory function (especially in those patients with previous memory problems).

NuLev™: Contains phenylalanine

Adverse Reactions Frequency not defined.
Cardiovascular: Palpitations, tachycardia
Central nervous system: Ataxia, dizziness, drowsiness, headache, insomnia, mental confusion/excitement, nervousness, speech disorder, weakness
Dermatologic: Urticaria
Endocrine & metabolic: Lactation suppression
Gastrointestinal: Bloating, constipation, dry mouth, loss of taste, nausea, vomiting
Genitourinary: Impotence, urinary hesitancy, urinary retention
Ocular: Blurred vision, cycloplegia, increased ocular tension, mydriasis
Miscellaneous: Allergic reactions, sweating decreased

Overdosage/Toxicology Symptoms include dilated, unreactive pupils; blurred vision; hot, dry, flushed skin; dry mucous membranes; difficulty swallowing, foul breath, diminished or absent bowel sounds, urinary retention, tachycardia, hyperthermia, hypertension, and increased respiratory rate. Anticholinergic toxicity is caused by strong binding of the drug to cholinergic receptors. Anticholinesterase inhibitors reduce acetylcholinesterase, the enzyme that breaks down acetylcholine and thereby allows acetylcholine to accumulate and compete for receptor binding with the offending anticholinergic. For anticholinergic overdose with severe life-threatening symptoms, physostigmine 1-2 mg (0.5 mg or 0.02 mg/kg for children) S.C. or slow I.V. may be given to reverse these effects.

Drug Interactions
Increased Effect/Toxicity: Increased toxicity with amantadine, antihistamines, antimuscarinics, haloperidol, phenothiazines, tricyclic antidepressants, and MAO inhibitors.
Decreased Effect: Decreased effect with antacids.

Stability Store at controlled room temperature. Protect NuLev™ from moisture.

Mechanism of Action Blocks the action of acetylcholine at parasympathetic sites in smooth muscle, secretory glands and the CNS; increases cardiac output, dries secretions, antagonizes histamine and serotonin

Pharmacodynamics/Kinetics
Onset of action: 2-3 minutes
Duration: 4-6 hours
Absorption: Well absorbed
Distribution: Crosses placenta; small amounts enter breast milk
Protein binding: 50%
Metabolism: Hepatic
Half-life elimination: 13% to 38%
Excretion: Urine

Usual Dosage
Oral: Children: Gastrointestinal disorders: Dose as listed, based on age and weight (kg) using 0.125 mg/mL drops; repeat dose every 4 hours as needed:
Children <2 years:
3.4 kg: 4 drops; maximum: 24 drops/24 hours
5 kg: 5 drops; maximum: 30 drops/24 hours
7 kg: 6 drops; maximum: 36 drops/24 hours
10 kg: 8 drops; maximum: 48 drops/24 hours
Oral, S.L.:
Children 2-12 years: Gastrointestinal disorders: Dose as listed, based on age and weight (kg); repeat dose every 4 hours as needed:
10 kg: 0.031-0.033 mg; maximum: 0.75 mg/24 hours
20 kg: 0.0625 mg; maximum: 0.75 mg/24 hours
40 kg: 0.0938 mg; maximum: 0.75 mg/24 hours
50 kg: 0.125 mg; maximum: 0.75 mg/24 hours
Children >12 years and Adults: Gastrointestinal disorders: 0.125-0.25 mg every 4 hours or as needed (before meals or food); maximum: 1.5 mg/24 hours
Cystospaz®: 0.15-0.3 mg up to 4 times/day
Oral (timed release): Children >12 years and Adults: Gastrointestinal disorders: 0.375-0.75 mg every 12 hours; maximum: 1.5 mg/24 hours
I.M., I.V., S.C.: Children >12 years and Adults: Gastrointestinal disorders: 0.25-0.5 mg; may repeat as needed up to 4 times/day, at 4-hour intervals
(Continued)

Hyoscyamine *(Continued)*

I.V.: Children >2 year and Adults: I.V.: Preanesthesia: 5 mcg/kg given 30-60 minutes prior to induction of anesthesia or at the time preoperative narcotics or sedatives are administered

I.V.: Adults: Diagnostic procedures: 0.25-0.5 mg given 5-10 minutes prior to procedure

To reduce drug-induced bradycardia during surgery: 0.125 mg; repeat as needed

To reverse neuromuscular blockade: 0.2 mg for every 1 mg neostigmine (or the physostigmine/pyridostigmine equivalent)

Dietary Considerations Should be taken before meals or food; NuLev™ contains phenylalanine

Administration

Oral: Tablets should be administered before meals or food.

Levbid®: Tablets are scored and may be broken in half for dose titration; do not crush or chew.

Levsin/SL®: Tablets may be used sublingually, chewed, or swallowed whole.

NuLev™: Tablet is placed on tongue and allowed to disintegrate before swallowing; may take with or without water.

Symax SL: Tablets may be used sublingually or swallowed whole.

I.M.: May be administered without dilution.

Inject over at least 1 minute. May be administered without dilution.

Patient Information Maintain good oral hygiene habits, because lack of saliva may increase chance of cavities. Observe caution while driving or performing other tasks requiring alertness, as may cause drowsiness, dizziness, or blurred vision. Notify physician if skin rash, flushing or eye pain occurs; or if difficulty in urinating, constipation or sensitivity to light becomes severe or persists.

Nursing Implications Observe for tachycardia if patient has cardiac problems. Do not crush or chew extended release forms.

Dosage Forms

Capsule, timed release, as sulfate (Cystospaz-M®, Levsinex®): 0.375 mg

Elixir, as sulfate (Hyosine, Levsin®): 0.125 mg/5 mL [orange flavor with alcohol 20%] (480 mL)

Injection, as sulfate (Levsin®): 0.5 mg/mL (1 mL)

Liquid, as sulfate (Spacol): 0.125 mg/5 mL [sugar free, alcohol free, simethicone based, bubble-gum flavor] (120 mL)

Solution, oral drops, as sulfate (Hyosine, Levsin®): 0.125 mg/mL [orange flavor with alcohol 5%] (15 mL)

Tablet (Cystospaz®): 0.15 mg

Tablet, as sulfate (Anaspaz®, ED-SPAZ®, Levsin®, Spacol): 0.125 mg

Tablet, extended release, as sulfate (Levbid®, Symax SR, Spacol T/S): 0.375 mg

Tablet, orally disintegrating, as sulfate (NuLev™): 0.125 mg [contains phenylalanine 1.7 mg/tablet, mint flavor]

Tablet, sublingual, as sulfate:

Levsin/SL®: 0.125 mg [peppermint flavor]

A-Spas® S/L, Symax SL: 0.125 mg

Hyoscyamine, Atropine, Scopolamine, and Phenobarbital

(hye oh SYE a meen, A troe peen, skoe POL a meen & fee noe BAR bi tal)

U.S. Brand Names Barbidonna®; Bellatal®; Donnatal®

Canadian Brand Names Donnatal®

Synonyms Atropine, Hyoscyamine, Scopolamine, and Phenobarbital; Phenobarbital, Hyoscyamine, Atropine, and Scopolamine; Scopolamine, Hyoscyamine, Atropine, and Phenobarbital

Therapeutic Category Anticholinergic Agent; Antispasmodic Agent, Gastrointestinal

Use Adjunct in treatment of peptic ulcer disease, irritable bowel, spastic colitis, spastic bladder, and renal colic

Pregnancy Risk Factor C

Contraindications Hypersensitivity to hyoscyamine, atropine, scopolamine, phenobarbital, or any component of the formulation; narrow-angle glaucoma, tachycardia, GI and GU obstruction, myasthenia gravis

Warnings/Precautions Use with caution in patients with hepatic or renal disease, hyperthyroidism, cardiovascular disease, hypertension, prostatic hyperplasia, autonomic neuropathy in the elderly; abrupt withdrawal may precipitate status epilepticus. Because of the anticholinergic effects of this product, it is not recommended for use in the elderly.

Adverse Reactions Frequency not defined.

Cardiovascular: Tachycardia, palpitations, hypotension

Central nervous system: Fatigue, delirium, restlessness, drowsiness, headache, ataxia, confusion, impairment of judgment and coordination

Dermatologic: Dry hot skin, skin rash

Gastrointestinal: Impaired GI motility, xerostomia, constipation

Genitourinary: Urinary hesitancy/retention

Neuromuscular & skeletal: Tremors

Ocular: Mydriasis, blurred vision, dry eyes

Respiratory: Respiratory depression (rare)

Overdosage/Toxicology Symptoms include unsteady gait, slurred speech, confusion, hypotension, respiratory collapse, dilated unreactive pupils, hot or flushed skin, diminished bowel sounds, and urinary retention. Anticholinergic toxicity is caused by strong binding of the drug to cholinergic receptors. Anticholinesterase inhibitors reduce acetylcholinesterase, the enzyme that breaks down acetylcholine and thereby allows acetylcholine to accumulate and compete for receptor binding with the offending anticholinergic. For anticholinergic overdose with severe life-threatening symptoms, physostigmine 1-2 mg (0.5 mg or 0.02 mg/kg for children) S.C. or slow I.V. may be given to reverse these effects.

Drug Interactions

Increased Effect/Toxicity: Toxicity of CNS depressants, coumarin anticoagulants, amantadine, antihistamine, phenothiazides, antidiarrheal suspensions, corticosteroids, digitalis, griseofulvin, tetracyclines, anticonvulsants, MAO inhibitors, and tricyclic antidepressants may be increased.

Mechanism of Action Refer to individual agents

Pharmacodynamics/Kinetics Absorption: Well absorbed

Usual Dosage Oral:

Children 2-12 years: Kinesed® dose: $^1/_2$ to 1 tablet 3-4 times/day

Children: Donnatal® elixir: 0.1 mL/kg/dose every 4 hours; maximum dose: 5 mL **OR** alternatively, dose (mL) based on weight (kg):

4.5 kg: 0.5 mL every 4 hours OR 0.75 mL every 6 hours

10 kg: 1 mL every 4 hours OR 1.5 mL every 6 hours

14 kg: 1.5 mL every 4 hours OR 2 mL every 6 hours

23 kg: 2.5 mL every 4 hours OR 3.8 mL every 6 hours

34 kg: 3.8 mL every 4 hours OR 5 mL every 6 hours

≥45 kg: 5 mL every 4 hours OR 7.5 mL every 6 hours

Adults: 1-2 capsules or tablets 3-4 times/day; or 1 Donnatal® Extentab® in sustained release form every 12 hours; or 5-10 mL elixir 3-4 times/day or every 8 hours

Dietary Considerations Should be taken 30-60 minutes before meals unless otherwise directed.

Patient Information Maintain good oral hygiene habits, because lack of saliva may increase chance of cavities. Observe caution while driving or performing other tasks requiring alertness, as may cause drowsiness, dizziness, or blurred vision. Notify physician if skin rash, flushing or eye pain occurs; or if difficulty in urinating, constipation, or sensitivity to light becomes severe or persists. Do not attempt tasks requiring mental alertness or physical coordination until you know the effects of the drug. Swallow extended release tablet whole, do not crush or chew.

Nursing Implications Do not crush extended release tablets

Dosage Forms

Capsule (Donnatal®): Hyoscyamine sulfate 0.1037 mg, atropine sulfate 0.0194 mg, scopolamine hydrobromide 0.0065 mg, and phenobarbital 16.2 mg

Elixir (Donnatal®): Hyoscyamine sulfate 0.1037 mg, atropine sulfate 0.0194 mg, scopolamine hydrobromide 0.0065 mg, and phenobarbital 16.2 mg per 5 mL (120 mL, 480 mL, 4000 mL)

Tablet:

Barbidonna®: Hyoscyamine hydrobromide 0.1286 mg, atropine sulfate 0.025 mg, scopolamine hydrobromide 0.0074 mg, and phenobarbital 16 mg

Barbidonna® No. 2: Hyoscyamine hydrobromide 0.1286 mg, atropine sulfate 0.025 mg, scopolamine hydrobromide 0.0074 mg, and phenobarbital 32 mg

Bellatal®, Donnatal®: Hyoscyamine sulfate 0.1037 mg, atropine sulfate 0.0194 mg, scopolamine hydrobromide 0.0065 mg, and phenobarbital 16.2 mg

Tablet, long-acting (Donnatal®): Hyoscyamine sulfate 0.3111 mg, atropine sulfate 0.0582 mg, scopolamine hydrobromide 0.0195 mg, and phenobarbital 48.6 mg

Ibritumomab (ib ri TYOO mo mab)

U.S. Brand Names Zevalin™

Synonyms Ibritumomab Tiuxetan; In-111 Zevalin; Y-90 Zevalin

Therapeutic Category Antineoplastic Agent, Monoclonal Antibody; Radiopharmaceutical

Use Treatment of relapsed or refractory low-grade, follicular, or transformed B-cell non-Hodgkin's lymphoma (including rituximab-refractory follicular non-Hodgkin's lymphoma) as part of a therapeutic regimen with rituximab (Zevalin™ therapeutic regimen); **not to be used as single-agent therapy**; must be radiolabeled prior to use

Pregnancy Risk Factor D

Pregnancy/Breast-Feeding Implications No adequate or well-controlled studies in pregnant women. Y-90 ibritumomab may cause fetal harm. Women of childbearing potential should avoid becoming pregnant during treatment with ibritumomab. Both males and females should use effective contraception for 12 months following treatment. The effect on future

(Continued)

695

Ibritumomab (Continued)

fertility is unknown. It is not known whether ibrutomomab is excreted in breast milk; women are advised to discontinue breast-feeding and substitute with formula feedings.

Contraindications Known type I hypersensitivity or anaphylactic reactions to murine proteins, rituximab, yttrium chloride, indium chloride, or any component of the formulation; ≥25% lymphoma marrow involvement; prior myeloablative therapies; platelet count <100,000 cells/mm³; neutrophil count <1,500 cells/mm³; hypocellular bone marrow (≤15% cellularity of marked reduction in bone marrow precursors); history of failed stem cell collection; pregnancy; breast-feeding. Y-90 ibritumomab should not be administered to patients with altered In-111 ibritumomab biodistribution.

Warnings/Precautions To be used as part of the Zevalin™ therapeutic regimen (in combination with rituximab). The contents of the kit are not radioactive until radiolabeling occurs. During and after radiolabeling, adequate shielding should be used with this product, in accordance with institutional radiation safety practices.

Severe, potentially-fatal infusion reactions (angioedema, bronchospasm, hypotension, hypoxia) have been reported, typically during the first rituximab infusion (during infusion or within 30-120 minutes of infusion). Patients should be screened for human antimouse antibodies (HAMA); may be at increased risk of allergic or serious hypersensitivity reactions. Interrupt infusion for severe reactions. Consult additional warnings for rituximab. Therapy is associated with severe hematologic adverse events (thrombocytopenia, neutropenia), severe infections, and hemorrhage (including fatal cerebral hemorrhage). Do not administer to patients with impaired bone marrow reserve (see Contraindications).

Safety and efficacy of repeated courses of the therapeutic regimen have not been established. Safety and efficacy have not been established in pediatric patients.

Adverse Reactions Severe, potentially life-threatening allergic reactions have occurred in association with infusions. Also refer to Rituximab monograph.

>10%:
  Central nervous system: Chills (24%), fever (17%), pain (13%), headache (12%)
  Gastrointestinal: Nausea (31%), abdominal pain (16%), vomiting (12%)
  Hematologic: Thrombocytopenia (95%), neutropenia (77%), anemia (61%)
    Myelosuppressive:
      WBC: Severe
      Platelets: Severe
      Nadir: 7-9 weeks
      Recovery: 22-35 days
  Neuromuscular & skeletal: Weakness (43%)
  Respiratory: Dyspnea (14%)
  Miscellaneous: Infection (29%)

1% to 10%:
  Cardiovascular: Peripheral edema (8%), hypotension (6%), flushing (6%), angioedema (5%)
  Central nervous system: Dizziness (10%), insomnia (5%), anxiety (4%)
  Dermatologic: Pruritus (9%), rash (8%), urticaria (4%), petechia (3%)
  Gastrointestinal: Diarrhea (9%), anorexia (8%), abdominal distension (5%), constipation (5%), dyspepsia (5%), melena (2%; life threatening in 1%), gastrointestinal hemorrhage (1%)
  Hematologic: Bruising (7%), pancytopenia (2%), secondary malignancies (2%)
  Neuromuscular & skeletal: Back pain (8%), arthralgia (7%), myalgia (7%)
  Respiratory: Cough (10%), throat irritation (10%), rhinitis (6%), bronchospasm (5%), epistaxis (3%), apnea (1%)
  Miscellaneous: Diaphoresis (4%), allergic reaction (2%; life-threatening in 1%)

<1%: Arthritis, encephalopathy, hematemesis, pulmonary edema, pulmonary embolism, stroke (hemorrhagic), subdural hematoma, tachycardia, urticaria, vaginal hemorrhage. Myeloid malignancies and dysplasia have also been reported in patients who had received treatment with ibritumomab.

Overdosage/Toxicology Symptoms may include severe hematological toxicity. Treatment is supportive. In early clinical experience with high dosages, some patients required autologous stem cell transplantation.

Drug Interactions

Increased Effect/Toxicity: Due to the high incidence of thrombocytopenia associated with ibritumomab, the use of agents which decrease platelet function may be associated with a higher risk of bleeding (includes aspirin, NSAIDs, glycoprotein IIb/IIIa antagonists, clopidogrel and ticlopidine). In addition, the risk of bleeding may be increased with anticoagulant agents, including heparin, low molecular weight heparins, thrombolytics, and warfarin. The safety of live viral vaccines has not been established.

Decreased Effect: Response to vaccination may be impaired.

Ethanol/Nutrition/Herb Interactions Herb/Nutraceutical: Avoid cat's claw, dong quai, evening primrose, feverfew, garlic, ginger, ginkgo, red clover, horse chestnut, green tea, ginseng (all have antiplatelet activity).

Stability Store at 2°C to 8°C (36°F to 46°F). Do not freeze. Kit is not radioactive.

To prepare radiolabeled injection, follow preparation guidelines provided by manufacturer. Should be done only by individuals trained in the preparation of radiopharmaceuticals in a facility which is designated for this purpose.

Mechanism of Action Ibritumomab is a monoclonal antibody directed against the CD20 antigen found on B lymphocytes (normal and malignant). Ibritumomab binding induces apoptosis in B lymphocytes *in vitro*. It is combined with the chelator tiuxetan, which acts as a specific chelation site for either Indium-111 (In-111) or Yttrium-90 (Y-90). The monoclonal antibody acts as a delivery system to direct the radioactive isotope to the targeted cells, however binding has been observed in lymphoid cells throughout the body and in lymphoid nodules in organs such as the large and small intestines. Indium-111 is a gamma-emitter used to assess biodistribution of ibritumomab, while Y-90 emits beta particles. Beta-emission induces cellular damage through the formation of free radicals (in both target cells and surrounding cells).

Pharmacodynamics/Kinetics

Duration: Beta cell recovery begins in ~12 weeks; generally in normal range within 9 months

Distribution: To lymphoid cells throughout the body and in lymphoid nodules in organs such as the large and small intestines, spleen, testes, and liver

Metabolism: Has not been characterized. The product of yttrium-90 radioactive decay is zirconium-90 (nonradioactive); Indium-111 decays to cadmium-111 (nonradioactive)

Half-life: Y-90 ibritumomab: 30 hours; Indium-111 decays with a physical half-life of 67 hours; Yttrium-90 decays with a physical half-life of 64 hours

Excretion: A median of 7.2% of the radiolabeled activity was excreted in urine over 7 days

Usual Dosage I.V.: Adults: Ibritumomab is administered **only** as part of the Zevalin™ therapeutic regimen (a combined treatment regimen with rituximab). The regimen consists of two steps:

Step 1:

Rituximab infusion: 250 mg/m² at an initial rate of 50 mg/hour. If hypersensitivity or infusion-related events do not occur, increase infusion in increments of 50 mg/hour every 30 minutes, to a maximum of 400 mg/hour. Infusions should be temporarily slowed or interrupted if hypersensitivity or infusion-related events occur. The infusion may be resumed at one-half the previous rate upon improvement of symptoms.

In-111 ibritumomab infusion: Within 4 hours of the completion of rituximab infusion, inject 5 mCi (1.6 mg total antibody dose) over 10 minutes.

Biodistribution of In-111 ibritumomab should be assessed by imaging at 2-24 hours and at 48-72 hours post-injection. An optional third imaging may be performed 90-120 hours following injection. If biodistribution is not acceptable, the patient should not proceed to Step 2.

Step 2 (initiated 7-9 days following Step 1):

Rituximab infusion: 250 mg/m² at an initial rate of 100 mg/hour (50 mg/hour if infusion-related events occurred with the first infusion). If hypersensitivity or infusion-related events do not occur, increase infusion in increments of 100 mg/hour every 30 minutes, to a maximum of 400 mg/hour, as tolerated.

Y-90 ibritumomab infusion: Within 4 hours of the completion of rituximab infusion:

Platelet count >150,000 cells/mm³: Inject 4 mCi (14.8 MBq/kg actual body weight) over 10 minutes

Platelet count between 100,000-149,000 cells/mm³: Inject 3 mCi (11.1 MBq/kg actual body weight) over 10 minutes

Platelet count <100,000 cells/mm³: Do **not** administer

Maximum dose: The prescribed, measured, and administered dose of Y-90 ibritumomab must not exceed 32 mCi (1184 MBq), regardless of the patient's body weight

Administration

Rituximab: Administer the first infusion of rituximab at an initial rate of 50 mg/hour. If hypersensitivity or infusion-related events do not occur, escalate the infusion rate in 50 mg/hour increments every 30 minutes, to a maximum of 400 mg/hour. If hypersensitivity or an infusion-related event develops, temporarily slow or interrupt the infusion (discontinue if reaction is severe). The infusion can continue at one-half the previous rate upon improvement of patient symptoms. Subsequent rituximab infusion can be administered at an initial rate of 100 mg/hour and increased in 100 mg/hour increments at 30-minute intervals, to a maximum of 400 mg/hour as tolerated.

Ibritumomab: Inject slowly, over 10 minutes. Use syringe shield. Appropriate measures should be undertaken to minimize radiation exposure to patients and medical personnel.

Monitoring Parameters Human antimurine antibody (HAMA) prior to treatment (if positive, may have an allergic or hypersensitivity reaction when treated with this or other murine or chimeric monoclonal antibodies).

Patients must be monitored for infusion-related allergic reactions (typically within 30-120 minutes of administration). Obtain complete blood counts and platelet counts at regular intervals during rituximab therapy (at least weekly and more frequently in patients who develop cytopenia). Platelet count must be obtained prior to step 2. Monitor for up to 3 months after use.

Biodistribution of In-111 ibritumomab should be assessed by imaging at 2-24 hours and at 48-72 hours post injection. An optional third imaging may be performed 90-120 hours following injection. If biodistribution is not acceptable, the patient should not proceed to Step 2.

Additional Information Ibritumomab tiuxetan is produced in Chinese hamster ovary cell cultures. Kit is not radioactive. Radiolabeling of ibritumomab with Yttrium-90 and Indium-111 (not included in kit) must be performed by appropriate personnel in a specialized facility.

Dosage Forms Each kit contains 4 vials for preparation of either In-111 or Y-90 conjugate (as indicated on container label)

Injection: 1.6 mg/mL (2 mL) [supplied with sodium acetate solution, formulation buffer vial (includes albumin 750 mg), and an empty reaction vial]

♦ **Ibritumomab Tiuxetan** see Ibritumomab on page 695

Ibuprofen (eye byoo PROE fen)

Related Information

Nonsteroidal Anti-Inflammatory Agents Comparison on page 1512

U.S. Brand Names Advil® [OTC]; Advil® Migraine Liqui-Gels [OTC]; Children's Advil® [OTC]; Children's Motrin® [OTC]; Genpril® [OTC]; Haltran® [OTC]; Junior Strength Motrin® [OTC]; Menadol® [OTC]; Midol® IB [OTC]; Motrin®; Motrin® IB [OTC]; Motrin® Migraine Pain [OTC]; Nuprin® [OTC]

Canadian Brand Names Advil®; Apo®-Ibuprofen; Motrin®; Motrin® (Children's); Motrin® IB; Novo-Profen®; Nu-Ibuprofen

Synonyms p-Isobutylhydratropic Acid

(Continued)

Ibuprofen *(Continued)*

Therapeutic Category Analgesic, Nonsteroidal Anti-inflammatory Drug; Anti-inflammatory Agent; Antimigraine Agent, Prophylactic; Antipyretic; Nonsteroidal Anti-inflammatory Drug (NSAID), Oral

Use Inflammatory diseases and rheumatoid disorders including juvenile rheumatoid arthritis, mild to moderate pain, fever, dysmenorrhea, gout, ankylosing spondylitis, acute migraine headache

Unlabeled/Investigational Use Cystic fibrosis

Pregnancy Risk Factor B/D (3rd trimester)

Pregnancy/Breast-Feeding Implications Limited data suggests minimal excretion in breast milk.

Contraindications Hypersensitivity to ibuprofen, any component of the formulation, aspirin, or other nonsteroidal anti-inflammatory drugs (NSAIDs); patients with "aspirin triad" (bronchial asthma, aspirin intolerance, rhinitis); pregnancy (3rd trimester)

Warnings/Precautions Use with caution in patients with congestive heart failure, hypertension, dehydration, decreased renal or hepatic function, history of GI disease (bleeding or ulcers), or those receiving anticoagulants. Elderly are at a high risk for adverse effects from nonsteroidal anti-inflammatory drugs. As many as 60% of elderly can develop peptic ulceration and/or hemorrhage asymptomatically. Fatal asthmatic and anaphylactoid reactions have occurred in patients with "aspirin triad" (see Contraindications).

Use lowest effective dose for shortest period possible. Use of NSAIDs can compromise existing renal function especially when Cl_{cr} is <30 mL/minute. CNS adverse effects such as confusion, agitation, and hallucination are generally seen in overdose or high-dose situations; however, elderly may demonstrate these adverse effects at lower doses than younger adults. Do not exceed 3200 mg/day. Withhold for at least 4-6 half-lives prior to surgical or dental procedures.

Adverse Reactions
1% to 10%:
Central nervous system: Headache (1% to 3%), nervousness (<3%), fatigue (<3%)
Dermatologic: Itching (1% to 3%), rash (3% to 9%), urticaria
Endocrine & metabolic: Fluid retention
Gastrointestinal: Dyspepsia (1% to 3%), vomiting (1% to 3%), abdominal pain/cramps/distress (1% to 3%), peptic ulcer, GI bleed, GI perforation, heartburn, nausea (3% to 9%), diarrhea (1% to 3%), constipation (1% to 3%), flatulence (1% to 3%), indigestion (1% to 3%)
Otic: Tinnitus

<1% (Limited to important or life-threatening): Acute renal failure, agranulocytosis, angioedema, aplastic anemia, arrhythmias, aseptic meningitis with fever and coma, bone marrow depression, congestive heart failure, dyspnea, eosinophilia, erythema multiforme, hemolytic anemia, Henoch-Schönlein vasculitis, hepatitis, hypertension, leukopenia, lupus erythematosus syndrome, neutropenia, Stevens-Johnson syndrome, thrombocytopenia, toxic epidermal necrolysis

Overdosage/Toxicology Symptoms include apnea, metabolic acidosis, coma, and nystagmus; leukocytosis, renal failure. Management of nonsteroidal anti-inflammatory drug (NSAID) intoxication is primarily supportive and symptomatic. Fluid therapy is commonly effective in managing hypotension that may occur following an acute NSAID overdose, except when due to acute blood loss. Seizures tend to be very short-lived and often do not require drug treatment, although recurrent seizures should be treated with I.V. diazepam. Since many of NSAIDs undergo enterohepatic cycling, multiple doses of charcoal may be needed to reduce the potential for delayed toxicities.

Drug Interactions

Cytochrome P450 Effect: CYP2C8 and 2C9 enzyme substrate

Increased Effect/Toxicity: Ibuprofen may increase cyclosporine, digoxin, lithium, and methotrexate serum concentrations. The renal adverse effects of ACE inhibitors may be potentiated by NSAIDs. Corticosteroids may increase the risk of GI ulceration.

Decreased Effect: Aspirin may decrease ibuprofen serum concentrations. Ibuprofen may decrease the effect of some antihypertensive agents (including ACE inhibitors and angiotensin antagonists) and diuretics.

Ethanol/Nutrition/Herb Interactions
Ethanol: Avoid ethanol (may enhance gastric mucosal irritation).
Food: Ibuprofen peak serum levels may be decreased if taken with food.
Herb/Nutraceutical: Avoid cat's claw, dong quai, evening primrose, feverfew, garlic, ginger, ginkgo, red clover, horse chestnut, green tea, ginseng (all have additional antiplatelet activity).

Mechanism of Action Inhibits prostaglandin synthesis by decreasing the activity of the enzyme, cyclo-oxygenase, which results in decreased formation of prostaglandin precursors

Pharmacodynamics/Kinetics
Onset of action: Analgesic: 30-60 minutes; Anti-inflammatory: ≤7 days
Peak effect: 1-2 weeks
Duration: 4-6 hours
Absorption: Oral: Rapid (85%)
Protein binding: 90% to 99%
Metabolism: Hepatic via oxidation
Half-life elimination: 2-4 hours; End-stage renal disease: Unchanged
Time to peak: ~1-2 hours
Excretion: Urine (1% as free drug); some feces

Usual Dosage Oral:
Children:
Antipyretic: 6 months to 12 years: Temperature <102.5°F (39°C): 5 mg/kg/dose; temperature >102.5°F: 10 mg/kg/dose given every 6-8 hours; maximum daily dose: 40 mg/kg/day
Juvenile rheumatoid arthritis: 30-70 mg/kg/24 hours divided every 6-8 hours
<20 kg: Maximum: 400 mg/day
20-30 kg: Maximum: 600 mg/day

30-40 kg: Maximum: 800 mg/day
>40 kg: Adult dosage
Start at lower end of dosing range and titrate upward; maximum: 2.4 g/day
Analgesic: 4-10 mg/kg/dose every 6-8 hours
Adults:
Inflammatory disease: 400-800 mg/dose 3-4 times/day; maximum dose: 3.2 g/day
Analgesia/pain/fever/dysmenorrhea: 200-400 mg/dose every 4-6 hours; maximum daily dose: 1.2 g (unless directed by physician)
Dosing adjustment/comments in severe hepatic impairment: Avoid use
Dietary Considerations Should be taken with food.
Administration Administer with food
Monitoring Parameters CBC; occult blood loss and periodic liver function tests; monitor response (pain, range of motion, grip strength, mobility, ADL function), inflammation; observe for weight gain, edema; monitor renal function (urine output, serum BUN and creatinine); observe for bleeding, bruising; evaluate gastrointestinal effects (abdominal pain, bleeding, dyspepsia); mental confusion, disorientation; with long-term therapy, periodic ophthalmic exams
Reference Range Plasma concentrations >200 µg/mL may be associated with severe toxicity
Patient Information Serious gastrointestinal bleeding can occur as well as ulceration and perforation. Pain may or may not be present. Avoid aspirin and aspirin-containing products while taking this medication. If gastric upset occurs, take with food, milk, or antacid. If gastric adverse effects persist, contact physician. May cause drowsiness, dizziness, blurred vision, and confusion. Use caution when performing tasks that require alertness (eg, driving). Do not take for more than 3 days for fever or 10 days for pain without physician's advice.
Nursing Implications Do not crush tablet
Additional Information Sucrose content of 5 mL (suspension): 2.5 g
Dosage Forms
Caplet: 200 mg [OTC]
Capsule (Advil® Migraine Liqui-Gel): 200 mg [OTC]
Suspension, oral: 100 mg/5 mL [OTC] (60 mL, 120 mL, 480 mL)
Suspension, oral [drops]: 40 mg/mL (15 mL) [OTC] [berry flavor]
Tablet: 100 mg [OTC], 200 mg [OTC], 300 mg, 400 mg, 600 mg, 800 mg
Tablet, chewable: 50 mg, 100 mg [OTC]

♦ **Ibuprofen and Hydrocodone** see Hydrocodone and Ibuprofen on page 680
♦ **Ibuprofen and Pseudoephedrine** see Pseudoephedrine and Ibuprofen on page 1157

Ibutilide (i BYOO ti lide)

Related Information
Antiarrhythmic Drugs Comparison on page 1478
U.S. Brand Names Corvert®
Synonyms Ibutilide Fumarate
Therapeutic Category Antiarrhythmic Agent, Class III
Use Acute termination of atrial fibrillation or flutter of recent onset; the effectiveness of ibutilide has not been determined in patients with arrhythmias >90 days in duration
Pregnancy Risk Factor C
Pregnancy/Breast-Feeding Implications
Clinical effects on the fetus: Teratogenic and embryocidal in rats; avoid use in pregnancy
Breast-feeding/lactation: Avoid breast-feeding during therapy
Contraindications Hypersensitivity to ibutilide or any component of the formulation; QT_c >440 msec
Warnings/Precautions Potentially fatal arrhythmias (eg, polymorphic ventricular tachycardia) can occur with ibutilide, **usually** in association with torsade de pointes (QT prolongation). Studies indicate a 1.7% incidence of arrhythmias in treated patients. The drug should be given in a setting of continuous EKG monitoring and by personnel trained in treating arrhythmias particularly polymorphic ventricular tachycardia. Patients with chronic atrial fibrillation may not be the best candidates for ibutilide since they often revert after conversion and the risks of treatment may not be justified when compared to alternative management. Dosing adjustments are not required in patients with renal or hepatic dysfunction since a maximum of only two 10-minute infusions are utilized. Drug distribution, rather than administration, is one of the primary mechanisms responsible for termination of the pharmacologic effect. Safety and efficacy in children have not been established. Avoid any drug that can prolong QT interval. Correct hyperkalemia and hypomagnesemia before using. Monitor for heart block.
Adverse Reactions
1% to 10%:
Cardiovascular: Sustained polymorphic ventricular tachycardia (ie, torsade de pointes) (2%, often requiring cardioversion), nonsustained polymorphic ventricular tachycardia (3%), nonsustained monomorphic ventricular tachycardia (5%), ventricular extrasystoles (5%), nonsustained monomorphic VT (5%), tachycardia/supraventricular tachycardia (3%), hypotension (2%), bundle branch block (2%), AV block (2%), bradycardia (1%), QT segment prolongation, hypertension (1%), palpitations (1%)
Central nervous system: Headache (4%)
Gastrointestinal: Nausea (>1%)
<1% (Limited to important or life-threatening): Congestive heart failure, erythematous bullous lesions, idioventricular rhythm, nodal arrhythmia, renal failure, supraventricular extrasystoles, sustained monomorphic ventricular tachycardia, syncope (0.3%, not > placebo)
Overdosage/Toxicology Symptoms include CNS depression, rapid gasping breathing, and convulsions; arrhythmias can occur. Treatment is supportive and should include measures appropriate for the condition. Antiarrhythmics are generally avoided. Pharmacologic therapies may include magnesium sulfate and correction of other electrolyte abnormalities. Overdrive cardiac pacing, electrical cardioversion, or defibrillaton may be required.
Drug Interactions
Increased Effect/Toxicity: Class Ia antiarrhythmic drugs (disopyramide, quinidine, and procainamide) and other class III drugs such as amiodarone and sotalol should not be
(Continued)

Ibutilide (Continued)

given concomitantly with ibutilide due to their potential to prolong refractoriness. Signs of digoxin toxicity may be masked when coadministered with ibutilide. Toxicity of ibutilide is potentiated by concurrent administration of other drugs which may prolong QT interval: phenothiazines, tricyclic and tetracyclic antidepressants, cisapride, sparfloxacin, gatifloxacin, moxifloxacin, erythromycin, terfenadine, and astemizole.

Stability Admixtures are chemically and physically stable for 24 hours at room temperature and for 48 hours at refrigerated temperatures

Mechanism of Action Exact mechanism of action is unknown; prolongs the action potential in cardiac tissue

Pharmacodynamics/Kinetics

Onset of action: ~90 minutes after start of infusion ($1/2$ of conversions to sinus rhythm occur during infusion)

Distribution: V_d: 11 L/kg

Protein binding: 40%

Metabolism: Extensively hepatic; oxidation

Half-life elimination: 2-12 hours (average: 6 hours)

Excretion: Urine (82%, 7% as unchanged drug and metabolites); feces (19%)

Usual Dosage I.V.: Initial:

Adults:

<60 kg: 0.01 mg/kg over 10 minutes

≥60 kg: 1 mg over 10 minutes

If the arrhythmia does not terminate within 10 minutes after the end of the initial infusion, a second infusion of equal strength may be infused over a 10-minute period

Elderly: Dose selection should be cautious, usually starting at the lower end of the dosing range.

Administration May be administered undiluted or diluted in 50 mL diluent (0.9% NS or D_5W); infuse over 10 minutes

Monitoring Parameters Observe patient with continuous EKG monitoring for at least 4 hours following infusion or until QT_c has returned to baseline; skilled personnel and proper equipment should be available during administration of ibutilide and subsequent monitoring of the patient

Nursing Implications See Monitoring Parameters; EKG, electrolytes

Dosage Forms Injection, as fumarate: 0.1 mg/mL (10 mL)

* **Ibutilide Fumarate** see Ibutilide on page 699
* **ICI 204, 219** see Zafirlukast on page 1430
* **ICRF-187** see Dexrazoxane on page 385
* **Idamycin®** see Idarubicin on page 700
* **Idamycin PFS®** see Idarubicin on page 700

Idarubicin (eye da ROO bi sin)

U.S. Brand Names Idamycin®; Idamycin PFS®

Canadian Brand Names Idamycin®

Synonyms 4-demethoxydaunorubicin; 4-dmdr; Idarubicin Hydrochloride

Therapeutic Category Antineoplastic Agent, Anthracycline; Antineoplastic Agent, Antibiotic; Vesicant

Use Treatment of acute leukemias (AML, ANLL, ALL), accelerated phase or blast crisis of chronic myelogenous leukemia (CML), breast cancer

Pregnancy Risk Factor D

Contraindications Hypersensitivity to idarubicin, daunorubicin, or any component of the formulation; bilirubin >5 mg/dL; pregnancy

Warnings/Precautions The U.S. Food and Drug Administration (FDA) currently recommends that procedures for proper handling and disposal of antineoplastic agents be considered. Administer I.V. slowly into a freely flowing I.V. infusion; do not administer I.M. or S.C., severe necrosis can result if extravasation occurs; can cause myocardial toxicity and is more common in patients who have previously received anthracyclines or have pre-existing cardiac disease; reduce dose in patients with impaired hepatic function; irreversible myocardial toxicity may occur as total dosage approaches 137.5 mg/m²; severe myelosuppression is also possible.

Adverse Reactions

>10%:

Cardiovascular: Transient EKG abnormalities (supraventricular tachycardia, S-T wave changes, atrial or ventricular extrasystoles); generally asymptomatic and self-limiting. Congestive heart failure, dose-related. The relative cardiotoxicity of idarubicin compared to doxorubicin is unclear. Some investigators report no increase in cardiac toxicity at cumulative oral idarubicin doses up to 540 mg/m²; other reports suggest a maximum cumulative intravenous dose of 150 mg/m².

Central nervous system: Headache

Dermatologic: Alopecia (25% to 30%), radiation recall, skin rash (11%), urticaria

Gastrointestinal: Nausea, vomiting (30% to 60%); diarrhea (9% to 22%); stomatitis (11%); GI hemorrhage (30%)

Emetic potential: Moderate (30% to 60%)

Genitourinary: Discoloration of urine (reddish)

Hematologic: Myelosuppression, primarily leukopenia; thrombocytopenia and anemia. Effects are generally less severe with oral dosing.

Nadir: 10-15 days

Recovery: 21-28 days

Hepatic: Elevations of bilirubin and transaminases (44%)

Local: Tissue necrosis upon extravasation, erythematous streaking

Vesicant chemotherapy

1% to 10%:

Central nervous system: Seizures

Neuromuscular & skeletal: Peripheral neuropathy

<1% (Limited to important or life-threatening): Hyperuricemia

Overdosage/Toxicology Symptoms include severe myelosuppression and increased GI toxicity. Treatment is supportive. It is unlikely that therapeutic efficacy or toxicity would be altered by conventional peritoneal or hemodialysis.

Drug Interactions

Decreased Effect: Patients may experience impaired immune response to vaccines; possible infection after administration of live vaccines in patients receiving immunosuppressants.

Stability Store intact vials of solution under refrigeration (2°C to 8°C/36°F to 46°F). Store intact vials of lyophilized powder at room temperature (15°C to 30°C/59°F to 86°F), protected from light. Reconstituted solutions may be stored under refrigeration for 7 days or at room temperature for 3 days. Solutions diluted in D_5W or NS for infusion are stable for 4 weeks at room temperature, protected from light. Syringe and IVPB solutions are stable for 72 hours at room temperature and 7 days under refrigeration.

Dilute powder with SWFI, NS, or D_5W to a concentration of 1 mg/mL. Further dilution in D_5W or NS is stable for 4 weeks at room temperature and protected from light

Incompatible with dexamethasone, etoposide, fluorouracil, heparin, hydrocortisone, methotrexate, vincristine

Standard I.V. dilution:

I.V. push: Dose/syringe (concentration: 1 mg/mL)

Maximum syringe size for IVP: 30 mL syringe and syringe should be ≤75% full

IVPB: Dose/100 mL D_5W or NS

Syringe and IVPB solutions are stable for 72 hours at room temperature and 7 days under refrigeration

Mechanism of Action Derivative of daunorubicin; the only structural difference between idarubicin and the parent compound, daunorubicin, is lack of the methoxyl group at the C4 position of the aglycone. Similar to daunorubicin, idarubicin exhibits inhibitory effects on DNA and RNA polymerase *in vitro*. Idarubicin has an affinity for DNA similar to the parent compound and somewhat higher efficacy than daunorubicin in stabilizing the DNA double helix against heat denaturation.

Pharmacodynamics/Kinetics

Distribution: Large V_d; extensive tissue binding; CSF

Protein binding: 94% to 97%

Metabolism: Hepatically to idarubicinol (pharmacologically active)

Half-life elimination: I.V.: 12-27 hours

Time to peak, serum: ~2-4 hours; varies considerably

Excretion: I.V.: Urine (~15% as idarubicin and idarubicinol); feces (similar amounts)

Usual Dosage Refer to individual protocols. I.V.:

Children:

Leukemia: 10-12 mg/m²/day for 3 days every 3 weeks

Solid tumors: 5 mg/m²/day for 3 days every 3 weeks

Adults:

Leukemia induction: 12 mg/m²/day for 3 days

Leukemia consolidation: 10-12 mg/m²/day for 2 days

Dosing adjustment in renal impairment: No specific dosage adjustment is recommended

Hemodialysis: Significant drug removal is unlikely based on physiochemical characteristics

Peritoneal dialysis: Significant drug removal is unlikely based on physiochemical characteristics

Dosing adjustment/comments in hepatic impairment: No specific dosage adjustment is recommended

Administration

Administer by intermittent infusion over 10-15 minutes into a free flowing I.V. solution of NS or D_5W

Avoid extravasation - potent vesicant

Monitoring Parameters CBC with differential, platelet count, ECHO, EKG, serum electrolytes, creatinine, uric acid, ALT, AST, bilirubin, signs of extravasation

Patient Information This drug can only be administered I.V. Maintain adequate nutrition and hydration (2-3 L/day of fluids unless instructed to restrict fluid intake). May cause hair loss (will grow back); nausea or vomiting (consult prescriber for antiemetic medication); you will be susceptible to infection (avoid crowds and exposure to infection); or urine may turn red-brown (normal). Report immediately any pain, burning, or stinging at infusion site; difficulty breathing; or swelling of extremities. Contraceptive measures are recommended during therapy.

Nursing Implications

Local erythematous streaking along the vein may indicate too rapid a rate of administration

Unless specific data available, do not mix with other drugs

Extravasation management:

Apply ice immediately for 30-60 minutes; then alternate off/on every 15 minutes for one day

Topical cooling may be achieved using ice packs or cooling pad with circulating ice water. Cooling of site for 24 hours as tolerated by the patient. Elevate and rest extremity 24-48 hours, then resume normal activity as tolerated. Application of cold inhibits vesicant's cytotoxicity.

Application of heat or sodium bicarbonate can be harmful and is contraindicated

If pain, erythema, and/or swelling persist beyond 48 hours, refer patient immediately to plastic surgeon for consultation and possible debridement

Dosage Forms

Injection, as hydrochloride [preservative free] (Idamycin PFS®): 1 mg/mL (5 mL, 10 mL, 20 mL)

Powder for injection, lyophilized, as hydrochloride (Idamycin®): 20 mg

♦ **Idarubicin Hydrochloride** *see* Idarubicin *on page 700*

♦ **Ifex®** *see* Ifosfamide *on page 702*

♦ **IFLrA** *see* Interferon Alfa-2a *on page 726*

Ifosfamide (eye FOSS fa mide)

U.S. Brand Names Ifex®

Canadian Brand Names Ifex®

Therapeutic Category Antineoplastic Agent, Alkylating Agent; Antineoplastic Agent, Nitrogen Mustard

Use Treatment of lung cancer, Hodgkin's and non-Hodgkin's lymphoma, breast cancer, acute and chronic lymphocytic leukemias, ovarian cancer, sarcomas, pancreatic and gastric carcinomas

Orphan drug: Treatment of testicular cancer

Pregnancy Risk Factor D

Contraindications Hypersensitivity to ifosfamide or any component of the formulation; patients with severely depressed bone marrow function; pregnancy

Warnings/Precautions The U.S. Food and Drug Administration (FDA) currently recommends that procedures for proper handling and disposal of antineoplastic agents be considered. May require therapy cessation if confusion or coma occurs; be aware of hemorrhagic cystitis and severe myelosuppression. Use with caution in patients with impaired renal function or those with compromised bone marrow reserve.

Adverse Reactions

>10%:

Central nervous system: Somnolence, confusion, hallucinations (12%)

Dermatologic: Alopecia (75% to 100%)

Endocrine & metabolic: Metabolic acidosis (31%)

Gastrointestinal: Nausea and vomiting (58%), may be more common with higher doses or bolus infusions; constipation

Genitourinary: Hemorrhagic cystitis (40% to 50%), patients should be vigorously hydrated (at least 2 L/day) and receive mesna

Hematologic: Myelosuppression, leukopenia (65% to 100%), thrombocytopenia (10%) - dose-related

Onset: 7-14 days

Nadir: 21-28 days

Recovery: 21-28 days

Renal: Hematuria (6% to 92%)

1% to 10%:

Central nervous system: Hallucinations, depressive psychoses, polyneuropathy

Dermatologic: Dermatitis, nail banding/ridging, hyperpigmentation

Endocrine & metabolic: SIADH, sterility, elevated transaminases (3%)

Hematologic: Anemia

Local: Phlebitis

Renal: Increased creatinine/BUN (6%)

Respiratory: Nasal stuffiness

<1% (Limited to important or life-threatening): Acute tubular necrosis, anorexia, cardiotoxicity, diarrhea, pulmonary fibrosis, stomatitis

Overdosage/Toxicology Symptoms include myelosuppression, nausea, vomiting, diarrhea, and alopecia, which is a direct extension of the drug's pharmacologic effect. Treatment is supportive.

Drug Interactions

Cytochrome P450 Effect: CYP2B6 and 3A3/4 enzyme substrate

Increased Effect/Toxicity: Activation by microsomal enzymes may be enhanced during therapy with enzyme inducers such as phenobarbital, carbamazepine, and phenytoin.

Ethanol/Nutrition/Herb Interactions Herb/Nutraceutical: St John's wort may decrease ifosfamide levels.

Stability

Store intact vials at room temperature or under refrigeration

Dilute powder with SWI or NS to a concentration of 50 mg/mL as follows. **Do not use bacteriostatic SWI or NS** - incompatible; solution is stable for 7 days at room temperature and 6 weeks under refrigeration

1 g vial = 20 mL

3 g vial = 60 mL

Further dilution in NS, D_5W or LR is stable for 7 days at room temperature and 6 weeks under refrigeration

Compatible with mesna in NS for up to 9 days at room temperature

Standard I.V. dilution:

I.V. push: Dose/syringe (concentration = 50 mg/mL)

Maximum syringe size for IVP is a 30 mL syringe and syringe should be ≤75% full

IVPB: Dose/100-1000 mL D_5W or NS

Syringe and IVPB are stable for 7 days at room temperature and 6 weeks under refrigeration

Mechanism of Action Causes cross-linking of strands of DNA by binding with nucleic acids and other intracellular structures; inhibits protein synthesis and DNA synthesis; an analogue of cyclophosphamide, and like cyclophosphamide, it undergoes activation by microsomal enzymes in the liver. Ifosfamide is metabolized to active compounds, ifosfamide mustard, and acrolein

Pharmacodynamics/Kinetics Pharmacokinetics are dose-dependent

Distribution: V_d: 5.7-49 L; does penetrate CNS, but not in therapeutic levels

Protein binding: Negligible

Metabolism: Hepatic to active species; requires biotransformation before it can act as an alkylating agent; metabolite acrolein is the toxic agent implicated in development of hemorrhagic cystitis

Half-life elimination: Beta: High dose: 11-15 hours (3800-5000 mg/m²); Lower dose: 4-7 hours (1800 mg/m²)

Time to peak, plasma: Oral: Within 1 hour

Excretion: Urine (15% to 50% as unchanged drug)

Usual Dosage Refer to individual protocols. To prevent bladder toxicity, ifosfamide should be given with the urinary protector mesna and hydration of at least 2 L of oral or I.V. fluid per day. I.V.:

Children:

1200-1800 mg/m^2/day for 3-5 days every 21-28 days **or**

5 g/m^2 once every 21-28 days **or**

3 g/m^2/day for 2 days every 21-28 days

Adults:

50 mg/kg/day or 700-2000 mg/m^2 for 5 days every 3-4 weeks

Alternatives: 2400 mg/m^2/day for 3 days or 5000 mg/m^2 as a single dose every 3-4 weeks

Dosing adjustment in renal impairment:

S_{cr} >3.0 mg/dL: Withhold drug

S_{cr} 2.1-3.0 mg/dL: Reduce dose by 25% to 50%

Dosing adjustment in hepatic impairment: Although no specific guidelines are available, it is possible that adjusted doses are indicated in hepatic disease. One author (Falkson G, et al, "An Extended Phase II Trial of Ifosfamide Plus Mesna in Malignant Mesothelioma," *Invest New Drugs*, 1992, 10:337-43.) recommended the following dosage adjustments: AST >300 or bilirubin >3.0 mg/dL: Decrease ifosfamide dose by 75%

Administration

Administer slow I.V. push, IVPB over 30 minutes or continuous I.V. over 5 days

Adequate hydration (at least 2 L/day) of the patient before and for 72 hours after therapy is recommended to minimize the risk of hemorrhagic cystitis

MESNA should be administered concomitantly (20% of the ifosfamide dose 15 minutes before, 4 hours after and 8 hours after ifosfamide administration)

Monitoring Parameters CBC with differential, hemoglobin, and platelet count, urine output, urinalysis, liver function, and renal function tests

Patient Information This drug can only be administered I.V. Report immediately any pain, stinging, or burning at infusion site. It is vital to maintain adequate hydration (2-3 L/day of fluids unless instructed to restrict fluid intake) for 3 days prior to infusion and each day of therapy. May cause hair loss (will grow back); nausea or vomiting (consult prescriber for antiemetic medication); and you will be susceptible to infection (avoid crowds and exposure to infection). Report immediately pain or irritation on urination, severe diarrhea, CNS changes (eg, hallucinations, confusion, somnolence), signs of opportunistic infection (eg, fever, chills, easy bruising or unusual bleeding), difficulty breathing, swelling of extremities, or any other adverse effects. Contraceptive measures are recommended during therapy.

Nursing Implications Mesna to be used concomitantly for prophylaxis against hemorrhagic cystitis

Dosage Forms

Powder for injection for I.V. infusion, parenteral kit:

Ifosfamide (Ifex®) 1 g and mesna (Mesnex®) 1 g

Ifosfamide (Ifex®) 3 g and mesna (Mesnex®) 1 g

♦ **IG** *see Immune Globulin (Intramuscular) on page 710*

♦ **IGIM** *see Immune Globulin (Intramuscular) on page 710*

♦ **IL-1Ra** *see Anakinra on page 98*

♦ **IL-2** *see Aldesleukin on page 43*

♦ **IL-11** *see Oprelvekin on page 1012*

♦ **Iletin® II Pork (Can)** *see Insulin Preparations on page 722*

♦ **Ilopan®** *see Dexpanthenol on page 385*

♦ **Ilosone® (Can)** *see Erythromycin (Systemic) on page 486*

Imatinib *eye MAT eh nib*

U.S. Brand Names Gleevec™

Synonyms CGP 57148B; Glivec; Imatinib Mesylate; STI571

Therapeutic Category Antineoplastic, Tyrosine Kinase Inhibitor

Use Treatment of patients with chronic myeloid leukemia (CML) in blast crisis, accelerated phase, or in chronic phase after failure of interferon-alpha therapy; treatment of Kit-positive (CD117) unresectable and/or (metastatic) malignant gastrointestinal stromal tumors (GIST)

Unlabeled/Investigational Use Philadelphia chromosome-positive leukemias

Pregnancy Risk Factor D

Pregnancy/Breast-Feeding Implications There are no adequate or well-controlled studies in pregnant women. Has been noted to be teratogenic in animal models. Women of child-bearing potential are advised not to become pregnant. Excretion in breast milk unknown; breast-feeding is not recommended.

Contraindications Hypersensitivity to imatinib or any component of the formulation; pregnancy

Warnings/Precautions Often associated with fluid retention, weight gain, and edema (probability increases with higher doses and age >65 years); occasionally leading to significant complications, including pleural effusion, pericardial effusion, pulmonary edema, and ascites. Use caution in patients where fluid accumulation may be poorly tolerated, such as in cardiovascular disease (congestive heart failure or hypertension) and pulmonary disease. Use with caution in renal impairment, hematologic impairment, or hepatic disease. May cause GI irritation, hepatotoxicity, or hematologic toxicity (neutropenia or thrombocytopenia). Median duration of neutropenia is 2-3 weeks; median duration of thrombocytopenia is 3-4 weeks. Hepatotoxic reactions may be severe. Has been associated with development of opportunistic infections. Use with caution in patients receiving concurrent therapy with drugs which alter cytochrome P450 activity or require metabolism by these isoenzymes. Review all medications, including OTC and herbal products, before initiating therapy. Safety and efficacy in patients <18 years of age have not been established. Long-term safety data is limited.

Adverse Reactions Adverse effect profile is based on limited data, established in patients with a wide variation in level of illness. Patients in blast crisis or accelerated disease reported a higher frequency of symptoms. In many cases, other medications were used concurrently. (Continued)

Imatinib *(Continued)*

>10%:

Cardiovascular: Fluid retention (superficial, 51% to 66%; other 2% to 16%)

Central nervous system: Headache (24% to 28%, severe <1% to 4%), fatigue (24% to 33%, severe <1% to 3%), fever (14% to 38%)

Dermatologic: Rash (32% to 39%, severe 3% to 4%)

Endocrine & metabolic: Hypokalemia (2% to 12%)

Gastrointestinal: Nausea (55% to 68%), diarrhea (33% to 49%, severe <1% to 4%), vomiting (28% to 54%, severe <1% to 4%), dyspepsia (9% to 19%), abdominal pain (20% to 26%), constipation (4% to 13%), weight gain (4% to 14%), anorexia (3% to 14%)

Hematologic: Hematologic toxicity (neutropenia, thrombocytopenia, anemia) is common (higher in blast crisis or accelerated phase in CML, up to 30% to 46%) and may require dosage adjustment, interruption, or discontinuation of therapy

Neuromuscular & skeletal: Muscle cramps (25% to 46%, severe <1%), musculoskeletal pain (27% to 39%, severe 1% to 8%), arthralgia (21% to 26%), myalgia (7% to 18%)

Respiratory: Cough (9% to 22%), dyspnea (5% to 16%), epistaxis (3% to 12%)

Miscellaneous: Night sweats (8% to 10%)

1% to 10%:

Cardiovascular: Edema (severe 1% to 5%; includes pleural effusion, pulmonary edema, pericardial effusion, anasarca, and ascites)

Central nervous system: CNS hemorrhage (<1% to 4%)

Dermatologic: Pruritus (6% to 10%), petechiae (<1% to 10%)

Gastrointestinal: Gastrointestinal hemorrhage (<1% to 5%), intratumoral hemorrhage

Hepatic: Hepatotoxicity (1% to 4%); elevated transaminases, bilirubin, and alkaline phosphatase

Neuromuscular & skeletal: Weakness (5% to 10%)

Renal: Increased serum creatinine

Respiratory: Nasopharyngitis (5% to 10%), pneumonia (1% to 10%)

Miscellaneous: Tumor lysis syndrome

Overdosage/Toxicology Experience with overdose is limited (>800 mg/day). Hematologic adverse effects are more common at dosages >750 mg/day. Treatment is symptomatic and supportive.

Drug Interactions

Cytochrome P450 Effect: CYP3A3/4 enzyme substrate; CYP3A3/4 enzyme inhibitor (potent); CYP2C9, 2D6 enzyme inhibitors

Increased Effect/Toxicity: Note: Drug interaction data is limited. Few clinical studies have been conducted. Many interactions listed below are derived by extrapolation from *in vitro* inhibition of cytochrome P450 isoenzymes.

Acetaminophen: Chronic use may increase potential for hepatotoxic reaction with imatinib (case report of hepatic failure with concurrent therapy).

Due to potent CYP3A3/4 inhibition, imatinib should not be used with cisapride, pimozide, thioridazine, and/or mesoridazine, may result in potential life-threatening toxicities. Imatinib may also inhibit the metabolism of benzodiazepines (alprazolam, diazepam, and triazolam), some beta-blockers, carbamazepine, carvedilol, clozapine, dextromethorphan, haloperidol, HMG-CoA reductase inhibitors (except pravastatin and fluvastatin), immunosuppressants (cyclosporine, sirolimus, and tacrolimus), methadone, nefazodone, phenothiazines (thioridazine and mesoridazine should be avoided), phenytoin, propafenone, quinidine, sibutramine, sildenafil, SSRIs, tricyclic antidepressants, trazodone, vinca alkaloids (vincristine, vinblastine), and warfarin. Increased toxicity leading to liver failure has been reported with regular concomitant acetaminophen use (case report).

Serum concentrations and/or toxicity of imatinib may be increased by drugs which inhibit CYP3A3/4. Established with ketoconazole; other inhibitors include amiodarone, cimetidine, clarithromycin, delavirdine, diltiazem, dirithromycin, disulfiram, erythromycin, fluoxetine, fluvoxamine, grapefruit juice, indinavir, itraconazole, nefazodone, nevirapine, propoxyphene, quinupristin-dalfopristin, ritonavir, saquinavir, verapamil, zafirlukast, and zileuton.

Decreased Effect: Metabolism of imatinib may be increased by CYP3A3/4 enzyme inducers, decreasing its therapeutic effect. An interaction has been established with phenytoin; other potential inducers include phenobarbital, carbamazepine, rifampin, and rifabutin.

Ethanol/Nutrition/Herb Interactions

Ethanol: Avoid ethanol.

Food: Food may reduce gastrointestinal irritation.

Herb/Nutraceutical: Avoid St John's wort (may increase metabolism and decrease imatinib plasma concentration).

Stability Store at 25°C (77°F); excursions permitted to 15°C to 30°C (59°F to 86°F)

Mechanism of Action Inhibits Bcr-Abl tyrosine kinase, the constitutive abnormal gene product of the Philadelphia chromosome in chronic myeloid leukemia (CML). Inhibition of this enzyme blocks proliferation and induces apoptosis in Bcr-Abl positive cell lines as well as in fresh leukemic cells in Philadelphia chromosome positive CML. Also inhibits tyrosine kinase for platelet-derived growth factor (PDGF), stem cell factor (SCF), c-kit, and events mediated by PDGF and SCF.

Pharmacodynamics/Kinetics

Protein binding: 95% to albumin and alpha$_1$-acid glycoprotein

Metabolism: Hepatic via CYP3A3/4 (minor metabolism via CYP1A2, CYP2D6, CYP2C9, CYP2C19); primary metabolite (active): N-demethylated piperazine derivative

Bioavailability: 98%

Half-life elimination: Parent drug: 18 hours; N-demethyl metabolite: 40 hours

Time to peak: 2-4 hours

Excretion: Feces (68%, primarily as metabolites, 20% as unchanged drug); urine (13%, primarily metabolites, 5% as unchanged drug)

Clearance: Highly variable; Mean: 8-14 L/hour (for 50 kg and 100 kg male, respectively)

Usual Dosage Oral: Adults: Dose should be taken with food and large glass of water:

Chronic myeloid leukemia (CML):

Chronic phase: 400 mg once daily; may be increased to 600 mg daily in the event of disease progression, loss of previously achieved response, or failure to achieve response after at least 3 months of therapy and in the absence of severe adverse reaction

Accelerated phase or blast crisis: 600 mg once daily; may be increased to 800 mg daily (400 mg twice daily) in the event of disease progression, loss of previously achieved response, or failure to achieve response after at least 3 months of therapy and in the absence of severe adverse reaction

Gastrointestinal stromal tumors: 400-600 mg/day

Dosage adjustment for hepatotoxicity or other nonhematologic adverse reactions:

Withhold therapy for any severe nonhematologic event (severe hepatotoxicity or severe fluid retention). May resume treatment, as appropriate, following resolution of acute event, depending on the initial severity of the event.

If elevations of bilirubin >3 times upper limit of normal (ULN) or transaminases (ALT/AST) >5 times ULN occur, withhold until bilirubin <1.5 times ULN or transaminases <2.5 times ULN. Resume treatment at reduced dose (if initial dose 400 mg/day, reduce to 300 mg/day, if initial dose 600 mg/day then reduce to 400 mg/day).

Dosage adjustment for hematologic adverse reactions:

Chronic phase (initial dose: 400 mg/day): If ANC <1.0 x 10^9/L and/or platelets <50 x 10^9/L: Discontinue until ANC ≥1.5 x 10^9/L and platelets ≥75 x 10^9/L; resume treatment at 400 mg/day. If depression in neutrophils or platelets recurs, withhold until recovery (as above), and re-institute treatment at 300 mg/day.

Accelerated phase or blast crisis (initial dose: 600 mg/day): If ANC <0.5 x 10^9/L and/or platelets <10 x 10^9/L: Check to establish whether cytopenia is related to leukemia (bone marrow aspirate). If unrelated to leukemia, reduce dose of imatinib to 400 mg daily. If cytopenia persists for an additional 2 weeks, further reduce dose to 300 mg/day. If cytopenia persists for 4 weeks and is still unrelated to leukemia, stop treatment until ANC ≥1.0 x 10^9/L and platelets ≥20 x 10^9/L, resume treatment at 300 mg/day.

Dietary Considerations Should be taken with food and a large glass of water to decrease gastrointestinal irritation.

Administration Should be administered with food and a large glass of water; vigorous hydration and administration of allopurinol are recommended.

Monitoring Parameters CBC (weekly for first month, biweekly for second month, then periodically thereafter), liver function tests (at baseline and monthly or as clinically indicated), renal function, weight, and edema/fluid status.

Patient Information Take exactly as directed; do not alter or discontinue dose without consulting prescriber. Take with food or a large glass of water. Avoid alcohol, chronic use of acetaminophen or aspirin, OTC or prescription medications, or herbal products unless approved by prescriber. Maintain adequate hydration (2-3 L/day) unless instructed to restrict fluids. You will be required to have regularly scheduled laboratory tests while on this medication. You will be more susceptible to infection (avoid crowds or contagious persons, and do not receive any vaccination unless approved by prescriber). You may experience headache or fatigue (use caution when driving or engaged in tasks requiring alertness until response to drug is known); loss of appetite, nausea, vomiting, or mouth sores (small frequent meals, frequent mouth care, chewing gum, or sucking lozenges may help); constipation (increased dietary fiber and fluids, exercise may help); or diarrhea (buttermilk, boiled milk, or yogurt may reduce diarrhea). Report chest pain, palpitations, or swelling of extremities; cough, difficulty breathing, or wheezing; weight gain greater than 5 lb; skin rash; muscle or bone pain, tremors, or cramping; persistent fatigue or weakness; easy bruising or unusual bleeding (eg, tarry stools, blood in vomitus, stool, urine, or mouth); persistent gastrointestinal problems or pain; or other adverse effects. Inform prescriber if you are pregnant. Do not get pregnant. Use appropriate contraception while on this medication. Breast-feeding is not recommended.

Additional Information Median time to hematologic response was one month; only short-term studies have been completed. Follow-up is insufficient to estimate duration of cytogenic response.

Dosage Forms Capsule, as mesylate: 100 mg

♦ **Imatinib Mesylate** see Imatinib on page 703

♦ **Imdur**® see Isosorbide Mononitrate on page 751

♦ **Imidazole Carboxamide** see Dacarbazine on page 354

Imiglucerase (i mi GLOO ser ace)

U.S. Brand Names Cerezyme®

Therapeutic Category Enzyme

Use Orphan drug: Long-term enzyme replacement therapy for patients with Type 1 Gaucher's disease

Pregnancy Risk Factor C

Contraindications Hypersensitivity to imiglucerase or any component of the formulation

Warnings/Precautions Anaphylactoid reactions have been reported (<1%). Most patients have continued treatment with pretreatment (antihistamines and/or corticosteroids) and a slower rate of infusion.

Adverse Reactions

1% to 10%:

Cardiovascular: Hypotension, cyanosis

Central nervous system: Headache, dizziness

Dermatologic: Rash, pruritus

Gastrointestinal: Nausea, abdominal discomfort

Genitourinary: Decreased urinary frequency

Miscellaneous: Hypersensitivity reaction (4.4%)

<1% (Limited to important or life-threatening): Anaphylactoid reaction, pulmonary hypertension

(Continued)

Imiglucerase *(Continued)*

Usual Dosage I.V.: 2.5 units/kg 3 times/week up to as much as 60 units/kg administered as frequently as once a week or as infrequently as every 4 weeks; 60 units/kg administered every 2 weeks is the most common dose

Administration Infuse over 1-2 hours; may be infused through an in-line, low protein-binding 0.2 micron filter. Do not use vials with discoloration or opaque particles.

Dosage Forms

Powder for injection, lyophilized [preservative free]:
212 units [equivalent to a withdrawal dose of 200 units]
424 units [equivalent to a withdrawal dose of 400 units]

♦ **Imipemide** *see* Imipenem and Cilastatin *on page 706*

Imipenem and Cilastatin (i mi PEN em & sye la STAT in)

Related Information

Antimicrobial Drugs of Choice *on page 1588*

U.S. Brand Names Primaxin®

Canadian Brand Names Primaxin®

Synonyms Imipemide

Therapeutic Category Antibiotic, Anaerobic; Antibiotic, Carbapenem

Use Treatment of respiratory tract, urinary tract, intra-abdominal, gynecologic, bone and joint, skin structure, and polymicrobic infections as well as bacterial septicemia and endocarditis. Antibacterial activity includes resistant gram-negative bacilli (*Pseudomonas aeruginosa* and *Enterobacter* sp), gram-positive bacteria (methicillin-sensitive *Staphylococcus aureus* and *Streptococcus* sp) and anaerobes.

Note: I.M. administration is not intended for severe or life-threatening infections (eg, septicemia, endocarditis, shock)

Pregnancy Risk Factor C

Pregnancy/Breast-Feeding Implications There are no well-controlled or adequate studies in pregnant women. Use during pregnancy only if the potential benefits outweigh the potential risks to mother and fetus.

Contraindications Hypersensitivity to imipenem/cilastatin or any component of the formulation; refer to Lidocaine monograph for Contraindications associated with I.M. dosing

Warnings/Precautions Dosage adjustment required in patients with impaired renal function; prolonged use may result in superinfection; has been associated with CNS adverse effects, including confusional states and seizures; use with caution in patients with a history of seizures or hypersensitivity to beta-lactams (including penicillins and cephalosporins); serious hypersensitivity reactions, including anaphylaxis, have been reported (some without a history of previous allergic reactions to beta-lactams); elderly patients often require lower doses; not recommended in pediatric CNS infections; refer to Lidocaine monograph for Warnings/Precautions associated with I.M. dosing

Adverse Reactions

1% to 10%:

Gastrointestinal: Nausea/diarrhea/vomiting (1% to 2%)

Local: Phlebitis (3%), pain at I.M. injection site (1%)

<1% (Limited to important or life-threatening): Anaphylaxis, angioneurotic edema, confusion (acute), drug fever, dyspnea, emergence of resistant strains of *P. aeruginosa*, encephalopathy, eosinophilia, erythema multiforme, hallucinations, hemolytic anemia, hemorrhagic colitis, hepatitis, hypersensitivity, hypotension, increased PT, jaundice, leukopenia, neutropenia (including agranulocytosis), pancytopenia, paresthesia, positive Coombs' test, pruritus, pseudomembranous colitis, psychic disturbances, rash, renal failure (acute), seizures, somnolence, Stevens-Johnson syndrome, thrombocytopenia, toxic epidermal necrolysis, urticaria, vertigo

Overdosage/Toxicology Symptoms include neuromuscular hypersensitivity and seizures. Hemodialysis may be helpful to aid in removal of the drug from the blood, otherwise most treatment is supportive or symptom directed.

Drug Interactions

Increased Effect/Toxicity: Beta-lactam antibiotics and probenecid may increase potential for toxicity.

Stability

Imipenem/cilastatin powder for injection should be stored at <30°C

Reconstituted solutions are stable 10 hours at room temperature and 48 hours at refrigeration (4°C) with NS

If reconstituted with 5% or 10% dextrose injection, 5% dextrose and sodium bicarbonate, 5% dextrose and 0.9% sodium chloride, is stable for 4 hours at room temperature and 24 hours when refrigerated

Imipenem/cilastatin is most stable at a pH of 6.5-7.5; imipenem is inactivated at acidic or alkaline pH

Standard diluent: 500 mg/100 mL NS; 1 g/250 mL NS

Comments: All IVPB should be prepared fresh; do not use dextrose as a diluent due to limited stability

Mechanism of Action Inhibits bacterial cell wall synthesis by binding to one or more of the penicillin binding proteins (PBPs); which in turn inhibits the final transpeptidation step of peptidoglycan synthesis in bacterial cell walls, thus inhibiting cell wall biosynthesis. Bacteria eventually lyse due to ongoing activity of cell wall autolytic enzymes (autolysins and murein hydrolases) while cell wall assembly is arrested. Cilastatin prevents renal metabolism of imipenem by competitive inhibition of dehydropeptidase along the brush border of the renal tubules.

Pharmacodynamics/Kinetics

Absorption: I.M.: Imipenem: 60% to 75%; cilastatin: 95% to 100%

Distribution: Rapidly and widely to most tissues and fluids including sputum, pleural fluid, peritoneal fluid, interstitial fluid, bile, aqueous humor, reproductive organs, and bone;

highest concentrations in pleural fluid, interstitial fluid, peritoneal fluid, and reproductive organs; low concentrations in CSF; crosses placenta; enters breast milk

Metabolism: Renally by dehydropeptidase; activity is blocked by cilastatin; cilastatin is partially metabolized renally

Half-life elimination: Both drugs: 60 minutes, extended with renal insufficiency

Excretion: Both drugs: Urine (~70% as unchanged drug)

Usual Dosage Dosage based on **imipenem** content:

Neonates: Non-CNS infections: I.V.:

<1 week: 25 mg/kg every 12 hours

1-4 weeks: 25 mg/kg every 8 hours

4 weeks to 3 months: 25 mg/kg every 6 hours

Children: >3 months: Non-CNS infections: I.V.: 15-25 mg/kg every 6 hours

Maximum dosage: Susceptible infections: 2 g/day; moderately susceptible organisms: 4 g/day

Children: Cystic fibrosis: I.V.: Doses up to 90 mg/kg/day have been used

Adults:

Mild infections:

I.M.: 500 mg every 12 hours; intra-abdominal infections: 750 mg every 12 hours

I.V.:

Fully-susceptible organisms: 250 mg every 6 hours (1g/day)

Moderately-susceptible organisms: 500 mg every 6 hours (2 g/day)

Moderate infections:

I.M.: 750 mg every 12 hours

I.V.:

Fully-susceptible organisms: 500 mg every 6-8 hours (1.5-2 g/day)

Moderately-susceptible organisms: 500 mg every 6 hours or 1 g every 8 hours (2-3 g/day)

Severe infections: I.V.: **Note:** I.M. administration is not intended for severe or life-threatening infections (eg, septicemia, endocarditis, shock):

Fully-susceptible organisms: 500 mg every 6 hours (2 g/day)

Moderately-susceptible organisms: 1 g every 6-8 hours (3-4 g/day)

Maximum daily dose should not exceed 50 mg/kg or 4 g/day, whichever is lower

Urinary tract infection, uncomplicated: I.V.: 250 mg every 6 hours (1 g/day)

Urinary tract infection, complicated: I.V.: 500 mg every 6 hours (2 g/day)

Dosage adjustment in renal impairment: I.V.: **Note:** Adjustments have not been established for I.M. dosing: See table.

Imipenem/Cilastatin

Creatinine Clearance (mL/min/1.73 m^2)	Frequency	Dose (mg)
30-70	q8h	500
20-30	q12h	500
5-20	q12h	250

Patients with a Cl$_{cr}$ <5 mL/minute/1.73 m^2 should not receive imipenem/cilastatin unless hemodialysis is instituted within 48 hours.

Patients weighing <30 kg with impaired renal function should not receive imipenem/cilastatin.

Hemodialysis: Use the dosing recommendation for patients with a Cl$_{cr}$ 6-20 mL/minute

Peritoneal dialysis: Dose as for Cl$_{cr}$ <10 mL/minute

Continuous arteriovenous or venovenous hemofiltration: Dose as for Cl$_{cr}$ 20-30 mL/minute; monitor for seizure activity; imipenem is well removed by CAVH but cilastatin is not; removes 20 mg of imipenem per liter of filtrate per day

Administration

I.M.: Prepare 500 mg vial with 2 mL 1% lidocaine; prepare 750 mg vial with 3 mL 1% lidocaine **(do not use lidocaine with epinephrine)**. Administer by deep injection into a large muscle (gluteal or lateral thigh). Aspiration is necessary to avoid inadvertent injection into a blood vessel.

I.V.: Not for direct infusion; vial contents must be transferred to 100 mL of infusion solution; final concentration should not exceed 5 mg/mL; infuse each 250-500 mg dose over 20-30 minutes; infuse each 1 g dose over 40-60 minutes; watch for convulsions. If nausea and/or vomiting occur during administration, decrease the rate of I.V. infusion; do not mix with or physically add to other antibiotics; however, may administer concomitantly

Monitoring Parameters Periodic renal, hepatic, and hematologic function tests; monitor for signs of anaphylaxis during first dose

Test Interactions Interferes with urinary glucose determination using Clinitest®

Nursing Implications Administer by I.V. intermittent infusion; final concentration for administration should not exceed 5 mg/mL; in fluid-restricted patients, a final concentration of 7 mg/mL has been administered; infuse over 20-60 minutes; if nausea and/or vomiting occur during administration, decrease the rate of I.V. infusion

Additional Information Sodium content of 1 g injection:

I.M.: 64.4 mg (2.8 mEq)

I.V.: 73.6 mg (3.2 mEq)

Dosage Forms

Powder for injection, I.M.:

Imipenem 500 mg and cilastatin 500 mg

Imipenem 750 mg and cilastatin 750 mg

Powder for injection, I.V.:

Imipenem 250 mg and cilastatin 250 mg

Imipenem 500 mg and cilastatin 500 mg

Imipramine (im IP ra meen)

Related Information

Antidepressant Agents Comparison *on page 1482*

U.S. Brand Names Tofranil®; Tofranil-PM®

Canadian Brand Names Apo®-Imipramine; Tofranil®

Synonyms Imipramine Hydrochloride; Imipramine Pamoate

Therapeutic Category Antidepressant, Tricyclic

Use Treatment of various forms of depression

Unlabeled/Investigational Use Enuresis in children; analgesic for certain chronic and neuro-pathic pain; panic disorder; attention-deficit/hyperactivity disorder (ADHD)

Pregnancy Risk Factor D

Contraindications Hypersensitivity to imipramine (cross-reactivity with other dibenzodiazepines may occur) or any component of the formulation; concurrent use of MAO inhibitors (within 14 days); in a patient during acute recovery phase of MI; pregnancy

Warnings/Precautions Use with caution in patients with cardiovascular disease, conduction disturbances, seizure disorders, urinary retention, hyperthyroidism or those receiving thyroid replacement. Do not discontinue abruptly in patients receiving long-term, high-dose therapy. Some oral preparations contain tartrazine and injection contains sulfites, both of which can cause allergic reactions. May cause sedation, resulting in impaired performance of tasks requiring alertness (ie, operating machinery or driving). Sedative effects may be additive with other CNS depressants and/or ethanol. The degree of sedation is high relative to other antidepressants. May worsen psychosis in some patients or precipitate a shift to mania or hypomania in patients with bipolar disease. May increase the risks associated with electro-convulsive therapy. This agent should be discontinued, when possible, prior to elective surgery. Therapy should not be abruptly discontinued in patients receiving high doses for prolonged periods.

Orthostatic hypotension is a concern with this agent, especially in patients taking other medications that may affect blood pressure; may precipitate arrhythmias in predisposed patients; may aggravate seizures. The degree of anticholinergic blockade produced by this agent is high relative to other cyclic antidepressants - use caution in patients with urinary retention, benign prostatic hyperplasia, narrow-angle glaucoma, xerostomia, visual problems, constipation, or history of bowel obstruction. A less anticholinergic antidepressant may be a better choice.

Adverse Reactions Frequency not defined.

Cardiovascular: Orthostatic hypotension, arrhythmias, tachycardia, hypertension, palpitations, myocardial infarction, heart block, EKG changes, CHF, stroke

Central nervous system: Dizziness, drowsiness, headache, agitation, insomnia, nightmares, hypomania, psychosis, fatigue, confusion, hallucinations, disorientation, delusions, anxiety, restlessness, seizures

Endocrine & metabolic: Gynecomastia, breast enlargement, galactorrhea, increase or decrease in libido, increase or decrease in blood sugar, SIADH

Gastrointestinal: Nausea, unpleasant taste, weight gain/loss, xerostomia, constipation, ileus, stomatitis, abdominal cramps, vomiting, anorexia, epigastric disorders, diarrhea, black tongue

Genitourinary: Urinary retention, impotence

Neuromuscular & skeletal: Weakness, numbness, tingling, paresthesias, incoordination, ataxia, tremor, peripheral neuropathy, extrapyramidal symptoms

Ocular: Blurred vision, disturbances of accommodation, mydriasis

Otic: Tinnitus

Miscellaneous: Diaphoresis

<1% (Limited to important or life-threatening): Agranulocytosis, alopecia, cholestatic jaundice, eosinophilia, increased liver enzymes, itching, petechiae, photosensitivity, purpura, rash, thrombocytopenia, urticaria

Overdosage/Toxicology Symptoms include confusion, hallucinations, constipation, cyanosis, tachycardia, urinary retention, ventricular tachycardia, and seizures. Following initiation of essential overdose management, toxic symptoms should be treated. Sodium bicarbonate is indicated when the QRS interval is >0.10 seconds or the QT_c interval is >0.42 seconds. Ventricular arrhythmias often respond to concurrent systemic alkalinization (sodium bicarbonate 0.5-2 mEq/kg I.V.). Ventricular arrhythmias unresponsive to this therapy may respond to lidocaine 1 mg/kg I.V., followed by a titrated infusion. Physostigmine (1-2 mg slow I.V. for adults or 0.5 mg slow I.V. for children) may be indicated in reversing life-threatening cardiac arrhythmias. Seizures usually respond to diazepam I.V. boluses (5-10 mg for adults up to 30 mg or 0.25-0.4 mg/kg/dose for children up to 10 mg/dose). If seizures are unresponsive or recur, phenytoin or phenobarbital may be required.

Drug Interactions

Cytochrome P450 Effect: CYP1A2, 2C9, 2C19, 2D6, and 3A3/4 enzyme substrate

Increased Effect/Toxicity: Imipramine increases the effects of amphetamines, anticholinergics, other CNS depressants (sedatives, hypnotics, or ethanol), chlorpropamide, tolazamide, and warfarin. When used with MAO inhibitors, hyperpyrexia, hypertension, tachycardia, confusion, seizures, and **deaths have been reported** (serotonin syndrome). Serotonin syndrome has also been reported with ritonavir (rare). The SSRIs (to varying degrees), cimetidine, grapefruit juice, indinavir, methylphenidate, ritonavir, quinidine, diltiazem, and verapamil inhibit the metabolism of TCAs and clinical toxicity may result. Use of lithium with a TCA may increase the risk for neurotoxicity. Phenothiazines may increase concentration of some TCAs and TCAs may increase concentration of phenothiazines. Pressor response to I.V. epinephrine, norepinephrine, and phenylephrine may be enhanced in patients receiving TCAs (**Note:** Effect is unlikely with epinephrine or levonordefrin dosages typically administered as infiltration in combination with local anesthetics). Combined use of beta-agonists or drugs which prolong QT_c (including quinidine, procainamide, disopyramide, cisapride, sparfloxacin, gatifloxacin, moxifloxacin) with TCAs may predispose patients to cardiac arrhythmias.

Decreased Effect: Carbamazepine, phenobarbital, and rifampin may increase the metabolism of imipramine resulting in decreased effect of imipramine. Imipramine inhibits the antihypertensive response to bethanidine, clonidine, debrisoquin, guanadrel, guanethidine, guanabenz, and guanfacine. Cholestyramine and colestipol may bind TCAs and reduce their absorption; monitor for altered response.

Ethanol/Nutrition/Herb Interactions
Ethanol: Avoid ethanol (may increase CNS depression).
Food: Grapefruit juice may inhibit the metabolism of some TCAs and clinical toxicity may result.
Herb/Nutraceutical: St John's wort may decrease imipramine levels. Avoid valerian, St John's wort, SAMe, kava kava (may increase risk of serotonin syndrome and/or excessive sedation).

Stability Solutions stable at a pH of 4-5; turns yellowish or reddish on exposure to light. Slight discoloration does not affect potency; marked discoloration is associated with loss of potency.

Mechanism of Action Traditionally believed to increase the synaptic concentration of serotonin and/or norepinephrine in the central nervous system by inhibition of their reuptake by the presynaptic neuronal membrane. However, additional receptor effects have been found including desensitization of adenyl cyclase, down regulation of beta-adrenergic receptors, and down regulation of serotonin receptors.

Pharmacodynamics/Kinetics
Onset of action: Peak antidepressant effect: Usually after ≥2 weeks
Absorption: Well absorbed
Distribution: Crosses placenta
Metabolism: Hepatically by microsomal enzymes to desipramine (active) and other metabolites; significant first-pass effect
Half-life elimination: 6-18 hours
Excretion: Urine (as metabolites)

Usual Dosage Oral:
Children:
Depression: 1.5 mg/kg/day with dosage increments of 1 mg/kg every 3-4 days to a maximum dose of 5 mg/kg/day in 1-4 divided doses; monitor carefully especially with doses ≥3.5 mg/kg/day
Enuresis: ≥6 years: Initial: 10-25 mg at bedtime, if inadequate response still seen after 1 week of therapy, increase by 25 mg/day; dose should not exceed 2.5 mg/kg/day or 50 mg at bedtime if 6-12 years of age or 75 mg at bedtime if ≥12 years of age
Adjunct in the treatment of cancer pain: Initial: 0.2-0.4 mg/kg at bedtime; dose may be increased by 50% every 2-3 days up to 1-3 mg/kg/dose at bedtime
Adolescents: Initial: 25-50 mg/day; increase gradually; maximum: 100 mg/day in single or divided doses
Adults: Initial: 25 mg 3-4 times/day, increase dose gradually, total dose may be given at bedtime; maximum: 300 mg/day
Elderly: Initial: 10-25 mg at bedtime; increase by 10-25 mg every 3 days for inpatients and weekly for outpatients if tolerated; average daily dose to achieve a therapeutic concentration: 100 mg/day; range: 50-150 mg/day

Monitoring Parameters Monitor blood pressure and pulse rate prior to and during initial therapy; EKG in older adults, CBC; evaluate mental status; blood levels are useful for therapeutic monitoring

Reference Range Therapeutic: Imipramine and desipramine: 150-250 ng/mL (SI: 530-890 nmol/L); desipramine: 150-300 ng/mL (SI: 560-1125 nmol/L); Toxic: >500 ng/mL (SI: 446-893 nmol/L); utility of serum level monitoring controversial

Patient Information May require 2-4 weeks to achieve desired effect; avoid alcohol; do not discontinue medication abruptly; may cause urine to turn blue-green; may cause drowsiness, avoid alcohol and other CNS depressants; dry mouth may be helped by sips of water, sugarless gum, or hard candy; rise slowly to avoid dizziness

Nursing Implications Raise bed rails, institute safety measures

Dosage Forms
Capsule, as pamoate (Tofranil-PM®): 75 mg, 100 mg, 125 mg, 150 mg
Tablet, as hydrochloride (Tofranil®): 10 mg, 25 mg, 50 mg

♦ **Imipramine Hydrochloride** *see* Imipramine *on page 708*
♦ **Imipramine Pamoate** *see* Imipramine *on page 708*

Imiquimod (i mi KWI mod)

U.S. Brand Names Aldara™
Canadian Brand Names Aldara™
Therapeutic Category Skin and Mucous Membrane Agent; Topical Skin Product
Use Treatment of external genital and perianal warts/condyloma acuminata in children ≥12 years of age and adults
Pregnancy Risk Factor B
Contraindications Hypersensitivity to imiquimod or any component of the formulation
Warnings/Precautions Imiquimod has not been evaluated for the treatment of urethral, intravaginal, cervical, rectal, or intra-anal human papilloma viral disease and is not recommended for these conditions. Topical imiquimod is not intended for ophthalmic use. Topical imiquimod administration is not recommended until genital/perianal tissue is healed from any previous drug or surgical treatment. Imiquimod has the potential to exacerbate inflammatory conditions of the skin.
Adverse Reactions
>10%: Local, mild/moderate: Erythema (54% to 61%), itching (22% to 32%), erosion (21% to 32%), burning (9% to 26%), excoriation/flaking (18% to 25%), edema (12% to 17%), scabbing (9% to 13%)
1% to 10%:
Central nervous system: Pain (2% to 8%), headache (4% to 5%)
Local, severe: Erythema (4%), erosion (1%), edema (1%)
Local, mild/moderate: Pain, induration, ulceration (5% to 7%), vesicles (2% to 3%), soreness (<1% to 3%)
(Continued)

Imiquimod *(Continued)*

Neuromuscular & skeletal: Myalgia (1%)

Miscellaneous: Influenza-like symptoms (1% to 3%), fungal infections (2% to 11%)

Overdosage/Toxicology Overdosage is unlikely because of minimal percutaneous absorption. Persistent topical overdosing of imiquimod could result in severe local skin reactions. The most clinically serious adverse event reported, following multiple oral imiquimod doses of ≥200 mg, was hypotension which resolved following oral or I.V. fluid administration. Treat symptomatically.

Stability Do not store at ≥30°C (86°F); avoid freezing

Mechanism of Action Mechanism of action is unknown; however, induces cytokines, including interferon-alpha and others

Pharmacodynamics/Kinetics

Absorption: Minimal

Excretion: Urine and feces (<0.9%)

Usual Dosage Children ≥12 years and Adults: Topical: Apply 3 times/week prior to normal sleeping hours and leave on the skin for 6-10 hours. Following treatment period, remove cream by washing the treated area with mild soap and water. Examples of 3 times/week application schedules are: Monday, Wednesday, Friday; or Tuesday, Thursday, Saturday. Continue imiquimod treatment until there is total clearance of the genital/perianal warts for ≤16 weeks. A rest period of several days may be taken if required by the patient's discomfort or severity of the local skin reaction. Treatment may resume once the reaction subsides.

Administration Nonocclusive dressings such as cotton gauze or cotton underwear may be used in the management of skin reactions. Handwashing before and after cream application is recommended. Imiquimod is packaged in single-use packets that contain sufficient cream to cover a wart area of up to 20 cm^2; avoid use of excessive amounts of cream. Instruct patients to apply imiquimod to external or perianal warts. Apply a thin layer to the wart area and rub in until the cream is no longer visible. Do not occlude the application site.

Monitoring Parameters Reduction in wart size is indicative of a therapeutic response; patients should be monitored for signs and symptoms of hypersensitivity to imiquimod

Patient Information Imiquimod may weaken condoms and vaginal diaphragms; therefore, concurrent use is not recommended. This medication is for external use only; avoid contact with eyes. Do not occlude the treatment area with bandages or other covers or wraps. Avoid sexual (genital, anal, oral) contact while the cream is on the skin. Wash the treatment area with mild soap and water 6-10 hours following application of imiquimod.

Patients commonly experience local skin reactions such as erythema, erosion, excoriation/flaking, and edema at the site of application or surrounding areas. Most skin reactions are mild to moderate. Severe skin reactions can occur; promptly report severe reactions to physician. Uncircumcised males treating warts under the foreskin should retract the foreskin and clean the area daily.

Imiquimod is not a cure; new warts may develop during therapy.

Nursing Implications Apply only to external or perianal warts; wash hands before and after application of the cream; cotton gauze or underwear may be used to manage treatment area; do not occlude treatment area; avoid sexual contact while cream is on skin; cream may weaken condoms or diaphragms, concurrent use is not recommended

Dosage Forms Cream, topical [single-dose packets in boxes of 12]: 5% (250 mg)

♦ **Imitrex®** *see* Sumatriptan Succinate *on page 1279*

♦ **ImmuCyst® (Can)** *see* BCG Vaccine *on page 148*

Immune Globulin (Intramuscular)

(i MYUN GLOB yoo lin, IN tra MUS kyoo ler)

Related Information

Immunization Recommendations *on page 1538*

U.S. Brand Names BayGam®

Canadian Brand Names Baygam™

Synonyms Gamma Globulin; IG; IGIM; Immune Serum Globulin; ISG

Therapeutic Category Immune Globulin

Use Household and sexual contacts of persons with hepatitis A, measles, varicella, and possibly rubella; travelers to high-risk areas outside tourist routes; staff, attendees, parents of diapered attendees in day-care center outbreaks

For travelers, IG is not an alternative to careful selection of foods and water; immune globulin can interfere with the antibody response to parenterally administered live virus vaccines. Frequent travelers should be tested for hepatitis A antibody, immune hemolytic anemia, and neutropenia (with ITP, I.V. route is usually used).

Pregnancy Risk Factor C

Contraindications Hypersensitivity to immune globulin, thimerosal, or any component of the formulation; IgA deficiency; I.M. injections in patients with thrombocytopenia or coagulation disorders

Warnings/Precautions Skin testing should not be performed as local irritation can occur and be misinterpreted as a positive reaction; IG should **not** be used to control outbreaks of measles. As a product of human plasma, this product may potentially transmit disease; screening of donors, as well as testing and/or inactivation of certain viruses reduces this risk. Epidemiologic and laboratory data indicate current IMIG products do not have a discernible risk of transmitting HIV. Use caution in patients with thrombocytopenia or coagulation disorders (I.M. injections may be contraindicated). Not for I.V. administration.

Adverse Reactions Frequency not defined.

Cardiovascular: Flushing, angioedema,

Central nervous system: Chills, lethargy, fever

Dermatologic: Urticaria, erythema

Gastrointestinal: Nausea, vomiting

Local: Pain, tenderness, muscle stiffness at I.M. site

Neuromuscular & skeletal: Myalgia

Miscellaneous: Hypersensitivity reactions

Drug Interactions

Increased Effect/Toxicity: Increased toxicity: Live virus, vaccines (measles, mumps, rubella); do not administer within 3 months after administration of these vaccines.

Stability Keep in refrigerator; do not freeze

Mechanism of Action Provides passive immunity by increasing the antibody titer and antigen-antibody reaction potential

Pharmacodynamics/Kinetics

Duration: Immune effect: Usually 3-4 weeks

Half-life elimination: 23 days

Time to peak, serum: I.M.: ~24-48 hours

Usual Dosage I.M.:

Hepatitis A:

Pre-exposure prophylaxis upon travel into endemic areas (hepatitis A vaccine preferred):

0.02 mL/kg for anticipated risk 1-3 months

0.06 mL/kg for anticipated risk >3 months

Repeat approximate dose every 4-6 months if exposure continues

Postexposure prophylaxis: 0.02 mL/kg given within 7 days of exposure

Measles:

Prophylaxis: 0.25 mL/kg/dose (maximum dose: 15 mL) given within 6 days of exposure followed by live attenuated measles vaccine in 3 months or at 15 months of age (whichever is later)

For patients with leukemia, lymphoma, immunodeficiency disorders, generalized malignancy, or receiving immunosuppressive therapy: 0.5 mL/kg (maximum dose: 15 mL)

Poliomyelitis: Prophylaxis: 0.3 mL/kg/dose as a single dose

Rubella: Prophylaxis: 0.55 mL/kg/dose within 72 hours of exposure

Varicella:: Prophylaxis: 0.6-1.2 mL/kg (varicella zoster immune globulin preferred) within 72 hours of exposure

IgG deficiency: 1.3 mL/kg, then 0.66 mL/kg in 3-4 weeks

Hepatitis B: Prophylaxis: 0.06 mL/kg/dose (HBIG preferred)

Administration Intramuscular injection only

Test Interactions Skin tests should **not** be done

Nursing Implications Do not mix with other medications; skin testing should not be performed as local irritation can occur and be misinterpreted as a positive reaction

Dosage Forms Injection: I.M.: 165 ±15 mg (of protein)/mL (2 mL, 10 mL)

Immune Globulin (Intravenous) (i MYUN GLOB yoo lin, IN tra VEE nus)

Related Information

Immunization Recommendations *on page 1538*

U.S. Brand Names Gamimune® N; Gammagard®; Gammagard® S/D; Gammar®-P I.V.; Polygam®; Polygam® S/D; Sandoglobulin®; Venoglobulin®-I; Venoglobulin®-S

Canadian Brand Names Gamimune® N; Gammagard® S/D; Iveegam Immuno®

Synonyms IVIG

Therapeutic Category Immune Globulin

Use Treatment of immunodeficiency syndromes (hypogammaglobulinemia, agammaglobulinemia, IgG subclass deficiencies, severe combined immunodeficiency syndromes (SCIDS), Wiskott-Aldrich syndrome), idiopathic thrombocytopenic purpura; used in conjunction with appropriate anti-infective therapy to prevent or modify acute bacterial or viral infections in patients with iatrogenically-induced or disease-associated immunodepression, chronic lymphocytic leukemia (CLL), chronic prophylaxis autoimmune neutropenia, bone marrow transplantation patients, autoimmune hemolytic anemia or neutropenia, refractory dermatomyositis/polymyositis, autoimmune diseases (myasthenia gravis, SLE, bullous pemphigoid, severe rheumatoid arthritis), Guillain-Barré syndrome; pediatric HIV infection to decrease frequency of serious bacterial infections; Kawasaki disease in combination with aspirin

Pregnancy Risk Factor C

Contraindications Hypersensitivity to immune globulin or any component of the formulation; IgA deficiency (except with the use of Gammagard®, Polygam®)

Adverse Reactions Frequency not defined.

Cardiovascular: Flushing of the face, tachycardia, hypotension, chest tightness, angioedema.

Central nervous system: Chills, dizziness, fever, headache, lethargy, aseptic meningitis syndrome

Dermatologic: Urticaria

Gastrointestinal: Nausea, vomiting

Neuromuscular & skeletal: Myalgia

Renal: Nephrotic syndrome

Respiratory: Dyspnea

Miscellaneous: Diaphoresis, hypersensitivity reactions, anaphylaxis

Drug Interactions

Increased Effect/Toxicity: Live virus, vaccines (measles, mumps, rubella); do not administer within 3 months after administration of these vaccines.

Stability Stability and dilution is dependent upon the manufacturer and brand; do not mix with other drugs

Mechanism of Action Replacement therapy for primary and secondary immunodeficiencies; interference with F_c receptors on the cells of the reticuloendothelial system for autoimmune cytopenias and ITP; possible role of contained antiviral-type antibodies

Pharmacodynamics/Kinetics

Onset of action: I.V.: Provides immediate antibody levels

Duration: Immune effect: 3-4 weeks

Half-life elimination: 21-24 days

Usual Dosage Children and Adults: I.V.:

Dosages should be based on ideal body weight and not actual body weight in morbidly obese patients; approved doses and regimens may vary between brands; check manufacturer guidelines

(Continued)

Immune Globulin (Intravenous) *(Continued)*

Primary immunodeficiency disorders: 200-400 mg/kg every 4 weeks or as per monitored serum IgG concentrations

Chronic lymphocytic leukemia (CLL): 400 mg/kg/dose every 3 weeks

Idiopathic thrombocytopenic purpura (ITP): Maintenance dose:

400 mg/kg/day for 2-5 consecutive days; or 1000 mg/kg every other day for 3 doses, if needed or

1000 mg/kg/day for 2 consecutive days; or up to 2000 mg/kg/day over 2-7 consecutive days

Chronic ITP: 400-2000 mg/kg/dose as needed to maintain appropriate platelet counts

Kawasaki disease: Initiate within 10 days of disease onset: In combination with aspirin 80-100 mg/kg/day in 4 divided doses for 14 days; when fever subsides, dose aspirin at 3-5 mg/kg once daily for ≥ 6-8 weeks

2 g/kg for one dose only

400 mg/kg/day for 4 days within 10 days of onset of fever

Acquired immunodeficiency syndrome (patients must be symptomatic):

200-250 mg/kg/dose every 2 weeks

400-500 mg/kg/dose every month or every 4 weeks

Pediatric HIV: 400 mg/kg every 28 days

Autoimmune hemolytic anemia and neutropenia: 1000 mg/kg/dose for 2-3 days

Autoimmune diseases: 400 mg/kg/day for 4 days

Bone marrow transplant: 500 mg/kg beginning on days 7 and 2 pretransplant, then 500 mg/kg/week for 90 days post-transplant

Adjuvant to severe cytomegalovirus infections: 500 mg/kg/dose every other day for 7 doses

Severe systemic viral and bacterial infections: Children: 500-1000 mg/kg/week

Prevention of gastroenteritis: Infants and Children: Oral: 50 mg/kg/day divided every 6 hours

Guillain-Barré syndrome:

400 mg/kg/day for 4 days

1000 mg/kg/day for 2 days

2000 mg/kg/day for one day

Refractory dermatomyositis: 2 g/kg/dose every month x 3-4 doses

Refractory polymyositis: 1 g/kg/day x 2 days every month x 4 doses

Chronic inflammatory demyelinating polyneuropathy:

400 mg/kg/day for 5 doses once each month

800 mg/kg/day for 3 doses once each month

1000 mg/kg/day for 2 days once each month

Dosing adjustment/comments in renal impairment: Cl_{cr} <10 mL/minute: Avoid use

Administration I.V. use only; for initial treatment, a lower concentration and/or a slower rate of infusion should be used

Nursing Implications

I.V. use only; for initial treatment, a lower concentration and/or a slower rate of infusion should be used

Monitor platelet count, vital signs

Stability: Parenteral admixture at room temperature (25°C): 30 days; parenteral admixture at refrigeration temperature (4°C): 36 months

Additional Information

Intravenous Immune Globulin Product Comparison:

Gamimune®N:

FDA indication: Primary immunodeficiency, ITP

Contraindication: IgA deficiency

IgA content: 270 mcg/mL

Adverse reactions (%): 5.2

Plasma source: >2000 paid donors

Half-life: 21 days

IgG subclass (%):

IgG_1 (60-70): 60

IgG_2 (19-31): 29.4

IgG_3 (5-8.4): 6.5

IgG_4 (0.7-4): 4.1

Monomers (%): >95

Gamma globulin (%): >98

Storage: Refrigerate

Recommendations for **initial** infusion rate: 0.01-0.02 mL/kg/minute

Maximum infusion rate: 0.08 mL/kg/minute

Maximum concentration for infusion (%):10

Gammagard®SD:

FDA indication: Primary immunodeficiency, ITP, CLL prophylaxis

Contraindication: None (caution with IgA deficiency)

IgA content: 0.92-1.6 mcg/mL

Adverse reactions (%): 6

Plasma source: 4000-5000 paid donors

Half-life: 24 days

IgG subclass (%):

IgG_1 (60-70): 67 (66.8)*

IgG_2 (19-31): 25 (25.4)

IgG_3 (5-8.4): 5 (7.4)

IgG_4 (0.7-4): 3 (0.3)

Monomers (%): >95

Gamma globulin (%): >90

Storage: Room temperature

Recommendations for **initial** infusion rate: 0.5 mL/kg/hour

Maximum infusion rate: 4 mL/kg/hour

Maximum concentration for infusion (%): 5

Gammar®-P I.V.:
  FDA indication: Primary immunodeficiency
  Contraindication: IgA deficiency
  IgA content: <20 mcg/mL
  Adverse reactions (%): 15
  Plasma source: >8000 paid donors
  Half-life: 21-24 days
  IgG subclass (%):
    IgG_1 (60-70): 69
    IgG_2 (19-31): 23
    IgG_3 (5-8.4): 6
    IgG_4 (0.7-4): 2
  Monomers (%): >98
  Gamma globulin (%): >98
  Storage: Room temperature
  Recommendations for **initial** infusion rate: 0.01-0.02 mL/kg/minute
  Maximum infusion rate: 0.06 mL/kg/minute
  Maximum concentration for infusion (%): 5

Polygram®:
  FDA indication: Primary immunodeficiency, ITP, CLL
  Contraindication: None (caution with IgA deficiency)
  IgA content: 0.74 ±0.33 mcg/mL
  Adverse reactions (%): 6
  Plasma source: 50,000 voluntary donors
  Half-life: 21-25 days
  IgG subclass (%):
    IgG_1 (60-70): 67
    IgG_2 (19-31): 25
    IgG_3 (5-8.4): 5
    IgG_4 (0.7-4): 3
  Monomers (%): >95
  Gamma globulin (%): >90
  Storage: Room temperature
  Recommendations for **initial** infusion rate: 0.5 mL/kg/hour
  Maximum infusion rate: 4 mL/kg/hour
  Maximum concentration for infusion (%): 10

Sandoglobulin®:
  FDA indication: Primary immunodeficiency, ITP
  Contraindication: IgA deficiency
  IgA content: 720 mcg/mL
  Adverse reactions (%): 2.5-6.6
  Plasma source: 8000-15,000 voluntary donors
  Half-life: 21-23 days
  IgG subclass (%):
    IgG_1 (60-70): 60.5 (55.3)*
    IgG_2 (19-31): 30.2 (35.7)
    IgG_3 (5-8.4): 6.6 (6.3)
    IgG_4 (0.7-4): 2.6 (2.6)
  Monomers (%): >92
  Gamma globulin (%): >96
  Storage: Room temperature
  Recommendations for **initial** infusion rate: 0.01-0.03 mL/kg/minute
  Maximum infusion rate: 2.5 mL/minute
  Maximum concentration for infusion (%): 12

Venoglobulin®-I:
  FDA indication: Primary immunodeficiency, ITP
  Contraindication: IgA deficiency
  IgA content: 20-24 mcg/mL
  Adverse reactions (%): 6
  Plasma source: 6000-9000 paid donors
  Half-life: 29 days
  IgG subclass (%):
    IgG_1 (60-70): 62.3**
    IgG_2 (19-31): 32.8
    IgG_3 (5-8.4): 2.9
    IgG_4 (0.7-4): 2
  Monomers (%): >98
  Gamma globulin (%): >98
  Storage: Room temperature
  Recommendations for **initial** infusion rate: 0.01-0.02 mL/kg/minute
  Maximum infusion rate: 0.04 mL/kg/minute
  Maximum concentration for infusion (%):10

*Skvaril F and Gardi A, "Differences Among Available Immunoglobulin Preparations for Intravenous Use," *Pediatr Infect Dis J*, 1988, 7:543-48.
**Roomer J, Morgenthaler JJ, Scherz R, et al, "Characterization of Various Immunoglobulin Preparations for Intravenous Application," *Vox Sang*, 1982, 42:62-73.

Dosage Forms
  Injection (Gamimune® N): 5% [50 mg/mL] (10 mL, 50 mL, 100 mL, 250 mL); 10% [100 mg/mL] (10 mL, 50 mL, 100 mL, 200 mL)
  Powder for injection, detergent treated:
    Gammagard® S/D: 2.5 g, 5 g, 10 g
    Polygam® S/D: 2.5 g, 5 g, 10 g
    Venoglobulin®-S: 5% [50 mg/mL] (50 mL, 100 mL, 200 mL); 10% [100 mg/mL] (50 mL, 100 mL, 200 mL)
  (Continued)

Immune Globulin (Intravenous) *(Continued)*

Powder for injection, lyophilized:
Gammar®-P I.V. (5% IgG and 3% albumin): 1 g, 2.5 g, 5 g, 10 g
Polygam®: 0.5 g, 2.5 g, 5 g, 10 g
Sandoglobulin®: 1 g, 3 g, 6 g, 12 g
Venoglobulin®-I: 0.5 g, 2.5 g, 5 g, 10 g

♦ **Immune Serum Globulin** *see Immune Globulin (Intramuscular) on page 710*
♦ **Immunine® VH (Can)** *see Factor IX (Purified/Human) on page 540*
♦ **Immunization Recommendations** *see page 1538*
♦ **Imodium®** *see Loperamide on page 816*
♦ **Imodium® A-D [OTC]** *see Loperamide on page 816*
♦ **Imogam® Rabies Immune Globulin (Human)** *see Rabies Immune Globulin (Human) on page 1174*
♦ **Imogam® Rabies Pasteurized (Can)** *see Rabies Immune Globulin (Human) on page 1174*
♦ **Imovax® Rabies (Can)** *see Rabies Virus Vaccine on page 1175*
♦ **Imovax® Rabies Vaccine** *see Rabies Virus Vaccine on page 1175*
♦ **Imuran®** *see Azathioprine on page 136*
♦ **In-111 Zevalin** *see Ibritumomab on page 695*

Inamrinone *(eye NAM ri none)*

Related Information
Adrenergic Agonists, Cardiovascular Comparison *on page 1469*
Adult ACLS Algorithms *on page 1632*

Synonyms Amrinone Lactate

Therapeutic Category Phosphodiesterase Enzyme Inhibitor

Use Infrequently used as a last resort, short-term therapy in patients with intractable heart failure

Pregnancy Risk Factor C

Contraindications Hypersensitivity to inamrinone, any component of the formulation, or bisulfites (contains sodium metabisulfite); patients with severe aortic or pulmonic valvular disease

Warnings/Precautions Due to a slight effect on AV conduction, may increase ventricular response rate in atrial fibrillation/atrial flutter; prior treatment with digoxin is recommended. Monitor liver function. Discontinue therapy if alteration in LFTs and clinical symptoms of hepatotoxicity occur. Observe for arrhythmias in this very high-risk patient population. Not recommended in acute MI treatment. Monitor fluid status closely; patients may require adjustment of diuretic and electrolyte replacement therapy. Can cause thrombocytopenia (dose-dependent). Correct hypokalemia before initiating therapy. Increase risk of hospitalization and death with long-term therapy.

Adverse Reactions
1% to 10%:
Cardiovascular: Arrhythmias (3%, especially in high-risk patients), hypotension (1% to 2%) (may be infusion rate-related)
Gastrointestinal: Nausea (1% to 2%)
Hematologic: Thrombocytopenia (may be dose-related)
<1% (Limited to important or life-threatening): Chest pain, fever, hepatotoxicity, hypersensitivity (especially with prolonged therapy), vomiting; contains sulfites resulting in allergic reactions in susceptible people

Drug Interactions
Increased Effect/Toxicity: Diuretics may cause significant hypovolemia and decrease filling pressure. Inotropic effects with digitalis are additive.

Stability May be administered undiluted for I.V. bolus doses. For continuous infusion: Dilute with 0.45% or 0.9% sodium chloride to final concentration of 1-3 mg/mL; use within 24 hours; do not directly dilute with dextrose-containing solutions, chemical interaction occurs; may be administered I.V. into running dextrose infusions. Furosemide forms a precipitate when injected in I.V. lines containing inamrinone.

Mechanism of Action Inhibits myocardial cyclic adenosine monophosphate (cAMP) phosphodiesterase activity and increases cellular levels of cAMP resulting in a positive inotropic effect and increased cardiac output; also possesses systemic and pulmonary vasodilator effects resulting in pre- and afterload reduction; slightly increases atrioventricular conduction

Pharmacodynamics/Kinetics
Onset of action: I.V.: 2-5 minutes
Peak effect: ~10 minutes
Duration: Dose dependent: Low dose: ~30 minutes; Higher doses: ~2 hours
Half-life elimination, serum: Adults, normal volunteers: 3.6 hours; Adults with CHF: 5.8 hours

Usual Dosage Dosage is based on clinical response (**Note:** Dose should not exceed 10 mg/kg/24 hours).
Infants, Children, and Adults: 0.75 mg/kg I.V. bolus over 2-3 minutes followed by maintenance infusion of 5-10 mcg/kg/minute; I.V. bolus may need to be repeated in 30 minutes.
Dosing adjustment in renal failure: Cl$_{cr}$ <10 mL/minute: Administer 50% to 75% of dose.

Administration May be administered undiluted for I.V. bolus doses. For continuous infusion: Dilute with 0.45% or 0.9% sodium chloride to final concentration of 1-3 mg/mL use within 24 hours.

Nursing Implications
Do **not** "Y" furosemide IVP into inamrinone solutions:
I.V. bolus doses: May be administered undiluted
Continuous infusion: Dilute with 0.45% or 0.9% sodium chloride to final concentration of 1-3 mg/mL use within 24 hours
Monitor cardiac index, stroke volume, systemic vascular resistance, and pulmonary vascular resistance (if Swan-Ganz catheter available); CVP, SBP, DBP, heart rate, platelet count, CBC, liver function and renal function tests

Additional Information To avoid confusion with similarly sounding medication names, the name "amrinone" was changed to "inamrinone" in July, 2000.

Dosage Forms Injection, solution, as lactate: 5 mg/mL (20 mL) [contains sodium metabisulfite]

◆ Inapsine® see Droperidol on page 451

Indapamide (in DAP a mide)
Related Information
Depression on page 1655
Sulfonamide Derivatives on page 1515
U.S. Brand Names Lozol®
Canadian Brand Names Apo®-Indapamide; Gen-Indapamide; Lozide®; Lozol®; Novo-Indapamide; Nu-Indapamide; PMS-Indapamide
Therapeutic Category Antihypertensive Agent; Diuretic, Miscellaneous
Use Management of mild to moderate hypertension; treatment of edema in congestive heart failure and nephrotic syndrome
Pregnancy Risk Factor B (manufacturer); D (expert analysis)
Contraindications Hypersensitivity to indapamide or any component of the formulation, thiazides, or sulfonamide-derived drugs; anuria; renal decompensation; pregnancy (based on expert analysis)
Warnings/Precautions Use with caution in severe renal disease. Electrolyte disturbances (hypokalemia, hypochloremic alkalosis, hyponatremia) can occur. Use with caution in severe hepatic dysfunction; hepatic encephalopathy can be caused by electrolyte disturbances. Gout can be precipitate in certain patients with a history of gout, a familial predisposition to gout, or chronic renal failure. Cautious use in diabetics; may see a change in glucose control. I.V. use is generally not recommended (but is available). Hypersensitivity reactions can occur. Can cause SLE exacerbation or activation. Use with caution in patients with moderate or high cholesterol concentrations. Photosensitization may occur. Correct hypokalemia before initiating therapy.

Chemical similarities are present among sulfonamides, sulfonylureas, carbonic anhydrase inhibitors, thiazides, and loop diuretics (except ethacrynic acid). Use in patients with thiazide or sulfonamide allergy is specifically contraindicated in product labeling, however a risk of cross-reaction exists in patients with allergy to any of these compounds; avoid use when previous reaction has been severe.
Adverse Reactions
1% to 10%:
Cardiovascular: Orthostatic hypotension, palpitations, flushing
Central nervous system: Dizziness, lightheadedness, vertigo, headache, weakness, restlessness, drowsiness, fatigue, lethargy, malaise, lassitude, anxiety, agitation, depression, nervousness
Gastrointestinal: Anorexia, gastric irritation, nausea, vomiting, abdominal pain, cramping, bloating, diarrhea, constipation, dry mouth, weight loss
Genitourinary: Nocturia, frequent urination, polyuria
Neuromuscular & skeletal: Muscle cramps, spasm
Ocular: Blurred vision
Respiratory: Rhinorrhea
<1% (Limited to important or life-threatening): Cutaneous vasculitis, glycosuria, hyperglycemia, hyperuricemia, impotency, necrotizing angiitis, purpura, reduced libido, vasculitis
Overdosage/Toxicology Symptoms include lethargy, diuresis, hypermotility, confusion, and muscle weakness. Following GI decontamination, therapy is supportive I.V. fluids, electrolytes, and I.V. pressors if needed.
Drug Interactions
Increased Effect/Toxicity: The diuretic effect of indapamide is synergistic with furosemide and other loop diuretics. Increased hypotension and/or renal adverse effects of ACE inhibitors may result in aggressively treated patients. Cyclosporine and thiazide-type diuretics can increase the risk of gout or renal toxicity. Digoxin toxicity can be exacerbated if a diuretic induces hypokalemia or hypomagnesemia. Lithium toxicity can occur with thiazide-type diuretics due to reduced renal excretion of lithium. Thiazide-type diuretics may prolong the duration of action of neuromuscular blocking agents.
Decreased Effect: Effects of oral hypoglycemics may be decreased. Decreased absorption of indapamide with cholestyramine and colestipol. NSAIDs can decrease the efficacy of thiazide-type diuretics, reducing the diuretic and antihypertensive effects.
Ethanol/Nutrition/Herb Interactions Herb/Nutraceutical: Avoid dong quai if using for hypertension (has estrogenic activity). Avoid ephedra, yohimbe, ginseng (may worsen hypertension). Avoid garlic (may have increased antihypertensive effect).
Mechanism of Action Diuretic effect is localized at the proximal segment of the distal tubule of the nephron; it does not appear to have significant effect on glomerular filtration rate nor renal blood flow; like other diuretics, it enhances sodium, chloride, and water excretion by interfering with the transport of sodium ions across the renal tubular epithelium
Pharmacodynamics/Kinetics
Onset of action: 1-2 hours
Duration: ≤36 hours
Absorption: Completely
Protein binding, plasma: 71% to 79%
Metabolism: Extensively hepatic
Half-life elimination: 14-18 hours
Time to peak: 2-2.5 hours
Excretion: Urine (~60%) within 48 hours; feces (~16% to 23%)
Usual Dosage Adults: Oral:
Edema: 2.5-5 mg/day. Note: There is little therapeutic benefit to increasing the dose >5 mg/day; there is, however, an increased risk of electrolyte disturbances
(Continued)

Indapamide *(Continued)*

Hypertension: 1.25 mg in the morning, may increase to 5 mg/day by increments of 1.25-2.5 mg; consider adding another antihypertensive and decreasing the dose if response is not adequate

Dietary Considerations May be taken with food or milk to decrease GI adverse effects.

Monitoring Parameters Blood pressure (both standing and sitting/supine), serum electrolytes, renal function, assess weight, I & O reports daily to determine fluid loss

Patient Information May be taken with food or milk; take early in day to avoid nocturia; take the last dose of multiple doses no later than 6 PM unless instructed otherwise. A few people who take this medication become more sensitive to sunlight and may experience skin rash, redness, itching, or severe sunburn, especially if sun block SPF ≥15 is not used on exposed skin areas.

Nursing Implications Take blood pressure with patient lying down and standing; may increase serum glucose in diabetic patients

Dosage Forms Tablet: 1.25 mg, 2.5 mg

- ◆ **Inderal**® *see Propranolol on page 1149*
- ◆ **Inderal**® **LA** *see Propranolol on page 1149*
- ◆ **Inderide**® *see Propranolol and Hydrochlorothiazide on page 1151*
- ◆ **Inderide**® **LA** *see Propranolol and Hydrochlorothiazide on page 1151*

Indinavir *(in DIN a veer)*

Related Information

Antiretroviral Agents Comparison *on page 1488*
Antiretroviral Therapy for HIV Infection *on page 1595*
Management of Healthcare Worker Exposures to HIV, HBV, HCV *on page 1555*

U.S. Brand Names Crixivan®

Canadian Brand Names Crixivan®

Therapeutic Category Antiretroviral Agent, Protease Inhibitor; Protease Inhibitor

Use Treatment of HIV infection; should always be used as part of a multidrug regimen (at least three antiretroviral agents)

Pregnancy Risk Factor C

Pregnancy/Breast-Feeding Implications Safety and pharmacokinetic studies are currently underway in pregnant women; hyperbilirubinemia may be exacerbated in neonates. Pregnancy and protease inhibitors are both associated with an increased risk of hyperglycemia. Glucose levels should be closely monitored. Healthcare professionals are encouraged to contact the antiretroviral pregnancy registry to monitor outcomes of pregnant women exposed to antiretroviral medications (1-800-258-4263).

Contraindications Hypersensitivity to indinavir or any component of the formulation; concurrent use of terfenadine, astemizole, cisapride, triazolam, midazolam, pimozide, or ergot alkaloids

Warnings/Precautions Because indinavir may cause nephrolithiasis/urolithiasis the drug should be discontinued if signs and symptoms occur; risk is substantially higher in pediatric patients versus adults. Indinavir should not be administered concurrently with lovastatin or simvastatin (caution with atorvastatin and cerivastatin) because of competition for metabolism of these drugs through the CYP3A4 system, and potential serious or life-threatening events. Use caution with other drugs metabolized by this enzyme (particular caution with sildenafil). Avoid concurrent use of St John's wort (may lead to loss of virologic response and/or resistance). Patients with hepatic insufficiency due to cirrhosis should have dose reduction. Warn patients about fat redistribution that can occur. Indinavir has been associated with hemolytic anemia (discontinue if diagnosed), hepatitis, and hyperglycemia (exacerbation or new-onset diabetes).

Adverse Reactions Protease inhibitors cause dyslipidemia which includes elevated cholesterol and triglycerides and a redistribution of body fat centrally to cause "protease paunch", buffalo hump, facial atrophy, and breast enlargement. These agents also cause hyperglycemia (exacerbation or new-onset diabetes).

10%:
Hepatic: Hyperbilirubinemia (14%)
Renal: Nephrolithiasis/urolithiasis (29%, pediatric patients)

1% to 10%:
Central nervous system: Headache (6%), insomnia (3%)
Gastrointestinal: Abdominal pain (9%), nausea (12%), diarrhea/vomiting (4% to 5%), taste perversion (3%)
Neuromuscular & skeletal: Weakness (4%), flank pain (3%)
Renal: Nephrolithiasis/urolithiasis (12%, adult patients), hematuria

<1% (Limited to important or life-threatening): Acute renal failure, alopecia, anaphylactoid reactions, angina, anorexia, crystalluria, decreased hemoglobin, depression, dizziness, dysuria, erythema multiforme, fever, hemolytic anemia, hepatic failure, hepatitis, hyperglycemia, increased serum cholesterol, interstitial nephritis, malaise, myocardial infarction, new-onset diabetes, pancreatitis, paresthesia (oral), pruritus, pyelonephritis, somnolence, Stevens-Johnson syndrome, urticaria, xerostomia

Drug Interactions

Cytochrome P450 Effect: CYP3A3/4 enzyme substrate; CYP3A3/4 enzyme inhibitor

Increased Effect/Toxicity: Levels of indinavir are increased by delavirdine, itraconazole, ketoconazole, nelfinavir, sildenafil, and ritonavir. Cisapride, terfenadine, pimozide, and astemizole should be avoided with indinavir due to life-threatening cardiotoxicity. Concurrent use of indinavir with lovastatin and simvastatin may increase the risk of myopathy or rhabdomyolysis. Cautious use of atorvastatin and cerivastatin may be possible. Benzodiazepines with indinavir may result in prolonged sedation and respiratory depression (midazolam and triazolam are contraindicated). Concurrent use of ergot alkaloids is contraindicated. Amprenavir and rifabutin concentrations are increased during concurrent therapy with indinavir. Other medications metabolized by cytochrome P450 isoenzyme

3A3/4 may be affected. Concurrent sildenafil is associated with increased risk of hypotension, visual changes, and priapism. Clarithromycin and quinidine may increase serum concentrations of indinavir. Serum concentrations of these drugs may also be increased. Other CYP3A3/4 inhibitors may have similar effects.

Decreased Effect: Concurrent use of efavirenz, rifampin, and rifabutin may decrease the effectiveness of indinavir (dosage increase of indinavir is recommended); concurrent use of rifampin is not recommended; dosage decrease of rifabutin is recommended. The efficacy of protease inhibitors may be decreased when given with nevirapine. Gastric pH is lowered and absorption may be decreased when didanosine and indinavir are taken <1 hour apart. Fluconazole may decrease serum concentration of indinavir.

Ethanol/Nutrition/Herb Interactions

Food: Indinavir bioavailability may be decreased if taken with food. Meals high in calories, fat, and protein result in a significant decrease in drug levels. Indinavir serum concentrations may be decreased by grapefruit juice.

Herb/Nutraceutical: St John's wort *(Hypericum)* appears to induce CYP3A enzymes and has lead to 57% reductions in indinavir AUCs and 81% reductions in trough serum concentrations, which may lead to treatment failures; concurrent use is contraindicated.

Stability Capsules are sensitive to moisture; medication should be stored and used in the original container and the desiccant should remain in the bottle

Mechanism of Action Indinavir is a human immunodeficiency virus protease inhibitor, binding to the protease activity site and inhibiting the activity of this enzyme. HIV protease is an enzyme required for the cleavage of viral polyprotein precursors into individual functional proteins found in infectious HIV. Inhibition prevents cleavage of these polyproteins resulting in the formation of immature noninfectious viral particles.

Pharmacodynamics/Kinetics

Absorption: Administration with a high fat, high calorie diet resulted in a reduction in AUC and in maximum serum concentration (77% and 84% respectively). Administration with a lighter meal resulted in little or no change in these parameters.

Protein binding, plasma: 60%

Metabolism: Hepatic via CYP450 3A4 enzymes; seven metabolites of indinavir identified

Bioavailability: Good

Half-life elimination: 1.8 ± 0.4 hour

Time to peak: 0.8 ± 0.3 hour

Excretion: Urine and feces

Usual Dosage

Children (investigational): 500 mg/m^2 every 8 hours (patients with smaller BSA may require lower doses of 300-400 mg/m^2 every 8 hours)

Adults: Oral: 800 mg every 8 hours

Note: Dosage adjustments for indinavir when administered in combination therapy:

Delavirdine, itraconazole, or ketoconazole: Reduce indinavir dose to 600 mg every 8 hours

Efavirenz: Increase indinavir dose to 1000 mg every 8 hours

Lopinavir and ritonavir (Kaletra™): Indinavir 600 mg twice daily

Nevirapine: Increase indinavir dose to 1000 mg every 8 hours

Rifabutin: Reduce rifabutin to $^1/_2$ the standard dose plus increase indinavir to 1000 mg every 8 hours

Ritonavir: Adjustments necessary for both agents:

Ritonavir 100-200 mg twice daily plus indinavir 800 mg twice daily **or**

Ritonavir 400 mg twice daily plus indinavir 400 mg twice daily

Dosage adjustment in hepatic impairment: Mild-moderate impairment due to cirrhosis: 600 mg every 8 hours or with ketoconazole coadministration

Dietary Considerations Should be taken without food but with water 1 hour before or 2 hours after a meal. Administration with lighter meals (eg, dry toast, skim milk, corn flakes) resulted in little/no change in indinavir concentration. If taking with ritonavir, may take with food. Patient should drink at least 48 oz of water daily.

Administration Drink at least 48 oz of water daily. Administer with water, 1 hour before or 2 hours after a meal. Administer around-the-clock to avoid significant fluctuation in serum levels.

Monitoring Parameters Monitor viral load, CD4 count, triglycerides, cholesterol, glucose, liver function tests, CBC

Patient Information Take with a full glass of water; any symptoms of kidney stones, including flank pain, dysuria, etc, indicates the drug should be discontinued and physician or pharmacist should be contacted. Drug should be administered on an empty stomach 1 hour before or 2 hours after a large meal. May take with a small, light meal. Do not take any prescription medications, over-the-counter products or herbal products, especially St John's wort, without consulting prescriber. Indinavir should be stored and used in the original container.

Nursing Implications Administer around-the-clock to avoid significant fluctuation in serum levels; administer with plenty of water

Dosage Forms Capsule: 100 mg, 200 mg, 333 mg, 400 mg

♦ **Indocid® (Can)** *see* Indomethacin *on page 717*

♦ **Indocid® P.D.A. (Can)** *see* Indomethacin *on page 717*

♦ **Indocin®** *see* Indomethacin *on page 717*

♦ **Indo-Lemmon (Can)** *see* Indomethacin *on page 717*

♦ **Indometacin** *see* Indomethacin *on page 717*

Indomethacin (in doe METH a sin)

Related Information

Antacid Drug Interactions *on page 1477*

Depression *on page 1655*

Nonsteroidal Anti-Inflammatory Agents Comparison *on page 1512*

U.S. Brand Names Indocin®

Canadian Brand Names Apo®-Indomethacin; Indocid®; Indocid® P.D.A.; Indocin®; Indo-Lemmon; Indotec; Novo-Methacin; Nu-Indo; Rhodacine®

(Continued)

Indomethacin *(Continued)*

Synonyms Indometacin; Indomethacin Sodium Trihydrate

Therapeutic Category Analgesic, Nonsteroidal Anti-inflammatory Drug; Anti-inflammatory Agent; Antipyretic; Nonsteroidal Anti-inflammatory Drug (NSAID), Oral; Nonsteroidal Anti-inflammatory Drug (NSAID), Parenteral

Use Management of inflammatory diseases and rheumatoid disorders; moderate pain; acute gouty arthritis, acute bursitis/tendonitis, moderate to severe osteoarthritis, rheumatoid arthritis, ankylosing spondylitis; I.V. form used as alternative to surgery for closure of patent ductus arteriosus in neonates

Pregnancy Risk Factor B/D (3rd trimester)

Contraindications Hypersensitivity to indomethacin, any component of the formulation, aspirin, or other nonsteroidal anti-inflammatory drugs (NSAIDs); patients in whom asthma, urticaria, or rhinitis are precipitated by NSAIDs/aspirin; active GI bleeding or ulcer disease; premature neonates with necrotizing enterocolitis; impaired renal function; active bleeding; thrombocytopenia; pregnancy (3rd trimester); suppositories are contraindicated in patients with a history of proctitis or recent rectal bleeding

Warnings/Precautions Use with caution in patients with congestive heart failure, hypertension, dehydration, decreased renal or hepatic function, history of GI disease (bleeding or ulcers), or those receiving anticoagulants. Elderly are at a high risk for adverse effects from nonsteroidal anti-inflammatory agents. As many as 60% of elderly can develop peptic ulceration and/or hemorrhage asymptomatically.

Use lowest effective dose for shortest period possible. Use of NSAIDs can compromise existing renal function especially when Cl_{cr} is <30 mL/minute.

CNS adverse effects such as confusion, agitation, and hallucination are generally seen in overdose or high-dose situations; but elderly may demonstrate these adverse effects at lower doses than younger adults. Withhold for at least 4-6 half-lives prior to surgical or dental procedures.

Adverse Reactions
>10%:
  Central nervous system: Headache (11%)
  Gastrointestinal: Nausea (3% to 9%), epigastric pain, abdominal pain/cramps/distress (<3%), anorexia, GI bleeding, ulcers, perforation, heartburn, indigestion
  Hematologic: Inhibition of platelet aggregation
1% to 10%:
  Central nervous system: Drowsiness (<3%), fatigue (<3%), vertigo (<3%), depression (<3%), malaise (<3%)
  Gastrointestinal: Constipation (<3%), diarrhea (<3%), dyspepsia (3% to 9%)
  Otic: Tinnitus (<3%)
<1% (Limited to important or life-threatening): Acute respiratory distress, agranulocytosis, anaphylaxis, angioedema, arrhythmias, aseptic meningitis, asthma, bone marrow suppression, bronchospasm, cholestatic jaundice, congestive heart failure, depression, dyspnea/bronchospasm, erythema multiforme, exfoliative dermatitis, GI ulceration, hallucinations, hemolytic anemia, hepatitis (including fatal cases), hypersensitivity reactions, hypertension, hypoglycemia (I.V.), inhibition of platelet aggregation, interstitial nephritis, nephrotic syndrome, peripheral neuropathy, proctitis, psychic disturbances, psychosis, rash, renal failure, retinal/macular disturbances, shock, somnolence, Stevens-Johnson syndrome, thrombocytopenia, toxic amblyopia, toxic epidermal necrolysis, urticaria

Overdosage/Toxicology Symptoms include drowsiness, lethargy, nausea, vomiting, seizures, paresthesias, headache, dizziness, GI bleeding, cerebral edema, tinnitus, leukocytosis, and renal failure. Management of nonsteroidal anti-inflammatory drug (NSAID) intoxication is primarily supportive and symptomatic. Fluid therapy is commonly effective in managing hypotension that may occur following an acute NSAID overdose, except when due to acute blood loss. Seizures tend to be very short-lived and often do not require drug treatment, although recurrent seizures should be treated with I.V. diazepam.

Drug Interactions
  Cytochrome P450 Effect: CYP2C9 enzyme substrate
  Increased Effect/Toxicity: Indomethacin may increase serum potassium with potassium-sparing diuretics. Probenecid may increase indomethacin serum concentrations. Other NSAIDs may increase GI adverse effects. May increase nephrotoxicity of cyclosporine and increase renal adverse effects of ACE inhibitors. Indomethacin may increase serum concentrations of digoxin, methotrexate, lithium, and aminoglycosides (reported with I.V. use in neonates).
  Decreased Effect: May decrease antihypertensive effects of beta-blockers, hydralazine, ACE inhibitors, and angiotensin II antagonists. Indomethacin may decrease the antihypertensive and diuretic effect of thiazides (hydrochlorothiazide, etc) and loop diuretics (furosemide, bumetanide).

Ethanol/Nutrition/Herb Interactions
  Ethanol: Avoid ethanol (may enhance gastric mucosal irritation).
  Food: Food may decrease the rate but not the extent of absorption. Indomethacin peak serum levels may be delayed if taken with food.
  Herb/Nutraceutical: Avoid cat's claw, dong quai, evening primrose, feverfew, garlic, ginger, ginkgo, red clover, horse chestnut, green tea, ginseng (all have additional antiplatelet activity).

Stability I.V.: Protect from light; not stable in alkaline solution; reconstitute just prior to administration; discard any unused portion; do not use preservative-containing diluents for reconstitution; suppositories do not require refrigeration

Mechanism of Action Inhibits prostaglandin synthesis by decreasing the activity of the enzyme, cyclo-oxygenase, which results in decreased formation of prostaglandin precursors

Pharmacodynamics/Kinetics
  Onset of action: ~30 minutes
  Duration: 4-6 hours
  Absorption: Prompt and extensive

Distribution: V_d: 0.34-1.57 L/kg; crosses placenta; enters breast milk

Protein binding: 90%

Metabolism: Hepatic; significant enterohepatic cycling

Half-life elimination: 4.5 hours, longer in neonates

Time to peak: Oral: ~3-4 hours

Excretion: Urine (primarily as glucuronide conjugates)

Usual Dosage

Patent ductus arteriosus:

Neonates: I.V.: Initial: 0.2 mg/kg, followed by 2 doses depending on postnatal age (PNA):

PNA **at time of first dose** <48 hours: 0.1 mg/kg at 12- to 24-hour intervals

PNA **at time of first dose** 2-7 days: 0.2 mg/kg at 12- to 24-hour intervals

PNA **at time of first dose** >7 days: 0.25 mg/kg at 12- to 24-hour intervals

In general, may use 12-hour dosing interval if urine output >1 mL/kg/hour after prior dose; use 24-hour dosing interval if urine output is <1 mL/kg/hour but >0.6 mL/kg/hour; doses should be withheld if patient has oliguria (urine output <0.6 mL/kg/hour) or anuria

Inflammatory/rheumatoid disorders:

Oral:

Children: 1-2 mg/kg/day in 2-4 divided doses; maximum dose: 4 mg/kg/day; not to exceed 150-200 mg/day

Adults: 25-50 mg/dose 2-3 times/day; maximum dose: 200 mg/day; extended release capsule should be given on a 1-2 times/day schedule

Rectal: Adults: Persistent night pain and/or morning stiffness: 50-100 mg at bedtime (as part of total daily dose maximum of 200 mg/day)

Dietary Considerations May cause GI upset, bleeding, ulceration, perforation; take with food or milk to minimize GI upset.

Administration

Oral: Administer with food, milk, or antacids to decrease GI adverse effects; extended release capsules must be swallowed whole, do not crush

I.V.: Administer over 20-30 minutes at a concentration over 0.5-1 mg/mL in preservative-free sterile water for injection or normal saline. Reconstitute I.V. formulation just prior to administration; discard any unused portion; avoid I.V. bolus administration or infusion via an umbilical catheter into vessels near the superior mesenteric artery as these may cause vasoconstriction and can compromise blood flow to the intestines. Do not administer intra-arterially.

Monitoring Parameters Monitor response (pain, range of motion, grip strength, mobility, ADL function), inflammation; observe for weight gain, edema; monitor renal function (serum creatinine, BUN); observe for bleeding, bruising; evaluate gastrointestinal effects (abdominal pain, bleeding, dyspepsia); mental confusion, disorientation, CBC, liver function tests

Test Interactions Positive direct Coombs'; increased sodium, chloride, prolonged bleeding time

Patient Information Take with food, milk, or with antacids; sustained release capsules must be swallowed whole/intact, can cause dizziness or drowsiness

Nursing Implications Extended release capsules must be swallowed intact; shake suspension well before use

Dosage Forms

Capsule (Indocin®): 25 mg, 50 mg

Capsule, sustained release (Indocin® SR): 75 mg

Powder for injection, as sodium trihydrate (Indocin® I.V.): 1 mg

Suppository, rectal (Indocin®): 50 mg

Suspension, oral (Indocin®): 25 mg/5 mL (5 mL, 10 mL, 237 mL, 500 mL)

+ **Indomethacin Sodium Trihydrate** see Indomethacin on page 717

+ **Indotec (Can)** see Indomethacin on page 717

+ **INF-alpha 2** see Interferon Alfa-2b on page 728

+ **Infanrix®** see Diphtheria, Tetanus Toxoids, and Acellular Pertussis Vaccine on page 418

+ **Infantaire [OTC]** see Acetaminophen on page 22

+ **Infants Tylenol® Cold [OTC]** see Acetaminophen and Pseudoephedrine on page 25

+ **Infants' Tylenol® Cold Plus Cough Concentrated Drops [OTC]** see Acetaminophen, Dextromethorphan, and Pseudoephedrine on page 27

+ **Infasurf®** see Calfactant on page 213

+ **INFeD®** see Iron Dextran Complex on page 745

+ **Infergen®** see Interferon Alfacon-1 on page 731

+ **Inflamase® Forte** see PrednisoLONE on page 1122

+ **Inflamase® Mild** see PrednisoLONE on page 1122

Infliximab (in FLIKS e mab)

U.S. Brand Names Remicade®

Synonyms Infliximab, Recombinant

Therapeutic Category Antirheumatic, Disease Modifying; Gastrointestinal Agent, Anti-TNF; Monoclonal Antibody

Use

Crohn's disease: Reduce the signs and symptoms of moderate to severe disease in patients who have an inadequate response to conventional therapy; reduce the number of draining enterocutaneous fistulas in fistulizing disease

Rheumatoid arthritis: Used with methotrexate in patients who have had an inadequate response to methotrexate alone; used with methotrexate to inhibit the progression of structural damage in patients with moderate to severe disease

Pregnancy Risk Factor B (manufacturer)

Pregnancy/Breast-Feeding Implications Reproduction studies have not been conducted. Use during pregnancy only if clearly needed.

It is not known whether infliximab is secreted in human milk. Because many immunoglobulins are secreted in milk and the potential for serious adverse reactions exists, a decision

(Continued)

Infliximab *(Continued)*

should be made whether to discontinue nursing or discontinue the drug, taking into account the importance of the drug to the mother.

Breast-feeding is not recommended

Contraindications Hypersensitivity to murine proteins or any component of the formulation; congestive heart failure

Warnings/Precautions Hypersensitivity reactions, including urticaria, dyspnea, and hypotension have occurred. Discontinue the drug if a reaction occurs. Medications for the treatment of hypersensitivity reactions should be available for immediate use. Autoimmune antibodies and a lupus-like syndrome have been reported. If antibodies to double-stranded DNA are confirmed in a patient with lupus-like symptoms, treatment should be discontinued. Rare cases of demyelinating disease have been reported, use with caution in patients with pre-existing or recent onset CNS demyelinating disorders. Treatment may lead to antibody development to infliximab. Chronic exposure to immunosuppressants in patients with Crohn's disease or rheumatoid arthritis has been associated with the increased risk of developing lymphomas; the effect of infliximab is not known.

Serious infections, including sepsis and fatal infections, have been reported in patients receiving TNF-blocking agents. Many of the serious infections in patients treated with infliximab have occurred in patients on concomitant immunosuppressive therapy. Caution should be exercised when considering the use of infliximab in patients with a chronic infection or history of recurrent infection. Infliximab should not be given to patients with a clinically-important, active infection. Patients should be evaluated for latent tuberculosis infection with a tuberculin skin test prior to infliximab therapy. Treatment of latent tuberculosis should be initiated before infliximab is used. Tuberculosis (may be disseminated or extrapulmonary) has been reactivated in patients previously exposed to TB while on infliximab. Most cases have been reported within the first 3-6 months of treatment. Other opportunistic infections (eg, invasive fungal infections, listeriosis, *Pneumocystis*) have occurred during therapy. The risk/benefit ratio should be weighed in patients who have resided in regions where histoplasmosis is endemic. Patients who develop a new infection while undergoing treatment with infliximab should be monitored closely. If a patient develops a serious infection or sepsis, infliximab should be discontinued.

Safety and efficacy for use in juvenile rheumatoid arthritis and in pediatric patients with Crohn's disease have not been established.

Increased mortality and hospitalization were seen in clinical trials where infliximab was used to treat congestive heart failure (CHF). As a result, infliximab is not recommended to treat Crohn's disease or rheumatoid arthritis in patients with existing CHF. The manufacturer recommends re-evaluation of patients with CHF who started treatment with infliximab for Crohn's disease or rheumatoid arthritis prior to this information, and treatment should be stopped if CHF worsens. In addition, consider discontinuing infliximab if significant clinical response is not attained, and monitor cardiac status closely if treatment is continued.

Adverse Reactions Note: Although profile is similar, frequency of effects may be different in specific populations (Crohn's disease vs rheumatoid arthritis).

>10%:
Central nervous system: Headache (22% to 23%), fatigue (8% to 11%), fever (8% to 10%)
Dermatologic: Rash (6% to 12%)
Gastrointestinal: Nausea (17%), diarrhea (3% to 13%), abdominal pain (10% to 12%)
Local: Infusion reactions (19%)
Respiratory: Upper respiratory tract infection (16% to 26%), cough (5% to 13%), sinusitis (5% to 13%), pharyngitis (9% to 11%)
Miscellaneous: Development of antinuclear antibodies (34%); infections (32%); Crohn's patients with fistulizing disease: Development of new abscess (12%, 8-16 weeks after the last infusion)

2% to 10%:
Cardiovascular: Chest pain (5% to 6%, similar to placebo)
Central nervous system: Pain (8% to 9%), dizziness (8% to 10%, similar to placebo)
Dermatologic: Pruritus (5% to 6%)
Gastrointestinal: Vomiting (7% to 9%), dyspepsia (5% to 6%)
Genitourinary: Urinary tract infection (3% to 8%, similar to placebo)
Neuromuscular & skeletal: Arthralgia (5% to 6%), back pain (5% to 6%)
Respiratory: Bronchitis (6% to 7%), rhinitis (6% to 10%)
Miscellaneous: Development of antibodies to double-stranded DNA (9%)

<2% (Limited to important or life-threatening): Arrhythmia, AV block, azotemia, basal cell carcinoma, bradycardia, brain infarction, breast cancer, cardiac arrest, cardiac failure, cholecystitis, cholelithiasis, delirium, depression, dyspnea, encephalopathy, gastrointestinal hemorrhage, hemarthrosis, hepatitis, hydronephrosis, hypertension, hypotension, injection site inflammation, intestinal obstruction, intestinal perforation, intestinal stenosis, kidney infarction, latent tuberculosis reactivation, leukopenia, lupus erythematosus syndrome, lymphangitis, lymphoma, myocardial ischemia, pancreatitis, peripheral ischemia, peritonitis, pleural effusion, pneumothorax, pulmonary edema, pulmonary embolism, pyelonephritis, renal failure, respiratory insufficiency, sepsis, splenic infarction, spinal stenosis, splenomegaly, syncope, thrombocytopenia, thrombophlebitis (deep), upper motor neuron lesion, worsening CHF

Overdosage/Toxicology Doses up to 20 mg/kg have been given without toxic effects. In case of overdose, treatment should be symptom directed and supportive.

Drug Interactions
Increased Effect/Toxicity: Specific drug interaction studies have not been conducted.
Decreased Effect: Specific drug interaction studies have not been conducted.

Decreased toxicity: Immunosuppressants: When used with infliximab, may decrease the risk of infusion related reactions, and may decrease development of anti-double-stranded DNA antibodies

Stability Store vials at 2°C to 8°C (36°F to 46°F); do not freeze; does not contain preservative. Reconstitute vials with 10 mL sterile water for injection; swirl vial gently to dissolve powder, do not shake, allow solution to stand for 5 minutes; total dose of reconstituted product should be further diluted to 250 mL of 0.9% sodium chloride injection; infusion of dose should begin within 3 hours of preparation

Mechanism of Action Infliximab is a chimeric monoclonal antibody that binds to human tumor necrosis factor alpha (TNFα) receptor sites, thereby interfering with endogenous TNFα activity. Biological activities of TNFα include the induction of pro-inflammatory cytokines (interleukins), enhancement of leukocyte migration, activation of neutrophils and eosinophils, and the induction of acute phase reactants and tissue degrading enzymes. Animal models have shown TNFα expression causes polyarthritis, and infliximab can prevent disease as well as allow diseased joints to heal.

Pharmacodynamics/Kinetics
  Onset of action: Crohn's disease: ~2 weeks
  Half-life elimination: 8-9.5 days

Usual Dosage I.V.: Adults:
  Crohn's disease:
    Moderately- to severely-active: 5 mg/kg as a single infusion over a minimum of 2 hours
    Fistulizing: 5 mg/kg as an infusion over a minimum of 2 hours; dose repeated at 2- and 6 weeks after the initial infusion
    Rheumatoid arthritis (in combination with methotrexate therapy): 3 mg/kg followed by an additional 3 mg/kg at 2- and 6 weeks after the first dose; then repeat every 8 weeks thereafter; doses have ranged from 3-10 mg/kg intravenous infusion repeated at 4-week intervals or 8-week intervals

  Dosage adjustment in renal impairment: No specific adjustment is recommended
  Dosage adjustment in hepatic impairment: No specific adjustment is recommended

Administration Infuse over at least 2 hours; must use an infusion set with an in-line filter (pore size ≤1.2 μm); infusion should begin within 3 hours of preparation; do not infuse with other agents

Monitoring Parameters Improvement of symptoms; signs of infection; place and read PPD before initiation.

Nursing Implications Do not shake reconstituted vials; infusion of dose should begin within 3 hours of preparation; infuse over at least 2 hours (must use an infusion set with an in-line filter); medications for the treatment of hypersensitivity reactions should be readily available

Dosage Forms Powder for injection: 100 mg

♦ **Infliximab, Recombinant** see Infliximab on page 719

Influenza Virus Vaccine (in floo EN za VYE rus vak SEEN)

Related Information
Immunization Recommendations on page 1538
Recommended Immunization Schedule for HIV-Infected Children on page 1543
USPHA/IDSA Guidelines for the Prevention of Opportunistic Infections in Persons With HIV on page 1574

U.S. Brand Names Fluogen®; FluShield®; Fluvirin®; Fluzone®

Canadian Brand Names Fluviral S/F®; Fluzone®; Vaxigrip®

Synonyms Influenza Virus Vaccine (inactivated whole-virus); Influenza Virus Vaccine (purified split-virus); Influenza Virus Vaccine (purified surface antigen); Influenza Virus Vaccine (split-virus)

Therapeutic Category Vaccine, Inactivated Virus

Use Provide active immunity to influenza virus strains contained in the vaccine; for high-risk persons, previous year vaccines should not be used to prevent present year influenza

Groups at Increased Risk for Influenza Related Complications:
- Persons ≥65 years of age
- Residents of nursing homes and other chronic-care facilities that house persons of any age with chronic medical conditions
- Adults and children with chronic disorders of the pulmonary or cardiovascular systems, including children with asthma
- Adults and children who have required regular medical follow-up or hospitalization during the preceding year because of chronic metabolic diseases (including diabetes mellitus), renal dysfunction, hemoglobinopathies, or immunosuppression (including immunosuppression caused by medications)
- Children and adolescents (6 months to 18 years of age) who are receiving long-term aspirin therapy and therefore, may be at risk for developing Reye's syndrome after influenza

Pregnancy Risk Factor C

Contraindications Hypersensitivity to thimerosal, influenza virus vaccine, or any component of the formulation; allergy history to eggs or egg products, chicken, chicken feathers or chicken dander; presence of acute respiratory disease or other active infections or illnesses; delay immunization in a patient with an active neurological disorder

Warnings/Precautions Although there is no evidence of maternal or fetal risk when vaccine is given in pregnancy, waiting until the 2nd or 3rd trimester to vaccinate the pregnant woman with a high-risk condition may be reasonable. Antigenic response may not be as great as expected in patients requiring immunosuppressive drug; hypersensitivity reactions may occur; because of potential for febrile reactions, risks and benefits must be carefully be considered in patients with history of febrile convulsions; influenza vaccines from previous seasons must not be used; patients with sulfite sensitivity may be affected by this product.

Adverse Reactions All serious adverse reactions must be reported to the U.S. Department of Health and Human Services (DHHS) Vaccine Adverse Event Reporting System (VAERS) 1-800-822-7967.
  1% to 10%:
    Central nervous system: Fever, malaise
    Local: Tenderness, redness, or induration at the site of injection (<33%)
(Continued)

Influenza Virus Vaccine *(Continued)*

<1% (Limited to important or life-threatening): Allergic reactions, anaphylactoid reactions (most likely to residual egg protein), angioedema, asthma, fever, Guillain-Barré syndrome, myalgia, urticaria

Stability Store between 2°C to 8°C (36°F to 46°F). Potency is destroyed by freezing; do not use if product has been frozen.

Mechanism of Action Promotes immunity to influenza virus by inducing specific antibody production. Each year the formulation is standardized according to the U.S. Public Health Service. Preparations from previous seasons must not be used.

Usual Dosage I.M.:

Children:

6-35 months: 1-2 doses of 0.25 mL with ≥4 weeks between doses and the last dose administered before December

3-8 years: 1-2 doses of 0.5 mL (in anterolateral aspect of thigh) with ≥4 weeks between doses and the last dose administered before December

Children ≥9 years and Adults: 0.5 mL each year of appropriate vaccine for the year, one dose is all that is necessary; administer in late fall to allow maximum titers to develop by peak epidemic periods usually occurring in early December

Note: The split virus or purified surface antigen is recommended for children ≤12 years of age; if the child has received at least one dose of the 1978-79 or later vaccine, one dose is sufficient

Administration Inspect for particulate matter and discoloration prior to administration.

For patients at risk of hemorrhage following intramuscular injection, the ACIP recommends "it should be administered intramuscularly if, in the opinion of the physician familiar with the patients bleeding risk, the vaccine can be administered with reasonable safety by this route. If the patient receives antihemophilia or other similar therapy, intramuscular vaccination can be scheduled shortly after such therapy is administered. A fine needle (23 gauge or smaller) can be used for the vaccination and firm pressure applied to the site (without rubbing) for at least 2 minutes. The patient should be instructed concerning the risk of hematoma from the injection."

Nursing Implications Inspect for particulate matter and discoloration prior to administration; for I.M. administration only

Additional Information Pharmacies will stock the formulations(s) standardized according to the USPHS requirements for the season. Influenza vaccines from previous seasons must not be used. Federal law requires that the date of administration, the vaccine manufacturer, lot number of vaccine, and the administering person's name, title, and address be entered into the patient's permanent medical record.

Dosage Forms

Injection, purified split virus (FluShield®): 0.5 mL, 5 mL
Injection, purified surface antigen (Fluvirin®): 0.5 mL, 5 mL
Injection, split-virus (Fluogen®, Fluzone®): 0.5 mL, 5 mL
Injection, whole-virus (Fluzone®): 5 mL

♦ **Influenza Virus Vaccine (inactivated whole-virus)** *see* Influenza Virus Vaccine *on page 721*

♦ **Influenza Virus Vaccine (purified split-virus)** *see* Influenza Virus Vaccine *on page 721*

♦ **Influenza Virus Vaccine (purified surface antigen)** *see* Influenza Virus Vaccine *on page 721*

♦ **Influenza Virus Vaccine (split-virus)** *see* Influenza Virus Vaccine *on page 721*

♦ **Infufer® (Can)** *see* Iron Dextran Complex *on page 745*

♦ **Infumorph™** *see* Morphine Sulfate *on page 936*

♦ **INH** *see* Isoniazid *on page 747*

♦ **Innohep®** *see* Tinzaparin *on page 1335*

Insulin Preparations *(IN su lin prep a RAY shuns)*

Related Information

Desensitization Protocols *on page 1525*
Diabetes Mellitus Treatment *on page 1657*

U.S. Brand Names Humalog®; Humalog® Mix 75/25™; Humulin®; Humulin® 50/50; Humulin® 70/30; Humulin® L; Humulin® N; Humulin® R; Humulin® R (Concentrated) U-500; Lantus®; Lente® Iletin® II; Novolin® 70/30; Novolin® L; Novolin® N; Novolin® R; NovoLog®; NPH Iletin® II; Regular Iletin® II; Velosulin® BR (Buffered)

Canadian Brand Names Humalog®; Humalog® Mix25™; Humulin®; Iletin® II Pork; Novolin®ge

Therapeutic Category Antidiabetic Agent, Parenteral; Antidote, Hyperglycemia

Use Treatment of type 1 diabetes mellitus (insulin dependent, IDDM); type 2 diabetes mellitus (noninsulin dependent, NIDDM) unresponsive to treatment with diet and/or oral hypoglycemics; adjunct to parenteral nutrition; hyperkalemia (regular insulin only; use with glucose to shift potassium into cells to lower serum potassium levels)

Pregnancy Risk Factor B; C (insulin glargine [Lantus®]; insulin aspart [NovoLog®])

Pregnancy/Breast-Feeding Implications

Clinical effects on the fetus: Does not cross the placenta. Insulin is the drug of choice for the control of diabetes mellitus during pregnancy. There are no well-controlled studies using insulin glargine (Lantus®) during pregnancy; use during pregnancy only if clearly needed.

Breast-feeding/lactation: The gastrointestinal tract destroys insulin when administered orally and therefore would not be expected to be absorbed intact by the breast-feeding infant.

Warnings/Precautions Hypoglycemia is the most common adverse effect of insulin. The timing of hypoglycemia differs among various insulin formulations. Any change of insulin should be made cautiously; changing manufacturers, type and/or method of manufacture, may result in the need for a change of dosage; human insulin differs from animal-source insulin; regular insulin is the only insulin to be used I.V.; hypoglycemia may result from increased work or exercise without eating; use of long-acting insulin preparations (insulin glargine, Ultralente®, insulin U) may delay recovery from hypoglycemia

In type 1 diabetes, insulin lispro (Humalog®) should be used in combination with a long-acting insulin. However, in type 2 diabetes it may be used without a long-acting insulin when used in combination with a sulfonylurea.

Use with caution in renal or hepatic impairment

Insulin aspart (NovoLog®): Safety and efficacy of use in children has not been established

Adverse Reactions Frequency not defined.

Cardiovascular: Palpitation, tachycardia, pallor

Central nervous system: Fatigue, mental confusion, loss of consciousness, headache, hypothermia

Dermatologic: Urticaria, redness

Endocrine & metabolic: Hypoglycemia

Gastrointestinal: Hunger, nausea, numbness of mouth

Local: Itching, edema, stinging, pain or warmth at injection site; atrophy or hypertrophy of S.C. fat tissue

Neuromuscular & skeletal: Muscle weakness, paresthesia, tremors

Ocular: Transient presbyopia or blurred vision

Miscellaneous: Diaphoresis, anaphylaxis

Overdosage/Toxicology Symptoms include tachycardia, anxiety, hunger, tremors, pallor, headache, motor dysfunction, speech disturbances, sweating, palpitations, coma, and death. Antidote includes glucose and glucagon, if necessary.

Drug Interactions

Increased Effect/Toxicity: Increased hypoglycemic effect of insulin with alcohol, alpha-blockers, anabolic steroids, beta-blockers (nonselective beta-blockers may delay recovery from hypoglycemic episodes and mask signs/symptoms of hypoglycemia; cardioselective beta-blocker agents may be alternatives), clofibrate, guanethidine, MAO inhibitors, pentamidine, phenylbutazone, salicylates, sulfinpyrazone, and tetracyclines.

Insulin increases the risk of hypoglycemia associated with oral hypoglycemic agents (including sulfonylureas, metformin, pioglitazone, rosiglitazone, and troglitazone).

Decreased Effect: Decreased hypoglycemic effect of insulin with corticosteroids, dextrothyroxine, diltiazem, dobutamine, epinephrine, niacin, oral contraceptives, thiazide diuretics, thyroid hormone, and smoking.

Ethanol/Nutrition/Herb Interactions

Ethanol: Caution with ethanol (may increase hypoglycemia).

Food: Insulin shifts potassium from extracellular to intracellular space. Decreases potassium serum concentration.

Herb/Nutraceutical: Use caution with chromium, garlic, gymnema (may increase hypoglycemia).

Stability

Newer neutral formulation of insulin is stable at room temperature up to one month (studies indicate up to 24-30 months)

Insulin aspart (NovoLog®): Can be infused S.C. by external insulin pump; do not dilute or mix with other insulins when used in an external pump for S.C. infusion; insulin in reservoir should be replaced every 48 hours. Do not expose to temperatures ≥37°C (98.6°F).

Insulin glargine (Lantus®): When refrigeration is unavailable, 10 mL vials and 3 mL cartridges may be stored at room temperature for up to 28 days, 5 mL vials may be stored at room temperature for 14 days; solution not used within these times must be discarded

Freezing causes more damage to insulin than room temperatures up to 100°F. Avoid direct sunlight.

Compatibility of insulin preparations:

Rapid-acting:

Insulin injection (regular): Compatible mixed with all types insulin

Lispro (Humalog®): Compatible mixed with Ultralente® / NPH

Insulin aspart (NovoLog®): Compatible mixed with NPH human insulin

Intermediate-acting: Isophane insulin suspension (NPH): Compatible mixed with regular insulin

Long-acting: When mixing with NPH insulin in any proportion, the excess protamine may combine with regular insulin and may reduce or delay activity of regular insulin (does not appear to be clinically significant); phosphate-buffered regular insulins bind with Lente® insulins forming short-acting insulin; excess protamine in PZI combines with regular insulin and prolongs its action, therefore, should not be mixed; administer as a separate injection; insulin glargine (Lantus®) cannot be diluted or mixed with any other insulin or solution

Stability of parenteral admixture of regular insulin at room temperature (25°C) and at refrigeration temperature (4°C): 24 hours

Standard diluent: 100 units/100 mL NS

Comments: All bags should be prepared fresh; tubing should be flushed 30 minutes prior to administration to allow adsorption as time permits

Mechanism of Action The principal hormone required for proper glucose utilization in normal metabolic processes; it is obtained from beef or pork pancreas or a biosynthetic process converting pork insulin to human insulin; insulins are categorized into 3 groups related to promptness, duration, and intensity of action

Pharmacodynamics/Kinetics

Onset and duration: Biosynthetic NPH human insulin shows a more rapid onset and shorter duration of action than corresponding porcine insulins; human insulin and purified porcine regular insulin are similarly efficacious following S.C. administration. The duration of action of highly purified porcine insulins is shorter than that of conventional insulin equivalents. Duration depends on type of preparation and route of administration as well as patient-related variables. In general, the larger the dose of insulin, the longer the duration of activity.

Absorption: Biosynthetic regular human insulin is absorbed from the S.C. injection site more rapidly than insulins of animal origin (60-90 minutes peak vs 120-150 minutes peak respectively) and lowers the initial blood glucose much faster. Human Ultralente® insulin is

(Continued)

Insulin Preparations (Continued)

absorbed about twice as quickly as its bovine equivalent, and bioavailability is also improved. Human Lente® insulin preparations are also absorbed more quickly than their animal equivalents. Insulin glargine (Lantus®) is designed to form microprecipitates when injected subcutaneously. Small amounts of insulin glargine are then released over a 24-hour period, with no pronounced peak. Insulin glargine (Lantus®) for the treatment of type 1 diabetes (insulin dependent, IDDM) and type 2 diabetes mellitus (noninsulin dependent, NIDDM) in patients who require basal (long-acting) insulin.

Bioavailability: Medium-acting S.C. Lente®-type human insulins did not differ from the corresponding porcine insulins

Lispro (Humalog®):
  Onset 0.25 hours; peak 0.5-1.5 hours; duration 6-8 hours

Insulin aspart (NovoLog®):
  Onset 0.5 hours; peak 1-3 hours; duration 3-5 hours

Insulin, regular (Novolin® R):
  Onset 0.5-1 hours; peak 2-3 hours; duration 8-12 hours

Isophane insulin suspension (NPH) (Novolin® N):
  Onset 1-1.5 hours; peak 4-12 hours; duration 24 hours

Insulin zinc suspension (Lente®):
  Onset 1-2.5 hours; peak 8-12 hours; duration 18-24 hours

Isophane insulin suspension and regular insulin injection (Novolin® 70/30):
  Onset 0.5 hours; peak 2-12 hours; duration 24 hours

Extended insulin zinc suspension (Ultralente®):
  Onset 4-8 hours; peak 16-18 hours; duration >36 hours

Insulin glargine (Lantus®):
  Duration 24 hours

Usual Dosage Dose requires continuous medical supervision; may administer I.V. (regular), I.M., S.C.

Diabetes mellitus: The number and size of daily doses, time of administration, and diet and exercise require continuous medical supervision. In addition, specific formulations may require distinct administration procedures.
  Lispro should be given within 15 minutes before or immediately after a meal
  Aspart should be given immediately before a meal (within 5-10 minutes of the start of a meal)
  Human regular insulin should be given within 30-60 minutes before a meal.
  Intermediate-acting insulins may be administered 1-2 times/day.
  Long-acting insulins may be administered once daily.
  Insulin glargine (Lantus®) should be administered subcutaneously once daily at bedtime. Maintenance doses should be administered subcutaneously and sites should be rotated to prevent lipodystrophy.
  Children and Adults: 0.5-1 unit/kg/day in divided doses
  Adolescents (growth spurts): 0.8-1.2 units/kg/day in divided doses
  Adjust dose to maintain premeal and bedtime blood glucose of 80-140 mg/dL (children <5 years: 100-200 mg/dL)
  Insulin glargine (Lantus®):
    Type 2 diabetes (patient not already on insulin): 10 units once daily, adjusted according to patient response (range in clinical study 2-100 units/day)
    Patients already receiving insulin: In clinical studies, when changing to insulin glargine from once-daily NPH or Ultralente® insulin, the initial dose was not changed; when changing from twice-daily NPH to once-daily insulin glargine, the total daily dose was reduced by 20% and adjusted according to patient response
Hyperkalemia: Administer calcium gluconate and $NaHCO_3$ first then 50% dextrose at 0.5-1 mL/kg and insulin 1 unit for every 4-5 g dextrose given
Diabetic ketoacidosis: Children and Adults: Regular insulin: I.V. loading dose: 0.1 unit/kg, then maintenance continuous infusion: 0.1 unit/kg/hour (range: 0.05-0.2 units/kg/hour depending upon the rate of decrease of serum glucose - too rapid decrease of serum glucose may lead to cerebral edema).
  Optimum rate of decrease (serum glucose): 80-100 mg/dL/hour
  Note: Newly diagnosed patients with IDDM presenting in DKA and patients with blood sugars <800 mg/dL may be relatively "sensitive" to insulin and should receive loading and initial maintenance doses approximately $\frac{1}{2}$ of those indicated above.
Dosing adjustment in renal impairment (regular): Insulin requirements are reduced due to changes in insulin clearance or metabolism
  Cl_{cr} 10-50 mL/minute: Administer at 75% of normal dose
  Cl_{cr} <10 mL/minute: Administer at 25% to 50% of normal dose and monitor glucose closely
Hemodialysis: Because of a large molecular weight (6000 daltons), insulin is not significantly removed by either peritoneal or hemodialysis
  Supplemental dose is not necessary
Peritoneal dialysis: Supplemental dose is not necessary
Continuous arteriovenous or venovenous hemofiltration effects: Supplemental dose is not necessary
Dietary Considerations Dietary modification based on ADA recommendations is a part of therapy. Monitor potassium serum concentration.
Administration
  Buffered insulin (Velosulin® BR) should not be mixed with any other form of insulin
  Insulin aspart (NovoLog®): Can be infused S.C. by external insulin pump; do not dilute or mix with other insulins when used in an external pump for S.C. infusion; should replace insulin in reservoir every 48 hours.
  Insulin glargine (Lantus®): Cannot be diluted or mixed with any other insulin or solution; should be administered S.C. only; use only if solution is clear and colorless

Insulin lispro (Humalog®): May be administered within 15 minutes before or immediately after a meal

Regular insulin may be administered by S.C., I.M., or I.V. routes

S.C. administration is usually made into the thighs, arms, buttocks, or abdomen, with sites rotated

When mixing regular insulin with other preparations of insulin, regular insulin should be drawn into syringe first

I.V. administration (requires use of an infusion pump): **Only regular insulin** may be administered I.V.

I.V. infusions: To minimize adsorption problems to I.V. solution bag:

If new tubing is **not** needed: Wait a minimum of 30 minutes between the preparation of the solution and the initiation of the infusion

If new tubing is needed: After receiving the insulin drip solution, the administration set should be attached to the I.V. container and the line should be flushed with the insulin solution. The nurse should then wait 30 minutes, then flush the line again with the insulin solution prior to initiating the infusion

If insulin is required prior to the availability of the insulin drip, regular insulin should be administered by I.V. push injection

Because of adsorption, the actual amount of insulin being administered could be substantially less than the apparent amount. Therefore, adjustment of the insulin drip rate should be based on effect and not solely on the apparent insulin dose. Furthermore, the apparent dose should not be used as the basis for determining the subsequent insulin dose upon discontinuing the insulin drip. Dose requires continuous medical supervision.

To be ordered as units/hour

Example: Standard diluent of regular insulin only: 100 units/100 mL NS (can be administered as a more diluted solution, ie, 100 units/250 mL NS)

Insulin rate of infusion (100 units regular/100 mL NS)

1 unit/hour: 1 mL/hour
2 units/hour: 2 mL/hour
3 units/hour: 3 mL/hour
4 units/hour: 4 mL/hour
5 units/hour: 5 mL/hour, etc

Monitoring Parameters Urine sugar and acetone, serum glucose, electrolytes, Hb A$_{1c}$, lipid profile

Reference Range

Therapeutic, serum insulin (fasting): 5-20 µIU/mL (SI: 35-145 pmol/L)

Glucose, fasting:

Newborns: 60-110 mg/dL
Adults: 60-110 mg/dL
Elderly: 100-180 mg/dL

Patient Information This medication is used to control diabetes; it is not a cure. Other components of treatment plan are important: follow prescribed diet, medication, and exercise regimen. Take exactly as directed. Do not change dose or discontinue unless so advised by prescriber. Inform prescriber of all other prescription or OTC medications you are taking; do not introduce new medication without consulting prescriber. If you experience hypoglycemic reaction, contact prescriber immediately. Maintain regular dietary intake and exercise routine and always carry quick source of sugar with you. Report adverse side effects, including chest pain or palpitations; persistent fatigue, confusion, headache; skin rash or redness; numbness of mouth, lips, or tongue; muscle weakness or tremors; changes in vision; difficulty breathing; or nausea, vomiting, or flu-like symptoms. With insulin aspart (NovoLog®), you must start eating within 5-10 minutes after injection.

Nursing Implications Patients using human insulin may be less likely to recognize hypoglycemia than if they use pork insulin, patients on pork insulin that have low blood sugar exhibit hunger and sweating; regular insulin is the only form for I.V. use. Patients who are unable to accurately draw up their dose will need assistance such as prefilled syringes. Patients using insulin aspart (NovoLog®) must start eating within 5-10 minutes following injection.

Additional Information The term "purified" refers to insulin preparations containing no more than 10 ppm proinsulin (purified and human insulins are less immunogenic). Buffering agent in Velosulin® BR may alter the activity of other insulin products.

Dosage Forms

Rapid-Acting:

Injection, solution, rapid-acting, aspart, human:

NovoLog®: 100 units/mL (10 mL vial)
NovoLog® PenFill: 100 units/mL (3 mL cartridge)

Injection, solution, rapid-acting, lispro, human (Humalog®): 100 units/mL (1.5 mL cartridge, 3 mL disposable pen, 10 mL vial)

Short-Acting:

Injection, solution, short-acting, regular, human:

Humlin® R: 100 units/mL (10 mL vial)
Novolin® R: 100 units/mL (10 mL vial)
Novolin R® PenFill: 100 units/mL (1.5 mL cartridge, 3 mL cartridge)
Novolin R® [prefilled syringe]: 100 units/mL (1.5 mL)

Injection, solution, short-acting, regular, human, buffered (Velosulin® BR): 100 units/mL (10 mL vial)

Injection, solution, short-acting, regular, human, concentrate (Humulin® R U-500): 500 units/mL (20 mL vial)

Injection, solution, short-acting, regular, purified pork (Regular Iletin® II): 100 units/mL (10 mL vial)

Intermediate-Acting:

Injection, suspension, intermediate-acting, lente, human (Humulin® L, Novolin® L): 100 units/mL (10 mL vial) [zinc]

Injection, suspension, intermediate-acting, lente, purified pork (Lente® Iletin II): 100 units/mL (10 mL vial) [zinc]

(Continued)

Insulin Preparations (Continued)

Injection, suspension, intermediate-acting, NPH, human [isophane]:
Humulin® N: 100 units/mL (3 mL disposable pen, 10 mL vial)
Novolin® N: 100 units/mL (10 mL vial)
Novolin® N PenFill: 100 units/mL (1.5 mL cartridge, 3 mL cartridge)
Novolin® N [prefilled syringe]: 100 units/mL (1.5 mL)
Injection, suspension, intermediate-acting, NPH, purified pork (NPH Iletin® II): 100 units/mL (10 mL vial) [isophane]

Long-Acting:

Injection, suspension, long-acting, Ultralente®, human (Humulin U Ultralente®): 100 units/mL (10 mL vial) [zinc]
Injection, solution, long-acting, glargine, human (Lantus®): 100 unit/mL (10 mL vial)

Combination:

Injection, combination, intermediate-acting, lispro human suspension 75% and rapid-acting lispro human solution 25% (Humalog® Mix 75/25®): 100 units/mL (3 mL disposable pen, 10 mL vial)
Injection, combination, intermediate-acting, NPH human insulin suspension 50% and short-acting regular human insulin solution 50% (Humulin® 50/50): 100 units/mL (10 mL vial)
Injection, combination, intermediate-acting, NPH human insulin suspension 70% and short-acting regular human insulin solution 30%:
Humulin® 70/30: 100 units/mL (3 ml disposable pen, 10 mL vial)
Novolin® 70/30: 100 units/mL (10 mL vial)
Novolin® 70/30 PenFill: 100 units/mL (1.5 mL cartridge, 3 mL cartridge)
Novolin® 70/30 [prefilled syringe]: 100 units/mL (1.5 mL)

♦ **Intal®** see Cromolyn Sodium on page 337
♦ **Integrilin®** see Eptifibatide on page 480
♦ **α-2-interferon** see Interferon Alfa-2b on page 728

Interferon Alfa-2a (in ter FEER on AL fa too aye)

U.S. Brand Names Roferon-A®
Canadian Brand Names Roferon-A®
Synonyms IFLrA; rIFN-A
Therapeutic Category Biological Response Modulator; Interferon
Use

Patients >18 years of age: Hairy cell leukemia, AIDS-related Kaposi's sarcoma, chronic hepatitis C
Children and Adults: Chronic myelogenous leukemia (CML), Philadelphia chromosome positive, within 1 year of diagnosis (limited experience in children)

Unlabeled/Investigational Use Adjuvant therapy for malignant melanoma, AIDS-related thrombocytopenia, cutaneous ulcerations of Behçet's disease, brain tumors, metastatic ileal carcinoid tumors, cervical and colorectal cancers, genital warts, idiopathic mixed cryoglobulinemia, hemangioma, hepatitis D, hepatocellular carcinoma, idiopathic hypereosinophilic syndrome, mycosis fungoides, Sézary syndrome, low-grade non-Hodgkin's lymphoma, macular degeneration, multiple myeloma, renal cell carcinoma, basal and squamous cell skin cancer, essential thrombocythemia, cutaneous T-cell lymphoma

Pregnancy Risk Factor C

Pregnancy/Breast-Feeding Implications Safety and efficacy for use during pregnancy have not been established. Interferon alpha has been shown to decrease serum estradiol and progesterone levels in humans. Menstrual irregularities and abortion have been reported in animals. Effective contraception is recommended during treatment.

Contraindications Hypersensitivity to alfa interferon, benzyl alcohol, or any component of the formulation; autoimmune disorders, including autoimmune hepatitis; transplant patients receiving therapeutic immunosuppression; visceral AIDS-related Kaposi's sarcoma associated with rapidly-progressing or life-threatening disease

Warnings/Precautions Use with caution in patients with seizure disorders, brain metastases, compromised CNS, multiple sclerosis, and patients with pre-existing cardiac disease (ischemic or thromboembolic), arrhythmias, renal impairment (Cl_{cr} <50 mL/minute) or hepatic impairment, or myelosuppression; may cause severe psychiatric adverse events (psychosis, mania, depression, suicidal behavior/ideation) in patients with and without previous psychiatric symptoms, avoid use in severe psychiatric disorders or in patients with a history of depression; careful neuropsychiatric monitoring is required during therapy. May cause thyroid dysfunction or hyperglycemia, use caution in patients with diabetes. Use caution in patients with pulmonary dysfunction. Treatment should be discontinued in patients with worsening or persistently severe signs/symptoms of autoimmune, infectious, ischemic (including radiographic changes or worsening hepatic function), or neuropsychiatric disorders (including depression and/or suicidal thoughts/behavior). Safety and efficacy in children <18 years of age have not been established. Higher doses in the elderly or in malignancies other than hairy cell leukemia may result in severe obtundation. Ophthalmologic disorders (including retinal hemorrhages, cotton wool spots, and retinal artery or vein obstruction) have occurred in patients receiving alpha interferons. **Due to differences in dosage, patients should not change brands of interferons.** Injection solution contains benzyl alcohol, do not use in neonates or infants.

Adverse Reactions Flu-like symptoms are common (up to 92%).
>10%:
Cardiovascular: Chest pain (4% to 11%), edema (11%), hypertension (11%)
Central nervous system: Psychiatric disturbances (including depression and suicidal behavior/ideation; reported incidence highly variable, generally >15%), fatigue (90%), headache (52%), dizziness (21%), irritability (15%), insomnia (14%), somnolence, lethargy, confusion, mental impairment, and motor weakness (most frequently seen at high doses [>100 million units], usually reverses within a few days); vertigo (19%); mental status changes (12%)

Dermatologic: Rash (usually maculopapular) on the trunk and extremities (7% to 18%), alopecia (19% to 22%), pruritus (13%), dry skin

Endocrine & metabolic: Hypocalcemia (10% to 51%), hyperglycemia (33% to 39%), elevation of transaminase levels (25% to 30%), elevation of alkaline phosphatase (48%)

Gastrointestinal: Loss of taste, anorexia (30% to 70%), nausea (28% to 53%), vomiting (10% to 30%, usually mild), diarrhea (22% to 34%, may be severe), taste change (13%), dry throat, xerostomia, abdominal cramps, abdominal pain

Hematologic (often due to underlying disease): Myelosuppression; neutropenia (32% to 70%); thrombocytopenia (22% to 70%); anemia (24% to 65%, may be dose-limiting, usually seen only during the first 6 months of therapy)

Onset: 7-10 days

Nadir: 14 days, may be delayed 20-40 days in hairy cell leukemia

Recovery: 21 days

Hepatic: Elevation of AST (SGOT) (77% to 80%), LDH (47%), bilirubin (31%)

Local: Injection site reaction (29%)

Neuromuscular & skeletal: Weakness (may be severe at doses >20,000,000 units/day); arthralgia and myalgia (5% to 73%, usually during the first 72 hours of treatment); rigors

Renal: Proteinuria (15% to 25%)

Respiratory: Cough (27%), irritation of oropharynx (14%)

Miscellaneous: Flu-like syndrome (up to 92% of patients), loss of taste, diaphoresis (15%)

1% to 10%:

Cardiovascular: Hypotension (6%), supraventricular tachyarrhythmias, palpitations (<3%), acute myocardial infarction (<1% to 1%)

Central nervous system: Confusion (10%), delirium

Dermatologic: Erythema (diffuse), urticaria

Endocrine & metabolic: Hyperphosphatemia (2%)

Gastrointestinal: Stomatitis, pancreatitis (<5%), flatulence, liver pain

Genitourinary: Impotence (6%), menstrual irregularities

Neuromuscular & skeletal: Leg cramps; peripheral neuropathy, paresthesias (7%), and numbness (4%) are more common in patients previously treated with vinca alkaloids or receiving concurrent vinblastine

Ocular: Conjunctivitis (4%)

Respiratory: Dyspnea (7.5%), epistaxis (4%), rhinitis (3%)

Miscellaneous: Antibody production to interferon (10%)

<1% (Limited to important or life-threatening): Acute renal failure, aplastic anemia, autoimmune reaction with worsening of liver disease, bronchospasm, cardiomyopathy, coma, congestive heart failure, GI hemorrhage, hallucinations, hemolytic anemia, hyponatremia (SIADH), mania, pneumonia, seizures, stroke, syncope, vasculitis

Overdosage/Toxicology Symptoms include CNS depression, obtundation, flu-like symptoms, and myelosuppression. Treatment is supportive.

Drug Interactions

Cytochrome P450 Effect: Inhibits metabolism by cytochrome P450 (isoenzyme profiles not defined)

Increased Effect/Toxicity: Cimetidine may augment the antitumor effects of interferon in melanoma. Theophylline clearance has been reported to be decreased in hepatitis patients receiving interferon. Vinblastine enhances interferon toxicity in several patients; increased incidence of paresthesia has also been noted. Interferons may increase the adverse/toxic effects of ACE inhibitors, specifically the development of granulocytopenia. Agranulocytosis has been reported with concurrent use of clozapine (case report). Interferons may increase the anticoagulant effects of warfarin, and interferons may increase serum levels of zidovudine.

Decreased Effect: Prednisone may decrease the therapeutic effects of interferon alpha. A decreased response to erythropoietin has been reported (case reports) in patients receiving interferons. Interferon alpha may decrease the serum concentrations of melphalan (may or may not decrease toxicity of melphalan).

Stability Refrigerate (2°C to 8°C/36°F to 46°F); do not freeze; do not shake; after reconstitution, the solution is stable for 24 hours at room temperature and for 1 month when refrigerated

Mechanism of Action Alpha interferons are a family of proteins, produced by nucleated cells, that have antiviral, antiproliferative, and immune-regulating activity. There are 16 known subtypes of alpha interferons. Interferons interact with cells through high affinity cell surface receptors. Following activation, multiple effects can be detected including induction of gene transcription. Inhibits cellular growth, alters the state of cellular differentiation, interferes with oncogene expression, alters cell surface antigen expression, increases phagocytic activity of macrophages, and augments cytotoxicity of lymphocytes for target cells

Pharmacodynamics/Kinetics

Absorption: Filtered and absorbed at the renal tubule

Distribution: V_d: 0.223-0.748 L/kg

Metabolism: Majority renal; filtered through glomeruli and undergoes rapid proteolytic degradation during tubular reabsorption

Bioavailability: I.M.: 83%; S.C.: 90%

Half-life elimination: I.V.: 3.7-8.5 hours (mean ~5 hours)

Time to peak, serum: I.M., S.C.: ~6-8 hours

Usual Dosage Refer to individual protocols

Children (limited data):

Chronic myelogenous leukemia (CML): I.M.: 2.5-5 million units/m^2/day; **Note:** In juveniles, higher dosages (30 million units/m^2/day) have been associated with severe adverse events, including death

Adults:

Hairy cell leukemia: S.C., I.M.: 3 million units/day for 16-24 weeks, then 3 million units 3 times/week for up to 6-24 months

Chronic myelogenous leukemia (CML): S.C., I.M.: 9 million units/day, continue treatment until disease progression

(Continued)

Interferon Alfa-2a *(Continued)*

AIDS-related Kaposi's sarcoma: S.C., I.M.: 36 million units/day for 10-12 weeks, then 36 million units 3 times/week; to minimize adverse reactions, can use escalating dose (3-, 9-, then 18 million units each day for 3 days, then 36 million units daily thereafter). If severe reactions occur, reduce dose by 50% or discontinue until reaction subsides.

Hepatitis C: S.C., I.M.: 3 million units 3 times/week for 12 months

Dosage adjustment in renal impairment: Not removed by hemodialysis

Dosage adjustment for toxicity: If severe adverse reactions occur, modify dosage (reduce dose by 50%) or temporarily discontinue treatment until reaction subsides.

Administration S.C. administration is suggested for those who are at risk for bleeding or are thrombocytopenic; rotate S.C. injection site; patient should be well hydrated

Monitoring Parameters

Chronic hepatitis C: Monitor ALT and HCV-RNA to assess response (particularly in first 3 months of therapy)

CML/hairy cell leukemia: Hematologic monitoring should be performed monthly

Patient Information Use as directed; do not change dosage or schedule of administration without consulting prescriber. Maintain adequate hydration (2-3 L/day of fluids unless instructed to restrict fluid intake). You may experience flu-like syndrome (acetaminophen may help); nausea, vomiting, dry mouth, or metallic taste (frequent small meals, frequent mouth care, sucking lozenges, or chewing gum may help); drowsiness, dizziness, agitation, abnormal thinking (use caution when driving or engaging in tasks requiring alertness until response to drug is known). Inform prescriber **immediately** if you feel depressed or have any thoughts of suicide. Report unusual bruising or bleeding; persistent abdominal disturbances; unusual fatigue; muscle pain or tremors; chest pain or palpitation; swelling of extremities or unusual weight gain; difficulty breathing; pain, swelling, or redness at injection site; or other unusual symptoms.

Nursing Implications Do not freeze or shake solution; a flu-like syndrome (fever, chills) occurs in the majority of patients 2-6 hours after a dose; pretreatment with nonsteroidal anti-inflammatory drug (NSAID) or acetaminophen can decrease fever and its severity and alleviate headache

Dosage Forms

Injection [single-dose vial]:

3 million units/1 mL

6 million units/1 mL

9 million units/0.9 mL

36 million units/1 mL

Injection [multidose vial]:

9 million units/vial (3 million units/0.3 mL)

18 million units/vial (3 million units/0.3 mL)

Injection, prefilled syringe [single-dose]:

3 million units/0.5 mL [S.C. only]

6 million units/0.5 mL [S.C. only]

9 million units/0.5 mL [S.C. only]

Interferon Alfa-2b *(in ter FEER on AL fa too bee)*

U.S. Brand Names Intron® A

Canadian Brand Names Intron® A

Synonyms INF-alpha 2; α-2-interferon; rLFN-α2

Therapeutic Category Antiviral Agent, Hepatitis; Biological Response Modulator; Interferon

Use

Patients >1 year of age: Chronic hepatitis B

Patients >18 years of age: Condyloma acuminata, chronic hepatitis C, hairy cell leukemia, malignant melanoma, AIDS-related Kaposi's sarcoma, follicular non-Hodgkin's lymphoma

Unlabeled/Investigational Use AIDS-related thrombocytopenia, cutaneous ulcerations of Behçet's disease, carcinoid syndrome, lymphomatoid granulomatosis, genital herpes, hepatitis D, chronic myelogenous leukemia (CML), non-Hodgkin's lymphomas (other than follicular lymphoma, see approved use), polycythemia vera, medullary thyroid carcinoma, multiple myeloma, renal cell carcinoma, basal and squamous cell skin cancers, essential thrombocytopenia, thrombocytopenic purpura

Pregnancy Risk Factor C

Pregnancy/Breast-Feeding Implications Safety and efficacy for use during pregnancy have not been established. Interferon alpha has been shown to decrease serum estradiol and progesterone levels in humans. Menstrual irregularities and abortion have been reported in animals. Effective contraception is recommended during treatment.

Contraindications Hypersensitivity to interferon alfa or any component of the formulation; patients with visceral AIDS-related Kaposi's sarcoma associated with rapidly-progressing or life-threatening disease; decompensated liver disease; autoimmune hepatitis; history of autoimmune disease; immunocompromised or transplant patients

Warnings/Precautions Use with caution in patients with a history of seizures, brain metastases, multiple sclerosis, cardiac disease (ischemic or thromboembolic), arrhythmias, myelosuppression, hepatic impairment, or renal dysfunction. Use caution in patients with a history of pulmonary disease, coagulopathy, thyroid disease, hypertension, or diabetes mellitus (particularly if prone to DKA). Avoid use in patient with autoimmune disorders; worsening of psoriasis and/or development of autoimmune disorders has been associated with alpha interferons. May cause severe psychiatric events (psychosis, mania, depression, suicidal behavior/ideation) in patients with and without previous psychiatric symptoms, avoid use in severe psychiatric disorders or in patients with a history of depression; careful neuropsychiatric monitoring is required during therapy. Higher doses in elderly patients, or diseases other than hairy cell leukemia, may result in increased CNS toxicity. Ophthalmologic disorders (including retinal hemorrhages, cotton wool spots, and retinal artery or vein obstruction) have occurred in patients receiving alpha interferons.

A transient increase in SGOT (>2x baseline) is common in patients treated with interferon alfa-2b for chronic hepatitis. Therapy generally may continue, however functional indicators (albumin, prothrombin time, bilirubin) should be monitored at 2-week intervals. Treatment should be discontinued in patients who develop severe pulmonary symptoms with chest x-ray changes, autoimmune disorders, worsening of hepatic function, psychiatric symptoms (including depression and/or suicidal thoughts/behaviors), severe or persistent infectious or ischemic disorders. Safety and efficacy in children <18 years of age have not been established (except in chronic hepatitis B). **Due to differences in dosage, patients should not change brands of interferons.**

Adverse Reactions Flu-like symptoms are common (up to 79%)

>10%:

Cardiovascular: Chest pain (2% to 28%)

Central nervous system: Fatigue (8% to 96%), headache (21% to 62%), fever (34% to 94%), depression (4% to 40%), somnolence (1% to 33%), irritability (1% to 22%), paresthesia (1% to 21%, more common in patients previously treated with vinca alkaloids or receiving concurrent vinblastine), dizziness (7% to 23%), confusion (1% to 12%), malaise (3% to 14%), pain (3% to 15%), insomnia (1% to 12%), impaired concentration (1% to 14%, usually reverses within a few days), amnesia (1% to 14%), chills (45% to 54%),

Dermatologic: Alopecia (8% to 38%), rash (usually maculopapular) on the trunk and extremities (1% to 25%), pruritus (3% to 11%), dry skin (1% to 10%)

Endocrine & metabolic: Hypocalcemia (10% to 51%), hyperglycemia (33% to 39%), amenorrhea (up to 12% in lymphoma)

Gastrointestinal: Anorexia (1% to 69%), nausea (19% to 66%), vomiting (2% to 32%, usually mild), diarrhea (2% to 45%, may be severe), taste change (2% to 24%), xerostomia (1% to 28%), abdominal pain (2% to 23%), gingivitis (2% to 14%), constipation (1% to 14%)

Hematologic: Myelosuppression; neutropenia (30% to 66%); thrombocytopenia (5% to 15%); anemia (15% to 32%, may be dose-limiting, usually seen only during the first 6 months of therapy)

Onset: 7-10 days

Nadir: 14 days, may be delayed 20-40 days in hairy cell leukemia

Recovery: 21 days

Hepatic: Increased transaminases (increased SGOT in up to 63%), elevation of alkaline phosphatase (48%), right upper quadrant pain (15% in hepatitis C)

Local: Injection site reaction (1% to 20%)

Neuromuscular & skeletal: Weakness (5% to 63%) may be severe at doses >20,000,000 units/day; mild arthralgia and myalgia (5% to 75% - usually during the first 72 hours of treatment), rigors (2% to 42%), back pain (1% to 19%), musculoskeletal pain (1% to 21%), paresthesia (1% to 21%)

Renal: Urinary tract infection (up to 5% in hepatitis C)

Respiratory: Dyspnea (1% to 34%), cough (1% to 31%), pharyngitis (1% to 31%),

Miscellaneous: Loss of smell, flu-like symptoms (5% to 79%), diaphoresis (2% to 21%)

5% to 10%:

Cardiovascular: Hypertension (9% in hepatitis C)

Central nervous system: Anxiety (1% to 9%), nervousness (1% to 3%), vertigo (up to 8% in lymphoma)

Dermatologic: Dermatitis (1% to 8%)

Endocrine & metabolic: Decreased libido (1% to 5%)

Gastrointestinal: Loose stools (1% to 21%), dyspepsia (2% to 8%)

Neuromuscular & skeletal: Hypoesthesia (1% to 10%)

Respiratory: Nasal congestion (1% to 10%)

<5% (Limited to important or life-threatening): Acute hypersensitivity reactions, allergic reactions, angina, aphasia, arrhythmia, ataxia, atrial fibrillation, Bell's palsy, bronchospasm, cardiomyopathy, CHF, coma, depression, epidermal necrolysis, extrapyramidal disorder, gastrointestinal hemorrhage, gingival hyperplasia, granulocytopenia, hallucinations, hemolytic anemia, hemoptysis, hepatic encephalopathy (rare), hepatic failure (rare), hepatotoxic reaction, hypoventilation, jaundice, lupus erythematosus, mania, myocardial infarction, nephrotic syndrome, pancreatitis, polyarteritis nodosa, psychosis, pulmonary embolism, pulmonary fibrosis, Raynaud's phenomenon, renal failure, seizures, stroke, suicidal ideation, suicide attempt, syncope, tendonitis, thrombocytopenic purpura, thrombosis, vasculitis

Overdosage/Toxicology Symptoms include CNS depression, obtundation, flu-like symptoms, and myelosuppression. Treatment is supportive.

Drug Interactions

Cytochrome P450 Effect: Inhibits metabolism by cytochrome P450 (isoenzyme profiles not defined)

Increased Effect/Toxicity: Cimetidine may augment the antitumor effects of interferon in melanoma. Theophylline clearance has been reported to be decreased in hepatitis patients receiving interferon. Vinblastine enhances interferon toxicity in several patients; increased incidence of paresthesia has also been noted. Interferons may increase the adverse/toxic effects of ACE inhibitors, specifically the development of granulocytopenia. Agranulocytosis has been reported with concurrent use of clozapine (case report). Interferons may increase the anticoagulant effects of warfarin, and interferons may increase serum levels of zidovudine.

Stability Store intact vials at refrigeration (2°C to 8°C); powder and premixed solutions are stable at room temperature for 7 days. Reconstitute vials with diluent; reconstituted solution is stable for 30 days under refrigeration (2°C to 8°C).

Mechanism of Action Alpha interferons are a family of proteins, produced by nucleated cells, that have antiviral, antiproliferative, and immune-regulating activity. There are 16 known subtypes of alpha interferons. Interferons interact with cells through high affinity cell surface receptors. Following activation, multiple effects can be detected including induction of gene transcription. Inhibits cellular growth, alters the state of cellular differentiation, interferes with oncogene expression, alters cell surface antigen expression, increases phagocytic activity of macrophages, and augments cytotoxicity of lymphocytes for target cells

(Continued)

Interferon Alfa-2b *(Continued)*

Pharmacodynamics/Kinetics

Distribution: V_d: 31 L; but has been noted to be much greater (370-720 L) in leukemia patients receiving continuous infusion IFN; IFN does not penetrate the CSF

Metabolism: Majority renally

Bioavailability: I.M.: 83%; S.C.: 90%

Half-life elimination: I.M., I.V.: 2 hours; S.C.: 3 hours

Time to peak, serum: I.M., S.C.: ~3-12 hours

Usual Dosage Refer to individual protocols

Children 1-17 years: Chronic hepatitis B: S.C.: 3 million units/m² 3 times/week for 1 week; then 6 million units/m² 3 times/week; maximum: 10 million units 3 times/week; total duration of therapy 16-24 weeks

Adults:

Hairy cell leukemia: I.M., S.C.: 2 million units/m² 3 times/week for 2-6 months

Lymphoma (follicular): S.C.: 5 million units 3 times/week for up to 18 months

Malignant melanoma: 20 million units/m² I.V. for 5 consecutive days per week for 4 weeks, then 10 million units/m² S.C. 3 times/week for 48 weeks

AIDS-related Kaposi's sarcoma: I.M., S.C.: 30 million units/m² 3 times/week

Chronic hepatitis B: I.M., S.C.: 5 million units/day or 10 million units 3 times/week for 16 weeks

Chronic hepatitis C: I.M., S.C.: 3 million units 3 times/week for 16 weeks. In patients with normalization of ALT at 16 weeks, continue treatment for 18-24 months; consider discontinuation if normalization does not occur at 16 weeks. **Note:** May be used in combination therapy with ribavirin in previously untreated patients or in patients who relapse following alpha interferon therapy; refer to Interferon Alfa-2b and Ribavirin Combination Pack monograph.

Condyloma acuminata: Intralesionally: 1 million units/lesion (maximum: 5 lesions/treatment) 3 times/week (on alternate days) for 3 weeks. Use 1 million unit per 0.1 mL concentration.

Dosage adjustment in renal impairment: Not removed by peritoneal or hemodialysis

Dosage adjustment for toxicity:

Reduce dose by 50% if WBC <1500 cells/mm³, granulocytes <750 cells/mm³ (<1000 cells/mm³ in children), or platelet count <50,000 cells/mm³ (<100,000 cells/mm³ in children)

Interrupt therapy if WBC <1200 cells/mm³, granulocytes <500 cells/mm³ (<750 cells/mm³ in children), or platelet count <30,000 cells/mm³ (<70,000 cells/mm³ in children)

Administration Do not use 3-, 5-, 18-, and 25 million unit strengths intralesionally, solutions are hypertonic; 50 million unit strength is not for use in condylomata, hairy cell leukemia, or chronic hepatitis.

Monitoring Parameters Baseline chest x-ray, EKG, CBC with differential, liver function tests, electrolytes, thyroid function tests, platelets, weight; patients with pre-existing cardiac abnormalities, or in advanced stages of cancer should have EKGs taken before and during treatment. Discontinue if neutrophils <0.5 x 10⁹/L, platelets <25 x 10⁹/L.

Patient Information Do not change brands of interferon as changes in dosage may result; do not operate heavy machinery while on therapy since changes in mental status may occur; report to physician any persistent or severe sore throat, fever, fatigue, unusual bleeding, or bruising

Nursing Implications Use acetaminophen to prevent or partially alleviate headache and fever; do not use 3, 5, 18, and 25 million unit strengths intralesionally, solutions are hypertonic; 50 million unit strength is not for use in condylomata, hairy cell leukemia, or chronic hepatitis.

Dosage Forms

Injection, albumin free:

3 million units (0.5 mL)

5 million units (0.5 mL) (10 million units/mL)

10 million units (1 mL) (10 million units/mL)

18 million units (3 mL) (6 million units/mL)

25 million units (2.5 mL) (10 million units/mL)

Pens [multidose]:

6 doses of 3 million units (18 million units)

6 doses of 5 million units (30 million units)

6 doses of 10 million units (60 million units)

Powder for injection, lyophilized:

3 million units

5 million units

10 million units

18 million units

25 million units

50 million units

See also Interferon Alfa-2b and Ribavirin Combination Pack monograph

Interferon Alfa-2b and Ribavirin Combination Pack

(in ter FEER on AL fa too bee & rye ba VYE rin com bi NAY shun pak)

U.S. Brand Names Rebetron™

Canadian Brand Names Rebetron®

Synonyms Interferon Alfa-2b and Ribavirin Combination Pack; Ribavirin and Interferon Alfa-2b Combination Pack

Therapeutic Category Antiviral Agent, Hepatitis; Biological Response Modulator

Use The combination therapy of oral ribavirin with interferon alfa-2b, recombinant (Intron® A) injection is indicated for the treatment of chronic hepatitis C in patients with compensated liver disease who have relapsed after alpha interferon therapy.

Pregnancy Risk Factor X

Usual Dosage

Children: Chronic hepatitis C: **Note:** Safety and efficacy have not been established; dosing based on pharmacokinetic profile: Recommended dosage of combination therapy (Intron® A with Rebetrol®):

Intron® A: S.C.:

25-61 kg: 3 million int. units/m² 3 times/week

>61 kg: Refer to adult dosing

Rebetol® capsule: Oral:

25-36 kg: 400 mg/day (200 mg twice daily)

37-49 kg: 600 mg/day (200 mg in morning and 400 mg in evening)

50-61 kg: 800 mg/day (400 mg twice daily)

>61 kg: Refer to adult dosing

Adults: Chronic hepatitis C: Recommended dosage of combination therapy:

Intron® A: S.C.: 3 million int. units 3 times/week **and**

Rebetol® capsule: Oral: Range: 1000-1200 mg in a divided daily (morning and evening) dose for 24 weeks

≤75 kg (165 pounds): 1000 mg/day (two 200 mg capsules in the morning and three 200 mg capsules in the evening)

>75 kg: 1200 mg/day (three 200 mg capsules in the morning and three 200 mg capsules in the evening)

Additional Information

Rebetron™ - Guidelines for Dosing Modifications

Hemoglobin:

<10 g/dL: Reduce dose of Rebetol® to 600 mg/day

<8.5 d/dL: Permanently discontinue Rebetol®/Intron® A combination therapy

Hemoglobin in patients with cardiac history:

≥2 g/dL decrease during any 4-week period during therapy: Reduce of Rebetol® to 600 mg/day, reduce dose of Intron® A to 1.5 million int. units 3 times/week

<12 g/dL after 4 weeks on reduced dose: Permanently discontinue Rebetol®/Intron® A combination therapy

White blood count:

<1.5 x 10⁹/L: Reduce Intron® A dose to 1.5 million int. units 3 times/week

<1.0 x 10⁹/L: Permanently discontinue Rebetol®/Intron® A combination therapy

Neutrophil count:

<0.75 x 10⁹/L: Reduce Intron® A dose to 1.5 million int. units 3 times/week

<0.5 x 10⁹/L: Permanently discontinue Rebetol®/Intron® A combination therapy

Platelet count:

<50 x 10⁹/L: Reduce Intron® A dose to 1.5 million int. units 3 times/week

<25 x 10⁹/L: Permanently discontinue Rebetol®/Intron® A combination therapy

Dosage Forms

Combination package:

Patients ≤75 kg (Rebetron™):

A box containing 6 vials of Intron® A (3 million int. units in 0.5 mL per vial) and 6 syringes and alcohol swabs; two boxes containing 35 Rebetol® 200 mg capsules each for a total of 70 capsules (5 capsules per blister card)

One 18 million int. units [multidose vial] of Intron® A injection (22.8 million int. units per 3.8 mL; 3 million int. units/0.5 mL) and 6 syringes and alcohol swabs; two boxes containing 35 Rebetol® 200 mg capsules each for a total of 70 capsules (5 capsules per blister card)

One 18 million int. units Intron® A injection [multidose pen] (22.5 million int. units per 1.5 mL; 3 million int. units/0.2 mL) and 6 disposable needles and alcohol swabs; two boxes containing 35 Rebetol® 200 mg capsules each for a total of 70 capsules (5 capsules per blister card)

Patients >75 kg:

A box containing 6 vials of Intron® A injection (3 million int. units in 0.5 mL per vial) and 6 syringes and alcohol swabs; two boxes containing 42 Rebetol® 200 mg capsules each for a total of 84 capsules (6 capsules per blister card)

One 18 million int. units [multidose vial] of Intron® A injection (22.5 million int. units per 3.8 mL; 3 million int. units/0.5 mL) and 6 syringes and alcohol swabs; two boxes containing 42 Rebetol® 200 mg capsules each for a total of 84 capsules (6 capsules per blister card)

One 18 million int. units Intron® A injection [multidose pen] (22.5 million int. units per 1.5 mL; 3 million int. units/0.2 mL) and 6 disposable needles and alcohol swabs; two boxes containing 42 Rebetol® 200 mg capsules each for a total of 84 capsules (6 capsules per blister card)

Rebetol® dose reduction:

A box containing 6 vials of Intron® A injection (3 million int. units in 0.5 mL per vial) and 6 syringes and alcohol swabs; one box containing 42 Rebetol® 200 mg capsules (6 capsules per blister card)

One 18 million int. units Intron® A injection [multidose vial] (22.8 million int. units per 3.8 mL; 3 million int. units/0.5 mL) and 6 syringes and alcohol swabs; one box containing 42 Rebetol® 200 mg capsules (6 capsules per blister card)

One 18 million int. units Intron® A injection [multidose pen] (22.5 million int. units per 1.5 mL; 3 million int. units/0.2 mL) and 6 disposable needles and alcohol swabs; one box containing 42 Rebetol® 200 mg capsules (6 capsules per blister card)

♦ **Interferon Alfa-2b (PEG Conjugate)** see Peginterferon Alfa-2b on page 1046

Interferon Alfacon-1 (in ter FEER on AL fa con one)

U.S. Brand Names Infergen®

Canadian Brand Names Infergen®

Therapeutic Category Antiviral Agent, Hepatitis; Biological Response Modulator; Interferon

Use Treatment of chronic hepatitis C virus (HCV) infection in patients ≥18 years of age with compensated liver disease and anti-HCV serum antibodies or HCV RNA.

Pregnancy Risk Factor C

(Continued)

Interferon Alfacon-1 *(Continued)*

Pregnancy/Breast-Feeding Implications There have been no well-controlled studies in pregnant women. Animal studies have shown embryolethal or abortifacient effects. Males and females who are being treated with interferon alfacon-1 should use effective contraception. It is unknown if interferon alfacon-1 is excreted in breast milk. Caution should be used if administered to a nursing woman.

Contraindications Hypersensitivity to interferon alfacon-1 or any component of the formulation, other alpha interferons, or *E. coli*-derived products

Warnings/Precautions Severe psychiatric adverse effects, including depression, suicidal ideation, and suicide attempt, may occur. Avoid use in severe psychiatric disorders. Use with caution in patients with a history of depression. Use with caution in patients with prior cardiac disease (ischemic or thromboembolic), arrhythmias, patients who are chronically immunosuppressed, and patients with endocrine disorders. Do not use in patients with hepatic decompensation. Ophthalmologic disorders (including retinal hemorrhages, cotton wool spots and retinal artery or vein obstruction) have occurred in patients using other alpha interferons. Prior to start of therapy, visual exams are recommended for patients with diabetes mellitus or hypertension. Treatment should be discontinued in patients with worsening or persistently severe signs/symptoms of autoimmune, infectious, ischemic (including radiographic changes or worsening hepatic function), or neuropsychiatric disorders (including depression and/or suicidal thoughts/behavior). Use caution in patients with autoimmune disorders; type-1 interferon therapy has been reported to exacerbate autoimmune diseases. Do not use interferon alfacon-1 in patients with autoimmune hepatitis. Use caution in patients with low peripheral blood counts or myelosuppression, including concurrent use of myelosuppressive therapy. Safety and efficacy have not been determined for patients <18 years of age.

Adverse Reactions Adverse reactions reported using 9 mcg/dose interferon alfacon-1 3 times/week. Reactions listed were reported in ≥5% of patients treated.

>10%:
  Central nervous system: Headache (82%), fatigue (69%), fever (61%), insomnia (39%), nervousness (31%), depression (26%), dizziness (22%), anxiety (19%), noncardiac chest pain (13%), emotional lability (12%), malaise (11%)
  Dermatologic: Alopecia (14%), pruritus (14%), rash (13%)
  Endocrine & metabolic: Hot flashes (13%)
  Gastrointestinal: Abdominal pain (41%), nausea (40%), diarrhea (29%), anorexia (24%), dyspepsia (21%), vomiting (12%)
  Hematologic: Granulocytopenia (23%), thrombocytopenia (19%), leukopenia (15%)
  Local: Injection site erythema (23%)
  Neuromuscular & skeletal: Myalgia (58%), body pain (54%), arthralgia (51%), back pain (42%), limb pain (26%), neck pain (14%), skeletal pain (14%), paresthesia (13%)
  Respiratory: Pharyngitis (34%), upper respiratory tract infection (31%), cough (22%), sinusitis (17%), rhinitis (13%), respiratory tract congestion (12%)
  Miscellaneous: Flu-like syndrome (15%), increased diaphoresis (12%)

1% to 10%:
  Cardiovascular: Peripheral edema (9%), hypertension (5%), tachycardia (4%), palpitations (3%)
  Central nervous system: Amnesia (10%), hypoesthesia (10%), abnormal thinking (8%), agitation (6%), confusion (4%), somnolence (4%)
  Dermatologic: Bruising (6%), erythema (6%), dry skin (6%), wound (4%)
  Endocrine & metabolic: Thyroid test abnormalities (9%), dysmenorrhea (9%), increased triglycerides (6%), menstrual disorder (6%), decreased libido (5%), hypothyroidism (4%)
  Gastrointestinal: Constipation (9%), flatulence (8%), toothache (7%), decreased salivation (6%), hemorrhoids (6%), weight loss (5%), taste perversion (4%)
  Genitourinary: Vaginitis (8%), genital moniliasis (2%)
  Hepatic: Hepatomegaly (5%), liver tenderness (5%), increased prothrombin time (3%)
  Local: Injection site pain (9%), access pain (8%), injection site bruising (6%)
  Neuromuscular & skeletal: Weakness (9%), hypertonia (7%), musculoskeletal disorder (4%)
  Ocular: Conjunctivitis (8%), eye pain (5%), vision abnormalities (3%)
  Otic: Tinnitus (6%), earache (5%), otitis (2%)
  Respiratory: Upper respiratory tract congestion (10%), epistaxis (8%), dyspnea (7%), bronchitis (6%)
  Miscellaneous: Allergic reaction (7%), lymphadenopathy (6%), lymphocytosis (5%), infection (3%)

Flu-like symptoms, which included headache, fatigue, fever, myalgia, rigors, arthralgia, and increased diaphoresis, were the most commonly reported adverse reaction. This was reported separately from flu-like syndrome. Most patients were treated symptomatically.

Other adverse reactions associated with interferon therapy include arrhythmia, autoimmune disorders, chest pain, hepatotoxic reactions, lupus erythematosus, myocardial infarction, neuropsychiatric disorders (including suicidal thoughts/behavior), pneumonia, pneumonitis, severe hypersensitivity reactions (rare), vasculitis

Overdosage/Toxicology One overdose has been reported. A patient received ten times the prescribed dose (150 mcg) for 3 days. In addition to an increase in anorexia, chills, fever, and myalgia, there was also an increase in ALT, AST, and LDH. Laboratory values reportedly returned to baseline within 30 days.

Drug Interactions
  Cytochrome P450 Effect: No drug interaction studies have been conducted. Use with caution in combination with medications metabolized by the cytochrome P450 pathway or with other medications known to cause myelosuppression.
  Increased Effect/Toxicity: Cimetidine may augment the antitumor effects of interferon in melanoma. Theophylline clearance has been reported to be decreased in hepatitis patients receiving interferon. Vinblastine enhances interferon toxicity in several patients; increased incidence of paresthesia has also been noted. Interferons may increase the adverse/toxic

effects of ACE inhibitors, specifically the development of granulocytopenia. Agranulocytosis has been reported with concurrent use of clozapine (case report). Interferons may increase the anticoagulant effects of warfarin, and interferons may increase serum levels of zidovudine.

Decreased Effect: Prednisone may decrease the therapeutic effects of interferon alpha. A decreased response to erythropoietin has been reported (case reports) in patients receiving interferons. Interferon alpha may decrease the serum concentrations of melphalan (may or may not decrease toxicity of melphalan).

Stability Store in refrigerator 2°C to 8°C (36°F to 46°F). Do not freeze. Avoid exposure to direct sunlight. Do not shake vigorously.

Mechanism of Action Alpha interferons are a family of proteins, produced by nucleated cells, that have antiviral, antiproliferative, and immune-regulating activity. There are at least 25 alpha interferons identified. Interferons interact with cells through high affinity cell surface receptors. Following activation, multiple effects can be detected. Interferons induce gene transcription, inhibit cellular growth, alter the state of cellular differentiation, interfere with oncogene expression, alter cell surface antigen expression, increase phagocytic activity of macrophages, and augment cytotoxicity of lymphocytes for target cells. Although all alpha interferons share similar properties, the actual biological effects vary between subtypes.

Pharmacodynamics/Kinetics Pharmacokinetic studies have not been done in patients with chronic hepatitis C.
Time to peak: Healthy volunteers: 24-36 hours

Usual Dosage Adults ≥18 years: S.C.:
Chronic HCV infection: 9 mcg 3 times/week for 24 weeks; allow 48 hours between doses
Patients who have previously tolerated interferon therapy but did not respond or relapsed: 15 mcg 3 times/week for 6 months
Dose reduction for toxicity: Dose should be held in patients who experience a severe adverse reaction, and treatment should be stopped or decreased if the reaction does not become tolerable.
Doses were reduced from 9 mcg to 7.5 mcg in the pivotal study.
For patients receiving 15 mcg/dose, doses were reduced in 3 mcg increments. Efficacy is decreased with doses <7.5 mcg
Dosage adjustment in renal impairment: No information available.
Dosage adjustment in hepatic impairment: Avoid use in decompensated hepatic disease.
Elderly: No information available.

Administration Interferon alfacon-1 is administered by S.C. injection, 3 times/week, with at least 48 hours between doses

Monitoring Parameters
Hemoglobin and hematocrit; white blood cell count; platelets; triglycerides; thyroid function. Laboratory tests should be taken 2 weeks prior to therapy, after therapy has begun, and periodically during treatment. HCV RNA, ALT to determine success/response to therapy.
The following guidelines were used during the clinical studies as acceptable baseline values:
Platelet count ≥75 x 10^9/L
Hemoglobin ≥100 g/L
ANC ≥1500 x 10^6/L
S_{cr} <180 μmol/L (<2 mg/dL) or Cl_{cr} >0.83 mL/second (>50 mL/minute)
Serum albumin ≥25 g/L
Bilirubin WNL
TSH and T_4 WNL
Patients should also be monitored for signs of depression. Patients with pre-existing diabetes mellitus or hypertension should have an ophthalmologic exam prior to treatment.

Patient Information There are many different types of interferon products. Do not change brands or change your dose without consulting with your prescriber. Promptly report any adverse effects to your prescriber, including flu-like symptoms, signs of infection, signs of depression, suicidal thoughts, or visual complaints. Flu-like symptoms include fatigue, fever, rigors, headache, arthralgia, myalgia, and increased sweating. Your prescriber may instruct you to use this medication in the evening, or to take a non-narcotic analgesic to help prevent or decrease these symptoms. Because interferon alfacon-1 may have hazardous effects to a fetus, males and females using this medication should use effective contraception. You will need periodic laboratory tests while on this medication. If you have diabetes or hypertension you should also have an eye exam prior to starting therapy. If self-administering this medication at home, follow procedures for proper disposal of your syringes and needles.

Nursing Implications Patients who will be using this at home should be taught proper administration techniques as well as instructions for proper syringe disposal. Medication should be stored under refrigeration; however, it may be allowed to reach room temperature prior to administration. Do not use if discolored or containing particulate matter.

Dosage Forms
Injection [single dose] [preservative free]:
Prefilled syringe: 30 mcg/mL (0.3 mL, 0.5 mL)
Vial: 30 mcg/mL (0.3 mL, 0.5 mL)

Interferon Alfa-n3 (in ter FEER on AL fa en three)

U.S. Brand Names Alferon® N
Canadian Brand Names Alferon® N
Therapeutic Category Biological Response Modulator; Interferon
Use Patients ≥18 years of age: Intralesional treatment of refractory or recurring genital or venereal warts (condylomata acuminata)
Pregnancy Risk Factor C
Pregnancy/Breast-Feeding Implications Safety and efficacy for use during pregnancy have not been established. Interferon alpha has been shown to decrease serum estradiol and progesterone levels in humans. Menstrual irregularities and abortion have been reported in animals. Effective contraception is recommended during treatment.
Contraindications Hypersensitivity to alpha interferon or any component of the formulation; anaphylactic sensitivity to mouse immunoglobulin, egg protein, or neomycin
(Continued)

Interferon Alfa-n3 *(Continued)*

Warnings/Precautions Use with caution in patients with pre-existing cardiac disease, including unstable angina, uncontrolled congestive heart failure, or arrhythmias; severe pulmonary disease; diabetes with ketoacidosis; coagulation disorders (such as thrombophlebitis, pulmonary embolism, hemophilia); severe myelosuppression; or seizure disorder. **Due to differences in dosage, patients should not change brands of interferons.** Safety and efficacy in patients <18 years of age have not been established.

Adverse Reactions Flu-like reactions, consisting of headache, fever, and/or myalgia, was reported in 30% of patients, and abated with repeated dosing.

>10%:
   Central nervous system: Chills, fatigue, fever, headache
   Hematologic: Decreased WBC
   Neuromuscular & skeletal: Myalgia
   Miscellaneous: Flu-like syndrome
1% to 10%
   Central nervous system: Depression, dizziness, insomnia, malaise, thirst
   Dermatologic: Pruritus
   Gastrointestinal: Diarrhea, dyspepsia, taste disturbance, tongue hyperesthesia, nausea, vomiting
   Genitourinary: Groin lymph node swelling
   Neuromuscular & skeletal: Arthralgia, back pain, cramps, paresthesia
   Ocular: Visual disturbance
   Respiratory: Nose bleed, pharyngitis, rhinitis
   Miscellaneous: Increased sweating, vasovagal reaction
<1% (Limited to important or life-threatening): Photosensitivity. Rare adverse reactions reported with other alfa-interferons include autoimmune disorders, depression, ophthalmic disorders, suicide.

Overdosage/Toxicology Symptoms include CNS depression, obtundation, flu-like symptoms, and myelosuppression. Treatment is supportive.

Drug Interactions
   Increased Effect/Toxicity: Interferons may increase the adverse/toxic effects of ACE inhibitors, specifically the development of granulocytopenia. Risk: Monitor A case report of agranulocytosis has been reported with concurrent use of clozapine. Case reports of decreased hematopoietic effect with erythropoietin. Interferon alpha may decrease the P450 isoenzyme metabolism of theophylline. Interferons may increase the anticoagulant effects of warfarin. Interferons may decrease the metabolism of zidovudine.
   Decreased Effect: Interferon alpha may decrease the serum concentrations of melphalan; this may or may not decrease the potential toxicity of melphalan. Prednisone may decrease the therapeutic effects of Interferon alpha.

Stability Store solution at 2°C to 8°C (36°F to 46°F); do not freeze or shake solution

Mechanism of Action Interferons interact with cells through high affinity cell surface receptors. Following activation, multiple effects can be detected including induction of gene transcription. Inhibits cellular growth, alters the state of cellular differentiation, interferes with oncogene expression, alters cell surface antigen expression, increases phagocytic activity of macrophages, and augments cytotoxicity of lymphocytes for target cells

Usual Dosage Adults: Inject 250,000 units (0.05 mL) in each wart twice weekly for a maximum of 8 weeks; therapy should not be repeated for at least 3 months after the initial 8-week course of therapy

Administration Inject into base of wart with a small 30-gauge needle

Patient Information Warts are highly contagious until they completely disappear, abstain from sexual activity or use barrier protection; inform nurse or physician if allergy exists to eggs, neomycin, mouse immunoglobulin, or to human interferon alpha; acetaminophen can be used to treat flu-like symptoms

Dosage Forms Injection: 5 million units (1 mL)

Interferon Beta-1a (in ter FEER on BAY ta won aye)

U.S. Brand Names Avonex®; Rebif®

Canadian Brand Names Avonex®; Rebif®

Synonyms rIFN beta-1a

Therapeutic Category Interferon

Use Treatment of relapsing forms of multiple sclerosis (MS), to slow the accumulation of physical disability and decrease the frequency of clinical exacerbations

Pregnancy Risk Factor C

Pregnancy/Breast-Feeding Implications Safety and efficacy in pregnant women have not been established. Treatment should be discontinued if a woman becomes pregnant, or plans to become pregnant during therapy. A dose-related abortifacient activity was reported in Rhesus monkeys. Because its use has not been evaluated during lactation, breast-feeding is not recommended

Contraindications Hypersensitivity to natural or recombinant interferons, human albumin, or any other component of the formulation

Warnings/Precautions Interferons have been associated with severe psychiatric adverse events (psychosis, mania, depression, suicidal behavior/ideation) in patients with and without previous psychiatric symptoms, avoid use in severe psychiatric disorders and use caution in patients with a history of depression; patients exhibiting depressive symptoms should be closely monitored and discontinuation of therapy should be considered. Due to high incidence of flu-like adverse effects, use caution in patients with pre-existing cardiovascular disease, pulmonary disease, seizure disorders, myelosuppression, renal impairment or hepatic impairment. Suspend treatment if jaundice or symptoms of hepatic dysfunction occur. Safety and efficacy in patients <18 years of age have not been established.

Adverse Reactions Note: Flu-like symptoms (including headache, fever, myalgia, and weakness) are the most common adverse reaction (up to 61%) and may diminish with repeated dosing. Frequencies noted here indicate the highest reported frequency for either product, either from placebo-controlled trials or comparative studies (some effects reported for only one product).

In a comparative study, the adverse effect profiles of Avonex® and Rebif® were noted to be similar, with the exception of three adverse events noted to occur more frequently in the Rebif® group: Transaminase elevations, local reactions, and reductions in white blood cell counts.

>10%:
  Central nervous system: Headache (30% to 70%), fever (23% to 28%), chills (21%), sleep disturbance (19%), dizziness (15%), depression (11% to 13%), insomnia (10% to 13%)
  Gastrointestinal: Nausea (33%), abdominal pain (9% to 22%) diarrhea (16%), dyspepsia (11%)
  Hematologic: Leukopenia (up to 36% in Rebif® patients), lymphadenopathy (12%)
  Hepatic: Transaminases increased (up to 27% with Rebif®; hepatic dysfunction noted in <10%)
  Local: Injection site disorders: A comparative trial noted events in 80% with Rebif® versus 24% with Avonex® (includes inflammation, pain, bruising, or site reaction)
  Neuromuscular & skeletal: Myalgia (25% to 34%), back pain (23% to 25%), skeletal pain (15%), weakness (21%)
  Ocular: Visual abnormalities (13%)
  Respiratory: Upper respiratory tract infection (31%), sinusitis (18%), rhinitis (15% to 17%)
  Miscellaneous; Flu-like symptoms (61%), infection (11%)

1% to 10%:
  Cardiovascular: Chest pain (8%), syncope (4%), vasodilation (4%)
  Central nervous system: Somnolence (5%), suicidal tendency (4%), malaise (5%), seizure (5%), ataxia (5%)
  Dermatologic: Urticaria (5%), alopecia (4%), rash (7%)
  Endocrine & metabolic: Thyroid abnormalities (up to 6% with Rebif®)
  Gastrointestinal: Abdominal pain (9%), anorexia (7%), xerostomia (5%)
  Genitourinary: Vaginitis (4%), ovarian cyst (3%), urinary frequency (7%), incontinence (4%)
  Hematologic: Thrombocytopenia (8%), anemia (8%), eosinophilia (5%)
  Hepatic: Hepatic function abnormalities (9%), hyperbilirubinemia (3%)
  Neuromuscular & skeletal: Arthralgia (9%), muscle spasm (7%), rigors (13%)
  Ocular: Dry eyes (3%)
  Otic: Otitis media (6%), hearing decreased (3%)
  Respiratory: Dyspnea (6%)
  Miscellaneous: Herpesvirus infection (3%), hypersensitivity reaction (3%)

<1% (Limited to important or life-threatening): Amnesia, anaphylaxis, arrhythmia, basal cell carcinoma, Bell's palsy, cardiac arrest, colitis, erythema multiforme, gastrointestinal hemorrhage, hepatic failure, hypothyroidism, injection site necrosis, intestinal perforation, myasthenia, osteonecrosis, pharyngeal edema, photosensitivity, psychosis, pulmonary embolism, rash, sepsis, Stevens-Johnson syndrome, vaginal hemorrhage

Overdosage/Toxicology Symptoms include CNS depression, obtundation, flu-like symptoms, and myelosuppression. Treatment is supportive.

Drug Interactions
  Cytochrome P450 Effect: Inhibits metabolism by cytochrome P450 (isoenzyme profiles not defined)
  Increased Effect/Toxicity: Interferons may increase the adverse/toxic effects of ACE inhibitors, specifically the development of granulocytopenia. Agranulocytosis has been reported with concurrent use of clozapine (case report). Interferons may increase the anticoagulant effects of warfarin, and interferons may increase serum levels of zidovudine.

Stability
  Avonex®: The reconstituted product contains no preservative and is for single-use only; discard unused portion; store unreconstituted vial or reconstituted vial at 2°C to 8°C (36°F to 46°F). If refrigeration is not available, may be stored at 25°C (77°F) for up to 30 days. Do not freeze. Use the reconstituted product within 6 hours.
  Rebif®: Store at 2°C to 8°C (36°F to 46°F). Do not freeze. Protect from light.

Mechanism of Action Interferon beta differs from naturally occurring human protein by a single amino acid substitution and the lack of carbohydrate side chains; alters the expression and response to surface antigens and can enhance immune cell activities. Properties of interferon beta that modify biologic responses are mediated by cell surface receptor interactions; mechanism in the treatment of MS is unknown.

Pharmacodynamics/Kinetics Limited data due to small doses used
  Half-life elimination: Avonex®: 10 hours; Rebif®: 69 hours
  Time to peak, serum: Avonex® (I.M.): 3-15 hours; Rebif® (S.C.): 14 hours

Usual Dosage Adults:
  I.M. (Avonex®): 30 mcg once weekly
  S.C. (Rebif®): Initial: 8.8 mcg 3 times/week, increasing over a 4-week period to the recommended dose of 44 mcg 3 times/week; doses should be separated by at least 48 hours

Administration
  Avonex®: Reconstitute with 1.1 mL of diluent and swirl gently to dissolve
  Rebif®: Administer at the same time of day on the same 3 days each week (ie, late afternoon/evening Mon, Wed, Fri)

Monitoring Parameters Hemoglobin, liver function, and blood chemistries
  Rebif®: CBC and liver function testing at 1-, 3-, and 6 months, then periodically thereafter. Thyroid function every 6 months (in patients with pre-existing abnormalities and/or clinical indications)

Patient Information Flu-like symptoms are not uncommon following initiation of therapy. Acetaminophen may reduce these symptoms. Do not change the dosage or schedule of administration without medical consultation. If self-injecting and you miss a dose, take it as soon as you remember, but 2 injections should not be given within 48 hours of each other. Report depression or suicide ideation to physicians. Avoid prolonged exposure to sunlight or sunlamps. Inform prescriber **immediately** if you feel depressed or have any thoughts of suicide.

(Continued)

Interferon Beta-1a *(Continued)*

Nursing Implications Patient should be informed of possible side effects, especially depression, suicidal ideations, and the risk of abortion; flu-like symptoms such as chills, fever, malaise, diaphoresis, and myalgia are common

Dosage Forms

Injection (Rebif®) [prefilled syringe; preservative free]: 44 mcg/mL (0.5 mL) (12s); 88 mcg/mL (0.5 mL)

Injection, powder for reconstitution (Avonex®): 33 mcg [6.6 million units]

Interferon Beta-1b *(in ter FEER on BAY ta won bee)*

U.S. Brand Names Betaseron®

Canadian Brand Names Betaseron®

Synonyms rIFN beta-1b

Therapeutic Category Interferon

Use Reduces the frequency of clinical exacerbations in ambulatory patients with relapsing-remitting multiple sclerosis (MS)

Pregnancy Risk Factor C

Pregnancy/Breast-Feeding Implications Safety and efficacy in pregnant women has not been established. Treatment should be discontinued if a woman becomes pregnant, or plans to become pregnant during therapy. A dose-related abortifacient activity was reported in Rhesus monkeys. Because its use has not been evaluated during lactation, breast-feeding is not recommended.

Contraindications Hypersensitivity to *E. coli* derived products, natural or recombinant interferon beta, albumin human or any other component of the formulation

Warnings/Precautions Interferons have been associated with severe psychiatric adverse events (psychosis, mania, depression, suicidal behavior/ideation) in patients with and without previous psychiatric symptoms, avoid use in severe psychiatric disorders and use caution in patients with a history of depression; patients exhibiting symptoms of depression should be closely monitored and discontinuation of therapy should be considered. Due to high incidence of flu-like adverse effects, use caution in patients with pre-existing cardiovascular disease, pulmonary disease, seizure disorders, myelosuppression, renal impairment or hepatic impairment. Severe injection site reactions (necrosis) may occur; patient and/or caregiver competency in injection technique should be confirmed and periodically re-evaluated. Safety and efficacy in patients with chronic progressive MS and in patients <18 years of age have not been established.

Adverse Reactions Note: Flu-like symptoms are reported in the majority of patients (76%).

>10%:

Central nervous system: Headache (84%), fever (59%), pain (52%), chills (46%), dizziness (35%), malaise (15%), anxiety (15%), migraine (12%)

Endocrine & metabolic: Dysmenorrhea (18%), menstrual disorder (17%), metrorrhagia (15%), hypoglycemia (15%)

Gastrointestinal: Diarrhea (35%), abdominal pain (32%), constipation (24%), vomiting (21%)

Hematologic: Lymphopenia (82%), neutropenia (18%), leukopenia (16%), lymphadenopathy (14%)

Hepatic: SGPT increased >5x baseline (19%), SGOT increased >5x baseline (4%)

Local: injection site reaction (85%)

Neuromuscular & skeletal: Weakness (49%), myalgia (44%). Hypertonia (26%), myasthenia (13%)

Ocular: Conjunctivitis (12%)

Respiratory: Sinusitis (36%)

Miscellaneous: Flu-like symptoms (76%), increased diaphoresis (23%)

1% to 10% (Limited to important or life-threatening):

Cardiovascular: Hypertension (7%), peripheral vascular disorder (5%), hemorrhage (3%)

Central nervous system: Somnolence (6%), confusion (4%), seizure (2%), suicide attempt (2%), amnesia (2%)

Dermatologic: Alopecia (4%)

Endocrine & metabolic: Menorrhagia (6%), fibrocystic breast (3%), breast neoplasm (2%), goiter (2%)

Hepatic: Bilirubin increased >2.5x baseline (6%), SGOT increased >5x baseline (4%)

Local: Injection site necrosis (5%)

Renal: Proteinuria (5%)

Respiratory: Dyspnea (8%), laryngitis (6%)

<1% (Limited to important or life-threatening): Apnea, arrhythmia, cardiac arrest, cardiomegaly, cerebral hemorrhage, coma, delirium, erythema nodosum, ethanol intolerance, exfoliative dermatitis, GI hemorrhage, hallucinations, heart failure, hematemesis, hepatitis, mania, myocardial infarction, pancreatitis, pericardial effusion, photosensitivity, psychosis, pulmonary embolism, rash, sepsis, shock, SIADH, skin necrosis, syncope, thrombocytopenia, vaginal hemorrhage

Overdosage/Toxicology Symptoms include CNS depression, obtundation, flu-like symptoms, and myelosuppression. Treatment is supportive.

Drug Interactions

Increased Effect/Toxicity: Interferons may increase the adverse/toxic effects of ACE inhibitors, specifically the development of granulocytopenia. Risk: Monitor A case report of agranulocytosis has been reported with concurrent use of clozapine. Case reports of decreased hematopoietic effect with erythropoietin. Interferon alpha may decrease the P450 isoenzyme metabolism of theophylline. Interferons may increase the anticoagulant effects of warfarin. Interferons may decrease the metabolism of zidovudine.

Stability Store solution at 2°C to 8°C (36°F to 46°F); do not freeze or shake solution; use product within 3 hours of reconstitution. If refrigeration is not possible, keep as cool as possible (30°C/86°F); protect from heat/light and use within 7 days.

Mechanism of Action Interferon beta-1b differs from naturally occurring human protein by a single amino acid substitution and the lack of carbohydrate side chains; alters the expression and response to surface antigens and can enhance immune cell activities. Properties of interferon beta-1b that modify biologic responses are mediated by cell surface receptor interactions; mechanism in the treatment of MS is unknown.

Pharmacodynamics/Kinetics Limited data due to small doses used

Half-life elimination: 8 minutes to 4.3 hours

Time to peak, serum: 1-8 hours

Usual Dosage S.C.:

Children <18 years: Not recommended

Adults >18 years: 0.25 mg (8 million units) every other day

Administration Withdraw 1 mL of reconstituted solution from the vial into a sterile syringe fitted with a 27-gauge needle and inject the solution subcutaneously; sites for self-injection include arms, abdomen, hips, and thighs

Monitoring Parameters Hemoglobin, liver function, and blood chemistries

Patient Information Instruct patients on self-injection technique and procedures. If possible, perform first injection under the supervision of an appropriately qualified healthcare professional. Injection site reactions may occur during therapy. They are usually transient and do not require discontinuation of therapy, but careful assessment of the nature and severity of all reported reactions. Flu-like symptoms are not uncommon following initiation of therapy. Acetaminophen may reduce these symptoms. Do not change the dosage or schedule of administration without medical consultation. Inform prescriber **immediately** if you feel depressed or have any thoughts of suicide. Report any broken skin or black-blue discoloration around the injection site. Avoid prolonged exposure to sunlight or sunlamps.

Nursing Implications Patient should be informed of possible side effects, especially depression, suicidal ideations, and the risk of abortion; flu-like symptoms such as chills, fever, malaise, sweating, and myalgia are common

Additional Information May be available only in small supplies; for information on availability and distribution, call the patient information line at 800-580-3837.

Dosage Forms Powder for injection, lyophilized: 0.3 mg [9.6 million units]

Interferon Gamma-1b (in ter FEER on GAM ah won bee)

U.S. Brand Names Actimmune®

Canadian Brand Names Actimmune®

Therapeutic Category Biological Response Modulator; Interferon

Use Reduce frequency and severity of serious infections associated with chronic granulomatous disease; delay time to disease progression in patients with severe, malignant osteopetrosis

Pregnancy Risk Factor C

Pregnancy/Breast-Feeding Implications Safety and efficacy in pregnant women has not been established. Treatment should be discontinued if a woman becomes pregnant, or plans to become pregnant during therapy. A dose-related abortifacient activity was reported in Rhesus monkeys. Because its use has not been evaluated during lactation, breast-feeding is not recommended.

Contraindications Hypersensitivity to interferon gamma, *E. coli* derived proteins, or any component of the formulation

Warnings/Precautions Patients with pre-existing cardiac disease, seizure disorders, CNS disturbances, or myelosuppression should be carefully monitored; long-term effects on growth and development are unknown; safety and efficacy in children <1 year of age have not been established.

Adverse Reactions Based on 50 mcg/m^2 dose administered 3 times weekly for chronic granulomatous disease

>10%:

Central nervous system: Fever (52%), headache (33%), chills (14%), fatigue (14%)

Dermatologic: Rash (17%)

Gastrointestinal: Diarrhea (14%), vomiting (13%)

Local: Injection site erythema or tenderness (14%)

1% to 10%:

Central nervous system: Depression (3%)

Gastrointestinal: Nausea (10%), abdominal pain (8%)

Neuromuscular & skeletal: Myalgia (6%), arthralgia (2%), back pain (2%)

Drug Interactions

Increased Effect/Toxicity: Interferon gamma-1b may increase hepatic enzymes or enhance myelosuppression when taken with other myelosuppressive agents. May decrease cytochrome P450 concentrations leading to increased serum concentrations of drugs metabolized by this pathway.

Ethanol/Nutrition/Herb Interactions Herb/Nutraceutical: Dietary supplements containing aristolochic acid (found most often in Chinese medicines/herbal therapies); cases of nephropathy and ESRD associated with their use.

Stability Store in refrigerator. Do not freeze. Do not shake. Discard if left unrefrigerated for >12 hours.

Pharmacodynamics/Kinetics

Absorption: I.M., S.C.: Slowly

Half-life elimination: I.V.: 38 minutes; I.M., S.C.: 3-6 hours

Time to peak, plasma: I.M.: 4 hours (1.5 ng/mL); S.C.: 7 hours (0.6 ng/mL)

Usual Dosage If severe reactions occur, modify dose (50% reduction) or therapy should be discontinued until adverse reactions abate.

Chronic granulomatous disease: Children >1 year and Adults: S.C.:

BSA ≤0.5 m^2: 1.5 mcg/kg/dose 3 times/week

BSA >0.5 m^2: 50 mcg/m^2 (1.5 million int. units/m^2) 3 times/week

Severe, malignant osteopetrosis: Children >1 year: S.C.:

BSA ≤0.5 m^2: 1.5 mcg/kg/dose 3 times/week

BSA >0.5 m^2: 50 mcg/m^2 (1.5 million int. units/m^2) 3 times/week

(Continued)

Interferon Gamma-1b *(Continued)*

Monitoring Parameters CBC with differential, platelets, LFTs, electrolytes, BUN, creatinine, and urinalysis prior to therapy and at 3-month intervals

Patient Information Use as directed; do not change the dosage or schedule of administration without consulting prescriber. Maintain adequate hydration (2-3 L/day of fluids unless instructed to restrict fluid intake). You may experience flu-like syndrome (acetaminophen may help or can administer dose at bedtime); nausea, vomiting, or loss of appetite (frequent small meals, frequent mouth care, sucking lozenges, or chewing gum may help); drowsiness, dizziness, agitation, or abnormal thinking (use caution when driving or engaging in tasks requiring alertness until response to drug is known). Report unusual bruising or bleeding; persistent abdominal disturbances; unusual fatigue; muscle pain or tremors; chest pain or palpitations; swelling of extremities; visual disturbances; pain, swelling, or redness at injection site; or other unusual symptoms.

Nursing Implications Single-dose vials only: discard unused portion; do not shake

Dosage Forms Injection: 100 mcg [3 million int. units] per 0.5 mL

- **Interleukin-1 Receptor antagonist** *see Anakinra on page 98*
- **Interleukin-2** *see Aldesleukin on page 43*
- **Interleukin-11** *see Oprelvekin on page 1012*
- **Intralipid®** *see Fat Emulsion on page 545*
- **Intravenous Fat Emulsion** *see Fat Emulsion on page 545*
- **Intrifiban** *see Eptifibatide on page 480*
- **Intron® A** *see Interferon Alfa-2b on page 728*
- **Intropin®** *see DOPamine on page 435*
- **Invanz™** *see Ertapenem on page 484*
- **Inversine®** *see Mecamylamine on page 844*
- **Invirase®** *see Saquinavir on page 1221*
- **Iobid DM®** *see Guaifenesin and Dextromethorphan on page 646*
- **Iodex® [OTC]** *see Povidone-Iodine on page 1114*
- **Iodex-p® [OTC]** *see Povidone-Iodine on page 1114*
- **Iodochlorhydroxyquin** *see Clioquinol on page 311*

Iodoquinol *(eye oh doe KWIN ole)*

U.S. Brand Names Yodoxin®

Canadian Brand Names Diodoquin®

Synonyms Diiodohydroxyquin

Therapeutic Category Amebicide

Use Treatment of acute and chronic intestinal amebiasis; asymptomatic cyst passers; *Blastocystis hominis* infections; ineffective for amebic hepatitis or hepatic abscess

Pregnancy Risk Factor C

Contraindications Hypersensitivity to iodine or iodoquinol or any component of the formulation; hepatic damage; pre-existing optic neuropathy

Warnings/Precautions Optic neuritis, optic atrophy, and peripheral neuropathy have occurred following prolonged use; avoid long-term therapy

Adverse Reactions Frequency not defined.

Central nervous system: Fever, chills, agitation, retrograde amnesia, headache

Dermatologic: Rash, urticaria, pruritus

Endocrine & metabolic: Thyroid gland enlargement

Gastrointestinal: Diarrhea, nausea, vomiting, stomach pain, abdominal cramps

Neuromuscular & skeletal: Peripheral neuropathy, weakness

Ocular: Optic neuritis, optic atrophy, visual impairment

Miscellaneous: Itching of rectal area

Overdosage/Toxicology Chronic overdose can result in vomiting, diarrhea, abdominal pain, metallic taste, paresthesias, paraplegia, and loss of vision. Can lead to destruction of the long fibers of the spinal cord and optic nerve. Acute overdose symptoms includes delirium, stupor, coma, and amnesia. Following GI decontamination, treatment is symptomatic.

Mechanism of Action Contact amebicide that works in the lumen of the intestine by an unknown mechanism

Pharmacodynamics/Kinetics

Absorption: Poor and erratic

Metabolism: Hepatic

Excretion: Feces (high percentage)

Usual Dosage Oral:

Children: 30-40 mg/kg/day (maximum: 650 mg/dose) in 3 divided doses for 20 days; not to exceed 1.95 g/day

Adults: 650 mg 3 times/day after meals for 20 days; not to exceed 1.95 g/day

Dietary Considerations Should be taken after meals.

Monitoring Parameters Ophthalmologic exam

Test Interactions May increase protein-bound serum iodine concentrations reflecting a decrease in ^{131}I uptake; false-positive ferric chloride test for phenylketonuria

Patient Information May take with food or milk to reduce stomach upset; complete full course of therapy

Nursing Implications Tablets may be crushed and mixed with applesauce or chocolate syrup

Dosage Forms

Powder: 25 g

Tablet: 210 mg, 650 mg

Iodoquinol and Hydrocortisone

(eye oh doe KWIN ole & hye droe KOR ti sone)

U.S. Brand Names Vytone®

Synonyms Hydrocortisone and Iodoquinol

IPECAC SYRUP

Therapeutic Category Antifungal/Corticosteroid
Use Treatment of eczema; infectious dermatitis; chronic eczematoid otitis externa; mycotic dermatoses
Pregnancy Risk Factor C
Usual Dosage Apply 3-4 times/day
Additional Information Complete prescribing information for this medication should be consulted for additional detail.
Dosage Forms Cream, topical: Iodoquinol 1% and hydrocortisone 1% (30 g)

♦ **Iofed®** see Brompheniramine and Pseudoephedrine on page 185
♦ **Iofed® PD** see Brompheniramine and Pseudoephedrine on page 185
♦ **Ionamin®** see Phentermine on page 1073
♦ **Iopidine®** see Apraclonidine on page 111
♦ **Iosopan® Plus** see Magaldrate and Simethicone on page 831

Ioxilan (eye OKS ee lan)
U.S. Brand Names Oxilan®
Therapeutic Category Radiopaque Agents
Use
Intra-arterial: Ioxilan 300 mgI/mL is indicated for cerebral arteriography. Ioxilan 350 mgI/mL is indicated for coronary arteriography and left ventriculography, visceral angiography, aortography, and peripheral arteriography
Intravenous: Both products are indicated for excretory urography and contrast enhanced computed tomographic (CECT) imaging of the head and body
Pregnancy Risk Factor B
Usual Dosage Adults:
Intra-arterial: Coronary arteriography and left ventriculography: For visualization of coronary arteries and left ventricle, ioxilan injection with a concentration of 350 mg iodine/mL is recommended
Usual injection volumes:
Left and right coronary: 2-10 mL (0.7-3.5 g iodine)
Left ventricle: 25-50 mL (8.75-17.5 g iodine)
Total doses should not exceed 250 mL; the injection rate of ioxilan should approximate the flow rate in the vessel injected
Cerebral arteriography: For evaluation of arterial lesions of the brain, a concentration of 300 mg iodine/mL is indicated
Recommended doses: 8-12 mL (2.4-3.6 g iodine)
Total dose should not exceed 150 mL
Additional Information Complete prescribing information for this medication should be consulted for additional detail.
Dosage Forms
Injection:
Oxilan® 300: 300 mgI/mL
Oxilan® 350: 350 mgI/mL

Ipecac Syrup (IP e kak SIR up)
Therapeutic Category Antidote, Emetic
Use Treatment of acute oral drug overdosage and in certain poisonings
Pregnancy Risk Factor C
Contraindications Hypersensitivity to ipecac or any component of the formulation; do not use in unconscious patients; patients with no gag reflex; following ingestion of strong bases, acids, or volatile oils; when seizures are likely
Warnings/Precautions Do not confuse ipecac syrup with ipecac fluid extract, which is 14 times more potent; use with caution in patients with cardiovascular disease and bulimics; may not be effective in antiemetic overdose
Adverse Reactions Frequency not defined.
Cardiovascular: Cardiotoxicity
Central nervous system: Lethargy
Gastrointestinal: Protracted vomiting, diarrhea
Neuromuscular & skeletal: Myopathy
Overdosage/Toxicology Ipecac syrup contains cardiotoxin. Symptoms include tachycardia, CHF, atrial fibrillation, depressed myocardial contractility, myocarditis, diarrhea, persistent vomiting, and hypotension. Treatment consists of activated charcoal and gastric lavage.
Drug Interactions
Increased Effect/Toxicity: Phenothiazines (chlorpromazine has been associated with serious dystonic reactions).
Decreased Effect: Activated charcoal, milk, carbonated beverages decrease the effect of ipecac syrup.
Ethanol/Nutrition/Herb Interactions Food: Milk, carbonated beverages may decrease effectiveness.
Mechanism of Action Irritates the gastric mucosa and stimulates the medullary chemoreceptor trigger zone to induce vomiting
Pharmacodynamics/Kinetics
Onset of action: 15-30 minutes
Duration: 20-25 minutes; 60 minutes in some cases
Absorption: Significant amounts, mainly when it does not produce emesis
Excretion: Urine; emetine (alkaloid component) may be detected in urine 60 days after excess dose or chronic use
Usual Dosage Oral:
Children:
6-12 months: 5-10 mL followed by 10-20 mL/kg of water; repeat dose one time if vomiting does not occur within 20 minutes
(Continued)

Ipecac Syrup *(Continued)*

1-12 years: 15 mL followed by 10-20 mL/kg of water; repeat dose one time if vomiting does not occur within 20 minutes

If emesis does not occur within 30 minutes after second dose, ipecac must be removed from stomach by gastric lavage

Adults: 15-30 mL followed by 200-300 mL of water; repeat dose one time if vomiting does not occur within 20 minutes

Patient Information Call Poison Center before administering. Patients should be kept active and moving following administration of ipecac; follow dose with 8 oz of water following initial episode; if vomiting, no food or liquids should be ingested for 1 hour

Nursing Implications Do **not** administer to unconscious patients; patients should be kept active and moving following administration of ipecac; if vomiting does not occur after second dose, gastric lavage may be considered to remove ingested substance

Dosage Forms Syrup: 70 mg/mL (15 mL, 30 mL)

♦ **I-Pentolate®** *see Cyclopentolate on page 341*

♦ **IPOL™** *see Poliovirus Vaccine (Inactivated) on page 1100*

Ipratropium (i pra TROE pee um)

U.S. Brand Names Atrovent®

Canadian Brand Names Alti-Ipratropium; Apo®-Ipravent; Atrovent®; Gen-Ipratropium; Novo-Ipramide; Novo-Ipramide; Nu-Ipratropium; PMS-Ipratropium

Synonyms Ipratropium Bromide

Therapeutic Category Anticholinergic Agent; Bronchodilator

Use Anticholinergic bronchodilator used in bronchospasm associated with COPD, bronchitis, and emphysema; symptomatic relief of rhinorrhea associated with the common cold and allergic and nonallergic rhinitis

Pregnancy Risk Factor B

Contraindications Hypersensitivity to atropine, its derivatives, or any component of the formulation

Warnings/Precautions Not indicated for the initial treatment of acute episodes of bronchospasm; use with caution in patients with narrow-angle glaucoma, prostatic hyperplasia, or bladder neck obstruction; ipratropium has not been specifically studied in the elderly, but it is poorly absorbed from the airways and appears to be safe in this population.

Adverse Reactions

Inhalation aerosol and inhalation solution:

1% to 10%:

Cardiovascular: Palpitations (2%)

Central nervous system: Nervousness (3%), dizziness (2%), fatigue, headache (6%), pain (4%)

Dermatologic: Rash (1%)

Gastrointestinal: Nausea, xerostomia, stomach upset, dry mucous membranes

Respiratory: Nasal congestion, dyspnea (10%), increased sputum (1%), bronchospasm (2%), pharyngitis (3%), rhinitis (2%), sinusitis (5%)

Miscellaneous: Influenza-like symptoms

<1% (Limited to important or life-threatening): Hypersensitivity reactions

Nasal spray: Epistaxis (8%) nasal, dryness (5%), nausea (2%)

Overdosage/Toxicology Symptoms include dry mouth, drying of respiratory secretions, cough, nausea, GI distress, blurred vision or impaired visual accommodation, headache, and nervousness. Acute overdose by inhalation is unlikely since it is so poorly absorbed. However, if poisoning occurs, it can be treated like any other anticholinergic toxicity. An anticholinergic overdose with severe life-threatening symptoms may be treated with physostigmine 1-2 mg (0.5 mg or 0.02 mg/kg for children) S.C. or slow I.V.

Drug Interactions

Increased Effect/Toxicity: Increased therapeutic effect with albuterol. Increased toxicity with anticholinergics or drugs with anticholinergic properties and dronabinol.

Stability Compatible for 1 hour when mixed with albuterol in a nebulizer

Mechanism of Action Blocks the action of acetylcholine at parasympathetic sites in bronchial smooth muscle causing bronchodilation

Pharmacodynamics/Kinetics

Onset of action: Bronchodilation: 1-3 minutes

Peak effect: 1.5-2 hours

Duration: ≤4-6 hours

Absorption: Negligible

Distribution: Inhalation: 15% of dose reaches lower airways

Usual Dosage

Nebulization:

Infants and Children ≤12 years: 125-250 mcg 3 times/day

Children >12 years and Adults: 500 mcg (one unit-dose vial) 3-4 times/day with doses 6-8 hours apart

Oral inhalation: MDI:

Children 3-12 years: 1-2 inhalations 3 times/day, up to 6 inhalations/24 hours

Children >12 years and Adults: 2 inhalations 4 times/day, up to 12 inhalations/24 hours

Intranasal: Nasal spray:

Symptomatic relief of rhinorrhea associated with the common cold (safety and efficacy of use beyond 4 days in patients with the common cold have not been established):

Children 5-11 years: 0.06%: 2 sprays in each nostril 3 times/day

Children ≥5 years and Adults: 0.06%: 2 sprays in each nostril 3-4 times/day

Symptomatic relief of rhinorrhea associated with allergic/nonallergic rhinitis: Children ≥6 years and Adults: 0.03%: 2 sprays in each nostril 2-3 times/day

Administration Shake inhaler before each use; rinsing mouth after each use decreases dry mouth side effect

Patient Information

Inhaler directions: Effects are enhanced by breath-holding 10 seconds after inhalation; temporary blurred vision may occur if sprayed into eyes; shake canister well before each use of the inhaler; follow instructions for use accompanying the product; close eyes when administering ipratropium; wait at least one full minute between inhalations

Nebulizer directions: Twist open the top of one unit dose vial and squeeze the contents into the nebulizer reservoir. Connect the nebulizer reservoir to the mouthpiece or face mask. Connect the nebulizer to the compressor. Sit in a comfortable, upright position; place the mouthpiece in your mouth or put on the face mask and turn on the compressor. If a face mask is used, care should be taken to avoid leakage around the mask as temporary blurring of vision, precipitation or worsening of narrow-angle glaucoma, or eye pain may occur if the solution comes into direct contact with the eyes. Breathe as calmly, deeply, and evenly as possible until no more mist is formed in the nebulizer chamber (about 5-15 minutes). At this point, the treatment is finished. Clean the nebulizer.

Nursing Implications Teach patients how to use the inhaler; shake inhaler before administering

Dosage Forms

Solution for nebulization, as bromide: 0.02% (2.5 mL)

Solution for oral inhalation, as bromide: 18 mcg/actuation (14 g)

Solution, intranasal, as bromide [spray]: 0.03% (30 mL); 0.06% (15 mL)

Ipratropium and Albuterol (i pra TROE pee um & al BYOO ter ole)

U.S. Brand Names Combivent®; DuoNeb™

Canadian Brand Names Combivent®

Synonyms Albuterol and Ipratropium

Therapeutic Category Bronchodilator

Use Treatment of chronic obstructive pulmonary disease (COPD) in those patients that are currently on a regular bronchodilator who continue to have bronchospasms and require a second bronchodilator

Pregnancy Risk Factor C

Usual Dosage Adults:

Inhalation: 2 inhalations 4 times/day (maximum: 12 inhalations/24 hours)

Inhalation via nebulization: Initial: 3 mL every 6 hours (maximum: 3 mL every 4 hours)

Additional Information Complete prescribing information for this medication should be consulted for additional detail.

Dosage Forms

Aerosol for oral inhalation: Ipratropium bromide 18 mcg and albuterol sulfate 103 mcg per actuation [200 doses] (14.7 g)

Solution for oral inhalation: Ipratropium bromide 0.5 mg [0.017%] and albuterol base 2.5 mg [0.083%] (3 mL)

- **Ipratropium Bromide** see Ipratropium on page 740
- **Iproveratril Hydrochloride** see Verapamil on page 1412
- **IPV** see Poliovirus Vaccine (Inactivated) on page 1100

Irbesartan (ir be SAR tan)

Related Information

Angiotensin Agents Comparison on page 1473

U.S. Brand Names Avapro®

Canadian Brand Names Avapro™

Therapeutic Category Angiotensin II Receptor Antagonist (ARB); Antihypertensive Agent

Use Treatment of hypertension alone or in combination with other antihypertensives

Pregnancy Risk Factor C/D (2nd and 3rd trimesters)

Pregnancy/Breast-Feeding Implications The drug should be discontinued as soon as possible after detection of pregnancy. Drugs which act directly on the renin-angiotensin system can cause fetal and neonatal morbidity and death.

Contraindications Hypersensitivity to irbesartan or any component of the formulation; hypersensitivity to other A-II receptor antagonists; primary hyperaldosteronism; bilateral renal artery stenosis; pregnancy (2nd and 3rd trimesters)

Warnings/Precautions Safety and efficacy have not been established in pediatric patients <6 years of age. Avoid use or use a much smaller dose in patients who are intravascularly volume-depleted; use caution in patients with unilateral or bilateral renal artery stenosis to avoid a decrease in renal function; AUCs of irbesartan (not the active metabolite) are about 50% greater in patients with Cl_{cr} <30 mL/minute and are doubled in hemodialysis patients

Adverse Reactions

1% to 10%:

Central nervous system: Fatigue (4%)

Gastrointestinal: Diarrhea (3%), dyspepsia (2%)

Respiratory: Upper respiratory infection (9%), cough (2.8% versus 2.7% in placebo)

<1% (Limited to important or life-threatening): Angina, angioedema, arrhythmia, cardiopulmonary arrest, conjunctivitis, decreased libido, depression, dyspnea, ecchymosis, edema, epistaxis, gout, heart failure, hyperkalemia, hypotension, increased transaminases, jaundice, myocardial infarction, orthostatic hypotension, paresthesia, sexual dysfunction, stroke, urticaria. May be associated with worsening of renal function in patients dependent on renin-angiotensin-aldosterone system.

Overdosage/Toxicology The most likely overdose manifestations would be hypotension and tachycardia. Bradycardia could occur from parasympathetic (vagal) stimulation. If symptomatic hypotension should occur, institute supportive treatment.

Drug Interactions

Cytochrome P450 Effect: CYP2C9 enzyme substrate

Increased Effect/Toxicity: Blood levels of irbesartan may be increased by inhibitors of cytochrome P450 isoenzyme 2C9 (eg, sulfaphenazole, tolbutamide, nifedipine). Potassium

(Continued)

Irbesartan *(Continued)*

salts/supplements, co-trimoxazole (high dose), ACE inhibitors, and potassium-sparing diuretics (amiloride, spironolactone, triamterene) may increase the risk of hyperkalemia.

Ethanol/Nutrition/Herb Interactions Herb/Nutraceutical: Avoid dong quai if using for hypertension (has estrogenic activity). Avoid ephedra, yohimbe, ginseng (may worsen hypertension). Avoid garlic (may have increased antihypertensive effect).

Mechanism of Action Irbesartan is an angiotensin receptor antagonist. Angiotensin II acts as a vasoconstrictor. In addition to causing direct vasoconstriction, angiotensin II also stimulates the release of aldosterone. Once aldosterone is released, sodium as well as water are reabsorbed. The end result is an elevation in blood pressure. Irbesartan binds to the AT1 angiotensin II receptor. This binding prevents angiotensin II from binding to the receptor thereby blocking the vasoconstriction and the aldosterone secreting effects of angiotensin II.

Pharmacodynamics/Kinetics

Onset of action: Peak effect: 1-2 hours

Duration: >24 hours

Distribution: V_d: 53-93 L

Protein binding, plasma: 90%

Metabolism: Hepatic

Bioavailability: 60% to 80%

Half-life elimination: Terminal: 11-15 hours

Time to peak, serum: 1.5-2 hours

Excretion: Feces (80%); urine (20%)

Usual Dosage Oral:

Children:

<6 years: Safety and efficacy have not been established.

≥6-12 years: Initial: 75 mg once daily; may be titrated to a maximum of 150 mg once daily

Children ≥13 years and Adults: 150 mg once daily; patients may be titrated to 300 mg once daily

Dietary Considerations May be taken with or without food.

Patient Information Patients of childbearing age should be informed about the consequences of 2nd and 3rd trimester exposure to drugs that act on the renin-angiotensin system, and that these consequences do not appear to have resulted from intrauterine drug exposure that has been limited to the 1st trimester. Patients should report pregnancy to their physician as soon as possible.

Dosage Forms Tablet: 75 mg, 150 mg, 300 mg

Irbesartan and Hydrochlorothiazide

(ir be SAR tan & hye droe klor oh THYE a zide)

U.S. Brand Names Avalide®

Canadian Brand Names Avalide®

Synonyms Avapro® HCT; Hydrochlorothiazide and Irbesartan

Therapeutic Category Angiotensin II Antagonist Combination; Antihypertensive Agent, Combination

Use Combination therapy for the management of hypertension

Pregnancy Risk Factor C/D (2nd and 3rd trimesters)

Usual Dosage Dose must be individualized. A patient who is not controlled with either agent alone may be switched to the combination product. Mean effect increases with the dose of each component. The lowest dosage available is irbesartan 150 mg/hydrochlorothiazide 12.5 mg. Dose increases should be made not more frequently than every 2-4 weeks.

Additional Information Complete prescribing information for this medication should be consulted for additional detail.

Dosage Forms

Tablet:

Irbesartan 150 mg and hydrochlorothiazide 12.5 mg

Irbesartan 300 mg and hydrochlorothiazide 12.5 mg

♦ Ircon® [OTC] *see* Ferrous Fumarate *on page 555*

Irinotecan (eye rye no TEE kan)

U.S. Brand Names Camptosar®

Canadian Brand Names Camptosar®

Synonyms Camptothecin-11; CPT-11

Therapeutic Category Antineoplastic Agent, Natural Source (Plant) Derivative

Use A component of first-line therapy in combination with 5-fluorouracil and leucovorin for the treatment of metastatic carcinoma of the colon or rectum; treatment of metastatic carcinoma of the colon or rectum which has recurred or progressed following fluorouracil-based therapy

Unlabeled/Investigational Use Lung cancer (small cell and nonsmall cell), cervical cancer, gastric cancer, pancreatic cancer, leukemia, lymphoma, breast cancer

Pregnancy Risk Factor D

Contraindications Hypersensitivity to irinotecan or any component of the formulation; pregnancy

Warnings/Precautions The U.S. Food and Drug Administration (FDA) currently recommends that procedures for proper handling and disposal of antineoplastic agents be considered

Deaths due to sepsis following severe myelosuppression have been reported. Therapy should be discontinued if neutropenic fever occurs or if the absolute neutrophil count is <500/mm³. The dose of irinotecan should be reduced if there is a clinically significant decrease in the total WBC (<200/mm³), neutrophil count (<1000/mm³), hemoglobin (<8 g/dL), or platelet count (<100,000/mm³). Routine administration of a colony-stimulating factor is generally not necessary. Avoid extravasation.

Patients with even modest elevations in total serum bilirubin levels (1.0-2.0 mg/dL) have a significantly greater likelihood of experiencing first-course grade 3 or 4 neutropenia than those with bilirubin levels that were <1.0 mg/dL. Patients with abnormal glucuronidation of bilirubin, such as those with Gilbert's syndrome, may also be at greater risk of myelosuppression when receiving therapy with irinotecan.

Adverse Reactions

>10%:

Cardiovascular: Vasodilation

Central nervous system: Insomnia, dizziness, fever (45.4%)

Dermatologic: Alopecia (60.5%), rash

Gastrointestinal: Irinotecan therapy may induce two different forms of diarrhea. Onset, symptoms, proposed mechanisms and treatment are different. Overall, 56.9% of patients treated experience abdominal pain and/or cramping during therapy. Anorexia, constipation, flatulence, stomatitis, and heartburn have also been reported.

Diarrhea: Dose-limiting toxicity with weekly dosing regimen

Early diarrhea (50.7% incidence) usually occurs during or within 24 hours of administration. May be accompanied by symptoms of cramping, vomiting, flushing, and diaphoresis. It is thought to be mediated by cholinergic effects which can be successfully managed with atropine (refer to Warnings/Precautions).

Late diarrhea (87.8% incidence) usually occurs >24 hours after treatment. National Cancer Institute (NCI) grade 3 or 4 diarrhea occurs in 30.6% of patients. Late diarrhea generally occurs with a median of 11 days after therapy and lasts approximately 3 days. Patients experiencing grade 3 or 4 diarrhea were noted to have symptoms a total of 7 days. Correlated with irinotecan or SN-38 levels in plasma and bile. Due to the duration, dehydration and electrolyte imbalances are significant clinical concerns. Loperamide therapy is recommended. The incidence of grade 3 or 4 late diarrhea is significantly higher in patients ≥ 65 years of age: close monitoring and prompt initiation of high-dose loperamide therapy is prudent (refer to Warnings/Precautions).

Emetic potential: Moderately high (86.2% incidence, however, only 12.5% grade 3 or 4 vomiting)

Hematologic: Myelosuppressive: Dose-limiting toxicity with 3 week dosing regimen

Grade 1-4 neutropenia occurred in 53.9% of patients. Patients who had previously received pelvic or abdominal radiation therapy or a bilirubin of ≥1.0 mg/dL were noted to have a significantly increased incidence of grade 3 or 4 neutropenia. White blood cell count nadir is 15 days after administration and is more frequent than thrombocytopenia. Recovery is usually within 24-28 days and cumulative toxicity has not been observed.

WBC: Mild to severe

Platelets: Mild

Onset: 10 days

Nadir: 14-16 days

Recovery: 21-28 days

Neuromuscular & skeletal: Weakness (75.7%)

Respiratory: Dyspnea (22%), coughing, rhinitis

Miscellaneous: Diaphoresis

1% to 10%: Local: **Irritant chemotherapy**; thrombophlebitis has been reported

Overdosage/Toxicology Symptoms include bone marrow suppression, leukopenia, thrombocytopenia, nausea, and vomiting. Treatment is supportive.

Drug Interactions

Increased Effect/Toxicity: Hold diuretics during dosing due to potential risk of dehydration secondary to vomiting and/or diarrhea induced by irinotecan. Prophylactic dexamethasone as an antiemetic may enhance lymphocytopenia. Prochlorperazine may increase incidence of akathisia. Adverse reactions such as myelosuppression and diarrhea would be expected to be exacerbated by other antineoplastic agents.

Stability

Store intact vials of injection at room temperature and protected from light

Doses should be diluted in D_5W or NS to a final concentration of 0.12-1.1 mg/mL. Due to the relatively acidic pH, irinotecan appears to be more stable in D_5W than NS. D_5W (500 mL) is the preferred diluent for most doses

Standardized dose: Dose/500 mL D_5W

Stability at room temperature (15°C to 30°C/59°F to 86°F): 24 hours

Stability at refrigeration (2°C to 8°C/36°F to 46°F): 48 hours

Standardized dose: Dose/500 mL NS

Stability at room temperature (15°C to 30°C/59°F to 86°F): 24 hours

Stability at refrigeration (2°C to 8°C/36°F to 46°F): NOT RECOMMENDED DUE TO THE OCCURRENCE OF VISIBLE PARTICULATES

Mechanism of Action Irinotecan and its active metabolite (SN-38) bind reversibly to topoisomerase I and stabilize the cleavable complex so that religation of the cleaved DNA strand cannot occur. This results in the accumulation of cleavable complexes and single-strand DNA breaks. This interaction results in double-stranded DNA breaks and cell death consistent with S-phase cell cycle specificity.

Pharmacodynamics/Kinetics

Distribution: V_d: 33-150 L/m²

Protein binding, plasma: Parent drug: 30% to 68%; SN-38 (active drug): 95%

Metabolism: Converted to SN-38 by carboxylesterase enzymes in intestinal mucosa, plasma, liver, and perhaps in some tumors. SN-38 is conjugated with glucuronide, the conjugate having much less activity than SN-38. Enterohepatic recirculation results in a second peak in the concentration of SN-38. The lactones of both irinotecan and SN-38 undergo hydrolysis to inactive hydroxy acid forms.

Half-life elimination: Parent drug: Alpha: 0.2 hours, beta: 2.5 hours, gamma: 14.2 hours; SN-38: 3-23.9 hours.

Time to peak: SN-38: 30-minute infusion: ~1 hour

Excretion: Urine (~20% of dose) within 24 hours; SN-38 excretion in 24 hours accounted for 0.25% of administered dose

Usual Dosage Refer to individual protocols; courses may be repeated indefinitely as long as the patient continues to experience clinical benefit: Adults: I.V.:

(Continued)

Irinotecan *(Continued)*

Single-agent therapy:

Weekly regimen: 125 mg/m^2 over 90 minutes on days 1, 8, 15, and 22, followed by a 2-week rest

Once-every-3-week regimen: 350 mg/m^2 over 90 minutes, once every 3 weeks

A reduction in the starting dose by one dose level may be considered for patients ≥65 years of age, prior pelvic/abdominal radiotherapy, performance status of 2, or increased bilirubin (dosing for patients with a bilirubin >2 mg/dL cannot be recommended based on lack of data per manufacturer)

Depending on the patient's ability to tolerate therapy, doses should be adjusted in increments of 25-50 mg/m^2. Irinotecan doses may range 50-150 mg/m^2.

Combination therapy with 5-FU and leucovorin: Six-week (42-day) cycle (next cycle beginning on day 45):

125 mg/m^2 over 90 minutes on days 1, 8, 15, and 22; to be given in combination with bolus leucovorin and 5-FU (leucovorin administered immediately following irinotecan; 5-FU immediately following leucovorin)

180 mg/m^2 over 90 minutes on days 1, 15, and 22; to be given in combination with infusional leucovorin and bolus/infusion 5-FU (leucovorin administered immediately following irinotecan; 5-FU immediately following leucovorin)

Note: For all regimens: It is recommended that new courses begin only after the granulocyte count recovers to ≥1500/mm^3, the platelet count recovers to ≥100,000/mm^3, and treatment-related diarrhea has fully resolved. Treatment should be delayed 1-2 weeks to allow for recovery from treatment-related toxicities. If the patient has not recovered after a 2-week delay, consideration should be given to discontinuing irinotecan.

Dosing adjustment in renal impairment: Effects have not been evaluated

Dosing adjustment in hepatic impairment:

AUC of irinotecan and SN-38 have been reported to be higher in patients with known hepatic tumor involvement. The manufacturer recommends that no change in dosage or administration be made for patients with liver metastases and normal hepatic function.

In patients with a combined history of prior pelvic/abdominal irradiation and modestly elevated total serum bilirubin levels (1.0-2.0 mg/dL) prior to treatment with irinotecan, there may be substantially increased likelihood of grade 3 or 4 neutropenia. Consideration may be given to starting irinotecan at a lower dose (eg, 100 mg/m^2) in such patients. Definite recommendations regarding the most appropriate starting dose in patients who have pretreatment total serum bilirubin elevations >2.0 mg/dL are not available, but it is likely that lower starting doses will need to be considered in such patients.

Dosage adjustment for toxicities: It is recommended that new courses begin only after the granulocyte count recovers to ≥1500/mm^3, the platelet counts recovers to ≥100,000/mm^3, and treatment-related diarrhea has fully resolved. Depending on the patient's ability to tolerate therapy, doses should be adjusted in increments of 50-50 mg/m^2. Irinotecan doses may range 50-150 mg/m^2. Treatment should be delayed 1-2 weeks to allow for recovery from treatment-related toxicities. If the patient has not recovered after a 2-week delay, consideration should be given to discontinuing irinotecan. See tables.

Combination Schedules: Recommended Dosage Modifications*

Toxicity NCI Grade (Value)	During a Course of Therapy	At the Start of the Next Courses of Therapy (After Adequate Recovery), Compared to the Starting Dose in the Previous Courses*
No toxicity	Maintain dose level	Maintain dose level
Neutropenia		
1 (1500-1999/mm^3)	Maintain dose level	Maintain dose level
2 (1000-1499/mm^3)	↓ 1 dose level	Maintain dose level
3 (500-999/mm^3)	Omit dose, then ↓ 1 dose level when resolved to ≤ grade 2	↓ 1 dose level
4 (<500/mm^3)	Omit dose, then ↓ 2 dose levels when resolved to ≤ grade 2	↓ 2 dose levels
Neutropenic Fever (grade 4 neutropenia and ≥ grade 2 fever)	Omit dose then ↓ 2 dose levels when resolved	↓ 2 dose levels
Other Hematologic Toxicities	Dose modifications for leukopenia or thrombocytopenia during a course of therapy and at the start of subsequent courses of therapy are also based on NCI toxicity criteria and are the same as recommended for neutropenia above.	
Diarrhea		
1 (2-3 stools/day > pretreatment)	Maintain dose level	Maintain dose level
2 (4-6 stools/day > pretreatment)	↓ 1 dose level	Maintain dose level
3 (7-9 stools/day > pretreatment)	Omit dose, then ↓ 1 dose level when resolved to ≤ grade 2	↓ 1 dose level
4 (≥10 stools/day > pretreatment)	Omit dose then ↓ 50 mg/m^2, when resolved to ≤ grade 2	↓ 2 dose levels
Other Nonhematologic Toxicities		
1	Maintain dose level	Maintain dose level
2	↓ 1 dose level	Maintain dose level
3	Omit dose, then ↓ 1 dose level when resolved to ≤ grade 2	↓ 1 dose level
4	Omit dose, then ↓ 2 dose levels when resolved to ≤ grade 2	↓ 2 dose levels
Mucositis and/or stomatitis	Decrease only 5-FU, not irinotecan	Decrease only 5-FU, not irinotecan

*All dose modifications should be based on the worst preceding toxicity.

Single-Agent Schedule: Recommended Dosage Modifications*

Toxicity NCI Grade (Value)	During a Course of Therapy	At the Start of the Next Courses of Therapy (After Adequate Recovery), Compared to the Starting Dose In the Previous Courses*	
	Weekly	Weekly	Once Every 3 Weeks
No toxicity	Maintain dose level	↑ 25 mg/m² up to a maximum dose of 150 mg/ m²	Maintain dose level
Neutropenia			
1 (1500-1999/mm³)	Maintain dose level	Maintain dose level	Maintain dose level
2 (1000-1499/mm³)	↓ 25 mg/m²	Maintain dose level	Maintain dose level
3 (500-999/mm³)	Omit dose, then ↓ 25 mg/m² when resolved to ≤ grade 2	↓ 25 mg/m²	↓ 50 mg/m²
4 (<500/mm³)	Omit dose, then ↓ 50 mg/m² when resolved to ≤ grade 2	↓ 50 mg/m²	↓ 50 mg/m²
Neutropenic Fever (grade 4 neutropenia and ≥ grade 2 fever)	Omit dose, then ↓ 50 mg/m² when resolved	↓ 50 mg/m²	↓ 50 mg/m²
Other Hematologic Toxicities	Dose modifications for leukopenia, thrombocytopenia, and anemia during a course of therapy and at the start of subsequent courses of therapy are also based on NCI toxicity criteria and are the same as recommended for neutropenia above.		
Diarrhea			
1 (2-3 stools/day > pretreatment)	Maintain dose level	Maintain dose level	Maintain dose level
2 (4-6 stools/day > pretreatment)	↓ 25 mg/m²	Maintain dose level	Maintain dose level
3 (7-9 stools/day > pretreatment)	Omit dose, then ↓ 25 mg/m² when resolved to ≤ grade 2	↓ 25 mg/m²	↓ 50 mg/m²
4 (≥10 stools/day > pretreatment)	Omit dose, then ↓ 50 mg/m², when resolved to ≤ grade 2	↓ 50 mg/m²	↓ 50 mg/m²
Other Nonhematologic Toxicities			
1	Maintain dose level	Maintain dose level	Maintain dose level
2	↓ 25 mg/m²	↓ 25 mg/m²	↓ 50 mg/m²
3	Omit dose, then ↓ 25 mg/m² when resolved to ≤ grade 2	↓ 25 mg/m²	↓ 50 mg/m²
4	Omit dose, then ↓ 50 mg/m² when resolved to ≤ grade 2	↓ 50 mg/m²	↓ 50 mg/m²

*All dose modifications should be based on the worst preceding toxicity.

Administration Dose of irinotecan is diluted in D_5W to a final concentration of 0.12-1.1 mg/mL (most commonly in 500 mL D_5W) and infused over 90 minutes. 0.9% NaCl can be used, but precipitation of irinotecan under refrigeration is more likely to occur with the latter solution, and D_5W is generally preferred.

Monitoring Parameters CBC with differential, platelet count, and hemoglobin with each dose

Patient Information

Patients and patients' caregivers should be informed of the expected toxic effects of irinotecan, particularly its gastrointestinal manifestations, such as nausea, vomiting, and diarrhea

Each patient should be instructed to have loperamide readily available and to begin treatment for late diarrhea (occurring >24 hours after administration of irinotecan) at the first episode of poorly formed or loose stools or the earliest onset of bowel movements more frequent than normally expected for the patient. Refer to Warnings/Precautions.

The patient should also be instructed to notify the physician if diarrhea occurs. Premedication with loperamide is not recommended. The use of drugs with laxative properties should be avoided because of the potential for exacerbation of diarrhea. Patients should be advised to contact their physician to discuss any laxative use.

Patients should consult their physician if vomiting occurs, fever or evidence of infection develops, or if symptoms of dehydration, such as fainting, lightheadedness, or dizziness, are noted following therapy

Nursing Implications Monitor infusion site for signs of inflammation and avoid extravasation

Extravasation treatment: Flush the site with sterile water and apply ice

Additional Information

Irinotecan can induce both early and late forms of diarrhea that appear to be mediated by different mechanisms. Early diarrhea (during or within 24 hours of administration) is cholinergic in nature. It can be preceded by complaints of diaphoresis and abdominal cramping and may be ameliorated by the administration of atropine. The elderly (≥65 years of age) are at particular risk for diarrhea. Late diarrhea (occurring >24 hours after administration) can be prolonged and may lead to dehydration and electrolyte imbalance, and can be life-threatening. Late diarrhea should be treated promptly with loperamide. If grade 3 diarrhea (7-9 stools daily, incontinence, or severe cramping) or grade 4 diarrhea (≥10 stools daily, grossly bloody stool, or need for parenteral support), the administration of irinotecan should be delayed until the patient recovers and subsequent doses should be decreased.

Early diarrhea treatment: 0.25-1 mg of intravenous atropine should be considered (unless clinically contraindicated) in patients experiencing diaphoresis, abdominal cramping, or early diarrhea

Late diarrhea treatment: High-dose loperamide: Oral: 4 mg at the first onset of late diarrhea and then 2 mg every 2 hours until the patient is diarrhea-free for at least 12 hours. During the night, the patient may take 4 mg of loperamide every 4 hours. **Premedication with loperamide is not recommended.**

Dosage Forms Injection: 20 mg/mL (5 mL)

Iron Dextran Complex (EYE ern DEKS tran KOM pleks)

Related Information

Antacid Drug Interactions *on page 1477*

U.S. Brand Names Dexferrum®; INFeD®

Canadian Brand Names Dexiron™; Infufer®

Therapeutic Category Iron Salt

Use Treatment of microcytic hypochromic anemia resulting from iron deficiency in patients in whom oral administration is infeasible or ineffective

(Continued)

Iron Dextran Complex *(Continued)*

Pregnancy Risk Factor C

Contraindications Hypersensitivity to iron dextran or any component of the formulation; all anemias that are not involved with iron deficiency; hemochromatosis; hemolytic anemia

Warnings/Precautions Use with caution in patients with history of asthma, hepatic impairment, rheumatoid arthritis; not recommended in children <4 months of age; deaths associated with parenteral administration following anaphylactic-type reactions have been reported; use only in patients where the iron deficient state is not amenable to oral iron therapy. A test dose of 0.5 mL I.V. or I.M. should be given to observe for adverse reactions. Anemia in the elderly is often caused by "anemia of chronic disease" or associated with inflammation rather than blood loss. Iron stores are usually normal or increased, with a serum ferritin >50 ng/mL and a decreased total iron binding capacity. I.V. administration of iron dextran is often preferred over I.M. in the elderly secondary to a decreased muscle mass and the need for daily injections.

Adverse Reactions

>10%:
  Cardiovascular: Flushing
  Central nervous system: Dizziness, fever, headache, pain
  Gastrointestinal: Nausea, vomiting, metallic taste
  Local: Staining of skin at the site of I.M. injection
  Miscellaneous: Diaphoresis

1% to 10%:
  Cardiovascular: Hypotension (1% to 2%)
  Dermatologic: Urticaria (1% to 2%), phlebitis (1% to 2%)
  Gastrointestinal: Diarrhea
  Genitourinary: Discoloration of urine

<1% (Limited to important or life-threatening): Anaphylactoid reaction, anaphylaxis, shock (cardiovascular collapse, respiratory difficulty; most frequently within minutes of administration)

Note: Diaphoresis, urticaria, arthralgia, fever, chills, dizziness, headache, and nausea may be delayed 24-48 hours after I.V. administration or 3-4 days after I.M. administration.

Overdosage/Toxicology Symptoms include erosion of GI mucosa, pulmonary edema, hyperthermia, convulsions, tachycardia, hepatic and renal impairment, coma, hematemesis, lethargy, tachycardia, and acidosis. Serum iron >300 mcg/mL requires overdose treatment, due to severe toxicity. Although rare, if a severe iron overdose (when the serum iron concentration exceeds the total iron-binding capacity) occurs, it may be treated with deferoxamine. Deferoxamine may be administered I.V. (80 mg/kg over 24 hours) or I.M. (40-90 mg/kg every 8 hours).

Drug Interactions

Decreased Effect: Decreased effect with chloramphenicol.

Ethanol/Nutrition/Herb Interactions Food: Iron bioavailability may be decreased if taken with dairy products.

Stability Store at room temperature
  Stability of parenteral admixture at room temperature (25°C): 3 months
  Standard diluent: Dose/250-1000 mL NS
  Minimum volume: 250 mL NS

Mechanism of Action The released iron, from the plasma, eventually replenishes the depleted iron stores in the bone marrow where it is incorporated into hemoglobin

Pharmacodynamics/Kinetics

Absorption:
  I.M.: 50% to 90% is promptly absorbed, the balance is slowly absorbed over month
  I.V.: Uptake of iron by the reticuloendothelial system appears to be constant at about 10-20 mg/hour

Excretion: Urine and feces via reticuloendothelial system

Usual Dosage I.M. (Z-track method should be used for I.M. injection), I.V.:

A 0.5 mL test dose (0.25 mL in infants) should be given prior to starting iron dextran therapy; total dose should be divided into a daily schedule for I.M., total dose may be given as a single continuous infusion

Iron-deficiency anemia: Dose (mL) = 0.0476 x LBW (kg) x (normal hemoglobin - observed hemoglobin) + (1 mL/5 kg of LBW to maximum of 14 mL for iron stores)
  LBW = Lean Body Weight

Iron replacement therapy for blood loss: Replacement iron (mg) = blood loss (mL) x hematocrit

Maximum daily dose (can administer total dose at one time I.V.):
  Infants <5 kg: 25 mg iron (0.5 mL)
  Children:
    5-10 kg: 50 mg iron (1 mL)
    10-50 kg: 100 mg iron (2 mL)
  Adults >50 kg: 100 mg iron (2 mL)

Administration Use Z-track technique for I.M. administration (deep into the upper outer quadrant of buttock); may be administered I.V. bolus at rate ≤50 mg/minute or diluted in 250-1000 mL NS and infused over 1-6 hours; infuse initial 25 mL slowly, observe for allergic reactions; have epinephrine nearby

Monitoring Parameters Hemoglobin, hematocrit, reticulocyte count, serum ferritin, serum iron, TIBC

Reference Range

Hemoglobin: Adults:
  Males: 13.5-16.5 g/dL
  Females: 12.0-15.0 g/dL
Serum iron: 40-160 µg/dL
Total iron binding capacity: 230-430 µg/dL
Transferrin: 204-360 mg/dL
Percent transferrin saturation: 20% to 50%

Test Interactions May cause falsely elevated values of serum bilirubin and falsely decreased values of serum calcium

Nursing Implications
I.M.: Use Z-track technique for I.M. administration (deep into the upper outer quadrant of buttock)
I.V.: Direct I.V. push administration is **not** recommended; dilute in normal saline (250-1000 mL) and infuse over 1-6 hours at a maximum rate of 50 mg/minute; avoid dilution in dextrose due to an increased incidence of local pain and phlebitis

Dosage Forms Injection: 50 mg/mL (2 mL, 10 mL)

♦ **ISD** see Isosorbide Dinitrate on page 750
♦ **ISDN** see Isosorbide Dinitrate on page 750
♦ **ISG** see Immune Globulin (Intramuscular) on page 710
♦ **Ismelin®** see Guanethidine on page 649
♦ **ISMN** see Isosorbide Mononitrate on page 751
♦ **Ismo®** see Isosorbide Mononitrate on page 751
♦ **Ismotic®** see Isosorbide on page 750
♦ **Isoamyl Nitrite** see Amyl Nitrite on page 97
♦ **Isobamate** see Carisoprodol on page 229
♦ **Isocaine® HCl** see Mepivacaine on page 861
♦ **Isoclor® Expectorant** see Guaifenesin, Pseudoephedrine, and Codeine on page 648

Isoetharine (eye soe ETH a reen)

Related Information
Antacid Drug Interactions on page 1477
Bronchodilators, Comparison of Inhaled Sympathomimetics on page 1493

U.S. Brand Names Arm-a-Med® Isoetharine; Beta-2®; Bronkometer®; Bronkosol®; Dey-Lute® Isoetharine

Canadian Brand Names Beta-2®; Bronkometer®; Bronkosol®

Synonyms Isoetharine Hydrochloride; Isoetharine Mesylate

Therapeutic Category Adrenergic Agonist Agent; Bronchodilator; Sympathomimetic

Use Bronchodilator in bronchial asthma and for reversible bronchospasm occurring with bronchitis and emphysema

Pregnancy Risk Factor C

Usual Dosage Treatments are not usually repeated more than every 4 hours, except in severe cases
Nebulizer: Children: 0.01 mL/kg; minimum dose 0.1 mL; maximum dose: 0.5 mL diluted in 2-3 mL normal saline

Additional Information Complete prescribing information for this medication should be consulted for additional detail.

Dosage Forms Solution for oral inhalation, as hydrochloride: 1% (10 mL, 30 mL)

♦ **Isoetharine Hydrochloride** see Isoetharine on page 747
♦ **Isoetharine Mesylate** see Isoetharine on page 747

Isoflurophate (eye soe FLURE oh fate)

Related Information
Glaucoma Drug Therapy Comparison on page 1499

U.S. Brand Names Floropryl®

Synonyms DFP; Diisopropyl Fluorophosphate; Dyflos; Fluostigmin

Therapeutic Category Cholinergic Agent, Ophthalmic; Ophthalmic Agent, Miotic

Use Treatment of primary open-angle glaucoma and conditions that obstruct aqueous outflow; treatment of accommodative convergent strabismus

Pregnancy Risk Factor X

Usual Dosage Adults: Ophthalmic:
Glaucoma: Instill 0.25" strip in eye every 8-72 hours
Strabismus: Instill 0.25" strip to each eye every night for 2 weeks then reduce to 0.25" every other night to once weekly for 2 months

Additional Information Complete prescribing information for this medication should be consulted for additional detail.

Dosage Forms Ointment, ophthalmic: 0.025% in polyethylene mineral oil gel (3.5 g)

♦ **Isollyl® Improved** see Butalbital Compound on page 197
♦ **Isometheptene, Acetaminophen, and Dichloralphenazone** see Acetaminophen, Isometheptene, and Dichloralphenazone on page 28
♦ **Isometheptene, Dichloralphenazone, and Acetaminophen** see Acetaminophen, Isometheptene, and Dichloralphenazone on page 28

Isoniazid (eye soe NYE a zid)

Related Information
Antacid Drug Interactions on page 1477
Tuberculosis Prophylaxis on page 1572
Tuberculosis Treatment Guidelines on page 1612
Tyramine Content of Foods on page 1737
USPHA/IDSA Guidelines for the Prevention of Opportunistic Infections in Persons With HIV on page 1574

U.S. Brand Names Nydrazid®

Canadian Brand Names Isotamine®; PMS-Isoniazid

Synonyms INH; Isonicotinic Acid Hydrazide

Therapeutic Category Antitubercular Agent

Use Treatment of susceptible tuberculosis infections; prophylactically in those individuals exposed to tuberculosis

Pregnancy Risk Factor C

(Continued)

Isoniazid *(Continued)*

Contraindications Hypersensitivity to isoniazid or any component of the formulation; acute liver disease; previous history of hepatic damage during isoniazid therapy

Warnings/Precautions Use with caution in patients with renal impairment and chronic liver disease. Severe and sometimes fatal hepatitis may occur or develop even after many months of treatment; patients must report any prodromal symptoms of hepatitis, such as fatigue, weakness, malaise, anorexia, nausea, or vomiting. Children with low milk and low meat intake should receive concomitant pyridoxine therapy. Periodic ophthalmic examinations are recommended even when usual symptoms do not occur; pyridoxine (10-50 mg/day) is recommended in individuals likely to develop peripheral neuropathies.

Adverse Reactions
>10%:
  Gastrointestinal: Loss of appetite, nausea, vomiting, stomach pain
  Hepatic: Mild increased LFTs (10% to 20%)
  Neuromuscular & skeletal: Weakness, peripheral neuropathy (dose-related incidence, 10% to 20% incidence with 10 mg/kg/day)
1% to 10%:
  Central nervous system: Dizziness, slurred speech, lethargy
  Hepatic: Progressive liver damage (increases with age; 2.3% in patients >50 years)
  Neuromuscular & skeletal: Hyper-reflexia
<1% (Limited to important or life-threatening): Blood dyscrasias, depression, psychosis, seizures

Overdosage/Toxicology Symptoms include nausea, vomiting, slurred speech, dizziness, blurred vision, hallucinations, stupor, coma, and intractable seizures. The onset of metabolic acidosis is 30 minutes to 3 hours. Because of severe morbidity and high mortality rates associated with isoniazid overdose, patients who are asymptomatic after an overdose should be monitored for 4-6 hours. Pyridoxine has been shown to be effective in the treatment of intoxication, especially when seizures occur. Pyridoxine I.V. is administered on a milligram to milligram dose. If the amount of isoniazid ingested is unknown, 5 g of pyridoxine should be given over 3-5 minutes and may be followed by an additional 5 g in 30 minutes. Treatment is supportive. Airway protection and ventilation may be required, with diazepam for seizures, and sodium bicarbonate for acidosis. Forced diuresis and hemodialysis can result in more rapid removal.

Drug Interactions
  Cytochrome P450 Effect: CYP2E1 enzyme substrate; CYP2E1 enzyme inducer; and CYP1A2, 2C, 2C9, 2C18, 2C19, and 3A3/4 enzyme inhibitor
  Increased Effect/Toxicity: Increased toxicity/levels of oral anticoagulants, carbamazepines, cycloserine, hydantoins, and hepatically metabolized benzodiazepines. Reaction with disulfiram.
  Decreased Effect: Decreased effect/levels of isoniazid with aluminum salts.

Ethanol/Nutrition/Herb Interactions
  Ethanol: Avoid ethanol (increases the risk of hepatitis).
  Food: Isoniazid serum levels may be decreased if taken with food. Clinically severe elevated blood pressure may occur if isoniazid is taken with tyramine-containing foods. Avoid foods with histamine or tyramine (cheese, broad beans, dry sausage, salami, nonfresh meat, liver pate, soy bean, liquid and powdered protein supplements, wine). Isoniazid decreases folic acid absorption. Isoniazid alters pyridoxine metabolism.

Stability Protect oral dosage forms from light

Mechanism of Action Unknown, but may include the inhibition of myocolic acid synthesis resulting in disruption of the bacterial cell wall

Pharmacodynamics/Kinetics
  Absorption: Rapid and complete; rate can be slowed with food
  Distribution: All body tissues and fluids including CSF; crosses placenta; enters breast milk
  Protein binding: 10% to 15%
  Metabolism: Hepatic with decay rate determined genetically by acetylation phenotype
  Half-life elimination: Fast acetylators: 30-100 minutes; Slow acetylators: 2-5 hours; may be prolonged with impaired hepatic function or severe renal impairment
  Time to peak, serum: 1-2 hours
  Excretion: Urine (75% to 95%); feces; saliva

Usual Dosage Recommendations often change due to resistant strains and newly developed information; consult *MMWR* for current CDC recommendations: **Oral** (injectable is available for patients who are unable to either take or absorb oral therapy):
  Note: A four-drug regimen (isoniazid, rifampin, pyrazinamide, and either streptomycin or ethambutol) is preferred for the initial, empiric treatment of TB. When the drug susceptibility results are available, the regimen should be altered as appropriate.
  Infants and Children:
    Prophylaxis: 10 mg/kg/day in 1-2 divided doses (maximum: 300 mg/day) 6 months in patients who do not have HIV infection and 12 months in patients who have HIV infection
    Treatment:
      Daily therapy: 10-20 mg/kg/day in 1-2 divided doses (maximum: 300 mg/day)
      Directly observed therapy (DOT): Twice weekly therapy: 20-40 mg/kg (maximum: 900 mg/day); 3 times/week therapy: 20-40 mg/kg (maximum: 900 mg)
  Adults:
    Prophylaxis: 300 mg/day for 6 months in patients who do not have HIV infection and 12 months in patients who have HIV infection
    Treatment:
      Daily therapy: 5 mg/kg/day given daily (usual dose: 300 mg/day); 10 mg/kg/day in 1-2 divided doses in patients with disseminated disease
      Directly observed therapy (DOT): Twice weekly therapy: 15 mg/kg (maximum: 900 mg); 3 times/week therapy: 15 mg/kg (maximum: 900 mg)
  Note: Concomitant administration of 6-50 mg/day pyridoxine is recommended in malnourished patients or those prone to neuropathy (eg, alcoholics, diabetics)
  Hemodialysis: Dialyzable (50% to 100%)

Administer dose postdialysis

Peritoneal dialysis effects: Dose for Cl$_{cr}$ <10 mL/minute

Continuous arteriovenous or venovenous hemofiltration: Dose for Cl$_{cr}$ <10 mL/minute

Dosing adjustment in hepatic impairment: Dose should be reduced in severe hepatic disease

Dietary Considerations Should be taken 1 hour before or 2 hours after meals on an empty stomach; increase dietary intake of folate, niacin, magnesium.

Monitoring Parameters Periodic liver function tests; monitoring for prodromal signs of hepatitis

Reference Range Therapeutic: 1-7 µg/mL (SI: 7-51 µmol/L); Toxic: 20-710 µg/mL (SI: 146-5176 µmol/L)

Test Interactions False-positive urinary glucose with Clinitest®

Patient Information Report any prodromal symptoms of hepatitis (fatigue, weakness, nausea, vomiting, dark urine, or yellowing of eyes) or any burning, tingling, or numbness in the extremities

Nursing Implications The AAP recommends that pyridoxine supplementation (1-2 mg/kg/day) should be administered to malnourished patients, children or adolescents on meat or milk-deficient diets, breast feeding infants, and those predisposed to neuritis to prevent peripheral neuropathy; administration of isoniazid syrup has been associated with diarrhea

Dosage Forms
Injection: 100 mg/mL (10 mL)
Syrup: 50 mg/5 mL (473 mL) [orange flavor]
Tablet: 100 mg, 300 mg

Extemporaneous Preparations A 10 mg/mL oral suspension was stable for 21 days when refrigerated when compounded as follows:
Triturate ten 10 mg tablets in a mortar, reduce to a fine powder, then add 10 mL of purified water U.S.P. to make a paste; then transfer to a graduate and qs to 100 mL with sorbitol (do not use sugar-based solutions)
Shake well before using and keep in refrigerator

Nahata MC and Hipple TF, *Pediatric Drug Formulations*, 3rd ed, Cincinnati, OH: Harvey Whitney Books Co, 1997.

♦ **Isonicotinic Acid Hydrazide** *see Isoniazid on page 747*
♦ **Isonipecaine Hydrochloride** *see Meperidine on page 858*

Isoproterenol (eye soe proe TER e nole)

Related Information
Adrenergic Agonists, Cardiovascular Comparison *on page 1469*
Adult ACLS Algorithms *on page 1632*
Antacid Drug Interactions *on page 1477*
Bronchodilators, Comparison of Inhaled Sympathomimetics *on page 1493*

U.S. Brand Names Isuprel®

Canadian Brand Names Isuprel®

Synonyms Isoproterenol Hydrochloride

Therapeutic Category Adrenergic Agonist Agent; Bronchodilator; Sympathomimetic

Use Ventricular arrhythmias due to AV nodal block; hemodynamically compromised bradyarrhythmias or atropine- and dopamine-resistant bradyarrhythmias (when transcutaneous/venous pacing is not available); temporary use in third-degree AV block until pacemaker insertion

Unlabeled/Investigational Use Temporizing measure before transvenous pacing for torsade de pointes; diagnostic aid (vasovagal syncope)

Pregnancy Risk Factor C

Contraindications Hypersensitivity to sulfites or isoproterenol, any component of the formulation, or other sympathomimetic amines; angina, pre-existing cardiac arrhythmias (ventricular); tachycardia or AV block caused by cardiac glycoside intoxication

Warnings/Precautions Use with extreme caution; not currently a treatment of choice. Elderly patients, diabetics, renal or cardiovascular disease, hyperthyroidism; excessive or prolonged use may result in decreased effectiveness

Adverse Reactions Frequency not defined.
Cardiovascular: Premature ventricular beats, bradycardia, hypertension, hypotension, chest pain, palpitations, tachycardia, ventricular arrhythmias, myocardial infarction size
Central nervous system: Headache, nervousness or restlessness
Gastrointestinal: Nausea, vomiting
Respiratory: Dyspnea

Overdosage/Toxicology Symptoms include tremors, nausea, vomiting, and hypotension. Beta-adrenergic stimulation can cause increased heart rate, decreased blood pressure, and CNS excitation. Increased heart rate can be treated with beta-blockers. Decreased blood pressure can be treated with pure alpha-adrenergic agents. Diazepam 0.07 mg/kg can be used for excitation and seizures.

Drug Interactions
Increased Effect/Toxicity: Sympathomimetic agents may cause headaches and elevate blood pressure. General anesthetics may cause arrhythmias.

Ethanol/Nutrition/Herb Interactions Herb/Nutraceutical: Avoid ephedra, yohimbe (may cause CNS stimulation).

Stability Isoproterenol solution should be stored at room temperature; it should not be used if a color or precipitate is present. Exposure to air, light, or increased temperature may cause a pink to brownish pink color to develop. Stability of parenteral admixture at room temperature (25°C) or at refrigeration (4°C) is 24 hours.
Standard diluent: 2 mg/500 mL D$_5$W; 4 mg/500 mL D$_5$W
Minimum volume: 1 mg/100 mL D$_5$W
Incompatible with alkaline solutions, aminophylline and furosemide
(Continued)

749

Isoproterenol *(Continued)*

Mechanism of Action Stimulates beta$_1$- and beta$_2$-receptors resulting in relaxation of bronchial, GI, and uterine smooth muscle, increased heart rate and contractility, vasodilation of peripheral vasculature

Pharmacodynamics/Kinetics

Onset of action: Bronchodilation: I.V.: Immediate

Duration: I.V.: 10-15 minutes

Metabolism: By conjugation in many tissues including hepatic and pulmonary

Half-life elimination: 2.5-5 minutes

Excretion: Urine (primarily as sulfate conjugates)

Usual Dosage I.V.: Cardiac arrhythmias:

Children: Initial: 0.1 mcg/kg/minute (usual effective dose 0.2-2 mcg/kg/minute)

Adults: Initial: 2 mcg/minute; titrate to patient response (2-10 mcg/minute)

Administration I.V. infusion administration requires the use of an infusion pump. To prepare for infusion: 1 mg isoproterenol to 500 mL D$_5$W, final concentration 2 mcg/mL

Monitoring Parameters EKG, heart rate, respiratory rate, arterial blood gas, arterial blood pressure, CVP

Patient Information Do not exceed recommended dosage; excessive use may lead to adverse effects or loss of effectiveness. Shake canister well before use. Administer pressurized inhalation during the second half of inspiration, as the airways are open wider and the aerosol distribution is more extensive. If more than one inhalation per dose is necessary, wait at least 1 full minute between inhalations - second inhalation is best delivered after 10 minutes. May cause nervousness, restlessness, insomnia; if these effects continue after dosage reduction, notify physician. Notify physician if palpitations, tachycardia, chest pain, muscle tremors, dizziness, headache, flushing or if breathing difficulty persists. Do not chew or swallow sublingual tablet.

Dosage Forms Injection: 0.02 mg/mL (10 mL); 0.2 mg/mL (1:5000) (1 mL, 5 mL, 10 mL)

- **Isoproterenol Hydrochloride** *see Isoproterenol on page 749*
- **Isoptin®** *see Verapamil on page 1412*
- **Isoptin® I.V. (Can)** *see Verapamil on page 1412*
- **Isoptin® SR** *see Verapamil on page 1412*
- **Isopto® Atropine** *see Atropine on page 131*
- **Isopto® Carbachol** *see Carbachol on page 221*
- **Isopto® Carpine** *see Pilocarpine on page 1083*
- **Isopto® Cetapred®** *see Sulfacetamide and Prednisolone on page 1269*
- **Isopto® Eserine (Can)** *see Physostigmine on page 1081*
- **Isopto® Homatropine** *see Homatropine on page 666*
- **Isopto® Hyoscine** *see Scopolamine on page 1225*
- **Isordil®** *see Isosorbide Dinitrate on page 750*

Isosorbide *(eye soe SOR bide)*

U.S. Brand Names Ismotic®

Synonyms OZIZ

Therapeutic Category Diuretic, Osmotic; Ophthalmic Agent, Osmotic

Use Short-term emergency treatment of acute angle-closure glaucoma and short-term reduction of intraocular pressure prior to and following intraocular surgery; may be used to interrupt an acute glaucoma attack; preferred agent when need to avoid nausea and vomiting

Pregnancy Risk Factor B

Usual Dosage Adults: Oral: Initial: 1.5 g/kg with a usual range of 1-3 g/kg 2-4 times/day as needed

Additional Information Complete prescribing information for this medication should be consulted for additional detail.

Dosage Forms Solution: 45% [450 mg/mL] (220 mL)

Isosorbide Dinitrate *(eye soe SOR bide dye NYE trate)*

Related Information

Heart Failure on page 1663

Nitrates Comparison on page 1511

U.S. Brand Names Dilatrate®-SR; Isordil®; Sorbitrate®

Canadian Brand Names Apo®-ISDN; Cedocard®-SR; Isordil®

Synonyms ISD; ISDN

Therapeutic Category Antianginal Agent; Nitrate; Vasodilator, Coronary

Use Prevention and treatment of angina pectoris; for congestive heart failure; to relieve pain, dysphagia, and spasm in esophageal spasm with GE reflux

Pregnancy Risk Factor C

Contraindications Hypersensitivity to isosorbide dinitrate or any component of the formulation; hypersensitivity to organic nitrates; concurrent use with sildenafil; angle-closure glaucoma (intraocular pressure may be increased); head trauma or cerebral hemorrhage (increase intracranial pressure); severe anemia

Warnings/Precautions Use with caution in patients with increased intracranial pressure, hypotension, hypovolemia, glaucoma; sustained release products may be absorbed erratically in patients with GI hypermotility or malabsorption syndrome; do not crush or chew sublingual dosage form; abrupt withdrawal may result in angina; tolerance may develop (adjust dose or change agent). Avoid use with sildenafil.

Adverse Reactions Frequency not defined.

Cardiovascular: Hypotension (infrequent), postural hypotension, crescendo angina (uncommon), rebound hypertension (uncommon), pallor, cardiovascular collapse, tachycardia, shock, flushing, peripheral edema

Central nervous system: Headache (most common), lightheadedness (related to blood pressure changes), syncope (uncommon), dizziness, restlessness

Gastrointestinal: Nausea, vomiting, bowel incontinence, xerostomia
Genitourinary: Urinary incontinence
Hematologic: Methemoglobinemia (rare, overdose)
Neuromuscular & skeletal: Weakness
Ocular: Blurred vision
Miscellaneous: Cold sweat

The incidence of hypotension and adverse cardiovascular events may be increased when used in combination with sildenafil (Viagra®).

Overdosage/Toxicology The most common symptoms of overdose include hypotension, throbbing headache, tachycardia, and flushing. Methemoglobinemia may occur with massive doses. Hypotension may aggravate symptoms of cardiac ischemia or cerebrovascular disease, and may even cause seizures (rare). Treatment consists of recumbent positioning and administration of fluids. Alpha-adrenergic vasopressors may be required. Treat methemoglobinemia with oxygen and methylene blue at a dose of 1-2 mg/kg slow I.V.

Drug Interactions
  Increased Effect/Toxicity: Combinations of sildenafil and nitrates has been associated with severe hypotensive reactions and death. Nitrate-induced hypotension may be exacerbated by ethanol and calcium channel blockers. Nitrates and aspirin may increase serum nitrate concentrations and therapeutic effect. Nitrates and dihydroergotamine may lead to elevated blood pressure or decrease antianginal effects.
  Decreased Effect: Nitrates may decrease the effect of heparin.

Ethanol/Nutrition/Herb Interactions Ethanol: Caution with ethanol (may increase risk of hypotension).

Mechanism of Action Stimulation of intracellular cyclic-GMP results in vascular smooth muscle relaxation of both arterial and venous vasculature. Increased venous pooling decreases left ventricular pressure (preload) and arterial dilatation decreases arterial resistance (afterload). Therefore, this reduces cardiac oxygen demand by decreasing left ventricular pressure and systemic vascular resistance by dilating arteries. Additionally, coronary artery dilation improves collateral flow to ischemic regions; esophageal smooth muscle is relaxed via the same mechanism.

Pharmacodynamics/Kinetics
  Onset of action: Sublingual tablet: 2-10 minutes; Chewable tablet: 3 minutes; Oral tablet: 45-60 minutes; Sustained release tablet: 30 minutes
  Duration: Sublingual tablet: 1-2 hours; Chewable tablet: 0.5-2 hours; Oral tablet: 4-6 hours; Sustained release tablet: 6-12 hours;
  Metabolism: Extensively hepatic to conjugated metabolites, including isosorbide 5-mononitrate (active) and 2-mononitrate (active)
  Half-life elimination: Parent drug: 1-4 hours; Metabolite (5-mononitrate): 4 hours
  Excretion: Urine and feces

Usual Dosage Adults (elderly should be given lowest recommended daily doses initially and titrate upward): Oral:
  Angina: 5-40 mg 4 times/day or 40 mg every 8-12 hours in sustained-release dosage form
  Congestive heart failure:
      Initial dose: 10 mg 3 times/day
      Target dose: 40 mg 3 times/day
      Maximum dose: 80 mg 3 times/day
  Sublingual: 2.5-10 mg every 4-6 hours
  Chewable tablet: 5-10 mg every 2-3 hours
  Tolerance to nitrate effects develops with chronic exposure
  Dose escalation does not overcome this effect. Short periods (14 hours) of nitrate withdrawal help minimize tolerance.
  Hemodialysis: During hemodialysis, administer dose postdialysis or administer supplemental 10-20 mg dose
  Peritoneal dialysis: Supplemental dose is not necessary

Administration Do not administer around-the-clock; the first dose of nitrates should be administered in a physician's office to observe for maximal cardiovascular dynamic effects and adverse effects (orthostatic blood pressure drop, headache); when immediate release products are prescribed twice daily - recommend 7 AM and noon; for 3 times/day dosing - recommend 7 AM, noon, and 5 PM; when sustained-release products are indicated, suggest once a day in morning or via twice daily dosing at 8 AM and 2 PM

Monitoring Parameters Monitor for orthostasis

Test Interactions ↓ cholesterol (S)

Patient Information Do not chew or crush sublingual or sustained release dosage form; do not change brands without consulting your pharmacist or physician; keep tablets or capsules in original container and keep container tightly closed; if no relief from sublingual tablets after 15 minutes, report to nearest emergency room or seek emergency help

Nursing Implications For isosorbide dinitrate, a 14-hour nitrate-free interval is recommended each day to prevent tolerance.

Dosage Forms
  Capsule, sustained release: 40 mg
  Tablet: 5 mg, 10 mg, 20 mg, 30 mg, 40 mg
  Tablet, chewable: 5 mg, 10 mg
  Tablet, sublingual: 2.5 mg, 5 mg, 10 mg
  Tablet, sustained release: 40 mg

Isosorbide Mononitrate (eye soe SOR bide mon oh NYE trate)

Related Information
  Nitrates Comparison on page 1511
U.S. Brand Names Imdur®; Ismo®; Monoket®
Canadian Brand Names Imdur®; ISMO®
Synonyms ISMN
Therapeutic Category Antianginal Agent; Nitrate; Vasodilator, Coronary
  (Continued)

Isosorbide Mononitrate *(Continued)*

Use Long-acting metabolite of the vasodilator isosorbide dinitrate used for the prophylactic treatment of angina pectoris

Pregnancy Risk Factor C

Contraindications Hypersensitivity to isosorbide or any component of the formulation; hypersensitivity to organic nitrates; concurrent use with sildenafil; angle-closure glaucoma (intraocular pressure may be increased); head trauma or cerebral hemorrhage (increase intracranial pressure); severe anemia

Warnings/Precautions Postural hypotension, transient episodes of weakness, dizziness, or syncope may occur even with small doses; ethanol accentuates these effects; tolerance and cross-tolerance to nitrate antianginal and hemodynamic effects may occur during prolonged isosorbide mononitrate therapy; (minimized by using the smallest effective dose, by alternating coronary vasodilators or offering drug-free intervals of as little as 12 hours). Excessive doses may result in severe headache, blurred vision, or dry mouth; increased anginal symptoms may be a result of dosage increases. Avoid use with sildenafil.

Adverse Reactions
>10%: Central nervous system: Headache (19% to 38%)
1% to 10%:
  Central nervous system: Dizziness (3% to 5%)
  Gastrointestinal: Nausea/vomiting (2% to 4%)
<1% (Limited to important or life-threatening): Angina pectoris, arrhythmias, atrial fibrillation, impotence, methemoglobinemia (rare), pruritus, rash, supraventricular tachycardia, syncope, vomiting

The incidence of hypotension and adverse cardiovascular events may be increased when used in combination with sildenafil (Viagra®).

Overdosage/Toxicology The most common symptoms of overdose include hypotension, throbbing headache, tachycardia, and flushing. Methemoglobinemia may occur with massive doses. Hypotension may aggravate symptoms of cardiac ischemia or cerebrovascular disease and may even cause seizures (rare). Treatment consists of placing patient in recumbent position and administering fluids; alpha-adrenergic vasopressors may be required; treat methemoglobinemia with oxygen and methylene blue at a dose of 1-2 mg/kg I.V. slowly.

Drug Interactions

Increased Effect/Toxicity: Combinations of sildenafil and nitrates has been associated with severe hypotensive reactions and death. Nitrate-induced hypotension may be exacerbated by ethanol and calcium channel blockers. Nitrates and aspirin may increase serum nitrate concentrations and therapeutic effect. Nitrates and dihydroergotamine may lead to elevated blood pressure or decrease antianginal effects.

Decreased Effect: Nitrates may decrease the effect of heparin.

Ethanol/Nutrition/Herb Interactions Ethanol: Caution with ethanol (may increase risk of hypotension).

Stability Tablets should be stored in a tight container at room temperature of 15°C to 30°C (59°F to 86°F)

Mechanism of Action Prevailing mechanism of action for nitroglycerin (and other nitrates) is systemic venodilation, decreasing preload as measured by pulmonary capillary wedge pressure and left ventricular end diastolic volume and pressure; the average reduction in left ventricular end diastolic volume is 25% at rest, with a corresponding increase in ejection fractions of 50% to 60%. This effect improves congestive symptoms in heart failure and improves the myocardial perfusion gradient in patients with coronary artery disease.

Pharmacodynamics/Kinetics
Onset of action: 30-60 minutes
Absorption: Nearly complete and low intersubject variability in its pharmacokinetic parameters and plasma concentrations
Half-life elimination: Mononitrate: ~4 hours

Usual Dosage Adults and Geriatrics (start with lowest recommended dose): Oral:
Regular tablet: 5-10 mg twice daily with the two doses given 7 hours apart (eg, 8 AM and 3 PM) to decrease tolerance development; then titrate to 10 mg twice daily in first 2-3 days.
Extended release tablet: Initial: 30-60 mg given in morning as a single dose; titrate upward as needed, giving at least 3 days between increases; maximum daily single dose: 240 mg

Dosing adjustment in renal impairment: Not necessary for elderly or patients with altered renal or hepatic function.

Tolerance to nitrate effects develops with chronic exposure. Dose escalation does not overcome this effect. Tolerance can only be overcome by short periods of nitrate absence from the body. Short periods (10-12 hours) of nitrate withdrawal help minimize tolerance. Recommended dosage regimens incorporate this interval. General recommendations are to take the last dose of short-acting agents no later than 7 PM; administer 2 times/day rather than 4 times/day. Administer sustained release tablet once daily in the morning.

Administration Do not administer around-the-clock; Monoket® and Ismo® should be scheduled twice daily with doses 7 hours apart (8 AM and 3 PM); Imdur® may be administered once daily

Monitoring Parameters Monitor for orthostasis, increased hypotension

Patient Information Dispense drug in easy-to-open container; do not change brands without consulting pharmacist or physician; keep tablets or capsules tightly closed in original container; extended release tablets should not be chewed or crushed and should be swallowed together with a half-glassful of fluid; the antianginal efficacy of tablets (Ismo®, Monoket®) can be maintained by carefully following the prescribed schedule of dosing (2 doses taken 7 hours apart); the extended-release (Imdur®) tablet should be given once daily; headaches are sometimes a marker of the activity of the drug

Nursing Implications Do not crush or chew extended release forms; 8- to 12-hour nitrate-free interval is needed each day to prevent tolerance (the recommended dosage regimens incorporate this interval)

Dosage Forms
Tablet:
  Ismo®: 20 mg

Monoket®: 10 mg
Tablet, extended release (Imdur®): 30 mg, 60 mg, 120 mg

♦ **Isotamine® (Can)** see Isoniazid on page 747

Isotretinoin (eye soe TRET i noyn)
U.S. Brand Names Accutane®
Canadian Brand Names Accutane®; Isotrex®
Synonyms 13-cis-Retinoic Acid
Therapeutic Category Acne Products; Retinoic Acid Derivative; Vitamin A Derivative
Use Treatment of severe recalcitrant nodular acne unresponsive to conventional therapy
Unlabeled/Investigational Use Investigational: Treatment of children with metastatic neuroblastoma or leukemia that does not respond to conventional therapy
Restrictions Prescriptions for Accutane® may not be dispensed unless they are affixed with a yellow self-adhesive Accutane® qualification sticker filled out by the prescriber. Telephone, fax, or computer-generated prescriptions are no longer valid. Prescriptions may not be written for more than a 1-month supply and must be dispensed with a patient education guide every month. In addition, prescriptions for females must be filled within 7 days of the date noted on the yellow sticker; prescriptions filled after 7 days of the noted date are considered to be expired and cannot be honored. Pharmacists may call the manufacturer to confirm the prescriber's authority to write for this medication, however, this is not mandatory.

Prescribers will be provided with Accutane® qualification stickers after they have read the details of the S.M.A.R.T. program and have signed and mailed to the manufacturer their agreement to participate. A half-day continuing education program is also available. Audits of pharmacies will be conducted to monitor program compliance.

Pregnancy Risk Factor X
Pregnancy/Breast-Feeding Implications Major fetal abnormalities (both internal and external), spontaneous abortion, premature births and low IQ scores in surviving infants have been reported. This medication is contraindicated in females of childbearing potential unless they are able to comply with the guidelines of pregnancy prevention programs put in place by the FDA and the manufacturer of Accutane®.
Contraindications Hypersensitivity to isotretinoin or any component of the formulation; sensitivity to parabens, vitamin A, or other retinoids; pregnancy
Warnings/Precautions This medication should only be prescribed by prescribers competent in treating severe recalcitrant nodular acne, are experienced in the use of systemic retinoids and are participating in the pregnancy prevention programs authorized by the FDA and product manufacturer. Use with caution in patients with diabetes mellitus, hypertriglyceridemia; acute pancreatitis and fatal hemorrhagic pancreatitis (rare) have been reported; not to be used in women of childbearing potential unless woman is capable of complying with effective contraceptive measures; therapy is begun after two negative pregnancy tests; effective contraception must be used for at least 1 month before beginning therapy, during therapy, and for 1 month after discontinuation of therapy. Prescriptions should be written for no more than a 1-month supply, and pregnancy testing and counseling should be repeated monthly. Because of the high likelihood of teratogenic effects (~20%), do not prescribe isotretinoin for women who are or who are likely to become pregnant while using the drug (see Additional Information for details). Male and female patients must be enrolled in the manufacturer sponsored and FDA approved monitoring programs. Depression, psychosis, and rarely suicidal thoughts and actions have been reported during isotretinoin usage. Discontinuation of treatment alone may not be sufficient, further evaluation may be necessary. Cases of pseudotumor cerebri (benign intracranial hypertension) have been reported, some with concomitant use of tetracycline (avoid using together). Patients with papilledema, headache, nausea, vomiting, and visual disturbances should be referred to a neurologist and treatment with isotretinoin discontinued. Hearing impairment, which can continue after therapy is discontinued, may occur. Clinical hepatitis, elevated liver enzymes, inflammatory bowel disease, skeletal hyperostosis, premature epiphyseal closure, vision impairment, corneal opacities, and decreased night vision have also been reported with the use of isotretinoin.
Adverse Reactions Frequency not defined.
Cardiovascular: Palpitation, tachycardia, vascular thrombotic disease, stroke, chest pain, syncope, flushing
Central nervous system: Edema, fatigue, pseudotumor cerebri, dizziness, drowsiness, headache, insomnia, lethargy, malaise, nervousness, paresthesias, seizures, stroke, suicidal ideation, suicide attempts, suicide, depression, psychosis, emotional instability
Dermatologic: Cutaneous allergic reactions, purpura, acne fulminans, alopecia, bruising, cheilitis, dry mouth, dry nose, dry skin, epistaxis, eruptive xanthomas, fragility of skin, hair abnormalities, hirsutism, hyperpigmentation, hypopigmentation, peeling of palms, peeling of soles, photoallergic reactions, photosensitizing reactions, pruritus, rash, dystrophy, paronychia, facial erythema, seborrhea, eczema, increased sunburn susceptibility, diaphoresis, urticaria, abnormal wound healing
Endocrine & metabolic: Increased triglycerides (25%), elevated blood glucose, increased HDL, increased cholesterol, abnormal menses
Gastrointestinal: Weight loss, inflammatory bowel disease, regional ileitis, pancreatitis, bleeding and inflammation of the gums, colitis, nausea, nonspecific gastrointestinal symptoms
Genitourinary: Nonspecific urogenital findings
Hematologic: Anemia, thrombocytopenia, neutropenia, agranulocytosis, pyogenic granuloma
Hepatic: Hepatitis
Neuromuscular & skeletal: Skeletal hyperostosis, calcification of tendons and ligaments, premature epiphyseal closure, arthralgia, CPK elevations, arthritis, tendonitis, bone abnormalities, weakness
Ocular: Corneal opacities, decreased night vision, cataracts, color vision disorder, conjunctivitis, dry eyes, eyelid inflammation, keratitis, optic neuritis, photophobia, visual disturbances
Otic: Hearing impairment, tinnitus
(Continued)

Isotretinoin *(Continued)*

Renal: Vasculitis, glomerulonephritis,

Respiratory: Bronchospasms, respiratory infection, voice alteration, Wegener's granulomatosis

Miscellaneous: Allergic reactions, anaphylactic reactions, lymphadenopathy, infection, disseminated herpes simplex

Overdosage/Toxicology Symptoms include headache, vomiting, flushing, abdominal pain, and ataxia. All signs and symptoms have been transient.

Drug Interactions

Increased Effect/Toxicity: Cases of pseudotumor cerebri have been reported in concurrent use; avoid combination.

Decreased Effect: Isotretinoin may increase clearance of carbamazepine resulting in reduced carbamazepine levels. Microdosed progesterone preparations ("mini-pills") may not be an adequate form of contraception.

Ethanol/Nutrition/Herb Interactions

Ethanol: Avoid or limit ethanol (may increase triglyceride levels if taken in excess).

Food: Isotretinoin bioavailability may be increased if taken with food or milk.

Herb/Nutraceutical: Avoid dong quai, St John's Wort (may also cause photosensitization and may decrease the effectiveness of birth control pills). Additional vitamin A supplements may lead to vitamin A toxicity (dry skin, irritation, arthralgias, myalgias, abdominal pain, hepatic changes); avoid use.

Stability Store at room temperature and protect from light

Mechanism of Action Reduces sebaceous gland size and reduces sebum production; regulates cell proliferation and differentiation

Pharmacodynamics/Kinetics

Absorption: Biphasic

Distribution: Crosses placenta; enters breast milk

Protein binding: 99% to 100%

Metabolism: Hepatic via CYP2B6, 2C8, 2C9, 2D6, 3A4; forms metabolites; major metabolite: 4-oxo-isotretinoin (active)

Half-life elimination: Terminal: Parent drug: 21 hours; Metabolite: 21-24 hours

Time to peak, serum: 3-5 hours

Excretion: Urine and feces (equal amounts)

Usual Dosage Oral:

Children: Maintenance therapy for neuroblastoma (investigational): 100-250 mg/m^2/day in 2 divided doses

Children and Adults: Severe recalcitrant nodular acne: 0.5-2 mg/kg/day in 2 divided doses (dosages as low as 0.05 mg/kg/day have been reported to be beneficial) for 15-20 weeks or until the total cyst count decreases by 70%, whichever is sooner. A second course of therapy may be initiated after a period of ≥2 months off therapy.

Dosing adjustment in hepatic impairment: Dose reductions empirically are recommended in hepatitis disease

Dietary Considerations Should be taken with food.

Administration Administer with food.

Monitoring Parameters CBC with differential and platelet count, baseline sedimentation rate, glucose, CPK

Pregnancy test (for all female patients of childbearing potential): Two negative tests with a sensitivity of at least 25 mIU/mL prior to beginning therapy (the second performed during the first five days of the menstrual period immediately preceding the start of therapy); monthly tests to rule out pregnancy prior to refilling prescription.

Lipids: Prior to treatment and at weekly or biweekly intervals until response to treatment is established. Test should not be performed <36 hours after consumption of ethanol.

Liver function tests: Prior to treatment and at weekly or biweekly intervals until response to treatment is established.

Patient Information Avoid pregnancy during therapy; effective contraceptive measures must be used since this drug may harm the fetus; there is information from manufacturers about this product that you should receive. Discontinue therapy if visual difficulties, abdominal pain, rectal bleeding, diarrhea; exacerbation of acne may occur during first weeks of therapy. Avoid use of other vitamin A products. Decreased tolerance to contact lenses may occur. Do not donate blood for at least 1 month following stopping of the drug. Loss of night vision may occur, avoid prolonged exposure to sunlight. Do not double next dose if dose is skipped. Isolated reports of depression, psychosis, and rarely suicidal thoughts and actions have been reported during isotretinoin usage.

Nursing Implications Capsules can be swallowed, or chewed and swallowed. The capsule may be opened with a large needle and the contents placed on applesauce or ice cream for patients unable to swallow the capsule.

Additional Information Females of childbearing potential must receive oral and written information reviewing the hazards of therapy and the effects that isotretinoin can have on a fetus. Therapy should not begin without two negative pregnancy tests, one to be performed in the physician's office when qualifying the patient for treatment, the second test performed on the second day of the next normal menstrual period or 11 days after the last unprotected intercourse, whichever is last. Two forms of contraception (a primary and secondary form as described in the pregnancy prevention program materials) must be used during treatment and limitations to their use must be explained. Prescriptions should be written for no more than a 1-month supply, and pregnancy testing and counseling should be repeated monthly. Urine pregnancy test kits (for monthly pregnancy testing) and a Pregnancy Prevention Program kit (to be given to the patient prior to therapy) are provided by the manufacturer. Any cases of accidental pregnancy should be reported to the manufacturer or the FDA MedWatch Program. All patients (male and female) must read and sign the informed consent material provided in the pregnancy prevention program. Prescriptions will not be honored unless they have the yellow qualification sticker affixed.

Dosage Forms Capsule: 10 mg, 20 mg, 40 mg

♦ **Isotrex® (Can)** *see* Isotretinoin *on page 753*

Isoxsuprine (eye SOKS syoo preen)
U.S. Brand Names Vasodilan®
Synonyms Isoxsuprine Hydrochloride
Therapeutic Category Vasodilator
Use Treatment of peripheral vascular diseases, such as arteriosclerosis obliterans and Raynaud's disease
Pregnancy Risk Factor C
Usual Dosage Adults: 10-20 mg 3-4 times/day; start with lower dose in elderly due to potential hypotension
Additional Information Complete prescribing information for this medication should be consulted for additional detail.
Dosage Forms Tablet, as hydrochloride: 10 mg, 20 mg

♦ **Isoxsuprine Hydrochloride** *see* Isoxsuprine *on page 755*

Isradipine (iz RA di peen)
Related Information
Calcium Channel Blockers Comparison *on page 1494*
U.S. Brand Names DynaCirc®; DynaCirc® CR
Canadian Brand Names DynaCirc®
Therapeutic Category Antihypertensive Agent; Antimigraine Agent; Calcium Channel Blocker
Use Treatment of hypertension
Pregnancy Risk Factor C
Pregnancy/Breast-Feeding Implications
Clinical effects on the fetus: No data on crossing the placenta
Breast-feeding/lactation: No data on crossing into breast milk. Not recommended due to potential harm to infant.
Contraindications Hypersensitivity to isradipine or any component of the formulation; hypotension (<90 mm Hg systolic)
Warnings/Precautions Avoid use in hypotension, congestive heart failure, cardiac conduction defects, PVCs, idiopathic hypertrophic subaortic stenosis; may cause platelet inhibition; do not abruptly withdraw (chest pain); may cause hepatic dysfunction or increased angina; increased intracranial pressure with cranial tumors; elderly may have greater hypotensive effect
Adverse Reactions
>10%: Central nervous system: Headache (dose-related 1.9% to 22%)
1% to 10%:
  Cardiovascular: Edema (dose-related 1.2% to 8.7%), palpitations (dose-related 0.8% to 5.1%), flushing (dose-related 0.8% to 5.1%), tachycardia (1% to 3.4%), chest pain (1.7% to 2.7%)
  Central nervous system: Dizziness (1.6% to 8%), fatigue (dose-related 0.4% to 8.5%), flushing (9%)
  Dermatologic: Rash (1.5% to 2%)
  Gastrointestinal: Nausea (1% to 5.1%), abdominal discomfort (0% to 3.3%), vomiting (0% to 1.3%), diarrhea (0% to 3.4%)
  Renal: Urinary frequency (1.3% to 3.4%)
  Respiratory: Dyspnea (0.5% to 3.4%)
0.5% to 1% (Limited to important or life-threatening): Atrial fibrillation, cough, cramps of legs and feet, depression, dyspnea, gingival hyperplasia (incidence unknown), heart failure, hypotension, impotence, insomnia, lethargy, leukopenia, myocardial infarction, paresthesias, pruritus, stroke, syncope, urticaria, ventricular fibrillation
Overdosage/Toxicology
Primary cardiac symptoms of calcium blocker overdose include hypotension and bradycardia. Hypotension is caused by peripheral vasodilation, myocardial depression, and bradycardia. Bradycardia results from sinus bradycardia, second- or third-degree atrioventricular block, or sinus arrest with junctional rhythm. Intraventricular conduction is usually not affected so the QRS duration is normal (verapamil prolongs the PR interval and bepridil prolongs the QT interval and may cause ventricular arrhythmias, including torsade de pointes).
Noncardiac symptoms include confusion, stupor, nausea, vomiting, metabolic acidosis and hyperglycemia. Following initial gastric decontamination, if possible, repeated calcium administration may promptly reverse depressed cardiac contractility (but not sinus node depression or peripheral vasodilation). Glucagon, epinephrine, and inamrinone (amrinone) may treat refractory hypotension. Glucagon and epinephrine also increase the heart rate (outside the U.S., 4-aminopyridine may be available as an antidote). Dialysis and hemoperfusion are not effective in enhancing elimination, although repeat-dose activated charcoal may serve as an adjunct with sustained-release preparations.
In a few reported cases, overdose with calcium channel blockers has been associated with hypotension and bradycardia, initially refractory to atropine, but becoming more responsive to this agent when larger doses (approaching 1 g/hour for more than 24 hours) of calcium chloride were administered.
Drug Interactions
Cytochrome P450 Effect: CYP3A3/4 enzyme substrate
Increased Effect/Toxicity: Isradipine may increase cardiovascular adverse effects of betablockers. Isradipine may minimally increase cyclosporine levels. Azole antifungals (and potentially other inhibitors of CYP3A3/4) may increase levels of isradipine; avoid this combination.
Decreased Effect: NSAIDs (diclofenac) may decrease the antihypertensive response of isradipine. Isradipine may cause a decrease in lovastatin effect. Rifampin may reduce blood levels and effects of isradipine due to enzyme induction (other enzyme inducers may share this effect).
(Continued)

Isradipine *(Continued)*

Ethanol/Nutrition/Herb Interactions
Food: Administration with food delays absorption, but does not affect availability

Herb/Nutraceutical: St John's wort may decrease isradipine levels. Avoid dong quai if using for hypertension (has estrogenic activity). Avoid ephedra, yohimbe, ginseng (may worsen hypertension). Avoid garlic (may have increased antihypertensive effect).

Mechanism of Action Inhibits calcium ion from entering the "slow channels" or select voltage-sensitive areas of vascular smooth muscle and myocardium during depolarization, producing a relaxation of coronary vascular smooth muscle and coronary vasodilation; increases myocardial oxygen delivery in patients with vasospastic angina

Pharmacodynamics/Kinetics
Duration: 8-16 hours

Absorption: 90% to 95%

Protein binding: 95%

Metabolism: Hepatic; extensive first-pass effect

Bioavailability: 15% to 24%

Half-life elimination: 8 hours

Time to peak, serum: 1-1.5 hours

Excretion: Urine (as metabolites)

Usual Dosage Adults: 2.5 mg twice daily; antihypertensive response occurs in 2-3 hours; maximal response in 2-4 weeks; increase dose at 2- to 4-week intervals at 2.5-5 mg increments; usual dose range: 5-20 mg/day. **Note:** Most patients show no improvement with doses >10 mg/day except adverse reaction rate increases

Dietary Considerations May be taken without regard to meals.

Administration May open capsule; avoid crushing contents

Patient Information Do not discontinue abruptly; report any dizziness, shortness of breath, palpitations, or edema

Nursing Implications Do not crush extended release tablets.

Dosage Forms
Capsule: 2.5 mg, 5 mg

Tablet, extended release: 5 mg, 10 mg

Extemporaneous Preparations A 1 mg/mL oral liquid was stable for 35 days when refrigerated when compounded as follows:

Dissolve the contents of ten 5 mg capsules in simple syrup, qs ad 50 mL

Shake well before using and keep in refrigerator

MacDonald JL, Johnson CE, and Jacobson P, "Stability of Isradipine in Extemporaneously Compounded Oral Liquids," *Am J Hosp Pharm*, 1994, 51(19):2409-11.

♦ **Isuprel**® *see Isoproterenol on page 749*

Itraconazole *(i tra KOE na zole)*

Related Information
Antifungal Agents Comparison *on page 1484*

USPHA/IDSA Guidelines for the Prevention of Opportunistic Infections in Persons With HIV *on page 1574*

U.S. Brand Names Sporanox®

Canadian Brand Names Sporanox®

Therapeutic Category Antifungal Agent, Imidazole Derivative; Antifungal Agent, Systemic

Use Treatment of susceptible fungal infections in immunocompromised and immunocompetent patients including blastomycosis and histoplasmosis; indicated for aspergillosis, and onychomycosis of the toenail; treatment of onychomycosis of the fingernail without concomitant toenail infection via a pulse-type dosing regimen; has activity against *Aspergillus, Candida, Coccidioides, Cryptococcus, Sporothrix,* tinea unguium

Oral: Useful in superficial mycoses including dermatophytoses (eg, tinea capitis), pityriasis versicolor, sebopsoriasis, vaginal and chronic mucocutaneous candidiases; systemic mycoses including candidiasis, meningeal and disseminated cryptococcal infections, paracoccidioidomycosis, coccidioidomycoses; miscellaneous mycoses such as sporotrichosis, chromomycosis, leishmaniasis, fungal keratitis, alternariosis, zygomycosis

Oral solution (not capsules): Marketed for oral and esophageal candidiasis

Intravenous solution: Indicated in the treatment of blastomycosis, histoplasmosis (nonmeningeal), and aspergillosis (in patients intolerant or refractory to amphotericin B therapy)

Pregnancy Risk Factor C

Pregnancy/Breast-Feeding Implications Should not be used to treat onychomycosis during pregnancy. Effective contraception should be used during treatment and for 2 months following treatment.

Contraindications Hypersensitivity to itraconazole, any component of the formulation, or to other azoles; concurrent administration with astemizole, cisapride, dofetilide, lovastatin, midazolam, pimozide, quinidine, or simvastatin; treatment of onychomycosis in patients with evidence of left ventricular dysfunction, CHF, or a history of CHF

Warnings/Precautions Rare cases of serious cardiovascular adverse events, including death, ventricular tachycardia and torsade de pointes have been observed due to increased terfenadine and cisapride concentrations induced by itraconazole. Patients who develop abnormal liver function tests during itraconazole therapy should be monitored and therapy discontinued if symptoms of liver disease develop. Itraconazole injection is not recommended in patients with Cl_{cr} <30 mL/minute. Discontinue if signs or symptoms of CHF occur during treatment. Use with caution in patients with left ventricular dysfunction or a history of CHF when itraconazole is being used for indications other than onychomycosis. Discontinue if signs or symptoms of CHF occur during treatment.

Adverse Reactions Listed incidences are for higher doses appropriate for systemic fungal infections.

>10%: Gastrointestinal: Nausea (11%)

1% to 10%:
  Cardiovascular: Edema (4%), hypertension (3%)
  Central nervous system: Headache (4%), fatigue (2% to 3%), malaise (1%), fever (3%), dizziness (2%)
  Dermatologic: Rash (9%), pruritus (3%)
  Endocrine & metabolic: Decreased libido (1%), hypertriglyceridemia, hypokalemia (2%)
  Gastrointestinal: Abdominal pain (2%), anorexia (1%), vomiting (5%), diarrhea (3%)
  Hepatic: Abnormal LFTs (3%), hepatitis
  Renal: Albuminuria (1%)
<1% (Limited to important or life-threatening): Adrenal suppression, allergic reactions (urticaria, angioedema), alopecia, anaphylaxis, arrhythmia, CHF, constipation, gastritis, gynecomastia, hepatic failure, impotence, neuropathy, neutropenia, somnolence, Stevens-Johnson syndrome, tinnitus

Overdosage/Toxicology Overdoses are well tolerated. Following decontamination, if possible, supportive measures only are required. Dialysis is not effective.

Drug Interactions
  Cytochrome P450 Effect: CYP3A3/4 enzyme substrate; CYP3A3/4 enzyme inhibitor
  Increased Effect/Toxicity: Due to inhibition of hepatic CYP3A3/4, itraconazole use is contraindicated with astemizole, cisapride, dofetilide, lovastatin, midazolam, pimozide, quinidine, simvastatin, and triazolam due to large substantial increases in the toxicity of these agents. Itraconazole may also increase the levels of benzodiazepines (alprazolam, diazepam, and others), buspirone, busulfan, calcium channel blockers (felodipine, nifedipine, verapamil), cyclosporine, digoxin, docetaxel, HMG-CoA reductase inhibitors (except fluvastatin, pravastatin), oral hypoglycemics (sulfonylureas), methylprednisolone, phenytoin, sirolimus, tacrolimus, trimetrexate, vincristine, vinblastine, warfarin, and zolpidem. Other medications metabolized by CYP3A3/4 should be used with caution. Amprenavir (and possibly other protease inhibitors), clarithromycin, and erythromycin may increase itraconazole concentrations.
  Decreased Effect: Decreased serum levels with carbamazepine, didanosine (oral solution only), isoniazid, phenobarbital, phenytoin, rifabutin, and rifampin. **Should not be administered concomitantly with rifampin.** Absorption requires gastric acidity; therefore, antacids, H₂ antagonists (cimetidine, famotidine, nizatidine, and ranitidine), proton pump inhibitors (omeprazole, lansoprazole, rabeprazole), and sucralfate may significantly reduce bioavailability resulting in treatment failures and should not be administered concomitantly. Oral contraceptive efficacy may be reduced (limited data).

Ethanol/Nutrition/Herb Interactions
  Food: Capsules: Enhanced by food and possibly by gastric acidity; avoid grapefruit juice. Solution: Decreased by food, time to peak concentration prolonged by food. Absorption of both products is increased when taken with a cola beverage.
  Herb/Nutraceutical: St John's wort may decrease itraconazole levels.

Stability Dilute with 0.9% sodium chloride only; do not dilute in dextrose or lactated Ringer's; may be stored refrigerated or at room temperature for 48 hours; use dedicated infusion line; do not mix with any other medication. A precise mixing ratio is required to maintain stability (3.33:1) and avoid precipitate formation. Add 25 mL (1 ampul) to 50 mL 0.9% sodium chloride. Mix and withdraw 15 mL of solution before infusing.

Mechanism of Action Interferes with cytochrome P450 activity, decreasing ergosterol synthesis (principal sterol in fungal cell membrane) and inhibiting cell membrane formation

Pharmacodynamics/Kinetics
  Absorption: Requires gastric acidity; capsule better absorbed with food, solution better absorbed on empty stomach; hypochlorhydria has been reported in HIV-infected patients; therefore, oral absorption in these patients may be decreased
  Distribution: V_d (average): 796 ± 185 L or 10 L/kg; highly lipophilic and tissue concentrations are higher than plasma concentrations. The highest concentrations: adipose, omentum, endometrium, cervical and vaginal mucus, and skin/nails. Aqueous fluids (eg, CSF and urine) contain negligible amounts.
  Protein binding, plasma: 99.9%; metabolite hydroxy-itraconazole: 99.5%
  Metabolism: Extensively hepatic into >30 metabolites including hydroxy-itraconazole (major metabolite); appears to have in vitro antifungal activity. The main metabolic pathway is oxidation; may undergo saturation metabolism with multiple dosing
  Bioavailability: 55%; Fasting: 40%; Postprandial: 100%
  Half-life elimination: Oral: After single 200 mg dose: 21 ± 5 hours; 64 hours at steady-state; I.V.: steady-state: 35 hours; steady-state concentrations are achieved in 13 days with multiple administration of itraconazole 100-400 mg/day.
  Excretion: Feces (~3% to 18%); urine (~0.03% as parent drug, 40% as metabolites)

Usual Dosage Note: Capsule: Absorption is best if taken with food, therefore, it is best to administer itraconazole after meals; Solution: Should be taken on an empty stomach. Absorption of both products is significantly increased when taken with a cola beverage.

  Children: Efficacy and safety have not been established; a small number of patients 3-16 years of age have been treated with 100 mg/day for systemic fungal infections with no serious adverse effects reported
  Adults:
    Oral:
      Blastomycosis/histoplasmosis: 200 mg once daily, if no obvious improvement or there is evidence of progressive fungal disease, increase the dose in 100 mg increments to a maximum of 400 mg/day; doses >200 mg/day are given in 2 divided doses; length of therapy varies from 1 day to >6 months depending on the condition and mycological response
      Aspergillosis: 200-400 mg/day
      Onychomycosis: 200 mg once daily for 12 consecutive weeks
      Life-threatening infections: Loading dose: 200 mg 3 times/day (600 mg/day) should be given for the first 3 days of therapy
      Oropharyngeal and esophageal candidiasis: Oral solution: 100-200 mg once daily
    I.V.: 200 mg twice daily for 4 doses, followed by 200 mg daily
  (Continued)

Itraconazole (Continued)

Dosing adjustment in renal impairment: Not necessary; itraconazole injection is not recommended in patients with Cl_{cr} <30 mL/minute

Hemodialysis: Not dialyzable

Dosing adjustment in hepatic impairment: May be necessary, but specific guidelines are not available. Risk-to-benefit evaluation should be undertaken in patients who develop liver function abnormalities during treatment.

Dietary Considerations

Capsule: Administer with food.

Solution: Take without food, if possible.

Administration

Oral: Doses >200 mg/day are administered in 2 divided doses; do not administer with antacids.

I.V.: Using a flow control device, infuse 60 mL of the dilute solution (3.33 mg/mL = 200 mg itraconazole, pH ~4.8) intravenously over 60 minutes, using an extension line and the infusion set provided. After administration, flush the infusion set with 15-20 mL of 0.9% sodium chloride over 30 seconds to 15 minutes, via the two-way stopcock. Do not use bacteriostatic sodium chloride injection, USP. The compatibility of Sporanox® injection with flush solutions other than 0.9% sodium chloride (normal saline) is not known. Discard the entire infusion line.

Monitoring Parameters Left ventricular function in patients with pre-existing hepatic dysfunction, and in all patients being treated for longer than 1 month

Patient Information Take capsule with food; take solution on an empty stomach; report any signs and symptoms that may suggest liver dysfunction so that the appropriate laboratory testing can be done; signs and symptoms may include unusual fatigue, anorexia, nausea and/or vomiting, jaundice, dark urine, or pale stool

Nursing Implications

Oral: Doses >200 mg/day are given in 2 divided doses; do not administer with antacids.

I.V.: Infuse over 1 hour

Additional Information Due to potential toxicity, the manufacturer recommends confirmation of diagnosis testing of nail specimens prior to treatment of onychomycosis.

Dosage Forms

Capsule: 100 mg

Injection [kit]: 10 mg/mL - 25 mL ampul, one 50 mL (100 mL capacity) bag 0.9% sodium chloride, one filtered infusion set

Solution, oral: 100 mg/10 mL (150 mL)

♦ Iveegam Immuno® (Can) *see* Immune Globulin (Intravenous) *on page 711*

Ivermectin (eye ver MEK tin)

U.S. Brand Names Stromectol®

Therapeutic Category Antibiotic, Miscellaneous

Use Treatment of the following infections: Strongyloidiasis of the intestinal tract due to the nematode parasite *Strongyloides stercoralis*. Onchocerciasis due to the nematode parasite *Onchocerca volvulus*. Ivermectin is only active against the immature form of *Onchocerca volvulus*, and the intestinal forms of *Strongyloides stercoralis*. Ivermectin has been used for other parasitic infections including *Ascaris lumbricoides*, Bancroftian filariasis, *Brugia malayi*, scabies, *Enterobius vermicularis*, *Mansonella ozzardi*, *Trichuris trichiura*.

Pregnancy Risk Factor C

Pregnancy/Breast-Feeding Implications Safety and efficacy have not been established in pregnant women. The WHO considers use after the first trimester as "probably acceptable."

Contraindications Hypersensitivity to ivermectin or any component of the formulation

Warnings/Precautions Data have shown that antihelmintic drugs like ivermectin may cause cutaneous and/or systemic reactions (Mazzoti reaction) of varying severity including ophthalmological reactions in patients with onchocerciasis. These reactions are probably due to allergic and inflammatory responses to the death of microfilariae. Patients with hyper-reactive onchodermatitis may be more likely than others to experience severe adverse reactions, especially edema and aggravation of the onchodermatitis. Repeated treatment may be required in immunocompromised patients (eg, HIV); control of extraintestinal strongyloidiasis may necessitate suppressive (once monthly) therapy. Pretreatment assessment for *Loa loa* infection is recommended in any patient with significant exposure to endemic areas (West and Central Africa); serious and/or fatal encephalopathy has been reported during treatment in patients with loiasis.

Adverse Reactions Frequency not defined.

Cardiovascular: Hypotension, mild EKG changes, peripheral and facial edema, transient tachycardia

Central nervous system: Dizziness, headache, hyperthermia, insomnia, somnolence, vertigo

Dermatologic: Pruritus, rash, urticaria

Gastrointestinal: Abdominal pain, diarrhea, nausea, vomiting

Hematologic: Eosinophilia, leukopenia

Hepatic: Increased ALT/AST

Neuromuscular & skeletal: Limbitis, myalgia, tremor, weakness

Ocular: Blurred vision, mild conjunctivitis, punctate opacity

Mazzotti reaction (with onchocerciasis): Edema, fever, lymphadenopathy, ocular damage, pruritus, rash

Overdosage/Toxicology Accidental intoxication with, or significant exposure to unknown quantities of veterinary formulations of ivermectin in humans, either by ingestion, inhalation, injection, or exposure to body surfaces, has resulted in the following adverse effects: rash, edema, headache, dizziness, asthenia, nausea, vomiting, and diarrhea. Other adverse effects that have been reported include seizure and ataxia. Treatment is supportive. The usual methods for decontamination are recommended.

Mechanism of Action Ivermectin is a semisynthetic antihelminthic agent; it binds selectively and with strong affinity to glutamate-gated chloride ion channels which occur in invertebrate nerve and muscle cells. This leads to increased permeability of cell membranes to chloride ions then hyperpolarization of the nerve or muscle cell, and death of the parasite.

Pharmacodynamics/Kinetics
Onset of action: Peak effect: 3-6 months
Absorption: Well absorbed
Distribution: Does not cross blood-brain barrier
Half-life elimination: 16-35 hours
Metabolism: Hepatic, >97%
Excretion: Urine (<1%); remainder in feces

Usual Dosage Oral:
Children ≥5 years: 150 mcg/kg as a single dose; treatment for onchocerciasis may need to be repeated every 3-12 months until the adult worms die
Adults:
Strongyloidiasis: 200 mcg/kg as a single dose; follow-up stool examinations
Onchocerciasis: 150 mcg/kg as a single dose; retreatment may be required every 3-12 months until the adult worms die

Monitoring Parameters Skin and eye microfilarial counts, periodic ophthalmologic exams

Patient Information If infected with strongyloidiasis, repeated stool examinations are required to document clearance of the organisms; repeated follow-up and retreatment is usually required in the treatment of onchocerciasis

Nursing Implications Ensure that patients take ivermectin with water

Dosage Forms Tablet: 3 mg, 6 mg

♦ **IVIG** *see* Immune Globulin (Intravenous) *on page 711*

♦ **IvyBlock® [OTC]** *see* Bentoquatam *on page 154*

Japanese Encephalitis Virus Vaccine (Inactivated)
(jap a NEESE en sef a LYE tis VYE rus vak SEEN, in ak ti VAY ted)

U.S. Brand Names JE-VAX®

Canadian Brand Names JE-VAX®

Therapeutic Category Vaccine, Live Virus

Use Active immunization against Japanese encephalitis for persons 1 year of age and older who plan to spend 1 month or more in endemic areas in Asia, especially persons traveling during the transmission season or visiting rural areas; consider vaccination for shorter trips to epidemic areas or extensive outdoor activities in rural endemic areas; elderly (>55 years of age) individuals should be considered for vaccination, since they have increased risk of developing symptomatic illness after infection; those planning travel to or residence in endemic areas should consult the Travel Advisory Service (Central Campus) for specific advice

Pregnancy Risk Factor C

Contraindications Serious adverse reaction (generalized urticaria or angioedema) to a prior dose of this vaccine; proven or suspected hypersensitivity to proteins or rodent or neural origin; hypersensitivity to thimerosal (used as a preservative). *CDC recommends that the following should not generally receive the vaccine, unless benefit to the individual clearly outweighs the risk:*
  • those acutely ill or with active infections
  • persons with heart, kidney, or liver disorders
  • persons with generalized malignancies such as leukemia or lymphoma
  • persons with a history of multiple allergies or hypersensitivity to components of the vaccine
  • pregnant women, unless there is a very high risk of Japanese encephalitis during the woman's stay in Asia

Warnings/Precautions Severe adverse reactions manifesting as generalized urticaria or angioedema may occur within minutes following vaccination, or up to 17 days later; most reactions occur within 10 days, with the majority within 48 hours; observe vaccinees for 30 minutes after vaccination; warn them of the possibility of delayed generalized urticaria and to remain where medical care is readily available for 10 days following any dose of the vaccine; because of the potential for severe adverse reactions, Japanese encephalitis vaccine is **not** recommended for all persons traveling to or residing in Asia; safety and efficacy in infants <1 year of age have not been established; therefore, immunization of infants should be deferred whenever possible; it is not known whether the vaccine is excreted in breast milk

Adverse Reactions Report allergic or unusual adverse reactions to the Vaccine Adverse Event Reporting System (VAERS) 1-800-822-7967.
Frequency not defined:
Common: Tenderness, redness, and swelling at injection site; systemic side effects (fever, headache, malaise, rash, chills, dizziness, myalgia, nausea, vomiting, abdominal pain, urticaria, itching with or without accompanying rash, and hypotension)
Rare: Anaphylactic reaction, angioedema, dyspnea, encephalitis, encephalopathy, erythema multiforme, erythema nodosum, joint swelling, peripheral neuropathy, seizure

Stability Refrigerate, discard 8 hours after reconstitution

Usual Dosage U.S. recommended primary immunization schedule:
Children 1-3 years: S.C.: Three 0.5 mL doses given on days 0, 7, and 30; abbreviated schedules should be used only when necessary due to time constraints
Children >3 years and Adults: S.C.: Three 1 mL doses given on days 0, 7, and 30. Give third dose on day 14 when time does not permit waiting; 2 doses a week apart produce immunity in about 80% of recipients; the longest regimen yields highest titers after 6 months.
Booster dose: Give after 2 years, or according to current recommendation
Note: Travel should not commence for at least 10 days after the last dose of vaccine, to allow adequate antibody formation and recognition of any delayed adverse reaction
Advise concurrent use of other means to reduce the risk of mosquito exposure when possible, including bed nets, insect repellents, protective clothing, avoidance of travel in endemic areas, and avoidance of outdoor activity during twilight and evening periods
(Continued)

Japanese Encephalitis Virus Vaccine (Inactivated) *(Continued)*

Administration The single-dose vial should only be reconstituted with the full 1.3 mL of diluent supplied; administer 1 mL of the resulting liquid as one standard adult dose; discard the unused portion

Patient Information Adverse reactions may occur shortly after vaccination or up to 17 days (usually within 10 days) after vaccination

Nursing Implications Adverse reactions may occur shortly after vaccination or up to 17 days (usually within 10 days) after vaccination

Additional Information Japanese encephalitis vaccine is currently available only from the Centers for Disease Control. Contact Centers for Disease Control at (404) 639-6370 (Mon-Fri) or (404) 639-2888 (nights, weekends, or holidays). Federal law requires that the date of administration, the vaccine manufacturer, lot number of vaccine, and the administering person's name, title and address be entered into the patient's permanent medical record.

Dosage Forms Powder for injection, lyophilized: 1 mL, 10 mL

- ◆ **Jenest™-28** *see Ethinyl Estradiol and Norethindrone on page 522*
- ◆ **JE-VAX®** *see Japanese Encephalitis Virus Vaccine (Inactivated) on page 759*
- ◆ **Junior Strength Motrin® [OTC]** *see Ibuprofen on page 697*
- ◆ **K+ 10®** *see Potassium Chloride on page 1108*
- ◆ **Kabikinase® (Can)** *see Streptokinase on page 1260*
- ◆ **Kadian™** *see Morphine Sulfate on page 936*
- ◆ **Kala® [OTC]** *see Lactobacillus on page 770*
- ◆ **Kaletra™** *see Lopinavir and Ritonavir on page 817*

Kanamycin *(kan a MYE sin)*

Related Information
Antimicrobial Drugs of Choice *on page 1588*
Tuberculosis Prophylaxis *on page 1572*
Tuberculosis Treatment Guidelines *on page 1612*

U.S. Brand Names Kantrex®

Canadian Brand Names Kantrex®

Synonyms Kanamycin Sulfate

Therapeutic Category Antibiotic, Aminoglycoside

Use

Oral: Preoperative bowel preparation in the prophylaxis of infections and adjunctive treatment of hepatic coma (oral kanamycin is not indicated in the treatment of systemic infections); treatment of susceptible bacterial infection including gram-negative aerobes, gram-positive *Bacillus* as well as some

Parenteral: Treatment of susceptible bacterial infection including gram-negative aerobes, gram-positive *Bacillus* as well as some mycobacteria

Intraperitoneal: Rarely used in irrigations during surgery

Aerosol: Management of bronchopulmonary infections, usually in cystic fibrosis patients

Pregnancy Risk Factor D

Usual Dosage

Children: Infections: I.M., I.V.: 15 mg/kg/day in divided doses every 8-12 hours

Adults:

Infections: I.M., I.V.: 5-7.5 mg/kg/dose in divided doses every 8-12 hours (<15 mg/kg/day)

Preoperative intestinal antisepsis: Oral: 1 g every 4-6 hours for 36-72 hours

Hepatic coma: Oral: 8-12 g/day in divided doses

Intraperitoneal: After contamination in surgery: 500 mg diluted in 20 mL distilled water; other irrigations: 0.25% solutions

Aerosol: 250 mg 2-4 times/day (250 mg diluted with 3 mL of NS and nebulized)

Dosing adjustment/interval in renal impairment:

Cl_{cr} 50-80 mL/minute: Administer 60% to 90% of dose or administer every 8-12 hours

Cl_{cr} 10-50 mL/minute: Administer 30% to 70% of dose or administer every 12 hours

Cl_{cr} <10 mL/minute: Administer 20% to 30% of dose or administer every 24-48 hours

Hemodialysis: Dialyzable (50% to 100%)

Additional Information Complete prescribing information for this medication should be consulted for additional detail.

Dosage Forms

Capsule, as sulfate: 500 mg

Injection, as sulfate:

Adults: 500 mg (2 mL); 1 g (3 mL)

Pediatrics: 75 mg (2 mL)

- ◆ **Kanamycin Sulfate** *see Kanamycin on page 760*
- ◆ **Kantrex®** *see Kanamycin on page 760*
- ◆ **Kaochlor®** *see Potassium Chloride on page 1108*
- ◆ **Kaochlor® SF** *see Potassium Chloride on page 1108*
- ◆ **Kaon®** *see Potassium Gluconate on page 1110*
- ◆ **Kaon-Cl®** *see Potassium Chloride on page 1108*
- ◆ **Kaon-Cl-10®** *see Potassium Chloride on page 1108*
- ◆ **Kaopectate® II [OTC]** *see Loperamide on page 816*
- ◆ **Karidium®** *see Fluoride on page 574*
- ◆ **Karigel®** *see Fluoride on page 574*
- ◆ **Karigel®-N** *see Fluoride on page 574*
- ◆ **Kay Ciel®** *see Potassium Chloride on page 1108*
- ◆ **Kayexalate®** *see Sodium Polystyrene Sulfonate on page 1249*
- ◆ **K+ Care®** *see Potassium Chloride on page 1108*
- ◆ **KCl** *see Potassium Chloride on page 1108*
- ◆ **K-Dur® (Can)** *see Potassium Chloride on page 1108*

- ♦ **K-Dur® 10** *see* Potassium Chloride *on page 1108*
- ♦ **K-Dur® 20** *see* Potassium Chloride *on page 1108*
- ♦ **Keflex®** *see* Cephalexin *on page 261*
- ♦ **Keftab®** *see* Cephalexin *on page 261*
- ♦ **Kefurox®** *see* Cefuroxime *on page 258*
- ♦ **Kefzol®** *see* Cefazolin *on page 240*
- ♦ **Kemadrin®** *see* Procyclidine *on page 1137*
- ♦ **Kenacort®** *see* Triamcinolone *on page 1366*
- ♦ **Kenaject-40®** *see* Triamcinolone *on page 1366*
- ♦ **Kenalog®** *see* Triamcinolone *on page 1366*
- ♦ **Kenalog-10®** *see* Triamcinolone *on page 1366*
- ♦ **Kenalog-40®** *see* Triamcinolone *on page 1366*
- ♦ **Kenalog® H** *see* Triamcinolone *on page 1366*
- ♦ **Kenalog® in Orabase®** *see* Triamcinolone *on page 1366*
- ♦ **Kenonel®** *see* Triamcinolone *on page 1366*
- ♦ **Keoxifene Hydrochloride** *see* Raloxifene *on page 1176*
- ♦ **Keppra®** *see* Levetiracetam *on page 787*
- ♦ **Kerlone®** *see* Betaxolol *on page 164*
- ♦ **Kestrone®** *see* Estrone *on page 502*
- ♦ **Ketalar®** *see* Ketamine *on page 761*

Ketamine (KEET a meen)

Related Information

Adult ACLS Algorithms *on page 1632*

U.S. Brand Names Ketalar®

Canadian Brand Names Ketalar®

Synonyms Ketamine Hydrochloride

Therapeutic Category General Anesthetic

Use Induction and maintenance of general anesthesia, especially when cardiovascular depression must be avoided (ie, hypotension, hypovolemia, cardiomyopathy, constrictive pericarditis); sedation; analgesia

Restrictions C-III

Pregnancy Risk Factor D

Contraindications Hypersensitivity to ketamine or any component of the formulation; elevated intracranial pressure; hypertension, aneurysms, thyrotoxicosis, congestive heart failure, angina, psychotic disorders

Warnings/Precautions Postanesthetic emergence reactions which can manifest as vivid dreams, hallucinations and/or frank delirium occur in 12% of patients; these reactions are less common in patients >65 and when given I.M.; emergence reactions, confusion, or irrational behavior may occur up to 24 hours postoperatively and may be reduced by pretreatment with a benzodiazepine. May cause dependence (withdrawal symptoms on discontinuation) and tolerance with prolonged use.

Adverse Reactions

>10%:
- Cardiovascular: Hypertension, increased cardiac output, paradoxical direct myocardial depression, tachycardia
- Central nervous system: Increased intracranial pressure, visual hallucinations, vivid dreams
- Neuromuscular & skeletal: Tonic-clonic movements, tremors
- Miscellaneous: Emergence reactions, vocalization

1% to 10%:
- Cardiovascular: Bradycardia, hypotension
- Dermatologic: Pain at injection site, skin rash
- Gastrointestinal: Anorexia, nausea, vomiting
- Ocular: Diplopia, nystagmus
- Respiratory: Respiratory depression

<1% (Limited to important or life-threatening): Anaphylaxis, cardiac arrhythmias, cough reflex may be depressed, decreased bronchospasm, fasciculations, hypersalivation, increased airway resistance, increased intraocular pressure, increased metabolic rate, increased skeletal muscle tone, laryngospasm, myocardial depression, respiratory depression or apnea with large doses or rapid infusions

Overdosage/Toxicology With excessive dosing or too-rapid administration, symptoms include respiratory depression. Supportive care is the treatment of choice. Mechanical respiratory support is preferred.

Drug Interactions

Cytochrome P450 Effect: CYP3A enzyme substrate

Increased Effect/Toxicity: Barbiturates, narcotics, hydroxyzine increase prolonged recovery; nondepolarizing neuromuscular blockers may increase effects. Muscle relaxants, thyroid hormones may increase blood pressure and heart rate. Halothane may decrease BP.

Stability Do not mix with barbiturates or diazepam (precipitation may occur).

Mechanism of Action Produces a cataleptic-like state in which the patient is dissociated from the surrounding environment by direct action on the cortex and limbic system. Releases endogenous catecholamines (epinephrine, norepinephrine) which maintain blood pressure and heart rate. Reduces polysynaptic spinal reflexes.

Pharmacodynamics/Kinetics

Onset of action:
- I.V.: General anesthesia: 1-2 minutes; Sedation: 1-2 minutes
- I.M.: General anesthesia: 3-8 minutes

Duration: I.V.: 5-15 minutes; I.M.: 12-25 minutes

(Continued)

Ketamine (Continued)

Metabolism: Hepatic via hydroxylation and N-demethylation; the metabolite norketamine is 25% as potent as parent compound

Half-life: 11-17 minutes; Elimination: 2.5-3.1 hours

Excretion: Clearance: 18 mL/kg/minute

Usual Dosage Used in combination with anticholinergic agents to decrease hypersalivation

Children:

Oral: 6-10 mg/kg for 1 dose (mixed in 0.2-0.3 mL/kg of cola or other beverage) given 30 minutes before the procedure

I.M.: 3-7 mg/kg

I.V.: Range: 0.5-2 mg/kg, use smaller doses (0.5-1 mg/kg) for sedation for minor procedures; usual induction dosage: 1-2 mg/kg

Continuous I.V. infusion: Sedation: 5-20 mcg/kg/minute

Adults:

I.M.: 3-8 mg/kg

I.V.: Range: 1-4.5 mg/kg; usual induction dosage: 1-2 mg/kg

Children and Adults: Maintenance: Supplemental doses of $^1/_3$ to $^1/_2$ of initial dose

Administration

Oral: Use 100 mg/mL I.V. solution and mix the appropriate dose in 0.2-0.3 mL/kg of cola or other beverage

Parenteral: I.V.: Do not exceed 0.5 mg/kg/minute or administer faster than 60 seconds; do not exceed final concentration of 2 mg/mL; dilute for I.V. administration with normal saline, sterile water, or D_5W

Monitoring Parameters Cardiovascular effects, heart rate, blood pressure, respiratory rate, transcutaneous O_2 saturation

Additional Information Produces emergence psychosis including auditory and visual hallucinations, restlessness, disorientation, vivid dreams, and irrational behavior in 15% to 30% of patients; pretreatment with a benzodiazepine reduces incidence of psychosis by >50%. Spontaneous involuntary movements, nystagmus, hypertonus, and vocalizations are also commonly seen.

The analgesia outlasts the general anesthetic component. Bronchodilation is beneficial in asthmatic or COPD patients. Laryngeal reflexes may remain intact or may be obtunded. The direct myocardial depressant action of ketamine can be seen in stressed, catecholamine-deficient patients. Ketamine increases cerebral metabolism and cerebral blood flow while producing a noncompetitive block of the neuronal postsynaptic NMDA receptor. It lowers seizure threshold and stimulates salivary secretions (atropine/scopolamine treatment is recommended).

Dosage Forms Injection, as hydrochloride: 10 mg/mL (20 mL, 25 mL, 50 mL); 50 mg/mL (10 mL); 100 mg/mL (5 mL)

♦ **Ketamine Hydrochloride** see Ketamine on page 761

Ketoconazole (kee toe KOE na zole)

Related Information

Antacid Drug Interactions on page 1477

Antifungal Agents Comparison on page 1484

USPHA/IDSA Guidelines for the Prevention of Opportunistic Infections in Persons With HIV on page 1574

U.S. Brand Names Nizoral®; Nizoral® A-D Shampoo [OTC]

Canadian Brand Names Apo®-Ketoconazole; Nizoral®; Novo-Ketoconazole

Therapeutic Category Antifungal Agent, Imidazole Derivative; Antifungal Agent, Systemic; Antifungal Agent, Topical

Use Treatment of susceptible fungal infections, including candidiasis, oral thrush, blastomycosis, histoplasmosis, paracoccidioidomycosis, coccidioidomycosis, chromomycosis, candiduria, chronic mucocutaneous candidiasis, as well as certain recalcitrant cutaneous dermatophytoses; used topically for treatment of tinea corporis, tinea cruris, tinea versicolor, and cutaneous candidiasis, seborrheic dermatitis

Pregnancy Risk Factor C

Contraindications Hypersensitivity to ketoconazole or any component of the formulation; CNS fungal infections (due to poor CNS penetration); coadministration with terfenadine, astemizole, or cisapride is contraindicated due to risk of potentially fatal cardiac arrhythmias

Warnings/Precautions Use with caution in patients with impaired hepatic function; has been associated with hepatotoxicity, including some fatalities; perform periodic liver function tests; high doses of ketoconazole may depress adrenocortical function.

Adverse Reactions

Oral:

1% to 10%:

Dermatologic: Pruritus (2%)

Gastrointestinal: Nausea/vomiting (3% to 10%), abdominal pain (1%)

<1% (Limited to important or life-threatening): Bulging fontanelles, chills, depression, diarrhea, dizziness, fever, gynecomastia, headache, hemolytic anemia, hepatotoxicity, impotence, leukopenia, photophobia, somnolence, thrombocytopenia

Cream: Severe irritation, pruritus, stinging (~5%)

Shampoo: Increases in normal hair loss, irritation (<1%), abnormal hair texture, scalp pustules, mild dryness of skin, itching, oiliness/dryness of hair

Overdosage/Toxicology Symptoms include dizziness, headache, nausea, vomiting, and diarrhea. Overdoses are well tolerated. Treatment includes supportive measures and gastric decontamination.

Drug Interactions

Cytochrome P450 Effect: CYP3A3/4 enzyme substrate; CYP1A2, 2C, 2C9, 2C19, 3A3/4, and 3A5-7 enzyme inhibitor

Increased Effect/Toxicity: Due to inhibition of hepatic CYP3A3/4, ketoconazole use is contraindicated with astemizole, cisapride, lovastatin, midazolam, simvastatin, terfenadine, and triazolam due to large substantial increases in the toxicity of these agents. Ketoconazole may also increase the levels of benzodiazepines (alprazolam. diazepam, and others), buspirone, busulfan, calcium channel blockers (felodipine, nifedipine, verapamil), cyclosporine, digoxin, docetaxel, HMG-CoA reductase inhibitors (except fluvastatin, pravastatin), oral hypoglycemics (sulfonylureas), methylprednisolone, phenytoin, quinolone, sirolimus, tacrolimus, trimetrexate, vincristine, vinblastine, warfarin, and zolpidem. Other medications metabolized by CYP3A3/4 should be used with caution. Amprenavir (and possibly other protease inhibitors), clarithromycin, and erythromycin may increase ketoconazole concentrations.

Decreased Effect: Oral: Decreased serum levels with carbamazepine, didanosine (oral solution only), isoniazid, phenobarbital, phenytoin, rifabutin, and rifampin. **Should not be administered concomitantly with rifampin.** Absorption requires gastric acidity; therefore, antacids, H$_2$ antagonists (cimetidine, famotidine, nizatidine, and ranitidine), proton pump inhibitors (omeprazole, lansoprazole, rabeprazole), and sucralfate may significantly reduce bioavailability resulting in treatment failures and should not be administered concomitantly. Oral contraceptive efficacy may be reduced (limited data).

Ethanol/Nutrition/Herb Interactions
Food: Ketoconazole peak serum levels may be prolonged if taken with food.
Herb/Nutraceutical: St John's wort may decrease ketoconazole levels.

Mechanism of Action Alters the permeability of the cell wall by blocking fungal cytochrome P450; inhibits biosynthesis of triglycerides and phospholipids by fungi; inhibits several fungal enzymes that results in a build-up of toxic concentrations of hydrogen peroxide

Pharmacodynamics/Kinetics
Absorption: Oral: Rapid (~75%); Shampoo: None
Distribution: Well into inflamed joint fluid, saliva, bile, urine, breast milk, sebum, cerumen, feces, tendons, skin and soft tissues, and testes; crosses blood-brain barrier poorly; only negligible amounts reach CSF
Protein binding: 93% to 96%
Metabolism: Partially hepatic via CYP3A3/4 to inactive compounds
Bioavailability: Decreases as gastric pH increases
Half-life elimination: Biphasic: Initial: 2 hours; Terminal: 8 hours
Time to peak, serum: 1-2 hours
Excretion: Primarily feces (57%); urine (13%)

Usual Dosage
Oral:
Children ≥2 years: 3.3-6.6 mg/kg/day as a single dose for 1-2 weeks for candidiasis, for at least 4 weeks in recalcitrant dermatophyte infections, and for up to 6 months for other systemic mycoses
Adults: 200-400 mg/day as a single daily dose for durations as stated above
Shampoo: Apply twice weekly for 4 weeks with at least 3 days between each shampoo
Topical: Rub gently into the affected area once daily to twice daily
Dosing adjustment in hepatic impairment: Dose reductions should be considered in patients with severe liver disease
Hemodialysis: Not dialyzable (0% to 5%)

Dietary Considerations May be taken with food or milk to decrease GI adverse effects.

Monitoring Parameters Liver function tests

Patient Information Cream is for topical application to the skin only; avoid contact with the eye; avoid taking antacids at the same time as ketoconazole; may take with food; may cause drowsiness, impair judgment or coordination. Notify physician of unusual fatigue, anorexia, vomiting, dark urine, or pale stools.

Nursing Implications Administer 2 hours prior to antacids to prevent decreased absorption due to the high pH of gastric contents

Dosage Forms
Cream, topical: 2% (15 g, 30 g, 60 g)
Shampoo, topical: 1% (120 mL, 207 mL); 2% (120 mL)
Tablet: 200 mg

Extemporaneous Preparations A 20 mg/mL suspension may be made by pulverizing twelve 200 mg ketoconazole tablets to a fine powder; add 40 mL Ora-Plus® in small portions with thorough mixing; incorporate Ora-Sweet® to make a final volume of 120 mL and mix thoroughly; refrigerate (no stability information is available)
Allen LV, "Ketoconazole Oral Suspension," *US Pharm*, 1993, 18(2):98-9, 101.

Ketoprofen (kee toe PROE fen)

Related Information
Nonsteroidal Anti-Inflammatory Agents Comparison *on page 1512*

U.S. Brand Names Actron® [OTC]; Orudis®; Orudis® KT [OTC]; Oruvail®

Canadian Brand Names Apo®-Keto; Apo®-Keto-E; Apo®-Keto SR; Novo-Keto; Novo-Keto-EC; Nu-Ketoprofen; Nu-Ketoprofen-E; Orafen; Orudis® SR; Oruvail®; Rhodis™; Rhodis-EC™; Rhodis SR™

Therapeutic Category Analgesic, Nonsteroidal Anti-inflammatory Drug; Anti-inflammatory Agent; Nonsteroidal Anti-inflammatory Drug (NSAID), Oral

Use Acute and long-term treatment of rheumatoid arthritis and osteoarthritis; primary dysmenorrhea; mild to moderate pain

Pregnancy Risk Factor B/D (3rd trimester)

Contraindications Hypersensitivity to ketoprofen, any component of the formulation, or other NSAIDs/aspirin; pregnancy (3rd trimester)

Warnings/Precautions Use with caution in patients with congestive heart failure, hypertension, dehydration, decreased renal or hepatic function, history of GI disease (bleeding or ulcers), or those receiving anticoagulants. Elderly are at a high risk for adverse effects from nonsteroidal anti-inflammatory agents. As many as 60% of elderly can develop peptic ulceration and/or hemorrhage asymptomatically.

Use lowest effective dose for shortest period possible. Use of NSAIDs can compromise existing renal function especially when Cl$_{cr}$ is <30 mL/minute. CNS adverse effects such as
(Continued)

Ketoprofen *(Continued)*

confusion, agitation, and hallucination are generally seen in overdose or high-dose situations; however, elderly may demonstrate these adverse effects at lower doses than younger adults. Withhold for at least 4-6 half-lives prior to surgical or dental procedures. Safety and efficacy in pediatric patients have not been established (per manufacturer).

Adverse Reactions

>10%:
  Central nervous system: Headache (11%)
  Gastrointestinal: Dyspepsia (11%)

1% to 10%:
  Central nervous system: Nervousness
  Dermatologic: Rash, itching
  Endocrine & metabolic: Fluid retention
  Gastrointestinal: Vomiting (>1%), diarrhea (3% to 9%), nausea (3% to 9%), constipation (3% to 9%), abdominal distress/cramping/pain (3% to 9%), flatulence (3% to 9%), anorexia (>1%), stomatitis (>1%)
  Genitourinary: Urinary tract infection (>1%)
  Otic: Tinnitus

<1% (Limited to important or life-threatening): Agranulocytosis, anemia, bronchospasm, bullous rash, congestive heart failure, dyspnea, exfoliative dermatitis, hematuria, hemolysis, hepatic dysfunction, hypercoagulability, hypertension, interstitial nephritis, nephrotic syndrome, palpitation, purpura, renal failure, tachycardia, thrombocytopenia

Overdosage/Toxicology Symptoms include apnea, metabolic acidosis, coma, and nystagmus; leukocytosis, renal failure. Management of nonsteroidal anti-inflammatory drug (NSAID) intoxication is primarily supportive and symptomatic. Fluid therapy is commonly effective in managing hypotension that may occur following an acute NSAID overdose, except when due to acute blood loss. Seizures tend to be very short-lived and often do not require drug treatment, although recurrent seizures should be treated with I.V. diazepam. Since many of NSAIDs undergo enterohepatic cycling, multiple doses of charcoal may be needed to reduce the potential for delayed toxicities.

Drug Interactions

Cytochrome P450 Effect: CYP2C and 2C9 enzyme inhibitor

Increased Effect/Toxicity: Increased effect/toxicity with probenecid, lithium, anticoagulants, and methotrexate.

Decreased Effect: Decreased effect of diuretics (loop and thiazides). May decrease effects of antihypertensives.

Ethanol/Nutrition/Herb Interactions

Ethanol: Avoid ethanol (due to GI irritation).

Food: Although food affects the bioavailability of ketoprofen, analgesic efficacy is not significantly diminished; food slows rate of absorption resulting in delayed and reduced peak serum concentrations.

Mechanism of Action Inhibits prostaglandin synthesis by decreasing the activity of the enzyme, cyclo-oxygenase, which results in decreased formation of prostaglandin precursors

Pharmacodynamics/Kinetics

Onset of action: Peak effect: 1-2 hours
Absorption: Almost completely
Metabolism: Hepatic
Half-life elimination: 1-4 hours
Time to peak, serum: 0.5-2 hours
Excretion: Urine (60% to 75% primarily as glucuronide conjugates)

Usual Dosage Oral:

Children 3 months to 14 years: Fever: 0.5-1 mg/kg every 6-8 hours
Children >12 years and Adults:
  Rheumatoid arthritis or osteoarthritis: 50-75 mg 3-4 times/day up to a maximum of 300 mg/day
  Mild to moderate pain: 25-50 mg every 6-8 hours up to a maximum of 300 mg/day

Dietary Considerations In order to minimize gastrointestinal effects, ketoprofen can be prescribed to be taken with food or milk.

Test Interactions ↑ chloride (S), ↑ sodium (S), ↑ bleeding time

Patient Information Take with food; may cause dizziness or drowsiness

Nursing Implications Dose must be lowest recommended in renal insufficiency and hypoalbuminemia. There are no clinical guidelines to predict which NSAID will give response in a particular patient. Trials with each must be initiated until response determined. Consider dose, patient convenience, and cost. Do not crush or break extended release capsules.

Dosage Forms

Capsule (Orudis®): 25 mg, 50 mg, 75 mg
Capsule, extended release:
  Actron®: 200 mg
  Oruvail®: 100 mg, 150 mg
Tablet (Orudis® KT): 12.5 mg

Ketorolac *(KEE toe role ak)*

Related Information

Nonsteroidal Anti-Inflammatory Agents Comparison *on page 1512*

U.S. Brand Names Acular®; Acular® PF; Toradol®

Canadian Brand Names Acular®; Apo®-Ketorolac; Novo-Ketorolac; Toradol®; Toradol® IM

Synonyms Ketorolac Tromethamine

Therapeutic Category Analgesic, Nonsteroidal Anti-inflammatory Drug; Anti-inflammatory Agent; Nonsteroidal Anti-inflammatory Drug (NSAID), Oral; Nonsteroidal Anti-inflammatory Drug (NSAID), Parenteral

Use

Oral, injection: Short-term (≤5 days) management of moderately-severe acute pain requiring analgesia at the opioid level

Ophthalmic: Temporary relief of ocular itching due to seasonal allergic conjunctivitis; postoperative inflammation following cataract extraction; reduction of ocular pain and photophobia following incisional refractive surgery

Pregnancy Risk Factor C/D (3rd trimester); ophthalmic: C

Pregnancy/Breast-Feeding Implications Ketorolac is contraindicated during labor and delivery (may inhibit uterine contractions and adversely affect fetal circulation). Avoid use of ketorolac ophthalmic solution during late pregnancy. Ketorolac enters breast milk; breast-feeding is contraindicated

Contraindications Hypersensitivity to ketorolac, aspirin, other NSAIDs, or any component of the formulation. In patients who have developed nasal polyps, angioedema, or bronchospastic reactions to other NSAIDs; active or history of peptic ulcer disease; recent or history of GI bleeding or perforation; patients with advanced renal disease or risk of renal failure, labor and delivery; nursing mothers; prophylaxis before major surgery; suspected or confirmed cerebrovascular bleeding; hemorrhagic diathesis; concurrent ASA or other NSAIDs; epidural or intrathecal administration, concomitant probenecid; pregnancy (3rd trimester)

Warnings/Precautions

Systemic: Treatment should be started with I.V./I.M. administration then changed to oral only as a continuation of treatment. Hypersensitivity reactions have occurred flowing the first dose of ketorolac injection, including patients without prior exposure to ketorolac, aspirin, or other NSAIDs. Use extra caution and reduce dosages in the elderly because it is cleared renally somewhat slower, and the elderly are also more sensitive to the renal effects of NSAIDs and have a greater risk of GI perforation and bleeding; use with caution in patients with congestive heart failure, hypertension, decreased renal or hepatic function, or those receiving anticoagulants. May prolong bleeding time; do not use when hemostasis is critical. Patients should be euvolemic prior to treatment. Withhold for at least 4-6 half-lives prior to surgical or dental procedures.

Ophthalmic: May increase bleeding time associated with ocular surgery. Use with caution in patients with known bleeding tendencies or those receiving anticoagulants. Do not administer while wearing soft contact lenses. Safety and efficacy in pediatric patients <3 years of age have not been established.

Adverse Reactions

>10%:

Systemic:

Central nervous system: Headache (17%)

Gastrointestinal: Gastrointestinal pain (13%), dyspepsia (12%), nausea (12%)

Ophthalmic solution: Ocular: Transient burning/stinging (Acular®: 40%; Acular® PF: 20%)

>1% to 10%:

Systemic:

Cardiovascular: Edema (4%), hypertension

Central nervous system: Dizziness (7%), drowsiness (6%)

Dermatologic: Pruritus, purpura, rash

Gastrointestinal: Diarrhea (7%), constipation, flatulence, gastrointestinal fullness, vomiting, stomatitis

Local: Injection site pain (2%)

Miscellaneous: Diaphoresis

Ophthalmic solution: Ocular: Ocular irritation, allergic reactions, superficial ocular infection, superficial keratitis, iritis, ocular inflammation

≤1% (Limited to important or life-threatening): Acute renal failure, anaphylactoid reaction, anaphylaxis, bronchospasm, convulsions, dyspnea, eosinophilia, extrapyramidal symptoms, GI hemorrhage, GI perforation, hemolytic uremic syndrome, hepatitis, hypersensitivity reactions, laryngeal edema, liver failure, rash, nephritis, peptic ulceration, pulmonary edema, stupor, syncope, Stevens-Johnson syndrome, thrombocytopenia, urinary retention, vertigo, toxic epidermal necrolysis, wound hemorrhage (postoperative)

Overdosage/Toxicology Symptoms include abdominal pain, peptic ulcers, and metabolic acidosis. Management of nonsteroidal anti-inflammatory (NSAID) intoxication is supportive and symptomatic. Dialysis is not effective.

Drug Interactions

Increased Effect/Toxicity: Increased toxicity: Lithium, methotrexate, probenecid increased drug level; increased effect/toxicity with salicylates, probenecid, anticoagulants, nondepolarizing muscle relaxants, alprazolam, fluoxetine, thiothixene

Decreased Effect: Decreased effect: Decreased antihypertensive effect seen with ACE inhibitors and angiotensin II antagonists; decreased antiepileptic effect seen with carbamazepine, phenytoin

Ethanol/Nutrition/Herb Interactions

Ethanol: Avoid ethanol (may enhance gastric mucosal irritation).

Food: Oral: High-fat meals may delay time to peak (by ~1 hour) and decrease peak concentrations.

Herb/Nutraceutical: Avoid cat's claw, dong quai, evening primrose, feverfew, garlic, ginger, ginkgo, red clover, horse chestnut, green tea, ginseng (all have additional antiplatelet activity).

Stability Ketorolac injection and ophthalmic solution should be stored at controlled room temperature and protected from light; injection is clear and has a slight yellow color; precipitation may occur at relatively low pH values. Store tablets at controlled room temperature. Compatible with NS, D_5W, D_5NS, LR

Incompatible with meperidine, morphine, promethazine, and hydroxyzine

Mechanism of Action Inhibits prostaglandin synthesis by decreasing the activity of the enzyme, cyclo-oxygenase, which results in decreased formation of prostaglandin precursors

Pharmacodynamics/Kinetics

Onset of action: Analgesic: I.M.: ~10 minutes

Peak effect: Analgesic: 2-3 hours

Duration: Analgesic: 6-8 hours

Absorption: Oral: Well absorbed

Distribution: Poor penetration into CSF; crosses placenta; enters breast milk

Protein binding: 99%

(Continued)

Ketorolac *(Continued)*

Metabolism: Hepatic

Half-life elimination: 2-8 hours; increased 30% to 50% in elderly

Time to peak, serum: I.M.: 30-60 minutes

Excretion: Urine (61% as unchanged drug)

Usual Dosage Note: The use of ketorolac in children <16 years of age is outside of product labeling

Children 2-16 years: Dosing guidelines are not established; **do not exceed adult doses**

Single-dose treatment:

I.M., I.V.: 0.4-1 mg/kg as a single dose; **Note:** Limited information exists. Single I.V. doses of 0.5 mg/kg, 0.75 mg/kg, 0.9 mg/kg and 1 mg/kg have been studied in children 2-16 years of age for postoperative analgesia. One study (Maunuksela, 1992) used a titrating dose starting with 0.2 mg/kg up to a total of 0.5 mg/kg (median dose required: 0.4 mg/kg).

Oral: One study used 1 mg/kg as a single dose for analgesia in 30 children (mean ± SD age: 3 ± 2.5 years) undergoing bilateral myringotomy

Multiple-dose treatment: I.M., I.V., Oral: No pediatric studies exist; one report (Buck, 1994) of the clinical experience with ketorolac in 112 children, 6 months to 19 years of age (mean: 9 years), described usual I.V. maintenance doses of 0.5 mg/kg every 6 hours (mean dose: 0.52 mg/kg; range: 0.17-1 mg/kg)

Adults (pain relief usually begins within 10 minutes with parenteral forms): **Note: The maximum combined duration of treatment (for parenteral and oral) is 5 days**; do not increase dose or frequency; supplement with low dose opioids if needed for breakthrough pain. For patients <50 kg and/or ≥65 years of age, see Elderly dosing.

I.M.: 60 mg as a single dose or 30 mg every 6 hours (maximum daily dose: 120 mg)

I.V.: 30 mg as a single dose or 30 mg every 6 hours (maximum daily dose: 120 mg)

Oral: 20 mg, followed by 10 mg every 4-6 hours; do not exceed 40 mg/day; oral dosing is intended to be a continuation of I.M. or I.V. therapy only

Ophthalmic: Children ≥3 years and Adults:

Allergic conjunctivitis (relief of ocular itching): Instill 1 drop (0.25 mg) 4 times/day for seasonal allergic conjunctivitis

Inflammation following cataract extraction: Instill 1 drop (0.25 mg) to affected eye(s) 4 times/day beginning 24 hours after surgery; continue for 2 weeks

Pain and photophobia following incisional refractive surgery: Instill 1 drop (0.25 mg) 4 times/day to affected eye for up to 3 days

Elderly >65 years: Renal insufficiency or weight <50 kg: **Note:** Ketorolac has decreased clearance and increased half-life in the elderly. In addition, the elderly have reported increased incidence of GI bleeding, ulceration, and perforation. The maximum combined duration of treatment (for parenteral and oral) is 5 days.

I.M.: 30 mg as a single dose or 15 mg every 6 hours (maximum daily dose: 60 mg)

I.V.: 15 mg as a single dose or 15 mg every 6 hours (maximum daily dose: 60 mg)

Oral: 10 mg every 4-6 hours; do not exceed 40 mg/day; oral dosing is intended to be a continuation of I.M. or I.V. therapy only

Dosage adjustment in renal impairment: Do not use in patients with advanced renal impairment. Patients with moderately-elevated serum creatinine should use half the recommended dose, not to exceed 60 mg/day I.M./I.V.

Dosage adjustment in hepatic impairment: Use with caution, may cause elevation of liver enzymes

Dietary Considerations Administer tablet with food or milk to decrease gastrointestinal distress.

Administration

Oral: May take with food to reduce GI upset

I.M.: Administer slowly and deeply into the muscle. Analgesia begins in 30 minutes and maximum effect within 2 hours

I.V.: Administer I.V. bolus over a minimum of 15 seconds; onset within 30 minutes; peak analgesia within 2 hours

Ophthalmic solution: Contact lenses should be removed before instillation.

Monitoring Parameters Monitor response (pain, range of motion, grip strength, mobility, ADL function), inflammation; observe for weight gain, edema; monitor renal function (serum creatinine, BUN, urine output); observe for bleeding, bruising; evaluate gastrointestinal effects (abdominal pain, bleeding, dyspepsia); mental confusion, disorientation, CBC, liver function tests

Reference Range Serum concentration: Therapeutic: 0.3-5 μg/mL; Toxic: >5 μg/mL

Patient Information Serious gastrointestinal bleeding can occur as well as ulceration and perforation. Pain may or may not be present. Avoid aspirin and aspirin-containing products while taking this medication. If gastric adverse effects persist, contact physician. May cause drowsiness, dizziness, blurred vision, and confusion. Use caution when performing tasks which require alertness (eg, driving).

Ophthalmic: Do not wear soft contact lenses.

Nursing Implications Monitor for signs of pain relief, such as an increased appetite and activity

Additional Information First parenteral NSAID for analgesia; 30 mg provides the analgesia comparable to 12 mg of morphine or 100 mg of meperidine.

Dosage Forms

Injection, as tromethamine: 15 mg/mL (1 mL); 30 mg/mL (1 mL, 2 mL)

Solution, ophthalmic, as tromethamine:

Acular®: 0.5% (3 mL, 5 mL, 10 mL) [contains benzalkonium chloride]

Acular® PF [preservative free]: 0.5% (0.4 mL)

Tablet, as tromethamine: 10 mg

♦ **Ketorolac Tromethamine** *see* Ketorolac *on page 764*

Ketotifen (kee toe TYE fen)

U.S. Brand Names Zaditor™

Canadian Brand Names Apo®-Ketotifen; Novo-Ketotifen; Zaditen®; Zaditor™

Synonyms Ketotifen Fumarate

Therapeutic Category Antihistamine, H₁ Blocker, Ophthalmic

Use Temporary prevention of eye itching due to allergic conjunctivitis

Pregnancy Risk Factor C

Pregnancy/Breast-Feeding Implications Oral treatment administered to pregnant animals have resulted in retarded ossification of the sternebrae, slight increase in postnatal mortality, and a decrease in weight gain in the first 4 days of life. Topical ocular administration has not been studied. Caution should be used when ketotifen is administered to a nursing mother.

Contraindications Hypersensitivity to ketotifen or any component of the formulation (the preservative is benzalkonium chloride)

Warnings/Precautions For topical ophthalmic use only. Not to treat contact lens-related irritation. After ketotifen use, soft contact lens wearers should wait at least 10 minutes before putting their lenses in. Do not wear contact lenses if eyes are red. Do not contaminate dropper tip or solution when placing drops in eyes. Safety and efficacy not established for children <3 years of age.

Adverse Reactions 1% to 10%:
Ocular: Allergic reactions, burning or stinging, conjunctivitis, discharge, dry eyes, eye pain, eyelid disorder, itching, keratitis, lacrimation disorder, mydriasis, photophobia, rash
Respiratory: Pharyngitis
Miscellaneous: Flu syndrome

Overdosage/Toxicology No serious signs or symptoms have been seen after ingestion up to 20 mg.

Stability Stable at room temperature

Mechanism of Action Relatively selective, noncompetitive H₁-receptor antagonist and mast cell stabilizer, inhibiting the release of mediators from cells involved in hypersensitivity reactions

Pharmacodynamics/Kinetics
Onset of action: Minutes
Duration: 8-12 hours
Absorption: Minimal systemic

Usual Dosage Children ≥3 years and Adults: Ophthalmic: Instill 1 drop into the affected eye(s) twice daily, every 8-12 hours

Patient Information For topical ophthalmic use only. Not to be used to treat contact lens-related irritation. After ketotifen's use, soft contact lens wearers should wait at least 10 minutes before putting their contact lenses in. Do not wear contact lenses if eyes are red. Do not contaminate dropper tip or solution when placing drops in eyes. Store at room temperature

Dosage Forms Solution, ophthalmic: 0.025% (5 mL)

- **Kondon's Nasal®** [OTC] *see Ephedrine on page 469*
- **Konsyl®** [OTC] *see Psyllium on page 1158*
- **Konsyl-D®** [OTC] *see Psyllium on page 1158*
- **Konÿne® 80** *see Factor IX Complex (Human) on page 539*
- **K-Phos® Neutral** *see Potassium Phosphate and Sodium Phosphate on page 1114*
- **K-Phos® Original** *see Potassium Acid Phosphate on page 1107*
- **Kristalose™** *see Lactulose on page 770*
- **K-Tab®** *see Potassium Chloride on page 1108*
- **Ku-Zyme® HP** *see Pancrelipase on page 1034*
- **Kwelcof®** *see Hydrocodone and Guaifenesin on page 679*
- **Kwellada-P™ (Can)** *see Permethrin on page 1065*
- **Kytril®** *see Granisetron on page 642*
- **L-3-Hydroxytyrosine** *see Levodopa on page 790*
- **L-749,345** *see Ertapenem on page 484*
- **LA-12®** *see Hydroxocobalamin on page 687*

Labetalol (la BET a lole)

Related Information
Beta-Blockers Comparison *on page 1491*
Hypertension *on page 1675*

U.S. Brand Names Normodyne®; Trandate®
Canadian Brand Names Normodyne®; Trandate®
Synonyms Ibidomide Hydrochloride; Labetalol Hydrochloride
Therapeutic Category Alpha-/Beta- Adrenergic Blocker; Antihypertensive Agent; Beta-Adrenergic Blocker
Use Treatment of mild to severe hypertension; I.V. for hypertensive emergencies
Pregnancy Risk Factor C (manufacturer); D (2nd and 3rd trimesters - expert analysis)
Pregnancy/Breast-Feeding Implications
Clinical effects on the fetus: Crosses the placenta. Bradycardia, hypotension, hypoglycemia, intrauterine growth rate (IUGR). IUGR probably related to maternal hypertension. Available evidence suggests safe use during pregnancy and breast-feeding. Monitor breast-fed infant for symptoms of beta-blockade.
Breast-feeding/lactation: Crosses into breast milk. AAP considers **compatible** with breast-feeding.
Contraindications Hypersensitivity to labetalol or any component of the formulation; sinus bradycardia; heart block greater than first degree (except in patients with a functioning artificial pacemaker); cardiogenic shock; bronchial asthma; uncompensated cardiac failure; pregnancy (2nd and 3rd trimesters)
Warnings/Precautions Paradoxical increase in blood pressure has been reported with treatment of pheochromocytoma or clonidine withdrawal syndrome; orthostatic hypotension may occur with I.V. administration; patient should remain supine during and for up to 3 hours after I.V. administration; use with caution in impaired hepatic function (discontinue if signs of liver dysfunction occur); may mask the signs and symptoms of hypoglycemia; a lower hemodynamic response rate and higher incidence of toxicity may be observed with administration to elderly patients.

Use only with extreme caution in compensated heart failure and monitor for a worsening of the condition. Avoid abrupt discontinuation in patients with a history of CAD; slowly wean while monitoring for signs and symptoms of ischemia. Use caution with concurrent use of beta-blockers and either verapamil or diltiazem; bradycardia or heart block can occur. Patients with bronchospastic disease should not receive beta-blockers. Labetalol may be used with caution in patients with nonallergic bronchospasm (chronic bronchitis, emphysema). Use cautiously in diabetics because it can mask prominent hypoglycemic symptoms. Can mask signs of thyrotoxicosis. Can cause fetal harm when administered in pregnancy. Use caution when using I.V. labetalol and halothane concurrently (significant myocardial depression).

Adverse Reactions
>10%:
Central nervous system: Dizziness (1% to 16%)
Gastrointestinal: Nausea (0% to 19%)
1% to 10%:
Cardiovascular: Edema (0% to 2%), hypotension (1% to 5%); with IV use, hypotension may occur in up to 58%
Central nervous system: Fatigue (1% to 10%), paresthesia (1% to 5%), headache (2%), vertigo (2%), weakness (1%)
Dermatologic: Rash (1%), scalp tingling (1% to 5%)
Gastrointestinal: Vomiting (<1% to 3%), dyspepsia (1% to 4%)
Genitourinary: Ejaculatory failure (0% to 5%), impotence (1% to 4%)
Hepatic: Increased transaminases (4%)
Respiratory: Nasal congestion (1% to 6%), dyspnea (2%)
Miscellaneous: Taste disorder (1%), abnormal vision (1%)
<1% (Limited to important or life-threatening): Alopecia (reversible), anaphylactoid reaction, angioedema, bradycardia, bronchospasm, cholestatic jaundice, congestive heart failure, diabetes insipidus, heart block, hepatic necrosis, hepatitis, hypersensitivity, hypotension, Peyronie's disease, positive ANA, pruritus, Raynaud's syndrome, syncope, systemic lupus erythematosus, toxic myopathy, urinary retention, urticaria, ventricular arrhythmias (I.V.).
Other adverse reactions noted with beta-adrenergic blocking agents include mental depression, catatonia, short-term memory loss, emotional lability, intensification of pre-existing AV block, laryngospasm, respiratory distress, agranulocytosis, thrombocytopenic purpura, nonthrombocytopenic purpura, mesenteric artery thrombosis, and ischemic colitis.

Overdosage/Toxicology Symptoms of intoxication include cardiac disturbances, CNS toxicity, bronchospasm, hypoglycemia and hyperkalemia. The most common cardiac symptoms include hypotension and bradycardia. Atrioventricular block, intraventricular conduction disturbances, cardiogenic shock, and asystole may occur with severe overdose, especially with membrane-depressant drugs (eg, propranolol). CNS effects include convulsions, coma, and respiratory arrest, commonly seen with propranolol and other membrane-depressant and lipid-soluble drugs. Treatment is symptomatic for seizures, hypotension, hyperkalemia and hypoglycemia. Bradycardia and hypotension resistant to atropine, isoproterenol or pacing may respond to glucagon. Wide QRS defects caused by membrane-depressant poisoning may respond to hypertonic sodium bicarbonate. Repeat-dose charcoal, hemoperfusion, or hemodialysis may be helpful in removal of only those beta-blockers with a small V_d, long half-life, or low intrinsic clearance (acebutolol, atenolol, nadolol, sotalol).

Drug Interactions
Cytochrome P450 Effect: CYP2D6 enzyme substrate; CYP2D6 enzyme inhibitor

Increased Effect/Toxicity: Inhibitors of CYP2D6 including quinidine, paroxetine, and propafenone are likely to increase blood levels of labetalol. Cimetidine increases the bioavailability of labetalol. Labetalol has additive hypotensive effects with other antihypertensive agents. Concurrent use with alpha-blockers (prazosin, terazosin) and beta-blockers increases the risk of orthostasis. Concurrent use with diltiazem, verapamil, or digoxin may increase the risk of bradycardia with beta-blocking agents. Halothane, enflurane, isoflurane, and potentially other inhalation anesthetics may cause synergistic hypotension. Beta-blockers may affect the action or levels of ethanol, disopyramide, nondepolarizing muscle relaxants, and theophylline although the effects are difficult to predict.

Decreased Effect: Decreased effect of beta-blockers with aluminum salts, barbiturates, calcium salts, cholestyramine, colestipol, NSAIDs, penicillins (ampicillin), rifampin, salicylates, and sulfinpyrazone due to decreased bioavailability and plasma levels. Beta-blockers may decrease the effect of sulfonylureas.

Ethanol/Nutrition/Herb Interactions
Food: Labetalol serum concentrations may be increased if taken with food.

Herb/Nutraceutical: Avoid dong quai if using for hypertension (has estrogenic activity). Avoid ephedra, yohimbe, ginseng (may worsen hypertension). Avoid natural licorice (causes sodium and water retention and increases potassium loss). Avoid garlic (may have increased antihypertensive effect).

Stability
Labetalol should be stored at room temperature or under refrigeration and should be protected from light and freezing; the solution is clear to slightly yellow

Stability of parenteral admixture at room temperature (25°C) and refrigeration temperature (4°C): 3 days

Standard diluent: 500 mg/250 mL D_5W

Minimum volume: 250 mL D_5W

Incompatible with sodium bicarbonate, most stable at pH of 2-4; **incompatible** with alkaline solutions

Mechanism of Action Blocks alpha-, beta$_1$-, and beta$_2$-adrenergic receptor sites; elevated renins are reduced

Pharmacodynamics/Kinetics
Onset of action: Oral: 20 minutes to 2 hours; I.V.: 2-5 minutes
Peak effect: Oral: 1-4 hours; I.V.: 5-15 minutes

Duration: Oral: 8-24 hours (dose dependent); I.V.: 2-4 hours

Distribution: V_d: Adults: 3-16 L/kg; mean: <9.4 L/kg; moderately lipid soluble, therefore, can enter CNS; crosses placenta; small amounts enter breast milk

Protein binding: 50%

Metabolism: Hepatic primarily via glucuronide conjugation; extensive first-pass effect

Bioavailability: Oral: 25%; increased with liver disease, elderly, and concurrent cimetidine

Half-life elimination: Normal renal function: 2.5-8 hours

Excretion: Urine (<5% as unchanged drug)
Clearance: Possibly decreased in neonates/infants

Usual Dosage Due to limited documentation of its use, labetalol should be initiated cautiously in pediatric patients with careful dosage adjustment and blood pressure monitoring.

Children:
Oral: Limited information regarding labetalol use in pediatric patients is currently available in literature. Some centers recommend initial oral doses of 4 mg/kg/day in 2 divided doses. Reported oral doses have started at 3 mg/kg/day and 20 mg/kg/day and have increased up to 40 mg/kg/day.

I.V., intermittent bolus doses of 0.3-1 mg/kg/dose have been reported.

For treatment of pediatric hypertensive emergencies, initial continuous infusions of 0.4-1 mg/kg/hour with a maximum of 3 mg/kg/hour have been used. Administration requires the use of an infusion pump.

Adults:
Oral: Initial: 100 mg twice daily, may increase as needed every 2-3 days by 100 mg until desired response is obtained; usual dose: 200-400 mg twice daily; may require up to 2.4 g/day.

I.V.: 20 mg (0.25 mg/kg for an 80 kg patient) IVP over 2 minutes; may administer 40-80 mg at 10-minute intervals, up to 300 mg total dose.

I.V. infusion: Initial: 2 mg/minute; titrate to response up to 300 mg total dose, if needed. Administration requires the use of an infusion pump.

I.V. infusion (500 mg/250 mL D_5W) rates:
1 mg/minute: 30 mL/hour
2 mg/minute: 60 mL/hour
3 mg/minute: 90 mL/hour
4 mg/minute: 120 mL/hour
5 mg/minute: 150 mL/hour
6 mg/minute: 180 mL/hour

Dialysis: Not removed by hemo- or peritoneal dialysis; supplemental dose is not necessary.

Dosage adjustment in hepatic impairment: Dosage reduction may be necessary.

Monitoring Parameters Blood pressure, standing and sitting/supine, pulse, cardiac monitor and blood pressure monitor required for I.V. administration
(Continued)

Labetalol *(Continued)*

Test Interactions False-positive urine catecholamines, VMA if measured by fluorometric or photometric methods; use HPLC or specific catecholamine radioenzymatic technique

Patient Information Do not stop medication without aid of physician; may mask signs and symptoms of diabetes

Nursing Implications Instruct patient regarding compliance; do **not** abruptly withdraw medication in patients with ischemic heart disease; IVP: Administer over 2-3 minutes

Dosage Forms
Injection, as hydrochloride: 5 mg/mL (20 mL, 40 mL, 60 mL)
Injection, prefilled syringe, as hydrochloride: 5 mg/mL (4 mL, 8 mL)
Tablet, as hydrochloride: 100 mg, 200 mg, 300 mg

Extemporaneous Preparations A mixture of labetalol 40 mg/mL plus hydrochlorothiazide 5 mg/mL was found stable for 60 days in the refrigerator when prepared in a 1:1 mixture of Ora-Sweet® and Ora-Plus®, or Ora-Sweet® SF and Ora-Plus®, and of cherry syrup

Allen LV and Erickson III MA, "Stability of Labetalol Hydrochloride, Metoprolol Tartrate, Verapamil Hydrochloride, and Spironolactone With Hydrochlorothiazide in Extemporaneously Compounded Oral Liquids," *Am J Health Syst Pharm*, 1996, 53:2304-9.

- ◆ **Labetalol Hydrochloride** *see Labetalol on page 768*
- ◆ **LaBID®** *see Theophylline Salts on page 1310*
- ◆ **LactiCare-HC®** *see Hydrocortisone on page 682*
- ◆ **Lactinex® [OTC]** *see Lactobacillus on page 770*

Lactobacillus *(lak toe ba SIL us)*

U.S. Brand Names Bacid® [OTC]; Kala® [OTC]; Lactinex® [OTC]; MoreDophilus® [OTC]; Pro-Bionate® [OTC]; Superdophilus® [OTC]

Canadian Brand Names Bacid®; Fermalac

Synonyms *Lactobacillus acidophilus*; *Lactobacillus acidophilus* and *Lactobacillus bulgaricus*

Therapeutic Category Antidiarrheal

Use Treatment of uncomplicated diarrhea particularly that caused by antibiotic therapy; re-establish normal physiologic and bacterial flora of the intestinal tract

Pregnancy Risk Factor Not available

Contraindications Allergy to milk or lactose

Warnings/Precautions Discontinue if high fever present; do not use in children <3 years of age

Adverse Reactions No data reported

Stability Store in the refrigerator

Mechanism of Action Creates an environment unfavorable to potentially pathogenic fungi or bacteria through the production of lactic acid, and favors establishment of an aciduric flora, thereby suppressing the growth of pathogenic microorganisms; helps re-establish normal intestinal flora

Pharmacodynamics/Kinetics
Absorption: Oral: None
Distribution: Local, primarily colon
Excretion: Feces

Usual Dosage Children >3 years and Adults: Oral:
Capsules: 2 capsules 2-4 times/day
Granules: 1 packet added to or taken with cereal, food, milk, fruit juice, or water, 3-4 times/day
Powder: 1 teaspoonful daily with liquid
Tablet, chewable: 4 tablets 3-4 times/day; may follow each dose with a small amount of milk, fruit juice, or water

Dietary Considerations Granules or contents of capsules may be added to or administered with cereal, food, milk, fruit juice, or water.

Administration Granules may be added to or administered with cereal, food, milk, fruit juice, or water

Patient Information Refrigerate; granules may be added to or taken with cereal, food, milk, fruit juice, or water

Dosage Forms
Capsule:
Bacid®: ≥500 million units [cultured strain *L. acidophilus*] (50s, 100s)
Pro-Bionate®: 2 billion units per g [strain NAS *L. acidophilus*] (30s, 60s)
Granules (Lactinex®): 1 g/packet [mixed culture *L. acidophilus, L. bulgaricus*] (12 packets/box)
Powder:
MoreDophilus®: 4 billion units per g [*L. acidophilus*-carrot derivative] (120 g)
Superdophilus®: 2 billion units per g [strain DDS-1 *L. acidophilus*] (37.5 g, 75 g, 135 g)
Tablet (Kala®): 200 million units [soy-based *L. acidophilus*] (100s, 250s, 500s)
Tablet, chewable (Lactinex®): Mixed culture *L. acidophilus, L. bulgaricus* (50s)

- ◆ **Lactobacillus acidophilus** *see Lactobacillus on page 770*
- ◆ **Lactobacillus acidophilus and Lactobacillus bulgaricus** *see Lactobacillus on page 770*
- ◆ **Lactoflavin** *see Riboflavin on page 1191*

Lactulose *(LAK tyoo lose)*

Related Information
Laxatives, Classification and Properties *on page 1504*

U.S. Brand Names Cholac®; Chronulac®; Constilac®; Constulose®; Duphalac®; Enulose®; Evalose®; Kristalose™

Canadian Brand Names Acilac; Laxilose; PMS-Lactulose

Therapeutic Category Ammonium Detoxicant; Laxative, Miscellaneous

Use Adjunct in the prevention and treatment of portal-systemic encephalopathy; treatment of chronic constipation

Pregnancy Risk Factor B

Contraindications Hypersensitivity to lactulose or any component of the formulation; galacto-semia (or patients requiring a low galactose diet)

Warnings/Precautions Use with caution in patients with diabetes mellitus; monitor periodically for electrolyte imbalance when lactulose is used >6 months or in patients predisposed to electrolyte abnormalities (eg, elderly); patients receiving lactulose and an oral anti-infective agent should be monitored for possible inadequate response to lactulose

Adverse Reactions Frequency not defined: Gastrointestinal: Flatulence, diarrhea (excessive dose), abdominal discomfort, nausea, vomiting, cramping

Overdosage/Toxicology Symptoms include diarrhea, abdominal pain, hypochloremic alkalosis, dehydration, hypotension, and hypokalemia. Treatment is supportive.

Drug Interactions

Decreased Effect: Oral neomycin, laxatives, antacids

Stability Keep solution at room temperature to reduce viscosity; discard solution if cloudy or very dark

Mechanism of Action The bacterial degradation of lactulose resulting in an acidic pH inhibits the diffusion of NH_3 into the blood by causing the conversion of NH_3 to NH_4+; also enhances the diffusion of NH_3 from the blood into the gut where conversion to NH_4+ occurs; produces an osmotic effect in the colon with resultant distention promoting peristalsis

Pharmacodynamics/Kinetics

Absorption: Not appreciable

Metabolism: By colonic flora to lactic acid and acetic acid, requires colonic flora for drug activation

Excretion: Primarily feces and urine (~3%)

Usual Dosage Diarrhea may indicate overdosage and responds to dose reduction

Prevention of portal systemic encephalopathy (PSE): Oral:

Infants: 2.5-10 mL/day divided 3-4 times/day; adjust dosage to produce 2-3 stools/day

Older Children: Daily dose of 40-90 mL divided 3-4 times/day; if initial dose causes diarrhea, then reduce it immediately; adjust dosage to produce 2-3 stools/day

Constipation: Oral:

Children: 5 g/day (7.5 mL) after breakfast

Adults: 15-30 mL/day increased to 60 mL/day if necessary

Acute PSE: Adults:

Oral: 20-30 g (30-45 mL) every 1-2 hours to induce rapid laxation; adjust dosage daily to produce 2-3 soft stools; doses of 30-45 mL may be given hourly to cause rapid laxation, then reduce to recommended dose; usual daily dose: 60-100 g (90-150 mL) daily

Rectal administration: 200 g (300 mL) diluted with 700 mL of H_2O or NS; administer rectally via rectal balloon catheter and retain 30-60 minutes every 4-6 hours

Dietary Considerations Contraindicated in patients on galactose-restricted diet; may be mixed with fruit juice, milk, water, or citrus-flavored carbonated beverages.

Monitoring Parameters Blood pressure, standing/supine; serum potassium, bowel movement patterns, fluid status, serum ammonia

Patient Information Lactulose can be taken "as is" or diluted with water, fruit juice or milk, or taken in a food; laxative results may not occur for 24-48 hours

Nursing Implications Dilute lactulose in water, usually 60-120 mL, prior to administering through a gastric or feeding tube. Syrup formulation has been used in preparation of rectal solution.

Dosage Forms

Crystals for reconstitution (Kristalose™): 10 g, 20 g,

Syrup: 10 g/15 mL (15 mL, 30 mL, 237 mL, 473 mL, 946 mL, 1890 mL, 3785 mL)

♦ **L-AmB** *see* Amphotericin B (Liposomal) *on page 91*

♦ **Lamictal®** *see* Lamotrigine *on page 773*

♦ **Lamisil®** *see* Terbinafine *on page 1298*

♦ **Lamisil® AT™** *see* Terbinafine *on page 1298*

♦ **Lamisil® Dermgel** *see* Terbinafine *on page 1298*

♦ **Lamisil® Solution** *see* Terbinafine *on page 1298*

Lamivudine (la MI vyoo deen)

Related Information

Antiretroviral Agents Comparison *on page 1488*

Antiretroviral Therapy for HIV Infection *on page 1595*

Management of Healthcare Worker Exposures to HIV, HBV, HCV *on page 1555*

U.S. Brand Names Epivir®; Epivir-HBV®

Canadian Brand Names Heptovir®; 3TC®

Synonyms 3TC

Therapeutic Category Antiretroviral Agent, Nucleoside Reverse Transcriptase Inhibitor (NRTI) [Cytadine Analog]

Use

Epivir®: Treatment of HIV infection when antiretroviral therapy is warranted; should always be used as part of a multidrug regimen (at least three antiretroviral agents)

Epivir-HBV®: Treatment of chronic hepatitis B associated with evidence of hepatitis B viral replication and active liver inflammation

Unlabeled/Investigational Use Prevention of HIV following needlesticks (with or without protease inhibitor)

Pregnancy Risk Factor C

Pregnancy/Breast-Feeding Implications Lamivudine crosses the placenta. It may be used in combination with zidovudine in HIV-infected women who are in labor, but have had no prior antiretroviral therapy, in order to reduce the maternal-fetal transmission of HIV. Cases of lactic acidosis/hepatic steatosis syndrome have been reported in pregnant women receiving nucleoside analogues. It is not known if pregnancy itself potentiates this known side effect; (Continued)

Lamivudine (Continued)

however, pregnant women may be at increased risk of lactic acidosis and liver damage. Hepatic enzymes and electrolytes should be monitored frequently during the 3rd trimester of pregnancy in women receiving nucleoside analogues. Health professionals are encouraged to contact the antiretroviral pregnancy registry to monitor outcomes of pregnant women exposed to antiretroviral medications (1-800-258-4263).

Contraindications Hypersensitivity to lamivudine or any component of the formulation

Warnings/Precautions A decreased dosage is recommended in patients with renal dysfunction; use with extreme caution in children with history of pancreatitis or risk factors for development of pancreatitis. Do not use as monotherapy in treatment of HIV. Treatment of HBV in patients with unrecognized/untreated HIV may lead to rapid HIV resistance. Treatment of HIV in patients with unrecognized/untreated HBV may lead to rapid HBV resistance.

Lactic acidosis and severe hepatomegaly with steatosis have been reported, including fatal cases. Use caution in hepatic impairment. Pregnancy, obesity, and/or prolonged therapy may increase the risk of lactic acidosis and liver damage.

Adverse Reactions (As reported in adults treated for HIV infection)

>10%:
  Central nervous system: Headache, fatigue
  Gastrointestinal: Nausea, diarrhea, vomiting, pancreatitis (range: 0.5% to 18%; higher percentage in pediatric patients)
  Neuromuscular & skeletal: Peripheral neuropathy, paresthesia, musculoskeletal pain

1% to 10%:
  Central nervous system: Dizziness, depression, fever, chills, insomnia
  Dermatologic: Rash
  Gastrointestinal: Anorexia, abdominal pain, heartburn, elevated amylase
  Hematologic: Neutropenia
  Hepatic: Elevated AST, ALT
  Neuromuscular & skeletal: Myalgia, arthralgia
  Respiratory: Nasal signs and symptoms, cough

<1% (Limited to important or life-threatening): Alopecia, anaphylaxis, anemia, hepatomegaly, hyperbilirubinemia, hyperglycemia, increased CPK, lactic acidosis, lymphadenopathy, peripheral neuropathy, pruritus, rhabdomyolysis, splenomegaly, steatosis, stomatitis, thrombocytopenia, urticaria, weakness

Overdosage/Toxicology Very limited information is available, although there have been no clinical signs or symptoms noted in overdose, and hematologic tests have remained normal as well. No antidote is available. Dialyzability is unknown.

Drug Interactions

Increased Effect/Toxicity: Zidovudine concentrations increase significantly (~39%) with lamivudine coadministration. Trimethoprim/sulfamethoxazole increases lamivudine's blood levels.

Decreased Effect: Zalcitabine and lamivudine may inhibit the intracellular phosphorylation of each other; concomitant use should be avoided.

Ethanol/Nutrition/Herb Interactions Food: Food decreases the rate of absorption and C_{max}; however there is no change in the systemic AUC. Therefore, may be taken with or without food.

Stability Store at 2°C to 25°C (68°F to 77°F) tightly closed.

Mechanism of Action After lamivudine is triphosphorylated, the principle mode of action is inhibition of HIV reverse transcription via viral DNA chain termination; inhibits RNA- and DNA-dependent DNA polymerase activities of reverse transcriptase. The monophosphate form of lamivudine is incorporated into the viral DNA by hepatitis B virus polymerase, resulting in DNA chain termination.

Pharmacodynamics/Kinetics

Absorption: Rapid
Distribution: V_d: 1.3 L/kg
Protein binding, plasma: <36%
Metabolism: 5.6% to trans-sulfoxide metabolite
Bioavailability: Absolute; Cp_{max} decreased with food although AUC not significantly affected
  Children: 66%
  Adults: 87%
Half-life elimination: Children: 2 hours; Adults: 5-7 hours
Excretion: Primarily urine (as unchanged drug)

Usual Dosage Note: The formulation and dosage of Epivir-HBV® are not appropriate for patients infected with both HBV and HIV. Use with at least two other antiretroviral agents when treating HIV

Oral:
  Children 3 months to 16 years: HIV: 4 mg/kg twice daily (maximum: 150 mg twice daily)
  Children 2-17 years: Treatment of hepatitis B (Epivir-HBV®): 3 mg/kg once daily (maximum: 100 mg/day)
  Adolescents and Adults: Prevention of HIV following needlesticks (unlabeled use): 150 mg twice daily (with zidovudine with or without a protease inhibitor, depending on risk)
  Adults:
    HIV: 150 mg twice daily; <50 kg: 2 mg/kg twice daily
    Treatment of hepatitis B (Epivir-HBV®): 100 mg/day

Dosing interval in renal impairment in pediatric patients: Insufficient data; however, dose reduction should be considered.

Dosing interval in renal impairment in patients >16 years for HIV:
  Cl_{cr} 30-49 mL/minute: Administer 150 mg once daily
  Cl_{cr} 15-29 mL/minute: Administer 150 mg first dose, then 100 mg once daily
  Cl_{cr} 5-14 mL/minute: Administer 150 mg first dose, then 50 mg once daily
  Cl_{cr} <5 mL/minute: Administer 50 mg first dose, then 25 mg once daily

Dosing interval in renal impairment in adult patients with hepatitis B:
  Cl_{cr} 30-49: Administer 100 mg first dose then 50 mg once daily
  Cl_{cr} 15-29: Administer 100 mg first dose then 25 mg once daily

Cl$_{cr}$ 5-14: Administer 35 mg first dose then 15 mg once daily
Cl$_{cr}$ <5: Administer 35 mg first dose then 10 mg once daily
Dialysis: No data available

Dietary Considerations May be taken with or without food.

Administration May be taken with or without food. Adjust dosage in renal failure.

Monitoring Parameters Amylase, bilirubin, liver enzymes, hematologic parameters, viral load, and CD4 count; signs and symptoms of pancreatitis

Patient Information Patients may still experience illnesses associated with HIV infection; lamivudine is not a cure for HIV infection nor has it been shown to reduce the risk of transmission to others; long-term effects are unknown; take exactly as prescribed; children should be monitored for symptoms of pancreatitis

Additional Information Lamivudine has been well studied in the treatment of chronic hepatitis B infection. Potential compliance problems, frequency of administration and adverse effects should be discussed with patients before initiating therapy to help prevent the emergence of resistance.

Dosage Forms
Solution, oral:
Epivir®: 10 mg/mL (240 mL) [strawberry banana flavor]
Epivir-HBV®: 5 mg/mL (240 mL) [strawberry banana flavor]
Tablet:
Epivir®: 150 mg
Epivir-HBV®: 100 mg

♦ **Lamivudine, Abacavir, and Zidovudine** see Abacavir, Lamivudine, and Zidovudine on page 17

♦ **Lamivudine and Zidovudine** see Zidovudine and Lamivudine on page 1437

Lamotrigine (la MOE tri jeen)

Related Information
Anticonvulsants by Seizure Type on page 1481
Epilepsy & Seizure Treatment on page 1659

U.S. Brand Names Lamictal®

Canadian Brand Names Lamictal®

Synonyms BW-430C; LTG

Therapeutic Category Anticonvulsant

Use Adjunctive therapy in the treatment of partial seizures in adults with epilepsy (safety and effectiveness in children <16 years of age have not been established); conversion to monotherapy in adults with partial seizures who are receiving treatment with a single enzyme-inducing antiepileptic drug

Orphan drug: Adjunctive therapy in the generalized seizures of Lennox-Gastaut syndrome in pediatrics and adults

Unlabeled/Investigational Use Bipolar disorder

Pregnancy Risk Factor C

Pregnancy/Breast-Feeding Implications Lamotrigine has been found to decrease folate concentrations in animal studies.

Contraindications Hypersensitivity to lamotrigine or any component of the formulation

Warnings/Precautions Use caution in patients with impaired renal, hepatic, or cardiac function. Avoid abrupt cessation, taper over at least 2 weeks if possible. Severe and potentially life-threatening skin rashes have been reported; this appears to occur most frequently in pediatric patients. Discontinue at first sign of rash unless rash is clearly not drug related. May cause CNS depression, which may impair physical or mental abilities. Patients must be cautioned about performing tasks which require mental alertness (ie, operating machinery or driving). Effects with other sedative drugs or ethanol may be potentiated. Binds to melanin and may accumulate in the eye and other melanin-rich tissues; the clinical significance of this is not known. Safety and efficacy has not been established for use as initial monotherapy, conversion to monotherapy from nonenzyme-inducing antiepileptic drugs (AED), or conversion to monotherapy from two or more AEDs. **Use caution in writing and/or interpreting prescriptions/orders; medication dispensing errors have occurred with similar-sounding medications (Lamisil®, Ludiomil®, lamivudine, labetalol, and Lomotil®).**

Adverse Reactions
>10%:
Central nervous system: Headache (29%), dizziness (7% to 38%), ataxia (7% to 22%), somnolence
Gastrointestinal: Nausea (7% to 19%)
Ocular: Diplopia (28%), blurred vision (16%)
Respiratory: Rhinitis (7% to 14%)
1% to 10%:
Central nervous system: Depression (4%), anxiety (4%), irritability, confusion, speech disorder, difficulty concentrating, emotional lability, malaise, seizure (3% to 4%), incoordination, insomnia (5% to 6%)
Dermatologic: Hypersensitivity rash (10%), pruritus (3%)
Gastrointestinal: Abdominal pain, vomiting (9%), diarrhea (6%), dyspepsia (5% to 7%), constipation (4%), anorexia (2%)
Genitourinary: Vaginitis (4%), dysmenorrhea (7%)
Neuromuscular & skeletal: Tremor (6%), arthralgia, joint pain
Ocular: Nystagmus (2%)
Miscellaneous: Flu syndrome (7%), fever (2% to 6%)
<1% (Limited to important or life-threatening): Acute renal failure, agranulocytosis, allergic reactions, alopecia, amnesia, angina, angioedema, aplastic anemia, apnea, atrial fibrillation, bronchospasm, depersonalization, disseminated intravascular coagulation (DIC), dysarthria, dysphagia, dyspnea, eosinophilia, erythema multiforme, esophagitis, GI hemorrhage, gingival hyperplasia, hemolytic anemia, hemorrhage, hepatitis, hypersensitivity reactions (including rhabdomyolysis), immunosuppression (progressive), impotence, leukopenia, lupus-like reaction, mania, movement disorder, multiorgan failure, neutropenia,
(Continued)

Lamotrigine *(Continued)*

pancreatitis, pancytopenia, paralysis, Parkinson's disease exacerbation, rash, red cell aplasia, Stevens-Johnson syndrome, stroke, suicidal ideation, urticaria, vasculitis

Overdosage/Toxicology Decontaminate using lavage/activated charcoal with cathartic. Multiple dosing of activated charcoal may be useful.

Drug Interactions

Cytochrome P450 Effect: Effects on CYP not characterized, may act as inducer.

Increased Effect/Toxicity: Lamotrigine may increase the epoxide metabolite of carbamazepine resulting in toxicity. Valproic acid increases blood levels of lamotrigine. Toxicity has been reported following addition of sertraline (limited documentation).

Decreased Effect: Acetaminophen, carbamazepine, phenytoin, phenobarbital may decrease concentrations of lamotrigine. Lamotrigine enhances the metabolism of valproic acid.

Ethanol/Nutrition/Herb Interactions

Ethanol: Avoid ethanol (may increase CNS depression).

Food: Has no effect on absorption.

Herb/Nutraceutical: Avoid evening primrose (seizure threshold decreased).

Stability Store at 25°C (77°F); excursions are permitted to 15°C to 30°C (59°F to 86°F); protect from light

Mechanism of Action A triazine derivative which inhibits release of glutamate (an excitatory amino acid) and inhibits voltage-sensitive sodium channels, which stabilizes neuronal membranes. Lamotrigine has weak inhibitory effect on the 5-HT_3 receptor; *in vitro* inhibits dihydrofolate reductase.

Pharmacodynamics/Kinetics

Distribution: V_d: 1.1 L/kg

Protein binding: 55%

Metabolism: Hepatic and renal

Half-life elimination: 24 hours; Concomitant valproic acid therapy: 59 hours; Concomitant phenytoin or carbamazepine therapy: 15 hours

Time to peak: 1-4 hours

Excretion: Urine (as glucuronide conjugate)

Usual Dosage Oral:

Children <6.7 kg: Not recommended

Children 2-12 years: Lennox-Gastaut (adjunctive): **Note:** Children 2-6 years will likely require maintenance doses at the higher end of recommended range; only whole tablets should be used for dosing, rounded down to the nearest whole tablet

Patients receiving AED regimens containing valproic acid:

Weeks 1 and 2: 0.15 mg/kg/day in 1-2 divided doses; round dose down to the nearest whole tablet. For patients >6.7 kg and <14 kg, dosing should be 2 mg every other day.

Weeks 3 and 4: 0.3 mg/kg/day in 1-2 divided doses; round dose down to the nearest whole tablet; may use combinations of 2 mg and 5 mg tablets. For patients >6.7 kg and <14 kg, dosing should be 2 mg/day.

Maintenance dose: Titrate dose to effect; after week 4, increase dose every 1-2 weeks by a calculated increment; calculate increment as 0.3 mg/kg/day rounded down to the nearest whole tablet; add this amount to the previously administered daily dose; usual maintenance: 1-5 mg/kg/day in 1-2 divided doses; maximum: 200 mg/day given in 1-2 divided doses

Patients receiving enzyme-inducing AED regimens without valproic acid:

Weeks 1 and 2: 0.6 mg/kg/day in 2 divided doses; round dose down to the nearest whole tablet

Weeks 3 and 4: 1.2 mg/kg/day in 2 divided doses; round dose down to the nearest whole tablet

Maintenance dose: Titrate dose to effect; after week 4, increase dose every 1-2 weeks by a calculated increment; calculate increment as 1.2 mg/kg/day rounded down to the nearest whole tablet; add this amount to the previously administered daily dose; usual maintenance: 5-15 mg/kg/day in 2 divided doses; maximum: 400 mg/day

Children >12 years: Lennox-Gastaut (adjunctive): See adult dosing

Children ≥16 years: Treatment of partial seizures (adjunctive) or conversion from single enzyme-inducing AED regimen to monotherapy: See adult dosing

Adults:

Lennox-Gastaut (adjunctive) or treatment of partial seizures (adjunctive):

Patients receiving AED regimens containing valproic acid:

Initial dose: 25 mg every other day for 2 weeks, then 25 mg every day for 2 weeks

Maintenance dose: 100-400 mg/day in 1-2 divided doses (usual range 100-200 mg/day). Dose may be increased by 25-50 mg every day for 1-2 weeks in order to achieve maintenance dose.

Patients receiving enzyme-inducing AED regimens without valproic acid:

Initial dose: 50 mg/day for 2 weeks, then 100 mg in 2 doses for 2 weeks; thereafter, daily dose can be increased by 100 mg every 1-2 weeks to be given in 2 divided doses

Usual maintenance dose: 300-500 mg/day in 2 divided doses; doses as high as 700 mg/day have been reported

Partial seizures (monotherapy) conversion from single enzyme-inducing AED regimen:

Initial dose: 50 mg/day for 2 weeks, then 100 mg in 2 doses for 2 weeks; thereafter, daily dose should be increased by 100 mg every 1-2 weeks to be given in 2 divided doses until reaching a dose of 500 mg/day. Concomitant enzyme inducing AED should then be withdrawn by 20% decrements each week over a 4-week period. Patients should be monitored for rash.

Bipolar disorder (unlabeled use): 25 mg/day for 2 weeks, followed by 50 mg/day for 2 weeks, followed by 100 mg/day for 1 week; thereafter, daily dosage may be increased by 100 mg/week, up to a maximum of 500 mg/day as clinically indicated

Dosage adjustment in renal impairment: Decreased dosage may be effective in patients with significant renal impairment; use with caution

Dietary Considerations Take without regard to meals; drug may cause GI upset.

Administration Doses should be rounded down to the nearest whole tablet. Dispersible tablets may be chewed, dispersed in water or swallowed whole. To disperse tablets, add to a small amount of liquid (just enough to cover tablet); let sit ~1 minute until dispersed; swirl solution and consume immediately. Do not administer partial amounts of liquid. If tablets are chewed, a small amount of water or diluted fruit juice should be used to aid in swallowing.

Monitoring Parameters Seizure, frequency and duration, serum levels of concurrent anticonvulsants, hypersensitivity reactions, especially rash

Reference Range Therapeutic range: 2-20 µg/mL; a serum concentration relationship has not been demonstrated.

Nursing Implications Doses should be rounded down to the nearest whole tablet. Chewable tablets may be swallowed whole, chewed, dispersed in water, or diluted in fruit juice. When tablets are chewed, follow with water or diluted fruit juice to aid in swallowing. To disperse chewable tablet, cover tablet with one teaspoonful of water and allow to dissolve for 1 minute; entire amount is then administered. Do not use partial amounts of dispersed tablets.

Serious adverse consequences have been associated with medication errors and the manufacturer recommends using caution when interpreting and administering orders for lamotrigine (Lamictal®) as there are a number of similar-sounding medications (Lamisil®, Ludiomil®, lamivudine, labetalol, and Lomotil®).

Dosage Forms
Tablet: 25 mg, 100 mg, 150 mg, 200 mg
Tablet, dispersible/chewable: 2 mg, 5 mg, 25 mg [black currant flavor]

Extemporaneous Preparations A 1 mg/mL oral suspension was stable for 28 days stored at room temperature when compounded as follows:
Triturate five 25 mg tablets in a mortar, reduce to a fine powder, then make a paste with a small amount of syrup, add the remaining syrup to almost desired volume, then transfer to a graduate and qs to 125 mL
Shake well before using and keep in refrigerator
Stability information from GlaxoWellcome Co.

♦ **Lamprene®** see Clofazimine on page 312
♦ **Lanacane® [OTC]** see Benzocaine on page 154
♦ **Lanacort® [OTC]** see Hydrocortisone on page 682
♦ **Lanaphilic® [OTC]** see Urea on page 1391
♦ **Lanorinal®** see Butalbital Compound on page 197
♦ **Lanoxicaps®** see Digoxin on page 403
♦ **Lanoxin®** see Digoxin on page 403

Lansoprazole (lan SOE pra zole)

Related Information
Helicobacter pylori Treatment on page 1668
U.S. Brand Names Prevacid®
Canadian Brand Names Prevacid®
Therapeutic Category Gastric Acid Secretion Inhibitor; Proton Pump Inhibitor
Use Short-term treatment of active duodenal ulcers; maintenance treatment of healed duodenal ulcers; as part of a multidrug regimen for H. pylori eradication to reduce the risk of duodenal ulcer recurrence; short-term treatment of active benign gastric ulcer; treatment of NSAID-associated gastric ulcer; to reduce the risk of NSAID-associated gastric ulcer in patients with a history of gastric ulcer who require an NSAID; short-term treatment of symptomatic GERD; short-term treatment for all grades of erosive esophagitis; to maintain healing of erosive esophagitis; long-term treatment of pathological hypersecretory conditions, including Zollinger-Ellison syndrome

Pregnancy Risk Factor B
Pregnancy/Breast-Feeding Implications Animal studies have not shown teratogenic effects to the fetus. However, there are no adequate and well-controlled studies in pregnant women; use during pregnancy only if clearly needed. It is not known if lansoprazole is excreted in human milk; breast-feeding is not recommended.

Contraindications Hypersensitivity to lansoprazole or any component of the formulation
Warnings/Precautions Severe liver dysfunction may require dosage reductions
Adverse Reactions
1% to 10%: Gastrointestinal: Abdominal pain (2%), diarrhea (4%, more likely at doses of 60 mg/day), constipation (1%), nausea (1%)
<1% (Limited to important or life-threatening): Abnormal vision, agitation, allergic reaction, ALT increased, anaphylactoid reaction, anemia, angina, anxiety, aplastic anemia, arrhythmia, AST increased, chest pain, convulsion, depression, dizziness, dry eyes, dry mouth, esophagitis, gastrin levels increased, gastrointestinal disorder, glucocorticoids increased, globulins increased, hemolysis, hepatotoxicity, hyperglycemia, LDH increased, maculopapular rash, photophobia, rash, RBC abnormal, taste perversion, tinnitus, tremor, vertigo, visual field defect, vomiting, WBC abnormal

Overdosage/Toxicology No toxicity has been observed in animal studies. There is limited human overdose experience. Treatment is symptomatic and supportive.

Drug Interactions
Cytochrome P450 Effect: CYP2C19 enzyme substrate, CYP3A3/4 enzyme substrate (minor)
Decreased Effect: Lansoprazole may decrease blood levels/absorption of ketoconazole, itraconazole, ampicillin esters, iron salts, digoxin and other drugs dependent upon acid for absorption. Lansoprazole may decrease theophylline levels (slightly). Sucralfate delays and reduces lansoprazole absorption by 30%.

Ethanol/Nutrition/Herb Interactions
Ethanol: Avoid ethanol (may cause gastric mucosal irritation).
Food: Lansoprazole serum concentrations may be decreased if taken with food.

Stability Store at 15°C to 30°C (59°F to 86°F); protect from light and moisture.
(Continued)

Lansoprazole (Continued)

Mechanism of Action A proton pump inhibitor which decreases acid secretion in gastric parietal cells

Pharmacodynamics/Kinetics

Duration: >1 day

Absorption: Rapid

Protein binding: 97%

Metabolism: Hepatic and in parietal cells to two inactive metabolites

Bioavailability: 80% (decreased 50% if given 30 minutes after food)

Half-life elimination: 2 hours; Elderly: 2.9 hours; Hepatic impairment: ≤7 hours

Time to peak, plasma: 1.7 hours

Excretion: Feces (67%); urine (33%)

Usual Dosage Oral:

Adults:

Duodenal ulcer: Short-term treatment: 15 mg once daily for 4 weeks; maintenance therapy: 15 mg once daily

Gastric ulcer: Short-term treatment: 30 mg once daily for up to 8 weeks

NSAID-associated gastric ulcer (healing): 30 mg once daily for 8 weeks; controlled studies did not extend past 8 weeks of therapy

NSAID-associated gastric ulcer (to reduce risk): Oral: 15 mg once daily for up to 12 weeks; controlled studies did not extend past 12 weeks of therapy

Symptomatic GERD: Short-term treatment: 15 mg once daily for up to 8 weeks

Erosive esophagitis: Short-term treatment: 30 mg once daily for up to 8 weeks; continued treatment for an additional 8 weeks may be considered for recurrence or for patients that do not heal after the first 8 weeks of therapy; maintenance therapy: 15 mg once daily

Hypersecretory conditions: Initial: 60 mg once daily; adjust dose based upon patient response and to reduce acid secretion to <10 mEq/hour (5 mEq/hour in patients with prior gastric surgery); doses of 90 mg twice daily have been used; administer doses >120 mg/day in divided doses

Helicobacter pylori eradication: Currently accepted recommendations (may differ from product labeling): Dose varies with regimen: 30 mg once daily or 60 mg/day in 2 divided doses; requires combination therapy with antibiotics

Elderly: No dosage adjustment is needed in elderly patients with normal hepatic function

Dosage adjustment in renal impairment: No dosage adjustment is needed

Dosing adjustment in hepatic impairment: Dose reduction is necessary for severe hepatic impairment

Dietary Considerations Should be taken before eating.

Administration

Oral: Administer before food. The intact granules should not be chewed or crushed; however, in addition to oral suspension, several options are available for those patients unable to swallow capsules:

Capsules may be opened and the intact granules sprinkled on 1 tablespoon of applesauce, Ensure® pudding, cottage cheese, yogurt, or strained pears. The granules should then be swallowed immediately.

Capsules may be opened and emptied into ~60 mL orange juice, apple juice, or tomato juice; mix and swallow immediately. Rinse the glass with additional juice and swallow to assure complete delivery of the dose.

Capsule granules may be mixed with apple, cranberry, grape, orange, pineapple, prune, tomato and V-8® juice and stored for up to 30 minutes.

Nasogastric tube administration: Capsules can be opened, the granules mixed (not crushed) with 40 mL of apple juice and then injected through the NG tube into the stomach, then flush tube with additional apple juice

Monitoring Parameters Patients with Zollinger-Ellison syndrome should be monitored for gastric acid output, which should be maintained at ≤10 mEq/hour during the last hour before the next lansoprazole dose; lab monitoring should include CBC, liver function, renal function, and serum gastrin levels

Patient Information Take before eating; do not crush or chew capsules or granules for oral suspension

Dosage Forms

Capsule, delayed release: 15 mg, 30 mg

Granules, for oral suspension, delayed release: 15 mg/packet (30s), 30 mg/packet (30s)

Extemporaneous Preparations A 3 mg/mL lansoprazole oral solution (Simplified Lansoprazole Solution) can be prepared with ten lansoprazole 30 mg capsules and 100 mL 8.4% sodium bicarbonate. Empty capsules into beaker. Add sodium bicarbonate solution. Gently stir (about 15 minutes) until dissolved. Transfer to amber-colored syringe or bottle. Stable for 8 hours at room temperature or for 14 days under refrigeration.

DiGiacinto JL, Olsen KM, Bergman KL, et al, "Stability of Suspension Formulations of Lansoprazole and Omeprazole Stored in Amber-Colored Plastic Oral Syringes," *Ann Pharmacother*, 2000, 34:600-5

Sharma V, "Comparison of 24-hour Intragastric pH Using Four Liquid Formulations of Lansoprazole and Omeprazole," *Am J Health Syst Pharm*, 1999, 56(Suppl 4):S18-21.

Sharma VK, Vasudeva R, and Howden CW, "Simplified Lansoprazole Suspension - Liquid Formulations of Lansoprazole - Effectively Suppresses Intragastric Acidity When Administered Through a Gastrostomy," *Am J Gastroenterol*, 1999, 94(7):1813-7.

Lansoprazole, Amoxicillin, and Clarithromycin

(lan SOE pra zole, a moks i SIL in, & kla RITH roe mye sin)

U.S. Brand Names Prevpac™

Canadian Brand Names Hp-PAC®; Prevpac™

Synonyms Amoxicillin, Lansoprazole, and Clarithromycin; Clarithromycin, Lansoprazole, and Amoxicillin

Therapeutic Category Antibiotic, Macrolide Combination; Antibiotic, Penicillin; Gastrointestinal Agent, H. pylori

Use Eradication of *H. pylori* to reduce the risk of recurrent duodenal ulcer

Pregnancy Risk Factor C (clarithromycin)

Usual Dosage Lansoprazole 30 mg, amoxicillin 1 g, and clarithromycin 50 mg taken together twice daily

Additional Information Complete prescribing information for this medication should be consulted for additional detail.

Dosage Forms The package contains:
Capsule:
Amoxicillin: 500 mg
Lansoprazole: 30 mg
Tablet: Clarithromycin: 500 mg

♦ **Lantus®** *see* Insulin Preparations *on page 722*
♦ **Lanvis® (Can)** *see* Thioguanine *on page 1318*
♦ **Largactil® (Can)** *see* ChlorproMAZINE *on page 282*
♦ **Lariam®** *see* Mefloquine *on page 851*
♦ **Larodopa®** *see* Levodopa *on page 790*
♦ **Lasix®** *see* Furosemide *on page 612*
♦ **Lasix® Special (Can)** *see* Furosemide *on page 612*
♦ **L-asparaginase** *see* Asparaginase *on page 118*

Latanoprost (la TA noe prost)

Related Information
Glaucoma Drug Therapy Comparison *on page 1499*

U.S. Brand Names Xalatan®

Canadian Brand Names Xalatan™

Therapeutic Category Prostaglandin, Ophthalmic

Use Reduction of elevated intraocular pressure in patients with open-angle glaucoma and ocular hypertension who are intolerant to the other IOP lowering medications or insufficiently responsive (failed to achieve target IOP determined after multiple measurements over time) to another IOP lowering medication

Pregnancy Risk Factor C

Usual Dosage Adults: Ophthalmic: 1 drop (1.5 mcg) in the affected eye(s) once daily in the evening; do not exceed the once daily dosage because it has been shown that more frequent administration may decrease the IOP lowering effect

Additional Information Complete prescribing information for this medication should be consulted for additional detail.

Dosage Forms Solution, ophthalmic: 0.005% (2.5 mL)

♦ **Laxatives, Classification and Properties** *see page 1504*
♦ **Laxilose (Can)** *see* Lactulose *on page 770*
♦ **l-Bunolol Hydrochloride** *see* Levobunolol *on page 788*
♦ **L-Carnitine** *see* Levocarnitine *on page 789*
♦ **LCR** *see* VinCRIStine *on page 1417*
♦ **L-Deprenyl** *see* Selegiline *on page 1228*
♦ **L-Dopa** *see* Levodopa *on page 790*

Leflunomide (le FLOO noh mide)

U.S. Brand Names Arava™

Canadian Brand Names Arava™

Therapeutic Category Antimetabolite; Antirheumatic, Disease Modifying

Use Treatment of active rheumatoid arthritis to reduce signs and symptoms and to retard structural damage as evidenced by x-ray erosions and joint space narrowing

Pregnancy Risk Factor X

Pregnancy/Breast-Feeding Implications Has been associated with teratogenic and embryolethal effects in animal models at low doses. Leflunomide is contraindicated in pregnant women or women of childbearing potential who are not using reliable contraception. Pregnancy must be excluded prior to initiating treatment. Following treatment, pregnancy should be avoided until the drug elimination procedure is completed.

Breast-feeding is contraindicated. It is not known whether leflunomide is secreted in human milk; however, there is a potential for serious adverse reactions in nursing infants. A decision should be made whether to discontinue nursing or discontinue the drug, taking into account the importance of the drug to the mother.

Contraindications Hypersensitivity to leflunomide or any component of the formulation; pregnancy

Warnings/Precautions Hepatic disease (including seropositive hepatitis B or C patients) may increase risk of hepatotoxicity; immunosuppression may increase the risk of lymphoproliferative disorders or other malignancies; women of childbearing potential should not receive leflunomide until pregnancy has been excluded, patients have been counseled concerning fetal risk and reliable contraceptive measures have been confirmed. Caution in renal impairment, immune deficiency, bone marrow dysplasia or severe, uncontrolled infection. Use of live vaccines is not recommended; will increase uric acid excretion.

Adverse Reactions
>10%:
Gastrointestinal: Diarrhea (17%)
Respiratory: Respiratory tract infection (15%)
1% to 10% (Limited to important or life-threatening):
Cardiovascular: Hypertension (10%), chest pain (2%), vasculitis, edema (peripheral)
Central nervous system: Headache (7%), dizziness (4%) paresthesia (2%), fever, neuralgia, neuritis, sleep disorder
Dermatologic: Alopecia (10%), rash (10%), pruritus (4%), dry skin (2%), eczema (2%), dermatitis, hair discoloration, subcutaneous nodule, skin disorder/discoloration
(Continued)

Leflunomide *(Continued)*

Endocrine & metabolic: Hypokalemia (1%), diabetes mellitus, hyperlipidemia, hyperthyroidism

Gastrointestinal: Nausea (9%), weight loss (4%), anorexia (3%), gastroenteritis (3%), stomatitis (3%), vomiting (3%), cholelithiasis, colitis, esophagitis, gingivitis, melena, candidiasis (oral)

Genitourinary: Urinary tract infection (5%), albuminuria, cystitis, dysuria, hematuria

Hematologic: Anemia

Neuromuscular & skeletal: Tenosynovitis (3%), arthralgia (1%), muscle cramps (1%), neck pain, pelvic pain, arthrosis, bursitis, myalgia, bone necrosis, bone pain, tendon rupture

Ocular: Cataract, conjunctivitis

Respiratory: Bronchitis (7%), cough (3%), pharyngitis (3%), pneumonia (2%), rhinitis (2%), sinusitis (2%), asthma, dyspnea

Miscellaneous: Infection (4%), allergic reactions (2%)

<1% (Limited to important or life-threatening): Anaphylaxis, eosinophilia, hepatotoxicity, hepatic failure, leukopenia, thrombocytopenia, urticaria

Overdosage/Toxicology There is no human overdose experience. Leflunomide is not dialyzable. Cholestyramine and/or activated charcoal enhance elimination of leflunomide's active metabolite (MI). In cases of significant overdose or toxicity, cholestyramine 8 g every 8 hours for 1-3 days may be administered to enhance elimination. Plasma levels are reduced by approximately 40% in 24 hours and 49% to 65% after 48 hours of cholestyramine dosing.

Drug Interactions

Cytochrome P450 Effect: CYP2C9 enzyme inhibitor (*in vitro* only)

Increased Effect/Toxicity: Theoretically, concomitant use of drugs metabolized by this enzyme, including many NSAIDs, may result in increased serum concentrations and possible toxic effects. Coadministration with methotrexate increases the risk of hepatotoxicity. Leflunomide may also enhance the hepatotoxicity of other drugs. Tolbutamide free fraction may be increased. Rifampin may increase serum concentrations of leflunomide. Leflunomide has uricosuric activity and may enhance activity of other uricosuric agents.

Decreased Effect: Administration of cholestyramine and activated charcoal enhance the elimination of leflunomide's active metabolite.

Ethanol/Nutrition/Herb Interactions Food: No interactions with food have been noted.

Stability Protect from light; store at 25°C (77°F).

Mechanism of Action Inhibits pyrimidine synthesis, resulting in antiproliferative and anti-inflammatory effects

Pharmacodynamics/Kinetics

Distribution: V_d: 0.13 L/kg

Metabolism: Hepatic, to A77 1726 (MI) which accounts for nearly all pharmacologic activity; further metabolism to multiple inactive metabolites; enterohepatic recycling occurs

Bioavailability: 80%

Half-life elimination: Mean: 14-15 days; enterohepatic recycling appears to contribute to the long half-life of this agent, since activated charcoal and cholestyramine substantially reduce plasma half-life

Time to peak: 6-12 hours

Excretion: Feces (48%); urine (43%)

Usual Dosage

Adults: Oral: Initial: 100 mg/day for 3 days, followed by 20 mg/day; dosage may be decreased to 10 mg/day in patients who have difficulty tolerating the 20 mg dose. Due to the long half-life of the active metabolite, plasma levels may require a prolonged period to decline after dosage reduction.

Dosing adjustment in renal impairment: No specific dosage adjustment is recommended. There is no clinical experience in the use of leflunomide in patients with renal impairment. The free fraction of MI is doubled in dialysis patients. Patients should be monitored closely for adverse effects requiring dosage adjustment.

Dosing adjustment in hepatic impairment: No specific dosage adjustment is recommended. Since the liver is involved in metabolic activation and subsequent metabolism/elimination of leflunomide, patients with hepatic impairment should be monitored closely for adverse effects requiring dosage adjustment.

Guidelines for dosage adjustment or discontinuation based on the severity and persistence of ALT elevation secondary to leflunomide have been developed. For ALT elevations >2 times the upper limit of normal, dosage reduction to 10 mg/day may allow continued administration (consider increased monitoring frequency - ie, weekly). Cholestyramine 8 g 3 times/day for 1-3 days may be administered to decrease plasma levels. If elevations >2 times but ≤3 times the upper limit of normal persist, liver biopsy is recommended. If elevations >3 times the upper limit of normal persist despite cholestyramine administration and dosage reduction, leflunomide should be discontinued and drug elimination should be enhanced with additional cholestyramine as indicated.

Elderly: Although hepatic function may decline with age, no specific dosage adjustment is recommended. Patients should be monitored closely for adverse effects which may require dosage adjustment.

Dietary Considerations Administer without regard to meals.

Monitoring Parameters Serum transaminase determinations at baseline and monthly during the initial phase of treatment; if stable, monitoring frequency may be decreased to intervals determined by the individual clinical situation. Monitor for abnormalities in hepatic function tests or symptoms of hepatotoxicity.

Patient Information Do not take leflunomide if pregnant

Additional Information To enhance elimination, a drug elimination procedure has been developed. Without this procedure, it may take up to 2 years to reach plasma concentrations <0.02 mg/L (a concentration expected to have minimal risk of teratogenicity based on animal models). The procedure consists of the following steps: Administer cholestyramine 8 g 3 times/day for 11 days (the 11 days do not need to be consecutive). Plasma levels <0.02 mg/L should be verified by two separate tests performed at least 14 days apart. If plasma levels are >0.02 mg/L, additional cholestyramine treatment should be considered.

Dosage Forms Tablet: 10 mg, 20 mg, 100 mg

♦ **Legatrin PM®** [OTC] *see* Acetaminophen and Diphenhydramine *on page 25*

♦ **Lenoltec (Can)** *see* Acetaminophen and Codeine *on page 24*

♦ **Lente® Iletin® II** *see* Insulin Preparations *on page 722*

Lepirudin (leh puh ROO din)

U.S. Brand Names Refludan®

Canadian Brand Names Refludan®

Synonyms Lepirudin (rDNA); Recombinant Hirudin

Therapeutic Category Anticoagulant

Use Indicated for anticoagulation in patients with heparin-induced thrombocytopenia (HIT) and associated thromboembolic disease in order to prevent further thromboembolic complications

Unlabeled/Investigational Use Investigational: Prevention or reduction of ischemic complications associated with unstable angina

Pregnancy Risk Factor B

Pregnancy/Breast-Feeding Implications Lepirudin crosses the placenta in pregnant rats; however, it is not known if lepirudin crosses the placenta in humans. It is not known if lepirudin is excreted in human milk.

Contraindications Hypersensitivity to hirudins or any component of the formulation

Warnings/Precautions

Hemorrhagic events: Intracranial bleeding following concomitant thrombolytic therapy with rt-PA or streptokinase may be life threatening. For patients with an increased risk of bleeding, a careful assessment weighing the risk of lepirudin administration versus its anticipated benefit has to be made by the treating physician. In particular, this includes the following conditions:

Recent puncture of large vessels or organ biopsy

Anomaly of vessels or organs

Recent cerebrovascular accident, stroke, intracerebral surgery, or other neuroaxial procedures

Severe uncontrolled hypertension

Bacterial endocarditis

Advanced renal impairment

Hemorrhagic diathesis

Recent major surgery

Recent major bleeding (eg, intracranial, gastrointestinal, intraocular, or pulmonary bleeding)

With renal impairment, relative overdose might occur even with standard dosage regimen. The bolus dose and rate of infusion must be reduced in patients with known or suspected renal insufficiency.

Formation of antihirudin antibodies was observed in ~40% of HIT patients treated with lepirudin. This may increase the anticoagulant effect of lepirudin possibly due to delayed renal elimination of active lepirudin-antihirudin complexes. Therefore, strict monitoring of aPTT is necessary also during prolonged therapy. No evidence of neutralization of lepirudin or of allergic reactions associated with positive antibody test results was found.

Serious liver injury (eg, liver cirrhosis) may enhance the anticoagulant effect of lepirudin due to coagulation defects secondary to reduced generation of vitamin K-dependent clotting factors

Clinical trials have provided limited information to support any recommendations for re-exposure to lepirudin

Adverse Reactions As with all anticoagulants, bleeding is the most common adverse event associated with lepirudin. Hemorrhage may occur at virtually any site. Risk is dependent on multiple variables.

HIT patients:

>10%: Hematologic: Anemia (12%), bleeding from puncture sites (11%), hematoma (11%)

1% to 10%:

Cardiovascular: Heart failure (3%), pericardial effusion (1%), ventricular fibrillation (1%)

Central nervous system: Fever (7%)

Dermatologic: Eczema (3%), maculopapular rash (4%)

Gastrointestinal: GI bleeding/rectal bleeding (5%)

Genitourinary: Vaginal bleeding (2%)

Hepatic: Increased transaminases (6%)

Renal: Hematuria (4%)

Respiratory: Epistaxis (4%)

<1% (Limited to important or life-threatening): Hemoperitoneum, hemoptysis, injection site reactions, liver bleeding, mouth bleeding, pruritus, pulmonary bleeding, retroperitoneal bleeding, thrombocytopenia, urticaria

Non-HIT populations (including those receiving thrombolytics and/or contrast media):

1% to 10%: Respiratory: Bronchospasm/stridor/dyspnea/cough

<1% (Limited to important or life-threatening): Allergic reactions (unspecified), anaphylactoid reactions, anaphylaxis, angioedema, intracranial bleeding (0.6%), laryngeal edema, thrombocytopenia, tongue edema

Overdosage/Toxicology In case of overdose (eg, suggested by excessively high aPTT values), the risk of bleeding is increased. No specific antidote for lepirudin is available. If life-threatening bleeding occurs and excessive plasma levels of lepirudin are suspected, the following steps should be followed:

Immediately STOP LEPIRUDIN administration

Determine aPTT and other coagulation levels as appropriate

Determine hemoglobin and prepare for blood transfusion

Follow current guidelines for treating patients with shock

(Continued)

Lepirudin *(Continued)*

Individual clinical case reports and *in vitro* data suggest that either hemofiltration or hemo-dialysis (using high-flux dialysis membranes with a cutoff point of 50,000 daltons, eg, AN/69) may be useful in this situation

Drug Interactions

Increased Effect/Toxicity: Thrombolytics may enhance anticoagulant properties of lepirudin on aPTT and can increase the risk of bleeding complications. Bleeding risk may also be increased by oral anticoagulants (warfarin) and platelet function inhibitors (nonsteroidal anti-inflammatory drugs, dipyridamole, ticlopidine, clopidogrel, IIb/IIIa antagonists, and aspirin).

Ethanol/Nutrition/Herb Interactions Herb/Nutraceutical: Avoid cat's claw, dong quai, evening primrose, feverfew, garlic, ginger, ginkgo, red clover, horse chestnut, green tea, ginseng (all have additional antiplatelet activity)

Stability

Intact vials should be stored at 2°C to 25°C (36°F to 77°F)

Intravenous bolus: Use a solution with a concentration of 5 mg/mL

Preparation of a lepirudin solution with a concentration of 5 mg/mL: Reconstitute one vial (50 mg) of lepirudin with 1 mL of sterile water for injection or 0.9% sodium chloride injection; the final concentration of 5 mg/mL is obtained by transferring the contents of the vial into a sterile, single-use syringe (of at least 10 mL capacity) and diluting the solution to a total volume of 10 mL using sterile water for injection, 0.9% sodium chloride, or 5% dextrose in water

Intravenous infusion: For continuous intravenous infusion, solutions with concentrations of 0.2 or 0.4 mg/mL may be used

Preparation of a lepirudin solution with a concentration of 0.2 mg/mL or 0.4 mg/mL: Reconstitute 2 vials (50 mg each) of lepirudin with 1 mL each using either sterile water for injection or 0.9% sodium chloride injection; the final concentration of 0.2 mg/mL or 0.4 mg/mL is obtained by transferring the contents of both vials into an infusion bag containing 500 mL or 250 mL of 0.9% sodium chloride injection or 5% dextrose injection

Reconstituted solutions of lepirudin are stable for 24 hours at room temperature

Mechanism of Action Lepirudin is a highly specific direct inhibitor of thrombin; lepirudin is a recombinant hirudin derived from yeast cells

Pharmacodynamics/Kinetics

Distribution: Two-compartment model; confined to extracellular fluids.

Metabolism: By release of amino acids via catabolic hydrolysis of parent drug

Half-life elimination: Initial: ~10 minutes; Terminal: Healthy volunteers: 1.3 hours; Marked renal insufficiency (Cl_{cr} <15 mL/minute and on hemodialysis: ≤2 days)

Excretion: Urine (~48%, 35% as unchanged drug and unchanged drug fragments of parent drug); systemic clearance is proportional to glomerular filtration rate or creatinine clearance

Usual Dosage Adults: Maximum dose: Do not exceed 0.21 mg/kg/hour unless an evaluation of coagulation abnormalities limiting response has been completed. **Dosing is weight-based, however patients weighing >110 kg should not receive doses greater than the recommended dose for a patient weighing 110 kg (44 mg bolus and initial maximal infusion rate of 16.5 mg/hour).**

Heparin-induced thrombocytopenia: Bolus dose: 0.4 mg/kg IVP (over 15-20 seconds), followed by continuous infusion at 0.15 mg/kg/hour; bolus and infusion must be reduced in renal insufficiency

Concomitant use with thrombolytic therapy: Bolus dose: 0.2 mg/kg IVP (over 15-20 seconds), followed by continuous infusion at 0.1 mg/kg/hour

Dosing adjustments during infusions: Monitor first aPTT 4 hours after the start of the infusion. Subsequent determinations of aPTT should be obtained at least once daily during treatment. More frequent monitoring is recommended in renally impaired patients. Any aPTT ratio measurement out of range (1.5-2.5) should be confirmed prior to adjusting dose, unless a clinical need for immediate reaction exists. If the aPTT is below target range, increase infusion by 20%. If the aPTT is in excess of the target range, decrease infusion rate by 50%. A repeat aPTT should be obtained 4 hours after any dosing change.

Use in patients scheduled for switch to oral anticoagulants: Reduce lepirudin dose gradually to reach aPTT ratio just above 1.5 before starting warfarin therapy; as soon as INR reaches 2.0, lepirudin therapy should be discontinued.

Dosing adjustment in renal impairment: All patients with a creatinine clearance of <60 mL/minute or a serum creatinine of >1.5 mg/dL should receive a reduction in lepirudin dosage; there is only limited information on the therapeutic use of lepirudin in HIT patients with significant renal impairment; the following dosage recommendations are mainly based on single-dose studies in a small number of patients with renal impairment.

Initial: Bolus dose: 0.2 mg/kg IVP (over 15-20 seconds), followed by adjusted infusion based on renal function; refer to the following infusion rate adjustments based on creatinine clearance (mL/minute) and serum creatinine (mg/dL):

Lepirudin infusion rates in patients with renal impairment: See table.

Lepirudin Infusion Rates in Patients With Renal Impairment

Creatinine Clearance (mL/minute)	Serum Creatinine (mg/dL)	Adjusted Infusion Rate	
		% of Standard Initial Infusion Rate	mg/kg/hour
45-60	1.6-2.0	50%	0.075
30-44	2.1-3.0	30%	0.045
15-29	3.1-6.0	15%	0.0225
<15	>6.0	Avoid or STOP infusion	

Note: **Acute renal failure or hemodialysis:** Infusion is to be avoided or stopped. Following the bolus dose, additional bolus doses of 0.1 mg/kg may be administered every other day (only if aPTT falls below lower therapeutic limit).

Administration Administer **only** intravenously; administer I.V. bolus over 15-20 seconds

Monitoring Parameters aPTT levels

Reference Range aPTT 1.5 to 2.5 times the control value

Dosage Forms Injection: 50 mg vials

♦ **Lepirudin (rDNA)** *see* Lepirudin *on page 779*

♦ **Lescol®** *see* Fluvastatin *on page 592*

♦ **Lescol® XL** *see* Fluvastatin *on page 592*

Letrozole (LET roe zole)

U.S. Brand Names Femara®

Canadian Brand Names Femara®

Therapeutic Category Antineoplastic Agent, Hormone Antagonist; Antineoplastic Agent, Hormone (Antiestrogen); Aromatase Inhibitor

Use First-line treatment of hormone receptor positive or hormone receptor unknown, locally advanced, or metastatic breast cancer in postmenopausal women; treatment of advanced breast cancer in postmenopausal women with disease progression following antiestrogen therapy

Pregnancy Risk Factor D

Pregnancy/Breast-Feeding Implications Clinical effects on the fetus: Letrozole may cause fetal harm when administered to pregnant women. Letrozole is embryotoxic and fetotoxic when administered to rats. There are no studies in pregnant women and letrozole is indicated for postmenopausal women.

Contraindications Hypersensitivity to letrozole or any component of the formulation; pregnancy

Warnings/Precautions Dose-related effects on hematologic or chemistry parameters have not been observed. Increases in transaminases ≥5 times the upper limit of normal and of bilirubin ≥1.5 times the upper limit of normal were most often, but not always, associated with metastatic liver disease. Safety and efficacy have not been established in pediatric patients.

Adverse Reactions

>10% :
  Cardiovascular: Hot flushes (5% to 18%)
  Central nervous system: Headache (8% to 12%), fatigue (6% to 11%)
  Gastrointestinal: Nausea (13% to 15%)
  Neuromuscular & skeletal: Musculoskeletal pain, bone pain (20%), back pain (17%), arthralgia (8% to 14%),
  Respiratory: Dyspnea (7% to 14%), cough (5% to 11%)

2% to 10%:
  Cardiovascular: Chest pain (3% to 8%), peripheral edema (5%), hypertension (5% to 7%)
  Central nervous system: Pain (5%), insomnia (6%), dizziness (3% to 5%), somnolence (2% to 3%), depression (<5%), anxiety (<5%), vertigo (<5%)
  Dermatologic: Rash (5%), alopecia (<5% to 5%), pruritus (1%)
  Endocrine & metabolic: Breast pain (5%), hypercholesterolemia (3%)
  Gastrointestinal: Vomiting (7%), constipation (6% to 9%), diarrhea (5% to 7%), abdominal pain (4% to 6%), anorexia (4%), dyspepsia (3% to 4%), weight loss (6%), weight gain (2%)
  Neuromuscular & skeletal: Weakness (4% to 5%)
  Miscellaneous: Flu (5% to 6%)

<2% (Limited to important or life-threatening): Angina, cardiac ischemia, coronary artery disease, hemiparesis, hemorrhagic stroke, myocardial infarction, portal vein thrombosis, pulmonary embolism, thrombocytopenia, thrombotic stroke, transient ischemic attack, venous thrombosis

Overdosage/Toxicology Firm recommendations for treatment are not possible. Emesis could be induced if the patient is alert. In general, supportive care and frequent monitoring of vital signs are appropriate.

Drug Interactions

Cytochrome P450 Effect: CYP3A3/4 and 2A6 enzyme substrate; CYP2A6 and 2C19 enzyme inhibitor

Increased Effect/Toxicity: Inhibitors of this enzyme may, in theory, increase letrozole blood levels. Letrozole inhibits cytochrome P450 isoenzyme 2A6 and 2C19 *in vitro* and may increase blood levels of drugs metabolized by these enzymes. Specific drug interaction studies have not been reported.

Stability Store at 15°C to 30°C (59°F to 86°F)

Mechanism of Action Nonsteroidal, competitive inhibitor of the aromatase enzyme system which binds to the heme group of aromatase, a cytochrome P450 enzyme which catalyzes conversion of androgens to estrogens (specifically, androstenedione to estrone and testosterone to estradiol). This leads to inhibition of the enzyme and a significant reduction in plasma estrogen levels. Does not affect synthesis of adrenal or thyroid hormones, aldosterone, or androgens.

Pharmacodynamics/Kinetics

  Absorption: Well absorbed; not affected by food
  Distribution: V_d: ~1.9 L/kg
  Protein binding, plasma: Weak
  Metabolism: Hepatic via CYP3A4 and CYP2A6 to a pharmacologically inactive carbinol metabolite
  Half-life elimination: Terminal: ~2 days
  Time to steady state, plasma: 2-6 weeks
  Excretion: Urine (6% as unchanged drug, 75% as glucuronide carbinol metabolite)

Usual Dosage Oral (refer to individual protocols):
  Children: Not recommended for use in pediatric patients
  (Continued)

Letrozole *(Continued)*

Adults: Breast cancer in postmenopausal women: 2.5 mg once daily without regard to meals; continue treatment until tumor progression is evident. Patients treated with letrozole do not require glucocorticoid or mineralocorticoid replacement therapy.

Elderly: No dosage adjustments required

Dosage adjustment in renal impairment: No dosage adjustment is required in patients with renal impairment if $Cl_{cr} \geq 10$ mL/minute

Dosage adjustment in hepatic impairment: No dosage adjustment is recommended for patients with mild-to-moderate hepatic impairment. Patients with severe impairment of liver function have not been studied; dose patients with severe impairment of liver function with caution.

Dietary Considerations May be taken without regard to meals.

Monitoring Parameters Clinical/radiologic evidence of tumor regression in advanced breast cancer patients. Until the toxicity has been defined in larger patient populations, monitor the following laboratory tests periodically during therapy: complete blood counts, thyroid function tests, serum electrolytes, serum transaminases, and serum creatinine.

Patient Information Report chest pain, pressure, palpitations, or swollen extremities; weakness, severe headache, numbness, or loss of strength in any part of the body, difficulty speaking; vaginal bleeding; unusual signs of bleeding or bruising; difficulty breathing; severe nausea, or muscle pain; or skin rash.

Dosage Forms Tablet: 2.5 mg

Leucovorin *(loo koe VOR in)*

Related Information

USPHA/IDSA Guidelines for the Prevention of Opportunistic Infections in Persons With HIV *on page 1574*

Synonyms Calcium Leucovorin; Citrovorum Factor; Folinic Acid; 5-Formyl Tetrahydrofolate; Leucovorin Calcium

Therapeutic Category Antidote, Methotrexate; Folic Acid Derivative

Use Antidote for folic acid antagonists (methotrexate >100 mg/m², trimethoprim, pyrimethamine); treatment of megaloblastic anemias when folate is deficient as in infancy, sprue, pregnancy, and nutritional deficiency when oral folate therapy is not possible; in combination with fluorouracil in the treatment of malignancy

Pregnancy Risk Factor C

Contraindications Hypersensitivity to leucovorin or any component of the formulation; pernicious anemia or vitamin B_{12} deficient megaloblastic anemias; should **NOT** be administered intrathecally/intraventricularly

Warnings/Precautions Use with caution in patients with a history of hypersensitivity

Adverse Reactions Limited to important or life-threatening symptoms: Seizures, thrombocytosis, wheezing, anaphylactoid reactions

Drug Interactions

Increased Effect/Toxicity: Increased toxicity of fluorouracil

Decreased Effect: May decrease efficacy of co-trimoxazole against *Pneumocystis carinii* pneumonitis

Stability

Leucovorin injection should be stored at room temperature and protected from light

Reconstituted solution is stated to be chemically stable for 7 days; reconstitutions with bacteriostatic water for injection, U.S.P., must be used within 7 days. Doses >10 mg/m² must be prepared using leucovorin reconstituted with sterile water for injection, U.S.P., and used immediately.

Stability of parenteral admixture at room temperature (25°C): 24 hours

Stability of parenteral admixture at refrigeration temperature (4°C): 4 days

Standard diluent: 50-100 mg/50 mL D_5W

Minimum volume: 50 mL D_5W

Concentrations of >2 mg/mL of leucovorin and >25 mg/mL of fluorouracil are **incompatible** (precipitation occurs)

Mechanism of Action A reduced form of folic acid, but does not require a reduction reaction by an enzyme for activation, allows for purine and thymidine synthesis, a necessity for normal erythropoiesis; leucovorin supplies the necessary cofactor blocked by MTX, enters the cells via the same active transport system as MTX

Pharmacodynamics/Kinetics

Onset of action: Oral: ~30 minutes; I.V.: ~5 minutes

Absorption: Oral, I.M.: Rapid and well

Metabolism: Intestinal mucosa and hepatically; to 5-methyl-tetrahydrofolate (5MTHF; active)

Bioavailability: 31% (following 200 mg dose)

Half-life elimination: Leucovorin: 15 minutes; 5MTHF: 33-35 minutes

Excretion: Primarily urine (80% to 90%); feces (5% to 8%)

Usual Dosage Children and Adults:

Treatment of folic acid antagonist overdosage (eg, pyrimethamine or trimethoprim): Oral: 2-15 mg/day for 3 days or until blood counts are normal or 5 mg every 3 days; doses of 6 mg/day are needed for patients with platelet counts <100,000/mm³

Folate-deficient megaloblastic anemia: I.M.: 1 mg/day

Megaloblastic anemia secondary to congenital deficiency of dihydrofolate reductase: I.M.: 3-6 mg/day

Rescue dose (rescue therapy should start within 24 hours of MTX therapy): I.V.: 10 mg/m² to start, then 10 mg/m² every 6 hours orally for 72 hours until serum MTX concentration is <10^{-8} molar; if serum creatinine 24 hours after methotrexate is elevated 50% or more above the pre-MTX serum creatinine **or** the serum MTX concentration is >5 x 10^{-6} molar (see graph), increase dose to 100 mg/m²/dose (preservative-free) every 3 hours until serum methotrexate level is <1 x 10^{-8} molar

Investigational: Post I.T. methotrexate: Oral, I.V.: 12 mg/m² as a single dose; post high-dose methotrexate: 100-1000 mg/m²/dose until the serum methotrexate level is less than 1 x 10^{-7} molar

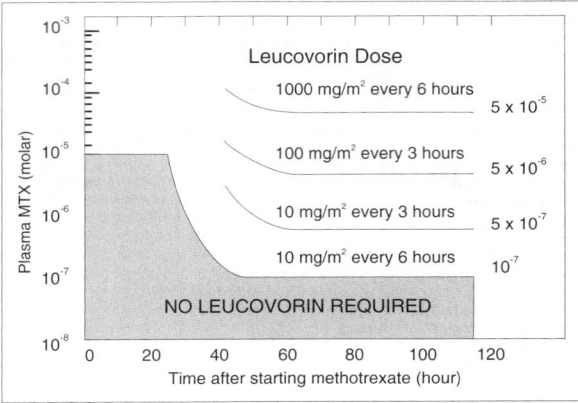

Time after starting methotrexate (hour)

The drug should be given parenterally instead of orally in patients with GI toxicity, nausea, vomiting, and when individual doses are >25 mg

Administration Leucovorin should not be administered concurrently with methotrexate. It is commonly initiated 24 hours after the start of methotrexate. Toxicity to normal tissues may be irreversible if leucovorin is not initiated by ~40 hours after the start of methotrexate. As a rescue after folate antagonists, leucovorin may be administered by I.V. bolus injection, I.M. injection, or orally. Doses >25 mg should be administered parenterally. In combination with 5-FU, leucovorin is given before or concurrent with 5-FU. Leucovorin is usually administered by I.V. bolus injection or short I.V. infusion. Other administration schedules have been used; refer to individual protocols.

Monitoring Parameters Plasma MTX concentration as a therapeutic guide to high-dose MTX therapy with leucovorin factor rescue

Leucovorin is continued until the plasma MTX level is <1 x 10^{-7} molar

Each dose of leucovorin is increased if the plasma MTX concentration is excessively high (see graph)

With 4- to 6-hour high-dose MTX infusions, plasma drug values in excess of 5 x 10^{-5} and 10^{-6} molar at 24 and 48 hours after starting the infusion, respectively, are often predictive of delayed MTX clearance; see graph.

Patient Information

Contact physician immediately, if you have an allergic reaction after taking leucovorin calcium (trouble breathing, wheezing, fainting, skin rash, or hives)

Let physician know if you are pregnant or are trying to get pregnant before taking leucovorin calcium

Leucovorin calcium can be taken with or without food

Take as directed, at evenly spaced intervals around-the-clock. Maintain hydration (2-3 L of water/day while taking for rescue therapy). For folic acid deficiency, eat foods high in folic acid (eg, meat proteins, bran, dried beans, asparagus, green leafy vegetables). Report respiratory difficulty, lethargy, or rash or itching.

Nursing Implications Parenteral: Reconstitute 50 mg or 100 mg powder for injection vials with 5-10 mL concentration (350 mg vial requires 17 mL diluent resulting in 20 mg/mL); infuse at a maximum rate of 160 mg/minute

Dosage Forms

Injection, as calcium: 3 mg/mL (1 mL)

Powder for injection, as calcium: 50 mg, 100 mg, 350 mg

Tablet, as calcium: 5 mg, 10 mg, 15 mg, 25 mg

♦ **Leucovorin Calcium** *see* Leucovorin *on page 782*

♦ **Leukeran**® *see* Chlorambucil *on page 271*

♦ **Leukine**™ *see* Sargramostim *on page 1223*

Leuprolide (loo PROE lide)

U.S. Brand Names Eligard™; Lupron®; Lupron Depot®; Lupron Depot-Ped®; Viadur™

Canadian Brand Names Lupron®; Lupron® Depot®; Viadur™

Synonyms Leuprolide Acetate; Leuprorelin Acetate

Therapeutic Category Gonadotropin Releasing Hormone Analog

Use Palliative treatment of advanced prostate carcinoma (alternative when orchiectomy or estrogen administration are not indicated or are unacceptable to the patient); combination therapy with flutamide for treating metastatic prostatic carcinoma; treatment of endometriosis as initial treatment and/or treatment of recurrent symptoms; central precocious puberty (may be used an agent to treat precocious puberty because of its effect in lowering levels of LH and FSH, testosterone, and estrogen).

Unlabeled/Investigational Use Treatment of breast, ovarian, and endometrial cancer; leiomyoma uteri; infertility; prostatic hyperplasia

Pregnancy Risk Factor X

Contraindications Hypersensitivity to leuprolide or any component of the formulation; spinal cord compression (orchiectomy suggested); undiagnosed abnormal vaginal bleeding; women who are or may be pregnant should not receive leuprolide

(Continued)

Leuprolide *(Continued)*

Warnings/Precautions Use with caution in patients hypersensitive to benzyl alcohol; after 6 months use of leuprolide, vertebral bone density decreased (average 13.5%); long-term safety of leuprolide in children has not been established; urinary tract obstruction may occur upon initiation of therapy. Closely observe patients for weakness, paresthesias, and urinary tract obstruction in first few weeks of therapy. Tumor flare and bone pain may occur at initiation of therapy; transient weakness and paresthesia of lower limbs, hematuria, and urinary tract obstruction in first week of therapy; animal studies have shown dose-related benign pituitary hyperplasia and benign pituitary adenomas after 2 years of use. Use caution in patients with a history of psychiatric illness; alteration in mood, memory impairment, and depression have been associated with use.

Adverse Reactions
Female:
>10%:
Endocrine & metabolic: Amenorrhea
Neuromuscular & skeletal: Changes in bone mineral density
1% to 10%:
Endocrine & metabolic: Libido decreased, breast tenderness
Miscellaneous: Deepening of voice
Male/Female:
>10%: Cardiovascular: Hot flashes
1% to 10%:
Cardiovascular: Arrhythmias, palpitations, edema
Central nervous system: Dizziness, headache, insomnia, paresthesias
Gastrointestinal: Weight gain, nausea, vomiting
Ocular: Blurred vision
Miscellaneous: Pain at injection site
Male:
1% to 10%:
Cardiovascular: Chest pain
Endocrine & metabolic: Gynecomastia, impotence or decreased libido
Gastrointestinal: Constipation, anorexia
Genitourinary: Testicle size decreased
All populations: <1% (Limited to important or life-threatening): Anaphylactoid reaction, asthma, depression, fibromyalgia, memory impairment, myocardial infarction, peripheral neuropathy, pulmonary embolism, rash, suicidal ideation/behavior, thrombophlebitis

Overdosage/Toxicology Treatment consists of general supportive care.

Stability
Store unopened vials of injection in refrigerator, vial in use can be kept at room temperature of ≤30°C (86°F) for several months with minimal loss of potency. Protect from light and store vial in carton until use. Do not freeze.
Eligard™: Store at 2°C to 8°C (36°F to 46°C). Allow to reach room temperature prior to using; once mixed, must be administered within 30 minutes.
Lupron Depot® may be stored at room temperature of 25°C, excursions permitted to 15°C to 30°C (59°F to 86°F). Upon reconstitution, the suspension is stable for 24 hours; does not contain a preservative.
Viadur™ may be stored at room temperature of 25°C.

Mechanism of Action Continuous daily administration results in suppression of ovarian and testicular steroidogenesis due to decreased levels of LH and FSH with subsequent decrease in testosterone (male) and estrogen (female) levels

Pharmacodynamics/Kinetics
Onset of action: Serum testosterone levels: Increase within 3 days
Duration: Levels decrease after 2-4 weeks with continued therapy
Distribution: 27 L
Protein binding: 43% to 49%
Metabolism: Destroyed within the GI tract
Bioavailability: Oral: None; S.C. and I.V.: Doses are comparable
Half-life elimination: 3-4.25 hours
Excretion: Not well defined

Usual Dosage Requires parenteral administration
Children: Precocious puberty:
S.C. (Lupron®): 20-45 mcg/kg/day
I.M. (Lupron Depot®): 0.3 mg/kg/dose given every 28 days
≤25 kg: 7.5 mg
>25-37.5 kg: 11.25 mg
>37.5 kg: 15 mg
Adults:
Advanced prostatic carcinoma:
S.C.:
Eligard™: 7.5 mg monthly
Lupron®: 1 mg/day
I.M.:
Lupron Depot®: 7.5 mg/dose given monthly (every 28-33 days) **or**
Lupron Depot-3®: 22.5 mg every 3 months **or**
Lupron Depot-4®: 30 mg every 4 months
Implant (Viadur™): One subcutaneous implant for 12 months. Must be removed after 12 months of hormonal therapy. Another implant may be inserted to continue therapy.
Endometriosis: I.M.:
Lupron Depot®: 3.75 mg/month for up to 6 months **or**
Lupron Depot-3®: 11.25 mg every 3 months for up to 2 doses (6 months total duration of treatment); may be combined with norethindrone acetate 5 mg/day for initial therapy or recurrence based on clinician's judgment
Uterine leiomyomata (fibroids): I.M.:
Lupron Depot®: 3.75 mg/month for up to 3 months **or**

Lupron Depot-3®: 11.25 mg as a single injection

Administration
Eligard™: Packaged in two syringes; one contains the Atrigel® polymer system, and the second contains leuprolide acetate powder; follow instructions for mixing; must be administered within 30 minutes of mixing
Lupron Depot®: Do not use needles smaller than 22 gauge; reconstitute only with diluent provided
Viadur™ implant: Requires surgical implantation and removal at 12-month intervals

Monitoring Parameters Precocious puberty: GnRH testing (blood LH and FSH levels), testosterone in males and estradiol in females; closely monitor patients with prostatic carcinoma for weakness, paresthesias, and urinary tract obstruction in first few weeks of therapy

Test Interactions Interferes with pituitary gonadotropic and gonadal function tests during and up to 4-8 weeks after therapy

Patient Information Do not discontinue medication without physician's advice. May cause depression; report changes in mood or memory immediately.

Nursing Implications Patient must be taught aseptic technique and S.C. injection technique. Rotate S.C. injection sites frequently. Disease flare (increased bone pain, urinary retention) can briefly occur with initiation of therapy.

Additional Information
Eligard™ Atrigel®: A nongelatin-based, biodegradable, polymer matrix
Viadur™: Leuprolide acetate implant containing 72 mg of leuprolide acetate, equivalent to 65 mg leuprolide free base. One Viadur™ implant delivers 120 mcg of leuprolide/day over 12 months.

Dosage Forms
Implant, as acetate (Viadur™): 65 mg leuprolide
Injection, as acetate (Lupron®): 5 mg/mL (2.8 mL)
Powder for injection (depot), as acetate:
Eligard™ Atrigel® Depot: 7.5 mg
Lupron Depot®: 3.75 mg, 7.5 mg
Lupron Depot®-3 Month: 11.25 mg, 22.5 mg
Lupron Depot®-4 Month: 30 mg
Lupron Depot-Ped®: 7.5 mg, 11.25 mg, 15 mg

♦ **Leuprolide Acetate** see Leuprolide on page 783
♦ **Leuprorelin Acetate** see Leuprolide on page 783
♦ **Leurocristine** see VinCRIStine on page 1417
♦ **Leustatin™** see Cladribine on page 305

Levalbuterol (leve al BYOO ter ole)

U.S. Brand Names Xopenex®
Canadian Brand Names Xopenex®
Synonyms R-albuterol
Therapeutic Category Beta₂-Adrenergic Agonist Agent

Use Treatment or prevention of bronchospasm in adults and adolescents ≥6 years of age with reversible obstructive airway disease

Pregnancy Risk Factor C

Pregnancy/Breast-Feeding Implications There are no studies in pregnant women. This drug should be used during pregnancy only if benefit exceeds risk. It is not known whether levalbuterol is excreted in human milk. Breast-feeding should be avoided or the drug should be discontinued.

Contraindications Hypersensitivity to levalbuterol, albuterol, or any component of the formulation

Adverse Reactions Immediate hypersensitivity reactions have occurred, including angioedema, oropharyngeal edema, urticaria, rash, and anaphylaxis. Events reported include those ≥2% with incidence higher than placebo in patients ≥12 years of age.

>10%:
Endocrine & metabolic: Increased serum glucose, decreased serum potassium
Respiratory: Viral infection (7% to 12%), rhinitis (3% to 11%)
>2% to <10%:
Central nervous system: Nervousness (3% to 10%), tremor (≤7%), anxiety (≤3%), dizziness (1% to 3%), migraine (≤3%), pain (1% to 3%)
Cardiovascular: Tachycardia (~3%)
Gastrointestinal: Dyspepsia (1% to 3%)
Neuromuscular & skeletal: Leg cramps (≤3%%)
Respiratory: Cough (1% to 4%), nasal edema (1% to 3%), sinusitis (1% to 4%)
Miscellaneous: Flu-like syndrome (1% to 4%), accidental injury (≤3%)
<2% (Limited to important or life-threatening): Abnormal EKG, anaphylaxis, angioedema, arrhythmias, asthma exacerbation, bronchospasm (paradoxical), hypesthesia (hand), paresthesia, rash, syncope, urticaria, vomiting, wheezing; immediate hypersensitivity reactions have occurred (including angioedema, oropharyngeal edema, urticaria, rash, and anaphylaxis)

Overdosage/Toxicology Symptoms include tachycardia, tremor, hypertension, angina, and seizures. Hypokalemia also may occur. Cardiac arrest and death may be associated with abuse of beta-agonist bronchodilators. Treatment includes immediate discontinuation, symptomatic and supportive therapies. Cautious use of beta-adrenergic blocking agents may be considered in severe cases.

Drug Interactions
Increased Effect/Toxicity: May add to effects of medications which deplete potassium (eg, loop or thiazide diuretics). Cardiac effects of levalbuterol may be potentiated in patients receiving MAO inhibitors, tricyclic antidepressants, sympathomimetics (eg, amphetamine, dobutamine), or inhaled anesthetics (eg, enflurane).
Decreased Effect: Beta-blockers (particularly nonselective agents) block the effect of levalbuterol. Digoxin levels may be decreased.
(Continued)

Levalbuterol *(Continued)*

Stability Store in protective foil pouch at room temperature of 20°C to 25°C (68°F to 77°F). Protect from light and excessive heat. Vials should be used within 2 weeks after opening protective pouch. Use within 1 week and protect from light if removed from pouch.

Mechanism of Action Relaxes bronchial smooth muscle by action on beta-2 receptors with little effect on heart rate

Pharmacodynamics/Kinetics
Onset of action: 10-17 minutes (measured as a 15% increase in FEV_1)
    Peak effect: 1.5 hours
Duration: 5-6 hours (up to 8 hours in some patients)
Absorption: A portion of inhaled dose is absorbed to systemic circulation
Half-life elimination: 3.3-4 hours
Time to peak, serum: 0.2 hours

Usual Dosage
Children 6-11 years: 0.31 mg 3 times/day via nebulization (maximum dose: 0.63 mg 3 times/day)
Children >12 years and Adults: Inhalation: 0.63 mg 3 times/day at intervals of 6-8 hours, via nebulization. Dosage may be increased to 1.25 mg 3 times/day with close monitoring for adverse effects. Most patients gain optimal benefit from regular use
Elderly: Only a small number of patients have been studied. Although greater sensitivity of some elderly patients cannot be ruled out, no overall differences in safety or effectiveness were observed. An initial dose of 0.63 mg should be used in all patients >65 years of age.

Administration Administered ONLY via nebulization. Safety and efficacy were established when administered with the following nebulizers: PARI LC Jet™, PARI LC Plus™, as well as the following compressors: PARI Master®, Dura-Neb® 2000, and Dura-Neb® 3000.

Monitoring Parameters Asthma symptoms, FEV_1 and/or peak expiratory flow rate, heart rate, blood pressure, CNS status, arterial blood gases (if condition warrants). In selected patients: Serum, glucose, and potassium

Patient Information Use only when necessary or as prescribed; tolerance may develop with overuse. First dose should not be used when you are alone. Avoid OTC medications without consulting prescriber. Maintain adequate hydration (unless instructed to restrict fluid intake). Stress or excessive exercising may exacerbate wheezing or bronchospasm. If diabetic, you will need to monitor serum glucose levels closely until response is known. You may experience tremor, anxiety, dizziness (use caution when driving or engaging in hazardous activities until response to drug is known). Paradoxical bronchospasm can occur; stop drug immediately and notify prescriber if any of the following occur: chest pain or tightness, palpitations; severe headache; difficulty breathing; increased nervousness, restlessness, or trembling; muscle cramps or weakness; seizures. Inform prescriber if you are or intend to be pregnant. Do not breast-feed.

Dosage Forms Solution for nebulization: 0.31 mg/3 mL (24s); 0.63 mg/3 mL (24s); 1.25 mg/3 mL (24s)

Levamisole *(lee VAM i sole)*

U.S. Brand Names Ergamisol®
Canadian Brand Names Ergamisol®; Novo-Levamisole
Synonyms Levamisole Hydrochloride
Therapeutic Category Immune Modulator
Use Adjuvant treatment with fluorouracil in Dukes stage C colon cancer
Pregnancy Risk Factor C
Contraindications Hypersensitivity to levamisole or any component of the formulation
Warnings/Precautions Agranulocytosis can occur asymptomatically and flu-like symptoms can occur without hematologic adverse effects; frequent hematologic monitoring is necessary

Adverse Reactions
>10%: Gastrointestinal: Nausea, diarrhea, metallic taste
1% to 10%:
    Cardiovascular: Edema
    Central nervous system: Fatigue, fever, dizziness, headache, somnolence, depression, nervousness
    Dermatologic: Dermatitis, alopecia
    Gastrointestinal: Stomatitis, vomiting, anorexia, abdominal pain, constipation
    Hematologic: Leukopenia
    Neuromuscular & skeletal: Rigors, arthralgia, myalgia, paresthesia
    Miscellaneous: Infection
<1% (Limited to important or life-threatening): Anemia, chest pain, encephalopathy-like syndrome, granulocytopenia, seizures, Stevens-Johnson syndrome (isolated cases), tardive dyskinesia, thrombocytopenia

Overdosage/Toxicology Treatment following decontamination is symptomatic and supportive.

Drug Interactions
Increased Effect/Toxicity: Increased toxicity/serum levels of phenytoin. Disulfiram-like reaction with alcohol.

Ethanol/Nutrition/Herb Interactions Ethanol: Avoid ethanol (due to GI irritation).

Mechanism of Action Clinically, combined therapy with levamisole and 5-fluorouracil has been effective in treating colon cancer patients, whereas demonstrable activity has been demonstrated. Due to the broad range of pharmacologic activities of levamisole, it has been suggested that the drug may act as a biochemical modulator (of fluorouracil, for example, in colon cancer), an effect entirely independent of immune modulation. Further studies are needed to evaluate the mechanisms of action of the drug in cancer patients.

Pharmacodynamics/Kinetics
Absorption: Well absorbed
Metabolism: Hepatic, >70%
Half-life elimination: 2-6 hours
Time to peak, serum: 1-2 hours

Excretion: Urine and feces; complete within 48 hours

Usual Dosage Adults: Oral: Initial: 50 mg every 8 hours for 3 days, then 50 mg every 8 hours for 3 days every 2 weeks (fluorouracil is always given concomitantly)

Dosing adjustment in hepatic impairment: May be necessary in patients with liver disease, but no specific guidelines are available

Monitoring Parameters CBC with platelet count prior to therapy and weekly prior to treatment; LFTs every 3 months

Patient Information Notify physician immediately if flu-like symptoms appear; may cause dizziness, drowsiness, impair judgment or coordination

Nursing Implications Monitor CBC with platelets prior to therapy and weekly prior to treatment; LFTs every 3 months

Dosage Forms Tablet, as base: 50 mg

- ◆ **Levamisole Hydrochloride** *see* Levamisole *on page 786*
- ◆ **Levaquin™** *see* Levofloxacin *on page 793*
- ◆ **Levarterenol Bitartrate** *see* Norepinephrine *on page 993*
- ◆ **Levbid®** *see* Hyoscyamine *on page 692*

Levetiracetam (lee va tye RA se tam)

Related Information
Anticonvulsants by Seizure Type *on page 1481*
Depression *on page 1655*
Epilepsy & Seizure Treatment *on page 1659*

U.S. Brand Names Keppra®

Canadian Brand Names Keppra®

Therapeutic Category Anticonvulsant

Use Indicated as adjunctive therapy in the treatment of partial onset seizures in adults with epilepsy

Pregnancy Risk Factor C

Contraindications Hypersensitivity to levetiracetam or any component of the formulation

Warnings/Precautions Associated with the occurrence of central nervous system adverse events; somnolence and fatigue, which were treated by discontinuation, reduction, or hospitalization; coordination difficulty was treated by reduction, and only one patient was hospitalized. Behavioral abnormalities, such as psychosis, hallucinations, psychotic depression and other behavioral symptoms (agitation, hostility, anxiety, apathy, emotional lability, depersonalization, and depression) were treated by reduction of dose and in some cases hospitalization. Levetiracetam should be withdrawn gradually to minimize the potential of increased seizure frequency.

Adverse Reactions

>10%:
Central nervous system: Somnolence (15% vs 8% with placebo)
Neuromuscular & skeletal: Weakness (15% vs 9% with placebo)

<10%:
Central nervous system: Psychotic symptoms (1%), amnesia (2% vs 1% with placebo), ataxia (3% vs 1% with placebo), depression (4% vs 2% with placebo), dizziness (9% vs 4% with placebo), emotional lability (2%), nervousness (4% vs 2% with placebo), vertigo (3% vs 1% with placebo)
Hematologic: Decreased erythrocyte counts (3%), decreased leukocytes (2% to 3%)
Neuromuscular & skeletal: Ataxia and other coordination difficulties (3% vs 2% with placebo), pain (7% vs 6% with placebo)
Ocular: Diplopia (2% vs 1% with placebo)

Drug Interactions

Increased Effect/Toxicity: No interaction was observed in pharmacokinetic trials with other anticonvulsants, including phenytoin, carbamazepine, valproic acid, phenobarbital, lamotrigine, gabapentin, and primidone.

Ethanol/Nutrition/Herb Interactions
Ethanol: Avoid ethanol (may increase CNS depression).
Food: Food may delay, but does not affect the extent of absorption.

Mechanism of Action The precise mechanism by which levetiracetam exerts its antiepileptic effect is unknown and does not appear to derive from any interaction with known mechanisms involved in inhibitory and excitatory neurotransmission

Pharmacodynamics/Kinetics
Onset of action: Peak effect: 1 hour
Absorption: Rapid and complete
Protein binding: <10%
Metabolism: Not extensive; primarily by enzymatic hydrolysis
Bioavailability: 100%
Half-life elimination: 6-8 hours
Excretion: Urine (66%)
Dialyzable: ~50% of pooled levetiracetam removed during standard 4-hour hemodialysis

Usual Dosage
Adults: Initial: 500 mg twice daily; additional dosing increments may be given (1000 mg/day additional every 2 weeks) to a maximum recommended daily dose of 3000 mg

Dosing adjustment in renal impairment:
Cl_{cr} >80 mL/minute: 500-1500 mg every 12 hours
Cl_{cr} 50-80 mL/minute: 500-1000 mg every 12 hours
Cl_{cr} 30-50 mL/minute: 250-750 mg every 12 hours
Cl_{cr} <30 mL/minute: 250-500 mg every 12 hours
End-stage renal disease patients using dialysis: 500-2000 mg every 24 hours

Patient Information Notify your physician and/or pharmacist if you become pregnant during therapy with levetiracetam; be advised that levetiracetam may cause dizziness and somnolence and accordingly, you should not drive or operate machinery or engage in other
(Continued)

Levetiracetam *(Continued)*

hazardous activities until sufficient experience has been gained on levetiracetam to gauge whether it adversely affects your performance of these activities

Dosage Forms Tablet: 250 mg, 500 mg, 750 mg

♦ **Levlen®** *see* Ethinyl Estradiol and Levonorgestrel *on page 518*

♦ **Levlite™** *see* Ethinyl Estradiol and Levonorgestrel *on page 518*

Levobetaxolol (lee voe be TAX oh lol)

Related Information

Glaucoma Drug Therapy Comparison *on page 1499*

U.S. Brand Names Betaxon®

Canadian Brand Names Betaxon®

Therapeutic Category Beta-Adrenergic Blocker, Ophthalmic

Use Lowering of intraocular pressure in patients with chronic open-angle glaucoma or ocular hypertension

Pregnancy Risk Factor C

Usual Dosage Adults: Ophthalmic: Instill 1 drop in affected eye(s) twice daily

Additional Information Complete prescribing information for this medication should be consulted for additional detail.

Dosage Forms Solution, ophthalmic: 0.5% (5 mL, 10 mL, 15 mL)

Levobunolol (lee voe BYOO noe lole)

Related Information

Glaucoma Drug Therapy Comparison *on page 1499*

U.S. Brand Names AKBeta®; Betagan® Liquifilm®

Canadian Brand Names Betagan®; Novo-Levobunolol; Optho-Bunolol®; PMS-Levobunolol

Synonyms *l*-Bunolol Hydrochloride; Levobunolol Hydrochloride

Therapeutic Category Beta-Adrenergic Blocker, Ophthalmic

Use To lower intraocular pressure in chronic open-angle glaucoma or ocular hypertension

Pregnancy Risk Factor C

Usual Dosage Adults: Ophthalmic: Instill 1 drop in the affected eye(s) 1-2 times/day

Additional Information Complete prescribing information for this medication should be consulted for additional detail.

Dosage Forms Solution, ophthalmic, as hydrochloride: 0.25% (5 mL, 10 mL, 15 mL); 0.5% (2 mL, 5 mL, 10 mL, 15 mL)

♦ **Levobunolol Hydrochloride** *see* Levobunolol *on page 788*

Levobupivacaine (LEE voe byoo PIV a kane)

U.S. Brand Names Chirocaine®

Canadian Brand Names Chirocaine®

Therapeutic Category Local Anesthetic, Injectable

Use Production of local or regional anesthesia for surgery and obstetrics, and for postoperative pain management

Pregnancy Risk Factor B

Usual Dosage Adults: **Note:** Rapid injection of a large volume of local anesthetic solution should be avoided. Fractional (incremental) doses are recommended.

Guidelines (individual response varies): See table.

	Concentration	Volume	Dose	Motor Block
Surgical Anesthesia				
Epidural for surgery	0.5%-0.75%	10-20 mL	50-150 mg	Moderate to complete
Epidural - C-section	0.5%	20-30 mL	100-150 mg	Moderate to complete
Peripheral nerve	0.25%-0.5%	0.4 mL/kg (30 mL)	1-2 mg/kg (75-150 mg)	Moderate to complete
Ophthalmic	0.75%	5-15 mL	37.5-112.5 mg	Moderate to complete
Local infiltration	0.25%	60 mL	150 mg	Not applicable
Pain Management				
Labor analgesia (epidural bolus)	0.25%	10-20 mL	25-50 mg	Minimal to moderate
Postoperative pain (epidural infusion)	0.125%*-0.25%	4-10 mL/h	5-25 mg/h	Minimal to moderate

* 0.125%: Adjunct therapy with fentanyl or clonidine

Maximum dosage: Epidural doses up to 375 mg have been administered incrementally to patients during a surgical procedure.

Intraoperative block and postoperative pain: 695 mg in 24 hours

Postoperative epidural infusion over 24 hours: 570 mg

Single-fractionated injection for brachial plexus block: 300 mg

Additional Information Complete prescribing information for this medication should be consulted for additional detail.

Dosage Forms Injection: 2.5 mg/mL (10 mL, 30 mL); 5 mg/mL (10 mL, 30 mL); 7.5 mg/mL (10 mL, 30 mL)

Levocabastine (LEE voe kab as teen)

U.S. Brand Names Livostin®

Canadian Brand Names Livostin®

Synonyms Levocabastine Hydrochloride

Therapeutic Category Antiallergic, Ophthalmic; Antihistamine, H₁ Blocker; Antihistamine, H₁ Blocker, Ophthalmic

Use Treatment of allergic conjunctivitis

Pregnancy Risk Factor C

Usual Dosage Children ≥12 years and Adults: Instill 1 drop in affected eye(s) 4 times/day for up to 2 weeks

Additional Information Complete prescribing information for this medication should be consulted for additional detail.

Dosage Forms Suspension, ophthalmic, as hydrochloride: 0.05% (2.5 mL, 5 mL, 10 mL)

♦ **Levocabastine Hydrochloride** *see Levocabastine on page 788*

Levocarnitine (lee voe KAR ni teen)

U.S. Brand Names Carnitor®; Vitacarn®

Canadian Brand Names Carnitor®

Synonyms L-Carnitine

Therapeutic Category Nutritional Supplement

Use Orphan drug:

Oral: Primary systemic carnitine deficiency; acute and chronic treatment of patients with an inborn error of metabolism which results in secondary carnitine deficiency

I.V.: Acute and chronic treatment of patients with an inborn error of metabolism which results in secondary carnitine deficiency; prevention and treatment of carnitine deficiency in patients with end-stage renal disease who are undergoing hemodialysis.

Pregnancy Risk Factor B

Pregnancy/Breast-Feeding Implications No adequate or well controlled studies in pregnant women. However, carnitine is a naturally occurring substance in mammalian metabolism. In breast-feeding women, use must be weighed against the potential exposure of the infant to increased carnitine intake. Use caution in breast-feeding women.

Warnings/Precautions Caution in patients with seizure disorders or in those at risk of seizures (CNS mass or medications which may lower seizure threshold). Both new-onset seizure activity as well as an increased frequency of seizures has been observed.

Adverse Reactions Frequencies noted with I.V. therapy (hemodialysis patients):

Cardiovascular: Hypertension (18% to 21%), peripheral edema (3% to 6%)

Central nervous system: Dizziness (10% to 18%), fever (5% to 12%), paresthesia (3% to 12%), depression (5% to 6%)

Endocrine & metabolic: Hypercalcemia (6% to 15%)

Gastrointestinal: Diarrhea (9% to 35%), abdominal pain (5% to 21%), vomiting (9% to 21%), nausea (5% to 12%)

Neuromuscular & skeletal: Weakness (9% to 12%)

Miscellaneous: Allergic reaction (2% to 6%)

Overdosage/Toxicology No reports of overdose. Easily removed by dialysis.

Stability Intravenous solution: Intact ampuls should be stored at controlled room temperature (25°C) and protected from light. Further dilutions in 0.9% sodium chloride or lactated Ringer's at a concentration ranging from 0.5-8 mg/mL are stable up to 24 hours in PVC at room temperature.

Mechanism of Action Carnitine is a naturally occurring metabolic compound which functions as a carrier molecule for long-chain fatty acids within the mitochondria, facilitating energy production. Carnitine deficiency is associated with accumulation of excess acyl CoA esters and disruption of intermediary metabolism. Carnitine supplementation increases carnitine plasma concentrations. The effects on specific metabolic alterations have not been evaluated. ESRD patients on maintenance HD may have low plasma carnitine levels because of reduced intake of meat and dairy products, reduced renal synthesis, and dialytic losses. Certain clinical conditions (malaise, muscle weakness, cardiomyopathy and arrhythmias) in HD patients may be related to carnitine deficiency.

Pharmacodynamics/Kinetics

Bioavailability: Tablet/solution: 15% to 16%

Half-life elimination: 17.4 hours

Time to peak: Tablet/solution: 3.3 hours

Excretion: Urine (76% as unchanged drug)

Usual Dosage

Oral:

Infants/Children: Initial: 50 mg/kg/day; titrate to 50-100 mg/kg/day in divided doses with a maximum dose of 3 g/day

Adults: 990 mg (oral tablets) 2-3 times/day or 1-3 g/day (oral solution)

I.V.:

Metabolic disorders: 50 mg/kg as a slow 2- to 3-minute I.V. bolus or by I.V. infusion

Severe metabolic crisis:

A loading dose of 50 mg/kg followed by an equivalent dose over the following 24 hours administered as every 3 hours or every 4 hours (never less than every 6 hours either by infusion or by intravenous injection)

All subsequent daily doses are recommended to be in the range of 50 mg/kg or as therapy may require

The highest dose administered has been 300 mg/kg

It is recommended that a plasma carnitine concentration be obtained prior to beginning parenteral therapy accompanied by weekly and monthly monitoring

ESRD patients on hemodialysis:

Predialysis levocarnitine concentrations below normal (40-50 µmol/L): 10-20 mg/kg dry body weight as a slow 2- to 3-minute bolus after each dialysis session

Dosage adjustments should be guided by predialysis trough levocarnitine concentrations and downward dose adjustments (to 5 mg/kg after dialysis) may be made as early as every 3rd or 4th week of therapy

Administration

Oral: Solution may be dissolved in either drink or liquid food, and should be consumed slowly. Doses should be spaced every 3 to 4 hours throughout the day, preferably during or following meals.

(Continued)

789

Levocarnitine *(Continued)*

    I.V.: Hemodialysis patients: Injection should be administered over 2-3 minutes into the venous return line after each dialysis session.

Monitoring Parameters Plasma concentrations should be obtained prior to beginning parenteral therapy, and should be monitored weekly to monthly. In metabolic disorders: monitor blood chemistry, vital signs, and plasma carnitine levels (maintain between 35-60 µmol/L). In ESRD patients on dialysis: Plasma levels below the normal range should prompt initiation of therapy. Monitor predialysis (trough) plasma carnitine levels.

Reference Range Normal carnitine levels are 40-50 µmol/L; levels should be maintained on therapy between 35-60 µmol/L

Patient Information The oral solution should be consumed slowly and spaced evenly throughout the day to improve tolerance

Nursing Implications

    Parenteral: May be administered by direct I.V. infusion over 2-3 minutes or as continuous infusion

    Monitor serum triglycerides, fatty acids, and carnitine levels

Additional Information Although supplemental carnitine has been shown to increase carnitine concentrations, effects on the signs and symptoms of carnitine deficiency have not been determined.

Dosage Forms

    Capsule: 250 mg

    Injection: 200 mg/mL ampul (5 mL)

    Solution, oral: 100 mg/mL (118 mL)

    Tablet: 330 mg

Levodopa *(lee voe DOE pa)*

Related Information

    Antacid Drug Interactions *on page 1477*

    Depression *on page 1655*

U.S. Brand Names Dopar®; Larodopa®

Canadian Brand Names Dopar®; Larodopa®

Synonyms *L*-3-Hydroxytyrosine; *L*-Dopa

Therapeutic Category Anti-Parkinson's Agent, Dopamine Agonist; Dopaminergic Agent (Antiparkinson's)

Use Treatment of Parkinson's disease

Unlabeled/Investigational Use Diagnostic agent for growth hormone deficiency

Pregnancy Risk Factor C

Contraindications Hypersensitivity to levodopa or any component of the formulation; narrow-angle glaucoma; use of MAO inhibitors within prior 14 days (however, may be administered concomitantly with the manufacturer's recommended dose of an MAO inhibitor with selectivity for MAO type B); history of melanoma or any undiagnosed skin lesions

Warnings/Precautions Use with caution in patients with history of cardiovascular disease (including myocardial infarction and arrhythmias); pulmonary diseases such as asthma, psychosis, wide-angle glaucoma, peptic ulcer disease; as well as in renal, hepatic, or endocrine disease. Sudden discontinuation of levodopa may cause a worsening of Parkinson's disease. Elderly may be more sensitive to CNS effects of levodopa. May cause or exacerbate dyskinesias. May cause orthostatic hypotension; Parkinson's disease patients appear to have an impaired capacity to respond to a postural challenge. Use with caution in patients at risk of hypotension (such as those receiving antihypertensive drugs) or where transient hypotensive episodes would be poorly tolerated (cardiovascular disease or cerebrovascular disease). Observe patients closely for development of depression with concomitant suicidal tendencies. Safety and effectiveness in pediatric patients have not been established. Some products may contain tartrazine. Dopaminergic agents have been associated with a syndrome resembling neuroleptic malignant syndrome on withdrawal or significant dosage reduction after long-term use. Pyridoxine may reverse effects of levodopa. Toxic reactions have occurred with dextromethorphan.

Adverse Reactions Frequency not defined.

    Cardiovascular: Orthostatic hypotension, arrhythmias, chest pain, hypertension, syncope, palpitations, phlebitis

    Central nervous system: Dizziness, anxiety, confusion, nightmares, headache, hallucinations, on-off phenomenon, decreased mental acuity, memory impairment, disorientation, delusions, euphoria, agitation, somnolence, insomnia, gait abnormalities, nervousness, ataxia, EPS, falling, psychosis

    Gastrointestinal: Anorexia, nausea, vomiting, constipation, GI bleeding, duodenal ulcer, diarrhea, dyspepsia, taste alterations, sialorrhea, heartburn

    Genitourinary: Discoloration of urine, urinary frequency

    Hematologic: Hemolytic anemia, agranulocytosis, thrombocytopenia, leukopenia, decreased hemoglobin and hematocrit, abnormalities in AST and ALT, LDH, bilirubin, BUN, Coombs' test

    Neuromuscular & skeletal: Choreiform and involuntary movements, paresthesia, bone pain, shoulder pain, muscle cramps, weakness

    Ocular: Blepharospasm

    Renal: Difficult urination

    Respiratory: Dyspnea, cough

    Miscellaneous: Hiccups, discoloration of sweat

Overdosage/Toxicology Symptoms include palpitations, dysrhythmias, spasms, and hypertension. Use fluids judiciously to maintain pressures. May precipitate a variety of arrhythmias.

Drug Interactions

    Increased Effect/Toxicity: Concurrent use of levodopa with nonselective MAO inhibitors may result in hypertensive reactions via an increased storage and release of dopamine, norepinephrine, or both. Use with carbidopa to minimize reactions if combination is necessary; otherwise avoid combination.

Decreased Effect: Antipsychotics, benzodiazepines, L-methionine, phenytoin, pyridoxine, spiramycin, and tacrine may inhibit the antiparkinsonian effects of levodopa; monitor for reduced effect. Antipsychotics may inhibit the antiparkinsonian effects of levodopa via dopamine receptor blockade. Use antipsychotics with low dopamine blockade (clozapine, olanzapine, quetiapine). High-protein diets may inhibit levodopa's efficacy; avoid high protein foods. Iron binds levodopa and reduces its bioavailability; separate doses of iron and levodopa.

Ethanol/Nutrition/Herb Interactions
Ethanol: Avoid ethanol (due to CNS depression).
Food: Avoid high protein diets and high intakes of vitamin B_6.
Herb/Nutraceutical: Pyridoxine in doses >10-25 mg (for levodopa alone) or higher doses >200 mg/day (for levodopa/carbidopa) may decrease efficacy.

Mechanism of Action Increases dopamine levels in the brain, then stimulates dopaminergic receptors in the basal ganglia to improve the balance between cholinergic and dopaminergic activity

Pharmacodynamics/Kinetics
Duration: Variable, usually 6-12 hours
Absorption: May be decreased if given with a high protein meal
Metabolism: Peripheral decarboxylation to dopamine; small amounts reach brain and are decarboxylated to active dopamine
Half-life elimination: 1.2-2.3 hours
Time to peak, serum: 1-2 hours
Excretion: Primarily urine (80% as dopamine, norepinephrine, and homovanillic acid)

Usual Dosage Oral:
Children (administer as a single dose to evaluate growth hormone deficiency [unlabeled use]):
0.5 g/m² **or**
<30 lb: 125 mg
30-70 lb: 250 mg
>70 lb: 500 mg
Adults: Parkinson's disease: 500-1000 mg/day in divided doses every 6-12 hours; increase by 100-750 mg/day every 3-7 days until response or total dose of 8000 mg is reached
A significant therapeutic response may not be obtained for 6 months

Dietary Considerations High-protein diets may decrease the efficacy of levodopa when used for parkinsonism via competition with amino acids in GI absorption .

Administration Administer with meals to decrease GI upset

Monitoring Parameters Serum growth hormone concentration

Test Interactions False-positive reaction for urinary glucose with Clinitest®; false-negative reaction using Clinistix®; false-positive urine ketones with Acetest®, Ketostix®, Labstix®

Patient Information Avoid vitamins with B_6 (pyridoxine); can take with food to prevent GI upset; do not stop taking this drug even if you do not think it is working; dizziness, lightheadedness, fainting may occur when you get up from a sitting or lying position.

Nursing Implications Sustained release product should not be crushed

Additional Information A single dose is not usually associated with the above adverse reactions.

Dosage Forms
Capsule: 100 mg, 250 mg, 500 mg
Tablet: 100 mg, 250 mg, 500 mg

Levodopa and Carbidopa (lee voe DOE pa & kar bi DOE pa)

Related Information
Parkinson's Agents *on page 1513*

U.S. Brand Names Sinemet®; Sinemet® CR

Canadian Brand Names Apo®-Levocarb; Endo®-Levodopa/Carbidopa; Nu-Levocarb; Sinemet®; Sinemet® CR

Synonyms Carbidopa and Levodopa

Therapeutic Category Anti-Parkinson's Agent, Dopamine Agonist; Dopaminergic Agent (Antiparkinson's)

Use Idiopathic Parkinson's disease; postencephalitic parkinsonism; symptomatic parkinsonism

Pregnancy Risk Factor C

Contraindications Hypersensitivity to levodopa, carbidopa, or any component of the formulation; narrow-angle glaucoma; use of MAO inhibitors within prior 14 days (however may be administered concomitantly with the manufacturer's recommended dose of an MAO inhibitor with selectivity for MAO type B); history of melanoma or undiagnosed skin lesions

Warnings/Precautions Use with caution in patients with history of cardiovascular disease (including myocardial infarction and arrhythmias); pulmonary diseases such as asthma, psychosis, wide-angle glaucoma, peptic ulcer disease; as well as in renal, hepatic, or endocrine disease. Sudden discontinuation of levodopa may cause a worsening of Parkinson's disease. Elderly may be more sensitive to CNS effects of levodopa. May cause or exacerbate dyskinesias. May cause orthostatic hypotension; Parkinson's disease patients appear to have an impaired capacity to respond to a postural challenge; use with caution in patients at risk of hypotension (such as those receiving antihypertensive drugs) or where transient hypotensive episodes would be poorly tolerated (cardiovascular disease or cerebrovascular disease). Observe patients closely for development of depression with concomitant suicidal tendencies. Some products may contain tartrazine. Has been associated with a syndrome resembling neuroleptic malignant syndrome on withdrawal or significant dosage reduction after long-term use. Toxic reactions have occurred with dextromethorphan. Protein in the diet should be distributed throughout the day to avoid fluctuations in levodopa absorption.

Adverse Reactions Frequency not defined.
Cardiovascular: Orthostatic hypotension, arrhythmias, chest pain, hypertension, syncope, palpitations, phlebitis
Central nervous system: Dizziness, anxiety, confusion, nightmares, headache, hallucinations, on-off phenomenon, decreased mental acuity, memory impairment, disorientation, (Continued)

Levodopa and Carbidopa (Continued)

delusions, euphoria, agitation, somnolence, insomnia, gait abnormalities, nervousness, ataxia, EPS, falling, psychosis, peripheral neuropathy, seizures (causal relationship not established)

Dermatologic: Rash, alopecia, malignant melanoma, hypersensitivity (angioedema, urticaria, pruritus, bullous lesions, Henoch-Schönlein purpura)

Endocrine & metabolic: Increased libido

Gastrointestinal: Anorexia, nausea, vomiting, constipation, GI bleeding, duodenal ulcer, diarrhea, dyspepsia, taste alterations, sialorrhea, heartburn

Genitourinary: Discoloration of urine, urinary frequency

Hematologic: Hemolytic anemia, agranulocytosis, thrombocytopenia, leukopenia; decreased hemoglobin and hematocrit; abnormalities in AST and ALT, LDH, bilirubin, BUN, Coombs' test

Neuromuscular & skeletal: Choreiform and involuntary movements, paresthesia, bone pain, shoulder pain, muscle cramps, weakness

Ocular: Blepharospasm, oculogyric crises (may be associated with acute dystonic reactions)

Renal: Difficult urination

Respiratory: Dyspnea, cough

Miscellaneous: Hiccups, discoloration of sweat, diaphoresis (increased)

Overdosage/Toxicology Symptoms include palpitations, arrhythmias, spasms, and hypotension. May cause hypertension or hypotension. Treatment is supportive. Initiate gastric lavage, administer I.V. fluids judiciously and monitor EKG. Use fluids judiciously to maintain pressures. May precipitate a variety of arrhythmias.

Drug Interactions

Increased Effect/Toxicity: Concurrent use of levodopa with nonselective MAO inhibitors may result in hypertensive reactions via an increased storage and release of dopamine, norepinephrine, or both. Use with carbidopa to minimize reactions if combination is necessary; otherwise avoid combination.

Decreased Effect: Antipsychotics, benzodiazepines, L-methionine, phenytoin, pyridoxine, spiramycin, and tacrine may inhibit the antiparkinsonian effects of levodopa; monitor for reduced effect. Antipsychotics may inhibit the antiparkinsonian effects of levodopa via dopamine receptor blockade. Use antipsychotics with low dopamine blockade (clozapine, olanzapine, quetiapine). High-protein diets may inhibit levodopa's efficacy; avoid high protein foods. Iron binds levodopa and reduces its bioavailability; separate doses of iron and levodopa.

Ethanol/Nutrition/Herb Interactions

Ethanol: Avoid ethanol (due to CNS depression).

Food: Avoid high protein diets and high intakes of vitamin B_6.

Herb/Nutraceutical: Avoid kava kava (may decrease effects). Pyridoxine in doses >10-25 mg (for levodopa alone) or higher doses >200 mg/day (for levodopa/carbidopa) may decrease efficacy.

Mechanism of Action Parkinson's symptoms are due to a lack of striatal dopamine; levodopa circulates in the plasma to the blood-brain-barrier (BBB), where it crosses, to be converted by striatal enzymes to dopamine; carbidopa inhibits the peripheral plasma breakdown of levodopa by inhibiting its decarboxylation, and thereby increases available levodopa at the BBB

Pharmacodynamics/Kinetics

Duration: Variable, 6-12 hours; longer with sustained release forms

See individual agents.

Usual Dosage Oral:

Adults: Initial: 25/100 2-4 times/day, increase as necessary to a maximum of 200/2000 mg/day

Elderly: Initial: 25/100 twice daily, increase as necessary

Conversion from Sinemet® to Sinemet® CR (50/200): (Sinemet® [total daily dose of levodopa] / Sinemet® CR)

300-400 mg / 1 tablet twice daily

500-600 mg / 1¹⁄₂ tablets twice daily or one 3 times/day

700-800 mg / 4 tablets in 3 or more divided doses

900-1000 mg / 5 tablets in 3 or more divided doses

Intervals between doses of Sinemet® CR should be 4-8 hours while awake

Dietary Considerations Levodopa peak serum concentrations may be decreased if taken with food. High protein diets (>2 g/kg) may decrease the efficacy of levodopa via competition with amino acids in crossing the blood-brain barrier.

Administration Administer with meals to decrease GI upset

Monitoring Parameters Blood pressure, standing and sitting/supine; symptoms of parkinsonism, dyskinesias, mental status

Test Interactions False-positive reaction for urinary glucose with Clinitest®; false-negative reaction using Clinistix®; false-positive urine ketones with Acetest®, Ketostix®, Labstix®

Patient Information Do not stop taking this drug even if you do not think it is working; take on an empty stomach if possible; if GI distress occurs, take with meals; rise carefully from lying or sitting position as dizziness, lightheadedness, or fainting may occur; do not crush or chew sustained release product

Nursing Implications Space doses evenly over the waking hours; sustained release product should not be crushed

Additional Information 50-100 mg/day of carbidopa is needed to block the peripheral conversion of levodopa to dopamine. "On-off" (a clinical syndrome characterized by sudden periods of drug activity/inactivity), can be managed by giving smaller, more frequent doses of Sinemet® or adding a dopamine agonist or selegiline; when adding a new agent, doses of Sinemet® can usually be decreased. Protein in the diet should be distributed throughout the day to avoid fluctuations in levodopa absorption. Levodopa is the drug of choice when rigidity is the predominant presenting symptom.

Dosage Forms

Tablet:

10/100: Carbidopa 10 mg and levodopa 100 mg

25/100: Carbidopa 25 mg and levodopa 100 mg
25/250: Carbidopa 25 mg and levodopa 250 mg
Tablet, sustained release:
  Carbidopa 25 mg and levodopa 100 mg
  Carbidopa 50 mg and levodopa 200 mg

♦ **Levo-Dromoran®** *see* Levorphanol *on page 799*

Levofloxacin (lee voe FLOKS a sin)

Related Information
Antacid Drug Interactions *on page 1477*
Antimicrobial Drugs of Choice *on page 1588*
Community-Acquired Pneumonia in Adults *on page 1603*
Tuberculosis Treatment Guidelines *on page 1612*

U.S. Brand Names Levaquin™; Quixin™ Ophthalmic

Canadian Brand Names Levaquin®

Therapeutic Category Antibiotic, Quinolone

Use
Systemic:
Acute bacterial exacerbation of chronic bronchitis and community-acquired pneumonia due to *S. aureus, S. pneumoniae* (including penicillin-resistant strains), *H. influenzae, H. parainfluenzae, M. catarrhalis, C. pneumoniae, L. pneumophila,* or *M. pneumoniae*
Acute maxillary sinusitis due to *S. pneumoniae, H. influenzae,* or *M. catarrhalis*
Acute pyelonephritis caused by *E. coli*
Skin or skin structure infections:
Complicated, due to methicillin-susceptible *S. aureus, Enterococcus fecalis, S. pyogenes,* or *Proteus mirabilis*
Uncomplicated, due to *S. aureus* or *S. pyogenes*
Urinary tract infections:
Complicated, due to gram-negative bacteria (*E. coli, Enterobacter cloacae, Klebsiella pneumoniae, Proteus mirabilis, Enterococcus fecalis,* or *Pseudomonas aeruginosa*)
Uncomplicated, due to *E. coli, K. pneumoniae,* or *S. saprophyticus*
Ophthalmic: Bacterial conjunctivitis due to *S. aureus* (methicillin-susceptible strains), *S. epidermidis* (methicillin-susceptible strains), *S. pneumoniae, Streptococcus* (groups C/F), *Streptococcus* (group G), Viridans group streptococci, *Corynebacterium* spp, *H. influenzae, Acinetobacter lwoffii,* or *Serratia marcescens*

Pregnancy Risk Factor C

Pregnancy/Breast-Feeding Implications
Clinical effects on the fetus: Avoid use in pregnant women unless the benefit justifies the potential risk to the fetus
Breast-feeding/lactation: Quinolones are known to distribute well into breast milk; consequently, use during lactation should be avoided, if possible

Contraindications Hypersensitivity to levofloxacin, any component of the formulation, or other quinolones

Warnings/Precautions
Systemic: Not recommended in children <18 years of age; CNS stimulation may occur (tremor, restlessness, confusion, and very rarely hallucinations or seizures); use with caution in patients with known or suspected CNS disorders or renal dysfunction; use caution to avoid possible photosensitivity reactions during and for several days following fluoroquinolone therapy
Rare cases of torsade de pointes have been reported in patients receiving levofloxacin. Use caution in patients with bradycardia, hypokalemia, hypomagnesemia, or in those receiving concurrent therapy with Class Ia or Class III antiarrhythmics.
Severe hypersensitivity reactions, including anaphylaxis, have occurred with quinolone therapy. If an allergic reaction occurs (itching, urticaria, dyspnea or facial edema, loss of consciousness, tingling, cardiovascular collapse), discontinue drug immediately. Prolonged use may result in superinfection; pseudomembranous colitis may occur and should be considered in all patients who present with diarrhea. Tendon inflammation and/or rupture has been reported; discontinue at first sign of tendon inflammation or pain. Quinolones may exacerbate myasthenia gravis.
Ophthalmic solution: For topical use only. Do not inject subconjunctivally or introduce into anterior chamber of the eye. Contact lenses should not be worn during treatment for bacterial conjunctivitis. Safety and efficacy in children <1 year of age have not been established.

Adverse Reactions
1% to 10%:
Central nervous system: Dizziness, fever, headache, insomnia
Gastrointestinal: Nausea, vomiting, diarrhea, constipation
Ocular (with ophthalmic solution use): Decreased vision (transient), foreign body sensation, transient ocular burning, ocular pain or discomfort, photophobia
Respiratory: Pharyngitis
<1% (Limited to important or life-threatening):
Systemic: Cardiac failure, hypertension, bradycardia, tachycardia, seizures, elevated transaminases, pseudomembraneous colitis, leukorrhea, granulocytopenia, leukopenia, leukocytosis, thrombocytopenia, jaundice, acute renal failure, arrhythmias (including ventricular tachycardia and torsade de pointes), tremor, arthralgia, photosensitivity (<0.1%), anaphylactoid reaction, allergic reaction (including pneumonitis and anaphylaxis), dysphonia, eosinophilia, erythema multiforme, Stevens-Johnson syndrome, hemolytic anemia, tendon rupture, QT_c prolongation
Ophthalmic solution: Allergic reaction, lid edema, ocular dryness, ocular itching

Overdosage/Toxicology Symptoms include acute renal failure and seizures. Treatment should include GI decontamination and supportive care. Not removed by peritoneal or hemodialysis.
(Continued)

Levofloxacin *(Continued)*

Drug Interactions
Cytochrome P450 Effect: CYP1A2 enzyme inhibitor (minor)

Increased Effect/Toxicity: Quinolones may cause increased levels of azlocillin, cyclosporine, and caffeine/theophylline (effect of levofloxacin on theophylline metabolism appears limited). Azlocillin, cimetidine, loop diuretics (furosemide, torsemide), and probenecid increase quinolone levels (decreased renal secretion). An increased incidence of seizures may occur with foscarnet or NSAIDs. The hypoprothrombinemic effect of warfarin is enhanced by some quinolone antibiotics. QT_c-prolonging agents (including Class Ia and Class III antiarrhythmics, erythromycin, cisapride, antipsychotics, and cyclic antidepressants) should be avoided with levofloxacin. Levofloxacin does not alter warfarin levels, but may alter the gastrointestinal flora. Monitor INR closely during therapy. Concurrent use of corticosteroids may increase risk of tendon rupture.

Decreased Effect: Metal cations (magnesium, aluminum, iron, and zinc) bind quinolones in the gastrointestinal tract and inhibit absorption (by up to 98%). Due to electrolyte content, antacids, electrolyte supplements, sucralfate, quinapril, and some didanosine formulations should be avoided. Levofloxacin should be administered 4 hours before or 8 hours (a minimum of 2 hours before and 2 hours after) after these agents. Antineoplastic agents may decrease the absorption of quinolones.

Stability
Injection: Stable for 72 hours when diluted to 5 mg/mL in a compatible I.V. fluid and stored at room temperature; stable for 14 days when stored under refrigeration; stable for 6 months when frozen, do not refreeze; do not thaw in microwave or by bath immersion; **incompatible** with mannitol and sodium bicarbonate

Ophthalmic solution: Store at 15°C to 25°C (59°F to 77°F)

Mechanism of Action As the S (-) enantiomer of the fluoroquinolone, ofloxacin, levofloxacin, inhibits DNA-gyrase in susceptible organisms thereby inhibits relaxation of supercoiled DNA and promotes breakage of DNA strands. DNA gyrase (topoisomerase II), is an essential bacterial enzyme that maintains the superhelical structure of DNA and is required for DNA replication and transcription, DNA repair, recombination, and transposition.

Pharmacodynamics/Kinetics
Absorption: Well absorbed

Distribution: V_d: 1.25 L/kg; CSF concentrations ~15% of serum levels; high concentrations are achieved in prostate and gynecological tissues, sinus, breast milk, and saliva

Protein binding: 50%

Metabolism: Hepatic, minimal

Bioavailability: 100%

Half-life elimination: 6 hours

Time to peak, serum: 1 hour

Excretion: Primarily urine (as unchanged drug)

Usual Dosage
Adults: Oral, I.V. (infuse I.V. solution over 60 minutes):

Acute bacterial exacerbation of chronic bronchitis: 500 mg every 24 hours for at least 7 days

Community-acquired pneumonia: 500 mg every 24 hours for 7-14 days

Acute maxillary sinusitis: 500 mg every 24 hours for 10-14 days

Uncomplicated skin infections: 500 mg every 24 hours for 7-10 days

Complicated skin infections: 750 mg every 24 hours for 7-14 days

Uncomplicated urinary tract infections: 250 mg once daily for 3 days

Complicated urinary tract infections, including acute pyelonephritis: 250 mg every 24 hours for 10 days

Children ≥1 year and Adults: Ophthalmic:

Treatment day 1 and day 2: Instill 1-2 drops into affected eye(s) every 2 hours while awake, up to 8 times/day

Treatment day 3 through day 7: Instill 1-2 drops into affected eye(s) every 4 hours while awake, up to 4 times/day

Dosing adjustment in renal impairment:
Chronic bronchitis, acute maxillary sinusitis, uncomplicated skin infection, community-acquired pneumonia

Cl_{cr} 20-49 mL/minute: Administer 250 mg every 24 hours (initial: 500 mg)

Cl_{cr} 10-19 mL/minute: Administer 250 mg every 48 hours (initial: 500 mg)

Complicated UTI, acute pyelonephritis:

Cl_{cr} 20-49 mL/minute: No dosage adjustment required required

Cl_{cr} 10-19 mL/minute: Administer 250 mg every 48 hours

Uncomplicated UTI: No dosage adjustment required

Complicated skin infection

Cl_{cr} 20-49 mL/minute: Administer 750 mg every 48 hours mg

Cl_{cr} 10-19 mL/minute: Administer 500 mg every 48 hours (initial: 750 mg)

Hemodialysis/CAPD: 250 mg every 48 hours (initial: 500 mg for most infections; initial: 750 mg for complicated skin/soft tissue infections followed by 500 mg every 48 hours)

Monitoring Parameters Evaluation of organ system functions (renal, hepatic, ophthalmologic, and hematopoietic) is recommended periodically during therapy; the possibility of crystalluria should be assessed; WBC and signs of infection

Patient Information
Oral: Take per recommended schedule, preferably on an empty stomach (1 hour before or 2 hours after meals). Maintain adequate hydration (2-3 L/day of fluids unless instructed to restrict fluid intake). Take complete prescription; do not skip doses. Do not take with antacids; separate by 2 hours. You may experience dizziness, lightheadedness, or confusion; use caution when driving or engaging in tasks that require alertness until response to drug is known. Small frequent meals and frequent mouth care may reduce nausea or vomiting. You may experience photosensitivity; use sunscreen, wear protective clothing and eyewear, and avoid direct sunlight. Report palpitations or chest pain, persistent diarrhea, GI disturbances or abdominal pain, muscle tremor or pain, yellowing of eyes or skin,

easy bruising or bleeding, unusual fatigue, fever, chills, signs of infection, or worsening of condition. Report immediately any rash, itching, unusual CNS changes, or any facial swelling. Report immediately any pain, inflammation, or rupture of tendon.

Ophthalmic: Wash hands before instilling solution. Sit or lie down to instill. Open eye, look at ceiling, and instill prescribed amount of solution. Close eye and roll eye in all directions, and apply gentle pressure to inner corner of eye. Do not let tip of applicator touch eye or contaminate tip of applicator. Temporary stinging or blurred vision may occur. Report persistent pain, burning, vision disturbances, swelling, itching, or worsening of condition. Discontinue medication and contact prescriber immediately if you develop a rash or allergic reaction. Do not wear contact lenses.

Nursing Implications Infuse I.V. solutions over 60 minutes

Additional Information Ophthalmic solution contains benzalkonium chloride 0.005% as a preservative.

Dosage Forms
Infusion [in D_5W]: 5 mg/mL (50 mL, 100 mL)
Injection: 25 mg/mL (20 mL)
Solution, ophthalmic: 0.5% (2.5 mL, 5 mL)
Tablet: 250 mg, 500 mg, 750 mg

Levomethadyl Acetate Hydrochloride
(lee voe METH a dil AS e tate hye droe KLOR ide)

U.S. Brand Names ORLAAM®

Therapeutic Category Analgesic, Narcotic

Use Management of opiate dependence; should be reserved for use in treatment of opiate-addicted patients who fail to show an acceptable response to other adequate treatments for addiction

Restrictions C-II; must be dispensed in a designated clinic setting only

Pregnancy Risk Factor C

Contraindications Hypersensitivity to levomethadyl or any component of the formulation; known or suspected QT_c prolongation (male: 430 msec, female: 450 msec); bradycardia (<50 bpm); significant cardiac disease; concurrent treatment with drugs known to prolong QT interval, including class I and III antiarrhythmics; concurrent treatment with MAO inhibitors; hypokalemia or hypomagnesemia

Warnings/Precautions May cause QT prolongation. Use of levomethadyl has been associated with rare, but serious cardiac arrhythmias. Perform EKG prior to treatment, 12-14 days after initiation, and periodically thereafter. Not recommended for use outside of the treatment of opiate addiction; shall be dispensed only by treatment programs approved by FDA, DEA, and the designated state authority. Approved treatment programs shall dispense and use levomethadyl in oral form only and according to the treatment requirements stipulated in federal regulations. Failure to abide by these requirements may result in injunction precluding operation of the program, seizure of the drug supply, revocation of the program approval, and possible criminal prosecution.

Use only with **extreme caution** in patients with head injury or increased intracranial pressure (ICP). Use with caution in patients with respiratory disease or asthma. Has been studied only in 3 times/week or every-other-day dosing; daily administration may lead to accumulation/risk of overdose. Use caution in the elderly and in patients with hepatic or renal dysfunctions. Safety and efficacy in pediatric patients have not been established.

Adverse Reactions
>10%:
Central nervous system: Malaise
Miscellaneous: Flu syndrome
1% to 10%:
Central nervous system: CNS depression, sedation, chills, abnormal dreams, anxiety, euphoria, headache, insomnia, nervousness, hypesthesia
Endocrine & metabolic: Hot flashes (males 2:1)
Gastrointestinal: Abdominal pain, constipation, diarrhea, xerostomia, nausea, vomiting
Genitourinary: Urinary tract spasm, difficult ejaculation, impotence, decreased sex drive
Neuromuscular & skeletal: Arthralgia, back pain, weakness
Ocular: Miosis, blurred vision
<1% (Limited to important or life-threatening): Apnea, breast enlargement, cardiac arrest, chest pain, dyspnea, hallucinations, migraine, myocardial infarction, postural hypotension, QT_c prolongation, seizures, syncope, torsade de pointes, ventricular tachycardia

Overdosage/Toxicology Consider the possibility of multiple drug ingestion. Treatment should be symptom directed and supportive. Naloxone may be used (as airway protection) and should be titrated to clinical effect. Due to duration of activity, repeated naloxone dosing may be needed.

Drug Interactions
Cytochrome P450 Effect: CYP3A3/4 enzyme substrate
Increased Effect/Toxicity: CNS depressants, including sedatives, tranquilizers, propoxyphene, antidepressants, benzodiazepines, and ethanol may result in serious overdose when used with levomethadyl. Enzyme inducers (carbamazepine, phenobarbital, rifampin, phenytoin) may enhance the metabolism of levomethadyl leading to an increase in levomethadyl peak effect (however duration of action is shortened). Enzyme inhibitors such as erythromycin, cimetidine, and ketoconazole may increase the risk of arrhythmia (including torsade de pointes) or may increase the duration of action of levomethadyl. Concurrent use of QT_c-prolonging agents is contraindicated (includes class I and III antiarrhythmics, cisapride, erythromycin, select quinolones, mesoridazine, thioridazine, zonisamide). Concurrent use of MAO inhibitors is contraindicated (per manufacturer), or drugs with MAO-blocking activity (linezolid). Safety of selegiline (selective MAO type B inhibitor) not established.
Decreased Effect: Levomethadyl used in combination with naloxone, naltrexone, pentazocine, nalbuphine, butorphanol, and buprenorphine may result in withdrawal symptoms. The
(Continued)

Levomethadyl Acetate Hydrochloride (Continued)

effect of meperidine may be decreased by levomethadyl. Enzyme inducers (carbamazepine, phenobarbital, rifampin, phenytoin) may shorten levomethadyl's duration of action. Enzyme inhibitors, such as erythromycin, cimetidine, and ketoconazole may slow the onset, lower the activity levomethadyl (may also increase duration of action).

Ethanol/Nutrition/Herb Interactions Ethanol: Avoid ethanol (may increase CNS depression, may lead to overdose).

Stability Store at room temperature.

Mechanism of Action A synthetic opioid agonist with actions similar to morphine; principal actions are analgesia and sedation. Its clinical effects in the treatment of opiate abuse occur through two mechanisms: 1) cross-sensitivity for opiates of the morphine type, suppressing symptoms of withdrawal in opiate-dependent persons; 2) with chronic oral administration, can produce sufficient tolerance to block the subjective high of usual doses of parenterally administered opiates

Usual Dosage Adults: Oral: 20-40 mg at 48- or 72-hour intervals, with ranges of 10 mg to as high as 140 mg 3 times/week; adjust dose in increments of 5-10 mg (too rapid induction may lead to overdose); always dilute before administration and mix with diluent prior to dispensing

Monitoring Parameters Patient adherence with regimen and avoidance of illicit substances; random drug testing is recommended; EKG prior to treatment, 12-14 days after initiation, and periodically thereafter

Nursing Implications Drug administration and dispensing is to take place in an authorized clinic setting only; can potentially cause QT prolongation on EKG (not dose related)

Additional Information The product labeling for ORLAAM® (levomethadyl acetate hydrochloride) has been changed to reflect reports of 10 cases of serious arrhythmias submitted through MedWatch (as of March 30, 2001). On April 18, 2001, the manufacturer (Roxane Laboratories, Inc) mailed a Dear Healthcare Professional letter to physicians licensed to treat narcotic addiction. A black box warning has been added to highlight the seriousness of these reactions. In addition, the approved indication for levomethadyl has been revised, indicating levomethadyl should be reserved for use in treatment of opiate-addicted patients who fail to show an acceptable response to other adequate treatments for addiction.

Dosage Forms Solution, oral: 10 mg/mL (474 mL)

Levonorgestrel (LEE voe nor jes trel)

U.S. Brand Names Mirena®; Norplant® Implant; Plan B™

Canadian Brand Names Norplant® Implant; Plan B™

Synonyms LNg 20

Therapeutic Category Contraceptive, Emergency; Contraceptive, Implant (Progestin); Contraceptive, Intrauterine

Use Prevention of pregnancy

Pregnancy Risk Factor X

Pregnancy/Breast-Feeding Implications Epidemiologic studies have not shown an increased risk of birth defects when used prior to pregnancy or inadvertently during early pregnancy, although rare reports of congenital anomalies have been reported.

Intrauterine system: Women who become pregnant with an IUD in place risk septic abortion (septic shock and death may occur); removal of IUD may result in pregnancy loss. In addition, miscarriage, premature labor, and premature delivery may occur if pregnancy is continued with IUD in place.

Contraindications Hypersensitivity to levonorgestrel or any component of the formulation; undiagnosed abnormal uterine bleeding, active hepatic disease or malignant tumors, active thrombophlebitis, or thromboembolic disorders (current or history of), known or suspected carcinoma of the breast; history of intracranial hypertension; renal impairment; pregnancy

Additional product-specific contraindications: Intrauterine system: Congenital or acquired uterine anomaly, acute pelvic inflammatory disease, history of pelvic inflammatory disease (unless there has been a subsequent intrauterine pregnancy), postpartum endometritis, infected abortion within past 3 months, known or suspected uterine or cervical neoplasia, unresolved/abnormal Pap smear, untreated acute cervicitis or vaginitis, patient or partner with multiple sexual partners, conditions which increase susceptibility to infections (ie, leukemia, AIDS, I.V. drug abuse), unremoved IUD, history of ectopic pregnancy, conditions which predispose to ectopic pregnancy

Warnings/Precautions Menstrual bleeding patterns may be altered, missed menstrual periods should not be used to identify early pregnancy. These products do not protect against HIV infection or other sexually-transmitted diseases. Patients presenting with lower abdominal pain should be evaluated for follicular atresia and ectopic pregnancy. Patients receiving enzyme-inducing medications should be evaluated for an alternative method of contraception. Levonorgestrel may affect glucose tolerance, monitor serum glucose in patients with diabetes. Safety and efficacy for use in renal or hepatic impairment have not been established. Use with caution in conditions that may be aggravated by fluid retention, depression, or history of migraine. Only for use in women of reproductive age.

Use of combination hormonal contraceptives increases the risk of cardiovascular side effects in women who smoke cigarettes, especially those who are >35 years of age; although this may be an estrogen-related effect, the risk with progestin-only contraceptives is not known and women should be strongly advised not to smoke. Combination hormonal contraceptives may lead to increased risk of myocardial infarction and should be used with caution in patients with risk factors for coronary artery disease; the actual risk with progestin-only contraceptives is not known, however there have been postmarketing reports of myocardial infarction in women using levonorgestrel-only contraception. May increase the risk of thromboembolism; discontinue therapy if this occurs. Combination hormonal contraceptives may have a dose-related risk of vascular disease and hypertension; strokes have also been reported with postmarketing use of levonorgestrel-only contraception. Women with hypertension should be encouraged to use a nonhormonal form of contraception. The use of combination hormonal contraceptives has been associated with a slight increase in frequency of breast cancer (studies are not consistent); studies with progestin only contraceptives have been similar. Retinal thrombosis has been reported (rarely) with combination hormonal contraceptives and may be related to the estrogen component, however, progestin-only therapy should also be discontinued with unexplained partial or complete loss of vision.

Additional formulation-specific warnings:

Intrauterine system: Increased incidence of group A streptococcal sepsis and pelvic inflammatory disease (may be asymptomatic); may perforate uterus or cervix; risk of perforation is increased in lactating women; partial penetration or embedment in the myometrium may decrease effectiveness and lead to difficult removal; postpartum insertion should be delayed until uterine involution is complete; use caution in patients with coagulopathy or receiving anticoagulants

Oral tablet: Not intended to be used for routine contraception and will not terminate an existing pregnancy

Subdermal capsules: Insertion-related complications may occur; expulsion of capsules, capsule displacement, thrombophlebitis, and superficial phlebitis have been reported. Insertion and removal are surgical procedures. To decrease risk of thromboembolic disease, consider removing capsules with prolonged immobilization. Idiopathic intracranial hypertension has been reported and may be more likely to occur in obese females.

Adverse Reactions

Intrauterine system:
>5%:
  Cardiovascular: Hypertension
  Central nervous system: Headache, depression, nervousness
  Dermatologic: Acne
  Endocrine & metabolic: Breast pain, dysmenorrhea, decreased libido, abnormal Pap smear, amenorrhea (20% at 1 year), enlarged follicles (12%)
  Gastrointestinal: Abdominal pain, nausea, weight gain
  Genitourinary: Leukorrhea, vaginitis
  Neuromuscular & skeletal: Back pain
  Respiratory: Upper respiratory tract infection, sinusitis
<3%: Alopecia, anemia, cervicitis, dyspareunia, eczema, failed insertion, migraine, sepsis, vomiting

Oral tablets:
>10%:
  Central nervous system: Fatigue (17%), headache (17%), dizziness (11%)
  Endocrine & metabolic: Heavier menstrual bleeding (14%), lighter menstrual bleeding (12%), breast tenderness (11%)
  Gastrointestinal: Nausea (23%), abdominal pain (18%)
1% to 10%: Gastrointestinal: Vomiting (6%), diarrhea (5%)

Subdermal capsules:
>10%: Endocrine & metabolic: Increased/prolonged bleeding (28%), spotting (17%)
1% to 10%:
  Endocrine & metabolic: Breast discharge (≥5%), menstrual irregularities
  Gastrointestinal: Abdominal discomfort (≥5%)
  Genitourinary: Cervicitis (≥5%), leukorrhea (≥5%), vaginitis (≥5%)
  Local: Pain/itching at implant site (4%, usually transient)
  Neuromuscular & skeletal: Musculoskeletal pain (≥5%)
  Miscellaneous: Removal difficulties (6%); these may include multiple incisions, remaining capsule fragments, pain, multiple visits, deep placement, lengthy procedure
<1% (Limited to important or life-threatening): Alopecia, breast cancer, deep vein thrombosis, emotional lability, hirsutism, hyperpigmentation, idiopathic intracranial hypertension, infection at implant site, myocardial infarction, pulmonary embolism, rash, stroke, superficial venous thrombosis, thrombotic thrombocytopenic purpura (TTP), urticaria, vomiting

Overdosage/Toxicology Can result if >6 capsules are *in situ*. Symptoms include uterine bleeding irregularities and fluid retention. Treatment includes removal of all implanted capsules.

Drug Interactions

Decreased Effect: Enzyme inducers: May increase the metabolism of levonorgestrel resulting in decreased effect; includes carbamazepine, phenobarbital, phenytoin, and rifampin; additional contraceptive measures may be needed with use of enzyme inducers or following their withdrawal

Ethanol/Nutrition/Herb Interactions Herb/Nutraceutical: St John's wort (an enzyme inducer) may decrease serum levels of levonorgestrel.

Stability Store at room temperature of 25°C (77°F).

Mechanism of Action Pregnancy may be prevented through several mechanisms: Thickening of cervical mucus, which inhibits sperm passage through the uterus and sperm survival; inhibition of ovulation, from a negative feedback mechanism on the hypothalamus, leading to reduced secretion of follicle stimulating hormone (FSH) and luteinizing hormone (LH); inhibition of implantation. Levonorgestrel is not effective once the implantation process has begun.

Pharmacodynamics/Kinetics

Duration: Subdermal capsules and intrauterine system: Up to 5 years
Absorption: Rapid and complete
Protein binding: Highly bound to albumin and sex hormone-binding globulin
Metabolism: To inactive metabolites
Bioavailability: 100%
Half-life: Oral tablet: ~24 hours
Elimination: Primarily urine

Usual Dosage Adults:

Long-term prevention of pregnancy:
  Subdermal capsules: Total administration doses (implanted): 216 mg in 6 capsules which should be implanted during the first 7 days of onset of menses subdermally in the upper arm; each Norplant® silastic capsule releases 80 mcg of levonorgestrel/day for 6-18

(Continued)

Levonorgestrel *(Continued)*

months, following which a rate of release of 25-30 mcg/day is maintained for ≤5 years; capsules should be removed by end of 5th year

Intrauterine system: To be inserted into uterine cavity; should be inserted within 7 days of onset of menstruation or immediately after 1st trimester abortion; releases 20 mcg levonorgestrel/day over 5 years. May be removed and replaced with a new unit at anytime during menstrual cycle; do not leave any one system in place for >5 years

Emergency contraception: Oral tablet: One 0.75 mg tablet as soon as possible within 72 hours of unprotected sexual intercourse; a second 0.75 mg tablet should be taken 12 hours after the first dose; may be used at any time during menstrual cycle

Dosage adjustment in renal impairment: Safety and efficacy have not been established
Dosage adjustment in hepatic impairment: Safety and efficacy have not been established

Elderly: Not intended for use in postmenopausal women

Administration

Intrauterine system: Inserted in the uterine cavity, to a depth of 6-9 cm, with the provided insertion device; should not be forced into the uterus

Subdermal capsules: Six capsules are subdermally inserted to the medial aspect of the upper arm (under local anesthetic). Capsules are inserted in a fan-like manner, ~8-10 cm above the elbow crease, with the instruments provided. Prior to removal, palpate the area to locate all 6 capsules. The removal may take more time and may be more painful than the insertion.

Monitoring Parameters Monitor for prolonged menstrual bleeding, amenorrhea, irregularity of menses, Pap smear, blood pressure, serum glucose in patients with diabetes, LDL levels in patients with hyperlipidemias

Reference Range Contraceptive protection usually with plasma levonorgestrel concentrations of 0.29-0.35 ng/mL. Due to variability in individual responses, blood levels alone are not predictive of pregnancy risk.

Test Interactions Decreased concentrations of sex hormone-binding globulin; decreased thyroxine concentrations (slight); increased triiodothyronine uptake

Patient Information This does not protect against HIV infection or other sexually-transmitted diseases. Cigarette smoking is not recommended. You may experience cramping, headache, abdominal discomfort, hair loss, weight changes, or unusual menses (breakthrough bleeding, irregularity, excessive bleeding). Report sudden acute headache or visual disturbance, unusual nausea or vomiting, any loss of feeling in arms or legs, or lower abdominal pain.

Intrauterine system: This method provides up to 5 years of birth control from a T-shaped device inserted into the uterus. It will be inserted and removed by your prescriber. Notify your prescriber if the system comes out by itself, if you have long-lasting or heavy bleeding, unusual vaginal discharge, low abdominal pain, painful sexual intercourse, chills or fever. There is an increased risk of ectopic pregnancy with this product. Thread placement should be checked following each menstrual cycle; do not pull thread.

Oral tablet: This method provides emergency contraception. It is used after your normal form of birth control has failed, or following unprotected sexual intercourse. It should be used within 72 hours. Contact prescriber if you vomit within 1 hour of taking either dose.

Subdermal capsules: This method consists of 6 capsules, which will be placed under the skin, on the inside of your upper arm. They can provide up to 5 years of birth control. The capsules must be inserted and removed by your prescriber, do not attempt to remove implants yourself. Following insertion, keep area dry and avoid heavy lifting for 2-3 days. Report irritation at insertion site.

Nursing Implications Caution patient about need for annual medical exams.

Additional Information

Intrauterine system: The cumulative 5-year pregnancy rate is ~0.7 pregnancies/100 users. Over 70% of women in the trials had previously used IUDs. The reported pregnancy rate after 12 months was ≤0.2 pregnancies/100 users. Approximately 80% of women who wish to conceive have become pregnant within 12 months of device removal. The recommended patient profile for this product: A woman who has at least one child, is in a stable and mutually-monogamous relationship, no history of pelvic inflammatory disease, and no history of ectopic pregnancy or predisposition to ectopic pregnancy.

Oral tablet: When used as directed for emergency contraception, the expected pregnancy rate is decreased from 8% to 1%. Approximately 87% of women have their next menstrual period at approximately the expected time. A rapid return to fertility following use is expected.

Subdermal capsules: The net cumulative 5-year pregnancy rate for levonorgestrel implant use has been reported to be from 1.5-3.9 pregnancies/100 users. This compares to a cumulative rate of 4.9 pregnancies/100 women with an IUD after 5 years. At the end of the first year of use, the pregnancy rate with levonorgestrel implants has been reported to be from 0.2-0.6 pregnancies/100 users. This compares quite favorably with the 2.3 pregnancies/100 users of oral contraceptives during the first year of use and 2.4 pregnancies/100 women with an IUD during the first year. Norplant® is a very efficient, yet reversible, method of contraception. The long duration of action may be particularly advantageous in women who desire an extended period of contraceptive protection without sacrificing the possibility of future fertility.

Dosage Forms

Capsule, subdermal implantation (Norplant®): 36 mg (6s)
Intrauterine device (Mirena®): 52 mg levonorgestrel/unit
Tablet (Plan B™): 0.75 mg

- **Levonorgestrel and Ethinyl Estradiol** *see* Ethinyl Estradiol and Levonorgestrel *on page 518*
- **Levophed®** *see* Norepinephrine *on page 993*
- **Levora®** *see* Ethinyl Estradiol and Levonorgestrel *on page 518*

Levorphanol (lee VOR fa nole)

Related Information
Narcotic Agonists Comparison *on page 1506*
U.S. Brand Names Levo-Dromoran®
Synonyms Levorphanol Tartrate; Levorphan Tartrate
Therapeutic Category Analgesic, Narcotic
Use Relief of moderate to severe pain; also used parenterally for preoperative sedation and an adjunct to nitrous oxide/oxygen anesthesia; 2 mg levorphanol produces analgesia comparable to that produced by 10 mg of morphine
Restrictions C-II
Pregnancy Risk Factor B/D (prolonged use or high doses at term)
Contraindications Hypersensitivity to levorphanol or any component of the formulation; pregnancy B/D (prolonged use or high doses at term)
Warnings/Precautions Use with caution in patients with hypersensitivity reactions to other phenanthrene derivative opioid agonists (morphine, hydrocodone, hydromorphone, levorphanol, oxycodone, oxymorphone); respiratory diseases including asthma, emphysema, COPD or severe liver or renal insufficiency; some preparations contain sulfites which may cause allergic reactions; tolerance or dependence may result from extended use; dextromethorphan has equivalent antitussive activity but has much lower toxicity in accidental overdose. Elderly may be particularly susceptible to the CNS depressant and constipating effects of narcotics.
Adverse Reactions Frequency not defined.
Cardiovascular: Palpitations, hypotension, bradycardia, peripheral vasodilation, cardiac arrest, shock, tachycardia
Central nervous system: CNS depression, fatigue, drowsiness, dizziness, nervousness, headache, restlessness, anorexia, malaise, confusion, coma, convulsion, insomnia, amnesia, mental depression, hallucinations, paradoxical CNS stimulation, intracranial pressure (increased),
Dermatologic: Pruritus, urticaria, rash
Endocrine & metabolic: Antidiuretic hormone release
Gastrointestinal: Nausea, vomiting, dyspepsia, stomach cramps, xerostomia, constipation, abdominal pain, dry mouth, biliary tract spasm, paralytic ileus
Genitourinary: Decreased urination, urinary tract spasm, urinary retention
Local: Pain at injection site
Neuromuscular & skeletal: Weakness
Ocular: Miosis, diplopia
Respiratory: Respiratory depression, apnea, hypoventilation, cyanosis
Miscellaneous: Histamine release, physical and psychological dependence
Overdosage/Toxicology Symptoms include CNS depression, respiratory depression, miosis, apnea, pulmonary edema, and convulsions. Treatment includes naloxone 2 mg I.V. (0.01 mg/kg for children), with repeat administration as necessary, up to a total of 10 mg.
Drug Interactions
Increased Effect/Toxicity: CNS depression is enhanced with coadministration of other CNS depressants.
Ethanol/Nutrition/Herb Interactions
Ethanol: Avoid or limit ethanol (may increase CNS depression). Watch for sedation.
Herb/Nutraceutical: Avoid valerian, St John's wort, kava kava, gotu kola (may increase CNS depression).
Stability Store at room temperature, protect from freezing; I.V. is **incompatible** when mixed with aminophylline, barbiturates, heparin, methicillin, phenytoin, sodium bicarbonate
Mechanism of Action Levorphanol tartrate is a synthetic opioid agonist that is classified as a morphinan derivative. Opioids interact with stereospecific opioid receptors in various parts of the central nervous system and other tissues. Analgesic potency parallels the affinity for these binding sites. These drugs do not alter the threshold or responsiveness to pain, but the perception of pain.
Pharmacodynamics/Kinetics
Onset of action: Oral: 10-60 minutes
Duration: 4-8 hours
Usual Dosage Adults:
Oral: 2 mg every 6-24 hours as needed
S.C.: 2 mg, up to 3 mg if necessary, every 6-8 hours
I.V.: Not recommended (if no alternative; dilute to 10 mL with NS and inject no faster than 1 mg/min)
Dosing adjustment in hepatic disease: Reduction is necessary in patients with liver disease
Monitoring Parameters Pain relief, respiratory and mental status, blood pressure
Patient Information Avoid alcohol, may cause drowsiness, impaired judgment or coordination; may cause physical and psychological dependence with prolonged use
Nursing Implications Observe patient for excessive sedation, respiratory depression; implement safety measures, assist with ambulation
Dosage Forms
Injection, as tartrate: 2 mg/mL (1 mL, 10 mL)
Tablet, as tartrate: 2 mg

♦ **Levorphanol Tartrate** *see* Levorphanol *on page 799*
♦ **Levorphan Tartrate** *see* Levorphanol *on page 799*
♦ **Levo-T™** *see* Levothyroxine *on page 799*
♦ **Levotabs®** *see* Levothyroxine *on page 799*
♦ **Levothroid®** *see* Levothyroxine *on page 799*

Levothyroxine (lee voe thye ROKS een)

U.S. Brand Names Levo-T™; Levotabs®; Levothroid®; Levoxyl®; Synthroid®; Thyrox®; Unithroid™
(Continued)

Levothyroxine *(Continued)*

Canadian Brand Names Eltroxin®; Synthroid®

Synonyms Levothyroxine Sodium; *L*-Thyroxine Sodium; T_4

Therapeutic Category Thyroid Product

Use Replacement or supplemental therapy in hypothyroidism; some clinicians suggest levothyroxine is the drug of choice for replacement therapy

Pregnancy Risk Factor A

Contraindications Hypersensitivity to levothyroxine sodium or any component of the formulation; recent myocardial infarction or thyrotoxicosis; uncorrected adrenal insufficiency

Warnings/Precautions Ineffective for weight reduction; high doses may produce serious or even life-threatening toxic effects particularly when used with some anorectic drugs. Use with caution and reduce dosage in patients with angina pectoris or other cardiovascular disease; levothyroxine tablets contain tartrazine dye which may cause allergic reactions in susceptible individuals; use cautiously in elderly since they may be more likely to have compromised cardiovascular functions. Patients with adrenal insufficiency, myxedema, diabetes mellitus and insipidus may have symptoms exaggerated or aggravated; thyroid replacement requires periodic assessment of thyroid status. Chronic hypothyroidism predisposes patients to coronary artery disease.

Adverse Reactions Frequency not defined.

Cardiovascular: Palpitations, cardiac arrhythmias, tachycardia, chest pain

Central nervous system: Nervousness, headache, insomnia, fever, ataxia

Dermatologic: Alopecia

Endocrine & metabolic: Changes in menstrual cycle, weight loss, increased appetite

Gastrointestinal: Diarrhea, abdominal cramps, constipation, vomiting

Neuromuscular & skeletal: Myalgia, hand tremors, tremor

Respiratory: Dyspnea

Miscellaneous: Diaphoresis, allergic skin reactions (rare)

Overdosage/Toxicology Chronic overdose is treated by withdrawal of the drug. Massive overdose may require beta-blockers for increased sympathomimetic activity. Chronic overdose may cause hyperthyroidism, weight loss, nervousness, sweating, tachycardia, insomnia, heat intolerance, menstrual irregularities, palpitations, psychosis, and fever. Acute overdose may cause fever, hypoglycemia, CHF, and unrecognized adrenal insufficiency. Reduce the dose or temporarily discontinue therapy. The hypothalamic-pituitary-thyroid axis will return to normal in 6-8 weeks. Serum T_4 levels do not correlate well with toxicity. In massive acute ingestion, reduce GI absorption and administer general supportive care. Treat congestive heart failure with digitalis glycosides. Excessive adrenergic activity (tachycardia) requires propranolol 1-3 mg I.V. over 10 minutes or 80-160 mg orally/day. Fever may be treated with acetaminophen.

Drug Interactions

Cytochrome P450 Effect: CYP enzyme substrate (T_3 and T_4); thyroid hormone may alter metabolic activity of cytochrome P450 enzymes

Increased Effect/Toxicity: Levothyroxine may potentiate the hypoprothrombinemic effect of warfarin (and other oral anticoagulants). Effect of warfarin may be dramatically increased when levothyroxine is added. However, the addition of warfarin in a patient previously receiving a stable dose of levothyroxine does not require a significantly different dosing strategy. Tricyclic antidepressants (TCAs) coadministered with levothyroxine may increase potential for toxicity of both drugs. Excessive thyroid replacement in patients receiving growth hormone may lead to accelerated epiphyseal closure; inadequate replacement interferes with growth response. Coadministration with ketamine may lead to hypertension and tachycardia.

Decreased Effect: Aluminum- and magnesium-containing antacids, iron preparations, sucralfate, cholestyramine, colestipol, and Kayexalate® may decrease levothyroxine absorption (separate administration by 8 hours). Enzyme inducers (phenytoin, phenobarbital, carbamazepine, and rifampin/rifabutin) may decrease levothyroxine levels. Levothyroxine may decrease effect of oral sulfonylureas. Dosage of levothyroxine may need to be increased when SSRIs are added. Serum levels of digoxin and theophylline may be altered by thyroid function.

Ethanol/Nutrition/Herb Interactions Food: Taking levothyroxine with enteral nutrition may cause reduced bioavailability and may lower serum thyroxine levels leading to signs or symptoms of hypothyroidism. Limit intake of goitrogenic foods (eg, asparagus, cabbage, peas, turnip greens, broccoli, spinach, Brussels sprouts, lettuce, soybeans). Soybean flour (infant formula), walnuts, and dietary fiber may decrease absorption of levothyroxine from the GI tract.

Stability Protect tablets from light; do not mix I.V. solution with other I.V. infusion solutions; reconstituted solutions should be used immediately and any unused portions discarded

Mechanism of Action Exact mechanism of action is unknown; however, it is believed the thyroid hormone exerts its many metabolic effects through control of DNA transcription and protein synthesis; involved in normal metabolism, growth, and development; promotes gluconeogenesis, increases utilization and mobilization of glycogen stores, and stimulates protein synthesis, increases basal metabolic rate

Pharmacodynamics/Kinetics

Onset of action: Therapeutic: Oral: 3-5 days; I.V. 6-8 hours

Peak effect: I.V.: ~24 hours

Absorption: Oral: Erratic

Metabolism: Hepatic to triiodothyronine (active)

Time to peak, serum: 2-4 hours

Half-life elimination: Euthyroid: 6-7 days; Hypothyroid: 9-10 days; Hyperthyroid: 3-4 days

Excretion: Urine and feces

Usual Dosage

Children: Congenital hypothyroidism:

Oral:

0-6 months: 8-10 mcg/kg/day **or** 25-50 mcg/day

6-12 months: 6-8 mcg/kg/day **or** 50-75 mcg/day

1-5 years: 5-6 mcg/kg/day **or** 75-100 mcg/day

6-12 years: 4-5 mcg/kg/day **or** 100-150 mcg/day

>12 years: 2-3 mcg/kg/day **or** ≥150 mcg/day

I.M., I.V.: 50% to 75% of the oral dose

Adults:

Oral: Initial: 0.05 mcg/day, then increase by increments of 25 mcg/day at intervals of 2-3 weeks; average adult dose: 100-200 mcg/day; maximum dose: 200 mcg/day

I.M., I.V.: 50% of the oral dose

Myxedema coma or stupor: I.V.: 200-500 mcg one time, then 100-300 mcg the next day if necessary

Thyroid suppression therapy: Oral: 2-6 mcg/kg/day for 7-10 days

Dietary Considerations Should be taken on an empty stomach.

Administration

Oral: Administer on an empty stomach

Parenteral: Dilute vial with 5 mL normal saline; use immediately after reconstitution; administer by direct I.V. infusion over 2- to 3-minute period. I.V. form must be prepared immediately prior to administration; should not be admixed with other solutions

Monitoring Parameters Thyroid function test (serum thyroxine, thyrotropin concentrations), resin triiodothyronine uptake (RT_3U), free thyroxine index (FTI), T_4, TSH, heart rate, blood pressure, clinical signs of hypo- and hyperthyroidism; TSH is the most reliable guide for evaluating adequacy of thyroid replacement dosage. TSH may be elevated during the first few months of thyroid replacement despite patients being clinically euthyroid. In cases where T_4 remains low and TSH is within normal limits, an evaluation of "free" (unbound) T_4 is needed to evaluate further increase in dosage

Reference Range Pediatrics: Cord T_4 and values in the first few weeks are much higher, falling over the first months and years. ≥10 years: ~5.8-11 µg/dL (SI: 75-142 nmol/L). Borderline low: ≤4.5-5.7 µg/dL (SI: 58-73 nmol/L); low: ≤4.4 µg/dL (SI: 57 nmol/L); results <2.5 µg/dL (SI: <32 nmol/L) are strong evidence for hypothyroidism.

Approximate adult normal range: 4-12 µg/dL (SI: 51-154 nmol/L). Borderline high: 11.1-13 µg/dL (SI: 143-167 nmol/L); high: ≥13.1 µg/dL (SI: 169 nmol/L). Normal range is increased in women on birth control pills (5.5-12 µg/dL); normal range in pregnancy: ~5.5-16 µg/dL (SI: ~71-206 nmol/L). TSH: 0.4-10 (for those ≥80 years) mIU/L; T_4: 4-12 µg/dL (SI: 51-154 nmol/L); T_3 (RIA) (total T_3): 80-230 ng/dL (SI: 1.2-3.5 nmol/L); T_4 free (free T_4): 0.7-1.8 ng/dL (SI: 9-23 pmol/L).

Patient Information Do not change brands without physician's knowledge; report immediately to physician any chest pain, increased pulse, palpitations, heat intolerances, excessive sweating; do not discontinue without notifying your physician

Nursing Implications I.V. form must be prepared immediately prior to administration; should not be mixed with other solutions

Additional Information Levothroid® tablets contain lactose and tartrazine dye

Equivalent doses: Thyroid USP 60 mg ~ levothyroxine 0.05-0.06 mg ~ liothyronine 0.015-0.0375 mg

50-60 mg thyroid ~ 50-60 mcg levothyroxine and 12.5-15 mcg liothyronine Liotrix®

Dosage Forms

Powder for injection, lyophilized, as sodium: 200 mcg/vial (6 mL, 10 mL); 500 mcg/vial (6 mL, 10 mL)

Tablet, as sodium: 25 mcg, 50 mcg, 75 mcg, 88 mcg, 100 mcg, 112 mcg, 125 mcg, 137 mcg, 150 mcg, 175 mcg, 200 mcg, 300 mcg

Lidocaine (LYE doe kane)

Related Information

Adult ACLS Algorithms *on page 1632*

Antiarrhythmic Drugs Comparison *on page 1478*

Pediatric ALS Algorithms *on page 1628*

U.S. Brand Names Anestacon®; Dermaflex® Gel; ELA-Max® [OTC]; Lidoderm®; LidoPen® Auto-Injector; Solarcaine® Aloe Extra Burn Relief [OTC]; Xylocaine®; Zilactin-L® [OTC]

Canadian Brand Names Lidodan™; Lidoderm®; Xylocaine®; Xylocard®; Zilactin®

Synonyms Lidocaine Hydrochloride; Lignocaine Hydrochloride

Therapeutic Category Antiarrhythmic Agent, Class I-B; Local Anesthetic, Injectable; Local Anesthetic, Topical

Use Local anesthetic and acute treatment of ventricular arrhythmias from myocardial infarction, cardiac manipulation, digitalis intoxication; drug of choice for ventricular ectopy, ventricular tachycardia (VT), ventricular fibrillation (VF); for pulseless VT or VF preferably administer **after** defibrillation and epinephrine; control of premature ventricular contractions, wide-complex paroxysmal supraventricular tachycardia (PSVT); control of hemodynamically compromising PVCs; hemodynamically stable VT

(Continued)

Lidocaine *(Continued)*

ELA-Max® is a topical local anesthetic for use in laser, cosmetic, and outpatient surgeries; minor burns, cuts, and abrasions of the skin

Orphan drug: Lidoderm® Patch: Relief of allodynia (painful hypersensitivity) and chronic pain in postherpetic neuralgia

Pregnancy Risk Factor B (manufacturer); C (expert analysis)

Contraindications Hypersensitivity to lidocaine or any component of the formulation; hypersensitivity to another local anesthetic of the amide type; Adam-Stokes syndrome; severe degrees of SA, AV, or intraventricular heart block (except in patients with a functioning artificial pacemaker)

Warnings/Precautions

Intravenous: Constant EKG monitoring is necessary during I.V. administration. Use cautiously in hepatic impairment, any degree of heart block, Wolff-Parkinson-White syndrome, CHF, marked hypoxia, severe respiratory depression, hypovolemia, history of malignant hyperthermia, or shock. Increased ventricular rate may be seen when administered to a patient with atrial fibrillation. Correct any underlying causes of ventricular arrhythmias. Monitor closely for signs and symptoms of CNS toxicity. The elderly may be prone to increased CNS and cardiovascular side effects. Reduce dose in hepatic dysfunction and CHF.

Injectable anesthetic: Follow appropriate administration techniques so as not to administer any intravascularly. Solutions containing antimicrobial preservatives should not be used for epidural or spinal anesthesia. Some solutions contain a bisulfite; avoid in patients who are allergic to bisulfite. Resuscitative equipment, medicine and oxygen should be available in case of emergency. Use products containing epinephrine cautiously in patients with significant vascular disease, compromised blood flow, or during or following general anesthesia (increased risk of arrhythmias). Adjust the dose for the elderly, pediatric, acutely ill, and debilitated patients.

Topical: ELA-Max® cream: Do not leave on large body areas for >2 hours. Observe young children closely to prevent accidental ingestion. Not for use ophthalmic use or for use on mucous membranes.

Adverse Reactions Effects vary with route of administration. Many effects are dose-related.

Frequency not defined:

Cardiovascular: Bradycardia, hypotension, heart block, arrhythmias, cardiovascular collapse, sinus node suppression, increase defibrillator threshold, vascular insufficiency (periarticular injections), arterial spasms

Central nervous system: Drowsiness after administration is usually a sign of a high blood level. Other effects may include lightheadedness, dizziness, tinnitus, blurred vision, vomiting, twitching, tremors, lethargy, coma, agitation, slurred speech, seizures, anxiety, euphoria, hallucinations, paresthesia, psychosis

Dermatologic: Itching, rash, edema of the skin, contact dermatitis

Gastrointestinal: Nausea, vomiting, taste disorder

Local: Thrombophlebitis

Neuromuscular & skeletal: Transient radicular pain (subarachnoid administration; up to 1.9%)

Ocular: Blurred vision, diplopia

Respiratory: Dyspnea, respiratory depression or arrest, bronchospasm

Miscellaneous: Allergic reactions, urticaria, edema, anaphylactoid reaction

Following spinal anesthesia positional headache (3%), shivering (2%) nausea, peripheral nerve symptoms, respiratory inadequacy and double vision (<1%), hypotension, cauda equina syndrome

Postmarketing and/or case reports: ARDS (inhalation), asystole, methemoglobinemia, severe back pain

Overdosage/Toxicology Has a narrow therapeutic index and severe toxicity may occur slightly above the therapeutic range, especially with other antiarrhythmic drugs. Symptoms include sedation, confusion, coma, seizures, respiratory arrest and cardiac toxicity (sinus arrest, A-V block, asystole, and hypotension). The QRS and QT intervals are usually normal, although they may be prolonged after massive overdose. Other effects include dizziness, paresthesias, tremor, ataxia, and GI disturbance. Treatment is supportive, using conventional therapies (fluids, positioning, vasopressors, antiarrhythmics, anticonvulsants). Sodium bicarbonate may reverse QRS prolongation, bradyarrhythmias and hypotension. Enhanced elimination with dialysis, hemoperfusion or repeat charcoal is not effective.

Drug Interactions

Cytochrome P450 Effect: CYP1A2, 2B6, and 3A3/4 enzyme substrate; CYP1A2 enzyme inhibitor

Increased Effect/Toxicity: Concomitant cimetidine or propranolol may result in increased serum concentrations of lidocaine resulting in toxicity. Serum concentrations/toxicity of lidocaine may be increased by inhibitors of CYP3A3/4, including amprenavir, cimetidine, ciprofloxacin, clarithromycin, clozapine, diltiazem, disulfiram, digoxin, erythromycin, ethanol, fluconazole, fluoxetine, fluvoxamine, grapefruit juice, isoniazid, itraconazole, ketoconazole, labetalol, levodopa, loxapine, metoprolol, metronidazole, miconazole, nefazodone, nelfinavir, omeprazole, phenytoin, rifabutin, rifampin, ritonavir, troleandomycin, valproic acid, and verapamil. Effect of succinylcholine may be enhanced by lidocaine.

Ethanol/Nutrition/Herb Interactions Herb/Nutraceutical: St John's wort may decrease lidocaine levels; avoid concurrent use.

Stability Lidocaine injection is stable at room temperature. Stability of parenteral admixture at room temperature (25°C) is the expiration date on premixed bag; out of overwrap stability is 30 days.

Standard diluent: 2 g/250 mL D_5W

Mechanism of Action Class Ib antiarrhythmic; suppresses automaticity of conduction tissue, by increasing electrical stimulation threshold of ventricle, HIS-Purkinje system, and spontaneous depolarization of the ventricles during diastole by a direct action on the tissues; blocks both the initiation and conduction of nerve impulses by decreasing the neuronal membrane's permeability to sodium ions, which results in inhibition of depolarization with resultant blockade of conduction

Pharmacodynamics/Kinetics

Onset of action: Single bolus dose: 45-90 seconds

Duration: 10-20 minutes

Distribution: V_d: 1.1-2.1 L/kg; alterable by many patient factors; decreased in CHF and liver disease; crosses blood-brain barrier

Protein binding: 60% to 80% to alpha$_1$ acid glycoprotein

Metabolism: 90% hepatic; active metabolites monoethylglycinexylidide (MEGX) and glycinexylidide (GX) can accumulate and may cause CNS toxicity

Half-life elimination: Biphasic: Increased with CHF, liver disease, shock, severe renal disease; Initial: 7-30 minutes; Terminal: Infants, premature: 3.2 hours, Adults: 1.5-2 hours

Usual Dosage

Topical: Apply to affected area as needed; maximum: 3 mg/kg/dose; do not repeat within 2 hours.

ELA-Max® cream; Apply $\frac{1}{4}$ inch thick layer to intact skin. Leave on until adequate anesthetic effect is obtained. Remove cream and cleanse area before beginning procedure.

Injectable local anesthetic: Varies with procedure, degree of anesthesia needed, vascularity of tissue, duration of anesthesia required, and physical condition of patient; maximum: 4.5 mg/kg/dose; do not repeat within 2 hours.

Patch: Postherpetic neuralgia: Apply patch to most painful area. Up to 3 patches may be applied in a single application. Patch may remain in place for up to 12 hours in any 24-hour period.

Antiarrhythmic:

I.V.: 1-1.5 mg/kg bolus over 2-3 minutes; may repeat doses of 0.5-0.75 mg/kg in 5-10 minutes up to a total of 3 mg/kg; continuous infusion: 1-4 mg/minute

I.V. (2 g/250 mL D$_5$W) infusion rates (infusion pump should be used for I.V. infusion administration):

1 mg/minute: 7.5 mL/hour

2 mg/minute: 15 mL/hour

3 mg/minute: 22.5 mL/hour

4 mg/minute: 30 mL/hour

Ventricular fibrillation (after defibrillation and epinephrine): Initial: 1-1.5 mg/kg. Repeat 0.5-0.75 mg/kg bolus may be given 3-5 minutes after initial dose. Total dose should not exceed 200-300 mg during a 1-hour period or 3 mg/kg total dose. Follow with continuous infusion after return of perfusion.

Endotracheal: 2-2.5 times the I.V. dose (2-4 mg/kg diluted with NS to a total volume of 10 mL)

Decrease dose in patients with CHF, shock, or hepatic disease.

Dosage adjustment in renal impairment: Not dialyzable (0% to 5%) by hemo- or peritoneal dialysis; supplemental dose is not necessary.

Dosage adjustment in hepatic impairment: Reduce dose in acute hepatitis and decompensated cirrhosis by 50%.

Administration

Endotracheal doses should be diluted to 10 mL with normal saline prior to E.T. administration

I.V.: Use microdrip (60 gtt/mL) or infusion pump to administer an accurate dose

Buffered lidocaine for injectable local anesthetic: Add 2 mL of sodium bicarbonate 8.4% to 18 mL of lidocaine 1%

Topical: Patch may be cut to appropriate size; remove immediately if burning sensation occurs; wash hands after application

Reference Range

Therapeutic: 1.5-5.0 µg/mL (SI: 6-21 µmol/L)

Potentially toxic: >6 µg/mL (SI: >26 µmol/L)

Toxic: >9 µg/mL (SI: >38 µmol/L)

Nursing Implications Local thrombophlebitis may occur in patients receiving prolonged I.V. infusions Patch may be cut to appropriate size. remove immediately if burning sensation occurs. Wash hands after application.

Dosage Forms

Cream, as hydrochloride: 2% (56 g); 4% (5 g, 30 g)

Gel, as hydrochloride: 0.5% (15 mL); 2.5% (15 mL)

Injection, I.M.: 10% [100 mg/mL] (3 mL)

Injection, as hydrochloride:

0.5% [5 mg/mL] (50 mL)

1% [10 mg/mL] (2 mL, 5 mL, 10 mL, 20 mL, 30 mL, 50 mL)

1.5% [15 mg/mL] (20 mL)

2% [20 mg/mL] (2 mL, 5 mL, 10 mL, 20 mL, 30 mL, 50 mL)

4% [40 mg/mL] (5 mL); 10% [100 mg/mL] (10 mL)

20% [200 mg/mL] (10 mL, 20 mL)

Injection, I.V. direct:

1% [10 mg/mL] (5 mL, 20 mL, 30 mL, 50 mL)

2% [20 mg/mL] (5 mL, 10 mL, 20 mL, 30 mL, 50 mL)

Injection, I.V. admixture [preservative free]:

4% [40 mg/mL] (5 mL, 25 mL, 50 mL)

10% [100 mg/mL] (10 mL)

20% [200 mg/mL] (5 mL, 10 mL)

Injection, I.V. infusion [in D$_5$W]:

0.2% [2 mg/mL] (500 mL)

0.4% [4 mg/mL] (250 mL, 500 mL, 1000 mL)

0.8% [8 mg/mL] (250 mL, 500 mL)

Jelly, topical, as hydrochloride: 2%

Liquid, topical, as hydrochloride: 2.5% (7.5 mL)

(Continued)

Lidocaine *(Continued)*

Liquid, viscous, as hydrochloride: 2% (20 mL, 100 mL)
Ointment, topical, as hydrochloride: 2.5% [OTC], 5% (35 g)
Patch, transdermal: 5%
Solution, topical, as hydrochloride: 2% (15 mL, 240 mL); 4% (50 mL)

Lidocaine and Epinephrine *(LYE doe kane & ep i NEF rin)*

U.S. Brand Names Xylocaine® With Epinephrine
Canadian Brand Names Xylocaine® With Epinephrine
Synonyms Epinephrine and Lidocaine
Therapeutic Category Local Anesthetic, Injectable
Use Local infiltration anesthesia; AVS for nerve block
Pregnancy Risk Factor B
Contraindications Hypersensitivity to local anesthetics of the amide type or any component
of the formulation; myasthenia gravis; shock; cardiac conduction disease; also see individual
agents
Warnings/Precautions Do not use solutions in distal portions of the body (digits, nose, ears,
penis). Use with caution in endocrine, heart, hepatic, or thyroid disease. Should be avoided in
patients with uncontrolled hyperthyroidism. Should be used in minimal amounts in patients
with significant cardiovascular problems (because of epinephrine component). Aspirate the
syringe after tissue penetration and before injection to minimize chance of direct vascular
injection.
Adverse Reactions Degree of adverse effects in the central nervous system and cardiovascular system are directly related to the blood levels of lidocaine. The effects below are more
likely to occur after systemic administration rather than infiltration.

Cardiovascular: Myocardial effects include a decrease in contraction force as well as a
decrease in electrical excitability and myocardial conduction rate resulting in bradycardia
and reduction in cardiac output.
Central nervous system: High blood levels result in anxiety, restlessness, disorientation,
confusion, dizziness, tremors and seizures. This is followed by depression of CNS resulting
in somnolence, unconsciousness and possible respiratory arrest. In some cases, symptoms of CNS stimulation may be absent and the primary CNS effects are somnolence and
unconsciousness.
Gastrointestinal: Nausea and vomiting may occur
Hypersensitivity reactions: Extremely rare, but may be manifest as dermatologic reactions
and edema at injection site. Asthmatic syndromes have occurred. Patients may exhibit
hypersensitivity to bisulfites contained in local anesthetic solution to prevent oxidation of
epinephrine. In general, patients reacting to bisulfites have a history of asthma and their
airways are hyper-reactive to asthmatic syndrome.
Psychogenic reactions: It is common to misinterpret psychogenic responses to local anesthetic injection as an allergic reaction. Intraoral injections are perceived by many patients
as a stressful procedure in dentistry. Common symptoms to this stress are diaphoresis,
palpitations, hyperventilation, generalized pallor and a fainting feeling
Overdosage/Toxicology Refer to Lidocaine monograph.
Drug Interactions
Increased Effect/Toxicity: Epinephrine (and other direct alpha-agonists): Pressor
response to I.V. epinephrine, norepinephrine, and phenylephrine may be enhanced in
patients receiving TCAs (**Note:** Effect is unlikely with epinephrine or levonordefrin dosages
typically administered as infiltration in combination with local anesthetics).
Stability Solutions with epinephrine should be protected from light.
Mechanism of Action Lidocaine blocks both the initiation and conduction of nerve impulses
via decreased permeability of sodium ions; epinephrine increases the duration of action of
lidocaine by causing vasoconstriction (via alpha effects) which slows the vascular absorption
of lidocaine
Pharmacodynamics/Kinetics
Onset of action: Peak effect: ~5 minutes
Duration: ~2 hours; dose and anesthetic procedure dependent
See individual agents.
Usual Dosage
Children: Use lidocaine concentrations of 0.5% to 1% (or even more diluted) to decrease
possibility of toxicity; lidocaine dose should not exceed 7 mg/kg/dose; do not repeat within
2 hours
Adults: Dosage varies with the anesthetic procedure, degree of anesthesia needed, vascu-
larity of tissue, duration of anesthesia required, and physical condition of patient
Administration Before injecting, withdraw syringe plunger to ensure injection is not into vein
or artery
Nursing Implications Before injecting, withdraw syringe plunger to ensure injection is not into
vein or artery
Additional Information Contains metabisulfites
Dosage Forms
Injection with epinephrine:
Epinephrine 1:200,000: Lidocaine hydrochloride 0.5% [5 mg/mL] (50 mL); 1% [10 mg/mL]
(30 mL); 1.5% [15 mg/mL] (5 mL, 10 mL, 30 mL); 2% [20 mg/mL] (20 mL)
Epinephrine 1:100,000: Lidocaine hydrochloride 1% [10 mg/mL] (20 mL, 50 mL); 2% [20
mg/mL] (1.8 mL, 20 mL, 30 mL, 50 mL)
Epinephrine 1:50,000: Lidocaine hydrochloride 2% [20 mg/mL] (1.8 mL)

Lidocaine and Prilocaine *(LYE doe kane & PRIL oh kane)*

U.S. Brand Names EMLA®
Canadian Brand Names EMLA®
Synonyms Prilocaine and Lidocaine
Therapeutic Category Analgesic, Topical; Anesthetic, Topical; Local Anesthetic, Topical

Use Topical anesthetic for use on normal intact skin to provide local analgesia for minor procedures such as I.V. cannulation or venipuncture; has also been used for painful procedures such as lumbar puncture and skin graft harvesting; for superficial minor surgery of genital mucous membranes and as an adjunct for local infiltration anesthesia in genital mucous membranes.

Pregnancy Risk Factor B

Contraindications
Hypersensitivity to amide type anesthetic agents [ie, lidocaine, prilocaine, dibucaine, mepivacaine, bupivacaine, etidocaine]; hypersensitivity to any component of the formulation selected; application on mucous membranes or broken or inflamed skin; infants <1 month of age if gestational age is <37 weeks; infants <12 months of age receiving therapy with methemoglobin-inducing agents; children with congenital or idiopathic methemoglobinemia, or in children who are receiving medications associated with drug-induced methemoglobinemia [ie, acetaminophen (overdosage), benzocaine, chloroquine, dapsone, nitrofurantoin, nitroglycerin, nitroprusside, phenazopyridine, phenelzine, phenobarbital, phenytoin, quinine, sulfonamides]

Warnings/Precautions Use with caution in patients receiving class I antiarrhythmic drugs, since systemic absorption occurs and synergistic toxicity is possible. Although the incidence of systemic adverse reactions with EMLA® is very low, caution should be exercised, particularly when applying over large areas and leaving on for longer than 2 hours.

Adverse Reactions Frequency not defined.
Cardiovascular: Hypotension, angioedema
Central nervous system: Shock
Dermatologic: Hyperpigmentation, erythema, itching, rash, burning, urticaria
Genitourinary: Blistering of foreskin (rare)
Local: Burning, stinging, edema
Respiratory: Bronchospasm
Miscellaneous: Alteration in temperature sensation, hypersensitivity reactions

Drug Interactions
Increased Effect/Toxicity: Class I antiarrhythmic drugs (tocainide, mexiletine): Effects are additive and potentially synergistic. Prilocaine may enhance the effect of other drugs known to induce methemoglobinemia.

Stability Store at room temperature

Mechanism of Action Local anesthetic action occurs by stabilization of neuronal membranes and inhibiting the ionic fluxes required for the initiation and conduction of impulses

Pharmacodynamics/Kinetics
EMLA®:
Onset of action: 1 hour
Peak effect: 2-3 hours
Duration: 1-2 hours after removal
Absorption: Related to duration of application and area where applied
3-hour application: 3.6% lidocaine and 6.1% prilocaine
24-hour application: 16.2% lidocaine and 33.5% prilocaine
See individual agents.

Usual Dosage Although the incidence of systemic adverse effects with EMLA® is very low, caution should be exercised, particularly when applying over large areas and leaving on for >2 hours
Children (intact skin): EMLA® should **not** be used in neonates with a gestation age <37 weeks nor in infants <12 months of age who are receiving treatment with methemoglobin-inducing agents
Dosing is based on child's age and weight:
Age 0-3 months or <5 kg: Apply a maximum of 1 g over no more than 10 cm^2 of skin; leave on for no longer than 1 hour
Age 3 months to 12 months and >5 kg: Apply no more than a maximum 2 g total over no more than 20 cm^2 of skin; leave on for no longer than 4 hours
Age 1-6 years and >10 kg: Apply no more than a maximum of 10 g total over no more than 100 cm^2 of skin; leave on for no longer than 4 hours.
Age 7-12 years and >20 kg: Apply no more than a maximum 20 g total over no more than 200 cm^2 of skin; leave on for no longer than 4 hours.
Note: If a patient greater than 3 months old does not meet the minimum weight requirement, the maximum total dose should be restricted to the corresponding maximum based on patient weight.

Adults (intact skin):
EMLA® cream and EMLA® anesthetic disc: A thick layer of EMLA® cream is applied to intact skin and covered with an occlusive dressing, or alternatively, an EMLA® anesthetic disc is applied to intact skin
Minor dermal procedures (eg, I.V. cannulation or venipuncture): Apply 2.5 g of cream (1/2 of the 5 g tube) over 20-25 cm of skin surface area, or 1 anesthetic disc (1 g over 10 cm^2) for at least 1 hour. **Note:** In clinical trials, 2 sites were usually prepared in case there was a technical problem with cannulation or venipuncture at the first site.
Major dermal procedures (eg, more painful dermatological procedures involving a larger skin area such as split thickness skin graft harvesting): Apply 2 g of cream per 10 cm^2 of skin and allow to remain in contact with the skin for at least 2 hours.
Adult male genital skin (eg, pretreatment prior to local anesthetic infiltration): Apply a thick layer of cream (1 g/10 cm^2) to the skin surface for 15 minutes. Local anesthetic infiltration should be performed immediately after removal of EMLA® cream.
Note: Dermal analgesia can be expected to increase for up to 3 hours under occlusive dressing and persist for 1-2 hours after removal of the cream
Adult females: Genital mucous membranes: Minor procedures (eg, removal of condylomata acuminata, pretreatment for local anesthetic infiltration): Apply 5-10 g (thick layer) of cream for 5-10 minutes

Patient Information Not for ophthalmic use; for external use only. EMLA® may block sensation in the treated skin.
(Continued)

Lidocaine and Prilocaine *(Continued)*

Nursing Implications In small infants and children, observe patient to prevent accidental ingestion of cream, disc, or dressing.

Dosage Forms

Cream: Lidocaine 2.5% and prilocaine 2.5% [2 Tegaderm® dressings] (5 g, 30 g)

Disc, anesthetic: 1 g (25 mg lidocaine and 25 mg prilocaine in each 10 square centimeter disc)

♦ **Lidocaine Hydrochloride** *see Lidocaine on page 801*

♦ **Lidodan™ (Can)** *see Lidocaine on page 801*

♦ **Lidoderm®** *see Lidocaine on page 801*

♦ **LidoPen® Auto-Injector** *see Lidocaine on page 801*

♦ **LID-Pack® (Can)** *see Bacitracin and Polymyxin B on page 143*

♦ **Lignocaine Hydrochloride** *see Lidocaine on page 801*

♦ **Limbitrol®** *see Amitriptyline and Chlordiazepoxide on page 78*

♦ **Limbitrol® DS** *see Amitriptyline and Chlordiazepoxide on page 78*

♦ **Lin-Amox (Can)** *see Amoxicillin on page 84*

♦ **Lin-Buspirone (Can)** *see BusPIRone on page 194*

Lindane *(LIN dane)*

U.S. Brand Names G-well®

Canadian Brand Names Hexit™; PMS-Lindane

Synonyms Benzene Hexachloride; Gamma Benzene Hexachloride; Hexachlorocyclohexane

Therapeutic Category Antiparasitic Agent, Topical; Pediculocide; Scabicidal Agent; Shampoos

Use Treatment of scabies (*Sarcoptes scabiei*), *Pediculus capitis* (head lice), and *Pediculus pubis* (crab lice); FDA recommends reserving lindane as a second-line agent or with inadequate response to other therapies

Pregnancy Risk Factor B

Pregnancy/Breast-Feeding Implications Clinical effects on the fetus: There are no well-controlled studies in pregnant women; treat no more than twice during a pregnancy

Contraindications Hypersensitivity to lindane or any component of the formulation; premature neonates; acutely inflamed skin or raw, weeping surfaces

Warnings/Precautions Not considered a drug of first choice; use with caution in infants and small children, and patients with a history of seizures; avoid contact with face, eyes, mucous membranes, and urethral meatus. Because of the potential for systemic absorption and CNS side effects, lindane should be used with caution; consider permethrin or crotamiton agent first.

Adverse Reactions <1% (Limited to important or life-threatening): Aplastic anemia, ataxia, burning and stinging, cardiac arrhythmia, contact dermatitis, dizziness, eczematous eruptions, headache, hematuria, hepatitis, nausea, pulmonary edema, restlessness, seizures, skin and adipose tissue may act as repositories, vomiting

Overdosage/Toxicology Symptoms include vomiting, restlessness, ataxia, seizures, arrhythmias, pulmonary edema, hematuria, and hepatitis. The drug is absorbed through skin, mucous membranes, and the GI tract. When used excessively for prolonged periods or when accidental ingestion has occurred, the drug has occasionally caused serious CNS, hepatic, and renal toxicity. If ingested, perform gastric lavage and general supportive measures. Diazepam 0.01 mg/kg can be used to control seizures.

Drug Interactions

Increased Effect/Toxicity: Oil-based hair dressing may increase potential for toxicity of lindane.

Mechanism of Action Directly absorbed by parasites and ova through the exoskeleton; stimulates the nervous system resulting in seizures and death of parasitic arthropods

Pharmacodynamics/Kinetics

Absorption: ≤13% systemically

Distribution: Stored in body fat; accumulates in brain; skin and adipose tissue may act as repositories

Metabolism: Hepatic

Half-life elimination: Children: 17-22 hours

Time to peak, serum: Children: 6 hours

Excretion: Urine and feces

Usual Dosage Children and Adults: Topical:

Scabies: Apply a thin layer of lotion and massage it on skin from the neck to the toes (head to toe in infants). For adults, bathe and remove the drug after 8-12 hours; for children, wash off 6-8 hours after application (for infants, wash off 6 hours after application); repeat treatment in 7 days if lice or nits are still present

Pediculosis, capitis and pubis: 15-30 mL of shampoo is applied and lathered for 4-5 minutes; rinse hair thoroughly and comb with a fine tooth comb to remove nits; repeat treatment in 7 days if lice or nits are still present

Administration Drug should not be administered orally, for topical use only; apply to dry, cool skin

Patient Information Topical use only, do not apply to face, avoid getting in eyes; do **not** apply lotion immediately after a hot, soapy bath. Clothing and bedding should be washed in hot water or by dry cleaning to kill the scabies mite. Combs and brushes may be washed with lindane shampoo then thoroughly rinsed with water. Notify physician if condition worsens; treat sexual contact simultaneously.

Nursing Implications Lindane lotion should be applied to dry, cool skin

Dosage Forms

Lotion, topical: 1% (60 mL, 473 mL, 4000 mL)

Shampoo, topical: 1% (60 mL, 473 mL, 4000 mL)

Linezolid (li NE zoh lid)

Related Information
Antimicrobial Drugs of Choice *on page 1588*
Community-Acquired Pneumonia in Adults *on page 1603*

U.S. Brand Names Zyvox™

Therapeutic Category Antibiotic, Oxazolidinone

Use Treatment of vancomycin-resistant *Enterococcus faecium* (VRE) infections, nosocomial pneumonia caused by *Staphylococcus aureus* including MRSA or *Streptococcus pneumoniae* (penicillin-susceptible strains only), complicated and uncomplicated skin and skin structure infections, and community-acquired pneumonia caused by susceptible gram-positive organisms.

Pregnancy Risk Factor C

Pregnancy/Breast-Feeding Implications Should be used in pregnancy only if the potential benefit justifies the risk to the fetus. It is unknown if excreted in human milk. Use cautiously if administered to a breast-feeding woman.

Contraindications Hypersensitivity to linezolid or any other component of the formulation

Warnings/Precautions Myelosuppression has been reported and may be dependent on duration of therapy (generally >2 weeks of treatment); use with caution in patients with pre-existing myelosuppression, in patients receiving other drugs which may cause bone marrow suppression, or in chronic infection (previous or concurrent antibiotic therapy). Weekly CBC monitoring is recommended. Discontinue linezolid in patients developing myelosuppression (or in whom myelosuppression worsens during treatment).

Linezolid has mild MAO inhibitor properties and has the potential to have the same interactions as other MAO inhibitors; use with caution in uncontrolled hypertension, pheochromocytoma, carcinoid syndrome, or untreated hyperthyroidism; avoid use with serotonergic agents such as TCAs, venlafaxine, trazodone, sibutramine, meperidine, dextromethorphan, and SSRIs; consider alternatives before initiating outpatient treatment (unnecessary use may lead the development of resistance to linezolid)

Adverse Reactions
1% to 10%:
Cardiovascular: Hypertension (1% to 3%)
Central nervous system: Headache (0.5% to 11%), insomnia (3%), dizziness (0.4% to 2%), fever (2%)
Dermatologic: Rash (2%)
Gastrointestinal: Nausea (3% to 10%), diarrhea (3% to 11%), vomiting (1% to 4%), constipation (2%), taste alteration (1% to 2%), tongue discoloration (0.2% to 1%), oral moniliasis (0.4% to 1%), pancreatitis
Genitourinary: Vaginal moniliasis (1% to 2%)
Hematologic: Thrombocytopenia (0.3% to 10%), anemia, leukopenia, neutropenia
Hepatic: Abnormal LFTs (0.4% to 1%)
Miscellaneous: Fungal infections (0.1% to 2%)
<1% (Limited to important or life-threatening): *C. difficile*-related complications, creatinine increased, dyspepsia, localized abdominal pain, pruritus. In addition to hematologic effects observed in trials, myelosuppression (including anemia, leukopenia, pancytopenia, and thrombocytopenia) has been reported, and may be more common in patients receiving linezolid for >2 weeks.

Overdosage/Toxicology Treatment is supportive. Hemodialysis may improve elimination (30% of a dose is removed during a 3-hour hemodialysis session).

Drug Interactions
Increased Effect/Toxicity: Linezolid is a reversible, nonselective inhibitor of MAO. Serotonergic agents (eg, TCAs, venlafaxine, trazodone, sibutramine, meperidine, dextromethorphan, and SSRIs) may cause a serotonin syndrome (eg, hyperpyrexia, cognitive dysfunction) when used concomitantly. Adrenergic agents (eg, phenylpropanolamine, pseudoephedrine, sympathomimetic agents, vasopressor or dopaminergic agents) may cause hypertension. Tramadol may increase the risk of seizures when used concurrently with linezolid. Myelosuppressive medications may increase risk of myelosuppression when used concurrently with linezolid.

Ethanol/Nutrition/Herb Interactions
Ethanol: Avoid ethanol (may contain tyramine, hypertensive crisis may result).
Food: Avoid foods (eg, cheese) and beverages containing tyramine in patients receiving linezolid (hypertensive crisis may result).

Stability Store at 25°C (77°F). Protect from light. Keep infusion bags in overwrap until ready for use. Protect infusion bags from freezing. Use reconstituted suspension within 21 days.

Mechanism of Action Inhibits bacterial protein synthesis by binding to bacterial 23S ribosomal RNA of the 50S subunit. This prevents the formation of a functional 70S initiation complex that is essential for the bacterial translation process. Linezolid is bacteriostatic against enterococci and staphylococci and bactericidal against most strains of streptococci.

Pharmacodynamics/Kinetics
Absorption: Rapid and extensive
Distribution: V_{dss}: 40-50 L
Protein binding: 31%
Metabolism: Hepatic via oxidation of the morpholine ring, resulting in two inactive metabolites (aminoethoxyacetic acid, hydroxyethyl glycine); does not involve CYP450 isoenzymes
Bioavailability: 100%
Half-life elimination: 4-5 hours
Time to peak: 1-2 hours
Excretion: Urine (30%); nonrenal (65%)

Usual Dosage Adults:
Oral, I.V.:
VRE infections: 600 mg every 12 hours for 14-28 days
Nosocomial pneumonia, complicated skin and skin structure infections, community-acquired pneumonia including concurrent bacteremia: 600 mg every 12 hours for 10-14 days
(Continued)

Linezolid (Continued)

Oral: Uncomplicated skin and skin structure infections: 400 mg every 12 hours for 10-14 days

Dosage adjustment in renal impairment: No specific adjustment recommended. The two primary metabolites may accumulate in patients with renal impairment but the clinical significance is unknown. Weigh the risk of accumulation of metabolites versus the benefit of therapy. Both linezolid and the two metabolites are eliminated by dialysis. Linezolid should be given after hemodialysis.

Dosage adjustment in hepatic impairment: No dosage adjustment required for mild to moderate hepatic insufficiency (Child-Pugh class A or B). Use in severe hepatic insufficiency has not been adequately evaluated.

Elderly: No dosage adjustment required

Dietary Considerations Take with or without food. Suspension contains 20 mg phenylalanine per teaspoonful.

Administration Administer intravenous infusion over 30-120 minutes. Do not mix or infuse with other medications. The yellow color of the injection may intensify over time without affecting potency.

Monitoring Parameters At least weekly CBC and platelet counts, particularly in patients at increased risk of bleeding, with pre-existing myelosuppression, on concomitant medications that cause bone marrow suppression, in those who require >2 weeks of therapy, or in those with chronic infection who have received previous or concomitant antibiotic therapy.

Patient Information Take with or without food. Take with food if medicine causes stomach upset. Tell your prescriber if you have hypertension or are taking any cold remedy or decongestant. Limit quantities of tyramine-containing foods. Gently mix suspension. Store at room temperature. Notify your prescriber if you feel very weak, have any bleeding problems, bruising, new signs/symptoms of infection, shortness of breath, rapid heartbeats, or weight loss.

Nursing Implications Administer intravenous infusion over 30-120 minutes. Do not mix or infuse with other medications. The yellow color of the injection may intensify over time without affecting potency.

Dosage Forms

Injection [premixed]: 200 mg (100 mL); 400 mg (200 mL); 600 mg (300 mL)

Suspension, oral: 20 mg/mL (150 mL) [orange flavor]

Tablet: 400 mg, 600 mg

♦ **Lin-Megestrol (Can)** see Megestrol on page 852

♦ **Lin-Pravastatin (Can)** see Pravastatin on page 1118

♦ **Lioresal®** see Baclofen on page 144

♦ **Liotec (Can)** see Baclofen on page 144

Liothyronine (lye oh THYE roe neen)

U.S. Brand Names Cytomel®; Triostat™

Canadian Brand Names Cytomel®

Synonyms Liothyronine Sodium; Sodium L-Triiodothyronine; T₃ Sodium

Therapeutic Category Thyroid Product

Use Replacement or supplemental therapy in hypothyroidism; management of nontoxic goiter, chronic lymphocytic thyroiditis, as an adjunct in thyrotoxicosis and as a diagnostic aid; **levothyroxine is recommended for chronic therapy;** although previously thought to benefit cardiac patients with severely reduced fractions, liothyronine injection is no longer considered beneficial

Orphan drug: Triostat™: Treatment of myxedema coma/precoma

Pregnancy Risk Factor A

Usual Dosage

Congenital hypothyroidism: Children: Oral: 5 mcg/day increase by 5 mcg every 3-4 days until the desired response is achieved. Usual maintenance dose: 20 mcg/day for infants, 50 mcg/day for children 1-3 years of age, and adult dose for children >3 years.

Hypothyroidism: Oral:

Adults: 25 mcg/day increase by increments of 12.5-25 mcg/day every 1-2 weeks to a maximum of 100 mcg/day; usual maintenance dose: 25-75 mcg/day

Elderly: Initial: 5 mcg/day, increase by 5 mcg/day every 1-2 weeks; usual maintenance dose: 25-75 mcg/day

T₃ suppression test: Oral: 75-100 mcg/day for 7 days; use lowest dose for elderly

Myxedema: Oral: Initial: 5 mcg/day; increase in increments of 5-10 mcg/day every 1-2 weeks. When 25 mcg/day is reached, dosage may be increased at intervals of 12.5-25 mcg/day every 1-2 weeks. Usual maintenance dose: 50-100 mcg/day.

Myxedema coma: I.V.: 25-50 mcg

Patients with known or suspected cardiovascular disease: 10-20 mcg

Note: Normally, at least 4 hours should be allowed between doses to adequately assess therapeutic response and no more than 12 hours should elapse between doses to avoid fluctuations in hormone levels. Oral therapy should be resumed as soon as the clinical situation has been stabilized and the patient is able to take oral medication. If levothyroxine rather than liothyronine sodium is used in initiating oral therapy, the physician should bear in mind that there is a delay of several days in the onset of levothyroxine activity and that I.V. therapy should be discontinued gradually.

Additional Information Complete prescribing information for this medication should be consulted for additional detail.

Dosage Forms

Injection, as sodium: 10 mcg/mL (1 mL)

Tablet, as sodium: 5 mcg, 25 mcg, 50 mcg

♦ **Liothyronine Sodium** see Liothyronine on page 808

Liotrix (LYE oh triks)

U.S. Brand Names Thyrolar®

Canadian Brand Names Thyrolar®

Synonyms T_3/T_4 Liotrix

Therapeutic Category Thyroid Product

Use Replacement or supplemental therapy in hypothyroidism (uniform mixture of T_4:T_3 in 4:1 ratio by weight); little advantage to this product exists and cost is not justified

Pregnancy Risk Factor A

Usual Dosage Oral:

Congenital hypothyroidism:

Children (dose of T_4 or levothyroxine/day):

0-6 months: 8-10 mcg/kg or 25-50 mcg/day

6-12 months: 6-8 mcg/kg or 50-75 mcg/day

1-5 years: 5-6 mcg/kg or 75-100 mcg/day

6-12 years: 4-5 mcg/kg or 100-150 mcg/day

>12 years: 2-3 mcg/kg or >150 mcg/day

Hypothyroidism (dose of thyroid equivalent):

Adults: 30 mg/day (15 mg/day if cardiovascular impairment), increasing by increments of 15 mg/day at 2- to 3-week intervals to a maximum of 180 mg/day (usual maintenance dose: 60-120 mg/day)

Elderly: Initial: 15 mg, adjust dose at 2- to 4-week intervals by increments of 15 mg

Additional Information Complete prescribing information for this medication should be consulted for additional detail.

Dosage Forms

Tablet (in mg of thyroid equivalent):

15 mg [levothyroxine sodium 12.5 mcg and liothyronine sodium 3.1 mcg]

30 mg [levothyroxine sodium 25 mcg and liothyronine sodium 6.25 mcg]

60 mg [levothyroxine sodium 50 mcg and liothyronine sodium 12.5 mcg]

120 mg [levothyroxine sodium 100 mcg and liothyronine sodium 25 mcg]

180 mg [levothyroxine sodium 150 mcg and liothyronine sodium 37.5 mcg]

- ◆ **Lipancreatin** see Pancrelipase on page 1034
- ◆ **Lipidil Micro® (Can)** see Fenofibrate on page 548
- ◆ **Lipidil Supra® (Can)** see Fenofibrate on page 548
- ◆ **Lipid-Lowering Agents** see page 1505
- ◆ **Lipitor®** see Atorvastatin on page 127
- ◆ **Liposyn®** see Fat Emulsion on page 545
- ◆ **Lipram®** see Pancrelipase on page 1034
- ◆ **Lipram® 4500** see Pancrelipase on page 1034
- ◆ **Lipram-CR®** see Pancrelipase on page 1034
- ◆ **Lipram-PN®** see Pancrelipase on page 1034
- ◆ **Lipram-UL®** see Pancrelipase on page 1034
- ◆ **Liquibid®** see Guaifenesin on page 645
- ◆ **Liqui-Char® [OTC]** see Charcoal on page 268
- ◆ **Liquid Antidote** see Charcoal on page 268
- ◆ **Liquid Pred®** see PredniSONE on page 1124
- ◆ **Liquiprin® for Children [OTC]** see Acetaminophen on page 22

Lisinopril (lyse IN oh pril)

Related Information

Angiotensin Agents Comparison on page 1473

Heart Failure on page 1663

U.S. Brand Names Prinivil®; Zestril®

Canadian Brand Names Apo®-Lisinopril; Prinivil®; Zestril®

Therapeutic Category Angiotensin-Converting Enzyme (ACE) Inhibitor; Antihypertensive Agent

Use Treatment of hypertension, either alone or in combination with other antihypertensive agents; adjunctive therapy in treatment of CHF (afterload reduction); treatment of hemodynamically stable patients within 24 hours of acute myocardial infarction, to improve survival; treatment of acute myocardial infarction within 24 hours in hemodynamically stable patients to improve survival; treatment of left ventricular dysfunction after myocardial infarction

Pregnancy Risk Factor C/D (2nd and 3rd trimesters)

Pregnancy/Breast-Feeding Implications

Clinical effects on the fetus: No data available on crossing the placenta. Cranial defects, hypocalvaria/acalvaria, oligohydramnios, persistent anuria following delivery, hypotension, renal defects, renal dysgenesis/dysplasia, renal failure, pulmonary hypoplasia, limb contractures secondary to oligohydramnios and stillbirth reported. ACE inhibitors should be avoided during pregnancy.

Breast-feeding/lactation: Crosses into breast milk; AAP considers **compatible** with breast-feeding.

Contraindications Hypersensitivity to lisinopril or any component of the formulation; angioedema related to previous treatment with an ACE inhibitor; bilateral renal artery stenosis; primary hyperaldosteronism; pregnancy (2nd and 3rd trimesters)

Warnings/Precautions Anaphylactic reactions can occur. Angioedema can occur at any time during treatment (especially following first dose). Careful blood pressure monitoring with first dose (hypotension can occur especially in volume depleted patients). Dosage adjustment needed in renal impairment. Use with caution in collagen vascular diseases; valvular stenosis (particularly aortic stenosis); hyperkalemia; or before, during, or immediately after anesthesia. Avoid rapid dosage escalation, which may lead to renal insufficiency. Neutropenia/agranulocytosis with myeloid hyperplasia can rarely occur. If patient has renal impairment then a baseline WBC with differential and serum creatinine should be evaluated and monitored closely during the first 3 months of therapy. Hypersensitivity reactions may be seen during hemodialysis with high-flux dialysis membranes (eg, AN69). Deterioration in renal (Continued)

Lisinopril *(Continued)*

function can occur with initiation. Use with caution in unilateral renal artery stenosis and pre-existing renal insufficiency.

Adverse Reactions Note: Frequency ranges include data from hypertension and heart failure trials. Higher rates of adverse reactions have generally been noted in patients with congestive heart failure. However, the frequency of adverse effects associated with placebo is also increased in this population.

1% to 10%:
    Cardiovascular: Orthostatic effects (1%), hypotension (1% to 4%)
    Central nervous system: Headache (4% to 6%), dizziness (5% to 12%), fatigue (3%), weakness (1%)
    Dermatologic: Rash (1% to 2%)
    Endocrine & metabolic: Hyperkalemia (2% to 5%)
    Gastrointestinal: Diarrhea (3% to 4%), nausea (2%), vomiting (1%), abdominal pain (2%)
    Genitourinary: Impotence (1%)
    Hematologic: Decreased hemoglobin (small)
    Neuromuscular & skeletal: Chest pain (3%)
    Renal: Increased serum creatinine (often transient), increased BUN (2%); deterioration in renal function (in patients with bilateral renal artery stenosis or hypovolemia)
    Respiratory: Cough (4% to 9%), upper respiratory infection (2% to 2%)
<1% (Limited to important or life-threatening): Acute renal failure, alopecia, anaphylactoid reactions, angioedema, anuria, arrhythmia, arthralgia, asthma, ataxia, azotemia, bone marrow suppression, bronchospasm, cardiac arrest, decreased libido, gout, hepatitis, hyperkalemia, hyponatremia, increased bilirubin, increased transaminases, infiltrates, jaundice (cholestatic), myocardial infarction, neutropenia, oliguria, orthostatic hypotension, pancreatitis, paresthesia, pemphigus, peripheral neuropathy, photosensitivity, pleural effusion, pulmonary embolism, Stevens-Johnson syndrome, stroke, systemic lupus erythematosus, thrombocytopenia, TIA, toxic epidermal necrolysis, tremor, urticaria, vasculitis, vertigo, vision loss. In addition, a syndrome which may include fever, myalgia, arthralgia, interstitial nephritis, vasculitis, rash, eosinophilia and positive ANA, and elevated ESR has been reported with ACE inhibitors.

Overdosage/Toxicology Mild hypotension has been the only toxic effect seen with acute overdose; bradycardia may also occur. Hyperkalemia occurs even with therapeutic doses, especially in patients with renal insufficiency and those taking NSAIDs. Following initiation of essential overdose management, toxic symptom and supportive treatment should be initiated. Hypotension usually responds to I.V. fluids or Trendelenburg positioning.

Drug Interactions
Increased Effect/Toxicity: Potassium supplements, co-trimoxazole (high dose), angiotensin II receptor antagonists (candesartan, losartan, irbesartan, etc), or potassium-sparing diuretics (amiloride, spironolactone, triamterene) may result in elevated serum potassium levels when combined with lisinopril. ACE inhibitor effects may be increased by phenothiazines or probenecid (increases levels of captopril). ACE inhibitors may increase serum concentrations/effects of digoxin, lithium, and sulfonylureas.

Diuretics have additive hypotensive effects with ACE inhibitors, and hypovolemia increases the potential for adverse renal effects of ACE inhibitors. In patients with compromised renal function, coadministration with nonsteroidal anti-inflammatory drugs may result in further deterioration of renal function. Allopurinol and ACE inhibitors may cause a higher risk of hypersensitivity reaction when taken concurrently.

Decreased Effect: Aspirin (high dose) may reduce the therapeutic effects of ACE inhibitors; at low dosages this does not appear to be significant. Rifampin may decrease the effect of ACE inhibitors. Antacids may decrease the bioavailability of ACE inhibitors (may be more likely to occur with captopril); separate administration times by 1-2 hours. NSAIDs, specifically indomethacin, may reduce the hypotensive effects of ACE inhibitors. More likely to occur in low renin or volume dependent hypertensive patients.

Ethanol/Nutrition/Herb Interactions Herb/Nutraceutical: Avoid dong quai if using for hypertension (has estrogenic activity). Avoid ephedra, yohimbe, ginseng (may worsen hypertension). Avoid garlic (may have increased antihypertensive effect).

Mechanism of Action Competitive inhibitor of angiotensin-converting enzyme (ACE); prevents conversion of angiotensin I to angiotensin II, a potent vasoconstrictor; results in lower levels of angiotensin II which causes an increase in plasma renin activity and a reduction in aldosterone secretion; a CNS mechanism may also be involved in hypotensive effect as angiotensin II increases adrenergic outflow from CNS; vasoactive kallikreins may be decreased in conversion to active hormones by ACE inhibitors, thus reducing blood pressure

Pharmacodynamics/Kinetics
    Onset of action: 1 hour
    Peak effect: Hypotensive: Oral: ~6 hours
    Duration: 24 hours
    Absorption: Well absorbed; unaffected by food
    Protein binding: 25%
    Half-life elimination: 11-12 hours
    Excretion: Primarily urine (as unchanged drug)

Usual Dosage
    Hypertension:
        Adults: Initial: 10 mg/day; increase doses 5-10 mg/day at 1- to 2-week intervals; maximum daily dose: 40 mg
        Elderly: Initial: 2.5-5 mg/day; increase doses 2.5-5 mg/day at 1- to 2-week intervals; maximum daily dose: 40 mg
        Patients taking diuretics should have them discontinued 2-3 days prior to initiating lisinopril if possible. Restart diuretic after blood pressure is stable if needed. If diuretic cannot be discontinued prior to therapy, begin with 5 mg with close supervision until stable blood pressure. In patients with hyponatremia (<130 mEq/L), start dose at 2.5 mg/day,
        Congestive heart failure: Adults: Oral: Initial: 5 mg; then increase by no more than 10 mg increments at intervals no less than 2 weeks to a maximum daily dose of 40 mg. Usual

maintenance: 5-40 mg/day as a single dose. Patients should start/continue standard therapy, including diuretics, beta-blockers, and digoxin, as indicated.

Acute myocardial infarction (within 24 hours in hemodynamically stable patients): Oral: 5 mg immediately, then 5 mg at 24 hours, 10 mg at 48 hours, and 10 mg every day thereafter for 6 weeks. Patients should continue to receive standard treatments such as thrombolytics, aspirin, and beta-blockers.

Dosing adjustment in renal impairment:
Cl$_{cr}$ 10-50 mL/minute: Administer 50% to 75% of normal dose.
Cl$_{cr}$ <10 mL/minute: Administer 25% to 50% of normal dose.
Hemodialysis: Dialyzable (50%)

Administration Watch for hypotensive effects within 1-3 hours of first dose or new higher dose.

Monitoring Parameters Serum calcium levels, BUN, serum creatinine, renal function, WBC, and potassium

Test Interactions May cause false-positive results in urine acetone determinations using sodium nitroprusside reagent; ↑ potassium (S); ↑ serum creatinine/BUN

Patient Information Notify physician if vomiting, diarrhea, excessive perspiration, or dehydration should occur; also if swelling of face, lips, tongue or difficulty in breathing occurs or if persistent cough develops; do not stop therapy without the advise of the prescriber; do not add a salt substitute (potassium) without physician advice

Nursing Implications May cause depression in some patients; discontinue if angioedema of the face, extremities, lips, tongue, or glottis occurs; watch for hypotensive effects within 1-3 hours of first dose or new higher dose

Dosage Forms Tablet: 2.5 mg, 5 mg, 10 mg, 20 mg, 30 mg, 40 mg

Lisinopril and Hydrochlorothiazide
(lyse IN oh pril & hye droe klor oh THYE a zide)

U.S. Brand Names Prinzide®; Zestoretic®
Canadian Brand Names Prinzide®; Zestoretic®
Synonyms Hydrochlorothiazide and Lisinopril
Therapeutic Category Angiotensin-Converting Enzyme (ACE) Inhibitor Combination; Antihypertensive Agent, Combination
Use Treatment of hypertension
Pregnancy Risk Factor C/D (2nd and 3rd trimesters)
Usual Dosage Adults: Oral: Dosage is individualized; see each component for appropriate dosing suggestions; doses >80 mg/day lisinopril or >50 mg/day hydrochlorothiazide are not recommended.
Additional Information Complete prescribing information for this medication should be consulted for additional detail.
Dosage Forms
Tablet:
Lisinopril 10 mg and hydrochlorothiazide 12.5 mg
Lisinopril 20 mg and hydrochlorothiazide 12.5 mg
Lisinopril 20 mg and hydrochlorothiazide 25 mg

♦ Lithane™ (Can) see Lithium on page 811

Lithium (LITH ee um)
Related Information
Antacid Drug Interactions on page 1477
U.S. Brand Names Eskalith®; Eskalith CR®; Lithobid®
Canadian Brand Names Carbolith™; Duralith®; Lithane™; PMS-Lithium Carbonate; PMS-Lithium Citrate
Synonyms Lithium Carbonate; Lithium Citrate
Therapeutic Category Antidepressant, Miscellaneous; Antimanic Agent
Use Management of bipolar disorders
Unlabeled/Investigational Use Potential augmenting agent for antidepressants; aggression, post-traumatic stress disorder, conduct disorder in children
Pregnancy Risk Factor D
Contraindications Hypersensitivity to lithium or any component of the formulation; severe cardiovascular or renal disease; severe debilitation, dehydration, or sodium depletion; pregnancy
Warnings/Precautions Lithium toxicity is closely related to serum levels and can occur at therapeutic doses; serum lithium determinations are required to monitor therapy. Use caution in patients with suicidal risk. Use with caution in patients with cardiovascular or thyroid disease, or in patients receiving medications which alter sodium excretion (eg, diuretics, ACE inhibitors, NSAIDs). Some elderly patients may be extremely sensitive to the effects of lithium, see Usual Dosage and Reference Range. Chronic therapy results in diminished renal concentrating ability (nephrogenic DI). Changes in renal function should be monitored, and re-evaluation of treatment may be necessary.

Use with caution in patients receiving neuroleptic medications - a syndrome resembling NMS has been associated with concurrent therapy. Lithium may impair the patient's alertness, affecting the ability to operate machinery or driving a vehicle. Neuromuscular blocking agents should be administered with caution - the response may be prolonged.

Higher serum concentrations may be required and tolerated during an acute manic phase; however, the tolerance decreases when symptoms subside. Normal fluid and salt intake must be maintained during therapy.

Adverse Reactions Frequency not defined.
Cardiovascular: Cardiac arrhythmias, hypotension, sinus node dysfunction, flattened or inverted T waves (reversible), edema
Central nervous system: Dizziness, vertigo, slurred speech, blackout spells, seizures, sedation, restlessness, confusion, psychomotor retardation, stupor, coma, dystonia, fatigue, lethargy, headache, pseudotumor cerebri
(Continued)

Lithium *(Continued)*

Dermatologic: Dry or thinning of hair, folliculitis, alopecia, exacerbation of psoriasis, rash

Endocrine & metabolic: Euthyroid goiter and/or hypothyroidism, hyperthyroidism, hyperglycemia, diabetes insipidus

Gastrointestinal: Polydipsia, anorexia, nausea, vomiting, diarrhea, xerostomia, metallic taste, weight gain

Genitourinary: Incontinence, polyuria, glycosuria, oliguria, albuminuria

Hematologic: Leukocytosis

Neuromuscular & skeletal: Tremor, muscle hyperirritability, ataxia, choreoathetoid movements, hyperactive deep tendon reflexes

Ocular: Nystagmus, blurred vision

Miscellaneous: Discoloration of fingers and toes

Overdosage/Toxicology Symptoms include sedation, confusion, tremors, joint pain, visual changes, seizures, and coma. There is no specific antidote for lithium poisoning. For acute ingestion, following initiation of essential overdose management, correction of fluid and electrolyte imbalance should be commenced. Hemodialysis and whole bowel irrigation are the treatments of choice for severe intoxications. Charcoal is ineffective.

Drug Interactions

Increased Effect/Toxicity: Concurrent use of lithium with carbamazepine, diltiazem, SSRIs (fluoxetine, fluvoxamine), haloperidol, methyldopa, metronidazole (rare), phenothiazines, phenytoin, TCAs, and verapamil may increase the risk for neurotoxicity. Lithium concentrations/toxicity may be increased by diuretics, NSAIDs (sulindac and aspirin may be exceptions), ACE inhibitors, angiotensin receptor antagonists (losartan), or tetracyclines.

Lithium and MAO inhibitors should generally be avoided due to use reports of fatal malignant hyperpyrexia; risk with selective MAO type B inhibitors (selegiline) appears to be lower. Potassium iodide may enhance the hypothyroid effects of lithium. Combined use of lithium with tricyclic antidepressants or sibutramine may increase the risk of serotonin syndrome; this combination is best avoided. Lithium may potentiate effect of neuromuscular blockers.

Decreased Effect: Combined use of lithium and chlorpromazine may lower serum concentrations of both drugs. Sodium bicarbonate and high sodium intake may reduce serum lithium concentrations via enhanced excretion. Lithium may blunt the pressor response to sympathomimetics (epinephrine, norepinephrine).

Ethanol/Nutrition/Herb Interactions Food: Lithium serum concentrations may be increased if taken with food. Limit caffeine.

Mechanism of Action Alters cation transport across cell membrane in nerve and muscle cells and influences reuptake of serotonin and/or norepinephrine; second messenger systems involving the phosphatidylinositol cycle are inhibited; postsynaptic D2 receptor supersensitivity is inhibited

Pharmacodynamics/Kinetics

Distribution: V_d: Initial: 0.3-0.4 L/kg; V_{dss}: 0.7-1 L/kg; crosses placenta; enters breast milk at 35% to 50% the concentrations in serum

Half-life elimination: 18-24 hours; can increase to more than 36 hours in elderly or with renal impairment

Time to peak, serum (nonsustained release product): ~0.5-2 hours

Excretion: Urine (90% to 98% as unchanged drug); feces (1%); sweat (4% to 5%)

Usual Dosage Oral: Monitor serum concentrations and clinical response (efficacy and toxicity) to determine proper dose

Children 6-12 years:

Bipolar disorder: 15-60 mg/kg/day in 3-4 divided doses; dose not to exceed usual adult dosage

Conduct disorder (unlabeled use): 15-30 mg/kg/day in 3-4 divided doses; dose not to exceed usual adult dosage

Adults: Bipolar disorder: 900-2400 mg/day in 3-4 divided doses or 900-1800 mg/day (sustained release) in 2 divided doses

Elderly: Bipolar disorder: Initial dose: 300 mg once or twice daily; increase weekly in increments of 300 mg/day, monitoring levels; rarely need >900-1200 mg/day

Dosing adjustment in renal impairment:

Cl_{cr} 10-50 mL/minute: Administer 50% to 75% of normal dose

Cl_{cr} <10 mL/minute: Administer 25% to 50% of normal dose

Hemodialysis: Dialyzable (50% to 100%)

Dietary Considerations May be taken with meals to avoid GI upset; have patient drink 2-3 L of water daily.

Administration Administer with meals to decrease GI upset

Monitoring Parameters Serum lithium every 4-5 days during initial therapy; draw lithium serum concentrations 12 hours postdose; renal, thyroid, and cardiovascular function; fluid status; serum electrolytes; CBC with differential, urinalysis; monitor for signs of toxicity; b-HCG pregnancy test for all females not known to be sterile

Reference Range Levels should be obtained twice weekly until both patient's clinical status and levels are stable then levels may be obtained every 1-2 months

Timing of serum samples: Draw trough just before next dose

Therapeutic levels:

Acute mania: 0.6-1.2 mEq/L (SI: 0.6-1.2 mmol/L)

Protection against future episodes in most patients with bipolar disorder: 0.8-1 mEq/L (SI: 0.8-1.0 mmol/L); a higher rate of relapse is described in subjects who are maintained at <0.4 mEq/L (SI: 0.4 mmol/L)

Elderly patients can usually be maintained at lower end of therapeutic range (0.6-0.8 mEq/L)

Toxic concentration: >2 mEq/L (SI: >2 mmol/L)

Adverse effect levels:

GI complaints/tremor: 1.5-2 mEq/L

Confusion/somnolence: 2-2.5 mEq/L

Seizures/death: >2.5 mEq/L
Patient Information Avoid tasks requiring psychomotor coordination until the CNS effects are known, blood level monitoring is required to determine the proper dose; maintain a steady salt and fluid intake especially during the summer months; do not crush or chew slow or extended release dosage form, swallow whole
Nursing Implications Avoid dehydration
Dosage Forms
    Capsule, as carbonate: 150 mg, 300 mg, 600 mg
    Syrup, as citrate: 300 mg/5 mL (5 mL, 10 mL, 480 mL)
    Tablet, as carbonate: 300 mg
    Tablet, controlled release, as carbonate: 450 mg
    Tablet, extended release, as carbonate: 300 mg

- **Lithium Carbonate** *see Lithium on page 811*
- **Lithium Citrate** *see Lithium on page 811*
- **Lithobid®** *see Lithium on page 811*
- **Livostin®** *see Levocabastine on page 788*
- **LMD®** *see Dextran on page 386*
- **LNg 20** *see Levonorgestrel on page 796*
- **LoCHOLEST®** *see Cholestyramine Resin on page 286*
- **LoCHOLEST® Light** *see Cholestyramine Resin on page 286*
- **Locoid®** *see Hydrocortisone on page 682*
- **Lodine®** *see Etodolac on page 532*
- **Lodine® XL** *see Etodolac on page 532*
- **Lodosyn®** *see Carbidopa on page 225*

Lodoxamide (loe DOKS a mide)
U.S. Brand Names Alomide®
Canadian Brand Names Alomide®
Synonyms Lodoxamide Tromethamine
Therapeutic Category Antiallergic, Ophthalmic
Use Treatment of vernal keratoconjunctivitis, vernal conjunctivitis, and vernal keratitis
Pregnancy Risk Factor B
Usual Dosage Children ≥2 years and Adults: Instill 1-2 drops in eye(s) 4 times/day for up to 3 months
Additional Information Complete prescribing information for this medication should be consulted for additional detail.
Dosage Forms Solution, ophthalmic: 0.1% (10 mL)

- **Lodoxamide Tromethamine** *see Lodoxamide on page 813*
- **Loestrin®** *see Ethinyl Estradiol and Norethindrone on page 522*
- **Loestrin™ 1.5.30 (Can)** *see Ethinyl Estradiol and Norethindrone on page 522*
- **Loestrin® Fe** *see Ethinyl Estradiol and Norethindrone on page 522*

Lomefloxacin (loe me FLOKS a sin)
Related Information
    Antacid Drug Interactions *on page 1477*
    Treatment of Sexually Transmitted Diseases *on page 1609*
U.S. Brand Names Maxaquin®
Synonyms Lomefloxacin Hydrochloride
Therapeutic Category Antibiotic, Quinolone
Use Lower respiratory infections, acute bacterial exacerbation of chronic bronchitis, and urinary tract infections caused by *E. coli, K. pneumoniae, P. mirabilis, P. aeruginosa*; also has gram-positive activity including *S. pneumoniae* and some staphylococci; surgical prophylaxis (transrectal prostate biopsy or transurethral procedures)
Unlabeled/Investigational Use Skin infections, sexually-transmitted diseases
Pregnancy Risk Factor C
Contraindications Hypersensitivity to lomefloxacin, any component of the formulation, or other members of the quinolone group (such as, nalidixic acid, oxolinic acid, cinoxacin, norfloxacin, and ciprofloxacin); avoid use in children <18 years of age due to association of other quinolones with transient arthropathies
Warnings/Precautions

Not recommended in children <18 years of age; CNS stimulation may occur (tremor, restlessness, confusion, and very rarely hallucinations or seizures); use with caution in patients with known or suspected CNS disorders or renal dysfunction; use caution to avoid possible photosensitivity reactions during and for several days following fluoroquinolone therapy

Severe hypersensitivity reactions, including anaphylaxis, have occurred with quinolone therapy. If an allergic reaction occurs (itching, urticaria, dyspnea or facial edema, loss of consciousness, tingling, cardiovascular collapse), discontinue drug immediately. Prolonged use may result in superinfection; pseudomembranous colitis may occur and should be considered in all patients who present with diarrhea. Tendon inflammation and/or rupture has been reported; discontinue at first sign of tendon inflammation or pain. Quinolones may exacerbate myasthenia gravis, use with caution (rare, potentially life-threatening weakness of respiratory muscles may occur).
Adverse Reactions
  1% to 10%:
    Central nervous system: Headache (3%), dizziness (2%)
    Dermatologic: Photosensitivity (2%)
    Gastrointestinal: Nausea (4%)
  <1% (Limited to important or life-threatening): Abdominal pain, abnormal taste, allergic reaction, angina pectoris, anuria, arrhythmia, back pain, bradycardia, cardiac failure, chest pain, chills, coma, constipation, convulsions, cough, cyanosis, decreased heat tolerance,
(Continued)

Lomefloxacin *(Continued)*

diaphoresis (increased), discoloration of tongue, dyspnea, dysuria, earache, edema, epistaxis, extrasystoles, facial edema, fatigue, flatulence, flu-like symptoms, flushing, gout, hematuria, hyperkinesia, hypertension, hypoglycemia, hypotension, increased fibrinolysis, leg cramps, malaise, myalgia, myocardial infarction; paresthesia, purpura, rash, syncope, tachycardia, thirst, thrombocytopenia, tremor, urinary disorders, vertigo, vomiting, weakness, xerostomia; quinolones have been associated with tendon rupture and tendonitis

Overdosage/Toxicology Symptoms include acute renal failure and seizures. Treatment consists of GI decontamination and supportive care. Administer diazepam for the treatment of seizures. Not removed by peritoneal or hemodialysis.

Drug Interactions

Cytochrome P450 Effect: CYP1A2 enzyme inhibitor (minor)

Increased Effect/Toxicity: Quinolones can cause elevated levels of caffeine, warfarin, cyclosporine, and theophylline. Azlocillin, imipenem, cimetidine, loop diuretics, and probenecid may increase lomefloxacin serum levels. Increased CNS stimulation may occur with caffeine, theophylline, NSAIDs. Foscarnet has been associated with seizures in patients receiving quinolones.

Decreased Effect: Decreased absorption with antacids containing aluminum, magnesium, and/or calcium (by up to 98% if given at the same time). Antineoplastic agents may decrease quinolone absorption.

Ethanol/Nutrition/Herb Interactions

Food: Lomefloxacin peak serum levels may be prolonged if taken with food.

Herb/Nutraceutical: Avoid dong quai, St John's wort (may cause photosensitization).

Mechanism of Action Inhibits DNA-gyrase in susceptible organisms thereby inhibits relaxation of supercoiled DNA and promotes breakage of DNA strands. DNA gyrase (topoisomerase II), is an essential bacterial enzyme that maintains the superhelical structure of DNA and is required for DNA replication and transcription, DNA repair, recombination, and transposition.

Pharmacodynamics/Kinetics

Absorption: Well absorbed

Distribution: V_d: 2.4-3.5 L/kg; into bronchus, prostatic tissue, and urine

Protein binding: 20%

Half-life elimination: 5-7.5 hours

Excretion: Primarily urine (as unchanged drug)

Usual Dosage Adults:

Lower respiratory and urinary tract infections (UTI): 400 mg once daily for 10-14 days

Urinary tract infection (UTI) due to susceptible organisms:

Females:

Uncomplicated cystitis caused by *Escherichia coli*: 400 mg once daily for 3 successive days

Uncomplicated cystitis caused by *Klebsiella pneumoniae*, *Proteus mirabilis*, or *Staphylococcus saprophyticus*: 400 mg once daily for 10 successive days

Complicated UTI caused by *Escherichia coli*, *Klebsiella pneumoniae*, *Proteus mirabilis*, or *Pseudomonas aeruginosa*: 400 mg once daily for 14 successive days

Surgical prophylaxis: 400 mg 2-6 hours before surgery

Uncomplicated gonorrhea: 400 mg as a single dose

Elderly: No dosage adjustment is needed for elderly patients with normal renal function

Dosing adjustment in renal impairment:

Cl_{cr} 11-39 mL/minute: Loading dose: 400 mg, then 200 mg every day

Hemodialysis: Same as above

Dietary Considerations May be taken without regard to meals.

Nursing Implications Monitor signs and symptoms of infection, urinalysis, appropriate cultures, and sensitivities; patients receiving warfarin concurrent therapy should have protimes/INR monitored

Dosage Forms Tablet, as hydrochloride: 400 mg

♦ **Lomefloxacin Hydrochloride** *see* Lomefloxacin *on page 813*

♦ **Lomine (Can)** *see* Dicyclomine *on page 397*

♦ **Lomocot**® *see* Diphenoxylate and Atropine *on page 416*

♦ **Lomotil**® *see* Diphenoxylate and Atropine *on page 416*

Lomustine *(loe MUS teen)*

U.S. Brand Names CeeNU®

Canadian Brand Names CeeNU®

Synonyms CCNU

Therapeutic Category Antineoplastic Agent, Alkylating Agent (Nitrosourea)

Use Treatment of brain tumors and Hodgkin's disease, non-Hodgkin's lymphoma, melanoma, renal carcinoma, lung cancer, colon cancer

Pregnancy Risk Factor D

Pregnancy/Breast-Feeding Implications May cause fetal harm when administered to a pregnant woman. Women of childbearing potential should be advised to avoid pregnancy and should be advised of the potential harm to the fetus.

Contraindications Hypersensitivity to lomustine, any component of the formulation, or other nitrosoureas; pregnancy

Warnings/Precautions The U.S. Food and Drug Administration (FDA) currently recommends that procedures for proper handling and disposal of antineoplastic agents are considered. Bone marrow suppression, notably thrombocytopenia and leukopenia, may lead to bleeding and overwhelming infections in an already compromised patient; will last for at least 6 weeks after a dose, do not administer courses more frequently than every 6 weeks because the toxicity is cumulative. Use with caution in patients with depressed platelet, leukocyte or erythrocyte counts, renal or hepatic impairment.

Adverse Reactions

>10%:

Gastrointestinal: Nausea, vomiting

Emetic potential:

<60 mg: Moderately high (60% to 90%)

≥60 mg: High (>90%)

Time course of nausea/vomiting: Onset: 2-6 hours; Duration: 4-6 hours

Hematologic: Leukopenia; Thrombocytopenia; Myelosuppression: Anemia; effects occur 4-6 weeks after a dose and may persist for 1-2 weeks

WBC: Moderate

Platelets: Severe

Onset (days): 14

Nadir (weeks): 4-5

Recovery (weeks): 6

1% to 10%:

Central nervous system: Neurotoxicity

Dermatologic: Skin rash, alopecia

Gastrointestinal: Stomatitis, diarrhea

Hematologic: Anemia

Renal: Renal failure

<1% (Limited to important or life-threatening): Hepatotoxicity, pulmonary fibrosis with cumulative doses >600 mg

Overdosage/Toxicology Symptoms include nausea, vomiting, and leukopenia. There are no known antidotes. Treatment is primarily symptomatic and supportive.

Drug Interactions

Cytochrome P450 Effect: CYP2D6 enzyme inhibitor

Increased Effect/Toxicity: Increased toxicity with cimetidine, reported to cause bone marrow depression or to potentiate the myelosuppressive effects of lomustine.

Decreased Effect: Decreased effect with phenobarbital, resulting in reduced efficacy of both drugs.

Ethanol/Nutrition/Herb Interactions Ethanol: Avoid ethanol (due to GI irritation).

Stability Refrigerate (<40°C/<104°F)

Mechanism of Action Inhibits DNA and RNA synthesis via carbamylation of DNA polymerase, alkylation of DNA, and alteration of RNA, proteins, and enzymes

Pharmacodynamics/Kinetics

Duration: Marrow recovery: ≤6 weeks

Absorption: Complete; appears in plasma within 3 minutes after administration

Distribution: Crosses blood-brain barrier to a greater degree than BCNU; CNS concentrations are equal to that of plasma

Protein binding: 50%

Metabolism: Rapidly hepatic via hydroxylation producing at least two active metabolites; enterohepatically recycled

Half-life elimination: Parent drug: 16-72 hours; Active metabolite: Terminal: 1.3-2 days

Time to peak, serum: Active metabolite: ~3 hours

Excretion: Urine; feces (<5%); expired air (<10%)

Usual Dosage Oral (refer to individual protocols):

Children: 75-150 mg/m^2 as a single dose every 6 weeks; subsequent doses are readjusted after initial treatment according to platelet and leukocyte counts

Adults: 100-130 mg/m^2 as a single dose every 6 weeks; readjust after initial treatment according to platelet and leukocyte counts

With compromised marrow function: Initial dose: 100 mg/m^2 as a single dose every 6 weeks

Repeat courses should only be administered after adequate recovery: WBC >4000 and platelet counts >100,000

Subsequent dosing adjustment based on nadir:

Leukocytes 2000-2900/mm^3, platelets 25,000-74,999/mm^3: Administer 70% of prior dose

Leukocytes <2000/mm^3, platelets <25,000/mm^3: Administer 50% of prior dose

Dosage adjustment in renal impairment:

Cl$_{cr}$ 10-50 mL/minute: Administer 75% of normal dose

Cl$_{cr}$ <10 mL/minute: Administer 50% of normal dose

Hemodialysis: Supplemental dose is not necessary

Peritoneal dialysis: Significant drug removal is unlikely based on physiochemical characteristics

Dietary Considerations Should be taken with fluids on an empty stomach; no food or drink for 2 hours after administration to decrease nausea.

Monitoring Parameters CBC with differential and platelet count, hepatic and renal function tests, pulmonary function tests

Test Interactions Liver function tests

Patient Information Take with fluids on an empty stomach; do not eat or drink for 2 hours following administration. Do not use alcohol, aspirin, or aspirin-containing medications and/or OTC medications without consulting prescriber. Maintain adequate fluid balance (2-3 L/day of fluids unless instructed to restrict fluid intake). May cause hair loss (reversible); easy bleeding or bruising (use soft toothbrush or cotton swabs and frequent mouth care, use electric razor, avoid sharp knives or scissors); increased susceptibility to infection (avoid crowds or exposure to infection - do not have any vaccinations unless approved by prescriber). Report unusual bleeding or bruising or persistent fever or sore throat; blood in urine, stool, or vomitus; delayed healing of any wounds; skin rash; yellowing of skin or eyes; changes in color of urine of stool. Contraceptive measures are recommended during therapy.

Dosage Forms

Capsule: 10 mg, 40 mg, 100 mg

Dose pack: 10 mg (2s); 40 mg (2s); 100 mg (2s)

♦ **Loniten**® see Minoxidil on page 919

♦ **Lonox**® see Diphenoxylate and Atropine on page 416

♦ **Lo/Ovral®** *see Ethinyl Estradiol and Norgestrel on page 528*

♦ **Loperacap (Can)** *see Loperamide on page 816*

Loperamide *(loe PER a mide)*

U.S. Brand Names Diar-Aid® [OTC]; Imodium®; Imodium® A-D [OTC]; Kaopectate® II [OTC]; Pepto® Diarrhea Control [OTC]

Canadian Brand Names Apo®-Loperamide; Diarr-Eze; Imodium®; Loperacap; Novo-Loperamide; PMS-Loperamine; Rho®-Loperamine; Riva-Loperamine

Synonyms Loperamide Hydrochloride

Therapeutic Category Antidiarrheal

Use Treatment of acute diarrhea and chronic diarrhea associated with inflammatory bowel disease; chronic functional diarrhea (idiopathic), chronic diarrhea caused by bowel resection or organic lesions; to decrease the volume of ileostomy discharge

Unlabeled/Investigational Use Treatment of traveler's diarrhea in combination with trimethoprim-sulfamethoxazole (co-trimoxazole) (3-day therapy)

Pregnancy Risk Factor B

Contraindications Hypersensitivity to loperamide or any component of the formulation; bloody diarrhea; patients who must avoid constipation; diarrhea resulting from some infections; pseudomembranous colitis

Warnings/Precautions Large first-pass metabolism, use with caution in hepatic dysfunction; should not be used if diarrhea accompanied by high fever, blood in stool

Adverse Reactions Frequency not defined.
Cardiovascular: Shock
Central nervous system: Dizziness, drowsiness, fatigue, sedation
Dermatologic: Rash, toxic epidermal necrolysis
Gastrointestinal: Abdominal cramping, abdominal distention, constipation, dry mouth, nausea, paralytic ileus, vomiting
Miscellaneous: Anaphylaxis

Overdosage/Toxicology Symptoms include CNS and respiratory depression, gastrointestinal cramping, constipation, GI irritation, nausea, and vomiting. Overdosage is noted when daily doses approximate 60 mg of loperamide. Treatment includes gastric lavage followed by 100 g of activated charcoal through a nasogastric tube. Monitor for signs of CNS depression; if they occur, administer naloxone 2 mg I.V. (0.01 mg/kg for children), with repeat administration as necessary, up to a total of 10 mg.

Drug Interactions
Increased Effect/Toxicity: Loperamide may potentiate the adverse effects of CNS depressants, phenothiazines, tricyclic antidepressants.

Mechanism of Action Acts directly on intestinal muscles to inhibit peristalsis and prolongs transit time enhancing fluid and electrolyte movement through intestinal mucosa; reduces fecal volume, increases viscosity, and diminishes fluid and electrolyte loss; demonstrates antisecretory activity; exhibits peripheral action

Pharmacodynamics/Kinetics
Onset of action: 0.5-1 hour
Absorption: <40%
Distribution: Low amounts enter breast milk
Protein binding: 97%
Metabolism: Hepatic (>50%) to inactive compounds
Half-life elimination: 7-14 hours
Excretion: Urine and feces (1% as metabolites, 30% to 40% as unchanged drug)

Usual Dosage Oral:
Children:
Acute diarrhea: Initial doses (in first 24 hours):
2-6 years: 1 mg 3 times/day
6-8 years: 2 mg twice daily
8-12 years: 2 mg 3 times/day
Maintenance: After initial dosing, 0.1 mg/kg doses after each loose stool, but not exceeding initial dosage
Chronic diarrhea: 0.08-0.24 mg/kg/day divided 2-3 times/day, maximum: 2 mg/dose
Adults:
Acute diarrhea: Initial: 4 mg (2 capsules), followed by 2 mg after each loose stool, up to 16 mg/day (8 capsules)
Chronic diarrhea: Initial: Follow acute diarrhea; maintenance dose should be slowly titrated downward to minimum required to control symptoms (typically, 4-8 mg/day in divided doses)
Traveler's diarrhea: Treat for no more than 2 days
6-8 years: 1 mg after first loose stool followed by 1 mg after each subsequent stool; maximum dose: 4 mg/day
9-11 years: 2 mg after first loose stool followed by 1 mg after each subsequent stool; maximum dose: 6 mg/day
12 years to Adults: 4 mg after first loose stool followed by 2 mg after each subsequent stool; maximum dose: 8 mg/day

Patient Information Do not take more than 8 capsules or 80 mL in 24 hours; may cause drowsiness; if acute diarrhea lasts longer than 48 hours, consult physician

Nursing Implications Therapy for chronic diarrhea should not exceed 10 days

Dosage Forms
Caplet, as hydrochloride: 2 mg
Capsule, as hydrochloride: 2 mg
Liquid, oral, as hydrochloride: 1 mg/5 mL (60 mL, 90 mL, 120 mL)
Tablet, as hydrochloride: 2 mg

♦ **Loperamide Hydrochloride** *see Loperamide on page 816*

♦ **Lopid®** *see Gemfibrozil on page 624*

♦ **Lopinavir** *see Lopinavir and Ritonavir on page 817*

Lopinavir and Ritonavir (loe PIN a veer & rit ON uh veer)

Related Information

Antiretroviral Agents Comparison *on page 1488*

Antiretroviral Therapy for HIV Infection *on page 1595*

Management of Healthcare Worker Exposures to HIV, HBV, HCV *on page 1555*

U.S. Brand Names Kaletra™

Synonyms Lopinavir

Therapeutic Category Antiretroviral Agent, Protease Inhibitor; Antiretroviral Agent, Reverse Transcriptase Inhibitor (Combination)

Use Treatment of HIV infection in combination with other antiretroviral agents

Pregnancy Risk Factor C

Pregnancy/Breast-Feeding Implications It is not known if lopinavir crosses the placenta; transfer of ritonavir is minimal based on preliminary data. Pregnancy and protease inhibitors are both associated with an increased risk of hyperglycemia. Glucose levels should be closely monitored. Health professionals are encouraged to contact the antiretroviral pregnancy registry to monitor outcomes of pregnant women exposed to antiretroviral medications (1-800-258-4263).

Contraindications Hypersensitivity to lopinavir, ritonavir, or any component of the formulation; administration with medications highly dependent upon CYP3A or CYP2D6 for clearance for which increased levels are associated with serious and/or life-threatening events. Ritonavir is contraindicated with astemizole, cisapride, dihydroergotamine, ergonovine, ergotamine, flecainide, lovastatin, methylergonovine, midazolam, pimozide, propafenone, simvastatin, terfenadine, triazolam.

Warnings/Precautions Cases of pancreatitis, some fatal, have been associated with lopinavir/ritonavir; use caution in patients with a history of pancreatitis. Patients with signs or symptoms of pancreatitis should be evaluated and therapy suspended as clinically appropriate. Diabetes mellitus and exacerbation of diabetes mellitus have been reported in patients taking protease inhibitors. Use caution in patients with hepatic impairment; patients with hepatitis or elevations in transaminases prior to the start of therapy may be at increased risk for further increases in transaminases. Large increases in total cholesterol and triglycerides have been reported; screening should be done prior to therapy and periodically throughout treatment. Avoid concurrent use of St John's wort (may lead to loss of virologic response and/or resistance). Hemophilia type A and type B have been reported with protease inhibitor use. Redistribution or accumulation of body fat has been observed in patients using antiretroviral therapy. The potential for cross-resistance with other protease inhibitors is currently under study. Safety and efficacy have not been established for children <6 months of age.

Adverse Reactions Protease inhibitors cause dyslipidemia which includes elevated cholesterol and triglycerides and a redistribution of body fat centrally to cause "protease paunch," buffalo hump, facial atrophy, and breast enlargement. These agents also cause hyperglycemia.

>10%:
  Endocrine & metabolic: Hypercholesterolemia (9% to 28%), triglycerides increased (9% to 28%)
  Gastrointestinal: Diarrhea (16% to 24%), nausea (3% to 15%)
  Hepatic: GGT increased (4% to 25%)

2% to 10%:
  Central nervous system: Headache (2% to 7%), pain (0% to 2%), insomnia (1% to 2%)
  Dermatologic: Rash (1% to 4%)
  Endocrine & metabolic: Hyperglycemia (1% to 4%), hyperuricemia (up to 4%), sodium decreased (3% children), organic phosphorus decreased (up to 2%), amylase increased (2% to 10%)
  Gastrointestinal: Abnormal stools (up to 6%), abdominal pain (2% to 4%), vomiting (2% to 5%), dyspepsia (0.5% to 2%)
  Hematologic: Platelets decreased (4% children), neutrophils decreased (1% to 3%)
  Hepatic: AST increased (2% to 9%), ALT increased (4% to 8%), bilirubin increased (children 3%)
  Neuromuscular & skeletal: Weakness (4% to 7%)

<2% (Limited to important or life-threatening): Alopecia, amnesia, ataxia, avitaminosis, cholecystitis, Cushing's syndrome, deep vein thrombosis, depression, diabetes mellitus, dyskinesia, dyspnea, exfoliative dermatitis, facial paralysis, flu-like syndrome, hepatic dysfunction, lactic hemorrhagic colitis, maculopapular rash, migraine, neuritis, pancreatitis, paresthesia, peripheral neuropathy, pulmonary edema, renal calculus, somnolence, tinnitus, vasculitis

Overdosage/Toxicology The solution contains 42.4% alcohol. Overdosage in a child may cause alcohol-related toxicity and may be potentially lethal. Treatment should be symptomatic and supportive. Activated charcoal may aid in the removal of unabsorbed medication.

Drug Interactions

Cytochrome P450 Effect: CYP2D6 and CYP3A3/4 enzyme inhibitors

Increased Effect/Toxicity:

Contraindicated drugs: Life-threatening arrhythmias may result from concurrent use of flecainide or propafenone. Concurrent use is contraindicated. Concurrent use of cisapride, pimozide, astemizole, terfenadine is also contraindicated. Some benzodiazepines (midazolam and triazolam) are contraindicated, due to the potential for increased response/respiratory depression. Concurrent use of ergot alkaloids is contraindicated, due to potential toxicity.

Serum levels of other antiarrhythmics, including amiodarone, bepridil, lidocaine (systemic), and quinidine may be increased with concurrent use. Serum levels of calcium channel blockers (including felodipine, nicardipine, and nifedipine), clarithromycin, immunosuppressants (cyclosporin, tacrolimus, sirolimus), HMG-CoA reductase inhibitors (lovastatin and simvastatin are not recommended, atorvastatin and cerivastatin should be used at lowest possible dose), itraconazole, ketoconazole, methadone, and rifabutin (decreased dose recommended) may be increased. Serum levels of protease inhibitors may be altered during concurrent therapy. Ritonavir may increase serum concentrations of

(Continued)

Lopinavir and Ritonavir *(Continued)*

amprenavir, indinavir, or saquinavir. Serum levels of sildenafil may be substantially increased (use caution at decreased dose of sildenafil, maximum of 25 mg in 48 hours). Warfarin serum levels may also be increased.

Delavirdine increases levels of lopinavir; dosing recommendations are not yet established. Lopinavir/ritonavir solution contains alcohol, concurrent use with disulfiram or metronidazole should be avoided. May cause disulfiram-like reaction.

Decreased Effect: Carbamazepine, dexamethasone, phenobarbital, phenytoin, and rifampin may decrease levels of lopinavir. Non-nucleoside reverse transcriptase inhibitors: Efavirenz, nevirapine may decrease levels of lopinavir. To avoid incompatibility with didanosine, administer didanosine 1 hour before or 2 hours after lopinavir/ritonavir. Decreased levels of ethinyl estradiol may result from concurrent use. Lopinavir/ritonavir may decrease levels of abacavir, atovaquone, or zidovudine.

Ethanol/Nutrition/Herb Interactions Herb/Nutraceutical: St John's wort may decrease levels of protease inhibitors and lead to possible resistance; concurrent use in not recommended.

Stability Oral solution and gelatin capsules: Store at 2°C to 8°C (36°F to 46°F). Avoid exposure to excessive heat. If stored at room temperature (25°C or 77°F), use within 2 months.

Mechanism of Action A coformulation of lopinavir and ritonavir. The lopinavir component is the active inhibitor of HIV protease. Lopinavir inhibits HIV protease and renders the enzyme incapable of processing polyprotein precursor which leads to production of noninfectious immature HIV particles. The ritonavir component inhibits the CYP3A metabolism of lopinavir, allowing increased plasma levels of lopinavir.

Pharmacodynamics/Kinetics
Ritonavir: See Ritonavir monograph.
Lopinavir:
Protein binding: 98% to 99%
Metabolism: Hepatic via CYP3A; 13 metabolites identified
Half-life elimination: 5-6 hours
Excretion: Urine (2%); feces (83%, 20% as unchanged drug)

Usual Dosage Oral (take with food):
Children 6 months to 12 years: Dosage based on weight, presented based on mg of lopinavir (maximum dose: Lopinavir 400 mg/ritonavir 100 mg)
7-<15 kg: 12 mg/kg twice daily
15-40 kg: 10 mg/kg twice daily
>40 kg: Refer to adult dosing
Children >12 years and Adults: Lopinavir 400 mg/ritonavir 100 mg twice daily
Dosage adjustment when taken with efavirenz or nevirapine:
Children 6 months to 12 years:
7-<15 kg: 13 mg/kg twice daily
15-50 kg: 11 mg/kg twice daily
>50 kg: Refer to adult dosing
Children >12 years and Adults: Lopinavir 533 mg/ritonavir 133 mg twice daily
Elderly: Initial studies did not include enough elderly patients to determine effects based on age. Use with caution due to possible decreased hepatic, renal, and cardiac function.

Dosage adjustment in renal impairment: Has not been studied in patients with renal impairment; however, a decrease in clearance is not expected

Dosage adjustment in hepatic impairment: Plasma levels may be increased in patients with hepatic impairment.

Dietary Considerations Should be taken with food.

Administration Take with food; if using didanosine, take didanosine 1 hour before or 2 hours after lopinavir/ritonavir

Monitoring Parameters Triglycerides, cholesterol, LFTs, electrolytes, basic HIV monitoring, viral load and CD4 count, glucose

Patient Information This medication will be used with other medications to treat HIV infection. Take medication daily as prescribed. Take with food. Do not change doses or discontinue without contacting prescriber. It is important to find out what other medications cannot be taken with this medication. Do not take any prescription medications, over-the-counter products or herbal products, especially St John's wort, without consulting prescriber. May interfere with certain oral contraceptives; alternate contraceptive measures may be needed.

Nursing Implications Should be given with food. Oral solution contains 42.4% alcohol.

Dosage Forms
Capsule: Lopinavir 133.3 mg and ritonavir 33.3 mg
Solution, oral: Lopinavir 80 mg and ritonavir 20 mg per mL [contains 42.4% alcohol]

♦ **Lopressor**® *see* Metoprolol *on page 902*

♦ **Loprox**® *see* Ciclopirox *on page 290*

♦ **Lorabid**™ *see* Loracarbef *on page 818*

Loracarbef *(lor a KAR bef)*

U.S. Brand Names Lorabid™
Canadian Brand Names Lorabid™
Therapeutic Category Antibiotic, Carbacephem
Use Infections caused by susceptible organisms involving the respiratory tract, acute otitis media, sinusitis, skin and skin structure, bone and joint, and urinary tract and gynecologic
Pregnancy Risk Factor B
Contraindications Hypersensitivity to loracarbef, any component of the formulation, or cephalosporins
Warnings/Precautions Modify dosage in patients with severe renal impairment; prolonged use may result in superinfection; use with caution in patients with a previous history of hypersensitivity to other beta-lactam antibiotics (eg, penicillins, cephalosporins)

Adverse Reactions

≥1%:
Central nervous system: Headache (1% to 3%), somnolence (<2%)
Dermatologic: Rash (1% to 3%)
Gastrointestinal: Diarrhea (4% to 6%), nausea (2%), vomiting (1% to 3%), anorexia (<2%), abdominal pain (1%)
Genitourinary: Vaginitis (1%)
Respiratory: Rhinitis (2% to 6%)
<1%: Anaphylaxis, arthralgia, candidiasis, cholestasis, eosinophilia, hemolytic anemia, interstitial nephritis, jaundice, nephrotoxicity with transient elevations of BUN/creatinine, nervousness, neutropenia, positive Coombs' test, pruritus, pseudomembranous colitis, seizures (with high doses and renal dysfunction), serum sickness-like reaction, slightly increased AST/ALT, Stevens-Johnson syndrome, thrombocytopenia, urticaria

Overdosage/Toxicology Symptoms include abdominal discomfort and diarrhea. Treatment is supportive only.

Drug Interactions

Increased Effect/Toxicity: Loracarbef serum levels are increased with coadministered probenecid.

Ethanol/Nutrition/Herb Interactions Food: Administration with food decreases and delays the peak plasma concentration.

Stability Suspension may be kept at room temperature for 14 days

Mechanism of Action Inhibits bacterial cell wall synthesis by binding to one or more of the penicillin binding proteins (PBPs); inhibits the final transpeptidation step of peptidoglycan synthesis in bacterial cell walls, thus inhibiting cell wall biosynthesis. It is thought that beta-lactam antibiotics inactivate transpeptidase via acylation of the enzyme with cleavage of the CO-N bond of the beta-lactam ring. Upon exposure to beta-lactam antibiotics, bacteria eventually lyse due to ongoing activity of cell wall autolytic enzymes (autolysins and murein hydrolases) while cell wall assembly is arrested.

Pharmacodynamics/Kinetics

Absorption: Rapid
Half-life elimination: ~1 hour
Time to peak, serum: ~1 hour
Excretion: Clearance: Plasma: ~200-300 mL/minute

Usual Dosage Oral:

Children:
Acute otitis media: 15 mg/kg twice daily for 10 days
Pharyngitis and impetigo: 7.5-15 mg/kg twice daily for 10 days
Adults:
Uncomplicated urinary tract infections: 200 mg once daily for 7 days
Skin and soft tissue: 200-400 mg every 12-24 hours
Uncomplicated pyelonephritis: 400 mg every 12 hours for 14 days
Upper/lower respiratory tract infection: 200-400 mg every 12-24 hours for 7-14 days

Dosing comments in renal impairment:
Cl_{cr} 10-49 mL/minute: 50% of usual dose at usual interval or usual dose given half as often
Cl_{cr} <10 mL/minute: Administer usual dose every 3-5 days
Hemodialysis: Doses should be administered after dialysis sessions

Dietary Considerations Should be taken on an empty stomach at least 1 hour before or 2 hours after meals.

Administration Shake suspension well before using

Patient Information Take as directed, preferably on an empty stomach (30 minutes before or 2 hours after meals). Take entire prescription even if feeling better. Shake suspension well before using. Maintain adequate hydration (2-3 L/day of fluids unless instructed to restrict fluid intake). Report immediately any signs of skin rash, joint or back pain, or difficulty breathing. Report unusual fever, chills, vaginal itching or foul-smelling vaginal discharge, or easy bruising or bleeding.

Nursing Implications Finish all medication; shake suspension well before using

Dosage Forms

Capsule: 200 mg, 400 mg
Suspension, oral: 100 mg/5 mL (50 mL, 100 mL); 200 mg/5 mL (50 mL, 100 mL)

Loratadine (lor AT a deen)

U.S. Brand Names Claritin®; Claritin® RediTabs®

Canadian Brand Names Claritin®

Therapeutic Category Antihistamine, H_1 Blocker

Use Relief of nasal and non-nasal symptoms of seasonal allergic rhinitis; treatment of chronic idiopathic urticaria

Pregnancy Risk Factor B

Pregnancy/Breast-Feeding Implications Loratadine was not found to be teratogenic in animal studies. There are no adequate and well-controlled studies in pregnant woman; use during pregnancy only if clearly needed. Loratadine is found in human milk; breast-feeding is not recommended.

Contraindications Hypersensitivity to loratadine or any component of the formulation

Warnings/Precautions Use with caution and modify dose in patients with liver or renal impairment; safety and efficacy in children <2 years of age have not been established

Adverse Reactions

Adults:
Central nervous system: Headache (12%), somnolence (8%), fatigue (4%)
Gastrointestinal: Xerostomia (3%)
Children:
Central nervous system: Nervousness (4% ages 6-12 years), fatigue (3% ages 6-12 years, 2% to 3% ages 2-5 years), malaise (2% ages 6-12 years)
Dermatologic: Rash (2% to 3% ages 2-5 years)

(Continued)

Loratadine *(Continued)*

Gastrointestinal: Abdominal pain (2% ages 6-12 years), stomatitis (2% to 3% ages 2-5 years)

Neuromuscular & skeletal: Hyperkinesia (3% ages 6-12 years)

Ocular: Conjunctivitis (2% ages 6-12 years)

Respiratory: Wheezing (4% ages 6-12 years), dysphonia (2% ages 6-12 years), upper respiratory infection (2% ages 6-12 years), epistaxis (2% to 3% ages 2-5 years), pharyngitis (2% to 3% ages 2-5 years), flu-like symptoms (2% to 3% ages 2-5 years)

Miscellaneous: Viral infection (2% to 3% ages 2-5 years)

Adults and Children: <2% (Limited to important or life-threatening): Abnormal hepatic function, agitation, alopecia, altered lacrimation, altered micturition, altered salivation, altered taste, amnesia, anaphylaxis, angioneurotic edema, anorexia, arthralgia, back pain, blepharospasm, blurred vision, breast enlargement, breast pain, bronchospasm, chest pain, confusion, depression, dizziness, dysmenorrhea, dyspnea, erythema multiforme, hemoptysis, hepatic necrosis, hepatitis, hypotension, impaired concentration, impotence, insomnia, irritability, jaundice, menorrhagia, migraine, nausea, palpitations, paresthesia, paroniria, peripheral edema, photosensitivity, pruritus, purpura, rigors, seizures, supraventricular tachyarrhythmia, syncope, tachycardia, tremor, urinary discoloration, urticaria, thrombocytopenia, vaginitis, vertigo, vomiting, weight gain

Overdosage/Toxicology Symptoms include somnolence, tachycardia, and headache. No specific antidote is available. Treatment is symptomatic and supportive. Loratadine is not eliminated by dialysis.

Drug Interactions

Cytochrome P450 Effect: CYP2D6 and 3A3/4 enzyme substrate

Increased Effect/Toxicity: Increased plasma concentrations of loratadine and its active metabolite with ketoconazole and erythromycin, however no change in QT_c interval was seen. Increased toxicity with procarbazine, other antihistamines, alcohol. Protease inhibitors (amprenavir, ritonavir, nelfinavir) may increase the serum levels of loratadine.

Ethanol/Nutrition/Herb Interactions

Ethanol: Avoid ethanol (although sedation is limited with loratadine, may increase risk of CNS depression).

Food: Increases bioavailability and delays peak.

Herb/Nutraceutical: St John's wort may decrease loratadine levels.

Stability Store at 2°C to 25°C (36°F to 77°F).

Rapidly disintegrating tablets: Use within 6 months of opening foil pouch, and immediately after opening individual tablet blister. Store in a dry place.

Mechanism of Action Long-acting tricyclic antihistamine with selective peripheral histamine H_1-receptor antagonistic properties

Pharmacodynamics/Kinetics

Onset of action: 1-3 hours

Peak effect: 8-12 hours

Duration: >24 hours

Absorption: Rapid

Distribution: Significant amounts enter breast milk

Metabolism: Extensive to an active metabolite via CYP2D6 and 3A3/4

Half-life elimination: 12-15 hours

Excretion: Urine (40%) and feces (40%) as metabolites

Usual Dosage Oral: Seasonal allergic rhinitis, chronic idiopathic urticaria:

Children 2-5 years: 5 mg once daily

Children ≥6 years and Adults: 10 mg once daily

Elderly: Peak plasma levels are increased; elimination half-life is slightly increased; specific dosing adjustments are not available

Dosage adjustment in renal impairment: Cl_{cr} ≤30 mL/minute:

Children 2-5 years: 5 mg every other day

Children ≥6 years and Adults: 10 mg every other day

Dosage adjustment in hepatic impairment: Elimination half-life increases with severity of disease

Children 2-5 years: 5 mg every other day

Children ≥6 years and Adults: 10 mg every other day

Dietary Considerations Take on an empty stomach.

Patient Information Drink plenty of water; may cause dry mouth, sedation, drowsiness, and can impair judgment and coordination. Notify prescriber if pregnant.

Rapidly-disintegrating tablets: Place tablet on tongue; it dissolves rapidly. May be used with or without water. Use within 6 months of opening foil pouch, and immediately after opening individual tablet blister.

Nursing Implications Encourage patient to drink plenty of water; may cause dry mouth, sedation, drowsiness, and can impair judgment and coordination

Dosage Forms

Syrup: 1 mg/mL (480 mL)

Tablet: 10 mg

Tablet, rapid-disintegrating (RediTabs®): 10 mg

Loratadine and Pseudoephedrine *(lor AT a deen & soo doe e FED rin)*

U.S. Brand Names Claritin-D® 12-Hour; Claritin-D® 24-Hour

Canadian Brand Names Chlor-Tripolon ND®; Claritin® Extra

Synonyms Pseudoephedrine and Loratadine

Therapeutic Category Antihistamine/Decongestant Combination

Use Temporary relief of symptoms of seasonal allergic rhinitis and nasal congestion

Pregnancy Risk Factor B

Usual Dosage Children ≥12 years and Adults: Oral:

Claritin-D® 12-Hour: 1 tablet every 12 hours

Claritin-D® 24-Hour: 1 tablet daily

Dosage adjustment in renal impairment:
Claritin-D® 12-Hour: 1 tablet daily
Claritin-D® 24-Hour: 1 tablet every other day
Additional Information Complete prescribing information for this medication should be consulted for additional detail.

Dosage Forms
Tablet:
Extended release, 12-hour: Loratadine 5 mg and pseudoephedrine sulfate 120 mg
Extended release, 24-hour: Loratadine 10 mg and pseudoephedrine sulfate 240 mg

Lorazepam (lor A ze pam)

Related Information
Antacid Drug Interactions *on page 1477*
Benzodiazepines Comparison *on page 1490*
Convulsive Status Epilepticus *on page 1661*

U.S. Brand Names Ativan®

Canadian Brand Names Apo®-Lorazepam; Ativan®; Novo-Lorazepam®; Nu-Loraz; Riva-Lorazepam

Therapeutic Category Antianxiety Agent; Anticonvulsant; Antiemetic; Benzodiazepine; Sedative

Use
Oral: Management of anxiety disorders or short-term relief of the symptoms of anxiety or anxiety associated with depressive symptoms
I.V.: Status epilepticus, preanesthesia for desired amnesia, antiemetic adjunct

Unlabeled/Investigational Use Ethanol detoxification; insomnia; psychogenic catatonia; partial complex seizures

Restrictions C-IV

Pregnancy Risk Factor D

Pregnancy/Breast-Feeding Implications
Clinical effects on the fetus: Crosses the placenta. Respiratory depression or hypotonia if administered near time of delivery.
Breast-feeding/lactation: Crosses into breast milk and no data on clinical effects on the infant. AAP states MAY BE OF CONCERN.

Contraindications Hypersensitivity to lorazepam or any component of the formulation (cross-sensitivity with other benzodiazepines may exist); acute narrow-angle glaucoma; sleep apnea (parenteral); intra-arterial injection of parenteral formulation; severe respiratory insufficiency (except during mechanical ventilation); pregnancy

Warnings/Precautions Use with caution in elderly or debilitated patients, patients with hepatic disease (including alcoholics) or renal impairment. Use with caution in patients with respiratory disease or impaired gag reflex. Initial doses in elderly or debilitated patients should not exceed 2 mg. Prolonged lorazepam use may have a possible relationship to GI disease, including esophageal dilation.

The parenteral formulation of lorazepam contains polyethylene glycol and propylene glycol. Each agent has been associated with specific toxicities when administered in prolonged infusions at high dosages. Also contains benzyl alcohol - avoid rapid injection in neonates or prolonged infusions. Intra-arterial injection or extravasation should be avoided. Concurrent administration with scopolamine results in an increased risk of hallucinations, sedation, and irrational behavior.

Causes CNS depression (dose-related) resulting in sedation, dizziness, confusion, or ataxia which may impair physical and mental capabilities. Patients must be cautioned about performing tasks which require mental alertness (ie, operating machinery or driving). Use with caution in patients receiving other CNS depressants or psychoactive agents. Effects with other sedative drugs or ethanol may be potentiated. Benzodiazepines have been associated with falls and traumatic injury and should be used with extreme caution in patients who are at risk of these events (especially the elderly).

Lorazepam may cause anterograde amnesia. Paradoxical reactions, including hyperactive or aggressive behavior have been reported with benzodiazepines, particularly in adolescent/pediatric or psychiatric patients. Does not have analgesic, antidepressant, or antipsychotic properties.

Use caution in patients with depression, particularly if suicidal risk may be present. Use with caution in patients with a history of drug dependence. Benzodiazepines have been associated with dependence and acute withdrawal symptoms on discontinuation or reduction in dose. Acute withdrawal, including seizures, may be precipitated after administration of flumazenil to patients receiving long-term benzodiazepine therapy.

As a hypnotic agent, should be used only after evaluation of potential causes of sleep disturbance. Failure of sleep disturbance to resolve after 7-10 days may indicate psychiatric or medical illness. A worsening of insomnia or the emergence of new abnormalities of thought or behavior may represent unrecognized psychiatric or medical illness and requires immediate and careful evaluation.

Adverse Reactions
>10%:
Central nervous system: Sedation
Respiratory: Respiratory depression
1% to 10%:
Cardiovascular: Hypotension
Central nervous system: Confusion, dizziness, akathisia, unsteadiness, headache, depression, disorientation, amnesia
Dermatologic: Dermatitis, rash
Gastrointestinal: Weight gain/loss, nausea, changes in appetite
Neuromuscular & skeletal: Weakness
Respiratory: Nasal congestion, hyperventilation, apnea
(Continued)

Lorazepam *(Continued)*

<1% (Limited to important or life-threatening): Menstrual irregularities, increased salivation, blood dyscrasias, reflex slowing, physical and psychological dependence with prolonged use, polyethylene glycol or propylene glycol poisoning (prolonged I.V. infusion)

Overdosage/Toxicology Symptoms include confusion, coma, hypoactive reflexes, dyspnea, and labored breathing. **Note:** Prolonged infusions have been associated with toxicity from propylene glycol and/or polyethylene glycol. Treatment for benzodiazepine overdose is supportive. Rarely is mechanical ventilation required. Flumazenil has been shown to selectively block the binding of benzodiazepines to CNS receptors, resulting in a reversal of benzodiazepine-induced CNS depression, but not respiratory depression. Treatment requires blood pressure and respiratory support until drug effects subside.

Drug Interactions
Increased Effect/Toxicity: Ethanol and other CNS depressants may increase the CNS effects of lorazepam. Scopolamine in combination with parenteral lorazepam may increase the incidence of sedation, hallucinations, and irrational behavior. There are rare reports of significant respiratory depression, stupor, and/or hypotension with concomitant use of loxapine and lorazepam. Use caution if concomitant administration of loxapine and CNS drugs is required.

Decreased Effect: Oral contraceptives may increase the clearance of lorazepam. Lorazepam may decrease the antiparkinsonian efficacy of levodopa. Theophylline and other CNS stimulants may antagonize the sedative effects of lorazepam.

Ethanol/Nutrition/Herb Interactions
Ethanol: Avoid or limit ethanol (may increase CNS depression).
Herb/Nutraceutical: Avoid valerian, St John's wort, kava kava, gotu kola (may increase CNS depression).

Stability
Intact vials should be refrigerated, protected from light; do not use discolored or precipitate containing solutions
May be stored at room temperature for up to 60 days
Stability of parenteral admixture at room temperature (25°C): 24 hours
Standard diluent: 1 mg/100 mL D_5W
I.V. is **incompatible** when administered in the same line with foscarnet, ondansetron, sargramostim

Mechanism of Action Binds to stereospecific benzodiazepine receptors on the postsynaptic GABA neuron at several sites within the central nervous system, including the limbic system, reticular formation. Enhancement of the inhibitory effect of GABA on neuronal excitability results by increased neuronal membrane permeability to chloride ions. This shift in chloride ions results in hyperpolarization (a less excitable state) and stabilization.

Pharmacodynamics/Kinetics
Onset of action: Hypnosis: I.M.: 20-30 minutes; Sedation, anticonvulsant: I.V.: 5 minutes; oral: 0.5-1 hour
Duration: 6-8 hours
Absorption: Oral, I.M.: Prompt
Distribution:
V_d: Neonates: 0.76 L/kg, Adults: 1.3 L/kg; crosses placenta; enters breast milk
Protein binding: 85%; free fraction may be significantly higher in elderly
Metabolism: Hepatic to inactive compounds
Half-life elimination: Neonates: 40.2 hours; Older children: 10.5 hours; Adults: 12.9 hours; Elderly: 15.9 hours; End-stage renal disease: 32-70 hours
Excretion: Urine; feces (minimal)

Usual Dosage
Antiemetic:
Children 2-15 years: I.V.: 0.05 mg/kg (up to 2 mg/dose) prior to chemotherapy
Adults: Oral, I.V.: 0.5-2 mg every 4-6 hours as needed
Anxiety and sedation:
Infants and Children: Oral, I.M., I.V.: Usual: 0.05 mg/kg/dose (range: 0.02-0.09 mg/kg) every 4-8 hours
I.V.: May use smaller doses (eg, 0.01-0.03 mg/kg) and repeat every 20 minutes, as needed to titrate to effect
Adults: Oral: 1-10 mg/day in 2-3 divided doses; usual dose: 2-6 mg/day in divided doses
Elderly: 0.5-4 mg/day; initial dose not to exceed 2 mg
Insomnia: Adults: Oral: 2-4 mg at bedtime
Preoperative: Adults:
I.M.: 0.05 mg/kg administered 2 hours before surgery (maximum: 4 mg/dose)
I.V.: 0.044 mg/kg 15-20 minutes before surgery (usual maximum: 2 mg/dose)
Operative amnesia: Adults: I.V.: Up to 0.05 mg/kg (maximum: 4 mg/dose)
Sedation (preprocedure): Infants and Children:
Oral, I.M., I.V.: Usual: 0.05 mg/kg (range: 0.02-0.09 mg/kg);
I.V.: May use smaller doses (eg, 0.01-0.03 mg/kg) and repeat every 20 minutes, as needed to titrate to effect
Status epilepticus: I.V.:
Infants and Children: 0.1 mg/kg slow I.V. over 2-5 minutes; do not exceed 4 mg/single dose; may repeat second dose of 0.05 mg/kg slow I.V. in 10-15 minutes if needed
Adolescents: 0.07 mg/kg slow I.V. over 2-5 minutes; maximum: 4 mg/dose; may repeat in 10-15 minutes
Adults: 4 mg/dose slow I.V. over 2-5 minutes; may repeat in 10-15 minutes; usual maximum dose: 8 mg
Rapid tranquilization of agitated patient (administer every 30-60 minutes):
Oral: 1-2 mg
I.M.: 0.5-1 mg
Average total dose for tranquilization: Oral, I.M.: 4-8 mg

Administration
Lorazepam may be administered by I.M. or I.V.
I.M.: Should be administered deep into the muscle mass

I.V.: Do not exceed 2 mg/minute or 0.05 mg/kg over 2-5 minutes

Dilute I.V. dose with equal volume of compatible diluent (D_5W, NS, SWI)

Injection must be made slowly with repeated aspiration to make sure the injection is not intra-arterial and that perivascular extravasation has not occurred

Monitoring Parameters Respiratory and cardiovascular status, blood pressure, heart rate, symptoms of anxiety

Reference Range Therapeutic: 50-240 ng/mL (SI: 156-746 nmol/L)

Patient Information Advise patient of potential for physical and psychological dependence with chronic use; advise patient of possible retrograde amnesia after I.V. or I.M. use; will cause drowsiness, impairment of judgment or coordination

Nursing Implications Keep injectable form in the refrigerator; **inadvertent intra-arterial injection may produce arteriospasm resulting in gangrene which may require amputation**; emergency resuscitative equipment should be available when administering by I.V.; prior to I.V. use, lorazepam injection must be diluted with an equal amount of compatible diluent; injection must be made slowly with repeated aspiration to make sure the injection is not intra-arterial and that perivascular extravasation has not occurred; provide safety measures (ie, side rails, night light, and call button); supervise ambulation

Additional Information Oral doses >0.09 mg/kg produced ↑ ataxia without ↑ sedative benefit vs lower doses; preferred anxiolytic when I.M. route needed. Abrupt discontinuation after sustained use (generally >10 days) may cause withdrawal symptoms.

Dosage Forms

Injection: 2 mg/mL (1 mL, 10 mL); 4 mg/mL (1 mL, 10 mL)

Solution, oral concentrate: 2 mg/mL (30 mL) [alcohol free, dye free]

Tablet: 0.5 mg, 1 mg, 2 mg

- **Lorcet® 10/650** *see* Hydrocodone and Acetaminophen *on page 676*
- **Lorcet®-HD** *see* Hydrocodone and Acetaminophen *on page 676*
- **Lorcet® Plus** *see* Hydrocodone and Acetaminophen *on page 676*
- **Lortab®** *see* Hydrocodone and Acetaminophen *on page 676*
- **Lortab® ASA** *see* Hydrocodone and Aspirin *on page 677*

Losartan (loe SAR tan)

Related Information

Angiotensin Agents Comparison *on page 1473*

U.S. Brand Names Cozaar®

Canadian Brand Names Cozaar®

Synonyms DuP 753; Losartan Potassium; MK594

Therapeutic Category Angiotensin II Receptor Antagonist (ARB); Antihypertensive Agent

Use Treatment of hypertension with or without concurrent use of thiazide diuretics

Pregnancy Risk Factor C/D (2nd and 3rd trimesters)

Pregnancy/Breast-Feeding Implications Breast-feeding/lactation: Avoid use in the nursing mother, if possible, since it is postulated that losartan is excreted in breast milk

Contraindications Hypersensitivity to losartan or any component of the formulation; hypersensitivity to other A-II receptor antagonists; primary hyperaldosteronism; bilateral renal artery stenosis; pregnancy (2nd and 3rd trimesters)

Warnings/Precautions Avoid use or use a much smaller dose in patients who are volume-depleted; correct depletion first. Use with caution in patients with pre-existing renal insufficiency or significant aortic/mitral stenosis. Use caution in patients with unilateral or bilateral renal artery stenosis to avoid a decrease in renal function. AUCs of losartan (not the active metabolite) are about 50% greater in patients with Cl_{cr} <30 mL/minute and are doubled in hemodialysis patients.

Adverse Reactions

1% to 10%:

Central nervous system: Dizziness (4%), insomnia (1%)

Cardiovascular: First dose hypotension (dose-related; <1% with 50 mg, 2% with 100 mg)

Gastrointestinal: Diarrhea (2.4%), dyspepsia (1.3%), abdominal pain (2%), nausea (2%)

Neuromuscular & skeletal: Back pain (2%), muscle cramps (1%), myalgia (1%), leg pain (1%)

Respiratory: Upper respiratory infection (8%), cough (3.4% versus 3.3% in placebo), nasal congestion (2%), sinus disorder (1%), sinusitis (1%)

<1% (Limited to important or life-threatening): Acute psychosis with paranoid delusions, ageusia, alopecia, anemia, angina, angioedema, arrhythmias, AV block (second degree), depression, dysgeusia, dyspnea, gout, Henoch-Schönlein purpura, hepatitis, hyperkalemia, impotence, maculopapular rash, myocardial infarction, orthostatic effects, panic disorder, pancreatitis, paresthesia, peripheral neuropathy, photosensitivity, renal impairment (patients dependent on renin-angiotensin-aldosterone system), stroke, syncope, urticaria, vasculitis, vertigo

Overdosage/Toxicology Symptoms including hypotension and tachycardia may occur with very significant overdoses. Treatment should be supportive.

Drug Interactions

Cytochrome P450 Effect: CYP2C9 and 3A3/4 enzyme substrate

Increased Effect/Toxicity: Potassium salts/supplements, co-trimoxazole (high dose), ACE inhibitors, and potassium-sparing diuretics (amiloride, spironolactone, triamterene) may increase the risk of hyperkalemia. Cimetidine may increase the absorption of losartan by 18% (clinical effect is unknown). Blood levels of losartan may be increased by inhibitors of cytochrome P450 isoenzymes 2C9 (amiodarone, fluoxetine, isoniazid, ritonavir, sulfonamides) and 3A4 (diltiazem, erythromycin, verapamil, ketoconazole, itraconazole). Potassium salts/supplements, co-trimoxazole (high dose), ACE inhibitors, and potassium-sparing diuretics (amiloride, spironolactone, triamterene) may increase the risk of hyperkalemia.

Decreased Effect: Phenobarbital caused a reduction of losartan in serum by 20%, clinical effect is unknown. Other enzyme inducers may affect serum concentrations of losartan.

(Continued)

Losartan *(Continued)*

Ethanol/Nutrition/Herb Interactions Herb/Nutraceutical: St John's wort may decrease levels. Avoid dong quai if using for hypertension (has estrogenic activity). Avoid ephedra, yohimbe, ginseng (may worsen hypertension). Avoid garlic (may have increased antihypertensive effect).

Mechanism of Action As a selective and competitive, nonpeptide angiotensin II receptor antagonist, losartan blocks the vasoconstrictor and aldosterone-secreting effects of angiotensin II; losartan interacts reversibly at the AT1 and AT2 receptors of many tissues and has slow dissociation kinetics; its affinity for the AT1 receptor is 1000 times greater than the AT2 receptor. Angiotensin II receptor antagonists may induce a more complete inhibition of the renin-angiotensin system than ACE inhibitors, they do not affect the response to bradykinin, and are less likely to be associated with nonrenin-angiotensin effects (eg, cough and angioedema). Losartan increases urinary flow rate and in addition to being natriuretic and kaliuretic, increases excretion of chloride, magnesium, uric acid, calcium, and phosphate.

Pharmacodynamics/Kinetics
Onset of action: 6 hours
Distribution: V_d: Losartan: 34 L; E-3174: 12 L; does not cross blood brain barrier
Protein binding, plasma: High
Metabolism: Hepatic: 14% metabolized by CYP450 enzymes to an active metabolite E-3174 (40 times more potent than losartan); extensive first-pass effect
Bioavailability: 25% to 33%; AUC of E-3174 is four times greater than that of losartan
Half-life elimination: Losartan: 1.5-2 hours; E-3174: 6-9 hours
Time to peak, serum: Losartan: 1 hour; E-3174: 3-4 hours
Excretion: Urine (35%, 3% to 8% as unchanged drug, E-3174); feces (60%)
Clearance: Plasma: Losartan: 600 mL/minute; Active metabolite: 50 mL/minute

Usual Dosage Oral: The usual starting dose is 50 mg once daily. Can be administered once or twice daily with total daily doses ranging from 25 mg to 100 mg.
Usual initial doses in patients receiving diuretics or those with intravascular volume depletion: 25 mg
Patients not receiving diuretics: 50 mg
Dosing adjustment in renal impairment: None necessary
Dosing adjustment in hepatic impairment or geriatric patients: Reduce the initial dose to 25 mg; divide dosage intervals into two.
Not removed via hemodialysis

Monitoring Parameters Supine blood pressure, electrolytes, serum creatinine, BUN, urinalysis, symptomatic hypotension and tachycardia, CBC

Patient Information Use caution standing or rising abruptly following a dosage increase; report any symptoms of difficulty breathing, swallowing, swelling of face, lips, extremities, or tongue immediately, as well as symptoms of fever or sore throat; do not use if pregnant

Nursing Implications Observe for symptomatic hypotension and tachycardia especially in patients with CHF; hyponatremia, high-dose diuretics, or severe volume depletion

Dosage Forms Tablet, film coated, as potassium: 25 mg, 50 mg, 100 mg

Losartan and Hydrochlorothiazide
(loe SAR tan & hye droe klor oh THYE a zide)
U.S. Brand Names Hyzaar®
Canadian Brand Names Hyzaar®; Hyzaar® DS
Synonyms Hydrochlorothiazide and Losartan
Therapeutic Category Angiotensin II Antagonist Combination; Antihypertensive Agent, Combination
Use Treatment of hypertension
Pregnancy Risk Factor C/D (2nd and 3rd trimesters)
Usual Dosage Adults: Oral: 1 tablet daily
Additional Information Complete prescribing information for this medication should be consulted for additional detail.
Dosage Forms
Tablet:
Losartan potassium 50 mg and hydrochlorothiazide 12.5 mg
Losartan potassium 100 mg and hydrochlorothiazide 25 mg

♦ **Losartan Potassium** *see Losartan on page 823*
♦ **Lotemax™** *see Loteprednol on page 824*
♦ **Lotensin®** *see Benazepril on page 152*
♦ **Lotensin® HCT** *see Benazepril and Hydrochlorothiazide on page 154*

Loteprednol *(loe te PRED nol)*
U.S. Brand Names Alrex™; Lotemax™
Canadian Brand Names Alrex™; Lotemax™
Synonyms Loteprednol Etabonate
Therapeutic Category Corticosteroid, Ophthalmic
Use
Suspension, 0.2% (Alrex™): Temporary relief of signs and symptoms of seasonal allergic conjunctivitis
Suspension, 0.5% (Lotemax™): Inflammatory conditions (treatment of steroid-responsive inflammatory conditions of the palpebral and bulbar conjunctiva, cornea, and anterior segment of the globe such as allergic conjunctivitis, acne rosacea, superficial punctate keratitis, herpes zoster keratitis, iritis, cyclitis, selected infective conjunctivitis, when the inherent hazard of steroid use is accepted to obtain an advisable diminution in edema and inflammation) and treatment of postoperative inflammation following ocular surgery
Pregnancy Risk Factor C
Usual Dosage Adults: Ophthalmic:
Suspension, 0.2% (Alrex™): Instill 1 drop into affected eye(s) 4 times/day

Suspension, 0.5% (Lotemax™):
    Inflammatory conditions: Apply 1-2 drops into the conjunctival sac of the affected eye(s) 4
        times/day. During the initial treatment within the first week, the dosing may be increased
        up to 1 drop every hour. Advise patients not to discontinue therapy prematurely. If signs
        and symptoms fail to improve after 2 days, re-evaluate the patient.
    Postoperative inflammation: Apply 1-2 drops into the conjunctival sac of the operated
        eye(s) 4 times/day beginning 24 hours after surgery and continuing throughout the first 2
        weeks of the postoperative period
Additional Information Complete prescribing information for this medication should be
consulted for additional detail.
Dosage Forms
    Suspension, ophthalmic, as etabonate:
        0.2% (Alrex™): 5 mL, 10 mL
        0.5% (Lotemax™): 2.5 mL, 5 mL, 10 mL, 15 mL

♦ **Loteprednol Etabonate** see Loteprednol on page 824
♦ **Lotrel®** see Amlodipine and Benazepril on page 80
♦ **Lotrel® (Can)** see Benazepril and Hydrochlorothiazide on page 154
♦ **Lotriderm® (Can)** see Betamethasone and Clotrimazole on page 163
♦ **Lotrimin®** see Clotrimazole on page 323
♦ **Lotrimin® AF [OTC]** see Clotrimazole on page 323
♦ **Lotrimin® AF Powder/Spray [OTC]** see Miconazole on page 908
♦ **Lotrisone®** see Betamethasone and Clotrimazole on page 163

Lovastatin (LOE va sta tin)
Related Information
    Hyperlipidemia Management on page 1670
    Lipid-Lowering Agents on page 1505
U.S. Brand Names Mevacor®
Canadian Brand Names Apo®-Lovastatin; Mevacor®
Synonyms Mevinolin; Monacolin K
Therapeutic Category Antilipemic Agent, HMG-CoA Reductase Inhibitor; HMG-CoA Reductase Inhibitor
Use
    Adjunct to dietary therapy to decrease elevated serum total and LDL cholesterol concentrations in primary hypercholesterolemia
    Primary prevention of coronary artery disease (patients without symptomatic disease with average to moderately elevated total and LDL cholesterol and below average HDL cholesterol)
    Adjunct to dietary therapy in adolescent patients (10-17 years of age, females >1 year postmenarche) with heterozygous familial hypercholesterolemia having LDL >189 mg/dL, **or** LDL >160 mg/dL with positive family history of premature cardiovascular disease (CVD), **or** LDL >160 mg/dL with the presence of at least two other CVD risk factors
Pregnancy Risk Factor X
Pregnancy/Breast-Feeding Implications Safety and efficacy have not been established for use during pregnancy (treatment should be discontinued if pregnancy is recognized). Administer to women of childbearing potential only if conception is unlikely; females should be counseled on appropriate contraceptive methods.
Contraindications Hypersensitivity to lovastatin or any component of the formulation; active liver disease; unexplained persistent elevations of serum transaminases; pregnancy; breast-feeding
Warnings/Precautions May elevate aminotransferases; LFTs should be performed before and every 4-6 weeks during the first 12-15 months of therapy and periodically thereafter. Can also cause myalgia and rhabdomyolysis. Rhabdomyolysis with acute renal failure has occurred. Risk is increased with concurrent use of clarithromycin, danazol, diltiazem, fluvoxamine, indinavir, nefazodone, nelfinavir, ritonavir, verapamil, troleandomycin, cyclosporine, fibric acid derivatives, erythromycin, niacin, azole antifungals, or large quantities of grapefruit juice. Weigh the risk versus benefit when combining any of these drugs with lovastatin. Temporarily discontinue in any patient experiencing an acute or serious condition predisposing to renal failure secondary to rhabdomyolysis. Use with caution in patients who consume large amounts of alcohol or have a history of liver disease. Safety and efficacy have not been evaluated in prepubertal patients, patients <10 years of age, or doses >40 mg/day in appropriately-selected adolescents.
Adverse Reactions
    >10%: Neuromuscular & skeletal: Increased CPK (>2x normal) (11%)
    1% to 10%:
        Central nervous system: Headache (2% to 3%), dizziness (0.5% to 1%)
        Dermatologic: Rash (0.8% to 1%)
        Gastrointestinal: Abdominal pain (2% to 3%), constipation (2% to 4%), diarrhea (2% to 3%), dyspepsia (1% to 2%), flatulence (4% to 5%), nausea (2% to 3%)
        Neuromuscular & skeletal: Myalgia (2% to 3%), weakness (1% to 2%), muscle cramps (0.6% to 1%)
        Ocular: Blurred vision (0.8% to 1%)
    <1% (Limited to important or life-threatening): Acid regurgitation, alopecia, arthralgia, chest pain, dermatomyositis, eye irritation, insomnia, leg pain, paresthesia, pruritus, vomiting, xerostomia
    Additional class-related events or case reports (not necessarily reported with lovastatin therapy): Alopecia, alteration in taste, anaphylaxis, angioedema, anorexia, anxiety, arthritis, cataracts, chills, cholestatic jaundice, cirrhosis, decreased libido, depression, dryness of skin/mucous membranes, dyspnea, elevated transaminases, eosinophilia, erectile dysfunction, erythema multiforme, facial paresis, fatty liver, fever, flushing, fulminant hepatic necrosis, gynecomastia, hemolytic anemia, hepatitis, hepatoma, hyperbilirubinemia, hypersensitivity reaction, impaired extraocular muscle movement, impotence, increased alkaline phosphatase, increased CPK (>10x normal), increased ESR, increased
(Continued)

Lovastatin *(Continued)*

GGT, leukopenia, malaise, memory loss, myopathy, nail changes, nodules, ophthalmoplegia, pancreatitis, paresthesia, peripheral nerve palsy, peripheral neuropathy, photosensitivity, polymyalgia rheumatica, positive ANA, pruritus, psychic disturbance, purpura, rash, renal failure (secondary to rhabdomyolysis), rhabdomyolysis, skin discoloration, Stevens-Johnson syndrome, systemic lupus erythematosus-like syndrome, thrombocytopenia, thyroid dysfunction, toxic epidermal necrolysis, tremor, urticaria, vasculitis, vertigo, vomiting

Overdosage/Toxicology Few adverse events have been reported. Treatment is symptomatic.

Drug Interactions

Cytochrome P450 Effect: CYP3A3/4 enzyme substrate

Increased Effect/Toxicity: Inhibitors of CYP3A3/4 (amprenavir, clarithromycin, cyclosporine, diltiazem, fluvoxamine, erythromycin, fluconazole, indinavir, itraconazole, ketoconazole, miconazole, nefazodone, nelfinavir, ritonavir, troleandomycin, and verapamil) increase lovastatin blood levels and may increase the risk of myopathy and rhabdomyolysis. Cyclosporine, clofibrate, fenofibrate, gemfibrozil, and niacin also may increase the risk of myopathy and rhabdomyolysis. The effect/toxicity of warfarin (elevated PT) and levothyroxine may be increased by lovastatin. Digoxin, norethindrone, and ethinyl estradiol levels may be increased. Effects are additive with other lipid-lowering therapies.

Decreased Effect: Cholestyramine taken with lovastatin reduces lovastatin absorption and effect.

Ethanol/Nutrition/Herb Interactions

Food: The therapeutic effect of lovastatin may be decreased if taken with food. Lovastatin serum concentrations may be increased if taken with grapefruit juice; avoid concurrent use. Herb/Nutraceutical: St John's wort may decrease lovastatin levels.

Mechanism of Action Lovastatin acts by competitively inhibiting 3-hydroxyl-3-methylglutaryl-coenzyme A (HMG-CoA) reductase, the enzyme that catalyzes the rate-limiting step in cholesterol biosynthesis

Pharmacodynamics/Kinetics

Onset of action: LDL cholesterol reductions: 3 days

Absorption: 30%

Protein binding: 95%

Metabolism: Hepatic; extensive first-pass effect; hydrolyzed to B-hydroxy acid (active)

Half-life elimination: 1.1-1.7 hours

Time to peak, serum: 2-4 hours

Excretion: Feces (~80% to 85%); urine (10%)

Usual Dosage Oral:

Adolescents 10-17 years:

LDL reduction <20%: Initial: 10 mg/day with evening meal

LDL reduction ≥20%: Initial: 20 mg/day with evening meal

Usual range: 10-40 mg with evening meal, then adjust dose at 4-week intervals

Adults: Initial: 20 mg with evening meal, then adjust at 4-week intervals; maximum dose: 80 mg/day; before initiation of therapy, patients should be placed on a standard cholesterol-lowering diet for 3-6 months and the diet should be continued during drug therapy

Dietary Considerations Before initiation of therapy, patients should be placed on a standard cholesterol-lowering diet for 6 weeks and the diet should be continued during drug therapy.

Administration Administer with meals

Monitoring Parameters Obtain baseline LFTs and total cholesterol profile. LFTs should be performed before initiation of therapy, at 6- and 12 weeks after initiation or first dose, and periodically thereafter.

Reference Range NCEP classification of pediatric patients with familial history of hypercholesterolemia or premature CVD: Acceptable total cholesterol: <170 mg/dL, LDL: <110 mg/dL

Test Interactions ↑ liver transaminases (S), altered thyroid function tests

Patient Information Promptly report any unexplained muscle pain, tenderness or weakness, especially if accompanied by malaise or fever; do not interrupt, increase, or decrease dose without advice of physician; take with meals

Nursing Implications Urge patient to adhere to cholesterol-lowering diet

Dosage Forms Tablet: 10 mg, 20 mg, 40 mg

◆ **Lovastatin and Niacin** *see Niacin and Lovastatin on page 976*

◆ **Lovenox®** *see Enoxaparin on page 465*

◆ **Low-Ogestrel®** *see Ethinyl Estradiol and Norgestrel on page 528*

◆ **Low Potassium Diet** *see page 1727*

◆ **Lowsium® Plus** *see Magaldrate and Simethicone on page 831*

◆ **Loxapac® (Can)** *see Loxapine on page 826*

Loxapine *(LOKS a peen)*

Related Information

Antipsychotic Agents Comparison *on page 1486*

U.S. Brand Names Loxitane®; Loxitane® C; Loxitane® I.M.

Canadian Brand Names Apo®-Loxapine; Loxapac®; Nu-Loxapine; PMS-Loxapine

Synonyms Loxapine Hydrochloride; Loxapine Succinate; Oxilapine Succinate

Therapeutic Category Antipsychotic Agent, Miscellaneous

Use Management of psychotic disorders

Pregnancy Risk Factor C

Contraindications Hypersensitivity to loxapine or any component of the formulation; severe CNS depression; coma

Warnings/Precautions Watch for hypotension when administering I.M.; should not be given I.V. Safety in children <6 months of age has not been established. Moderately sedating, use with caution in disorders where CNS depression is a feature. Use with caution in Parkinson's disease. Caution in patients with hemodynamic instability; bone marrow suppression; predisposition to seizures; subcortical brain damage; severe cardiac, hepatic, renal or respiratory disease. Esophageal dysmotility and aspiration have been associated with antipsychotic use - use with caution in patients at risk of pneumonia (ie, Alzheimer's disease). Caution in breast cancer or other prolactin-dependent tumors (may elevate prolactin levels). May alter temperature regulation or mask toxicity of other drugs due to antiemetic effects. May alter cardiac conduction; life-threatening arrhythmias have occurred with therapeutic doses of phenothiazines. May cause orthostatic hypotension - use with caution in patients at risk of this effect or those who would tolerate transient hypotensive episodes (cerebrovascular disease, cardiovascular disease, or other medications which may predispose). Safety and effectiveness of loxapine in pediatric patients have not been established.

Phenothiazines may cause anticholinergic effects (confusion, agitation, constipation, dry mouth, blurred vision, urinary retention); therefore, they should be used with caution in patients with decreased gastrointestinal motility, urinary retention, BPH, xerostomia, or visual problems. Conditions which also may be exacerbated by cholinergic blockade include narrow-angle glaucoma (screening is recommended) and worsening of myasthenia gravis. Relative to other antipsychotics, loxapine has a low potency of cholinergic blockade.

May cause extrapyramidal reactions, including pseudoparkinsonism, acute dystonic reactions, akathisia, and tardive dyskinesia (risk of these reactions is moderate-high relative to other neuroleptics). May be associated with neuroleptic malignant syndrome (NMS) or pigmentary retinopathy.

Adverse Reactions Frequency not defined.

Cardiovascular: Orthostatic hypotension, tachycardia, arrhythmias, abnormal T waves with prolonged ventricular repolarization, hypertension, hypotension, lightheadedness, syncope

Central nervous system: Drowsiness, extrapyramidal reactions (dystonia, akathisia, pseudoparkinsonism, tardive dyskinesia, akinesia), dizziness, faintness, ataxia, insomnia, agitation, tension, seizures, slurred speech, confusion, headache, neuroleptic malignant syndrome (NMS), altered central temperature regulation

Dermatologic: Rash, pruritus, photosensitivity, dermatitis, alopecia, seborrhea

Endocrine & metabolic: Enlargement of breasts, galactorrhea, amenorrhea, gynecomastia, menstrual irregularity

Gastrointestinal: Xerostomia, constipation, nausea, vomiting, nasal congestion, weight gain/loss, adynamic ileus, polydipsia

Genitourinary: Urinary retention, sexual dysfunction

Hematologic: Agranulocytosis, leukopenia, thrombocytopenia

Neuromuscular & skeletal: Weakness

Ocular: Blurred vision

Overdosage/Toxicology Symptoms include deep sleep, dystonia, agitation, dysrhythmias, extrapyramidal symptoms, hypotension, and seizures. Following initiation of essential overdose management, toxic symptom and supportive treatment should be initiated. Hypotension usually responds to I.V. fluids or Trendelenburg positioning. If unresponsive to these measures, the use of a parenteral inotrope may be required (eg, norepinephrine 0.1-0.2 mcg/kg/minute titrated to response). Seizures commonly respond to diazepam (I.V. 5-10 mg bolus in adults every 15 minutes, if needed, up to a total of 30 mg; I.V. 0.25-0.4 mg/dose up to a total of 10 mg in children) or to phenytoin or phenobarbital. Critical cardiac arrhythmias often respond to I.V. phenytoin (15 mg/kg up to 1 g), while other antiarrhythmics can be used. Neuroleptics often cause extrapyramidal symptoms (eg, dystonic reactions) requiring management with diphenhydramine 1-2 mg/kg (adults), up to a maximum of 50 mg I.M. or slow I.V. push, followed by a maintenance dose for 48-72 hours. When these reactions are unresponsive to diphenhydramine, anticholinergic agents such as benztropine mesylate I.V. 1-2 mg (adults) may be effective. These agents are generally effective within 2-5 minutes.

Drug Interactions

Increased Effect/Toxicity: Loxapine concentrations may be increased by chloroquine, propranolol, sulfadoxine-pyrimethamine. Loxapine may increased the effect and/or toxicity of antihypertensives, lithium, TCAs, CNS depressants (ethanol, narcotics), and trazodone. There are rare reports of significant respiratory depression, stupor, and/or hypotension with the concomitant use of loxapine and lorazepam. Use caution if the concomitant administration of loxapine and CNS drugs is required.

Decreased Effect: Antipsychotics inhibit the activity of bromocriptine and levodopa. Benztropine (and other anticholinergics) may inhibit the therapeutic response to loxapine and excess anticholinergic effects may occur. Barbiturates and cigarette smoking may enhance the hepatic metabolism of loxapine. Loxapine and possibly other low potency antipsychotic may reverse the pressor effects of epinephrine.

Ethanol/Nutrition/Herb Interactions

Ethanol: Avoid ethanol (may increase CNS depression).

Herb/Nutraceutical: Avoid kava kava, gotu kola, valerian, St John's wort (may increase CNS depression).

Stability Protect from light; dispense in amber or opaque vials

Mechanism of Action Blocks postsynaptic mesolimbic D_1 and D_2 receptors in the brain, and also possesses serotonin 5-HT_2 blocking activity

Pharmacodynamics/Kinetics

Onset of action: Neuroleptic: Oral: 20-30 minutes

Peak effect: 1.5-3 hours

Duration: ~12 hours

Metabolism: Hepatic to glucuronide conjugates

Half-life elimination: Biphasic: Initial: 5 hours; Terminal: 12-19 hours

Excretion: Urine; feces (small amounts)

Usual Dosage Adults:

Oral: 10 mg twice daily, increase dose until psychotic symptoms are controlled; usual dose range: 20-100 mg/day in divided doses 2-4 times/day; dosages >250 mg/day are not recommended

Elderly: 20-60 mg/day

(Continued)

Loxapine *(Continued)*

I.M.: 12.5-50 mg every 4-6 hours or longer as needed and change to oral therapy as soon as possible

Administration Injectable is for I.M. use only

Monitoring Parameters EKG, CBC, blood pressure, electrolytes, pH

Test Interactions False-positives for phenylketonuria, amylase, uroporphyrins, urobilinogen

Patient Information May cause drowsiness; avoid alcohol; may impair judgment or coordination; may cause photosensitivity; avoid excessive sunlight; do not stop taking without consulting physician

Nursing Implications

Injectable is for I.M. use only; dilute the oral concentrate with water or juice before administration; avoid skin contact with oral suspension or solution; may cause contact dermatitis

Monitor orthostatic blood pressures 3-5 days after initiation of therapy or a dose increase; observe for tremor and abnormal movement or posturing (extrapyramidal symptoms)

Dosage Forms

Capsule, as succinate (Loxitane®): 5 mg, 10 mg, 25 mg, 50 mg

Injection, as hydrochloride (Loxitane® IM): 50 mg/mL (1 mL)

Solution, oral concentrate, as hydrochloride (Loxitane® C): 25 mg/mL (120 mL dropper bottle)

- **Loxapine Hydrochloride** *see* Loxapine *on page 826*
- **Loxapine Succinate** *see* Loxapine *on page 826*
- **Loxitane®** *see* Loxapine *on page 826*
- **Loxitane® C** *see* Loxapine *on page 826*
- **Loxitane® I.M.** *see* Loxapine *on page 826*
- **Lozide® (Can)** *see* Indapamide *on page 715*
- **Lozol®** *see* Indapamide *on page 715*
- **L-PAM** *see* Melphalan *on page 854*
- **LRH** *see* Gonadorelin *on page 640*
- **L-Sarcolysin** *see* Melphalan *on page 854*
- **LTG** *see* Lamotrigine *on page 773*
- **L-Thyroxine Sodium** *see* Levothyroxine *on page 799*
- **Ludiomil®** *see* Maprotiline *on page 839*
- **Lugol's Solution** *see* Potassium Iodide *on page 1111*
- **Lumigan™** *see* Bimatoprost *on page 169*
- **Luminal® Sodium** *see* Phenobarbital *on page 1070*
- **Lumitene™** *see* Beta-Carotene *on page 161*
- **Lunelle™** *see* Estradiol Cypionate and Medroxyprogesterone Acetate *on page 495*
- **Lupron®** *see* Leuprolide *on page 783*
- **Lupron Depot®** *see* Leuprolide *on page 783*
- **Lupron Depot-Ped®** *see* Leuprolide *on page 783*
- **Luride®** *see* Fluoride *on page 574*
- **Luride® Lozi-Tab®** *see* Fluoride *on page 574*
- **Luride®-SF Lozi-Tabs®** *see* Fluoride *on page 574*
- **Luteinizing Hormone Releasing Hormone** *see* Gonadorelin *on page 640*
- **Lutrepulse®** *see* Gonadorelin *on page 640*
- **Luvox®** *see* Fluvoxamine *on page 593*
- **Luxiq™** *see* Betamethasone *on page 161*
- **LY170053** *see* Olanzapine *on page 1006*
- **Lyderm® (Can)** *see* Fluocinonide *on page 573*
- **Lydonide® (Can)** *see* Fluocinonide *on page 573*
- **Lyme Disease Vaccine (Recombinant OspA)** *see* Lyme Disease Vaccine *Voluntarily Withdrawn From Market 2/02 on page 828*

Lyme Disease Vaccine *Voluntarily Withdrawn From Market 2/02*

(LIME dee seas vak SEEN)

U.S. Brand Names LYMErix™

Canadian Brand Names LYMErix™

Synonyms Lyme Disease Vaccine (Recombinant OspA)

Therapeutic Category Vaccine

Use Active immunization against Lyme disease in individuals between 15-70 years of age. Individuals most at risk are those who live, work, or travel to *B. burgdorferi*-infected, tick-infested, grassy/wooded areas.

Pregnancy Risk Factor C

Pregnancy/Breast-Feeding Implications It is not known whether Lyme disease vaccine is excreted in human milk. Because many drugs are excreted in milk, caution should be exercised when the vaccine is given to nursing mothers. Healthcare professionals are encouraged to register pregnant women who receive the vaccine with the SKB vaccination pregnancy registry (1-800-366-8900, ext 5231).

Contraindications Hypersensitivity to any component of the vaccine. Vaccination should be postponed during acute moderate to severe febrile illness (minor illness is generally not a contraindication). Safety and efficacy in patients <15 years of age have not been established.

Warnings/Precautions Do not administer to patients with treatment-resistant Lyme arthritis. Will not prevent disease in patients with prior infection and offers no protection against other tick-borne diseases. Immunosuppressed patients or those receiving immunosuppressive therapy (vaccine may not be effective) - defer vaccination until 3 months after therapy. Avoid in patients receiving anticoagulant therapy (due to intramuscular injection). The physician should take all known precautions for prevention of allergic or other reactions. Administer with caution to patients with known or suspected latex allergy (applies only to the LYMErix Tip-

Lok™ syringe, vaccine vial does not contain natural rubber). Duration of immunity has not been established.

Adverse Reactions (Limited to overall self-reported events occurring within 30 days following a dose)

>10%: Local: Injection site pain (21.9%)

1% to 10%:

Central nervous system: Headache (5.6%), fatigue (3.9%), fever (2.6%), chills (2%), dizziness (1%)

Dermatologic: Rash (1.4%)

Gastrointestinal: Nausea (1.1%)

Neuromuscular & skeletal: Arthralgia (6.8%), myalgia (4.8%), muscle aches (2.8%), back pain (1.9%), stiffness (1%)

Respiratory: Upper respiratory tract infection (4.4%), sinusitis (3.2%), pharyngitis (2.5%), rhinitis (2.4%), cough (1.5%), bronchitis (1.1%)

Miscellaneous: Viral infection (2.8%), flu-like syndrome (2.5%)

Solicited adverse event rates were higher than unsolicited event rates (above). These included local reactions of soreness (93.5%), redness (41.8%), and swelling (29.9%). In addition, general systemic symptoms included fatigue (40.8%), headache (38.6%), arthralgia (25.6%), rash (11.7%), and fever (3.5%).

Patients with a history of Lyme disease were noted to experience a higher frequency of early musculoskeletal reactions. Other differences in the observed rate of adverse reactions were not significantly different between vaccine and placebo recipients.

Stability Store between 2°C and 8°C (36°F and 46°F)

Mechanism of Action Lyme disease vaccine is a recombinant, noninfectious lipoprotein (OspA) derived from the outer surface of *Borrelia burgdorferi*, the causative agent of Lyme disease. Vaccination stimulates production of antibodies directed against this organism, including antibodies against the LA-2 epitope, which have bactericidal activity. Since OspA expression is down-regulated after inoculation into the human host, at least part of the vaccine's efficacy may be related to neutralization of bacteria within the midgut of the tick vector, preventing transmission to the human host.

Usual Dosage Adults: I.M.: Vaccination with 3 doses of 30 mcg (0.5 mL), administered at 0, 1, and 12 months, is recommended for optimal protection

Administration Intramuscular injection into the deltoid region is recommended. Do not administer intravenously, intradermally, or subcutaneously. The vaccine should be used as supplied without dilution. Shake well before withdrawal and use.

For patients at risk of hemorrhage following intramuscular injection, the ACIP recommends "it should be administered intramuscularly if, in the opinion of the physician familiar with the patients bleeding risk, the vaccine can be administered with reasonable safety by this route. If the patient receives antihemophilia or other similar therapy, intramuscular vaccination can be scheduled shortly after such therapy is administered. A fine needle (23 gauge or smaller) can be used for the vaccination and firm pressure applied to the site (without rubbing) for at least 2 minutes. The patient should be instructed concerning the risk of hematoma from the injection."

Test Interactions Vaccination will result in a positive *B. burgdorferi* IgG via ELISA (Western blot testing is recommended)

Patient Information Vaccination consists of a series of three injections over 12 months. Failure to complete the sequence may result in suboptimal protection. The vaccine may not provide 100% protection against Lyme disease, nor does it protect against other tick-borne disease. Individuals at risk should continue to use standard protective measures.

Additional Information Federal law requires that the date of administration, the vaccine manufacturer, lot number of vaccine, and the administering person's name, title and address be entered into the patient's permanent medical record.

Dosage Forms Injection:

Prefilled syringe (Tip-Lok™): 30 mcg/0.5 mL

Vial: 30 mcg/0.5 mL

♦ **LYMErix**™ *see* Lyme Disease Vaccine *Voluntarily Withdrawn From Market 2/02 on* *page 828*

Lymphocyte Immune Globulin (LIM foe site i MYUN GLOB yoo lin)

U.S. Brand Names Atgam®

Canadian Brand Names Atgam®

Synonyms Antithymocyte Globulin (Equine); Antithymocyte Immunoglobulin; ATG; Horse Antihuman Thymocyte Gamma Globulin

Therapeutic Category Immunosuppressant Agent

Use Prevention and treatment of acute renal and other solid organ allograft rejection; treatment of moderate to severe aplastic anemia in patients not considered suitable candidates for bone marrow transplantation; prevention of graft-versus-host disease following bone marrow transplantation

Pregnancy Risk Factor C

Contraindications Hypersensitivity to lymphocytic immune globulin, any component of the formulation, thimerosal, or other equine gamma globulins; severe, unremitting leukopenia and/or thrombocytopenia

Warnings/Precautions Must be administered via central line due to chemical phlebitis; should only be used by physicians experienced in immunosuppressive therapy or management of solid organ or bone marrow transplant patients; adequate laboratory and supportive medical resources must be readily available in the facility for patient management; rash, dyspnea, hypotension, or anaphylaxis precludes further administration of the drug. Dose must be administered over at least 4 hours; patient may need to be pretreated with an antipyretic, antihistamine, and/or corticosteroid. Intradermal skin testing is recommended prior to first-dose administration.

(Continued)

Lymphocyte Immune Globulin *(Continued)*

Adverse Reactions

>10%:
  Central nervous system: Fever, chills
  Dermatologic: Rash
  Hematologic: Leukopenia, thrombocytopenia
  Miscellaneous: Systemic infection

1% to 10%:
  Cardiovascular: Hypotension, hypertension, tachycardia, edema, chest pain
  Central nervous system: Headache, malaise, pain
  Gastrointestinal: Diarrhea, nausea, stomatitis, GI bleeding
  Local: Edema or redness at injection site, thrombophlebitis
  Neuromuscular & skeletal: Myalgia, back pain
  Renal: Abnormal renal function tests
  Respiratory: Dyspnea
  Miscellaneous: Sensitivity reactions: Anaphylaxis may be indicated by hypotension, respiratory distress, serum sickness, viral infection

<1% (Limited to important or life-threatening): Acute renal failure, anemia, hemolysis, lymphadenopathy, seizures

Stability

Ampuls must be refrigerated
Dose must be diluted in 0.45% or 0.9% sodium chloride
Diluted solution is stable for 12 hours (including infusion time) at room temperature and 24 hours (including infusion time) at refrigeration
The use of dextrose solutions is not recommended (precipitation may occur)
Standard diluent: Dose/1000 mL NS or 0.45% sodium chloride
Minimum volume: Concentration should not exceed 1 mg/mL for a peripheral line or 4 mg/mL for a central line

Mechanism of Action May involve elimination of antigen-reactive T-lymphocytes (killer cells) in peripheral blood or alteration of T-cell function

Pharmacodynamics/Kinetics

Distribution: Poorly into lymphoid tissues; binds to circulating lymphocytes, granulocytes, platelets, bone marrow cells
Half-life elimination, plasma: 1.5-12 days
Excretion: Urine (~1%)

Usual Dosage An intradermal skin test is recommended prior to administration of the initial dose of ATG; use 0.1 mL of a 1:1000 dilution of ATG in normal saline. A positive skin reaction consists of a wheal ≥10 mm in diameter. If a positive skin test occurs, the first infusion should be administered in a controlled environment with intensive life support immediately available. A systemic reaction precludes further administration of the drug. The absence of a reaction does **not** preclude the possibility of an immediate sensitivity reaction.

First dose: Premedicate with diphenhydramine 50 mg orally 30 minutes prior to and hydrocortisone 100 mg I.V. 15 minutes prior to infusion and acetaminophen 650 mg 2 hours after start of infusion

Children: I.V.:
  Aplastic anemia protocol: 10-20 mg/kg/day for 8-14 days; then administer every other day for 7 more doses; addition doses may be given every other day for 21 total doses in 28 days
  Renal allograft: 5-25 mg/kg/day

Adults: I.V.:
  Aplastic anemia protocol: 10-20 mg/kg/day for 8-14 days, then administer every other day for 7 more doses
  Renal allograft:
    Rejection prophylaxis: 15 mg/kg/day for 14 days followed by 14 days of alternative day therapy at the same dose; the first dose should be administered within 24 hours before or after transplantation
    Rejection treatment: 10-15 mg/kg/day for 14 days, then administer every other day for 10-14 days up to 21 doses in 28 days

Administration For I.V. use only; administer via central line; use of high flow veins will minimize the occurrence of phlebitis and thrombosis; administer by slow I.V. infusion through an inline filter with pore size of 0.2-1 micrometer over 4-8 hours at a final concentration not to exceed 4 mg ATG/mL

Monitoring Parameters Lymphocyte profile, CBC with differential and platelet count, vital signs during administration

Nursing Implications For I.V. use only; mild itching and erythema can be treated with antihistamines; infuse dose over at least 4 hours; any severe systemic reaction to the skin test such as generalized rash, tachycardia, dyspnea, hypotension, or anaphylaxis should preclude further therapy; **epinephrine and resuscitative equipment should be nearby.** Patient may need to be pretreated with an antipyretic, antihistamine, and/or corticosteroid.

Dosage Forms Injection: 50 mg of equine IgG/mL (5 mL)

- ◆ **Lymphocyte Mitogenic Factor** *see* Aldesleukin *on page 43*
- ◆ **Lyphocin**® *see* Vancomycin *on page 1403*
- ◆ **Lysodren**® *see* Mitotane *on page 924*
- ◆ **Lyteprep**™ **(Can)** *see* Polyethylene Glycol-Electrolyte Solution *on page 1101*
- ◆ **Maalox**® **[OTC]** *see* Aluminum Hydroxide and Magnesium Hydroxide *on page 64*
- ◆ **Maalox**® **Fast Release Liquid [OTC]** *see* Aluminum Hydroxide, Magnesium Hydroxide, and Simethicone *on page 64*
- ◆ **Maalox**® **Max [OTC]** *see* Aluminum Hydroxide, Magnesium Hydroxide, and Simethicone *on page 64*
- ◆ **Maalox**® **TC (Therapeutic Concentrate) [OTC]** *see* Aluminum Hydroxide and Magnesium Hydroxide *on page 64*
- ◆ **Macrobid**® *see* Nitrofurantoin *on page 987*

♦ **Macrodantin**® *see* Nitrofurantoin *on page 987*

♦ **Macrodex**® *see* Dextran *on page 386*

Mafenide (MA fe nide)

Related Information
Sulfonamide Derivatives *on page 1515*

U.S. Brand Names Sulfamylon®

Synonyms Mafenide Acetate

Therapeutic Category Antibacterial, Topical; Antibiotic, Topical

Use Adjunct in the treatment of second- and third-degree burns to prevent septicemia caused by susceptible organisms such as *Pseudomonas aeruginosa*
Orphan drug: Prevention of graft loss of meshed autografts on excised burn wounds

Pregnancy Risk Factor C

Contraindications Hypersensitivity to mafenide, sulfites, or any component of the formulation

Warnings/Precautions Use with caution in patients with renal impairment and in patients with G6PD deficiency; prolonged use may result in superinfection

Adverse Reactions Frequency not defined.
Cardiovascular: Facial edema
Central nervous system: Pain
Dermatologic: Rash, erythema
Endocrine & metabolic: Hyperchloremia, metabolic acidosis
Hematologic: Porphyria, bone marrow suppression, hemolytic anemia, bleeding
Local: Burning sensation, excoriation
Respiratory: Hyperventilation, tachypnea, dyspnea
Miscellaneous: Hypersensitivity

Stability
Mafenide 5% topical solution preparation:
Dissolve the 50 g mafenide acetate (Sulfamylon®) packet in 200 mL of either sterile water for irrigation or sterile saline for irrigation; (minimum solubility of 50 g of mafenide is in 200 mL of either solution)
Sterilize this solution by pushing through a 0.22 micron filter
Further dissolve this 200 mL of sterile Sulfamylon® solution in 800 mL of the initial diluent (either sterile water for irrigation or normal saline for irrigation)
This solution is stable and sterile for a total of 48 hours at room temperature

Note: Mafenide acetate topical solution CANNOT be mixed with nystatin due to reduced activity of mafenide
Note: Pilot *in vitro* studies: Silvadene® and Furacin® cream combined with nystatin cream were equally effective against the microorganisms as were the individual drugs. However, Sulfamylon® cream combined with nystatin lost its antimicrobial capability. [J Burn Care Rehabil 1989, 109:508-11.]

Mechanism of Action Interferes with bacterial folic acid synthesis through competitive inhibition of para-aminobenzoic acid

Pharmacodynamics/Kinetics
Absorption: Diffuses through devascularized areas and is rapidly absorbed from burned surface
Metabolism: To para-carboxybenzene sulfonamide, a carbonic anhydrase inhibitor
Time to peak, serum: 2-4 hours
Excretion: Urine (as metabolites)

Usual Dosage Children and Adults: Topical: Apply once or twice daily with a sterile gloved hand; apply to a thickness of approximately 16 mm; the burned area should be covered with cream at all times

Monitoring Parameters Acid base balance

Patient Information Discontinue and call physician immediately if rash, blisters, or swelling appear while using cream; discontinue if condition persists or worsens while using this product; for external use only

Nursing Implications For external use only; monitor acid base balance

Dosage Forms
Cream, topical, as acetate: 85 mg/g (56.7 g, 113.4 g, 411 g)
Powder, topical: 5% (50 g)

♦ **Mafenide Acetate** *see* Mafenide *on page 831*

Magaldrate and Simethicone (MAG al drate & sye METH i kone)

U.S. Brand Names Iosopan® Plus; Lowsium® Plus; Riopan Plus® [OTC]; Riopan Plus® Double Strength [OTC]

Canadian Brand Names Riopan Plus®

Synonyms Simethicone and Magaldrate

Therapeutic Category Antacid; Antiflatulent

Use Relief of hyperacidity associated with peptic ulcer, gastritis, peptic esophagitis and hiatal hernia which are accompanied by symptoms of gas

Pregnancy Risk Factor C

Usual Dosage Adults: Oral: 540-1080 mg magaldrate between meals and at bedtime

Additional Information Complete prescribing information for this medication should be consulted for additional detail.

Dosage Forms
Suspension, oral:
Magaldrate 540 mg and simethicone 20 mg per 5 mL (360 mL, 420 mL)
Magaldrate 540 mg and simethicone 40 mg per 5 mL (360 mL)
Magaldrate 1080 mg and simethicone 40 mg per 5 mL (360 mL)
Tablet, chewable:
Magaldrate 540 mg and simethicone 20 mg
Magaldrate 1080 mg and simethicone 20 mg

♦ **Mag-Gel**® **600** *see* Magnesium Oxide *on page 834*

* Maginex™ [OTC] *see Magnesium L-aspartate Hydrochloride on page 834*
* Maginex™ DS [OTC] *see Magnesium L-aspartate Hydrochloride on page 834*
* Magnesia Magma *see Magnesium Hydroxide on page 832*
* Magnesium Carbonate and Aluminum Hydroxide *see Aluminum Hydroxide and Magnesium Carbonate on page 63*
* Magnesium Chloride *see Magnesium Salts (Other) on page 835*

Magnesium Citrate (mag NEE zhum SIT rate)
Related Information
Laxatives, Classification and Properties *on page 1504*
Canadian Brand Names Citro-Mag®
Synonyms Citrate of Magnesia
Therapeutic Category Laxative, Saline
Use Evacuation of bowel prior to certain surgical and diagnostic procedures or overdose situations
Pregnancy Risk Factor B
Contraindications Renal failure, appendicitis, abdominal pain, intestinal impaction, obstruction or perforation, diabetes mellitus, complications in gastrointestinal tract, patients with colostomy or ileostomy, ulcerative colitis or diverticulitis
Warnings/Precautions Use with caution in patients with impaired renal function, especially if Cl_{cr} <30 mL/minute (accumulation of magnesium which may lead to magnesium intoxication); use with caution in digitalized patients (may alter cardiac conduction leading to heart block); use with caution in patients with lithium administration; use with caution with neuromuscular blocking agents, CNS depressants
Adverse Reactions 1% to 10%:
Cardiovascular: Hypotension
Endocrine & metabolic: Hypermagnesemia
Gastrointestinal: Abdominal cramps, diarrhea, gas formation
Respiratory: Respiratory depression
Overdosage/Toxicology
Due to diarrhea, serious potentially life-threatening electrolyte disturbances may occur with long-term use or overdose; hypermagnesemia may occur, as well as, CNS depression, confusion, hypotension, muscle weakness, and blockage of peripheral neuromuscular transmission.
Serum level >4 mEq/L (4.8 mg/dL): Deep tendon reflexes may be depressed
Serum level ≥10 mEq/L (12 mg/dL): Deep tendon reflexes may disappear, respiratory paralysis may occur, heart block may occur
I.V. calcium (5-10 mEq) will reverse respiratory depression or heart block. In extreme cases, peritoneal dialysis or hemodialysis may be required.
Serum level >12 mEq/L may be fatal, serum level ≥10 mEq/L may cause complete heart block
Mechanism of Action Promotes bowel evacuation by causing osmotic retention of fluid which distends the colon with increased peristaltic activity
Pharmacodynamics/Kinetics
Absorption: Oral: 15% to 30%
Excretion: Urine
Usual Dosage Cathartic: Oral:
Children:
<6 years: 0.5 mL/kg up to a maximum of 200 mL repeated every 4-6 hours until stools are clear
6-12 years: 100-150 mL
Children ≥12 years and Adults: ½ to 1 full bottle (120-300 mL)
Reference Range Serum magnesium:
Children: 1.5-1.9 mg/dL ~1.2-1.6 mEq/L
Adults: 2.2-2.8 mg/dL ~1.8-2.3 mEq/L
Test Interactions ↑ magnesium; ↓ protein, ↓ calcium (S), ↓ potassium (S)
Patient Information Take with a glass of water, fruit juice, or citrus flavored carbonated beverage to improve taste, chill before using; report severe abdominal pain to physician
Nursing Implications To increase palatability, manufacturer suggests chilling the solution prior to administration
Additional Information Magnesium content of 5 mL: 3.85-4.71 mEq
Dosage Forms Solution, oral: 300 mL (1.75 g/30 mL)

* Magnesium Gluconate *see Magnesium Salts (Other) on page 835*

Magnesium Hydroxide (mag NEE zhum hye DROKS ide)
Related Information
Laxatives, Classification and Properties *on page 1504*
U.S. Brand Names Phillips'® Milk of Magnesia [OTC]
Synonyms Magnesia Magma; Milk of Magnesia; MOM
Therapeutic Category Antacid; Laxative, Saline; Magnesium Salt
Use Short-term treatment of occasional constipation and symptoms of hyperacidity, magnesium replacement therapy
Pregnancy Risk Factor B
Contraindications Hypersensitivity to any component of the formulation; patients with colostomy or an ileostomy, intestinal obstruction, fecal impaction, renal failure, appendicitis
Warnings/Precautions Use with caution in patients with severe renal impairment (especially when doses are >50 mEq magnesium/day); hypermagnesemia and toxicity may occur due to decreased renal clearance of absorbed magnesium. Decreased renal function (Cl_{cr} <30 mL/minute) may result in toxicity; monitor for toxicity.
Adverse Reactions Frequency not defined.
Cardiovascular: Hypotension
Endocrine & metabolic: Hypermagnesemia

Gastrointestinal: Diarrhea, abdominal cramps
Neuromuscular & skeletal: Muscle weakness
Respiratory: Respiratory depression

Overdosage/Toxicology Magnesium antacids are also laxatives and may cause diarrhea and hypokalemia. In patients with renal failure, magnesium may accumulate to toxic levels. I.V. calcium (5-10 mEq) will reverse respiratory depression or heart block. In extreme cases, peritoneal dialysis or hemodialysis may be required.

Drug Interactions
Decreased Effect: Absorption of tetracyclines, digoxin, iron salts, isoniazid, or quinolones may be decreased.

Mechanism of Action Promotes bowel evacuation by causing osmotic retention of fluid which distends the colon with increased peristaltic activity; reacts with hydrochloric acid in stomach to form magnesium chloride

Pharmacodynamics/Kinetics
Onset of action: Laxative: 4-8 hours
Excretion: Urine (up to 30% as absorbed magnesium ions); feces (as unabsorbed drug)

Usual Dosage Oral:
Average daily intakes of dietary magnesium have declined in recent years due to processing of food; the latest estimate of the average American dietary intake was 349 mg/day
Laxative:
Liquid:
Children
<2 years: 0.5 mL/kg/dose
2-5 years: 5-15 mL/day (2.5-7.5 mL/day of liquid concentrate) or in divided doses
6-12 years: 15-30 mL/day (7.5-15 mL/day of liquid concentrate) or in divided doses
Children ≥12 years and Adults: 30-60 mL/day (15-30 mL/day of liquid concentrate) or in divided doses
Tablet:
Children:
2-5 years: 1-2 tablets before bedtime
6-11 years: 3-4 tablets before bedtime
Children ≥12 years and Adults: 6-8 tablets before bedtime
Antacid:
Liquid:
Children: 2.5-5 mL as needed up to 4 times/day
Adults: 5-15 mL (2.5-7.5 mL of liquid concentrate) as needed up to 4 times/day
Tablet:
Children 7-14 years: 1 tablet up to 4 times/day
Adults: 2-4 tablets up to 4 times/day

Dosing in renal impairment: Patients in severe renal failure should not receive magnesium due to toxicity from accumulation. Patients with a Cl_cr <25 mL/minute receiving magnesium should be monitored by serum magnesium levels.

Dietary Considerations Should be followed by 8 ounces of water; taste can be improved by following each dose with citrus fruit juice.

Reference Range Serum magnesium:
Children: 1.5-1.9 mg/dL (1.2-1.6 mEq/L)
Adults: 1.5-2.5 mg/dL (1.2-2.0 mEq/L)

Test Interactions ↑ magnesium; ↓ protein, calcium (S), ↓ potassium (S)

Patient Information Dilute dose in water or juice, shake well

Nursing Implications MOM concentrate is 3 times as potent as regular strength product

Additional Information Magnesium content of 30 mL: 1.05 g (87 mEq)

Dosage Forms
Liquid, oral: 400 mg/5 mL (15 mL, 30 mL, 100 mL, 120 mL, 180 mL, 360 mL, 720 mL)
Liquid, oral concentrate: 800 mg/5 mL (240 mL) [10 mL equivalent to 30 mL milk of magnesia USP]
Tablet: 300 mg, 600 mg

♦ **Magnesium Hydroxide, Aluminum Hydroxide, and Simethicone** *see* Aluminum Hydroxide, Magnesium Hydroxide, and Simethicone *on page 64*

♦ **Magnesium Hydroxide and Aluminum Hydroxide** *see* Aluminum Hydroxide and Magnesium Hydroxide *on page 64*

♦ **Magnesium Hydroxide and Calcium Carbonate** *see* Calcium Carbonate and Magnesium Hydroxide *on page 208*

Magnesium Hydroxide and Mineral Oil Emulsion
(mag NEE zhum hye DROKS ide & MIN er al oyl e MUL shun)

U.S. Brand Names Haley's M-O® [OTC]

Synonyms MOM/Mineral Oil Emulsion

Therapeutic Category Laxative

Use Short-term treatment of occasional constipation

Pregnancy Risk Factor B

Usual Dosage Adults: Oral: 5-45 mL at bedtime
Product labeling:
Children 6-11 years: 5-15 mL at bedtime or upon rising
Children ≥12 years and Adults: 30-60 mL at bedtime or upon rising

Additional Information Complete prescribing information for this medication should be consulted for additional detail.

Dosage Forms Suspension, oral: Magnesium hydroxide 300 mg and mineral oil 1.25 mL per 5 mL (12 oz, 29 oz) [equivalent to magnesium hydroxide 24 mL/mineral oil emulsion 6 mL]

♦ **Magnesium Hydroxide, Famotidine, and Calcium Carbonate** *see* Famotidine, Calcium Carbonate, and Magnesium Hydroxide *on page 544*

Magnesium L-aspartate Hydrochloride
(mag NEE zhum el as PAR tate hye droe KLOR ide)

U.S. Brand Names Maginex™ [OTC]; Maginex™ DS [OTC]

Synonyms MAH™

Therapeutic Category Electrolyte Supplement, Oral

Use Dietary supplement

Contraindications Hypersensitivity to any component of the formulation

Warnings/Precautions Hypermagnesemia and toxicity may occur due to decreased renal clearance (Cl$_{cr}$<30 mL/minute) of absorbed magnesium; use with caution in digitalized patients (may alter cardiac conduction leading heart block); use with caution in patients with lithium administration; elderly, due to disease or drug therapy, may be predisposed to diarrhea; diarrhea may result in electrolyte imbalance; monitor for toxicity.

Adverse Reactions Frequency not defined: Gastrointestinal: Diarrhea, loose stools

Usual Dosage Adults:

Recommended dietary allowance (RDA) of magnesium:

Male: 400-420 mg

Female: 310-320 mg

During pregnancy: 360 mg

During lactation: 320 mg

Dietary supplement: Oral: Magnesium-L-aspartate 1230 mg (magnesium 122 mg) up to 3 times/day

Dosage adjustment in renal impairment: Patients with severe renal failure should not receive magnesium due to toxicity from accumulation.

Dietary Considerations Take with food.

Administration

Granules: Mix each packet in 4 ounces of water or juice prior to administration

Tablet, enteric coated: Do not crush or chew

Patient Information Not for use in patients with kidney/renal disease.

Dosage Forms

Granules (Maginex™ DS): 1230 mg [10 mEq; equivalent to 122 mg magnesium] [lemon flavored]

Tablet (Maginex™): 615 mg [5 mEq; equivalent to 61 mg magnesium]

Magnesium Oxide (mag NEE zhum OKS ide)

U.S. Brand Names Mag-Gel® 600; Mag-Ox® 400 [OTC]; Uro-Mag® [OTC]

Therapeutic Category Antacid; Electrolyte Supplement, Oral; Laxative, Saline; Magnesium Salt

Use Electrolyte replacement

Pregnancy Risk Factor B

Contraindications Patients with colostomy or an ileostomy, appendicitis, ulcerative colitis, diverticulitis, heart block, myocardial damage, serious renal impairment, hepatitis, Addison's disease, hypersensitivity to any component

Warnings/Precautions Hypermagnesemia and toxicity may occur due to decreased renal clearance (Cl$_{cr}$ <30 mL/minute) of absorbed magnesium; monitor serum magnesium level, respiratory rate, deep tendon reflex, renal function when MgSO$_4$ is administered parenterally; use with caution in digitalized patients (may alter cardiac conduction leading heart block); use with caution in patients with lithium administration; elderly, due to disease or drug therapy, may be predisposed to diarrhea; diarrhea may result in electrolyte imbalance; monitor for toxicity

Adverse Reactions

>10%: Gastrointestinal: Diarrhea

1% to 10%:

Cardiovascular: Hypotension, EKG changes

Central nervous system: Mental depression, coma

Gastrointestinal: Nausea, vomiting

Respiratory: Respiratory depression

Overdosage/Toxicology Magnesium antacids are also laxatives and may cause diarrhea and hypokalemia. In patients with renal failure, magnesium may accumulate to toxic levels. I.V. calcium (5-10 mEq) will reverse respiratory depression or heart block. In extreme cases, peritoneal dialysis or hemodialysis may be required.

Drug Interactions

Increased Effect/Toxicity: Nondepolarizing neuromuscular blockers

Decreased Effect: Decreased absorption of aminoquinolones, digoxin, nitrofurantoin, penicillamine, and tetracyclines may occur with magnesium salts

Pharmacodynamics/Kinetics

Onset of action: Laxative: 4-8 hours

Excretion: Urine (up to 30% as absorbed magnesium ions); feces (as unabsorbed drug)

Usual Dosage The recommended dietary allowance (RDA) of magnesium is 4.5 mg/kg which is a total daily allowance of 350-400 mg for adult men and 280-300 mg for adult women. During pregnancy the RDA is 300 mg and during lactation the RDA is 355 mg.

Adults: Oral: Dietary supplement: 20-40 mEq (1-2 tablets) 2-3 times

Product labeling:

Mag-Ox 400®: 1-2 tablets daily with food

Uro-Mag®: 1-2 tablets 3 times/day with food

Dosing in renal impairment: Patients in severe renal failure should not receive magnesium due to toxicity from accumulation. Patients with a Cl$_{cr}$ <25 mL/minute should be monitored by serum magnesium levels.

Note: Oral magnesium is not generally adequate for repletion in patients with serum magnesium concentrations <1.5 mEq/L

Dietary Considerations Should be taken with food.

Reference Range Serum magnesium:

Children: 1.5-1.9 mg/dL (1.2-1.6 mEq/L)

Adults: 1.5-2.5 mg/dL (1.2-2.0 mEq/L)

Test Interactions ↑ magnesium; ↓ protein, calcium (S), ↓ potassium (S)

Patient Information Chew tablets before swallowing; take with full glass of water; notify physician if relief not obtained or if any signs of bleeding occur (black tarry stools, "coffee ground" vomit)

Nursing Implications Monitor for diarrhea and signs of hypermagnesemia

Additional Information Contains 60% elemental magnesium; 49.6 mEq magnesium/g; 25 mmol magnesium/g

Dosage Forms

Capsule: 140 mg [elemental magnesium 84.5 mg]

Tablet: 400 mg [elemental magnesium 241.3 mg]

Magnesium Salts (Other) (mag NEE zhum salts OTH er)

Related Information

Antiarrhythmic Drugs Comparison *on page 1478*

U.S. Brand Names Almora® (Gluconate); Magonate® (Gluconate) [OTC]; Magtrate® (Gluconate); Slow-Mag® (Chloride)

Synonyms Magnesium Chloride; Magnesium Gluconate

Therapeutic Category Magnesium Salt

Use Dietary supplement for treatment of magnesium deficiencies

Contraindications Patients with heart block, severe renal disease

Warnings/Precautions Use with caution in patients with impaired renal function; hypermagnesemia and toxicity may occur due to decreased renal clearance of absorbed magnesium

Adverse Reactions

1% to 10%: Gastrointestinal: Diarrhea (excessive dose)

<1%: Abdominal cramps, hypermagnesemia, hypotension, muscle weakness, respiratory depression

Drug Interactions

Increased Effect/Toxicity: Increased effect of nondepolarizing neuromuscular blockers

Decreased Effect: Decreased absorption of aminoquinolones, digoxin, nitrofurantoin, penicillamine, and tetracyclines may occur with magnesium salts

Mechanism of Action Magnesium is important as a cofactor in many enzymatic reactions in the body involving protein synthesis and carbohydrate metabolism, (at least 300 enzymatic reactions require magnesium). Actions on lipoprotein lipase have been found to be important in reducing serum cholesterol and on sodium/potassium ATPase in promoting polarization (ie, neuromuscular functioning).

Pharmacodynamics/Kinetics

Absorption: Oral: 15% to 30%

Elimination: Renal

Usual Dosage Oral:

Average daily intakes of dietary magnesium have declined in recent years due to processing of food; the latest estimate of the average American dietary intake was 349 mg/day

Adequate intakes:

Infants:

0-6 months: 30 mg

7-12 months: 75 mg

Recommended dietary allowance:

Children:

1-3 years: 80 mg/day

4-8 years: 130 mg/day

Male:

9-13 years: 240 mg/day

14-18 years: 130 mg/day

19-30 years: 400 mg/day

≥31 years: 420 mg/day

Female:

9-13 years: 240 mg/day

14-18 years: 360 mg/day

19-30 years: 310 mg/day

≥31 years: 320 mg/day

Female: Pregnancy:

≤18 years: 400 mg/day

19-30 years: 350 mg/day

31-50 years: 360 mg/day

Female: Lactation:

≤18 years: 360 mg/day

19-30 years: 310 mg/day

31-50 years: 320 mg/day

Hypomagnesemia: There are no specific dosage recommendations for this product in replacement of magnesium. Extrapolation from dosage recommendations of magnesium sulfate are as follows:

Children: 10-20 mg/kg/dose **elemental** magnesium 4 times/day

Adults: 300 mg **elemental** magnesium 4 times/day

The recommended dietary allowance (RDA) of magnesium is 4.5 mg/kg which is a total daily allowance of 350-400 mg for adult men and 280-300 mg for adult women. During pregnancy the RDA is 300 mg and during lactation the RDA is 355 mg.

Dietary supplement: Oral:

Children: 3-6 mg/kg/day in divided doses 3-4 times/day; maximum: 400 mg/day

Adults: 54-483 mg/day in divided doses; refer to product labeling

Dosing in renal impairment: Patients in severe renal failure should not receive magnesium due to toxicity from accumulation. Patients with a Cl_{cr} <25 mL/minute receiving magnesium should be monitored by serum magnesium levels.

Reference Range Serum magnesium:

Children: 1.5-1.9 mg/dL ~1.2-1.6 mEq/L

(Continued)

Magnesium Salts (Other) *(Continued)*

Adults: 2.2-2.8 mg/dL ~1.8-2.3 mEq/L

Additional Information Note: 1 g magnesium = 83.3 mEq (4.11 mmol)

Dosage Forms

Gluconate:

Liquid: 54 mg/5 mL as magnesium

Tablet: 500 mg (elemental magnesium 27 mg)

Chloride: Tablet, sustained release: 535 mg (64 mg magnesium)

Amino acids chelate: Tablet: 500 mg (100 mg magnesium)

Magnesium Sulfate (mag NEE zhum SUL fate)

Related Information

Adult ACLS Algorithms *on page 1632*

Synonyms Epsom Salts

Therapeutic Category Antacid; Antiarrhythmic Agent, Miscellaneous; Anticonvulsant; Electrolyte Supplement, Parenteral; Laxative, Saline; Magnesium Salt

Use Treatment and prevention of hypomagnesemia and in seizure prevention in severe pre-eclampsia or eclampsia, pediatric acute nephritis; also used as short-term treatment of constipation and torsade de pointes; treatment of cardiac arrhythmias (VT/VF) caused by hypomagnesemia

Pregnancy Risk Factor B

Contraindications Heart block, serious renal impairment, myocardial damage, hepatitis, Addison's disease

Warnings/Precautions Use with caution in patients with impaired renal function (accumulation of magnesium which may lead to magnesium intoxication); use with caution in digitalized patients (may alter cardiac conduction leading to heart block); monitor serum magnesium level, respiratory rate, deep tendon reflex, renal function when $MgSO_4$ is administered parenterally

Adverse Reactions Hypotension and asystole may occur with rapid administration. Frequency not defined:

Serum magnesium levels >3 mg/dL:

Central nervous system: Depressed CNS

Gastrointestinal: Diarrhea

Neuromuscular & skeletal: Depressed neuromuscular transmission and deep tendon reflexes

Serum magnesium levels >5 mg/dL:

Cardiovascular: Flushing

Central nervous system: Somnolence

Serum magnesium levels >12.5 mg/dL:

Cardiovascular: Complete heart block

Respiratory: Respiratory depression

Overdosage/Toxicology

Symptoms of overdose usually present with serum level >4 mEq/L

Serum magnesium >4: Deep tendon reflexes may be depressed

Serum magnesium ≥10: Deep tendon reflexes may disappear, respiratory paralysis may occur, heart block may occur

Serum level >12 mEq/L may be fatal, serum level ≥10 mEq/L may cause complete heart block

I.V. calcium (5-10 mEq) 1-2 g calcium gluconate will reverse respiratory depression or heart block. In extreme cases, peritoneal dialysis or hemodialysis may be required.

Stability Refrigeration of intact ampuls may result in precipitation or crystallization. Parenteral admixture is stable at room temperature (25°C) for 60 days.

I.V. is **incompatible** when mixed with fat emulsion (flocculation), calcium gluceptate, clindamycin, dobutamine, hydrocortisone (same syringe), nafcillin, polymyxin B, procaine hydrochloride, tetracyclines, thiopental.

Mechanism of Action Promotes bowel evacuation by causing osmotic retention of fluid which distends the colon with increased peristaltic activity when taken orally; parenterally, decreases acetylcholine in motor nerve terminals and acts on myocardium by slowing rate of S-A node impulse formation and prolonging conduction time

Pharmacodynamics/Kinetics

Onset of action: Oral: Cathartic: 1-2 hours; I.M.: 1 hour; I.V.: Immediate

Duration: I.M.: 3-4 hours; I.V.: 30 minutes

Excretion: Urine (as magnesium)

Usual Dosage The recommended dietary allowance (RDA) of magnesium is 4.5 mg/kg which is a total daily allowance of 350-400 mg for adult men and 280-300 mg for adult women. During pregnancy the RDA is 300 mg and during lactation the RDA is 355 mg. Average daily intakes of dietary magnesium have declined in recent years due to processing of food. The latest estimate of the average American dietary intake was 349 mg/day. Dose represented as $MgSO_4$ unless stated otherwise.

Note: Serum magnesium is poor reflection of repletional status as the majority of magnesium is intracellular; serum levels may be transiently normal for a few hours after a dose is given, therefore, aim for consistently high normal serum levels in patients with normal renal function for most efficient repletion

Hypomagnesemia:

Neonates: I.V.: 25-50 mg/kg/dose (0.2-0.4 mEq/kg/dose) every 8-12 hours for 2-3 doses

Children: I.M., I.V.: 25-50 mg/kg/dose (0.2-0.4 mEq/kg/dose) every 4-6 hours for 3-4 doses, maximum single dose: 2000 mg (16 mEq), may repeat if hypomagnesemia persists (higher dosage up to 100 mg/kg/dose $MgSO_4$ I.V. has been used); maintenance: I.V.: 30-60 mg/kg/day (0.25-0.5 mEq/kg/day)

Adults:

Oral: 3 g every 6 hours for 4 doses as needed

I.M., I.V.: 1 g every 6 hours for 4 doses; for severe hypomagnesemia: 8-12 g $MgSO_4$/day in divided doses has been used

Management of seizures and hypertension: Children: I.M., I.V.: 20-100 mg/kg/dose every 4-6 hours as needed; in severe cases doses as high as 200 mg/kg/dose have been used

Eclampsia, pre-eclampsia: Adults:

I.M.: 1-4 g every 4 hours

I.V.: Initial: 4 g, then switch to I.M. or 1-4 g/hour by continuous infusion

Note: Maximum dose not to exceed 30-40 g/day; maximum rate of infusion: 1-2 g/hour

Life-threatening arrhythmia: I.V.: 1-2 g (8-16 mEq) in 100 mL D$_5$W, administered over 5-60 minutes followed by an infusion of 0.5-1 g/hour, **or**

1-6 g administered over several minutes, followed by (in some cases) I.V. infusion of 3-20 mg/minute for 5-48 hours (depending on patient response and serum magnesium levels)

Maintenance electrolyte requirements:

Daily requirements: 0.2-0.5 mEq/kg/24 hours or 3-10 mEq/1000 kcal/24 hours

Maximum: 8-16 mEq/24 hours

Cathartic: Oral:

Children: 0.25 g/kg every 4-6 hours

Adults: 10-15 g in a glass of water

Dosing adjustment/comments in renal impairment: Cl$_{cr}$ <25 mL/minute: Do not administer or monitor serum magnesium levels carefully

Dietary Considerations MgSO$_4$ oral solution: Mix with water and administer on an empty stomach.

Administration Magnesium sulfate may be administered I.M. or I.V.

I.M.: A 25% or 50% concentration may be used for adults and a 20% solution is recommended for children

I.V.: Magnesium may be administered IVP, IVPB or I.V. infusion in an auxiliary medication infusion solution (eg, TPN); when giving I.V. push, must dilute first and should not be given any faster than 150 mg/minute

Maximal rate of infusion: 2 g/hour to avoid hypotension; doses of 4 g/hour have been given in emergencies (eclampsia, seizures); optimally, should add magnesium to I.V. fluids or to IVH, bolus doses are also effective

For I.V., a concentration <20% (200 mg/mL) should be used and the rate of injection should not exceed 1.5 mL of a 10% solution (or equivalent) per minute (150 mg/minute)

Monitoring Parameters Monitor blood pressure when administering MgSO$_4$ I.V.; serum magnesium levels should be monitored to avoid overdose; monitor for diarrhea; monitor for arrhythmias, hypotension, respiratory and CNS depression during rapid I.V. administration

Reference Range Serum magnesium:

Children: 1.5-1.9 mg/dL (1.2-1.6 mEq/L)

Adults: 1.5-2.5 mg/dL (1.2-2.0 mEq/L)

Note: Serum magnesium is poor reflection of repletional status as the majority of magnesium is intracellular; serum levels may be transiently normal for a few hours after a dose is given, therefore, aim for consistently high normal serum levels in patients with normal renal function for most efficient repletion

Test Interactions ↑ magnesium; ↓ protein, calcium (S), ↓ potassium (S)

Nursing Implications

Dilute to a maximum concentration of 100 mg/mL and infuse over 2-4 hours; do not exceed 125 mg/kg/hour (1 mEq/kg/hour)

Monitor arrhythmias, hypotension, diarrhea, respiratory and CNS depression during rapid I.V. administration; monitor serum magnesium level to avoid overdosages

Additional Information 10% elemental magnesium; 8.1 mEq magnesium/g; 4 mmol magnesium/g

500 mg MgSO$_4$ = 4.06 mEq magnesium = 49.3 mg elemental magnesium

Dosage Forms

Granules: ~40 mEq magnesium/5 g (120 g, 240 g)

Injection: 100 mg/mL (20 mL); 125 mg/mL (8 mL); 200 mg/mL (50 mL); 500 mg/mL (2 mL, 5 mL, 10 mL, 50 mL)

♦ **Magnesium Trisilicate and Aluminum Hydroxide** *see* Aluminum Hydroxide and Magnesium Trisilicate *on page 64*

♦ **Magonate® (Gluconate) [OTC]** *see* Magnesium Salts (Other) *on page 835*

♦ **Mag-Ox® 400 [OTC]** *see* Magnesium Oxide *on page 834*

♦ **Magtrate® (Gluconate)** *see* Magnesium Salts (Other) *on page 835*

♦ **MAH™** *see* Magnesium L-aspartate Hydrochloride *on page 834*

♦ **Malaria Treatment** *see page 1607*

♦ **Malarone™** *see* Atovaquone and Proguanil *on page 129*

Malathion (mal a THYE on)

U.S. Brand Names Ovide™

Therapeutic Category Pediculocide

Use Treatment of head lice and their ova

Pregnancy Risk Factor B

Contraindications Hypersensitivity to malathion or any component of the formulation

Usual Dosage Sprinkle Ovide™ lotion on dry hair and rub gently until the scalp is thoroughly moistened; pay special attention to the back of the head and neck. Allow to dry naturally - use no heat and leave uncovered. After 8-12 hours, the hair should be washed with a nonmedicated shampoo; rinse and use a fine-toothed comb to remove dead lice and eggs. If required, repeat with second application in 7-9 days. Further treatment is generally not necessary. Other family members should be evaluated to determine if infested and if so, receive treatment.

Patient Information Topical use only

Nursing Implications Topical use only

Dosage Forms Lotion, topical: 0.5% (59 mL)

♦ **Mallamint® [OTC]** *see* Calcium Carbonate *on page 207*

♦ **Mallisol® [OTC]** *see* Povidone-Iodine *on page 1114*

+ **Management of Healthcare Worker Exposures to HIV, HBV, HCV** *see page 1555*
+ **Management of Overdosages** *see page 1688*
+ **Mandelamine® (Can)** *see Methenamine on page 881*
+ **Mandol®** *see Cefamandole on page 239*
+ **Mandrake** *see Podophyllum Resin on page 1099*

Manganese (MAN ga nees)

U.S. Brand Names Chelated Manganese® [OTC]

Synonyms Manganese Chloride; Manganese Sulfate

Therapeutic Category Trace Element; Trace Element, Parenteral

Use Trace element added to TPN (total parenteral nutrition) solution to prevent manganese deficiency; orally as a dietary supplement

Pregnancy Risk Factor C

Contraindications High manganese levels; severe liver dysfunction or cholestasis (conjugated bilirubin >2 mg/dL) due to reduced biliary excretion

Overdosage/Toxicology Acute poisoning due to ingestion of manganese or manganese salts is rare, owing to poor absorption. In chronic poisoning, either from injection, or usually, from inhalation of manganese dust or fumes in the air, symptoms are mainly extrapyramidal and toxicity can lead to progressive CNS deterioration.

Stability Compatible with electrolytes usually present in amino acid/dextrose solution used for TPN solutions

Mechanism of Action Cofactor in many enzyme systems, stimulates synthesis of cholesterol and fatty acids in liver, and influences mucopolysaccharide synthesis

Pharmacodynamics/Kinetics

Distribution: Concentrated in mitochondria of pituitary gland, pancreas, liver, kidney, and bone

Excretion: Primarily feces; urine (negligible)

Usual Dosage

Infants: I.V.: 2-10 mcg/kg/day usually administered in TPN solutions

Adults:

Oral: 20-50 mg/day

I.V.: 150-800 mcg/day usually administered in TPN solutions

Administration Do not administer I.M. or by direct I.V. injection since the acidic pH of the solution may cause tissue irritations and it is hypotonic

Monitoring Parameters Periodic manganese plasma level

Reference Range 4-14 µg/L

Dosage Forms

Injection, as chloride: 0.1 mg/mL (10 mL)

Injection, as sulfate: 0.1 mg/mL (10 mL, 30 mL)

Tablet: 20 mg, 50 mg

+ **Manganese Chloride** *see Manganese on page 838*
+ **Manganese Sulfate** *see Manganese on page 838*

Mannitol (MAN i tole)

U.S. Brand Names Osmitrol®; Resectisol® Irrigation Solution

Canadian Brand Names Osmitrol®

Synonyms *D*-Mannitol

Therapeutic Category Diuretic, Osmotic

Use Reduction of increased intracranial pressure associated with cerebral edema; promotion of diuresis in the prevention and/or treatment of oliguria or anuria due to acute renal failure; reduction of increased intraocular pressure; promoting urinary excretion of toxic substances; genitourinary irrigant in transurethral prostatic resection or other transurethral surgical procedures

Pregnancy Risk Factor C

Contraindications Hypersensitivity to mannitol or any component or the formulation; severe renal disease (anuria); dehydration; active intracranial bleeding; severe pulmonary edema or congestion

Warnings/Precautions Should not be administered until adequacy of renal function and urine flow is established; cardiovascular status should also be evaluated; do not administer electrolyte-free mannitol solutions with blood

Adverse Reactions Frequency not defined.

Cardiovascular: Circulatory overload, congestive heart failure

Central nervous system: Headache, convulsions, headache, chills, dizziness

Dermatologic: Rash

Endocrine & metabolic: Fluid and electrolyte imbalance, water intoxication, dehydration and hypovolemia secondary to rapid diuresis, hyponatremia

Gastrointestinal: Nausea, vomiting, xerostomia

Genitourinary: Polyuria, dysuria

Local: Tissue necrosis

Ocular: Blurred vision

Respiratory: Pulmonary edema

Miscellaneous: Allergic reactions

Overdosage/Toxicology Symptoms include polyuria, hypotension, cardiovascular collapse, pulmonary edema, hyponatremia, hypokalemia, oliguria, and seizures. Increased electrolyte excretion and fluid overload can occur. Hemodialysis will clear mannitol and reduce osmolality.

Drug Interactions

Increased Effect/Toxicity: Lithium toxicity (with diuretic-induced hyponatremia).

Stability Should be stored at room temperature (15°C to 30°C) and protected from freezing; crystallization may occur at low temperatures; do not use solutions that contain crystals, heating in a hot water bath and vigorous shaking may be utilized for resolubilization; cool solutions to body temperature before using

Mechanism of Action Increases the osmotic pressure of glomerular filtrate, which inhibits tubular reabsorption of water and electrolytes and increases urinary output

Pharmacodynamics/Kinetics
Onset of action: Diuresis: Injection: 1-3 hours; Reduction in intracerebral pressure: ~15 minutes

Duration: Reduction in intracerebral pressure: 3-6 hours

Distribution: Remains confined to extracellular space (except in extreme concentrations); does not penetrate the blood-brain barrier

Metabolism: Minimal hepatic to glycogen

Half-life elimination: 1.1-1.6 hours

Excretion: Primarily urine (as unchanged drug)

Usual Dosage I.V.:
Children:
Test dose (to assess adequate renal function): 200 mg/kg over 3-5 minutes to produce a urine flow of at least 1 mL/kg for 1-3 hours

Initial: 0.5-1 g/kg

Maintenance: 0.25-0.5 g/kg given every 4-6 hours

Adults:
Test dose (to assess adequate renal function): 12.5 g (200 mg/kg) over 3-5 minutes to produce a urine flow of at least 30-50 mL of urine per hour over the next 2-3 hours

Initial: 0.5-1 g/kg

Maintenance: 0.25-0.5 g/kg every 4-6 hours; usual adult dose: 20-200 g/24 hours

Intracranial pressure: Cerebral edema: 1.5-2 g/kg/dose I.V. as a 15% to 20% solution over ≥30 minutes; maintain serum osmolality 310-320 mOsm/kg

Preoperative for neurosurgery: 1.5-2 g/kg administered 1-1.5 hours prior to surgery

Transurethral irrigation: Use urogenital solution as required for irrigation

Administration In-line 5-micron filter set should always be used for mannitol infusion with concentrations ≥20%; administer test dose (for oliguria) I.V. push over 3-5 minutes; for cerebral edema or elevated ICP, administer over 20-30 minutes

Monitoring Parameters Renal function, daily fluid I & O, serum electrolytes, serum and urine osmolality; for treatment of elevated intracranial pressure, maintain serum osmolality 310-320 mOsm/kg

Nursing Implications Avoid extravasation; crenation and agglutination of red blood cells may occur if administered with whole blood

Additional Information May autoclave or heat to redissolve crystals; mannitol 20% has an approximate osmolarity of 1100 mOsm/L and mannitol 25% has an approximate osmolarity of 1375 mOsm/L

Dosage Forms
Injection: 5% [50 mg/mL] (1000 mL); 10% [100 mg/mL] (500 mL, 1000 mL); 15% [150 mg/mL] (500 mL); 20% [200 mg/mL] (250 mL, 500 mL); 25% [250 mg/mL] (50 mL)

Solution, urogenital: 0.5% [5 mg/mL] (2000 mL); 0.54% [5.4 mg/mL with sorbitol 2.7 g/mL] (1500 mL, 3000 mL)

- ◆ **Mantoux** see Tuberculin Tests on page 1386
- ◆ **Mapap® [OTC]** see Acetaminophen on page 22
- ◆ **Mapap® Children's [OTC]** see Acetaminophen on page 22
- ◆ **Mapap® Extra Strength [OTC]** see Acetaminophen on page 22
- ◆ **Mapap® Infants [OTC]** see Acetaminophen on page 22

Maprotiline (ma PROE ti leen)

Related Information
Antidepressant Agents Comparison on page 1482

U.S. Brand Names Ludiomil®

Canadian Brand Names Ludiomil®; Novo-Maprotiline

Synonyms Maprotiline Hydrochloride

Therapeutic Category Antidepressant, Tetracyclic

Use Treatment of depression and anxiety associated with depression

Unlabeled/Investigational Use Bulimia; duodenal ulcers; enuresis; urinary symptoms of multiple sclerosis; pain; panic attacks; tension headache; cocaine withdrawal

Pregnancy Risk Factor B

Usual Dosage Oral:
Children 6-14 years: Depression/anxiety: 10 mg/day; increase to a maximum daily dose of 75 mg

Adults: Depression/anxiety: 75 mg/day to start, increase by 25 mg every 2 weeks up to 150-225 mg/day; given in 3 divided doses or in a single daily dose

Elderly: Depression/anxiety: Initial: 25 mg at bedtime, increase by 25 mg every 3 days for inpatients and weekly for outpatients if tolerated; usual maintenance dose: 50-75 mg/day, higher doses may be necessary in nonresponders

Additional Information Complete prescribing information for this medication should be consulted for additional detail.

Dosage Forms Tablet, as hydrochloride: 25 mg, 50 mg, 75 mg

- ◆ **Maprotiline Hydrochloride** see Maprotiline on page 839
- ◆ **Marcaine®** see Bupivacaine on page 190
- ◆ **Marcaine® Spinal** see Bupivacaine on page 190
- ◆ **Marcillin®** see Ampicillin on page 93
- ◆ **Margesic®** see Butalbital Compound on page 197
- ◆ **Margesic® H** see Hydrocodone and Acetaminophen on page 676
- ◆ **Marinol®** see Dronabinol on page 450
- ◆ **Marnal®** see Butalbital Compound on page 197
- ◆ **Marvelon® (Can)** see Ethinyl Estradiol and Desogestrel on page 510

Masoprocol (ma SOE pro kole)

U.S. Brand Names Actinex®

Therapeutic Category Topical Skin Product, Acne

Use Treatment of actinic keratosis

Pregnancy Risk Factor B

Contraindications Hypersensitivity to masoprocol or any component of the formulation

Adverse Reactions
>10%:
  Dermatologic: Erythema, flaking, dryness, itching
  Local: Burning
1% to 10%:
  Dermatologic: Soreness, rash, blistering, excoriation, skin roughness, wrinkling
  Neuromuscular & skeletal: Paresthesia
  Ocular: Eye irritation

Mechanism of Action Antiproliferative activity against keratinocytes

Pharmacodynamics/Kinetics Absorption: Topical: <1% to 2%

Usual Dosage Adults: Topical: Wash and dry area; gently massage into affected area every morning and evening for 28 days

Patient Information For external use only. Apply with gloves in thin film to thoroughly clean/dry skin; avoid area around eyes or mouth. Do not cover with occlusive dressing. Results make take some time to appear. May stain clothing or fabrics. You may experience transient stinging or burning after application. Report worsening of condition; eye irritation; or skin redness, dryness, peeling, or burning that persists between applications. Consult prescriber if breast-feeding.

Nursing Implications For external use only; may stain clothing or fabrics; avoid eyes and mucous membranes; do not use occlusive dressings; transient local burning sensation may occur immediately after application; contact physician if oozing or blistering occurs; wash hands immediately after use.

Dosage Forms Cream, topical: 10% (30 g)

Measles and Rubella Vaccines (Combined)
(MEE zels & roo BEL a vak SEENS, kom BINED)

Related Information
Adverse Events and Vaccination *on page 1553*
Immunization Recommendations *on page 1538*

U.S. Brand Names M-R-VAX® II

Canadian Brand Names MoRu-Viraten Berna™

Synonyms Rubella and Measles Vaccines, Combined

Therapeutic Category Vaccine

Use Simultaneous immunization against measles and rubella
  Note: Trivalent measles - mumps - rubella (MMR) vaccine is the preferred immunizing agent for most children and many adults. Adults born before 1957 are generally considered to be immune and need not be revaccinated.

Pregnancy Risk Factor C

Contraindications Hypersensitivity to neomycin or any component of the formulation; immune deficiency condition; pregnancy

Warnings/Precautions Immunocompromised persons, history of anaphylactic reaction following receipt of neomycin

Adverse Reactions All serious adverse reactions must be reported to the U.S. Department of Health and Human Services (DHHS) Vaccine Adverse Event Reporting System (VAERS) 1-800-822-7967.
>10%:
  Cardiovascular: Edema
  Central nervous system: Fever (<100°F)
  Local: Burning or stinging, induration

1% to 10%:
Central nervous system: Fever between 100°F and 103°F usually between 5th and 12th days postvaccination
Dermatologic: Rash (rarely generalized)

<1% (Limited to important or life-threatening): Allergic reactions, ataxia, confusion, convulsions, coryza, cough, diarrhea, diplopia, dyspnea, encephalitis, erythema multiforme, fatigue, fever (>103°F - prolonged), Guillain-Barré syndrome, headache (severe), itching, lymphadenopathy, palsies, reddening of skin (especially around ears and eyes), rhinitis, sore throat, stiff neck, thrombocytopenic purpura, urticaria, vomiting

Stability Refrigerate prior to use, use as soon as possible; discard if not used within 8 hours of reconstitution

Mechanism of Action Promotes active immunity to measles and rubella by inducing specific antibodies including measles-specific IgG and IgM and rubella hemagglutination-inhibiting antibodies.

Usual Dosage Children at 15 months and Adults: S.C.: Inject 0.5 mL into outer aspect of upper arm; no routine booster for rubella

Administration Not for I.V. administration

Test Interactions May temporarily depress tuberculin skin test sensitivity and reduce the seroconversion.

Patient Information Parents should monitor children closely for fever 5-11 days after vaccination; females should not become pregnant within 3 months of vaccination

Additional Information Contains 25 mcg neomycin per dose

Federal law requires that the date of administration, the vaccine manufacturer, lot number of vaccine, and the administering person's name, title, and address be entered into the patient's permanent medical record

Adults born before 1957 are generally considered to be immune to measles; all born in or after 1957 without documentation of live vaccine on or after first birthday, physician-diagnosed measles, or laboratory evidence of immunity should be vaccinated with two doses separated by or less than 1 month. For those previously vaccinated with one dose of measles vaccine, revaccination is indicated for students entering institutions of higher learning, for healthcare workers at time of employment, and for travelers to endemic areas. Guidelines for rubella vaccination are the same with the exception of birth year. All adults should be vaccinated against rubella. A booster dose of rubella vaccine is not necessary. Women who are pregnant when vaccinated or become pregnant within 3 months of vaccination should be consulted on the risks to the fetus; although the risks appear negligible. MMR is the vaccine of choice if recipients are likely to be susceptible to mumps as well as measles and rubella.

Dosage Forms Injection: 1000 TCID$_{50}$ each of live attenuated measles virus vaccine and live rubella virus vaccine

Measles, Mumps, and Rubella Vaccines (Combined)
(MEE zels, mumpz & roo BEL a vak SEENS, kom BINED)

Related Information
Adverse Events and Vaccination *on page 1553*
Immunization Recommendations *on page 1538*
Recommendations of the Advisory Committee on Immunization Practices (ACIP) *on page 1540*
Recommended Childhood Immunization Schedule - US - 2002 *on page 1539*
Recommended Immunization Schedule for HIV-Infected Children *on page 1543*
USPHA/IDSA Guidelines for the Prevention of Opportunistic Infections in Persons With HIV *on page 1574*

U.S. Brand Names M-M-R® II

Canadian Brand Names M-M-R® II; Priorix™

Synonyms MMR; Mumps, Measles and Rubella Vaccines, Combined; Rubella, Measles and Mumps Vaccines, Combined

Therapeutic Category Vaccine

Use Measles, mumps, and rubella prophylaxis

Pregnancy Risk Factor C

Pregnancy/Breast-Feeding Implications Animal reproduction studies have not been conducted. It is not known whether the drug can cause fetal harm or affect reproduction capacity (contracting natural measles during pregnancy can increase fetal risk). Do not administer to pregnant females, and avoid pregnancy for 28 days following vaccination. It is not known if measles or mumps virus vaccines enter breast milk; use caution in breast-feeding. Rubella virus vaccine enters breast milk; use caution in breast-feeding.

Contraindications Hypersensitivity to measles, mumps, and rubella vaccine or any component of the formulation; hypersensitivity to neomycin or gelatin; current febrile respiratory illness or other febrile infection; severely immunocompromised persons; blood dyscrasias, cancers affecting the bone marrow or lymphatic systems; children with active untreated tuberculosis; pregnancy

Warnings/Precautions
Females should not become pregnant within 28 days of vaccination
MMR vaccine should not be given within 3 months of immune globulin or whole blood
MMR vaccine should not be administered to severely immunocompromised persons with the exception of asymptomatic children with HIV (ACIP and AAP recommendation)
Severely immunocompromised patients and symptomatic HIV-infected patients who are exposed to measles should receive immune globulin, regardless of prior vaccination status
The immunogenicity of measles virus vaccine is decreased if vaccine is administered <6 months after immune globulin
Defer immunization during any acute illness
Use caution with history of cerebral injury, convulsions, or other conditions where stress due to fever should be avoided. Use caution in patients with thrombocytopenia and those who develop thrombocytopenia after first dose; thrombocytopenia may worsen.
(Continued)

Measles, Mumps, and Rubella Vaccines (Combined) *(Continued)*

Adverse Reactions All serious adverse reactions must be reported to the U.S. Department of Health and Human Services (DHHS) Vaccine Adverse Event Reporting System (VAERS) 1-800-822-7967.

Frequency not defined:

Cardiovascular: Syncope, vasculitis

Central nervous system: Ataxia, dizziness, febrile convulsions, fever, encephalitis, encephalopathy, Guillain-Barré syndrome, headache, irritability, malaise, measles inclusion body encephalitis, polyneuritis, polyneuropathy, seizures, subacute sclerosing panencephalitis,

Dermatologic: Angioneurotic edema, erythema multiforme, purpura, rash, Stevens-Johnson syndrome, urticaria

Endocrine & metabolic: Diabetes mellitus

Gastrointestinal: Diarrhea, nausea, orchitis, pancreatitis, parotitis, sore throat, vomiting

Hematologic: Leukocytosis, thrombocytopenia

Local: Injection site reactions which include burning, induration, redness, stinging, swelling, tenderness, wheal and flare, vesiculation

Neuromuscular & skeletal: Arthralgia/arthritis (variable; highest rates in women, 12% to 26% versus children, up to 3%), myalgia, paresthesia

Ocular: Ocular palsies

Otic: Otitis media

Renal: Conjunctivitis, retinitis, optic neuritis, papillitis, retrobulbar neuritis

Respiratory: Bronchospasm, cough, pneumonitis, rhinitis

Miscellaneous: Anaphylactoid reactions, anaphylaxis, atypical measles, panniculitis, regional lymphadenopathy

Drug Interactions

Decreased Effect: The effect of the vaccine may be decreased in individuals who are receiving immunosuppressant drugs (including high dose systemic corticosteroids). Effect of vaccine may be decreased when given with immune globulin; do not administer with vaccine. Effectiveness of MMR may be decreased if given within 30 days of varicella vaccine (effectiveness not decreased when administered simultaneously).

Stability Prior to reconstitution, store the powder at 2°C to 8°C (36°F to 46°F) or colder (freezing does not affect potency). Protect from light. Diluent may be stored with powder or at room temperature. Use entire contents of the provided diluent to reconstitute vaccine. Gently agitate to mix thoroughly. Discard if powder does not dissolve. Use as soon as possible following reconstitution (may be stored at 2°C to 8°C/36°F to 46°F; protect from light); discard if not used within 8 hours.

Mechanism of Action As a live, attenuated vaccine, MMR vaccine offers active immunity to disease caused by the measles, mumps, and rubella viruses.

Usual Dosage S.C.:

Infants <12 months: If there is risk of exposure to measles, single-antigen measles vaccine should be administered at 6-11 months of age with a second dose (of MMR) at >12 months of age.

Children ≥12 months: 0.5 mL at 12 months and then repeated at 4-6 years of age. If the second dose was not received, the schedule should be completed by the 11- to 12-year old visit. Administer in outer aspect of the upper arm. Recommended age of primary immunization is 12-15 months; revaccination is recommended prior to elementary school.

Administration Administer S.C. in outer aspect of the upper arm. **Not for I.V. administration.** Federal law requires that the date of administration, the vaccine manufacturer, lot number of vaccine, and the administering person's name, title and address be entered into the patient's permanent medical record.

Test Interactions Temporary suppression of TB skin test reactivity with onset approximately 3 days after administration

Patient Information Females should not become pregnant within 28 days of vaccination

Nursing Implications Federal law requires that the date of administration, the vaccine manufacturer, lot number of vaccine, and the administering person's name, title and address be entered into the patient's permanent medical record

Additional Information Adults born before 1957 are generally considered to be immune to measles and mumps; all born in or after 1957 without documentation of live vaccine on or after first birthday, physician-diagnosed measles or mumps, or laboratory evidence of immunity should be vaccine with two doses separated by no less than 1 month; for those previously vaccinated with one dose of measles vaccine, revaccination is indicated for students entering institutions of higher learning, healthcare workers at time of employment, and for travelers to endemic areas. Guidelines for rubella vaccination are the same with the exception of birth year; all adults should be vaccinated against rubella. Booster doses of mumps and rubella are not necessary; women who are pregnant when vaccinated or become pregnant within 28 days should be counseled on the risks to the fetus; although the risks appear negligible.

Using separate sites and syringes, MMR may be administered concurrently with DTaP or *Haemophilus* b conjugate vaccine (PedvaxHIB®). Varicella vaccine may be administered with MMR using separate sites and syringes; however, if not administered simultaneously, doses should be separated by at least 30 days. Unless otherwise specified, MMR should be given 1 month before or 1 month after live viral vaccines.

Dosage Forms Powder for injection [preservative free]: 1000 TCID$_{50}$ each of measles virus and rubella virus, and 20,000 TCID$_{50}$ mumps virus [contains neomycin 25 mcg, gelatin, human albumin; produced in chick embryo cell culture]

Measles Virus Vaccine (Live) (MEE zels VYE rus vak SEEN, live)

Related Information

Adverse Events and Vaccination *on page 1553*

Immunization Recommendations *on page 1538*

U.S. Brand Names Attenuvax®

Synonyms More Attenuated Enders Strain; Rubeola Vaccine

Therapeutic Category Vaccine, Live Virus

Use Adults born before 1957 are generally considered to be immune. All those born in or after 1957 without documentation of live vaccine on or after first birthday, physician-diagnosed measles, or laboratory evidence of immunity should be vaccinated, ideally with two doses of vaccine separated by no less than 1 month. For those previously vaccinated with one dose of measles vaccine, revaccination is recommended for students entering colleges and other institutions of higher education, for healthcare workers at the time of employment, and for international travelers who visit endemic areas.

MMR is the vaccine of choice if recipients are likely to be susceptible to rubella and/or mumps as well as to measles. Persons vaccinated between 1963 and 1967 with a killed measles vaccine, followed by live vaccine within 3 months, or with a vaccine of unknown type should be revaccinated with live measles virus vaccine.

Pregnancy Risk Factor X

Contraindications Hypersensitivity to neomycin or any component of the formulation; acute respiratory infections, activated tuberculosis, immunosuppressed patients; pregnancy; known anaphylactoid reaction to eggs

Warnings/Precautions Avoid use in immunocompromised patients; defer administration in presence of acute respiratory or other active infections or inactive, untreated tuberculosis; avoid pregnancy for 3 months following vaccination; history of febrile seizures, hypersensitivity reactions may occur

Adverse Reactions All serious adverse reactions must be reported to the U.S. Department of Health and Human Services (DHHS) Vaccine Adverse Event Reporting System (VAERS) 1-800-822-7967.

>10%:
  Cardiovascular: Edema
  Central nervous system: Fever (<100°F)
  Local: Burning or stinging, induration
1% to 10%:
  Central nervous system: Fever between 100°F and 103°F usually between 5th and 12th days postvaccination
  Dermatologic: Rash (rarely generalized)
<1% (Limited to important or life-threatening): Allergic reactions, ataxia, confusion, convulsions, coryza, cough, diarrhea, diplopia, dyspnea, encephalitis, erythema multiforme, fatigue, fever (>103°F - prolonged), Guillain-Barré syndrome, headache (severe), itching, lymphadenopathy, palsies, reddening of skin (especially around ears and eyes), rhinitis, sore throat, stiff neck, thrombocytopenic purpura, urticaria, vomiting

Stability Refrigerate at 2°C to 8°C (36°F to 46°F); discard if left at room temperature for over 8 hours; protect from light

Mechanism of Action Promotes active immunity to measles virus by inducing specific measles IgG and IgM antibodies.

Usual Dosage Children ≥15 months and Adults: S.C.: 0.5 mL in outer aspect of the upper arm, no routine boosters

Administration Vaccine should not be administered I.V.; S.C. injection preferred

Test Interactions May temporarily depress tuberculin skin test sensitivity

Patient Information Parents should monitor children closely for fever for 5-11 days after vaccination; females should not become pregnant within 3 months of vaccination

Nursing Implications Vaccine should not be administered I.V.; S.C. injection preferred with a 25-gauge ⅝" needle

Additional Information Contains 25 mcg neomycin per dose. Federal law requires that the date of administration, the vaccine manufacturer, lot number of vaccine, and the administering person's name, title, and address be entered into the patient's permanent medical record.

Dosage Forms Injection: 1000 TCID$_{50}$ per dose

♦ **Mebaral**® *see* Mephobarbital *on page 860*

Mebendazole (me BEN da zole)

U.S. Brand Names Vermox®

Canadian Brand Names Vermox®

Therapeutic Category Anthelmintic

Use Treatment of pinworms (*Enterobius vermicularis*), whipworms (*Trichuris trichiura*), roundworms (*Ascaris lumbricoides*), and hookworms (*Ancylostoma duodenale*)

Pregnancy Risk Factor C

Contraindications Hypersensitivity to mebendazole or any component of the formulation

Warnings/Precautions Pregnancy and children <2 years of age are relative contraindications since safety has not been established; not effective for hydatid disease

Adverse Reactions Frequency not defined.
  Cardiovascular: Angioedema
  Central nervous system: Fever, dizziness, headache, seizures
  Dermatologic: Rash, itching, alopecia (with high doses)
  Gastrointestinal: Abdominal pain, diarrhea, nausea, vomiting
  Hematologic: Neutropenia (sore throat, unusual fatigue)
  Neuromuscular & skeletal: Unusual weakness

Overdosage/Toxicology Symptoms include abdominal pain and altered mental status. Treatment is GI decontamination and supportive care.

Drug Interactions
  Decreased Effect: Anticonvulsants such as carbamazepine and phenytoin may increase metabolism of mebendazole

Ethanol/Nutrition/Herb Interactions Food: Mebendazole serum levels may be increased if taken with food.

Mechanism of Action Selectively and irreversibly blocks glucose uptake and other nutrients in susceptible adult intestine-dwelling helminths

(Continued)

Mebendazole *(Continued)*

Pharmacodynamics/Kinetics

Absorption: 2% to 10%

Distribution: To serum, cyst fluid, liver, omental fat, and pelvic, pulmonary, and hepatic cysts; highest concentrations found in liver; relatively high concentrations found in muscle-encysted *Trichinella spiralis* larvae; crosses placenta

Protein binding: 95%

Metabolism: Extensively hepatic

Half-life elimination: 1-11.5 hours

Time to peak, serum: 2-4 hours

Excretion: Primarily feces; urine (5% to 10%)

Usual Dosage Children and Adults: Oral:

Pinworms: 100 mg as a single dose; may need to repeat after 2 weeks; treatment should include family members in close contact with patient

Whipworms, roundworms, hookworms: One tablet twice daily, morning and evening on 3 consecutive days; if patient is not cured within 3-4 weeks, a second course of treatment may be administered

Capillariasis: 200 mg twice daily for 20 days

Dosing adjustment in hepatic impairment: Dosage reduction may be necessary in patients with liver dysfunction

Hemodialysis: Not dialyzable (0% to 5%)

Dietary Considerations Tablet can be crushed and mixed with food, swallowed whole, or chewed.

Monitoring Parameters Check for helminth ova in feces within 3-4 weeks following the initial therapy

Patient Information Tablets may be chewed, swallowed whole, or crushed and mixed with food; hygienic precautions should be taken to prevent reinfection such as wearing shoes and washing hands

Nursing Implications Monitor for helminth ova in feces within 3-4 weeks following the initial therapy

Dosage Forms Tablet, chewable: 100 mg

Mecamylamine (mek a MIL a meen)

U.S. Brand Names Inversine®

Canadian Brand Names Inversine®

Synonyms Mecamylamine Hydrochloride

Therapeutic Category Antihypertensive Agent; Ganglionic Blocking Agent

Use Treatment of moderately severe to severe hypertension and in uncomplicated malignant hypertension

Unlabeled/Investigational Use Tourette's syndrome

Pregnancy Risk Factor C

Contraindications Coronary insufficiency, pyloric stenosis, glaucoma, uremia, recent myocardial infarction, unreliable, uncooperative patients

Warnings/Precautions Use with caution in patients receiving sulfonamides or antibiotics that cause neuromuscular blockade; use with caution in patients with impaired renal function, previous CNS abnormalities, prostatic hyperplasia, bladder obstruction, or urethral strictive; do not abruptly discontinue

Adverse Reactions Frequency not defined.

Cardiovascular: Postural hypotension

Central nervous system: Drowsiness, convulsions, confusion, mental depression

Endocrine & metabolic: Sexual ability decreased

Gastrointestinal: Xerostomia, loss of appetite, nausea, vomiting, bloating; frequent stools followed by severe constipation

Genitourinary: Dysuria

Neuromuscular & skeletal: Uncontrolled movements of hands, arms, legs, or face; trembling

Ocular: Blurred vision; enlarged pupils

Respiratory: Dyspnea

Overdosage/Toxicology Symptoms include hypotension, nausea, vomiting, urinary retention, and constipation. Signs and symptoms are a directly result of ganglionic blockade. Treatment is supportive. Pressor amines may be used to correct hypotension. Use caution as patients will be unusually sensitive to these agents.

Drug Interactions

Increased Effect/Toxicity: Sulfonamides and antibiotics that cause neuromuscular blockade may increase effect of mecamylamine. The action of mecamylamine may be increased by anesthesia, other antihypertensives, and alcohol.

Mechanism of Action Mecamylamine is a ganglionic blocker. This agent inhibits acetylcholine at the autonomic ganglia, causing a decrease in blood pressure. Mecamylamine also blocks central nicotinic cholinergic receptors, which inhibits the effects of nicotine and may suppress the desire to smoke.

Usual Dosage Adults: Oral: 2.5 mg twice daily after meals for 2 days; increased by increments of 2.5 mg at intervals ≥2 days until desired blood pressure response is achieved; average daily dose: 25 mg (usually in 3 divided doses)

Note: Reduce dosage of other antihypertensives when combined with mecamylamine with exception of thiazide diuretics which may be maintained at usual dose while decreasing mecamylamine by 50%

Dosing adjustment/comments in renal impairment: Use with caution, if at all, although no specific guidelines are available

Dietary Considerations Should be taken after meals.

Patient Information Take after meals at the same time each day; notify physician immediately if frequent loose bowel movements occur; rise slowly from sitting or lying for prolonged periods; do not restrict salt intake

Nursing Implications Check frequently for orthostatic hypotension; aid with ambulation

Dosage Forms Tablet, as hydrochloride: 2.5 mg

♦ **Mecamylamine Hydrochloride** *see* Mecamylamine *on page 844*

Mechlorethamine (me klor ETH a meen)

U.S. Brand Names Mustargen®
Canadian Brand Names Mustargen®
Synonyms HN$_2$; Mechlorethamine Hydrochloride; Mustine; Nitrogen Mustard
Therapeutic Category Antineoplastic Agent, Alkylating Agent; Antineoplastic Agent, Nitrogen Mustard; Vesicant
Use Combination therapy of Hodgkin's disease and malignant lymphomas; non-Hodgkin's lymphoma; palliative treatment of bronchogenic, breast and ovarian carcinoma; may be used by intracavitary injection for treatment of metastatic tumors; pleural and other malignant effusions; topical treatment of mycosis fungoides
Pregnancy Risk Factor D
Contraindications Hypersensitivity to mechlorethamine or any component of the formulation; pre-existing profound myelosuppression or infection; pregnancy
Warnings/Precautions The U.S. Food and Drug Administration (FDA) currently recommends that procedures for proper handling and disposal of antineoplastic agents be considered. Extravasation of the drug into subcutaneous tissues results in painful inflammation and induration; sloughing may occur. Patients with lymphoma should receive prophylactic allopurinol 2-3 days prior to therapy to prevent complications resulting from tumor lysis.
Adverse Reactions
>10%:
  Endocrine & metabolic: Delayed menses, oligomenorrhea, temporary or permanent amenorrhea, impaired spermatogenesis; spermatogenesis may return in patients in remission several years after the discontinuation of chemotherapy, chromosomal abnormalities
  Gastrointestinal: Nausea and vomiting usually occur in nearly 100% of patients and onset is within 30 minutes to 2 hours after administration
  Emetic potential: High (>90%)
  Time course of nausea/vomiting: Onset: 1-3 hours; duration 2-8 hours
  Genitourinary: Azoospermia
  Hematologic: Myelosuppressive: Leukopenia and thrombocytopenia can be severe; caution should be used with patients who are receiving radiotherapy, secondary leukemia
    WBC: Severe
    Platelets: Severe
    Onset (days): 4-7
    Nadir (days): 14
    Recovery (days): 21
  Otic: Ototoxicity
  Miscellaneous: Precipitation of herpes zoster
1% to 10%:
  Central nervous system: Fever, vertigo
  Dermatologic: Alopecia
  Endocrine & metabolic: Hyperuricemia
  Gastrointestinal: Diarrhea, anorexia, metallic taste
  Local: Thrombophlebitis/extravasation: May cause local vein discomfort which may be relieved by warm soaks and pain medication. A brown discoloration of veins may occur. Mechlorethamine is a strong vesicant and can cause tissue necrosis and sloughing.
    Vesicant chemotherapy
  Secondary malignancies: Have been reported after several years in 1% to 6% of patients treated
  Neuromuscular & skeletal: Weakness
  Otic: Tinnitus
  Miscellaneous: Hypersensitivity, anaphylaxis
<1% (Limited to important or life-threatening): Hemolytic anemia, hepatotoxicity, myelosuppression, peripheral neuropathy
Overdosage/Toxicology Signs and symptoms include suppression of all formed elements of the blood, uric acid crystals, nausea, vomiting, and diarrhea. Sodium thiosulfate is the specific antidote for nitrogen mustard extravasations. Treatment of systemic overdose is supportive.
Drug Interactions
  Decreased Effect: Patients may experience impaired immune response to vaccines; possible infection after administration of live vaccines in patients receiving immunosuppressants.
Ethanol/Nutrition/Herb Interactions Ethanol: Avoid ethanol (due to GI irritation).
Stability Store intact vials at room temperature (15°C to 30°C/59°F to 86°F). The manufacturer reports that reconstituted solutions are stable for 15 minutes; other sources suggest the drug may be stable for 1-4 hours, particularly in nonacidic solutions. Extemporaneous formulations for topical use have been reported to retain biologic activity for 30 days.

  Standard I.V. dilution:
    I.V. push: Dose/syringe (concentration is 1 mg/mL)
      Maximum syringe for IVP is 30 mL and syringe should be ≤75% full
    Must be prepared fresh; solution is stable for only 1 hour after dilution and must be administered within that time period
Mechanism of Action Alkylating agent that inhibits DNA and RNA synthesis via formation of carbonium ions; cross-links strands of DNA, causing miscoding, breakage, and failure of replication; produces interstrand and intrastrand cross-links in DNA resulting in miscoding, breakage, and failure of replication
Pharmacodynamics/Kinetics
  Duration: Unchanged drug is undetectable in blood within a few minutes
  Absorption: Intracavitary administration: Incomplete secondary to rapid deactivation by body fluids
(Continued)

845

Mechlorethamine *(Continued)*

Metabolism: Rapid hydrolysis and demethylation, possibly in plasma

Half-life elimination: <1 minute

Excretion: Urine (<0.01% as unchanged drug)

Usual Dosage Refer to individual protocols.

Children and Adults: I.V.: 6 mg/m^2 on days 1 and 8 of a 28-day cycle (MOPP regimen)

Adults:

I.V.: 0.4 mg/kg **or** 12-16 mg/m^2 for one dose **or** divided into 0.1 mg/kg/day for 4 days, repeated at 4- to 6-week intervals

Intracavitary: 0.2-0.4 mg/kg (10-20 mg) as a single dose; may be repeated if fluid continues to accumulate.

Intrapericardially: 0.2-0.4 mg/kg as a single dose; may be repeated if fluid continues to accumulate.

Topical: 0.01% to 0.02% solution, lotion, or ointment

Hemodialysis: Not removed; supplemental dosing is not required.

Peritoneal dialysis: Not removed; supplemental dosing is not required.

Administration I.V. as a slow push through the side of a freely flowing saline or dextrose solution. Due to the limited stability of the drug, and the increased risk of phlebitis and venous irritation and blistering with increased contact time, infusions of the drug are not recommended.

Monitoring Parameters CBC with differential, hemoglobin, and platelet count

Patient Information This medication can only be given by infusion, usually in cycles of therapy. You will need frequent laboratory and medical monitoring during treatment. Do not use alcohol, aspirin or aspirin-containing medications, and/or OTC medications without consulting prescriber. Maintain adequate fluid balance (2-3 L/day of fluids unless instructed to restrict fluid intake) and adequate nutrition (small frequent meals, frequent mouth care, sucking lozenges, or chewing gum may reduce anorexia and nausea). May cause discoloration (brown color) of veins used for infusion; hair loss (reversible); easy bleeding or bruising (use soft toothbrush or cotton swabs and frequent mouth care, use electric razor, avoid sharp knives or scissors); increased susceptibility to infection (avoid crowds or exposure to infection - do not have any vaccinations unless approved by prescriber). This drug may cause menstrual irregularities, permanent sterility, and birth defects. Report changes in auditory or visual acuity; unusual bleeding or bruising or persistent fever or sore throat; blood in urine, stool, or vomitus; delayed healing of any wounds; skin rash; yellowing of skin or eyes; changes in color of urine of stool; acute or unresolved nausea or vomiting; diarrhea; or loss of appetite. The drug may be excreted in breast milk, therefore, an alternative form of feeding your baby should be used. Contraceptive measures are recommended during therapy.

Nursing Implications Use within 1 hour of preparation; avoid extravasation since mechlorethamine is a potent vesicant

Extravasation treatment: Sodium thiosulfate $\frac{1}{8}$ molar solution is the specific antidote for nitrogen mustard extravasations and should be used as follows: Mix 4 mL of 10% sodium thiosulfate with 6 mL of sterile water for injection; inject 5-6 mL of this solution into the existing I.V. line; remove the needle; inject 2-3 mL of the solution S.C. clockwise into the infiltrated area using a 25-gauge needle; change the needle with each new injection; apply ice immediately for 6-12 hours.

Dosage Forms Powder for injection, as hydrochloride: 10 mg

♦ **Mechlorethamine Hydrochloride** *see Mechlorethamine on page 845*

Meclizine *(MEK li zeen)*

U.S. Brand Names Antivert®; Antrizine®; Bonine® [OTC]; Dizmiss® [OTC]; Dramamine® II [OTC]; Meni-D®; Vergon® [OTC]

Canadian Brand Names Antivert®; Bonamine™; Bonine®

Synonyms Meclizine Hydrochloride; Meclozine Hydrochloride

Therapeutic Category Antiemetic; Antihistamine, H$_1$ Blocker

Use Prevention and treatment of symptoms of motion sickness; management of vertigo with diseases affecting the vestibular system

Pregnancy Risk Factor B

Pregnancy/Breast-Feeding Implications

Clinical effects on the fetus: No data available on crossing the placenta. Probably no effect on the fetus (insufficient data). Available evidence suggests safe use during pregnancy.

Breast-feeding/lactation: No data available

Contraindications Hypersensitivity to meclizine or any component of the formulation

Warnings/Precautions Use with caution in patients with angle-closure glaucoma, prostatic hyperplasia, pyloric or duodenal obstruction, or bladder neck obstruction; use with caution in hot weather, and during exercise; elderly may be at risk for anticholinergic side effects such as glaucoma, prostatic hyperplasia, constipation, gastrointestinal obstructive disease; if vertigo does not respond in 1-2 weeks, it is advised to discontinue use

Adverse Reactions

>10%:

Central nervous system: Slight to moderate drowsiness

Respiratory: Thickening of bronchial secretions

1% to 10%:

Central nervous system: Headache, fatigue, nervousness, dizziness

Gastrointestinal: Appetite increase, weight gain, nausea, diarrhea, abdominal pain, dry mouth

Neuromuscular & skeletal: Arthralgia

Respiratory: Pharyngitis

<1% (Limited to important or life-threatening): Bronchospasm, hepatitis, hypotension, palpitations

Overdosage/Toxicology Symptoms include CNS depression, confusion, nervousness, hallucinations, dizziness, blurred vision, nausea, vomiting, and hyperthermia. There is no specific treatment for antihistamine overdose, however, clinical toxicity is mostly due to anticholinergic effects. For anticholinergic overdose with severe life-threatening symptoms, physostigmine 1-2 mg (0.5 mg or 0.02 mg/kg for children) slow I.V. may be given to reverse these effects.

Drug Interactions
  Increased Effect/Toxicity: Increased toxicity with CNS depressants, neuroleptics, and anticholinergics.

Ethanol/Nutrition/Herb Interactions Ethanol: Avoid ethanol (may increase CNS depression).

Mechanism of Action Has central anticholinergic action by blocking chemoreceptor trigger zone; decreases excitability of the middle ear labyrinth and blocks conduction in the middle ear vestibular-cerebellar pathways

Pharmacodynamics/Kinetics
  Onset of action: ~1 hour
  Duration: 8-24 hours
  Metabolism: Hepatic
  Half-life elimination: 6 hours
  Excretion: Urine (as metabolites); feces (as unchanged drug)

Usual Dosage Children >12 years and Adults: Oral:
  Motion sickness: 12.5-25 mg 1 hour before travel, repeat dose every 12-24 hours if needed; doses up to 50 mg may be needed
  Vertigo: 25-100 mg/day in divided doses

Patient Information Take after meals; do not discontinue drug abruptly; notify physician if adverse GI effects, fever, or heat intolerance occurs; may cause drowsiness; avoid alcohol; adequate fluid intake, sugar free gum, or hard candy may help dry mouth; adequate fluid and exercise may help constipation; may impair ability to perform hazardous tasks

Dosage Forms
  Capsule, as hydrochloride: 25 mg, 30 mg
  Tablet, as hydrochloride: 12.5 mg, 25 mg, 50 mg
  Tablet, chewable, as hydrochloride: 25 mg

♦ **Meclizine Hydrochloride** *see* Meclizine *on page 846*

Meclocycline (me kloe SYE kleen)
Synonyms Meclocycline Sulfosalicylate
Therapeutic Category Antibiotic, Topical; Topical Skin Product, Acne
Use Topical treatment of inflammatory acne vulgaris
Pregnancy Risk Factor B
Contraindications Hypersensitivity to tetracyclines or any component of the formulation
Warnings/Precautions Use with caution in patients allergic to formaldehyde; for external use only

Adverse Reactions
  >10%: Topical: Follicular staining, yellowing of the skin, burning/stinging feeling
  1% to 10%: Topical: Pain, redness, skin irritation, dermatitis

Mechanism of Action Inhibits bacterial protein synthesis by binding with the 30S and possibly the 50S ribosomal subunit(s) of susceptible bacteria; may also cause alterations in the cytoplasmic membrane

Pharmacodynamics/Kinetics Absorption: Very little

Usual Dosage Children >11 years and Adults: Topical: Apply generously to affected areas twice daily

Patient Information Apply generously until skin is wet; avoid contact with eyes, nose, and mouth; stinging may occur with application, but soon stops; if skin is discolored yellow, washing will remove the color

Nursing Implications Apply generously until skin is wet; avoid contact with eyes, nose, and mouth; stinging may occur with application, but soon stops; if skin is discolored yellow, washing will remove the color

Dosage Forms Cream, topical, as sulfosalicylate: 1% (20 g, 45 g)

♦ **Meclocycline Sulfosalicylate** *see* Meclocycline *on page 847*

Meclofenamate (me kloe fen AM ate)
Related Information
  Nonsteroidal Anti-Inflammatory Agents Comparison *on page 1512*
Canadian Brand Names Meclomen®
Synonyms Meclofenamate Sodium
Therapeutic Category Analgesic, Nonsteroidal Anti-inflammatory Drug; Anti-inflammatory Agent; Nonsteroidal Anti-inflammatory Drug (NSAID), Oral
Use Treatment of inflammatory disorders, arthritis, mild to moderate pain, dysmenorrhea
Pregnancy Risk Factor B/D (3rd trimester)
Contraindications Hypersensitivity to nonsteroidal anti-inflammatory drugs (NSAIDs) including aspirin, meclofenamate, or any component of the formulation; active GI bleeding, ulcer disease; pregnancy (3rd trimester)
Warnings/Precautions Use with caution in patients with congestive heart failure, hypertension, dehydration, decreased renal or hepatic function, history of GI disease (bleeding or ulcers), or those receiving anticoagulants. Elderly are at a high risk for adverse effects from nonsteroidal anti-inflammatory agents. As many as 60% of elderly can develop peptic ulceration and/or hemorrhage asymptomatically.

Use lowest effective dose for shortest period possible. Use of NSAIDs can compromise existing renal function especially when Cl_{cr} is <30 mL/minute. CNS adverse effects such as confusion, agitation, and hallucination are generally seen in overdose or high-dose situations; however, elderly may demonstrate these adverse effects at lower doses than younger adults. Withhold for at least 4-6 half-lives prior to surgical or dental procedures. May have adverse effects on fetus. Use with caution with dehydration. Use in children is not recommended.
(Continued)

Meclofenamate *(Continued)*

Adverse Reactions
>10%:
  Central nervous system: Dizziness
  Dermatologic: Skin rash
  Gastrointestinal: Abdominal cramps, heartburn, indigestion, nausea
1% to 10%:
  Central nervous system: Headache, nervousness
  Dermatologic: Itching
  Endocrine & metabolic: Fluid retention
  Gastrointestinal: Vomiting
  Otic: Tinnitus
<1% (Limited to important or life-threatening): Acute renal failure, agranulocytosis, angioe-
    dema, arrhythmias, aseptic meningitis, bone marrow suppression, confusion, congestive
    heart failure, dyspnea, erythema multiforme, GI ulceration, hallucinations, hemolytic
    anemia, hepatitis, leukopenia, mental depression, peripheral neuropathy, somnolence,
    Stevens-Johnson syndrome, tachycardia, thrombocytopenia, toxic amblyopia, toxic
    epidermal necrolysis, urticaria

Overdosage/Toxicology Symptoms include drowsiness, lethargy, nausea, vomiting,
  seizures, paresthesia, headache, dizziness, GI bleeding, cerebral edema, cardiac arrest, and
  tinnitus. Management of nonsteroidal anti-inflammatory drug (NSAID) intoxication is primarily
  supportive and symptomatic. Fluid therapy is commonly effective in managing hypotension
  that may occur following an acute NSAID overdose, except when due to acute blood loss.
  Seizures tend to be very short-lived and often do not require drug treatment, although
  recurrent seizures should be treated with I.V. diazepam. Since many of NSAIDs undergo
  enterohepatic cycling, multiple doses of charcoal may be needed to reduce the potential for
  delayed toxicities.

Drug Interactions
Increased Effect/Toxicity: Anticoagulants (warfarin, heparin, LMWHs) in combination with
  NSAIDs can cause increased risk of bleeding. Other antiplatelet drugs (ticlopidine,
  clopidogrel, aspirin, abciximab, dipyridamole, eptifibatide, tirofiban) can cause an
  increased risk of bleeding. NSAIDs may increase serum creatinine, potassium, blood
  pressure, and cyclosporine levels during concurrent therapy; monitor cyclosporine levels
  and renal function carefully. Lithium levels can be increased; avoid concurrent use if
  possible or monitor lithium levels and adjust dose. Sulindac may have the least effect.
  When NSAID is stopped, lithium will need adjustment again. Corticosteroids may increase
  the risk of GI ulceration; avoid concurrent use.

Decreased Effect: Antihypertensive effects of ACE-inhibitors, angiotensin antagonists,
  diuretics, and hydralazine may be decreased by concurrent therapy with NSAIDs; monitor
  blood pressure. Cholestyramine and colestipol reduce the bioavailability of diclofenac;
  separate administration times.

Ethanol/Nutrition/Herb Interactions Ethanol: Avoid ethanol (due to GI irritation).

Mechanism of Action Inhibits prostaglandin synthesis by decreasing the activity of the
  enzyme, cyclo-oxygenase, which results in decreased formation of prostaglandin precursors

Pharmacodynamics/Kinetics
Duration: 2-4 hours
Distribution: Crosses placenta
Protein binding: 99%
Half-life elimination: 2-3.3 hours
Time to peak, serum: 0.5-1.5 hours
Excretion: Primarily urine and feces (as metabolites)

Usual Dosage Children >14 years and Adults: Oral:
  Mild to moderate pain: 50 mg every 4-6 hours, not to exceed 400 mg/day
  Rheumatoid arthritis/osteoarthritis: 200-400 mg/day in 3-4 equal doses

Dietary Considerations May be taken with food, milk, or antacids.

Test Interactions ↑ chloride (S), ↑ sodium (S)

Patient Information Take with food, milk, or with antacids

Nursing Implications Should be used for short-term only (<7 days); advise patient to report
  persistent GI discomfort, sore throat, fever, or malaise

Dosage Forms Capsule, as sodium: 50 mg, 100 mg

- ♦ **Meclofenamate Sodium** *see* Meclofenamate *on page 847*
- ♦ **Meclomen® (Can)** *see* Meclofenamate *on page 847*
- ♦ **Meclozine Hydrochloride** *see* Meclizine *on page 846*
- ♦ **Medicinal Carbon** *see* Charcoal *on page 268*
- ♦ **Medicinal Charcoal** *see* Charcoal *on page 268*
- ♦ **Medigesic®** *see* Butalbital Compound *on page 197*
- ♦ **Medi-Lice® [OTC]** *see* Permethrin *on page 1065*
- ♦ **Medipain 5®** *see* Hydrocodone and Acetaminophen *on page 676*
- ♦ **Medi-Synal [OTC]** *see* Acetaminophen and Pseudoephedrine *on page 25*
- ♦ **Medralone®** *see* MethylPREDNISolone *on page 896*
- ♦ **Medrol®** *see* MethylPREDNISolone *on page 896*

MedroxyPROGESTERone *(me DROKS ee proe JES te rone)*

U.S. Brand Names Depo-Provera®; Provera®

Canadian Brand Names Alti-MPA; Depo-Prevera®; Gen-Medroxy; Novo-Medrone; Provera®

Synonyms Acetoxymethylprogesterone; Medroxyprogesterone Acetate; Methylacetoxyprogesterone

Therapeutic Category Contraceptive, Parenteral (Estrogen/Progestin); Progestin

Use Endometrial carcinoma or renal carcinoma as well as secondary amenorrhea or abnormal uterine bleeding due to hormonal imbalance; reduction of endometrial hyperplasia in post-menopausal women receiving 0.625 mg conjugated estrogens for 12-14 consecutive days per month; Depo-Provera® injection is used for the prevention of pregnancy

Unlabeled/Investigational Use Hypoventilation disorders, advanced breast cancer

Pregnancy Risk Factor X

Contraindications Hypersensitivity to medroxyprogesterone or any component of the formulation; cerebral apoplexy, undiagnosed vaginal bleeding, liver dysfunction; thrombophlebitis; pregnancy

Warnings/Precautions Use with caution in patients with depression, diabetes, epilepsy, asthma, migraines, renal or cardiac dysfunction; pretreatment exams should include PAP smear, physical exam of breasts and pelvic areas. May increase serum cholesterol, LDL, decrease HDL and triglycerides; use of any progestin during the first 4 months of pregnancy is not recommended; monitor patient closely for loss of vision, sudden onset of proptosis, diplopia, migraine, and signs and symptoms of thromboembolic disorders.

Adverse Reactions Frequency not defined.

Cardiovascular: Edema, embolism, central thrombosis

Central nervous system: Mental depression, fever, insomnia, somnolence, headache (rare), dizziness

Dermatologic: Melasma or chloasma, allergic rash with or without pruritus, acne, hirsutism, angioneurotic edema

Endocrine & metabolic: Breakthrough bleeding, spotting, changes in menstrual flow, amenorrhea, increased breast tenderness, changes in cervical erosion and secretions

Gastrointestinal: Weight gain/loss, anorexia, nausea

Hepatic: Cholestatic jaundice

Local: Pain at injection site, sterile abscess, thrombophlebitis

Neuromuscular & skeletal: Weakness

Respiratory: Pulmonary embolism

Miscellaneous: Anaphylaxis

Overdosage/Toxicology Toxicity is unlikely following single exposures of excessive doses. Supportive treatment is adequate in most cases.

Drug Interactions

Decreased Effect: Aminoglutethimide may decrease effects by increasing hepatic metabolism.

Mechanism of Action Inhibits secretion of pituitary gonadotropins, which prevents follicular maturation and ovulation, stimulates growth of mammary tissue

Pharmacodynamics/Kinetics

Absorption: Oral: Well absorbed; I.M.: Slow

Bioavailability: 0.6% to 10%

Protein binding: 90% primarily to albumin; not to sex-hormone-binding globulin

Metabolism: Oral: Hepatic; hydroxylated and conjugated

Time to peak: Oral: 2-4 hours

Half-life elimination: Oral: 38-46 hours; I.M.: Acetate: 50 days

Excretion: Oral: Urine and feces

Usual Dosage

Adolescents and Adults: Oral:

Amenorrhea: 5-10 mg/day for 5-10 days or 2.5 mg/day

Abnormal uterine bleeding: 5-10 mg for 5-10 days starting on day 16 or 21 of cycle

Accompanying cyclic estrogen therapy, postmenopausal: 2.5-10 mg the last 10-13 days of estrogen dosing each month

Hypoventilation syndromes (unlabeled use): 20 mg 3 times/day

Adults:

I.M.:

Endometrial or renal carcinoma: 400-1000 mg/week

Contraception: 150 mg every 3 months

Dosing adjustment in hepatic impairment: Dose needs to be lowered in patients with alcoholic cirrhosis

Monitoring Parameters Monitor patient closely for loss of vision, sudden onset of proptosis, diplopia, migraine, and signs and symptoms of thromboembolic disorders

Test Interactions Altered thyroid and liver function tests

Patient Information Follow dosage schedule and do not take more than prescribed. You may experience sensitivity to sunlight (use sunblock, wear protective clothing and eyewear, and avoid extensive exposure to direct sunlight); dizziness, anxiety, depression (use caution when driving or engaging in tasks that require alertness until response to drug is known); changes in appetite (maintain adequate hydration and diet - 2-3 L/day of fluids unless instructed to restrict fluid intake); decreased libido or increased body hair (reversible when drug is discontinued); hot flashes (cool clothes and environment may help). May cause discoloration of stool (green). Report swelling of face, lips, or mouth; absent or altered menses; abdominal pain; vaginal itching, irritation, or discharge; heat, warmth, redness, or swelling of extremities; or sudden change in vision.

Nursing Implications Patients should receive a copy of the patient labeling for the drug

Dosage Forms

Injection, suspension, as acetate (Depot-Provera®): 150 mg/mL (1 mL); 400 mg/mL (1 mL, 2.5 mL, 10 mL)

Tablet, as acetate (Provera®): 2.5 mg, 5 mg, 10 mg

♦ **Medroxyprogesterone Acetate** *see* MedroxyPROGESTERone *on page 848*

♦ **Medroxyprogesterone Acetate and Estradiol Cypionate** *see* Estradiol Cypionate and Medroxyprogesterone Acetate *on page 495*

♦ **Medroxyprogesterone and Estrogens (Conjugated)** *see* Estrogens (Conjugated) and Medroxyprogesterone *on page 497*

Medrysone (ME dri sone)

U.S. Brand Names HMS Liquifilm®

Therapeutic Category Anti-inflammatory Agent, Ophthalmic; Corticosteroid, Ophthalmic

Use Treatment of allergic conjunctivitis, vernal conjunctivitis, episcleritis, ophthalmic epinephrine sensitivity reaction

Pregnancy Risk Factor C

Contraindications Hypersensitivity to medrysone or any component of the formulation; fungal, viral, or untreated pus-forming bacterial ocular infections; not for use in iritis and uveitis

Warnings/Precautions Prolonged use has been associated with the development of corneal or scleral perforation and posterior subcapsular cataracts; may mask or enhance the establishment of acute purulent untreated infections of the eye; effectiveness and safety have not been established in children. Medrysone is a synthetic corticosteroid; structurally related to progesterone; if no improvement after several days of treatment, discontinue medrysone and institute other therapy; duration of therapy: 3-4 days to several weeks dependent on type and severity of disease; taper dose to avoid disease exacerbation.

Adverse Reactions

1% to 10%: Ocular: Temporary mild blurred vision

<1% (Limited to important or life-threatening): Burning/stinging eyes, cataracts, corneal thinning, damage to the optic nerve, defects in visual activity, glaucoma, intraocular pressure increased, secondary ocular infection

Overdosage/Toxicology Systemic toxicity is unlikely from the ophthalmic preparation.

Mechanism of Action Decreases inflammation by suppression of migration of polymorphonuclear leukocytes and reversal of increased capillary permeability

Pharmacodynamics/Kinetics

Absorption: Through aqueous humor

Metabolism: Hepatic if absorbed

Excretion: Urine and feces

Usual Dosage Children and Adults: Ophthalmic: Instill 1 drop in conjunctival sac 2-4 times/day up to every 4 hours; may use every 1-2 hours during first 1-2 days

Monitoring Parameters Intraocular pressure and periodic examination of lens (with prolonged use)

Patient Information Shake well before using, do not touch dropper to the eye

Nursing Implications

Shake well before using; do not touch dropper to the eye

Monitor intraocular pressure and periodic examination of lens (with prolonged use)

Dosage Forms Solution, ophthalmic: 1% (5 mL, 10 mL)

Mefenamic Acid (me fe NAM ik AS id)

Related Information

Nonsteroidal Anti-Inflammatory Agents Comparison *on page 1512*

U.S. Brand Names Ponstel®

Canadian Brand Names Apo®-Mefenamic; Nu-Mefenamic; PMS-Mefenamic Acid; Ponstan®; Ponstel®

Therapeutic Category Analgesic, Nonsteroidal Anti-inflammatory Drug; Anti-inflammatory Agent; Nonsteroidal Anti-inflammatory Drug (NSAID), Oral

Use Short-term relief of mild to moderate pain including primary dysmenorrhea

Pregnancy Risk Factor C/D (3rd trimester)

Contraindications Hypersensitivity to nonsteroidal anti-inflammatory drugs (NSAIDs) including aspirin or any component of the formulation; pregnancy (3rd trimester)

Warnings/Precautions May have adverse effects on fetus. Withhold for at least 4-6 half-lives prior to surgical or dental procedures.

Adverse Reactions

1% to 10%:

Central nervous system: Headache, nervousness, dizziness (3% to 9%)

Dermatologic: Itching, rash

Endocrine & metabolic: Fluid retention

Gastrointestinal: Abdominal cramps, heartburn, indigestion, nausea (1% to 10%), vomiting (1% to 10%), diarrhea (1% to 10%), constipation (1% to 10%), abdominal distress/cramping/pain (1% to 10%), dyspepsia (1% to 10%), flatulence (1% to 10%), gastric or duodenal ulcer with bleeding or perforation (1% to 10%), gastritis (1% to 10%)

Hematologic: Bleeding (1% to 10%)

Hepatic: Elevated LFTs (1% to 10%)

Otic: Tinnitus (1% to 10%)

<1%: Congestive heart failure, hypertension, arrhythmias, tachycardia, confusion, hallucinations, aseptic meningitis, mental depression, drowsiness, insomnia, urticaria, erythema multiforme, toxic epidermal necrolysis, Stevens-Johnson syndrome, angioedema, polydipsia, hot flashes, gastritis, GI ulceration, cystitis, polyuria, agranulocytosis, anemia, hemolytic anemia, bone marrow suppression, leukopenia, thrombocytopenia, hepatitis, peripheral neuropathy, toxic amblyopia, blurred vision, conjunctivitis, dry eyes, decreased hearing, acute renal failure, dyspnea, allergic rhinitis, epistaxis, stomatitis

Overdosage/Toxicology Symptoms include CNS stimulation, agitation, and seizures. Management of nonsteroidal anti-inflammatory drug (NSAID) intoxication is primarily supportive and symptomatic. Fluid therapy is commonly effective in managing hypotension that may occur following an acute NSAID overdose, except when due to acute blood loss. Seizures tend to be very short-lived and often do not require drug treatment, although recurrent seizures should be treated with I.V. diazepam. Since many of the NSAIDs undergo enterohepatic cycling, multiple doses of charcoal may be needed to reduce the potential for delayed toxicities.

Drug Interactions

Increased Effect/Toxicity: Anticoagulants (warfarin, heparin, LMWHs) in combination with NSAIDs can cause increased risk of bleeding. Other antiplatelet drugs (ticlopidine, clopidogrel, aspirin, abciximab, dipyridamole, eptifibatide, tirofiban) can cause an increased risk of bleeding. NSAIDs may increase serum creatinine, potassium, blood pressure, and cyclosporine levels during concurrent therapy; monitor cyclosporine levels and renal function carefully. Lithium levels can be increased; avoid concurrent use if possible or monitor lithium levels and adjust dose. Sulindac may have the least effect. When NSAID is stopped, lithium will need adjustment again. Corticosteroids may increase the risk of GI ulceration; avoid concurrent use.

Decreased Effect: Antihypertensive effects of ACE-inhibitors, angiotensin antagonists, diuretics, and hydralazine may be decreased by concurrent therapy with NSAIDs; monitor blood pressure. Cholestyramine and colestipol reduce the bioavailability of diclofenac; separate administration times.

Ethanol/Nutrition/Herb Interactions Ethanol: Avoid ethanol (due to GI irritation).

Mechanism of Action Inhibits prostaglandin synthesis by decreasing the activity of the enzyme, cyclo-oxygenase, which results in decreased formation of prostaglandin precursors

Pharmacodynamics/Kinetics
Onset of action: Peak effect: 2-4 hours
Duration: ≤6 hours
Protein binding: High
Metabolism: Conjugated hepatically
Half-life elimination: 3.5 hours
Excretion: Urine (50%) and feces as unchanged drug and metabolites

Usual Dosage Children >14 years and Adults: Oral: 500 mg to start then 250 mg every 4 hours as needed; maximum therapy: 1 week

Dosing adjustment/comments in renal impairment: Not recommended for use

Dietary Considerations May be taken with food, milk, or antacids.

Test Interactions ↑ chloride (S), ↑ sodium (S), positive Coombs' [direct], false-positive urinary bilirubin

Patient Information Take with food, milk, or with antacids; extended release capsules must be swallowed intact

Nursing Implications Should be taken with food, milk, or antacids; monitor for bleeding

Dosage Forms Capsule: 250 mg

Mefloquine (ME floe kwin)

Related Information
Malaria Treatment *on page 1607*
Prevention of Malaria *on page 1552*

U.S. Brand Names Lariam®

Canadian Brand Names Lariam®

Synonyms Mefloquine Hydrochloride

Therapeutic Category Antimalarial Agent

Use Treatment of acute malarial infections and prevention of malaria

Pregnancy Risk Factor C

Contraindications Hypersensitivity mefloquine or any component of the formulation; epilepsy; cardiac conduction abnormalities; severe psychotic illness

Warnings/Precautions Caution is warranted with lactation; discontinue if unexplained neuro-psychiatric disturbances occur, caution in epilepsy patients or in patients with significant cardiac disease. If mefloquine is to be used for a prolonged period, periodic evaluations including liver function tests and ophthalmic examinations should be performed. In cases of life-threatening, serious, or overwhelming malaria infections due to *Plasmodium falciparum*, patients should be treated with intravenous antimalarial drug. Mefloquine may be given orally to complete the course. Caution should be exercised with regard to driving, piloting airplanes, and operating machines since dizziness, disturbed sense of balance; neuropsychiatric reactions have been reported with mefloquine. In patients with epilepsy, mefloquine may increase the risk of convulsions. Administration of mefloquine with quinine or quinidine may produce electrocardiographic change; when administered with halofantrine, life-threatening prolongation of QT interval may occur.

Adverse Reactions
1% to 10%:
Central nervous system: Difficulty concentrating, headache, insomnia, lightheadedness, vertigo
Gastrointestinal: Vomiting (3%), diarrhea, stomach pain, nausea
Ocular: Visual disturbances
Otic: Tinnitus
<1% (Limited to important or life-threatening): Anxiety, bradycardia, confusion, dizziness, extrasystoles, hallucinations, mental depression, psychosis, seizures, syncope

Overdosage/Toxicology Symptoms include vomiting and diarrhea. Mefloquine is cardiotoxic. Following GI contamination care is supportive only.

Drug Interactions
Cytochrome P450 Effect: Unknown; potentially similar to quinidine.
Increased Effect/Toxicity: Increased bradycardia possible with beta-blockers; caution with other drugs that alter cardiac conduction; increased toxicity with chloroquine, quinine, and quinidine (hold treatment until at least 12 hours after these later drugs)
Decreased Effect: Mefloquine may decrease the effect of valproic acid.

Mechanism of Action Mefloquine is a quinoline-methanol compound structurally similar to quinine; mefloquine's effectiveness in the treatment and prophylaxis of malaria is due to the destruction of the asexual blood forms of the malarial pathogens that affect humans, *Plasmodium falciparum*, *P. vivax*, *P. malariae*, *P. ovale*

Pharmacodynamics/Kinetics
Absorption: Well absorbed
Distribution: V_d: 19 L/kg; blood, urine, CSF, tissues; enters breast milk
Protein binding: 98%
Half-life elimination: 21-22 days
Excretion: Urine (~1.5% to 9% as unchanged drug)
(Continued)

Mefloquine (Continued)

Usual Dosage Oral:

Children:

Malaria treatment: 15-25 mg/kg in a single dose (maximum: 1250 mg)

Malaria prophylaxis:

15-19 kg: 1/4 tablet

20-30 kg: 1/2 tablet

31-45 kg: 3/4 tablet

>45 kg: 1 tablet

Administer weekly starting 1 week before travel, continuing weekly during travel and for 4 weeks after leaving endemic area

Adults:

Treatment of mild to moderate malaria infection: 5 tablets (1250 mg) as a single dose with at least 8 oz of water

Malaria prophylaxis: 1 tablet (250 mg) weekly starting 1 week before travel, continuing weekly during travel and for 4 weeks after leaving endemic area

Monitoring Parameters LFTS; ocular examination

Patient Information Begin therapy before trip and continue after; do not take drug on empty stomach; take with food and at least 8 oz of water; women of childbearing age should use reliable contraception during prophylaxis treatment and for 2 months after the last dose; be aware of signs and symptoms of malaria when traveling to an endemic area. Caution should be exercised with regard to driving, piloting airplanes, and operating machines since dizziness, disturbed sense of balance, or neuropsychiatric reactions have been reported with mefloquine.

Nursing Implications Monitor LFTS; ocular examination

Dosage Forms Tablet, as hydrochloride: 250 mg

- ◆ **Mefloquine Hydrochloride** see Mefloquine on page 851
- ◆ **Mefoxin**® see Cefoxitin on page 249
- ◆ **Megace**® see Megestrol on page 852
- ◆ **Megace**® **OS (Can)** see Megestrol on page 852

Megestrol (me JES trole)

U.S. Brand Names Megace®

Canadian Brand Names Apo®-Megestrol; Lin-Megestrol; Megace®; Megace® OS; Nu-Megestrol

Synonyms Megestrol Acetate

Therapeutic Category Antineoplastic Agent, Hormone; Progestin

Use Palliative treatment of breast and endometrial carcinoma

Orphan drug: Treatment of anorexia, cachexia, or significant weight loss (≥10% baseline body weight); treatment of AIDS

Pregnancy Risk Factor X

Contraindications Hypersensitivity to megestrol or any component of the formulation; pregnancy

Warnings/Precautions The U.S. Food and Drug Administration (FDA) currently recommends that procedures for proper handling and disposal of antineoplastic agents be considered. Use during the first few months of pregnancy is not recommended. Use with caution in patients with a history of thrombophlebitis. Elderly females may have vaginal bleeding or discharge and need to be forewarned of this side effect and inconvenience.

Adverse Reactions

Cardiovascular: Edema, hypertension (≤8%), cardiomyopathy, palpitations

Central nervous system: Insomnia, depression (≤6%), fever (2% to 6%), headache (≤10%), pain (≤6%, similar to placebo), confusion (1% to 3%), convulsions (1% to 3%), depression (1% to 3%)

Dermatologic: Allergic rash (2% to 12%) with or without pruritus, alopecia

Endocrine & metabolic: Breakthrough bleeding and amenorrhea, spotting, changes in menstrual flow, changes in cervical erosion and secretions, increased breast tenderness, changes in vaginal bleeding pattern, edema, fluid retention, hyperglycemia (≤6%)

Gastrointestinal: Weight gain (not attributed to edema or fluid retention), nausea (≤5%, less than placebo), vomiting, diarrhea (8% to 15%, similar to placebo), flatulence (≤10%), constipation (1% to 3%)

Genitourinary: Impotence (4% to 14%), decreased libido (≤5%)

Hepatic: Cholestatic jaundice, hepatotoxicity, hepatomegaly (1% to 3%)

Local: Thrombophlebitis

Neuromuscular & skeletal: Carpal tunnel syndrome, weakness, paresthesia (1% to 3%)

Respiratory: Hyperpnea, dyspnea (1% to 3%), cough (1% to 3%)

Miscellaneous: Diaphoresis

Overdosage/Toxicology Toxicity is unlikely following single exposures of excessive doses.

Ethanol/Nutrition/Herb Interactions Herb/Nutraceutical: Avoid black cohosh, dong quai in estrogen-dependent tumors.

Stability Store at 25°C (77°F), excursions permitted at 15°C to 30°C (59°F to 86°F). Megestrol acetate (Megace®) oral suspension is compatible with water, orange juice, apple juice, or Sustacal H.C. for immediate consumption.

Mechanism of Action A synthetic progestin with antiestrogenic properties which disrupt the estrogen receptor cycle. Megace® interferes with the normal estrogen cycle and results in a lower LH titer. May also have a direct effect on the endometrium. Megestrol is an antineoplastic progestin thought to act through an antileutenizing effect mediated via the pituitary.

Pharmacodynamics/Kinetics

Onset of action: ≥2 months of continuous therapy

Absorption: Well absorbed

Metabolism: Completely hepatic to free steroids and glucuronide conjugates

Time to peak, serum: 1-3 hours

Half-life elimination: 15-20 hours

Excretion: Urine (as steroid metabolites and inactive compound); feces (minor amounts)

Usual Dosage Adults: Oral (refer to individual protocols):

Female:

Breast carcinoma: 40 mg 4 times/day

Endometrial: 40-320 mg/day in divided doses; use for 2 months to determine efficacy; maximum doses used have been up to 800 mg/day

Uterine bleeding: 40 mg 2-4 times/day

Male/Female: HIV-related cachexia: Initial dose: 800 mg/day; daily doses of 400 and 800 mg/day were found to be clinically effective

Dosing adjustment in renal impairment: No data available; however, the urinary excretion of megestrol acetate administered in doses of 4-90 mg ranged from 56% to 78% within 10 days

Hemodialysis: Megestrol acetate has not been tested for dialyzability; however, due to its low solubility, it is postulated that dialysis would not be an effective means of treating an overdose

Monitoring Parameters Monitor for tumor response; observe for signs of thromboembolic phenomena; monitor for thromboembolism

Test Interactions Altered thyroid and liver function tests

Patient Information Follow dosage schedule and do not take more than prescribed. You may experience sensitivity to sunlight (use sunblock, wear protective clothing, and avoid extended exposure to direct sunlight); dizziness, anxiety, depression (use caution when driving or engaging in tasks that require alertness until response to drug is known); change in appetite (maintain adequate hydration and diet - 2-3 L/day of fluids unless instructed to restrict fluid intake); decreased libido or increased body hair (reversible when drug is discontinued); hot flashes (cool clothes and environment may help). Report swelling of face, lips, or mouth; absence or altered menses; abdominal pain; vaginal itching, irritation, or discharge; heat, warmth, redness, or swelling of extremities; or sudden onset change in vision.

Nursing Implications Monitor tumor response; observe for signs of thromboembolic phenomena

Dosage Forms

Suspension, oral, as acetate: 40 mg/mL with alcohol 0.06% (240 mL)

Tablet, as acetate: 20 mg, 40 mg

♦ **Megestrol Acetate** *see Megestrol on page 852*

♦ **Melanex®** *see Hydroquinone on page 686*

♦ **Mellaril®** *see Thioridazine on page 1321*

Meloxicam (mel OKS i kam)

Related Information

Nonsteroidal Anti-Inflammatory Agents Comparison *on page 1512*

U.S. Brand Names MOBIC®

Canadian Brand Names MOBIC®; Mobicox®

Therapeutic Category Nonsteroidal Anti-inflammatory Drug (NSAID), Oral

Use Relief of signs and symptoms of osteoarthritis

Pregnancy Risk Factor C/D (3rd trimester)

Pregnancy/Breast-Feeding Implications May cause premature closure of the ductus arteriosus in the 3rd trimester of pregnancy. It is not known whether meloxicam is excreted in human milk. Due to a potential for serious adverse reactions, the manufacturer recommends that a decision be made whether to discontinue nursing or discontinue the drug, taking into account the importance of the drug to the mother.

Contraindications Hypersensitivity to meloxicam or any component, aspirin, or other nonsteroidal anti-inflammatory drugs (NSAIDs); pregnancy C/D (3rd trimester)

Warnings/Precautions Gastrointestinal irritation, ulceration, bleeding, and perforation may occur with NSAIDs. Serious complications may occur without prior symptoms of gastrointestinal distress. Use with caution in patients with a history of GI disease (bleeding or ulcers), decreased renal function, hepatic disease, congestive heart failure, dehydration, hypertension, or asthma. Use with caution in elderly patients. Anaphylactoid reactions may occur, even with no prior exposure to meloxicam. Use in advanced renal disease is not recommended. May alter platelet function; use with caution in patients receiving anticoagulants or with hemostatic disorders. Safety and efficacy in pediatric patients have not been established. Withhold for at least 4-6 half-lives prior to surgical or dental procedures.

Adverse Reactions

1% to 10%:

Cardiovascular: Edema (2% to 5%)

Central nervous system: Headache and dizziness occurred in 2% to 8% of patients, but occurred less frequently than placebo in controlled trials

Dermatologic: Rash (1% to 3%)

Gastrointestinal: Diarrhea (3% to 8%), dyspepsia (5%), nausea (4%), flatulence (3%), abdominal pain (2% to 3%)

Respiratory: Upper respiratory infection (2% to 3%), pharyngitis (1% to 3%)

Miscellaneous: Flu-like symptoms (4% to 5%), falls (3%)

<2% (Limited to important or life-threatening): Agranulocytosis, allergic reaction, alopecia, anaphylactic reaction, angina, angioedema, anxiety, arrhythmia, bronchospasm, bullous eruption, cardiac failure, colitis, confusion, depression, duodenal perforation, duodenal ulcer, dyspnea, erythema multiforme, gastric perforation, gastric ulcer, gastritis, gastroesophageal reflux, gastrointestinal hemorrhage, hematemesis, hematuria, hepatic failure, hepatitis, hypertension, hypotension, interstitial nephritis, intestinal perforation, jaundice, leukopenia, melena, myocardial infarction, pancreatitis, paresthesia, photosensitivity reaction, pruritus, purpura, renal failure, seizures, shock, somnolence, Stevens-Johnson syndrome, syncope, thrombocytopenia, tinnitus, toxic epidermal necrolysis, tremor, ulcerative stomatitis, urticaria, vasculitis, vertigo

Overdosage/Toxicology Symptoms include lethargy, drowsiness, nausea, vomiting, and epigastric pain. Rarely, severe symptoms have been associated with NSAID overdose including apnea, metabolic acidosis, coma, nystagmus, seizures, leukocytosis, and renal

(Continued)

Meloxicam (Continued)

failure. Management of nonsteroidal anti-inflammatory (NSAID) intoxication is supportive and symptomatic. Since meloxicam undergoes enterohepatic cycling, multiple doses of charcoal may be needed to reduce the potential for delayed toxicities. Cholestyramine has been shown to increase meloxicam clearance.

Drug Interactions

Increased Effect/Toxicity:

Anticoagulants (warfarin, heparin, LMWHs) in combination with NSAIDs can cause increased risk of bleeding.

Antiplatelet drugs (ticlopidine, clopidogrel, aspirin, abciximab, dipyridamole, eptifibatide, tirofiban) can cause an increased risk of bleeding.

Aspirin increases serum concentrations (AUC) of meloxicam (in addition to potential for additive adverse effects); concurrent use is not recommended.

Corticosteroids may increase the risk of GI ulceration; avoid concurrent use.

Cyclosporine: NSAIDs may increase serum creatinine, potassium, blood pressure, and cyclosporine levels; monitor cyclosporine levels and renal function carefully.

Lithium levels can be increased; avoid concurrent use if possible or monitor lithium levels and adjust dose. When NSAID is stopped, lithium will need adjustment again.

Warfarin INRs may be increased by meloxicam. Monitor INR closely, particularly during initiation or change in dose. May increase risk of bleeding. Use lowest possible dose for shortest duration possible.

Decreased Effect:

Cholestyramine (and possibly colestipol) increases the clearance of meloxicam.

Hydralazine's antihypertensive effect is decreased; avoid concurrent use.

Loop diuretic efficacy (diuretic and antihypertensive effect) may be reduced by NSAIDs.

Antihypertensive effects of thiazide diuretics are decreased; avoid concurrent use.

Ethanol/Nutrition/Herb Interactions Ethanol: Avoid ethanol (may enhance gastric mucosal irritation).

Stability Store at 25°C (77°F)

Mechanism of Action Inhibits prostaglandin synthesis by decreasing the activity of the enzyme, cyclo-oxygenase, which results in decreased formation of prostaglandin precursors

Pharmacodynamics/Kinetics

Distribution: 10 L

Protein binding: 99.4%

Metabolism: Hepatic, including metabolism by CYP2C9 and CYP3A4 (minor)

Bioavailability: 89%

Half-life elimination: 15-20 hours

Time to peak: 5-10 hours

Excretion: Urine and feces (as inactive metabolites)

Usual Dosage Adult: Oral: Initial: 7.5 mg once daily; some patients may receive additional benefit from an increased dose of 15 mg once daily; maximum dose: 15 mg/day

Dosage adjustment in renal impairment: No specific dosage adjustment is recommended for mild to moderate renal impairment; avoid use in significant renal impairment

Dosage adjustment in hepatic impairment: No specific adjustment is recommended in hepatic impairment; patients with severe hepatic impairment have not been adequately studied

Elderly: Increased concentrations may occur in elderly patients (particularly in females); however, no specific dosage adjustment is recommended

Dietary Considerations Should be taken with food or milk to minimize gastrointestinal irritation.

Monitoring Parameters CBC, periodic liver function, renal function (serum BUN, and creatinine)

Patient Information If self-administered, use exactly as directed (do not increase dose or frequency); adverse reactions can occur with overuse. Take with food or milk. While using this medication, do not use alcohol, excessive amounts of vitamin C, or salicylate-containing foods (curry powder, prunes, raisins, tea, or licorice), other prescription or OTC medications containing aspirin or salicylate, or other NSAIDs without consulting prescriber. Maintain adequate hydration (2-3 L/day of fluids unless instructed to restrict fluid intake). You may experience nausea, vomiting, gastric discomfort (frequent mouth care, small frequent meals, chewing gum, sucking lozenges may help). GI bleeding, ulceration, or perforation can occur with or without pain. Stop taking medication and report ringing in ears; persistent cramping or pain in stomach; unresolved nausea or vomiting; difficulty breathing or shortness of breath; unusual bruising or bleeding (mouth, urine, stool); skin rash; unusual swelling of extremities; chest pain; or palpitations.

Dosage Forms Tablet: 7.5 mg, 15 mg

♦ Melpaque HP® see Hydroquinone on page 686

Melphalan (MEL fa lan)

U.S. Brand Names Alkeran®

Canadian Brand Names Alkeran®

Synonyms L-PAM; L-Sarcolysin; Phenylalanine Mustard

Therapeutic Category Antineoplastic Agent, Alkylating Agent; Antineoplastic Agent, Nitrogen Mustard

Use Palliative treatment of multiple myeloma and nonresectable epithelial ovarian carcinoma; neuroblastoma, rhabdomyosarcoma, breast cancer

Pregnancy Risk Factor D

Contraindications Hypersensitivity to melphalan or any component of the formulation; severe bone marrow suppression; patients whose disease was resistant to prior therapy; pregnancy

Warnings/Precautions The U.S. Food and Drug Administration (FDA) currently recommends that procedures for proper handling and disposal for antineoplastic agents are considered. Is potentially mutagenic, carcinogenic, and teratogenic; produces amenorrhea. Reduce dosage or discontinue therapy if leukocyte count <3000/mm^3 or platelet count <100,000/mm^3; use with caution in patients with bone marrow suppression, impaired renal function, or who have received prior chemotherapy or irradiation; will cause amenorrhea. Toxicity to immunosuppressives is increased in elderly. Start with lowest recommended adult doses. Signs of infection, such as fever and WBC rise, may not occur. Lethargy and confusion may be more prominent signs of infection.

Adverse Reactions

>10%: Hematologic: Myelosuppressive: Leukopenia and thrombocytopenia are the most common effects of melphalan. Irreversible bone marrow failure has been reported.

WBC: Moderate

Platelets: Moderate

Onset (days): 7

Nadir (days): 8-10 and 27-32

Recovery (days): 42-50

1% to 10%:

Cardiovascular: Vasculitis

Dermatologic: Vesiculation of skin, alopecia, pruritus, rash

Endocrine & metabolic: SIADH, sterility and amenorrhea

Gastrointestinal: Nausea and vomiting are mild; stomatitis and diarrhea are infrequent

Emetic potential: Low (<10%): <100 mg/m^2; high (>90%): >100 mg/m^2

Genitourinary: Bladder irritation, hemorrhagic cystitis

Hematologic: Anemia, agranulocytosis, hemolytic anemia

Hepatic: Transaminases increased (hepatitis, jaundice have been reported)

Respiratory: Pulmonary fibrosis, interstitial pneumonitis

Miscellaneous: Hypersensitivity, secondary malignancies

BMT:

Dermatologic: Alopecia

Gastrointestinal: Mucositis (severity increases with Cl$_{cr}$ ≤40 mL/minute), nausea and vomiting (moderate), diarrhea

Hematologic: Myelosuppression, secondary leukemia

Renal: Increased serum creatinine and azotemia possible without adequate hydration

Rare side effects: Abnormal LFTs, interstitial pneumonitis, secondary leukemia, SIADH, vasculitis

Overdosage/Toxicology Symptoms include hypocalcemia, pulmonary fibrosis, nausea, vomiting, and bone marrow suppression.

Drug Interactions

Increased Effect/Toxicity: Cyclosporine: Risk of nephrotoxicity is increased by melphalan.

Decreased Effect: Cimetidine and other H$_2$ antagonists: The reduction in gastric pH has been reported to decrease bioavailability of melphalan by 30%.

Ethanol/Nutrition/Herb Interactions

Ethanol: Avoid ethanol (due to GI irritation).

Food: Food interferes with oral absorption.

Stability

Tablets/injection: Protect from light, store at room temperature (15°C to 30°C)

The time between reconstitution/dilution and administration of parenteral melphalan must be kept to a minimum (<60 minutes) because reconstituted and diluted solutions are unstable.

Injection: Preparation:

Dissolve powder initially with 10 mL of diluent to a concentration of 5 mg/mL. This solution is chemically and physically stable for at least 90 minutes when stored at 25°C (77°F).

Immediately dilute dose in 0.9% sodium chloride to a concentration of 0.1-0.45 mg/mL. This solution is physically and chemically stable for at least 60 minutes at 25°C (77°F). HIGHLY UNSTABLE SOLUTION; administration should occur within 1 hour of dissolution. Do not refrigerate solution; precipitation occurs.

Standard I.V. dilution:

Dose/250-500 mL NS (concentration of 0.1-0.45 mg/mL)

MUST BE PREPARED FRESH; solution is stable for 1 hour after dilution and must be administered within that time period

Mechanism of Action Alkylating agent which is a derivative of mechlorethamine that inhibits DNA and RNA synthesis via formation of carbonium ions; cross-links strands of DNA

Pharmacodynamics/Kinetics

Absorption: Oral: Variable and incomplete

Distribution: V$_d$: 0.5-0.6 L/kg throughout total body water

Bioavailability: Unpredictable, decreasing from 85% to 58% with repeated doses

Half-life elimination: Terminal: 1.5 hours

Time to peak, serum: ~2 hours

Excretion: Oral: Urine (10% to 30% as unchanged drug); feces (20% to 50%)

Usual Dosage Refer to individual protocols.

Oral: Dose should always be adjusted to patient response and weekly blood counts:

Children: 4-20 mg/m^2/day for 1-21 days

Adults:

Multiple myeloma: 6 mg/day initially adjusted as indicated **or** 0.15 mg/kg/day for 7 days **or** 0.25 mg/kg/day for 4 days; repeat at 4- to 6-week intervals.

Ovarian carcinoma: 0.2 mg/kg/day for 5 days, repeat every 4-5 weeks.

I.V.:

Children:

Pediatric rhabdomyosarcoma: 10-35 mg/m^2/dose every 21-28 days

High-dose melphalan with bone marrow transplantation for neuroblastoma: I.V.: 100-220 mg/m^2 as a single dose or divided into 2-5 daily doses. Infuse over 20-60 minutes.

Adults: Multiple myeloma: 16 mg/m^2 administered at 2-week intervals for 4 doses, then repeat monthly as per protocol for multiple myeloma.

Dosing adjustment in renal impairment:

Cl$_{cr}$ 10-50 mL/minute: Administer at 75% of normal dose

Cl$_{cr}$ <10 mL/minute: Administer at 50% of normal dose

or

(Continued)

Melphalan *(Continued)*

BUN >30 mg/dL: Reduce dose by 50%

Serum creatinine >1.5 mg/dL: Reduce dose by 50%

Hemodialysis: Unknown

CAPD effects: Unknown

CAVH effects: Dose for GFR 10-50 mL/minute

Dietary Considerations Should be taken on an empty stomach (1 hour prior to or 2 hours after meals).

Administration

Oral: Administer on an empty stomach (1 hour prior to or 2 hours after meals)

Parenteral: Due to limited stability, complete administration of I.V. dose should occur within 60 minutes of reconstitution

I.V. infusion: I.V. dose is FDA-approved for administration as a single infusion over 15-20 minutes

I.V. bolus: I.V. may be administered via central line and via peripheral vein as a rapid I.V. bolus; there have not been any unexpected or serious adverse events specifically related to rapid I.V. bolus administration; the most common adverse events were transient mild symptoms of hot flush and tingling sensation over the body

Central line: I.V. bolus doses of 17-200 mg/m^2 (reconstituted and not diluted) have been infused over 2-20 minutes

Peripheral line: I.V. bolus doses of 2-23 mg/m^2 (reconstituted and not diluted) have been infused over 1-4 minutes

Monitoring Parameters CBC with differential and platelet count, serum electrolytes, serum uric acid

Test Interactions False-positive Coombs' test [direct]

Patient Information

Infusion: Report promptly any pain, irritation, or redness at infusion site

Oral: Preferable to take on an empty stomach, 1 hour prior to or 2 hours after meals

Do not take alcohol, aspirin or aspirin-containing medications, and/or OTC medications without consulting prescriber. Inform prescriber of all prescription medication you are taking. Maintain adequate fluid balance (2-3 L/day of fluids unless instructed to restrict fluid intake). May cause hair loss (reversible); easy bleeding or bruising (use a soft toothbrush or cotton swabs and frequent mouth care, use electric razor, avoid sharp knives or scissors); increased susceptibility to infection (avoid crowds or exposure to infection - do not have any vaccinations unless approved by prescriber). Report unusual bleeding or bruising or persistent fever or sore throat; blood in urine, stool, or vomitus; delayed healing of any wounds; skin rash; yellowing of skin or eyes; changes in color of urine or black stool; pain or burning on urination; respiratory difficulty; or other severe adverse reactions. Contraceptive measures should be used during therapy. The drug may be excreted in breast milk, therefore, an alternative form of feeding your baby should be used.

Nursing Implications Avoid skin contact with I.V. formulation

Dosage Forms

Powder for injection: 50 mg

Tablet: 2 mg

♦ **Melquin HP**® **Melquin-3**® **[OTC]** *see* Hydroquinone *on page 686*

♦ **Menadol**® **[OTC]** *see* Ibuprofen *on page 697*

♦ **Menest**® *see* Estrogens (Esterified) *on page 500*

♦ **Meni-D**® *see* Meclizine *on page 846*

Meningococcal Polysaccharide Vaccine (Groups A / C / Y and W-135)

(me NIN joe kok al pol i SAK a ride vak SEEN groops aye, see, why & dubl yoo won thur tee fyve)

Related Information

Immunization Recommendations *on page 1538*

U.S. Brand Names Menomune®-A/C/Y/W-135

Therapeutic Category Vaccine, Inactivated Bacteria

Use

Immunization of persons ≥2 years of age in epidemic or endemic areas as might be determined in a population delineated by neighborhood, school, dormitory, or other reasonable boundary. The prevalent serogroup in such a situation should match a serogroup in the vaccine. Individuals at particular high-risk include persons with terminal component complement deficiencies and those with anatomic or functional asplenia.

Travelers visiting areas of a country that are recognized as having hyperendemic or epidemic meningococcal disease

Vaccinations should be considered for household or institutional contacts of persons with meningococcal disease as an adjunct to appropriate antibiotic chemoprophylaxis as well as medical and laboratory personnel at risk of exposure to meningococcal disease

Pregnancy Risk Factor C

Pregnancy/Breast-Feeding Implications Excretion in breast milk unknown/use caution

Contraindications Hypersensitivity to any component of the formulation (10-dose vial contains thimerosal); defer immunization during acute illness; children <2 years of age

Warnings/Precautions Patients who undergo splenectomy secondary to trauma or nonlymphoid tumors respond well; however, those asplenic patients with lymphoid tumors who receive either chemotherapy or irradiation respond poorly; pregnancy, unless there is substantial risk of infection. Safety and efficacy in pediatric patients <2 years of age have not been established. Use with caution in patients with latex sensitivity; the stopper to the vial contains dry, natural latex rubber. Should not be administered with whole-cell pertussis or whole-cell typhoid vaccines due to combined endotoxin content.

Adverse Reactions All serious adverse reactions must be reported to the U.S. Department of Health and Human Services (DHHS) Vaccine Adverse Event Reporting System

(VAERS) 1-800-822-7967. Incidence of erythema, swelling, or tenderness may be higher in children

>10%: Local: Tenderness (9% to 36% as reported in adults)

1% to 10%:
   Central nervous system: Headache (2% to 5%), malaise (2%), fever (100°F to 106°F: 3%), chills (2%)
   Local: Pain at injection site (2% to 3%), erythema (1% to 4%), induration (1% to 4%)

Stability Store at 2°C to 8°C (35°F to 46°F). Use single-dose vial within 30 minutes of reconstitution. Use multidose vial within 10 days of reconstitution.

Mechanism of Action Induces the formation of bactericidal antibodies to meningococcal antigens; the presence of these antibodies is strongly correlated with immunity to meningococcal disease caused by *Neisseria meningitidis* groups A, C, Y and W-135.

Pharmacodynamics/Kinetics
   Onset of action: Antibody levels: 10-14 days
   Duration: Antibodies against group A and C polysaccharides decline markedly (to prevaccination levels) over the first 3 years following a single dose of vaccine, especially in children <4 years of age

Usual Dosage One dose S.C. (0.5 mL); the need for booster is unknown; **Note:** Individuals who are sensitive to thimerosal should receive single-dose pack (reconstituted with 0.78 mL vial without preservative).

Administration Administer by S.C. injection; do not administer intradermally, I.M., or I.V.

Nursing Implications Epinephrine 1:1000 should be available to control allergic reaction

Additional Information Federal law requires that the date of administration, the vaccine manufacturer, lot number of vaccine, and the administering person's name, title and address be entered into the patient's permanent medical record.

Dosage Forms Powder for injection: Polysaccharide antigen groups A, C, Y, and W-135 (50 mcg of each antigen/0.5 mL following reconstitution) (1 mL, 6 mL) [contains lactose; 6 mL vial contains thimerosal; vial stoppers contain dry, natural latex rubber]

♦ **Menomune®-A/C/Y/W-135** *see* Meningococcal Polysaccharide Vaccine (Groups A / C / Y and W-135) *on page 856*

Menotropins (men oh TROE pins)

U.S. Brand Names Humegon™; Pergonal®; Repronex®

Canadian Brand Names Pergonal®

Therapeutic Category Gonadotropin; Ovulation Stimulator

Use Sequentially with hCG to induce ovulation and pregnancy in the infertile woman with functional anovulation or in patients who have previously received pituitary suppression; stimulation of multiple follicle development in ovulatory patients as part of an *in vitro* fertilization program; used with hCG in men to stimulate spermatogenesis in those with primary hypogonadotropic hypogonadism

Pregnancy Risk Factor X

Pregnancy/Breast-Feeding Implications Ectopic pregnancy and congenital abnormalities have been reported. The incidence of congenital abnormality is similar during natural conception. It is unknown if menotropins are excreted in human milk, use caution if administered to a nursing woman.

Contraindications Hypersensitivity to menotropins or any component of the formulation; primary ovarian failure as indicated by a high follicle-stimulating hormone (FSH) level; uncontrolled thyroid and adrenal dysfunction; abnormal bleeding of undetermined origin; intracranial lesion (ie, pituitary tumor); ovarian cyst or enlargement not due to polycystic ovary syndrome; infertility due to any cause other than anovulation (except candidates for *in vitro* fertilization); men with normal urinary gonadotropin concentrations, elevated gonadotropin levels indicating primary testicular failure; pregnancy

Warnings/Precautions For use by infertility specialists. Advise patient of frequency and potential hazards of multiple pregnancy. May cause ovarian hyperstimulation syndrome (OHSS); if severe, treatment should be discontinued and patient should be hospitalized (may become more severe if pregnancy occurs). Monitor for ovarian enlargement; to minimize the hazard of abnormal ovarian enlargement, use the lowest possible dose. Serious pulmonary conditions (atelectasis, acute respiratory distress syndrome) and arterial thromboembolism have been reported. Safety and efficacy in pediatric and geriatric patients have not been established.

Adverse Reactions
   Male:
   >10%: Endocrine & metabolic: Gynecomastia
   1% to 10%: Erythrocytosis (dyspnea, dizziness, anorexia, syncope, epistaxis)
   Female:
   1% to 10%:
      Central nervous system: Headache
      Endocrine & metabolic: Breast tenderness
      Gastrointestinal: Abdominal cramping, abdominal pain, diarrhea, enlarged abdomen, nausea, vomiting
      Genitourinary: Ectopic pregnancy, OHSS (% is dose related), ovarian disease, vaginal hemorrhage
      Local: Injection site edema/reaction
      Miscellaneous: Infection, pelvic pain
   Frequency not defined:
      Cardiovascular: Stroke, tachycardia, thrombosis (venous or arterial)
      Central nervous system: Dizziness
      Dermatologic: Angioedema, urticaria
      Genitourinary: Adnexal torsion, hemoperitoneum, ovarian enlargement
      Neuromuscular & skeletal: Limb necrosis
      Respiratory: Acute respiratory distress syndrome, atelectasis, dyspnea, embolism, laryngeal edema pulmonary infarction tachypnea
      Miscellaneous: Allergic reactions, anaphylaxis, rash

(Continued)

Menotropins *(Continued)*

Overdosage/Toxicology Symptoms include ovarian hyperstimulation.

Drug Interactions

Increased Effect/Toxicity: Clomiphene may decrease the amount of human menopausal gonadotropin (HMG) needed to induce ovulation (Gonadorelin, Factrel®); should not be used with drugs that stimulate ovulation.

Stability Lyophilized powder may be refrigerated or stored at room temperature; after reconstitution inject immediately, discard any unused portion; protect from light

Mechanism of Action Actions occur as a result of both follicle stimulating hormone (FSH) effects and luteinizing hormone (LH) effects; menotropins stimulate the development and maturation of the ovarian follicle (FSH), cause ovulation (LH), and stimulate the development of the corpus luteum (LH); in males it stimulates spermatogenesis (LH)

Pharmacodynamics/Kinetics Excretion: Urine (~10% as unchanged drug)

Usual Dosage Adults: I.M.:

Spermatogenesis (Male): Following pretreatment with hCG, 1 ampul 3 times/week and hCG 2000 units twice weekly until sperm is detected in the ejaculate (4-6 months) then may be increased to 2 ampuls of menotropins (150 units FSH/150 units LH) 3 times/week

Induction of ovulation (Female): 1 ampul/day (75 units of FSH and LH) for 9-12 days followed by 10,000 units hCG 1 day after the last dose; repeated at least twice at same level before increasing dosage to 2 ampuls (150 units FSH/150 units LH)

Repronex®: I.M., S.C.:

Infertile patients with oligo-anovulation: Initial: 150 int. units daily for the first 5 days of treatment. Adjustments should not be made more frequently than once every 2 days and should not exceed 75-150 int. units per adjustment. Maximum daily dose should not exceed 450 int. units and dosing beyond 12 days is not recommended. If patient's response to Repronex® is appropriate, hCG 5000-10,000 units should be given one day following the last dose of Repronex®. Hold dose if serum estradiol is >2000 pg/mL, if the ovaries are abnormally enlarged, or if abdominal pain occurs; the patient should also be advised to refrain from intercourse.

Assisted reproductive technologies: Initial (in patients who have received GnRH agonist or antagonist pituitary suppression): 225 int. units; adjustments in dose should not be made more frequently than once every 2 days and should not exceed more than 75-50 int. units per adjustment. The maximum daily doses of Repronex® given should not exceed 450 int. units and dosing beyond 12 days is not recommended. Once adequate follicular development is evident, hCG (5000-10,000 units) should be administered to induce final follicular maturation in preparation for oocyte retrieval. Withhold treatment when ovaries are abnormally enlarged on last day of therapy (to reduce chance of developing OHSS).

Administration I.M. or S.C. (Repronex® ONLY) administration. The lower abdomen (alternating sides) should be used for subcutaneous administration.

Monitoring Parameters hCG levels, serum estradiol; vaginal ultrasound; in cases of suspected OHSS, monitor fluid intake and output, weight, hematocrit, serum and urinary electrolytes, urine specific gravity, BUN and creatinine, and abdominal girth

Patient Information Multiple ovulations resulting in plural gestations have been reported

Nursing Implications Female: Assess knowledge/teach appropriate method for measuring basal body temperature to indicate ovulation. Stress importance of following prescriber's instructions for timing intercourse. If self-administered, assess/teach appropriate injection technique and needle disposal.

Dosage Forms

Injection:

Follicle stimulating hormone activity 75 units and luteinizing hormone activity 75 units per 2 mL ampul

Follicle stimulating hormone activity 150 units and luteinizing hormone activity 150 units per 2 mL ampul

♦ **Mentax**® *see Butenafine on page 198*

♦ 292 **MEP**® (Can) *see Aspirin and Meprobamate on page 124*

♦ **Mepergan**® *see Meperidine and Promethazine on page 860*

Meperidine *(me PER i deen)*

Related Information

Adult ACLS Algorithms *on page 1632*
Narcotic Agonists Comparison *on page 1506*

U.S. Brand Names Demerol®; Meperitab®

Canadian Brand Names Demerol®

Synonyms Isonipecaine Hydrochloride; Meperidine Hydrochloride; Pethidine Hydrochloride

Therapeutic Category Analgesic, Narcotic

Use Management of moderate to severe pain; adjunct to anesthesia and preoperative sedation

Restrictions C-II

Pregnancy Risk Factor B/D (prolonged use or high doses at term)

Contraindications Hypersensitivity to meperidine or any component of the formulation; patients receiving MAO inhibitors presently or in the past 14 days; pregnancy (prolonged use or high doses near term)

Warnings/Precautions Use with caution in patients with pulmonary, hepatic, renal disorders, or increased intracranial pressure; use with caution in patients with renal failure or seizure disorders or those receiving high-dose meperidine; normeperidine (an active metabolite and CNS stimulant) may accumulate and precipitate twitches, tremors, or seizures; some preparations contain sulfites which may cause allergic reaction; not recommended as a drug of first choice for the treatment of chronic pain in the elderly due to the accumulation of normeperidine; for acute pain, its use should be limited to 1-2 doses; tolerance or drug dependence may result from extended use

Adverse Reactions Frequency not defined.

Cardiovascular: Hypotension

Central nervous system: Fatigue, drowsiness, dizziness, nervousness, headache, restlessness, malaise, confusion, mental depression, hallucinations, paradoxical CNS stimulation, increased intracranial pressure, seizures (associated with metabolite accumulation)

Dermatologic: Rash, urticaria

Gastrointestinal: Nausea, vomiting, constipation, anorexia, stomach cramps, xerostomia, biliary spasm, paralytic ileus

Genitourinary: Ureteral spasms, decreased urination

Local: Pain at injection site

Neuromuscular & skeletal: Weakness

Respiratory: Dyspnea

Miscellaneous: Histamine release, physical and psychological dependence

Overdosage/Toxicology Symptoms include CNS depression, respiratory depression, mydriasis, bradycardia, pulmonary edema, chronic tremors, CNS excitability, and seizures. Treatment of overdose includes airway support, establishment of an I.V. line, and administration of naloxone 2 mg I.V. (0.01 mg/kg for children), with repeat administration as necessary, up to a total of 10 mg.

Drug Interactions

Cytochrome P450 Effect: CYP2D6 enzyme substrate

Increased Effect/Toxicity: Meperidine may aggravate the adverse effects of isoniazid. MAO inhibitors, fluoxetine, and other serotonin uptake inhibitors greatly potentiate the effects of meperidine, severe toxic reactions may occur. CNS depressants, tricyclic antidepressants, and phenothiazines may potentiate the effects of meperidine. Ritonavir may increase the risk of CNS toxicity and seizures of meperidine (increased formation of normeperidine).

Decreased Effect: Phenytoin may decrease the analgesic effects of meperidine.

Ethanol/Nutrition/Herb Interactions

Ethanol: Avoid or limit ethanol (may increase CNS depression). Watch for sedation.

Food: Glucose may cause hyperglycemia; monitor blood glucose concentrations.

Herb/Nutraceutical: Avoid valerian, St John's wort, kava kava, gotu kola (may increase CNS depression).

Stability Meperidine injection should be stored at room temperature and protected from light and freezing; protect oral dosage forms from light

Incompatible with aminophylline, heparin, phenobarbital, phenytoin, and sodium bicarbonate

Mechanism of Action Binds to opiate receptors in the CNS, causing inhibition of ascending pain pathways, altering the perception of and response to pain; produces generalized CNS depression

Pharmacodynamics/Kinetics

Onset of action: Analgesic: Oral, S.C., I.M.: 10-15 minutes; I.V.: ~5 minutes

Peak effect: Oral, S.C., I.M.: ~1 hour

Duration: Oral, S.C., I.M.: 2-4 hours

Distribution: Crosses placenta; enters breast milk

Protein binding: 65% to 75%

Metabolism: Hepatic; active metabolite (normeperidine)

Bioavailability: ~50% to 60%; increased with liver disease

Half-life elimination:

Parent drug: Terminal phase: Neonates: 23 hours; range: 12-39 hours; Adults: 2.5-4 hours; Adults with liver disease: 7-11 hours

Normeperidine (active metabolite): 15-30 hours; can accumulate with high doses or with decreased renal function

Usual Dosage Doses should be titrated to appropriate analgesic effect; when changing route of administration, note that oral doses are about half as effective as parenteral dose; in addition, oral route may result in a greater accumulation of normeperidine; chronic oral therapy is not generally advised

Children: Oral, I.M., I.V., S.C.: 1-1.5 mg/kg/dose every 3-4 hours as needed; 1-2 mg/kg as a single dose preoperative medication may be used; maximum 100 mg/dose

Adults: Oral, I.M., I.V.: S.C.: 50-150 mg/dose every 3-4 hours as needed

Elderly:

Oral: 50 mg every 4 hours

I.M.: 25 mg every 4 hours

Dosing adjustment in renal impairment: Avoid repeated administration of meperidine in renal dysfunction:

Cl_{cr} 10-50 mL/minute: Administer at 75% of normal dose

Cl_{cr} <10 mL/minute: Administer at 50% of normal dose

Dosing adjustment/comments in hepatic disease: Increased narcotic effect in cirrhosis; reduction in dose more important for oral than I.V. route

Administration

Meperidine may be administered I.M. (preferably), S.C., or I.V.

I.V. push should be administered slowly, use of a 10 mg/mL concentration has been recommended

Monitoring Parameters Pain relief, respiratory and mental status, blood pressure; observe patient for excessive sedation, CNS depression, seizures, respiratory depression

Reference Range Therapeutic: 70-500 ng/mL (SI: 283-2020 nmol/L); Toxic: >1000 ng/mL (SI: >4043 nmol/L)

Test Interactions ↑ amylase (S), ↑ BSP retention, ↑ CPK (I.M. injections)

Patient Information Avoid alcohol, may cause drowsiness

Nursing Implications If I.V. administration is required, inject very slowly using a diluted solution; administer over at least 5 minutes; intermittent infusion: dilute to 1 mg/mL and administer over 15-30 minutes; dilute to ≤10 mg/mL for intermittent I.V. use

Dosage Forms

Infusion, as hydrochloride: 10 mg/mL (30 mL) [via compatible infusion device only]

Injection, as hydrochloride [multidose vial]: 50 mg/mL (30 mL); 100 mg/mL (20 mL)

Injection as hydrochloride [single-dose]: 25 mg/dose (1 mL); 50 mg/dose (1 mL); 75 mg/dose (1 mL); 100 mg/dose (1 mL)

(Continued)

Meperidine *(Continued)*

Syrup, as hydrochloride: 50 mg/5 mL (500 mL)
Tablet, as hydrochloride: 50 mg, 100 mg

Meperidine and Promethazine *(me PER i deen & proe METH a zeen)*

U.S. Brand Names Mepergan®
Synonyms Promethazine and Meperidine
Therapeutic Category Analgesic, Narcotic
Use Management of moderate to severe pain
Restrictions C-II
Pregnancy Risk Factor B/D (prolonged use or high doses at term)
Usual Dosage Adults:

Oral: One (1) capsule every 4-6 hours
I.M.: Inject 1-2 mL every 3-4 hours

Additional Information Complete prescribing information for this medication should be consulted for additional detail.
Dosage Forms

Capsule: Meperidine hydrochloride 50 mg and promethazine hydrochloride 25 mg
Injection: Meperidine hydrochloride 25 mg and promethazine hydrochloride 25 per mL (2 mL, 10 mL)

♦ **Meperidine Hydrochloride** *see Meperidine on page 858*
♦ **Meperitab®** *see Meperidine on page 858*

Mephobarbital *(me foe BAR bi tal)*

U.S. Brand Names Mebaral®
Canadian Brand Names Mebaral®
Synonyms Methylphenobarbital
Therapeutic Category Anticonvulsant; Barbiturate; Sedative
Use Sedative; treatment of grand mal and petit mal epilepsy
Restrictions C-IV
Pregnancy Risk Factor D
Contraindications Hypersensitivity to mephobarbital, other barbiturates, or any component of the formulation; pre-existing CNS depression; respiratory depression; severe uncontrolled pain; history of porphyria; pregnancy
Adverse Reactions

>10%: Central nervous system: Dizziness, "hangover" effect, lightheadedness, somnolence
1% to 10%:

Central nervous system: Confusion, faint feeling, headache, insomnia, mental depression, nervousness, nightmares, unusual excitement
Gastrointestinal: Constipation, nausea, vomiting

<1% (Limited to important or life-threatening): Agranulocytosis, angioedema, dependence, exfoliative dermatitis, hallucinations, hypotension, megaloblastic anemia, respiratory depression, skin rash, Stevens-Johnson syndrome, thrombocytopenia, thrombophlebitis

Drug Interactions

Cytochrome P450 Effect: CYP2C, 2C8, and 2C19 enzyme substrate
Increased Effect/Toxicity: When combined with other CNS depressants, ethanol, narcotic analgesics, antidepressants, or benzodiazepines, additive respiratory and CNS depression may occur. Barbiturates may enhance the hepatotoxic potential of acetaminophen overdoses. Chloramphenicol, MAO inhibitors, valproic acid, and felbamate may inhibit barbiturate metabolism. Barbiturates may impair the absorption of griseofulvin, and may enhance the nephrotoxic effects of methoxyflurane. Concurrent use of phenobarbital with meperidine may result in increased CNS depression.
Decreased Effect: Barbiturates are hepatic enzyme inducers, and may increase the metabolism of antipsychotics, some beta-blockers (unlikely with atenolol and nadolol), calcium channel blockers, chloramphenicol, cimetidine, corticosteroids, cyclosporine, disopyramide, doxycycline, ethosuximide, felbamate, furosemide, griseofulvin, lamotrigine, phenytoin, propafenone, quinidine, tacrolimus, TCAs, and theophylline. Barbiturates may increase the metabolism of estrogens and reduce the efficacy of oral contraceptives; an alternative method of contraception should be considered. Barbiturates inhibit the hypoprothrombinemic effects of oral anticoagulants via increased metabolism. Barbiturates may enhance the metabolism of methadone resulting in methadone withdrawal.

Mechanism of Action Increases seizure threshold in the motor cortex; depresses monosynaptic and polysynaptic transmission in the CNS
Pharmacodynamics/Kinetics

Onset of action: 20-60 minutes
Duration: 6-8 hours
Absorption: ~50%
Half-life elimination, serum: 34 hours

Usual Dosage Oral:

Epilepsy:

Children: 6-12 mg/kg/day in 2-4 divided doses
Adults: 200-600 mg/day in 2-4 divided doses

Sedation:

Children:

<5 years: 16-32 mg 3-4 times/day
>5 years: 32-64 mg 3-4 times/day

Adults: 32-100 mg 3-4 times/day

Dosing adjustment in renal or hepatic impairment: Use with caution and reduce dosages
Dietary Considerations High doses of pyridoxine may decrease drug effect; barbiturates may increase the metabolism of vitamin D & K; dietary requirements of vitamin D, K, C, B$_{12}$, folate and calcium may be increased with long-term use.
Nursing Implications High doses of pyridoxine may decrease drug effect

Dosage Forms Tablet: 32 mg, 50 mg, 100 mg

♦ **Mephyton**® *see* Phytonadione *on page 1082*

Mepivacaine (me PIV a kane)
U.S. Brand Names Carbocaine®; Isocaine® HCl; Polocaine®
Canadian Brand Names Carbocaine®; Polocaine®
Synonyms Mepivacaine Hydrochloride
Therapeutic Category Local Anesthetic, Injectable
Use Local anesthesia by nerve block; **not** for use in spinal anesthesia
Pregnancy Risk Factor C
Contraindications Hypersensitivity to mepivacaine, any component of the formulation, or other amide anesthetics; allergy to sodium bisulfate
Warnings/Precautions Use with caution in patients with cardiac disease, renal disease, and hyperthyroidism; convulsions due to systemic toxicity leading to cardiac arrest have been reported presumably due to intravascular injection
Adverse Reactions Degree of adverse effects in the CNS and cardiovascular system are directly related to the blood levels of mepivacaine. The effects below are more likely to occur after systemic administration rather than infiltration.

Cardiovascular: Bradycardia, cardiovascular collapse, edema, heart block, hypotension, myocardial depression, ventricular arrhythmias, angioneurotic edema
Central nervous system: High blood levels result in anxiety, restlessness, disorientation, confusion, dizziness, and seizures. This is followed by depression of CNS resulting in somnolence, unconsciousness, and possible respiratory arrest. In some cases, symptoms of CNS stimulation may be absent and the primary CNS effects are somnolence and unconsciousness.
Dermatologic: Cutaneous lesions, urticaria
Gastrointestinal: Nausea, vomiting
Local: Transient stinging or burning at injection site
Ophthalmic: Blurred vision
Otic: Tinnitus
Respiratory: Respiratory arrest
Miscellaneous: Anaphylactoid reactions

Overdosage/Toxicology Symptoms include dizziness, cyanosis, tremors, and bronchial spasm. Treatment is primarily symptomatic and supportive. Termination of anesthesia by pneumatic tourniquet inflation should be attempted when the agent is administered by infiltration or regional injection. Seizures commonly respond to diazepam, while hypotension responds to I.V. fluids and Trendelenburg positioning. Bradyarrhythmias (when the heart rate is <60) can be treated with I.V., I.M., or S.C. atropine 15 mcg/kg. With the development of metabolic acidosis, I.V. sodium bicarbonate 0.5-2 mEq/kg and ventilatory assistance should be instituted.
Drug Interactions
   Increased Effect/Toxicity: Beta-blockers could theoretically decrease clearance.
Mechanism of Action Mepivacaine is an amino amide local anesthetic similar to lidocaine; like all local anesthetics, mepivacaine acts by preventing the generation and conduction of nerve impulses
Pharmacodynamics/Kinetics
   Onset of action: Epidural: 7-15 minutes
   Duration: 2-2.5 hours; similar onset and duration following infiltration
   Protein binding: 70% to 85%
   Metabolism: Primarily hepatic via N-demethylation, hydroxylation, and glucuronidation
   Half-life elimination: 1.9 hours
   Excretion: Urine (95% as metabolites)
Usual Dosage Children and Adults: Injectable local anesthetic: Varies with procedure, degree of anesthesia needed, vascularity of tissue, duration of anesthesia required, and physical condition of patient
Administration Before injecting, withdraw syringe plunger to ensure injection is not into vein or artery
Nursing Implications Before injecting, withdraw syringe plunger to ensure injection is not into vein or artery
Additional Information
   Peripheral nerve block, caudal/epidural, therapeutic block: 1% or 2% solution
   Transvaginal, paracervical block: 1% solution
   Infiltration: 0.5% solution
   Dental procedures: Mepivacaine 3% or mepivacaine 2% solution with levonordefrin
Dosage Forms Injection, as hydrochloride: 1% [10 mg/mL] (30 mL, 50 mL); 1.5% [15 mg/mL] (30 mL); 2% [20 mg/mL] (20 mL, 50 mL); 3% [30 mg/mL] (1.8 mL)

♦ **Mepivacaine Hydrochloride** *see* Mepivacaine *on page 861*

Meprobamate (me proe BA mate)
U.S. Brand Names Equanil®; Miltown®
Canadian Brand Names Apo®-Meprobamate
Therapeutic Category Antianxiety Agent
Use Management of anxiety disorders
Unlabeled/Investigational Use Demonstrated value for muscle contraction, headache, premenstrual tension, external sphincter spasticity, muscle rigidity, opisthotonos-associated with tetanus
Restrictions C-IV
Pregnancy Risk Factor D
Contraindications Hypersensitivity to meprobamate, related compounds (including carisoprodol), or any component of the formulation; acute intermittent porphyria; pre-existing CNS depression; narrow-angle glaucoma; severe uncontrolled pain; pregnancy
(Continued)

Meprobamate *(Continued)*

Warnings/Precautions Physical and psychological dependence and abuse may occur; abrupt cessation may precipitate withdrawal. Use with caution in patients with depression or suicidal tendencies, or in patients with a history of drug abuse. May cause CNS depression, which may impair physical or mental abilities. Patients must be cautioned about performing tasks which require mental alertness (ie, operating machinery or driving). Effects with other sedative drugs or ethanol may be potentiated. Not recommended in children <6 years of age; allergic reaction may occur in patients with history of dermatological condition (usually by fourth dose). Use with caution in patients with renal or hepatic impairment, or with a history of seizures. Use caution in the elderly as it may cause confusion, cognitive impairment, or excessive sedation.

Adverse Reactions Frequency not defined.

Cardiovascular: Syncope, peripheral edema, palpitations, tachycardia, arrhythmia

Central nervous system: Drowsiness, ataxia, dizziness, paradoxical excitement, confusion, slurred speech, headache, euphoria, chills, vertigo, paresthesia, overstimulation

Dermatologic: Rashes, purpura, dermatitis, Stevens-Johnson syndrome, petechiae, ecchymosis

Gastrointestinal: Diarrhea, vomiting, nausea

Hematologic: Leukopenia, eosinophilia, agranulocytosis, aplastic anemia

Neuromuscular & skeletal: Weakness

Ocular: Blurred vision, impairment of accommodation

Renal: Renal failure

Respiratory: Wheezing, dyspnea, bronchospasm, angioneurotic edema

Overdosage/Toxicology Symptoms include drowsiness, lethargy, ataxia, coma, hypotension, shock, and death. Treatment is supportive following attempts to enhance drug elimination. Hypotension should be treated with I.V. fluids and/or Trendelenburg positioning. Dialysis and hemoperfusion have not demonstrated significant reductions in blood drug concentrations.

Drug Interactions

Increased Effect/Toxicity: CNS depressants (ethanol) may increase CNS depression.

Ethanol/Nutrition/Herb Interactions

Ethanol: Avoid ethanol (may increase CNS depression).

Herb/Nutraceutical: Avoid valerian, St John's wort, kava kava, gotu kola (may increase CNS depression).

Mechanism of Action Affects the thalamus and limbic system; also appears to inhibit multineuronal spinal reflexes

Pharmacodynamics/Kinetics

Onset of action: Sedation: ~1 hour

Distribution: Crosses placenta; enters breast milk

Metabolism: Hepatic

Half-life elimination: 10 hours

Excretion: Urine (8% to 20% as unchanged drug); feces (10% as metabolites)

Usual Dosage Oral:

Children 6-12 years: Anxiety: 100-200 mg 2-3 times/day

Adults: Anxiety: 400 mg 3-4 times/day, up to 2400 mg/day

Dosing interval in renal impairment:

Cl_{cr} 10-50 mL/minute: Administer every 9-12 hours

Cl_{cr} <10 mL/minute: Administer every 12-18 hours

Hemodialysis: Moderately dialyzable (20% to 50%)

Dosing adjustment in hepatic impairment: Probably necessary in patients with liver disease

Monitoring Parameters Mental status

Reference Range Therapeutic: 6-12 μg/mL (SI: 28-55 μmol/L); Toxic: >60 μg/mL (SI: >275 μmol/L)

Patient Information May cause drowsiness; avoid alcohol

Nursing Implications Assist with ambulation; monitor mental status

Additional Information Withdrawal should be gradual over 1-2 weeks. Benzodiazepine and buspirone are better choices for treatment of anxiety disorders.

Dosage Forms Tablet: 200 mg, 400 mg

♦ **Meprobamate and Aspirin** *see* Aspirin and Meprobamate *on page 124*

♦ **Mepron™** *see* Atovaquone *on page 128*

Mequinol and Tretinoin *(ME kwi nole & TRET i noyn)*

U.S. Brand Names Solagé™

Canadian Brand Names Solagé™

Therapeutic Category Retinoic Acid Derivative; Vitamin A Derivative

Use Treatment of solar lentigines; the efficacy of using Solagé™ daily for >24 weeks has not been established. The local cutaneous safety of Solagé™ in non-Caucasians has not been adequately established.

Pregnancy Risk Factor X

Pregnancy/Breast-Feeding Implications May cause fetal harm when administered to a pregnant woman. It is unknown if mequinol or tretinoin are excreted in breast milk. Use caution in breast-feeding.

Contraindications Hypersensitivity to mequinol, tretinoin, or any component of the formulation; pregnancy, women of childbearing potential

Warnings/Precautions Discontinue if hypersensitivity is noted. Use extreme caution in eczematous skin conditions. Safety and efficacy have not been established in moderately or heavily pigmented skin. Not to be taken with photosensitizing drugs (eg, thiazides, tetracyclines, fluoroquinolones, phenothiazines, sulfonamides). Avoid sun (including sun lamps) or use protective clothing. Do not use in sunburned patients until they have fully recovered. Use extreme caution in patients who have significant exposure to the sun through their occupation. Use caution in patient with history or family history of vitiligo. For external use only.

Weather extremes (wind, cold) may be irritating to users of Solagé™. Do not use in pediatric patients. No bathing or showering for at least 6 hours after application. Effects of chronic use (>52 weeks) are unknown.

Adverse Reactions
>10%: Dermatologic: Erythema (49%), burning, stinging or tingling (26%), desquamation (14%), pruritus (12%),
1% to 10%: Dermatologic: Skin irritation (5%), hypopigmentation (5%), halo hypopigmentation (7%), rash (3%), dry skin (3%), crusting (3%), vesicular bullae rash (2%), contact allergic reaction (1%)

Overdosage/Toxicology Excessive topical application will lead to marked redness, peeling, discomfort, or hypopigmentation. Oral ingestion may lead to the adverse events seen in vitamin A overdose. If oral ingestion occurs, the patient should be monitored and appropriate supportive measures used as necessary. In rats who ingested 5 mL/kg, the signs of toxicity were of alcohol (high alcohol content in formulation).

Drug Interactions
Increased Effect/Toxicity:
Topical products with skin drying effects (eg, those containing alcohol, astringents, spices, or lime; medicated soaps or shampoos; permanent wave solutions; hair depilatories or waxes; and others) may increase skin irritation. Avoid concurrent use.
Photosensitizing drugs (eg, thiazides, tetracyclines, fluoroquinolones, phenothiazines, sulfonamides) can further increase sun sensitivity. Avoid concurrent use.

Stability Store at controlled room temperature of 15°C to 30°C (59°F to 86°F); flammable, keep away from heat and open flame

Mechanism of Action Solar lentigines are localized, pigmented, macular lesions of the skin on areas of the body chronically exposed to the sun. Mequinol is a substrate for the enzyme tyrosinase and acts as a competitive inhibitor of the formation of melanin precursors. The mechanisms of depigmentation for both drugs is unknown.

Pharmacodynamics/Kinetics
Absorption: Percutaneous absorption was 4.4% of tretinoin when applied as 0.8 mL of Solagé™ to a 400 cm^2 area of the back
Time to peak: Mequinol: 2 hours

Usual Dosage Solar lentigines: Topical: Apply twice daily to solar lentigines using the applicator tip while avoiding application to the surrounding skin. Separate application by at least 8 hours or as directed by physician.

Administration Avoid eyes, mouth, paranasal creases, and mucous membranes when applying

Patient Information No bathing or showering for at least 6 hours after application. Avoid eyes, mouth, paranasal creases, and mucous membranes when applying. Application of larger amounts or more frequently will not result in more rapid or better results. Follow application directions closely. Wait 30 minutes after use before applying cosmetics. Avoid sun exposure (including sun lamps) or use protective clothing. Some reappearance of freckles may occur after discontinuation. After application, short-term stinging, burning, or irritation may occur.

Nursing Implications Educate patient about sun avoidance or use of protective clothing. If patient experiences significant local irritation (redness, burning, stinging, peeling, or itching) then direct patient to use less medication, decrease frequency of use, discontinue temporarily, or discontinue altogether.

Dosage Forms Liquid, topical: Mequinol 2% and tretinoin 0.01% (30 mL)

Mercaptopurine (mer kap toe PYOOR een)

U.S. Brand Names Purinethol®
Canadian Brand Names Purinethol®
Synonyms 6-Mercaptopurine; 6-MP
Therapeutic Category Antineoplastic Agent, Antimetabolite (Purine)
Use Maintenance therapy in acute lymphoblastic leukemia (ALL); other (less common) uses include chronic granulocytic leukemia, induction therapy in ALL, and treatment of non-Hodgkin's lymphomas
Pregnancy Risk Factor D
Contraindications Hypersensitivity to mercaptopurine or any component of the formulation; patients whose disease showed prior resistance to mercaptopurine or thioguanine; severe liver disease, severe bone marrow suppression; pregnancy
Warnings/Precautions The U.S. Food and Drug Administration (FDA) currently recommends that procedures for proper handling and disposal of antineoplastic agents be considered. Mercaptopurine may cause birth defects; potentially carcinogenic; adjust dosage in patients with renal impairment or hepatic failure; use with caution in patients with prior bone marrow suppression; patients may be at risk for pancreatitis. Toxicity to immunosuppressives is increased in elderly. Start with lowest recommended adult doses. Signs of infection, such as fever and WBC rise, may not occur. Lethargy and confusion may be more prominent signs of infection.

To avoid potentially serious dosage errors, the terms "6-mercaptopurine" or "6-MP" should be avoided; use of these terms has been associated with sixfold overdosages.

Adverse Reactions
>10%:
Hematologic: Myelosuppression; leukopenia, thrombocytopenia, anemia
Onset: 7-10 days
Nadir: 14-16 days
Recovery: 21-28 days
Hepatic: Intrahepatic cholestasis and focal centralobular necrosis (40%), characterized by hyperbilirubinemia, increased alkaline phosphatase and AST, jaundice, ascites, encephalopathy; more common at doses >2.5 mg/kg/day. Usually occurs within 2 months of therapy but may occur within 1 week, or be delayed up to 8 years.
1% to 10%:
Central nervous system: Drug fever
(Continued)

Mercaptopurine *(Continued)*

Dermatologic: Hyperpigmentation, rash

Endocrine & metabolic: Hyperuricemia

Gastrointestinal: Nausea, vomiting, diarrhea, stomatitis, anorexia, stomach pain, mucositis

Renal: Renal toxicity

<1% (Limited to important or life-threatening): Dry and scaling rash, eosinophilia, glossitis, tarry stools

Overdosage/Toxicology Immediate symptoms are nausea and vomiting. Delayed symptoms include bone marrow suppression, hepatic necrosis, and gastroenteritis.

Drug Interactions

Increased Effect/Toxicity: Allopurinol can cause increased levels of 6-MP by inhibition of xanthine oxidase. Decrease dose of 6-MP by 75% when both drugs are used concomitantly. Seen only with oral 6-MP usage, not with I.V. May potentiate effect of bone marrow suppression (reduce 6-MP to 25% of dose).

Doxorubicin: Synergistic liver toxicity with 6-MP in >50% of patients, which resolved with discontinuation of the 6-MP.

Hepatotoxic drugs: Any agent which could potentially alter the metabolic function of the liver could produce higher drug levels and greater toxicities from either 6-MP or thioguanine (6-TG).

Decreased Effect: 6-MP inhibits the anticoagulation effect of warfarin by an unknown mechanism.

Stability Store at room temperature.

Mechanism of Action Purine antagonist which inhibits DNA and RNA synthesis; acts as false metabolite and is incorporated into DNA and RNA, eventually inhibiting their synthesis. 6-MP is substituted for hypoxanthine; must be metabolized to active nucleotides once inside the cell.

Pharmacodynamics/Kinetics

Absorption: Variable and incomplete (16% to 50%)

Distribution: V_d = total body water; CNS penetration is poor

Protein binding: 30%

Metabolism: Hepatic (first-pass effect) and in GI mucosa; hepatically via xanthine oxidase and methylation to sulfate conjugates, 6-thiouric acid, and other inactive compounds

Half-life elimination: Age dependent: Children: 21 minutes; Adults: 47 minutes

Time to peak, serum: ~2 hours

Excretion: Urine; following high (1 g/m^2) I.V. doses, 20% to 40% excreted unchanged; at lower doses renal elimination minor

Usual Dosage Oral (refer to individual protocols):

Children: Maintenance: 75 mg/m^2/day given once daily

Adults:

Induction: 2.5-5 mg/kg/day (100-200 mg)

Maintenance: 1.5-2.5 mg/kg/day OR 80-100 mg/m^2/day given once daily

Elderly: Due to renal decline with age, start with lower recommended doses for adults

Dosing adjustment in renal or hepatic impairment: Dose should be reduced to avoid accumulation, but specific guidelines are not available

Hemodialysis: Removed; supplemental dosing is usually required

Dietary Considerations Should not be administered with meals.

Administration Further dilute the 10 mg/mL reconstituted solution in normal saline or D_5W to a final concentration for administration of 1-2 mg/mL; administer by slow I.V. continuous infusion

Monitoring Parameters CBC with differential and platelet count, liver function tests, uric acid, urinalysis

Patient Information Take daily dose at the same time each day. Preferable to take an on empty stomach (1 hour before or 2 hours after meals). Maintain adequate hydration (2-3 L/ day of fluids unless instructed to restrict fluid intake). You may experience nausea and vomiting, diarrhea, or loss of appetite (frequent small meals may help/request medication) or weakness or lethargy (use caution when driving or engaging in tasks that require alertness until response to drug is known). Use good oral care to reduce incidence of mouth sores. You may be more susceptible to infection (avoid crowds or exposure to infection). May cause headache (request medication). Report signs of opportunistic infection (eg, fever, chills, sore throat, burning urination, fatigue); bleeding (eg, tarry stools, easy bruising); unresolved mouth sores, nausea, or vomiting; swelling of extremities, difficulty breathing, or unusual weight gain. The drug may be excreted in breast milk, therefore, an alternative form of feeding your baby should be used. Contraceptive measures are recommended during therapy.

Nursing Implications Adjust dosage in patients with renal insufficiency to lowest recommended dose; monitor dose response with WBC and platelet counts; observe for signs of infection and bleeding or bruising; further dilute the 10 mg/mL reconstituted solution in normal saline or D_5W to a final concentration for administration to 1-2 mg/mL; administer by slow I.V. continuous infusion

Dosage Forms Tablet, scored: 50 mg

Extemporaneous Preparations A 50 mg/mL oral suspension was made by crushing the tablets, mixing with a volume of Cologel® suspending agent equal to $^1/_3$ the final volume, and adding a 2:1 mixture of simple syrup and cherry syrup to make the final volume; stable for 14 days when stored in an amber glass bottle at room temperature

Dressman JB and Poust RI, "Stability of Allopurinol and of Five Antineoplastics in Suspension," *Am J Hosp Pharm*, 1983, 40:616-8.

+ **6-Mercaptopurine** *see* Mercaptopurine *on page 863*

+ **Mercapturic Acid** *see* Acetylcysteine *on page 32*

+ **Meridia®** *see* Sibutramine *on page 1234*

Meropenem (mer oh PEN em)

Related Information
Antimicrobial Drugs of Choice *on page 1588*
Community-Acquired Pneumonia in Adults *on page 1603*

U.S. Brand Names Merrem® I.V.

Canadian Brand Names Merrem®

Therapeutic Category Antibiotic, Anaerobic; Antibiotic, Carbapenem

Use Intra-abdominal infections (complicated appendicitis and peritonitis) caused by viridans group streptococci, *E. coli*, *K. pneumoniae*, *P. aeruginosa*, *B. fragilis*, *B. thetaiotaomicron*, and *Peptostreptococcus* sp; also indicated for bacterial meningitis in pediatric patients >3 months of age caused by *S. pneumoniae*, *H. influenzae*, and *N. meningitidis*; meropenem has also been used to treat soft tissue infections, febrile neutropenia, and urinary tract infections

Pregnancy Risk Factor B

Pregnancy/Breast-Feeding Implications Although no teratogenic or infant harm has been found in studies, excretion in breast milk is not known and this drug should be used during pregnancy and lactation only if clearly indicated

Contraindications Hypersensitivity to meropenem, any component of the formulation, or other carbapenems (eg, imipenem); patients who have experienced anaphylactic reactions to other beta-lactams

Warnings/Precautions Pseudomembranous colitis and hypersensitivity reactions have occurred and often require immediate drug discontinuation; thrombocytopenia has been reported in patients with significant renal dysfunction; seizures have occurred in patients with underlying neurologic disorders (less frequent than with imipenem and cilastatin); safety and efficacy have not been established for children <3 months of age; superinfection possible with long courses of therapy

Adverse Reactions
1% to 10%:
Central nervous system: Headache (2%)
Dermatologic: Rash (2% to 3%, includes diaper-area moniliasis in pediatrics), pruritus (1%)
Gastrointestinal: Diarrhea (4% to 5%), nausea/vomiting (1% to 4%), constipation (1%), oral moniliasis (up to 2% in pediatric patients), glossitis
Local: Inflammation at the injection site (2%), phlebitis/thrombophlebitis (1%), injection site reaction (1%)
Respiratory: Apnea (1%)
Miscellaneous: Sepsis (2%), septic shock (1%)
<1% (Limited to important or life-threatening): Agitation/delirium, agranulocytosis, angioedema, anorexia, arrhythmias, cholestatic jaundice/jaundice, decreased prothrombin time, dyspepsia, dyspnea, eosinophilia, epistaxis, erythema multiforme, gastrointestinal hemorrhage, hallucinations, heart failure, hemoperitoneum, hepatic failure, hypotension, ileus, leukopenia, melena, myocardial infarction, neutropenia, paresthesia, pleural effusion, pulmonary edema, renal failure, seizures, Stevens-Johnson syndrome, toxic epidermal necrolysis, urticaria, vaginal moniliasis

Overdosage/Toxicology No cases of acute overdosage are reported which have resulted in symptoms. Supportive therapy is recommended. Meropenem and its metabolite are removable by dialysis.

Drug Interactions
Decreased Effect: Probenecid interferes with renal excretion of meropenem. Serum concentrations of valproic acid may be reduced during meropenem therapy (potentially to subtherapeutic levels).

Stability Store at room temperature; when vials are reconstituted with NaCl/D_5W, they are stable for 2 hours/1 hour at room temperature or for 18 hours/8 hours when refrigerated; when diluted in minibags, they are stable for up to 24 hours refrigerated in NaCl and 6 hours in D_5W

Mechanism of Action Inhibits bacterial cell wall synthesis by binding to several of the penicillin-binding proteins, which in turn inhibit the final transpeptidation step of peptidoglycan synthesis in bacterial cell walls, thus inhibiting cell wall biosynthesis; bacteria eventually lyse due to ongoing activity of cell wall autolytic enzymes (autolysins and murein hydrolases) while cell wall assembly is arrested

Pharmacodynamics/Kinetics
Distribution: V_d: Adults: ~0.3 L/kg, Children: 0.4-0.5 L/kg; penetrates well into most body fluids and tissues; CSF concentrations approximate those of the plasma
Protein binding: 2%
Metabolism: Hepatic; metabolizes to open beta-lactam form (inactive)
Half-life elimination:
Normal renal function: 1-1.5 hours
Cl_{cr} 30-80 mL/minute: 1.9-3.3 hours
Cl_{cr} 2-30 mL/minute: 3.82-5.7 hours
Time to peak, tissue: 1 hour following infusion
Excretion: Urine (~25% as inactive metabolites)

Usual Dosage I.V.:
Neonates:
Preterm: 20 mg/kg/dose every 12 hours (may be increased to 40 mg/kg/dose if treating a highly resistant organism such as *Pseudomonas aeruginosa*)
Full-term (<3 months of age): 20 mg/kg/dose every 8 hours (may be increased to 40 mg/kg/dose if treating a highly resistant organism such as *Pseudomonas aeruginosa*)
Children >3 months (<50 kg):
Intra-abdominal infections: 20 mg/kg every 8 hours (maximum dose: 1 g every 8 hours)
Meningitis: 40 mg/kg every 8 hours (maximum dose: 2 g every 8 hours)
Children >50 kg:
Intra-abdominal infections: 1 g every 8 hours
Meningitis: 2 g every 8 hours
Adults: 1 g every 8 hours
(Continued)

Meropenem *(Continued)*

Elderly: No differences in safety or efficacy have been reported. However, increased sensitivity may occur in some elderly patients; adjust dose based on renal function; see Warnings/Precautions

Dosing adjustment in renal impairment: Adults:
Cl_{cr} 26-50 mL/minute: Administer 1 g every 12 hours
Cl_{cr} 10-25 mL/minute: Administer 500 mg every 12 hours
Cl_{cr} <10 mL/minute: Administer 500 mg every 24 hours
Dialysis: Meropenem and its metabolites are readily dialyzable
Continuous arteriovenous or venovenous hemodiafiltration effects: Dose as Cl_{cr} 10-50 mL/minute

Administration Administer I.V. infusion over 15-30 minutes; I.V. bolus injection over 3-5 minutes

Monitoring Parameters Monitor for signs of anaphylaxis during first dose

Additional Information 1 g of meropenem contains 90.2 mg of sodium as sodium carbonate (3.92 mEq)

Dosage Forms
Powder for injection: 500 mg, 1 g
ADD-Vantage®: 500 mg, 1 g

◆ **Merrem® (Can)** *see Meropenem on page 865*
◆ **Merrem® I.V.** *see Meropenem on page 865*
◆ **Meruvax® II** *see Rubella Virus Vaccine (Live) on page 1217*

Mesalamine *(me SAL a meen)*

U.S. Brand Names Asacol®; Canasa™; Pentasa®; Rowasa®
Canadian Brand Names Asacol®; Mesasal®; Novo-5 ASA; Pentasa®; Quintasa®; Rowasa®; Salofalk®
Synonyms 5-Aminosalicylic Acid; 5-ASA; Fisalamine; Mesalazine
Therapeutic Category 5-Aminosalicylic Acid Derivative; Anti-inflammatory Agent; Anti-inflammatory Agent, Rectal
Use
Oral: Treatment and maintenance of remission of mildly to moderately active ulcerative colitis
Rectal: Treatment of active mild to moderate distal ulcerative colitis, proctosigmoiditis, or proctitis
Pregnancy Risk Factor B
Contraindications Hypersensitivity to mesalamine, sulfasalazine, salicylates, or any component of the formulation
Warnings/Precautions May cause an acute intolerance syndrome (cramping, acute abdominal pain, bloody diarrhea; sometimes fever, headache, rash); discontinue if this occurs. Patients with pyloric stenosis may have prolonged gastric retention of tablets, delaying the release of mesalamine in the colon. Pericarditis should be considered in patients with chest pain; pancreatitis should be considered in patients with new abdominal complaints. Use caution in patients with impaired renal or hepatic function. Renal impairment (including minimal change nephropathy and acute/chronic interstitial nephritis) has been reported; use caution with other medications converted to mesalamine. Postmarketing reports suggest an increased incidence of blood dyscrasias in patients >65 years of age. In addition, elderly may have difficulty administering and retaining rectal suppositories and decreased renal function; use with caution and monitor. Safety and efficacy in pediatric patients have not been established.

Rowasa® enema: Contains potassium metabisulfite; may cause severe hypersensitivity reactions (ie, anaphylaxis) in patients with sulfite allergies.

Adverse Reactions Adverse effects vary depending upon dosage form. Effects as reported with tablets, unless otherwise noted:
>10%:
Central nervous system: Pain (14%)
Gastrointestinal: Abdominal pain (18%; enema: 8%)
Genitourinary: Eructation (16%)
Respiratory: Pharyngitis (11%)
1% to 10%:
Cardiovascular: Chest pain (3%), peripheral edema (3%)
Central nervous system: Chills (3%), dizziness (suppository: 3%), fever (enema: 3%; suppository: 1%), insomnia (2%), malaise (2%)
Dermatologic: Rash (6%; suppository: 1%), pruritus (3%; enema: 1%), acne (2%; suppository: 1%)
Gastrointestinal: Dyspepsia (6%), constipation (5%), vomiting (5%), colitis exacerbation (3%; suppository: 1%), nausea (capsule: 3%), flatulence (enema: 6%), hemorrhoids (enema: 1%), nausea and vomiting (capsule: 1%), rectal pain (enema: 1%; suppository: 2%)
Local: Pain on insertion of enema tip (enema: 1%)
Neuromuscular & skeletal: Back pain (7%; enema: 1%), arthralgia (5%), hypertonia (5%), myalgia (3%), arthritis (2%), leg/joint pain (enema: 2%),
Ocular: Conjunctivitis (2%)
Respiratory: Flu-like syndrome (3%; enema: 5%), diaphoresis (3%), cough increased (2%)
<1% (Limited to important or life-threatening): Agranulocytosis, alopecia, aplastic anemia, cholestatic jaundice, cholecystitis, edema, elevated liver enzymes, erythema nodosum, fibrosing alveolitis, gout, Guillain-Barré syndrome, hepatitis, hepatocellular damage, hepatotoxicity, interstitial nephritis, Kawasaki-like syndrome, liver failure, liver necrosis, lupus-like syndrome, minimal change nephrotic syndrome, myocarditis, nephropathy, pancreatitis, pancytopenia, pericarditis, thrombocytopenia, vertigo
Overdosage/Toxicology Symptoms include decreased motor activity, diarrhea, vomiting, and renal function impairment. Treatment is supportive following emesis, gastric lavage, and activated charcoal slurry.

Drug Interactions
Decreased Effect: Decreased digoxin bioavailability.

Ethanol/Nutrition/Herb Interactions Food: Oral: Mesalamine serum levels may be decreased if taken with food.

Stability
Enema: Store at controlled room temperature. Use promptly once foil wrap is removed; contents may darken with time (do not use if dark brown)

Suppository: Store at controlled room temperature away from direct heat, light, and humidity; do not refrigerate

Tablet: Store at controlled room temperature

Mechanism of Action Mesalamine (5-aminosalicylic acid) is the active component of sulfa-salazine; the specific mechanism of action of mesalamine is unknown; however, it is thought that it modulates local chemical mediators of the inflammatory response, especially leukotri-enes; action appears topical rather than systemic

Pharmacodynamics/Kinetics
Absorption: Rectal: Variable and dependent upon retention time, underlying GI disease, and colonic pH; Oral: Tablet: ~28%, capsule: ~20% to 30%

Metabolism: Hepatic to acetyl-5-aminosalicylic acid (intestinal metabolism may also occur)

Half-life elimination: 5-ASA: 0.5-1.5 hours; acetyl-5-ASA: 5-10 hours

Time to peak, serum: 4-7 hours

Excretion: Urine (as metabolites); feces (<2%)

Usual Dosage
Adults (usual course of therapy is 3-8 weeks):
Oral:
Treatment of ulcerative colitis:
Capsule: 1 g 4 times/day
Tablet: Initial: 800 mg (2 tablets) 3 times/day for 6 weeks
Maintenance of remission of ulcerative colitis:
Capsule: 1 g 4 times/day
Tablet: 1.6 g/day in divided doses
Rectal:
Retention enema: 60 mL (4 g) at bedtime, retained overnight, approximately 8 hours
Rectal suppository: Insert 1 suppository in rectum twice daily; retain suppositories for at least 1-3 hours to achieve maximum benefit
Canasa™: May increase to 3 times/day if inadequate response is seen after 2 weeks.
Note: Some patients may require rectal and oral therapy concurrently.
Elderly: See adult dosing; use with caution

Administration Swallow capsules or tablets whole, do not chew or crush

Monitoring Parameters CBC and renal function, particularly in elderly patients

Patient Information Retain enemas for 8 hours or as long as practical; shake bottle well; do not chew or break oral tablets; for suppositories, remove foil wrapper, avoid excessive handling

Nursing Implications Provide patient with copy of mesalamine administration instructions and discuss proper use.

Dosage Forms
Capsule, controlled release (Pentasa®): 250 mg
Suppository, rectal (Canasa™, Rowasa®): 500 mg
Suspension, rectal (Rowasa®): 4 g/60 mL [contains potassium metabisulphite] (7s)
Tablet, delayed release, enteric coated (Asacol®): 400 mg

♦ **Mesalazine** see Mesalamine on page 866
♦ **Mesasal® (Can)** see Mesalamine on page 866
♦ **M-Eslon® (Can)** see Morphine Sulfate on page 936

Mesna (MES na)
U.S. Brand Names Mesnex™
Canadian Brand Names Mesnex™; Uromitexan™
Synonyms Sodium 2-Mercaptoethane Sulfonate
Therapeutic Category Antidote, Cyclophosphamide-induced Hemorrhagic Cystitis; Anti-dote, Ifosfamide-induced Hemorrhagic Cystitis
Use Orphan drug: Mesna is a uroprotectant used to prevent hemorrhagic cystitis induced by ifosfamide and cyclophosphamide; mesna is always given in conjunction with ifosfamide, and is often given in conjunction with cyclophosphamide
Pregnancy Risk Factor B
Contraindications Hypersensitivity to mesna or other thiol compounds, or any component of the formulation
Warnings/Precautions Examine morning urine specimen for hematuria prior to ifosfamide or cyclophosphamide treatment; if hematuria (>50 RBC/HPF) develops, reduce the ifosfamide/cyclophosphamide dose or discontinue the drug; will not prevent or alleviate other toxicities associated with ifosfamide or cyclophosphamide and will not prevent hemorrhagic cystitis in all patients. Allergic reactions have been reported; patients with autoimmune disorders may be at increased risk. Symptoms ranged from mild hypersensitivity to systemic anaphylactic reactions. I.V. formulation contains benzyl alcohol; do not use in neonates or infants.
Adverse Reactions It is difficult to distinguish reactions from those caused by concomitant chemotherapy.
>10%: Gastrointestinal: Bad taste in mouth with oral administration (100%), vomiting (secondary to the bad taste after oral administration, or with high I.V. doses)
<1% (Limited to important or life-threatening): Anaphylaxis, hypersensitivity, hypertonia, injection site reaction, limb pain, myalgia, platelet count decreased, tachycardia, tachypnea

Drug Interactions
Decreased Effect: Warfarin: Questionable alterations in coagulation control.

Stability Store unopened vials at controlled room temperature of 20°C to 25°C (68°F to 77°F). Diluted solutions are chemically and physically stable for 24 hours at room temperature; (Continued)

Mesna *(Continued)*

polypropylene syringes are stable for 9 days at refrigeration or room temperature; injection diluted for oral administration is stable 24 hours at refrigeration

Standard dose: Dose/100-1,000 mL D_5W or NS to a final concentration of 1-20 mg/mL
Incompatible with cisplatin
Compatible with bleomycin, cyclophosphamide, dexamethasone, etoposide, lorazepam, potassium chloride
Mechanism of Action In blood, mesna is oxidized to dimesna which is chemically less reactive than mesna; dimesna is reduced in the kidney back to mesna, supplying a free thiol group which binds to and inactivates acrolein, the urotoxic metabolite of ifosfamide and cyclophosphamide

Pharmacodynamics/Kinetics
Distribution: No tissue penetration
Protein binding: 69% to 75%
Metabolism: Rapidly oxidized intravascularly to mesna disulfide; mesna disulfide is reduced in renal tubules back to mesna following glomerular filtration.
Bioavailability: 45% to 79% (oral)
Half-life elimination: Parent drug: 24 minutes; Mesna disulfide: 72 minutes
Time to peak, plasma: 2-3 hours
Excretion: Urine; as unchanged drug (18% to 26%) and metabolites

Usual Dosage Refer to individual protocols.
Children and Adults:
I.V. regimen: Recommended dose is 60% of the ifosfamide dose given in 3 divided doses, with ifosfamide, and 4 hours and 8 hours after the ifosfamide dose.
Note: Other I.V. doses/regimens include 4 divided doses of mesna (0, 3, 6, and 9 hours after the start of ifosfamide) and continuous infusions. Continuous infusions commonly employ doses equal to the dose of ifosfamide or cyclophosphamide. It has been suggested that continuous infusions provide more consistent urinary free thiol levels. Infusions are continued for 8-24 hours after completion of ifosfamide or cyclophosphamide.
I.V./Oral regimen: Commonly, the first dose is I.V. and the 2-hour and 6-hour doses are oral. I.V. dose is 20% of the ifosfamide dose at the time of ifosfamide dosing. Oral doses are 40% of the ifosfamide dose and are given 2 hours and 6 hours after the ifosfamide dose. **Note:** Total dose equal 100% of the ifosfamide dose.

Administration
Oral: For oral administration (if tablets are not used), injection may be diluted in 1:1, 1:2, 1:10, 1:100 concentrations in carbonated beverages (cola, ginger ale, Pepsi®, Sprite®, Dr Pepper®, etc), juices (apple or orange), or whole milk (chocolate or white), and is stable 24 hours at refrigeration; used in conjunction with ifosfamide; examine morning urine specimen for hematuria prior to ifosfamide or cyclophosphamide treatment. Patients who vomit within 2 hours of taking oral mesna should repeat the dose or receive I.V. mesna.
I.V.: Administer by I.V. infusion over 15-30 minutes or per protocol; mesna can be diluted in D_5W or NS to a final concentration of 1-20 mg/mL

Monitoring Parameters Urinalysis

Test Interactions False-positive urinary ketones with Multistix® or Labstix®

Nursing Implications Used concurrent with and/or following high-dose ifosfamide or cyclophosphamide; mesna also has been administered orally with carbonated beverages or juice (most palatable in grape juice); administer by I.V. infusion over 15-30 minutes or per protocol; mesna can be diluted in D_5W or NS to a final concentration of 1-20 mg/mL

Dosage Forms
Injection: 100 mg/mL (2 mL, 4 mL, 10 mL)
Tablet: 400 mg

♦ Mesnex™ *see Mesna on page 867*

Mesoridazine *(mez oh RID a zeen)*
Related Information
Antacid Drug Interactions *on page 1477*
Antipsychotic Agents Comparison *on page 1486*
U.S. Brand Names Serentil®
Canadian Brand Names Serentil®
Synonyms Mesoridazine Besylate
Therapeutic Category Antipsychotic Agent, Phenothiazine; Phenothiazine Derivative
Use Management of schizophrenic patients who fail to respond adequately to treatment with other antipsychotic drugs, either because of insufficient effectiveness or the inability to achieve an effective dose due to intolerable adverse effects from these drugs
Unlabeled/Investigational Use Psychosis
Pregnancy Risk Factor C
Contraindications Hypersensitivity to mesoridazine or any component of the formulation (cross-reactivity between phenothiazines may occur); severe CNS depression and coma; prolonged QT interval (>450 msec), including prolongation due to congenital causes; history of arrhythmias; concurrent use of medications which prolong QT_c (including type Ia and type III antiarrhythmics, cyclic antidepressants, some fluoroquinolones, cisapride); concurrent use of mesoridazine with fluvoxamine, fluoxetine, paroxetine, pindolol, or propranolol
Warnings/Precautions Safety in children <6 months of age has not been established; use with caution in patients with cardiovascular disease or seizures; benefits of therapy must be weighed against risks of therapy; doses >1 g/day frequently cause pigmentary retinopathy; some products contain sulfites and/or tartrazine; use with caution in patients with narrow-angle glaucoma, bone marrow suppression, severe liver disease.

Has been shown to prolong QT_c interval in a dose-dependent manner (associated with an increased risk of torsade de pointes). Patients should have a baseline EKG prior to initiation, and should not receive mesoridazine if baseline QT_c >450 msec. Mesoridazine should be discontinued in patients with a QT_c interval >500 msec. Potassium levels must be evaluated and normalized prior to and throughout treatment.

May cause hypotension, particularly with I.M. administration. Highly sedating, use with caution in disorders where CNS depression is a feature. Use with caution in Parkinson's disease. Caution in patients with hemodynamic instability; bone marrow suppression; predisposition to seizures; subcortical brain damage; severe cardiac, hepatic, renal, or respiratory disease. Esophageal dysmotility and aspiration have been associated with antipsychotic use; use with caution in patients at risk of pneumonia (ie, Alzheimer's disease). Caution in breast cancer or other prolactin-dependent tumors (may elevate prolactin levels). May alter temperature regulation or mask toxicity of other drugs due to antiemetic effects. May cause orthostatic hypotension - use with caution in patients at risk of this effect or those who would tolerate transient hypotensive episodes (cerebrovascular disease, cardiovascular disease, or other medications which may predispose).

Phenothiazines may cause anticholinergic effects (confusion, agitation, constipation, dry mouth, blurred vision, urinary retention). Therefore, they should be used with caution in patients with decreased gastrointestinal motility, urinary retention, BPH, xerostomia, or visual problems. Conditions which also may be exacerbated by cholinergic blockade include narrow-angle glaucoma (screening is recommended) and worsening of myasthenia gravis. Relative to other antipsychotics, mesoridazine has a high potency of cholinergic blockade.

May cause extrapyramidal reactions, including pseudoparkinsonism, acute dystonic reactions, akathisia, and tardive dyskinesia (risk of these reactions is low relative to other neuroleptics). May be associated with neuroleptic malignant syndrome (NMS) or pigmentary retinopathy (particularly at doses >1 g/day).

Adverse Reactions Frequency not defined.
    Cardiovascular: Hypotension, orthostatic hypotension, tachycardia, QT prolongation (dose-dependent, up to 100% of patients at higher dosages), syncope, edema
    Central nervous system: Pseudoparkinsonism, akathisia, dystonias, tardive dyskinesia, dizziness, drowsiness, restlessness, ataxia, slurred speech, neuroleptic malignant syndrome (NMS), impairment of temperature regulation, lowering of seizure threshold
    Dermatologic: Increased sensitivity to sun, rash, itching, angioneurotic edema, dermatitis, discoloration of skin (blue-gray)
    Endocrine & metabolic: Changes in menstrual cycle, changes in libido, gynecomastia, lactation, galactorrhea
    Gastrointestinal: Constipation, xerostomia, weight gain, nausea, vomiting, stomach pain
    Genitourinary: Difficulty in urination, ejaculatory disturbances, impotence, enuresis, incontinence, priapism, urinary retention
    Hematologic: Agranulocytosis, leukopenia, eosinophilia, thrombocytopenia, anemia, aplastic anemia
    Hepatic: Cholestatic jaundice, hepatotoxicity
    Neuromuscular & skeletal: Weakness, tremor, rigidity
    Ocular: Pigmentary retinopathy, photophobia, blurred vision, cornea and lens changes
    Respiratory: Nasal congestion
    Miscellaneous: Diaphoresis (decreased), lupus-like syndrome

Overdosage/Toxicology Symptoms include deep sleep, coma, extrapyramidal symptoms, abnormal involuntary muscle movements, and hypotension. Monitor for cardiac arrhythmias and avoid use of drugs which prolong the QT interval. Following initiation of essential overdose management, toxic symptom supportive treatment should be initiated. Hypotension usually responds to I.V. fluids or Trendelenburg positioning. If unresponsive to these measures, the use of a parenteral inotrope may be required. Seizures commonly respond to diazepam (I.V. 5-10 mg bolus in adults every 15 minutes, if needed, up to a total of 30 mg; I.V. 0.25-0.4 mg/kg/dose up to a total of 10 mg in children) or to phenytoin or phenobarbital. Critical cardiac arrhythmias often respond to I.V. phenytoin (15 mg/kg up to 1 g), while other antiarrhythmics can be used. Extrapyramidal symptoms (eg, dystonic reactions) can be managed with benztropine mesylate I.V. 1-2 mg (adults).

Drug Interactions
    Cytochrome P450 Effect: CYP1A2, 2D6, and 3A3/4 enzyme substrate; CYP2D6 enzyme inhibitor
    Increased Effect/Toxicity: Concurrent use with inhibitors of CYP2D6 or CYP3A3/4 is contraindicated, due to the potential to increase mesoridazine concentrations. In addition, use of mesoridazine with other agents known to prolong QT_c may increase the risk of malignant arrhythmias; concurrent use is contraindicated - includes type I and type III antiarrhythmics, TCAs, and some quinolone antibiotics (sparfloxacin, moxifloxacin, gatifloxacin). Mesoridazine concentrations may be increased by chloroquine, propranolol, and sulfadoxine-pyrimethamine (propranolol is contraindicated). Mesoridazine may increase the effect and/or toxicity of antihypertensives, anticholinergics, lithium, CNS depressants (ethanol, narcotics), and trazodone.
    Decreased Effect: Mesoridazine may inhibit the activity of bromocriptine and levodopa. Benztropine (and other anticholinergics) may inhibit the therapeutic response to mesoridazine and excess anticholinergic effects may occur. Barbiturates and cigarette smoking may enhance the hepatic metabolism of mesoridazine. Mesoridazine and possibly other low potency antipsychotic may reverse the pressor effects of epinephrine.

Ethanol/Nutrition/Herb Interactions
    Ethanol: Avoid ethanol (may increase CNS depression).
    Herb/Nutraceutical: Avoid valerian, St John's wort, kava kava, gotu kola (may increase CNS depression).

Stability Protect all dosage forms from light; clear or slightly yellow solutions may be used; should be dispensed in amber or opaque vials/bottles. Solutions may be diluted or mixed with fruit juices or other liquids but must be administered immediately after mixing; do not prepare bulk dilutions or store bulk dilutions.

Mechanism of Action Blockade of postsynaptic CNS dopamine$_2$ receptors in the mesolimbic and mesocortical areas

Pharmacodynamics/Kinetics
    Duration: 4-6 hours
    (Continued)

Mesoridazine *(Continued)*

Absorption: Tablet: Erratic; Liquid: More dependable

Protein binding: 91% to 99%

Half-life elimination: 24-48 hours

Time to peak, serum: 2-4 hours; Steady-state serum: 4-7 days

Excretion: Urine

Usual Dosage Concentrate may be diluted just prior to administration with distilled water, acidified tap water, orange or grape juice; do not prepare and store bulk dilutions

Adults: Schizophrenia/psychoses:

Oral: 25-50 mg 3 times/day; maximum: 100-400 mg/day

I.M.: Initial: 25 mg, repeat in 30-60 minutes as needed; optimal dosage range: 25-200 mg/day

Elderly: Behavioral symptoms associated with dementia:

Oral: Initial: 10 mg 1-2 times/day; if <10 mg/day is desired, consider administering 10 mg every other day (qod). Increase dose at 4- to 7-day intervals by 10-25 mg/day; increase dose intervals (bid, tid, etc) as necessary to control response or side effects. Maximum daily dose: 250 mg. Gradual increases (titration) may prevent some side effects or decrease their severity.

I.M.: Initial: 25 mg; repeat doses in 30-60 minutes if necessary. Dose range: 25-200 mg/day. Elderly usually require less than maximal daily dose.

Hemodialysis: Not dialyzable (0% to 5%)

Administration When administering I.M. or I.V., watch for hypotension. Dilute oral concentrate just prior to administration with distilled water, acidified tap water, orange or grape juice. Do not prepare and store bulk dilutions. Do not mix oral solutions of mesoridazine and lithium, these oral liquids are incompatible when mixed. **Note:** Avoid skin contact with oral medication; may cause contact dermatitis.

Monitoring Parameters Orthostatic blood pressures; tremors, gait changes, abnormal movement in trunk, neck, buccal area or extremities; monitor target behaviors for which the agent is given; monitor hepatic function (especially if fever with flu-like symptoms); baseline EKG, baseline (and periodic) serum potassium; do not initiate if QT_c >450 msec (discontinue in any patient with a QT_c >500 msec)

Patient Information May cause drowsiness or restlessness, avoid alcohol and other CNS depressants; do not alter dosage or discontinue without consulting physician; avoid excessive sunlight, yearly ophthalmic examinations are necessary

Nursing Implications

Dilute oral concentrate with water or juice before administration; avoid skin contact with oral suspension or solution; may cause contact dermatitis; monitor orthostatic blood pressures 3-5 days after initiation of therapy or a dose increase

Monitor orthostatic blood pressures; tremors, gait changes, abnormal movement in trunk, neck, buccal area or extremities; monitor target behaviors for which the agent is administered; monitor hepatic function (especially if fever with flu-like symptoms); watch for hypotension when administering I.M. or I.V.

Additional Information Coadministration of two or more antipsychotics does not improve clinical response and may increase the potential for adverse effects.

Dosage Forms

Injection, as besylate: 25 mg/mL (1 mL)

Liquid, oral, as besylate: 25 mg/mL (118 mL)

Tablet, as besylate: 10 mg, 25 mg, 50 mg, 100 mg

- ♦ **Mesoridazine Besylate** *see Mesoridazine on page 868*
- ♦ **Mestinon®** *see Pyridostigmine on page 1161*
- ♦ **Mestinon®-SR (Can)** *see Pyridostigmine on page 1161*
- ♦ **Mestinon® Timespan®** *see Pyridostigmine on page 1161*

Mestranol and Norethindrone *(MES tra nole & nor eth IN drone)*

U.S. Brand Names Necon® 1/50; Norinyl® 1+50; Ortho-Novum® 1/50

Canadian Brand Names Ortho-Novum® 1/50

Synonyms Norethindrone and Mestranol

Therapeutic Category Contraceptive, Oral (Low Potency Estrogen, Low Potency Progestin); Contraceptive, Oral (Monophasic); Estrogen Derivative, Oral; Progestin

Use Prevention of pregnancy

Unlabeled/Investigational Use Treatment of hypermenorrhea, endometriosis, female hypogonadism

Pregnancy Risk Factor X

Pregnancy/Breast-Feeding Implications Breast-feeding is not recommended; excreted in breast milk; combination oral contraceptives decrease the quality and quantity of breast milk.

Pregnancy should be ruled out prior to treatment and discontinued if pregnancy occurs. In general, the use of combination hormonal contraceptives when inadvertently taken early in pregnancy have not been associated with teratogenic effects. Due to increased risk of thromboembolism postpartum, combination hormonal contraceptives should not be started earlier than 4-6 weeks following delivery.

Contraindications Hypersensitivity to mestranol, norethindrone, or any component of the formulation; thrombophlebitis or thromboembolic disorders (current or history of), cerebral vascular disease, coronary artery disease, valvular heart disease with complications, severe hypertension; diabetes mellitus with vascular involvement; severe headache with focal neurological symptoms; known or suspected breast carcinoma, endometrial cancer, estrogen-dependent neoplasms, undiagnosed abnormal genital bleeding; hepatic dysfunction or tumor, cholestatic jaundice of pregnancy, jaundice with prior combination hormonal contraceptive use; major surgery with prolonged immobilization; heavy smoking (≥15 cigarettes/day) in patients >35 years of age; pregnancy

Warnings/Precautions Combination hormonal contraceptives do not protect against HIV infection or other sexually-transmitted diseases. The risk of cardiovascular side effects increases in women who smoke cigarettes, especially those who are >35 years of age; women who use combination hormonal contraceptives should be strongly advised not to smoke. Combination hormonal contraceptives may lead to increased risk of myocardial infarction, use with caution in patients with risk factors for coronary artery disease. May increase the risk of thromboembolism. Combination hormonal contraceptives may have a dose-related risk of vascular disease, hypertension, and gallbladder disease. Women with hypertension should be encouraged to use a nonhormonal form of contraception. The use of combination hormonal contraceptives has been associated with a slight increase in frequency of breast cancer, however, studies are not consistent. Combination hormonal contraceptives may cause glucose intolerance. Retinal thrombosis has been reported (rarely). Use with caution in patients with renal disease, conditions that may be aggravated by fluid retention, depression, or history of migraine. Not for use prior to menarche.

The minimum dosage combination of estrogen/progestin that will effectively treat the individual patient should be used. New patients should be started on products containing <50 mcg of estrogen per tablet.

Adverse Reactions Frequency not defined.

Cardiovascular: Arterial thromboembolism, cerebral hemorrhage, cerebral thrombosis, edema, hypertension, mesenteric thrombosis, myocardial infarction

Central nervous system: Depression, dizziness, headache, migraine, nervousness, premenstrual syndrome, stroke

Dermatologic: Acne, erythema multiforme, erythema nodosum, hirsutism, loss of scalp hair, melasma (may persist), rash (allergic)

Endocrine & metabolic: Amenorrhea, breakthrough bleeding, breast enlargement, breast secretion, breast tenderness, carbohydrate intolerance, lactation decreased (postpartum), glucose tolerance decreased, libido changes, menstrual flow changes, sex hormone-binding globulins (SHBG) increased, spotting, temporary infertility (following discontinuation), thyroid-binding globulin increased, triglycerides increased

Gastrointestinal: Abdominal cramps, appetite changes, bloating, cholestasis, colitis, gallbladder disease, jaundice, nausea, vomiting, weight gain/loss

Genitourinary: Cervical erosion changes, cervical secretion changes, cystitis-like syndrome, vaginal candidiasis, vaginitis

Hematologic: Antithrombin III decreased, folate levels decreased, hemolytic uremic syndrome, norepinephrine induced platelet aggregability increased, porphyria, prothrombin increased; factors VII, VIII, IX, and X increased

Hepatic: Benign liver tumors, Budd-Chiari syndrome, cholestatic jaundice, hepatic adenomas

Local: Thrombophlebitis

Ocular: Cataracts, change in corneal curvature (steepening), contact lens intolerance, optic neuritis, retinal thrombosis

Renal: Impaired renal function

Respiratory: Pulmonary thromboembolism

Miscellaneous: Hemorrhagic eruption

Overdosage/Toxicology Toxicity is unlikely following single exposures of excessive doses. Treatment following emesis and charcoal administration should be supportive and symptomatic.

Drug Interactions

Cytochrome P450 Effect: Ethinyl estradiol: CYP3A3/4 enzyme substrate; mestranol: CYP2C9 enzyme substrate

Increased Effect/Toxicity: Acetaminophen and ascorbic acid may increase plasma levels of estrogen component. Atorvastatin and indinavir increase plasma levels of combination hormonal contraceptives. Combination hormonal contraceptives increase the plasma levels of alprazolam, chlordiazepoxide, cyclosporine, diazepam, prednisolone, selegiline, theophylline, tricyclic antidepressants. Combination hormonal contraceptives may increase (or decrease) the effects of coumarin derivatives.

Decreased Effect: Combination hormonal contraceptives may decrease plasma levels of acetaminophen, clofibric acid, lorazepam, morphine, oxazepam, salicylic acid, temazepam. Contraceptive effect decreased by acitretin, aminoglutethimide, amprenavir, anticonvulsants, griseofulvin, lopinavir, nelfinavir, nevirapine, penicillins (effect not consistent), rifampin, ritonavir, tetracyclines (effect not consistent) troglitazone. Combination hormonal contraceptives may decrease (or increase) the effects of coumarin derivatives.

Ethanol/Nutrition/Herb Interactions

Food: CNS effects of caffeine may be enhanced if oral contraceptives are used concurrently with caffeine. Grapefruit juice increases ethinyl estradiol concentrations and would be expected to increase progesterone serum levels as well; clinical implications are unclear.

Herb/Nutraceutical: St John's wort may decrease the effectiveness of combination hormonal contraceptives by inducing hepatic enzymes. Avoid dong quai and black cohosh (have estrogen activity). Avoid saw palmetto, red clover, ginseng.

Stability Store at controlled room temperature of 25°C (77°F).

Mechanism of Action Combination oral contraceptives inhibit ovulation via a negative feed-back mechanism on the hypothalamus, which alters the normal pattern of gonadotropin secretion of a follicle-stimulating hormone (FSH) and luteinizing hormone by the anterior pituitary. The follicular phase FSH and midcycle surge of gonadotropins are inhibited. In addition, combination hormonal contraceptives produce alterations in the genital tract, including changes in the cervical mucus, rendering it unfavorable for sperm penetration even if ovulation occurs. Changes in the endometrium may also occur, producing an unfavorable environment for nidation. Combination hormonal contraceptive drugs may alter the tubal transport of the ova through the fallopian tubes. Progestational agents may also alter sperm fertility.

Pharmacodynamics/Kinetics

Mestranol: Metabolism: Hepatic via demethylation to ethinyl estradiol via CYP2C9

Norethindrone: See Norethindrone monograph.

See Ethinyl Estradiol monograph for additional information.

Usual Dosage Oral: Adults: Female: Contraception:

Schedule 1 (Sunday starter): Dose begins on first Sunday after onset of menstruation; if the menstrual period starts on Sunday, take first tablet that very same day. **With a Sunday**

(Continued)

Mestranol and Norethindrone (Continued)

start, an additional method of contraception should be used until after the first 7 days of consecutive administration.

For 21-tablet package: Dosage is 1 tablet daily for 21 consecutive days, followed by 7 days off of the medication; a new course begins on the 8th day after the last tablet is taken.

For 28-tablet package: Dosage is 1 tablet daily without interruption.

Schedule 2 (Day 1 starter): Dose starts on first day of menstrual cycle taking 1 tablet daily.

For 21-tablet package: Dosage is 1 tablet daily for 21 consecutive days, followed by 7 days off of the medication; a new course begins on the 8th day after the last tablet is taken.

For 28-tablet package: Dosage is 1 tablet daily without interruption.

If all doses have been taken on schedule and one menstrual period is missed, continue dosing cycle. If two consecutive menstrual periods are missed, pregnancy test is required before new dosing cycle is started.

Missed doses **monophasic formulations** (refer to package insert for complete information):

One dose missed: Take as soon as remembered or take 2 tablets next day

Two consecutive doses missed in the first 2 weeks: Take 2 tablets as soon as remembered or 2 tablets next 2 days. **An additional method of contraception should be used for 7 days after missed dose.**

Two consecutive doses missed in week 3 or three consecutive doses missed at any time: **An additional method of contraception must be used for 7 days after a missed dose:**

Schedule 1 (Sunday starter): Continue dose of 1 tablet daily until Sunday, then discard the rest of the pack, and a new pack should be started that same day.

Schedule 2 (Day 1 starter): Current pack should be discarded, and a new pack should be started that same day.

Dosage adjustment in renal impairment: Specific guidelines not available; use with caution

Dosage adjustment in hepatic impairment: Contraindicated in patients with hepatic impairment

Dietary Considerations Should be taken at same time each day.

Administration Administer at the same time each day.

Monitoring Parameters Blood pressure, breast exam, Pap smear, and pregnancy; lipid profiles in patients being treated for hyperlipidemias

Patient Information Take exactly as directed; use additional method of birth control during first week of administration of first cycle

Women should inform their physicians if signs or symptoms of any of the following occur thromboembolic or thrombotic disorders including sudden severe headache or vomiting, disturbance of vision or speech, loss of vision, numbness or weakness in an extremity, sharp or crushing chest pain, calf pain, shortness of breath, severe abdominal pain or mass, mental depression or unusual bleeding. Women should discontinue taking the medication if they suspect they are pregnant or become pregnant.

Nursing Implications Administer at bedtime to minimize occurrence of adverse effects

Dosage Forms Tablet, monophasic formulations:

Necon® 1/50-21: Norethindrone 1 mg and mestranol 0.05 mg [light blue tablets] (21s)

Necon® 1/50-28: Norethindrone 1 mg and mestranol 0.05 mg [21 light blue tablets] and 7 white inactive tablets (28s)

Norinyl® 1+50: Norethindrone 1 mg and mestranol 0.05 mg [21 white tablets] and 7 orange inactive tablets (28s)

Ortho-Novum® 1/50: Norethindrone 1 mg and mestranol 0.05 mg [21 yellow tablets] and 7 green inactive tablets (28s)

- ♦ **Metacortandralone** see PrednisoLONE on page 1122
- ♦ **Metadate® CD** see Methylphenidate on page 894
- ♦ **Metadate™ ER** see Methylphenidate on page 894
- ♦ **Metadol™ (Can)** see Methadone on page 877
- ♦ **Metahydrin®** see Trichlormethiazide on page 1371
- ♦ **Metamucil® [OTC]** see Psyllium on page 1158
- ♦ **Metamucil® Smooth Texture [OTC]** see Psyllium on page 1158

Metaproterenol (met a proe TER e nol)

Related Information

Antacid Drug Interactions on page 1477

Bronchodilators, Comparison of Inhaled Sympathomimetics on page 1493

U.S. Brand Names Alupent®

Synonyms Metaproterenol Sulfate; Orciprenaline Sulfate

Therapeutic Category Beta$_2$-Adrenergic Agonist Agent; Bronchodilator; Sympathomimetic

Use Bronchodilator in reversible airway obstruction due to asthma or COPD; because of its delayed onset of action (1 hour) and prolonged effect (4 or more hours), this may not be the drug of choice for assessing response to a bronchodilator

Pregnancy Risk Factor C

Pregnancy/Breast-Feeding Implications

Clinical effects on the fetus: No data on crossing the placenta. Reported association with polydactyly in 1 study; may be secondary to severe maternal disease or chance.

Breast-feeding/lactation: No data on crossing into breast milk or clinical effects on the infant

Contraindications Hypersensitivity to metaproterenol or any component of the formulation; pre-existing cardiac arrhythmias associated with tachycardia

Warnings/Precautions Use with caution in patients with hypertension, CHF, hyperthyroidism, CAD, diabetes, or sensitivity to sympathomimetics; excessive prolonged use may result in decreased efficacy or increased toxicity and death; use caution in patients with pre-existing cardiac arrhythmias associated with tachycardia. Metaproterenol has more beta$_1$ activity than other sympathomimetics such as albuterol and, therefore, may no longer be the beta agonist of first choice. All patients should utilize a spacer device when using a metered dose inhaler. Oral use should be avoided due to the increased incidence of adverse effects.

Adverse Reactions
>10%:
  Cardiovascular: Tachycardia (<17%)
  Central nervous system: Nervousness (3% to 14%)
  Neuromuscular & skeletal: Tremor (1% to 33%)
1% to 10%:
  Cardiovascular: Palpitations (<4%)
  Central nervous system: Headache (<4%), dizziness (1% to 4%), insomnia (2%)
  Gastrointestinal: Nausea, vomiting, bad taste, heartburn (≥4%), xerostomia
  Neuromuscular & skeletal: Trembling, muscle cramps, weakness (1%)
  Respiratory: Coughing, pharyngitis (≤4%)
  Miscellaneous: Diaphoresis (increased) (≤4%)
<1% (Limited to important or life-threatening): Angina, chest pain, diarrhea, drowsiness, hypertension, paradoxical bronchospasm, taste change

Overdosage/Toxicology Symptoms include angina, arrhythmias, tremor, dry mouth, and insomnia. Beta-adrenergic stimulation can increase and cause increased heart rate, decreased blood pressure, and decreased CNS excitation. In cases of overdose, supportive therapy should be instituted, and prudent use of a cardioselective beta-adrenergic blocker (eg, atenolol or metoprolol) should be considered, keeping in mind the potential for induction of bronchoconstriction in an asthmatic individual. Dialysis has not been shown to be of value in the treatment of an overdose with this agent. Diazepam 0.07 mg/kg can be used for excitation seizures.

Drug Interactions
  Increased Effect/Toxicity: Sympathomimetics, TCAs, MAO inhibitors taken with metaproterenol may result in toxicity. Inhaled ipratropium may increase duration of bronchodilation. Halothane may increase risk of malignant arrhythmias; avoid concurrent use.
  Decreased Effect: Decreased effect of beta-blockers.

Stability Store in tight, light-resistant container; do not use if brown solution or contains a precipitate

Mechanism of Action Relaxes bronchial smooth muscle by action on beta$_2$-receptors with very little effect on heart rate

Pharmacodynamics/Kinetics
  Onset of action: Bronchodilation: Oral: ~15 minutes; Inhalation: ~60 seconds
    Peak effect: Oral: ~1 hour
  Duration: ~1-5 hours

Usual Dosage
  Oral:
    Children:
      <2 years: 0.4 mg/kg/dose given 3-4 times/day; in infants, the dose can be given every 8-12 hours
      2-6 years: 1-2.6 mg/kg/day divided every 6 hours
      6-9 years: 10 mg/dose 3-4 times/day
    Children >9 years and Adults: 20 mg 3-4 times/day
    Elderly: Initial: 10 mg 3-4 times/day, increasing as necessary up to 20 mg 3-4 times/day
  Inhalation: Children >12 years and Adults: 2-3 inhalations every 3-4 hours, up to 12 inhalations in 24 hours
  Nebulizer:
    Infants and Children: 0.01-0.02 mL/kg of 5% solution; minimum dose: 0.1 mL; maximum dose: 0.3 mL diluted in 2-3 mL normal saline every 4-6 hours (may be given more frequently according to need)
    Adolescents and Adults: 5-20 breaths of full strength 5% metaproterenol **or** 0.2 to 0.3 mL 5% metaproterenol in 2.5-3 mL normal saline until nebulized every 4-6 hours (can be given more frequently according to need)

Administration
  Inhalation: Do not use solutions for nebulization if they are brown or contain a precipitate. Shake inhaler well before using.
  Oral: Administer around-the-clock to promote less variation in peak and trough serum levels

Monitoring Parameters Assess lung sounds, pulse, and blood pressure before administration and during peak of medication; observe patient for wheezing after administration, if this occurs, call physician; monitor heart rate, respiratory rate, blood pressure, and arterial or capillary blood gases if applicable

Test Interactions ↑ potassium (S)

Patient Information Do not exceed recommended dosage - excessive use may lead to adverse effects or loss of effectiveness. Shake canister well before use. Administer pressurized inhalation during the second half of inspiration, as the airways are open wider and the aerosol distribution is more extensive. If more than one inhalation per dose is necessary, wait at least 1 full minute between inhalations - second inhalation is best delivered after 10 minutes for Alupent®. May cause nervousness, restlessness, insomnia - if these effects continue after dosage reduction, notify physician. Also notify physician if palpitations, tachycardia, chest pain, muscle tremors, dizziness, headache, flushing, or if breathing difficulty persists.

Nursing Implications Do not use solutions for nebulization if they are brown or contain a precipitate; before using, the inhaler must be shaken well

Additional Information Use with caution perioperatively due to beta$_1$ effect of agent. Hypertension and tachycardia are increased with exogenous sympathomimetics. During endotracheal intubation, beta$_2$-specific agent is more appropriate for perioperative use.

Dosage Forms
  Aerosol for oral inhalation, as sulfate: 0.65 mg/dose (14 g) [200 actuations]
  Solution for oral inhalation, as sulfate [preservative free]: 0.4% [4 mg/mL] (2.5 mL); 0.6% [6 mg/mL] (2.5 mL); 5% [50 mg/mL] (10 mL, 30 mL)
  Syrup, as sulfate: 10 mg/5 mL (120 mL, 480 mL)
  Tablet, as sulfate: 10 mg, 20 mg

♦ **Metaproterenol Sulfate** see Metaproterenol on page 872

Metaraminol (met a RAM i nole)

Related Information

Adrenergic Agonists, Cardiovascular Comparison *on page 1469*

Antacid Drug Interactions *on page 1477*

U.S. Brand Names Aramine®

Canadian Brand Names Aramine®

Synonyms Metaraminol Bitartrate

Therapeutic Category Adrenergic Agonist Agent; Sympathomimetic

Use Acute hypotensive crisis in the treatment of shock

Pregnancy Risk Factor D

Contraindications Hypersensitivity to metaraminol or any component of the formulation; cyclopropane or halothane anesthesia, or MAO inhibitors

Warnings/Precautions Can cause cardiac arrhythmias; use with caution in patients with a previous myocardial infarction, hypertension, hyperthyroidism; prolonged use may produce cumulative effects

Adverse Reactions Frequency not defined.

Cardiovascular: Tachycardia, hypertension, cardiac arrhythmias, flushing, palpitations, hypotension, angina

Central nervous system: Tremors, nervousness, headache, dizziness, weakness

Dermatologic: Sloughing of tissue

Gastrointestinal: Nausea

Local: Blanching of skin, abscess formation

Miscellaneous: Diaphoresis

Overdosage/Toxicology Symptoms include hypertension, cerebral hemorrhage, cardiac arrest, and seizures.

Drug Interactions

Increased Effect/Toxicity: Increased toxicity with cyclopropane, halothane, MAO inhibitors (hypertensive crisis), digoxin, oxytocin, rauwolfia alkaloids, reserpine

Decreased Effect: Effect may be decreased by TCAs

Stability Infusion solutions are stable for 24 hours; I.V. metaraminol is **incompatible** when mixed with amphotericin B, dexamethasone, erythromycin, hydrocortisone, methicillin, penicillin G, prednisolone, thiopental

Mechanism of Action Stimulates alpha-adrenergic receptors to cause vasoconstriction, reflex bradycardia, inhibits GI smooth muscle and vascular smooth muscle supplying skeletal muscle, increases heart rate and force of heart muscle contraction

Pharmacodynamics/Kinetics

Onset of action: Pressor effect: I.M.: ~10 minutes; I.V.: 1-2 minutes; S.C.: 5-20 minutes

Excretion: Not yet fully elucidated

Usual Dosage

Children:

I.M.: 0.01 mg/kg as a single dose

I.V.: 0.01 mg/kg as a single dose or intravenous infusion of 5 mcg/kg/minute

Adults:

Prevention of hypotension: I.M., S.C.: 2-10 mg

Adjunctive treatment of hypotension: I.V.: 15-100 mg in 250-500 mL NS or 5% dextrose in water

Severe shock: I.V.: 0.5-5 mg direct I.V. injection followed by intravenous infusion of 15-100 mg in 250-500 mL NS or D_5W; may also be administered endotracheally

Administration May be administered I.M., I.V., S.C.; however, I.V. is the preferred route because extravasation or local injection can cause necrosis; to prevent necrosis infiltrate area with 10-15 mL of saline containing 5-10 mg of phentolamine

Monitoring Parameters Blood pressure, EKG, PCWP, CVP, pulse, and urine output

Dosage Forms Injection, as bitartrate: 10 mg/mL (10 mL)

♦ **Metaraminol Bitartrate** *see Metaraminol on page 874*

♦ **Metastron®** *see Strontium-89 on page 1263*

♦ **Metatensin® (Can)** *see Trichlormethiazide on page 1371*

Metaxalone (me TAKS a lone)

U.S. Brand Names Skelaxin®

Canadian Brand Names Skelaxin®

Therapeutic Category Skeletal Muscle Relaxant

Use Relief of discomfort associated with acute, painful musculoskeletal conditions

Pregnancy Risk Factor C

Contraindications Hypersensitivity to metaxalone or any component of the formulation; impaired hepatic or renal function, history of drug-induced hemolytic anemias or other anemias

Warnings/Precautions Use with caution in patients with impaired hepatic function

Adverse Reactions Frequency not defined.

Central nervous system: Paradoxical stimulation, headache, drowsiness, dizziness, irritability

Dermatologic: Allergic dermatitis

Gastrointestinal: Nausea, vomiting, stomach cramps

Hematologic: Leukopenia, hemolytic anemia

Hepatic: Hepatotoxicity

Miscellaneous: Anaphylaxis

Overdosage/Toxicology No major toxicities have been reported.

Drug Interactions

Increased Effect/Toxicity: Additive effects with ethanol or CNS depressants

Ethanol/Nutrition/Herb Interactions Ethanol: Avoid ethanol (may increase CNS depression).

Mechanism of Action Does not have a direct effect on skeletal muscle; most of its therapeutic effect comes from actions on the central nervous system

Pharmacodynamics/Kinetics
Onset of action: ~1 hour
Duration: ~4-6 hours
Half-life elimination: 2-3 hours
Excretion: Urine (as metabolites)

Usual Dosage Children >12 years and Adults: Oral: 800 mg 3-4 times/day

Test Interactions False-positive Benedict's test

Patient Information Avoid alcohol and other CNS depressants; may cause drowsiness, impairment of judgment, or coordination; notify physician of dark urine, pale stools, yellowing of eyes, severe nausea, vomiting, or abdominal pain

Nursing Implications Raise bed rails, institute safety measures, assist with ambulation

Dosage Forms Tablet: 400 mg

Metformin (met FOR min)

Related Information
Diabetes Mellitus Treatment *on page 1657*
Hypoglycemic Drugs & Thiazolidinedione Information *on page 1502*

U.S. Brand Names Glucophage®; Glucophage® XR

Canadian Brand Names Apo®-Metformin; Gen-Metformin; Glucophage®; Glycon; Novo-Metformin; Nu-Metformin; Rho®-Metformin

Synonyms Metformin Hydrochloride

Therapeutic Category Antidiabetic Agent, Biguanide; Hypoglycemic Agent, Oral

Use Management of type 2 diabetes mellitus (noninsulin dependent, NIDDM) as monotherapy when hyperglycemia cannot be managed on diet alone. May be used concomitantly with a sulfonylurea or insulin to improve glycemic control.

Unlabeled/Investigational Use Treatment of HIV lipodystrophy syndrome

Pregnancy Risk Factor B

Pregnancy/Breast-Feeding Implications Abnormal blood glucose levels are associated with a higher incidence of congenital abnormalities. Insulin is the drug of choice for the control of diabetes mellitus during pregnancy. It is not known if metformin is excreted in human breast milk (excretion occurs in animal models); insulin therapy should be considered in breast-feeding women.

Contraindications Hypersensitivity to metformin or any component of the formulation; renal disease or renal dysfunction (serum creatinine ≥1.5 mg/dL in males or ≥1.4 mg/dL in females or abnormal clearance); clinical situations predisposing to hypoxemia, including conditions such as cardiovascular collapse, respiratory failure, acute myocardial infarction, acute congestive heart failure, and septicemia; acute or chronic metabolic acidosis with or without coma (including diabetic ketoacidosis); should be temporarily discontinued for 48 hours in patients undergoing radiologic studies involving the intravascular administration of iodinated contrast materials (potential for acute alteration in renal function).

Warnings/Precautions Administration of oral antidiabetic drugs has been reported to be associated with increased cardiovascular mortality as compared to treatment with diet alone or diet plus insulin.

Lactic acidosis is a rare, but potentially severe consequence of therapy with metformin. Withhold therapy in hypoxemia, dehydration or sepsis. The risk of lactic acidosis is increased in any patient with CHF requiring pharmacologic management. This risk is particularly high during acute or unstable congestive heart failure (see Contraindications) because of the risk of hypoperfusion and hypoxemia.

Metformin is substantially excreted by the kidney. The risk of accumulation and lactic acidosis increases with the degree of impairment of renal function. Patients with renal function below the limit of normal for their age should not receive metformin. In elderly patients, renal function should be monitored regularly. should not be used in any patient 80 years of age or older unless measurement of creatinine clearance verifies normal renal function. Use of concomitant medications that may affect renal function (ie, affect tubular secretion) may also affect metformin disposition. Therapy should be suspended for any surgical procedures - resume only after normal intake resumed and normal renal function is verified. Avoid use in patients with impaired liver function. Patient must be instructed to avoid excessive acute or chronic ethanol use.

Lactic acidosis should be suspected in any diabetic patient receiving metformin who has evidence of acidosis when evidence of ketoacidosis is lacking.

Adverse Reactions
>10%:
· Gastrointestinal: Nausea/vomiting (6% to 25%), diarrhea (10% to 53%), flatulence (12%)
Neuromuscular & skeletal: Weakness (9%)
1% to 10%:
Cardiovascular: Chest discomfort, flushing, palpitation
Central nervous system: Headache (6%), chills, dizziness, lightheadedness
Dermatologic: Rash
Endocrine & metabolic: Hypoglycemia
Gastrointestinal: Indigestion (7%), abdominal discomfort (6%), abdominal distention, abnormal stools, constipation, dyspepsia/ heartburn, taste disorder
Neuromuscular & skeletal: Myalgia
Respiratory: Dyspnea, upper respiratory tract infection
Miscellaneous: Decreased vitamin B_{12} levels (7%), increased diaphoresis, flu-like syndrome, nail disorder
<1% (Limited to important or life-threatening): Lactic acidosis, megaloblastic anemia

Overdosage/Toxicology Hypoglycemia has not been observed with ingestions up to 85 g of metformin, although lactic acidosis has occurred in such circumstances. Metformin is dialyzable with a clearance of up to 170 mL/minute. Hemodialysis may be useful for removal of accumulated drug from patients in whom metformin overdose is suspected.
(Continued)

Metformin *(Continued)*

Drug Interactions

Increased Effect/Toxicity: Furosemide and cimetidine may increase metformin blood levels. Cationic drugs (eg, amiloride, digoxin, morphine, procainamide, quinidine, quinine, ranitidine, triamterene, trimethoprim, and vancomycin) which are eliminated by renal tubular secretion have the potential to increase metformin levels by competing for common renal tubular transport systems.

Decreased Effect: Drugs which tend to produce hyperglycemia (eg, diuretics, corticosteroids, phenothiazines, thyroid products, estrogens, oral contraceptives, phenytoin, nicotinic acid, sympathomimetics, calcium channel blocking drugs, isoniazid) may lead to a loss of glucose control.

Ethanol/Nutrition/Herb Interactions

Ethanol: Avoid or limit ethanol (incidence of lactic acidosis may be increased; may cause hypoglycemia).

Food: Food decreases the extent and slightly delays the absorption. May decrease absorption of vitamin B_{12} and/or folic acid.

Herb/Nutraceutical: Caution with chromium, garlic, gymnema (may cause hypoglycemia).

Stability Store at 20°C to 25°C (68°F to 77°F).

Mechanism of Action Decreases hepatic glucose production, decreasing intestinal absorption of glucose and improves insulin sensitivity (increases peripheral glucose uptake and utilization).

Pharmacodynamics/Kinetics

Onset of action: Within days; maximum effects up to 2 weeks

Distribution: V_d: 654 ± 358 L

Protein binding: 92% to 99%; Plasma: negligible

Bioavailability, absolute: 50% to 60% under fasting conditions

Half-life elimination, plasma: 6.2 hours

Excretion: Urine (90% as unchanged drug)

Usual Dosage Note: Allow 1-2 weeks between dose titrations: Generally, clinically significant responses are not seen at doses <1500 mg daily; however, a lower recommended starting dose and gradual increased dosage is recommended to minimize gastrointestinal symptoms

Children 10-16 years: Management of type 2 diabetes mellitus: Oral: 500 mg tablets: Initial: 500 mg twice daily (give with the morning and evening meals); dosage increases should be made in increments of 1 tablet every week, given in divided doses, up to a maximum of 2000 mg/day

Adults: ≥17 years: Management of type 2 diabetes mellitus: Oral:

500 mg tablets: Initial: 500 mg twice daily (give with the morning and evening meals); dosage increases should be made in increments of 1 tablet every week, given in divided doses, up to a maximum of 2500 mg/day. Doses of up to 2000 mg/day may be given twice daily; if a dose of 2500 mg/day is required, it may be better tolerated 3 times/day (with meals).

850 mg tablets: Initial: 850 mg once daily (give with the morning meal); dosage increases should be made in increments of 1 tablet every *other* week, given in divided doses, up to a maximum of 2550 mg/day. Usual maintenance dose: 850 mg twice daily (with the morning and evening meals). Some patients may be given 850 mg 3 times/day (with meals).

Extended release tablets: Initial: 500 mg once daily (with the evening meal); dosage may be increased by 500 mg weekly; maximum dose: 2000 mg once daily. If glycemic control is not achieved at maximum dose, may divide dose to 1000 mg twice daily; if doses >2000 mg/day are needed, switch to regular release tablets and titrate to maximum dose of 2550 mg/day

Elderly: The initial and maintenance dosing should be conservative, due to the potential for decreased renal function. Generally, elderly patients should not be titrated to the maximum dose of metformin. Do not use in patients ≥80 years of age unless normal renal function has been established.

Transfer from other antidiabetic agents: No transition period is generally necessary except when transferring from chlorpropamide. When transferring from chlorpropamide, care should be exercised during the first 2 weeks because of the prolonged retention of chlorpropamide in the body, leading to overlapping drug effects and possible hypoglycemia.

Concomitant metformin and oral sulfonylurea therapy: If patients have not responded to 4 weeks of the maximum dose of metformin monotherapy, consider a gradual addition of an oral sulfonylurea, even if prior primary or secondary failure to a sulfonylurea has occurred. Continue metformin at the maximum dose.

Failed sulfonylurea therapy: Patients with prior failure on glyburide may be treated by gradual addition of metformin. Initiate with glyburide 20 mg and metformin 500 mg daily. Metformin dosage may be increased by 500 mg/day at weekly intervals, up to a maximum of 2500 mg/day (dosage of glyburide maintained at 20 mg/day).

Concomitant metformin and insulin therapy: Initial: 500 mg metformin once daily, continue current insulin dose; increase by 500 mg metformin weekly until adequate glycemic control is achieved

Maximum dose: 2500 mg metformin; 2000 mg metformin extended release

Decrease insulin dose 10% to 25% when FPG <120 mg/dL; monitor and make further adjustments as needed

Dosing adjustment/comments in renal impairment: The plasma and blood half-life of metformin is prolonged and the renal clearance is decreased in proportion to the decrease in creatinine clearance. Metformin is contraindicated in the presence of renal dysfunction defined as a serum creatinine >1.5 mg/dL in males or >1.4 mg/dL in females or a creatinine clearance <60 mL/minute.

Dosing adjustment in hepatic impairment: Avoid metformin; liver disease is a risk factor for the development of lactic acidosis during metformin therapy.

Dietary Considerations Drug may cause GI upset; take with food (to decrease GI upset). Take at the same time each day. Dietary modification based on ADA recommendations is a part of therapy. Monitor for signs and symptoms of vitamin B_{12} and/or folic acid deficiency; supplementation may be required.

Administration Extended release dosage form should be swallowed whole; do not crush, break, or chew

Monitoring Parameters Urine for glucose and ketones, fasting blood glucose, and hemoglobin A_{1c}. Initial and periodic monitoring of hematologic parameters (eg, hemoglobin/hematocrit and red blood cell indices) and renal function should be performed, at least annually. Check vitamin B_{12} and folate if anemia is present.

Reference Range Target range: Adults:
Fasting blood glucose: <120 mg/dL
Glycosylated hemoglobin: <7%

Patient Information Patients must be counseled by someone experienced in diabetes education, signs and symptoms of hyper- and hypoglycemia, exercise and diet, blood glucose monitoring, and other related topics; eat regularly, do not skip meals; carry quick source of sugar; medical alert bracelet. Patients should be counselled against excessive alcohol intake while receiving metformin. Metformin alone does not usually cause hypoglycemia, although it may occur in conjunction with oral sulfonylureas.

Nursing Implications Patients who are NPO may need to have their dose held to avoid hypoglycemia. Extended release tablets: Inert components of the tablet may be found excreted in the stool.

Dosage Forms
Tablet, as hydrochloride: 500 mg, 850 mg, 1000 mg
Tablet, extended release, as hydrochloride: 500 mg

♦ **Metformin Hydrochloride** *see Metformin on page 875*

Methacholine (meth a KOLE leen)

U.S. Brand Names Provocholine®
Canadian Brand Names Provocholine®
Synonyms Methacholine Chloride
Therapeutic Category Cholinergic Agent; Diagnostic Agent, Bronchial Airway Hyperactivity
Use Diagnosis of bronchial airway hyperactivity
Pregnancy Risk Factor C
Usual Dosage Before inhalation challenge, perform baseline pulmonary function tests; the patient must have an FEV_1 of at least 70% of the predicted value. The following is a suggested schedule for administration of methacholine challenge. Calculate cumulative units by multiplying number of breaths by concentration given. Total cumulative units is the sum of cumulative units for each concentration given. See table.

Methacholine

Vial	Serial Concentration (mg/mL)	No. of Breaths	Cumulative Units per Concentration	Total Cumulative Units
E	0.025	5	0.125	0.125
D	0.25	5	1.25	1.375
C	2.5	5	12.5	13.88
B	10	5	50	63.88
A	25	5	125	188.88

Determine FEV_1 within 5 minutes of challenge, a positive challenge is a 20% reduction in FEV_1

Additional Information Complete prescribing information for this medication should be consulted for additional detail.

Dosage Forms Powder for oral inhalation, as chloride: 100 mg/5 mL [when reconstituted]

♦ **Methacholine Chloride** *see Methacholine on page 877*

Methadone (METH a done)

Related Information
Narcotic Agonists Comparison *on page 1506*
U.S. Brand Names Dolophine®; Methadose®
Canadian Brand Names Dolophine®; Metadol™; Methadose®
Synonyms Methadone Hydrochloride
Therapeutic Category Analgesic, Narcotic
Use Management of severe pain; detoxification and maintenance treatment of narcotic addiction (if used for detoxification and maintenance treatment of narcotic addiction, it must be part of an FDA-approved program)
Restrictions C-II
Pregnancy Risk Factor B/D (prolonged use or high doses at term)
Contraindications Hypersensitivity to methadone or any component of the formulation; pregnancy (prolonged use or high doses near term)
Warnings/Precautions Tablets are to be used only for oral administration and **must not** be used for injection; use with caution in patients with respiratory diseases including asthma, emphysema, or COPD and in patients with severe liver disease; because methadone's effects on respiration last much longer than its analgesic effects, the dose must be titrated slowly; because of its long half-life and risk of accumulation, it is not considered a drug of first choice in the elderly, who may be particularly susceptible to its CNS depressant and constipating effects; tolerance or drug dependence may result from extended use
Adverse Reactions Frequency not defined.
Cardiovascular: Bradycardia, peripheral vasodilation, cardiac arrest, syncope, faintness
Central nervous system: Euphoria, dysphoria, headache, insomnia, agitation, disorientation, drowsiness, dizziness, lightheadedness, sedation
(Continued)

Methadone (Continued)

Dermatologic: Pruritus, urticaria, rash

Endocrine & metabolic: Decreased libido

Gastrointestinal: Nausea, vomiting, constipation, anorexia, stomach cramps, xerostomia, biliary tract spasm

Genitourinary: Urinary retention or hesitancy, antidiuretic effect, impotence

Neuromuscular & skeletal: Weakness

Ocular: Miosis, visual disturbances

Respiratory: Respiratory depression, respiratory arrest

Miscellaneous: Physical and psychological dependence

Overdosage/Toxicology Symptoms include respiratory depression, CNS depression, miosis, hypothermia, circulatory collapse, and convulsions. Treatment includes naloxone 2 mg I.V. (0.01 mg/kg for children), with repeat administration as necessary, up to a total of 10 mg.

Drug Interactions

Cytochrome P450 Effect: CYP1A2, 2D6, and 3A3/4 enzyme substrate; CYP2D6 enzyme inhibitor

Increased Effect/Toxicity: Fluconazole, itraconazole, and ketoconazole increase serum methadone concentrations via CYP3A3/4 inhibition; an increased narcotic effect may be experienced. Similar effects may be seen with ritonavir, nelfinavir, amiodarone, erythromycin, clarithromycin, diltiazem, verapamil, paroxetine, fluoxetine, and other inhibitors of CYP2D6 or CYP3A3/4.

Decreased Effect: Barbiturates, carbamazepine, nevirapine, phenytoin, primidone, rifampin and ritonavir may decrease serum methadone concentrations via enhanced hepatic metabolism; monitor for methadone withdrawal. Larger doses of methadone may be required.

Ethanol/Nutrition/Herb Interactions

Ethanol: Avoid ethanol (may increase CNS effects). Watch for sedation.

Herb/Nutraceutical: Avoid St John's wort (may decrease methadone levels; may increase CNS depression). Avoid valerian, kava kava, gotu kola (may increase CNS depression). Methadone is metabolized by CYP3A4 in the intestines; avoid concurrent use of grapefruit juice.

Stability Highly **incompatible** with all other I.V. agents when mixed together

Mechanism of Action Binds to opiate receptors in the CNS, causing inhibition of ascending pain pathways, altering the perception of and response to pain; produces generalized CNS depression

Pharmacodynamics/Kinetics

Onset of action: Oral: Analgesic: 0.5-1 hour; Parenteral: 10-20 minutes

Peak effect: Parenteral: 1-2 hours

Duration: Oral: 6-8 hours, increases to 22-48 hours with repeated doses

Distribution: Crosses placenta; enters breast milk

Protein binding: 80% to 85%

Metabolism: Hepatic; N-demethylation

Half-life elimination: 15-29 hours; may be prolonged with alkaline pH

Excretion: Urine (<10% as unchanged drug); increased with urine pH <6

Usual Dosage Doses should be titrated to appropriate effects

Children:

Analgesia:

Oral, I.M., S.C.: 0.7 mg/kg/24 hours divided every 4-6 hours as needed or 0.1-0.2 mg/kg every 4-12 hours as needed; maximum: 10 mg/dose

I.V.: 0.1 mg/kg every 4 hours initially for 2-3 doses, then every 6-12 hours as needed; maximum: 10 mg/dose

Iatrogenic narcotic dependency: Oral: General guidelines: Initial: 0.05-0.1 mg/kg/dose every 6 hours; increase by 0.05 mg/kg/dose until withdrawal symptoms are controlled; after 24-48 hours, the dosing interval can be lengthened to every 12-24 hours; to taper dose, wean by 0.05 mg/kg/day; if withdrawal symptoms recur, taper at a slower rate

Adults:

Analgesia: Oral, I.M., S.C.: 2.5-10 mg every 3-8 hours as needed, up to 5-20 mg every 6-8 hours. Higher doses may be required in patients with severe, debilitating pain or in patients who have become narcotic tolerant.

Detoxification: Oral: 15-40 mg/day

Maintenance treatment of opiate dependence: Oral: 20-120 mg/day

Dosing adjustment in renal impairment: Cl_cr <10 mL/minute: Administer at 50% to 75% of normal dose

Dosing adjustment/comments in hepatic disease: Avoid in severe liver disease

Important note: Methadone accumulates with repeated doses and dosage may need to be adjusted downward after 3-5 days to prevent toxic effects. Some patients may benefit from every 8- to 12-hour dosing interval (pain control).

Monitoring Parameters Pain relief, respiratory and mental status, blood pressure

Reference Range Therapeutic: 100-400 ng/mL (SI: 0.32-1.29 µmol/L); Toxic: >2 µg/mL (SI: >6.46 µmol/L)

Patient Information May cause drowsiness, avoid alcohol and other CNS depressants

Nursing Implications Observe patient for excessive sedation, respiratory depression, implement safety measures, assist with ambulation

Additional Information Methadone accumulates with repeated doses and dosage may need to be adjusted downward after 3-5 days to prevent toxic effects. Some patients may benefit from every 8- to 12-hour dosing interval (pain control). Oral dose for detoxification and maintenance may be administered in Tang®, Kool-Aid®, apple juice, grape Crystal Light®.

Dosage Forms

Injection, as hydrochloride: 10 mg/mL (20 mL)

Solution, oral, as hydrochloride: 5 mg/5 mL (5 mL, 500 mL); 10 mg/5 mL (500 mL)

Solution, oral concentrate, as hydrochloride: 10 mg/mL (30 mL)

Tablet, as hydrochloride: 5 mg, 10 mg
Tablet, dispersible, as hydrochloride: 40 mg

♦ **Methadone Hydrochloride** *see* Methadone *on page 877*
♦ **Methadose®** *see* Methadone *on page 877*
♦ **Methaminodiazepoxide Hydrochloride** *see* Chlordiazepoxide *on page 274*

Methamphetamine (meth am FET a meen)

Related Information
Obesity Treatment Guidelines for Adults *on page 1685*
U.S. Brand Names Desoxyn®; Desoxyn® Gradumet®
Canadian Brand Names Desoxyn®
Synonyms Desoxyephedrine Hydrochloride; Methamphetamine Hydrochloride
Therapeutic Category Amphetamine; Central Nervous System Stimulant, Amphetamine
Use Treatment of attention-deficit/hyperactivity disorder (ADHD); exogenous obesity (short-term adjunct)
Unlabeled/Investigational Use Narcolepsy
Restrictions C-II
Pregnancy Risk Factor C
Contraindications Hypersensitivity or idiosyncrasy to amphetamines or other sympathomimetic amines; patients with advanced arteriosclerosis, symptomatic cardiovascular disease, moderate to severe hypertension (stage II or III), hyperthyroidism, glaucoma, agitated states; patients with a history of drug abuse; use during or within 14 days following MAO inhibitor therapy; stimulant medications are contraindicated for use in children with attention-deficit/hyperactivity disorders and concomitant Tourette's syndrome or tics
Warnings/Precautions Use with caution in patients with bipolar disorder, diabetes mellitus, cardiovascular disease, seizure disorders, insomnia, porphyria, or mild hypertension (stage I). May exacerbate symptoms of behavior and thought disorder in psychotic patients. Potential for drug dependency exists - avoid abrupt discontinuation in patients who have received for prolonged periods. Use in weight reduction programs only when alternative therapy has been ineffective. Products may contain tartrazine - use with caution in potentially sensitive individuals. Stimulant use in children has been associated with growth suppression. Stimulants may unmask tics in individuals with coexisting Tourette's syndrome.
Adverse Reactions Frequency not defined.
Cardiovascular: Hypertension, tachycardia, palpitations
Central nervous system: Restlessness, headache, exacerbation of motor and phonic tics and Tourette's syndrome, dizziness, psychosis, dysphoria, overstimulation, euphoria, insomnia
Dermatologic: Rash, urticaria
Endocrine & metabolic: Change in libido
Gastrointestinal: Diarrhea, nausea, vomiting, stomach cramps, constipation, anorexia, weight loss, xerostomia, unpleasant taste
Genitourinary: Impotence
Neuromuscular & skeletal: Tremor
Miscellaneous: Suppression of growth in children, tolerance and withdrawal with prolonged use
Overdosage/Toxicology Symptoms include seizures, hyperactivity, coma, and hypertension. There is no specific antidote for amphetamine intoxication and the bulk of treatment is supportive. Hyperactivity and agitation usually respond to reduced sensory input, however, with extreme agitation haloperidol (2-5 mg I.M. for adults) may be required. Hyperthermia is best treated with external cooling measures, or when severe or unresponsive, muscle paralysis with pancuronium may be needed. Hypertension is usually transient and generally does not require treatment unless severe. For diastolic blood pressures >110 mm Hg, a nitroprusside infusion should be initiated. Seizures usually respond to diazepam IVP and/or phenytoin maintenance regimens.
Drug Interactions
Cytochrome P450 Effect: CYP2D6 enzyme substrate
Increased Effect/Toxicity: Amphetamines may precipitate hypertensive crisis or serotonin syndrome in patients receiving MAO inhibitors (selegiline >10 mg/day, isocarboxazid, phenelzine, tranylcypromine, furazolidone). Serotonin syndrome has also been associated with combinations of amphetamines and SSRIs; these combinations should be avoided. TCAs may enhance the effects of amphetamines, potentially leading to hypertensive crisis. Large doses of antacids or urinary alkalinizers increase the half-life and duration of action of amphetamines. May precipitate arrhythmias in patients receiving general anesthetics. Inhibitors of CYP2D6 may increase the effects of amphetamines (includes amiodarone, cimetidine, delavirdine, fluoxetine, paroxetine, propafenone, quinidine, and ritonavir).
Decreased Effect: Amphetamines inhibit the antihypertensive response to guanethidine and guanadrel. Urinary acidifiers decrease the half-life and duration of action of amphetamines. Enzyme inducers (barbiturates, carbamazepine, phenytoin, and rifampin) may decrease serum concentrations of amphetamines.
Ethanol/Nutrition/Herb Interactions
Ethanol: Avoid ethanol (may cause CNS depression).
Food: Amphetamine serum levels may be altered if taken with acidic food, juices, or vitamin C. Avoid caffeine.
Herb/Nutraceutical: Avoid ephedra (may cause hypertension or arrhythmias).
Mechanism of Action A sympathomimetic amine related to ephedrine and amphetamine with CNS stimulant activity; peripheral actions include elevation of systolic and diastolic blood pressure and weak bronchodilator and respiratory stimulant action
Pharmacodynamics/Kinetics Duration: 12-24 hours
Usual Dosage
Children >6 years and Adults: ADHD: 2.5-5 mg 1-2 times/day; may increase by 5 mg increments at weekly intervals until optimum response is achieved, usually 20-25 mg/day
Children >12 years and Adults: Exogenous obesity: 5 mg 30 minutes before each meal; long-acting formulation: 10-15 mg in morning; treatment duration should not exceed a few weeks
(Continued)

Methamphetamine *(Continued)*

Dietary Considerations Should be taken 30 minutes before meals.

Monitoring Parameters Heart rate, respiratory rate, blood pressure, and CNS activity

Patient Information Take during day to avoid insomnia; do not discontinue abruptly, may cause physical and psychological dependence with prolonged use; do not crush or chew extended release tablet

Nursing Implications Dose should not be given in evening or at bedtime; do not crush extended release tablet

Additional Information Illicit methamphetamine may contain lead; alkalinizing urine can result in longer methamphetamine half-life and elevated blood level; ephedrine is a precursor in the illicit manufacture of methamphetamine; ephedrine is extracted by dissolving ephedrine tablets in water or alcohol (50,000 tablets can result in 1 kg of ephedrine); conversion to methamphetamine occurs at a rate of 50% to 70% of the weight of ephedrine. 3,4-methylene dioxymethamphetamine (slang: XTC, Ecstasy, Adam) affects the serotonergic, dopaminergic, and noradrenergic pathways. As such, it can cause the serotonin syndrome associated with malignant hyperthermia and rhabdomyolysis.

Dosage Forms
Tablet, as hydrochloride: 5 mg

Tablet, extended release, as hydrochloride (Desoxyn® Gradumet®): 5 mg, 10 mg, 15 mg

♦ **Methamphetamine Hydrochloride** *see* Methamphetamine *on page 879*

Methazolamide *(meth a ZOE la mide)*

Related Information
Glaucoma Drug Therapy Comparison *on page 1499*
Sulfonamide Derivatives *on page 1515*

U.S. Brand Names Neptazane®

Canadian Brand Names Neptazane®

Therapeutic Category Carbonic Anhydrase Inhibitor; Diuretic, Carbonic Anhydrase Inhibitor

Use Adjunctive treatment of open-angle or secondary glaucoma; short-term therapy of narrow-angle glaucoma when delay of surgery is desired

Pregnancy Risk Factor C

Contraindications Hypersensitivity to methazolamide or any component of the formulation; marked kidney or liver dysfunction; severe pulmonary obstruction

Warnings/Precautions Sulfonamide-type reactions, melena, anorexia, nausea, vomiting, constipation, hematuria, glycosuria, urinary frequency, renal colic, renal calculi, crystalluria, polyuria, hepatic insufficiency, various CNS effects, transient myopia, bone marrow suppression, thrombocytopenia/purpura, hemolytic anemia, leukopenia, pancytopenia, agranulocytosis, urticaria, pruritus, rash, Stevens-Johnson syndrome, weight loss, fever, acidosis; use with caution in patients with respiratory acidosis and diabetes mellitus; impairment of mental alertness and/or physical coordination. Malaise and complaints of tiredness and myalgia are signs of excessive dosing and acidosis in the elderly.

Chemical similarities are present among sulfonamides, sulfonylureas, carbonic anhydrase inhibitors, thiazides, and loop diuretics (except ethacrynic acid). In patients with allergy to one of these compounds, a risk of cross-reaction exists; avoid use when previous reaction has been severe.

Adverse Reactions Frequency not defined.
Central nervous system: Malaise, fever, mental depression, drowsiness, dizziness, nervousness, headache, confusion, seizures, fatigue, trembling, unsteadiness
Dermatologic: Urticaria, pruritus, photosensitivity, rash, Stevens-Johnson syndrome
Endocrine & metabolic: Hyperchloremic metabolic acidosis, hypokalemia, hyperglycemia
Gastrointestinal: Metallic taste, anorexia, nausea, vomiting, diarrhea, constipation, weight loss, GI irritation, xerostomia, black tarry stools
Genitourinary: Polyuria, crystalluria, hematuria, polyuria, renal calculi, impotence
Hematologic: Bone marrow depression, thrombocytopenia, thrombocytopenic purpura, hemolytic anemia, leukopenia, pancytopenia, agranulocytosis
Hepatic: Hepatic insufficiency
Neuromuscular & skeletal: Weakness, ataxia, paresthesias
Miscellaneous: Hypersensitivity

Drug Interactions
Increased Effect/Toxicity: Methazolamide may induce hypokalemia which would sensitize a patient to digitalis toxicity. Hypokalemia may be compounded with concurrent diuretic use or steroids. Methazolamide may increase the potential for salicylate toxicity. Primidone absorption may be delayed.

Decreased Effect: Increased lithium excretion and altered excretion of other drugs by alkalinization of the urine, such as amphetamines, quinidine, procainamide, methenamine, phenobarbital, and salicylates.

Mechanism of Action Noncompetitive inhibition of the enzyme carbonic anhydrase; thought that carbonic anhydrase is located at the luminal border of cells of the proximal tubule. When the enzyme is inhibited, there is an increase in urine volume and a change to an alkaline pH with a subsequent decrease in the excretion of titratable acid and ammonia.

Pharmacodynamics/Kinetics
Onset of action: Slow in comparison with acetazolamide (2-4 hours)
Peak effect: 6-8 hours
Duration: 10-18 hours
Absorption: Slowly
Distribution: Well into tissue
Protein binding: ~55%
Half-life elimination: ~14 hours
Excretion: Urine (~25% as unchanged drug)

Usual Dosage Adults: Oral: 50-100 mg 2-3 times/day

Patient Information Take with food, report any numbness or tingling in extremities to physician; may cause drowsiness, impaired judgment or coordination

Nursing Implications May cause an alteration in taste, especially when drinking carbonated beverages

Dosage Forms Tablet: 25 mg, 50 mg

Methenamine (meth EN a meen)

U.S. Brand Names Hiprex®; Urex®

Canadian Brand Names Dehydral®; Hiprex®; Mandelamine®; Urasal®; Urex®

Synonyms Hexamethylenetetramine; Methenamine Hippurate; Methenamine Mandelate

Therapeutic Category Antibiotic, Miscellaneous

Use Prophylaxis or suppression of recurrent urinary tract infections; urinary tract discomfort secondary to hypermotility

Pregnancy Risk Factor C

Contraindications Hypersensitivity to methenamine or any component of the formulation; severe dehydration, renal insufficiency, hepatic insufficiency in patients receiving hippurate salt; patients receiving sulfonamides

Warnings/Precautions Use with caution in patients with hepatic disease, gout, and the elderly; doses of 8 g/day for 3-4 weeks may cause bladder irritation, some products may contain tartrazine; methenamine should not be used to treat infections outside of the lower urinary tract. Use care to maintain an acid pH of the urine, especially when treating infections due to urea splitting organisms (eg, *Proteus* and strains of *Pseudomonas*); reversible increases in LFTs have occurred during therapy especially in patients with hepatic dysfunction. Hiprex® contains tartrazine dye.

Adverse Reactions

1% to 10%:

Dermatologic: Rash (4%)

Gastrointestinal: Nausea, dyspepsia (4%)

Genitourinary: Dysuria (4%)

<1% (Limited to important or life-threatening): Bladder irritation, crystalluria (especially with large doses), increased AST/ALT (reversible, rare)

Overdosage/Toxicology Well tolerated. Treatment includes GI decontamination, if possible, and supportive care.

Drug Interactions

Increased Effect/Toxicity: Sulfonamides may precipitate in the urine.

Decreased Effect: Sodium bicarbonate and acetazolamide will decrease effect secondary to alkalinization of urine.

Ethanol/Nutrition/Herb Interactions Food: Foods/diets which alkalinize urine pH >5.5 decrease therapeutic effect of methenamine.

Stability Protect from excessive heat

Mechanism of Action Methenamine is hydrolyzed to formaldehyde and ammonia in acidic urine; formaldehyde has nonspecific bactericidal action

Pharmacodynamics/Kinetics

Absorption: Readily

Metabolism: Gastric juices: Hydrolyze 10% to 30% unless protected via enteric coating; Hepatic: ~10% to 25%

Half-life elimination: 3-6 hours

Excretion: Urine (~70% to 90% as unchanged drug) within 24 hours

Usual Dosage Oral:

Children:

<6 years: 0.25 g/30 lb 4 times/day

6-12 years:

Hippurate: 25-50 mg/kg/day divided every 12 hours or 0.5-1 g twice daily

Mandelate: 50-75 mg/kg/day divided every 6 hours or 0.5 g 4 times/day

Children >12 years and Adults:

Hippurate: 1 g twice daily

Mandelate: 1 g 4 times/day after meals and at bedtime

Dosing adjustment/comments in renal impairment: Cl$_{cr}$ <50 mL/minute: Avoid use

Dietary Considerations Foods/diets which alkalinize urine pH >5.5 decrease activity of methenamine; cranberry juice can be used to acidify urine and increase activity of methenamine. Hiprex® contains tartrazine dye.

Monitoring Parameters Urinalysis, periodic liver function tests in patients

Test Interactions ↑ catecholamines and VMA (U); ↓ HIAA (U)

Patient Information Take with food to minimize GI upset; take with ascorbic acid to acidify urine; drink sufficient fluids to ensure adequate urine flow. Avoid excessive intake of alkalinizing foods (citrus fruits and milk products) or medication (bicarbonate, acetazolamide); notify physician if skin rash, painful urination or excessive abdominal pain occur.

Nursing Implications Urine should be acidic (pH <5.5) for maximum effect

Additional Information Should not be used to treat infections outside of the lower urinary tract. Methenamine has little, if any, role in the treatment or prevention of infections in patients with indwelling urinary (Foley) catheters. Furthermore, in noncatheterized patients, more effective antibiotics are available for the prevention or treatment of urinary tract infections. The influence of decreased renal function on the pharmacologic effects of methenamine results are unknown.

Dosage Forms

Suspension, oral, as mandelate: 0.5 g/5 mL (480 mL)

Tablet, as hippurate (Hiprex®, Urex®): 1 g [Hiprex® contains tartrazine dye]

Tablet, enteric coated, as mandelate: 500 mg, 1 g

♦ **Methenamine Hippurate** see Methenamine on page 881

♦ **Methenamine Mandelate** see Methenamine on page 881

Methenamine, Sodium Biphosphate, Phenyl Salicylate, Methylene Blue, and Hyoscyamine

(meth EN a meen, SOW dee um bye FOS fate, fen nil sa LIS i late, METH i leen bloo, & hye oh SYE a meen)

U.S. Brand Names Urimax™

Synonyms Hyoscyamine, Methenamine, Sodium Biphosphate, Phenyl Salicylate, and Methylene Blue; Methylene Blue, Methenamine, Sodium Biphosphate, Phenyl Salicylate, and Hyoscyamine; Phenyl Salicylate, Methenamine, Methylene Blue, Sodium Biphosphate, and Hyoscyamine; Sodium Biphosphate, Methenamine, Methylene Blue, Phenyl Salicylate, and Hyoscyamine

Therapeutic Category Antibiotic, Miscellaneous

Use Treatment of symptoms of irritative voiding; relief of local symptoms associated with urinary tract infections; relief of urinary tract symptoms caused by diagnostic procedures

Pregnancy Risk Factor C

Contraindications Hypersensitivity to methenamine, hyoscyamine, methylene blue, or any component of the formulation

Warnings/Precautions Use caution in patients with a history of intolerance to belladonna alkaloids or salicylates. Use caution in patients with cardiovascular disease (cardiac arrhythmias, congestive heart failure, coronary heart disease, mitral stenosis), gastrointestinal tract obstruction, glaucoma, myasthenia gravis, or obstructive uropathy (bladder neck obstruction or prostatic hypertrophy). Discontinue use immediately if tachycardia, dizziness, or blurred vision occur. Elderly may be more sensitive to anticholinergic effects of hyoscyamine; use caution. May cause urinary discoloration (blue). Safety and efficacy have not been established in children ≤6 years of age.

Adverse Reactions Frequency not defined.
Cardiovascular: Tachycardia, flushing
Central nervous system: Dizziness
Gastrointestinal: Xerostomia, nausea, vomiting
Genitourinary: Urinary retention (acute), micturition difficulty, discoloration of urine (blue)
Ocular: Blurred vision
Respiratory: Dyspnea, shortness of breath

Drug Interactions
Increased Effect/Toxicity: Refer to individual monographs for Hyoscyamine and Methenamine.
Decreased Effect: Refer to individual monographs for Hyoscyamine and Methenamine.

Stability Store at controlled room temperature of 15°C to 30°C (59°F to 86°F).

Usual Dosage Oral:
Children >6 years: Dosage must be individualized
Adults: One tablet 4 times daily (followed by liberal fluid intake)

Dosage Forms Tablet, delayed release, film-coated: Methenamine 81.6 mg, sodium biphosphate 40.8 mg, phenyl salicylate 36.2 mg, methylene blue 10.8 mg, hyoscyamine sulfate 0.12 mg

◆ **Methergine®** see Methylergonovine on page 893

Methimazole (meth IM a zole)

U.S. Brand Names Tapazole®
Canadian Brand Names Tapazole®
Synonyms Thiamazole
Therapeutic Category Antithyroid Agent

Use Palliative treatment of hyperthyroidism, return the hyperthyroid patient to a normal metabolic state prior to thyroidectomy, and to control thyrotoxic crisis that may accompany thyroidectomy. The use of antithyroid thioamides is as effective in elderly as they are in younger adults; however, the expense, potential adverse effects, and inconvenience (compliance, monitoring) make them undesirable. The use of radioiodine due to ease of administration and less concern for long-term side effects and reproduction problems (some older males) makes it a more appropriate therapy.

Pregnancy Risk Factor D

Pregnancy/Breast-Feeding Implications Hypothyroidism and congenital defects (rare) may occur.

Contraindications Hypersensitivity to methimazole or any component of the formulation; nursing mothers (per manufacturer; however, expert analysis and the AAP state this drug may be used with caution in nursing mothers); pregnancy

Warnings/Precautions Use with extreme caution in patients receiving other drugs known to cause myelosuppression particularly agranulocytosis, patients >40 years of age; avoid doses >40 mg/day (↑ myelosuppression); may cause acneiform eruptions or worsen the condition of the thyroid

Adverse Reactions Frequency not defined.
Cardiovascular: Edema
Central nervous system: Headache, vertigo, drowsiness, CNS stimulation, depression
Dermatologic: Skin rash, urticaria, pruritus, erythema nodosum, skin pigmentation, exfoliative dermatitis, alopecia
Endocrine & metabolic: Goiter
Gastrointestinal: Nausea, vomiting, stomach pain, abnormal taste, constipation, weight gain, salivary gland swelling
Hematologic: Leukopenia, agranulocytosis, granulocytopenia, thrombocytopenia, aplastic anemia, hypoprothrombinemia
Hepatic: Cholestatic jaundice, jaundice, hepatitis
Neuromuscular & skeletal: Arthralgia, paresthesia
Renal: Nephrotic syndrome
Miscellaneous: SLE-like syndrome

Overdosage/Toxicology Symptoms include nausea, vomiting, epigastric distress, headache, fever, arthralgia, pruritus, edema, pancytopenia, and signs of hypothyroidism. Management of overdose is supportive.

Drug Interactions
Increased Effect/Toxicity: Increased toxicity with lithium or potassium iodide. Anticoagulant effect of warfarin may be increased. Dosage of some drugs (including beta-blockers, digoxin, and theophylline) require adjustment during treatment of hyperthyroidism.

Stability Protect from light

Mechanism of Action Inhibits the synthesis of thyroid hormones by blocking the oxidation of iodine in the thyroid gland, blocking iodine's ability to combine with tyrosine to form thyroxine and triiodothyronine (T_3), does not inactivate circulating T_4 and T_3

Pharmacodynamics/Kinetics
Onset of action: Antithyroid: Oral: 12-18 hours
Duration: 36-72 hours
Distribution: Concentrated in thyroid gland; crosses placenta; enters breast milk (1:1)
Protein binding, plasma: None
Metabolism: Hepatic
Bioavailability: 80% to 95%
Half-life elimination: 4-13 hours
Excretion: Urine (80%)

Usual Dosage Oral: Administer in 3 equally divided doses at approximately 8-hour intervals
Children: Initial: 0.4 mg/kg/day in 3 divided doses; maintenance: 0.2 mg/kg/day in 3 divided doses up to 30 mg/24 hours maximum
Alternatively: Initial: 0.5-0.7 mg/kg/day **or** 15-20 mg/m^2/day in 3 divided doses
Maintenance: $^1/_3$ to $^2/_3$ of the initial dose beginning when the patient is euthyroid
Maximum: 30 mg/24 hours
Adults: Initial: 15 mg/day for mild hyperthyroidism; 30-40 mg/day in moderately severe hyperthyroidism; 60 mg/day in severe hyperthyroidism; maintenance: 5-15 mg/day
Adjust dosage as required to achieve and maintain serum T_3, T_4, and TSH levels in the normal range. An elevated T_3 may be the sole indicator of inadequate treatment. An elevated TSH indicates excessive antithyroid treatment.
Dosing adjustment in renal impairment: Adjustment is not necessary

Dietary Considerations Should be taken consistently in relation to meals every day.

Monitoring Parameters Monitor for signs of hypothyroidism, hyperthyroidism, T_4, T_3; CBC with differential, liver function (baseline and as needed), serum thyroxine, free thyroxine index

Patient Information Take with meals, take at regular intervals around-the-clock; notify physician if persistent fever, sore throat, fatigue, unusual bleeding or bruising occurs

Dosage Forms Tablet: 5 mg, 10 mg

Methocarbamol (meth oh KAR ba mole)

U.S. Brand Names Robaxin®
Canadian Brand Names Robaxin®
Therapeutic Category Skeletal Muscle Relaxant
Use Treatment of muscle spasm associated with acute painful musculoskeletal conditions, supportive therapy in tetanus
Pregnancy Risk Factor C
Contraindications Hypersensitivity to methocarbamol or any component of the formulation; renal impairment
Warnings/Precautions Rate of injection should not exceed 3 mL/minute; solution is hypertonic; avoid extravasation; use with caution in patients with a history of seizures
Adverse Reactions Frequency not defined.
Cardiovascular: Flushing of face, bradycardia, hypotension
Central nervous system: Drowsiness, dizziness, lightheadedness, syncope, convulsion, vertigo, headache, fever
Dermatologic: Allergic dermatitis, urticaria, pruritus, rash
Gastrointestinal: Nausea, vomiting, metallic taste
Hematologic: Leukopenia
Local: Pain at injection site, thrombophlebitis
Ocular: Nystagmus, blurred vision, diplopia, conjunctivitis
Renal: Renal impairment
Respiratory: Nasal congestion
Miscellaneous: Allergic manifestations, anaphylactic reaction

Overdosage/Toxicology Symptoms include cardiac arrhythmias, nausea, vomiting, drowsiness, and coma. Treatment is supportive following attempts to enhance drug elimination. Hypotension should be treated with I.V. fluids and/or Trendelenburg positioning. Dialysis, hemoperfusion, and osmotic diuresis have all been useful in reducing serum drug concentrations. The patient should be observed for possible relapses due to incomplete gastric emptying.

Drug Interactions
Increased Effect/Toxicity: Increased effect/toxicity with CNS depressants.

Ethanol/Nutrition/Herb Interactions
Ethanol: Avoid ethanol (may increase CNS depression).
Herb/Nutraceutical: Avoid valerian, St John's wort, kava kava, gotu kola (may increase CNS depression).

Stability Injection when diluted to 4 mg/mL in sterile water, 5% dextrose, or 0.9% saline is stable for 6 days at room temperature; do **not** refrigerate after dilution

Mechanism of Action Causes skeletal muscle relaxation by reducing the transmission of impulses from the spinal cord to skeletal muscle

Pharmacodynamics/Kinetics
Onset of action: Muscle relaxation: Oral: ~30 minutes
Metabolism: Hepatic
Half-life elimination: 1-2 hours
(Continued)

Methocarbamol *(Continued)*

Time to peak, serum: ~2 hours
Excretion: Urine (as metabolites)

Usual Dosage

Children: Recommended **only** for use in tetanus: I.V.: 15 mg/kg/dose or 500 mg/m²/dose, may repeat every 6 hours if needed; maximum dose: 1.8 g/m²/day for 3 days only

Adults: Muscle spasm:

Oral: 1.5 g 4 times/day for 2-3 days, then decrease to 4-4.5 g/day in 3-6 divided doses

I.M., I.V.: 1 g every 8 hours if oral not possible

Dosing adjustment/comments in renal impairment: Do not administer parenteral formulation to patients with renal dysfunction

Administration Maximum rate: 3 mL/minute

Patient Information May cause drowsiness, impair judgment or coordination; avoid alcohol or other CNS depressants; may turn urine brown, black, or green; notify physician of rash, itching, or nasal congestion

Nursing Implications Monitor closely for extravasation of I.V. injection

Dosage Forms

Injection: 100 mg/mL in polyethylene glycol 50% (10 mL)
Tablet: 500 mg, 750 mg

Methocarbamol and Aspirin *(meth oh KAR ba mole & AS pir in)*

U.S. Brand Names Robaxisal®

Canadian Brand Names Aspirin® Backache; Methoxisal; Methoxisal-C; Robaxisal®; Robaxisal® Extra Strength

Synonyms Aspirin and Methocarbamol

Therapeutic Category Skeletal Muscle Relaxant

Use Adjunct to rest, physical therapy, and other measures for the relief of discomfort associated with acute, painful musculoskeletal disorders

Pregnancy Risk Factor C/D (full-dose aspirin in 3rd trimester)

Usual Dosage Children >12 years and Adults: Oral: 2 tablets 4 times/day

Additional Information Complete prescribing information for this medication should be consulted for additional detail.

Dosage Forms Tablet: Methocarbamol 400 mg and aspirin 325 mg

Methohexital *(meth oh HEKS i tal)*

Related Information

Adult ACLS Algorithms *on page 1632*

U.S. Brand Names Brevital® Sodium

Canadian Brand Names Brevital®; Brietal Sodium®

Synonyms Methohexital Sodium

Therapeutic Category Barbiturate; General Anesthetic

Use Induction and maintenance of general anesthesia for short procedures

Can be used in pediatric patients >1 month of age as follows: For rectal or intramuscular induction of anesthesia prior to the use of other general anesthetic agents, as an adjunct to subpotent inhalational anesthetic agents for short surgical procedures, or for short surgical, diagnostic, or therapeutic procedures associated with minimal painful stimuli

Restrictions C-IV

Pregnancy Risk Factor C

Usual Dosage Doses must be titrated to effect

Children 3-12 years:

I.M.: Preop: 5-10 mg/kg/dose

I.V.: Induction: 1-2 mg/kg/dose

Rectal: Preop/induction: 20-35 mg/kg/dose; usual 25 mg/kg/dose; administer as 10% aqueous solution

Adults: I.V.: Induction: 50-120 mg to start; 20-40 mg every 4-7 minutes

Dosing adjustment/comments in hepatic impairment: Lower dosage and monitor closely

Additional Information Complete prescribing information for this medication should be consulted for additional detail.

Dosage Forms Injection, as sodium: 500 mg, 2.5 g, 5 g

♦ **Methohexital Sodium** *see Methohexital on page 884*

Methotrexate *(meth oh TREKS ate)*

U.S. Brand Names Rheumatrex®; Trexall™

Synonyms Amethopterin; Methotrexate Sodium; MTX

Therapeutic Category Antineoplastic Agent, Antimetabolite; Antineoplastic Agent, Folate Antagonist; Antineoplastic Agent, Irritant; Immunosuppressant Agent

Use Treatment of trophoblastic neoplasms; leukemias; psoriasis; rheumatoid arthritis (RA), including polyarticular-course juvenile rheumatoid arthritis (JRA); breast, head and neck, and lung carcinomas; osteosarcoma; sarcomas; carcinoma of gastric, esophagus, testes; lymphomas; mycosis fungoides (cutaneous T-cell lymphoma)

Pregnancy Risk Factor D

Contraindications Hypersensitivity to methotrexate or any component of the formulation; severe renal or hepatic impairment; pre-existing profound bone marrow suppression in patients with psoriasis or rheumatoid arthritis, alcoholic liver disease, AIDS, pre-existing blood dyscrasias; pregnancy

Warnings/Precautions The U.S. Food and Drug Administration (FDA) currently recommends that procedures for proper handling and disposal of antineoplastic agents be considered

Bone and soft tissue necrosis may occur following radiation treatment. Painful plaque erosions may occur with psoriasis treatment.

May cause photosensitivity-type reaction. Reduce dosage in patients with renal or hepatic impairment. Methotrexate penetrates slowly into 3rd space fluids, such as pleural effusions or ascites, and exits slowly from these compartments (slower than from plasma). Drain ascites and pleural effusions prior to treatment. Use with caution in patients with peptic ulcer disease, ulcerative colitis, pre-existing bone marrow suppression. Monitor closely for pulmonary disease; use with caution in the elderly. Safety and efficacy in pediatric patients have been established only in cancer chemotherapy and polyarticular-course JRA.

Because of the possibility of severe toxic reactions, fully inform patient of the risks involved. Do not use in women of childbearing age unless benefit outweighs risks; may cause hepato-toxicity, fibrosis, and cirrhosis, along with marked bone marrow depression. Death from intestinal perforation may occur.

Severe bone marrow suppression, aplastic anemia, and GI toxicity have occurred during concomitant administration with nonsteroidal anti-inflammatory drugs (NSAIDs).

Patients should receive 1-2 L of I.V. fluid prior to initiation of high-dose methotrexate. Patients should receive sodium bicarbonate to alkalinize their urine during and after high-dose metho-trexate (urine SG <1.010 and pH >7 should be maintained for at least 24 hours after infusion).

Toxicity to methotrexate or any immunosuppressive is increased in elderly; must monitor carefully. For rheumatoid arthritis and psoriasis, immunosuppressive therapy should only be used when disease is active and less toxic, traditional therapy is ineffective. Recommended doses should be reduced when initiating therapy in elderly due to possible decreased metab-olism, reduced renal function, and presence of interacting diseases and drugs. Methotrexate formulations and/or diluents containing preservatives should not be used for intrathecal or high-dose therapy. Methotrexate injection may contain benzyl alcohol and should not be used in neonates.

Adverse Reactions Frequencies vary widely with dose (chemotherapy versus immune modu-lation).

>10%:
  Cardiovascular: Vasculitis
  Central nervous system (with I.T. administration only):
    Arachnoiditis: Acute reaction manifested as severe headache, nuchal rigidity, vomiting, and fever; may be alleviated by reducing the dose
    Subacute toxicity: 10% of patients treated with 12-15 mg/m² of I.T. MTX may develop this in the second or third week of therapy; consists of motor paralysis of extremities, cranial nerve palsy, seizures, or coma. This has also been seen in pediatric cases receiving very high-dose I.V. MTX (when enough MTX can get across into the CSF).
    Demyelinating encephalopathy: Seen months or years after receiving MTX; usually in association with cranial irradiation or other systemic chemotherapy
  Dermatologic: Reddening of skin
  Endocrine & metabolic: Hyperuricemia, defective oogenesis or spermatogenesis
  Gastrointestinal: Ulcerative stomatitis, glossitis, gingivitis, nausea, vomiting, diarrhea, anorexia, intestinal perforation, mucositis (dose-dependent; appears in 3-7 days after therapy, resolving within 2 weeks)
    Emetic potential:
    <100 mg: Moderately low (10% to 30%)
    ≥100 mg or <250 mg: Moderate (30% to 60%)
    ≥250 mg: Moderately high (60% to 90%)
  Hematologic: Leukopenia, thrombocytopenia
  Renal: Renal failure, azotemia, nephropathy
  Respiratory: Pharyngitis
1% to 10%:
  Central nervous system: Dizziness, malaise, encephalopathy, seizures, fever, chills
  Dermatologic: Alopecia, rash, photosensitivity, depigmentation or hyperpigmentation of skin
  Endocrine & metabolic: Diabetes
  Genitourinary: Cystitis
  Hematologic: Hemorrhage
    Myelosuppressive: This is the primary dose-limiting factor (along with mucositis) of MTX; occurs about 5-7 days after MTX therapy, and should resolve within 2 weeks
      WBC: Mild
      Platelets: Moderate
      Onset: 7 days
      Nadir: 10 days
      Recovery: 21 days
  Hepatic: Cirrhosis and portal fibrosis have been associated with chronic MTX therapy; acute elevation of liver enzymes are common after high-dose MTX, and usually resolve within 10 days.
  Neuromuscular & skeletal: Arthralgia
  Ocular: Blurred vision
  Renal: Renal dysfunction: Manifested by an abrupt rise in serum creatinine and BUN and a fall in urine output; more common with high-dose MTX, and may be due to precipitation of the drug. The best treatment is prevention: Aggressively hydrate with 3 L/m²/day starting 12 hours before therapy and continue for 24-36 hours; alkalinize the urine by adding 50 mEq of bicarbonate to each liter of fluid; keep urine flow over 100 mL/hour and urine pH >7.
  Respiratory: Pneumonitis: Associated with fever, cough, and interstitial pulmonary infil-trates; treatment is to withhold MTX during the acute reaction; interstitial pneumonitis has been reported to occur with an incidence of 1% in patients with RA (dose 7.5-15 mg/week)
<1% (Limited to important or life-threatening): Anaphylaxis, decreased resistance to infection, osteonecrosis and soft tissue necrosis (with radiotherapy), plaque erosions (psoriasis)

Overdosage/Toxicology Symptoms include nausea, vomiting, alopecia, melena, and renal failure.
  Antidote: Leucovorin; administer as soon as toxicity is seen. Administer 10 mg/m² orally or parenterally; follow with 10 mg/m² orally every 6 hours for 72 hours. After 24 hours following methotrexate administration, if the serum creatinine is ≥50% of premethotrexate
(Continued)

Methotrexate *(Continued)*

serum creatinine, increase leucovorin dose to 100 mg/m^2 every 3 hours until serum MTX level is <5 x 10^{-8} M. Hydration and alkalinization may be used to prevent precipitation of MTX or MTX metabolites in the renal tubules. Toxicity in low dose range is negligible, but may present mucositis and mild bone marrow suppression. Severe bone marrow toxicity can result from overdose. Generally, neither peritoneal nor hemodialysis have been shown to increase elimination. However, effective clearance of methotrexate has been reported with acute, intermittent hemodialysis using a high-flux dialyzer. Leucovorin should be administered intravenously, never intrathecally, for overdoses of intrathecal methotrexate.

Drug Interactions

Cytochrome P450 Effect: Involvement with CYP isoenzymes not defined; may act as inhibitor of some isoenzymes.

Increased Effect/Toxicity:

Live virus vaccines → vaccinia infections.

Vincristine: Inhibits MTX efflux from the cell, leading to increased and prolonged MTX levels in the cell; the dose of VCR needed to produce this effect is not achieved clinically.

Organic acids: Salicylates, sulfonamides, probenecid, and high doses of penicillins compete with MTX for transport and reduce renal tubular secretion. Salicylates and sulfonamides may also displace MTX from plasma proteins, increasing MTX levels.

Ara-C: Increased formation of the Ara-C nucleotide can occur when MTX precedes Ara-C, thus promoting the action of Ara-C.

Cyclosporine: CSA and MTX interfere with each other's renal elimination, which may result in increased toxicity.

Nonsteroidal anti-inflammatory drugs (NSAIDs): Severe bone marrow suppression, aplastic anemia, and GI toxicity have been reported with concomitant therapy. Should not be used during moderate or high-dose methotrexate due to increased and prolonged methotrexate levels (may increase toxicity). NSAID use during treatment of rheumatoid arthritis has not been fully explored, but continuation of prior regimen has been allowed in some circumstances, with cautious monitoring.

Patients receiving concomitant therapy with methotrexate and other potential hepatotoxins (eg, azathioprine, retinoids, sulfasalazine) should be closely monitored for possible increased risk of hepatotoxicity.

Decreased Effect: Corticosteroids have been reported to decrease methotrexate entry into leukemia cells. Administration should be separated by 12 hours. Dexamethasone has been reported to not affect methotrexate entry. May decrease phenytoin and 5-FU activity.

Ethanol/Nutrition/Herb Interactions

Ethanol: Avoid ethanol (may be associated with increased liver injury).

Food: Methotrexate peak serum levels may be decreased if taken with food. Milk-rich foods may decrease MTX absorption. Folate may decrease drug response.

Herb/Nutraceutical: Avoid echinacea (has immunostimulant properties).

Stability

Store intact vials at room temperature (15°C to 25°C) and protect from light

Use preservative-free preparations for high-dose and intrathecal administration

Dilute powder with D$_5$W or NS to a concentration of ≤25 mg/mL (20 mg and 50 mg vials) and 50 mg/mL (1 g vial) as follows; solution is stable for 7 days at room temperature

20 mg = 20 mL (1 mg/mL)

50 mg = 5 mL (10 mg/mL)

1 g = 19.4 mL (50 mg/mL)

Further dilution in D$_5$W or NS is stable for 24 hours at room temperature (21°C to 25°C)

Standard I.V. dilution:

Maximum syringe size for IVP is a 30 mL syringe and syringe should be ≤75% full

Doses <149 mg: Administer slow I.V. push

Dose/syringe (concentration ≤25 mg/mL)

Doses of 150-499 mg: Administer IVPB over 20-30 minutes

Dose/50 mL D$_5$W or NS

Doses of 500-1500 mg: Administer IVPB over ≥60 minutes

Dose/250 mL D$_5$W or NS

Doses of >1500 mg: Administer IVPB over 1-6 hours

Dose/1000 mL D$_5$W or NS

Standard I.M. dilution: Dose/syringe (concentration = 25 mg/mL)

I.V. dilutions are stable for 8 days at room temperature (25°C)

Intrathecal solutions in 3-20 mL LR are stable for 7 days at room temperature (30°C); compatible with cytarabine and hydrocortisone in LR or NS for 7 days at room temperature (25°C)

Standard intrathecal dilution: Dose/3-5 mL LR +/- methotrexate (12 mg) +/- hydrocortisone (15-25 mg)

Intrathecal dilutions are stable for 7 days at room temperature (25°C) but due to sterility issues, use within 24 hours

Mechanism of Action An antimetabolite that inhibits DNA synthesis and cell reproduction in malignant cells

Cytotoxicity is determined by both drug concentration and duration of cell exposure; extracellular drug concentrations of 1 x 10^{-8} M are required to inhibit thymidylate synthesis; reduced folates are able to rescue cells and reverse MTX toxicity if given within 40 hours of the MTX dose

Folates must be in the reduced form (FH$_4$) to be active

Folates are activated by dihydrofolate reductase (DHFR)

DHFR is inhibited by MTX (by binding irreversibly), causing an increase in the intracellular dihydrofolate pool (the inactive cofactor) and inhibition of both purine and thymidylate synthesis (TS)

MTX enters the cell through an energy-dependent and temperature-dependent process which is mediated by an intramembrane protein; this carrier mechanism is also used by naturally occurring reduced folates, including folinic acid (leucovorin), making this a competitive process

At high drug concentrations (>20 μM), MTX enters the cell by a second mechanism which is not shared by reduced folates; the process may be passive diffusion or a specific, saturable process, and provides a rationale for high-dose MTX

A small fraction of MTX is converted intracellularly to polyglutamates, which leads to a prolonged inhibition of DHFR

The MOA in the treatment of rheumatoid arthritis is unknown, but may affect immune function

In psoriasis, methotrexate is thought to target rapidly proliferating epithelial cells in the skin

Pharmacodynamics/Kinetics

Onset of action: Antirheumatic: 3-6 weeks; additional improvement may continue longer than 12 weeks

Absorption: Oral: Rapid; well absorbed at low doses (<30 mg/m²), incomplete after large doses; I.M. injection: Complete

Distribution: Penetrates slowly into 3rd space fluids (eg, pleural effusions, ascites), exits slowly from these compartments (slower than from plasma); crosses placenta; small amounts enter breast milk; does not achieve therapeutic concentrations in CSF; must be given intrathecally if given for CNS prophylaxis or treatment; sustained concentrations retained in kidney and liver

Protein binding: 50%

Metabolism: <10%; degraded by intestinal flora to DAMPA by carboxypeptidase; hepatic aldehyde oxidase converts MTX to 7-OH MTX; polyglutamates are produced intracellularly and are just as potent as MTX; their production is dose and duration dependent and are slowly eliminated by the cell once formed

Half-life elimination: Low dose: 3-10 hours; High dose: 8-12 hours

Time to peak, serum: Oral: 1-2 hours; Parenteral: 30-60 minutes

Excretion: Primarily urine (44% to 100%); feces (small amounts)

Usual Dosage Refer to individual protocols. May be administered orally, I.M., intra-arterially, intrathecally, or I.V.

Leucovorin may be administered concomitantly or within 24 hours of methotrexate - refer to Leucovorin *on page 782* for details

Children:

Dermatomyositis: Oral: 15-20 mg/m²/week as a single dose once weekly or 0.3-1 mg/kg/dose once weekly

Juvenile rheumatoid arthritis: Oral, I.M.: Recommended starting dose: 10 mg/m² once weekly (at higher doses, gastrointestinal side effects may be decreased with I.M. administration); 5-15 mg/m²/week as a single dose **or** as 3 divided doses given 12 hours apart

Antineoplastic dosage range:

Oral, I.M.: 7.5-30 mg/m²/week **or** every 2 weeks

I.V.: 10-18,000 mg/m² bolus dosing **or** continuous infusion over 6-42 hours

See table for dosing schedules:

Methotrexate Dosing Schedules

Dose	Route	Frequency
Conventional		
15-20 mg/m²	P.O.	Twice weekly
30-50 mg/m²	P.O., I.V.	Weekly
15 mg/day for 5 days	P.O., I.M.	Every 2-3 weeks
Intermediate		
50-150 mg/m²	I.V. push	Every 2-3 weeks
240 mg/m²*	I.V. infusion	Every 4-7 days
0.5-1 g/m²*	I.V. infusion	Every 2-3 weeks
High		
1-12 g/m²*	I.V. infusion	Every 1-3 weeks

*Followed with leucovorin rescue - refer to Leucovorin monograph for details.

Pediatric solid tumors (high-dose): I.V.:

<12 years: 12 g/m² (dosage range: 12-18 g)

≥12 years: 8 g/m² (maximum: 18 g)

Acute lymphocytic leukemia (intermediate-dose): I.V.: Loading: 100 mg/m² over 1 hour, followed by a 35-hour infusion of 900 mg/m²/day

Meningeal leukemia: I.T.: 10-15 mg/m² (maximum dose: 15 mg) **or**

≤3 months: 3 mg/dose

4-11 months: 6 mg/dose

1 year: 8 mg/dose

2 years: 10 mg/dose

≥3 years: 12 mg/dose

I.T. doses are prepared with preservative-free MTX only. Hydrocortisone may be added to the I.T. preparation; total volume should range from 3-6 mL. Doses should be repeated at 2- to 5-day intervals until CSF counts return to normal followed by a dose once weekly for 2 weeks then monthly thereafter.

Adults: I.V.: Range is wide from 30-40 mg/m²/week to 100-12,000 mg/m² with leucovorin rescue

Doses **not** requiring leucovorin rescue range from 30-40 mg/m² I.V. or I.M. repeated weekly, or oral regimens of 10 mg/m² twice weekly

High-dose MTX is considered to be >100 mg/m² and can be as high as 1500-7500 mg/m². These doses **require** leucovorin rescue. Patients receiving doses ≥1000 mg/m² should have their urine alkalinized with bicarbonate or Bicitra® prior to and following MTX therapy.

(Continued)

Methotrexate *(Continued)*

Trophoblastic neoplasms: Oral, I.M.: 15-30 mg/day for 5 days; repeat in 7 days for 3-5 courses

Head and neck cancer: Oral, I.M., I.V.: 25-50 mg/m² once weekly

Rheumatoid arthritis: Oral: 7.5 mg once weekly **OR** 2.5 mg every 12 hours for 3 doses/week; not to exceed 20 mg/week

Bone marrow suppression is increased at dosages >20 mg/week; absorption and GI effects may be improved with I.M. administration at higher end of dosage range

Psoriasis: Oral: 2.5-5 mg/dose every 12 hours for 3 doses given weekly **or** Oral, I.M.: 10-25 mg/dose given once weekly

Ectopic pregnancy: I.M./I.V.: 50 mg/m² single-dose without leucovorin rescue

Elderly: Rheumatoid arthritis/psoriasis: Oral: Initial: 5 mg once weekly; if nausea occurs, split dose to 2.5 mg every 12 hours for the day of administration; dose may be increased to 7.5 mg/week based on response, not to exceed 20 mg/week

Dosing adjustment in renal impairment:
Cl_{cr} 61-80 mL/minute: Reduce dose to 75% of usual dose
Cl_{cr} 51-60 mL/minute: Reduce dose to 70% of usual dose
Cl_{cr} 10-50 mL/minute: Reduce dose to 30% to 50% of usual dose
Cl_{cr} <10 mL/minute: Avoid use
Hemodialysis: Not dialyzable (0% to 5%); supplemental dose is not necessary
Peritoneal dialysis: Supplemental dose is not necessary

Dosage adjustment in hepatic impairment:
Bilirubin 3.1-5 mg/dL **or** AST >180 units: Administer 75% of usual dose
Bilirubin >5 mg/dL: Do not use

Administration

Methotrexate may be administered I.M., I.V., or I.T.; refer to Stability section for I.V. administration recommendations based on dosage

I.V. administration rates:
Doses <149 mg: Administer slow I.V. push
Doses of 150-499 mg: Administer IVPB over 20-30 minutes
Doses of 500-1500 mg: Administer IVPB over ≥60 minutes
Doses of >1500 mg: Administer IVPB over 1-6 hours

Specific dosing schemes vary, but high dose should be followed by leucovorin calcium 24-36 hours after initiation of therapy to prevent toxicity

Renal toxicity can be minimized/prevented by alkalinizing the urine (with sodium bicarbonate) and increasing urine flow (hydration therapy)

Monitoring Parameters For prolonged use (especially rheumatoid arthritis, psoriasis) a baseline liver biopsy, repeated at each 1-1.5 g cumulative dose interval, should be performed; WBC and platelet counts every 4 weeks; CBC and creatinine, LFTs every 3-4 months; chest x-ray

Reference Range Refer to chart in Leucovorin Calcium monograph. Therapeutic levels: Variable; Toxic concentration: Variable; therapeutic range is dependent upon therapeutic approach.

High-dose regimens produce drug levels that are between 10^{-6} Molar and 10^{-7} Molar 24-72 hours after drug infusion

10^{-6} **Molar unit = 1 microMolar unit**

Toxic: Low-dose therapy: >9.1 ng/mL; high-dose therapy: >454 ng/mL

Patient Information Avoid alcohol to prevent serious side effects. Avoid intake of extra dietary folic acid, maintain adequate hydration (2-3 L/day of fluids unless instructed to restrict fluid intake) and adequate nutrition (frequent small meals may help). You may experience nausea and vomiting (small frequent meals may help or request antiemetic from prescriber); drowsiness, tingling, numbness, or blurred vision (avoid driving or engaging in tasks that require alertness until response to drug is known); mouth sores (frequent oral care is necessary); loss of hair; skin rash; photosensitivity (use sunscreen, wear protective clothing and eyewear, and avoid direct sunlight). Report black or tarry stools, fever, chills, unusual bleeding or bruising, shortness of breath or difficulty breathing, yellowing of skin or eyes, dark or bloody urine, or acute joint pain or other side effects you may experience. The drug may cause permanent sterility and may cause birth defects; contraceptive measures are recommended during therapy. Pregnancy should be avoided for a minimum of 3 months after completion of therapy in male patients, and at least one ovulatory cycle in female patients. The drug is excreted in breast milk, therefore, an alternative form of feeding your baby should be used.

Nursing Implications

For intrathecal use, mix methotrexate without preservatives with normal saline or lactated Ringer's to a concentration no greater than 2 mg/mL; can be administered I.V. push, I.V. intermittent infusion, or I.V. continuous infusion at a concentration <25 mg/mL; doses >100-300 mg/m² are usually administered by I.V. continuous infusion and are followed by a course of leucovorin rescue

Monitor CBC with differential and platelet count, creatinine clearance, serum creatinine, BUN, and hepatic function tests, LFTs every 3-4 months, chest x-ray; for prolonged use (especially rheumatoid arthritis, psoriasis) a baseline liver biopsy, repeated at each 1-1.5 g cumulative dose interval, should be performed

Additional Information

Sodium content of 100 mg injection: 20 mg (0.86 mEq)
Sodium content of 100 mg (low sodium) injection: 15 mg (0.65 mEq)
Latex-free products: 50 mg/2 mL, 100 mg/4 mL, and 250 mg/10 mL vials with and without preservatives by Immunex

Dosage Forms

Injection, as sodium: 25 mg/mL (2 mL, 10 mL) [with benzyl alcohol 0.9%]
Injection, as sodium [preservative free]: 25 mg/mL (2 mL, 4 mL, 8 mL, 10 mL)
Powder for injection: 20 mg, 1 g
Tablet, as sodium: 2.5 mg

Rheumatrex®: 25 mg

Trexall™: 5 mg, 7.5 mg, 10 mg, 15 mg

Tablet, dose pack, as sodium (Rheumatrex® Dose Pack): 2.5 mg (4 cards with 2, 3, 4, 5, or 6 tablets each)

♦ **Methotrexate Sodium** *see* Methotrexate *on page 884*

♦ **Methoxisal (Can)** *see* Methocarbamol and Aspirin *on page 884*

♦ **Methoxisal-C (Can)** *see* Methocarbamol and Aspirin *on page 884*

Methoxsalen (meth OKS a len)

U.S. Brand Names 8-MOP®; Oxsoralen®; Oxsoralen-Ultra®; Uvadex®

Canadian Brand Names 8-MOP®; Oxsoralen™; Oxsoralen-Ultra™; Ultramop™; Uvadex®

Synonyms Methoxypsoralen; 8-Methoxypsoralen; 8-MOP

Therapeutic Category Psoralen

Use

Oral: Symptomatic control of severe, recalcitrant disabling psoriasis, not responsive to other therapy when the diagnosis has been supported by biopsy. Administer only in conjunction with a schedule of controlled doses of long wave ultraviolet (UV) radiation; also used with long wave ultraviolet (UV) radiation for repigmentation of idiopathic vitiligo.

Topical: Repigmenting agent in vitiligo, used in conjunction with controlled doses of UVA or sunlight

Orphan drug: Uvadex®: Palliative treatment of skin manifestations of cutaneous T-cell lymphoma

Pregnancy Risk Factor C

Contraindications Hypersensitivity to methoxsalen (psoralens) or any component of the formulation; children <12 years of age; diseases associated with photosensitivity; cataract; invasive squamous cell cancer

Warnings/Precautions Family history of sunlight allergy or chronic infections; lotion should only be applied under direct supervision of a physician and should not be dispensed to the patient; for use only if inadequate response to other forms of therapy, serious burns may occur from UVA or sunlight even through glass if dose and or exposure schedule is not maintained; some products may contain tartrazine; use caution in patients with hepatic or cardiac disease

Adverse Reactions Frequency not always defined.

Cardiovascular: Severe edema, hypotension

Central nervous system: Nervousness, vertigo, depression

Dermatologic: Painful blistering, burning, and peeling of skin; pruritus (10%), freckling, hypopigmentation, rash, cheilitis, erythema, itching

Gastrointestinal: Nausea (10%)

Neuromuscular & skeletal: Loss of muscle coordination

Overdosage/Toxicology Symptoms include nausea and severe burns. Follow accepted treatment of severe burns. Keep room darkened until reaction subsides (8-24 hours or more).

Drug Interactions

Increased Effect/Toxicity: Concomitant therapy with other photosensitizing agents such as anthralin, coal tar, griseofulvin, phenothiazines, nalidixic acid, sulfanilamides, tetracyclines, and thiazide diuretics.

Ethanol/Nutrition/Herb Interactions Food: Methoxsalen serum concentrations may be increased if taken with food. Avoid furocoumarin-containing foods (limes, figs, parsley, celery, cloves, lemon, mustard, carrots).

Mechanism of Action Bonds covalently to pyrimidine bases in DNA, inhibits the synthesis of DNA, and suppresses cell division. The augmented sunburn reaction involves excitation of the methoxsalen molecule by radiation in the long-wave ultraviolet light (UVA), resulting in transference of energy to the methoxsalen molecule producing an excited state ("triplet electronic state"). The molecule, in this "triplet state", then reacts with cutaneous DNA.

Pharmacodynamics/Kinetics

Metabolism: Hepatic

Bioavailability: May be less with capsule than with gelcap

Time to peak, serum: Oral: 2-4 hours

Excretion: Urine (>90% as metabolites)

Usual Dosage

Children >12 years and Adults: Vitiligo:

Oral: 20 mg 2-4 hours before exposure to UVA light or sunlight; limit exposure to 15-40 minutes based on skin basic color and exposure

Topical: Apply lotion 1-2 hours before exposure to UVA light, no more than once weekly

Adults: Oral: Psoriasis: 10-70 mg 1½-2 hours before exposure to UVA light, 2-3 times at least 48 hours apart; dosage is based upon patient's body weight and skin type

<30 kg: 10 mg

30-50 kg: 20 mg

51-65 kg: 30 mg

66-80 kg: 40 mg

81-90 kg: 50 mg

91-115 kg: 60 mg

>115 kg: 70 mg

Uvadex® sterile solution is used in conjunction with UVAR® Photopheresis System (consult user's guide): Treatment schedule: Two consecutive days every 4 weeks for a minimum of seven treatment cycles

Dietary Considerations To reduce nausea, oral drug can be administered with food or milk or in 2 divided doses 30 minutes apart.

Patient Information To reduce nausea, oral drug can be taken with food or milk or in 2 divided doses 30 minutes apart. If burning or blistering or intractable pruritus occurs, discontinue therapy until effects subside. Do not sunbathe for at least 24 hours prior to therapy or 48 hours after PUVA therapy. Avoid direct and indirect sunlight for 8 hours after oral and 12-48 hours after topical therapy. **If sunlight cannot be avoided, protective clothing and/or sunscreens must be worn.** Following oral therapy, wraparound sunglasses with UVA-
(Continued)

889

Methoxsalen (Continued)

absorbing properties must be worn for 24 hours. Avoid furocoumarin-containing foods (limes, figs, parsley, celery, cloves, lemon, mustard, carrots); do not exceed prescribed dose or exposure times.

Dosage Forms
Capsule (8-MOP®): 10 mg
Gelcap (Oxsoralen-Ultra®): 10 mg
Lotion (Oxsoralen®): 1% (30 mL)
Solution, sterile (Uvadex®): 20 mcg/mL (10 mL) [**not for injection**]

◆ **Methoxypsoralen** *see Methoxsalen on page 889*
◆ **8-Methoxypsoralen** *see Methoxsalen on page 889*

Methsuximide (meth SUKS i mide)

Related Information
Epilepsy & Seizure Treatment *on page 1659*
U.S. Brand Names Celontin®
Canadian Brand Names Celontin®
Therapeutic Category Anticonvulsant
Use Control of absence (petit mal) seizures that are refractory to other drugs
Unlabeled/Investigational Use Partial complex (psychomotor) seizures
Pregnancy Risk Factor C
Usual Dosage Oral:
Children: Anticonvulsant: Initial: 10-15 mg/kg/day in 3-4 divided doses; increase weekly up to maximum of 30 mg/kg/day
Adults: Anticonvulsant: 300 mg/day for the first week; may increase by 300 mg/day at weekly intervals up to 1.2 g/day in 2-4 divided doses/day
Additional Information Complete prescribing information for this medication should be consulted for additional detail.
Dosage Forms Capsule: 150 mg, 300 mg

Methyclothiazide (meth i kloe THYE a zide)

Related Information
Sulfonamide Derivatives *on page 1515*
U.S. Brand Names Aquatensen®; Enduron®
Canadian Brand Names Aquatensen®; Enduron®
Therapeutic Category Antihypertensive Agent; Diuretic, Thiazide
Use Management of mild to moderate hypertension; treatment of edema in congestive heart failure and nephrotic syndrome
Pregnancy Risk Factor B
Contraindications Hypersensitivity to methyclothiazide or any component, thiazides, or sulfonamide-derived drugs; anuria; renal decompensation
Warnings/Precautions Use with caution in renal disease, hepatic disease, gout, lupus erythematosus, diabetes mellitus; some products may contain tartrazine

Chemical similarities are present among sulfonamides, sulfonylureas, carbonic anhydrase inhibitors, thiazides, and loop diuretics (except ethacrynic acid). Use in patients with thiazide or sulfonamide allergy is specifically contraindicated in product labeling, however a risk of cross-reaction exists in patients with allergy to any of these compounds; avoid use when previous reaction has been severe.

Adverse Reactions
1% to 10%:
Cardiovascular: Orthostatic hypotension
Dermatologic: Photosensitivity
Endocrine & metabolic: Hypokalemia
Gastrointestinal: Anorexia, epigastric distress
<1% (Limited to important or life-threatening): Agranulocytosis, aplastic anemia, cutaneous vasculitis, erythema multiforme, hemolytic anemia, hepatic function impairment, leukopenia, necrotizing angiitis, respiratory distress, Stevens-Johnson syndrome, thrombocytopenia, vasculitis

Overdosage/Toxicology Symptoms include hypermotility, diuresis, and lethargy. Treatment includes GI decontamination and supportive care; fluids for hypovolemia.

Drug Interactions
Increased Effect/Toxicity: Increased effect of methyclothiazide with furosemide and other loop diuretics. Increased hypotension and/or renal adverse effects of ACE inhibitors may result in aggressively diuresed patients. Beta-blockers increase hyperglycemic effects of thiazides in Type 2 diabetes mellitus. Cyclosporine and thiazides can increase the risk of gout or renal toxicity. Digoxin toxicity can be exacerbated if a thiazide induces hypokalemia or hypomagnesemia. Lithium toxicity can occur with thiazides due to reduced renal excretion of lithium. Thiazides may prolong the duration of action with neuromuscular blocking agents.
Decreased Effect: Effects of oral hypoglycemics may be decreased. Decreased absorption of thiazides with cholestyramine and colestipol. NSAIDs can decrease the efficacy of thiazides, reducing the diuretic and antihypertensive effects.
Ethanol/Nutrition/Herb Interactions Herb/Nutraceutical: Avoid dong quai if using for hypertension (has estrogenic activity). Avoid dong quai, St John's wort (may also cause photosensitization). Avoid ephedra, yohimbe, ginseng (may worsen hypertension). Avoid garlic (may have increased antihypertensive effect).
Mechanism of Action Inhibits sodium reabsorption in the distal tubules causing increased excretion of sodium and water, as well as, potassium and hydrogen ions
Pharmacodynamics/Kinetics
Onset of action: Diuresis: 2 hours
Peak effect: 6 hours

Duration: ~1 day
Distribution: Crosses placenta; enters breast milk
Excretion: Urine (as unchanged drug)
Usual Dosage Adults: Oral:
Edema: 2.5-10 mg/day
Hypertension: 2.5-5 mg/day; may add another antihypertensive if 5 mg is not adequate after a trial of 8-12 weeks of therapy
Monitoring Parameters Blood pressure, fluids, weight loss, serum potassium
Patient Information May be taken with food or milk; take early in day to avoid nocturia; take the last dose of multiple doses no later than 6 PM unless instructed otherwise. A few people who take this medication become more sensitive to sunlight and may experience skin rash, redness, itching, or severe sunburn, especially if sun block SPF ≥15 is not used on exposed skin areas.
Nursing Implications Assess weight, I & O reports daily to determine fluid loss; take blood pressure with patient lying down and standing
Dosage Forms Tablet: 2.5 mg, 5 mg

Methyclothiazide and Deserpidine
(meth i kloe THYE a zide & de SER pi deen)
U.S. Brand Names Enduronyl®; Enduronyl® Forte
Canadian Brand Names Enduronyl®; Enduronyl® Forte
Synonyms Deserpidine and Methyclothiazide
Therapeutic Category Antihypertensive Agent, Combination
Use Management of mild to moderately severe hypertension
Pregnancy Risk Factor C
Usual Dosage Oral: Individualized, normally 1-4 tablets/day
Additional Information Complete prescribing information for this medication should be consulted for additional detail.
Dosage Forms Tablet: Methyclothiazide 5 mg and deserpidine 0.25 mg; methyclothiazide 5 mg and deserpidine 0.5 mg

◆ **Methylacetoxyprogesterone** *see* MedroxyPROGESTERone *on page 848*

Methyldopa (meth il DOE pa)
Related Information
Depression *on page 1655*
Hypertension *on page 1675*
U.S. Brand Names Aldomet®
Canadian Brand Names Aldomet®; Apo®-Methyldopa; Novo-Medopa®; Nu-Medopa
Synonyms Methyldopate Hydrochloride
Therapeutic Category Alpha-Adrenergic Inhibitor; Antihypertensive Agent
Use Management of moderate to severe hypertension
Pregnancy Risk Factor B
Pregnancy/Breast-Feeding Implications
Clinical effects on the fetus: Crosses the placenta. Hypotension reported. A large amount of clinical experience with the use of these drugs for the management of hypertension during pregnancy is available. Available evidence suggests safe use during pregnancy and breast-feeding.
Breast-feeding/lactation: Crosses into breast milk at extremely low levels. AAP considers **compatible** with breast-feeding.
Contraindications Hypersensitivity to methyldopa or any component of the formulation; active hepatic disease; liver disorders previously associated with use of methyldopa; on MAO inhibitors; bisulfite allergy if using oral suspension or injectable
Warnings/Precautions May rarely produce hemolytic anemia and liver disorders; positive Coombs' test occurs in 10% to 20% of patients (perform periodic CBCs); sedation usually transient may occur during initial therapy or whenever the dose is increased. Use with caution in patients with previous liver disease or dysfunction, the active metabolites of methyldopa accumulate in uremia. Patients with impaired renal function may respond to smaller doses. Elderly patients may experience syncope (avoid by giving smaller doses). Tolerance may occur usually between the second and third month of therapy. Adding a diuretic or increasing the dosage of methyldopa frequently restores blood pressure control. Because of its CNS effects, methyldopa is not considered a drug of first choice in the elderly.
Adverse Reactions
>10%: Cardiovascular: Peripheral edema
1% to 10%:
Central nervous system: Drug fever, mental depression, anxiety, nightmares, drowsiness, headache
Gastrointestinal: Dry mouth
<1% (Limited to important or life-threatening): Bradycardia (sinus), cholestasis or hepatitis and heptocellular injury, cirrhosis, dyspnea, gynecomastia, hemolytic anemia, hyperprolactinemia, increased liver enzymes, jaundice, leukopenia, orthostatic hypotension, positive Coombs' test, sexual dysfunction, SLE-like syndrome, sodium retention, thrombocytopenia, transient leukopenia or granulocytopenia
Overdosage/Toxicology Symptoms include hypotension, sedation, bradycardia, dizziness, constipation or diarrhea, flatus, nausea, and vomiting. Hypotension usually responds to I.V. fluids, Trendelenburg positioning, or vasoconstrictors. Treatment is primarily supportive and symptomatic; can be removed by hemodialysis.
Drug Interactions
Increased Effect/Toxicity: Beta-blockers, MAO inhibitors, phenothiazines, and sympathomimetics (including epinephrine) may result in hypertension (sometimes severe) when combined with methyldopa. Methyldopa may increase lithium serum levels resulting in lithium toxicity. Levodopa may cause enhanced blood pressure lowering; methyldopa may
(Continued)

Methyldopa *(Continued)*

also potentiate the effect of levodopa. Tolbutamide, haloperidol, and anesthetics effects/toxicity are increased with methyldopa.

Decreased Effect: Iron supplements can interact and cause a significant **increase** in blood pressure. Ferrous sulfate and ferrous gluconate decrease bioavailability. Barbiturates and TCAs may reduce response to methyldopa.

Ethanol/Nutrition/Herb Interactions Herb/Nutraceutical: Avoid dong quai if using for hypertension (has estrogenic activity). Avoid ephedra, yohimbe, ginseng (may worsen hypertension). Avoid valerian, St John's wort, kava kava, gotu kola (may increase CNS depression). Avoid natural licorice (causes sodium and water retention and increases potassium loss). Avoid garlic (may have increased antihypertensive effect).

Stability Injectable dosage form is most stable at acid to neutral pH; stability of parenteral admixture at room temperature (25°C): 24 hours; stability of parenteral admixture at refrigeration temperature (4°C): 4 days; standard diluent: 250-500 mg/100 mL D_5W

Mechanism of Action Stimulation of central alpha-adrenergic receptors by a false transmitter that results in a decreased sympathetic outflow to the heart, kidneys, and peripheral vasculature

Pharmacodynamics/Kinetics
Onset of action: Peak effect: Hypotensive: Oral/parenteral: 3-6 hours
Duration: 12-24 hours
Distribution: Crosses placenta; enters breast milk
Protein binding: <15%
Metabolism: Intestinal and hepatic
Half-life elimination: 75-80 minutes; End-stage renal disease: 6-16 hours
Excretion: Urine (85% as metabolites) within 24 hours

Usual Dosage
Children:
Oral: Initial: 10 mg/kg/day in 2-4 divided doses; increase every 2 days as needed to maximum dose of 65 mg/kg/day; do not exceed 3 g/day.
I.V.: 5-10 mg/kg/dose every 6-8 hours up to a total dose of 65 mg/kg/24 hours or 3 g/24 hours
Adults:
Oral: Initial: 250 mg 2-3 times/day; increase every 2 days as needed; usual dose 1-1.5 g/day in 2-4 divided doses; maximum dose: 3 g/day.
I.V.: 250-500 mg every 6-8 hours; maximum dose: 1 g every 6 hours
Dosing interval in renal impairment:
Cl_{cr} >50 mL/minute: Administer every 8 hours.
Cl_{cr} 10-50 mL/minute: Administer every 8-12 hours.
Cl_{cr} <10 mL/minute: Administer every 12-24 hours.
Hemodialysis: Slightly dialyzable (5% to 20%)

Dietary Considerations Dietary requirements for vitamin B_{12} and folate may be increased with high doses of methyldopa.

Administration When methyldopa is administered with antihypertensives other than thiazides, limit initial doses to 500 mg/day

Monitoring Parameters Blood pressure, standing and sitting/lying down, CBC, liver enzymes, Coombs' test (direct); blood pressure monitor required during I.V. administration

Test Interactions Methyldopa interferes with the following laboratory tests: urinary uric acid, serum creatinine (alkaline picrate method), AST (colorimetric method), and urinary catecholamines (falsely high levels)

Patient Information May cause transient drowsiness; may cause urine discoloration; notify physician of unexplained prolonged general tiredness, fever, or jaundice; rise slowly from prolonged sitting or lying position

Nursing Implications Transient sedation or depression may be common for first 72 hours of therapy; usually disappears over time; infuse over 30 minutes; assist with ambulation

Dosage Forms
Injection, as methyldopate hydrochloride: 50 mg/mL (5 mL, 10 mL)
Suspension, oral: 250 mg/5 mL (5 mL, 473 mL)
Tablet: 125 mg, 250 mg, 500 mg

Methyldopa and Hydrochlorothiazide

(meth il DOE pa & hye droe klor oh THYE a zide)
U.S. Brand Names Aldoril®
Canadian Brand Names Apo®-Methazide
Synonyms Hydrochlorothiazide and Methyldopa
Therapeutic Category Antihypertensive Agent, Combination
Use Management of moderate to severe hypertension
Pregnancy Risk Factor C
Usual Dosage Oral: Dosage titrated on individual components, then switch to combination product; no more than methyldopa 3 g/day and/or hydrochlorothiazide 50 mg/day; maintain initial dose for first 48 hours, then decrease or increase at intervals of not less than 2 days until an adequate response is achieved
Methyldopa 250 mg and hydrochlorothiazide 15 mg: 2-3 times/day
Methyldopa 250 mg and hydrochlorothiazide 25 mg: Twice daily
Methyldopa 500 mg and hydrochlorothiazide 30 mg: Once daily
Methyldopa 500 mg and hydrochlorothiazide 50 mg: Once daily

Additional Information Complete prescribing information for this medication should be consulted for additional detail.

Dosage Forms
Tablet:
Aldoril® 15: Methyldopa 250 mg and hydrochlorothiazide 15 mg
Aldoril® 25: Methyldopa 250 mg and hydrochlorothiazide 25 mg
Aldoril® D30: Methyldopa 500 mg and hydrochlorothiazide 30 mg
Aldoril® D50: Methyldopa 500 mg and hydrochlorothiazide 50 mg

♦ **Methyldopate Hydrochloride** *see* Methyldopa *on page 891*

Methylene Blue (METH i leen bloo)
U.S. Brand Names Urolene Blue®
Therapeutic Category Antidote, Cyanide; Antidote, Drug-induced Methemoglobinemia
Use Antidote for cyanide poisoning and drug-induced methemoglobinemia, indicator dye
Unlabeled/Investigational Use Has been used topically (0.1% solutions) in conjunction with polychromatic light to photoinactivate viruses such as herpes simplex; has been used alone or in combination with vitamin C for the management of chronic urolithiasis
Pregnancy Risk Factor C/D (injected intra-amniotically)
Contraindications Hypersensitivity to methylene blue or any component of the formulation; intraspinal injection; renal insufficiency; pregnancy (injected intra-amniotically)
Warnings/Precautions Do not inject S.C. or intrathecally; use with caution in young patients and in patients with G6PD deficiency; continued use can cause profound anemia
Adverse Reactions Frequency not defined.
  Cardiovascular: Hypertension, precordial pain
  Central nervous system: Dizziness, mental confusion, headache, fever
  Dermatologic: Staining of skin
  Gastrointestinal: Fecal discoloration (blue-green), nausea, vomiting, abdominal pain
  Genitourinary: Discoloration of urine (blue-green), bladder irritation
  Hematologic: Anemia
  Miscellaneous: Diaphoresis
Overdosage/Toxicology Symptoms include nausea, vomiting, precordial pain, hypertension, methemoglobinemia, and cyanosis. Overdosage has resulted in methemoglobinemia and cyanosis. Treatment is symptomatic and supportive.
Mechanism of Action Weak germicide in low concentrations, hastens the conversion of methemoglobin to hemoglobin; has opposite effect at high concentrations by converting ferrous ion of reduced hemoglobin to ferric ion to form methemoglobin; in cyanide toxicity, it combines with cyanide to form cyanmethemoglobin preventing the interference of cyanide with the cytochrome system
Pharmacodynamics/Kinetics
  Absorption: Oral: 53% to 97%
  Excretion: Urine and feces
Usual Dosage
  Children: NADPH-methemoglobin reductase deficiency: Oral: 1-1.5 mg/kg/day (maximum: 300 mg/day) given with 5-8 mg/kg/day of ascorbic acid
  Children and Adults: Methemoglobinemia: I.V.: 1-2 mg/kg or 25-50 mg/m^2 over several minutes; may be repeated in 1 hour if necessary
  Adults: Genitourinary antiseptic: Oral: 65-130 mg 3 times/day with a full glass of water (maximum: 390 mg/day)
Administration Administer I.V. undiluted by direct I.V. injection over several minutes
Patient Information May discolor urine and feces blue-green; take oral formulation after meals with a glass of water; skin stains may be removed using a hypochlorite solution
Nursing Implications Parenteral: Administer undiluted by direct I.V. injection over several minutes
Additional Information Skin stains may be removed using a hypochlorite solution.
Dosage Forms
  Injection: 10 mg/mL (1 mL, 10 mL)
  Tablet: 65 mg

♦ **Methylene Blue, Methenamine, Sodium Biphosphate, Phenyl Salicylate, and Hyoscyamine** *see* Methenamine, Sodium Biphosphate, Phenyl Salicylate, Methylene Blue, and Hyoscyamine *on page 882*
♦ **Methylergometrine Maleate** *see* Methylergonovine *on page 893*

Methylergonovine (meth il er goe NOE veen)
U.S. Brand Names Methergine®
Canadian Brand Names Methergine®
Synonyms Methylergometrine Maleate; Methylergonovine Maleate
Therapeutic Category Ergot Alkaloid and Derivative
Use Prevention and treatment of postpartum and postabortion hemorrhage caused by uterine atony or subinvolution
Pregnancy Risk Factor C
Pregnancy/Breast-Feeding Implications Prolonged constriction of the uterine vessels and/or increased myometrial tone may lead to reduced placental blood flow. This has contributed to fetal growth retardation in animals. Excreted in breast milk, breast-feeding is not recommended.
Contraindications Hypersensitivity to methylergonovine or any component of the formulation; induction of labor; threatened spontaneous abortion; hypertension; toxemia
Warnings/Precautions Use caution in patients with sepsis, obliterative vascular disease, hepatic, or renal involvement, hypertension; administer with extreme caution if using I.V.
Adverse Reactions Frequency not defined.
  Cardiovascular: Hypertension, temporary chest pain, palpitations
  Central nervous system: Hallucinations, dizziness, seizures, headache
  Endocrine & metabolic: Water intoxication
  Gastrointestinal: Nausea, vomiting, diarrhea, foul taste
  Local: Thrombophlebitis
  Neuromuscular & skeletal: Leg cramps
  Otic: Tinnitus
  Renal: Hematuria
  Respiratory: Dyspnea, nasal congestion
  Miscellaneous: Diaphoresis
  (Continued)

Methylergonovine *(Continued)*

Overdosage/Toxicology Symptoms include vasospastic effects, nausea, vomiting, lassitude, impaired mental function, hypotension, hypertension, unconsciousness, seizures, shock, and death. Treatment includes general supportive therapy, gastric lavage or induction of emesis, activated charcoal, and saline cathartic. Keep extremities warm. Activated charcoal is effective at binding certain chemicals, and this is especially true for ergot alkaloids. Treatment is symptomatic with heparin and vasodilators (nitroprusside). Vasodilators should be used with caution to avoid exaggerating any pre-existing hypotension.

Drug Interactions

Increased Effect/Toxicity: Avoid use of 5-HT_1 receptor antagonists (sumatriptan) within 24 hours (per manufacturer). Erythromycin, clarithromycin, and troleandomycin may increase levels of ergot alkaloids, resulting in toxicity (ischemia, vasospasm). Rare toxicity (peripheral vasoconstriction) has been reported with propranolol. Ritonavir, amprenavir, and nelfinavir increase blood levels of ergot alkaloids; avoid concurrent use. Concurrent use of sibutramine may cause serotonin syndrome; avoid concurrent use. Rarely, weakness and incoordination have been noted when SSRIs are used concurrently with 5-HT_1 agonists. The effects of vasoconstrictors may be increased by ergot derivatives.

Stability Ampuls must be protected from light and stored at temperatures 25°C (<77°F).

Mechanism of Action Similar smooth muscle actions as seen with ergotamine; however, it affects primarily uterine smooth muscles producing sustained contractions and thereby shortens the third stage of labor

Pharmacodynamics/Kinetics

Onset of action: Oxytocic: Oral: 5-10 minutes; I.M.: 2-5 minutes; I.V.: Immediately

Duration: Oral: ~3 hours; I.M.: ~3 hours; I.V.: 45 minutes

Absorption: Rapid

Distribution: Rapid; primarily to plasma and extracellular fluid following I.V. administration; tissues

Metabolism: Hepatic

Half-life elimination: Biphasic: Initial: 1-5 minutes; Terminal: 0.5-2 hours

Time to peak, serum: 0.5-3 hours

Excretion: Urine and feces

Usual Dosage Adults:

Oral: 0.2 mg 3-4 times/day for 2-7 days

I.M.: 0.2 mg after delivery of anterior shoulder, after delivery of placenta, or during puerperium; may be repeated as required at intervals of 2-4 hours

I.V.: Same dose as I.M., but should not be routinely administered I.V. because of possibility of inducing sudden hypertension and cerebrovascular accident

Administration Administer over no less than 60 seconds

Patient Information May cause nausea, vomiting, dizziness, increased blood pressure, headache, ringing in the ears, chest pain, or shortness of breath

Nursing Implications Ampuls containing discolored solution should not be used

Dosage Forms

Injection, as maleate: 0.2 mg/mL (1 mL)

Tablet, as maleate: 0.2 mg

♦ **Methylergonovine Maleate** *see* Methylergonovine *on page 893*

♦ **Methylin™** *see* Methylphenidate *on page 894*

♦ **Methylin™ ER** *see* Methylphenidate *on page 894*

♦ **Methylmorphine** *see* Codeine *on page 328*

Methylphenidate *(meth il FEN i date)*

U.S. Brand Names Concerta™; Metadate® CD; Metadate™ ER; Methylin™; Methylin™ ER; Ritalin®; Ritalin-SR®

Canadian Brand Names PMS-Methylphenidate; Riphenidate; Ritalin®; Ritalin® SR

Synonyms Methylphenidate Hydrochloride

Therapeutic Category Central Nervous System Stimulant, Nonamphetamine

Use Treatment of attention-deficit/hyperactivity disorder (ADHD); symptomatic management of narcolepsy

Unlabeled/Investigational Use Depression (especially elderly or medically ill)

Restrictions C-II

Pregnancy Risk Factor C

Pregnancy/Breast-Feeding Implications There are no well-controlled studies establishing safety in pregnant women. Animal studies have shown teratogenic effects to the fetus. Do not use in women of childbearing age unless the potential benefit outweighs the possible risk. It is unknown if methylphenidate is excreted in human milk. Use caution if administering to a nursing woman.

Contraindications Hypersensitivity to methylphenidate, any component of the formulation, or idiosyncrasy to sympathomimetic amines; marked anxiety, tension, and agitation; glaucoma; use during or within 14 days following MAO inhibitor therapy; Tourette's syndrome or tics

Warnings/Precautions Methylphenidate has a high potential for abuse; avoid abrupt discontinuation in patients who have received for prolonged periods. Has demonstrated value as part of a comprehensive treatment program for ADHD. May have value in selected patients as an antidepressant.

Safety and efficacy in children <6 years of age not established. Use with caution in patients with bipolar disorder, diabetes mellitus, cardiovascular disease, seizure disorders, insomnia, porphyria, or mild hypertension (stage I). May exacerbate symptoms of behavior and thought disorder in psychotic patients. Do not use to treat severe depression or fatigue states. Stimulant use has been associated with growth suppression. Concerta™ should not be used in patients with pre-existing severe gastrointestinal narrowing (small bowel disease, short gut syndrome, history of peritonitis, cystic fibrosis, chronic intestinal pseudo-obstruction, Meckel's diverticulum)

Adverse Reactions Frequency not defined.

Cardiovascular: Angina, cardiac arrhythmias, cerebral arteritis, cerebral occlusion, hypertension, hypotension, palpitations, pulse increase/decrease, tachycardia

Central nervous system: Depression, dizziness, drowsiness, fever, headache, insomnia, nervousness, neuroleptic malignant syndrome (NMS), Tourette's syndrome, toxic psychosis

Dermatologic: Erythema multiforme, exfoliative dermatitis, hair loss, rash, urticaria

Endocrine & metabolic: Growth retardation

Gastrointestinal: Abdominal pain, anorexia, nausea, vomiting, weight loss

Hematologic: Anemia, leukopenia, thrombocytopenic purpura

Hepatic: Abnormal liver function tests, hepatic coma, transaminase elevation

Neuromuscular & skeletal: Arthralgia, dyskinesia

Ocular: Blurred vision

Renal: Necrotizing vasculitis

Respiratory: Cough increased, pharyngitis, sinusitis, upper respiratory tract infection

Miscellaneous: Hypersensitivity reactions

Overdosage/Toxicology Symptoms include vomiting, agitation, tremors, hyperpyrexia, muscle twitching, hallucinations, tachycardia, mydriasis, sweating, and palpitations. There is no specific antidote for methylphenidate intoxication and the bulk of the treatment is supportive. Hyperactivity and agitation usually respond to reduced sensory input or benzodiazepines, however, with extreme agitation haloperidol (2-5 mg I.M. for adults) may be required. Hyperthermia is best treated with external cooling measures, or when severe or unresponsive, muscle paralysis with pancuronium may be needed. Hypertension is usually transient and generally does not require treatment unless severe. For diastolic blood pressures >110 mm Hg, a nitroprusside infusion should be initiated. Seizures usually respond to diazepam I.V. and/or phenytoin maintenance regimens.

Drug Interactions

Cytochrome P450 Effect: May inhibit CYP isoenzymes (profile not defined).

Increased Effect/Toxicity: Methylphenidate may cause hypertensive effects when used in combination with MAO inhibitors or drugs with MAO-inhibiting activity (linezolid). Risk may be less with selegiline (MAO type B selective at low doses); it is best to avoid this combination. NMS has been reported in a patient receiving methylphenidate and venlafaxine. Methylphenidate may increase levels of phenytoin, phenobarbital, TCAs, and warfarin. Increased toxicity with clonidine and sibutramine.

Decreased Effect: Effectiveness of antihypertensive agents may be decreased. Carbamazepine may decrease the effect of methylphenidate.

Ethanol/Nutrition/Herb Interactions

Ethanol: Avoid ethanol (may cause CNS depression).

Food: Food may increase oral absorption; Concerta™ formulation is not affected. Food delays early peak and high-fat meals increase C_{max} and AUC of Metadate® CD formulation.

Herb/Nutraceutical: Avoid ephedra (may cause hypertension or arrhythmias) and yohimbe (also has CNS stimulatory activity).

Stability

Tablet: Do not store above 30°C (86°F); protect from light

Extended release capsule: Store in dose pack provided at 25°C (77°F)

Sustained release tablet: Do not store above 30°C (86°F); protect from moisture

Osmotic controlled release tablet (Concerta™): Store at 25°C (77°F); protect from humidity

Mechanism of Action Mild CNS stimulant; blocks the reuptake mechanism of dopaminergic neurons; appears to stimulate the cerebral cortex and subcortical structures similar to amphetamines

Pharmacodynamics/Kinetics

Onset of action: Peak effect:

Immediate release tablet: Cerebral stimulation: ~2 hours

Extended release capsule (Metadate® CD): Biphasic; initial peak similar to immediate release product, followed by second rising portion (corresponding to extended release portion)

Sustained release tablet: 4-7 hours

Osmotic release tablet (Concerta™): Initial: 1-2 hours

Duration: Immediate release tablet: 3-6 hours; Sustained release tablet: 8 hours

Absorption: Readily

Metabolism: Hepatic via de-esterification to active metabolite

Half-life elimination: 2-4 hours

Time to peak: C_{max}: 6-8 hours

Excretion: Urine (90% as metabolites and unchanged drug)

Usual Dosage Oral (discontinue periodically to re-evaluate or if no improvement occurs within 1 month):

Children ≥6 years: ADHD: Initial: 0.3 mg/kg/dose or 2.5-5 mg/dose given before breakfast and lunch; increase by 0.1 mg/kg/dose or by 5-10 mg/day at weekly intervals; usual dose: 0.5-1 mg/kg/day; maximum dose: 2 mg/kg/day or 90 mg/day

Extended release products:

Metadate™ ER, Methylin™ ER, Ritalin® SR: Duration of action is 8 hours. May be given in place of regular tablets, once the daily dose is titrated using the regular tablets and the titrated 8-hour dosage corresponds to sustained release tablet size.

Metadate® CD: Initial: 20 mg once daily; may be adjusted in 20 mg increments at weekly intervals; maximum: 60 mg/day

Concerta™: Duration of action is 12 hours:

Children not currently taking methylphenidate:

Initial: 18 mg once daily in the morning

Adjustment: May increase to 54 mg/day; dose may be adjusted at weekly intervals

Children currently taking methylphenidate: **Note:** Dosing based on current regimen and clinical judgment; suggested dosing listed below:

Patients taking methylphenidate 5 mg 2-3 times/day or 20 mg/day sustained release formulation: Initial dose: 18 mg once every morning (maximum: 54 mg/day)

Patients taking methylphenidate 10 mg 2-3 times/day or 40 mg/day sustained release formulation: Initial dose: 36 mg once every morning (maximum: 54 mg/day)

(Continued)

Methylphenidate *(Continued)*

Patients taking methylphenidate 15 mg 2-3 times/day or 60 mg/day sustained release formulation: Initial dose: 54 mg once every morning (maximum: 54 mg/day)

Adults:

Narcolepsy: 10 mg 2-3 times/day, up to 60 mg/day

Depression (unlabeled use): Initial: 2.5 mg every morning before 9 AM; dosage may be increased by 2.5-5 mg every 2-3 days as tolerated to a maximum of 20 mg/day; may be divided (ie, 7 AM and 12 noon), but should not be given after noon; do not use sustained release product

Dietary Considerations Should be taken 30-45 minutes before meals. Concerta™ is not affected by food and may be taken with or without meals. Metadate® CD should be taken before breakfast. Metadate™ ER should be taken before breakfast and lunch.

Administration Do not crush or allow patient to chew sustained release dosage form. To effectively avoid insomnia, dosing should be completed by noon.

Concerta™: Administer dose once daily in the morning. May be taken with or without food, but must be taken with water, milk, or juice.

Monitoring Parameters Blood pressure, heart rate, signs and symptoms of depression, CBC, differential and platelet counts, growth rate in children, signs of central nervous system stimulation

Patient Information Take exactly as directed; do not change dosage or discontinue without consulting prescriber. Response may take some time. Do not crush or chew sustained release dosage forms. Tablets and sustained release tablets should be taken 30-45 minutes before meals. Concerta™ may be taken with or without food, but must be taken with water, milk, or juice. Avoid alcohol, caffeine, or other stimulants. Maintain adequate fluid intake (2-3 L/day of fluids unless instructed to restrict fluid intake). You may experience decreased appetite or weight loss (small frequent meals may help maintain adequate nutrition); restlessness, impaired judgment, or dizziness, especially during early therapy (use caution when driving or engaging in tasks requiring alertness until response to drug is known). Report unresolved rapid heartbeat; excessive agitation, nervousness, insomnia, tremors, or dizziness; blackened stool; skin rash or irritation; or altered gait or movement. Concerta™ tablet shell may appear intact in stool; this is normal.

Nursing Implications Do not crush or allow patient to chew sustained release dosage forms; to effectively avoid insomnia, dosing should be completed by noon.

Concerta™ tablet shell may appear intact in stool; this is normal. Must be taken with water, milk, or juice.

Additional Information Treatment with methylphenidate should include "drug holidays" or periodic discontinuation in order to assess the patient's requirements and to decrease tolerance and limit suppression of linear growth and weight. Specific patients may require 3 doses/day for treatment of ADHD (ie, additional dose at 4 PM).

Concerta™ is an osmotic controlled release formulation (OROS®) of methylphenidate. The tablet has an immediate-release overcoat that provides an initial dose of methylphenidate within 1 hour. The overcoat covers a trilayer core. The trilayer core is composed of two layers containing the drug and excipients, and one layer of osmotic components. As water from the gastrointestinal tract enters the core, the osmotic components expand and methylphenidate is released.

Metadate® CD capsules contain a mixture of immediate release and extended release beads, designed to release 30% of the dose (6 mg) immediately and 70% (14 mg) over an extended period.

Dosage Forms

Capsule, extended release, as hydrochloride (Metadate® CD): 20 mg
Tablet, as hydrochloride: 5 mg, 10 mg, 20 mg
Methylin™, Ritalin®: 5 mg, 10 mg, 20 mg
Tablet, extended release, as hydrochloride (Metadate™ ER): 10 mg, 20 mg
Tablet, osmotic controlled release, as hydrochloride (Concerta™): 18 mg, 36 mg, 54 mg
Tablet, sustained release, as hydrochloride: 20 mg
Methylin™ ER: 10 mg, 20 mg
Ritalin-SR®: 20 mg

- **Methylphenidate Hydrochloride** *see* Methylphenidate *on page 894*
- **Methylphenobarbital** *see* Mephobarbital *on page 860*
- **Methylphenyl Isoxazolyl Penicillin** *see* Oxacillin *on page 1016*
- **Methylphytyl Napthoquinone** *see* Phytonadione *on page 1082*

MethylPREDNISolone *(meth il pred NIS oh lone)*

Related Information

Contrast Media Reactions, Premedication for Prophylaxis *on page 1653*
Corticosteroids Comparison *on page 1495*

U.S. Brand Names A-methaPred®; depMedalone®; Depoject®; Depo-Medrol®; Depopred®; Duralone®; Medralone®; Medrol®; M-Prednisol®; Solu-Medrol®

Canadian Brand Names Depo-Medrol®; Medrol®; Solu-Medrol®

Synonyms 6-α-Methylprednisolone; Methylprednisolone Acetate; Methylprednisolone Sodium Succinate

Therapeutic Category Anti-inflammatory Agent; Corticosteroid, Systemic; Glucocorticoid

Use Primarily as an anti-inflammatory or immunosuppressant agent in the treatment of a variety of diseases including those of hematologic, allergic, inflammatory, neoplastic, and autoimmune origin. Prevention and treatment of graft-versus-host disease following allogeneic bone marrow transplantation.

Unlabeled/Investigational Use Treatment of fibrosing-alveolitis phase of adult respiratory distress syndrome (ARDS)

Pregnancy Risk Factor C

Contraindications Hypersensitivity to methylprednisolone or any component of the formulation; viral, fungal, or tubercular skin lesions; administration of live virus vaccines; serious infections, except septic shock or tuberculous meningitis. Methylprednisolone formulations containing benzyl alcohol preservative are contraindicated in infants.

Warnings/Precautions Use with caution in patients with hyperthyroidism, cirrhosis, nonspecific ulcerative colitis, hypertension, osteoporosis, thromboembolic tendencies, CHF, convulsive disorders, myasthenia gravis, thrombophlebitis, peptic ulcer, diabetes, glaucoma, cataracts, or tuberculosis. Use caution in hepatic impairment. Because of the risk of adverse effects, systemic corticosteroids should be used cautiously in the elderly, in the smallest possible dose, and for the shortest possible time

Acute adrenal insufficiency may occur with abrupt withdrawal after long-term therapy or with stress; young pediatric patients may be more susceptible to adrenal axis suppression from topical therapy

Adverse Reactions Frequency not defined.

Cardiovascular: Edema, hypertension, arrhythmias

Central nervous system: Insomnia, nervousness, vertigo, seizures, psychoses, pseudotumor cerebri, headache, mood swings, delirium, hallucinations, euphoria

Dermatologic: Hirsutism, acne, skin atrophy, bruising, hyperpigmentation

Endocrine & metabolic: Diabetes mellitus, adrenal suppression, hyperlipidemia, Cushing's syndrome, pituitary-adrenal axis suppression, growth suppression, glucose intolerance, hypokalemia, alkalosis, amenorrhea, sodium and water retention, hyperglycemia

Gastrointestinal: Increased appetite, indigestion, peptic ulcer, nausea, vomiting, abdominal distention, ulcerative esophagitis, pancreatitis

Hematologic: Transient leukocytosis

Neuromuscular & skeletal: Arthralgia, muscle weakness, osteoporosis, fractures

Ocular: Cataracts, glaucoma

Miscellaneous: Infections, hypersensitivity reactions, avascular necrosis, secondary malignancy, intractable hiccups

Overdosage/Toxicology Arrhythmias and cardiovascular collapse are possible with rapid intravenous infusion of high dose methylprednisolone. Symptoms include cushingoid appearance (systemic), muscle weakness (systemic), and osteoporosis (systemic) - all with long-term use only. When consumed in excessive quantities for prolonged periods, systemic hypercorticism and adrenal suppression may occur; in those cases, discontinuation and withdrawal of the corticosteroid should be done judiciously.

Drug Interactions

Cytochrome P450 Effect: CYP3A3/4 enzyme inducer

Increased Effect/Toxicity: Methylprednisolone may increase circulating glucose levels; may need adjustments of insulin or oral hypoglycemics. Methylprednisolone increases cyclosporine and tacrolimus blood levels. Itraconazole increases corticosteroid levels.

Decreased Effect: Phenytoin, phenobarbital, rifampin increase clearance of methylprednisolone. Potassium-depleting diuretics enhance potassium depletion. Skin test antigens, immunizations decrease antibody response and increase potential infections.

Ethanol/Nutrition/Herb Interactions

Ethanol: Avoid ethanol (may increase gastric mucosal irritation).

Food: Methylprednisolone interferes with calcium absorption. Limit caffeine.

Herb/Nutraceutical: St John's wort may decrease methylprednisolone levels. Avoid cat's claw, echinacea (have immunostimulant properties).

Stability

Intact vials of methylprednisolone sodium succinate should be stored at controlled room temperature

Reconstituted solutions of methylprednisolone sodium succinate should be stored at room temperature (15°C to 30°C) and used within 48 hours

Stability of parenteral admixture at room temperature (25°C) and at refrigeration temperature (4°C): 48 hours

Standard diluent (Solu-Medrol®): 40 mg/50 mL D_5W; 125 mg/50 mL D_5W

Minimum volume (Solu-Medrol®): 50 mL D_5W

Mechanism of Action In a tissue-specific manner, corticosteroids regulate gene expression subsequent to binding specific intracellular receptors and translocation into the nucleus. Corticosteroids exert a wide array of physiologic effects including modulation of carbohydrate, protein, and lipid metabolism and maintenance of fluid and electrolyte homeostasis. Moreover cardiovascular, immunologic, musculoskeletal, endocrine, and neurologic physiology are influenced by corticosteroids. Decreases inflammation by suppression of migration of polymorphonuclear leukocytes and reversal of increased capillary permeability.

Pharmacodynamics/Kinetics

Onset of action: Peak effect (route dependent): Oral: 1-2 hours; I.M.: 4-8 days; Intra-articular: 1 week; methylprednisolone sodium succinate is highly soluble and has a rapid effect by I.M. and I.V. routes

Duration (route dependent): Oral: 30-36 hours; I.M.: 1-4 weeks; Intra-articular: 1-5 weeks; methylprednisolone acetate has a low solubility and has a sustained I.M. effect

Distribution: V_d: 0.7-1.5 L/kg

Half-life elimination: 3-3.5 hours; reduced in obese

Excretion: Clearance: Reduced in obese

Usual Dosage Dosing should be based on the lesser of ideal body weight or actual body weight

Only sodium succinate may be given I.V.; methylprednisolone sodium succinate is highly soluble and has a rapid effect by I.M. and I.V. routes. Methylprednisolone acetate has a low solubility and has a sustained I.M. effect.

Children:

Anti-inflammatory or immunosuppressive: Oral, I.M., I.V. (sodium succinate): 0.5-1.7 mg/kg/day **or** 5-25 mg/m²/day in divided doses every 6-12 hours; "Pulse" therapy: 15-30 mg/kg/dose over ≥30 minutes given once daily for 3 days

Status asthmaticus: I.V. (sodium succinate): Loading dose: 2 mg/kg/dose, then 0.5-1 mg/kg/dose every 6 hours for up to 5 days

Acute spinal cord injury: I.V. (sodium succinate): 30 mg/kg over 15 minutes, followed in 45 minutes by a continuous infusion of 5.4 mg/kg/hour for 23 hours

(Continued)

MethylPREDNISolone *(Continued)*

Lupus nephritis: I.V. (sodium succinate): 30 mg/kg over ≥30 minutes every other day for 6 doses

Adults: **Only sodium succinate may be given I.V.;** methylprednisolone sodium succinate is highly soluble and has a rapid effect by I.M. and I.V. routes. Methylprednisolone acetate has a low solubility and has a sustained I.M. effect.

Acute spinal cord injury: I.V. (sodium succinate): 30 mg/kg over 15 minutes, followed in 45 minutes by a continuous infusion of 5.4 mg/kg/hour for 23 hours

Anti-inflammatory or immunosuppressive:

Oral: 2-60 mg/day in 1-4 divided doses to start, followed by gradual reduction in dosage to the lowest possible level consistent with maintaining an adequate clinical response.

I.M. (sodium succinate): 10-80 mg/day once daily

I.M. (acetate): 10-80 mg every 1-2 weeks

I.V. (sodium succinate): 10-40 mg over a period of several minutes and repeated I.V. or I.M. at intervals depending on clinical response; when high dosages are needed, give 30 mg/kg over a period ≥30 minutes and may be repeated every 4-6 hours for 48 hours.

Status asthmaticus: I.V. (sodium succinate): Loading dose: 2 mg/kg/dose, then 0.5-1 mg/kg/dose every 6 hours for up to 5 days

High-dose therapy for acute spinal cord injury: I.V. bolus: 30 mg/kg over 15 minutes, followed 45 minutes later by an infusion of 5.4 mg/kg/hour for 23 hours

Lupus nephritis: High-dose "pulse" therapy: I.V. (sodium succinate): 1 g/day for 3 days

Aplastic anemia: I.V. (sodium succinate): 1 mg/kg/day or 40 mg/day (whichever dose is higher), for 4 days. After 4 days, change to oral and continue until day 10 or until symptoms of serum sickness resolve, then rapidly reduce over approximately 2 weeks.

Pneumocystis pneumonia in AIDs patients: I.V.: 40-60 mg every 6 hours for 7-10 days

Intra-articular (acetate): Administer every 1-5 weeks.

Large joints: 20-80 mg

Small joints: 4-10 mg

Intralesional (acetate): 20-60 mg every 1-5 weeks

Dietary Considerations Should be taken after meals or with food or milk; need diet rich in pyridoxine, vitamin C, vitamin D, folate, calcium, phosphorus, and protein.

Administration

Oral: Administer after meals or with food or milk

Parenteral: Methylprednisolone sodium succinate may be administered I.M. or I.V.; I.V. administration may be IVP over one to several minutes or IVPB or continuous I.V. infusion

I.V.: Succinate:

Low dose: ≤1.8 mg/kg or ≤125 mg/dose: I.V. push over 3-15 minutes

Moderate dose: ≥2 mg/kg or 250 mg/dose: I.V. over 15-30 minutes

High dose: 15 mg/kg or ≥500 mg/dose: I.V. over ≥30 minutes

Doses >15 mg/kg or ≥1 g: Administer over 1 hour

Do **not** administer high-dose I.V. push; hypotension, cardiac arrhythmia, and sudden death have been reported in patients given high-dose methylprednisolone I.V. push over <20 minutes; intermittent infusion over 15-60 minutes; maximum concentration: I.V. push 125 mg/mL

Monitoring Parameters Blood pressure, blood glucose, electrolytes

Test Interactions Interferes with skin tests

Patient Information Do not discontinue or decrease the drug without contacting your physician; carry an identification card or bracelet advising that you are on steroids; may take with meals to decrease GI upset

Nursing Implications Acetate salt should not be given I.V.

Additional Information Sodium content of 1 g sodium succinate injection: 2.01 mEq; 53 mg of sodium succinate salt is equivalent to 40 mg of methylprednisolone base

Methylprednisolone acetate: Depo-Medrol®

Methylprednisolone sodium succinate: Solu-Medrol®

Dosage Forms

Injection, as acetate: 20 mg/mL (5 mL, 10 mL); 40 mg/mL (1 mL, 5 mL, 10 mL); 80 mg/mL (1 mL, 5 mL)

Injection, as sodium succinate: 40 mg (1 mL, 3 mL); 125 mg (2 mL, 5 mL); 500 mg (1 mL, 4 mL, 8 mL, 20 mL); 1000 mg (1 mL, 8 mL, 50 mL); 2000 mg (30.6 mL)

Tablet: 2 mg, 4 mg, 8 mg, 16 mg, 24 mg, 32 mg

Tablet, dose pack: 4 mg (21s)

♦ **6-α-Methylprednisolone** *see* MethylPREDNISolone *on page 896*

♦ **Methylprednisolone Acetate** *see* MethylPREDNISolone *on page 896*

♦ **Methylprednisolone Sodium Succinate** *see* MethylPREDNISolone *on page 896*

♦ **4-Methylpyrazole** *see* Fomepizole *on page 599*

♦ **Methylrosaniline Chloride** *see* Gentian Violet *on page 630*

MethylTESTOSTERone *(meth il tes TOS te rone)*

U.S. Brand Names Android®; Oreton® Methyl; Testred®; Virilon®

Therapeutic Category Androgen

Use

Male: Hypogonadism; delayed puberty; impotence and climacteric symptoms

Female: Palliative treatment of metastatic breast cancer

Restrictions C-III

Pregnancy Risk Factor X

Contraindications Hypersensitivity to methyltestosterone or any component of the formulation; in males, known or suspected carcinoma of the breast or the prostate; pregnancy

Warnings/Precautions Use with extreme caution in patients with liver or kidney disease or serious heart disease; may accelerate bone maturation without producing compensatory gain in linear growth

Adverse Reactions Frequency not defined.

Male: Virilism, priapism, prostatic hyperplasia, prostatic carcinoma, impotence, testicular atrophy, gynecomastia

Female: Virilism, menstrual problems (amenorrhea), breast soreness, hirsutism (increase in pubic hair growth) atrophy

Cardiovascular: Edema

Central nervous system: Headache, anxiety, depression

Dermatologic: Acne, "male pattern" baldness, seborrhea

Endocrine & metabolic: Hypercalcemia, hypercholesterolemia

Gastrointestinal: GI irritation, nausea, vomiting

Hematologic: Leukopenia, polycythemia

Hepatic: Hepatic dysfunction, hepatic necrosis, cholestatic hepatitis

Miscellaneous: Hypersensitivity reactions

Overdosage/Toxicology Abnormal liver function tests.

Drug Interactions

Increased Effect/Toxicity: Effects of oral anticoagulants and hypoglycemic agents may be increased. Toxicity may occur with cyclosporine; avoid concurrent use.

Decreased Effect: Decreased oral anticoagulant effect

Mechanism of Action Stimulates receptors in organs and tissues to promote growth and development of male sex organs and maintains secondary sex characteristics in androgen-deficient males

Pharmacodynamics/Kinetics

Metabolism: Hepatic

Excretion: Urine

Usual Dosage Adults (buccal absorption produces twice the androgenic activity of oral tablets):

Male:

Hypogonadism, male climacteric and impotence: Oral: 10-40 mg/day

Androgen deficiency:

Oral: 10-50 mg/day

Buccal: 5-25 mg/day

Postpubertal cryptorchidism: Oral: 30 mg/day

Female:

Breast pain/engorgement:

Oral: 80 mg/day for 3-5 days

Buccal: 40 mg/day for 3-5 days

Breast cancer:

Oral: 50-200 mg/day

Buccal: 25-100 mg/day

Patient Information Men should report overly frequent or persistent penile erections; women should report menstrual irregularities; all patients should report persistent GI distress, diarrhea, or jaundice; buccal tablet should not be chewed or swallowed

Nursing Implications In prepubertal children, perform radiographic examination of the hand and wrist every 6 months to determine the rate of bone maturation and to assess the effect of treatment on the epiphyseal centers

Dosage Forms

Capsule: 10 mg

Tablet: 10 mg, 25 mg

Methysergide (meth i SER jide)

U.S. Brand Names Sansert®

Canadian Brand Names Sansert®

Synonyms Methysergide Maleate

Therapeutic Category Ergot Alkaloid and Derivative

Use Prophylaxis of vascular headache

Pregnancy Risk Factor X

Usual Dosage Adults: Oral: 4-8 mg/day with meals; if no improvement is noted after 3 weeks, drug is unlikely to be beneficial; must not be given continuously for longer than 6 months, and a drug-free interval of 3-4 weeks must follow each 6-month course

Additional Information Complete prescribing information for this medication should be consulted for additional detail.

Dosage Forms Tablet, as maleate: 2 mg

♦ **Methysergide Maleate** see Methysergide on page 899

♦ **Meticorten®** see PredniSONE on page 1124

♦ **Metimyd®** see Sulfacetamide and Prednisolone on page 1269

Metipranolol (met i PRAN oh lol)

Related Information

Glaucoma Drug Therapy Comparison on page 1499

U.S. Brand Names OptiPranolol®

Canadian Brand Names OptiPranolol®

Synonyms Metipranolol Hydrochloride

Therapeutic Category Beta-Adrenergic Blocker, Ophthalmic

Use Agent for lowering intraocular pressure in patients with chronic open-angle glaucoma

Pregnancy Risk Factor C

Usual Dosage Ophthalmic: Adults: Instill 1 drop in the affected eye(s) twice daily

Additional Information Complete prescribing information for this medication should be consulted for additional detail.

Dosage Forms Solution, ophthalmic, as hydrochloride: 0.3% (5 mL, 10 mL)

♦ **Metipranolol Hydrochloride** see Metipranolol on page 899

Metoclopramide (met oh kloe PRA mide)

U.S. Brand Names Reglan®

Canadian Brand Names Apo®-Metoclop; Nu-Metoclopramide; Reglan®

Therapeutic Category Antiemetic; Gastroprokinetic Agent

Use Prevention and/or treatment of nausea and vomiting associated with chemotherapy, radiation therapy, or postsurgery; symptomatic treatment of diabetic gastric stasis; gastroesophageal reflux; facilitation of intubation of the small intestine

Pregnancy Risk Factor B

Pregnancy/Breast-Feeding Implications

Clinical effects on the fetus: Crosses the placenta. Available evidence suggests safe use during pregnancy.

Breast-feeding/lactation: Crosses into breast milk

Clinical effects on the infant: Increased milk production; 2 reports of mild intestinal discomfort; AAP states MAY BE OF CONCERN

Contraindications Hypersensitivity to metoclopramide or any component of the formulation; GI obstruction, perforation or hemorrhage; pheochromocytoma; history of seizure disorder

Warnings/Precautions Use with caution in patients with Parkinson's disease and in patients with a history of mental illness; has been associated with extrapyramidal symptoms, depression; may exacerbate seizures; to prevent extrapyramidal symptoms, patients may be pretreated with diphenhydramine; elderly are more likely to develop dystonic reactions than younger adults; use lowest recommended doses initially; may cause transient increase in serum aldosterone; use caution in patients who are at risk of fluid overload (CHF, cirrhosis); dosage and/or frequency of administration should be modified in response to degree of renal impairment

Adverse Reactions Adverse reactions are more common/severe at dosages used for prophylaxis of chemotherapy-induced emesis.

>10%:

Central nervous system: Restlessness, drowsiness, extrapyramidal symptoms (high-dose, up to 34%) - may be more severe in the elderly

Gastrointestinal: Diarrhea (may be dose-limiting)

Neuromuscular & skeletal: Weakness

1% to 10%:

Central nervous system: Insomnia, depression

Dermatologic: Rash

Endocrine & metabolic: Breast tenderness, prolactin stimulation

Gastrointestinal: Nausea, xerostomia

<1% (Limited to important or life-threatening): Agranulocytosis, allergic reaction, AV block, CHF, gynecomastia, hepatotoxicity, hypertension or hypotension, jaundice, methemoglobinemia, neuroleptic malignant syndrome (NMS), sulfhemoglobinemia, tachycardia, tardive dyskinesia

Overdosage/Toxicology Symptoms include drowsiness, ataxia, extrapyramidal symptoms, seizures, methemoglobinemia (in infants), disorientation, muscle hypertonia, irritability, and agitation. Metoclopramide often causes extrapyramidal symptoms (eg, dystonic reactions) requiring management with diphenhydramine 1-2 mg/kg (adults), up to a maximum of 50 mg I.M. or slow I.V. push, followed by a maintenance dose for 48-72 hours. When these reactions are unresponsive to diphenhydramine, anticholinergic agents such as benztropine mesylate I.V. 1-2 mg (adults) may be effective. These agents are generally effective within 2-5 minutes.

Drug Interactions

Cytochrome P450 Effect: CYP1A2 and 2D6 enzyme substrate

Increased Effect/Toxicity: Opiate analgesics may increase CNS depression.

Decreased Effect: Anticholinergic agents antagonize metoclopramide's actions.

Ethanol/Nutrition/Herb Interactions Ethanol: Avoid ethanol (may increase CNS depression).

Stability Injection is a clear, colorless solution and should be stored at controlled room temperature and protected from freezing; injection is photosensitive and should be protected from light during storage; dilutions do not require light protection if used within 24 hours

Stability of parenteral admixture at room temperature (25°C) and at refrigeration temperature (4°C): 24 hours

Standard diluent: 10-150 mg/50 mL D_5W or NS

Minimum volume: 50 mL D_5W or NS; send 10 mg unmixed to nursing unit

Compatible with diphenhydramine

Mechanism of Action Blocks dopamine receptors in chemoreceptor trigger zone of the CNS; enhances the response to acetylcholine of tissue in upper GI tract causing enhanced motility and accelerated gastric emptying without stimulating gastric, biliary, or pancreatic secretions

Pharmacodynamics/Kinetics

Onset of action: Oral: 0.5-1 hour; I.V.: 1-3 minutes

Duration: Therapeutic: 1-2 hours, regardless of route

Distribution: Crosses placenta; enters breast milk

Protein binding: 30%

Half-life elimination: Normal renal function: 4-7 hours (may be dose dependent)

Excretion: Primarily urine and feces (as unchanged drug)

Usual Dosage

Children:

Gastroesophageal reflux: Oral: 0.1-0.2 mg/kg/dose up to 4 times/day; efficacy of continuing metoclopramide beyond 12 weeks in reflux has not been determined; total daily dose should not exceed 0.5 mg/kg/day

Gastrointestinal hypomotility (gastroparesis): Oral, I.M., I.V.: 0.1 mg/kg/dose up to 4 times/day, not to exceed 0.5 mg/kg/day

Antiemetic (chemotherapy-induced emesis): I.V.: 1-2 mg/kg 30 minutes before chemotherapy and every 2-4 hours

Facilitate intubation: I.V.:

<6 years: 0.1 mg/kg

6-14 years: 2.5-5 mg
Adults:
Gastroesophageal reflux: Oral: 10-15 mg/dose up to 4 times/day 30 minutes before meals or food and at bedtime; single doses of 20 mg are occasionally needed for provoking situations; efficacy of continuing metoclopramide beyond 12 weeks in reflux has not been determined
Gastrointestinal hypomotility (gastroparesis):
Oral: 10 mg 30 minutes before each meal and at bedtime for 2-8 weeks
I.V. (for severe symptoms): 10 mg over 1-2 minutes; 10 days of I.V. therapy may be necessary for best response
Antiemetic (chemotherapy-induced emesis): I.V.: 1-2 mg/kg 30 minutes before chemotherapy and every 2-4 hours to every 4-6 hours (and usually given with diphenhydramine 25-50 mg I.V./oral)
Postoperative nausea and vomiting: I.M.: 10 mg near end of surgery; 20 mg doses may be used
Facilitate intubation: I.V.: 10 mg
Elderly:
Gastroesophageal reflux: Oral: 5 mg 4 times/day (30 minutes before meals and at bedtime); increase dose to 10 mg 4 times/day if no response at lower dose
Gastrointestinal hypomotility:
Oral: Initial: 5 mg 30 minutes before meals and at bedtime for 2-8 weeks; increase if necessary to 10 mg doses
I.V.: Initiate at 5 mg over 1-2 minutes; increase to 10 mg if necessary
Postoperative nausea and vomiting: I.M.: 5 mg near end of surgery; may repeat dose if necessary
Dosing adjustment in renal impairment:
Cl$_{cr}$ 10-40 mL/minute: Administer at 50% of normal dose
Cl$_{cr}$ <10 mL/minute: Administer at 25% of normal dose
Hemodialysis: Not dialyzable (0% to 5%); supplemental dose is not necessary
Administration Lower doses of metoclopramide can be given I.V. push undiluted over 1-2 minutes; parenteral doses of up to 10 mg should be given I.V. push; higher doses to be given IVPB; infuse over at least 15 minutes
Monitoring Parameters Periodic renal function test; monitor for dystonic reactions; monitor for signs of hypoglycemia in patients using insulin and those being treated for gastroparesis; monitor for agitation and irritable confusion
Test Interactions ↑ aminotransferase [ALT (SGPT)/AST (SGOT)] (S), ↑ amylase (S)
Patient Information May impair mental alertness or physical coordination; avoid alcohol, barbiturates or other CNS depressants; take 30 minutes before meals; notify physician if involuntary movements occur
Nursing Implications
Parenteral doses of up to 10 mg should be administered I.V. push over 1-2 minutes; rapid boluses cause transient anxiety and restlessness followed by drowsiness; higher doses to be administered IVPB; dilute to 0.2 mg/mL (maximum concentration: 5 mg/mL) and infuse over 15-30 minutes (maximum rate of infusion: 5 mg/minute); rapid I.V. administration is associated with a transient but intense feeling of anxiety and restlessness, followed by drowsiness
Monitor periodic renal function test
Dosage Forms
Injection: 5 mg/mL (2 mL, 10 mL, 30 mL, 50 mL, 100 mL)
Solution, oral concentrate: 10 mg/mL (10 mL, 30 mL)
Syrup: 5 mg/5 mL (10 mL, 480 mL) [sugar free]
Tablet: 5 mg, 10 mg

Metolazone (me TOLE a zone)
Related Information
Heart Failure on page 1663
Sulfonamide Derivatives on page 1515
U.S. Brand Names Mykrox®; Zaroxolyn®
Canadian Brand Names Mykrox®; Zaroxolyn®
Therapeutic Category Antihypertensive Agent; Diuretic, Miscellaneous
Use Management of mild to moderate hypertension; treatment of edema in congestive heart failure and nephrotic syndrome, impaired renal function
Pregnancy Risk Factor B (manufacturer); D (expert analysis)
Contraindications Hypersensitivity to metolazone, any component of the formulation, other thiazides, and sulfonamide derivatives; anuria; hepatic coma; pregnancy
Warnings/Precautions Use with caution in renal disease, hepatic disease, gout, lupus erythematosus, diabetes mellitus; some products may contain tartrazine. **Mykrox® is not bioequivalent to Zaroxolyn® and should not be interchanged for one another.** Electrolyte disturbances (hypokalemia, hypochloremic alkalosis, hyponatremia) can occur. Orthostatic hypotension may occur (potentiated by alcohol, barbiturates, narcotics, other antihypertensive drugs).

Chemical similarities are present among sulfonamides, sulfonylureas, carbonic anhydrase inhibitors, thiazides, and loop diuretics (except ethacrynic acid). Use in patients with thiazide or sulfonamide allergy is specifically contraindicated in product labeling, however a risk of cross-reaction exists in patients with allergy to any of these compounds; avoid use when previous reaction has been severe.
Adverse Reactions
>10%: Central nervous system: Dizziness
1% to 10%:
Cardiovascular: Orthostatic hypotension, palpitations, chest pain, cold extremities (rapidly acting), edema (rapidly acting), venous thrombosis (slow acting), syncope (slow acting)
Central nervous system: Headache, fatigue, lethargy, malaise, lassitude, anxiety, depression, nervousness, "weird" feeling (rapidly acting), chills (slow acting)
(Continued)

Metolazone *(Continued)*

Dermatologic: Rash, pruritus, dry skin (rapidly acting)

Endocrine & metabolic: Hypokalemia, impotence, reduced libido, excessive volume depletion (slow acting), hemoconcentration (slow acting), acute gouty attach (slow acting), weakness

Gastrointestinal: Nausea, vomiting, abdominal pain, cramping, bloating, diarrhea or constipation, dry mouth

Genitourinary: Nocturia

Neuromuscular & skeletal: Muscle cramps, spasm

Ocular: Eye itching (rapidly acting)

Otic: Tinnitus (rapidly acting)

Respiratory: Cough (rapidly acting), epistaxis (rapidly acting), sinus congestion (rapidly acting), sore throat (rapidly acting),

<1% (Limited to important or life-threatening): Agranulocytosis, aplastic anemia, glycosuria, hepatitis, hyperglycemia, leukopenia, purpura, Stevens-Johnson syndrome, thrombocytopenia, toxic epidermal necrolysis

Overdosage/Toxicology Symptoms include hypermotility, diuresis, lethargy, confusion, and muscle weakness. Following GI decontamination, therapy is supportive with I.V. fluids, electrolytes, and I.V. pressors if needed.

Drug Interactions

Increased Effect/Toxicity: Increased diuretic effect of metolazone with furosemide and other loop diuretics. Increased hypotension and/or renal adverse effects of ACE inhibitors may result in aggressively diuresed patients. Cyclosporine and thiazide-type diuretics can increase the risk of gout or renal toxicity. Digoxin toxicity can be exacerbated if a diuretic induces hypokalemia or hypomagnesemia. Lithium toxicity can occur with thiazide-type diuretics due to reduced renal excretion of lithium. Thiazide-type diuretics may prolong the duration of action of neuromuscular blocking agents.

Decreased Effect: Effects of oral hypoglycemics may be decreased. Decreased absorption of metolazone with cholestyramine and colestipol. NSAIDs can decrease the efficacy of thiazide-type diuretics, reducing the diuretic and antihypertensive effects.

Ethanol/Nutrition/Herb Interactions Herb/Nutraceutical: Avoid dong quai if using for hypertension (has estrogenic activity). Avoid dong quai, St John's wort (may also cause photosensitization). Avoid ephedra, yohimbe, ginseng (may worsen hypertension). Avoid natural licorice. Avoid garlic (may have increased antihypertensive effect).

Mechanism of Action Inhibits sodium reabsorption in the distal tubules causing increased excretion of sodium and water, as well as, potassium and hydrogen ions

Pharmacodynamics/Kinetics

Onset of action: Diuresis: ~60 minutes

Duration: 12-24 hours

Absorption: Incomplete

Distribution: Crosses placenta; enters breast milk

Protein binding: 95%

Metabolism: Enterohepatic recycling

Bioavailability: Mykrox® reportedly has highest

Half-life elimination: 6-20 hours, renal function dependent

Excretion: Urine (80% to 95%)

Usual Dosage Adults: Oral:

Edema: 5-20 mg/dose every 24 hours

Hypertension: 2.5-5 mg/dose every 24 hours

Hypertension (Mykrox®): 0.5 mg/day; if response is not adequate, increase dose to maximum of 1 mg/day

Dialysis: Not dialyzable (0% to 5%) via hemo- or peritoneal dialysis; supplemental dose is not necessary

Dietary Considerations Should be taken after breakfast; may require potassium supplementation

Administration May be taken with food or milk. Take early in day to avoid nocturia. Take the last dose of multiple doses no later than 6 PM unless instructed otherwise.

Monitoring Parameters Serum electrolytes (potassium, sodium, chloride, bicarbonate), renal function, blood pressure (standing, sitting/supine)

Patient Information May be taken with food or milk; take early in day to avoid nocturia; take the last dose of multiple doses no later than 6 PM unless instructed otherwise. A few people who take this medication become more sensitive to sunlight and may experience skin rash, redness, itching, or severe sunburn, especially if sun block SPF ≥15 is not used on exposed skin areas.

Nursing Implications Assess weight, I & O reports daily to determine fluid loss; take blood pressure with patient lying down and standing

Additional Information Metolazone 5 mg is approximately equivalent to hydrochlorothiazide 50 mg. When taken the day of surgery, it may cause hypovolemia and the hypertensive patient undergoing general anesthesia to have labile blood pressure; use with caution prior to surgery or perioperatively.

Dosage Forms

Tablet, rapid acting (Mykrox®): 0.5 mg

Tablet, slow acting (Zaroxolyn®): 2.5 mg, 5 mg, 10 mg

Extemporaneous Preparations A 1 mg/mL suspension can be made by crushing twenty-four 5 mg tablets. Add a small amount of distilled water. Add 30 mL Cologel® and mix well. Add a sufficient amount of 2:1 simple syrup/cherry syrup mixture to make a final volume of 120 mL. Label "shake well". Stability is 2 weeks refrigerated.

Handbook on Extemporaneous Formulations, Bethesda MD: American Society of Hospital Pharmacists, 1987.

Metoprolol *(me toe PROE lole)*

Related Information

Beta-Blockers Comparison *on page 1491*

Heart Failure *on page 1663*
Hypertension *on page 1675*

U.S. Brand Names Lopressor®; Toprol XL®

Canadian Brand Names Apo®-Metoprolol; Betaloc®; Betaloc® Durules®; Gen-Metoprolol; Lopressor®; Novo-Metoprolol; Nu-Metop; PMS-Metoprolol; Toprol-XL®

Synonyms Metoprolol Tartrate

Therapeutic Category Antihypertensive Agent; Beta-Adrenergic Blocker

Use Treatment of hypertension and angina pectoris; prevention of myocardial infarction, atrial fibrillation, flutter, symptomatic treatment of hypertrophic subaortic stenosis; to reduce mortality/hospitalization in patients with congestive heart failure (stable NYHA class II or III) in patients already receiving ACE inhibitors, diuretics, and/or digoxin (sustained-release only)

Unlabeled/Investigational Use Treatment of ventricular arrhythmias, atrial ectopy, migraine prophylaxis, essential tremor, aggressive behavior

Pregnancy Risk Factor C (manufacturer); D (2nd and 3rd trimesters - expert analysis)

Pregnancy/Breast-Feeding Implications
Clinical effects on the fetus: Crosses the placenta. None; mild IUGR probably secondary to maternal hypertension. Available evidence suggests safe use during pregnancy and breast-feeding. Monitor breast-fed infant for symptoms of beta-blockade.
Breast-feeding/lactation: Crosses into breast milk. AAP considers **compatible** with breast-feeding.

Contraindications Hypersensitivity to metoprolol or any component of the formulation; sinus bradycardia; heart block greater than first degree (except in patients with a functioning artificial pacemaker); cardiogenic shock; uncompensated cardiac failure; pregnancy (2nd and 3rd trimesters)

Warnings/Precautions Abrupt withdrawal of the drug should be avoided (may result in an exaggerated cardiac beta-adrenergic response, tachycardia, hypertension, ischemia, angina, myocardial infarction, and sudden death), drug should be discontinued over 1-2 weeks. Must use care in compensated heart failure and monitor closely for a worsening of the condition (efficacy has not been established for metoprolol). Avoid abrupt discontinuation in patients with a history of CAD; slowly wean while monitoring for signs and symptoms of ischemia. Use caution in patients with PVD (can aggravate arterial insufficiency). Use caution with concurrent use of beta-blockers and either verapamil or diltiazem; bradycardia or heart block can occur. Avoid concurrent I.V. use of both agents. In general, beta-blockers should be avoided in patients with bronchospastic disease. Metoprolol, with B1 selectivity, should be used cautiously in bronchospastic disease with close monitoring, since selectivity can be lost with higher doses. Use cautiously in diabetics because it can mask prominent hypoglycemic symptoms. Can mask signs of thyrotoxicosis. Can cause fetal harm when administered in pregnancy. Use cautiously in the hepatically impaired. Use care with anesthetic agents which decrease myocardial function.

Adverse Reactions
>10%:
Central nervous system: Drowsiness, insomnia
Endocrine & metabolic: Decreased sexual ability
1% to 10%:
Cardiovascular: Bradycardia, palpitations, edema, congestive heart failure, reduced peripheral circulation
Central nervous system: Mental depression
Gastrointestinal: Diarrhea or constipation, nausea, vomiting, stomach discomfort
Respiratory: Bronchospasm
Miscellaneous: Cold extremities
<1% (Limited to important or life-threatening): Arrhythmias, chest pain, confusion (especially in the elderly), depression, dyspnea, hallucinations, headache, hepatic dysfunction, hepatitis, jaundice, leukopenia, nervousness, orthostatic hypotension, thrombocytopenia

Overdosage/Toxicology Symptoms of intoxication include cardiac disturbances, CNS toxicity, bronchospasm, hypoglycemia and hyperkalemia. The most common cardiac symptoms include hypotension and bradycardia. Atrioventricular block, intraventricular conduction disturbances, cardiogenic shock, and asystole may occur with severe overdose, especially with membrane-depressant drugs (eg, propranolol). CNS effects include convulsions, coma, and respiratory arrest. Treatment is symptomatic for seizures, hypotension, hyperkalemia and hypoglycemia. Bradycardia and hypotension resistant to atropine, isoproterenol, or pacing may respond to glucagon. Wide QRS defects caused by membrane-depressant poisoning may respond to hypertonic sodium bicarbonate. Repeat-dose charcoal, hemoperfusion, or hemodialysis may be helpful in removal of only those beta-blockers with a small V_d, long half-life, or low intrinsic clearance (acebutolol, atenolol, nadolol, sotalol).

Drug Interactions
Cytochrome P450 Effect: CYP2D6 enzyme substrate
Increased Effect/Toxicity: Metoprolol may increase the effects of other drugs which slow AV conduction (digoxin, verapamil, diltiazem), alpha-blockers (prazosin, terazosin), and alpha-adrenergic stimulants (epinephrine, phenylephrine). Metoprolol may mask the tachycardia from hypoglycemia caused by insulin and oral hypoglycemics. In patients receiving concurrent therapy, the risk of hypertensive crisis is increased when either clonidine or the beta-blocker is withdrawn. Reserpine has been shown to enhance the effect of beta-blockers. Beta-blockers may increase the action or levels of ethanol, disopyramide, nondepolarizing muscle relaxants, and theophylline although the effects are difficult to predict.
Decreased Effect: Decreased effect of beta-blockers with aluminum salts, barbiturates, calcium salts, cholestyramine, colestipol, NSAIDs, penicillins (ampicillin), rifampin, salicylates, and sulfinpyrazone due to decreased bioavailability and plasma levels. Beta-blockers may decrease the effect of sulfonylureas.

Ethanol/Nutrition/Herb Interactions
Food: Food increases absorption. Metoprolol serum levels may be increased if taken with food.
Herb/Nutraceutical: Avoid dong quai if using for hypertension (has estrogenic activity). Avoid ephedra, yohimbe, ginseng (may worsen hypertension). Avoid garlic (may have increased antihypertensive effect).
(Continued)

Metoprolol *(Continued)*

Mechanism of Action Selective inhibitor of beta$_1$-adrenergic receptors; competitively blocks beta$_1$-receptors, with little or no effect on beta$_2$-receptors at doses <100 mg; does not exhibit any membrane stabilizing or intrinsic sympathomimetic activity

Pharmacodynamics/Kinetics

Onset of action: Peak effect: antihypertensive: Oral: 1.5-4 hours

Duration: 10-20 hours

Absorption: 95%

Protein binding: 8%

Metabolism: Extensively hepatic; significant first-pass effect

Bioavailability: Oral: 40% to 50%

Half-life elimination: 3-4 hours; End-stage renal disease: 2.5-4.5 hours

Excretion: Urine (3% to 10% as unchanged drug)

Usual Dosage

Children: Oral: 1-5 mg/kg/24 hours divided twice daily; allow 3 days between dose adjustments

Adults:

Hypertension, angina, SVT, MI prophylaxis: Oral: 100-450 mg/day in 2-3 divided doses, begin with 50 mg twice daily and increase doses at weekly intervals to desired effect

Extended release: Same daily dose administered as a single dose

I.V.: Hypertension: Has been given in dosages 1.25-5 mg every 6-12 hours in patients unable to take oral medications

Congestive heart failure: Oral (extended release): Initial: 25 mg once daily (reduce to 12.5 mg once daily in NYHA class higher than class II); may double dosage every 2 weeks as tolerated, up to 200 mg/day

Myocardial infarction (acute): I.V.: 5 mg every 2 minutes for 3 doses in early treatment of myocardial infarction; thereafter give 50 mg orally every 6 hours 15 minutes after last I.V. dose and continue for 48 hours; then administer a maintenance dose of 100 mg twice daily.

Elderly: Oral: Initial: 25 mg/day; usual range: 25-300 mg/day

Hemodialysis: Administer dose posthemodialysis or administer 50 mg supplemental dose; supplemental dose is not necessary following peritoneal dialysis

Dosing adjustment/comments in hepatic disease: Reduced dose probably necessary

Dietary Considerations Regular tablets should be taken with food. Sustained release tablets may be taken without regard to meals.

Administration Administer I.V. push, inject slowly over 1 minute

Monitoring Parameters Blood pressure, apical and radial pulses, fluid I & O, daily weight, respirations, mental status, and circulation in extremities before and during therapy

Patient Information Do not discontinue medication abruptly, sudden stopping of medication may precipitate or cause angina; consult pharmacist or physician before taking with other adrenergic drugs (eg, cold medications); use with caution while driving or performing tasks requiring alertness; may mask signs of hypoglycemia in diabetics; regular tablets may be taken with food; sustained release tablets may be taken without regard to meals

Nursing Implications Monitor hemodynamic status carefully after acute MI, monitor orthostatic blood pressures, apical and peripheral pulse and mental status changes (ie, confusion, depression)

Dosage Forms

Injection, as tartrate: 1 mg/mL (5 mL)

Tablet, as tartrate: 25 mg, 50 mg, 100 mg

Tablet, sustained release, as succinate [equivalent to tartrate]: 25 mg, 50 mg, 100 mg, 200 mg

Extemporaneous Preparations A mixture of metoprolol 10 mg/mL plus hydrochlorothiazide 5 mg/mL was found to be stable for 60 days in a refrigerator in a 1:1 preparation of Ora-Sweet® and Ora-Plus®, in Ora-Sweet® SF and Ora-Plus®, and in cherry syrup

Allen LV and Erickson III MA, "Stability of Labetalol Hydrochloride, Metoprolol Tartrate, Verapamil Hydrochloride, and Spironolactone With Hydrochlorothiazide in Extemporaneously Compounded Oral Liquids," *Am J Health Syst Pharm*, 1996, 53:2304-9.

♦ **Metoprolol Tartrate** *see Metoprolol on page 902*

♦ **MetroCream®** *see Metronidazole on page 904*

♦ **Metrodin®** *see Urofollitropin on page 1391*

♦ **Metrogel® (Can)** *see Metronidazole on page 904*

♦ **MetroGel® Topical** *see Metronidazole on page 904*

♦ **MetroGel®-Vaginal** *see Metronidazole on page 904*

♦ **Metro I.V.®** *see Metronidazole on page 904*

♦ **MetroLotion®** *see Metronidazole on page 904*

Metronidazole *(me troe NI da zole)*

Related Information

Antimicrobial Drugs of Choice *on page 1588*

Community-Acquired Pneumonia in Adults *on page 1603*

Helicobacter pylori Treatment *on page 1668*

Treatment of Sexually Transmitted Diseases *on page 1609*

U.S. Brand Names Flagyl®; Flagyl ER®; MetroCream®; MetroGel® Topical; MetroGel®-Vaginal; Metro I.V.®; MetroLotion®; Noritate™; Protostat® Oral

Canadian Brand Names Apo®-Metronidazole; Flagyl®; MetroCream™; Metrogel®; Nidagel™; Noritate®; Novo-Nidazol

Synonyms Metronidazole Hydrochloride

Therapeutic Category Amebicide; Antibiotic, Anaerobic; Antibiotic, Topical; Antibiotic, Miscellaneous; Antiprotozoal

Use Treatment of susceptible anaerobic bacterial and protozoal infections in the following conditions: Amebiasis, symptomatic and asymptomatic trichomoniasis; skin and skin structure infections; CNS infections; intra-abdominal infections (as part of combination regimen); systemic anaerobic infections; treatment of antibiotic-associated pseudomembranous colitis (AAPC), bacterial vaginosis; as part of a multidrug regimen for *H. pylori* eradication to reduce the risk of duodenal ulcer recurrence; also used in Crohn's disease and hepatic encephalopathy

Orphan drug: MetroGel® Topical: Treatment of acne rosacea

Pregnancy Risk Factor B (may be contraindicated in 1st trimester)

Pregnancy/Breast-Feeding Implications Found to be carcinogenic in rats

Contraindications Hypersensitivity to metronidazole or any component of the formulation; 1st trimester of pregnancy since found to be carcinogenic in rats

Warnings/Precautions Use with caution in patients with liver impairment due to potential accumulation, blood dyscrasias; history of seizures, congestive heart failure, or other sodium retaining states; reduce dosage in patients with severe liver impairment, CNS disease, and severe renal failure; seizures and neuropathies have been reported especially with increased doses and chronic treatment; if this occurs, discontinue therapy

Adverse Reactions

Systemic:

>10%:
Central nervous system: Dizziness, headache
Gastrointestinal (12%): Nausea, diarrhea, loss of appetite, vomiting

<1% (Limited to important or life-threatening): Ataxia, change in taste sensation, dark urine, disulfiram-type reaction with alcohol, furry tongue, hypersensitivity, leukopenia, metallic taste, neuropathy, pancreatitis, seizures, thrombophlebitis, vaginal candidiasis, xerostomia

Vaginal:

>10%: Genitourinary: *Candida* cervicitis or vaginitis

1% to 10%:
Central nervous system: Dry mouth, furry tongue, diarrhea, nausea, vomiting, anorexia
Gastrointestinal: Altered taste sensation
Genitourinary: Burning or irritation of penis of sexual partner; burning or increased frequency of urination, vulvitis, dark urine

Overdosage/Toxicology Symptoms include nausea, vomiting, ataxia, seizures, and peripheral neuropathy. Treatment is symptomatic and supportive.

Drug Interactions

Cytochrome P450 Effect: CYP2C9 enzyme substrate; CYP2C9, 3A3/4, and 3A5-7 enzyme inhibitor

Increased Effect/Toxicity: Ethanol may cause a disulfiram-like reaction. Warfarin and metronidazole may increase bleeding times (PT) which may result in bleeding. Cimetidine may increase metronidazole levels. Metronidazole may inhibit metabolism of cisapride, causing potential arrhythmias; avoid concurrent use. Metronidazole may increase lithium levels/toxicity.

Decreased Effect: Phenytoin, phenobarbital (potentially other enzyme inducers) may decrease metronidazole half-life and effects.

Ethanol/Nutrition/Herb Interactions

Ethanol: Metronidazole inhibits ethanol's usual metabolism. Avoid all ethanol or any ethanol-containing drugs (may cause disulfiram-like reaction characterized by flushing, headache, nausea, vomiting, sweating or tachycardia). Patients should be warned to avoid ethanol during and 72 hours after therapy.

Food: Peak antibiotic serum concentration lowered and delayed, but total drug absorbed not affected.

Stability Metronidazole injection should be stored at 15°C to 30°C and protected from light. Product may be refrigerated but crystals may form; crystals redissolve on warming to room temperature. Prolonged exposure to light will cause a darkening of the product. However, short-term exposure to normal room light does not adversely affect metronidazole stability. Direct sunlight should be avoided. Stability of parenteral admixture at room temperature (25°C): Out of overwrap stability: 30 days.

Standard diluent: 500 mg/100 mL NS

Mechanism of Action Reduced to a product which interacts with DNA to cause a loss of helical DNA structure and strand breakage resulting in inhibition of protein synthesis and cell death in susceptible organisms

Pharmacodynamics/Kinetics

Absorption: Oral: Well absorbed; Topical: Concentrations achieved systemically after application of 1 g topically are 10 times less than those obtained after a 250 mg oral dose

Distribution: To saliva, bile, seminal fluid, breast milk, bone, liver, and liver abscesses, lung and vaginal secretions; crosses placenta and blood-brain barrier

CSF:blood level ratio: Normal meninges: 16% to 43%; Inflamed meninges: 100%

Protein binding: <20%

Metabolism: Hepatic, 30% to 60%

Half-life elimination: Neonates: 25-75 hours; Others: 6-8 hours, increases with hepatic impairment; End-stage renal disease: 21 hours

Time to peak, serum: Oral: Immediate release: 1-2 hours

Excretion: Urine (20% to 40% as unchanged drug); feces (6% to 15%)

Usual Dosage

Infants and Children:

Amebiasis: Oral: 35-50 mg/kg/day in divided doses every 8 hours for 10 days

Trichomoniasis: Oral: 15-30 mg/kg/day in divided doses every 8 hours for 7 days

Anaerobic infections:

Oral: 15-35 mg/kg/day in divided doses every 8 hours

I.V.: 30 mg/kg/day in divided doses every 6 hours

Clostridium difficile (antibiotic-associated colitis): Oral: 20 mg/kg/day divided every 6 hours

Maximum dose: 2 g/day

Adults:

Amebiasis: Oral: 500-750 mg every 8 hours for 5-10 days

(Continued)

Metronidazole *(Continued)*

Trichomoniasis: Oral: 250 mg every 8 hours for 7 days or 2 g as a single dose

Anaerobic infections: Oral, I.V.: 500 mg every 6-8 hours, not to exceed 4 g/day

Antibiotic-associated pseudomembranous colitis: Oral: 250-500 mg 3-4 times/day for 10-14 days

Helicobacter pylori eradication: 250 mg with meals and at bedtime for 14 days; requires combination therapy with at least one other antibiotic and an acid-suppressing agent (proton pump inhibitor or H_2 blocker)

Vaginosis: 1 applicatorful (~37.5 mg metronidazole) intravaginally once or twice daily for 5 days; apply once in morning and evening if using twice daily, if daily, use at bedtime

Elderly: Use lower end of dosing recommendations for adults, do not administer as a single dose

Topical (acne rosacea therapy): Apply and rub a thin film twice daily, morning and evening, to entire affected areas after washing. Significant therapeutic results should be noticed within 3 weeks. Clinical studies have demonstrated continuing improvement through 9 weeks of therapy.

Dosing adjustment in renal impairment: Cl_{cr} <10 mL/minute: Administer every 12 hours

Hemodialysis: Extensively removed by hemodialysis and peritoneal dialysis (50% to 100%); administer dose posthemodialysis

Peritoneal dialysis: Dose as for Cl_{cr} <10 mL/minute

Continuous arteriovenous or venovenous hemofiltration: Administer usual dose

Dosing adjustment/comments in hepatic disease: Unchanged in mild liver disease; reduce dosage in severe liver disease

Dietary Considerations Take on an empty stomach. Drug may cause GI upset; if GI upset occurs, take with food.

Administration

Oral: May be taken with food to minimize stomach upset.

I.V.: Avoid contact between the drug and aluminum in the infusion set.

Topical: No disulfiram-like reactions have been reported after **topical** application, although metronidazole can be detected in the blood.

Test Interactions May interfere with AST, ALT, triglycerides, glucose, and LDH testing

Patient Information Urine may be discolored to a dark or reddish-brown; do not take alcohol for at least 24 hours after the last dose; avoid beverage alcohol or any topical products containing alcohol during therapy; may cause metallic taste; may be taken with food to minimize stomach upset; notify physician if numbness or tingling in extremities; avoid contact of the topical product with the eyes; cleanse areas to be treated well before application

Nursing Implications No disulfiram-like reactions have been reported after **topical** application, although metronidazole can be detected in the blood; avoid contact between the drug and aluminum in the infusion set

Additional Information Sodium content of 500 mg (I.V.): 322 mg (14 mEq)

Dosage Forms

Capsule: 375 mg

Cream, topical: 0.75% (45 g), 1% (30 g)

Gel, topical: 0.75% [7.5 mg/mL] (30 g)

Gel, vaginal: 0.75% (5 g applicator delivering 37.5 mg; 70 g tube)

Injection, ready-to-use: 5 mg/mL (100 mL)

Lotion, topical: 0.75%

Powder for injection, as hydrochloride: 500 mg

Tablet: 250 mg, 500 mg

Tablet, extended release: 750 mg

Extemporaneous Preparations To prepare metronidazole suspension 50 mg/mL, pulverize ten 250 mg tablets; levigate with a small amount of distilled water; add 10 mL Cologel® and levigate; add sufficient quantity of cherry syrup to total 50 mL and levigate until a uniform mixture is obtained; stable for 30 days if refrigerated

Committee on Extemporaneous Formulations, ASHP Special Interest Group (SIG) on Pediatric Pharmacy Practice, *Handbook on Extemporaneous Formulations*, 1987.

♦ **Metronidazole, Bismuth Subsalicylate, and Tetracycline** *see* Bismuth Subsalicylate, Metronidazole, and Tetracycline *on page 172*

♦ **Metronidazole Hydrochloride** *see* Metronidazole *on page 904*

♦ **Metronidazole, Tetracycline, and Bismuth Subsalicylate** *see* Bismuth Subsalicylate, Metronidazole, and Tetracycline *on page 172*

Metyrosine *(me TYE roe seen)*

U.S. Brand Names Demser®

Canadian Brand Names Demser®

Synonyms AMPT; OGMT

Therapeutic Category Tyrosine Hydroxylase Inhibitor

Use Short-term management of pheochromocytoma before surgery, long-term management when surgery is contraindicated or when chronic malignant pheochromocytoma exists

Pregnancy Risk Factor C

Usual Dosage Children >12 years and Adults: Oral: Initial: 250 mg 4 times/day, increased by 250-500 mg/day up to 4 g/day; maintenance: 2-3 g/day in 4 divided doses; for preoperative preparation, administer optimum effective dosage for 5-7 days

Dosing adjustment in renal impairment: Adjustment should be considered

Additional Information Complete prescribing information for this medication should be consulted for additional detail.

Dosage Forms Capsule: 250 mg

♦ **Mevacor®** *see* Lovastatin *on page 825*

♦ **Mevinolin** *see* Lovastatin *on page 825*

Mexiletine (MEKS i le teen)

Related Information
Antiarrhythmic Drugs Comparison *on page 1478*

U.S. Brand Names Mexitil®

Canadian Brand Names Mexitil®; Novo-Mexiletine

Therapeutic Category Antiarrhythmic Agent, Class I-B

Use Management of serious ventricular arrhythmias; suppression of PVCs

Unlabeled/Investigational Use Diabetic neuropathy

Pregnancy Risk Factor C

Contraindications Hypersensitivity to mexiletine or any component of the formulation; cardiogenic shock; second- or third-degree AV block (except in patients with a functioning artificial pacemaker)

Warnings/Precautions Exercise extreme caution in patients with pre-existing sinus node dysfunction; mexiletine can worsen CHF, bradycardias, and other arrhythmias; mexiletine, like other antiarrhythmic agents, is proarrhythmic; CAST study indicates a trend toward increased mortality with antiarrhythmics in the face of cardiac disease (myocardial infarction); leukopenia, agranulocytopenia, and thrombocytopenia; seizures; alterations in urinary pH may change urinary excretion; may cause acute hepatic injury; use caution in patients with significant hepatic dysfunction; electrolyte disturbances alter response; rare hepatic toxicity may occur; electrolyte abnormalities should be corrected before initiating therapy (can worsen CHF)

Adverse Reactions
>10%:
Central nervous system: Lightheadedness (11% to 25%), dizziness (20% to 25%), nervousness (5% to 10%), incoordination (10%)
Gastrointestinal: GI distress (41%), nausea/vomiting (40%)
Neuromuscular & skeletal: Trembling, unsteady gait, tremor (13%), ataxia (10% to 20%)
1% to 10%:
Cardiovascular: Chest pain (3% to 8%), premature ventricular contractions (1% to 2%), palpitations (4% to 8%), angina (2%), proarrhythmic (10% to 15% in patients with malignant arrhythmias)
Central nervous system: Confusion, headache, insomnia (5% to 7%), depression (2%)
Dermatologic: Rash (4%)
Gastrointestinal: Constipation or diarrhea (4% to 5%), xerostomia (3%), abdominal pain (1%)
Neuromuscular & skeletal: Weakness (5%), numbness of fingers or toes (2% to 4%), paresthesias (2%), arthralgias (1%)
Ocular: Blurred vision (5% to 7%), nystagmus (6%)
Otic: Tinnitus (2% to 3%)
Respiratory: Dyspnea (3%)
<1% (Limited to important or life-threatening): Agranulocytosis, alopecia, AV block, cardiogenic shock, congestive heart failure, dysphagia, exfoliative dermatitis, hallucinations, hepatic necrosis, hepatitis, hypotension, impotence, leukopenia, myelofibrosis, pancreatitis (rare), psychosis, pulmonary fibrosis, seizures, sinus arrest, SLE syndrome, Stevens-Johnson syndrome, syncope, thrombocytopenia, torsade de pointes, upper GI bleeding, urinary retention, urticaria

Overdosage/Toxicology Has a narrow therapeutic index and severe toxicity may occur slightly above the therapeutic range, especially with other antiarrhythmic drugs. Acute ingestion of twice the daily therapeutic dose is potentially life-threatening. Symptoms include sedation, confusion, coma, seizures, respiratory arrest, and cardiac toxicity (sinus arrest, A-V block, asystole, hypotension). The QRS and QT intervals are usually normal, although they may be prolonged after massive overdose. Other effects include dizziness, paresthesias, tremor, ataxia, and GI disturbance. Treatment is supportive, using conventional therapies (fluids, positioning, vasopressors, antiarrhythmics, anticonvulsants). Sodium bicarbonate may reverse QRS prolongation, bradyarrhythmias. and hypotension. Enhanced elimination with dialysis, hemoperfusion, or repeat charcoal is not effective.

Drug Interactions
Cytochrome P450 Effect: CYP2D6 enzyme substrate; CYP1A2 enzyme inhibitor
Increased Effect/Toxicity: Mexiletine and caffeine or theophylline may result in elevated levels of theophylline and caffeine. Quinidine, fluvoxamine, and urinary alkalinizers (antacids, sodium bicarbonate, acetazolamide) may increase mexiletine blood levels.
Decreased Effect: Decreased mexiletine plasma levels when used with phenobarbital, phenytoin, rifampin, cimetidine, or other hepatic enzyme inducers. Urinary acidifying agents may decrease mexiletine levels.

Ethanol/Nutrition/Herb Interactions Food: Food may decrease the rate, but not the extent of oral absorption; diets which affect urine pH can increase or decrease excretion of mexiletine. Avoid dietary changes that alter urine pH.

Mechanism of Action Class IB antiarrhythmic, structurally related to lidocaine, which inhibits inward sodium current, decreases rate of rise of phase 0, increases effective refractory period/action potential duration ratio

Pharmacodynamics/Kinetics
Absorption: Elderly have a slightly slower rate, but extent of absorption is the same as young adults
Distribution: V_d: 5-7 L/kg
Protein binding: 50% to 70%
Metabolism: Hepatic; low first-pass effect
Half-life elimination: Adults: 10-14 hours (average: 14.4 hours elderly, 12 hours in younger adults); increase in half-life with hepatic or heart failure
Time to peak: 2-3 hours
Excretion: Urine (10% to 15% as unchanged drug); urinary acidification increases excretion, alkalinization decreases excretion

Usual Dosage Adults: Oral: Initial: 200 mg every 8 hours (may load with 400 mg if necessary); adjust dose every 2-3 days; usual dose: 200-300 mg every 8 hours; maximum dose: 1.2 g/
(Continued)

Mexiletine *(Continued)*

day (some patients respond to every 12-hour dosing). When switching from another antiarrhythmic, initiate a 200 mg dose 6-12 hours after stopping former agents, 3-6 hours after
stopping procainamide.

Dosage adjustment in hepatic impairment: Reduce dose to 25% to 30% of usual dose

Administration Administer around-the-clock rather than 3 times/day to promote less variation
in peak and trough serum levels; administer with food

Reference Range Therapeutic range: 0.5-2 µg/mL; potentially toxic: >2 µg/mL

Test Interactions Abnormal liver function test, positive ANA, thrombocytopenia

Patient Information Take with food or antacid; notify physician of severe or persistent
abdominal pain, nausea, vomiting, yellowing of eyes or skin, pale stools, dark urine, or if
persistent fever, sore throat, bleeding, or bruising occurs

Nursing Implications Administer around-the-clock rather than 3 times/day to promote less
variation in peak and trough serum levels

Dosage Forms Capsule: 150 mg, 200 mg, 250 mg

♦ **Mexitil**® *see Mexiletine on page 907*
♦ **Miacalcin**® *see Calcitonin on page 204*
♦ **Miacalcin**® **NS (Can)** *see Calcitonin on page 204*
♦ **Micanol**® *see Anthralin on page 100*
♦ **Micardis**® *see Telmisartan on page 1290*
♦ **Micardis**® **HCT** *see Telmisartan and Hydrochlorothiazide on page 1291*
♦ **Micatin**® **[OTC]** *see Miconazole on page 908*

Miconazole *(mi KON a zole)*

Related Information
Antifungal Agents Comparison *on page 1484*
Treatment of Sexually Transmitted Diseases *on page 1609*

U.S. Brand Names Aloe Vesta® 2-n-1 Antifungal [OTC]; Baza® Antifungal [OTC]; Carrington
Antifungal [OTC]; Fungoid® Tincture [OTC]; Lotrimin® AF Powder/Spray [OTC]; Micatin®
[OTC]; Micro-Guard® [OTC]; Mitrazol® [OTC]; Monistat® 1 Combination Pack [OTC];
Monistat® 3 [OTC]; Monistat® 7 [OTC]; Monistat-Derm®; Zeasorb®-AF [OTC]

Canadian Brand Names Micatin®; Micozole; Monazole-7; Monistat®

Synonyms Miconazole Nitrate

Therapeutic Category Antifungal Agent, Imidazole Derivative; Antifungal Agent, Systemic;
Antifungal Agent, Topical; Antifungal Agent, Vaginal

Use Treatment of vulvovaginal candidiasis and a variety of skin and mucous membrane fungal
infections

Pregnancy Risk Factor C

Contraindications Hypersensitivity to miconazole or any component of the formulation

Warnings/Precautions For external use only; discontinue if sensitivity or irritation develop.
Petrolatum-based vaginal products may damage rubber or latex condoms or diaphragms.
Separate use by 3 days.

Adverse Reactions Frequency not defined.
Topical: Allergic contact dermatitis, burning, maceration
Vaginal: Abdominal cramps, burning, irritation, itching

Drug Interactions
Cytochrome P450 Effect: CYP3A3/4 enzyme substrate; CYP2C9 enzyme inhibitor,
CYP3A3/4 enzyme inhibitor

Increased Effect/Toxicity: Note: The majority of reported drug interactions were observed
following intravenous miconazole administration. Although systemic absorption following
topical and/or vaginal administration is low, potential interactions due to CYP isoenzyme
inhibition may occur (rarely). This may be particularly true in situations where topical
absorption may be increased (ie, inflamed tissue).
Miconazole coadministered with warfarin has increased the anticoagulant effect of warfarin
(including reports associated with vaginal miconazole therapy of as little as 3 days).
Phenytoin levels may be increased. Miconazole may inhibit the metabolism of oral
sulfonylureas. Concurrent administration of cisapride is contraindicated due to an
increased risk of cardiotoxicity.

Decreased Effect: Amphotericin B may decrease antifungal effect of both agents.

Ethanol/Nutrition/Herb Interactions Herb/Nutraceutical: St John's wort may decrease
miconazole levels.

Mechanism of Action Inhibits biosynthesis of ergosterol, damaging the fungal cell wall
membrane, which increases permeability causing leaking of nutrients

Pharmacodynamics/Kinetics
Absorption: Topical: Negligible
Distribution: Widely to body tissues; penetrates well into inflamed joints, vitreous humor of
eye, and peritoneal cavity, but poorly into saliva and sputum; crosses blood-brain barrier
but only to a small extent
Protein binding: 91% to 93%
Metabolism: Hepatic
Half-life elimination: Multiphasic: Initial: 40 minutes; Secondary: 126 minutes; Terminal: 24
hours
Excretion: Feces (~50%); urine (<1% as unchanged drug)

Usual Dosage
Topical: Children and Adults: **Note:** Not for OTC use in children <2 years:
Tinea pedis and tinea corporis: Apply twice daily for 4 weeks
Tinea cruris: Apply twice daily for 2 weeks
Vaginal: Adults: Vulvovaginal candidiasis:
Cream, 2%: Insert 1 applicatorful at bedtime for 7 days
Cream, 4%: Insert 1 applicatorful at bedtime for 3 days
Suppository, 100 mg: Insert 1 suppository at bedtime for 7 days

Suppository, 200 mg: Insert 1 suppository at bedtime for 3 days

Suppository, 1200 mg: Insert 1 suppository at bedtime (a one-time dose)

Note: Many products are available as a combination pack, with a suppository for vaginal instillation and cream to relieve external symptoms.

Patient Information Take full course of therapy as directed; do not discontinue without consulting prescriber. Some infections may require long periods of therapy. Practice good hygiene measures to prevent reinfection.

Topical: Wash and dry area before applying medication; apply thinly. Do not get in or near eyes.

Vaginal: Insert high in vagina. Refrain from intercourse during treatment. OTC products, even if administered topically, may not mix well with certain prescription medications (which may lead to drug interactions). Consult with your prescriber.

If you are diabetic you should test serum glucose regularly at the same time of day. You may experience nausea and vomiting (small, frequent meals may help) or headache, dizziness (use caution when driving). Report unresolved headache, rash, burning, itching, anorexia, unusual fatigue, diarrhea, nausea, or vomiting.

Dosage Forms

Combination products:

Monistat® 1 Combination Pack: Miconazole nitrate vaginal insert 1200 mg (1) and micona-zole external cream 2% (5 g) [Note: Do not confuse with 1-Day™ (formerly Monistat® 1) which contains tioconazole]

Monistat® 3 Combination Pack: Miconazole nitrate vaginal suppository 200 mg (3s) and miconazole nitrate external cream 2%

Monistat® 3 Cream Combination Pack: Miconazole nitrate vaginal cream 4% and micona-zole nitrate external cream 2%

Monistat® 7 Combination Pack: Miconazole nitrate vaginal suppository 100 mg (7s) and miconazole nitrate external cream (2%)

Cream, topical, as nitrate:

Baza® Antifungal: 2% (4 g, 57 g, 142 g) [zinc oxide based formula]

Carrington Antifungal: 2% (150 g)

Micatin® [OTC], Monistat-Derm® [Rx]: 2% (15 g, 30g)

Micro-Guard®: 2% (60 g)

Triple Care Antifungal: 2% (60 g, 98 g)

Cream, vaginal, as nitrate [available in prefilled applicators or single refillable applicator]:

Monistat® 3: 4% (15 g, 25g)

Monistat® 7: 2% (45 g)

Liquid spray, topical, as nitrate (Micatin®): 2% (90 mL, 105 mL)

Lotion powder, topical, as nitrate (Zeasorb®-AF): 2% (60 g)

Ointment, topical, as nitrate: (Aloe Vesta® 2-n-1 Antifungal): 2% (60 g, 150 g)

Powder, topical, as nitrate:

Lotrimin® AF, Micatin®, Micro-Guard®: 2% (90 g)

Zeasorb®-AF: 2% (70 g)

Powder spray, topical, as nitrate (Lotrimin® AF): 2% (100 g)

Suppository, vaginal, as nitrate:

Monistat® 3: 200 mg (3s)

Monistat® 7: 100 mg (7s)

Tincture, topical, as nitrate (Fungoid®): 2% (30 mL, 473 mL)

♦ **Miconazole Nitrate** *see* Miconazole *on page 908*

♦ **Micozole (Can)** *see* Miconazole *on page 908*

♦ **MICRhoGAM**™ *see* Rh₀(D) Immune Globulin (Intramuscular) *on page 1187*

Microfibrillar Collagen Hemostat (mye kro FI bri lar KOL la jen HEE moe stat)

U.S. Brand Names Avitene®; Helistat®; Hemotene®

Synonyms Collagen; MCH

Therapeutic Category Hemostatic Agent

Use Adjunct to hemostasis when control of bleeding by ligature is ineffective or impractical

Pregnancy Risk Factor C

Usual Dosage Apply dry directly to source of bleeding

Additional Information Complete prescribing information for this medication should be consulted for additional detail.

Dosage Forms

Fibrous: 1 g

Nonwoven web: 2.5 cm x 5 cm; 5 cm x 8 cm; 8 cm x 10 cm; 35 mm x 35 mm x 1 mm; 70 mm x 70 mm x 1 mm; 70 mm x 35 mm x 1 mm

♦ **Microgestin**™ **Fe** *see* Ethinyl Estradiol and Norethindrone *on page 522*

♦ **Micro-Guard® [OTC]** *see* Miconazole *on page 908*

♦ **Micro-K® 10 Extencaps®** *see* Potassium Chloride *on page 1108*

♦ **Micro-K® Extencaps** *see* Potassium Chloride *on page 1108*

♦ **Micro-K® LS** *see* Potassium Chloride *on page 1108*

♦ **Micronase®** *see* GlyBURIDE *on page 635*

♦ **Microzide**™ *see* Hydrochlorothiazide *on page 674*

♦ **Midamor®** *see* Amiloride *on page 69*

Midazolam (MID aye zoe lam)

Related Information

Adult ACLS Algorithms *on page 1632*

Antacid Drug Interactions *on page 1477*

Benzodiazepines Comparison *on page 1490*

U.S. Brand Names Versed®

Canadian Brand Names Versed®

(Continued)

Midazolam *(Continued)*

Synonyms Midazolam Hydrochloride

Therapeutic Category Benzodiazepine; Hypnotic; Sedative

Use Preoperative sedation and provides conscious sedation prior to diagnostic or radiographic procedures; ICU sedation (continuous infusion); intravenous anesthesia (induction); intravenous anesthesia (maintenance)

Unlabeled/Investigational Use Anxiety, status epilepticus

Restrictions C-IV

Pregnancy Risk Factor D

Pregnancy/Breast-Feeding Implications Midazolam has been found to cross the placenta; not recommended for use during pregnancy

Contraindications Hypersensitivity to midazolam or any component of the formulation, including benzyl alcohol (cross-sensitivity with other benzodiazepines may exist); parenteral form is not for intrathecal or epidural injection; narrow-angle glaucoma; pregnancy

Warnings/Precautions May cause severe respiratory depression, respiratory arrest, or apnea. Use with extreme caution, particularly in noncritical care settings. Appropriate resuscitative equipment and qualified personnel must be available for administration and monitoring. Initial dosing must be cautiously titrated and individualized, particularly in elderly or debilitated patients, patients with hepatic impairment (including alcoholics), or in renal impairment, particularly if other CNS depressants (including opiates) are used concurrently. Initial doses in elderly or debilitated patients should not exceed 2.5 mg. Use with caution in patients with respiratory disease or impaired gag reflex. Use during upper airway procedures may increase risk of hypoventilation. Prolonged responses have been noted following extended administration by continuous infusion (possibly due to metabolite accumulation) or in the presence of drugs which inhibit midazolam metabolism.

May cause hypotension - hemodynamic events are more common in pediatric patients or patients with hemodynamic instability. Hypotension and/or respiratory depression may occur more frequently in patients who have received narcotic analgesics. Use with caution in obese patients, chronic renal failure, and CHF. Parenteral form contains benzyl alcohol - avoid rapid injection in neonates or prolonged infusions. Does not protect against increases in heart rate or blood pressure during intubation. Should not be used in shock, coma, or acute alcohol intoxication. Avoid intra-arterial administration or extravasation of parenteral formulation.

Causes CNS depression (dose-related) resulting in sedation, dizziness, confusion, or ataxia which may impair physical and mental capabilities. Patients must be cautioned about performing tasks which require mental alertness (ie, operating machinery or driving). A minimum of 1 day should elapse after midazolam administration before attempting these tasks. Use with caution in patients receiving other CNS depressants or psychoactive agents. Effects with other sedative drugs or ethanol may be potentiated. Benzodiazepines have been associated with falls and traumatic injury and should be used with extreme caution in patients who are at risk of these events (especially the elderly).

Midazolam causes anterograde amnesia. Paradoxical reactions, including hyperactive or aggressive behavior have been reported with benzodiazepines, particularly in adolescent/pediatric or psychiatric patients. Does not have analgesic, antidepressant, or antipsychotic properties.

Benzodiazepines have been associated with dependence and acute withdrawal symptoms on discontinuation or reduction in dose. Acute withdrawal, including seizures, may be precipitated after administration of flumazenil to patients receiving long-term benzodiazepine therapy.

Adverse Reactions As reported in adults unless otherwise noted:

>10%: Respiratory: Decreased tidal volume and/or respiratory rate decrease, apnea (3% children)

1% to 10%:

Cardiovascular: Hypotension (3% children)

Central nervous system: Drowsiness (1%), oversedation, headache (1%), seizure-like activity (1% children)

Gastrointestinal: Nausea (3%), vomiting (3%)

Local: Pain and local reactions at injection site (4% I.M., 5% I.V.; severity less than diazepam)

Ocular: Nystagmus (1% children)

Respiratory: Cough (1%)

Miscellaneous: Physical and psychological dependence with prolonged use, hiccups (4%, 1% children), paradoxical reaction (2% children)

<1% (Limited to important or life-threatening): Agitation, amnesia, bigeminy, bronchospasm, emergence delirium, euphoria, hallucinations, laryngospasm, rash

Overdosage/Toxicology Symptoms include respiratory depression, hypotension, coma, stupor, confusion, and apnea. Treatment for benzodiazepine overdose is supportive. Rarely is mechanical ventilation required. Flumazenil has been shown to selectively block the binding of benzodiazepines to CNS receptors, resulting in a reversal of benzodiazepine-induced CNS depression. Respiratory reaction to hypoxia may not be restored.

Drug Interactions

Cytochrome P450 Effect: CYP3A3/4 enzyme substrate

Increased Effect/Toxicity: Midazolam levels/effects may be increased by inhibitors of CYP3A3/4, including delavirdine, indinavir, saquinavir, quinupristin-dalfopristin, zafirlukast, zileuton, verapamil, troleandomycin, miconazole, itraconazole, nifedipine, grapefruit juice, diltiazem, fluconazole, ketoconazole, clarithromycin, and erythromycin. Use is contraindicated with amprenavir and ritonavir. **If narcotics or other CNS depressants are administered concomitantly, the midazolam dose should be reduced by 30% if <65 years of age, or by at least 50% if >65 years of age.**

Decreased Effect: Carbamazepine, phenytoin, and rifampin may reduce the effects of midazolam.

Ethanol/Nutrition/Herb Interactions
Ethanol: Avoid ethanol (may increase CNS depression).

Food: Grapefruit juice may increase serum concentrations of midazolam; avoid concurrent use with oral form.

Herb/Nutraceutical: Avoid concurrent use with St John's wort (may decrease midazolam levels, may increase CNS depression). Avoid concurrent use with valerian, kava kava, gotu kola (may increase CNS depression).

Stability Stable for 24 hours at room temperature/refrigeration; at a final concentration of 0.5 mg/mL, stable for up to 24 hours when diluted with D_5W or NS, or for up to 4 hours when diluted with lactated Ringer's; admixtures do not require protection from light for short-term storage

Mechanism of Action Binds to stereospecific benzodiazepine receptors on the postsynaptic GABA neuron at several sites within the central nervous system, including the limbic system, reticular formation. Enhancement of the inhibitory effect of GABA on neuronal excitability results by increased neuronal membrane permeability to chloride ions. This shift in chloride ions results in hyperpolarization (a less excitable state) and stabilization.

Pharmacodynamics/Kinetics
Onset of action: I.M.: Sedation: ~15 minutes; I.V.: 1-5 minutes

Peak effect: I.M.: 0.5-1 hour

Duration: I.M.: Up to 6 hours; Mean: 2 hours

Absorption: Oral: Rapid

Distribution: V_d: 0.8-2.5 L/kg; increased with congestive heart failure (CHF) and chronic renal failure

Protein binding: 95%

Metabolism: Extensively hepatic; CYP3A3/4 substrate

Bioavailability: Mean: 45%

Half-life elimination: 1-4 hours, increased with cirrhosis, CHF, obesity, elderly

Excretion: Urine (as glucuronide conjugated metabolites); feces (~2% to 10%)

Usual Dosage The dose of midazolam needs to be individualized based on the patient's age, underlying diseases, and concurrent medications. Decrease dose (by ~30%) if narcotics or other CNS depressants are administered concomitantly. **Personnel and equipment needed for standard respiratory resuscitation should be immediately available during midazolam administration.**

Children <6 years may require higher doses and closer monitoring than older children; calculate dose on ideal body weight

Conscious sedation for procedures or preoperative sedation:
Oral: 0.25-0.5 mg/kg as a single dose preprocedure, up to a maximum of 20 mg; administer 30-45 minutes prior to procedure. Children <6 years or less cooperative patients may require as much as 1 mg/kg as a single dose; 0.25 mg/kg may suffice for children 6-16 years of age.

Intranasal (not an approved route): 0.2 mg/kg (up to 0.4 mg/kg in some studies), to a maximum of 15 mg; may be administered 30-45 minutes prior to procedure

I.M.: 0.1-0.15 mg/kg 30-60 minutes before surgery or procedure; range 0.05-0.15 mg/kg; doses up to 0.5 mg/kg have been used in more anxious patients; maximum total dose: 10 mg

I.V.:
Infants <6 months: Limited information is available in nonintubated infants; dosing recommendations not clear; infants <6 months are at higher risk for airway obstruction and hypoventilation; titrate dose in small increments to desired effect; monitor carefully

Infants 6 months to Children 5 years: Initial: 0.05-0.1 mg/kg; titrate dose carefully; total dose of 0.6 mg/kg may be required; usual maximum total dose: 6 mg

Children 6-12 years: Initial: 0.025-0.05 mg/kg; titrate dose carefully; total doses of 0.4 mg/kg may be required; usual maximum total dose: 10 mg

Children 12-16 years: Dose as adults; usual maximum total dose: 10 mg

Conscious sedation during mechanical ventilation: Children: Loading dose: 0.05-0.2 mg/kg, followed by initial continuous infusion: 0.06-0.12 mg/kg/hour (1-2 mcg/kg/minute); titrate to the desired effect; usual range: 0.4-6 mcg/kg/minute

Status epilepticus refractory to standard therapy (unlabeled use): Infants >2 months and Children: Loading dose: 0.15 mg/kg followed by a continuous infusion of 1 mcg/kg/minute; titrate dose upward very 5 minutes until clinical seizure activity is controlled; mean infusion rate required in 24 children was 2.3 mcg/kg/minute with a range of 1-18 mcg/kg/minute

Adults:
Preoperative sedation:
I.M.: 0.07-0.08 mg/kg 30-60 minutes prior to surgery/procedure; usual dose: 5 mg; **Note:** Reduce dose in patients with COPD, high-risk patients, patients ≥60 years of age, and patients receiving other narcotics or CNS depressants

I.V.: 0.02-0.04 mg/kg; repeat every 5 minutes as needed to desired effect or up to 0.1-0.2 mg/kg

Intranasal (not an approved route): 0.2 mg/kg (up to 0.4 mg/kg in some studies); administer 30-45 minutes prior to surgery/procedure

Conscious sedation: I.V.: Initial: 0.5-2 mg slow I.V. over at least 2 minutes; slowly titrate to effect by repeating doses every 2-3 minutes if needed; usual total dose: 2.5-5 mg; use decreased doses in elderly

Healthy Adults <60 years: Some patients respond to doses as low as 1 mg; no more than 2.5 mg should be administered over a period of 2 minutes. Additional doses of midazolam may be administered after a 2-minute waiting period and evaluation of sedation after each dose increment. A total dose >5 mg is generally not needed. If narcotics or other CNS depressants are administered concomitantly, the midazolam dose should be reduced by 30%.

Anesthesia: I.V.:
Induction:
Unpremedicated patients: 0.3-0.35 mg/kg (up to 0.6 mg/kg in resistant cases)
Premedicated patients: 0.15-0.35 mg/kg

(Continued)

911

Midazolam *(Continued)*

Maintenance: 0.05-0.3 mg/kg as needed, or continuous infusion 0.25-1.5 mcg/kg/minute

Sedation in mechanically-ventilated patients: I.V. continuous infusion: 100 mg in 250 mL D₅W or NS (if patient is fluid-restricted, may concentrate up to a maximum of 0.5 mg/mL); initial dose: 0.01-0.05 mg/kg (~0.5-4 mg for a typical adult) initially and either repeated at 10-15 minute intervals until adequate sedation is achieved or continuous infusion rates of 0.02-0.1 mg/kg/hour (1-7 mg/hour) and titrate to reach desired level of sedation

Elderly: I.V.: Conscious sedation: Initial: 0.5 mg slow I.V.; give no more than 1.5 mg in a 2-minute period; if additional titration is needed, give no more than 1 mg over 2 minutes, waiting another 2 or more minutes to evaluate sedative effect; a total dose of >3.5 mg is rarely necessary

Dosage adjustment in renal impairment:

Hemodialysis: Supplemental dose is not necessary

Peritoneal dialysis: Significant drug removal is unlikely based on physiochemical characteristics

Dietary Considerations Sodium content of 1 mL: 0.14 mEq

Administration

Intranasal: Administer using a 1 mL needleless syringe into the nares over 15 seconds; use the 5 mg/mL injection; ½ of the dose may be administered to each nare

Oral: Do not mix with any liquid (such as grapefruit juice) prior to administration

Parenteral:

I.M.: Administer deep I.M. into large muscle.

I.V.: Administer by slow I.V. injection over at least 2-5 minutes at a concentration of 1-5 mg/mL or by I.V. infusion. Continuous infusions should be administered via an infusion pump.

Monitoring Parameters Respiratory and cardiovascular status, blood pressure, blood pressure monitor required during I.V. administration

Nursing Implications Midazolam is a short-acting benzodiazepine; recovery occurs within 2 hours in most patients, however, may require up to 6 hours in some cases

Additional Information Abrupt discontinuation after sustained use (generally >10 days) may cause withdrawal symptoms. For neonates, since both concentrations of the injection contain 1% benzyl alcohol, use the 5 mg/mL injection and dilute to 0.5 mg/mL with SWI without preservatives to decrease the amount of benzyl alcohol delivered to the neonate; with continuous infusion, midazolam may accumulate in peripheral tissues; use lowest effective infusion rate to reduce accumulation effects; midazolam is 3-4 times as potent as diazepam; paradoxical reactions associated with midazolam use in children (eg, agitation, restlessness, combativeness) have been successfully treated with flumazenil (see Massanari, 1997).

Dosage Forms

Injection, as hydrochloride: 1 mg/mL (2 mL, 5 mL, 10 mL); 5 mg/mL (1 mL, 2 mL, 5 mL, 10 mL)

Syrup, as hydrochloride: 2 mg/mL (118 mL)

♦ **Midazolam Hydrochloride** *see Midazolam on page 909*

Midodrine *(MI doe dreen)*

U.S. Brand Names ProAmatine®

Canadian Brand Names Amatine®

Synonyms Midodrine Hydrochloride

Therapeutic Category Alpha-Adrenergic Agonist

Use Orphan drug: Treatment of symptomatic orthostatic hypotension

Unlabeled/Investigational Use Investigational: Management of urinary incontinence

Pregnancy Risk Factor C

Pregnancy/Breast-Feeding Implications Clinical effects on the fetus: No studies are available; use during pregnancy and lactation should be avoided unless the potential benefit outweighs the risk to the fetus

Contraindications Hypersensitivity to midodrine or any component of the formulation; severe organic heart disease; urinary retention; pheochromocytoma; thyrotoxicosis; persistent and significant supine hypertension; concurrent use of fludrocortisone

Warnings/Precautions Only indicated for patients for whom orthostatic hypotension significantly impairs their daily life. Use is not recommended with supine hypertension and caution should be exercised in patients with diabetes, visual problems, urinary retention (reduce initial dose) or hepatic dysfunction; monitor renal and hepatic function prior to and periodically during therapy; safety and efficacy has not been established in children; discontinue and re-evaluate therapy if signs of bradycardia occur.

Adverse Reactions

>10%:

Dermatologic: Piloerection (13%), pruritus (12%)

Genitourinary: Urinary urgency, retention, or polyuria, dysuria (up to 13%)

Neuromuscular & skeletal: Paresthesia (18.3%)

1% to 10%:

Cardiovascular: Supine hypertension (7%), facial flushing

Central nervous system: Confusion, anxiety, dizziness, chills (5%)

Dermatologic: Rash, dry skin (2%)

Gastrointestinal: Xerostomia, nausea, abdominal pain

Neuromuscular & skeletal: Pain (5%)

<1% (Limited to important or life-threatening): Headache, insomnia

Overdosage/Toxicology Symptoms include hypertension, piloerection, and urinary retention. Treatment is symptomatic following gastric decontamination. Alpha-sympatholytics and/or dialysis may be helpful.

Drug Interactions

Increased Effect/Toxicity: Concomitant fludrocortisone results in hypernatremia or an increase in intraocular pressure and glaucoma. Bradycardia may be accentuated with concomitant administration of cardiac glycosides, psychotherapeutics, and beta-blockers. Alpha agonists may increase the pressure effects and alpha antagonists may negate the effects of midodrine.

Mechanism of Action Midodrine forms an active metabolite, desglymidodrine, that is an alpha$_1$-agonist. This agent increases arteriolar and venous tone resulting in a rise in standing, sitting, and supine systolic and diastolic blood pressure in patients with orthostatic hypotension. See table.

Causes of Orthostatic Hypotension

Primary Autonomic Causes
Pure autonomic failure (Bradbury-Eggleston syndrome, idiopathic orthostatic hypotension)
Autonomic failure with multiple system atrophy (Shy-Drager syndrome)
Familial dysautonomia (Riley-Day syndrome)
Dopamine beta-hydroxylase deficiency
Secondary Autonomic Causes
Chronic alcoholism
Parkinson's disease
Diabetes mellitus
Porphyria
Amyloidosis
Various carcinomas
Vitamin B$_1$ or B$_{12}$ deficiency
Nonautonomic Causes
Hypovolemia (such as associated with hemorrhage, burns, or hemodialysis) and dehydration
Diminished homeostatic regulation (such as associated with aging, pregnancy, fever, or prolonged best rest)
Medications (eg, antihypertensives, insulin, tricyclic antidepressants)

Pharmacodynamics/Kinetics
Onset of action: ~1 hour
Duration: 2-3 hours
Absorption: Rapid
Distribution: V_d (desglymidodrine): <1.6 L/kg; poorly across membrane (eg, blood brain barrier)
Protein binding: Minimal
Metabolism: Rapid deglycination to desglymidodrine occurs in many tissues and plasma; hepatic
Bioavailability: Absolute, 93%
Half-life elimination: ~3-4 hours (active drug); 25 minutes (prodrug)
Time to peak, serum: Active drug: 1-2 hours; Prodrug: 30 minutes
Excretion: Urine (2% to 4%)
Clearance: Desglymidodrine: 385 mL/minute (predominantly by renal secretion)

Usual Dosage Adults: Oral: 10 mg 3 times/day during daytime hours (every 3-4 hours) when patient is upright (maximum: 40 mg/day)

Dosing adjustment in renal impairment: 2.5 mg 3 times/day, gradually increasing as tolerated

Monitoring Parameters Blood pressure, renal and hepatic parameters

Patient Information Use caution with over-the-counter medications which may affect blood pressure (cough and cold, diet, stay-awake medications); avoid taking a particular dose if you are to be supine for any length of time; take your last daily dose 3-4 hours before bedtime to minimize nighttime supine hypertension

Nursing Implications Doses may be given in approximately 3- to 4-hour intervals (eg, shortly before or upon rising in the morning, at midday, in the late afternoon not later than 6 PM); avoid dosing after the evening meal or within 4 hours of bedtime; continue therapy only in patients who appear to attain symptomatic improvement during initial treatment; standing systolic blood pressure may be elevated 15-30 mm Hg at 1 hour after a 10 mg dose; some effect may persist for 2-3 hours

Dosage Forms Tablet, as hydrochloride: 2.5 mg, 5 mg

◆ **Midodrine Hydrochloride** *see* Midodrine *on page 912*

◆ **Midol® IB [OTC]** *see* Ibuprofen *on page 697*

◆ **Midrin®** *see* Acetaminophen, Isometheptene, and Dichloralphenazone *on page 28*

◆ **Mifeprex™** *see* Mifepristone *on page 913*

Mifepristone (mi FE pris tone)

U.S. Brand Names Mifeprex™

Synonyms RU-486; RU-38486

Therapeutic Category Abortifacient; Antineoplastic Agent; Hormone Antagonist; Antiprogestin

Use Medical termination of intrauterine pregnancy, through day 49 of pregnancy. Patients may need treatment with misoprostol and possibly surgery to complete therapy

Unlabeled/Investigational Use Treatment of unresectable meningioma; has been studied in the treatment of breast cancer, ovarian cancer, and adrenal cortical carcinoma

Restrictions There are currently no clinical trials with mifepristone in oncology open in the U.S.; investigators wishing to obtain the agent for use in oncology patients must apply for a patient-specific IND from the FDA. Mifepristone will be supplied only to licensed physicians (Continued)

Mifepristone *(Continued)*

who sign and return a "Prescriber's Agreement." Distribution of mifepristone will be subject to specific requirements imposed by the distributor. Mifepristone will **not** be available to the public through licensed pharmacies.

Pregnancy Risk Factor X

Pregnancy/Breast-Feeding Implications This medication is used to terminate pregnancy; there are no approved treatment indications for its use during pregnancy. Prostaglandins (including mifepristone and misoprostol) may have teratogenic effects when used during pregnancy. It is unknown if mifepristone is excreted in human milk; breast-feeding is not recommended. Breast milk should be discarded for a few days following use of this medication.

Contraindications Hypersensitivity to mifepristone, misoprostol, other prostaglandins, or any component of the formulation; chronic adrenal failure; porphyrias; hemorrhagic disorder or concurrent anticoagulant therapy; pregnancy termination >49 days; intrauterine device (IUD) in place; ectopic pregnancy or undiagnosed adnexal mass; concurrent long-term corticosteroid therapy; inadequate or lack of access to emergency medical services; inability to understand effects and/or comply with treatment

Warnings/Precautions Patient must be instructed of the treatment procedure and expected effects. A signed agreement form must be kept in the patient's file. Physicians may obtain patient agreement forms, physician enrollment forms, and medical consultation directly from Danco Laboratories at 1-877-432-7596. Adverse effects (including blood transfusions, hospitalization, ongoing pregnancy, and other major complications) must be reported in writing to the medication distributor. To be administered only by physicians who can date pregnancy, diagnose ectopic pregnancies, provide access to surgical abortion (if needed), and can provide access to emergency care. Medication will be distributed directly to these physicians following signed agreement with the distributor. Must be administered under supervision by the qualified physician. Pregnancy is dated from day 1 of last menstrual period (presuming a 28-day cycle, ovulation occurring mid-cycle). Pregnancy duration can be determined using menstrual history and clinical examination. Ultrasound should be used if an ectopic pregnancy is suspected or if duration of pregnancy is uncertain. Bleeding occurs and should be expected (average 9-16 days, may be ≥30 days). Bleeding may require blood transfusion (rare), curettage, saline infusions, and/or vasoconstrictors. Use caution in patients with severe anemia. Confirmation of pregnancy termination by clinical exam or ultrasound must be made 14 days following treatment. Manufacturer recommends surgical termination of pregnancy when medical termination fails or is not completed. Prescriber should determine in advance whether they will provide such care themselves or through other providers. Preventative measures to prevent rhesus immunization must be taken prior to surgical abortion. Prescriber should also give the patient clear instructions on whom to call and what to do in the event of an emergency following administration of mifepristone.

Safety and efficacy have not been established for use in women with chronic cardiovascular, hypertensive, respiratory, or renal disease, diabetes mellitus, severe anemia, or heavy smokers. Women >35 years of age and smokers (>10 cigarettes/day) were excluded from clinical trials. Safety and efficacy in pediatric patients have not been established.

Adverse Reactions Vaginal bleeding and uterine cramping are expected to occur when this medication is used to terminate a pregnancy; 90% of women using this medication for this purpose also report adverse reactions

>10%:
  Central nervous system: Headache (2% to 31%), dizziness (1% to 12%)
  Gastrointestinal: Abdominal pain (cramping) (96%), nausea (43% to 61%), vomiting (18% to 26%), diarrhea (12% to 20%)
  Genitourinary: Uterine cramping (83%)
1% to 10%:
  Cardiovascular: Syncope (1%)
  Central nervous system: Fatigue (10%), fever (4%), insomnia (3%), anxiety (2%), fainting (2%)
  Gastrointestinal: Dyspepsia (3%)
  Genitourinary: Uterine hemorrhage (5%), vaginitis (3%), pelvic pain (2%)
  Hematologic: Decreased hemoglobin >2 g/dL (6%), anemia (2%), leukorrhea (2%)
  Neuromuscular & skeletal: Back pain (9%), rigors (3%), leg pain (2%), weakness (2%)
  Respiratory: Sinusitis (2%)
  Miscellaneous: Viral infection (4%)
<1% (Limited to important or life-threatening): Significant elevations of hepatic enzymes (rare)

In trials for unresectable meningioma, the most common adverse effects included fatigue, hot flashes, gynecomastia or breast tenderness, hair thinning, and rash. In premenopausal women, vaginal bleeding may be seen shortly after beginning therapy and cessation of menses is common. Thyroiditis and effects related to antiglucocorticoid activity have also been noted.

Overdosage/Toxicology In studies using 3 times the recommended dose for termination of pregnancy, no serious maternal adverse effects were reported. This medication is supplied in single-dose containers to be given under physician supervision, therefore, the risk of overdose should be low. In case of massive ingestion, treat symptomatically and monitor for signs of adrenal failure.

Drug Interactions
  Cytochrome P450 Effect: CYP3A3/4 enzyme substrate; CYP3A3/4 enzyme inhibitor
  Increased Effect/Toxicity:
    There are no reported interactions. It might be anticipated that the effects of one or both agents would be minimized if mifepristone were administered concurrently with a progestin (exogenous). During concurrent use of CYP3A3/4 inhibitors, serum level and/or toxicity of mifepristone may be increased; inhibitors include amiodarone, cimetidine, clarithromycin, erythromycin, delavirdine, diltiazem, dirithromycin, disulfiram, fluoxetine, fluvoxamine, grapefruit juice, indinavir, itraconazole, ketoconazole, nefazodone,

nevirapine, propoxyphene, quinupristin-dalfopristin, ritonavir, saquinavir, verapamil, zafirlukast, zileuton; monitor for altered response

Decreased Effect: Enzyme inducers may increase the metabolism of mifepristone resulting in decreased effect; includes carbamazepine, dexamethasone, phenobarbital, phenytoin, and rifampin. St John's wort may induce mifepristone metabolism, leading to decreased levels.

Ethanol/Nutrition/Herb Interactions

Food: Do not take with grapefruit juice; grapefruit juice may inhibit mifepristone metabolism leading to increased levels.

Herb/Nutraceutical: Avoid St John's wort (may induce mifepristone metabolism, leading to decreased levels).

Stability Store at room temperature, 25°C (77°F)

Mechanism of Action Mifepristone, a synthetic steroid, competitively binds to the intracellular progesterone receptor, blocking the effects of progesterone. When used for the termination of pregnancy, this leads to contraction-inducing activity in the myometrium. In the absence of progesterone, mifepristone acts as a partial progesterone agonist. Mifepristone also has weak antiglucocorticoid and antiandrogenic properties; it blocks the feedback effect of cortisol on corticotropin secretion.

Pharmacodynamics/Kinetics

Protein binding: 98% to albumin and α_1-acid glycoprotein

Metabolism: Hepatic via CYP450 3A4 to three metabolites (may possess some antiprogestin and antiglucocorticoid activity)

Bioavailability: 69%

Half-life elimination: Terminal: 18 hours following a slower phase where 50% eliminated between 12-72 hours

Time to peak: 90 minutes

Excretion: Feces (83%); urine (9%)

Usual Dosage Oral:

Adults: Termination of pregnancy: Treatment consists of three office visits by the patient; the patient must read medication guide and sign patient agreement prior to treatment:

Day 1: 600 mg (three 200 mg tablets) taken as a single dose under physician supervision

Day 3: Patient must return to the healthcare provider 2 days following administration of mifepristone; if termination of pregnancy cannot be confirmed using ultrasound or clinical examination: 400 mcg (two 200 mcg tablets) of misoprostol; patient may need treatment for cramps or gastrointestinal symptoms at this time

Day 14: Patient must return to the healthcare provider ~14 days after administration of mifepristone; confirm complete termination of pregnancy by ultrasound or clinical exam. Surgical termination is recommended to manage treatment failures.

Elderly: Safety and efficacy have not been established

Dosage adjustment in renal impairment: Safety and efficacy have not been established

Dosage adjustment in hepatic impairment: Safety and efficacy have not been established; use with caution due to CYP3A4 metabolism

Unlabeled use: Refer to individual protocols. The dose used in meningioma is usually 200 mg/day, continued based on toxicity and response.

Monitoring Parameters Clinical exam and/or ultrasound to confirm complete termination of pregnancy; hemoglobin, hematocrit, and red blood cell count in cases of heavy bleeding

Test Interactions hCG levels will not be useful to confirm pregnancy termination until at least 10 days following mifepristone treatment

Patient Information This medication is used to terminate pregnancy. It is not to be used for pregnancies >49 days (7 weeks). Vaginal bleeding and cramping are expected to occur and may require medical treatment if severe. Most women report that this is heavier bleeding than experienced during a heavy menstrual period. Other side effects that may be expected include abdominal pain, nausea, vomiting, and diarrhea. Follow-up with physician at approximately 3 days and 14 days following initial treatment. Surgical termination of pregnancy may be required if medication fails. There is a risk of fetal malformation if treatment fails. Your physician will give you a phone number to call for problems, questions, or emergencies; you should not use this medication if you do not have access to emergency care. It is possible to become pregnant again following treatment with this medication but before your next period starts. Contraception should be started once the pregnancy's end has been proven and before resuming sexual intercourse. You will be given a medication guide to help you understand this medication and its effects. It is important to review this carefully. Ask any questions you may have. You will also be required to sign a form saying that you understand the effects of this treatment and are able to return to the physician for follow-up appointments. Do not breast feed while using this medication.

Nursing Implications Clinical exam and/or ultrasound are needed to confirm complete termination of pregnancy. Vaginal bleeding and cramping are expected to occur and may require medical treatment. Hemoglobin, hematocrit, and red blood cell count should be monitored in cases of heavy bleeding. Patients must be instructed of the treatment procedure and expected effects. A signed agreement must be kept on file. Adverse effects (including blood transfusions, hospitalization, ongoing pregnancy, and other major complications) must be reported in writing to the medication distributor.

Additional Information Medication will be distributed directly to qualified physicians following signed agreement with the distributor, Danco Laboratories. It will not be available through pharmacies.

Dosage Forms Tablet: 200 mg

Miglitol (MIG li tol)

Related Information

Diabetes Mellitus Treatment *on page 1657*

Hypoglycemic Drugs & Thiazolidinedione Information *on page 1502*

U.S. Brand Names Glyset™

Canadian Brand Names Glyset™

(Continued)

Miglitol *(Continued)*

Therapeutic Category Alpha-Glucosidase Inhibitor; Antidiabetic Agent, Alpha-glucosidase Inhibitor; Hypoglycemic Agent, Oral

Use Type 2 diabetes mellitus (noninsulin-dependent, NIDDM):

Monotherapy adjunct to diet to improve glycemic control in patients with type 2 diabetes mellitus (noninsulin-dependent, NIDDM) whose hyperglycemia cannot be managed with diet alone

Combination therapy with a sulfonylurea when diet plus either miglitol or a sulfonylurea alone do not result in adequate glycemic control. The effect of miglitol to enhance glycemic control is additive to that of sulfonylureas when used in combination.

Pregnancy Risk Factor B

Pregnancy/Breast-Feeding Implications Abnormal blood glucose levels are associated with a higher incidence of congenital abnormalities. Insulin is the drug of choice for the control of diabetes mellitus during pregnancy.

Contraindications Hypersensitivity to miglitol or any of component of the formulation; diabetic ketoacidosis; inflammatory bowel disease; colonic ulceration; partial intestinal obstruction or predisposition to intestinal obstruction; chronic intestinal diseases associated with marked disorders of digestion or absorption or with conditions that may deteriorate as a result of increased gas formation in the intestine

Warnings/Precautions GI symptoms are the most common reactions. The incidence of abdominal pain and diarrhea tend to diminish considerably with continued treatment. Long-term clinical trials in diabetic patients with significant renal dysfunction (serum creatinine >2 mg/dL) have not been conducted. Treatment of these patients is not recommended. Because of its mechanism of action, miglitol administered alone should not cause hypoglycemia in the fasting of postprandial state. In combination with a sulfonylurea will cause a further lowering of blood glucose and may increase the hypoglycemic potential of the sulfonylurea.

Adverse Reactions

>10%: Gastrointestinal: Flatulence (41.5%), diarrhea (28.7%), abdominal pain (11.7%)

1% to 10%: Dermatologic: Rash (4.3%)

Overdosage/Toxicology An overdose of miglitol will not result in hypoglycemia. An overdose may result in transient increases in flatulence, diarrhea, and abdominal discomfort. No serious systemic reactions are expected in the event of an overdose.

Drug Interactions

Decreased Effect: Miglitol may decrease the absorption and bioavailability of digoxin, propranolol, and ranitidine. Digestive enzymes (amylase, pancreatin, charcoal) may reduce the effect of miglitol and should **not** be taken concomitantly.

Mechanism of Action In contrast to sulfonylureas, miglitol does not enhance insulin secretion; the antihyperglycemic action of miglitol results from a reversible inhibition of membrane-bound intestinal alpha-glucosidases which hydrolyze oligosaccharides and disaccharides to glucose and other monosaccharides in the brush border of the small intestine; in diabetic patients, this enzyme inhibition results in delayed glucose absorption and lowering of postprandial hyperglycemia

Pharmacodynamics/Kinetics

Absorption: Saturable at high doses: 25 mg dose: Completely absorbed; 100 mg dose: 50% to 70% absorbed

Distribution: V_d: 0.18 L/kg

Protein binding: Negligible (<4%)

Metabolism: None

Half-life elimination: ~2 hours

Time to peak: 2-3 hours

Excretion: Urine (as unchanged drug)

Usual Dosage Adults: Oral: 25 mg 3 times/day with the first bite of food at each meal; the dose may be increased to 50 mg 3 times/day after 4-8 weeks; maximum recommended dose: 100 mg 3 times/day

Dosing adjustment in renal impairment: Miglitol is primarily excreted by the kidneys; there is little information of miglitol in patients with a Cl_{cr} <25 mL/minute

Dosing adjustment in hepatic impairment: No adjustment necessary

Administration Should be taken orally at the start (with the first bite) of each main meal

Monitoring Parameters Monitor therapeutic response by periodic blood glucose tests; measurement of glycosylated hemoglobin is recommended for the monitoring of long-term glycemic control

Reference Range Target range: Adults:

Fasting blood glucose: <120 mg/dL

Glycosylated hemoglobin: <7%

Patient Information Take orally 3 times/day with the first bite of each main meal. It is important to continue to adhere to dietary instructions, a regular exercise program, and regular testing of urine or blood glucose. If side effects occur, they usually develop during the first few weeks of therapy. They are most commonly mild-to-moderate dose-related GI effects, such as flatulence, soft stools, diarrhea, or abdominal discomfort, and they generally diminish in frequency and intensity with time. Discontinuation of drug usually results in rapid resolution of these GI symptoms.

Dosage Forms Tablet: 25 mg, 50 mg, 100 mg

Milrinone (MIL ri none)

Related Information
Adrenergic Agonists, Cardiovascular Comparison *on page 1469*

U.S. Brand Names Primacor®

Canadian Brand Names Primacor®

Synonyms Milrinone Lactate

Therapeutic Category Phosphodiesterase Enzyme Inhibitor

Use Short-term I.V. therapy of congestive heart failure; calcium antagonist intoxication

Pregnancy Risk Factor C

Contraindications Hypersensitivity to milrinone, inamrinone, or any component of the formulation; concurrent use of inamrinone

Warnings/Precautions Avoid in severe obstructive aortic or pulmonic valvular disease, history of ventricular arrhythmias; atrial fibrillation, flutter. Life-threatening arrhythmias were infrequent and have been associated with pre-existing arrhythmias, metabolic abnormalities, abnormal digoxin levels, and catheter insertion. It may aggravate outflow tract obstruction in hypertrophic subaortic stenosis. Monitor closely during the infusion. Ensure that ventricular rate controlled in atrial fibrillation/flutter before initiating. Not recommended for use in acute MI patients. Monitor and correct fluid and electrolyte problems. Adjust dose in renal dysfunction.

Adverse Reactions
1% to 10%:
Cardiovascular: Arrhythmias, hypotension
Central nervous system: Headache
<1% (Limited to important or life-threatening): Atrial fibrillation, chest pain, hypokalemia, myocardial infarction, thrombocytopenia, ventricular fibrillation

Overdosage/Toxicology Hypotension should respond to I.V. fluids and Trendelenburg position. Use of vasopressors may be required.

Stability Colorless to pale yellow solution; store at room temperature and protect from light; stable at 0.2 mg/mL in 0.9% sodium chloride or D₅W for 72 hours at room temperature in normal light

Incompatible with furosemide and procainamide; **compatible** with atropine, calcium chloride, digoxin, epinephrine, lidocaine, morphine, propranolol, and sodium bicarbonate

Standardized dose: 20 mg in 80 mL of 0.9% sodium chloride or D₅W (0.2 mg/mL)

Mechanism of Action Phosphodiesterase inhibitor resulting in vasodilation

Pharmacodynamics/Kinetics
Onset of action: I.V.: 5-15 minutes
Serum level: I.V.: Following a 125 mcg/kg dose, peak plasma concentrations ~1000 ng/mL were observed at 2 minutes postinjection, decreasing to <100 ng/mL in 2 hours
Drug concentration levels:
Therapeutic:
Serum levels of 166 ng/mL, achieved during I.V. infusions of 0.25-1 mcg/kg/minute, were associated with sustained hemodynamic benefit in severe congestive heart failure patients over a 24-hour period
Maximum beneficial effects on cardiac output and pulmonary capillary wedge pressure following I.V. infusion have been associated with plasma milrinone concentrations of 150-250 ng/mL
Toxic: Serum concentrations >250-300 ng/mL have been associated with marked reductions in mean arterial pressure and tachycardia; however, more studies are required to determine the toxic serum levels for milrinone
Distribution: V$_{dss}$: 0.32 L/kg; Severe CHF: V$_d$: 0.33-0.47 L/kg; not significantly bound to tissues; excretion in breast milk unknown
Protein binding, plasma: ~70%
Metabolism: Hepatic: 12%
Half-life elimination: I.V.: 136 minutes in patients with CHF; patients with severe CHF have a more prolonged half-life, with values ranging from 1.7-2.7 hours. Patients with CHF have a reduction in the systemic clearance of milrinone, resulting in a prolonged elimination half-life. Alternatively, one study reported that 1 month of therapy with milrinone did not change the pharmacokinetic parameters for patients with CHF despite improvement in cardiac function.
Excretion: I.V.: Urine (85% as unchanged drug) within 24 hours; active tubular secretion is a major elimination pathway for milrinone
Clearance: Bolus doses of I.V. milrinone produced systemic clearance values of 25.9 ± 5.7 L/hour (0.37 L/hour/kg); however, in patients with severe congestive heart failure, the clearance is reduced to 0.11-0.13 L/hour/kg. The reduction in clearance may be a result of reduced renal function. Creatinine clearance values were ¹/₂ those reported for healthy adults in patients with severe congestive heart failure (52 vs 119 mL/minute).

Usual Dosage Adults: I.V.: Loading dose: 50 mcg/kg administered over 10 minutes followed by a maintenance dose titrated according to the hemodynamic and clinical response; see following table:

Maintenance Dosage	Dose Rate (mcg/kg/min)	Total Dose (mg/kg/24 h)
Minimum	0.375	0.59
Standard	0.500	0.77
Maximum	0.750	1.13

Dosing adjustment in renal impairment:
Cl$_{cr}$ 50 mL/minute/1.73 m²: Administer 0.43 mcg/kg/minute.
Cl$_{cr}$ 40 mL/minute/1.73 m²: Administer 0.38 mcg/kg/minute.
Cl$_{cr}$ 30 mL/minute/1.73 m²: Administer 0.33 mcg/kg/minute.
Cl$_{cr}$ 20 mL/minute/1.73 m²: Administer 0.28 mcg/kg/minute.
(Continued)

Milrinone *(Continued)*

Cl$_{cr}$ 10 mL/minute/1.73 m^2: Administer 0.23 mcg/kg/minute.
Cl$_{cr}$ 5 mL/minute/1.73 m^2: Administer 0.2 mcg/kg/minute.

Administration Requires an infusion pump; continuous I.V. infusion; 20 mg/100 mL 0.9% sodium chloride or D$_5$W (0.2 mg/mL); see table.

Dose (mcg/kg/min)	Rate (mL/kg/h)
0.375	0.11
0.400	0.12
0.500	0.15
0.600	0.18
0.700	0.21
0.750	0.22

Monitoring Parameters Cardiac monitor and blood pressure monitor required; serum potassium

Therapeutic: Patients should be monitored for improvement in the clinical signs and symptoms of congestive heart failure

Toxic: Patients should be monitored for ventricular arrhythmias and exacerbation of anginal symptoms; during I.V. therapy with milrinone, blood pressure and heart rate should be monitored

Nursing Implications Monitor closely, titrate to blood pressure cardiac index

Dosage Forms
Infusion, as lactate [in D$_5$W]: 200 mcg/mL (100 mL, 200 mL)
Injection, as lactate: 1 mg/mL (5 mL, 10 mL, 20 mL, 50 mL)

- **Milrinone Lactate** *see Milrinone on page 917*
- **Miltown®** *see Meprobamate on page 861*
- **Minestrin™ 1/20 (Can)** *see Ethinyl Estradiol and Norethindrone on page 522*
- **Minidyne® [OTC]** *see Povidone-Iodine on page 1114*
- **Minipress®** *see Prazosin on page 1120*
- **Minitran™ Patch** *see Nitroglycerin on page 989*
- **Minitrans™ (Can)** *see Nitroglycerin on page 989*
- **Minizide®** *see Prazosin and Polythiazide on page 1121*
- **Minocin®** *see Minocycline on page 918*
- **Minocin® IV [DSC]** *see Minocycline on page 918*

Minocycline *(mi noe SYE kleen)*

Related Information
Antimicrobial Drugs of Choice *on page 1588*
Community-Acquired Pneumonia in Adults *on page 1603*

U.S. Brand Names Dynacin®; Minocin®; Minocin® IV [DSC]; Vectrin® [DSC]

Canadian Brand Names Alti-Minocycline; Apo®-Minocycline; Gen-Minocycline; Minocin®; Novo-Minocycline; Rhoxal-minocycline; Scheinpharm™ Minocycline

Synonyms Minocycline Hydrochloride

Therapeutic Category Antibiotic, Tetracycline Derivative

Use Treatment of susceptible bacterial infections of both gram-negative and gram-positive organisms; treatment of anthrax (inhalational, cutaneous, and gastrointestinal); acne, meningococcal carrier state

Pregnancy Risk Factor D

Pregnancy/Breast-Feeding Implications May cause permanent discoloration (brown-grey) of teeth. Animal studies indicate possible embryotoxicity.

Contraindications Hypersensitivity to minocycline, other tetracyclines, or any component of the formulation; pregnancy

Warnings/Precautions Avoid use during tooth development (children ≤8 years of age) unless other drugs are not likely to be effective or are contraindicated. May be associated with increases in BUN secondary to anti-anabolic effects. Avoid in renal insufficiency (associated with hepatotoxicity). CNS effects (lightheadedness, vertigo) may occur, potentially affecting a patient's ability to drive or operate heavy machinery. Has been associated (rarely) with pseudotumor cerebri. May cause photosensitivity.

Adverse Reactions
>10%: Miscellaneous: Discoloration of teeth (in children)
1% to 10%:
Central nervous system: Lightheadedness, vertigo
Dermatologic: Photosensitivity
Gastrointestinal: Nausea, diarrhea
<1%: Acute renal failure, anaphylaxis, angioedema, diabetes insipidus, eosinophilia, erythema multiforme, esophagitis, exfoliative dermatitis, hemolytic anemia, hepatitis, hepatic failure, neutropenia, paresthesia, pericarditis, pigmentation of nails, pseudotumor cerebri, rash, Stevens-Johnson syndrome, superinfections, thrombocytopenia, thyroid dysfunction (extremely rare), tinnitus, vomiting

Overdosage/Toxicology Symptoms include diabetes insipidus, nausea, anorexia, and diarrhea. Following GI decontamination, care is supportive only. Fluid support may be required.

Drug Interactions
Increased Effect/Toxicity: Minocycline may increase the effect of warfarin.
Decreased Effect: Decreased effect with antacids (aluminum, calcium, zinc, or magnesium), bismuth salts, sodium bicarbonate, barbiturates, carbamazepine, hydantoins. Decreased effect of oral contraceptives.

Ethanol/Nutrition/Herb Interactions
Food: Minocycline serum concentrations are not altered if taken with dairy products.
Herb/Nutraceutical: Avoid dong quai, St John's wort (may also cause photosensitization).

Mechanism of Action Inhibits bacterial protein synthesis by binding with the 30S and possibly the 50S ribosomal subunit(s) of susceptible bacteria; cell wall synthesis is not affected

Pharmacodynamics/Kinetics
Absorption: Well absorbed
Distribution: Majority deposits for extended periods in fat; crosses placenta; enters breast milk
Protein binding: 70% to 75%
Half-life elimination: 15 hours
Excretion: Urine

Usual Dosage
Children >8 years: Oral, I.V.: Initial: 4 mg/kg followed by 2 mg/kg/dose every 12 hours
Adults:
Infection: Oral, I.V.: 200 mg stat, 100 mg every 12 hours not to exceed 400 mg/24 hours
Acne: Oral: 50 mg 1-3 times/day
Hemodialysis: Not dialyzable (0% to 5%)

Dietary Considerations May be taken with food or milk.

Administration
Oral: May be taken with food or milk.
I.V.: Infuse slowly, usually over a 4- to 6-hour period.

Test Interactions May cause interference with fluorescence test for urinary catecholamines (false elevations)

Patient Information Avoid unnecessary exposure to sunlight; do not take with antacids, iron products, or dairy products; finish all medication; do not skip doses; take 1 hour before or 2 hours after meals

Nursing Implications Infuse I.V. minocycline slowly, usually over a 4- to 6-hour period.

Dosage Forms
Capsule, as hydrochloride: 50 mg, 100 mg
Dynacin®: 50 mg, 75 mg, 100 mg
Vectrin® [DSC]: 50 mg, 100 mg
Capsule, pellet-filled, as hydrochloride (Minocin®): 50 mg, 100 mg
Injection, powder for reconstitution, as hydrochloride (Minocin® IV [DSC]): 100 mg

♦ **Minocycline Hydrochloride** *see* Minocycline *on page 918*

♦ **Min-Ovral® (Can)** *see* Ethinyl Estradiol and Levonorgestrel *on page 518*

♦ **Minox (Can)** *see* Minoxidil *on page 919*

Minoxidil (mi NOKS i dil)

Related Information
Hypertension *on page 1675*

U.S. Brand Names Loniten®; Rogaine® Extra Strength for Men [OTC]; Rogaine® for Men [OTC]; Rogaine® for Women [OTC]

Canadian Brand Names Apo®-Gain; Minox; Rogaine®

Therapeutic Category Antihypertensive Agent; Vasodilator

Use Management of severe hypertension (usually in combination with a diuretic and beta-blocker); treatment (topical formulation) of alopecia androgenetica in males and females

Pregnancy Risk Factor C

Contraindications Hypersensitivity to minoxidil or any component of the formulation; pheochromocytoma; acute MI; dissecting aortic aneurysm

Warnings/Precautions Note: Minoxidil can cause pericardial effusion, occasionally progressing to tamponade and it can exacerbate angina pectoris; use with caution in patients with pulmonary hypertension, significant renal failure, or congestive heart failure; use with caution in patients with coronary artery disease or recent myocardial infarction; renal failure or dialysis patients may require smaller doses; usually used with a beta-blocker (to treat minoxidil-induced tachycardia) and a diuretic (for treatment of water retention/edema); may take 1-6 months for hypertrichosis to totally reverse after minoxidil therapy is discontinued.

Adverse Reactions
>10%:
Cardiovascular: Congestive heart failure, edema, EKG (transient change in T-wave amplitude and direction), tachycardia
Dermatologic: Hypertrichosis (commonly occurs within 1-2 months of therapy)
1% to 10%: Endocrine & metabolic: Fluid and electrolyte imbalance
<1% (Limited to important or life-threatening): Angina, coarsening facial features, leukopenia, pericardial effusion tamponade, rashes, Stevens-Johnson syndrome, thrombocytopenia, weight gain

Overdosage/Toxicology Symptoms include hypotension, tachycardia, headache, nausea, dizziness, weakness syncope, warm flushed skin and palpitations. Lethargy and ataxia may occur in children. Hypotension usually responds to I.V. fluids, Trendelenburg positioning or vasoconstrictor. Treatment is primarily supportive and symptomatic.

Drug Interactions
Increased Effect/Toxicity: Concurrent use of guanethidine can cause severe orthostasis; avoid concurrent use - discontinue 1-3 weeks prior to initiating minoxidil. Effects of other antihypertensives may be additive with minoxidil.

Ethanol/Nutrition/Herb Interactions Herb/Nutraceutical: Avoid natural licorice (causes sodium and water retention and increases potassium loss).

Mechanism of Action Produces vasodilation by directly relaxing arteriolar smooth muscle, with little effect on veins; effects may be mediated by cyclic AMP; stimulation of hair growth is secondary to vasodilation, increased cutaneous blood flow and stimulation of resting hair follicles
(Continued)

Minoxidil (Continued)

Pharmacodynamics/Kinetics

Onset of action: Hypotensive: Oral: ~30 minutes
  Peak effect: 2-8 hours
Duration: 2-5 days
Protein binding: None
Metabolism: 88% primarily via glucuronidation
Bioavailability: Oral: 90%
Half-life elimination: Adults: 3.5-4.2 hours
Excretion: Urine (12% as unchanged drug)

Usual Dosage

Children <12 years: Hypertension: Oral: Initial: 0.1-0.2 mg/kg once daily; maximum: 5 mg/day; increase gradually every 3 days; usual dosage: 0.25-1 mg/kg/day in 1-2 divided doses; maximum: 50 mg/day

Children >12 years and Adults: Hypertension: Oral: Initial: 5 mg once daily, increase gradually every 3 days; usual dose: 10-40 mg/day in 1-2 divided doses; maximum: 100 mg/day

Adults: Alopecia: Topical: Apply twice daily; 4 months of therapy may be necessary for hair growth.

Elderly: Initial: 2.5 mg once daily; increase gradually.

Note: Dosage adjustment is needed when added to concomitant therapy.

Dialysis: Supplemental dose is not necessary via hemo- or peritoneal dialysis.

Monitoring Parameters Blood pressure, standing and sitting/supine; fluid and electrolyte balance and body weight should be monitored

Patient Information Topical product must be used every day. Hair growth usually takes 4 months. Notify physician if any of the following occur: Heart rate ≥20 beats per minute over normal; rapid weight gain >5 lb (2 kg); unusual swelling of extremities, face, or abdomen; breathing difficulty, especially when lying down; rise slowly from prolonged lying or sitting; new or aggravated angina symptoms (chest, arm, or shoulder pain); severe indigestion; dizziness, lightheadedness, or fainting; nausea or vomiting may occur. Do not make up for missed doses.

Nursing Implications May cause hirsutism or hypertrichosis; observe for fluid retention and orthostatic hypotension

Dosage Forms

Solution, topical: 2% [20 mg/metered dose] (60 mL); 5% [50 mg/metered dose] (60 mL)
Tablet: 2.5 mg, 10 mg

- **Mintezol®** see Thiabendazole on page 1315
- **Minute-Gel®** see Fluoride on page 574
- **Miocarpine® (Can)** see Pilocarpine on page 1083
- **Miochol-E®** see Acetylcholine on page 32
- **Miostat® (Can)** see Carbachol on page 221
- **Miostat® Intraocular** see Carbachol on page 221
- **MiraLax™** see Polyethylene Glycol-Electrolyte Solution on page 1101
- **Mirapex®** see Pramipexole on page 1116
- **Mircette®** see Ethinyl Estradiol and Desogestrel on page 510
- **Mirena®** see Levonorgestrel on page 796

Mirtazapine (mir TAZ a peen)

Related Information

Antidepressant Agents Comparison on page 1482

U.S. Brand Names Remeron®; Remeron® SolTab™

Therapeutic Category Antidepressant, Alpha-2 Antagonist

Use Treatment of depression

Pregnancy Risk Factor C

Pregnancy/Breast-Feeding Implications Animal studies did not show teratogenic effects, however there was an increase in fetal loss and decrease in birth weight; use during pregnancy only if clearly needed. Excretion in human breast milk unknown; breast-feeding is not recommended

Contraindications Hypersensitivity to mirtazapine or any component of the formulation; use of MAO inhibitors within 14 days

Warnings/Precautions Discontinue immediately if signs and symptoms of neutropenia/agranulocytosis occur. May cause sedation, resulting in impaired performance of tasks requiring alertness (ie, operating machinery or driving). Sedative effects may be additive with other CNS depressants and/or ethanol. The degree of sedation is moderate-high relative to other antidepressants. May worsen psychosis in some patients or precipitate a shift to mania or hypomania in patients with bipolar disease. The risks of orthostatic hypotension or anticholinergic effects are low relative to other antidepressants. The incidence of sexual dysfunction with mirtazapine is generally lower than with SSRIs.

May increase appetite and stimulate weight gain, may increase serum cholesterol and triglyceride levels. Use caution in patients with depression, particularly if suicidal risk may be present. Use caution in patients with a previous seizure disorder or condition predisposing to seizures such as brain damage, alcoholism, or concurrent therapy with other drugs which lower the seizure threshold. Use with caution in patients with hepatic or renal dysfunction and in elderly patients.

SolTab™ formulation contains phenylalanine

Adverse Reactions

>10%:
  Central nervous system: Somnolence (54%)
  Endocrine & metabolic: Increased cholesterol
  Gastrointestinal: Constipation (13%), xerostomia (25%), increased appetite (17%), weight gain (12%)

1% to 10%:
  Cardiovascular: Hypertension, vasodilatation, peripheral edema (2%), edema (1%)
  Central nervous system: Dizziness (7%), abnormal dreams (4%), abnormal thoughts (3%), confusion (2%), malaise
  Endocrine & metabolic: Increased triglycerides
  Gastrointestinal: Vomiting, anorexia, abdominal pain
  Genitourinary: Urinary frequency (2%)
  Neuromuscular & skeletal: Myalgia (2%), back pain (2%), arthralgias, tremor (2%), weakness (8%)
  Respiratory: Dyspnea (1%)
  Miscellaneous: Flu-like symptoms (5%), thirst (<1%)
<1% (Limited to important or life-threatening): Agranulocytosis, dehydration, liver function test increases, lymphadenopathy, neutropenia, orthostatic hypotension, seizures (1 case reported), torsade de pointes (1 case reported), weight loss

Drug Interactions
  Cytochrome P450 Effect: CYP1A2, 2C9, 2D6, and 3A3/4 enzyme substrate
  Increased Effect/Toxicity: Increased sedative effect seen with CNS depressants, CYP inhibitors, linezolid, MAO inhibitors, selegiline, sibutramine
  Decreased Effect: Decreased effect seen with clonidine, CYP inducers

Ethanol/Nutrition/Herb Interactions
  Ethanol: Avoid ethanol (may increase CNS depression).
  Herb/Nutraceutical: Avoid St John's wort (may decrease mirtazapine levels). Avoid valerian, St John's wort, SAMe, kava kava (may increase CNS depression).

Stability Store at controlled room temperature
  SolTab™: Protect from light and moisture; use immediately upon opening tablet blister

Mechanism of Action Mirtazapine is a tetracyclic antidepressant that works by its central presynaptic alpha$_2$-adrenergic antagonist effects, which results in increased release of norepinephrine and serotonin. It is also a potent antagonist of 5-HT$_2$ and 5-HT$_3$ serotonin receptors and H1 histamine receptors and a moderate peripheral alpha$_1$-adrenergic and muscarinic antagonist; it does not inhibit the reuptake of norepinephrine or serotonin.

Pharmacodynamics/Kinetics
  Onset of action: Therapeutic: >2 weeks
  Protein binding: 85%
  Metabolism: Extensively hepatic via CYP1A2, 2C9, 2D6, 3A3/4 and via demethylation and hydroxylation
  Bioavailability: 50%
  Half-life elimination: 20-40 hours; hampered with renal or hepatic dysfunction
  Time to peak, serum: 2 hours
  Excretion: Primarily urine (75%) and feces (15%) as metabolites

Usual Dosage
  Children: Safety and efficacy in children have not been established
  Treatment of depression: Adults: Oral: Initial: 15 mg nightly, titrate up to 15-45 mg/day with dose increases made no more frequently than every 1-2 weeks; there is an inverse relationship between dose and sedation
  Elderly: Decreased clearance seen (40% males, 10% females); no specific dosage adjustment recommended by manufacturer

  Dosage adjustment in renal impairment:
    Cl$_{cr}$ 11-39 mL/minute: 30% decreased clearance
    Cl$_{cr}$ <10 mL/minute: 50% decreased clearance
  Dosage adjustment in hepatic impairment: Clearance decreased by 30%

Dietary Considerations Remeron® SolTab™ contains phenylalanine: 2.6 mg per 15 mg tablet; 5.2 mg per 30 mg tablet; 7.8 mg per 45 mg tablet

Administration SolTab™: Open blister pack and place tablet on the tongue. Do not split tablet. Tablet is formulated to dissolve on the tongue without water.

Monitoring Parameters Patients should be monitored for signs of agranulocytosis or severe neutropenia such as sore throat, stomatitis or other signs of infection or a low WBC; monitor for improvement in clinical signs and symptoms of depression, improvement may be observed within 1-4 weeks after initiating therapy

Patient Information Be aware of the risk of developing agranulocytosis; contact physician if any indication of infection occurs (ie, fever, chills, sore throat, mucous membrane ulceration, and especially flu-like symptoms); may impair judgment, thinking, and particularly motor skills; may impair ability to drive, use machinery, or perform tasks that require you remain alert; avoid concurrent alcohol use
  SolTab™: Open blister pack and place tablet on the tongue. Do not split tablet. Tablet is formulated to dissolve on the tongue without water.

Additional Information Note: At least 14 days should elapse between discontinuation of an MAO inhibitor and initiation of therapy with mirtazapine; at least 14 days should be allowed after discontinuing mirtazapine before starting an MAO inhibitor.

Dosage Forms
  Tablet: 15 mg, 30 mg, 45 mg
  Tablet, orally disintegrating:
    15 mg [phenylalanine 2.6 mg/tablet] [orange flavor]
    30 mg [phenylalanine 5.2 mg/tablet] [orange flavor]
    45 mg [phenylalanine 7.8 mg/tablet] [orange flavor]

Misoprostol (mye soe PROST ole)

U.S. Brand Names Cytotec®
Canadian Brand Names Cytotec®
Therapeutic Category Prostaglandin
Use Prevention of NSAID-induced gastric ulcers
Unlabeled/Investigational Use Cervical ripening and labor induction, NSAID-induced nephropathy, fat malabsorption in cystic fibrosis
Pregnancy Risk Factor X
(Continued)

Misoprostol *(Continued)*

Pregnancy/Breast-Feeding Implications Misoprostol is an abortifacient. During pregnancy, administration by any route is contraindicated by the manufacturer. Reports of fetal death and congenital anomalies have been received after the use of misoprostol as an abortifacient. Excretion in breast milk is unknown; breast-feeding is contraindicated.

Contraindications Hypersensitivity to misoprostol, prostaglandins, or any component of the formulation; pregnancy

Warnings/Precautions Safety and efficacy have not been established in children <18 years of age; use with caution in patients with renal impairment and the elderly; not to be used in pregnant women or women of childbearing potential unless woman is capable of complying with effective contraceptive measures; therapy is normally begun on the second or third day of next normal menstrual period. Uterine perforation and/or rupture have been reported in association with intravaginal use to induce labor or with combined oral/intravaginal use to induce abortion. Should not be used as a cervical-ripening agent for induction of labor or termination of pregnancy. However, The American College of Obstetricians and Gynecologists (ACOG) continues to support this off-label use.

Adverse Reactions
>10%: Gastrointestinal: Diarrhea, abdominal pain
1% to 10%:
  Central nervous system: Headache
  Gastrointestinal: Constipation, flatulence, nausea, dyspepsia, vomiting
<1% (Limited to important or life-threatening): Anaphylaxis, anxiety, appetite changes, arrhythmia, bronchospasm, confusion, depression, drowsiness, edema, fetal or infant death (when used during pregnancy), fever, GI bleeding, GI inflammation, gingivitis, gout, hypertension, hypotension, impotence, loss of libido, neuropathy, neurosis, purpura, rash, reflux, rigors, thrombocytopenia, uterine rupture, weakness, weight changes

Overdosage/Toxicology Symptoms include sedation, tremor, convulsions, dyspnea, abdominal pain, diarrhea, hypotension, and bradycardia.

Drug Interactions
  Decreased Effect: Antacids may diminish absorption (not clinically significant)

Ethanol/Nutrition/Herb Interactions Food: Misoprostol peak serum concentrations may be decreased if taken with food (not clinically significant).

Stability Store at or below 25°C (77°F).

Mechanism of Action Misoprostol is a synthetic prostaglandin E_1 analog that replaces the protective prostaglandins consumed with prostaglandin-inhibiting therapies eg, nonsteroidal anti-inflammatory drugs

Pharmacodynamics/Kinetics
Absorption: Rapid
Metabolism: Hepatic; rapidly de-esterified to misoprostol acid (active)
Half-life elimination: Metabolite: 20-40 minutes
Time to peak, serum: Active metabolite: 15-30 minutes (fasting)
Excretion: Urine (64% to 73%) and feces (15%) within 24 hours

Usual Dosage
Oral:
  Children 8-16 years: Fat absorption in cystic fibrosis (unlabeled use): 100 mcg 4 times/day
  Adults: Prevention of NSAID-induced gastric ulcers: 200 mcg 4 times/day with food; if not tolerated, may decrease dose to 100 mcg 4 times/day with food or 200 mcg twice daily with food; last dose of the day should be taken at bedtime
Intravaginal: Adult: Labor induction or cervical ripening (unlabeled use): 25 mcg (¹/₄ of 100 mcg tablet); may repeat at intervals no more frequent than every 3-6 hours. Do not use in patients with previous cesarean delivery or prior major uterine surgery.

Dietary Considerations Should be taken with food; incidence of diarrhea may be lessened by having patient take dose right after meals.

Administration Incidence of diarrhea may be lessened by having patient take dose right after meals. Therapy is usually begun on the second or third day of the next normal menstrual period.

Patient Information May cause diarrhea when first being used; take after meals and at bedtime; avoid taking with magnesium-containing antacids

Nursing Implications Incidence of diarrhea may be lessened by having patient take dose right after meals.

Dosage Forms Tablet: 100 mcg, 200 mcg

♦ **Misoprostol and Diclofenac** *see Diclofenac and Misoprostol on page 395*
♦ **Mithracin®** *see Plicamycin on page 1095*
♦ **Mithramycin** *see Plicamycin on page 1095*

Mitomycin *(mye toe MYE sin)*

U.S. Brand Names Mutamycin®
Canadian Brand Names Mutamycin®
Synonyms Mitomycin-C; MTC
Therapeutic Category Antineoplastic Agent, Antibiotic; Antineoplastic Agent, Vesicant; Vesicant
Use Therapy of disseminated adenocarcinoma of stomach or pancreas in combination with other approved chemotherapeutic agents; bladder cancer, colorectal cancer
Pregnancy Risk Factor D
Contraindications Hypersensitivity to mitomycin or any component of the formulation; platelet counts <75,000/mm³; leukocyte counts <3000/mm³ or serum creatinine >1.7 mg/dL; thrombocytopenia; pregnancy
Warnings/Precautions The U.S. Food and Drug Administration (FDA) currently recommends that procedures for proper handling and disposal of antineoplastic agents be considered. Use with caution in patients who have received radiation therapy or in the presence of hepatobiliary dysfunction; reduce dosage in patients who are receiving radiation therapy simultaneously. Hemolytic-uremic syndrome, potentially fatal, occurs in some patients

receiving long-term therapy. It is correlated with total dose (single doses ≥60 mg or cumulative doses ≥50 mg/m^2) and total duration of therapy (>5-11 months). **Mitomycin is a potent vesicant, may cause ulceration, necrosis, cellulitis, and tissue sloughing if infiltrated.**

Adverse Reactions
>10%:
    Cardiovascular: Congestive heart failure (3% to 15%) (doses >30 mg/m^2)
    Dermatologic: Alopecia, nail banding/discoloration
    Gastrointestinal: Nausea, vomiting and anorexia (14%)
    Hematologic: Anemia (19% to 24%); myelosuppression, common, dose-limiting, delayed
        Onset: 3 weeks
        Nadir: 4-6 weeks
        Recovery: 6-8 weeks
1% to 10%:
    Dermatologic: Rash
    Gastrointestinal: Stomatitis
    Neuromuscular: Paresthesias
    Respiratory: Interstitial pneumonitis, infiltrates, dyspnea, cough (7%)
<1% (Limited to important or life-threatening): Extravasation reactions, fever, hemolytic uremic syndrome, malaise, pruritus, renal failure

Overdosage/Toxicology Symptoms include bone marrow suppression, nausea, vomiting, and alopecia.

Drug Interactions
Increased Effect/Toxicity: *Vinca* alkaloids or doxorubicin may enhance cardiac toxicity when coadministered with mitomycin.

Ethanol/Nutrition/Herb Interactions Herb/Nutraceutical: Avoid black cohosh, dong quai in estrogen-dependent tumors.

Stability
Store intact vials of lyophilized powder at room temperature
Dilute powder with SWI to a concentration of 0.5 mg/mL as follows: Solution is stable for 7 days at room temperature and 14 days at refrigeration if protected from light
    5 mg = 10 mL
    20 mg = 40 mL
    40 mg = 80 mL
    Further dilution to 20-40 mcg/mL:
        In normal saline: Stable for 12 hours at room temperature
        In D$_5$: Stable for 3 hours at room temperature
        In sodium lactate: Stable for 12 hours at room temperature

Standard I.V. dilution:
    I.V. push: Dose/syringe (concentration = 0.5 mg/mL)
        Maximum syringe size for IVP is a 30 mL syringe and syringe should be ≤75% full
        Syringe is stable for 7 days at room temperature and 14 days at refrigeration if protected from light
    IVPB: Dose/100 mL NS
    IVPB solution is stable for 24 hours at room temperature

Mechanism of Action Isolated from *Streptomyces caespitosus*; acts primarily as an alkylating agent and produces DNA cross-linking (primarily with guanine and cytosine pairs); cell-cycle nonspecific; inhibits DNA and RNA synthesis by alkylation and cross-linking the strands of DNA

Pharmacodynamics/Kinetics
Distribution: V$_d$: 22 L/m^2; high drug concentrations found in kidney, tongue, muscle, heart, and lung tissue; probably not distributed into the CNS
Metabolism: Hepatic
Half-life elimination: 23-78 minutes; Terminal: 50 minutes
Excretion: In urine, when serum concentrations are elevated.

Usual Dosage Refer to individual protocols. Children and Adults: I.V.:
Single agent therapy: 20 mg/m^2 every 6-8 weeks
Combination therapy: 10 mg/m^2 every 6-8 weeks
Bladder carcinoma: 20-40 mg/dose (1 mg/mL in sterile aqueous solution) instilled into the bladder for 3 hours repeated up to 3 times/week for up to 20 procedures per course
Dosage adjustment in renal impairment: Varying approaches to dosing adjustments have been published. Consult individual protocols.
    Cl$_{cr}$ <10 mL/minute: Administer 75% of normal dose
    OR
    S$_{cr}$ 1.6-2.4 mg/dL: Administer 50% of dose
    S$_{cr}$ >2.4 mg/dL: Do not administer drug
Hemodialysis: Unknown
CAPD effects: Unknown
CAVH effects: Unknown
Dosage adjustment in hepatic impairment: Varying approaches to dosing adjustments have been published. Consult individual protocols.
    Bilirubin 1.5-3 mg/dL: Administer 50% of dose
    Bilirubin >3.1 mg/dL: Administer 25% of dose
    OR
    Bilirubin >3 mg/dL **or** hepatic enzymes >3 times normal: Administer 50% of dose

Administration
Administer slow I.V. push by **central line only**
    Administer mitomycin doses of 10 mg/m^2 over 5-10 minutes
    Administer mitomycin doses of 10-20 mg/m^2 over 10-20 minutes
Avoid extravasation; severe local tissue necrosis occurs. Flush with 5-10 mL of I.V. solution before and after drug administration; IVPB infusions should be closely monitored for adequate vein patency.

Monitoring Parameters Platelet count, CBC with differential, hemoglobin, prothrombin time, renal and pulmonary function tests
(Continued)

Mitomycin *(Continued)*

Patient Information This drug can only be given I.V. Make note of scheduled return dates. Maintain adequate hydration (2-3 L/day of fluids unless instructed to restrict fluid intake) and nutrition. You may experience, rash, skin lesions, loss of hair, or permanent sterility. Small frequent meals may help if you experience nausea, vomiting, or loss of appetite. Frequent mouth care will help reduce the incidence of mouth sores. Use caution when driving or engaging in tasks that require alertness because you may experience dizziness, drowsiness, syncope, or blurred vision. Report difficulty breathing, swelling of extremities, or sudden weight gain; burning, pain, or redness at infusion site; unusual bruising or bleeding; pain on urination; or other adverse effects. The drug may be excreted in breast milk, therefore, an alternative form of feeding your baby should be used. Contraceptive measures are recommended during therapy.

Nursing Implications

Extravasation management:

Care should be taken to avoid extravasation. If extravasation occurs, the site should be observed closely; these injuries frequently cause necrosis; a plastic surgery consult may be required.

Few agents have been effective as antidotes, but there are reports in the literature of some benefit with dimethylsulfoxide (DMSO). Delayed dermal reactions with mitomycin are possible, even in patients who are asymptomatic at time of drug administration.

Dosage Forms Powder for injection: 5 mg, 20 mg, 40 mg

♦ **Mitomycin-C** *see* Mitomycin *on page 922*

Mitotane *(MYE toe tane)*

U.S. Brand Names Lysodren®

Canadian Brand Names Lysodren®

Synonyms o,p′-DDD

Therapeutic Category Antiadrenal Agent; Antineoplastic Agent, Miscellaneous

Use Treatment of adrenocortical carcinoma

Unlabeled/Investigational Use Treatment of Cushing's syndrome

Pregnancy Risk Factor C

Contraindications Hypersensitivity to mitotane or any component of the formulation

Warnings/Precautions The U.S. Food and Drug Administration (FDA) currently recommends that procedures for proper handling and disposal of antineoplastic agents be considered. Patients should be hospitalized when mitotane therapy is initiated until a stable dose regimen is established. Discontinue temporarily following trauma or shock since the prime action of mitotane is adrenal suppression; exogenous steroids may be indicated since adrenal function may not start immediately. Administer with care to patients with severe hepatic impairment; observe patients for neurotoxicity with prolonged (2 years) use.

Adverse Reactions The following reactions are reversible:

Central nervous system: CNS depression (32%), dizziness (15%), headache (5%), confusion (3%)

Dermatologic: Skin rash (12%)

Gastrointestinal: Anorexia (24%), nausea (39%), vomiting (37%), diarrhea (13%)

Neuromuscular & skeletal: Muscle tremor (3%), weakness (12%)

Overdosage/Toxicology Symptoms include diarrhea, vomiting, numbness of limbs, and weakness.

Drug Interactions

Increased Effect/Toxicity: CNS depressants taken with mitotane may enhance CNS depression.

Decreased Effect: Mitotane may enhance the clearance of barbiturates and warfarin by induction of the hepatic microsomal enzyme system resulting in a decreased effect. Coadministration of spironolactone has resulted in negation of mitotane's effect. Mitotane may increase clearance of phenytoin by microsomal enzyme stimulation.

Ethanol/Nutrition/Herb Interactions Ethanol: Avoid ethanol (may increase CNS depression).

Stability Protect from light, store at room temperature

Mechanism of Action Causes adrenal cortical atrophy; drug affects mitochondria in adrenal cortical cells and decreases production of cortisol; also alters the peripheral metabolism of steroids

Pharmacodynamics/Kinetics

Absorption: Oral: ~35% to 40%

Distribution: Stored mainly in fat tissue but is found in all body tissues

Metabolism: Hepatically and by other tissues

Half-life elimination: 18-159 days

Time to peak, serum: 3-5 hours

Excretion: Urine and feces (as metabolites)

Usual Dosage Oral:

Children: 0.1-0.5 mg/kg or 1-2 g/day in divided doses increasing gradually to a maximum of 5-7 g/day

Adults: Start at 1-6 g/day in divided doses, then increase incrementally to 8-10 g/day in 3-4 divided doses; dose is changed on basis of side effect with aim of giving as high a dose as tolerated; maximum daily dose: 18 g

Dosing adjustment in hepatic impairment: Dose may need to be decreased in patients with liver disease

Patient Information Desired effects of this drug may not be seen for 2-3 months. Wear identification that alerts medical personnel that you are taking this drug in event of shock or trauma. Maintain adequate hydration (2-3 L/day of fluids unless instructed to restrict fluid intake) and nutrition. Avoid alcohol or OTC medications unless approved by prescriber. May cause dizziness and vertigo (avoid driving or performing tasks requiring alertness until response to drug is known); nausea, vomiting, or loss of appetite (small frequent meals, frequent mouth care, sucking lozenges, or chewing gum may help); orthostatic hypotension (use caution when rising from sitting or lying position or climbing stairs); muscle aches or pain (if severe, request medication from prescriber). Report severe vomiting or acute loss of appetite, muscular twitching, fever or infection, blood in urine or pain on urinating, or darkening of skin. Contraceptive measures are recommended during therapy.

Nursing Implications Patients should be warned that mitotane may impair ability to operate hazardous equipment or drive; ethanol and other CNS depressants should be avoided; physician should be notified if rash or darkening of skin, severe nausea, vomiting, depression, flushing, or fever occurs; contraceptive measures are recommended during therapy

Dosage Forms Tablet, scored: 500 mg

Mitoxantrone (mye toe ZAN trone)

U.S. Brand Names Novantrone®

Canadian Brand Names Novantrone®

Synonyms DHAD; Mitoxantrone Hydrochloride

Therapeutic Category Antineoplastic Agent, Anthracycline; Antineoplastic Agent, Antibiotic; Antineoplastic Agent, Irritant; Vesicant

Use Treatment of acute nonlymphocytic leukemia (ANLL) in adults in combination with other agents; very active against various leukemias, lymphoma, and breast cancer; moderately active against pediatric sarcoma; treatment of secondary (chronic) progressive, progressive relapsing, or worsening relapsing-remitting multiple sclerosis; treatment of pain related to advanced hormone-refractory prostate cancer (in combination with corticosteroids)

Pregnancy Risk Factor D

Pregnancy/Breast-Feeding Implications May cause fetal harm if administered to a pregnant woman. Women with multiple sclerosis and who are biologically capable of becoming pregnant should have a pregnancy test prior to each dose. Mitoxantrone is excreted in human milk and significant concentrations (180 mg/mL) have been reported for 28 days after the last administration. Because of the potential for serious adverse reactions in infants from mitoxantrone, breast-feeding should be discontinued before starting treatment.

Contraindications Hypersensitivity to mitoxantrone or any component of the formulation; multiple sclerosis with left ventricular ejection fraction (LVEF) <50% or clinically significant decrease in LVEF; pregnancy

Warnings/Precautions The FDA currently recommends that procedures for proper handling and disposal of antineoplastic agents be considered. Dosage should be reduced in patients with impaired hepatobiliary function; not for treatment of multiple sclerosis in patients with concurrent hepatic impairment. Treatment may lead to severe myelosuppression; use with caution in patients with pre-existing myelosuppression. Do not use if baseline neutrophil count <1500 cells/mm^3 (except for treatment of ANLL). May cause myocardial toxicity and potentially-fatal congestive heart failure; risk increases with cumulative dosing. Predisposing factors for mitoxantrone-induced cardiotoxicity include prior anthracycline therapy, prior cardiovascular disease, and mediastinal irradiation. The risk of developing cardiotoxicity is <3% when the cumulative doses are <100-120 mg/m^2 in patients with predisposing factors and <160 mg/m^2 in patients with no predisposing factors. Monitor for cardiac toxicity throughout treatment and prior to each dose once cumulative dose of 100 mg/m^2 is reached in patients with multiple sclerosis, and once cumulative dose of 140 mg/m^2 is reached for patients with cancer. Not for treatment of primary progressive multiple sclerosis. Has been associated with the development of secondary acute myelogenous leukemia and myelodysplasia when used in combination with other antineoplastic agents. For I.V. use only. May cause urine, saliva, tears, and sweat to turn blue-green for 24 hours postinfusion. Whites of eyes may have blue-green tinge (this is normal).

Adverse Reactions

>10%:

Central nervous system: Headache

Dermatologic: Alopecia

Gastrointestinal: Nausea, vomiting, diarrhea, abdominal pain, mucositis, stomatitis, GI bleeding

Emetic potential: Moderate (31% to 72%)

Genitourinary: Discoloration of urine (blue-green)

Hepatic: Abnormal LFTs

Respiratory: Coughing, dyspnea

1% to 10%:

Cardiovascular: Cardiotoxicity (primarily in patients who have received prior anthracycline therapy), congestive heart failure, hypotension

Central nervous system: Seizures, fever

Dermatologic: Pruritus, skin desquamation

Hematologic: Myelosuppressive effects of chemotherapy:

WBC: Mild

Platelets: Mild

Onset: 7-10 days

Nadir: 14 days

Recovery: 21 days

Hepatic: Transient elevation of liver enzymes, jaundice

Ocular: Conjunctivitis

Renal: Renal failure

Miscellaneous: Development of secondary leukemia (~1% to 2%)

<1% (Limited to important or life-threatening): Anaphylactoid reactions, anaphylaxis, interstitial pneumonitis (has occurred during combination chemotherapy), **irritant chemotherapy** with blue skin discoloration, tissue necrosis following extravasation, pain or redness at injection site, phlebitis

Overdosage/Toxicology Symptoms include leukopenia, tachycardia, and marrow hypoplasia. There is no known antidote.

(Continued)

Mitoxantrone *(Continued)*

Drug Interactions
Cytochrome P450 Effect: CYP2E1 enzyme inducer (weak)

Decreased Effect: Patients may experience impaired immune response to vaccines; possible infection after administration of live vaccines in patients receiving immunosuppressants.

Ethanol/Nutrition/Herb Interactions
Herb/Nutraceutical: Avoid black cohosh, dong quai in estrogen-dependent tumors.

Stability
Store intact vials at 15°C to 25°C (59°F to 77°F); do not freeze

Dilute in at least 50 mL of NS or D_5W; solution is stable for 7 days at room temperature or refrigeration

Incompatible with heparin and hydrocortisone

Standard I.V. dilution: IVPB: Dose/100 mL D_5W or NS

Mechanism of Action
Analogue of the anthracyclines, but different in mechanism of action, cardiac toxicity, and potential for tissue necrosis; mitoxantrone does intercalate DNA; binds to nucleic acids and inhibits DNA and RNA synthesis by template disordering and steric obstruction; replication is decreased by binding to DNA topoisomerase II (enzyme responsible for DNA helix supercoiling); active throughout entire cell cycle; does not appear to produce free radicals

Pharmacodynamics/Kinetics
Distribution: V_d: 1000 L/m^2; distributes into pleural fluid, kidney, thyroid, liver, heart, and red blood cells

Protein binding: 78%, mostly to albumin

Metabolism: Hepatic; pathway not determined, weak inducer of CYP2E1 *(in vitro)*

Half-life elimination: Terminal: 23-215 hours; may be prolonged with liver impairment

Excretion: Slowly in urine (6% to 11%) and feces as unchanged drug and metabolites

Usual Dosage
Refer to individual protocols. I.V. (dilute in D_5W or NS):

ANLL leukemias:
Children ≤2 years: 0.4 mg/kg/day once daily for 3-5 days
Children >2 years and Adults: 12 mg/m^2/day once daily for 3 days; acute leukemia in relapse: 8-12 mg/m^2/day once daily for 4-5 days

Solid tumors:
Children: 18-20 mg/m^2 every 3-4 weeks **OR** 5-8 mg/m^2 every week
Adults: 12-14 mg/m^2 every 3-4 weeks **OR** 2-4 mg/m^2/day for 5 days every 4 weeks
Maximum total dose: 80-120 mg/m^2 in patients with predisposing factor and <160 mg in patients with no predisposing factor

Hormone-refractory prostate cancer: Adults: 12-14 mg/m^2 over 5-15 minutes via intravenous infusion every 21 days

Multiple sclerosis: Adults: 12 mg/m^2 over 5-15 minutes via intravenous infusion every 3 months; do **not** use if LVEF <50% (or following significant reduction); cumulative lifetime dose should not exceed ≥140 mg/m^2

Dosing adjustment in renal impairment: Safety and efficacy have not been established
Hemodialysis: Supplemental dose is not necessary
Peritoneal dialysis: Supplemental dose is not necessary

Dosing adjustment in hepatic impairment: Official dosage adjustment recommendations have not been established; not indicated for patients with multiple sclerosis who are hepatically impaired. Use with caution when used to treat other indications.
Moderate dysfunction (bilirubin 1.5-3 mg/dL): Some clinicians recommend a 50% dosage reduction
Severe dysfunction (bilirubin >3.0 mg/dL) have a lower total body clearance and may require a dosage adjustment to 8 mg/m^2; some clinicians recommend a dosage reduction to 25% of dose

Dose modifications based on degree of leukopenia or thrombocytopenia: See table.

Granulocyte Count Nadir (cells/mm²)	Platelet Count Nadir (cells/mm²)	Total Bilirubin (mg/dL)	Dose Adjustment
>2000	>150,000	<1.5	Increase by 1 mg/m^2
1000-2000	75,000-150,000	<1.5	Maintain same dose
<1000	<75,000	1.5-3	Decrease by 1 mg/m^2

Elderly: Clearance is decreased in elderly patients; use with caution

Administration Must be diluted prior to administration; should only be administered into a free-flowing intravenous infusion; do **not** administer S.C., I.M., intra-arterially, or intrathecally; do **not** administer I.V. bolus over <3 minutes; can be administered I.V. intermittent infusion over 15-30 minutes; **avoid extravasation** (although has not generally been proven to be a vesicant)

Monitoring Parameters CBC, serum uric acid (for treatment of leukemia), liver function tests, signs and symptoms of CHF; evaluate LVEF prior to start of therapy and regularly during treatment. In addition, for the treatment of multiple sclerosis, monitor LVEF prior to all doses following cumulative dose of ≥100 mg/m^2.

Patient Information This drug can only be given I.V. Make note of scheduled return dates. Your urine may turn blue-green for 24 hours after infusion and the whites of your eyes may have a blue-green tinge; this is normal. Maintain adequate hydration (2-3 L/day of fluids unless instructed to restrict fluid intake). You may experience rash, skin lesions, or loss of hair. Small frequent meals may help if you experience nausea, vomiting, or loss of appetite. Frequent mouth care will help reduce the incidence of mouth sores. Use caution when driving or engaging in tasks that require alertness because you may experience dizziness, drowsiness, syncope, or blurred vision. Report chest pain or heart palpitations; difficulty breathing or constant cough; swelling of extremities or sudden weight gain; burning, pain, or redness at the I.V. infusion site; persistent fever or chills; unusual bruising or bleeding; twitching or tremors; or pain on urination. Contraceptive measures are recommended during therapy.

Nursing Implications Vesicant; avoid extravasation. Must be diluted prior to administration; for I.V. use **only**; do **not** administer S.C., I.M., intra-arterially, or intrathecally; should only be administered into a free-flowing intravenous infusion

Mitoxantrone is excreted in human milk and significant concentrations (180 mg/mL) have been reported for 28 days after the last administration. Because of the potential for serious adverse reactions in infants from mitoxantrone, breast-feeding should be discontinued before starting treatment.

Dosage Forms Injection, as base: 2 mg/mL (10 mL, 12.5 mL, 15 mL)

♦ **Mitoxantrone Hydrochloride** *see* Mitoxantrone *on page 925*

♦ **Mitrazol**® **[OTC]** *see* Miconazole *on page 908*

♦ **Mivacron**® *see* Mivacurium *on page 927*

Mivacurium (mye va KYOO ree um)

Related Information
Neuromuscular Blocking Agents Comparison *on page 1508*

U.S. Brand Names Mivacron®

Canadian Brand Names Mivacron®

Synonyms Mivacurium Chloride

Therapeutic Category Neuromuscular Blocker Agent, Nondepolarizing; Skeletal Muscle Relaxant

Use Adjunct to general anesthesia to facilitate endotracheal intubation and to relax skeletal muscles during surgery; to facilitate mechanical ventilation in ICU patients; does not relieve pain or produce sedation

Pregnancy Risk Factor C

Contraindications Hypersensitivity to mivacurium chloride, any component of the formulation, or other benzylisoquinolinium agents; use of multidose vials in patients with allergy to benzyl alcohol; pre-existing tachycardia

Warnings/Precautions Ventilation must be supported during neuromuscular blockade; does not counteract bradycardia produced by anesthetics/vagal stimulation; prolonged neuromuscular block may be seen in patients with reduced or atypical plasma cholinesterase activity (eg, pregnancy, liver or kidney disease, infections, peptic ulcer, anemia); patients homozygous for the atypical plasma cholinesterase gene are extremely sensitive to the neuromuscular blocking effect of mivacurium (use extreme caution if at all in those patients); duration prolonged in patients with renal and/or hepatic impairment; reduce initial dosage and inject slowly (over 60 seconds) in patients in whom substantial histamine release would be potentially hazardous; certain clinical conditions may result in potentiation or antagonism of neuromuscular blockade:

Potentiation: Electrolyte abnormalities, severe hyponatremia, severe hypocalcemia, severe hypokalemia, hypermagnesemia, neuromuscular diseases, acidosis, acute intermittent porphyria, renal failure, hepatic failure

Antagonism: Alkalosis, hypercalcemia, demyelinating lesions, peripheral neuropathies, diabetes mellitus

Increased sensitivity in patients with myasthenia gravis, Eaton-Lambert syndrome, resistance in burn patients (>30% of body) for period of 5-70 days postinjury; resistance in patients with muscle trauma, denervation, immobilization, infection.

Adverse Reactions

>10%: Cardiovascular: Flushing of face

1% to 10%: Cardiovascular: Hypotension

<1% (Limited to important or life-threatening): Anaphylactoid reaction, anaphylaxis, bradycardia, bronchospasm, cutaneous erythema, dizziness, endogenous histamine release, hypersensitivity reactions, hypoxemia, injection site reaction, muscle spasms, rash, tachycardia, wheezing

Drug Interactions

Increased Effect/Toxicity: Increased effects are possible with aminoglycosides, betablockers, clindamycin, calcium channel blockers, halogenated anesthetics, imipenem, ketamine, lidocaine, loop diuretics (furosemide), macrolides (case reports), magnesium sulfate, procainamide, quinidine, quinolones, tetracyclines, and vancomycin. May increase risk of myopathy when used with high-dose corticosteroids for extended periods. Drugs which inhibit acetylcholinesterase may prolong effect of mivacurium.

Decreased Effect: Effect of nondepolarizing neuromuscular blockers may be reduced by carbamazepine (chronic use), corticosteroids (also associated with myopathy - see increased effect), phenytoin (chronic use), sympathomimetics, and theophylline.

Stability Store at room temperature of 15°C to 25°C (59°F to 77°F); protect from direct ultraviolet light

Mechanism of Action Mivacurium is a short-acting, nondepolarizing, neuromuscular-blocking agent. Like other nondepolarizing drugs, mivacurium antagonizes acetylcholine by competitively binding to cholinergic sites on motor endplates in skeletal muscle. This inhibits contractile activity in skeletal muscle leading to muscle paralysis. This effect is reversible with cholinesterase inhibitors such as edrophonium, neostigmine, and physostigmine.

Pharmacodynamics/Kinetics

Onset of action: Neuromuscular blockade: I.V.: 1.5-3 minutes (dose dependent)

Duration: Short due to rapid hydrolysis by plasma cholinesterases; clinically effective block may last for 12-20 minutes; spontaneous recovery may be 95% complete in 25-30 minutes; duration shorter in children and may be slightly longer in elderly

Metabolism: By plasma cholinesterase

Half-life elimination: 2 minutes (more active isomers only)

Usual Dosage Continuous infusion requires an infusion pump; dose to effect; doses will vary due to interpatient variability; use ideal body weight for obese patients

(Continued)

Mivacurium *(Continued)*

Children 2-12 years (duration of action is shorter and dosage requirements are higher): 0.2 mg/kg I.V. followed by average infusion rate of 14 mcg/kg/minute (range: 5-31 mcg/kg/minute) upon evidence of spontaneous recovery from initial dose

Adults: Initial: I.V.: 0.15-0.25 mg/kg bolus followed by maintenance doses of 0.1 mg/kg at approximately 15-minute intervals; for prolonged neuromuscular block, initial infusion of 9-10 mcg/kg/minute is used upon evidence of spontaneous recovery from initial dose, usual infusion rate of 6-7 mcg/kg/minute (1-15 mcg/kg/minute) under balanced anesthesia; initial dose after succinylcholine for intubation (balanced anesthesia): Adults: 0.1 mg/kg

Pretreatment/priming: 10% of intubating dose given 3-5 minutes before initial dose

Dosing adjustment in renal impairment: 0.15 mg/kg I.V. bolus; duration of action of blockade: 1.5 times longer in ESRD, may decrease infusion rates by as much as 50%, dependent on degree of renal impairment

Dosing adjustment in hepatic impairment: 0.15 mg/kg I.V. bolus; duration of blockade: 3 times longer in ESLD, may decrease rate of infusion by as much as 50% in ESLD, dependent on the degree of impairment

Administration Children require higher mivacurium infusion rates than adults; during opioid/nitrous oxide/oxygen anesthesia, the infusion rate required to maintain 89% to 99% neuromuscular block averages 14 mcg/kg/minute (range: 5-31). For adults and children, the amount of infusion solution required per hour depends upon the clinical requirements of the patient, the concentration of mivacurium in the infusion solution, and the patient's weight. The contribution of the infusion solution to the fluid requirements of the patient must be considered.

Nursing Implications Use with caution in patients in whom histamine release would be detrimental (eg, patients with severe cardiovascular disease or asthma)

Additional Information Mivacurium is classified as a short-duration neuromuscular-blocking agent. Do not mix with barbiturates in the same syringe. Mivacurium does not appear to have a cumulative effect on the duration of blockade. It does not relieve pain or produce sedation.

Dosage Forms

Infusion, as chloride [in D$_5$W]: 0.5 mg/mL (50 mL)

Injection, as chloride: 2 mg/mL (5 mL, 10 mL)

♦ **Mivacurium Chloride** *see* Mivacurium *on page 927*

♦ **MK383** *see* Tirofiban *on page 1338*

♦ **MK462** *see* Rizatriptan *on page 1207*

♦ **MK594** *see* Losartan *on page 823*

♦ **MK-0826** *see* Ertapenem *on page 484*

♦ **MMR** *see* Measles, Mumps, and Rubella Vaccines (Combined) *on page 841*

♦ **M-M-R® II** *see* Measles, Mumps, and Rubella Vaccines (Combined) *on page 841*

♦ **Moban®** *see* Molindone *on page 931*

♦ **MOBIC®** *see* Meloxicam *on page 853*

♦ **Mobicox® (Can)** *see* Meloxicam *on page 853*

Modafinil *(moe DAF i nil)*

U.S. Brand Names Provigil®

Canadian Brand Names Alertec®; Provigil®

Therapeutic Category Central Nervous System Stimulant, Nonamphetamine

Use Improve wakefulness in patients with excessive daytime sleepiness associated with narcolepsy

Unlabeled/Investigational Use Attention-deficit/hyperactivity disorder (ADHD); treatment of fatigue in MS and other disorders

Restrictions C-IV

Pregnancy Risk Factor C

Pregnancy/Breast-Feeding Implications Currently, there are no studies in humans evaluating its teratogenicity. Embryotoxicity of modafinil has been observed in animal models at dosages above those employed therapeutically. As a result, it should be used cautiously during pregnancy and should be used only when the potential risk of drug therapy is outweighed by the drug's benefits. It remains unknown if modafinil is secreted into human milk and, therefore, should be used cautiously in nursing women.

Contraindications Hypersensitivity to modafinil or any component of the formulation

Warnings/Precautions History of angina, ischemic EKG changes, left ventricular hypertrophy, or clinically significant mitral valve prolapse in association with CNS stimulant use; caution should be exercised when modafinil is given to patients with a history of psychosis, recent history of myocardial infarction, and because it has not yet been adequately studied in patients with hypertension, periodic monitoring of hypertensive patients receiving modafinil may be appropriate; caution is warranted when operating machinery or driving, although functional impairment has not been demonstrated with modafinil, all CNS-active agents may alter judgment, thinking and/or motor skills. Efficacy of oral contraceptives may be reduced, therefore, use of alternative contraception should be considered. Stimulants may unmask tics in individuals with coexisting Tourette's syndrome.

Adverse Reactions Limited to reports equal to or greater than placebo-related events.

<10%:

Cardiovascular: Chest pain (2%), hypertension (2%), hypotension (2%), vasodilation (1%), arrhythmia (1%), syncope (1%)

Central nervous system: Headache (50%, compared to 40% with placebo), nervousness (8%), dizziness (5%), depression (4%), anxiety (4%), cataplexy (3%), insomnia (3%), chills (2%), fever (1%), confusion (1%), amnesia (1%), emotional lability (1%), ataxia (1%)

Dermatologic: Dry skin (1%)

Endocrine & metabolic: Hyperglycemia (1%), albuminuria (1%)

Gastrointestinal: Diarrhea (8%), nausea (13%, compared to 4% with placebo), xerostomia (5%), anorexia (5%), vomiting (1%), mouth ulceration (1%), gingivitis (1%)

Genitourinary: Abnormal urine (1%), urinary retention (1%), ejaculatory disturbance (1%)

Hematologic: Eosinophilia (1%)

Hepatic: Abnormal LFTs (3%)

Neuromuscular & skeletal: Paresthesias (3%), dyskinesia (2%), neck pain (2%), hypertonia (2%), neck rigidity (1%), joint disorder (1%), tremor (1%)

Ocular: Amblyopia (2%), abnormal vision (2%)

Respiratory: Pharyngitis (6%), rhinitis (11%, compared to 8% with placebo), lung disorder (4%), dyspnea (2%), asthma (1%), epistaxis (1%)

Overdosage/Toxicology Signs and symptoms of overdose include agitation, irritability, aggressiveness, confusion, nervousness, tremor, sleep disturbance, palpitations, decreased prothrombin time, and slight-to-moderate elevations of hemodynamic parameters. Treatment is symptomatic and supportive. There is no data to suggest the utility of dialysis or urinary pH alteration in enhancing elimination. Cardiac monitoring is warranted.

Drug Interactions

Cytochrome P450 Effect: CYP3A3/4 enzyme substrate; CYP1A2, 2B6, and 3A3/4 enzyme inducer (weak); CYP2C19 enzyme inhibitor

Increased Effect/Toxicity: Modafinil may increase levels of diazepam, mephenytoin, phenytoin, propranolol, and warfarin. In populations deficient in the CYP2D6 isoenzyme, where CYP2C19 acts as a secondary metabolic pathway, concentrations of tricyclic antidepressants and selective serotonin reuptake inhibitors may be increased during coadministration.

Decreased Effect: Modafinil may decrease serum concentrations of oral contraceptives, cyclosporine, and to a lesser degree, theophylline. Agents that induce CYP3A4, including phenobarbital, carbamazepine, and rifampin may result in decreased modafinil levels. There is also evidence to suggest that modafinil may induce its own metabolism.

Mechanism of Action The exact mechanism of action is unclear, it does not appear to alter the release of dopamine or norepinephrine, it may exert its stimulant effects by decreasing GABA-mediated neurotransmission, although this theory has not yet been fully evaluated; several studies also suggest that an intact central alpha-adrenergic system is required for modafinil's activity; the drug increases high-frequency alpha waves while decreasing both delta and theta wave activity, and these effects are consistent with generalized increases in mental alertness

Pharmacodynamics/Kinetics Modafinil is a racemic compound (10% *d*-isomer and 90% *l*-isomer at steady state), whose enantiomers have different pharmacokinetics

Distribution: V_d: 0.9 L/kg

Protein binding: 60%, mostly to albumin

Metabolism: Hepatic; multiple pathways including CYP3A3/4

Half-life elimination: Effective half-life: 15 hours; time to steady-state: 2-4 days

Time to peak, serum: 2-4 hours

Excretion: Urine (as metabolites, <10% as unchanged drug)

Usual Dosage

Children: ADHD (unlabeled use): 50-100 mg once daily

Adults:

ADHD (unlabeled use): 100-300 mg once daily

Narcolepsy: Initial: 200 mg as a single daily dose in the morning

Doses of 400 mg/day, given as a single dose, have been well tolerated, but there is no consistent evidence that this dose confers additional benefit

Elderly: Elimination of modafinil and its metabolites may be reduced as a consequence of aging and as a result, lower doses should be considered

Dosing adjustment in renal impairment: Inadequate data to determine safety and efficacy in severe renal impairment

Dosing adjustment in hepatic impairment: Dose should be reduced to one-half of that recommended for patients with normal liver function

Patient Information Take during the day to avoid insomnia; may cause dependence with prolonged use; patients should be reminded to notify their physician if they become pregnant, intend to become pregnant, or are breast-feeding an infant; patients should be advised that combined use with alcohol has not been studied and that it is prudent to avoid this combination. Patients should notify their physician and/or pharmacist of any concomitant medications they are taking, due to the drug interaction potential this might represent.

Dosage Forms Tablet: 100 mg, 200 mg

♦ **Modane® Bulk [OTC]** *see* Psyllium *on page 1158*

♦ **Modane® Soft [OTC]** *see* Docusate *on page 430*

♦ **Modecate® (Can)** *see* Fluphenazine *on page 581*

♦ **Modicon®** *see* Ethinyl Estradiol and Norethindrone *on page 522*

♦ **Modified Dakin's Solution** *see* Sodium Hypochlorite Solution *on page 1248*

♦ **Modified Shohl's Solution** *see* Sodium Citrate and Citric Acid *on page 1246*

♦ **Moditen® Enanthate (Can)** *see* Fluphenazine *on page 581*

♦ **Moditen® HCl (Can)** *see* Fluphenazine *on page 581*

♦ **Moduret® (Can)** *see* Amiloride and Hydrochlorothiazide *on page 71*

♦ **Moduretic®** *see* Amiloride and Hydrochlorothiazide *on page 71*

Moexipril (mo EKS i pril)

Related Information

Angiotensin Agents Comparison *on page 1473*

U.S. Brand Names Univasc®

Synonyms Moexipril Hydrochloride

Therapeutic Category Angiotensin-Converting Enzyme (ACE) Inhibitor; Antihypertensive Agent

Use Treatment of hypertension, alone or in combination with thiazide diuretics; treatment of left ventricular dysfunction after myocardial infarction

Pregnancy Risk Factor C/D (2nd and 3rd trimesters)

(Continued)

Moexipril *(Continued)*

Contraindications Hypersensitivity to moexipril, moexiprilat, or any component of the formulation; hypersensitivity or allergic reactions or angioedema related to previous treatment with an ACE inhibitor; pregnancy (2nd or 3rd trimester)

Warnings/Precautions Do not administer in pregnancy; use with caution and modify dosage in patients with renal impairment especially renal artery stenosis, severe congestive heart failure, or with coadministered diuretic therapy; experience in children is limited. Severe hypotension may occur in patients who are sodium and/or volume depleted; initiate lower doses and monitor closely when starting therapy in these patients; ACE inhibitors may be preferred agents in elderly patients with congestive heart failure and diabetes mellitus (diabetic proteinuria is reduced, minimal CNS effects, and enhanced insulin sensitivity), however due to decreased renal function, tolerance must be carefully monitored; if possible, discontinue the diuretic 2-3 days prior to initiating moexipril in patients receiving them to reduce the risk of symptomatic hypotension.

Anaphylactic reactions can occur. Angioedema can occur at any time during treatment (especially following first dose). Use with caution in collagen vascular diseases; valvular stenosis (particularly aortic stenosis); hyperkalemia; or before, during, or immediately after anesthesia. Avoid rapid dosage escalation which may lead to renal insufficiency. Neutropenia/agranulocytosis with myeloid hyperplasia can rarely occur. If patient has renal impairment then a baseline WBC with differential and serum creatinine should be evaluated and monitored closely during the first 3 months of therapy. Hypersensitivity reactions may be seen during hemodialysis with high-flux dialysis membranes (eg, AN69). Deterioration in renal function can occur with initiation.

Adverse Reactions
1% to 10%:
Cardiovascular: Hypotension, peripheral edema
Central nervous system: Headache, dizziness, fatigue
Dermatologic: Rash, alopecia, flushing, rash
Endocrine & metabolic: Hyperkalemia, hyponatremia
Gastrointestinal: Diarrhea, nausea, heartburn
Genitourinary: Polyuria
Neuromuscular & skeletal: Myalgia
Renal: Reversible increases in creatinine or BUN
Respiratory: Cough, pharyngitis, upper respiratory infection, sinusitis
<1% (Limited to important or life-threatening): Alopecia, anemia, arrhythmias, bronchospasm, cerebrovascular accident, chest pain, dyspnea, elevated LFTs, eosinophilic pneumonitis, hepatitis, hypercholesterolemia, myocardial infarction, oliguria, orthostatic hypotension, palpitations, proteinuria, syncope

Overdosage/Toxicology Mild hypotension has been the only toxic effect seen with acute overdose; bradycardia may also occur. Hyperkalemia occurs even with therapeutic doses, especially in patients with renal insufficiency and those taking NSAIDs. Following initiation of essential overdose management, toxic symptom and supportive treatment should be initiated. Hypotension usually responds to I.V. fluids or Trendelenburg positioning.

Drug Interactions
Increased Effect/Toxicity: Potassium supplements, co-trimoxazole (high dose), angiotensin II receptor antagonists (candesartan, losartan, irbesartan, etc) or potassium-sparing diuretics (amiloride, spironolactone, triamterene) may result in elevated serum potassium levels when combined with moexipril. ACE inhibitor effects may be increased by probenecid (increases levels of captopril). ACE inhibitors may increase serum concentrations/effects of digoxin, lithium, and sulfonlyureas.

Diuretics have additive hypotensive effects with ACE inhibitors, and hypovolemia increases the potential for adverse renal effects of ACE inhibitors. In patients with compromised renal function, coadministration with nonsteroidal anti-inflammatory drugs may result in further deterioration of renal function. Allopurinol and ACE inhibitors may cause a higher risk of hypersensitivity reaction when taken concurrently.

Decreased Effect: Aspirin (high dose) may reduce the therapeutic effects of ACE inhibitors; at low dosages this does not appear to be significant. Rifampin may decrease the effect of ACE inhibitors. Antacids may decrease the bioavailability of ACE inhibitors (may be more likely to occur with captopril); separate administration times by 1-2 hours. NSAIDs, specifically indomethacin, may reduce the hypotensive effects of ACE inhibitors. More likely to occur in low renin or volume dependent hypertensive patients.

Ethanol/Nutrition/Herb Interactions
Food: Food may delay and reduce peak serum levels.
Herb/Nutraceutical: Avoid dong quai if using for hypertension (has estrogenic activity). Avoid ephedra, yohimbe, ginseng (may worsen hypertension). Avoid garlic (may have increased antihypertensive effect).

Mechanism of Action Competitive inhibitor of angiotensin-converting enzyme (ACE); prevents conversion of angiotensin I to angiotensin II, a potent vasoconstrictor; results in lower levels of angiotensin II which causes an increase in plasma renin activity and a reduction in aldosterone secretion

Pharmacodynamics/Kinetics
Onset of action: Peak effect: 1-2 hours
Duration: >24 hours
Distribution: V_d (moexiprilat): 180 L
Protein binding, plasma: Moexipril: 90%; Moexiprilat: 50% to 70%
Metabolism: Parent drug: Hepatic and small intestine to moexiprilat, 1000 times more potent than parent
Bioavailability (moexiprilat): 13%; food decreases bioavailability (AUC decreased by ~40%)
Half-life elimination: Moexipril: 1 hour; Moexiprilat: 2-9 hours
Time to peak: 1.5 hours
Excretion: Feces (50%)

Usual Dosage Adults: Oral: Initial: 7.5 mg once daily (in patients **not** receiving diuretics), 1 hour prior to a meal **or** 3.75 mg once daily (when combined with thiazide diuretics); maintenance dose: 7.5-30 mg/day in 1 or 2 divided doses 1 hour before meals

Dosing adjustment in renal impairment: $Cl_{cr} \leq 40$ mL/minute: Patients may be cautiously placed on 3.75 mg once daily, then upwardly titrated to a maximum of 15 mg/day.

Dietary Considerations Administer on an empty stomach.

Monitoring Parameters Blood pressure, heart rate, electrolytes, CBC, symptoms of hypotension

Test Interactions Increases BUN, creatinine, potassium, positive Coombs' [direct]; decreases cholesterol (S); may cause false-positive results in urine acetone determinations using sodium nitroprusside reagent

Patient Information Food may delay and reduce peak serum levels; take on an empty stomach, if possible. Report swelling of the face, mouth, or tongue, rash, or difficulty breathing to your physician immediately; bothersome side effects such as cough, dizziness, diarrhea, tiredness, rash, headache, irregular heartbeat, anxiety, and flu-like symptoms should also be reported; avoid use of this medication if you are pregnant or have had a previous reaction to other ACE inhibitors.

Nursing Implications Observe for symptoms of severe hypotension, especially within the first 2 hours following the initial dose or subsequent increases in dose as well as for signs of hyperkalemia or cough; administer on an empty stomach

Dosage Forms Tablet, as hydrochloride: 7.5 mg, 15 mg

Moexipril and Hydrochlorothiazide
(mo EKS i pril & hye droe klor oh THYE a zide)

U.S. Brand Names Uniretic™

Canadian Brand Names Uniretic™

Synonyms Hydrochlorothiazide and Moexipril

Therapeutic Category Angiotensin-Converting Enzyme (ACE) Inhibitor Combination; Antihypertensive Agent, Combination; Diuretic, Thiazide

Use Combination therapy for hypertension, however, not indicated for initial treatment of hypertension; replacement therapy in patients receiving separate dosage forms (for patient convenience); when monotherapy with one component fails to achieve desired antihypertensive effect, or when dose-limiting adverse effects limit upward titration of monotherapy

Pregnancy Risk Factor C/D (2nd and 3rd trimesters)

Usual Dosage Adults: Oral: 7.5-30 mg of moexipril, taken either in a single or divided dose one hour before meals; hydrochlorothiazide dose should be ≤ 50 mg/day

Additional Information Complete prescribing information for this medication should be consulted for additional detail.

Dosage Forms
Tablet:
Moexipril hydrochloride 7.5 mg and hydrochlorothiazide 12.5 mg
Moexipril hydrochloride 15 mg and hydrochlorothiazide 25 mg

♦ **Moexipril Hydrochloride** *see* Moexipril *on page 929*

Molindone (moe LIN done)
Related Information
Antipsychotic Agents Comparison *on page 1486*

U.S. Brand Names Moban®

Canadian Brand Names Moban®

Synonyms Molindone Hydrochloride

Therapeutic Category Antipsychotic Agent, Miscellaneous

Use Management of schizophrenia

Unlabeled/Investigational Use Management of psychotic disorders

Pregnancy Risk Factor C

Contraindications Hypersensitivity to molindone or any component of the formulation (cross-reactivity between phenothiazines may occur); severe CNS depression; coma

Warnings/Precautions May be sedating, use with caution in disorders where CNS depression is a feature. Use with caution in Parkinson's disease. Caution in patients with hemodynamic instability; bone marrow suppression; predisposition to seizures; subcortical brain damage; severe cardiac, hepatic, renal, or respiratory disease. Esophageal dysmotility and aspiration have been associated with antipsychotic use - use with caution in patients at risk of pneumonia (ie, Alzheimer's disease). Caution in breast cancer or other prolactin-dependent tumors (may elevate prolactin levels). May alter temperature regulation or mask toxicity of other drugs due to antiemetic effects. May alter cardiac conduction; life-threatening arrhythmias have occurred with therapeutic doses of neuroleptics. May cause orthostatic hypotension - use with caution in patients at risk of this effect or those who would tolerate transient hypotensive episodes (cerebrovascular disease, cardiovascular disease, or other medications which may predispose).

May cause anticholinergic effects (confusion, agitation, constipation, dry mouth, blurred vision, urinary retention); therefore, they should be used with caution in patients with decreased gastrointestinal motility, urinary retention, BPH, xerostomia, or visual problems. Conditions which also may be exacerbated by cholinergic blockade include narrow-angle glaucoma (screening is recommended) and worsening of myasthenia gravis. Relative to other neuroleptics, molindone has a low potency of cholinergic blockade.

May cause extrapyramidal reactions, including pseudoparkinsonism, acute dystonic reactions, akathisia, and tardive dyskinesia (risk of these reactions is moderate-high relative to other neuroleptics). May be associated with neuroleptic malignant syndrome (NMS) or pigmentary retinopathy.

Adverse Reactions Frequency not defined.
Cardiovascular: Orthostatic hypotension, tachycardia, arrhythmias
(Continued)

931

Molindone *(Continued)*

Central nervous system: Extrapyramidal reactions (akathisia, pseudoparkinsonism, dystonia, tardive dyskinesia), mental depression, altered central temperature regulation, sedation, drowsiness, restlessness, anxiety, hyperactivity, euphoria, seizures, neuroleptic malignant syndrome (NMS)

Dermatologic: Pruritus, rash, photosensitivity

Endocrine & metabolic: Change in menstrual periods, edema of breasts, amenorrhea, galactorrhea, gynecomastia

Gastrointestinal: Constipation, xerostomia, nausea, salivation, weight gain (minimal compared to other antipsychotics), weight loss

Genitourinary: Urinary retention, priapism

Hematologic: Leukopenia, leukocytosis

Ocular: Blurred vision, retinal pigmentation

Miscellaneous: Diaphoresis (decreased)

Overdosage/Toxicology Symptoms include deep sleep, extrapyramidal symptoms, cardiac arrhythmias, seizures, and hypotension. Following initiation of essential overdose management, toxic symptom and supportive treatment should be initiated. Hypotension usually responds to I.V. fluids or Trendelenburg positioning. If unresponsive to these measures, the use of a parenteral inotrope may be required (eg, norepinephrine 0.1-0.2 mcg/kg/minute titrated to response). Seizures commonly respond to diazepam (I.V. 5-10 mg bolus in adults every 15 minutes, if needed up to a total of 30 mg; I.V. 0.25-0.4 mg/kg/dose up to a total of 10 mg in children) or to phenytoin or phenobarbital. Critical cardiac arrhythmias often respond to I.V. phenytoin (15 mg/kg up to 1 g), while other antiarrhythmics can be used. Neuroleptics often cause extrapyramidal symptoms (eg, dystonic reactions) requiring management with diphenhydramine 1-2 mg/kg (adults), up to a maximum of 50 mg I.M. or slow I.V. push, followed by a maintenance dose for 48-72 hours. When these reactions are unresponsive to diphenhydramine, anticholinergic agents such as benztropine mesylate I.V. 1-2 mg (adults) may be effective. These agents are generally effective within 2-5 minutes.

Drug Interactions

Cytochrome P450 Effect: CYP2D6 enzyme substrate

Increased Effect/Toxicity: Molindone concentrations may be increased by chloroquine, propranolol, sulfadoxine-pyrimethamine. Molindone may increase the effect and/or toxicity of antihypertensives, lithium, TCAs, CNS depressants (ethanol, narcotics), and trazodone.

Decreased Effect: Antipsychotics inhibit the activity of bromocriptine and levodopa. Benztropine (and other anticholinergics) may inhibit the therapeutic response to molindone and excess anticholinergic effects may occur. Barbiturates and cigarette smoking may enhance the hepatic metabolism of molindone. Molindone and possibly other low potency antipsychotic may reverse the pressor effects of epinephrine.

Ethanol/Nutrition/Herb Interactions

Ethanol: Avoid ethanol (may increase CNS depression).

Herb/Nutraceutical: Avoid kava kava, gotu kola, valerian, St John's wort (may increase CNS depression).

Stability Protect from light; dispense in amber or opaque vials

Mechanism of Action Mechanism of action mimics that of chlorpromazine; however, it produces more extrapyramidal symptoms and less sedation than chlorpromazine

Pharmacodynamics/Kinetics

Metabolism: Hepatic

Half-life elimination: 1.5 hours

Time to peak, serum: ~1.5 hours

Excretion: Primarily urine and feces (90%) within 24 hours

Usual Dosage Oral:

Children: Schizophrenia/psychoses:

3-5 years: 1-2.5 mg/day in 4 divided doses

5-12 years: 0.5-1 mg/kg/day in 4 divided doses

Adults: Schizophrenia/psychoses: 50-75 mg/day increase at 3- to 4-day intervals up to 225 mg/day

Elderly: Behavioral symptoms associated with dementia: Initial: 5-10 mg 1-2 times/day; increase at 4- to 7-day intervals by 5-10 mg/day; increase dosing intervals (bid, tid, etc) as necessary to control response or side effects.

Monitoring Parameters Monitor blood pressure and pulse rate prior to and during initial therapy; evaluate mental status

Patient Information Dry mouth may be helped by sips of water, sugarless gum or hard candy; avoid alcohol; very important to maintain established dosage regimen; photosensitivity to sunlight can occur, do not discontinue abruptly; full effect may not occur for 3-4 weeks; full dosage may be taken at bedtime to avoid daytime sedation; report to physician any involuntary movements or feelings of restlessness

Nursing Implications May increase appetite and possibly a craving for sweets; recognize signs of neuroleptic malignant syndrome and tardive dyskinesia

Additional Information Coadministration of two or more antipsychotics does not improve clinical response and may increase the potential for adverse effects.

Dosage Forms

Solution, oral concentrate, as hydrochloride: 20 mg/mL (120 mL)

Tablet, as hydrochloride: 5 mg, 10 mg, 25 mg, 50 mg, 100 mg

♦ **Molindone Hydrochloride** *see* Molindone *on page 931*

♦ **Mollifene® Ear Wax Removing Formula [OTC]** *see* Carbamide Peroxide *on page 224*

♦ **MOM** *see* Magnesium Hydroxide *on page 832*

Mometasone Furoate *(moe MET a sone FYOOR oh ate)*

Related Information

Corticosteroids Comparison *on page 1495*

U.S. Brand Names Elocon®; Nasonex®

Canadian Brand Names Elocom®; Nasonex®

Therapeutic Category Corticosteroid, Topical (Medium Potency)
Use Relief of the inflammatory and pruritic manifestations of corticosteroid-responsive dermatoses (medium potency topical corticosteroid); treatment of nasal symptoms of seasonal and
perennial rhinitis in adults and children ≥3 years of age; prevention of nasal symptoms
associated with seasonal allergic rhinitis in children ≥12 years of age and adults
Pregnancy Risk Factor C
Contraindications Hypersensitivity to mometasone or any component of the formulation;
fungal, viral, or tubercular skin lesions, herpes simplex or zoster
Warnings/Precautions Adverse systemic effects may occur when used on large areas of the
body, denuded areas, for prolonged periods of time, with an occlusive dressing, and/or in
infants or small children
Adverse Reactions <1% (Limited to important or life-threatening): Allergic dermatitis,
anaphylaxis and angioedema (reported with inhalation), Cushing's syndrome, growth retardation, HPA suppression, hypopigmentation, maceration of the skin, skin atrophy
Mechanism of Action May depress the formation, release, and activity of endogenous
chemical mediators of inflammation (kinins, histamine, liposomal enzymes, prostaglandins).
Leukocytes and macrophages may have to be present for the initiation of responses mediated by the above substances. Inhibits the margination and subsequent cell migration to the
area of injury, and also reverses the dilatation and increased vessel permeability in the area
resulting in decreased access of cells to the sites of injury.
Usual Dosage
    Nasal spray:
        Children 3-12 years: 1 spray in each nostril daily
        Children ≥12 years and Adults: 2 sprays in each nostril daily
    Topical: Adults: Apply sparingly to area once daily, do not use occlusive dressings. Therapy
        should be discontinued when control is achieved; if no improvement is seen, reassessment
        of diagnosis may be necessary.
Patient Information Before applying, gently wash area to reduce risk of infection; apply a thin
film to cleansed area and rub in gently and thoroughly until medication vanishes; avoid
exposure to sunlight, severe sunburn may occur
Nursing Implications For external use only; do not use on open wounds; should not be used
in the presence of open or weeping lesions; use sparingly
Dosage Forms
    Cream, topical: 0.1% (15 g, 45 g)
    Lotion, topical: 0.1% (30 mL, 60 mL)
    Ointment, topical: 0.1% (15 g, 45 g)
    Suspension, intranasal [spray]: 50 mcg/spray (17 g)

- **MOM/Mineral Oil Emulsion** *see* Magnesium Hydroxide and Mineral Oil Emulsion *on page 833*
- **Monacolin K** *see* Lovastatin *on page 825*
- **Monafed®** *see* Guaifenesin *on page 645*
- **Monafed® DM** *see* Guaifenesin and Dextromethorphan *on page 646*
- **Monarc® M** *see* Antihemophilic Factor (Human) *on page 102*
- **Monazole-7 (Can)** *see* Miconazole *on page 908*
- **Monistat® (Can)** *see* Miconazole *on page 908*
- **Monistat® 1 Combination Pack [OTC]** *see* Miconazole *on page 908*
- **Monistat® 3 [OTC]** *see* Miconazole *on page 908*
- **Monistat® 7 [OTC]** *see* Miconazole *on page 908*
- **Monistat-Derm®** *see* Miconazole *on page 908*
- **Monitan® (Can)** *see* Acebutolol *on page 21*
- **Monoclate-P®** *see* Antihemophilic Factor (Human) *on page 102*
- **Monoclonal Antibody** *see* Muromonab-CD3 *on page 941*
- **Monocor® (Can)** *see* Bisoprolol *on page 172*
- **Monodox®** *see* Doxycycline *on page 448*
- **Monoethanolamine** *see* Ethanolamine Oleate *on page 508*
- **Mono-Gesic®** *see* Salsalate *on page 1220*
- **Monoket®** *see* Isosorbide Mononitrate *on page 751*
- **Mononine®** *see* Factor IX (Purified/Human) *on page 540*
- **Monopril®** *see* Fosinopril *on page 607*

Montelukast (mon te LOO kast)

U.S. Brand Names Singulair®
Canadian Brand Names Singulair®
Synonyms Montelukast Sodium
Therapeutic Category Leukotriene Receptor Antagonist
Use Prophylaxis and chronic treatment of asthma in adults and children ≥2 years of age
Pregnancy Risk Factor B
Contraindications Hypersensitivity to montelukast or any component of the formulation
Warnings/Precautions Montelukast is not indicated for use in the reversal of bronchospasm
in acute asthma attacks, including status asthmaticus. Should not be used as monotherapy
for the treatment and management of exercise-induced bronchospasm. Advise patients to
have appropriate rescue medication available. Appropriate clinical monitoring and caution are
recommended when systemic corticosteroid reduction is considered in patients receiving
montelukast. Inform phenylketonuric patients that the chewable tablet contains phenylalanine.

In rare cases, patients on therapy with montelukast may present with systemic eosinophilia,
sometimes presenting with clinical features of vasculitis consistent with Churg-Strauss
syndrome, a condition which is often treated with systemic corticosteroid therapy. See
Adverse Reactions.
(Continued)

Montelukast *(Continued)*

Adverse Reactions

>10%: Central nervous system: Headache (18%)

1% to 10%:

Central nervous system: Dizziness (2%), fatigue (2%), fever (2%)

Dermatologic: Rash (2%)

Gastrointestinal: Dyspepsia (2%), dental pain (2%), gastroenteritis (2%), abdominal pain (3%)

Neuromuscular & skeletal: Weakness (2%)

Respiratory: Cough (3%), nasal congestion (2%)

Miscellaneous: Flu-like symptoms (4%), trauma (1%)

<1% (Limited to important or life-threatening): Anaphylaxis, angioedema, Churg-Strauss syndrome (systemic eosinophilia vasculitis), hepatic eosinophilic infiltration (rare), myalgia, pancreatitis, pruritus, seizures

Overdosage/Toxicology There is no specific antidote. Remove unabsorbed material from the GI tract, employ clinical monitoring and institute supportive therapy if required.

Drug Interactions

Cytochrome P450 Effect: CYP2A6, 2C9, and 3A3/4 enzyme substrate

Decreased Effect: Phenobarbital decreases montelukast area under the curve by 40%. Clinical significance is uncertain. Rifampin may increase the metabolism of montelukast similar to phenobarbital. No dosage adjustment is recommended when taking phenobarbital with montelukast.

Ethanol/Nutrition/Herb Interactions Herb/Nutraceutical: St John's wort may decrease montelukast levels.

Mechanism of Action Selective leukotriene receptor antagonist that inhibits the cysteinyl leukotriene receptor. Cysteinyl leukotrienes and leukotriene receptor occupation have been correlated with the pathophysiology of asthma, including airway edema, smooth muscle contraction, and altered cellular activity associated with the inflammatory process, which contribute to the signs and symptoms of asthma.

Pharmacodynamics/Kinetics

Duration: >24 hours

Distribution: V_d: 8-11 L

Protein binding, plasma: >99%

Metabolism: Extensively hepatic via CYP3A4 and 2C9

Bioavailability: Tablet: 10 mg: Mean: 64%; 5 mg: 63% to 73%

Half-life elimination, plasma: Mean: 2.7-5.5 hours

Time to peak, serum: Tablet: 10 mg: 3-4 hours; 5 mg: 2-2.5 hours

Excretion: Feces (86%); urine (<0.2%)

Usual Dosage Oral:

Children:

<2 years: Safety and efficacy have not been established

2-5 years: Chew one 4 mg chewable tablet/day, taken in the evening

6 to 14 years: Chew one 5 mg chewable tablet/day, taken in the evening

Children ≥15 years and Adults: 10 mg/day, taken in the evening

Dosing adjustment in hepatic impairment: Mild moderate: No adjustment necessary

Dietary Considerations Tablet, chewable: 4 mg strength contains phenylalanine 0.674 mg; 5 mg strength contains phenylalanine 0.842 mg

Patient Information Advise patients to take montelukast daily as prescribed, even when they are symptomatic, as well as during periods of worsening asthma, and to contact physician if the asthma is not well controlled. Advise patients that oral tablets of montelukast are not for the treatment of acute asthma attacks. Patients should have appropriate short-acting inhaled beta-agonist medication available to treat asthma exacerbations.

Advise patients using montelukast to seek medical attention if short-acting inhaled bronchodilators are needed more often than usual or if more than the maximum number of inhalations of short-acting bronchodilator treatment prescribed for a 24-hour period are needed. Instruct patients receiving montelukast not to decrease the dose or to stop taking any other antiasthma medications unless instructed by a physician.

Instruct patients who have exacerbations of asthma after exercise to continue to use their usual regimen of inhaled beta-agonists as prophylaxis unless otherwise instructed by a physician. All patients should have a short-acting inhaled beta-agonist available for rescue.

Phenylketonurics: Chewable tablets contain phenylalanine.

Dosage Forms

Tablet, as sodium: 10 mg

Tablet, chewable, as sodium: 4 mg [cherry flavor] [contains phenylalanine 0.674 mg]; 5 mg [cherry flavor] [contains phenylalanine 0.842 mg]

♦ **Montelukast Sodium** *see Montelukast on page 933*

♦ **Monurol™** *see Fosfomycin on page 606*

♦ **8-MOP®** *see Methoxsalen on page 889*

♦ **More Attenuated Enders Strain** *see Measles Virus Vaccine (Live) on page 842*

♦ **MoreDophilus® [OTC]** *see Lactobacillus on page 770*

Moricizine *(mor I siz een)*

Related Information

Antiarrhythmic Drugs Comparison *on page 1478*

U.S. Brand Names Ethmozine®

Canadian Brand Names Ethmozine®

Synonyms Moricizine Hydrochloride

Therapeutic Category Antiarrhythmic Agent, Class I

Use Treatment of ventricular tachycardia and life-threatening ventricular arrhythmias

Unlabeled/Investigational Use PVCs, complete and nonsustained ventricular tachycardia, atrial arrhythmias

Pregnancy Risk Factor B

Contraindications Hypersensitivity to moricizine or any component of the formulation; pre-existing second- or third-degree AV block (except in patients with a functioning artificial pacemaker); right bundle branch block when associated with left hemiblock or bifascicular block (unless functional pacemaker in place); cardiogenic shock

Warnings/Precautions Considering the known proarrhythmic properties and lack of evidence of improved survival for any antiarrhythmic drug in patients without life-threatening arrhythmias, it is prudent to reserve the use for patients with life-threatening ventricular arrhythmias; CAST II trial demonstrated a trend towards decreased survival for patients treated with moricizine; proarrhythmic effects occur as with other antiarrhythmic agents; hypokalemia, hyperkalemia, hypomagnesemia may effect response to class I agents; use with caution in patients with sick-sinus syndrome, hepatic, and renal impairment; safety and efficacy have not been established in pediatric patients

Adverse Reactions

>10%: Central nervous system: Dizziness

1% to 10%:

Cardiovascular: Proarrhythmia, palpitations, cardiac death, EKG abnormalities, congestive heart failure

Central nervous system: Headache, fatigue, insomnia

Endocrine & metabolic: Decreased libido

Gastrointestinal: Nausea, diarrhea, ileus

Ocular: Blurred vision, periorbital edema

Respiratory: Dyspnea

<1% (Limited to important or life-threatening): Apnea, cardiac chest pain, hypotension or hypertension, myocardial infarction, supraventricular arrhythmias, syncope, ventricular tachycardia

Overdosage/Toxicology Has a narrow therapeutic index and severe toxicity may occur slightly above the therapeutic range, especially if combined with other antiarrhythmic drugs. Acute single ingestion of twice the daily therapeutic dose is life-threatening. Symptoms include increased PR, QRS, and QT intervals, amplitude of the T wave, A-V block, bradycardia, hypotension, ventricular arrhythmias (monomorphic or polymorphic ventricular tachycardia), and asystole. Other symptoms include dizziness, blurred vision, headache, and GI upset. Treatment is supportive, using conventional treatment (fluids, positioning, anticonvulsants, antiarrhythmics). **Note:** Type Ia antiarrhythmic agents should not be used to treat cardiotoxicity caused by type 1c antiarrhythmic drugs. Sodium bicarbonate may reverse QRS prolongation, bradycardia and hypotension. Ventricular pacing may be needed.

Drug Interactions

Cytochrome P450 Effect: May act an inhibitor of CYP1A2; may be a substrate for CYP isoenzymes

Increased Effect/Toxicity: Moricizine levels may be increased by cimetidine and diltiazem. Digoxin may result in additive prolongation of the PR interval when combined with moricizine (but not rate of second- and third-degree AV block). Drugs which may prolong QT interval (including cisapride, erythromycin, phenothiazines, cyclic antidepressants, and some quinolones) are contraindicated with type Ia antiarrhythmics. Moricizine has some type Ia activity, and caution should be used.

Decreased Effect: Moricizine may decrease levels of theophylline (50%) and diltiazem.

Ethanol/Nutrition/Herb Interactions Food: Moricizine peak serum concentrations may be decreased if taken with food.

Mechanism of Action Class I antiarrhythmic agent; reduces the fast inward current carried by sodium ions, shortens Phase I and Phase II repolarization, resulting in decreased action potential duration and effective refractory period

Pharmacodynamics/Kinetics

Protein binding, plasma: 95%

Metabolism: Significant first-pass effect; some enterohepatic recycling

Bioavailability: 38%

Half-life elimination: Normal patients: 3-4 hours; Cardiac disease: 6-13 hours

Excretion: Feces (56%); urine (39%)

Usual Dosage Adults: Oral: 200-300 mg every 8 hours, adjust dosage at 150 mg/day at 3-day intervals.

Recommendations for transferring patients from other antiarrhythmic agents to Ethmozine®: See table.

Moricizine

Transferred From	Start Ethmozine®
Encainide, propafenone, tocainide, or mexiletine	8-12 hours after last dose
Flecainide	12-24 hours after last dose
Procainamide	3-6 hours after last dose
Quinidine, disopyramide	6-12 hours after last dose

Dosing interval in renal or hepatic impairment: Start at 600 mg/day or less.

Dietary Considerations Best if taken on an empty stomach.

Patient Information Take as directed; do not change dose except from advice of your physician; report any chest pain and irregular heartbeats

Nursing Implications Administering 30 minutes after a meal delays the rate of absorption, resulting in lower peak plasma concentrations

Dosage Forms Tablet, as hydrochloride: 200 mg, 250 mg, 300 mg

♦ **Moricizine Hydrochloride** see Moricizine on page 934

♦ **Morning After Pill** see Ethinyl Estradiol and Norgestrel on page 528

♦ **Morphine HP® (Can)** see Morphine Sulfate on page 936

Morphine Sulfate (MOR feen SUL fate)

Related Information

Adult ACLS Algorithms *on page 1632*

Narcotic Agonists Comparison *on page 1506*

U.S. Brand Names Astramorph™ PF; Duramorph®; Infumorph™; Kadian™; MS Contin®; MSIR®; Oramorph SR™; RMS®; Roxanol™; Roxanol 100™; Roxanol Rescudose™; Roxanol™-T

Canadian Brand Names Kadian®; M-Eslon®; Morphine HP®; M.O.S.-Sulfate®; MS Contin®; MS-IR®; Oramorph SR®; Statex®

Synonyms MS

Therapeutic Category Analgesic, Narcotic

Use Relief of moderate to severe acute and chronic pain; relief of pain of myocardial infarction; relief of dyspnea of acute left ventricular failure and pulmonary edema; preanesthetic medication

Orphan drug: Infumorph™: Used in microinfusion devices for intraspinal administration in treatment of intractable chronic pain

Restrictions C-II

Pregnancy Risk Factor B/D (prolonged use or high doses at term)

Contraindications Hypersensitivity to morphine sulfate or any component of the formulation; increased intracranial pressure; severe respiratory depression (in absence of resuscitative equipment or ventilatory support); acute or severe asthma; known or suspected paralytic ileus (sustained release products only); sustained release products are not recommended in acute/postoperative pain; pregnancy (prolonged use or high doses at term)

Warnings/Precautions Some preparations contain sulfites which may cause allergic reactions; infants <3 months of age are more susceptible to respiratory depression, use with caution and generally in reduced doses in this age group; use with caution in patients with impaired respiratory function or severe hepatic dysfunction and in patients with hypersensitivity reactions to other phenanthrene derivative opioid agonists (codeine, hydrocodone, hydromorphone, levorphanol, oxycodone, oxymorphone). Morphine shares the toxic potential of opiate agonists and usual precautions of opiate agonist therapy should be observed; may cause hypotension in patients with acute myocardial infarction. Tolerance or drug dependence may result from extended use. MS Contin® 200 mg tablets are for use only in opioid-tolerant patients requiring >400 mg/day.

Elderly may be particularly susceptible to the CNS depressant and constipating effects of narcotics

Adverse Reactions Note: Percentages are based on a study in 19 chronic cancer pain patients (*J Pain Symptom Manage*, 1995, 10:416-22). Chronic use of various opioids in cancer pain is accompanied by similar adverse reactions; individual patient differences are unpredictable, and percentage may differ in acute pain (surgical) treatment.

Frequency not defined: Flushing, CNS depression, sedation, antidiuretic hormone release, physical and psychological dependence, diaphoresis

>10%:

Cardiovascular: Palpitations, hypotension, bradycardia

Central nervous system: Drowsiness (48%, tolerance usually develops to drowsiness with regular dosing for 1-2 weeks); dizziness (20%); confusion

Dermatologic: Pruritus (may be secondary to histamine release)

Gastrointestinal: Nausea (28%, tolerance usually develops to nausea and vomiting with chronic use); vomiting (9%); constipation (40%, tolerance develops very slowly if at all); xerostomia (78%)

Genitourinary: Urinary retention (16%)

Local: Pain at injection site

Neuromuscular & skeletal: Weakness

Miscellaneous: Histamine release

1% to 10%:

Central nervous system: Restlessness, headache, false feeling of well being

Gastrointestinal: Anorexia, GI irritation, paralytic ileus

Genitourinary: Decreased urination

Neuromuscular & skeletal: Trembling

Ocular: Vision problems

Respiratory: Respiratory depression, dyspnea

<1% (Limited to important or life-threatening): Anaphylaxis, biliary tract spasm, hallucinations, insomnia, intestinal obstruction, intracranial pressure increased, increased liver function tests, mental depression, miosis, muscle rigidity, paradoxical CNS stimulation, peripheral vasodilation, urinary tract spasm

Overdosage/Toxicology Symptoms include respiratory depression, miosis, hypotension, bradycardia, apnea, and pulmonary edema. Treatment includes airway support, establishment of an I.V. line, and administration of naloxone 2 mg I.V. (0.01 mg/kg for children), with repeat administration as necessary, up to a total of 10 mg. Primary attention should be directed to ensuring adequate respiratory exchange.

Drug Interactions

Cytochrome P450 Effect: CYP2D6 enzyme substrate

Increased Effect/Toxicity: CNS depressants (phenothiazines, tranquilizers, anxiolytics, sedatives, hypnotics, or alcohol), tricyclic antidepressants may potentiate the effects of morphine and other opiate agonists. Dextroamphetamine may enhance the analgesic effect of morphine and other opiate agonists. Concurrent use of MAO inhibitors and meperidine has been associated with significant adverse effects. Use caution with morphine. Some manufacturers recommend avoiding use within 14 days of MAO inhibitors.

Decreased Effect: Phenothiazines may antagonize the analgesic effect of morphine and other opiate agonists. Diuretic effects may be decreased (due to antidiuretic hormone release).

Ethanol/Nutrition/Herb Interactions

Ethanol: Avoid ethanol (may increase CNS depression).

Food: Administration of oral morphine solution with food may increase bioavailability (ie, a report of 34% increase in morphine AUC when morphine oral solution followed a high-fat meal). The bioavailability of Oramorph SR™ does not appear to be affected by food.

Herb/Nutraceutical: Avoid valerian, St John's wort, kava kava, gotu kola (may increase CNS depression).

Stability

Suppositories: Refrigerate suppositories; do not freeze.

Injection: Degradation depends on pH and presence of oxygen; relatively stable in pH ≤4; darkening of solutions indicate degradation. Usual concentration for continuous I.V. infusion = 0.1-1 mg/mL in D_5W

Mechanism of Action Binds to opiate receptors in the CNS, causing inhibition of ascending pain pathways, altering the perception of and response to pain; produces generalized CNS depression

Pharmacodynamics/Kinetics

Onset of action: Oral: 1 hour; I.V.: 5-10 minutes

Duration: Pain relief (not sustained/controlled/extended release forms): 4 hours

Bioavailability: Oral: 17% to 33% (first-pass effect limits oral bioavailability; oral:parenteral effectiveness reportedly varies from 1:6 in opioid naive patients to 1:3 with chronic use)

Distribution: Binds to opioid receptors in the CNS and periphery (eg, GI tract)

Metabolism: Hepatic via conjugation with glucuronic acid to morphine-3-glucuronide (inactive), morphine-6-glucuronide (active), and in lesser amounts, morphine-3-6-diglucuronide; other minor metabolites include normorphine (active) and the 3-ethereal sulfate

Half-life elimination: Adults: 2-4 hours (not sustained/controlled/extended release forms)

Excretion: Urine (primarily as morphine-3-glucuronide, ~2% to 12% excreted unchanged); feces (~7% to 10%). It has been suggested that accumulation of morphine-6-glucuronide might cause toxicity with renal insufficiency. All of the metabolites (ie, morphine-3-glucuronide, morphine-6-glucuronide, and normorphine) have been suggested as possible causes of neurotoxicity (eg, myoclonus).

Usual Dosage Doses should be titrated to appropriate effect; when changing routes of administration in chronically treated patients, please note that oral doses are approximately one-half as effective as parenteral dose

Infants and Children:

Oral: Tablet and solution (prompt release): 0.2-0.5 mg/kg/dose every 4-6 hours as needed; tablet (controlled release): 0.3-0.6 mg/kg/dose every 12 hours

I.M., I.V., S.C.: 0.1-0.2 mg/kg/dose every 2-4 hours as needed; usual maximum: 15 mg/dose; may initiate at 0.05 mg/kg/dose

I.V., S.C. continuous infusion: Sickle cell or cancer pain: 0.025-2 mg/kg/hour; postoperative pain: 0.01-0.04 mg/kg/hour

Sedation/analgesia for procedures: I.V.: 0.05-0.1 mg/kg 5 minutes before the procedure

Adolescents >12 years: Sedation/analgesia for procedures: I.V.: 3-4 mg and repeat in 5 minutes if necessary

Adults:

Oral: Prompt release: 10-30 mg every 4 hours as needed; controlled release: 15-30 mg every 8-12 hours

I.M., I.V., S.C.: 2.5-20 mg/dose every 2-6 hours as needed; usual: 10 mg/dose every 4 hours as needed

I.V., S.C. continuous infusion: 0.8-10 mg/hour; may increase depending on pain relief/adverse effects; usual range: up to 80 mg/hour

Epidural: Initial: 5 mg in lumbar region; if inadequate pain relief within 1 hour, administer 1-2 mg, maximum dose: 10 mg/24 hours

Intrathecal ($^1/_{10}$ of epidural dose): 0.2-1 mg/dose; repeat doses **not** recommended

Rectal: 10-20 mg every 4 hours

Elderly or debilitated patients: Use with caution; may require dose reduction

Dosing adjustment in renal impairment:

Cl_{cr} 10-50 mL/minute: Administer at 75% of normal dose

Cl_{cr} <10 mL/minute: Administer at 50% of normal dose

Dosing adjustment/comments in hepatic disease: Unchanged in mild liver disease; substantial extrahepatic metabolism may occur; excessive sedation may occur in cirrhosis

Dietary Considerations Morphine may cause GI upset; take with food if GI upset occurs. Be consistent when taking morphine with or without meals.

Administration

Oral: Do not crush controlled release drug product, swallow whole. Kadian™ can be opened and sprinkled on applesauce. Administration of oral morphine solution with food may increase bioavailability (not observed with Oramorph SR™).

I.V.: When giving morphine I.V. push, it is best to first dilute in 4-5 mL of sterile water, and then to administer slowly (eg, 15 mg over 3-5 minutes)

Epidural or intrathecal: Use preservative-free solutions

Monitoring Parameters Pain relief, respiratory and mental status, blood pressure

Reference Range Therapeutic: Surgical anesthesia: 65-80 ng/mL (SI: 227-280 nmol/L); Toxic: 200-5000 ng/mL (SI: 700-17,500 nmol/L)

Patient Information Avoid alcohol, may cause drowsiness, impaired judgment or coordination; may cause physical and psychological dependence with prolonged use

Nursing Implications Do not crush controlled release drug product; observe patient for excessive sedation, respiratory depression; implement safety measures, assist with ambulation; use preservative-free solutions for intrathecal or epidural use

Dosage Forms

Capsule (MSIR®): 15 mg, 30 mg

Capsule, sustained release (Kadian™): 20 mg, 30 mg, 50 mg, 60 mg, 100 mg

Injection: 0.5 mg/mL (30 mL); 1 mg/mL (10 mL, 30 mL, 50 mL, 60 mL); 2 mg/mL (1 mL, 60 mL); 4 mg/mL (1 mL); 5 mg/mL (1 mL, 30 mL, 50 mL); 8 mg/mL (1 mL); 10 mg/mL (1 mL, 10 mL, 20 mL); 15 mg/mL (1 mL, 20 mL); 25 mg/mL (4 mL, 10 mL, 20 mL, 40 mL, 50 mL); 50 mg/mL (10 mL, 20 mL, 40 mL, 50 mL)

Astramorph™ PF [preservative free]: 0.5 mg/mL (2 mL, 10 mL); 1 mg/mL (2 mL, 10 mL)

Infumorph™: 10 mg/mL (20 mL); 25 mg/mL (20 mL)

(Continued)

Morphine Sulfate *(Continued)*

    Duramorph® [preservative free]: 0.5 mg/mL (2 mL, 10 mL); 1 mg/mL (2 mL, 10 mL)
    Injection, I.V. infusion preparation: 25 mg/mL (4 mL, 10 mL, 20 mL)
    Injection, I.V. via PCA pump: 1 mg/mL (10 mL, 30 mL, 60 mL); 5 mg/mL (30 mL)
    Infusion: 0.2 mg/mL in D₅W (250 mL, 500 mL); 1 mg/mL in D₅W (100 mL, 250 mL, 500 mL)
    Solution, oral: 10 mg/5 mL (5 mL, 100 mL, 500 mL); 20 mg/5 mL (5 mL, 100 mL, 120 mL, 500 mL)
        MSIR®: 10 mg/5 mL (5 mL, 120 mL); 20 mg/5 mL (5 mL, 120 mL); 20 mg/mL (30 mL, 120 mL)
        Roxanol™: 20 mg/mL (30 mL, 120 mL)
        Roxanol™ T: 20 mg/mL (30 mL, 120 mL) [flavored] [tinted]
        Roxanol 100™: 100 mg/5 mL (240 mL) [with calibrated spoon]
    Suppository, rectal: 5 mg, 10 mg, 20 mg, 30 mg
        MS/S®, RMS®, Roxanol™: 5 mg, 10 mg, 20 mg, 30 mg
    Tablet: 15 mg, 30 mg
        MSIR®: 15 mg, 30 mg
    Tablet, controlled release: MS Contin®: 15 mg, 30 mg, 60 mg, 100 mg, 200 mg
    Tablet, extended release: 15 mg, 30 mg, 60 mg
    Tablet, sustained release (Oramorph SR™): 15 mg, 30 mg, 60 mg, 100 mg

Morrhuate Sodium *(MOR yoo ate SOW dee um)*

U.S. Brand Names Scleromate™

Therapeutic Category Sclerosing Agent

Use Treatment of small, uncomplicated varicose veins of the lower extremities

Pregnancy Risk Factor C

Contraindications Hypersensitivity to morrhuate sodium or any component of the formulation; arterial disease, thrombophlebitis

Warnings/Precautions Sloughing and necrosis of tissue may occur following extravasation; anaphylactoid and allergic reactions have occurred; this drug should only be administered by a physician familiar with proper injection techniques; a test dose of 0.25-5 mL of a 5% injection should be given 24 hours before full-dose treatment

Adverse Reactions Frequency not defined.
    Cardiovascular: Thrombosis, valvular incompetency, vascular collapse
    Central nervous system: Drowsiness, headache, dizziness
    Dermatologic: Urticaria
    Gastrointestinal: Nausea, vomiting
    Local: Burning at the site of injection, severe extravasation effects
    Neuromuscular & skeletal: Weakness
    Respiratory: Asthma
    Miscellaneous: Anaphylaxis, hypersensitivity reactions

Stability Refrigerate

Mechanism of Action Both varicose veins and esophageal varices are treated by the thrombotic action of morrhuate sodium. By causing inflammation of the vein's intima, a thrombus is formed. Occlusion secondary to the fibrous tissue and the thrombus results in the obliteration of the vein.

Pharmacodynamics/Kinetics
    Onset of action: ~5 minutes
    Absorption: Most stays at site of injection
    Distribution: Esophageal varices treatment: ~20% of dose to lungs

Usual Dosage Adults: I.V.: 50-250 mg, repeated at 5- to 7-day intervals (50-100 mg for small veins, 150-250 mg for large veins)

Administration For I.V. use only

Nursing Implications Avoid extravasation; use only clear solutions, solution should become clear when warmed

Dosage Forms Injection: 50 mg/mL (30 mL)

- ◆ **MoRu-Viraten Berna™ (Can)** *see* Measles and Rubella Vaccines (Combined) *on page 840*
- ◆ **M.O.S.-Sulfate® (Can)** *see* Morphine Sulfate *on page 936*
- ◆ **Motofen®** *see* Difenoxin and Atropine *on page 400*
- ◆ **Motrin®** *see* Ibuprofen *on page 697*
- ◆ **Motrin® (Children's) (Can)** *see* Ibuprofen *on page 697*
- ◆ **Motrin® IB [OTC]** *see* Ibuprofen *on page 697*
- ◆ **Motrin® Migraine Pain [OTC]** *see* Ibuprofen *on page 697*
- ◆ **Motrin® Sinus [OTC]** *see* Pseudoephedrine and Ibuprofen *on page 1157*

Moxifloxacin *(moxs i FLOKS a sin)*

Related Information
    Antacid Drug Interactions *on page 1477*
    Antimicrobial Drugs of Choice *on page 1588*
    Community-Acquired Pneumonia in Adults *on page 1603*

U.S. Brand Names ABC Pack™ (Avelox®); Avelox®

Canadian Brand Names Avelox®

Synonyms Moxifloxacin Hydrochloride

Therapeutic Category Antibiotic, Quinolone

Use Treatment of mild to moderate community-acquired pneumonia, acute bacterial exacerbation of chronic bronchitis, acute bacterial sinusitis, uncomplicated skin infections

Pregnancy Risk Factor C

Pregnancy/Breast-Feeding Implications No adequate or well-controlled studies in pregnant women. Should be used during pregnancy only when the potential benefit justifies the potential risk to the fetus. Moxifloxacin may be excreted in human breast milk. Breast-feeding is not recommended.

Contraindications Hypersensitivity to moxifloxacin, other quinolone antibiotics, or any component of the formulation

Warnings/Precautions Use with caution in patients with significant bradycardia or acute myocardial ischemia. Moxifloxacin causes a dose-dependent QT prolongation. Coadministration of moxifloxacin with other drugs that also prolong the QT interval or induce bradycardia (eg, beta-blockers, amiodarone) should be avoided. Careful consideration should be given in the use of moxifloxacin in patients with cardiovascular disease, particularly in those with conduction abnormalities. Use with caution in individuals at risk of seizures (CNS disorders or concurrent therapy with medications which may lower seizure threshold). Discontinue in patients who experience significant CNS adverse effects (dizziness, hallucinations, suicidal ideation or actions). Not recommended in patients with moderate to severe hepatic insufficiency. Use with caution in diabetes; glucose regulation may be altered.

Severe hypersensitivity reactions, including anaphylaxis, have occurred with quinolone therapy. If an allergic reaction occurs (itching, urticaria, dyspnea or facial edema, loss of consciousness, tingling, cardiovascular collapse) discontinue drug immediately. Prolonged use may result in superinfection; pseudomembranous colitis may occur and should be considered in all patients who present with diarrhea. Quinolones may exacerbate myasthenia gravis.

Adverse Reactions

3% to 10%:
Central nervous system: Dizziness (3%)
Gastrointestinal: Nausea (7%), diarrhea (6%)

<3% (Limited to important or life-threatening): Allergic reactions, anaphylactic reaction, anaphylactic shock, anxiety, confusion, convulsions, EKG abnormalities, hallucinations, hyperglycemia, hypoglycemia, hypertension, hypotension, injection site reaction, peripheral edema, prothrombin time increased/decreased, QT prolongation, tachycardia, tendon disorders, tongue discoloration, tremor, vertigo, vision abnormalities

Overdosage/Toxicology Potential symptoms of overdose may include CNS excitation, seizures, QT prolongation, and arrhythmias (including torsade de pointes). Patients should be monitored by continuous EKG in the event of an overdose. Management is supportive and symptomatic.

Drug Interactions

Increased Effect/Toxicity: Drugs which prolong QT interval (including Class Ia and Class III antiarrhythmics, erythromycin, cisapride, antipsychotics, and cyclic antidepressants) are contraindicated with moxifloxacin. Cimetidine and probenecid increase quinolone levels. An increased incidence of seizures may occur with foscarnet or NSAIDs. Serum levels of some quinolones are increased by loop diuretic administration. Digoxin levels may be increased in some patients by quinolones. The hypoprothrombinemic effect of warfarin is enhanced by some quinolone antibiotics. Monitoring of the INR during concurrent therapy is recommended by the manufacturer.

Decreased Effect: Metal cations (magnesium, aluminum, iron, and zinc) bind quinolones in the gastrointestinal tract and inhibit absorption (by up to 98%). Antacids, multivitamins with minerals, sucralfate, and some didanosine formulations should be avoided. Moxifloxacin should be administered 4 hours before or 8 hours (a minimum of 2 hours before and 2 hours after) after these agents. Antineoplastic agents may decrease the absorption of quinolones.

Ethanol/Nutrition/Herb Interactions Food: Absorption is not affected by administration with a high-fat meal or yogurt.

Stability Store at 25°C (77°F). I.V.: Do not refrigerate

Mechanism of Action Moxifloxacin is a DNA gyrase inhibitor, and also inhibits topoisomerase IV. DNA gyrase (topoisomerase II) is an essential bacterial enzyme that maintains the superhelical structure of DNA. DNA gyrase is required for DNA replication and transcription, DNA repair, recombination, and transposition; inhibition is bactericidal.

Pharmacodynamics/Kinetics

Absorption: Well absorbed; not affected by high fat meal or yogurt

Distribution: V_d: 1.7 to 2.7 L/kg; tissue concentrations often exceed plasma concentrations in respiratory tissues, alveolar macrophages, and sinus tissues

Protein binding: 50%

Metabolism: Hepatic via glucuronide (14%) and sulfate (38%) conjugation

Bioavailability: 90%

Half-life elimination: Oral: 12 hours; I.V.: 15 hours

Excretion: Urine (20%) and feces (25%) as unchanged drug; sulfate conjugates in feces, glucuronide conjugates in urine

Usual Dosage Oral, I.V.:

Adults:
Acute bacterial sinusitis: 400 mg every 24 hours for 10 days
Chronic bronchitis, acute bacterial exacerbation: 400 mg every 24 hours for 5 days
Note: Avelox® ABC Pack™ (Avelox® Bronchitis Course) contains five tablets of 400 mg each.
Community-acquired pneumonia: 400 mg every 24 hours for 7-14 days
Uncomplicated skin infections: 400 mg every 24 hours for 7 days
Elderly: No dosage adjustments are required based on age

Dosage adjustment in renal impairment: No dosage adjustment is required.

Dosage adjustment in hepatic impairment: No dosage adjustment is required in mild to moderate hepatic insufficiency (Child-Pugh Classes A and B). Not recommended in patients with severe hepatic insufficiency.

Dietary Considerations May be taken with or without food. Take 4 hours before or 8 hours after multiple vitamins, antacids, or other products containing magnesium, aluminum, iron, or zinc.

Administration I.V.: Infuse over 60 minutes; do not infuse by rapid or bolus intravenous infusion

Monitoring Parameters WBC, signs of infection

(Continued)

Moxifloxacin *(Continued)*

Patient Information May be taken with or without food. Drink plenty of fluids. Do not take antacids within 4 hours before or 8 hours after dosing. Contact your physician immediately if signs of allergy occur. Contact your physician immediately if signs of tendon inflammation or pain occur. Do not discontinue therapy until your course has been completed. Take a missed dose as soon as possible, unless it is almost time for your next dose.

Dosage Forms
Solution for infusion, as hydrochloride [premixed in sodium chloride 0.8%]: 400 mg/250 mL
Tablet, as hydrochloride: 400 mg
Tablet, dose pack, as hydrochloride (Avelox® ABC Pack™): 400 mg (one 5-tablet card)

◆ **Moxifloxacin Hydrochloride** *see Moxifloxacin on page 938*
◆ **Moxilin®** *see Amoxicillin on page 84*
◆ **4-MP** *see Fomepizole on page 599*
◆ **6-MP** *see Mercaptopurine on page 863*
◆ **MPA and Estrogens (Conjugated)** *see Estrogens (Conjugated) and Medroxyprogesterone on page 497*
◆ **M-Prednisol®** *see MethylPREDNISolone on page 896*
◆ **M-R-VAX® II** *see Measles and Rubella Vaccines (Combined) on page 840*
◆ **MS** *see Morphine Sulfate on page 936*
◆ **MS Contin®** *see Morphine Sulfate on page 936*
◆ **MSIR®** *see Morphine Sulfate on page 936*
◆ **MTC** *see Mitomycin on page 922*
◆ **MTX** *see Methotrexate on page 884*
◆ **Muco-Fen-DM®** *see Guaifenesin and Dextromethorphan on page 646*
◆ **Muco-Fen-LA®** *see Guaifenesin on page 645*
◆ **Mucomyst®** *see Acetylcysteine on page 32*
◆ **Mucosil™** *see Acetylcysteine on page 32*
◆ **Multiple Sulfonamides** *see Sulfadiazine, Sulfamethazine, and Sulfamerazine on page 1271*
◆ **Multiple Vitamins** *see Vitamins (Multiple) on page 1424*
◆ **Multitest CMI®** *see Skin Test Antigens (Multiple) on page 1242*
◆ **Multivitamins, Fluoride** *see Vitamins (Multiple) on page 1424*
◆ **Mumps, Measles and Rubella Vaccines, Combined** *see Measles, Mumps, and Rubella Vaccines (Combined) on page 841*
◆ **Mumpsvax®** *see Mumps Virus Vaccine (Live/Attenuated) on page 940*

Mumps Virus Vaccine (Live/Attenuated)

(mumpz VYE rus vak SEEN, live, a ten YOO ate ed)

Related Information
Immunization Recommendations *on page 1538*
Skin Tests *on page 1533*

U.S. Brand Names Mumpsvax®
Canadian Brand Names Mumpsvax®
Therapeutic Category Vaccine, Live Virus
Use Mumps prophylaxis by promoting active immunity

Note: Trivalent measles-mumps-rubella (MMR) vaccine is the preferred agent for most children and many adults; persons born prior to 1957 are generally considered immune and need not be vaccinated

Pregnancy Risk Factor X

Pregnancy/Breast-Feeding Implications Although mumps virus can infect the placenta and fetus, there is not good evidence that it causes congenital malformations

Warnings/Precautions Pregnancy, immunocompromised persons, history of anaphylactic reaction following egg ingestion or receipt of neomycin

Adverse Reactions All serious adverse reactions must be reported to the U.S. Department of Health and Human Services (DHHS) Vaccine Adverse Event Reporting System (VAERS) 1-800-822-7967.
>10%: Local: Burning or stinging at injection site
1% to 10%:
Central nervous system: Fever (≤100°F)
Dermatologic: Rash
Endocrine & metabolic: Parotitis
<1%: Anaphylactic reactions, confusion, convulsions, fever (>103°F), severe or continuing headache, orchitis in postpubescent and adult males, thrombocytopenia, purpura

Stability Refrigerate, protect from light, discard within 8 hours after reconstitution
Mechanism of Action Promotes active immunity to mumps virus by inducing specific antibodies.
Usual Dosage Children ≥15 months and Adults: 0.5 mL S.C. in outer aspect of the upper arm, no booster

Administration Reconstitute only with diluent provided; administer only S.C. on outer aspect of upper arm

Test Interactions Temporary suppression of tuberculosis skin test
Patient Information Pregnancy should be avoided for 3 months following vaccination; a little swelling of the glands in the cheeks and under the jaw may occur that lasts for a few days; this could happen from 1-2 weeks after getting the mumps vaccine; this happens rarely

Nursing Implications Federal law requires that the date of administration, the vaccine manufacturer, lot number of vaccine, and the administering person's name, title and address be entered into the patient's permanent medical record

Additional Information Federal law requires that the date of administration, the vaccine manufacturer, lot number of vaccine, and the administering person's name, title and address be entered into the patient's permanent medical record. All adults without documentation of live vaccine on or after the first birthday or physician-diagnosed mumps, or laboratory evidence or immunity (particularly males and young adults who work in or congregate in hospitals, colleges, and on military bases) should be vaccinated. It is reasonable to consider persons born before 1957 immune, but there is no contraindication to vaccination of older persons. Susceptible travelers should be vaccinated.

Dosage Forms Powder for injection [single dose]: 20,000 TCID$_{50}$ [with diluent]

Mupirocin (myoo PEER oh sin)
U.S. Brand Names Bactroban®; Bactroban® Nasal
Canadian Brand Names Bactroban®
Synonyms Mupirocin Calcium; Pseudomonic Acid A
Therapeutic Category Antibiotic, Topical
Use
   Intranasal: Eradication of nasal colonization with MRSA in adult patients and healthcare workers
   Topical treatment of impetigo due to *Staphylococcus aureus*, beta-hemolytic *Streptococcus*, and *S. pyogenes*
Pregnancy Risk Factor B
Pregnancy/Breast-Feeding Implications There are no adequate and well-controlled studies in pregnant women; use during pregnancy only if clearly needed.
Contraindications Hypersensitivity to mupirocin, polyethylene glycol, or any component of the formulation
Warnings/Precautions Potentially toxic amounts of polyethylene glycol contained in the vehicle may be absorbed percutaneously in patients with extensive burns or open wounds; prolonged use may result in over growth of nonsusceptible organisms; for external use only; not for treatment of pressure sores
Adverse Reactions 1% to 10%:
   Dermatologic: Pruritus, rash, erythema, dry skin
   Local: Burning, stinging, tenderness, edema, pain
Stability Do not mix with Aquaphor®, coal tar solution, or salicylic acid
Mechanism of Action Binds to bacterial isoleucyl transfer-RNA synthetase resulting in the inhibition of protein and RNA synthesis
Pharmacodynamics/Kinetics
   Absorption: Topical: Penetrates the outer layers of skin; systemic absorption minimal through intact skin
   Protein binding: 95%
   Metabolism: Skin: 3% to monic acid
   Half-life elimination: 17-36 minutes
   Excretion: Urine
Usual Dosage
   Children ≥12 years and Adults: Intranasal: Approximately one-half of the ointment from the single-use tube should be applied into one nostril and the other half into the other nostril twice daily for 5 days
   Children ≥3 months and Adults: Topical: Apply small amount to affected area 2-5 times/day for 5-14 days
Patient Information For topical use only; do not apply into the eye; discontinue if rash, itching, or irritation occurs; improvement should be seen in 5 days
Nursing Implications Not for treatment of pressure sores in elderly patients; contains polyethylene glycol vehicle
Additional Information Not for treatment of pressure sores; contains polyethylene glycol vehicle.
Dosage Forms
   Cream, topical, as calcium: 2% (15 g, 30 g)
   Ointment, topical: 2% (22 g)
   Ointment, intranasal, topical, as calcium [single-use tube]: 2% (1 g)
   Ointment, topical, as calcium: 2% (15 g, 30 g)

♦ **Mupirocin Calcium** *see* Mupirocin *on page 941*
♦ **Murine® Ear Drops [OTC]** *see* Carbamide Peroxide *on page 224*
♦ **Muro 128® [OTC]** *see* Sodium Chloride *on page 1245*
♦ **Murocoll-2®** *see* Phenylephrine and Scopolamine *on page 1076*

Muromonab-CD3 (myoo roe MOE nab see dee three)
U.S. Brand Names Orthoclone OKT® 3
Canadian Brand Names Orthoclone OKT® 3
Synonyms Monoclonal Antibody; OKT3
Therapeutic Category Immunosuppressant Agent
Use Treatment of acute allograft rejection in renal transplant patients; treatment of acute hepatic, kidney, and pancreas rejection episodes resistant to conventional treatment. Acute graft-versus-host disease following bone marrow transplantation resistant to conventional treatment.
Pregnancy Risk Factor C
Contraindications Hypersensitivity to OKT3 or any murine product; patients in fluid overload or those with >3% weight gain within 1 week prior to start of OKT3; mouse antibody titers >1:1000
Warnings/Precautions It is imperative, especially prior to the first few doses, that there be no clinical evidence of volume overload, uncontrolled hypertension, or uncompensated heart failure, including a clear chest x-ray and weight restriction of ≤3% above the patient's minimum weight during the week prior to injection.

May result in an increased susceptibility to infection; dosage of concomitant immunosuppressants should be reduced during OKT3 therapy; cyclosporine should be decreased to 50% usual maintenance dose and maintenance therapy resumed about 4 days before stopping OKT3.
(Continued)

Muromonab-CD3 *(Continued)*

Severe pulmonary edema has occurred in patients with fluid overload.

First dose effect (flu-like symptoms, anaphylactic-type reaction): may occur within 30 minutes to 6 hours up to 24 hours after the first dose and may be minimized by using the recommended regimens. See table.

Suggested Prevention/Treatment of Muromonab-CD3 First-Dose Effects

Adverse Reaction	Effective Prevention or Palliation	Supportive Treatment
Severe pulmonary edema	Clear chest x-ray within 24 hours preinjection; weight restriction to ≤3% gain over 7 days preinjection	Prompt intubation and oxygenation 24 hours close observation
Fever, chills	15 mg/kg methylprednisolone sodium succinate 1 hour preinjection; fever reduction to <37.8°C (100°F) 1 hour preinjection; acetaminophen (1 g orally) and diphenhydramine (50 mg orally) 1 hour preinjection	Cooling blanket Acetaminophen prn
Respiratory effects	100 mg hydrocortisone sodium succinate 30 minutes postinjection	Additional 100 mg hydrocortisone sodium succinate prn for wheezing; if respiratory distress, give epinephrine 1:1000 (0.3 mL S.C.)

Cardiopulmonary resuscitation may be needed. If the patient's temperature is >37.8°C, reduce before administering OKT3

Adverse Reactions First-dose effect (cytokine release syndrome), onset 1-3 hours after dose, duration 12-16 hours, severity mild to life-threatening, signs and symptoms include fever, chilling, dyspnea, wheezing, chest pain, chest tightness, nausea, vomiting, and diarrhea. Hypervolemic pulmonary edema, nephrotoxicity, meningitis, and encephalopathy are possible. Reactions tend to decrease with repeated doses.

>10%:
Cardiovascular: Tachycardia (including ventricular)
Central nervous system: Dizziness, faintness
Gastrointestinal: Diarrhea, nausea, vomiting
Hematologic: Transient lymphopenia
Neuromuscular & skeletal: Trembling
Respiratory: Dyspnea

1% to 10%:
Central nervous system: Headache
Neuromuscular & skeletal: Stiff neck
Ocular: Photophobia
Respiratory: Pulmonary edema

<1% (Limited to important or life-threatening): BUN increased, chest pain or tightness, creatinine increased, dyspnea, hypertension, hypotension, pancytopenia, secondary lymphoproliferative disorder or lymphoma, thrombosis of major vessels in renal allograft, wheezing

Drug Interactions
Increased Effect/Toxicity: Recommend decreasing dose of prednisone to 0.5 mg/kg, azathioprine to 0.5 mg/kg (approximate 50% decrease in dose), and discontinuing cyclosporine while patient is receiving OKT3.
Decreased Effect: Decreased effect with immunosuppressive drugs.

Stability Refrigerate; do not shake or freeze; stable in Becton Dickinson syringe for 16 hours at room temperature or refrigeration

Mechanism of Action Reverses graft rejection by binding to T cells and interfering with their function by binding T-cell receptor-associated CD3 glycoprotein

Pharmacodynamics/Kinetics
Duration: 7 days after discontinuation
Time to peak: Steady-state: Trough: 3-14 days

Usual Dosage I.V. (refer to individual protocols):
Children <30 kg: 2.5 mg/day once daily for 7-14 days
Children >30 kg: 5 mg/day once daily for 7-14 days
OR
Children <12 years: 0.1 mg/kg/day once daily for 10-14 days
Children ≥12 years and Adults: 5 mg/day once daily for 10-14 days
Hemodialysis: Molecular size of OKT3 is 150,000 daltons; not dialyzed by most standard dialyzers; however, may be dialyzed by high flux dialysis; OKT3 will be removed by plasmapheresis; administer following dialysis treatments
Peritoneal dialysis: Significant drug removal is unlikely based on physiochemical characteristics

Administration Filter each dose through a low protein-binding 0.22 micron filter (Millex GV) before administration; administer I.V. push over <1 minute at a final concentration of 1 mg/mL

Children and Adults:
Methylprednisolone sodium succinate 15 mg/kg I.V. administered prior to first muromonab-CD3 administration and I.V. hydrocortisone sodium succinate 50-100 mg given 30 minutes after administration are strongly recommended to decrease the incidence of reactions to the first dose
Patient temperature should not exceed 37.8°C (100°F) at time of administration

Monitoring Parameters Chest x-ray, weight gain, CBC with differential, temperature, vital signs (blood pressure, temperature, pulse, respiration); immunologic monitoring of T cells, serum levels of OKT3

Reference Range

OKT3 serum concentrations:

Serum level monitoring should be performed in conjunction with lymphocyte subset determinations; Trough concentration sampling best correlates with clinical outcome. Serial monitoring may provide a better early indicator of inadequate dosing during induction or rejection.

Mean serum trough levels rise during the first 3 days, then average 0.9 mcg/mL on days 3-14

Circulating levels ≥0.8 mcg/mL block the function of cytotoxic T cells *in vitro* and *in vivo*

Several recent analysis have suggested appropriate dosage adjustments of OKT3 induction course are better determined with OKT3 serum levels versus lymphocyte subset determination; however, no prospective controlled trials have been performed to validate the equivalency of these tests in predicting clinical outcome.

Lymphocyte subset monitoring: CD3+ cells: Trough sample measurement is preferable and reagent utilized defines reference range.

OKT3-FITC: <10-50 cells/mm^3 or <3% to 5%

CD3(IgG1)-FITC: similar to OKT3-FITC

Leu-4a: Higher number of CD3+ cells appears acceptable

Dosage adjustments should be made in conjunction with clinical response and based upon trends over several consecutive days

Patient Information Inform patient of expected first dose effects which are markedly reduced with subsequent treatments

Nursing Implications Do not administer I.M., monitor patient closely for 24 hours after the first dose; drugs and equipment for treating pulmonary edema and anaphylaxis should be on hand

Dosage Forms Injection: 1 mg/mL (5 mL)

- ◆ **Muse® Pellet** *see* Alprostadil *on page 57*
- ◆ **Mustargen®** *see* Mechlorethamine *on page 845*
- ◆ **Mustine** *see* Mechlorethamine *on page 845*
- ◆ **Mutacol Berna® (Can)** *see* Cholera Vaccine *on page 285*
- ◆ **Mutamycin®** *see* Mitomycin *on page 922*
- ◆ **Myambutol®** *see* Ethambutol *on page 507*
- ◆ **Mycelex®** *see* Clotrimazole *on page 323*
- ◆ **Mycelex®-3 [OTC]** *see* Butoconazole *on page 199*
- ◆ **Mycelex®-3** *see* Clotrimazole *on page 323*
- ◆ **Mycelex®-7 [OTC]** *see* Clotrimazole *on page 323*
- ◆ **Mycelex® Twin Pack [OTC]** *see* Clotrimazole *on page 323*
- ◆ **Mycifradin® Sulfate** *see* Neomycin *on page 967*
- ◆ **Mycinettes® [OTC]** *see* Benzocaine *on page 154*
- ◆ **Mycitracin® [OTC]** *see* Bacitracin, Neomycin, and Polymyxin B *on page 143*
- ◆ **Mycobutin®** *see* Rifabutin *on page 1192*
- ◆ **Mycogen II** *see* Nystatin and Triamcinolone *on page 1002*
- ◆ **Mycolog®-II** *see* Nystatin and Triamcinolone *on page 1002*

Mycophenolate (mye koe FEN oh late)

Related Information

Antacid Drug Interactions *on page 1477*

U.S. Brand Names CellCept®

Canadian Brand Names CellCept®

Synonyms Mycophenolate Mofetil

Therapeutic Category Immunosuppressant Agent

Use Prophylaxis of organ rejection concomitantly with cyclosporine and corticosteroids in patients receiving allogenic renal, cardiac, or hepatic transplants. Intravenous formulation is an alternative dosage form to oral capsules, suspension, and tablets.

Unlabeled/Investigational Use Treatment of rejection in liver transplant patients unable to tolerate tacrolimus or cyclosporine due to neurotoxicity; mild rejection in heart transplant patients; treatment of moderate-severe psoriasis

Pregnancy Risk Factor C (manufacturer)

Pregnancy/Breast-Feeding Implications There are no adequate and well-controlled studies using mycophenolate in pregnant women, however, it may cause fetal harm. Women of childbearing potential should have a negative pregnancy test prior to beginning therapy. Two reliable forms of contraception should be used prior to, during, and for 6 weeks after therapy. It is unknown if mycophenolate is excreted in human milk. Due to potentially serious adverse reactions, the decision to discontinue the drug or discontinue breast-feeding should be considered.

Contraindications Hypersensitivity to mycophenolate mofetil, mycophenolic acid, or any component of the formulation; intravenous is contraindicated in patients who are allergic to polysorbate 80

Warnings/Precautions Increased risk for infection and development of lymphoproliferative disorders. Patients should be monitored appropriately and given supportive treatment should these conditions occur. Increased toxicity in patients with renal impairment. Should be used with caution in patients with active peptic ulcer disease.

Because mycophenolate mofetil has demonstrated teratogenic effects in rats and rabbits, tablets should not be crushed, and capsules should not be opened or crushed. Avoid inhalation or direct contact with skin or mucous membranes of the powder contained in the capsules and the powder for oral suspension. Caution should be exercised in the handling and preparation of solutions of intravenous mycophenolate. Avoid skin contact with the intravenous solution and reconstituted suspension. If such contact occurs, wash thoroughly with soap and water, rinse eyes with plain water.

(Continued)

943

Mycophenolate (Continued)

Theoretically, use should be avoided in patients with the rare hereditary deficiency of hypo-xanthine-guanine phosphoribosyl-transferase (such as Lesch-Nyhan or Kelley-Seegmiller syndrome). Oral suspension contains 0.56 mg phenylalanine/mL, use caution if administered to patients with phenylketonuria. Intravenous solutions should be given over at least 2 hours; **never** administer intravenous solution by rapid or bolus injection.

Adverse Reactions Reported following oral dosing of mycophenolate alone in renal, cardiac, and hepatic allograft rejection studies. In general, lower doses used in renal rejection patients had less adverse effects than higher doses. Rates of adverse effects were similar for each indication, except for those unique to the specific organ involved.

>10%:

Cardiovascular: Hypertension (28% to 77%), peripheral edema (27% to 64%), hypotension (18% to 32%), edema (12% to 28%), cardiovascular disorder (26%), chest pain (13% to 26%), tachycardia (20% to 22%), arrhythmia (19%), bradycardia (17%), hypervolemia (17%), pericardial effusion (16%), heart failure (12%)

Central nervous system: Pain (31% to 76%), headache (16% to 54%), fever (21% to 52%), insomnia (9% to 52%), tremor (11% to 34%), anxiety (19% to 28%), dizziness (6% to 28%), depression (16% to 17%), confusion (13% to 17%), agitation (13%), chills (11%), somnolence (11%), nervousness (10% to 11%)

Dermatologic: Rash (18% to 22%), pruritus (14%), skin disorder (12%), diaphoresis (11%), acne (10% to 12%)

Endocrine & metabolic: Hyperglycemia (9% to 47%), hypercholesterolemia (8% to 41%), hypomagnesemia (18% to 39%), hypokalemia (10% to 37%), hypocalcemia (30%), elevated LDH (23%), hyperkalemia (9% to 22%), elevated AST (17%), elevated ALT (16%), hyperuricemia (16%), hypophosphatemia (12% to 16%), acidosis (14%), hypo-proteinemia (13%), hyponatremia (11%)

Gastrointestinal: Abdominal pain (25% to 62%), nausea (20% to 54%), diarrhea (31% to 51%), constipation (18% to 41%), vomiting (12% to 34%), anorexia (25%), dyspepsia (13% to 22%), abdominal enlargement (19%), weight gain (16%), flatulence (13% to 14%), oral moniliasis (10% to 12%), nausea and vomiting (10% to 11%)

Genitourinary: Urinary tract infection (13% to 37%), urinary tract disorder

Hematologic: Leukopenia (23% to 46%), anemia (26% to 43%), leukocytosis (7% to 40%), thrombocytopenia (8% to 38%), hypochromic anemia (7% to 25%), ecchymosis (17%)

Hepatic: Abnormal liver function tests (25%), ascites (24%), bilirubinemia (14% to 18%), cholangitis (14%), hepatitis (13%), cholestatic jaundice (12%)

Neuromuscular & skeletal: Back pain (12% to 47%), weakness (14% to 43%), paresthesia (15% to 21%), leg cramps (17%), hypertonia (16%), myasthenia (12%), myalgia (12%)

Ocular: Amblyopia (15%)

Renal: Elevated creatinine (20% to 40%), elevated BUN (10% to 35%), abnormal kidney function (22% to 27%), oliguria (14% to 17%), hematuria (12% to 14%), kidney tubular necrosis (6% to 10%)

Respiratory: Respiratory infection (16% to 37%), dyspnea (15% to 37%), pleural effusion (17% to 34%), increased cough (13% to 31%), lung disorder (22% to 30%), sinusitis (11% to 26%), rhinitis (19%), pharyngitis (9% to 18%), pneumonia (11% to 14%), atelectasis (13%), asthma (11%), bronchitis

Miscellaneous: Infection (18% to 27%), sepsis (18% to 27%), herpes simplex (10% to 21%), accidental injury (11% to 19%), mucocutaneous *Candida* (15% to 18%), CMV viremia/syndrome (12% to 14%), hernia (12%), CMV tissue invasive disease (6% to 11%), herpes zoster cutaneous disease (6% to 11%)

1% to 10%:

Cardiovascular: I.V.: Thrombosis (4%)

Dermatologic: Nonmelanoma skin carcinomas (2% to 4%)

Endocrine & metabolic: Hypoglycemia (10%)

Hematologic: Severe neutropenia (2% to 4%), lymphoproliferative disease/lymphoma (0.4% to 1%)

Local: I.V.: Phlebitis (4%)

Miscellaneous: Abnormal healing (10%), peritonitis (10%), fatal sepsis (2% to 5%), other systemic/opportunistic infections (see above), malignancy (0.7% to 2%)

<1% (Limited to important or life-threatening): Colitis, infectious endocarditis, interstitial lung disorders, meningitis, pancreatitis, pulmonary fibrosis (rare, fatalities reported)

Overdosage/Toxicology There are no reported overdoses with mycophenolate. At plasma concentrations >100 mcg/mL, small amounts of the inactive metabolite MPAG are removed by hemodialysis. Excretion of the active metabolite, MPA, may be increased by using bile acid sequestrants (cholestyramine).

Drug Interactions

Increased Effect/Toxicity: Acyclovir and ganciclovir levels may increase due to competi-tion for tubular secretion of these drugs. Probenecid may increase mycophenolate levels due to inhibition of tubular secretion. High doses of salicylates may increase free fraction of mycophenolic acid. Azathioprine's bone marrow suppression may be potentiated; do not administer together.

Decreased Effect: Antacids decrease serum levels (C$_{max}$ and AUC); **do not administer together**. Cholestyramine resin decreases serum levels; **do not administer together**. Avoid use of live vaccines; vaccinations may be less effective. During concurrent use of oral contraceptives, progesterone levels are not significantly affected, however, effect on estrogen component varies; an additional form of contraception should be used.

Ethanol/Nutrition/Herb Interactions

Food: Decreases C$_{max}$ of MPA by 40% however the extent of absorption is not changed

Herb/Nutraceutical: Avoid cat's claw, echinacea (have immunostimulant properties)

Stability Tablets/capsules/powder for oral suspension should be stored at room temperature (15°C to 39°C/59°F to 86°F). Tablets should also be protected from light. Intact vials of injection should be stored at room temperature (15°C to 30°C/59°F to 86°F).

Stability of the infusion solution: 4 hours from reconstitution and dilution of the product. Store solutions at 15°C to 30°C (59°F to 86°F)

Once reconstituted, the oral solution may be stored at room temperature or under refrigeration. Do not freeze. The mixed solution is stable for 60 days.

Reconstitution:

Mycophenolate injection does not contain an antibacterial preservative; therefore, reconstitution and dilution of the product must be done under aseptic conditions. Preparation of intravenous formulation should take place in a vertical laminar flow hood with the same precautions as antineoplastic agents.

Intravenous preparation procedure:

Step 1:
a. Two vials of mycophenolate injection are used for preparing a 1 g dose, whereas 3 vials are needed for each 1.5 g dose. Reconstitute the contents of each vial by injecting 14 mL of 5% dextrose injection.
b. Gently shake the vial to dissolve the drug
c. Inspect the resulting slightly yellow solution for particulate matter and discoloration prior to further dilution. Discard the vial if particulate matter or discoloration is observed.

Step 2:
a. To prepare a 1 g dose, further dilute the contents of the two reconstituted vials into 140 mL of 5% dextrose in water. To prepare a 1.5 g dose, further dilute the contents of the three reconstituted vials into 210 mL of 5% dextrose in water. The final concentration of both solutions is 6 mg mycophenolate mofetil per mL.
b. Inspect the infusion solution for particulate matter or discoloration. Discard the infusion solution if particulate matter or discoloration is observed.

Oral Suspension: Should be constituted by a pharmacist prior to dispensing to the patient and **not** mixed with any other medication. Closed bottle should be tapped to loosen the powder. Add 47 mL of water to the bottle and shake well for ~1 minute. Add another 47 mL of water to the bottle and shake well for an additional minute. Remove child-resistant cap and push bottle adapter into neck of the bottle; close bottle with child-resistant cap tightly to assure proper placement of adapter and status of child-resistant cap. Final concentration is 200 mg/mL of mycophenolate mofetil.

Mechanism of Action Inhibition of purine synthesis of human lymphocytes and proliferation of human lymphocytes

Pharmacodynamics/Kinetics

Onset of action: Peak effect: Correlation of toxicity or efficacy is still being developed, however, one study indicated that 12-hour AUCs >40 mcg/mL/hour were correlated with efficacy and decreased episodes of rejection

Absorption: The AUC values for MPA are lower in the early post-transplant period versus the later (>3 months) post-transplant period. The extent of absorption in pediatrics is similar to that seen in adults, although there was wide variability reported.

Distribution: Oral: 4 L/kg; I.V.: 3.6 L/kg

Protein binding: MPA: 97%, MPAG 82%

Metabolism: Hepatic and via gastrointestinal tract; hydrolyzed to mycophenotic acid (MPA; active metabolite); enterohepatic cycling of MPA may occur; MPA is glucuronidated to MPAG (inactive metabolite)

Bioavailability: Oral: 94%

Half-life elimination: Oral: 17 hours; I.V.: 18 hours

Excretion: MPAG: Urine and feces; MPA: Urine (87% as inactive MPAG)

Usual Dosage

Children: Renal transplant: Oral:
Suspension: 600 mg/m²/dose twice daily; maximum dose: 1 g twice daily
Alternatively, may use solid dosage forms according to BSA as follows:
BSA 1.25-1.5 m²: 750 mg capsule twice daily
BSA >1.5 m²: 1 g capsule or tablet twice daily

Adults: The initial dose should be given as soon as possible following transplantation; intravenous solution may be given until the oral medication can be tolerated (up to 14 days)
Renal transplant:
Oral: 1 g twice daily. Although a dose of 1.5 g twice daily was used in clinical trials and shown to be effective, no efficacy advantage was established. Patients receiving 2 g/day demonstrated an overall better safety profile than patients receiving 3 g/day. Doses >2 g/day are not recommended in these patients because of the possibility for enhanced immunosuppression as well as toxicities.
I.V.: 1 g twice daily
Cardiac transplantation:
Oral: 1.5 g twice daily
I.V.: 1.5 g twice daily
Hepatic transplantation:
Oral: 1.5 g twice daily
I.V.: 1 g twice daily

Dosing adjustment in renal impairment:
Renal transplant: GFR <25 mL/minute in patients outside the immediate post-transplant period: Doses of >1 g administered twice daily should be avoided; patients should also be carefully observed; no dose adjustments are needed in renal transplant patients experiencing delayed graft function postoperatively
Cardiac or liver transplant: No data available; mycophenolate may be used in cardiac or hepatic transplant patients with severe chronic renal impairment if the potential benefit outweighs the potential risk
Hemodialysis: Not removed; supplemental dose is not necessary
Peritoneal dialysis: Supplemental dose is not necessary

Dosage adjustment in hepatic impairment: No dosage adjustment is recommended for renal patients with severe hepatic parenchymal disease; however, it is not currently known whether dosage adjustments are necessary for hepatic disease with other etiologies

Elderly: Dosage is the same as younger patients, however, dosing should be cautious due to possibility of increased hepatic, renal or cardiac dysfunction; elderly patients may be at an

(Continued)

Mycophenolate *(Continued)*

increased risk of certain infections, gastrointestinal hemorrhage, and pulmonary edema, as compared to younger patients

Dosing adjustment for toxicity (neutropenia): ANC <1.3 x 10³/μL: Dosing should be interrupted or the dose reduced, appropriate diagnostic tests performed and patients managed appropriately

Dietary Considerations Oral dosage formulations should be taken on an empty stomach. However, in stable renal transplant patients, may be administered with food if necessary.

Administration

Oral dosage formulations (tablet, capsule, suspension) should be administered as soon as possible following transplantation. Oral dosage forms should be administered on an empty stomach. The oral solution may be administered via a nasogastric tube (minimum 8 French, 1.7 mm interior diameter) and cannot be mixed with other medications.

Intravenous solutions should be administered over at least 2 hours (either peripheral or central vein); do **not** administer intravenous solution by rapid or bolus injection. Following reconstitution, dilute to a concentration of 6 mg/mL using D₅W; mycophenolate is not compatible with other solutions.

Monitoring Parameters Complete blood count

Patient Information Take as directed, preferably 1 hour before or 2 hours after meals. Do not take within 1 hour before or 2 hours after antacids or cholestyramine medications. Do not alter dose and do not discontinue without consulting prescriber. Maintain adequate hydration (2-3 L/day of fluids unless instructed to restrict fluid intake) during entire course of therapy. You will be susceptible to infection (avoid crowds and people with infections or contagious diseases). If you are diabetic, monitor glucose levels closely (may alter glucose levels). You may experience dizziness or trembling (use caution until response to medication is known); nausea or vomiting (frequent small meals, frequent mouth care may help); diarrhea (boiled milk, yogurt, or buttermilk may help); sores or white plaques in mouth (frequent rinsing of mouth and frequent mouth care may help); or muscle or back pain (mild analgesics may be recommended). Report chest pain; acute headache or dizziness; symptoms of respiratory infection, cough, or difficulty breathing; unresolved gastrointestinal effects; fatigue, chills, fever unhealed sores, white plaques in mouth; irritation in genital area or unusual discharge; unusual bruising or bleeding; or other unusual effects related to this medication. May be at increased risk for skin cancer; wear protective clothing and use sunscreen with high protective factor to help limit exposure to sunlight and UV light. Two reliable forms of contraception should be used prior to, during, and for 6 weeks after therapy.

Nursing Implications Increased risk for infection and development of lymphoproliferative disorders. Patients should be monitored appropriately and given supportive treatment should these conditions occur. Increased toxicity in patients with renal impairment. Intravenous solutions should be given over at least 2 hours. Do not administer intravenous solution by rapid or bolus injection. The oral suspension cannot be mixed with other medications.

Dosage Forms

Capsule, as mofetil: 250 mg

Injection: 500 mg

Suspension for reconstitution, oral, as mofetil: 200 mg/mL (225 mL)

Tablet, film coated, as mofetil: 500 mg

♦ **Nabi-HB®** *see* Hepatitis B Immune Globulin *on page 661*

Nabumetone (na BYOO me tone)

Related Information
Nonsteroidal Anti-Inflammatory Agents Comparison *on page 1512*

U.S. Brand Names Relafen®

Canadian Brand Names Apo®-Nabumetone; Relafen™

Therapeutic Category Analgesic, Nonsteroidal Anti-inflammatory Drug; Anti-inflammatory Agent; Nonsteroidal Anti-inflammatory Drug (NSAID), Oral

Use Management of osteoarthritis and rheumatoid arthritis

Unlabeled/Investigational Use Sunburn, mild to moderate pain

Pregnancy Risk Factor C/D (3rd trimester)

Contraindications Hypersensitivity to nonsteroidal anti-inflammatory drugs (NSAIDs) including aspirin, or any component of the formulation; should not be administered to patients with active peptic ulceration and those with severe hepatic impairment or in patients in whom nabumetone, aspirin, or other NSAIDs have induced asthma, urticaria, or other allergic-type reactions; fatal asthmatic reactions have occurred following NSAID administration; pregnancy (3rd trimester)

Warnings/Precautions Elderly patients may sometimes require lower doses; patients with impaired renal function may need a dose reduction; use with caution in patients with severe hepatic impairment; dehydration. Withhold for at least 4-6 half-lives prior to surgical or dental procedures.

Adverse Reactions
>10%:
  Central nervous system: Dizziness
  Dermatologic: Rash
  Gastrointestinal: Abdominal cramps, abdominal pain (12%), diarrhea (14%), dyspepsia (13%), heartburn, indigestion, nausea

1% to 10%:
  Cardiovascular: Edema
  Central nervous system: Dizziness, headache, fatigue, insomnia, nervousness, somnolence
  Dermatologic: Pruritus, rash
  Gastrointestinal: Constipation, flatulence, nausea, guaiac postive stool, stomatitis, gastritis, dry mouth, vomiting
  Otic: Tinnitus

<1% (Limited to important or life-threatening): Albuminuria, alopecia, anaphylactoid reaction, anaphylaxis, angina, angioneurotic edema, arrhythmia, asthma, azotemia, bullous eruptions, cholestatic jaundice, confusion, congestive heart failure, depression, duodenal ulcer, dysphagia, dyspnea, eosinophilic pneumonia, erythema multiforme, gastric ulcer, GI bleeding, granulocytopenia, hepatic failure, hepatitis, hypersensitivity pneumonitis, hypertension, hyperuricemia, impotence, interstitial nephritis, interstitial pneumonitis, leukopenia, myocardial infarction, nephrotic syndrome, nightmares, pancreatitis, paresthesia, photosensitivity, pseudoporphyria cutanea tarda, renal failure, Stevens-Johnson syndrome, syncope, thrombocytopenia, toxic epidermal necrolysis, urticaria, vasculitis

Drug Interactions
Increased Effect/Toxicity: NSAIDs may increase digoxin, methotrexate, and lithium serum concentrations. The renal adverse effects of ACE inhibitors may be potentiated by NSAIDs. Potential for bleeding may be increased with anticoagulants or antiplatelet agents. Concurrent use of corticosteroids may increase the risk of GI ulceration.

Decreased Effect: NSAIDs may decrease the effect of some antihypertensive agents, including ACE inhibitors, angiotensin receptor antagonists, and hydralazine. The efficacy of diuretics (loop and/or thiazide) may be decreased.

Ethanol/Nutrition/Herb Interactions
Ethanol: Avoid ethanol (may enhance gastric mucosal irritation).
Food: Nabumetone peak serum concentrations may be increased if taken with food or dairy products.
Herb/Nutraceutical: Avoid cat's claw, dong quai, evening primrose, feverfew, garlic, ginger, ginkgo, red clover, horse chestnut, green tea, ginseng (all have additional antiplatelet activity).

Mechanism of Action Nabumetone is a nonacidic, nonsteroidal anti-inflammatory drug that is rapidly metabolized after absorption to a major active metabolite, 6-methoxy-2-naphthylacetic acid. As found with previous nonsteroidal anti-inflammatory drugs, nabumetone's active metabolite inhibits the cyclo-oxygenase enzyme which is indirectly responsible for the production of inflammation and pain during arthritis by way of enhancing the production of endoperoxides and prostaglandins E_2 and I_2 (prostacyclin). The active metabolite of nabumetone is felt to be the compound primarily responsible for therapeutic effect. Comparatively, the parent drug is a poor inhibitor of prostaglandin synthesis.

Pharmacodynamics/Kinetics
Onset of action: Several days
Distribution: Diffusion occurs readily into synovial fluid
Protein binding: >99%
Metabolism: A prodrug being rapidly metabolized to an active metabolite (6-methoxy-2-naphthylacetic acid); extensive first-pass hepatic effect
Half-life elimination: Major metabolite: 24 hours
Time to peak, serum: Metabolite: Oral: 3-6 hours; Synovial fluid: 4-12 hours
Excretion: Urine (80%) and feces (10%) with little as unchanged drug

Usual Dosage Adults: Oral: 1000 mg/day; an additional 500-1000 mg may be needed in some patients to obtain more symptomatic relief; may be administered once or twice daily

Dosing adjustment in renal impairment: None necessary; however, adverse effects due to accumulation of inactive metabolites of nabumetone that are renally excreted have not been studied and should be considered

(Continued)

Nabumetone (Continued)

Monitoring Parameters Patients with renal insufficiency: Baseline renal function followed by repeat test within weeks (to determine if renal function has deteriorated)

Patient Information Take this medication at meal times or with food or milk to minimize gastric irritation; inform your physician if you develop stomach disturbances, blurred vision, or other eye symptoms, rash, weight gain, or edema; inform your physician if you pass dark-colored or tarry stools; concomitant use of alcohol should be avoided, if possible, since it may add to the irritant action of nabumetone in the stomach; aspirin should be avoided

Nursing Implications Advise patient to inform physician if stomach disturbances, blurred vision, or other eye symptoms, rash, weight gain, edema, or passing of dark-colored or tarry stools occurs; concomitant use of ethanol should be avoided if possible since it may add to the irritant action of nabumetone in the stomach; aspirin should be avoided

Dosage Forms Tablet: 500 mg, 750 mg

♦ **NAC** see Acetylcysteine on page 32

♦ **N-Acetylcysteine** see Acetylcysteine on page 32

♦ **N-Acetyl-L-cysteine** see Acetylcysteine on page 32

♦ **N-Acetyl-P-Aminophenol** see Acetaminophen on page 22

♦ **NaCl** see Sodium Chloride on page 1245

Nadolol (nay DOE lole)

Related Information
Beta-Blockers Comparison on page 1491

U.S. Brand Names Corgard®

Canadian Brand Names Alti-Nadolol; Apo®-Nadol; Corgard®; Novo-Nadolol

Therapeutic Category Antianginal Agent; Antihypertensive Agent; Antimigraine Agent; Beta-Adrenergic Blocker

Use Treatment of hypertension and angina pectoris; prophylaxis of migraine headaches

Pregnancy Risk Factor C

Pregnancy/Breast-Feeding Implications
Clinical effects on the fetus: No data available on crossing the placenta. Bradycardia, hypotension, hypoglycemia, respiratory depression, hypothermia, IUGR reported. IUGR probably related to maternal hypertension. Alternative beta-blockers are preferred for use during pregnancy due to limited data. Monitor breast-fed infant for symptoms of beta-blockade.

Breast-feeding/lactation: Crosses into breast milk. AAP considers **compatible** with breast-feeding.

Contraindications Hypersensitivity to nadolol or any component of the formulation; bronchial asthma; sinus bradycardia; sinus node dysfunction; heart block greater than first degree (except in patients with a functioning artificial pacemaker); cardiogenic shock; uncompensated cardiac failure

Warnings/Precautions Administer only with extreme caution in patients with compensated heart failure, monitor for a worsening of the condition. Efficacy in heart failure has not been established for nadolol. Avoid abrupt discontinuation in patients with a history of CAD; slowly wean while monitoring for signs and symptoms of ischemia. Use caution with concurrent use of beta-blockers and either verapamil or diltiazem; bradycardia or heart block can occur. In general, patients with bronchospastic disease should not receive beta-blockers. Nadolol, if used at all, should be used cautiously in bronchospastic disease with close monitoring. Use cautiously in diabetics because it can mask prominent hypoglycemic symptoms. Can mask signs of thyrotoxicosis. Can cause fetal harm when administered in pregnancy. Use cautiously in the renally impaired (dosage adjustments are required). Use care with anesthetic agents which decrease myocardial function.

Adverse Reactions
>10%:
Central nervous system: Drowsiness, insomnia
Endocrine & metabolic: Decreased sexual ability

1% to 10%:
Cardiovascular: Bradycardia, palpitations, edema, congestive heart failure, reduced peripheral circulation
Central nervous system: Mental depression
Gastrointestinal: Diarrhea or constipation, nausea, vomiting, stomach discomfort
Respiratory: Bronchospasm
Miscellaneous: Cold extremities

<1% (Limited to important or life-threatening): Arrhythmias, chest pain, confusion (especially in the elderly), depression, dyspnea, hallucinations, leukopenia, orthostatic hypotension, thrombocytopenia

Overdosage/Toxicology Symptoms of intoxication include cardiac disturbances, CNS toxicity, bronchospasm, hypoglycemia, and hyperkalemia. The most common cardiac symptoms include hypotension and bradycardia. Atrioventricular block, intraventricular conduction disturbances, cardiogenic shock, and asystole may occur with severe overdose, especially with membrane-depressant drugs (eg, propranolol). CNS effects include convulsions, coma, and respiratory arrest (commonly seen with propranolol and other membrane-depressant and lipid-soluble drugs). Treatment is symptomatic for seizures, hypotension, hyperkalemia, and hypoglycemia. Bradycardia and hypotension resistant to atropine, isoproterenol, or pacing may respond to glucagon. Wide QRS defects caused by membrane-depressant poisoning may respond to hypertonic sodium bicarbonate. Repeat-dose charcoal, hemoperfusion, or hemodialysis may be helpful in removal of only those beta-blockers with a small V_d, long half-life, or low intrinsic clearance (acebutolol, atenolol, nadolol, sotalol).

Drug Interactions
Increased Effect/Toxicity: The heart rate lowering effects of nadolol are additive with other drugs which slow AV conduction (digoxin, verapamil, diltiazem). Concurrent use of alpha-blockers (prazosin, terazosin) with beta-blockers may increase risk of orthostasis.

Nadolol may mask the tachycardia from hypoglycemia caused by insulin and oral hypoglycemics. In patients receiving concurrent therapy, the risk of hypertensive crisis is increased when either clonidine or the beta-blocker is withdrawn. Reserpine has been shown to enhance the effect of beta-blockers. Avoid using with alpha-adrenergic stimulants (phenylephrine, epinephrine, etc) which may have exaggerated hypertensive responses. Beta-blockers may affect the action or levels of ethanol, disopyramide, nondepolarizing muscle relaxants, and theophylline although the effects are difficult to predict. The vasoconstrictive effects of ergot alkaloids may be enhanced.

Decreased Effect: Decreased effect of beta-blockers with aluminum salts, barbiturates, calcium salts, cholestyramine, colestipol, NSAIDs, penicillins (ampicillin), rifampin, salicylates, and sulfinpyrazone due to decreased bioavailability and plasma levels. Beta-blockers may decrease the effect of sulfonylureas (possibly hyperglycemia). Nonselective beta-blockers blunt the effect of beta-2 adrenergic agonists (albuterol).

Ethanol/Nutrition/Herb Interactions Herb/Nutraceutical: Avoid dong quai if using for hypertension (has estrogenic activity). Avoid ephedra, garlic, yohimbe, ginseng (may worsen hypertension). Avoid natural licorice (causes sodium and water retention and increases potassium loss).

Mechanism of Action Competitively blocks response to beta$_1$- and beta$_2$-adrenergic stimulation; does not exhibit any membrane stabilizing or intrinsic sympathomimetic activity

Pharmacodynamics/Kinetics
Duration: 17-24 hours
Absorption: 30% to 40%
Distribution: Concentration in human breast milk is 4.6 times higher than serum
Protein binding: 28%
Half-life elimination: Adults: 10-24 hours; increased half-life with decreased renal function; End-stage renal disease: 45 hours
Time to peak, serum: 2-4 hours
Excretion: Urine (as unchanged drug)

Usual Dosage Oral:
Adults: Initial: 40 mg/day, increase dosage gradually by 40-80 mg increments at 3- to 7-day intervals until optimum clinical response is obtained with profound slowing of heart rate; doses up to 160-240 mg/day in angina and 240-320 mg/day in hypertension may be necessary.
Elderly: Initial: 20 mg/day; increase doses by 20 mg increments at 3- to 7-day intervals; usual dosage range: 20-240 mg/day.

Dosing adjustment in renal impairment:
Cl$_{cr}$ 31-40 mL/minute: Administer every 24-36 hours or administer 50% of normal dose.
Cl$_{cr}$ 10-30 mL/minute: Administer every 24-48 hours or administer 50% of normal dose.
Cl$_{cr}$ <10 mL/minute: Administer every 40-60 hours or administer 25% of normal dose.
Hemodialysis: Moderately dialyzable (20% to 50%); administer dose postdialysis or administer 40 mg supplemental dose.
Peritoneal dialysis: Supplemental dose is not necessary.

Dosing adjustment/comments in hepatic disease: Reduced dose probably necessary.

Dietary Considerations May be taken without regard to meals.

Patient Information Check pulse daily prior to taking medication. If pulse is <50, hold medication and consult prescriber. Do not adjust dosage without consulting prescriber. May cause dizziness, fatigue, blurred vision; change position slowly (lying/sitting to standing) and use caution when driving or engaging in tasks that require alertness until response to drug is known. Exercise and increasing bulk or fiber in diet may help resolve constipation. If diabetic, monitor serum glucose closely (the drug may mask symptoms of hypoglycemia). Report swelling in feet or legs, difficulty breathing or persistent cough, unresolved fatigue, unusual weight gain >5 lb/week, or unresolved constipation.

Nursing Implications Patient's therapeutic response may be evaluated by looking at blood pressure, apical and radial pulses

Dosage Forms Tablet: 20 mg, 40 mg, 80 mg, 120 mg, 160 mg

♦ **Nadopen-V® (Can)** see Penicillin V Potassium on page 1055

Nafarelin (NAF a re lin)

U.S. Brand Names Synarel®
Canadian Brand Names Synarel®
Synonyms Nafarelin Acetate
Therapeutic Category Hormone, Posterior Pituitary; Luteinizing Hormone-Releasing Hormone Analog
Use Treatment of endometriosis, including pain and reduction of lesions; treatment of central precocious puberty (gonadotropin-dependent precocious puberty) in children of both sexes
Pregnancy Risk Factor X
Contraindications Hypersensitivity to GnRH, GnRH-agonist analogs, or any component of the formulation; undiagnosed abnormal vaginal bleeding; pregnancy
Warnings/Precautions Use with caution in patients with risk factors for decreased bone mineral content, nafarelin therapy may pose an additional risk; hypersensitivity reactions occur in 0.2% of the patients; safety and efficacy in children have not been established

Adverse Reactions
>10%:
Central nervous system: Headache, emotional lability
Dermatologic: Acne
Endocrine & metabolic: Hot flashes, breakthrough bleeding, spotting, menorrhagia, decreased libido, decreased breast size, amenorrhea, hypoestrogenism
Genitourinary: Vaginal dryness
Respiratory: Nasal irritation
1% to 10%:
Cardiovascular: Edema, chest pain
Central nervous system: Insomnia, mental depression
Dermatologic: Urticaria, rash, pruritus, seborrhea
Respiratory: Dyspnea, rhinitis
(Continued)

949

Nafarelin *(Continued)*

Stability Store at room temperature; protect from light

Mechanism of Action Potent synthetic decapeptide analogue of gonadotropin-releasing hormone (GnRH; LHRH) which is approximately 200 times more potent than GnRH in terms of pituitary release of luteinizing hormone (LH) and follicle-stimulating hormone (FSH). Effects on the pituitary gland and sex hormones are dependent upon its length of administration. After acute administration, an initial stimulation of the release of LH and FSH from the pituitary is observed; an increase in androgens and estrogens subsequently follows. Continued administration of nafarelin, however, suppresses gonadotrope responsiveness to endogenous GnRH resulting in reduced secretion of LH and FSH and, secondarily, decreased ovarian and testicular steroid production.

Pharmacodynamics/Kinetics
Protein binding, plasma: 80%
Time to peak, serum: 10-45 minutes

Usual Dosage
Endometriosis: Adults: Female: 1 spray (200 mcg) in 1 nostril each morning and the other nostril each evening starting on days 2-4 of menstrual cycle for 6 months
Central precocious puberty: Children: Males/Females: 2 sprays (400 mcg) into each nostril in the morning 2 sprays (400 mcg) into each nostril in the evening. If inadequate suppression, may increase dose to 3 sprays (600 mcg) into alternating nostrils 3 times/day.

Patient Information Begin treatment between days 2 and 4 of menstrual cycle; usually menstruation will stop (as well as ovulation), but is not a reliable contraceptive, use of a nonhormonal contraceptive is suggested; full compliance with taking the medicine is very important; do not use nasal decongestant for at least 30 minutes after using nafarelin spray; notify physician if regular menstruation persists

Nursing Implications Do not administer to pregnant or breast-feeding patients; topical nasal decongestant should be used at least 30 minutes after nafarelin use

Additional Information Each spray delivers 200 mcg

Dosage Forms Solution, intranasal, as acetate [spray]: 2 mg/mL (10 mL) [200 mcg/spray]

♦ **Nafarelin Acetate** *see Nafarelin on page 949*

Nafcillin *(naf SIL in)*

Related Information
Antibiotic Treatment of Adults With Infective Endocarditis *on page 1585*
Community-Acquired Pneumonia in Adults *on page 1603*

U.S. Brand Names Nallpen® [DSC]

Canadian Brand Names Nallpen®; Unipen®

Synonyms Ethoxynaphthamido Penicillin Sodium; Nafcillin Sodium; Sodium Nafcillin

Therapeutic Category Antibiotic, Penicillin

Use Treatment of infections such as osteomyelitis, septicemia, endocarditis, and CNS infections caused by susceptible strains of staphylococci species

Pregnancy Risk Factor B

Contraindications Hypersensitivity to nafcillin, or any component of the formulation, or penicillins

Warnings/Precautions Extravasation of I.V. infusions should be avoided; modification of dosage is necessary in patients with both severe renal and hepatic impairment; elimination rate will be slow in neonates; use with caution in patients with cephalosporin hypersensitivity

Adverse Reactions Frequency not defined.
Central nervous system: Pain, fever
Dermatologic: Rash
Gastrointestinal: Nausea, diarrhea
Hematologic: Neutropenia
Local: Thrombophlebitis; oxacillin (less likely to cause phlebitis) is often preferred in pediatric patients
Renal: Interstitial nephritis (acute)
Miscellaneous: Hypersensitivity reactions

Overdosage/Toxicology Symptoms of penicillin overdose include neuromuscular hypersensitivity (agitation, hallucinations, asterixis, encephalopathy, confusion, and seizures) and electrolyte imbalance (with potassium or sodium salts), especially in renal failure. Hemodialysis may be helpful to aid in the removal of the drug from the blood, otherwise most treatment is supportive or symptom directed.

Drug Interactions
Cytochrome P450 Effect: CYP3A3/4 enzyme inducer
Increased Effect/Toxicity: Probenecid may cause an increase in nafcillin levels.
Decreased Effect: Chloramphenicol may decrease nafcillin efficacy. Oral contraceptives may have a decreased contraceptive effect when taken with nafcillin. If taken concomitantly with warfarin, nafcillin may inhibit the anticoagulant response to warfarin. This effect may persist for up to 30 days after nafcillin has been discontinued. Subtherapeutic cyclosporine levels may result when taken concomitantly with nafcillin.

Stability Reconstituted parenteral solution is stable for 3 days at room temperature and 7 days when refrigerated or 12 weeks when frozen; for I.V. infusion in NS or D_5W, solution is stable for 24 hours at room temperature and 96 hours when refrigerated

Mechanism of Action Interferes with bacterial cell wall synthesis during active multiplication, causing cell wall death and resultant bactericidal activity against susceptible bacteria

Pharmacodynamics/Kinetics
Distribution: Widely distributed; CSF penetration is poor but enhanced by meningeal inflammation; crosses placenta
Metabolism: Primarily hepatic; undergoes enterohepatic circulation
Half-life elimination:
Neonates: <3 weeks: 2.2-5.5 hours; 4-9 weeks: 1.2-2.3 hours
Children 3 months to 14 years: 0.75-1.9 hours

Adults: 30 minutes to 1.5 hours with normal renal and hepatic function
Time to peak, serum: I.M.: 30-60 minutes
Excretion: Primarily feces; urine (10% to 30% as unchanged drug)

Usual Dosage
Neonates:
    <2000 g, <7 days: 50 mg/kg/day divided every 12 hours
    <2000 g, >7 days: 75 mg/kg/day divided every 8 hours
    >2000 g, <7 days: 50 mg/kg/day divided every 8 hours
    >2000 g, >7 days: 75 mg/kg/day divided every 6 hours
Children:
    I.M.: 25 mg/kg twice daily
    I.V.:
        Mild to moderate infections: 50-100 mg/kg/day in divided doses every 6 hours
        Severe infections: 100-200 mg/kg/day in divided doses every 4-6 hours
    Maximum dose: 12 g/day
Adults:
    I.M.: 500 mg every 4-6 hours
    I.V.: 500-2000 mg every 4-6 hours
Dosing adjustment in renal impairment: Not necessary
Dialysis: Not dialyzable (0% to 5%) via hemodialysis; supplemental dosage not necessary with hemo- or peritoneal dialysis or continuous arteriovenous or venovenous hemofiltration
Dietary Considerations Should be taken on an empty stomach.
Administration
I.M.: Rotate injection sites
I.V.: Vesicant. Administer around-the-clock to promote less variation in peak and trough serum levels; infuse over 30-60 minutes
Monitoring Parameters Periodic CBC, urinalysis, BUN, serum creatinine, AST and ALT; observe for signs and symptoms of anaphylaxis during first dose
Test Interactions Positive Coombs' test (direct), false-positive urinary and serum proteins; may inactivate aminoglycosides *in vitro*
Nursing Implications
Extravasation: Use cold packs
    Hyaluronidase (Wydase®): Add 1 mL NS to 150 unit vial to make 150 units/mL of concentration; mix 0.1 mL of above with 0.9 mL NS in 1 mL syringe to make final concentration = 15 units/mL
Additional Information Sodium content of 1 g: 66.7 mg (2.9 mEq); other penicillinase-resistant penicillins (ie, dicloxacillin or cloxacillin) are preferred for oral therapy.
Dosage Forms Powder for injection, as sodium: 1 g, 2 g, 10 g

♦ **Nafcillin Sodium** *see* Nafcillin *on page 950*

Naftifine (NAF ti feen)
U.S. Brand Names Naftin®
Synonyms Naftifine Hydrochloride
Therapeutic Category Antifungal Agent, Topical
Use Topical treatment of tinea cruris (jock itch), tinea corporis (ringworm), and tinea pedis (athlete's foot)
Pregnancy Risk Factor B
Contraindications Hypersensitivity to any component
Warnings/Precautions For external use only
Adverse Reactions
>10%: Local: Burning, stinging
1% to 10%:
    Dermatologic: Erythema, itching
    Local: Dryness, irritation
Mechanism of Action Synthetic, broad-spectrum antifungal agent in the allylamine class; appears to have both fungistatic and fungicidal activity. Exhibits antifungal activity by selectively inhibiting the enzyme squalene epoxidase in a dose-dependent manner which results in the primary sterol, ergosterol, within the fungal membrane not being synthesized.
Pharmacodynamics/Kinetics
Absorption: Systemic: Cream: 6%; Gel: ≤4%
Half-life elimination: 2-3 days
Excretion: Urine and feces (as metabolites)
Usual Dosage Adults: Topical: Apply cream once daily and gel twice daily (morning and evening) for up to 4 weeks
Patient Information External use only; avoid eyes, mouth, and other mucous membranes; do not use occlusive dressings unless directed to do so; discontinue if irritation or sensitivity develops; wash hands after application
Nursing Implications External use only; avoid eyes, mouth, and other mucous membranes; do not use occlusive dressings unless directed to do so; discontinue if irritation or sensitivity develops; wash hands after application
Dosage Forms
Cream, topical, as hydrochloride: 1% (15 g, 30 g, 60 g)
Gel, topical, as hydrochloride: 1% (20 g, 40 g, 60 g)

♦ **Naftifine Hydrochloride** *see* Naftifine *on page 951*
♦ **Naftin®** *see* Naftifine *on page 951*
♦ **NaHCO$_3$** *see* Sodium Bicarbonate *on page 1243*

Nalbuphine (NAL byoo feen)
Related Information
    Narcotic Agonists Comparison *on page 1506*
U.S. Brand Names Nubain®
Canadian Brand Names Nubain®
(Continued)

Nalbuphine *(Continued)*

Synonyms Nalbuphine Hydrochloride

Therapeutic Category Analgesic, Narcotic

Use Relief of moderate to severe pain; preoperative analgesia, postoperative and surgical anesthesia, and obstetrical analgesia during labor and delivery

Pregnancy Risk Factor B/D (prolonged use or high doses at term)

Contraindications Hypersensitivity to nalbuphine or any component, including sulfites; pregnancy (prolonged use or high dosages at term)

Warnings/Precautions Use with caution in patients with recent myocardial infarction, biliary tract surgery, or sulfite sensitivity; may produce respiratory depression; use with caution in women delivering premature infants; use with caution in patients with a history of drug dependence, head trauma or increased intracranial pressure, decreased hepatic or renal function, or pregnancy; tolerance or drug dependence may result from extended use

Adverse Reactions

>10%:
   Central nervous system: Fatigue, drowsiness
   Miscellaneous: Histamine release

1% to 10%:
   Cardiovascular: Hypotension
   Central nervous system: Headache, nightmares, dizziness
   Gastrointestinal: Anorexia, nausea, vomiting, dry mouth
   Local: Pain at injection site
   Neuromuscular & skeletal: Weakness

<1% (Limited to important or life-threatening): Bradycardia, dyspnea, hypertension, tachycardia

Overdosage/Toxicology Symptoms include CNS depression, respiratory depression, miosis, hypotension, and bradycardia. Treatment of overdose includes airway support, establishment of an I.V. line, and administration of naloxone 2 mg I.V. (0.01 mg/kg for children), with repeat administration as necessary, up to a total of 10 mg.

Drug Interactions

Increased Effect/Toxicity: Barbiturate anesthetics may increase CNS depression.

Ethanol/Nutrition/Herb Interactions

Ethanol: Avoid ethanol (may increase CNS depression).

Herb/Nutraceutical: Avoid valerian, St John's wort, kava kava, gotu kola (may increase CNS depression).

Mechanism of Action Binds to opiate receptors in the CNS, causing inhibition of ascending pain pathways, altering the perception of and response to pain; produces generalized CNS depression

Pharmacodynamics/Kinetics

Onset of action: Peak effect: I.M.: 30 minutes; I.V.: 1-3 minutes
Metabolism: Hepatic
Half-life elimination: 3.5-5 hours
Excretion: Feces; urine (~7% as metabolites)

Usual Dosage I.M., I.V., S.C.:

Children 10 months to 14 years: Premedication: 0.2 mg/kg; maximum: 20 mg/dose
Adults: 10 mg/70 kg every 3-6 hours; maximum single dose: 20 mg; maximum daily dose: 160 mg

Dosing adjustment/comments in hepatic impairment: Use with caution and reduce dose

Administration Administer I.M., S.C., or I.V.

Monitoring Parameters Relief of pain, respiratory and mental status, blood pressure

Patient Information Avoid alcohol, may cause drowsiness, impaired judgment or coordination; may cause physical and psychological dependence with prolonged use; will cause withdrawal in patients currently dependent on narcotics

Nursing Implications Observe patient for excessive sedation, respiratory depression, implement safety measures, assist with ambulation; observe for narcotic withdrawal

Dosage Forms Injection, as hydrochloride: 1.5 mg/mL (30 mL); 10 mg/mL (1 mL, 10 mL); 20 mg/mL (1 mL, 10 mL)

- ◆ **Nalbuphine Hydrochloride** *see Nalbuphine on page 951*
- ◆ **Nalcrom® (Can)** *see Cromolyn Sodium on page 337*
- ◆ **Naldecon® Senior DX [OTC]** *see Guaifenesin and Dextromethorphan on page 646*
- ◆ **Naldecon® Senior EX [OTC]** *see Guaifenesin on page 645*
- ◆ **Nalfon®** *see Fenoprofen on page 550*

Nalidixic Acid *(nal i DIKS ik AS id)*

Related Information

Antacid Drug Interactions *on page 1477*

U.S. Brand Names NegGram®

Canadian Brand Names NegGram®

Synonyms Nalidixinic Acid

Therapeutic Category Antibiotic, Quinolone

Use Treatment of urinary tract infections

Pregnancy Risk Factor B

Contraindications Hypersensitivity to nalidixic acid or any component of the formulation; infants <3 months of age

Warnings/Precautions Use with caution in patients with impaired hepatic or renal function and prepubertal children; has been shown to cause cartilage degeneration in immature animals; may induce hemolysis in patients with G6PD deficiency. Tendon inflammation and/or rupture have been reported with other quinolone antibiotics. Discontinue at first sign of tendon inflammation or pain. Quinolones may exacerbate myasthenia gravis.

Adverse Reactions Frequency not defined.

Central nervous system: Dizziness, drowsiness, headache, increased intracranial pressure, malaise, vertigo, confusion, toxic psychosis, convulsions, fever, chills

Dermatologic: Rash, urticaria, photosensitivity reactions

Endocrine & metabolic: Metabolic acidosis

Gastrointestinal: Nausea, vomiting

Hematologic: Leukopenia, thrombocytopenia

Hepatic: Hepatotoxicity

Ocular: Visual disturbances

Miscellaneous: Quinolones have been associated with tendonitis and tendon rupture

Overdosage/Toxicology Symptoms include nausea, vomiting, toxic psychosis, convulsions, increased intracranial pressure, and metabolic acidosis. Severe overdose, intracranial hypertension, increased pressure, and seizures have occurred. After GI decontamination, treatment is symptomatic.

Drug Interactions

Cytochrome P450 Effect: CYP1A2 enzyme inhibitor (minor)

Increased Effect/Toxicity: Nalidixic acid increases the levels/effect of cyclosporine, caffeine, theophylline, and warfarin. The CNS-stimulating effect of some quinolones may be enhanced by NSAIDs, and foscarnet has been associated with an increased risk of seizures with some quinolones. Serum levels of some quinolones are increased by loop diuretics, probenecid, and cimetidine (and possibly other H_2-blockers) due to altered renal elimination. This effect may be more important for quinolones with high percentage of renal elimination than with nalidixic acid.

Decreased Effect: Enteral feedings may decrease plasma concentrations of nalidixic acid probably by >30% inhibition of absorption. Aluminum/magnesium products, didanosine, quinapril, and sucralfate may decrease absorption of nalidixic acid by ≥90% if administered concurrently. (Administer nalidixic acid at least 4 hours and preferably 6 hours after the dose of these agents.) Calcium, iron, zinc, and multivitamins with minerals products may decrease absorption of nalidixic acid significantly if administered concurrently. (Administer nalidixic acid 2 hours before dose or at least 2 hours after the dose of these agents.) Antineoplastic agents may decrease quinolone absorption.

Mechanism of Action Inhibits DNA polymerization in late stages of chromosomal replication

Pharmacodynamics/Kinetics

Distribution: Achieves significant antibacterial concentrations only in the urinary tract; crosses placenta; enters breast milk

Protein binding: 90%

Metabolism: Partially hepatic

Half-life elimination: 6-7 hours; increases significantly with renal impairment

Time to peak, serum: 1-2 hours

Excretion: Urine (as unchanged drug, 80% as metabolites); feces (small amounts)

Usual Dosage Oral:

Children 3 months to 12 years: 55 mg/kg/day divided every 6 hours; suppressive therapy is 33 mg/kg/day divided every 6 hours

Adults: 1 g 4 times/day for 2 weeks; then suppressive therapy of 500 mg 4 times/day

Dosing comments in renal impairment: Cl_{cr} <50 mL/minute: Avoid use

Dietary Considerations May administer with food to minimize GI upset

Test Interactions False-positive urine glucose with Clinitest®, false increase in urinary VMA

Patient Information Avoid undue exposure to direct sunlight or use a sunscreen; take 1 hour before meals, but can take with food to decrease GI upset, finish all medication, do not skip doses; if persistent cough occurs, notify physician

Nursing Implications

Administer around-the-clock rather than 4 times/day, 3 times/day, etc (ie, 12-6-12-6, not 9-1-5-9) to promote less variation in peak and trough serum levels

Monitor urinalysis, urine culture; CBC, renal and hepatic function tests

Dosage Forms

Suspension, oral: 250 mg/5 mL (473 mL) [raspberry flavor]

Tablet: 250 mg, 500 mg, 1 g

♦ **Nalidixinic Acid** see Nalidixic Acid on page 952

♦ **Nallpen® [DSC]** see Nafcillin on page 950

♦ **N-allylnoroxymorphine Hydrochloride** see Naloxone on page 954

Nalmefene (NAL me feen)

U.S. Brand Names Revex®

Synonyms Nalmefene Hydrochloride

Therapeutic Category Antidote for Narcotic Agonists

Use Complete or partial reversal of opioid drug effects, including respiratory depression induced by natural or synthetic opioids; reversal of postoperative opioid depression; management of known or suspected opioid overdose

Pregnancy Risk Factor B

Pregnancy/Breast-Feeding Implications Limited information available; do not use in pregnant or lactating women if possible

Contraindications Hypersensitivity to nalmefene, naltrexone, or any component of the formulation

Warnings/Precautions May induce symptoms of acute withdrawal in opioid-dependent patients; recurrence of respiratory depression is possible if the opioid involved is long-acting; observe patients until there is no reasonable risk of recurrent respiratory depression. Safety and efficacy have not been established in children. Avoid abrupt reversal of opioid effects in patients of high cardiovascular risk or who have received potentially cardiotoxic drugs. Pulmonary edema and cardiovascular instability have been reported in association with abrupt reversal with other narcotic antagonists.

Adverse Reactions

>10%: Gastrointestinal: Nausea

1% to 10%:

Cardiovascular: Tachycardia, hypertension, hypotension, vasodilation

(Continued)

Nalmefene *(Continued)*

Central nervous system: Fever, dizziness, headache, chills
Gastrointestinal: Vomiting
Miscellaneous: Postoperative pain

<1% (Limited to important or life-threatening): Agitation, arrhythmia, bradycardia, confusion, depression, diarrhea, myoclonus, nervousness, pharyngitis, pruritus, somnolence, tremor, urinary retention, xerostomia

Overdosage/Toxicology There are no known symptoms in significant overdose. However, large doses of opioids, administered to overcome a full blockade of opioid antagonists, have resulted in adverse respiratory and circulatory reactions.

Drug Interactions

Increased Effect/Toxicity: Potential increased risk of seizures may exist with use of flumazenil and nalmefene coadministration.

Mechanism of Action As a 6-methylene analog of naltrexone, nalmefene acts as a competitive antagonist at opioid receptor sites, preventing or reversing the respiratory depression, sedation, and hypotension induced by opiates; no pharmacologic activity of its own (eg, opioid agonist activity) has been demonstrated

Pharmacodynamics/Kinetics

Onset of action: I.M., S.C.: 5-15 minutes
Distribution: V_d: 8.6 L/kg; rapid
Protein binding: 45%
Metabolism: Hepatic via glucuronide conjugation to metabolites with little or no activity
Bioavailability: I.M., I.V., S.C.: 100%
Half-life elimination: 10.8 hours
Time to peak, serum: I.M.: 2.3 hours; I.V.: <2 minutes; S.C.: 1.5 hours
Excretion: Urine (<5% as unchanged drug); feces (17%)
Clearance: 0.8 L/hour/kg

Usual Dosage

Reversal of postoperative opioid depression: Blue labeled product (100 mcg/mL): Titrate to reverse the undesired effects of opioids; initial dose for nonopioid dependent patients: 0.25 mcg/kg followed by 0.25 mcg/kg incremental doses at 2- to 5-minute intervals; after a total dose >1 mcg/kg, further therapeutic response is unlikely

Management of known/suspected opioid overdose: Green labeled product (1000 mcg/mL): Initial dose: 0.5 mg/70 kg; may repeat with 1 mg/70 kg in 2-5 minutes; further increase beyond a total dose of 1.5 mg/70 kg will not likely result in improved response and may result in cardiovascular stress and precipitated withdrawal syndrome. (If opioid dependency is suspected, administer a challenge dose of 0.1 mg/70 kg; if no withdrawal symptoms are observed in 2 minutes, the recommended doses can be administered.)

Note: If recurrence of respiratory depression is noted, dose may again be titrated to clinical effect using incremental doses.

Note: If I.V. access is lost or not readily obtainable, a single S.C. or I.M. dose of 1 mg may be effective in 5-15 minutes.

Dosing adjustment in renal or hepatic impairment: Not necessary with single uses, however, slow administration (over 60 seconds) of incremental doses is recommended to minimize hypertension and dizziness

Administration Dilute drug (1:1) with diluent and use smaller doses in patients known to be at increased cardiovascular risk; may be administered via I.M. or S.C. routes if I.V. access is not feasible

Nursing Implications Check dosage strength carefully before use to avoid error (labeling is color-coded; postoperative reversal - blue, overdose management - green); monitor patients for signs of withdrawal, especially those physically dependent who are in pain or at high cardiovascular risk

Additional Information Proper steps should be used to prevent use of the incorrect dosage strength. The goal of treatment in the postoperative setting is to achieve reversal of excessive opioid effects without inducing a complete reversal and acute pain.

If opioid dependence is suspected, nalmefene should only be used in opioid overdose if the likelihood of overdose is high based on history or the clinical presentation of respiratory depression with concurrent pupillary constriction is present.

Dosage Forms Injection, as hydrochloride: 100 mcg/mL [blue label] (1 mL); 1000 mcg/mL [green label] (2 mL)

♦ **Nalmefene Hydrochloride** *see Nalmefene on page 953*

Naloxone *(nal OKS one)*

Related Information
Narcotic Agonists Comparison *on page 1506*

U.S. Brand Names Narcan®

Canadian Brand Names Narcan®

Synonyms *N*-allylnoroxymorphine Hydrochloride; Naloxone Hydrochloride

Therapeutic Category Antidote for Narcotic Agonists

Use

Complete or partial reversal of opioid depression, including respiratory depression, induced by natural and synthetic opioids, including propoxyphene, methadone, and certain mixed agonist-antagonist analgesics: nalbuphine, pentazocine, and butorphanol

Diagnosis of suspected opioid tolerance or acute opioid overdose

Adjunctive agent to increase blood pressure in the management of septic shock

Unlabeled/Investigational Use PCP and ethanol ingestion

Pregnancy Risk Factor B

Contraindications Hypersensitivity to naloxone or any component

Warnings/Precautions Use with caution in patients with cardiovascular disease; excessive dosages should be avoided after use of opiates in surgery, because naloxone may cause an increase in blood pressure and reversal of anesthesia; may precipitate withdrawal symptoms in patients addicted to opiates, including pain, hypertension, sweating, agitation, irritability, shrill cry, failure to feed

Adverse Reactions Frequency not defined.
Cardiovascular: Hypertension, hypotension, tachycardia, ventricular arrhythmias, cardiac arrest
Central nervous system: Irritability, anxiety, narcotic withdrawal, restlessness, seizures
Gastrointestinal: Nausea, vomiting, diarrhea
Neuromuscular & skeletal: Tremulousness
Respiratory: Dyspnea, pulmonary edema, runny nose, sneezing
Miscellaneous: Diaphoresis

Overdosage/Toxicology Naloxone is the drug of choice for respiratory depression that is known or suspected to be caused by an opiate or opioid overdose.

Caution: Naloxone's effects are due to its action on narcotic reversal, not due to direct effect upon opiate receptors. Therefore, adverse events occur secondarily to reversal (withdrawal) of narcotic analgesia and sedation, which can cause severe reactions.

Drug Interactions
Decreased Effect: Decreased effect of narcotic analgesics.

Stability Protect from light; stable in 0.9% sodium chloride and D$_5$W at 4 mcg/mL for 24 hours; do not mix with alkaline solutions

Mechanism of Action Pure opioid antagonist that competes and displaces narcotics at opioid receptor sites

Pharmacodynamics/Kinetics
Onset of action: Endotracheal, I.M., S.C.: 2-5 minutes; I.V.: ~2 minutes
Duration: 20-60 minutes; since shorter than that of most opioids, repeated doses are usually needed
Distribution: Crosses placenta
Metabolism: Primarily hepatic via glucuronidation
Half-life elimination: Neonates: 1.2-3 hours; Adults: 1-1.5 hours
Excretion: Urine (as metabolites)

Usual Dosage I.M., I.V. (preferred), intratracheal, S.C.:
Postanesthesia narcotic reversal: Infants and Children: 0.01 mg/kg; may repeat every 2-3 minutes, as needed based on response
Opiate intoxication:
Children:
Birth (including premature infants) to 5 years or <20 kg: 0.1 mg/kg; repeat every 2-3 minutes if needed; may need to repeat doses every 20-60 minutes
>5 years or ≥20 kg: 2 mg/dose; if no response, repeat every 2-3 minutes; may need to repeat doses every 20-60 minutes
Children and Adults: Continuous infusion: I.V.: If continuous infusion is required, calculate dosage/hour based on effective intermittent dose used and duration of adequate response seen, titrate dose 0.04-0.16 mg/kg/hour for 2-5 days in children, adult dose typically 0.25-6.25 mg/hour (short-term infusions as high as 2.4 mg/kg/hour have been tolerated in adults during treatment for septic shock); alternatively, continuous infusion utilizes ⅔ of the initial naloxone bolus on an hourly basis; add 10 times this dose to each liter of D$_5$W and infuse at a rate of 100 mL/hour; ½ of the initial bolus dose should be readministered 15 minutes after initiation of the continuous infusion to prevent a drop in naloxone levels; increase infusion rate as needed to assure adequate ventilation
Narcotic overdose: Adults: I.V.: 0.4-2 mg every 2-3 minutes as needed; may need to repeat doses every 20-60 minutes, if no response is observed after 10 mg, question the diagnosis.
Note: Use 0.1-0.2 mg increments in patients who are opioid dependent and in postoperative patients to avoid large cardiovascular changes.

Administration
Endotracheal: Dilute to 1-2 mL with normal saline
I.V. push: Administer over 30 seconds as undiluted preparation
I.V. continuous infusion: Dilute to 4 mcg/mL in D$_5$W or normal saline

Monitoring Parameters Respiratory rate, heart rate, blood pressure

Nursing Implications The use of neonatal naloxone (0.02 mg/mL) is no longer recommended because unacceptable fluid volumes will result, especially to small neonates; the 0.4 mg/mL preparation is available and can be accurately dosed with appropriately sized syringes (1 mL)

Additional Information May contain methyl and propylparabens

Dosage Forms
Injection, as hydrochloride: 0.4 mg/mL (1 mL, 2 mL, 10 mL); 1 mg/mL (2 mL, 10 mL)
Injection, neonatal, as hydrochloride: 0.02 mg/mL (2 mL)

♦ **Naloxone Hydrochloride** *see* Naloxone *on page 954*

Naltrexone (nal TREKS one)
U.S. Brand Names ReVia®
Canadian Brand Names ReVia®
Synonyms Naltrexone Hydrochloride
Therapeutic Category Antidote for Narcotic Agonists
Use Treatment of ethanol dependence; blockade of the effects of exogenously administered opioids
Pregnancy Risk Factor C
Contraindications Hypersensitivity to naltrexone or any component of the formulation; narcotic dependence or current use of opioid analgesics; acute opioid withdrawal; failure to pass Narcan® challenge or positive urine screen for opioids; acute hepatitis; liver failure
Warnings/Precautions Dose-related hepatocellular injury is possible; the margin of separation between the apparent safe and hepatotoxic doses appear to be only fivefold or less
Adverse Reactions
>10%:
Central nervous system: Insomnia, nervousness, headache, low energy
(Continued)

Naltrexone *(Continued)*

Gastrointestinal: Abdominal cramping, nausea, vomiting
Neuromuscular & skeletal: Arthralgia

1% to 10%:

Central nervous system: Increased energy, feeling down, irritability, dizziness, anxiety, somnolence
Dermatologic: Rash
Endocrine & metabolic: Polydipsia
Gastrointestinal: Diarrhea, constipation
Genitourinary: Delayed ejaculation, impotency

<1% (Limited to important or life-threatening): Depression, disorientation, hallucinations, narcotic withdrawal, paranoia, restlessness, suicide attempts

Overdosage/Toxicology Symptoms include clonic-tonic convulsions and respiratory failure. Patients receiving up to 800 mg/day for 1 week have shown no toxicity. Seizures and respiratory failure have been seen in animals.

Drug Interactions

Increased Effect/Toxicity: Lethargy and somnolence have been reported with the combination of naltrexone and thioridazine.

Decreased Effect: Naltrexone decreases effects of opioid-containing products.

Mechanism of Action Naltrexone (a pure opioid antagonist) is a cyclopropyl derivative of oxymorphone similar in structure to naloxone and nalorphine (a morphine derivative); it acts as a competitive antagonist at opioid receptor sites

Pharmacodynamics/Kinetics

Duration: 50 mg: 24 hours; 100 mg: 48 hours; 150 mg: 72 hours
Absorption: Almost completely
Distribution: V_d: 19 L/kg; widely throughout the body but considerable interindividual variation exists
Protein binding: 21%
Metabolism: Extensive first-pass effect to 6-β-naltrexol
Half-life elimination: 4 hours; 6-β-naltrexol: 13 hours
Time to peak, serum: ~60 minutes
Excretion: Primarily urine (as metabolites and unchanged drug)

Usual Dosage Do not give until patient is opioid-free for 7-10 days as determined by urine analysis

Adults: Oral: 25 mg; if no withdrawal signs within 1 hour give another 25 mg; maintenance regimen is flexible, variable and individualized (50 mg/day to 100-150 mg 3 times/week for 12 weeks); up to 800 mg/day has been tolerated in adults without an adverse effect

Dosing cautions in renal/hepatic impairment: Caution in patients with renal and hepatic impairment. An increase in naltrexone AUC of approximately five- and tenfold in patients with compensated or decompensated liver cirrhosis respectively, compared with normal liver function has been reported.

Administration If there is any question of occult opioid dependence, perform a naloxone challenge test; do not attempt treatment until naloxone challenge is negative

Naltrexone is administered orally; to minimize adverse gastrointestinal effects, administer with food or antacids or after meals; advise patient not to self-administer opiates while receiving naltrexone therapy

Monitoring Parameters For narcotic withdrawal; liver function tests

Patient Information Will cause narcotic withdrawal; serious overdose can occur after attempts to overcome the blocking effect of naltrexone

Nursing Implications Monitor for narcotic withdrawal

Dosage Forms Tablet, as hydrochloride: 50 mg

- ♦ **Naltrexone Hydrochloride** *see* Naltrexone *on page 955*
- ♦ **Names Alka-Seltzer Plus® Cold and Sinus [OTC]** *see* Acetaminophen and Pseudoephedrine *on page 25*

Nandrolone *(NAN droe lone)*

U.S. Brand Names Deca-Durabolin®; Hybolin™ Decanoate; Hybolin™ Improved Injection
Canadian Brand Names Deca-Durabolin®; Durabolin®
Synonyms Nandrolone Decanoate; Nandrolone Phenpropionate
Therapeutic Category Anabolic Steroid; Androgen
Use Control of metastatic breast cancer; management of anemia of renal insufficiency
Restrictions C-III
Pregnancy Risk Factor X
Contraindications Hypersensitivity to nandrolone or any component of the formulation; carcinoma of breast or prostate; nephrosis; pregnancy; not for use in infants
Warnings/Precautions Monitor diabetic patients carefully; anabolic steroids may cause peliosis hepatis, liver cell tumors, and blood lipid changes with increased risk of arteriosclerosis; use with caution in elderly patients, they may be at greater risk for prostatic hyperplasia; use with caution in patients with cardiac, renal, or hepatic disease or epilepsy
Adverse Reactions

Male: Postpubertal:

>10%:

Dermatologic: Acne
Endocrine & metabolic: Gynecomastia
Genitourinary: Bladder irritability, priapism

1% to 10%:

Central nervous system: Insomnia, chills
Endocrine & metabolic: Decreased libido, hepatic dysfunction,
Gastrointestinal: Nausea, diarrhea
Genitourinary: Prostatic hyperplasia (elderly)
Hematologic: Iron-deficiency anemia, suppression of clotting factors

<1% (Limited to important or life-threatening): Hepatic necrosis, hepatocellular carcinoma

Male: Prepubertal:
>10%:
  Dermatologic: Acne
  Endocrine & metabolic: Virilism
1% to 10%:
  Central nervous system: Chills, insomnia, factors
  Dermatologic: Hyperpigmentation
  Gastrointestinal: Diarrhea, nausea
  Hematologic: Iron deficiency anemia, suppression of clotting
<1% (Limited to important or life-threatening): Hepatocellular carcinoma, necrosis
Female:
>10%: Endocrine & metabolic: Virilism
1% to 10%:
  Central nervous system: Chills, insomnia
  Endocrine & metabolic: Hypercalcemia
  Gastrointestinal: Nausea, diarrhea
  Hematologic: Iron deficiency anemia, suppression of clotting factors
  Hepatic: Hepatic dysfunction
<1% (Limited to important or life-threatening): Hepatic necrosis, hepatocellular carcinoma
Drug Interactions
  Increased Effect/Toxicity: Nandrolone may increase the effect of oral anticoagulants, insulin, oral hypoglycemic agents, adrenal steroids, or ACTH when taken together.
Mechanism of Action Promotes tissue-building processes, increases production of erythropoietin, causes protein anabolism; increases hemoglobin and red blood cell volume
Pharmacodynamics/Kinetics
  Onset of action: 3-6 months
  Duration: Up to 30 days
  Absorption: I.M.: 77%
  Metabolism: Hepatic
  Excretion: Urine
Usual Dosage Deep I.M. (into gluteal muscle):
  Children 2-13 years (decanoate): 25-50 mg every 3-4 weeks
  Adults:
    Male:
      Breast cancer (phenpropionate): 50-100 mg/week
      Anemia of renal insufficiency (decanoate): 100-200 mg/week
    Female: 50-100 mg/week
      Breast cancer (phenpropionate): 50-100 mg/week
      Anemia of renal insufficiency (decanoate): 50-100 mg/week
Administration Inject deeply I.M., preferably into the gluteal muscle
Test Interactions Altered glucose tolerance tests
Patient Information Virilization may occur in female patients; report menstrual irregularities; male patients report persistent penile erections; all patients should report persistent GI distress, diarrhea, dark urine, pale stools, yellow coloring of skin or sclera; diabetic patients should monitor glucose closely
Nursing Implications Inject deeply I.M., preferably into the gluteal muscle
Additional Information Both phenpropionate and decanoate are injections in oil.
Dosage Forms
  Injection, in oil, as decanoate: 50 mg/mL (1 mL, 2 mL); 100 mg/mL (1 mL, 2 mL); 200 mg/mL (1 mL)
  Injection, repository, as decanoate: 50 mg/mL (2 mL); 100 mg/mL (2 mL); 200 mg/mL (2 mL)

♦ **Nandrolone Decanoate** *see* Nandrolone *on page 956*
♦ **Nandrolone Phenpropionate** *see* Nandrolone *on page 956*

Naphazoline (naf AZ oh leen)

U.S. Brand Names AK-Con®; Albalon® Liquifilm®; Allersol®; Clear Eyes® [OTC]; Clear Eyes® ACR [OTC]; Naphcon® [OTC]; Ocu-Zoline®; Privine® Nasal [OTC]; VasoClear® [OTC]; Vasocon Regular®
Canadian Brand Names Naphcon Forte®; Vasocon®
Synonyms Naphazoline Hydrochloride
Therapeutic Category Adrenergic Agonist Agent, Ophthalmic; Decongestant, Nasal; Nasal Agent, Vasoconstrictor; Ophthalmic Agent, Vasoconstrictor
Use Topical ocular vasoconstrictor; will temporarily relieve congestion, itching, and minor irritation, and to control hyperemia in patients with superficial corneal vascularity; treatment of nasal congestion; adjunct for sinusitis
Pregnancy Risk Factor C
Contraindications Hypersensitivity to naphazoline or any component of the formulation; narrow-angle glaucoma, prior to peripheral iridectomy (in patients susceptible to angle block)
Warnings/Precautions Rebound congestion may occur with extended use; use with caution in the presence of hypertension, diabetes, hyperthyroidism, heart disease, coronary artery disease, cerebral arteriosclerosis, or long-standing bronchial asthma
Adverse Reactions Frequency not defined.
  Cardiovascular: Systemic cardiovascular stimulation
  Central nervous system: Dizziness, headache, nervousness
  Gastrointestinal: Nausea
  Local: Transient stinging, nasal mucosa irritation, dryness, rebound congestion
  Ocular: Mydriasis, increased intraocular pressure, blurring of vision
  Respiratory: Sneezing
Overdosage/Toxicology Symptoms include CNS depression, hypothermia, bradycardia, cardiovascular collapse, apnea, and coma. Following initiation of essential overdose management, toxic symptoms should be treated. The patient should be kept warm and monitored for alterations in vital functions. Seizures commonly respond to diazepam (5-10 mg I.V. bolus in adults every 15 minutes, if needed, up to a total of 30 mg; I.V. 0.25-0.4 mg/
(Continued)

Naphazoline *(Continued)*

kg/dose up to a total of 10 mg for children) or to phenytoin or phenobarbital. Hypotension should be treated with fluids.

Stability Store in tight, light-resistant containers

Mechanism of Action Stimulates alpha-adrenergic receptors in the arterioles of the conjunctiva and the nasal mucosa to produce vasoconstriction

Pharmacodynamics/Kinetics
Onset of action: Decongestant: Topical: ~10 minutes
Duration: 2-6 hours

Usual Dosage
Nasal:
Children:
<6 years: Intranasal: Not recommended (especially infants) due to CNS depression
6-12 years: 1 spray of 0.05% into each nostril every 6 hours if necessary; therapy should not exceed 3-5 days
Children >12 years and Adults: 0.05%, instill 1-2 drops or sprays every 6 hours if needed; therapy should not exceed 3-5 days
Ophthalmic:
Children <6 years: Not recommended for use due to CNS depression (especially in infants)
Children >6 years and Adults: Instill 1-2 drops into conjunctival sac of affected eye(s) every 3-4 hours; therapy generally should not exceed 3-4 days

Patient Information Do not use discolored solutions; discontinue eye drops if visual changes or ocular pain occur; notify physician of insomnia, tremor, or irregular heartbeat; stinging, burning, or drying of the nasal mucosa may occur; do not use beyond 72 hours

Nursing Implications Rebound congestion can result with continued use

Dosage Forms
Solution, intranasal, as hydrochloride [drops] (Privine®): 0.05% (25 mL)
Solution, intranasal, as hydrochloride [spray] (Privine®): 0.05% (20 mL, 480 mL)
Solution, ophthalmic, as hydrochloride:
AK-Con®, Albalon® Liquifilm®, Vasocon®: 0.1% (15 mL)
Clear Eyes®, Clear Eyes® ACR, Naphcon®: 0.012% (6 mL, 15 mL, 30 mL)
VasoClear®: 0.02% (15 mL)

Naphazoline and Antazoline *(naf AZ oh leen & an TAZ oh leen)*
U.S. Brand Names Vasocon-A® [OTC]
Canadian Brand Names Albalon®-A Liquifilm; Vasocon-A®
Synonyms Antazoline and Naphazoline
Therapeutic Category Ophthalmic Agent, Vasoconstrictor
Use Topical ocular congestion, irritation and itching
Pregnancy Risk Factor C
Usual Dosage 1-2 drops every 3-4 hours
Additional Information Complete prescribing information for this medication should be consulted for additional detail.
Dosage Forms Solution, ophthalmic: Naphazoline hydrochloride 0.05% and antazoline phosphate 0.5% (5 mL, 15 mL)

Naphazoline and Pheniramine *(naf AZ oh leen & fen NIR a meen)*
U.S. Brand Names Naphcon-A® [OTC]
Canadian Brand Names Naphcon®-A
Synonyms Pheniramine and Naphazoline
Therapeutic Category Ophthalmic Agent, Vasoconstrictor
Use Topical ocular vasoconstrictor
Pregnancy Risk Factor C
Usual Dosage 1-2 drops every 3-4 hours
Additional Information Complete prescribing information for this medication should be consulted for additional detail.
Dosage Forms Solution, ophthalmic: Naphazoline hydrochloride 0.025% and pheniramine 0.3% (15 mL)

♦ **Naphazoline Hydrochloride** *see Naphazoline on page 957*
♦ **Naphcon® [OTC]** *see Naphazoline on page 957*
♦ **Naphcon-A® [OTC]** *see Naphazoline and Pheniramine on page 958*
♦ **Naphcon Forte® (Can)** *see Naphazoline on page 957*
♦ **Naprelan®** *see Naproxen on page 958*
♦ **Naprosyn®** *see Naproxen on page 958*

Naproxen *(na PROKS en)*
Related Information
Antacid Drug Interactions on page 1477
Nonsteroidal Anti-Inflammatory Agents Comparison on page 1512
U.S. Brand Names Aleve® [OTC]; Anaprox®; EC-Naprosyn®; Naprelan®; Naprosyn®
Canadian Brand Names Anaprox®; Anaprox® DS; Apo®-Napro-Na; Apo®-Napro-Na DS; Apo®-Naproxen; Apo®-Naproxen SR; Gen-Naproxen EC; Naprosyn®; Naxen®; Novo-Naprox; Novo-Naprox Sodium; Novo-Naprox Sodium DS; Novo-Naprox SR; Nu-Naprox; Riva-Naproxen; Synflex®; Synflex® DS
Synonyms Naproxen Sodium
Therapeutic Category Analgesic, Nonsteroidal Anti-inflammatory Drug; Anti-inflammatory Agent; Antimigraine Agent; Antipyretic; Nonsteroidal Anti-inflammatory Drug (NSAID), Oral
Use Management of inflammatory disease and rheumatoid disorders (including juvenile rheumatoid arthritis); acute gout; mild to moderate pain; dysmenorrhea; fever, migraine headache
Pregnancy Risk Factor B/D (3rd trimester)

Contraindications Hypersensitivity to naproxen, aspirin, other nonsteroidal anti-inflammatory drugs (NSAIDs), or any component of the formulation; pregnancy (3rd trimester)

Warnings/Precautions Use with caution in patients with GI disease (bleeding or ulcers), cardiovascular disease (CHF, hypertension), dehydration, renal or hepatic impairment, and patients receiving anticoagulants; perform ophthalmologic evaluation for those who develop eye complaints during therapy (blurred vision, diminished vision, changes in color vision, retinal changes); NSAIDs may mask signs/symptoms of infections; photosensitivity reported; elderly are at especially high-risk for adverse effects (including gastrointestinal and CNS adverse effects) from nonsteroidal anti-inflammatory agents. As many as 60% of elderly can develop peptic ulceration and/or hemorrhage asymptomatically. Use lowest effective dose for shortest period possible. Use of NSAIDs can compromise existing renal function especially when Cl_{cr} is <30 mL/minute. Withhold for at least 4-6 half-lives prior to surgical or dental procedures.

Adverse Reactions
1% to 10%:
Central nervous system: Headache (11%), nervousness, malaise (<3%), somnolence (3% to 9%)
Dermatologic: Itching, pruritus, rash, ecchymosis (3% to 9%)
Endocrine & metabolic: Fluid retention (3% to 9%)
Gastrointestinal: Abdominal discomfort, nausea (3% to 9%), heartburn, constipation (3% to 9%), GI bleeding, ulcers, perforation, indigestion, diarrhea (<3%), abdominal distress/cramps/pain (3% to 9%), dyspepsia (<3%), stomatitis (<3%), heartburn (<3%)
Hematologic: Hemolysis (3% to 9%), ecchymosis (3% to 9%)
Otic: Tinnitus (3% to 9%)
Respiratory: Dyspnea (3% to 9%)
<1% (Limited to important or life-threatening): Acute renal failure, agranulocytosis, allergic rhinitis, anemia, angioedema, arrhythmias, aseptic meningitis, bone marrow suppression, bronchospasm, congestive heart failure, erythema multiforme, GI ulceration, hallucinations, hemolytic anemia, hepatitis, hypertension, leukopenia, mental depression, peripheral neuropathy, renal dysfunction, Stevens-Johnson syndrome, thrombocytopenia, toxic amblyopia, toxic epidermal necrolysis, urticaria, vomiting

Overdosage/Toxicology Symptoms include drowsiness, heartburn, vomiting, CNS depression, leukocytosis, and renal failure. Management of nonsteroidal anti-inflammatory drug (NSAID) intoxication is primarily supportive and symptomatic. Fluid therapy is commonly effective in managing hypotension that may occur following an acute NSAID overdose, except when due to acute blood loss. Seizures tend to be very short-lived and often do not require drug treatment, although recurrent seizures should be treated with I.V. diazepam. Since many of NSAIDs undergo enterohepatic cycling, multiple doses of charcoal may be needed to reduce the potential for delayed toxicities.

Drug Interactions
Cytochrome P450 Effect: CYP2C8, 2C9, and 2C18 enzyme substrate
Increased Effect/Toxicity: Naproxen could displace other highly protein-bound drugs, increasing the effect of oral anticoagulants, hydantoins, salicylates, sulfonamides, and first-generation sulfonylureas. Naproxen and warfarin may cause a slight increase in free warfarin. Naproxen and probenecid may cause increased levels of naproxen. Naproxen and methotrexate may significantly increase and prolong blood methotrexate concentration, which may be severe or fatal. May increase lithium or cyclosporine levels. Corticosteroids may increase risk of GI ulceration.
Decreased Effect: NSAIDs may decrease the effect of some antihypertensive agents, including ACE inhibitors, angiotensin receptor antagonists, and hydralazine. The efficacy of diuretics (loop and/or thiazide) may be decreased.

Ethanol/Nutrition/Herb Interactions
Ethanol: Avoid or limit ethanol (may enhance gastric mucosal irritation).
Food: Naproxen absorption rate may be decreased if taken with food.
Herb/Nutraceutical: Avoid cat's claw, dong quai, evening primrose, feverfew, garlic, ginger, ginkgo, red clover, horse chestnut, green tea, ginseng (all have additional antiplatelet activity).

Mechanism of Action Inhibits prostaglandin synthesis by decreasing the activity of the enzyme, cyclo-oxygenase, which results in decreased formation of prostaglandin precursors

Pharmacodynamics/Kinetics
Onset of action: Analgesic: 1 hour; Anti-inflammatory: ~2 weeks
Peak effect: Anti-inflammatory: 2-4 weeks
Duration: Analgesic: ≤7 hours; Anti-inflammatory: ≤12 hours
Absorption: Almost 100%
Protein binding: >90%; increased free fraction in elderly
Half-life elimination: Normal renal function: 12-15 hours; End-stage renal disease: Unchanged
Time to peak, serum: 1-2 hours

Usual Dosage Oral:
Children >2 years:
Fever: 2.5-10 mg/kg/dose; maximum: 10 mg/kg/day
Juvenile arthritis: 10 mg/kg/day in 2 divided doses
Adults:
Rheumatoid arthritis, osteoarthritis, and ankylosing spondylitis: 500-1000 mg/day in 2 divided doses; may increase to 1.5 g/day of naproxen base for limited time period
Mild to moderate pain or dysmenorrhea: Initial: 500 mg, then 250 mg every 6-8 hours; maximum: 1250 mg/day naproxen base
Dosing adjustment in hepatic impairment: Reduce dose to 50%

Dietary Considerations Drug may cause GI upset, bleeding, ulceration, perforation; take with food or milk to minimize GI upset.

Administration Administer with food, milk, or antacids to decrease GI adverse effects

Monitoring Parameters Occult blood loss, periodic liver function test, CBC, BUN, serum creatinine
(Continued)

Naproxen *(Continued)*

Patient Information Serious gastrointestinal bleeding can occur as well as ulceration and perforation. Pain may or may not be present. Avoid aspirin and aspirin-containing products while taking this medication. If gastric upset occurs, take with food, milk, or antacid. If gastric adverse effects persist, contact physician. May cause drowsiness, dizziness, blurred vision, and confusion. Use caution when performing tasks which require alertness (eg, driving). Do not take for more than 3 days for fever or 10 days for pain without physician's advice.

Nursing Implications Monitor occult blood loss, periodic liver function test, hemoglobin, CBC, BUN, serum creatinine

Additional Information Naproxen: Naprosyn®; naproxen sodium: Anaprox®; 275 mg of Anaprox® equivalent to 250 mg of Naprosyn®

Dosage Forms
    Caplet, as sodium (Aleve®): 220 mg (200 mg base)
    Gelcap, as sodium (Aleve®): 220 mg (200 mg base)
    Suspension, oral: 125 mg/5 mL (15 mL, 30 mL, 480 mL)
    Tablet (Naprosyn®): 250 mg, 375 mg, 500 mg
    Tablet, as sodium:
      Aleve®: 220 mg (200 mg base)
      Anaprox®: 275 mg (250 mg base); 550 mg (500 mg base)
    Tablet, delayed release (EC-Naprosyn®): 375 mg, 500 mg
    Tablet, extended release, as sodium: 375 mg, 500 mg, 750 mg
      Naprelan®: 375 mg (421.5 mg base); 500 mg (550 mg base)

♦ **Naproxen Sodium** *see* Naproxen *on page 958*

♦ **Naqua**® *see* Trichlormethiazide *on page 1371*

Naratriptan *(NAR a trip tan)*

Related Information
    Antimigraine Drugs Comparison *on page 1485*

U.S. Brand Names Amerge®

Canadian Brand Names Amerge®

Synonyms Naratriptan Hydrochloride

Therapeutic Category Antimigraine Agent, Serotonin 5-HT$_{1D}$ Agonist; Serotonin Agonist

Use Treatment of acute migraine headache with or without aura

Pregnancy Risk Factor C

Contraindications Hypersensitivity to naratriptan or any component of the formulation; cerebrovascular, peripheral vascular disease (ischemic bowel disease), ischemic heart disease (angina pectoris, history of myocardial infarction, or proven silent ischemia); or in patients with symptoms consistent with ischemic heart disease, coronary artery vasospasm, or Prinzmetal's angina; uncontrolled hypertension or patients who have received within 24 hours another 5-HT agonist (sumatriptan, zolmitriptan) or ergotamine-containing product; patients with known risk factors associated with coronary artery disease; patients with severe hepatic or renal disease (Cl$_{cr}$ <15 mL/minute); do not administer naratriptan to patients with hemiplegic or basilar migraine

Warnings/Precautions Use only if there is a clear diagnosis of migraine. Patients who are at risk of CAD but have had a satisfactory cardiovascular evaluation may receive naratriptan but with extreme caution (ie, in a physician's office where there are adequate precautions in place to protect the patient). Blood pressure may increase with the administration of naratriptan. Monitor closely, especially with the first administration of the drug. If the patient does not respond to the first dose, re-evaluate the diagnosis of migraine before trying a second dose.

Adverse Reactions
    1% to 10%:
      Central nervous system: Dizziness, drowsiness, malaise/fatigue, paresthesias
      Gastrointestinal: Nausea, vomiting
      Miscellaneous: Pain or pressure in throat or neck
    <1% (Limited to important or life-threatening): Allergic reaction, atrial fibrillation, atrial flutter, coronary artery vasospasm, hallucinations, myocardial infarction, PR prolongation, premature ventricular contractions, QT$_c$ prolongation, seizure, ventricular fibrillation, ventricular tachycardia

Drug Interactions
    Increased Effect/Toxicity: Ergot-containing drugs (dihydroergotamine or methysergide) may cause vasospastic reactions when taken with naratriptan. Avoid concomitant use with ergots; separate dose of naratriptan and ergots by at least 24 hours. Oral contraceptives taken with naratriptan reduced the clearance of naratriptan ~30% which may contribute to adverse effects. Selective serotonin reuptake inhibitors (SSRIs) (eg, fluoxetine, fluvoxamine, paroxetine, sertraline) may cause lack of coordination, hyper-reflexia, or weakness and should be avoided when taking naratriptan.

    Decreased Effect: Smoking increases the clearance of naratriptan.

Mechanism of Action The therapeutic effect for migraine is due to serotonin agonist activity

Pharmacodynamics/Kinetics
    Onset of action: 30 minutes
    Protein binding, plasma: 28% to 31%
    Metabolism: Hepatic, CYP450 isoenzymes
    Bioavailability: 70%
    Time to peak: 2-3 hours
    Excretion: Urine

Usual Dosage
    Adults: Oral: 1-2.5 mg at the onset of headache; it is recommended to use the lowest possible dose to minimize adverse effects. If headache returns or does not fully resolve, the dose may be repeated after 4 hours; do not exceed 5 mg in 24 hours.
    Elderly: Not recommended for use in the elderly

Dosing in renal impairment:
Cl$_{cr}$: 18-39 mL/minute: Initial: 1 mg; do not exceed 2.5 mg in 24 hours
Cl$_{cr}$: <15 mL/minute: Do not use
Dosing in hepatic impairment: Contraindicated in patients with severe liver failure; maximum dose: 2.5 mg in 24 hours for patients with mild or moderate liver failure; recommended starting dose: 1 mg

Patient Information Do not crush or chew tablet; swallow whole with water. This drug is to be used to reduce migraine, not to prevent or reduce the number of attacks. If headache returns or is not fully resolved, the dose may be repeated after 4 hours. If no relief with first dose, do not take a second dose without consulting prescriber. Do not exceed 5 mg in 24 hours. Do not take within 24 hours of any other migraine medication without first consulting prescriber. May experience some dizziness, fatigue, or drowsiness; use caution when driving or engaging in tasks that require alertness. Frequent mouth care and sucking on lozenges may relieve dry mouth. Report immediately any chest pain, heart throbbing, tightness in throat, skin rash or hives, hallucinations, anxiety, or panic. Inform prescriber if they are or intend to become pregnant. Breast-feeding is not recommended.

Dosage Forms Tablet: 1 mg, 2.5 mg

Natamycin (na ta MYE sin)

U.S. Brand Names Natacyn®
Canadian Brand Names Natacyn®
Synonyms Pimaricin
Therapeutic Category Antifungal Agent, Ophthalmic
Use Treatment of blepharitis, conjunctivitis, and keratitis caused by susceptible fungi (*Aspergillus*, *Candida*, *Cephalosporium*, *Curvularia*, *Fusarium*, *Penicillium*, *Microsporum*, *Epidermophyton*, *Blastomyces dermatitidis*, *Coccidioides immitis*, *Cryptococcus neoformans*, *Histoplasma capsulatum*, *Sporothrix schenckii*, and *Trichomonas vaginalis*
Pregnancy Risk Factor C
Contraindications Hypersensitivity to natamycin or any component of the formulation
Warnings/Precautions Failure to improve (keratitis) after 7-10 days of administration suggests infection caused by a microorganism not susceptible to natamycin; inadequate as a single agent in fungal endophthalmitis
Adverse Reactions Frequency not defined (limited to important or life-threatening): Blurred vision, eye irritation not present before therapy, eye pain, photophobia
Drug Interactions
Increased Effect/Toxicity: Topical corticosteroids (concomitant use contraindicated).
Stability Store at room temperature (8°C to 24°C/46°F to 75°F); protect from excessive heat and light; do not freeze
Mechanism of Action Increases cell membrane permeability in susceptible fungi
Pharmacodynamics/Kinetics
Absorption: Ophthalmic: Systemic, <2%
Distribution: Adheres to cornea, retained in conjunctival fornices
Usual Dosage Adults: Ophthalmic: Instill 1 drop in conjunctival sac every 1-2 hours, after 3-4 days reduce to one drop 6-8 times/day; usual course of therapy is 2-3 weeks.
Patient Information Shake well before using, do not touch dropper to eye; notify physician if condition worsens or does not improve after 3-4 days
Nursing Implications Shake suspension before using
Dosage Forms Suspension, ophthalmic: 5% (15 mL)

Nateglinide (na te GLYE nide)

Related Information
Diabetes Mellitus Treatment on page 1657
Hypoglycemic Drugs & Thiazolidinedione Information on page 1502
U.S. Brand Names Starlix®
Therapeutic Category Antidiabetic Agent, Miscellaneous; Meglitinide
Use Management of type 2 diabetes mellitus (noninsulin dependent, NIDDM) as monotherapy when hyperglycemia cannot be managed by diet and exercise alone; in combination with metformin to lower blood glucose in patients whose hyperglycemia cannot be controlled by exercise, diet, and metformin alone.
Pregnancy Risk Factor C
Pregnancy/Breast-Feeding Implications Safety and efficacy in pregnant women have not been established. Do not use during pregnancy. Abnormal blood glucose levels are associated with a higher incidence of congenital abnormalities. Insulin is the drug of choice for the control of diabetes mellitus during pregnancy.
(Continued)

Nateglinide *(Continued)*

Contraindications Hypersensitivity to nateglinide or any component of the formulation; diabetic ketoacidosis, with or without coma (treat with insulin); type 1 diabetes mellitus (insulin dependent, IDDM); patients not adequately controlled on oral agents which stimulate insulin release (eg, glyburide)

Warnings/Precautions Use with caution in patients with moderate to severe hepatic impairment. All oral hypoglycemic agents are capable of producing hypoglycemia. Proper patient selection, dosage, and instructions to the patients are important to avoid hypoglycemic episodes. It may be necessary to discontinue nateglinide and administer insulin if the patient is exposed to stress (ie, fever, trauma, infection, surgery). Indicated for adjunctive therapy with metformin; not to be used as a substitute for metformin monotherapy. Combination treatment with sulfonylureas is not recommended (no additional benefit). Safety and efficacy in pediatric patients have not been established.

Adverse Reactions As reported with nateglinide monotherapy:

1% to 10%:

Central nervous system: Dizziness (4%)

Endocrine & metabolic: Hypoglycemia (2%), increased uric acid

Gastrointestinal: Weight gain

Neuromuscular & skeletal: Arthropathy (3%)

Respiratory: Upper respiratory infection (10%)

Miscellaneous: Flu-like symptoms (4%)

Overdosage/Toxicology In case of overdose, hypoglycemic symptoms would be expected. Severe hypoglycemic reactions should be treated with intravenous glucose. Dialysis is not effective.

Drug Interactions

Cytochrome P450 Effect: CYP2C9 and CYP3A4 substrate; CYP2C9 inhibitor

Increased Effect/Toxicity: Increased hypoglycemic effect: Possible increased hypoglycemic effect may be seen with NSAIDs, salicylates, MAO inhibitors, and nonselective beta-adrenergic blocking agents. Monitor glucose closely when agents are initiated, modified, or discontinued. Drugs which are highly protein bound may increase effect (theoretical, *in vitro* studies have not documented this effect)

Decreased Effect: Decreased hypoglycemic effect: Possible decreased hypoglycemic effect may be seen with thiazides, corticosteroids, thyroid products, and sympathomimetic drugs. Monitor glucose closely when agents are initiated, modified, or discontinued.

Ethanol/Nutrition/Herb Interactions

Ethanol: Avoid ethanol (increased risk of hypoglycemia).

Food: Rate of absorption is decreased and time to T_{max} is delayed when taken with food. Food does not affect AUC. Multiple peak plasma concentrations may be observed if fasting. Not affected by composition of meal.

Stability Store at 25°C (77°F)

Mechanism of Action A phenylalanine derivative, nonsulfonylurea hypoglycemic agent used in the management of type 2 diabetes mellitus (noninsulin dependent, NIDDM); stimulates insulin release from the pancreatic beta cells to reduce postprandial hyperglycemia; amount of insulin release is dependent upon existing glucose levels

Pharmacodynamics/Kinetics

Onset of action: Insulin secretion: ~20 minutes

Peak effect: 1 hour

Duration: 4 hours

Absorption: Rapid

Distribution: 10 L

Protein binding: 98%, primarily to albumin

Metabolism: Hepatic via hydroxylation followed by glucuronide conjugation via CYP2C9 (70%) and CYP3A4 (30%) to metabolites

Bioavailability: 73%

Half-life elimination: 1.5 hours

Time to peak: ≤1 hour

Excretion: Urine (83%, 16% as unchanged drug); feces (10%)

Usual Dosage

Children: Safety and efficacy have not been established

Adults: Management of type 2 diabetes mellitus: Oral: Initial and maintenance dose: 120 mg 3 times/day, 1-30 minutes before meals; may be given alone or in combination with metformin; patients close to Hb A_{1c} goal may be started at 60 mg 3 times/day

Elderly: No changes in safety and efficacy were seen in patients ≥65 years; however, some elderly patients may show increased sensitivity to dosing

Dosage adjustment in renal impairment: No specific dosage adjustment is recommended for patients with mild to severe renal disease; patients on dialysis showed reduced medication exposure and plasma protein binding

Dosage adjustment in hepatic impairment: Increased serum levels seen with mild hepatic insufficiency; no dosage adjustment is needed. Has not been studied in patients with moderate to severe liver disease; use with caution.

Dietary Considerations Nateglinide should be taken 1-30 minutes prior to meals. Scheduled dose should not be taken if meal is missed. Dietary modification based on ADA recommendations is a part of therapy. Decreases blood glucose concentration. Hypoglycemia may occur. Must be able to recognize symptoms of hypoglycemia (palpitations, sweaty palms, lightheadedness).

Monitoring Parameters Glucose and Hb A_{1c} levels, weight, lipid profile

Reference Range Target range: Adults:

Fasting blood glucose: <110 mg/dL

Glycosylated hemoglobin: <6%

Patient Information Take this medication exactly as directed, 3 times/day, 1-30 minutes prior to a meal. If you skip a meal, skip the dose for that meal. Do not change dosage or discontinue without first consulting prescriber. It is important to follow dietary and lifestyle recommendations of prescriber. You will be instructed in signs of hypo-/hyperglycemia by prescriber or diabetic educator; be alert for adverse hypoglycemia (tachycardia, profuse perspiration, tingling of lips and tongue, seizures, or change in sensorium) and follow prescriber's instructions for intervention. The risk of hypoglycemia may be increased by strenuous physical exercise, alcohol ingestion, or insufficient calorie intake. You may experience dizziness or joint pain; if these do not diminish, notify prescriber.

Nursing Implications Patients who are anorexic or NPO will need to have their dose held to avoid hypoglycemia.

Additional Information An increase in weight was seen in nateglinide monotherapy, which was not seen when used in combination with metformin.

Dosage Forms Tablet: 60 mg, 120 mg

- ♦ **Natrecor®** see Nesiritide on page 971
- ♦ **Natriuretic Peptide** see Nesiritide on page 971
- ♦ **Natulan® (Can)** see Procarbazine on page 1133
- ♦ **Natural Lung Surfactant** see Beractant on page 160
- ♦ **Nature-Throid® NT** see Thyroid on page 1326
- ♦ **Navane®** see Thiothixene on page 1324
- ♦ **Navelbine®** see Vinorelbine on page 1418
- ♦ **Naxen® (Can)** see Naproxen on page 958
- ♦ **Na-Zone® [OTC]** see Sodium Chloride on page 1245
- ♦ **n-Docosanol** see Docosanol on page 430
- ♦ **Nebcin®** see Tobramycin on page 1340
- ♦ **NebuPent™** see Pentamidine on page 1056
- ♦ **Necon® 0.5/35** see Ethinyl Estradiol and Norethindrone on page 522
- ♦ **Necon® 1/35** see Ethinyl Estradiol and Norethindrone on page 522
- ♦ **Necon® 1/50** see Mestranol and Norethindrone on page 870
- ♦ **Necon® 10/11** see Ethinyl Estradiol and Norethindrone on page 522

Nedocromil (ne doe KROE mil)

Related Information
Asthma on page 1645

U.S. Brand Names Alocril™; Tilade®

Canadian Brand Names Alocril™; Tilade®

Synonyms Nedocromil Sodium

Therapeutic Category Antiallergic, Inhalation; Antiallergic, Ophthalmic

Use
Aerosol: Maintenance therapy in patients with mild to moderate bronchial asthma
Ophthalmic: Treatment of itching associated with allergic conjunctivitis

Pregnancy Risk Factor B

Contraindications Hypersensitivity to nedocromil or any component of the formulation

Warnings/Precautions
Aerosol: Safety and efficacy in children <6 years of age have not been established; if systemic or inhaled steroid therapy is at all reduced, monitor patients carefully; nedocromil is **not** a bronchodilator and, therefore, should not be used for reversal of acute bronchospasm
Ophthalmic solution: Users of contact lenses should not wear them during periods of symptomatic allergic conjunctivitis

Adverse Reactions
Inhalation:
>10%: Gastrointestinal: Unpleasant taste after inhalation
1% to 10%:
Cardiovascular: Chest pain
Central nervous system: Dizziness, dysphonia, headache, fatigue
Dermatologic: Rash
Gastrointestinal: Nausea, vomiting, heartburn, diarrhea, abdominal pain, dry mouth
Hepatic: Increased ALT
Neuromuscular & skeletal: Arthritis, tremor
Respiratory: Cough, pharyngitis, rhinitis, bronchitis, upper respiratory infection, bronchospasm, increased sputum production
Ophthalmic solution
>10%:
Central nervous system: Headache
Gastrointestinal: Unpleasant taste
Ocular: Burning, irritation, stinging
Respiratory: nasal congestion
1% to 10%
Ocular: Conjunctivitis, eye redness, photophobia
Respiratory: Asthma, rhinitis

Stability Store at 2°C to 30°C/36°F to 86°F; do not freeze

Mechanism of Action Inhibits the activation of and mediator release from a variety of inflammatory cell types associated with asthma including eosinophils, neutrophils, macrophages, mast cells, monocytes, and platelets; it inhibits the release of histamine, leukotrienes, and slow-reacting substance of anaphylaxis; it inhibits the development of early and late bronchoconstriction responses to inhaled antigen

Pharmacodynamics/Kinetics
Duration: Therapeutic effect: 2 hours
Protein binding, plasma: 89%
Bioavailability: 7% to 9%
Half-life elimination: 1.5-2 hours
Excretion: Urine (as unchanged drug)
(Continued)

Nedocromil *(Continued)*

Usual Dosage

Inhalation: Children >6 years and Adults: 2 inhalations 4 times/day; may reduce dosage to 2-3 times/day once desired clinical response to initial dose is observed

Ophthalmic: 1-2 drops in each eye twice daily

Nursing Implications Nedocromil is **not** a bronchodilator and, therefore, should not be used for reversal of acute bronchospasm.

Additional Information Nedocromil has no known therapeutic systemic activity when delivered by inhalation.

Dosage Forms

Aerosol for inhalation, as sodium (Tilade®): 1.75 mg/activation (16.2 g)

Solution, ophthalmic, as sodium (Alocril™): 2% (5 mL)

♦ **Nedocromil Sodium** *see* Nedocromil *on page 963*

Nefazodone *(nef AY zoe done)*

Related Information

Antidepressant Agents Comparison *on page 1482*

U.S. Brand Names Serzone®

Canadian Brand Names Serzone-5HT$_2$®

Synonyms Nefazodone Hydrochloride

Therapeutic Category Antidepressant, Miscellaneous

Use Treatment of depression

Unlabeled/Investigational Use Post-traumatic stress disorder

Pregnancy Risk Factor C

Contraindications Hypersensitivity to nefazodone, related compounds (phenylpiperazines), or any component of the formulation; liver injury due to previous nefazodone treatment, active liver disease, or elevated serum transaminases; concurrent use or use of MAO inhibitors within previous 14 days; use in a patient during the acute recovery phase of MI; concurrent use with astemizole, carbamazepine, cisapride, or pimozide; concurrent therapy with triazolam or alprazolam is generally contraindicated (dosage must be reduced by 75% for triazolam and 50% for alprazolam; such reductions may not be possible with available dosage forms).

Warnings/Precautions Cases of life-threatening hepatic failure have been reported; discontinue if clinical signs or symptoms suggest liver failure. Safety and efficacy in children <18 years of age have not been established. May cause sedation, resulting in impaired performance of tasks requiring alertness (ie, operating machinery or driving). Sedative effects may be additive with other CNS depressants. Does not potentiate ethanol but use is not advised. The degree of sedation is low relative to other antidepressants. May worsen psychosis in some patients or precipitate a shift to mania or hypomania in patients with bipolar disease. May increase the risks associated with electroconvulsive therapy. This agent should be discontinued, when possible, prior to elective surgery. Therapy should not be abruptly discontinued in patients receiving high doses for prolonged periods. Rare reports of priapism have occurred. The incidence of sexual dysfunction with nefazodone is generally lower than with SSRIs.

Use with caution in patients at risk of hypotension or in patients where transient hypotensive episodes would be poorly tolerated (cardiovascular disease or cerebrovascular disease). The risk of postural hypotension is low relative to other antidepressants. Use with caution in patients with urinary retention, benign prostatic hypertrophy, narrow-angle glaucoma, xerostomia, visual problems, constipation, or history of bowel obstruction (due to anticholinergic effects). The degree of anticholinergic blockade produced by this agent is very low relative to other cyclic antidepressants.

Use caution in patients with suicidal risk. Use caution in patients with a previous seizure disorder or condition predisposing to seizures such as brain damage, alcoholism, or concurrent therapy with other drugs which lower the seizure threshold. Use with caution in patients with hepatic or renal dysfunction and in elderly patients. Use with caution in patients with a history of cardiovascular disease (including previous MI, stroke, tachycardia, or conduction abnormalities). However, the risk of conduction abnormalities with this agent is very low relative to other antidepressants.

Adverse Reactions

>10%:

Central nervous system: Headache, drowsiness, insomnia, agitation, dizziness

Gastrointestinal: Xerostomia, nausea, constipation

Neuromuscular & skeletal: Weakness

1% to 10%:

Cardiovascular: Bradycardia, hypotension, peripheral edema, postural hypotension, vasodilation

Central nervous system: Chills, fever, incoordination, lightheadedness, confusion, memory impairment, abnormal dreams, decreased concentration, ataxia, psychomotor retardation, tremor

Dermatologic: Pruritus, rash

Endocrine & metabolic: Breast pain, impotence, libido decreased

Gastrointestinal: Gastroenteritis, vomiting, dyspepsia, diarrhea, increased appetite, thirst, taste perversion

Genitourinary: Urinary frequency, urinary retention

Hematologic: Hematocrit decreased

Neuromuscular & skeletal: Arthralgia, hypertonia, paresthesia, neck rigidity, tremor

Ocular: Blurred vision (9%), abnormal vision (7%), eye pain, visual field defect

Otic: Tinnitus

Respiratory: Bronchitis, cough, dyspnea, pharyngitis

Miscellaneous: Flu syndrome, infection

<1% (Limited to important or life-threatening): Allergic reaction, angioedema, AV block, galactorrhea, gynecomastia, hallucinations, hepatic failure, hepatic necrosis, hyponatremia, impotence, increased prolactin, leukopenia, liver function tests (abnormal), liver failure, liver necrosis, photosensitivity, priapism, rhabdomyolysis (with lovastatin/simvastatin), seizures, serotonin syndrome, Stevens-Johnson syndrome, thrombocytopenia

Overdosage/Toxicology Symptoms include drowsiness, vomiting, hypotension, tachycardia, incontinence, and coma. Following initiation of essential overdose management, toxic symptoms should be treated. Ventricular arrhythmias often respond to lidocaine 1.5 mg/kg bolus followed by a 2 mg/minute infusion with concurrent systemic alkalinization (sodium bicarbonate 0.5-2 mEq/kg I.V.). Seizures usually respond to diazepam I.V. boluses (5-10 mg for adults up to 30 mg or 0.25-0.4 mg/kg/dose for children up to 10 mg/dose). If seizures are unresponsive or recur, phenytoin or phenobarbital may be required. Hypotension is best treated by I.V. fluids and by Trendelenburg positioning.

Drug Interactions

Cytochrome P450 Effect: CYP3A3/4 enzyme substrate; CYP3A3/4 enzyme inhibitor

Increased Effect/Toxicity:

CYP3A3/4 substrates: Serum concentrations of drugs metabolized by CYP3A3/4 may be elevated by nefazodone; cisapride, pimozide, and triazolam are contraindicated. Nefazodone may increase the serum levels/effects of antiarrhythmics (amiodarone, lidocaine, propafenone, quinidine), some antipsychotics (clozapine, haloperidol, mesoridazine, quetiapine, and risperidone), some benzodiazepines (triazolam is contraindicated; decrease alprazolam dose by 50%), buspirone (limit buspirone dose to <2.5 mg/day), calcium channel blockers, cyclosporine, digoxin, donepezil, HMG-CoA reductase inhibitors (lovastatin, simvastatin - increased risk of myositis), methadone, oral contraceptives, protease inhibitors (ritonavir, saquinavir), sibutramine, sildenafil, tacrolimus, tricyclic antidepressants, vinca alkaloids, and zolpidem.

CYP3A3/4 inhibitors: Serum level and/or toxicity of nefazodone may be increased; inhibitors include amiodarone, cimetidine, clarithromycin, erythromycin, delavirdine, diltiazem, dirithromycin, disulfiram, fluoxetine, fluvoxamine, grapefruit juice, indinavir, itraconazole, ketoconazole, metronidazole, nevirapine, propoxyphene, quinupristin-dalfopristin, ritonavir, saquinavir, verapamil, zafirlukast, zileuton

MAO inhibitors: Concurrent use may lead to serotonin syndrome; avoid concurrent use or use within 14 days (includes phenelzine, isocarboxazid, and linezolid). Selegiline may increase the risk of serotonin syndrome, particularly at higher doses (>10 mg/day, where selectivity for MAO type B is decreased).

Theoretically, concurrent use of buspirone, meperidine, serotonin agonists (sumatriptan, rizatriptan), SSRIs, and venlafaxine may result in serotonin syndrome.

Decreased Effect: Carbamazepine may reduce serum concentrations of nefazodone - concurrent administration should be avoided.

Ethanol/Nutrition/Herb Interactions

Ethanol: Avoid ethanol (may increase CNS depression).

Food: Nefazodone absorption may be delayed and bioavailability may be decreased if taken with food.

Herb/Nutraceutical: Avoid valerian, St John's wort, SAMe, kava kava (may increase risk of serotonin syndrome and/or excessive sedation).

Stability Store at room temperature, below 40°C (104°F) in a tight container.

Mechanism of Action Inhibits neuronal reuptake of serotonin and norepinephrine; also blocks 5-HT$_2$ and alpha$_1$ receptors; has no significant affinity for alpha$_2$, beta-adrenergic, 5-HT$_{1A}$, cholinergic, dopaminergic, or benzodiazepine receptors

Pharmacodynamics/Kinetics

Onset of action: Therapeutic: Up to 6 weeks

Metabolism: Hepatic to three active metabolites: triazoledione, hydroxynefazodone, and m-chlorophenylpiperazine (mCPP)

Half-life elimination: Parent drug: 2-4 hours; active metabolites persist longer

Time to peak, serum: 30 minutes; prolonged in presence of food

Excretion: Primarily urine (as metabolites); feces

Usual Dosage Oral:

Children and Adolescents: Depression: Target dose: 300-400 mg/day (mean: 3.4 mg/kg)

Adults: Depression: 200 mg/day, administered in 2 divided doses initially, with a range of 300-600 mg/day in 2 divided doses thereafter

Administration Dosing after meals may decrease lightheadedness and postural hypotension, but may also decrease absorption and therefore effectiveness.

Reference Range Therapeutic plasma levels have not yet been defined

Patient Information Take shortly after a meal or light snack; can be given at bedtime if drowsiness occurs; optimum effect may take 2-4 weeks to be achieved; avoid alcohol; may cause painful erections (contact physician if this should occur); avoid sudden changes in position; report signs/symptoms of liver failure immediately (jaundice, gastrointestinal complaints, malaise)

Nursing Implications Dosing after meals may decrease lightheadedness and postural hypotension, but may also decrease absorption and therefore effectiveness; use side rails on bed if administered to the elderly; observe patient's activity and compare with admission level; assist with ambulation; sitting and standing blood pressure and pulse

Additional Information May cause less sexual dysfunction than other antidepressants. Women and elderly receiving single doses attain significant higher peak concentrations than male volunteers.

Dosage Forms Tablet, as hydrochloride: 50 mg, 100 mg, 150 mg, 200 mg, 250 mg

♦ **Nefazodone Hydrochloride** see Nefazodone on page 964

♦ **NegGram®** see Nalidixic Acid on page 952

Nelfinavir (nel FIN a veer)

Related Information

Antiretroviral Agents Comparison on page 1488
Antiretroviral Therapy for HIV Infection on page 1595

(Continued)

Nelfinavir *(Continued)*

Management of Healthcare Worker Exposures to HIV, HBV, HCV *on page 1555*

U.S. Brand Names Viracept®

Canadian Brand Names Viracept®

Therapeutic Category Antiretroviral Agent, Protease Inhibitor; Protease Inhibitor

Use In combination with other antiretroviral therapy in the treatment of HIV infection

Pregnancy Risk Factor B

Pregnancy/Breast-Feeding Implications Preliminary data show that nelfinavir pharmacokinetics may be affected by pregnancy; studies are not yet complete. Pregnancy and protease inhibitors are both associated with an increased risk of hyperglycemia. Glucose levels should be closely monitored. Health professionals are encouraged to contact the antiretroviral pregnancy registry to monitor outcomes of pregnant women exposed to antiretroviral medications (1-800-258-4263).

Contraindications Hypersensitivity to nelfinavir or any component of the formulation; phenylketonuria; concurrent therapy with amiodarone, astemizole, cisapride, ergot derivatives, lovastatin, midazolam, quinidine, simvastatin, terfenadine, triazolam

Warnings/Precautions Avoid use of powder in phenylketonurics since contains phenylalanine; use extreme caution when administered to patients with hepatic insufficiency since nelfinavir is metabolized in the liver and excreted predominantly in the feces. Avoid concurrent use of St John's wort. New onset diabetes mellitus, exacerbation of diabetes, and hyperglycemia have been reported in HIV-infected patients receiving protease inhibitors.

Adverse Reactions Protease inhibitors cause hyperglycemia and dyslipidemia (elevated cholesterol/triglycerides) and a redistribution of fat (protease paunch, buffalo hump, facial atrophy and breast engorgement)

>10%: Gastrointestinal: Diarrhea

1% to 10%:

Central nervous system: Impaired concentration

Dermatologic: Rash

Gastrointestinal: Nausea, flatulence, abdominal pain

Neuromuscular & skeletal: Weakness

<1% (Limited to important or life-threatening): Allergic reaction, arthralgia, dyspnea, elevated LFTs, fever, GI bleeding, hepatitis, hyperlipidemia, hyperuricemia, hypoglycemia, kidney calculus, leukopenia, migraine, pancreatitis, seizures, suicidal ideation, thrombocytopenia, vomiting

Overdosage/Toxicology No data are available. However, unabsorbed drug should be removed via gastric lavage and activated charcoal. Significant symptoms beyond gastrointestinal disturbances are likely following acute overdose. Hemodialysis will not be effective due to the high protein binding of nelfinavir.

Drug Interactions

Cytochrome P450 Effect: CYP3A3/4 enzyme substrate; CYP3A3/4 enzyme inducer; CYP3A3/4 enzyme inhibitor

Increased Effect/Toxicity: Nelfinavir inhibits the metabolism of cisapride, terfenadine, astemizole, amiodarone, quinidine, lovastatin, simvastatin - should not be administered concurrently due to risk of life-threatening cardiac arrhythmias. Concentrations of atorvastatin and cerivastatin may be increased by nelfinavir. Do not administer with ergot alkaloids. Rifabutin plasma levels (AUC) are increased when coadministered with nelfinavir (decrease rifabutin dose by 50%). Nelfinavir increases levels of ketoconazole and indinavir. An increase in midazolam and triazolam serum levels may occur resulting in significant oversedation when administered with nelfinavir. Indinavir and ritonavir may increase nelfinavir plasma concentrations resulting in potential increases in side effects (the safety of these combinations have not been established). Concentrations of nelfinavir may be doubled during therapy with delavirdine. Sildenafil serum concentration may be substantially increased (do not exceed single doses of 25 mg in 48 hours).

Decreased Effect: Rifampin decreases nelfinavir's blood levels (AUC decreased by ~82%); the two drugs should not be administered concurrently. Serum levels of ethinyl estradiol and norethindrone (including many oral contraceptives) may decrease significantly with administration of nelfinavir. Patients should use alternative methods of contraceptives during nelfinavir therapy. Phenobarbital, phenytoin, and carbamazepine may decrease serum levels and consequently effectiveness of nelfinavir. Delavirdine concentrations may be decreased by up to 50% during nelfinavir treatment. Nelfinavir's effectiveness may be decreased with concomitant nevirapine use.

Ethanol/Nutrition/Herb Interactions

Food: Nelfinavir taken with food increases plasma concentration time curve (AUC) by two- to threefold. Do not administer with acidic food or juice (orange juice, apple juice, or applesauce) since the combination may have a bitter taste.

Herb/Nutraceutical: St John's wort may decrease nelfinavir serum concentrations; avoid concurrent use.

Stability Store at room temperature. Oral powder (or dissolved tablets) diluted in nonacidic liquid is stable for 6 hours at room temperature.

Mechanism of Action Inhibits the HIV-1 protease; inhibition of the viral protease prevents cleavage of the gag-pol polyprotein resulting in the production of immature, noninfectious virus

Pharmacodynamics/Kinetics

Absorption: Food increases plasma concentration-time curve (AUC) by two- to threefold

Distribution: V_d: 2-7 L/kg

Protein binding: 98%

Metabolism: Hepatic via CYP3A3/4; major metabolite has activity comparable to the parent drug

Half-life elimination: 3.5-5 hours

Time to peak, serum: 2-4 hours

Excretion: Feces (98% to 99%, 78% as metabolites, 22% as unchanged drug); urine (1% to 2%)

Usual Dosage Oral:
 Children 2-13 years (labeled dose): 20-30 mg/kg 3 times/day with a meal or light snack; if tablets are unable to be taken, use oral powder in small amount of water, milk, formula, or dietary supplements; do not use acidic food/juice or store for >6 hours
  Note: Clinically, dosages as high as 45 mg/kg every 8 hours are used; twice-daily dosages of 50-55 mg/kg are under investigation in older children (>6 years)
 Adults: 750 mg 3 times/day with meals or 1250 mg twice daily with meals in combination with other antiretroviral therapies
  Note: Dosage adjustments for nelfinavir when administered in combination with ritonavir: Nelfinavir 500-750 mg twice daily plus ritonavir 400 mg twice daily
 Dosing adjustment in renal impairment: No adjustment needed
 Dosing adjustment in hepatic impairment: Use caution when administering to patients with hepatic impairment since eliminated predominantly by the liver
Dietary Considerations Should be taken as scheduled with food.
Administration Oral powder: Mix powder or tablets in a small amount of water, milk, formula, soy milk, soy formula, or dietary supplement. Be sure entire contents is consumed to receive full dose. Do not use acidic food/juice to dilute due to bitter taste. Do not store dilution for longer than 6 hours.
Monitoring Parameters Liver function tests, viral load, CD4 count, triglycerides, cholesterol, blood glucose, CBC with differential
Patient Information Nelfinavir should be taken with food to increase its absorption; it is not a cure for HIV infection and the long-term effects of the drug are unknown at this time; the drug has not demonstrated a reduction in the risk of transmitting HIV to others. Take the drug as prescribed; if you miss a dose, take it as soon as possible and then return to your usual schedule (never double a dose, however). If tablets are unable to be taken, use oral powder in small amount of water, milk, formula, or dietary supplement; do not use acidic food/juice of store dilution for >6 hours (refrigerate). Do not take any prescription medications, over-the-counter products or herbal products, especially St John's wort, without consulting prescriber. Use an alternative method of contraception from birth control pills during nelfinavir therapy.
Nursing Implications If diarrhea occurs, it may be treated with OTC antidiarrheals
Dosage Forms
 Powder, oral: 50 mg/g (contains 11.2 mg phenylalanine) [144 g]
 Tablet, film coated: 250 mg

- **Nemasol® Sodium (Can)** *see* Aminosalicylate Sodium *on page 73*
- **Nembutal®** *see* Pentobarbital *on page 1059*
- **Nembutal® Sodium (Can)** *see* Pentobarbital *on page 1059*
- **Neo-Calglucon® [OTC]** *see* Calcium Glubionate *on page 210*
- **Neo-Cortef® (Can)** *see* Neomycin and Hydrocortisone *on page 968*
- **NeoDecadron®** *see* Neomycin and Dexamethasone *on page 968*
- **Neo-Dexameth®** *see* Neomycin and Dexamethasone *on page 968*
- **Neo-Fradin®** *see* Neomycin *on page 967*

Neomycin (nee oh MYE sin)

Related Information
 Prevention of Wound Infection & Sepsis in Surgical Patients *on page 1569*
U.S. Brand Names Mycifradin® Sulfate; Neo-Fradin®; Neo-Tabs®
Synonyms Neomycin Sulfate
Therapeutic Category Ammonium Detoxicant; Antibiotic, Aminoglycoside; Antibiotic, Irrigation; Antibiotic, Topical
Use Orally to prepare GI tract for surgery; topically to treat minor skin infections; treatment of diarrhea caused by *E. coli*; adjunct in the treatment of hepatic encephalopathy
Pregnancy Risk Factor C
Contraindications Hypersensitivity to neomycin or any component of the formulation, or other aminoglycosides; intestinal obstruction
Warnings/Precautions Use with caution in patients with renal impairment, pre-existing hearing impairment, neuromuscular disorders; neomycin is more toxic than other aminoglycosides when given parenterally; **do not administer parenterally**; topical neomycin is a contact sensitizer with sensitivity occurring in 5% to 15% of patients treated with the drug; symptoms include itching, reddening, edema, and failure to heal; **do not use as peritoneal lavage** due to significant systemic adsorption of the drug
Adverse Reactions
 Oral:
 >10%: Gastrointestinal: Nausea, diarrhea, vomiting, irritation or soreness of the mouth or rectal area
 <1% (Limited to important or life-threatening): Dyspnea, eosinophilia, nephrotoxicity, neurotoxicity, ototoxicity (auditory), ototoxicity (vestibular)
 Topical: >10%: Dermatologic: Contact dermatitis
Overdosage/Toxicology Symptoms of overdose are rare, due to poor oral bioavailability, but include ototoxicity, nephrotoxicity, and neuromuscular toxicity. The treatment of choice following a single acute overdose appears to be the maintenance of urine output of at least 3 mL/kg/hour. Dialysis is of questionable value in enhancing aminoglycoside elimination. If required, hemodialysis is preferred over peritoneal dialysis in patients with normal renal function. Chelation with penicillin may be of benefit.
Drug Interactions
 Increased Effect/Toxicity: Oral neomycin may potentiate the effects of oral anticoagulants. Neomycin may increase the adverse effects with other neurotoxic, ototoxic, or nephrotoxic drugs.
 Decreased Effect: May decrease GI absorption of digoxin and methotrexate.
Mechanism of Action Interferes with bacterial protein synthesis by binding to 30S ribosomal subunits
Pharmacodynamics/Kinetics
 Absorption: Oral, percutaneous: Poor (3%)
 (Continued)

Neomycin *(Continued)*

Distribution: V$_d$: 0.36 L/kg

Metabolism: Slightly hepatic

Half-life elimination: 3 hours (age and renal function dependent)

Time to peak, serum: Oral: 1-4 hours; I.M.: ~2 hours

Excretion: Urine (30% to 50% of absorbed drug as unchanged drug); feces (97% oral dose as unchanged drug)

Usual Dosage

Children: Oral:

Preoperative intestinal antisepsis: 90 mg/kg/day divided every 4 hours for 2 days; or 25 mg/kg at 1 PM, 2 PM, and 11 PM on the day preceding surgery as an adjunct to mechanical cleansing of the intestine and in combination with erythromycin base

Hepatic coma: 50-100 mg/kg/day in divided doses every 6-8 hours or 2.5-7 g/m^2/day divided every 4-6 hours for 5-6 days not to exceed 12 g/day

Children and Adults: Topical: Apply ointment 1-4 times/day; topical solutions containing 0.1% to 1% neomycin have been used for irrigation

Adults: Oral:

Preoperative intestinal antisepsis: 1 g each hour for 4 doses then 1 g every 4 hours for 5 doses; or 1 g at 1 PM, 2 PM, and 11 PM on day preceding surgery as an adjunct to mechanical cleansing of the bowel and oral erythromycin; or 6 g/day divided every 4 hours for 2-3 days

Hepatic coma: 500-2000 mg every 6-8 hours or 4-12 g/day divided every 4-6 hours for 5-6 days

Chronic hepatic insufficiency: 4 g/day for an indefinite period

Monitoring Parameters Renal function tests, audiometry in symptomatic patients

Patient Information Notify physician if redness, burning, itching, ringing in the ears, hearing impairment, or dizziness occurs of if condition does not improve in 3-4 days

Dosage Forms

Cream, as sulfate: 0.5% (15 g)

Ointment, topical, as sulfate: 0.5% (15 g, 30 g, 120 g)

Solution, oral, as sulfate: 125 mg/5 mL (480 mL)

Tablet, as sulfate: 500 mg [base 300 mg]

Neomycin and Dexamethasone *(nee oh MYE sin & deks a METH a sone)*

U.S. Brand Names AK-Neo-Dex®; NeoDecadron®; Neo-Dexameth®

Synonyms Dexamethasone and Neomycin

Therapeutic Category Antibiotic/Corticosteroid, Ophthalmic

Use Treatment of steroid responsive inflammatory conditions of the palpebral and bulbar conjunctiva, lid, cornea, and anterior segment of the globe

Pregnancy Risk Factor C

Usual Dosage Ophthalmic: Instill 1-2 drops in eye(s) every 3-4 hours

Additional Information Complete prescribing information for this medication should be consulted for additional detail.

Dosage Forms Solution, ophthalmic: Neomycin sulfate 0.35% [3.5 mg/mL] and dexamethasone 0.1% [1 mg/mL] (5 mL)

Neomycin and Hydrocortisone *(nee oh MYE sin & hye droe KOR ti sone)*

Canadian Brand Names Neo-Cortef®

Synonyms Hydrocortisone and Neomycin

Therapeutic Category Antibiotic/Corticosteroid, Topical

Use Treatment of susceptible topical bacterial infections with associated inflammation

Pregnancy Risk Factor C

Usual Dosage Topical: Apply to area in a thin film 2-4 times/day

Additional Information Complete prescribing information for this medication should be consulted for additional detail.

Dosage Forms Ointment, topical: Neomycin sulfate 0.5% and hydrocortisone 1% (20 g)

Neomycin and Polymyxin B *(nee oh MYE sin & pol i MIKS in bee)*

U.S. Brand Names Neosporin® Cream [OTC]; Neosporin® G.U. Irrigant

Canadian Brand Names Cortimyxin®; Neosporin® Irrigating Solution

Synonyms Polymyxin B and Neomycin

Therapeutic Category Antibiotic, Topical; Antibiotic, Urinary Irrigation

Use Short-term as a continuous irrigant or rinse in the urinary bladder to prevent bacteriuria and gram-negative rod septicemia associated with the use of indwelling catheters; to help prevent infection in minor cuts, scrapes, and burns

Pregnancy Risk Factor C/D (for G.U. irrigant)

Usual Dosage Children and Adults:

Bladder irrigation: **Not for injection;** add 1 mL irrigant to 1 liter isotonic saline solution and connect container to the inflow of lumen of 3-way catheter. Continuous irrigant or rinse in the urinary bladder for up to a maximum of 10 days with administration rate adjusted to patient's urine output; usually no more than 1 L of irrigant is used per day.

Topical: Apply cream 1-4 times/day to affected area

Additional Information Complete prescribing information for this medication should be consulted for additional detail.

Dosage Forms

Cream, topical: Neomycin sulfate 3.5 mg and polymyxin B sulfate 10,000 units per g (0.94 g, 15 g)

Solution, irrigant, topical: Neomycin sulfate 40 mg and polymyxin B sulfate 200,000 units per mL (1 mL, 20 mL)

◆ **Neomycin, Bacitracin, and Polymyxin B** *see* Bacitracin, Neomycin, and Polymyxin B *on page 143*

- **Neomycin, Bacitracin, Polymyxin B, and Hydrocortisone** *see* Bacitracin, Neomycin, Polymyxin B, and Hydrocortisone *on page 143*
- **Neomycin, Colistin, and Hydrocortisone** *see* Colistin, Neomycin, and Hydrocortisone *on page 334*

Neomycin, Polymyxin B, and Dexamethasone
(nee oh MYE sin, pol i MIKS in bee, & deks a METH a sone)

U.S. Brand Names AK-Trol®; Dexacidin®; Dexasporin®; Maxitrol®

Canadian Brand Names Dioptrol®; Maxitrol®

Synonyms Dexamethasone, Neomycin, and Polymyxin B; Polymyxin B, Neomycin, and Dexamethasone

Therapeutic Category Antibiotic, Ophthalmic; Corticosteroid, Ophthalmic

Use Steroid-responsive inflammatory ocular conditions in which a corticosteroid is indicated and where bacterial infection or a risk of bacterial infection exists

Pregnancy Risk Factor C

Usual Dosage Children and Adults: Ophthalmic:
  Ointment: Place a small amount ($\sim^1\!/_2$") in the affected eye 3-4 times/day or apply at bedtime as an adjunct with drops
  Suspension: Instill 1-2 drops into affected eye(s) every 3-4 hours; in severe disease, drops may be used hourly and tapered to discontinuation

Additional Information Complete prescribing information for this medication should be consulted for additional detail.

Dosage Forms
  Ointment, ophthalmic: Neomycin sulfate 3.5 mg, polymyxin B sulfate 10,000 units, and dexamethasone 0.1% per g (3.5 g, 5 g)
  Suspension, ophthalmic: Neomycin sulfate 3.5 mg, polymyxin B sulfate 10,000 units, and dexamethasone 0.1% per mL (5 mL, 10 mL)

Neomycin, Polymyxin B, and Gramicidin
(nee oh MYE sin, pol i MIKS in bee, & gram i SYE din)

U.S. Brand Names AK-Spore® Ophthalmic Solution; Neosporin® Ophthalmic Solution

Canadian Brand Names Neosporin®; Optimyxin Plus®

Synonyms Gramicidin, Neomycin, and Polymyxin B; Polymyxin B, Neomycin, and Gramicidin

Therapeutic Category Antibiotic, Ophthalmic

Use Treatment of superficial ocular infection, infection prophylaxis in minor skin abrasions

Pregnancy Risk Factor C

Contraindications Hypersensitivity to neomycin, polymyxin B, gramicidin or any component of the formulation

Warnings/Precautions Symptoms of neomycin sensitization include itching, reddening, edema, failure to heal; prolonged use may result in glaucoma, defects in visual acuity, posterior subcapsular cataract formation, and secondary ocular infections

Adverse Reactions Frequency not defined: Ocular: Transient irritation, burning, stinging, itching, inflammation, angioneurotic edema, urticaria, vesicular and maculopapular dermatitis

Drug Interactions
  Increased Effect/Toxicity: Refer to individual agents.
  Decreased Effect: Refer to individual agents.

Mechanism of Action Interferes with bacterial protein synthesis by binding to 30S ribosomal subunits; binds to phospholipids, alters permeability, and damages the bacterial cytoplasmic membrane permitting leakage of intracellular constituents

Usual Dosage Children and Adults: Ophthalmic: Instill 1-2 drops 4-6 times/day or more frequently as required for severe infections

Patient Information Tilt head back, place medication in conjunctival sac, and close eyes; apply finger pressure on lacrimal sac for 1 minute following instillation

Nursing Implications Tilt head back, place medication in conjunctival sac, and close eyes; apply finger pressure on lacrimal sac for 1 minute following instillation

Dosage Forms Solution, ophthalmic: Neomycin sulfate 1.75 mg, polymyxin B sulfate 10,000 units, and gramicidin 0.025 mg per mL (2 mL, 10 mL)

Neomycin, Polymyxin B, and Hydrocortisone
(nee oh MYE sin, pol i MIKS in bee, & hye droe KOR ti sone)

U.S. Brand Names AK-Spore® H.C. Otic; AntibiOtic® Otic; Cortatrigen® Otic; Cortisporin®; Cortisporin® Ophthalmic Suspension; Octicair® Otic; Otic-Care®; Otocort®; Otosporin®; Pedi-Otic®; UAD Otic®

Canadian Brand Names Cortimyxin®; Cortisporin®

Synonyms Hydrocortisone, Neomycin, and Polymyxin B; Polymyxin B, Neomycin, and Hydrocortisone

Therapeutic Category Antibiotic, Ophthalmic; Antibiotic, Otic; Antibiotic, Topical; Anti-inflammatory Agent; Corticosteroid, Ophthalmic; Corticosteroid, Otic; Corticosteroid, Topical (Low Potency)

Use Steroid-responsive inflammatory condition for which a corticosteroid is indicated and where bacterial infection or a risk of bacterial infection exists

Pregnancy Risk Factor C

Usual Dosage Duration of use should be limited to 10 days unless otherwise directed by the physician
  Otic solution is used **only** for swimmer's ear (infections of external auditory canal)
  Otic:
    Children: Instill 3 drops into affected ear 3-4 times/day
    Adults: Instill 4 drops 3-4 times/day; otic suspension is the preferred otic preparation
  Children and Adults:
    Ophthalmic: Drops: Instill 1-2 drops 2-4 times/day, or more frequently as required for severe infections; in acute infections, instill 1-2 drops every 15-30 minutes gradually reducing the frequency of administration as the infection is controlled

(Continued)

Neomycin, Polymyxin B, and Hydrocortisone *(Continued)*

Topical: Apply a thin layer 1-4 times/day. Therapy should be discontinued when control is achieved; if no improvement is seen, reassessment of diagnosis may be necessary.

Additional Information Complete prescribing information for this medication should be consulted for additional detail.

Dosage Forms

Cream, topical: Neomycin sulfate 5 mg, polymyxin B sulfate 10,000 units, and hydrocortisone 5 mg per g (7.5 g)

Solution, otic: Neomycin sulfate 5 mg, polymyxin B sulfate 10,000 units, and hydrocortisone 10 mg per mL (10 mL)

Suspension, ophthalmic: Neomycin sulfate 5 mg, polymyxin B sulfate 10,000 units, and hydrocortisone 10 mg per mL (10 mL)

Cortisporin®: Neomycin sulfate 5 mg, polymyxin B sulfate 10,000 units, and hydrocortisone 10 mg per mL (7.5 mL) [with thimerosal 0.001% as preservative]

Suspension, otic: Neomycin sulfate 5 mg, polymyxin B sulfate 10,000 units, and hydrocortisone 10 mg per mL (10 mL)

Neomycin, Polymyxin B, and Prednisolone

(nee oh MYE sin, pol i MIKS in bee, & pred NIS oh lone)

U.S. Brand Names Poly-Pred®

Synonyms Polymyxin B, Neomycin, and Prednisolone; Prednisolone, Neomycin, and Polymyxin B

Therapeutic Category Antibiotic, Ophthalmic; Corticosteroid, Ophthalmic

Use Steroid-responsive inflammatory ocular condition in which bacterial infection or a risk of bacterial ocular infection exists

Pregnancy Risk Factor C

Usual Dosage Children and Adults: Ophthalmic: Instill 1-2 drops every 3-4 hours; acute infections may require every 30-minute instillation initially with frequency of administration reduced as the infection is brought under control. To treat the lids: Instill 1-2 drops every 3-4 hours, close the eye and rub the excess on the lids and lid margins.

Additional Information Complete prescribing information for this medication should be consulted for additional detail.

Dosage Forms Suspension, ophthalmic: Neomycin sulfate 0.35%, polymyxin B sulfate 10,000 units, and prednisolone acetate 0.5% per mL (5 mL, 10 mL)

♦ **Neomycin Sulfate** *see Neomycin on page 967*

♦ **Neoral®** *see CycloSPORINE on page 345*

♦ **Neosar®** *see Cyclophosphamide on page 342*

♦ **Neosporin® (Can)** *see Neomycin, Polymyxin B, and Gramicidin on page 969*

♦ **Neosporin® Cream [OTC]** *see Neomycin and Polymyxin B on page 968*

♦ **Neosporin® G.U. Irrigant** *see Neomycin and Polymyxin B on page 968*

♦ **Neosporin® Irrigating Solution (Can)** *see Neomycin and Polymyxin B on page 968*

♦ **Neosporin® Ophthalmic Ointment** *see Bacitracin, Neomycin, and Polymyxin B on page 143*

♦ **Neosporin® Ophthalmic Solution** *see Neomycin, Polymyxin B, and Gramicidin on page 969*

♦ **Neosporin® Topical [OTC]** *see Bacitracin, Neomycin, and Polymyxin B on page 143*

Neostigmine (nee oh STIG meen)

U.S. Brand Names Prostigmin®

Canadian Brand Names Prostigmin®

Synonyms Neostigmine Bromide; Neostigmine Methylsulfate

Therapeutic Category Antidote, Neuromuscular Blocking Agent; Cholinergic Agent; Diagnostic Agent, Myasthenia Gravis

Use Diagnosis and treatment of myasthenia gravis; prevention and treatment of postoperative bladder distention and urinary retention; reversal of the effects of nondepolarizing neuromuscular-blocking agents after surgery

Pregnancy Risk Factor C

Contraindications Hypersensitivity to neostigmine, bromides, or any component of the formulation; GI or GU obstruction

Warnings/Precautions Does **not** antagonize and may prolong the phase I block of depolarizing muscle relaxants (eg, succinylcholine); use with caution in patients with epilepsy, asthma, bradycardia, hyperthyroidism, cardiac arrhythmias, or peptic ulcer; adequate facilities should be available for cardiopulmonary resuscitation when testing and adjusting dose for myasthenia gravis; have atropine and epinephrine ready to treat hypersensitivity reactions; overdosage may result in cholinergic crisis, this must be distinguished from myasthenic crisis; anticholinesterase insensitivity can develop for brief or prolonged periods

Adverse Reactions Frequency not defined.

Cardiovascular: Arrhythmias (especially bradycardia), hypotension, decreased carbon monoxide, tachycardia, AV block, nodal rhythm, nonspecific EKG changes, cardiac arrest, syncope, flushing

Central nervous system: Convulsions, dysarthria, dysphonia, dizziness, loss of consciousness, drowsiness, headache

Dermatologic: Skin rash, thrombophlebitis (I.V.), urticaria

Gastrointestinal: Hyperperistalsis, nausea, vomiting, salivation, diarrhea, stomach cramps, dysphagia, flatulence

Genitourinary: Urinary urgency

Neuromuscular & skeletal: Weakness, fasciculations, muscle cramps, spasms, arthralgias

Ocular: Small pupils, lacrimation

Respiratory: Increased bronchial secretions, laryngospasm, bronchiolar constriction, respiratory muscle paralysis, dyspnea, respiratory depression, respiratory arrest, bronchospasm

Miscellaneous: Diaphoresis (increased), anaphylaxis, allergic reactions

Overdosage/Toxicology Symptoms include muscle weakness, blurred vision, excessive sweating, tearing and salivation, nausea, vomiting, diarrhea, hypertension, bradycardia, muscle weakness, and paralysis. Atropine sulfate injection should be readily available as an antagonist for the effects of neostigmine.

Drug Interactions

Increased Effect/Toxicity: Neuromuscular blocking agent effects are increased when combined with neostigmine.

Decreased Effect: Antagonizes effects of nondepolarizing muscle relaxants (eg, pancuronium, tubocurarine). Atropine antagonizes the muscarinic effects of neostigmine.

Mechanism of Action Inhibits destruction of acetylcholine by acetylcholinesterase which facilitates transmission of impulses across myoneural junction

Pharmacodynamics/Kinetics

Onset of action: I.M.: 20-30 minutes; I.V.: 1-20 minutes

Duration: I.M.: 2.5-4 hours; I.V.: 1-2 hours

Absorption: Oral: Poor, <2%

Metabolism: Hepatic

Half-life elimination: Normal renal function: 0.5-2.1 hours; End-stage renal disease: Prolonged

Excretion: Urine (50% as unchanged drug)

Usual Dosage

Myasthenia gravis: Diagnosis: I.M.:

Children: 0.04 mg/kg as a single dose

Adults: 0.02 mg/kg as a single dose

Myasthenia gravis: Treatment:

Children:

Oral: 2 mg/kg/day divided every 3-4 hours

I.M., I.V., S.C.: 0.01-0.04 mg/kg every 2-4 hours

Adults:

Oral: 15 mg/dose every 3-4 hours up to 375 mg/day maximum

I.M., I.V., S.C.: 0.5-2.5 mg every 1-3 hours up to 10 mg/24 hours maximum

Reversal of nondepolarizing neuromuscular blockade after surgery in conjunction with atropine: I.V.:

Infants: 0.025-0.1 mg/kg/dose

Children: 0.025-0.08 mg/kg/dose

Adults: 0.5-2.5 mg; total dose not to exceed 5 mg

Bladder atony: Adults: I.M., S.C.:

Prevention: 0.25 mg every 4-6 hours for 2-3 days

Treatment: 0.5-1 mg every 3 hours for 5 doses after bladder has emptied

Dosing adjustment in renal impairment:

Cl_{cr} 10-50 mL/minute: Administer 50% of normal dose

Cl_{cr} <10 mL/minute: Administer 25% of normal dose

Administration May be administered undiluted by slow I.V. injection over several minutes

Patient Information Side effects are generally due to exaggerated pharmacologic effects; most common are salivation and muscle fasciculations; notify physician if nausea, vomiting, muscle weakness, severe abdominal pain, or difficulty breathing occurs

Nursing Implications In the diagnosis of myasthenia gravis, all anticholinesterase medications should be discontinued for at least 8 hours before administering neostigmine

Dosage Forms

Injection, as methylsulfate: 0.5 mg/mL (1 mL, 10 mL); 1 mg/mL (10 mL)

Tablet, as bromide: 15 mg

Nesiritide (ni SIR i tide)

U.S. Brand Names Natrecor®

Synonyms B-type Natriuretic Peptide (Human); hBNP; Natriuretic Peptide

Therapeutic Category Natriuretic Peptide, B-type, Human; Vasodilator

Use Treatment of acutely decompensated congestive heart failure (CHF) in patients with dyspnea at rest or with minimal activity

Pregnancy Risk Factor C

Pregnancy/Breast-Feeding Implications Excretion in breast milk is unknown; use caution in breast-feeding women.

Contraindications Hypersensitivity to natriuretic peptide or any component of the formulation; cardiogenic shock (when used as primary therapy); hypotension (systolic blood pressure <90 mm Hg)

(Continued)

Nesiritide *(Continued)*

Warnings/Precautions May cause hypotension; administer in clinical situations when blood pressure may be closely monitored. Use caution in patients with systolic blood pressure <100 mm Hg (contraindicated if <90 mm Hg); more likely to experience hypotension. Effects may be additive with other agents capable of causing hypotension. Hypotensive effects may last for several hours.

Should not be used in patients with low filling pressures, or in patients with conditions which depend on venous return including significant valvular stenosis, restrictive or obstructive cardiomyopathy, constrictive pericarditis, and pericardial tamponade. May be associated with development of azotemia; use caution in patients with renal impairment or in patients where renal perfusion is dependent on renin-angiotensin-aldosterone system.

Atrial natriuretic peptide (ANP), a related peptide, has been associated with increased vascular permeability and decreased intravascular volume. This has not been observed in clinical trials with nesiritide, however patients should be monitored for this effect.

Monitor for allergic or anaphylactic reactions. Use caution with prolonged infusions; limited experience for infusions >48 hours. Safety and efficacy in pediatric patients have not been established.

Adverse Reactions Note: Frequencies cited below were recorded in VMAC trial at dosages similar to approved labeling. Higher frequencies have been observed in trials using higher dosages of nesiritide.

>10%:
  Cardiovascular: Hypotension (total: 11%; symptomatic: 4% at recommended dose, up to 17% at higher doses)
  Renal: Increased serum creatinine (28% with >0.5 mg/dL increase over baseline)

1% to 10%:
  Cardiovascular: Ventricular tachycardia (3%)*, ventricular extrasystoles (3%)*, angina (2%)*, bradycardia (1%), tachycardia, atrial fibrillation, AV node conduction abnormalities
  Central nervous system: Headache (8%)*, dizziness (3%)*, insomnia (2%), anxiety (3%), fever, confusion, paresthesia, somnolence, tremor
  Dermatologic: Pruritus, rash
  Gastrointestinal: Nausea (4%)*, abdominal pain (1%)*, vomiting (1%)*
  Hematologic: Anemia
  Local: Injection site reaction
  Neuromuscular & skeletal: Back pain (4%), leg cramps
  Ocular: Amblyopia
  Respiratory: Cough (increased), hemoptysis, apnea
  Miscellaneous: Increased diaphoresis
*Frequency less than or equal to placebo or other standard therapy

Drug Interactions
  Increased Effect/Toxicity: An increased frequency of symptomatic hypotension was observed with concurrent administration of ACE inhibitors. Other hypotensive agents are likely to have additive effects on hypotension. In patients receiving diuretic therapy leading to depletion of intravascular volume, the risk of hypotension and/or renal impairment may be increased. Nesiritide should be avoided in patients with low filling pressures.

Stability Vials may be stored at controlled room temperature of 20°C to 25°C (68°F to 77 °F) or under refrigeration at 2°C to 8°C (36°F to 46°F). Following reconstitution, vials are stable under these conditions for up to 24 hours.

Reconstitute 1.5 mg vial with 5 mL of diluent removed from a premixed plastic I.V. bag (compatible with 5% dextrose, 0.9% sodium chloride, 5% dextrose and 0.45% sodium chloride, or 5% dextrose and 0.2% sodium chloride). Do not shake vial to dissolve (roll gently). Withdraw entire contents of vial and add to 250 mL I.V. bag. Resultant concentration of solution approximately 6 mcg/mL.

Mechanism of Action Binds to guanylate cyclase receptor on vascular smooth muscle and endothelial cells, increasing intracellular cyclic GMP, resulting in smooth muscle cell relaxation. Has been shown to produce dose-dependent reductions in pulmonary capillary wedge pressure (PCWP) and systemic arterial pressure.

Pharmacodynamics/Kinetics
  Onset of action: 15 minutes (60% of 3-hour effect achieved)
  Duration: >60 minutes (up to several hours) for systolic blood pressure; hemodynamic effects persist longer than serum half-life would predict
  Distribution: V_{ss}: 0.19 L/kg
  Metabolism: Proteolytic cleavage by vascular endopeptidases and proteolysis following receptor binding and cellular internalization
  Half-life elimination: Initial (distribution) 2 minutes; Terminal: 18 minutes
  Time to peak: 1 hour
  Excretion: Urine

Usual Dosage Adults: I.V.: Initial: 2 mcg/kg (bolus); followed by continuous infusion at 0.01 mcg/kg/minute; **Note:** Should not be initiated at a dosage higher than initial recommended dose. At intervals of ≥3 hours, the dosage may be increased by 0.005 mcg/kg/minute (preceded by a bolus of 1 mcg/kg), up to a maximum of 0.03 mcg/kg/minute. Increases beyond the initial infusion rate should be limited to selected patients and accompanied by hemodynamic monitoring.

Patients experiencing hypotension during the infusion: Infusion should be interrupted. May attempt to restart at a lower dose (reduce initial infusion dose by 30% and omit bolus).

Dosage adjustment in renal impairment: No adjustment required

Administration Do not administer through a heparin-coated catheter (concurrent administration of heparin via a separate catheter is acceptable, per manufacturer).

Prime I.V. tubing with 25 mL of infusion prior to connection with vascular access port and prior to administering bolus or starting the infusion. Withdraw bolus from the prepared infusion bag and administer over 60 seconds. Begin infusion immediately following administration of the bolus. Using a standard 6 mcg/mL concentration, bolus volume in mL = patient weight in kg x 0.33.

Physically incompatible with heparin, insulin, ethacrynate sodium, bumetanide, enalaprilat, hydralazine, and furosemide. Do not administer through the same catheter. Do not administer with any solution containing sodium metabisulfite. Catheter must be flushed between administration of nesiritide and physically incompatible drugs.

Monitoring Parameters Blood pressure, hemodynamic responses (PCWP, RAP, CI)

Patient Information This medication can only be administered I.V. You will be closely monitored during and following infusion. Remain in bed until advised otherwise. Do not make sudden turns or changes in position; call for assistance to change position. Immediately report any acute headache, dizziness, chest pain or palpitations, abdominal pain or nausea, back pain, or increase in breathing difficulty. Inform prescriber if you are or intend to be pregnant. Consult prescriber if breast-feeding.

Additional Information The duration of symptomatic improvement with nesiritide following discontinuation of the infusion has been limited (generally lasting several days). Atrial natriuretic peptide, which is related to nesiritide, has been associated with increased vascular permeability. This has not been observed in clinical trials with nesiritide, but patients should be monitored for this effect.

Dosage Forms Powder for injection: 1.5 mg

Nevirapine (ne VYE ra peen)

Related Information
Antiretroviral Agents Comparison *on page 1488*
Antiretroviral Therapy for HIV Infection *on page 1595*
Management of Healthcare Worker Exposures to HIV, HBV, HCV *on page 1555*
Prevention of Perinatal HIV Transmission *on page 1567*

U.S. Brand Names Viramune®

Canadian Brand Names Viramune®

Therapeutic Category Antiretroviral Agent, Non-nucleoside Reverse Transcriptase Inhibitor (NNRTI)

Use In combination therapy with other antiretroviral agents for the treatment of HIV-1 in adults

Pregnancy Risk Factor C

Pregnancy/Breast-Feeding Implications Nevirapine crosses the placenta. It may be used in combination with zidovudine in HIV-infected women who are in labor, but have had no prior antiretroviral therapy, in order to reduce the maternal-fetal transmission of HIV. Health professionals are encouraged to contact the antiretroviral pregnancy registry to monitor outcomes of pregnant women exposed to antiretroviral medications (1-800-258-4263).

Contraindications Hypersensitivity to nevirapine or any component of the formulation; manufacturer recommends against concurrent administration of ketoconazole or oral contraceptives

Warnings/Precautions Consider alteration of antiretroviral therapies if disease progression occurs while patients are receiving nevirapine. Safety and efficacy have not been established in neonates.

Severe life-threatening skin reactions (eg, Stevens-Johnson syndrome, toxic epidermal necrolysis, hypersensitivity reactions with rash and organ dysfunction) have occurred. Nevirapine must be initiated with a 14-day lead-in dosing period to decrease the incidence of adverse effects. Severe hepatotoxic reactions may also occur (fulminant and cholestatic hepatitis, hepatic necrosis), and in some cases have resulted in hepatic failure and death. Intensive monitoring is required during the initial 12 weeks of therapy to detect potentially life-threatening dermatologic, hypersensitivity, and hepatic reactions. Patients with a history of chronic hepatitis (B or C) or increased transaminase levels (AST or ALT) may be at increased risk of hepatotoxic reactions.

If a severe dermatologic or hypersensitivity reaction occurs, or if signs and symptoms of hepatitis occur, nevirapine should be permanently discontinued. These may include a severe rash, or a rash associated with fever, blisters, oral lesions, conjunctivitis, facial edema, muscle or joint aches, general malaise, hepatitis, eosinophilia, granulocytopenia, lymphadenopathy or renal dysfunction.

Adverse Reactions
>10%:
  Central nervous system: Headache (11%), fever (8% to 11%)
  Dermatologic: Rash (15% to 20%)
  Gastrointestinal: Diarrhea (15% to 20%)
  Hematologic: Neutropenia (10% to 11%)
1% to 10%:
  Gastrointestinal: Ulcerative stomatitis (4%), nausea, abdominal pain (2%)
  Hematologic: Anemia
  Hepatic: Hepatitis, increased LFTs (2% to 4%)
  Neuromuscular & skeletal: Peripheral neuropathy, paresthesia (2%), myalgia
<1% (Limited to important or life-threatening): Hepatic necrosis, hepatotoxicity, severe hypersensitivity/dermatologic reactions (may include severe rash, fever, blisters, oral lesions, (Continued)

Nevirapine *(Continued)*

conjunctivitis, facial edema, muscle or joint aches, general malaise, hepatitis, eosinophilia, granulocytopenia, lymphadenopathy, or renal dysfunction), Stevens-Johnson syndrome. If a severe hypersensitivity reaction occurs, nevirapine should be permanently discontinued.

Overdosage/Toxicology No toxicities have been reported with acute ingestions of large sums of tablets.

Drug Interactions

Cytochrome P450 Effect: CYP3A3/4 enzyme substrate; CYP3A3/4 enzyme inducer; CYP3A3/4 enzyme inhibitor

Increased Effect/Toxicity: Cimetidine, itraconazole, ketoconazole, and some macrolide antibiotics may increase nevirapine plasma concentrations. Increased toxicity when used concomitantly with protease inhibitors or oral contraceptives. Ketoconazole should NOT be coadministered. Concurrent administration of prednisone for the initial 14 days of nevirapine therapy was associated with an increased incidence and severity of rash.

Decreased Effect: Rifampin and rifabutin may decrease nevirapine concentrations due to induction of CYP3A; since nevirapine may decrease concentrations of protease inhibitors (eg, indinavir, saquinavir), they should not be administered concomitantly or doses should be increased. Nevirapine may decrease the effectiveness of oral contraceptives - suggest alternate method of birth control. Nevirapine also decreases the effect of ketoconazole and methadone. Nevirapine may decrease serum concentrations of some protease inhibitors (AUC of indinavir and saquinavir may be decreased - no effect noted with ritonavir), specific dosage adjustments have not been recommended (no adjustment recommended for ritonavir).

Ethanol/Nutrition/Herb Interactions Herb/Nutraceutical: Nevirapine serum concentration may be decreased by St John's wort; avoid concurrent use.

Stability Store at room temperature

Mechanism of Action As a non-nucleoside reverse transcriptase inhibitor, nevirapine has activity against HIV-1 by binding to reverse transcriptase. It consequently blocks the RNA-dependent and DNA-dependent DNA polymerase activities including HIV-1 replication. It does not require intracellular phosphorylation for antiviral activity.

Pharmacodynamics/Kinetics

Absorption: >90%

Distribution: Widely; V_d: 1.2-1.4 L/kg; crosses placenta; enters breast milk; CSF penetration approximates 50% of plasma

Protein binding, plasma: 50% to 60%

Metabolism: Extensively hepatic via CYP3A3/4 (hydroxylation to inactive compounds); may undergo enterohepatic recycling

Half-life elimination: Decreases over 2- to 4-week time with chronic dosing due to autoinduction (ie, half-life = 45 hours initially and decreases to 23 hours)

Time to peak, serum: 2-4 hours

Excretion: Urine (as metabolites, <3% as unchanged drug)

Usual Dosage Oral:

Children 2 months to <8 years: Initial: 4 mg/kg/dose once daily for 14 days; increase dose to every 12 hours if no rash or other adverse effects occur; maintenance dose: 7 mg/kg/dose every 12 hours; maximum dose: 200 mg/dose every 12 hours

Children ≥8 years: Initial: 4 mg/kg/dose once daily for 14 days; increase dose to 4 mg/kg/dose every 12 hours if no rash or other adverse effects occur; maximum dose: 200 mg/dose every 12 hours

Note: Alternative pediatric dosing (unlabeled): 120-200 mg/m² every 12 hours; this dosing has been proposed due to the fact that dosing based on mg/kg may result in an abrupt decrease in dose at the 8th birthday, which may be inappropriate.

Adults: Initial: 200 mg once daily for 14 days; maintenance: 200 mg twice daily (in combination with an additional antiretroviral agent)

Note: If therapy is interrupted for >7 days, restart with initial dose for 14 days

Administration Oral: May be administered with or without food; may be administered with an antacid or didanosine; shake suspension gently prior to administration

Monitoring Parameters Liver function tests should be monitored at baseline, and intensively during the first 12 weeks of therapy (optimal frequency not established, recommendations recommend more often than once a month, including prior to dose escalation, and at 2 weeks following dose escalation), then periodically throughout therapy; observe for CNS side effects

Patient Information Report any right upper quadrant pain, jaundice, or rash to your physician immediately

Nursing Implications May be given with food, antacids, or didanosine; if therapy is interrupted for >7 days, the dose should be decreased to the initial regimen and increased after 14 days.

Suspension: Shake gently prior to use. Use oral syringe for volumes of 5 mL or less. When using dosing cups, rinse cup with water and give to patient as well.

Additional Information Potential compliance problems, frequency of administration, and adverse effects should be discussed with patients before initiating therapy to help prevent the emergence of resistance.

Dosage Forms

Suspension, oral: 50 mg/5 mL (240 mL)

Tablet: 200 mg

♦ **Nexium**™ *see* Esomeprazole *on page 490*

♦ **N.G.A.**® *see* Nystatin and Triamcinolone *on page 1002*

Niacin *(NYE a sin)*

Related Information

Hyperlipidemia Management *on page 1670*

Lipid-Lowering Agents *on page 1505*

U.S. Brand Names Niacor®; Niaspan®; Nicolar® [OTC]; Nicotinex [OTC]; Slo-Niacin® [OTC]

Canadian Brand Names Niaspan®

Synonyms Nicotinic Acid; Vitamin B_3

Therapeutic Category Antilipemic Agent, Miscellaneous; Vitamin, Water Soluble

Use Adjunctive treatment of hyperlipidemias; peripheral vascular disease and circulatory disorders; treatment of pellagra; dietary supplement; use in elevating HDL in patients with dyslipidemia

Pregnancy Risk Factor A/C (dose exceeding RDA recommendation)

Contraindications Hypersensitivity to niacin, nicotinamide, or any component of the formulation; liver disease; active peptic ulcer; severe hypotension; arterial hemorrhage

Warnings/Precautions Monitor liver function tests, blood glucose; may elevate uric acid levels; use with caution in patients predisposed to gout; large doses should be administered with caution to patients with gallbladder disease, jaundice, liver disease, or diabetes; some products may contain tartrazine

Adverse Reactions
1% to 10%:
  Cardiovascular: Generalized flushing
  Central nervous system: Headache
  Gastrointestinal: Bloating, flatulence, nausea
  Hepatic: Abnormalities of hepatic function tests, jaundice
  Neuromuscular & skeletal: Paresthesia in extremities
  Miscellaneous: Increased sebaceous gland activity, sensation of warmth
<1% (Limited to important or life-threatening): Blurred vision, dizziness, liver damage (dose-related incidence), rash, syncope, tachycardia, vasovagal attacks, wheezing

Overdosage/Toxicology Symptoms of acute overdose include flushing, GI distress, and pruritus. Chronic excessive use has been associated with hepatitis. Antihistamines may relieve niacin-induced histamine release, otherwise, treatment is symptomatic.

Drug Interactions
  Increased Effect/Toxicity: Niacin increase the potential for myopathy and/or rhabdomyolysis with lovastatin (and possibly other HMG-CoA reductase inhibitors). Use with adrenergic blocking agents may result in additive vasodilating effect and postural hypotension.
  Decreased Effect: The effect of oral hypoglycemics may be decreased by niacin. Niacin may inhibit uricosuric effects of sulfinpyrazone and probenecid. Aspirin (or other NSAIDs) decreases niacin-induced flushing.

Mechanism of Action Component of two coenzymes which is necessary for tissue respiration, lipid metabolism, and glycogenolysis; inhibits the synthesis of very low density lipoproteins

Pharmacodynamics/Kinetics
  Metabolism: Niacin converts to niacinamide (dose-dependent); niacinamide is 30% hepatically metabolized
  Half-life elimination: 45 minutes
  Time to peak, serum: ~45 minutes
  Excretion: Urine; with larger doses, greater percentage as unchanged drug

Usual Dosage
  Children: Oral:
    Pellagra: 50-100 mg/dose 3 times/day
    Recommended daily allowances:
      0-0.5 years: 5 mg/day
      0.5-1 year: 6 mg/day
      1-3 years: 9 mg/day
      4-6 years: 12 mg/day
      7-10 years: 13 mg/day
  Children and Adolescents: Recommended daily allowances:
    Male:
      11-14 years: 17 mg/day
      15-18 years: 20 mg/day
      19-24 years: 19 mg/day
    Female: 11-24 years: 15 mg/day
  Adults: Oral:
    Recommended daily allowances:
      Male: 25-50 years: 19 mg/day; >51 years: 15 mg/day
      Female: 25-50 years: 15 mg/day; >51 years: 13 mg/day
    Hyperlipidemia: Usual target dose: 1.5-6 g/day in 3 divided doses with or after meals using a dosage titration schedule; extended release: 375 mg to 2 g once daily at bedtime
      Regular release formulation (Niacor®): Initial: 250 mg once daily (with evening meal); increase frequency and/or dose every 4-7 days to desired response or first-level therapeutic dose (1.5-2 g/day in 2-3 divided doses); after 2 months, may increase at 2- to 4-week intervals to 3 g/day in 3 divided doses
      Extended release formulation (Niaspan®): 500 mg at bedtime for 4 weeks, then 1 g at bedtime for 4 weeks; adjust dose to response and tolerance; can increase to a maximum of 2 g/day, but only at 500 mg/day at 4-week intervals
    Pellagra: 50-100 mg 3-4 times/day, maximum: 500 mg/day
    Niacin deficiency: 10-20 mg/day, maximum: 100 mg/day

Dietary Considerations Should be taken after meals.

Administration Administer with food

Monitoring Parameters Blood glucose, liver function tests (with large doses or prolonged therapy), serum cholesterol

Test Interactions False elevations in some fluorometric determinations of urinary catecholamines; false-positive urine glucose (Benedict's reagent)

Patient Information May experience transient cutaneous flushing and sensation of warmth, especially of face and upper body; itching or tingling, and headache may occur, these adverse effects may be decreased by increasing the dose slowly or by taking aspirin or a NSAID 30 minutes to 1 hour prior to taking niacin; may cause GI upset, take with food; if dizziness occurs, avoid sudden changes in posture; report any persistent nausea, vomiting, abdominal pain, dark urine, or pale stools to the physician; do not crush sustained release capsule
(Continued)

Niacin *(Continued)*

Nursing Implications Monitor closely for signs of hepatotoxicity and myositis; avoid sudden changes in posture. Do not crush timed release forms.

Dosage Forms
Capsule, timed release: 125 mg, 250 mg, 400 mg, 500 mg
Elixir: 50 mg/5 mL (473 mL, 4000 mL)
Tablet: 50 mg, 100 mg, 250 mg, 500 mg
Tablet, extended release: 500 mg, 750 mg, 1000 mg
Tablet, timed release: 150 mg, 250 mg, 500 mg, 750 mg

Niacinamide (nye a SIN a mide)

Synonyms Nicotinamide; Vitamin B_3

Therapeutic Category Vitamin, Water Soluble

Use Prophylaxis and treatment of pellagra

Pregnancy Risk Factor A/C (dose exceeding RDA recommendation)

Contraindications Hypersensitivity to niacin, niacinamide, or any component of the formulation; liver disease; active peptic ulcer; severe hypotension; arterial hemorrhage

Warnings/Precautions Large doses should be administered with caution to patients with gallbladder disease or diabetes; monitor blood glucose; may elevate uric acid levels; use with caution in patients predisposed to gout; some products may contain tartrazine

Adverse Reactions Frequency not defined.
Cardiovascular: Tachycardia
Dermatologic: Increased sebaceous gland activity, rash
Gastrointestinal: Bloating, flatulence, nausea
Neuromuscular & skeletal: Paresthesia in extremities
Ocular: Blurred vision
Respiratory: Wheezing

Overdosage/Toxicology Symptoms include GI distress. Treatment is supportive.

Mechanism of Action Used by the body as a source of niacin; is a component of two coenzymes which is necessary for tissue respiration, lipid metabolism, and glycogenolysis; inhibits the synthesis of very low density lipoproteins; does not have hypolipidemia or vasodilating effects

Pharmacodynamics/Kinetics
Absorption: Rapid
Metabolism: Hepatic
Half-life elimination: 45 minutes
Time to peak, serum: 20-70 minutes
Excretion: Urine

Usual Dosage Oral:
Children: Pellagra: 100-300 mg/day in divided doses
Adults: 50 mg 3-10 times/day
Pellagra: 300-500 mg/day
Recommended daily allowance: 13-19 mg/day

Test Interactions False elevations of urinary catecholamines in some fluorometric determinations

Dosage Forms Tablet: 50 mg, 100 mg, 500 mg

Niacin and Lovastatin (NYE a sin & LOE va sta tin)

U.S. Brand Names Advicor™

Synonyms Lovastatin and Niacin

Therapeutic Category Antilipemic Agent, HMG-CoA Reductase Inhibitor; Antilipemic Agent, Miscellaneous

Use Treatment of primary hypercholesterolemia (heterozygous familial and nonfamilial) and mixed dyslipidemia (Fredrickson types IIa and IIb) in patients previously treated with either agent alone (patients who require further lowering of triglycerides or increase in HDL cholesterol from addition of niacin or further lowering of LDL cholesterol from addition of lovastatin). Combination product; not intended for initial treatment.

Pregnancy Risk Factor X

Usual Dosage Dosage forms are a fixed combination of niacin and lovastatin.
Oral: Adults: Lowest dose: Niacin 500 mg/lovastatin 20 mg; may increase by not more than 500 mg (niacin) at 4-week intervals (maximum dose: Niacin 2000 mg/lovastatin 40 mg daily); should be taken at bedtime with a low-fat snack
Not for use as initial therapy of dyslipidemias. May be substituted for equivalent dose of Niaspan®, however manufacturer does not recommend direct substitution with other niacin products.

Dosage Forms Tablet, extended release (niacin) and immediate release (lovastatin): Niacin 500 mg and lovastatin 20 mg; niacin 750 mg and lovastatin 20 mg; niacin 1000 mg and lovastatin 20 mg

♦ **Niacor**® *see Niacin on page 974*
♦ **Niaspan**® *see Niacin on page 974*

NiCARdipine (nye KAR de peen)

Related Information
Calcium Channel Blockers Comparison *on page 1494*
Hypertension *on page 1675*

U.S. Brand Names Cardene®; Cardene® I.V.; Cardene® SR

Synonyms Nicardipine Hydrochloride

Therapeutic Category Antianginal Agent; Antihypertensive Agent; Antimigraine Agent; Calcium Channel Blocker

Use Chronic stable angina (immediate-release product only); management of essential hypertension (immediate and sustained release; parenteral only for short time that oral treatment is not feasible)

Unlabeled/Investigational Use Congestive heart failure

Pregnancy Risk Factor C

Pregnancy/Breast-Feeding Implications

Clinical effects on the fetus: Crosses the placenta; may exhibit tocolytic effect

Breast-feeding/lactation: No data available

Contraindications Hypersensitivity to nicardipine or any component of the formulation; advanced aortic stenosis; severe hypotension; cardiogenic shock; ventricular tachycardia

Warnings/Precautions Blood pressure lowering should be done at a rate appropriate for the patient's condition. Rapid drops in blood pressure can lead to arterial insufficiency. Use with caution in CAD (can cause increase in angina), CHF (can worsen heart failure symptoms), and pheochromocytoma (limited clinical experience). Peripheral infusion sites (for I.V. therapy) should be changed ever 12 hours. Titrate I.V. dose cautiously in patients with CHF, renal, or hepatic dysfunction. Use the I.V. form cautiously in patients with portal hypertension (can cause increase in hepatic pressure gradient). Safety and efficacy have not been demonstrated in pediatric patients. Abrupt withdrawal may cause rebound angina in patients with CAD.

Adverse Reactions

1% to 10%:

Cardiovascular: Flushing (6% to 10%), palpitations (3% to 4%), tachycardia (1% to 3%), peripheral edema (dose-related 7% to 8%), increased angina (dose-related 5.6%)

Central nervous system: Headache (6% to 8%), dizziness (4% to 7%), somnolence (4% to 6%), paresthesia (1%)

Dermatologic: Rash (1%)

Gastrointestinal: Nausea (2% to 5%), dry mouth (1%)

Neuromuscular & skeletal: Weakness (4% to 6%), myalgia (1%)

<1% (Limited to important or life-threatening): Abnormal EKG, dyspnea, gingival hyperplasia, nervousness, parotitis, sustained tachycardia, syncope

Overdosage/Toxicology

Primary cardiac symptoms of calcium blocker overdose include hypotension and brady-cardia. Hypotension is caused by peripheral vasodilation, myocardial depression, and bradycardia. Bradycardia results from sinus bradycardia, second- or third-degree atrioventricular block, or sinus arrest with junctional rhythm. Intraventricular conduction is usually not affected so the QRS duration is normal (verapamil prolongs the P-R interval and bepridil prolongs the QT interval and may cause ventricular arrhythmias, including torsade de pointes).

Noncardiac symptoms include confusion, stupor, nausea, vomiting, metabolic acidosis, and hyperglycemia. Following initial gastric decontamination, if possible, repeated calcium administration may promptly reverse depressed cardiac contractility (but not sinus node depression or peripheral vasodilation). Glucagon, epinephrine, and inamrinone (amrinone) may treat refractory hypotension. Glucagon and epinephrine also increase the heart rate (outside the U.S., 4-aminopyridine may be available as an antidote). Dialysis and hemoperfusion are not effective in enhancing elimination, although repeat-dose activated charcoal may serve as an adjunct with sustained-release preparations.

In a few reported cases, overdose with calcium channel blockers has been associated with hypotension and bradycardia, initially refractory to atropine, but becoming more responsive to this agent when larger doses (approaching 1 g/hour for more than 24 hours) of calcium chloride were administered.

Drug Interactions

Cytochrome P450 Effect: CYP3A3/4 enzyme substrate; CYP2C8/9, 2C19, 2D6, 3A3/4 enzyme inhibitor

Increased Effect/Toxicity: H_2 blockers (cimetidine) may increase the bioavailability of nicardipine. Serum concentrations/toxicity of nicardipine may be increased by inhibitors of CYP3A3/4, including amprenavir, cimetidine, ciprofloxacin, clarithromycin, clozapine, diltiazem, disulfiram, digoxin, erythromycin, ethanol, fluconazole, fluoxetine, fluvoxamine, grapefruit juice, isoniazid, itraconazole, ketoconazole, labetalol, levodopa, loxapine, metoprolol, metronidazole, miconazole, nefazodone, nelfinavir, omeprazole, phenytoin, propranolol, rifabutin, rifampin, ritonavir, troleandomycin, valproic acid, and verapamil. Calcium may reduce the calcium channel blocker's effects, particularly hypotension. Cyclosporine levels (and possibly tacrolimus) may be increased by nicardipine. May increase effect of vecuronium (reduce dose 25%) and increase serum levels of metoprolol.

Decreased Effect: Rifampin (and potentially other enzyme inducers) increase the metabolism of calcium channel blockers.

Ethanol/Nutrition/Herb Interactions

Ethanol: Avoid ethanol (may increase CNS depression).

Food: Nicardipine average peak concentrations may be decreased if taken with food. Serum concentrations/toxicity of nicardipine may be increased by grapefruit juice; avoid concurrent use.

Herb/Nutraceutical: St John's wort may decrease levels. Avoid dong quai if using for hypertension (has estrogenic activity). Avoid ephedra, yohimbe, ginseng (may worsen hypertension). Avoid garlic (may have increased antihypertensive effect).

Stability Compatible with D_5W, $D_5\frac{1}{2}NS$, D_5NS, and D_5W with 40 mEq potassium chloride; 0.45% and 0.9% NS; **do not** mix with 5% sodium bicarbonate and lactated Ringer's solution; store at room temperature; protect from light; stable for 24 hours at room temperature

Mechanism of Action Inhibits calcium ion from entering the "slow channels" or select voltage-sensitive areas of vascular smooth muscle and myocardium during depolarization, producing a relaxation of coronary vascular smooth muscle and coronary vasodilation; increases myocardial oxygen delivery in patients with vasospastic angina

Pharmacodynamics/Kinetics

Onset of action: Oral: 1-2 hours; I.V.: 10 minutes; Hypotension: ~20 minutes

Duration: 2-6 hours

Absorption: Oral: ~100%

Protein binding: 95%

Metabolism: Hepatic; extensive first-pass effect

Bioavailability: 35%

(Continued)

NiCARdipine *(Continued)*

Half-life elimination: 2-4 hours
Time to peak, serum: 20-120 minutes
Excretion: Urine (as metabolites)

Usual Dosage Note: The total daily dose of immediate-release product may not automatically be equivalent to the daily sustained-release dose; use caution in converting: Adults:

Oral:
Immediate release: Initial: 20 mg 3 times/day; usual: 20-40 mg 3 times/day (allow 3 days between dose increases)
Sustained release: Initial: 30 mg twice daily, titrate up to 60 mg twice daily
I.V. (dilute to 0.1 mg/mL): Initial: 5 mg/hour increased by 2.5 mg/hour every 15 minutes to a maximum of 15 mg/hour

Dosing adjustment in renal impairment: Titrate dose beginning with 20 mg 3 times/day (immediate release) or 30 mg twice daily (sustained release).

Dosing adjustment in hepatic impairment: Starting dose: 20 mg twice daily (immediate release) with titration.

Equivalent oral vs I.V. infusion doses:
20 mg every 8 hours oral, equivalent to 0.5 mg/hour I.V. infusion
30 mg every 8 hours oral, equivalent to 1.2 mg/hour I.V. infusion
40 mg every 8 hours oral, equivalent to 2.2 mg/hour I.V. infusion

Administration

Oral: The total daily dose of immediate-release product may not automatically be equivalent to the daily sustained-release dose; use caution in converting. Do not chew or crush the sustained release formulation, swallow whole. Do not open or cut capsules.
I.V.: Ampuls must be diluted before use. Administer as a slow continuous infusion.

Patient Information Sustained release products should be taken with food (not fatty meal); do not crush; limit caffeine intake; avoid alcohol; notify physician if angina pain is not reduced when taking this drug, irregular heartbeat, shortness of breath, swelling, dizziness, constipation, nausea, or hypotension occur; do not stop therapy without advice of physician

Nursing Implications Monitor closely for orthostasis; ampuls must be diluted before use; do not crush sustained release product; to assess adequacy of blood pressure response, measure blood pressure 8 hours after dosing

Dosage Forms
Capsule: 20 mg, 30 mg
Capsule, sustained release: 30 mg, 45 mg, 60 mg
Injection: 2.5 mg/mL (10 mL)

♦ **Nicardipine Hydrochloride** *see* NiCARdipine *on page 976*

♦ **Niclocide®** *see* Niclosamide *Not available in the U.S. on page 978*

Niclosamide *Not available in the U.S.* (ni KLOE sa mide)

U.S. Brand Names Niclocide®
Therapeutic Category Anthelmintic
Use Treatment of intestinal beef and fish tapeworm infections and dwarf tapeworm infections
Pregnancy Risk Factor B
Contraindications Hypersensitivity to niclosamide or any component of the formulation
Warnings/Precautions Affects cestodes of the intestine only; it is without effect in cysticercosis

Adverse Reactions
1% to 10%:
Central nervous system: Drowsiness, dizziness, headache
Gastrointestinal: Nausea, vomiting, loss of appetite, diarrhea
<1% (Limited to important or life-threatening): Alopecia, backache, bad taste in mouth, constipation, diaphoresis, edema in the arm, fever, oral irritation, palpitations, pruritus ani, rash, rectal bleeding, weakness

Overdosage/Toxicology Signs and symptoms of overdose include nausea, vomiting, and anorexia. In the event of an overdose, do not administer ipecac.

Mechanism of Action Inhibits the synthesis of ATP through inhibition of oxidative phosphorylation in the mitochondria of cestodes

Pharmacodynamics/Kinetics
Absorption: Insignificant
Metabolism: Not appreciably metabolized by mammalian host, but may be metabolized in GI tract by the worm
Excretion: Feces

Usual Dosage Oral:
Beef and fish tapeworm:
Children:
11-34 kg: 1 g (2 tablets) as a single dose
>34 kg: 1.5 g (3 tablets) as a single dose
Adults: 2 g (4 tablets) in a single dose
May require a second course of treatment 7 days later
Dwarf tapeworm:
Children:
11-34 g: 1 g (2 tablets) chewed thoroughly in a single dose the first day, then 500 mg/day (1 tablet) for next 6 days
>34 g: 1.5 g (3 tablets) in a single dose the first day, then 1 g/day for 6 days
Adults: 2 g (4 tablets) in a single daily dose for 7 days

Monitoring Parameters Stool cultures

Patient Information Chew tablets thoroughly; tablets can be pulverized and mixed with water to form a paste for administration to children; can be taken with food; a mild laxative can be used for constipation

Nursing Implications Administer a laxative 2-3 hours after the niclosamide dose if treating *Taenia solium* infections to prevent the development of cysticercosis

Dosage Forms Tablet, chewable: 500 mg [vanilla flavor]

♦ **Nicoderm® (Can)** see Nicotine on page 979
♦ **NicoDerm® CQ® Patch** see Nicotine on page 979
♦ **Nicolar® [OTC]** see Niacin on page 974
♦ **Nicorette® (Can)** see Nicotine on page 979
♦ **Nicorette® DS Gum** see Nicotine on page 979
♦ **Nicorette® Gum** see Nicotine on page 979
♦ **Nicorette® Plus (Can)** see Nicotine on page 979
♦ **Nicotinamide** see Niacinamide on page 976

Nicotine (nik oh TEEN)

Related Information
Nicotine Products Comparison on page 1510
U.S. Brand Names Habitrol™ Patch; NicoDerm® CQ® Patch; Nicorette® DS Gum; Nicorette® Gum; Nicotrol® NS; Nicotrol® Patch [OTC]; ProStep® Patch
Canadian Brand Names Habitrol®; Nicoderm®; Nicorette®; Nicorette® Plus; Nicotrol®
Therapeutic Category Smoking Deterrent
Use Treatment to aid smoking cessation for the relief of nicotine withdrawal symptoms (including nicotine craving)
Unlabeled/Investigational Use Management of ulcerative colitis (transdermal)
Pregnancy Risk Factor D (transdermal); X (chewing gum)
Contraindications Hypersensitivity to nicotine or any component of the formulation; patients who are smoking during the postmyocardial infarction period; patients with life-threatening arrhythmias, or severe or worsening angina pectoris; active temporomandibular joint disease (gum); pregnancy; not for use in nonsmokers
Warnings/Precautions Use with caution in oropharyngeal inflammation and in patients with history of esophagitis, peptic ulcer, coronary artery disease, vasospastic disease, angina, hypertension, hyperthyroidism, diabetes, and hepatic dysfunction; nicotine is known to be one of the most toxic of all poisons; while the gum is being used to help the patient overcome a health hazard, it also must be considered a hazardous drug vehicle.
Adverse Reactions
  Chewing gum:
    >10%:
      Cardiovascular: Tachycardia
      Central nervous system: Headache (mild)
      Gastrointestinal: Nausea, vomiting, indigestion, excessive salivation, belching, increased appetite
      Miscellaneous: Mouth or throat soreness, jaw muscle ache, hiccups
    1% to 10%:
      Central nervous system: Insomnia, dizziness, nervousness
      Endocrine & metabolic: Dysmenorrhea
      Gastrointestinal: GI distress, eructation
      Neuromuscular & skeletal: Muscle pain
      Respiratory: Hoarseness
      Miscellaneous: Hiccups
    <1% (Limited to important or life-threatening): Atrial fibrillation, erythema, hypersensitivity reactions, itching
  Transdermal systems:
    >10%:
      Central nervous system: Insomnia, abnormal dreams
      Dermatologic: Pruritus, erythema
      Local: Application site reaction
      Respiratory: Rhinitis, cough, pharyngitis, sinusitis
    1% to 10%:
      Cardiovascular: Chest pain
      Central nervous system: Dysphoria, anxiety, difficulty concentrating, dizziness, somnolence
      Dermatologic: Rash
      Gastrointestinal: Diarrhea, dyspepsia, nausea, xerostomia, constipation, anorexia, abdominal pain
      Neuromuscular & skeletal: Arthralgia, myalgia
    <1% (Limited to important or life-threatening): Atrial fibrillation, hypersensitivity reactions, itching, nervousness, taste perversion, thirst, tremor
Overdosage/Toxicology Symptoms include nausea, vomiting, abdominal pain, mental confusion, diarrhea, salivation, tachycardia, respiratory and cardiovascular collapse. Treatment after decontamination is symptomatic and supportive. Remove the patch, rinse the area with water and dry; do not use soap as this may increase absorption.
Drug Interactions
  Cytochrome P450 Effect: CYP2B6 and 2A6 enzyme substrate; CYP1A2 enzyme inducer
  Increased Effect/Toxicity: Nicotine increases the hemodynamic and AV blocking effects of adenosine; monitor. Cimetidine increases nicotine concentrations; therefore, may decrease amount of gum or patches needed. Monitor for treatment-emergent hypertension in patients treated with the combination of nicotine patch and bupropion.
Stability Store inhaler cartridge at room temperature not to exceed 30°C (86°F); protect cartridges from light
Mechanism of Action Nicotine is one of two naturally-occurring alkaloids which exhibit their primary effects via autonomic ganglia stimulation. The other alkaloid is lobeline which has many actions similar to those of nicotine but is less potent. Nicotine is a potent ganglionic and central nervous system stimulant, the actions of which are mediated via nicotine-specific receptors. Biphasic actions are observed depending upon the dose administered. The main effect of nicotine in small doses is stimulation of all autonomic ganglia; with larger doses, initial stimulation is followed by blockade of transmission. Biphasic effects are also evident in
(Continued)

Nicotine *(Continued)*

the adrenal medulla; discharge of catecholamines occurs with small doses, whereas prevention of catecholamines release is seen with higher doses as a response to splanchnic nerve stimulation. Stimulation of the central nervous system (CNS) is characterized by tremors and respiratory excitation. However, convulsions may occur with higher doses, along with respiratory failure secondary to both central paralysis and peripheral blockade to respiratory muscles.

Pharmacodynamics/Kinetics

Onset of action: Intranasal: More closely approximate the time course of plasma nicotine levels observed after cigarette smoking than other dosage forms

Duration: Transdermal: 24 hours

Absorption: Transdermal: Slow

Metabolism: Hepatic, primarily to cotinine ($\frac{1}{5}$ as active)

Half-life elimination: 4 hours

Time to peak, serum: Transdermal: 8-9 hours

Excretion: Urine

Clearance: Renal: pH-dependent

Usual Dosage

Gum: Chew 1 piece of gum when urge to smoke, up to 30 pieces/day; most patients require 10-12 pieces of gum/day

Transdermal patch:

Smoking deterrent: Patients should be advised to completely stop smoking upon initiation of therapy; Apply new patch every 24 hours to nonhairy, clean, dry skin on the upper body or upper outer arm; each patch should be applied to a different site. **Note:** Adjustment may be required during initial treatment (move to higher dose if experiencing withdrawal symptoms; lower dose if side effects are experienced).

Habitrol®, NicoDerm CQ®:

Patients smoking ≥10 cigarettes/day: Begin with **step 1** (21 mg/day) for 4-6 weeks, followed by **step 2** (14 mg/day) for 2 weeks; finish with **step 3** (7 mg/day) for 2 weeks

Patients smoking <10 cigarettes/day: Begin with **step 2** (14 mg/day) for 6 weeks, followed by **step 3** (7 mg/day) for 2 weeks

Note: Initial starting dose for patients <100 pounds, history of cardiovascular disease: 14 mg/day for 4-6 weeks, followed by 7 mg/day for 2-4 weeks

Note: Patients receiving >600 mg/day of cimetidine: Decrease to the next lower patch size

Nicotrol®: One patch daily for 6 weeks

ProStep®:

Patients smoking >15 cigarettes/day: One 22 mg patch daily for 6 weeks

Patients smoking ≤15 cigarettes/day: One 11 mg patch daily for 6 weeks

Note: Benefits of use of nicotine transdermal patches beyond 3 months have not been demonstrated.

Ulcerative colitis (unlabeled use): Titrated to 22-25 mg/day

Spray: 1-2 sprays/hour; do not exceed more than 5 doses (10 sprays) per hour; each dose (2 sprays) contains 1 mg of nicotine. **Warning:** A dose of 40 mg can cause fatalities.

Monitoring Parameters Heart rate and blood pressure periodically during therapy; discontinue therapy if signs of nicotine toxicity occur (eg, severe headache, dizziness, mental confusion, disturbed hearing and vision, abdominal pain; rapid, weak and irregular pulse; salivation, nausea, vomiting, diarrhea, cold sweat, weakness); therapy should be discontinued if rash develops; discontinuation may be considered if other adverse effects of patch occur such as myalgia, arthralgia, abnormal dreams, insomnia, nervousness, dry mouth, sweating

Patient Information Notify physician if persistent rash, itching, or burning may occur with the patch; do not smoke while wearing patches

Nursing Implications

Chew gum formulation: Patient should be instructed to chew slowly to avoid jaw ache and to maximize benefit

Transdermal patch: Patches cannot be cut; use of an aerosol corticosteroid may diminish local irritation under patches; instructions for the proper use of the patch should be given to the patient

Additional Information A cigarette has 10-25 mg nicotine. Use of an aerosol corticosteroid may diminish local irritation under patches.

Dosage Forms

Gum, chewing pieces, as polacrilex: 2 mg/square [OTC] (96 pieces/box); 4 mg/square (96 pieces/box) [original flavor, mint flavor, orange flavor]

Liquid for oral inhalation (Nicotrol® Inhaler): 10 mg cartridge [delivering 4 mg] (42s); each unit consists of one mouthpiece, 7 storage trays each containing 6 cartridges and one storage case

Patch, transdermal:

Habitrol™: 21 mg/day; 14 mg/day; 7 mg/day (30 systems/box)

NicoDerm® CQ® [OTC]: 21 mg/day; 14 mg/day; 7 mg/day (14 systems/box) [clear or tan patch]

Nicotrol® [OTC]: 15 mg/day (gradually released over 16 hours)

ProStep®: 22 mg/day; 11 mg/day (7 systems/box)

Solution, intranasal [spray] (Nicotrol® NS): 0.5 mg/actuation [10 mg/mL - 200 actuations] (10 mL)

- **Nicotine Products Comparison** *see page 1510*
- **Nicotinex [OTC]** *see Niacin on page 974*
- **Nicotinic Acid** *see Niacin on page 974*
- **Nicotrol® (Can)** *see Nicotine on page 979*
- **Nicotrol® NS** *see Nicotine on page 979*
- **Nicotrol® Patch [OTC]** *see Nicotine on page 979*

♦ Nidagel™ **(Can)** *see* Metronidazole *on page 904*

NIFEdipine (nye FED i peen)

Related Information
Calcium Channel Blockers Comparison *on page 1494*

U.S. Brand Names Adalat® CC; Procardia®; Procardia XL®

Canadian Brand Names Adalat® PA; Adalat® XL®; Apo®-Nifed; Apo®-Nifed PA; Novo-Nifedin; Nu-Nifed; Procardia®

Therapeutic Category Antianginal Agent; Antihypertensive Agent; Antimigraine Agent; Calcium Channel Blocker

Use Angina and hypertension (sustained release only), pulmonary hypertension

Pregnancy Risk Factor C

Pregnancy/Breast-Feeding Implications
Clinical effects on the fetus: Use in pregnancy only when clearly needed and when the benefits outweigh the potential hazard to the fetus. No data on crossing the placenta. Hypotension, IUGR reported. IUGR probably related to maternal hypertension. May exhibit tocolytic effects. Available evidence suggests safe use during pregnancy and breast-feeding.

Breast-feeding/lactation: Crosses into breast milk. AAP considers **compatible** with breast-feeding.

Contraindications Hypersensitivity to nifedipine or any component of the formulation; immediate release preparation for treatment of urgent or emergent hypertension; acute MI

Warnings/Precautions The routine use of short-acting nifedipine capsules in hypertensive emergencies and pseudoemergencies is not recommended. **The use of sublingual short-acting nifedipine in hypertensive emergencies is neither safe or effective and SHOULD BE ABANDONED!** Serious adverse events (cerebrovascular ischemia, syncope, heart block, stroke, sinus arrest, severe hypotension, acute myocardial infarction, EKG changes, and fetal distress) have been reported in relation to the administration of short-acting nifedipine in hypertensive emergencies.

Increased angina may be seen upon starting or increasing doses; may increase frequency, duration, and severity of angina during initiation of therapy; use with caution in patients with congestive heart failure or aortic stenosis (especially with concomitant beta-adrenergic blocker); severe left ventricular dysfunction, hepatic or renal impairment, hypertrophic cardiomyopathy (especially obstructive), concomitant therapy with beta-blockers or digoxin, edema

Mild and transient elevations in liver function enzymes may be apparent within 8 weeks of therapy initiation.

Therapeutic potential of sustained-release formulation (elementary osmotic pump, gastrointestinal therapeutic system [GITS]) may be decreased in patients with certain GI disorders that accelerate intestinal transit time (eg, short bowel syndrome, inflammatory bowel disease, severe diarrhea).

Note: Elderly patients may experience a greater hypotensive response and the use of the immediate release formulation in patients >71 years of age has been associated with a nearly fourfold increased risk for all-cause mortality when compared to beta-blockers, ACE inhibitors, or other classes of calcium channel blockers

Adverse Reactions
>10%:
Cardiovascular: Flushing (10% to 25%), peripheral edema (dose-related 7% to 10%; up to 50%)
Central nervous system: Dizziness/lightheadedness/giddiness (10% to 27%), headache (10% to 23%)
Gastrointestinal: Nausea/heartburn (10% to 11%)
Neuromuscular & skeletal: Weakness (10% to 12%)

≥1% to 10%:
Cardiovascular: Palpitations (≤2% to 7%), transient hypotension (dose-related 5%), CHF (2%)
Central nervous system: Nervousness/mood changes (≤2% to 7%), shakiness (≤2%), jitteriness (≤2%), sleep disturbances (≤2%), difficulties in balance (≤2%), fever (≤2%), chills (≤2%)
Dermatologic: Dermatitis (≤2%), pruritus (≤2%), urticaria (≤2%)
Endocrine & metabolic: Sexual difficulties (≤2%)
Gastrointestinal: Diarrhea (≤2%), constipation (≤2%), cramps (≤2%), flatulence (≤2%), gingival hyperplasia (≤10%)
Neuromuscular & skeletal: Muscle cramps/tremor (≤2% to 8%), weakness (10%), inflammation (≤2%), joint stiffness (≤2%)
Ocular: Blurred vision (≤2%)
Respiratory: Cough/wheezing (6%), nasal congestion/sore throat (≤2% to 6%), chest congestion (≤2%), dyspnea (≤2%)
Miscellaneous: Diaphoresis (≤2%)

<1% (Limited to important or life-threatening): Agranulocytosis, allergic hepatitis, angina, angioedema, aplastic anemia, arthritis with positive ANA, bezoars (sustained-release preparations), cerebral ischemia, depression, erythema multiforme, erythromelalgia, exfoliative dermatitis, extrapyramidal symptoms, fever, gingival hyperplasia, gynecomastia, leukopenia, memory dysfunction, paranoid syndrome, phototoxicity, purpura, Stevens-Johnson syndrome, syncope, thrombocytopenia, tinnitus, transient blindness

Reported with use of sublingual short-acting nifedipine: Acute myocardial infarction, cerebrovascular ischemia, EKG changes, fetal distress, heart block, severe hypotension, sinus arrest, stroke, syncope

Overdosage/Toxicology
Primary cardiac symptoms of calcium blocker overdose include hypotension and bradycardia. Hypotension is caused by peripheral vasodilation, myocardial depression, and
(Continued)

NIFEdipine *(Continued)*

bradycardia. Bradycardia results from sinus bradycardia, second- or third-degree atrioventricular block, or sinus arrest with junctional rhythm. Intraventricular conduction is usually not affected so the QRS duration is normal.

Noncardiac symptoms include confusion, stupor, nausea, vomiting, metabolic acidosis and hyperglycemia. Following initial gastric decontamination, if possible, repeated calcium administration may promptly reverse depressed cardiac contractility (but not sinus node depression or peripheral vasodilation). Glucagon, epinephrine, and inamrinone (amrinone) may treat refractory hypotension. Glucagon and epinephrine also increase the heart rate (outside the U.S., 4-aminopyridine may be available as an antidote). Dialysis and hemoperfusion are not effective in enhancing elimination although repeat-dose activated charcoal may serve as an adjunct with sustained-release preparations.

In a few reported cases, overdose with calcium channel blockers has been associated with hypotension and bradycardia, initially refractory to atropine, but becoming more responsive to this agent when larger doses (approaching 1 g/hour for more than 24 hours) of calcium chloride were administered.

Drug Interactions

Cytochrome P450 Effect: CYP3A3/4 and 3A5-7 enzyme substrate

Increased Effect/Toxicity: H_2-blockers may increase bioavailability and serum concentrations of nifedipine. Serum concentrations/toxicity of nifedipine may be increased by inhibitors of CYP3A3/4, including amprenavir, cimetidine, ciprofloxacin, clarithromycin, clozapine, diltiazem, disulfiram, digoxin, erythromycin, ethanol, fluconazole, fluoxetine, fluvoxamine, grapefruit juice, isoniazid, itraconazole, ketoconazole, labetalol, levodopa, loxapine, metoprolol, metronidazole, miconazole, nefazodone, nelfinavir, omeprazole, phenytoin, rifabutin, rifampin, ritonavir, troleandomycin, valproic acid, and verapamil. Nifedipine may increase serum levels of digoxin, phenytoin, theophylline, and vincristine.

Decreased Effect: Phenobarbital and nifedipine may decrease nifedipine levels. Quinidine and nifedipine may decrease quinidine serum levels. Rifampin and nifedipine may decrease nifedipine serum levels. Calcium may reduce the hypotension from of calcium channel blockers.

Ethanol/Nutrition/Herb Interactions

Ethanol: Avoid ethanol (may increase CNS depression).

Food: Nifedipine serum levels may be decreased if taken with food. Food may decrease the rate but not the extent of absorption of Procardia XL®. Increased therapeutic and vasodilator side effects, including severe hypotension and myocardial ischemia, may occur if nifedipine is taken by patients ingesting grapefruit.

Herb/Nutraceutical: St John's wort may decrease nifedipine levels. Avoid dong quai if using for hypertension (has estrogenic activity). Avoid ephedra, yohimbe, ginseng (may worsen hypertension). Avoid garlic (may have increased antihypertensive effect).

Mechanism of Action
Inhibits calcium ion from entering the "slow channels" or select voltage-sensitive areas of vascular smooth muscle and myocardium during depolarization, producing a relaxation of coronary vascular smooth muscle and coronary vasodilation; increases myocardial oxygen delivery in patients with vasospastic angina

Pharmacodynamics/Kinetics

Onset of action: ~20 minutes

Protein binding (concentration dependent): 92% to 98%

Metabolism: Hepatic to inactive metabolites

Bioavailability: Capsules: 45% to 75%; Sustained release: 65% to 86%

Half-life elimination: Adults, normal: 2-5 hours; Adults with cirrhosis: 7 hours

Excretion: Urine

Usual Dosage
Oral:

Children: Hypertrophic cardiomyopathy: 0.6-0.9 mg/kg/24 hours in 3-4 divided doses

Adolescents and Adults: (**Note:** When switching from immediate release to sustained release formulations, total daily dose will start the same)

Initial: 30 mg once daily as sustained release formulation, or if indicated, 10 mg 3 times/day as capsules

Usual dose: 10-30 mg 3 times/day as capsules or 30-60 mg once daily as sustained release

Maximum dose: 120-180 mg/day

Increase sustained release at 7- to 14-day intervals

Hemodialysis: Supplemental dose is not necessary.

Peritoneal dialysis effects: Supplemental dose is not necessary.

Dosing adjustment in hepatic impairment: Reduce oral dose by 50% to 60% in patients with cirrhosis.

Dietary Considerations
Capsule is rapidly absorbed orally if it is administered without food, but may result in vasodilator side effects; administration with low-fat meals may decrease flushing. Avoid grapefruit juice.

Administration
Sustained release tablets should be swallowed whole; do not crush or chew.

Monitoring Parameters
Heart rate, blood pressure, signs and symptoms of CHF, peripheral edema

Patient Information
Sustained release products should not be crushed or chewed; Adalat® CC should be taken on an empty stomach; limit caffeine intake; avoid alcohol; notify physician if angina pain is not reduced when taking this drug, irregular heartbeat, shortness of breath, swelling, dizziness, constipation, nausea, or hypotension occurs; do not stop therapy without advice of physician; the shell of the sustained-release tablet may appear intact in the stool, this is no cause for concern

Nursing Implications
May cause some patients to urinate frequently at night; may cause inflamed gums; do not crush or chew tablets or capsules

Additional Information
When measuring smaller doses from the liquid-filled capsules, consider the following concentrations (for Procardia®) 10 mg capsule = 10 mg/0.34 mL; 20 mg capsule = 20 mg/0.45 mL; may be used preoperative to treat hypertensive urgency.

Considerable attention has been directed to potential increases in mortality and morbidity when short-acting nifedipine is used in treating hypertension. The rapid reduction in blood pressure may precipitate adverse cardiovascular events. At this time, there is no indication for the use of short-acting calcium channel blocker therapy. Nifedipine also has potent negative inotropic effects and can worsen heart failure.

Dosage Forms
Capsule, liquid-filled (Procardia®): 10 mg, 20 mg
Tablet, extended release (Adalat® CC): 30 mg, 60 mg, 90 mg
Tablet, sustained release (Procardia XL®): 30 mg, 60 mg, 90 mg

◆ **Niferex® [OTC]** *see* Polysaccharide-Iron Complex *on page 1104*

◆ **Niferex®-PN** *see* Vitamins (Multiple) *on page 1424*

◆ **Nilandron™** *see* Nilutamide *on page 983*

◆ **Nilstat®** *see* Nystatin *on page 1001*

Nilutamide (ni LOO ta mide)

U.S. Brand Names Nilandron™
Canadian Brand Names Anandron®
Therapeutic Category Antiandrogen; Antineoplastic Agent, Miscellaneous
Use Treatment of metastatic prostate cancer
Pregnancy Risk Factor C
Contraindications Hypersensitivity to nilutamide or any component of the formulation; severe hepatic impairment; severe respiratory insufficiency
Warnings/Precautions The U.S. Food and Drug Administration (FDA) currently recommends that procedures for proper handling and disposal of antineoplastic agents be considered.

Interstitial pneumonitis has been reported in 2% of patients exposed to nilutamide. Patients typically experienced progressive exertional dyspnea, and possibly cough, chest pain and fever. X-rays showed interstitial or alveolar-interstitial changes. The suggestive signs of pneumonitis most often occurred within the first 3 months of nilutamide treatment.

Hepatitis or marked increases in liver enzymes leading to drug discontinuation occurred in 1% of nilutamide patients. There has been a report of elevated hepatic enzymes followed by death in a 65 year old patient treated with nilutamide.

Foreign postmarketing surveillance has revealed isolated cases of aplastic anemia in which a causal relationship with nilutamide could not be ascertained.

13% to 57% of patients receiving nilutamide reported a delay in adaptation to the dark, ranging from seconds to a few minutes. This effect sometimes does not abate as drug treatment is continued. Caution patients who experience this effect about driving at night or through tunnels. This effect can be alleviated by wearing tinted glasses.

Adverse Reactions
>10%:
Central nervous system: Pain, insomnia
Endocrine & metabolic: Hot flashes (60% to 80%), gynecomastia (4% to 44%); higher incidence in patients receiving the drug as a single agent
Gastrointestinal: Nausea, mild (10% to 32%); constipation, anorexia
Genitourinary: Decreased libido, impotence, sexual dysfunction (50%)
Hepatic: Transient elevation in serum transaminases (13%)
Ocular: Impaired dark adaptation (13% to 57%, up to 90%), usually reversible with dose reduction, may require discontinuation of the drug in 1% to 2% of patients; blurred vision
1% to 10%:
Cardiovascular: Hypertension
Central nervous system: Dizziness, drowsiness, malaise, headache, hypesthesia
Dermatologic: Disulfiram-like reaction (hot flashes, rashes) (20%); pruritus (<5%), alopecia, dry skin
Endocrine & metabolic: Flu-like syndrome, fever
Gastrointestinal: Vomiting, diarrhea, abdominal cramps
Genitourinary: Hematuria, nocturia
Hepatic: Hepatitis (1%)
Respiratory: Interstitial pneumonitis, pulmonary fibrosis (1% to 3%), usually reversible
<1% (Limited to important or life-threatening): Aplastic anemia, diaphoresis
Overdosage/Toxicology One case of massive overdose has been published. A 79-year-old man attempted suicide by ingesting 13 g of nilutamide. There were no clinical signs or symptoms, or changes in parameters such as transaminases or chest x-ray. Maintenance treatment (150 mg/day) was resumed 30 days later. Management is supportive and there is no benefit from dialysis. Induce vomiting if the patient is alert. Administer general supportive care (including frequent monitoring of vital signs and close observation).
Ethanol/Nutrition/Herb Interactions
Ethanol: Avoid ethanol. Up to 5% of patients may experience a systemic reaction (flushing, hypotension, malaise) when combined with nilutamide.
Herb/Nutraceutical: St John's wort may decrease nilutamide levels.
Stability Store at room temperature (15°C to 30°C/59°F to 86°F); protect from light
Mechanism of Action Nonsteroidal antiandrogen that inhibits androgen uptake or inhibits binding of androgen in target tissues
Pharmacodynamics/Kinetics
Absorption: Well absorbed
Protein binding, plasma: 80% to 84%; some to erythrocytes
Metabolism: Hepatic (1% to 7%)
Half-life elimination: Variable; Mean: 50 hours (range: 23-87 hours)
Time to peak, serum: 1-4 hours
Excretion: Urine (67% to 78% as metabolites, 1% to 2% as unchanged drug)
Usual Dosage Refer to individual protocols.
Adults: Oral: 300 mg daily for 30 days, then 150 mg/day
Dietary Considerations Can be taken without regard to food.
(Continued)

Nilutamide *(Continued)*

Monitoring Parameters

Perform routine chest x-rays before treatment, and tell patients to report immediately any dyspnea or aggravation of pre-existing dyspnea. At the onset of dyspnea or worsening of pre-existing dyspnea any time during therapy, interrupt nilutamide until it can be determined if respiratory symptoms are drug-related. Obtain a chest x-ray, and if there are findings suggestive of interstitial pneumonitis, discontinue treatment with nilutamide. The pneumonitis is almost always reversible when treatment is discontinued. If the chest x-ray appears normal, perform pulmonary function tests.

Measure serum hepatic enzyme levels at baseline and at regular intervals (3 months); if transaminases increase over 2-3 times the upper limit of normal, discontinue treatment. Perform appropriate laboratory testing at the first symptom/sign of liver injury (eg, jaundice, dark urine, fatigue, abdominal pain or unexplained GI symptoms) and nilutamide treatment must be discontinued immediately if transaminases exceed 3 times the upper limit of normal.

Dosage Forms Tablet: 50 mg

♦ **Nimbex**® see Cisatracurium *on page 300*

Nimodipine *(nye MOE di peen)*

Related Information

Calcium Channel Blockers Comparison *on page 1494*

U.S. Brand Names Nimotop®

Canadian Brand Names Nimotop®

Therapeutic Category Calcium Channel Blocker

Use Spasm following subarachnoid hemorrhage from ruptured intracranial aneurysms regardless of the patients neurological condition postictus (Hunt and Hess grades I-V)

Pregnancy Risk Factor C

Pregnancy/Breast-Feeding Implications

Clinical effects on the fetus: Use in pregnancy only when clearly needed and when the benefits outweigh the potential hazard to the fetus. Teratogenic and embryotoxic effects have been demonstrated in small animals. No well controlled studies have been conducted in pregnant women.

Breast milk/lactation: It is unknown if nimodipine appears in human breast milk. Breast-feeding is not recommended while using this medication.

Contraindications Hypersensitivity to nimodipine or any component of the formulation

Warnings/Precautions Use with caution and titrate dosages for patients with impaired renal or hepatic function; use caution when treating patients with congestive heart failure, sick-sinus syndrome, PVCs, severe left ventricular dysfunction, hypertrophic cardiomyopathy (especially obstructive, IHSS), concomitant therapy with beta-blockers or digoxin, edema, or increased intracranial pressure with cranial tumors; do not abruptly withdraw (may cause chest pain); elderly may experience hypotension and constipation more readily; intestinal pseudo-obstruction and ileus have been reported during the use of nimodipine; use caution in patients with decreased GI motility of a history of bowel obstruction

Adverse Reactions

1% to 10%:

Cardiovascular: Reductions in systemic blood pressure (1% to 8%)

Central nervous system: Headache (1% to 4%)

Dermatologic: Rash (1% to 2%)

Gastrointestinal: Diarrhea (2% to 4%), abdominal discomfort (2%)

<1% (Limited to important or life-threatening): Anemia, congestive heart failure, deep vein thrombosis, depression, disseminated intravascular coagulation, dyspnea, EKG abnormalities, GI hemorrhage, hepatitis, jaundice, neurological deterioration, rebound vasospasm, thrombocytopenia, vomiting

Overdosage/Toxicology

Primary cardiac symptoms of calcium blocker overdose include hypotension and bradycardia. Hypotension is caused by peripheral vasodilation, myocardial depression, and bradycardia. Bradycardia results from sinus bradycardia, second- or third-degree atrioventricular block, or sinus arrest with junctional rhythm. Intraventricular conduction is usually not affected so the QRS duration is normal.

Noncardiac symptoms include confusion, stupor, nausea, vomiting, metabolic acidosis and hyperglycemia. Following initial gastric decontamination, if possible, repeated calcium administration may promptly reverse the depressed cardiac contractility (but not sinus node depression or peripheral vasodilation). Glucagon, epinephrine, and inamrinone (amrinone) may treat refractory hypotension. Glucagon and epinephrine also increase the heart rate (outside the U.S., 4-aminopyridine may be available as an antidote). Dialysis and hemoperfusion are not effective in enhancing elimination although repeat-dose activated charcoal may serve as an adjunct with sustained-release preparations.

In a few reported cases, overdose with calcium channel blockers has been associated with hypotension and bradycardia, initially refractory to atropine, but becoming more responsive to this agent when larger doses (approaching 1 g/hour for more than 24 hours) of calcium chloride were administered.

Drug Interactions

Cytochrome P450 Effect: CYP3A3/4 enzyme substrate

Increased Effect/Toxicity: Calcium channel blockers and nimodipine may result in enhanced cardiovascular effects of other calcium channel blockers. Cimetidine, omeprazole, and valproic acid may increase serum nimodipine levels. The effects of antihypertensive agents may be increased by nimodipine. Azole antifungals (itraconazole, ketoconazole, fluconazole), erythromycin, protease inhibitors (amprenavir, nelfinavir, ritonavir) and other inhibitors of cytochrome P450 isoenzyme 3A4 may inhibit calcium channel blocker metabolism.

Decreased Effect: Rifampin (and potentially other enzyme inducers) increase the metabolism of calcium channel blockers.

Ethanol/Nutrition/Herb Interactions
  Food: Nimodipine has shown a 1.5 fold increase in bioavailability when taken with grapefruit juice; avoid concurrent use.
  Herb/Nutraceutical: St John's wort may decrease levels. Avoid dong quai if using for hypertension (has estrogenic activity). Avoid ephedra, yohimbe, ginseng (may worsen hypertension). Avoid garlic (may have increased antihypertensive effect).
Mechanism of Action Nimodipine shares the pharmacology of other calcium channel blockers; animal studies indicate that nimodipine has a greater effect on cerebral arterials than other arterials; this increased specificity may be due to the drug's increased lipophilicity and cerebral distribution as compared to nifedipine; inhibits calcium ion from entering the "slow channels" or select voltage sensitive areas of vascular smooth muscle and myocardium during depolarization
Pharmacodynamics/Kinetics
  Protein binding: >95%
  Metabolism: Extensively hepatic
  Bioavailability: 13%
  Half-life elimination: 3 hours, increases with reduced renal function
  Time to peak, serum: ~1 hour
  Excretion: Feces (32%) and urine (50%) within 4 days
Usual Dosage Adults: Oral: 60 mg every 4 hours for 21 days, start therapy within 96 hours after subarachnoid hemorrhage.
  Dialysis: Not removed by hemo- or peritoneal dialysis; supplemental dose is not necessary.
  Dosing adjustment in hepatic impairment: Reduce dosage to 30 mg every 4 hours in patients with liver failure.
Administration If the capsules cannot be swallowed, the liquid may be removed by making a hole in each end of the capsule with an 18-gauge needle and extracting the contents into a syringe. If administered via NG tube, follow with a flush of 30 mL NS.
Nursing Implications If the capsules cannot be swallowed, the liquid may be removed by making a hole in each end of the capsule with an 18-gauge needle and extracting the contents into a syringe; if given via NG tube, follow with a flush of 30 mL NS
Dosage Forms Capsule, liquid filled: 30 mg

♦ **Nimotop**® see Nimodipine on page 984
♦ **Nipent**® see Pentostatin on page 1061

Nisoldipine (NYE sole di peen)
Related Information
  Calcium Channel Blockers Comparison on page 1494
U.S. Brand Names Sular®
Therapeutic Category Antihypertensive Agent; Calcium Channel Blocker
Use Management of hypertension, alone or in combination with other antihypertensive agents
Pregnancy Risk Factor C
Contraindications Hypersensitivity to nisoldipine, any component of the formulation, or other dihydropyridine calcium channel blockers
Warnings/Precautions Increased angina and/or myocardial infarction in patients with coronary artery disease. Use with caution in patients with hypotension, congestive heart failure, and hepatic impairment. Blood pressure lowering must be done at a rate appropriate for the patient's condition.
Adverse Reactions
  >10%:
    Cardiovascular: Peripheral edema (dose-related 7% to 29%)
    Central nervous system: Headache (22%)
  1% to 10%:
    Cardiovascular: Chest pain (2%), palpitations (3%), vasodilation (4%)
    Central nervous system: Dizziness (3% to 10%)
    Dermatologic: Rash (2%)
    Gastrointestinal: Nausea (2%)
    Respiratory: Pharyngitis (5%), sinusitis (3%), dyspnea (3%), cough (5%)
  <1% (Limited to important or life-threatening): Alopecia, amblyopia, angina, anxiety, ataxia, atrial fibrillation, cerebral ischemia, cholestatic jaundice, confusion, congestive heart failure, depression, dyspnea, exfoliative dermatitis, first-degree AV block, GI hemorrhage, gingival hyperplasia, gout, impotence, leukopenia, migraine, myasthenia, myocardial infarction, paresthesia, pruritus, pulmonary edema, rash, somnolence, stroke, supraventricular tachycardia, syncope, temporary unilateral loss of vision, tinnitus, T-wave abnormalities on EKG (flattening, inversion, nonspecific changes), urticaria, vaginal hemorrhage, ventricular extrasystoles, vertigo
Overdosage/Toxicology
  Primary cardiac symptoms of calcium blocker overdose include hypotension and bradycardia. Hypotension is caused by peripheral vasodilation, myocardial depression, and bradycardia. Bradycardia results from sinus bradycardia, second- or third-degree atrioventricular block, or sinus arrest with junctional rhythm. Intraventricular conduction is usually not affected so the QRS duration is normal.
  Noncardiac symptoms include confusion, stupor, nausea, vomiting, metabolic acidosis and hyperglycemia. Following initial gastric decontamination, if possible, repeated calcium administration may promptly reverse the depressed cardiac contractility (but not sinus node depression or peripheral vasodilation). Glucagon, epinephrine, and inamrinone (amrinone) may treat refractory hypotension. Glucagon and epinephrine also increase the heart rate (outside the U.S., 4-aminopyridine may be available as an antidote). Dialysis and hemoperfusion are not effective in enhancing elimination although repeat-dose activated charcoal may serve as an adjunct with sustained release preparations.
  In a few reported cases, overdose with calcium channel blockers has been associated with hypotension and bradycardia, initially refractory to atropine, but becoming more responsive to this agent when larger doses (approaching 1 g/hour for more than 24 hours) of calcium chloride were administered.
  (Continued)

Nisoldipine *(Continued)*

Drug Interactions

Cytochrome P450 Effect: CYP3A3/4 enzyme substrate

Increased Effect/Toxicity: H_2-antagonists or omeprazole may cause an increase in the serum concentrations of nisoldipine. Digoxin and nisoldipine may increase digoxin effect. Azole antifungals (itraconazole, ketoconazole, fluconazole), erythromycin, and other inhibitors of cytochrome P450 isoenzyme 3A4 may inhibit calcium channel blocker metabolism. Calcium may reduce the calcium channel blocker's effects, particularly hypotension.

Decreased Effect: Rifampin, phenytoin, and potentially other enzyme inducers decrease the levels of nisoldipine. Calcium may decrease the hypotension from calcium channel blockers.

Ethanol/Nutrition/Herb Interactions

Food: Nisoldipine bioavailability may be increased if taken with high-lipid foods or with grapefruit juice. Avoid grapefruit products before and after dosing.

Herb/Nutraceutical: St John's wort may decrease nisoldipine levels. Avoid dong quai if using for hypertension (has estrogenic activity). Avoid ephedra, yohimbe, ginseng (may worsen hypertension). Avoid garlic (may have increased antihypertensive effect).

Mechanism of Action As a dihydropyridine calcium channel blocker, structurally similar to nifedipine, nisoldipine impedes the movement of calcium ions into vascular smooth muscle and cardiac muscle. Dihydropyridines are potent vasodilators and are not as likely to suppress cardiac contractility and slow cardiac conduction as other calcium antagonists such as verapamil and diltiazem; nisoldipine is 5-10 times as potent a vasodilator as nifedipine.

Pharmacodynamics/Kinetics

Duration: >24 hours

Absorption: Well absorbed

Metabolism: Extensively hepatic; hepatically to inactive metabolites; first-pass effect

Bioavailability: 5%

Half-life elimination: 7-12 hours

Time to peak: 6-12 hours

Excretion: Urine

Usual Dosage Adults: Oral: Initial: 20 mg once daily, then increase by 10 mg/week (or longer intervals) to attain adequate control of blood pressure; doses >60 mg once daily are not recommended. A starting dose not exceeding 10 mg/day is recommended for the elderly and those with hepatic impairment.

Administration Administer at the same time each day to ensure minimal fluctuation of serum levels. Avoid high-fat diet.

Patient Information Avoid grapefruit products before and after dosing; administration with a high fat meal can lead to excessive peak drug concentrations and should be avoided

Nursing Implications Administer at the same time each day to ensure minimal fluctuation of serum levels

Dosage Forms Tablet, extended release: 10 mg, 20 mg, 30 mg, 40 mg

♦ **Nitalapram** *see Citalopram on page 304*

Nitisinone *(ni TIS i known)*

U.S. Brand Names Orfadin®

Therapeutic Category 4-Hydroxyphenylpyruvate Dioxygenase Inhibitor

Use Treatment of hereditary tyrosinemia type 1 (HT-1); to be used with dietary restriction of tyrosine and phenylalanine

Restrictions Distributed by Rare Disease Therapeutics, Inc (contact 615-399-0700)

Pregnancy Risk Factor C

Pregnancy/Breast-Feeding Implications Safety and efficacy have not been established for pregnant women; use only if potential benefit to the mother outweighs possible risk to the fetus. Excretion in breast milk is unknown; use caution if breast-feeding.

Contraindications Hypersensitivity to nitisinone or any component of the formulation

Warnings/Precautions For use by physicians experienced in treating HT-1. Must be used with dietary restriction of tyrosine and phenylalanine; inadequate restriction can result in toxic effects to the eyes, skin, and nervous system (nutritional consultation required). Patients should have slit-lamp examination of the eyes prior to beginning treatment. Careful monitoring of liver, platelet and white blood cell counts, plasma tyrosine levels and other recommended laboratory parameters are required.

Adverse Reactions

1% to 10%:

Dermatologic: Alopecia (1%), dry skin (1%), exfoliative dermatitis (1%), maculopapular rash (1%), pruritus (1%)

Hematologic: Thrombocytopenia (3%), leukopenia (3%), porphyria (1%), epistaxis (1%)

Hepatic: Hepatic neoplasm (8%), hepatic failure (7%)

Ocular: Conjunctivitis (2%), corneal opacity (2%), keratitis, (2%), photophobia (2%), cataracts (1%), blepharitis (1%), eye pain (1%)

<1% (Limited to important or life-threatening): Abdominal pain, amenorrhea, brain tumor, bronchitis, cyanosis, dehydration, diarrhea, enanthema, encephalopathy, gastritis, gastroenteritis, gastrointestinal hemorrhage, headache, hepatic dysfunction, hepatomegaly, hyperkinesias, infection, liver enzyme elevation, melena, nervousness, otitis, pathologic fracture, respiratory insufficiency, seizures, septicemia, somnolence, thirst, tooth discoloration

Overdosage/Toxicology In the event of an overdose, elevated tyrosine levels would be expected. High plasma tyrosine levels (>500 µmol/L) can cause toxic effects to the eyes (corneal ulcers, corneal opacities, keratitis, conjunctivitis, eye pain and photophobia), the skin (painful hyperkeratotic plaques on soles and palms) and the nervous system (mental retardation, developmental delay). Treatment should be symptom directed and supportive and dietary tyrosine and phenylalanine should be limited. Tyrosine elevation and toxicity may also occur in the event of dietary indiscretion.

Ethanol/Nutrition/Herb Interactions Food: Effect of taking with food is unknown. Tyrosine toxicity can occur without proper dietary restriction of tyrosine and phenylalanine.

Stability Store under refrigeration at 2°C to 8°C (36°F to 46°F).

Mechanism of Action In patients with HT-1, tyrosine metabolism is interrupted due to a lack of the enzyme (fumarylacetoacetate hydrolase) needed in the last step of tyrosine degradation. Toxic metabolites of tyrosine accumulate and cause liver and kidney toxicity. Nitisinone competitively inhibits 4-hydroxyphenyl-pyruvate dioxygenase, an enzyme needed earlier in the tyrosine degradation pathway, and therefore prevents the build-up of the damaging metabolites.

Pharmacodynamics/Kinetics Limited pharmacokinetic studies in children or HT-1 patients.
Bioavailability: >90% (animal studies)
Half-life: Terminal: 54 hours (healthy males)
Time to peak: 3 hours
Excretion: Urine (animal studies)

Usual Dosage Oral: **Note:** Must be used in conjunction with a low protein diet restricted in tyrosine and phenylalanine.
Infants: See dosing for Children and Adults; infants may require maximal dose once liver function has improved
Children and Adults: Initial: 1 mg/kg/day in divided doses, given in the morning and evening, 1 hour before meals; doses do not need to be divided evenly
Dose adjustment: If biochemical parameters (see Monitoring Parameters) are not normalized within in 1-month period, dose may be increased to 1.5 mg/kg/day (maximum dose: 2 mg/kg/day).

Dietary Considerations Because the effect of food is unknown, nitisinone should be taken 1 hour prior to a meal. Dietary restriction of tyrosine and phenylalanine is required.

Administration Administer 1 hour prior to a meal. Capsules may be opened and contents suspended in a small quantity of water, formula, or apple sauce; use immediately.

Monitoring Parameters
Dietary tyrosine and phenylalanine
Liver: Ultrasound, computerized tomography, magnetic resonance imaging
Ophthalmic exam: Slit-lamp examination prior to treatment; repeat during therapy in patients with photophobia, eye pain, redness, swelling, or burning of the eyes.
Plasma tyrosine: Levels should be kept <500 μmol/L to avoid toxicity.
Plasma succinylacetone: May take up to 3 months to normalize after start of therapy
Platelets, white blood cell counts
Serum alpha-fetoprotein: To monitor effectiveness of treatment and potential liver neoplasia.
Serum phosphate in patients with renal dysfunction
Urine succinylacetone: Should not be detectable during treatment; dose should be increased if detectable after the first month of treatment.

Patient Information Must follow a low protein diet restricted in tyrosine and phenylalanine. Report immediately rash, excessive bleeding, eye pain, sensitivity to light, skin changes on feet or hands, yellowing of skin or eyes to prescriber. Notify prescriber if pregnant or breast-feeding.

Additional Information Use has been associated with increased 2- to 4-year survival probabilities of HT-1 and lower risk of early onset hepatic failure.

Dosage Forms Capsule: 2 mg, 5 mg, 10 mg

♦ **Nitrates Comparison** see page 1511
♦ **Nitrek® Patch** see Nitroglycerin on page 989
♦ **Nitro-Bid® Ointment** see Nitroglycerin on page 989
♦ **Nitrodisc® Patch** see Nitroglycerin on page 989
♦ **Nitro-Dur® (Can)** see Nitroglycerin on page 989
♦ **Nitro-Dur® Patch** see Nitroglycerin on page 989
♦ **Nitrofural** see Nitrofurazone on page 988

Nitrofurantoin (nye troe fyoor AN toyn)

Related Information
Antacid Drug Interactions on page 1477
Antimicrobial Drugs of Choice on page 1588

U.S. Brand Names Furadantin®; Macrobid®; Macrodantin®

Canadian Brand Names Apo®-Nitrofurantoin; MacroBID®; Macrodantin®; Novo-Furantoin

Therapeutic Category Antibiotic, Miscellaneous

Use Prevention and treatment of urinary tract infections caused by susceptible gram-negative and some gram-positive organisms; *Pseudomonas*, *Serratia*, and most species of *Proteus* are generally resistant to nitrofurantoin

Pregnancy Risk Factor B

Contraindications Hypersensitivity to nitrofurantoin or any component of the formulation; renal impairment; infants <1 month (due to the possibility of hemolytic anemia)

Warnings/Precautions Use with caution in patients with G6PD deficiency, patients with anemia, vitamin B deficiency, diabetes mellitus or electrolyte abnormalities; therapeutic concentrations of nitrofurantoin are not attained in urine of patients with Cl_{cr} <40 mL/minute; acute, subacute, or chronic (usually after 6 months of therapy) pulmonary reactions have been observed in patients treated with nitrofurantoin; if these occur, discontinue therapy; monitor closely for malaise, dyspnea, cough, fever, radiologic evidence of diffuse interstitial pneumonitis or fibrosis

Adverse Reactions Frequency not defined.
Cardiovascular: Chest pains
Central nervous system: Chills, dizziness, drowsiness, fatigue, fever, headache
Dermatologic: Exfoliative dermatitis, itching, rash
Gastrointestinal: *C. difficile*-colitis, diarrhea, loss of appetite/vomiting/nausea (most common), sore throat, stomach upset
Hematologic: Hemolytic anemia
Hepatic: Hepatitis, increased LFTs
(Continued)

Nitrofurantoin *(Continued)*

Neuromuscular & skeletal: Arthralgia, numbness, paresthesia, weakness
Respiratory: Cough, dyspnea, pneumonitis, pulmonary fibrosis
Miscellaneous: Hypersensitivity, lupus-like syndrome

Overdosage/Toxicology Symptoms include vomiting. Treatment is supportive care only.

Drug Interactions
Increased Effect/Toxicity: Probenecid decreases renal excretion of nitrofurantoin.
Decreased Effect: Antacids decrease absorption of nitrofurantoin.

Ethanol/Nutrition/Herb Interactions
Ethanol: Avoid ethanol (may increase CNS depression).
Food: Nitrofurantoin serum concentrations may be increased if taken with food.

Mechanism of Action Inhibits several bacterial enzyme systems including acetyl coenzyme A interfering with metabolism and possibly cell wall synthesis

Pharmacodynamics/Kinetics
Absorption: Well absorbed; macrocrystalline form is absorbed more slowly due to slower dissolution (causes less GI distress)
Distribution: V_d: 0.8 L/kg; crosses placenta; enters breast milk
Protein binding: ~40%
Metabolism: Body tissues (except plasma) metabolize 60% of drug to inactive metabolites
Bioavailability: Increased by presence of food
Half-life elimination: 20-60 minutes; prolonged with renal impairment
Excretion: Urine (40%) and feces (small amounts) as metabolites and unchanged drug

Usual Dosage Oral:
Children >1 month: 5-7 mg/kg/day in divided doses every 6 hours; maximum: 400 mg/day
Chronic therapy: 1-2 mg/kg/day in divided doses every 12-24 hours; maximum dose: 100 mg/day
Adults: 50-100 mg/dose every 6 hours
Macrocrystal/monohydrate: 100 mg twice daily
Prophylaxis or chronic therapy: 50-100 mg/dose at bedtime
Dosing adjustment in renal impairment: Cl_{cr} <50 mL/minute: Avoid use
Avoid use in hemo and peritoneal dialysis and continuous arteriovenous or venovenous hemofiltration

Administration Administer with meals to slow the rate of absorption and decrease adverse effects; suspension may be mixed with water, milk, fruit juice, or infant formula

Monitoring Parameters Signs of pulmonary reaction, signs of numbness or tingling of the extremities, periodic liver function tests

Test Interactions Causes false-positive urine glucose with Clinitest®

Patient Information Take with food or milk; may discolor urine to a dark yellow or brown color; notify physician if fever, chest pain, persistent, nonproductive cough, or difficulty breathing occurs; avoid alcohol

Nursing Implications
Higher peak serum levels may cause increased GI upset; administer around-the-clock rather than 4 times/day, 3 times/day, etc (ie, 12-6-12-6, not 9-1-5-9) to promote less variation in peak and trough serum levels; therapeutic concentrations of nitrofurantoin are not attained in the urine of patients with Cl_{cr} <40 mL/minute
Monitor for signs of pulmonary reaction, signs of numbness or tingling of the extremities, periodic liver function tests

Additional Information Nitrofurantoin macrocrystal/monohydrate is Macrobid®

Dosage Forms
Capsule, macrocrystal: 25 mg, 50 mg, 100 mg
Capsule, macrocrystal/monohydrate: 100 mg
Suspension, oral: 25 mg/5 mL (60 mL, 470 mL)

Nitrofurazone *(nye troe FYOOR a zone)*

U.S. Brand Names Furacin®

Synonyms Nitrofural

Therapeutic Category Antibacterial, Topical

Use Antibacterial agent in second and third degree burns and skin grafting

Pregnancy Risk Factor C

Contraindications Hypersensitivity to nitrofurazone or any component of the formulation

Warnings/Precautions Use with caution in patients with renal impairment and patients with G6PD deficiency

Adverse Reactions <1% (Limited to important or life-threatening): Dermatologic reactions, rash

Drug Interactions
Decreased Effect: Sutilains decrease activity of nitrofurazone.

Stability Avoid exposure to direct sunlight, excessive heat, strong fluorescent lighting, and alkaline materials

Mechanism of Action A broad antibacterial spectrum; it acts by inhibiting bacterial enzymes involved in carbohydrate metabolism; effective against a wide range of gram-negative and gram-positive organisms; bactericidal against most bacteria commonly causing surface infections including *Staphylococcus aureus*, *Streptococcus*, *Escherichia coli*, *Enterobacter cloacae*, *Clostridium perfringens*, *Aerobacter aerogenes*, and *Proteus* sp; not particularly active against most *Pseudomonas aeruginosa* strains and does not inhibit viruses or fungi. Topical preparations of nitrofurazone are readily soluble in blood, pus, and serum and are nonmacerating.

Usual Dosage Adults: Topical: Apply once daily or every few days to lesion or place on gauze

Patient Information Notify physician if condition worsens or if irritation develops

Nursing Implications Discoloration does not appreciably affect potency of the drug

Dosage Forms
Cream, topical: 0.2% (28 g)
Ointment, soluble dressing, topical: 0.2% (28 g, 56 g, 454 g, 480 g)

Solution, topical: 0.2% (480 mL, 4000 mL)

- **Nitrogard® Buccal** *see* Nitroglycerin *on page 989*
- **Nitrogen Mustard** *see* Mechlorethamine *on page 845*

Nitroglycerin (nye troe GLI ser in)

Related Information

Adrenergic Agonists, Cardiovascular Comparison *on page 1469*
Adult ACLS Algorithms *on page 1632*
Hypertension *on page 1675*
Nitrates Comparison *on page 1511*

U.S. Brand Names Deponit® Patch; Minitran™ Patch; Nitrek® Patch; Nitro-Bid® Ointment; Nitrodisc® Patch; Nitro-Dur® Patch; Nitrogard® Buccal; Nitroglyn® Oral; Nitrolingual® Pump-spray; Nitrol® Ointment; Nitrong® Oral; Nitrostat® Sublingual; Transderm-Nitro® Patch; Tridil®

Canadian Brand Names Minitrans™; Nitro-Dur®; Nitrol®; Nitrong® SR; Nitrostat™; Trans-derm-Nitro®

Synonyms Glyceryl Trinitrate; Nitroglycerol; NTG

Therapeutic Category Antianginal Agent; Antihypertensive Agent; Nitrate; Vasodilator; Vasodilator, Coronary

Use Treatment of angina pectoris; I.V. for congestive heart failure (especially when associated with acute myocardial infarction); pulmonary hypertension; hypertensive emergencies occurring perioperatively (especially during cardiovascular surgery)

Pregnancy Risk Factor C

Contraindications Hypersensitivity to organic nitrates; hypersensitivity to isosorbide, nitroglycerin, or any component of the formulation; concurrent use with sildenafil; angle-closure glaucoma (intraocular pressure may be increased); head trauma or cerebral hemorrhage (increase intracranial pressure); severe anemia; allergy to adhesive (transdermal product)

I.V. product: Hypotension; uncorrected hypovolemia; inadequate cerebral circulation; increased intracranial pressure; constrictive pericarditis; pericardial tamponade

Warnings/Precautions Do not use extended release preparations in patients with GI hypermotility or malabsorptive syndrome; use with caution in patients with hepatic impairment, CHF, or acute myocardial infarction; available preparations of I.V. nitroglycerin differ in concentration or volume; pay attention to dilution and dosing; I.V. preparations contain alcohol and/or propylene glycol; avoid loss of nitroglycerin in standard PVC tubing; dosing instructions must be followed with care when the appropriate infusion sets are used

Hypotension may occur, use with caution in patients who are volume-depleted, are hypotensive, have inadequate circulation; nitrate therapy may aggravate angina caused by hypertrophic cardiomyopathy

Adverse Reactions

Spray or patch:

>10%: Central nervous system: Headache (patch 63%, spray 50%)

1% to 10%:
 Cardiovascular: Hypotension (patch 4%), increased angina (patch 2%)
 Central nervous system: Lightheadedness (patch 6%), syncope (patch 4%)

<1% (Limited to important or life-threatening): Allergic reactions, application site irritation (patch), collapse, dizziness, exfoliative dermatitis, methemoglobinemia (rare, overdose), pallor, palpitations, perspiration, rash, restlessness, vertigo, weakness

Topical, sublingual, intravenous: Frequency not defined:
 Cardiovascular: Hypotension (infrequent), postural hypotension, crescendo angina (uncommon), rebound hypertension (uncommon), pallor, cardiovascular collapse, tachycardia, shock, flushing, peripheral edema
 Central nervous system: Headache (most common), lightheadedness (related to blood pressure changes), syncope (uncommon), dizziness, restlessness
 Gastrointestinal: Nausea, vomiting, bowel incontinence, xerostomia
 Genitourinary: Urinary incontinence
 Hematologic: Methemoglobinemia (rare, overdose)
 Neuromuscular & skeletal: Weakness
 Ocular: Blurred vision
 Miscellaneous: Cold sweat

Overdosage/Toxicology Symptoms include hypotension, flushing, syncope, throbbing headache with reflex tachycardia, and methemoglobinemia with extremely large overdoses. I.V. overdose may additionally be associated with increased intracranial pressure, confusion, vertigo, palpitations, nausea, vomiting, dyspnea, diaphoresis, heart block, bradycardia, coma, seizures, and death. After gastric decontamination, treatment is supportive and symptomatic. Hypotension is treated with positioning, fluids, and careful use of low-dose pressors, if needed. Methylene blue may treat methemoglobinemia.

Drug Interactions

Increased Effect/Toxicity: Has been associated with severe reactions and death when sildenafil is given concurrently with nitrites. Ethanol can cause hypotension when nitrates are taken 1 hour or more after ethanol ingestion.

Decreased Effect: I.V. nitroglycerin may antagonize the anticoagulant effect of heparin (possibly only at high nitroglycerin dosages); monitor closely. May need to decrease heparin dosage when nitroglycerin is discontinued. Alteplase (tissue plasminogen activator) has a lesser effect when used with I.V. nitroglycerin; avoid concurrent use. Ergot alkaloids may cause an increase in blood pressure and decrease in antianginal effects; avoid concurrent use.

Stability Doses should be made in glass bottles, Excell® or PAB® containers; adsorption occurs to soft plastic (ie, PVC)

Nitroglycerin diluted in D_5W or NS in glass containers is physically and chemically stable for 48 hours at room temperature and 7 days under refrigeration; in D_5W or NS in Excell®/PAB® containers is physically and chemically stable for 24 hours at room temperature and 14 days under refrigeration
Premixed bottles are stable according to the manufacturer's expiration dating

(Continued)

989

Nitroglycerin (Continued)

Standard diluent: 50 mg/250 mL D₅W; 50 mg/500 mL D₅W

Minimum volume: 100 mg/250 mL D₅W; concentration should not exceed 400 mcg/mL

Store sublingual tablets and ointment in tightly closed containers at 15°C to 30°C

Mechanism of Action Reduces cardiac oxygen demand by decreasing left ventricular pressure and systemic vascular resistance; dilates coronary arteries and improves collateral flow to ischemic regions

Pharmacodynamics/Kinetics

Onset of action: Sublingual tablet: 1-3 minutes; Translingual spray: 2 minutes; Buccal tablet: 2-5 minutes; Sustained release: 20-45 minutes; Topical: 15-60 minutes; Transdermal: 40-60 minutes; I.V. drip: Immediate

Peak effect: Sublingual tablet: 4-8 minutes; Translingual spray: 4-10 minutes; Buccal tablet: 4-10 minutes; Sustained release: 45-120 minutes; Topical: 30-120 minutes; Transdermal: 60-180 minutes; I.V. drip: Immediate

Duration: Sublingual tablet: 30-60 minutes; Translingual spray: 30-60 minutes; Buccal tablet: 2 hours; Sustained release: 4-8 hours; Topical: 2-12 hours; Transdermal: 18-24 hours; I.V. drip: 3-5 minutes

Protein binding: 60%

Metabolism: Extensive first-pass effect

Half-life elimination: 1-4 minutes

Excretion: Urine (as inactive metabolites)

Usual Dosage Note: Hemodynamic and antianginal tolerance often develop within 24-48 hours of continuous nitrate administration

Children: Pulmonary hypertension: Continuous infusion: Start 0.25-0.5 mcg/kg/minute and titrate by 1 mcg/kg/minute at 20- to 60-minute intervals to desired effect; usual dose: 1-3 mcg/kg/minute; maximum: 5 mcg/kg/minute

Adults:

Buccal: Initial: 1 mg every 3-5 hours while awake (3 times/day); titrate dosage upward if angina occurs with tablet in place

Oral: 2.5-9 mg 2-4 times/day (up to 26 mg 4 times/day)

I.V.: 5 mcg/minute, increase by 5 mcg/minute every 3-5 minutes to 20 mcg/minute; if no response at 20 mcg/minute increase by 10 mcg/minute every 3-5 minutes, up to 200 mcg/minute

Ointment: ½" upon rising and ½" 6 hours later; the dose may be doubled and even doubled again as needed

Patch, transdermal: Initial: 0.2-0.4 mg/hour, titrate to doses of 0.4-0.8 mg/hour; tolerance is minimized by using a patch-on period of 12-14 hours and patch-off period of 10-12 hours

Sublingual: 0.2-0.6 mg every 5 minutes for maximum of 3 doses in 15 minutes; may also use prophylactically 5-10 minutes prior to activities which may provoke an attack

Translingual: 1-2 sprays into mouth under tongue every 3-5 minutes for maximum of 3 doses in 15 minutes, may also be used 5-10 minutes prior to activities which may provoke an attack prophylactically

Hemodialysis: Supplemental dose is not necessary

Peritoneal dialysis: Supplemental dose is not necessary

May need to use nitrate-free interval (10-12 hours/day) to avoid tolerance development; gradually decrease dose in patients receiving NTG for prolonged period to avoid withdrawal reaction

Elderly: In general, dose selection should be cautious, usually starting at the low end of the dosing range

Monitoring Parameters Blood pressure, heart rate

Patient Information Go to hospital if no relief after 3 sublingual doses; do not swallow or chew sublingual form; do not change brands without notifying your physician or pharmacist; take oral nitrates on an empty stomach; keep tablets and capsules in original container; keep tightly closed; use spray only when lying down; highly flammable; do not inhale spray; do not chew sustained release products; a treatment-free interval of 8-12 hours is recommended each day; take 3 times/day rather than every 8 hours

Nursing Implications

I.V. must be prepared in glass bottles and use special sets intended for nitroglycerin; NTG infusions should be administered only via a pump that can maintain a constant infusion rate

S.L.: Do not crush sublingual drug product

Transdermal patches are labeled as mg/hour; a 10-12 hour nitrate-free interval is recommended to prevent the development of tolerance

Additional Information I.V. preparations contain alcohol and/or propylene glycol; may need to use nitrate-free interval (10-12 hours/day) to avoid tolerance development. Tolerance may possibly be reversed with acetylcysteine; gradually decrease dose in patients receiving NTG for prolonged period to avoid withdrawal reaction.

Concomitant use of sildenafil (Viagra®) may precipitate acute hypotension, myocardial infarction, or death. Nitrates used in right ventricular infarction may induce acute hypotension. Nitrate use in severe pericardial effusion may reduce cardiac filling pressure and precipitate cardiac tamponade. In the management of heart failure, the combination of isosorbide dinitrate and hydralazine confers beneficial effects on disease progression and cardiac outcomes.

Dosage Forms

Aerosol, translingual (Nitrolingual® Pumpspray): 0.4 mg/metered spray (5.7 g - 75 metered sprays, 12 g - 200 metered sprays) [20% ethanol]

Capsule, sustained release: 2.5 mg, 6.5 mg, 9 mg, 13 mg

Injection: 0.5 mg/mL (10 mL); 5 mg/mL (1 mL, 5 mL, 10 mL, 20 mL)

Injection, solution [in D₅W]: 25 mg (250 mL); 50 mg (250 mL, 500 mL); 100 mg (250 mL); 200 mg (500 mL)

Ointment, topical (Nitro-Bid®, Nitrol®): 2% [20 mg/g] (30 g, 60 g)

Patch, transdermal, topical: Systems designed to deliver 0.1 mg/hour, 0.2 mg/hour, 0.4 mg/hour, 0.6 mg/hour

Tablet, buccal, controlled release: 2 mg, 3 mg

Tablet, sublingual (Nitrostat®, NitroTab®): 0.3 mg, 0.4 mg, 0.6 mg
Tablet, sustained release: 2.6 mg, 6.5 mg, 9 mg

◆ **Nitroglycerol** *see Nitroglycerin on page 989*
◆ **Nitroglyn® Oral** *see Nitroglycerin on page 989*
◆ **Nitrol® (Can)** *see Nitroglycerin on page 989*
◆ **Nitrolingual® Pumpspray** *see Nitroglycerin on page 989*
◆ **Nitrol® Ointment** *see Nitroglycerin on page 989*
◆ **Nitrong® Oral** *see Nitroglycerin on page 989*
◆ **Nitrong® SR (Can)** *see Nitroglycerin on page 989*
◆ **Nitropress®** *see Nitroprusside on page 991*

Nitroprusside (nye troe PRUS ide)

Related Information
Adrenergic Agonists, Cardiovascular Comparison *on page 1469*
Adult ACLS Algorithms *on page 1632*
Hypertension *on page 1675*
U.S. Brand Names Nitropress®
Synonyms Nitroprusside Sodium; Sodium Nitroferricyanide; Sodium Nitroprusside
Therapeutic Category Antihypertensive Agent; Vasodilator
Use Management of hypertensive crises; congestive heart failure; used for controlled hypotension to reduce bleeding during surgery
Pregnancy Risk Factor C
Contraindications Hypersensitivity to nitroprusside or any component of the formulation; treatment of compensatory hypertension (aortic coarctation, arteriovenous shunting); high output failure; congenital optic atrophy or tobacco amblyopia
Warnings/Precautions Use with caution in patients with increased intracranial pressure (head trauma, cerebral hemorrhage); severe renal impairment, hepatic failure, hypothyroidism; use only as an infusion with 5% dextrose in water; continuously monitor patient's blood pressure; excessive amounts of nitroprusside can cause cyanide toxicity (usually in patients with decreased liver function) or thiocyanate toxicity (usually in patients with decreased renal function, or in patients with normal renal function but prolonged nitroprusside use)
Adverse Reactions 1% to 10%:
Cardiovascular: Excessive hypotensive response, palpitations, substernal distress
Central nervous system: Disorientation, psychosis, headache, restlessness
Endocrine & metabolic: Thyroid suppression
Gastrointestinal: Nausea, vomiting
Neuromuscular & skeletal: Weakness, muscle spasm
Otic: Tinnitus
Respiratory: Hypoxia
Miscellaneous: Diaphoresis, thiocyanate toxicity
Overdosage/Toxicology Symptoms include hypotension, vomiting, hyperventilation, tachycardia, muscular twitching, hypothyroidism, cyanide or thiocyanate toxicity. Thiocyanate toxicity includes psychosis, hyper-reflexia, confusion, weakness, tinnitus, seizures, and coma. Cyanide toxicity includes acidosis (decreased HCO_3, decreased pH, increased lactate), increase in mixed venous blood oxygen tension, tachycardia, altered consciousness, coma, convulsions, and almond smell on breath. Nitroprusside has been shown to release cyanide *in vivo* with hemoglobin. Cyanide toxicity does not usually occur because of the rapid uptake of cyanide by erythrocytes and its eventual incorporation into cyanocobalamin. However, prolonged administration of nitroprusside or its reduced elimination can lead to cyanide intoxication. In these situations, airway support with oxygen therapy is germane, followed closely with antidotal therapy of amyl nitrate perles, sodium nitrate 300 mg I.V. for adults (range based on hemoglobin concentration: 6-12 mg/kg for children), and sodium thiosulfate 12.5 g I.V. for adults (range based on hemoglobin concentration: 0.95-1.95 mL/kg of the 25% solution for children). Nitrates should not be administered to neonates and small children. Thiocyanate is dialyzable. May be mixed with sodium thiosulfate in I.V. to prevent cyanide toxicity.
Stability
Nitroprusside sodium should be reconstituted freshly by diluting 50 mg in 250-1000 mL of D_5W
Use only clear solutions; solutions of nitroprusside exhibit a color described as brownish, brown, brownish-pink, light orange, and straw. Solutions are highly sensitive to light. Exposure to light causes decomposition, resulting in a highly colored solution of orange, dark brown or blue. **A blue color indicates almost complete degradation and breakdown to cyanide.**
Solutions should be wrapped with aluminum foil or other opaque material to protect from light (do as soon as possible)
Stability of parenteral admixture at room temperature (25°C) and at refrigeration temperature (4°C): 24 hours
Mechanism of Action Causes peripheral vasodilation by direct action on venous and arteriolar smooth muscle, thus reducing peripheral resistance; will increase cardiac output by decreasing afterload; reduces aortal and left ventricular impedance
Pharmacodynamics/Kinetics
Onset of action: BP reduction <2 minutes
Duration: 1-10 minutes
Metabolism: Nitroprusside is converted to cyanide ions in the bloodstream; decomposes to prussic acid which in the presence of sulfur donor is converted to thiocyanate (hepatic and renal rhodanase systems)
Half-life elimination: Parent drug: <10 minutes; Thiocyanate: 2.7-7 days
Excretion: Urine (as thiocyanate)
Usual Dosage Administration requires the use of an infusion pump. Average dose: 5 mcg/kg/minute.
(Continued)

Nitroprusside *(Continued)*

Children: Pulmonary hypertension: I.V.: Initial: 1 mcg/kg/minute by continuous I.V. infusion; increase in increments of 1 mcg/kg/minute at intervals of 20-60 minutes; titrating to the desired response; usual dose: 3 mcg/kg/minute, rarely need >4 mcg/kg/minute; maximum: 5 mcg/kg/minute.

Adults: I.V.: Initial: 0.3-0.5 mcg/kg/minute; increase in increments of 0.5 mcg/kg/minute, titrating to the desired hemodynamic effect or the appearance of headache or nausea; usual dose: 3 mcg/kg/minute; rarely need >4 mcg/kg/minute; maximum: 10 mcg/kg/minute. When administered by prolonged infusion faster than 2 mcg/kg/minute, cyanide is generated faster than an unaided patient can handle.

Administration I.V. infusion only, not for direct injection

Monitoring Parameters Blood pressure, heart rate; monitor for cyanide and thiocyanate toxicity; monitor acid-base status as acidosis can be the earliest sign of cyanide toxicity; monitor thiocyanate levels if requiring prolonged infusion (>3 days) or dose ≥4 mcg/kg/minute or patient has renal dysfunction; monitor cyanide blood levels in patients with decreased hepatic function; cardiac monitor and blood pressure monitor required

Reference Range Monitor thiocyanate levels if requiring prolonged infusion (>4 days) or ≥4 µg/kg/minute; not to exceed 100 µg/mL (or 10 mg/dL) plasma thiocyanate

Thiocyanate:
  Therapeutic: 6-29 µg/mL
  Toxic: 35-100 µg/mL
  Fatal: >200 µg/mL
Cyanide: Normal <0.2 µg/mL; normal (smoker): <0.4 µg/mL
  Toxic: >2 µg/mL
  Potentially lethal: >3 µg/mL

Nursing Implications Brownish solution is usable, discard if bluish in color

Dosage Forms Injection, as sodium: 10 mg/mL (5 mL); 25 mg/mL (2 mL)

♦ **Nitroprusside Sodium** *see Nitroprusside on page 991*

♦ **Nitrostat™ (Can)** *see Nitroglycerin on page 989*

♦ **Nitrostat® Sublingual** *see Nitroglycerin on page 989*

♦ **Nix® (Can)** *see Permethrin on page 1065*

♦ **Nix™ Creme Rinse** *see Permethrin on page 1065*

Nizatidine *(ni ZA ti deen)*

U.S. Brand Names Axid®; Axid® AR [OTC]

Canadian Brand Names Apo®-Nizatidine; Axid®; Novo-Nizatidine

Therapeutic Category Antihistamine, H_2 Blocker; Histamine H_2 Antagonist

Use Treatment and maintenance of duodenal ulcer; treatment of benign gastric ulcer; treatment of gastroesophageal reflux disease (GERD); OTC tablet used for the prevention of meal-induced heartburn, acid indigestion, and sour stomach

Unlabeled/Investigational Use Part of a multidrug regimen for *H. pylori* eradication to reduce the risk of duodenal ulcer recurrence

Pregnancy Risk Factor C

Contraindications Hypersensitivity to nizatidine or any component of the formulation; hypersensitivity to other H_2 antagonists (cross-sensitivity has been observed)

Warnings/Precautions Use with caution in children <12 years of age; use with caution in patients with liver and renal impairment; dosage modification required in patients with renal impairment

Adverse Reactions

>10%: Central nervous system: Headache (16%)

1% to 10%:
  Central nervous system: Dizziness, insomnia, somnolence, nervousness, anxiety
  Dermatologic: Rash, pruritus
  Gastrointestinal: Abdominal pain, constipation, diarrhea, nausea, flatulence, vomiting, heartburn, dry mouth, anorexia

<1% (Limited to important or life-threatening): Alkaline phosphatase increased, anemia, AST/ALT increased, bronchospasm, eosinophilia, hepatitis, jaundice, laryngeal edema, thrombocytopenic purpura, ventricular tachycardia

Overdosage/Toxicology Symptoms include muscular tremors, vomiting, rapid respiration. LD_{50}: ~80 mg/kg. Treatment is primarily symptomatic and supportive.

Drug Interactions

Decreased Effect: May decrease the absorption of itraconazole or ketoconazole.

Ethanol/Nutrition/Herb Interactions Ethanol: Avoid ethanol (may cause gastric mucosal irritation).

Mechanism of Action Nizatidine is an H_2-receptor antagonist. In healthy volunteers, nizatidine has been effective in suppressing gastric acid secretion induced by pentagastrin infusion or food. Nizatidine reduces gastric acid secretion by 30% to 78%. This compares with a 60% reduction by cimetidine. Nizatidine 100 mg is reported to provide equivalent acid suppression as cimetidine 300 mg.

Usual Dosage Adults: Oral:

Active duodenal ulcer:
  Treatment: 300 mg at bedtime or 150 mg twice daily
  Maintenance: 150 mg/day
Gastric ulcer: 150 mg twice daily or 300 mg at bedtime
GERD: 150 mg twice daily
Meal-induced heartburn, acid indigestion, and sour stomach: 75 mg tablet [OTC] twice daily, 30 to 60 minutes prior to consuming food or beverages
Helicobacter pylori eradication (unlabeled use): 150 mg twice daily; requires combination therapy

Dosing adjustment in renal impairment:
Cl_{cr} 50-80 mL/minute: Administer 75% of normal dose

Cl$_{cr}$ 10-50 mL/minute: Administer 50% of normal dose or 150 mg/day for active treatment and 150 mg every other day for maintenance treatment

Cl$_{cr}$ <10 mL/minute: Administer 25% of normal dose or 150 mg every other day for treatment and 150 mg every 3 days for maintenance treatment

Test Interactions False-positive urine protein using Multistix®, gastric acid secretion test, skin tests allergen extracts, serum creatinine and serum transaminase concentrations, urine protein test

Patient Information May take several days before medication begins to relieve stomach pain; antacids may be taken with nizatidine unless physician has instructed you not to use them; wait 30-60 minutes between taking the antacid and nizatidine; avoid aspirin, cough and cold preparations; avoid use of black pepper, caffeine, alcohol, and harsh spices; may cause drowsiness or impair coordination and judgment

Nursing Implications Giving dose at 6 PM may better suppress nocturnal acid secretion than 10 PM

Dosage Forms
Capsule: 150 mg, 300 mg
Tablet [OTC]: 75 mg

Norepinephrine (nor ep i NEF rin)

Related Information
Adrenergic Agonists, Cardiovascular Comparison *on page 1469*
Adult ACLS Algorithms *on page 1632*
Antacid Drug Interactions *on page 1477*

U.S. Brand Names Levophed®

Canadian Brand Names Levophed®

Synonyms Levarterenol Bitartrate; Noradrenaline; Noradrenaline Acid Tartrate; Norepinephrine Bitartrate

Therapeutic Category Adrenergic Agonist Agent; Sympathomimetic

Use Treatment of shock which persists after adequate fluid volume replacement

Pregnancy Risk Factor C

Contraindications Hypersensitivity to norepinephrine, bisulfites (contains metabisulfite), or any component of the formulation; hypotension from hypovolemia except as an emergency measure to maintain coronary and cerebral perfusion until volume could be replaced; mesenteric or peripheral vascular thrombosis unless it is a lifesaving procedure; during anesthesia with cyclopropane or halothane anesthesia (risk of ventricular arrhythmias)

Warnings/Precautions Assure adequate circulatory volume to minimize need for vasoconstrictors. Avoid hypertension; monitor blood pressure closely and adjust infusion rate. Infuse into a large vein if possible. Avoid infusion into leg veins. Watch I.V. site closely. Avoid extravasation. Never use leg veins for infusion sites.

Adverse Reactions Frequency not defined.
Cardiovascular: Bradycardia, arrhythmias, peripheral (digital) ischemia
Central nervous system: Headache (transient), anxiety
Local: Skin necrosis (with extravasation)
Respiratory: Dyspnea, respiratory difficulty

Overdosage/Toxicology Symptoms include hypertension, sweating, cerebral hemorrhage, and convulsions. For treatment of extravasation, infiltrate the area of extravasation with phentolamine 5-10 mg in 10-15 mL of saline solution.

Drug Interactions
Increased Effect/Toxicity: The effects of norepinephrine may be increased by tricyclic antidepressants, MAO inhibitors, antihistamines (diphenhydramine, tripelennamine), beta-blockers (nonselective), guanethidine, ergot alkaloids, reserpine, and methyldopa. Atropine sulfate may block the reflex bradycardia caused by norepinephrine and enhances the vasopressor response.

Decreased Effect: Alpha blockers may blunt response to norepinephrine.

Stability Readily oxidized, protect from light, do not use if brown coloration; dilute with D$_5$W or D$_5$NS, but not recommended to dilute in normal saline; not stable with alkaline solutions; stability of parenteral admixture at room temperature (25°C): 24 hours

Mechanism of Action Stimulates beta$_1$-adrenergic receptors and alpha-adrenergic receptors causing increased contractility and heart rate as well as vasoconstriction, thereby increasing systemic blood pressure and coronary blood flow; clinically alpha effects (vasoconstriction) are greater than beta effects (inotropic and chronotropic effects)

Pharmacodynamics/Kinetics
Onset of action: I.V.: Very rapid-acting
Duration: Limited
(Continued)

Norepinephrine *(Continued)*

Metabolism: By catechol-o-methyltransferase (COMT) and monoamine oxidase (MAO)
Excretion: Urine (84% to 96% as inactive metabolites)

Usual Dosage Administration requires the use of an infusion pump!

Note: Norepinephrine dosage is stated in terms of norepinephrine base and intravenous formulation is norepinephrine bitartrate

Norepinephrine bitartrate 2 mg = Norepinephrine base 1 mg

Continuous I.V. infusion:

Children: Initial: 0.05-0.1 mcg/kg/minute; titrate to desired effect; maximum dose: 1-2 mcg/kg/minute

Adults: Initial: 0.5-1 mcg/minute and titrate to desired response; 8-30 mcg/minute is usual range; range used in clinical trials: 0.01-3 mcg/kg/minute; ACLS dosage range: 0.5-30 mcg/minute

Administration Administer into large vein to avoid the potential for extravasation; potent drug, must be diluted prior to use. Rate (mL/hour) = dose (mcg/kg/minute) x weight (kg) x 60 minutes/hour divided by concentration (mcg/mL)

To prepare for infusion:

$$\frac{6 \times weight~(kg) \times desired~dose~(mcg/kg/min)}{I.V.~infusion~rate~(mL/h)} = \begin{array}{l} mg~of~drug~to~be~added~to \\ 100~mL~of~I.V.~fluid \end{array}$$

"Rule of 6" method for infusion preparation:

Simplified equation: 0.6 x weight (kg) = amount (mg) of drug to be added to 100 mL of I.V. fluid

When infused at 1 mL/hour, then it will deliver the drug at a rate of 0.1 mcg/kg/minute

Complex equation: 6 x desired dose (mcg/minute) x body weight (kg) divided by desired rate (mL/hour) is the mg added to make 100 mL of solution

Nursing Implications Central line administration required; do not administer NaHCO$_3$ through an I.V. line containing norepinephrine; administer into large vein to avoid the potential for extravasation; potent drug, must be diluted prior to use

Extravasation: Use phentolamine as antidote; mix 5 mg with 9 mL of NS; inject a small amount of this dilution into extravasated area; blanching should reverse immediately. Monitor site; if blanching should recur, additional injections of phentolamine may be needed.

Dosage Forms Injection, as bitartrate: 1 mg/mL (4 mL)

♦ **Norepinephrine Bitartrate** *see Norepinephrine on page 993*
♦ **Norethindrone Acetate and Ethinyl Estradiol** *see Ethinyl Estradiol and Norethindrone on page 522*
♦ **Norethindrone and Estradiol** *see Estradiol and Norethindrone on page 494*
♦ **Norethindrone and Mestranol** *see Mestranol and Norethindrone on page 870*
♦ **Norflex™** *see Orphenadrine on page 1014*

Norfloxacin *(nor FLOKS a sin)*

Related Information

Antacid Drug Interactions *on page 1477*
Treatment of Sexually Transmitted Diseases *on page 1609*

U.S. Brand Names Chibroxin™; Noroxin®

Canadian Brand Names Apo®-Norflox; Noroxin® Ophthalmic; Noroxin® Tablet; Novo-Norfloxacin; Riva-Norfloxacin

Therapeutic Category Antibiotic, Ophthalmic; Antibiotic, Quinolone

Use Uncomplicated urinary tract infections and cystitis caused by susceptible gram-negative and gram-positive bacteria; sexually-transmitted disease (eg, uncomplicated urethral and cervical gonorrhea) caused by *N. gonorrhoeae*; prostatitis due to *E. coli*; ophthalmic solution for conjunctivitis

Pregnancy Risk Factor C

Contraindications Hypersensitivity to norfloxacin, quinolones, or any component of the formulation

Warnings/Precautions Not recommended in children <18 years of age; other quinolones have caused transient arthropathy in children; CNS stimulation may occur which may lead to tremor, restlessness, confusion, and very rarely to hallucinations or convulsive seizures; use with caution in patients with known or suspected CNS disorders. Tendon inflammation and/or rupture have been reported with other quinolone antibiotics. Discontinue at first sign of tendon inflammation or pain. Quinolones may exacerbate myasthenia gravis.

Severe hypersensitivity reactions, including anaphylaxis, have occurred with quinolone therapy. If an allergic reaction occurs (itching, urticaria, dyspnea, facial edema, loss of consciousness, tingling, cardiovascular collapse), discontinue drug immediately. Prolonged use may result in superinfection; pseudomembranous colitis may occur and should be considered in all patients who present with diarrhea.

Adverse Reactions

Ophthalmic:

>10%: Ocular: Burning or other discomfort of the eye, crusting or crystals in corner of eye

1% to 10%:

Gastrointestinal: Bad taste instillation

Ocular: Foreign body sensation, conjunctival hyperemia, itching of eye, corneal deposits

Systemic:

>10%:

Central nervous system: Dizziness or lightheadedness, headache, nervousness, drowsiness, insomnia

Gastrointestinal: Nausea, diarrhea, vomiting, abdominal pain

1% to 10%: Dermatologic: Photosensitivity

<1% (Limited to important or life-threatening): Anemia, ataxia, diplopia, dyspnea, erythema multiforme, hemolytic anemia (sometimes associated with glucose-6-phosphate deficiency), exacerbation of myasthenia gravis, interstitial nephritis, psychic disturbances,

seizures, Stevens-Johnson syndrome, tendon rupture, tendonitis, tinnitus, toxic epidermal necrolysis, tremor

Overdosage/Toxicology Symptoms include acute renal failure and seizures. Following GI decontamination, use supportive measures.

Drug Interactions

Cytochrome P450 Effect: CYP1A2 and 3A3/4 enzyme inhibitor

Increased Effect/Toxicity: Quinolones cause increased levels of caffeine, warfarin, cyclosporine, and theophylline. Cimetidine and probenecid may increase norfloxacin serum levels.

Decreased Effect: Decreased absorption with antacids containing aluminum, magnesium, and/or calcium (by up to 98% if given at the same time). Didanosine (chewable/buffered or pediatric powder) may decrease quinolone absorption.

Ethanol/Nutrition/Herb Interactions

Food: Norfloxacin average peak serum concentrations may be decreased if taken with dairy products.

Herb/Nutraceutical: Avoid dong quai, St John's wort (may also cause photosensitization).

Mechanism of Action Norfloxacin is a DNA gyrase inhibitor. DNA gyrase is an essential bacterial enzyme that maintains the superhelical structure of DNA. DNA gyrase is required for DNA replication and transcription, DNA repair, recombination, and transposition; bactericidal

Pharmacodynamics/Kinetics

Absorption: Oral: Rapid, up to 40%

Distribution: Crosses placenta; small amounts enter breast milk

Protein binding: 15%

Metabolism: Hepatic

Half-life elimination: 4.8 hours; prolonged in renal impairment

Time to peak, serum: 1-2 hours

Excretion: Urine; feces (30%)

Usual Dosage

Ophthalmic: Children >1 year and Adults: Instill 1-2 drops in affected eye(s) 4 times/day for up to 7 days

Oral: Adults:

Urinary tract infections: 400 mg twice daily for 3-21 days depending on severity of infection or organism sensitivity; maximum: 800 mg/day

Uncomplicated gonorrhea: 800 mg as a single dose (CDC recommends as an alternative regimen to ciprofloxacin or ofloxacin)

Prostatitis: 400 mg every 12 hours for 4 weeks

Dosing interval in renal impairment:

Cl$_{cr}$ 10-30 mL/minute: Administer every 24 hours

Cl$_{cr}$ <10 mL/minute: Do not use

Dietary Considerations Oral formulations should be administered on an empty stomach with water.

Administration Hold antacids or sucralfate for 3-4 hours after giving norfloxacin; do not administer together. Best taken on an empty stomach with water.

Patient Information Tablets should be taken at least 1 hour before or at least 2 hours after a meal with a glass of water; patients receiving norfloxacin should be well hydrated; take all the medication, do not skip doses; do not take with antacids; contact your physician immediately with inflammation or tendon pain

Nursing Implications Hold antacids, sucralfate for 3-4 hours after giving

Dosage Forms

Solution, ophthalmic (Chibroxin®): 0.3% [3 mg/mL] (5 mL)

Tablet (Noroxin®): 400 mg

♦ **Norgesic™** see Orphenadrine, Aspirin, and Caffeine on page 1015

♦ **Norgesic™ Forte** see Orphenadrine, Aspirin, and Caffeine on page 1015

♦ **Norgestimate and Ethinyl Estradiol** see Ethinyl Estradiol and Norgestimate on page 525

Norgestrel (nor JES trel)

U.S. Brand Names Ovrette®

Canadian Brand Names Ovrette®

Therapeutic Category Contraceptive, Emergency; Contraceptive, Oral (Progestin); Progestin

Use Prevention of pregnancy; **progestin only products have higher risk of failure in contraceptive use**

Pregnancy Risk Factor X

Contraindications Hypersensitivity to norgestrel or any component of the formulation; hypersensitivity to tartrazine; thromboembolic disorders; severe hepatic disease; breast cancer; undiagnosed vaginal bleeding; pregnancy

Warnings/Precautions Discontinue if sudden loss of vision or if diplopia or proptosis occur; use with caution in patients with a history of mental depression.

Adverse Reactions Frequency not defined.

Cardiovascular: Embolism, central thrombosis, edema

Central nervous system: Mental depression, fever, insomnia

Dermatologic: Melasma or chloasma, allergic rash with or without pruritus

Endocrine & metabolic: Breakthrough bleeding, spotting, changes in menstrual flow, amenorrhea, changes in cervical erosion and secretions, increased breast tenderness

Gastrointestinal: Weight gain/loss, anorexia

Hepatic: Cholestatic jaundice

Local: Thrombophlebitis

Neuromuscular & skeletal: Weakness

Overdosage/Toxicology Toxicity is unlikely following single exposures of excessive doses. Supportive treatment is adequate in most cases.

(Continued)

Norgestrel *(Continued)*

Drug Interactions

Increased Effect/Toxicity: Oral contraceptives may increase toxicity of acetaminophen, anticoagulants, benzodiazepines, caffeine, corticosteroids, metoprolol, theophylline, and tricyclic antidepressants.

Decreased Effect: Azole antifungals (ketoconazole, itraconazole, fluconazole), barbiturates, hydantoins (phenytoin), carbamazepine, and rifampin decrease oral contraceptive efficacy due to increased metabolism. Antibiotics (penicillins, tetracyclines, griseofulvin) may decrease efficacy of oral contraceptives.

Ethanol/Nutrition/Herb Interactions

Food: CNS effects of caffeine may be enhanced if oral contraceptives are used concurrently with caffeine.

Herb/Nutraceutical: St John's wort may decrease levels. Avoid dong quai and black cohosh (have estrogen activity). Avoid saw palmetto, red clover, ginseng.

Mechanism of Action Inhibits secretion of pituitary gonadotropin (LH) which prevents follicular maturation and ovulation

Pharmacodynamics/Kinetics

Absorption: Oral: Well absorbed

Protein binding: >97% to sex-hormone-binding globulin

Metabolism: Primarily hepatic via reduction and conjugation

Half-life elimination: ~20 hours

Excretion: Urine (as metabolites)

Usual Dosage Administer daily, starting the first day of menstruation, take 1 tablet at the same time each day, every day of the year. If one dose is missed, take as soon as remembered, then next tablet at regular time; if two doses are missed, take 1 tablet as soon as it is remembered, followed by an additional dose that same day at the usual time. When one or two doses are missed, additional contraceptive measures should be used until 14 consecutive tablets have been taken. If three doses are missed, discontinue norgestrel and use an additional form of birth control until menses or pregnancy is ruled out.

Dietary Considerations Should be taken with food at same time each day.

Test Interactions Thyroid function tests, metyrapone test, liver function tests

Patient Information Take this medicine only as directed; do not take more of it and do not take it for a longer period of time; if you suspect you may have become pregnant, stop taking this medicine; report any loss of vision or vision changes immediately; avoid excessive exposure to sunlight

Nursing Implications Patients should receive a copy of the patient labeling

Dosage Forms Tablet: 0.075 mg

- ◆ **Norgestrel and Ethinyl Estradiol** *see Ethinyl Estradiol and Norgestrel on page 528*
- ◆ **Norinyl® 1+35** *see Ethinyl Estradiol and Norethindrone on page 522*
- ◆ **Norinyl® 1+50** *see Mestranol and Norethindrone on page 870*
- ◆ **Noritate™** *see Metronidazole on page 904*
- ◆ **Normal Human Serum Albumin** *see Albumin on page 40*
- ◆ **Normal Saline** *see Sodium Chloride on page 1245*
- ◆ **Normal Serum Albumin (Human)** *see Albumin on page 40*
- ◆ **Normodyne®** *see Labetalol on page 768*
- ◆ **Noroxin®** *see Norfloxacin on page 994*
- ◆ **Noroxin® Ophthalmic (Can)** *see Norfloxacin on page 994*
- ◆ **Noroxin® Tablet (Can)** *see Norfloxacin on page 994*
- ◆ **Norpace®** *see Disopyramide on page 424*
- ◆ **Norpace® CR** *see Disopyramide on page 424*
- ◆ **Norplant® Implant** *see Levonorgestrel on page 796*
- ◆ **Norpramin®** *see Desipramine on page 376*
- ◆ **Nortrel™** *see Ethinyl Estradiol and Norethindrone on page 522*

Nortriptyline *(nor TRIP ti leen)*

Related Information

Antidepressant Agents Comparison *on page 1482*

U.S. Brand Names Aventyl®; Pamelor®

Canadian Brand Names Alti-Nortriptyline; Apo®-Nortriptyline; Aventyl®; Gen-Nortriptyline; Norventyl; Novo-Nortriptyline; Nu-Nortriptyline; PMS-Nortriptyline

Synonyms Nortriptyline Hydrochloride

Therapeutic Category Antidepressant, Tricyclic

Use Treatment of symptoms of depression

Unlabeled/Investigational Use Chronic pain, anxiety disorders, enuresis, attention-deficit/hyperactivity disorder (ADHD)

Pregnancy Risk Factor D

Contraindications Hypersensitivity to nortriptyline and similar chemical class, or any component of the formulation; use of MAO inhibitors within 14 days; use in a patient during the acute recovery phase of MI; pregnancy

Warnings/Precautions May cause sedation, resulting in impaired performance of tasks requiring alertness (ie, operating machinery or driving). Sedative effects may be additive with other CNS depressants and/or ethanol. The degree of sedation is low-moderate relative to other antidepressants. May worsen psychosis in some patients or precipitate a shift to mania or hypomania in patients with bipolar disease. May increase the risks associated with electroconvulsive therapy. This agent should be discontinued, when possible, prior to elective surgery. Therapy should not be abruptly discontinued in patients receiving high doses for prolonged periods. May alter glucose regulation - use caution in patients with diabetes.

May cause orthostatic hypotension (risk is low relative to other antidepressants) - use with caution in patients at risk of hypotension or in patients where transient hypotensive episodes would be poorly tolerated (cardiovascular disease or cerebrovascular disease). The degree of anticholinergic blockade produced by this agent is moderate relative to other cyclic antidepressants, however, caution should still be used in patients with urinary retention, benign prostatic hypertrophy, narrow-angle glaucoma, xerostomia, visual problems, constipation, or history of bowel obstruction.

Use caution in patients with suicidal risk. Use with caution in patients with a history of cardiovascular disease (including previous MI, stroke, tachycardia, or conduction abnormalities). The risk conduction abnormalities with this agent is moderate relative to other antidepressants. Use caution in patients with a previous seizure disorder or condition predisposing to seizures such as brain damage, alcoholism, or concurrent therapy with other drugs which lower the seizure threshold. Use with caution in hyperthyroid patients or those receiving thyroid supplementation. Use with caution in patients with hepatic or renal dysfunction and in elderly patients.

Adverse Reactions Frequency not defined.
Cardiovascular: Postural hypotension, arrhythmias, hypertension, heart block, tachycardia, palpitations, myocardial infarction
Central nervous system: Confusion, delirium, hallucinations, restlessness, insomnia, disorientation, delusions, anxiety, agitation, panic, nightmares, hypomania, exacerbation of psychosis, incoordination, ataxia, extrapyramidal symptoms, seizures
Dermatologic: Alopecia, photosensitivity, rash, petechiae, urticaria, itching
Endocrine & metabolic: Sexual dysfunction, gynecomastia, breast enlargement, galactorrhea, increase or decrease in libido, increase in blood sugar, SIADH
Gastrointestinal: Xerostomia, constipation, vomiting, anorexia, diarrhea, abdominal cramps, black tongue, nausea, unpleasant taste, weight gain/loss
Genitourinary: Urinary retention, delayed micturition, impotence, testicular edema
Hematologic: Rarely agranulocytosis, eosinophilia, purpura, thrombocytopenia
Hepatic: Increased liver enzymes, cholestatic jaundice
Neuromuscular & skeletal: Tremor, numbness, tingling, paresthesias, peripheral neuropathy
Ocular: Blurred vision, eye pain, disturbances in accommodation, mydriasis
Otic: Tinnitus
Miscellaneous: Diaphoresis, allergic reactions

Overdosage/Toxicology Signs and symptoms include agitation, confusion, hallucinations, urinary retention, hypothermia, hypotension, seizures, ventricular and tachycardia. Following initiation of essential overdose management, toxic symptoms should be treated. Ventricular arrhythmias often respond to phenytoin 15-20 mg/kg (adults) with concurrent systemic alkalinization (sodium bicarbonate 0.5-2 mEq/kg I.V.). Arrhythmias unresponsive to this therapy may respond to lidocaine 1 mg/kg I.V. followed by a titrated infusion. Physostigmine (1-2 mg slow I.V. for adults or 0.5 mg slow I.V. for children) may be indicated in reversing life-threatening cardiac arrhythmias. Seizures usually respond to diazepam I.V. boluses (5-10 mg for adults up to 30 mg or 0.25-0.4 mg/kg/dose for children up to 10 mg/dose). If seizures are unresponsive or recur, phenytoin or phenobarbital may be required.

Drug Interactions
Cytochrome P450 Effect: CYP1A2 and 2D6 enzyme substrate
Increased Effect/Toxicity: Nortriptyline increases the effects of amphetamines, anticholinergics, other CNS depressants (sedatives, hypnotics, ethanol), chlorpropamide, tolazamide, and warfarin. When used with MAO inhibitors, hyperpyrexia, hypertension, tachycardia, confusion, seizures, and **deaths have been reported** (serotonin syndrome). Serotonin syndrome has also been reported with ritonavir (rare). The SSRIs (to varying degrees), cimetidine, grapefruit juice, indinavir, methylphenidate, ritonavir, quinidine, diltiazem, and verapamil inhibit the metabolism of TCAs and clinical toxicity may result. Use of lithium with a TCA may increase the risk for neurotoxicity. Phenothiazines may increase concentration of some TCAs and TCAs may increase concentration of phenothiazines. Pressor response to I.V. epinephrine, norepinephrine, and phenylephrine may be enhanced in patients receiving TCAs (**Note:** Effect is unlikely with epinephrine or levonordefrin dosages typically administered as infiltration in combination with local anesthetics). Combined use of beta-agonists or drugs which prolong QT_c (including quinidine, procainamide, disopyramide, cisapride, sparfloxacin, gatifloxacin, moxifloxacin) with TCAs may predispose patients to cardiac arrhythmias. Use with altretamine may cause orthostatic hypotension.
Decreased Effect: Carbamazepine, phenobarbital, and rifampin may increase the metabolism of nortriptyline resulting in decreased effect of nortriptyline. Nortriptyline inhibits the antihypertensive response to bethanidine, clonidine, debrisoquin, guanadrel, guanethidine, guanabenz, or guanfacine. Cholestyramine and colestipol may bind TCAs and reduce their absorption; monitor for altered response.

Ethanol/Nutrition/Herb Interactions
Ethanol: Avoid ethanol (may increase CNS depression).
Food: Grapefruit juice may inhibit the metabolism of some TCAs and clinical toxicity may result.
Herb/Nutraceutical: Avoid valerian, St John's wort, SAMe, kava kava (may increase risk of serotonin syndrome and/or excessive sedation).

Stability Protect from light
Mechanism of Action Traditionally believed to increase the synaptic concentration of serotonin and/or norepinephrine in the central nervous system by inhibition of their reuptake by the presynaptic neuronal membrane. However, additional receptor effects have been found including desensitization of adenyl cyclase, down regulation of beta-adrenergic receptors, and down regulation of serotonin receptors.
Pharmacodynamics/Kinetics
Onset of action: Therapeutic: 1-3 weeks
Distribution: V_d: 21 L/kg
Protein binding: 93% to 95%
Metabolism: Primarily hepatic; extensive first-pass effect
Half-life elimination: 28-31 hours
Time to peak, serum: 7-8.5 hours
Excretion: Urine (as metabolites and small amounts of unchanged drug); feces (small amounts)
(Continued)

Nortriptyline (Continued)

Usual Dosage Oral:

Nocturnal enuresis:

Children:

6-7 years (20-25 kg): 10 mg/day

8-11 years (25-35 kg): 10-20 mg/day

>11 years (35-54 kg): 25-35 mg/day

Depression or ADHD (unlabeled use):

Children 6-12 years: 1-3 mg/kg/day or 10-20 mg/day in 3-4 divided doses

Adolescents: 30-100 mg/day in divided doses

Depression:

Adults: 25 mg 3-4 times/day up to 150 mg/day

Elderly (**Note:** Nortriptyline is one of the best tolerated TCAs in the elderly)

Initial: 10-25 mg at bedtime

Dosage can be increased by 25 mg every 3 days for inpatients and weekly for outpatients if tolerated

Usual maintenance dose: 75 mg as a single bedtime dose or 2 divided doses; however, lower or higher doses may be required to stay within the therapeutic window

Dosing adjustment in hepatic impairment: Lower doses and slower titration dependent on individualization of dosage is recommended

Monitoring Parameters Blood pressure and pulse rate (EKG, cardiac monitoring) prior to and during initial therapy in older adults; weight; blood levels are useful for therapeutic monitoring

Reference Range

Plasma levels do not always correlate with clinical effectiveness

Therapeutic: 50-150 ng/mL (SI: 190-570 nmol/L)

Toxic: >500 ng/mL (SI: >1900 nmol/L)

Patient Information Avoid alcohol; do not discontinue medication abruptly; may cause urine to turn blue-green; may cause drowsiness; full effect may not occur for 3-6 weeks; dry mouth may be helped by sips of water, sugarless gum, or hard candy

Nursing Implications May increase appetite and possibly a craving for sweets

Dosage Forms

Capsule, as hydrochloride: 10 mg, 25 mg, 50 mg, 75 mg

Solution, as hydrochloride: 10 mg/5 mL (473 mL)

- **Novo-Cycloprine**® **(Can)** *see* Cyclobenzaprine *on page 340*
- **Novo-Desipramine (Can)** *see* Desipramine *on page 376*
- **Novo-Difenac**® **(Can)** *see* Diclofenac *on page 393*
- **Novo-Difenac K (Can)** *see* Diclofenac *on page 393*
- **Novo-Difenac-SR**® **(Can)** *see* Diclofenac *on page 393*
- **Novo-Diflunisal (Can)** *see* Diflunisal *on page 401*
- **Novo-Diltazem (Can)** *see* Diltiazem *on page 409*
- **Novo-Diltazem SR (Can)** *see* Diltiazem *on page 409*
- **Novo-Dipiradol (Can)** *see* Dipyridamole *on page 422*
- **Novo-Divalproex (Can)** *see* Valproic Acid and Derivatives *on page 1398*
- **Novo-Doxazosin (Can)** *see* Doxazosin *on page 439*
- **Novo-Doxepin (Can)** *see* Doxepin *on page 440*
- **Novo-Doxylin (Can)** *see* Doxycycline *on page 448*
- **Novo-Famotidine (Can)** *see* Famotidine *on page 543*
- **Novo-Fluoxetine (Can)** *see* Fluoxetine *on page 578*
- **Novo-Flurprofen (Can)** *see* Flurbiprofen *on page 585*
- **Novo-Flutamide (Can)** *see* Flutamide *on page 586*
- **Novo-Fluvoxamine (Can)** *see* Fluvoxamine *on page 593*
- **Novo-Furantoin (Can)** *see* Nitrofurantoin *on page 987*
- **Novo-Gemfibrozil (Can)** *see* Gemfibrozil *on page 624*
- **Novo-Glyburide (Can)** *see* GlyBURIDE *on page 635*
- **Novo-Hydroxyzin (Can)** *see* HydrOXYzine *on page 691*
- **Novo-Hylazin (Can)** *see* HydrALAZINE *on page 671*
- **Novo-Indapamide (Can)** *see* Indapamide *on page 715*
- **Novo-Ipramide (Can)** *see* Ipratropium *on page 740*
- **Novo-Keto (Can)** *see* Ketoprofen *on page 763*
- **Novo-Ketoconazole (Can)** *see* Ketoconazole *on page 762*
- **Novo-Keto-EC (Can)** *see* Ketoprofen *on page 763*
- **Novo-Ketorolac (Can)** *see* Ketorolac *on page 764*
- **Novo-Ketotifen (Can)** *see* Ketotifen *on page 767*
- **Novo-Levamisole (Can)** *see* Levamisole *on page 786*
- **Novo-Levobunolol (Can)** *see* Levobunolol *on page 788*
- **Novo-Lexin**® **(Can)** *see* Cephalexin *on page 261*
- **Novolin**® **70/30** *see* Insulin Preparations *on page 722*
- **Novolin**®**ge (Can)** *see* Insulin Preparations *on page 722*
- **Novolin**® **L** *see* Insulin Preparations *on page 722*
- **Novolin**® **N** *see* Insulin Preparations *on page 722*
- **Novolin**® **R** *see* Insulin Preparations *on page 722*
- **NovoLog**® *see* Insulin Preparations *on page 722*
- **Novo-Loperamide (Can)** *see* Loperamide *on page 816*
- **Novo-Lorazepam**® **(Can)** *see* Lorazepam *on page 821*
- **Novo-Maprotiline (Can)** *see* Maprotiline *on page 839*
- **Novo-Medopa**® **(Can)** *see* Methyldopa *on page 891*
- **Novo-Medrone (Can)** *see* MedroxyPROGESTERone *on page 848*
- **Novo-Metformin (Can)** *see* Metformin *on page 875*
- **Novo-Methacin (Can)** *see* Indomethacin *on page 717*
- **Novo-Metoprolol (Can)** *see* Metoprolol *on page 902*
- **Novo-Mexiletine (Can)** *see* Mexiletine *on page 907*
- **Novo-Minocycline (Can)** *see* Minocycline *on page 918*
- **Novo-Mucilax (Can)** *see* Psyllium *on page 1158*
- **Novo-Nadolol (Can)** *see* Nadolol *on page 948*
- **Novo-Naprox (Can)** *see* Naproxen *on page 958*
- **Novo-Naprox Sodium (Can)** *see* Naproxen *on page 958*
- **Novo-Naprox Sodium DS (Can)** *see* Naproxen *on page 958*
- **Novo-Naprox SR (Can)** *see* Naproxen *on page 958*
- **Novo-Nidazol (Can)** *see* Metronidazole *on page 904*
- **Novo-Nifedin (Can)** *see* NIFEdipine *on page 981*
- **Novo-Nizatidine (Can)** *see* Nizatidine *on page 992*
- **Novo-Norfloxacin (Can)** *see* Norfloxacin *on page 994*
- **Novo-Nortriptyline (Can)** *see* Nortriptyline *on page 996*
- **Novo-Oxybutynin (Can)** *see* Oxybutynin *on page 1023*
- **Novo-Pen-VK**® **(Can)** *see* Penicillin V Potassium *on page 1055*
- **Novo-Peridol (Can)** *see* Haloperidol *on page 654*
- **Novo-Pindol (Can)** *see* Pindolol *on page 1086*
- **Novo-Pirocam**® **(Can)** *see* Piroxicam *on page 1093*
- **Novo-Poxide**® **(Can)** *see* Chlordiazepoxide *on page 274*
- **Novo-Prazin (Can)** *see* Prazosin *on page 1120*
- **Novo-Prednisolone**® **(Can)** *see* PrednisoLONE *on page 1122*
- **Novo-Profen**® **(Can)** *see* Ibuprofen *on page 697*
- **Novo-Ranidine (Can)** *see* Ranitidine *on page 1178*
- **Novo-Rythro Encap (Can)** *see* Erythromycin (Systemic) *on page 486*
- **Novo-Salmol (Can)** *see* Albuterol *on page 41*
- **Novo-Selegiline (Can)** *see* Selegiline *on page 1228*
- **Novo-Sertraline (Can)** *see* Sertraline *on page 1231*

- **Novo-Seven**® *see* Factor VIIa (Recombinant) *on page 538*
- **Novo-Sotalol (Can)** *see* Sotalol *on page 1252*
- **Novo-Soxazole**® **(Can)** *see* SulfiSOXAZOLE *on page 1277*
- **Novo-Spiroton (Can)** *see* Spironolactone *on page 1256*
- **Novo-Spirozine (Can)** *see* Hydrochlorothiazide and Spironolactone *on page 675*
- **Novo-Sucralate (Can)** *see* Sucralfate *on page 1266*
- **Novo-Sundac (Can)** *see* Sulindac *on page 1278*
- **Novo-Tamoxifen (Can)** *see* Tamoxifen *on page 1286*
- **Novo-Temazepam (Can)** *see* Temazepam *on page 1292*
- **Novo-Terazosin (Can)** *see* Terazosin *on page 1298*
- **Novo-Tetra (Can)** *see* Tetracycline *on page 1306*
- **Novo-Timol (Can)** *see* Timolol *on page 1334*
- **Novo-Tolmetin (Can)** *see* Tolmetin *on page 1346*
- **Novo-Trazodone (Can)** *see* Trazodone *on page 1362*
- **Novo-Triamzide (Can)** *see* Hydrochlorothiazide and Triamterene *on page 675*
- **Novo-Trimel (Can)** *see* Sulfamethoxazole and Trimethoprim *on page 1273*
- **Novo-Trimel D.S. (Can)** *see* Sulfamethoxazole and Trimethoprim *on page 1273*
- **Novo-Tripramine (Can)** *see* Trimipramine *on page 1378*
- **Novo-Veramil (Can)** *see* Verapamil *on page 1412*
- **Novo-Veramil SR (Can)** *see* Verapamil *on page 1412*
- **NP-27**® **[OTC]** *see* Tolnaftate *on page 1347*
- **NPH Iletin**® **II** *see* Insulin Preparations *on page 722*
- **NSC-13875** *see* Altretamine *on page 62*
- **NSC-26271** *see* Cyclophosphamide *on page 342*
- **NSC-106977 (Erwinia)** *see* Asparaginase *on page 118*
- **NSC-109229 (E. coli)** *see* Asparaginase *on page 118*
- **NSC-125066** *see* Bleomycin *on page 176*
- **NSC-373364** *see* Aldesleukin *on page 43*
- **NTG** *see* Nitroglycerin *on page 989*
- **Nu-Acebutolol (Can)** *see* Acebutolol *on page 21*
- **Nu-Acyclovir (Can)** *see* Acyclovir *on page 34*
- **Nu-Alprax (Can)** *see* Alprazolam *on page 55*
- **Nu-Amilzide (Can)** *see* Amiloride and Hydrochlorothiazide *on page 71*
- **Nu-Amoxi (Can)** *see* Amoxicillin *on page 84*
- **Nu-Ampi (Can)** *see* Ampicillin *on page 93*
- **Nu-Atenol (Can)** *see* Atenolol *on page 125*
- **Nu-Baclo (Can)** *see* Baclofen *on page 144*
- **Nubain**® *see* Nalbuphine *on page 951*
- **Nu-Beclomethasone (Can)** *see* Beclomethasone *on page 149*
- **Nu-Buspirone (Can)** *see* BusPIRone *on page 194*
- **Nu-Capto**® **(Can)** *see* Captopril *on page 218*
- **Nu-Carbamazepine**® **(Can)** *see* Carbamazepine *on page 221*
- **Nu-Cefaclor (Can)** *see* Cefaclor *on page 237*
- **Nu-Cephalex**® **(Can)** *see* Cephalexin *on page 261*
- **Nu-Cimet**® **(Can)** *see* Cimetidine *on page 293*
- **Nu-Clonazepam (Can)** *see* Clonazepam *on page 316*
- **Nu-Clonidine**® **(Can)** *see* Clonidine *on page 318*
- **Nu-Cloxi**® **(Can)** *see* Cloxacillin *on page 324*
- **Nucofed**® *see* Guaifenesin, Pseudoephedrine, and Codeine *on page 648*
- **Nucofed**® **Pediatric Expectorant** *see* Guaifenesin, Pseudoephedrine, and Codeine *on page 648*
- **Nu-Cotrimox**® **(Can)** *see* Sulfamethoxazole and Trimethoprim *on page 1273*
- **Nucotuss**® *see* Guaifenesin, Pseudoephedrine, and Codeine *on page 648*
- **Nu-Cromolyn (Can)** *see* Cromolyn Sodium *on page 337*
- **Nu-Cyclobenzaprine (Can)** *see* Cyclobenzaprine *on page 340*
- **Nu-Desipramine (Can)** *see* Desipramine *on page 376*
- **Nu-Diclo (Can)** *see* Diclofenac *on page 393*
- **Nu-Diclo-SR (Can)** *see* Diclofenac *on page 393*
- **Nu-Diflunisal (Can)** *see* Diflunisal *on page 401*
- **Nu-Diltiaz (Can)** *see* Diltiazem *on page 409*
- **Nu-Diltiaz-CD (Can)** *see* Diltiazem *on page 409*
- **Nu-Divalproex (Can)** *see* Valproic Acid and Derivatives *on page 1398*
- **Nu-Doxycycline (Can)** *see* Doxycycline *on page 448*
- **Nu-Erythromycin-S (Can)** *see* Erythromycin (Systemic) *on page 486*
- **Nu-Famotidine (Can)** *see* Famotidine *on page 543*
- **Nu-Fenofibrate (Can)** *see* Fenofibrate *on page 548*
- **Nu-Fluoxetine (Can)** *see* Fluoxetine *on page 578*
- **Nu-Flurprofen (Can)** *see* Flurbiprofen *on page 585*
- **Nu-Fluvoxamine (Can)** *see* Fluvoxamine *on page 593*
- **Nu-Gemfibrozil (Can)** *see* Gemfibrozil *on page 624*
- **Nu-Glyburide (Can)** *see* GlyBURIDE *on page 635*
- **Nu-Hydral (Can)** *see* HydrALAZINE *on page 671*
- **Nu-Ibuprofen (Can)** *see* Ibuprofen *on page 697*
- **Nu-Indapamide (Can)** *see* Indapamide *on page 715*

- **Nu-Indo (Can)** *see Indomethacin on page 717*
- **Nu-Ipratropium (Can)** *see Ipratropium on page 740*
- **Nu-Iron® [OTC]** *see Polysaccharide-Iron Complex on page 1104*
- **Nu-Ketoprofen (Can)** *see Ketoprofen on page 763*
- **Nu-Ketoprofen-E (Can)** *see Ketoprofen on page 763*
- **NuLev™** *see Hyoscyamine on page 692*
- **Nu-Levocarb (Can)** *see Levodopa and Carbidopa on page 791*
- **Nu-Loraz (Can)** *see Lorazepam on page 821*
- **Nu-Loxapine (Can)** *see Loxapine on page 826*
- **NuLytely®** *see Polyethylene Glycol-Electrolyte Solution on page 1101*
- **Nu-Medopa (Can)** *see Methyldopa on page 891*
- **Nu-Mefenamic (Can)** *see Mefenamic Acid on page 850*
- **Nu-Megestrol (Can)** *see Megestrol on page 852*
- **Nu-Metformin (Can)** *see Metformin on page 875*
- **Nu-Metoclopramide (Can)** *see Metoclopramide on page 900*
- **Nu-Metop (Can)** *see Metoprolol on page 902*
- **Numorphan®** *see Oxymorphone on page 1027*
- **Nu-Naprox (Can)** *see Naproxen on page 958*
- **Nu-Nifed (Can)** *see NIFEdipine on page 981*
- **Nu-Nortriptyline (Can)** *see Nortriptyline on page 996*
- **Nu-Oxybutyn (Can)** *see Oxybutynin on page 1023*
- **Nu-Pen-VK® (Can)** *see Penicillin V Potassium on page 1055*
- **Nu-Pindol (Can)** *see Pindolol on page 1086*
- **Nu-Pirox (Can)** *see Piroxicam on page 1093*
- **Nu-Prazo (Can)** *see Prazosin on page 1120*
- **Nuprin® [OTC]** *see Ibuprofen on page 697*
- **Nu-Prochlor (Can)** *see Prochlorperazine on page 1134*
- **Nu-Propranolol (Can)** *see Propranolol on page 1149*
- **Nuquin® Gel** *see Hydroquinone on page 686*
- **Nuquin HP® Cream** *see Hydroquinone on page 686*
- **Nu-Ranit (Can)** *see Ranitidine on page 1178*
- **Nuromax®** *see Doxacurium on page 438*
- **Nu-Selegiline (Can)** *see Selegiline on page 1228*
- **Nu-Sotalol (Can)** *see Sotalol on page 1252*
- **Nu-Sucralate (Can)** *see Sucralfate on page 1266*
- **Nu-Sulfinpyrazone (Can)** *see Sulfinpyrazone on page 1276*
- **Nu-Sundac (Can)** *see Sulindac on page 1278*
- **Nu-Temazepam (Can)** *see Temazepam on page 1292*
- **Nu-Terazosin (Can)** *see Terazosin on page 1298*
- **Nu-Tetra (Can)** *see Tetracycline on page 1306*
- **Nu-Ticlopidine (Can)** *see Ticlopidine on page 1331*
- **Nu-Timolol (Can)** *see Timolol on page 1334*
- **Nutracort®** *see Hydrocortisone on page 682*
- **Nutraplus® [OTC]** *see Urea on page 1391*
- **Nu-Trazodone (Can)** *see Trazodone on page 1362*
- **Nu-Triazide (Can)** *see Hydrochlorothiazide and Triamterene on page 675*
- **Nutrilipid®** *see Fat Emulsion on page 545*
- **Nu-Trimipramine (Can)** *see Trimipramine on page 1378*
- **Nutropin®** *see Human Growth Hormone on page 667*
- **Nutropin AQ ®** *see Human Growth Hormone on page 667*
- **Nutropin Depot®** *see Human Growth Hormone on page 667*
- **Nutropine® (Can)** *see Human Growth Hormone on page 667*
- **NuvaRing®** *see Ethinyl Estradiol and Etonogestrel on page 516*
- **Nu-Verap (Can)** *see Verapamil on page 1412*
- **Nyaderm (Can)** *see Nystatin on page 1001*
- **Nydrazid®** *see Isoniazid on page 747*

Nystatin (nye STAT in)

Related Information

Antifungal Agents Comparison *on page 1484*
Treatment of Sexually Transmitted Diseases *on page 1609*
USPHA/IDSA Guidelines for the Prevention of Opportunistic Infections in Persons With HIV *on page 1574*

U.S. Brand Names Bio-Statin®; Mycostatin®; Nilstat®; Nystex®; Peri-Dri®

Canadian Brand Names Candistatin®; Mycostatin®; Nilstat; Nyaderm; PMS-Nystatin

Therapeutic Category Antifungal Agent, Oral Nonabsorbed; Antifungal Agent, Topical; Antifungal Agent, Vaginal

Use Treatment of susceptible cutaneous, mucocutaneous, and oral cavity fungal infections normally caused by the *Candida* species

Pregnancy Risk Factor B/C (oral)

Contraindications Hypersensitivity to nystatin or any component of the formulation

Adverse Reactions

Frequency not defined: Dermatologic: Contact dermatitis, Stevens-Johnson syndrome
1% to 10%: Gastrointestinal: Nausea, vomiting, diarrhea, stomach pain
<1% (Limited to important or life-threatening): Hypersensitivity reactions
(Continued)

Nystatin *(Continued)*

Overdosage/Toxicology Symptoms include nausea, vomiting, and diarrhea. Treatment is supportive.

Stability Keep vaginal inserts in refrigerator; protect from temperature extremes, moisture, and light

Mechanism of Action Binds to sterols in fungal cell membrane, changing the cell wall permeability allowing for leakage of cellular contents

Pharmacodynamics/Kinetics

Onset of action: Symptomatic relief from candidiasis: 24-72 hours

Absorption: Topical: None through mucous membranes or intact skin; Oral: Poorly absorbed

Excretion: Feces (as unchanged drug)

Usual Dosage

Oral candidiasis:

Suspension (swish and swallow orally):

Premature infants: 100,000 units 4 times/day

Infants: 200,000 units 4 times/day or 100,000 units to each side of mouth 4 times/day

Children and Adults: 400,000-600,000 units 4 times/day

Troche: Children and Adults: 200,000-400,000 units 4-5 times/day

Powder for compounding: Children and Adults: ⅛ teaspoon (500,000 units) to equal approximately ½ cup of water; give 4 times/day

Mucocutaneous infections: Children and Adults: Topical: Apply 2-3 times/day to affected areas; very moist topical lesions are treated best with powder

Intestinal infections: Adults: Oral: 500,000-1,000,000 units every 8 hours

Vaginal infections: Adults: Vaginal tablets: Insert 1 tablet/day at bedtime for 2 weeks

Patient Information The oral suspension should be swished about the mouth and retained in the mouth for as long as possible (several minutes) before swallowing. For neonates and infants, paint nystatin suspension into recesses of the mouth. Troches must be allowed to dissolve slowly and should not be chewed or swallowed whole. If topical irritation occurs, discontinue; for external use only; do not discontinue therapy even if symptoms are gone

Nursing Implications Administer around-the-clock rather than 4 times/day, 3 times/day etc (ie, 12-6-12-6, not 9-1-5-9) to promote less variation in peak and trough serum levels

Dosage Forms

Capsule: 500,000 units, 1 million units

Cream: 100,000 units/g (15 g, 30 g)

Ointment, topical: 100,000 units/g (15 g, 30 g)

Powder for oral suspension: 50 million units, 1 billion units, 2 billion units, 5 billion units

Powder, topical: 100,000 units/g (15 g, 56.7 g)

Suspension, oral: 100,000 units/mL (5 mL, 60 mL, 480 mL)

Tablet: 500,000 units

Tablet, vaginal: 100,000 units (15 and 30/box with applicator)

Troche: 200,000 units

Nystatin and Triamcinolone *(nye STAT in & trye am SIN oh lone)*

U.S. Brand Names Mycogen II; Mycolog®-II; Myco-Triacet® II; Mytrex® F; N.G.A.®; Quenalog®

Synonyms Triamcinolone and Nystatin

Therapeutic Category Antifungal Agent, Topical; Corticosteroid, Topical (Medium Potency)

Use Treatment of cutaneous candidiasis

Pregnancy Risk Factor C

Usual Dosage Children and Adults: Topical: Apply sparingly 2-4 times/day. Therapy should be discontinued when control is achieved; if no improvement is seen, reassessment of diagnosis may be necessary.

Additional Information Complete prescribing information for this medication should be consulted for additional detail.

Dosage Forms

Cream, topical: Nystatin 100,000 units and triamcinolone acetonide 0.1% (1.5 g, 15 g, 30 g, 60 g, 120 g)

Ointment, topical: Nystatin 100,000 units and triamcinolone acetonide 0.1% (15 g, 30 g, 60 g, 120 g)

- ◆ **Nystex®** *see Nystatin on page 1001*
- ◆ **Nytol® [OTC]** *see DiphenhydrAMINE on page 414*
- ◆ **Nytol™ Extra Strength (Can)** *see DiphenhydrAMINE on page 414*
- ◆ **Obesity Treatment Guidelines for Adults** *see page 1685*
- ◆ **Ocean® [OTC]** *see Sodium Chloride on page 1245*
- ◆ **OCL®** *see Polyethylene Glycol-Electrolyte Solution on page 1101*
- ◆ **Octicair® Otic** *see Neomycin, Polymyxin B, and Hydrocortisone on page 969*
- ◆ **Octostim® (Can)** *see Desmopressin on page 378*

Octreotide *(ok TREE oh tide)*

U.S. Brand Names Sandostatin®; Sandostatin LAR®

Canadian Brand Names Sandostatin®; Sandostatin LAR®

Synonyms Octreotide Acetate

Therapeutic Category Antidiarrheal; Antisecretory Agent; Somatostatin Analog

Use Control of symptoms in patients with metastatic carcinoid and vasoactive intestinal peptide-secreting tumors (VIPomas); pancreatic tumors, gastrinoma, secretory diarrhea, acromegaly

Unlabeled/Investigational Use AIDS-associated secretory diarrhea, control of bleeding of esophageal varices, breast cancer, cryptosporidiosis, Cushing's syndrome, insulinomas, small bowel fistulas, postgastrectomy dumping syndrome, chemotherapy-induced diarrhea, graft-versus-host disease (GVHD) induced diarrhea, Zollinger-Ellison syndrome, congenital hyperinsulinism

Pregnancy Risk Factor B

Contraindications Hypersensitivity to octreotide or any component of the formulation

Warnings/Precautions Dosage adjustment may be required to maintain symptomatic control; insulin requirements may be reduced as well as sulfonylurea requirements; monitor patients for cholelithiasis, hyper- or hypoglycemia; use with caution in patients with renal impairment

Adverse Reactions

>10%:

Cardiovascular: Sinus bradycardia (19% to 25%)

Endocrine & metabolic: Hyperglycemia (15% acromegaly, 27% carcinoid)

Gastrointestinal: Diarrhea (36% to 58% acromegaly), abdominal pain (30% to 44% acromegaly), flatulence (13% to 26% acromegaly), constipation (9% to 19% acromegaly), nausea (10% to 30%)

1% to 10%:

Cardiovascular: Flushing, edema, conduction abnormalities (9% to 10%), arrhythmias (3% to 9%)

Central nervous system: Fatigue, headache, dizziness, vertigo, anorexia, depression

Endocrine & metabolic: Hypoglycemia (2% acromegaly, 4% carcinoid), hyperglycemia (1%), hypothyroidism, galactorrhea

Gastrointestinal: Nausea, vomiting, diarrhea, constipation, abdominal pain, cramping, discomfort, fat malabsorption, loose stools, flatulence, tenesmus

Hepatic: Jaundice, hepatitis, increase LFTs, cholelithiasis has occurred, presumably by altering fat absorption and decreasing the motility of the gallbladder

Local: Pain at injection site (dose-related)

Neuromuscular & skeletal: Weakness

<1% (Limited to important or life-threatening): Alopecia, Bell's palsy, chest pain, dyspnea, gallstones, hypertensive reaction, thrombophlebitis

Overdosage/Toxicology Symptoms include hypo- or hyperglycemia, blurred vision, dizziness, drowsiness, and loss of motor function. Well tolerated bolus doses up to 1000 mcg have failed to produce adverse effects.

Drug Interactions

Cytochrome P450 Effect: CYP2D6 (high dose) and 3A enzyme inhibitor

Increased Effect/Toxicity: Octreotide may increase the effect of insulin or sulfonylurea agents which may result in hypoglycemia.

Decreased Effect: Octreotide may lower cyclosporine serum levels (case report of a transplant rejection due to reduction of serum cyclosporine levels). Codeine effect may be reduced.

Stability Octreotide is a clear solution and should be stored under refrigeration; ampuls may be stored at room temperature for up to 14 days when protected from light

Stability of parenteral admixture in NS at room temperature (25°C) and at refrigeration temperature (4°C): 48 hours

Common diluent: 50-100 mcg/50 mL NS; common diluent for continuous I.V. infusion: 1200 mcg/250 mL NS

Minimum volume: 50 mL NS

Mechanism of Action Mimics natural somatostatin by inhibiting serotonin release, and the secretion of gastrin, VIP, insulin, glucagon, secretin, motilin, and pancreatic polypeptide. Decreases growth hormone and IGF-1 in acromegaly.

Pharmacodynamics/Kinetics

Duration: S.C.: 6-12 hours

Absorption: S.C.: Rapid

Distribution: V_d: 14 L

Protein binding: 65% to lipoproteins

Metabolism: Extensively hepatic

Bioavailability: S.C.: 100%

Half-life elimination: 60-110 minutes

Excretion: Urine (32%)

Usual Dosage Adults: S.C.: Initial: 50 mcg 1-2 times/day and titrate dose based on patient tolerance and response

Carcinoid: 100-600 mcg/day in 2-4 divided doses

VIPomas: 200-300 mcg/day in 2-4 divided doses

Diarrhea: Initial: I.V.: 50-100 mcg every 8 hours; increase by 100 mcg/dose at 48-hour intervals; maximum dose: 500 mcg every 8 hours

Esophageal varices bleeding: I.V. bolus: 25-50 mcg followed by continuous I.V. infusion of 25-50 mcg/hour

Acromegaly: Initial: S.C.: 50 mcg 3 times/day; titrate to achieve growth hormone levels <5 ng/mL or IGF-I (somatomedin C) levels <1.9 U/mL in males and <2.2 U/mL in females; usual effective dose 100 mcg 3 times/day; range 300-1500 mcg/day

Note: Should be withdrawn yearly for a 4-week interval in patients who have received irradiation. Resume if levels increase and signs/symptoms recur.

Acromegaly, carcinoid tumors, and VIPomas (depot injection): Patients must be stabilized on subcutaneous octreotide for at least 2 weeks before switching to the long-acting depot: Upon switch: 20 mg I.M. intragluteally every 4 weeks for 2-3 months, then the dose may be modified based upon response

Dosage adjustment for acromegaly: After 3 months of depot injections the dosage may be continued or modified as follows:

GH ≤1 ng/mL, IGF-1 is normal, symptoms controlled: Reduce octreotide LAR® to 10 mg I.M. every 4 weeks

GH ≤2.5 ng/mL, IGF-1 is normal, symptoms controlled: Maintain octreotide LAR® at 20 mg I.M. every 4 weeks

GH >2.5 ng/mL, IGF-1 is elevated, and/or symptoms uncontrolled: Increase octreotide LAR® to 30 mg I.M. every 4 weeks

Dosages >40 mg are not recommended

Dosage adjustment for carcinoid tumors and VIPomas: After 2 months of depot injections the dosage may be continued or modified as follows:

Increase to 30 mg I.M. every 4 weeks if symptoms are inadequately controlled

(Continued)

Octreotide *(Continued)*

Decrease to 10 mg I.M. every 4 weeks, for a trial period, if initially responsive to 20 mg dose

Dosage >30 mg is not recommended

Dietary Considerations Schedule injections between meals to decrease GI effects.

Administration

Regular injection formulation (do not use if solution contains particles or is discolored): Administer S.C. or I.V.; I.V. administration may be IVP, IVPB, or continuous I.V. infusion:

IVP should be administered undiluted over 3 minutes

IVPB should be administered over 15-30 minutes

Continuous I.V. infusion rates have ranged from 25-50 mcg/hour for the treatment of esophageal variceal bleeding

Depot formulation: Administer I.M. intragluteal; must be administered immediately after mixing

Reference Range Vasoactive intestinal peptide: <75 ng/L; levels vary considerably between laboratories

Dosage Forms

Injection, as acetate (Sandostatin®): 0.05 mg/mL (1 mL); 0.1 mg/mL (1 mL); 0.2 mg/mL (5 mL); 0.5 mg/mL (1 mL); 1 mg/mL (5 mL)

Injection, powder for suspension, depot, as acetate [with diluent and syringe] (Sandostatin LAR®): 10 mg, 20 mg, 30 mg

- ◆ **Octreotide Acetate** *see Octreotide on page 1002*
- ◆ **Ocu-Carpine®** *see Pilocarpine on page 1083*
- ◆ **Ocu-Chlor®** *see Chloramphenicol on page 272*
- ◆ **Ocufen™ (Can)** *see Flurbiprofen on page 585*
- ◆ **Ocufen® Ophthalmic** *see Flurbiprofen on page 585*
- ◆ **Ocuflox®** *see Ofloxacin on page 1004*
- ◆ **Ocupress® Ophthalmic** *see Carteolol on page 232*
- ◆ **Ocusert Pilo-20®** *see Pilocarpine on page 1083*
- ◆ **Ocusert Pilo-40®** *see Pilocarpine on page 1083*
- ◆ **Ocu-Sul®** *see Sulfacetamide on page 1268*
- ◆ **Ocu-Zoline®** *see Naphazoline on page 957*
- ◆ **Oesclim® (Can)** *see Estradiol on page 491*
- ◆ **Oestrilin (Can)** *see Estrone on page 502*

Ofloxacin *(oh FLOKS a sin)*

Related Information

Antacid Drug Interactions *on page 1477*

Antimicrobial Drugs of Choice *on page 1588*

Treatment of Sexually Transmitted Diseases *on page 1609*

Tuberculosis Treatment Guidelines *on page 1612*

U.S. Brand Names Floxin®; Ocuflox®

Canadian Brand Names Apo®-Oflox; Floxin®; Ocuflox®

Therapeutic Category Antibiotic, Quinolone

Use Quinolone antibiotic for skin and skin structure, lower respiratory, and urinary tract infections and sexually-transmitted diseases. Active against many gram-positive and gram-negative aerobic bacteria.

Ophthalmic: Treatment of superficial ocular infections involving the conjunctiva or cornea due to strains of susceptible organisms

Otic: Otitis externa, chronic suppurative otitis media (patients >12 years of age); acute otitis media

Pregnancy Risk Factor C

Contraindications Hypersensitivity to ofloxacin or other members of the quinolone group such as nalidixic acid, oxolinic acid, cinoxacin, norfloxacin, and ciprofloxacin; hypersensitivity to any component of the formulation

Warnings/Precautions Use with caution in patients with epilepsy or other CNS diseases which could predispose seizures; use with caution in patients with renal impairment; failure to respond to an ophthalmic antibiotic after 2-3 days may indicate the presence of resistant organisms, or another causative agent; use caution with systemic preparation in children <18 years of age due to association of other quinolones with transient arthropathy. Tendon inflammation and/or rupture have been reported with other quinolone antibiotics. Discontinue at first sign of tendon inflammation or pain. Quinolones may exacerbate myasthenia gravis.

Severe hypersensitivity reactions, including anaphylaxis, have occurred with quinolone therapy. If an allergic reaction occurs (itching, urticaria, dyspnea, facial edema, loss of consciousness, tingling, cardiovascular collapse), discontinue drug immediately. Prolonged use may result in superinfection; pseudomembranous colitis may occur and should be considered in all patients who present with diarrhea.

Adverse Reactions

Ophthalmic:

>10%: Ocular: Burning or other discomfort of the eye, crusting or crystals in corner of eye

1% to 10%:

Gastrointestinal: Bad taste instillation

Ocular: Foreign body sensation, conjunctival hyperemia, itching of eye, ocular or facial edema, redness, stinging, photophobia

<1% (Limited to important or life-threatening): Dizziness, nausea

Otic: Local reactions (3%), earache (1%), tinnitus, otorrhagia

Systemic:

1% to 10%:

Cardiovascular: Chest pain (1% to 3%)

Central nervous system: Headache (1% to 9%), insomnia (3% to 7%), dizziness (1% to 5%), fatigue (1% to 3%), somnolence (1% to 3%), sleep disorders, nervousness (1% to 3%), pyrexia (1% to 3%), pain

Dermatologic: Rash/pruritus (1% to 3%)

Gastrointestinal: Diarrhea (1% to 4%), vomiting (1% to 3%), GI distress, cramps, abdominal cramps (1% to 3%), flatulence (1% to 3%), abnormal taste (1% to 3%), xerostomia (1% to 3%), decreased appetite, nausea (3% to 10%)

Genitourinary: Vaginitis (1% to 3%), external genital pruritus in women

Local: Pain at injection site

Ocular: Superinfection (ophthalmic), photophobia, lacrimation, dry eyes, stinging, visual disturbances (1% to 3%)

Miscellaneous: Trunk pain

<1% (Limited to important or life-threatening): Anxiety, cognitive change, depression, euphoria, hallucinations, hepatitis, interstitial nephritis, paresthesia, photosensitivity, seizures, Stevens-Johnson syndrome, syncope, tinnitus, Tourette's syndrome, vasculitis, vertigo; quinolones have been associated with tendonitis and tendon rupture

Overdosage/Toxicology Symptoms include acute renal failure, seizures, nausea, and vomiting. Treatment includes GI decontamination, if possible, and supportive care.

Drug Interactions

Increased Effect/Toxicity: Quinolones can cause increased caffeine, warfarin, cyclosporine, and theophylline levels (unlikely to occur with ofloxacin). Azlocillin, cimetidine, and probenecid may increase ofloxacin serum levels. Foscarnet and NSAIDs have been associated with an increased risk of seizures with some quinolones. Serum levels of some quinolones are increased by loop diuretic administration. The hypoprothrombinemic effect of warfarin is enhanced by some quinolone antibiotics. Ofloxacin does not alter warfarin levels, but may alter the gastrointestinal flora which may increase warfarin's effect.

Decreased Effect: Metal cations (magnesium, aluminum, iron, and zinc) bind quinolones in the gastrointestinal tract and inhibit absorption (as much as 98%). Antacids, electrolyte supplements, sucralfate, quinapril, and some didanosine formulations should be avoided. Ofloxacin should be administered 4 hours before or 8 hours after these agents. Antineoplastic agents may decrease the absorption of quinolones.

Ethanol/Nutrition/Herb Interactions

Food: Ofloxacin average peak serum concentrations may be decreased by 20% if taken with food.

Herb/Nutraceutical: Avoid dong quai, St John's wort (may also cause photosensitization).

Mechanism of Action Ofloxacin is a DNA gyrase inhibitor. DNA gyrase is an essential bacterial enzyme that maintains the superhelical structure of DNA. DNA gyrase is required for DNA replication and transcription, DNA repair, recombination, and transposition; bactericidal

Pharmacodynamics/Kinetics

Absorption: Well absorbed; taking with food causes only minor alterations

Distribution: V_d: 2.4-3.5 L/kg

Protein binding: 20%

Half-life elimination: 5-7.5 hours; prolonged in renal impairment

Excretion: Primarily urine (as unchanged drug)

Usual Dosage

Oral, I.V.: Adults:

Lower respiratory tract infection: 400 mg every 12 hours for 10 days

Epididymitis (gonorrhea): 300 mg twice daily for 10 days

Cervicitis due to *C. trachomatis* and/or *N. gonorrhoeae*: 300 mg every 12 hours for 7 days

Skin/skin structure: 400 mg every 12 hours for 10 days

Urinary tract infection: 200-400 mg every 12 hours for 3-10 days

Prostatitis: 300 mg every 12 hours for 6 weeks

Ophthalmic: Children >1 year and Adults:

Conjunctivitis: Instill 1-2 drops in affected eye(s) every 2-4 hours for the first 2 days, then use 4 times/day for an additional 5 days

Corneal ulcer: Instill 1-2 drops every 30 minutes while awake and every 4-6 hours after retiring for the first 2 days; beginning on day 3, instill 1-2 drops every hour while awake for 4-6 additional days; thereafter, 1-2 drops 4 times/day until clinical cure.

Otic:

Children >1-12 years: Otitis externa or acute otitis media with tympanostomy tubes: Instill 5 drops into affected ear(s) twice daily for 10 days

Children >12 years and Adults:

Chronic otitis media with perforated tympanic membranes: Otic: 10 drops into affected ear twice daily for 14 days

Chronic suppurative otitis media: Instill 10 drops into affected ear(s) twice daily for 14 days

Otitis externa: Instill 10 drops into affected ear(s) twice daily for 10 days

Dosing adjustment/interval in renal impairment: Adults: I.V., Oral:

Cl_{cr} 10-50 mL/minute: Administer 200-400 mg every 24 hours

Cl_{cr} <10 mL/minute: Administer 100-200 mg every 24 hours

Continuous arteriovenous or venovenous hemodiafiltration effects: Administer 300 mg every 24 hours

Administration

Oral: Do not take within 2 hours of food or any antacids which contain zinc, magnesium, or aluminum.

I.V.: Administer over at least 60 minutes. Infuse separately. Do not infuse though lines containing solutions with magnesium or calcium.

Patient Information Report any skin rash or other allergic reactions; avoid excessive sunlight; do not take with food; do not take within 2 hours of any products including antacids which contain calcium, magnesium, or aluminum; contact your physician immediately with signs of inflammation or tendon pain

Nursing Implications Hold antacids for 2-4 hours before and after administering dose

(Continued)

Ofloxacin *(Continued)*

Dosage Forms

Injection, flexible containers [premixed in D₅W] [single-use dose] (Floxin®): 4 mg/mL (50 mL, 100 mL)

Injection [single-dose vial] (Floxin®): 40 mg/mL (10 mL)

Solution, ophthalmic (Ocuflox®): 0.3% (5 mL)

Solution, otic (Floxin®[): 0.3% (5 mL)

Tablet (Floxin®): 200 mg, 300 mg, 400 mg

- ◆ **Ogen®** *see Estropipate on page 503*
- ◆ **Ogestrel®** *see Ethinyl Estradiol and Norgestrel on page 528*
- ◆ **OGMT** *see Metyrosine on page 906*
- ◆ **OKT3** *see Muromonab-CD3 on page 941*

Olanzapine *(oh LAN za peen)*

Related Information

Antipsychotic Agents Comparison *on page 1486*

U.S. Brand Names Zyprexa®; Zyprexa® Zydis®

Canadian Brand Names Zyprexa®

Synonyms LY170053

Therapeutic Category Antipsychotic Agent, Atypical

Use Treatment of the manifestations of schizophrenia; short-term treatment of acute mania episodes associated with bipolar mania

Unlabeled/Investigational Use Treatment of psychotic symptoms

Pregnancy Risk Factor C

Contraindications Hypersensitivity to olanzapine or any component of the formulation

Warnings/Precautions Moderate to highly sedating, use with caution in disorders where CNS depression is a feature. Use with caution in Parkinson's disease and Alzheimer's disease. Caution in patients with hemodynamic instability; bone marrow suppression; predisposition to seizures; subcortical brain damage; severe cardiac, hepatic, renal, or respiratory disease. Esophageal dysmotility and aspiration have been associated with antipsychotic use - use with caution in patients at risk of pneumonia (ie, Alzheimer's disease). Caution in breast cancer or other prolactin-dependent tumors (may elevate prolactin levels). May alter temperature regulation or mask toxicity of other drugs due to antiemetic effects. Life-threatening arrhythmias have occurred with therapeutic doses of some neuroleptics. Significant weight gain may occur.

May cause anticholinergic effects (constipation, dry mouth, blurred vision, urinary retention); therefore, they should be used with caution in patients with decreased gastrointestinal motility, urinary retention, BPH, xerostomia, or visual problems. Conditions which also may be exacerbated by cholinergic blockade include narrow-angle glaucoma (screening is recommended) and worsening of myasthenia gravis. Relative to other neuroleptics, olanzapine has a moderate potency of cholinergic blockade.

May cause extrapyramidal reactions, including pseudoparkinsonism, acute dystonic reactions, akathisia, and tardive dyskinesia (risk of these reactions is very low relative to other neuroleptics). May be associated with neuroleptic malignant syndrome (NMS).

Adverse Reactions

>10%: Central nervous system: Headache, somnolence, insomnia, agitation, nervousness, hostility, dizziness

1% to 10%:

Cardiovascular: Postural hypotension, tachycardia, hypotension, peripheral edema

Central nervous system: Dystonic reactions, parkinsonian events, amnesia, euphoria, stuttering, akathisia, anxiety, personality changes, fever

Dermatologic: Rash

Gastrointestinal: Xerostomia, constipation, abdominal pain, weight gain, increased appetite

Genitourinary: Premenstrual syndrome

Neuromuscular & skeletal: Arthralgia, neck rigidity, twitching, hypertonia, tremor

Ocular: Amblyopia

Respiratory: Rhinitis, cough, pharyngitis

<1% (Limited to important or life-threatening): Diabetes mellitus, hyperglycemia, neuroleptic malignant syndrome, priapism, seizures, tardive dyskinesia

Drug Interactions

Cytochrome P450 Effect: CYP1A2 enzyme substrate, CYP2C19 enzyme substrate (minor), and CYP2D6 enzyme substrate (minor)

Increased Effect/Toxicity: Olanzapine levels may be increased by CYP1A2 inhibitors such as cimetidine and fluvoxamine. Sedations from olanzapine is increased with ethanol or other CNS depressants. The risk of hypotension and orthostatic hypotension from olanzapine is increased by concurrent antihypertensives.

Decreased Effect: Olanzapine levels may be decreased by cytochrome P450 enzyme inducers such as rifampin, omeprazole, and carbamazepine (also cigarette smoking). Olanzapine may antagonize the effects of levodopa and dopamine agonists.

Ethanol/Nutrition/Herb Interactions

Ethanol: Avoid ethanol (may increase CNS depression).

Herb/Nutraceutical: Avoid dong quai, St John's wort (may also cause photosensitization). Avoid kava kava, gotu kola, valerian, St John's wort (may increase CNS depression).

Stability Store at room temperature (20°C to 25°C); protect from light

Mechanism of Action Olanzapine is a thienobenzodiazepine neuroleptic; thought to work by antagonizing dopamine and serotonin activities. It is a selective monoaminergic antagonist with high affinity binding to serotonin 5-HT$_{2A}$ and 5-HT$_{2C}$, dopamine D$_{1-4}$, muscarinic M$_{1-5}$, histamine H$_1$- and alpha$_1$-adrenergic receptor sites. Olanzapine binds weakly to GABA-A, BZD, and beta-adrenergic receptors.

Pharmacodynamics/Kinetics Tablets and orally-disintegrating tablets are bioequivalent

Onset of action: Therapeutic: ≥1 week

Absorption: Readily absorbed
Protein binding: 93%
Metabolism: Extensively hepatic (40%); first-pass effect
Half-life elimination: 21-54 hours
Time to peak: ~6 hours
Excretion: Urine (57%); feces (30%)

Usual Dosage Oral:
Children: Schizophrenia/bipolar disorder: Initial: 2.5 mg/day; titrate as necessary to 20 mg/day (0.12-0.29 mg/kg/day)
Adults:
Schizophrenia: Usual starting dose: 5-10 mg once daily; increase to 10 mg once daily within 5-7 days, thereafter adjust by 5-10 mg/day at 1-week intervals, up to a maximum of 20 mg/day; doses of 30-50 mg/day have been used; typical dosage range: 10-30 mg/day
Bipolar mania: Usual starting dose: 10-15 mg once daily; increase by 5 mg/day at intervals of not less than 24 hours; maximum dose: 20 mg/day
Elderly: Schizophrenia: Usual starting dose: 2.5 mg/day, increase as clinically indicated and monitor blood pressure; typical dosage range: 2.5-10 mg/day

Administration Orally-disintegrating tablets: Remove from foil blister by peeling back (do not push tablet through the foil); place tablet in mouth immediately upon removal; tablet dissolves rapidly in saliva and may be swallowed with or without liquid

Dosage Forms
Tablet (Zyprexa®): 2.5 mg, 5 mg, 7.5 mg, 10 mg, 15 mg, 20 mg
Tablet, orally-disintegrating (Zyprexa® Zydis®): 5 mg, 10 mg, 15 mg, 20 mg

♦ **Oleovitamin A** see Vitamin A on page 1421

Olopatadine (oh loe pa TA deen)

U.S. Brand Names Patanol®
Canadian Brand Names Patanol®
Therapeutic Category Antihistamine; Ophthalmic Agent, Miscellaneous
Use Treatment of the signs and symptoms of allergic conjunctivitis
Pregnancy Risk Factor C
Contraindications Hypersensitivity to olopatadine hydrochloride or any component of the formulation
Adverse Reactions
>5%: Central nervous system: Headache (7%)
<5%:
Central nervous system: Weakness, cold syndrome
Gastrointestinal: Taste perversion
Ocular: Burning, stinging, dry eyes, foreign body sensation, hyperemia, keratitis, eyelid edema, itching
Respiratory: Pharyngitis, rhinitis, sinusitis
Usual Dosage Adults: Ophthalmic: 1 to 2 drops in affected eye(s) twice daily every 6 to 8 hours; results from an environmental study demonstrated that olopatadine was effective when dosed twice daily for up to 6 weeks
Dosage Forms Solution, ophthalmic: 0.1% (5 mL)

Olsalazine (ole SAL a zeen)

U.S. Brand Names Dipentum®
Canadian Brand Names Dipentum®
Synonyms Olsalazine Sodium
Therapeutic Category 5-Aminosalicylic Acid Derivative; Anti-inflammatory Agent
Use Maintenance of remission of ulcerative colitis in patients intolerant to sulfasalazine
Pregnancy Risk Factor C
Contraindications Hypersensitivity to olsalazine, salicylates, or any component of the formulation
Warnings/Precautions Diarrhea is a common adverse effect of olsalazine; use with caution in patients with hypersensitivity to salicylates, sulfasalazine, or mesalamine
Adverse Reactions
>10%: Gastrointestinal: Diarrhea, cramps, abdominal pain
1% to 10%:
Central nervous system: Headache, fatigue, depression
Dermatologic: Rash, itching
Gastrointestinal: Nausea, heartburn, bloating, anorexia
Neuromuscular & skeletal: Arthralgia
<1% (Limited to important or life-threatening): Blood dyscrasias, cholestatic jaundice, cirrhosis, hepatic necrosis, hepatitis, jaundice, Kawasaki-like syndrome
Overdosage/Toxicology Symptoms include decreased motor activity and diarrhea.
Drug Interactions
Increased Effect/Toxicity: Olsalazine has been reported to increase the prothrombin time in patients taking warfarin.
Mechanism of Action The mechanism of action appears to be topical rather than systemic
Pharmacodynamics/Kinetics
Absorption: <3%; very little intact olsalazine is systemically absorbed
Protein binding, plasma: >99%
Metabolism: Mostly by colonic bacteria to active drug, 5-aminosalicylic acid
Half-life elimination: Olsalazine: 56 minutes
Time to peak: ~1 hour
Excretion: Primarily feces
Usual Dosage Adults: Oral: 1 g/day in 2 divided doses
Dietary Considerations Administer with food, increases residence of drug in body.
Test Interactions ↑ ALT, AST (S)
(Continued)

Olsalazine (Continued)

Patient Information Take with food in evenly divided doses; report any sign of allergic reaction including rash

Nursing Implications Monitor stool frequency

Dosage Forms Capsule, as sodium: 250 mg

♦ **Olsalazine Sodium** *see* Olsalazine *on page 1007*

♦ **Olux™** *see* Clobetasol *on page 311*

Omeprazole (oh ME pray zol)

Related Information

Helicobacter pylori Treatment *on page 1668*

U.S. Brand Names Prilosec®

Canadian Brand Names Prilosec®

Therapeutic Category Gastric Acid Secretion Inhibitor; Proton Pump Inhibitor

Use Short-term (4-8 weeks) treatment of active duodenal ulcer disease or active benign gastric ulcer; treatment of heartburn and other symptoms associated with gastroesophageal reflux disease (GERD); short-term (4-8 weeks) treatment of endoscopically-diagnosed erosive esophagitis; maintenance healing of erosive esophagitis; long-term treatment of pathological hypersecretory conditions; as part of a multidrug regimen for *H. pylori* eradication to reduce the risk of duodenal ulcer recurrence

Unlabeled/Investigational Use Healing NSAID-induced ulcers; prevention of NSAID-induced ulcers

Pregnancy Risk Factor C

Pregnancy/Breast-Feeding Implications Clinical effects on the fetus: Crosses the placenta. Excretion in breast milk is unknown; use caution.

Contraindications Hypersensitivity to omeprazole or any component of the formulation

Warnings/Precautions In long-term (2-year) studies in rats, omeprazole produced a dose-related increase in gastric carcinoid tumors. While available endoscopic evaluations and histologic examinations of biopsy specimens from human stomachs have not detected a risk from short-term exposure to omeprazole, further human data on the effect of sustained hypochlorhydria and hypergastrinemia are needed to rule out the possibility of an increased risk for the development of tumors in humans receiving long-term therapy. Bioavailability may be increased in the elderly.

Adverse Reactions

1% to 10%:

Central nervous system: Headache (7%), dizziness (2%)

Dermatologic: Rash (2%)

Gastrointestinal: Diarrhea (3%), abdominal pain (2%), nausea (2%), vomiting (2%), constipation (1%)

Neuromuscular & skeletal: Weakness (1%), back pain (1%)

Respiratory: Upper respiratory infection (2%), cough (1%)

<1% (Limited to important or life-threatening): Agranulocytosis, alopecia, angina, angioedema, erythema multiforme, esophageal candidiasis, gynecomastia, hallucinations, hemifacial dysesthesia, hemolytic anemia, hepatic encephalopathy, hepatic failure, hepatic necrosis, hyponatremia, interstitial nephritis, jaundice, leukocytosis, mucosal atrophy (tongue), neutropenia, pancreatitis, pancytopenia, paresthesia, psychic disturbance, somnolence, Stevens-Johnson syndrome, thrombocytopenia, toxic epidermal necrolysis, urticaria, vertigo

Overdosage/Toxicology Limited experience with human overdose. Symptoms include confusion, drowsiness, blurred vision, tachycardia, nausea, flushing, diaphoresis, headache, and dry mouth. Treatment is symptom directed and supportive.

Drug Interactions

Cytochrome P450 Effect: CYP2C8, 2C9, 2C18, 2C19, and 3A3/4 enzyme substrate; CYP1A2 enzyme inducer; CYP2C8, 2C9, and 2C19 enzyme inhibitor; CYP3A3/4 enzyme inhibitor (weak)

Increased Effect/Toxicity: Omeprazole may increase the half-life of diazepam, digoxin, phenytoin, warfarin, and other drugs metabolized by the liver.

Decreased Effect: The clinical effect of ketoconazole, itraconazole, and other drugs dependent upon acid for absorption is reduced. Theophylline clearance is increased slightly.

Ethanol/Nutrition/Herb Interactions

Ethanol: Avoid ethanol (may cause gastric mucosal irritation).

Food: Food delays absorption.

Herb/Nutraceutical: St John's wort may decrease omeprazole levels.

Stability Omeprazole stability is a function of pH; it is rapidly degraded in acidic media, but has acceptable stability under alkaline conditions. Prilosec® is supplied as capsules for oral administration; each capsule contains omeprazole in the form of enteric coated granules to inhibit omeprazole degradation by gastric acidity; therefore, the manufacturer recommends against extemporaneously preparing it in an oral liquid form for administration via an NG tube.

Mechanism of Action Suppresses gastric acid secretion by inhibiting the parietal cell H+/K+ ATP pump

Pharmacodynamics/Kinetics

Onset of action: Antisecretory: ~1 hour

Peak effect: 2 hours

Duration: 72 hours

Protein binding: 95%

Metabolism: Extensively hepatic

Half-life elimination: 0.5-1 hour

Usual Dosage Adults: Oral:

Active duodenal ulcer: 20 mg/day for 4-8 weeks

Gastric ulcers: 40 mg/day for 4-8 weeks

Symptomatic GERD: 20 mg/day for up to 4 weeks

Erosive esophagitis: 20 mg/day for 4-8 weeks

Helicobacter pylori eradication: Dose varies with regimen: 20 mg once daily **or** 40 mg/day as single dose or in 2 divided doses; requires combination therapy with antibiotics

Pathological hypersecretory conditions: Initial: 60 mg once daily; doses up to 120 mg 3 times/day have been administered; administer daily doses >80 mg in divided doses

Dietary Considerations Should be on an empty stomach.

Administration Capsule should be swallowed whole. Do not chew, crush, or open. May be opened and contents added to applesauce. Administration via NG tube should be in an acidic juice.

Patient Information Take before eating; do not chew, crush, or open capsule

Nursing Implications Capsule should be swallowed whole; not chewed, crushed, or opened

Dosage Forms Capsule, delayed release: 10 mg, 20 mg, 40 mg

Extemporaneous Preparations A 2 mg/mL oral omeprazole solution (Simplified Omeprazole Solution) can be prepared with five omeprazole 20 mg capsules and 50 mL 8.4% sodium bicarbonate. Empty capsules into beaker. Add sodium bicarbonate solution. Gently stir (about 15 minutes) until a white suspension is formed. Transfer to amber-colored syringe or bottle. Stable for 14 days at room temperature or for 30 days under refrigeration.

DiGiancinto JL, Olsen KM, Bergman KL, et al, "Stability of Suspension Formulations of Lansoprazole and Omeprazole Stored in Amber-Colored Plastic Oral Syringes," *Ann Pharmacother*, 2000, 34:600-5.

Quercia R, Fan C, Liu X, et al, "Stability of Omeprazole in an Extemporaneously Prepared Oral Liquid," *Am J Health Syst Pharm*, 1997, 54:1833-6.

Sharma V, "Comparison of 24-hour Intragastric pH Using Four Liquid Formulations of Lansoprazole and Omeprazole," *Am J Health Syst Pharm*, 1999, 56(Suppl 4):S18-21.

♦ **Omnicef**® *see* Cefdinir *on page 241*

♦ **Oncaspar**® *see* Pegaspargase *on page 1043*

♦ **Oncotice™ (Can)** *see* BCG Vaccine *on page 148*

♦ **Oncovin**® *see* VinCRIStine *on page 1417*

Ondansetron (on DAN se tron)

U.S. Brand Names Zofran®; Zofran® ODT

Canadian Brand Names Zofran®; Zofran® ODT

Synonyms Ondansetron Hydrochloride

Therapeutic Category Antiemetic, Serotonin Antagonist; 5-HT$_3$ Receptor Antagonist; Serotonin Antagonist

Use Prevention of nausea and vomiting associated with moderately to highly emetogenic cancer chemotherapy; radiotherapy in patients receiving total body irradiation or fractions to the abdomen; postoperatively, when nausea and vomiting should be avoided

Unlabeled/Investigational Use Treatment of early-onset alcoholism

Pregnancy Risk Factor B

Pregnancy/Breast-Feeding Implications Clinical effects on the fetus: No data available on crossing the placenta; no effects on the fetus from two case reports. Excretion in breast milk unknown; opportunity for use is minimal.

Contraindications Hypersensitivity to ondansetron, other selective 5-HT$_3$ antagonists, or any component of the formulation

Warnings/Precautions Ondansetron should be used on a scheduled basis, not on an "as needed" (PRN) basis, since data supports the use of this drug in the prevention of nausea and vomiting and not in the rescue of nausea and vomiting. Ondansetron should only be used in the first 24-48 hours of receiving chemotherapy. Data does not support any increased efficacy of ondansetron in delayed nausea and vomiting. Does not stimulate gastric or intestinal peristalsis; may mask progressive ileus and/or gastric distension. Orally-disintegrating tablets contain phenylalanine.

Adverse Reactions

>10%:

Cardiovascular: Malaise/fatigue (9% to 13%)

Central nervous system: Headache (9% to 27%)

1% to 10%:

Central nervous system: Drowsiness (8%), fever (2% to 8%), dizziness (4% to 7%), anxiety (6%), cold sensation (2%)

Dermatologic: Pruritus (2% to 5%), rash (1%)

Gastrointestinal: Constipation (6% to 9%), diarrhea (3% to 7%)

Genitourinary: Gynecological disorder (7%), urinary retention (5%)

Hepatic: Increased ALT/AST (1% to 2%)

Local: Injection site reaction (4%)

Neuromuscular & skeletal: Paresthesia (2%)

Respiratory: Hypoxia (9%)

<1% (Limited to important or life-threatening): Angioedema, anaphylaxis, angina, bronchospasm, cardiopulmonary arrest, dyspnea, dystonic reactions, EKG changes, extrapyramidal reactions, grand mal seizures, hiccups, hypersensitivity reactions, hypokalemia, hypotension, laryngeal edema, laryngospasm, oculogyric crisis, shock, stridor, tachycardia, vascular occlusive events

Overdosage/Toxicology Sudden transient blindness, severe constipation, hypotension, and vasovagal episode with transient secondary heart block have been reported in some cases of overdose. I.V. doses up to 252 mg/day have been inadvertently given without adverse effects. There is no specific antidote. Treatment is symptom directed and supportive.

Drug Interactions

Cytochrome P450 Effect: CYP1A2, 2D6, 2E1, and 3A3/4 enzyme substrate

Increased Effect/Toxicity: Increased toxicity: CYP1A2, 2D6, 2E1, and 3A3/4 enzyme inhibitors (eg, cimetidine, allopurinol, and disulfiram) may change the clearance of ondansetron; monitor

(Continued)

ONDANSETRON

Ondansetron *(Continued)*

Decreased Effect: Decreased effect: CYP1A2, 2D6, 2E1, and 3A3/4 enzyme inducers (eg, barbiturates, carbamazepine, rifampin, phenytoin, and phenylbutazone) may change the clearance of ondansetron; monitor

Ethanol/Nutrition/Herb Interactions

Food: Food increases the extent of absorption. The C_{max} and T_{max} do not change much.

Herb/Nutraceutical: St John's wort may decrease ondansetron levels.

Stability

Oral solution: Store between 15°C and 30°C (59°F and 86°F); protect from light

Tablet: Store between 2°C and 30°C (36°F and 86°F)

Vial: Store between 2°C and 30°C (36°F and 86°F); protect from light

Reconstitution: Vial: Prior to I.V. infusion, dilute in 50 mL D_5W or NS; solution is stable for 48 hours at room temperature; does not need protection from light

Do not mix injection with alkaline solutions; precipitate may form

Mechanism of Action Selective 5-HT$_3$-receptor antagonist, blocking serotonin, both peripherally on vagal nerve terminals and centrally in the chemoreceptor trigger zone

Pharmacodynamics/Kinetics

Onset of action: ~30 minutes

Protein binding, plasma: 70% to 76%

Metabolism: Extensively hepatic via hydroxylation, followed by glucuronide or sulfate conjugation; CYP1A2, CYP2D6 and CYP3A4 substrate

Bioavailability: Oral: 56%

Half-life elimination: Children <15 years: 2-3 hours, adults: 3-6 hours

Time to peak: Oral: ~2 hours

Excretion: Urine (<10% as unchanged drug); feces

Usual Dosage

Children:

I.V.:

Chemotherapy-induced emesis: 4-18 years: 0.15 mg/kg/dose administered 30 minutes prior to chemotherapy, 4 and 8 hours after the first dose

Postoperative nausea and vomiting: 2-12 years:

≤40 kg: 0.1 mg/kg

>40 kg: 4 mg

Oral: Chemotherapy-induced emesis of moderately-emetogenic agents:

4-11 years: 4 mg 30 minutes before chemotherapy; repeat 4 and 8 hours after initial dose, then 4 mg every 8 hours for 1-2 days after chemotherapy completed

≥12 years: Refer to adult dosing.

Adults:

I.V.: Chemotherapy-induced emesis: Administer either three 0.15 mg/kg doses or a single 32 mg dose:

Three-dose regimen: Initial dose is given 30 minutes prior to chemotherapy with subsequent doses administered 4 and 8 hours after the first dose

Single-dose regimen: 32 mg is infused over 15 minutes beginning 30 minutes before the start of emetogenic chemotherapy

I.M., I.V.: Postoperative nausea and vomiting: 4 mg as a single dose approximately 30 minutes before the end of anesthesia, or as treatment if vomiting occurs after surgery

Oral:

Chemotherapy-induced emesis:

Highly-emetogenic agents/single-day therapy: 24 mg given 30 minutes prior to the start of therapy

Moderately-emetogenic agents: 8 mg every 8 hours for 2 doses beginning 30 minutes before chemotherapy, then 8 mg every 12 hours for 1-2 days after chemotherapy completed

Total body irradiation: 8 mg 1-2 hours before each fraction of radiotherapy administered each day

Single high-dose fraction radiotherapy to abdomen: 8 mg 1-2 hours before irradiation, then 8 mg every 8 hours after first dose for 1-2 days after completion of radiotherapy

Daily fractionated radiotherapy to abdomen: 8 mg 1-2 hours before irradiation, then 8 mg every 8 hours after first dose for each day of radiotherapy

Postoperative nausea and vomiting: 16 mg given 1 hour prior to induction of anesthesia

Elderly: No dosing adjustment required

Dosage adjustment in renal impairment: No dosing adjustment required

Dosage adjustment in hepatic impairment: Maximum daily dose: 8 mg in patients with severe liver disease (Child-Pugh score ≥10)

Dietary Considerations Take without regard to meals.

Potassium: Hypokalemia; monitor potassium serum concentration

Orally-disintegrating tablet contains <0.03 mg phenylalanine

Administration

Oral: Oral dosage forms should be administered 30 minutes prior to chemotherapy; 1-2 hours before radiotherapy; 1 hour prior to the induction of anesthesia

Orally-disintegrating tablets: Do not remove from blister until needed. Peel backing off the blister, do not push tablet through. Using dry hands, place tablet on tongue and allow to dissolve. Swallow with saliva.

I.M.: Should be administered undiluted

I.V. push: Administer undiluted over 2-5 minutes; the I.V. preparation has been successful when administered orally

IVPB: Infuse diluted solution over 15 minutes

Patient Information Orally-disintegrating tablets: Do not remove from blister until needed. Peel backing off the blister, do not push tablet through. Using dry hands, place tablet on tongue and allow to dissolve. Swallow with saliva. Contains <0.03 mg phenylalanine/tablet.

Nursing Implications Oral dosage forms should be given 30 minutes prior to chemotherapy; 1-2 hours before radiotherapy; 1 hour prior to the induction of anesthesia

Dosage Forms
Injection, as hydrochloride (Zofran®): 2 mg/mL (2 mL, 20 mL)
Injection, as hydrochloride [premixed] (Zofran®): 32 mg/50 mL
Solution, as hydrochloride (Zofran®): 4 mg/5 mL (50 mL) [strawberry flavor]
Tablet, as hydrochloride (Zofran®): 4 mg, 8 mg, 24 mg
Tablet, orally disintegrating (Zofran® ODT): 4 mg, 8 mg [contains <0.03 mg phenylalanine/tablet]

Extemporaneous Preparations A 0.8 mg/mL syrup may be made by crushing ten 8 mg tablets; flaking of the tablet coating occurs. Mix thoroughly with 50 mL of the suspending vehicle, Ora-Plus® (Paddock), in 5 mL increments. Add sufficient volume of any of the following syrups: Cherry syrup USP, Syrpalta® (Humco), Ora-Sweet® (Paddock), or Ora-Sweet® Sugar-Free (Paddock) to make a final volume of 100 mL. Stability is 42 days refrigerated.

Trissel LA, "Trissel's Stability of Compounded Formulations," American Pharmaceutical Association, 1996.

- ◆ **Ondansetron Hydrochloride** *see Ondansetron on page 1009*
- ◆ **ONTAK®** *see Denileukin Diftitox on page 374*
- ◆ **OPC13013** *see Cilostazol on page 292*
- ◆ **o,p'-DDD** *see Mitotane on page 924*
- ◆ **Operand® [OTC]** *see Povidone-Iodine on page 1114*
- ◆ **Ophthetic®** *see Proparacaine on page 1144*
- ◆ **Ophthifluor®** *see Fluorescein Sodium on page 573*
- ◆ **Ophtho-Dipivefrin™ (Can)** *see Dipivefrin on page 422*
- ◆ **Ophtho-Tate® (Can)** *see PrednisoLONE on page 1122*
- ◆ **Opium and Belladonna** *see Belladonna and Opium on page 151*

Opium Tincture (OH pee um TING chur)
Synonyms DTO; Opium Tincture, Deodorized
Therapeutic Category Analgesic, Narcotic; Antidiarrheal
Use Treatment of diarrhea or relief of pain
Restrictions C-II
Pregnancy Risk Factor B/D (prolonged use or high doses at term)
Contraindications Hypersensitivity to morphine sulfate or any component of the formulation; increased intracranial pressure; severe respiratory depression; severe hepatic or renal insufficiency; pregnancy (prolonged use or high dosages near term)
Warnings/Precautions Opium shares the toxic potential of opiate agonists, and usual precautions of opiate agonist therapy should be observed; some preparations contain sulfites which may cause allergic reactions; infants <3 months of age are more susceptible to respiratory depression, use with caution and generally in reduced doses in this age group; this is **not** paregoric, dose accordingly
Adverse Reactions Frequency not defined.
Cardiovascular: Palpitations, hypotension, bradycardia, peripheral vasodilation,
Central nervous system: Drowsiness, dizziness, restlessness, headache, malaise, CNS depression, increased intracranial pressure, insomnia, mental depression
Gastrointestinal: Nausea, vomiting, constipation, anorexia, stomach cramps, biliary tract spasm
Genitourinary: Decreased urination, urinary tract spasm
Neuromuscular & skeletal: Weakness
Ocular: Miosis
Respiratory: Respiratory depression
Miscellaneous: Histamine release, physical and psychological dependence
Overdosage/Toxicology Primary attention should be directed to ensuring adequate respiratory exchange; opiate agonist-induced respiratory depression may be reversed with parenteral naloxone hydrochloride. Treatment includes naloxone 2 mg I.V. (0.01 mg/kg for children), with repeat administration as necessary, up to a total of 10 mg.
Drug Interactions
Increased Effect/Toxicity: Opium tincture and CNS depressants, MAO inhibitors, tricyclic antidepressants may potentiate the effects of opiate agonists (eg, codeine, morphine, etc). Dextroamphetamine may enhance the analgesic effect of opiate agonists.
Decreased Effect: Phenothiazines may antagonize the analgesic effect of opiate agonists.
Ethanol/Nutrition/Herb Interactions Ethanol: Avoid ethanol (may increase CNS depression).
Stability Protect from light
Mechanism of Action Contains many narcotic alkaloids including morphine; its mechanism for gastric motility inhibition is primarily due to this morphine content; it results in a decrease in digestive secretions, an increase in GI muscle tone, and therefore a reduction in GI propulsion
Pharmacodynamics/Kinetics
Duration: 4-5 hours
Absorption: Variable
Metabolism: Hepatic
Excretion: Urine
Usual Dosage Oral:
Children:
Diarrhea: 0.005-0.01 mL/kg/dose every 3-4 hours for a maximum of 6 doses/24 hours
Analgesia: 0.01-0.02 mL/kg/dose every 3-4 hours
Adults:
Diarrhea: 0.3-1 mL/dose every 2-6 hours to maximum of 6 mL/24 hours
Analgesia: 0.6-1.5 mL/dose every 3-4 hours
Monitoring Parameters Observe patient for excessive sedation, respiratory depression, implement safety measures, assist with ambulation
(Continued)

Opium Tincture *(Continued)*

Test Interactions ↑ aminotransferase [ALT (SGPT)/AST (SGOT)] (S)

Patient Information Avoid alcohol, may cause drowsiness, impair judgment, or coordination; may cause physical and psychological dependence with prolonged use

Nursing Implications Monitor patient for excessive sedation, respiratory depression, implement safety measures, assist with ambulation

Dosage Forms Liquid: 10% [0.6 mL equivalent to morphine 6 mg - with alcohol 19%]

♦ **Opium Tincture, Deodorized** *see* Opium Tincture *on page 1011*

Oprelvekin (oh PREL ve kin)

U.S. Brand Names Neumega®

Synonyms IL-11; Interleukin-11; Recombinant Human Interleukin-11; Recombinant Interleukin-11; rhIL-11; rIL-11

Therapeutic Category Platelet Growth Factor

Use Prevention of severe thrombocytopenia and the reduction of the need for platelet transfusions following myelosuppressive chemotherapy in patients with nonmyeloid malignancies who are at high risk of severe thrombocytopenia.

Pregnancy Risk Factor C

Contraindications Hypersensitivity to oprelvekin or any component of the formulation

Warnings/Precautions Oprelvekin should be used cautiously in patients with conditions where expansion of plasma volume should be avoided (eg, left ventricular dysfunction, congestive heart failure, hypertension); cardiac arrhythmias or conduction defects, respiratory disease; history of thromboembolic problems; hepatic or renal dysfunction; not indicated following myeloablative chemotherapy. Per the manufacturer, should not be used in children, particularly those <12 years of age, except as part of a controlled clinical trial.

Adverse Reactions

>10%:

Cardiovascular: Atrial arrhythmias (12%), palpitations (14% to 24%), peripheral edema (60% to 75%), tachycardia (19% to 30%)

Central nervous system: Dizziness (38%), fatigue (30%), fever (36%), headache (41%), insomnia (33%)

Dermatologic: Rash (25%)

Endocrine & metabolic: Fluid retention

Gastrointestinal: Anorexia, nausea (50% to 77%), vomiting

Hematologic: Anemia (100%), probably a dilutional phenomena; appears within 3 days of initiation of therapy, resolves in about 2 weeks after cessation of oprelvekin

Neuromuscular & skeletal: Arthralgia, myalgias

Respiratory: Dyspnea (48%), pleural effusions (10%)

1% to 10%:

Cardiovascular: Syncope (6% to 13%)

Gastrointestinal: Weight gain (5%)

Overdosage/Toxicology Doses of oprelvekin >50 mcg/kg may be associated with an increased incidence of cardiovascular events. If an overdose is administered, discontinue oprelvekin and closely observe for signs of toxicity. Base reinstitution of therapy on individual patient factors (evidence of toxicity and continued need for therapy).

Stability Store vials of lyophilized oprelvekin and diluent under refrigeration (2°C to 8°C/36°F to 46°F); do not freeze.

Reconstitute oprelvekin with 1 mL of sterile water for injection, USP (without preservative). Direct at the side of vial and swirl the contents gently. Avoid excessive or vigorous agitation. Reconstituted solution contains 5 mg/mL of oprelvekin. Use reconstituted oprelvekin within 3 hours of reconstitution and store in the vial at either 2°C to 8°C/36°F to 46°F or room temperature (≤25°C/70°F). Do not freeze or shake reconstituted solution.

Mechanism of Action Oprelvekin stimulates multiple stages of megakaryocytopoiesis and thrombopoiesis, resulting in proliferation of megakaryocyte progenitors and megakaryocyte maturation

Pharmacodynamics/Kinetics

Metabolism: Uncertain

Half-life elimination: Terminal: 5-8 hours

Time to peak, serum: 1-6 hours

Excretion: Urine (primarily as metabolites)

Usual Dosage S.C.:

Children: 75-100 mcg/kg once daily for 10-21 days (until postnadir platelet count ≥50,000 cells/μL)

Note: The manufacturer states that, until efficacy/toxicity parameters are established, the use of oprelvekin in pediatric patients (particularly those <12 years of age) should be restricted to use in controlled clinical trials.

Adults: 50 mcg/kg once daily for 10-21 days (until postnadir platelet count ≥50,000 cells/μL)

Administration Subcutaneously in either the abdomen, thigh, or hip (or upper arm if not self-injected). Initiate dosing 6-24 hours after the completion of chemotherapy. Discontinue treatment with oprelvekin ≥2 days before starting the next planned cycle of chemotherapy.

Monitoring Parameters Monitor fluid balance during therapy, appropriate medical management is advised. If a diuretic is used, carefully monitor fluid and electrolyte balance. Obtain a CBC prior to chemotherapy and at regular intervals during therapy. Monitor platelet counts during the time of the expected nadir and until adequate recovery has occurred (postnadir counts ≥50,000 cells/μL).

Test Interactions Decrease in hemoglobin concentration, serum concentration of albumin and other proteins (result of expansion of plasma volume)

Patient Information Report any swelling in the arms or legs (peripheral edema), shortness of breath (congestive failure, anemia), irregular heartbeat, headaches

Dosage Forms Powder for injection, lyophilized: 5 mg

♦ **Optho-Bunolol® (Can)** *see* Levobunolol *on page 788*

- **Opticrom**® *see* Cromolyn Sodium *on page 337*
- **Opticyl**® *see* Tropicamide *on page 1384*
- **Optimine**® *see* Azatadine *on page 135*
- **Optimyxin**® **(Can)** *see* Bacitracin and Polymyxin B *on page 143*
- **Optimyxin Plus**® **(Can)** *see* Bacitracin and Polymyxin B *on page 143*
- **Optimyxin Plus**® **(Can)** *see* Neomycin, Polymyxin B, and Gramicidin *on page 969*
- **OptiPranolol**® *see* Metipranolol *on page 899*
- **Optivar**™ *see* Azelastine *on page 137*
- **Orabase**®**-B [OTC]** *see* Benzocaine *on page 154*
- **Orabase**® **HCA** *see* Hydrocortisone *on page 682*
- **Orabase**® **Plain [OTC]** *see* Gelatin, Pectin, and Methylcellulose *on page 622*
- **Orabase**® **With Benzocaine [OTC]** *see* Benzocaine, Gelatin, Pectin, and Sodium Carboxy-methylcellulose *on page 156*
- **Oracit**® *see* Sodium Citrate and Citric Acid *on page 1246*
- **Oracort (Can)** *see* Triamcinolone *on page 1366*
- **Orafen (Can)** *see* Ketoprofen *on page 763*
- **Orajel**® **[OTC]** *see* Benzocaine *on page 154*
- **Orajel**® **Baby [OTC]** *see* Benzocaine *on page 154*
- **Orajel**® **Baby Nighttime [OTC]** *see* Benzocaine *on page 154*
- **Orajel**® **Maximum Strength [OTC]** *see* Benzocaine *on page 154*
- **Orajel**® **Perioseptic**® **[OTC]** *see* Carbamide Peroxide *on page 224*
- **Oramorph SR**™ *see* Morphine Sulfate *on page 936*
- **Orap**™ *see* Pimozide *on page 1085*
- **Orasol**® **[OTC]** *see* Benzocaine *on page 154*
- **Orasone**® *see* PredniSONE *on page 1124*
- **Orazinc**® **[OTC]** *see* Zinc Supplements *on page 1439*
- **Orciprenaline Sulfate** *see* Metaproterenol *on page 872*
- **Oretic**® *see* Hydrochlorothiazide *on page 674*
- **Oreton**® **Methyl** *see* MethylTESTOSTERone *on page 898*
- **Orfadin**® *see* Nitisinone *on page 986*
- **ORG 946** *see* Rocuronium *on page 1209*
- **Organidin**® **NR** *see* Guaifenesin *on page 645*
- **Orgaran**® *see* Danaparoid *on page 360*
- **ORG NC 45** *see* Vecuronium *on page 1409*
- **Orinase Diagnostic**® *see* TOLBUTamide *on page 1344*
- **ORLAAM**® *see* Levomethadyl Acetate Hydrochloride *on page 795*

Orlistat (OR li stat)

Related Information
Obesity Treatment Guidelines for Adults *on page 1685*

U.S. Brand Names Xenical®

Canadian Brand Names Xenical®

Therapeutic Category Lipase Inhibitor

Use Management of obesity, including weight loss and weight management when used in conjunction with a reduced-calorie diet; reduce the risk of weight regain after prior weight loss; indicated for obese patients with an initial body mass index (BMI) ≥30 kg/m² or ≥27 kg/m² in the presence of other risk factors

Pregnancy Risk Factor B

Pregnancy/Breast-Feeding Implications There are no adequate and well-controlled studies of orlistat in pregnant women. Because animal reproductive studies are not always predictive of human response, orlistat is not recommended for use during pregnancy. Teratogenicity studies were conducted in rats and rabbits at doses up to 800 mg/kg/day. Neither study showed embryotoxicity or teratogenicity. This dose is 23 and 47 times the daily human dose calculated on a body surface area basis for rats and rabbits, respectively. It is not know if orlistat is secreted in human milk. Therefore, it should not be taken by nursing women.

Contraindications Hypersensitivity to orlistat or any component of the formulation; chronic malabsorption syndrome or cholestasis

Warnings/Precautions Patients should be advised to adhere to dietary guidelines; gastrointestinal adverse events may increase if taken with a diet high in fat (>30% total daily calories from fat). The daily intake of fat should be distributed over three main meals. If taken with any one meal very high in fat, the possibility of gastrointestinal effects increases. Patients should be counseled to take a multivitamin supplement that contains fat-soluble vitamins to ensure adequate nutrition because orlistat has been shown to reduce the absorption of some fat-soluble vitamins and beta-carotene. The supplement should be taken once daily at least 2 hours before or after the administration of orlistat (ie, bedtime). Some patients may develop increased levels of urinary oxalate following treatment; caution should be exercised when prescribing it to patients with a history of hyperoxaluria or calcium oxalate nephrolithiasis. As with any weight-loss agent, the potential exists for misuse in appropriate patient populations (eg, patients with anorexia nervosa or bulimia). Write and fill prescriptions carefully; confusion has occurred between Xenical® and Xeloda®.

Adverse Reactions
>10%:
  Central nervous system: Headache (31%)
  Gastrointestinal: Oily spotting (27%), abdominal pain/discomfort (26%), flatus with discharge (24%), fatty/oily stool (20%), fecal urgency (22%), oily evacuation (12%), increased defecation (11%)
  Neuromuscular & skeletal: Back pain (14%)
  Respiratory: Upper respiratory infection (38%)

(Continued)

Orlistat (Continued)

1% to 10%:
Central nervous system: Fatigue (7%), anxiety (5%), sleep disorder (4%)
Dermatologic: Dry skin (2%)
Endocrine & metabolic: Menstrual irregularities (10%)
Gastrointestinal: Fecal incontinence (8%), nausea (8%), infectious diarrhea (5%), rectal pain/discomfort (5%), vomiting (4%)
Neuromuscular & skeletal: Arthritis (5%), myalgia (4%)
Otic: Otitis (4%)
<1% (Limited to important or life-threatening): Allergic reactions, anaphylaxis, angioedema, pruritus, rash, urticaria

Overdosage/Toxicology Single doses of 800 mg and multiple doses up to 400 mg 3 times daily for 15 days have been studied in normal weight and obese patients, without significant adverse findings. In significant overdose, observation of the patient is recommended for 24 hours.

Drug Interactions
Decreased Effect: Vitamin K absorption may be decreased when taken with orlistat. Coadministration with cyclosporine may decrease plasma levels of cyclosporine.

Usual Dosage Oral: Adults: 120 mg 3 times/day with each main meal containing fat (during or up to 1 hour after the meal); omit dose if meal is occasionally missed or contains no fat. **Note:** A once-daily multivitamin containing the fat-soluble vitamins (A, D, E, and K) should be administered at least 2 hours prior to orlistat.

Monitoring Parameters Changes in coagulation parameters

Patient Information Patient should be on a nutritionally balanced, reduced-calorie diet that contains approximately 30% of calories from fat; daily intake of fat, carbohydrate, and protein should be distributed over the three main meals

Dosage Forms Capsule: 120 mg

♦ **Ornex® [OTC]** see Acetaminophen and Pseudoephedrine on page 25
♦ **Ornex® Maximum Strength [OTC]** see Acetaminophen and Pseudoephedrine on page 25

Orphenadrine (or FEN a dreen)

U.S. Brand Names Norflex™
Canadian Brand Names Norflex™; Rhoxal-orphendrine
Synonyms Orphenadrine Citrate
Therapeutic Category Anti-Parkinson's Agent, Anticholinergic; Skeletal Muscle Relaxant
Use Treatment of muscle spasm associated with acute painful musculoskeletal conditions; supportive therapy in tetanus
Pregnancy Risk Factor C
Contraindications Hypersensitivity to orphenadrine or any component of the formulation; glaucoma; GI obstruction; cardiospasm; myasthenia gravis
Warnings/Precautions Use with caution in patients with CHF or cardiac arrhythmias; some products contain sulfites

Adverse Reactions
>10%:
Central nervous system: Drowsiness, dizziness
Ocular: Blurred vision
1% to 10%:
Cardiovascular: Flushing of face, tachycardia, syncope
Dermatologic: Rash
Gastrointestinal: Nausea, vomiting, constipation
Genitourinary: Decreased urination
Neuromuscular & skeletal: Weakness
Ocular: Nystagmus, increased intraocular pressure
Respiratory: Nasal congestion
<1% (Limited to important or life-threatening): Aplastic anemia, hallucinations

Overdosage/Toxicology Symptoms include blurred vision, tachycardia, confusion, seizures, respiratory arrest, and dysrhythmias. There is no specific treatment for an antihistamine overdose, however, clinical toxicity is mostly due to anticholinergic effects. Anticholinesterase inhibitors may be useful by reducing acetylcholinesterase. Anticholinesterase inhibitors include physostigmine, neostigmine, pyridostigmine and edrophonium. For anticholinergic overdose with severe life-threatening symptoms, physostigmine 1-2 mg (0.5 mg or 0.02 mg/kg for children) slow I.V. may be given to reverse these effects. Lethal dose: 2-3 g. Treatment is symptomatic.

Drug Interactions
Cytochrome P450 Effect: CYP2B6, 2D6, and 3A3/4 enzyme substrate; CYP2B6 enzyme inhibitor
Increased Effect/Toxicity: Orphenadrine may increase potential for anticholinergic adverse effects of anticholinergic agents; includes drugs with high anticholinergic activity (diphenhydramine, TCAs, phenothiazines). Sedative effects of may be additive in concurrent use of orphenadrine and CNS depressants (monitor). Effects of levodopa may be decreased by orphenadrine. Monitor.

Ethanol/Nutrition/Herb Interactions
Ethanol: Avoid ethanol (may increase CNS depression).
Herb/Nutraceutical: St John's wort may decrease orphenadrine levels. Avoid valerian, St John's wort, kava kava, gotu kola (may increase CNS depression).

Mechanism of Action Indirect skeletal muscle relaxant thought to work by central atropine-like effects; has some euphorigenic and analgesic properties

Pharmacodynamics/Kinetics
Onset of effect: Peak effect: Oral: 2-4 hours
Duration: 4-6 hours
Protein binding: 20%
Metabolism: Extensive

Half-life elimination: 14-16 hours
Excretion: Primarily urine (8% as unchanged drug)
Usual Dosage Adults:
  Oral: 100 mg twice daily
  I.M., I.V.: 60 mg every 12 hours
Patient Information May cause drowsiness; swallow whole, do not crush or chew sustained release product; avoid alcohol, may impair coordination and judgment
Nursing Implications Do not crush sustained release drug product; raise bed rails, institute safety measures, assist with ambulation
Dosage Forms
  Injection, as citrate: 30 mg/mL (2 mL, 10 mL)
  Tablet, sustained release, as citrate: 100 mg

Orphenadrine, Aspirin, and Caffeine (or FEN a dreen, AS pir in, & KAF een)
U.S. Brand Names Norgesic™; Norgesic™ Forte
Canadian Brand Names Norgesic™; Norgesic™ Forte
Synonyms Aspirin, Orphenadrine, and Caffeine; Caffeine, Orphenadrine, and Aspirin
Therapeutic Category Skeletal Muscle Relaxant
Use Relief of discomfort associated with skeletal muscular conditions
Pregnancy Risk Factor D
Usual Dosage Oral: 1-2 tablets 3-4 times/day
Additional Information Complete prescribing information for this medication should be consulted for additional detail.
Dosage Forms
  Tablet:
    Norgesic™: Orphenadrine citrate 25 mg, aspirin 385 mg, and caffeine 30 mg
    Norgesic™ Forte: Orphenadrine citrate 50 mg, aspirin 770 mg, and caffeine 60 mg

Oseltamivir (oh sel TAM i vir)
U.S. Brand Names Tamiflu™
Canadian Brand Names Tamiflu™
Therapeutic Category Antiviral Agent, Influenza; Neuraminidase Inhibitor
Use Treatment of uncomplicated acute illness due to influenza (A or B) infection in adults and children >1 year of age who have been symptomatic for no more than 2 days; prophylaxis against influenza (A or B) infection in adults and adolescents ≥13 years of age
Pregnancy Risk Factor C
Pregnancy/Breast-Feeding Implications There are insufficient human data to determine the risk to a pregnant woman or developing fetus. Studies evaluating the effects on embryo-fetal development in rats and rabbits showed a dose-dependent increase in the rates of minor skeleton abnormalities in exposed offspring. The rate of each abnormality remained within the background rate of occurrence in the species studied. Oseltamivir and its metabolite are excreted in the breast milk of lactating rats. It is unknown if they appear in human milk.
Contraindications Hypersensitivity to oseltamivir or any component of the formulation
Warnings/Precautions Oseltamivir is not a substitute for the flu shot. Dosage adjustment is required for creatinine clearance between 10-30 mL/minute. Safety and efficacy in children (<1 year of age) have not been established for treatment regimens. Safety and efficacy have not been established for prophylactic use in patients <13 years of age. Also consider primary or concomitant bacterial infections. Safety and efficacy for treatment or prophylaxis in immunocompromised patients have not been established.
Adverse Reactions
As seen with **treatment** doses: 1% to 10%:
  Central nervous system: Insomnia (adults 1%), vertigo (1%)
  Gastrointestinal: Nausea (10%), vomiting (9%)
  Similar adverse effects were seen in **prophylactic** use, however, the incidence was generally less. The following reactions were seen more commonly with prophylactic use: Headache (20%), fatigue (8%), cough (6%), diarrhea (3%)
  <1% (Limited to important or life-threatening): Aggravation of diabetes, arrhythmia, confusion, hepatitis, pseudomembranous colitis, pyrexia, rash, seizure, swelling of face or tongue, toxic epidermal necrolysis, unstable angina.
Overdosage/Toxicology Single doses of 1000 mg resulted in nausea and vomiting.
  (Continued)

Oseltamivir *(Continued)*

Drug Interactions
Increased Effect/Toxicity: Cimetidine and amoxicillin have no effect on plasma concentrations. Probenecid increases oseltamivir carboxylate serum concentration by twofold. Dosage adjustments are not required.

Stability Capsules and powder for suspension: Store at 25°C (77°F). Once reconstituted, the suspension may be stored at room temperature or under refrigeration (2°C to 8°C / 36°F to 46°F); do not freeze; use within 10 days of preparation

Mechanism of Action Oseltamivir, a prodrug, is hydrolyzed to the active form, oseltamivir carboxylate. It is thought to inhibit influenza virus neuraminidase, with the possibility of alteration of virus particle aggregation and release. In clinical studies of the influenza virus, 1.3% of post-treatment isolates had decreased neuraminidase susceptibility to oseltamivir carboxylate.

Pharmacodynamics/Kinetics
Absorption: Well absorbed

Distribution: V_d: 23-26 L (oseltamivir carboxylate)

Protein binding, plasma: Oseltamivir carboxylate: 3%; Oseltamivir: 42%

Metabolism: Hepatic, (90%) to oseltamivir carboxylate; neither the parent drug nor active metabolite has any effect on the P450 system.

Bioavailability: 75% reaches systemic circulation in active form

Half-life elimination: Oseltamivir carboxylate: 6-10 hours; similar in geriatrics (68-78 years)

Time to peak: C_{max}: Oseltamivir: 65 ng/mL; Oseltamivir carboxylate: 348 ng/mL

Excretion: Urine (as carboxylate metabolite)

Usual Dosage Oral:
Treatment: Initiate treatment within 2 days of onset of symptoms; duration of treatment: 5 days:

Children: 1-12 years:
≤15 kg: 30 mg twice daily
>15 kg - ≤23 kg: 45 mg twice daily
>23 kg - ≤40 kg: 60 mg twice daily
>40 kg: 75 mg twice daily

Adolescents and Adults: 75 mg twice daily

Prophylaxis: Adolescents and Adults: 75 mg once daily for at least 7 days; treatment should begin within 2 days of contact with an infected individual. During community outbreaks, dosing is 75 mg once daily. May be used for up to 6 weeks; duration of protection lasts for length of dosing period

Dosage adjustment in renal impairment:
Cl_{cr} 10-30 mL/minute:
Treatment: Reduce dose to 75 mg once daily for 5 days
Prophylaxis: 75 mg every other day
Cl_{cr} <10 mL/minute: Has not been studied

Dosage adjustment in hepatic impairment: Has not been evaluated

Elderly: No adjustments required

Dietary Considerations Take with or without food; take with food to improve tolerance.

Patient Information When used as treatment of influenza infection, take within 2 days of onset of flu symptoms (fever, cough, headache, fatigue, muscular weakness, and sore throat). When used as prevention of influenza infection, take every day during the "flu season" as instructed by your prescriber. This is not a substitute for the flu shot. Not recommended for pregnant or nursing women. For best results, do not miss doses.

Suspension: Shake well before using; may be stored under refrigeration or at room temperature. Use the oral syringe provided to measure appropriate dose.

Nursing Implications Have patient take with food to decrease the nausea associated with this medicine; administer at breakfast and dinner when used for treatment (dosing is once daily when used for prophylaxis). Shake suspension well before using; may be stored under refrigeration or at room temperature.

Dosage Forms
Capsule, as phosphate: 75 mg (blister package 10)
Powder for oral suspension: 12 mg/mL (100 mL) [tutti-frutti flavor]

- ◆ Osmitrol® *see Mannitol on page 838*
- ◆ Ostoforte® (Can) *see Ergocalciferol on page 481*
- ◆ Otic-Care® *see Neomycin, Polymyxin B, and Hydrocortisone on page 969*
- ◆ Otic Domeboro® *see Aluminum Acetate and Acetic Acid on page 62*
- ◆ Otobiotic® *see Polymyxin B and Hydrocortisone on page 1103*
- ◆ Otocort® *see Neomycin, Polymyxin B, and Hydrocortisone on page 969*
- ◆ Otosporin® *see Neomycin, Polymyxin B, and Hydrocortisone on page 969*
- ◆ Ovcon® *see Ethinyl Estradiol and Norethindrone on page 522*
- ◆ Over-the-Counter Products *see page 1729*
- ◆ Ovide™ *see Malathion on page 837*
- ◆ Ovidrel® *see Chorionic Gonadotropin (Recombinant) on page 289*
- ◆ Ovral® *see Ethinyl Estradiol and Norgestrel on page 528*
- ◆ Ovrette® *see Norgestrel on page 995*

Oxacillin (oks a SIL in)
Related Information
Antibiotic Treatment of Adults With Infective Endocarditis *on page 1585*
Community-Acquired Pneumonia in Adults *on page 1603*

U.S. Brand Names Bactocill®
Canadian Brand Names Bactocill®
Synonyms Methylphenyl Isoxazolyl Penicillin; Oxacillin Sodium
Therapeutic Category Antibiotic, Penicillin

Use Treatment of infections such as osteomyelitis, septicemia, endocarditis, and CNS infections caused by susceptible strains of *Staphylococcus*

Pregnancy Risk Factor B

Contraindications Hypersensitivity to oxacillin or other penicillins or any component of the formulation

Warnings/Precautions Elimination rate will be slow in neonates; modify dosage in patients with renal impairment and in the elderly; use with caution in patients with cephalosporin hypersensitivity

Adverse Reactions

1% to 10%: Gastrointestinal: Nausea, diarrhea

<1% (Limited to important or life-threatening): Acute interstitial nephritis, agranulocytosis, eosinophilia, fever, hematuria, hepatotoxicity, increased AST, leukopenia, neutropenia, rash, serum sickness-like reactions, thrombocytopenia, vomiting

Overdosage/Toxicology Symptoms of penicillin overdose include neuromuscular hypersensitivity (agitation, hallucinations, asterixis, encephalopathy, confusion, and seizures) and electrolyte imbalance (with potassium or sodium salts), especially in renal failure. Hemodialysis may be helpful to aid in the removal of the drug from the blood, otherwise most treatment is supportive or symptom directed.

Drug Interactions

Increased Effect/Toxicity: Probenecid increases penicillin levels. Penicillins and anticoagulants may increase the effect of anticoagulants.

Decreased Effect: Efficacy of oral contraceptives may be reduced when taken with oxacillin.

Ethanol/Nutrition/Herb Interactions Food: Oxacillin serum levels may be decreased if taken with food.

Stability Reconstituted parenteral solution is stable for 3 days at room temperature and 7 days when refrigerated; for I.V. infusion in NS or D_5W, solution is stable for 24 hours at room temperature

Mechanism of Action Inhibits bacterial cell wall synthesis by binding to one or more of the penicillin binding proteins (PBPs); which in turn inhibits the final transpeptidation step of peptidoglycan synthesis in bacterial cell walls, thus inhibiting cell wall biosynthesis. Bacteria eventually lyse due to ongoing activity of cell wall autolytic enzymes (autolysins and murein hydrolases) while cell wall assembly is arrested.

Pharmacodynamics/Kinetics

Absorption: Oral: 35% to 67%

Distribution: Into bile, synovial and pleural fluids, bronchial secretions, peritoneal, and pericardial fluids; crosses placenta; enters breast milk; penetrates the blood-brain barrier only when meninges are inflamed

Metabolism: Hepatic to active metabolites

Half-life elimination: Children 1 week to 2 years: 0.9-1.8 hours; Adults: 23-60 minutes; prolonged with reduced renal function and in neonates

Time to peak, serum: Oral: ~2 hours; I.M.: 30-60 minutes

Excretion: Urine and feces (small amounts as unchanged drug and metabolites)

Usual Dosage

Neonates: I.M., I.V.:

Postnatal age <7 days:

<2000 g: 25 mg/kg/dose every 12 hours

>2000 g: 25 mg/kg/dose every 8 hours

Postnatal age >7 days:

<1200 g: 25 mg/kg/dose every 12 hours

1200-2000 g: 30 mg/kg/dose every 8 hours

>2000 g: 37.5 mg/kg/dose every 6 hours

Infants and Children:

Oral: 50-100 mg/kg/day divided every 6 hours

I.M., I.V.: 150-200 mg/kg/day in divided doses every 6 hours; maximum dose: 12 g/day

Adults:

Oral: 500-1000 mg every 4-6 hours for at least 5 days

I.M., I.V.: 250 mg to 2 g/dose every 4-6 hours

Dosing adjustment in renal impairment: Cl_{cr} <10 mL/minute: Use lower range of the usual dosage

Hemodialysis: Not dialyzable (0% to 5%)

Dietary Considerations Should be taken orally on an empty stomach 1 hour before meals or 2 hours after meals. Sodium content of 1 g: 64.4-71.3 mg (2.8-3.1 mEq).

Administration Administer around-the-clock to promote less variation in peak and trough serum levels.

Oral: Take on an empty stomach 1 hour before meals or 2 hours after meals. Take all medication; do not skip doses.

I.V.: Administer IVP over 10 minutes. Administer IVPB over 30 minutes.

Monitoring Parameters Observe for signs and symptoms of anaphylaxis during first dose

Test Interactions May interfere with urinary glucose tests using cupric sulfate (Benedict's solution, Clinitest®); may inactivate aminoglycosides *in vitro*; false-positive urinary and serum proteins

Patient Information Take orally on an empty stomach 1 hour before meals or 2 hours after meals; take all medication, do not skip doses

Nursing Implications

Administer around-the-clock rather than 4 times/day, 3 times/day, etc (ie, 12-6-12-6, not 9-1-5-9) to promote less variation in peak and trough serum levels; I.M. injections should be administered deep into a large muscle mass such as the gluteus maximus; can be administered by I.V. push over 10 minutes at a maximum concentration of 100 mg/mL or by I.V. intermittent infusion over 15-30 minutes at a final concentration ≤40 mg/mL

Monitor periodic CBC, urinalysis, BUN, serum creatinine, AST and ALT

Dosage Forms

Capsule, as sodium: 250 mg, 500 mg

Powder for injection, as sodium: 250 mg, 500 mg, 1 g, 2 g, 4 g, 10 g

Powder for or oral solution, as sodium: 250 mg/5 mL (100 mL)

♦ **Oxacillin Sodium** *see* Oxacillin *on page 1016*

Oxamniquine (oks AM ni kwin)
U.S. Brand Names Vansil™
Canadian Brand Names Vansil™
Therapeutic Category Anthelmintic
Use Treatment of all stages of *Schistosoma mansoni* infection
Pregnancy Risk Factor C
Warnings/Precautions Rare epileptiform convulsions have been observed within the first few hours of administration, especially in patients with a history of CNS pathology
Adverse Reactions
>10%: Central nervous system: Dizziness, drowsiness, headache
<10%:
Central nervous system: Insomnia, malaise, hallucinations, behavior changes
Dermatologic: Rash, urticaria, pruritus
Gastrointestinal: GI effects, orange/red discoloration of urine
Hepatic: Elevated LFTs
Renal: Proteinuria
Drug Interactions
Increased Effect/Toxicity: May be synergistic with praziquantel.
Mechanism of Action Not fully elucidated; causes worms to dislodge from their usual site of residence (mesenteric veins to the liver) by paralysis and contraction of musculature and subsequently phagocytized
Pharmacodynamics/Kinetics
Absorption: Well absorbed
Metabolism: Extensive in GI tract via oxidation
Half-life elimination: 1-2.5 hours
Time to peak: 1-3 hours
Excretion: Urine (<2% as unchanged drug, ≤75% as metabolites)
Usual Dosage Oral:
Children <30 kg: 20 mg/kg in 2 divided doses of 10 mg/kg at 2- to 8-hour intervals
Adults: 12-15 mg/kg as a single dose
Dietary Considerations May be taken with food.
Test Interactions May interfere with spectrometric or color reaction urinalysis
Patient Information Take with food
Additional Information Strains other than from the western hemisphere may require higher doses.
Dosage Forms Capsule: 250 mg

♦ **Oxandrin®** *see* Oxandrolone *on page 1018*

Oxandrolone (oks AN droe lone)
U.S. Brand Names Oxandrin®
Therapeutic Category Androgen
Use Adjunctive therapy to promote weight gain after weight loss following extensive surgery, chronic infections, or severe trauma, and in some patients who, without definite pathophysiologic reasons, fail to gain or to maintain normal weight
Restrictions C-III
Pregnancy Risk Factor X
Contraindications Hypersensitivity to oxandrolone or any component of the formulation; nephrosis; carcinoma of breast or prostate; pregnancy
Warnings/Precautions May stunt bone growth in children; anabolic steroids may cause peliosis hepatis, liver cell tumors, and blood lipid changes with increased risk of arteriosclerosis; monitor diabetic patients carefully; use with caution in elderly patients, they may be at greater risk for prostatic hyperplasia; use with caution in patients with cardiac, renal, or hepatic disease or epilepsy
Adverse Reactions
Male:
Postpubertal:
>10%:
Dermatologic: Acne
Endocrine & metabolic: Gynecomastia
Genitourinary: Bladder irritability, priapism
1% to 10%:
Central nervous system: Insomnia, chills
Endocrine & metabolic: Decreased libido, hepatic dysfunction
Gastrointestinal: Nausea, diarrhea
Genitourinary: Prostatic hyperplasia (elderly)
Hematologic: Iron-deficiency anemia, suppression of clotting factors
<1% (Limited to important or life-threatening): Hepatic necrosis, hepatocellular carcinoma
Prepubertal:
>10%:
Dermatologic: Acne
Endocrine & metabolic: Virilism
1% to 10%:
Central nervous system: Chills, insomnia,
Dermatologic: Hyperpigmentation
Gastrointestinal: Diarrhea, nausea
Hematologic: Iron deficiency anemia, suppression of clotting factors
<1% (Limited to important or life-threatening): Hepatic necrosis, hepatocellular carcinoma

Female:
>10%: Endocrine & metabolic: Virilism
1% to 10%:
Central nervous system: Chills, insomnia
Endocrine & metabolic: Hypercalcemia
Gastrointestinal: Nausea, diarrhea
Hematologic: Iron deficiency anemia, suppression of clotting factors
Hepatic: Hepatic dysfunction
<1% (Limited to important or life-threatening): Hepatic necrosis, hepatocellular carcinoma

Drug Interactions
Increased Effect/Toxicity: ACTH, adrenal steroids may increase risk of edema and acne. Stanozolol enhances the hypoprothrombinemic effects of oral anticoagulants, enhances the hypoglycemic effects of insulin and sulfonylureas (oral hypoglycemics).

Mechanism of Action Synthetic testosterone derivative with similar androgenic and anabolic actions

Pharmacodynamics/Kinetics
Onset of action: 1 month
Absorption: High
Distribution: V_d: 0.578 L/kg
Protein binding, plasma: 94% to 97%
Metabolism: Hepatic
Excretion: Urine (60%); feces (3%)

Usual Dosage
Children: Total daily dose: ≤0.1 mg/kg **or** ≤0.045 mg/lb
Adults: 2.5 mg 2-4 times/day; however, since the response of individuals to anabolic steroids varies, a daily dose of as little as 2.5 mg or as much as 20 mg may be required to achieve the desired response. A course of therapy of 2-4 weeks is usually adequate. This may be repeated intermittently as needed.
Dosing adjustment in renal impairment: Caution is recommended because of the propensity of oxandrolone to cause edema and water retention
Dosing adjustment in hepatic impairment: Caution is advised but there are not specific guidelines for dosage reduction

Patient Information High protein, high caloric diet is suggested, restrict salt intake; glucose tolerance may be altered in diabetics

Dosage Forms Tablet: 2.5 mg

Oxaprozin (oks a PROE zin)

Related Information
Nonsteroidal Anti-Inflammatory Agents Comparison *on page 1512*

U.S. Brand Names Daypro™
Canadian Brand Names Daypro™
Therapeutic Category Anti-inflammatory Agent; Nonsteroidal Anti-inflammatory Drug (NSAID), Oral
Use Acute and long-term use in the management of signs and symptoms of osteoarthritis and rheumatoid arthritis; juvenile rheumatoid arthritis
Pregnancy Risk Factor C/D (3rd trimester)
Contraindications Hypersensitivity to oxaprozin, aspirin, other NSAIDs, or any component of the formulation; history of GI disease; renal or hepatic dysfunction; bleeding disorders; cardiac failure; use in elderly or debilitated patients; pregnancy (3rd trimester)
Warnings/Precautions GI toxicity (bleeding, ulceration, perforation); CNS effects may occur (headaches, confusion, depression); dehydration, hypersensitivity, anaphylactoid reactions (intermittent tolmetin use more often); renal function decline, acute renal insufficiency, interstitial nephritis, dysuria, cystitis, hematuria, nephrotic syndrome, hyperkalemia in acute renal insufficiency, hyponatremia, papillary necrosis, hepatic function impairment; elderly have increased risk for adverse reactions to NSAIDs. Withhold for at least 4-6 half-lives prior to surgical or dental procedures.

Adverse Reactions
1% to 10%:
Central nervous system: Sleep disturbance, CNS inhibition
Dermatologic: Rash
Gastrointestinal: nausea, vomiting, abdominal cramps, dyspepsia, anorexia, flatulence
Genitourinary: Dysuria, frequency
Otic: Tinnitus
<1% (Limited to important or life-threatening): Acute interstitial nephritis, agranulocytosis, anaphylaxis, anemia, bronchospasm, dyspnea, erythema multiforme, exfoliative dermatitis, GI bleeding, leukopenia, nephrotic syndrome, pancreatitis, pancytopenia, peptic ulcer, photosensitivity, pruritus, renal insufficiency, serum sickness, Stevens-Johnson syndrome, thrombocytopenia, toxic epidermal necrolysis, urticaria

Overdosage/Toxicology Symptoms include acute renal failure, vomiting, drowsiness, and leukocytosis. Management of nonsteroidal anti-inflammatory drug (NSAID) intoxication is primarily supportive and symptomatic. Fluid therapy is commonly effective in managing hypotension that may occur following an acute NSAID overdose, except when due to acute blood loss. Seizures tend to be very short-lived and often do not require drug treatment, although recurrent seizures should be treated with I.V. diazepam. Since many of NSAIDs undergo enterohepatic cycling, multiple doses of charcoal may be needed to reduce the potential for delayed toxicities.

Drug Interactions
Cytochrome P450 Effect: CYP2C9 enzyme inhibitor
Increased Effect/Toxicity: Oxaprozin may increase cyclosporine, digoxin, lithium, and methotrexate serum concentrations. The renal adverse effects of ACE inhibitors may be potentiated by NSAIDs. Corticosteroids may increase the risk of GI ulceration. The risk of bleeding with anticoagulants (warfarin, antiplatelet agents, low molecular weight heparins) may be increased.
(Continued)

Oxaprozin *(Continued)*

Decreased Effect: Oxaprozin may decrease the effect of some antihypertensive agents (including ACE inhibitors and angiotensin antagonists) and diuretics.

Ethanol/Nutrition/Herb Interactions
Ethanol: Avoid ethanol (may enhance gastric mucosal irritation).
Herb/Nutraceutical: Avoid cat's claw, dong quai, evening primrose, feverfew, garlic, ginger, ginkgo, red clover, horse chestnut, green tea, ginseng (all have additional antiplatelet activity).

Mechanism of Action Inhibits prostaglandin synthesis by decreasing the activity of the enzyme, cyclo-oxygenase, which results in decreased formation of prostaglandin precursors

Pharmacodynamics/Kinetics
Absorption: Almost completely
Protein binding: >99%
Half-life elimination: 40-50 hours
Time to peak: 2-4 hours

Usual Dosage Oral (individualize dosage to lowest effective dose to minimize adverse effects):
Children: Juvenile rheumatoid arthritis: Maximum daily dose: 1200 mg or 26 mg/kg (whichever is lower) in divided doses
Adults:
Osteoarthritis: 600-1200 mg once daily
Rheumatoid arthritis: 1200 mg once daily; a one-time loading dose of up to 1800 mg/day or 26 mg/kg (whichever is lower) may be given
Maximum daily dose: 1800 mg or 26 mg/kg (whichever is lower) in divided doses

Monitoring Parameters Monitor CBC; hepatic, renal, and ocular function
Dosage Forms Tablet: 600 mg

Oxazepam *(oks A ze pam)*

Related Information
Antacid Drug Interactions *on page 1477*
Benzodiazepines Comparison *on page 1490*
U.S. Brand Names Serax®
Canadian Brand Names Apo®-Oxazepam; Serax®
Therapeutic Category Antianxiety Agent; Anticonvulsant; Benzodiazepine
Use Treatment of anxiety; management of ethanol withdrawal
Unlabeled/Investigational Use Anticonvulsant in management of simple partial seizures; hypnotic
Restrictions C-IV
Pregnancy Risk Factor D
Contraindications Hypersensitivity to oxazepam or any component of the formulation (cross-sensitivity with other benzodiazepines may exist); narrow-angle glaucoma (not in product labeling, however, benzodiazepines are contraindicated); not indicated for use in the treatment of psychosis; pregnancy

Warnings/Precautions May cause hypotension (rare) - use with caution in patients with cardiovascular or cerebrovascular disease, or in patients who would not tolerate transient decreases in blood pressure. Serax® 15 contains tartrazine; use is not recommended in pediatric patients <6 years of age; dose has not been established between 6-12 years of age.

Use with caution in elderly or debilitated patients, patients with hepatic disease (including alcoholics), or renal impairment. Use with caution in patients with respiratory disease or impaired gag reflex. Avoid use in patients with sleep apnea.

Causes CNS depression (dose-related) resulting in sedation, dizziness, confusion, or ataxia which may impair physical and mental capabilities. Patients must be cautioned about performing tasks which require mental alertness (ie, operating machinery or driving). Use with caution in patients receiving other CNS depressants or psychoactive agents. Effects with other sedative drugs or ethanol may be potentiated. Benzodiazepines have been associated with falls and traumatic injury and should be used with extreme caution in patients who are at risk of these events (especially the elderly).

Use caution in patients with suicidal risk. Use with caution in patients with a history of drug dependence. Benzodiazepines have been associated with dependence and acute withdrawal symptoms on discontinuation or reduction in dose. Acute withdrawal, including seizures, may be precipitated after administration of flumazenil to patients receiving long-term benzodiazepine therapy.

Benzodiazepines have been associated with anterograde amnesia. Paradoxical reactions, including hyperactive or aggressive behavior have been reported with benzodiazepines, particularly in adolescent/pediatric or psychiatric patients. Does not have analgesic, antidepressant, or antipsychotic properties.

Adverse Reactions Frequency not defined.
Cardiovascular: Syncope (rare), edema
Central nervous system: Drowsiness, ataxia, dizziness, vertigo, memory impairment, headache, paradoxical reactions (excitement, stimulation of effect), lethargy, amnesia, euphoria
Dermatologic: Rash
Endocrine & metabolic: Decreased libido, menstrual irregularities
Genitourinary: Incontinence
Hematologic: Leukopenia, blood dyscrasias
Hepatic: Jaundice
Neuromuscular & skeletal: Dysarthria, tremor, reflex slowing
Ocular: Blurred vision, diplopia
Miscellaneous: Drug dependence

Overdosage/Toxicology Symptoms include somnolence, confusion, coma, hypoactive reflexes, dyspnea, hypotension, slurred speech, and impaired coordination. Treatment for benzodiazepine overdose is supportive. Rarely is mechanical ventilation required. Flumazenil has been shown to selectively block the binding of benzodiazepines to CNS receptors, resulting in reversal of benzodiazepine-induced CNS depression, but not respiratory depression due to toxicity.

Drug Interactions

Increased Effect/Toxicity: Ethanol and other CNS depressants may increase the CNS effects of oxazepam. Oxazepam may decrease the antiparkinsonian efficacy of levodopa. Flumazenil may cause seizures if administered following long-term benzodiazepine treatment.

Decreased Effect: Oral contraceptives may increase the clearance of oxazepam. Theophylline and other CNS stimulants may antagonize the sedative effects of oxazepam. Phenytoin may increase the clearance of oxazepam.

Ethanol/Nutrition/Herb Interactions

Ethanol: Avoid ethanol (may increase CNS depression).

Herb/Nutraceutical: Avoid valerian, St John's wort, kava kava, gotu kola (may increase CNS depression).

Mechanism of Action Binds to stereospecific benzodiazepine receptors on the postsynaptic GABA neuron at several sites within the central nervous system, including the limbic system, reticular formation. Enhancement of the inhibitory effect of GABA on neuronal excitability results by increased neuronal membrane permeability to chloride ions. This shift in chloride ions results in hyperpolarization (a less excitable state) and stabilization.

Pharmacodynamics/Kinetics

Absorption: Almost completely

Protein binding: 86% to 99%

Metabolism: Hepatic to inactive compounds (primarily as glucuronides)

Half-life elimination: 2.8-5.7 hours

Time to peak, serum: 2-4 hours

Excretion: Urine (as unchanged drug (50%) and metabolites)

Usual Dosage Oral:

Children: Anxiety: 1 mg/kg/day has been administered

Adults:

Anxiety: 10-30 mg 3-4 times/day

Ethanol withdrawal: 15-30 mg 3-4 times/day

Hypnotic: 15-30 mg

Elderly: Oral: Anxiety: 10 mg 2-3 times/day; increase gradually as needed to a total of 30-45 mg/day. Dose titration should be slow to evaluate sensitivity.

Hemodialysis: Not dialyzable (0% to 5%)

Administration Administer orally in divided doses

Monitoring Parameters Respiratory and cardiovascular status

Reference Range Therapeutic: 0.2-1.4 µg/mL (SI: 0.7-4.9 µmol/L)

Patient Information Avoid alcohol and other CNS depressants; avoid activities needing good psychomotor coordination until CNS effects are known; drug may cause physical or psychological dependence; avoid abrupt discontinuation after prolonged use

Nursing Implications Provide safety measures (ie, side rails, night light, and call button); remove smoking materials from area; supervise ambulation

Additional Information Not intended for management of anxieties and minor distresses associated with everyday life. Treatment longer than 4 months should be re-evaluated to determine the patient's need for the drug. Abrupt discontinuation after sustained use (generally >10 days) may cause withdrawal symptoms.

Dosage Forms

Capsule: 10 mg, 15 mg, 30 mg

Tablet: 15 mg

Oxcarbazepine (ox car BAZ e peen)

Related Information

Anticonvulsants by Seizure Type on page 1481

Epilepsy & Seizure Treatment on page 1659

U.S. Brand Names Trileptal®

Canadian Brand Names Trileptal®

Synonyms GP 47680

Therapeutic Category Anticonvulsant

Use Monotherapy or adjunctive therapy in the treatment of partial seizures in adults with epilepsy; adjunctive therapy in the treatment of partial seizures in children (4-16 years of age) with epilepsy

Unlabeled/Investigational Use Antimanic

Pregnancy Risk Factor C

Pregnancy/Breast-Feeding Implications Although many epidemiological studies of congenital anomalies in infants born to women treated with various anticonvulsants during pregnancy have been reported, none of these investigations includes enough women treated with oxcarbazepine to assess possible teratogenic effects of this drug. Given that teratogenic effects have been observed in animal studies, and that oxcarbazepine is structurally related to carbamazepine (teratogenic in humans), use during pregnancy only if the benefit to the mother outweighs the potential risk to the fetus. Nonhormonal forms of contraception should be used during therapy.

Contraindications Hypersensitivity to oxcarbazepine or any component of the formulation

Warnings/Precautions Clinically significant hyponatremia (sodium <125 mmol/L) can develop during oxcarbazepine use. As with all antiepileptic drugs, oxcarbazepine should be withdrawn gradually to minimize the potential of increased seizure frequency. Use of oxcarbazepine has been associated with CNS related adverse events, most significant of these were cognitive symptoms including psychomotor slowing, difficulty with concentration, and speech or language problems, somnolence or fatigue, and coordination abnormalities, including ataxia and gait disturbances. Use caution in patients with previous hypersensitivity to carbamazepine (cross-sensitivity occurs in 25% to 30%). May reduce the efficacy of oral contraceptives (nonhormonal contraceptive measures are recommended).

(Continued)

Oxcarbazepine *(Continued)*

Adverse Reactions As reported in adults with doses of up to 2400 mg/day (includes patients on monotherapy, adjunctive therapy, and those not previously on AEDs); incidence in children was similar.

>10%:
  Central nervous system: Dizziness (22% to 49%), somnolence (20% to 36%), headache (13% to 32%, placebo 23%), ataxia (5% to 31%), fatigue (12% to 15%), vertigo (6% to 15%)
  Gastrointestinal: Vomiting (7% to 36%), nausea (15% to 29%), abdominal pain (10% to 13%)
  Neuromuscular & skeletal: Abnormal gait (5% to 17%), tremor (3% to 16%)
  Ocular: Diplopia (14% to 40%), nystagmus (7% to 26%), abnormal vision (4% to 14%)
1% to 10%:
  Cardiovascular: Hypotension (1% to 2%)
  Central nervous system: Nervousness (2% to 5%), amnesia (4%), agitation (1% to 2%)
  Dermatologic: Rash (4%)
  Endocrine & metabolic: Hyponatremia (1% to 3%)
  Gastrointestinal: Diarrhea (5% to 7%), gastritis (1% to 2%)
  Neuromuscular & skeletal: Weakness (3% to 6%), back pain (4%), falls (4%), abnormal coordination (1% to 4%), muscle weakness (1% to 2%)
  Ocular: Abnormal accommodation (2%)
  Respiratory: Upper respiratory tract infection (7%)
<1% (Limited to important or life-threatening): Aggressive reaction, alopecia, amnesia, angioedema, aphasia, asthma, blood in stool, cardiac failure, cataract, cerebral hemorrhage, cholelithiasis, convulsions aggravated, delirium, duodenal ulcer, dysphagia, dysphonia, dyspnea, dystonia, erythema multiforme, eosinophilia, extrapyramidal disorder, gastric ulcer, genital pruritus, gingival hyperplasia, hematemesis, hematuria, hemianopia, hemiplegia, hypersensitivity reaction, intermenstrual bleeding, laryngismus, leukopenia, maculopapular rash, malaise, manic reaction, menorrhagia, migraine, muscle contractions (involuntary), neuralgia, oculogyric crisis, paralysis, photosensitivity reaction, postural hypotension, priapism, purpura, psychosis, scotoma, sialoadenitis, Stevens-Johnson syndrome, stupor, syncope, systemic lupus erythematosus, tetany, thrombocytopenia, toxic epidermal necrolysis

Overdosage/Toxicology Symptoms may include CNS depression (somnolence, ataxia). Treatment is symptomatic and supportive.

Drug Interactions
  Cytochrome P450 Effect: CYP2C19 enzyme inhibitor; CYP3A4/5 enzyme inducer
  Increased Effect/Toxicity: Serum concentrations of phenytoin and phenobarbital are increased by oxcarbazepine.
  Decreased Effect: Oxcarbazine serum concentrations may be reduced by carbamazepine, phenytoin, phenobarbital, valproic acid and verapamil (decreases levels of active oxcarbazepine metabolite). Oxcarbazepine reduces the serum concentrations of felodipine (similar effects may be anticipated with other dihydropyridines), oral contraceptives (use alternative contraceptive measures), and verapamil.

Ethanol/Nutrition/Herb Interactions
  Ethanol: Avoid ethanol (may increase CNS depression).
  Herb/Nutraceutical: St John's wort may decrease oxcarbazepine levels. Avoid evening primrose (seizure threshold decreased). Avoid valerian, St John's wort, kava kava, gotu kola.

Stability Store tablets and suspension at 25°C (77°F). Use suspension within 7 weeks of first opening container.

Mechanism of Action Pharmacological activity results from both oxcarbazepine and its monohydroxy metabolite (MHD). Precise mechanism of anticonvulsant effect has not been defined. Oxcarbazepine and MHD block voltage sensitive sodium channels, stabilizing hyperexcited neuronal membranes, inhibiting repetitive firing, and decreasing the propagation of synaptic impulses. These actions are believed to prevent the spread of seizures. Oxcarbazepine and MHD also increase potassium conductance and modulate the activity of high-voltage activated calcium channels.

Pharmacodynamics/Kinetics
  Absorption: Completely; food has no affect on rate or extent
  Distribution: MHD: V_d: 49 L
  Protein binding, serum: 40%
  Metabolism: Hepatic, to 10-monohydroxy metabolite (active); MHD which is further conjugated to DHD (inactive)
  Bioavailability: Decreased in children <8 years; increased in elderly >60 years
  Half-life elimination: Parent drug: 2 hours; MHD: 9 hours; Cl_{cr} 30 mL/minute: 19 hours
  Excretion: Urine (95%, <1% as unchanged oxcarbazepine, 27% as unchanged MHD, 49% as MHD glucuronides); feces (<4%)

Usual Dosage Oral:
  Children:
    Adjunctive therapy: 8-10 mg/kg/day, not to exceed 600 mg/day, given in 2 divided daily doses. Maintenance dose should be achieved over 2 weeks, and is dependent upon patient weight, according to the following:
      20-29 kg: 900 mg/day in 2 divided doses
      29.1-39 kg: 1200 mg/day in 2 divided doses
      >39 kg: 1800 mg/day in 2 divided doses
  Adults:
    Adjunctive therapy: Initial: 300 mg twice daily; dose may be increased by as much as 600 mg/day at weekly intervals; recommended daily dose: 1200 mg/day in 2 divided doses. Although daily doses >1200 mg/day demonstrated greater efficacy, most patients were unable to tolerate 2400 mg/day (due to CNS effects).
    Conversion to monotherapy: Oxcarbazepine 600 mg/day in twice daily divided doses while simultaneously initiating the reduction of the dose of the concomitant antiepileptic drug. The concomitant dosage should be withdrawn over 3-6 weeks, while the maximum dose of

oxcarbazepine should be reached in about 2-4 weeks. Recommended daily dose: 2400 mg/day.

Initiation of monotherapy: Oxcarbazepine should be initiated at a dose of 600 mg/day in twice daily divided doses; doses may be titrated upward by 300 mg/day every third day to a final dose of 1200 mg/day given in 2 daily divided doses

Dosing adjustment in renal impairment: Therapy should be initiated at one-half the usual starting dose (300 mg/day) and increased slowly to achieve the desired clinical response

Dietary Considerations May be taken with or without food.

Administration Suspension: Prior to using for the first time, firmly insert the plastic adapter provided with the bottle. Cover adapter with child-resistant cap when not in use. Shake bottle for at least 10 seconds, remove child-resistant cap and insert the oral dosing syringe provided to withdraw appropriate dose. Dose may be taken directly from oral syringe or may be mixed in a small glass of water immediately prior to swallowing. Rinse syringe with warm water after use and allow to dry thoroughly. Discard any unused portion after 7 weeks of first opening bottle.

Monitoring Parameters Serum sodium

Patient Information Hormonal contraceptives may be less effective when used with oxcarbazepine; caution should be exercised if alcohol is taken with oxcarbazepine, due to the possible additive sedative effects and that it may cause dizziness and somnolence; therefore, early in therapy be advised not to drive or operate machinery

Nursing Implications Inform those patients who have exhibited hypersensitivity reactions to carbamazepine that there is the possibility of cross-sensitivity reactions with oxcarbazepine. Inform patients of childbearing age that hormonal contraceptives may be less effective when used with oxcarbazepine. Caution should be exercised if ethanol is taken with oxcarbazepine, due to the possible additive sedative effects. Advise patients that oxcarbazepine may cause dizziness and somnolence and that early in therapy they are advised not to drive or operate machinery

Dosage Forms
Suspension, oral: 300 mg/5 mL (250 mL)
Tablet: 150 mg, 300 mg, 600 mg

♦ **Oxeze® Turbuhaler® (Can)** see Formoterol on page 603

Oxiconazole (oks i KON a zole)

U.S. Brand Names Oxistat®
Canadian Brand Names Oxistat®; Oxizole®
Synonyms Oxiconazole Nitrate
Therapeutic Category Antifungal Agent, Topical
Use Treatment of tinea pedis (athlete's foot), tinea cruris (jock itch), and tinea corporis (ringworm)
Pregnancy Risk Factor B
Contraindications Hypersensitivity to oxiconazole or any component of the formulation; not for ophthalmic use
Warnings/Precautions May cause irritation during therapy; if a sensitivity to oxiconazole occurs, therapy should be discontinued; avoid contact with eyes or vagina
Adverse Reactions 1% to 10%:
Dermatologic: Itching, erythema
Local: Transient burning, local irritation, stinging, dryness
Mechanism of Action The cytoplasmic membrane integrity of fungi is destroyed by oxiconazole which exerts a fungicidal activity through inhibition of ergosterol synthesis. Effective for treatment of tinea pedis, tinea cruris, and tinea corporis. Active against *Trichophyton rubrum*, *Trichophyton mentagrophytes*, *Trichophyton violaceum*, *Microsporum canis*, *Microsporum audouini*, *Microsporum gypseum*, *Epidermophyton floccosum*, *Candida albicans*, and *Malassezia furfur*.
Pharmacodynamics/Kinetics
Absorption: In each layer of the dermis; very little systemically after one topical dose
Distribution: To each layer of the dermis; enters breast milk
Excretion: Urine (<0.3%)
Usual Dosage Children and Adults: Topical: Apply once to twice daily to affected areas for 2 weeks (tinea corporis/tinea cruris) to 1 month (tinea pedis)
Patient Information External use only; discontinue if sensitivity or chemical irritation occurs, contact physician if condition fails to improve in 3-4 days
Nursing Implications External use only; discontinue if sensitivity or chemical irritation occurs, contact physician if condition fails to improve in 3-4 days
Dosage Forms
Cream, topical, as nitrate: 1% (15 g, 30 g, 60 g)
Lotion, topical, as nitrate: 1% (30 mL)

♦ **Oxiconazole Nitrate** see Oxiconazole on page 1023
♦ **Oxilan®** see Ioxilan on page 739
♦ **Oxilapine Succinate** see Loxapine on page 826
♦ **Oxistat®** see Oxiconazole on page 1023
♦ **Oxizole® (Can)** see Oxiconazole on page 1023
♦ **Oxpentifylline** see Pentoxifylline on page 1061
♦ **Oxsoralen®** see Methoxsalen on page 889
♦ **Oxsoralen-Ultra®** see Methoxsalen on page 889
♦ **Oxtriphylline** see Theophylline Salts on page 1310

Oxybutynin (oks i BYOO ti nin)

U.S. Brand Names Ditropan®; Ditropan® XL
Canadian Brand Names Albert® Oxybutynin; Ditropan®; Gen-Oxybutynin; Novo-Oxybutynin; Nu-Oxybutyn; PMS-Oxybutynin
Synonyms Oxybutynin Chloride
(Continued)

Oxybutynin *(Continued)*

Therapeutic Category Antispasmodic Agent, Urinary

Use Antispasmodic for neurogenic bladder (urgency, frequency, urge incontinence) and uninhibited bladder

Pregnancy Risk Factor B

Contraindications Hypersensitivity to oxybutynin or any component of the formulation; glaucoma, myasthenia gravis; partial or complete GI obstruction; GU obstruction; ulcerative colitis; intestinal atony; megacolon; toxic megacolon

Warnings/Precautions Use with caution in patients with urinary tract obstruction, angle-closure glaucoma, hyperthyroidism, reflux esophagitis, heart disease, hepatic or renal disease, prostatic hyperplasia, autonomic neuropathy, ulcerative colitis (may cause ileus and toxic megacolon), hypertension, hiatal hernia. Caution should be used in elderly due to anticholinergic activity (eg, confusion, constipation, blurred vision, and tachycardia).

Adverse Reactions
>10%:
  Central nervous system: Drowsiness
  Gastrointestinal: Dry mouth, constipation
  Miscellaneous: Diaphoresis (decreased)
1% to 10%:
  Cardiovascular: Tachycardia, palpitations
  Central nervous system: Dizziness, insomnia, fever, headache
  Dermatologic: Rash
  Endocrine & metabolic: Decreased flow of breast milk, decreased sexual ability, hot flashes
  Gastrointestinal: Nausea, vomiting
  Genitourinary: Urinary hesitancy or retention
  Neuromuscular & skeletal: Weakness
  Ocular: Blurred vision, mydriatic effect
<1% (Limited to important or life-threatening): Increased intraocular pressure

Overdosage/Toxicology Symptoms include hypotension, circulatory failure, psychotic behavior, flushing, respiratory failure, paralysis, tremor, irritability, seizures, delirium, hallucinations, and coma. Treatment is symptomatic and supportive. Induce emesis or perform gastric lavage followed by charcoal and a cathartic. Physostigmine may be required. Treat hyperpyrexia with cooling techniques (ice bags, cold applications, alcohol sponges).

Drug Interactions
  Increased Effect/Toxicity: Additive sedation with CNS depressants and alcohol. Additive anticholinergic effects with antihistamines and anticholinergic agents.

Mechanism of Action Direct antispasmodic effect on smooth muscle, also inhibits the action of acetylcholine on smooth muscle (exhibits $1/5$ the anticholinergic activity of atropine, but is 4-10 times the antispasmodic activity); does not block effects at skeletal muscle or at autonomic ganglia; increases bladder capacity, decreases uninhibited contractions, and delays desire to void; therefore, decreases urgency and frequency

Pharmacodynamics/Kinetics
  Onset of action: 30-60 minutes
    Peak effect: 3-6 hours
  Duration: 6-10 hours
  Absorption: Rapid and well absorbed
  Metabolism: Hepatic
  Half-life elimination: 1-2.3 hours
  Time to peak, serum: ~60 minutes
  Excretion: Urine

Usual Dosage Oral:
  Children:
    1-5 years: 0.2 mg/kg/dose 2-4 times/day
    >5 years: 5 mg twice daily, up to 5 mg 4 times/day maximum
  Adults: 5 mg 2-3 times/day up to 5 mg 4 times/day maximum
    Extended release: Initial: 5 mg once daily, may increase in 5-10 mg increments; maximum: 30 mg daily
  Elderly: 2.5-5 mg twice daily; increase by 2.5 mg increments every 1-2 days
  Note: Should be discontinued periodically to determine whether the patient can manage without the drug and to minimize resistance to the drug

Dietary Considerations Should be taken on an empty stomach with water.

Monitoring Parameters Incontinence episodes, postvoid residual (PVR)

Test Interactions May suppress the wheal and flare reactions to skin test antigens

Patient Information May impair ability to perform activities requiring mental alertness or physical coordination; alcohol or other sedating drugs may enhance drowsiness; swallow extended release tablets whole, do not crush, chew, or break

Nursing Implications Raise bed rails, institute safety measures, assist with ambulation; do not crush extended release tablets.

Dosage Forms
  Syrup, as chloride: 5 mg/5 mL (473 mL)
  Tablet, as chloride: 5 mg
  Tablet, extended release, as chloride: 5 mg, 10 mg, 15 mg

♦ **Oxybutynin Chloride** *see* Oxybutynin *on page 1023*
♦ **Oxycocet® (Can)** *see* Oxycodone and Acetaminophen *on page 1026*
♦ **Oxycodan® (Can)** *see* Oxycodone and Aspirin *on page 1026*

Oxycodone *(oks i KOE done)*

U.S. Brand Names Endocodone™; OxyContin®; OxyIR™; Percolone®; Roxicodone™; Roxicodone™ Intensol™

Canadian Brand Names OxyContin®; Oxy.IR®; Supeudol®

Synonyms Dihydrohydroxycodeinone; Oxycodone Hydrochloride

Therapeutic Category Analgesic, Narcotic

Use Management of moderate to severe pain, normally used in combination with non-narcotic analgesics

OxyContin® is indicated for around-the-clock management of moderate to severe pain when an analgesic is needed for an extended period of time. **Note:** OxyContin® is not intended for use as an "as needed" analgesic or for immediately-postoperative pain management (should be used postoperatively only if the patient has received it prior to surgery or if severe, persistent pain is anticipated).

Restrictions C-II

Pregnancy Risk Factor B/D (prolonged use or high doses at term)

Pregnancy/Breast-Feeding Implications Should be used in pregnancy only if clearly needed.

Contraindications Hypersensitivity to oxycodone or any component of the formulation; significant respiratory depression; hypercarbia; acute or severe bronchial asthma; OxyContin® is also contraindicated in paralytic ileus (known or suspected); pregnancy (prolonged use or high doses at term)

Warnings/Precautions Use with caution in patients with hypersensitivity reactions to other phenanthrene derivative opioid agonists (morphine, hydrocodone, hydromorphone, levorphanol, oxycodone, oxymorphone); respiratory diseases including asthma, emphysema, COPD, or severe liver or renal insufficiency; some preparations contain sulfites which may cause allergic reactions; dextromethorphan has equivalent antitussive activity but has much lower toxicity in accidental overdose; tolerance or drug dependence may result from extended use.

Use with caution in the elderly, debilitated, severe hepatic or renal function, hypothyroidism, Addison's disease, prostatic hyperplasia, or urethral stricture. Respiratory depressant effects and capacity to elevate CSF pressure may be exaggerated in presence of head injury, other intracranial lesion, or pre-existing intracranial pressure. Tolerance or drug dependence may result from extended use. Healthcare provider should be alert to problems of abuse, misuse, and diversion. Do NOT crush controlled-release tablets.

Adverse Reactions

>10%:
  Cardiovascular: Hypotension
  Central nervous system: Fatigue, drowsiness, dizziness
  Gastrointestinal: Nausea, vomiting
  Neuromuscular & skeletal: Weakness

1% to 10%:
  Central nervous system: Nervousness, headache, restlessness, malaise
  Gastrointestinal: Stomach cramps, dry mouth, biliary spasm, constipation
  Genitourinary: Ureteral spasms, decreased urination
  Ocular: Blurred vision
  Miscellaneous: Histamine release

<1% (Limited to important or life-threatening): Dyspnea

Note: Deaths due to overdose have been reported due to misuse/abuse after crushing the sustained release tablets.

Overdosage/Toxicology Symptoms include CNS depression, respiratory depression, and miosis. Treatment consists of naloxone 2 mg I.V. (0.01 mg/kg for children), with repeat administration as necessary, up to a total of 10 mg.

Drug Interactions

Cytochrome P450 Effect: CYP2D6 enzyme substrate

Increased Effect/Toxicity: MAO inhibitors may increase adverse symptoms. Cimetidine may increase narcotic analgesic serum levels resulting in toxicity. CNS depressants (barbiturates, ethanol) and TCAs may potentiate the sedative and respiratory depressive effects of morphine and other opiate agonists. Dextroamphetamine may enhance the analgesic effect of morphine and other opiate agonists.

Decreased Effect: Phenothiazines may antagonize the analgesic effect of opiate agonists.

Ethanol/Nutrition/Herb Interactions

Ethanol: Avoid ethanol (may increase CNS depression).

Herb/Nutraceutical: Avoid valerian, St John's wort, kava kava, gotu kola (may increase CNS depression).

Stability Tablets should be stored at room temperature.

Mechanism of Action Binds to opiate receptors in the CNS, causing inhibition of ascending pain pathways, altering the perception of and response to pain; produces generalized CNS depression

Pharmacodynamics/Kinetics

Onset of action: Pain relief: 10-15 minutes
  Peak effect: 0.5-1 hour
Duration: 3-6 hours; Controlled release: ≤12 hours
Metabolism: Hepatic
Half-life elimination: 2-3 hours
Excretion: Urine

Usual Dosage Oral:

Immediate release:
  Children:
    6-12 years: 1.25 mg every 6 hours as needed
    >12 years: 2.5 mg every 6 hours as needed
  Adults: 5 mg every 6 hours as needed

Controlled release: Adults:
  Opioid naive (not currently on opioid): 10 mg every 12 hours
  Currently on opioid/ASA or acetaminophen or NSAID combination:
    1-5 tablets: 10-20 mg every 12 hours
    6-9 tablets: 20-30 mg every 12 hours
    10-12 tablets: 30-40 mg every 12 hours
  May continue the nonopioid as a separate drug.

(Continued)

Oxycodone *(Continued)*

Currently on opioids: Use standard conversion chart to convert daily dose to oxycodone equivalent. Divide daily dose in 2 (for every 12-hour dosing) and round down to nearest dosage form.

Dosing adjustment in hepatic impairment: Reduce dosage in patients with severe liver disease

Administration Do not crush controlled-release tablets.

Monitoring Parameters Pain relief, respiratory and mental status, blood pressure

Reference Range Blood level of 5 mg/L associated with fatality

Patient Information Avoid alcohol; may cause drowsiness, impaired judgment or coordination; may be addicting if used for prolonged periods; do not crush or chew the controlled-release product

Nursing Implications Observe patient for excessive sedation, respiratory depression, implement safety measures, assist with ambulation. Do not crush controlled-release tablets.

Additional Information Prophylactic use of a laxative should be considered. OxyContin® 80 mg and 160 mg tablets are for use in opioid-tolerant patients only.

Dosage Forms

Capsule, immediate release, as hydrochloride (OxyIR™): 5 mg

Liquid, oral, as hydrochloride (Roxicodone™): 5 mg/5 mL (500 mL)

Solution, oral concentrate, as hydrochloride (Roxicodone™ Intensol™): 20 mg/mL (30 mL)

Tablet, as hydrochloride:

Endocodone™, Percolone®: 5 mg

Roxicodone™: 5 mg, 15 mg, 30 mg

Tablet, controlled release, as hydrochloride (OxyContin®): 10 mg, 20 mg, 40 mg, 80 mg, 160 mg

Oxycodone and Acetaminophen (oks i KOE done & a seet a MIN oh fen)

Related Information

Narcotic Agonists Comparison *on page 1506*

U.S. Brand Names Endocet®; Percocet® 2.5/325; Percocet® 5/325; Percocet® 7.5/325; Percocet® 7.5/500; Percocet® 10/325; Percocet® 10/650; Roxicet®; Roxicet® 5/500; Roxilox®; Tylox®

Canadian Brand Names Endocet®; Oxycocet®; Percocet®; Percocet®-Demi

Synonyms Acetaminophen and Oxycodone

Therapeutic Category Analgesic, Narcotic

Use Management of moderate to severe pain

Restrictions C-II

Pregnancy Risk Factor C (D if used for prolonged periods or high doses at term)

Usual Dosage Oral: Doses should be given every 4-6 hours as needed and titrated to appropriate analgesic effects. **Note:** Initial dose is based on the **oxycodone** content; however, the maximum daily dose is based on the **acetaminophen** content.

Children: Maximum acetaminophen dose: Children <45 kg: 90 mg/kg/day; children >45 kg: 4 g/day

Mild to moderate pain: Initial dose, **based on oxycodone content:** 0.05-0.1 mg/kg/dose

Severe pain: Initial dose, **based on oxycodone content:** 0.3 mg/kg/dose

Adults:

Mild to moderate pain: Initial dose, **based on oxycodone content:** 5 mg

Severe pain: Initial dose, **based on oxycodone content:** 15-30 mg. Do not exceed acetaminophen 4 g/day.

Elderly: Doses should be titrated to appropriate analgesic effects: Initial dose, **based on oxycodone content:** 2.5-5 mg every 6 hours. Do not exceed acetaminophen 4 g/day.

Dosage adjustment in hepatic impairment: Dose should be reduced in patients with severe liver disease.

Additional Information Complete prescribing information for this medication should be consulted for additional detail.

Dosage Forms

Caplet (Roxicet® 5/500): Oxycodone hydrochloride 5 mg and acetaminophen 500 mg

Capsule:

Roxilox®: Oxycodone hydrochloride 5 mg and acetaminophen 500 mg

Tylox®: Oxycodone hydrochloride 5 mg and acetaminophen 500 mg [contains sodium metabisulfite]

Solution, oral (Roxicet®): Oxycodone hydrochloride 5 mg and acetaminophen 325 mg per 5 mL (5 mL, 500 mL) [mint flavor]

Tablet:

Endocet®, Percocet® 5/325, Roxicet®: Oxycodone hydrochloride 5 mg and acetaminophen 325 mg

Percocet® 2.5/325: Oxycodone hydrochloride 2.5 mg and acetaminophen 325 mg

Percocet® 7.5/325: Oxycodone hydrochloride 7.5 mg and acetaminophen 325 mg

Endocet®, Percocet® 7.5/500: Oxycodone hydrochloride 7.5 mg and acetaminophen 500 mg

Percocet® 10/325: Oxycodone hydrochloride 10 mg and acetaminophen 325 mg

Endocet®, Percocet® 10/650: Oxycodone hydrochloride 10 mg and acetaminophen 650 mg

Oxycodone and Aspirin (oks i KOE done & AS pir in)

Related Information

Narcotic Agonists Comparison *on page 1506*

U.S. Brand Names Endodan®; Percodan®; Percodan®-Demi

Canadian Brand Names Endodan®; Oxycodan®; Percodan®; Percodan®-Demi

Synonyms Aspirin and Oxycodone

Therapeutic Category Analgesic, Narcotic

Use Management of moderate to severe pain

Restrictions C-II

Pregnancy Risk Factor D

Usual Dosage Oral (based on oxycodone combined salts):

Children: 0.05-0.15 mg/kg/dose every 4-6 hours as needed; maximum: 5 mg/dose (1 tablet Percodan® or 2 tablets Percodan®-Demi/dose)

Adults: Percodan®: 1 tablet every 6 hours as needed for pain or Percodan®-Demi: 1-2 tablets every 6 hours as needed for pain

Dosing adjustment in hepatic impairment: Dose should be reduced in patients with severe liver disease

Additional Information Complete prescribing information for this medication should be consulted for additional detail.

Dosage Forms

Tablet:

Endodan®, Percodan®: Oxycodone hydrochloride 4.5 mg, oxycodone terephthalate 0.38 mg, and aspirin 325 mg

Percodan®-Demi: Oxycodone hydrochloride 2.25 mg, oxycodone terephthalate 0.19 mg, and aspirin 325 mg

♦ **Oxycodone Hydrochloride** *see* Oxycodone *on page 1024*

♦ **OxyContin**® *see* Oxycodone *on page 1024*

♦ **OxyIR**™ *see* Oxycodone *on page 1024*

Oxymetholone (oks i METH oh lone)

U.S. Brand Names Anadrol®

Therapeutic Category Anabolic Steroid; Androgen

Use Anemias caused by the administration of myelotoxic drugs

Restrictions C-III

Pregnancy Risk Factor X

Usual Dosage Adults: Erythropoietic effects: Oral: 1-5 mg/kg/day in one daily dose; usual effective dose: 1-2 mg/kg/day; give for a minimum trial of 3-6 months because response may be delayed

Dosing adjustment in hepatic impairment:

Mild to moderate hepatic impairment: Oxymetholone should be used with caution in patients with liver dysfunction because of it's hepatotoxic potential

Severe hepatic impairment: Oxymetholone should **not** be used

Additional Information Complete prescribing information for this medication should be consulted for additional detail.

Dosage Forms Tablet: 50 mg

Oxymorphone (oks i MOR fone)

Related Information

Narcotic Agonists Comparison *on page 1506*

U.S. Brand Names Numorphan®

Canadian Brand Names Numorphan®

Synonyms Oxymorphone Hydrochloride

Therapeutic Category Analgesic, Narcotic

Use Management of moderate to severe pain and preoperatively as a sedative and a supplement to anesthesia

Restrictions C-II

Pregnancy Risk Factor B/D (prolonged use or high doses at term)

Contraindications Hypersensitivity to oxymorphone or any component of the formulation; increased intracranial pressure; severe respiratory depression; pregnancy (prolonged use or high doses at term)

Warnings/Precautions Some preparations contain sulfites which may cause allergic reactions; infants <3 months of age are more susceptible to respiratory depression, use with caution and generally in reduced doses in this age group; use with caution in patients with impaired respiratory function or severe hepatic dysfunction and in patients with hypersensitivity reactions to other phenanthrene derivative opioid agonists (codeine, hydrocodone, hydromorphone, levorphanol, oxycodone, oxymorphone); tolerance or drug dependence may result from extended use

Adverse Reactions

>10%:

Cardiovascular: Hypotension

Central nervous system: Fatigue, drowsiness, dizziness

Gastrointestinal: Nausea, vomiting

Neuromuscular & skeletal: Weakness

1% to 10%:

Cardiovascular: Tachycardia or bradycardia

Central nervous system: Nervousness, headache, restlessness, malaise, confusion, false sense of well-being

Gastrointestinal: Anorexia, stomach cramps, dry mouth, biliary spasm, constipation

Genitourinary: Ureteral spasms, decreased urination

Local: Pain at injection site

Neuromuscular & skeletal: Trembling

Ocular: Blurred vision

Respiratory: Dyspnea

Miscellaneous: Histamine release

Overdosage/Toxicology Symptoms include respiratory depression, miosis, hypotension, bradycardia, apnea, and pulmonary edema. Treatment of overdose includes airway support, establishment of an I.V. line, and administration of naloxone 2 mg I.V. (0.01 mg/kg for children), with repeat administration as necessary, up to a total of 10 mg.

(Continued)

Oxymorphone *(Continued)*

Drug Interactions

Increased Effect/Toxicity: Increased effect/toxicity with CNS depressants (phenothiazines, tranquilizers, anxiolytics, sedatives, hypnotics, alcohol), tricyclic antidepressants, and dextroamphetamine.

Decreased Effect: Decreased effect with phenothiazines.

Ethanol/Nutrition/Herb Interactions

Ethanol: Avoid ethanol (may increase CNS depression).

Herb/Nutraceutical: Avoid valerian, St John's wort, kava kava, gotu kola (may increase CNS depression).

Stability Refrigerate suppository

Mechanism of Action Oxymorphone hydrochloride (Numorphan®) is a potent narcotic analgesic with uses similar to those of morphine. The drug is a semisynthetic derivative of morphine (phenanthrene derivative) and is closely related to hydromorphone chemically (Dilaudid®).

Pharmacodynamics/Kinetics

Onset of action: Analgesic: I.V., I.M., S.C.: 5-10 minutes; Rectal: 15-30 minutes

Duration: Analgesic: Parenteral, rectal: 3-4 hours

Metabolism: Conjugated with glucuronic acid

Excretion: Urine

Usual Dosage Adults:

I.M., S.C.: 0.5 mg initially, 1-1.5 mg every 4-6 hours as needed

I.V.: 0.5 mg initially

Rectal: 5 mg every 4-6 hours

Monitoring Parameters Respiratory rate, heart rate, blood pressure, CNS activity

Patient Information Avoid alcohol, may cause drowsiness, impaired judgment or coordination; may cause physical and psychological dependence with prolonged use

Nursing Implications Observe patient for excessive sedation, respiratory depression, implement safety measures, assist with ambulation

Dosage Forms

Injection, as hydrochloride: 1 mg (1 mL); 1.5 mg/mL (1 mL, 10 mL)

Suppository, rectal, as hydrochloride: 5 mg

♦ **Oxymorphone Hydrochloride** *see Oxymorphone on page 1027*

Oxytetracycline *(oks i tet ra SYE kleen)*

U.S. Brand Names Terramycin® I.M.

Canadian Brand Names Terramycin®

Synonyms Oxytetracycline Hydrochloride

Therapeutic Category Antibiotic, Tetracycline Derivative

Use Treatment of susceptible bacterial infections; both gram-positive and gram-negative, as well as, *Rickettsia* and *Mycoplasma* organisms

Pregnancy Risk Factor D

Contraindications Hypersensitivity to tetracycline or any component of the formulation

Warnings/Precautions Avoid in children ≤8 years of age, pregnant and nursing women; photosensitivity can occur with oxytetracycline

Adverse Reactions

>10%: Miscellaneous: Discoloration of teeth and enamel hypoplasia (infants)

1% to 10%:

Dermatologic: Photosensitivity

Gastrointestinal: Nausea, diarrhea

<1% (Limited to important or life-threatening): Acute renal failure, anaphylaxis, bulging fontanels in infants, diabetes insipidus, exfoliative dermatitis, hepatotoxicity, hypersensitivity reactions, increased intracranial pressure, paresthesia, pericarditis, pigmentation of nails, pseudomembranous colitis, pseudotumor cerebri, superinfections

Overdosage/Toxicology Symptoms include nausea, anorexia, and diarrhea. Treatment following GI decontamination is supportive care only.

Drug Interactions

Increased Effect/Toxicity: Oral anticoagulant (warfarin) effects may be increased.

Decreased Effect: Antacids containing aluminum, calcium or magnesium, as well as iron and bismuth subsalicylate may decrease bioavailability of tetracyclines. Barbiturates, phenytoin, and carbamazepine decrease serum levels of tetracyclines.

Ethanol/Nutrition/Herb Interactions Food: Oxytetracycline serum concentrations may be decreased if taken with dairy products.

Mechanism of Action Inhibits bacterial protein synthesis by binding with the 30S and possibly the 50S ribosomal subunit(s) of susceptible bacteria, cell wall synthesis is not affected

Pharmacodynamics/Kinetics

Absorption: Oral: ~75%; I.M.: Poor

Distribution: Crosses placenta

Metabolism: Hepatic, small amounts

Half-life elimination: 8.5-9.6 hours; increases with renal impairment

Time to peak, serum: 2-4 hours

Excretion: Urine; feces (higher amounts)

Usual Dosage

Oral:

Children >8 years: 40-50 mg/kg/day in divided doses every 6 hours (maximum: 2 g/24 hours)

Adults: 250-500 mg/dose every 6-12 hours depending on severity of the infection

I.M.:

Children >8 years: 15-25 mg/kg/day (maximum: 250 mg/dose) in divided doses every 8-12 hours

Adults: 250 mg every 24 hours or 300 mg/day divided every 8-12 hours

Syphilis: 30-40 g in divided doses over 10-15 days
Gonorrhea: 1.5 g, then 500 mg every 6 hours for total of 9 g
Uncomplicated chlamydial infections: 500 mg every 6 hours for 7 days
Severe acne: 1 g/day then decrease to 125-500 mg/day
Dosing interval in renal impairment:
 Cl$_{cr}$ <10 mL/minute: Administer every 24 hours or avoid use if possible
Dosing adjustment/comments in hepatic impairment: Avoid use in patients with severe liver disease
Administration Injection for intramuscular use only; do not administer with antacids, iron products, or dairy products; administer 1 hour before or 2 hours after meals
Patient Information Avoid unnecessary exposure to sunlight; do not take with antacids, iron products, or dairy products; finish all medication; do not skip doses; take 1 hour before or 2 hours after meals
Nursing Implications Injection for intramuscular use only; reduce dose in renal insufficiency
Dosage Forms
 Capsule, as hydrochloride: 250 mg
 Injection, with lidocaine 2%, as hydrochloride: 5% [50 mg/mL] (2 mL, 10 mL); 12.5% [125 mg/mL] (2 mL)

Oxytetracycline and Polymyxin B (oks i tet ra SYE kleen & pol i MIKS in bee)
U.S. Brand Names Terramycin® w/Polymyxin B Ophthalmic
Synonyms Polymyxin B and Oxytetracycline
Therapeutic Category Antibiotic, Ophthalmic
Use Treatment of superficial ocular infections involving the conjunctiva and/or cornea
Pregnancy Risk Factor D
Usual Dosage Topical: Apply ½" of ointment onto the lower lid of affected eye 2-4 times/day
Additional Information Complete prescribing information for this medication should be consulted for additional detail.
Dosage Forms Ointment, ophthalmic/otic: Oxytetracycline hydrochloride 5 mg and polymyxin B 10,000 units per g (3.5 g)

♦ **Oxytetracycline Hydrochloride** see Oxytetracycline on page 1028

Oxytocin (oks i TOE sin)
U.S. Brand Names Pitocin®
Canadian Brand Names Pitocin®; Syntocinon®
Synonyms Pit
Therapeutic Category Oxytocic Agent
Use Induces labor at term; controls postpartum bleeding
Pregnancy Risk Factor X
Contraindications Hypersensitivity to oxytocin or any component of the formulation; significant cephalopelvic disproportion; unfavorable fetal positions; fetal distress; hypertonic or hyperactive uterus; contraindicated vaginal delivery; prolapse, total placenta previa, and vasa previa
Warnings/Precautions To be used for medical rather than elective induction of labor; may produce antidiuretic effect (ie, water intoxication and excess uterine contractions); high doses or hypersensitivity to oxytocin may cause uterine hypertonicity, spasm, tetanic contraction, or rupture of the uterus; severe water intoxication with convulsions, coma, and death is associated with a slow oxytocin infusion over 24 hours
Adverse Reactions
 Fetal: <1% (Limited to important or life-threatening): Arrhythmias, bradycardia, brain damage, death, hypoxia, intracranial hemorrhage, neonatal jaundice
 Maternal: <1% (Limited to important or life-threatening): Anaphylactic reactions, arrhythmias, coma, death, fatal afibrinogenemia, hypotension, increased blood loss, increased uterine motility, nausea, pelvic hematoma, postpartum hemorrhage, premature ventricular contractions, seizures, SIADH with hyponatremia, tachycardia, vomiting
Overdosage/Toxicology Symptoms include tetanic uterine contractions, impaired uterine blood flow, amniotic fluid embolism, uterine rupture, SIADH, and seizures. Treat SIADH via fluid restriction, diuresis, saline administration, and anticonvulsants, if needed.
Stability Oxytocin should be stored at 2°C to 8°C and protected from freezing; **incompatible** with norepinephrine, prochlorperazine
Mechanism of Action Produces the rhythmic uterine contractions characteristic to delivery
Pharmacodynamics/Kinetics
 Onset of action: Uterine contractions: I.V.: ~1 minute
 Duration: <30 minutes
 Metabolism: Rapidly hepatic and via plasma (by oxytocinase) and to a smaller degree the mammary gland
 Half-life elimination: 1-5 minutes
 Excretion: Urine
Usual Dosage I.V. administration requires the use of an infusion pump. Adults:
 Induction of labor: I.V.: 0.001-0.002 units/minute; increase by 0.001-0.002 units every 15-30 minutes until contraction pattern has been established; maximum dose should not exceed 20 milliunits/minute
 Postpartum bleeding:
  I.M.: Total dose of 10 units after delivery
  I.V.: 10-40 units by I.V. infusion in 1000 mL of intravenous fluid at a rate sufficient to control uterine atony
Administration Sodium chloride 0.9% (NS) and dextrose 5% in water (D$_5$W) have been recommended as diluents; dilute 10-40 units to 1 L in NS, LR, or D$_5$W.
Monitoring Parameters Fluid intake and output during administration; fetal monitoring
Dosage Forms Injection: 10 units/mL (1 mL, 10 mL)

♦ **Oyst-Cal 500 [OTC]** see Calcium Carbonate on page 207
♦ **Oystercal® 500** see Calcium Carbonate on page 207

♦ **OZIZ** *see* Isosorbide *on page 750*

♦ **P-071** *see* Cetirizine *on page 265*

♦ **Pacerone®** *see* Amiodarone *on page 74*

♦ **Pacis™ (Can)** *see* BCG Vaccine *on page 148*

Paclitaxel (PAK li taks el)

U.S. Brand Names Taxol®

Canadian Brand Names Taxol™

Therapeutic Category Antineoplastic Agent, Antimicrotubular; Antineoplastic Agent, Miscellaneous

Use Treatment of advanced carcinoma of the ovary in combination with cisplatin; treatment of metastatic carcinoma of the ovary after failure of first-line or subsequent chemotherapy; adjuvant treatment of node-positive breast cancer administered sequentially to standard doxorubicin-containing chemotherapy; treatment of metastatic breast cancer after failure of combination chemotherapy or relapse within 6 months of adjuvant chemotherapy; treatment of nonsmall cell lung cancer; second-line treatment of AIDS-related Kaposi's sarcoma

Pregnancy Risk Factor D

Contraindications Hypersensitivity to paclitaxel or any component of the formulation; pregnancy

Warnings/Precautions Severe hypersensitivity reactions have been reported with the first or later infusions. Current evidence indicates that prolongation of the infusion (to ≥6 hours) plus premedication may minimize this effect. When administered as sequential infusions, taxane derivatives (docetaxel, paclitaxel) should be administered before platinum derivatives (carboplatin, cisplatin) to limit myelosuppression and to enhance efficacy.

Adverse Reactions

>10%:

Allergic: Appear to be primarily nonimmunologically mediated release of histamine and other vasoactive substances; almost always seen within the first hour of an infusion (~75% occur within 10 minutes of starting the infusion); incidence is significantly reduced by premedication

Cardiovascular: Bradycardia, transient (25%)

Hematologic: Myelosuppression, leukopenia, neutropenia (6% to 21%), thrombocytopenia
Onset: 8-11 days
Nadir: 15-21 days
Recovery: 21 days

Dermatologic: Alopecia, venous erythema, tenderness, discomfort, phlebitis (2%)

Neurotoxicity: Sensory and/or autonomic neuropathy (numbness, tingling, burning pain), myopathy or myopathic effects (25% to 55%), and central nervous system toxicity. May be cumulative and dose-limiting.

Gastrointestinal: Severe, potentially dose-limiting mucositis, stomatitis (15%), most common at doses >390 mg/m^2

Hepatic: Mild increases in liver enzymes

Neuromuscular & skeletal: Arthralgia, myalgia

1% to 10%:

Cardiovascular: Myocardial infarction

Gastrointestinal: Mild nausea and vomiting (5% to 6%), diarrhea (5% to 6%)

Hematologic: Anemia

<1% (Limited to important or life-threatening): Pruritus, radiation pneumonitis, rash

Drug Interactions

Cytochrome P450 Effect: CYP2C8 and 3A3/4 enzyme substrate

Increased Effect/Toxicity: In Phase I trials, myelosuppression was more profound when given after cisplatin than with alternative sequence. Pharmacokinetic data demonstrates a decrease in clearance of ~33% when administered following cisplatin. Possibility of an inhibition of metabolism in patients treated with ketoconazole. When administered as sequential infusions, observational studies indicate a potential for increased toxicity when platinum derivatives (carboplatin, cisplatin) are administered before taxane derivatives (docetaxel, paclitaxel).

Decreased Effect: Paclitaxel metabolism is dependent on cytochrome P450 isoenzymes. Inducers of these enzymes may decrease the effect of paclitaxel.

Ethanol/Nutrition/Herb Interactions Herb/Nutraceutical: Avoid black cohosh, dong quai in estrogen-dependent tumors. Avoid valerian, St John's wort, kava kava, gotu kola (may increase CNS depression).

Stability Store intact vials at room temperature of 20°C to 25°C (68°F to 77°F). Further dilution in NS or D$_5$W to a concentration of 0.3-1.2 mg/mL is stable for up to 27 hours at room temperature (25°C) and ambient light conditions.

Paclitaxel should be administered in either glass or Excel™/PAB™ containers. Should also use **nonpolyvinyl** (non-PVC) tubing (eg, polyethylene) to minimize leaching. Formulated in a vehicle known as Cremophor® EL (polyoxyethylated castor oil). Cremophor® EL has been found to leach the plasticizer DEHP from polyvinyl chloride infusion bags or administration sets. Contact of the undiluted concentrate with plasticized polyvinyl chloride (PVC) equipment or devices is not recommended. Administer through I.V. tubing containing an in-line (NOT >0.22 μ) filter; administration through IVEX-2® filters (which incorporate short inlet and outlet polyvinyl chloride-coated tubing) has not resulted in significant leaching of DEHP.

Visually **compatible** via Y-site: Acyclovir, amikacin, bleomycin, calcium chloride, carboplatin, ceftazidime, ceftriaxone, cimetidine, cisplatin, cyclophosphamide, cytarabine, dexamethasone sodium phosphate, diphenhydramine hydrochloride, doxorubicin, etoposide, famotidine, fluconazole, fluorouracil, ganciclovir, gentamicin, haloperidol lactate, heparin, hydrocortisone sodium succinate, hydrocortisone phosphate hydromorphone, lorazepam, magnesium sulfate, mannitol, meperidine, mesna, methotrexate sodium, metoclopramide hydrochloride, morphine sulfate, ondansetron, potassium chloride, prochlorperazine edisylate, ranitidine hydrochloride, sodium bicarbonate, vancomycin hydrochloride

Visually/chemically **incompatible** via Y-site: amphotericin B, chlorpromazine, hydroxyzine, methylprednisolone, mitoxantrone

Standard I.V. dilution: IVPB: Dose/500-1000 mL D_5W or NS
Solutions are stable for 27 hours at room temperature (25°C)

Mechanism of Action Paclitaxel exerts its effects on microtubules and their protein subunits, tubulin dimers. Microtubules serve as facilitators of intracellular transport and maintain the integrity and function of cells. Paclitaxel promotes microtubule assembly by enhancing the action of tubulin dimers, stabilizing existing microtubules, and inhibiting their disassembly. Maintaining microtubule assembly inhibits mitosis and cell death. The G_2- and M-phases of the cell cycle are affected. In addition, the drug can distort mitotic spindles, resulting in the breakage of chromosomes.

Pharmacodynamics/Kinetics

Distribution: V_{dss}: 42-162 L/m^2, indicating extensive extravascular distribution and/or tissue binding; initial rapid decline represents distribution to the peripheral compartment and significant elimination of the drug; later phase is due to a relatively slow efflux of paclitaxel from the peripheral compartment

Protein binding: 89% to 98% (concentrations of 0.1-50 mcg/mL)

Metabolism: Hepatic in animals; evidence suggests hepatic in humans

Half-life elimination: Mean: Terminal: 5.3-17.4 hours after 1- and 6-hour infusions at dosing levels of 15-275 mg/m^2

Excretion: Urine (as unchanged drug); 1.3% to 12.6% following 1-, 6-, and 24-hour infusions of 15-275 mg/m^2

Clearance: Mean: Total body: After 1- and 6-hour infusions: 5.8-16.3 L/hour/m^2; After 24-hour infusions: 14.2-17.2 L/hour/m^2

Usual Dosage Premedication with dexamethasone (20 mg orally or I.V. at 12 and 6 hours **or** 14 and 7 hours before the dose), diphenhydramine (50 mg I.V. 30-60 minutes prior to the dose), and cimetidine, famotidine or ranitidine (I.V. 30-60 minutes prior to the dose) is recommended

Adults: I.V.: Refer to individual protocols
Ovarian carcinoma:
First-line therapy: 175 mg/m^2 over 3 hours every 3 weeks
or 135 mg/m^2 over 24 hours every 3 weeks
After failure of first-line therapy: 135-175 mg/m^2 over 3 hours every 3 weeks (doses up to 350 mg/m^2 have been studied, but are not generally recommended)
or 50-80 mg/m^2 over 1-3 hours weekly
or 1.4-4 mg/m^2/day continuous infusion for 14 days every 4 weeks
Metastatic breast cancer:
Adjuvant treatment of node-positive breast cancer: 175 mg/m^2 over 3 hours every 3 weeks for 4 courses
Metastatic or recurrent disease: 175 mg/m^2 over 3 hours every 3 weeks
Nonsmall cell lung carcinoma: 135 mg/m^2 over 24 hours, followed by cisplatin 75 mg/m^2; repeat every 3 weeks
AIDS-related Kaposi's sarcoma: 135 mg/m^2 over 3 hours every 3 weeks
or 100 mg/m^2 over 3 hours every 2 weeks

Dosage modification for toxicity (solid tumors, including ovary, breast, and lung carcinoma): Courses of paclitaxel should not be repeated until the neutrophil count is ≥1500 cells/mm^3 and the platelet count is ≥100,000 cells/mm^3; reduce dosage by 20% for patients experiencing severe peripheral neuropathy or severe neutropenia (neutrophil <500 cells/mm^3 for a week or longer)

Dosage modification for immunosuppression in advanced HIV disease: Paclitaxel should not be given to patients with HIV if the baseline or subsequent neutrophil count is <1000 cells/mm^3. Additional modifications include: Reduce dosage of dexamethasone in premedication to 10 mg orally; reduce dosage by 20% in patients experiencing severe peripheral neuropathy or severe neutropenia (neutrophil <500 cells/mm^3 for a week or longer); initiate concurrent hematopoietic growth factor (G-CSF) as clinically indicated

Hemodialysis: Significant drug removal is unlikely based on physiochemical characteristics

Peritoneal dialysis: Significant drug removal is unlikely based on physiochemical characteristics

Dosage adjustment in hepatic impairment:
Total bilirubin ≤1.5 mg/dL and AST >2 times normal limits: Total dose <135 mg/m^2
Total bilirubin 1.6-3.0 mg/dL: Total dose ≤75 mg/m^2
Total bilirubin ≥3.1 mg/dL: Total dose ≤50 mg/m^2

Administration

Anaphylactoid-like reactions have been reported: Corticosteroids (dexamethasone), H_1-antagonists (diphenhydramine), and H_2-antagonists (famotidine), should be administered prior to paclitaxel administration to minimize potential for anaphylaxis

Administer I.V. infusion over 1-24 hours; use of a 0.22 micron in-line filter is recommended during the infusion

Monitoring Parameters Monitor for hypersensitivity reactions

Reference Range Mean maximum serum concentrations: 435-802 ng/mL following 24-hour infusions of 200-275 mg/m^2 and were approximately 10% to 30% of those following 6-hour infusions of equivalent doses

Patient Information This medication can only be administered by I.V. infusion, usually on a cyclic basis. Maintain adequate hydration (2-3 L/day of fluids unless instructed to restrict fluid intake) and nutrition (small frequent meals will help). You will most likely lose your hair (will grow back after therapy); experience some nausea or vomiting (request antiemetic); feel weak or lethargic (use caution when driving or engaging in tasks that require alertness until response to drug is known). Use good oral care to reduce incidence of mouth sores. You will be more susceptible to infection; avoid crowds or exposure to infection. Report numbness or tingling in fingers or toes (use care to prevent injury); signs of infection (fever, chills, sore throat, burning urination, fatigue); unusual bleeding (tarry stools, easy bruising, or blood in stool, urine, or mouth); unresolved mouth sores; nausea or vomiting; or skin rash or itching. Contraceptive measures are recommended during therapy.

(Continued)

Paclitaxel *(Continued)*

Additional Information Sensory neuropathy is almost universal at doses >250 mg/m²; motor neuropathy is uncommon at doses <250 mg/m². Myopathic effects are common with doses >200 mg/m², generally occur within 2-3 days of treatment, and resolve over 5-6 days. Patients with pre-existing neuropathies from chemotherapy or coexisting conditions (eg, diabetes mellitus) may be at a higher risk.

Dosage Forms Injection: 6 mg/mL (5 mL, 16.7 mL, 50 mL)

♦ **Palafer® (Can)** *see* Ferrous Fumarate *on page 555*

Palivizumab *(pah li VIZ u mab)*

U.S. Brand Names Synagis®

Therapeutic Category Monoclonal Antibody

Use Prevention of serious lower respiratory tract disease caused by respiratory syncytial virus (RSV) in infants and children <2 years of age with chronic lung disease who have required medical therapy for their chronic lung disease within 6 months before the anticipated RSV season; prevention of serious RSV disease in patients with a history of prematurity (≤28 weeks gestation) up to 12 months of age or infants born at 29-32 weeks of gestation up to 6 months of age; prophylaxis of infants with severe immune deficiency exposed to RSV

Pregnancy Risk Factor C

Pregnancy/Breast-Feeding Implications Not for adult use; reproduction studies have not been conducted

Contraindications History of severe prior reaction to palivizumab or any component of the formulation; not recommended for children with cyanotic congenital heart disease

Warnings/Precautions Anaphylactoid reactions have not been observed following palivizumab administration; however, can occur after administration of proteins. Safety and efficacy of palivizumab have not been demonstrated in the treatment of established RSV disease.

Adverse Reactions The incidence of adverse events was similar between the palivizumab and placebo groups.

>1%:
Central nervous system: Nervousness
Dermatologic: Fungal dermatitis, eczema, seborrhea, rash
Gastrointestinal: Diarrhea, vomiting, gastroenteritis
Hematologic: Anemia
Hepatic: ALT increase, abnormal LFTs
Local: Injection site reaction, erythema, induration
Ocular: Conjunctivitis
Otic: Otitis media
Respiratory: Cough, wheezing, bronchiolitis, pneumonia, bronchitis, asthma, croup, dyspnea, sinusitis, apnea, upper respiratory infection, rhinitis
Miscellaneous: Oral moniliasis, failure to thrive, viral infection, flu syndrome

Overdosage/Toxicology No data from clinical studies are available.

Stability Store in refrigerator at a temperature between 2°C to 8°C (35.6°F to 46.4°F) in original container; do not freeze

Use aseptic technique when reconstituting; add 1 mL of sterile water for injection to a 100 mg vial; swirl vial gently for 30 seconds to avoid foaming. Do not shake vial. Allow to stand at room temperature for 20 minutes until the solution clarifies; solution should be administered within 6 hours of reconstitution.

Mechanism of Action Exhibits neutralizing and fusion-inhibitory activity against RSV; these activities inhibit RSV replication in laboratory and clinical studies

Pharmacodynamics/Kinetics

Half-life elimination: Children <24 months: 20 days; Adults: 18 days
Time to peak, serum: 48 hours

Usual Dosage I.M.: Infants and Children: 15 mg/kg of body weight, monthly throughout RSV season (First dose administered prior to commencement of RSV season)

Administration Injection should (preferably) be in the anterolateral aspect of the thigh; gluteal muscle should not be used routinely; injection volume over 1 mL should be administered as divided doses

Additional Information RSV prophylaxis should be initiated at the onset of the RSV season. In most areas of the United States, onset of RSV outbreaks is October to December, and termination is March to May, but regional differences occur.

Dosage Forms Injection, lyophilized: 50 mg, 100 mg

♦ **Palmitate-A® [OTC]** *see* Vitamin A *on page 1421*
♦ **2-PAM** *see* Pralidoxime *on page 1115*
♦ **Pamelor®** *see* Nortriptyline *on page 996*

Pamidronate *(pa mi DROE nate)*

U.S. Brand Names Aredia®

Canadian Brand Names Aredia®

Synonyms Pamidronate Disodium

Therapeutic Category Antidote, Hypercalcemia; Bisphosphonate Derivative

Use Treatment of hypercalcemia associated with malignancy; treatment of osteolytic bone lesions associated with multiple myeloma or metastatic breast cancer; moderate to severe Paget's disease of bone

Pregnancy Risk Factor C

Pregnancy/Breast-Feeding Implications Pamidronate has been shown to cross the placenta and cause embryo/fetal effects in animals. There are no adequate and well-controlled studies in pregnant women; use is not recommended during pregnancy.

Contraindications Hypersensitivity to pamidronate, other biphosphonates, or any component of the formulation

Warnings/Precautions Use caution in patients with renal impairment as nephropathy was seen in animal studies. However, in contrast to reports of renal failure with other biphosphonates, impairment of renal function has not been reported with pamidronate in studies to date. However, further experience is needed to assess the nephrotoxic potential with higher doses and prolonged administration. Use caution in patients who are pregnant or in the breast-feeding period; leukopenia has been observed with oral pamidronate and monitoring of white blood cell counts is suggested. Vein irritation and thrombophlebitis may occur with infusions. Has not been studied exclusively in the elderly; monitor serum electrolytes periodically since elderly are often receiving diuretics which can result in decreases in serum calcium, potassium, and magnesium.

Adverse Reactions As reported with hypercalcemia of malignancy; percentage of adverse effect varies upon dose and duration of infusion.

>10%:
 Central nervous system: Fever (18% to 26%), fatigue (12%)
 Endocrine & metabolic: Hypophosphatemia (9% to 18%), hypokalemia (4% to 18%), hypomagnesemia (4% to 12%), hypocalcemia (1% to 12%)
 Gastrointestinal: Nausea (0% to 18%), anorexia (1% to 12%)
 Local: Infusion site reaction (0% to 18%)

1% to 10%:
 Cardiovascular: Atrial fibrillation (0% to 6%), hypertension (0% to 6%), syncope (0% to 6%), tachycardia (0% to 6%), atrial flutter (0% to 1%), cardiac failure (0% to 1%)
 Central nervous system: Somnolence (1% to 6%), psychosis (0% to 4%), insomnia (0% to 1%)
 Endocrine & metabolic: Hypothyroidism (6%)
 Gastrointestinal: Constipation (4% to 6%), stomatitis (0% to 1%)
 Hematologic: Leukopenia (0% to 4%), neutropenia (0% to 1%), thrombocytopenia (0% to 1%)
 Neuromuscular & skeletal: Myalgia (0% to 1%)
 Renal: Uremia (0% to 4%)
 Respiratory: Rales (0% to 6%), rhinitis (0% to 6%), upper respiratory tract infection (0% to 3%)

<1% (Limited to important or life-threatening): Allergic reaction, anaphylactic shock, angioedema, episcleritis, hypotension, iritis, scleritis, uveitis

Overdosage/Toxicology Symptoms include hypocalcemia, EKG changes, seizures, bleeding, paresthesias, carpopedal spasm, and fever. Treat with I.V. calcium gluconate and general supportive care. Fever and hypotension can be treated with corticosteroids.

Stability Do not store powder for reconstitution at temperatures above 30°C (86°F). Reconstitute by adding 10 mL of sterile water for injection to each vial of lyophilized pamidronate disodium powder, the resulting solution will be 30 mg/10 mL or 90 mg/10 mL. The reconstituted solution is stable under refrigeration at 2°C to 8°C (36°F to 46°F) for 24 hours.

Pamidronate may be further diluted in 250-1000 mL of 0.45% or 0.9% sodium chloride or 5% dextrose; pamidronate should not be mixed with calcium-containing solutions (eg, Ringer's solution). Pamidronate solution for infusion is stable at room temperature for up to 24 hours.

Mechanism of Action A biphosphonate which inhibits bone resorption via actions on osteoclasts or on osteoclast precursors. Does not appear to produce any significant effects on renal tubular calcium handling and is poorly absorbed following oral administration (high oral doses have been reported effective); therefore, I.V. therapy is preferred.

Pharmacodynamics/Kinetics
Onset of action: 24-48 hours
 Peak effect: Maximum: 5-7 days
Absorption: Poor; pharmacokinetic studies lacking
Half-life elimination: 21-35 hours Bone: Terminal: ~300 days
Excretion: Biphasic; urine (~50% as unchanged drug) within 120 hours

Usual Dosage Drug must be diluted properly before administration and infused intravenously slowly. I.V.: Adults:
Hypercalcemia of malignancy:
 Moderate cancer-related hypercalcemia (corrected serum calcium: 12-13.5 mg/dL): 60-90 mg, as a single dose, given as a slow infusion over 2-24 hours; dose should be diluted in 1000 mL 0.45% NaCl, 0.9% NaCl, or D$_5$W
 Severe cancer-related hypercalcemia (corrected serum calcium: >13.5 mg/dL): 90 mg, as a single dose, as a slow infusion over 2-24 hours; dose should be diluted in 1000 mL 0.45% NaCl, 0.9% NaCl, or D$_5$W
 A period of 7 days should elapse before the use of second course; repeat infusions every 2-3 weeks have been suggested, however, could be administered every 2-3 months according to the degree of and severity of hypercalcemia and/or the type of malignancy.
 Note: Some investigators have suggested a lack of a dose-response relationship. Courses of pamidronate for hypercalcemia may be repeated at varying intervals, depending on the duration of normocalcemia (median 2-3 weeks), but the manufacturer recommends a minimum interval between courses of 7 days. Oral etidronate at a dose of 20 mg/kg/day has been used to maintain the calcium lowering effect following I.V. bisphosphonates, although it is of limited effectiveness.
Osteolytic bone lesions with multiple myeloma: 90 mg in 500 mL D$_5$W, 0.45% NaCl or 0.9% NaCl administered over 4 hours on a monthly basis
Osteolytic bone lesions with metastatic breast cancer: 90 mg in 250 mL D$_5$W, 0.45% NaCl or 0.9% NaCl administered over 2 hours, repeated every 3-4 weeks
Paget's disease: 30 mg in 500 mL 0.45% NaCl, 0.9% NaCl or D$_5$W administered over 4 hours for 3 consecutive days
Dosing adjustment in renal impairment: Adjustment is not necessary. Pamidronate was not studied in patients with serum creatinine >5 mg/dL, and only in a few multiple myeloma patients with serum creatinine ≥3 mg/dL.

Administration Drug must be properly diluted before administration and slowly infused intravenously (over at least 2 hours).
(Continued)

Pamidronate *(Continued)*

Monitoring Parameters Serum electrolytes, monitor for hypocalcemia for at least 2 weeks after therapy; serum calcium, phosphate, magnesium, potassium, serum creatinine, CBC with differential

Reference Range Calcium (total): Adults: 9.0-11.0 mg/dL (SI: 2.05-2.54 mmol/L), may slightly decrease with aging; Phosphorus: 2.5-4.5 mg/dL (SI: 0.81-1.45 mmol/L)

Patient Information This medication can only be administered I.V. Avoid foods high in calcium, or vitamins with minerals, during infusion or for 2-3 hours after completion. You may experience nausea or vomiting (small frequent meals and good mouth care may help); or recurrent bone pain (consult prescriber for analgesic). Report unusual muscle twitching or spasms, severe diarrhea/constipation, or acute bone pain.

Dosage Forms Powder for injection, lyophilized, as disodium: 30 mg, 90 mg

♦ **Pamidronate Disodium** *see Pamidronate on page 1032*

♦ **p-Aminoclonidine** *see Apraclonidine on page 111*

♦ **Pancrease®** *see Pancrelipase on page 1034*

♦ **Pancrease® MT** *see Pancrelipase on page 1034*

♦ **Pancrecarb MS®** *see Pancrelipase on page 1034*

Pancrelipase *(pan kre LI pase)*

U.S. Brand Names Creon®; Ku-Zyme® HP; Lipram®; Lipram® 4500; Lipram-CR®; Lipram-PN®; Lipram-UL®; Pancrease®; Pancrease® MT; Pancrecarb MS®; Pangestyme™ CN; Pangestyme™ EC; Pangestyme™ MT; Pangestyme™ UL; Ultrase®; Ultrase® MT; Viokase®; Zymase® [DSC]

Canadian Brand Names Cotazym®; Creon® 5; Creon® 10; Creon® 20; Creon® 25; Pancrease®; Pancrease® MT; Ultrase®; Ultrase® MT; Viokase®

Synonyms Lipancreatin

Therapeutic Category Enzyme, Pancreatic; Pancreatic Enzyme

Use Replacement therapy in symptomatic treatment of malabsorption syndrome caused by pancreatic insufficiency

Unlabeled/Investigational Use Treatment of occluded feeding tubes

Pregnancy Risk Factor B/C (product specific)

Contraindications Hypersensitivity to pork protein or any component of the formulation; acute pancreatitis or acute exacerbations of chronic pancreatic disease

Warnings/Precautions Pancrelipase is inactivated by acids; use microencapsulated products whenever possible, since these products permit better dissolution of enzymes in the duodenum and protect the enzyme preparations from acid degradation in the stomach. Fibrotic strictures in the colon, some requiring surgery, have been reported with high doses; use caution, especially in children with cystic fibrosis. Use caution when adjusting doses or changing brands. Avoid inhalation of powder, may cause nasal and respiratory tract irritation.

Adverse Reactions Frequency not defined; occurrence of events may be dose related.

Central nervous system: Pain

Dermatologic: Rash

Endocrine & metabolic: Hyperuricemia

Gastrointestinal: Nausea, cramps, constipation, diarrhea, perianal irritation/inflammation (large doses), irritation of the mouth, abdominal pain, intestinal obstruction, vomiting, flatulence, melena, weight loss, fibrotic strictures, greasy stools

Ocular: Lacrimation

Renal: Hyperuricosuria

Respiratory: Sneezing, dyspnea, bronchospasm

Miscellaneous: Allergic reactions

Overdosage/Toxicology Symptoms include diarrhea, other transient intestinal upset, hyperuricosuria, and hyperuricemia.

Ethanol/Nutrition/Herb Interactions Food: Avoid placing contents of opened capsules on alkaline food (pH >5.5); pancrelipase may impair absorption of oral iron and folic acid.

Stability Store between 15°C to 25°C (59°F to 77°F); keep in a dry place, do not refrigerate

Mechanism of Action Pancrelipase is a natural product harvested from the hog pancreas. It contains a combination of lipase, amylase, and protease. Products are formulated to dissolve in the more basic pH of the duodenum so that they may act locally to break down fats, protein, and starch.

Pharmacodynamics/Kinetics

Absorption: None, acts locally in GI tract

Excretion: Feces

Usual Dosage Oral:

Powder: Actual dose depends on the condition being treated and the digestive requirements of the patient

Children <1 year: Start with ⅛ teaspoonful with feedings

Adults: 0.7 g (¼ teaspoonful) with meals

Capsules/tablets: The following dosage recommendations are only an approximation for initial dosages. The actual dosage will depend on the condition being treated and the digestive requirements of the individual patient. Adjust dose based on body weight and stool fat content. Total daily dose reflects ~3 meals/day and 2-3 snacks/day, with half the mealtime dose given with a snack. Older patients may need less units/kg due to increased weight, but decreased ingestion of fat/kg. Maximum dose: 2500 units of lipase/kg/meal (10,000 units of lipase/kg/day)

Children:

<1 year: 2000 units of lipase with meals

1-6 years: 4000-8000 units of lipase with meals and 4000 units with snacks

7-12 years: 4000-12,000 units of lipase with meals and snacks

Adults: 4000-48,000 units of lipase with meals and with snacks

Occluded feeding tubes: One tablet of Viokase® crushed with one 325 mg tablet of sodium bicarbonate (to activate the Viokase®) in 5 mL of water can be instilled into the nasogastric tube and clamped for 5 minutes; then, flushed with 50 mL of tap water

Dietary Considerations Should be used as part of a high-calorie diet, appropriate for age and clinical status. Administer with meals or snacks and swallow whole with a generous amount of liquid. Do not crush or chew. Delayed-release capsules containing enteric coated microspheres or microtablets may also be opened and the contents sprinkled on soft food with a low pH such as applesauce, gelatin; apricot, banana, or sweet potato baby food; baby formula. Dairy products such as milk, custard or ice cream may have a high pH and should be avoided.

Administration Oral: Administer with meals or snacks and swallow whole with a generous amount of liquid. Do not crush or chew; retention in the mouth before swallowing may cause mucosal irritation and stomatitis. Delayed-release capsules containing enteric-coated microspheres or microtablets may also be opened and the contents sprinkled on soft food with a low pH that does not require chewing, such as applesauce, gelatin; apricot, banana, or sweet potato baby food; baby formula. Dairy products such as milk, custard, or ice cream may have a high pH and should be avoided. Avoid inhalation of powder, may cause nasal and respiratory tract irritation.

Monitoring Parameters Abdominal symptoms, nutritional intake, growth (in children), stool character, fecal fat

Patient Information To be taken with a meal or a snack. Swallow tablets and capsules whole, do not chew, crush, or dissolve. Swallow with a generous amount of liquid; do not let dissolve in mouth. Capsules may also be opened and sprinkled on soft food with a low pH such as applesauce; gelatin; apricot, banana, or sweet potato baby food; baby formula. Do not sprinkle on dairy products such as milk, custard, or ice cream as they may have a high pH. Do not change brands, increase or decrease dosage without consulting prescriber. May experience nausea, vomiting, cramps, or constipation. Notify prescriber if experiencing abdominal pain, ongoing diarrhea or poor weight gain, especially if using large doses, are <12 years of age, or have cystic fibrosis. Inform prescriber if you are or intend to be pregnant; notify prescriber if breast-feeding.

Nursing Implications Monitor stool fat content

Dosage Forms
Capsule: Ku-Zyme® HP: Lipase 8000 units, protease 30,000 units, amylase 30,000 units
Capsule, delayed release:
    Lipram 4500: Lipase 4500 units, protease 25000 units, amylase 20000 units
    Pangestyme™ CN-10: Lipase 10,000 units, protease 37,500 units, amylase 33,200 units
    Pangestyme™ CN-20: Lipase 20,000 units, protease 75,000 units, amylase 66,400 units
Capsule, delayed release, enteric coated microspheres:
    Creon® 5: Lipase 5000 units, protease 18,750 units, amylase 16,600 units
    Creon® 10, Lipram-CR10®: Lipase 10,000 units, protease 37,500 units, amylase 33,200 units
    Creon® 20, Lipram-CR20®: Lipase 20,000 units, protease 75,000 units, amylase 66,400 units
    Lipram-PN10®: Lipase 10,000 units, protease 30,000 units, amylase 39,000 units
    Lipram-PN16®: Lipase 16,000 units, protease 48,000 units, amylase 48,000 units
    Lipram-UL12®: Lipase 12,000 units, protease 39,000 units, amylase 39,000 units
    Lipram-UL18®: Lipase 18,000 units, protease 58,500 units, amylase 58,500 units
    Lipram-UL20®: Lipase 20,000 units, protease 65,000 units, amylase 65,000 units
    Pancrecarb MS-4®: Lipase 4000 units, protease 25,000 units, amylase 25,000 units
    Pancrecarb MS-8®: Lipase 8000 units, protease 45,000 units, amylase 40,000 units
Capsule, delayed release, enteric coated spheres: Zymase®: Lipase 12,000 units, protease 24,000 units, amylase 24,000 units [DSC]
Capsule, enteric-coated microspheres
    Pancrease®, Pangestyme™ EC: Lipase 4500 units, protease 25,000 units, amylase 20,000 units
    Ultrase®: Lipase 4500 units, protease 25,000 units, amylase 20,000 units
Capsule, enteric coated microtablets:
    Pancrease® MT 4: Lipase 4000 units, protease 12,000 units, amylase 12,000 units
    Pancrease® MT 10: Lipase 10,000 units, protease 30,000 units, amylase 30,000 units
    Pancrease® MT 16, Pangestyme™ MT 16: Lipase 16,000 units, protease 48,000 units, amylase 48,000 units
    Pancrease® MT 20: Lipase 20,000 units, protease 44,000 units, amylase 56,000 units
    Pangestyme™ UL 12: Lipase 12,000 units, protease 39,000 units, amylase 39,000 units
    Pangestyme™ UL 18: Lipase 18,000 units, protease 58,500 units, amylase 58,500 units
    Pangestyme™ UL 20: Lipase 20,000 units, protease 65,000 units, amylase 65,000 units
Capsule, enteric coated minitablets:
    Ultrase® MT12: Lipase 12,000 units, protease 39,000 units, amylase 39,000 units
    Ultrase® MT18: Lipase 18,000 units, protease 58,500 units, amylase 58,500 units
    Ultrase® MT20: Lipase 20,000 units, protease 65,000 units, amylase 65,000 units
Powder (Viokase®): Lipase 16,800 units, protease 70,000 units, amylase 70,000 units per 0.7 g (227 g)
Tablet:
    Viokase® 8: Lipase 8000 units, protease 30,000 units, amylase 30,000 units
    Viokase® 16: Lipase 16,000 units, protease 60,000 units, amylase 60,000 units

Pancuronium (pan kyoo ROE nee um)

Related Information
    Neuromuscular Blocking Agents Comparison *on page 1508*

U.S. Brand Names Pavulon®

Synonyms Pancuronium Bromide

Therapeutic Category Neuromuscular Blocker Agent, Nondepolarizing; Skeletal Muscle Relaxant

Use Adjunct to general anesthesia to facilitate endotracheal intubation and to relax skeletal muscles during surgery; to facilitate mechanical ventilation in ICU patients; does not relieve pain or produce sedation
(Continued)

Pancuronium *(Continued)*

Drug of choice for neuromuscular blockade except in patients with renal failure, hepatic failure, or cardiovascular instability or in situations not suited for pancuronium's long duration of action

Pregnancy Risk Factor C

Contraindications Hypersensitivity to pancuronium, bromide, or any component of the formulation

Warnings/Precautions Ventilation must be supported during neuromuscular blockade; use with caution in patients with renal and/or hepatic impairment (adjust dose appropriately); certain clinical conditions may result in potentiation or antagonism of neuromuscular blockade:

Potentiation: Electrolyte abnormalities, severe hyponatremia, severe hypocalcemia, severe hypokalemia, hypermagnesemia, neuromuscular diseases, acidosis, acute intermittent porphyria, renal failure, hepatic failure

Antagonism: Alkalosis, hypercalcemia, demyelinating lesions, peripheral neuropathies, diabetes mellitus

Increased sensitivity in patients with myasthenia gravis, Eaton-Lambert syndrome; resistance in burn patients (>30% of body) for period of 5-70 days postinjury; resistance in patients with muscle trauma, denervation, immobilization, infection.

Adverse Reactions Frequency not defined.

Cardiovascular: Elevation in pulse rate, elevated blood pressure and cardiac output, tachycardia, edema, skin flushing, circulatory collapse

Dermatologic: Rash, itching, erythema, burning sensation along the vein

Gastrointestinal: Excessive salivation

Neuromuscular & skeletal: Profound muscle weakness

Respiratory: Wheezing, bronchospasm

Miscellaneous: Hypersensitivity reaction

Overdosage/Toxicology Symptoms include apnea, respiratory depression, and cardiovascular collapse. Pyridostigmine, neostigmine, or edrophonium in conjunction with atropine will usually antagonize the action of pancuronium.

Drug Interactions

Increased Effect/Toxicity: Increased effects are possible with aminoglycosides, beta-blockers, clindamycin, calcium channel blockers, halogenated anesthetics, imipenem, ketamine, lidocaine, loop diuretics (furosemide), macrolides (case reports), magnesium sulfate, procainamide, quinidine, quinolones, tetracyclines, and vancomycin. May increase risk of myopathy when used with high-dose corticosteroids for extended periods.

Decreased Effect: Effect of nondepolarizing neuromuscular blockers may be reduced by carbamazepine (chronic use), corticosteroids (also associated with myopathy - see increased effect), phenytoin (chronic use), sympathomimetics, and theophylline.

Stability Refrigerate; however, is stable for up to 6 months at room temperature; I.V. form is **incompatible** when mixed with diazepam at a Y-site injection

Mechanism of Action Blocks neural transmission at the myoneural junction by binding with cholinergic receptor sites

Pharmacodynamics/Kinetics

Onset of effect: Peak effect: I.V.: 2-3 minutes

Duration: 40-60 minutes (dose dependent)

Metabolism: Hepatic, 30% to 45%

Half-life elimination: 110 minutes

Excretion: Urine (55% to 70% as unchanged drug)

Usual Dosage Administer I.V.; dose to effect; doses will vary due to interpatient variability; use ideal body weight for obese patients

Surgery:

Neonates <1 month:

Test dose: 0.02 mg/kg to measure responsiveness

Initial: 0.03 mg/kg/dose repeated twice at 5- to 10-minute intervals as needed; maintenance: 0.03-0.09 mg/kg/dose every 30 minutes to 4 hours as needed

Infants >1 month, Children, and Adults: Initial: 0.06-0.1 mg/kg or 0.05 mg/kg after initial dose of succinylcholine for intubation; maintenance dose: 0.01 mg/kg 60-100 minutes after initial dose and then 0.01 mg/kg every 25-60 minutes

Pretreatment/priming: 10% of intubating dose given 3-5 minutes before initial dose

ICU: 0.05-0.1 mg/kg bolus followed by 0.8-1.7 mcg/kg/minute once initial recovery from bolus observed or 0.1-0.2 mg/kg every 1-3 hours; **continuous I.V. infusions are not recommended due to case reports of prolonged paralysis**

Dosing adjustment in renal impairment: Elimination half-life is doubled, plasma clearance is reduced and rate of recovery is sometimes much slower

Cl_{cr} 10-50 mL/minute: Administer 50% of normal dose

Cl_{cr} <10 mL/minute: Do not use

Dosing adjustment/comments in hepatic/biliary tract disease: Elimination half-life is doubled, plasma clearance is reduced, recovery time is prolonged, volume of distribution is increased (50%) and results in a slower onset, higher total initial dosage and prolongation of neuromuscular blockade

Administration May be administered undiluted by rapid I.V. injection

Monitoring Parameters Heart rate, blood pressure, assisted ventilation status; cardiac monitor, blood pressure monitor, and ventilator required

Nursing Implications Does not alter the patient's state of consciousness; addition of sedation and analgesia are recommended; may be administered undiluted by rapid I.V. injection

Additional Information Pancuronium is classified as a long-duration neuromuscular-blocking agent. Neuromuscular blockade will be prolonged in patients with decreased renal function. Pancuronium does not relieve pain or produce sedation. It may produce cumulative effect on duration of blockade. It produces tachycardia secondary to vagolytic activity and sympathetic stimulation.

Dosage Forms Injection, as bromide: 1 mg/mL (10 mL); 2 mg/mL (2 mL, 5 mL)

- **Pancuronium Bromide** *see Pancuronium on page 1035*
- **Pandel®** *see Hydrocortisone on page 682*
- **Pangestyme™ CN** *see Pancrelipase on page 1034*
- **Pangestyme™ EC** *see Pancrelipase on page 1034*
- **Pangestyme™ MT** *see Pancrelipase on page 1034*
- **Pangestyme™ UL** *see Pancrelipase on page 1034*
- **Panretin®** *see Alitretinoin on page 51*
- **Panthoderm® Cream [OTC]** *see Dexpanthenol on page 385*
- **Panto™ IV (Can)** *see Pantoprazole on page 1037*
- **Pantoloc™ (Can)** *see Pantoprazole on page 1037*

Pantoprazole (pan TOE pra zole)

U.S. Brand Names Protonix®

Canadian Brand Names Panto™ IV; Pantoloc™; Protonix®

Therapeutic Category Gastric Acid Secretion Inhibitor; Proton Pump Inhibitor

Use

Oral: Treatment and maintenance of healing of erosive esophagitis associated with GERD; reduction in relapse rates of daytime and nighttime heartburn symptoms in GERD

I.V.: As an alternative to oral therapy in patients unable to continue oral pantoprazole; hypersecretory disorders associated with Zollinger-Ellison syndrome or other neoplastic disorders

Unlabeled/Investigational Use Hypersecretory disorders (oral), peptic ulcer disease, active ulcer bleeding with parenterally-administered pantoprazole; adjunct treatment with antibiotics for *Helicobacter pylori*

Pregnancy Risk Factor B

Pregnancy/Breast-Feeding Implications No adequate and well-controlled studies have been done in pregnant women. Use in pregnancy only if clearly needed. Pantoprazole and its metabolites are excreted in the milk of rats. It is unknown if pantoprazole is excreted in human milk. Do not use in women who are breast-feeding.

Contraindications Hypersensitivity to pantoprazole or any component of the formulation

Warnings/Precautions Symptomatic response does not preclude gastric malignancy; not indicated for maintenance therapy; safety and efficacy for use beyond 16 weeks have not been established; safety and efficacy in pediatric patients have not been established

Adverse Reactions

1% to 10%:

Cardiovascular: Chest pain (I.V. ≤6%)

Central nervous system: Pain, migraine, anxiety, dizziness, headache (I.V. >1%)

Dermatologic: Rash (I.V. 6%), pruritus (I.V. 4%)

Endocrine & metabolic: Hyperglycemia (1%), hyperlipidemia

Gastrointestinal: Diarrhea (4%), constipation, dyspepsia, gastroenteritis, nausea, rectal disorder, vomiting, abdominal pain (I.V. 12%)

Genitourinary: Urinary frequency, urinary tract infection

Hepatic: Liver function test abnormality, increased SGPT

Local: Injection site pain (>1%)

Neuromuscular & skeletal: Weakness, back pain, neck pain, arthralgia, hypertonia

Respiratory: Bronchitis, increased cough, dyspnea, pharyngitis, rhinitis, sinusitis, upper respiratory tract infection

Miscellaneous: Flu syndrome, infection

<1% (Limited to important or life-threatening): Allergic reaction, anaphylaxis, anemia, angina pectoris, angioedema, anterior ischemic optic neuropathy, arrhythmia, asthma, blurred vision, cholecystitis, cholelithiasis, cholestatic jaundice, congestive heart failure, convulsion, depression, diabetes mellitus, erythema multiforme, extraocular palsy, gastrointestinal carcinoma, gastrointestinal hemorrhage, glaucoma, gout, hepatic failure, hepatitis, hypokinesia, hypotension, increased salivation, myocardial ischemia, pancreatitis, pancytopenia, retinal vascular disorder, rhabdomyolysis, speech disorder, Stevens-Johnson syndrome, syncope, thrombophlebitis (I.V.), thrombosis, tinnitus, toxic epidermal necrolysis

Overdosage/Toxicology Treatment of an overdose would include appropriate supportive treatment. No adverse events were seen with ingestions of 400 mg and 600 mg. Pantoprazole is not removed by hemodialysis.

Drug Interactions

Cytochrome P450 Effect: CYP2C19 and 3A3/4 enzyme substrate

Decreased Effect: Drugs (eg, itraconazole, ketoconazole, and other azole antifungals, ampicillin esters, iron salts) where absorption is determined by an acidic gastric pH, may have decreased absorption when used concurrently. Monitor for change in effectiveness.

Ethanol/Nutrition/Herb Interactions Ethanol: Avoid ethanol (may cause gastric mucosal irritation).

Stability

Oral: Store tablet at 15°C to 30°C (59°F to 77°F)

I.V.: Store at 2°C to 8°C (36°F to 46°F); protect from light; reconstitute with 10 mL 0.9% sodium chloride; add to 100 mL D_5W or 0.9% sodium chloride; use within 12 hours

Mechanism of Action Suppresses gastric acid secretin by inhibiting the parietal cell H^+/K^+ ATP pump

Pharmacodynamics/Kinetics

Absorption: Well absorbed

Distribution: V_d: 11-24 L

Protein binding: 98%, primarily to albumin

Metabolism: Extensively hepatic; CYP2C19 (demethylation), CYP3A4; no evidence that metabolites have pharmacologic activity

Bioavailability: 77%

Half-life elimination: 1 hour

Time to peak: Oral: 2.5 hours

Excretion: Urine (71%); feces (18%)

(Continued)

Pantoprazole (Continued)

Usual Dosage Adults:

Oral:

Erosive esophagitis associated with GERD:

Treatment: 40 mg once daily for up to 8 weeks; an additional 8 weeks may be used in patients who have not healed after an 8-week course

Maintenance of healing: 40 mg once daily

Note: Lower doses (20 mg once daily) have been used successfully in mild GERD treatment and maintenance of healing

Hypersecretory disorders (unlabeled use): Doses of 40-160 mg/day have been used; adjust dose based on acid output measurements

I.V.:

Erosive esophagitis associated with GERD: 40 mg once daily (infused over 15 minutes) for 7-10 days

Helicobacter pylori eradication (unlabeled use): Doses up to 40 mg twice daily have been used as part of combination therapy

Hypersecretory disorders: 80 mg twice daily; adjust dose based on acid output measurements; 160-240 mg/day in divided doses has been used for a limited period (up to 7 days)

Elderly: Dosage adjustment not required

Dosage adjustment in renal impairment: Not required; pantoprazole is not removed by hemodialysis

Dosage adjustment in hepatic impairment: Not required

Dietary Considerations Oral: May be taken with or without food.

Administration

I.V.: Infuse over 15 minutes at a rate not to exceed 3 mg/minute; use in-line filter (positioned below Y-site if used)

Oral: Tablets should be swallowed whole, do not crush or chew. Do not administer via nasogastric or feeding tube.

Monitoring Parameters Hypersecretory disorders: Acid output measurements, target level <10 mEq/hour (<5 mEq/hour if prior gastric acid-reducing surgery)

Patient Information Take with or without food. Do not split, chew or crush tablet; take at a similar time every day; inform prescriber if you are or intend to be pregnant; discontinue breast-feeding prior to starting this medicine.

Nursing Implications

Tablets should be swallowed whole; not chewed, crushed, or split. Do not administer via a nasogastric or feeding tube. Assess other medications the patient may be taking where absorption may be altered by a change in gastric pH (itraconazole, ketoconazole, iron salts, ampicillin esters).

Injection should be used only as an alternative to oral therapy and should be discontinued when patient is able to take tablets. Infuse over 15 minutes.

Dosage Forms

Powder for injection: 40 mg

Tablet, enteric coated: 20 mg, 40 mg

♦ **Pantothenyl Alcohol** *see* Dexpanthenol *on page 385*

♦ **Papacon®** *see* Papaverine *on page 1038*

Papaverine (pa PAV er een)

U.S. Brand Names Papacon®; Para-Time S.R.®; Pavabid® [DSC]; Pavacot®

Synonyms Papaverine Hydrochloride

Therapeutic Category Vasodilator

Use Oral: Relief of peripheral and cerebral ischemia associated with arterial spasm and myocardial ischemia complicated by arrhythmias

Unlabeled/Investigational Use Investigational: Parenteral: Various vascular spasms associated with muscle spasms as in myocardial infarction, angina, peripheral and pulmonary embolism, peripheral vascular disease, angiospastic states, and visceral spasm (ureteral, biliary, and GI colic); testing for impotence

Pregnancy Risk Factor C

Usual Dosage

I.M., I.V.:

Children: 6 mg/kg/day in 4 divided doses

Adults: 30-65 mg (rarely up to 120 mg); may repeat every 3 hours

Oral, sustained release: Adults: 150-300 mg every 12 hours; in difficult cases: 150 mg every 8 hours

Additional Information Complete prescribing information for this medication should be consulted for additional detail.

Dosage Forms

Capsule, sustained release, as hydrochloride: 150 mg

Injection, as hydrochloride: 30 mg/mL (2 mL, 10 mL)

♦ **Papaverine Hydrochloride** *see* Papaverine *on page 1038*

♦ **Para-Aminosalicylate Sodium** *see* Aminosalicylate Sodium *on page 73*

♦ **Paracetamol** *see* Acetaminophen *on page 22*

♦ **Parafon Forte® (Can)** *see* Chlorzoxazone *on page 285*

♦ **Parafon Forte® DSC** *see* Chlorzoxazone *on page 285*

♦ **Paraplatin®** *see* Carboplatin *on page 226*

♦ **Paraplatin-AQ (Can)** *see* Carboplatin *on page 226*

♦ **Para-Time S.R.®** *see* Papaverine *on page 1038*

♦ **Parcaine®** *see* Proparacaine *on page 1144*

Paregoric (par e GOR ik)

Synonyms Camphorated Tincture of Opium

Therapeutic Category Analgesic, Narcotic; Antidiarrheal

Use Treatment of diarrhea or relief of pain; neonatal opiate withdrawal

Restrictions C-III

Pregnancy Risk Factor B/D (prolonged use or high doses)

Contraindications Hypersensitivity to opium or any component of the formulation; diarrhea caused by poisoning until the toxic material has been removed; pregnancy (long-term prolonged use or high doses)

Warnings/Precautions Use with caution in patients with respiratory, hepatic or renal dysfunction, severe prostatic hyperplasia, or history of narcotic abuse; opium shares the toxic potential of opiate agonists, and usual precautions of opiate agonist therapy should be observed; some preparations contain sulfites which may cause allergic reactions; infants <3 months of age are more susceptible to respiratory depression, use with caution and generally in reduced doses in this age group; tolerance or drug dependence may result from extended use

Adverse Reactions Frequency not defined.

Cardiovascular: Hypotension, peripheral vasodilation

Central nervous system: Drowsiness, dizziness, insomnia, CNS depression, mental depression, increased intracranial pressure, restlessness, headache, malaise

Gastrointestinal: Constipation, anorexia, stomach cramps, nausea, vomiting, biliary tract spasm

Genitourinary: Ureteral spasms, decreased urination, urinary tract spasm

Hepatic: Increased liver function tests

Neuromuscular & skeletal: Weakness

Ocular: Miosis

Respiratory: Respiratory depression

Miscellaneous: Physical and psychological dependence, histamine release

Overdosage/Toxicology Symptoms include hypotension, drowsiness, seizures, and respiratory depression. Treatment consists of naloxone 2 mg I.V. (0.01 mg/kg for children), with repeat administration as necessary, up to a total of 10 mg.

Drug Interactions

Increased Effect/Toxicity: Increased effect/toxicity with CNS depressants (eg, alcohol, narcotics, benzodiazepines, tricyclic antidepressants, MAO inhibitors, phenothiazine).

Ethanol/Nutrition/Herb Interactions Ethanol: Avoid ethanol (may increase CNS depression).

Stability Store in light-resistant, tightly closed container

Mechanism of Action Increases smooth muscle tone in GI tract, decreases motility and peristalsis, diminishes digestive secretions

Pharmacodynamics/Kinetics In terms of opium

Metabolism: Hepatic

Excretion: Urine (primarily as morphine glucuronide conjugates and as unchanged drug - morphine, codeine, papaverine, etc)

Usual Dosage Oral:

Neonatal opiate withdrawal: 3-6 drops every 3-6 hours as needed, or initially 0.2 mL every 3 hours; increase dosage by approximately 0.05 mL every 3 hours until withdrawal symptom's are controlled; it is rare to exceed 0.7 mL/dose. Stabilize withdrawal symptoms for 3-5 days, then gradually decrease dosage over a 2- to 4-week period.

Children: 0.25-0.5 mL/kg 1-4 times/day

Adults: 5-10 mL 1-4 times/day

Patient Information Avoid alcohol, may cause drowsiness, impaired judgment or coordination; may cause physical and psychological dependence with prolonged use

Nursing Implications Observe patient for excessive sedation, respiratory depression, implement safety measures, assist with ambulation

Additional Information Contains morphine 0.4 mg/mL and alcohol 45%. Do **not** confuse this product with opium tincture which is 25 times **more** potent; each 5 mL of paregoric contains 2 mg morphine equivalent, 0.02 mL anise oil, 20 mg benzoic acid, 20 mg camphor, 0.2 mL glycerin and alcohol; final alcohol content 45%; paregoric also contains papaverine and noscapine; because all of these additives may be harmful to neonates, **a 25-fold dilution of opium tincture** is often preferred for treatment of neonatal abstinence syndrome (opiate withdrawal).

Dosage Forms Liquid: 2 mg morphine equivalent/5 mL [equivalent to 20 mg opium powder] (473 mL)

♦ **Parenteral Multiple Vitamins** see Vitamins (Multiple) on page 1424

♦ **Parenteral Nutrition, Calculations for Therapy - Adult Patients** see page 1626

Paricalcitol (pah ri KAL si tole)

U.S. Brand Names Zemplar™

Canadian Brand Names Zemplar™

Therapeutic Category Vitamin D Analog

Use Prevention and treatment of secondary hyperparathyroidism associated with chronic renal failure. Has been evaluated only in hemodialysis patients.

Pregnancy Risk Factor C

Contraindications Hypersensitivity to paricalcitol or any component of the formulation; patients with evidence of vitamin D toxicity; hypercalcemia

Warnings/Precautions The most frequently reported adverse reactions with paricalcitol include nausea, vomiting, and edema. Chronic administration can place patients at risk of hypercalcemia, elevated calcium-phosphorus product and metastatic calcification; it should not be used in patients with evidence of hypercalcemia or vitamin D toxicity.

Adverse Reactions The three most frequently reported events in clinical studies were nausea, vomiting, and edema, which are commonly seen in hemodialysis patients.

(Continued)

Paricalcitol (Continued)

>10%: Gastrointestinal: Nausea (13%)

1% to 10%:

Cardiovascular: Palpitations, peripheral edema (7%)

Central nervous system: Chills, malaise, fever, lightheadedness (5%)

Gastrointestinal: Vomiting (8%), GI bleeding (5%), xerostomia (3%)

Respiratory: Pneumonia (5%)

Miscellaneous: Flu-like symptoms, sepsis

Overdosage/Toxicology Acute overdose may cause hypercalcemia. Monitor serum calcium and phosphorus closely during titration of paricalcitol. Dosage reduction/interruption may be required if hypercalcemia develops. Chronic use may predispose to metastatic calcification. Bone lesions may develop if parathyroid hormone is suppressed below normal.

Drug Interactions

Increased Effect/Toxicity: Phosphate or vitamin D-related compounds should not be taken concurrently. Digitalis toxicity is potentiated by hypercalcemia.

Mechanism of Action Synthetic vitamin D analog which has been shown to reduce PTH serum concentrations

Pharmacodynamics/Kinetics

Protein binding: >99%

Excretion: Feces (74%) in healthy subjects; urine (16%); metabolites represent 51% to 59%

Usual Dosage Adults: I.V.: 0.04-0.1 mcg/kg (2.8-7 mcg) given as a bolus dose no more frequently than every other day at any time during dialysis; doses as high as 0.24 mcg/kg (16.8 mcg) have been administered safely; usually start with 0.04 mcg/kg 3 times/week by I.V. bolus, increased by 0.04 mcg/kg every 2 weeks; the dose of paricalcitol should be adjusted based on serum PTH levels, as follows:

Same or increasing serum PTH level: Increase paricalcitol dose

Serum PTH level decreased by <30%: Increase paricalcitol dose

Serum PTH level decreased by >30% and <60%: Maintain paricalcitol dose

Serum PTH level decrease by >60%: Decrease paricalcitol dose

Serum PTH level 1.5-3 times upper limit of normal: Maintain paricalcitol dose

Monitoring Parameters Serum calcium and phosphorus should be monitored closely (eg, twice weekly) during dose titration; monitor for signs and symptoms of vitamin D intoxication; serum PTH; in trials, a mean PTH level reduction of 30% was achieved within 6 weeks

Patient Information To ensure effectiveness of therapy, it is important to adhere to a dietary regimen of calcium supplementation and phosphorous restriction; avoid excessive use of aluminum-containing compounds

Dosage Forms Injection: 5 mcg/mL (1 mL, 2 mL, 5 mL)

♦ **Pariprazole** *see Rabeprazole on page 1173*

♦ **Parkinson's Agents** *see page 1513*

♦ **Parlodel®** *see Bromocriptine on page 184*

♦ **Parnate®** *see Tranylcypromine on page 1358*

Paromomycin (par oh moe MYE sin)

U.S. Brand Names Humatin®

Canadian Brand Names Humatin®

Synonyms Paromomycin Sulfate

Therapeutic Category Amebicide

Use Treatment of acute and chronic intestinal amebiasis; preoperatively to suppress intestinal flora; tapeworm infestations; treatment of *Cryptosporidium*

Pregnancy Risk Factor C

Contraindications Hypersensitivity to paromomycin or any component of the formulation; intestinal obstruction, renal failure

Warnings/Precautions Use with caution in patients with impaired renal function or possible or proven ulcerative bowel lesions

Adverse Reactions

1% to 10%: Gastrointestinal: Diarrhea, abdominal cramps, nausea, vomiting, heartburn

<1% (Limited to important or life-threatening): Eosinophilia, exanthema, headache, ototoxicity, pruritus, rash, secondary enterocolitis, steatorrhea, vertigo

Overdosage/Toxicology Symptoms include nausea, vomiting, and diarrhea. Treatment following GI decontamination, if possible, is supportive and symptomatic.

Ethanol/Nutrition/Herb Interactions Food: Paromomycin may cause malabsorption of xylose, sucrose, and fats.

Mechanism of Action Acts directly on ameba; has antibacterial activity against normal and pathogenic organisms in the GI tract; interferes with bacterial protein synthesis by binding to 30S ribosomal subunits

Pharmacodynamics/Kinetics

Absorption: None

Excretion: Feces (100% as unchanged drug)

Usual Dosage Oral:

Intestinal amebiasis: Children and Adults: 25-35 mg/kg/day in 3 divided doses for 5-10 days

Dientamoeba fragilis: Children and Adults: 25-30 mg/kg/day in 3 divided doses for 7 days

Cryptosporidium: Adults with AIDS: 1.5-2.25 g/day in 3-6 divided doses for 10-14 days (occasionally courses of up to 4-8 weeks may be needed)

Tapeworm (fish, dog, bovine, porcine):

Children: 11 mg/kg every 15 minutes for 4 doses

Adults: 1 g every 15 minutes for 4 doses

Hepatic coma: Adults: 4 g/day in 2-4 divided doses for 5-6 days

Dwarf tapeworm: Children and Adults: 45 mg/kg/dose every day for 5-7 days

Patient Information Take full course of therapy; do not skip doses; notify physician if ringing in ears, hearing loss, or dizziness occurs

Nursing Implications Monitor hearing loss before and during therapy

Dosage Forms Capsule, as sulfate: 250 mg

♦ **Paromomycin Sulfate** *see Paromomycin on page 1040*

Paroxetine (pa ROKS e teen)

Related Information
Antidepressant Agents Comparison *on page 1482*
Selective Serotonin Reuptake Inhibitor (SSRIs) Pharmacokinetics *on page 1514*

U.S. Brand Names Paxil®; Paxil® CR™
Canadian Brand Names Paxil®; Paxil® CR™
Therapeutic Category Antidepressant, Serotonin Reuptake Inhibitor
Use Treatment of depression in adults; treatment of panic disorder with or without agoraphobia; obsessive-compulsive disorder (OCD) in adults; social anxiety disorder (social phobia); generalized anxiety disorder (GAD); post-traumatic stress disorder (PTSD)

Paxil® CR™: Treatment of depression; treatment of panic disorder
Unlabeled/Investigational Use May be useful in eating disorders, impulse control disorders, self-injurious behavior; premenstrual disorders, vasomotor symptoms of menopause; treatment of depression and obsessive-compulsive disorder (OCD) in children
Pregnancy Risk Factor C
Pregnancy/Breast-Feeding Implications Enters breast milk; use caution in breast-feeding
Contraindications Hypersensitivity to paroxetine or any component of the formulation; use of MAO inhibitors or within 14 days; concurrent use with thioridazine or mesoridazine
Warnings/Precautions Use cautiously in children or during breast-feeding in lactating women. Upon discontinuation of paroxetine therapy, gradually taper dose. Potential for severe reaction when used with MAO inhibitors - serotonin syndrome (hyperthermia, muscular rigidity, mental status changes/agitation, autonomic instability) may occur. May precipitate a shift to mania or hypomania in patients with bipolar disease. Has a low potential to impair cognitive or motor performance - caution operating hazardous machinery or driving. Low potential for sedation or anticholinergic effects relative to cyclic antidepressants. Use caution in patients with suicidal risk. Use caution in patients with a previous seizure disorder or condition predisposing to seizures such as brain damage, alcoholism, or concurrent therapy with other drugs which lower the seizure threshold. Use with caution in patients with hepatic or dysfunction and in elderly patients. May cause hyponatremia/SIADH. Use with caution in patients at risk of bleeding or receiving anticoagulant therapy - may cause impairment in platelet aggregation. Use with caution in patients with renal insufficiency or other concurrent illness (due to limited experience). May cause or exacerbate sexual dysfunction.

Adverse Reactions
>10%:
Central nervous system: Headache, somnolence, dizziness, insomnia
Gastrointestinal: Nausea, xerostomia, constipation, diarrhea
Genitourinary: Ejaculatory disturbances
Neuromuscular & skeletal: Weakness
Miscellaneous: Diaphoresis
1% to 10%:
Cardiovascular: Palpitations, vasodilation, postural hypotension
Central nervous system: Nervousness, anxiety, yawning, abnormal dreams
Dermatologic: Rash
Endocrine & metabolic: Decreased libido, delayed ejaculation
Gastrointestinal: Anorexia, flatulence, vomiting, dyspepsia, taste perversion
Genitourinary: Urinary frequency, impotence
Neuromuscular & skeletal: Tremor, paresthesia, myopathy, myalgia
<1% (Limited to important or life-threatening: Acute renal failure, agranulocytosis, akinesia, allergic alveolitis, alopecia, amenorrhea, anaphylactoid reaction, anaphylaxis, angioedema, aplastic anemia, asthma, atrial fibrillation, bone marrow aplasia, bruxism, bundle branch block, colitis, dysphasia, eclampsia, EPS, erythema multiforme, exfoliative dermatitis, Guillain-Barré syndrome, hemolytic anemia, hepatic necrosis, hypotension, laryngismus, leukopenia, mania, migraine, myasthenia, neuroleptic malignant syndrome (NMS), optic neuritis, pancreatitis, pancytopenia, porphyria, priapism, pulmonary hypertension, seizures (including status epilepticus), serotonin syndrome, SIADH, thrombocytopenia, torsade de pointes, toxic epidermal necrolysis, ventricular fibrillation, ventricular tachycardia, withdrawal reactions (dizziness; sensory disturbances - eg, paresthesias such as electric shock sensations; agitation; anxiety; nausea; diaphoresis - particularly following abrupt withdrawal)

Overdosage/Toxicology Symptoms include somnolence, nausea, vomiting, hepatic dysfunction, drowsiness, sinus tachycardia, urinary retention, renal failure (acute), and dilated pupils. Convulsions, status epilepticus, and ventricular arrhythmias (including torsade de pointes) have been reported, as well as serotonin syndrome and manic reaction. There are no specific antidotes. Following attempts at decontamination, treatment is supportive and symptomatic. Forced diuresis, dialysis, and hemoperfusion are unlikely to be beneficial.

Drug Interactions
Cytochrome P450 Effect: CYP2D6 enzyme substrate (minor); CYP2D6 and 1A2 enzyme inhibitor, and CYP3A3/4 enzyme inhibitor (weak)
Increased Effect/Toxicity:
MAO inhibitors: Paroxetine should not be used with nonselective MAO inhibitors (phenelzine, isocarboxazid) or other drugs with MAO inhibition (linezolid); fatal reactions have been reported. Wait 5 weeks after stopping fluoxetine before starting a nonselective MAO inhibitor and 2 weeks after stopping an MAO inhibitor before starting paroxetine. Concurrent selegiline has been associated with mania, hypertension, or serotonin syndrome (risk may be reduced relative to nonselective MAO inhibitors).
Phenothiazines: Paroxetine may inhibit the metabolism of thioridazine or mesoridazine, resulting in increased plasma levels and increasing the risk of QT_c interval prolongation. This may lead to serious ventricular arrhythmias, such as torsade de pointes-type arrhythmias and sudden death. Do not use together. Wait at least 5 weeks after discontinuing paroxetine prior to starting thioridazine.

(Continued)

Paroxetine *(Continued)*

Combined used of SSRIs and amphetamines, buspirone, meperidine, nefazodone, serotonin agonists (such as sumatriptan), sibutramine, other SSRIs, sympathomimetics, ritonavir, tramadol, and venlafaxine may increase the risk of serotonin syndrome. Paroxetine may increase serum levels/effects of benzodiazepines (alprazolam and diazepam), carbamazepine, carvedilol, clozapine, cyclosporine (and possibly tacrolimus), dextromethorphan, digoxin, haloperidol, HMG-CoA reductase inhibitors (lovastatin and simvastatin - increasing the risk of rhabdomyolysis), phenytoin, propafenone, theophylline, trazodone, tricyclic antidepressants, and valproic acid. Concurrent lithium may increase risk of nephrotoxicity. Risk of hyponatremia may increase with concurrent use of loop diuretics (bumetanide, furosemide, torsemide). Paroxetine may increase the hypoprothrombinemic response to warfarin.

Combined use of sumatriptan (and other serotonin agonists) may result in toxicity; weakness, hyper-reflexia, and incoordination have been observed with sumatriptan and SSRIs. In addition, concurrent use may theoretically increase the risk of serotonin syndrome; includes sumatriptan, naratriptan, rizatriptan, and zolmitriptan.

Decreased Effect: Cyproheptadine, a serotonin antagonist, may inhibit the effects of serotonin reuptake inhibitors (paroxetine).

Ethanol/Nutrition/Herb Interactions
Ethanol: Avoid ethanol.
Food: Peak concentration is increased, but bioavailability is not significantly altered by food.
Herb/Nutraceutical: Avoid valerian, St John's wort, SAMe, kava kava.

Stability
Suspension: Store at ≤25°C (≤77°F)
Tablet: Store at 15°C to 30°C (59°F to 86°F)

Mechanism of Action Paroxetine is a selective serotonin reuptake inhibitor, chemically unrelated to tricyclic, tetracyclic, or other antidepressants; presumably, the inhibition of serotonin reuptake from brain synapse stimulated serotonin activity in the brain

Pharmacodynamics/Kinetics
Onset of action: Therapeutic: >2 weeks
Metabolism: Extensive following absorption by CYP450 enzymes
Half-life elimination: 21 hours; Steady-state: 10 days
Excretion: Feces and urine (as metabolites)

Usual Dosage Oral:
Children:
Depression (unlabeled use): Initial: 10 mg/day and adjusted upward on an individual basis to 20 mg/day
OCD (unlabeled use): Initial: 10 mg/day and titrate up as necessary to 60 mg/day
Self-Injurious behavior (unlabeled use): 20 mg/day
Adults:
Depression: Initial: 20 mg once daily, preferably in the morning; increase if needed by 10 mg/day increments at intervals of at least 1 week; maximum dose: 50 mg/day
Paxil® CR™: Initial: 25 mg once daily; increase if needed by 12.5 mg/day increments at intervals of at least 1 week; maximum dose: 62.5 mg/day
GAD: Initial: 20 mg once daily, preferably in the morning; doses of 20-50 mg/day were used in clinical trials, however, no greater benefit was seen with doses >20 mg. If dose is increased, adjust in increments of 10 mg/day at 1-week intervals.
OCD: Initial: 20 mg once daily, preferably in the morning; increase if needed by 10 mg/day increments at intervals of at least 1 week; recommended: 40 mg/day; range: 20-60 mg/day; maximum dose: 60 mg/day
Panic disorder: Initial: 10 mg once daily, preferably in the morning; increase if needed by 10 mg/day increments at intervals of at least 1 week; recommended dose: 40 mg/day; range: 10-60 mg/day; maximum dose: 60 mg/day
Paxil® CR™: Initial: 12 mg once daily; increase if needed by 12.5 mg/day at intervals of at least 1 week; maximum dose: 75 mg/day
PTSD: Initial: 20 mg once daily, preferably in the morning; increase if needed by 10 mg/day increments at intervals of at least 1 week; range: 20-50 mg
Social anxiety disorder: Initial: 20 mg once daily, preferably in the morning; recommended dose: 20 mg/day; range: 20-60 mg/day; doses >20 mg may not have additional benefit
Elderly: Initial: 10 mg/day; increase if needed by 10 mg/day increments at intervals of at least 1 week; maximum dose: 40 mg/day
Paxil® CR™: Initial: 12.5 mg/day; increase if needed by 12.5 mg/day increments at intervals of at least 1 week; maximum dose: 50 mg/day

Note: Upon discontinuation of paroxetine therapy, gradually taper dose (taper-phase regimen used in PTSD/GAD clinical trials involved an incremental decrease in the daily dose by 10 mg/day at weekly intervals; when 20 mg/day dose was reached, this dose was continued for 1 week before treatment was stopped).

Dosage adjustment in severe renal/hepatic impairment: Adults: Initial: 10 mg/day; increase if needed by 10 mg/day increments at intervals of at least 1 week; maximum dose: 40 mg/day
Paxil® CR™: Initial: 12.5 mg/day; increase if needed by 12.5 mg/day increments at intervals of at least 1 week; maximum dose: 50 mg/day

Dietary Considerations May be taken with or without food.

Administration May be administered with or without food. Do not crush, break, or chew controlled release tablets.

Monitoring Parameters Hepatic and renal function tests, blood pressure, heart rate

Nursing Implications Monitor hepatic and renal function tests, blood pressure, heart rate

Additional Information Has properties similar to fluvoxamine maleate; buspirone (15-60 mg/day) may be useful in treatment of sexual dysfunction during treatment with a selective serotonin reuptake inhibitor. Paxil® CR™ incorporates a multi-layer formulation (Geomatrix™) to control dissolution and absorption.

Dosage Forms
Suspension, oral (Paxil®): 10 mg/5 mL (250 mL) [orange flavor]

Tablet (Paxil®): 10 mg, 20 mg, 30 mg, 40 mg
Tablet, controlled release (Paxil® CR™): 12.5 mg, 25 mg, 37.5 mg

◆ **Parvolex® (Can)** see Acetylcysteine on page 32
◆ **PAS** see Aminosalicylate Sodium on page 73
◆ **Patanol®** see Olopatadine on page 1007
◆ **Pathocil®** see Dicloxacillin on page 396
◆ **Pavabid® [DSC]** see Papaverine on page 1038
◆ **Pavacot®** see Papaverine on page 1038
◆ **Pavulon®** see Pancuronium on page 1035
◆ **Paxil®** see Paroxetine on page 1041
◆ **Paxil® CR™** see Paroxetine on page 1041
◆ **Paxipam®** see Halazepam on page 652
◆ **PBZ®** see Tripelennamine on page 1380
◆ **PBZ-SR®** see Tripelennamine on page 1380
◆ **PCA** see Procainamide on page 1130
◆ **PC-Cap®** see Propoxyphene and Aspirin on page 1148
◆ **PCE®** see Erythromycin (Systemic) on page 486
◆ **PCV7** see Pneumococcal Conjugate Vaccine (7-Valent) on page 1097
◆ **PediaCare® Decongestant Infants [OTC]** see Pseudoephedrine on page 1155
◆ **Pediacof®** see Chlorpheniramine, Phenylephrine, and Codeine With Potassium Iodide on page 280
◆ **Pediaflor®** see Fluoride on page 574
◆ **Pediamist® [OTC]** see Sodium Chloride on page 1245
◆ **Pediapred®** see PrednisoLONE on page 1122
◆ **Pediatric ALS Algorithms** see page 1628
◆ **Pediatrix (Can)** see Acetaminophen on page 22
◆ **Pediazole®** see Erythromycin and Sulfisoxazole on page 485
◆ **Pedi-Boro® [OTC]** see Aluminum Sulfate and Calcium Acetate on page 64
◆ **PediOtic®** see Neomycin, Polymyxin B, and Hydrocortisone on page 969
◆ **Pedituss®** see Chlorpheniramine, Phenylephrine, and Codeine With Potassium Iodide on page 280
◆ **PedvaxHIB®** see Haemophilus b Conjugate Vaccine on page 651

Pegademase Bovine (peg A de mase BOE vine)

U.S. Brand Names Adagen™
Canadian Brand Names Adagen™
Therapeutic Category Enzyme, Replacement Therapy
Use Orphan drug: Enzyme replacement therapy for adenosine deaminase (ADA) deficiency in patients with severe combined immunodeficiency disease (SCID) who can not benefit from bone marrow transplant; not a cure for SCID, unlike bone marrow transplants, injections must be used the rest of the child's life, therefore is not really an alternative
Pregnancy Risk Factor C
Contraindications Hypersensitivity to pegademase bovine or any component of the formulation; not to be used as preparatory or support therapy for bone marrow transplantation
Warnings/Precautions Use with caution in patients with thrombocytopenia.
Adverse Reactions <1% (Limited to important or life-threatening): Headache, pain at injection site
Stability Refrigerate at 2°C to 8°C (36°F to 46°F); do not freeze.
Mechanism of Action Adenosine deaminase is an enzyme that catalyzes the deamination of both adenosine and deoxyadenosine. Hereditary lack of adenosine deaminase activity results in severe combined immunodeficiency disease, a fatal disorder of infancy characterized by profound defects of both cellular and humoral immunity. It is estimated that 25% of patients with the autosomal recessive form of severe combined immunodeficiency lack adenosine deaminase.
Pharmacodynamics/Kinetics
Absorption: Rapid
Half-life elimination: 48-72 hours
Time to peak: Plasma adenosine deaminase activity: 2-3 weeks
Usual Dosage Children: I.M.: Dose given every 7 days, 10 units/kg the first dose, 15 units/kg the second dose, and 20 units/kg the third dose; maintenance dose: 20 units/kg/week is recommended depending on patient's ADA level; maximum single dose: 30 units/kg
Patient Information Not a cure for SCID; unlike bone marrow transplants, injections must be used the rest of the child's life; frequent blood tests are necessary to monitor effect and adjust the dose as needed
Dosage Forms Injection: 250 units/mL (1.5 mL)

Pegaspargase (peg AS par jase)

U.S. Brand Names Oncaspar®
Canadian Brand Names Oncaspar®
Synonyms PEG-L-asparaginase
Therapeutic Category Antineoplastic Agent, Protein Synthesis Inhibitor
Use Treatment of acute lymphocytic leukemia, blast crisis of chronic lymphocytic leukemia (CLL), salvage therapy of non-Hodgkin's lymphoma; may be used in some patients who have had hypersensitivity reactions to E. coli asparaginase
Pregnancy Risk Factor C
Pregnancy/Breast-Feeding Implications Clinical effects on the fetus: Based on limited reports in humans, the use of asparaginase does not seem to pose a major risk to the fetus when used in the 2nd and 3rd trimesters, or when exposure occurs prior to conception in either females or males. Because of the teratogenicity observed in animals and the lack of
(Continued)

Pegaspargase *(Continued)*

human data after 1st trimester exposure, asparaginase should be used cautiously, if at all, during this period.

Contraindications Hypersensitivity to pegaspargase or any component of the formulation; pancreatitis or a history of pancreatitis; patients who have had significant hemorrhagic events associated with prior asparaginase therapy; previous serious allergic reactions, such as generalized urticaria, bronchospasm, laryngeal edema, hypotension, or other unacceptable adverse reactions to pegaspargase

Warnings/Precautions The U.S. Food and Drug Administration (FDA) currently recommends that procedures for proper handling and disposal of antineoplastic agents be considered

Hypersensitivity reactions to pegaspargase, including life-threatening anaphylaxis, may occur during therapy, especially in patients with known hypersensitivity to the other forms of asparaginase. As a routine precaution, keep patients under observation for 1 hour with resuscitation equipment and other agents necessary to treat anaphylaxis (eg, epinephrine, oxygen, I.V. steroids) available. Use caution when treating patients with pegaspargase in combination with hepatotoxic agents, especially when liver dysfunction is present

Adverse Reactions In general, pegaspargase toxicities tend to be less frequent and appear somewhat later than comparable toxicities of asparaginase. Intramuscular rather than intravenous injection may decrease the incidence of coagulopathy; GI, hepatic, and renal toxicity.

>10%:

Cardiovascular: Edema

Central nervous system: Fatigue, disorientation (10%)

Gastrointestinal: Nausea, vomiting (50% to 60%), generally mild to moderate, but may be severe and protracted in some patients; anorexia (33%); abdominal pain (38%); diarrhea (28%); increased serum lipase and amylase

Hematologic: Hypofibrinogenemia and depression of clotting factors V and VII, variable decreases in factors VII and IX, severe protein C deficiency and decrease in antithrombin III - overt bleeding is uncommon, but may be dose-limiting, or fatal in some patients

Neuromuscular & skeletal: Weakness (33%)

Miscellaneous: Acute allergic reactions, including fever, rash, urticaria, arthralgia, hypotension, angioedema, bronchospasm, anaphylaxis (10% to 30%) - dose-limiting in some patients

1% to 10%:

Cardiovascular: Hypotension, tachycardia, thrombosis

Dermatologic: Urticaria, erythema, lip edema

Endocrine & metabolic: Hyperglycemia (3%)

Gastrointestinal: Acute pancreatitis (1%)

<1% (Limited to important or life-threatening): Agitation, bronchospasm, coma, convulsions, depression, dyspnea, hallucinations, paresthesias, parkinsonian symptoms (tremor, increased muscle tone), seizures, somnolence; transient elevations of transaminases, bilirubin, and alkaline phosphatase

Mild to moderate myelosuppression, leukopenia, anemia, thrombocytopenia; onset: 7 days, nadir: 14 days, recovery: 21 days

Overdosage/Toxicology Symptoms include nausea and diarrhea.

Drug Interactions

Increased Effect/Toxicity:

Aspirin, dipyridamole, heparin, warfarin, NSAIDs: Imbalances in coagulation factors have been noted with the use of pegaspargase - use with caution.

Vincristine and prednisone: An increased toxicity has been noticed when asparaginase is administered with VCR and prednisone.

Cyclophosphamide (decreased metabolism)

Mercaptopurine (increased hepatotoxicity)

Vincristine (increased neuropathy)

Prednisone (hyperglycemia)

Decreased Effect: Asparaginase terminates methotrexate action by inhibition of protein synthesis and prevention of cell entry into the S Phase.

Stability Avoid excessive agitation; do **not** shake; refrigerate at 2°C to 8°C (36°F to 46°F); single-use vial; discard unused portions

Do not use if cloudy or if precipitate is present; do not use if stored at room temperature for >48 hours; do **not** freeze; do not use product if it is known to have been frozen

Standard I.M. dilution: Usually no >2 mL/injection site

Standard I.V. dilution: Dose/100 mL NS or D_5W; stable for 48 hours at room temperature

Mechanism of Action Pegaspargase is a modified version of the enzyme L-asparaginase; the L-asparaginase used in the manufacture of pegaspargase is derived from *Escherichia coli*

Some malignant cells (ie, lymphoblastic leukemia cells and those of lymphocyte derivation) must acquire the amino acid asparagine from surrounding fluid such as blood, whereas normal cells can synthesize their own asparagine. Asparaginase is an enzyme that deaminates asparagine to aspartic acid and ammonia in the plasma and extracellular fluid and therefore deprives tumor cells of the amino acid for protein synthesis.

Pharmacodynamics/Kinetics

Duration: Asparaginase was measurable for at least 15 days following initial treatment with pegaspargase

Distribution: V_d: 4-5 L/kg; 70% to 80% of plasma volume; does not penetrate the CSF

Metabolism: Systemically degraded

Half-life elimination: 5.73 days; unaffected by age, renal function, or hepatic function

Excretion: Urine (trace amounts)

Usual Dosage Refer to individual protocols; dose must be individualized based upon clinical response and tolerance of the patient

I.M. administration is **preferred** over I.V. administration; I.M. administration may decrease the incidence of hepatotoxicity, coagulopathy, and GI and renal disorders

Children: I.M., I.V.:
  Body surface area <0.6 m^2: 82.5 international units/kg every 14 days
  Body surface area ≥0.6 m^2: 2500 international units/m^2 every 14 days

Adults: I.M., I.V.: 2500 international units/m^2 every 14 days

Hemodialysis: Significant drug removal is unlikely based on physiochemical characteristics

Peritoneal dialysis: Significant drug removal is unlikely based on physiochemical characteristics

Administration

I.M.: Must only be administered as a deep intramuscular injection into a large muscle; limit the volume of a single injection site to 2 mL; if the volume to be administered is >2 mL, use multiple injection sites

May be administered as a 1- to 2-hour I.V. infusion; **do not administer I.V. push.** Some institutions recommend the following precautions for pegaspargase administration:
  Have parenteral epinephrine, diphenhydramine, and hydrocortisone available at the bedside
  Have a freely running I.V. in place
  Have a physician readily accessible
  Monitor the patient closely for 30-60 minutes

Monitoring Parameters Vital signs during administration, CBC, urinalysis, amylase, liver enzymes, prothrombin time, renal function tests, urine dipstick for glucose, blood glucose

Patient Information This drug can only be given I.M. or I.V. Make note of scheduled return dates. Inform prescriber if you are using any other medications that may increase risk of bleeding. Possibility of hypersensitivity reactions includes anaphylaxis. Maintain adequate hydration (2-3 L/day of fluids unless instructed to restrict fluid intake) and nutrition (small frequent meals may help if you experience nausea, vomiting, or loss of appetite). Frequent mouth care may help reduce the incidence of mouth sores. You may experience dizziness, drowsiness, syncope, or blurred vision (use caution when driving or engaging in tasks that require alertness until response to drug is known). You may experience increased sweating, decreased sexual drive, or cough. Report immediately chest pain or heart palpitations; difficulty breathing or constant cough; rash, hives, or swelling of lips or mouth; or abdominal pain. Report swelling of extremities or sudden weight gain; burning, pain, or redness at infusion site; persistent fever or chills; unusual bruising or bleeding; twitching or tremors; pain on urination; or persistent nausea or diarrhea.

Nursing Implications Do not filter solution; appropriate agents for maintenance of an adequate airway and treatment of a hypersensitivity reaction (antihistamine, epinephrine, oxygen, I.V. corticosteroids) should be readily available. Be prepared to treat anaphylaxis at each administration; monitor for onset of abdominal pain and mental status changes.

Additional Information Not commercially available in the U.S.; obtain from Olsten Health Services 1-888-276-2217.

Dosage Forms Injection [preservative free]: 750 units/mL

Pegfilgrastim (peg fil GRA stim)

U.S. Brand Names Neulasta™

Synonyms G-CSF (PEG Conjugate); Granulocyte Colony Stimulating Factor (PEG Conjugate)

Therapeutic Category Colony-Stimulating Factor

Use Decrease the incidence of infection, by stimulation of granulocyte production, in patients with nonmyeloid malignancies receiving myelosuppressive therapy associated with a significant risk of febrile neutropenia

Pregnancy Risk Factor C

Pregnancy/Breast-Feeding Implications No adequate or well-controlled studies in pregnant women; use only if potential benefit to mother justifies risk to the fetus. Excretion in breast milk is unknown; use caution in breast-feeding.

Contraindications Hypersensitivity to pegfilgrastim, filgrastim, E. coli-derived proteins, or any component of the formulation; concurrent myelosuppressive, chemotherapy, or radiation therapy

Warnings/Precautions Complete blood count and platelet count should be obtained prior to chemotherapy. Do not use pegfilgrastim in the period 14 days before to 24 hours after administration of cytotoxic chemotherapy because of the potential sensitivity of rapidly dividing myeloid cells to cytotoxic chemotherapy. Pegfilgrastim can potentially act as a growth factor for any tumor type, particularly myeloid malignancies. Precaution should be exercised in the usage of pegfilgrastim in any malignancy with myeloid characteristics. Tumors of nonhematopoietic origin may have surface receptors for pegfilgrastim.

Allergic-type reactions have occurred in patients receiving the parent compound, filgrastim (G-CSF) with first or later doses. Reactions tended to occur more frequently with intravenous administration and within 30 minutes of infusion. Rare cases of splenic rupture or adult respiratory distress syndrome have been reported in association with filgrastim; patients must be instructed to report left upper quadrant pain or shoulder tip pain or respiratory distress. Use caution in patients with sickle cell diseases; sickle cell crises have been reported following filgrastim therapy. Safety and efficacy in pediatric patients have not been established; not for use in adolescents weighing <45 kg.

Adverse Reactions

>10%
  Neuromuscular & skeletal: Bone pain (medullary, 26%)
  Hepatic: Increased LDH (19%)

1% to 10%
  Endocrine & metabolic: Uric acid increased (8%)
  Hepatic: Alkaline phosphatase increased (9%)

<1% (Limited to important or life-threatening): Leukocytosis, hypoxia. **Note:** Rare adverse reactions reported for filgrastim include adult respiratory distress syndrome, allergic reactions (including urticaria, rash or anaphylaxis), sickle cell crisis (in patients with sickle cell

(Continued)

Pegfilgrastim (Continued)

disease), and splenic rupture (following use for peripheral blood progenitor cell [PBPC] mobilization). Cytopenias resulting from an antibody response to exogenous growth factors have been reported on rare occasions in patients treated with other recombinant growth factors.

Overdosage/Toxicology No clinical adverse effects have been seen with high doses producing ANC >10,000/mm³. The duration of leukocytosis has ranged from 6-13 days. Leukapheresis may be considered in symptomatic individuals.

Drug Interactions

Increased Effect/Toxicity: No formal drug interactions studies have been conducted. Lithium may potentiate release of neutrophils.

Stability Store under refrigeration 2°C to 8°C (36°F to 46°F). Protect from light. Allow to reach room temperature prior to injection. May be kept at room temperature for 48 hours. Do not freeze. If inadvertently frozen, allow to thaw in refrigerator; discard if frozen more than one time.

Mechanism of Action Stimulates the production, maturation, and activation of neutrophils, pegfilgrastim activates neutrophils to increase both their migration and cytotoxicity. Pegfilgrastim has a prolonged duration of effect relative to filgrastim and a reduced renal clearance.

Pharmacodynamics/Kinetics Half-life: S.C.: 15-80 hours

Usual Dosage S.C.: Adolescents >45 kg and Adults: 6 mg once per chemotherapy cycle; do not administer in the period between 14 days before and 24 hours after administration of cytotoxic chemotherapy; do not use in patients infants, children and smaller adolescents weighing <45 kg

Administration Do not use 6 mg fixed dose in infants, children, or adolescents <45 kg. Engage/activate needle guard following use to prevent accidental needlesticks.

Monitoring Parameters Complete blood count and platelet count should be obtained prior to chemotherapy. Leukocytosis (white blood cell counts 100,000/mm³) has been observed in <1% of patients receiving pegfilgrastim. Monitor platelets and hematocrit regularly.

Reference Range No clinical benefit seen with ANC >10,000/mm³.

Patient Information Follow directions for proper storage and administration of S.C. medication. Never reuse syringes or needles. You may experience bone pain (request analgesic). Report unusual fever or chills; unhealed sores; severe bone pain; pain, redness, or swelling at injection site; pain in the upper abdomen or shoulder tip; unusual swelling of extremities or difficulty breathing; or chest pain and palpitations.

Dosage Forms Injection, solution [preservative free]: 10 mg/mL (0.6 mL) [prefilled syringe]

Peginterferon Alfa-2b (peg in ter FEER on AL fa too bee)

U.S. Brand Names PEG-Intron™

Synonyms Interferon Alfa-2b (PEG Conjugate)

Therapeutic Category Antiviral Agent, Hepatitis; Interferon

Use Treatment of chronic hepatitis C (as monotherapy or in combination with ribavirin) in adult patients who have never received interferon alpha and have compensated liver disease

Restrictions Patients must have an Access Assurance ID number (obtained by calling Schering-Plough at 1-888-437-2608). Pharmacists should receive the ID number from the patient, and must obtain an order authorization number from the manufacturer prior to placing an order with their wholesaler (effective October 22, 2001). The patient's authorization number will be retained throughout therapy. This number may be inactivated if the patient fails to fill the prescription over any 60-day period, and access will no longer be assured by the manufacturer.

Pregnancy Risk Factor C (manufacturer) as monotherapy; X in combination with ribavirin

Pregnancy/Breast-Feeding Implications Very high doses are abortifacient in Rhesus monkeys. Assumed to have abortifacient potential in humans. Case reports of use in pregnant women (usually interferon alfa-2a) did not result in adverse effects in the fetus or newborn. There are no adequate or well-controlled studies in pregnant women. Risk of maternal-infant transmission of hepatitis C is <5%. Reliable contraception should be used in women of childbearing potential. Not recommended for use in pregnancy (per manufacturer).

Contraindications Hypersensitivity to polyethylene glycol (PEG), interferon alfa, or any component of the formulation; autoimmune hepatitis; decompensated liver disease; previous treatment with interferon; severe psychiatric disorder

Warnings/Precautions Severe psychiatric adverse effects, including depression, suicidal ideation, and suicide attempt, may occur. Avoid use in severe psychiatric disorders. Use with caution in patients with a history of depression. Use caution in patients with cardiovascular disease, endocrine disorders, autoimmune disorders, and pulmonary dysfunction. Avoid use in renal dysfunction (Cl_cr <50 mL/minute). Use caution in geriatric patients, patients with chronic immunosuppression, low peripheral blood counts or myelosuppression, including concurrent use of myelosuppressive therapy. Discontinue therapy when significant decreases in neutrophil (<0.5 x 10⁹/L) or platelet counts (<50,000/mm³); colitis develops; known or suspected pancreatitis develops. Treatment should be discontinued in patients with worsening or persistently severe signs/symptoms of autoimmune, infectious, ischemic (including radiographic changes or worsening hepatic function), or neuropsychiatric disorders (including depression and/or suicidal thoughts/behavior). Visual exams are recommended for patients with diabetes mellitus or hypertension. Safety and efficacy have not been established in children.

Adverse Reactions

>10%:

Central nervous system: Headache (56%), fatigue (52%), depression (16% to 29%), anxiety/emotional liability/irritability (28%), insomnia (23%), fever (22%), dizziness (12%), impaired concentration (5% to 12%), pain (12%)

Dermatologic: Alopecia (22%), pruritus (12%), dry skin (11%)

Gastrointestinal: Nausea (26%), anorexia (20%), diarrhea (18%), abdominal pain (15%), weight loss (11%)

Local: Injection site inflammation/reaction (47%),

Neuromuscular & skeletal: Musculoskeletal pain (56%), myalgia (38% to 42%), rigors (23% to 45%)
Respiratory: Epistaxis (14%), nasopharyngitis (11%)
Miscellaneous: Flu-like syndrome (46%), viral infection (11%)
>1% to 10%:
Cardiovascular: Flushing (6%)
Central nervous system: Malaise (8%)
Dermatologic: Rash (6%), dermatitis (7%)
Endocrine & metabolic: Hypothyroidism (5%)
Gastrointestinal: Vomiting (7%), dyspepsia (6%), taste perversion
Hematologic: Neutropenia, thrombocytopenia
Hepatic: Transient increase in transaminases (10%), hepatomegaly (6%)
Local: Injection site pain (2%)
Neuromuscular & skeletal: Hypertonia (5%)
Respiratory: Pharyngitis (10%), sinusitis (7%), cough (6%)
Miscellaneous: Diaphoresis (6%)
≤1% (Limited to important or life-threatening): Anaphylaxis, angioedema, aplastic anemia, arrhythmias, autoimmune disorder (eg, thyroiditis, thrombocytopenia, rheumatoid arthritis, interstitial nephritis, systemic lupus erythematosus, psoriasis), diabetes mellitus, dyspnea, facial oculomotor nerve palsy, hallucinations, hemorrhagic colitis, homicidal ideation, hyperthyroidism, hypotension, myocardial infarction, nerve palsy, neutralizing antibodies, pancreatitis, pneumonia, pneumonitis, psychosis, pulmonary infiltrates, retinal hemorrhage, retinal ischemia, severe depression, severe neutropenia (<0.5 x 10^9/L), severe thrombocytopenia (<50,000/mm^3), suicidal behavior, suicidal ideation, supraventricular arrhythmias, tachycardia, transient ischemic attack, urticaria

Overdosage/Toxicology Limited experience with accidental doses ≥2.5 times the intended dose. No serious side effects have been noted. Treatment is symptom directed and supportive.

Drug Interactions
Cytochrome P450 Effect: Does not inhibit CYP1A2, 2C8/9, 2D6, 3A4 after a single dose in healthy subjects. Interferons, including alfa, have been shown to depress (to varying degrees) the CYP enzyme system.
Increased Effect/Toxicity: ACE inhibitors, clozapine, erythropoietin may increase risk of bone marrow suppression. Fluorouracil, theophylline, zidovudine concentrations may increase. Warfarin's anticoagulant effect may increase.
Decreased Effect: Melphalan concentrations may decrease. Prednisone may decrease effects of interferon alpha.

Ethanol/Nutrition/Herb Interactions Ethanol: Avoid use in patients with hepatitis C virus.

Stability Store vials at 15°C to 30°C (59°F to 86°F). Once reconstituted use immediately or store for <24 hours at 2°C to 8°C (36°F to 46°F). To reconstitute, add 0.7 mL of sterile water for injection, USP (supplied diluent) to the vial. Gently swirl. Do not re-enter vial after dose removed. Discard unused portion. Does not contain preservative. Do not freeze.

Mechanism of Action Alpha interferons are a family of proteins, produced by nucleated cells, that have antiviral, antiproliferative, and immune-regulating activity. There are 16 known subtypes of alpha interferons. Interferons interact with cells through high affinity cell surface receptors. Following activation, multiple effects can be detected including induction of gene transcription. Inhibits cellular growth, alters the state of cellular differentiation, interferes with oncogene expression, alters cell surface antigen expression, increases phagocytic activity of macrophages, and augments cytotoxicity of lymphocytes for target cells.

Pharmacodynamics/Kinetics
Bioavailability: Increases with chronic dosing
Half-life elimination: 40 hours
Time to peak: 15-44 hours
Excretion: Urine (30%)

Usual Dosage S.C.:
Children: Safety and efficacy have not been established
Adults: Chronic hepatitis C: Administer dose once weekly; **Note:** Usual duration is for 1 year; after 24 weeks of treatment, if serum HCV RNA is not below the limit of detection of the assay, consider discontinuation:
Monotherapy: Initial:
≤45 kg: 40 mcg
46-56 kg: 50 mcg
57-72 kg: 64 mcg
73-88 kg: 80 mcg
89-106 kg: 96 mcg
107-136 kg: 120 mcg
137-160 kg: 150 mcg
Combination therapy with ribavirin (400 mg twice daily): Initial: 1.5 mcg/kg/week
<40 kg: 50 mcg
40-50 kg: 64 mcg
51-60 kg: 80 mcg
61-75 kg: 96 mcg
76-85 kg: 120 mcg
>95 kg: 150 mcg
Elderly: May require dosage reduction based upon renal dysfunction, but no established guidelines are available.

Dosage adjustment if serious adverse event occurs: Depression (severity based upon DSM-IV criteria):
Mild depression: No dosage adjustment required; evaluate once weekly by visit/phone call. If depression remains stable, continue weekly visits. If depression improves, resume normal visit schedule.
Moderate depression: Decrease interferon dose by 50%; evaluate once weekly with an office visit at least every other week. If depression remains stable, consider psychiatric evaluation and continue with reduced dosing. If symptoms improve and remain stable for
(Continued)

Peginterferon Alfa-2b *(Continued)*

4 weeks, resume normal visit schedule; continue reduced dosing or return to normal dose.

Severe depression: Discontinue interferon and ribavirin permanently. Obtain immediate psychiatric consultation.

Dosage adjustment in renal impairment: Monitor for signs and symptoms of toxicity and if toxicity occurs then adjust dose. Do not use patients with Cl$_{cr}$ <50 mL/minute. Patients were excluded from the clinical trials if serum creatinine >1.5 times the upper limits of normal.

Dosage adjustment in hepatic impairment: Contraindicated in decompensated liver disease

Dosage adjustment in hematologic toxicity:

Hemoglobin:

Hemoglobin <10 g/dL: Continue current peginterferon alfa-2b dose; decrease ribavirin dose by 200 mg/day.

Hemoglobin <8.5 g/dL: Permanently discontinue peginterferon alfa-2b and ribavirin.

Hemoglobin decrease >2 g/dL in any 4-week period and stable cardiac disease: Decrease peginterferon alfa-2b dose by half; decrease ribavirin dose by 200 mg per day. Hemoglobin <12 g/dL after ribavirin dose is decreased: Permanently discontinue both peginterferon alfa-2b and ribavirin.

White blood cells:

WBC <1.5 x 10^9/L: Decrease peginterferon alfa-2b dose by half.

WBC <1.0 x 10^9/L: Permanently discontinue peginterferon alfa-2b and ribavirin.

Neutrophils:

Neutrophils <0.75 x 10^9/L: Decrease peginterferon alfa-2b dose by half.

Neutrophils <0.5 x 10^9/L: Permanently discontinue peginterferon alfa-2b and ribavirin.

Platelets:

Platelet count <80 x 10^9/L: Decrease peginterferon alfa-2b dose by half.

Platelet count <50 x 10^9/L: Permanently discontinue peginterferon alfa-2b and ribavirin.

Administration For S.C. administration; rotate injection site

Monitoring Parameters Baseline and periodic TSH, hematology (including CBC with differential, platelets), and chemistry (including LFTs) testing. Evaluate for depression and other psychiatric symptoms before and after initiation of therapy; baseline eye examination in diabetic and hypertensive patients; baseline echocardiogram in patients with cardiac disease; serum HCV RNA levels after 24 weeks of treatment

Patient Information Blood work will be done before the start of this medicine and during its use. Maintain adequate hydration (2-3 L/day of fluids unless instructed to restrict fluid intake). You may experience flu-like syndrome (giving the medicine at bedtime or using acetaminophen may help), nausea and vomiting (frequent small meals, frequent mouth care, sucking lozenges, or chewing gum may help), feeling tired (use caution when driving or engaging in tasks requiring alertness until response to drug is known), or headache. Report persistent abdominal pain, bloody diarrhea, and fever; symptoms of depression, suicidal ideas; unusual bruising or bleeding, any signs or symptoms of infection, unusual fatigue, chest pain or palpitations, difficulty breathing, wheezing, severe nausea or vomiting.

Nursing Implications Monitor laboratory results on a regular basis. Monitor for effectiveness of therapy and possible adverse reactions. Assess knowledge and instruct patient/caregiver on appropriate reconstitution, injection and needle disposal, possible side effects, and symptoms to report. Contraceptive teaching may be appropriate.

Dosage Forms Powder for injection: 50 mcg/0.5 mL, 80 mcg/0.5 mL, 120 mcg/0.5 mL, 150 mcg/0.5 mL

- ◆ **PEG-Intron**™ *see* Peginterferon Alfa-2b *on page 1046*
- ◆ **PEG-L-asparaginase** *see* Pegaspargase *on page 1043*
- ◆ **PegLyte® (Can)** *see* Polyethylene Glycol-Electrolyte Solution *on page 1101*
- ◆ **PemADD®** *see* Pemoline *on page 1048*
- ◆ **PemADD® CT** *see* Pemoline *on page 1048*

Pemirolast *(pe MIR oh last)*

U.S. Brand Names Alamast™

Canadian Brand Names Alamast™

Therapeutic Category Antiallergic, Ophthalmic

Use Prevention of itching of the eye due to allergic conjunctivitis

Pregnancy Risk Factor C

Usual Dosage Children >3 years and Adults: 1-2 drops instilled in affected eye(s) 4 times/day

Additional Information Complete prescribing information for this medication should be consulted for additional detail.

Dosage Forms Solution, ophthalmic: 0.1% (10 mL)

Pemoline *(PEM oh leen)*

U.S. Brand Names Cylert®; PemADD®; PemADD® CT

Synonyms Phenylisohydantoin; PIO

Therapeutic Category Central Nervous System Stimulant, Nonamphetamine

Use Treatment of attention-deficit/hyperactivity disorder (ADHD) (not first-line)

Unlabeled/Investigational Use Narcolepsy

Restrictions C-IV

Pregnancy Risk Factor B

Contraindications Hypersensitivity to pemoline or any component of the formulation; hepatic impairment (including abnormalities on baseline liver function tests); children <6 years of age; Tourette's syndrome; psychosis

Warnings/Precautions Not considered first-line therapy for ADHD due to association with hepatic failure. The manufacturer has recommended that signed informed consent following a discussion of risks and benefits must or should be obtained prior to the initiation of therapy.

Therapy should be discontinued if a response is not evident after 3 weeks of therapy. Pemoline should not be started in patients with abnormalities in baseline liver function tests, and should be discontinued if clinically significant liver function test abnormalities are revealed at any time during therapy. Use with caution in patients with renal dysfunction or psychosis. In general, stimulant medications should be used with caution in patients with bipolar disorder, diabetes mellitus, cardiovascular disease, seizure disorders, insomnia, porphyria, or hypertension (although pemoline has been demonstrated to have a low potential to elevated blood pressure relative to other stimulants). May exacerbate symptoms of behavior and thought disorder in psychotic patients. Potential for drug dependency exists - avoid abrupt discontinuation in patients who have received for prolonged periods. Stimulant use has been associated with growth suppression, and careful monitoring is recommended. Stimulants may unmask tics in individuals with coexisting Tourette's syndrome.

Adverse Reactions Frequency not defined.

Central nervous system: Insomnia, dizziness, drowsiness, mental depression, increased irritability, seizures, precipitation of Tourette's syndrome, hallucinations, headache, movement disorders

Dermatologic: Rash

Endocrine & metabolic: Suppression of growth in children

Gastrointestinal: Anorexia, weight loss, stomach pain, nausea

Hematologic: Aplastic anemia

Hepatic: Increased liver enzyme (usually reversible upon discontinuation), hepatitis, jaundice, hepatic failure

Overdosage/Toxicology Symptoms include tachycardia, hallucinations, and agitation. There is no specific antidote for intoxication and the bulk of the treatment is supportive. Hyperactivity and agitation usually respond to reduced sensory input or benzodiazepines, however, with extreme agitation haloperidol (2-5 mg I.M. for adults) may be required. Hyperthermia is best treated with external cooling measures, or when severe or unresponsive, muscle paralysis with pancuronium may be needed.

Drug Interactions

Increased Effect/Toxicity: Use caution when pemoline is used with other CNS-acting medications.

Decreased Effect: Pemoline in combination with antiepileptic medications may decrease seizure threshold.

Ethanol/Nutrition/Herb Interactions Ethanol: Avoid ethanol (may increase CNS depression).

Mechanism of Action Blocks the reuptake mechanism of dopaminergic neurons, appears to act at the cerebral cortex and subcortical structures; CNS and respiratory stimulant with weak sympathomimetic effects; actions may be mediated via increase in CNS dopamine

Pharmacodynamics/Kinetics

Onset of action: Peak effect: 4 hours

Duration: 8 hours

Protein binding: 50%

Metabolism: Partially hepatic

Half-life elimination: Children: 7-8.6 hours; Adults: 12 hours

Time to peak, serum: 2-4 hours

Excretion: Urine; feces (negligible amounts)

Usual Dosage Children ≥6 years: Oral: Initial: 37.5 mg given once daily in the morning, increase by 18.75 mg/day at weekly intervals; usual effective dose range: 56.25-75 mg/day; maximum: 112.5 mg/day; dosage range: 0.5-3 mg/kg/24 hours; significant benefit may not be evident until third or fourth week of administration

Dosing adjustment/comments in renal impairment: Cl_{cr} <50 mL/minute: Avoid use

Administration Administer medication in the morning.

Monitoring Parameters Liver enzymes (baseline and every 2 weeks)

Patient Information Avoid caffeine; avoid alcohol; last daily dose should be given several hours before retiring; do not abruptly discontinue; prolonged use may cause dependence

Nursing Implications Administer medication in the morning

Additional Information Treatment of ADHD should include "Drug Holidays" or periodic discontinuation of stimulant medication in order to assess the patient's requirements and to decrease tolerance and limit suppression of linear growth and weight. The labeling for Cylert® includes recommendations for liver function monitoring and a Patient Information Consent Form.

Dosage Forms

Tablet: 18.75 mg, 37.5 mg, 75 mg

Tablet, chewable: 37.5 mg

Penciclovir (pen SYE kloe veer)

U.S. Brand Names Denavir™

Therapeutic Category Antiviral Agent, Nonantiretroviral; Antiviral Agent, Topical

Use Topical treatment of herpes simplex labialis (cold sores); potentially used for Epstein-Barr virus infections

Pregnancy Risk Factor B

Contraindications Hypersensitivity to the penciclovir or any component of the formulation; previous and significant adverse reactions to famciclovir

Warnings/Precautions Penciclovir should only be used on herpes labialis on the lips and face; because no data are available, application to mucous membranes is not recommended. Avoid application in or near eyes since it may cause irritation. The effect of penciclovir has not been established in immunocompromised patients.

Adverse Reactions

>10%: Dermatologic: Erythema (mild) (50%)

1% to 10%: Central nervous system: Headache (5.3%)

<1% (Limited to important or life-threatening): Local anesthesia

Stability Store at or below 30°C; do not freeze

(Continued)

Penciclovir (Continued)

Mechanism of Action In cells infected with HSV-1 or HSV-2, viral thymidine kinase phospho-rylates penciclovir to a monophosphate form which, in turn, is converted to penciclovir triphosphate by cellular kinases. Penciclovir triphosphate inhibits HSV polymerase competi-tively with deoxyguanosine triphosphate. Consequently, herpes viral DNA synthesis and, therefore, replication are selectively inhibited

Pharmacodynamics/Kinetics Absorption: Topical: None

Usual Dosage Apply cream at the first sign or symptom of cold sore (eg, tingling, swelling); apply every 2 hours during waking hours for 4 days

Monitoring Parameters Reduction in virus shedding, negative cultures for herpes virus; resolution of pain and healing of cold sore lesion

Patient Information Inform your physician if you experience significant burning, itching, stinging, or redness when using this medication

Additional Information Penciclovir is the active metabolite of the prodrug famciclovir. Penciclovir is an alternative to topical acyclovir for HSV-1 and HSV-2 infections. Neither drug will prevent recurring HSV attacks.

Dosage Forms Cream: 1% [10 mg/g] (1.5 g)

♦ Penecort® *see* Hydrocortisone *on page 682*

Penicillamine (pen i SIL a meen)

Related Information

Antacid Drug Interactions *on page 1477*

U.S. Brand Names Cuprimine®; Depen®

Canadian Brand Names Cuprimine®; Depen®

Synonyms D-3-Mercaptovaline; β,β-Dimethylcysteine; D-Penicillamine

Therapeutic Category Antidote, Copper Toxicity; Antidote, Lead Toxicity; Chelating Agent, Oral

Use Treatment of Wilson's disease, cystinuria, adjunct in the treatment of rheumatoid arthritis; lead, mercury, copper, and possibly gold poisoning. (**Note:** Oral DMSA is preferable for lead or mercury poisoning); primary biliary cirrhosis; as adjunctive therapy following initial treat-ment with calcium EDTA or BAL

Pregnancy Risk Factor D

Contraindications Hypersensitivity to penicillamine or any component of the formulation; renal insufficiency; patients with previous penicillamine-related aplastic anemia or agranulo-cytosis; concomitant administration with other hematopoietic-depressant drugs (eg, gold, immunosuppressants, antimalarials, phenylbutazone); pregnancy

Warnings/Precautions Cross-sensitivity with penicillin is possible; therefore, should be used cautiously in patients with a history of penicillin allergy. Patients on penicillamine for Wilson's disease or cystinuria should receive pyridoxine supplementation 25 mg/day; once instituted for Wilson's disease or cystinuria, continue treatment on a daily basis; interruptions of even a few days have been followed by hypersensitivity with reinstitution of therapy. Penicillamine has been associated with fatalities due to agranulocytosis, aplastic anemia, thrombocyto-penia, Goodpasture's syndrome, and myasthenia gravis; patients should be warned to report promptly any symptoms suggesting toxicity; approximately 33% of patients will experience an allergic reaction; since toxicity may be dose related, it is recommended not to exceed 750 mg/day in elderly.

Adverse Reactions

>10%:

Dermatologic: Rash, urticaria, itching (44% to 50%)

Gastrointestinal: Hypogeusia (25% to 33%)

Neuromuscular & skeletal: Arthralgia

1% to 10%:

Cardiovascular: Edema of the face, feet, or lower legs

Central nervous system: Fever, chills

Gastrointestinal: Weight gain, sore throat

Genitourinary: Bloody or cloudy urine

Hematologic: Aplastic or hemolytic anemia, leukopenia (2%), thrombocytopenia (4%)

Miscellaneous: White spots on lips or mouth, positive ANA

<1% (Limited to important or life-threatening): Allergic reactions, anorexia, cholestatic jaun-dice, hepatitis, increased friability of the skin, lymphadenopathy, myasthenia gravis syndrome, nephrotic syndrome, pancreatitis, pemphigus, optic neuritis, SLE-like syndrome, toxic epidermal necrolysis, vomiting

Overdosage/Toxicology Symptoms include nausea and vomiting. Following GI decontami-nation, treatment is supportive.

Drug Interactions

Increased Effect/Toxicity: Increased effect or toxicity of gold, antimalarials, immunosup-pressants, and phenylbutazone (hematologic, renal toxicity).

Decreased Effect: Decreased effect of penicillamine when taken with iron and zinc salts, antacids (magnesium, calcium, aluminum), and food. Digoxin levels may be decreased when taken with penicillamine.

Ethanol/Nutrition/Herb Interactions

Ethanol: Avoid or limit ethanol.

Food: Penicillamine serum levels may be decreased if taken with food. Do not administer with milk. Iron and zinc may decrease drug action.

Stability Store in tight, well-closed containers

Mechanism of Action Chelates with lead, copper, mercury and other heavy metals to form stable, soluble complexes that are excreted in urine; depresses circulating IgM rheumatoid factor, depresses T-cell but not B-cell activity; combines with cystine to form a compound which is more soluble, thus cystine calculi are prevented

Pharmacodynamics/Kinetics

Absorption: 40% to 70%

Metabolism: Hepatic, small amounts

Protein binding: 80% to albumin
Half-life elimination: 1.7-3.2 hours
Time to peak, serum: ~2 hours
Excretion: Primarily urine (30% to 60% as unchanged drug)

Usual Dosage Oral:

Rheumatoid arthritis:

Children: Initial: 3 mg/kg/day (≤250 mg/day) for 3 months, then 6 mg/kg/day (≤500 mg/day) in divided doses twice daily for 3 months to a maximum of 10 mg/kg/day in 3-4 divided doses

Adults: 125-250 mg/day, may increase dose at 1- to 3-month intervals up to 1-1.5 g/day

Wilson's disease (doses titrated to maintain urinary copper excretion >1 mg/day):

Infants <6 months: 250 mg/dose once daily

Children <12 years: 250 mg/dose 2-3 times/day

Adults: 250 mg 4 times/day

Cystinuria:

Children: 30 mg/kg/day in 4 divided doses

Adults: 1-4 g/day in divided doses every 6 hours

Lead poisoning (continue until blood lead level is <60 µg/dL): Children and Adults: 25-35 mg/kg/d, administered in 3-4 divided doses; initiating treatment at 25% of this dose and gradually increasing to the full dose over 2-3 weeks may minimize adverse reactions

Primary biliary cirrhosis: 250 mg/day to start, increase by 250 mg every 2 weeks up to a maintenance dose of 1 g/day, usually given 250 mg 4 times/day

Arsenic poisoning: Children: 100 mg/kg/day in divided doses every 6 hours for 5 days; maximum: 1 g/day

Dosing adjustment/comments in renal impairment: Cl_{cr} <50 mL/minute: Avoid use

Dietary Considerations Should be taken at least 1 hour before a meal on an empty stomach. Iron and zinc may decrease drug action; increase dietary intake of pyridoxine. For Wilson's disease, decrease copper in diet and omit chocolate, nuts, shellfish, mushrooms, liver, raisins, broccoli, and molasses. For lead poisoning, decrease calcium in diet.

Administration Administer on an empty stomach (1 hour before meals and at bedtime). Patients unable to swallow capsules may mix contents of capsule with fruit juice or chilled puréed fruit.

Monitoring Parameters Urinalysis, CBC with differential, platelet count, liver function tests; weekly measurements of urinary and blood concentration of the intoxicating metal is indicated (3 months has been tolerated)

CBC: WBC <3500/mm^3, neutrophils <2000/mm^3 or monocytes >500/mm^3 indicate need to stop therapy immediately; quantitative 24-hour urine protein at 1- to 2-week intervals initially (first 2-3 months); urinalysis, LFTs occasionally; platelet counts <100,000/mm^3 indicate need to stop therapy until numbers of platelets increase

Patient Information Take at least 1 hour before a meal on an empty stomach; patients with cystinuria should drink copious amounts of water; notify physician if unusual bleeding or bruising, or persistent fever, sore throat, or fatigue occurs; report any unexplained cough, shortness of breath, or rash; loss of taste may occur; do not skip or miss doses or discontinue without notifying physician

Nursing Implications For patients who cannot swallow capsules, contents of capsules may be administered in 15-30 mL of chilled puréed fruit or fruit juice; patients should be warned to report promptly any symptoms suggesting toxicity

Dosage Forms

Capsule: 125 mg, 250 mg

Tablet: 250 mg

Extemporaneous Preparations A 50 mg/mL suspension may be made by mixing twenty 250 mg capsules with 1 g carboxymethylcellulose, 50 g sucrose, 100 mg citric acid, parabens, and purified water to a total volume of 100 mL; cherry flavor may be added. Stability is 30 days refrigerated.

Nahata MC and Hipple TF, *Pediatric Drug Formulations*, 1st ed, Cincinnati, OH: Harvey Whitney Books Co, 1990.

Penicillin G Benzathine (pen i SIL in jee BENZ a theen)

Related Information

Treatment of Sexually Transmitted Diseases *on page 1609*

U.S. Brand Names Bicillin® L-A; Permapen®

Canadian Brand Names Bicillin® L-A

Synonyms Benzathine Benzylpenicillin; Benzathine Penicillin G; Benzylpenicillin Benzathine

Therapeutic Category Antibiotic, Penicillin

Use Active against some gram-positive organisms, few gram-negative organisms such as *Neisseria gonorrhoeae*, and some anaerobes and spirochetes; used in the treatment of syphilis; used only for the treatment of mild to moderately severe infections caused by organisms susceptible to low concentrations of penicillin G or for prophylaxis of infections caused by these organisms

Pregnancy Risk Factor B

Contraindications Hypersensitivity to penicillin or any component of the formulation

Warnings/Precautions Use with caution in patients with impaired renal function, seizure disorder, or history of hypersensitivity to other beta-lactams; CDC and AAP do not currently recommend the use of penicillin G benzathine to treat congenital syphilis or neurosyphilis due to reported treatment failures and lack of published clinical data on its efficacy

Adverse Reactions Frequency not defined.

Central nervous system: Convulsions, confusion, drowsiness, myoclonus, fever

Dermatologic: Rash

Endocrine & metabolic: Electrolyte imbalance

Hematologic: Positive Coombs' reaction, hemolytic anemia

Local: Pain, thrombophlebitis

Renal: Acute interstitial nephritis

Miscellaneous: Anaphylaxis, hypersensitivity reactions, Jarisch-Herxheimer reaction

(Continued)

Penicillin G Benzathine *(Continued)*

Overdosage/Toxicology Symptoms of penicillin overdose include neuromuscular hypersensitivity (agitation, hallucinations, asterixis, encephalopathy, confusion, seizures) and electrolyte imbalance with potassium or sodium salts, especially in renal failure. Hemodialysis may be helpful to aid in removal of the drug from the blood, otherwise, most treatment is supportive or symptom directed.

Drug Interactions

Increased Effect/Toxicity: Probenecid increases penicillin levels. Aminoglycosides may lead to synergistic efficacy.

Decreased Effect: Tetracyclines may decrease penicillin effectiveness. Efficacy of oral contraceptives may be reduced when taken with penicillins.

Stability Store in refrigerator

Mechanism of Action Interferes with bacterial cell wall synthesis during active multiplication, causing cell wall death and resultant bactericidal activity against susceptible bacteria

Pharmacodynamics/Kinetics

Duration: 1-4 weeks (dose dependent); larger doses result in more sustained levels

Absorption: I.M.: Slow

Time to peak, serum: 12-24 hours

Usual Dosage I.M.: Administer undiluted injection; higher doses result in more sustained rather than higher levels. Use a penicillin G benzathine-penicillin G procaine combination to achieve early peak levels in acute infections.

Infants and Children:

Group A streptococcal upper respiratory infection: 25,000-50,000 units/kg as a single dose; maximum: 1.2 million units

Prophylaxis of recurrent rheumatic fever: 25,000-50,000 units/kg every 3-4 weeks; maximum: 1.2 million units/dose

Early syphilis: 50,000 units/kg as a single injection; maximum: 2.4 million units

Syphilis of more than 1-year duration: 50,000 units/kg every week for 3 doses; maximum: 2.4 million units/dose

Adults:

Group A streptococcal upper respiratory infection: 1.2 million units as a single dose

Prophylaxis of recurrent rheumatic fever: 1.2 million units every 3-4 weeks or 600,000 units twice monthly

Early syphilis: 2.4 million units as a single dose in 2 injection sites

Syphilis of more than 1-year duration: 2.4 million units in 2 injection sites once weekly for 3 doses

Not indicated as single drug therapy for neurosyphilis, but may be given 1 time/week for 3 weeks following I.V. treatment; refer to Penicillin G Parenteral/Aqueous monograph for dosing

Administration Administer by deep I.M. injection in the upper outer quadrant of the buttock do **not** administer I.V., intra-arterially, or S.C.; in children <2 years of age, I.M. injections should be made into the midlateral muscle of the thigh, not the gluteal region; when doses are repeated, rotate the injection site

Monitoring Parameters Observe for signs and symptoms of anaphylaxis during first dose

Test Interactions Positive Coombs' [direct], false-positive urinary and/or serum proteins; false-positive or negative urinary glucose using Clinitest®

Patient Information Report any rash

Nursing Implications Monitor CBC, urinalysis, renal function tests

Dosage Forms Injection: 300,000 units/mL (10 mL); 600,000 units/mL (1 mL, 2 mL, 4 mL)

Penicillin G Benzathine and Procaine Combined

(pen i SIL in jee BENZ a theen & PROE kane KOM bined)

U.S. Brand Names Bicillin® C-R; Bicillin® C-R 900/300

Synonyms Penicillin G Procaine and Benzathine Combined

Therapeutic Category Antibiotic, Penicillin

Use May be used in specific situations in the treatment of streptococcal infections

Pregnancy Risk Factor B

Contraindications Hypersensitivity to penicillin or any component of the formulation

Warnings/Precautions Use with caution in patients with impaired renal function, impaired cardiac function or seizure disorder

Adverse Reactions Frequency not defined.

Central nervous system: CNS toxicity (convulsions, confusion, drowsiness, myoclonus)

Hematologic: Positive Coombs' reaction, hemolytic anemia

Renal: Interstitial nephritis

Miscellaneous: Hypersensitivity reactions, Jarisch-Herxheimer reaction

Overdosage/Toxicology Many beta-lactam-containing antibiotics have the potential to cause neuromuscular hyperirritability or convulsive seizures. Hemodialysis may be helpful to aid in removal of the drug from the blood, otherwise, most treatment is supportive or symptom directed.

Drug Interactions

Increased Effect/Toxicity: Probenecid increases penicillin levels. Aminoglycosides may lead to synergistic efficacy. Warfarin effects may be increased.

Decreased Effect: Tetracyclines may decrease penicillin effectiveness. Efficacy of oral contraceptives may be reduced when taken with penicillins.

Stability Store in refrigerator.

Mechanism of Action Inhibits bacterial cell wall synthesis by binding to one or more of the penicillin binding proteins (PBPs); which in turn inhibits the final transpeptidation step of peptidoglycan synthesis in bacterial cell walls, thus inhibiting cell wall biosynthesis. Bacteria eventually lyse due to ongoing activity of cell wall autolytic enzymes (autolysins and murein hydrolases) while cell wall assembly is arrested.

Usual Dosage I.M.:
  Children:
    <30 lb: 600,000 units in a single dose
    30-60 lb: 900,000 units to 1.2 million units in a single dose
  Children >60 lb and Adults: 2.4 million units in a single dose

Administration Administer by deep I.M. injection in the upper outer quadrant of the buttock; administered around-the-clock rather than 4 times/day, 3 times/day, etc (ie, 12-6-12-6, not 9-1-5-9) to promote less variation in peak and trough serum levels; do **not** administer I.V., intravascularly, or intra-arterially. In infants and children, I.M. injections should be made into the midlateral muscle of the thigh.

Monitoring Parameters Observe for signs and symptoms of anaphylaxis during first dose

Test Interactions May interfere with urinary glucose tests using cupric sulfate (Benedict's solution, Clinitest®); may inactivate aminoglycosides *in vitro*; positive Coombs' [direct], increased protein

Nursing Implications Administer by deep I.M. injection in the upper outer quadrant of the buttock

Dosage Forms
  Injection:
    300,000 units [150,000 units each of penicillin G benzathine and penicillin G procaine] (10 mL)
    600,000 units [300,000 units each penicillin G benzathine and penicillin G procaine] (1 mL)
    900,000 units penicillin G benzathine and 300,000 units penicillin G procaine per dose (2 mL)

Penicillin G (Parenteral/Aqueous)
  (pen i SIL in jee, pa REN ter al, AYE kwee us)

Related Information
  Antibiotic Treatment of Adults With Infective Endocarditis *on page 1585*
  Antimicrobial Drugs of Choice *on page 1588*
  Desensitization Protocols *on page 1525*
  Treatment of Sexually Transmitted Diseases *on page 1609*

U.S. Brand Names Pfizerpen®

Canadian Brand Names Pfizerpen®

Synonyms Benzylpenicillin Potassium; Benzylpenicillin Sodium; Crystalline Penicillin; Penicillin G Potassium; Penicillin G Sodium

Therapeutic Category Antibiotic, Penicillin

Use Active against some gram-positive organisms, generally not *Staphylococcus aureus*; some gram-negative organisms such as *Neisseria gonorrhoeae*, and some anaerobes and spirochetes

Pregnancy Risk Factor B

Contraindications Hypersensitivity to penicillin or any component of the formulation

Warnings/Precautions Avoid intra-arterial administration or injection into or near major peripheral nerves or blood vessels since such injections may cause severe and/or permanent neurovascular damage; use with caution in patients with renal impairment (dosage reduction required), pre-existing seizure disorders, or with a history of hypersensitivity to cephalosporins

Adverse Reactions Frequency not defined.
  Central nervous system: Convulsions, confusion, drowsiness, myoclonus, fever
  Dermatologic: Rash
  Endocrine & metabolic: Electrolyte imbalance
  Hematologic: Positive Coombs' reaction, hemolytic anemia
  Local: Thrombophlebitis
  Renal: Acute interstitial nephritis
  Miscellaneous: Anaphylaxis, hypersensitivity reactions, Jarisch-Herxheimer reaction

Overdosage/Toxicology Symptoms of penicillin overdose include neuromuscular hypersensitivity (agitation, hallucinations, asterixis, encephalopathy, confusion, seizures) and electrolyte imbalance with potassium or sodium salts, especially in renal failure. Hemodialysis may be helpful to aid in removal of the drug from the blood, otherwise, most treatment is supportive or symptom directed.

Drug Interactions
  Increased Effect/Toxicity: Probenecid increases penicillin levels. Aminoglycosides may lead to synergistic efficacy.
  Decreased Effect: Tetracyclines may decrease penicillin effectiveness. Efficacy of oral contraceptives may be reduced when taken with penicillins.

Stability
  Penicillin G potassium is stable at room temperature
  Reconstituted parenteral solution is stable for 7 days when refrigerated (2°C to 15°C)
  Penicillin G potassium for I.V. infusion in NS or D₅W, solution is stable for 24 hours at room temperature
  Incompatible with aminoglycosides; inactivated in acidic or alkaline solutions

Mechanism of Action Interferes with bacterial cell wall synthesis during active multiplication, causing cell wall death and resultant bactericidal activity against susceptible bacteria

Pharmacodynamics/Kinetics
  Distribution: Poor penetration across blood-brain barrier, despite inflamed meninges; crosses placenta; enters breast milk
    Relative diffusion from blood into CSF: Good only with inflammation (exceeds usual MICs)
    CSF:blood level ratio: Normal meninges: <1%; Inflamed meninges: 3% to 5%
  Protein binding: 65%
  Metabolism: Hepatic (30%) to penicilloic acid
  Half-life elimination:
    Neonates: <6 days old: 3.2-3.4 hours; 7-13 days old: 1.2-2.2 hours; >14 days old: 0.9-1.9 hours
    Children and adults: Normal renal function: 20-50 minutes
  (Continued)

Penicillin G (Parenteral/Aqueous) *(Continued)*

End-stage renal disease: 3.3-5.1 hours

Time to peak, serum: I.M.: ~30 minutes; I.V. ~1 hour

Excretion: Urine

Usual Dosage I.M., I.V.:

Infants:

<7 days, <2000 g: 50,000 units/kg/day in divided doses every 12 hours

<7 days, >2000 g: 50,000 units/kg/day in divided doses every 8 hours

>7 days, <2000 g: 75,000 units/kg/day in divided doses every 8 hours

>7 days, >2000 g: 100,000 units/kg/day in divided doses every 6 hours

Infants and Children (sodium salt is preferred in children): 100,000-250,000 units/kg/day in divided doses every 4 hours

Severe infections: Up to 400,000 units/kg/day in divided doses every 4 hours; maximum dose: 24 million units/day

Congenital syphilis:

Newborns: 50,000 units/kg/day I.V. every 8-12 hours for 10-14 days

Infants: 50,000 units/kg every 4-6 hours for 10-14 days

Disseminated gonococcal infections or gonococcus ophthalmia (if organism proven sensitive): 100,000 units/kg/day in 2 equal doses (4 equal doses/day for infants >1 week)

Gonococcal meningitis: 150,000 units/kg in 2 equal doses (4 doses/day for infants >1 week)

Adults: 2-24 million units/day in divided doses every 4 hours depending on sensitivity of the organism and severity of the infection

Neurosyphilis: 18-24 million units/day in divided doses every 3-4 hours for 10-14 days

Dosing interval in renal impairment:

Cl_{cr} 30-50 mL/minute: Administer every 6 hours

Cl_{cr} 10-30 mL/minute: Administer every 8 hours

Cl_{cr} <10 mL/minute: Administer every 12 hours

Hemodialysis: Moderately dialyzable (20% to 50%)

Continuous arteriovenous or venovenous hemodiafiltration effects: Dose as for Cl_{cr} 10-50 mL/minute

Administration Administer I.M. by deep injection in the upper outer quadrant of the buttock

Monitoring Parameters Observe for signs and symptoms of anaphylaxis during first dose

Test Interactions False-positive or negative urinary glucose determination using Clinitest®; positive Coombs' [direct]; false-positive urinary and/or serum proteins

Patient Information Report any rash or shortness of breath

Nursing Implications Dosage modification required in patients with renal insufficiency

Additional Information 1 million units is approximately equal to 625 mg.

Penicillin G potassium: 1.7 mEq of potassium and 0.3 mEq of sodium per 1 million units of penicillin G

Penicillin G sodium: 2 mEq of sodium per 1 million units of penicillin G

Dosage Forms

Injection, penicillin G potassium [premixed, frozen]: 1 million units, 2 million units, 3 million units

Injection, penicillin G potassium, powder: 1 million units, 5 million units, 10 million units, 20 million units

Injection, penicillin G sodium: 5 million units

♦ **Penicillin G Potassium** *see* Penicillin G (Parenteral/Aqueous) *on page 1053*

Penicillin G Procaine *(pen i SIL in jee PROE kane)*

Related Information

Treatment of Sexually Transmitted Diseases *on page 1609*

U.S. Brand Names Wycillin®

Canadian Brand Names Pfizerpen-AS®; Wycillin®

Synonyms APPG; Aqueous Procaine Penicillin G; Procaine Benzylpenicillin; Procaine Penicillin G

Therapeutic Category Antibiotic, Penicillin

Use Moderately severe infections due to *Treponema pallidum* and other penicillin G-sensitive microorganisms that are susceptible to low, but prolonged serum penicillin concentrations; anthrax due to *Bacillus anthracis* (postexposure) to reduce the incidence or progression of disease following exposure to aerolized *Bacillus anthracis*

Pregnancy Risk Factor B

Contraindications Hypersensitivity to penicillin, procaine, or any component of the formulation

Warnings/Precautions May need to modify dosage in patients with severe renal impairment, seizure disorders, or history of hypersensitivity to cephalosporins; avoid I.V., intravascular, or intra-arterial administration of penicillin G procaine since severe and/or permanent neurovascular damage may occur; use of penicillin for longer than 2 weeks may be associated with an increased risk for some adverse reactions (neutropenia, serum sickness)

Adverse Reactions Frequency not defined.

Cardiovascular: Myocardial depression, vasodilation, conduction disturbances

Central nervous system: Confusion, drowsiness, myoclonus, CNS stimulation, seizures

Hematologic: Positive Coombs' reaction, hemolytic anemia, neutropenia

Local: Pain at injection site, thrombophlebitis, sterile abscess at injection site

Renal: Interstitial nephritis

Miscellaneous: Pseudoanaphylactic reactions, hypersensitivity reactions, Jarisch-Herxheimer reaction, serum sickness

Overdosage/Toxicology Symptoms of penicillin overdose include neuromuscular hypersensitivity (agitation, hallucinations, asterixis, encephalopathy, confusion, seizures) and electrolyte imbalance with potassium or sodium salts, especially in renal failure. Hemodialysis may be helpful to aid in removal of the drug from the blood, otherwise, most treatment is supportive or symptom directed.

Drug Interactions
    Increased Effect/Toxicity: Probenecid increases penicillin levels. Aminoglycosides may lead to synergistic efficacy.
    Decreased Effect: Tetracyclines may decrease penicillin effectiveness. Efficacy of oral contraceptives may be reduced when taken with penicillins.
Stability Store in refrigerator
Mechanism of Action Inhibits bacterial cell wall synthesis by binding to one or more of the penicillin binding proteins (PBPs); which in turn inhibits the final transpeptidation step of peptidoglycan synthesis in bacterial cell walls, thus inhibiting cell wall biosynthesis. Bacteria eventually lyse due to ongoing activity of cell wall autolytic enzymes (autolysins and murein hydrolases) while cell wall assembly is arrested.
Pharmacodynamics/Kinetics
    Duration: Therapeutic: 15-24 hours
    Absorption: I.M.: Slow
    Distribution: Penetration across the blood-brain barrier is poor, despite inflamed meninges; enters breast milk
    Protein binding: 65%
    Metabolism: ~30% hepatically inactivated
    Time to peak, serum: 1-4 hours
    Excretion: Urine (60% to 90% as unchanged drug)
    Clearance: Renal: Delayed in neonates, young infants, and with impaired renal function
Usual Dosage I.M.:
    Children: 25,000-50,000 units/kg/day in divided doses 1-2 times/day; not to exceed 4.8 million units/24 hours
        Anthrax, inhalational (postexposure prophylaxis): 25,000 units/kg every 12 hours (maximum: 1,200,000 units every 12 hours); see "Note" in Adults dosing
        Congenital syphilis: 50,000 units/kg/day for 10-14 days
    Adults: 0.6-4.8 million units/day in divided doses every 12-24 hours
        Anthrax:
            Inhalational (postexposure prophylaxis): 1,200,000 units every 12 hours
            Note: Overall treatment duration should be 60 days. Available safety data suggest continued administration of penicillin G procaine for longer than 2 weeks may incur additional risk for adverse reactions. Clinicians may consider switching to effective alternative treatment for completion of therapy beyond 2 weeks.
            Cutaneous (treatment): 600,000-1,200,000 units/day; alternative therapy is recommended in severe cutaneous or other forms of anthrax infection
        Endocarditis caused by susceptible viridans *Streptococcus* (when used in conjunction with an aminoglycoside): 1.2 million units every 6 hours for 2-4 weeks
        Neurosyphilis: I.M.: 2-4 million units/day with 500 mg probenecid by mouth 4 times/day for 10-14 days; **penicillin G aqueous I.V. is the preferred agent**
    Hemodialysis: Moderately dialyzable (20% to 50%)
Administration Procaine suspension for deep I.M. injection only; rotate the injection site avoid I.V., intravascular, or intra-arterial administration of penicillin G procaine since severe and/or permanent neurovascular damage may occur
Monitoring Parameters Periodic renal and hematologic function tests with prolonged therapy; fever, mental status, WBC count
Test Interactions Positive Coombs' [direct], false-positive urinary and/or serum proteins
Patient Information Notify physician if skin rash, itching, hives, or severe diarrhea occurs
Nursing Implications Renal and hematologic systems should be evaluated periodically during prolonged therapy; do not inject in gluteal muscle in children <2 years of age
Dosage Forms Injection, suspension: 300,000 units/mL (10 mL); 600,000 units/mL (1 mL, 2 mL, 4 mL)

♦ **Penicillin G Procaine and Benzathine Combined** *see* Penicillin G Benzathine and Procaine Combined *on page 1052*
♦ **Penicillin G Sodium** *see* Penicillin G (Parenteral/Aqueous) *on page 1053*

Penicillin V Potassium (pen i SIL in vee poe TASS ee um)

Related Information
    Animal and Human Bites Guidelines *on page 1584*
    Antimicrobial Drugs of Choice *on page 1588*
    Desensitization Protocols *on page 1525*
U.S. Brand Names Suspen®; Truxcillin®; Veetids®
Canadian Brand Names Apo®-Pen VK; Nadopen-V®; Novo-Pen-VK®; Nu-Pen-VK®; PVF® K
Synonyms Pen VK; Phenoxymethyl Penicillin
Therapeutic Category Antibiotic, Penicillin
Use Treatment of infections caused by susceptible organisms involving the respiratory tract, otitis media, sinusitis, skin, and urinary tract; prophylaxis in rheumatic fever
Pregnancy Risk Factor B
Contraindications Hypersensitivity to penicillin or any component of the formulation
Warnings/Precautions Use with caution in patients with severe renal impairment (modify dosage), history of seizures, or hypersensitivity to cephalosporins
Adverse Reactions
    >10%: Gastrointestinal: Mild diarrhea, vomiting, nausea, oral candidiasis
    <1% (Limited to important or life-threatening): Acute interstitial nephritis, convulsions, hemolytic anemia, positive Coombs' reaction
Overdosage/Toxicology Symptoms of penicillin overdose include neuromuscular hypersensitivity (agitation, hallucinations, asterixis, encephalopathy, confusion, seizures) and electrolyte imbalance with potassium or sodium salts, especially in renal failure. Hemodialysis may be helpful to aid in removal of the drug from the blood, otherwise, most treatment is supportive or symptom directed.
Drug Interactions
    Increased Effect/Toxicity: Probenecid increases penicillin levels. Aminoglycosides may cause synergistic efficacy.
(Continued)

Penicillin V Potassium *(Continued)*

Decreased Effect: Tetracyclines may decrease penicillin effectiveness. Efficacy of oral contraceptives may be reduced when taken with penicillins.

Ethanol/Nutrition/Herb Interactions Food: Decreases drug absorption rate; decreases drug serum concentration.

Stability Refrigerate suspension after reconstitution; discard after 14 days

Mechanism of Action Inhibits bacterial cell wall synthesis by binding to one or more of the penicillin binding proteins (PBPs); which in turn inhibits the final transpeptidation step of peptidoglycan synthesis in bacterial cell walls, thus inhibiting cell wall biosynthesis. Bacteria eventually lyse due to ongoing activity of cell wall autolytic enzymes (autolysins and murein hydrolases) while cell wall assembly is arrested.

Pharmacodynamics/Kinetics

Absorption: 60% to 73%

Distribution: Enters breast milk

Protein binding, plasma: 80%

Half-life elimination: 0.5 hours; prolonged with renal impairment

Time to peak, serum: 0.5-1 hour

Excretion: Urine (as unchanged drug and metabolites)

Usual Dosage Oral:

Systemic infections:

Children <12 years: 25-50 mg/kg/day in divided doses every 6-8 hours; maximum dose: 3 g/day

Children ≥12 years and Adults: 125-500 mg every 6-8 hours

Prophylaxis of pneumococcal infections:

Children <5 years: 125 mg twice daily

Children ≥5 years and Adults: 250 mg twice daily

Prophylaxis of recurrent rheumatic fever:

Children <5 years: 125 mg twice daily

Children ≥5 years and Adults: 250 mg twice daily

Dosing interval in renal impairment: Cl_{cr} <10 mL/minute: Administer 250 mg every 6 hours

Dietary Considerations Take on an empty stomach 1 hour before or 2 hours after meals.

Administration Administer on an empty stomach to increase oral absorption

Monitoring Parameters Periodic renal and hematologic function tests during prolonged therapy; monitor for signs of anaphylaxis during first dose

Test Interactions False-positive or negative urinary glucose determination using Clinitest®; positive Coombs' [direct]; false-positive urinary and/or serum proteins

Patient Information Take on an empty stomach 1 hour before or 2 hours after meals, take until gone, do not skip doses, report any rash or shortness of breath; shake liquid well before use

Nursing Implications Administer around-the-clock rather than 4 times/day, 3 times/day, etc (ie, 12-6-12-6, not 9-1-5-9) to promote less variation in peak and trough serum levels; dosage modification required in patients with renal insufficiency

Additional Information 0.7 mEq of potassium per 250 mg penicillin V; 250 mg equals 400,000 units of penicillin

Dosage Forms 250 mg = 400,000 units

Powder for oral solution: 125 mg/5 mL (80 mL, 100 mL, 150 mL, 200 mL); 250 mg/5 mL (80 mL, 100 mL, 150 mL, 200 mL)

Tablet: 250 mg, 500 mg

♦ **Penicilloyl-polylysine** *see Benzylpenicilloyl-polylysine on page 158*

♦ **Penlac™** *see Ciclopirox on page 290*

♦ **Pentacarinat®** *see Pentamidine on page 1056*

♦ **Pentacel™ (Can)** *see Diphtheria, Tetanus Toxoids, and Whole-Cell Pertussis Vaccine on page 420*

♦ **Pentam-300®** *see Pentamidine on page 1056*

Pentamidine *(pen TAM i deen)*

Related Information

USPHA/IDSA Guidelines for the Prevention of Opportunistic Infections in Persons With HIV on page 1574

U.S. Brand Names NebuPent™; Pentacarinat®; Pentam-300®

Canadian Brand Names Pentacarinat®

Synonyms Pentamidine Isethionate

Therapeutic Category Antibiotic, Miscellaneous

Use Treatment and prevention of pneumonia caused by *Pneumocystis carinii*; treatment of trypanosomiasis and visceral leishmaniasis

Pregnancy Risk Factor C

Contraindications Hypersensitivity to pentamidine isethionate or any component of the formulation (inhalation and injection)

Warnings/Precautions Use with caution in patients with diabetes mellitus, renal or hepatic dysfunction; hypertension or hypotension; leukopenia, thrombocytopenia, asthma, hypo/hyperglycemia

Adverse Reactions

Inhalation:

>10%:

Cardiovascular: Chest pain

Dermatologic: Rash

Respiratory: Wheezing, dyspnea, coughing, pharyngitis

1% to 10%: Gastrointestinal: Bitter or metallic taste

<1% (Limited to important or life-threatening): Hypoglycemia, renal insufficiency

Systemic:

>10%:

Cardiovascular: Hypotension

Dermatologic: Rash
Endocrine & metabolic: Hyperglycemia or hypoglycemia
Gastrointestinal: Nausea, vomiting, anorexia, diarrhea
Hematologic: Leukopenia or neutropenia, thrombocytopenia
Hepatic: Elevated LFTs
Renal: Nephrotoxicity
1% to 10%:
Hematologic: Anemia
Cardiovascular: Cardiac arrhythmias
Gastrointestinal: Pancreatitis, metallic taste
Local: Local reactions at injection site
<1% (Limited to important or life-threatening): Arrhythmias

Overdosage/Toxicology Symptoms include hypotension, hypoglycemia, and cardiac arrhythmias. Treatment is supportive.

Drug Interactions
Cytochrome P450 Effect: CYP2C19 enzyme substrate
Increased Effect/Toxicity: Pentamidine may potentiate the effect of other drugs which prolong QT interval (cisapride, terfenadine, astemizole, sparfloxacin, gatifloxacin, moxifloxacin, and type Ia and type III antiarrhythmics).

Ethanol/Nutrition/Herb Interactions Ethanol: Avoid ethanol (may increase CNS depression or aggravate hypoglycemia).

Stability Do not refrigerate due to the possibility of crystallization; do not use NS as a diluent, NS is **incompatible** with pentamidine; reconstituted solutions (60-100 mg/mL) are stable for 48 hours at room temperature and do not require light protection; diluted solutions (1-2.5 mg/mL) in D_5W are stable for at least 24 hours at room temperature

Mechanism of Action Interferes with RNA/DNA, phospholipids and protein synthesis, through inhibition of oxidative phosphorylation and/or interference with incorporation of nucleotides and nucleic acids into RNA and DNA, in protozoa

Pharmacodynamics/Kinetics
Absorption: I.M.: Well absorbed; Inhalation: Limited systemic absorption
Half-life elimination: Terminal: 6.4-9.4 hours; may be prolonged with severe renal impairment
Excretion: Urine (33% to 66% as unchanged drug)

Usual Dosage
Children:
Treatment: I.M., I.V. (I.V. preferred): 4 mg/kg/day once daily for 10-14 days
Prevention:
I.M., I.V.: 4 mg/kg monthly or every 2 weeks
Inhalation (aerosolized pentamidine in children ≥5 years): 300 mg/dose given every 3-4 weeks via Respirgard® II inhaler (8 mg/kg dose has also been used in children <5 years)
Treatment of trypanosomiasis: I.V.: 4 mg/kg/day once daily for 10 days
Adults:
Treatment: I.M., I.V. (I.V. preferred): 4 mg/kg/day once daily for 14-21 days
Prevention: Inhalation: 300 mg every 4 weeks via Respirgard® II nebulizer
Dialysis: Not removed by hemo or peritoneal dialysis or continuous arteriovenous or venovenous hemofiltration; supplemental dosage is not necessary
Dosing adjustment in renal impairment: Adults: I.V.:
Cl_{cr} 10-50 mL/minute: Administer 4 mg/kg every 24-36 hours
Cl_{cr} <10 mL/minute: Administer 4 mg/kg every 48 hours

Administration Infuse I.V. slowly over a period of at least 60 minutes or administer deep I.M.; patients receiving I.V. or I.M. pentamidine should be lying down and blood pressure should be monitored closely during administration of drug and several times thereafter until it is stable

Monitoring Parameters Liver function tests, renal function tests, blood glucose, serum potassium and calcium, EKG, blood pressure

Patient Information PCP pneumonia may still occur despite pentamidine use; notify physician of fever, shortness of breath, or coughing up blood; maintain adequate fluid intake

Nursing Implications Virtually undetectable amounts are transferred to healthcare personnel during aerosol administration; **do not use NS as a diluent**

Dosage Forms
Powder for injection, lyophilized, as isethionate: 300 mg
Powder for nebulization, as isethionate: 300 mg

♦ **Pentamidine Isethionate** *see* Pentamidine *on page 1056*

♦ **Pentamycetin® (Can)** *see* Chloramphenicol *on page 272*

♦ **Pentasa®** *see* Mesalamine *on page 866*

Pentazocine (pen TAZ oh seen)

Related Information
Depression *on page 1655*
Narcotic Agonists Comparison *on page 1506*

U.S. Brand Names Talwin®; Talwin® NX

Canadian Brand Names Talwin®

Synonyms Pentazocine Hydrochloride; Pentazocine Lactate

Therapeutic Category Analgesic, Narcotic; Sedative

Use Relief of moderate to severe pain; has also been used as a sedative prior to surgery and as a supplement to surgical anesthesia

Restrictions C-IV

Pregnancy Risk Factor B/D (prolonged use or high doses at term)

Contraindications Hypersensitivity to pentazocine or any component of the formulation; increased intracranial pressure (unless the patient is mechanically ventilated); pregnancy (prolonged use or high doses at term)
(Continued)

Pentazocine *(Continued)*

Warnings/Precautions Use with caution in seizure-prone patients, acute myocardial infarction, patients undergoing biliary tract surgery, patients with renal and hepatic dysfunction, head trauma, increased intracranial pressure, and patients with a history of prior opioid dependence or abuse; pentazocine may precipitate opiate withdrawal symptoms in patients who have been receiving opiates regularly; injection contains sulfites which may cause allergic reaction; tolerance or drug dependence may result from extended use. Talwin® NX is intended for oral administration **only** - severe vascular reactions have resulted from misuse by injection.

Adverse Reactions Frequency not defined.

Cardiovascular: Hypotension, palpitations, peripheral vasodilation

Central nervous system: Malaise, headache, restlessness, nightmares, insomnia, CNS depression, sedation, hallucinations, confusion, disorientation, dizziness, euphoria, drowsiness

Dermatologic: Rash, pruritus

Gastrointestinal: Nausea, vomiting, xerostomia, constipation, anorexia, diarrhea, GI irritation, biliary tract spasm

Genitourinary: Urinary tract spasm

Local: Tissue damage and irritation with I.M./S.C. use

Neuromuscular & skeletal: Weakness

Ocular: Blurred vision, miosis

Respiratory: Dyspnea, respiratory depression (rare)

Miscellaneous: Histamine release, physical and psychological dependence

Overdosage/Toxicology Symptoms include drowsiness, sedation, respiratory depression, and coma. Treatment consists of naloxone 2 mg I.V. (0.01 mg/kg for children), with repeat administration as necessary, up to a total of 10 mg.

Drug Interactions

Cytochrome P450 Effect: CYP2D6 enzyme substrate

Increased Effect/Toxicity: Increased effect/toxicity with tripelennamine (can be lethal), CNS depressants (eg, phenothiazines, tranquilizers, anxiolytics, sedatives, hypnotics, alcohol).

Decreased Effect: May potentiate or reduce analgesic effect of opiate agonist (eg, morphine) depending on patients tolerance to opiates; can precipitate withdrawal in narcotic addicts.

Ethanol/Nutrition/Herb Interactions Ethanol: Avoid ethanol (may increase CNS depression).

Stability Store at room temperature, protect from heat and from freezing; I.V. form is **incompatible** with aminophylline, amobarbital (and all other I.V. barbiturates), glycopyrrolate (same syringe), heparin (same syringe), nafcillin (Y-site)

Mechanism of Action Binds to opiate receptors in the CNS, causing inhibition of ascending pain pathways, altering the perception of and response to pain; produces generalized CNS depression; partial agonist-antagonist

Pharmacodynamics/Kinetics

Onset of action: Oral, I.M., S.C.: 15-30 minutes; I.V.: 2-3 minutes

Duration: Oral: 4-5 hours; Parenteral: 2-3 hours

Protein binding: 60%

Metabolism: Hepatically via oxidative and glucuronide conjugation pathways; large first-pass effect

Bioavailability: Oral: ~20%; increased to 60% to 70% with cirrhosis

Half-life elimination: 2-3 hours; increased with decreased hepatic function

Excretion: Urine (small amounts as unchanged drug)

Usual Dosage

Children: I.M., S.C.:

5-8 years: 15 mg

8-14 years: 30 mg

Children >12 years and Adults: Oral: 50 mg every 3-4 hours; may increase to 100 mg/dose if needed, but should not exceed 600 mg/day

Adults:

I.M., S.C.: 30-60 mg every 3-4 hours, not to exceed total daily dose of 360 mg

I.V.: 30 mg every 3-4 hours

Elderly: Elderly patients may be more sensitive to the analgesic and sedating effects. The elderly may also have impaired renal function. If needed, dosing should be started at the lower end of dosing range and adjust dose for renal function.

Dosing adjustment in renal impairment:

Cl_{cr} 10-50 mL/minute: Administer 75% of normal dose

Cl_{cr} <10 mL/minute: Administer 50% of normal dose

Dosing adjustment in hepatic impairment: Reduce dose or avoid use in patients with liver disease

Administration Rotate injection site for I.M., S.C. use; avoid intra-arterial injection

Monitoring Parameters Relief of pain, respiratory and mental status, blood pressure

Patient Information Avoid alcohol, may cause drowsiness, impaired judgment or coordination; may cause physical and psychological dependence with prolonged use; will cause withdrawal in patients currently dependent on narcotics

Nursing Implications Observe patient for excessive sedation, respiratory depression, implement safety measures, assist with ambulation; observe for narcotic withdrawal

Additional Information Pentazocine hydrochloride: Talwin® NX tablet (with naloxone); naloxone is used to prevent abuse by dissolving tablets in water and using as injection.

Dosage Forms

Injection, as lactate: 30 mg/mL (1 mL, 1.5 mL, 2 mL, 10 mL)

Tablet: Pentazocine hydrochloride 50 mg and naloxone hydrochloride 0.5 mg

♦ **Pentazocine Hydrochloride** *see* Pentazocine *on page 1057*

♦ **Pentazocine Lactate** *see* Pentazocine *on page 1057*

Pentobarbital (pen toe BAR bi tal)

U.S. Brand Names Nembutal®
Canadian Brand Names Nembutal® Sodium
Synonyms Pentobarbital Sodium
Therapeutic Category Anticonvulsant; Barbiturate; Sedative
Use Sedative/hypnotic; preanesthetic; high-dose barbiturate coma for treatment of increased intracranial pressure or status epilepticus unresponsive to other therapy
Unlabeled/Investigational Use Tolerance test during withdrawal of sedative hypnotics
Restrictions C-II (capsules, injection); C-III (suppositories)
Pregnancy Risk Factor D
Contraindications Hypersensitivity to barbiturates or any component of the formulation; marked hepatic impairment; dyspnea or airway obstruction; porphyria; pregnancy
Warnings/Precautions Tolerance to hypnotic effect can occur; do not use for >2 weeks to treat insomnia. Potential for drug dependency exists, abrupt cessation may precipitate withdrawal, including status epilepticus in epileptic patients. Do not administer to patients in acute pain. Use caution in elderly, debilitated, renally impaired, hepatic dysfunction, or pediatric patients. May cause paradoxical responses, including agitation and hyperactivity, particularly in acute pain and pediatric patients. Use with caution in patients with depression or suicidal tendencies, or in patients with a history of drug abuse. Tolerance, psychological and physical dependence may occur with prolonged use.

May cause CNS depression, which may impair physical or mental abilities. Patients must be cautioned about performing tasks which require mental alertness (ie, operating machinery or driving). Effects with other sedative drugs or ethanol may be potentiated. Use of this agent as a hypnotic in the elderly is not recommended due to its long half-life and potential for physical and psychological dependence.

May cause respiratory depression or hypotension, particularly when administered intravenously. Use with caution in hemodynamically unstable patients or patients with respiratory disease. High doses (loading doses of 15-35 mg/kg given over 1-2 hours) have been utilized to induce pentobarbital coma, but these higher doses often cause hypotension requiring vasopressor therapy.

Adverse Reactions Frequency not defined.
Cardiovascular: Bradycardia, hypotension, syncope
Central nervous system: Drowsiness, lethargy, CNS excitation or depression, impaired judgment, "hangover" effect, confusion, somnolence, agitation, hyperkinesia, ataxia, nervousness, headache, insomnia, nightmares, hallucinations, anxiety, dizziness
Dermatologic: Rash, exfoliative dermatitis, Stevens-Johnson syndrome
Gastrointestinal: Nausea, vomiting, constipation
Hematologic: Agranulocytosis, thrombocytopenia, megaloblastic anemia
Local: Pain at injection site, thrombophlebitis with I.V. use
Renal: Oliguria
Respiratory: Laryngospasm, respiratory depression, apnea (especially with rapid I.V. use), hypoventilation, apnea
Miscellaneous: Gangrene with inadvertent intra-arterial injection
Overdosage/Toxicology Symptoms include unsteady gait, slurred speech, confusion, jaundice, hypothermia, hypotension, respiratory depression, and coma. If hypotension occurs, administer I.V. fluids and place in the Trendelenburg position. If unresponsive, an I.V. vasopressor (eg, dopamine, epinephrine) may be required. Forced alkaline diuresis is of no value in the treatment of intoxications with short-acting barbiturates. Charcoal hemoperfusion or hemodialysis may be useful in harder-to-treat intoxications, especially in the presence of very high serum barbiturate levels when the patient is in a coma, shock, or renal failure.

Drug Interactions
Cytochrome P450 Effect: Note: Barbiturates are enzyme inducers; patients should be monitored when these drugs are started or stopped for a decreased or increased therapeutic effect respectively
Increased Effect/Toxicity: When combined with other CNS depressants, ethanol, narcotic analgesics, antidepressants, or benzodiazepines, additive respiratory and CNS depression may occur. Chronic use of barbiturates may enhance the hepatotoxic potential of acetaminophen overdoses. Chloramphenicol, MAO inhibitors, valproic acid, and felbamate may inhibit barbiturate metabolism. Barbiturates may impair the absorption of griseofulvin, and may enhance the nephrotoxic effects of methoxyflurane.
Decreased Effect: Barbiturates such as pentobarbital are hepatic enzyme inducers, and (only with chronic use) may increase the metabolism of antipsychotics, some beta-blockers (unlikely with atenolol and nadolol), calcium channel blockers, chloramphenicol, cimetidine, corticosteroids, cyclosporine, disopyramide, doxycycline, ethosuximide, felbamate, furosemide, griseofulvin, lamotrigine, phenytoin, propafenone, quinidine, tacrolimus, TCAs, and theophylline. Barbiturates may increase the metabolism of estrogens and reduce the efficacy of oral contraceptives; an alternative method of contraception should be considered. Barbiturates inhibit the hypoprothrombinemic effects of oral anticoagulants via increased metabolism. Barbiturates may enhance the metabolism of methadone resulting in methadone withdrawal.
Ethanol/Nutrition/Herb Interactions
Ethanol: Avoid ethanol (may increase CNS depression).
Food: Food may decrease the rate but not the extent of oral absorption.
Stability Protect from freezing; aqueous solutions are not stable, commercially available vehicle (containing propylene glycol) is more stable; low pH may cause precipitate; use only clear solution
Mechanism of Action Short-acting barbiturate with sedative, hypnotic, and anticonvulsant properties. Barbiturates depress the sensory cortex, decrease motor activity, alter cerebellar function, and produce drowsiness, sedation, and hypnosis. In high doses, barbiturates exhibit anticonvulsant activity; barbiturates produce dose-dependent respiratory depression.
Pharmacodynamics/Kinetics
Onset of action: Oral, rectal: 15-60 minutes; I.M.: 10-15 minutes; I.V.: ~1 minute
(Continued)

Pentobarbital *(Continued)*

Duration: Oral, rectal: 1-4 hours; I.V.: 15 minutes

Distribution: V_d: Children: 0.8 L/kg; Adults: 1 L/kg

Protein binding: 35% to 55%

Metabolism: Extensively hepatic via hydroxylation and oxidation pathways

Half-life elimination: Terminal: Children: 25 hours; Adults, normal: 22 hours; range: 35-50 hours

Excretion: Urine (<1% as unchanged drug)

Usual Dosage

Children:

Sedative: Oral: 2-6 mg/kg/day divided in 3 doses; maximum: 100 mg/day

Hypnotic: I.M.: 2-6 mg/kg; maximum: 100 mg/dose

Sedative/hypnotic: Rectal:

2 months to 1 year (10-20 lb): 30 mg

1-4 years (20-40 lb): 30-60 mg

5-12 years (40-80 lb): 60 mg

12-14 years (80-110 lb): 60-120 mg

or

<4 years: 3-6 mg/kg/dose

>4 years: 1.5-3 mg/kg/dose

Preoperative/preprocedure sedation: ≥6 months:

Oral, I.M., rectal: 2-6 mg/kg; maximum: 100 mg/dose

I.V.: 1-3 mg/kg to a maximum of 100 mg until asleep

Conscious sedation prior to a procedure: Children 5-12 years: I.V.: 2 mg/kg 5-10 minutes before procedures, may repeat one time

Adolescents: Conscious sedation: Oral, I.V.: 100 mg prior to a procedure

Children and Adults: Barbiturate coma in head injury patients: I.V.: Loading dose: 5-10 mg/kg given slowly over 1-2 hours; monitor blood pressure and respiratory rate; Maintenance infusion: Initial: 1 mg/kg/hour; may increase to 2-3 mg/kg/hour; maintain burst suppression on EEG

Status epilepticus: I.V.: **Note**: Intubation required; monitor hemodynamics

Children: Loading dose: 5-15 mg/kg given slowly over 1-2 hours; maintenance infusion: 0.5-5 mg/kg/hour

Adults: Loading dose: 2-15 mg/kg given slowly over 1-2 hours; maintenance infusion: 0.5-3 mg/kg/hour

Adults:

Hypnotic:

Oral: 100-200 mg at bedtime or 20 mg 3-4 times/day for daytime sedation

I.M.: 150-200 mg

I.V.: Initial: 100 mg, may repeat every 1-3 minutes up to 200-500 mg total dose

Rectal: 120-200 mg at bedtime

Preoperative sedation: I.M.: 150-200 mg

Tolerance testing (unlabeled use): 200 mg every 2 hours until signs of intoxication are exhibited at any time during the 2 hours after the dose; maximum dose: 1000 mg

Dosing adjustment in hepatic impairment: Reduce dosage in patients with severe liver dysfunction

Administration Pentobarbital may be administered by deep I.M. or slow I.V. injection. I.M.: No more than 5 mL (250 mg) should be injected at any one site because of possible tissue irritation. I.V. push doses can be given undiluted, but should be administered no faster than 50 mg/minute; parenteral solutions are highly alkaline; avoid extravasation; avoid rapid I.V. administration >50 mg/minute; avoid intra-arterial injection

Monitoring Parameters Respiratory status (for conscious sedation, includes pulse oximetry), cardiovascular status, CNS status; cardiac monitor and blood pressure monitor required

Reference Range

Therapeutic:

Hypnotic: 1-5 µg/mL (SI: 4-22 µmol/L)

Coma: 10-50 µg/mL (SI: 88-221 µmol/L)

Toxic: >10 µg/mL (SI: >44 µmol/L)

Patient Information Avoid alcohol and other CNS depressants; avoid driving and other hazardous tasks; avoid abrupt discontinuation; may cause physical and psychological dependence; do not alter dose without notifying physician

Nursing Implications Avoid extravasation; institute safety measures to avoid injuries; has many incompatibilities when given I.V.; monitor blood pressure closely with I.V. administration

Additional Information Sodium content of 1 mL injection: 5 mg (0.2 mEq)

Dosage Forms

Capsule, as sodium (C-II): 50 mg, 100 mg

Injection, as sodium (C-II): 50 mg/mL (20 mL, 50 mL)

Suppository, rectal (C-III): 60 mg, 200 mg

♦ **Pentobarbital Sodium** *see Pentobarbital on page 1059*

Pentosan Polysulfate Sodium *(PEN toe san pol i SUL fate SOW dee um)*

U.S. Brand Names Elmiron®

Canadian Brand Names Elmiron™

Synonyms PPS

Therapeutic Category Analgesic, Urinary

Use Orphan drug: Relief of bladder pain or discomfort due to interstitial cystitis

Pregnancy Risk Factor B

Usual Dosage Adults: Oral: 100 mg 3 times/day taken with water 1 hour before or 2 hours after meals

Patients should be evaluated at 3 months and may be continued an additional 3 months if there has been no improvement and if there are no therapy-limiting side effects. **The risks** and benefits of continued use beyond 6 months in patients who have not responded is not yet known.

Additional Information Complete prescribing information for this medication should be consulted for additional detail.

Dosage Forms Capsule: 100 mg

Pentostatin (PEN toe stat in)

U.S. Brand Names Nipent®

Canadian Brand Names Nipent®

Synonyms DCF; Deoxycoformycin; 2'-deoxycoformycin

Therapeutic Category Antineoplastic Agent, Antimetabolite (Purine)

Use Treatment of adult patients with alpha-interferon-refractory hairy cell leukemia; non-Hodgkin's lymphoma, cutaneous T-cell lymphoma

Pregnancy Risk Factor D

Contraindications Hypersensitivity to pentostatin or any component; pregnancy

Warnings/Precautions The FDA currently recommends that procedures for proper handling and disposal of antineoplastic agents be considered. Pregnant women or women of child-bearing age should be apprised of the potential risk to the fetus; use extreme caution in the presence of renal insufficiency; use with caution in patients with signs or symptoms of impaired hepatic function.

Adverse Reactions

>10%:

Central nervous system: Fever, chills, infection (57%), severe, life-threatening (35%); headache, lethargy, seizures, coma (10% to 15%), potentially dose-limiting, uncommon at doses 4 mg/m^2

Dermatologic: Skin rashes (25% to 30%), alopecia (10%)

Gastrointestinal: Mild to moderate nausea, vomiting (60%), controlled with non-5-HT$_3$ antagonist antiemetics; stomatitis, diarrhea (13%), anorexia

Genitourinary: Acute renal failure (35%)

Hematologic: Thrombocytopenia (50%), dose-limiting in 25% of patients; anemia (40% to 45%), neutropenia, mild to moderate, not dose-limiting (11%)

Nadir: 7 days

Recovery: 10-14 days

Hepatic: Mild to moderate increases in transaminase levels (30%), usually transient; hepatitis (19%), usually reversible

Respiratory: Pulmonary edema (15%), may be exacerbated by fludarabine

1% to 10%:

Cardiovascular: Chest pain, arrhythmia, peripheral edema

Central nervous system: Opportunistic infections (8%); anxiety, confusion, depression, dizziness, insomnia, nervousness, somnolence, myalgias, malaise

Dermatologic: Dry skin, eczema, pruritus

Gastrointestinal: Constipation, flatulence, weight loss

Neuromuscular & skeletal: Paresthesia, weakness

Ocular: Moderate to severe keratoconjunctivitis, abnormal vision, eye pain

Otic: Ear pain

Respiratory: Dyspnea, pneumonia, bronchitis, pharyngitis, rhinitis, epistaxis, sinusitis (3% to 7%)

<1% (Limited to important or life-threatening): Abnormal EKG arrhythmias, dysuria, hematuria, hypersensitivity reactions, increased BUN, thrombophlebitis

Overdosage/Toxicology Symptoms include severe renal, hepatic, pulmonary, and CNS toxicity. Treatment is supportive.

Drug Interactions

Increased Effect/Toxicity: Increased toxicity with vidarabine, fludarabine, and allopurinol.

Stability Vials are stable under refrigeration at 2°C to 8°C; reconstituted vials, or further dilutions, may be stored at room temperature exposed to ambient light; diluted solutions are stable for 24 hours in D$_5$W or 48 hours in NS or lactated Ringer's at room temperature; infusion with 5% dextrose injection USP or 0.9% sodium chloride injection USP does not interact with PVC-containing administration sets or containers

Mechanism of Action Pentostatin is a purine antimetabolite that inhibits adenosine deaminase, preventing the deamination of adenosine to inosine. Accumulation of deoxyadenosine (dAdo) and deoxyadenosine 5'-triphosphate (dATP) results in a reduction of purine metabolism and DNA synthesis and cell death.

Pharmacodynamics/Kinetics

Distribution: I.V.: V$_d$: 36.1 L (20.1 L/m^2); rapidly to body tissues and may obtain plasma concentrations ranging from 12-36 ng following doses of 250 mcg/kg for 4-5 days

Half-life elimination: Terminal: 5-15 hours

Excretion: Urine (~50% to 96%) within 24 hours

Usual Dosage Refractory hairy cell leukemia: Adults (refer to individual protocols): 4 mg/m^2 every other week; I.V. bolus over ≥3-5 minutes in D$_5$W or NS at concentrations ≥2 mg/mL

Dosing interval in renal impairment:

Cl$_{cr}$ <60 mL/minute: Use extreme caution

Cl$_{cr}$ 50-60 mL/minute: 2 mg/m^2/dose

Dosage Forms Powder for injection: 10 mg/vial

♦ **Pentothal® (Can)** see Thiopental on page 1319

♦ **Pentothal® Sodium** see Thiopental on page 1319

Pentoxifylline (pen toks I fi leen)

U.S. Brand Names Trental®

Canadian Brand Names Albert® Pentoxifylline; Apo®-Pentoxifylline SR Nu-Pentoxifylline SR; Trental®

Synonyms Oxpentifylline

Therapeutic Category Blood Viscosity Reducer Agent; Hemorheologic Agent

(Continued)

Pentoxifylline *(Continued)*

Use Treatment of intermittent claudication on the basis of chronic occlusive arterial disease of the limbs; may improve function and symptoms, but not intended to replace more definitive therapy

Unlabeled/Investigational Use AIDS patients with increased TNF, CVA, cerebrovascular diseases, diabetic atherosclerosis, diabetic neuropathy, gangrene, hemodialysis shunt thrombosis, vascular impotence, cerebral malaria, septic shock, sickle cell syndromes, and vasculitis

Pregnancy Risk Factor C

Contraindications Hypersensitivity to pentoxifylline, xanthines, or any component of the formulation; recent cerebral and/or retinal hemorrhage

Warnings/Precautions Use with caution in patients with renal impairment

Adverse Reactions

1% to 10%:
Central nervous system: Dizziness, headache
Gastrointestinal: Heartburn, nausea, vomiting
<1% (Limited to important or life-threatening): Angioedema, arrhythmias, chest pain, cholecystitis, congestion, dyspnea, hallucinations, hepatitis, jaundice, rash, tremor

Overdosage/Toxicology Symptoms include hypotension, flushing, convulsions, deep sleep, agitation, bradycardia, and A-V block. Treatment is supportive. Seizures can be treated with diazepam 5-10 mg (0.25-0.4 mg/kg in children). Arrhythmias respond to lidocaine.

Drug Interactions

Increased Effect/Toxicity: Pentoxifylline levels may be increased with cimetidine and other H_2 antagonists. May increase anticoagulation with warfarin. Pentoxifylline may increase the serum levels of theophylline.

Decreased Effect: Blood pressure changes (decreases) have been observed with the addition of pentoxifylline therapy in patients receiving antihypertensives.

Ethanol/Nutrition/Herb Interactions Food: Food may decrease rate but not extent of absorption. Pentoxifylline peak serum levels may be decreased if taken with food.

Mechanism of Action Mechanism of action remains unclear; is thought to reduce blood viscosity and improve blood flow by altering the rheology of red blood cells

Pharmacodynamics/Kinetics

Absorption: Well absorbed
Metabolism: Hepatic and via erythrocytes; extensive first-pass effect
Half-life elimination: Parent drug: 24-48 minutes; Metabolites: 60-96 minutes
Time to peak, serum: 2-4 hours
Excretion: Primarily urine

Usual Dosage Adults: Oral: 400 mg 3 times/day with meals; may reduce to 400 mg twice daily if GI or CNS side effects occur

Dietary Considerations May be taken with meals or food.

Test Interactions ↓ calcium (S), ↓ magnesium (S), false-positive theophylline levels

Patient Information Take with food or meals; if GI or CNS side effects continue, contact physician; while effects may be seen in 2-4 weeks, continue treatment for at least 8 weeks

Nursing Implications Do not crush or chew

Dosage Forms Tablet, controlled release: 400 mg

- ◆ **Pen VK** *see Penicillin V Potassium on page 1055*
- ◆ **Pepcid®** *see Famotidine on page 543*
- ◆ **Pepcid® AC [OTC]** *see Famotidine on page 543*
- ◆ **Pepcid® Complete [OTC]** *see Famotidine, Calcium Carbonate, and Magnesium Hydroxide on page 544*
- ◆ **Pepcid® I.V. (Can)** *see Famotidine on page 543*
- ◆ **Pepcid RPD™** *see Famotidine on page 543*
- ◆ **Pepto-Bismol® [OTC]** *see Bismuth on page 170*
- ◆ **Pepto-Bismol® Maximum Strength [OTC]** *see Bismuth on page 170*
- ◆ **Pepto® Diarrhea Control [OTC]** *see Loperamide on page 816*
- ◆ **Percocet® (Can)** *see Oxycodone and Acetaminophen on page 1026*
- ◆ **Percocet® 2.5/325** *see Oxycodone and Acetaminophen on page 1026*
- ◆ **Percocet® 5/325** *see Oxycodone and Acetaminophen on page 1026*
- ◆ **Percocet® 7.5/325** *see Oxycodone and Acetaminophen on page 1026*
- ◆ **Percocet® 7.5/500** *see Oxycodone and Acetaminophen on page 1026*
- ◆ **Percocet® 10/325** *see Oxycodone and Acetaminophen on page 1026*
- ◆ **Percocet® 10/650** *see Oxycodone and Acetaminophen on page 1026*
- ◆ **Percocet®-Demi (Can)** *see Oxycodone and Acetaminophen on page 1026*
- ◆ **Percodan®** *see Oxycodone and Aspirin on page 1026*
- ◆ **Percodan®-Demi** *see Oxycodone and Aspirin on page 1026*
- ◆ **Percogesic® [OTC]** *see Acetaminophen and Phenyltoloxamine on page 25*
- ◆ **Percolone®** *see Oxycodone on page 1024*
- ◆ **Perdiem® Plain [OTC]** *see Psyllium on page 1158*

Pergolide *(PER go lide)*

Related Information
Parkinson's Agents *on page 1513*

U.S. Brand Names Permax®

Canadian Brand Names Permax®

Synonyms Pergolide Mesylate

Therapeutic Category Anti-Parkinson's Agent, Dopamine Agonist; Dopaminergic Agent (Antiparkinson's); Ergot Alkaloid and Derivative

Use Adjunctive treatment to levodopa/carbidopa in the management of Parkinson's disease

Unlabeled/Investigational Use Tourette's disorder, chronic motor or vocal tic disorder

Pregnancy Risk Factor B

Contraindications Hypersensitivity to pergolide mesylate, other ergot derivatives, or any component of the formulation

Warnings/Precautions Symptomatic hypotension occurs in 10% of patients; use with caution in patients with a history of cardiac arrhythmias, hallucinations, or mental illness

Adverse Reactions

>10%:
   Central nervous system: Dizziness, somnolence, confusion, hallucinations, dystonia
   Gastrointestinal: Nausea, constipation
   Neuromuscular & skeletal: Dyskinesia
   Respiratory: Rhinitis

1% to 10%:
   Cardiovascular: Myocardial infarction, postural hypotension, syncope, arrhythmias, peripheral edema, vasodilation, palpitations, chest pain, hypertension
   Central nervous system: Chills, insomnia, anxiety, psychosis, EPS, incoordination
   Dermatologic: Rash
   Gastrointestinal: Diarrhea, abdominal pain, xerostomia, anorexia, weight gain, dyspepsia, taste perversion
   Hematologic: Anemia
   Neuromuscular & skeletal: Weakness, myalgia, tremor, NMS (with rapid dose reduction), pain
   Ocular: Abnormal vision, diplopia
   Respiratory: Dyspnea, epistaxis
   Miscellaneous: Flu syndrome, hiccups

<1% (Limited to important or life-threatening): Pericarditis, pericardial effusion, pleural effusion, pleural fibrosis, pleuritis, pneumothorax, retroperitoneal fibrosis, vasculitis

Overdosage/Toxicology Symptoms include vomiting, hypotension, agitation, hallucinations, ventricular extrasystoles, and possible seizures. Data on overdose are limited. Treatment is supportive and may require antiarrhythmics and/or neuroleptics for agitation. Hypotension, when unresponsive to I.V. fluids or Trendelenburg positioning, often responds to norepinephrine infusions started at 0.1-0.2 mcg/kg/minute, followed by a titrated infusion. If signs of CNS stimulation are present, a neuroleptic may be indicated. Monitor EKG. Activated charcoal is useful in preventing further absorption and hastening elimination.

Drug Interactions

   Increased Effect/Toxicity: Use caution with other highly plasma protein bound drugs.

   Decreased Effect: Dopamine antagonists (ie, antipsychotics, metoclopramide) may diminish the effects of pergolide; these combinations should generally be avoided.

Ethanol/Nutrition/Herb Interactions Ethanol: Avoid ethanol (may cause CNS depression).

Mechanism of Action Pergolide is a semisynthetic ergot alkaloid similar to bromocriptine but stated to be more potent (10-1000 times) and longer-acting; it is a centrally-active dopamine agonist stimulating both D_1 and D_2 receptors. Pergolide is believed to exert its therapeutic effect by directly stimulating postsynaptic dopamine receptors in the nigrostriatal system.

Pharmacodynamics/Kinetics

Absorption: Well absorbed
Protein binding, plasma: 90%
Metabolism: Extensively hepatic
Half-life elimination: 27 hours
Excretion: Urine (~50%); feces (50%)

Usual Dosage When adding pergolide to levodopa/carbidopa, the dose of the latter can usually and should be decreased. Patients no longer responsive to bromocriptine may benefit by being switched to pergolide. Oral:

Children and Adolescents: Tourette's disorder, chronic motor or vocal disorder (unlabeled uses): Up to 300 mcg/day

Adults: Parkinson's disease: Start with 0.05 mg/day for 2 days, then increase dosage by 0.1 or 0.15 mg/day every 3 days over next 12 days, increase dose by 0.25 mg/day every 3 days until optimal therapeutic dose is achieved, up to 5 mg/day maximum; usual dosage range: 2-3 mg/day in 3 divided doses

Monitoring Parameters Blood pressure (both sitting/supine and standing), symptoms of parkinsonism, dyskinesias, mental status

Patient Information Take with food or milk; rise slowly from sitting or lying down; report any confusion or change in mental status

Nursing Implications Monitor closely for orthostasis and other adverse effects; raise bed rails and institute safety measures; aid patient with ambulation, may cause postural hypotension and drowsiness

Dosage Forms Tablet, as mesylate: 0.05 mg, 0.25 mg, 1 mg

♦ **Pergolide Mesylate** see Pergolide on page 1062

♦ **Pergonal®** see Menotropins on page 857

♦ **Periactin®** see Cyproheptadine on page 349

♦ **Peridex® Oral Rinse** see Chlorhexidine Gluconate on page 275

♦ **Peridol (Can)** see Haloperidol on page 654

♦ **Peri-Dri®** see Nystatin on page 1001

Perindopril Erbumine (per IN doe pril er BYOO meen)

Related Information

Angiotensin Agents Comparison on page 1473

U.S. Brand Names Aceon®

Canadian Brand Names Coversyl®

Therapeutic Category Angiotensin-Converting Enzyme (ACE) Inhibitor; Antihypertensive Agent

Use Treatment of stage I or II hypertension and congestive heart failure; treatment of left ventricular dysfunction after myocardial infarction

Pregnancy Risk Factor D (especially 2nd and 3rd trimesters)

(Continued)

Perindopril Erbumine *(Continued)*

Pregnancy/Breast-Feeding Implications Breast-feeding/lactation: Only small amounts are excreted in breast milk

Contraindications Hypersensitivity to perindopril or any component of the formulation; angio-edema related to previous treatment with an ACE inhibitor; bilateral renal artery stenosis; primary hyperaldosteronism; pregnancy (2nd and 3rd trimesters)

Warnings/Precautions Anaphylactic reactions can occur. Angioedema can occur at any time during treatment (especially following first dose). Careful blood pressure monitoring with first dose (hypotension can occur especially in volume depleted patients). Dosage adjustment needed in renal impairment. Use with caution in hypovolemia; collagen vascular diseases; valvular stenosis (particularly aortic stenosis); hyperkalemia; or before, during, or immediately after anesthesia. Avoid rapid dosage escalation, which may lead to renal insufficiency. Neutropenia/agranulocytosis with myeloid hyperplasia can rarely occur. If patient has renal impairment then a baseline WBC with differential and serum creatinine should be evaluated and monitored closely during the first 3 months of therapy. Hypersensitivity reactions may be seen during hemodialysis with high-flux dialysis membranes (eg, AN69). Use with caution in unilateral renal artery stenosis and pre-existing renal insufficiency.

Adverse Reactions

>10% Central nervous system: Headache (23%)

1% to 10%:

Cardiovascular: edema (4%), chest pain (2%)

Central nervous system: Dizziness (8%), sleep disorders (3%), depression (2%), fever (2%), weakness (8%), nervousness (1%)

Dermatologic: Rash (2%)

Endocrine & metabolic: Hyperkalemia (1%), increased triglycerides (1%)

Gastrointestinal: Nausea (2%), diarrhea (4%), vomiting (2%), dyspepsia (2%), abdominal pain (3%), flatulence (1%)

Genitourinary: Sexual dysfunction (male: 1%)

Hepatic: Increased ALT (2%)

Neuromuscular & skeletal: Back pain (6%), upper extremity pain (3%), lower extremity pain (5%), paresthesia (2%), joint pain (1%), myalgia (1%), arthritis (1%)

Renal: Proteinuria (2%)

Respiratory: Cough (incidence is higher in women, 3:1) (12%), sinusitis (5%), rhinitis (5%), pharyngitis (3%)

Otic: Tinnitus (2%)

Miscellaneous: Viral infection (3%)

Note: Some reactions occurred at an incidence >1% but ≤ placebo.

<1% (Limited to important or life-threatening): Amnesia, anaphylaxis, angioedema, anxiety, dyspnea, erythema, gout, migraine, myocardial infarction, nephrolithiasis, orthostatic hypotension, pruritus, psychosocial disorder, pulmonary fibrosis, purpura, stroke, syncope, urinary retention, vertigo

Additional adverse effects associated with **ACE inhibitors** include agranulocytosis, neutropenia, decreases in creatinine clearance in some elderly hypertensive patients or those with chronic renal failure, and worsening of renal function in patients with bilateral renal artery stenosis or hypovolemic patients (diuretic therapy). In addition, a syndrome which may include fever, myalgia, arthralgia, interstitial nephritis, vasculitis, rash, eosinophilia and positive ANA, and elevated ESR has been reported with ACE inhibitors.

Overdosage/Toxicology Mild hypotension has been the primary toxic effect seen with acute overdose. Bradycardia may also occur. Hyperkalemia occurs even with therapeutic doses, especially in patients with renal insufficiency and those taking NSAIDs. Treatment is symptom directed and supportive.

Drug Interactions

Increased Effect/Toxicity: Potassium supplements, co-trimoxazole (high dose), angiotensin II receptor antagonists (candesartan, losartan, irbesartan, etc), or potassium-sparing diuretics (amiloride, spironolactone, triamterene) may result in elevated serum potassium levels when combined with perindopril. ACE inhibitor effects may be increased by phenothiazines or probenecid (increases levels of captopril). ACE inhibitors may increase serum concentrations/effects of digoxin, lithium, and sulfonlyureas.

Diuretics have additive hypotensive effects with ACE inhibitors, and hypovolemia increases the potential for adverse renal effects of ACE inhibitors. In patients with compromised renal function, coadministration with nonsteroidal anti-inflammatory drugs may result in further deterioration of renal function. Allopurinol and ACE inhibitors may cause a higher risk of hypersensitivity reaction when taken concurrently.

Decreased Effect: Aspirin (high dose) may reduce the therapeutic effects of ACE inhibitors; at low dosages this does not appear to be significant. Rifampin may decrease the effect of ACE inhibitors. Antacids may decrease the bioavailability of ACE inhibitors (may be more likely to occur with captopril); separate administration times by 1-2 hours. NSAIDs, specifically indomethacin, may reduce the hypotensive effects of ACE inhibitors. More likely to occur in low renin or volume dependent hypertensive patients.

Ethanol/Nutrition/Herb Interactions

Food: Perindopril active metabolite concentrations may be lowered if taken with food.

Herb/Nutraceutical: Avoid dong quai if using for hypertension (has estrogenic activity). Avoid ephedra, yohimbe, ginseng (may worsen hypertension). Avoid garlic (may have increased antihypertensive effect).

Mechanism of Action Competitive inhibitor of angiotensin-converting enzyme (ACE); prevents conversion of angiotensin I to angiotensin II, a potent vasoconstrictor; results in lower levels of angiotensin II which, in turn, causes an increase in plasma renin activity and a reduction in aldosterone secretion

Pharmacodynamics/Kinetics

Onset of action: Peak effect: 1-2 hours

Distribution: Small amounts enter breast milk

Protein binding: Perindopril: 60%; Perindoprilat: 10% to 20%

Metabolism: Perindopril is hydrolyzed hepatically to active metabolite, perindoprilat (~17% to 20% of a dose) and other inactive metabolites

Bioavailability: Perindopril: 65% to 95%

Half-life elimination: Parent drug: 1.5-3 hours; Metabolite: Effective: 3-10 hours, Terminal: 30-120 hours

Time to peak: Chronic therapy: Perindopril: 1 hour; Perindoprilat: 3-4 hours (maximum perindoprilat serum levels are 2-3 times higher and T_{max} is shorter following chronic therapy); CHF: Perindopril: 6 hours

Elimination: Urine (75%, 10% as unchanged drug)

Usual Dosage Adults: Oral:

Congestive heart failure: 4 mg once daily

Hypertension: Initial: 4 mg/day but may be titrated to response; usual range: 4-8 mg/day, maximum: 16 mg/day

Dosing adjustment in renal impairment:

Cl_{cr} >60 mL/minute: Administer 4 mg/day.

Cl_{cr} 30-60 mL/minute: Administer 2 mg/day.

Cl_{cr} 15-29 mL/minute: Administer 2 mg every other day.

Cl_{cr} <15 mL/minute: Administer 2 mg on the day of dialysis.

Hemodialysis: Perindopril and its metabolites are dialyzable

Dosing adjustment in hepatic impairment: None needed

Dosing adjustment in geriatric patients: Due to greater bioavailability and lower renal clearance of the drug in elderly subjects, dose reduction of 50% is recommended.

Monitoring Parameters Serum creatinine, electrolytes, and WBC with differential initially and repeated at 2-week intervals for at least 90 days; urinalysis for protein

Patient Information This medication does not replace the need to follow exercise and diet recommendations for hypertension. Take as directed; do not miss doses, alter dosage, or discontinue without consulting prescriber. Consult prescriber for appropriate diet. Change position slowly when rising from sitting or lying. May cause transient drowsiness; avoid driving or engaging in tasks that require alertness until response to drug is known. May be taken consistently either with or without food; however, small frequent meals may help reduce any nausea, vomiting, or epigastric pain. Notify physician of persistent cough or other side effects. Do not end therapy except under prescriber advice; especially in first week of therapy may experience dizziness, fainting, and lightheadedness. Have blood pressure monitored regularly.

Nursing Implications A reduction in clinical signs of congestive heart failure (dyspnea, orthopnea, cough) and an improvement in exercise duration are indicative of therapeutic response; a reduction of supine diastolic blood pressure of 10 mm Hg or to 90 mm Hg is indicative of excellent therapeutic response in patients with hypertension; observe for cough, difficulty breathing/swallowing, perioral swelling and signs and symptoms of agranulocytosis; monitor for 6 hours after initial dosing for profound hypotension or first-dose phenomenon

Dosage Forms Tablet: 2 mg, 4 mg, 8 mg

♦ **PerioChip**® *see* Chlorhexidine Gluconate *on page 275*

♦ **PerioGard**® *see* Chlorhexidine Gluconate *on page 275*

♦ **Periostat**® *see* Doxycycline *on page 448*

♦ **Permapen**® *see* Penicillin G Benzathine *on page 1051*

♦ **Permax**® *see* Pergolide *on page 1062*

Permethrin (per METH rin)

U.S. Brand Names A200® Lice [OTC]; Acticin®; Elimite™; Medi-Lice® [OTC]; Nix™ Creme Rinse; R&C® Lice

Canadian Brand Names Kwellada-P™; Nix®

Therapeutic Category Antiparasitic Agent, Topical; Scabicidal Agent; Shampoos

Use Single-application treatment of infestation with *Pediculus humanus capitis* (head louse) and its nits or *Sarcoptes scabiei* (scabies); indicated for prophylactic use during epidemics of lice

Pregnancy Risk Factor B

Contraindications Hypersensitivity to pyrethroid, pyrethrin, chrysanthemums, or any component of the formulation; lotion is contraindicated for use in infants <2 months of age

Warnings/Precautions Treatment may temporarily exacerbate the symptoms of itching, redness, swelling; for external use only; use during pregnancy only if clearly needed

Adverse Reactions 1% to 10%:

Dermatologic: Pruritus, erythema, rash of the scalp

Local: Burning, stinging, tingling, numbness or scalp discomfort, edema

Mechanism of Action Inhibits sodium ion influx through nerve cell membrane channels in parasites resulting in delayed repolarization and thus paralysis and death of the pest

Pharmacodynamics/Kinetics

Absorption: <2%

Metabolism: Hepatic via ester hydrolysis to inactive metabolites

Excretion: Urine

Usual Dosage Topical:

Head lice: Children >2 months and Adults: After hair has been washed with shampoo, rinsed with water, and towel dried, apply a sufficient volume of topical liquid (lotion or cream rinse) to saturate the hair and scalp. Leave on hair for 10 minutes before rinsing off with water; remove remaining nits; may repeat in 1 week if lice or nits still present.

Scabies: Apply cream from head to toe; leave on for 8-14 hours before washing off with water; for infants, also apply on the hairline, neck, scalp, temple, and forehead; may reapply in 1 week if live mites appear

Permethrin 5% cream was shown to be safe and effective when applied to an infant <1 month of age with neonatal scabies; time of application was limited to 6 hours before rinsing with soap and water

Administration

Cream: Apply from neck to toes. Bathe to remove drug after 8-14 hours. Repeat in 7 days if lice or nits are still present. Report if condition persists or infection occurs.

(Continued)

Permethrin (Continued)

Cream rinse/lotion: Apply immediately after hair is shampooed, rinsed, and towel-dried. Apply enough to saturate hair and scalp (especially behind ears and on nape of neck). Leave on hair for 10 minutes before rinsing with water. Remove nits with fine-tooth comb. May repeat in 1 week if lice or nits are still present.

Patient Information Avoid contact with eyes and mucous membranes during application; shake well before using; notify physician if irritation persists; clothing and bedding should be washed in hot water or dry cleaned to kill the scabies mite

Nursing Implications Because scabies and lice are so contagious, use caution to avoid spreading or infecting oneself; wear gloves when applying

Dosage Forms
Cream, topical: 5% (60 g)
Liquid, topical [cream rinse]: 1% (60 mL)
Lotion, topical: 1% (59 mL)
Solution, topical [spray]: 0.4% (150 mL, 300 mL); 0.5% (5 mL, 142 g, 170 g, 300 mL)

♦ **Permitil**® see Fluphenazine on page 581

Perphenazine (per FEN a zeen)

Related Information
Antacid Drug Interactions on page 1477
Antipsychotic Agents Comparison on page 1486

U.S. Brand Names Trilafon®

Canadian Brand Names Apo®-Perphenazine; Trilafon®

Therapeutic Category Antipsychotic Agent, Phenothiazine; Phenothiazine Derivative

Use Treatment of severe schizophrenia; nausea and vomiting

Unlabeled/Investigational Use Ethanol withdrawal; dementia in elderly; Tourette's syndrome; Huntington's chorea; spasmodic torticollis; Reye's syndrome; psychosis

Pregnancy Risk Factor C

Contraindications Hypersensitivity to perphenazine or any component of the formulation (cross-reactivity between phenothiazines may occur); severe CNS depression; subcortical brain damage; bone marrow suppression; blood dyscrasias; coma

Warnings/Precautions Safety in children <6 months of age has not been established. May cause hypotension, particularly with parenteral administration. May be sedating, use with caution in disorders where CNS depression is a feature. Use with caution in Parkinson's disease. Caution in patients with hemodynamic instability; predisposition to seizures; severe cardiac, hepatic, renal, or respiratory disease. Esophageal dysmotility and aspiration have been associated with antipsychotic use - use with caution in patients at risk of pneumonia (ie, Alzheimer's disease). Caution in breast cancer or other prolactin-dependent tumors (may elevate prolactin levels). May alter temperature regulation or mask toxicity of other drugs due to antiemetic effects. May alter cardiac conduction - life-threatening arrhythmias have occurred with therapeutic doses of phenothiazines. May cause orthostatic hypotension - use with caution in patients at risk of this effect or those who would tolerate transient hypotensive episodes (cerebrovascular disease, cardiovascular disease, or other medications which may predispose).

Phenothiazines may cause anticholinergic effects (confusion, agitation, constipation, dry mouth, blurred vision, urinary retention); therefore, they should be used with caution in patients with decreased gastrointestinal motility, urinary retention, BPH, xerostomia, or visual problems. Conditions which also may be exacerbated by cholinergic blockade include narrow-angle glaucoma (screening is recommended) and worsening of myasthenia gravis. Relative to other neuroleptics, perphenazine has a low potency of cholinergic blockade.

May cause extrapyramidal reactions, including pseudoparkinsonism, acute dystonic reactions, akathisia, and tardive dyskinesia (risk of these reactions is moderate-high relative to other neuroleptics). May be associated with neuroleptic malignant syndrome (NMS) or pigmentary retinopathy.

Adverse Reactions Frequency not defined.
Cardiovascular: Hypotension, orthostatic hypotension, hypertension, tachycardia, bradycardia, dizziness, cardiac arrest
Central nervous system: Extrapyramidal symptoms (pseudoparkinsonism, akathisia, dystonias, tardive dyskinesia), dizziness, cerebral edema, seizures, headache, drowsiness, paradoxical excitement, restlessness, hyperactivity, insomnia, neuroleptic malignant syndrome (NMS), impairment of temperature regulation
Dermatologic: Increased sensitivity to sun, rash, discoloration of skin (blue-gray)
Endocrine & metabolic: Hypoglycemia, hyperglycemia, galactorrhea, lactation, breast enlargement, gynecomastia, menstrual irregularity, amenorrhea, SIADH, changes in libido
Gastrointestinal: Constipation, weight gain, vomiting, stomach pain, nausea, xerostomia, salivation, diarrhea, anorexia, ileus
Genitourinary: Difficulty in urination, ejaculatory disturbances, incontinence, polyuria, ejaculating dysfunction, priapism
Hematologic: Agranulocytosis, leukopenia, eosinophilia, hemolytic anemia, thrombocytopenic purpura, pancytopenia
Hepatic: Cholestatic jaundice, hepatotoxicity
Neuromuscular & skeletal: Tremor
Ocular: Pigmentary retinopathy, blurred vision, cornea and lens changes
Respiratory: Nasal congestion
Miscellaneous: Diaphoresis

Overdosage/Toxicology Symptoms include deep sleep, dystonia, agitation, coma, abnormal involuntary muscle movements, hypotension, and arrhythmias. Following initiation of essential overdose management, toxic symptom and supportive treatment should be initiated. Hypotension usually responds to I.V. fluids or Trendelenburg positioning. If unresponsive to these measures, the use of a parenteral inotrope may be required (eg, norepinephrine 0.1-0.2 mcg/kg/minute titrated to response). Seizures commonly respond to diazepam (I.V. 5-10 mg bolus in adults every 15 minutes, if needed, up to a total of 30 mg; I.V. 0.25-0.4 mg/kg/

dose up to a total of 10 mg in children) or to phenytoin or phenobarbital. Extrapyramidal symptoms (eg, dystonic reactions) may be managed with diphenhydramine. When these reactions are unresponsive to diphenhydramine, benztropine mesylate may be effective.

Drug Interactions

Cytochrome P450 Effect: CYP2D6 enzyme substrate; CYP2D6 enzyme inhibitor

Increased Effect/Toxicity: Effects on CNS depression may be additive when perphenazine is combined with CNS depressants (narcotic analgesics, ethanol, barbiturates, cyclic antidepressants, antihistamines, or sedative-hypnotics). Perphenazine may increase the effects/toxicity of anticholinergics, antihypertensives, lithium (rare neurotoxicity), trazodone, or valproic acid. Concurrent use with TCA may produce increased toxicity or altered therapeutic response. Chloroquine and propranolol may increase perphenazine concentrations. Hypotension may occur when perphenazine is combined with epinephrine. May increase the risk of arrhythmia when combined with antiarrhythmics, cisapride, pimozide, sparfloxacin, or other drugs which prolong QT interval.

Decreased Effect: Phenothiazines inhibit the ability of bromocriptine to lower serum prolactin concentrations. Benztropine (and other anticholinergics) may inhibit the therapeutic response to perphenazine and excess anticholinergic effects may occur. Cigarette smoking and barbiturates may enhance the hepatic metabolism of chlorpromazine. Antihypertensive effects of guanethidine and guanadrel may be inhibited by perphenazine. Perphenazine may inhibit the antiparkinsonian effect of levodopa. Perphenazine and possibly other low potency antipsychotics may reverse the pressor effects of epinephrine.

Ethanol/Nutrition/Herb Interactions

Ethanol: Avoid ethanol (may increase CNS depression).

Herb/Nutraceutical: Avoid kava kava, gotu kola, valerian, St John's wort (may increase CNS depression).

Stability Do not mix with beverages containing caffeine (coffee, cola), tannins (tea), or pectinates (apple juice) since physical incompatibility exists; use ~60 mL diluent for each 5 mL of concentrate; protect all dosage forms from light; clear or slightly yellow solutions may be used; should be dispensed in amber or opaque vials/bottles. Solutions may be diluted or mixed with fruit juices or other liquids but must be administered immediately after mixing; do not prepare bulk dilutions or store bulk dilutions.

Mechanism of Action Blocks postsynaptic mesolimbic dopaminergic receptors in the brain; exhibits alpha-adrenergic blocking effect and depresses the release of hypothalamic and hypophyseal hormones

Pharmacodynamics/Kinetics

Absorption: Oral: Well absorbed

Distribution: Crosses placenta

Metabolism: Hepatic

Half-life elimination: 9 hours

Time to peak, serum: 4-8 hours

Excretion: Urine and feces

Usual Dosage

Children:

Schizophrenia/psychoses:

Oral:

1-6 years: 4-6 mg/day in divided doses

6-12 years: 6 mg/day in divided doses

>12 years: 4-16 mg 2-4 times/day

I.M.: 5 mg every 6 hours

Nausea/vomiting: I.M.: 5 mg every 6 hours

Adults:

Schizophrenia/psychoses:

Oral: 4-16 mg 2-4 times/day not to exceed 64 mg/day

I.M.: 5 mg every 6 hours up to 15 mg/day in ambulatory patients and 30 mg/day in hospitalized patients

Nausea/vomiting:

Oral: 8-16 mg/day in divided doses up to 24 mg/day

I.M.: 5-10 mg every 6 hours as necessary up to 15 mg/day in ambulatory patients and 30 mg/day in hospitalized patients

I.V. (severe): 1 mg at 1- to 2-minute intervals up to a total of 5 mg

Elderly: Behavioral symptoms associated with dementia: Oral: Initial: 2-4 mg 1-2 times/day; increase at 4- to 7-day intervals by 2-4 mg/day. Increase dose intervals (bid, tid, etc) as necessary to control behavior response or side effects. Maximum daily dose: 32 mg; gradual increase (titration) and bedtime administration may prevent some side effects or decrease their severity.

Hemodialysis: Not dialyzable (0% to 5%)

Dosing adjustment in hepatic impairment: Dosage reductions should be considered in patients with liver disease although no specific guidelines are available

Administration Dilute oral concentration to at least 2 oz with water, juice, or milk; for I.V. use, injection should be diluted to at least 0.5 mg/mL with NS and administered at a rate of 1 mg/minute; observe for tremor and abnormal movements or posturing

Monitoring Parameters Cardiac, blood pressure (hypotension when administering I.M. or I.V.); respiratory status

Reference Range 2-6 nmol/L

Patient Information May cause drowsiness, impair judgment and coordination; report any feelings of restlessness or any involuntary movements; avoid alcohol and other CNS depressants; do not alter dose or discontinue without consulting physician

Nursing Implications Monitor for hypotension when administering I.M. or I.V. during the first 3-5 days after initiating therapy or making a dosage adjustment

Dosage Forms

Injection: 5 mg/mL (1 mL)

Solution, oral concentrate: 16 mg/5 mL (118 mL) [berry flavored]

Tablet: 2 mg, 4 mg, 8 mg, 16 mg

- **Perphenazine and Amitriptyline** *see Amitriptyline and Perphenazine on page 78*
- **Persantine®** *see Dipyridamole on page 422*
- **Pethidine Hydrochloride** *see Meperidine on page 858*
- **Pexicam® (Can)** *see Piroxicam on page 1093*
- **PFA** *see Foscarnet on page 604*
- **Pfizerpen®** *see Penicillin G (Parenteral/Aqueous) on page 1053*
- **Pfizerpen-AS® (Can)** *see Penicillin G Procaine on page 1054*
- **PGE₁** *see Alprostadil on page 57*
- **PGE₂** *see Dinoprostone on page 412*
- **PGI₂** *see Epoprostenol on page 477*
- **PGX** *see Epoprostenol on page 477*
- **Phanatuss® Cough Syrup [OTC]** *see Guaifenesin and Dextromethorphan on page 646*
- **Pharmaflur®** *see Fluoride on page 574*
- **Pharmorubicin® (Can)** *see Epirubicin on page 472*
- **Phenadex® Senior [OTC]** *see Guaifenesin and Dextromethorphan on page 646*
- **Phenameth® DM** *see Promethazine and Dextromethorphan on page 1141*
- **Phenaphen® With Codeine** *see Acetaminophen and Codeine on page 24*
- **Phenazo™ (Can)** *see Phenazopyridine on page 1068*

Phenazopyridine (fen az oh PEER i deen)

U.S. Brand Names Azo-Dine® [OTC]; Azo-Gesic® [OTC]; Azo-Standard®; Baridium®; Prodium™ [OTC]; Pyridiate®; Pyridium®; Uristat® [OTC]; Urodol® [OTC]; Urofemme® [OTC]; Urogesic®

Canadian Brand Names Phenazo™; Pyridium®

Synonyms Phenazopyridine Hydrochloride; Phenylazo Diamino Pyridine Hydrochloride

Therapeutic Category Analgesic, Urinary; Local Anesthetic, Urinary

Use Symptomatic relief of urinary burning, itching, frequency and urgency in association with urinary tract infection or following urologic procedures

Pregnancy Risk Factor B

Contraindications Hypersensitivity to phenazopyridine or any component of the formulation; kidney or liver disease; patients with a Cl$_{cr}$ <50 mL/minute

Warnings/Precautions Does not treat infection, acts only as an analgesic; drug should be discontinued if skin or sclera develop a yellow color; use with caution in patients with renal impairment. Use of this agent in the elderly is limited since accumulation of phenazopyridine can occur in patients with renal insufficiency. It should not be used in patients with a Cl$_{cr}$ <50 mL/minute.

Adverse Reactions

1% to 10%:

Central nervous system: Headache, dizziness

Gastrointestinal: Stomach cramps

<1% (Limited to important or life-threatening): Acute renal failure, hemolytic anemia, hepatitis, methemoglobinemia

Overdosage/Toxicology Symptoms include methemoglobinemia, hemolytic anemia, skin pigmentation, and renal and hepatic impairment. The antidote for methemoglobinemia is methylene blue 1-2 mg/kg I.V.

Mechanism of Action An azo dye which exerts local anesthetic or analgesic action on urinary tract mucosa through an unknown mechanism

Pharmacodynamics/Kinetics

Metabolism: Hepatic and via other tissues

Excretion: Urine (65% as unchanged drug)

Usual Dosage Oral:

Children: 12 mg/kg/day in 3 divided doses administered after meals for 2 days

Adults: 100-200 mg 3 times/day after meals for 2 days when used concomitantly with an antibacterial agent

Dosing interval in renal impairment:

Cl$_{cr}$ 50-80 mL/minute: Administer every 8-16 hours

Cl$_{cr}$ <50 mL/minute: Avoid use

Dietary Considerations Should be taken after meals.

Test Interactions Phenazopyridine may cause delayed reactions with glucose oxidase reagents (Clinistix®, Tes-Tape®); occasional false-positive tests occur with Tes-Tape®; cupric sulfate tests (Clinitest®) are not affected; interference may also occur with urine ketone tests (Acetest®, Ketostix®) and urinary protein tests; tests for urinary steroids and porphyrins may also occur

Patient Information Take after meals; tablets may color urine orange or red and may stain clothing

Nursing Implications Colors urine orange or red; stains clothing and is difficult to remove

Dosage Forms Tablet, as hydrochloride: 95 mg, 97.2 mg, 100 mg, 200 mg

Extemporaneous Preparations A 10 mg/mL suspension may be made by crushing three 200 mg tablets. Mix with a small amount of distilled water or glycerin. Add 20 mL Cologel® and levigate until a uniform mixture is obtained. Add sufficient 2:1 simple syrup/cherry syrup mixture to make a final volume of 60 mL. Store in an amber container. Label "shake well". Stability is 60 days refrigerated.

Handbook on Extemporaneous Formulations, Bethesda MD: American Society of Hospital Pharmacists, 1987.

- **Phenazopyridine Hydrochloride** *see Phenazopyridine on page 1068*

Phenelzine (FEN el zeen)

Related Information

Antidepressant Agents Comparison *on page 1482*

Tyramine Content of Foods *on page 1737*

U.S. Brand Names Nardil®
Canadian Brand Names Nardil®
Synonyms Phenelzine Sulfate
Therapeutic Category Antidepressant, Monoamine Oxidase Inhibitor
Use Symptomatic treatment of atypical, nonendogenous, or neurotic depression
Unlabeled/Investigational Use Selective mutism
Pregnancy Risk Factor C
Contraindications Hypersensitivity to phenelzine or any component of the formulation; uncontrolled hypertension; pheochromocytoma; hepatic disease; congestive heart failure; concurrent use of sympathomimetics (and related compounds), CNS depressants, ethanol, meperidine, bupropion, buspirone, guanethidine, serotonergic drugs (including SSRIs) - do not use within 5 weeks of fluoxetine discontinuation or 2 weeks of other antidepressant discontinuation; general anesthesia, local vasoconstrictors; spinal anesthesia (hypotension may be exaggerated); foods with a high content of tyramine, tryptophan, or dopamine, chocolate, or caffeine (may cause hypertensive crisis)
Warnings/Precautions Safety in children <16 years of age has not been established; use with caution in patients who are hyperactive, hyperexcitable, or who have glaucoma; avoid use of meperidine within 2 weeks of phenelzine use. Hypertensive crisis may occur with tyramine. See "Tyramine Content of Foods" *on page 1737* in Appendix.

Should not be used in combination with other antidepressants. Hypotensive effects of antihypertensives (beta-blockers, thiazides) may be exaggerated. Use with caution in depressed patients at risk of suicide. May cause orthostatic hypotension - use with caution in patients with hypotension or patients who would not tolerate transient hypotensive episodes (cardiovascular or cerebrovascular disease) - effects may be additive with other agents which cause orthostasis. Has been associated with activation of hypomania and/or mania in bipolar patients. May worsen psychotic symptoms in some patients. Use with caution in patients at risk of seizures, or in patients receiving other drugs which may lower seizure threshold. Toxic reactions have occurred with dextromethorphan. Discontinue at least 48 hours prior to myelography.

The MAO inhibitors are effective and generally well tolerated by older patients. It is the potential interactions with tyramine or tryptophan-containing foods and other drugs, and their effects on blood pressure that have limited their use.
Adverse Reactions Frequency not defined.
Cardiovascular: Orthostatic hypotension, edema
Central nervous system: Dizziness, headache, drowsiness, sleep disturbances, fatigue, hyper-reflexia, twitching, ataxia, mania
Dermatologic: Rash, pruritus
Endocrine & metabolic: Decreased sexual ability (anorgasmia, ejaculatory disturbances, impotence), hypernatremia, hypermetabolic syndrome
Gastrointestinal: Xerostomia, constipation, weight gain
Genitourinary: Urinary retention
Hematologic: Leukopenia
Hepatic: Hepatitis
Neuromuscular & skeletal: Weakness, tremor, myoclonus
Ocular: Blurred vision, glaucoma
Miscellaneous: Diaphoresis
Overdosage/Toxicology Symptoms include tachycardia, palpitations, muscle twitching, seizures, insomnia, restlessness, transient hypertension, hypotension, drowsiness, hyperpyrexia, and coma. Competent supportive care is the most important treatment for overdose with a monoamine oxidase (MAO) inhibitor. Both hypertension or hypotension can occur with intoxication. Hypotension may respond to I.V. fluids or vasopressors and hypertension usually responds to an alpha-adrenergic blocker. While treating the hypertension, care is warranted to avoid sudden drops in blood pressure, since this may worsen MAO inhibitor toxicity. Muscle irritability and seizures often respond to diazepam, while hyperthermia is best treated with antipyretics and cooling blankets. Cardiac arrhythmias are best treated with phenytoin or procainamide.
Drug Interactions
  Increased Effect/Toxicity: In general, the combined use of phenelzine with TCAs, venlafaxine, trazodone, dexfenfluramine, sibutramine, lithium, meperidine, fenfluramine, dextromethorphan, and SSRIs should be avoided due to the potential for severe adverse reactions (serotonin syndrome, death). MAO inhibitors (including phenelzine) may inhibit the metabolism of barbiturates and prolong their effect. Phenelzine in combination with amphetamines, other stimulants (methylphenidate), levodopa, metaraminol, reserpine, and decongestants (pseudoephedrine) may result in severe hypertensive reactions. Foods (eg, cheese) and beverages (eg, ethanol) containing tyramine should be avoided; hypertensive crisis may result. Phenelzine may increase the pressor response of norepinephrine and may prolong neuromuscular blockade produced by succinylcholine. Tramadol may increase the risk of seizures and serotonin syndrome in patients receiving an MAO inhibitor. Phenelzine may produce additive hypoglycemic effect in patients receiving hypoglycemic agents and may produce delirium in patients receiving disulfiram.
  Decreased Effect: Phenelzine (and other MAO inhibitors) inhibits the antihypertensive response to guanadrel or guanethidine.
Ethanol/Nutrition/Herb Interactions
  Ethanol: Avoid ethanol (alcoholic beverages containing tyramine may induce a severe hypertensive response).
  Food: Clinically-severe elevated blood pressure may occur if phenelzine is taken with tyramine-containing foods. Avoid foods containing tryptophan, dopamine, chocolate, or caffeine.
Stability Protect from light
Mechanism of Action Thought to act by increasing endogenous concentrations of norepinephrine, dopamine, and serotonin through inhibition of the enzyme (monoamine oxidase) responsible for the breakdown of these neurotransmitters
(Continued)

Phenelzine *(Continued)*

Pharmacodynamics/Kinetics

Onset of action: Therapeutic: 2-4 weeks

Absorption: Well absorbed

Duration: May continue to have a therapeutic effect and interactions 2 weeks after discontinuing therapy

Excretion: Urine (primarily as metabolites and unchanged drug)

Usual Dosage Oral:

Children: Selective mutism (unlabeled use): 30-60 mg/day

Adults: Depression: 15 mg 3 times/day; may increase to 60-90 mg/day during early phase of treatment, then reduce dose for maintenance therapy slowly after maximum benefit is obtained; takes 2-4 weeks for a significant response to occur

Elderly: Depression: Initial: 7.5 mg/day; increase by 7.5-15 mg/day every 3-4 days as tolerated; usual therapeutic dose: 15-60 mg/day in 3-4 divided doses

Monitoring Parameters
Blood pressure, heart rate, diet, weight, mood (if depressive symptoms)

Patient Information
Avoid tyramine-containing foods: Red wine, cheese (except cottage, ricotta, and cream), smoked or pickled fish, beef or chicken liver, dried sausage, fava or broad bean pods, yeast vitamin supplements; do not begin any prescription or OTC medications without consulting your physician or pharmacist; may take as long as 3 weeks to see effects; report any severe headaches, irregular heartbeats, skin rash, insomnia, sedation, changes in strength; sensations of pain, burning, touch, or vibration; or any other unusual symptoms to your physician; avoid alcohol; get up slowly from chair or bed

Nursing Implications
Watch for postural hypotension; monitor blood pressure carefully, especially at therapy onset or if other CNS drugs or cardiovascular drugs are added; check for dietary and drug restriction

Additional Information
Pyridoxine deficiency has occurred; symptoms include numbness and edema of hands; may respond to supplementation.

The MAO inhibitors are usually reserved for patients who do not tolerate or respond to other antidepressants. The brain activity of monoamine oxidase increases with age and even more so in patients with Alzheimer's disease. Therefore, the MAO inhibitors may have an increased role in patients with Alzheimer's disease who are depressed. Phenelzine is less stimulating than tranylcypromine.

Dosage Forms
Tablet, as sulfate: 15 mg

* **Phenelzine Sulfate** *see Phenelzine on page 1068*
* **Phenergan®** *see Promethazine on page 1139*
* **Phenergan® VC** *see Promethazine and Phenylephrine on page 1142*
* **Phenergan® VC With Codeine** *see Promethazine, Phenylephrine, and Codeine on page 1142*
* **Phenergan® With Codeine** *see Promethazine and Codeine on page 1141*
* **Phenergan® With Dextromethorphan** *see Promethazine and Dextromethorphan on page 1141*
* **Phenhist® Expectorant** *see Guaifenesin, Pseudoephedrine, and Codeine on page 648*
* **Pheniramine and Naphazoline** *see Naphazoline and Pheniramine on page 958*

Phenobarbital *(fee noe BAR bi tal)*

Related Information

Anticonvulsants by Seizure Type *on page 1481*
Convulsive Status Epilepticus *on page 1661*
Epilepsy & Seizure Treatment *on page 1659*
Febrile Seizures *on page 1660*

U.S. Brand Names Luminal® Sodium

Synonyms Phenobarbital Sodium; Phenobarbitone; Phenylethylmalonylurea

Therapeutic Category Anticonvulsant; Barbiturate; Hypnotic; Sedative

Use Management of generalized tonic-clonic (grand mal) and partial seizures; sedative

Unlabeled/Investigational Use Febrile seizures in children; may also be used for prevention and treatment of neonatal hyperbilirubinemia and lowering of bilirubin in chronic cholestasis; neonatal seizures; management of sedative/hypnotic withdrawal

Restrictions C-IV

Pregnancy Risk Factor D

Pregnancy/Breast-Feeding Implications

Clinical effects on the fetus: Crosses the placenta. Cardiac defect reported; hemorrhagic disease of newborn due to fetal vitamin K depletion may occur; may induce maternal folic acid deficiency; withdrawal symptoms observed in infant following delivery. Epilepsy itself, number of medications, genetic factors, or a combination of these probably influence the teratogenicity of anticonvulsant therapy. Benefit:risk ratio usually favors continued use during pregnancy and breast-feeding.

Breast-feeding/Lactation: Crosses into breast milk

Clinical effects on the infant: Sedation; withdrawal with abrupt weaning reported. AAP recommends USE WITH CAUTION.

Contraindications Hypersensitivity to barbiturates or any component of the formulation; marked hepatic impairment; dyspnea or airway obstruction; porphyria; pregnancy

Warnings/Precautions Use with caution in patients with hypovolemic shock, congestive heart failure, hepatic impairment, respiratory dysfunction or depression, previous addiction to the sedative/hypnotic group, chronic or acute pain, renal dysfunction, and the elderly, due to its long half-life and risk of dependence, phenobarbital is not recommended as a sedative in the elderly; tolerance or psychological and physical dependence may occur with prolonged use. Use with caution in patients with depression or suicidal tendencies, or in patients with a history of drug abuse. **Abrupt withdrawal in patients with epilepsy may precipitate status epilepticus.**

Adverse Reactions Frequency not defined.

Cardiovascular: Bradycardia, hypotension, syncope

Central nervous system: Drowsiness, lethargy, CNS excitation or depression, impaired judgment, "hangover" effect, confusion, somnolence, agitation, hyperkinesia, ataxia, nervousness, headache, insomnia, nightmares, hallucinations, anxiety, dizziness

Dermatologic: Rash, exfoliative dermatitis, Stevens-Johnson syndrome

Gastrointestinal: Nausea, vomiting, constipation

Hematologic: Agranulocytosis, thrombocytopenia, megaloblastic anemia

Local: Pain at injection site, thrombophlebitis with I.V. use

Renal: Oliguria

Respiratory: Laryngospasm, respiratory depression, apnea (especially with rapid I.V. use), hypoventilation, apnea

Miscellaneous: Gangrene with inadvertent intra-arterial injection

Overdosage/Toxicology Symptoms include unsteady gait, slurred speech, confusion, jaundice, hypothermia, hypotension, respiratory depression, and coma. If hypotension occurs, administer I.V. fluids and place in Trendelenburg position. If unresponsive, an I.V. vasopressor (eg, dopamine, epinephrine) may be required. Repeat oral doses of activated charcoal significantly reduce the half-life of phenobarbital resulting from enhancement of nonrenal elimination. The usual dose is 0.1-1 g/kg every 4-6 hours for 3-4 days, unless the patient has no bowel movement, causing charcoal to remain in the GI tract. Assure adequate hydration and renal function. Urinary alkalinization with I.V. sodium bicarbonate also helps enhance elimination. Hemodialysis or hemoperfusion is of uncertain value. Patients in stage IV coma, due to high serum barbiturate levels, may require charcoal hemoperfusion.

Drug Interactions

Cytochrome P450 Effect: CYP1A2, 2B6, 2C, 2C8, 2C9, 2C18, 2C19, 3A3/4, and 3A5-7 enzyme inducer

Increased Effect/Toxicity: When combined with other CNS depressants, ethanol, narcotic analgesics, antidepressants, or benzodiazepines, additive respiratory and CNS depression may occur. Barbiturates may enhance the hepatotoxic potential of acetaminophen overdoses. Chloramphenicol, MAO inhibitors, valproic acid, and felbamate may inhibit barbiturate metabolism. Barbiturates may impair the absorption of griseofulvin, and may enhance the nephrotoxic effects of methoxyflurane. Concurrent use of phenobarbital with meperidine may result in increased CNS depression. Concurrent use of phenobarbital with primidone may result in elevated phenobarbital serum concentrations.

Decreased Effect: Barbiturates are hepatic enzyme inducers, and may increase the metabolism of antipsychotics, some beta-blockers (unlikely with atenolol and nadolol), calcium channel blockers, chloramphenicol, cimetidine, corticosteroids, cyclosporine, disopyramide, doxycycline, ethosuximide, felbamate, furosemide, griseofulvin, lamotrigine, phenytoin, propafenone, quinidine, tacrolimus, TCAs, and theophylline. Barbiturates may increase the metabolism of estrogens and reduce the efficacy of oral contraceptives; an alternative method of contraception should be considered. Barbiturates inhibit the hypoprothrombinemic effects of oral anticoagulants via increased metabolism. Barbiturates may enhance the metabolism of methadone resulting in methadone withdrawal.

Ethanol/Nutrition/Herb Interactions

Ethanol: Avoid ethanol (may increase CNS depression).

Food: May cause decrease in vitamin D and calcium.

Herb/Nutraceutical: Avoid evening primrose (seizure threshold decreased). Avoid valerian, St John's wort, kava kava, gotu kola (may increase CNS depression).

Stability Protect elixir from light; not stable in aqueous solutions; use only clear solutions; do not add to acidic solutions, precipitation may occur; I.V. form is **incompatible** with benzquinamide (in syringe), cephalothin, chlorpromazine, hydralazine, hydrocortisone, hydroxyzine, insulin, levorphanol, meperidine, methadone, morphine, norepinephrine, pentazocine, prochlorperazine, promazine, promethazine, ranitidine (in syringe), vancomycin

Mechanism of Action Short-acting barbiturate with sedative, hypnotic, and anticonvulsant properties. Barbiturates depress the sensory cortex, decrease motor activity, alter cerebellar function, and produce drowsiness, sedation, and hypnosis. In high doses, barbiturates exhibit anticonvulsant activity; barbiturates produce dose-dependent respiratory depression;

Pharmacodynamics/Kinetics

Onset of action: Oral: Hypnosis: 20-60 minutes; I.V.: ~5 minutes

Peak effect: I.V.: ~30 minutes

Duration: Oral: 6-10 hours; I.V.: 4-10 hours

Absorption: Oral: 70% to 90%

Protein binding: 20% to 45%; decreased in neonates

Metabolism: Hepatic via hydroxylation and glucuronide conjugation

Half-life elimination: Neonates: 45-500 hours; Infants: 20-133 hours; Children: 37-73 hours; Adults: 53-140 hours

Time to peak, serum: Oral: 1-6 hours

Excretion: Urine (20% to 50% as unchanged drug)

Usual Dosage

Children:

Sedation: Oral: 2 mg/kg 3 times/day

Hypnotic: I.M., I.V., S.C.: 3-5 mg/kg at bedtime

Preoperative sedation: Oral, I.M., I.V.: 1-3 mg/kg 1-1.5 hours before procedure

Adults:

Sedation: Oral, I.M.: 30-120 mg/day in 2-3 divided doses

Hypnotic: Oral, I.M., I.V., S.C.: 100-320 mg at bedtime

Preoperative sedation: I.M.: 100-200 mg 1-1.5 hours before procedure

Anticonvulsant: Status epilepticus: **Loading dose:** I.V.:

Infants and Children: 10-20 mg/kg in a single or divided dose; in select patients may administer additional 5 mg/kg/dose every 15-30 minutes until seizure is controlled or a total dose of 40 mg/kg is reached

Adults: 300-800 mg initially followed by 120-240 mg/dose at 20-minute intervals until seizures are controlled or a total dose of 1-2 g

Anticonvulsant maintenance dose: Oral, I.V.:

Infants: 5-8 mg/kg/day in 1-2 divided doses

(Continued)

Phenobarbital *(Continued)*

Children:
1-5 years: 6-8 mg/kg/day in 1-2 divided doses
5-12 years: 4-6 mg/kg/day in 1-2 divided doses
Children >12 years and Adults: 1-3 mg/kg/day in divided doses or 50-100 mg 2-3 times/day
Sedative/hypnotic withdrawal (unlabeled use): Initial daily requirement is determined by substituting phenobarbital 30 mg for every 100 mg pentobarbital used during tolerance testing; then daily requirement is decreased by 10% of initial dose

Dosing interval in renal impairment: Cl_{cr} <10 mL/minute: Administer every 12-16 hours
Hemodialysis: Moderately dialyzable (20% to 50%)
Dosing adjustment/comments in hepatic disease: Increased side effects may occur in severe liver disease; monitor plasma levels and adjust dose accordingly
Dietary Considerations Vitamin D: Loss in vitamin D due to malabsorption; increase intake of foods rich in vitamin D. Supplementation of vitamin D and/or calcium may be necessary.
Administration Avoid rapid I.V. administration >50 mg/minute; avoid intra-arterial injection
Monitoring Parameters Phenobarbital serum concentrations, mental status, CBC, LFTs, seizure activity
Reference Range
Therapeutic:
Infants and children: 15-30 µg/mL (SI: 65-129 µmol/L)
Adults: 20-40 µg/mL (SI: 86-172 µmol/L)
Toxic: >40 µg/mL (SI: >172 µmol/L)
Toxic concentration: Slowness, ataxia, nystagmus: 35-80 µg/mL (SI: 150-344 µmol/L)
Coma with reflexes: 65-117 µg/mL (SI: 279-502 µmol/L)
Coma without reflexes: >100 µg/mL (SI: >430 µmol/L)
Test Interactions Assay interference of LDH
Patient Information Avoid alcohol and other CNS depressants; avoid driving and other hazardous tasks; avoid abrupt discontinuation; may cause physical and psychological dependence; do not alter dose without notifying physician
Nursing Implications Parenteral solutions are highly alkaline; avoid extravasation; institute safety measures to avoid injuries; observe patient for excessive sedation and respiratory depression
Additional Information Injectable solutions contain propylene glycol; sodium content of injection (65 mg, 1 mL): 6 mg (0.3 mEq).
Dosage Forms
Elixir: 20 mg/5 mL (5 mL, 7.5 mL, 15 mL, 120 mL, 473 mL, 946 mL, 4000 mL)
Injection, as sodium: 30 mg/mL (1 mL); 60 mg/mL (1 mL); 65 mg/mL (1 mL); 130 mg/mL (1 mL)
Luminal®: 60 mg/mL (1 mL); 130 mg/mL (1 mL);
Tablet: 15 mg, 16 mg, 30 mg, 32 mg, 60 mg, 65 mg, 100 mg

♦ **Phenobarbital, Belladonna, and Ergotamine Tartrate** *see* Belladonna, Phenobarbital, and Ergotamine Tartrate *on page 152*
♦ **Phenobarbital, Hyoscyamine, Atropine, and Scopolamine** *see* Hyoscyamine, Atropine, Scopolamine, and Phenobarbital *on page 694*
♦ **Phenobarbital Sodium** *see* Phenobarbital *on page 1070*
♦ **Phenobarbitone** *see* Phenobarbital *on page 1070*

Phenoxybenzamine *(fen oks ee BEN za meen)*

U.S. Brand Names Dibenzyline®
Canadian Brand Names Dibenzyline®
Synonyms Phenoxybenzamine Hydrochloride
Therapeutic Category Alpha-Adrenergic Blocking Agent, Oral; Antihypertensive Agent
Use Symptomatic management of pheochromocytoma; treatment of hypertensive crisis caused by sympathomimetic amines
Unlabeled/Investigational Use Micturition problems associated with neurogenic bladder, functional outlet obstruction, and partial prostate obstruction
Pregnancy Risk Factor C
Contraindications Hypersensitivity to phenoxybenzamine or any component of the formulation; conditions in which a fall in blood pressure would be undesirable (eg, shock)
Warnings/Precautions Use with caution in patients with renal impairment, cerebral, or coronary arteriosclerosis, can exacerbate symptoms of respiratory tract infections. Because of the risk of adverse effects, avoid the use of this medication in the elderly if possible.
Adverse Reactions Frequency not defined.
Cardiovascular: Postural hypotension, tachycardia, syncope, shock
Central nervous system: Lethargy, headache, confusion, fatigue
Gastrointestinal: Vomiting, nausea, diarrhea, xerostomia
Genitourinary: Inhibition of ejaculation
Neuromuscular & skeletal: Weakness
Ocular: Miosis
Respiratory: Nasal congestion
Overdosage/Toxicology Symptoms include hypotension, tachycardia, lethargy, dizziness, and shock. Hypotension and shock should be treated with fluids and Trendelenburg positioning. Only alpha-adrenergic pressors, such as norepinephrine should be used. Mixed agents such as epinephrine, may cause more hypotension.
Drug Interactions
Increased Effect/Toxicity: Beta-blockers may result in increased toxicity (hypotension, tachycardia).
Decreased Effect: Alpha adrenergic agonists decrease the effect of phenoxybenzamine.
Ethanol/Nutrition/Herb Interactions Ethanol: Avoid ethanol.

Mechanism of Action Produces long-lasting noncompetitive alpha-adrenergic blockade of postganglionic synapses in exocrine glands and smooth muscle; relaxes urethra and increases opening of the bladder

Pharmacodynamics/Kinetics

Onset of action: ~2 hours
  Peak effect: 4-6 hours
Duration: ≥4 days
Half-life elimination: 24 hours
Excretion: Primarily urine and feces

Usual Dosage Oral:

Children: Initial: 0.2 mg/kg (maximum: 10 mg) once daily, increase by 0.2 mg/kg increments; usual maintenance dose: 0.4-1.2 mg/kg/day every 6-8 hours, higher doses may be necessary

Adults: Initial: 10 mg twice daily, increase by 10 mg every other day until optimum dose is achieved; usual range: 20-40 mg 2-3 times/day

Administration GI irritation may be reduced by giving in divided doses

Monitoring Parameters Blood pressure, pulse, urine output, orthostasis

Patient Information Avoid alcohol; if dizziness occurs, avoid sudden changes in posture; may cause nasal congestion and constricted pupils; may inhibit ejaculation; avoid cough, cold or allergy medications containing sympathomimetics

Nursing Implications Monitor for orthostasis; assist with ambulation

Dosage Forms Capsule, as hydrochloride: 10 mg

- ◆ **Phenoxybenzamine Hydrochloride** *see* Phenoxybenzamine *on page 1072*
- ◆ **Phenoxymethyl Penicillin** *see* Penicillin V Potassium *on page 1055*

Phentermine (FEN ter meen)

Related Information

Antacid Drug Interactions *on page 1477*
Obesity Treatment Guidelines for Adults *on page 1685*

U.S. Brand Names Adipex-P®; Ionamin®

Canadian Brand Names Ionamin®

Synonyms Phentermine Hydrochloride

Therapeutic Category Anorexiant

Use Short-term adjunct in a regimen of weight reduction based on exercise, behavioral modification, and caloric reduction in the management of exogenous obesity for patients with an initial body mass index ≥30 kg/m^2 or ≥27 kg/m^2 in the presence of other risk factors (diabetes, hypertension)

Restrictions C-IV

Pregnancy Risk Factor C

Contraindications Hypersensitivity or idiosyncrasy to sympathomimetic amines or any component of the formulation; patients with advanced arteriosclerosis, symptomatic cardiovascular disease, moderate to severe hypertension (stage II or III), hyperthyroidism, glaucoma, agitated states; patients with a history of drug abuse; use during or within 14 days following MAO inhibitor therapy; children <16 years of age (per manufacturer)

Warnings/Precautions Use with caution in patients with bipolar disorder, diabetes mellitus, cardiovascular disease, seizure disorders, insomnia, porphyria, or mild hypertension (stage I). May exacerbate symptoms of behavior and thought disorder in psychotic patients. Stimulants may unmask tics in individuals with coexisting Tourette's syndrome. Potential for drug dependency exists - avoid abrupt discontinuation in patients who have received for prolonged periods. Use in weight reduction programs only when alternative therapy has been ineffective. Stimulant use has been associated with growth suppression, and careful monitoring is recommended.

Primary pulmonary hypertension (PPH), a rare and frequently fatal pulmonary disease, has been reported to occur in patients receiving a combination of phentermine and fenfluramine or dexfenfluramine. The possibility of an association between PPH and the use of phentermine alone cannot be ruled out.

Adverse Reactions Frequency not defined.

Cardiovascular: Hypertension, palpitations, tachycardia, primary pulmonary hypertension and/or regurgitant cardiac valvular disease

Central nervous system: Euphoria, insomnia, overstimulation, dizziness, dysphoria, headache, restlessness, psychosis

Dermatologic: Urticaria

Endocrine & metabolic: Changes in libido, impotence

Gastrointestinal: Nausea, constipation, xerostomia, unpleasant taste, diarrhea

Hematologic: Blood dyscrasias

Neuromuscular & skeletal: Tremor

Ocular: Blurred vision

Overdosage/Toxicology Symptoms include hyperactivity, agitation, hyperthermia, hypertension, and seizures. There is no specific antidote for phentermine intoxication and the bulk of the treatment is supportive. Hyperactivity and agitation usually respond to reduced sensory input; however, with extreme agitation haloperidol (2-5 mg I.M. for adults) may be required. Hyperthermia is best treated with external cooling measures, or when severe or unresponsive, muscle paralysis with pancuronium may be needed. Hypertension is usually transient and generally does not require treatment unless severe. For diastolic blood pressures >110 mm Hg, a nitroprusside infusion should be initiated. Seizures usually respond to diazepam IVP and/or phenytoin maintenance regimens.

Drug Interactions

Increased Effect/Toxicity: Dosage of hypoglycemic agents may need to be adjusted when phentermine is used in a diabetic receiving a special diet. Concurrent use of MAO inhibitors and drugs with MAO activity (furazolidone, linezolid) may be associated with hypertensive episodes. Concurrent use of SSRIs may be associated with a risk of serotonin syndrome.

(Continued)

Phentermine (Continued)

Decreased Effect: Phentermine may decrease the effect of antihypertensive medications The efficacy of anorexiants may be decreased by antipsychotics; in addition, amphetamines or related compounds may induce an increase in psychotic symptoms in some patients. Amphetamines (and related compounds) inhibit the antihypertensive response to guanethidine; probably also may occur with guanadrel.

Mechanism of Action Phentermine is structurally similar to dextroamphetamine and is comparable to dextroamphetamine as an appetite suppressant, but is generally associated with a lower incidence and severity of CNS side effects. Phentermine, like other anorexiants, stimulates the hypothalamus to result in decreased appetite; anorexiant effects are most likely mediated via norepinephrine and dopamine metabolism. However, other CNS effects or metabolic effects may be involved.

Pharmacodynamics/Kinetics
Duration: Resin produces more prolonged clinical effects
Absorption: Well absorbed; resin absorbed slower
Half-life elimination: 20 hours
Excretion: Primarily urine (as unchanged drug)

Usual Dosage Oral: Adults: Obesity: 8 mg 3 times/day 30 minutes before meals or food or 15-37.5 mg/day before breakfast or 10-14 hours before retiring

Monitoring Parameters CNS

Patient Information Take during day to avoid insomnia; do not discontinue abruptly, may cause physical and psychological dependence with prolonged use

Nursing Implications Dose should not be given in evening or at bedtime

Dosage Forms
Capsule, as hydrochloride: 15 mg, 18.75 mg, 30 mg, 37.5 mg
Adipex-P®: 37.5 mg
Capsule, resin complex, as hydrochloride (Ionamin®): 15 mg, 30 mg
Tablet, as hydrochloride: 8 mg, 37.5 mg
Adipex-P®: 37.5 mg

♦ **Phentermine Hydrochloride** *see Phentermine on page 1073*

Phentolamine (fen TOLE a meen)

Related Information
Hypertension *on page 1675*

U.S. Brand Names Regitine®

Canadian Brand Names Regitine®

Synonyms Phentolamine Mesylate

Therapeutic Category Alpha-Adrenergic Blocking Agent, Parenteral; Antidote, Extravasation; Antihypertensive Agent; Diagnostic Agent, Pheochromocytoma

Use Diagnosis of pheochromocytoma and treatment of hypertension associated with pheochromocytoma or other caused by excess sympathomimetic amines; as treatment of dermal necrosis after extravasation of drugs with alpha-adrenergic effects (norepinephrine, dopamine, epinephrine, dobutamine)

Pregnancy Risk Factor C

Contraindications Hypersensitivity to phentolamine or any component of the formulation; renal impairment; coronary or cerebral arteriosclerosis

Warnings/Precautions Myocardial infarction, cerebrovascular spasm and cerebrovascular occlusion have occurred following administration; use with caution in patients with gastritis or peptic ulcer, tachycardia, or a history of cardiac arrhythmias

Adverse Reactions Frequency not defined.
Cardiovascular: Hypotension, tachycardia, arrhythmia, flushing, orthostatic hypotension
Central nervous system: Weakness, dizziness
Gastrointestinal: Nausea, vomiting, diarrhea
Respiratory: Nasal congestion
Postmarketing and/or case reports: Pulmonary hypertension

Overdosage/Toxicology Symptoms include tachycardia, shock, vomiting, and dizziness. Hypotension and shock should be treated with fluids and Trendelenburg positioning. Only alpha-adrenergic pressors, such as norepinephrine should be used. Mixed agents such as epinephrine, may cause more hypotension. Take care not to cause so much swelling of the extremity or digit that a compartment syndrome would occur.

Drug Interactions
Increased Effect/Toxicity: Phentolamine's toxicity is increased with ethanol (disulfiram reaction).
Decreased Effect: Decreased effect of phentolamine with epinephrine and ephedrine.

Stability Reconstituted solution is stable for 48 hours at room temperature and 1 week when refrigerated

Mechanism of Action Competitively blocks alpha-adrenergic receptors to produce brief antagonism of circulating epinephrine and norepinephrine to reduce hypertension caused by alpha effects of these catecholamines; also has a positive inotropic and chronotropic effect on the heart

Pharmacodynamics/Kinetics
Onset of action: I.M.: 15-20 minutes; I.V.: Immediate
Duration: I.M.: 30-45 minutes; I.V.: 15-30 minutes
Metabolism: Hepatic
Half-life elimination: 19 minutes
Excretion: Urine (10% as unchanged drug)

Usual Dosage
Treatment of alpha-adrenergic drug extravasation: S.C.:
Children: 0.1-0.2 mg/kg diluted in 10 mL 0.9% sodium chloride infiltrated into area of extravasation within 12 hours

Adults: Infiltrate area with small amount of solution made by diluting 5-10 mg in 10 mL
0.9% sodium chloride within 12 hours of extravasation; do not exceed 0.1-0.2 mg/kg or 5
mg total

If dose is effective, normal skin color should return to the blanched area within 1 hour

Diagnosis of pheochromocytoma: I.M., I.V.:
Children: 0.05-0.1 mg/kg/dose, maximum single dose: 5 mg
Adults: 5 mg

Surgery for pheochromocytoma: Hypertension: I.M., I.V.:
Children: 0.05-0.1 mg/kg/dose given 1-2 hours before procedure; repeat as needed every
2-4 hours until hypertension is controlled; maximum single dose: 5 mg
Adults: 5 mg given 1-2 hours before procedure and repeated as needed every 2-4 hours

Hypertensive crisis: Adults: 5-20 mg

Administration Infiltrate the area of dopamine extravasation with multiple small injections
using only 27- or 30-gauge needles and changing the needle between each skin entry; take
care not to cause so much swelling of the extremity or digit that a compartment syndrome
occurs

Monitoring Parameters Blood pressure, heart rate; area of infiltration

Test Interactions ↑ LFTs rarely

Nursing Implications Monitor patient for orthostasis; assist with ambulation; if infiltration is
severe, may also need to consult vascular surgeon

Dosage Forms Injection, as mesylate: 5 mg/mL (1 mL)

- ♦ **Phentolamine Mesylate** *see* Phentolamine *on page 1074*
- ♦ **Phenylalanine Mustard** *see* Melphalan *on page 854*
- ♦ **Phenylazo Diamino Pyridine Hydrochloride** *see* Phenazopyridine *on page 1068*

Phenylephrine *(fen il EF rin)*

Related Information
Adrenergic Agonists, Cardiovascular Comparison *on page 1469*
Antacid Drug Interactions *on page 1477*

U.S. Brand Names AK-Dilate® Ophthalmic; AK-Nefrin® Ophthalmic; Alconefrin® Nasal [OTC];
Children's Nostril®; Mydfrin® Ophthalmic; Neo-Synephrine® Injection; Neo-Synephrine® Nasal
[OTC]; Neo-Synephrine® Ophthalmic; Nostril® Nasal [OTC]; Prefrin™ Ophthalmic; Relief®
Ophthalmic; Rhinall® Nasal [OTC]; Vicks Sinex® Nasal [OTC]

Canadian Brand Names Dionephrine®; Mydfrin®; Neo-Synephrine®

Synonyms Phenylephrine Hydrochloride

Therapeutic Category Adrenergic Agonist Agent; Adrenergic Agonist Agent, Ophthalmic;
Alpha-Adrenergic Agonist; Nasal Agent, Vasoconstrictor; Ophthalmic Agent, Mydriatic;
Sympathomimetic

Use Treatment of hypotension, vascular failure in shock; as a vasoconstrictor in regional
analgesia; symptomatic relief of nasal and nasopharyngeal mucosal congestion; as a mydriatic in ophthalmic procedures and treatment of wide-angle glaucoma; supraventricular tachycardia

Pregnancy Risk Factor C

Contraindications Hypersensitivity to phenylephrine, bisulfite (some products contain metabisulfite), or any component of the formulation; hypertension; ventricular tachycardia

Warnings/Precautions Use with caution in the elderly, patients with hyperthyroidism, bradycardia, partial heart block, myocardial disease, or severe CAD. Not a substitute for volume
replacement. Avoid hypertension; monitor blood pressure closely and adjust infusion rate.
Infuse into a large vein if possible. Watch I.V. site closely. Avoid extravasation. The elderly
can be more sensitive to side effects from the nasal decongestant form. Rebound congestion
can occur when the drug is discontinued after chronic use.

Adverse Reactions Frequency not defined.
Cardiovascular: Reflex bradycardia, excitability, restlessness, arrhythmias (rare), precordial
pain or discomfort, pallor, hypertension, severe peripheral and visceral vasoconstriction,
decreased cardiac output
Central nervous system: Headache, anxiety, weakness, dizziness, tremor, paresthesia, rest-
lessness
Endocrine & metabolic: Metabolic acidosis
Local: Extravasation which may lead to necrosis and sloughing of surrounding tissue,
blanching of skin
Neuromuscular & skeletal: Pilomotor response, weakness
Renal: Decreased renal perfusion, reduced urine output, reduced urine output
Respiratory: Respiratory distress

Overdosage/Toxicology Symptoms include vomiting, hypertension, palpitations, paresthesia, and ventricular extrasystoles. Treatment is supportive. In extreme cases, I.V. phentolamine may be used.

Drug Interactions
Increased Effect/Toxicity: Phenylephrine, taken with sympathomimetics, may induce
tachycardia or arrhythmias. If taken with MAO inhibitors or oxytocic agents, actions may be
potentiated.
Decreased Effect: Alpha- and beta-adrenergic blocking agents may have a decreased
effect if taken with phenylephrine.

Ethanol/Nutrition/Herb Interactions Herb/Nutraceutical: Avoid ephedra, yohimbe (may
cause CNS stimulation).

Stability Stable for 48 hours in 5% dextrose in water at pH 3.5-7.5; do not use brown colored
solutions

Mechanism of Action Potent, direct-acting alpha-adrenergic stimulator with weak beta-
adrenergic activity; causes vasoconstriction of the arterioles of the nasal mucosa and
conjunctiva; activates the dilator muscle of the pupil to cause contraction; produces vasoconstriction of arterioles in the body; produces systemic arterial vasoconstriction

Pharmacodynamics/Kinetics
Onset of action: I.M., S.C.: 10-15 minutes; I.V.: Immediate
Duration: I.M.: 0.5-2 hours; I.V.: 15-30 minutes; S.C.: 1 hour
(Continued)

Phenylephrine *(Continued)*

Metabolism: To phenolic conjugates; hepatically and via intestinal monoamine oxidase
Half-life elimination: 2.5 hours (increased after long-term infusion)
Excretion: Urine (90%)

Usual Dosage

Ophthalmic procedures:
Infants <1 year: Instill 1 drop of 2.5% 15-30 minutes before procedures
Children and Adults: Instill 1 drop of 2.5% or 10% solution, may repeat in 10-60 minutes as needed

Nasal decongestant (therapy should not exceed 3 continuous days):
Children:
2-6 years: Instill 1 drop every 2-4 hours of 0.125% solution as needed
6-12 years: Instill 1-2 sprays or instill 1-2 drops every 4 hours of 0.25% solution as needed
Children >12 years and Adults: Instill 1-2 sprays or instill 1-2 drops every 4 hours of 0.25% to 0.5% solution as needed; 1% solution may be used in adult in cases of extreme nasal congestion; do not use nasal solutions more than 3 days

Hypotension/shock:
Children:
I.M., S.C.: 0.1 mg/kg/dose every 1-2 hours as needed (maximum: 5 mg)
I.V. bolus: 5-20 mcg/kg/dose every 10-15 minutes as needed
I.V. infusion: 0.1-0.5 mcg/kg/minute
Adults:
I.M., S.C.: 2-5 mg/dose every 1-2 hours as needed (initial dose should not exceed 5 mg)
I.V. bolus: 0.1-0.5 mg/dose every 10-15 minutes as needed (initial dose should not exceed 0.5 mg)
I.V. infusion: 10 mg in 250 mL D_5W or NS (1:25,000 dilution) (40 mcg/mL); start at 100-180 mcg/minute (2-5 mL/minute; 50-90 drops/minute) initially; when blood pressure is stabilized, maintenance rate: 40-60 mcg/minute (20-30 drops/minute); rates up to 360 mg/minutes have been reported; dosing range: 0.4-9.1 mcg/kg/minute
Note: Concentrations up to 100-500 mg in 250 mL have been used.

Paroxysmal supraventricular tachycardia: I.V.:
Children: 5-10 mcg/kg/dose over 20-30 seconds
Adults: 0.25-0.5 mg/dose over 20-30 seconds

Administration Concentration and rate of infusion can be calculated using the following formulas: Dilute 0.6 mg x weight (kg) to 100 mL; then the dose in mcg/kg/minute = 0.1 x the infusion rate in mL/hour

Monitoring Parameters Blood pressure, heart rate, arterial blood gases, central venous pressure

Patient Information Nasal decongestant should not be used for >3 days in a row, thereby reducing problems of rebound congestion; notify physician of insomnia, dizziness, tremor, or irregular heartbeat; if symptoms do not improve within 7 days or are accompanied by signs of infection, consult physician

Nursing Implications May cause necrosis or sloughing tissue if extravasation occurs during I.V. administration or S.C. administration

Extravasation: Use phentolamine as antidote; mix 5 mg with 9 mL of NS; inject a small amount of this dilution into extravasated area; blanching should reverse immediately. Monitor site; if blanching should recur, additional injections of phentolamine may be needed.

Additional Information Phenylephrine allows for close titration of blood pressure and should be used in patients with hypotension or shock due to peripheral vasodilation. Phenylephrine should not constitute sole therapy in patients with hypotension due to aortic dysfunction or hypovolemia. An important benefit of this drug is the short half-life, allowing rapid changes in dosage with prompt appropriate blood pressure responses. When administered intravenously, it should be used in intensive care settings or under very close monitoring.

Dosage Forms

Injection, as hydrochloride (Neo-Synephrine®): 1% [10 mg/mL] (1 mL)
Solution, intranasal, as hydrochloride [drops]:
Alconefrin®, Neo-Synephrine®: 0.5% (15 mL, 30 mL)
Alconefrin® 12: 0.16% (30 mL)
Alconefrin® 25, Neo-Synephrine®, Children's Nostril®, Rhinall®: 0.25% (15 mL, 30 mL, 40 mL)
Neo-Synephrine®: 0.125% (15 mL)
Solution, intranasal, as hydrochloride [spray]:
Alconefrin® 25, Neo-Synephrine®, Rhinall®: 0.25% (15 mL, 30 mL, 40 mL)
Neo-Synephrine®: 1% (15 mL)
Neo-Synephrine®, Nostril®, Sinex®: 0.5% (15 mL, 30 mL)
Solution, ophthalmic, as hydrochloride:
AK-Dilate®, Mydfrin®, Neo-Synephrine®, Phenoptic®: 2.5% (2 mL, 3 mL, 5 mL, 15 mL)
AK-Dilate®, Neo-Synephrine®, Neo-Synephrine® Viscous: 10% (1 mL, 2 mL, 5 mL, 15 mL)
AK-Nefrin®, Prefrin™ Liquifilm®, Relief®: 0.12% (0.3 mL, 15 mL, 20 mL)

♦ **Phenylephrine and Chlorpheniramine** see Chlorpheniramine and Phenylephrine on page 279

♦ **Phenylephrine and Cyclopentolate** see Cyclopentolate and Phenylephrine on page 341

♦ **Phenylephrine and Guaifenesin** see Guaifenesin and Phenylephrine on page 647

♦ **Phenylephrine and Promethazine** see Promethazine and Phenylephrine on page 1142

Phenylephrine and Scopolamine *(fen il EF rin & skoe POL a meen)*

U.S. Brand Names Murocoll-2®
Synonyms Scopolamine and Phenylephrine
Therapeutic Category Anticholinergic/Adrenergic Agonist
Use Mydriasis, cycloplegia, and to break posterior synechiae in iritis
Pregnancy Risk Factor C

Usual Dosage Instill 1-2 drops into eye(s); repeat in 5 minutes
Additional Information Complete prescribing information for this medication should be consulted for additional detail.
Dosage Forms Solution, ophthalmic: Phenylephrine hydrochloride 10% and scopolamine hydrobromide 0.3% (7.5 mL)

Phenylephrine and Zinc Sulfate (fen il EF rin & zingk SUL fate)
U.S. Brand Names Zincfrin® [OTC]
Canadian Brand Names Zincfrin®
Synonyms Zinc Sulfate and Phenylephrine
Therapeutic Category Adrenergic Agonist Agent
Use Soothe, moisturize, and remove redness due to minor eye irritation
Usual Dosage Instill 1-2 drops in eye(s) 2-4 times/day as needed
Additional Information Complete prescribing information for this medication should be consulted for additional detail.
Dosage Forms Solution, ophthalmic: Phenylephrine hydrochloride 0.12% and zinc sulfate 0.25% (15 mL)

- ◆ **Phenylephrine Hydrochloride** see Phenylephrine on page 1075
- ◆ **Phenylephrine, Hydrocodone, Chlorpheniramine, Acetaminophen, and Caffeine** see Hydrocodone, Chlorpheniramine, Phenylephrine, Acetaminophen, and Caffeine on page 682
- ◆ **Phenylephrine, Promethazine, and Codeine** see Promethazine, Phenylephrine, and Codeine on page 1142
- ◆ **Phenylethylmalonylurea** see Phenobarbital on page 1070
- ◆ **Phenylgesic® [OTC]** see Acetaminophen and Phenyltoloxamine on page 25
- ◆ **Phenylisohydantoin** see Pemoline on page 1048

Phenylpropanolamine *Withdrawn From Market 11/00*
(fen il proe pa NOLE a meen)
Warnings/Precautions On November 6, 2000, the FDA issued a public health advisory concerning the risk of hemorrhagic stroke associated with the use of phenylpropanolamine hydrochloride (PPA). An increased risk of hemorrhagic stroke has been identified in women following the first dose of PPA when used as an appetite suppressant, and within the first 3 days of use when used as a decongestant. Men may also be at risk. The FDA has asked all drug companies to discontinue the marketing of products containing phenylpropanolamine.

- ◆ **Phenyl Salicylate, Methenamine, Methylene Blue, Sodium Biphosphate, and Hyoscyamine** see Methenamine, Sodium Biphosphate, Phenyl Salicylate, Methylene Blue, and Hyoscyamine on page 882
- ◆ **Phenyltoloxamine and Acetaminophen** see Acetaminophen and Phenyltoloxamine on page 25

Phenytoin (FEN i toyn)
Related Information
Antacid Drug Interactions on page 1477
Anticonvulsants by Seizure Type on page 1481
Convulsive Status Epilepticus on page 1661
Epilepsy & Seizure Treatment on page 1659
Fosphenytoin and Phenytoin, Parenteral Comparison on page 1498
U.S. Brand Names Dilantin®
Canadian Brand Names Dilantin®
Synonyms Diphenylhydantoin; DPH; Phenytoin Sodium; Phenytoin Sodium, Extended; Phenytoin Sodium, Prompt
Therapeutic Category Antiarrhythmic Agent, Class I-B; Anticonvulsant
Use Management of generalized tonic-clonic (grand mal), complex partial seizures; prevention of seizures following head trauma/neurosurgery
Unlabeled/Investigational Use Ventricular arrhythmias, including those associated with digitalis intoxication, prolonged QT interval and surgical repair of congenital heart diseases in children; epidermolysis bullosa
Pregnancy Risk Factor D
Pregnancy/Breast-Feeding Implications
Clinical effects on the fetus: Crosses the placenta. Cardiac defects and multiple other malformations reported; characteristic pattern of malformations called "fetal hydantoin syndrome"; hemorrhagic disease of newborn due to fetal vitamin K depletion, maternal folic acid deficiency may occur. Epilepsy itself, number of medications, genetic factors, or a combination of these probably influence the teratogenicity of anticonvulsant therapy. Benefit:risk ratio usually favors continued use during pregnancy and breast-feeding.
Breast-feeding/lactation: Crosses into breast milk
Clinical effects on the infant: Methemoglobinemia, drowsiness and decreased sucking reported in 1 case. AAP considers **compatible** with breast-feeding.
Contraindications Hypersensitivity to phenytoin, other hydantoins, or any component of the formulation; pregnancy
Warnings/Precautions May increase frequency of petit mal seizures; I.V. form may cause hypotension, skin necrosis at I.V. site; avoid I.V. administration in small veins; use with caution in patients with porphyria; discontinue if rash or lymphadenopathy occurs; use with caution in patients with hepatic dysfunction, sinus bradycardia, S-A block, or A-V block; use with caution in elderly or debilitated patients, or in any condition associated with low serum albumin levels, which will increase the free fraction of phenytoin in the serum and, therefore, the pharmacologic response. Sedation, confusional states, or cerebellar dysfunction (loss of motor coordination) may occur at higher total serum concentrations, or at lower total serum concentrations when the free fraction of phenytoin is increased. Abrupt withdrawal may precipitate status epilepticus.
Adverse Reactions I.V. effects: Hypotension, bradycardia, cardiac arrhythmias, cardiovascular collapse (especially with rapid I.V. use), venous irritation and pain, thrombophlebitis
(Continued)

Phenytoin (Continued)

Effects not related to plasma phenytoin concentrations: Hypertrichosis, gingival hypertrophy, thickening of facial features, carbohydrate intolerance, folic acid deficiency, peripheral neuropathy, vitamin D deficiency, osteomalacia, systemic lupus erythematosus

Concentration-related effects: Nystagmus, blurred vision, diplopia, ataxia, slurred speech, dizziness, drowsiness, lethargy, coma, rash, fever, nausea, vomiting, gum tenderness confusion, mood changes, folic acid depletion, osteomalacia, hyperglycemia

Related to elevated concentrations:

>20 mcg/mL: Far lateral nystagmus

>30 mcg/mL: 45° lateral gaze nystagmus and ataxia

>40 mcg/mL: Decreased mentation

>100 mcg/mL: Death

Cardiovascular: Hypotension, bradycardia, cardiac arrhythmias, cardiovascular collapse

Central nervous system: Psychiatric changes, slurred speech, dizziness, drowsiness, headache, insomnia

Dermatologic: Rash

Gastrointestinal: Constipation, nausea, vomiting, gingival hyperplasia, enlargement of lips

Hematologic: Leukopenia, thrombocytopenia, agranulocytosis

Hepatic: Hepatitis

Local: Thrombophlebitis

Neuromuscular & skeletal: Tremor, peripheral neuropathy, paresthesia

Ocular: Diplopia, nystagmus, blurred vision

Rarely seen effects: Blood dyscrasias, coarsening of facial features, dyskinesias, hepatitis, hypertrichosis, lymphadenopathy, lymphoma, pseudolymphoma, SLE-like syndrome, Stevens-Johnson syndrome, venous irritation and pain

Overdosage/Toxicology Symptoms include unsteady gait, slurred speech, confusion, nausea, hypothermia, fever, hypotension, respiratory depression, and coma. Treatment is supportive for hypotension. Treat with I.V. fluids and place in Trendelenburg position. Seizures may be controlled with diazepam 5-10 mg (0.25-0.4 mg/kg in children).

Drug Interactions

Cytochrome P450 Effect: CYP2C9 and 2C19 enzyme substrate; CYP1A2, 2B6, 2C8, 2C9, 2C18, 2C19, 3A3/4, and 3A5-7 enzyme inducer

Increased Effect/Toxicity: Phenytoin serum concentrations may be increased by isoniazid, chloramphenicol, ticlopidine, or fluconazole. In addition, trimethoprim, sulfamethoxazole, valproic acid, sulfamethizole, sulfaphenazole, nifedipine, omeprazole, phenylbutazone, phenobarbital, amiodarone, chloramphenicol, cimetidine, ciprofloxacin, disulfiram, enoxacin, norfloxacin, felbamate, fluconazole, fluoxetine, influenza vaccine, isoniazid, and metronidazole inhibit the metabolism of phenytoin resulting in increased serum phenytoin concentrations. Valproic acid may increase, decrease, or have no effect on phenytoin serum concentrations. Phenytoin may increase the effect of dopamine (enhanced hypotension), warfarin (transiently enhanced anticoagulation), or increase the rate of conversion of primidone to phenobarbital resulting in increased phenobarbital serum concentrations. Phenytoin may enhance the hepatotoxic potential of acetaminophen. Concurrent use of acetazolamide and phenytoin may result in an increased risk of osteomalacia. Concurrent use of phenytoin and lithium has resulted in lithium intoxication. Phenytoin enhances the conversion of primidone to phenobarbital resulting in elevated phenobarbital serum concentrations. Valproic acid and sulfisoxazole may displace phenytoin from binding sites, transiently increasing phenytoin free levels.

Decreased Effect: The blood levels of phenytoin may be decreased by carbamazepine, rifampin, amiodarone, cisplatin, disulfiram, vinblastine, bleomycin, folic acid, phenobarbital, ethanol (chronic), pyridoxine, vigabatrin, and theophylline. Sucralfate and continuous NG feedings may decrease absorption of phenytoin. Phenytoin induces hepatic enzymes, and may decrease the effect of oral contraceptives, itraconazole, mebendazole, methadone, oral midazolam, valproic acid, cyclosporine, theophylline, doxycycline, quinidine, mexiletine, disopyramide. Phenytoin also may increase the metabolism of alprazolam, amiodarone, bromfenac, carbamazepine, clozapine, cyclosporine, diazepam, disopyramide, doxycycline, felbamate, furosemide, itraconazole, lamotrigine, mebendazole, meperidine, methadone, metyrapone, mexiletine, midazolam, oral contraceptives, quetiapine, quinidine, tacrolimus, teniposide, theophylline, thyroid hormones, triazolam, and valproic acid resulting in decreased levels/effect. Phenytoin may inhibit the anti-Parkinson effect of levodopa. Long-term concurrent use of phenytoin may inhibit hypoprothrombinemic response to warfarin. Phenytoin may reduce the effectiveness of some nondepolarizing neuromuscular blocking agents.

Ethanol/Nutrition/Herb Interactions

Ethanol:

Acute use: Avoid or limit ethanol (inhibits metabolism of phenytoin). Watch for sedation.

Chronic use: Avoid or limit ethanol (stimulates metabolism of phenytoin).

Food: Phenytoin serum concentrations may be altered if taken with food. If taken with enteral nutrition, phenytoin serum concentrations may be decreased. Tube feedings decrease bioavailability; hold tube feedings 2 hours before and 2 hours after phenytoin administration. May decrease calcium, folic acid, and vitamin D levels.

Herb/Nutraceutical: Avoid evening primrose (seizure threshold decreased). Avoid valerian, St John's wort, kava kava, gotu kola (may increase CNS depression).

Stability Phenytoin is stable as long as it remains free of haziness and precipitation. Use only clear solutions; parenteral solution may be used as long as there is no precipitate and it is not hazy, slightly yellowed solution may be used. Refrigeration may cause precipitate, sometimes the precipitate is resolved by allowing the solution to reach room temperature again. Drug may precipitate at a pH <11.5. May dilute with normal saline for I.V. infusion; stability is concentration dependent. Standard diluent: Dose/100 mL NS

Minimum volume: Concentration should be maintained at 1-10 mg/mL secondary to stability problems (stable for 4 hours)

Comments: Maximum rate of infusion: 50 mg/minute

IVPB dose should be administered via an in-line 0.22-5 micron filter because of high potential for precipitation I.V. form is highly **incompatible** with many drugs and solutions such as dextrose in water, some saline solutions, amikacin, bretylium, cephapirin, dobutamine, heparin, insulin, levorphanol, lidocaine, meperidine, metaraminol, morphine, norepinephrine, potassium chloride, vitamin B complex with C

Mechanism of Action Stabilizes neuronal membranes and decreases seizure activity by increasing efflux or decreasing influx of sodium ions across cell membranes in the motor cortex during generation of nerve impulses; prolongs effective refractory period and suppresses ventricular pacemaker automaticity, shortens action potential in the heart

Pharmacodynamics/Kinetics

Onset of action: I.V.: ~0.5-1 hour

Absorption: Oral: Slow

Distribution: V_d:
  Neonates: Premature: 1-1.2 L/kg; Full-term: 0.8-0.9 L/kg
  Infants: 0.7-0.8 L/kg
  Children: 0.7 L/kg
  Adults: 0.6-0.7 L/kg

Protein binding:
  Neonates: ≥80% (≤20% free)
  Infants: ≥85% (≤15% free)
  Adults: 90% to 95%
  Others: Decreased protein binding
    Disease states resulting in a decrease in serum albumin concentration: Burns, hepatic cirrhosis, nephrotic syndrome, pregnancy, cystic fibrosis
    Disease states resulting in an apparent decrease in affinity of phenytoin for serum albumin: Renal failure, jaundice (severe), other drugs (displacers), hyperbilirubinemia (total bilirubin >15 mg/dL), Cl_{cr} <25 mL/minute (unbound fraction is increased two- to threefold in uremia)

Metabolism: Follows dose-dependent capacity-limited (Michaelis-Menten) pharmacokinetics with increased V_{max} in infants >6 months of age and children versus adults; major metabolite (via oxidation) HPPA undergoes enterohepatic recycling

Bioavailability: Form dependent

Time to peak, serum: (form dependent) Oral: Extended-release capsule: 4-12 hours; Immediate release preparation: 2-3 hours

Excretion: Urine (<5% as unchanged drug); as glucuronides
  Clearance: Highly variable, dependent upon intrinsic hepatic function and dose administered; increased clearance and decreased serum concentrations with febrile illness

Usual Dosage

Status epilepticus: I.V.:
  Infants and Children: Loading dose: 15-20 mg/kg in a single or divided dose; maintenance dose: Initial: 5 mg/kg/day in 2 divided doses; usual doses:
    6 months to 3 years: 8-10 mg/kg/day
    4-6 years: 7.5-9 mg/kg/day
    7-9 years: 7-8 mg/kg/day
    10-16 years: 6-7 mg/kg/day, some patients may require every 8 hours dosing
  Adults: Loading dose: Manufacturer recommends 10-15 mg/kg, however 15-25 mg/kg has been used clinically; maintenance dose: 300 mg/day or 5-6 mg/kg/day in 3 divided doses or 1-2 divided doses using extended release

Anticonvulsant: Children and Adults: Oral:
  Loading dose: 15-20 mg/kg; based on phenytoin serum concentrations and recent dosing history; administer oral loading dose in 3 divided doses given every 2-4 hours to decrease GI adverse effects and to ensure complete oral absorption; maintenance dose: same as I.V.
  Neurosurgery (prophylactic): 100-200 mg at approximately 4-hour intervals during surgery and during the immediate postoperative period

Dosing adjustment/comments in renal impairment or hepatic disease: Safe in usual doses in mild liver disease; clearance may be substantially reduced in cirrhosis and plasma level monitoring with dose adjustment advisable. Free phenytoin levels should be monitored closely.

Dietary Considerations

Folic acid: Phenytoin may decrease mucosal uptake of folic acid; to avoid folic acid deficiency and megaloblastic anemia, some clinicians recommend giving patients on anticonvulsants prophylactic doses of folic acid and cyanocobalamin. However, folate supplementation may increase seizures in some patients (dose dependent). Discuss with healthcare provider prior to using any supplements.

Calcium: Hypocalcemia has been reported in patients taking prolonged high-dose therapy with an anticonvulsant. Some clinicians have given an additional 4000 units/week of vitamin D (especially in those receiving poor nutrition and getting no sun exposure) to prevent hypocalcemia.

Vitamin D: Phenytoin interferes with vitamin D metabolism and osteomalacia may result; may need to supplement with vitamin D

Tube feedings: Tube feedings decrease phenytoin absorption. To avoid decreased serum levels with continuous NG feeds, hold feedings for 2 hours prior to and 2 hours after phenytoin administration, if possible. There is a variety of opinions on how to administer phenytoin with enteral feedings. Be **consistent** throughout therapy.

Administration

Phenytoin may be administered by IVP or IVPB administration

I.M. administration is not recommended due to erratic absorption, pain on injection and precipitation of drug at injection site

S.C. administration is not recommended because of the possibility of local tissue damage

The maximum rate of I.V. administration is 50 mg/minute; highly sensitive patients (eg, elderly, patients with pre-existing cardiovascular conditions) should receive phenytoin more slowly (eg, 20 mg/minute)

(Continued)

Phenytoin (Continued)

An in-line 0.22-5 micron filter is recommended for IVPB solutions due to the high potential for precipitation of the solution; avoid extravasation; following I.V. administration, NS should be injected through the same needle or I.V. catheter to prevent irritation

Monitoring Parameters Blood pressure, vital signs (with I.V. use), plasma phenytoin level, CBC, liver function tests

Reference Range Timing of serum samples: Because it is slowly absorbed, peak blood levels may occur 4-8 hours after ingestion of an oral dose. The serum half-life varies with the dosage and the drug follows Michaelis-Menten kinetics. The average adult half-life is about 24 hours. Steady-state concentrations are reached in 5-10 days.

Children and Adults: Toxicity is measured clinically, and some patients require levels outside the suggested therapeutic range

Therapeutic range:

Total phenytoin: 10-20 µg/mL (children and adults), 8-15 µg/mL (neonates)

Concentrations of 5-10 µg/mL may be therapeutic for some patients but concentrations <5 µg/mL are not likely to be effective

50% of patients show decreased frequency of seizures at concentrations >10 µg/mL

86% of patients show decreased frequency of seizures at concentrations >15 µg/mL

Add another anticonvulsant if satisfactory therapeutic response is not achieved with a phenytoin concentration of 20 µg/mL

Free phenytoin: 1-2.5 µg/mL

Toxic: <30-50 µg/mL (SI: <120-200 µmol/L)

Lethal: >100 µg/mL (SI: >400 µmol/L)

When to draw levels: This is dependent on the disease state being treated and the clinical condition of the patient

Key points:

Slow absorption of extended capsules and prolonged half-life minimize fluctuations between peak and trough concentrations, timing of sampling not crucial

Trough concentrations are generally recommended for routine monitoring. Daily levels are not necessary and may result in incorrect dosage adjustments. If it is determined essential to monitor free phenytoin concentrations, concomitant monitoring of total phenytoin concentrations is not necessary and expensive.

After a loading dose: Draw level within 48-96 hours

Rapid achievement: Draw within 2-3 days of therapy initiation to ensure that the patient's metabolism is not remarkably different from that which would be predicted by average literature-derived pharmacokinetic parameters; early levels should be used cautiously in design of new dosing regimens

Second concentration: Draw within 6-7 days with subsequent doses of phenytoin adjusted accordingly

If plasma concentrations have not changed over a 3- to 5-day period, monitoring interval may be increased to once weekly in the acute clinical setting

In stable patients requiring long-term therapy, generally monitor levels at 3- to 12-month intervals

Adjustment of serum concentration: See tables.

Adjustment of Serum Concentration in Patients With Low Serum Albumin

Measured Total Phenytoin Concentration (mcg/mL)	Patient's Serum Albumin (g/dL)			
	3.5	3	2.5	2
	Adjusted Total Phenytoin Concentration (mcg/mL)*			
5	6	7	8	10
10	13	14	17	20
15	19	21	25	30

*Adjusted concentration = measured total concentration ÷ [(0.2 x albumin) + 0.1].

Adjustment of Serum Concentration in Patients With Renal Failure (Cl$_{cr}$ ≤10 mL/min)

Measured Total Phenytoin Concentration (mcg/mL)	Patient's Serum Albumin (g/dL)				
	4	3.5	3	2.5	2
	Adjusted Total Phenytoin Concentration (mcg/mL)*				
5	10	11	13	14	17
10	20	22	25	29	33
15	30	33	38	43	50

*Adjusted concentration = measured total concentration ÷ [(0.1 x albumin) + 0.1].

Patient Information Shake oral suspension well prior to each dose; do not change brand or dosage form without consulting physician; do not skip doses, may cause drowsiness, dizziness, ataxia, loss of coordination or judgment; take with food; maintain good oral hygiene; do not crush or open extended capsules

Nursing Implications Maintenance doses usually start 12 hours after loading dose; shake oral suspension well prior to each dose; do not exceed I.V. infusion rate of 1-3 mg/kg/minute or 50 mg/minute; I.V. injections should be followed by normal saline flushes through the same needle or I.V. catheter to avoid local irritation of the vein; avoid extravasation; avoid I.M. use due to erratic absorption, pain on injection, and precipitation of drug at injection site

Additional Information Sodium content of 1 g injection: 88 mg (3.8 mEq)

Dosage Forms
Capsule, extended, as sodium: 30 mg, 100 mg
Capsule, prompt, as sodium: 100 mg
Injection, as sodium: 50 mg/mL (2 mL, 5 mL)
Suspension, oral: 125 mg/5 mL (5 mL, 240 mL)
Tablet, chewable: 50 mg

- **Phenytoin Sodium** *see Phenytoin on page 1077*
- **Phenytoin Sodium, Extended** *see Phenytoin on page 1077*
- **Phenytoin Sodium, Prompt** *see Phenytoin on page 1077*
- **Phillips'® Milk of Magnesia [OTC]** *see Magnesium Hydroxide on page 832*
- **pHisoHex®** *see Hexachlorophene on page 665*
- **Phos-Flur®** *see Fluoride on page 574*
- **PhosLo®** *see Calcium Acetate on page 206*
- **Phosphate, Potassium** *see Potassium Phosphate on page 1112*
- **Phospholine Iodide®** *see Echothiophate Iodide on page 455*
- **Phosphonoformate** *see Foscarnet on page 604*
- **Phosphonoformic Acid** *see Foscarnet on page 604*
- **Photofrin®** *see Porfimer on page 1104*
- **Phoxal-timolol (Can)** *see Timolol on page 1334*
- **Phrenilin®** *see Butalbital Compound on page 197*
- **Phrenilin® Forte** *see Butalbital Compound on page 197*
- **p-Hydroxyampicillin** *see Amoxicillin on page 84*
- **Phyllocontin®** *see Theophylline Salts on page 1310*
- **Phylloquinone** *see Phytonadione on page 1082*

Physostigmine (fye zoe STIG meen)

Related Information
Depression *on page 1655*
Glaucoma Drug Therapy Comparison *on page 1499*
U.S. Brand Names Antilirium®
Canadian Brand Names Eserine®; Isopto® Eserine
Synonyms Eserine Salicylate; Physostigmine Salicylate; Physostigmine Sulfate
Therapeutic Category Antidote, Anticholinergic Agent; Antidote, Belladonna Alkaloids;
Cholinergic Agent; Cholinergic Agent, Ophthalmic; Ophthalmic Agent, Miotic
Use Reverse toxic CNS effects caused by anticholinergic drugs; used as miotic in treatment of glaucoma
Pregnancy Risk Factor C
Contraindications Hypersensitivity to physostigmine or any component of the formulation; GI or GU obstruction; physostigmine therapy of drug intoxications should be used with extreme caution in patients with asthma, gangrene, severe cardiovascular disease, or mechanical obstruction of the GI tract or urogenital tract. In these patients, physostigmine should be used only to treat life-threatening conditions.
Warnings/Precautions Use with caution in patients with epilepsy, asthma, diabetes, gangrene, cardiovascular disease, bradycardia. Discontinue if excessive salivation or emesis, frequent urination or diarrhea occur. Reduce dosage if excessive sweating or nausea occurs. Administer I.V. slowly or at a controlled rate not faster than 1 mg/minute. Due to the possibility of hypersensitivity or overdose/cholinergic crisis, atropine should be readily available; ointment may delay corneal healing, may cause loss of dark adaptation; not intended as a first-line agent for anticholinergic toxicity or Parkinson's disease.
Adverse Reactions Frequency not defined.
Ophthalmic:
Central nervous system: Headache, browache
Dermatologic: Burning, redness
Ocular: Lacrimation, marked miosis, blurred vision, eye pain
Miscellaneous: Diaphoresis
Systemic:
Cardiovascular: Palpitations, bradycardia
Central nervous system: Restlessness, nervousness, hallucinations, seizures
Gastrointestinal: Nausea, salivation, diarrhea, stomach pains
Genitourinary: Frequent urge to urinate
Neuromuscular & skeletal: Muscle twitching
Ocular: Lacrimation, miosis
Respiratory: Dyspnea, bronchospasm, respiratory paralysis, pulmonary edema
Miscellaneous: Diaphoresis
Overdosage/Toxicology Symptoms include muscle weakness, blurred vision, excessive sweating, tearing and salivation, nausea, vomiting, bronchospasm, and seizures. If physostigmine is used in excess or in the absence of an anticholinergic overdose, patients may manifest signs of cholinergic toxicity. At this point a cholinergic agent (eg, atropine 0.015-0.05 mg/kg) may be necessary.
Drug Interactions
Increased Effect/Toxicity: Increased toxicity with bethanechol, methacholine. Succinylcholine may increase neuromuscular blockade with systemic administration.
Stability Do not use solution if cloudy or dark brown
Mechanism of Action Inhibits destruction of acetylcholine by acetylcholinesterase which facilitates transmission of impulses across myoneural junction and prolongs the central and peripheral effects of acetylcholine
Pharmacodynamics/Kinetics
Onset of action: Ophthalmic: ~2 minutes; Parenteral: ~5 minutes
Duration: Ophthalmic: 12-48 hours; Parenteral: 0.5-5 hours
Absorption: I.M., ophthalmic, S.C.: Readily absorbed
(Continued)

Physostigmine *(Continued)*

Distribution: Crosses blood-brain barrier readily and reverses both central and peripheral anticholinergic effects

Metabolism: Hepatic and via hydrolysis by cholinesterases

Half-life elimination: 15-40 minutes

Usual Dosage

Children: Anticholinergic drug overdose: Reserve for life-threatening situations only: I.V.: 0.01-0.03 mg/kg/dose (maximum: 0.5 mg/minute); may repeat after 5-10 minutes to a maximum total dose of 2 mg or until response occurs or adverse cholinergic effects occur

Adults: Anticholinergic drug overdose:

I.M., I.V., S.C.: 0.5-2 mg to start, repeat every 20 minutes until response occurs or adverse effect occurs

Repeat 1-4 mg every 30-60 minutes as life-threatening signs (arrhythmias, seizures, deep coma) recur; maximum I.V. rate: 1 mg/minute

Ophthalmic: Ointment: Instill a small quantity to lower fornix up to 3 times/day

Administration

Injection: Infuse slowly I.V. at a maximum rate of 0.5 mg/minute in children or 1 mg/minute in adults

Ophthalmic: Apply thin ribbon of ointment inside lower eyelid. Close eye and roll eyeball in all directions. Do not blink for $1/2$ minute. Do not use any other eye preparation for at least 10 minutes.

Test Interactions ↑ aminotransferase [ALT (SGPT)/AST (SGOT)] (S), ↑ amylase (S)

Patient Information Burning or stinging may occur with application; may cause loss of dark adaptation; notify physician if abdominal cramps, sweating, salivation, or cramps occur

Nursing Implications

Too rapid administration (I.V. rate not to exceed 1 mg/minute) can cause bradycardia, hypersalivation leading to respiratory difficulties and seizures

Monitor heart rate, respiratory rate

Dosage Forms

Injection, as salicylate: 1 mg/mL (2 mL)

Ointment, ophthalmic, as sulfate: 0.25% (3.5 g, 3.75 g)

♦ **Physostigmine Salicylate** *see Physostigmine on page 1081*

♦ **Physostigmine Sulfate** *see Physostigmine on page 1081*

♦ **Phytomenadione** *see Phytonadione on page 1082*

Phytonadione *(fye toe na DYE one)*

U.S. Brand Names AquaMEPHYTON®; Mephyton®

Canadian Brand Names AquaMEPHYTON®; Konakion; Mephyton®

Synonyms Methylphytyl Napthoquinone; Phylloquinone; Phytomenadione; Vitamin K₁

Therapeutic Category Vitamin, Fat Soluble

Use Prevention and treatment of hypoprothrombinemia caused by drug-induced or anticoagulant-induced vitamin K deficiency, hemorrhagic disease of the newborn; phytonadione is more effective and is preferred to other vitamin K preparations in the presence of impending hemorrhage; oral absorption depends on the presence of bile salts

Pregnancy Risk Factor C

Contraindications Hypersensitivity to phytonadione or any component of the formulation

Warnings/Precautions Severe reactions resembling anaphylaxis or hypersensitivity have occurred rarely during or immediately after I.V. administration (even with proper dilution and rate of administration), as well as I.M. administration; restrict I.V. administration for emergency use only; allergic reactions have also occurred with I.M. and S.C. injection; ineffective in hereditary hypoprothrombinemia, hypoprothrombinemia caused by severe liver disease; severe hemolytic anemia has been reported rarely in neonates following large doses (10-20 mg) of phytonadione

Adverse Reactions <1% (Limited to important or life-threatening): Anaphylaxis, cyanosis, diaphoresis, dizziness (rarely), dyspnea, hemolysis in neonates and in patients with G6PD deficiency, hypersensitivity reactions, hypotension (rare)

Drug Interactions

Decreased Effect: The anticoagulant effects of warfarin, dicumarol, anisindione are reversed by phytonadione.

Stability Protect injection from light at all times; may be autoclaved

Mechanism of Action Promotes liver synthesis of clotting factors (II, VII, IX, X); however, the exact mechanism as to this stimulation is unknown. Menadiol is a water soluble form of vitamin K; phytonadione has a more rapid and prolonged effect than menadione; menadiol sodium diphosphate (K₄) is half as potent as menadione (K₃).

Pharmacodynamics/Kinetics

Onset of action: Increased coagulation factors: Oral: 6-12 hours; Parenteral: 1-2 hours; prothrombin may become normal after 12-14 hours

Absorption: Oral: From intestines in presence of bile

Metabolism: Rapidly hepatic

Excretion: Urine and feces

Usual Dosage S.C. is the preferred (per manufacturer) parenteral route; I.V. route should be restricted for emergency use only

Minimum daily requirement: Not well established

Infants: 1-5 mcg/kg/day

Adults: 0.03 mcg/kg/day

Hemorrhagic disease of the newborn:

Prophylaxis: I.M.: 0.5-1 mg within 1 hour of birth

Treatment: I.M., S.C.: 1-2 mg/dose/day

Oral anticoagulant overdose:

Infants: I.M., S.C.: 1-2 mg/dose every 4-8 hours

Children and Adults: Oral, I.V.: 1-10 mg/dose depending on degree of INR elevation

Serious bleeding or major overdose: 10 mg I.V. (slow infusion); may repeat every 12 hours

Vitamin K deficiency: Due to drugs, malabsorption, or decreased synthesis of vitamin K

Infants and Children:

Oral: 2.5-5 mg/24 hours

I.M., I.V.: 1-2 mg/dose as a single dose

Adults:

Oral: 5-25 mg/24 hours

I.M., I.V.: 10 mg

Administration I.V. administration: Dilute in normal saline, D_5W or D_5NS and infuse slowly; rate of infusion should not exceed 1 mg/minute. **This route should be used only if administration by another route is not feasible.** The parenteral preparation has been administered orally to neonates. I.V. administration should not exceed 1 mg/minute; for I.V. infusion, dilute in PF (preservative free) D_5W or normal saline.

Monitoring Parameters PT

Nursing Implications I.V. administration: Dilute in normal saline, D_5W or D_5NS and infuse slowly; rate of infusion should not exceed 1 mg/minute. **This route should be used only if administration by another route is not feasible for phytonadione;** I.V. administration should not exceed 1 mg/minute; for I.V. infusion, dilute in PF (preservative free) D_5W or normal saline.

Additional Information Injection contains benzyl alcohol 0.9% as preservative

Dosage Forms

Injection, aqueous colloidal: 2 mg/mL (0.5 mL)

Injection, aqueous, I.M. only: 10 mg/mL (1 mL)

Tablet: 5 mg

Extemporaneous Preparations A 1 mg/mL oral suspension was stable for only 3 days when refrigerated when compounded as follows:

Triturate six 5 mg tablets in a mortar, reduce to a fine powder, then add 5 mL each of water and methylcellulose 1% while mixing; then transfer to a graduate and qs to 30 mL with sorbitol

Shake well before using and keep in refrigerator

Nahata MC and Hipple TF, *Pediatric Drug Formulations*, 3rd ed, Cincinnati, OH: Harvey Whitney Books Co, 1997.

♦ **Pilagan**® *see Pilocarpine on page 1083*

♦ **Pilocar**® *see Pilocarpine on page 1083*

Pilocarpine (pye loe KAR peen)

Related Information

Glaucoma Drug Therapy Comparison *on page 1499*

U.S. Brand Names Adsorbocarpine®; Akarpine®; Isopto® Carpine; Ocu-Carpine®; Ocusert Pilo-20®; Ocusert Pilo-40®; Pilagan®; Pilocar®; Pilopine HS®; Piloptic®; Pilostat®; Salagen®

Canadian Brand Names Diocarpine; Isopto® Carpine; Miocarpine®; Pilopine HS®; Salagen®; Scheinpharm Pilocarpine

Synonyms Pilocarpine Hydrochloride; Pilocarpine Nitrate

Therapeutic Category Cholinergic Agent; Cholinergic Agent, Ophthalmic; Ophthalmic Agent, Miotic

Use

Ophthalmic: Management of chronic simple glaucoma, chronic and acute angle-closure glaucoma; counter effects of cycloplegics

Orphan drug: Oral: Symptomatic treatment of xerostomia caused by salivary gland hypofunction resulting from radiotherapy for cancer of the head and neck

Pregnancy Risk Factor C

Contraindications Hypersensitivity to pilocarpine or any component of the formulation; acute inflammatory disease of the anterior chamber; tablets are contraindicated in patients with uncontrolled asthma, acute iritis, angle-closure glaucoma

Warnings/Precautions Use with caution in patients with corneal abrasion, CHF, asthma, peptic ulcer, urinary tract obstruction, Parkinson's disease, or narrow-angle glaucoma

Adverse Reactions

Ophthalmic:

>10%: Ocular: Blurred vision, miosis, decrease in night vision

1% to 10%:

Central nervous system: Headache

Genitourinary: Polyuria

Local: Stinging, burning

Ocular: Ciliary spasm, retinal detachment, browache, photophobia, acute iritis, lacrimation, conjunctival and ciliary congestion early in therapy

Miscellaneous: Hypersensitivity reactions

<1% (Limited to important or life-threatening): Hypertension, tachycardia

Systemic: >10%: Miscellaneous: Diaphoresis

1% to 10%:

Cardiovascular: Edema, flushing, hypertension, tachycardia

Central nervous system: Muscle weakness, headache, tremors, chills

Gastrointestinal: Nausea, vomiting, heartburn, dysphagia

Genitourinary: Polyuria

Ocular: Amblyopia

Respiratory: Epistaxis, rhinitis, voice change

Overdosage/Toxicology Symptoms include bronchospasm, bradycardia, involuntary urination, vomiting, hypotension, and tremors. Atropine is the treatment of choice for intoxications manifesting with significant muscarinic symptoms. Atropine I.V. 2-4 mg every 3-60 minutes (or 0.04-0.08 mg I.V. every 5-60 minutes, if needed, for children) should be repeated to control symptoms and then continued as needed for 1-2 days following acute ingestion. Epinephrine 0.1-1 mg S.C. may be useful in reversing severe cardiovascular or pulmonary sequelae.

(Continued)

Pilocarpine (Continued)

Ethanol/Nutrition/Herb Interactions Food: Avoid administering oral formulation with high fat meal; fat decreases the rate of absorption, maximum concentration and increases the time it takes to reach maximum concentration.

Stability Refrigerate gel; store solution at room temperature of 8°C to 30°C (46°F to 86°F) and protect from light. Ocusert® Pilo should be refrigerated.

Mechanism of Action Directly stimulates cholinergic receptors in the eye causing miosis (by contraction of the iris sphincter), loss of accommodation (by constriction of ciliary muscle), and lowering of intraocular pressure (with decreased resistance to aqueous humor outflow)

Pharmacodynamics/Kinetics

Onset of action:

Ophthalmic: Miosis: 10-30 minutes; Intraocular pressure reduction: 1 hour

Ocusert® Pilo: Miosis: 1.5-2 hours; Reduced intraocular pressure: 1.5-2 hours

Oral: 20 minutes

Duration:

Ophthalmic: Miosis: 4-8 hours; Intraocular pressure reduction: 4-12 hours

Ocusert® Pilo: Intraocular pressure reduction: ~1 week

Oral: 3-5 hours

Half-life elimination: Oral: 0.76-1.35 hours

Usual Dosage Adults:

Ophthalmic:

Nitrate solution: Shake well before using; instill 1-2 drops 2-4 times/day

Hydrochloride solution:

Instill 1-2 drops up to 6 times/day; adjust the concentration and frequency as required to control elevated intraocular pressure

To counteract the mydriatic effects of sympathomimetic agents: Instill 1 drop of a 1% solution in the affected eye

Gel: Instill 0.5" ribbon into lower conjunctival sac once daily at bedtime

Ocular systems: Systems are labeled in terms of mean rate of release of pilocarpine over 7 days; begin with 20 mcg/hour at night and adjust based on response

Oral: 5 mg 3 times/day, titration up to 10 mg 3 times/day may be considered for patients who have not responded adequately

Administration

Oral: Avoid administering with high fat meal. Fat decreases the rate of absorption, maximum concentration, and increases the time it takes to reach maximum concentration.

If both solution and gel are used, the solution should be applied first, then the gel at least 5 minutes later. Following administration of the solution, finger pressure should be applied on the lacrimal sac for 1-2 minutes.

Monitoring Parameters Intraocular pressure, funduscopic exam, visual field testing

Patient Information May sting on instillation; notify physician of sweating, urinary retention; usually causes difficulty in dark adaptation; advise patients to use caution while night driving or performing hazardous tasks in poor illumination; after topical instillation, finger pressure should be applied to lacrimal sac to decrease drainage into the nose and throat and minimize possible systemic absorption

Nursing Implications Usually causes difficulty in dark adaptation; advise patients to use caution while night driving or performing hazardous tasks in poor illumination; finger pressure should be applied to lacrimal sac for 1-2 minutes after instillation to decrease risk of absorption and systemic reactions. Assure the patient or a caregiver can adequately administer ophthalmic medication dosage form.

Additional Information Ophthalmic:

Ocusert® 20 mcg is approximately equivalent to 0.5% or 1% drops

Ocusert® 40 mcg is approximately equivalent to 2% or 3% drops

Dosage Forms

Gel, ophthalmic, as hydrochloride (Pilopine HS®): 4% (3.5 g)

Ocular therapeutic system:

Ocusert Pilo-20®: Releases 20 mcg/hour for 1 week (8's)

Ocusert Pilo-40®: Releases 40 mcg/hour for 1 week (8's)

Solution, ophthalmic, as hydrochloride (Adsorbocarpine®, Isopto® Carpine, Pilagan®, Pilocar®, Piloptic®, Pilostat®): 0.25% (15 mL); 0.5% (15 mL, 30 mL); 1% (1 mL, 2 mL, 15 mL, 30 mL); 2% (1 mL, 2 mL, 15 mL, 30 mL); 3% (15 mL, 30 mL); 4% (1 mL, 2 mL, 15 mL, 30 mL); 5% (15 mL); 6% (15 mL, 30 mL); 8% (2 mL); 10% (15 mL)

Solution, ophthalmic, as nitrate (Pilagan®): 1% (15 mL); 2% (15 mL); 4% (15 mL)

Tablet (Salagen®): 5 mg

Pilocarpine and Epinephrine (pye loe KAR peen & ep i NEF rin)

U.S. Brand Names E-Pilo-x®; P$_x$E$_x$®

Canadian Brand Names E-Pilo®

Synonyms Epinephrine and Pilocarpine

Therapeutic Category Cholinergic Agent

Use Treatment of glaucoma; counter effect of cycloplegics

Pregnancy Risk Factor C

Usual Dosage Instill 1-2 drops up to 6 times/day

Additional Information Complete prescribing information for this medication should be consulted for additional detail.

Dosage Forms Solution, ophthalmic: Epinephrine bitartrate 1% and pilocarpine hydrochloride 1%, 2%, 3%, 4%, 6% (10 mL, 15 mL)

♦ **Pimaricin** *see Natamycin on page 961*

Pimozide (PI moe zide)

Related Information
Antipsychotic Agents Comparison *on page 1486*

U.S. Brand Names Orap™

Canadian Brand Names Orap®

Therapeutic Category Antipsychotic Agent, Miscellaneous

Use Suppression of severe motor and phonic tics in patients with Tourette's disorder who have failed to respond satisfactorily to standard treatment

Unlabeled/Investigational Use Psychosis; reported use in individuals with delusions focused on physical symptoms (ie, preoccupation with parasitic infestation); Huntington's chorea

Pregnancy Risk Factor C

Contraindications Hypersensitivity to pimozide or any component of the formulation; severe CNS depression; coma; history of dysrhythmia; prolonged QT syndrome; concurrent use of drugs that are inhibitors of CYP3A3/4, including concurrent use of azole antifungals, macrolide antibiotics (such as clarithromycin or erythromycin), mesoridazine, nefazodone, protease inhibitors (ie, indinavir, nelfinavir, ritonavir, saquinavir), thioridazine, zileuton, and ziprasidone; simple tics other than Tourette's

Warnings/Precautions Sudden, unexpected deaths have been known to occur in patients taking high doses (>10 mg) of pimozide. One possible explanation is prolongation of QT intervals predisposing the patients to arrhythmias. May alter cardiac conduction - life-threatening arrhythmias have occurred with therapeutic doses of phenothiazines. May cause hypotension, use with caution in patients with autonomic instability. Moderately sedating, use with caution in disorders where CNS depression is a feature. Use with caution in Parkinson's disease. Caution in patients with hemodynamic instability; bone marrow suppression; predisposition to seizures; subcortical brain damage; severe cardiac, hepatic, renal, or respiratory disease. Esophageal dysmotility and aspiration have been associated with antipsychotic use - use with caution in patients at risk of pneumonia (ie, Alzheimer's disease). Caution in breast cancer or other prolactin-dependent tumors (may elevate prolactin levels). May alter temperature regulation or mask toxicity of other drugs due to antiemetic effects. May cause orthostatic hypotension - use with caution in patients at risk of this effect or those who would tolerate transient hypotensive episodes (cerebrovascular disease, cardiovascular disease, or other medications which may predispose).

May cause anticholinergic effects (confusion, agitation, constipation, dry mouth, blurred vision, urinary retention); therefore, use with caution in patients with decreased gastrointestinal motility, urinary retention, BPH, xerostomia, or visual problems. Conditions which also may be exacerbated by cholinergic blockade include narrow-angle glaucoma (screening is recommended) and worsening of myasthenia gravis. Relative to neuroleptics, pimozide has a moderate potency of cholinergic blockade.

May cause extrapyramidal symptoms, including pseudoparkinsonism, acute dystonic reactions, akathisia, and tardive dyskinesia (risk of these reactions is high relative to other neuroleptics). May be associated with neuroleptic malignant syndrome (NMS) or pigmentary retinopathy.

Avoid concurrent grapefruit juice, macrolide antibiotics, azole antifungal agents, protease inhibitors, nefazodone, and zileuton due to their potential inhibition of pimozide metabolism, leading to the accumulation of active compound and the increased chance of serious arrhythmias

Adverse Reactions Frequency not defined.
Cardiovascular: Facial edema, tachycardia, orthostatic hypotension, chest pain, hypertension, palpitations, ventricular arrhythmias, QT prolongation
Central nervous system: Extrapyramidal symptoms (akathisia, akinesia, dystonia, pseudoparkinsonism, tardive dyskinesia), drowsiness, NMS, headache, dizziness, excitement
Dermatologic: Rash
Endocrine & metabolic: Edema of breasts, decreased libido
Gastrointestinal: Constipation, xerostomia, weight gain/loss, nausea, salivation, vomiting, anorexia
Genitourinary: Impotence
Hematologic: Blood dyscrasias
Hepatic: Jaundice
Neuromuscular & skeletal: Weakness, tremor
Ocular: Visual disturbance, decreased accommodation, blurred vision
Miscellaneous: Diaphoresis

Overdosage/Toxicology Symptoms include hypotension, respiratory depression, EKG abnormalities, and extrapyramidal symptoms. Following attempts at decontamination, treatment is supportive and symptomatic. Seizures can be treated with diazepam, phenytoin, or phenobarbital.

Drug Interactions
Cytochrome P450 Effect: CYP1A2 enzyme substrate (minor), CYP3A3/4 enzyme substrate
Increased Effect/Toxicity: Pimozide levels/toxicity may be increased by macrolide antibiotics (clarithromycin, erythromycin, dirithromycin, troleandomycin), azole antifungals (fluconazole, itraconazole), protease inhibitors (amprenavir, nelfinavir, ritonavir), nefazodone, ziprasidone, mesoridazine, thioridazine, and zileuton; may predispose to life-threatening arrhythmias. Chloroquine, propranolol, and sulfadoxine-pyrimethamine also may increase pimozide concentrations. Concurrent use with TCA may produce increased toxicity or altered therapeutic response. Pimozide plus lithium may (rarely) produce neurotoxicity. Pimozide and CNS depressants (ethanol, narcotics) may produce additive CNS depressant effects. Pimozide with fluoxetine has been associated with the development of bradycardia (case report).
(Continued)

Pimozide *(Continued)*

Decreased Effect: Barbiturates and carbamazepine may increase the metabolism of pimozide, lowering its serum levels. Benztropine (and other anticholinergics) may inhibit the therapeutic response to pimozide. Antipsychotics such as pimozide inhibit the ability of bromocriptine to lower serum prolactin concentrations. The antihypertensive effects of guanethidine and guanadrel may be inhibited by pimozide. Pimozide may inhibit the antiparkinsonian effect of levodopa. Pimozide (and possibly other low potency antipsychotics) may reverse the pressor effects of epinephrine.

Ethanol/Nutrition/Herb Interactions

Food: Pimozide serum concentration may be increased when taken with grapefruit juice; avoid concurrent use.

Ethanol: Avoid ethanol (may increase CNS depression).

Herb/Nutraceutical: St John's wort may decrease pimozide levels. Avoid kava kava, gotu kola, valerian, St John's wort (may increase CNS depression).

Mechanism of Action A potent centrally-acting dopamine-receptor antagonist resulting in its characteristic neuroleptic effects

Pharmacodynamics/Kinetics

Absorption: 50%

Protein binding: 99%

Metabolism: Hepatic; significant first-pass effect

Half-life elimination: 50 hours

Time to peak, serum: 6-8 hours

Excretion: Urine

Usual Dosage Oral:

Children ≤12 years: Tourette's disorder: Initial: 1-2 mg/day in divided doses; usual range: 2-4 mg/day; do not exceed 10 mg/day (0.2 mg/kg/day)

Children >12 years and Adults: Tourette's disorder: Initial: 1-2 mg/day in divided doses, then increase dosage as needed every other day; range is usually 7-16 mg/day, maximum dose: 20 mg/day or 0.3 mg/kg/day should not be exceeded.

Note: Sudden unexpected deaths have occurred in patients taking doses >10 mg. Therefore, dosages exceeding 10 mg/day are generally not recommended.

Dosing adjustment in hepatic impairment: Reduction of dose is necessary in patients with liver disease

Patient Information Treatment with pimozide exposes the patient to serious risks; a decision to use pimozide chronically in Tourette's disorder is one that deserves full consideration by the patient (or patient's family) as well as by the treating physician. Because the goal of treatment is symptomatic improvement, the patient's view of the need for treatment and assessment of response are critical in evaluating the impact of therapy and weighing its benefits against the risks. Avoid grapefruit juice.

Nursing Implications Perform EKG at baseline and periodically thereafter, and with dose increases; refer to Contraindications for medicines which may predispose patients to fatal cardiac arrhythmias

Additional Information Less sedation but pimozide is more likely to cause acute extrapyramidal symptoms than chlorpromazine.

Dosage Forms Tablet: 1 mg, 2 mg

Pindolol *(PIN doe lole)*

Related Information

Beta-Blockers Comparison *on page 1491*

U.S. Brand Names Visken®

Canadian Brand Names Apo®-Pindol; Gen-Pindolol; Novo-Pindol; Nu-Pindol; PMS-Pindolol; Visken®

Therapeutic Category Antihypertensive Agent; Beta-Adrenergic Blocker

Use Management of hypertension

Unlabeled/Investigational Use Potential augmenting agent for antidepressants; ventricular arrhythmias/tachycardia, antipsychotic-induced akathisia, situational anxiety; aggressive behavior associated with dementia

Pregnancy Risk Factor B

Contraindications Hypersensitivity to pindolol, beta-blockers, or any component of the formulation; uncompensated congestive heart failure; cardiogenic shock; bradycardia, sinus node dysfunction, or heart block (2nd or 3rd degree) except in patients with a functioning artificial pacemaker; pulmonary edema; severe hyperactive airway disease (asthma or COPD); Raynaud's disease

Warnings/Precautions Use with caution in patients with inadequate myocardial function, undergoing anesthesia, bronchospastic disease, diabetes mellitus, hyperthyroidism, impaired hepatic function; abrupt withdrawal of the drug should be avoided (may exacerbate symptoms; discontinue over 1-2 weeks); do not use in pregnant or nursing women; may potentiate hypoglycemia in a diabetic patient and mask signs and symptoms; beta-blockers with intrinsic sympathomimetic activity (including pindolol) do not appear to be of benefit in congestive heart failure

Adverse Reactions

1% to 10%:

Cardiovascular: Chest pain (3%), edema (6%)

Central nervous system: Nightmares/vivid dreams (5%), dizziness (9%), insomnia (10%), fatigue (8%), nervousness (7%), anxiety (<2%)

Dermatologic: Rash, itching (4%)

Gastrointestinal: Nausea (5%), abdominal discomfort (4%)

Neuromuscular & skeletal: Weakness (4%), paresthesia (3%), arthralgia (7%), muscle pain (10%)

Respiratory: Dyspnea (5%)

<1% (Limited to important or life-threatening): Bradycardia, CHF, confusion, hallucinations, hypotension, mental depression, thrombocytopenia

Overdosage/Toxicology Symptoms of intoxication include cardiac disturbances, CNS toxicity, bronchospasm, hypoglycemia, and hyperkalemia. The most common cardiac symptoms include hypotension and bradycardia. Atrioventricular block, intraventricular conduction disturbances, cardiogenic shock, and asystole may occur with severe overdose, especially with membrane-depressant drugs (eg, propranolol). CNS effects include convulsions, coma, and respiratory arrest and are commonly seen with propranolol and other membrane-depressant and lipid-soluble drugs. Treatment is symptomatic for seizures, hypotension, hyperkalemia and hypoglycemia; bradycardia and hypotension resistant to atropine, isoproterenol or pacing may respond to glucagon. Wide QRS defects caused by membrane-depressant poisoning may respond to hypertonic sodium bicarbonate. Repeat-dose charcoal, hemoperfusion, or hemodialysis may be helpful in removal of only those beta-blockers with a small V_d, long half-life, or low intrinsic clearance (acebutolol, atenolol, nadolol, sotalol).

Drug Interactions

Cytochrome P450 Effect: CYP2D6 enzyme substrate

Increased Effect/Toxicity: Pindolol may increase the effects of other drugs which slow AV conduction (digoxin, verapamil, diltiazem), alpha-blockers (prazosin, terazosin), and alpha-adrenergic stimulants (epinephrine, phenylephrine). Pindolol may mask the tachycardia from hypoglycemia caused by insulin and oral hypoglycemics. In patients receiving concurrent therapy, the risk of hypertensive crisis is increased when either clonidine or the beta-blocker is withdrawn. Reserpine has been shown to enhance the effect of beta-blockers. Beta-blockers may increase the action or levels of ethanol, disopyramide, nondepolarizing muscle relaxants, and theophylline although the effects are difficult to predict.

Decreased Effect: Decreased levels/effect of pindolol with aluminum salts, barbiturates, calcium salts, cholestyramine, colestipol, NSAIDs, penicillins (ampicillin), rifampin, salicylates, and sulfinpyrazone due to decreased bioavailability and plasma levels. Beta-blockers may decrease the effect of sulfonylureas (possibly hyperglycemia). Nonselective beta-blockers blunt the effect of beta-2 adrenergic agonists (albuterol).

Ethanol/Nutrition/Herb Interactions Herb/Nutraceutical: Avoid dong quai if using for hypertension (has estrogenic activity). Avoid ephedra, yohimbe, ginseng (may worsen hypertension).

Stability Protect from light

Mechanism of Action Blocks both beta$_1$- and beta$_2$-receptors and has mild intrinsic sympathomimetic activity; pindolol has negative inotropic and chronotropic effects and can significantly slow AV nodal conduction. Augmentive action of antidepressants thought to be mediated via a serotonin 1A autoreceptor antagonism.

Pharmacodynamics/Kinetics

Duration: ~12 hours
Absorption: Rapid, 50% to 95%
Protein binding: 50%
Metabolism: Hepatic, 60% to 65%, to conjugates
Half-life elimination: 2.5-4 hours; increased with renal insufficiency, age, and cirrhosis
Time to peak, serum: 1-2 hours
Excretion: Urine (35% to 50% as unchanged drug)

Usual Dosage Oral:

Adults:
Hypertension: Initial: 5 mg twice daily, increase as necessary by 10 mg/day every 3-4 weeks; maximum daily dose: 60 mg
Antidepressant augmentation: 2.5 mg 3 times/day
Elderly: Initial: 5 mg once daily, increase as necessary by 5 mg/day every 3-4 weeks

Dosing adjustment in renal and hepatic impairment: Reduction is necessary in severely impaired

Dietary Considerations May be taken without regard to meals.

Monitoring Parameters Blood pressure, standing and sitting/supine, pulse, respiratory function

Patient Information Adhere to dosage regimen; watch for postural hypotension; abrupt withdrawal of the drug should be avoided; take at the same time each day; may mask diabetes symptoms; do not discontinue medication abruptly; consult pharmacist or physician before taking over-the-counter cold preparations

Nursing Implications Evaluate blood pressure, apical and radial pulses; do not discontinue abruptly

Dosage Forms Tablet: 5 mg, 10 mg

♦ **Pink Bismuth** see Bismuth on page 170
♦ **Pin-Rid® [OTC]** see Pyrantel Pamoate on page 1159
♦ **Pin-X® [OTC]** see Pyrantel Pamoate on page 1159
♦ **PIO** see Pemoline on page 1048

Pioglitazone (pye oh GLI ta zone)

Related Information
Hypoglycemic Drugs & Thiazolidinedione Information on page 1502

U.S. Brand Names Actos™

Canadian Brand Names Actos™

Therapeutic Category Antidiabetic Agent, Thiazolidinedione; Hypoglycemic Agent, Oral

Use
Type 2 diabetes mellitus (noninsulin dependent, NIDDM), monotherapy: Adjunct to diet and exercise, to improve glycemic control
Type 2 diabetes mellitus (noninsulin dependent, NIDDM), combination therapy with sulfonylurea, metformin, or insulin: When diet, exercise, and a single agent alone does not result in adequate glycemic control

Pregnancy Risk Factor C

Pregnancy/Breast-Feeding Implications Treatment during mid-late gestation was associated with delayed parturition, embryotoxicity and postnatal growth retardation in animal models. Abnormal blood glucose levels are associated with a higher incidence of congenital

(Continued)

Pioglitazone *(Continued)*

abnormalities. Insulin is the drug of choice for the control of diabetes mellitus during pregnancy. In animal studies, pioglitazone has been found to be excreted in milk. It is not known whether pioglitazone is excreted in human milk. Should not be administered to a nursing woman.

Contraindications Hypersensitivity to pioglitazone or any component of the formulation; active liver disease (transaminases >2.5 times the upper limit of normal at baseline); patients who have experienced jaundice during troglitazone therapy

Warnings/Precautions Should not be used in diabetic ketoacidosis. Mechanism requires the presence of insulin, therefore use in type 1 diabetes is not recommended. May potentiate hypoglycemia when used in combination with sulfonylureas or insulin. Use with caution in premenopausal, anovulatory women - may result in a resumption of ovulation, increasing the risk of pregnancy. Use with caution in patients with anemia (may reduce hemoglobin and hematocrit). Use with caution in patients with heart failure or edema - may increase plasma volume and/or increase cardiac hypertrophy. In general, use should be avoided in patients with NYHA class III or IV heart failure. Use with caution in patients with minor elevations in transaminases (AST or ALT) - see Contraindications and Monitoring Parameters. Idiosyncratic hepatotoxicity has been reported with another thiazolidinedione agent (troglitazone) and postmarketing case reports of hepatitis (with rare hepatic failure) have been received for pioglitazone. Monitoring should include periodic determinations of liver function.

Adverse Reactions

>10%:

Endocrine & metabolic: Decreased serum triglycerides, increased HDL cholesterol

Gastrointestinal: Weight gain

Respiratory: Upper respiratory tract infection (13%)

1% to 10%:

Cardiovascular: Edema (5%) (in combination trials with sulfonylureas or insulin, the incidence of edema was as high as 15%)

Central nervous system: Headache (9%), fatigue (4%)

Endocrine & metabolic: Aggravation of diabetes mellitus (5%), hypoglycemia (range 2% to 15% when used in combination with sulfonylureas or insulin)

Hematologic; Anemia (1%)

Neuromuscular & skeletal: Myalgia (5%)

Respiratory: Sinusitis (6%), pharyngitis (5%)

<1% (Limited to important or life-threatening): Congestive heart failure, elevated CPK, elevated transaminases, hepatic failure (very rare), hepatitis

Overdosage/Toxicology Experience in overdose is limited. Symptoms may include hypoglycemia. Treatment is supportive.

Drug Interactions

Cytochrome P450 Effect: CYP2C8 and CYP3A4 substrate

Increased Effect/Toxicity: Ketoconazole (*in vitro*) inhibits metabolism of pioglitazone. Other inhibitors of CYP3A4, including itraconazole, are likely to decrease pioglitazone metabolism. Patients receiving inhibitors of CYP3A4 should have their glycemic control evaluated more frequently.

Decreased Effect: Effects of oral contraceptives may be decreased, based on data from a related compound. This has not been specifically evaluated for pioglitazone. CYP3A3/4 inducers may decrease the therapeutic effect of pioglitazone.

Ethanol/Nutrition/Herb Interactions

Ethanol: Caution with ethanol (may cause hypoglycemia).

Food: Peak concentrations are delayed when administered with food, but the extent of absorption is not affected. Pioglitazone may be taken without regard to meals.

Herb/Nutraceutical: St John's wort may decrease levels. Caution with chromium, garlic, gymnema (may cause hypoglycemia).

Mechanism of Action Thiazolidinedione antidiabetic agent that lowers blood glucose by improving target cell response to insulin, without increasing pancreatic insulin secretion. It has a mechanism of action that is dependent on the presence of insulin for activity. Pioglitazone is a potent and selective agonist for peroxisome proliferator-activated receptor-gamma (PPARgamma). Activation of nuclear PPARgamma receptors influences the production of a number of gene products involved in glucose and lipid metabolism.

Pharmacodynamics/Kinetics

Onset of action: Delayed

Peak effect: Glucose control: Several weeks

Distribution: V_{ss} (apparent): 0.63 L/kg

Protein binding: 99.8%

Metabolism: Hepatic (99%) via CYP2C8 and 3A4 to both active and inactive metabolites

Half-life elimination: Parent drug: 3-7 hours; Total: 16-24 hours

Time to peak: ~2 hours

Excretion: Urine (15% to 30%) and feces as metabolites

Usual Dosage Adults: Oral:

Monotherapy: Initial: 15-30 mg once daily; if response is inadequate, the dosage may be increased in increments up to 45 mg once daily; maximum recommended dose: 45 mg once daily

Combination therapy:

With sulfonylureas: Initial: 15-30 mg once daily; dose of sulfonylurea should be reduced if the patient reports hypoglycemia

With metformin: Initial: 15-30 mg once daily; it is unlikely that the dose of metformin will need to be reduced due to hypoglycemia

With insulin: Initial: 15-30 mg once daily; dose of insulin should be reduced by 10% to 25% if the patient reports hypoglycemia or if the plasma glucose falls to <100 mg/dL. Doses >30 mg/day have not been evaluated in combination regimens.

A 1-week washout period is recommended in patients with normal liver enzymes who are changed from troglitazone to pioglitazone therapy.

Elderly: No dosage adjustment is recommended in elderly patients.

Dosage adjustment in renal impairment: No dosage adjustment is required.

Dosage adjustment in hepatic impairment: Clearance is significantly lower in hepatic impairment. Therapy should not be initiated if the patient exhibits active liver disease or increased transaminases (>2.5 times the upper limit of normal) at baseline.

Dietary Considerations Management of type 2 diabetes mellitus (noninsulin dependent, NIDDM) should include diet control. May be taken without regard to meals.

Administration May be administered without regard to meals

Monitoring Parameters Hemoglobin A$_{1c}$, liver enzymes (prior to initiation and every 2 months for the first year of treatment, then periodically). If the ALT is increased to >2.5 times the upper limit of normal, liver function testing should be performed more frequently until the levels return to normal or pretreatment values. Patients with an elevation in ALT >3 times the upper limit of normal should be rechecked as soon as possible. If the ALT levels remain >3 times the upper limit of normal, therapy with pioglitazone should be discontinued.

Patient Information May be taken without regard to meals. Follow directions of prescriber. Monitor urine or serum glucose as recommended by prescriber. More frequent monitoring is required during periods of stress, trauma, surgery, pregnancy, increased activity or exercise. Avoid alcohol. Report chest pain, rapid heartbeat or palpitations, abdominal pain, fever, rash, hypoglycemia reactions, yellowing of skin or eyes, dark urine or light stool, unusual fatigue, or nausea/vomiting.

Dosage Forms Tablet: 15 mg, 30 mg, 45 mg

Pipecuronium (pi pe kure OH nee um)

Related Information
Neuromuscular Blocking Agents Comparison *on page 1508*

U.S. Brand Names Arduan®

Canadian Brand Names Arduan®

Synonyms Pipecuronium Bromide

Therapeutic Category Neuromuscular Blocker Agent, Nondepolarizing; Skeletal Muscle Relaxant

Use Adjunct to general anesthesia to facilitate endotracheal intubation and to relax skeletal muscles during surgery; to facilitate mechanical ventilation in ICU patients; does not relieve pain or produce sedation

Pregnancy Risk Factor C

Contraindications Hypersensitivity to pipecuronium, bromide, or any component of the formulation

Warnings/Precautions Ventilation must be supported during neuromuscular blockade; use with caution in patients with renal impairment (adjust dosage appropriately); certain clinical conditions may result in potentiation or antagonism of neuromuscular blockade:

Potentiation: Electrolyte abnormalities, severe hyponatremia, severe hypocalcemia, severe hypokalemia, hypermagnesemia, neuromuscular diseases, acidosis, acute intermittent porphyria, renal failure, hepatic failure

Antagonism: Alkalosis, hypercalcemia, demyelinating lesions, peripheral neuropathies, diabetes mellitus

Increased sensitivity in patients with myasthenia gravis, Eaton-Lambert syndrome; resistance in burn patients (>30% of body) for period of 5-70 days postinjury; resistance in patients with muscle trauma, denervation, immobilization, infection; does not counteract bradycardia produced by anesthetics/vagal stimulation. Do not reconstitute with bacteriostatic water for injection for use in newborns (contains benzyl alcohol).

Adverse Reactions
1% to 10%: Cardiovascular: Hypotension, bradycardia
<1% (Limited to important or life-threatening): Anuria, atrial fibrillation, CNS depression, dyspnea, hyperkalemia, hypertension, hypoglycemia, muscle atrophy, myocardial ischemia, respiratory depression, thrombosis, urticaria, ventricular extrasystole

Overdosage/Toxicology Symptoms include paralysis, including cessation of respiration. Treatment includes supporting ventilation by artificial means.

Drug Interactions
Increased Effect/Toxicity: Increased effects are possible with aminoglycosides, beta-blockers, clindamycin, calcium channel blockers, halogenated anesthetics, imipenem, ketamine, lidocaine, loop diuretics (furosemide), macrolides (case reports), magnesium sulfate, procainamide, quinidine, quinolones, tetracyclines, and vancomycin. May increase risk of myopathy if used with high- dose corticosteroids for extended periods.

Decreased Effect: Effect of nondepolarizing neuromuscular blockers may be reduced by carbamazepine (chronic use), corticosteroids (also associated with myopathy - see increased effect), phenytoin (chronic use), sympathomimetics, and theophylline. Anticholinesterases (can prolong the effects of acetylcholine) may decrease effect.

Stability Compatible with D$_5$W, 0.9% sodium chloride, D$_5$ 0.9% sodium chloride, LR, sterile and bacteriostatic water for injection

Mechanism of Action Pipecuronium bromide is a nondepolarizing neuromuscular blocking agent structurally related to pancuronium and vecuronium. Studies in adult patients have demonstrated that pipecuronium is ~20% to 50% more potent than pancuronium as a neuromuscular blocking agent. The neuromuscular effects and pharmacokinetics of pipecuronium appears to lack vagolytic or autonomic activity and produces minimal cardiovascular effects.

Pharmacodynamics/Kinetics
Onset of action (dose dependent): 3-5 minutes
Duration: Clinically effective block: 60-120 minutes following initial dose of 0.07-0.085 mg/kg
Metabolism: Hepatic, primarily to 3-desacetyl-pipecuronium (40% to 50% activity of parent drug)
Half-life elimination: 120-180 minutes
Excretion: Primarily urine (41% as unchanged drug)

Usual Dosage Administer I.V.; dose to effect; doses will vary due to interpatient variability; use ideal body weight for obese patients
(Continued)

Pipecuronium *(Continued)*

Surgery:
Children:
3 months to 1 year: Similar to adult dosage (mg/kg)
1-14 years: May be less sensitive to effects
Adults: Initial: 0.07-0.085 mg/kg or 0.05-0.085 mg/kg after initial dose of succinylcholine for intubation; maintenance: 0.01-0.015 mg/kg 60-120 minutes after initial dose, then 0.01-0.015 mg/kg every 50 minutes
Pretreatment/priming: 10% of intubating dose given 3-5 minutes before initial dose
ICU: Adults: 0.085-0.1 mg/kg bolus followed by 0.5-2 mcg/kg/minute once initial recovery from bolus observed or 0.085-0.1 mg/kg every 90-100 minutes

Dosing adjustment in renal impairment:
Cl_{cr} 81-100 mL/minute: 85 mcg/kg
Cl_{cr} 61-80 mL/minute: 70 mcg/kg
Cl_{cr} 41-60 mL/minute: 55 mcg/kg
Cl_{cr} <40 mL/minute: 50 mcg/kg
Extended duration should be expected

Administration Administer undiluted I.V. injection as a single bolus or via continuous infusion using an infusion pump; not recommended for dilution into or administration from large volume I.V. solutions

Nursing Implications Not recommended for dilution into or administration from large volume I.V. solutions

Additional Information Classified as a long duration neuromuscular blocking agent; produces minimal, if any, histamine release; does not relieve pain or produce sedation; may produce cumulative effect on duration of blockade; recommended for procedures anticipated to last ≥90 minutes

Dosage Forms Injection, as bromide: 10 mg (10 mL)

◆ **Pipecuronium Bromide** *see Pipecuronium on page 1089*

Piperacillin *(pi PER a sil in)*

Related Information
Antimicrobial Drugs of Choice *on page 1588*
Community-Acquired Pneumonia in Adults *on page 1603*
U.S. Brand Names Pipracil®
Canadian Brand Names Pipracil®
Synonyms Piperacillin Sodium
Therapeutic Category Antibiotic, Penicillin
Use Treatment of susceptible infections such as septicemia, acute and chronic respiratory tract infections, skin and soft tissue infections, and urinary tract infections due to susceptible strains of *Pseudomonas*, *Proteus*, and *Escherichia coli* and *Enterobacter*; active against some streptococci and some anaerobic bacteria; febrile neutropenia (as part of combination regimen)
Pregnancy Risk Factor B
Contraindications Hypersensitivity to piperacillin, other penicillins, or any component of the formulation
Warnings/Precautions Dosage modification required in patients with impaired renal function; history of seizure activity; use with caution in patients with a history of beta-lactam allergy
Adverse Reactions Frequency not defined.
Central nervous system: Confusion, convulsions, drowsiness, fever, Jarisch-Herxheimer reaction
Dermatologic: Rash
Endocrine & metabolic: Electrolyte imbalance
Hematologic: Abnormal platelet aggregation and prolonged PT (high doses), hemolytic anemia, Coombs' reaction (positive)
Local: Thrombophlebitis
Neuromuscular & skeletal: Myoclonus
Renal: Acute interstitial nephritis
Miscellaneous: Anaphylaxis, hypersensitivity reactions
Overdosage/Toxicology Symptoms of penicillin overdose include neuromuscular hypersensitivity (agitation, hallucinations, asterixis, encephalopathy, confusion, and seizures) and electrolyte imbalance (with potassium or sodium salts), especially in renal failure. Hemodialysis may be helpful to aid in the removal of the drug from the blood, otherwise, most treatment is supportive or symptom directed.
Drug Interactions
Increased Effect/Toxicity: Probenecid may increase penicillin levels. Neuromuscular blockers may increase duration of blockade.
Decreased Effect: Tetracyclines may decrease penicillin effectiveness. Efficacy of oral contraceptives may be reduced when taken with piperacillin. High concentrations of piperacillin may cause physical inactivation of aminoglycosides and lead to potential toxicity in patients with mild-moderate renal dysfunction.
Stability Reconstituted solution is stable (I.V. infusion) in NS or D_5W for 24 hours at room temperature, 7 days when refrigerated or 4 weeks when frozen; after freezing, thawed solution is stable for 24 hours at room temperature or 48 hours when refrigerated; 40 g bulk vial should **not** be frozen after reconstitution; **incompatible** with aminoglycosides
Mechanism of Action Inhibits bacterial cell wall synthesis by binding to one or more of the penicillin binding proteins (PBPs); which in turn inhibits the final transpeptidation step of peptidoglycan synthesis in bacterial cell walls, thus inhibiting cell wall biosynthesis. Bacteria eventually lyse due to ongoing activity of cell wall autolytic enzymes (autolysins and murein hydrolases) while cell wall assembly is arrested.
Pharmacodynamics/Kinetics
Absorption: I.M.: 70% to 80%
Distribution: Crosses placenta; low concentrations enter breast milk

Protein binding: 22%

Half-life elimination (dose dependent; prolonged with moderately severe renal or hepatic impairment):

Neonates: 1-5 days old: 3.6 hours; >6 days old: 2.1-2.7 hours

Children: 1-6 months: 0.79 hour; 6 months to 12 years: 0.39-0.5 hour

Adults: 36-80 minutes

Time to peak, serum: I.M.: 30-50 minutes

Excretion: Primarily urine; partially feces

Usual Dosage

Neonates: 100 mg/kg every 12 hours

Infants and Children: I.M., I.V.: 200-300 mg/kg/day in divided doses every 4-6 hours

Higher doses have been used in cystic fibrosis: 350-500 mg/kg/day in divided doses every 4-6 hours

Adults: I.M., I.V.:

Moderate infections (urinary tract infections): 2-3 g/dose every 6-12 hours; maximum: 2 g I.M./site

Serious infections: 3-4 g/dose every 4-6 hours; maximum: 24 g/24 hours

Uncomplicated gonorrhea: 2 g I.M. in a single dose accompanied by 1 g probenecid 30 minutes prior to injection

Dosing adjustment in renal impairment: Adults: I.V.:

Cl_{cr} 20-40 mL/minute: Administer 3-4 g every 8 hours

Cl_{cr} <20 mL/minute: Administer 3-4 g every 12 hours

Moderately dialyzable (20% to 50%)

Continuous arteriovenous or venovenous hemodiafiltration effects: Dose as for Cl_{cr} 10-50 mL/minute

Dietary Considerations Sodium content of 1 g: 1.85 mEq

Administration Administer at least 1 hour apart from aminoglycosides

Monitoring Parameters Observe for signs and symptoms for anaphylaxis during first dose

Test Interactions May interfere with urinary glucose tests using cupric sulfate (Benedict's solution, Clinitest®); may inactivate aminoglycosides *in vitro*; false-positive urinary and serum proteins, positive Coombs' test [direct]

Nursing Implications

Administer one hour apart from aminoglycosides; extended spectrum includes *Pseudomonas aeruginosa*; dosage modification required in patients with impaired renal function; can be administered I.V. push over 3-5 minutes at a maximum concentration of 200 mg/mL or I.V. intermittent infusion over 30-60 minutes at a final concentration ≤20 mg/mL

Monitor serum electrolytes, bleeding time especially in patients with renal impairment, periodic tests of renal, hepatic and hematologic function

Dosage Forms Powder for injection, as sodium: 2 g, 3 g, 4 g, 40 g

Piperacillin and Tazobactam Sodium

(pi PER a sil in & ta zoe BAK tam SOW dee um)

Related Information

Antimicrobial Drugs of Choice *on page 1588*

Community-Acquired Pneumonia in Adults *on page 1603*

U.S. Brand Names Zosyn®

Canadian Brand Names Tacozin®

Synonyms Piperacillin Sodium and Tazobactam Sodium

Therapeutic Category Antibiotic, Anaerobic; Antibiotic, Penicillin; Antibiotic, Penicillin & Beta-lactamase Inhibitor

Use Treatment of infections of lower respiratory tract, urinary tract, skin and skin structures, gynecologic, bone and joint infections, and septicemia caused by susceptible organisms. Tazobactam expands activity of piperacillin to include beta-lactamase producing strains of *S. aureus, H. influenzae, Bacteroides*, and other gram-negative bacteria.

Pregnancy Risk Factor B

Pregnancy/Breast-Feeding Implications Breast-feeding/lactation: Use by the breast-feeding mother may result in diarrhea, candidiasis, or allergic response in the infant

Contraindications Hypersensitivity to penicillins, beta-lactamase inhibitors, or any component of the formulation

Warnings/Precautions Due to sodium load and to the adverse effects of high serum concentrations of penicillins, dosage modification is required in patients with impaired or underdeveloped renal function; use with caution in patients with seizures or in patients with history of beta-lactam allergy; safety and efficacy have not been established in children <12 years of age

Adverse Reactions

>10%: Gastrointestinal: Diarrhea (11%)

1% to 10%:

Cardiovascular: Hypertension (2%)

Central nervous system: Insomnia (7%), headache (7% to 8%), agitation (2%), fever (2%), dizziness (1%)

Dermatologic: Rash (4%), pruritus (3%)

Gastrointestinal: Constipation (7% to 8%), nausea (7%), vomiting/dyspepsia (3%)

Respiratory: Rhinitis/dyspnea (~1%)

Miscellaneous: Serum sickness-like reaction

<1% (Limited to important or life-threatening): *Clostridium difficile* colitis, eosinophilia, hepatotoxicity, interstitial nephritis, jaundice, leukopenia, neutropenia, positive direct Coombs' test, prolonged PT and PTT, seizures, thrombocytopenia

Overdosage/Toxicology Symptoms of penicillin overdose include neuromuscular hypersensitivity (agitation, hallucinations, asterixis, encephalopathy, confusion, and seizures) and electrolyte imbalance (with potassium or sodium salts), especially in renal dysfunction. Hemodialysis may be helpful to aid in the removal of the drug from the blood, otherwise, most treatment is supportive or symptom directed.

(Continued)

Piperacillin and Tazobactam Sodium *(Continued)*

Drug Interactions

Increased Effect/Toxicity: Probenecid may increase penicillin levels. Neuromuscular blockers may increase duration of blockade.

Decreased Effect: Tetracyclines may decrease penicillin effectiveness. Efficacy of oral contraceptives may be reduced when taken with piperacillin and tazobactam sodium. Aminoglycosides may cause physical inactivation of aminoglycosides in the presence of high concentrations of piperacillin and potential toxicity in patients with mild-moderate renal dysfunction.

Stability Store at controlled room temperature; after reconstitution, solution is stable in NS or D_5W for 24 hours at room temperature and 7 days when refrigerated; use single-dose vials immediately after reconstitution (discard unused portions after 24 hours at room temperature and 48 hours if refrigerated)

Mechanism of Action Inhibits bacterial cell wall synthesis by binding to one or more of the penicillin binding proteins (PBPs); which in turn inhibits the final transpeptidation step of peptidoglycan synthesis in bacterial cell walls, thus inhibiting cell wall biosynthesis. Bacteria eventually lyse due to ongoing activity of cell wall autolytic enzymes (autolysins and murein hydrolases) while cell wall assembly is arrested. Tazobactam inhibits many beta-lactamases, including staphylococcal penicillinase and Richmond and Sykes types II, III, IV, and V, including extended spectrum enzymes; it has only limited activity against class I beta-lactamases other than class Ic types.

Pharmacodynamics/Kinetics Both AUC and peak concentrations are dose proportional; hepatic impairment does not affect kinetics

Distribution: Well into lungs, intestinal mucosa, skin, muscle, uterus, ovary, prostate, gall-bladder, and bile; penetration into CSF is low in subject with noninflamed meninges

Metabolism: Piperacillin: 6% to 9%; Tazobactam: ~26%; hepatic impairment does not affect the kinetics of piperacillin or tazobactam significantly

Protein binding: Piperacillin: ~26% to 33%; Tazobactam: 31% to 32%

Half-life elimination: Piperacillin: 1 hour; Metabolite: 1-1.5 hours; Tazobactam: 0.7-0.9 hour

Excretion: Both piperacillin and tazobactam are directly proportional to renal function

Piperacillin: Urine (50% to 70%), feces (10% to 20%)

Tazobactam: Urine (26% as inactive metabolite) within 24 hours

Usual Dosage

Children <12 years: Not recommended due to lack of data

Children >12 years and Adults:

Severe infections: I.V.: Piperacillin/tazobactam 4/0.5 g every 8 hours or 3/0.375 g every 6 hours

Moderate infections: I.M.: Piperacillin/tazobactam 2/0.25 g every 6-8 hours; treatment should be continued for ≥7-10 days depending on severity of disease (**Note:** I.M. route not FDA-approved)

Dosing interval in renal impairment:

Cl_{cr} 20-40 mL/minute: Administer 2/0.25 g every 6 hours

Cl_{cr} <20 mL/minute: Administer 2/0.25 g every 8 hours

Hemodialysis: Administer 2/0.25 g every 8 hours with an additional dose of 0.75 g after each dialysis

Continuous arteriovenous or venovenous hemodiafiltration effects: Dose as for Cl_{cr} 10-50 mL/minute

Administration Administer by I.V. infusion over 30 minutes; reconstitute with 5 mL of diluent per 1 g of piperacillin and then further dilute; **compatible** diluents include NS, SW, dextran 6%, D_5W, D_5W with potassium chloride 40 mEq, bacteriostatic saline and water; **incompatible** with lactated Ringer's solution

Monitoring Parameters LFTs, creatinine, BUN, CBC with differential, serum electrolytes, urinalysis, PT, PTT; monitor for signs of anaphylaxis during first dose

Test Interactions Positive Coombs' [direct] test 3.8%, ALT, AST, bilirubin, and LDH

Nursing Implications Discontinue primary infusion, if possible, during infusion and administer aminoglycosides separately from Zosyn®

Additional Information Sodium content of 1 g injection: 54 mg (2.35 mEq)

Dosage Forms Vials at an 8:1 ratio of piperacillin sodium/tazobactam sodium

Injection:

Piperacillin sodium 2 g and tazobactam sodium 0.25 g

Piperacillin sodium 3 g and tazobactam sodium 0.375 g

Piperacillin sodium 4 g and tazobactam sodium 0.5 g

♦ **Piperacillin Sodium** *see* Piperacillin *on page 1090*

♦ **Piperacillin Sodium and Tazobactam Sodium** *see* Piperacillin and Tazobactam Sodium *on page 1091*

♦ **Piperazine Estrone Sulfate** *see* Estropipate *on page 503*

♦ **Pipracil®** *see* Piperacillin *on page 1090*

Pirbuterol *(peer BYOO ter ole)*

Related Information

Bronchodilators, Comparison of Inhaled Sympathomimetics *on page 1493*

U.S. Brand Names Maxair™; Maxair™ Autohaler™

Synonyms Pirbuterol Acetate

Therapeutic Category Beta$_2$-Adrenergic Agonist Agent; Bronchodilator

Use Prevention and treatment of reversible bronchospasm including asthma

Pregnancy Risk Factor C

Contraindications Hypersensitivity to pirbuterol, albuterol, or any component of the formulation

Warnings/Precautions Excessive use may result in tolerance; use with caution in patients with hyperthyroidism, diabetes mellitus; cardiovascular disorders including coronary insufficiency or hypertension or sensitivity to sympathomimetic amines

Adverse Reactions
>10%:
Central nervous system: Nervousness, restlessness
Neuromuscular & skeletal: Trembling
1% to 10%:
Cardiovascular: Tachycardia, pounding heartbeat
Central nervous system: Headache, dizziness, lightheadedness
Gastrointestinal: Taste changes, vomiting, nausea
<1% (Limited to important or life-threatening): Arrhythmias, chest pain, hypertension, insomnia, paradoxical bronchospasm

Overdosage/Toxicology Symptoms include hypertension, tachycardia, angina, and hypokalemia. In cases of overdose, supportive therapy should be instituted and prudent use of a cardioselective beta-adrenergic blocker (eg, atenolol or metoprolol) should be considered, keeping in mind the potential for induction of bronchoconstriction in an asthmatic individual. Dialysis has not been shown to be of value in the treatment of an overdose with this agent.

Drug Interactions
Increased Effect/Toxicity: Increased toxicity with other beta agonists, MAO inhibitors, tricyclic antidepressants.
Decreased Effect: Decreased effect with beta-blockers.

Stability Store between 15°C and 30°C (59°F and 86°F).

Mechanism of Action Pirbuterol is a beta$_2$-adrenergic agonist with a similar structure to albuterol, specifically a pyridine ring has been substituted for the benzene ring in albuterol. The increased beta$_2$ selectivity of pirbuterol results from the substitution of a tertiary butyl group on the nitrogen of the side chain, which additionally imparts resistance of pirbuterol to degradation by monoamine oxidase and provides a lengthened duration of action in comparison to the less selective previous beta-agonist agents.

Pharmacodynamics/Kinetics
Onset of action: Peak effect: Therapeutic: Oral: 2-3 hours with peak serum concentration of 6.2-9.8 mcg/L; Inhalation: 0.5-1 hour
Half-life elimination: 2-3 hours
Metabolism: Hepatic
Excretion: Urine (10% as unchanged drug)

Usual Dosage Children ≥12 years and Adults: 2 inhalations every 4-6 hours for prevention; two inhalations at an interval of at least 1-3 minutes, followed by a third inhalation in treatment of bronchospasm, not to exceed 12 inhalations/day

Administration Inhalation: Shake inhaler well before use.

Monitoring Parameters Respiratory rate, heart rate, and blood pressure

Patient Information Patient instructions are available with product. Do not exceed recommended dosage; rinse mouth with water following each inhalation to help with dry throat and mouth.

Nursing Implications Before using, the inhaler must be shaken well; assess lung sounds, pulse, and blood pressure before administration and during peak of medication; observe patient for wheezing after administration, if this occurs, call prescriber.

Dosage Forms Aerosol for oral inhalation, as acetate:
Maxair™ Autohaler™: 0.2 mg per actuation (2.8 g - 80 inhalations, 14 g - 400 inhalations)
Maxair™: 0.2 mg per actuation (25.6 g - 300 inhalations)

♦ **Pirbuterol Acetate** see Pirbuterol on page 1092

Piroxicam (peer OKS i kam)
Related Information
Nonsteroidal Anti-Inflammatory Agents Comparison on page 1512
U.S. Brand Names Feldene®
Canadian Brand Names Alti-Piroxicam; Apo®-Piroxicam; Feldene™; Gen-Piroxicam; Novo-Pirocam; Nu-Pirox; Pexicam®
Therapeutic Category Analgesic, Nonsteroidal Anti-inflammatory Drug; Anti-inflammatory Agent; Nonsteroidal Anti-inflammatory Drug (NSAID), Oral
Use Management of inflammatory disorders; symptomatic treatment of acute and chronic rheumatoid arthritis, osteoarthritis, and ankylosing spondylitis; also used to treat sunburn
Pregnancy Risk Factor B/D (3rd trimester or near term)
Contraindications Hypersensitivity to piroxicam, aspirin, other nonsteroidal anti-inflammatory drugs (NSAIDs) or any component of the formulation; active GI bleeding; pregnancy (3rd trimester or near term)
Warnings/Precautions Use with caution in patients with impaired cardiac function, dehydration, hypertension, impaired renal function, GI disease (bleeding or ulcers) and patients receiving anticoagulants; elderly have increased risk for adverse reactions to NSAIDs. As many as 60% of elderly can develop peptic ulceration and/or hemorrhage asymptomatically.

Use lowest effective dose for shortest period possible. Use of NSAIDs can compromise existing renal function especially when Cl$_{cr}$ is <30 mL/minute. Withhold for at least 4-6 half-lives prior to surgical or dental procedures. May have adverse effects on fetus. Use with caution with dehydration. Use in children is not recommended.

Adverse Reactions
1% to 10%:
Cardiovascular: Edema
Central nervous system: Headache, dizziness, somnolence, vertigo
Dermatologic: Pruritus, rash
Gastrointestinal: Stomatitis, anorexia, epigastric distress, nausea, constipation, abdominal discomfort, flatulence, diarrhea, indigestion
Hematologic: Decreases in hemoglobin and hematocrit, anemia, leukopenia, eosinophilia
Renal: Elevated BUN, elevated serum creatinine, Polyuria, acute renal failure
Otic: Tinnitus
(Continued)

Piroxicam *(Continued)*

<1% (Limited to important or life-threatening): Abnormal LFTs, aplastic anemia, bone marrow depression, bronchospasm, chest pain, congestive heart failure, dyspnea, erythema multiforme, hemolytic anemia, hepatitis, hyperglycemia, hypertension, hypoglycemia, jaundice, Stevens-Johnson syndrome, thrombocytopenia, toxic epidermal necrolysis

Overdosage/Toxicology Symptoms include nausea, epigastric distress, CNS depression, leukocytosis, and renal failure. Management of nonsteroidal anti-inflammatory drug (NSAID) intoxication is primarily supportive and symptomatic. Fluid therapy is commonly effective in managing hypotension that may occur following an acute NSAID overdose, except when due to acute blood loss. Seizures tend to be very short-lived and often do not require drug treatment; although, recurrent seizures should be treated with I.V. diazepam. Since many of the NSAIDs undergo enterohepatic cycling, multiple doses of charcoal may be needed to reduce the potential for delayed toxicities.

Drug Interactions

Cytochrome P450 Effect: CYP2C9 and 2C18 enzyme substrate

Increased Effect/Toxicity: Increased effect/toxicity of lithium, warfarin, and methotrexate (controversial).

Decreased Effect: Decreased effect of diuretics, beta-blockers. Decreased effect with aspirin, antacids, and cholestyramine.

Ethanol/Nutrition/Herb Interactions

Ethanol: Avoid ethanol (may enhance gastric mucosal irritation).

Food: Onset of effect may be delayed if piroxicam is taken with food.

Herb/Nutraceutical: Avoid cat's claw, dong quai, evening primrose, feverfew, garlic, red clover, horse chestnut, green tea, ginseng, ginkgo (all have additional antiplatelet activity).

Mechanism of Action Inhibits prostaglandin synthesis, acts on the hypothalamus heat-regulating center to reduce fever, blocks prostaglandin synthetase action which prevents formation of the platelet-aggregating substance thromboxane A_2; decreases pain receptor sensitivity. Other proposed mechanisms of action for salicylate anti-inflammatory action are lysosomal stabilization, kinin and leukotriene production, alteration of chemotactic factors, and inhibition of neutrophil activation. This latter mechanism may be the most significant pharmacologic action to reduce inflammation.

Pharmacodynamics/Kinetics

Onset of action: Analgesic: ~1 hour

Peak effect: 3-5 hours

Protein binding: 99%

Metabolism: Hepatic

Half-life elimination: 45-50 hours

Excretion: Primarily urine and feces (small amounts) as unchanged drug (5%) and metabolites

Usual Dosage Oral:

Children: 0.2-0.3 mg/kg/day once daily; maximum dose: 15 mg/day

Adults: 10-20 mg/day once daily; although associated with increase in GI adverse effects, doses >20 mg/day have been used (ie, 30-40 mg/day)

Dosing adjustment in hepatic impairment: Reduction of dosage is necessary

Dietary Considerations May be taken with food to decrease GI adverse effect.

Monitoring Parameters Occult blood loss, hemoglobin, hematocrit, and periodic renal and hepatic function tests; periodic ophthalmologic exams with chronic use

Test Interactions ↑ chloride (S), ↑ sodium (S), ↑ bleeding time

Patient Information Take with food, may cause drowsiness or dizziness

Nursing Implications Monitor occult blood loss, hemoglobin, hematocrit, and periodic renal and hepatic function tests; periodic ophthalmologic exams with chronic use

Dosage Forms Capsule: 10 mg, 20 mg

- ◆ *p*-Isobutylhydratropic Acid *see Ibuprofen on page 697*
- ◆ **Pit** *see Oxytocin on page 1029*
- ◆ **Pitocin**® *see Oxytocin on page 1029*
- ◆ **Pitressin**® *see Vasopressin on page 1408*
- ◆ **Pitrex (Can)** *see Tolnaftate on page 1347*
- ◆ **Placidyl**® *see Ethchlorvynol on page 509*

Plague Vaccine *(plaig vak SEEN)*

Therapeutic Category Vaccine, Inactivated Bacteria

Use Selected travelers to countries reporting cases for whom avoidance of rodents and fleas is impossible; all laboratory and field personnel working with *Yersinia pestis* organisms possibly resistant to antimicrobials; those engaged in *Yersinia pestis* aerosol experiments or in field operations in areas with enzootic plague where regular exposure to potentially infected wild rodents, rabbits, or their fleas cannot be prevented. Prophylactic antibiotics may be indicated following definite exposure, whether or not the exposed persons have been vaccinated.

Pregnancy Risk Factor C

Contraindications Hypersensitivity to any of the vaccine constituents (see manufacturer's label); patients who have had severe local or systemic reactions to a previous dose; defer immunization in patients with a febrile illness until resolved

Warnings/Precautions Pregnancy, unless there is substantial and unavoidable risk of exposure; the expected immune response may not be obtained if plague vaccine is administered to immunosuppressed persons or patients receiving immunosuppressive therapy; be prepared with epinephrine injection (1:1000) in cases of anaphylaxis

Adverse Reactions All serious adverse reactions must be reported to the U.S. Department of Health and Human Services (DHHS) Vaccine Adverse Event Reporting System (VAERS) 1-800-822-7967.

1% to 10%:

Central nervous system: Malaise (10%), fever, headache (7% to 20%)

Dermatologic: Tenderness (20% to 80%)

<1% (Limited to important or life-threatening): Local erythema (5%), nausea (3% to 13%), sterile abscess, tachycardia, vomiting

Mechanism of Action Promotes active immunity to plague in high-risk individuals.

Usual Dosage Three I.M. doses: First dose 1 mL, second dose (0.2 mL) 1 month later, third dose (0.2 mL) 5 months after the second dose; booster doses (0.2 mL) at 1- to 2-year intervals if exposure continues

Administration For patients at risk of hemorrhage following intramuscular injection, the ACIP recommends "it should be administered intramuscularly if, in the opinion of the physician familiar with the patients bleeding risk, the vaccine can be administered with reasonable safety by this route. If the patient receives antihemophilia or other similar therapy, intramuscular vaccination can be scheduled shortly after such therapy is administered. A fine needle (23 gauge or smaller) can be used for the vaccination and firm pressure applied to the site (without rubbing) for at least 2 minutes. The patient should be instructed concerning the risk of hematoma from the injection."

Test Interactions Temporary suppression of tuberculosis skin test

Nursing Implications Federal law requires that the date of administration, the vaccine manufacturer, lot number of vaccine, and the administering person's name, title and address be entered into the patient's permanent medical record

Additional Information Federal law requires that the date of administration, the vaccine manufacturer, lot number of vaccine, and the administering person's name, title, and address be entered into the patient's permanent medical record.

Dosage Forms Injection: 2 mL, 20 mL

- ◆ **Plan B**™ see Levonorgestrel on page 796
- ◆ **Plantago Seed** see Psyllium on page 1158
- ◆ **Plantain Seed** see Psyllium on page 1158
- ◆ **Plaquase**® see Collagenase on page 334
- ◆ **Plaquenil**® see Hydroxychloroquine on page 687
- ◆ **Plasbumin**® see Albumin on page 40
- ◆ **Plasbumin**®**-5 (Can)** see Albumin on page 40
- ◆ **Plasbumin**®**-25 (Can)** see Albumin on page 40
- ◆ **Platinol**® see Cisplatin on page 301
- ◆ **Platinol**®**-AQ** see Cisplatin on page 301
- ◆ **Plavix**® see Clopidogrel on page 321
- ◆ **Plendil**® see Felodipine on page 547
- ◆ **Pletal**® see Cilostazol on page 292

Plicamycin (plye kay MYE sin)

U.S. Brand Names Mithracin®

Canadian Brand Names Mithracin®

Synonyms Mithramycin

Therapeutic Category Antidote, Hypercalcemia; Antineoplastic Agent, Vesicant; Antineoplastic Agent, Miscellaneous; Vesicant

Use Malignant testicular tumors, in the treatment of hypercalcemia and hypercalciuria of malignancy unresponsive to conventional treatment; Paget's disease; blast crisis of chronic granulocytic leukemia

Pregnancy Risk Factor X

Contraindications Hypersensitivity to plicamycin or any component of the formulation; thrombocytopenia; thrombocytopathy; coagulation disorders or any other condition where a bleeding tendency is increased; bone marrow function impaired; pregnancy

Warnings/Precautions The U.S. Food and Drug Administration (FDA) currently recommends that procedures for proper handling and disposal of antineoplastic agents be considered. Use with caution in patients with hepatic or renal impairment; reduce dosage in patients with renal impairment; discontinue if bleeding or epistaxis occurs. Plicamycin may cause permanent sterility and may cause birth defects. **Note:** Dosing of plicamycin is in **micrograms**.

Adverse Reactions

>10%: Gastrointestinal: Anorexia, stomatitis, nausea, vomiting, diarrhea

Nausea and vomiting occur in almost 100% of patients within the first 6 hours after treatment; incidence increases with rapid injection; stomatitis has also occurred

Time course for nausea/vomiting: Onset 4-6 hours; Duration: 4-24 hours

1% to 10%:

Cardiovascular: Facial flushing

Central nervous system: Fever, headache, depression, drowsiness

Endocrine & metabolic: Hypocalcemia

Hematologic: Myelosuppressive: Mild leukopenia and thrombocytopenia

WBC: Moderate, but uncommon

Platelets: Moderate, rapid onset

Onset: 7-10 days

Nadir: 14 days

Recovery: 21 days

Clotting disorders: May also depress hepatic synthesis of clotting factors, leading to a form of coagulopathy; petechiae, increased prothrombin time, epistaxis, and thrombocytopenia may be seen and may require discontinuation of the drug. Epistaxis is frequently the first sign of this bleeding disorder.

Hepatic: Hepatotoxicity

Local: Pain at injection site

Irritant chemotherapy

Renal: Azotemia, nephrotoxicity

Miscellaneous: Hemorrhagic diathesis

Overdosage/Toxicology Symptoms include bone marrow suppression, bleeding syndrome, and thrombocytopenia. Treatment is supportive. Treatment of hemorrhagic episodes should include transfusion of fresh whole blood or packed red blood cells and fresh frozen plasma, vitamin K, and corticosteroids.

(Continued)

Plicamycin *(Continued)*

Drug Interactions

Increased Effect/Toxicity: Calcitonin, etidronate, or glucagon taken with plicamycin may result in additive hypoglycemic effects.

Ethanol/Nutrition/Herb Interactions Ethanol: Avoid ethanol (due to GI irritation).

Stability Store intact vials under refrigeration (2°C to 8°C); vials are stable at room temperature (<25°C) for up to 3 months. Dilute powder in 4.9 mL SWI to result in a concentration of 500 mcg/mL which is stable for 24 hours at room temperature (25°C) and 48 hours under refrigeration (4°C). Further dilution in 1000 mL D$_5$W or NS is stable for 24 hours at room temperature.

Standard I.V. dilution: Dose/1000 mL D$_5$W or NS; solution is stable for 24 hours at room temperature (25°C)

Mechanism of Action Potent osteoclast inhibitor; may inhibit parathyroid hormone effect on osteoclasts; inhibits bone resorption; forms a complex with DNA in the presence of magnesium or other divalent cations inhibiting DNA-directed RNA synthesis

Pharmacodynamics/Kinetics

Onset of action: Decreasing calcium levels: ~24 hours
   Peak effect: Decreasing calcium levels: 48-72 hours
Duration: Decreasing calcium levels: 5-15 days
Distribution: Crosses blood-brain barrier in low concentrations
Protein binding: 0%
Half-life elimination, plasma: 1 hour
Excretion: Urine (90%) within 24 hours

Usual Dosage Refer to individual protocols. Dose should be diluted in 1 L of D$_5$W or NS and administered over 4-6 hours. Dosage should be based on the patient's body weight. If a patient has abnormal fluid retention (ie, edema, hydrothorax or ascites), the patient's ideal weight rather than actual body weight should be used to calculate the dose.

Adults: I.V.:
  Testicular cancer: 25-30 mcg/kg/day for 8-10 days
  Blastic chronic granulocytic leukemia: 25 mcg/kg over 2-4 hours every other day for 3 weeks
  Paget's disease: 15 mcg/kg/day once daily for 10 days
  Hypercalcemia:
    25 mcg/kg single dose which may be repeated in 48 hours if no response occurs
    OR 25 mcg/kg/day for 3-4 days
    OR 25-50 mcg/kg/dose every other day for 3-8 doses

Dosing adjustment in renal impairment:
Cl$_{cr}$ 10-50 mL/minute: Decrease dosage to 75% of normal dose
Cl$_{cr}$ <10 mL/minute: Decrease dosage to 50% of normal dose
Hemodialysis: Unknown
CAPD effects: Unknown
CAVH effects: Unknown

Dosing in hepatic impairment: In the treatment of hypercalcemia in patients with hepatic dysfunction: Reduce dose to 12.5 mcg/kg/day

Administration Administer I.V. infusion over 4-7 hours via central line

Avoid extravasation; local tissue irritation and cellulitis has been reported

Monitoring Parameters Hepatic and renal function tests, CBC, platelet count, prothrombin time, serum electrolytes

Patient Information This medication can only be administered I.V. and frequent blood tests will be necessary to monitor effects of the drug. Report pain, swelling, or irritation at infusion site. Do not take alcohol, prescription, and/or OTC medications containing aspirin or ibuprofen without consulting prescriber. Maintain adequate hydration (2-3 L/day of fluids unless instructed to restrict fluid intake). Maintain good oral hygiene (use a soft toothbrush or cotton applicators several times a day and rinse mouth frequently). You will be susceptible to infection; avoid crowds and infected persons and do not receive any vaccinations unless approved by prescriber. Report persistent fever or chills, unhealed sores, oral or vaginal sores, foul-smelling urine, easy bruising or bleeding, yellowing of eyes or skin, or change in color of urine or stool. The drug may cause permanent sterility and may cause birth defects. Contraception should be used during therapy. The drug may be excreted in breast milk, therefore, an alternative form of feeding your baby should be used.

Nursing Implications Rapid I.V. infusion has been associated with an increased incidence of nausea and vomiting; an antiemetic given prior to and during plicamycin infusion may be helpful. Avoid extravasation since plicamycin is a strong vesicant.

Dosage Forms Powder for injection: 2.5 mg

- **PMS-Dexamethasone (Can)** *see* Dexamethasone *on page 380*
- **PMS-Dicitrate™ (Can)** *see* Sodium Citrate and Citric Acid *on page 1246*
- **PMS-Diclofenac (Can)** *see* Diclofenac *on page 393*
- **PMS-Diclofenac SR (Can)** *see* Diclofenac *on page 393*
- **PMS-Diphenhydramine (Can)** *see* DiphenhydrAMINE *on page 414*
- **PMS-Dipivefrin (Can)** *see* Dipivefrin *on page 422*
- **PMS-Docusate Calcium (Can)** *see* Docusate *on page 430*
- **PMS-Docusate Sodium (Can)** *see* Docusate *on page 430*
- **PMS-Erythromycin (Can)** *see* Erythromycin (Systemic) *on page 486*
- **PMS-Fenofibrate Micro (Can)** *see* Fenofibrate *on page 548*
- **PMS-Fluoxetine (Can)** *see* Fluoxetine *on page 578*
- **PMS-Fluphenazine Decanoate (Can)** *see* Fluphenazine *on page 581*
- **PMS-Flutamide (Can)** *see* Flutamide *on page 586*
- **PMS-Fluvoxamine (Can)** *see* Fluvoxamine *on page 593*
- **PMS-Gemfibrozil (Can)** *see* Gemfibrozil *on page 624*
- **PMS-Glyburide (Can)** *see* GlyBURIDE *on page 635*
- **PMS-Haloperidol LA (Can)** *see* Haloperidol *on page 654*
- **PMS-Hydromorphone (Can)** *see* Hydromorphone *on page 685*
- **PMS-Hydroxyzine (Can)** *see* HydrOXYzine *on page 691*
- **PMS-Indapamide (Can)** *see* Indapamide *on page 715*
- **PMS-Ipratropium (Can)** *see* Ipratropium *on page 740*
- **PMS-Isoniazid (Can)** *see* Isoniazid *on page 747*
- **PMS-Lactulose (Can)** *see* Lactulose *on page 770*
- **PMS-Levobunolol (Can)** *see* Levobunolol *on page 788*
- **PMS-Lindane (Can)** *see* Lindane *on page 806*
- **PMS-Lithium Carbonate (Can)** *see* Lithium *on page 811*
- **PMS-Lithium Citrate (Can)** *see* Lithium *on page 811*
- **PMS-Loperamine (Can)** *see* Loperamide *on page 816*
- **PMS-Loxapine (Can)** *see* Loxapine *on page 826*
- **PMS-Mefenamic Acid (Can)** *see* Mefenamic Acid *on page 850*
- **PMS-Methylphenidate (Can)** *see* Methylphenidate *on page 894*
- **PMS-Metoprolol (Can)** *see* Metoprolol *on page 902*
- **PMS-Nortriptyline (Can)** *see* Nortriptyline *on page 996*
- **PMS-Nystatin (Can)** *see* Nystatin *on page 1001*
- **PMS-Oxybutynin (Can)** *see* Oxybutynin *on page 1023*
- **PMS-Pindolol (Can)** *see* Pindolol *on page 1086*
- **PMS-Polytrimethoprim (Can)** *see* Trimethoprim and Polymyxin B *on page 1377*
- **PMS-Pseudoephedrine (Can)** *see* Pseudoephedrine *on page 1155*
- **PMS-Sodium Polystyrene Sulfonate (Can)** *see* Sodium Polystyrene Sulfonate *on page 1249*
- **PMS-Sotalol (Can)** *see* Sotalol *on page 1252*
- **PMS-Sucralate (Can)** *see* Sucralfate *on page 1266*
- **PMS-Tamoxifen (Can)** *see* Tamoxifen *on page 1286*
- **PMS-Temazepam (Can)** *see* Temazepam *on page 1292*
- **PMS-Terbinafine (Can)** *see* Terbinafine *on page 1298*
- **PMS-Timolol (Can)** *see* Timolol *on page 1334*
- **PMS-Tobramycin (Can)** *see* Tobramycin *on page 1340*
- **PMS-Trazodone (Can)** *see* Trazodone *on page 1362*
- **PMS-Valproic Acid (Can)** *see* Valproic Acid and Derivatives *on page 1398*
- **PMS-Valproic Acid E.C. (Can)** *see* Valproic Acid and Derivatives *on page 1398*
- **Pneumo 23™ (Can)** *see* Pneumococcal Polysaccharide Vaccine (Polyvalent) *on page 1098*
- **Pneumococcal 7-Valent Conjugate Vaccine** *see* Pneumococcal Conjugate Vaccine (7-Valent) *on page 1097*

Pneumococcal Conjugate Vaccine (7-Valent)
(noo moe KOK al KON ju gate vak SEEN, seven vay lent)

U.S. Brand Names Prevnar®

Synonyms Diphtheria CRM₁₉₇ Protein; PCV7; Pneumococcal 7-Valent Conjugate Vaccine

Therapeutic Category Vaccine

Use Immunization of infants and toddlers against *Streptococcus pneumoniae* infection caused by serotypes included in the vaccine

Advisory Committee on Immunization Practices (ACIP) guidelines also recommend PCV7 for use in:

All children ≥23 months

Children ages 24-59 months with: Sickle cell disease (including other sickle cell hemoglobinopathies, asplenia, splenic dysfunction), HIV infection, immunocompromising conditions (congenital immunodeficiencies, renal failure, nephrotic syndrome, diseases associated with immunosuppressive or radiation therapy, solid organ transplant), chronic illnesses (cardiac disease, cerebrospinal fluid leaks, diabetes mellitus, pulmonary disease excluding asthma unless on high dose corticosteroids)

Consider use in all children 24-59 months with priority given to:

Children 24-35 months

Children 24-59 months who are of Alaska native, American Indian, or African-American descent

Children 24-59 months who attend group day care centers

Pregnancy Risk Factor C

(Continued)

Pneumococcal Conjugate Vaccine (7-Valent) *(Continued)*

Contraindications Hypersensitivity to pneumococcal vaccine or any component of the formulation, including diphtheria toxoid; current or recent severe or moderate febrile illness; thrombocytopenia; any contraindication to I.M. injection; not for I.V. use

Warnings/Precautions Caution in latex sensitivity. Children with impaired immune responsiveness may have a reduced response to active immunization. Safety and efficacy have not been established in children <6 weeks of age. Not for I.V. use.

Adverse Reactions All serious adverse reactions must be reported to the U.S. Department of Health and Human Services (DHHS) Vaccine Adverse Event Reporting System (VAERS) 1-800-822-7967.

>10%:
    Central nervous system: Fever, irritability, drowsiness, restlessness
    Dermatologic: Erythema
    Gastrointestinal: Decreased appetite, vomiting, diarrhea
    Local: Induration, tenderness, nodule
1% to 10%: Dermatologic: Rash (0.5% to 1.4%)

Stability Store refrigerated at 2°C to 8°C (36°F to 46°F).

Mechanism of Action Contains saccharides of capsular antigens of serotypes 4, 6B, 9V, 18C, 19F, and 23F, individually conjugated to CRM197 protein

Usual Dosage I.M.:

Infants: 2-6 months: 0.5 mL at approximately 2-month intervals for 3 consecutive doses, followed by a fourth dose of 0.5 mL at 12-15 months of age; first dose may be given as young as 6 weeks of age, but is typically given at 2 months of age. In case of a moderate shortage of vaccine, defer the fourth dose until shortage is resolved; in case of a severe shortage of vaccine, defer third and fourth doses until shortage is resolved.

Previously Unvaccinated Infants and Children:

7-11 months: 0.5 mL for a total of 3 doses; 2 doses at least 4 weeks apart, followed by a third dose after the 1-year birthday (12-15 months), separated from the second dose by at least 2 months. In case of a severe shortage of vaccine, defer the third dose until shortage is resolved.

12-23 months: 0.5 mL for a total of 2 doses, separated by at least 2 months. In case of a severe shortage of vaccine, defer the second dose until shortage is resolved.

24-59 months:

    Healthy Children: 0.5 mL as a single dose. In case of a severe shortage of vaccine, defer dosing until shortage is resolved.

    Children with sickle cell disease, asplenia, HIV infection, chronic illness or immunocompromising conditions (not including bone marrow transplants - results pending; use PPV23 [pneumococcal polysaccharide vaccine, polyvalent] at 12- and 24-months until studies are complete): 0.5 mL for a total of 2 doses, separated by 2 months

Previously Vaccinated Children with a lapse in vaccine administration:

7-11 months: Previously received 1 or 2 doses PCV7: 0.5 mL dose at 7-11 months of age, followed by a second dose ≥2 months later at 12-15 months of age

12-23 months:

    Previously received 1 dose before 12 months of age: 0.5 mL dose, followed by a second dose ≥2 months later

    Previously received 2 doses before age 12 months: 0.5 mL dose ≥2 months after the most recent dose

24-59 months: Any incomplete schedule: 0.5 mL as a single dose; **Note:** Patients with chronic diseases or immunosuppressing conditions should receive 2 doses ≥2 months apart

Administration Do not inject I.V.; avoid intradermal route; administer I.M. (deltoid muscle or lateral mid thigh)

For patients at risk of hemorrhage following intramuscular injection, the ACIP recommends "it should be administered intramuscularly if, in the opinion of the physician familiar with the patients bleeding risk, the vaccine can be administered with reasonable safety by this route. If the patient receives antihemophilia or other similar therapy, intramuscular vaccination can be scheduled shortly after such therapy is administered. A fine needle (23 gauge or smaller) can be used for the vaccination and firm pressure applied to the site (without rubbing) for at least 2 minutes. The patient should be instructed concerning the risk of hematoma from the injection."

Additional Information Children 24-59 months of age at high risk for pneumococcal disease but that have already received pneumococcal polysaccharide vaccine (PPV23) may benefit from the immunologic response induced by PCV7. Suggested dosing: Starting ≥2 months after last PPV23 dose: 0.5 mL dose of PCV7, followed by a second dose ≥2 months later. (**Note:** Although it is believed that this will provide additional protection, safety data is limited.)

Federal law requires that the date of administration, the vaccine manufacturer, lot number of vaccine, and the administering person's name, title and address be entered into the patient's permanent medical record.

Dosage Forms Injection: 2 mcg of each saccharide for each of six serotypes and 4 mcg of a seventh serotype; also 20 mcg of CRM197 carrier protein and 0.125 mg of aluminum phosphate adjuvant per 0.5 mL per dose

Pneumococcal Polysaccharide Vaccine (Polyvalent)

(noo moe KOK al pol i SAK a ride vak SEEN, pol i VAY lent)

Related Information

Immunization Recommendations *on page 1538*
USPHA/IDSA Guidelines for the Prevention of Opportunistic Infections in Persons With HIV *on page 1574*

U.S. Brand Names Pneumovax® 23; Pnu-Imune® 23

Canadian Brand Names Pneumo 23™; Pneumovax® 23; Pnu-Imune® 23

Synonyms PPV23; 23PS; 23-Valent Pneumococcal Polysaccharide Vaccine

Therapeutic Category Vaccine, Inactivated Bacteria

Use Children >2 years of age and adults who are at increased risk of pneumococcal disease and its complications because of underlying health conditions; older adults, including all those ≥65 years of age

Current Advisory Committee on Immunization Practices (ACIP) guidelines recommend **pneumococcal 7-valent conjugate vaccine (PCV7)** be used for children 2-23 months of age and, in certain situations, children up to 59 months of age

Pregnancy Risk Factor C

Pregnancy/Breast-Feeding Implications The safety of vaccine in pregnant women has not been evaluated; it should not be given during pregnancy unless the risk of infection is high

Contraindications Hypersensitivity to pneumococcal vaccine or any component of the formulation; active infection, Hodgkin's disease patients, <10 days prior to or during treatment with immunosuppressive drugs or radiation; <2 years of age (children <5 years of age do not respond satisfactorily to the capsular types of 23-capsular pneumococcal vaccine); pregnancy (the safety of vaccine in pregnant women has not been evaluated; it should not be given during pregnancy unless the risk of infection is high)

Warnings/Precautions Epinephrine injection (1:1000) must be immediately available in the case of anaphylaxis; use caution in individuals who have had episodes of pneumococcal infection within the preceding 3 years (pre-existing pneumococcal antibodies may result in increased reactions to vaccine); may cause relapse in patients with stable idiopathic thrombocytopenia purpura

Adverse Reactions All serious adverse reactions must be reported to the U.S. Department of Health and Human Services (DHHS) Vaccine Adverse Event Reporting System (VAERS) 1-800-822-7967.

>10%: Local: Induration and soreness at the injection site (~72%) (2-3 days)

<1% (Limited to important or life-threatening): Anaphylaxis, arthralgia, erythema, Guillain-Barré syndrome, low-grade fever, myalgia, paresthesia, rash

Stability Refrigerate

Mechanism of Action Although there are more than 80 known pneumococcal capsular types, pneumococcal disease is mainly caused by only a few types of pneumococci. Pneumococcal vaccine contains capsular polysaccharides of 23 pneumococcal types which represent at least 98% of pneumococcal disease isolates in the United States and Europe. The pneumococcal vaccine with 23 pneumococcal capsular polysaccharide types became available in 1983. The 23 capsular pneumococcal vaccine contains purified capsular polysaccharides of pneumococcal types 1, 2, 3, 4, 5, 8, 9, 12, 14, 17, 19, 20, 22, 23, 26, 34, 43, 51, 56, 57, 67, 70 (American Classification). These are the main pneumococcal types associated with serious infections in the United States.

Usual Dosage I.M., S.C.:

Children >2 years and Adults: 0.5 mL

Previously vaccinated with PCV7 vaccine: Children ≥2 years and Adults:

With sickle cell disease, asplenia, immunocompromised or HIV infection: 0.5 mL at ≥2 years of age and ≥2 months after last dose of PCV7; revaccination with PPV23 should be given ≥5 years for children >10 years of age and every 3-5 years for children ≤10 years of age; revaccination should not be administered <3 years after the previous PPV23 dose

With chronic illness: 0.5 mL at ≥2 years of age and ≥2 months after last dose of PCV7; revaccination with PPV23 is not recommended

Following bone marrow transplant (use of PCV7 under study): Administer one dose PPV23 at 12- and 24-months following BMT

Revaccination should be considered:
1. If ≥6 years since initial vaccination has elapsed, or
2. In patients who received 14-valent pneumococcal vaccine and are at highest risk (asplenic) for fatal infection or
3. At ≥6 years in patients with nephrotic syndrome, renal failure, or transplant recipients, or
4. 3-5 years in children with nephrotic syndrome, asplenia, or sickle cell disease

Administration Do not inject I.V., avoid intradermal, administer S.C. or I.M. (deltoid muscle or lateral midthigh)

For patients at risk of hemorrhage following intramuscular injection, the ACIP recommends "it should be administered intramuscularly if, in the opinion of the physician familiar with the patients bleeding risk, the vaccine can be administered with reasonable safety by this route. If the patient receives antihemophilia or other similar therapy, intramuscular injection can be scheduled shortly after such therapy is administered. A fine needle (23 gauge or smaller) can be used for the vaccination and firm pressure applied to the site (without rubbing) for at least 2 minutes. The patient should be instructed concerning the risk of hematoma from the injection."

Additional Information Inactivated bacteria vaccine. Federal law requires that the date of administration, the vaccine manufacturer, lot number of vaccine, and the administering person's name, title, and address be entered into the patient's permanent medical record.

Dosage Forms Injection: 25 mcg each of 23 polysaccharide isolates/0.5 mL dose (0.5 mL, 1 mL, 5 mL)

- **Pneumomist®** *see* Guaifenesin *on page 645*
- **Pneumovax® 23** *see* Pneumococcal Polysaccharide Vaccine (Polyvalent) *on page 1098*
- **Pnu-Imune® 23** *see* Pneumococcal Polysaccharide Vaccine (Polyvalent) *on page 1098*
- **Podocon-25™** *see* Podophyllum Resin *on page 1099*
- **Podofilm® (Can)** *see* Podophyllum Resin *on page 1099*
- **Podofin®** *see* Podophyllum Resin *on page 1099*
- **Podophyllin** *see* Podophyllum Resin *on page 1099*

Podophyllum Resin (po DOF fil um REZ in)

U.S. Brand Names Podocon-25™; Podofin®

Canadian Brand Names Podofilm®

Synonyms Mandrake; May Apple; Podophyllin

Therapeutic Category Keratolytic Agent

(Continued)

Podophyllum Resin (Continued)

Use Topical treatment of benign growths including external genital and perianal warts, papillomas, fibroids; compound benzoin tincture generally is used as the medium for topical application

Pregnancy Risk Factor X

Contraindications Not to be used on birthmarks, moles, or warts with hair growth; cervical, urethral, oral warts; not to be used by diabetic patient or patient with poor circulation; pregnancy

Warnings/Precautions Use of large amounts of drug should be avoided; avoid contact with the eyes as it can cause severe corneal damage; do not apply to moles, birthmarks, or unusual warts; to be applied by a physician only; for external use only; 25% solution should not be applied to or near mucous membranes

Adverse Reactions
1% to 10%:
Dermatologic: Pruritus
Gastrointestinal: Nausea, vomiting, abdominal pain, diarrhea
<1% (Limited to important or life-threatening): Hepatotoxicity, leukopenia, peripheral neuropathy, renal failure, thrombocytopenia

Mechanism of Action Directly affects epithelial cell metabolism by arresting mitosis through binding to a protein subunit of spindle microtubules (tubulin)

Usual Dosage Topical:
Children and Adults: 10% to 25% solution in compound benzoin tincture; apply drug to dry surface, use 1 drop at a time allowing drying between drops until area is covered; total volume should be limited to <0.5 mL per treatment session
Condylomata acuminatum: 25% solution is applied daily; use a 10% solution when applied to or near mucous membranes
Verrucae: 25% solution is applied 3-5 times/day directly to the wart

Patient Information Notify physician if undue skin irritation develops; should be applied by a physician

Nursing Implications Shake well before using; solution should be washed off within 1-4 hours for genital and perianal warts and within 1-2 hours for accessible meatal warts; use protective occlusive dressing around warts to prevent contact with unaffected skin

Dosage Forms Liquid, topical: 25% in benzoin tincture (15 mL)

♦ **Point-Two**® *see* Fluoride *on page 574*
♦ **Polaramine**® *see* Dexchlorpheniramine *on page 383*

Poliovirus Vaccine (Inactivated)

(POE lee oh VYE rus vak SEEN, in ak ti VAY ted)

Related Information
Adverse Events and Vaccination *on page 1553*
Immunization Recommendations *on page 1538*
Recommendations of the Advisory Committee on Immunization Practices (ACIP) *on page 1540*
Recommended Childhood Immunization Schedule - US - 2002 *on page 1539*
Recommended Immunization Schedule for HIV-Infected Children *on page 1543*
USPHA/IDSA Guidelines for the Prevention of Opportunistic Infections in Persons With HIV *on page 1574*

U.S. Brand Names IPOL™

Canadian Brand Names IPOL™

Synonyms Enhanced-potency Inactivated Poliovirus Vaccine; IPV; Salk Vaccine

Therapeutic Category Vaccine, Live Virus and Inactivated Virus

Use
As the global eradication of poliomyelitis continues, the risk for importation of wild-type poliovirus into the United States decreases dramatically. To eliminate the risk for vaccine-associated paralytic poliomyelitis (VAPP), an all-IPV schedule is recommended for routine childhood vaccination in the United States. All children should receive four doses of IPV (at age 2 months, age 4 months, between ages 6-18 months, and between ages 4-6 years). Oral poliovirus vaccine (OPV), if available, may be used only for the following special circumstances:
Mass vaccination campaigns to control outbreaks of paralytic polio
Unvaccinated children who will be traveling within 4 weeks to areas where polio is endemic or epidemic
Children of parents who do not accept the recommended number of vaccine injections; these children may receive OPV only for the third or fourth dose or both. In this situation, healthcare providers should administer OPV only after discussing the risk for VAPP with parents or caregivers.
OPV supplies are expected to be very limited in the United States after inventories are depleted. ACIP reaffirms its support for the global eradication initiative and use of OPV as the vaccine of choice to eradicate polio where it is endemic.

Pregnancy Risk Factor C

Contraindications Hypersensitivity to any component including neomycin, streptomycin, or polymyxin B; defer vaccination for persons with acute febrile illness until recovery

Warnings/Precautions Although there is no convincing evidence documenting adverse effects of either OPV or E-IPV on the pregnant woman or developing fetus, it is prudent on theoretical grounds to avoid vaccinating pregnant women. However, if immediate protection against poliomyelitis is needed, OPV is recommended. OPV should not be given to immunocompromised individuals or to persons with known or possibly immunocompromised family members; E-IPV is recommended in such situations.

Adverse Reactions All serious adverse reactions must be reported to the U.S. Department of Health and Human Services (DHHS) Vaccine Adverse Event Reporting System (VAERS) 1-800-822-7967.
1% to 10%:
Central nervous system: Fever (>101.3°F)

Dermatologic: Rash

Local: Tenderness or pain at injection site

<1% (Limited to important or life-threatening): Crying, decreased appetite, dyspnea, erythema, fatigue, fussiness, Guillain-Barré, reddening of skin, sleepiness, weakness

Stability Refrigerate

Usual Dosage S.C.: **Enhanced-potency inactivated poliovirus vaccine (E-IPV) is preferred for primary vaccination of adults**, two doses S.C. 4-8 weeks apart, a third dose 6-12 months after the second. For adults with a completed primary series and for whom a booster is indicated, either OPV or E-IPV can be given (E-IPV preferred). If immediate protection is needed, either OPV or E-IPV is recommended.

Administration Do not administer I.V.

Nursing Implications Do not administer I.V.

Additional Information Federal law requires that the date of administration, the vaccine manufacturer, lot number of vaccine, and the administering person's name, title, and address be entered into the patient's permanent medical record.

Dosage Forms Injection (E-IPV, Enhanced-Potency Inactivated Poliovirus Vaccine, IPOL™, Poliomyelitis Vaccine, Salk): Suspension of three types of poliovirus (Types 1, 2, and 3) grown in human diploid cell cultures (0.5 mL)

◆ **Polocaine®** *see* Mepivacaine *on page 861*

◆ **Polycidin® Ophthalmic Ointment (Can)** *see* Bacitracin and Polymyxin B *on page 143*

◆ **Polycitra®** *see* Sodium Citrate and Potassium Citrate Mixture *on page 1247*

◆ **Polycitra®-K** *see* Potassium Citrate and Citric Acid *on page 1110*

◆ **Polydine® [OTC]** *see* Povidone-Iodine *on page 1114*

Polyethylene Glycol-Electrolyte Solution

(pol i ETH i leen GLY kol ee LEK troe lite soe LOO shun)

Related Information

Laxatives, Classification and Properties *on page 1504*

U.S. Brand Names Colyte®; GoLYTELY®; MiraLax™; NuLytely®; OCL®

Canadian Brand Names Colyte™; Klean-Prep®; Klean-Prep®; Lyteprep™; PegLyte®; Peglyte™

Synonyms Electrolyte Lavage Solution

Therapeutic Category Cathartic; Laxative, Bowel Evacuant

Use Bowel cleansing prior to GI examination or following toxic ingestion (electrolyte containing solutions only); treatment of occasional constipation (MiraLax™)

Pregnancy Risk Factor C

Pregnancy/Breast-Feeding Implications Reproduction studies have not been conducted in animals or in humans.

Contraindications Hypersensitivity to polyethylene glycol or any component of the formulation; gastrointestinal obstruction, gastric retention, bowel perforation, toxic colitis, megacolon

Warnings/Precautions Do not add flavorings as additional ingredients before use; observe unconscious or semiconscious patients with impaired gag reflex or those who are otherwise prone to regurgitation or aspiration during administration; use with caution in ulcerative colitis, caution against the use of hot loop polypectomy. Evaluate patients with symptoms of bowel obstruction (nausea, vomiting, abdominal pain or distension) prior to use. Do not use MiraLax™ for longer than 2 weeks.

Adverse Reactions Frequency not defined.

Dermatologic: Dermatitis, rash, urticaria

Gastrointestinal: Nausea, abdominal fullness, bloating, abdominal cramps, vomiting, anal irritation, diarrhea, flatulence

Postmarketing and/or case reports: Anaphylaxis, asystole, dehydration and hypokalemia (reported in children), dyspnea (acute), esophageal perforation, Mallory-Weiss tear, pulmonary edema, upper GI bleeding, vomiting with aspiration of PEG

Drug Interactions

Decreased Effect: Oral medications should not be administered within 1 hour of start of therapy.

Stability Store at 15°C to 30°C (59°F to 86°F) before reconstitution.

Powder for solution (with electrolytes): Use within 48 hours of preparation; refrigerate reconstituted solution; tap water may be used for preparation of the solution; shake container vigorously several times to ensure dissolution of powder. Do not add additional flavorings to solution.

MiraLax™: Dissolve powder in 8 ounces of water, juice, cola, or tea

Mechanism of Action Induces catharsis by strong electrolyte and osmotic effects

Pharmacodynamics/Kinetics Onset of effect: Oral: Bowel cleansing: ~1-2 hours; Constipation: 48-96 hours

Usual Dosage

Oral:

Children ≥6 months: Bowel cleansing prior to GI exam (solutions with electrolytes only): 25-40 mL/kg/hour for 4-10 hours (until rectal effluent is clear). Ideally, patients should fast for ~3-4 hours prior to administration; absolutely no solid food for at least 2 hours before the solution is given. The solution may be given via nasogastric tube to patients who are unwilling or unable to drink the solution. Patients <2 years should be monitored closely.

Adults:

Bowel cleansing prior to GI exam (solutions with electrolytes only): 240 mL (8 oz) every 10 minutes, until 4 L are consumed or the rectal effluent is clear; rapid drinking of each portion is preferred to drinking small amounts continuously. Ideally, patients should fast for ~3-4 hours prior to administration; absolutely no solid food for at least 2 hours before the solution is given. The solution may be given via nasogastric tube to patients who are unwilling or unable to drink the solution.

Occasional constipation (MiraLax™): 17 g of powder (~1 heaping tablespoon) dissolved in 8 oz of water; once daily; do not use for >2 weeks.

(Continued)

Polyethylene Glycol-Electrolyte Solution (Continued)

Nasogastric tube:

Children ≥6 months: Bowel cleansing prior to GI exam (solutions with electrolytes only): 25 mL/kg/hour until rectal effluent is clear. Ideally, patients should fast for ~3-4 hours prior to administration; absolutely no solid food for at least 2 hours before the solution is given.

Adults: Bowel cleansing prior to GI exam (solutions with electrolytes only): 20-30 mL/minute (1.2-1.8 L/hour); the first bowel movement should occur ~1 hour after the start of administration. Ideally, patients should fast for ~3-4 hours prior to administration; absolutely no solid food for at least 2 hours before the solution is given.

Dietary Considerations Bowel cleansing prior to GI exam: Ideally, the patient should fast for ~3-4 hours prior to administration, but in no case should solid food be given for at least 2 hours before the solution is given.

Administration Bowel cleansing prior to GI exam (solutions with electrolytes only): Oral: Rapid drinking of each portion is preferred to drinking small amounts continuously. Do not add flavorings as additional ingredients before use. Chilled solution often more palatable.

Monitoring Parameters Electrolytes, serum glucose, BUN, urine osmolality; children <2 years of age should be monitored for hypoglycemia, dehydration, hypokalemia

Patient Information Chilled solution is often more palatable

Nursing Implications Bowel cleansing prior to GI exam (solutions with electrolytes only): Rapid drinking of each portion is preferred over small amounts continuously; first bowel movement should occur in 1 hour; chilled solution often more palatable; do not add flavorings as additional ingredients before use

Dosage Forms

Powder, for oral solution:

Colyte®:

PEG 3350 240 g, sodium sulfate 22.72 g, sodium bicarbonate 6.72 g, sodium chloride 5.84 g, and potassium chloride 2.98 g (to make 4000 mL) [with citrus berry, lemon lime, cherry, and pineapple flavor packets]

PEG 3350 227.1 g, sodium sulfate 21.5 g, sodium bicarbonate 6.36 g, sodium chloride 5.53 g, and potassium chloride 2.82 g (to make 4000 mL) [regular and pineapple flavor]

GoLYTELY®:

Disposable jug: PEG 3350 236 g, sodium sulfate 22.74 g, sodium bicarbonate 6.74 g, sodium chloride 5.86 g, and potassium chloride 2.97 g (to make 4000 mL) [regular and pineapple flavor]

Packets: PEG 3350 227.1 g, sodium sulfate 21.5 g, sodium bicarbonate 6.36 g, sodium chloride 5.53 g, and potassium chloride 2.82 g (to make 4000 mL) [regular flavor]

MiraLax™: PEG 3350 255 g (to make 14 oz); PEG 3350 527 g (to make 26 oz)

NuLytely®: PEG 3350 420 g, sodium bicarbonate 5.72 g, sodium chloride 11.2 g, and potassium chloride 1.48 (to make 4000 mL) [cherry flavor, lemon-lime flavor, and orange flavor]

Solution, oral (OCL®): PEG 3350 6 g, sodium sulfate decahydrate 1.29 g, sodium bicarbonate 168 mg, potassium chloride 75 mg, and polysorbate 80 30 mg per 100 mL (1500 mL)

♦ **Polygam®** see Immune Globulin (Intravenous) on page 711

♦ **Polygam® S/D** see Immune Globulin (Intravenous) on page 711

Polymyxin B (pol i MIKS in bee)

Synonyms Polymyxin B Sulfate

Therapeutic Category Antibiotic, Irrigation; Antibiotic, Miscellaneous

Use Treatment of acute infections caused by susceptible strains of *Pseudomonas aeruginosa*; used occasionally for gut decontamination; parenteral use of polymyxin B has mainly been replaced by less toxic antibiotics, reserved for life-threatening infections caused by organisms resistant to the preferred drugs (eg, pseudomonal meningitis - intrathecal administration)

Pregnancy Risk Factor B (per expert opinion)

Pregnancy/Breast-Feeding Implications Safety and efficacy for use in pregnant women have not been established.

Contraindications Hypersensitivity to polymyxin B or any component of the formulation; concurrent use of neuromuscular blockers

Warnings/Precautions Use with caution in patients with impaired renal function (modify dosage); polymyxin B-induced nephrotoxicity may be manifested by albuminuria, cellular casts, and azotemia. Discontinue therapy with decreasing urinary output and increasing BUN; neurotoxic reactions are usually associated with high serum levels, often in patients with renal dysfunction. Avoid concurrent or sequential use of other nephrotoxic and neurotoxic drugs (eg, aminoglycosides). The drug's neurotoxicity can result in respiratory paralysis from neuromuscular blockade, especially when the drug is given soon after anesthesia or muscle relaxants. Polymyxin B sulfate is most toxic when given parenterally; avoid parenteral use whenever possible.

Adverse Reactions Frequency not defined (limited to important or life-threatening):

Central nervous system: Neurotoxicity (irritability, drowsiness, ataxia, perioral paresthesia, numbness of the extremities, and blurring of vision); dizziness

Neuromuscular & skeletal: Neuromuscular blockade

Renal: Nephrotoxicity

Respiratory: Respiratory arrest

Overdosage/Toxicology Symptoms include respiratory paralysis, ototoxicity, and nephrotoxicity. Supportive care is indicated. Ventilatory support may be necessary.

Drug Interactions

Increased Effect/Toxicity: Increased/prolonged effect of neuromuscular blocking agents.

Stability Prior to reconstitution, store at room temperature of 15°C to 30°C (59°F to 86°F); protect from light. After reconstitution, store under refrigeration at 2°C to 8°C (36°F to 46°F); discard any unused solution after 72 hours. **Incompatible** with strong acids/alkalies, calcium, magnesium, cephalothin, cefazolin, chloramphenicol, heparin, penicillins.

Mechanism of Action Binds to phospholipids, alters permeability, and damages the bacterial cytoplasmic membrane permitting leakage of intracellular constituents

Pharmacodynamics/Kinetics

Absorption: Well absorbed from peritoneum; minimal from GI tract (except in neonates) from mucous membranes or intact skin

Distribution: Minimal into CSF; does not cross placenta

Half-life elimination: 4.5-6 hours, increased with reduced renal function

Time to peak, serum: I.M.: ~2 hours

Excretion: Urine (>60% primarily as unchanged drug)

Usual Dosage

Otic (in combination with other drugs): 1-2 drops, 3-4 times/day; should be used sparingly to avoid accumulation of excess debris

Infants <2 years:

I.M.: Up to 40,000 units/kg/day divided every 6 hours (not routinely recommended due to pain at injection sites)

I.V.: Up to 40,000 units/kg/day divided every 12 hours

Intrathecal: 20,000 units/day for 3-4 days, then 25,000 units every other day for at least 2 weeks after CSF cultures are negative and CSF (glucose) has returned to within normal limits

Children ≥2 years and Adults:

I.M.: 25,000-30,000 units/kg/day divided every 4-6 hours (not routinely recommended due to pain at injection sites)

I.V.: 15,000-25,000 units/kg/day divided every 12 hours

Intrathecal: 50,000 units/day for 3-4 days, then every other day for at least 2 weeks after CSF cultures are negative and CSF (glucose) has returned to within normal limits

Total daily dose should not exceed 2,000,000 units/day

Bladder irrigation: Continuous irrigant or rinse in the urinary bladder for up to 10 days using 20 mg (equal to 200,000 units) added to 1 L of normal saline; usually no more than 1 L of irrigant is used per day unless urine flow rate is high; administration rate is adjusted to patient's urine output

Topical irrigation or topical solution: 500,000 units/L of normal saline; topical irrigation should not exceed 2 million units/day in adults

Gut sterilization: Oral: 15,000-25,000 units/kg/day in divided doses every 6 hours

Clostridium difficile enteritis: Oral: 25,000 units every 6 hours for 10 days

Ophthalmic: A concentration of 0.1% to 0.25% is administered as 1-3 drops every hour, then increasing the interval as response indicates to 1-2 drops 4-6 times/day

Dosing adjustment/interval in renal impairment:

Cl_{cr} 20-50 mL/minute: Administer 75% to 100% of normal dose every 12 hours

Cl_{cr} 5-20 mL/minute: Administer 50% of normal dose every 12 hours

Cl_{cr} <5 mL/minute: Administer 15% of normal dose every 12 hours

Administration Dissolve 500,000 units in 300-500 mL D_5W for continuous I.V. drip; dissolve 500,000 units in 2 mL water for injection, saline, or 1% procaine solution for I.M. injection; dissolve 500,000 units in 10 mL physiologic solution for intrathecal administration

Monitoring Parameters Neurologic symptoms and signs of superinfection; renal function (decreasing urine output and increasing BUN may require discontinuance of therapy)

Reference Range Serum concentrations >5 μg/mL are toxic in adults

Patient Information Report any dizziness or sensations of ringing in the ear, loss of hearing, or any muscle weakness

Nursing Implications Parenteral use is indicated only in life-threatening infections caused by organisms not susceptible to other agents

Additional Information 1 mg = 10,000 units

Dosage Forms Powder for reconstitution: 500,000 units/vial

♦ **Polymyxin B and Bacitracin** *see* Bacitracin and Polymyxin B *on page 143*

Polymyxin B and Hydrocortisone (pol i MIKS in bee & hye droe KOR ti sone)

U.S. Brand Names Otobiotic®

Synonyms Hydrocortisone and Polymyxin B

Therapeutic Category Antibiotic/Corticosteroid, Otic

Use Treatment of superficial bacterial infections of external ear canal

Pregnancy Risk Factor C

Usual Dosage Instill 4 drops 3-4 times/day

Additional Information Complete prescribing information for this medication should be consulted for additional detail.

Dosage Forms Solution, otic: Polymyxin B sulfate 10,000 units and hydrocortisone 0.5% [5 mg/mL] per mL (15 mL)

♦ **Polymyxin B and Neomycin** *see* Neomycin and Polymyxin B *on page 968*

♦ **Polymyxin B and Oxytetracycline** *see* Oxytetracycline and Polymyxin B *on page 1029*

♦ **Polymyxin B and Trimethoprim** *see* Trimethoprim and Polymyxin B *on page 1377*

♦ **Polymyxin B, Bacitracin, and Neomycin** *see* Bacitracin, Neomycin, and Polymyxin B *on page 143*

♦ **Polymyxin B, Bacitracin, Neomycin, and Hydrocortisone** *see* Bacitracin, Neomycin, Polymyxin B, and Hydrocortisone *on page 143*

♦ **Polymyxin B, Neomycin, and Dexamethasone** *see* Neomycin, Polymyxin B, and Dexamethasone *on page 969*

♦ **Polymyxin B, Neomycin, and Gramicidin** *see* Neomycin, Polymyxin B, and Gramicidin *on page 969*

♦ **Polymyxin B, Neomycin, and Hydrocortisone** *see* Neomycin, Polymyxin B, and Hydrocortisone *on page 969*

♦ **Polymyxin B, Neomycin, and Prednisolone** *see* Neomycin, Polymyxin B, and Prednisolone *on page 970*

♦ **Polymyxin B Sulfate** *see* Polymyxin B *on page 1102*

♦ **Poly-Pred®** *see* Neomycin, Polymyxin B, and Prednisolone *on page 970*

Polysaccharide-Iron Complex (pol i SAK a ride-EYE ern KOM pleks)
U.S. Brand Names Hytinic® [OTC]; Niferex® [OTC]; Nu-Iron® [OTC]
Therapeutic Category Iron Salt
Use Prevention and treatment of iron-deficiency anemias
Pregnancy Risk Factor A
Adverse Reactions
>10%: Gastrointestinal: Stomach cramping, constipation, nausea, vomiting, dark stools, GI irritation, epigastric pain, nausea
1% to 10%:
Gastrointestinal: Heartburn, diarrhea
Genitourinary: Discolored urine
Miscellaneous: Staining of teeth
<1% (Limited to important or life-threatening): Contact irritation
Usual Dosage
Children ≥6 years: Tablets/elixir: 50-100 mg/day; may be given in divided doses
Adults:
Tablets/elixir: 50-100 mg twice daily
Capsules: 150-300 mg/day
Patient Information May color stool black, take between meals for maximum absorption; may take with food if GI upset occurs, do not take with milk or antacids; keep out of reach of children
Nursing Implications 100% elemental iron
Dosage Forms
Capsule: Elemental iron 150 mg
Elixir: Elemental iron 100 mg/5 mL (240 mL)
Tablet: Elemental iron 50 mg

◆ **Polysporin® Ophthalmic** see Bacitracin and Polymyxin B on page 143
◆ **Polysporin® Topical [OTC]** see Bacitracin and Polymyxin B on page 143

Polythiazide (pol i THYE a zide)
Related Information
Sulfonamide Derivatives on page 1515
U.S. Brand Names Renese®
Therapeutic Category Antihypertensive Agent; Diuretic, Thiazide
Use Adjunctive therapy in treatment of edema and hypertension
Pregnancy Risk Factor D
Usual Dosage Adults: Oral:
Edema: 1-4 mg/day
Hypertension: 2-4 mg/day
Additional Information Complete prescribing information for this medication should be consulted for additional detail.
Dosage Forms Tablet: 1 mg, 2 mg, 4 mg

◆ **Polythiazide and Prazosin** see Prazosin and Polythiazide on page 1121
◆ **Polytrim®** see Trimethoprim and Polymyxin B on page 1377
◆ **Ponstan® (Can)** see Mefenamic Acid on page 850
◆ **Ponstel®** see Mefenamic Acid on page 850
◆ **Pontocaine®** see Tetracaine on page 1306
◆ **Porcelana® [OTC]** see Hydroquinone on page 686
◆ **Porcelana® Sunscreen [OTC]** see Hydroquinone on page 686

Porfimer (POR fi mer)
U.S. Brand Names Photofrin®
Canadian Brand Names Photofrin®
Synonyms CL184116; Dihematoporphyrin Ether; Porfimer Sodium
Therapeutic Category Antineoplastic Agent, Miscellaneous
Use Orphan drug: Photodynamic therapy (PDT) with porfimer for palliation of patients with completely obstructing esophageal cancer, or of patients with partially obstructing esophageal cancer who cannot be satisfactorily treated with Nd:YAG laser therapy; completely- or partially-obstructing endobronchial nonsmall cell lung cancer; microinvasive endobronchial nonsmall cell lung cancer
Pregnancy Risk Factor C
Contraindications Hypersensitivity to porfimer, porphyrins, or any component of the formulation; porphyria; tracheoesophageal or bronchoesophageal fistula; tumors eroding into a major blood vessel
Warnings/Precautions The U.S. Food and Drug Administration (FDA) currently recommends that procedures for proper handling and disposal of antineoplastic agents be considered. If the esophageal tumor is eroding into the trachea or bronchial tree, the likelihood of tracheoesophageal or bronchoesophageal fistula resulting from treatment is sufficiently high that PDT is not recommended. All patients who receive porfimer sodium will be photosensitive and must observe precautions to avoid exposure of skin and eyes to direct sunlight or bright indoor light for at least 30 days. Some patients remain photosensitive for up to 90 days or more. The photosensitivity is due to residual drug which will be present in all parts of the skin. Exposure of the skin to ambient indoor light is, however, beneficial because the remaining drug will be inactivated gradually and safely through a photobleaching reaction. Patients should not stay in a darkened room during this period and should be encouraged to expose their skin to ambient indoor light. Ocular discomfort has been reported; for at least 30 days, when outdoors, patients should wear dark sunglasses which have an average white light transmittance of <4%. Conventional UV sunscreens are not protective against photosensitivity.

Adverse Reactions
>10%:
  Cardiovascular: Atrial fibrillation, chest pain
  Central nervous system: Fever, pain, insomnia
  Dermatologic: Photosensitivity reaction
  Gastrointestinal: abdominal pain, constipation, dysphagia, nausea, vomiting
    Emetic potential: Low (10% to 30%)
  Hematologic: Anemia
  Neuromuscular & skeletal: Back pain
  Respiratory: Dyspnea, pharyngitis, pleural effusion, pneumonia, respiratory insufficiency
1% to 10%:
  Cardiovascular: Hypertension, hypotension, edema, cardiac failure, tachycardia, chest pain (substernal)
  Central nervous system: Anxiety, confusion
  Endocrine & metabolic: Dehydration
  Gastrointestinal: Diarrhea, heartburn, eructation, esophageal edema, esophageal tumor bleeding, esophageal stricture, esophagitis, hematemesis, melena, weight loss, anorexia
  Genitourinary: Urinary tract infection
  Neuromuscular & skeletal: Weakness
  Respiratory: Coughing, tracheoesophageal fistula
  Miscellaneous: Moniliasis, surgical complication

Overdosage/Toxicology Overdose of laser light following porfimer injection: Increased symptoms and damage to normal tissue might be expected following an overdose of light. Effects of overdosage on the duration of photosensitivity are unknown. Laser treatment should not be given if an overdose of porfimer is administered. In the event of an overdose, patients should protect their eyes and skin from direct sunlight or bright indoor lights for 30 days. At this time, patients should test for residual photosensitivity. Porfimer is not dialyzable.

Drug Interactions
  Increased Effect/Toxicity: Concomitant administration of other photosensitizing agents (eg, tetracyclines, sulfonamides, phenothiazines, sulfonylureas, thiazide diuretics, griseofulvin) could increase the photosensitivity reaction.
  Decreased Effect: Compounds that quench active oxygen species or scavenge radicals (eg, dimethyl sulfoxide, beta-carotene, ethanol, mannitol) would be expected to decrease photodynamic therapy (PDT) activity. Allopurinol, calcium channel blockers, and some prostaglandin synthesis inhibitors could interfere with porfimer. Drugs that decrease clotting, vasoconstriction, or platelet aggregation could decrease the efficacy of PDT. Glucocorticoid hormones may decrease the efficacy of the treatment.

Stability Store intact vials at controlled room temperature of 20°C to 25°C/68°F to 77°F

Reconstitute each vial of porfimer with 31.8 mL of either 5% dextrose injection or 0.9% sodium chloride injection resulting in a final concentration of 2.5 mg/mL and a pH of 7-8. Shake well until dissolved. Do not mix porfimer with other drugs in the same solution. Protect the reconstituted product from bright light and use immediately. Reconstituted porfimer is an opaque solution in which detection of particulate matter by visual inspection is extremely difficult.

Mechanism of Action Photosensitizing agent used in the photodynamic therapy (PDT) of tumors: cytotoxic and antitumor actions of porfimer are light and oxygen dependent. Cellular damage caused by porfimer PDT is a consequence of the propagation of radical reactions.

Pharmacodynamics/Kinetics
  Distribution: V_{dss}: 0.49 L/kg
  Protein binding, plasma: 90%
  Half-life elimination: 250 hours
  Time to peak, serum: ~2 hours
  Excretion: Clearance: Plasma: Total: 0.051 mL/minute/kg

Usual Dosage I.V. (refer to individual protocols):
  Children: Safety and efficacy have not been established
  Adults: I.V.: 2 mg/kg over 3-5 minutes
    Photodynamic therapy is a two-stage process requiring administration of both drug and light. The first stage of PDT is the I.V. injection of porfimer. Illumination with laser light 40-50 hours following the injection with porfimer constitutes the second stage of therapy. A second laser light application may be given 90-120 hours after injection, preceded by gentle debridement of residual tumor.
    Patients may receive a second course of PDT a minimum of 30 days after the initial therapy; up to three courses of PDT (each separated by a minimum of 30 days) can be given. Before each course of treatment, evaluate patients for the presence of a tracheoesophageal or bronchoesophageal fistula.

Administration Administer slow I.V. injection over 3-5 minutes; avoid extravasation; if extravasation occurs, take care to protect the area from light. There is no known benefit from injecting the extravasation site with another substance. Wipe up spills with a damp cloth. Avoid skin and eye contact due to the potential for photosensitivity reactions upon exposure to light; use of rubber gloves and eye protection is recommended. The laser light is administered 40-50 hours following porfimer. Occasionally, a second light application is administered 96-120 hours after the drug.

Patient Information This medication can only be administered I.V. and will be followed by laser light therapy. Avoid any exposure to sunlight or bright indoor light for 30 days following therapy (cover skin with protective clothing and wear dark sunglasses with light transmittance <4% when outdoors - severe blistering, burning, and skin/eye damage can result). After 30 days, test a small area of skin (not face) for remaining sensitivity. Retest sensitivity if traveling to a different geographic area with greater sunshine. Exposure to indoor normal light is beneficial since it will help dissipate photosensitivity gradually. Maintain adequate hydration (2-3 L/day of fluids unless instructed to restrict fluid intake); maintain good oral hygiene (use a soft toothbrush or cotton applicators several times a day and rinse mouth frequently). Small frequent meals, frequent mouth care, sucking lozenges, or chewing gum may reduce nausea or vomiting. Report rapid heart rate, chest pain or palpitations, difficulty breathing or air
(Continued)

Porfimer (Continued)

hunger, persistent fever or chills, foul-smelling urine or burning on urination, swelling of extremities, increased anxiety, confusion, or hallucination.

Dosage Forms Powder for injection, as sodium: 75 mg

♦ **Porfimer Sodium** see Porfimer on page 1104

♦ **Postexposure Prophylaxis for Hepatitis B** see page 1549

♦ **Potasalan®** see Potassium Chloride on page 1108

Potassium Acetate (poe TASS ee um AS e tate)

Therapeutic Category Electrolyte Supplement, Parenteral; Potassium Salt; Vesicant

Use Potassium deficiency; to avoid chloride when high concentration of potassium is needed, source of bicarbonate

Pregnancy Risk Factor C

Contraindications Severe renal impairment; hyperkalemia

Warnings/Precautions Use with caution in patients with renal disease, hyperkalemia, cardiac disease, metabolic alkalosis; must be administered in patients with adequate urine flow

Adverse Reactions

1% to 10%:
  Cardiovascular: Bradycardia
  Endocrine & metabolic: Hyperkalemia
  Neuromuscular & skeletal: Weakness
  Respiratory: Dyspnea
  Local: Local tissue necrosis with extravasation

<1% (Limited to important or life-threatening): Abdominal pain, alkalosis, chest pain, mental confusion, paralysis, paresthesia, phlebitis, throat pain

Overdosage/Toxicology Symptoms include muscle weakness, paralysis, peaked T waves, flattened P waves, prolongation of chloride, QRS complex, and ventricular arrhythmias. Removal of potassium can be accomplished by various means such as removal through the GI tract with Kayexalate® administration, by way of the kidney through diuresis, mineralocorticoid administration or increased sodium intake, by hemodialysis or peritoneal dialysis, or by shifting potassium back into the cells by insulin and glucose infusion or administration of sodium bicarbonate. Calcium chloride will reverse cardiac effects.

Drug Interactions

Increased Effect/Toxicity: Potassium-sparing diuretics, salt substitutes, and ACE inhibitors

Mechanism of Action Potassium is the major cation of intracellular fluid and is essential for the conduction of nerve impulses in heart, brain, and skeletal muscle; contraction of cardiac, skeletal and smooth muscles; maintenance of normal renal function, acid-base balance, carbohydrate metabolism, and gastric secretion

Pharmacodynamics/Kinetics

Distribution: Enters cells via active transport from extracellular fluid

Excretion: Primarily urine; skin and feces (small amounts); most intestinal potassium reabsorbed

Usual Dosage I.V. doses should be incorporated into the patient's maintenance I.V. fluids, intermittent I.V. potassium administration should be reserved for severe depletion situations and requires EKG monitoring; doses listed as mEq of potassium

Treatment of hypokalemia: I.V.:
  Children: 2-5 mEq/kg/day
  Adults: 40-100 mEq/day

I.V. intermittent infusion (must be diluted prior to administration):
  Children: 0.5-1 mEq/kg/dose (maximum: 30 mEq/dose) to infuse at 0.3-0.5 mEq/kg/hour (maximum: 1 mEq/kg/hour)
  Adults: 5-10 mEq/dose (maximum: 40 mEq/dose) to infuse over 2-3 hours (maximum: 40 mEq over 1 hour)

Note: Continuous cardiac monitor recommended for rates >0.5 mEq/hour

Potassium dosage/rate of infusion guidelines:
  Serum potassium >2.5 mEq/L: Maximum infusion rate: 10 mEq/hour; maximum concentration: 40 mEq/L; maximum 24-hour dose: 200 mEq
  Serum potassium <2.5 mEq/L: Maximum infusion rate: 40 mEq/hour; maximum concentration: 80 mEq/L; maximum 24-hour dose: 400 mEq

Administration Potassium must be diluted prior to parenteral administration; maximum recommended concentration (peripheral line): 80 mEq/L; maximum recommended concentration (central line): 150 mEq/L or 15 mEq/100 mL; in severely fluid-restricted patients (with central lines): 200 mEq/L or 20 mEq/100 mL has been used; maximum rate of infusion, see Usual Dosage, I.V. intermittent infusion

Nursing Implications Supplements usually not needed with adequate diet; EKG should be monitored continuously during the course of highly concentrate potassium solutions

Additional Information 1 mEq of acetate is equivalent to the alkalinizing effect of 1 mEq of bicarbonate.

Dosage Forms Injection: 2 mEq/mL (20 mL, 50 mL, 100 mL); 4 mEq/mL (50 mL)

Potassium Acetate, Potassium Bicarbonate, and Potassium Citrate

(poe TASS ee um AS e tate, poe TASS ee um bye KAR bun ate, & poe TASS ee um SIT rate)

U.S. Brand Names Tri-K®

Synonyms Potassium Acetate, Potassium Citrate, and Potassium Bicarbonate; Potassium Bicarbonate, Potassium Acetate, and Potassium Citrate; Potassium Bicarbonate, Potassium Citrate, and Potassium Acetate; Potassium Citrate, Potassium Acetate, and Potassium Bicarbonate; Potassium Citrate, Potassium Bicarbonate, and Potassium Acetate

Therapeutic Category Electrolyte Supplement, Oral

Use Treatment or prevention of hypokalemia

Pregnancy Risk Factor C

Usual Dosage Oral:

Children: 1-4 mEq/kg/24 hours in divided doses as required to maintain normal serum potassium

Adults:

Prevention: 16-24 mEq/day in 2-4 divided doses

Treatment: 40-100 mEq/day in 2-4 divided doses

Additional Information Complete prescribing information for this medication should be consulted for additional detail.

Dosage Forms Solution, oral: 45 mEq/15 mL from potassium acetate 1500 mg, potassium bicarbonate 1500 mg, and potassium citrate 1500 mg per 15 mL

♦ **Potassium Acetate, Potassium Citrate, and Potassium Bicarbonate** *see* Potassium Acetate, Potassium Bicarbonate, and Potassium Citrate *on page 1106*

Potassium Acid Phosphate (poe TASS ee um AS id FOS fate)

U.S. Brand Names K-Phos® Original

Therapeutic Category Potassium Salt; Urinary Acidifying Agent

Use Acidifies urine and lowers urinary calcium concentration; reduces odor and rash caused by ammoniacal urine; increases the antibacterial activity of methenamine

Pregnancy Risk Factor C

Contraindications Severe renal impairment; hyperkalemia, hyperphosphatemia; infected magnesium ammonium phosphate stones

Warnings/Precautions Use with caution in patients receiving other potassium supplementation and in patients with renal insufficiency, or severe tissue breakdown (eg, chemotherapy or hemodialysis)

Adverse Reactions

>10%: Gastrointestinal: Diarrhea, nausea, stomach pain, flatulence, vomiting

1% to 10%:

Cardiovascular: Bradycardia

Endocrine & metabolic: Hyperkalemia

Local: Local tissue necrosis with extravasation

Neuromuscular & skeletal: Weakness

Respiratory: Dyspnea

<1% (Limited to important or life-threatening): Arrhythmia, dyspnea, edema, hyperphosphatemia, hypocalcemia, mental confusion, paralysis, paresthesia, tetany

Overdosage/Toxicology Symptoms include muscle weakness, paralysis, peaked T waves, flattened P waves, prolongation of QRS complex, and ventricular arrhythmias. Removal of potassium can be accomplished by various means such as through the GI tract with Kayexalate® administration, by way of the kidney through diuresis, mineralocorticoid administration or increased sodium intake, by hemodialysis or peritoneal dialysis, or by shifting potassium back into the cells by insulin and glucose infusion or sodium bicarbonate. Calcium chloride will reverse cardiac effects.

Drug Interactions

Increased Effect/Toxicity: Potassium-sparing diuretics, salt substitutes, salicylates, and ACE inhibitors

Decreased Effect: Antacids containing magnesium, calcium or aluminum (bind phosphate and decreased its absorption)

Mechanism of Action The principal intracellular cation; involved in transmission of nerve impulses, muscle contractions, enzyme activity, and glucose utilization

Pharmacodynamics/Kinetics

Absorption: Well absorbed from upper GI tract

Distribution: Enters cells via active transport from extracellular fluid

Excretion: Primarily urine; skin and feces (small amounts); most intestinal potassium reabsorbed

Usual Dosage Adults: Oral: 1000 mg dissolved in 6-8 oz of water 4 times/day with meals and at bedtime; for best results, soak tablets in water for 2-5 minutes, then stir and swallow

Dietary Considerations May be taken with meals.

Monitoring Parameters Serum potassium, sodium, phosphate, calcium; serum salicylates (if taking salicylates)

Test Interactions ↓ ammonia (B)

Patient Information Dissolve tablets completely before drinking; avoid taking magnesium, calcium, or aluminum antacids at the same time; patients may pass old kidney stones when starting therapy; notify physician if experiencing nausea, vomiting, or abdominal pain

Nursing Implications Monitor renal function, electrolytes, calcium, phosphorus, serum potassium

Dosage Forms Tablet: 500 mg [potassium 3.67 mEq] [sodium free]

Potassium Bicarbonate and Potassium Chloride (Effervescent)

(poe TASS ee um bye KAR bun ate & poe TASS ee um KLOR ide, ef er VES ent)

U.S. Brand Names Klorvess® Effervescent; K-Lyte/Cl®

Synonyms Potassium Bicarbonate and Potassium Chloride (Effervescent)

Therapeutic Category Electrolyte Supplement, Oral

Use Treatment or prevention of hypokalemia

Pregnancy Risk Factor C

Usual Dosage Oral:

Children: 1-4 mEq/kg/24 hours in divided doses as required to maintain normal serum potassium

Adults:

Prevention: 16-24 mEq/day in 2-4 divided doses

Treatment: 40-100 mEq/day in 2-4 divided doses

(Continued)

Potassium Bicarbonate and Potassium Chloride (Effervescent)
(Continued)

Additional Information Complete prescribing information for this medication should be consulted for additional detail.

Dosage Forms
Tablet for oral solution, effervescent:
Klorvess®: 20 mEq per packet
K-Lyte/Cl®: 25 mEq, 50 mEq per packet

Potassium Bicarbonate and Potassium Citrate (Effervescent)
(poe TASS ee um bye KAR bun ate & poe TASS ee um SIT rate, ef er VES ent)

U.S. Brand Names Effer-K™; Klor-Con®/EF; K-Lyte®

Synonyms Potassium Bicarbonate and Potassium Citrate (Effervescent)

Therapeutic Category Potassium Salt

Use Treatment or prevention of hypokalemia

Pregnancy Risk Factor C

Contraindications Severe renal impairment, hyperkalemia

Warnings/Precautions Use with caution in patients with renal disease, cardiac disease

Adverse Reactions
>10%: Gastrointestinal: Diarrhea, nausea, stomach pain, flatulence, vomiting
1% to 10%:
Cardiovascular: Bradycardia
Endocrine & metabolic: Hyperkalemia
Local: Local tissue necrosis with extravasation
Neuromuscular & skeletal: Weakness
Respiratory: Dyspnea
<1% (Limited to important or life-threatening): Abdominal pain, alkalosis, chest pain, mental confusion, paralysis, paresthesias, phlebitis, throat pain

Overdosage/Toxicology Symptoms include muscle weakness, paralysis, peaked T waves, flattened P waves, prolongation of QRS complex, and ventricular arrhythmias. Removal of potassium can be accomplished by various means such as through the GI tract with Kayexalate® administration, by way of the kidney through diuresis, mineralocorticoid administration or increased sodium intake, by hemodialysis or peritoneal dialysis, or by shifting potassium back into the cells by insulin and glucose infusion or sodium bicarbonate. Calcium chloride will reverse cardiac effects.

Drug Interactions
Increased Effect/Toxicity: Potassium-sparing diuretics, salt substitutes, ACE inhibitors

Mechanism of Action Needed for the conduction of nerve impulses in heart, brain, and skeletal muscle; contraction of cardiac, skeletal and smooth muscles; maintenance of normal renal function

Pharmacodynamics/Kinetics
Absorption: Well absorbed from upper GI tract
Distribution: Enters cells via active transport from extracellular fluid
Excretion: Primarily urine; skin and feces (small amounts); most intestinal potassium reabsorbed

Usual Dosage Oral:
Children: 1-4 mEq/kg/24 hours in divided doses as required to maintain normal serum potassium
Adults:
Prevention: 16-24 mEq/day in 2-4 divided doses
Treatment: 40-100 mEq/day in 2-4 divided doses

Monitoring Parameters Serum potassium

Test Interactions ↓ ammonia (B)

Patient Information Dissolve completely in 3-8 oz cold water, juice, or other suitable beverage and drink slowly

Nursing Implications Monitor serum potassium

Dosage Forms Tablet, effervescent: 25 mEq

♦ **Potassium Bicarbonate, Potassium Acetate, and Potassium Citrate** *see* Potassium Acetate, Potassium Bicarbonate, and Potassium Citrate *on page 1106*

♦ **Potassium Bicarbonate, Potassium Citrate, and Potassium Acetate** *see* Potassium Acetate, Potassium Bicarbonate, and Potassium Citrate *on page 1106*

Potassium Chloride (poe TASS ee um KLOR ide)

U.S. Brand Names Cena-K®; Gen-K®; K+ 10®; Kaochlor®; Kaochlor® SF; Kaon-Cl®; Kaon-Cl-10®; Kay Ciel®; K+ Care®; K-Dur® 10; K-Dur® 20; K-Lease®; K-Lor™; Klor-Con®; Klor-Con® 8; Klor-Con® 10; Klor-Con®/25; Klorvess®; Klotrix®; K-Norm®; K-Tab®; Micro-K® 10 Extencaps®; Micro-K® Extencaps; Micro-K® LS; Potasalan®; Rum-K®; Slow-K®; Ten-K®

Canadian Brand Names Apo®-K; K-10®; Kaochlor®; K-Dur®; K-Lor®; K-Lyte®/Cl; Micro-k Extencaps®; Roychlor®; Slow-K®

Synonyms KCl

Therapeutic Category Electrolyte Supplement, Oral; Electrolyte Supplement, Parenteral; Potassium Salt; Vesicant

Use Treatment or prevention of hypokalemia

Pregnancy Risk Factor A

Contraindications Severe renal impairment, untreated Addison's disease, heat cramps, hyperkalemia, severe tissue trauma; solid oral dosage forms are contraindicated in patients in whom there is a structural, pathological, and/or pharmacologic cause for delay or arrest in passage through the GI tract; an oral liquid potassium preparation should be used in patients with esophageal compression or delayed gastric emptying time

Warnings/Precautions Use with caution in patients with cardiac disease, severe renal impairment, hyperkalemia

Adverse Reactions
>10%: Gastrointestinal: Diarrhea, nausea, stomach pain, flatulence, vomiting (oral)

1% to 10%:
Cardiovascular: Bradycardia
Endocrine & metabolic: Hyperkalemia
Local: Local tissue necrosis with extravasation, pain at the site of injection
Neuromuscular & skeletal: Weakness
Respiratory: Dyspnea

<1% (Limited to important or life-threatening): Abdominal pain, alkalosis, arrhythmias, chest pain, heart block, hypotension, mental confusion, phlebitis, paresthesias, paralysis, throat pain

Overdosage/Toxicology Symptoms include muscle weakness, paralysis, peaked T waves, flattened P waves, prolongation of QRS complex, and ventricular arrhythmias. Removal of potassium can be accomplished by various means such as through the GI tract with Kayexalate® administration, by way of the kidney through diuresis, mineralocorticoid administration or increased sodium intake, by hemodialysis or peritoneal dialysis, or by shifting potassium back into the cells by insulin and glucose infusion or sodium bicarbonate. Calcium chloride reverses cardiac effects.

Drug Interactions
Increased Effect/Toxicity: Potassium-sparing diuretics, salt substitutes, ACE inhibitors

Stability Store at room temperature, protect from freezing; use only clear solutions; use admixtures within 24 hours

Mechanism of Action Potassium is the major cation of intracellular fluid and is essential for the conduction of nerve impulses in heart, brain, and skeletal muscle; contraction of cardiac, skeletal and smooth muscles; maintenance of normal renal function, acid-base balance, carbohydrate metabolism, and gastric secretion

Pharmacodynamics/Kinetics
Absorption: Well absorbed from upper GI tract
Distribution: Enters cells via active transport from extracellular fluid
Excretion: Primarily urine; skin and feces (small amounts); most intestinal potassium reabsorbed

Usual Dosage I.V. doses should be incorporated into the patient's maintenance I.V. fluids; intermittent I.V. potassium administration should be reserved for severe depletion situations in patients undergoing EKG monitoring.

Normal daily requirements: Oral, I.V.:
Premature infants: 2-6 mEq/kg/24 hours
Term infants 0-24 hours: 0-2 mEq/kg/24 hours
Infants >24 hours: 1-2 mEq/kg/24 hours
Children: 2-3 mEq/kg/day
Adults: 40-80 mEq/day

Prevention during diuretic therapy: Oral:
Children: 1-2 mEq/kg/day in 1-2 divided doses
Adults: 20-40 mEq/day in 1-2 divided doses

Treatment of hypokalemia: Children:
Oral: 1-2 mEq/kg initially, then as needed based on frequently obtained lab values. If deficits are severe or ongoing losses are great, I.V. route should be considered.
I.V.: 1 mEq/kg over 1-2 hours initially, then repeated as needed based on frequently obtained lab values; severe depletion or ongoing losses may require >200% of normal limit needs
I.V. intermittent infusion: Dose should not exceed 1 mEq/kg/hour, or 40 mEq/hour; if it exceeds 0.5 mEq/kg/hour, physician should be at bedside and patient should have continuous EKG monitoring; usual pediatric maximum: 3 mEq/kg/day or 40 mEq/m²/day

Treatment of hypokalemia: Adults:
I.V. intermittent infusion: 5-10 mEq/hour (continuous cardiac monitor recommended for rates >5 mEq/hour), not to exceed 40 mEq/hour; usual adult maximum per 24 hours: 400 mEq/day.
Potassium dosage/rate of infusion guidelines:
Serum potassium >2.5 mEq/L: Maximum infusion rate: 10 mEq/hour; maximum concentration: 40 mEq/L; maximum 24-hour dose: 200 mEq
Serum potassium <2.5 mEq/L: Maximum infusion rate: 40 mEq/hour; maximum concentration: 80 mEq/L; maximum 24-hour dose: 400 mEq
Potassium >2.5 mEq/L:
Oral: 60-80 mEq/day plus additional amounts if needed
I.V.: 10 mEq over 1 hour with additional doses if needed
Potassium <2.5 mEq/L:
Oral: Up to 40-60 mEq initial dose, followed by further doses based on lab values
I.V.: Up to 40 mEq over 1 hour, with doses based on frequent lab monitoring; deficits at a plasma level of 2 mEq/L may be as high as 400-800 mEq of potassium

Dietary Considerations Administer with plenty of fluid and/or food because of stomach irritation and discomfort.

Administration Potassium must be diluted prior to parenteral administration; maximum recommended concentration (peripheral line): 80 mEq/L; maximum recommended concentration (central line): 150 mEq/L or 15 mEq/100 mL; in severely fluid-restricted patients (with central lines): 200 mEq/L or 20 mEq/100 mL has been used; maximum rate of infusion, see Usual Dosage, I.V. intermittent infusion

Monitoring Parameters Serum potassium, glucose, chloride, pH, urine output (if indicated), cardiac monitor (if intermittent infusion or potassium infusion rates >0.25 mEq/kg/hour)

Patient Information Sustained release and wax matrix tablets should be swallowed whole, do not crush or chew; effervescent tablets must be dissolved in water before use; take with food; liquid and granules can be diluted or dissolved in water or juice

Nursing Implications Wax matrix tablets must be swallowed and not allowed to dissolve in mouth

Dosage Forms
Capsule, controlled release, microcapsulated: 600 mg [8 mEq]; 750 mg [10 mEq]
(Continued)

Potassium Chloride *(Continued)*

K-Lease®, K-Norm®, Micro-K® 10 Extencaps®: 750 mg [10 mEq]
Micro-K® Extencaps®: 600 mg [8 mEq]
Crystals for oral suspension, extended release (Micro-K® LS®): 20 mEq per packet
Liquid: 10% [20 mEq/15 mL] (480 mL, 4000 mL); 20% [40 mEq/15 mL] (480 mL, 4000 mL)
Cena-K®, Kaochlor®, Kaochlor® SF, Kay Ciel®, Klorvess®, Potasalan®: 10% [20 mEq/15 mL] (480 mL, 4000 mL)
Cena-K®, Kaon-Cl® 20%: 20% [40 mEq/15 mL] (480 mL, 4000 mL)
Rum-K®: 15% [30 mEq/15 mL] (480 mL, 4000 mL)
Infusion: 0.1 mEq/mL (100 mL); 0.2 mEq/mL (50 mL, 100 mL); 0.3 mEq/mL (100 mL); 0.4 mEq/mL (50 mL, 100 mL); 0.6 mEq/mL (50 mL); 0.8 mEq/mL (50 mL)
Injection, concentrate: 2 mEq/mL
Powder:
Gen-K®, K+ Care®, Kay Ciel®, K-Lor™, Klor-Con®: 20 mEq per packet (30s, 100s)
K+ Care®: 15 mEq per packet (30s, 100s)
K+ Care®, Klor-Con®/25: 25 mEq per packet (30s, 100s)
Tablet, controlled release, microencapsulated:
K-Dur® 10, Ten-K®: 750 mg [10 mEq]
K-Dur® 20: 1500 mg [20 mEq]
Tablet, controlled release, wax matrix: 600 mg [8 mEq]; 750 mg [10 mEq]
K+ 10®, Kaon-Cl-10®, Klor-Con® 10, Klotrix®, K-Tab®: 750 mg [10 mEq]
Kaon-Cl®: 500 mg [6.7 mEq]
Klor-Con® 8, Slow-K®: 600 mg [8 mEq]

Potassium Citrate and Citric Acid *(poe TASS ee um SIT rate & SI trik AS id)*

U.S. Brand Names Polycitra®-K

Synonyms Citric Acid and Potassium Citrate

Therapeutic Category Alkalinizing Agent, Oral

Use Treatment of metabolic acidosis; alkalinizing agent in conditions where long-term maintenance of an alkaline urine is desirable

Pregnancy Risk Factor A

Usual Dosage Oral:
Mild to moderate hypocitraturia: 10 mEq 3 times/day with meals
Severe hypocitraturia: Initial: 20 mEq 3 times/day or 15 mEq 4 times/day with meals or within 30 minutes after meals; do not exceed 100 mEq/day

Additional Information Complete prescribing information for this medication should be consulted for additional detail.

Dosage Forms
Crystals for reconstitution: Potassium citrate 3300 mg and citric acid 1002 mg per packet
Solution, oral: Potassium citrate 1100 mg and citric acid 334 mg per 5 mL

Potassium Citrate and Potassium Gluconate

(poe TASS ee um SIT rate & poe TASS ee um GLOO coe nate)

U.S. Brand Names Twin-K®

Synonyms Potassium Gluconate and Potassium Citrate

Therapeutic Category Electrolyte Supplement, Oral

Use Treatment or prevention of hypokalemia

Pregnancy Risk Factor C

Usual Dosage Oral:
Children: 1-4 mEq/kg/24 hours in divided doses as required to maintain normal serum potassium
Adults:
Prevention: 16-24 mEq/day in 2-4 divided doses
Treatment: 40-100 mEq/day in 2-4 divided doses

Additional Information Complete prescribing information for this medication should be consulted for additional detail.

Dosage Forms Solution, oral: 20 mEq/5 mL from potassium citrate 170 mg and potassium gluconate 170 mg per 5 mL

♦ **Potassium Citrate Mixture and Sodium Citrate** *see* Sodium Citrate and Potassium Citrate Mixture *on page 1247*
♦ **Potassium Citrate, Potassium Acetate, and Potassium Bicarbonate** *see* Potassium Acetate, Potassium Bicarbonate, and Potassium Citrate *on page 1106*
♦ **Potassium Citrate, Potassium Bicarbonate, and Potassium Acetate** *see* Potassium Acetate, Potassium Bicarbonate, and Potassium Citrate *on page 1106*

Potassium Gluconate *(poe TASS ee um GLOO coe nate)*

U.S. Brand Names Glu-K® [OTC]; Kaon®; K-G®

Canadian Brand Names Kaon®

Therapeutic Category Potassium Salt

Use Treatment or prevention of hypokalemia

Pregnancy Risk Factor A

Contraindications Severe renal impairment, untreated Addison's disease, heat cramps, hyperkalemia, severe tissue trauma; solid oral dosage forms are contraindicated in patients in whom there is a structural, pathological, and/or pharmacologic cause for delay or arrest in passage through the GI tract; an oral liquid potassium preparation should be used in patients with esophageal compression or delayed gastric emptying time

Warnings/Precautions Use with caution in patients with cardiac disease, severe renal impairment, hyperkalemia; patients must be on a cardiac monitor during intermittent infusions

Adverse Reactions
>10%: Gastrointestinal: Diarrhea, nausea, stomach pain, flatulence, vomiting (oral)
1% to 10%:
Cardiovascular: Bradycardia

Endocrine & metabolic: Hyperkalemia
Neuromuscular & skeletal: Weakness
Respiratory: Dyspnea
<1% (Limited to important or life-threatening): Mental confusion, paralysis, paresthesias, phlebitis

Overdosage/Toxicology Symptoms include muscle weakness, paralysis, peaked T waves, flattened P waves, prolongation of QRS complex, and ventricular arrhythmias. Removal of potassium can be accomplished by various means such as through the GI tract with Kayexalate® administration, by way of the kidney through diuresis, mineralocorticoid administration or increased sodium intake, by hemodialysis or peritoneal dialysis, or by shifting potassium back into the cells by insulin, glucose infusion, or sodium bicarbonate. Calcium chloride reverses cardiac effects.

Drug Interactions
Increased Effect/Toxicity: Potassium-sparing diuretics, salt substitutes, ACE inhibitors; increased effect of digitalis

Stability Store at room temperature, protect from freezing; use only clear solutions

Mechanism of Action Potassium is the major cation of intracellular fluid and is essential for the conduction of nerve impulses in heart, brain, and skeletal muscle; contraction of cardiac, skeletal and smooth muscles; maintenance of normal renal function, acid-base balance, carbohydrate metabolism, and gastric secretion

Pharmacodynamics/Kinetics
Absorption: Well absorbed from upper GI tract
Distribution: Enters cells via active transport from extracellular fluid
Excretion: Primarily urine; skin and feces (small amounts); most intestinal potassium reabsorbed

Usual Dosage Oral (doses listed as mEq of potassium):
Normal daily requirement:
Children: 2-3 mEq/kg/day
Adults: 40-80 mEq/day
Prevention of hypokalemia during diuretic therapy:
Children: 1-2 mEq/kg/day in 1-2 divided doses
Adults: 16-24 mEq/day in 1-2 divided doses
Treatment of hypokalemia:
Children: 2-5 mEq/kg/day in 2-4 divided doses
Adults: 40-100 mEq/day in 2-4 divided doses

Administration Liquid potassium preparation should be used in patients with esophageal compression or delayed gastric-emptying time

Monitoring Parameters Serum potassium, chloride, glucose, pH, urine output (if indicated)

Test Interactions ↓ ammonia (B)

Patient Information Take with food, water, or fruit juice; swallow tablets whole; do not crush or chew

Nursing Implications Do not administer liquid full strength, must be diluted in 2-6 parts of water or juice

Additional Information 9.4 g potassium gluconate is approximately equal to 40 mEq potassium (4.3 mEq potassium/g potassium gluconate).

Dosage Forms
Elixir (K-G®, Kaon®): 20 mEq/15 mL
Tablet (Glu-K®): 2 mEq

♦ **Potassium Gluconate and Potassium Citrate** *see* Potassium Citrate and Potassium Gluconate *on page 1110*

Potassium Iodide (poe TASS ee um EYE oh dide)
U.S. Brand Names Pima®; SSKI®
Canadian Brand Names Thyro-Block®
Synonyms KI; Lugol's Solution; Strong Iodine Solution
Therapeutic Category Antithyroid Agent; Cough Preparation; Expectorant
Use Expectorant for the symptomatic treatment of chronic pulmonary diseases complicated by mucous; reduce thyroid vascularity prior to thyroidectomy and management of thyrotoxic crisis; block thyroidal uptake of radioactive isotopes of iodine in a radiation emergency or other exposure to radioactive iodine
Unlabeled/Investigational Use Lymphocutaneous and cutaneous sporotrichosis
Pregnancy Risk Factor D
Pregnancy/Breast-Feeding Implications Iodide crosses the placenta (may cause hypothyroidism and goiter in fetus/newborn). Use as an expectorant during pregnancy is contraindicated by the AAP. Use for protection against thyroid cancer secondary to radioactive iodine exposure is considered acceptable based upon risk/benefit, keeping in mind the dose and duration. Enters breast milk; use caution in breast-feeding (AAP rates "compatible").
Contraindications Hypersensitivity to iodine or any component of the formulation; hyperkalemia; pulmonary edema; impaired renal function; hyperthyroidism; iodine-induced goiter; pregnancy (see Pregnancy Implications)
Warnings/Precautions Prolonged use can lead to hypothyroidism; cystic fibrosis patients have an exaggerated response; can cause acne flare-ups, can cause dermatitis; use with caution in patients with a history of thyroid disease, Addison's disease, cardiac disease, myotonia congenita, tuberculosis, acute bronchitis
Adverse Reactions Frequency not defined.
Cardiovascular: Irregular heart beat
Central nervous system: Confusion, tiredness, fever
Dermatologic: Skin rash
Endocrine & metabolic: Goiter, salivary gland swelling/tenderness, thyroid adenoma, swelling of neck/throat, myxedema, lymph node swelling
Gastrointestinal: Diarrhea, gastrointestinal bleeding, metallic taste, nausea, stomach pain, stomach upset, vomiting
Neuromuscular & skeletal: Numbness, tingling, weakness
(Continued)

Potassium Iodide (Continued)

Miscellaneous: Chronic iodine poisoning (with prolonged treatment/high doses); iodism, hypersensitivity reactions (angioedema, cutaneous and mucosal hemorrhage, serum sickness-like symptoms)

Overdosage/Toxicology Symptoms include angioedema, laryngeal edema in patients with hypersensitivity; muscle weakness, paralysis, peaked T waves, flattened P waves, prolongation of QRS complex, ventricular arrhythmias. Removal of potassium can be accomplished by various means such as through the GI tract with Kayexalate® administration, by way of the kidney through diuresis, mineralocorticoid administration or increased sodium intake, by hemodialysis or peritoneal dialysis, or by shifting potassium back into the cells by insulin and glucose infusion.

Drug Interactions

Increased Effect/Toxicity: Lithium may cause additive hypothyroid effects; ACE-inhibitors, potassium-sparing diuretics, and potassium/potassium-containing products may lead to hyperkalemia, cardiac arrhythmias, or cardiac arrest

Stability Store at controlled room temperature of 25°C (77°F) excursions permitted to 15°C to 30°C (59°F to 86°F); protect from light, keep tightly closed.

SSKI®: If exposed to cold, crystallization may occur. Warm and shake to redissolve. If solution becomes brown/yellow, it should be discarded. May be mixed in water, fruit juice, or milk.

Mechanism of Action Reduces viscosity of mucus by increasing respiratory tract secretions; inhibits secretion of thyroid hormone, fosters colloid accumulation in thyroid follicles

Pharmacodynamics/Kinetics

Onset of action: 24-48 hours

Peak effect: 10-15 days after continuous therapy

Duration: May persist for up to 6 weeks

Excretion: Clearance: Euthyroid patient: Renal: 2 times that of thyroid

Usual Dosage Oral:

Adults: RDA: 150 mcg (iodide)

Expectorant:

Children (Pima®):

<3 years: 162 mg 3 times day

>3 years: 325 mg 3 times/day

Adults:

Pima®: 325-650 mg 3 times/day

SSKI®: 300-600 mg 3-4 times/day

Preoperative thyroidectomy: Children and Adults: 50-250 mg (1-5 drops SSKI®) 3 times/day **or** 0.1-0.3 mL (3-5 drops) of strong iodine (Lugol's solution) 3 times/day; administer for 10 days before surgery

Radiation protectant to radioactive isotopes of iodine (Pima®):

Children:

Infants up to 1 year: 65 mg once daily for 10 days; start 24 hours prior to exposure

>1 year: 130 mg once daily for 10 days; start 24 hours prior to exposure

Adults: 195 mg once daily for 10 days; start 24 hours prior to exposure

To reduce risk of thyroid cancer following nuclear accident (dosing should continue until risk of exposure has passed or other measures are implemented):

Children (see adult dose for children >68 kg):

Infants <1 month: 16 mg once daily

1 month to 3 years: 32 mg once daily

3-18 years: 65 mg once daily

Children >68 kg and Adults (including pregnant/lactating women): 130 mg once daily

Thyrotoxic crisis:

Infants <1 year: 150-250 mg (3-5 drops SSKI®) 3 times/day

Children and Adults: 300-500 mg (6-10 drops SSKI®) 3 times/day or 1 mL strong iodine (Lugol's solution) 3 times/day

Sporotrichosis (cutaneous, lymphocutaneous): Adults: Oral: Initial: 5 drops (SSKI®) 3 times/day; increase to 40-50 drops (SSKI®) 3 times/day as tolerated for 3-6 months

Dietary Considerations SSKI®: Take with food to decrease gastric irritation.

Administration

Pima®: When used as an expectorant, take each dose with at least 4-6 ounces of water

SSKI®: Dilute in a glassful of water, fruit juice or milk. Take with food to decrease gastric irritation

Monitoring Parameters Thyroid function tests, signs/symptoms of hyperthyroidism

Test Interactions May alter thyroid function tests.

Patient Information SSKI®: Take after meals. Dilute in 6 oz of water, fruit juice, or milk. Do not exceed recommended dosage. You may experience a metallic taste. Discontinue use and report stomach pain, severe nausea or vomiting, black or tarry stools, or unresolved weakness. Notify prescriber if pregnant or breast-feeding; do not get pregnant while taking this medication.

Additional Information 10 drops of SSKI® = potassium iodide 500 mg

Dosage Forms

Solution, oral:

SSKI®: 1 g/mL (30 mL, 240 mL) [contains sodium thiosulfate]

Lugol's solution, strong iodine: Potassium iodide 100 mg/mL with iodine 50 mg/mL

Syrup (Pima®): 325 mg/5 mL [equivalent to iodide 249 mg/5 mL] (473 mL) [black raspberry flavor]

Potassium Phosphate (poe TASS ee um FOS fate)

U.S. Brand Names Neutra-Phos®-K

Synonyms Phosphate, Potassium

Therapeutic Category Electrolyte Supplement, Oral; Electrolyte Supplement, Parenteral; Phosphate Salt; Potassium Salt; Vesicant

Use Treatment and prevention of hypophosphatemia or hypokalemia

Pregnancy Risk Factor C

Contraindications Hyperphosphatemia, hyperkalemia, hypocalcemia, hypomagnesemia, renal failure

Warnings/Precautions Use with caution in patients with renal insufficiency, cardiac disease, metabolic alkalosis; admixture of phosphate and calcium in I.V. fluids can result in calcium phosphate precipitation

Adverse Reactions

>10%: Gastrointestinal: Diarrhea, nausea, stomach pain, flatulence, vomiting

1% to 10%:

Cardiovascular: Bradycardia

Endocrine & metabolic: Hyperkalemia

Neuromuscular & skeletal: Weakness

Respiratory: Dyspnea

<1% (Limited to important or life-threatening): Acute renal failure, arrhythmia, chest pain, decreased urine output, dyspnea, edema, mental confusion, paralysis, paresthesias, phlebitis, tetany (with large doses of phosphate)

Overdosage/Toxicology Symptoms include muscle weakness, paralysis, peaked T waves, flattened P waves, prolongation of QRS complex, ventricular arrhythmias, tetany, and calcium-phosphate precipitation. Removal of potassium can be accomplished by various means such as through the GI tract with Kayexalate® administration, by way of the kidney through diuresis, mineralocorticoid administration or increased sodium intake, by hemodialysis or peritoneal dialysis, or by shifting potassium back into the cells by insulin, glucose infusion, or sodium bicarbonate. Calcium chloride reverses cardiac effects.

Drug Interactions

Increased Effect/Toxicity: Potassium-sparing diuretics, salt substitutes, or ACE inhibitors; increased effect of digitalis

Decreased Effect: Aluminum and magnesium-containing antacids or sucralfate can act as phosphate binders

Ethanol/Nutrition/Herb Interactions Food: Avoid administering with oxalate (berries, nuts, chocolate, beans, celery, tomato) or phytate-containing foods (bran, whole wheat).

Stability Store at room temperature, protect from freezing; use only clear solutions; up to 10-15 mEq of calcium may be added per liter before precipitate may occur

Stability of parenteral admixture at room temperature (25°C): 24 hours

Phosphate salts may precipitate when mixed with calcium salts; solubility is improved in amino acid parenteral nutrition solutions; check with a pharmacist to determine compatibility

Usual Dosage I.V. doses should be incorporated into the patient's maintenance I.V. fluids; intermittent I.V. infusion should be reserved for severe depletion situations in patients undergoing continuous EKG monitoring. It is difficult to determine total body phosphorus deficit; the following dosages are empiric guidelines:

Normal requirements elemental phosphorus: Oral:

0-6 months: 240 mg

6-12 months: 360 mg

1-10 years: 800 mg

>10 years: 1200 mg

Pregnancy lactation: Additional 400 mg/day

Adults: 800 mg

Treatment: It is difficult to provide concrete guidelines for the treatment of severe hypophosphatemia because the extent of total body deficits and response to therapy are difficult to predict. Aggressive doses of phosphate may result in a transient serum elevation followed by redistribution into intracellular compartments or bone tissue. It is recommended that repletion of severe hypophosphatemia (<1 mg/dL in adults) be done I.V. because large doses of oral phosphate may cause diarrhea and intestinal absorption may be unreliable

Pediatric I.V. phosphate repletion:

Children: 0.25-0.5 mmol/kg **administer over 4-6 hours and repeat if symptomatic hypophosphatemia persists**; to assess the need for further phosphate administration, obtain serum inorganic phosphate after administration of the first dose and base further doses on serum levels and clinical status

Adult I.V. phosphate repletion:

Initial dose: 0.08 mmol/kg if recent uncomplicated hypophosphatemia

Initial dose: 0.16 mmol/kg if prolonged hypophosphatemia with presumed total body deficits; increase dose by 25% to 50% if patient symptomatic with severe hypophosphatemia

Do not exceed 0.24 mmol/kg/day; administer over 6 hours by I.V. infusion

With orders for I.V. phosphate, there is considerable confusion associated with the use of millimoles (mmol) versus milliequivalents (mEq) to express the phosphate requirement. Because inorganic phosphate exists as monobasic and dibasic anions, with the mixture of valences dependent on pH, ordering by mEq amounts is unreliable and may lead to large dosing errors. In addition, I.V. phosphate is available in the sodium and potassium salt; therefore, the content of these cations must be considered when ordering phosphate. The most reliable method of ordering I.V. phosphate is by millimoles, then specifying the potassium or sodium salt. For example, an order for 15 mmol of phosphate as potassium phosphate in one liter of normal saline. The dosing of phosphate should be 0.2-0.3 mmol/kg with a usual daily requirement of 30-60 mmol/day or 15 mmol of phosphate per liter of TPN or 15 mmol phosphate per 1000 calories of dextrose. Would also provide 22 mEq of potassium.

Maintenance:

I.V. solutions:

Children: 0.5-1.5 mmol/kg/24 hours I.V. or 2-3 mmol/kg/24 hours orally in divided doses

Adults: 15-30 mmol/24 hours I.V. or 50-150 mmol/24 hours orally in divided doses

Oral:

Children <4 years: 1 capsule (250 mg phosphorus/8 mmol) 4 times/day; dilute as instructed

(Continued)

Potassium Phosphate (Continued)

Children >4 years and Adults: 1-2 capsules (250-500 mg phosphorus/8-16 mmol) 4 times/day; dilute as instructed

Administration Injection must be diluted in appropriate I.V. solution and volume prior to administration and administered over a minimum of 4 hours

Monitoring Parameters Serum potassium, calcium, phosphate, sodium, cardiac monitor (when intermittent infusion or high-dose I.V. replacement needed)

Test Interactions ↓ ammonia (B)

Patient Information Do not swallow the capsule; empty contents of capsule into 3-4 oz of water before taking; take with food to reduce the risk of diarrhea

Nursing Implications Capsule must be emptied into 3-4 oz of water before administration

Dosage Forms

Injection (per mL): Phosphate 3 mmol, potassium 4.4 mEq

Powder [capsule] (Neutra-Phos®-K): Elemental phosphorus 250 mg, phosphate 8 mmol, potassium 14.2 mEq

Potassium Phosphate and Sodium Phosphate

(poe TASS ee um FOS fate & SOW dee um FOS fate)

U.S. Brand Names K-Phos® Neutral; Neutra-Phos®; Uro-KP-Neutral®

Synonyms Sodium Phosphate and Potassium Phosphate

Therapeutic Category Phosphate Salt; Potassium Salt

Use Treatment of conditions associated with excessive renal phosphate loss or inadequate GI absorption of phosphate; to acidify the urine to lower calcium concentrations; to increase the antibacterial activity of methenamine; reduce odor and rash caused by ammonia in urine

Pregnancy Risk Factor C

Contraindications Addison's disease, hyperkalemia, hyperphosphatemia, infected urolithiasis or struvite stone formation, patients with severely impaired renal function

Warnings/Precautions Use with caution in patients with renal disease, hyperkalemia, cardiac disease and metabolic alkalosis

Adverse Reactions

>10%: Gastrointestinal: Diarrhea, nausea, stomach pain, flatulence, vomiting

1% to 10%:

Cardiovascular: Bradycardia

Endocrine & metabolic: Hyperkalemia

Neuromuscular & skeletal: Weakness

Respiratory: Dyspnea

<1% (Limited to important or life-threatening): Acute renal failure, arrhythmia, chest pain, decreased urine output, dyspnea, edema, mental confusion, paralysis, paresthesias, phlebitis, tetany (with large doses of phosphate)

Overdosage/Toxicology Symptoms include muscle weakness, paralysis, peaked T waves, flattened P waves, prolongation of QRS complex, ventricular arrhythmias, tetany, and calcium phosphate precipitation. Removal of potassium can be accomplished by various means such as through the GI tract with Kayexalate® administration, by way of the kidney through diuresis, mineralocorticoid administration or increased sodium intake, by hemodialysis or peritoneal dialysis, or by shifting potassium back into the cells by insulin and glucose infusion. Calcium chloride reverses cardiac effects.

Drug Interactions

Increased Effect/Toxicity: Potassium-sparing diuretics, salt substitutes, or ACE inhibitors; increased effect of digitalis

Decreased Effect: Aluminum and magnesium-containing antacids or sucralfate can act as phosphate binders

Usual Dosage All dosage forms to be mixed in 6-8 oz of water prior to administration

Children: 2-3 mmol phosphate/kg/24 hours given 4 times/day **or** 1 capsule 4 times/day

Adults: 1-2 capsules (250-500 mg phosphorus/8-16 mmol) 4 times/day after meals and at bedtime

Dietary Considerations Should be taken after meals.

Monitoring Parameters Serum potassium, sodium, calcium, phosphate, EKG

Patient Information Do not swallow, open capsule and dissolve in 6-8 oz of water; powder packets are to be mixed in 6-8 oz of water; tablets should be crushed and mixed in 6-8 oz of water

Nursing Implications Tablets may be crushed and stirred vigorously to speed dissolution

Dosage Forms

Liquid: Whole cow's milk per mL: Phosphate 0.29 mmol, sodium 0.025 mEq, potassium 0.035 mEq

Powder, concentrated [capsule] (Neutra-Phos®): Elemental phosphorus 250 mg, phosphate 8 mmol, sodium 7.1 mEq, potassium 7.1 mEq

Tablet:

K-Phos® MF: Elemental phosphorus 125.6 mg, phosphate 4 mmol, sodium 2.9 mEq, potassium 1.1 mEq

K-Phos® Neutral: Elemental phosphorus 250 mg, phosphate 8 mmol, sodium 13 mEq, potassium 1.1 mEq

K-Phos® No. 2: Elemental phosphorus 250 mg, phosphate 8 mmol, sodium 5.8 mEq, potassium 2.3 mEq

K-Phos® Original: Elemental phosphorus 114 mg, phosphate 3.6 mmol, potassium 3.7 mEq

Uro-KP-Neutral®: Elemental phosphorus 250 mg, phosphate 8 mmol, sodium 10.8 mEq, potassium 1.3 mEq

Povidone-Iodine (POE vi done EYE oh dyne)

U.S. Brand Names ACU-dyne® [OTC]; Aerodine® [OTC]; Betadine® [OTC]; Betadine® 5% Sterile Ophthalmic Prep Solution; Betagan® [OTC]; Biodine [OTC]; Etodine® [OTC]; Iodex® [OTC]; Iodex-p® [OTC]; Mallisol® [OTC]; Massengill® Medicated Douche w/Cepticin [OTC];

Minidyne® [OTC]; Operand® [OTC]; Polydine® [OTC]; Summer's Eve® Medicated Douche [OTC]; Yeast-Gard® Medicated Douche [OTC]

Canadian Brand Names Betadine®; Proviodine

Therapeutic Category Antibacterial, Topical; Antifungal Agent, Topical; Antiviral Agent, Nonantiretroviral; Antiviral Agent, Topical; Shampoos

Use External antiseptic with broad microbicidal spectrum against bacteria, fungi, viruses, protozoa, and yeasts

Pregnancy Risk Factor D

Contraindications Hypersensitivity to iodine or any component of the formulation

Warnings/Precautions Highly toxic if ingested; sodium thiosulfate is the most effective chemical antidote; avoid contact with eyes; use with caution in infants and nursing women

Adverse Reactions
1% to 10%:
Dermatologic: Rash, pruritus
Local: Local edema
<1% (Limited to important or life-threatening): Metabolic acidosis, renal impairment, systemic absorption in extensive burns causing iododerma

Mechanism of Action Povidone-iodine is known to be a powerful broad spectrum germicidal agent effective against a wide range of bacteria, viruses, fungi, protozoa, and spores.

Pharmacodynamics/Kinetics Absorption: Normal individuals: Topical: Little systemic absorption; Vaginal: Rapid, serum concentrations of total iodine and inorganic iodide are increased significantly

Usual Dosage
Shampoo: Apply 2 teaspoons to hair and scalp, lather and rinse; repeat application 2 times/ week until improvement is noted, then shampoo weekly
Topical: Apply as needed for treatment and prevention of susceptible microbial infections

Patient Information Do not swallow; avoid contact with eyes

Nursing Implications Avoid contact with eyes

Dosage Forms
Aerosol, topical: 5% (88.7 mL, 90 mL)
Antiseptic gauze pads, topical: 10% (3" x 9")
Cleanser, topical: 60 mL, 240 mL
Cleanser, skin, topical: 7.5% (30 mL, 118 mL)
Cleanser, skin, foam, topical: 7.5% (170 g)
Cream, topical: 5% (14 g)
Foam, topical (10%): 250 g
Gel, lubricating, topical: 5% (5 g)
Gel, vaginal (10%): 18 g, 90 g
Liquid, concentrate [whirlpool]: 3840 mL
Liquid, topical: 473 mL
Ointment, topical: 1% (30 g, 454 g); 10% (0.94 g, 3.8 g, 28 g, 30 g, 454 g); 1 g, 1.2 g, 2.7 g packets
Shampoo, topical: 7.5% (118 mL)
Solution, douche: 10%: 0.5 oz/packet (6 packets/box), 240 mL
Solution, douche, concentrate: 10% (240 mL); 20% (120 mL, 240 mL)
Solution, douche, diluted: 0.3% (135 mL, 180 mL)
Solution, mouthwash (0.5%): 177 mL
Solution, ophthalmic, sterile prep: 5% (50 mL)
Solution, prep: 10% (30 mL, 60 mL, 240 mL, 473 mL, 1000 mL, 4000 mL)
Solution, swab aid: 1%
Solution, swabsticks: 10%
Solution, topical: 1% (480 mL, 4000 mL); 10% (15 mL, 30 mL, 120 mL, 237 mL, 473 mL, 480 mL, 1000 mL, 4000 mL)
Solution, topical, concentrate [perineal wash], : 1% (240 mL); 10% (236 mL)
Solution [surgical scrub]: 7.5% (15 mL, 473 mL, 946 mL)
Suppositories, vaginal: 10% (7s)

♦ **PPD** see Tuberculin Tests on page 1386
♦ **PPL** see Benzylpenicilloyl-polylysine on page 158
♦ **PPS** see Pentosan Polysulfate Sodium on page 1060
♦ **PPV23** see Pneumococcal Polysaccharide Vaccine (Polyvalent) on page 1098

Pralidoxime (pra li DOKS eem)

U.S. Brand Names Protopam®

Canadian Brand Names Protopam®

Synonyms 2-PAM; Pralidoxime Chloride; 2-Pyridine Aldoxime Methochloride

Therapeutic Category Antidote, Ambenonium; Antidote, Anticholinesterase; Antidote, Neostigmine; Antidote, Organophosphate Poisoning; Antidote, Pyridostigmine

Use Reverse muscle paralysis with toxic exposure to organophosphate anticholinesterase pesticides and chemicals; control of overdose of drugs used to treat myasthenia gravis (ambenonium, neostigmine, pyridostigmine)

Pregnancy Risk Factor C

Contraindications Hypersensitivity to pralidoxime or any component of the formulation; poisonings due to phosphorus, inorganic phosphates, or organic phosphates without anticholinesterase activity

Warnings/Precautions Use with caution in patients with myasthenia gravis; dosage modification required in patients with impaired renal function may not be effective for treating carbamate intoxication; use with caution in patients receiving theophylline, succinylcholine, phenothiazines, respiratory depressants (eg, narcotics, barbiturates)

Adverse Reactions
>10%: Local: Pain at injection site after I.M. administration
1% to 10%:
Cardiovascular: Tachycardia, hypertension
(Continued)

Pralidoxime *(Continued)*

Central nervous system: Dizziness, headache, drowsiness
Dermatologic: Rash
Gastrointestinal: Nausea
Neuromuscular & skeletal: Muscle rigidity, weakness
Ocular: Blurred vision, diplopia
Respiratory: Hyperventilation, laryngospasm

Overdosage/Toxicology Symptoms include blurred vision, nausea, tachycardia, and dizziness. Therapy is supportive. Mechanical ventilation may be required.

Drug Interactions
Increased Effect/Toxicity: Increased effect with barbiturates (potentiated). Avoid morphine, theophylline, succinylcholine, reserpine, and phenothiazines in patients with organophosphate poisoning.
Decreased Effect: Atropine is often used concurrently with pralidoxime to blunt excessive cholinergic stimulation. However, the onset of atropine's effect may be unpredictable, and may occur earlier than anticipated, diminishing the therapeutic response to pralidoxime

Mechanism of Action Reactivates cholinesterase that had been inactivated by phosphorylation due to exposure to organophosphate pesticides by displacing the enzyme from its receptor sites; removes the phosphoryl group from the active site of the inactivated enzyme

Pharmacodynamics/Kinetics
Protein binding: None
Metabolism: Hepatic
Half-life elimination: 0.8-2.7 hours
Time to peak, serum: I.V.: 5-15 minutes
Excretion: Urine (80% to 90% as metabolites and unchanged drug)

Usual Dosage Poisoning: I.M. (use in conjunction with atropine; atropine effects should be established before pralidoxime is administered), I.V.:
Children: 20-50 mg/kg/dose; repeat in 1-2 hours if muscle weakness has not been relieved, then at 10- to 12-hour intervals if cholinergic signs recur
Adults: 1-2 g; repeat in 1-2 hours if muscle weakness has not been relieved, then at 10- to 12-hour intervals if cholinergic signs recur
Treatment of acetylcholinesterase inhibitor toxicity: Initial: 1-2 g followed by increments of 250 mg every 5 minutes until response is observed
Dosing adjustment in renal impairment: Dose should be reduced

Administration Infuse over 15-30 minutes at a rate not to exceed 200 mg/minute; may administer I.M. or S.C. if I.V. is not accessible; reconstitute with 20 mL sterile water (preservative free) resulting in 50 mg/mL solution; dilute in normal saline 20 mg/mL and infuse over 15-30 minutes; if a more rapid onset of effect is desired or in a fluid-restricted situation, the maximum concentration is 50 mg/mL; the maximum rate of infusion is over 5 minutes

Monitoring Parameters Heart rate, respiratory rate, blood pressure, continuous EKG; cardiac monitor and blood pressure monitor required for I.V. administration

Nursing Implications
Parenteral: Reconstitute with 20 mL sterile water (preservative free) resulting in 50 mg/mL solution; dilute in normal saline 20 mg/mL and infuse over 15-30 minutes; if a more rapid onset of effect is desired or in a fluid restricted situation, the maximum concentration is 50 mg/mL; the maximum rate of infusion is over 5 minutes
Monitor heart rate, respiratory rate, blood pressure, continuous EKG

Dosage Forms
Injection: 20 mL vial containing 1 g each pralidoxime chloride with one 20 mL ampul diluent, disposable syringe, needle, and alcohol swab
Injection, as chloride: 300 mg/mL (2 mL)

♦ **Pralidoxime Chloride** *see Pralidoxime on page 1115*

Pramipexole *(pra mi PEKS ole)*

Related Information
Parkinson's Agents *on page 1513*
U.S. Brand Names Mirapex®
Canadian Brand Names Mirapex®
Therapeutic Category Anti-Parkinson's Agent, Dopamine Agonist; Dopaminergic Agent (Antiparkinson's)
Use Treatment of the signs and symptoms of idiopathic Parkinson's disease
Unlabeled/Investigational Use Treatment of depression
Pregnancy Risk Factor C
Contraindications Hypersensitivity to pramipexole or any component of the formulation
Warnings/Precautions Caution should be taken in patients with renal insufficiency and in patients with pre-existing dyskinesias. May cause orthostatic hypotension; Parkinson's disease patients appear to have an impaired capacity to respond to a postural challenge. Use with caution in patients at risk of hypotension (such as those receiving antihypertensive drugs) or where transient hypotensive episodes would be poorly tolerated (cardiovascular disease or cerebrovascular disease). Parkinson's patients being treated with dopaminergic agonists ordinarily require careful monitoring for signs and symptoms of postural hypotension, especially during dose escalation, and should be informed of this risk. May cause hallucinations, particularly in older patients.

Although not reported for pramipexole, other dopaminergic agents have been associated with a syndrome resembling neuroleptic malignant syndrome on withdrawal or significant dosage reduction after long-term use. Dopaminergic agents from the ergot class have also been associated with fibrotic complications, such as retroperitoneum, lungs, and pleura.

Pramipexole has been associated with somnolence, particularly at higher dosages (>1.5 mg/day). In addition, patients have been reported to fall asleep during activities of daily living, including driving, while taking this medication. Whether these patients exhibited somnolence prior to these events is not clear. Patients should be advised of this issue and factors which may increase risk (sleep disorders, other sedating medications, or concomitant medications which increase pramipexole concentrations) and instructed to report daytime somnolence or sleepiness to the prescriber. Patients should use caution in performing activities which require alertness (driving or operating machinery), and to avoid other medications which may cause CNS depression, including ethanol.

Adverse Reactions
Frequency not defined, dose-related: Falling asleep during activities of daily living
>10%:
Cardiovascular: Postural hypotension
Central nervous system: Asthenia, dizziness, somnolence, insomnia, hallucinations, abnormal dreams
Gastrointestinal: Nausea, constipation
Neuromuscular & skeletal: Weakness, dyskinesia, EPS
1% to 10%:
Cardiovascular: Edema, postural hypotension, syncope, tachycardia, chest pain
Central nervous system: Malaise, confusion, amnesia, dystonias, akathisia, thinking abnormalities, myoclonus, myesthesia, gait abnormalities, hypertonia, paranoia
Endocrine & metabolic: Decreased libido
Gastrointestinal: Anorexia, weight loss, xerostomia
Genitourinary: Urinary frequency (up to 6%), impotence
Neuromuscular & skeletal: Muscle twitching, leg cramps, arthritis, bursitis
Ocular: Vision abnormalities (3%)
Respiratory: Dyspnea, rhinitis
<1% (Limited to important or life-threatening): Liver transaminases increased

Drug Interactions
Increased Effect/Toxicity: Cimetidine in combination with pramipexole produced a 50% increase in AUC and a 40% increase in half-life. Drugs secreted by the cationic transport system (diltiazem, triamterene, verapamil, quinidine, quinine, ranitidine) decrease the clearance of pramipexole by ~20%.
Decreased Effect: Dopamine antagonists (antipsychotics, metoclopramide) may decrease the efficiency of pramipexole.

Ethanol/Nutrition/Herb Interactions
Ethanol: Avoid ethanol (may increase CNS depression).
Food: Food intake does not affect the extent of drug absorption, although the time to maximal plasma concentration is delayed by 60 minutes when taken with a meal.
Herb/Nutraceutical: Avoid valerian, St John's wort, SAMe, kava kava (may increase risk of serotonin syndrome and/or excessive sedation).

Mechanism of Action Pramipexole is a nonergot dopamine agonist with specificity for the D_2 subfamily dopamine receptor, and has also been shown to bind to D_3 and D_4 receptors. By binding to these receptors, it is thought that pramipexole can stimulate dopamine activity on the nerves of the striatum and substantia nigra.

Pharmacodynamics/Kinetics
Protein binding: 15%
Bioavailability: 90%
Half-life elimination: ~8 hours; Elderly: 12-14 hours
Time to peak, serum: ~2 hours
Excretion: Urine (90% as unchanged drug)

Usual Dosage Adults: Oral: Initial: 0.375 mg/day given in 3 divided doses, increase gradually by 0.125 mg/dose every 5-7 days; range: 1.5-4.5 mg/day

Administration Doses should be titrated gradually in all patients to avoid the onset of intolerable side effects. The dosage should be increased to achieve a maximum therapeutic effect, balanced against the side effects of dyskinesia, hallucinations, somnolence, and dry mouth.

Monitoring Parameters Monitor for improvement in symptoms of Parkinson's disease (eg, mentation, behavior, daily living activities, motor examinations), blood pressure, body weight changes, and heart rate

Patient Information Ask your physician or pharmacist before taking any other medicine, including over-the-counter products; especially important are other medicines that could make you sleepy such as sleeping pills, tranquilizers, some cold and allergy medicines, narcotic pain killers, or medicines that relax muscles. Avoid alcohol; use caution in performing activities that require alertness (driving or operating machinery); can cause significant drowsiness.

Dosage Forms Tablet: 0.125 mg, 0.25 mg, 0.5 mg, 1 mg, 1.5 mg

♦ **Pramosone®** *see* Pramoxine and Hydrocortisone *on page 1117*
♦ **Pramox® HC (Can)** *see* Pramoxine and Hydrocortisone *on page 1117*

Pramoxine and Hydrocortisone (pra MOKS een & hye droe KOR ti sone)
U.S. Brand Names Analpram-HC®; Enzone®; Epifoam®; Pramosone®; ProctoFoam®-HC; Zone-A Forte®
Canadian Brand Names Pramox® HC; Proctofoam™-HC
Synonyms Hydrocortisone and Pramoxine
Therapeutic Category Anesthetic/Corticosteroid
Use Treatment of severe anorectal or perianal swelling
Pregnancy Risk Factor C
Usual Dosage Apply to affected areas 3-4 times/day
Additional Information Complete prescribing information for this medication should be consulted for additional detail.
Dosage Forms
Cream, topical: Pramoxine hydrochloride 1% and hydrocortisone acetate 1%; pramoxine hydrochloride 1% and hydrocortisone acetate 2.5%
Foam, rectal: Pramoxine hydrochloride 1% and hydrocortisone acetate 1% (10 g)
Lotion, topical: Pramoxine hydrochloride 1% and hydrocortisone 1%; pramoxine hydrochloride 2.5% and hydrocortisone 1% (37.5 mL, 120 mL, 240 mL)

- ◆ **Prandase®** (Can) *see* Acarbose *on page 19*
- ◆ **Prandin®** *see* Repaglinide *on page 1183*
- ◆ **Pravachol®** *see* Pravastatin *on page 1118*

Pravastatin (PRA va stat in)

Related Information
Hyperlipidemia Management *on page 1670*
Lipid-Lowering Agents *on page 1505*

U.S. Brand Names Pravachol®

Canadian Brand Names Lin-Pravastatin; Pravachol®

Synonyms Pravastatin Sodium

Therapeutic Category Antilipemic Agent, HMG-CoA Reductase Inhibitor; HMG-CoA Reductase Inhibitor

Use
Primary prevention of coronary events: In combination with dietary therapy in hypercholesterolemic patients without established coronary heart disease, to reduce cardiovascular morbidity (myocardial infarction, coronary revascularization procedures) and mortality.

Secondary prevention of coronary events:

In combination with dietary therapy in hypercholesterolemic patients with established coronary heart disease, to slow the progression of coronary atherosclerosis, to reduce cardiovascular morbidity (myocardial infarction, coronary vascular procedures) and to reduce mortality; to reduce the risk of stroke and transient ischemic attacks

In combination with dietary therapy in patients with a history of prior myocardial infarction or unstable angina and "normal" cholesterol concentrations (total cholesterol ~219 mg/dL, LDL-C ~150 mg/dL); pravastatin may reduce cardiovascular mortality, the risk for recurrent myocardial infarction, stroke, and TIA, and the risk for undergoing coronary revascularization procedures.

Hyperlipidemias: As an adjunct to diet to reduce elevations in total cholesterol, LDL-C, apolipoprotein B, and triglycerides (elevations of one or more components are present in Fredrickson type IIa, IIb, III, and IV hyperlipidemias).

Pregnancy Risk Factor X

Contraindications Hypersensitivity to pravastatin or any component of the formulation; active liver disease; unexplained persistent elevations of serum transaminases; pregnancy; breast-feeding

Warnings/Precautions Use with caution in patients who consume large amounts of ethanol or have a history of liver disease. May elevate aminotransferases; LFTs should be performed before therapy, prior to elevation of dose, and periodically thereafter. Can also cause myalgia and rhabdomyolysis. Risk is increased with concurrent use of clarithromycin, danazol, diltiazem, fluvoxamine, indinavir, nefazodone, nelfinavir, ritonavir, verapamil, troleandomycin, cyclosporine, fibric acid derivatives, erythromycin, niacin, or azole antifungals. The risk of combining any of these drugs with pravastatin is minimal. Temporarily discontinue in any patient experiencing an acute or serious condition predisposing to renal failure secondary to rhabdomyolysis. Safety and efficacy in patients <18 years of age have not been established.

Adverse Reactions
1% to 10%:

Cardiovascular: Chest pain (4%)

Central nervous system: Headache (2% to 6%), fatigue (4%), dizziness (1% to 3%)

Dermatologic: Rash (4%)

Gastrointestinal: Nausea/vomiting (7%), diarrhea (6%), heartburn (3%)

Hepatic: Increased transaminases (>3x normal on two occasions - 1%)

Neuromuscular & skeletal: Myalgia (2%)

Respiratory: Cough (3%)

Miscellaneous: Influenza (2%)

<1% (Limited to important or life-threatening): Lichenoid eruption, myopathy, neuropathy, porphyria cutanea tarda

Additional class-related events or case reports (not necessarily reported with pravastatin therapy): Alopecia, anaphylaxis, angioedema, arthritis, cataracts, cholestatic jaundice, dermatomyositis, dyspnea, eosinophilia, erythema multiforme, facial or ocular paresis, fulminant hepatic necrosis, gynecomastia, hemolytic anemia, hepatitis, hepatoma, impotence, increased ESR, leukopenia, memory loss, ophthalmoplegia, pancreatitis, paresthesia, peripheral nerve palsy, peripheral neuropathy, photosensitivity, polymyalgia rheumatica, positive ANA, pruritus, psychic disturbance, purpura, rash, renal failure (secondary to rhabdomyolysis), rhabdomyolysis, Stevens-Johnson syndrome, systemic lupus erythematosus-like syndrome, thrombocytopenia, thyroid dysfunction, toxic epidermal necrolysis, tremor, urticaria, vasculitis, vertigo

Overdosage/Toxicology Few adverse events have been reported. Treatment is symptomatic.

Drug Interactions
Cytochrome P450 Effect: CYP3A3/4 enzyme substrate

Increased Effect/Toxicity: Clofibrate, fenofibrate, gemfibrozil, and niacin may increase the risk of myopathy and rhabdomyolysis. Imidazole antifungals (itraconazole, ketoconazole), P-glycoprotein inhibitors may increase pravastatin concentrations.

Decreased Effect: Concurrent administration of cholestyramine or colestipol can decrease pravastatin absorption.

Ethanol/Nutrition/Herb Interactions
Ethanol: Consumption of large amounts of ethanol may increase the risk of liver damage with HMG-CoA reductase inhibitors.

Herb/Nutraceutical: St John's wort may decrease pravastatin levels.

Stability Store at <30°C (86°F). Protect from moisture and light.

Mechanism of Action Pravastatin is a competitive inhibitor of 3-hydroxy-3-methylglutaryl coenzyme A (HMG-CoA) reductase, which is the rate-limiting enzyme involved in *de novo* cholesterol synthesis.

Pharmacodynamics/Kinetics
 Onset of action: Several days
   Peak effect: 4 weeks
 Absorption: Poor
 Protein binding: 50%
 Metabolism: Hepatic to at least two metabolites
 Bioavailability: 17%
 Half-life elimination: ~2-3 hours
 Time to peak, serum: 1-1.5 hours
 Excretion: Urine (≤20%, 8% as unchanged drug)
Usual Dosage Oral:
 Adults: Initial: 40 mg once daily (10 mg in patients with renal/hepatic dysfunction or receiving immunosuppressants, such as cyclosporine); titrate dosage to response (usual range: 10-80 mg); maximum dose: 80 mg once daily (maximum dose of 20 mg once daily recommended in patients receiving immunosuppressants, such as cyclosporine)
 Elderly: No specific dosage recommendations. Clearance is reduced in the elderly, resulting in an increase in AUC between 25% to 50%. However, substantial accumulation is not expected.
 Dosing adjustment in renal impairment: 10 mg/day
 Dosing adjustment in hepatic impairment: 10 mg/day
Dietary Considerations May be taken without regard to meals. Before initiation of therapy, patients should be placed on a standard cholesterol-lowering diet for 6 weeks and the diet should be continued during drug therapy.
Administration May be taken without regard to meals.
Monitoring Parameters Obtain baseline LFTs and total cholesterol profile; creatine phosphokinase due to possibility of myopathy. Repeat LFTs prior to elevation of dose. May be measured when clinically indicated and/or periodically thereafter.
Patient Information Promptly report any unexplained muscle pain, tenderness or weakness, especially if accompanied by malaise or fever
Nursing Implications Liver enzyme elevations may be observed during therapy with pravastatin; diet, weight reduction, and exercise should be attempted prior to therapy with pravastatin
Dosage Forms Tablet, as sodium: 10 mg, 20 mg, 40 mg, 80 mg

◆ **Pravastatin Sodium** *see* Pravastatin *on page 1118*

Prazepam *Not Available in U.S.* (PRA ze pam)

 Therapeutic Category Benzodiazepine
 Use Treatment of anxiety
 Unlabeled/Investigational Use Ethanol withdrawal; duodenal ulcer; narcotic addiction; spasticity; partial seizures
 Pregnancy Risk Factor D
 Contraindications Hypersensitivity to prazepam or any component of the formulation (cross-sensitivity with other benzodiazepines may exist); narrow-angle glaucoma; pregnancy
 Warnings/Precautions Use with caution in elderly or debilitated patients, patients with hepatic disease (including alcoholics), or renal impairment. Use with caution in patients with respiratory disease or impaired gag reflex. Avoid use in patients with sleep apnea.

 Causes CNS depression (dose-related) resulting in sedation, dizziness, confusion, or ataxia which may impair physical and mental capabilities. Patients must be cautioned about performing tasks which require mental alertness (operating machinery or driving). Use with caution in patients receiving other CNS depressants or psychoactive agents. Effects with other sedative drugs or ethanol may be potentiated. Benzodiazepines have been associated with falls and traumatic injury and should be used with extreme caution in patients who are at risk of these events (especially the elderly).

 Use caution in patients with depression, particularly if suicidal risk may be present. Use with caution in patients with a history of drug dependence. Benzodiazepines have been associated with dependence and acute withdrawal symptoms on discontinuation or reduction in dose. Acute withdrawal, including seizures, may be precipitated after administration of flumazenil to patients receiving long-term benzodiazepine therapy.

 Benzodiazepines have been associated with anterograde amnesia. Paradoxical reactions, including hyperactive or aggressive behavior have been reported with benzodiazepines, particularly in adolescent/pediatric or psychiatric patients. Does not have analgesic, antidepressant, or antipsychotic properties.
 Adverse Reactions Frequency not defined.
 Cardiovascular: Hypotension
 Central nervous system: Drowsiness, fatigue, impaired coordination, lightheadedness, memory impairment, insomnia, depression, headache, anxiety, confusion, nervousness, syncope, dizziness, akathisia, drowsiness, ataxia, lightheadedness, vivid dreams
 Dermatologic: Rash, pruritus
 Endocrine & metabolic: Decreased libido, menstrual irregularities
 Gastrointestinal: Xerostomia, constipation, diarrhea, decreased salivation, nausea, vomiting, increased or decreased appetite, increased salivation, weight gain/loss
 Hematologic: Blood dyscrasias
 Neuromuscular & skeletal: Dysarthria, tremor, muscle cramps, rigidity, weakness, reflex slowing
 Ocular: Blurred vision, increased lenticular pressure
 Otic: Tinnitus
 Respiratory: Nasal congestion, hyperventilation
 Miscellaneous: Diaphoresis, drug dependence
 Ethanol/Nutrition/Herb Interactions
 Ethanol: Avoid ethanol (may increase CNS depression).
 Herb/Nutraceutical: Avoid valerian, St John's wort, kava kava, gotu kola (may increase CNS depression).
 (Continued)

Prazepam *Not Available in U.S.* (Continued)

Mechanism of Action Binds to stereospecific benzodiazepine receptors on the postsynaptic GABA neuron at several sites within the central nervous system, including the limbic system, reticular formation. Enhancement of the inhibitory effect of GABA on neuronal excitability results by increased neuronal membrane permeability to chloride ions. This shift in chloride ions results in hyperpolarization (a less excitable state) and stabilization.

Pharmacodynamics/Kinetics
Duration: 48 hours
Half-life elimination, serum: Parent drug: 78 minutes; Desmethyldiazepam: 30-100 hours

Usual Dosage Adults: Oral: 30 mg/day in divided doses, may increase gradually to a maximum of 60 mg/day

Monitoring Parameters Respiratory and cardiovascular status

Patient Information Avoid alcohol and other CNS depressants; avoid activities needing good psychomotor coordination until CNS effects are known; drug may cause physical or psychological dependence; avoid abrupt discontinuation after prolonged use

Additional Information Prazepam offers no significant advantage over other benzodiazepines.

Dosage Forms
Capsule: 5 mg, 10 mg, 20 mg
Tablet: 5 mg, 10 mg

Praziquantel (pray zi KWON tel)

U.S. Brand Names Biltricide®
Canadian Brand Names Biltricide®
Therapeutic Category Anthelmintic
Use All stages of schistosomiasis caused by all *Schistosoma* species pathogenic to humans; clonorchiasis and opisthorchiasis
Unlabeled/Investigational Use Cysticercosis, flukes, and many intestinal tapeworms
Pregnancy Risk Factor B
Contraindications Hypersensitivity to praziquantel or any component of the formulation; ocular cysticercosis
Warnings/Precautions Use caution in patients with severe hepatic disease; patients with cerebral cysticercosis require hospitalization
Adverse Reactions
1% to 10%:
Central nervous system: Dizziness, drowsiness, headache, malaise
Gastrointestinal: Abdominal pain, loss of appetite, nausea, vomiting
Miscellaneous: Diaphoresis
<1% (Limited to important or life-threatening): CSF reaction syndrome in patients being treated for neurocysticercosis, diarrhea, fever, itching, rash, urticaria
Overdosage/Toxicology Symptoms include dizziness, drowsiness, headache, and liver function impairment. Treatment is supportive following GI decontamination. Administer fast-acting laxative.
Mechanism of Action Increases the cell permeability to calcium in schistosomes, causing strong contractions and paralysis of worm musculature leading to detachment of suckers from the blood vessel walls and to dislodgment
Pharmacodynamics/Kinetics
Absorption: Oral: ~80%
Distribution: CSF concentration is 14% to 20% of plasma concentration; enters breast milk
Protein binding: ~80%
Metabolism: Extensive first-pass effect
Half-life elimination: Parent drug: 0.8-1.5 hours; Metabolites: 4.5 hours
Time to peak, serum: 1-3 hours
Excretion: Urine (99% as metabolites)
Usual Dosage Children >4 years and Adults: Oral:
Schistosomiasis: 20 mg/kg/dose 2-3 times/day for 1 day at 4- to 6-hour intervals
Flukes: 25 mg/kg/dose every 8 hours for 1-2 days
Cysticercosis: 50 mg/kg/day divided every 8 hours for 14 days
Tapeworms: 10-20 mg/kg as a single dose (25 mg/kg for *Hymenolepis nana*)
Clonorchiasis/opisthorchiasis: 3 doses of 25 mg/kg as a 1-day treatment
Patient Information Do not chew tablets due to bitter taste; take with food; caution should be used when performing tasks requiring mental alertness, may impair judgment and coordination
Nursing Implications Tablets can be halved or quartered
Dosage Forms Tablet, tri-scored: 600 mg

Prazosin (PRA zoe sin)

Related Information
Depression *on page 1655*
U.S. Brand Names Minipress®
Canadian Brand Names Alti-Prazosin; Apo®-Prazo; Minipress™; Novo-Prazin; Nu-Prazo
Synonyms Furazosin; Prazosin Hydrochloride
Therapeutic Category Alpha-Adrenergic Blocking Agent, Oral; Antihypertensive Agent
Use Treatment of hypertension
Unlabeled/Investigational Use Benign prostatic hyperplasia; Raynaud's syndrome
Pregnancy Risk Factor C
Contraindications Hypersensitivity to quinazolines (doxazosin, prazosin, terazosin) or any component of the formulation
Warnings/Precautions Marked orthostatic hypotension, syncope, and loss of consciousness may occur with first dose ("first dose phenomenon") occurs more often in patients receiving beta-blockers, diuretics, low sodium diets, or larger first doses (ie, >1 mg/dose in adults);

avoid rapid increase in dose; use with caution in patients with renal impairment; use cautiously in patients with a known sensitivity to other quinazolines (eg, terazosin, doxazosin)

Adverse Reactions
>10%: Central nervous system: Dizziness (10%)
1% to 10%:
 Cardiovascular: Palpitations (5%), edema, orthostatic hypotension, syncope (1%)
 Central nervous system: Headache (8%), drowsiness (8%), weakness (7%), vertigo, depression, nervousness
 Dermatologic: Rash (1% to 4%)
 Endocrine & metabolic: Decreased energy (7%)
 Gastrointestinal: Nausea (5%), vomiting, diarrhea, constipation
 Genitourinary: Urinary frequency (1% to 5%)
 Ocular: Blurred vision, reddened sclera, xerostomia
 Respiratory: Dyspnea, epistaxis, nasal congestion
<1% (Limited to important or life-threatening): Allergic reaction, alopecia, angina, cataplexy, cataracts (both development and disappearance have been reported), hallucinations, impotence, leukopenia, lichen planus, myocardial infarction, narcolepsy (worsened), pancreatitis, paresthesia, pigmentary mottling and serous retinopathy, priapism, pruritus, systemic lupus erythematosus, tinnitus, urticaria, vasculitis

Overdosage/Toxicology Symptoms include hypotension and drowsiness. Hypotension usually responds to I.V. fluids, Trendelenburg positioning, or vasoconstrictors. Treatment is otherwise supportive and symptomatic.

Drug Interactions
 Increased Effect/Toxicity: Prazosin's hypotensive effect may be increased with beta-blockers, diuretics, ACE inhibitors, calcium channel blockers, and other antihypertensive medications. Concurrent use with tricyclic antidepressants (TCAs) and low-potency anti-psychotics may increase risk of orthostasis.
 Decreased Effect: Decreased antihypertensive effect if taken with NSAIDs.

Ethanol/Nutrition/Herb Interactions
 Ethanol: Avoid ethanol (may increase vasodilation).
 Food: Food has variable effects on absorption.
 Herb/Nutraceutical: Avoid dong quai if using for hypertension (has estrogenic activity). Avoid ephedra, yohimbe, ginseng (may worsen hypertension). Avoid saw palmetto (due to limited experience with this combination). Avoid garlic (may have increased antihypertensive effect).

Stability Store in airtight container; protect from light

Mechanism of Action Competitively inhibits postsynaptic alpha-adrenergic receptors which results in vasodilation of veins and arterioles and a decrease in total peripheral resistance and blood pressure

Pharmacodynamics/Kinetics
 Onset of action: BP reduction: ~2 hours
  Maximum decrease: 2-4 hours
 Duration: 10-24 hours
 Distribution: Hypertensive adults: V_d: 0.5 L/kg
 Protein binding: 92% to 97%
 Metabolism: Extensively hepatic
 Bioavailability: 43% to 82%
 Half-life elimination: 2-4 hours; increased with congestive heart failure
 Excretion: Urine (6% to 10% as unchanged drug)

Usual Dosage Oral:
 Children: Initial: 5 mcg/kg/dose (to assess hypotensive effects); usual dosing interval: every 6 hours; increase dosage gradually up to maximum of 25 mcg/kg/dose every 6 hours
 Adults:
  Hypertension: Initial: 1 mg/dose 2-3 times/day; usual maintenance dose: 3-15 mg/day in divided doses 2-4 times/day; maximum daily dose: 20 mg
  Hypertensive urgency: 10-20 mg once, may repeat in 30 minutes
  Raynaud's (unlabeled use): 0.5-3 mg twice daily
  Benign prostatic hyperplasia (unlabeled use): 2 mg twice daily

Monitoring Parameters Blood pressure, standing and sitting/supine

Test Interactions Increased urinary UMA 17%, norepinephrine metabolite 42%

Patient Information Rise from sitting/lying carefully; take first dose at bedtime; may cause dizziness; report if painful, persistent erection occurs; avoid alcohol

Nursing Implications Syncope may occur (usually within 90 minutes of the initial dose)

Dosage Forms Capsule, as hydrochloride: 1 mg, 2 mg, 5 mg

Prazosin and Polythiazide (PRA zoe sin & pol i THYE a zide)

U.S. Brand Names Minizide®
Synonyms Polythiazide and Prazosin
Therapeutic Category Antihypertensive Agent, Combination
Use Management of mild to moderate hypertension
Pregnancy Risk Factor C
Usual Dosage Adults: Oral: 1 capsule 2-3 times/day
Additional Information Complete prescribing information for this medication should be consulted for additional detail.
Dosage Forms
 Capsule:
  1: Prazosin 1 mg and polythiazide 0.5 mg
  2: Prazosin 2 mg and polythiazide 0.5 mg
  5: Prazosin 5 mg and polythiazide 0.5 mg

♦ **Prazosin Hydrochloride** see Prazosin on page 1120
♦ **Precedex™** see Dexmedetomidine on page 383
♦ **Precose®** see Acarbose on page 19

♦ **Pred Forte®** *see* PrednisoLONE *on page 1122*

♦ **Pred-G®** *see* Prednisolone and Gentamicin *on page 1124*

♦ **Pred Mild®** *see* PrednisoLONE *on page 1122*

Prednicarbate (PRED ni kar bate)

Related Information
Corticosteroids Comparison *on page 1495*

U.S. Brand Names Dermatop®

Therapeutic Category Corticosteroid, Topical (Medium Potency)

Use Relief of the inflammatory and pruritic manifestations of corticosteroid-responsive dermatoses (medium potency topical corticosteroid)

Pregnancy Risk Factor C

Contraindications Hypersensitivity to prednicarbate or any component of the formulation; fungal, viral, or tubercular skin lesions, herpes simplex or zoster

Warnings/Precautions Systemic absorption of topical corticosteroids has produced reversible HPA axis suppression. This is more likely to occur when the preparation is used on large surface or denuded areas for prolonged periods of time or with an occlusive dressing.

Adverse Reactions
1% to 10%: Dermatologic: Skin atrophy, shininess, thinness, mild telangiectasia

<1% (Limited to important or life-threatening): Acneiform eruptions, allergic contact dermatitis and rash, burning, edema, folliculitis, hypopigmentation, miliaria, paresthesia, perioral dermatitis, pruritus, secondary infection, striae, urticaria

Mechanism of Action Topical corticosteroids have anti-inflammatory, antipruritic, vasoconstrictive, and antiproliferative actions

Usual Dosage Adults: Topical: Apply a thin film to affected area twice daily. Therapy should be discontinued when control is achieved; if no improvement is seen, reassessment of diagnosis may be necessary.

Monitoring Parameters Relief of symptoms

Patient Information Use only as prescribed and for no longer than the period prescribed; apply sparingly in a thin film and rub in lightly; avoid contact with eyes; do not apply to the face, underarms, or groin areas; notify physician if condition persists or worsens

Nursing Implications Use sparingly

Additional Information Has been shown that the atrophic activity of prednicarbate is many times less than agents with similar clinical potency, nevertheless, avoid use on the face.

Dosage Forms
Cream, topical: 0.1% (15 g, 60 g)

Ointment, topical: 0.1% (15 g, 60 g)

PrednisoLONE (pred NISS oh lone)

Related Information
Corticosteroids Comparison *on page 1495*

U.S. Brand Names AK-Pred®; Delta-Cortef®; Econopred®; Econopred® Plus; Inflamase® Forte; Inflamase® Mild; Key-Pred®; Key-Pred-SP®; Pediapred®; Pred Forte®; Pred Mild®; Prednisol® TBA; Prelone®

Canadian Brand Names Diopred®; Hydeltra T.B.A.®; Inflamase® Forte; Inflamase® Mild; Novo-Prednisolone®; Ophtho-Tate®; Ophtho-tate®; Pediapred®; Pred Forte®; Pred Mild®

Synonyms Deltahydrocortisone; Metacortandralone; Prednisolone Acetate; Prednisolone Acetate, Ophthalmic; Prednisolone Sodium Phosphate; Prednisolone Sodium Phosphate, Ophthalmic; Prednisolone Tebutate

Therapeutic Category Anti-inflammatory Agent; Anti-inflammatory Agent, Ophthalmic; Corticosteroid, Ophthalmic; Corticosteroid, Systemic; Glucocorticoid

Use Treatment of palpebral and bulbar conjunctivitis; corneal injury from chemical, radiation, thermal burns, or foreign body penetration; endocrine disorders, rheumatic disorders, collagen diseases, dermatologic diseases, allergic states, ophthalmic diseases, respiratory diseases, hematologic disorders, neoplastic diseases, edematous states, and gastrointestinal diseases; useful in patients with inability to activate prednisone (liver disease)

Pregnancy Risk Factor C

Contraindications Hypersensitivity to prednisolone or any component of the formulation; acute superficial herpes simplex keratitis; systemic fungal infections; varicella

Warnings/Precautions Use with caution in patients with hyperthyroidism, cirrhosis, nonspecific ulcerative colitis, hypertension, osteoporosis, thromboembolic tendencies, CHF, convulsive disorders, myasthenia gravis, thrombophlebitis, peptic ulcer, diabetes; acute adrenal insufficiency may occur with abrupt withdrawal after long-term therapy or with stress; young pediatric patients may be more susceptible to adrenal axis suppression from topical therapy. Because of the risk of adverse effects, systemic corticosteroids should be used cautiously in the elderly, in the smallest possible dose, and for the shortest possible time.

Adverse Reactions Systemic:
>10%:

Central nervous system: Insomnia, nervousness

Gastrointestinal: Increased appetite, indigestion

1% to 10%:

Central nervous system: Dizziness or lightheadedness, headache

Dermatologic: Hirsutism, hypopigmentation

Endocrine & metabolic: Diabetes mellitus

Neuromuscular & skeletal: Arthralgia

Ocular: Cataracts, glaucoma

Respiratory: Epistaxis

Miscellaneous: Diaphoresis

<1% (Limited to important or life-threatening): Cushing's syndrome, edema, fractures, hallucinations, hypersensitivity reactions, hypertension, muscle wasting, osteoporosis, pancreatitis, pituitary-adrenal axis suppression, pseudotumor cerebri, seizures

Overdosage/Toxicology When consumed in excessive quantities for prolonged periods, systemic hypercorticism and adrenal suppression may occur; in those cases, discontinuation and withdrawal of the corticosteroid should be done judiciously.

Drug Interactions

Cytochrome P450 Effect: CYP3A3/4 enzyme substrate; inducer of cytochrome P450 enzymes

Increased Effect/Toxicity: Systemic: The combined use of cyclosporine and prednisolone may result in elevated levels of both agents. Oral contraceptives may enhance the effect of prednisolone.

Decreased Effect: Systemic: Decreased effect or corticosteroids with barbiturates, aminoglutethimide, phenytoin, and rifampin. Decreased effect of salicylates, vaccines, and toxoids. Prednisolone may decrease the effect of isoniazid. Corticosteroids may decrease the effect of warfarin or IUD contraceptives.

Ethanol/Nutrition/Herb Interactions

Ethanol: Avoid ethanol (may increase gastric mucosal irritation).

Food: Prednisolone interferes with calcium absorption. Limit caffeine.

Herb/Nutraceutical: St John's wort may decrease prednisolone levels. Avoid cat's claw, echinacea (have immunostimulant properties).

Mechanism of Action Decreases inflammation by suppression of migration of polymorphonuclear leukocytes and reversal of increased capillary permeability; suppresses the immune system by reducing activity and volume of the lymphatic system

Pharmacodynamics/Kinetics

Duration: 18-36 hours

Protein binding (concentration dependent): 65% to 91%

Metabolism: Primarily hepatic, but also metabolized in most tissues, to inactive compounds

Half-life elimination: 3.6 hours; Biological: 18-36 hours; End-stage renal disease: 3-5 hours

Excretion: Primarily urine (as glucuronides, sulfates, and unconjugated metabolites)

Usual Dosage Dose depends upon condition being treated and response of patient; dosage for infants and children should be based on severity of the disease and response of the patient rather than on strict adherence to dosage indicated by age, weight, or body surface area. Consider alternate day therapy for long-term therapy. Discontinuation of long-term therapy requires gradual withdrawal by tapering the dose.

Children:

Acute asthma:

Oral: 1-2 mg/kg/day in divided doses 1-2 times/day for 3-5 days

I.V. (sodium phosphate salt): 2-4 mg/kg/day divided 3-4 times/day

Anti-inflammatory or immunosuppressive dose: Oral, I.V., I.M. (sodium phosphate salt): 0.1-2 mg/kg/day in divided doses 1-4 times/day

Nephrotic syndrome: Oral:

Initial (first 3 episodes): 2 mg/kg/day **or** 60 mg/m^2/day (maximum: 80 mg/day) in divided doses 3-4 times/day until urine is protein free for 3 consecutive days (maximum: 28 days); followed by 1-1.5 mg/kg/dose **or** 40 mg/m^2/dose given every other day for 4 weeks

Maintenance (long-term maintenance dose for frequent relapses): 0.5-1 mg/kg/dose given every other day for 3-6 months

Adults:

Oral, I.V., I.M. (sodium phosphate salt): 5-60 mg/day

Multiple sclerosis (sodium phosphate): Oral: 200 mg/day for 1 week followed by 80 mg every other day for 1 month

Rheumatoid arthritis: Oral: Initial: 5-7.5 mg/day; adjust dose as necessary

Elderly: Use lowest effective dose

Dosing adjustment in hyperthyroidism: Prednisolone dose may need to be increased to achieve adequate therapeutic effects

Hemodialysis: Slightly dialyzable (5% to 20%); administer dose posthemodialysis

Peritoneal dialysis: Supplemental dose is not necessary

Intra-articular, intralesional, soft-tissue administration:

Tebutate salt: 4-40 mg/dose

Sodium phosphate salt: 2-30 mg/dose

Ophthalmic suspension/solution: Children and Adults: Instill 1-2 drops into conjunctival sac every hour during day, every 2 hours at night until favorable response is obtained, then use 1 drop every 4 hours

Dietary Considerations Should be taken after meals or with food or milk to decrease GI effects; increase dietary intake of pyridoxine, vitamin C, vitamin D, folate, calcium, and phosphorus.

Administration Administer oral formulation with food or milk to decrease GI effects

Monitoring Parameters Blood pressure, blood glucose, electrolytes

Test Interactions Response to skin tests

Patient Information Notify surgeon or dentist before surgical repair; may cause GI upset, take orally with food; notify physician if any sign of infection occurs; avoid abrupt withdrawal when on long-term therapy

Nursing Implications Do not administer acetate or tebutate salt I.V.

Additional Information

Sodium phosphate injection: For I.V., I.M., intra-articular, intralesional, or soft tissue administration

Tebutate injection: For intra-articular, intralesional, or soft tissue administration only

Dosage Forms

Injection, solution, as sodium phosphate (for I.M., I.V., intra-articular, intralesional, or soft tissue administration): 20 mg/mL (2 mL, 5 mL, 10 mL)

Injection, suspension, as acetate (for I.M., intralesional, intra-articular, or soft tissue administration only): 25 mg/mL (10 mL, 30 mL); 50 mg/mL (10 mL, 30 mL)

Injection, suspension, as tebutate (for intra-articular, intralesional, soft tissue administration only): 20 mg/mL (10 mL)

Liquid, oral, as sodium phosphate: 5 mg/5 mL (120 mL)

(Continued)

PrednisoLONE *(Continued)*

Solution, ophthalmic, as sodium phosphate: 0.125% (5 mL, 10 mL); 1% (5 mL, 10 mL, 15 mL)
Suspension, ophthalmic, as acetate: 0.12% (5 mL, 10 mL); 0.125% (5 mL, 10 mL, 15 mL);
    1% (1 mL, 5 mL, 10 mL, 15 mL)
Syrup: 5 mg/5 mL (120 mL); 15 mg/5 mL (240 mL)
Tablet: 5 mg

◆ **Prednisolone Acetate** *see PrednisoLONE on page 1122*
◆ **Prednisolone Acetate, Ophthalmic** *see PrednisoLONE on page 1122*

Prednisolone and Gentamicin *(pred NIS oh lone & jen ta MYE sin)*
U.S. Brand Names Pred-G®
Synonyms Gentamicin and Prednisolone
Therapeutic Category Antibiotic/Corticosteroid, Ophthalmic
Use Treatment of steroid responsive inflammatory conditions and superficial ocular infections
    due to strains of microorganisms susceptible to gentamicin such as *Staphylococcus, E. coli,*
    H. influenzae, Klebsiella, Neisseria, Pseudomonas, Proteus, and *Serratia* species
Pregnancy Risk Factor C
Usual Dosage Children and Adults: Ophthalmic: 1 drop 2-4 times/day; during the initial 24-48
    hours, the dosing frequency may be increased if necessary
Additional Information Complete prescribing information for this medication should be
    consulted for additional detail.
Dosage Forms
Ointment, ophthalmic: Prednisolone acetate 0.6% and gentamicin sulfate 0.3% (3.5 g)
Suspension, ophthalmic: Prednisolone acetate 1% and gentamicin sulfate 0.3% (2 mL, 5 mL,
    10 mL)

◆ **Prednisolone and Sulfacetamide** *see Sulfacetamide and Prednisolone on page 1269*
◆ **Prednisolone, Neomycin, and Polymyxin B** *see Neomycin, Polymyxin B, and Prednisolone*
    on page 970
◆ **Prednisolone Sodium Phosphate** *see PrednisoLONE on page 1122*
◆ **Prednisolone Sodium Phosphate, Ophthalmic** *see PrednisoLONE on page 1122*
◆ **Prednisolone Tebutate** *see PrednisoLONE on page 1122*
◆ **Prednisol® TBA** *see PrednisoLONE on page 1122*

PredniSONE *(PRED ni sone)*
Related Information
Contrast Media Reactions, Premedication for Prophylaxis *on page 1653*
Corticosteroids Comparison *on page 1495*
U.S. Brand Names Deltasone®; Liquid Pred®; Meticorten®; Orasone®
Canadian Brand Names Apo®-Prednisone; Winpred™
Synonyms Deltacortisone; Deltadehydrocortisone
Therapeutic Category Anti-inflammatory Agent; Corticosteroid, Systemic; Glucocorticoid
Use Treatment of a variety of diseases including adrenocortical insufficiency, hypercalcemia,
    rheumatic, and collagen disorders; dermatologic, ocular, respiratory, gastrointestinal, and
    neoplastic diseases; organ transplantation and a variety of diseases including those of
    hematologic, allergic, inflammatory, and autoimmune in origin; not available in injectable
    form, prednisolone must be used
Unlabeled/Investigational Use Investigational: Prevention of postherpetic neuralgia and
    relief of acute pain in the early stages
Pregnancy Risk Factor B
Pregnancy/Breast-Feeding Implications
Clinical effects on the fetus: Crosses the placenta. Immunosuppression reported in 1 infant
    exposed to high-dose prednisone plus azathioprine throughout gestation. One report of
    congenital cataracts. Available evidence suggests safe use during pregnancy.
Breast-feeding/lactation: Crosses into breast milk. No data on clinical effects on the infant.
    AAP considers **compatible** with breast-feeding.
Contraindications Hypersensitivity to prednisone or any component of the formulation;
    serious infections, except tuberculous meningitis; systemic fungal infections; varicella
Warnings/Precautions Withdraw therapy with gradual tapering of dose, may retard bone
    growth. Use with caution in patients with hypothyroidism, cirrhosis, congestive heart failure,
    ulcerative colitis, thromboembolic disorders, and patients at increased risk for peptic ulcer
    disease. Corticosteroids should be used with caution in patients with diabetes, hypertension,
    osteoporosis, glaucoma, cataracts, or tuberculosis. Use caution in hepatic impairment.
    Because of the risk of adverse effects, systemic corticosteroids should be used cautiously in
    the elderly, in the smallest possible dose, and for the shortest possible time.
Adverse Reactions In chronic, long-term use, may result in cushingoid appearance, osteopo-
    rosis, muscle weakness (proximal), and suppression of the adrenal-hypothalmic pituitary
    axis.

>10%:
    Central nervous system: Insomnia, nervousness
    Gastrointestinal: Increased appetite, indigestion
1% to 10%:
    Central nervous system: Dizziness or lightheadedness, headache
    Dermatologic: Hirsutism, hypopigmentation
    Endocrine & metabolic: Diabetes mellitus, glucose intolerance, hyperglycemia
    Neuromuscular & skeletal: Arthralgia
    Ocular: Cataracts, glaucoma
    Respiratory: Epistaxis
    Miscellaneous: Diaphoresis
<1% (Limited to important or life-threatening): Cushing's syndrome, edema, fractures, halluci-
    nations, hypertension, muscle-wasting, osteoporosis, pancreatitis, pituitary-adrenal axis
    suppression, seizures

Overdosage/Toxicology When consumed in excessive quantities for prolonged periods, systemic hypercorticism and adrenal suppression may occur; in those cases, discontinuation and withdrawal of the corticosteroid should be done judiciously.

Drug Interactions

Cytochrome P450 Effect: CYP3A3/4 enzyme substrate

Increased Effect/Toxicity: Concurrent use with NSAIDs may increase the risk of GI ulceration.

Decreased Effect: Decreased effect with barbiturates, phenytoin, rifampin; decreased effect of salicylates, vaccines, and toxoids.

Ethanol/Nutrition/Herb Interactions

Ethanol: Avoid ethanol (may increase gastric mucosal irritation).

Food: Prednisone interferes with calcium absorption, Limit caffeine.

Herb/Nutraceutical: St John's wort may decrease prednisone levels. Avoid cat's claw, echinacea (have immunostimulant properties).

Mechanism of Action Decreases inflammation by suppression of migration of polymorphonuclear leukocytes and reversal of increased capillary permeability; suppresses the immune system by reducing activity and volume of the lymphatic system; suppresses adrenal function at high doses. Antitumor effects may be related to inhibition of glucose transport, phosphorylation, or induction of cell death in immature lymphocytes. Antiemetic effects are thought to occur due to blockade of cerebral innervation of the emetic center via inhibition of prostaglandin synthesis.

Pharmacodynamics/Kinetics

Protein binding (concentration dependent): 65% to 91%

Metabolism: Converted rapidly from prednisone (inactive) to prednisolone (active); may be impaired with hepatic dysfunction

Half-life elimination: Normal renal function: 2.5-3.5 hours

See Prednisolone monograph for complete information.

Usual Dosage Oral: Dose depends upon condition being treated and response of patient; dosage for infants and children should be based on severity of the disease and response of the patient rather than on strict adherence to dosage indicated by age, weight, or body surface area. Consider alternate day therapy for long-term therapy. Discontinuation of long-term therapy requires gradual withdrawal by tapering the dose.

Children:

Anti-inflammatory or immunosuppressive dose: 0.05-2 mg/kg/day divided 1-4 times/day

Acute asthma: 1-2 mg/kg/day in divided doses 1-2 times/day for 3-5 days

Alternatively (for 3- to 5-day "burst"):

<1 year: 10 mg every 12 hours

1-4 years: 20 mg every 12 hours

5-13 years: 30 mg every 12 hours

>13 years: 40 mg every 12 hours

Asthma long-term therapy (alternative dosing by age):

<1 year: 10 mg every other day

1-4 years: 20 mg every other day

5-13 years: 30 mg every other day

>13 years: 40 mg every other day

Nephrotic syndrome:

Initial (first 3 episodes): 2 mg/kg/day **or** 60 mg/m^2/day (maximum: 80 mg/day) in divided doses 3-4 times/day until urine is protein free for 3 consecutive days (maximum: 28 days); followed by 1-1.5 mg/kg/dose **or** 40 mg/m^2/dose given every other day for 4 weeks

Maintenance dose (long-term maintenance dose for frequent relapses): 0.5-1 mg/kg/dose given every other day for 3-6 months

Children and Adults: Physiologic replacement: 4-5 mg/m^2/day

Children ≥5 years and Adults: Asthma:

Moderate persistent: Inhaled corticosteroid (medium dose) or inhaled corticosteroid (low-medium dose) with a long-acting bronchodilator

Severe persistent: Inhaled corticosteroid (high dose) and corticosteroid tablets or syrup long term: 2 mg/kg/day, generally not to exceed 60 mg/day

Adults:

Immunosuppression/chemotherapy adjunct: Range: 5-60 mg/day in divided doses 1-4 times/day

Allergic reaction (contact dermatitis):

Day 1: 30 mg divided as 10 mg before breakfast, 5 mg at lunch, 5 mg at dinner, 10 mg at bedtime

Day 2: 5 mg at breakfast, 5 mg at lunch, 5 mg at dinner, 10 mg at bedtime

Day 3: 5 mg 4 times/day (with meals and at bedtime)

Day 4: 5 mg 3 times/day (breakfast, lunch, bedtime)

Day 5: 5 mg 2 times/day (breakfast, bedtime)

Day 6: 5 mg before breakfast

Pneumocystis carinii pneumonia (PCP):

40 mg twice daily for 5 days **followed by**

40 mg once daily for 5 days **followed by**

20 mg once daily for 11 days or until antimicrobial regimen is completed

Thyrotoxicosis: Oral: 60 mg/day

Chemotherapy (refer to individual protocols): Oral: Range: 20 mg/day to 100 mg/m^2/day

Rheumatoid arthritis: Oral: Use lowest possible daily dose (often ≤7.5 mg/day)

Idiopathic thrombocytopenia purpura (ITP): Oral: 60 mg daily for 4-6 weeks, gradually tapered over several weeks

Systemic lupus erythematosus (SLE): Oral:

Acute: 1-2 mg/kg/day in 2-3 divided doses

Maintenance: Reduce to lowest possible dose, usually <1 mg/kg/day as single dose (morning)

Elderly: Use the lowest effective dose

(Continued)

PredniSONE *(Continued)*

Dosing adjustment in hepatic impairment: Prednisone is inactive and must be metabolized by the liver to prednisolone. This conversion may be impaired in patients with liver disease, however, prednisolone levels are observed to be higher in patients with severe liver failure than in normal patients. Therefore, compensation for the inadequate conversion of prednisone to prednisolone occurs.

Dosing adjustment in hyperthyroidism: Prednisone dose may need to be increased to achieve adequate therapeutic effects

Hemodialysis: Supplemental dose is not necessary

Peritoneal dialysis: Supplemental dose is not necessary

Dietary Considerations Should be taken after meals or with food or milk; increase dietary intake of pyridoxine, vitamin C, vitamin D, folate, calcium, and phosphorus.

Administration Administer with meals to decrease gastrointestinal upset

Monitoring Parameters Blood pressure, blood glucose, electrolytes

Test Interactions Response to skin tests

Patient Information Notify surgeon or dentist before surgical repair; may cause GI upset, take with food; notify physician if any sign of infection occurs; avoid abrupt withdrawal when on long-term therapy; do not discontinue or decrease drug without contacting physician, carry an identification card or bracelet advising that you are on steroids

Nursing Implications Withdraw therapy with gradual tapering of dose

Additional Information Tapering of corticosteroids after a short course of therapy (<7-10 days) is generally not required unless the disease/inflammatory process is slow to respond. Tapering after prolonged exposure is dependent upon the individual patient, duration of corticosteroid treatments, and size of steroid dose. Recovery of the HPA axis may require several months. Subtle but important HPA axis suppression may be present for as long as several months after a course of as few as 10-14 days duration. Testing of HPA axis (cosyntropin) may be required, and signs/symptoms of adrenal insufficiency should be monitored in patients with a history of use.

Dosage Forms

Solution, oral: 1 mg/mL (5 mL, 120 mL, 500 mL) [alcohol 5%]
Solution, oral concentrate: 5 mg/mL (30 mL) [alcohol 30%]
Syrup: 1 mg/mL (120 mL, 240 mL)
Tablet: 1 mg, 2.5 mg, 5 mg, 10 mg, 20 mg, 50 mg

Primaquine *(PRIM a kween)*

Related Information

Malaria Treatment *on page 1607*
Prevention of Malaria *on page 1552*

Synonyms Primaquine Phosphate; Prymaccone

Therapeutic Category Antimalarial Agent

Use Provides radical cure of *P. vivax* or *P. ovale* malaria after a clinical attack has been confirmed by blood smear or serologic titer and postexposure prophylaxis

Pregnancy Risk Factor C

Contraindications Hypersensitivity to primaquine, similar alkaloids, or any component of the formulation; acutely ill patients who have a tendency to develop granulocytopenia (rheumatoid arthritis, SLE); patients receiving other drugs capable of depressing the bone marrow (eg, quinacrine and primaquine)

Warnings/Precautions Use with caution in patients with G6PD deficiency, NADH methemo-globin reductase deficiency, acutely ill patients who have a tendency to develop granulocyto-penia; patients receiving other drugs capable of depressing the bone marrow; do not exceed recommended dosage

Adverse Reactions
>10%:
Gastrointestinal: Abdominal pain, nausea, vomiting
Hematologic: Hemolytic anemia
1% to 10%: Hematologic: Methemoglobinemia
<1% (Limited to important or life-threatening): Agranulocytosis, arrhythmias, leukocytosis, leukopenia

Overdosage/Toxicology Symptoms of acute overdose include abdominal cramps, vomiting, cyanosis, methemoglobinemia (possibly severe), leukopenia, acute hemolytic anemia (often significant), and granulocytopenia. With chronic overdose, symptoms include ototoxicity and retinopathy. Following GI decontamination, treatment is supportive (fluids, anticonvulsants, blood transfusions, methylene blue if methemoglobinemia is severe - 1-2 mg/kg over several minutes).

Drug Interactions
Cytochrome P450 Effect: CYP2D6 enzyme inhibitor
Increased Effect/Toxicity: Increased toxicity/levels with quinacrine.
Ethanol/Nutrition/Herb Interactions Ethanol: Avoid ethanol (due to GI irritation).
Mechanism of Action Eliminates the primary tissue exoerythrocytic forms of *P. falciparum*; disrupts mitochondria and binds to DNA

Pharmacodynamics/Kinetics
Absorption: Well absorbed
Metabolism: Hepatic to carboxyprimaquine (active)
Half-life elimination: 3.7-9.6 hours
Time to peak, serum: 1-2 hours
Excretion: Urine (small amounts as unchanged drug)

Usual Dosage Oral:
Children: 0.3 mg base/kg/day once daily for 14 days (not to exceed 15 mg/day) or 0.9 mg base/kg once weekly for 8 weeks not to exceed 45 mg base/week
Adults: 15 mg/day (base) once daily for 14 days or 45 mg base once weekly for 8 weeks
CDC treatment recommendations: Begin therapy during last 2 weeks of, or following a course of, suppression with chloroquine or a comparable drug

Monitoring Parameters Periodic CBC, visual color check of urine, glucose, electrolytes; if hemolysis suspected - CBC, haptoglobin, peripheral smear, urinalysis dipstick for occult blood

Patient Information Take with meals to decrease adverse GI effects; drug has a bitter taste; notify physician if a darkening of urine occurs or if shortness of breath, weakness or skin discoloration (chocolate cyanosis) occurs; complete full course of therapy

Nursing Implications Monitor periodic CBC, visual color check of urine
Dosage Forms Tablet, as phosphate: 26.3 mg [15 mg base]

♦ **Primaquine Phosphate** *see* Primaquine *on page 1126*
♦ **Primatene® Mist [OTC]** *see* Epinephrine *on page 470*
♦ **Primaxin®** *see* Imipenem and Cilastatin *on page 706*

Primidone (PRI mi done)

Related Information
Anticonvulsants by Seizure Type *on page 1481*
Epilepsy & Seizure Treatment *on page 1659*

U.S. Brand Names Mysoline®
Canadian Brand Names Apo®-Primidone; Mysoline®
Synonyms Desoxyphenobarbital; Primaclone
Therapeutic Category Anticonvulsant; Barbiturate
Use Management of grand mal, psychomotor, and focal seizures
Unlabeled/Investigational Use Benign familial tremor (essential tremor)
Pregnancy Risk Factor D
Pregnancy/Breast-Feeding Implications
Clinical effects on the fetus: Crosses the placenta. Dysmorphic facial features; hemorrhagic disease of newborn due to fetal vitamin K depletion, maternal folic acid deficiency may occur. Epilepsy itself, number of medications, genetic factors, or a combination of these probably influence the teratogenicity of anticonvulsant therapy. Benefit:risk ratio usually favors continued use during pregnancy and breast-feeding.
Breast-feeding/lactation: Crosses into breast milk
Clinical effects on the infant: Sedation; feeding problems reported. AAP recommends USE WITH CAUTION.

Contraindications Hypersensitivity to primidone, phenobarbital, or any component of the formulation; porphyria; pregnancy

Warnings/Precautions Use with caution in patients with renal or hepatic impairment, pulmonary insufficiency; abrupt withdrawal may precipitate status epilepticus. Potential for drug dependency exists. Do not administer to patients in acute pain. Use caution in elderly, debilitated, or pediatric patients - may cause paradoxical responses. May cause CNS depres-sion, which may impair physical or mental abilities. Patients must cautioned about performing tasks which require mental alertness (ie, operating machinery or driving). Effects with other sedative drugs or ethanol may be potentiated. Use with caution in patients with depression or suicidal tendencies, or in patients with a history of drug abuse. Tolerance or psychological and physical dependence may occur with prolonged use. Primidone's metabolite, phenobar-bital, has been associated with cognitive deficits in children. Use with caution in patients with hypoadrenalism.

Adverse Reactions Frequency not defined.
(Continued)

Primidone *(Continued)*

Central nervous system: Drowsiness, vertigo, ataxia, lethargy, behavior change, fatigue, hyperirritability

Dermatologic: Rash

Gastrointestinal: Nausea, vomiting, anorexia

Genitourinary: Impotence

Hematologic: Agranulocytopenia, agranulocytosis, anemia

Ocular: Diplopia, nystagmus

Overdosage/Toxicology Symptoms include unsteady gait, slurred speech, confusion, jaundice, hypothermia, fever, hypotension, coma, and respiratory arrest. Assure adequate hydration and renal function. Urinary alkalinization with I.V. sodium bicarbonate also helps enhance elimination. Repeat oral doses of activated charcoal significantly reduce the half-life of primidone resulting from enhancement of nonrenal elimination. The usual dose is 0.1-1 g/kg every 4-6 hours for 3-4 days, unless the patient has no bowel movement, causing charcoal to remain in the GI tract. Hemodialysis or hemoperfusion is of uncertain value. Patients in stage IV coma, due to high serum drug levels, may require charcoal hemoperfusion.

Drug Interactions

Cytochrome P450 Effect: CYP1A2, 2B6, 2C, 2C8, 3A3/4, and 3A5-7 enzyme inducer

Note: Primidone is metabolically converted to phenobarbital. Barbiturates are cytochrome P450 enzyme inducers. Patients should be monitored when these drugs are started or stopped for a decreased or increased therapeutic effect respectively.

Increased Effect/Toxicity: Central nervous system depression (and possible respiratory depression) may be increased when combined with other CNS depressants, benzodiazepines, valproic acid, chloramphenicol, or antidepressants. MAO inhibitors may prolong the effect of primidone.

Decreased Effect: Primidone may induce the hepatic metabolism of many drugs due to enzyme induction, and may reduce the efficacy of beta-blockers, chloramphenicol, cimetidine, clozapine, corticosteroids, cyclosporine, disopyramide, doxycycline, ethosuximide, furosemide, griseofulvin, haloperidol, lamotrigine, methadone, nifedipine, oral contraceptives, phenothiazine, phenytoin, propafenone, quinidine, tacrolimus, TCAs, theophylline, warfarin, and verapamil.

Ethanol/Nutrition/Herb Interactions

Ethanol: Avoid ethanol (may increase CNS depression).

Food: Protein-deficient diets increase duration of action of primidone.

Herb/Nutraceutical: Avoid valerian, St John's wort, kava kava, gotu kola (may increase CNS depression).

Stability Protect from light

Mechanism of Action Decreases neuron excitability, raises seizure threshold similar to phenobarbital; primidone has two active metabolites, phenobarbital and phenylethylmalonamide (PEMA); PEMA may enhance the activity of phenobarbital

Pharmacodynamics/Kinetics

Distribution: Adults: V_d: 2-3 L/kg

Protein binding: 99%

Metabolism: Hepatic to phenobarbital (active) and phenylethylmalonamide (PEMA)

Bioavailability: 60% to 80%

Half-life elimination (age dependent): Primidone: 10-12 hours; PEMA: 16 hours; Phenobarbital: 52-118 hours

Time to peak, serum: ~4 hours

Excretion: Urine (15% to 25% as unchanged drug and active metabolites)

Usual Dosage Oral:

Children <8 years: Initial: 50-125 mg/day given at bedtime; increase by 50-125 mg/day increments every 3-7 days; usual dose: 10-25 mg/kg/day in divided doses 3-4 times/day

Children ≥8 years and Adults: Initial: 125-250 mg/day at bedtime; increase by 125-250 mg/day every 3-7 days; usual dose: 750-1500 mg/day in divided doses 3-4 times/day with maximum dosage of 2 g/day

Dosing interval in renal impairment:

Cl_{cr} 50-80 mL/minute: Administer every 8 hours

Cl_{cr} 10-50 mL/minute: Administer every 8-12 hours

Cl_{cr} <10 mL/minute: Administer every 12-24 hours

Hemodialysis: Moderately dialyzable (20% to 50%); administer dose postdialysis or administer supplemental 30% dose

Dietary Considerations Folic acid: Low erythrocyte and CSF folate concentrations. Megaloblastic anemia has been reported. To avoid folic acid deficiency and megaloblastic anemia, some clinicians recommend giving patients on anticonvulsants prophylactic doses of folic acid and cyanocobalamin.

Monitoring Parameters Serum primidone and phenobarbital concentration, CBC, neurological status. Due to CNS effects, monitor closely when initiating drug in elderly. Monitor CBC at 6-month intervals to compare with baseline obtained at start of therapy. Since elderly metabolize phenobarbital at a slower rate than younger adults, it is suggested to measure both primidone and phenobarbital together.

Reference Range Therapeutic: Children <5 years: 7-10 µg/mL (SI: 32-46 µmol/L); Adults: 5-12 µg/mL (SI: 23-55 µmol/L); toxic effects rarely present with levels <10 µg/mL (SI: 46 µmol/L) if phenobarbital concentrations are low. Dosage of primidone is adjusted with reference mostly to the phenobarbital level; Toxic: >15 µg/mL (SI: >69 µmol/L)

Patient Information May cause drowsiness, impair judgment and coordination; do not abruptly discontinue or change dosage without notifying physician; can take with food to avoid GI upset

Nursing Implications Observe patient for excessive sedation; institute safety measures

Dosage Forms

Suspension, oral: 250 mg/5 mL (240 mL)

Tablet: 50 mg, 250 mg

♦ **Primsol**® *see* Trimethoprim *on page 1376*

- **Principen**® *see* Ampicillin *on page 93*
- **Prinivil**® *see* Lisinopril *on page 809*
- **Prinzide**® *see* Lisinopril and Hydrochlorothiazide *on page 811*
- **Priorix**™ **(Can)** *see* Measles, Mumps, and Rubella Vaccines (Combined) *on page 841*
- **Priscoline**® *see* Tolazoline *on page 1344*
- **Pristinamycin** *see* Quinupristin and Dalfopristin *on page 1172*
- **Privine**® **Nasal [OTC]** *see* Naphazoline *on page 957*
- **ProAmatine**® *see* Midodrine *on page 912*

Probenecid (proe BEN e sid)

Related Information
Treatment of Sexually Transmitted Diseases *on page 1609*

U.S. Brand Names Benemid® [DSC]

Canadian Brand Names Benuryl™

Therapeutic Category Uricosuric Agent

Use Prevention of gouty arthritis; hyperuricemia; prolongation of beta-lactam effect (ie, serum levels)

Pregnancy Risk Factor B

Contraindications Hypersensitivity to probenecid or any component of the formulation; high-dose aspirin therapy; moderate to severe renal impairment; children <2 years of age

Warnings/Precautions Use with caution in patients with peptic ulcer; use extreme caution in the use of probenecid with penicillin in patients with renal insufficiency; probenecid may not be effective in patients with a creatinine clearance <30-50 mL/minute; may cause exacerbation of acute gouty attack

Adverse Reactions Frequency not defined.
Cardiovascular: Flushing of face
Central nervous system: Headache, dizziness
Dermatologic: Rash, itching
Gastrointestinal: Anorexia, nausea, vomiting, sore gums
Genitourinary: Painful urination
Hematologic: Aplastic anemia, hemolytic anemia, leukopenia
Hepatic: Hepatic necrosis
Neuromuscular & skeletal: Gouty arthritis (acute)
Renal: Renal calculi, nephrotic syndrome, urate nephropathy
Miscellaneous: Anaphylaxis

Overdosage/Toxicology Symptoms include nausea, vomiting, clonic-tonic seizures, and coma. Activated charcoal is especially effective at binding probenecid and for GI decontamination.

Drug Interactions
Increased Effect/Toxicity: Increases methotrexate toxic potential. Probenecid increases the serum concentrations of quinolones and beta-lactams such as penicillins and cephalosporins. Also increases levels/toxicity of acyclovir, diflunisal, ketorolac, thiopental, benzodiazepines, dapsone, fluoroquinolones, methotrexate, NSAIDs, sulfonylureas, zidovudine.

Decreased Effect: Salicylates (high-dose) may decrease uricosuria. Decreased urinary levels of nitrofurantoin may decrease efficacy.

Mechanism of Action Competitively inhibits the reabsorption of uric acid at the proximal convoluted tubule, thereby promoting its excretion and reducing serum uric acid levels; increases plasma levels of weak organic acids (penicillins, cephalosporins, or other beta-lactam antibiotics) by competitively inhibiting their renal tubular secretion

Pharmacodynamics/Kinetics
Onset of action: Effect on penicillin levels: 2 hours
Absorption: Rapid and complete
Metabolism: Hepatic
Half-life elimination (dose dependent): Normal renal function: 6-12 hours
Time to peak, serum: 2-4 hours
Excretion: Urine

Usual Dosage Oral:
Children:
<2 years: Not recommended
2-14 years: Prolong penicillin serum levels: 25 mg/kg starting dose, then 40 mg/kg/day given 4 times/day
Gonorrhea: <45 kg: 25 mg/kg x 1 (maximum: 1 g/dose) 30 minutes before penicillin, ampicillin or amoxicillin
Adults:
Hyperuricemia with gout: 250 mg twice daily for one week; increase to 250-500 mg/day; may increase by 500 mg/month, if needed, to maximum of 2-3 g/day (dosages may be increased by 500 mg every 6 months if serum urate concentrations are controlled)
Prolong penicillin serum levels: 500 mg 4 times/day
Gonorrhea: 1 g 30 minutes before penicillin, ampicillin, procaine, or amoxicillin
Pelvic inflammatory disease: Cefoxitin 2 g I.M. plus probenecid 1 g orally as a single dose
Neurosyphilis: Aqueous procaine penicillin 2.4 million units/day I.M. plus probenecid 500 mg 4 times/day for 10-14 days
Dosing adjustment in renal impairment: Cl_{cr} <50 mL/minute: Avoid use

Dietary Considerations Drug may cause GI upset; take with food if GI upset. Drink plenty of fluids.

Administration Administer with food or antacids to minimize GI effects

Monitoring Parameters Uric acid, renal function, CBC

Test Interactions False-positive glucosuria with Clinitest®, a falsely high determination of theophylline has occurred and the renal excretion of phenolsulfonphthalein 17-ketosteroids and bromsulfophthalein (BSP) may be inhibited
(Continued)

Probenecid *(Continued)*

Patient Information Take with food or antacids; drink plenty of fluids to reduce the risk of uric acid stones; the frequency of acute gouty attacks may increase during the first 6-12 months of therapy; avoid taking large doses of aspirin or other salicylates

Nursing Implications An alkaline urine is recommended to avoid crystallization of urates; use of sodium bicarbonate or potassium citrate is suggested until serum uric acid normalizes and tophaceous deposits disappear

Additional Information Avoid fluctuation in uric acid (increase or decrease); may precipitate gout attack.

Dosage Forms Tablet: 500 mg

♦ **Probenecid and Colchicine** *see Colchicine and Probenecid on page 331*
♦ **Pro-Bionate® [OTC]** *see Lactobacillus on page 770*

Procainamide *(proe kane A mide)*

Related Information
Adult ACLS Algorithms *on page 1632*
Antiarrhythmic Drugs Comparison *on page 1478*
Depression *on page 1655*

U.S. Brand Names Procanbid®; Pronestyl®; Pronestyl-SR®

Canadian Brand Names Apo®-Procainamide; Procan® SR; Pronestyl®; Pronestyl®-SR

Synonyms PCA; Procainamide Hydrochloride; Procaine Amide Hydrochloride

Therapeutic Category Antiarrhythmic Agent, Class I-A

Use Treatment of ventricular tachycardia (VT), premature ventricular contractions, paroxysmal atrial tachycardia (PSVT), and atrial fibrillation (AF); prevent recurrence of ventricular tachycardia, paroxysmal supraventricular tachycardia, atrial fibrillation or flutter

Unlabeled/Investigational Use ACLS guidelines:
Intermittent/recurrent VF or pulseless VT not responsive to earlier interventions
Monomorphic VT (EF >40%, no CHF)
Polymorphic VT with normal baseline QT interval
Wide complex tachycardia of unknown type (EF >40%, no CHF, patient stable)
Refractory paroxysmal SVT
Atrial fibrillation or flutter (EF >40%, no CHF) including pre-excitation syndrome

Pregnancy Risk Factor C

Contraindications Hypersensitivity to procaine, other ester-type local anesthetics, or any component of the formulation; complete heart block (except in patients with a functioning artificial pacemaker); second-degree AV block (without a functional pacemaker); various types of hemiblock (without a functional pacemaker); SLE; torsade de pointes; concurrent cisapride use; QT prolongation

Warnings/Precautions Use with caution in patients with marked AV conduction disturbances, myasthenia gravis, bundle-branch block, or severe cardiac glycoside intoxication, ventricular arrhythmias with organic heart disease or coronary occlusion, CHF supraventricular tachyarrhythmias unless adequate measures are taken to prevent marked increases in ventricular rates; concurrent therapy with other class Ia drugs may accumulate in patients with renal or hepatic dysfunction; some tablets contain tartrazine; injection may contain bisulfite (allergens). Long-term administration leads to the development of a positive antinuclear antibody (ANA) test in 50% of patients which may result in a lupus erythematosus-like syndrome (in 20% to 30% of patients); discontinue procainamide with SLE symptoms and choose an alternative agent; elderly have reduced clearance and frequent drug interactions. Potentially fatal blood dyscrasias have occurred with therapeutic doses; close monitoring is recommended during the first 3 months of therapy.

Adverse Reactions
>1%:
Cardiovascular: Hypotension (I.V., up to 5%)
Dermatologic: Rash
Gastrointestinal: Diarrhea (3% to 4%), nausea, vomiting, taste disorder, GI complaints (3% to 4%)
<1% (Limited to important or life-threatening): Agranulocytosis, angioneurotic edema, aplastic anemia, arrhythmia (proarrhythmic effect, new or worsened), bone marrow suppression, cerebellar ataxia, cholestasis, demyelinating polyradiculoneuropathy, depressed myocardial contractility, depression, disorientation, drug fever, granulomatous hepatitis, hallucinations, hemolytic anemia, hepatic failure, hypoplastic anemia, leukopenia, mania, myasthenia gravis (worsened), myocarditis, myopathy, neuromuscular blockade, neutropenia, pancreatitis, pancytopenia, paradoxical increase in ventricular rate in atrial fibrillation/flutter, pericarditis, peripheral neuropathy, pleural effusion, positive ANA, positive Coombs' test, pruritus, pseudo-obstruction, psychosis, pulmonary embolism, QT prolongation (excessive), rash, respiratory failure due to myopathy, second-degree heart block, SLE-like syndrome, thrombocytopenia (0.5%), torsade de pointes, tremor, urticaria, vasculitis, ventricular arrhythmias

Overdosage/Toxicology
Has a low toxic:therapeutic ratio and may easily produce fatal intoxication (acute toxic dose: 5 g in adults). Symptoms of include sinus bradycardia, sinus node arrest or asystole; PR, QRS or QT interval prolongation; torsade de pointes (polymorphous ventricular tachycardia); and depressed myocardial contractility, which along with alpha-adrenergic or ganglionic blockade, may result in hypotension and pulmonary edema. Other effects are seizures, coma, and respiratory arrest.
Treatment is primarily symptomatic and effects usually respond to conventional therapies (fluids, positioning, vasopressors, anticonvulsants, antiarrhythmics). **Note:** Do not use other type 1a or 1c antiarrhythmic agents to treat ventricular tachycardia. Sodium bicarbonate may treat wide QRS intervals or hypotension. Markedly impaired conduction or high degree A-V block, unresponsive to bicarbonate, indicates consideration of a pacemaker is needed.

Drug Interactions

Increased Effect/Toxicity: Amiodarone, cimetidine, ofloxacin (and potentially other renally eliminated quinolones), ranitidine, and trimethoprim increase procainamide and NAPA blood levels; consider reducing procainamide dosage by 25% with concurrent use. Cisapride and procainamide may increase the risk of malignant arrhythmia; concurrent use is contraindicated. Neuromuscular blocking agents: Procainamide may potentiate neuro-muscular blockade.

Drugs which may prolong the QT interval include amiodarone, amitriptyline, astemizole, bepridil, cisapride, disopyramide, erythromycin, haloperidol, imipramine, pimozide, quini-dine, sotalol, mesoridazine, thioridazine, and some quinolone antibiotics (sparfloxacin, gatifloxacin, moxifloxacin); concurrent use may result in additional prolongation of the QT interval.

Ethanol/Nutrition/Herb Interactions

Ethanol: Avoid ethanol (acute ethanol administration reduces procainamide serum concen-trations).

Herb/Nutraceutical: Avoid ephedra (may worsen arrhythmia).

Stability Procainamide may be stored at room temperature up to 27°C; however, refrigeration retards oxidation, which causes color formation. The solution is initially colorless but may turn slightly yellow on standing. Injection of air into the vial causes the solution to darken. Solutions darker than a light amber should be discarded.

Minimum volume: 1 g/250 mL NS/D_5W

Stability of admixture at room temperature in D_5W or NS: 24 hours

Some information indicates that procainamide may be subject to greater decomposition in D_5W unless the admixture is refrigerated or the pH is adjusted. Procainamide is believed to form an association complex with dextrose - the bioavailability of procainamide in this complex is not known and the complex formation is reversible.

Mechanism of Action Decreases myocardial excitability and conduction velocity and may depress myocardial contractility, by increasing the electrical stimulation threshold of ventricle, HIS-Purkinje system and through direct cardiac effects

Pharmacodynamics/Kinetics

Onset of action: I.M. 10-30 minutes

Distribution: V_d: Children: 2.2 L/kg; Adults: 2 L/kg; Congestive heart failure or shock: Decreased V_d

Protein binding: 15% to 20%

Metabolism: By hepatic acetylation to produce N-acetyl procainamide (NAPA) (active metab-olite)

Bioavailability: Oral: 75% to 95%

Half-life elimination:

Procainamide (dependent upon hepatic acetylator, phenotype, cardiac function, and renal function):

Children: 1.7 hours; Adults: 2.5-4.7 hours; Anephric: 11 hours

NAPA (dependent upon renal function):

Children: 6 hours; Adults: 6-8 hours; Anephric: 42 hours

Time to peak, serum: Capsule: 45 minutes to 2.5 hours; I.M.: 15-60 minutes

Excretion: Urine (25% as NAPA)

Usual Dosage Must be titrated to patient's response

Children:

Oral: 15-50 mg/kg/24 hours divided every 3-6 hours

I.M.: 50 mg/kg/24 hours divided into doses of $^1/_8$ to $^1/_4$ every 3-6 hours in divided doses until oral therapy is possible

I.V. (infusion requires use of an infusion pump):

Load: 3-6 mg/kg/dose over 5 minutes not to exceed 100 mg/dose; may repeat every 5-10 minutes to maximum of 15 mg/kg/load

Maintenance as continuous I.V. infusion: 20-80 mcg/kg/minute; maximum: 2 g/24 hours

Adults:

Oral: 250-500 mg/dose every 3-6 hours or 500 mg to 1 g every 6 hours sustained release; usual dose: 50 mg/kg/24 hours; maximum: 4 g/24 hours (**Note:** Twice daily dosing approved for Procanbid®)

I.M.: 0.5-1 g every 4-8 hours until oral therapy is possible

I.V. (infusion requires use of an infusion pump): Loading dose: 15-18 mg/kg administered as slow infusion over 25-30 minutes or 100-200 mg/dose repeated every 5 minutes as needed to a total dose of 1 g; maintenance dose: 1-4 mg/minute by continuous infusion

Infusion rate: **2 g/250 mL** D_5W/NS (I.V. infusion requires use of an infusion pump):

1 mg/minute: 7.5 mL/hour

2 mg/minute: 15 mL/hour

3 mg/minute: 22.5 mL/hour

4 mg/minute: 30 mL/hour

5 mg/minute: 37.5 mL/hour

6 mg/minute: 45 mL/hour

Intermittent/recurrent VF or pulseless VT:

Initial: 20-30 mg/minute (maximum: 50 mg/minute if necessary), up to a total of 17 mg/kg. ACLS guidelines: I.V.: Infuse 20 mg/minute until arrhythmia is controlled, hypoten-sion occurs, QRS complex widens by 50% of its original width, or total of 17 mg/kg is given.

Note: Reduce to 12 mg/kg in setting of cardiac or renal dysfunction

I.V. maintenance infusion: 1-4 mg/minute; monitor levels and do not exceed 3 mg/minute for >24 hours in adults with renal failure.

Dosing interval in renal impairment:

Cl_{cr} 10-50 mL/minute: Administer every 6-12 hours.

Cl_{cr} <10 mL/minute: Administer every 8-24 hours.

Dialysis:

Procainamide: Moderately hemodialyzable (20% to 50%): 200 mg supplemental dose posthemodialysis is recommended.

(Continued)

Procainamide *(Continued)*

N-acetylprocainamide: Not dialyzable (0% to 5%)

Procainamide/N-acetylprocainamide: Not peritoneal dialyzable (0% to 5%)

Procainamide/N-acetylprocainamide: Replace by blood level during continuous arteriovenous or venovenous hemofiltration

Dosing adjustment in hepatic impairment: Reduce dose by 50%.

Dietary Considerations Should be taken with water on an empty stomach.

Administration Dilute I.V. with D_5W; maximum rate: 50 mg/minute; administer around-the-clock rather than 4 times/day to promote less variation in peak and trough serum levels

Monitoring Parameters EKG, blood pressure, CBC with differential, platelet count; cardiac monitor and blood pressure monitor required during I.V. administration; blood levels in patients with renal failure or receiving constant infusion >3 mg/minute for longer than 24 hours

Reference Range

Timing of serum samples: Draw trough just before next oral dose; draw 6-12 hours after I.V. infusion has started; half-life is 2.5-5 hours

Therapeutic levels: Procainamide: 4-10 µg/mL; NAPA 15-25 µg/mL; Combined: 10-30 µg/mL

Toxic concentration: Procainamide: >10-12 µg/mL

Patient Information Do not discontinue therapy unless instructed by physician; notify physician or pharmacist if soreness of mouth, throat or gums, unexplained fever, or symptoms of upper respiratory tract infection occur. Do not chew sustained release tablets; some sustained release tablets contain a wax core that slowly releases the drug; when this process is complete, the empty, nonabsorbable wax core is eliminated and may be visible in feces; some sustained release tablets may be broken in half.

Nursing Implications Do not crush sustained release drug product

Dosage Forms

Capsule, as hydrochloride: 250 mg, 375 mg, 500 mg

Injection, as hydrochloride: 100 mg/mL (10 mL); 500 mg/mL (2 mL)

Tablet, as hydrochloride: 250 mg, 375 mg, 500 mg

Tablet, sustained release, as hydrochloride: 250 mg, 500 mg, 750 mg, 1000 mg

Procanbid®: 500 mg, 1000 mg

Extemporaneous Preparations Note: Several formulations have been described, some being more complex; for all formulations, the pH must be 4-6 to prevent degradation; some preparations require adjustment of pH; shake well before use

A suspension of 50 mg/mL can be made with the capsules, distilled water, and a 2:1 simple syrup/cherry syrup mixture; stability 2 weeks under refrigeration; (ASHP, 1987)

Concentrations of 5, 50, and 100 mg/mL oral liquid preparations (made with the capsules, sterile water for irrigation and cherry syrup) stored at 4°C to 6°C (pH 6) were stable for at least 6 months (Metras, 1992).

A sucrose-based syrup (procainamide 50 mg/mL) made with capsules, distilled water, simple syrup, parabens, and cherry flavoring had a calculated stability of 456 days at 25°C and measured stability of 42 days at 40°C (pH ~5) while a maltitol-based syrup (procainamide 50 mg/mL) made with capsules, distilled water, Lycasin® (a syrup vehicle with 75% w/w maltitol), parabens, sodium bisulfate, saccharin, sodium acetate, pineapple and apricot flavoring, FD & C yellow number 6 (pH adjusted to 5 with glacial acetic acid) had a calculated stability of 97 days at 25°C and a measured stability of 94 days at 40°C. The maltitol-based syrup was more stable than the sucrose-based syrup when temperature was >37°C, but the sucrose-based syrup was more stable at temperatures <37°C (Alexander, 1993).

Alexander KS, Pudipeddi M, and Parker GA, "Stability of Procainamide Hydrochloride Syrups Compounded From Capsules," *Am J Hosp Pharm*, 1993, 50(4):693-8.

Handbook in Extemporaneous Formulations, Bethesda, MD: American Society of Hospital Pharmacists, 1987.

Metras JI, Swenson CF, and MacDermott MP, "Stability of Procainamide Hydrochloride in an Extemporaneously Compounded Oral Liquid," *Am J Hosp Pharm*, 1992, 49(7):1720-4.

Swenson CF, "Importance of Following Instructions When Compounding," *Am J Hosp Pharm*, 1993, 50(2):261.

♦ **Procainamide Hydrochloride** see Procainamide on page 1130

Procaine *(PROE kane)*

U.S. Brand Names Novocain®

Canadian Brand Names Novocain®

Synonyms Procaine Hydrochloride

Therapeutic Category Local Anesthetic, Injectable

Use Produces spinal anesthesia and epidural and peripheral nerve block by injection and infiltration methods

Pregnancy Risk Factor C

Contraindications Hypersensitivity to procaine, PABA, parabens, other ester local anesthetics, or any component of the formulation

Warnings/Precautions Patients with cardiac diseases, hyperthyroidism, or other endocrine diseases may be more susceptible to toxic effects of local anesthetics; some preparations contain metabisulfite

Adverse Reactions

1% to 10%: Local: Burning sensation at site of injection, tissue irritation, pain at injection site

<1% (Limited to important or life-threatening): Aseptic meningitis resulting in paralysis, chills, CNS stimulation followed by CNS depression

Overdosage/Toxicology Treatment is primarily symptomatic and supportive. Termination of anesthesia by pneumatic tourniquet inflation should be attempted when the agent is administered by infiltration or regional injection. Seizures commonly respond to diazepam, while hypotension responds to I.V. fluids and Trendelenburg positioning. Bradyarrhythmias (heart rate <60) can be treated with I.V., I.M., or S.C. atropine 15 mcg/kg. With the development of metabolic acidosis, I.V. sodium bicarbonate 0.5-2 mEq/kg and ventilatory assistance should be instituted.

Drug Interactions

Decreased Effect: Decreased effect of sulfonamides with the PABA metabolite of procaine, chloroprocaine, and tetracaine. Decreased/increased effect of vasopressors, ergot alkaloids, and MAO inhibitors on blood pressure when using anesthetic solutions with a vasoconstrictor.

Mechanism of Action Blocks both the initiation and conduction of nerve impulses by decreasing the neuronal membrane's permeability to sodium ions, which results in inhibition of depolarization with resultant blockade of conduction

Pharmacodynamics/Kinetics

Onset of action: 2-5 minutes

Duration (dependent upon patient, type of block, concentration, and method of anesthesia); 0.5-1.5 hours

Metabolism: Rapidly hydrolyzed by plasma enzymes to para-aminobenzoic acid and diethylaminoethanol (80% conjugated before elimination)

Half-life elimination: 7.7 minutes

Excretion: Urine (as metabolites and some unchanged drug)

Usual Dosage Dose varies with procedure, desired depth, and duration of anesthesia, desired muscle relaxation, vascularity of tissues, physical condition, and age of patient

Nursing Implications Prior to instillation of anesthetic agent, withdraw plunger to ensure needle is not in artery or vein; resuscitative equipment should be available when local anesthetics are administered

Dosage Forms Injection, as hydrochloride: 1% [10 mg/mL] (2 mL, 6 mL, 30 mL, 100 mL); 2% [20 mg/mL] (30 mL, 100 mL); 10% (2 mL)

♦ **Procaine Amide Hydrochloride** see Procainamide on page 1130

♦ **Procaine Benzylpenicillin** see Penicillin G Procaine on page 1054

♦ **Procaine Hydrochloride** see Procaine on page 1132

♦ **Procaine Penicillin G** see Penicillin G Procaine on page 1054

♦ **Procanbid®** see Procainamide on page 1130

♦ **Procan® SR (Can)** see Procainamide on page 1130

Procarbazine (proe KAR ba zeen)

Related Information

Tyramine Content of Foods on page 1737

U.S. Brand Names Matulane®

Canadian Brand Names Matulane®; Natulan®

Synonyms Benzmethyzin; N-Methylhydrazine; Procarbazine Hydrochloride

Therapeutic Category Antineoplastic Agent, Alkylating Agent

Use Treatment of Hodgkin's disease; other uses include non-Hodgkin's lymphoma, brain tumors, melanoma, lung cancer, multiple myeloma

Pregnancy Risk Factor D

Contraindications Hypersensitivity to procarbazine or any component of the formulation; pre-existing bone marrow aplasia; ethanol ingestion; pregnancy

Warnings/Precautions The U.S. Food and Drug Administration (FDA) currently recommends that procedures for proper handling and disposal of antineoplastic agents be considered; use with caution in patients with pre-existing renal or hepatic impairment; modify dosage in patients with renal or hepatic impairment, or marrow disorders; reduce dosage with serum creatinine >2 mg/dL or total bilirubin >3 mg/dL; procarbazine possesses MAO inhibitor activity. Procarbazine is a carcinogen which may cause acute leukemia; procarbazine may cause infertility.

Adverse Reactions

>10%:

Central nervous system: Mental depression, manic reactions, hallucinations, dizziness, headache, nervousness, insomnia, nightmares, ataxia, disorientation, confusion, seizure, CNS stimulation

Endocrine & metabolic: Amenorrhea

Gastrointestinal: Severe nausea and vomiting occur frequently and may be dose-limiting; anorexia, abdominal pain, stomatitis, dysphagia, diarrhea, and constipation; use a nonphenothiazine antiemetic, when possible

Emetic potential: Moderately high (60% to 90%)

Time course of nausea/vomiting: Onset: 24-27 hours; Duration: variable

Hematologic: Thrombocytopenia, hemolytic anemia, anemia

Myelosuppressive: May be dose-limiting toxicity; procarbazine should be discontinued if leukocyte count is <4000/mm^3 or platelet count <100,000/mm^3

WBC: Moderate

Platelets: Moderate

Onset (days): 14

Nadir (days): 21

Recovery (days): 28

Neuromuscular & skeletal: Weakness, paresthesia, neuropathies, decreased reflexes, foot drop, tremors

Ocular: Nystagmus

Respiratory: Pleural effusion, cough

1% to 10%:

Dermatologic: Alopecia, hyperpigmentation

Gastrointestinal: Diarrhea, stomatitis, constipation

Hepatic: Hepatotoxicity

Neuromuscular & skeletal: Peripheral neuropathy

<1% (Limited to important or life-threatening): Disulfiram-like reactions, hypertensive crisis, orthostatic hypotension, pneumonitis

(Continued)

Procarbazine *(Continued)*

Overdosage/Toxicology Symptoms include arthralgia, alopecia, paresthesias, bone marrow suppression, hallucinations, nausea, vomiting, diarrhea, seizures, and coma. Treatment is supportive. Adverse effects such as marrow toxicity may begin as late as 2 weeks after exposure.

Drug Interactions

Increased Effect/Toxicity: Procarbazine exhibits weak MAO inhibitor activity. Foods containing high amounts of tyramine should, therefore, be avoided. When an MAO inhibitor is given with food high in tyramine, hypertensive crisis, intracranial bleeding, and headache have been reported.

Sympathomimetic amines (epinephrine and amphetamines) and antidepressants (tricyclics) should be used cautiously with procarbazine. Barbiturates, narcotics, phenothiazines, and other CNS depressants can cause somnolence, ataxia, and other symptoms of CNS depression. Ethanol has caused a disulfiram-like reaction with procarbazine. May result in headache, respiratory difficulties, nausea, vomiting, sweating, thirst, hypotension, and flushing.

Ethanol/Nutrition/Herb Interactions

Ethanol: Avoid ethanol and ethanol-containing products.

Food: Clinically severe and possibly life-threatening elevations in blood pressure may occur if procarbazine is taken with tyramine-containing foods.

Stability Protect from light

Mechanism of Action Mechanism of action is not clear, methylating of nucleic acids; inhibits DNA, RNA, and protein synthesis; may damage DNA directly and suppresses mitosis; metabolic activation required by host

Pharmacodynamics/Kinetics

Absorption: Rapid and complete

Distribution: Crosses blood-brain barrier; distributes into CSF

Metabolism: Hepatic and renal

Half-life elimination: 1 hour

Excretion: Urine and respiratory tract (<5% as unchanged drug, 70% as metabolites)

Usual Dosage Refer to individual protocols. Dose based on patient's ideal weight if the patient is obese or has abnormal fluid retention. Oral:

Children:

BMT aplastic anemia conditioning regimen: 12.5 mg/kg/dose every other day for 4 doses

Hodgkin's disease: MOPP/IC-MOPP regimens: 100 mg/m^2/day for 14 days and repeated every 4 weeks

Neuroblastoma and medulloblastoma: Doses as high as 100-200 mg/m^2/day once daily have been used

Adults: Initial: 2-4 mg/kg/day in single or divided doses for 7 days then increase dose to 4-6 mg/kg/day until response is obtained or leukocyte count decreased <4000/mm^3 or the platelet count decreased <100,000/mm^3; maintenance: 1-2 mg/kg/day

In MOPP, 100 mg/m^2/day on days 1-14 of a 28-day cycle

Dosing in renal/hepatic impairment: Use with caution, may result in increased toxicity

Monitoring Parameters CBC with differential, platelet and reticulocyte count, urinalysis, liver function test, renal function test.

Patient Information Take as directed. Maintain adequate hydration (2-3 L/day of fluids unless instructed to restrict fluid intake). Avoid aspirin and aspirin-containing substances; avoid alcohol, may cause acute disulfiram-like reaction - flushing, headache, acute vomiting, chest and/or abdominal pain; avoid tyramine-containing foods (aged cheese, chocolate, pickles, aged meat, wine, etc). You may experience mental depression, nervousness, insomnia, nightmares, dizziness, confusion, or lethargy (use caution when driving or engaging in tasks that require alertness until response to drug is known); photosensitivity (use sunscreen, wear protective clothing and eyewear, and avoid direct sunlight). You may experience rash or hair loss (reversible), loss of libido, increased sensitivity to infection (avoid crowds and infected persons). Report persistent fever, chills, sore throat; unusual bleeding; blood in urine, stool (black stool), or vomitus; unresolved depression; mania; hallucinations; nightmares; disorientation; seizures; chest pain or palpitations; or difficulty breathing.

Dosage Forms Capsule, as hydrochloride: 50 mg

- ◆ **Procarbazine Hydrochloride** *see Procarbazine on page 1133*
- ◆ **Procardia®** *see NIFEdipine on page 981*
- ◆ **Procardia XL®** *see NIFEdipine on page 981*
- ◆ **Procetofene** *see Fenofibrate on page 548*

Prochlorperazine *(proe klor PER a zeen)*

Related Information

Antacid Drug Interactions *on page 1477*

U.S. Brand Names Compazine®; Compro™

Canadian Brand Names Compazine®; Nu-Prochlor; Stemetil®

Synonyms Prochlorperazine Edisylate; Prochlorperazine Maleate

Therapeutic Category Antiemetic; Antipsychotic Agent, Phenothiazine; Phenothiazine Derivative

Use Management of nausea and vomiting; psychosis; anxiety

Unlabeled/Investigational Use Dementia behavior

Pregnancy Risk Factor C

Pregnancy/Breast-Feeding Implications

Clinical effects on the fetus: Crosses the placenta. Isolated reports of congenital anomalies, however some included exposures to other drugs. Available evidence with use of occasional low doses suggests safe use during pregnancy.

Breast-feeding/lactation: No data available. AAP considers **compatible** with breast-feeding.

Contraindications Hypersensitivity to prochlorperazine or any component of the formulation (cross-reactivity between phenothiazines may occur); severe CNS depression; coma; bone marrow suppression; should not be used in children <2 years of age or <10 kg

Warnings/Precautions Injection contains sulfites which may cause allergic reactions; may impair ability to perform hazardous tasks requiring mental alertness or physical coordination; some products contain tartrazine dye, avoid use in sensitive individuals

Tardive dyskinesia: Prevalence rate may be 40% in elderly; development of the syndrome and the irreversible nature are proportional to duration and total cumulative dose over time. May be reversible if diagnosed early in therapy.

High incidence of extrapyramidal symptoms, especially in children or the elderly, so reserve use in children <5 years of age to those who are unresponsive to other antiemetics; incidence of extrapyramidal symptoms is increased with acute illnesses such as chicken pox, measles, CNS infections, gastroenteritis, and dehydration

Drug-induced **Parkinson's syndrome** occurs often. **Akathisia** is the most common extrapyramidal symptom in elderly.

Increased confusion, memory loss, psychotic behavior, and agitation frequently occur as a consequence of anticholinergic effects

Lowers seizure threshold, use cautiously in patients with seizure history

Orthostatic hypotension is due to alpha-receptor blockade, the elderly are at greater risk for orthostatic hypotension

Antipsychotic associated sedation in nonpsychotic patients is extremely unpleasant due to feelings of depersonalization, derealization, and dysphoria

Life-threatening arrhythmias have occurred at therapeutic doses of antipsychotics

Adverse Reactions Frequency not defined.

Cardiovascular: Hypotension, orthostatic hypotension, hypertension, tachycardia, bradycardia, dizziness, cardiac arrest

Central nervous system: Extrapyramidal symptoms (pseudoparkinsonism, akathisia, dystonias, tardive dyskinesia), dizziness, cerebral edema, seizures, headache, drowsiness, paradoxical excitement, restlessness, hyperactivity, insomnia, neuroleptic malignant syndrome (NMS), impairment of temperature regulation

Dermatologic: Increased sensitivity to sun, rash, discoloration of skin (blue-gray)

Endocrine & metabolic: Hypoglycemia, hyperglycemia, galactorrhea, lactation, breast enlargement, gynecomastia, menstrual irregularity, amenorrhea, SIADH, changes in libido

Gastrointestinal: Constipation, weight gain, vomiting, stomach pain, nausea, xerostomia, salivation, diarrhea, anorexia, ileus

Genitourinary: Difficulty in urination, ejaculatory disturbances, incontinence, polyuria, ejaculating dysfunction, priapism

Hematologic: Agranulocytosis, leukopenia, eosinophilia, hemolytic anemia, thrombocytopenic purpura, pancytopenia

Hepatic: Cholestatic jaundice, hepatotoxicity

Neuromuscular & skeletal: Tremor

Ocular: Pigmentary retinopathy, blurred vision, cornea and lens changes

Respiratory: Nasal congestion

Miscellaneous: Diaphoresis

Overdosage/Toxicology Symptoms include deep sleep, coma, extrapyramidal symptoms, abnormal involuntary muscle movements, and hypotension. Following initiation of essential overdose management, toxic symptom and supportive treatment should be initiated. Hypotension usually responds to I.V. fluids or Trendelenburg positioning. If unresponsive to these measures, the use of a parenteral inotrope may be required (eg, norepinephrine 0.1-0.2 mcg/kg/minute titrated to response). Seizures commonly respond to diazepam (I.V. 5-10 mg bolus in adults every 15 minutes, if needed, up to a total of 30 mg; I.V. 0.25-0.4 mg/dose up to a total of 10 mg in children) or to phenytoin or phenobarbital. Critical cardiac arrhythmias often respond to I.V. phenytoin (15 mg/kg up to 1 g), while other antiarrhythmics can be used. Extrapyramidal symptoms (eg, dystonic reactions) may require management with diphenhydramine 1-2 mg/kg (adults) up to a maximum of 50 mg I.M. or slow I.V. push followed by a maintenance dose for 48-72 hours. When these reactions are unresponsive to diphenhydramine, anticholinergic agents such as benztropine mesylate I.V. 1-2 mg (adults) may be effective. These agents are generally effective within 2-5 minutes.

Drug Interactions

Cytochrome P450 Effect: Possible CYP2D6 enzyme substrate

Increased Effect/Toxicity: Chloroquine, propranolol, and sulfadoxine-pyrimethamine may increase prochlorperazine concentrations. Concurrent use with TCA may produce increased toxicity or altered therapeutic response. Prochlorperazine plus lithium may rarely produce neurotoxicity. Prochlorperazine may produce additive CNS depressant effects with CNS depressants (ethanol, narcotics).

Decreased Effect: Barbiturates and carbamazepine may increase the metabolism of prochlorperazine, lowering its serum levels. Benztropine (and other anticholinergics) may inhibit the therapeutic response to prochlorperazine. Antipsychotics such as prochlorperazine inhibit the activity of bromocriptine to lower serum prolactin concentrations. The antihypertensive effects of guanethidine and guanadrel may be inhibited by prochlorperazine. Prochlorperazine may inhibit the antiparkinsonian effect of levodopa. Prochlorperazine (and possibly other low potency antipsychotics) may reverse the pressor effects of epinephrine.

Ethanol/Nutrition/Herb Interactions

Ethanol: Avoid ethanol (may increase CNS depression).

Food: Limit caffeine.

Herb/Nutraceutical: Avoid dong quai, St John's wort (may also cause photosensitization). Avoid kava kava, gotu kola, valerian, St John's wort (may increase CNS depression).

Stability Protect from light; clear or slightly yellow solutions may be used; **incompatible** when mixed with aminophylline, amphotericin B, ampicillin, calcium salts, cephalothin, foscarnet (Y-site), furosemide, hydrocortisone, hydromorphone, methohexital, midazolam, penicillin G, pentobarbital, phenobarbital, thiopental

Mechanism of Action Blocks postsynaptic mesolimbic dopaminergic D_1 and D_2 receptors in the brain, including the medullary chemoreceptor trigger zone; exhibits a strong alpha-

(Continued)

Prochlorperazine (Continued)

adrenergic and anticholinergic blocking effect and depresses the release of hypothalamic and hypophyseal hormones; believed to depress the reticular activating system, thus affecting basal metabolism, body temperature, wakefulness, vasomotor tone and emesis

Pharmacodynamics/Kinetics

Onset of action: Oral: 30-40 minutes; I.M.: 10-20 minutes; Rectal: ~60 minutes

Duration: I.M., oral extended-release: 12 hours; Rectal, immediate release: 3-4 hours

Distribution: Crosses placenta; enters breast milk

Metabolism: Primarily hepatic

Half-life elimination: 23 hours

Usual Dosage

Antiemetic: Children (not recommended in children <10 kg or <2 years):

Oral, rectal:

>10 kg: 0.4 mg/kg/24 hours in 3-4 divided doses; **or**

9-14 kg: 2.5 mg every 12-24 hours as needed; maximum: 7.5 mg/day

14-18 kg: 2.5 mg every 8-12 hours as needed; maximum: 10 mg/day

18-39 kg: 2.5 mg every 8 hours or 5 mg every 12 hours as needed; maximum: 15 mg/day

I.M.: 0.1-0.15 mg/kg/dose; usual: 0.13 mg/kg/dose; change to oral as soon as possible

Antiemetic: Adults:

Oral:

Tablet: 5-10 mg 3-4 times/day; usual maximum: 40 mg/day

Capsule, sustained action: 15 mg upon arising or 10 mg every 12 hours

I.M.: 5-10 mg every 3-4 hours; usual maximum: 40 mg/day

I.V.: 2.5-10 mg; maximum 10 mg/dose or 40 mg/day; may repeat dose every 3-4 hours as needed

Rectal: 25 mg twice daily

Surgical nausea/vomiting: Adults:

I.M.: 5-10 mg 1-2 hours before induction; may repeat once if necessary

I.V.: 5-10 mg 15-30 minutes before induction; may repeat once if necessary

Antipsychotic:

Children 2-12 years (not recommended in children <10 kg or <2 years):

Oral, rectal: 2.5 mg 2-3 times/day; increase dosage as needed to maximum daily dose of 20 mg for 2-5 years and 25 mg for 6-12 years

I.M.: 0.13 mg/kg/dose; change to oral as soon as possible

Adults:

Oral: 5-10 mg 3-4 times/day; doses up to 150 mg/day may be required in some patients for treatment of severe disturbances

I.M.: 10-20 mg every 4-6 hours may be required in some patients for treatment of severe disturbances; change to oral as soon as possible

Nonpsychotic anxiety: Oral: Adults: Usual dose: 15-20 mg/day in divided doses; do not give doses >20 mg/day or for longer than 12 weeks

Elderly: Behavioral symptoms associated with dementia: Initial: 2.5-5 mg 1-2 times/day; increase dose at 4- to 7-day intervals by 2.5-5 mg/day; increase dosing intervals (twice daily, 3 times/day, etc) as necessary to control response or side effects; maximum daily dose should probably not exceed 75 mg in elderly; gradual increases (titration) may prevent some side effects or decrease their severity

Hemodialysis: Not dialyzable (0% to 5%)

Dietary Considerations Increase dietary intake of riboflavin; should be administered with food or water.

Administration May be administered orally, I.M., or I.V.:

Oral: Avoid skin contact with oral solution; contact dermatitis has occurred.

I.M. should be administered into the upper outer quadrant of the buttock; avoid skin contact with injection solution; contact dermatitis has occurred

I.V. may be administered IVP or IVPB; IVP should be administered at a concentration of 5 mg/mL at a rate not to exceed 5 mg/minute; avoid skin contact with injection solution; contact dermatitis has occurred

Monitoring Parameters CBC with differential and periodic ophthalmic exams (if chronically used)

Test Interactions False-positives for phenylketonuria, urinary amylase, uroporphyrins, urobilinogen

Patient Information May cause drowsiness, impair judgment and coordination; may cause photosensitivity; avoid excessive sunlight; notify physician of involuntary movements or feelings of restlessness

Nursing Implications Avoid skin contact with oral solution or injection, contact dermatitis has occurred; observe for extrapyramidal symptoms

Additional Information Not recommended as an antipsychotic due to inferior efficacy compared to other phenothiazines.

Dosage Forms

Capsule, sustained action, as maleate: 10 mg, 15 mg, 30 mg

Injection, as edisylate: 5 mg/mL (2 mL, 10 mL)

Suppository, rectal: 2.5 mg, 5 mg, 25 mg (12/box)

Syrup, as edisylate: 5 mg/5 mL (120 mL)

Tablet, as maleate: 5 mg, 10 mg, 25 mg

Procyclidine (proe SYE kli deen)

U.S. Brand Names Kemadrin®

Canadian Brand Names Kemadrin®; Procyclid™

Synonyms Procyclidine Hydrochloride

Therapeutic Category Anticholinergic Agent; Anti-Parkinson's Agent, Anticholinergic

Use Relieves symptoms of parkinsonian syndrome and drug-induced extrapyramidal symptoms

Pregnancy Risk Factor C

Contraindications Angle-closure glaucoma; safe use in children not established

Warnings/Precautions Use with caution in hot weather or during exercise. Elderly patients frequently develop increased sensitivity and require strict dosage regulation - side effects may be more severe in elderly patients with atherosclerotic changes. Use with caution in patients with tachycardia, cardiac arrhythmias, hypertension, hypotension, prostatic hyperplasia (especially in the elderly) or any tendency toward urinary retention, liver or kidney disorders and obstructive disease of the GI or GU tract. When given in large doses or to susceptible patients, may cause weakness and inability to move particular muscle groups.

Adverse Reactions Frequency not defined.

   Cardiovascular: Tachycardia, palpitations

   Central nervous system: Confusion, drowsiness, headache, loss of memory, fatigue, ataxia, giddiness, lightheadedness

   Dermatologic: Dry skin, increased sensitivity to light, rash

   Gastrointestinal: Constipation, xerostomia, dry throat, nausea, vomiting, epigastric distress

   Genitourinary: Difficult urination

   Neuromuscular & skeletal: Weakness

   Ocular: Increased intraocular pain, blurred vision, mydriasis

   Respiratory: Dry nose

   Miscellaneous: Diaphoresis (decreased)

Overdosage/Toxicology Symptoms include disorientation, hallucinations, delusions, blurred vision, dysphagia, absent bowel sounds, hyperthermia, hypertension, and urinary retention. Anticholinergic toxicity is caused by strong binding of the drug to cholinergic receptors. Anticholinesterase inhibitors reduce acetylcholinesterase, the enzyme that breaks down acetylcholine and thereby allows acetylcholine to accumulate and compete for receptor binding with the offending anticholinergic. For anticholinergic overdose with severe life-threatening symptoms, physostigmine 1-2 mg (0.5 mg or 0.02 mg/kg for children) S.C. or slow I.V. may be given to reverse these effects.

Drug Interactions

   Increased Effect/Toxicity: Central and/or peripheral anticholinergic syndrome can occur when administered with amantadine, rimantadine, narcotic analgesics, phenothiazines and other antipsychotics (especially with high anticholinergic activity), tricyclic antidepressants, quinidine and some other antiarrhythmics, and antihistamines.

   Decreased Effect: May increase gastric degradation of levodopa and decrease the amount of levodopa absorbed by delaying gastric emptying; the opposite may be true for digoxin. Therapeutic effects of cholinergic agents (tacrine, donepezil) and neuroleptics may be antagonized.

Ethanol/Nutrition/Herb Interactions Ethanol: Avoid ethanol.

Mechanism of Action Thought to act by blocking excess acetylcholine at cerebral synapses; many of its effects are due to its pharmacologic similarities with atropine; it exerts an antispasmodic effect on smooth muscle, is a potent mydriatic; inhibits salivation

Pharmacodynamics/Kinetics

   Onset of action: 30-40 minutes

   Duration: 4-6 hours

Usual Dosage Adults: Oral: 2.5 mg 3 times/day after meals; if tolerated, gradually increase dose, maximum of 20 mg/day if necessary

   Dosing adjustment in hepatic impairment: Decrease dose to a twice daily dosing regimen

Dietary Considerations Should be taken after meals to minimize stomach upset.

Administration Should be administered after meals to minimize stomach upset.

Monitoring Parameters Symptoms of EPS or Parkinson's disease, pulse, anticholinergic effects (ie, CNS, bowel and bladder function)

Patient Information Take after meals; do not discontinue drug abruptly; notify physician if adverse GI effects, fever or heat intolerance occurs; may cause drowsiness; avoid alcohol; adequate fluid intake or sugar free gum or hard candy may help dry mouth; adequate fluid and exercise may help constipation

Nursing Implications Do not discontinue drug abruptly

Dosage Forms Tablet, as hydrochloride: 5 mg

Progesterone (proe JES ter one)

Related Information

   Depression *on page 1655*

U.S. Brand Names Crinone®; Progestasert®; Prometrium®

Canadian Brand Names Crinone®; Prometrium®

Synonyms Pregnenedione; Progestin

Therapeutic Category Progestin

(Continued)

Progesterone *(Continued)*

Use
Oral: Prevention of endometrial hyperplasia in nonhysterectomized, postmenopausal women who are receiving conjugated estrogen tablets; secondary amenorrhea

I.M.: Amenorrhea; abnormal uterine bleeding due to hormonal imbalance

Intrauterine device (IUD): Contraception in women who have had at least one child, are in a stable and mutually-monogamous relationship, and have no history of pelvic inflammatory disease; amenorrhea; functional uterine bleeding

Intravaginal gel: Part of assisted reproductive technology (ART) for infertile women with progesterone deficiency

Pregnancy Risk Factor
B (Prometrium®, per manufacturer); none established for gel (Crinone®), injection (contraindicated), or intrauterine device (contraindicated)

Pregnancy/Breast-Feeding Implications
There is an increased risk of minor birth defects in children whose mothers take progesterones during the first 4 months of pregnancy. Hypospadias has been reported in male and mild masculinization of the external genitalia has been reported in female babies exposed during the first trimester. Crinone® is indicated for use in ART. Excreted in breast milk; use caution in breast-feeding women.

Contraindications
Hypersensitivity to progesterone or any component of the formulation; thrombophlebitis; undiagnosed vaginal bleeding; carcinoma of the breast; cerebral apoplexy; severe liver dysfunction; missed abortion; diagnostic test for pregnancy; pregnancy (see Pregnancy Risk Factor)

Capsule: Contains peanut oil; contraindicated in patients with allergy to peanuts

IUD: Should also not be used in patients with current or history of ectopic pregnancy, pelvic inflammatory disease, sexually-transmitted disease, postpartum endometritis, incomplete involution of uterus; vaginitis or cervicitis, genital actinomycosis, uterus <6 cm or >10 cm, cervical cancer, or conditions associated with increased susceptibility to infection.

Warnings/Precautions
Use with caution in patients with impaired liver function, depression, diabetes, and epilepsy. Except when used as indicated in ART, use of any progestin during the first 4 months of pregnancy is not recommended. Monitor closely for loss of vision, proptosis, diplopia, migraine, and signs or symptoms of embolic disorders. Not a progestin of choice in the elderly for hormonal cycling. May cause some degree of fluid retention, use with caution in conditions which may be aggravated by this factor, including CHF, renal dysfunction, epilepsy, migraine, or asthma. Patients should be warned that progesterone may cause transient dizziness or drowsiness during initial therapy.

Use of the IUD is associated with increased risk of ectopic pregnancy if pregnancy occurs. In addition, women should be informed that the IUD does not protect against HIV infection, pelvic inflammatory disease, or other sexually-transmitted diseases.

Adverse Reactions Oral capsule:
>10%:
  Central nervous system: Dizziness (16%)
  Endocrine & metabolic: Breast pain (11%)
5% to 10%:
  Central nervous system: Headache (10%), fatigue (7%), emotional lability (6%), irritability (5%)
  Gastrointestinal: Abdominal pain (10%), abdominal distention (6%)
  Neuromuscular & skeletal: Musculoskeletal pain (6%)
  Respiratory: Upper respiratory tract infection (5%)
  Miscellaneous: Viral infection (7%)
<5% (Limited to important or life-threatening): Angina pectoris, anxiety, arthritis, bronchitis, chest pain, edema, gastroenteritis, hemorrhagic rectum, hepatitis (reversible), hypertension, hypertonia, hypotension, leukorrhea, lymphadenopathy, myalgia, pneumonitis, somnolence, syncope, uterine fibroid, vaginal dryness, vaginitis, verruca, vomiting

Overdosage/Toxicology
Toxicity is unlikely following single exposures of excessive doses. Supportive treatment is adequate in most cases.

Drug Interactions
Cytochrome P450 Effect: CYP2C19, 3A3/4, and 3A5 enzyme substrate

Increased Effect/Toxicity: Ketoconazole may increase the bioavailability of progesterone. Progesterone may increase concentrations of estrogenic compounds during concurrent therapy with conjugated estrogens.

Decreased Effect: Aminoglutethimide may decrease effect by increasing hepatic metabolism.

Ethanol/Nutrition/Herb Interactions
Food: Food increases oral bioavailability.

Herb/Nutraceutical: St John's wort may decrease progesterone levels.

Stability
Store at controlled room temperature.

Mechanism of Action
Natural steroid hormone that induces secretory changes in the endometrium, promotes mammary gland development, relaxes uterine smooth muscle, blocks follicular maturation and ovulation, and maintains pregnancy

Pharmacodynamics/Kinetics
Duration: 24 hours
Protein binding: 96% to 99%
Metabolism: Hepatic
Half-life elimination: 5 minutes
Time to peak: Oral: 1.5-2.3 hours
Excretion: Urine (50% to 60%); feces (~10%)

Usual Dosage
I.M.: Adults: Female:
  Amenorrhea: 5-10 mg/day for 6-8 consecutive days
  Functional uterine bleeding: 5-10 mg/day for 6 doses
IUD: Adults: Female: Contraception: Insert a single system into the uterine cavity; contraceptive effectiveness is retained for 1 year and system must be replaced 1 year after insertion

Oral: Adults: Female:

Prevention of endometrial hyperplasia (in postmenopausal women with a uterus who are receiving daily conjugated estrogen tablets): 200 mg as a single daily dose every evening for 12 days sequentially per 28-day cycle

Amenorrhea: 400 mg every evening for 10 days

Intravaginal gel: Adults: Female:

ART in women who require progesterone supplementation: 90 mg (8% gel) once daily; if pregnancy occurs, may continue treatment for up to 10-12 weeks

ART in women with partial or complete ovarian failure: 90 mg (8% gel) intravaginally twice daily; if pregnancy occurs, may continue up to 10-12 weeks

Secondary amenorrhea: 45 mg (4% gel) intravaginally every other day for up to 6 doses; women who fail to respond may be increased to 90 mg (8% gel) every other day for up to 6 doses

Administration

I.M.: Administer deep I.M. only

Intravaginal: Vaginal gel: (A small amount of gel will remain in the applicator following insertion): Administer into the vagina directly from sealed applicator. Remove applicator from wrapper; holding applicator by thickest end, shake down to move contents to thin end; while holding applicator by flat section of thick end, twist off tab; gently insert into vagina and squeeze thick end of applicator.

For use at altitudes above 2500 feet: Remove applicator from wrapper; hold applicator on both sides of bubble in the thick end; using a lancet, make a single puncture in the bubble to relieve air pressure; holding applicator by thickest end, shake down to move contents to thin end; while holding applicator by flat section of thick end, twist off tab; gently insert into vagina and squeeze thick end of applicator.

Monitoring Parameters Before starting therapy, a physical exam including the breasts and pelvis are recommended, also a Pap smear; signs or symptoms of depression, glucose in diabetics

Test Interactions Thyroid function, metyrapone, liver function, coagulation tests, endocrine function tests

Patient Information Notify physician if sudden loss of vision or migraine headache occur or if you suspect you may have become pregnant; may cause photosensitivity, wear protective clothing or sunscreen

Nursing Implications Patients should receive a copy of the patient labeling for the drug; administer deep I.M. only; monitor patient closely for loss of vision, sudden onset of proptosis, diplopia, migraine, and signs and symptoms of embolic disorders

Dosage Forms

Capsule (Prometrium®): 100 mg, 200 mg [contains peanut oil]

Gel, vaginal (Crinone®): 4% (45 mg); 8% (90 mg)

Injection, in oil: 50 mg/mL (10 mL) [products may contain benzyl alcohol, sesame oil]

Intrauterine system, reservoir (Progestasert®): 38 mg in silicone fluid [delivers progesterone 65 mcg/day over 1 year]

- ◆ **Progestin** *see* Progesterone *on page 1137*
- ◆ **Proglycem®** *see* Diazoxide *on page 393*
- ◆ **Prograf®** *see* Tacrolimus *on page 1283*
- ◆ **Proguanil and Atovaquone** *see* Atovaquone and Proguanil *on page 129*
- ◆ **Proleukin®** *see* Aldesleukin *on page 43*
- ◆ **Prolixin®** *see* Fluphenazine *on page 581*
- ◆ **Prolixin Decanoate®** *see* Fluphenazine *on page 581*
- ◆ **Prolixin Enanthate®** *see* Fluphenazine *on page 581*
- ◆ **Proloprim®** *see* Trimethoprim *on page 1376*
- ◆ **Promatussin® DM (Can)** *see* Promethazine and Dextromethorphan *on page 1141*

Promazine (PROE ma zeen)

Related Information

Antacid Drug Interactions *on page 1477*

Antipsychotic Agents Comparison *on page 1486*

U.S. Brand Names Sparine®

Canadian Brand Names Sparine®

Synonyms Promazine Hydrochloride

Therapeutic Category Antiemetic; Antipsychotic Agent, Phenothiazine; Phenothiazine Derivative

Use Management of manifestations of psychotic disorders

Unlabeled/Investigational Use Nausea and vomiting; preoperative sedation

Pregnancy Risk Factor C

Usual Dosage Oral, I.M.:

Children >12 years: Psychosis: 10-25 mg every 4-6 hours

Adults:

Psychosis: 10-200 mg every 4-6 hours not to exceed 1000 mg/day

Antiemetic (unlabeled use): 25-50 mg every 4-6 hours as needed

Hemodialysis: Not dialyzable (0% to 5%)

Additional Information Complete prescribing information for this medication should be consulted for additional detail.

Dosage Forms

Injection, as hydrochloride: 50 mg/mL (10 mL)

Tablet, as hydrochloride: 25 mg, 50 mg

- ◆ **Promazine Hydrochloride** *see* Promazine *on page 1139*

Promethazine (proe METH a zeen)

Related Information

Antacid Drug Interactions *on page 1477*

(Continued)

Promethazine (Continued)

U.S. Brand Names Anergan®; Phenergan®

Canadian Brand Names Phenergan®

Synonyms Promethazine Hydrochloride

Therapeutic Category Antihistamine, H₁ Blocker; Phenothiazine Derivative; Sedative

Use Symptomatic treatment of various allergic conditions; antiemetic; motion sickness; sedative; analgesic adjunct for control of postoperative pain; anesthetic adjunct

Pregnancy Risk Factor C

Pregnancy/Breast-Feeding Implications

Clinical effects on the fetus: Crosses the placenta. Possible respiratory depression if drug is administered near time of delivery; behavioral changes, EEG alterations, impaired platelet aggregation reported with use during labor. Available evidence with use of occasional low doses suggests safe use during pregnancy.

Breast-feeding/lactation: No data available. AAP makes NO RECOMMENDATION.

Contraindications Hypersensitivity to promethazine or any component of the formulation (cross-reactivity between phenothiazines may occur); severe CNS depression; coma; intra-arterial or subcutaneous injection

Warnings/Precautions Do not administer S.C. or intra-arterially, necrotic lesions may occur; injection may contain sulfites which may cause allergic reactions in some patients; use with caution in patients with cardiovascular disease, impaired liver function, asthma, sleep apnea, seizures. Rapid I.V. administration may produce a transient fall in blood pressure, rate of administration should not exceed 25 mg/minute; slow I.V. administration may produce a slightly elevated blood pressure. Because promethazine is a phenothiazine (and can, therefore, cause side effects such as extrapyramidal symptoms), it is not considered an antihistamine of choice in the elderly.

Adverse Reactions Frequency not defined.

Cardiovascular: Postural hypotension, tachycardia, dizziness, nonspecific QT changes

Central nervous system: Drowsiness, dystonias, akathisia, pseudoparkinsonism, tardive dyskinesia, neuroleptic malignant syndrome, seizures

Dermatologic: Photosensitivity, dermatitis, skin pigmentation (slate gray)

Endocrine & metabolic: Lactation, breast engorgement, false-positive pregnancy test, amenorrhea, gynecomastia, hyper- or hypoglycemia

Gastrointestinal: Xerostomia, constipation, nausea

Genitourinary: Urinary retention, ejaculatory disorder, impotence

Hematologic: Agranulocytosis, eosinophilia, leukopenia, hemolytic anemia, aplastic anemia, thrombocytopenic purpura

Hepatic: Jaundice

Ocular: Blurred vision, corneal and lenticular changes, epithelial keratopathy, pigmentary retinopathy

Overdosage/Toxicology Symptoms include CNS depression, respiratory depression, possible CNS stimulation, dry mouth, fixed and dilated pupils, and hypotension. Following initiation of essential overdose management, toxic symptom and supportive treatment should be initiated. Hypotension usually responds to I.V. fluids or Trendelenburg positioning. If unresponsive to these measures, norepinephrine 0.1-0.2 mcg/kg/minute titrated to response may be tried. Seizures commonly respond to diazepam (I.V. 5-10 mg bolus in adults every 15 minutes if needed up to a total of 30 mg; I.V. 0.25-0.4 mg/kg/dose up to a total of 10 mg in children) or to phenytoin or phenobarbital. Critical cardiac arrhythmias often respond to I.V. phenytoin (15 mg/kg up to 1 g), while other antiarrhythmics can be used. Neuroleptics often cause extrapyramidal symptoms (eg, dystonic reactions) requiring management with diphenhydramine 1-2 mg/kg (adults) up to a maximum of 50 mg I.M. or slow I.V. push followed by a maintenance dose for 48-72 hours. When these reactions are unresponsive to diphenhydramine, anticholinergic agents such as benztropine mesylate I.V. 1-2 mg (adults) may be effective. These agents are generally effective within 2-5 minutes.

Drug Interactions

Cytochrome P450 Effect: CYP2D6 enzyme substrate

Increased Effect/Toxicity: Chloroquine, propranolol, and sulfadoxine-pyrimethamine also may increase promethazine concentrations. Concurrent use with TCA may produce increased toxicity or altered therapeutic response. Promethazine plus lithium may rarely produce neurotoxicity. Concurrent use of promethazine and CNS depressants (ethanol, narcotics) may produce additive depressant effects.

Decreased Effect: Barbiturates and carbamazepine may increase the metabolism of promethazine, lowering its serum levels. Benztropine (and other anticholinergics) may inhibit the therapeutic response to promethazine. Promethazine may inhibit the ability of bromocriptine to lower serum prolactin concentrations. The antihypertensive effects of guanethidine and guanadrel may be inhibited by promethazine. Promethazine may inhibit the antiparkinsonian effect of levodopa. Promethazine (and possibly other low potency antipsychotics) may reverse the pressor effects of epinephrine.

Ethanol/Nutrition/Herb Interactions

Ethanol: Avoid ethanol (may increase CNS depression).

Herb/Nutraceutical: Avoid valerian, St John's wort, kava kava, gotu kola (may increase CNS depression).

Stability Protect from light and from freezing; **compatible** (when comixed in the same syringe) with atropine, chlorpromazine, diphenhydramine, droperidol, fentanyl, glycopyrrolate, hydromorphone, hydroxyzine hydrochloride, meperidine, midazolam, nalbuphine, pentazocine, prochlorperazine, scopolamine; **incompatible** when mixed with aminophylline, cefoperazone (Y-site), chloramphenicol, dimenhydrinate (same syringe), foscarnet (Y-site), furosemide, heparin, hydrocortisone, methohexital, penicillin G, pentobarbital, phenobarbital, thiopental

Mechanism of Action Blocks postsynaptic mesolimbic dopaminergic receptors in the brain; exhibits a strong alpha-adrenergic blocking effect and depresses the release of hypothalamic and hypophyseal hormones; competes with histamine for the H₁-receptor; reduces stimuli to the brainstem reticular system

Pharmacodynamics/Kinetics

Onset of action: I.M.: ~20 minutes; I.V.: 3-5 minutes

Duration: 2-6 hours
Metabolism: Hepatic
Excretion: Primarily urine and feces (as inactive metabolites)

Usual Dosage

Children:
  Antihistamine: Oral, rectal: 0.1 mg/kg/dose every 6 hours during the day and 0.5 mg/kg/dose at bedtime as needed
  Antiemetic: Oral, I.M., I.V., rectal: 0.25-1 mg/kg 4-6 times/day as needed
  Motion sickness: Oral, rectal: 0.5 mg/kg/dose 30 minutes to 1 hour before departure, then every 12 hours as needed
  Sedation: Oral, I.M., I.V., rectal: 0.5-1 mg/kg/dose every 6 hours as needed

Adults:
  Antihistamine (including allergic reactions to blood or plasma):
    Oral, rectal: 12.5 mg 3 times/day and 25 mg at bedtime
    I.M., I.V.: 25 mg, may repeat in 2 hours when necessary; switch to oral route as soon as feasible
  Antiemetic: Oral, I.M., I.V., rectal: 12.5-25 mg every 4 hours as needed
  Motion sickness: Oral, rectal: 25 mg 30-60 minutes before departure, then every 12 hours as needed
  Sedation: Oral, I.M., I.V., rectal: 25-50 mg/dose

Hemodialysis: Not dialyzable (0% to 5%)

Dietary Considerations Increase dietary intake of riboflavin; should be administered with food or water.

Administration Avoid I.V. use; if necessary, may dilute to a maximum concentration of 25 mg/mL and infuse at a maximum rate of 25 mg/minute; rapid I.V. administration may produce a transient fall in blood pressure

Monitoring Parameters Relief of symptoms, mental status

Test Interactions Alters the flare response in intradermal allergen tests

Patient Information May cause drowsiness, impair judgment and coordination; may cause photosensitivity; avoid excessive sunlight; notify physician of involuntary movements or feelings of restlessness

Nursing Implications Avoid S.C. administration, promethazine is a chemical irritation which may produce necrosis; avoid I.V. use; if necessary, may dilute to a maximum concentration of 25 mg/mL and infuse at a maximum rate of 25 mg/minute

Dosage Forms
Injection, as hydrochloride: 25 mg/mL (1 mL, 10 mL); 50 mg/mL (1 mL, 10 mL)
Suppository, rectal, as hydrochloride: 12.5 mg, 25 mg, 50 mg
Syrup, as hydrochloride: 6.25 mg/5 mL (5 mL, 120 mL, 480 mL, 4000 mL); 25 mg/5 mL (120 mL, 480 mL, 4000 mL)
Tablet, as hydrochloride: 12.5 mg, 25 mg, 50 mg

Promethazine and Codeine (proe METH a zeen & KOE deen)

U.S. Brand Names Phenergan® With Codeine; Prothazine-DC®

Synonyms Codeine and Promethazine

Therapeutic Category Antihistamine/Antitussive

Use Temporary relief of coughs and upper respiratory symptoms associated with allergy or the common cold

Restrictions C-V

Pregnancy Risk Factor C

Usual Dosage Oral (in terms of codeine):
  Children: 1-1.5 mg/kg/day every 4 hours as needed; maximum: 30 mg/day **or**
    2-6 years: 1.25-2.5 mL every 4-6 hours or 2.5-5 mg/dose every 4-6 hours as needed; maximum: 30 mg codeine/day
    6-12 years: 2.5-5 mL every 4-6 hours as needed or 5-10 mg/dose every 4-6 hours as needed; maximum: 60 mg codeine/day
  Adults: 10-20 mg/dose every 4-6 hours as needed; maximum: 120 mg codeine/day; or 5-10 mL every 4-6 hours as needed

Additional Information Complete prescribing information for this medication should be consulted for additional detail.

Dosage Forms Syrup: Promethazine hydrochloride 6.25 mg and codeine phosphate 10 mg per 5 mL (120 mL, 180 mL, 473 mL)

Promethazine and Dextromethorphan
(proe METH a zeen & deks troe meth OR fan)

U.S. Brand Names Phenameth® DM; Phenergan® With Dextromethorphan

Canadian Brand Names Promatussin® DM

Synonyms Dextromethorphan and Promethazine

Therapeutic Category Antihistamine/Antitussive

Use Temporary relief of coughs and upper respiratory symptoms associated with allergy or the common cold

Pregnancy Risk Factor C

Usual Dosage Oral:
  Children:
    2-6 years: 1.25-2.5 mL every 4-6 hours up to 10 mL in 24 hours
    6-12 years: 2.5-5 mL every 4-6 hours up to 20 mL in 24 hours
  Adults: 5 mL every 4-6 hours up to 30 mL in 24 hours

Additional Information Complete prescribing information for this medication should be consulted for additional detail.

Dosage Forms Syrup: Promethazine hydrochloride 6.25 mg and dextromethorphan hydrobromide 15 mg per 5 mL with alcohol 7% (120 mL, 480 mL, 4000 mL)

♦ **Promethazine and Meperidine** see Meperidine and Promethazine on page 860

Promethazine and Phenylephrine (proe METH a zeen & fen il EF rin)
U.S. Brand Names Phenergan® VC; Promethazine VC; Promethazine VC Plain; Prometh VC Plain
Synonyms Phenylephrine and Promethazine
Therapeutic Category Antihistamine/Decongestant Combination
Use Temporary relief of upper respiratory symptoms associated with allergy or the common cold
Pregnancy Risk Factor C
Usual Dosage Oral:
Children:
2-6 years: 1.25 mL every 4-6 hours, not to exceed 7.5 mL in 24 hours
6-12 years: 2.5 mL every 4-6 hours, not to exceed 15 mL in 24 hours
Children >12 years and Adults: 5 mL every 4-6 hours, not to exceed 30 mL in 24 hours
Additional Information Complete prescribing information for this medication should be consulted for additional detail.
Dosage Forms Liquid: Promethazine hydrochloride 6.25 mg and phenylephrine hydrochloride 5 mg per 5 mL (120 mL, 240 mL, 473 mL)

♦ **Promethazine Hydrochloride** see Promethazine on page 1139

Promethazine, Phenylephrine, and Codeine
(proe METH a zeen, fen il EF rin, & KOE deen)
U.S. Brand Names Phenergan® VC With Codeine; Promethist® With Codeine; Prometh® VC With Codeine
Synonyms Codeine, Promethazine, and Phenylephrine; Phenylephrine, Promethazine, and Codeine
Therapeutic Category Antihistamine/Decongestant/Antitussive
Use Temporary relief of coughs and upper respiratory symptoms including nasal congestion
Restrictions C-V
Pregnancy Risk Factor C
Usual Dosage Oral:
Children (expressed in terms of codeine dosage): 1-1.5 mg/kg/day every 4 hours, maximum: 30 mg/day **or**
<2 years: Not recommended
2-6 years:
Weight 25 lb: 1.25-2.5 mL every 4-6 hours, not to exceed 6 mL/24 hours
Weight 30 lb: 1.25-2.5 mL every 4-6 hours, not to exceed 7 mL/24 hours
Weight 35 lb: 1.25-2.5 mL every 4-6 hours, not to exceed 8 mL/24 hours
Weight 40 lb: 1.25-2.5 mL every 4-6 hours, not to exceed 9 mL/24 hours
6 to <12 years: 2.5-5 mL every 4-6 hours, not to exceed 15 mL/24 hours
Adults: 5 mL every 4-6 hours, not to exceed 30 mL/24 hours
Additional Information Complete prescribing information for this medication should be consulted for additional detail.
Dosage Forms Liquid: Promethazine hydrochloride 6.25 mg, phenylephrine hydrochloride 5 mg, and codeine phosphate 10 mg per 5 mL with alcohol 7% (120 mL, 240 mL, 480 mL, 4000 mL)

♦ **Promethazine VC** see Promethazine and Phenylephrine on page 1142
♦ **Promethazine VC Plain** see Promethazine and Phenylephrine on page 1142
♦ **Promethist® With Codeine** see Promethazine, Phenylephrine, and Codeine on page 1142
♦ **Prometh VC Plain** see Promethazine and Phenylephrine on page 1142
♦ **Prometh® VC With Codeine** see Promethazine, Phenylephrine, and Codeine on page 1142
♦ **Prometrium®** see Progesterone on page 1137
♦ **Promit®** see Dextran 1 on page 387
♦ **Pronap-100®** see Propoxyphene and Acetaminophen on page 1148
♦ **Pronestyl®** see Procainamide on page 1130
♦ **Pronestyl-SR®** see Procainamide on page 1130
♦ **Pronto® [OTC]** see Pyrethrins and Piperonyl Butoxide on page 1160
♦ **Propaderm® (Can)** see Beclomethasone on page 149

Propafenone (proe pa FEEN one)
Related Information
Antiarrhythmic Drugs Comparison on page 1478
U.S. Brand Names Rythmol®
Canadian Brand Names Rythmol®
Synonyms Propafenone Hydrochloride
Therapeutic Category Antiarrhythmic Agent, Class I-C
Use Life-threatening ventricular arrhythmias
Unlabeled/Investigational Use Supraventricular tachycardias, including those patients with Wolff-Parkinson-White syndrome
Pregnancy Risk Factor C
Contraindications Hypersensitivity to propafenone or any component of the formulation; sinoatrial, AV, and intraventricular disorders of impulse generation and/or conduction (except in patients with a functioning artificial pacemaker); sinus bradycardia; cardiogenic shock; uncompensated cardiac failure; hypotension; bronchospastic disorders; uncorrected electrolyte abnormalities; concurrent use of amprenavir, cimetidine, metoprolol, propranolol quinidine, and ritonavir (see Drug Interactions)
Warnings/Precautions Until evidence to the contrary, propafenone should be considered acceptable only for the treatment of life-threatening arrhythmias; propafenone may cause new or worsened arrhythmias, worsen CHF, decrease AV conduction and alter pacemaker thresholds; use with caution in patients with recent myocardial infarction, congestive heart failure, hepatic or renal dysfunction; elderly may be at greater risk for toxicity

Adverse Reactions

1% to 10%:

Cardiovascular: New or worsened arrhythmias (proarrhythmic effect) (2% to 10%), angina (2% to 5%), congestive heart failure (1% to 4%), ventricular tachycardia (1% to 3%), palpitations (1% to 3%), AV block (first-degree) (1% to 3%), syncope (1% to 2%), increased QRS interval (1% to 2%), chest pain (1% to 2%), PVCs (1% to 2%), bradycardia (1% to 2%), edema (0% to 1%), bundle branch block (0% to 1%), atrial fibrillation (1%), hypotension (0% to 1%), intraventricular conduction delay (0% to 1%)

Central nervous system: Dizziness (4% to 15%), fatigue (2% to 6%), headache (2% to 5%), weakness (1% to 2%), ataxia (0% to 2%), insomnia (0% to 2%), anxiety (1% to 2%), drowsiness (1%)

Dermatologic: Rash (1% to 3%)

Gastrointestinal: Nausea/vomiting (2% to 11%), unusual taste (3% to 23%), constipation (2% to 7%), dyspepsia (1% to 3%), diarrhea (1% to 3%), xerostomia (1% to 2%), anorexia (1% to 2%), abdominal pain (1% to 2%), flatulence (0% to 1%)

Neuromuscular & skeletal: Tremor (0% to 1%), arthralgia (0% to 1%)

Ocular: Blurred vision (1% to 6%)

Respiratory: Dyspnea (2% to 5%)

Miscellaneous: Diaphoresis (1%)

<1% (Limited to important or life-threatening): Agranulocytosis, alopecia, amnesia, anemia, apnea, AV block (second or third degree), AV dissociation, cardiac arrest, cholestasis (0.1%), coma, confusion, congestive heart failure, depression, granulocytopenia, hepatitis (0.03%), hyperglycemia, impotence, increased bleeding time, leukopenia, lupus erythematosus, mania, memory loss, nephrotic syndrome, paresthesia, peripheral neuropathy, pruritus, psychosis, purpura, renal failure, seizures (0.3%), SIADH, sinus node dysfunction, thrombocytopenia, tinnitus, vertigo

Overdosage/Toxicology Has a narrow therapeutic index and severe toxicity may occur slightly above the therapeutic range, especially if combined with other antiarrhythmic drugs. Acute single ingestion of twice the daily therapeutic dose is life-threatening. Symptoms include increases in PR, QRS, QT intervals and amplitude of the T wave, as well as A-V block, bradycardia, hypotension, ventricular arrhythmias (monomorphic or polymorphic ventricular tachycardia), and asystole. Other symptoms include dizziness, blurred vision, headache, and GI upset. Treatment is supportive, using conventional treatment (fluids, positioning, anticonvulsants, antiarrhythmics). **Note:** Type Ia antiarrhythmic agents should not be used to treat cardiotoxicity caused by type 1c antiarrhythmic drugs. Sodium bicarbonate may reverse QRS prolongation, bradycardia and hypotension; ventricular pacing may be needed. Hemodialysis is only of possible benefit for tocainide or flecainide overdose in patients with renal failure.

Drug Interactions

Cytochrome P450 Effect: CYP1A2, 2D6, 3A3/4 enzyme substrate; CYP2D6 enzyme inhibitor

Increased Effect/Toxicity: Amprenavir, cimetidine, metoprolol, propranolol, quinidine, and ritonavir may increase propafenone levels; concurrent use is contraindicated. Digoxin (reduce dose by 25%), cyclosporine, local anesthetics, theophylline, and warfarin blood levels are increased by propafenone.

Decreased Effect: Enzyme inducers (phenobarbital, phenytoin, rifabutin, rifampin) may decrease propafenone blood levels.

Ethanol/Nutrition/Herb Interactions

Food: Propafenone serum concentrations may be increased if taken with food.

Herb/Nutraceutical: St John's wort may decrease propafenone levels. Avoid ephedra (may worsen arrhythmia).

Mechanism of Action Propafenone is a class 1c antiarrhythmic agent which possesses local anesthetic properties, blocks the fast inward sodium current, and slows the rate of increase of the action potential. Prolongs conduction and refractoriness in all areas of the myocardium, with a slightly more pronounced effect on intraventricular conduction; it prolongs effective refractory period, reduces spontaneous automaticity and exhibits some beta-blockade activity.

Pharmacodynamics/Kinetics

Absorption: Well absorbed

Metabolism: Hepatic; two genetically determined metabolism groups exist: fast or slow metabolizers; 10% of Caucasians are slow metabolizers; exhibits nonlinear pharmacokinetics; when dose is increased from 300-900 mg/day, serum concentrations increase tenfold; this nonlinearity is thought to be due to saturable first-pass hepatic enzyme effect

Half-life elimination: Single dose (100-300 mg): 2-8 hours; Chronic dosing: 10-32 hours

Time to peak: 2 hours with 150 mg dose, 3 hours after 300 mg dose

Usual Dosage Adults: Oral: 150 mg every 8 hours, increase at 3- to 4-day intervals up to 300 mg every 8 hours. **Note:** Patients who exhibit significant widening of QRS complex or second- or third-degree AV block may need dose reduction.

Dosing adjustment in hepatic impairment: Reduction is necessary.

Dietary Considerations Administer at the same time in relation to meals each day, either always with meals or always between meals.

Monitoring Parameters EKG, blood pressure, pulse (particularly at initiation of therapy)

Patient Information Take dose the same way each day, either with or without food; do not double the next dose if present dose is missed; do not discontinue drug or change dose without advice of physician; report any severe or persistent fatigue, sore throat, or any unusual bleeding or bruising; may cause drowsiness and impair coordination and judgment

Nursing Implications Patients should be on a cardiac monitor during initiation of therapy or when dosage is increased; monitor heart sounds and pulses for rate, rhythm and quality

Dosage Forms Tablet, as hydrochloride: 150 mg, 225 mg, 300 mg

- ◆ **Propafenone Hydrochloride** *see* Propafenone *on page 1142*
- ◆ **Propanthel™ (Can)** *see* Propantheline *on page 1144*

Propantheline (proe PAN the leen)
Canadian Brand Names Propanthel™
Synonyms Propantheline Bromide
Therapeutic Category Anticholinergic Agent; Antispasmodic Agent, Gastrointestinal; Antispasmodic Agent, Urinary
Use Adjunctive treatment of peptic ulcer, irritable bowel syndrome, pancreatitis, ureteral and urinary bladder spasm; reduce duodenal motility during diagnostic radiologic procedures
Pregnancy Risk Factor C
Usual Dosage Oral:
Antisecretory:
Children: 1-2 mg/kg/day in 3-4 divided doses
Adults: 15 mg 3 times/day before meals or food and 30 mg at bedtime
Elderly: 7.5 mg 3 times/day before meals and at bedtime
Antispasmodic:
Children: 2-3 mg/kg/day in divided doses every 4-6 hours and at bedtime
Adults: 15 mg 3 times/day before meals or food and 30 mg at bedtime
Additional Information Complete prescribing information for this medication should be consulted for additional detail.
Dosage Forms Tablet, as bromide: 15 mg

♦ **Propantheline Bromide** see Propantheline on page 1144

Proparacaine (proe PAR a kane)
U.S. Brand Names Alcaine®; Ophthetic®; Parcaine®
Canadian Brand Names Alcaine®; Diocaine®
Synonyms Proparacaine Hydrochloride; Proxymetacaine
Therapeutic Category Local Anesthetic, Ophthalmic
Use Anesthesia for tonometry, gonioscopy; suture removal from cornea; removal of corneal foreign body; cataract extraction, glaucoma surgery; short operative procedure involving the cornea and conjunctiva
Pregnancy Risk Factor C
Contraindications Hypersensitivity to proparacaine or any component of the formulation
Warnings/Precautions Use with caution in patients with cardiac disease, hyperthyroidism; for typical ophthalmic use only; prolonged use not recommended
Adverse Reactions
1% to 10%: Local: Burning, stinging, redness
<1% (Limited to important or life-threatening): Allergic contact dermatitis, arrhythmia, blurred vision, CNS depression, conjunctival congestion and hemorrhage, corneal opacification, diaphoresis (increased), epithelium, erosion of the corneal iritis, irritation, keratitis, lacrimation, sensitization
Drug Interactions
Increased Effect/Toxicity: Effects of phenylephrine and tropicamide (ophthalmics) are increased
Stability Store in tight, light-resistant containers
Mechanism of Action Prevents initiation and transmission of impulse at the nerve cell membrane by decreasing ion permeability through stabilizing
Pharmacodynamics/Kinetics
Onset of action: ~20 seconds
Duration: 15-20 minutes
Usual Dosage Children and Adults:
Ophthalmic surgery: Instill 1 drop of 0.5% solution in eye every 5-10 minutes for 5-7 doses
Tonometry, gonioscopy, suture removal: Instill 1-2 drops of 0.5% solution in eye just prior to procedure
Patient Information May slow wound healing; use sparingly, avoid touching or rubbing the eye until anesthesia has worn off
Nursing Implications Do not use if discolored; protect eye from irritating chemicals, foreign bodies, and blink reflex; use eye patch if necessary
Dosage Forms Solution, ophthalmic, as hydrochloride: 0.5% (2 mL, 15 mL)

Proparacaine and Fluorescein (proe PAR a kane & FLURE e seen)
U.S. Brand Names Fluoracaine®
Therapeutic Category Diagnostic Agent, Ophthalmic Dye; Local Anesthetic, Ester Derivative (Ophthalmic); Local Anesthetic, Ophthalmic
Use Anesthesia for tonometry, gonioscopy; suture removal from cornea; removal of corneal foreign body; cataract extraction, glaucoma surgery
Pregnancy Risk Factor C
Usual Dosage
Ophthalmic surgery: Children and Adults: Instill 1 drop in each eye every 5-10 minutes for 5-7 doses
Tonometry, gonioscopy, suture removal: Adults: Instill 1-2 drops in each eye just prior to procedure
Additional Information Complete prescribing information for this medication should be consulted for additional detail.
Dosage Forms Solution: Proparacaine hydrochloride 0.5% and fluorescein sodium 0.25% (5 mL)

♦ **Proparacaine Hydrochloride** see Proparacaine on page 1144
♦ **Propecia®** see Finasteride on page 562
♦ **Propine®** see Dipivefrin on page 422
♦ **Proplex® T** see Factor IX Complex (Human) on page 539

Propofol (PROE po fole)

U.S. Brand Names Diprivan®

Canadian Brand Names Diprivan®

Therapeutic Category General Anesthetic; Sedative

Use Induction of anesthesia for inpatient or outpatient surgery in patients ≥3 years of age; maintenance of anesthesia for inpatient or outpatient surgery in patients >2 months of age; in adults, for the induction and maintenance of monitored anesthesia care sedation during diagnostic procedures; may be used (for patients >18 years of age who are intubated and mechanically ventilated) as an alternative to benzodiazepines for the treatment of agitation in the intensive care unit

Unlabeled/Investigational Use Postoperative antiemetic; refractory delirium tremens (case reports)

Pregnancy Risk Factor B

Pregnancy/Breast-Feeding Implications Propofol is not recommended for obstetrics, including cesarean section deliveries. Propofol crosses the placenta and may be associated with neonatal depression. Excreted in breast milk; breast-feeding is contraindicated.

Contraindications

Absolute contraindications:

Patients with a hypersensitivity to propofol or any component of the formulation

Patients who are not intubated or mechanically ventilated

Patients who are pregnant or nursing

When general anesthesia or sedation is contraindicated

Relative contraindications:

Pediatric intensive care unit patients: Safety and efficacy of propofol are not established

Patients with severe cardiac disease (ejection fraction <50%) or respiratory disease - propofol may have more profound adverse cardiovascular responses

Patients with a history of epilepsy or seizures; risk of seizure during recovery phase

Patients with increased intracranial pressure or impaired cerebral circulation - substantial decreases in mean arterial pressure and subsequent decreases in cerebral perfusion pressure may occur

Patients with hyperlipidemia as evidenced by increased serum triglyceride levels or serum turbidity

Patients who are hypotensive, hypovolemic, hemodynamically unstable, or abnormally low vascular tone (eg, sepsis)

Warnings/Precautions Use slower rate of induction in the elderly; transient local pain may occur during I.V. injection; perioperative myoclonia has occurred; do not administer with blood or blood products through the same I.V. catheter; not for obstetrics, including cesarean section deliveries. Abrupt discontinuation prior to weaning or daily wake up assessments should be avoided. Abrupt discontinuation can result in rapid awakening, anxiety, agitation, and resistance to mechanical ventilation. Several deaths associated with severe metabolic acidosis have been reported in pediatric ICU patients on long-term propofol infusion. Propofol emulsion contains soybean oil, egg phosphatide, and glycerol.

Adverse Reactions

>10%:

Cardiovascular: Hypotension (3% to 26% adults, 17% children)

Central nervous system: Movement (17% children)

Local: Injection site burning, stinging, or pain (adults 18%, children 10%)

Respiratory: Apnea, lasting 30-60 seconds (24% adults, 10% children); Apnea, lasting >60 seconds (12% adults, 5% children)

3% to 10%:

Cardiovascular: Hypertension (8% children)

Central nervous system: Movement (adults)

Dermatologic: Pruritus (adults), rash

Endocrine & metabolic: Hyperlipidemia

Respiratory: Respiratory acidosis during weaning

1% to 3%:

Cardiovascular: Arrhythmia, bradycardia, decreased cardiac output, tachycardia

Dermatologic: Pruritus (children)

<1% (Limited to important or life-threatening): Anaphylaxis, anaphylactoid reaction, anticholinergic syndrome, bigeminy, cardiac arrest, delirium; discoloration (green) of urine, hair, or nailbed; dystonia, EKG abnormal, hemorrhage, hypoxia, infusion site reactions, laryngospasm, pancreatitis, perioperative myoclonia (rarely including convulsions and opisthotonos), premature atrial contractions, premature pulmonary edema, rhabdomyolysis, syncope, thrombosis, increased serum triglycerides, tissue necrosis following accidental extravasation

Overdosage/Toxicology Symptoms include hypotension, bradycardia, and cardiovascular collapse. Treatment is symptomatic and supportive. Hypotension usually responds to I.V. fluids and/or Trendelenburg positioning. Parenteral inotropes may be needed.

Drug Interactions

Increased Effect/Toxicity: Increased toxicity:

Neuromuscular blockers:

Atracurium: Anaphylactoid reactions (including bronchospasm) have been reported in patients who have received concomitant atracurium and propofol.

Vecuronium: Propofol may potentiate the neuromuscular blockade of vecuronium.

Central nervous system depressants: Additive CNS depression and respiratory depression may necessitate dosage reduction when used with anesthetics, benzodiazepines, opiates, ethanol, narcotics, phenothiazines.

Decreased Effect: Theophylline may antagonize the effect of propofol, requiring dosage increases.

Ethanol/Nutrition/Herb Interactions Food: EDTA, an ingredient of propofol emulsion, may lead to decreased zinc levels in patients on prolonged therapy (>5 days) or those predisposed to deficiency (burns, diarrhea, and/or major sepsis).

(Continued)

Propofol *(Continued)*

Stability Store at room temperature 4°C to 22°C (40°F to 72°F), refrigeration is not recommended; protect from light. If transferred to a syringe or other container prior to administration, use within 6 hours. If used directly from vial/prefilled syringe, use within 12 hours. Shake well before use. Do not use if there is evidence of separation of phases of emulsion.

Does not need to be diluted; however, propofol may be further diluted in 5% dextrose in water to a concentration of 2 mg/mL and is stable for 8 hours at room temperature.

Y-site administration compatible with D_5LR, D_5W, lactated Ringer's, lidocaine, 5% dextrose and 0.45% sodium chloride, 5% dextrose and 0.2% sodium chloride. Do not mix with other therapeutic agents.

Mechanism of Action Propofol is a hindered phenolic compound with intravenous general anesthetic properties. The drug is unrelated to any of the currently used barbiturate, opioid, benzodiazepine, arylcyclohexylamine, or imidazole intravenous anesthetic agents.

Pharmacodynamics/Kinetics

Onset of action: Anesthetic: Bolus infusion (dose-dependent): 9-51 seconds (average 30 seconds)

Duration (dose and rate dependent): 3-10 minutes

Distribution: V_d: 2-10 L/kg; highly lipophilic

Protein binding: 97% to 99%

Metabolism: Hepatic to water-soluble sulfate and glucuronide conjugates

Half-life elimination: Biphasic: Initial: 40 minutes; Terminal: 4-7 hours (up to 1-3 days)

Excretion: Urine (~88% as metabolites, 40% as glucuronide metabolite); feces (<2%)

Clearance: 20-30 mL/kg/minute; total body clearance exceeds liver blood flow

Usual Dosage Dosage must be individualized based on total body weight and titrated to the desired clinical effect; wait at least 3-5 minutes between dosage adjustments to clinically assess drug effects; smaller doses are required when used with narcotics; the following are general dosing guidelines:

General anesthesia:

Induction: I.V.:

Children 3-16 years, ASA I or II: 2.5-3.5 mg/kg over 20-30 seconds; use a lower dose for children ASA III or IV

Adults, ASA I or II, <55 years: 2-2.5 mg/kg (~40 mg every 10 seconds until onset of induction)

Elderly, debilitated, hypovolemic, or ASA III or IV: 1-1.5 mg/kg (~20 mg every 10 seconds until onset of induction)

Cardiac anesthesia: 0.5-1.5 mg/kg (~20 mg every 10 seconds until onset of induction)

Neurosurgical patients: 1-2 mg/kg (~20 mg every 10 seconds until onset of induction)

Maintenance: I.V. infusion:

Children 2 months to 16 years, ASA I or II: Initial: 200-300 mcg/kg/minute; decrease dose after 30 minutes if clinical signs of light anesthesia are absent; usual infusion rate: 125-150 mcg/kg/minute (range: 125-300 mcg/kg/minute; 7.5-18 mg/kg/hour); children ≤5 years may require larger infusion rates compared to older children

Adults, ASA I or II, <55 years: Initial: 150-200 mcg/kg/minute for 10-15 minutes; decrease by 30% to 50% during first 30 minutes of maintenance; usual infusion rate: 100-200 mcg/kg/minute (6-12 mg/kg/hour)

Elderly, debilitated, hypovolemic, ASA III or IV: 50-100 mcg/kg/minute (3-6 mg/kg/ hour)

Cardiac anesthesia:

Low-dose propofol with primary opioid: 50-100 mcg/kg/minute (see manufacturer's labeling)

Primary propofol with secondary opioid: 100-150 mcg/kg/minute

Neurosurgical patients: 100-200 mcg/kg/minute (6-12 mg/kg/hour)

Maintenance: I.V. intermittent bolus: Adults, ASA I or II, <55 years: 20-50 mg increments as needed

Monitored anesthesia care sedation:

Initiation:

Adults, ASA I or II, <55 years: Slow I.V. infusion: 100-150 mcg/kg/minute for 3-5 minutes **or** slow injection: 0.5 mg/kg over 3-5 minutes

Elderly, debilitated, neurosurgical, or ASA III or IV patients: Use similar doses to healthy adults; avoid rapid I.V. boluses

Maintenance:

Adults, ASA I or II, <55 years: I.V. infusion using variable rates (preferred over intermittent boluses): 25-75 mcg/kg/minute **or** incremental bolus doses: 10 mg or 20 mg

Elderly, debilitated, neurosurgical, or ASA III or IV patients: Use 80% of healthy adult dose; **do not** use rapid bolus doses (single or repeated)

ICU sedation in intubated mechanically-ventilated patients: Avoid rapid bolus injection; individualize dose and titrate to response

Adults: Continuous infusion: Initial: 0.3 mg/kg/hour; increase by 0.3-0.6 mg/kg/hour every 5-10 minutes until desired sedation level is achieved; usual maintenance: 0.3-3 mg/kg/ hour or higher; reduce dose by 80% in elderly, debilitated, and ASA III or IV patients; reduce dose after adequate sedation established and adjust to response (ie, evaluate frequently to use minimum dose for sedation). Some clinicians recommend daily interruption of infusion to perform clinical evaluation.

Dietary Considerations Propofol is formulated in an oil-in-water emulsion. If on parenteral nutrition, may need to adjust the amount of lipid infused. Propofol emulsion contains 1.1 kcal/mL.

Administration To reduce pain associated with injection, use larger veins of forearm or antecubital fossa; lidocaine I.V. (1 mL of a 1% solution) may also be used prior to administration. Do not use filter with <5 micron for administration. Soybean fat emulsion is used as a vehicle for propofol. Strict aseptic technique must be maintained in handling although a preservative has been added. Do not administer through the same I.V. catheter with blood or plasma. The American College of Critical Care Medicine recommends the use of a central vein for administration in an ICU setting.

Monitoring Parameters Cardiac monitor, blood pressure monitor, and ventilator required; serum triglyceride levels should be obtained prior to initiation of therapy (ICU setting) and every 3-7 days thereafter; daily sedation levels using standardized scale

Vital signs: Blood pressure, heart rate, cardiac output, pulmonary capillary wedge pressure should be monitored

Monitor zinc levels in patients predisposed to deficiency (burns, diarrhea, major sepsis). In patients at risk for renal impairment, urinalysis and urine sediment should be monitored prior to treatment and every other day of sedation.

Test Interactions ↓ cholesterol (S); ↑ porphyrin (U); ↓ cortisol (S), but does not appear to inhibit adrenal responsiveness to ACTH

Nursing Implications Changes urine color to green; abrupt discontinuation of infusion may result in rapid awakening of the patient associated with anxiety, agitation, and resistance to mechanical ventilation, making weaning from mechanical ventilation difficult; use a light level of sedation throughout the weaning process until 10-15 minutes before extubation; titrate the infusion rate so the patient awakens slowly. Tubing and any unused portions of propofol vials should be discarded after 12 hours. Soybean fat emulsion is used as a vehicle for propofol. Strict aseptic technique must be maintained in handling although a preservative has been added.

Additional Information On March 26, 2001, a specific warning was issued concerning the use of propofol in pediatric ICU patients. In the opinion of the FDA, a clinical trial evaluating the use of propofol as a sedative agent in this population was associated with a higher number of deaths as compared to standard sedative agents. The warning reminded health-care professionals that propofol is not approved in the U.S. for sedation in pediatric ICU patients. A new clinical trial is planned to evaluate differences in safety within this population.

Dosage Forms Injection: 10 mg/mL (20 mL, 50 mL, 100 mL) [with EDTA preservative]

Propoxyphene (proe POKS i feen)

Related Information
Narcotic Agonists Comparison *on page 1506*

U.S. Brand Names Darvon®; Darvon-N®

Canadian Brand Names Darvon-N®; 642® Tablet

Synonyms Dextropropoxyphene; Propoxyphene Hydrochloride; Propoxyphene Napsylate

Therapeutic Category Analgesic, Narcotic

Use Management of mild to moderate pain

Restrictions C-IV

Pregnancy Risk Factor C/D (prolonged use)

Contraindications Hypersensitivity to propoxyphene or any component of the formulation; pregnancy (prolonged use)

Warnings/Precautions Administer with caution in patients dependent on opiates, substitution may result in acute opiate withdrawal symptoms, use with caution in patients with severe renal or hepatic dysfunction; when given in excessive doses, either alone or in combination with other CNS depressants or propoxyphene products, propoxyphene is a major cause of drug-related deaths; **do not exceed recommended dosage**; tolerance or drug dependence may result from extended use

Adverse Reactions Frequency not defined.

Cardiovascular: Hypotension, bundle branch block

Central nervous system: Dizziness, lightheadedness, sedation, paradoxical excitement and insomnia, fatigue, drowsiness, mental depression, hallucinations, paradoxical CNS stimulation, increased intracranial pressure, nervousness, headache, restlessness, malaise, confusion

Dermatologic: Rash, urticaria

Endocrine & metabolic: May decrease glucose, urinary 17-OHCS

Gastrointestinal: Anorexia, stomach cramps, xerostomia, biliary spasm, nausea, vomiting, constipation, paralytic ileus

Genitourinary: Decreased urination, ureteral spasms

Neuromuscular & skeletal: Weakness

Hepatic: Increased liver enzymes (may increase LFTs)

Respiratory: Dyspnea

Miscellaneous: Psychologic and physical dependence with prolonged use, histamine release

Overdosage/Toxicology Symptoms include CNS and respiratory depression, hypotension, pulmonary edema, and seizures. Treatment includes airway support, establishment of an I.V. line, and administration of naloxone 2 mg I.V. (0.01 mg/kg for children), with repeat administration as necessary, up to a total of 10 mg. Emesis is not indicated as overdose may cause seizures. Charcoal is very effective (>95%) at binding propoxyphene.

Drug Interactions

Cytochrome P450 Effect: CYP2C9, 2D6, 3A4, and 3A7 enzyme inhibitor

Increased Effect/Toxicity: CNS depressants (phenothiazines, tranquilizers, anxiolytics, sedatives, hypnotics, or alcohol) may potentiate pharmacologic effects. Propoxyphene may inhibit the metabolism and increase the serum concentrations of carbamazepine, phenobarbital, MAO inhibitors, tricyclic antidepressants, and warfarin.

Decreased Effect: Decreased effect with cigarette smoking.

Ethanol/Nutrition/Herb Interactions

Ethanol: Avoid or limit ethanol (may increase CNS depression). Watch for sedation.

Food: May decrease rate of absorption, but may slightly increase bioavailability. Glucose may cause hyperglycemia; monitor blood glucose concentrations.

Mechanism of Action Propoxyphene is a weak narcotic analgesic which acts through binding to opiate receptors to inhibit ascending pain pathways. Propoxyphene, as with other narcotic (opiate) analgesics, blocks pain perception in the cerebral cortex by binding to specific receptor molecules (opiate receptors) within the neuronal membranes of synapses. This binding results in a decreased synaptic chemical transmission throughout the CNS thus inhibiting the flow of pain sensations into the higher centers. Mu and kappa are the two subtypes of the opiate receptor which propoxyphene binds to to cause analgesia.

(Continued)

Propoxyphene *(Continued)*

Pharmacodynamics/Kinetics

Onset of action: 0.5-1 hour

Duration: 4-6 hours

Metabolism: Hepatic to an active metabolite (norpropoxyphene) and inactive metabolites, first-pass effect

Bioavailability: 30% to 70%

Half-life elimination: Adults: Parent drug: 8-24 hours (mean: ~15 hours); Norpropoxyphene: 34 hours

Excretion: Urine (20% to 25%)

Usual Dosage Oral:

Children: Doses for children are not well established; doses of the hydrochloride of 2-3 mg/kg/d divided every 6 hours have been used

Adults:

Hydrochloride: 65 mg every 3-4 hours as needed for pain; maximum: 390 mg/day

Napsylate: 100 mg every 4 hours as needed for pain; maximum: 600 mg/day

Dosing comments in renal impairment: Cl_{cr} <10 mL/minute: Avoid use

Hemodialysis: Not dialyzable (0% to 5%)

Dosing adjustment in hepatic impairment: Reduced doses should be used

Dietary Considerations May administer with food if gastrointestinal distress occurs.

Administration Should be administered with glass of water on an empty stomach. Food may decrease rate of absorption, but may slightly increase bioavailability.

Monitoring Parameters Pain relief, respiratory and mental status, blood pressure

Reference Range

Therapeutic: Ranges published vary between laboratories and may not correlate with clinical effect

Therapeutic concentration: 0.1-0.4 µg/mL (SI: 0.3-1.2 µmol/L)

Toxic: >0.5 µg/mL (SI: >1.5 µmol/L)

Test Interactions False-positive methadone test

Patient Information May cause drowsiness, dizziness, or blurring of vision; avoid alcohol and other sedatives; may take with food; can impair judgment and coordination

Nursing Implications Monitor pain relief, respiratory and mental status, blood pressure, excessive sedation

Additional Information 100 mg of napsylate = 65 mg of hydrochloride

Propoxyphene hydrochloride: Darvon®

Propoxyphene napsylate: Darvon-N®

Dosage Forms

Capsule, as hydrochloride: 65 mg

Tablet, as napsylate: 100 mg

Propoxyphene and Acetaminophen

(proe POKS i feen & a seet a MIN oh fen)

U.S. Brand Names Darvocet-N® 50; Darvocet-N® 100; Pronap-100®; Wygesic®

Canadian Brand Names Darvocet-N® 50; Darvocet-N® 100

Synonyms Propoxyphene Hydrochloride and Acetaminophen; Propoxyphene Napsylate and Acetaminophen

Therapeutic Category Analgesic, Narcotic

Use Management of mild to moderate pain

Restrictions C-IV

Pregnancy Risk Factor C

Usual Dosage Adults: Oral:

Darvocet-N® 50: 1-2 tablets every 4 hours as needed; maximum: 600 mg propoxyphene napsylate/day

Darvocet-N® 100: 1 tablet every 4 hours as needed; maximum: 600 mg propoxyphene napsylate/day

Note: Dosage of acetaminophen should not exceed 4 g/day (6 tablets of Darvocet-N® 100); possibly less in patients with ethanol

Additional Information Complete prescribing information for this medication should be consulted for additional detail.

Dosage Forms

Tablet:

Darvocet-N® 50: Propoxyphene napsylate 50 mg and acetaminophen 325 mg

Darvocet-N® 100, Pronap-100®: Propoxyphene napsylate 100 mg and acetaminophen 650 mg

Wygesic®: Propoxyphene hydrochloride 65 mg and acetaminophen 650 mg

Propoxyphene and Aspirin (proe POKS i feen & AS pir in)

U.S. Brand Names Darvon® Compound-65 Pulvules®; PC-Cap®

Synonyms Propoxyphene Hydrochloride and Aspirin; Propoxyphene Napsylate and Aspirin

Therapeutic Category Analgesic, Narcotic

Use Management of mild to moderate pain

Restrictions C-IV

Pregnancy Risk Factor D

Usual Dosage Oral:

Children: Not recommended

Adults: 1-2 capsules every 4 hours as needed

Additional Information Complete prescribing information for this medication should be consulted for additional detail.

Dosage Forms Capsule (Darvon® Compound-65, PC-Cap®): Propoxyphene hydrochloride 65 mg and aspirin 389 mg with caffeine 32.4 mg

♦ **Propoxyphene Hydrochloride** *see* Propoxyphene *on page 1147*

♦ **Propoxyphene Hydrochloride and Acetaminophen** *see* Propoxyphene and Acetaminophen *on page 1148*

♦ **Propoxyphene Hydrochloride and Aspirin** *see* Propoxyphene and Aspirin *on page 1148*

♦ **Propoxyphene Napsylate** *see* Propoxyphene *on page 1147*

♦ **Propoxyphene Napsylate and Acetaminophen** *see* Propoxyphene and Acetaminophen *on page 1148*

♦ **Propoxyphene Napsylate and Aspirin** *see* Propoxyphene and Aspirin *on page 1148*

Propranolol (proe PRAN oh lole)

Related Information
Antiarrhythmic Drugs Comparison *on page 1478*
Beta-Blockers Comparison *on page 1491*
Depression *on page 1655*

U.S. Brand Names Inderal®; Inderal® LA

Canadian Brand Names Apo®-Propranolol; Inderal®; Inderal®-LA; Nu-Propranolol

Synonyms Propranolol Hydrochloride

Therapeutic Category Antianginal Agent; Antiarrhythmic Agent, Class II; Antihypertensive Agent; Antimigraine Agent; Beta-Adrenergic Blocker

Use Management of hypertension; angina pectoris; pheochromocytoma; essential tremor; tetralogy of Fallot cyanotic spells; arrhythmias (such as atrial fibrillation and flutter, AV nodal re-entrant tachycardias, and catecholamine-induced arrhythmias); prevention of myocardial infarction; migraine headache; symptomatic treatment of hypertrophic subaortic stenosis

Unlabeled/Investigational Use Tremor due to Parkinson's disease; ethanol withdrawal; aggressive behavior; antipsychotic-induced akathisia; prevention of bleeding esophageal varices; anxiety; schizophrenia; acute panic; gastric bleeding in portal hypertension

Pregnancy Risk Factor C (manufacturer); D (2nd and 3rd trimesters - expert analysis)

Pregnancy/Breast-Feeding Implications
Clinical effects on the fetus: Crosses the placenta. IUGR, hypoglycemia, bradycardia, respiratory depression, hyperbilirubinemia, polycythemia, polydactyly reported. IUGR probably related to maternal hypertension. Preterm labor has been reported. Available evidence suggests safe use during pregnancy and breast-feeding. Monitor breast-fed infant for symptoms of beta-blockade.
Breast-feeding/lactation: Crosses into breast milk. AAP considers **compatible** with breast-feeding.

Contraindications Hypersensitivity to propranolol, beta-blockers, or any component of the formulation; uncompensated congestive heart failure (unless the failure is due to tachyarrhythmias being treated with propranolol); cardiogenic shock, bradycardia or heart block (2nd or 3rd degree); pulmonary edema, severe hyperactive airway disease (asthma or COPD), Raynaud's disease; pregnancy (2nd and 3rd trimesters)

Warnings/Precautions Administer cautiously in compensated heart failure and monitor for a worsening of the condition (efficacy of propranolol in CHF has not been demonstrated). Avoid abrupt discontinuation in patients with a history of CAD; slowly wean while monitoring for signs and symptoms of ischemia. Use caution in patient with PVD. Use caution with concurrent use of beta-blockers and either verapamil or diltiazem; bradycardia or heart block can occur. Avoid concurrent I.V. use of both agents. Use cautiously in diabetics because it can mask prominent hypoglycemic symptoms. Can mask signs of thyrotoxicosis. Can cause fetal harm when administered in pregnancy. Use cautiously in hepatic dysfunction (dosage adjustment required). Use care with anesthetic agents which decrease myocardial function.

Adverse Reactions Frequency not defined.
Cardiovascular: Bradycardia, congestive heart failure, reduced peripheral circulation, chest pain, hypotension, impaired myocardial contractility, worsening of AV conduction disturbance, cardiogenic shock, Raynaud's syndrome, mesenteric thrombosis (rare)
Central nervous system: Mental depression, lightheadedness, amnesia, emotional lability, confusion, hallucinations, dizziness, insomnia, fatigue, vivid dreams, lethargy, cold extremities, vertigo, syncope, cognitive dysfunction, psychosis, hypersomnolence
Dermatologic: Rash, alopecia, exfoliative dermatitis, psoriasiform eruptions, eczematous eruptions, hyperkeratosis, nail changes, pruritus, urticaria, ulcerative lichenoid, contact dermatitis
Endocrine & metabolic: Hypoglycemia, hyperglycemia, hyperlipidemia, hyperkalemia
Gastrointestinal: Diarrhea, nausea, vomiting, stomach discomfort, constipation, anorexia
Genitourinary: Impotence, proteinuria (rare), oliguria (rare), interstitial nephritis (rare), Peyronie's disease
Hematologic: Agranulocytosis, thrombocytopenia, thrombocytopenic purpura
Neuromuscular & skeletal: Weakness, carpal tunnel syndrome (rare), paresthesias, myotonus, polyarthritis, arthropathy
Respiratory: Wheezing, pharyngitis, bronchospasm, pulmonary edema
Ocular: Hyperemia of the conjunctiva, decreased tear production, decreased visual acuity, mydriasis
Miscellaneous: Lupus-like syndrome (rare)

Overdosage/Toxicology Symptoms of intoxication include cardiac disturbances, CNS toxicity, bronchospasm, hypoglycemia, and hyperkalemia. The most common cardiac symptoms include hypotension and bradycardia. Atrioventricular block, intraventricular conduction disturbances, cardiogenic shock, and asystole may occur with severe overdose, especially with membrane-depressant drugs (eg, propranolol). CNS effects include convulsions, coma, and respiratory arrest and are commonly seen with propranolol and other membrane-depressant and lipid-soluble drugs. Treatment is symptomatic for seizures, hypotension, hyperkalemia, and hypoglycemia. Bradycardia and hypotension resistant to atropine, isoproterenol, or pacing may respond to glucagon. Wide QRS defects caused by membrane-depressant poisoning may respond to hypertonic sodium bicarbonate. Repeat-dose charcoal, hemoperfusion, or hemodialysis may be helpful in removal of only those beta-blockers with a small V_d, long half-life, or low intrinsic clearance (acebutolol, atenolol, nadolol, sotalol).
(Continued)

Propranolol (Continued)

Drug Interactions

Cytochrome P450 Effect: CYP1A2, 2C18, 2C19, and 2D6 enzyme substrate

Increased Effect/Toxicity: The heart rate lowering effects of propranolol are additive with other drugs which slow AV conduction (digoxin, verapamil, diltiazem). Reserpine increases the effects of propranolol. Concurrent use of propranolol may increase the effects of alpha-blockers (prazosin, terazosin), alpha-adrenergic stimulants (epinephrine, phenylephrine), and the vasoconstrictive effects of ergot alkaloids. Propranolol may mask the tachycardia from hypoglycemia caused by insulin and oral hypoglycemics. In patients receiving concurrent therapy, the risk of hypertensive crisis is increased when either clonidine or the beta-blocker is withdrawn. Beta-blockers may increase the action or levels of ethanol, disopyramide, nondepolarizing muscle relaxants, and theophylline although the effects are difficult to predict.

Beta-blocker effects may be enhanced by oral contraceptives, flecainide, haloperidol (hypotensive effects), H_2-antagonists (cimetidine, possibly ranitidine), hydralazine, loop diuretics, possibly MAO inhibitors, phenothiazines, propafenone, quinidine (in extensive metabolizers), ciprofloxacin, thyroid hormones (when hypothyroid patient is converted to euthyroid state). Beta-blockers may increase the effect/toxicity of flecainide, haloperidol (hypotensive effects), hydralazine, phenothiazines, acetaminophen, anticoagulants (warfarin), and benzodiazepines.

Decreased Effect: Aluminum salts, barbiturates, calcium salts, cholestyramine, colestipol, NSAIDs, penicillins (ampicillin), rifampin, salicylates, and sulfinpyrazone decrease effect of beta-blockers due to decreased bioavailability and plasma levels. Beta-blockers may decrease the effect of sulfonylureas. Ascorbic acid decreases propranolol Cp_{max} and AUC and increases the T_{max} significantly resulting in a greater decrease in the reduction of heart rate, possibly due to decreased absorption and first pass metabolism (n=5). Nefazodone decreased peak plasma levels and AUC of propranolol and increases time to reach steady-state; monitoring of clinical response is recommended. Nonselective beta-blockers blunt the response to beta-2 adrenergic agonists (albuterol).

Ethanol/Nutrition/Herb Interactions

Food: Propranolol serum levels may be increased if taken with food. Protein-rich foods may increase bioavailability; a change in diet from high carbohydrate/low protein to low carbohydrate/high protein may result in increased oral clearance.

Herb/Nutraceutical: Avoid dong quai if using for hypertension (has estrogenic activity). Avoid ephedra, yohimbe, ginseng (may worsen hypertension or arrhythmia). Avoid natural licorice (causes sodium and water retention and increases potassium loss). Avoid garlic (may have increased antihypertensive effect).

Stability Compatible in saline, **incompatible** with HCO_3^-; protect injection from light; solutions have maximum stability at pH of 3 and decompose rapidly in alkaline pH; propranolol is stable for 24 hours at room temperature in D_5W or NS

Mechanism of Action Nonselective beta-adrenergic blocker (class II antiarrhythmic); competitively blocks response to beta$_1$- and beta$_2$-adrenergic stimulation which results in decreases in heart rate, myocardial contractility, blood pressure, and myocardial oxygen demand

Pharmacodynamics/Kinetics

Onset of action: Beta-blockade: Oral: 1-2 hours

Duration: ~6 hours

Distribution: V_d: 3.9 L/kg in adults; crosses placenta; small amounts enter breast milk

Protein binding: Newborns: 68%; Adults: 93%

Metabolism: Hepatic to active and inactive compounds; extensive first-pass effect

Bioavailability: 30% to 40%; may be increased in Down syndrome children

Half-life elimination: Neonates and Infants: Possible increased half-life; Children: 3.9-6.4 hours; Adults: 4-6 hours

Excretion: Primarily urine (96% to 99%)

Usual Dosage

Tachyarrhythmias:

Oral:

Children: Initial: 0.5-1 mg/kg/day in divided doses every 6-8 hours; titrate dosage upward every 3-7 days; usual dose: 2-4 mg/kg/day; higher doses may be needed; do not exceed 16 mg/kg/day or 60 mg/day

Adults: 10-30 mg/dose every 6-8 hours

Elderly: Initial: 10 mg twice daily; increase dosage every 3-7 days; usual dosage range: 10-320 mg given in 2 divided doses

I.V.:

Children: 0.01-0.1 mg/kg slow IVP over 10 minutes; maximum dose: 1 mg

Adults: 1 mg/dose slow IVP; repeat every 5 minutes up to a total of 5 mg

Hypertension: Oral:

Children: Initial: 0.5-1 mg/kg/day in divided doses every 6-12 hours; increase gradually every 3-7 days; maximum: 2 mg/kg/24 hours

Adults: Initial: 40 mg twice daily; increase dosage every 3-7 days; usual dose: ≤320 mg divided in 2-3 doses/day; maximum daily dose: 640 mg

Long-acting formulation: Initial: 80 mg once daily; usual maintenance: 120-160 mg once daily; maximum daily dose: 640 mg

Migraine headache prophylaxis: Oral:

Children: 0.6-1.5 mg/kg/day **or**

≤35 kg: 10-20 mg 3 times/day

>35 kg: 20-40 mg 3 times/day

Adults: Initial: 80 mg/day divided every 6-8 hours; increase by 20-40 mg/dose every 3-4 weeks to a maximum of 160-240 mg/day given in divided doses every 6-8 hours; if satisfactory response not achieved within 6 weeks of starting therapy, drug should be withdrawn gradually over several weeks

Long-acting formulation: Initial: 80 mg once daily; effective dose range: 160-240 mg once daily

Tetralogy spells: Children:
Oral: 1-2 mg/kg/day every 6 hours as needed, may increase by 1 mg/kg/day to a maximum of 5 mg/kg/day, or if refractory may increase slowly to a maximum of 10-15 mg/kg/day
I.V.: 0.15-0.25 mg/kg/dose slow IVP; may repeat in 15 minutes

Thyrotoxicosis:
Adolescents and Adults: Oral: 10-40 mg/dose every 6 hours
Adults: I.V.: 1-3 mg/dose slow IVP as a single dose

Adults: Oral:
Akathisia: 30-120 mg/day in 2-3 divided doses
Angina: 80-320 mg/day in doses divided 2-4 times/day
Long-acting formulation: Initial: 80 mg once daily; maximum dose: 320 mg once daily
Essential tremor: 20-40 mg twice daily initially; maintenance doses: usually 120-320 mg/day
Hypertrophic subaortic stenosis: 20-40 mg 3-4 times/day
Long-acting formulation: 80-160 mg once daily
Myocardial infarction prophylaxis: 180-240 mg/day in 3-4 divided doses
Pheochromocytoma: 30-60 mg/day in divided doses

Dosing adjustment in renal impairment:
Cl_{cr} 31-40 mL/minute: Administer every 24-36 hours or administer 50% of normal dose
Cl_{cr} 10-30 mL/minute: Administer every 24-48 hours or administer 50% of normal dose
Cl_{cr} <10 mL/minute: Administer every 40-60 hours or administer 25% of normal dose
Hemodialysis: Not dialyzable (0% to 5%); supplemental dose is not necessary
Peritoneal dialysis: Supplemental dose is not necessary

Dosing adjustment/comments in hepatic disease: Marked slowing of heart rate may occur in cirrhosis with conventional doses; low initial dose and regular heart rate monitoring

Dietary Considerations Administer with food.

Administration I.V. administration should not exceed 1 mg/minute; I.V. dose much smaller than oral dose

Monitoring Parameters Blood pressure, EKG, heart rate, CNS and cardiac effects

Reference Range Therapeutic: 50-100 ng/mL (SI: 190-390 nmol/L) at end of dose interval

Patient Information Do not discontinue abruptly; notify physician if CHF symptoms become worse or side effects develop; take at the same time each day; may mask diabetes symptoms; consult pharmacist or physician before taking with other adrenergic drugs (eg, cold medications); use with caution while driving or performing tasks requiring alertness

Nursing Implications Patient's therapeutic response may be evaluated by looking at blood pressure, apical and radial pulses, fluid I & O, daily weight, respirations, and circulation in extremities before and during therapy. Do not crush long acting forms.

Additional Information Not indicated for hypertensive emergencies. Do not abruptly discontinue therapy, taper dosage gradually over 2 weeks.

Dosage Forms
Capsule, long-acting, as hydrochloride: 60 mg, 80 mg, 120 mg, 160 mg
Injection, as hydrochloride: 1 mg/mL (1 mL)
Solution, oral, as hydrochloride: 4 mg/mL (5 mL, 500 mL); 8 mg/mL (5 mL, 500 mL) [strawberry-mint flavor]
Solution, oral concentrate, as hydrochloride: 80 mg/mL (30 mL)
Tablet, as hydrochloride: 10 mg, 20 mg, 40 mg, 60 mg, 80 mg, 90 mg

Propranolol and Hydrochlorothiazide
(proe PRAN oh lole & hye droe klor oh THYE a zide)

U.S. Brand Names Inderide®; Inderide® LA

Canadian Brand Names Inderide®

Synonyms Hydrochlorothiazide and Propranolol

Therapeutic Category Antihypertensive Agent, Combination

Use Management of hypertension

Pregnancy Risk Factor C

Usual Dosage Oral: Adults: Hypertension: Dose is individualized; typical dosages of **hydrochlorothiazide**: 12.5-50 mg/day; initial dose of **propranolol**: 80 mg/day
Daily dose of tablet form should be divided into 2 daily doses; may be used to maximum dosage of up to 160 mg of propranolol; higher dosages would result in higher than optimal thiazide dosages.
Long acting capsules may be given once daily.

Additional Information Complete prescribing information for this medication should be consulted for additional detail.

Dosage Forms
Capsule, long-acting (Inderide® LA):
80/50 Propranolol hydrochloride 80 mg and hydrochlorothiazide 50 mg
120/50 Propranolol hydrochloride 120 mg and hydrochlorothiazide 50 mg
160/50 Propranolol hydrochloride 160 mg and hydrochlorothiazide 50 mg
Tablet (Inderide®):
40/25 Propranolol hydrochloride 40 mg and hydrochlorothiazide 25 mg
80/25 Propranolol hydrochloride 80 mg and hydrochlorothiazide 25 mg

♦ **Propranolol Hydrochloride** *see Propranolol on page 1149*
♦ **Propulsid**® *see Cisapride **U.S. - Available Via Limited-Access Protocol Only** on page 298*
♦ **Propylene Glycol Diacetate, Acetic Acid, and Hydrocortisone** *see Acetic Acid, Propylene Glycol Diacetate, and Hydrocortisone on page 31*
♦ **Propylene Glycol Diacetate, Hydrocortisone, and Acetic Acid** *see Acetic Acid, Propylene Glycol Diacetate, and Hydrocortisone on page 31*
♦ **2-Propylpentanoic Acid** *see Valproic Acid and Derivatives on page 1398*

Propylthiouracil (proe pil thye oh YOOR a sil)

Canadian Brand Names Propyl-Thyracil®

Synonyms PTU

(Continued)

Propylthiouracil *(Continued)*

Therapeutic Category Antithyroid Agent

Use Palliative treatment of hyperthyroidism as an adjunct to ameliorate hyperthyroidism in preparation for surgical treatment or radioactive iodine therapy; management of thyrotoxic crisis

Pregnancy Risk Factor D

Pregnancy/Breast-Feeding Implications Crosses the placenta and may induce goiter and hypothyroidism in the developing fetus (cretinism). May need to monitor infant's thyroid function periodically. Enters breast milk/use caution (AAP rates "compatible").

Contraindications Hypersensitivity to propylthiouracil or any component of the formulation; pregnancy

Warnings/Precautions Use with caution in patients >40 years of age because PTU may cause hypoprothrombinemia and bleeding; use with extreme caution in patients receiving other drugs known to cause agranulocytosis; may cause agranulocytosis, thyroid hyperplasia, thyroid carcinoma (usage >1 year). Discontinue in the presence of agranulocytosis, aplastic anemia, ANCA-positive vasculitis, hepatitis, unexplained fever, or exfoliative dermatitis. Safety and efficacy have not been established in children <6 years of age.

Adverse Reactions Frequency not defined.

Cardiovascular: Edema, cutaneous vasculitis, leukocytoclastic vasculitis, ANCA-positive vasculitis

Central nervous system: Fever, drowsiness, vertigo, headache, drug fever, dizziness, neuritis

Dermatologic: Skin rash, urticaria, pruritus, exfoliative dermatitis, alopecia, erythema nodosum

Endocrine & metabolic: Goiter, weight gain, swollen salivary glands

Gastrointestinal: Nausea, vomiting, loss of taste perception, stomach pain, constipation

Hematologic: Leukopenia, agranulocytosis, thrombocytopenia, bleeding, aplastic anemia

Hepatic: Cholestatic jaundice, hepatitis

Neuromuscular & skeletal: Arthralgia, paresthesia

Renal: Nephritis, glomerulonephritis, acute renal failure

Respiratory: Interstitial pneumonitis, alveolar hemorrhage

Miscellaneous: SLE-like syndrome

Overdosage/Toxicology Symptoms include nausea, vomiting, epigastric pain, headache, fever, arthralgia, pruritus, edema, pancytopenia, epigastric distress, headache, fever, CNS stimulation or depression. Treatment is supportive and includes monitoring bone marrow response, forced diuresis, peritoneal and hemodialysis, as well as charcoal hemoperfusion.

Drug Interactions

Increased Effect/Toxicity: Propylthiouracil may increase the anticoagulant activity of warfarin.

Decreased Effect: Oral anticoagulant activity is increased only until metabolic effect stabilizes. Anticoagulants may be potentiated by anti-vitamin K effect of propylthiouracil. Correction of hyperthyroidism may alter disposition of beta-blockers, digoxin, and theophylline, necessitating a dose reduction of these agents.

Ethanol/Nutrition/Herb Interactions Food: Propylthiouracil serum levels may be altered if taken with food.

Mechanism of Action Inhibits the synthesis of thyroid hormones by blocking the oxidation of iodine in the thyroid gland; blocks synthesis of thyroxine and triiodothyronine

Pharmacodynamics/Kinetics

Onset of action: Therapeutic: 24-36 hours

Peak effect: Remission: 4 months of continued therapy

Duration: 2-3 hours

Distribution: Concentrated in the thyroid gland

Protein binding: 75% to 80%

Metabolism: Hepatic

Bioavailability: 80% to 95%

Half-life elimination: 1.5-5 hours; End-stage renal disease: 8.5 hours

Time to peak, serum: ~1 hour

Excretion: Urine (35%)

Usual Dosage Oral: Administer in 3 equally divided doses at approximately 8-hour intervals. Adjust dosage to maintain T_3, T_4, and TSH levels in normal range; elevated T_3 may be sole indicator of inadequate treatment. Elevated TSH indicates excessive antithyroid treatment.

Children: Initial: 5-7 mg/kg/day **or** 150-200 mg/m^2/day in divided doses every 8 hours

or

6-10 years: 50-150 mg/day

>10 years: 150-300 mg/day

Maintenance: Determined by patient response **or** $^1/_3$ to $^2/_3$ of the initial dose in divided doses every 8-12 hours. This usually begins after 2 months on an effective initial dose.

Adults: Initial: 300 mg/day in divided doses every 8 hours. In patients with severe hyperthyroidism, very large goiters, or both, the initial dosage is usually 450 mg/day; an occasional patient will require 600-900 mg/day; maintenance: 100-150 mg/day in divided doses every 8-12 hours

Elderly: Use lower dose recommendations; Initial: 150-300 mg/day

Withdrawal of therapy: Therapy should be withdrawn gradually with evaluation of the patient every 4-6 weeks for the first 3 months then every 3 months for the first year after discontinuation of therapy to detect any reoccurrence of a hyperthyroid state.

Dosing adjustment in renal impairment: Adjustment is not necessary

Dietary Considerations Administer at the same time in relation to meals each day, either always with meals or always between meals.

Monitoring Parameters CBC with differential, prothrombin time, liver function tests, thyroid function tests (TSH, T_3, T_4); periodic blood counts are recommended chronic therapy

Reference Range Normal laboratory values:

Total T_4: 5-12 mcg/dL

Serum T_3: 90-185 ng/dL

Free thyroxine index (FT$_4$ I): 6-10.5

TSH: 0.5-4.0 microU/mL

Patient Information Do not exceed prescribed dosage; take at regular intervals around-the-clock; notify physician or pharmacist if fever, sore throat, unusual bleeding or bruising, headache, or general malaise occurs

Nursing Implications Monitor CBC with differential, prothrombin time, liver function tests, thyroid function tests (T_4, T_3, TSH); periodic blood counts are recommended chronic therapy.

Additional Information Preferred over methimazole in thyroid storm due to inhibition of peripheral conversion as well as synthesis of thyroid hormone.

Dosage Forms Tablet: 50 mg

Extemporaneous Preparations A 5 mg/mL oral suspension was stable for 10 days when refrigerated when compounded as follows:

Triturate six 50 mg tablets in a mortar, reduce to a fine powder, add 30 mL of carboxymethyl-cellulose 1.5%, transfer to a graduate and qs to 60 mL

Shake well before using and keep in refrigerator; protect from light

Nahata MC and Hipple TF, *Pediatric Drug Formulations*, 3rd ed, Cincinnati, OH: Harvey Whitney Books Co, 1997.

Protamine Sulfate (PROE ta meen SUL fate)

Therapeutic Category Antidote, Heparin

Use Treatment of heparin overdosage; neutralize heparin during surgery or dialysis procedures

Pregnancy Risk Factor C

Contraindications Hypersensitivity to protamine or any component of the formulation

Warnings/Precautions May not be totally effective in some patients following cardiac surgery despite adequate doses; may cause hypersensitivity reaction in patients with a history of allergy to fish (have epinephrine 1:1000 available) and in patients sensitized to protamine (via protamine zinc insulin); too rapid administration can cause severe hypotensive and anaphylactoid-like reactions. Heparin rebound associated with anticoagulation and bleeding has been reported to occur occasionally; symptoms typically occur 8-9 hours after protamine administration, but may occur as long as 18 hours later.

Adverse Reactions Frequency not defined.

Cardiovascular: Sudden fall in blood pressure, bradycardia, flushing, hypotension

Central nervous system: Lassitude

Gastrointestinal: Nausea, vomiting

Hematologic: Hemorrhage

Respiratory: Dyspnea, pulmonary hypertension

Miscellaneous: Hypersensitivity reactions

Overdose/Toxicology Symptoms include hypertension; may cause hemorrhage. Doses exceeding 100 mg may cause paradox anticoagulation.

Stability Refrigerate, avoid freezing; remains stable for at least 2 weeks at room temperature; **incompatible** with cephalosporins and penicillins; preservative-free formulation does not require refrigeration

Mechanism of Action Combines with strongly acidic heparin to form a stable complex (salt) neutralizing the anticoagulant activity of both drugs

Pharmacodynamics/Kinetics Onset of action: I.V.: Heparin neutralization: ~5 minutes

Usual Dosage Protamine dosage is determined by the dosage of heparin; 1 mg of protamine neutralizes 90 USP units of heparin (lung) and 115 USP units of heparin (intestinal); maximum dose: 50 mg

In the situation of heparin overdosage, since blood heparin concentrations decrease rapidly **after** administration, adjust the protamine dosage depending upon the duration of time since heparin administration as follows: See table.

Time Elapsed	Dose of Protamine (mg) to Neutralize 100 units of Heparin
Immediate	1-1.5
30-60 min	0.5-0.75
>2 h	0.25-0.375

If heparin administered by deep S.C. injection, use 1-1.5 mg protamine per 100 units heparin; this may be done by a portion of the dose (eg, 25-50 mg) given slowly I.V. followed by the remaining portion as a continuous infusion over 8-16 hours (the expected absorption time of the S.C. heparin dose)

Administration For I.V. use only; **incompatible** with cephalosporins and penicillins; administer slow IVP (50 mg over 10 minutes); rapid I.V. infusion causes hypotension; reconstitute vial with 5 mL sterile water; if using protamine in neonates, reconstitute with preservative-free sterile water for injection; resulting solution equals 10 mg/mL; inject without further dilution over 1-3 minutes; maximum of 50 mg in any 10-minute period

(Continued)

Protamine Sulfate *(Continued)*

Monitoring Parameters Coagulation test, aPTT or ACT, cardiac monitor and blood pressure monitor required during administration

Nursing Implications Parenteral: Reconstitute vial with 5 mL sterile water; if using protamine in neonates, reconstitute with preservative-free sterile water for injection; resulting solution equals 10 mg/mL; inject without further dilution over 1-3 minutes; maximum of 50 mg in any 10-minute period

Dosage Forms Injection: 10 mg/mL (5 mL, 25 mL)

- ♦ **Protein C (Activated), Human, Recombinant** *see* Drotrecogin Alfa *on page 453*
- ♦ **Prothazine-DC**® *see* Promethazine and Codeine *on page 1141*
- ♦ **Prothrombin Complex Concentrate** *see* Factor IX Complex (Human) *on page 539*
- ♦ **Protonix**® *see* Pantoprazole *on page 1037*
- ♦ **Protopam**® *see* Pralidoxime *on page 1115*
- ♦ **Protopic**® *see* Tacrolimus *on page 1283*
- ♦ **Protostat**® **Oral** *see* Metronidazole *on page 904*

Protriptyline *(proe TRIP ti leen)*

Related Information
Antidepressant Agents Comparison *on page 1482*

U.S. Brand Names Vivactil®

Canadian Brand Names Triptil®

Synonyms Protriptyline Hydrochloride

Therapeutic Category Antidepressant, Tricyclic

Use Treatment of depression

Pregnancy Risk Factor C

Contraindications Hypersensitivity to protriptyline (cross-reactivity to other cyclic antidepressants may occur) or any component of the formulation; use of MAO inhibitors within 14 days; use of cisapride; use in a patient during the acute recovery phase of MI

Warnings/Precautions May cause sedation, resulting in impaired performance of tasks requiring alertness (ie, operating machinery or driving). Sedative effects may be additive with other CNS depressants and/or ethanol. May worsen psychosis in some patients or precipitate a shift to mania or hypomania in patients with bipolar disease. May aggravate aggressive behavior. May increase the risks associated with electroconvulsive therapy. This agent should be discontinued, when possible, prior to elective surgery. Therapy should not be abruptly discontinued in patients receiving high doses for prolonged periods. May alter glucose regulation - use with caution in patients with diabetes.

May cause orthostatic hypotension (risk is moderate relative to other antidepressants) - use with caution in patients at risk of hypotension or in patients where transient hypotensive episodes would be poorly tolerated (cardiovascular disease or cerebrovascular disease). The degree of anticholinergic blockade produced by this agent is moderate relative to other cyclic antidepressants, however, caution should still be used in patients with urinary retention, benign prostatic hypertrophy, narrow-angle glaucoma, xerostomia, visual problems, constipation, or history of bowel obstruction.

Use caution in patients with suicidal risk. Use with caution in patients with a history of cardiovascular disease (including previous MI, stroke, tachycardia, or conduction abnormalities). The risk of conduction abnormalities with this agent is moderate-high relative to other antidepressants. Use caution in patients with a previous seizure disorder or condition predisposing to seizures such as brain damage, alcoholism, or concurrent therapy with other drugs which lower the seizure threshold. Use with caution in hyperthyroid patients or those receiving thyroid supplementation. Use with caution in patients with hepatic or renal dysfunction and in elderly patients.

Adverse Reactions Frequency not defined.

Cardiovascular: Arrhythmias, hypotension, myocardial infarction, stroke, heart block, hypertension, tachycardia, palpitations

Central nervous system: Dizziness, drowsiness, headache, confusion, delirium, hallucinations, restlessness, insomnia, nightmares, fatigue, delusions, anxiety, agitation, hypomania, exacerbation of psychosis, panic, seizures, incoordination, ataxia, EPS

Dermatologic: Alopecia, photosensitivity, rash, petechiae, urticaria, itching

Endocrine & metabolic: Breast enlargement, galactorrhea, SIADH, gynecomastia, increased or decreased libido

Gastrointestinal: Xerostomia, constipation, unpleasant taste, weight gain, increased appetite, nausea, diarrhea, heartburn, vomiting, anorexia, weight loss, trouble with gums, decreased lower esophageal sphincter tone may cause GE reflux

Genitourinary: Difficult urination, impotence, testicular edema

Hematologic: Agranulocytosis, leukopenia, eosinophilia, thrombocytopenia, purpura

Hepatic: Cholestatic jaundice, increased liver enzymes

Neuromuscular & skeletal: Fine muscle tremors, weakness, tremor, numbness, tingling

Ocular: Blurred vision, eye pain, increased intraocular pressure

Otic: Tinnitus

Miscellaneous: Diaphoresis (excessive), allergic reactions

Overdosage/Toxicology Symptoms include confusion, hallucinations, urinary retention, hypotension, tachycardia, seizures, and hyperthermia. Following initiation of essential overdose management, toxic symptoms should be treated. Sodium bicarbonate is indicated when the QRS interval is >0.10 seconds or the QT_c >0.42 seconds. Ventricular arrhythmias often respond to systemic alkalinization (sodium bicarbonate 0.5-2 mEq/kg I.V.). Arrhythmias unresponsive to this therapy may respond to lidocaine 1 mg/kg I.V. followed by a titrated infusion. Physostigmine (1-2 mg I.V. slowly for adults or 0.5 mg slow I.V. for children) may be indicated in reversing life-threatening cardiac arrhythmias. Seizures usually respond to diazepam I.V. boluses (5-10 mg for adults up to 30 mg or 0.25-0.4 mg/kg/dose for children up to 10 mg/dose). If seizures are unresponsive or recur, phenytoin or phenobarbital may be required.

Drug Interactions

Cytochrome P450 Effect: CYP2D6 enzyme substrate

Increased Effect/Toxicity: Protriptyline increases the effects of amphetamines, anticholinergics, other CNS depressants (sedatives, hypnotics, or ethanol), chlorpropamide, tolazamide, and warfarin. When used with MAO inhibitors, hyperpyrexia, hypertension, tachycardia, confusion, seizures, and **deaths have been reported** (serotonin syndrome). The SSRIs (to varying degrees), cimetidine, grapefruit juice, indinavir, methylphenidate, ritonavir, quinidine, diltiazem, and verapamil inhibit the metabolism of TCAs and clinical toxicity may result. Use of lithium with a TCA may increase the risk for neurotoxicity. Phenothiazines may increase concentration of some TCAs and TCAs may increase concentration of phenothiazines. Pressor response to I.V. epinephrine, norepinephrine, and phenylephrine may be enhanced in patients receiving TCAs (**Note:** Effect is unlikely with epinephrine or levonordefrin dosages typically administered as infiltration in combination with local anesthetics). Combined use of beta-agonists or drugs which prolong QT$_c$ (including quinidine, procainamide, disopyramide, cisapride, sparfloxacin, gatifloxacin, moxifloxacin) with TCAs may predispose patients to cardiac arrhythmias.

Decreased Effect: Carbamazepine, phenobarbital, and rifampin may increase the metabolism of protriptyline, decreasing its effects. Protriptyline inhibits the antihypertensive response to bethanidine, clonidine, debrisoquin, guanadrel, guanethidine, guanabenz, guanfacine. Cimetidine and methylphenidate may decrease the metabolism of protriptyline. Cholestyramine and colestipol may bind TCAs and reduce their absorption.

Ethanol/Nutrition/Herb Interactions

Ethanol: Avoid ethanol (may increase CNS depression).

Food: Grapefruit juice may inhibit the metabolism of some TCAs and clinical toxicity may result.

Herb/Nutraceutical: Avoid valerian, St John's wort, SAMe, kava kava (may increase risk of serotonin syndrome and/or excessive sedation).

Mechanism of Action Increases the synaptic concentration of serotonin and/or norepinephrine in the central nervous system by inhibition of their reuptake by the presynaptic neuronal membrane

Pharmacodynamics/Kinetics

Onset of action: Peak effect: Antidepressant effect: 2 weeks of continuous therapy

Distribution: Crosses placenta

Protein binding: 92%

Metabolism: Extensively hepatic via N-oxidation, hydroxylation, and glucuronidation; first-pass effect (10% to 25%)

Half-life elimination: 54-92 hours (average 74 hours)

Time to peak, serum: 24-30 hours

Excretion: Urine

Usual Dosage Oral:

Adolescents: 15-20 mg/day

Adults: 15-60 mg in 3-4 divided doses

Elderly: 15-20 mg/day

Dietary Considerations May be taken with food to decrease GI distress.

Administration Make any dosage increase in the morning dose

Monitoring Parameters Monitor for cardiac abnormalities in elderly patients receiving doses >20 mg

Reference Range Therapeutic: 70-250 ng/mL (SI: 266-950 nmol/L); Toxic: >500 ng/mL (SI: >1900 nmol/L)

Patient Information Avoid unnecessary exposure to sunlight; do not discontinue abruptly; take dose in morning to avoid insomnia

Nursing Implications Offer patient sugarless hard candy or gum for dry mouth

Dosage Forms Tablet, as hydrochloride: 5 mg, 10 mg

Pseudoephedrine (soo doe e FED rin)

Related Information

Antacid Drug Interactions on page 1477

U.S. Brand Names Cenafed® [OTC]; Children's Silfedrine® [OTC]; Children's Sudafed® Nasal Decongestant [OTC]; Decofed® [OTC]; Dimetapp® Decongestant Liqui-Gels® [OTC]; Efidac/24® [OTC]; Genaphed® [OTC]; PediaCare® Decongestant Infants [OTC]; Sudafed® [OTC]; (Continued)

Pseudoephedrine *(Continued)*

Sudafed® 12 Hour [OTC]; Triaminic® AM Decongestant Formula [OTC]; Triaminic® Infant Decongestant [OTC]

Canadian Brand Names Balminil® Decongestant; Contac® Cold 12 Hour Relief Non Drowsy; Eltor®; PMS-Pseudoephedrine; Pseudofrin; Robidrine®; Sudafed® Decongestant

Synonyms *d*-Isoephedrine Hydrochloride; Pseudoephedrine Hydrochloride; Pseudoephedrine Sulfate

Therapeutic Category Adrenergic Agonist Agent; Decongestant; Sympathomimetic

Use Temporary symptomatic relief of nasal congestion due to common cold, upper respiratory allergies, and sinusitis; also promotes nasal or sinus drainage

Pregnancy Risk Factor C

Contraindications Hypersensitivity to pseudoephedrine or any component of the formulation; MAO inhibitor therapy

Warnings/Precautions Use with caution in patients >60 years of age; administer with caution to patients with hypertension, hyperthyroidism, diabetes mellitus, cardiovascular disease, ischemic heart disease, increased intraocular pressure, or prostatic hyperplasia. Elderly patients are more likely to experience adverse reactions to sympathomimetics. Overdosage may cause hallucinations, seizures, CNS depression, and death. Avoid prolonged use; generally limited to not more than 5 days.

Adverse Reactions Frequency not defined.

Cardiovascular: Tachycardia, palpitations, arrhythmias

Central nervous system: Nervousness, transient stimulation, insomnia, excitability, dizziness, drowsiness, convulsions, hallucinations, headache

Gastrointestinal: Nausea, vomiting

Genitourinary: Dysuria

Neuromuscular & skeletal: Weakness, tremor

Respiratory: Dyspnea

Miscellaneous: Diaphoresis

Overdosage/Toxicology Symptoms include seizures, nausea, vomiting, cardiac arrhythmias, hypertension, and agitation. There is no specific antidote. The bulk of treatment is supportive. Hyperactivity and agitation usually respond to reduced sensory input; however, with extreme agitation, haloperidol (2-5 mg I.M. for adults) may be required. Hyperthermia is best treated with external cooling measures; or when severe or unresponsive, muscle paralysis with pancuronium may be needed. Hypertension is usually transient and generally does not require treatment unless severe. For diastolic blood pressures >110 mm Hg, a nitroprusside infusion should be initiated. Seizures usually respond to diazepam I.V. and/or phenytoin maintenance regimens.

Drug Interactions

Increased Effect/Toxicity: MAO inhibitors may increase blood pressure effects of pseudoephedrine. Sympathomimetic agents may increase toxicity.

Decreased Effect: Decreased effect of methyldopa, reserpine.

Ethanol/Nutrition/Herb Interactions

Food: Onset of effect may be delayed if pseudoephedrine is taken with food.

Herb/Nutraceutical: Avoid ephedra, yohimbe (may cause hypertension).

Mechanism of Action Directly stimulates alpha-adrenergic receptors of respiratory mucosa causing vasoconstriction; directly stimulates beta-adrenergic receptors causing bronchial relaxation, increased heart rate and contractility

Pharmacodynamics/Kinetics

Onset of action: Decongestant: Oral: 15-30 minutes

Duration: Immediate release tablet: 4-6 hours; Extended release: ≤12 hours

Absorption: Rapid

Metabolism: Partially hepatic

Half-life elimination: 9-16 hours

Excretion: Urine (70% to 90% as unchanged drug, 1% to 6% as active norpseudoephedrine); dependent on urine pH and flow rate; alkaline urine decreases renal elimination of pseudoephedrine

Usual Dosage Oral:

Children:

<2 years: 4 mg/kg/day in divided doses every 6 hours

2-5 years: 15 mg every 6 hours; maximum: 60 mg/24 hours

6-12 years: 30 mg every 6 hours; maximum: 120 mg/24 hours

Adults: 30-60 mg every 4-6 hours, sustained release: 120 mg every 12 hours; maximum: 240 mg/24 hours

Dosing adjustment in renal impairment: Reduce dose

Dietary Considerations Should be taken with water or milk to decrease GI distress.

Test Interactions Interferes with urine detection of amphetamine (false-positive)

Patient Information Do not exceed recommended dosage and do not use for more than 3-5 days; may cause wakefulness or nervousness; take last dose 4-6 hours before bedtime; do not crush sustained release product; consult pharmacist or physician before using

Nursing Implications Do not crush extended release drug product; patients should be counseled about the proper use of over-the-counter cough and cold preparations

Dosage Forms

Gelcap, as hydrochloride: 30 mg

Liquid, as hydrochloride: 15 mg/5 mL (120 mL); 30 mg/5 mL (120 mL, 240 mL, 473 mL)

Solution, oral, as hydrochloride [drops]: 7.5 mg/0.8 mL (15 mL)

Syrup, as hydrochloride: 15 mg/5 mL (118 mL); 30 mg/mL (480 mL, 4000 mL)

Tablet, as hydrochloride: 30 mg, 60 mg

Tablet, chewable: 15 mg

Tablet, extended release, as sulfate: 120 mg, 240 mg

* **Pseudoephedrine, Acetaminophen, and Chlorpheniramine** *see* Acetaminophen, Chlorpheniramine, and Pseudoephedrine *on page 27*

♦ **Pseudoephedrine, Acetaminophen, and Dextromethorphan** *see Acetaminophen, Dextro-methorphan, and Pseudoephedrine on page 27*
♦ **Pseudoephedrine and Acetaminophen** *see Acetaminophen and Pseudoephedrine on page 25*
♦ **Pseudoephedrine and Acrivastine** *see Acrivastine and Pseudoephedrine on page 34*
♦ **Pseudoephedrine and Azatadine** *see Azatadine and Pseudoephedrine on page 136*
♦ **Pseudoephedrine and Brompheniramine** *see Brompheniramine and Pseudoephedrine on page 185*
♦ **Pseudoephedrine and Carbinoxamine** *see Carbinoxamine and Pseudoephedrine on page 225*
♦ **Pseudoephedrine and Chlorpheniramine** *see Chlorpheniramine and Pseudoephedrine on page 279*
♦ **Pseudoephedrine and Dexbrompheniramine** *see Dexbrompheniramine and Pseudoephed-rine on page 383*

Pseudoephedrine and Dextromethorphan
(soo doe e FED rin & deks troe meth OR fan)
U.S. Brand Names Children's Sudafed® Cough & Cold; Robitussin® Maximum Strength Cough & Cold; Robitussin® Pediatric Cough & Cold; Vicks® 44D Cough & Head Congestion
Canadian Brand Names Balminil DM D; Benylin® DM-D; Koffex DM-D; Novahistex® DM Decongestant; Novahistine® DM Decongestant; Robitussin® Childrens Cough & Cold
Synonyms Dextromethorphan and Pseudoephedrine
Therapeutic Category Antitussive/Decongestant
Use Temporary symptomatic relief of nasal congestion due to common cold, upper respiratory allergies, and sinusitis; also promotes nasal or sinus drainage; symptomatic relief of coughs caused by minor viral upper respiratory tract infections or inhaled irritants; most effective for a chronic nonproductive cough
Usual Dosage Oral:
Children: Dose should be based on pseudoephedrine component
Adults: 5-10 mL every 6 hours
Additional Information Complete prescribing information for this medication should be consulted for additional detail.
Dosage Forms
Liquid:
Children's Sudafed® Cold & Cough: Pseudoephedrine hydrochloride 15 mg and dextro-methorphan hydrobromide 5 mg per 5 mL
Robitussin® Maximum Strength Cough & Cold: Pseudoephedrine hydrochloride 30 mg and dextromethorphan hydrobromide 15 mg per 5 mL
Robitussin® Pediatric Cough & Cold: Pseudoephedrine hydrochloride 15 mg and dextro-methorphan hydrobromide 7.5 mg per 5 mL
Vicks® 44D Cough & Head Congestion: Pseudoephedrine hydrochloride 20 mg and dextro-methorphan hydrobromide 10 mg per 5 mL

♦ **Pseudoephedrine and Diphenhydramine** *see Diphenhydramine and Pseudoephedrine on page 415*
♦ **Pseudoephedrine and Fexofenadine** *see Fexofenadine and Pseudoephedrine on page 560*
♦ **Pseudoephedrine and Guaifenesin** *see Guaifenesin and Pseudoephedrine on page 647*
♦ **Pseudoephedrine and Hydrocodone** *see Hydrocodone and Pseudoephedrine on page 681*

Pseudoephedrine and Ibuprofen (soo doe e FED rin & eye byoo PROE fen)
U.S. Brand Names Advil® Cold & Sinus Caplets [OTC]; Dristan® Sinus Caplets; Motrin® Sinus [OTC]
Canadian Brand Names Advil® Cold & Sinus; Dristan® Sinus
Synonyms Ibuprofen and Pseudoephedrine
Therapeutic Category Decongestant/Analgesic
Use Temporary symptomatic relief of nasal congestion due to common cold, upper respiratory allergies, and sinusitis; also promotes nasal or sinus drainage; sinus headaches and pains
Pregnancy Risk Factor Ibuprofen: B/D (3rd trimester)
Usual Dosage Oral: Adults:
Based on pseudoephedrine: Decongestant: 60 mg every 4 hours; do not exceed 360 mg/day
Based on ibuprofen: Analgesic: 200-400 mg every 4-6 hours

Product labeling:
Children ≥12 years and Adults:
Advil® Cold & Sinus: One tablet every 4-6 hours as needed; may increase to 2 tablets every 4-6 hours if necessary
Motrin® Sinus/Headache: One caplet every 4-6 hours as needed
Additional Information Complete prescribing information for this medication should be consulted for additional detail.
Dosage Forms
Caplet: Pseudoephedrine hydrochloride 30 mg and ibuprofen 200 mg
Tablet: Pseudoephedrine hydrochloride 30 mg and ibuprofen 200 mg

♦ **Pseudoephedrine and Loratadine** *see Loratadine and Pseudoephedrine on page 820*
♦ **Pseudoephedrine and Triprolidine** *see Triprolidine and Pseudoephedrine on page 1380*
♦ **Pseudoephedrine, Carbinoxamine, and Dextromethorphan** *see Carbinoxamine, Pseudoe-phedrine, and Dextromethorphan on page 225*
♦ **Pseudoephedrine, Chlorpheniramine, and Acetaminophen** *see Acetaminophen, Chlor-pheniramine, and Pseudoephedrine on page 27*
♦ **Pseudoephedrine, Dextromethorphan, and Acetaminophen** *see Acetaminophen, Dextro-methorphan, and Pseudoephedrine on page 27*

- **Pseudoephedrine, Dextromethorphan, and Carbinoxamine** *see* Carbinoxamine, Pseudoephedrine, and Dextromethorphan *on page 225*
- **Pseudoephedrine, Dextromethorphan, and Guaifenesin** *see* Guaifenesin, Pseudoephedrine, and Dextromethorphan *on page 648*
- **Pseudoephedrine, Guaifenesin, and Codeine** *see* Guaifenesin, Pseudoephedrine, and Codeine *on page 648*
- **Pseudoephedrine Hydrochloride** *see* Pseudoephedrine *on page 1155*
- **Pseudoephedrine Sulfate** *see* Pseudoephedrine *on page 1155*
- **Pseudoephedrine, Triprolidine, and Codeine Pseudoephedrine, Codeine, and Triprolidine** *see* Triprolidine, Pseudoephedrine, and Codeine *on page 1381*
- **Pseudofrin (Can)** *see* Pseudoephedrine *on page 1155*
- **Pseudo-Gest Plus® [OTC]** *see* Chlorpheniramine and Pseudoephedrine *on page 279*
- **Pseudomonic Acid A** *see* Mupirocin *on page 941*
- **Psorcon™** *see* Diflorasone *on page 401*
- **Psorcon™ E** *see* Diflorasone *on page 401*

Psyllium (SIL i yum)

Related Information
Laxatives, Classification and Properties *on page 1504*

U.S. Brand Names Fiberall® Powder [OTC]; Fiberall® Wafer [OTC]; Hydrocil® [OTC]; Konsyl® [OTC]; Konsyl-D® [OTC]; Metamucil® [OTC]; Metamucil® Smooth Texture [OTC]; Modane® Bulk [OTC]; Perdiem® Plain [OTC]; Reguloid® [OTC]; Serutan® [OTC]; Syllact® [OTC]

Canadian Brand Names Metamucil®; Novo-Mucilax

Synonyms Plantago Seed; Plantain Seed; Psyllium Hydrophilic Mucilloid

Therapeutic Category Laxative, Bulk-Producing

Use Treatment of chronic atonic or spastic constipation and in constipation associated with rectal disorders; management of irritable bowel syndrome

Pregnancy Risk Factor B

Contraindications Hypersensitivity to psyllium or any component of the formulation; fecal impaction; GI obstruction

Warnings/Precautions May contain aspartame which is metabolized in the GI tract to phenylalanine which is contraindicated in individuals with phenylketonuria; use with caution in patients with esophageal strictures, ulcers, stenosis, or intestinal adhesions; elderly may have insufficient fluid intake which may predispose them to fecal impaction and bowel obstruction.

Adverse Reactions Frequency not defined.
Gastrointestinal: Esophageal or bowel obstruction, diarrhea, constipation, abdominal cramps
Respiratory: Bronchospasm
Miscellaneous: Anaphylaxis upon inhalation in susceptible individuals, rhinoconjunctivitis

Overdosage/Toxicology Symptoms include abdominal pain, diarrhea, and constipation.

Drug Interactions
Decreased Effect: Decreased effect of warfarin, digitalis, potassium-sparing diuretics, salicylates, tetracyclines, nitrofurantoin when taken together. Separate administration times to reduce potential for drug-drug interaction.

Mechanism of Action Adsorbs water in the intestine to form a viscous liquid which promotes peristalsis and reduces transit time

Pharmacodynamics/Kinetics
Onset of action: 12-24 hours; full effect may take 2-3 days
Peak effect: 2-3 days
Absorption: None; small amounts of grain extracts present in the preparation have been reportedly absorbed following colonic hydrolysis

Usual Dosage Oral (administer at least 3 hours before or after other drugs):
Children 6-11 years (approximately ½ adult dosage): ½ to 1 rounded teaspoonful in 4 oz glass of liquid 1-3 times/day
Adults: 1-2 rounded teaspoonfuls or 1-2 packets or 1-2 wafers in 8 oz glass of liquid 1-3 times/day

Dietary Considerations Should be taken with large amount of fluids. Some products contain aspartame, dextrose, or sucrose, as well as additional ingredients. Check individual product information for caloric and nutritional value.

Administration Inhalation of psyllium dust may cause sensitivity to psyllium (eg, runny nose, watery eyes, wheezing). Must be mixed in a glass of water or juice. Drink a full glass of liquid with each dose. Separate dose from other drug therapies.

Patient Information Must be mixed in a glass of water or juice; drink a full glass of liquid with each dose; do not use for longer than 1 week without the advice of a physician

Nursing Implications Inhalation of psyllium dust may cause sensitivity to psyllium (runny nose, watery eyes, wheezing)

Additional Information 3.4 g psyllium hydrophilic mucilloid per 7 g powder is equivalent to a rounded teaspoonful or one packet.

Dosage Forms
Granules: 4.03 g per rounded teaspoon (100 g, 250 g); 2.5 g per rounded teaspoon
Powder, psyllium hydrophilic: 3.4 g per rounded teaspoon (210 g, 300 g, 420 g, 630 g)
Wafers: 3.4 g

- **Psyllium Hydrophilic Mucilloid** *see* Psyllium *on page 1158*
- **Pteroylglutamic Acid** *see* Folic Acid *on page 595*
- **PTU** *see* Propylthiouracil *on page 1151*
- **Pulmicort® (Can)** *see* Budesonide *on page 186*
- **Pulmicort Respules®** *see* Budesonide *on page 186*
- **Pulmicort Turbuhaler®** *see* Budesonide *on page 186*
- **Pulmozyme®** *see* Dornase Alfa *on page 437*
- **Puregon™ (Can)** *see* Follitropins *on page 596*

◆ **Purinethol®** *see* Mercaptopurine *on page 863*
◆ **PVF® K (Can)** *see* Penicillin V Potassium *on page 1055*
◆ **PₓEₓ®** *see* Pilocarpine and Epinephrine *on page 1084*
◆ **Pylorid® (Can)** *see* Ranitidine Bismuth Citrate *on page 1180*

Pyrantel Pamoate (pi RAN tel PAM oh ate)

U.S. Brand Names Antiminth® [OTC]; Pin-Rid® [OTC]; Pin-X® [OTC]; Reese's® Pinworm Medicine [OTC]

Canadian Brand Names Combantrin™

Therapeutic Category Anthelmintic

Use Treatment of pinworms (*Enterobius vermicularis*), whipworms (*Trichuris trichiura*), roundworms (*Ascaris lumbricoides*), and hookworms (*Ancylostoma duodenale*)

Pregnancy Risk Factor C

Contraindications Hypersensitivity to pyrantel pamoate or any component of the formulation

Warnings/Precautions Use with caution in patients with liver impairment, anemia, malnutrition, or pregnancy. Since pinworm infections are easily spread to others, treat all family members in close contact with the patient.

Adverse Reactions Frequency not defined.
Central nervous system: Dizziness, drowsiness, insomnia, headache
Dermatologic: Rash
Gastrointestinal: Anorexia, nausea, vomiting, abdominal cramps, diarrhea, tenesmus
Hepatic: Elevated liver enzymes
Neuromuscular & skeletal: Weakness

Overdosage/Toxicology Symptoms include anorexia, nausea, vomiting, cramps, diarrhea, and ataxia. Treatment is supportive following GI decontamination.

Drug Interactions
Decreased Effect: Decreased effect with piperazine

Stability Protect from light

Mechanism of Action Causes the release of acetylcholine and inhibits cholinesterase; acts as a depolarizing neuromuscular blocker, paralyzing the helminths

Pharmacodynamics/Kinetics
Absorption: Oral: Poor
Metabolism: Partially hepatic
Time to peak, serum: 1-3 hours
Excretion: Feces (50% as unchanged drug); urine (7% as unchanged drug)

Usual Dosage Children and Adults (purgation is not required prior to use): Oral:
Roundworm, pinworm, or trichostrongyliasis: 11 mg/kg administered as a single dose; maximum dose: 1 g. (**Note:** For pinworm infection, dosage should be repeated in 2 weeks and all family members should be treated.)
Hookworm: 11 mg/kg administered once daily for 3 days

Administration May be mixed with milk or fruit juice

Monitoring Parameters Stool for presence of eggs, worms, and occult blood, serum AST and ALT

Patient Information May mix drug with milk or fruit juice; strict hygiene is essential to prevent reinfection

Nursing Implications Shake well before pouring to assure accurate dosage; protect from light

Dosage Forms
Capsule: 180 mg
Liquid: 50 mg/mL (30 mL)
Suspension, oral: 50 mg/mL (60 mL) [caramel-currant flavor]

Pyrazinamide (peer a ZIN a mide)

Related Information
Antimicrobial Drugs of Choice *on page 1588*
Tuberculosis Treatment Guidelines *on page 1612*

Canadian Brand Names Tebrazid™

Synonyms Pyrazinoic Acid Amide

Therapeutic Category Antitubercular Agent

Use Adjunctive treatment of tuberculosis in combination with other antituberculosis agents in combination with rifampin or rifabutin for prevention of tuberculosis (as an alternative to isoniazid monotherapy)

Pregnancy Risk Factor C

Contraindications Hypersensitivity to pyrazinamide or any component of the formulation; acute gout; severe hepatic damage

Warnings/Precautions Use with caution in patients with renal failure, chronic gout, diabetes mellitus, or porphyria

Adverse Reactions
1% to 10%:
Central nervous system: Malaise
Gastrointestinal: Nausea, vomiting, anorexia
Neuromuscular & skeletal: Arthralgia, myalgia
<1% (Limited to important or life-threatening): Hepatotoxicity, interstitial nephritis, porphyria, thrombocytopenia

Overdosage/Toxicology Symptoms include gout, gastric upset, and hepatic damage (mild). Treatment following GI decontamination is supportive.

Drug Interactions
Increased Effect/Toxicity: Combination therapy with rifampin and pyrazinamide has been associated with severe and fatal hepatotoxic reactions.

Mechanism of Action Converted to pyrazinoic acid in susceptible strains of *Mycobacterium* which lowers the pH of the environment; exact mechanism of action has not been elucidated
(Continued)

Pyrazinamide *(Continued)*

Pharmacodynamics/Kinetics Bacteriostatic or bactericidal depending on drug's concentration at infection site

Absorption: Well absorbed

Distribution: Widely into body tissues and fluids including liver, lung, and CSF

    Relative diffusion from blood into CSF: Adequate with or without inflammation (exceeds usual MICs)

    CSF:blood level ratio: Inflamed meninges: 100%

Protein binding: 50%

Metabolism: Hepatic

Half-life elimination: 9-10 hours

Time to peak, serum: Within 2 hours

Excretion: Urine (4% as unchanged drug)

Usual Dosage Oral (calculate dose on ideal body weight rather than total body weight): **Note:** A four-drug regimen (isoniazid, rifampin, pyrazinamide, and either streptomycin or ethambutol) is preferred for the initial, empiric treatment of TB. When the drug susceptibility results are available, the regimen should be altered as appropriate.

Children and Adults:

    Daily therapy: 15-30 mg/kg/day (maximum: 2 g/day)

    Directly observed therapy (DOT):

        Twice weekly: 50-70 mg/kg (maximum: 4 g)

        Three times/week: 50-70 mg/kg (maximum: 3 g)

    Prevention of tuberculosis (in combination with rifampin or rifabutin): 15-30 mg/kg/day for 2 months

Elderly: Start with a lower daily dose (15 mg/kg) and increase as tolerated

Dosing adjustment in renal impairment: Cl_{cr} <50 mL/minute: Avoid use or reduce dose to 12-20 mg/kg/day

Dosing adjustment in hepatic impairment: Reduce dose

Monitoring Parameters Periodic liver function tests, serum uric acid, sputum culture, chest x-ray 2-3 months into treatment and at completion

Test Interactions Reacts with Acetest® and Ketostix® to produce pinkish-brown color

Patient Information Notify physician if fever, loss of appetite, malaise, nausea, vomiting, darkened urine, pale stools occur; do not stop taking without consulting a physician

Nursing Implications Monitor periodic liver function tests, serum uric acid

Dosage Forms Tablet: 500 mg

Extemporaneous Preparations Pyrazinamide suspension can be compounded with simple syrup or 0.5% methylcellulose with simple syrup at a concentration of 100 mg/mL; the suspension is stable for 2 months at 4°C or 25°C when stored in glass or plastic bottles

To prepare pyrazinamide suspension in 0.5% methylcellulose with simple syrup: Crush 200 pyrazinamide 500 mg tablets and mix with a suspension containing 500 mL of 1% methylcellulose and 500 mL simple syrup. Add to this a suspension containing 140 crushed pyrazinamide tablets in 350 mL of 1% methylcellulose and 350 mL of simple syrup to make 1.7 L of suspension containing pyrazinamide 100 mg/mL in 0.5% methylcellulose with simple syrup.

Nahata MC, Morosco RS, and Peritre SP, "Stability of Pyrazinamide in Two Suspensions," *Am J Health Syst Pharm,* 1995, 52:1558-60.

♦ **Pyrazinoic Acid Amide** *see* Pyrazinamide *on page 1159*

Pyrethrins and Piperonyl Butoxide *(pye RE thrins)*

U.S. Brand Names A-200™ [OTC]; End Lice® [OTC]; Pronto® [OTC]; Pyrinex® Pediculicide [OTC]; Pyrinyl® [OTC]; Pyrinyl Plus® [OTC]; R & C® [OTC]; RID® [OTC]; Tisit® [OTC]; Tisit® Blue Gel [OTC]

Canadian Brand Names R & C™ II; R & C™ Shampoo/Conditioner; RID® Mousse

Therapeutic Category Antiparasitic Agent, Topical; Pediculocide; Shampoo, Pediculocide

Use Treatment of *Pediculus humanus* infestations (head lice, body lice, pubic lice and their eggs)

Pregnancy Risk Factor C

Contraindications Hypersensitivity to pyrethrins, ragweed, or chrysanthemums

Warnings/Precautions For external use only; do not use in eyelashes or eyebrows

Adverse Reactions Frequency not defined.

Dermatologic: Pruritus

Local: Burning, stinging, irritation with repeat use

Mechanism of Action Pyrethrins are derived from flowers that belong to the chrysanthemum family. The mechanism of action on the neuronal membranes of lice is similar to that of DDT. Piperonyl butoxide is usually added to pyrethrin to enhance the product's activity by decreasing the metabolism of pyrethrins in arthropods.

Pharmacodynamics/Kinetics

Onset of action: ~30 minutes

Absorption: Minimal

Metabolism: By ester hydrolysis and hydroxylation

Usual Dosage Application of pyrethrins: Topical:

Apply enough solution to completely wet infested area, including hair

Allow to remain on area for 10 minutes

Wash and rinse with large amounts of warm water

Use fine-toothed comb to remove lice and eggs from hair

Shampoo hair to restore body and luster

Treatment may be repeated if necessary once in a 24-hour period

Repeat treatment in 7-10 days to kill newly hatched lice

Administration For external use only; avoid touching eyes, mouth, or other mucous membranes.

Patient Information For external use only; avoid touching eyes, mouth, or other mucous membranes; do not use in eyelashes or eyebrows; contact physician if irritation occurs or if condition does not improve in 2-3 days

Dosage Forms All in combination with piperonyl butoxide

Gel, topical: 0.3% (30 g)

Liquid, topical: 0.2% (60 mL, 120 mL); 0.3% (60 mL, 118 mL, 120 mL, 177 mL, 237 mL, 240 mL)

Shampoo, topical: 0.3% (59 mL, 60 mL, 118 mL, 120 mL, 240 mL); 0.33% (120 mL)

♦ **Pyridiate®** *see* Phenazopyridine *on page 1068*

♦ **2-Pyridine Aldoxime Methochloride** *see* Pralidoxime *on page 1115*

♦ **Pyridium®** *see* Phenazopyridine *on page 1068*

Pyridostigmine (peer id oh STIG meen)

U.S. Brand Names Mestinon®; Mestinon® Timespan®; Regonol®
Canadian Brand Names Mestinon®; Mestinon®-SR
Synonyms Pyridostigmine Bromide
Therapeutic Category Antidote, Neuromuscular Blocking Agent; Cholinergic Agent
Use Symptomatic treatment of myasthenia gravis; also used as an antidote for nondepolarizing neuromuscular blockers
Pregnancy Risk Factor C
Pregnancy/Breast-Feeding Implications Safety has not been established for use during pregnancy. The potential benefit to the mother should outweigh the potential risk to the fetus. When pyridostigmine is needed in myasthenic mothers, giving dose parenterally 1 hour before completion of the second stage of labor may facilitate delivery and protect the neonate during the immediate postnatal state.
Contraindications Hypersensitivity to pyridostigmine, bromides, or any component of the formulation; GI or GU obstruction
Warnings/Precautions Use with caution in patients with epilepsy, asthma, bradycardia, hyperthyroidism, cardiac arrhythmias, or peptic ulcer; adequate facilities should be available for cardiopulmonary resuscitation when testing and adjusting dose for myasthenia gravis; have atropine and epinephrine ready to treat hypersensitivity reactions; overdosage may result in cholinergic crisis, this must be distinguished from myasthenic crisis; anticholinesterase insensitivity can develop for brief or prolonged periods. Safety and efficacy in pediatric patients have not been established. Regonol® injection contains 1% benzyl alcohol as the preservative (not intended for use in newborns).
Adverse Reactions Frequency not defined.

Cardiovascular: Arrhythmias (especially bradycardia), hypotension, decreased carbon monoxide, tachycardia, AV block, nodal rhythm, nonspecific EKG changes, cardiac arrest, syncope, flushing

Central nervous system: Convulsions, dysarthria, dysphonia, dizziness, loss of consciousness, drowsiness, headache

Dermatologic: Skin rash, thrombophlebitis (I.V.), urticaria

Gastrointestinal: Hyperperistalsis, nausea, vomiting, salivation, diarrhea, stomach cramps, dysphagia, flatulence

Genitourinary: Urinary urgency

Neuromuscular & skeletal: Weakness, fasciculations, muscle cramps, spasms, arthralgias

Ocular: Small pupils, lacrimation

Respiratory: Increased bronchial secretions, laryngospasm, bronchiolar constriction, respiratory muscle paralysis, dyspnea, respiratory depression, respiratory arrest, bronchospasm

Miscellaneous: Diaphoresis (increased), anaphylaxis, allergic reactions

Overdosage/Toxicology Symptoms include muscle weakness, blurred vision, excessive sweating, tearing and salivation, nausea, vomiting, diarrhea, hypertension, bradycardia, and paralysis. Atropine is the treatment of choice for intoxications manifesting with significant muscarinic symptoms. Atropine I.V. 2-4 mg every 3-60 minutes (or 0.04-0.08 mg I.V. every 5-60 minutes if needed for children) should be repeated to control symptoms and then continued as needed for 1-2 days following the acute ingestion.

Drug Interactions

Increased Effect/Toxicity: Increased effect of depolarizing neuromuscular blockers (succinylcholine). Increased toxicity with edrophonium. Increased bradycardia/hypotension with beta-blockers.

Decreased Effect: Neuromuscular blockade reversal effect of pyridostigmine may be decreased by aminoglycosides, quinolones, tetracyclines, bacitracin, colistin, polymyxin B, sodium colistimethate, quinidine, elevated serum magnesium concentrations.

Stability Pyridostigmine 25 mg in 100 mL D_5W was stable for 12 hours as judged by visual compatibility.
Mechanism of Action Inhibits destruction of acetylcholine by acetylcholinesterase which facilitates transmission of impulses across myoneural junction
Pharmacodynamics/Kinetics

Onset of action: Oral, I.M.: 15-30 minutes; I.V. injection: 2-5 minutes

Duration: Oral: Up to 6-8 hours (due to slow absorption); I.V.: 2-3 hours

Absorption: Oral: Very poor (10% to 20%)

Metabolism: Hepatic

Half-life elimination: 1-2 hours; Renal failure: ≤6 hours

Excretion: Urine (80% to 90% as unchanged drug)

Usual Dosage

Myasthenia gravis:

Oral:

Children: 7 mg/kg/24 hours divided into 5-6 doses

Adults: Highly individualized dosing ranges: 60-1500 mg/day, usually 600 mg/day divided into 5-6 doses, spaced to provide maximum relief

Sustained release formulation: Highly individualized dosing ranges: 180-540 mg once or twice daily (doses separated by at least 6 hours); **Note:** Most clinicians reserve sustained release dosage form for bedtime dose only.

(Continued)

Pyridostigmine *(Continued)*

I.M., slow I.V. push:

Children: 0.05-0.15 mg/kg/dose

Adults: To supplement oral dosage pre- and postoperatively during labor and post-partum, during myasthenic crisis, or when oral therapy is impractical: ~1/30th of oral dose; observe patient closely for cholinergic reactions

or

I.V. infusion: Initial: 2 mg/hour with gradual titration in increments of 0.5-1 mg/hour, up to a maximum rate of 4 mg/hour

Reversal of nondepolarizing muscle relaxants: **Note:** Atropine sulfate (0.6-1.2 mg) I.V. immediately prior to pyridostigmine to minimize side effects: I.V.:

Children: Dosing range: 0.1-0.25 mg/kg/dose*

Adults: 0.1-0.25 mg/kg/dose; 10-20 mg is usually sufficient*

*Full recovery usually occurs ≤15 minutes, but ≥30 minutes may be required

Dosage adjustment in renal dysfunction: Lower dosages may be required due to prolonged elimination; no specific recommendations have been published

Administration Do **not** crush sustained release drug product.

Test Interactions ↑ aminotransferase [ALT (SGPT)/AST (SGOT)] (S), ↑ amylase (S)

Patient Information Side effects are generally due to exaggerated pharmacologic effects; most common side effects are salivation and muscle fasciculations; notify physician if nausea, vomiting, muscle weakness, severe abdominal pain, or difficulty breathing occurs

Nursing Implications Do not crush sustained release drug product; observe for cholinergic reactions, particularly when administered I.V.

Dosage Forms

Injection, as bromide:

Mestinon®: 5 mg/mL (2 mL)

Regonol®: 5 mg/mL (2 mL, 5 mL) [contains benzyl alcohol 1%]

Syrup, as bromide (Mestinon®): 60 mg/5 mL (480 mL) [raspberry flavor; contains alcohol 5%]

Tablet, as bromide (Mestinon®): 60 mg

Tablet, sustained release, as bromide (Mestinon® Timespan®): 180 mg

♦ **Pyridostigmine Bromide** *see Pyridostigmine on page 1161*

Pyridoxine *(peer i DOKS een)*

Related Information

Anticonvulsants by Seizure Type *on page 1481*

Epilepsy & Seizure Treatment *on page 1659*

USPHA/IDSA Guidelines for the Prevention of Opportunistic Infections in Persons With HIV *on page 1574*

U.S. Brand Names Aminoxin® [OTC]; Nestrex® [OTC]

Synonyms Pyridoxine Hydrochloride; Vitamin B_6

Therapeutic Category Antidote, Cycloserine Toxicity; Antidote, Hydralazine Toxicity; Antidote, Isoniazid Toxicity; Vitamin, Water Soluble

Use Prevention and treatment of vitamin B_6 deficiency, pyridoxine-dependent seizures in infants; adjunct to treatment of acute toxicity from isoniazid, cycloserine, or hydralazine overdose

Pregnancy Risk Factor A/C (dose exceeding RDA recommendation)

Pregnancy/Breast-Feeding Implications

Clinical effects on the fetus: Crosses the placenta; available evidence suggests safe use during pregnancy and breast-feeding

Breast-feeding/lactation: Crosses into breast milk; possible inhibition of lactation at doses >600 mg/day. AAP considers **compatible** with breast-feeding.

Contraindications Hypersensitivity to pyridoxine or any component of the formulation

Warnings/Precautions Dependence and withdrawal may occur with doses >200 mg/day

Adverse Reactions Frequency not defined.

Central nervous system: Headache, seizures (following very large I.V. doses), sensory neuropathy

Endocrine & metabolic: Decreased serum folic acid secretions

Gastrointestinal: Nausea

Hepatic: Increased AST

Neuromuscular & skeletal: Paresthesia

Miscellaneous: Allergic reactions

Overdosage/Toxicology Symptoms include ataxia and sensory neuropathy with doses of 50 mg to 2 g daily over prolonged periods. Acute doses of 70-357 mg/kg have been well tolerated.

Drug Interactions

Decreased Effect: Pyridoxine may decrease serum levels of levodopa, phenobarbital, and phenytoin (patients taking levodopa without carbidopa should avoid supplemental vitamin B_6 >5 mg per day, which includes multivitamin preparations).

Stability Protect from light

Mechanism of Action Precursor to pyridoxal, which functions in the metabolism of proteins, carbohydrates, and fats; pyridoxal also aids in the release of liver and muscle-stored glycogen and in the synthesis of GABA (within the central nervous system) and heme

Pharmacodynamics/Kinetics

Absorption: Enteral, parenteral: Well absorbed

Metabolism: Metabolized in 4-pyridoxic acid (active form) and other metabolites

Half-life elimination: 15-20 days

Usual Dosage

Recommended daily allowance (RDA):

Children:

1-3 years: 0.9 mg

4-6 years: 1.3 mg

7-10 years: 1.6 mg
Adults:
  Male: 1.7-2.0 mg
  Female: 1.4-1.6 mg
Pyridoxine-dependent Infants:
  Oral: 2-100 mg/day
  I.M., I.V., S.C.: 10-100 mg
Dietary deficiency: Oral:
  Children: 5-25 mg/24 hours for 3 weeks, then 1.5-2.5 mg/day in multiple vitamin product
  Adults: 10-20 mg/day for 3 weeks
Drug-induced neuritis (eg, isoniazid, hydralazine, penicillamine, cycloserine): Oral:
  Children:
    Treatment: 10-50 mg/24 hours
    Prophylaxis: 1-2 mg/kg/24 hours
  Adults:
    Treatment: 100-200 mg/24 hours
    Prophylaxis: 25-100 mg/24 hours
Treatment of seizures and/or coma from acute isoniazid toxicity, a dose of pyridoxine hydro-
chloride equal to the amount of INH ingested can be given I.M./I.V. in divided doses
together with other anticonvulsants; if the amount INH ingested is not known, administer 5
g I.V. pyridoxine
Treatment of acute hydralazine toxicity, a pyridoxine dose of 25 mg/kg in divided doses I.M./
I.V. has been used

Reference Range Over 50 ng/mL (SI: 243 nmol/L) (varies considerably with method). A broad
range is ~25-80 ng/mL (SI: 122-389 nmol/L). HPLC method for pyridoxal phosphate has
normal range of 3.5-18 ng/mL (SI: 17-88 ng/mL).

Test Interactions Urobilinogen

Patient Information Dietary sources of pyridoxine include red meats, bananas, potatoes,
yeast, lima beans, whole grain cereals; do not exceed recommended doses

Nursing Implications Burning may occur at the injection site after I.M. or S.C. administration;
seizures have occurred following I.V. administration of very large doses

Dosage Forms
  Injection, as hydrochloride: 100 mg/mL (10 mL, 30 mL)
  Tablet, as hydrochloride: 25 mg, 50 mg, 100 mg, 250 mg, 500 mg
  Tablet, enteric coated, as hydrochloride: 20 mg

Extemporaneous Preparations A 1 mg/mL oral solution was stable for 30 days when
refrigerated when compounded as follows:
  Withdraw 100 mg (1 mL of a 100 mg/mL injection) from a vial with a needle and syringe, add
  to 99 mL of simple syrup in an amber bottle
  Keep in refrigerator

  Nahata MC and Hipple TF, *Pediatric Drug Formulations*, 3rd ed, Cincinnati, OH: Harvey
  Whitney Books Co, 1997.

• **Pyridoxine, Folic Acid, and Cyanocobalamin** *see* Folic Acid, Cyanocobalamin, and Pyridoxine *on page 596*

• **Pyridoxine Hydrochloride** *see* Pyridoxine *on page 1162*

Pyrimethamine (peer i METH a meen)
Related Information
Malaria Treatment *on page 1607*
Prevention of Malaria *on page 1552*
USPHA/IDSA Guidelines for the Prevention of Opportunistic Infections in Persons With HIV
on page 1574

U.S. Brand Names Daraprim®

Canadian Brand Names Daraprim®

Therapeutic Category Antimalarial Agent

Use Prophylaxis of malaria due to susceptible strains of plasmodia; used in conjunction with
quinine and sulfadiazine for the treatment of uncomplicated attacks of chloroquine-resistant
P. falciparum malaria; used in conjunction with fast-acting schizonticide to initiate transmission control and suppression cure; synergistic combination with sulfonamide in treatment of
toxoplasmosis

Pregnancy Risk Factor C

Contraindications Hypersensitivity to pyrimethamine or any component of the formulation;
chloroguanide; resistant malaria; megaloblastic anemia secondary to folate deficiency

Warnings/Precautions When used for more than 3-4 days, it may be advisable to administer
leucovorin to prevent hematologic complications; monitor CBC and platelet counts every 2
weeks; use with caution in patients with impaired renal or hepatic function or with possible
G6PD

Adverse Reactions Frequency not defined.
  Cardiovascular: Arrhythmias (large doses)
  Central nervous system: Depression, fever, insomnia, lightheadedness, malaise, seizures
  Dermatologic: Abnormal skin pigmentation, dermatitis, erythema multiforme, rash, Stevens-
    Johnson syndrome
  Gastrointestinal: Anorexia, abdominal cramps, vomiting, diarrhea, xerostomia, atrophic glos-
    sitis
  Hematologic: Megaloblastic anemia, leukopenia, pancytopenia, thrombocytopenia,
    pulmonary eosinophilia
  Miscellaneous: Anaphylaxis

Overdosage/Toxicology Symptoms include megaloblastic anemia, leukopenia, thrombocytopenia, anorexia, CNS stimulation, seizures, nausea, vomiting, and hematemesis. Following
GI decontamination, leucovorin should be administered in a dosage of 5-15 mg/day I.M., I.V.,
or oral for 5-7 days, or as required to reverse symptoms of folic acid deficiency. Diazepam
0.1-0.25 mg/kg can be used to treat seizures.
(Continued)

Pyrimethamine *(Continued)*

Drug Interactions

Increased Effect/Toxicity: Increased effect with sulfonamides (synergy), methotrexate, and TMP/SMZ.

Decreased Effect: Pyrimethamine effectiveness is decreased by acid.

Mechanism of Action Inhibits parasitic dihydrofolate reductase, resulting in inhibition of vital tetrahydrofolic acid synthesis

Pharmacodynamics/Kinetics

Onset of action: ~1 hour

Absorption: Well absorbed

Distribution: Widely, mainly in blood cells, kidneys, lungs, liver, and spleen; crosses into CSF; crosses placenta; enters breast milk

Metabolism: Hepatic

Half-life elimination: 80-95 hours

Time to peak, serum: 1.5-8 hours

Excretion: Urine (20% to 30% as unchanged drug)

Usual Dosage

Malaria chemoprophylaxis (for areas where chloroquine-resistant *P. falciparum* exists): Begin prophylaxis 2 weeks before entering endemic area:

Children: 0.5 mg/kg once weekly; not to exceed 25 mg/dose

or

Children:

<4 years: 6.25 mg once weekly

4-10 years: 12.5 mg once weekly

Children >10 years and Adults: 25 mg once weekly

Dosage should be continued for all age groups for at least 6-10 weeks after leaving endemic areas

Chloroquine-resistant *P. falciparum* malaria (when used in conjunction with quinine and sulfadiazine):

Children:

<10 kg: 6.25 mg/day once daily for 3 days

10-20 kg: 12.5 mg/day once daily for 3 days

20-40 kg: 25 mg/day once daily for 3 days

Adults: 25 mg twice daily for 3 days

Toxoplasmosis:

Infants for congenital toxoplasmosis: Oral: 1 mg/kg once daily for 6 months with sulfadiazine then every other month with sulfa, alternating with spiramycin.

Children: Loading dose: 2 mg/kg/day divided into 2 equal daily doses for 1-3 days (maximum: 100 mg/day) followed by 1 mg/kg/day divided into 2 doses for 4 weeks; maximum: 25 mg/day

With sulfadiazine or trisulfapyrimidines: 2 mg/kg/day divided every 12 hours for 3 days followed by 1 mg/kg/day once daily or divided twice daily for 4 weeks given with trisulfapyrimidines or sulfadiazine

Adults: 50-75 mg/day together with 1-4 g of a sulfonamide for 1-3 weeks depending on patient's tolerance and response, then reduce dose by 50% and continue for 4-5 weeks **or** 25-50 mg/day for 3-4 weeks

Prophylaxis for first episode of *Toxoplasma gondii*:

Children ≥1 month of age: 1 mg/kg/day once daily with dapsone, plus oral folinic acid 5 mg every 3 days

Adolescents and Adults: 50 mg once weekly with dapsone, plus oral folinic acid 25 mg once weekly

Prophylaxis to prevent recurrence of *Toxoplasma gondii*:

Children ≥1 month of age: 1 mg/kg/day once daily given with sulfadiazine or clindamycin, plus oral folinic acid 5 mg every 3 days

Adolescents and Adults: 25-50 mg once daily in combination with sulfadiazine or clindamycin, plus oral folinic acid 10-25 mg daily **or** with atovaquone, plus oral folinic acid 10 mg daily

Monitoring Parameters CBC, including platelet counts

Patient Information Take with meals to minimize vomiting; begin malaria prophylaxis at least 1-2 weeks prior to departure; discontinue at first sign of skin rash; notify physician if persistent fever, sore throat, bleeding or bruising occurs; regular blood work may be necessary in patients taking high doses

Nursing Implications Leucovorin may be administered in a dosage of 3-9 mg/day for 3 days or 5 mg every 3 days or as required to reverse symptoms or to prevent hematologic problems due to folic acid deficiency

Dosage Forms Tablet: 25 mg

Extemporaneous Preparations Pyrimethamine tablets may be crushed to prepare oral suspensions of the drug in water, cherry syrup or sucrose-containing solutions at a concentration of 1 mg/mL; stable at room temperature for 5-7 days

AHFS Drug Information, McEvoy G, ed, Bethesda, MD: American Society of Heath-System Pharmacists, 1996.

* **Pyrimethamine and Sulfadoxine** *see* Sulfadoxine and Pyrimethamine *on page 1271*
* **Pyrinex® Pediculicide [OTC]** *see* Pyrethrins and Piperonyl Butoxide *on page 1160*
* **Pyrinyl® [OTC]** *see* Pyrethrins and Piperonyl Butoxide *on page 1160*
* **Pyrinyl Plus® [OTC]** *see* Pyrethrins and Piperonyl Butoxide *on page 1160*
* **Quaternium-18 Bentonite** *see* Bentoquatam *on page 154*

Quazepam *(KWAY ze pam)*

Related Information

Antacid Drug Interactions *on page 1477*

Benzodiazepines Comparison *on page 1490*

U.S. Brand Names Doral®

Canadian Brand Names Doral®
Therapeutic Category Benzodiazepine; Hypnotic; Sedative
Use Treatment of insomnia
Restrictions C-IV
Pregnancy Risk Factor X
Usual Dosage Adults: Oral: Initial: 15 mg at bedtime, in some patients the dose may be reduced to 7.5 mg after a few nights
Dosing adjustment in hepatic impairment: Dose reduction may be necessary
Additional Information Complete prescribing information for this medication should be consulted for additional detail.
Dosage Forms Tablet: 7.5 mg, 15 mg

Quetiapine (kwe TYE a peen)

Related Information
Antipsychotic Agents Comparison on page 1486
U.S. Brand Names Seroquel®
Canadian Brand Names Seroquel®
Synonyms Quetiapine Fumarate
Therapeutic Category Antipsychotic Agent, Atypical
Use Treatment of schizophrenia
Unlabeled/Investigational Use Treatment of mania, bipolar disorder (children and adults); autism, psychosis (children)
Pregnancy Risk Factor C
Contraindications Hypersensitivity to quetiapine or any component of the formulation; severe CNS depression; bone marrow suppression; blood dyscrasias; severe hepatic disease, coma
Warnings/Precautions May induce orthostatic hypotension associated with dizziness, tachycardia, and, in some cases, syncope, especially during the initial dose titration period. Should be used with particular caution in patients with known cardiovascular disease (history of MI or ischemic heart disease, heart failure, or conduction abnormalities), cerebrovascular disease, or conditions that predispose to hypotension. Development of cataracts has been observed in animal studies, therefore, lens examinations should be made upon initiation of therapy and every 6 months thereafter.

Neuroleptic malignant syndrome (NMS) is a potentially fatal symptom complex that has been reported in association with administration of antipsychotic drugs. Clinical manifestations of NMS are hyperpyrexia, muscle rigidity, altered mental status, and evidence of autonomic instability (irregular pulse or blood pressure, tachycardia, diaphoresis, and cardiac dysrhythmia). Management of NMS should include immediate discontinuation of antipsychotic drugs and other drugs not essential to concurrent therapy, intensive symptomatic treatment and medication monitoring, and treatment of any concomitant medical problems for which specific treatment are available.

Tardive dyskinesia; caution in patients with a history of seizures, decreases in total free thyroxine, pre-existing hyperprolactinemia, elevations of liver enzymes, cholesterol levels and/or triglyceride increases.

Adverse Reactions
>10%:
  Central nervous system: Headache, somnolence
  Gastrointestinal: Weight gain
1% to 10%:
  Cardiovascular: Postural hypotension, tachycardia, palpitations
  Central nervous system: Dizziness
  Dermatologic: Rash
  Gastrointestinal: Abdominal pain, constipation, xerostomia, dyspepsia, anorexia
  Hematologic: Leukopenia
  Neuromuscular & skeletal: Dysarthria, back pain, weakness
  Respiratory: Rhinitis, pharyngitis, cough, dyspnea
  Miscellaneous: Diaphoresis
<1% (Limited to important or life-threatening): Diabetes mellitus, hyperglycemia, hyperlipidemia, hypothyroidism, increased appetite, increased salivation, involuntary movements, leukocytosis, QT prolongation, rash, tardive dyskinesia, vertigo

Drug Interactions
  Cytochrome P450 Effect: CYP3A3/4 enzyme substrate; CYP2D6 enzyme substrate (minor); CYP2C9 enzyme substrate (minor)
  Increased Effect/Toxicity: Quetiapine reduces the metabolism of lorazepam (by 20%). The effects of other centrally-acting drugs, sedatives, or ethanol may be potentiated by quetiapine. Quetiapine may enhance the effects of antihypertensive agents. Although data is not yet available, caution is advised with inhibitors of CYP3A4 (eg, ketoconazole, erythromycin), which may increase levels of quetiapine. Cimetidine increases blood levels of quetiapine (quetiapine's clearance is reduced by 20%).
  Decreased Effect: The metabolism of quetiapine may be increased when administered with enzyme-inducing drugs (phenytoin, rifampin, barbiturates, carbamazepine). Thioridazine increases quetiapine's clearance (by 65%).

Ethanol/Nutrition/Herb Interactions
  Ethanol: Avoid ethanol (may cause excessive impairment in cognition/motor function).
  Food: In healthy volunteers, administration of quetiapine with food resulted in an increase in the peak serum concentration and AUC (each by ~15%) compared to the fasting state.
(Continued)

Quetiapine (Continued)

Herb/Nutraceutical: St John's wort may decrease quetiapine levels. Avoid valerian, St John's wort, kava kava, gotu kola (may increase CNS depression).

Mechanism of Action Mechanism of action of quetiapine, as with other antipsychotic drugs, is unknown. However, it has been proposed that this drug's antipsychotic activity is mediated through a combination of dopamine type 2 (D_2) and serotonin type 2 (5-HT_2) antagonism. However, it is an antagonist at multiple neurotransmitter receptors in the brain: serotonin 5-HT_{1A} and 5-HT_2, dopamine D_1 and D_2, histamine H_1, and adrenergic alpha$_1$- and alpha$_2$-receptors; but appears to have no appreciable affinity at cholinergic muscarinic and benzodiazepine receptors.

Antagonism at receptors other than dopamine and 5-HT_2 with similar receptor affinities may explain some of the other effects of quetiapine. The drug's antagonism of histamine H_1-receptors may explain the somnolence observed with it. The drug's antagonism of adrenergic alpha$_1$-receptors may explain the orthostatic hypotension observed with it.

Pharmacodynamics/Kinetics

Absorption: Accumulation is predictable upon multiple dosing

Distribution: V_{dss}: ~2 days; unlikely to interfere with the metabolism of drugs dependent upon CYP450 enzymes

Metabolism: Primarily Hepatic; both metabolites are pharmacologically inactive

Half-life elimination: Mean: Terminal: ~6 hours

Time to peak, plasma: 1.5 hours

Excretion: Urine (73% as metabolites, <1% as unchanged drug); feces (20%)

Usual Dosage Oral:

Children and Adolescents:

Autism (unlabeled use): 100-350 mg/day (1.6-5.2 mg/kg/day)

Psychosis and mania (unlabeled use): Initial: 25 mg twice daily; titrate as necessary to 450 mg/day

Adults: Schizophrenia/psychoses: Initial: 25 mg twice daily; increase in increments of 25-50 mg 2-3 times/day on the second and third day, if tolerated, to a target dose of 300-400 mg in 2-3 divided doses by day 4. Make further adjustments as needed at intervals of at least 2 days in adjustments of 25-50 mg twice daily. Usual maintenance range: 300-800 mg/day

Elderly: 40% lower mean oral clearance of quetiapine in adults >65 years of age; higher plasma levels expected and, therefore, dosage adjustment may be needed; elderly patients usually require 50-200 mg/day

Dosing comments in hepatic insufficiency: 30% lower mean oral clearance of quetiapine than normal subjects; higher plasma levels expected in hepatically impaired subjects; dosage adjustment may be needed

Dietary Considerations Can be taken with or without food.

Monitoring Parameters Patients should have eyes checked for cataracts every 6 months while on this medication

Patient Information May cause headache, drowsiness, dizziness, and/or lightheadedness, especially when the patient stands up or gets up from lying down. If this happens, the patient should sit or lie down immediately. This agent might increase the risk of cataracts; avoid alcohol, overheating, dehydration.

Additional Information Quetiapine has a very low incidence of extrapyramidal symptoms such as restlessness and abnormal movement, and is at least as effective as conventional antipsychotics.

Dosage Forms Tablet: 25 mg, 100 mg, 200 mg, 300 mg

- ♦ **Quetiapine Fumarate** see Quetiapine on page 1165
- ♦ **Quibron®** see Theophylline and Guaifenesin on page 1310
- ♦ **Quibron®-T/SR** see Theophylline Salts on page 1310
- ♦ **Quinaglute® Dura-Tabs®** see Quinidine on page 1168
- ♦ **Quinalbarbitone Sodium** see Secobarbital on page 1227

Quinapril (KWIN a pril)

Related Information

Angiotensin Agents Comparison on page 1473

Heart Failure on page 1663

U.S. Brand Names Accupril®

Canadian Brand Names Accupril™

Synonyms Quinapril Hydrochloride

Therapeutic Category Angiotensin-Converting Enzyme (ACE) Inhibitor; Antihypertensive Agent

Use Management of hypertension; treatment of congestive heart failure

Unlabeled/Investigational Use Treatment of left ventricular dysfunction after myocardial infarction

Pregnancy Risk Factor C/D (2nd and 3rd trimesters)

Contraindications Hypersensitivity to quinapril or any component of the formulation; angioedema related to previous treatment with an ACE inhibitor; bilateral renal artery stenosis; primary hyperaldosteronism; patients with idiopathic or hereditary angioedema; pregnancy (2nd and 3rd trimesters)

Warnings/Precautions Use with caution in patients with renal insufficiency, autoimmune disease, renal artery stenosis; excessive hypotension may be more likely in volume-depleted patients, the elderly, and following the first dose (first dose phenomenon); quinapril should be discontinued if laryngeal stridor or angioedema of the face, tongue, or glottis is observed

Adverse Reactions Note: Frequency ranges include data from hypertension and heart failure trials. Higher rates of adverse reactions have generally been noted in patients with congestive heart failure. However, the frequency of adverse effects associated with placebo is also increased in this population.

1% to 10%:

Cardiovascular: Hypotension (3%), chest pain (2%), first-dose hypotension (up to 3%)

Central nervous system: Dizziness (4% to 8%), headache (2% to 6%), fatigue (3%)

Dermatologic: Rash (1%)

Endocrine & metabolic: Hyperkalemia (2%)

Gastrointestinal: Vomiting/nausea (1% to 2%), diarrhea (1.7%)

Neuromuscular & skeletal: Myalgias (2% to 5%), back pain (1%)

Renal: Increased BUN/serum creatinine (2%, transient elevations may occur with a higher frequency), worsening of renal function (in patients with bilateral renal artery stenosis or hypovolemia)

Respiratory: Upper respiratory symptoms, cough (2% to 4%; up to 13% in some studies), dyspnea (2%)

<1% (Limited to important or life-threatening): Acute renal failure, agranulocytosis, alopecia, amblyopia, angina, angioedema, arrhythmia, arthralgia, depression, dermatopolymyositis, edema, eosinophilic pneumonitis, exfoliative dermatitis, hemolytic anemia, hepatitis, hyperkalemia, hypertensive crisis, impotence, insomnia, myocardial infarction, orthostatic hypotension, pancreatitis, paresthesia, pemphigus, photosensitivity, pruritus, shock, somnolence, stroke, syncope, thrombocytopenia, vertigo

A syndrome which may include fever, myalgia, arthralgia, interstitial nephritis, vasculitis, rash, eosinophilia and positive ANA, and elevated ESR has been reported with ACE inhibitors. In addition, pancreatitis, hepatic necrosis, neutropenia, and/or agranulocytosis (particularly in patients with collagen-vascular disease or renal impairment) have been associated with many ACE inhibitors.

Overdosage/Toxicology Mild hypotension has been the only toxic effect seen with acute overdose; bradycardia may also occur. Hyperkalemia occurs even with therapeutic doses, especially in patients with renal insufficiency and those taking NSAIDs. Following initiation of essential overdose management, toxic symptom and supportive treatment should be initiated. Hypotension usually responds to I.V. fluids or Trendelenburg positioning.

Drug Interactions

Increased Effect/Toxicity: Potassium supplements, co-trimoxazole (high dose), angiotensin II receptor antagonists (candesartan, losartan, irbesartan, etc), or potassium-sparing diuretics (amiloride, spironolactone, triamterene) may result in elevated serum potassium levels when combined with quinapril. ACE inhibitor effects may be increased by phenothiazines or probenecid (increases levels of captopril). ACE inhibitors may increase serum concentrations/effects of digoxin, lithium, and sulfonylureas.

Diuretics have additive hypotensive effects with ACE inhibitors, and hypovolemia increases the potential for adverse renal effects of ACE inhibitors. In patients with compromised renal function, coadministration with nonsteroidal anti-inflammatory drugs may result in further deterioration of renal function. Allopurinol and ACE inhibitors may cause a higher risk of hypersensitivity reaction when taken concurrently.

Decreased Effect: Quinapril may reduce the absorption of quinolones and tetracycline antibiotics. Aspirin (high dose) may reduce the therapeutic effects of ACE inhibitors; at low dosages this does not appear to be significant. Rifampin may decrease the effect of ACE inhibitors. Antacids may decrease the bioavailability of ACE inhibitors (may be more likely to occur with captopril); separate administration times by 1-2 hours. NSAIDs, specifically indomethacin, may reduce the hypotensive effects of ACE inhibitors.

Ethanol/Nutrition/Herb Interactions Herb/Nutraceutical: Avoid dong quai if using for hypertension (has estrogenic activity). Avoid ephedra, yohimbe, ginseng (may worsen hypertension). Avoid garlic (may have increased antihypertensive effect).

Stability Store at room temperature; unstable in aqueous solutions; to prepare solution for oral administration, mix prior to administration and use within 10 minutes

Mechanism of Action Competitive inhibitor of angiotensin-converting enzyme (ACE); prevents conversion of angiotensin I to angiotensin II, a potent vasoconstrictor; results in lower levels of angiotensin II which causes an increase in plasma renin activity and a reduction in aldosterone secretion; a CNS mechanism may also be involved in hypotensive effect as angiotensin II increases adrenergic outflow from CNS; vasoactive kallikreins may be decreased in conversion to active hormones by ACE inhibitors, thus reducing blood pressure

Pharmacodynamics/Kinetics

Onset of action: 1 hour

Duration: 24 hours

Absorption: Quinapril: ≥60%

Protein binding: Quinapril: 97%; Quinaprilat: 97%

Metabolism: Rapidly hydrolyzed to quinaprilat, the active metabolite

Half-life elimination: Quinapril: 0.8 hours; Quinaprilat: 3 hours; increases as Cl_{cr} decreases

Time to peak, serum: Quinapril: 1 hour; Quinaprilat: ~2 hours

Excretion: Urine (50% to 60% primarily as quinaprilat)

Usual Dosage

Adults: Oral:

Hypertension: Initial: 10-20 mg once daily, adjust according to blood pressure response at peak and trough blood levels; initial dose may be reduced to 5 mg in patients receiving diuretic therapy if the diuretic is continued (normal dosage range is 20-80 mg/day for hypertension)

Congestive heart failure or post-MI: Initial: 5 mg once daily, titrated at weekly intervals to 20-40 mg daily in 2 divided doses

Elderly: Initial: 2.5-5 mg/day; increase dosage at increments of 2.5-5 mg at 1- to 2-week intervals.

Dosing adjustment in renal impairment: Lower initial doses should be used; after initial dose (if tolerated), administer initial dose twice daily; may be increased at weekly intervals to optimal response:

Hypertension: Initial:

Cl_{cr} >60 mL/minute: Administer 10 mg/day

Cl_{cr} 30-60 mL/minute: Administer 5 mg/day

Cl_{cr} 10-30 mL/minute: Administer 2.5 mg/day

Congestive heart failure: Initial:

Cl_{cr} >30 mL/minute: Administer 5 mg/day

Cl_{cr} 10-30 mL/minute: Administer 2.5 mg/day

(Continued)

Quinapril *(Continued)*

Dosing comments in hepatic impairment: In patients with alcoholic cirrhosis, hydrolysis of quinapril to quinaprilat is impaired; however, the subsequent elimination of quinaprilat is unaltered.

Patient Information Do not discontinue medication without advice of physician; notify physician if sore throat, swelling, palpitations, cough, chest pains, difficulty swallowing, swelling of face, eyes, tongue, lips; hoarseness, sweating, vomiting, or diarrhea occurs; may cause dizziness, lightheadedness during first few days; may also cause changes in taste perception

Nursing Implications May cause depression in some patients; discontinue if angioedema of the face, extremities, lips, tongue, or glottis occurs; watch for hypotensive effects within 1-3 hours of first dose or new higher dose

Dosage Forms Tablet, as hydrochloride: 5 mg, 10 mg, 20 mg, 40 mg

Quinapril and Hydrochlorothiazide

(KWIN a pril & hye droe klor oh THYE a zide)

U.S. Brand Names Accuretic™

Canadian Brand Names Accuretic™

Synonyms Hydrochlorothiazide and Quinapril

Therapeutic Category Angiotensin-Converting Enzyme (ACE) Inhibitor; Diuretic, Thiazide

Use Treatment of hypertension (not for initial therapy)

Pregnancy Risk Factor C (1st trimester)/D (2nd and 3rd trimesters)

Usual Dosage Oral:

Children: Safety and efficacy have not been established.

Adults: Initial:

Patients who have failed quinapril monotherapy:

Quinapril 10 mg/hydrochlorothiazide 12.5 mg **or**

Quinapril 20 mg/hydrochlorothiazide 12.5 mg once daily

Patients with adequate blood pressure control on hydrochlorothiazide 25 mg/day, but significant potassium loss:

Quinapril 10 mg/hydrochlorothiazide 12.5 mg **or**

Quinapril 20 mg/hydrochlorothiazide 12.5 mg once daily

Note: Clinical trials of quinapril/hydrochlorothiazide combinations used quinapril doses of 2.5-40 mg/day and hydrochlorothiazide doses of 6.25-25 mg/day.

Dosage adjustment in renal impairment: Cl_{cr} <30 mL/minute/1.73 m² or serum creatinine ≤3 mg/dL: Use is not recommended.

Additional Information Complete prescribing information for this medication should be consulted for additional detail.

Dosage Forms Tablet: Quinapril hydrochloride 10 mg and hydrochlorothiazide 12.5 mg; quinapril hydrochloride 20 mg and hydrochlorothiazide 12.5 mg; quinapril hydrochloride 20 mg and hydrochlorothiazide 25 mg

♦ **Quinapril Hydrochloride** *see* Quinapril *on page 1166*

Quinethazone *(kwin ETH a zone)*

Related Information

Sulfonamide Derivatives *on page 1515*

U.S. Brand Names Hydromox®

Canadian Brand Names Hydromox®

Therapeutic Category Antihypertensive Agent; Diuretic, Thiazide

Use Adjunctive therapy in treatment of edema and hypertension

Pregnancy Risk Factor D

Usual Dosage Adults: Oral: 50-100 mg once daily; usual maximum: 200 mg/day

Additional Information Complete prescribing information for this medication should be consulted for additional detail.

Dosage Forms Tablet: 50 mg

♦ **Quinidex® Extentabs®** *see* Quinidine *on page 1168*

Quinidine *(KWIN i deen)*

Related Information

Adult ACLS Algorithms *on page 1632*

Antacid Drug Interactions *on page 1477*

Antiarrhythmic Drugs Comparison *on page 1478*

Malaria Treatment *on page 1607*

U.S. Brand Names Cardioquin®; Quinaglute® Dura-Tabs®; Quinidex® Extentabs®

Canadian Brand Names Apo®-Quinidine; Cardioquin®; Quinidex Extentabs®

Synonyms Quinidine Gluconate; Quinidine Polygalacturonate; Quinidine Sulfate

Therapeutic Category Antiarrhythmic Agent, Class I-A

Use Prophylaxis after cardioversion of atrial fibrillation and/or flutter to maintain normal sinus rhythm; prevent recurrence of paroxysmal supraventricular tachycardia, paroxysmal AV junctional rhythm, paroxysmal ventricular tachycardia, paroxysmal atrial fibrillation, and atrial or ventricular premature contractions; has activity against *Plasmodium falciparum* malaria

Pregnancy Risk Factor C

Contraindications Hypersensitivity to quinidine or any component of the formulation; thrombocytopenia; thrombocytopenic purpura; myasthenia gravis; heart block greater than first degree; idioventricular conduction delays (except in patients with a functioning artificial pacemaker); those adversely affected by anticholinergic activity; concurrent use of quinolone antibiotics which prolong QT interval, cisapride, amprenavir, or ritonavir

Warnings/Precautions Monitor and adjust dose to prevent QT_c prolongation; watch for proarrhythmic effects. May precipitate or exacerbate CHF. Reduce dosage in hepatic impairment. In patients with atrial fibrillation or flutter, block the AV node before initiating. Correct hypokalemia before initiating therapy. Hypokalemia may worsen toxicity. Use may cause digoxin-induced toxicity (adjust digoxin's dose). Use caution with concurrent use of other antiarrhythmics. Hypersensitivity reactions can occur. Can unmask sick sinus syndrome (causes bradycardia). Has been associated with severe hepatotoxic reactions, including granulomatous hepatitis, increased serum AST and alkaline phosphatase concentrations, and jaundice may occur; use with caution in nursing women and elderly. Hemolysis may occur in patients with G6PD (glucose-6-phosphate dehydrogenase) deficiency.

Adverse Reactions

Frequency not defined: Hypotension, syncope

>10%:
Cardiovascular: QT$_c$ prolongation (modest prolongation is common, however excessive prolongation is rare and indicates toxicity)

Central nervous system: Lightheadedness (15%)

Gastrointestinal: Diarrhea (35%), upper GI distress, bitter taste, diarrhea, anorexia, nausea, vomiting, stomach cramping (22%)

1% to 10%:
Cardiovascular: Angina (6%), palpitation (7%), new or worsened arrhythmias (proarrhythmic effect)

Central nervous system: Syncope (1% to 8%), headache (7%), fatigue (7%), weakness (5%), sleep disturbance (3%), tremor (2%), nervousness (2%), incoordination (1%)

Dermatologic: Rash (5%)

Ocular: Blurred vision

Otic: Tinnitus

Respiratory: Wheezing

<1% (Limited to important or life-threatening): Abnormal pigmentation, acute psychotic reactions, agranulocytosis, angioedema, arthralgia, bronchospasm, cerebral hypoperfusion (possibly resulting in ataxia, apprehension, and seizures), cholestasis, confusion, delirium, depression, drug-induced lupus-like syndrome, eczematous dermatitis, esophagitis, exacerbated bradycardia (in sick sinus syndrome), exfoliative rash, fever, flushing, granulomatous hepatitis, hallucinations, heart block, hemolytic anemia, hepatotoxic reaction (rare), impaired hearing, increased CPK, lichen planus, livedo reticularis, lymphadenopathy, melanin pigmentation of the hard palate, myalgia, mydriasis, nephropathy, optic neuritis, pancytopenia, paradoxical increase in ventricular rate during atrial fibrillation/flutter, photosensitivity, pneumonitis, pruritus, psoriaform rash, QT$_c$ prolongation (excessive), respiratory depression, sicca syndrome, tachycardia, thrombocytopenia, thrombocytopenic purpura, torsade de pointes, urticaria, uveitis, vascular collapse, vasculitis, ventricular fibrillation, ventricular tachycardia, vertigo, visual field loss

Note: Cinchonism, a syndrome which may include tinnitus, high-frequency hearing loss, deafness, vertigo, blurred vision, diplopia, photophobia, headache, confusion, and delirium has been associated with quinidine use. Usually associated with chronic toxicity, this syndrome has also been described after brief exposure to a moderate dose in sensitive patients. Vomiting and diarrhea may also occur as isolated reactions to therapeutic quinidine levels.

Overdosage/Toxicology

Has a low toxic:therapeutic ratio and may easily produce fatal intoxication (acute toxic dose: 1 g in adults); symptoms include sinus bradycardia, sinus node arrest or asystole, PR, QRS, or QT interval prolongation, torsade de pointes (polymorphous ventricular tachycardia) and depressed myocardial contractility, which along with alpha-adrenergic or ganglionic blockade, may result in hypotension and pulmonary edema. Other effects are anticholinergic (dry mouth, dilated pupils, and delirium) as well as seizures, coma and respiratory arrest.

Treatment is primarily symptomatic and effects usually respond to conventional therapies (fluids, positioning, vasopressors, anticonvulsants, antiarrhythmics). **Note:** Do not use other type 1a or 1c antiarrhythmic agents to treat ventricular tachycardia. Sodium bicarbonate may treat wide QRS intervals or hypotension. Markedly impaired conduction or high degree A-V block, unresponsive to bicarbonate, indicates consideration of a pacemaker is needed.

Drug Interactions

Cytochrome P450 Effect: CYP3A3/4 enzyme substrate; CYP2D6 (potent) and 3A3/4 (weak) enzyme inhibitor

Increased Effect/Toxicity: Quinidine potentiates nondepolarizing and depolarizing muscle relaxants. Quinidine may increase plasma concentration of digoxin; closely monitor digoxin concentrations. Digoxin dosage may need to be reduced (by 50%) when quinidine is initiated; new steady-state digoxin plasma concentrations occur in 5-7 days. When combined with quinidine, amiloride may cause prolonged ventricular conduction leading to arrhythmias. Urinary alkalinizers (antacids, sodium bicarbonate, acetazolamide) increase quinidine blood levels. Warfarin effects may be increased by quinidine.

Amprenavir, amiodarone, cimetidine, clarithromycin, diltiazem, erythromycin, itraconazole, ketoconazole, nelfinavir, ritonavir, troleandomycin, and verapamil (as well as other inhibitors of cytochrome P450 isoenzyme 3A3/4 may increase quinidine blood levels). Quinidine may increase blood levels of metoprolol mexiletine, nifedipine, propafenone, propranolol, and timolol.

Effects may be additive with drugs which prolong the QT interval, including amiodarone, amitriptyline, astemizole, bepridil, cisapride (use is contraindicated), disopyramide, erythromycin, haloperidol, imipramine, pimozide, procainamide, sotalol, thioridazine, and some quinolones (sparfloxacin, gatifloxacin, moxifloxacin - concurrent use is contraindicated).

Decreased Effect: Analgesic efficacy of codeine may be reduced. Enzyme inducers (aminoglutethimide, carbamazepine, phenobarbital, phenytoin, primidone, rifabutin, rifampin) may decrease quinidine blood levels.

Ethanol/Nutrition/Herb Interactions

Food: Dietary salt intake may alter the rate and extent of quinidine absorption. A decrease in dietary salt may lead to an increase in quinidine serum concentrations. Avoid changes in dietary salt intake. Quinidine serum levels may be increased if taken with food. Food has a variable effect on absorption of sustained release formulation. The rate of absorption of quinidine may be decreased following the ingestion of grapefruit juice. In addition,
(Continued)

Quinidine *(Continued)*

CYP3A3/4 metabolism of quinidine may be reduced by grapefruit juice. Grapefruit juice should be avoided. Excessive intake of fruit juices or vitamin C may decrease urine pH and result in increased clearance of quinidine with decreased serum concentration. Alkaline foods may result in increased quinidine serum concentrations.

Herb/Nutraceutical: St John's wort may decrease quinidine levels. Avoid ephedra (may worsen arrhythmia).

Stability Do not use discolored parenteral solution.

Mechanism of Action Class 1a antiarrhythmic agent; depresses phase O of the action potential; decreases myocardial excitability and conduction velocity, and myocardial contractility by decreasing sodium influx during depolarization and potassium efflux in repolarization; also reduces calcium transport across cell membrane

Pharmacodynamics/Kinetics

Distribution: V_d: Adults: 2-3.5 L/kg, decreased with congestive heart failure, malaria; increased with cirrhosis; crosses placenta; enters breast milk

Protein binding:

Newborns: 60% to 70%; decreased protein binding with cyanotic congenital heart disease, cirrhosis, or acute myocardial infarction

Adults: 80% to 90%

Metabolism: Extensively hepatic (50% to 90%) to inactive compounds

Bioavailability: Sulfate: 80%; Gluconate: 70%

Half-life elimination, plasma: Children: 2.5-6.7 hours; Adults: 6-8 hours; increased half-life with elderly, cirrhosis, and congestive heart failure

Excretion: Urine (15% to 25% as unchanged drug)

Usual Dosage Dosage expressed in terms of the salt: 267 mg of quinidine gluconate = 200 mg of quinidine sulfate.

Children: Test dose for idiosyncratic reaction (sulfate, oral or gluconate, I.M.): 2 mg/kg or 60 mg/m²

Oral (quinidine sulfate): 15-60 mg/kg/day in 4-5 divided doses or 6 mg/kg every 4-6 hours; usual 30 mg/kg/day or 900 mg/m²/day given in 5 daily doses

I.V. **not** recommended (quinidine gluconate): 2-10 mg/kg/dose given at a rate ≤10 mg/minute every 3-6 hours as needed

Adults: Test dose: Oral, I.M.: 200 mg administered several hours before full dosage (to determine possibility of idiosyncratic reaction)

Oral (for malaria):

Sulfate: 100-600 mg/dose every 4-6 hours; begin at 200 mg/dose and titrate to desired effect (maximum daily dose: 3-4 g)

Gluconate: 324-972 mg every 8-12 hours

I.M.: 400 mg/dose every 2-6 hours; initial dose: 600 mg (gluconate)

I.V.: 200-400 mg/dose diluted and given at a rate ≤10 mg/minute; may require as much as 500-750 mg

Dosing adjustment in renal impairment: Cl_{cr} <10 mL/minute: Administer 75% of normal dose.

Hemodialysis: Slightly hemodialyzable (5% to 20%); 200 mg supplemental dose posthemodialysis is recommended.

Peritoneal dialysis: Not dialyzable (0% to 5%)

Dosing adjustment/comments in hepatic impairment: Larger loading dose may be indicated, reduce maintenance doses by 50% and monitor serum levels closely.

Dietary Considerations Administer with food or milk to decrease gastrointestinal irritation. Avoid changes in dietary salt intake.

Administration Administer around-the-clock to promote less variation in peak and trough serum levels

Oral: Do not crush, chew, or break sustained release dosage forms.

Parenteral: When injecting I.M., aspirate carefully to avoid injection into a vessel; maximum I.V. infusion rate: 10 mg/minute

Monitoring Parameters Cardiac monitor required during I.V. administration; CBC, liver and renal function tests, should be routinely performed during long-term administration

Reference Range Therapeutic: 2-5 µg/mL (SI: 6.2-15.4 µmol/L). Patient dependent therapeutic response occurs at levels of 3-6 µg/mL (SI: 9.2-18.5 µmol/L). Optimal therapeutic level is method dependent; >6 µg/mL (SI: >18 µmol/L).

Patient Information Do not crush or chew sustained release preparations. Patients should notify their physician if rash, fever, unusual bleeding or bruising, ringing in the ears, visual disturbances, or syncope occurs; seek emergency help if palpitations occur.

Dosage Forms

Injection, as gluconate: 80 mg/mL (10 mL)

Tablet, as polygalacturonate: 275 mg

Tablet, as sulfate: 200 mg, 300 mg

Tablet, sustained action, as sulfate: 300 mg

Tablet, sustained release, as gluconate: 324 mg

Extemporaneous Preparations

A 10 mg/mL oral liquid preparation made from tablets and 3 different vehicles (cherry syrup, a 1:1 mixture of Ora-Sweet® and Ora-Plus®, or a 1:1 mixture of Ora-Sweet® SF and Ora-Plus®) was stable for 60 days when stored in amber plastic prescription bottles in the dark at room temperature (25°C) or under refrigeration (5°C); Grind six 200 mg tablets in a mortar into a fine powder; add 15 mL of the vehicle and mix well to form a uniform paste; mix while adding the vehicle in geometric proportions to **almost** 120 mL; transfer to a calibrated bottle and qsad to 120 mL; label "shake well" and "protect from light" (Allen 1998).

Allen LV and Erickson MA, "Stability of Bethanechol Chloride, Pyrazinamide, Quinidine Sulfate, Rifampin, and Tetracycline in Extemporaneously Compounded Oral Liquids," *Am J Health Syst Pharm*, 1998, 55(17):1804-9.

♦ **Quinidine Gluconate** *see* Quinidine *on page 1168*

♦ **Quinidine Polygalacturonate** *see* Quinidine *on page 1168*
♦ **Quinidine Sulfate** *see* Quinidine *on page 1168*

Quinine (KWYE nine)

Related Information
Malaria Treatment *on page 1607*

Canadian Brand Names Quinine-Odan™

Synonyms Quinine Sulfate

Therapeutic Category Antimalarial Agent

Use In conjunction with other antimalarial agents, suppression or treatment of chloroquine-resistant *P. falciparum* malaria; treatment of *Babesia microti* infection in conjunction with clindamycin

Unlabeled/Investigational Use Prevention and treatment of nocturnal recumbency leg muscle cramps

Pregnancy Risk Factor X

Contraindications Hypersensitivity to quinine or any component of the formulation; tinnitus, optic neuritis, G6PD deficiency; history of black water fever; thrombocytopenia with quinine or quinidine; pregnancy

Warnings/Precautions Use with caution in patients with cardiac arrhythmias (quinine has quinidine-like activity) and in patients with myasthenia gravis

Adverse Reactions
Frequency not defined:
Central nervous system: Severe headache
Gastrointestinal: Nausea, vomiting, diarrhea
Ocular: Blurred vision
Otic: Tinnitus
Miscellaneous: Cinchonism (risk of cinchonism is directly related to dose and duration of therapy)
<1% (Limited to important or life-threatening): Anginal symptoms, diplopia, epigastric pain, fever, flushing of the skin, hemolysis in G6PD deficiency, hepatitis, hypersensitivity reactions, hypoglycemia, impaired hearing, nightblindness, optic atrophy, pruritus, rash, thrombocytopenia

Overdosage/Toxicology Symptoms of mild toxicity include nausea, vomiting, and cinchonism. Severe intoxication may cause ataxia, obtundation, convulsions, coma, and respiratory arrest. With massive intoxication quinidine-like cardiotoxicity (hypotension, QRS and QT interval prolongation, A-V block, and ventricular arrhythmias) may be fatal. Retinal toxicity occurs 9-10 hours after ingestion (blurred vision, impaired color perception, constriction of visual fields, blindness). Other toxic effects include hypokalemia, hypoglycemia, hemolysis, and congenital malformations when taken during pregnancy. Treatment includes symptomatic therapy with conventional agents (anticonvulsants, fluids, positioning, vasoconstrictors, antiarrhythmics). **Note:** Avoid type 1a and 1c antiarrhythmic drugs. Treat cardiotoxicity with sodium bicarbonate. Dialysis and hemoperfusion procedures are ineffective in enhancing elimination.

Drug Interactions
Cytochrome P450 Effect: CYP3A3/4 enzyme substrate; CYP3A3/4 enzyme inhibitor
Increased Effect/Toxicity: Beta-blockers + quinine may increase bradycardia. Quinine may enhance warfarin anticoagulant effect. Quinine potentiates nondepolarizing and depolarizing muscle relaxants. Quinine may increase plasma concentration of digoxin. Closely monitor digoxin concentrations. Digoxin dosage may need to be reduced (by one-half) when quinine is initiated. New steady-state digoxin plasma concentrations occur in 5-7 days. Verapamil, amiodarone, alkalinizing agents, and cimetidine may increase quinine serum concentrations.
Decreased Effect: Phenobarbital, phenytoin, and rifampin may decrease quinine serum concentrations.

Ethanol/Nutrition/Herb Interactions Herb/Nutraceutical: St John's wort may decrease quinine levels.

Stability Protect from light

Mechanism of Action Depresses oxygen uptake and carbohydrate metabolism; intercalates into DNA, disrupting the parasite's replication and transcription; affects calcium distribution within muscle fibers and decreases the excitability of the motor end-plate region; cardiovascular effects similar to quinidine

Pharmacodynamics/Kinetics
Absorption: Readily absorbed, mainly from upper small intestine
Protein binding: 70% to 95%
Metabolism: Primarily hepatic
Half-life elimination: Children: 6-12 hours; Adults: 8-14 hours
Time to peak, serum: 1-3 hours
Excretion: Feces and saliva; urine (<5% as unchanged drug)

Usual Dosage Oral:
Children:
Treatment of chloroquine-resistant malaria: 25-30 mg/kg/day in divided doses every 8 hours for 3-7 days with tetracycline (consider risk versus benefit in children <8 years of age)
Babesiosis: 25 mg/kg/day divided every 8 hours for 7 days
Adults:
Treatment of chloroquine-resistant malaria: 650 mg every 8 hours for 3-7 days with tetracycline
Suppression of malaria: 325 mg twice daily and continued for 6 weeks after exposure
Babesiosis: 650 mg every 6-8 hours for 7 days
Leg cramps: 200-300 mg at bedtime
Dosing interval/adjustment in renal impairment:
Cl_{cr} 10-50 mL/minute: Administer every 8-12 hours or 75% of normal dose
Cl_{cr} <10 mL/minute: Administer every 24 hours or 30% to 50% of normal dose
(Continued)

Quinine *(Continued)*

Dialysis: Not removed

Peritoneal dialysis: Dose as for Cl$_{cr}$ <10 mL/minute

Continuous arteriovenous or venovenous hemodiafiltration effects: Dose for Cl$_{cr}$ 10-50 mL/minute

Dietary Considerations May be taken with food.

Reference Range Toxic: >10 µg/mL

Test Interactions Positive Coombs' [direct]; false elevation of urinary steroids and catecholamines

Patient Information Avoid use of aluminum-containing antacids because of drug absorption problems; swallow dose whole to avoid bitter taste; may cause night blindness. Patients should notify their physician if rash, fever, unusual bleeding or bruising, ringing in the ears, visual disturbances, or syncope occur; seek emergency help if palpitations occur.

Nursing Implications

Do not crush tablets or capsule to avoid bitter taste

Monitor CBC with platelet count, liver function tests, blood glucose, ophthalmologic examination

Dosage Forms

Capsule, as sulfate: 200 mg, 260 mg, 325 mg

Tablet, as sulfate: 260 mg

♦ **Quinine-Odan™ (Can)** *see* Quinine *on page 1171*

♦ **Quinine Sulfate** *see* Quinine *on page 1171*

♦ **Quinol** *see* Hydroquinone *on page 686*

♦ **Quinsana Plus® [OTC]** *see* Tolnaftate *on page 1347*

♦ **Quintasa® (Can)** *see* Mesalamine *on page 866*

Quinupristin and Dalfopristin *(kwi NYOO pris tin & dal FOE pris tin)*

Related Information

Antimicrobial Drugs of Choice *on page 1588*

U.S. Brand Names Synercid®

Canadian Brand Names Synercid®

Synonyms Pristinamycin; RP59500

Therapeutic Category Antibiotic, Streptogramin

Use Treatment of serious or life-threatening infections associated with vancomycin-resistant *Enterococcus faecium* bacteremia; treatment of complicated skin and skin structure infections caused by methicillin-susceptible *Staphylococcus aureus* or *Streptococcus pyogenes*

Has been studied in the treatment of a variety of infections caused by *Enterococcus faecium* (not *E. fecalis*) including vancomycin-resistant strains. May also be effective in the treatment of serious infections caused by *Staphylococcus* species including those resistant to methicillin.

Pregnancy Risk Factor B

Pregnancy/Breast-Feeding Implications No evidence of impaired fertility or harm to the fetus in animal reproductive studies. Excretion in human breast milk is unknown, use caution in breast-feeding women.

Contraindications Hypersensitivity to quinupristin, dalfopristin, pristinamycin, or virginiamycin, or any component of the formulation

Warnings/Precautions Use with caution in patients with hepatic or renal dysfunction. May cause pain and phlebitis when infused through a peripheral line (not relieved by hydrocortisone or diphenhydramine). Superinfection may occur. As with many antibiotics, antibiotic-associated colitis and pseudomembranous colitis may occur. May cause arthralgias, myalgias, and hyperbilirubinemia. May inhibit the metabolism of many drugs metabolized by CYP3A4. Concurrent therapy with astemizole, terfenadine, and cisapride (which may prolong QT$_c$ interval and lead to arrhythmias) should be avoided.

Adverse Reactions

>10%:

Hepatic: Hyperbilirubinemia (3% to 35%)

Local: Inflammation at infusion site (38% to 42%), local pain (40% to 44%), local edema (17% to 18%), infusion site reaction (12% to 13%)

Note: High baseline values were noted in many patients, contributing to the high incidence of this reaction in some studies.

1% to 10%:

Central nervous system: Pain (2% to 3%), headache (2%)

Dermatologic: Pruritus (2%), rash (3%)

Endocrine & metabolic: Hyperglycemia (1%)

Gastrointestinal: Nausea (3% to 5%), diarrhea (3%), vomiting (3% to 4%)

Hematologic: Anemia (3%)

Hepatic: Increased LDH (3%), increased GGT (2%)

Local: Thrombophlebitis (2%)

Neuromuscular & skeletal: Arthralgia (<1% to 8%), myalgia (<1% to 5%), Increased CPK (2%)

<1% (Limited to important or life-threatening): Allergic reaction, anaphylactoid reaction, angina, apnea, arrhythmia, cardiac arrest, coagulation disorder, dysautonomia, dyspnea, encephalopathy, gout, hematuria, hemolytic anemia, hepatitis, hyperkalemia, hypotension, maculopapular rash, mesenteric artery occlusion, myasthenia, neuropathy, pancreatitis, pancytopenia, paraplegia, paresthesia, pericarditis, pleural effusion, pseudomembranous colitis, respiratory distress, seizures, shock, stomatitis, syncope, thrombocytopenia, urticaria

Overdosage/Toxicology Symptoms may include dyspnea, emesis, tremors, and ataxia. Treatment is supportive. Not removed by hemodialysis or peritoneal dialysis.

Drug Interactions
Cytochrome P450 Effect: CYP3A3/4 enzyme inhibitor

Increased Effect/Toxicity: Astemizole, terfenadine, and cisapride (which may prolong QT$_c$ interval and lead to arrhythmias) should be avoided. The metabolism of midazolam, nifedipine, and terfenadine have been demonstrated to be inhibited *in vitro*. An increase in cyclosporine levels has been documented in patients receiving concomitant therapy. Other medications metabolized by CYP3A4, including protease inhibitors, non-nucleoside reverse transcriptase inhibitors, benzodiazepines, calcium channel blockers, some HMG-CoA reductase inhibitors, immunosuppressive agents, corticosteroids, carbamazepine, quinidine, lidocaine, and disopyramide are predicted to have increased plasma concentrations during concurrent dosing.

Stability Store unopened vials under refrigeration (2°C to 8°C/36°F to 46°F). Reconstitute single dose vial with 5 mL of 5% dextrose in water or sterile water for injection. Swirl gently to dissolve, do not shake (to limit foam formation). After reconstitution, stability is ~5 hours at room temperature and 54 hours if refrigerated at 2°C to 8°C. Reconstituted solution should be added to at least 250 mL of 5% dextrose in water for peripheral administration (increase to 500 mL or 750 mL if necessary to limit venous irritation). An infusion volume of 100 mL may be used for central line infusions. Do not freeze solution.

Mechanism of Action Quinupristin/dalfopristin inhibits bacterial protein synthesis by binding to different sites on the 50S bacterial ribosomal subunit thereby inhibiting protein synthesis

Pharmacodynamics/Kinetics
Distribution: Quinupristin: 0.45 L/kg; Dalfopristin: 0.24 L/kg

Protein binding: Moderate

Metabolism: To active metabolites via nonenzymatic reactions.

Half-life elimination: Quinupristin: 0.85 hour; Dalfopristin: 0.7 hour (mean elimination half-lives, including metabolites: 3 and 1 hours, respectively)

Excretion: Feces (75% to 77% as unchanged drug and metabolites); urine (15% to 19%)

Usual Dosage I.V.:
Children (limited information): Dosages similar to adult dosing have been used in the treatment of complicated skin/soft tissue infections and infections caused by vancomycin-resistant *Enterococcus faecium*

CNS shunt infection due to vancomycin-resistant *Enterococcus faecium*: 7.5 mg/kg/dose every 8 hours; concurrent intrathecal doses of 1-2 mg/day have been administered for up to 68 days

Adults:
Vancomycin-resistant *Enterococcus faecium*: 7.5 mg/kg every 8 hours
Complicated skin and skin structure infection: 7.5 mg/kg every 12 hours

Dosage adjustment in renal impairment: No adjustment required in renal failure, hemodialysis, or peritoneal dialysis

Dosage adjustment in hepatic impairment: Pharmacokinetic data suggest dosage adjustment may be necessary; however, specific recommendations have not been proposed

Elderly: No dosage adjustment is required

Administration Line should be flushed with 5% dextrose in water prior to and following administration. Incompatible with saline. Infusion should be completed over 60 minutes (toxicity may be increased with shorter infusion). Compatible (Y-site injection) with aztreonam, ciprofloxacin, haloperidol, metoclopramide or potassium chloride when admixed in 5% dextrose in water. Also compatible (Y-site injection) with fluconazole (used as undiluted solution). If severe venous irritation occurs following peripheral administration of quinupristin/dalfopristin diluted in 250 mL 5% dextrose in water, consideration should be given to increasing the infusion volume to 500 mL or 750 mL, changing the infusion site, or infusing by a peripherally inserted central catheter (PICC) or a central venous catheter.

Nursing Implications Monitor infusion site closely. If severe venous irritation occurs following peripheral administration of quinupristin/dalfopristin, consider changes to infusion volume, site, or administration via central line. Following infusion, flush with 5% dextrose in water to reduce vein irritation.

Dosage Forms Powder for injection: 500 mg (350 mg dalfopristin and 150 mg quinupristin)

♦ **Quixin™ Ophthalmic** *see* Levofloxacin *on page 793*

♦ **QVAR™** *see* Beclomethasone *on page 149*

Rabeprazole (ra BE pray zole)
U.S. Brand Names Aciphex™

Canadian Brand Names Aciphex™

Synonyms Pariprazole

Therapeutic Category Gastric Acid Secretion Inhibitor; Proton Pump Inhibitor

Use Short-term (4-8 weeks) treatment and maintenance of erosive or ulcerative gastroesophageal reflux disease (GERD); symptomatic GERD; short-term (up to 4 weeks) treatment of duodenal ulcers; long-term treatment of pathological hypersecretory conditions, including Zollinger-Ellison syndrome

Unlabeled/Investigational Use *H. pylori* eradication; maintenance of duodenal ulcer

Pregnancy Risk Factor B

Pregnancy/Breast-Feeding Implications Not recommended

Contraindications Hypersensitivity to rabeprazole, substituted benzimidazoles, or any component of the formulation

Warnings/Precautions Severe hepatic impairment; relief of symptoms with rabeprazole does not preclude the presence of a gastric malignancy

Adverse Reactions
1% to 10%: Central nervous system: Headache (2.4%)

<1% (Limited to important or life-threatening): Anaphylaxis, agranulocytosis, allergic reactions, alopecia, amnesia, angina, angioedema, apnea, asthma, bradycardia, bundle branch block, cholecystitis, coma, delirium, depression, dysphagia, dyspnea, extrapyramidal reaction, gout, hemolytic anemia, interstitial pneumonia, jaundice, leukopenia, myocardial infarction, neuralgia, neuropathy, pancreatitis, pancytopenia, paresthesia, photosensitivity,
(Continued)

Rabeprazole *(Continued)*

pulmonary embolus, QT prolongation, rash, renal calculus, retinal degeneration, rhabdo-myolysis, seizures, strabismus, syncope, tachycardia, thrombocytopenia, ventricular tachy-cardia, vertigo

Overdosage/Toxicology There has been no experience with large overdoses. Seven reports of accidental overdosage have been reported. The maximum reported overdose was 80 mg. There were no clinical signs or symptoms associated with any reported overdose. Patients with Zollinger-Ellison syndrome have been treated with up to 120 mg/day. No specific anti-dote is known. A single oral dose of 2000 mg/kg was not lethal to dogs.

Drug Interactions

Cytochrome P450 Effect: CYP3A3/4 and 2C19 (minor) enzyme substrate

Increased Effect/Toxicity: Rabeprazole (in extremely high concentrations) may increase serum levels of digoxin and cyclosporine.

Decreased Effect: Rabeprazole may decrease bioavailability of ketoconazole or itraconazole.

Ethanol/Nutrition/Herb Interactions Ethanol: Avoid ethanol (may cause gastric mucosal irritation).

Stability Rapidly degraded in acid conditions; may give antacid with rabeprazole

Mechanism of Action Potent proton pump inhibitor; suppresses gastric acid secretion by inhibiting the parietal cell H+/K+ ATP pump

Pharmacodynamics/Kinetics

Onset of action: 1 hour

Peak effect, plasma: ~2-5 hours

Duration: 24 hours

Absorption: Oral: Well absorbed within 1 hour

Distribution: 96.3%

Protein binding, serum: 94.8% to 97.5%

Metabolism: Hepatic via CYP3A and 2C19 to inactive metabolites

Bioavailability: Oral: 52%

Half-life elimination: 0.85-2 hours (dose-dependent)

Time to peak, serum: 2-5 hours

Excretion: Urine (90% primarily as thioether carboxylic acid); feces (remainder)

Usual Dosage Adults >18 years and Elderly:

GERD: 20 mg once daily for 4-8 weeks; maintenance: 20 mg once daily

Duodenal ulcer: 20 mg/day after breakfast for 4 weeks

Hypersecretory conditions: 60 mg once daily; dose may need to be adjusted as necessary. Doses as high as 100 mg and 60 mg twice daily have been used.

Patient Information Swallow whole - do not crush, chew, or split tablet; take before eating

Nursing Implications Do not crush tablet

Dosage Forms Tablet, delayed release, enteric coated: 20 mg

Rabies Immune Globulin (Human)

(RAY beez i MYUN GLOB yoo lin, HYU man)

Related Information

Immunization Recommendations *on page 1538*

U.S. Brand Names BayRab®; Imogam®

Canadian Brand Names BayRab™; Imogam® Rabies Pasteurized

Synonyms RIG

Therapeutic Category Immune Globulin

Use Part of postexposure prophylaxis of persons with rabies exposure who lack a history of pre-exposure or postexposure prophylaxis with rabies vaccine or a recently documented neutralizing antibody response to previous rabies vaccination; although it is preferable to administer RIG with the first dose of vaccine, it can be given up to 8 days after vaccination

Pregnancy Risk Factor C

Contraindications Hypersensitivity to thimerosal or any component of the formulation

Warnings/Precautions Have epinephrine 1:1000 available for anaphylactic reactions. As a product of human plasma, this product may potentially transmit disease; screening of donors, as well as testing and/or inactivation of certain viruses reduces this risk. Use caution in patients with thrombocytopenia or coagulation disorders (I.M. injections may be contraindi-cated), in patients with isolated IgA deficiency, or in patients with previous systemic hyper-sensitivity to human immunoglobulins. Not for intravenous administration.

Adverse Reactions

1% to 10%:

Central nervous system: Fever (mild)

Local: Soreness at injection site

<1% (Limited to important or life-threatening): Anaphylactic shock, angioedema, soreness of muscles, stiffness, urticaria

Stability Refrigerate

Mechanism of Action Rabies immune globulin is a solution of globulins dried from the plasma or serum of selected adult human donors who have been immunized with rabies vaccine and have developed high titers of rabies antibody. It generally contains 10% to 18% of protein of which not less than 80% is monomeric immunoglobulin G.

Usual Dosage Children and Adults: I.M.: 20 units/kg in a single dose (RIG should always be administered as part of rabies vaccine (HDCV)) regimen (as soon as possible after the first dose of vaccine, up to 8 days); infiltrate 1/2 of the dose locally around the wound; administer the remainder I.M.

Note: Persons known to have an adequate titer or who have been completely immunized with rabies vaccine should not receive RIG, only booster doses of HDCV

Administration Intramuscular injection only; injection should be made into the gluteal muscle

Nursing Implications Severe adverse reactions can occur if patient receives RIG I.V.

Dosage Forms Injection: 150 units/mL (2 mL, 10 mL)

Rabies Virus Vaccine (RAY beez VYE rus vak SEEN)

Related Information
Immunization Recommendations *on page 1538*

U.S. Brand Names Imovax® Rabies Vaccine

Canadian Brand Names Imovax® Rabies

Synonyms HDCV; Human Diploid Cell Cultures Rabies Vaccine

Therapeutic Category Vaccine, Inactivated Virus

Use Pre-exposure immunization: Vaccinate persons with greater than usual risk due to occupation or avocation including veterinarians, rangers, animal handlers, certain laboratory workers, and persons living in or visiting countries for longer than 1 month where rabies is a constant threat.

Postexposure prophylaxis: If a bite from a carrier animal is unprovoked, if it is not captured and rabies is present in that species and area, administer rabies immune globulin (RIG) and the vaccine as indicated

Pregnancy Risk Factor C

Contraindications Hypersensitivity to neomycin, gentamicin, or amphotericin B or any component of the formulation; developing febrile illness (during pre-exposure therapy only); life-threatening allergic reactions to rabies vaccine or any components of the formulation (however, carefully consider a patient's risk of rabies before continuing therapy)

Warnings/Precautions Report serious reactions to the State Health Department or the manufacturer/distributor, an immune complex reaction is possible 2-21 days following booster doses of HDCV; hypersensitivity reactions may be treated with antihistamines or epinephrine, if severe.

Use care to administer Imovax® rabies vaccine, human and rabies vaccine adsorbed (RDA) only by I.M. route; diploid cell (HDCV) (in the **deltoid only**)

Adverse Reactions All serious adverse reactions must be reported to the U.S. Department of Health and Human Services (DHHS) Vaccine Adverse Event Reporting System (VAERS) 1-800-822-7967. Mild systemic reactions occur at an incidence of ~8% to 10% with RVA and 20% with HDCV.

Frequency not defined.

Cardiovascular: Edema

Central nervous system: Dizziness, malaise, encephalomyelitis, transverse myelitis, fever, pain, headache, neuroparalytic reactions

Dermatologic: Itching, erythema

Gastrointestinal: Nausea, abdominal pain

Local: Local discomfort, pain at injection site

Neuromuscular & skeletal: Myalgia

Note: Serum sickness reaction is much less frequent with RVA (<1%) vs the HDCV (6%).

Stability Refrigerate dried vaccine; HDCV can presumably tolerate 30 days at room temperature; reconstituted vaccine should be used immediately

Mechanism of Action Rabies vaccine is an inactivated virus vaccine which promotes immunity by inducing an active immune response. The production of specific antibodies requires about 7-10 days to develop. Rabies immune globulin or antirabies serum, equine (ARS) is given in conjunction with rabies vaccine to provide immune protection until an antibody response can occur.

Pharmacodynamics/Kinetics
Onset of action: I.M.: Rabies antibody: ~7-10 days

Peak effect: ~30-60 days

Duration: ≥1 year

Usual Dosage
Pre-exposure prophylaxis: 1 mL I.M. on days 0, 7, and 21 to 28. **Note:** Prolonging the interval between doses does not interfere with immunity achieved after the concluding dose of the basic series.

Postexposure prophylaxis: All postexposure treatment should begin with immediate cleansing of the wound with soap and water

Persons not previously immunized as above: Rabies immune globulin 20 units/kg body weight, half infiltrated at bite site if possible, remainder I.M.; and 5 doses of rabies vaccine, 1 mL I.M., one each on days 0, 3, 7, 14, 28

Persons who have previously received postexposure prophylaxis with rabies vaccine, received a recommended I.M. pre-exposure series of rabies vaccine or have a previously documented rabies antibody titer considered adequate: 1 mL of either vaccine I.M. only on days 0 and 3; do not administer RIG

Booster (for occupational or other continuing risk): 1 mL I.M. every 2-5 years or based on antibody titers

Administration HDCV and RVA administered I.M.; administer I.M. injections in the deltoid muscle, not the gluteal, in adults and older children; for younger children, use the outer aspect of the thigh.

For patients at risk of hemorrhage following intramuscular injection, the ACIP recommends "it should be administered intramuscularly if, in the opinion of the physician familiar with the patients bleeding risk, the vaccine can be administered with reasonable safety by this route. If the patient receives antihemophilia or other similar therapy, intramuscular vaccination can be scheduled shortly after such therapy is administered. A fine needle (23 gauge or smaller) can be used for the vaccination and firm pressure applied to the site (without rubbing) for at least 2 minutes. The patient should be instructed concerning the risk of hematoma from the injection."

Reference Range Antibody titers ≥115 as determined by rapid fluorescent-focus inhibition test are indicative of adequate response; collect titers on day 28 postexposure

Nursing Implications For intramuscular injection only; this rabies vaccine product must not be administered intradermally; in older children and adults it should be given in deltoid area for best response

(Continued)

Rabies Virus Vaccine *(Continued)*

Additional Information Federal law requires that the date of administration, the vaccine manufacturer, lot number of vaccine, and the administering person's name, title, and address be entered into the patient's permanent medical record.

Dosage Forms

Injection:

Human diploid cell vaccine (HDCV): Rabies antigen 2.5 units/mL (1 mL)

Rabies vaccine, adsorbed: 1 mL

♦ **rAHF** *see* Antihemophilic Factor (Recombinant) *on page 105*

♦ **R-albuterol** *see* Levalbuterol *on page 785*

Raloxifene (ral OKS i feen)

U.S. Brand Names Evista®

Canadian Brand Names Evista®

Synonyms Keoxifene Hydrochloride; Raloxifene Hydrochloride

Therapeutic Category Selective Estrogen Receptor Modulator (SERM)

Use Prevention and treatment of osteoporosis in postmenopausal women

Pregnancy Risk Factor X

Pregnancy/Breast-Feeding Implications Raloxifene should not be used by pregnant women or by women planning to become pregnant in the immediate future

Contraindications Hypersensitivity to raloxifene or any component of the formulation; active thromboembolic disorder; pregnancy (not intended for use in premenopausal women)

Warnings/Precautions History of venous thromboembolism/pulmonary embolism; patients with cardiovascular disease; history of cervical/uterine carcinoma; renal/hepatic insufficiency (however, pharmacokinetic data are lacking); concurrent use of estrogens; women with a history of elevated triglycerides in response to treatment with oral estrogens (or estrogen/progestin)

Adverse Reactions Note: Has been associated with increased risk of thromboembolism (DVT, PE) and superficial thrombophlebitis; risk is similar to reported risk of HRT

>10%:

Cardiovascular: Hot flashes

Neuromuscular & skeletal: Arthralgia

Respiratory: Sinusitis

Miscellaneous: Flu syndrome, infection

1% to 10%:

Cardiovascular: Chest pain

Central nervous system: Fever, migraine, depression, insomnia

Dermatologic: Rash, diaphoresis

Endocrine & metabolic: Peripheral edema

Gastrointestinal: Nausea, dyspepsia, vomiting, flatulence, GI disorder, gastroenteritis, weight gain

Genitourinary: Urinary tract infection, vaginitis, cystitis, leukorrhea, endometrial disorder

Neuromuscular & skeletal: Myalgia, leg cramps, arthritis

Respiratory: Pharyngitis, cough, pneumonia, laryngitis

<1% (Limited to important or life-threatening): Hypertriglyceridemia, retinal vein occlusion (very rare)

Overdosage/Toxicology Incidence of overdose in humans has not been reported. In an 8-week study of postmenopausal women, a dose of raloxifene 600 mg/day was safely tolerated. No mortality was seen after a single oral dose in rats or mice (at 810 times the human dose for rats and 405 times the human dose for mice). There is no specific antidote for raloxifene.

Drug Interactions

Increased Effect/Toxicity: Raloxifene has the potential to interact with highly protein-bound drugs (increase effects of either agent). Use caution with highly protein-bound drugs, warfarin, clofibrate, indomethacin, naproxen, ibuprofen, diazepam, phenytoin, or tamoxifen.

Decreased Effect: Ampicillin and cholestyramine reduce raloxifene absorption/blood levels.

Mechanism of Action A selective estrogen receptor modulator, meaning that it affects some of the same receptors that estrogen does, but not all, and in some instances, it antagonizes or blocks estrogen; it acts like estrogen to prevent bone loss and improve lipid profiles (decreases total and LDL cholesterol but does not raise triglycerides), but it has the potential to block some estrogen effects such as those that lead to breast cancer and uterine cancer

Pharmacodynamics/Kinetics

Onset of action: 8 weeks

Distribution: 2348 L/kg

Protein binding: >95% to albumin and α-glycoprotein

Metabolism: Extensive first-pass effect

Bioavailability: ~2%

Half-life elimination: 27.7-32.5 hours

Excretion: Primarily feces; urine (0.2%)

Usual Dosage Adults: Female: Oral: 60 mg/day which may be administered any time of the day without regard to meals

Monitoring Parameters Radiologic evaluation of bone mineral density (BMD) is the best measure of the treatment of osteoporosis; to monitor for the potential toxicities of raloxifene, complete blood counts should be evaluated periodically.

Additional Information The decrease in estrogen-related adverse effects with the selective estrogen-receptor modulators in general and raloxifene in particular should improve compliance and decrease the incidence of cardiovascular events and fractures while not increasing breast cancer.

Dosage Forms Tablet, as hydrochloride: 60 mg

♦ **Raloxifene Hydrochloride** *see* Raloxifene *on page 1176*

Ramipril (ra MI pril)

Related Information

Angiotensin Agents Comparison *on page 1473*
Heart Failure *on page 1663*

U.S. Brand Names Altace®

Canadian Brand Names Altace®

Therapeutic Category Angiotensin-Converting Enzyme (ACE) Inhibitor; Antihypertensive Agent

Use Treatment of hypertension, alone or in combination with thiazide diuretics; treatment of congestive heart failure; treatment of left ventricular dysfunction after myocardial infarction; to reduce risk of heart attack, stroke, and death in patients at increased risk for these problems

Pregnancy Risk Factor C/D (2nd and 3rd trimesters)

Contraindications Hypersensitivity to ramipril or any component of the formulation; angioedema related to previous treatment with an ACE inhibitor; bilateral renal artery stenosis; primary hyperaldosteronism; pregnancy (2nd and 3rd trimesters)

Warnings/Precautions Anaphylactic or anaphylactoid reactions can occur. Use with caution and modify dosage in patients with renal impairment (especially renal artery stenosis), severe congestive heart failure. Severe hypotension may occur in the elderly and patients who are sodium and/or volume depleted, initiate lower doses and monitor closely when starting therapy in these patients. Should be discontinued if laryngeal stridor or angioedema of the face, tongue, or glottis is observed. Angioedema can occur at any time during treatment (especially following first dose). Careful blood pressure monitoring with first dose (hypotension can occur especially in volume depleted patients). Use with caution in hypovolemia; collagen vascular diseases; valvular stenosis (particularly aortic stenosis); hyperkalemia; or before, during, or immediately after anesthesia. Avoid rapid dosage escalation, which may lead to renal insufficiency. Neutropenia/agranulocytosis with myeloid hyperplasia can rarely occur. If patient has renal impairment then a baseline WBC with differential and serum creatinine should be evaluated and monitored closely during the first 3 months of therapy. Hypersensitivity reactions may be seen during hemodialysis with high-flux dialysis membranes (eg, AN69).

Adverse Reactions Note: Frequency ranges include data from hypertension and heart failure trials. Higher rates of adverse reactions have generally been noted in patients with congestive heart failure. However, the frequency of adverse effects associated with placebo is also increased in this population.

>10%: Respiratory: Cough (increased) (7% to 12%)

1% to 10%:
  Cardiovascular: Hypotension (11%), angina (3%), postural hypotension (2%), syncope (2%)
  Central nervous system: Headache (1% to 5%), dizziness (2% to 4%), fatigue (2%), vertigo (2%)
  Endocrine & metabolic: Hyperkalemia (1% to 10%)
  Gastrointestinal: Nausea/vomiting (1% to 2%)
  Neuromuscular & skeletal: Chest pain (noncardiac) (1%)
  Renal: Renal dysfunction (1%), elevation in serum creatinine (1% to 2%), increased BUN (<1% to 3%); transient elevations of creatinine and/or BUN may occur more frequently
  Respiratory: Cough (estimated 1% to 10%)

<1% (Limited to important or life-threatening): Agitation, amnesia, anaphylactoid reaction, angina, angioedema, arrhythmia, convulsions, depression, dysphagia, dyspnea, edema, eosinophilia, erythema multiforme, hearing loss, hemolytic anemia, hepatitis, hypersensitivity reactions (urticaria, rash, fever), impotence, insomnia, myalgia, myocardial infarction, neuropathy, pancreatitis, pancytopenia, paresthesia, pemphigus, photosensitivity, proteinuria, somnolence, symptomatic hypotension, syncope, thrombocytopenia, vertigo

Worsening of renal function may occur in patients with bilateral renal artery stenosis or in hypovolemia. In addition, a syndrome which may include fever, myalgia, arthralgia, interstitial nephritis, vasculitis, rash, eosinophilia and positive ANA, and elevated ESR has been reported with ACE inhibitors. Pancreatitis and agranulocytosis (particularly in patients with collagen vascular disease or renal impairment) have been associated with ACE inhibitors.

Overdosage/Toxicology Mild hypotension has been the only toxic effect seen with acute overdose; bradycardia may also occur. Mild hyperkalemia may occur even with therapeutic doses, especially in patients with renal insufficiency and those taking NSAIDs. Following initiation of essential overdose management, toxic symptom and supportive treatment should be initiated. Hypotension usually responds to I.V. fluids or Trendelenburg positioning.

Drug Interactions

Increased Effect/Toxicity: Potassium supplements, co-trimoxazole (high dose), angiotensin II receptor antagonists (candesartan, losartan, irbesartan, etc), or potassium-sparing diuretics (amiloride, spironolactone, triamterene) may result in elevated serum potassium levels when combined with ramipril. ACE inhibitor effects may be increased by phenothiazines or probenecid (increases levels of captopril). ACE inhibitors may increase serum concentrations/effects of digoxin, lithium, and sulfonylureas.

Diuretics have additive hypotensive effects with ACE inhibitors, and hypovolemia increases the potential for adverse renal effects of ACE inhibitors. In patients with compromised renal function, coadministration with nonsteroidal anti-inflammatory drugs may result in further deterioration of renal function. Allopurinol and ACE inhibitors may cause a higher risk of hypersensitivity reaction when taken concurrently.

Decreased Effect: Aspirin (high dose) may reduce the therapeutic effects of ACE inhibitors; at low dosages this does not appear to be significant. Rifampin may decrease the effect of ACE inhibitors. Antacids may decrease the bioavailability of ACE inhibitors (may be more likely to occur with captopril); separate administration times by 1-2 hours. NSAIDs, specifically indomethacin, may reduce the hypotensive effects of ACE inhibitors. More likely to occur in low renin or volume dependent hypertensive patients.

Ethanol/Nutrition/Herb Interactions Herb/Nutraceutical: Avoid dong quai if using for hypertension (has estrogenic activity). Avoid ephedra, yohimbe, ginseng (may worsen hypertension). Avoid garlic (may have increased antihypertensive effect).

(Continued)

Ramipril (Continued)

Stability Stable for 24 hours at room temperature or 48 hours under refrigeration.

Mechanism of Action Ramipril is an angiotensin-converting enzyme (ACE) inhibitor which prevents the formation of angiotensin II from angiotensin I and exhibits pharmacologic effects that are similar to captopril. Ramipril must undergo enzymatic saponification by esterases in the liver to its biologically active metabolite, ramiprilat. The pharmacodynamic effects of ramipril result from the high-affinity, competitive, reversible binding of ramiprilat to angiotensin-converting enzyme thus preventing the formation of the potent vasoconstrictor angiotensin II. This isomerized enzyme-inhibitor complex has a slow rate of dissociation, which results in high potency and a long duration of action; a CNS mechanism may also be involved in the hypotensive effect as angiotensin II increases adrenergic outflow from CNS; vasoactive kallikreins may be decreased in conversion to active hormones by ACE inhibitors, thus reducing blood pressure

Pharmacodynamics/Kinetics

Onset of action: 1-2 hours

Duration: 24 hours

Absorption: Well absorbed (50% to 60%)

Distribution: Plasma levels decline in a triphasic fashion; rapid decline is a distribution phase to peripheral compartment, plasma protein and tissue ACE (half-life 2-4 hours); 2nd phase is an apparent elimination phase representing the clearance of free ramiprilat (half-life: 9-18 hours); and final phase is the terminal elimination phase representing the equilibrium phase between tissue binding and dissociation

Metabolism: Hepatic to the active form, ramiprilat

Half-life elimination: Ramiprilat: Effective: 13-17 hours; Terminal: >50 hours

Time to peak, serum: ~1 hour

Excretion: Urine (60%) and feces (40%) as parent drug and metabolites

Usual Dosage Adults: Oral:

Hypertension: 2.5-5 mg once daily, maximum: 20 mg/day

Reduction in risk of MI, stroke, and death from cardiovascular causes: Initial: 2.5 mg once daily for 1 week, then 5 mg once daily for the next 3 weeks, then increase as tolerated to 10 mg once daily (may be given as divided dose)

Heart failure postmyocardial infarction: Initial: 2.5 mg twice daily titrated upward, if possible, to 5 mg twice daily.

Note: The dose of any concomitant diuretic should be reduced. If the diuretic cannot be discontinued, initiate therapy with 1.25 mg. After the initial dose, the patient should be monitored carefully until blood pressure has stabilized.

Dosing adjustment in renal impairment:

Cl_{cr} <40 mL/minute: Administer 25% of normal dose.

Renal failure and hypertension: Administer 1.25 mg once daily, titrated upward as possible.

Renal failure and heart failure: Administer 1.25 mg once daily, increasing to 1.25 mg twice daily up to 2.5 mg twice daily as tolerated.

Test Interactions Increases BUN, creatinine, potassium, positive Coombs' [direct]; decreases cholesterol (S); may cause false-positive results in urine acetone determinations using sodium nitroprusside reagent

Patient Information Notify physician if vomiting, diarrhea, excessive perspiration, or dehydration should occur; also if sore throat, fever, swelling of face, lips, tongue, or difficulty in breathing occurs or if persistent cough develops; may cause lightheadedness during first few days of therapy; if a cough develops which is bothersome, consult a physician. Capsule is usually swallowed whole but may be sprinkled on applesauce or mixed in water or juice.

Nursing Implications May cause depression in some patients; discontinue if angioedema of the face, extremities, lips, tongue, or glottis occurs; watch for hypotensive effects within 1-3 hours of first dose or new higher dose; may be mixed in water, apple juice, or applesauce and will remain stable for 48 hours if refrigerated or 24 hours at room temperature

Dosage Forms Capsule: 1.25 mg, 2.5 mg, 5 mg, 10 mg

Ranitidine (ra NI ti deen)

Related Information

Antacid Drug Interactions on page 1477

U.S. Brand Names Zantac®; Zantac® 75 [OTC]

Canadian Brand Names Alti-Ranitidine; Apo®-Ranitidine; Gen-Ranidine; Novo-Ranidine; Nu-Ranit; Scheinpharm™ Ranitidine; Zantac®; Zantac 75®

Synonyms Ranitidine Hydrochloride

Therapeutic Category Antihistamine, H_2 Blocker; Histamine H_2 Antagonist

Use

Zantac®: Short-term and maintenance therapy of duodenal ulcer, gastric ulcer, gastroesophageal reflux, active benign ulcer, erosive esophagitis, and pathological hypersecretory conditions; as part of a multidrug regimen for H. pylori eradication to reduce the risk of duodenal ulcer recurrence

Zantac® 75 [OTC]: Relief of heartburn, acid indigestion, and sour stomach

Unlabeled/Investigational Use Recurrent postoperative ulcer, upper GI bleeding, prevention of acid-aspiration pneumonitis during surgery, and prevention of stress-induced ulcers

Pregnancy Risk Factor B

Pregnancy/Breast-Feeding Implications Ranitidine crosses the placenta, teratogenic effects to the fetus have not been reported. Use with caution during pregnancy.

Contraindications Hypersensitivity to ranitidine or any component of the formulation

Warnings/Precautions Use with caution in patients with hepatic impairment; use with caution in renal impairment, dosage modification required; avoid use in patients with history of acute porphyria (may precipitate attacks); long-term therapy may be associated with vitamin B_{12} deficiency; EFFERdose® formulations contain phenylalanine; safety and efficacy have not been established for pediatric patients <1 month of age

Adverse Reactions Frequency not defined (limited to important or life-threatening):

Cardiovascular: Arrhythmias, vasculitis

Central nervous system: Dizziness, hallucinations, headache, mental confusion, somnolence, vertigo

Dermatologic: Erythema multiforme, rash

Gastrointestinal: Pancreatitis

Hematologic: Acquired hemolytic anemia, agranulocytosis, aplastic anemia, granulocytopenia, leukopenia, pancytopenia, thrombocytopenia

Hepatic: Hepatic failure

Miscellaneous: Anaphylaxis, hypersensitivity reactions

Overdosage/Toxicology Symptoms include abnormal gait, hypotension, and adverse effects seen with normal use. Treatment is primarily symptomatic and supportive.

Drug Interactions

Cytochrome P450 Effect: CYP2D6 and 3A3/4 enzyme inhibitor

Increased Effect/Toxicity: Increased the effect/toxicity of cyclosporine (increased serum creatinine), gentamicin (neuromuscular blockade), glipizide, glyburide, midazolam (increased concentrations), metoprolol, pentoxifylline, phenytoin, quinidine, and triazolam.

Decreased Effect:

Decreased effect: Variable effects on warfarin; antacids may decrease absorption of ranitidine; ketoconazole and itraconazole absorptions are decreased; may produce altered serum levels of procainamide and ferrous sulfate; decreased effect of nondepolarizing muscle relaxants, cefpodoxime, cyanocobalamin (decreased absorption), diazepam, oxaprozin

Decreased toxicity of atropine

Ethanol/Nutrition/Herb Interactions

Ethanol: Avoid ethanol (may cause gastric mucosal irritation).

Food: Does not interfere with absorption of ranitidine.

Stability

Injection: Vials: Store between 4°C to 30°C (39°F to 86°F); protect from light; solution is a clear, colorless to yellow solution; slight darkening does not affect potency

Premixed bag: Store between 2°C to 25°C (36°F to 77°F); protect from light

EFFERdose® formulations: Store between 2°C to 30°C (36°F to 86°F)

Syrup: Store between 4°C to 25°C (39°F to 77°F); protect from light

Tablet: Store in dry place, between 15°C to 30°C (59°F to 86°F); protect from light

Vials can be mixed with NS or D_5W; solutions are stable for 48 hours at room temperature

Intermittent bolus injection: Dilute to maximum of 2.5 mg/mL

Intermittent infusion: Dilute to maximum of 0.5 mg/mL

Do not add other medications to premixed bag

Mechanism of Action Competitive inhibition of histamine at H_2-receptors of the gastric parietal cells, which inhibits gastric acid secretion, gastric volume, and hydrogen ion concentration are reduced. Does not affect pepsin secretion, pentagastrin-stimulated intrinsic factor secretion, or serum gastrin.

Pharmacodynamics/Kinetics

Absorption: Oral: 50%

Distribution: Normal renal function: V_d: 1.7 L/kg; Cl_{cr} 25-35 mL/minute: 1.76 L/kg minimally penetrates the blood-brain barrier; enters breast milk

Protein binding: 15%

Metabolism: Hepatic; to N-oxide, S-oxide, and N-desmethyl metabolites

Bioavailability: Oral: 48%

Half-life elimination:

Oral: Normal renal function: 2.5-3 hours; Cl_{cr} 25-35 mL/minute: 4.8 hours

I.V.: Normal renal function: 2-2.5 hours

Time to peak, serum: Oral: 2-3 hours; I.M.: ≤15 minutes

Excretion: Urine: Oral: 30%, I.V.: 70% as unchanged drug; feces (as metabolites)

Usual Dosage

Children 1 month to 16 years:

Duodenal and gastric ulcer:

Oral:

Treatment: 2-4 mg/kg/day divided twice daily; maximum treatment dose: 300 mg/day

Maintenance: 2-4 mg/kg once daily; maximum maintenance dose: 150 mg/day

I.V.: 2-4 mg/kg/day divided every 6-8 hours; maximum: 150 mg/day

GERD and erosive esophagitis:

Oral: 5-10 mg/kg/day divided twice daily; maximum: GERD: 300 mg/day, erosive esophagitis: 600 mg/day

I.V.: 2-4 mg/kg/day divided every 6-8 hours; maximum: 150 mg/day **or as an alternative**

Continuous infusion: Initial: 1 mg/kg/dose for one dose followed by infusion of 0.08-0.17 mg/kg/hour or 2-4 mg/kg/day

Children ≥12 years: Prevention of heartburn: Oral: Zantac® 75 [OTC]: 75 mg 30-60 minutes before eating food or drinking beverages which cause heartburn; maximum: 150 mg/24 hours; do not use for more than 14 days

Adults:

Duodenal ulcer: Oral: Treatment: 150 mg twice daily, or 300 mg once daily after the evening meal or at bedtime; maintenance: 150 mg once daily at bedtime

Helicobacter pylori eradication: 150 mg twice daily; requires combination therapy

Pathological hypersecretory conditions:

Oral: 150 mg twice daily; adjust dose or frequency as clinically indicated; doses of up to 6 g/day have been used

I.V.: Continuous infusion for Zollinger-Ellison: 1 mg/kg/hour; measure gastric acid output at 4 hours, if >10 mEq or if patient is symptomatic, increase dose in increments of 0.5 mg/kg/hour; doses of up to 2.5 mg/kg/hour have been used

Gastric ulcer, benign: Oral: 150 mg twice daily; maintenance: 150 mg once daily at bedtime

Erosive esophagitis: Oral: Treatment: 150 mg 4 times/day; maintenance: 150 mg twice daily

(Continued)

Ranitidine *(Continued)*

Prevention of heartburn: Oral: Zantac® 75 [OTC]: 75 mg 30-60 minutes before eating food or drinking beverages which cause heartburn; maximum: 150 mg in 24 hours; do not use for more than 14 days

Patients not able to take oral medication:
I.M.: 50 mg every 6-8 hours
I.V.: Intermittent bolus or infusion: 50 mg every 6-8 hours
Continuous I.V. infusion: 6.25 mg/hour

Elderly: Ulcer healing rates and incidence of adverse effects are similar in the elderly, when compared to younger patients; dosing adjustments not necessary based on age alone

Dosing adjustment in renal impairment: Adults: Cl_{cr} <50 mL/minute: 150 mg every 24 hours; adjust dose cautiously if needed

Hemodialysis: Adjust dosing schedule so that dose coincides with the end of hemodialysis

Dosing adjustment/comments in hepatic disease: Patients with hepatic impairment may have minor changes in ranitidine half-life, distribution, clearance, and bioavailability; dosing adjustments not necessary, monitor

Dietary Considerations Oral dosage forms may be taken with or without food.

Administration

Ranitidine injection may be administered I.M. or I.V.:
I.M.: Injection is administered undiluted
I.V.: Must be diluted; may be administered IVP or IVPB or continuous I.V. infusion
IVP: Ranitidine (usually 50 mg) should be diluted to a total of 20 mL with NS or D_5W and administered over at least 5 minutes
IVPB: Administer over 15-20 minutes
Continuous I.V. infusion: Administer at 6.25 mg/hour and titrate dosage based on gastric pH by continuous infusion over 24 hours

EFFERdose® formulations: Dissolve each dose in 6-8 ounces of water before drinking

Monitoring Parameters AST, ALT, serum creatinine; when used to prevent stress-related GI bleeding, measure the intragastric pH and try to maintain pH >4; signs and symptoms of peptic ulcer disease, occult blood with GI bleeding, monitor renal function to correct dose; monitor for side effects

Test Interactions False-positive urine protein using Multistix®, gastric acid secretion test, skin test allergen extracts, serum creatinine, urine protein test

Patient Information It may take several days before this medicine begins to relieve stomach pain; antacids may be taken with ranitidine unless your physician has told you not to use them; wait 30-60 minutes between taking the antacid and ranitidine; may cause drowsiness, impair judgment, or coordination

Nursing Implications I.M. solution does not need to be diluted before use; monitor creatinine clearance for renal impairment; observe caution in patients with renal function impairment and hepatic function impairment

Dosage Forms

Granules, effervescent, as hydrochloride (EFFERdose®): 150 mg [contains 7.55 mEq sodium and 16.84 mg phenylalanine per 150 mg]

Infusion, as hydrochloride, in NaCl 0.45% [preservative free]: 1 mg/mL (50 mL)

Injection, as hydrochloride: 25 mg/mL (2 mL, 10 mL, 40 mL) [with phenol 0.5% as preservative]

Syrup, as hydrochloride: 15 mg/mL (473 mL) [contains 7.5% alcohol] [peppermint flavor]

Tablet, as hydrochloride: 75 mg [OTC]; 150 mg, 300 mg

Tablet, effervescent, as hydrochloride (EFFERdose®): 150 mg [contains 7.96 mEq sodium and 16.84 mg phenylalanine per 150 mg]

Ranitidine Bismuth Citrate *(ra NI ti deen BIZ muth SIT rate)*

Related Information
Helicobacter pylori Treatment *on page 1668*

U.S. Brand Names Tritec®

Canadian Brand Names Pylorid®

Synonyms GR1222311X; RBC

Therapeutic Category Antihistamine, H_2 Blocker; Histamine H_2 Antagonist

Use In combination with clarithromycin for the treatment of active duodenal ulcer associated with *H. pylori* infection; not to be used as monotherapy

Pregnancy Risk Factor C

Contraindications Hypersensitivity to ranitidine, bismuth compounds, or any component of the formulation; acute porphyria

Warnings/Precautions Avoid use in patients with Cl_{cr} <25 mL/minute; do not use for maintenance therapy or for >16 weeks/year

Adverse Reactions

>10%:
Central nervous system: Headache (14%)
Gastrointestinal: Darkening of the tongue and/or stool (60% to 70%), taste disturbance (11%)

>1%:
Central nervous system: Dizziness (1% to 2%)
Gastrointestinal: Diarrhea (5%), nausea/vomiting (3%), constipation (2%), abdominal pain, gastric upset (<10%)
Miscellaneous: Flu-like symptoms (2%)

<1% (Limited to important or life-threatening): Pruritus, rash, thrombocytopenia

Drug Interactions

Increased Effect/Toxicity: Refer to individual agents.

Decreased Effect: Refer to individual agents.

Ethanol/Nutrition/Herb Interactions Ethanol: Avoid ethanol (may cause gastric mucosal irritation).

Mechanism of Action As a complex of ranitidine and bismuth citrate, gastric acid secretion is inhibited by histamine-blocking activity at the parietal cell and the structural integrity of *H. pylori* organisms is disrupted; additionally bismuth reduces the adherence of *H. pylori* to epithelial cells of the stomach and may exert a cytoprotectant effect, inhibiting pepsin, as well. Adequate eradication of *H. pylori* is achieved with the combination of clarithromycin.

Pharmacodynamics/Kinetics See individual agents.

Absorption: Bismuth: Minimal systemic absorption (≤1%); Ranitidine: 50% to 60% (dose-dependent)

Distribution: Ranitidine: 1.7 L/kg

Protein binding: Bismuth: 90%; Ranitidine: 15%

Metabolism: Ranitidine: Metabolized to N-oxide, S-oxide, and N-desmethyl metabolites

Half-life elimination: Complex: 5-8 days; Bismuth: 11-28 days; Ranitidine: 3 hours

Time to peak, serum: Bismuth: 0.25-1 hour; Ranitidine: 0.5-5 hours; Time to peak effect of complex: 1 week

Excretion: Urine: Ranitidine (~30%); Bismuth (<1%)

Clearance: Ranitidine: 530 mL/minute; Bismuth: 50 mL/minute

Usual Dosage Adults: Oral: 400 mg twice daily for 4 weeks with clarithromycin 500 mg 2 times/day for first 2 week

Dosing adjustment in renal impairment: Not recommended with Cl$_{cr}$ <25 mL/minute

Dosing adjustment in hepatic impairment: No dosage change necessary

Note: Most patients not eradicated of *H. pylori* following an adequate course of therapy that includes clarithromycin will have clarithromycin-resistant isolates and should be treated with an alternative multiple drug regimen

Dietary Considerations May be taken without regard to food; however, optimal effects are seen when taken with food.

Monitoring Parameters (13) C-urea breath tests to detect *H. pylori*, endoscopic evidence of ulcer healing, CBCs, LFTs, renal function tests

Patient Information Inform your physician immediately if signs of allergy occur; take medication with food, if possible

Dosage Forms Tablet: 400 mg (ranitidine 162 mg, trivalent bismuth 128 mg, and citrate 110 mg)

◆ **Ranitidine Hydrochloride** *see* Ranitidine *on page 1178*

◆ **Rapamune**® *see* Sirolimus *on page 1240*

◆ **RBC** *see* Ranitidine Bismuth Citrate *on page 1180*

◆ **R & C**® **[OTC]** *see* Pyrethrins and Piperonyl Butoxide *on page 1160*

◆ **R & C**™ **II (Can)** *see* Pyrethrins and Piperonyl Butoxide *on page 1160*

◆ **R&C**® **Lice** *see* Permethrin *on page 1065*

◆ **R & C**™ **Shampoo/Conditioner (Can)** *see* Pyrethrins and Piperonyl Butoxide *on page 1160*

◆ **Reactine**™ **(Can)** *see* Cetirizine *on page 265*

◆ **Rea-Lo**® **[OTC]** *see* Urea *on page 1391*

◆ **Rebetol**® *see* Ribavirin *on page 1189*

◆ **Rebetron**™ *see* Interferon Alfa-2b and Ribavirin Combination Pack *on page 730*

◆ **Rebif**® *see* Interferon Beta-1a *on page 734*

◆ **Recombinant Hirudin** *see* Lepirudin *on page 779*

◆ **Recombinant Human Deoxyribonuclease** *see* Dornase Alfa *on page 437*

◆ **Recombinant Human Follicle Stimulating Hormone** *see* Follitropins *on page 596*

◆ **Recombinant Human Interleukin-11** *see* Oprelvekin *on page 1012*

◆ **Recombinant Human Platelet-Derived Growth Factor B** *see* Becaplermin *on page 148*

◆ **Recombinant Interleukin-11** *see* Oprelvekin *on page 1012*

◆ **Recombinant Plasminogen Activator** *see* Reteplase *on page 1186*

◆ **Recombinate**™ *see* Antihemophilic Factor (Recombinant) *on page 105*

◆ **Recombivax HB**® *see* Hepatitis B Vaccine *on page 662*

◆ **Recommendations of the Advisory Committee on Immunization Practices (ACIP)** *see page 1540*

◆ **Recommended Childhood Immunization Schedule - US - 2002** *see page 1539*

◆ **Recommended Immunization Schedule for HIV-Infected Children** *see page 1543*

◆ **Redutemp**® **[OTC]** *see* Acetaminophen *on page 22*

◆ **Reese's**® **Pinworm Medicine [OTC]** *see* Pyrantel Pamoate *on page 1159*

◆ **ReFacto**® *see* Antihemophilic Factor (Recombinant) *on page 105*

◆ **Refludan**® *see* Lepirudin *on page 779*

◆ **Regitine**® *see* Phentolamine *on page 1074*

◆ **Reglan**® *see* Metoclopramide *on page 900*

◆ **Regonol**® *see* Pyridostigmine *on page 1161*

◆ **Regranex**® *see* Becaplermin *on page 148*

◆ **Regular Iletin**® **II** *see* Insulin Preparations *on page 722*

◆ **Regulax SS**® **[OTC]** *see* Docusate *on page 430*

◆ **Regulex**® **(Can)** *see* Docusate *on page 430*

◆ **Reguloid**® **[OTC]** *see* Psyllium *on page 1158*

◆ **Rejuva-A**® **(Can)** *see* Tretinoin (Topical) *on page 1365*

◆ **Relafen**® *see* Nabumetone *on page 947*

◆ **Relenza**® *see* Zanamivir *on page 1434*

◆ **Relief**® **Ophthalmic** *see* Phenylephrine *on page 1075*

◆ **Remeron**® *see* Mirtazapine *on page 920*

◆ **Remeron**® **SolTab**™ *see* Mirtazapine *on page 920*

◆ **Remicade**® *see* Infliximab *on page 719*

Remifentanil (rem i FEN ta nil)

Related Information
Narcotic Agonists Comparison *on page 1506*

U.S. Brand Names Ultiva™

Canadian Brand Names Ultiva®

Synonyms GI87084B

Therapeutic Category Analgesic, Narcotic

Use Analgesic for use during general anesthesia for continued analgesia in children ≥2 years of age and adults

Restrictions C-II

Pregnancy Risk Factor C

Contraindications Not for intrathecal or epidural administration, due to the presence of glycine in the formulation; hypersensitivity to remifentanil, fentanyl, or fentanyl analogs, or any component of the formulation; interruption of an infusion will result in offset of effects within 5-10 minutes; the discontinuation of remifentanil infusion should be preceded by the establishment of adequate postoperative analgesia orders, especially for patients in whom postoperative pain is anticipated

Warnings/Precautions Remifentanil is not recommended as the sole agent in general anesthesia, because the loss of consciousness cannot be assured and due to the high incidence of apnea, hypotension, tachycardia and muscle rigidity; it should be administered by individuals specifically trained in the use of anesthetic agents and should not be used in diagnostic or therapeutic procedures outside the monitored anesthesia setting; resuscitative and intubation equipment should be readily available

Adverse Reactions
>10%: Gastrointestinal: Nausea, vomiting
1% to 10%:
Cardiovascular: Hypotension, bradycardia, tachycardia, hypertension
Central nervous system: Dizziness, headache, agitation, fever
Dermatologic: Pruritus
Ocular: Visual disturbances
Respiratory: Respiratory depression, apnea, hypoxia
Miscellaneous: Shivering, postoperative pain

Overdosage/Toxicology Symptoms include apnea, chest wall rigidity, seizures, hypoxemia, hypotension, and bradycardia. Treatment includes airway support, establishment of an I.V. line, administration of I.V. fluids and naloxone 2 mg I.V. (0.01 mg/kg for children) with repeat administration as needed up to a total of 10 mg. Glycopyrrolate or atropine may be useful for the treatment of bradycardia or hypotension.

Drug Interactions
Increased Effect/Toxicity: Additive effects with other CNS depressants.

Stability Stable for 24 hours at room temperature after reconstitution and further dilution to concentrations of 20-250 mcg/mL

Mechanism of Action Binds with stereospecific mu-opioid receptors at many sites within the CNS, increases pain threshold, alters pain reception, inhibits ascending pain pathways

Pharmacodynamics/Kinetics
Onset of action: I.V.: 1-3 minutes
Protein binding: 92%
Metabolism: Rapid by blood and tissue esterases
Half-life elimination (dose dependent): 10 minutes
Excretion: Urine

Usual Dosage I.V. continuous infusion:
Children ≥2 years: Per kg doses are the same as for adult patients
Adults:
During induction: 0.5-1 mcg/kg/minute
During maintenance:
With nitrous oxide (66%): 0.4 mcg/kg/minute (range: 0.1-2 mcg/kg/min)
With isoflurane: 0.25 mcg/kg/minute (range: 0.05-2 mcg/kg/min)
With propofol: 0.25 mcg/kg/minute (range: 0.05-2 mcg/kg/min)
Continuation as an analgesic in immediate postoperative period: 0.1 mcg/kg/minute (range: 0.025-0.2 mcg/kg/min)
Elderly: Elderly patients have an increased sensitivity to effect of remifentanil, doses should be decreased by ¹/₂ and titrated

Administration Inject slowly over 3-5 minutes. For final concentration of 50 mcg/mL, may dilute 1 mg in 20 mL, 2 mg in 40 mL, or 5 mg in 100 mL; for final concentration of 25 mcg/mL, dilute 1 mg in 40 mL or 2 mg in 80 mL.

Monitoring Parameters Respiratory and cardiovascular status, blood pressure, heart rate

Additional Information Ultra short-acting narcotic that is unique compared to other short-acting narcotics. This agent is not considered suitable as the sole agent for induction; remifentanil should be used in combination with other induction agents. Bolus doses are not recommended for sedation cases and in treatment of postoperative pain due to risk of respiratory depression and muscle rigidity. Due to remifentanil's short duration of action, when postoperative pain is anticipated, discontinuation of an infusion of remifentanil should be preceded by an adequate postoperative analgesic (ie, fentanyl, morphine).

Dosage Forms Powder for injection, lyophilized: 1 mg/3 mL vial, 2 mg/5 mL vial, 5 mg/10 mL vial

- **Reminyl**® *see Galantamine on page 616*
- **Renagel**® *see Sevelamer on page 1233*
- **Renedil**® **(Can)** *see Felodipine on page 547*
- **Renese**® *see Polythiazide on page 1104*
- **Renova**® *see Tretinoin (Topical) on page 1365*
- **Rentamine**® **[OTC]** *see Chlorpheniramine, Ephedrine, Phenylephrine, and Carbetapentane on page 262*
- **ReoPro**® *see Abciximab on page 17*

Repaglinide (re pa GLI nide)

Related Information
Diabetes Mellitus Treatment *on page 1657*
Hypoglycemic Drugs & Thiazolidinedione Information *on page 1502*

U.S. Brand Names Prandin®

Canadian Brand Names GlucoNorm®; Prandin®

Therapeutic Category Antidiabetic Agent, Miscellaneous; Hypoglycemic Agent, Oral; Meglitinide

Use Management of type 2 diabetes mellitus (noninsulin dependent, NIDDM)
An adjunct to diet and exercise to lower the blood glucose in patients with type 2 diabetes mellitus whose hyperglycemia cannot be controlled satisfactorily by diet and exercise alone
In combination with metformin to lower blood glucose in patients whose hyperglycemia cannot be controlled by exercise, diet and either agent alone

Pregnancy Risk Factor C

Pregnancy/Breast-Feeding Implications Clinical effects on the fetus: Safety in pregnant women has not been established. Use during pregnancy only if clearly needed. Abnormal blood glucose levels are associated with a higher incidence of congenital abnormalities. Insulin is the drug of choice for the control of diabetes mellitus during pregnancy. It is not known whether repaglinide is excreted in breast milk. Because the potential for hypoglycemia in nursing infants may exist, decide whether to discontinue repaglinide or discontinue breast-feeding. If repaglinide is discontinued and if diet alone is inadequate for controlling blood glucose, consider insulin therapy.

Contraindications Hypersensitivity to repaglinide or any component of the formulation; diabetic ketoacidosis, with or without coma (treat with insulin); type 1 diabetes (insulin dependent, IDDM)

Warnings/Precautions Use with caution in patients with hepatic or renal impairment. All oral hypoglycemic agents are capable of producing hypoglycemia. Proper patient selection, dosage, and instructions to the patients are important to avoid hypoglycemic episodes. It may be necessary to discontinue repaglinide and administer insulin if the patient is exposed to stress (fever, trauma, infection, surgery). Safety and efficacy have not been established in pediatric patients.

Adverse Reactions
>10%:
  Central nervous system: Headache (9% to 11%)
  Endocrine & metabolic: Hypoglycemia (16% to 31%)
1% to 10%:
  Cardiovascular: Chest pain (2% to 3%)
  Gastrointestinal: Nausea (3% to 5%), heartburn (2% to 4%), vomiting (2% to 3%) constipation (2% to 3%), diarrhea (4% to 5%), tooth disorder (<1% to 2%)
  Genitourinary: Urinary tract infection (2% to 3%)
  Neuromuscular & skeletal: Arthralgia (3% to 6%), back pain (5% to 6%), paresthesia (2% to 3%)
  Respiratory: Upper respiratory tract infection (10% to 16%), sinusitis (3% to 6%), rhinitis (3% to 7%), bronchitis (2% to 6%)
  Miscellaneous: Allergy (1% to 2%)
<1% (Limited to important or life-threatening): Alopecia, anaphylactoid reaction, hemolytic anemia, hepatic dysfunction (severe), leukopenia, liver function tests increased, pancreatitis, Stevens-Johnson syndrome, thrombocytopenia

Overdosage/Toxicology Symptoms include severe hypoglycemia, seizures, cerebral damage, tingling of lips and tongue, nausea, yawning, confusion, agitation, tachycardia, sweating, convulsions, stupor, and coma. Intoxications are best managed with glucose administration (oral for milder hypoglycemia or by injection in more severe forms) and symptomatic management.

Drug Interactions
Cytochrome P450 Effect: CYP2C9 and CYP3A3/4 enzyme substrate
Increased Effect/Toxicity: Agents that inhibit CYP3A3/4 (eg, ketoconazole, miconazole, erythromycin) may increase repaglinide concentrations. The effect of repaglinide may be potentiated when given concomitantly with other highly protein-bound drugs (ie, phenylbutazone, oral anticoagulants, hydantoins, salicylates, NSAIDs, sulfonamides). Concurrent use of other hypoglycemic agents may increase risk of hypoglycemia.
Decreased Effect: Drugs which induce cytochrome P450 isoenzyme 3A4 may increase metabolism of repaglinide (phenytoin, rifampin, barbiturates, carbamazepine). Certain drugs (thiazides, diuretics, corticosteroids, phenothiazines, thyroid products, estrogens, oral contraceptives, phenytoin, nicotinic acid, sympathomimetics, calcium channel blockers, isoniazid) tend to produce hyperglycemia and may lead to loss of glycemic control.

Ethanol/Nutrition/Herb Interactions
Ethanol: Avoid ethanol (may cause hypoglycemia).
Food: When given with food, the AUC of repaglinide is decreased.
Herb/Nutraceutical: St John's wort may decrease repaglinide levels. Avoid gymnema, garlic (may cause hypoglycemia).

Stability Do not store above 25°C (77°F). Protect from moisture.

Mechanism of Action Nonsulfonylurea hypoglycemic agent of the meglitinide class (the nonsulfonylurea moiety of glyburide) used in the management of type 2 diabetes mellitus; stimulates insulin release from the pancreatic beta cells

Pharmacodynamics/Kinetics
Onset of action: Single dose: Increased insulin levels: ~15-60 minutes
Duration: 4-6 hours
Absorption: Rapidly and completely
Distribution: V_d: 31 L
Protein binding, plasma: >98%
(Continued)

Repaglinide *(Continued)*

Metabolism: Completely by oxidative biotransformation and direct conjugation with glucuronic acid. The CYP450 enzyme system (specifically 3A4) is involved in metabolism (inactive metabolites)

Bioavailability: Mean absolute: ~56%

Time to peak, plasma: ~1 hour

Excretion: Feces (~90%); ~8% within 96 hours

Usual Dosage Adults: Oral: Should be taken within 15 minutes of the meal, but time may vary from immediately preceding the meal to as long as 30 minutes before the meal

Initial: For patients not previously treated or whose Hb A_{1c} is <8%, the starting dose is 0.5 mg. For patients previously treated with blood glucose-lowering agents whose Hb A_{1c} is ≥8%, the initial dose is 1 or 2 mg before each meal.

Dose adjustment: Determine dosing adjustments by blood glucose response, usually fasting blood glucose. Double the preprandial dose up to 4 mg until satisfactory blood glucose response is achieved. At least 1 week should elapse to assess response after each dose adjustment.

Dose range: 0.5-4 mg taken with meals. Repaglinide may be dosed preprandial 2, 3 or 4 times/day in response to changes in the patient's meal pattern. Maximum recommended daily dose: 16 mg.

Patients receiving other oral hypoglycemic agents: When repaglinide is used to replace therapy with other oral hypoglycemic agents, it may be started the day after the final dose is given. Observe patients carefully for hypoglycemia because of potential overlapping of drug effects. When transferred from longer half-life sulfonylureas (eg, chlorpropamide), close monitoring may be indicated for up to ≥1 week.

Combination therapy: If repaglinide monotherapy does not result in adequate glycemic control, metformin may be added. Or, if metformin therapy does not provide adequate control, repaglinide may be added. The starting dose and dose adjustments for combination therapy are the same as repaglinide monotherapy. Carefully adjust the dose of each drug to determine the minimal dose required to achieve the desired pharmacologic effect. Failure to do so could result in an increase in the incidence of hypoglycemic episodes. Use appropriate monitoring of FPG and Hb A_{1c} measurements to ensure that the patient is not subjected to excessive drug exposure or increased probability of secondary drug failure. If glucose is not achieved after a suitable trial of combination therapy, consider discontinuing these drugs and using insulin.

Dosing adjustment in renal impairment:

Cl_{cr} 40-80 mL/minute (mild to moderate renal dysfunction): Initial dosage adjustment does not appear to be necessary.

Cl_{cr} 20-40 mL/minute: Initiate 0.5 mg with meals; titrate carefully.

Dosing adjustment in hepatic impairment: Use conservative initial and maintenance doses. Use longer intervals between dosage adjustments.

Dietary Considerations Administer repaglinide before meals. Dietary modification based on ADA recommendations is a part of therapy. May cause hypoglycemia. Must be able to recognize symptoms of hypoglycemia (palpitations, tachycardia, sweaty palms, diaphoresis, lightheadedness).

Monitoring Parameters Periodically monitor fasting blood glucose and glycosylated hemoglobin (Hb A_{1c}) levels with a goal of decreasing these levels towards the normal range. During dose adjustment, fasting glucose can be used to determine response.

Reference Range Target range: Adults:

Fasting blood glucose: <120 mg/dL

Glycosylated hemoglobin: <7%

Patient Information Inform patients about the importance of adherence to dietary instructions, of a regular exercise program, and of regular testing of blood glucose and Hb A_{1c}

Explain the risks of hypoglycemia, its symptoms and treatment, and conditions that predispose to its development and concomitant administration of other glucose-lowering drugs to patients and responsible family members

Instruct patients to take repaglinide before meals (2, 3, or 4 times/day preprandial). Doses are usually taken within 15 minutes of the meal, but time may vary from immediately preceding the meal to as long as 30 minutes before the meal. Instruct patients who skip a meal (or add an extra meal) to skip (or add) a dose for that meal.

Nursing Implications Patients who are anorexic or NPO, may need to have their dose held to avoid hypoglycemia

Dosage Forms Tablet: 0.5 mg, 1 mg, 2 mg

- **Repan®** *see* Butalbital Compound *on page 197*
- **Repronex®** *see* Menotropins *on page 857*
- **Requip®** *see* Ropinirole *on page 1211*
- **Rescriptor®** *see* Delavirdine *on page 371*
- **Rescula®** *see* Unoprostone *on page 1389*
- **Resectisol®** Irrigation Solution *see* Mannitol *on page 838*

Reserpine *(re SER peen)*

Related Information

Depression *on page 1655*

Hypertension *on page 1675*

U.S. Brand Names Serpalan®

Therapeutic Category Antihypertensive Agent; Rauwolfia Alkaloid

Use Management of mild to moderate hypertension

Unlabeled/Investigational Use Management of tardive dyskinesia, schizophrenia

Pregnancy Risk Factor C

Usual Dosage Note: When used for management of hypertension, full antihypertensive effects may take as long as 3 weeks.

Oral:
  Children: Hypertension: 0.01-0.02 mg/kg/24 hours divided every 12 hours; maximum dose: 0.25 mg/day (not recommended in children)
  Adults:
    Hypertension: 0.1-0.25 mg/day in 1-2 doses; initial: 0.5 mg/day for 1-2 weeks; maintenance: reduce to 0.1-0.25 mg/day;
    Tardive dyskinesia/schizophrenia: Initial: 0.5 mg/day; usual range: 0.1-1 mg
  Elderly: Initial: 0.05 mg once daily, increasing by 0.05 mg every week as necessary
  Dosing adjustment in renal impairment: Cl_{cr} <10 mL/minute: Avoid use
  Dialysis: Not removed by hemo or peritoneal dialysis; supplemental dose is not necessary
Additional Information Complete prescribing information for this medication should be consulted for additional detail.
Dosage Forms Tablet: 0.1 mg, 0.25 mg

- ♦ **Reserpine, Hydralazine, and Hydrochlorothiazide** *see* Hydralazine, Hydrochlorothiazide, and Reserpine *on page 673*
- ♦ **Respa-1st®** *see* Guaifenesin and Pseudoephedrine *on page 647*
- ♦ **Respa®-DM** *see* Guaifenesin and Dextromethorphan *on page 646*
- ♦ **Respa-GF®** *see* Guaifenesin *on page 645*
- ♦ **Respaire®-60 SR** *see* Guaifenesin and Pseudoephedrine *on page 647*
- ♦ **Respaire®-120 SR** *see* Guaifenesin and Pseudoephedrine *on page 647*
- ♦ **Respbid®** *see* Theophylline Salts *on page 1310*
- ♦ **RespiGam™** *see* Respiratory Syncytial Virus Immune Globulin (Intravenous) *on page 1185*

Respiratory Syncytial Virus Immune Globulin (Intravenous)
(RES peer rah tor ee sin SISH al VYE rus i MYUN GLOB yoo lin in tra VEE nus)

U.S. Brand Names RespiGam™

Synonyms RSV-IGIV

Therapeutic Category Immune Globulin

Use Orphan drug: Prevention of serious lower respiratory infection caused by respiratory syncytial virus (RSV) in children <24 months of age with bronchopulmonary dysplasia (BPD) or a history of premature birth (≤35 weeks gestation)

Pregnancy Risk Factor C

Contraindications Hypersensitivity to any component of the formulation; selective IgA deficiency; history of severe prior reaction to any immunoglobulin preparation

Warnings/Precautions Use caution to avoid fluid overload in patients, particularly infants with bronchopulmonary dysplasia (BPD), when administering RSV-IGIV; hypersensitivity including anaphylaxis or angioneurotic edema may occur; rare occurrences of aseptic meningitis syndrome have been associated with IGIV treatment, particularly with high doses; observe carefully for signs and symptoms of such and treat promptly

Adverse Reactions
1% to 10%:
  Cardiovascular: Tachycardia (1%), hypertension (1%), hypotension
  Central nervous system: Fever (6%)
  Dermatologic: Rash (1%)
  Endocrine & metabolic: Fluid overload (1%)
  Gastrointestinal: Vomiting (2%), diarrhea (1%), gastroenteritis (1%)
  Local: Injection site inflammation (1%)
  Respiratory: Respiratory distress (2%), wheezing (2%), rales, hypoxia (1%), tachypnea (1%)
<1% (Limited to important or life-threatening): Abdominal cramps, anxiety, arthralgia, chest tightness, cough, cyanosis, dizziness, dyspnea, eczema, edema, flushing, heart murmur, myalgia, pallor, palpitations, pruritus, rhinorrhea

Overdosage/Toxicology Likely symptoms of overdose include those associated with fluid overload. Treatment is supportive (eg, diuretics).

Stability Store between 2°C and 8°C; do not freeze or shake vial; avoid foaming; discard after single use since it is preservative free

Mechanism of Action RSV-IGIV is a sterile liquid immunoglobulin G containing neutralizing antibody to respiratory syncytial virus. It is effective in reducing the incidence and duration of RSV hospitalization and the severity of RSV illness in high risk infants.

Usual Dosage I.V.: 750 mg/kg/month according to the following infusion schedule:
  1.5 mL/kg/hour for 15 minutes, then at 3 mL/kg/hour for the next 15 minutes if the clinical condition does not contraindicate a higher rate, and finally, administer at 6 mL/kg/hour until completion of dose

Monitoring Parameters Monitor for symptoms of allergic reaction; check vital signs, cardiopulmonary status after each rate increase and thereafter at 30-minute intervals until 30 minutes following completion of the infusion

Nursing Implications Begin infusion within 6 hours and complete within 12 hours after entering vial. Observe for signs of intolerance during and after infusion; administer through an I.V. line using a constant infusion pump and through a separate I.V. line, if possible; if needed, RSV-IGIV may be "piggybacked" into dextrose with or without saline solutions, avoiding dilutions >2:1 with such line configurations. Filters are not necessary, but an in-line filter with a pore size >15 micrometers may be used.

Monitor vital signs frequently; adverse reactions may be related to the rate of administration; RSV-IGIV is made from human plasma and carries the possibility for transmission of bloodborne pathogenic agents

Additional Information Each vial contains 1 to 1.5 mEq sodium.

Dosage Forms Injection: RSV immunoglobulin 1000 mg/20 mL vial; RSV immunoglobulin 2500 mg/50 mL vial

- ♦ **Resporal®** *see* Dexbrompheniramine and Pseudoephedrine *on page 383*
- ♦ **Restall®** *see* HydrOXYzine *on page 691*
- ♦ **Restoril®** *see* Temazepam *on page 1292*

♦ **Retavase**® *see Reteplase on page 1186*

Reteplase (RE ta plase)

U.S. Brand Names Retavase®

Canadian Brand Names Retavase®

Synonyms Recombinant Plasminogen Activator; r-PA

Therapeutic Category Fibrinolytic Agent

Use Management of acute myocardial infarction (AMI); improvement of ventricular function; reduction of the incidence of CHF and the reduction of mortality following AMI

Pregnancy Risk Factor C

Contraindications Hypersensitivity to reteplase or any component of the formulation; active internal bleeding; history of cerebrovascular accident; recent intracranial or intraspinal surgery or trauma; intracranial neoplasm, arteriovenous malformations, or aneurysm; known bleeding diathesis; severe uncontrolled hypertension

Warnings/Precautions Concurrent heparin anticoagulation can contribute to bleeding; careful attention to all potential bleeding sites. I.M. injections and nonessential handling of the patient should be avoided. Venipunctures should be performed carefully and only when necessary. If arterial puncture is necessary, use an upper extremity vessel that can be manually compressed. If serious bleeding occurs then the infusion of anistreplase and heparin should be stopped.

For the following conditions the risk of bleeding is higher with use of reteplase and should be weighed against the benefits of therapy: recent major surgery (eg, CABG, obstetrical delivery, organ biopsy, previous puncture of noncompressible vessels), cerebrovascular disease, recent gastrointestinal or genitourinary bleeding, recent trauma including CPR, hypertension (systolic BP >180 mm Hg and/or diastolic BP >110 mm Hg), high likelihood of left heart thrombus (eg, mitral stenosis with atrial fibrillation), acute pericarditis, subacute bacterial endocarditis, hemostatic defects including ones caused by severe renal or hepatic dysfunction, significant hepatic dysfunction, pregnancy, diabetic hemorrhagic retinopathy or other hemorrhagic ophthalmic conditions, septic thrombophlebitis or occluded AV cannula at seriously infected site, advanced age (eg, >75 years), patients receiving oral anticoagulants, any other condition in which bleeding constitutes a significant hazard or would be particularly difficult to manage because of location.

Coronary thrombolysis may result in reperfusion arrhythmias. Follow standard MI management. Rare anaphylactic reactions can occur. Safety and efficacy in pediatric patients have not been established.

Adverse Reactions Bleeding is the most frequent adverse effect associated with reteplase. Heparin and aspirin have been administered concurrently with reteplase in clinical trials. The incidence of adverse events is a reflection of these combined therapies, and are comparable with comparison thrombolytics.

>10%: Local: Injection site bleeding (4.6% to 48.6%)

1% to 10%:
  Gastrointestinal: Bleeding (1.8% to 9.0%)
  Genitourinary: Bleeding (0.9% to 9.5%)
  Hematologic: Anemia (0.9% to 2.6%)

<1% (Limited to important or life-threatening): Allergic/anaphylactoid reactions, cholesterol embolization, intracranial hemorrhage (0.8%)

Other adverse effects noted are frequently associated with myocardial infarction (and therefore may or may not be attributable to Retavase®) and include arrhythmias, arrest, cardiac reinfarction, cardiogenic shock, embolism, hypotension, pericarditis, pulmonary edema, tamponade, thrombosis

Overdosage/Toxicology Symptoms include increased incidence of intracranial bleeding.

Drug Interactions

Increased Effect/Toxicity: The risk of bleeding associated with reteplase may be increased by oral anticoagulants (warfarin), heparin, low molecular weight heparins, and drugs which affect platelet function (eg, NSAIDs, dipyridamole, ticlopidine, clopidogrel, IIb/ IIIa antagonists). Concurrent use with aspirin and heparin may increase the risk of bleeding; however, aspirin and heparin were used concomitantly with reteplase in the majority of patients in clinical studies.

Decreased Effect: Aminocaproic acid (antifibrinolytic agent) may decrease effectiveness of thrombolytic agents.

Stability Dosage kits should be stored at 2°C to 25°C (36°F to 77°F) and remain sealed until use in order to protect from light

Mechanism of Action Reteplase is a nonglycosylated form of tPA produced by recombinant DNA technology using *E. coli*; it initiates local fibrinolysis by binding to fibrin in a thrombus (clot) and converts entrapped plasminogen to plasmin

Pharmacodynamics/Kinetics

Onset of action: Thrombolysis: 30-90 minutes

Half-life elimination: 13-16 minutes

Excretion: Feces and urine

Clearance: Plasma: 250-450 mL/minute

Usual Dosage

Children: Not recommended

Adults: 10 units I.V. over 2 minutes, followed by a second dose 30 minutes later of 10 units I.V. over 2 minutes

Withhold second dose if serious bleeding or anaphylaxis occurs

Administration Reteplase should be reconstituted using the diluent, syringe, needle and dispensing pin provided with each kit and the each reconstituted dose should be administered I.V. over 2 minutes; no other medication should be added to the injection solution

Monitoring Parameters Monitor for signs of bleeding (hematuria, GI bleeding, gingival bleeding)

Dosage Forms Powder for injection [preservative free] [with 2 mL diluent]: Each vial contains reteplase 10.4 units [equivalent to 18.1 mg reteplase]

- **Retin-A**® *see* Tretinoin (Topical) *on page 1365*
- **Retin-A**® **Micro** *see* Tretinoin (Topical) *on page 1365*
- **Retinoic Acid** *see* Tretinoin (Topical) *on page 1365*
- **Retinova**® **(Can)** *see* Tretinoin (Topical) *on page 1365*
- **Retrovir**® *see* Zidovudine *on page 1435*
- **Reversol**® *see* Edrophonium *on page 458*
- **Revex**® *see* Nalmefene *on page 953*
- **Rēv-Eyes**™ *see* Dapiprazole *on page 364*
- **ReVia**® *see* Naltrexone *on page 955*
- **Revitalose C-1000**® **(Can)** *see* Ascorbic Acid *on page 116*
- **rFSH-alpha** *see* Follitropins *on page 596*
- **rFSH-beta** *see* Follitropins *on page 596*
- **rFVIIa** *see* Factor VIIa (Recombinant) *on page 538*
- **R-Gene**® *see* Arginine *on page 114*
- **rGM-CSF** *see* Sargramostim *on page 1223*
- **r-hCG** *see* Chorionic Gonadotropin (Recombinant) *on page 289*
- **Rheomacrodex**® *see* Dextran *on page 386*
- **Rheumatrex**® *see* Methotrexate *on page 884*
- **rhFSH-alpha** *see* Follitropins *on page 596*
- **rhFSH-beta** *see* Follitropins *on page 596*
- **rhIL-11** *see* Oprelvekin *on page 1012*
- **Rhinalar**® **(Can)** *see* Flunisolide *on page 572*
- **Rhinall**® **Nasal [OTC]** *see* Phenylephrine *on page 1075*
- **Rhinatate**® *see* Chlorpheniramine, Pyrilamine, and Phenylephrine *on page 282*
- **Rhinocort**® *see* Budesonide *on page 186*
- **Rhinocort**® **Aqua**™ *see* Budesonide *on page 186*
- **Rhinocort**® **Turbuhaler**® **(Can)** *see* Budesonide *on page 186*
- **Rhinosyn**® **[OTC]** *see* Chlorpheniramine and Pseudoephedrine *on page 279*
- **Rhinosyn-DMX**® **[OTC]** *see* Guaifenesin and Dextromethorphan *on page 646*
- **Rhinosyn-PD**® **[OTC]** *see* Chlorpheniramine and Pseudoephedrine *on page 279*
- **Rhinosyn-X**® **Liquid [OTC]** *see* Guaifenesin, Pseudoephedrine, and Dextromethorphan *on page 648*
- **Rho-Clonazepam (Can)** *see* Clonazepam *on page 316*
- **Rhodacine**® **(Can)** *see* Indomethacin *on page 717*

Rh$_0$(D) Immune Globulin (Intramuscular)

(ar aych oh (dee) i MYUN GLOB yoo lin in tra MUS kue lar)

U.S. Brand Names BayRho-D®; BayRho-D® Mini-Dose; MICRhoGAM™; RhoGAM™

Therapeutic Category Immune Globulin

Use Prevention of isoimmunization in Rh-negative individuals exposed to Rh-positive blood during delivery of an Rh-positive infant, as a result of an abortion, following amniocentesis or abdominal trauma, or following a transfusion accident; prevention of hemolytic disease of the newborn if there is a subsequent pregnancy with an Rh-positive fetus

Pregnancy Risk Factor C

Contraindications Hypersensitivity to immune globulins or to thimerosal, or to any component of the formulation; Rh$_0$(D)-positive patient; transfusion of Rh$_0$(D)-positive blood in previous 3 months; prior sensitization to Rh$_0$(D)

Warnings/Precautions May cause anaphylactic reaction. Use with caution in patients with IgA deficiency; do not administer to neonates. As a product of human plasma, this product may potentially transmit disease; screening of donors, as well as testing and/or inactivation of certain viruses reduces this risk. Use caution in patients with thrombocytopenia or coagulation disorders (I.M. injections may be contraindicated). Not for intravenous administration.

Adverse Reactions <1% (Limited to important or life-threatening): Elevated bilirubin, lethargy, myalgia, pain at the injection site, splenomegaly, temperature elevation

Stability Reconstituted solution should be refrigerated and will remain stable for 30 days; solution that has been frozen should be discarded

Mechanism of Action Suppresses the immune response and antibody formation of Rh-negative individuals to Rh-positive red blood cells

Pharmacodynamics/Kinetics
Distribution: Enters breast milk; however, not absorbed by the nursing infant
Half-life elimination: 23-26 days

Usual Dosage Adults (administered I.M. to mothers **not** to infant) I.M.:
Obstetrical usage: 1 vial (300 mcg) prevents maternal sensitization if fetal packed red blood cell volume that has entered the circulation is <15 mL; if it is more, give additional vials. The number of vials = RBC volume of the calculated fetomaternal hemorrhage divided by 15 mL
Postpartum prophylaxis: 300 mcg within 72 hours of delivery
Antepartum prophylaxis: 300 mcg at approximately 26-28 weeks gestation; followed by 300 mcg within 72 hours of delivery if infant is Rh-positive
Following miscarriage, abortion, or termination of ectopic pregnancy at up to 13 weeks of gestation: 50 mcg ideally within 3 hours, but may be given up to 72 hours after; if pregnancy has been terminated at 13 or more weeks of gestation, administer 300 mcg

Administration Administer I.M. in deltoid muscle; do **not** administer I.V.; the total volume can be administered in divided doses at different sites at one time or may be divided and given at intervals, provided the total dosage is given within 72 hours of the fetomaternal hemorrhage or transfusion.

Patient Information Acetaminophen may be taken to ease minor discomfort after vaccination

Dosage Forms
Injection [single dose]: 300 mcg Rh$_0$(D) immune globulin
Injection [single dose of microdose]: 50 mcg Rh$_0$(D) immune globulin

Rho(D) Immune Globulin (Intravenous-Human)

(ar aych oh (dee) i MYUN GLOB yoo lin in tra VEE nus HYU man)

U.S. Brand Names WinRho SDF®

Canadian Brand Names WinRho SDF™

Synonyms RhoIGIV

Therapeutic Category Immune Globulin

Use

Prevention of Rh isoimmunization in nonsensitized Rho(D) antigen-negative women within 72 hours after spontaneous or induced abortion, amniocentesis, chorionic villus sampling, ruptured tubal pregnancy, abdominal trauma, transplacental hemorrhage, or in the normal course of pregnancy unless the blood type of the fetus or father is known to be Rho(D) antigen-negative.

Suppression of Rh isoimmunization in Rho(D) antigen-negative female children and female adults in their childbearing years transfused with Rho(D) antigen-positive RBCs or blood components containing Rho(D) antigen-positive RBCs

Orphan drug: Treatment of idiopathic thrombocytopenic purpura (ITP) in nonsplenectomized Rho(D) antigen-positive patients

Pregnancy Risk Factor C

Contraindications Hypersensitivity to immune globulin or any component of the formulation; IgA deficiency

Warnings/Precautions Anaphylactic hypersensitivity reactions can occur; studies indicate that there is no discernible risk of transmitting HIV or hepatitis B; do not administer by S.C. route; use only the I.V. route when treating ITP. Rho(D)-positive ITP patients should be monitored for signs and/or symptoms of intravascular hemolysis, clinically compromising anemia, and renal insufficiency

Adverse Reactions 1% to 10%:

Central nervous system: Headache (2%), fever (1%), chills (<2%)

Hematologic: Hemolysis (Hgb decrease of >2 g/dL in 5% to 10% of ITP patients)

Local: Slight edema and pain at the injection site

Overdosage/Toxicology Overdose symptoms are not likely, however, high doses have been associated with mild, transient hemolytic anemia. Treatment is supportive.

Stability Store at 2°C to 8°C; do not freeze; if not used immediately, store the product at room temperature for 4 hours; do not freeze the reconstituted product; use within 4 hours; discard unused portions

Mechanism of Action The Rho(D) antigen is responsible for most cases of Rh sensitization, which occurs when Rh-positive fetal RBCs enter the maternal circulation of an Rh-negative woman. Injection of anti-D globulin results in opsonization of the fetal RBCs, which are then phagocytized in the spleen, preventing immunization of the mother. Injection of anti-D into an Rh-positive patient with ITP coats the patient's own D-positive RBCs with antibody and, as they are cleared by the spleen, they saturate the capacity of the spleen to clear antibody-coated cells, sparing antibody-coated platelets. Other proposed mechanisms involve the generation of cytokines following the interaction between antibody-coated RBCs and macrophages.

Pharmacodynamics/Kinetics

Half-life elimination: I.V.: 24 days; I.M.: 30 days

Time to peak, serum: I.V.: 2 hours; I.M.: 5-10 days

Usual Dosage

Prevention of Rh isoimmunization: I.V.: 1500 units (300 mcg) at 28 weeks gestation or immediately after amniocentesis if before 34 weeks gestation or after chorionic villus sampling; repeat this dose every 12 weeks during the pregnancy. Administer 600 units (120 mcg) at delivery (within 72 hours) and after invasive intrauterine procedures such as abortion, amniocentesis, or any other manipulation if at >34 weeks gestation. **Note:** If the Rh status of the baby is not known at 72 hours, administer Rho(D) immune globulin to the mother at 72 hours after delivery. If >72 hours have elapsed, do not withhold Rho(D) immune globulin, but administer as soon as possible, up to 28 days after delivery.

I.M.: Reconstitute vial with 1.25 mL and administer as above

Transfusion: Administer within 72 hours after exposure for treatment of incompatible blood transfusions or massive fetal hemorrhage as follows:

I.V.: 3000 units (600 mcg) every 8 hours until the total dose is administered (45 units [9 mcg] of Rh-positive blood/mL blood; 90 units [18 mcg] Rh-positive red cells/mL cells)

I.M.: 6000 units [1200 mcg] every 12 hours until the total dose is administered (60 units [12 mcg] of Rh-positive blood/mL blood; 120 units [24 mcg] Rh-positive red cells/mL cells)

Treatment of ITP: I.V.: Initial: 25-50 mcg/kg depending on the patient's Hgb concentration; maintenance: 25-60 mcg/kg depending on the clinical response

Administration The product should not be shaken when reconstituting or transporting; reconstitute the product shortly before use with NS, according to the manufacturer's guidelines; do not administer with other products

Nursing Implications Pretreatment with acetaminophen, diphenhydramine, or prednisone can prevent the fever/chill reaction; increasing the time of infusion from 1-3 minutes to 15-20 minutes may also help

Additional Information Rho(D) is IgA-depleted and is unlikely to cause an anaphylactic reaction in women with IgA deficiency and anti-IgA antibodies. Although immune globulins for I.M. use, manufactured in the U.S. have never been found to transmit any viral infection, Rho(D) is the only Rho(D) preparation treated with highly effective solvent detergent method of viral inactivation for hepatitis C, HIV, and hepatitis B; treatment of ITP in Rh-positive patients with an intact spleen appears to be about as effective as IVIG.

Dosage Forms Injection [with 2.5 mL diluent]: 600 units [120 mcg]; 1500 units [300 mcg]

♦ **Rhodis™ (Can)** see Ketoprofen on page 763

♦ **Rhodis-EC™ (Can)** see Ketoprofen on page 763

- **Rhodis SR™ (Can)** *see* Ketoprofen *on page 763*
- **Rho®-Fluphenazine Decanoate (Can)** *see* Fluphenazine *on page 581*
- **RhoGAM™** *see* Rh₀(D) Immune Globulin (Intramuscular) *on page 1187*
- **Rho®-Haloperidol Decanoate (Can)** *see* Haloperidol *on page 654*
- **RholGIV** *see* Rh₀(D) Immune Globulin (Intravenous-Human) *on page 1188*
- **Rho®-Loperamine (Can)** *see* Loperamide *on page 816*
- **Rho®-Metformin (Can)** *see* Metformin *on page 875*
- **Rho®-Sotalol (Can)** *see* Sotalol *on page 1252*
- **Rhotral (Can)** *see* Acebutolol *on page 21*
- **Rhotrimine® (Can)** *see* Trimipramine *on page 1378*
- **Rhoxal-atenolol (Can)** *see* Atenolol *on page 125*
- **Rhoxal-diltiazem SR (Can)** *see* Diltiazem *on page 409*
- **Rhoxal-famotidine (Can)** *see* Famotidine *on page 543*
- **Rhoxal-fluoxetine (Can)** *see* Fluoxetine *on page 578*
- **Rhoxal-minocycline (Can)** *see* Minocycline *on page 918*
- **Rhoxal-orphenadrine (Can)** *see* Orphenadrine *on page 1014*
- **Rhoxal-ticlopidine (Can)** *see* Ticlopidine *on page 1331*
- **Rhoxal-valproic (Can)** *see* Valproic Acid and Derivatives *on page 1398*
- **rHuEPO-α** *see* Epoetin Alfa *on page 474*

Ribavirin (rye ba VYE rin)

U.S. Brand Names Rebetol®; Virazole® Aerosol

Canadian Brand Names Virazole™

Synonyms RTCA; Tribavirin

Therapeutic Category Antiviral Agent, Hepatitis; Antiviral Agent, Inhalation Therapy; Antiviral Agent, Nonantiretroviral

Use

Inhalation: Treatment of patients with respiratory syncytial virus (RSV) infections; may also be used in other viral infections including influenza A and B and adenovirus; specially indicated for treatment of severe lower respiratory tract RSV infections in patients with an underlying compromising condition (prematurity, bronchopulmonary dysplasia and other chronic lung conditions, congenital heart disease, immunodeficiency, immunosuppression), and recent transplant recipients

Oral capsules: The combination therapy of oral ribavirin with interferon alfa-2b, recombinant (Intron® A) injection is indicated for the treatment of chronic hepatitis C in patients with compensated liver disease who have relapsed after alpha interferon therapy or were previously untreated with alpha interferons

Unlabeled/Investigational Use Treatment of West Nile virus; hemorrhagic fever virus infections with renal syndrome (Lassa, Venezuelan, Korean hemorrhagic fever, Sabia, Argentian hemorrhagic fever, Bolivian hemorrhagic fever, Junin, Machupa)

Pregnancy Risk Factor X

Pregnancy/Breast-Feeding Implications Produced significant embryocidal and/or teratogenic effects in all animal studies at ~0.01 times the maximum recommended daily human dose. Use is contraindicated in pregnancy. May cause birth defects and/or death of the exposed fetus. Avoid pregnancy during therapy and for 6 months after completion of therapy in female patients and in female partners of male patients. If pregnancy occurs during use or within 6 months after treatment, report to company (800-727-7064).

Contraindications Hypersensitivity to ribavirin or any component of the formulation; women of childbearing age who will not use contraception reliably; pregnancy

Additional contraindications for oral formulation: Male partners of pregnant women; Cl_cr< 50 mL/minute; hemoglobinopathies (eg, thalassemia major, sickle cell anemia); as monotherapy for treatment of chronic hepatitis C; patients with autoimmune hepatitis, anemia, severe heart disease

Warnings/Precautions

Inhalation: Use with caution in patients requiring assisted ventilation or who have COPD or asthma. Monitor for anemia 1-2 weeks post-treatment. Pregnant healthcare workers may consider unnecessary occupational exposure. Healthcare professions or family members who are pregnant or may become pregnant should be counseled about potential risks of exposure and counseled about risk reduction strategies.

Oral: Monitor for anemia 1-2 weeks after initiation. Use caution in cardiac, pulmonary, and elderly patients. Severe psychiatric events have occurred during combination therapy; avoid use in patients with a psychiatric history. Negative pregnancy test required before initiation and monthly thereafter. Avoid pregnancy in female patients and female partners of patients during therapy by using two effective forms of birth control. Continue birth control measures for at least 6 months after completion of therapy. If patient or female partner becomes pregnant during treatment, she should be counseled about risks. Discontinue therapy in suspected/confirmed pancreatitis. Take renal function into consideration before initiating. Safety and efficacy not established in organ transplant patients, decompensated liver disease, concurrent hepatitis B virus or HIV exposure or pediatric patients.

Adverse Reactions

Inhalation:

1% to 10%:

Central nervous system: Fatigue, headache, insomnia

Gastrointestinal: Nausea, anorexia

Hematologic: Anemia

<1%: Apnea, bronchospasm, cardiac arrest, conjunctivitis, digitalis toxicity, hypotension, mild worsening of respiratory function

Note: Incidence of adverse effects (approximate) in healthcare workers: Headache (51%); conjunctivitis (32%); rhinitis, nausea, rash, dizziness, pharyngitis, and lacrimation (10% to 20%)

(Continued)

Ribavirin *(Continued)*

Oral (all adverse reactions are documented while receiving combination therapy with interferon alpha-2b):

>10%:

Central nervous system: Dizziness (17% to 26%), headache (63% to 66%)*, fatigue (60% to 70%)*, fever (32% to 41%)*, insomnia (26% to 39%), irritability (23% to 32%), depression (23% to 36%)*, emotional lability (7% to 12%)*, impaired concentration (10% to 14%)*

Dermatologic: Alopecia (27% to 32%), rash (20% to 28%), pruritus (13% to 21%)

Gastrointestinal: Nausea (38% to 47%), anorexia (21% to 27%), dyspepsia (14% to 16%), vomiting (9% to 12%)*

Hematologic: Decreased hemoglobin (25% to 36%), decreased WBC, absolute neutrophil count <0.5 x 10⁹/L (5% to 11%), thrombocytopenia (6% to 14%), hyperbilirubinemia (24% to 34%), hemolysis

Neuromuscular & skeletal: Myalgia (61% to 64%)*, arthralgia (29% to 33%)*, musculoskeletal pain (20% to 28%), rigors (40% to 43%)

Respiratory: Dyspnea (17% to 19%), sinusitis (9% to 12%)*, nasal congestion

Miscellaneous: Flu-like syndrome (13% to 18%)*

*Similar to interferon alone

1% to 10%:

Cardiovascular: Chest pain (5% to 9%)*

Central nervous system: Nervousness (~5%)*

Gastrointestinal: Taste perversion (6% to 8%)

Hematologic: Hemolytic anemia (~10%)

Neuromuscular & skeletal: Weakness (9% to 10%)

*Similar to interferon alone

<1% (Limited to important or life-threatening): Diabetes mellitus, gout, hearing disorder, pancreatitis, pulmonary dysfunction, suicidal ideation, thyroid function test abnormalities, vertigo

Drug Interactions

Decreased Effect: Decreased effect of zidovudine.

Ethanol/Nutrition/Herb Interactions Food: Oral formulation: High-fat meal (54 g fat) increases the AUC and C_{max} by 70%.

Stability

Inhalation: Store vials in a dry place at 15°C to 25°C (59°F to 78°F). Do not use any water containing an antimicrobial agent to reconstitute drug; reconstituted solution is stable for 24 hours at room temperature. Should not be mixed with other aerosolized medication.

Oral: Store at 15°C to 30°C (59°F to 86°F).

Mechanism of Action Inhibits replication of RNA and DNA viruses; inhibits influenza virus RNA polymerase activity and inhibits the initiation and elongation of RNA fragments resulting in inhibition of viral protein synthesis

Pharmacodynamics/Kinetics

Absorption: Systemically from respiratory tract following nasal and oral inhalation; dependent upon respiratory factors and method of drug delivery; maximal absorption occurs with the use of aerosol generator via endotracheal tube; highest concentrations in respiratory tract and erythrocytes

Distribution: Oral: V_d 2825 L (single dose)

Protein binding: Oral: None

Metabolism: Hepatically and intracellularly; may be necessary for drug action

Bioavailability: Oral: 64%

Half-life elimination, plasma:

Children: 6.5-11 hours

Adults: 24 hours, much longer in the erythrocyte (16-40 days), which can be used as a marker for intracellular metabolism

Time to peak, serum: Inhalation: At end of inhalation period; Oral: 3 hours (multiple dose)

Excretion: Inhalation: Urine (40% as unchanged drug and metabolites); Oral: Urine (61%) and feces (12%)

Usual Dosage

Aerosol inhalation: Infants and children: Use with Viratek® small particle aerosol generator (SPAG-2) at a concentration of 20 mg/mL (6 g reconstituted with 300 mL of sterile water without preservatives). Continuous aerosol administration: 12-18 hours/day for 3 days, up to 7 days in length

Oral:

Children: Chronic hepatitis C (in combination with interferon alfa-2b): **Note:** Safety and efficacy have not been established; dosing based on pharmacokinetic profile:

25-36 kg: 400 mg/day (200 mg twice daily)

37-49 kg: 600 mg/day (200 mg in morning and 400 mg in evening)

50-61 kg: 800 mg/day (400 mg twice daily)

>61 kg: Refer to adult dosing

Note: Also refer to Interferon Alfa-2B and Ribavirin Combination Pack monograph.

Adults:

Chronic hepatitis C (in combination with interferon alfa-2b):

≤75 kg: 400 mg in the morning, then 600 mg in the evening

>75 kg: 600 mg in the morning, then 600 mg in the evening

Note: If HCV-RNA is undetectable at 24 weeks, duration of therapy is 48 weeks. In patients who relapse following interferon therapy, duration of dual therapy is 24 weeks.

Note: Also refer to Interferon Alfa-2B and Ribavirin Combination Pack monograph.

Chronic hepatitis C (in combination with peginterferon alfa-2b): 400 mg twice daily; duration of therapy is 1 year; after 24 weeks of treatment, if serum HCV-RNA is not below the limit of detection of the assay, consider discontinuation.

Dosage adjustment in renal impairment: Cl_{cr} <50 mL/minute: Oral route is contraindicated

Dosage adjustment for toxicity: Oral:

Patient **without** cardiac history:

Hemoglobin <10 g/dL: Decrease dose to 600 mg/day

Hemoglobin <8.5 g/dL: Permanently discontinue treatment

Patient **with** cardiac history:

Hemoglobin has ≥2 g/dL decrease during any 4-week period of treatment: Decrease dose to 600 mg/day

Hemoglobin <12 g/dL after 4 weeks of reduced dose: Permanently discontinue treatment

Dietary Considerations Take oral formulation without regard to food, but always in a consistent manner with respect to food intake (ie, always take with food or always take on an empty stomach).

Administration

Inhalation: Ribavirin should be administered in well-ventilated rooms (at least 6 air changes/ hour). In mechanically-ventilated patients, ribavirin can potentially be deposited in the ventilator delivery system depending on temperature, humidity, and electrostatic forces; this deposition can lead to malfunction or obstruction of the expiratory valve, resulting in inadvertently high positive end-expiratory pressures. The use of one-way valves in the inspiratory lines, a breathing circuit filter in the expiratory line, and frequent monitoring and filter replacement have been effective in preventing these problems. Solutions in SPAG-2 unit should be discarded at least every 24 hours and when the liquid level is low before adding newly reconstituted solution. Should not be mixed with other aerosolized medication.

Oral: Administer concurrently with interferon alfa-2b

Monitoring Parameters

Inhalation: Respiratory function, hemoglobin, reticulocyte count, CBC, I & O

Oral: CBC with differential (pretreatment, 2- and 4 weeks after initiation); pretreatment and monthly pregnancy test for women of childbearing age; LFTs, TSH, HCV-RNA after 24 weeks of therapy

Patient Information Do not use if pregnant

Nursing Implications

Inhalation: Keep accurate I & O record; discard solutions placed in the SPAG-2 unit at least every 24 hours and before adding additional fluid; healthcare workers who are pregnant or who may become pregnant should be advised of the potential risks of exposure and counseled about risk reduction strategies including alternate job responsibilities; ribavirin may adsorb to contact lenses

Oral: Educate female patients about prevention of pregnancy and need for monthly pregnancy testing. Educate male patients about protection of female sexual partners from pregnancy.

Dosage Forms

Capsule: 200 mg;

Powder for aerosol: 6 g (100 mL)

♦ **Ribavirin and Interferon Alfa-2b Combination Pack** *see* Interferon Alfa-2b and Ribavirin Combination Pack *on page 730*

Riboflavin (RYE boe flay vin)

Synonyms Lactoflavin; Vitamin B$_2$; Vitamin G

Therapeutic Category Vitamin, Water Soluble

Use Prevention of riboflavin deficiency and treatment of ariboflavinosis

Pregnancy Risk Factor A/C (dose exceeding RDA recommendation)

Warnings/Precautions Riboflavin deficiency often occurs in the presence of other B vitamin deficiencies

Adverse Reactions Frequency not defined: Genitourinary: Discoloration of urine (yellow-orange)

Drug Interactions

Decreased Effect: Decreased absorption with probenecid.

Mechanism of Action Component of flavoprotein enzymes that work together, which are necessary for normal tissue respiration; also needed for activation of pyridoxine and conversion of tryptophan to niacin

Pharmacodynamics/Kinetics

Absorption: Readily via GI tract, however, food increases extent; decreased with hepatitis, cirrhosis, or biliary obstruction

Metabolism: None

Half-life elimination: Biologic: 66-84 minutes

Excretion: Urine (9%) as unchanged drug

Usual Dosage Oral:

Riboflavin deficiency:

Children: 2.5-10 mg/day in divided doses

Adults: 5-30 mg/day in divided doses

Recommended daily allowance:

Children: 0.4-1.8 mg

Adults: 1.2-1.7 mg

Test Interactions Large doses may interfere with urinalysis based on spectrometry; may cause false elevations in fluorometric determinations of catecholamines and urobilinogen

Patient Information Take with food; large doses may cause bright yellow or orange urine

Nursing Implications Monitor CBC and reticulocyte counts (if anemic when treating deficiency)

Additional Information Dietary sources of riboflavin include liver, kidney, dairy products, green vegetables, eggs, whole grain cereals, yeast, and mushroom.

Dosage Forms Tablet: 50 mg, 100 mg

♦ **RID® [OTC]** *see* Pyrethrins and Piperonyl Butoxide *on page 1160*

♦ **Ridaura®** *see* Auranofin *on page 133*

♦ **Ridifed® [OTC]** *see* Triprolidine and Pseudoephedrine *on page 1380*

♦ **RID® Mousse (Can)** see Pyrethrins and Piperonyl Butoxide on page 1160

Rifabutin (rif a BYOO tin)

Related Information
Antimicrobial Drugs of Choice on page 1588
Tuberculosis Prophylaxis on page 1572
Tuberculosis Treatment Guidelines on page 1612
USPHA/IDSA Guidelines for the Prevention of Opportunistic Infections in Persons With HIV on page 1574

U.S. Brand Names Mycobutin®

Canadian Brand Names Mycobutin®

Synonyms Ansamycin

Therapeutic Category Antibiotic, Miscellaneous; Antitubercular Agent

Use Prevention of disseminated Mycobacterium avium complex (MAC) in patients with advanced HIV infection; also utilized in multiple drug regimens for treatment of MAC

Pregnancy Risk Factor B

Contraindications Hypersensitivity to rifabutin, any other rifamycins, or any component of the formulation; rifabutin is contraindicated in patients with a WBC <1000/mm^3 or a platelet count <50,000/mm^3

Warnings/Precautions Rifabutin as a single agent must not be administered to patients with active tuberculosis since its use may lead to the development of tuberculosis that is resistant to both rifabutin and rifampin; rifabutin should be discontinued in patients with AST >500 units/L or if total bilirubin is >3 mg/dL. Use with caution in patients with liver impairment; modification of dosage should be considered in patients with renal impairment.

Adverse Reactions
>10%:
  Dermatologic: Rash
  Gastrointestinal: Vomiting, nausea, discolored feces, saliva (reddish orange)
  Genitourinary: Discolored urine (reddish orange)
  Miscellaneous: Discolored sputum, sweat, tears (reddish orange)
1% to 10%:
  Central nervous system: Headache
  Gastrointestinal: Abdominal pain, diarrhea, anorexia, flatulence, eructation
  Hematologic: Anemia, thrombocytopenia
<1% (Limited to important or life-threatening): Chest pain, dyspnea, leukopenia, neutropenia, uveitis

Overdosage/Toxicology Symptoms include nausea, vomiting, hepatotoxicity, lethargy, and CNS depression. Treatment is supportive. Hemodialysis will remove rifabutin, its effect on outcome is unknown.

Drug Interactions
Cytochrome P450 Effect: CYP3A3/4 enzyme inducer

Increased Effect/Toxicity: Concentrations of rifabutin are increased by indinavir (reduce rifabutin to 50% of standard dose) and ritonavir (reduce rifabutin dose to 150 mg every other day). Fluconazole increases rifabutin concentrations.

Decreased Effect: Rifabutin may decreased plasma concentrations (due to induction of liver enzymes) of verapamil, methadone, digoxin, cyclosporine, corticosteroids, oral anticoagulants, theophylline, barbiturates, chloramphenicol, itraconazole, ketoconazole, oral contraceptives, quinidine, protease inhibitors (indinavir, nelfinavir, ritonavir, saquinavir), non-nucleoside reverse transcriptase inhibitors, halothane, and clarithromycin.

Ethanol/Nutrition/Herb Interactions Food: High-fat meal may decrease the rate but not the extent of absorption.

Mechanism of Action Inhibits DNA-dependent RNA polymerase at the beta subunit which prevents chain initiation

Pharmacodynamics/Kinetics
Absorption: Readily, 53%
Distribution: V_d: 9.32 L/kg; distributes to body tissues including the lungs, liver, spleen, eyes, and kidneys
Protein binding: 85%
Metabolism: To active and inactive metabolites
Bioavailability: Absolute, 20% in HIV patients
Half-life elimination: Terminal: 45 hours (range: 16-69 hours)
Time to peak, serum: 2-4 hours
Excretion: Urine (10% as unchanged drug, 53% as metabolites); feces (10% as unchanged drug, 30% as metabolites)

Usual Dosage Oral:
Children >1 year:
  Treatment: Patients not receiving NNRTIs or protease inhibitors:
    Initial phase (2 weeks to 2 months): 10-20 mg/kg daily (maximum: 300 mg).
    Second phase: 10-20 mg/kg daily (maximum: 300 mg) or twice weekly
  Prophylaxis: 5 mg/kg daily; higher dosages have been used in limited trials
Adults:
  Treatment:
    Patients not receiving NNRTIs or protease inhibitors:
      Initial phase: 5 mg/kg daily (maximum: 300 mg)
      Second phase: 5 mg/kg daily or twice weekly
    Patients receiving nelfinavir, amprenavir, indinavir: Reduce dose to 150 mg/day; no change in dose if administered twice weekly
  Prophylaxis: 300 mg once daily (alone or in combination with azithromycin)

Dosage adjustment in renal impairment: Cl_{cr} <30 mL/minute: Reduce dose by 50%

Dietary Considerations May be taken with meals or without food or mix with applesauce.

Monitoring Parameters Periodic liver function tests, CBC with differential, platelet count

Patient Information May discolor urine, tears, sweat, or other body fluids to a red-orange color; take 1 hour before or 2 hours after a meal on an empty stomach; soft contact lenses may be permanently stained; report to physician any severe or persistent flu-like symptoms, nausea, vomiting, dark urine or pale stools, unusual bleeding or bruising, or any eye problems; can be taken with meals or sprinkled on applesauce

Nursing Implications Monitor periodic liver function tests, CBC with differential, platelet count, hemoglobin, hematocrit

Dosage Forms Capsule: 150 mg

♦ **Rifadin®** see Rifampin on page 1193

♦ **Rifampicin** see Rifampin on page 1193

Rifampin (RIF am pin)

Related Information

Antibiotic Treatment of Adults With Infective Endocarditis on page 1585
Antimicrobial Drugs of Choice on page 1588
Desensitization Protocols on page 1525
Tuberculosis Prophylaxis on page 1572
Tuberculosis Treatment Guidelines on page 1612
USPHA/IDSA Guidelines for the Prevention of Opportunistic Infections in Persons With HIV on page 1574

U.S. Brand Names Rifadin®; Rimactane®

Canadian Brand Names Rifadin®; Rofact™

Synonyms Rifampicin

Therapeutic Category Antibiotic, Miscellaneous; Antitubercular Agent

Use Management of active tuberculosis in combination with other agents; eliminate meningococci from asymptomatic carriers; prophylaxis of *Haemophilus influenzae* type b infection; used in combination with other anti-infectives in the treatment of staphylococcal infections; *Legionella* pneumonia

Pregnancy Risk Factor C

Pregnancy/Breast-Feeding Implications Clinical effects on the fetus: Teratogenicity has occurred in rodents given many times the adult human dose

Contraindications Hypersensitivity to rifampin, any rifamycins, or any component of the formulation; concurrent use of amprenavir (possibly other protease inhibitors)

Warnings/Precautions Use with caution and modify dosage in patients with liver impairment; observe for hyperbilirubinemia; discontinue therapy if this in conjunction with clinical symptoms or any signs of significant hepatocellular damage develop; since rifampin has enzyme-inducing properties, porphyria exacerbation is possible; use with caution in patients with porphyria; do not use for meningococcal disease, only for short-term treatment of asymptomatic carrier states

Monitor for compliance and effects including hypersensitivity, thrombocytopenia in patients on intermittent therapy; urine, feces, saliva, sweat, tears, and CSF may be discolored to red/orange; do not administer I.V. form via I.M. or S.C. routes; restart infusion at another site if extravasation occurs; remove soft contact lenses during therapy since permanent staining may occur; regimens of 600 mg once or twice weekly have been associated with a high incidence of adverse reactions including a flu-like syndrome

Adverse Reactions

Frequency not defined:

Cardiovascular: Flushing, edema

Central nervous system: Headache, drowsiness, dizziness, confusion, numbness, behavioral changes, ataxia

Dermatologic: Pruritus, urticaria, pemphigoid reaction

Hematologic: Eosinophilia, leukopenia, hemolysis, hemolytic anemia, thrombocytopenia (especially with high-dose therapy)

Hepatic: Hepatitis (rare)

Neuromuscular & skeletal: Myalgia, weakness, osteomalacia

Ocular: Visual changes, exudative conjunctivitis

1% to 10%:

Dermatologic: Rash (1% to 5%)

Gastrointestinal (1% to 2%): Epigastric distress, anorexia, nausea, vomiting, diarrhea, cramps, pseudomembranous colitis, pancreatitis

Hepatic: Increased LFTs (up to 14%)

Overdosage/Toxicology Symptoms include nausea, vomiting, and hepatotoxicity. Treatment is supportive. Lavage with activated charcoal is preferred to ipecac, as emesis is frequently present with overdose. Hemodialysis will remove rifampin, but its effect on outcome is unknown.

Drug Interactions

Cytochrome P450 Effect: CYP3A3/4 enzyme substrate; CYP1A2, 2C, 2C8, 2C9, 2C18, 2C19, 3A3/4, and 3A5-7 enzyme inducer

Increased Effect/Toxicity: Rifampin levels may be increased when given with co-trimoxazole, probenecid, or ritonavir. Rifampin given with halothane or isoniazid increases the potential for hepatotoxicity. Combination therapy with rifampin and pyrazinamide has been associated with severe and fatal hepatotoxic reactions.

Decreased Effect: Rifampin induces liver enzymes which may decrease the plasma concentration of calcium channel blockers (verapamil, diltiazem, nifedipine), methadone, digoxin, cyclosporine, corticosteroids, haloperidol, oral anticoagulants, theophylline, barbiturates, chloramphenicol, imidazole antifungals (ketoconazole), oral contraceptives, acetaminophen, benzodiazepines, hydantoins, sulfa drugs, enalapril, beta-blockers, clofibrate, dapsone, antiarrhythmics (disopyramide, mexiletine, quinidine, tocainide), doxycycline, fluoroquinolones, levothyroxine, nortriptyline, tacrolimus, zidovudine, protease inhibitors (ie, amprenavir), and non-nucleoside reverse transcriptase inhibitors.

Ethanol/Nutrition/Herb Interactions

Ethanol: Avoid ethanol (may increase risk of hepatotoxicity).

Food: Food decreases the extent of absorption; rifampin concentrations may be decreased if taken with food.

Herb/Nutraceutical: St John's wort may decrease rifampin levels.

(Continued)

Rifampin *(Continued)*

Stability Rifampin powder is reddish brown. Intact vials should be stored at room temperature and protected from excessive heat and light. Reconstituted vials are stable for 24 hours at room temperature

Stability of parenteral admixture at room temperature (25°C) is 4 hours for D$_5$W and 24 hours for NS

Mechanism of Action Inhibits bacterial RNA synthesis by binding to the beta subunit of DNA-dependent RNA polymerase, blocking RNA transcription

Pharmacodynamics/Kinetics

Duration: ≤24 hours

Absorption: Oral: Well absorbed; food may delay or slightly reduce peak

Distribution: Highly lipophilic; crosses blood-brain barrier well

Relative diffusion from blood into CSF: Adequate with or without inflammation (exceeds usual MICs)

CSF:blood level ratio: Inflamed meninges: 25%

Protein binding: 80%

Metabolism: Hepatic, undergoes enterohepatic recycling

Half-life elimination: 3-4 hours; prolonged with hepatic impairment; End-stage renal disease: 1.8-11 hours

Time to peak, serum: Oral: 2-4 hours

Excretion: Primarily feces (60% to 65%) and urine (~30%) as unchanged drug

Usual Dosage Oral (I.V. infusion dose is the same as for the oral route):

Tuberculosis therapy: Note: A four-drug regimen (isoniazid, rifampin, pyrazinamide, and either streptomycin or ethambutol) is preferred for the initial, empiric treatment of TB. When the drug susceptibility results are available, the regimen should be altered as appropriate.

Infants and Children <12 years:

Daily therapy: 10-20 mg/kg/day usually as a single dose (maximum: 600 mg/day)

Directly observed therapy (DOT): Twice weekly: 10-20 mg/kg (maximum: 600 mg); 3 times/week: 10-20 mg/kg (maximum: 600 mg)

Adults:

Daily therapy: 10 mg/kg/day (maximum: 600 mg/day)

Directly observed therapy (DOT): Twice weekly: 10 mg/kg (maximum: 600 mg); 3 times/week: 10 mg/kg (maximum: 600 mg)

Tuberculosis prevention: As an alternative to isoniazid:

Children: 10-20 mg/kg/day (maximum: 600 mg/day)

Adults: 10 mg/kg/day (maximum: 600 mg/day) for 2 months in combination with pyrazinamide

H. influenzae prophylaxis:

Infants and Children: 20 mg/kg/day every 24 hours for 4 days, not to exceed 600 mg/dose

Adults: 600 mg every 24 hours for 4 days

Leprosy: Adults:

Multibacillary: 600 mg once monthly for 24 months in combination with ofloxacin and minocycline

Paucibacillary: 600 mg once monthly for 6 months in combination with dapsone

Single lesion: 600 mg as a single dose in combination with ofloxacin 400 mg and minocycline 100 mg

Meningococcal meningitis prophylaxis:

Infants <1 month: 10 mg/kg/day in divided doses every 12 hours for 2 days

Infants ≥1 month and Children: 20 mg/kg/day in divided doses every 12 hours for 2 days

Adults: 600 mg every 12 hours for 2 days

Nasal carriers of *Staphylococcus aureus*:

Children: 15 mg/kg/day divided every 12 hours for 5-10 days in combination with other antibiotics

Adults: 600 mg/day for 5-10 days in combination with other antibiotics

Synergy for *Staphylococcus aureus* infections: Adults: 300-600 mg twice daily with other antibiotics

Dosing adjustment in hepatic impairment: Dose reductions may be necessary to reduce hepatotoxicity

Hemodialysis or peritoneal dialysis: Plasma rifampin concentrations are not significantly affected by hemodialysis or peritoneal dialysis.

Dietary Considerations Rifampin is best taken on an empty stomach.

Administration Administer on an empty stomach (ie, 1 hour prior to, or 2 hours after meals or antacids) to increase total absorption

Monitoring Parameters Periodic (baseline and every 2-4 weeks during therapy) monitoring of liver function (AST, ALT, bilirubin), CBC; hepatic status and mental status, sputum culture, chest x-ray 2-3 months into treatment

Test Interactions Positive Coombs' reaction [direct], rifampin inhibits standard assay's ability to measure serum folate and B$_{12}$; transient increase in LFTs and decreased biliary excretion of contrast media

Patient Information May discolor urine, tears, sweat, or other body fluids to a red-orange color; take 1 hour before or 2 hours after a meal on an empty stomach; soft contact lenses may be permanently stained; report to physician any severe or persistent flu-like symptoms, nausea, vomiting, dark urine or pale stools, or unusual bleeding or bruising; utilize an alternate form from oral/other systemic contraceptives during therapy; compliance and completion with course of therapy is very important; if you are a diabetic taking oral medications or if you regularly take oral anticoagulant therapy, your medication may need special and careful adjustment.

Nursing Implications The compounded oral suspension must be shaken well before using; may mix contents of capsule with applesauce or jelly; administer I.V. preparation once daily by slow I.V. infusion over 30 minutes to 3 hours at a final concentration not to exceed 6 mg/mL

Dosage Forms

Capsule (Rifadin®, Rimactane®): 150 mg, 300 mg

Powder for injection (Rifadin®): 600 mg

Extemporaneous Preparations For pediatric and adult patients with difficulty swallowing or where lower doses are needed, the package insert lists an extemporaneous liquid suspension as follows:

Rifampin 1% w/v suspension (10 mg/mL) can be compounded using one of four syrups (Syrup NF, simple syrup, Syrpalta® syrup, or raspberry syrup)
Empty contents of four 300 mg capsules or eight 150 mg capsules onto a piece of weighing paper
If necessary, crush contents to produce a fine powder
Transfer powder blend to a 4 oz amber glass or plastic prescription bottle
Rinse paper and spatula with 20 mL of syrup and add the rinse to bottle; shake vigorously
Add 100 mL of syrup to the bottle and shake vigorously
This compounding procedure results in a 1% w/v suspension containing 10 mg rifampin/mL; stability studies indicate suspension is stable at room temperature (25°C ±3°C) or in refrigerator (2°C to 8°C) for 4 weeks; shake well prior to administration

Rifapentine (RIF a pen teen)
U.S. Brand Names Priftin®
Canadian Brand Names Priftin®
Therapeutic Category Antitubercular Agent
Use Treatment of pulmonary tuberculosis; rifapentine must always be used in conjunction with at least one other antituberculosis drug to which the isolate is susceptible; it may also be necessary to add a third agent (either streptomycin or ethambutol) until susceptibility is known.
Pregnancy Risk Factor C
Pregnancy/Breast-Feeding Implications Has been shown to be teratogenic in rats and rabbits. Rat offspring showed cleft palates, right aortic arch, and delayed ossification and increased number of ribs. Rabbits displayed ovarian agenesis, pes varus, arhinia, microphthalmia, and irregularities of the ossified facial tissues. Rat studies also show decreased fetal weight, increased number of stillborns, and decreased gestational survival. No adequate well-controlled studies in pregnant women are available. Rifapentine should be used during pregnancy only if the potential benefits justifies the potential risk to the fetus. Excreted in breast milk; may discolor breast milk; use with caution in breast-feeding women
Contraindications Hypersensitivity to rifapentine, rifampin, rifabutin, any rifamycin analog, or any component of the formulation
Warnings/Precautions Patients with abnormal liver tests and/or liver disease should only be given rifapentine when absolutely necessary and under strict medical supervision. If signs of liver disease occur or worsen, rifapentine should be discontinued. Experience in treating TB in HIV-infected patients is limited.

Rifapentine may produce a red-orange discoloration of body tissues/fluids including skin, teeth, tongue, urine, feces, saliva, sputum, tears, sweat, and cerebral spinal fluid. Contact lenses may become permanently stained. All patients treated with rifapentine should have baseline measurements of liver function tests and enzymes, bilirubin, and a complete blood count. Patients should be seen and monitored monthly and specifically questioned regarding symptoms associated with adverse reactions. Routine laboratory monitoring in people with normal baseline measurements is generally not necessary.
Adverse Reactions
>10%: Endocrine & metabolic: Hyperuricemia (most likely due to pyrazinamide from initiation phase combination therapy)
1% to 10%:
Cardiovascular: Hypertension
Central nervous system: Headache, dizziness
Dermatologic: Rash, pruritus, acne
Gastrointestinal: Anorexia, nausea, vomiting, dyspepsia, diarrhea
Genitourinary: Pyuria, proteinuria, hematuria, urinary casts
Hematologic: Neutropenia, lymphopenia, anemia, leukopenia, thrombocytosis
Hepatic: Increased ALT, AST
Neuromuscular & skeletal: Arthralgia, pain
Respiratory: Hemoptysis
<1% (Limited to important or life-threatening): Aggressive reaction, arthrosis, gout, hepatitis, hyperkalemia, pancreatitis, purpura, thrombocytopenia
Overdosage/Toxicology There is no experience with treatment of acute overdose. Experience with other rifamycins suggests that gastric lavage, followed by activated charcoal, may help adsorb any remaining drug from the GI tract. Hemodialysis or forced diuresis is not expected to enhance elimination of unchanged rifapentine in an overdose.
Drug Interactions
Cytochrome P450 Effect: CYP3A3/4, 2C8, and 2C9 enzyme inducer
Increased Effect/Toxicity: Rifapentine metabolism is mediated by esterase activity, therefore, there is minimal potential for rifapentine metabolism to be affected by other drug therapy.
Decreased Effect: Rifapentine may increase the metabolism of coadministered drugs that are metabolized by these enzymes. Enzymes are induced within 4 days after the first dose and returned to baseline 14 days after discontinuation of rifapentine. The magnitude of enzyme induction is dose and frequency dependent.

Rifampin has been shown to accelerate the metabolism and may reduce activity of the following drugs (therefore, rifapentine may also do the same): Phenytoin, disopyramide, mexiletine, quinidine, tocainide, chloramphenicol, clarithromycin, dapsone, doxycycline, fluoroquinolones, warfarin, fluconazole, itraconazole, ketoconazole, barbiturates, benzodiazepines, beta-blockers, diltiazem, nifedipine, verapamil, corticosteroids, cardiac glycoside preparations, clofibrate, oral or other systemic hormonal contraceptives, haloperidol, HIV protease inhibitors, sulfonylureas, cyclosporine, tacrolimus, levothyroxine, methadone, progestins, quinine, delavirdine, zidovudine, sildenafil, theophylline, amitriptyline, and nortriptyline.
(Continued)

Rifapentine *(Continued)*

Rifapentine should be used with extreme caution, if at all, in patients who are also taking protease inhibitors.

Patients using oral or other systemic hormonal contraceptives should be advised to change to nonhormonal methods of birth control when receiving concomitant rifapentine.

Ethanol/Nutrition/Herb Interactions Food: Food increases AUC and maximum serum concentration by 43% and 44% respectively as compared to fasting conditions.

Stability Store at room temperature (15°C to 30°C; 59°F to 86°F); protect from excessive heat and humidity

Mechanism of Action Inhibits DNA-dependent RNA polymerase in susceptible strains of *Mycobacterium tuberculosis* (but not in mammalian cells). Rifapentine is bactericidal against both intracellular and extracellular MTB organisms. MTB resistant to other rifamycins including rifampin are likely to be resistant to rifapentine. Cross-resistance does not appear between rifapentine and other nonrifamycin antimycobacterial agents.

Pharmacodynamics/Kinetics

Absorption: Food increases AUC and C_{max} by 43% and 44% respectively.

Distribution: V_d: ~70.2 L; rifapentine and metabolite accumulate in human monocyte-derived macrophages with intracellular/extracellular ratios of 24:1 and 7:1 respectively

Metabolism: Hepatic; hydrolyzed by an esterase and esterase enzyme to form the active metabolite 25-desacetyl rifapentine

Protein binding: Rifapentine and 25-desacetyl metabolite: 97.7% and 93.2% (mainly to albumin)

Bioavailability: ~70%

Half-life elimination: Rifapentine: 14-17 hours; 25-desacetyl rifapentine: 13 hours

Time to peak, serum: 5-6 hours

Excretion: Urine (17% mostly as metabolites)

Usual Dosage

Children: No dosing information available

Adults: **Rifapentine should not be used alone**; initial phase should include a 3- to 4-drug regimen

Intensive phase of short-term therapy: 600 mg (four 150 mg tablets) given weekly (every 72 hours); following the intensive phase, treatment should continue with rifapentine 600 mg once weekly for 4 months in combination with INH or appropriate agent for susceptible organisms

Dosing adjustment in renal or hepatic impairment: Unknown

Monitoring Parameters Patients with pre-existing hepatic problems should have liver function tests monitored every 2-4 weeks during therapy

Test Interactions Rifampin has been shown to inhibit standard microbiological assays for serum folate and vitamin B_{12}; this should be considered for rifapentine; therefore, alternative assay methods should be considered.

Patient Information May produce a reddish coloration of urine, sweat, sputum, tears, and contact lenses may be permanently stained. Oral or other systemic hormonal contraceptives may not be effective while taking rifapentine; alternative contraceptive measures should be used. Administration of rifapentine with food may decrease GI intolerance. Notify physician if experiencing fever, decreased appetite, malaise, nausea/vomiting, darkened urine, yellowish discoloration of skin or eyes, chest pain, palpitations, and pain or swelling of the joints. Adherence with the full course of therapy is essential; no doses of therapy should be missed.

Additional Information Rifapentine has only been studied in patients with tuberculosis receiving a 6-month short-course intensive regimen approval. Outcomes have been based on 6-month follow-up treatment observed in clinical trial 008 as a surrogate for the 2-year follow-up generally accepted as evidence for efficacy in the treatment of pulmonary tuberculosis.

Dosage Forms Tablet, film coated: 150 mg

♦ **rIFN-A** *see* Interferon Alfa-2a *on page 726*
♦ **rIFN beta-1a** *see* Interferon Beta-1a *on page 734*
♦ **rIFN beta-1b** *see* Interferon Beta-1b *on page 736*
♦ **RIG** *see* Rabies Immune Globulin (Human) *on page 1174*
♦ **rIL-11** *see* Oprelvekin *on page 1012*
♦ **Rilutek®** *see* Riluzole *on page 1196*

Riluzole *(RIL yoo zole)*

U.S. Brand Names Rilutek®

Synonyms 2-Amino-6-Trifluoromethoxy-benzothiazole; RP54274

Therapeutic Category Amyotrophic Lateral Sclerosis (ALS) Agent; Glutamate Inhibitor

Use Orphan drug: Treatment of amyotrophic lateral sclerosis (ALS); riluzole can extend survival or time to tracheostomy

Pregnancy Risk Factor C

Contraindications Severe hypersensitivity reactions to riluzole or any component of the formulation

Warnings/Precautions Among 4000 patients given riluzole for ALS, there were 3 cases of marked neutropenia (ANC <500/mm³), all seen within the first 2 months of treatment. Use with caution in patients with concomitant renal insufficiency. Use with caution in patients with current evidence or history of abnormal liver function. Monitor liver chemistries.

Adverse Reactions

>10%:

Gastrointestinal: Nausea (10% to 21%)

Neuromuscular & skeletal: Weakness (15% to 20%)

Respiratory: Decreased lung function (10% to 16%)

1% to 10%:

Cardiovascular: Hypertension, tachycardia, postural hypotension, edema

Central nervous system: headache, dizziness, somnolence, insomnia, malaise, depression, vertigo, agitation, tremor, circumoral paresthesia

Dermatologic: Pruritus, eczema, alopecia
Gastrointestinal: Abdominal pain, diarrhea, anorexia, dyspepsia, vomiting, stomatitis
Neuromuscular & skeletal: Arthralgia, back pain
Respiratory: Rhinitis, increased cough
Miscellaneous: Aggravation reaction
<1% (Limited to important or life-threatening): Exfoliative dermatitis, neutropenia, seizures

Overdosage/Toxicology No specific antidote or treatment information is available. Treatment should be supportive and directed toward alleviating symptoms.

Drug Interactions
Cytochrome P450 Effect: CYP1A2 enzyme substrate
Increased Effect/Toxicity: Inhibitors of CYP1A2 (eg, caffeine, theophylline, amitriptyline, quinolones) could decrease the rate of riluzole elimination resulting in accumulation of riluzole.
Decreased Effect: Drugs that induce CYP1A2 (eg, cigarette smoke, charbroiled food, rifampin, omeprazole) could increase the rate of riluzole elimination.

Ethanol/Nutrition/Herb Interactions
Ethanol: Avoid ethanol (due to CNS depression).
Food: A high-fat meal decreases absorption of riluzole (decreasing AUC by 20% and peak blood levels by 45%).

Stability Protect from bright light

Mechanism of Action Inhibitory effect on glutamate release, inactivation of voltage-dependent sodium channels; and ability to interfere with intracellular events that follow transmitter binding at excitatory amino acid receptors

Pharmacodynamics/Kinetics
Absorption: 90%; high fat meal decreases AUC by 20%, peak blood levels by 45%
Protein binding, plasma: 96%, mainly to albumin and lipoproteins
Metabolism: Extensively to six major and a number of minor metabolites; primarily hepatic, consisting of CYP450 dependent hydroxylation and glucuronidation; principle isozyme is CYP 1A2
Bioavailability: Oral: Absolute (50%)

Usual Dosage Adults: Oral: 50 mg every 12 hours; no increased benefit can be expected from higher daily doses, but adverse events are increased

Dosage adjustment in smoking: Cigarette smoking is known to induce CYP1A2; patients who smoke cigarettes would be expected to eliminate riluzole faster. There is no information, however, on the effect of, or need for, dosage adjustment in these patients.

Dosage adjustment in special populations: Females and Japanese patients may possess a lower metabolic capacity to eliminate riluzole compared with male and Caucasian subjects, respectively

Dosage adjustment in renal impairment: Use with caution in patients with concomitant renal insufficiency

Dosage adjustment in hepatic impairment: Use with caution in patients with current evidence or history of abnormal liver function indicated by significant abnormalities in serum transaminase, bilirubin or GGT levels. Baseline elevations of several LFTs (especially elevated bilirubin) should preclude use of riluzole.

Monitoring Parameters Monitor serum aminotransferases including ALT levels before and during therapy. Evaluate serum ALT levels every month during the first 3 months of therapy, every 3 months during the remainder of the first year and periodically thereafter. Evaluate ALT levels more frequently in patients who develop elevations. Maximum increases in serum ALT usually occurred within 3 months after the start of therapy and were usually transient when <5 x ULN (upper limits of normal).

In trials, if ALT levels were <5 x ULN, treatment continued and ALT levels usually returned to below 2 x ULN within 2-6 months. Treatment in studies was discontinued, however, if ALT levels exceed 5 x ULN, so that there is no experience with continued treatment of ALS patients once ALT values exceed 5 x ULN.

If a decision is made to continue treatment in patients when the ALT exceeds 5 x ULN, frequent monitoring (at least weekly) of complete liver function is recommended. Discontinue treatment if ALT exceeds 10 x ULN or if clinical jaundice develops.

Patient Information Take at least 1 hour before or 2 hours after a meal to avoid decreased bioavailability. Report any febrile illness to your physician. Take riluzole at the same time of the day each day. If a dose is missed, take the next tablet as originally planned.

Nursing Implications Warn patients about the potential for dizziness, vertigo or somnolence and advise them not to drive or operate machinery until they have gained sufficient experience on riluzole to gauge whether or not it affects their mental or motor performance adversely. Whether ethanol increases the risk of serious hepatotoxicity with riluzole is unknown; discourage riluzole-treated patients from drinking ethanol in excess.

Additional Information May be obtained through Rhone-Poulenc Rorer Inc (Collegeville, PA) for compassionate use (through treatment IND process) by calling 800-727-6737 for treatment of amyotrophic lateral sclerosis. May be more effective for amyotrophic lateral sclerosis of bulbar onset. In animal models, riluzole was a potent inhibitor of seizures induced by ouabain.

Dosage Forms Tablet: 50 mg

♦ **Rimactane®** *see* Rifampin *on page 1193*

Rimantadine (ri MAN ta deen)

Related Information
USPHA/IDSA Guidelines for the Prevention of Opportunistic Infections in Persons With HIV *on page 1574*
U.S. Brand Names Flumadine®
Canadian Brand Names Flumadine®
Synonyms Rimantadine Hydrochloride
Therapeutic Category Antiviral Agent, Oral
(Continued)

Rimantadine (Continued)

Use Prophylaxis (adults and children >1 year of age) and treatment (adults) of influenza A viral infection

Pregnancy Risk Factor C

Pregnancy/Breast-Feeding Implications
Clinical effects on the fetus: Embryotoxic in high dose rat studies
Breast-feeding/lactation: Avoid use in nursing mothers due to potential adverse effect in infants; rimantadine is concentrated in milk

Contraindications Hypersensitivity to drugs of the adamantine class, including rimantadine and amantadine, or any component of the formulation

Warnings/Precautions Use with caution in patients with renal and hepatic dysfunction; avoid use, if possible, in patients with recurrent and eczematoid dermatitis, uncontrolled psychosis, or severe psychoneurosis. An increase in seizure incidence may occur in patients with seizure disorders; discontinue drug if seizures occur; consider the development of resistance during rimantadine treatment of the index case as likely if failure of rimantadine prophylaxis among family contact occurs and if index case is a child; viruses exhibit cross-resistance between amantadine and rimantadine.

Adverse Reactions 1% to 10%:
Cardiovascular: Orthostatic hypotension, edema
Central nervous system: Dizziness (2%), confusion, headache (1%), insomnia (2%), difficulty in concentrating, anxiety (1%), restlessness, irritability, hallucinations; incidence of CNS side effects may be less than that associated with amantadine
Gastrointestinal: Nausea (3%), vomiting (2%), xerostomia (2%), abdominal pain (1%), anorexia (2%)
Genitourinary: Urinary retention

Overdosage/Toxicology Agitation, hallucinations, ventricular cardiac arrhythmias (torsade de pointes and PVCs), slurred speech, anticholinergic effects (dry mouth, urinary retention and mydriasis), ataxia, tremor, myoclonus, seizures, and death have been reported with amantadine (a related drug). Treatment is symptomatic (do not use physostigmine). Tachyarrhythmias may be treated with beta-blockers such as propranolol. Dialysis is not recommended except possibly in renal failure.

Drug Interactions
Increased Effect/Toxicity: Cimetidine increases blood levels/toxicity of rimantadine.
Decreased Effect: Acetaminophen may cause a small reduction in AUC and peak concentration of rimantadine. Peak plasma and AUC concentrations of rimantadine are slightly reduced by aspirin.

Ethanol/Nutrition/Herb Interactions Food: Food does not affect rate or extent of absorption

Mechanism of Action Exerts its inhibitory effect on three antigenic subtypes of influenza A virus (H1N1, H2N2, H3N2) early in the viral replicative cycle, possibly inhibiting the uncoating process; it has no activity against influenza B virus and is two- to eightfold more active than amantadine

Pharmacodynamics/Kinetics
Onset of action: Antiviral activity: No data exist establishing a correlation between plasma concentration and antiviral effect
Absorption: Tablet and syrup formulations are equally absorbed
Metabolism: Extensively hepatic
Half-life elimination: 25.4 hours (increased in elderly)
Time to peak: 6 hours
Excretion: Urine (<25% as unchanged drug)
Clearance: Hemodialysis does not contribute to clearance

Usual Dosage Oral:
Prophylaxis:
Children <10 years: 5 mg/kg once daily; maximum: 150 mg
Children >10 years and Adults: 100 mg twice daily; decrease to 100 mg/day in elderly or in patients with severe hepatic or renal impairment (Cl_{cr} ≤10 mL/minute)
Treatment: Adults: 100 mg twice daily; decrease to 100 mg/day in elderly or in patients with severe hepatic or renal impairment (Cl_{cr} ≤10 mL/minute)

Administration Initiation of rimantadine within 48 hours of the onset of influenza A illness halves the duration of illness and significantly reduces the duration of viral shedding and increased peripheral airways resistance; continue therapy for 5-7 days after symptoms begin

Monitoring Parameters Monitor for CNS or GI effects in elderly or patients with renal or hepatic impairment

Nursing Implications Avoid use in pregnant or breast-feeding women

Dosage Forms
Syrup, as hydrochloride: 50 mg/5 mL (240 mL)
Tablet, as hydrochloride: 100 mg

♦ **Rimantadine Hydrochloride** see Rimantadine on page 1197

Rimexolone (ri MEKS oh lone)

U.S. Brand Names Vexol®

Canadian Brand Names Vexol®

Therapeutic Category Anti-inflammatory Agent, Ophthalmic; Corticosteroid, Ophthalmic

Use Treatment of inflammation after ocular surgery and the treatment of anterior uveitis

Pregnancy Risk Factor C

Contraindications Hypersensitivity to rimexolone or any component of the formulation; fungal, viral, or untreated pus-forming bacterial ocular infections

Warnings/Precautions Prolonged use has been associated with the development of corneal or scleral perforation and posterior subcapsular cataracts; may mask or enhance the establishment of acute purulent untreated infections of the eye; effectiveness and safety have not been established in children

Adverse Reactions
1% to 10%: Ocular: Temporary mild blurred vision

<1% (Limited to important or life-threatening): Burning or stinging eyes, cataracts, corneal thinning, glaucoma, increased intraocular pressure, optic nerve damage, secondary ocular infection, visual acuity defects

Mechanism of Action Decreases inflammation by suppression of migration of polymorphonuclear leukocytes and reversal of increased capillary permeability

Pharmacodynamics/Kinetics
Absorption: Through aqueous humor
Metabolism: Hepatic for any amount of drug absorbed
Excretion: Urine and feces

Usual Dosage Adults: Ophthalmic: Instill 1 drop in conjunctival sac 2-4 times/day up to every 4 hours; may use every 1-2 hours during first 1-2 days

Monitoring Parameters Intraocular pressure and periodic examination of lens (with prolonged use)

Dosage Forms Suspension, ophthalmic: 1% (5 mL, 10 mL)

♦ **Riopan Plus® [OTC]** *see* Magaldrate and Simethicone *on page 831*

♦ **Riopan Plus® Double Strength [OTC]** *see* Magaldrate and Simethicone *on page 831*

♦ **Riphenidate (Can)** *see* Methylphenidate *on page 894*

Risedronate (ris ED roe nate)

U.S. Brand Names Actonel™

Canadian Brand Names Actonel®

Synonyms Risedronate Sodium

Therapeutic Category Bisphosphonate Derivative

Use Paget's disease of the bone; treatment and prevention of glucocorticoid-induced osteoporosis; treatment and prevention of osteoporosis in postmenopausal women

Pregnancy Risk Factor C

Contraindications Hypersensitivity to risedronate, bisphosphonates, or any component of the formulation; hypocalcemia; abnormalities of the esophagus which delay esophageal emptying such as stricture or achalasia; inability to stand or sit upright for at least 30 minutes

Warnings/Precautions Bisphosphonates may cause upper gastrointestinal disorders such as dysphagia, esophageal ulcer, and gastric ulcer. Use caution in patients with renal impairment; hypocalcemia must be corrected before therapy initiation with alendronate; ensure adequate calcium and vitamin D intake, especially for patients with Paget's disease in whom the pretreatment rate of bone turnover may be greatly elevated.

Adverse Reactions
Seen in patients taking 30 mg/day for Paget's disease:
>10%:
Central nervous system: Headache (18%)
Dermatologic: Rash (11%)
Gastrointestinal: Diarrhea (20%), abdominal pain (11%)
Neuromuscular & skeletal: Arthralgia (33%)
Miscellaneous: Flu-like syndrome (10%)
1% to 10%:
Cardiovascular: Peripheral edema (8%)
Central nervous system: Chest pain (7%), dizziness (7%)
Gastrointestinal: Nausea (10%), constipation (7%), belching (3%), colitis (3%, placebo 3%)
Neuromuscular & skeletal: Weakness (5%), bone pain (5%, placebo 5%), leg cramps (3%, placebo 3%), myasthenia (3%)
Ocular: Amblyopia (3%, placebo 3%), dry eye (3%)
Otic: Tinnitus (3%, placebo 3%)
Respiratory: Sinusitis (5%), bronchitis (3%, placebo 5%) <1%: Acute iritis
Miscellaneous: Neoplasm (3%)

Events observed in patients taking 5 mg/day for osteoporosis were similar to those seen with placebo

Overdosage/Toxicology Symptoms include hypophosphatemia and upper GI adverse events (upset stomach, heartburn, esophagitis, gastritis, or ulcer). Signs and symptoms of hypocalcemia may also occur in some patients. Milk or antacids containing calcium should be given to bind Actonel™ and reduce absorption of the drug. Decreases in serum calcium and phosphorus following substantial overdose may be expected in some patients. In cases of substantial overdose, gastric lavage may be considered to remove unabsorbed drug. Standard procedures that are effective for treating hypocalcemia, including the administration of calcium intravenously, would be expected to restore physiologic amounts of ionized calcium and to relieve signs and symptoms of hypocalcemia.

Drug Interactions
Decreased Effect: Calcium supplements and antacids interfere with absorption of risedronate.

Ethanol/Nutrition/Herb Interactions Food: Food may reduce absorption (similar to other bisphosphonates); mean oral bioavailability is decreased when given with food.

Mechanism of Action A bisphosphonate which inhibits bone resorption via actions on osteoclasts or on osteoclast precursors; decreases the rate of bone resorption direction, leading to an indirect decrease in bone formation

Pharmacodynamics/Kinetics
Onset of action: May require weeks
Absorption: Rapid
Distribution: V_d: 6.3 L/kg
Protein binding: ~24%
Bioavailability: Poor, ~0.54% to 0.75%
Metabolism: None
Half-life elimination: Terminal: 220 hours
Excretion: Urine (up to 80%); feces (as unabsorbed drug)
(Continued)

Risedronate (Continued)

Usual Dosage Risedronate should be taken at least 30 minutes before the first food or drink of the day other than water. Oral:

Adults (patients should receive supplemental calcium and vitamin D if dietary intake is inadequate):

Paget's disease of bone: 30 mg once daily for 2 months

Retreatment may be considered (following post-treatment observation of at least 2 months) if relapse occurs, or if treatment fails to normalize serum alkaline phosphatase. For retreatment, the dose and duration of therapy are the same as for initial treatment. No data are available on more than one course of retreatment.

Osteoporosis prevention and treatment (postmenopausal or glucocorticoid-induced): 5 mg once daily; efficacy for use longer than 1 year has not been established; **alternatively**, a dose of 35 mg once weekly has been demonstrated to be effective

Dosage adjustment in elderly: Dosage adjustment is not necessary except in patients who have severe renal impairment (Cl_{cr} <30 mL/minute)

Dosage adjustment in renal impairment: Cl_{cr} <30 mL/minute: Not recommended for use

Dietary Considerations Take ≥30 minutes before the first food or drink of the day other than water.

Administration It is imperative to administer risedronate 30-60 minutes before the patient takes any food, drink, or other medications orally to avoid interference with absorption. The patient should take risedronate on an empty stomach with a full glass (8 oz) of **plain water** (not mineral water) and avoid lying down for 30 minutes after swallowing tablet to help delivery to stomach.

Monitoring Parameters Alkaline phosphatase should be periodically measured; serum calcium, phosphorus, and possibly potassium due to its drug class; use of absorptiometry may assist in noting benefit in osteoporosis; monitor pain and fracture rate

Reference Range Calcium (total): Adults: 9.0-11.0 mg/dL (2.05-2.54 mmol/L), may slightly decrease with aging; phosphorus: 2.5-4.5 mg/dL (0.81-1.45 mmol/L)

Patient Information The expected benefits of risedronate may only be obtained when each tablet is taken with plain water the first thing in the morning and at least 30 minutes before the first food, beverage, or medication of the day. Wait >30 minutes to improve risedronate absorption. Even dosing with orange juice or coffee markedly reduces the absorption of risedronate.

Take risedronate with a full glass of water (6-8 oz/180-240 mL) and do not lie down (stay fully upright sitting or standing) for at least 30 minutes following administration to facilitate delivery to the stomach and reduce the potential for esophageal irritation.

You may experience headache (request analgesic), skin rash, abdominal pain, diarrhea, or constipation (report if persistent). Report unresolved muscle or bone pain, leg cramps, acute abdominal pain, chest pain, palpitations, swollen extremities, disturbed vision, excessively dry eyes, ringing in the ears, or persistent flu-like symptoms. Also notify prescriber if experiencing difficulty swallowing, pain when swallowing, or severe or persistent heartburn.

Take supplemental calcium and vitamin D if dietary intake is inadequate. Consider weight-bearing exercise along with the modification of certain behavioral factors, such as excessive cigarette smoking or alcohol consumption if these factors exist.

Dosage Forms Tablet, as sodium: 5 mg, 30 mg

♦ **Risedronate Sodium** see Risedronate on page 1199

♦ **Risperdal**® see Risperidone on page 1200

Risperidone (ris PER i done)

Related Information

Antipsychotic Agents Comparison on page 1486

U.S. Brand Names Risperdal®

Canadian Brand Names Risperdal®

Therapeutic Category Antipsychotic Agent, Atypical

Use Management of psychotic disorders (eg, schizophrenia)

Unlabeled/Investigational Use Behavioral symptoms associated with dementia in elderly; treatment of bipolar disorder, mania, Tourette's disorder; treatment of pervasive developmental disorder and autism in children and adolescents

Pregnancy Risk Factor C

Contraindications Hypersensitivity to risperidone or any component of the formulation

Warnings/Precautions Low to moderately sedating, use with caution in disorders where CNS depression is a feature. Use with caution in Parkinson's disease. Caution in patients with hemodynamic instability; bone marrow suppression; predisposition to seizures; subcortical brain damage; severe cardiac, hepatic, or respiratory disease. Use with caution in renal dysfunction. Esophageal dysmotility and aspiration have been associated with antipsychotic use - use with caution in patients at risk of aspiration pneumonia (ie, Alzheimer's disease). Caution in breast cancer or other prolactin-dependent tumors (may elevate prolactin levels). May alter temperature regulation or mask toxicity of other drugs due to antiemetic effects. May alter cardiac conduction (low risk relative to other neuroleptics) - life-threatening arrhythmias have occurred with therapeutic doses of neuroleptics. Use with caution in elderly patients or in patients who would not tolerate transient hypotensive episodes (cerebrovascular or cardiovascular disease) due to potential for orthostasis.

May cause anticholinergic effects (confusion, agitation, constipation, dry mouth, blurred vision, urinary retention); therefore, they should be used with caution in patients with decreased gastrointestinal motility, urinary retention, BPH, xerostomia, or visual problems. Conditions which also may be exacerbated by cholinergic blockade include narrow-angle glaucoma (screening is recommended) and worsening of myasthenia gravis. Relative to other neuroleptics, risperidone has a low potency of cholinergic blockade.

May cause extrapyramidal symptoms, including pseudoparkinsonism, acute dystonic reactions, akathisia, and tardive dyskinesia (risk of these reactions is low relative to other neuroleptics, and is dose-dependent). May be associated with neuroleptic malignant syndrome (NMS). May rarely cause hyperglycemia - use with caution in patients with diabetes or other disorders of glucose regulation.

Adverse Reactions

Frequency not defined: Gastrointestinal: Dysphagia, esophageal dysmotility

>10%: Central nervous system: Insomnia, agitation, anxiety, headache

1% to 10%:

Cardiovascular: Hypotension (especially orthostatic), tachycardia

Central nervous system: Sedation, dizziness, restlessness, extrapyramidal reactions (dose dependent), dystonic reactions, pseudoparkinson, tardive dyskinesia, neuroleptic malignant syndrome, altered central temperature regulation

Dermatologic: Photosensitivity (rare), rash, dry skin

Endocrine & metabolic: Amenorrhea, galactorrhea, gynecomastia, sexual dysfunction

Gastrointestinal: Constipation, GI upset, xerostomia, dyspepsia, vomiting, abdominal pain, nausea, anorexia, weight gain

Genitourinary: Polyuria

Ocular: Abnormal vision

Respiratory: Rhinitis, coughing, sinusitis, pharyngitis, dyspnea

<1% (Limited to important or life-threatening): Diabetes mellitus, hyperglycemia

Drug Interactions

Cytochrome P450 Effect: CYP2D6 enzyme substrate and weak inhibitor; CYP3A3/4 substrate

Increased Effect/Toxicity: Risperidone may enhance the hypotensive effects of antihypertensive agents. Clozapine decreases clearance of risperidone.

Decreased Effect: Risperidone may antagonize effects of levodopa. Carbamazepine decreases risperidone serum concentrations.

Ethanol/Nutrition/Herb Interactions

Ethanol: Avoid ethanol (may increase CNS depression).

Food: Risperidone serum concentration may be increased if taken with grapefruit juice.

Herb/Nutraceutical: Avoid kava kava, gotu kola, valerian, St John's wort (may increase CNS depression).

Mechanism of Action Risperidone is a benzisoxazole derivative, mixed serotonin-dopamine antagonist; binds to 5-HT$_2$-receptors in the CNS and in the periphery with a very high affinity; binds to dopamine-D$_2$ receptors with less affinity. The binding affinity to the dopamine-D$_2$ receptor is 20 times lower than the 5-HT$_2$ affinity. The addition of serotonin antagonism to dopamine antagonism (classic neuroleptic mechanism) is thought to improve negative symptoms of psychoses and reduce the incidence of extrapyramidal side effects. Alpha$_1$, alpha$_2$ adrenergic, and histaminergic receptors are also antagonized with high affinity. Risperidone has low to moderate affinity for 5-HT$_{1C}$, 5-HT$_{1D}$, and 5-HT$_{1A}$ receptors, weak affinity for D$_1$ and no affinity for muscarinics or beta$_1$ and beta$_2$ receptors

Pharmacodynamics/Kinetics

Absorption: Rapid; well absorbed; food does not affect either the rate or extent

Metabolism: Extensive by CYP2D6 to 9-hydroxyrisperidone (equi-effective with risperidone); N-dealkylation is a second minor pathway

Protein binding, plasma: Risperidone 90%; 9-hydroxyrisperidone: 77%

Bioavailability: Tablet: 70%; solution: 74.5%

Half-life elimination: 20 hours (risperidone and its active metabolite 9-hydroxyrisperidone)

Time to peak, plasma: Risperidone: Within 1 hour; 9-hydroxyrisperidone: 3 hours in extensive metabolizers and 17 hours in poor metabolizers

Usual Dosage Oral:

Children and Adolescents:

Pervasive developmental disorder (unlabeled use): Initial: 0.25 mg twice daily; titrate up 0.25 mg/day every 5-7 days; optimal dose range: 0.75-3 mg/day

Autism (unlabeled use): Initial: 0.25 mg at bedtime; titrate to 1 mg/day (0.1 mg/kg/day)

Schizophrenia: Initial: 0.5 mg twice daily; titrate as necessary up to 2-6 mg/day

Bipolar disorder (unlabeled use): Initial: 0.5 mg; titrate to 0.5-3 mg/day

Tourette's disorder (unlabeled use): Initial: 0.5 mg; titrate to 2-4 mg/day

Adults: Recommended starting dose: 0.5-1 mg twice daily; slowly increase to the optimum range of 3-6 mg/day; may be given as a single daily dose once maintenance dose is achieved; daily dosages >10 mg does not appear to confer any additional benefit, and the incidence of extrapyramidal symptoms is higher than with lower doses

Elderly: A starting dose of 0.25-1 mg in 1-2 divided doses, and titration should progress slowly. Additional monitoring of renal function and orthostatic blood pressure may be warranted. If once-a-day dosing in the elderly or debilitated patient is considered, a twice daily regimen should be used to titrate to the target dose, and this dose should be maintained for 2-3 days prior to attempts to switch to a once-daily regimen.

Dosing adjustment in renal, hepatic impairment: Starting dose of 0.25-0.5 mg twice daily is advisable

Dietary Considerations May be taken with or without food.

Administration Oral solution can be mixed with water, coffee, orange juice, or low-fat milk, but is **not compatible** with cola, grapefruit juice, or tea. May be administered with or without food.

Monitoring Parameters Monitor for extrapyramidal symptoms, orthostatic blood pressure changes for 3-5 days after starting or increasing dose

Patient Information Use exactly as directed (do not increase dose or frequency). It may take several weeks to achieve desired results; do not discontinue without consulting prescriber. Dilute solution with water, milk, or orange juice; do not dilute with grapefruit juice or beverages containing tannin, or pectinate (eg, colas, tea). Avoid concurrent grapefruit juice. Avoid alcohol or caffeine and other prescription or OTC medications not approved by prescriber. Maintain adequate hydration (2-3 L/day of fluids unless instructed to restrict fluid intake). You may experience excess sedation, drowsiness, restlessness, dizziness, or blurred vision (use caution driving or when engaging in tasks requiring alertness until response to drug is (Continued)

Risperidone *(Continued)*

known); dry mouth, nausea, or GI upset (small frequent meals, frequent mouth care, chewing gum, or sucking lozenges may help); postural hypotension (use caution climbing stairs or when changing position from lying or sitting to standing); or urinary retention (void before taking medication). Report persistent CNS effects (eg, trembling fingers, altered gait or balance, excessive sedation, seizures, unusual muscle or skeletal movements, anxiety, abnormal thoughts, confusion, personality changes); chest pain, palpitations, rapid heartbeat, severe dizziness; swelling or pain in breasts (male and female), altered menstrual pattern, sexual dysfunction; pain or difficulty on urination; vision changes; skin rash or yellowing of skin; difficulty breathing; or worsening of condition. Inform prescriber if you are or intend to be pregnant. Do not breast-feed.

Nursing Implications Monitor and observe for extrapyramidal symptoms, orthostatic blood pressure changes for 3-5 days after starting or increasing dose

Dosage Forms
Solution, oral: 1 mg/mL (30 mL)
Tablet: 0.25 mg, 0.5 mg, 1 mg, 2 mg, 3 mg, 4 mg

- ♦ **Ritalin®** *see Methylphenidate on page 894*
- ♦ **Ritalin-SR®** *see Methylphenidate on page 894*
- ♦ **Ritifed® [OTC]** *see Triprolidine and Pseudoephedrine on page 1380*

Ritodrine *(RI toe dreen)*

Related Information
Antacid Drug Interactions *on page 1477*

Synonyms Ritodrine Hydrochloride

Therapeutic Category Adrenergic Agonist Agent; Beta$_2$-Adrenergic Agonist Agent; Sympathomimetic; Tocolytic Agent

Use Inhibits uterine contraction in preterm labor

Pregnancy Risk Factor B (contraindicated before 20th week)

Contraindications Cardiac arrhythmias; pheochromocytoma; pregnancy (before 20th week)

Warnings/Precautions Monitor hydration status and blood glucose concentrations; fatal maternal pulmonary edema has been reported, sometimes after delivery; fluid overload must be avoided, hydration levels should be monitored closely; if pulmonary edema occurs, the drug should be discontinued; use with caution in patients with moderate pre-eclampsia, diabetes, or migraine; some products may contain sulfites; maternal deaths have been reported in patients treated with ritodrine and concurrent corticosteroids (pulmonary edema)

Adverse Reactions
>10%:
   Cardiovascular: Increases in maternal and fetal heart rates and maternal hypertension, palpitations, chest pain
   Central nervous system: Headache
   Dermatologic: Erythema
   Endocrine & metabolic: Temporary hyperglycemia (maternal)
   Gastrointestinal: Nausea, vomiting
   Neuromuscular & skeletal: Tremor (trembling)
   Respiratory: Pulmonary edema
1% to 10%:
   Central nervous system: Nervousness, anxiety, restlessness
   Dermatologic: Rash
<1% (Limited to important or life-threatening): Agranulocytosis, impaired liver function, ketoacidosis, leukopenia

Overdosage/Toxicology Symptoms include tachycardia, palpitations, hypotension, nervousness, nausea, vomiting, and tremor. Use an appropriate beta-blocker as an antidote.

Drug Interactions
Increased Effect/Toxicity: Increased effect/toxicity with meperidine, sympathomimetics, diazoxide, magnesium, betamethasone (pulmonary edema), potassium-depleting diuretics, and general anesthetics.
Decreased Effect: Decreased effect with beta-blockers.

Stability Stable for 48 hours at room temperature after dilution in 500 mL of NS, D$_5$W, or LR I.V. solutions

Mechanism of Action Tocolysis due to its uterine beta$_2$-adrenergic receptor stimulating effects; this agent's beta$_2$ effects can also cause bronchial relaxation and vascular smooth muscle stimulation

Pharmacodynamics/Kinetics
Distribution: Crosses placenta
Protein binding: 32%
Metabolism: Hepatic
Half-life elimination: 15 hours
Time to peak, serum: 0.5-1 hour
Excretion: Urine (as unchanged drug and inactive conjugates)

Usual Dosage Adults: I.V.: 50-100 mcg/minute; increase by 50 mcg/minute every 10 minutes; continue for 12 hours after contractions have stopped
Hemodialysis: Removed by hemodialysis

Administration Monitor amount of I.V. fluid administered to prevent fluid overload; place patient in left lateral recumbent position to reduce risk of hypotension; use microdrip chamber or I.V. pump to control infusion rate

Monitoring Parameters Hematocrit, serum potassium, glucose, colloidal osmotic pressure, heart rate, and uterine contractions

Patient Information Remain in bed during infusion

Dosage Forms
Infusion [in D$_5$W]: 0.3 mL (500 mL)
Injection, as hydrochloride: 10 mg/mL (5 mL); 15 mg/mL (10 mL)

♦ **Ritodrine Hydrochloride** see Ritodrine *on page 1202*

Ritonavir (ri TOE na veer)

Related Information
Antiretroviral Agents Comparison *on page 1488*
Antiretroviral Therapy for HIV Infection *on page 1595*
Management of Healthcare Worker Exposures to HIV, HBV, HCV *on page 1555*

U.S. Brand Names Norvir®

Canadian Brand Names Norvir®; Norvir® SEC

Therapeutic Category Antiretroviral Agent, Protease Inhibitor; Protease Inhibitor

Use Treatment of HIV infection; should always be used as part of a multidrug regimen (at least 3 antiretroviral agents)

Pregnancy Risk Factor B

Pregnancy/Breast-Feeding Implications According to preliminary data, placental passage of ritonavir is minimal. Pregnancy and protease inhibitors are both associated with an increased risk of hyperglycemia. Glucose levels should be closely monitored. Healthcare professionals are encouraged to contact the antiretroviral pregnancy registry to monitor outcomes of pregnant women exposed to antiretroviral medications (1-800-258-4263).

Contraindications Hypersensitivity to ritonavir or any component of the formulation; concurrent amiodarone, astemizole, bepridil, cisapride, dihydroergotamine, ergonovine, ergotamine, flecainide, lovastatin, methylergonovine, midazolam, pimozide, propafenone, quinidine, simvastatin, St John's wort, terfenadine, triazolam

Warnings/Precautions Use caution in patients with hepatic insufficiency; safety and efficacy have not been established in children <2 years of age; use caution with benzodiazepines, rifabutin, sildenafil, and certain analgesics (meperidine, piroxicam, propoxyphene). Selected HMG-CoA reductase inhibitors are contraindicated (see Contraindications); atorvastatin should be used at the lowest possible dose, while fluvastatin or pravastatin may be safer alternatives. Avoid concurrent use of St John's wort (may lead to loss of virologic response and/or resistance). Ritonavir may interact with many medications. Careful review is required.

Adverse Reactions
Protease inhibitors cause hyperglycemia and dyslipidemia (elevated cholesterol/triglycerides) and a redistribution of fat (protease paunch, buffalo hump, facial atrophy and breast engorgement).

>10%:
Endocrine & metabolic: Increased GGT, increased triglycerides
Gastrointestinal: Diarrhea, nausea, vomiting, taste perversion
Hematologic: Anemia, decreased WBCs
Neuromuscular & skeletal: Weakness

1% to 10%:
Cardiovascular: Vasodilation
Central nervous system: Headache, fever, malaise, paresthesia, dizziness, insomnia, somnolence, thinking abnormally
Dermatologic: Rash
Endocrine & metabolic: Hyperlipidemia, increased glucose, increased uric acid, increased CPK, increased potassium, increased calcium
Gastrointestinal: Abdominal pain, anorexia, constipation, heartburn, flatulence, local throat irritation, increased CPK
Hematologic: Decreased neutrophils, increased eosinophils, increased, neutrophils, increased prothrombin time, increased WBC
Hepatic: Increased LFTs
Neuromuscular & skeletal: Myalgia
Respiratory: Pharyngitis
Miscellaneous: Diaphoresis

Overdosage/Toxicology Human experience is limited. There is no specific antidote for overdose with ritonavir. The oral solution contains 43% ethanol by volume, potentially causing significant ethanol-related toxicity in younger patients. Dialysis is unlikely to be beneficial in significant removal of the drug. Charcoal or gastric lavage may be useful to remove unabsorbed drug.

Drug Interactions
Cytochrome P450 Effect: CYP1A2, 2A6, 2C9, 2C19, 2E1, and 3A3/4 enzyme substrate, CYP2D6 enzyme substrate (minor); CYP1A2 enzyme inducer; CYP1A2, 2A6, 2C9, 2C19, 2D6, 2E1, and 3A3/4 enzyme inhibitor

Increased Effect/Toxicity: Concurrent use of amiodarone, bepridil, cisapride, flecainide, pimozide, propafenone, and quinidine is contraindicated. Serum concentrations/toxicity of many benzodiazepines may be increased; midazolam and triazolam are contraindicated. Concurrent use of ergot alkaloids (dihydroergotamine, ergotamine, ergonovine, methylergonovine) with ritonavir is also contraindicated (may cause vasospasm and peripheral ischemia). HMG-CoA reductase inhibitors serum concentrations may be increased by ritonavir, increasing the risk of myopathy/rhabdomyolysis; lovastatin and simvastatin are contraindicated; fluvastatin and pravastatin may be safer alternatives. Serum concentrations of meperidine's neuroexcitatory metabolite (normeperidine) are increased by ritonavir, which may increase the risk of CNS toxicity/seizures. Rifabutin and rifabutin metabolite serum concentrations may be increased by ritonavir; reduce rifabutin dose to 150 mg every other day. Sildenafil serum concentrations may be increased by ritonavir; when used concurrently, do not exceed a maximum sildenafil dose of 25 mg in a 48-hour period. Saquinavir's serum concentrations are increased by ritonavir; the dosage of both agents should be reduced to 400 mg twice daily. Concurrent therapy with amprenavir may result in increased serum concentrations: dosage adjustment is recommended. Metronidazole or disulfiram may cause disulfiram reaction (oral solution contains 43% ethanol).

Ritonavir may also increase the serum concentrations of the following drugs (dose decrease may be needed): Benzodiazepines, beta-blockers (metoprolol, timolol), bupropion, calcium channel blockers (diltiazem, nifedipine, verapamil), carbamazepine, clarithromycin, clonazepam, clorazepate, clozapine, cyclosporin, dexamethasone, disopyramide, dronabinol, ethosuximide, fluoxetine (and other SSRIs), indinavir, ketoconazole, lidocaine,

(Continued)

Ritonavir *(Continued)*

methamphetamine, mexiletine, nefazodone, perphenazine, prednisone, propoxyphene, piroxicam, quinine, risperidone, tacrolimus, tramadol, thioridazine, tricyclic antidepressants (including desipramine), and zolpidem. Serum concentrations of rifabutin may be increased by ritonavir; dosage adjustment required.

Decreased Effect: The administration of didanosine (buffered formulation) should be separated from ritonavir by 2.5 hours to limit interaction with ritonavir. Concurrent use of rifampin, rifabutin, dexamethasone, and many anticonvulsants may lower serum concentration of ritonavir. Ritonavir may reduce the concentration of ethinyl estradiol which may result in loss of contraception (including combination products). Theophylline concentrations may be reduced in concurrent therapy. Levels of didanosine and zidovudine may be decreased by ritonavir, however, no dosage adjustment is necessary. In addition, ritonavir may decrease the serum concentrations of the following drugs: Atovaquone, divalproex, lamotrigine, methadone, phenytoin, warfarin.

Ethanol/Nutrition/Herb Interactions
Food: Food enhances absorption.
Herb/Nutraceutical: St John's wort may decrease ritonavir serum levels. Avoid use.

Stability
Capsule: Store under refrigeration at 2°C to 80°C (36°F to 46°F); may be left out at room temperature of <25°C (<77°F) if used within 30 days. Protect from light. Avoid exposure to excessive heat.
Solution: Store at room temperature at 20°C to 25°C (68°F to 77°F). Do not refrigerate.

Mechanism of Action Ritonavir inhibits HIV protease and renders the enzyme incapable of processing of polyprotein precursor which leads to production of noninfectious immature HIV particles

Pharmacodynamics/Kinetics
Absorption: Variable, with or without food
Distribution: High concentrations in serum and lymph nodes
Protein binding: 98% to 99%
Metabolism: Hepatic; five metabolites, low concentration of an active metabolite achieved in plasma (oxidative); see Drug Interactions
Half-life elimination: 3-5 hours
Excretion: Urine (negligible amounts)

Usual Dosage Oral:
Children ≥2 years: 250 mg/m² twice daily; titrate dose upward to 400 mg/m² twice daily (maximum: 600 mg twice daily)
Adults: 600 mg twice daily; dose escalation tends to avoid nausea that many patients experience upon initiation of full dosing. Escalate the dose as follows: 300 mg twice daily for 1 day, 400 mg twice daily for 2 days, 500 mg twice daily for 1 day, then 600 mg twice daily. Ritonavir may be better tolerated when used in combination with other antiretrovirals by initiating the drug alone and subsequently adding the second agent within 2 weeks.
Note: Dosage adjustments for ritonavir when administered in combination therapy:
Amprenavir: Adjustments necessary for each agent:
Amprenavir 1200 mg with ritonavir 200 mg once daily **or**
Amprenavir 600 mg with ritonavir 100 mg twice daily
Amprenavir plus efavirenz (3-drug regimen): Amprenavir 1200 mg twice daily plus ritonavir 200 mg twice daily plus efavirenz at standard dose
Indinavir: Adjustments necessary for both agents:
Indinavir 800 mg twice daily plus ritonavir 100-200 mg twice daily **or**
Indinavir 400 mg twice daily plus ritonavir 400 mg twice daily
Nelfinavir or saquinavir: Ritonavir 400 mg twice daily
Dosing adjustment in renal impairment: None necessary
Dosing adjustment in hepatic impairment: No adjustment required in mild impairment; insufficient data in moderate-severe impairment; caution advised with severe impairment

Dietary Considerations Oral solution contains 43% ethanol by volume.

Administration Take with food. Liquid formulations usually have an unpleasant taste. Consider mixing it with chocolate milk or a liquid nutritional supplement.

Monitoring Parameters Triglycerides, cholesterol, CBC, LFTs, CPK, uric acid, basic HIV monitoring, viral load, and CD4 count, glucose

Patient Information Take with food. Mix liquid formulation with chocolate milk or liquid nutritional supplement. You may experience headache or confusion; if these persist notify prescriber. Diarrhea may be moderate to severe. Notify prescriber if problematic. Report swelling, numbness of tongue, mouth, lips, unresolved vomiting, fever, chills, or extreme fatigue. Do not take any prescription medications, over-the-counter products or herbal products, especially St John's wort, without consulting prescriber.

Additional Information Potential compliance problems, frequency of administration and adverse effects should be discussed with patients before initiating therapy to help prevent the emergence of resistance.

Dosage Forms
Capsule: 100 mg
Solution: 80 mg/mL (240 mL)

♦ **Rituxan**® see Rituximab *on page 1204*

Rituximab *(ri TUK si mab)*

U.S. Brand Names Rituxan®
Canadian Brand Names Rituxan®
Synonyms C2B8
Therapeutic Category Antineoplastic Agent, Natural Source (Plant) Derivative; Monoclonal Antibody
Use Treatment of patients with relapsed or refractory low-grade or follicular, CD20 positive, B-cell non-Hodgkin's lymphoma; treatment (as part of combination therapy with radiolabeled ibritumomab) of patients with relapsed or refractory low-grade, follicular, or transformed B-cell non-Hodgkin's lymphoma (including rituximab refractory follicular non-Hodgkin's lymphoma)

Pregnancy Risk Factor C

Contraindications Type I hypersensitivity or anaphylactic reactions to murine proteins or any component of the formulation; breast-feeding

Warnings/Precautions Rituximab is associated with hypersensitivity reactions which may respond to adjustments in the infusion rate. Hypotension, bronchospasm, and angioedema have occurred as part of an infusion-related symptom complex. Interrupt rituximab infusion for severe reactions and resume at a 50% reduction in rate (eg, from 100 to 50 mg/hour) when symptoms have completely resolved. Treatment of these symptoms with diphenhydramine and acetaminophen is recommended; additional treatment with bronchodilators or I.V. saline may be indicated. In most cases, patients who have experienced nonlife-threatening reactions have been able to complete the full course of therapy. Medications for the treatment of hypersensitivity reactions (eg, epinephrine, antihistamines, corticosteroids) should be available for immediate use in the event of such a reaction during administration.

Discontinue infusions in the event of serious or life-threatening cardiac arrhythmias. Patients who develop clinically significant arrhythmias should undergo cardiac monitoring during and after subsequent infusions of rituximab. Patients with pre-existing cardiac conditions including arrhythmias and angina have had recurrences of these events during rituximab therapy; monitor these patients throughout the infusion and immediate postinfusion periods.

Adverse Reactions Infusion-related symptoms are common. The incidence of infusion-related events decreased from 80% during the first infusion to ~40% with subsequent infusions. Fever, chills/rigors, and other infusion-related events occurred in the majority of patients during the first rituximab infusion. Angioedema may occur in up to 13% of patients. These reactions generally occurred within 30 minutes to 2 hours of beginning the first infusion, and resolved with slowing or interruption of the infusion and with supportive care.

>10%:
　Central nervous system: Headache (14%)
　Gastrointestinal: Nausea (18%)
　Hematologic: Leukopenia (11%)
　Miscellaneous: Fever (49%), chills (32%), asthenia (16%), angioedema (13%)
　Immunologic: Rituximab-induced B-cell depletion (70% to 80%)

1% to 10%:
　Cardiovascular: Hypotension (10%)
　Central nervous system: Myalgia (7%), dizziness (7%)
　Dermatologic: Pruritus (10%), rash (10%), urticaria (8%)
　Gastrointestinal: Vomiting (7%), abdominal pain (6%)
　Hematologic: During the treatment period (up to 30 days following the last dose), the following occurred: Severe thrombocytopenia, severe neutropenia, and severe anemia
　Respiratory: Bronchospasm occurred in 8%; 25% of these patients were treated with bronchodilators; rhinitis (8%)
　Miscellaneous: Throat irritation (6%)

<1% (Limited to important or life-threatening): Angina, aplastic anemia (pure red-cell aplasia), arrhythmia (ventricular and supraventricular), hemolytic anemia, myocardial infarction

Note: The following adverse events were reported more frequently in retreated patients: Anemia, anorexia, asthenia, depression, dizziness, flushing, leukopenia, night sweats, peripheral edema, pruritus, respiratory symptoms, tachycardia, throat irritation, thrombocytopenia

Stability

Store vials at refrigeration at 2°C to 8°C (36°F to 46°F); protect vials from direct sunlight

Withdraw the necessary amount of rituximab and dilute to a final concentration of 1-4 mg/mL into an infusion bag containing either 0.9% sodium chloride or 5% dextrose in water. Gently invert the bag to mix the solution. Solutions for infusion are stable at 2°C to 8°C (36°F to 46°F) for 24 hours and at room temperature for an additional 12 hours.

Mechanism of Action Rituximab is a monoclonal antibody directed against the CD20 antigen on B-lymphocytes. CD20 regulates cell cycle initiation; and, possibly, functions as a calcium channel. Rituximab binds to the antigen on the cell surface, activating complement-dependent cytotoxicity; and to human Fc receptors, mediating cell killing through an antibody-dependent cellular toxicity. The CD20 antigen is also expressed on >90% of B-cell non-Hodgkin's lymphomas (NHL) but is not found on hematopoietic stem cells, pro-B cells, normal plasma cells, or other normal tissues.

Pharmacodynamics/Kinetics

Duration: Detectable in serum 3-6 months after completion of treatment; B-cell recovery begins ~6 months following completion of treatment; median B-cell levels return to normal by 12 months following completion of treatment

Absorption: I.V.: Immediate and results in a rapid and sustained depletion of circulating and tissue-based B cells

Half-life elimination:
　>100 mg/m^2: 4.4 days (range 1.6-10.5 days)
　375 mg/m^2: 50 hours (following first dose) to 174 hours (following fourth dose)

Excretion: Uncertain; may undergo phagocytosis and catabolism in the reticuloendothelial system (RES)

Usual Dosage Adults: I.V. (refer to individual protocols): **Do not administer I.V. push or bolus** (hypersensitivity reactions may occur). Consider premedication (consisting of acetaminophen and diphenhydramine) before each infusion of rituximab. Premedication may attenuate infusion-related events. Because transient hypotension may occur during infusion, give consideration to withholding antihypertensive medications 12 hours prior to rituximab infusion.

I.V. infusion: 375 mg/m^2 once weekly for 4 doses (days 1, 8, 15, and 22).

As part of combination therapy with ibritumomab (Zevalin™ therapeutic regimen): Two infusions of rituximab are completed, separated by 7-9 days (corresponding to two infusions of ibritumomab with differing radiolabels).

Rituximab dose (also see Ibritumomab monograph):
　Step 1: 250 mg/m^2 at an initial rate of 50 mg/hour. If hypersensitivity or infusion-related events do not occur, increase infusion in increments of 50 mg/hour every 30 minutes,

(Continued)

Rituximab *(Continued)*

to a maximum of 400 mg/hour. Infusions should be temporarily slowed or interrupted if hypersensitivity or infusion related events occur. The infusion may be resumed at $^1/_2$ the previous rate upon improvement of symptoms.

Step 2: 250 mg/m^2 at an initial rate of 100 mg/hour (50 mg/hour if infusion-related events occurred with the first infusion). If hypersensitivity or infusion-related events do not occur, increase infusion in increments of 100 mg/hour every 30 minutes, to a maximum of 400 mg/hour, as tolerated.

Administration Administer the first infusion at an initial rate of 50 mg/hour. If hypersensitivity or infusion-related events do not occur, escalate the infusion rate in 50 mg/hour increments every 30 minutes, to a maximum of 400 mg/hour. If hypersensitivity or an infusion-related event develops, temporarily slow or interrupt the infusion. The infusion can continue at one-half the previous rate upon improvement of patient symptoms. Subsequent rituximab infusion can be administered at an initial rate of 100 mg/hour and increased by 100 mg/hour increments at 30-minute intervals, to a maximum of 400 mg/hour as tolerated.

Monitoring Parameters Obtain complete blood counts and platelet counts at regular intervals during rituximab therapy and more frequently in patients who develop cytopenia. Human antimurine antibody (HAMA) was not detected in 57 patients evaluated. Less than 1% of patients evaluated for human antichimeric antibody (HACA) was positive. Patients who develop HAMA/HACA titers may have an allergic or hypersensitivity reaction when treated with this or other murine or chimeric monoclonal antibodies. Monitor peripheral CD20+ cells.

Reference Range Peripheral CD20+ cells: High level pretreatment (500-1600 cells/µL, malignant or normal) may indicate risk of more severe infusional reactions

Additional Information Rapid infusion or bolus administration are associated with a high incidence of infusion-related reactions.

Dosage Forms Injection [preservative free]: 10 mg/mL (10 mL, 50 mL)

- ◆ **Riva-Diclofenac (Can)** *see Diclofenac on page 393*
- ◆ **Riva-Diclofenac-K (Can)** *see Diclofenac on page 393*
- ◆ **Riva-Loperamine (Can)** *see Loperamide on page 816*
- ◆ **Riva-Lorazepam (Can)** *see Lorazepam on page 821*
- ◆ **Riva-Naproxen (Can)** *see Naproxen on page 958*
- ◆ **Rivanase AQ (Can)** *see Beclomethasone on page 149*
- ◆ **Riva-Norfloxacin (Can)** *see Norfloxacin on page 994*

Rivastigmine *(ri va STIG meen)*

U.S. Brand Names Exelon®

Canadian Brand Names Exelon®

Synonyms ENA 713; SDZ ENA 713

Therapeutic Category Acetylcholinesterase Inhibitor; Cholinergic Agent

Use Mild to moderate dementia from Alzheimer's disease

Pregnancy Risk Factor B

Pregnancy/Breast-Feeding Implications There are no adequate studies in pregnant women. Should be used only if the benefit outweighs the potential risk to the fetus. It is unknown if rivastigmine is excreted in human breast milk. There is no indication for use in nursing mothers.

Contraindications Hypersensitivity to rivastigmine, other carbamate derivatives, or any component of the formulation

Warnings/Precautions Significant nausea, vomiting, anorexia, and weight loss are associated with use; occurs more frequently in women and during the titration phase. If treatment is interrupted for more than several days, reinstate at the lowest daily dose. Use caution in patients with a history of peptic ulcer disease or concurrent NSAID use. Caution in patients undergoing anesthesia who will receive succinylcholine-type muscle relaxation, patients with sick sinus syndrome, bradycardia or supraventricular conduction conditions, urinary obstruction, seizure disorders, or pulmonary conditions such as asthma or COPD. There are no trials evaluating the safety and efficacy in children.

Adverse Reactions

>10%:

Central nervous system: Dizziness (21%), headache(17%)

Gastrointestinal: Nausea (47%), vomiting (31%), diarrhea (19%), anorexia (17%), abdominal pain (13%)

2% to 10%:

Central nervous system: Fatigue (9%), insomnia (9%), confusion (8%), depression (6%), anxiety (5%), malaise (5%), somnolence (5%), hallucinations (4%), aggressiveness (3%)

Cardiovascular: Syncope (3%), hypertension (3%)

Gastrointestinal: Dyspepsia (9%), constipation (5%), flatulence (4%), weight loss (3%), eructation (2%)

Genitourinary: Urinary tract infection (7%)

Neuromuscular & skeletal: Weakness (6%), tremor (4%)

Respiratory: Rhinitis (4%)

Miscellaneous: Increased diaphoresis (4%), flu-like syndrome (3%)

<2% (Limited to important or life-threatening; reactions may be at a similar frequency to placebo): Acute renal failure, allergic reaction, angina pectoris, aphasia, apnea, apraxia, ataxia, atrial fibrillation, AV block, bradycardia, bronchospasm, bundle branch block, cardiac arrest, cardiac failure, cholecystitis, convulsions, delirium, dysphonia, GI hemorrhage, intestinal obstruction, intracranial hemorrhage, migraine, myocardial infarction, pancreatitis, peripheral ischemia, peripheral neuropathy, postural hypotension, psychosis, pulmonary embolism, rash, sick sinus syndrome, Stevens-Johnson syndrome, supraventricular tachycardia, thrombocytopenia, thrombophlebitis, thrombosis, urticaria, vomiting (severe) with esophageal rupture (following inappropriate reinitiation of dose)

Overdosage/Toxicology In cases of asymptomatic overdoses, rivastigmine should be held for 24 hours. Cholinergic crisis, caused by significant acetylcholinesterase inhibition, is characterized by severe nausea, vomiting, salivation, sweating, bradycardia, hypotension, respiratory depression, cardiovascular collapse, and convulsions. Treatment is supportive and symptomatic. Dialysis would not be helpful.

Drug Interactions

Increased Effect/Toxicity:

Beta-blockers without ISA activity may increase risk of bradycardia.

Calcium channel blockers (diltiazem or verapamil) may increase risk of bradycardia.

Cholinergic agonists effects may be increased with rivastigmine.

Cigarette use increases the clearance of rivastigmine by 23%.

Depolarizing neuromuscular blocking agents effects may be increased with rivastigmine.

Digoxin may increase risk of bradycardia.

Decreased Effect: Anticholinergic agents effects may be reduced with rivastigmine.

Ethanol/Nutrition/Herb Interactions

Cigarette use: Increases the clearance of rivastigmine by 23%.

Ethanol: Avoid ethanol (due to risk of sedation; may increase GI irritation).

Food: Food delays absorption by 90 minutes, lowers C_{max} by 30% and increases AUC by 30%.

Stability Store below 25°C (77°F); store solution in an upright position and protect from freezing

Mechanism of Action A deficiency of cortical acetylcholine is thought to account for some of the symptoms of Alzheimer's disease; rivastigmine increases acetylcholine in the central nervous system through reversible inhibition of its hydrolysis by cholinesterase

Pharmacodynamics/Kinetics

Absorption: Fasting: Rapid and complete within 1 hour

Distribution: V_d: 1.8-2.7 L/kg

Protein binding: 40%

Metabolism: Extensively via cholinesterase-mediated hydrolysis in the brain; metabolite undergoes N-demethylation and/or sulfate conjugation hepatically; CYP450 minimally involved; linear kinetics at 3 mg twice daily, but nonlinear at higher doses

Bioavailability: 40%

Half-life elimination: 1.5 hours

Time to peak: 1 hour

Excretion: Urine (97% as metabolites); feces (0.4%)

Usual Dosage Adults: Mild to moderate Alzheimer's dementia: Oral: Initial: 1.5 mg twice daily to start; if dose is tolerated for at least 2 weeks then it may be increased to 3 mg twice daily; increases to 4.5 mg twice daily and 6 mg twice daily should only be attempted after at least 2 weeks at the previous dose; maximum dose: 6 mg twice daily. If adverse events such as nausea, vomiting, abdominal pain, or loss of appetite occur, the patient should be instructed to discontinue treatment for several doses then restart at the same or next lower dosage level; antiemetics have been used to control GI symptoms. If treatment is interrupted for longer than several days, restart the treatment at the lowest dose and titrate as previously described.

Elderly: Clearance is significantly lower in patients older than 60 years of age, but dosage adjustments are not recommended. Titrate dose to individual's tolerance.

Dosage adjustment in renal impairment: Dosage adjustments are not recommended, however, titrate the dose to the individual's tolerance.

Dosage adjustment in hepatic impairment: Clearance is significantly reduced in mild to moderately impaired patients. Although dosage adjustments are not recommended, use lowest possible dose and titrate according to individual's tolerance. May consider waiting >2 weeks between dosage adjustments.

Dietary Considerations Take with meals.

Monitoring Parameters Cognitive function at periodic intervals

Patient Information Take with meals at breakfast and dinner. Swallow capsule whole. Do not chew, break, or crush capsule. A liquid (solution) is available for patients who cannot swallow capsules. Monitor for nausea, vomiting, loss of appetite, or weight loss; notify prescriber if any of these occur. See instructions for use of oral solution. Can swallow solution directly from syringe or mix with water, juice, or soda. Stir well and drink all of mixture within 4 hours of mixing. Do not mix with other liquids. Avoid concurrent ethanol use.

Nursing Implications Educate patient or caregiver about medicine.

Dosage Forms

Capsule, as tartrate: 1.5 mg, 3 mg, 4.5 mg, 6 mg

Solution, oral, as tartrate: 2 mg/mL (120 mL)

♦ **Rivotril® (Can)** see Clonazepam on page 316

Rizatriptan (rye za TRIP tan)

Related Information

Antimigraine Drugs Comparison on page 1485

U.S. Brand Names Maxalt®; Maxalt-MLT™

Canadian Brand Names Maxalt™; Maxalt RPD™

Synonyms MK462

Therapeutic Category Antimigraine Agent, Serotonin 5-HT$_{1D}$ Agonist; Serotonin Agonist

Use Acute treatment of migraine with or without aura

Pregnancy Risk Factor C

Contraindications Hypersensitivity to rizatriptan or any component of the formulation; documented ischemic heart disease or Prinzmetal's angina; uncontrolled hypertension; basilar or hemiplegic migraine; during or within 2 weeks of MAO inhibitors; during or within 24 hours of treatment with another 5-HT$_1$ agonist, or an ergot-containing or ergot-type medication (eg, methysergide, dihydroergotamine)

Warnings/Precautions Use only in patients with a clear diagnosis of migraine; use with caution in elderly or patients with hepatic or renal impairment, history of hypersensitivity to sumatriptan or adverse effects from sumatriptan, and in patients at risk of coronary artery

(Continued)

Rizatriptan *(Continued)*

disease (as predicted by presence of risk factors) unless cardiovascular evaluation provides evidence that the patient is free of cardiovascular disease. In patients with risk factors for coronary artery disease, following adequate evaluation to establish the absence of coronary artery disease, the initial dose should be administered in a setting where response may be evaluated (physician's office or similarly staffed setting). EKG monitoring may be considered. Do not use with ergotamines. May increase blood pressure transiently; may cause coronary vasospasm (less than sumatriptan); avoid in patients with signs/symptoms suggestive of reduced arterial flow (ischemic bowel, Raynaud's) which could be exacerbated by vaso-spasm. Phenylketonurics (tablets contain phenylalanine).

Patients who experience sensations of chest pain/pressure/tightness or symptoms sugges-tive of angina following dosing should be evaluated for coronary artery disease or Prinzmetal's angina before receiving additional doses.

Caution in dialysis patients or hepatically impaired. Reconsider diagnosis of migraine if no response to initial dose. Long-term effects on vision have not been evaluated.

Adverse Reactions

1% to 10%:

Cardiovascular: Systolic/diastolic blood pressure increases (5-10 mm Hg), chest pain (5%), palpitation

Central nervous system: Dizziness, drowsiness, fatigue (13% to 30%, dose related)

Dermatologic: Skin flushing

Endocrine & metabolic: Mild increase in growth hormone, hot flashes

Gastrointestinal: Nausea, abdominal pain, dry mouth (<5%)

Respiratory: Dyspnea

<1% (Limited to important or life-threatening): Akinesia, angina, arrhythmia, bradycardia, bradykinesia, decreased mental activity, myalgia, myocardial ischemia, myocardial infarc-tion, neck pain/stiffness, neurological/psychiatric abnormalities, pruritus, stroke, syncope, tachycardia, tinnitus, toxic epidermal necrolysis

Drug Interactions

Increased Effect/Toxicity: Use within 24 hours of another selective 5-HT$_1$ antagonist or ergot-containing drug should be avoided due to possible additive vasoconstriction. Use with propranolol increased plasma concentration of rizatriptan by 70%. Rarely, concurrent use with SSRIs results in weakness and incoordination; monitor closely. MAO inhibitors and nonselective MAO inhibitors increase concentration of rizatriptan.

Ethanol/Nutrition/Herb Interactions Food: Food delays absorption.

Stability Store in blister pack until administration

Mechanism of Action Selective agonist for serotonin (5-HT$_{1D}$ receptor) in cranial arteries to cause vasoconstriction and reduce sterile inflammation associated with antidromic neuronal transmission correlating with relief of migraine

Pharmacodynamics/Kinetics

Onset of action: ~30 minutes

Duration: 14-16 hours

Protein binding: 14%

Metabolism: Via monoamine oxidase-A; first-pass effect

Bioavailability: 40% to 50%

Half-life elimination: 2-3 hours

Time to peak: 1-1.5 hours

Excretion: Urine (82%, 8% to 16% as unchanged drug); feces (12%)

Usual Dosage Note: In patients with risk factors for coronary artery disease, following adequate evaluation to establish the absence of coronary artery disease, the initial dose should be administered in a setting where response may be evaluated (physician's office or similarly staffed setting). EKG monitoring may be considered.

Oral: 5-10 mg, repeat after 2 hours if significant relief is not attained; maximum: 30 mg in a 24-hour period (use 5 mg dose in patients receiving propranolol with a maximum of 15 mg in 24 hours)

Note: For orally-disintegrating tablets (Maxalt-MLT™): Patient should be instructed to place tablet on tongue and allow to dissolve. Dissolved tablet will be swallowed with saliva.

Dietary Considerations Orally-disintegrating tablet contains phenylalanine (1.05 mg per 5 mg tablet, 2.10 mg per 10 mg tablet).

Monitoring Parameters Headache severity, signs/symptoms suggestive of angina; consider monitoring blood pressure, heart rate, and/or EKG with first dose in patients with likelihood of unrecognized coronary disease, such as patients with significant hypertension, hypercholes-terolemia, obese patients, diabetics, smokers with other risk factors or strong family history of coronary artery disease

Patient Information For orally disintegrating tablets: Do not remove blister from outer pouch until just before dosing; open blister with dry hands, place tablet on tongue and allow to dissolve. Dissolved tablet will be swallowed with saliva.

For all dosage forms: May repeat dose anytime after 2 hours of the first dose. Do not take a second dose without first consulting your physician. Do not take more than 30 mg in a 24-hour period (15 mg maximum in 24 hours if taking propranolol).

Dosage Forms

Tablet, as benzoate (Maxalt®): 5 mg, 10 mg

Tablet, orally disintegrating (Maxalt-MLT™): 5 mg, 10 mg

- **rLFN-α2** *see* Interferon Alfa-2b *on page 728*
- **RMS®** *see* Morphine Sulfate *on page 936*
- **Robafen® AC** *see* Guaifenesin and Codeine *on page 646*
- **Robafen DM® [OTC]** *see* Guaifenesin and Dextromethorphan *on page 646*
- **Robaxin®** *see* Methocarbamol *on page 883*
- **Robaxisal®** *see* Methocarbamol and Aspirin *on page 884*
- **Robaxisal® Extra Strength (Can)** *see* Methocarbamol and Aspirin *on page 884*
- **Robidrine® (Can)** *see* Pseudoephedrine *on page 1155*

Rocuronium (roe kyoor OH nee um)

Related Information
Neuromuscular Blocking Agents Comparison *on page 1508*

U.S. Brand Names Zemuron®

Canadian Brand Names Zemuron®

Synonyms ORG 946; Rocuronium Bromide

Therapeutic Category Neuromuscular Blocker Agent, Nondepolarizing; Skeletal Muscle Relaxant

Use Adjunct to general anesthesia to facilitate both rapid sequence and routine endotracheal intubation and to relax skeletal muscles during surgery; to facilitate mechanical ventilation in ICU patients; does not relieve pain or produce sedation

Pregnancy Risk Factor C

Pregnancy/Breast-Feeding Implications No adequate or well-controlled studies in pregnant women; use only when potential benefit justifies potential risk to the fetus.

Contraindications Hypersensitivity to rocuronium or any component of the formulation

Warnings/Precautions Use with caution in patients with valvular heart disease, pulmonary disease, hepatic impairment; ventilation must be supported during neuromuscular blockade; certain clinical conditions may result in potentiation or antagonism of neuromuscular blockade:

Potentiation: Electrolyte abnormalities, severe hyponatremia, severe hypocalcemia, severe hypokalemia, hypermagnesemia, neuromuscular diseases, acidosis, acute intermittent porphyria, renal failure, hepatic failure

Antagonism: Alkalosis, hypercalcemia, demyelinating lesions, peripheral neuropathies, diabetes mellitus

Increased sensitivity in patients with myasthenia gravis, Eaton-Lambert syndrome; resistance in burn patients (>30% of body) for period of 5-70 days postinjury; resistance in patients with muscle trauma, denervation, immobilization, infection

Adverse Reactions
>1%: Cardiovascular: Transient hypotension and hypertension

<1% (Limited to important or life-threatening): Abnormal EKG, anaphylaxis, arrhythmia, bronchospasm, edema, hiccups, injection site pruritus, nausea, rash, rhonchi, shock, tachycardia, vomiting, wheezing

Overdosage/Toxicology Symptoms include prolonged skeletal muscle block, muscle weakness and apnea. Treatment consists of airway support and controlled ventilation until recovery of normal neuromuscular block is observed. Further recovery may be facilitated by administering an anticholinesterase agent (eg, neostigmine, edrophonium, or pyridostigmine) with atropine, to antagonize skeletal muscle relaxation. Support of the cardiovascular system with fluids and pressors may be necessary.

Drug Interactions
Increased Effect/Toxicity: Increased effects are possible with aminoglycosides, betablockers, clindamycin, calcium channel blockers, halogenated anesthetics, imipenem, ketamine, lidocaine, loop diuretics (furosemide), macrolides (case reports), magnesium sulfate, procainamide, quinidine, quinolones, tetracyclines, and vancomycin. May increase risk of myopathy when used with high- dose corticosteroids for extended periods.

Decreased Effect: Effect of nondepolarizing neuromuscular blockers may be reduced by carbamazepine (chronic use), corticosteroids (also associated with myopathy - see increased effect), phenytoin (chronic use), sympathomimetics, and theophylline.

Stability Store under refrigeration (2°C to 8°C), do not freeze; when stored at room temperature, it is stable for 30 days; unlike vecuronium, it is stable in 0.9% sodium chloride and 5% dextrose in water, this mixture should be used within 24 hours of preparation

Mechanism of Action Blocks acetylcholine from binding to receptors on motor endplate inhibiting depolarization

Pharmacodynamics/Kinetics
Onset of action: Good intubation conditions in 1-2 minutes; maximum neuromuscular blockade within 4 minutes

Duration: ~30 minutes (with standard doses, increases with higher doses)

Metabolism: Minimally hepatic

Excretion: Feces

Usual Dosage Administer I.V.; dose to effect; doses will vary due to interpatient variability; use ideal body weight for obese patients

(Continued)

Rocuronium *(Continued)*

Children:

Initial: 0.6 mg/kg under halothane anesthesia produce excellent to good intubating conditions within 1 minute and will provide a median time of 41 minutes of clinical relaxation in children 3 months to 1 year of age, and 27 minutes in children 1-12 years

Maintenance: 0.075-0.125 mg/kg administered upon return of T_1 to 25% of control provides clinical relaxation for 7-10 minutes

Adults:

Tracheal intubation: I.V.:

Initial: 0.6 mg/kg is expected to provide approximately 31 minutes of clinical relaxation under opioid/nitrous oxide/oxygen anesthesia with neuromuscular block sufficient for intubation attained in 1-2 minutes; lower doses (0.45 mg/kg) may be used to provide 22 minutes of clinical relaxation with median time to neuromuscular block of 1-3 minutes; maximum blockade is achieved in <4 minutes

Maximum: 0.9-1.2 mg/kg may be given during surgery under opioid/nitrous oxide/oxygen anesthesia without adverse cardiovascular effects and is expected to provide 58-67 minutes of clinical relaxation; neuromuscular blockade sufficient for intubation is achieved in <2 minutes with maximum blockade in <3 minutes

Maintenance: 0.1, 0.15, and 0.2 mg/kg administered at 25% recovery of control T_1 (defined as 3 twitches of train-of-four) provides a median of 12, 17, and 24 minutes of clinical duration under anesthesia

Rapid sequence intubation: 0.6-1.2 mg/kg in appropriately premedicated and anesthetized patients with excellent or good intubating conditions within 2 minutes

Continuous infusion: 0.01-0.012 mg/kg/minute only after early evidence of spontaneous recovery of neuromuscular function is evident; infusion rates have ranged from 4-16 mcg/kg/minute

ICU: 10 mcg/kg/minute; adjust dose to maintain appropriate degree of neuromuscular blockade (eg, 1 or 2 twitches on train-of-four)

Dosing adjustment in hepatic impairment: Reductions are necessary in patients with liver disease

Administration Administer I.V. only; may be administered undiluted as a bolus injection or via a continuous infusion using an infusion pump

Monitoring Parameters Peripheral nerve stimulator measuring twitch response, heart rate, blood pressure, assisted ventilation status

Nursing Implications Concurrent sedation and analgesia are needed

Additional Information Rocuronium is classified as an intermediate-duration neuromuscular-blocking agent. Do not mix in the same syringe with barbiturates. Rocuronium does not relieve pain or produce sedation.

Dosage Forms Injection, as bromide: 10 mg/mL (5 mL, 10 mL)

♦ **Rocuronium Bromide** *see* Rocuronium *on page 1209*

♦ **Rofact™ (Can)** *see* Rifampin *on page 1193*

Rofecoxib *(roe fe COX ib)*

Related Information

Antacid Drug Interactions *on page 1477*

Nonsteroidal Anti-Inflammatory Agents Comparison *on page 1512*

U.S. Brand Names Vioxx®

Canadian Brand Names Vioxx®

Therapeutic Category Analgesic, COX-2 Inhibitor; Nonsteroidal Anti-inflammatory Drug (NSAID), COX-2 Selective

Use Relief of the signs and symptoms of osteoarthritis; management of acute pain in adults; treatment of primary dysmenorrhea

Pregnancy Risk Factor C/D (3rd trimester)

Pregnancy/Breast-Feeding Implications In late pregnancy may cause premature closure of the ductus arteriosus. In animal studies, rofecoxib has been found to be excreted in milk. It is not known whether rofecoxib is excreted in human milk. Because many drugs are excreted in milk, and the potential for serious adverse reactions exists, a decision should be made whether to discontinue nursing or discontinue the drug, taking into account the importance of the drug to the mother.

Contraindications Hypersensitivity to rofecoxib or any component of the formulation, aspirin, or other nonsteroidal anti-inflammatory drugs (NSAIDs); pregnancy (3rd trimester)

Warnings/Precautions Gastrointestinal irritation, ulceration, bleeding, and perforation may occur with NSAIDs (it is unclear whether rofecoxib is associated with rates of these events which are similar to nonselective NSAIDs). Use with caution in patients with a history of GI disease (bleeding or ulcers), decreased renal function, hepatic disease, congestive heart failure, hypertension, or asthma. Anaphylactoid reactions may occur, even with no prior exposure to rofecoxib.

Adverse Reactions

2% to 10%:

Cardiovascular: Peripheral edema (4%), hypertension (4%)

Central nervous system: Headache (5%), dizziness (3%), weakness (2%)

Gastrointestinal: Diarrhea (7%), nausea (5%), heartburn (4%), epigastric discomfort (4%), dyspepsia (4%), abdominal pain (3%)

Genitourinary: Urinary tract infection (3%)

Neuromuscular & skeletal: Back pain (3%)

Respiratory: Upper respiratory infection (9%), bronchitis (2%), sinusitis (3%)

Miscellaneous: Flu-like syndrome (3%)

<2% (Limited to important or life-threatening): Allergy, alopecia, angina, arrhythmia, asthma, atopic dermatitis, atrial fibrillation, blurred vision, decreased mental acuity, depression, dyspnea, esophageal reflux, esophagitis, fluid retention, gastritis, hematochezia, hematoma, hemorrhoids, muscle cramps, neuropathy, paresthesia, pruritus, rash, somnolence, syncope, tendonitis, tinnitus, urinary retention, urticaria, venous insufficiency, vertigo

<0.1% (Limited to important or life-threatening): Breast cancer, cholecystitis, colitis, colonic neoplasm, congestive heart failure, deep vein thrombosis, duodenal ulcer, gastrointestinal bleeding, intestinal obstruction, lymphoma, myocardial infarction, pancreatitis, prostatic cancer, stroke, transient ischemic attack, unstable angina, urolithiasis

Overdosage/Toxicology Symptoms may include epigastric pain, drowsiness, lethargy, nausea, and vomiting. Gastrointestinal bleeding may occur. Rare manifestations include hypertension, respiratory depression, coma, and acute renal failure. Treatment is symptomatic and supportive. Hemodialysis does not remove rofecoxib.

Drug Interactions

Cytochrome P450 Effect: May be a mild inducer of CYP3A4 (CYP3A3/4)

Increased Effect/Toxicity: Cimetidine increases AUC of rofecoxib by 23%. Rofecoxib may increase plasma concentrations of methotrexate and lithium. Rofecoxib may be used with low-dose aspirin, however, rates of gastrointestinal bleeding may be increased with coadministration. Rofecoxib may increase the INR in patients receiving warfarin and may increase the risk of bleeding complications.

Decreased Effect: Efficacy of thiazide diuretics, loop diuretics (furosemide), or ACE-inhibitors may be diminished by rofecoxib. Rifampin reduces the serum concentration of rofecoxib by approximately 50%. Antacids may reduce rofecoxib absorption.

Ethanol/Nutrition/Herb Interactions

Ethanol: Avoid ethanol (may increase gastric mucosal irritation)

Food: Time to peak concentrations are delayed when taken with a high-fat meal, however peak concentration and AUC are unchanged.

Mechanism of Action Inhibits prostaglandin synthesis by decreasing the activity of the enzyme, cyclooxygenase-2 (COX-2), which results in decreased formation of prostaglandin precursors. Rofecoxib does not inhibit cyclooxygenase-1 (COX-1) at therapeutic concentrations.

Pharmacodynamics/Kinetics

Onset of action: 45 minutes

Duration: Up to >24 hours

Distribution: V_{dss} (apparent): 86-91 L

Protein binding: 87%

Metabolism: Hepatic (99%), minor metabolism via CYP3A4 isoenzyme

Half-life elimination: 17 hours

Time to peak: 2-3 hours

Excretion: Urine (as metabolites, <1% as unchanged drug)

Usual Dosage Adult: Oral:

Osteoarthritis: 12.5 mg once daily; may be increased to a maximum of 25 mg once daily

Acute pain and management of dysmenorrhea: 50 mg once daily as needed (use for longer than 5 days has not been studied)

Dosing comment in renal impairment: Use in advanced renal disease is not recommended

Dosing adjustment in hepatic impairment: No specific dosage adjustment is recommended (AUC may be increased by 69%)

Elderly: No specific adjustment is recommended. However, the AUC in elderly patients may be increased by 34% as compared to younger subjects. Use the lowest recommended dose.

Dietary Considerations May be taken without regard to meals.

Patient Information Patients should be informed of the signs and symptoms of gastrointestinal bleeding; gastrointestinal bleeding may occur as well as ulceration and perforation; pain may or may not be present. If gastric upset occurs, take with food, milk, or antacid. If gastric upset persists, contact physician.

Dosage Forms

Suspension, oral: 12.5 mg/5 mL, 25 mg/5 mL

Tablet: 12.5 mg, 25 mg, 50 mg

♦ **Roferon-A®** *see* Interferon Alfa-2a *on page 726*

♦ **Rogaine® (Can)** *see* Minoxidil *on page 919*

♦ **Rogaine® Extra Strength for Men [OTC]** *see* Minoxidil *on page 919*

♦ **Rogaine® for Men [OTC]** *see* Minoxidil *on page 919*

♦ **Rogaine® for Women [OTC]** *see* Minoxidil *on page 919*

♦ **Rolaids® [OTC]** *see* Calcium Carbonate and Magnesium Hydroxide *on page 208*

♦ **Rolaids® Calcium Rich [OTC]** *see* Calcium Carbonate *on page 207*

♦ **Rolatuss® Plain** *see* Chlorpheniramine and Phenylephrine *on page 279*

♦ **Romazicon™** *see* Flumazenil *on page 570*

♦ **Rondamine-DM® Drops** *see* Carbinoxamine, Pseudoephedrine, and Dextromethorphan *on page 225*

♦ **Rondec®-DM** *see* Carbinoxamine, Pseudoephedrine, and Dextromethorphan *on page 225*

♦ **Rondec® Drops** *see* Carbinoxamine and Pseudoephedrine *on page 225*

♦ **Rondec® Filmtab®** *see* Carbinoxamine and Pseudoephedrine *on page 225*

♦ **Rondec-TR®** *see* Carbinoxamine and Pseudoephedrine *on page 225*

Ropinirole (roe PIN i role)

Related Information

Parkinson's Agents *on page 1513*

U.S. Brand Names Requip®

Canadian Brand Names ReQuip™

Synonyms Ropinirole Hydrochloride

Therapeutic Category Anti-Parkinson's Agent, Dopamine Agonist; Dopaminergic Agent (Antiparkinson's)

Use Treatment of idiopathic Parkinson's disease; in patients with early Parkinson's disease who were not receiving concomitant levodopa therapy as well as in patients with advanced disease on concomitant levodopa

Pregnancy Risk Factor C

(Continued)

Ropinirole *(Continued)*

Contraindications Hypersensitivity to ropinirole or any component of the formulation

Warnings/Precautions Syncope, sometimes associated with bradycardia, was observed in association with ropinirole in both early Parkinson's disease (without levodopa) patients and advanced Parkinson's disease (with levodopa) patients. Dopamine agonists appear to impair the systemic regulation of blood pressure resulting in postural hypotension, especially during dose escalation. Parkinson's disease patients appear to have an impaired capacity to respond to a postural challenge; use with caution in patients at risk of hypotension (ie, those receiving antihypertensive drugs) or where transient hypotensive episodes would be poorly tolerated (cardiovascular disease or cerebrovascular disease). Parkinson's patients being treated with dopaminergic agonists ordinarily require careful monitoring for signs and symptoms of postural hypotension, especially during dose escalation, and should be informed of this risk. May cause hallucinations. Use with caution in patients with pre-existing dyskinesia, severe hepatic or renal dysfunction.

Patients treated with ropinirole have reported falling asleep while engaging in activities of daily living. Discontinue if significant daytime sleepiness or episodes of falling asleep occur. Pathologic degenerative changes were observed in the retinas of albino rats during studies with this agent, but were not observed in the retinas of albino mice or in other species. The significance of these data for humans remains uncertain.

Although not reported for ropinirole, other dopaminergic agents have been associated with a syndrome resembling neuroleptic malignant syndrome on withdrawal or significant dosage reduction after long-term use. Dopaminergic agents from the ergot class have been associated with fibrotic complications, such as retroperitoneum, lungs, and pleura. No clear association with non-ergot agents (ropinirole) has been established.

Adverse Reactions

Early Parkinson's disease (without levodopa):

>10%:
  Cardiovascular: Syncope (12%)
  Central nervous system: Dizziness (40%), somnolence (40%), fatigue (11%)
  Gastrointestinal: Nausea (60%), vomiting (12%)
  Miscellaneous: Viral infection (11%)

1% to 10%:
  Cardiovascular: Dependent/leg edema (6% to 7%), orthostasis (6%), hypertension (5%), chest pain (4%), flushing (3%), palpitations (3%), peripheral ischemia (3%), hypotension (2%), tachycardia (2%),
  Central nervous system: Pain (8%), confusion (5%), hallucinations (5%, dose related), hypoesthesia (4%), amnesia (3%), malaise (3%), vertigo (2%), yawning (3%)
  Gastrointestinal: Constipation (>5%), dyspepsia (10%), abdominal pain (6%), xerostomia (5%), anorexia (4%), flatulence (3%)
  Genitourinary: Urinary tract infection (5%), impotence (3%)
  Hepatic: Elevated alkaline phosphatase (3%)
  Neuromuscular & skeletal: Weakness (6%)
  Ocular: Abnormal vision (6%), xerophthalmia (2%)
  Respiratory: Pharyngitis (6%), rhinitis (4%), sinusitis (4%), dyspnea (3%)
  Miscellaneous: Diaphoresis (increased) (6%)

Advanced Parkinson's disease (with levodopa):

>10%:
  Central nervous system: Dizziness (26%), somnolence (20%), headache (17%)
  Gastrointestinal: Nausea (30%)
  Neuromuscular & skeletal: Dyskinesias (34%)

1% to 10%:
  Cardiovascular: Syncope (3%), hypotension (2%)
  Central nervous system: Hallucinations (10%, dose related), aggravated parkinsonism, confusion (9%), pain (5%), paresis (3%), amnesia (5%), anxiety (6%), abnormal dreaming (3%), insomnia
  Gastrointestinal: Abdominal pain (9%), vomiting (7%), constipation (6%), diarrhea (5%), dysphagia (2%), flatulence (2%), increased salivation (2%), xerostomia, weight loss (2%)
  Genitourinary: Urinary tract infections
  Hematologic: Anemia (2%)
  Neuromuscular & skeletal: Falls (10%), arthralgia (7%), tremor (6%), hypokinesia (5%), paresthesia (5%), arthritis (3%)
  Respiratory: Upper respiratory tract infection (9%), dyspnea (3%)
  Miscellaneous: Injury, increased diaphoresis (7%), viral infection, increased drug level (7%)

Other adverse effects (all phase 2/3 trials):

<1% (Limited to important or life-threatening): Acute renal failure, aphasia, asthma, bradycardia, bundle branch block, cardiac arrest, cardiac failure, cholecystitis, coma, delirium, dementia, eosinophilia, extrapyramidal symptoms, gangrene, gastrointestinal hemorrhage, gastrointestinal ulceration, leukopenia, lymphopenia, manic reaction, pancreatitis, paralysis, paranoid reaction, peripheral neuropathy, photosensitivity, pleural effusion, pulmonary edema, pulmonary embolism, rash, renal calculus, renal failure (acute), seizures, SIADH, stupor, suicide attempt, thrombocytopenia, thrombosis, torticollis, urticaria, ventricular tachycardia

Overdosage/Toxicology There have been no reports of intentional overdose. Symptoms reported with accidental overdosage included agitation, increased dyskinesia, sedation, orthostatic hypotension, chest pain, confusion, nausea, and vomiting. It is anticipated that the symptoms of overdose will be related to its dopaminergic activity. General supportive measures are recommended. Vital signs should be maintained, if necessary. Removal of any unabsorbed material (eg, by gastric lavage) should be considered.

Drug Interactions

Cytochrome P450 Effect: CYP1A2 enzyme substrate

Increased Effect/Toxicity: Inhibitors of CYP1A2 inhibitors may increase serum concentrations of ropinirole; inhibitors include cimetidine, ciprofloxacin, erythromycin, fluvoxamine, isoniazid, ritonavir, and zileuton. Estrogens may also reduce the metabolism of ropinirole; dosage adjustments may be needed.

Decreased Effect: Antipsychotics, enzyme inducers (barbiturates, carbamazepine, phenytoin, rifampin, rifabutin), cigarette smoking, and metoclopramide may reduce the effect or serum concentrations of ropinirole.

Ethanol/Nutrition/Herb Interactions

Ethanol: Avoid ethanol (may increase CNS depression).

Herb/Nutraceutical: Avoid kava kava, gotu kola, valerian, St John's wort (may increase CNS depression).

Mechanism of Action Ropinirole has a high relative *in vitro* specificity and full intrinsic activity at the D_2 and D_3 dopamine receptor subtypes, binding with higher affinity to D_3 than to D_2 or D_4 receptor subtypes; relevance of D_3 receptor binding in Parkinson's disease is unknown. Ropinirole has moderate *in vitro* affinity for opioid receptors. Ropinirole and its metabolites have negligible *in vitro* affinity for dopamine D_1, 5-HT_1, 5-HT_2, benzodiazepine, GABA, muscarinic, alpha$_1$-, alpha$_2$-, and beta-adrenoreceptors. Although precise mechanism of action of ropinirole is unknown, it is believed to be due to stimulation of postsynaptic dopamine D_2-type receptors within the caudate-putamen in the brain. Ropinirole caused decreases in systolic and diastolic blood pressure at doses >0.25 mg. The mechanism of ropinirole-induced postural hypotension is believed to be due to D_2-mediated blunting of the noradrenergic response to standing and subsequent decrease in peripheral vascular resistance.

Pharmacodynamics/Kinetics

Absorption: Not affected by food

Distribution: V_d: 525 L

Metabolism: Extensively hepatic via CYP1A2 to inactive metabolites; first-pass effect

Bioavailability: Absolute 55%

Half-life elimination: ~6 hours

Time to peak: ~1-2 hours; T_{max} increased by 2.5 hours when drug taken with a meal

Excretion: Clearance: Reduced by 30% in patients >65 years of age

Usual Dosage Adults: Oral: The dosage should be increased to achieve a maximum therapeutic effect, balanced against the principal side effects of nausea, dizziness, somnolence and dyskinesia

Recommended starting dose is 0.25 mg 3 times/day; based on individual patient response, the dosage should be titrated with weekly increments as described below:

- Week 1: 0.25 mg 3 times/day; total daily dose: 0.75 mg
- Week 2: 0.5 mg 3 times/day; total daily dose: 1.5 mg
- Week 3: 0.75 mg 3 times/day; total daily dose: 2.25 mg
- Week 4: 1 mg 3 times/day; total daily dose: 3 mg

After week 4, if necessary, daily dosage may be increased by 1.5 mg per day on a weekly basis up to a dose of 9 mg/day, and then by up to 3 mg/day weekly to a total of 24 mg/day

Removal by hemodialysis is unlikely.

Dietary Considerations May be taken with or without food.

Patient Information Ropinirole can be taken with or without food. Hallucinations can occur and elderly are at a higher risk than younger patients with Parkinson's disease. Postural hypotension may develop with or without symptoms such as dizziness, nausea, syncope, and sometimes sweating. Hypotension and/or orthostatic symptoms may occur more frequently during initial therapy or with an increase in dose at any time. Use caution when rising rapidly after sitting or lying down, especially after having done so for prolonged periods and especially at the initiation of treatment with ropinirole. Because of additive sedative effects, caution should be used when taking CNS depressants (eg, benzodiazepines, antipsychotics, antidepressants) in combination with ropinirole.

Nursing Implications Hallucinations can occur and elderly are at a higher risk than younger patients with Parkinson's disease. Postural hypotension may develop with or without symptoms such as dizziness, nausea, syncope, and sometimes sweating. Hypotension and/or orthostatic symptoms may occur more frequently during initial therapy or with an increase in dose at any time. Use caution when rising rapidly after sitting or lying down, especially after having done so for prolonged periods and especially at the initiation of treatment with ropinirole. Because of additive sedative effects, caution should be used when taking CNS depressants (eg, benzodiazepines, antipsychotics, antidepressants) in combination with ropinirole.

Additional Information If therapy with a drug known to be a potent inhibitor of CYP1A2 is stopped or started during treatment with ropinirole, adjustment of ropinirole dose may be required. Ropinirole binds to melanin-containing tissues (ie, eyes, skin) in pigmented rats. After a single dose, long-term retention of drug was demonstrated, with a half-life in the eye of 20 days; not known if ropinirole accumulates in these tissues over time.

Dosage Forms Tablet: 0.25 mg, 0.5 mg, 1 mg, 2 mg, 4 mg, 5 mg

♦ **Ropinirole Hydrochloride** *see* Ropinirole *on page 1211*

Ropivacaine (roe PIV a kane)

U.S. Brand Names Naropin™

Canadian Brand Names Naropin®

Synonyms Ropivacaine Hydrochloride

Therapeutic Category Local Anesthetic, Injectable

Use Local anesthetic (injectable) for use in surgery, postoperative pain management, and obstetrical procedures when local or regional anesthesia is needed. It can be administered via local infiltration, epidural block and epidural infusion, or intermittent bolus.

Pregnancy Risk Factor B

(Continued)

Ropivacaine *(Continued)*

Contraindications Hypersensitivity to amide-type local anesthetics (eg, bupivacaine, mepivacaine, lidocaine) or any component of the formulation; septicemia, severe hypotension and for spinal anesthesia, in the presence of complete heart block

Warnings/Precautions Use with caution in patients with liver disease, cardiovascular disease, neurological or psychiatric disorders; it is not recommended for use in emergency situations where rapid administration is necessary

Adverse Reactions

1% to 10%: Cardiovascular: Hypotension

<1% (Limited to important or life-threatening): Cardiovascular collapse, dizziness, drowsiness, lightheadedness, methemoglobinemia, myocardial depression, nausea, seizures, tinnitus, vomiting

Overdosage/Toxicology Treatment is primarily symptomatic and supportive. Termination of anesthesia by pneumatic tourniquet inflation should be attempted when the agent is administered by infiltration or regional injection. Seizures commonly respond to diazepam, while hypotension responds to I.V. fluids and Trendelenburg positioning. Bradyarrhythmias (when the heart rate is <60) can be treated with I.V., or S.C. atropine 15 mcg/kg. With the development of metabolic acidosis, I.V. sodium bicarbonate 0.5-2 mEq/kg and ventilatory assistance should be instituted. Methemoglobinemia should be treated with methylene blue 1-2 mg/kg in a 1% sterile aqueous solution, given I.V. push over 4-6 minutes and repeated up to a total dose of 7 mg/kg.

Drug Interactions

Cytochrome P450 Effect: CYP1A2 enzyme substrate

Increased Effect/Toxicity: Other local anesthetics or agents structurally related to the amide-type anesthetics. Increased toxicity possible (but not yet reported) with drugs that decrease cytochrome P450 1A enzyme function. SSRIs may increase ropivacaine levels.

Stability Epidural infusions can be used ≤24 hours

Mechanism of Action Blocks both the initiation and conduction of nerve impulses by decreasing the neuronal membrane's permeability to sodium ions, which results in inhibition of depolarization with resultant blockade of conduction

Pharmacodynamics/Kinetics

Onset of action: Anesthesia (route dependent): 3-15 minutes

Duration (dose and route dependent): 3-15 hours

Metabolism: Hepatic

Half-life elimination: Epidural: 5-7 hours; I.V.: 2.4 hours

Excretion: Urine (86% as metabolites)

Usual Dosage Dose varies with procedure, onset and depth of anesthesia desired, vascularity of tissues, duration of anesthesia, and condition of patient: Adults:

Surgical anesthesia:

Lumbar epidural: 15-30 mL of 0.5% to 1% solution

Lumbar epidural block for cesarean section:

20-30 mL dose of 0.5% solution

15-20 mL dose of 0.75% solution

Thoracic epidural block: 5-15 mL dose of 0.5% to 0.75% solution

Major nerve block:

35-50 mL dose of 0.5% solution (175-250 mg)

10-40 mL dose of 0.75% solution (75-300 mg)

Field block: 1-40 mL dose of 0.5% solution (5-200 mg)

Labor pain management: Lumbar epidural: Initial: 10-20 mL 0.2% solution; continuous infusion dose: 6-14 mL/hour of 0.2% solution with incremental injections of 10-15 mL/hour of 0.2% solution

Postoperative pain management:

Lumbar or thoracic epidural: Continuous infusion dose: 6-14 mL/hour of 0.2% solution

Infiltration/minor nerve block:

1-100 mL dose of 0.2% solution

1-40 mL dose of 0.5% solution

Dosage Forms

Infusion, as hydrochloride: 2 mg/mL (100 mL, 200 mL)

Injection, as hydrochloride [single dose]: 2 mg/mL (20 mL); 5 mg/mL (30 mL); 7.5 mg/mL (10 mL, 20 mL); 10 mg/mL (10 mL, 20 mL)

- **Ropivacaine Hydrochloride** *see Ropivacaine on page 1213*

Rosiglitazone *(roh si GLI ta zone)*

Related Information

Hypoglycemic Drugs & Thiazolidinedione Information *on page 1502*

U.S. Brand Names Avandia®

Canadian Brand Names Avandia™

Therapeutic Category Antidiabetic Agent, Thiazolidinedione; Hypoglycemic Agent, Oral

Use Type 2 diabetes mellitus (noninsulin dependent, NIDDM):

Monotherapy: Improve glycemic control as an adjunct to diet and exercise

Combination therapy: In combination with metformin or a sulfonylurea when diet, exercise, and metformin or a sulfonylurea alone do not result in adequate glycemic control; **or** when diet, exercise, and rosiglitazone alone do not result in adequate glycemic control

Pregnancy Risk Factor C

Pregnancy/Breast-Feeding Implications Treatment during mid to late gestation was associated with fetal death and growth retardation in animal models. Abnormal blood glucose levels are associated with a higher incidence of congenital abnormalities. Insulin is the drug of choice for the control of diabetes mellitus during pregnancy. In animal studies, rosiglitazone has been found to be excreted in milk. It is not known whether rosiglitazone is excreted in human milk. Should not be administered to a nursing woman.

Contraindications Hypersensitivity to rosiglitazone or any component of the formulation; active liver disease (transaminases >2.5 times the upper limit of normal at baseline); contraindicated in patients who previously experienced jaundice during troglitazone therapy

Warnings/Precautions Should not be used in diabetic ketoacidosis. Mechanism requires the presence of insulin, therefore use in type 1 diabetes is not recommended. Use with caution in premenopausal, anovulatory women; may result in resumption of ovulation, increasing the risk of pregnancy. May result in hormonal imbalance; development of menstrual irregularities should prompt reconsideration of therapy. Use with caution in patients with anemia or depressed leukocyte counts (may reduce hemoglobin, hematocrit, and/or WBC). Use with caution in patients with heart failure or edema; may increase in plasma volume and/or increase cardiac hypertrophy. In general, use should be avoided in patients with NYHA class 3 or 4 heart failure. Use with caution in patients with elevated transaminases (AST or ALT); see Contraindications and Monitoring. Idiosyncratic hepatotoxicity has been reported with another thiazolidinedione agent (troglitazone). Monitoring should include periodic determinations of liver function.

Adverse Reactions
>10%:
  Endocrine & metabolic: Increased total cholesterol, increased LDL cholesterol, increased HDL cholesterol
  Gastrointestinal: Weight gain
1% to 10%:
  Cardiovascular: Edema (5%)
  Central nervous system: Headache (6%), fatigue (4%)
  Endocrine & metabolic: Hyperglycemia (4%), hypoglycemia (<1% to 2%)
  Gastrointestinal: Diarrhea (2%)
  Hematologic: Anemia (2%)
  Neuromuscular & skeletal: Back pain (4%)
  Respiratory: Upper respiratory tract infection (10%), sinusitis (3%)
  Miscellaneous: Injury (8%)
<1% (Limited to important or life-threatening): Congestive heart failure or exacerbation of CHF, elevated transaminases, increased bilirubin, pulmonary edema
Isolated case reports of hepatotoxic reactions have been reported in patients receiving rosiglitazone; causality not established

Overdosage/Toxicology Experience in overdose is limited. Symptoms may include hypoglycemia. Treatment is supportive.

Drug Interactions
  Cytochrome P450 Effect: CYP2C8 enzyme substrate; minor metabolism by CYP2C9
  Increased Effect/Toxicity: When rosiglitazone was coadministered with glyburide, metformin, digoxin, warfarin, ethanol, or ranitidine, no significant pharmacokinetic alterations were observed.

Ethanol/Nutrition/Herb Interactions
  Ethanol: Avoid ethanol (may cause hypoglycemia).
  Food: Peak concentrations are lower by 28% and delayed when administered with food, but these effects are not believed to be clinically significant.
  Herb/Nutraceutical: Avoid garlic, gymnema (may cause hypoglycemia).

Mechanism of Action Thiazolidinedione antidiabetic agent that lowers blood glucose by improving target cell response to insulin, without increasing pancreatic insulin secretion. It has a mechanism of action that is dependent on the presence of insulin for activity.

Pharmacodynamics/Kinetics
  Onset of action: Delayed; Maximum effect: Up to 12 weeks
  Distribution: V_{dss} (apparent): 17.6 L
  Protein binding: 99.8%
  Metabolism: Hepatic (99%), metabolism via CYP2C8, minor metabolism via CYP2C9
  Bioavailability: 99%
  Half-life elimination: 3.15-3.59 hours
  Time to peak: 1 hour
  Excretion: Urine (64%) and feces (23%) as metabolites

Usual Dosage Oral:
  Adults: Initial: 4 mg daily as a single daily dose or in divided doses twice daily. If response is inadequate after 12 weeks of treatment, the dosage may be increased to 8 mg daily as a single daily dose or in divided doses twice daily. In clinical trials, the 4 mg twice-daily regimen resulted in the greatest reduction in fasting plasma glucose and Hb A_{1c}. (**Note:** Doses >4 mg in combination with sulfonylureas have not been evaluated in clinical trials.)
  Elderly: No dosage adjustment is recommended
  Dosage adjustment in renal impairment: No dosage adjustment is required
  Dosage comment in hepatic impairment: Clearance is significantly lower in hepatic impairment. Therapy should not be initiated if the patient exhibits active liver disease of increased transaminases (>2.5 times the upper limit of normal) at baseline.

Dietary Considerations Management of type 2 diabetes mellitus (noninsulin dependent, NIDDM) should include diet control. May be taken without regard to meals.

Monitoring Parameters Hemoglobin A_{1c} liver enzymes (prior to initiation of therapy, every 2 months for the first year of therapy, then periodically thereafter). Patients with an elevation in ALT >3 times the upper limit of normal should be rechecked as soon as possible. If the ALT levels remain >3 times the upper limit of normal, therapy with rosiglitazone should be discontinued. Monitor serum glucose as recommended by prescriber.

Patient Information May be taken without regard to meals. Follow directions of prescriber. Monitor urine or serum glucose as recommended by prescriber. More frequent monitoring is required during periods of stress, trauma, surgery, pregnancy, increased activity, or exercise. Avoid alcohol. Report chest pain, rapid heartbeat or palpitations, abdominal pain, fever, rash, hypoglycemia reactions, yellowing of skin or eyes, dark urine or light stool, unusual fatigue, or nausea/vomiting. In anovulatory, premenopausal women, ovulation may occur, increasing the risk of pregnancy. Adequate contraception is recommended. Use alternate means of contraception if using oral contraceptives.

Dosage Forms Tablet: 2 mg, 4 mg, 8 mg

- **Rowasa®** *see* Mesalamine *on page 866*
- **Roxanol™** *see* Morphine Sulfate *on page 936*
- **Roxanol 100™** *see* Morphine Sulfate *on page 936*
- **Roxanol Rescudose™** *see* Morphine Sulfate *on page 936*
- **Roxanol™-T** *see* Morphine Sulfate *on page 936*
- **Roxicet®** *see* Oxycodone and Acetaminophen *on page 1026*
- **Roxicet® 5/500** *see* Oxycodone and Acetaminophen *on page 1026*
- **Roxicodone™** *see* Oxycodone *on page 1024*
- **Roxicodone™ Intensol™** *see* Oxycodone *on page 1024*
- **Roxilox®** *see* Oxycodone and Acetaminophen *on page 1026*
- **Roychlor® (Can)** *see* Potassium Chloride *on page 1108*
- **RP54274** *see* Riluzole *on page 1196*
- **RP59500** *see* Quinupristin and Dalfopristin *on page 1172*
- **r-PA** *see* Reteplase *on page 1186*
- **rPDGF-BB** *see* Becaplermin *on page 148*
- **RSV-IGIV** *see* Respiratory Syncytial Virus Immune Globulin (Intravenous) *on page 1185*
- **R-Tannamine®** *see* Chlorpheniramine, Pyrilamine, and Phenylephrine *on page 282*
- **R-Tannate®** *see* Chlorpheniramine, Pyrilamine, and Phenylephrine *on page 282*
- **RTCA** *see* Ribavirin *on page 1189*
- **RU-486** *see* Mifepristone *on page 913*
- **RU-38486** *see* Mifepristone *on page 913*
- **Rubella and Measles Vaccines, Combined** *see* Measles and Rubella Vaccines (Combined) *on page 840*

Rubella and Mumps Vaccines (Combined)
(rue BEL a & mumpz vak SEENS, kom BINED)

Related Information
Adverse Events and Vaccination *on page 1553*
Immunization Recommendations *on page 1538*

U.S. Brand Names Biavax®₂

Therapeutic Category Vaccine

Use Promote active immunity to rubella and mumps by inducing production of antibodies
Note: Routine vaccination with trivalent MMR is recommended by ACIP as children enter kindergarten or first grade. AAP recommends a routine second vaccination as children enter into middle or junior high school.

Pregnancy Risk Factor C

Pregnancy/Breast-Feeding Implications Women who are pregnant when vaccinated or who become pregnant within 3 months of vaccination should be counseled on the theoretical risks to the fetus. The risk of rubella-associated malformations in these women is so small as to be negligible. MMR is the vaccine of choice if recipients are likely to be susceptible to measles or mumps as well as to rubella.

Contraindications Known hypersensitivity to neomycin, eggs; children <1 year, pregnant women, primary immunodeficient patients, patients receiving immunosuppressant drugs except corticosteroids

Warnings/Precautions Women planning on becoming pregnant in the next 3 months should not be vaccinated

Adverse Reactions All serious adverse reactions must be reported to the U.S. Department of Health and Human Services (DHHS) Vaccine Adverse Event Reporting System (VAERS) 1-800-822-7967.
>10%:
  Dermatologic: Local tenderness and erythema, urticaria, rash
  Neuromuscular & skeletal: Arthralgia
1% to 10%:
  Central nervous system: Malaise, moderate fever, headache
  Gastrointestinal: Sore throat
  Miscellaneous: Lymphadenopathy
<1%: Allergic reactions to the vaccine, encephalitis, erythema multiforme, high fever (>103°F), hypersensitivity, optic neuritis, polyneuropathy

Drug Interactions
Decreased Effect: Whole blood, interferon immune globulin, radiation therapy, and immunosuppressive drugs (eg, corticosteroids) may result in insufficient response to immunization; may temporarily depress tuberculin skin test sensitivity and reduce the seroconversion. DTP, OPV, MMR, Hib, and hepatitis B may be given concurrently; other virus vaccine administration should be separated by ≥1 month.

Stability Refrigerate, discard unused portion within 8 hours, protect from light

Usual Dosage Children >12 months (preferably at 15 months) and Adults: 1 vial (0.5 mL) in outer aspect of the upper arm; children vaccinated before 12 months of age should be revaccinated

Administration Administer S.C. only

Test Interactions Temporary suppression of TB skin test

Patient Information Patient may experience burning or stinging at the injection site; joint pain usually occurs 1-10 weeks after vaccination and persists 1-3 days

Nursing Implications Children immunized before 12 months of age should be reimmunized

Additional Information Federal law requires that the date of administration, the vaccine manufacturer, lot number of vaccine, and the administering person's name, title and address be entered into the patient's permanent medical record

Dosage Forms Injection (mixture of 2 viruses):
1. Wistar RA 27/3 strain of rubella virus
2. Jeryl Lynn (B level) mumps strain grown cell cultures of chick embryo

♦ **Rubella, Measles and Mumps Vaccines, Combined** *see* Measles, Mumps, and Rubella Vaccines (Combined) *on page 841*

Rubella Virus Vaccine (Live) (rue BEL a VYE rus vak SEEN, live)

Related Information
Adverse Events and Vaccination *on page 1553*
Immunization Recommendations *on page 1538*

U.S. Brand Names Meruvax® II

Synonyms German Measles Vaccine

Therapeutic Category Vaccine, Live Virus

Use Selective active immunization against rubella; vaccination is routinely recommended for persons from 12 months of age to puberty. All adults, both male and female, lacking documentation of live vaccine on or after first birthday, or laboratory evidence of immunity (particularly women of childbearing age and young adults who work in or congregate in hospitals, colleges, and on military bases) should be vaccinated. Susceptible travelers should be vaccinated.

Note: Trivalent measles - mumps - rubella (MMR) vaccine is the preferred immunizing agent for most children and many adults.

Pregnancy Risk Factor C

Pregnancy/Breast-Feeding Implications Women who are pregnant when vaccinated or who become pregnant within 28 days of vaccination should be counseled on the theoretical risks to the fetus. The risk of rubella-associated malformations in these women is so small as to be negligible. MMR is the vaccine of choice if recipients are likely to be susceptible to measles or mumps as well as to rubella. Enters breast milk; use caution in breast-feeding.

Contraindications Hypersensitivity to gelatin or any other component of the vaccine; history of anaphylactic reactions to neomycin; individuals with blood dyscrasias, leukemia, lymphomas, or other malignant neoplasms affecting the bone marrow or lymphatic systems; concurrent immunosuppressive therapy; primary and acquired immunodeficiency states; family history of congenital or hereditary immunodeficiency; active/untreated tuberculosis; current febrile illness or active febrile infection; pregnancy

Warnings/Precautions Immediate treatment for anaphylactic/anaphylactoid reaction should be available during vaccine use. Use with caution in patients with thrombocytopenia and those who develop thrombocytopenia after first dose; thrombocytopenia may worsen. Defer vaccine following blood, plasma, or immune globulin (human) administration; children with HIV infection, who are asymptomatic and not immunosuppressed may be vaccinated.

Adverse Reactions All serious adverse reactions must be reported to the U.S. Department of Health and Human Services (DHHS) Vaccine Adverse Event Reporting System (VAERS) 1-800-822-7967.

Frequency not defined.

Cardiovascular: Syncope, vasculitis

Central nervous system: Dizziness, encephalitis, fever, Guillain-Barré syndrome, headache, irritability, malaise, polyneuritis, polyneuropathy

Dermatologic: Angioneurotic edema, erythema multiforme, purpura, rash, Stevens-Johnson syndrome, urticaria

Gastrointestinal: Diarrhea, nausea, sore throat, vomiting

Hematologic: Leukocytosis, thrombocytopenia

Local: Injection site reactions which include burning, induration, pain, redness, stinging, wheal and flare

Neuromuscular & skeletal: Arthralgia/arthritis (variable; highest rates in women, 12% to 26% versus children, up to 3%), myalgia, paresthesia

Ocular: Conjunctivitis, optic neuritis, papillitis, retrobulbar neuritis

Otic: Nerve deafness, otitis media

Respiratory: Bronchial spasm, cough, rhinitis

Miscellaneous: Anaphylactoid reactions, anaphylaxis, regional lymphadenopathy

Drug Interactions

Decreased Effect: The effect of the vaccine may be decreased in individuals who are receiving immunosuppressant drugs (including high-dose systemic corticosteroids). Effect of vaccine may be decreased if given with immune globulin, whole blood or plasma; do not administer with vaccine. Effectiveness may be decreased if given within 30 days of varicella vaccine (effectiveness not decreased when administered simultaneously).

Stability Refrigerate, discard reconstituted vaccine after 8 hours; store at 2°C to 8°C (36°F to 46°F); ship vaccine at 10°C; may use dry ice, protect from light

Mechanism of Action Rubella vaccine is a live attenuated virus that contains the Wistar Institute RA 27/3 strain, which is adapted to and propagated in human diploid cell culture. Promotes active immunity by inducing rubella hemagglutination-inhibiting antibodies.

Pharmacodynamics/Kinetics Onset of action: Antibodies to vaccine: 2-4 weeks

Usual Dosage Children ≥12 months and Adults: S.C.: 0.5 mL in outer aspect of upper arm; children vaccinated before 12 months of age should be revaccinated. Recommended age for primary immunization is 12-15 months; revaccination with MMR-II is recommended prior to elementary school.

Administration S.C. injection only in outer aspect of upper arm; avoid injection into blood vessel. **Not for I.V. administration.** Federal law requires that the date of administration, the vaccine manufacturer, lot number of vaccine, and the administering person's name, title and address be entered into the patient's permanent medical record.

Test Interactions May depress tuberculin skin test sensitivity

Patient Information Patient may experience burning or stinging at the injection site; joint pain usually occurs 1-10 weeks after vaccination and persists 1-3 days

Nursing Implications Reconstituted vaccine should be used within 8 hours; S.C. injection only

Additional Information Live virus vaccine. Federal law requires that the date of administration, the vaccine manufacturer, lot number of vaccine, and the administering person's name, title, and address be entered into the patient's permanent record.

(Continued)

Rubella Virus Vaccine (Live) *(Continued)*

Using separate sites and syringes, rubella virus vaccine may be administered concurrently with DTaP, *Haemophilus* b conjugate vaccine (PedvaxHIB®), or hepatitis B vaccine. Unless otherwise specified, rubella virus vaccine should be given 1 month before or 1 month after other live viral vaccines. OPV and rubella virus vaccines may be administered together. Rubella virus vaccine and varicella virus vaccine may be administered together (using separate sites and syringes); however, if vaccines are not administered simultaneously, doses should be separated by at least 30 days.

Dosage Forms Injection [single dose]: 1000 $TCID_{50}$ (Wistar RA 27/3 Strain) [contains gelatin, human albumin and neomycin]

- ◆ **Rubeola Vaccine** *see* Measles Virus Vaccine (Live) *on page 842*
- ◆ **Rubex®** *see* DOXOrubicin *on page 443*
- ◆ **Rubidomycin Hydrochloride** *see* DAUNOrubicin Hydrochloride *on page 368*
- ◆ **Rum-K®** *see* Potassium Chloride *on page 1108*
- ◆ **Ru-Tuss®** *see* Chlorpheniramine and Phenylephrine *on page 279*
- ◆ **Ru-Tuss® DE** *see* Guaifenesin and Pseudoephedrine *on page 647*
- ◆ **Ru-Tuss® Expectorant [OTC]** *see* Guaifenesin, Pseudoephedrine, and Dextromethorphan *on page 648*
- ◆ **Rymed®** *see* Guaifenesin and Pseudoephedrine *on page 647*
- ◆ **Ryna® [OTC]** *see* Chlorpheniramine and Pseudoephedrine *on page 279*
- ◆ **Ryna-C®** *see* Chlorpheniramine, Pseudoephedrine, and Codeine *on page 281*
- ◆ **Ryna-CX®** *see* Guaifenesin, Pseudoephedrine, and Codeine *on page 648*
- ◆ **Rynatan® Pediatric Suspension** *see* Chlorpheniramine, Pyrilamine, and Phenylephrine *on page 282*
- ◆ **Rynatan® Tablet** *see* Azatadine and Pseudoephedrine *on page 136*
- ◆ **Rynatuss® [OTC]** *see* Chlorpheniramine, Ephedrine, Phenylephrine, and Carbetapentane *on page 280*
- ◆ **Rynatuss® Pediatric Suspension [OTC]** *see* Chlorpheniramine, Ephedrine, Phenylephrine, and Carbetapentane *on page 280*
- ◆ **Rythmodan® (Can)** *see* Disopyramide *on page 424*
- ◆ **Rythmodan®-LA (Can)** *see* Disopyramide *on page 424*
- ◆ **Rythmol®** *see* Propafenone *on page 1142*

Sacrosidase *(sak ROE si dase)*

U.S. Brand Names Sucraid®

Canadian Brand Names Sucraid®

Therapeutic Category Enzyme, Gastrointestinal

Use Orphan drug: Oral replacement therapy in sucrase deficiency, as seen in congenital sucrase-isomaltase deficiency (CSID)

Pregnancy Risk Factor C

Pregnancy/Breast-Feeding Implications Animal studies have not been conducted. Should be administered to a pregnant woman only when indicated; **compatible** with breast-feeding

Contraindications Hypersensitivity to yeast, yeast products, or glycerin

Warnings/Precautions Hypersensitivity reactions to sacrosidase, including bronchospasm, have been reported. Administer initial doses in a setting where acute hypersensitivity reactions may be treated within a few minutes. Skin testing for hypersensitivity may be performed prior to administration to identify patients at risk.

Adverse Reactions

1% to 10%: Gastrointestinal: Abdominal pain, vomiting, nausea, diarrhea, constipation

<1% (Limited to important or life-threatening symptoms): Bronchospasm, dehydration, headache, hypersensitivity reaction, insomnia, nervousness

Overdosage/Toxicology Symptoms may include epigastric pain, drowsiness, lethargy, nausea, and vomiting. Gastrointestinal bleeding may occur. Rare manifestations include hypertension, respiratory depression, coma, and acute renal failure. Treatment is symptomatic and supportive. Forced diuresis, hemodialysis, and/or urinary alkalinization are not likely to be useful.

Drug Interactions

Increased Effect/Toxicity: Drug-drug interactions have not been evaluated.

Ethanol/Nutrition/Herb Interactions Food: May be inactivated or denatured if administered with fruit juice, warm or hot food or liquids. Since isomaltase deficiency is not addressed by supplementation of sacrosidase, adherence to a low-starch diet may be required.

Stability Store under refrigeration at 4°C to 8°C (36°F to 46°F); protect from heat or light

Mechanism of Action Sacrosidase is a naturally-occurring gastrointestinal enzyme which breaks down the disaccharide sucrose to its monosaccharide components. Hydrolysis is necessary to allow absorption of these nutrients.

Pharmacodynamics/Kinetics

Absorption: Amino acids

Metabolism: GI tract to individual amino acids

Usual Dosage Oral:

Infants ≥5 months and Children <15 kg: 8500 int. units (1 mL) per meal or snack

Children >15 kg and Adults: 17,000 int. units (2 mL) per meal or snack

Doses should be diluted with 2-4 oz of water, milk, or formula with each meal or snack. Approximately one-half of the dose may be taken before, and the remainder of a dose taken at the completion of each meal or snack.

Administration Do not administer with fruit juices, warm or hot liquids; the solution is fully soluble with water, milk, or formula

Additional Information Oral solution contains 50% glycerol.

Dosage Forms Solution, oral: 8500 int. units per mL (118 mL)

- ◆ **Safe Tussin® 30 [OTC]** *see* Guaifenesin and Dextromethorphan *on page 646*
- ◆ **Saizen®** *see* Human Growth Hormone *on page 667*

- **Salagen**® *see* Pilocarpine *on page 1083*
- **Salazopyrin**® **(Can)** *see* Sulfasalazine *on page 1275*
- **Salazopyrin En-Tabs**® **(Can)** *see* Sulfasalazine *on page 1275*
- **Salbutamol** *see* Albuterol *on page 41*
- **Salflex**® *see* Salsalate *on page 1220*
- **Salicylates** *see page 1692*
- **Salicylazosulfapyridine** *see* Sulfasalazine *on page 1275*
- **Salicylsalicylic Acid** *see* Salsalate *on page 1220*
- **SalineX**® **[OTC]** *see* Sodium Chloride *on page 1245*
- **Salk Vaccine** *see* Poliovirus Vaccine (Inactivated) *on page 1100*

Salmeterol (sal ME te role)

Related Information
Bronchodilators, Comparison of Inhaled Sympathomimetics *on page 1493*

U.S. Brand Names Serevent®; Serevent® Diskus®

Canadian Brand Names Serevent®

Synonyms Salmeterol Xinafoate

Therapeutic Category Adrenergic Agonist Agent; Beta$_2$-Adrenergic Agonist Agent; Bronchodilator

Use

Inhalation aerosol: Maintenance treatment of asthma and in prevention of bronchospasm in patients >12 years of age with reversible obstructive airway disease, including patients with symptoms of nocturnal asthma, who require regular treatment with inhaled, short-acting beta$_2$ agonists; prevention of exercise-induced bronchospasm; maintenance treatment of bronchospasm associated with COPD

Inhalation powder: Maintenance treatment of asthma and in prevention of bronchospasm in patients ≥4 years of age with reversible obstructive airway disease, including patients with symptoms of nocturnal asthma, who require regular treatment with inhaled, short-acting beta$_2$ agonists; prevention of exercise-induced bronchospasm; maintenance treatment of bronchospasm associated with COPD

Pregnancy Risk Factor C

Contraindications Hypersensitivity to salmeterol, adrenergic amines, or any component of the formulation; need for acute bronchodilation; within 2 weeks of MAO inhibitor use

Warnings/Precautions Salmeterol is not meant to relieve acute asthmatic symptoms. Acute episodes should be treated with short-acting beta$_2$ agonist. Do not increase the frequency of salmeterol. Cardiovascular effects are not common with salmeterol when used in recommended doses. All beta agonists may cause elevation in blood pressure, heart rate, and result in excitement (CNS). Use with caution in patients with prostatic hyperplasia, diabetes, cardiovascular disorders, convulsive disorders, thyrotoxicosis, or others who are sensitive to the effects of sympathomimetic amines. Paroxysmal bronchospasm (which can be fatal) has been reported with this and other inhaled agents. If this occurs, discontinue treatment. The elderly may be at greater risk of cardiovascular side effects; safety and efficacy have not been established in children <4 years of age.

Adverse Reactions

>10%:
  Central nervous system: Headache
  Respiratory: Pharyngitis

1% to 10%:
  Cardiovascular: Tachycardia, palpitations, elevation or depression of blood pressure, cardiac arrhythmias
  Central nervous system: Nervousness, CNS stimulation, hyperactivity, insomnia, malaise, dizziness
  Gastrointestinal: GI upset, diarrhea, nausea
  Neuromuscular & skeletal: Tremors (may be more common in the elderly), myalgias, back pain, arthralgia
  Respiratory: Upper respiratory infection, cough, bronchitis

<1% (Limited to important or life-threatening): Arrhythmias, atrial fibrillation, hypertension, immediate hypersensitivity reactions (rash, urticaria, bronchospasm), laryngeal spasm, paradoxical bronchospasms

Overdosage/Toxicology Decontaminate using lavage and activated charcoal. Beta-blockers can be used for hyperadrenergic signs (use with caution in patients with bronchospasm). Prudent use of a cardioselective beta-adrenergic blocker (eg, atenolol or metoprolol). Keep in mind the potential for induction of bronchoconstriction in an asthmatic. Dialysis has not been shown to be of value in the treatment of an overdose with this agent.

Drug Interactions

Cytochrome P450 Effect: CYP3A3/4 enzyme substrate

Increased Effect/Toxicity:
Increased toxicity (cardiovascular): MAO inhibitors, tricyclic antidepressants
Increased effect: Inhaled corticosteroids: The addition of salmeterol has been demonstrated to improve response to inhaled corticosteroids (as compared to increasing steroid dosage).

Decreased Effect: Beta-adrenergic blockers (eg, propranolol)

Stability
Aerosol: Store at 15°C to 30°C (59°F to 86°F); store canister with nozzle down; shake well before each use. Protect from freezing temperature. The therapeutic effect may decrease when the canister is cold therefore the canister should remain at room temperature. Do not store at temperatures >120°F.
Inhalation powder: Store at controlled room temperature 20°C to 25°C (68°F to 77°F) in a dry place away from direct heat or sunlight. Stable for 6 weeks after removal from foil pouch.

Mechanism of Action Relaxes bronchial smooth muscle by selective action on beta$_2$-receptors with little effect on heart rate; because salmeterol acts locally in the lung, therapeutic effect is not predicted by plasma levels

(Continued)

Salmeterol *(Continued)*

Pharmacodynamics/Kinetics

Onset of action: 5-20 minutes (average 10 minutes)

Peak effect: 2-4 hours

Duration: 12 hours

Protein binding: 94% to 98%

Metabolism: Hepatically hydroxylated

Half-life elimination: 3-4 hours

Usual Dosage

Note: Do **not** use spacer with inhalation powder

Asthma, maintenance and prevention:

Inhalation, aerosol: Children ≥12 years and Adults: 42 mcg (2 puffs) twice daily (12 hours apart)

Inhalation, powder (Serevent® Diskus®): Children ≥4 years and Adults: One inhalation (50 mcg) twice daily

Exercise-induced asthma, prevention:

Inhalation, aerosol: Children ≥12 years and Adults: 42 mcg (2 puffs) 30-60 minutes prior to exercise; additional doses should not be used for 12 hours

Inhalation, powder (Serevent® Diskus®): Children ≥4 years and Adults: One inhalation (50 mcg) at least 30 minutes prior to exercise; additional doses should not be used for 12 hours

COPD (maintenance treatment of associated bronchospasm):

Inhalation, aerosol: Adults: 42 micrograms (2 puffs) twice daily (morning and evening, 12 hours apart)

Inhalation, powder (Serevent® Diskus®): Adults: One inhalation (50 mcg) twice daily, ~12 hours apart

Administration Inhalation: Shake well before use. **Not** to be used for the relief of acute attacks.

Monitoring Parameters Pulmonary function tests, blood pressure, pulse, CNS stimulation

Patient Information Do not use to treat acute symptoms; do not exceed the prescribed dose of salmeterol. Do not stop using inhaled or oral corticosteroids without medical advice even if you "feel better". Shake well before using; avoid spraying in eyes. Remove the canister and rinse the plastic case and cap under warm water and dry daily. Store canister with nozzle end down.

Nursing Implications Not to be used for the relief of acute attacks. Monitor lung sounds, pulse, blood pressure. Before using, the inhaler must be shaken well. Observe for wheezing after administration; if this occurs, call physician.

Dosage Forms

Aerosol for oral inhalation, as xinafoate (Serevent®): 21 mcg/spray [60 inhalations] (6.5 g), [120 inhalations] (13 g)

Powder for oral inhalation (Serevent® Diskus®): 50 mcg [46 mcg/inhalation] (60 doses)

- **Salmeterol and Fluticasone** *see* Fluticasone and Salmeterol *on page 590*
- **Salmeterol Xinafoate** *see* Salmeterol *on page 1219*
- **Salofalk® (Can)** *see* Mesalamine *on page 866*

Salsalate *(SAL sa late)*

Related Information

Antacid Drug Interactions *on page 1477*

Salicylates *on page 1692*

U.S. Brand Names Amigesic®; Argesic®-SA; Disalcid®; Mono-Gesic®; Salflex®

Canadian Brand Names Amigesic®; Disalcid™; Salflex®

Synonyms Disalicylic Acid; Salicylsalicylic Acid

Therapeutic Category Analgesic, Salicylate; Anti-inflammatory Agent; Antipyretic; Nonsteroidal Anti-inflammatory Drug (NSAID), Oral; Salicylate

Use Treatment of minor pain or fever; arthritis

Pregnancy Risk Factor C/D (3rd trimester)

Contraindications Hypersensitivity to salsalate or any component of the formulation; GI ulcer or bleeding; pregnancy (3rd trimester)

Warnings/Precautions Use with caution in patients with platelet and bleeding disorders, dehydration, renal dysfunction, erosive gastritis, or peptic ulcer disease, previous nonreaction does not guarantee future safe taking of medication; do not use aspirin in children <16 years of age for chickenpox or flu symptoms due to the association with Reye's syndrome

Adverse Reactions

>10%: Gastrointestinal: Nausea, heartburn, stomach pains, heartburn

1% to 10%:

Central nervous system: Drowsiness

Dermatologic: Rash

Gastrointestinal: Gastrointestinal ulceration

Hematologic: Hemolytic anemia

Neuromuscular & skeletal: Weakness

Respiratory: Dyspnea

Miscellaneous: Anaphylactic shock

<1% (Limited to important or life-threatening): Bronchospasm, does not appear to inhibit platelet aggregation, hepatotoxicity, impaired renal function, iron-deficiency anemia, leukopenia, occult bleeding, thrombocytopenia

Overdosage/Toxicology Symptoms include respiratory alkalosis, hyperpnea, tachypnea, tinnitus, headache, hyperpyrexia, metabolic acidosis, hypoglycemia, and coma. The "Done" nomogram is very helpful for estimating the severity of aspirin poisoning and directing treatment using serum salicylate levels. Treatment can also be based upon symptomatology. See "Salicylates" *on page 1692* in the Appendix.

Drug Interactions
Increased Effect/Toxicity: Increased effect/toxicity of oral anticoagulants, hypoglycemics, and methotrexate.

Decreased Effect: Decreased effect with urinary alkalinizers, antacids, and corticosteroids. Decreased effect of uricosurics and spironolactone.

Ethanol/Nutrition/Herb Interactions
Ethanol: Avoid ethanol (may enhance gastric mucosal irritation).

Food: Salsalate peak serum levels may be delayed if taken with food.

Herb/Nutraceutical: Avoid cat's claw, dong quai, evening primrose, feverfew, garlic, ginger, ginkgo, red clover, horse chestnut, green tea, ginseng (all have additional antiplatelet activity).

Mechanism of Action Inhibits prostaglandin synthesis, acts on the hypothalamus heat-regulating center to reduce fever, blocks prostaglandin synthetase action which prevents formation of the platelet-aggregating substance thromboxane A_2

Pharmacodynamics/Kinetics
Onset of action: Therapeutic: 3-4 days of continuous dosing

Absorption: Completely from small intestine

Metabolism: Hepatically hydrolyzed to two moles of salicylic acid (active)

Half-life elimination: 7-8 hours

Excretion: Primarily urine

Usual Dosage Adults: Oral: 3 g/day in 2-3 divided doses

Dosing comments in renal impairment: In patients with end-stage renal disease undergoing hemodialysis: 750 mg twice daily with an additional 500 mg after dialysis

Dietary Considerations May be taken with food to decrease GI distress.

Test Interactions False-negative results for glucose oxidase urinary glucose tests (Clinistix®); false-positives using the cupric sulfate method (Clinitest®); also, interferes with Gerhardt test, VMA determination; 5-HIAA, xylose tolerance test and T_3 and T_4

Patient Information Do not self-medicate with other drug products containing aspirin; use antacids to relieve upset stomach; watch for bleeding gums or any signs of GI bleeding; take with food or milk to minimize GI distress, notify physician if ringing in ears or persistent GI pain occurs

Nursing Implications Does not appear to inhibit platelet aggregation

Dosage Forms
Capsule: 500 mg

Tablet: 500 mg, 750 mg

Saquinavir (sa KWIN a veer)
Related Information

Antiretroviral Agents Comparison on page 1488

Antiretroviral Therapy for HIV Infection on page 1595

U.S. Brand Names Fortovase®; Invirase®

Canadian Brand Names Fortovase™; Invirase®

Synonyms Saquinavir Mesylate

Therapeutic Category Antiretroviral Agent, Protease Inhibitor; Protease Inhibitor

Use Treatment of HIV infection in selected patients; used in combination with at least two other antiretroviral agents

Pregnancy Risk Factor B

Pregnancy/Breast-Feeding Implications Preliminary data show that saquinavir pharmacokinetics may be affected by pregnancy; studies are not yet complete. Pregnancy and protease inhibitors are both associated with an increased risk of hyperglycemia. Glucose levels should be closely monitored. Health professionals are encouraged to contact the antiretroviral pregnancy registry to monitor outcomes of pregnant women exposed to antiretroviral medications (1-800-258-4263).

Contraindications Hypersensitivity to saquinavir or any component of the formulation; exposure to direct sunlight without sunscreen or protective clothing; coadministration with terfenadine, cisapride, astemizole, triazolam, midazolam, or ergot derivatives

Warnings/Precautions The indication for saquinavir for the treatment of HIV infection is based on changes in surrogate markers. At present, there are no results from controlled clinical trials evaluating its effect on patient survival or the clinical progression of HIV infection (ie, occurrence of opportunistic infections or malignancies); use caution in patients with hepatic insufficiency; safety and efficacy have not been established in children <16 years of age. May exacerbate pre-existing hepatic dysfunction; use with caution in patients with hepatitis B or C and in cirrhosis. Not recommended for use in patients receiving lovastatin or simvastatin; use caution with atorvastatin or cerivastatin. May be associated with fat redistribution (buffalo hump, protease paunch, breast engorgement, facial atrophy). Avoid concurrent use of St John's wort (may lead to loss of virologic response and/or resistance).

Adverse Reactions Protease inhibitors cause dyslipidemia which includes elevated cholesterol and triglycerides and a redistribution of body fat centrally to cause "protease paunch", (Continued)

Saquinavir *(Continued)*

buffalo hump, facial atrophy, and breast enlargement. These agents also cause hyperglycemia.

1% to 10%:
Dermatologic: Rash
Endocrine & metabolic: Hyperglycemia
Gastrointestinal: Diarrhea, abdominal discomfort, nausea, abdominal pain, buccal mucosa ulceration
Neuromuscular & skeletal: Paresthesia, weakness, increased CPK
<1% (Limited to important or life-threatening): Acute myeloblastic leukemia, ascites, ataxia, bullous skin eruption, exacerbation of chronic liver disease, hemolytic anemia, jaundice, polyarthritis, portal hypertension, seizures, Stevens-Johnson syndrome, thrombocytopenia, thrombophlebitis

Drug Interactions
Cytochrome P450 Effect: CYP3A3/4 enzyme substrate; CYP3A3/4 enzyme inhibitor
Increased Effect/Toxicity: CYP3A3/4 enzyme substrate; CYP3A3/4 enzyme inhibitor
Decreased effect: Rifampin may decrease saquinavir's plasma levels and AUC by 40% to 80%; other enzyme inducers may induce saquinavir's metabolism (eg, phenobarbital, phenytoin, dexamethasone, carbamazepine); may decrease delavirdine concentrations
Increased effect: Ketoconazole significantly increases plasma levels and AUC of saquinavir; as a known, although not potent inhibitor of the cytochrome P450 system, saquinavir may decrease the metabolism of terfenadine and astemizole, as well as cisapride and ergot derivatives (and result in rare but serious effects including cardiac arrhythmias); other drugs which may have increased adverse effects if coadministered with saquinavir include benzodiazepines (midazolam and triazolam), calcium channel blockers, clindamycin, dapsone, ergot alkaloids, and quinidine. Both clarithromycin and saquinavir levels/effects may be increased with coadministration. Delavirdine may increase concentration; ritonavir may increase AUC >17-fold; concurrent administration of nelfinavir results in increase in nelfinavir (18%) and saquinavir (mean: 392%).
Saquinavir increased serum concentrations of simvastatin, lovastatin, and atorvastatin; risk of myopathy/rhabdomyolysis may be increased. Use cautiously with HMG-CoA reductase inhibitors. Avoid use with simvastatin and lovastatin. Use caution with atorvastatin and cerivastatin (fluvastatin and pravastatin are not metabolized by CYP3A3/4).
Sildenafil serum concentrations are increased in concurrent therapy (limit sildenafil dosage to 25 mg).
Decreased Effect: Nevirapine, rifabutin, rifampin, phenobarbital, phenytoin, dexamethasone, and carbamazepine may decrease saquinavir concentrations. Saquinavir may decrease delavirdine concentrations.

Ethanol/Nutrition/Herb Interactions
Food: A high-fat meal maximizes bioavailability. Saquinavir levels may increase if taken with grapefruit juice.
Herb/Nutraceutical: Saquinavir serum concentrations may be decreased by St John's wort; avoid concurrent use.

Mechanism of Action As an inhibitor of HIV protease, saquinavir prevents the cleavage of viral polyprotein precursors which are needed to generate functional proteins in and maturation of HIV-infected cells

Pharmacodynamics/Kinetics
Absorption: Poor, increased with high fat meal; Fortovase® has improved absorption over Invirase®
Distribution: V_d: 700 L; does not distribute into CSF
Protein binding, plasma: ~98%
Metabolism: Widely; extensive first-pass effect
Bioavailability: ~4% (Invirase®); 12% to 15% (Fortovase®)

Usual Dosage Oral:
Children and Adolescents <16 years: Safety and efficacy have not been established; dosages of 33-50 mg/kg/dose 3 times/day are under study
Adults: **Note:** Fortovase® and Invirase® are not bioequivalent and should not be used interchangeably; only Fortovase® should be used to initiate therapy:
Fortovase®: Six 200 mg capsules (1200 mg) 3 times/day within 2 hours after a meal in combination with a nucleoside analog
Invirase®: Three 200 mg capsules (600 mg) 3 times/day within 2 hours after a full meal in combination with a nucleoside analog
Note: Dosage adjustment of either Fortovase® or Invirase® in combination with ritonavir: 400 mg twice daily
Note: Dosage adjustments of Fortovase® when administered in combination therapy:
Delavirdine: Fortovase® 800 mg 3 times/day
Lopinavir and ritonavir (Kaletra™): Fortovase® 800 mg twice daily
Nelfinavir: Fortovase® 800 mg 3 times/day or 1200 mg twice daily
Elderly: Clinical studies did not include sufficient numbers of patients ≥65 years of age; use caution due to increased frequency of organ dysfunction

Dietary Considerations Administer within 2 hours of a meal.

Monitoring Parameters Monitor viral load, CD4 count, triglycerides, cholesterol, glucose

Patient Information Saquinavir is not a cure for HIV infection nor has it been found to reduce the transmission of HIV; opportunistic infections and other illnesses associated with AIDS may still occur; take saquinavir within 2 hours after a full meal; avoid direct sunlight when taking saquinavir. Do not take any prescription medications, over-the-counter products or herbal products, especially St John's wort, without consulting prescriber.

Nursing Implications Observe for signs of opportunistic infections and other illnesses associated with HIV; administer on a full stomach, if possible

Additional Information The indication for saquinavir for the treatment of HIV infection is based on changes in surrogate markers. At present, there are no results from controlled clinical trials evaluating the effect of regimens containing saquinavir on patient survival or the clinical progression of HIV infection, such as the occurrence of opportunistic infections or malignancies; in cell culture, saquinavir is additive to synergistic with AZT, ddC, and DDI without enhanced toxicity. According to the manufacturer, Invirase® will be phased out over time and completely replaced by Fortovase®. Potential compliance problems, frequency of administration and adverse effects should be discussed with patients before initiating therapy to help prevent the emergence of resistance.

Dosage Forms
Capsule, as mesylate (Invirase®): 200 mg
Capsule, soft gelatin (Fortovase®): 200 mg

♦ **Saquinavir Mesylate** *see* Saquinavir *on page 1221*
♦ **Sarafem**™ *see* Fluoxetine *on page 578*

Sargramostim (sar GRAM oh stim)

Related Information
Filgrastim *on page 561*
U.S. Brand Names Leukine™
Canadian Brand Names Leukine™
Synonyms GM-CSF; Granulocyte-Macrophage Colony Stimulating Factor; rGM-CSF
Therapeutic Category Colony-Stimulating Factor

Use
Myeloid reconstitution after autologous bone marrow transplantation: Non-Hodgkin's lymphoma (NHL), acute lymphoblastic leukemia (ALL), Hodgkin's lymphoma, metastatic breast cancer
Myeloid reconstitution after allogeneic bone marrow transplantation
Peripheral stem cell transplantation: Metastatic breast cancer, non-Hodgkin's lymphoma, Hodgkin's lymphoma, multiple myeloma
Orphan drug:
Acute myelogenous leukemia (AML) following induction chemotherapy in older adults to shorten time to neutrophil recovery and to reduce the incidence of severe and life-threatening infections and infections resulting in death
Bone marrow transplant (allogeneic or autologous) failure or engraftment delay
Safety and efficacy of GM-CSF given simultaneously with cytotoxic chemotherapy have not been established. Concurrent treatment may increase myelosuppression.

Pregnancy Risk Factor C
Pregnancy/Breast-Feeding Implications Clinical effects to the fetus: Animal reproduction studies have not been conducted. It is not known whether sargramostim can cause fetal harm when administered to a pregnant woman or can affect reproductive capability. Sargramostim should be given to a pregnant woman only if clearly needed.
Contraindications Hypersensitivity to sargramostim, yeast-derived products, or any component of the formulation; concurrent myelosuppressive chemotherapy or radiation therapy. The solution for injection contains benzyl alcohol and should not be used in neonates.
Warnings/Precautions Simultaneous administration, or administration 24 hours preceding/following cytotoxic chemotherapy or radiotherapy is not recommended. Use with caution in patients with pre-existing cardiac problems, hypoxia, fluid retention, pulmonary infiltrates or congestive heart failure, renal or hepatic impairment.

Rapid increase in peripheral blood counts: If ANC >20,000/mm³ or platelets >500,000/mm³, decrease dose by 50% or discontinue drug (counts will fall to normal within 3-7 days after discontinuing drug)

Growth factor potential: Use with caution with myeloid malignancies. Precaution should be exercised in the usage of GM-CSF in any malignancy with myeloid characteristics. GM-CSF can potentially act as a growth factor for any tumor type, particularly myeloid malignancies. Tumors of nonhematopoietic origin may have surface receptors for GM-CSF.

There is a "first-dose effect" (refer to Adverse Reactions for details) which is rarely seen with the first dose and does not usually occur with subsequent doses.

Adverse Reactions
>10%:
Cardiovascular: Hypotension, tachycardia, flushing, and syncope may occur with the first dose of a cycle ("first-dose effect"); peripheral edema (11%)
Central nervous system: Headache (26%)
Dermatologic: Rash, alopecia
Endocrine & metabolic: Polydypsia
Gastrointestinal: Diarrhea (52% to 89%), stomatitis, mucositis
Local: Local reactions at the injection site (~50%)
Neuromuscular & skeletal: Myalgia (18%), arthralgia (21%), bone pain
Renal: Increased serum creatinine (14%)
Respiratory: Dyspnea (28%)
1% to 10%:
Cardiovascular: Transient supraventricular arrhythmias; chest pain; capillary leak syndrome; pericardial effusion (4%)
Central nervous system: Headache
Gastrointestinal: Nausea, vomiting
Hematologic: Leukocytosis, thrombocytopenia
Neuromuscular & skeletal: Weakness
Respiratory: Cough; pleural effusion (1%)
<1% (Limited to important or life-threatening): Anaphylaxis, anorexia, arrhythmia, constipation, eosinophilia, fever, lethargy, malaise, pericarditis, rigors, sore throat, thrombophlebitis, thrombosis
Overdosage/Toxicology The maximum amount that can be safely administered in single or multiple doses has not been determined. Symptoms include dyspnea, malaise, nausea, fever, rash, sinus tachycardia, headache, and chills. All of these adverse events were reversible after discontinuation of sargramostim. Discontinue therapy and carefully monitor the patient for WBC increase and respiratory symptoms.
(Continued)

Sargramostim *(Continued)*

Drug Interactions
Increased Effect/Toxicity: Lithium, corticosteroids may potentiate myeloproliferative effects.

Stability The manufacturer currently recommends that solutions which are reconstituted with sterile water should be used within 6 hours (due to a lack of a preservative) and that solution reconstituted with bacteriostatic water should be used within 20 days. The manufacturer recommends that further diluted solutions be discarded if not used within 6 hours

Sargramostim is available as a sterile, white, preservative-free, lyophilized powder

Sargramostim should be stored at 2°C to 8°C (36°F to 46°F)

Vials should not be frozen or shaken

Sargramostim is stable after dilution in 1 mL of bacteriostatic or nonbacteriostatic sterile water for injection for 30 days at 2°C to 8°C or 25°C

Sargramostim may also be further diluted in 0.9% sodium chloride to a concentration of ≥10 mcg/mL for I.V. infusion administration; this diluted solution is stable for 48 hours at room temperature and refrigeration

If the final concentration of sargramostim is <10 mcg/mL, human albumin should be added to the saline prior to the addition of sargramostim to prevent absorption of the components to the delivery system

It is recommended that 1 mg of human albumin/1 mL of 0.9% sodium chloride (eg, 1 mL of 5% human albumin/50 mL of 0.9% sodium chloride) be added

Standard diluent: Dose ≥250 mcg/25 mL NS

Incompatible with dextrose-containing solutions

Mechanism of Action Stimulates proliferation, differentiation and functional activity of neutrophils, eosinophils, monocytes, and macrophages, as indicated: See table.

Comparative Effects — G-CSF vs. GM-CSF

Proliferation/Differentiation	G-CSF (Filgrastim)	GM-CSF (Sargramostim)
Neutrophils	Yes	Yes
Eosinophils	No	Yes
Macrophages	No	Yes
Neutrophil migration	Enhanced	Inhibited

Pharmacodynamics/Kinetics
Onset of action: Increase in WBC: 7-14 days

Duration: WBCs return to baseline within 1 week of discontinuing drug

Half-life elimination: 2 hours

Time to peak, serum: S.C.: 1-2 hours

Usual Dosage
Children and Adults: I.V. infusion over ≥2 hours or S.C.

Existing clinical data suggest that starting GM-CSF between 24 and 72 hours subsequent to chemotherapy may provide optimal neutrophil recover; continue therapy until the occurrence of an absolute neutrophil count of 10,000/µL after the neutrophil nadir

The available data suggest that rounding the dose to the nearest vial size may enhance patient convenience and reduce costs without clinical detriment

Myeloid reconstitution after peripheral stem cell, allogeneic or autologous bone marrow transplant: I.V.: 250 mcg/m^2/day for 21 days to begin 2-4 hours after the marrow infusion on day 0 of autologous bone marrow transplant or ≥24 hours after chemotherapy or 12 hours after last dose of radiotherapy

If a severe adverse reaction occurs, reduce or temporarily discontinue the dose until the reaction abates

If blast cells appear or progression of the underlying disease occurs, disrupt treatment Interrupt or reduce the dose by half if ANC is >20,000 cells/mm^3

Patients should not receive sargramostim until the postmarrow infusion ANC is <500 cells/mm^3

Neutrophil recovery following chemotherapy in AML: I.V.: 250 mcg/m^2/day over a 4-hour period starting approximately day 11 or 4 days following the completion of induction chemotherapy, if day 10 bone marrow is hypoblastic with <5% blasts

If a second cycle of chemotherapy is necessary, administer ~4 days after the completion of chemotherapy if the bone marrow is hypoblastic with <5% blasts

Continue sargramostim until ANC is >1500 cells/mm^3 for consecutive days or a maximum of 42 days

Discontinue sargramostim immediately if leukemic regrowth occurs

If a severe adverse reaction occurs, reduce the dose by 50% or temporarily discontinue the dose until the reaction abates

Mobilization of peripheral blood progenitor cells: I.V.: 250 mcg/m^2/day over 24 hours or S.C. once daily

Continue the same dose through the period of PBPC collection

The optimal schedule for PBPC collection has not been established (usually begun by day 5 and performed daily until protocol specified targets are achieved)

If WBC >50,000 cells/mm^3, reduce the dose by 50%

If adequate numbers of progenitor cells are not collected, consider other mobilization therapy

Postperipheral blood progenitor cell transplantation: I.V.: 250 mcg/m^2/day over 24 hours or S.C. once daily beginning immediately following infusion of progenitor cells and continuing until ANC is >1500 for 3 consecutive days is attained

BMT failure or engraftment delay: I.V.: 250 mcg/m^2/day for 14 days as a 2-hour infusion

The dose can be repeated after 7 days off therapy if engraftment has not occurred

If engraftment still has not occurred, a third course of 500 mcg/m^2/day for 14 days may be tried after another 7 days off therapy; if there is still no improvement, it is unlikely that further dose escalation will be beneficial

If a severe adverse reaction occurs, reduce or temporarily discontinue the dose until the reaction abates

If blast cells appear or disease progression occurs, discontinue treatment

Administration Sargramostim is administered as a subcutaneous injection or intravenous infusion; intravenous infusion should be over at least 2 hours; continuous infusions may be more effective than short infusion or bolus injection

Monitoring Parameters Vital signs, weight, CBC with differential, platelets, renal/liver function tests, especially with previous dysfunction, WBC with differential, pulmonary function

Reference Range Excessive leukocytosis: ANC >20,000/mm^3 or WBC >50,000 cells/mm^3

Patient Information You may experience bone pain (request analgesic), nausea and vomiting (small frequent meals may help), hair loss (reversible). Report fever, chills, unhealed sores, severe bone pain, difficulty breathing, swelling or pain at infusion site. Avoid crowds or exposure to infected persons; you will be susceptible to infection.

Nursing Implications Can premedicate with analgesics and antipyretics; control bone pain with non-narcotic analgesics; do not shake solution; when administering GM-CSF subcutaneously, rotate injection sites

Additional Information
Reimbursement Hotline (Leukine™): 1-800-321-4669
Professional Services (Immunex): 1-800-334-6273

Dosage Forms Injection: 250 mcg, 500 mcg

- **Sarna® HC (Can)** *see* Hydrocortisone *on page 682*
- **S.A.S.™ (Can)** *see* Sulfasalazine *on page 1275*
- **Scalpicin®** *see* Hydrocortisone *on page 682*
- **Scheinpharm™ Amoxicillin (Can)** *see* Amoxicillin *on page 84*
- **Scheinpharm™ Atenolol (Can)** *see* Atenolol *on page 125*
- **Scheinpharm B12 (Can)** *see* Cyanocobalamin *on page 339*
- **Scheinpharm Cefaclor (Can)** *see* Cefaclor *on page 237*
- **Scheinpharm™ Clotrimazole (Can)** *see* Clotrimazole *on page 323*
- **Scheinpharm™ Desonide (Can)** *see* Desonide *on page 379*
- **Scheinpharm™ Fluoxetine (Can)** *see* Fluoxetine *on page 578*
- **Scheinpharm Gentamicin (Can)** *see* Gentamicin *on page 627*
- **Scheinpharm™ Minocycline (Can)** *see* Minocycline *on page 918*
- **Scheinpharm™ Pilocarpine (Can)** *see* Pilocarpine *on page 1083*
- **Scheinpharm™ Ranitidine (Can)** *see* Ranitidine *on page 1178*
- **Scleromate™** *see* Morrhuate Sodium *on page 938*
- **Scopace®** *see* Scopolamine *on page 1225*

Scopolamine (skoe POL a meen)

Related Information
Cycloplegic Mydriatics Comparison *on page 1498*

U.S. Brand Names Isopto® Hyoscine; Scopace®; Transderm Scōp®

Canadian Brand Names Transderm-V®

Synonyms Hyoscine; Scopolamine Hydrobromide

Therapeutic Category Anticholinergic Agent; Anticholinergic Agent, Ophthalmic; Anticholinergic Agent, Transdermal; Ophthalmic Agent, Mydriatic

Use Preoperative medication to produce amnesia and decrease salivary and respiratory secretions; to produce cycloplegia and mydriasis; treatment of iridocyclitis; prevention of motion sickness; prevention of nausea/vomiting associated with anesthesia or opiate analgesia (patch); symptomatic treatment of postencephalitic parkinsonism and paralysis agitans (oral); inhibits excessive motility and hypertonus of the gastrointestinal tract in such conditions as the irritable colon syndrome, mild dysentery, diverticulitis, pylorospasm, and cardiospasm

Pregnancy Risk Factor C

Pregnancy/Breast-Feeding Implications Crosses the placenta; except when used prior to cesarean section, use during pregnancy only if the benefit to the mother outweighs the potential risk to the fetus.

Contraindications Hypersensitivity to scopolamine or any component of the formulation; narrow-angle glaucoma; acute hemorrhage, gastrointestinal or genitourinary obstruction, thyrotoxicosis, tachycardia secondary to cardiac insufficiency, paralytic ileus

Warnings/Precautions Use with caution with hepatic or renal impairment since adverse CNS effects occur more often in these patients; use with caution in infants and children since they may be more susceptible to adverse effects of scopolamine; use with caution in patients with GI obstruction; anticholinergic agents are not well tolerated in the elderly and their use should be avoided when possible

Adverse Reactions Frequency not defined.
Ophthalmic: Note: Systemic adverse effects have been reported following ophthalmic administration.
Cardiovascular: Vascular congestion, edema
Central nervous system: Drowsiness,
Dermatologic: Eczematoid dermatitis,
Ocular: Blurred vision, photophobia, local irritation, increased intraocular pressure, follicular conjunctivitis, exudate
Respiratory: Congestion
Systemic:
Cardiovascular: Orthostatic hypotension, ventricular fibrillation, tachycardia, palpitations
Central nervous system: Confusion, drowsiness, headache, loss of memory, ataxia, fatigue
Dermatologic: Dry skin, increased sensitivity to light, rash
Endocrine & metabolic: Decreased flow of breast milk
Gastrointestinal: Constipation, xerostomia, dry throat, dysphagia, bloated feeling, nausea, vomiting
Genitourinary: Dysuria
Local: Irritation at injection site
(Continued)

Scopolamine *(Continued)*

Neuromuscular & skeletal: Weakness
Ocular: Increased intraocular pain, blurred vision
Respiratory: Dry nose, diaphoresis (decreased)
Postmarketing and/or case reports (Limited to important or life-threatening): Hallucinations, restlessness

Overdosage/Toxicology Symptoms include dilated pupils, flushed skin, tachycardia, hypertension, EKG abnormalities, and CNS manifestations resembling acute psychosis. CNS depression, circulatory collapse, respiratory failure, and death can occur. Pure scopolamine intoxication is extremely rare. However, for a scopolamine overdose with severe life-threatening symptoms, physostigmine 1-2 mg (0.5 mg or 0.02 mg/kg for children) S.C. or slow I.V. should be given to reverse the toxic effects.

Drug Interactions
Increased Effect/Toxicity: Additive adverse effects with other anticholinergic agents.
Decreased Effect: Decreased effect of acetaminophen, levodopa, ketoconazole, digoxin, riboflavin, and potassium chloride in wax matrix preparations.

Ethanol/Nutrition/Herb Interactions Ethanol: Avoid ethanol (may increase CNS depression).

Stability Avoid acid solutions, because hydrolysis occurs at pH <3; **physically compatible** when mixed in the same syringe with atropine, butorphanol, chlorpromazine, dimenhydrinate, diphenhydramine, droperidol, fentanyl, glycopyrrolate, hydromorphone, hydroxyzine, meperidine, metoclopramide, morphine, pentazocine, pentobarbital, perphenazine, prochlorperazine, promazine, promethazine, or thiopental

Mechanism of Action Blocks the action of acetylcholine at parasympathetic sites in smooth muscle, secretory glands and the CNS; increases cardiac output, dries secretions, antagonizes histamine and serotonin

Pharmacodynamics/Kinetics
Onset of action: Oral, I.M.: 0.5-1 hour; I.V.: 10 minutes
Peak effect: 20-60 minutes; may take 3-7 days for full recovery; transdermal: 24 hours
Duration: Oral, I.M.: 4-6 hours; I.V.: 2 hours
Absorption: Well absorbed from all routes
Protein binding, plasma: Reversible
Metabolism: Hepatic
Excretion: Urine

Usual Dosage
Preoperatively:
Children: I.M., S.C.: 6 mcg/kg/dose (maximum: 0.3 mg/dose) or 0.2 mg/m^2 may be repeated every 6-8 hours **or** alternatively:
4-7 months: 0.1 mg
7 months to 3 years: 0.15 mg
3-8 years: 0.2 mg
8-12 years: 0.3 mg
Adults:
I.M., I.V., S.C.: 0.3-0.65 mg; may be repeated every 4-6 hours
Transdermal patch: Apply 2.5 cm^2 patch to hairless area behind ear the night before surgery or 1 hour prior to cesarean section (the patch should be applied no sooner than 1 hour before surgery for best results and removed 24 hours after surgery)
Motion sickness: Transdermal: Children >12 years and Adults: Apply 1 disc behind the ear at least 4 hours prior to exposure and every 3 days as needed; effective if applied as soon as 2-3 hours before anticipated need, best if 12 hours before
Ophthalmic:
Refraction:
Children: Instill 1 drop of 0.25% to eye(s) twice daily for 2 days before procedure
Adults: Instill 1-2 drops of 0.25% to eye(s) 1 hour before procedure
Iridocyclitis:
Children: Instill 1 drop of 0.25% to eye(s) up to 3 times/day
Adults: Instill 1-2 drops of 0.25% to eye(s) up to 4 times/day
Oral: Parkinsonism, spasticity, motion sickness: 0.4-0.8 mg as a range; the dosage may be cautiously increased in parkinsonism and spastic states.

Administration
I.V.: Dilute with an equal volume of sterile water and administer by direct I.V. injection over 2-3 minutes
Transdermal: Topical disc is programmed to deliver *in vivo* 1 mg over 3 days. Once applied, do not remove the patch for 3 full days. Apply to hairless area of skin behind the ear.

Patient Information Report any changes of vision; wait 5 minutes after instilling ophthalmic preparation before using any other drops, do not blink excessively, after instilling ophthalmic preparation, apply pressure to the side of the nose near the eye to minimize systemic absorption; put patch on day before traveling; once applied, do not remove the patch for 3 full days; may cause drowsiness, dizziness, and blurred vision; may impair coordination and judgment; report to physician any CNS effects; apply patch behind ear

Nursing Implications Topical disc is programmed to deliver *in vivo* 1 mg over 3 days; wash hands before and after applying the disc to avoid drug contact with eyes

Dosage Forms
Injection, as hydrobromide: 0.4 mg/mL (0.5 mL, 1 mL)
Solution, ophthalmic, as hydrobromide (Isopto® Hyoscine, Scopace®): 0.25% (5 mL, 15 mL)
Tablet, as hydrobromide: 0.4 mg
Transdermal system (Transderm Scōp®): 0.33 mg/24 hours [2.5 cm^2] total scopolamine 1.5 mg per patch (releases ~1 mg over 72 hours)

♦ **Scopolamine and Phenylephrine** *see* Phenylephrine and Scopolamine *on page 1076*
♦ **Scopolamine Hydrobromide** *see* Scopolamine *on page 1225*
♦ **Scopolamine, Hyoscyamine, Atropine, and Phenobarbital** *see* Hyoscyamine, Atropine, Scopolamine, and Phenobarbital *on page 694*

- **Scot-Tussin® [OTC]** *see* Guaifenesin *on page 645*
- **Scot-Tussin® Senior Clear [OTC]** *see* Guaifenesin and Dextromethorphan *on page 646*
- **SDZ ENA 713** *see* Rivastigmine *on page 1206*
- **SeaMist® [OTC]** *see* Sodium Chloride *on page 1245*
- **Sebizon®** *see* Sulfacetamide *on page 1268*

Secobarbital (see koe BAR bi tal)

U.S. Brand Names Seconal™

Synonyms Quinalbarbitone Sodium; Secobarbital Sodium

Therapeutic Category Barbiturate; Hypnotic; Sedative

Use Preanesthetic agent; short-term treatment of insomnia

Restrictions C-II

Pregnancy Risk Factor D

Contraindications Hypersensitivity to barbiturates or any component of the formulation; marked hepatic impairment; dyspnea or airway obstruction; porphyria; pregnancy

Warnings/Precautions Should be used only after evaluation of potential causes of sleep disturbance. Failure of sleep disturbance to resolve after 7-10 days may indicate psychiatric or medical illness. Potential for drug dependency exists, abrupt cessation may precipitate withdrawal, including status epilepticus in epileptic patients. Do not administer to patients in acute pain. Use caution in elderly, debilitated, renally impaired, or pediatric patients. May cause paradoxical responses, including agitation and hyperactivity, particularly in acute pain and pediatric patients. Use with caution in patients with depression or suicidal tendencies, or in patients with a history of drug abuse. Tolerance, psychological and physical dependence may occur with prolonged use. Use with caution in patients with hepatic function impairment. May cause CNS depression, which may impair physical or mental abilities. Patients must cautioned about performing tasks which require mental alertness (ie, operating machinery or driving). Effects with other sedative drugs or ethanol may be potentiated. May cause respiratory depression or hypotension, Use with caution in hemodynamically unstable patients or patients with respiratory disease.

Adverse Reactions Frequency not defined.

Cardiovascular: Hypotension

Central nervous system: Dizziness, lightheadedness, "hangover" effect, drowsiness, CNS depression, fever, confusion, mental depression, unusual excitement, nervousness, faint feeling, headache, insomnia, nightmares, hallucinations

Dermatologic: Exfoliative dermatitis, rash, Stevens-Johnson syndrome

Gastrointestinal: Nausea, vomiting, constipation

Hematologic: Agranulocytosis, megaloblastic anemia, thrombocytopenia, thrombophlebitis, urticaria apnea

Local: Pain at injection site

Respiratory: Respiratory depression, laryngospasm

Drug Interactions

Cytochrome P450 Effect: CYP2C9, 3A3/4, and 3A5-7 enzyme inducer

Increased Effect/Toxicity: Increased toxicity when combined with other CNS depressants, antidepressants, benzodiazepines, chloramphenicol, or valproic acid; respiratory and CNS depression may be additive. MAO inhibitors may prolong the effect of secobarbital. Barbiturates may enhance the hepatotoxic potential of acetaminophen (due to an increased formation of toxic metabolites). Chloramphenicol may inhibit the metabolism of barbiturates.

Decreased Effect: Barbiturates, such as secobarbital, are hepatic enzyme inducers, and may increase the metabolism of antipsychotics, some beta-blockers (unlikely with atenolol and nadolol), calcium channel blockers, chloramphenicol, cimetidine, corticosteroids, cyclosporine, disopyramide, doxycycline, ethosuximide, felbamate, furosemide, griseofulvin, lamotrigine, phenytoin, propafenone, quinidine, tacrolimus, TCAs, and theophylline. Barbiturates may increase the metabolism of estrogens and reduce the efficacy of oral contraceptives; an alternative method of contraception should be considered. Barbiturates inhibit the hypoprothrombinemic effects of oral anticoagulants via increased metabolism. Barbiturates may enhance the metabolism of methadone resulting in methadone withdrawal.

Ethanol/Nutrition/Herb Interactions

Ethanol: Avoid ethanol (may increase CNS depression).

Herb/Nutraceutical: Avoid valerian, St John's wort, kava kava, gotu kola (may increase CNS depression).

Mechanism of Action Depresses CNS activity by binding to barbiturate site at GABA-receptor complex enhancing GABA activity, depressing reticular activity system; higher doses may be gabamimetic

Pharmacodynamics/Kinetics

Onset of action: Hypnosis: Oral: 1-3 minutes

Duration: ~15 minutes

Absorption: 90%

Half-life elimination, serum: 25 hours

Time to peak, serum: 2-4 hours

Usual Dosage Oral:

Children:

Preoperative sedation: 2-6 mg/kg (maximum dose: 100 mg/dose) 1-2 hours before procedure

Sedation: 6 mg/kg/day divided every 8 hours

Adults:

Hypnotic: Usual: 100 mg/dose at bedtime; range 100-200 mg/dose

Preoperative sedation: 100-300 mg 1-2 hours before procedure

Monitoring Parameters Blood pressure, heart rate, respiratory rate, CNS status

Dosage Forms Capsule, as sodium: 100 mg

- **Secobarbital and Amobarbital** *see* Amobarbital and Secobarbital *on page 82*

- **Secobarbital Sodium** *see Secobarbital on page 1227*
- **Seconal™** *see Secobarbital on page 1227*
- **Secran®** *see Vitamins (Multiple) on page 1424*
- **Sectral®** *see Acebutolol on page 21*
- **Sedapap-10®** *see Butalbital Compound on page 197*
- **Selax® (Can)** *see Docusate on page 430*
- **Select™ 1/35 (Can)** *see Ethinyl Estradiol and Norethindrone on page 522*
- **Selective Serotonin Reuptake Inhibitor (SSRIs) Pharmacokinetics** *see page 1514*

Selegiline (se LE ji leen)
Related Information
Parkinson's Agents *on page 1513*
Tyramine Content of Foods *on page 1737*

U.S. Brand Names Atapryl®; Eldepryl®; Selpak®

Canadian Brand Names Apo®-Selegiline; Eldepryl®; Gen-Selegiline; Novo-Selegiline; Nu-Selegiline

Synonyms Deprenyl; L-Deprenyl; Selegiline Hydrochloride

Therapeutic Category Anti-Parkinson's Agent, MAO Type B Inhibitor

Use Adjunct in the management of parkinsonian patients in which levodopa/carbidopa therapy is deteriorating

Unlabeled/Investigational Use Early Parkinson's disease; attention-deficit/hyperactivity disorder (ADHD); negative symptoms of schizophrenia; extrapyramidal symptoms; depression; Alzheimer's disease (studies have shown some improvement in behavioral and cognitive performance)

Pregnancy Risk Factor C

Contraindications Hypersensitivity to selegiline or any component of the formulation; concomitant use of meperidine

Warnings/Precautions Increased risk of nonselective MAO inhibition occurs with doses >10 mg/day; it is a monoamine oxidase inhibitor type "B", there should not be a problem with tyramine-containing products as long as the typical doses are employed, however, rare reactions have been reported. Use with tricyclic antidepressants and SSRIs has also been associated with rare reactions and should generally be avoided. Addition to levodopa therapy may result in exacerbation of levodopa adverse effects, requiring a reduction in levodopa dosage.

Adverse Reactions Frequency not defined.
Cardiovascular: Orthostatic hypotension, hypertension, arrhythmias, palpitations, angina, tachycardia, peripheral edema, bradycardia, syncope
Central nervous system: Hallucinations, dizziness, confusion, anxiety, depression, drowsiness, behavior/mood changes, dreams/nightmares, fatigue, delusions
Dermatologic: Rash, photosensitivity
Gastrointestinal: Xerostomia, nausea, vomiting, constipation, weight loss, anorexia, diarrhea, heartburn
Genitourinary: Nocturia, prostatic hyperplasia, urinary retention, sexual dysfunction
Neuromuscular & skeletal: Tremor, chorea, loss of balance, restlessness, bradykinesia
Ocular: Blepharospasm, blurred vision
Miscellaneous: Diaphoresis (increased)

Overdosage/Toxicology Symptoms include tachycardia, palpitations, muscle twitching, and seizures. Competent supportive care is the most important treatment. Both hypertension or hypotension can occur with intoxication. Hypotension may respond to I.V. fluids or vasopressors, and hypertension usually responds to an alpha-adrenergic blocker. While treating the hypertension, care is warranted to avoid sudden drops in blood pressure, since this may worsen MAO inhibitor toxicity. Muscle irritability and seizures often respond to diazepam, while hyperthermia is best treated with antipyretics and cooling blankets. Cardiac arrhythmias are best treated with phenytoin or procainamide.

Drug Interactions
Cytochrome P450 Effect: CYP2D6 enzyme substrate
Increased Effect/Toxicity: Concurrent use of selegiline (high dose) in combination with amphetamines, methylphenidate, dextromethorphan, fenfluramine, meperidine, nefazodone, sibutramine, tramadol, trazodone, tricyclic antidepressants, and venlafaxine may result in serotonin syndrome; these combinations are best avoided. Concurrent use of selegiline with an SSRI may result in mania or hypertension; it is generally best to avoid these combinations. Selegiline (>10 mg/day) in combination with tyramine (cheese, ethanol) may increase the pressor response; avoid high tyramine-containing foods in patients receiving >10 mg/day of selegiline. The toxicity of levodopa (hypertension), lithium (hyperpyrexia), and reserpine may be increased by MAO inhibitors.

Ethanol/Nutrition/Herb Interactions
Ethanol: Avoid ethanol. Avoid beverages containing tyramine (wine [Chianti and hearty red] and beer).
Food: Selegiline may cause sudden and severe high blood pressure when taken with food high in tyramine (cheeses, sour cream, yogurt, pickled herring, chicken liver, canned figs, raisins, bananas, avocados, soy sauce, broad bean pods, yeast extracts, meats prepared with tenderizers, and many foods aged to improve flavor). Small amounts of caffeine may produce irregular heartbeat or high blood pressure and can interact with this medication for up to 2 weeks after stopping its use.
Herb/Nutraceutical: Avoid valerian, St John's wort, SAMe, kava kava (may increase risk of serotonin syndrome and/or excessive sedation).

Mechanism of Action Potent monoamine oxidase (MAO) type-B inhibitor; MAO type B plays a major role in the metabolism of dopamine; selegiline may also increase dopaminergic activity by interfering with dopamine reuptake at the synapse

Pharmacodynamics/Kinetics
Onset of action: Therapeutic: Within 1 hour
Duration: 24-72 hours
Half-life elimination: 9 minutes

Metabolism: Hepatic to amphetamine and methamphetamine

Usual Dosage Oral:

Children and Adolescents: ADHD (unlabeled use): 5-15 mg/day

Adults: Parkinson's disease: 5 mg twice daily with breakfast and lunch or 10 mg in the morning

Elderly: Parkinson's disease: Initial: 5 mg in the morning, may increase to a total of 10 mg/day

Monitoring Parameters Blood pressure, symptoms of parkinsonism

Patient Information Do not exceed daily doses of 10 mg; report to physician any involuntary movements or CNS agitation; explain the tyramine reaction to patients and tell them to report severe headaches or other unusual symptoms to physician

Nursing Implications MAO type B inhibitor; there should **not** be a problem with tyramine-containing products as long as the typical doses are employed

Additional Information When adding selegiline to levodopa/carbidopa, the dose of the latter can usually be decreased. Studies are investigating the use of selegiline in early Parkinson's disease to slow the progression of the disease.

Dosage Forms

Capsule, as hydrochloride (Eldepryl®): 5 mg

Tablet, as hydrochloride: 5 mg

♦ **Selegiline Hydrochloride** *see Selegiline on page 1228*

Selenium (se LEE nee um)

U.S. Brand Names Selepen®

Therapeutic Category Trace Element, Parenteral

Use Trace metal supplement

Pregnancy Risk Factor C

Contraindications Hypersensitivity to selenium or any component of the formulation

Adverse Reactions Frequency not defined.

Central nervous system: Lethargy

Dermatologic: Alopecia or hair discoloration

Gastrointestinal: Vomiting following long-term use on damaged skin; abdominal pain, garlic breath

Local: Irritation

Neuromuscular & skeletal: Tremor

Miscellaneous: Diaphoresis

Overdosage/Toxicology Symptoms include nausea, vomiting, and diarrhea.

Mechanism of Action Part of glutathione peroxidase which protects cell components from oxidative damage due to peroxidases produced in cellular metabolism

Pharmacodynamics/Kinetics Excretion: Urine, feces, lungs, skin

Usual Dosage I.V. in TPN solutions:

Children: 3 mcg/kg/day

Adults:

Metabolically stable: 20-40 mcg/day

Deficiency from prolonged TPN support: 100 mcg/day for 24 and 21 days

Dosage Forms Injection: 40 mcg/mL (10 mL, 30 mL)

Selenium Sulfide (se LEE nee um SUL fide)

U.S. Brand Names Exsel®; Head & Shoulders® Intensive Treatment [OTC]; Selsun®; Selsun Blue® [OTC]; Selsun Gold® for Women [OTC]

Canadian Brand Names Versel®

Therapeutic Category Antiseborrheic Agent, Topical; Shampoos

Use Treatment of itching and flaking of the scalp associated with dandruff, to control scalp seborrheic dermatitis; treatment of tinea versicolor

Pregnancy Risk Factor C

Contraindications Hypersensitivity to selenium or any component of the formulation

Warnings/Precautions Do not use on damaged skin to avoid any systemic toxicity; avoid topical use in very young children; safety of topical in infants has not been established

Adverse Reactions Frequency not defined.

Central nervous system: Lethargy

Dermatologic: Alopecia or hair discoloration, unusual dryness or oiliness of scalp

Gastrointestinal: Vomiting following long-term use on damaged skin, abdominal pain, garlic breath

Local: Irritation

Neuromuscular & skeletal: Tremor

Miscellaneous: Diaphoresis

Overdosage/Toxicology Symptoms include nausea, vomiting, and diarrhea.

Mechanism of Action May block the enzymes involved in growth of epithelial tissue

Pharmacodynamics/Kinetics

Absorption: Topical: Not absorbed through intact skin, but can be absorbed through damaged skin

Excretion: Urine, feces, lungs, skin

Usual Dosage Topical:

Dandruff, seborrhea: Massage 5-10 mL into wet scalp, leave on scalp 2-3 minutes, rinse thoroughly, and repeat application; shampoo twice weekly for 2 weeks initially, then use once every 1-4 weeks as indicated depending upon control

Tinea versicolor: Apply the 2.5% lotion to affected area and lather with small amounts of water; leave on skin for 10 minutes, then rinse thoroughly; apply every day for 7 days

Patient Information Topical formulations are for external use only; notify physician if condition persists or worsens; avoid contact with eyes; thoroughly rinse after application

Nursing Implications Notify physician if condition persists or worsens

Dosage Forms

Lotion, topical: 1% (120 mL, 210 mL, 240 mL); 2.5% (120 mL)

Shampoo, topical: 1% (120 mL, 210 mL, 330 mL)

Sermorelin Acetate (ser moe REL in AS e tate)

U.S. Brand Names Geref®; Geref® Diagnostic

Therapeutic Category Diagnostic Agent, Pituitary Function

Use

> Geref® Diagnostic: For the evaluation of short children whose height is at least 2 standard deviations below the mean height for their chronological age and sex, presenting with low basal serum levels of IGF-1 and IGF-1-BP3. A single intravenous injection of sermorelin is indicated for evaluating the ability of the somatotroph of the pituitary gland to secrete growth hormone (GH). A normal plasma GH response demonstrates that the somatotroph is intact.

> Geref® injection: Treatment of idiopathic growth hormone deficiency

> **Orphan drug**: Sermorelin has been designated an orphan product for AIDS-associated catabolism or weight loss, and as an adjunct to gonadotropin on ovulation induction.

Pregnancy Risk Factor C

Pregnancy/Breast-Feeding Implications Clinical effects on the fetus: Sermorelin has been shown to produce minor variations in fetuses of rats and rabbits when given in S.C. doses of 50, 150, and 500 mcg/kg. In the rat teratology study, external malformations (thin tail) were observed in the higher dose groups, and there was an increase in minor skeletal variants at the high dose. Some visceral malformations (hydroureter) were observed in all treatment groups, with the incidence greatest in the high-dose group. In rabbits, minor skeletal anomalies were significantly greater in the treated animals than in the controls. There are no adequate and well-controlled studies in pregnant women.

Contraindications Hypersensitivity to sermorelin acetate, mannitol, or albumin, or any component of the formulation

Warnings/Precautions Not used for the diagnosis of acromegaly; subnormal GH response may cause obesity, hyperglycemia, and elevated plasma fatty acids. Not recommended for the treatment of GH deficiency due to intracranial lesions. Thyroid status should be evaluated prior to treatment and periodically during therapy with sermorelin.

Adverse Reactions

> 1% to 10%:
> > Cardiovascular: Tightness in the chest
> > Central nervous system: Headache
> > Dermatologic: Transient flushing of the face
> > Gastrointestinal: Nausea, vomiting
> > Local: Pain, redness, and/or swelling at the injection site

> <1% (Limited to important or life-threatening): Dysphagia, dizziness, hyperactivity, somnolence, urticaria

Overdosage/Toxicology Changes of heart rate and blood pressure have been reported with sermorelin in I.V. doses exceeding 10 mcg/kg. Cardiovascular collapse is a conceivable, but as of yet, unreported, complication of overdosage with sermorelin.

Drug Interactions

> **Decreased Effect:** The test should not be conducted in the presence of drugs that directly affect the pituitary secretion of somatotropin. These include preparations that contain or release somatostatin, insulin, glucocorticoids, or cyclo-oxygenase inhibitors such as ASA or indomethacin. Somatotropin levels may be transiently elevated by clonidine, levodopa, and insulin-induced hypoglycemia. Response to sermorelin may be blunted in patients who are receiving muscarinic antagonists (atropine) or who are hypothyroid or being treated with antithyroid medications such as propylthiouracil. Obesity, hyperglycemia, and elevated plasma fatty acids generally are associated with subnormal GH responses to sermorelin. Exogenous growth hormone therapy should be discontinued at least 1 week before administering the test.

Stability Lyophilized preparation must be stored in the refrigerator; use immediately after reconstitution; each ampul should be reconstituted with a minimum of 0.5 mL of the accompanying sterile diluent.

Pharmacodynamics/Kinetics Peak effect: In a study of 71 children, the growth hormone peak plasma response to a bolus injection of sermorelin occurred at 30 ± 27 minutes; however, the response following subsequent injections is smaller and gradually diminishes; continuous infusion does not lead to sustained increases in growth hormone secretion

Usual Dosage
Children and Adults: Diagnostic: I.V.: As a single dose in the morning following an overnight fast:
    <50 kg: Draw venous blood samples for GH determinations 15 minutes before and immediately prior to administration, then administer 1 mcg/kg followed by a 3 mL normal saline flush, draw blood samples again at 15, 30, 45, and 60 minutes for GH determinations
    >50 kg: Determine the number of ampuls needed based on a dose of 1 mcg/kg, draw venous blood samples for GH determinations 15 minutes before and immediately prior to administration, then administer 1 mcg/kg followed by a 3 mL normal saline flush, draw blood samples again at 15, 30, 45, and 60 minutes for GH determinations

Children: Treatment of idiopathic growth hormone deficiency: S.C.: 30 mcg/kg at bedtime; discontinue when epiphyses are fused
Administration Venous blood samples for growth hormone determinations should be drawn 15 minutes before and immediately prior to sermorelin administration. Administer a bolus of 1 mcg/kg/body weight sermorelin I.V. over 1-3 minutes at a final concentration not to exceed 100 mcg/mL followed by a 3 mL normal saline flush. Draw venous blood samples for growth hormone determinations at 15, 30, 45, and 60 minutes after sermorelin administration.
Monitoring Parameters Height (every 6 months)
Reference Range Peak growth hormone levels of >7-10 mcg/L are rarely achieved upon provocation in patients with classic growth hormone deficiency; a marked growth hormone response in time (>10-12 mcg/L) is strongly suggestive of hypothalamic dysfunction, as opposed to pituitary dysfunction
Test Interactions See Drug Interactions
Dosage Forms
Powder for injection, lyophilized:
    Geref®: 0.5 mg, 1 mg
    Geref® Diagnostic: 50 mcg

♦ **Seromycin® Pulvules®** see CycloSERINE on page 344
♦ **Serophene®** see ClomiPHENE on page 314
♦ **Seroquel®** see Quetiapine on page 1165
♦ **Serostim®** see Human Growth Hormone on page 667
♦ **Serpalan®** see Reserpine on page 1184

Sertraline (SER tra leen)

Related Information
Antidepressant Agents Comparison on page 1482
Selective Serotonin Reuptake Inhibitor (SSRIs) Pharmacokinetics on page 1514
U.S. Brand Names Zoloft®
Canadian Brand Names Apo®-Sertraline; Novo-Sertraline; Zoloft™
Synonyms Sertraline Hydrochloride
Therapeutic Category Antidepressant, Serotonin Reuptake Inhibitor
Use Treatment of major depression; obsessive-compulsive disorder (OCD); panic disorder; post-traumatic stress disorder
Unlabeled/Investigational Use Eating disorders; anxiety disorders; premenstrual disorders; impulse control disorders
Pregnancy Risk Factor C
Contraindications Hypersensitivity to sertraline or any component of the formulation; use of MAO inhibitors within 14 days; concurrent use of sertraline oral concentrate with disulfiram is contraindicated
Warnings/Precautions Do not use in combination with MAO inhibitor or within 14 days of discontinuing treatment or initiating treatment with a MAO inhibitor due to the risk of serotonin syndrome; use with caution in patients with pre-existing seizure disorders, patients in whom weight loss is undesirable, patients with recent myocardial infarction, unstable heart disease, hepatic or renal impairment, patients taking other psychotropic medications, agitated or hyperactive patients as drug may produce or activate mania or hypomania; because the risk of suicide is inherent in depression, patient should be closely monitored until depressive symptoms remit and prescriptions should be written for minimum quantities to reduce the risk of overdose. Use oral concentrate formulation with caution in patients with latex sensitivity; dropper dispenser contains dry natural rubber.
Adverse Reactions
>10%:
    Central nervous system: Insomnia, somnolence, dizziness, headache, fatigue
    Gastrointestinal: Xerostomia, diarrhea, nausea
    Genitourinary: Ejaculatory disturbances
1% to 10%:
    Cardiovascular: Palpitations
    Central nervous system: Agitation, anxiety, nervousness
    Dermatologic: Rash
    Endocrine & metabolic: Decreased libido
    Gastrointestinal: Constipation, anorexia, dyspepsia, flatulence, vomiting, weight gain
    Genitourinary: Micturition disorders
    Neuromuscular & skeletal: Tremors, paresthesia
    Ocular: Visual difficulty, abnormal vision
    Otic: Tinnitus
    Miscellaneous: Diaphoresis (increased)
<1% (Limited to important or life-threatening): Acute renal failure, agranulocytosis, angioedema, aplastic anemia, atrial arrhythmias, AV block, blindness, extrapyramidal symptoms, hepatic failure, hypothyroidism, jaundice, lupus-like syndrome, neuroleptic malignant syndrome, oculogyric crisis, optic neuritis, pancreatitis (rare), photosensitivity, psychosis, pulmonary hypertension, QT_c prolongation, serotonin syndrome, serum sickness, SIADH, Stevens-Johnson syndrome (and other severe dermatologic reactions), thrombocytopenia, vasculitis, ventricular tachycardia (including torsade de pointes)
(Continued)

Sertraline *(Continued)*

Overdosage/Toxicology Symptoms include somnolence, vomiting, tachycardia, nausea, dizziness, agitation, and tremor. Treatment is symptomatic and supportive.

Drug Interactions

Cytochrome P450 Effect: CYP3A3/4 enzyme substrate, CYP2D6 enzyme substrate (minor); CYP1A2 and 2D6 enzyme inhibitor (weak); CYP2C9, 2C19, and 3A3/4 enzyme inhibitor

Increased Effect/Toxicity:

MAO inhibitors: Sertraline should not be used with nonselective MAO inhibitors (phenelzine, isocarboxazid) or other drugs with MAO inhibition (linezolid); fatal reactions have been reported. Wait 5 weeks after stopping sertraline before starting a nonselective MAO inhibitor and 2 weeks after stopping an MAO inhibitor before starting sertraline. Concurrent selegiline has been associated with mania, hypertension, or serotonin syndrome (risk may be reduced relative to nonselective MAO inhibitors).

Combined used of SSRIs and amphetamines, buspirone, meperidine, nefazodone, serotonin agonists (such as sumatriptan), sibutramine, other SSRIs, sympathomimetics, ritonavir, tramadol, and venlafaxine may increase the risk of serotonin syndrome. Sertraline may increase serum levels/effects of benzodiazepines (alprazolam and diazepam), carbamazepine, carvedilol, clozapine, cyclosporine (and possibly tacrolimus), dextromethorphan, digoxin, haloperidol, HMG-CoA reductase inhibitors (lovastatin and simvastatin - increasing the risk of rhabdomyolysis, despite sertraline's weak inhibition), phenytoin, propafenone, trazodone, tricyclic antidepressants, and valproic acid. Concurrent lithium may increase risk of nephrotoxicity. Risk of hyponatremia may increase with concurrent use of loop diuretics (bumetanide, furosemide, torsemide). Sertraline may increase the hypoprothrombinemic response to warfarin.

Combined use of sumatriptan (and other serotonin agonists) may result in toxicity; weakness, hyper-reflexia, and incoordination have been observed with sumatriptan and SSRIs. In addition, concurrent use may theoretically increase the risk of serotonin syndrome; includes sumatriptan, naratriptan, rizatriptan, and zolmitriptan.

Phenothiazines: CYP3A3/4 inhibitors (including sertraline) may inhibit the metabolism of thioridazine or mesoridazine, resulting in increased plasma levels and increasing the risk of QT_c interval prolongation. This may lead to serious ventricular arrhythmias, such as torsade de pointes-type arrhythmias and sudden death. Do not use together. Wait at least 5 weeks after discontinuing sertraline prior to starting thioridazine.

Ethanol/Nutrition/Herb Interactions

Ethanol: Avoid ethanol (may increase CNS depression).

Food: Sertraline average peak serum levels may be increased if taken with food.

Herb/Nutraceutical: Avoid valerian, St John's wort, kava kava, gotu kola (may increase CNS depression).

Stability Tablets should be stored at controlled room temperature of 15°C to 30°C (59°F to 86°F).

Mechanism of Action Antidepressant with selective inhibitory effects on presynaptic serotonin (5-HT) reuptake and only very weak effects on norepinephrine and dopamine neuronal uptake

Pharmacodynamics/Kinetics

Onset of action: Steady-state: 7 days; Therapeutic effect: >2 weeks

Absorption: Slow

Protein binding: High

Metabolism: Extensive

Half-life elimination: Parent drug: 24 hours; Metabolites: 66 hours

Excretion: Urine and feces

Usual Dosage Oral:

Children and Adolescents: Depression/OCD:

6-12 years: Initial: 25 mg once daily

13-17 years: Initial: 50 mg once daily

May increase by 50 mg/day increments at intervals of not less than 1 week if tolerated to 100 mg/day; additional increases may be necessary; maximum: 200 mg/day. If somnolence is noted, give at bedtime.

Adults:

Depression/OCD: Oral: Initial: 50 mg/day (see "Note")

Panic disorder/post-traumatic stress disorder: Oral: Initial 25 mg once daily; increased after 1 week to 50 mg once daily (see "Note")

Note: May increase by 50 mg/day increments at intervals of not less than 1 week if tolerated to 100 mg/day; additional increases may be necessary; maximum: 200 mg/day. If somnolence is noted, give at bedtime.

Elderly: Depression/OCD: Start treatment with 25 mg/day in the morning and increase by 25 mg/day increments every 2-3 days if tolerated to 50-100 mg/day; additional increases may be necessary; maximum dose: 200 mg/day

Hemodialysis: Not removed by hemodialysis

Dosage comments in hepatic impairment: Sertraline is extensively metabolized by the liver; caution should be used in patients with hepatic impairment

Administration Oral concentrate: Must be diluted before use. Immediately before administration, use the dropper provided to measure the required amount of concentrate; mix with 4 ounces (¹/₂ cup) of water, ginger ale, lemon/lime soda, lemonade, or orange juice **only**. Do not mix with any other liquids than these. The dose should be taken immediately after mixing; do not mix in advance. A slight haze may appear after mixing; this is normal. **Note:** Use with caution in patients with latex sensitivity; dropper dispenser contains dry natural rubber.

Monitoring Parameters Uric acid, liver function, CBC; monitor nutritional intake and weight

Patient Information If you are currently on another antidepressant drug, please notify your physician. Although sertraline has not been shown to increase the effects of alcohol, it is recommended that you refrain from drinking while on this medication. If you are pregnant or intend becoming pregnant while on this drug, please alert your physician to this fact. You may experience some weight loss, but it is usually minimal.

Nursing Implications If patient becomes anxious or overstimulated, notify physician; if somnolent, administer dose at bedtime; offer hard, sugarless candy or ice chips for dry mouth. Monitor nutritional intake and weight

Additional Information Buspirone (15-60 mg/day) may be useful in treatment of sexual dysfunction during treatment with a selective serotonin reuptake inhibitor. May exacerbate tics in Tourette's syndrome.

Dosage Forms
Solution, oral concentrate: 20 mg/mL (60 mL)
Tablet, as hydrochloride: 25 mg, 50 mg, 100 mg

◆ **Sertraline Hydrochloride** *see Sertraline on page 1231*

◆ **Serutan® [OTC]** *see Psyllium on page 1158*

◆ **Serzone®** *see Nefazodone on page 964*

◆ **Serzone-5HT₂® (Can)** *see Nefazodone on page 964*

Sevelamer (se VEL a mer)

U.S. Brand Names Renagel®
Canadian Brand Names Renagel®
Synonyms Sevelamer Hydrochloride
Therapeutic Category Antidote, Hyperphosphatemia; Phosphate Binder
Use Reduction of serum phosphorous in patients with end-stage renal disease
Pregnancy Risk Factor C
Pregnancy/Breast-Feeding Implications It is not known whether sevelamer is excreted in human milk. Because sevelamer may cause a reduction in the absorption of some vitamins, it should be used with caution in pregnant and/or nursing women.
Contraindications Hypersensitivity to sevelamer or any component of the formulation; hypophosphatemia; bowel obstruction
Warnings/Precautions Use with caution in patients with gastrointestinal disorders including dysphagia, swallowing disorders, severe gastrointestinal motility disorders, or major gastrointestinal surgery. May cause reductions in vitamin D, E, K, and folic acid absorption. Long-term studies of carcinogenic potential have not been completed. Capsules should not be taken apart or chewed.

Adverse Reactions
>10%:
Cardiovascular: Hypotension (11%), thrombosis (10%)
Central nervous system: Headache (10%)
Endocrine & metabolic: Decreased absorption of vitamins D, E, K and folic acid
Gastrointestinal: Diarrhea (16%), dyspepsia (5% to 11%), vomiting (12%)
Neuromuscular & skeletal: Pain (13%)
Miscellaneous: Infection (15%)
1% to 10%:
Cardiovascular: Hypertension (9%)
Gastrointestinal: Nausea (7%), flatulence (4%), diarrhea (4%), constipation (2%)
Respiratory: Cough (4%)

Overdosage/Toxicology Sevelamer is not absorbed systemically. There are no reports of overdosage in patients.

Drug Interactions
Decreased Effect: Sevelamer may bind to some drugs in the gastrointestinal tract and decrease their absorption. When changes in absorption of oral medications may have significant clinical consequences (such as antiarrhythmic and antiseizure medications), these medications should be taken at least 1 hour before or 3 hours after a dose of sevelamer.

Stability Store at controlled room temperature.
Mechanism of Action Sevelamer (a polymeric compound) binds phosphate within the intestinal lumen, limiting absorption and decreasing serum phosphate concentrations without altering calcium, aluminum, or bicarbonate concentrations
Pharmacodynamics/Kinetics
Absorption: None
Excretion: Feces
Usual Dosage Adults: Oral: Patients not taking a phosphate binder: 800-1600 mg 3 times/day with meals; the initial dose may be based on serum phosphorous:
(Phosphorous: Initial Dose:)
>6.0 mg/dL and <7.5 mg/dL: 800 mg 3 times/day
≥7.5 mg/dL and <9.0 mg/dL: 1200-1600 mg 3 times/day
≥9.0 mg/dL: 1600 mg 3 times/day
Dosage should be adjusted based on serum phosphorous concentration, with a goal of lowering to <6.0 mg/dL; maximum daily dose studied was equivalent to 30 capsules/day

Administration Must be administered with meals
Monitoring Parameters Serum phosphorus
Patient Information Take as directed, with meals. Do not break or chew capsules or tablets (contents will expand in water). You may experience headache or dizziness (use caution when driving or engaging in tasks requiring alertness until response to drug is known); upset stomach, nausea, or vomiting (frequent small meals, frequent mouth care, or sucking hard candy may help); diarrhea (yogurt or buttermilk may help); hypotension (use caution when rising from sitting or lying position or when climbing stairs or bending over); or mild neuromuscular pain or stiffness (mild analgesic may help). Report persistent adverse reactions.
Additional Information Switching patients from calcium acetate to sevelamer: 667 mg of calcium acetate is equivalent to 800 mg sevelamer

Dosage Forms
Capsule: 403 mg
Tablet: 400 mg, 800 mg

◆ **Sevelamer Hydrochloride** *see Sevelamer on page 1233*

Sevoflurane (see voe FLOO rane)

U.S. Brand Names Ultane®

Canadian Brand Names Sevorane™

Therapeutic Category General Anesthetic

Use Induction and maintenance of general anesthesia in pediatric and adult patients (inhalation); sevoflurane is less irritating to the airway and therefore is useful to induce general anesthesia

Pregnancy Risk Factor B

Contraindications Previous hypersensitivity to sevoflurane, other halogenated anesthetics, or any component of the formulation; known or suspected susceptibility to malignant hyperthermia

Warnings/Precautions Decrease in blood pressure is dose-dependent. Respiration is depressed; hypoxic pulmonary vasoconstriction is blunted which may lead to increased pulmonary shunt. Hypoxemia induced increase in ventilation is abolished at low concentration of sevoflurane. It dilates the cerebral vasculature which can, in certain conditions, increase intracranial pressure. Sevoflurane may trigger malignant hyperthermia. Sevoflurane is degraded in CO_2 absorbers to produce an olefin concentration (compound A), which has caused nephrotoxicity in rats. It is recommended that sevoflurane exposure not exceed 2 MAC-hours at flow rates of 1 to <2 L/minute. Fresh gas flow rates <1 L/minute are not recommended. Use with caution in patients at risk for seizures; seizures have been reported in children and young adults.

Adverse Reactions

≥1%:
  Cardiovascular: Bradycardia, hypotension, tachycardia, hypertension
  Central nervous system: Agitation, headache, somnolence, dizziness, fever, early emergence movement, hypothermia
  Gastrointestinal: Nausea (25%) and vomiting (18%), increased salivation
  Respiratory: Laryngospasm, airway obstruction, breath holding, increased cough
  Miscellaneous: Shivering

<1% (Limited to important or life-threatening): Albuminuria, alkaline phosphate increased, ALT increased, apnea, arrhythmia, AST increased, AV block, bilirubinemia, bronchospasm, BUN increased, creatinine increased, dyspnea, fluorosis, glycosuria, hemorrhage, hiccups, hyperglycemia, hypoxia, insomnia, LDH increased, leukocytosis, malignant hyperthermia (rare), pain, postoperative hepatic dysfunction (hepatitis, jaundice), pruritus, rash, seizures, syncope, thrombocytopenia, urination impaired, weakness, wheezing

Drug Interactions

Cytochrome P450 Effect: CYP2E1 enzyme substrate

Increased Effect/Toxicity: Administration of 50% N_2O reduces the minimum alveolar concentration (MAC) equivalent dose of sevoflurane by 50% in adults and 25% in children; benzodiazepines and opioids also reduce the MAC of sevoflurane. Sevoflurane may increase the nephrotoxicity of aminoglycosides. Excessive hypotension may occur when combined with antihypertensive drugs. Sevoflurane potentiates the actions of nondepolarizing, neuromuscular-blocking agents.

Stability Store at controlled room temperature (15°C to 30°C); use cautiously in low-flow or closed-circuit systems, since sevoflurane is unstable, potentially toxic breakdown products have been liberated

Pharmacodynamics/Kinetics Sevoflurane has a low blood/gas partition coefficient and therefore is associated with a rapid onset of anesthesia and recovery

Onset of action: Time to induction: Within 2 minutes

Duration: 4-14 minutes

Metabolism: 3% to 5% producing an increase in plasma and urinary fluoride concentration (rarely associated with hepatic or renal injury)

Excretion: Exhaled gases (97%)

Usual Dosage Minimum alveolar concentration (MAC), the concentration at which 50% of patients do not respond to surgical incision, is 2.6% (25 years of age) for sevoflurane. The concentration at which amnesia and loss of awareness occur (MAC - awake) is 0.6%. MAC is reduced in the elderly (50% reduction by age 80).

Dosage adjustment in renal impairment: Safety for use in patients with creatinine >15 mg/dL has not been established.

Dosage adjustment in hepatic impairment: Safety and efficacy have not been established in patients with severe hepatic dysfunction.

Administration Via sevoflurane-specific calibrated vaporizers

Monitoring Parameters Blood pressure, temperature, heart rate, neuromuscular function, oxygen saturation, end-tidal CO_2 and end-tidal sevoflurane concentrations should be monitored prior to and throughout anesthesia.

Dosage Forms Liquid for inhalation: 250 mL

♦ **Sevorane™ (Can)** see Sevoflurane on page 1234

Sibutramine (si BYOO tra meen)

Related Information

  Antacid Drug Interactions on page 1477
  Obesity Treatment Guidelines for Adults on page 1685

U.S. Brand Names Meridia®

Canadian Brand Names Meridia®

Synonyms Sibutramine Hydrochloride Monohydrate

Therapeutic Category Anorexiant

Use Management of obesity, including weight loss and maintenance of weight loss, and should be used in conjunction with a reduced calorie diet

Restrictions C-IV; recommended only for obese patients with a body mass index ≥30 kg/m² or ≥27 kg/m² in the presence of other risk factors such as hypertension, diabetes, and/or dyslipidemia

Pregnancy Risk Factor C

Contraindications Hypersensitivity to sibutramine or any component of the formulation; during or within 2 weeks of MAO inhibitors (eg, phenelzine, selegiline) or concomitant centrally-acting appetite suppressants; anorexia nervosa; uncontrolled or poorly controlled hypertension; congestive heart failure; coronary heart disease; conduction disorders (arrhythmias); stroke; concurrent use of serotonergic agents (eg, SSRIs sumatriptan, dihydroergotamine, dextromethorphan, meperidine, pentazocine, fentanyl, lithium)

Warnings/Precautions Use with caution in severe renal impairment or severe hepatic dysfunction, seizure disorder, hypertension, gallstones, narrow-angle glaucoma, nursing mothers, elderly patients. Primary pulmonary hypertension (PPH), a rare and frequently fatal pulmonary disease, has been reported to occur in patients receiving other agents with serotonergic activity which have been used as anorexiants. Although not reported in clinical trials, it is possible that sibutramine may share this potential, and patients should be monitored closely. Stimulants may unmask tics in individuals with coexisting Tourette's syndrome.

Adverse Reactions
>10%
    Central nervous system: Headache, insomnia
    Gastrointestinal: Anorexia, xerostomia, constipation
    Respiratory: Rhinitis
1% to 10%
    Cardiovascular: Tachycardia, vasodilation, hypertension, palpitations, chest pain, edema
    Central nervous system: Migraine, dizziness, nervousness, anxiety, depression, somnolence, CNS stimulation, emotional liability
    Dermatologic: Rash
    Endocrine & metabolic: Dysmenorrhea
    Gastrointestinal: Increased appetite, nausea, dyspepsia, gastritis, vomiting, taste perversion, abdominal pain
    Neuromuscular & skeletal: Weakness, arthralgia, back pain
    Respiratory: Pharyngitis, sinusitis, cough, laryngitis
    Miscellaneous: Diaphoresis, flu-like syndrome, allergic reactions, thirst
Postmarketing and/or reports (frequency not defined; limited to important or life-threatening): Alopecia, anaphylactic shock, anaphylactoid reaction, angina, arrhythmia, atrial fibrillation, cardiac arrest, cholecystitis, cholelithiasis, congestive heart failure, GI hemorrhage, goiter, hyperthyroidism, hypothyroidism, impotence, increased intraocular pressure, intestinal obstruction, mania, photosensitivity, serotonin syndrome, stroke, syncope, torsade de pointes, transient ischemic attack, vascular headache, ventricular dysrhythmias

Overdosage/Toxicology There is no specific antidote. Treatment should consist of general supportive measures employed in the management of overdosage. Cautious use of beta-blockers to control elevated blood pressure and tachycardia may be indicated. The benefits of forced diuresis and hemodialysis remain unknown.

Drug Interactions
    Cytochrome P450 Effect: CYP3A3/4 enzyme substrate
    Increased Effect/Toxicity: Serotonergic agents such as buspirone, selective serotonin reuptake inhibitors (eg, citalopram, fluoxetine, fluvoxamine, paroxetine, sertraline), sumatriptan (and similar serotonin agonists), dihydroergotamine, lithium, tryptophan, some opioid/analgesics (eg, meperidine, tramadol), and venlafaxine, when combined with sibutramine may result in serotonin syndrome. Dextromethorphan, MAO inhibitors and other drugs that can raise the blood pressure (eg decongestants, centrally-acting weight loss products, amphetamines, and amphetamine-like compounds) can increase the possibility of sibutramine-associated cardiovascular complications. Sibutramine may increase serum levels of tricyclic antidepressants. Theoretically, inhibitors of CYP3A4 (including ketoconazole, itraconazole, erythromycin) may increase sibutramine levels.
    Decreased Effect: Inducers of CYP3A4 (including phenytoin, phenobarbital, carbamazepine, and rifampin) theoretically may reduce sibutramine serum concentrations.

Ethanol/Nutrition/Herb Interactions
    Ethanol: Avoid excess ethanol ingestion.
    Herb/Nutraceutical: St John's wort may decrease sibutramine levels.

Mechanism of Action Sibutramine blocks the neuronal uptake of norepinephrine and, to a lesser extent, serotonin and dopamine

Usual Dosage Adults ≥16 years: Initial: 10 mg once daily; after 4 weeks may titrate up to 15 mg once daily as needed and tolerated (may be used for up to 2 years, per manufacturer labeling)

Dietary Considerations Sibutramine, as an appetite suppressant, is the most effective when combined with a low calorie diet and behavior modification counseling.

Monitoring Parameters Do initial blood pressure and heart rate evaluation and then monitor regularly during therapy. If patient has sustained increases in either blood pressure or pulse rate, consider discontinuing or reducing the dose of the drug.

Patient Information Maintain proper medical follow-up and inform physician of any potential concomitant medications including over-the-counter products you are taking, especially weight loss products, antidepressants, antimigraine drugs, decongestants, lithium, tryptophan, antitussives, or ergot derivatives

Additional Information Physicians should carefully evaluate patients for history of drug abuse and follow such patients closely, observing them for signs of misuse or abuse (eg, development of tolerance, excessive increases of doses, drug seeking behavior).

Unlike dexfenfluramine and fenfluramine, the medication does not cause the release of serotonin from neurons. Tests done on humans show no evidence of valvular heart disease and experiments done on animals show no evidence of the neurotoxicity which was found in similar testing using animals treated with fenfluramine and dexfenfluramine; has minimal potential for abuse.

Dosage Forms Capsule, as hydrochloride: 5 mg, 10 mg, 15 mg

♦ **Silapap® Infants [OTC]** *see* Acetaminophen *on page 22*

Sildenafil (sil DEN a fil)

U.S. Brand Names Viagra®
Canadian Brand Names Viagra™
Synonyms UK 92480
Therapeutic Category Phosphodiesterase (Type 5) Enzyme Inhibitor
Use Treatment of erectile dysfunction
Unlabeled/Investigational Use Psychotropic-induced sexual dysfunction
Pregnancy Risk Factor B
Contraindications Hypersensitivity to sildenafil or any component of the formulation; concurrent use of organic nitrates (nitroglycerin) in any form (potentiates the hypotensive effects)
Warnings/Precautions There is a degree of cardiac risk associated with sexual activity; therefore, physicians may wish to consider the cardiovascular status of their patients prior to initiating any treatment for erectile dysfunction. Agents for the treatment of erectile dysfunction should be used with caution in patients with anatomical deformation of the penis (angulation, cavernosal fibrosis, or Peyronie's disease), or in patients who have conditions which may predispose them to priapism (sickle cell anemia, multiple myeloma, leukemia).

The safety and efficacy of sildenafil with other treatments for erectile dysfunction have not been studied and are, therefore, not recommended as combination therapy.

A minority of patients with retinitis pigmentosa have generic disorders of retinal phosphodiesterases. There is no safety information on the administration of sildenafil to these patients and sildenafil should be administered with caution.

Adverse Reactions
>10%:
    Central nervous system: Headache
    Note: Dyspepsia and abnormal vision (blurred or increased sensitivity to light) occurred at an incidence of >10% with doses of 100 mg.
1% to 10%:
    Cardiovascular: Flushing
    Central nervous system: Dizziness
    Dermatologic: Rash
    Genitourinary: Urinary tract infection
    Ophthalmic: Abnormal vision (blurred or increased sensitivity to light)
    Respiratory: Nasal congestion
<2% (Limited to important of life-threatening): Allergic reaction, angina pectoris, anorgasmia, asthma, AV block, cardiac arrest, cardiomyopathy, cataract, cerebral thrombosis, colitis, dyspnea, edema, exfoliative dermatitis, eye hemorrhage, gout, heart failure, hyperglycemia, hypotension, migraine, myocardial ischemia, neuralgia, postural hypotension, priapism, rectal hemorrhage, seizures, shock, syncope, vertigo
Overdosage/Toxicology In studies of healthy volunteers with single doses up to 800 mg, adverse events were similar to those seen at lower doses, but incidence rates were increased.

Drug Interactions
Cytochrome P450 Effect: CYP3A3/4 enzyme substrate (major); CYP2C9 enzyme substrate (minor)
Increased Effect/Toxicity: Sildenafil potentiates the hypotensive effects of nitrates (amyl nitrate, isosorbide dinitrate, isosorbide mononitrate, nitroglycerin); severe reactions have occurred and concurrent use is contraindicated. Sildenafil may potentiate the effect of other antihypertensives. Serum concentrations/toxicity of sildenafil may be increased by inhibitors of CYP3A3/4, including amprenavir, cimetidine, ciprofloxacin, clarithromycin, clozapine, diltiazem, disulfiram, digoxin, erythromycin, ethanol, fluconazole, fluoxetine, fluvoxamine, grapefruit juice, ritonavir, isoniazid, itraconazole, ketoconazole, labetalol, levodopa, loxapine, metoprolol, metronidazole, miconazole, nefazodone, nelfinavir, omeprazole, phenytoin, rifabutin, rifampin, ritonavir, troleandomycin, valproic acid, and verapamil. Sildenafil may potentiate bleeding in patients receiving heparin. A reduction in sildenafil's dose is recommended when used with ritonavir or indinavir (no more than 25 mg/dose; no more than 25 mg in 48 hours).
Decreased Effect: Enzyme inducers (including phenytoin, carbamazepine, phenobarbital, rifampin) may decrease the serum concentration and efficacy of sildenafil.

Ethanol/Nutrition/Herb Interactions
Food: Amount and rate of absorption of sildenafil is reduced when taken with a high-fat meal. Serum concentrations/toxicity may be increased with grapefruit juice; avoid concurrent use.
Herb/Nutraceutical: St John's wort may decrease sildenafil levels.

Stability Store tablets at controlled room temperature of 15°C to 30°C (59°F to 86°F).
Mechanism of Action Does not directly cause penile erections, but affects the response to sexual stimulation. The physiologic mechanism of erection of the penis involves release of nitric oxide (NO) in the corpus cavernosum during sexual stimulation. NO then activates the enzyme guanylate cyclase, which results in increased levels of cyclic guanosine monophosphate (cGMP), producing smooth muscle relaxation and inflow of blood to the corpus cavernosum. Sildenafil enhances the effect of NO by inhibiting phosphodiesterase type 5 (PDE5), which is responsible for degradation of cGMP in the corpus cavernosum; when sexual stimulation causes local release of NO, inhibition of PDE5 by sildenafil causes increased levels of cGMP in the corpus cavernosum, resulting in smooth muscle relaxation and inflow of blood to the corpus cavernosum; at recommended doses, it has no effect in the absence of sexual stimulation.

Pharmacodynamics/Kinetics
Onset of action: ~60 minutes
Duration: 2-4 hours
Bioavailability: 40%
Protein binding, plasma: ~96%
Metabolism: Hepatic via CYP3A4 (major) and CYP2C9 (minor route)
Half-life elimination: 4 hours
Time to peak: 30-120 minutes

Excretion: Feces (80%); urine (13%)

Usual Dosage Adults: Oral: For most patients, the recommended dose is 50 mg taken as needed, approximately 1 hour before sexual activity. However, sildenafil may be taken anywhere from 30 minutes to 4 hours before sexual activity. Based on effectiveness and tolerance, the dose may be increased to a maximum recommended dose of 100 mg or decreased to 25 mg. The maximum recommended dosing frequency is once daily.

> **Dosage adjustment for patients >65 years of age, hepatic impairment (cirrhosis), severe renal impairment (creatinine clearance <30 mL/minute), or concomitant use of potent cytochrome P450 3A4 inhibitors (erythromycin, ketoconazole, itraconazole, ritonavir, amprenavir):** Higher plasma levels have been associated which may result in increase in efficacy and adverse effects and a starting dose of 25 mg should be considered

Administration Administer 30 minutes to 4 hours before sexual activity (optimally 1 hour before)

Patient Information Discuss with your physician the contraindication of sildenafil citrate with concurrent organic nitrates. The use of sildenafil offers no protection against sexually transmitted diseases. Counseling of patients about the protective measures necessary to guard against transmitted diseases, including the human immunodeficiency virus (HIV), may be considered.

Dosage Forms Tablet, as citrate: 25 mg, 50 mg, 100 mg

♦ **Silphen® Cough [OTC]** *see* DiphenhydrAMINE *on page 414*

♦ **Siltussin® [OTC]** *see* Guaifenesin *on page 645*

♦ **Siltussin DM® [OTC]** *see* Guaifenesin and Dextromethorphan *on page 646*

♦ **Silvadene®** *see* Silver Sulfadiazine *on page 1238*

Silver Nitrate (SIL ver NYE trate)

Synonyms AgNO₃

Therapeutic Category Antibiotic, Ophthalmic; Antibiotic, Topical; Cauterizing Agent, Topical; Topical Skin Product, Antibacterial

Use Prevention of gonococcal ophthalmia neonatorum; cauterization of wounds and sluggish ulcers, removal of granulation tissue and warts; aseptic prophylaxis of burns

Pregnancy Risk Factor C

Contraindications Hypersensitivity to silver nitrate or any component of the formulation; not for use on broken skin or cuts

Warnings/Precautions Do not use applicator sticks on the eyes; repeated applications of the ophthalmic solution into the eye can cause cauterization of the cornea and blindness

Adverse Reactions
>10%:
Dermatologic: Burning and skin irritation
Ocular: Chemical conjunctivitis
1% to 10%:
Dermatologic: Staining of the skin
Hematologic: Methemoglobinemia
Ocular: Cauterization of the cornea, blindness

Overdosage/Toxicology Symptoms include pain and burning of the mouth, salivation, vomiting, diarrhea, shock, coma, convulsions, death and blackening of skin and mucous membranes. Absorbed nitrate can cause methemoglobinemia. Fatal dose is as low as 2 g. Administer sodium chloride in water (10 g/L) to cause precipitation of silver.

Drug Interactions
Decreased Effect: Sulfacetamide preparations are incompatible.

Stability Must be stored in a dry place; exposure to light causes silver to oxidize and turn brown, dipping in water causes oxidized film to readily dissolve

Mechanism of Action Free silver ions precipitate bacterial proteins by combining with chloride in tissue forming silver chloride; coagulates cellular protein to form an eschar; silver ions or salts or colloidal silver preparations can inhibit the growth of both gram-positive and gram-negative bacteria. This germicidal action is attributed to the precipitation of bacterial proteins by liberated silver ions. Silver nitrate coagulates cellular protein to form an eschar, and this mode of action is the postulated mechanism for control of benign hematuria, rhinitis, and recurrent pneumothorax.

Pharmacodynamics/Kinetics
Absorption: Because silver ions readily combine with protein, there is minimal GI and cutaneous absorption of the 0.5% and 1% preparations
Excretion: Highest amounts of silver noted on autopsy have been in kidneys, excretion in urine is minimal

Usual Dosage
Neonates: Ophthalmic: Instill 2 drops immediately after birth (no later than 1 hour after delivery) into conjunctival sac of each eye as a single dose, allow to sit for ≥30 seconds; do not irrigate eyes following instillation of eye drops
Children and Adults:
Ointment: Apply in an apertured pad on affected area or lesion for approximately 5 days
Sticks: Apply to mucous membranes and other moist skin surfaces only on area to be treated 2-3 times/week for 2-3 weeks
Topical solution: Apply a cotton applicator dipped in solution on the affected area 2-3 times/week for 2-3 weeks

Monitoring Parameters With prolonged use, monitor methemoglobin levels

Patient Information Discontinue topical preparation if redness or irritation develop

Nursing Implications Silver nitrate solutions stain skin and utensils

Additional Information Applicators are **not** for ophthalmic use.

Dosage Forms
Applicator sticks: 75% with potassium nitrate 25% (6")
Ointment: 10% (30 g)
Solution, ophthalmic: 1% (wax ampuls)
Solution, topical: 10% (30 mL); 25% (30 mL); 50% (30 mL)

Silver Sulfadiazine (SIL ver sul fa DYE a zeen)

Related Information
Sulfonamide Derivatives *on page 1515*

U.S. Brand Names Silvadene®; SSD® AF; SSD® Cream; Thermazene®

Canadian Brand Names Dermazin™; Flamazine®; SSD™

Therapeutic Category Antibacterial, Topical

Use Prevention and treatment of infection in second and third degree burns

Pregnancy Risk Factor B

Contraindications Hypersensitivity to silver sulfadiazine or any component of the formulation; premature infants or neonates <2 months of age (sulfonamides may displace bilirubin and cause kernicterus); pregnancy (approaching or at term)

Warnings/Precautions Use with caution in patients with G6PD deficiency, renal impairment, or history of allergy to other sulfonamides; sulfadiazine may accumulate in patients with impaired hepatic or renal function; fungal superinfection may occur; use of analgesic might be needed before application; systemic absorption is significant and adverse reactions may occur

Adverse Reactions Frequency not defined.
Dermatologic: Itching, rash, erythema multiforme, discoloration of skin, photosensitivity
Hematologic: Hemolytic anemia, leukopenia, agranulocytosis, aplastic anemia
Hepatic: Hepatitis
Renal: Interstitial nephritis
Miscellaneous: Allergic reactions may be related to sulfa component

Drug Interactions
Decreased Effect: Topical proteolytic enzymes are inactivated by silver sulfadiazine.

Stability Silvadene® cream will occasionally darken either in the jar or after application to the skin. This color change results from a light catalyzed reaction which is a common characteristic of all silver salts. A similar analogy is the oxidation of silverware. The product of this color change reaction is silver oxide which ranges in color from gray to black. Silver oxide has rarely been associated with permanent skin discoloration. Additionally, the antimicrobial activity of the product is not substantially diminished because the color change reaction involves such a small amount of the active drug and is largely a surface phenomenon.

Mechanism of Action Acts upon the bacterial cell wall and cell membrane. Bactericidal for many gram-negative and gram-positive bacteria and is effective against yeast. Active against *Pseudomonas aeruginosa*, *Pseudomonas maltophilia*, *Enterobacter* species, *Klebsiella* species, *Serratia* species, *Escherichia coli*, *Proteus mirabilis*, *Morganella morganii*, *Providencia rettgeri*, *Proteus vulgaris*, *Providencia* species, *Citrobacter* species, *Acinetobacter calcoaceticus*, *Staphylococcus aureus*, *Staphylococcus epidermidis*, *Enterococcus* species, *Candida albicans*, *Corynebacterium diphtheriae*, and *Clostridium perfringens*

Pharmacodynamics/Kinetics
Absorption: Significant percutaneous absorption of silver sulfadiazine can occur especially when applied to extensive burns
Half-life elimination: 10 hours; prolonged with renal insufficiency
Time to peak, serum: 3-11 days of continuous therapy
Excretion: Urine (~50% as unchanged drug)

Usual Dosage Children and Adults: Topical: Apply once or twice daily with a sterile-gloved hand; apply to a thickness of $^1/_{16}$"; burned area should be covered with cream at all times

Monitoring Parameters Serum electrolytes, urinalysis, renal function tests, CBC in patients with extensive burns on long-term treatment

Patient Information For external use only; bathe daily to aid in debridement (if not contraindicated); apply liberally to burned areas; for external use only; notify physician if condition persists or worsens

Nursing Implications Evaluate the development of granulation

Additional Information Contains methylparaben and propylene glycol

Dosage Forms Cream, topical: 1% [10 mg/g] (20 g, 50 g, 85 g, 100 g, 400 g, 1000 g)

♦ **Simethicone, Aluminum Hydroxide, and Magnesium Hydroxide** *see* Aluminum Hydroxide, Magnesium Hydroxide, and Simethicone *on page 64*

♦ **Simethicone and Magaldrate** *see* Magaldrate and Simethicone *on page 831*

♦ **Simulect®** *see* Basiliximab *on page 146*

Simvastatin (SIM va stat in)

Related Information
Hyperlipidemia Management *on page 1670*
Lipid-Lowering Agents *on page 1505*

U.S. Brand Names Zocor®

Canadian Brand Names Zocor®

Therapeutic Category Antilipemic Agent, HMG-CoA Reductase Inhibitor; HMG-CoA Reductase Inhibitor

Use Adjunct to dietary therapy to decrease elevated serum total and LDL cholesterol, apolipoprotein B (apo-B), and triglyceride levels, and to increase HDL cholesterol in patients with primary hypercholesterolemia (heterozygous, familial and nonfamilial) and mixed dyslipidemia (Fredrickson types IIa and IIb); treatment of homozygous familial hypercholesterolemia; treatment of isolated hypertriglyceridemia (Fredrickson type IV) and type III hyperlipoproteinemia

"Secondary prevention" in patients with coronary heart disease and hypercholesterolemia to reduce the risk of total mortality by reducing coronary death; reduce the risk of nonfatal myocardial infarction; reduce the risk of undergoing myocardial revascularization procedures; and reduce the risk of stroke or transient ischemic attack

Pregnancy Risk Factor X

Contraindications Hypersensitivity to simvastatin or any component of the formulation; acute liver disease; unexplained persistent elevations of serum transaminases; pregnancy

Warnings/Precautions Liver function must be monitored by periodic laboratory assessment. Rhabdomyolysis with acute renal failure has occurred. Risk is increased with concurrent use of clarithromycin, danazol, diltiazem, fluvoxamine, indinavir, nefazodone, nelfinavir, ritonavir, verapamil, troleandomycin, cyclosporine, fibric acid derivatives, erythromycin, niacin, or azole antifungals. Weigh the risk versus benefit when combining any of these drugs with simvastatin. Temporarily discontinue in any patient experiencing an acute or serious condition predisposing to renal failure secondary to rhabdomyolysis.

Adverse Reactions

1% to 10%:

Gastrointestinal: Constipation (2%), dyspepsia (1%), flatulence (2%)

Neuromuscular & skeletal: CPK elevation (>3x normal on one or more occasions - 5%)

Respiratory: Upper respiratory infection (2%)

<1% (Limited to important or life-threatening): Depression, lichen planus, photosensitivity, thrombocytopenia, vertigo

Additional class-related events: Alopecia, anaphylaxis, angioedema, anxiety, cataracts, cholestatic jaundice, depression, dermatomyositis, dyspnea, eosinophilia, erythema multiforme, facial paresis, fulminant hepatic necrosis, gynecomastia, hemolytic anemia, hepatitis, hypersensitivity reaction, impotence, leukopenia, myopathy, ophthalmoplegia, pancreatitis, paresthesia, peripheral nerve palsy, peripheral neuropathy, photosensitivity, polymyalgia rheumatica, psychic disturbance, rash, renal failure (secondary to rhabdomyolysis), rhabdomyolysis, Stevens-Johnson syndrome, systemic lupus erythematosus-like syndrome, thrombocytopenia, thyroid dysfunction, toxic epidermal necrolysis, urticaria, vasculitis, vertigo

Overdosage/Toxicology Very few adverse events. Treatment is symptomatic.

Drug Interactions

Cytochrome P450 Effect: CYP3A3/4 enzyme substrate

Increased Effect/Toxicity: Simvastatin may increased the effect or toxicity of warfarin, erythromycin, niacin, cyclosporine, gemfibrozil, or digoxin. Inhibitors of CYP3A3/4 (amprenavir, clarithromycin, cyclosporine, diltiazem, fluvoxamine, erythromycin, fluconazole, indinavir, itraconazole, ketoconazole, miconazole, nefazodone, nelfinavir, ritonavir, troleandomycin, and verapamil) increase simvastatin blood levels and may increase the risk of myopathy and rhabdomyolysis. Cyclosporine, clofibrate, fenofibrate, gemfibrozil, and niacin also may increase the risk of myopathy and rhabdomyolysis. The effect/toxicity of levothyroxine may be increased by cerivastatin. Digoxin, norethindrone, and ethinyl estradiol levels may be increased. Effects are additive with other lipid-lowering therapies.

Decreased Effect: When taken within 1 before or up to 2 hours after cholestyramine, a decrease in absorption of simvastatin can occur.

Ethanol/Nutrition/Herb Interactions

Food: Simvastatin serum concentration may be increased when taken with grapefruit juice; avoid concurrent use.

Herb/Nutraceutical: St John's wort may decrease simvastatin levels.

Stability Tablets should be stored in well closed containers at temperatures between 5°C to 30°C (41°F to 86°F)

Mechanism of Action Simvastatin is a methylated derivative of lovastatin that acts by competitively inhibiting 3-hydroxy-3-methylglutaryl-coenzyme A (HMG-CoA) reductase, the enzyme that catalyzes the rate-limiting step in cholesterol biosynthesis

Pharmacodynamics/Kinetics

Onset of action: >3 days

Peak effect: 2 weeks

Absorption: 85%

Protein binding: ~95%

Metabolism: Hepatic via CYP3A4;; extensive first-pass effect

Bioavailability: <5%

Half-life elimination: Unknown

Time to peak: 1.3-2.4 hours

Excretion: Feces (60%); urine (13%)

Usual Dosage Oral:

Adults:

Initial: 20 mg once daily in the evening

Patients who require only a moderate reduction of LDL cholesterol may be started at 10 mg once daily

Patients who require a reduction of >45% in low-density lipoprotein (LDL) cholesterol may be started at 40 mg once daily in the evening

Maintenance: Recommended dosage range: 5-80 mg/day as a single dose in the evening; doses should be individualized according to the baseline LDL cholesterol levels, the recommended goal of therapy, and the patient's response.

Adjustments: Should be made at intervals of 4 weeks or more.

Patients with homozygous familial hypercholesteremia: Adults: 40 mg in the evening or 80 mg/day in 3 divided doses of 20 mg, 20 mg, and an evening dose of 40 mg.

Patients who are concomitantly receiving cyclosporine: Initial: 5 mg, should not exceed 10 mg/day.

Patients receiving concomitant fibrates or niacin: Dose should **not** exceed 10 mg/day.

Dosing adjustment/comments in renal impairment: Because simvastatin does not undergo significant renal excretion, modification of dose should not be necessary in patients with mild to moderate renal insufficiency.

Severe renal impairment: Cl_{cr} <10 mL/minute: Initial: 5 mg/day with close monitoring.

Administration May be taken without regard to meals.

Monitoring Parameters Creatine phosphokinase levels due to possibility of myopathy; serum cholesterol (total and fractionated)

Patient Information Promptly report any unexplained muscle pain, tenderness or weakness, especially if accompanied by malaise or fever; follow prescribed diet; take with meals

(Continued)

Simvastatin *(Continued)*

Nursing Implications Liver enzyme elevations may be observed during simvastatin therapy; combination therapy with other hypolipidemic agents may be required to achieve optimal reductions of LDL cholesterol; diet, weight reduction, and exercise should be attempted to control hypercholesterolemia before the institution of simvastatin therapy

Dosage Forms Tablet: 5 mg, 10 mg, 20 mg, 40 mg, 80 mg

- ♦ **Sinemet®** *see* Levodopa and Carbidopa *on page 791*
- ♦ **Sinemet® CR** *see* Levodopa and Carbidopa *on page 791*
- ♦ **Sinequan®** *see* Doxepin *on page 440*
- ♦ **Singulair®** *see* Montelukast *on page 933*
- ♦ **Sinufed® Timecelles®** *see* Guaifenesin and Pseudoephedrine *on page 647*
- ♦ **Sinumist®-SR Capsulets®** *see* Guaifenesin *on page 645*
- ♦ **Sinupan®** *see* Guaifenesin and Phenylephrine *on page 647*
- ♦ **Sinus-Relief® [OTC]** *see* Acetaminophen and Pseudoephedrine *on page 25*
- ♦ **Sinutab® Non Drowsy (Can)** *see* Acetaminophen and Pseudoephedrine *on page 25*
- ♦ **Sinutab® Sinus & Allergy (Can)** *see* Acetaminophen, Chlorpheniramine, and Pseudoephedrine *on page 27*
- ♦ **Sinutab® Sinus Allergy Maximum Strength [OTC]** *see* Acetaminophen, Chlorpheniramine, and Pseudoephedrine *on page 27*
- ♦ **Sinutab® Sinus Maximum Strength Without Drowsiness [OTC]** *see* Acetaminophen and Pseudoephedrine *on page 25*
- ♦ **Sirdalud®** *see* Tizanidine *on page 1339*

Sirolimus *(sir OH li mus)*

U.S. Brand Names Rapamune®

Canadian Brand Names Rapamune®

Therapeutic Category Immunosuppressant Agent

Use Prophylaxis of organ rejection in patients receiving renal transplants, in combination with cyclosporine and corticosteroids

Unlabeled/Investigational Use Prophylaxis of organ rejection in solid organ transplant patients in combination with tacrolimus and corticosteroids

Pregnancy Risk Factor C

Pregnancy/Breast-Feeding Implications Embryotoxicity and fetotoxicity may occur, as evidenced by increased mortality, reduced fetal weights and delayed ossification. Effective contraception must be initiated before therapy with sirolimus and continued for 12 weeks after discontinuation. Excretion in breast milk unknown. Breast-feeding is not recommended.

Contraindications Hypersensitivity to sirolimus or any component of the formulation

Warnings/Precautions Immunosuppressive agents, including sirolimus, increase the risk of infection and may be associated with the development of lymphoma. Only physicians experienced in the management of organ transplant patients should prescribe sirolimus. May increase serum lipids (cholesterol and triglycerides). Use with caution in patients with hyperlipidemia. May decrease GFR and increase serum creatinine. Use caution in patients with renal impairment, or when used concurrently with medications which may alter renal function. Has been associated with an increased risk of lymphocele. Avoid concurrent use of ketoconazole.

Adverse Reactions Incidence of many adverse effects are dose related

>20%:

Cardiovascular: Hypertension (39% to 49%), peripheral edema (54% to 64%), edema (16% to 24%), chest pain (16% to 24%)

Central nervous system: Fever (23% to 34%), headache (23% to 34%), pain (24% to 33%), insomnia (13% to 22%)

Dermatologic: Acne (20% to 31%), rash (10% to 20%)

Endocrine & metabolic: Hypercholesterolemia (38% to 46%), hyperkalemia (12% to 17%), hypokalemia (11% to 21%), hypophosphatemia (15% to 23%), hyperlipidemia (38% to 57%)

Gastrointestinal: Abdominal pain (28% to 36%), nausea (25% to 36%), vomiting (19% to 25%), diarrhea (25% to 42%), constipation (28% to 38%), dyspepsia (17% to 25%), weight gain (8% to 21%)

Genitourinary: Urinary tract infection (20% to 33%)

Hematologic: Anemia (23% to 37%), leukopenia (9% to 15%), thrombocytopenia (13% to 40%)

Neuromuscular & skeletal: Arthralgia (25% to 31%), weakness (22% to 40%), back pain (16% to 26%), tremor (21% to 31%)

Renal: Increased serum creatinine (35% to 40%)

Respiratory: Dyspnea (22% to 30%), upper respiratory infection (20% to 26%), pharyngitis (16% to 21%)

3% to 20% (Limited to important or life-threatening):

Cardiovascular: Atrial fibrillation, congestive heart failure, postural hypotension, syncope, thrombosis

Central nervous system: Anxiety, confusion, depression, emotional lability, neuropathy, somnolence

Dermatologic: Hirsutism, pruritus, skin hypertrophy

Endocrine & metabolic: Cushing's syndrome, diabetes mellitus, hypercalcemia, hyperglycemia, hyperphosphatemia, hypocalcemia, hypoglycemia, hypomagnesemia, hyponatremia

Gastrointestinal: Esophagitis, gastritis, gingival hyperplasia, ileus

Genitourinary: Impotence

Hematologic: TTP, hemolytic-uremic syndrome, hemorrhage

Hepatic: Increased transaminases, ascites

Neuromuscular & skeletal: Increased CPK, bone necrosis, tetany, paresthesia

Otic: Deafness

Renal: Acute tubular necrosis, nephropathy (toxic), urinary retention
Respiratory: Asthma, pulmonary edema, pleural effusion
Miscellaneous: Flu-like syndrome, infection, peritonitis, sepsis

Overdosage/Toxicology Experience with overdosage has been limited. Dose-limiting toxicities include immune suppression. Reported symptoms of overdose include atrial fibrillation. Treatment is supportive and dialysis is not likely to facilitate removal.

Drug Interactions

Cytochrome P450 Effect: CYP3A3/4 enzyme substrate and P-glycoprotein substrate

Increased Effect/Toxicity: Cyclosporine increases sirolimus concentrations during concurrent therapy, and cyclosporine levels may be increased. Diltiazem, ketoconazole, and rifampin increase serum concentrations of sirolimus. Other inhibitors of CYP3A4 (eg, calcium channel blockers, antifungal agents, macrolide antibiotics, gastrointestinal prokinetic agents, HIV-protease inhibitors) are likely to increase sirolimus concentrations

Decreased Effect: Inducers of CYP3A4 (eg, rifampin, phenobarbital, carbamazepine, rifabutin, phenytoin) are likely to decrease serum concentrations of sirolimus.

Ethanol/Nutrition/Herb Interactions

Food: Do not administer with grapefruit juice; may decrease clearance of sirolimus. Ingestion with high-fat meals decreases peak concentrations but increases AUC by 35%. Sirolimus should be taken consistently either with or without food to minimize variability.

Herb/Nutraceutical: St John's wort may decrease sirolimus levels; avoid concurrent use. Avoid cat's claw, echinacea (have immunostimulant properties).

Stability

Oral solution: Protect from light and store under refrigeration, 2°C to 8°C (36°F to 46°F); stable for 24 months under these conditions. A slight haze may develop in refrigerated solutions, but the quality of the product is not affected. After opening, solution should be used in 1 month. If necessary, may be stored at temperatures up to 25°C (77°F) for several days after opening (not longer than 30 days). Product may be stored in amber syringe for a maximum of 24 hours (at room temperature or refrigerated). Discard syringe after use. Solution should be used immediately following dilution.

Tablet: Store at room temperature, 20°C to 25°C (68°F to 77°F); protect from light

Mechanism of Action Sirolimus inhibits T-lymphocyte activation and proliferation in response to antigenic and cytokine stimulation. Its mechanism differs from other immunosuppressants. It inhibits acute rejection of allografts and prolongs graft survival.

Pharmacodynamics/Kinetics

Absorption: Rapid
Distribution: 12 L/kg (± 7.52 L/kg)
Protein binding: 92%, primarily to albumin
Metabolism: Extensively hepatic via CYP3A4 and P-glycoprotein
Bioavailability: 14%
Half-life elimination: Mean, 62 hours
Time to peak: 1-3 hours
Excretion: Feces (91%); urine (2.2%)

Usual Dosage Oral:

Adults ≥40 kg: Loading dose: For *de novo* transplant recipients, a loading dose of 3 times the daily maintenance dose should be administered on day 1 of dosing. Maintenance dose: 2 mg/day. Doses should be taken 4 hours after cyclosporine, and should be taken consistently either with or without food.

Children ≥13 years or Adults <40 kg: Loading dose: 3 mg/m^2 (day 1); followed by a maintenance of 1 mg/m^2/day.

Dosage adjustment in renal impairment: No dosage adjustment is necessary in renal impairment

Dosage adjustment in hepatic impairment: Reduce maintenance dose by approximately 33% in hepatic impairment. Loading dose is unchanged.

Administration Amber oral dose syringe should be used to withdraw solution from the bottle. Syringe should then be emptied, or, if a pouch is used, the entire contents should be squeezed out into a glass or plastic cup. The solution in the cup should be mixed with at least 2 ounces of water or orange juice. No other liquids should be used for dilution. Patient should drink diluted solution immediately. The cup should then be refilled with an additional 4 ounces of water or orange juice, stirred vigorously, and the patient should drink the contents at once. Sirolimus should be taken 4 hours after cyclosporine oral solution (modified) or cyclosporine capsules (modified)

Monitoring Parameters Monitor sirolimus levels in pediatric patients, patients with hepatic impairment, or on concurrent inhibitors or inducers of CYP3A4, and/or if cyclosporine dosing is markedly reduced or discontinued. Also monitor serum cholesterol and triglycerides, blood pressure, and serum creatinine. Routine therapeutic drug level monitoring is not required in most patients.

Reference Range Mean serum trough concentrations: 9 ng/mL for the 2 mg/day treatment groups and 17 ng/mL in the 5 mg/day group

Patient Information Do not get pregnant while taking this medication. Use reliable contraception while on this medication and for 3 months after discontinuation. May be taken with or without food but take medication consistently with respect to meals (always take with food or always take on an empty stomach). Wear protective clothing and use sunscreen to limit exposure to sunlight and UV light; decreases risk of skin cancer.

Dosage Forms

Solution, oral: 1 mg/mL (1 mL, 2 mL, 5 mL, 60 mL, 150 mL)
Tablet: 1 mg

♦ **SK** *see* Streptokinase *on page 1260*
♦ **SK and F 104864** *see* Topotecan *on page 1350*
♦ **Skelaxin**® *see* Metaxalone *on page 874*
♦ **Skelid**® *see* Tiludronate *on page 1333*
♦ **SKF 104864** *see* Topotecan *on page 1350*
♦ **SKF 104864-A** *see* Topotecan *on page 1350*

Skin Test Antigens (Multiple) (skin test AN tee gens, MUL ti pul)

U.S. Brand Names Multitest CMI®

Canadian Brand Names Multitest® CMI

Therapeutic Category Diagnostic Agent, Hypersensitivity Skin Testing

Use Detection of nonresponsiveness to antigens by means of delayed hypersensitivity skin testing

Pregnancy Risk Factor C

Contraindications Hypersensitivity to skin test antigens; infected or inflamed skin; do not apply at sites involving acneiform, infected or inflamed skin; although severe systemic reactions are rare to diphtheria and tetanus antigens, persons known to have a history of systemic reactions should be tested with this test only after the test heads containing these antigens have been removed

Warnings/Precautions Epinephrine should be available is case of severe reactions. Safety and effectiveness in children <17 years of age have not been established; discard applicator after use, do not reuse.

Adverse Reactions 1% to 10%: Local: Irritation

Stability Keep in refrigerator at 2°C to 8°C (35°F to 46°F).

Usual Dosage Select only test sites that permit sufficient surface area and subcutaneous tissue to allow adequate penetration of all eight points, avoid hairy areas. Press loaded unit into the skin with sufficient pressure to puncture the skin and allow adequate penetration of all points, maintain firm contact for at least 5 seconds, during application the device should not be "rocked" back and forth and side to side without removing any of the test heads from the skin sites.

If adequate pressure is applied it will be possible to observe:
1. The puncture marks of the nine tines on each of the eight test heads
2. An imprint of the circular platform surrounding each test head
3. Residual antigen and glycerin at each of the eight sites

If any of the above three criteria are not fully followed, the test results may not be reliable.

Reading should be done in good light, read the test sites at both 24 and 48 hours, the largest reaction recorded from the two readings at each test site should be used. If two readings are not possible, a single 48 hour is recommended. A positive reaction from any of the seven delayed hypersensitivity skin test antigens is **induration ≥2 mm** providing there is no induration at the negative control site. The size of the induration reactions with this test may be smaller than those obtained with other intradermal procedures.

Nursing Implications Patients should be informed of the types of test site reactions that may be expected. Remove tests from refrigeration approximately 1 hour before use; select only test sites that permit sufficient surface area and subcutaneous tissue to allow adequate penetration of all points on all eight test heads; avoid hairy areas when possible because interpretation of reactions will be more difficult

Additional Information Contains disposable plastic applicator consisting of 8 sterile test heads preloaded with the following 7 delayed-hypersensitivity skin test antigens and glycerin negative control for percutaneous administration.

Test Head No. 1 = Tetanus toxoid antigen
Test Head No. 2 = Diphtheria toxoid antigen
Test Head No. 3 = *Streptococcus* antigen
Test Head No. 4 = Tuberculin, old
Test Head No. 5 = Glycerin negative control
Test Head No. 6 = *Candida* antigen
Test Head No. 7 = *Trichophyton* antigen
Test Head No. 8 = *Proteus* antigen

Dosage Forms Individual carton containing one preloaded skin test antigen for cellular hypersensitivity

- **Skin Tests** *see page 1533*
- **Sleep-eze 3® Oral [OTC]** *see DiphenhydrAMINE on page 414*
- **Sleepinal® [OTC]** *see DiphenhydrAMINE on page 414*
- **Sleepwell 2-nite® [OTC]** *see DiphenhydrAMINE on page 414*
- **Slo-bid™** *see Theophylline Salts on page 1310*
- **Slo-Niacin® [OTC]** *see Niacin on page 974*
- **Slo-Phyllin®** *see Theophylline Salts on page 1310*
- **Slo-Phyllin® GG** *see Theophylline and Guaifenesin on page 1310*
- **Slow FE® [OTC]** *see Ferrous Sulfate on page 557*
- **Slow-K®** *see Potassium Chloride on page 1108*
- **Slow-Mag® (Chloride)** *see Magnesium Salts (Other) on page 835*

Smallpox Vaccine (SMAL poks vak SEEN)

Therapeutic Category Vaccine, Inactivated Virus

Use There are no indications for the use of smallpox vaccine in the general civilian population. Laboratory workers involved with Orthopoxvirus or in the production and testing of smallpox vaccines should receive regular smallpox vaccinations. For advice on vaccine administration and contraindications, contact the Division of Immunization, CDC, Atlanta, GA 30333 (404-639-3356).

Pregnancy Risk Factor X

- **SMZ-TMP** *see Sulfamethoxazole and Trimethoprim on page 1273*
- **Sodium 2-Mercaptoethane Sulfonate** *see Mesna on page 867*

Sodium Acetate (SOW dee um AS e tate)

Therapeutic Category Alkalinizing Agent, Parenteral; Electrolyte Supplement, Parenteral; Sodium Salt

Use Sodium source in large volume I.V. fluids to prevent or correct hyponatremia in patients with restricted intake; used to counter acidosis through conversion to bicarbonate

Pregnancy Risk Factor C

Contraindications Alkalosis, hypocalcemia, low sodium diets, edema, cirrhosis

Warnings/Precautions Avoid extravasation, use with caution in patients with hepatic failure

Adverse Reactions 1% to 10%:

Cardiovascular: Thrombosis, hypervolemia

Dermatologic: Chemical cellulitis at injection site (extravasation)

Endocrine & metabolic: Hypernatremia, dilution of serum electrolytes, overhydration, hypokalemia, metabolic alkalosis, hypocalcemia

Gastrointestinal: Gastric distension, flatulence

Local: Phlebitis

Respiratory: Pulmonary edema

Miscellaneous: Congestive conditions

Stability Protect from light, heat, and from freezing; **incompatible** with acids, acidic salts, alkaloid salts, calcium salts, catecholamines, atropine

Usual Dosage Sodium acetate is metabolized to bicarbonate on an equimolar basis outside the liver; administer in large volume I.V. fluids as a sodium source. Refer to Sodium Bicarbonate monograph.

Maintenance electrolyte requirements of sodium in parenteral nutrition solutions:

Daily requirements: 3-4 mEq/kg/24 hours or 25-40 mEq/1000 kcal/24 hours

Maximum: 100-150 mEq/24 hours

Administration Must be diluted prior to I.V. administration; infusion hypertonic solutions (>154 mEq/L) via a central line; maximum rate of administration: 1 mEq/kg/hour

Additional Information Sodium and acetate content of 1 g: 7.3 mEq

Dosage Forms Injection: 2 mEq/mL (20 mL, 50 mL, 100 mL); 4 mEq/mL (50 mL, 100 mL)

♦ **Sodium Acid Carbonate** see Sodium Bicarbonate on page 1243

Sodium Ascorbate (SOW dee um a SKOR bate)

U.S. Brand Names Cenolate®

Therapeutic Category Urinary Acidifying Agent; Vitamin, Water Soluble

Use Prevention and treatment of scurvy and to acidify urine

Pregnancy Risk Factor C

Usual Dosage Oral, I.V., S.C.:

Infants:

Daily protective requirement: 30 mg

Treatment: 100-300 mg/day (75-100 mg in premature infants)

Children:

Scurvy: 100-300 mg/day in divided doses for at least 2 weeks

Urinary acidification: 500 mg every 6-8 hours

Dietary supplement: 35-45 mg/day

Adults:

Scurvy: 100-250 mg 1-2 times/day for at least 2 weeks

Urinary acidification: 4-12 g/day in divided doses

Dietary supplement: 50-60 mg/day (RDA: 60 mg)

Prevention and treatment of cold: 1-3 g/day

Additional Information Complete prescribing information for this medication should be consulted for additional detail.

Dosage Forms Injection: 562.5 mg/mL [ascorbic acid 500 mg/mL] (1 mL, 2 mL)

♦ **Sodium Benzoate and Caffeine** see Caffeine and Sodium Benzoate on page 202

♦ **Sodium Benzoate and Sodium Phenylacetate** see Sodium Phenylacetate and Sodium Benzoate on page 1248

Sodium Bicarbonate (SOW dee um bye KAR bun ate)

Related Information

Adult ACLS Algorithms on page 1632

U.S. Brand Names Neut®

Synonyms Baking Soda; NaHCO₃; Sodium Acid Carbonate; Sodium Hydrogen Carbonate

Therapeutic Category Alkalinizing Agent, Oral; Alkalinizing Agent, Parenteral; Antacid; Electrolyte Supplement, Oral; Electrolyte Supplement, Parenteral; Sodium Salt

Use Management of metabolic acidosis; gastric hyperacidity; as an alkalinization agent for the urine; treatment of hyperkalemia; management of overdose of certain drugs, including tricyclic antidepressants and aspirin

Pregnancy Risk Factor C

Contraindications Alkalosis, hypernatremia, severe pulmonary edema, hypocalcemia, unknown abdominal pain

Warnings/Precautions Rapid administration in neonates and children <2 years of age has led to hypernatremia, decreased CSF pressure and intracranial hemorrhage. **Use of I.V. NaHCO₃ should be reserved for documented metabolic acidosis and for hyperkalemia-induced cardiac arrest.** Routine use in cardiac arrest is not recommended. Avoid extravasation, tissue necrosis can occur due to the hypertonicity of NaHCO₃. May cause sodium retention especially if renal function is impaired; not to be used in treatment of peptic ulcer; use with caution in patients with CHF, edema, cirrhosis, or renal failure. Not the antacid of choice for the elderly because of sodium content and potential for systemic alkalosis.

Adverse Reactions Frequency not defined.

Cardiovascular: Cerebral hemorrhage, congestive heart failure (aggravated), edema

Central nervous system: Tetany

Gastrointestinal: Belching

Endocrine & metabolic: Hypernatremia, hyperosmolality, hypocalcemia, hypokalemia, increased affinity of hemoglobin for oxygen-reduced pH in myocardial tissue necrosis when extravasated, intracranial acidosis, metabolic alkalosis, milk-alkali syndrome (especially with renal dysfunction)

(Continued)

Sodium Bicarbonate *(Continued)*

Gastrointestinal: Flatulence (with oral), gastric distension
Respiratory: Pulmonary edema

Overdosage/Toxicology Symptoms include hypocalcemia, hypokalemia, hypernatremia, and seizures. Seizures can be treated with diazepam 0.1-0.25 mg/kg. Hypernatremia is resolved through the use of diuretics and free water replacement.

Drug Interactions

Increased Effect/Toxicity: Increased toxicity/levels of amphetamines, ephedrine, pseudo-ephedrine, flecainide, quinidine, and quinine due to urinary alkalinization.

Decreased Effect: Decreased effect/levels of lithium, chlorpropamide, and salicylates due to urinary alkalinization.

Ethanol/Nutrition/Herb Interactions Herb/Nutraceutical: Concurrent doses with iron may decrease iron absorption.

Stability Store injection at room temperature; protect from heat and from freezing; use only clear solutions; Advise patient of milk-alkali syndrome if use is long-term; observe for extravasation when giving I.V.; **incompatible** with acids, acidic salts, alkaloid salts, atropine, calcium salts, catecholamines

Mechanism of Action Dissociates to provide bicarbonate ion which neutralizes hydrogen ion concentration and raises blood and urinary pH

Pharmacodynamics/Kinetics
Onset of action: Oral: Rapid; I.V.: 15 minutes
Duration: Oral: 8-10 minutes; I.V.: 1-2 hours
Absorption: Oral: Well absorbed
Excretion: Urine (<1%)

Usual Dosage
Cardiac arrest: **Routine use of NaHCO$_3$ is not recommended and should be given only after adequate alveolar ventilation has been established and effective cardiac compressions are provided**

Infants and Children: I.V.: 0.5-1 mEq/kg/dose repeated every 10 minutes or as indicated by arterial blood gases; rate of infusion should not exceed 10 mEq/minute; neonates and children <2 years of age should receive 4.2% (0.5 mEq/mL) solution

Adults: I.V.: Initial: 1 mEq/kg/dose one time; maintenance: 0.5 mEq/kg/dose every 10 minutes or as indicated by arterial blood gases

Metabolic acidosis: Dosage should be based on the following formula if blood gases and pH measurements are available:

Infants and Children:
HCO_3^-(mEq) = 0.3 x weight (kg) x base deficit (mEq/L) **or**
HCO_3^-(mEq) = 0.5 x weight (kg) x [24 - serum HCO_3^- (mEq/L)]

Adults:
HCO_3^-(mEq) = 0.2 x weight (kg) x base deficit (mEq/L) **or**
HCO_3^-(mEq) = 0.5 x weight (kg) x [24 - serum HCO_3^- (mEq/L)]

If acid-base status is not available: Dose for older Children and Adults: 2-5 mEq/kg I.V. infusion over 4-8 hours; subsequent doses should be based on patient's acid-base status

Chronic renal failure: Oral: Initiate when plasma HCO_3^- <15 mEq/L
Children: 1-3 mEq/kg/day
Adults: Start with 20-36 mEq/day in divided doses, titrate to bicarbonate level of 18-20 mEq/L

Hyperkalemia: Adults: I.V.: 1 mEq/kg over 5 minutes

Renal tubular acidosis: Oral:
Distal:
Children: 2-3 mEq/kg/day
Adults: 0.5-2 mEq/kg/day in 4-5 divided doses
Proximal: Children: Initial: 5-10 mEq/kg/day; maintenance: Increase as required to maintain serum bicarbonate in the normal range

Urine alkalinization: Oral:
Children: 1-10 mEq (84-840 mg)/kg/day in divided doses every 4-6 hours; dose should be titrated to desired urinary pH
Adults: Initial: 48 mEq (4 g), then 12-24 mEq (1-2 g) every 4 hours; dose should be titrated to desired urinary pH; doses up to 16 g/day (200 mEq) in patients <60 years and 8 g (100 mEq) in patients >60 years

Antacid: Adults: Oral: 325 mg to 2 g 1-4 times/day

Dietary Considerations Oral product should be administered 1-3 hours after meals.

Administration For I.V. administration to infants, use the 0.5 mEq/mL solution or dilute the 1 mEq/mL solution 1:1 with **sterile water**; for direct I.V. infusion in emergencies, administer slowly (maximum rate in infants: 10 mEq/minute); for infusion, dilute to a maximum concentration of 0.5 mEq/mL in dextrose solution and infuse over 2 hours (maximum rate of administration: 1 mEq/kg/hour)

Patient Information Avoid chronic use as an antacid (<2 weeks)

Nursing Implications Advise patient of milk-alkali syndrome if use is long-term; observe for extravasation when giving I.V.

Additional Information
Sodium content of injection 50 mL, 8.4% = 1150 mg = 50 mEq; each 6 mg of NaHCO$_3$ contains 12 mEq sodium; 1 mEq NaHCO$_3$ = 84 mg.
Each 84 mg of sodium bicarbonate provides 1 mEq of sodium and bicarbonate ions; each gram of sodium bicarbonate provides 12 mEq of sodium and bicarbonate ions.

Dosage Forms
Injection:
4% [40 mg/mL = 2.4 mEq/5 mL] (5 mL)
4.2% [42 mg/mL = 5 mEq/10 mL] (10 mL)
5% [50 mg/mL = 5.95 mEq/10 mL] (500 mL)
7.5% [75 mg/mL = 8.92 mEq/10 mL] (10 mL, 50 mL)
8.4% [84 mg/mL = 10 mEq/10 mL] (10 mL, 50 mL)

Powder: 120 g, 480 g
Tablet: 325 mg [3.8 mEq]; 520 mg [6.3 mEq]; 650 mg [7.6 mEq]

♦ **Sodium Biphosphate, Methenamine, Methylene Blue, Phenyl Salicylate, and Hyoscyamine** *see* Methenamine, Sodium Biphosphate, Phenyl Salicylate, Methylene Blue, and Hyoscyamine *on page 882*

Sodium Chloride (SOW dee um KLOR ide)

U.S. Brand Names Adsorbonac® [DSC]; Altamist [OTC]; Ayr® Saline [OTC]; Breathe Free® [OTC]; Breathe Right® Saline [OTC]; Broncho Saline®; Entsol® [OTC]; Muro 128® [OTC]; NāSal™[OTC]; Nasal Moist® [OTC]; Na-Zone® [OTC]; Ocean® [OTC]; Pediamist® [OTC]; Pretz® [OTC]; SalineX® [OTC]; SeaMist® [OTC]; Wound Wash Saline™ [OTC]

Synonyms NaCl; Normal Saline; Salt

Therapeutic Category Electrolyte Supplement, Oral; Electrolyte Supplement, Parenteral; Lubricant, Ocular; Sodium Salt

Use
Parenteral: Restores sodium ion in patients with restricted oral intake (especially hyponatremia states or low salt syndrome). In general, parenteral saline uses:
Bacteriostatic sodium chloride: Dilution or dissolving drugs for I.M., I.V., or S.C. injections
Concentrated sodium chloride: Additive for parenteral fluid therapy
Hypertonic sodium chloride: For severe hyponatremia and hypochloremia
Hypotonic sodium chloride: Hydrating solution
Normal saline: Restores water/sodium losses
Pharmaceutical aid/diluent for infusion of compatible drug additives
Ophthalmic: Reduces corneal edema
Oral: Restores sodium losses
Inhalation: Restores moisture to pulmonary system; loosens and thins congestion caused by colds or allergies; diluent for bronchodilator solutions that require dilution before inhalation
Intranasal: Restores moisture to nasal membranes
Irrigation: Wound cleansing, irrigation, and flushing

Pregnancy Risk Factor C

Contraindications Hypersensitivity to sodium chloride or any component of the formulation; hypertonic uterus, hypernatremia, fluid retention

Warnings/Precautions Use with caution in patients with congestive heart failure, renal insufficiency, liver cirrhosis, hypertension, edema; sodium toxicity is almost exclusively related to how fast a sodium deficit is corrected; both rate and magnitude are extremely important; do not use bacteriostatic sodium chloride in newborns since benzyl alcohol preservatives have been associated with toxicity

Adverse Reactions Frequency not defined.
Cardiovascular: Congestive conditions
Endocrine & metabolic: Extravasation, hypervolemia, hypernatremia, dilution of serum electrolytes, overhydration, hypokalemia
Local: Thrombosis, phlebitis, extravasation
Respiratory: Pulmonary edema

Overdosage/Toxicology Symptoms include nausea, vomiting, diarrhea, abdominal cramps, hypocalcemia, hypokalemia, and hypernatremia. Hypernatremia is resolved through the use of diuretics and free water replacement.

Drug Interactions
Decreased Effect: Lithium serum concentrations may be decreased.

Stability Store injection at room temperature; protect from heat and from freezing; use only clear solutions

Mechanism of Action Principal extracellular cation; functions in fluid and electrolyte balance, osmotic pressure control, and water distribution

Pharmacodynamics/Kinetics
Absorption: Oral, I.V.: Rapid
Distribution: Widely distributed
Excretion: Primarily urine; also sweat, tears, saliva

Usual Dosage
Children: I.V.: Hypertonic solutions (>0.9%) should only be used for the initial treatment of acute serious symptomatic hyponatremia; maintenance: 3-4 mEq/kg/day; maximum: 100-150 mEq/day; dosage varies widely depending on clinical condition
Replacement: Determined by laboratory determinations mEq
Sodium deficiency (mEq/kg) = [% dehydration (L/kg)/100 x 70 (mEq/L)] + [0.6 (L/kg) x (140 - serum sodium) (mEq/L)]

Children ≥2 years and Adults:
Intranasal: 2-3 sprays in each nostril as needed
Irrigation: Spray affected area

Children and Adults: Inhalation: Bronchodilator diluent: 1-3 sprays (1-3 mL) to dilute bronchodilator solution in nebulizer prior to administration

Adults:
GU irrigant: 1-3 L/day by intermittent irrigation
Heat cramps: Oral: 0.5-1 g with full glass of water, up to 4.8 g/day
Replacement I.V.: Determined by laboratory determinations mEq
Sodium deficiency (mEq/kg) = [% dehydration (L/kg)/100 x 70 (mEq/L)] + [0.6 (L/kg) x (140 - serum sodium) (mEq/L)]
To correct acute, serious hyponatremia: mEq sodium = [desired sodium (mEq/L) - actual sodium (mEq/L)] x [0.6 x wt (kg)]; for acute correction use 125 mEq/L as the desired serum sodium; acutely correct serum sodium in 5 mEq/L/dose increments; more gradual correction in increments of 10 mEq/L/day is indicated in the asymptomatic patient
Chloride maintenance electrolyte requirement in parenteral nutrition: 2-4 mEq/kg/24 hours or 25-40 mEq/1000 kcals/24 hours; maximum: 100-150 mEq/24 hours
Sodium maintenance electrolyte requirement in parenteral nutrition: 3-4 mEq/kg/24 hours or 25-40 mEq/1000 kcals/24 hours; maximum: 100-150 mEq/24 hours.

(Continued)

Sodium Chloride (Continued)

Approximate Deficits of Water and Electrolytes in Moderately Severe Dehydration*

Condition	Water (mL/kg)	Sodium (mEq/kg)
Fasting and thirsting	100-120	5-7
Diarrhea		
isonatremic	100-120	8-10
hypernatremic	100-120	2-4
hyponatremic	100-120	10-12
Pyloric stenosis	100-120	8-10
Diabetic acidosis	100-120	9-10

*A **negative** deficit indicates total body **excess** prior to treatment.

Adapted from Behrman RE, Kleigman RM, Nelson WE, et al, eds, *Nelson Textbook of Pediatrics*, 14th ed, WB Saunders Co, 1992.

Ophthalmic:
Ointment: Apply once daily or more often
Solution: Instill 1-2 drops into affected eye(s) every 3-4 hours
Administration Infuse hypertonic solutions (>NaCl 0.9%) via central line only; maximum rate of administration: 1 mEq/kg/hour
Monitoring Parameters Serum sodium, potassium, chloride, and bicarbonate levels; I & O, weight
Reference Range Serum/plasma sodium levels:
Neonates:
Full-term: 133-142 mEq/L
Premature: 132-140 mEq/L
Children ≥2 months to Adults: 135-145 mEq/L
Patient Information Blurred vision is common with ophthalmic ointment; may sting eyes when first applied
Nursing Implications Bacteriostatic NS should not be used for diluting or reconstituting drugs for administration in neonates; I.V. infusion of 3% or 5% sodium chloride should not exceed 100 mL/hour and should be administered in a central line only
Dosage Forms
Gel, intranasal (Nasal Moist®): 0.65% (30 g)
Ointment, ophthalmic: 5% (3.5 g)
Muro-128®: 5% (3.5g)
Powder, for solution (Entsol®) 3% (10.5 g)
Solution, for inhalation: 0.45% (3 mL, 5 mL); 0.9% (3 mL, 5 mL); 3% (15 mL); 10% (15 mL)
Broncho Saline®: 0.9% (90 mL, 240 mL)
Solution for injection: 0.45% (25 mL, 50mL, 100 mL, 250 mL, 500 mL, 1000 mL, 1500 mL, 2000 mL); 0.9% (2 mL, 3 mL, 5 mL, 10 mL, 20 mL, 25 mL, 30 mL, 50 mL, 100 mL, 150 mL, 250 mL, 500 mL, 1000 mL); 2.5 % (250 mL); 3% (500 mL); 5% (500 mL)
Solution for injection [preservative free]: 0.9% (2mL, 5 mL, 10 mL, 20 mL, 50 mL, 100 mL)
Solution for injection, bacteriostatic: 0.9% (10 mL, 20 mL, 30 mL)
Solution for injection, concentrate: 14.6% (20 mL, 40 mL, 250 mL); 23.4% (30 mL 50 mL, 100 mL, 200 mL, 250 mL)
Solution, intranasal: 0.65% (45 mL, 90 mL)
Salinex®: 0.4% (15 mL, 50 mL)
Pediamist®: 0.5% (15 mL)
Altamist: 0.65% (60 mL)
Ayr® Baby Saline: 0.65% (30 mL)
Ayr® Saline, Ayr® Saline Mist: 0.65% (50 mL)
Breathe Free®, Breathe Right® Saline: 0.65% (44 mL)
NaSal™: 0.65% (15 mL, 30 mL)
Nasal Moist®: 0.65% (15 mL, 45 mL)
Ocean®: 0.65% (45 mL)
Sea Mist®: 0.65% (15 mL)
Pretz® Irrigation: 0.75% (240 mL)
Na-Zone®: 0.75% (60 mL)
Entsol®: 3% (100 mL)
Entsol® Mist: 3% (30 mL)
Enstol® Single Use [preservative free nasal wash]: 3% (240 mL)
Solution for irrigation: 0.45% (2000 mL); 0.9% (250 mL, 500 mL, 1000 mL, 2000 mL, 3000 mL, 4000 mL)
Wound Wash Saline™: 0.9% (90 mL, 210 mL)
Solution, ophthalmic: 5% (15 mL)
Muro-128®: 2% (15 mL), 5% (15 mL, 30 mL)
Tablet: 1 g

Sodium Citrate and Citric Acid (SOW dee um SIT rate & SI trik AS id)

U.S. Brand Names Bicitra®; Oracit®
Canadian Brand Names PMS-Dicitrate™
Synonyms Modified Shohl's Solution
Therapeutic Category Alkalinizing Agent, Oral
Use Treatment of metabolic acidosis; alkalinizing agent in conditions where long-term maintenance of an alkaline urine is desirable
Pregnancy Risk Factor Not established
Contraindications Severe renal insufficiency, sodium-restricted diet

Warnings/Precautions Conversion to bicarbonate may be impaired in patients with hepatic failure, in shock, or who are severely ill

Adverse Reactions Frequency not defined.
Central nervous system: Tetany
Endocrine & metabolic: Metabolic alkalosis, hyperkalemia
Gastrointestinal: Diarrhea, nausea, vomiting

Overdosage/Toxicology Symptoms include hypokalemia, hypernatremia, tetany, and seizures. Hypernatremia is resolved through the use of diuretics and free water replacement.

Drug Interactions
Increased Effect/Toxicity: Increased toxicity/levels of amphetamines, ephedrine, pseudoephedrine, flecainide, quinidine, and quinine due to urinary alkalinization.
Decreased Effect: Decreased effect/levels of lithium, chlorpropamide, and salicylates due to urinary alkalinization.

Usual Dosage Oral:
Infants and Children: 2-3 mEq/kg/day in divided doses 3-4 times/day **or** 5-15 mL with water after meals and at bedtime
Adults: 15-30 mL with water after meals and at bedtime

Dietary Considerations Should be taken after meals to avoid laxative effect.

Administration Administer after meals

Patient Information Palatability is improved by chilling solution, dilute each dose with 1-3 oz of water and follow with additional water; take after meals to prevent saline laxative effect

Nursing Implications May be ordered as modified Shohl's solution; dilute with 30-90 mL of chilled water to enhance taste

Additional Information 1 mL of Bicitra® contains 1 mEq of sodium and the equivalent of 1 mEq of bicarbonate.

Dosage Forms
Solution, oral:
Bicitra®: Sodium citrate 500 mg and citric acid 334 mg per 5 mL (15 mL unit dose, 480 mL)
Oracit®: Sodium citrate 490 mg and citric acid 640 mg per 5 mL

Sodium Citrate and Potassium Citrate Mixture
(SOW dee um SIT rate & poe TASS ee um SIT rate MIKS chur)

U.S. Brand Names Polycitra®

Synonyms Potassium Citrate Mixture and Sodium Citrate

Therapeutic Category Alkalinizing Agent, Oral

Use Conditions where long-term maintenance of an alkaline urine is desirable as in control and dissolution of uric acid and cystine calculi of the urinary tract

Pregnancy Risk Factor Not established

Usual Dosage Oral:
Children: 5-15 mL diluted in water after meals and at bedtime
Adults: 15-30 mL diluted in water after meals and at bedtime

Additional Information Complete prescribing information for this medication should be consulted for additional detail.

Dosage Forms
Solution, oral (Polycitra®-LC): Sodium citrate 500 mg and citric acid 334 mg with potassium citrate 550 mg per 5 mL [sugar free]
Syrup, oral (Polycitra®): Sodium citrate 500 mg and citric acid 334 mg with potassium citrate 550 mg per 5 mL

- **Sodium Edetate** *see* Edetate Disodium *on page 457*
- **Sodium Etidronate** *see* Etidronate Disodium *on page 531*
- **Sodium Ferric Gluconate** *see* Ferric Gluconate *on page 554*
- **Sodium Fluoride** *see* Fluoride *on page 574*

Sodium Hyaluronate (SOW dee um hye al yoor ON ate)

U.S. Brand Names AMO Vitrax®; Amvisc®; Amvisc® Plus; Healon®; Healon® GV; Hyalgan®

Canadian Brand Names Biolon™; Cystistat®; Eyestil®; Healon®; Healon® GV; Suplasyn®

Synonyms Hyaluronic Acid

Therapeutic Category Ophthalmic Agent, Viscoelastic

Use Surgical aid in cataract extraction, intraocular implantation, corneal transplant, glaucoma filtration, and retinal attachment surgery

Intra-articular injection (Hyalgan®): Treatment of pain in osteoarthritis in knee in patients who have failed nonpharmacologic treatment and simple analgesics

Pregnancy Risk Factor C

Contraindications Hypersensitivity to hyaluronate or any component of the formulation

Warnings/Precautions Do not overfill the anterior chamber; carefully monitor intraocular pressure; risk of hypersensitivity exists

Adverse Reactions 1% to 10%: Ocular: Postoperative inflammatory reactions (iritis, hypopyon), corneal edema, corneal decompensation, transient postoperative increase in IOP

Stability Store in refrigerator (2°C to 8°C); do not freeze

Mechanism of Action Functions as a tissue lubricant and is thought to play an important role in modulating the interactions between adjacent tissues. Sodium hyaluronate is a polysaccharide which is distributed widely in the extracellular matrix of connective tissue in man. (Vitreous and aqueous humor of the eye, synovial fluid, skin, and umbilical cord.) Sodium hyaluronate forms a viscoelastic solution in water (at physiological pH and ionic strength) which makes it suitable for aqueous and vitreous humor in ophthalmic surgery.

Pharmacodynamics/Kinetics
Distribution: Following intravitreous injection, diffusion occurs slowly
Excretion: Via Canal of Schlemm

Usual Dosage Depends upon procedure (slowly introduce a sufficient quantity into eye)
(Continued)

Sodium Hyaluronate *(Continued)*

Administration The drug may become cloudy or form a slight precipitate after administration; clinical significance unknown, but cloudy or precipitated material should be removed by irrigation or aspiration

Hyalgan® is injected directly into the knee joint

Monitoring Parameters Intraocular pressure

Dosage Forms

Injection, intra-articular (Hyalgan®): 10 mg/mL (2 mL)

Injection, intraocular:

AMO Vitrax®: 30 mg/mL (0.65 mL)

Amvisc®: 12 mg/mL (0.5 mL, 0.8 mL)

Amvisc® Plus: 16 mg/mL (0.5 mL, 8 mL)

Healon®: 10 mg/mL (0.4 mL, 0.55 mL, 0.85 mL, 2 mL)

Healon® GV: 14 mg/mL (0.55 mL, 0.85 mL)

♦ **Sodium Hyaluronate-Chrondroitin Sulfate** *see Chondroitin Sulfate-Sodium Hyaluronate on page 289*

♦ **Sodium Hydrogen Carbonate** *see Sodium Bicarbonate on page 1243*

Sodium Hypochlorite Solution

(SOW dee um hye poe KLOR ite soe LOO shun)

U.S. Brand Names Dakin's Solution

Synonyms Modified Dakin's Solution

Therapeutic Category Disinfectant, Antibacterial (Topical)

Use Treatment of athlete's foot (0.5%); wound irrigation (0.5%); disinfection of utensils and equipment (5%)

Pregnancy Risk Factor C

Contraindications Hypersensitivity to any component of the formulation

Warnings/Precautions For external use only; avoid eye or mucous membrane contact; do not use on open wounds

Adverse Reactions Frequency not defined.

Dermatologic: Irritating to skin

Hematologic: Dissolves blood clots, delays clotting

Stability Use prepared solution within 7 days.

Usual Dosage Topical irrigation

Administration For external use only; do **not** ingest.

Patient Information External use only

Nursing Implications Dakin's solution may hinder wound healing

Dosage Forms

Solution, topical: 5% (4000 mL)

Solution, topical (Dakin's):

Full strength: 0.5% (1000 mL)

Half strength: 0.25% (1000 mL)

Quarter strength: 0.125% (1000 mL)

♦ **Sodium *L*-Triiodothyronine** *see Liothyronine on page 808*

♦ **Sodium Nafcillin** *see Nafcillin on page 950*

♦ **Sodium Nitroferricyanide** *see Nitroprusside on page 991*

♦ **Sodium Nitroprusside** *see Nitroprusside on page 991*

Sodium Phenylacetate and Sodium Benzoate

(SOW dee um fen il AS e tate & SOW dee um BENZ oh ate)

U.S. Brand Names Ucephan®

Synonyms Sodium Benzoate and Sodium Phenylacetate

Therapeutic Category Ammonium Detoxicant

Use Orphan drug: Adjunctive therapy to prevention/treatment of hyperammonemia in patients with urea cycle enzymopathy involving partial or complete deficiencies of carbamoyl-phosphate synthetase, ornithine transcarbamoylase, or argininosuccinate synthetase

Pregnancy Risk Factor C

Usual Dosage Infants and Children: Oral: 2.5 mL (250 mg sodium benzoate and 250 mg sodium phenylacetate)/kg/day divided 3-6 times/day; total daily dose should not exceed 100 mL

Additional Information Complete prescribing information for this medication should be consulted for additional detail.

Dosage Forms Solution: Sodium phenylacetate 100 mg and sodium benzoate 100 mg per mL (100 mL)

Sodium Phenylbutyrate (SOW dee um fen il BYOO ti rate)

U.S. Brand Names Buphenyl®

Synonyms Ammonapse

Therapeutic Category Urea Cycle Disorder (UCD) Treatment Agent

Use Orphan drug: Adjunctive therapy in the chronic management of patients with urea cycle disorder involving deficiencies of carbamoylphosphate synthetase, ornithine transcarbamylase, or argininosuccinic acid synthetase

Pregnancy Risk Factor C

Usual Dosage

Powder: Patients weighing <20 kg: 450-600 mg/kg/day or 9.9-13 g/m^2/day, administered in equally divided amounts with each meal or feeding, four to six times daily; safety and efficacy of doses >20 g/day has not been established

Tablet: Children >20 kg and Adults: 450-600 mg/kg/day or 9.9-13 g/m^2/day, administered in equally divided amounts with each meal; safety and efficacy of doses >20 g/day have not been established

Additional Information Complete prescribing information for this medication should be consulted for additional detail.

Dosage Forms
Powder: 3.2 g [sodium phenylbutyrate 3 g] per **teaspoon** (500 mL, 950 mL)
Tablet: 500 mg

♦ **Sodium Phosphate and Potassium Phosphate** see Potassium Phosphate and Sodium Phosphate on page 1114

Sodium Polystyrene Sulfonate (SOW dee um pol ee STYE reen SUL fon ate)

Related Information
Antacid Drug Interactions on page 1477

U.S. Brand Names Kayexalate®; Kionex™; SPS®

Canadian Brand Names Kayexalate®; PMS-Sodium Polystyrene Sulfonate

Therapeutic Category Antidote, Hyperkalemia; Antidote, Potassium

Use Treatment of hyperkalemia

Pregnancy Risk Factor C

Contraindications Hypersensitivity to sodium polystyrene sulfonate or any component of the formulation; hypernatremia

Warnings/Precautions Use with caution in patients with severe congestive heart failure, hypertension, edema, or renal failure; avoid using the commercially available liquid product in neonates due to the preservative content; large oral doses may cause fecal impaction (especially in elderly); enema will reduce the serum potassium faster than oral administration, but the oral route will result in a greater reduction over several hours.

Adverse Reactions Frequency not defined.
Endocrine & metabolic: Hypokalemia, hypocalcemia, hypomagnesemia, sodium retention
Gastrointestinal: Fecal impaction, constipation, loss of appetite, nausea, vomiting

Overdosage/Toxicology Symptoms include hypokalemia including cardiac dysrhythmias, confusion, irritability, EKG changes, muscle weakness, and gastrointestinal effects. Treatment is supportive and is limited to management of fluid and electrolytes.

Drug Interactions
Increased Effect/Toxicity: Systemic alkalosis and seizure has occurred after cation-exchange resins were administered with nonabsorbable cation-donating antacids and laxatives (eg, magnesium hydroxide, aluminum carbonate).

Stability Store prepared suspensions at 15°C to 30°C (59°F to 86°F); store repackaged product in refrigerator and use within 14 days; freshly prepared suspensions should be used within 24 hours; do not heat resin suspension

Mechanism of Action Removes potassium by exchanging sodium ions for potassium ions in the intestine before the resin is passed from the body

Pharmacodynamics/Kinetics
Onset of action: 2-24 hours
Absorption: None
Excretion: Completely feces (primarily as potassium polystyrene sulfonate)

Usual Dosage
Children:
Oral: 1 g/kg/dose every 6 hours
Rectal: 1 g/kg/dose every 2-6 hours (In small children and infants, employ lower doses by using the practical exchange ratio of 1 mEq K+/g of resin as the basis for calculation)
Adults: Hyperkalemia:
Oral: 15 g (60 mL) 1-4 times/day
Rectal: 30-50 g every 6 hours

Dietary Considerations Do **not** mix in orange juice.

Monitoring Parameters Exchange capacity is 1 mEq/g in vivo, and in vitro capacity is 3.1 mEq/g, therefore, a wide range of exchange capacity exists such that close monitoring of serum electrolytes (potassium, sodium, calcium, magnesium) is necessary; EKG

Reference Range Serum potassium: Adults: 3.5-5.2 mEq/L

Patient Information Mix well in full glass of liquid prior to drinking

Nursing Implications Administer oral (or NG) as ~25% sorbitol solution, never mix in orange juice; enema route is less effective than oral administration; retain enema in colon for at least 30-60 minutes and for several hours, if possible; chilling the oral mixture will increase palatability; enema should be followed by irrigation with normal saline to prevent necrosis

Additional Information 1 g of resin binds approximately 1 mEq of potassium; sodium content of 1 g: 31 mg (1.3 mEq)

Dosage Forms
Powder for suspension, oral/rectal: 454 g
Suspension, oral/rectal: 1.25 g/5 mL with sorbitol 33% and alcohol 0.3% (60 mL, 120 mL, 200 mL, 500 mL)

♦ **Sodium Sulamyd®** see Sulfacetamide on page 1268

♦ **Sodium Sulfacetamide** see Sulfacetamide on page 1268

Sodium Tetradecyl (SOW dee um tetra DEK il)

U.S. Brand Names Sotradecol®

Canadian Brand Names Trombovar®

Synonyms Sodium Tetradecyl Sulfate

Therapeutic Category Sclerosing Agent

Use Treatment of small, uncomplicated varicose veins of the lower extremities; endoscopic sclerotherapy in the management of bleeding esophageal varices

Pregnancy Risk Factor C

Contraindications Hypersensitivity to sodium tetradecyl or any component of the formulation; arterial disease, thrombophlebitis; valvular or deep vein incompetence, phlebitis, migraines, cellulitis, acute infections; bedridden patients; patients with uncontrolled systemic disease such as diabetes, toxic hyperthyroidism, tuberculosis, asthma, neoplasm, sepsis, blood dyscrasias, and acute respiratory or skin diseases

(Continued)

Sodium Tetradecyl *(Continued)*

Warnings/Precautions Buerger's disease, peripheral arteriosclerosis, avoid extravasation; observe for hypersensitivity/anaphylactic reaction

Adverse Reactions Frequency not defined.

Central nervous system: Headache

Dermatologic: Discoloration at site of injection, sloughing and tissue necrosis following extravasation, ulceration at site, urticaria

Gastrointestinal: Esophageal perforation, mucosal lesions, nausea, vomiting

Local: Pain at injection site

Respiratory: Asthma, pulmonary edema

Stability Store at controlled room temperature in a well-closed container; protect from light

Mechanism of Action Acts by irritation of the vein intimal endothelium

Usual Dosage I.V.: Test dose: 0.5 mL given several hours prior to administration of larger dose; 0.5-2 mL in each vein, maximum: 10 mL per treatment session; 3% solution reserved for large varices

Administration Inject slowly.

Patient Information Notify physician if chest pain, shortness of breath, or heat, pain, or tenderness in lower extremities

Nursing Implications Observe for signs and symptoms of embolism

Dosage Forms Injection, as sulfate: 1% [10 mg/mL] (2 mL); 3% [30 mg/mL] (2 mL)

♦ **Sodium Tetradecyl Sulfate** *see* Sodium Tetradecyl *on page 1249*

Sodium Thiosulfate *(SOW dee um thye oh SUL fate)*

U.S. Brand Names Tinver®

Therapeutic Category Antidote, Arsenic Toxicity; Antidote, Cyanide; Antifungal Agent, Topical

Use

Parenteral: Used alone or with sodium nitrite or amyl nitrite in cyanide poisoning or arsenic poisoning; reduce the risk of nephrotoxicity associated with cisplatin therapy

Topical: Treatment of tinea versicolor

Pregnancy Risk Factor C

Pregnancy/Breast-Feeding Implications Safety has not been established in pregnant women. Use only when potential benefit to the mother outweighs the possible risk to the fetus.

Contraindications Hypersensitivity to sodium thiosulfate or any component of the formulation

Warnings/Precautions Safety in pregnancy has not been established; discontinue topical use if irritation or sensitivity occurs; rapid I.V. infusion has caused transient hypotension and EKG changes in dogs; can increase risk of thiocyanate intoxication

Adverse Reactions 1% to 10%:

Cardiovascular: Hypotension

Central nervous system: Coma, CNS depression secondary to thiocyanate intoxication, psychosis, confusion

Dermatologic: Contact dermatitis, local irritation

Neuromuscular & skeletal: Weakness

Otic: Tinnitus

Mechanism of Action

Cyanide toxicity: Increases the rate of detoxification of cyanide by the enzyme rhodanese by providing an extra sulfur

Cisplatin toxicity: Complexes with cisplatin to form a compound that is nontoxic to either normal or cancerous cells

Pharmacodynamics/Kinetics

Half-life elimination: 0.65 hour

Excretion: Urine (28.5% as unchanged drug)

Usual Dosage

Cyanide and nitroprusside antidote: I.V.:

Children <25 kg: 50 mg/kg after receiving 4.5-10 mg/kg sodium nitrite; a half dose of each may be repeated if necessary

Children >25 kg and Adults: 12.5 g after 300 mg of sodium nitrite; a half dose of each may be repeated if necessary

Cyanide poisoning: I.V.: Dose should be based on determination as with nitrite, at rate of 2.5-5 mL/minute to maximum of 50 mL.

Variation of sodium nitrate and sodium thiosulfate dose, based on hemoglobin concentration*: See table.

Variation of Sodium Nitrite and Sodium Thiosulfate Dose With Hemoglobin Concentration*

Hemoglobin (g/dL)	Initial Dose Sodium Nitrite (mg/kg)	Initial Dose Sodium Nitrite 3% (mL/kg)	Initial Dose Sodium Thiosulfate 25% (mL/kg)
7	5.8	0.19	0.95
8	6.6	0.22	1.10
9	7.5	0.25	1.25
10	8.3	0.27	1.35
11	9.1	0.30	1.50
12	10.0	0.33	1.65
13	10.8	0.36	1.80
14	11.6	0.39	1.95

*Adapted from Berlin DM Jr, "The Treatment of Cyanide Poisoning in Children," *Pediatrics*, 1970, 46:793.

Cisplatin rescue should be given before or during cisplatin administration: I.V. infusion (in sterile water): 12 g/m² over 6 hours or 9 g/m² I.V. push followed by 1.2 g/m² continuous infusion for 6 hours

Arsenic poisoning: I.V.: 1 mL first day, 2 mL second day, 3 mL third day, 4 mL fourth day, 5 mL on alternate days thereafter

Children and Adults: Topical: 20% to 25% solution: Apply a thin layer to affected areas twice daily

Administration I.V.: Inject slowly, over at least 10 minutes; rapid administration may cause hypotension

Monitoring Parameters Monitor for signs of thiocyanate toxicity

Patient Information Avoid topical application near the eyes, mouth, or other mucous membranes; notify physician if condition worsens or burning or irritation occurs; shake well before using

Nursing Implications
Do not apply topically to or near eyes; inject I.V. slowly, over at least 10 minutes; rapid administration may cause hypotension
Monitor for signs of thiocyanate toxicity

Dosage Forms
Injection: 100 mg/mL (10 mL); 250 mg/mL (50 mL)
Lotion: 25% with salicylic acid 1% and isopropyl alcohol 10% (120 mL, 180 mL)

- ◆ **Soflax™ (Can)** see Docusate on page 430
- ◆ **Solagé™** see Mequinol and Tretinoin on page 862
- ◆ **Solaquin® [OTC]** see Hydroquinone on page 686
- ◆ **Solaquin Forte®** see Hydroquinone on page 686
- ◆ **Solaraze™** see Diclofenac on page 393
- ◆ **Solarcaine® [OTC]** see Benzocaine on page 154
- ◆ **Solarcaine® Aloe Extra Burn Relief [OTC]** see Lidocaine on page 801
- ◆ **Solganal®** see Aurothioglucose on page 134
- ◆ **Soluble Fluorescein** see Fluorescein Sodium on page 573
- ◆ **Solu-Cortef®** see Hydrocortisone on page 682
- ◆ **Solu-Medrol®** see MethylPREDNISolone on page 896
- ◆ **Solurex®** see Dexamethasone on page 380
- ◆ **Solurex L.A.®** see Dexamethasone on page 380
- ◆ **Soma®** see Carisoprodol on page 229
- ◆ **Soma® Compound** see Carisoprodol and Aspirin on page 229
- ◆ **Soma® Compound w/Codeine** see Carisoprodol, Aspirin, and Codeine on page 230
- ◆ **Somatrem** see Human Growth Hormone on page 667
- ◆ **Somatropin** see Human Growth Hormone on page 667
- ◆ **Sominex® [OTC]** see DiphenhydrAMINE on page 414
- ◆ **Somnol® (Can)** see Flurazepam on page 584
- ◆ **Sonata®** see Zaleplon on page 1433

Sorbitol (SOR bi tole)

Related Information
Laxatives, Classification and Properties on page 1504

Therapeutic Category Genitourinary Irrigant; Laxative, Miscellaneous

Use Genitourinary irrigant in transurethral prostatic resection or other transurethral resection or other transurethral surgical procedures; diuretic; humectant; sweetening agent; hyperosmotic laxative; facilitate the passage of sodium polystyrene sulfonate through the intestinal tract

Contraindications Anuria

Warnings/Precautions Use with caution in patients with severe cardiopulmonary or renal impairment and in patients unable to metabolize sorbitol

Adverse Reactions Frequency not defined.
Cardiovascular: Edema
Endocrine & metabolic: Fluid and electrolyte losses, lactic acidosis
Gastrointestinal: Diarrhea, nausea, vomiting, abdominal discomfort, dry mouth

Overdosage/Toxicology Symptoms include nausea, diarrhea, fluid and electrolyte loss. Treatment is supportive to ensure fluid and electrolyte balance.

Stability Protect from freezing; avoid storage in temperatures >150°F

Mechanism of Action A polyalcoholic sugar with osmotic cathartic actions

Pharmacodynamics/Kinetics
Onset of action: 0.25-1 hour
Absorption: Oral, rectal: Poor
Metabolism: Primarily hepatic to fructose

Usual Dosage Hyperosmotic laxative (as single dose, at infrequent intervals):
Children 2-11 years:
Oral: 2 mL/kg (as 70% solution)
Rectal enema: 30-60 mL as 25% to 30% solution
Children >12 years and Adults:
Oral: 30-150 mL (as 70% solution)
Rectal enema: 120 mL as 25% to 30% solution
Adjunct to sodium polystyrene sulfonate: 15 mL as 70% solution orally until diarrhea occurs (10-20 mL/2 hours) or 20-100 mL as an oral vehicle for the sodium polystyrene sulfonate resin
When administered with charcoal:
Oral:
Children: 4.3 mL/kg of 35% sorbitol with 1 g/kg of activated charcoal
Adults: 4.3 mL/kg of 70% sorbitol with 1 g/kg of activated charcoal every 4 hours until first stool containing charcoal is passed
Topical: 3% to 3.3% as transurethral surgical procedure irrigation
(Continued)

Sorbitol *(Continued)*

Nursing Implications Do not use unless solution is clear

Dosage Forms
Solution: 70% (480 mL, 3840 mL)
Solution, genitourinary irrigation: 3% (1500 mL, 3000 mL); 3.3% (2000 mL)

♦ **Sorbitrate®** *see* Isosorbide Dinitrate *on page 750*

♦ **Sorine™** *see* Sotalol *on page 1252*

♦ **Sotacor® (Can)** *see* Sotalol *on page 1252*

Sotalol (SOE ta lole)

Related Information
Antiarrhythmic Drugs Comparison *on page 1478*
Beta-Blockers Comparison *on page 1491*

U.S. Brand Names Betapace®; Betapace AF™; Sorine™

Canadian Brand Names Alti-Sotalol; Apo®-Sotalol; Betapace AF™; Gen-Sotalol; Novo-Sotalol; Nu-Sotalol; PMS-Sotalol; Rho®-Sotalol; Sotacor®

Synonyms Sotalol Hydrochloride

Therapeutic Category Antiarrhythmic Agent, Class III; Beta-Adrenergic Blocker

Use Treatment of documented ventricular arrhythmias (ie, sustained ventricular tachycardia), that in the judgment of the physician are life-threatening; maintenance of normal sinus rhythm in patients with symptomatic atrial fibrillation and atrial flutter who are currently in sinus rhythm. Manufacturer states substitutions should not be made for Betapace AF™ since Betapace AF™ is distributed with a patient package insert specific for atrial fibrillation/flutter.

Pregnancy Risk Factor B

Pregnancy/Breast-Feeding Implications Clinical effects on the fetus: Although there are no adequate and well controlled studies in pregnant women, sotalol has been shown to cross the placenta, and is found in amniotic fluid. There has been a report of subnormal birth weight with sotalol, therefore, sotalol should be used during pregnancy only if the potential benefit outweighs the potential risk.

Contraindications Hypersensitivity to sotalol or any component of the formulation; bronchial asthma; sinus bradycardia; second- and third-degree AV block (unless a functioning pacemaker is present); congenital or acquired long QT syndromes; cardiogenic shock; uncontrolled congestive heart failure; concurrent use with cisapride, gatifloxacin, moxifloxacin, or sparfloxacin. Betapace AF® is contraindicated in patients with significantly reduced renal filtration (Cl_{cr} <40 mL/minute).

Warnings/Precautions Must be initiated (or reinitiated) in a setting with continuous monitoring and staff familiar with the recognition and treatment of life-threatening arrhythmias. Patients must be monitored with continuous EKG for a minimum of 3 days (on their maintenance dose). Use cautiously in the renally-impaired (dosage adjustment required). Creatinine clearance must be calculated prior to dosing.

Monitor and adjust dose to prevent QT_c prolongation. Watch for proarrhythmic effects. Correct electrolyte imbalances before initiating (especially hypokalemia and hyperkalemia). Consider pre-existing conditions such as sick sinus syndrome before initiating. Conduction abnormalities can occur particularly sinus bradycardia. Use cautiously within the first 2 weeks post-MI (experience limited). Administer cautiously in compensated heart failure and monitor for a worsening of the condition. Use caution in patients with PVD (can aggravate arterial insufficiency). Avoid abrupt discontinuation in patients with a history of CAD; slowly wean while monitoring for signs and symptoms of ischemia. Use caution with concurrent use of beta-blockers and either verapamil or diltiazem; bradycardia or heart block can occur. Use cautiously in diabetics because it can mask prominent hypoglycemic symptoms. Can mask signs of thyrotoxicosis. Use care with anesthetic agents which decrease myocardial function.

Adverse Reactions
>10%:
Cardiovascular: Bradycardia (16%), chest pain (16%), palpitations (14%)
Central nervous system: Fatigue (20%), dizziness (20%), lightheadedness (12%)
Neuromuscular & skeletal: Weakness (13%)
Respiratory: Dyspnea (21%)

1% to 10%:
Cardiovascular: Congestive heart failure (5%), peripheral vascular disorders (3%), edema (8%), abnormal EKG (7%), hypotension (6%), proarrhythmia (5% in ventricular arrhythmia patients; less than 1% in atrial fibrillation/flutter), syncope (5%)
Central nervous system: Mental confusion (6%), anxiety (4%), headache (8%), sleep problems (8%), depression (4%)
Dermatologic: Itching/rash (5%)
Endocrine & metabolic: Decreased sexual ability (3%)
Gastrointestinal: Diarrhea (7%), nausea/vomiting (10%), stomach discomfort (3% to 6%), flatulence (2%)
Genitourinary: Impotence (2%)
Hematologic: Bleeding (2%)
Neuromuscular & skeletal: Paresthesia (4%), extremity pain (7%), back pain (3%)
Ocular: Visual problems (5%)
Respiratory: Upper respiratory problems (5% to 8%), asthma (2%)

<1% (Limited to important or life-threatening): Alopecia, bronchiolitis obliterans with organized pneumonia (BOOP), cold extremities, diaphoresis, eosinophilia, leukocytoclastic vasculitis, leukopenia, paralysis, phlebitis, photosensitivity reaction, pruritus, pulmonary edema, Raynaud's phenomenon, red crusted skin, retroperitoneal fibrosis, serum transaminases increased, skin necrosis after extravasation, thrombocytopenia, vertigo

Overdosage/Toxicology Symptoms of intoxication include cardiac disturbances, CNS toxicity, bronchospasm, hypoglycemia and hyperkalemia. The most common cardiac symptoms include hypotension and bradycardia. Atrioventricular block, intraventricular conduction disturbances, cardiogenic shock, and asystole may occur with severe overdose, especially with membrane-depressant drugs (eg, propranolol). CNS effects include convulsions, coma, and respiratory arrest and are commonly seen with propranolol and other membrane-depressant and lipid-soluble drugs. Treatment is symptomatic for seizures, hypotension, hyperkalemia and hypoglycemia. Bradycardia and hypotension resistant to atropine, isoproterenol or pacing may respond to glucagon. Wide QRS defects caused by membrane-depressant poisoning may respond to hypertonic sodium bicarbonate. Repeat-dose charcoal, hemoperfusion, or hemodialysis may be helpful in removal of only those beta-blockers with a small V_d, long half-life, or low intrinsic clearance (acebutolol, atenolol, nadolol, sotalol).

Drug Interactions

Increased Effect/Toxicity: Increased effect/toxicity of beta-blockers with calcium blockers since there may be additive effects on AV conduction or ventricular function. Sotalol in combination with amiodarone. Other agents which prolong QT interval, including Class I antiarrhythmic agents, bepridil, cisapride (use is contraindicated), erythromycin, haloperidol, pimozide, phenothiazines, tricyclic antidepressants, specific quinolones (sparfloxacin, gatifloxacin, moxifloxacin), terfenadine, or astemizole may increase the effect of sotalol on the prolongation of the QT interval. When used concurrently with clonidine, sotalol may increase the risk of rebound hypertension after or during withdrawal of either agent. Beta-blocker and catecholamine depleting agents (reserpine or guanethidine) may result in additive hypotension or bradycardia. Beta-blockers may increase the action or levels of ethanol, nondepolarizing muscle relaxants, and theophylline although the effects are difficult to predict.

Decreased Effect: Decreased effect of sotalol may occur with aluminum-magnesium antacids (if taken within 2 hours), aluminum salts, barbiturates, calcium salts, cholestyramine, colestipol, NSAIDs, penicillins (ampicillin), rifampin, salicylates, and sulfinpyrazone due to decreased bioavailability and plasma levels. Beta-blockers may decrease the effect of sulfonylureas. Beta-agonists such as albuterol, terbutaline may have less of a therapeutic effect when administered concomitantly.

Ethanol/Nutrition/Herb Interactions

Food: Sotalol peak serum concentrations may be decreased if taken with food.

Herb/Nutraceutical: Avoid ephedra (may worsen arrhythmia).

Stability Store at 25°C (77°F); excursions permitted to 15°C to 30°C (59°F to 86°F)

Mechanism of Action

Beta-blocker which contains both beta-adrenoreceptor-blocking (Vaughan Williams Class II) and cardiac action potential duration prolongation (Vaughan Williams Class III) properties

Class II effects: Increased sinus cycle length, slowed heart rate, decreased AV nodal conduction, and increased AV nodal refractoriness

Class III effects: Prolongation of the atrial and ventricular monophasic action potentials, and effective refractory prolongation of atrial muscle, ventricular muscle, and atrioventricular accessory pathways in both the antegrade and retrograde directions

Sotalol is a racemic mixture of *d*- and *l*-sotalol; both isomers have similar Class III antiarrhythmic effects while the *l*-isomer is responsible for virtually all of the beta-blocking activity

Sotalol has both beta$_1$- and beta$_2$-receptor blocking activity

The beta-blocking effect of sotalol is a noncardioselective [half maximal at about 80 mg/day and maximal at doses of 320-640 mg/day]. Significant beta-blockade occurs at oral doses as low as 25 mg/day.

The Class III effects are seen only at oral doses ≥160 mg/day

Pharmacodynamics/Kinetics

Onset of action: Rapid, 1-2 hours

Peak effect: 2.5-4 hours

Duration: 8-16 hours

Absorption: Decreased 20% to 30% by meals compared to fasting

Bioavailability: 90% to 100%

Distribution: Low lipid solubility; enters milk of laboratory animals and is reported to be present in human milk

Protein binding: None

Metabolism: None

Half-life elimination: 12 hours; Children: 9.5 hours; terminal half-life decreases with age <2 years (may by ≥1 week in neonates)

Excretion: Urine (as unchanged drug)

Usual Dosage Sotalol should be initiated and doses increased in a hospital with facilities for cardiac rhythm monitoring and assessment. Proarrhythmic events can occur after initiation of therapy and with each upward dosage adjustment.

Children: Oral: The safety and efficacy of sotalol in children have not been established

Note: Dosing per manufacturer, based on pediatric pharmacokinetic data; wait at least 36 hours between dosage adjustments to allow monitoring of QT intervals

≤2 years: Dosage should be adjusted (decreased) by plotting of the child's age on a logarithmic scale; see graph on next page or refer to manufacturer's package labeling.

>2 years: Initial: 90 mg/m²/day in 3 divided doses; may be incrementally increased to a maximum of 180 mg/m²/day

Adults: Oral:

Ventricular arrhythmias (Betapace®, Sorine™):

Initial: 80 mg twice daily

Dose may be increased gradually to 240-320 mg/day; allow 3 days between dosing increments in order to attain steady-state plasma concentrations and to allow monitoring of QT intervals

Most patients respond to a total daily dose of 160-320 mg/day in 2-3 divided doses.

Some patients, with life-threatening refractory ventricular arrhythmias, may require doses as high as 480-640 mg/day; however, these doses should only be prescribed when the potential benefit outweighs the increased of adverse events.

Atrial fibrillation or atrial flutter (Betapace AF™): Initial: 80 mg twice daily

If the initial dose does not reduce the frequency of relapses of atrial fibrillation/flutter and is tolerated without excessive QT prolongation (not >520 msec) after 3 days, the dose may be increased to 120 mg twice daily. This may be further increased to 160 mg twice daily if response is inadequate and QT prolongation is not excessive.

(Continued)

Sotalol *(Continued)*

Age Factor Nomogram

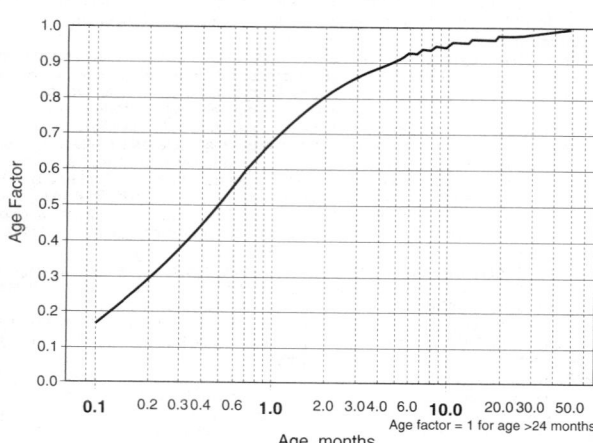

Age factor = 1 for age >24 months

Adapted from U.S. Food and Drug Administration.
http://www.fda.gov/cder/foi/label/2001/2115s3lbl.PDF

Elderly: Age does not significantly alter the pharmacokinetics of sotalol, but impaired renal function in elderly patients can increase the terminal half-life, resulting in increased drug accumulation

Dosage adjustment in renal impairment:
Children: Safety and efficacy in children with renal impairment have not been established.
Adults: Impaired renal function can increase the terminal half-life, resulting in increased drug accumulation. Sotalol (Betapace AF™) is contraindicated per the manufacturer for treatment of atrial fibrillation/flutter in patients with a Cl_{cr} <40 mL/minute.
Ventricular arrhythmias (Betapace®, Sorine™):
Cl_{cr} >60 mL/minute: Administer every 12 hours
Cl_{cr} 30-60 mL/minute: Administer every 24 hours
Cl_{cr} 10-30 mL/minute: Administer every 36-48 hours
Cl_{cr} <10 mL/minute: Individualize dose
Atrial fibrillation/flutter (Betapace AF™):
Cl_{cr} >60 mL/minute: Administer every 12 hours
Cl_{cr} 40-60 mL/minute: Administer every 24 hours
Cl_{cr} <40 mL/minute: Use is contraindicated
Dialysis: Hemodialysis would be expected to reduce sotalol plasma concentrations because sotalol is not bound to plasma proteins and does not undergo extensive metabolism; administer dose postdialysis or administer supplemental 80 mg dose; peritoneal dialysis does not remove sotalol; supplemental dose is not necessary

Dietary Considerations Administer on an empty stomach.

Administration Food may decrease adsorption

Monitoring Parameters Serum magnesium, potassium, EKG

Patient Information Seek emergency help if palpitations occur; do not discontinue abruptly or change dose without notifying physician; take on an empty stomach

Nursing Implications Initiation of therapy and dose escalation should be done in a hospital with cardiac monitoring; lidocaine and other resuscitative measures should be available

Additional Information Pharmacokinetics in children are more relevant for BSA than age.

Dosage Forms Tablet, as hydrochloride:
Betapace® [light blue]: 80 mg, 120 mg, 160 mg, 240 mg
Betapace AF™ [white]: 80 mg, 120 mg, 160 mg
Sorine™ [white]: 80 mg, 120 mg, 160 mg, 240 mg

Extemporaneous Preparations To make a 5 mg/mL oral solution, using a 6-ounce amber plastic prescription bottle, add five sotalol 120 mg tablets to 120 mL of simple syrup containing 0.1% sodium benzoate (tablets do not need to be crushed). Shake well. Allow tablets to hydrate for ~2 hours; shake intermittently until tablets completely disintegrate. Store at room temperature; shake well before use. Stable for 3 months. (Refer to manufacturer's current labeling.)

♦ **Sotalol Hydrochloride** *see* Sotalol *on page 1252*
♦ **Sotradecol®** *see* Sodium Tetradecyl *on page 1249*
♦ **Soyacal®** *see* Fat Emulsion *on page 545*
♦ **SPA** *see* Albumin *on page 40*
♦ **Spacol** *see* Hyoscyamine *on page 692*
♦ **Spacol T/S** *see* Hyoscyamine *on page 692*
♦ **Span-FF®** *see* Ferrous Fumarate *on page 555*

Sparfloxacin (spar FLOKS a sin)

Related Information
Antacid Drug Interactions *on page 1477*
Antimicrobial Drugs of Choice *on page 1588*

U.S. Brand Names Zagam®

Therapeutic Category Antibiotic, Quinolone

Use Treatment of adults with community-acquired pneumonia caused by *C. pneumoniae*, *H. influenzae*, *H. parainfluenzae*, *M. catarrhalis*, *M. pneumoniae* or *S. pneumoniae*; treatment of acute bacterial exacerbations of chronic bronchitis caused by *C. pneumoniae*, *E. cloacae*, *H. influenzae*, *H. parainfluenzae*, *K. pneumoniae*, *M. catarrhalis*, *S. aureus* or *S. pneumoniae*

Pregnancy Risk Factor C

Pregnancy/Breast-Feeding Implications
Clinical effects on the fetus: Avoid use in pregnant women unless the benefit justifies the potential risk to the fetus
Breast-feeding/lactation: Quinolones are known to distribute well into breast milk; consequently use during lactation should be avoided if possible

Contraindications Hypersensitivity to sparfloxacin, any component of the formulation, or other quinolones; a concurrent administration with drugs which increase the QT interval including: amiodarone, bepridil, bretylium, cisapride, disopyramide, furosemide, procainamide, quinidine, sotalol, albuterol, astemizole, chloroquine, halofantrine, phenothiazines, prednisone, terfenadine, and tricyclic antidepressants

Warnings/Precautions Not recommended in children <18 years of age; other quinolones have caused transient arthropathy in children; CNS stimulation may occur (tremor, restlessness, confusion, and very rarely hallucinations or seizures); use with caution in patients with known or suspected CNS disorder or renal dysfunction; prolonged use may result in superinfection; may cause photosensitivity (severe reactions reported rarely); pseudomembranous colitis may occur and should be considered in patients who present with diarrhea. Tendon inflammation and/or rupture have been reported with other quinolone antibiotics. Discontinue at first sign of tendon inflammation or pain.

Severe hypersensitivity reactions, including anaphylaxis, have occurred with quinolone therapy. If an allergic reaction occurs (itching, urticaria, dyspnea, facial edema, loss of consciousness, tingling, cardiovascular collapse), discontinue drug immediately. Although quinolones may exacerbate myasthenia gravis, sparfloxacin appears to be an exception; caution is still warranted.

Adverse Reactions
1% to 10%:
Cardiovascular: QT_c interval prolongation (1.3%)
Central nervous system: Insomnia, dizziness, headache, agitation, sleep disorders, anxiety, delirium
Dermatologic: Photosensitivity reaction, pruritus, vasodilatation
Gastrointestinal: Diarrhea, dyspepsia, nausea, abdominal pain, vomiting, flatulence, taste perversion, dry mouth
Hematologic: Leukopenia, eosinophilia, anemia
Hepatic: Increased LFTs
<1% (Limited to important or life-threatening): Angina pectoris, angioedema, arrhythmia, asthma, atrial fibrillation, atrial flutter, complete AV block, dyspnea, ecchymosis, exfoliative dermatitis, migraine, postural hypotension; quinolones have been associated with tendonitis and tendon rupture

Overdosage/Toxicology Symptoms include acute renal failure and seizures. Treatment consists of GI decontamination and supportive care; not removed by peritoneal or hemodialysis.

Drug Interactions
Increased Effect/Toxicity: Quinolones cause increased levels of caffeine, warfarin, cyclosporine, and theophylline (although one study indicates that sparfloxacin may not affect theophylline metabolism). Cimetidine, and probenecid increase quinolone levels. An increased incidence of seizures may occur with foscarnet and NSAIDs. Sparfloxacin does not appear to alter warfarin levels, but warfarin effect may be increased due possible effects on gastrointestinal flora.

Decreased Effect: Decreased absorption with antacids containing aluminum, didanosine (chewable/buffered tablets or pediatric powder for oral solution), magnesium, zinc, iron and/or calcium (by up to 98% if given at the same time). Phenytoin serum levels may be reduced by quinolones. Antineoplastic agents may also decrease serum levels of fluoroquinolones.

Ethanol/Nutrition/Herb Interactions Herb/Nutraceutical: Avoid dong quai, St John's wort (may also cause photosensitization).

Mechanism of Action Inhibits DNA-gyrase in susceptible organisms; inhibits relaxation of supercoiled DNA and promotes breakage of double-stranded DNA

Pharmacodynamics/Kinetics
Absorption: Unaffected by food or milk; reduced by ~50% by concurrent administration of aluminum- and magnesium-containing antacids
Distribution: Widely throughout the body
Metabolism: Hepatic, but does not utilize the CYP450 system
Half-life elimination: Mean terminal: 20 hours (range: 16-30 hours)
Excretion: Urine (~10% as unchanged drug) and feces (equal amounts)

Usual Dosage Adults: Oral:
Loading dose: 2 tablets (400 mg) on day 1
Maintenance: 1 tablet (200 mg) daily for 10 days total therapy (total 11 tablets)
Dosing adjustment in renal impairment: Cl_{cr} <50 mL/minute: Administer 400 mg on day 1, then 200 mg every 48 hours for a total of 9 days of therapy (total 6 tablets)

Dietary Considerations May be taken without regard to meals; should be taken at the same time each day.
(Continued)

Sparfloxacin *(Continued)*

Administration May be taken without regard to meals, however, should be administered at the same time each day. Antacids containing magnesium and aluminum or sucralfate, didanosine (chewable/buffered tablets or pediatric oral solution) should be taken 4 hours after sparfloxacin.

Monitoring Parameters Evaluation of organ system functions (renal, hepatic, ophthalmologic, and hematopoietic) is recommended periodically during therapy; the possibility of crystalluria should be assessed; WBC and signs and symptoms of infection

Patient Information May take with or without food; drink with plenty of fluids; avoid exposure to direct sunlight during therapy and for several days following; do not take antacids within 4 hours before or 2 hours after dosing; contact your physician immediately if signs of allergy occur; do not discontinue therapy until your course has been completed; take a missed dose as soon as possible, unless it is almost time for your next dose

Dosage Forms Tablet: 200 mg

♦ **Sparine**® *see* Promazine *on page 1139*

♦ **Spectazole**™ *see* Econazole *on page 455*

Spectinomycin *(spek ti noe MYE sin)*

Related Information
Treatment of Sexually Transmitted Diseases *on page 1609*

U.S. Brand Names Trobicin®

Synonyms Spectinomycin Hydrochloride

Therapeutic Category Antibiotic, Miscellaneous

Use Treatment of uncomplicated gonorrhea

Pregnancy Risk Factor B

Contraindications Hypersensitivity to spectinomycin or any component of the formulation

Adverse Reactions <1% (Limited to important or life-threatening): Abdominal cramps, chills, dizziness, headache, nausea, vomiting

Overdosage/Toxicology Symptoms include paresthesias, dizziness, blurred vision, ototoxicity, renal damage, nausea, sleeplessness, and decreased hemoglobin.

Stability Use reconstituted solutions within 24 hours; reconstitute with supplied diluent only

Mechanism of Action A bacteriostatic antibiotic that selectively binds to the 30s subunits of ribosomes, and thereby inhibiting bacterial protein synthesis

Pharmacodynamics/Kinetics
Duration: Up to 8 hours
Absorption: I.M.: Rapid and almost completely
Distribution: Concentrates in urine; does not distribute well into the saliva
Half-life elimination: 1.7 hours
Time to peak: ~1 hour
Excretion: Primarily urine (70% to 100% as unchanged drug)

Usual Dosage I.M.:
Children:
<45 kg: 40 mg/kg/dose 1 time (ceftriaxone preferred)
≥45 kg: Refer to adult dosing.
Children >8 years who are allergic to PCNS/cephalosporins may be treated with oral tetracycline
Adults:
Uncomplicated urethral, cervical, pharyngeal, or rectal gonorrhea: 2 g deep I.M. or 4 g where antibiotic resistance is prevalent 1 time; 4 g (10 mL) dose should be given as two 5 mL injections, followed by adequate chlamydial treatment (doxycycline 100 mg twice daily for 7 days)
Disseminated gonococcal infection: 2 g every 12 hours
Dosing adjustment in renal impairment: None necessary
Hemodialysis: 50% removed by hemodialysis

Administration For I.M. use only

Dosage Forms Powder for injection, as hydrochloride: 2 g

♦ **Spectinomycin Hydrochloride** *see* Spectinomycin *on page 1256*

♦ **Spectracef**™ *see* Cefditoren *on page 242*

♦ **Spectrocin Plus**® [OTC] *see* Bacitracin, Neomycin, Polymyxin B, and Lidocaine *on page 144*

Spironolactone *(speer on oh LAK tone)*

Related Information
Heart Failure *on page 1663*

U.S. Brand Names Aldactone®

Canadian Brand Names Aldactone®; Novo-Spiroton

Therapeutic Category Antihypertensive Agent; Diuretic, Potassium Sparing

Use Management of edema associated with excessive aldosterone excretion; hypertension; primary hyperaldosteronism; hypokalemia; treatment of hirsutism; cirrhosis of liver accompanied by edema or ascites. The benefits of spironolactone were additive to the benefits of angiotensin-converting enzyme inhibition in patients with severe CHF (further reducing mortality by 30% over 2 years) in RALES - a large controlled clinical trial.

Pregnancy Risk Factor D

Pregnancy/Breast-Feeding Implications
Clinical effects on the fetus: No data available on crossing the placenta. 1 report of oral cleft. Generally, use of diuretics during pregnancy is avoided due to risk of decreased placental perfusion.
Breast-feeding/lactation: Crosses into breast milk. AAP considers **compatible** with breast-feeding.

Contraindications Hypersensitivity to spironolactone or any component of the formulation; anuria; acute renal insufficiency; significant impairment of renal excretory function; hyperkalemia; pregnancy

Warnings/Precautions Avoid potassium supplements, potassium-containing salt substitutes, a diet rich in potassium, or other drugs that can cause hyperkalemia. Monitor for fluid and electrolyte imbalances. Gynecomastia is related to dose and duration of therapy. Diuretic therapy should be carefully used in severe hepatic dysfunction; electrolyte and fluid shifts can cause or exacerbate encephalopathy. Discontinue use prior to adrenal vein catheterization.

Adverse Reactions Incidence of adverse events is not always reported (mean daily dose 26 mg).

Cardiovascular: Edema (2%, placebo 2%)

Central nervous system: Disorders (23%, placebo 21%) which may include drowsiness, lethargy, headache, mental confusion, drug fever, ataxia, fatigue

Dermatologic: Maculopapular, erythematous cutaneous eruptions, urticaria, hirsutism, eosinophilia

Endocrine & metabolic: Gynecomastia (men 9%; placebo 1%), breast pain (men 2%; placebo 0.1%), serious hyperkalemia (2%, placebo 1%), hyponatremia, dehydration, hyperchloremic metabolic acidosis (in decompensated hepatic cirrhosis), impotence, menstrual irregularities, amenorrhea, postmenopausal bleeding

Gastrointestinal: Disorders (29%, placebo 29%) which may include anorexia, nausea, cramping, diarrhea, gastric bleeding, ulceration, gastritis, vomiting

Hematologic: Agranulocytosis

Hepatic: Cholestatic/hepatocellular toxicity

Renal: Increased BUN concentration

Miscellaneous: Deepening of the voice, anaphylactic reaction, breast cancer

Overdosage/Toxicology Symptoms include drowsiness, confusion, clinical signs of dehydration and electrolyte imbalance, and hyperkalemia. Ingestion of large amounts of potassium-sparing diuretics, may result in life-threatening hyperkalemia. This can be treated with I.V. glucose, with concurrent regular insulin. Sodium bicarbonate may also be used as a temporary measure. If needed, Kayexalate® oral or rectal solutions in sorbitol may also be used.

Drug Interactions

Increased Effect/Toxicity: Concurrent use of spironolactone with other potassium-sparing diuretics, potassium supplements, angiotensin-receptor antagonists, co-trimoxazole (high dose), and angiotensin-converting enzyme inhibitors can increase the risk of hyperkalemia, especially in patients with renal impairment. Cholestyramine can cause hyperchloremic acidosis in cirrhotic patients; avoid concurrent use.

Decreased Effect: The effects of digoxin (loss of positive inotropic effect) and mitotane may be reduced by spironolactone. Salicylates and NSAIDs (indomethacin) may decrease the natriuretic effect of spironolactone.

Ethanol/Nutrition/Herb Interactions

Food: Food increases absorption.

Herb/Nutraceutical: Avoid natural licorice (due to mineralocorticoid activity)

Stability Protect from light

Mechanism of Action Competes with aldosterone for receptor sites in the distal renal tubules, increasing sodium chloride and water excretion while conserving potassium and hydrogen ions; may block the effect of aldosterone on arteriolar smooth muscle as well

Pharmacodynamics/Kinetics

Protein binding: 91% to 98%

Metabolism: Hepatic to multiple metabolites, including canrenone (active)

Half-life elimination: 78-84 minutes

Time to peak, serum: 1-3 hours (primarily as the active metabolite)

Excretion: Urine and feces

Usual Dosage To reduce delay in onset of effect, a loading dose of 2 or 3 times the daily dose may be administered on the first day of therapy. Oral:

Neonates: Diuretic: 1-3 mg/kg/day divided every 12-24 hours

Children:

Diuretic, hypertension: 1.5-3.5 mg/kg/day **or** 60 mg/m^2/day in divided doses every 6-24 hours

Diagnosis of primary aldosteronism: 125-375 mg/m^2/day in divided doses

Vaso-occlusive disease: 7.5 mg/kg/day in divided doses twice daily (not FDA approved)

Adults:

Edema, hypertension, hypokalemia: 25-200 mg/day in 1-2 divided doses

Diagnosis of primary aldosteronism: 100-400 mg/day in 1-2 divided doses

Hirsutism in women: 50-200 mg/day in 1-2 divided doses

CHF, severe (with ACE inhibitor and a loop diuretic ± digoxin): 25 mg/day, increased or reduced depending on individual response and evidence of hyperkalemia

Elderly: Initial: 25-50 mg/day in 1-2 divided doses, increasing by 25-50 mg every 5 days as needed.

Dosing interval in renal impairment:

Cl_{cr} 10-50 mL/minute: Administer every 12-24 hours.

Cl_{cr} <10 mL/minute: Avoid use.

Dietary Considerations Should be taken with food to decrease gastrointestinal irritation and to increase absorption.

Monitoring Parameters Blood pressure, serum electrolytes (potassium, sodium), renal function, I & O ratios and daily weight throughout therapy

Test Interactions May cause false elevation in serum digoxin concentrations measured by RIA

Patient Information Avoid hazardous activity such as driving, until response to drug is known; take with meals or milk; avoid excessive ingestion of foods high in potassium or use of salt substitutes

Nursing Implications Diuretic effect may be delayed 2-3 days and maximum hypertensive may be delayed 2-3 weeks; monitor I & O ratios and daily weight throughout therapy

Dosage Forms Tablet: 25 mg, 50 mg, 100 mg

(Continued)

Spironolactone *(Continued)*

Extemporaneous Preparations A 5 mg/mL suspension may be made by crushing tablets, levigating with a small amount of distilled water or glycerin; dilute with 1 part Cologel® and 2 parts simple syrup and/or cherry syrup to make the final concentration; spironolactone 5 mg/mL plus hydrochlorothiazide 5 mg/mL were found stable for 60 days in refrigerator in a 1:1 preparation in Ora-Sweet®/Ora-Plus®, in Ora-Sweet® SF/Ora-Plus®, and in cherry syrup

A 1 mg/mL suspension may be compounded by crushing ten 25 mg tablets, add a small amount of water and soak for 5 minutes; add 50 mL 1.5% carboxymethylcellulose, 100 mL syrup NF, and mix; use a sufficient quantity of purified water to a total volume of 250 mL; stable at room temperature or refrigerated for 3 months

Allen LV and Erickson III MA, "Stability of Labetalol Hydrochloride, Metoprolol Tartrate, Verapamil Hydrochloride, and Spironolactone With Hydrochlorothiazide in Extemporaneously Compounded Oral Liquids," *Am J Health Syst Pharm*, 1996, 53:2304-9.

Handbook on Extemporaneous Formulations, Bethesda, MD: American Society of Hospital Pharmacists, 1987.

Nahata MC, Morosco RS, and Hipple TF, "Stability of Spironolactone in an Extemporaneously Prepared Suspension at Two Temperatures," *Ann Pharmacother*, 1993, 27:1198-9.

♦ **Spironolactone and Hydrochlorothiazide** *see* Hydrochlorothiazide and Spironolactone *on page 675*

♦ **Sporanox®** *see* Itraconazole *on page 756*

♦ **SPS®** *see* Sodium Polystyrene Sulfonate *on page 1249*

♦ **SSD™ (Can)** *see* Silver Sulfadiazine *on page 1238*

♦ **SSD® AF** *see* Silver Sulfadiazine *on page 1238*

♦ **SSD® Cream** *see* Silver Sulfadiazine *on page 1238*

♦ **SSKI®** *see* Potassium Iodide *on page 1111*

♦ **Stadol®** *see* Butorphanol *on page 199*

♦ **Stadol® NS** *see* Butorphanol *on page 199*

♦ **Stagesic®** *see* Hydrocodone and Acetaminophen *on page 676*

♦ **Stannous Fluoride** *see* Fluoride *on page 574*

Stanozolol *(stan OH zoe lole)*

U.S. Brand Names Winstrol®

Therapeutic Category Anabolic Steroid; Androgen

Use Prophylactic use against hereditary angioedema

Restrictions C-III

Pregnancy Risk Factor X

Contraindications Hypersensitivity to stanozolol or any component of the formulation; nephrosis; carcinoma of breast or prostate; pregnancy

Warnings/Precautions May stunt bone growth in children; anabolic steroids may cause peliosis hepatis, liver cell tumors, and blood lipid changes with increased risk of arteriosclerosis; monitor diabetic patients carefully; use with caution in elderly patients, they may be at greater risk for prostatic hyperplasia; use with caution in patients with cardiac, renal, or hepatic disease or epilepsy

Adverse Reactions

Male: Postpubertal:

>10%:

Dermatologic: Acne

Endocrine & metabolic: Gynecomastia

Genitourinary: Bladder irritability, priapism

1% to 10%:

Central nervous system: Insomnia, chills

Endocrine & metabolic: Decreased libido, hepatic dysfunction,

Gastrointestinal: Nausea, diarrhea

Genitourinary: Prostatic hyperplasia (elderly)

Hematologic: Iron-deficiency anemia, suppression of clotting factors

<1% (Limited to important or life-threatening): Hepatic necrosis, hepatocellular carcinoma

Female:

>10%: Endocrine & metabolic: Virilism

1% to 10%:

Central nervous system: Chills, insomnia

Endocrine & metabolic: Hypercalcemia

Gastrointestinal: Nausea, diarrhea

Hematologic: Iron deficiency anemia, suppression of clotting factors

Hepatic: Hepatic dysfunction

<1% (Limited to important or life-threatening): Hepatic necrosis, hepatocellular carcinoma

Drug Interactions

Increased Effect/Toxicity: ACTH, adrenal steroids may increase risk of edema and acne. Stanozolol enhances the hypoprothrombinemic effects of oral anticoagulants and enhances the hypoglycemic effects of insulin and sulfonylureas (oral hypoglycemics).

Mechanism of Action Synthetic testosterone derivative with similar androgenic and anabolic actions

Pharmacodynamics/Kinetics

Metabolism: Hepatic

Excretion: Urine (90%); feces (6%)

Usual Dosage

Children: Acute attacks:

<6 years: 1 mg/day

6-12 years: 2 mg/day

Adults: Oral: Initial: 2 mg 3 times/day, may then reduce to a maintenance dose of 2 mg/day or 2 mg every other day after 1-3 months

Dosing adjustment in hepatic impairment: Stanozolol is **not** recommended for patients with severe liver dysfunction

Patient Information High protein, high caloric diet is suggested, restrict salt intake; glucose tolerance may be altered in diabetics

Dosage Forms Tablet: 2 mg

◆ **Starlix**® *see* Nateglinide *on page 961*
◆ **Starnoc**® **(Can)** *see* Zaleplon *on page 1433*
◆ **Statex**® **(Can)** *see* Morphine Sulfate *on page 936*

Stavudine (STAV yoo deen)

Related Information
Antiretroviral Agents Comparison *on page 1488*
Antiretroviral Therapy for HIV Infection *on page 1595*

U.S. Brand Names Zerit®
Canadian Brand Names Zerit™
Synonyms d4T
Therapeutic Category Antiretroviral Agent, Nucleoside Reverse Transcriptase Inhibitor (NRTI) [Thymidine Analog]
Use Treatment of adults with HIV infection in combination with other antiretroviral agents
Pregnancy Risk Factor C
Pregnancy/Breast-Feeding Implications Cases of fatal and nonfatal lactic acidosis, with or without pancreatitis, have been reported in pregnant women. It is not known if pregnancy itself potentiates this known side effect; however, pregnant women may be at increased risk of lactic acidosis and liver damage. Hepatic enzymes and electrolytes should be monitored frequently during the 3rd trimester of pregnancy. Use during pregnancy only if the potential benefit to the mother outweighs the potential risk of this complication. Stavudine crosses the placenta *ex vivo*. Health professionals are encouraged to contact the antiretroviral pregnancy registry to monitor outcomes of pregnant women exposed to antiretroviral medications (1-800-258-4263).
Contraindications Hypersensitivity to stavudine or any component of the formulation
Warnings/Precautions Use with caution in patients who demonstrate previous hypersensitivity to zidovudine, didanosine, zalcitabine, pre-existing bone marrow suppression, renal insufficiency, or peripheral neuropathy. Peripheral neuropathy may be the dose-limiting side effect. Zidovudine should not be used in combination with stavudine. Lactic acidosis and severe hepatomegaly with steatosis have been reported with stavudine use, including fatal cases. Risk may be increased in obesity, prolonged nucleoside exposure, or in female patients. Suspend therapy in patients with suspected lactic acidosis; consider discontinuation of stavudine if lactic acidosis is confirmed. Pregnant women may be at increased risk of lactic acidosis and liver damage. Severe motor weakness (resembling Guillain-Barré syndrome) has also been reported (including fatal cases, usually in association with lactic acidosis); manufacturer recommends discontinuation if motor weakness develops (with or without lactic acidosis). Pancreatitis (including some fatal cases) has occurred during combination therapy (didanosine with or without hydroxyurea). Risk increased when used in combination regimen with didanosine and hydroxyurea. Suspend therapy with agents toxic to the pancreas (including stavudine, didanosine, or hydroxyurea) in patients with suspected pancreatitis.
Adverse Reactions All adverse reactions reported below were similar to comparative agent (zidovudine), except for peripheral neuropathy, which was greater with stavudine

>10%:
Neuromuscular & skeletal: Peripheral neuropathy (dose related)
Central nervous system: Headache, chills/fever, malaise, insomnia, anxiety, depression, pain
Gastrointestinal: Nausea, vomiting, anorexia, diarrhea, abdominal pain

1% to 10%
Hematologic: Neutropenia, thrombocytopenia
Hepatic: increased bilirubin
Neuromuscular & skeletal: Myalgia, arthralgia, back pain, weakness

Postmarketing and/or case reports (limited to important or life-threatening): Allergic reaction, anemia, anorexia, hepatomegaly, hepatic failure, hepatic steatosis, insomnia, lactic acidosis, leukopenia, motor weakness (severe), pancreatitis, redistribution/accumulation of body fat

Drug Interactions
Increased Effect/Toxicity: Drugs associated with peripheral neuropathy (chloramphenicol, cisplatin, dapsone, ethionamide, gold, hydralazine, iodoquinol, isoniazid, lithium, metronidazole, nitrofurantoin, pentamidine, phenytoin, ribavirin, vincristine) may increase risk for stavudine peripheral neuropathy. Risk of neuropathy, pancreatitis, or lactic acidosis and severe hepatomegaly is increased with concurrent use of didanosine and hydroxyurea.
Stability Reconstituted oral solution should be refrigerated and is stable for 30 days.
Mechanism of Action Stavudine is a thymidine analog which interferes with HIV viral DNA dependent DNA polymerase resulting in inhibition of viral replication; nucleoside reverse transcriptase inhibitor
Pharmacodynamics/Kinetics
Distribution: V_d: 0.5 L/kg
Bioavailability: 86.4%
Half-life elimination: 1-1.6 hours
Time to peak, serum: 1 hour
Excretion: Urine (40%)
Usual Dosage Oral:
Children: 2 mg/kg/day
Adults:
≥60 kg: 40 mg every 12 hours
<60 kg: 30 mg every 12 hours
Dose may be cut in half if symptoms of peripheral neuropathy occur
(Continued)

Stavudine *(Continued)*

Dosing adjustment in renal impairment:
Cl_{cr} >50 mL/minute:

Cl_{cr} >50 mL/minute:
≥60 kg: 40 mg every 12 hours
<60 kg: 30 mg every 12 hours
Cl_{cr} 26-50 mL/minute:
≥60 kg: 20 mg every 12 hours
<60 kg: 15 mg every 12 hours
Hemodialysis:
≥60 kg: 20 mg every 24 hours
<60 kg: 15 mg every 24 hours

Elderly: Older patients should be closely monitored for signs and symptoms of peripheral neuropathy; dosage should be carefully adjusted to renal function

Dietary Considerations May be taken without regard to meals.

Administration Take without regard to meals.

Monitoring Parameters Monitor liver function tests and signs and symptoms of peripheral neuropathy; monitor viral load and CD4 count

Patient Information Take as directed take for full length of prescription. Maintain adequate hydration and nutrition. Report immediately any tingling, unusual pain, or numbness in extremities. Report fever, chills, unusual fatigue or acute depression, acute abdominal or back pain, persistent muscle pain or weakness, nausea, vomiting, or unusual bruising or bleeding. Risk of adverse reactions may be increased with some combination therapies.

Nursing Implications Monitor liver function tests and signs and symptoms of peripheral neuropathy

Additional Information Potential compliance problems, frequency of administration and adverse effects should be discussed with patients before initiating therapy to help prevent the emergence of resistance.

Dosage Forms
Capsule: 15 mg, 20 mg, 30 mg, 40 mg
Powder for oral solution: 1 mg/mL (200 mL)

- ◆ **S-T Cort**® *see* Hydrocortisone *on page 682*
- ◆ **Stelazine**® *see* Trifluoperazine *on page 1372*
- ◆ **Stemetil**® **(Can)** *see* Prochlorperazine *on page 1134*
- ◆ **STI571** *see* Imatinib *on page 703*
- ◆ **Stilbestrol** *see* Diethylstilbestrol *on page 400*
- ◆ **Stilphostrol**® *see* Diethylstilbestrol *on page 400*
- ◆ **Stimate**™ *see* Desmopressin *on page 378*
- ◆ **St. Joseph**® **Pain Reliever [OTC]** *see* Aspirin *on page 120*
- ◆ **Stop**® **[OTC]** *see* Fluoride *on page 574*
- ◆ **Streptase**® *see* Streptokinase *on page 1260*

Streptokinase *(strep toe KYE nase)*

U.S. Brand Names Streptase®

Canadian Brand Names Kabikinase®; Streptase®

Synonyms SK

Therapeutic Category Fibrinolytic Agent

Use Thrombolytic agent used in treatment of recent severe or massive deep vein thrombosis, pulmonary emboli, myocardial infarction, and occluded arteriovenous cannulas

Pregnancy Risk Factor C

Contraindications Hypersensitivity to anistreplase, streptokinase, or any component of the formulation; active internal bleeding; history of CVA; recent (within 2 months) intracranial or intraspinal surgery or trauma; intracranial neoplasm, arteriovenous malformation, or aneurysm; known bleeding diathesis; severe uncontrolled hypertension

Warnings/Precautions Concurrent heparin anticoagulation can contribute to bleeding; careful attention to all potential bleeding sites. I.M. injections and nonessential handling of the patient should be avoided. Venipunctures should be performed carefully and only when necessary. If arterial puncture is necessary, use an upper extremity vessel that can be manually compressed. If serious bleeding occurs then the infusion of streptokinase and heparin should be stopped. Use with caution in patients >75 years of age, patients with a history of cardiac arrhythmias, septic thrombophlebitis or occluded AV cannula at seriously infected site, patients with a high likelihood of left heart thrombus (eg, mitral stenosis with atrial fibrillation), major surgery within last 10 days, GI bleeding, diabetic hemorrhagic retinopathy, subacute bacterial endocarditis, cerebrovascular disease, recent trauma including cardiopulmonary resuscitation, or severe hypertension (systolic BP >180 mm Hg and/or diastolic BP >110 mm Hg); antibodies to streptokinase remain for 3-6 months after initial dose, use another thrombolytic enzyme (ie, alteplase) if thrombolytic therapy is indicated in patients with prior streptokinase therapy

Coronary thrombolysis may result in reperfusion arrhythmias. Hypotension, occasionally severe, can occur (not from bleeding or anaphylaxis). Follow standard MI management. Rare anaphylactic reactions can occur. Cautious repeat administration in patients who have received anistreplase or streptokinase within 1 year (streptokinase antibody may decrease effectiveness or risk of allergic reactions). Safety and efficacy in pediatric patients have not been established.

Streptokinase is not indicated for restoration of patency of intravenous catheters. Serious adverse events relating to the use of streptokinase in the restoration of patency of occluded intravenous catheters have involved the use of high doses of streptokinase in small volumes (250,000 international units in 2 mL). Uses of lower doses of streptokinase in infusions over several hours, generally into partially occluded catheters, or local instillation into the catheter lumen and subsequent aspiration, have been described in the medical literature. Healthcare providers should consider the risk for potentially life-threatening reactions (eg, hypotension, hypersensitivity reactions, apnea, bleeding) associated with the use of streptokinase in the management of occluded intravenous catheters.

Adverse Reactions As with all drugs which may affect hemostasis, bleeding is the major adverse effect associated with streptokinase. Hemorrhage may occur at virtually any site. Risk is dependent on multiple variables, including the dosage administered, concurrent use of multiple agents which alter hemostasis, and patient predisposition (including hypertension). Rapid lysis of coronary artery thrombi by thrombolytic agents may be associated with reperfusion-related atrial and/or ventricular arrhythmias.

>10%:
  Cardiovascular: Hypotension
  Local: Injection site bleeding

1% to 10%:
  Central nervous system: Fever (1% to 4%)
  Dermatologic: Bruising, rash, pruritus
  Gastrointestinal: Gastrointestinal hemorrhage, nausea, vomiting
  Genitourinary: Genitourinary hemorrhage
  Hematologic: Anemia
  Neuromuscular & skeletal: Muscle pain
  Ocular: Eye hemorrhage, periorbital edema
  Respiratory: Bronchospasm, epistaxis
  Miscellaneous: Diaphoresis

<1% (Limited to important or life-threatening): Acute tubular necrosis, allergic reactions, anaphylactic shock, anaphylactoid reactions, anaphylaxis, angioneurotic edema, ARDS, back pain (during infusion), cholesterol embolization, elevated transaminases, erysipelas-like rash, Guillain-Barré syndrome, hemarthrosis, intracranial hemorrhage, laryngeal edema, morbilliform, Parsonage-Turner syndrome, pericardial hemorrhage, respiratory depression, retroperitoneal hemorrhage, splenic rupture, urticaria

Additional cardiovascular events associated with use in myocardial infarction: Asystole, AV block, cardiac arrest, cardiac tamponade, cardiogenic shock, electromechanical dissociation, heart failure, mitral regurgitation, myocardial rupture, pericardial effusion, pericarditis, pulmonary edema, recurrent ischemia/infarction, thromboembolism, ventricular tachycardia

Overdosage/Toxicology Symptoms include epistaxis, bleeding gums, hematoma, spontaneous ecchymoses, and oozing at catheter site. If uncontrollable bleeding occurs, discontinue infusion; whole blood or blood products may be used to reverse bleeding.

Drug Interactions
  Increased Effect/Toxicity: The risk of bleeding with streptokinase is increased by oral anticoagulants (warfarin), heparin, low molecular weight heparins, and drugs which affect platelet function (eg, NSAIDs, dipyridamole, ticlopidine, clopidogrel, IIb/IIIa antagonists). Although concurrent use with aspirin and heparin may increase the risk of bleeding. Aspirin and heparin were used concomitantly with streptokinase in the majority of patients in clinical studies of MI.
  Decreased Effect: Antifibrinolytic agents (aminocaproic acid) may decrease effectiveness to thrombolytic agents.

Ethanol/Nutrition/Herb Interactions Herb/Nutraceutical: Avoid cat's claw, dong quai, evening primrose, feverfew, red clover, horse chestnut, garlic, green tea, ginseng, ginkgo (all have additional antiplatelet activity).

Stability Streptokinase, a white lyophilized powder, may have a slight yellow color in solution due to the presence of albumin; intact vials should be stored at room temperature; reconstituted solutions should be refrigerated and are stable for 24 hours

Stability of parenteral admixture at room temperature (25°C): 8 hours; at refrigeration (4°C): 24 hours

Mechanism of Action Activates the conversion of plasminogen to plasmin by forming a complex, exposing plasminogen-activating site, and cleaving a peptide bond that converts plasminogen to plasmin; plasmin degrades fibrin, fibrinogen and other procoagulant proteins into soluble fragments; effective both outside and within the formed thrombus/embolus

Pharmacodynamics/Kinetics
  Onset of action: Activation of plasminogen occurs almost immediately
  Duration: Fibrinolytic effect: Several hours; Anticoagulant effect: 12-24 hours
  Half-life elimination: 83 minutes
  Excretion: By circulating antibodies and the reticuloendothelial system

Usual Dosage I.V.:
  Children: Safety and efficacy have not been not established. Limited studies have used 3500-4000 units/kg over 30 minutes followed by 1000-1500 units/kg/hour.
  Clotted catheter: I.V.: **Note:** Not recommended due to possibility of allergic reactions with repeated doses: 10,000-25,000 units diluted in NS to a final volume equivalent to catheter volume; instill into catheter and leave in place for 1 hour, then aspirate contents out of catheter and flush catheter with normal saline.
  Adults: Antibodies to streptokinase remain for at least 3-6 months after initial dose: Administration requires the use of an infusion pump.
    An intradermal skin test of 100 units has been suggested to predict allergic response to streptokinase. If a positive reaction is not seen after 15-20 minutes, a therapeutic dose may be administered.
  Guidelines for acute myocardial infarction (AMI): 1.5 million units over 60 minutes
    Administration:
      Dilute two 750,000 unit vials of streptokinase with 5 mL dextrose 5% in water (D$_5$W) each, gently swirl to dissolve.
      Add this dose of the 1.5 million units to 150 mL D$_5$W.
      This should be infused over 60 minutes; an in-line filter ≥0.45 micron should be used.
      Monitor for the first few hours for signs of anaphylaxis or allergic reaction. **Infusion should be slowed if blood pressure falls by 25 mm Hg or terminated if asthmatic symptoms appear**.

(Continued)

Streptokinase *(Continued)*

Following completion of streptokinase, initiate heparin, if directed, when aPTT returns to less than 2 times the upper limit of control; do not use a bolus, but initiate infusion adjusted to a target aPTT of 1.5-2 times the upper limit of control. If prolonged (>48 hours) heparin is required, infusion may be switched to subcutaneous therapy.

Guidelines for acute pulmonary embolism (APE): 3 million unit dose over 24 hours

Administration:

Dilute four 750,000 unit vials of streptokinase with 5 mL dextrose 5% in water (D_5W) each, gently swirl to dissolve.

Add this dose of 3 million units to 250 mL D_5W, an in-line filter ≥0.45 micron should be used.

Administer 250,000 units (23 mL) over 30 minutes followed by 100,000 units/hour (9 mL/hour) for 24 hours.

Monitor for the first few hours for signs of anaphylaxis or allergic reaction. **Infusion should be slowed if blood pressure is lowered by 25 mm Hg or if asthmatic symptoms appear**.

Begin heparin 1000 units/hour about 3-4 hours after completion of streptokinase infusion or when PTT is <100 seconds.

Monitor PT, PTT, and fibrinogen levels during therapy.

Thromboses: 250,000 units to start, then 100,000 units/hour for 24-72 hours depending on location.

Cannula occlusion: 250,000 units into cannula, clamp for 2 hours, then aspirate contents and flush with normal saline; **Not recommended; see Warnings/Precautions**

Administration Avoid I.M. injections

Monitoring Parameters Blood pressure, PT, aPTT, platelet count, hematocrit, fibrinogen concentration, signs of bleeding

Reference Range

Partial thromboplastin time (aPTT) activated: 20.4-33.2 seconds

Prothrombin time (PT): 10.9-13.7 seconds (same as control)

Fibrinogen: 200-400 mg/dL

Nursing Implications For I.V. or intracoronary use only; monitor for bleeding every 15 minutes for the first hour of therapy; do not mix with other drugs

Dosage Forms Powder for injection: 250,000 units, 750,000 units, 1,500,000 units

Streptomycin *(strep toe MYE sin)*

Related Information

Antimicrobial Drugs of Choice *on page 1588*

Tuberculosis Treatment Guidelines *on page 1612*

Synonyms Streptomycin Sulfate

Therapeutic Category Antibiotic, Aminoglycoside; Antitubercular Agent

Use Part of combination therapy of active tuberculosis; used in combination with other agents for treatment of streptococcal or enterococcal endocarditis, mycobacterial infections, plague, tularemia, and brucellosis

Pregnancy Risk Factor D

Contraindications Hypersensitivity to streptomycin or any component of the formulation; pregnancy

Warnings/Precautions Use with caution in patients with pre-existing vertigo, tinnitus, hearing loss, neuromuscular disorders, or renal impairment; modify dosage in patients with renal impairment; aminoglycosides are associated with significant nephrotoxicity or ototoxicity; the ototoxicity is directly proportional to the amount of drug given and the duration of treatment; tinnitus or vertigo are indications of vestibular injury and impending bilateral irreversible damage; renal damage is usually reversible

Adverse Reactions Frequency not defined.

Cardiovascular: Hypotension

Central nervous system: Neurotoxicity, drowsiness, headache, drug fever, paresthesia

Dermatologic: Skin rash

Gastrointestinal: Nausea, vomiting

Hematologic: Eosinophilia, anemia

Neuromuscular & skeletal: Arthralgia, weakness, tremor

Otic: Ototoxicity (auditory), ototoxicity (vestibular)

Renal: Nephrotoxicity

Respiratory: Difficulty in breathing

Overdosage/Toxicology Symptoms include ototoxicity, nephrotoxicity, and neuromuscular toxicity. The treatment of choice following a single acute overdose appears to be the maintenance of urine output of at least 3 mL/kg/hour. Dialysis is of questionable value in the enhancement of aminoglycoside elimination. If required, hemodialysis is preferred over peritoneal dialysis in patients with normal renal function. Careful hydration may be all that is required to promote diuresis and therefore enhance elimination.

Drug Interactions

Increased Effect/Toxicity: Increased/prolonged effect with depolarizing and nondepolarizing neuromuscular blocking agents. Concurrent use with amphotericin or loop diuretics may increase nephrotoxicity.

Stability Depending upon manufacturer, reconstituted solution remains stable for 2-4 weeks when refrigerated; exposure to light causes darkening of solution without apparent loss of potency

Mechanism of Action Inhibits bacterial protein synthesis by binding directly to the 30S ribosomal subunits causing faulty peptide sequence to form in the protein chain

Pharmacodynamics/Kinetics

Absorption: I.M.: Well absorbed

Distribution: To extracellular fluid including serum, abscesses, ascitic, pericardial, pleural, synovial, lymphatic, and peritoneal fluids; crosses placenta; small amounts enter breast milk

Half-life elimination: Newborns: 4-10 hours; Adults: 2-4.7 hours, prolonged with renal impairment

Excretion: Primarily urine (90% as unchanged drug); feces, saliva, sweat, and tears (<1%)

Usual Dosage

Children:

Tuberculosis:

Daily therapy: 20-40 mg/kg/day (maximum: 1 g/day)

Directly observed therapy (DOT): Twice weekly: 20-40 mg/kg (maximum: 1 g)

DOT: 3 times/week: 25-30 mg/kg (maximum: 1 g)

Adults:

Tuberculosis:

Daily therapy: 15 mg/kg/day (maximum: 1 g)

Directly observed therapy (DOT): Twice weekly: 25-30 mg/kg (maximum: 1.5 g)

DOT: 3 times/week: 25-30 mg/kg (maximum: 1 g)

Enterococcal endocarditis: 1 g every 12 hours for 2 weeks, 500 mg every 12 hours for 4 weeks in combination with penicillin

Streptococcal endocarditis: 1 g every 12 hours for 1 week, 500 mg every 12 hours for 1 week

Tularemia: 1-2 g/day in divided doses for 7-10 days or until patient is afebrile for 5-7 days

Plague: 2-4 g/day in divided doses until the patient is afebrile for at least 3 days

Elderly: 10 mg/kg/day, not to exceed 750 mg/day; dosing interval should be adjusted for renal function; some authors suggest not to give more than 5 days/week or give as 20-25 mg/kg/dose twice weekly

Dosing interval in renal impairment:

Cl_{cr} 10-50 mL/minute: Administer every 24-72 hours

Cl_{cr} <10 mL/minute: Administer every 72-96 hours

Removed by hemo and peritoneal dialysis: Administer dose postdialysis

Administration Inject deep I.M. into large muscle mass; may be administered I.V. over 30-60 minutes

Monitoring Parameters Hearing (audiogram), BUN, creatinine; serum concentration of the drug should be monitored in all patients; eighth cranial nerve damage is usually preceded by high-pitched tinnitus, roaring noises, sense of fullness in ears, or impaired hearing and may persist for weeks after drug is discontinued

Reference Range Therapeutic: Peak: 20-30 µg/mL; Trough: <5 µg/mL; Toxic: Peak: >50 µg/mL; Trough: >10 µg/mL

Test Interactions False-positive urine glucose with Benedict's solution or Clinitest®; penicillin may decrease aminoglycoside serum concentrations *in vitro*

Patient Information Report any unusual symptom of hearing loss, dizziness, roaring noises, or fullness in ears

Dosage Forms Injection, as sulfate: 400 mg/mL (2.5 mL) [1 g vial]

♦ **Streptomycin Sulfate** *see* Streptomycin *on page 1262*

♦ **Stresstabs® 600 Advanced Formula [OTC]** *see* Vitamins (Multiple) *on page 1424*

♦ **Strifon Forte® (Can)** *see* Chlorzoxazone *on page 285*

♦ **Stromectol®** *see* Ivermectin *on page 758*

♦ **Strong Iodine Solution** *see* Potassium Iodide *on page 1111*

Strontium-89 (STRON shee um atey nine)

U.S. Brand Names Metastron®

Canadian Brand Names Metastron®

Synonyms Strontium-89 Chloride

Therapeutic Category Radiopharmaceutical

Use Relief of bone pain in patients with skeletal metastases

Pregnancy Risk Factor D

Contraindications Hypersensitivity to any strontium-containing compounds or any other component of the formulation; pregnancy, lactation

Warnings/Precautions Use caution in patients with bone marrow compromise; incontinent patients may require urinary catheterization. Body fluids may remain radioactive up to one week after injection. Not indicated for use in patients with cancer not involving bone and should be used with caution in patients whose platelet counts fall <60,000 or whose white blood cell counts fall <2400. A small number of patients have experienced a transient increase in bone pain at 36-72 hours postdose; this reaction is generally mild and self-limiting. It should be handled cautiously, in a similar manner to other radioactive drugs. Appropriate safety measures to minimize radiation to personnel should be instituted.

Adverse Reactions Most severe reactions of marrow toxicity can be managed by conventional means

Frequency not defined:

Cardiovascular: Flushing (most common after rapid injection)

Central nervous system: Fever and chills (rare)

Hematologic: Thrombocytopenia, leukopenia

Neuromuscular & skeletal: Increase in bone pain may occur (10% to 20% of patients)

Stability Store vial and its contents inside its transportation container at room temperature.

Usual Dosage Adults: I.V.: 148 megabecquerel (4 millicurie) administered by slow I.V. injection over 1-2 minutes or 1.5-2.2 megabecquerel (40-60 microcurie)/kg; repeated doses are generally not recommended at intervals <90 days; measure the patient dose by a suitable radioactivity calibration system immediately prior to administration

Monitoring Parameters Routine blood tests

Patient Information Eat and drink normally, there is no need to avoid alcohol or caffeine unless already advised to do so; may be advised to take analgesics until Metastron® begins to become effective; the effect lasts for several months, if pain returns before that, notify medical personnel

Nursing Implications During the first week after injection, strontium-89 will be present in the blood and urine, therefore, the following common sense precautions should be instituted:

(Continued)

Strontium-89 *(Continued)*

1. Where a normal toilet is available, use in preference to a urinal, flush the toilet twice
2. Wipe away any spilled urine with a tissue and flush it away
3. Have patient wash hands after using the toilet
4. Immediately wash any linen or clothes that become stained with blood or urine
5. Wash away any spilled blood if a cut occurs

Dosage Forms Injection, as chloride: 10.9-22.6 mg/mL [148 megabecquerel, 4 millicurie] (10 mL)

♦ **Strontium-89 Chloride** *see* Strontium-89 *on page 1263*

♦ **Sublimaze®** *see* Fentanyl *on page 551*

Succimer *(SUKS si mer)*

U.S. Brand Names Chemet®
Canadian Brand Names Chemet®
Therapeutic Category Antidote, Lead Toxicity; Chelating Agent, Oral
Use Orphan drug: Treatment of lead poisoning in children with blood levels >45 μg/dL. It is not indicated for prophylaxis of lead poisoning in a lead-containing environment. Following oral administration, succimer is generally well tolerated and produces a linear dose-dependent reduction in serum lead concentrations. This agent appears to offer advantages over existing lead chelating agents.
Pregnancy Risk Factor C
Contraindications Hypersensitivity to succimer or any component of the formulation
Warnings/Precautions Caution in patients with renal or hepatic impairment; adequate hydration should be maintained during therapy
Adverse Reactions
>10%:
　Central nervous system: Fever
　Gastrointestinal: Nausea, vomiting, diarrhea, appetite loss, hemorrhoidal symptoms, metallic taste
　Neuromuscular & skeletal: Back pain
1% to 10%:
　Central nervous system: Drowsiness, dizziness
　Dermatologic: Rash
　Endocrine & metabolic: Serum cholesterol
　Gastrointestinal: Sore throat
　Hepatic: Elevated AST/ALT, alkaline phosphatase
　Respiratory: Nasal congestion, cough
　Miscellaneous: Flu-like symptoms
<1% (Limited to important or life-threatening): Arrhythmias
Overdosage/Toxicology Symptoms include anorexia, vomiting, nephritis, hepatotoxicity, renal tubular necrosis, and GI bleeding.
Drug Interactions
Decreased Effect: Not recommended for concomitant administration with edetate calcium disodium or penicillamine.
Mechanism of Action Succimer is an analog of dimercaprol. It forms water soluble chelates with heavy metals which are subsequently excreted renally. Initial data have shown encouraging results in the treatment of mercury and arsenic poisoning. Succimer binds heavy metals; however, the chemical form of these chelates is not known.
Pharmacodynamics/Kinetics
Absorption: Rapid but incomplete
Metabolism: Rapidly and extensively to mixed succimer cysteine disulfides
Half-life elimination: 2 days
Time to peak, serum: ~1-2 hours
Excretion: Urine (~25%) with peak urinary excretion between 2-4 hours (90% as mixed succimer-cysteine disulfide conjugates, 10% as unchanged drug); feces (as unabsorbed drug)
Usual Dosage Children and Adults: Oral: 10 mg/kg/dose every 8 hours for 5 days followed by 10 mg/kg/dose every 12 hours for 14 days

Dosing adjustment in renal/hepatic impairment: Administer with caution and monitor closely
Concomitant iron therapy has been reported in a small number of children without the formation of a toxic complex with iron (as seen with dimercaprol); courses of therapy may be repeated if indicated by weekly monitoring of blood lead levels; lead levels should be stabilized <15 μg/dL; 2 weeks between courses is recommended unless more timely treatment is indicated by lead levels
Monitoring Parameters Blood lead levels, serum aminotransferases
Test Interactions False-positive ketones (U) using nitroprusside methods, falsely elevated serum CPK; falsely decreased uric acid measurement
Patient Information Maintain adequate fluid intake; notify physician if rash occurs; capsules may be opened and contents sprinkled on food or put on a spoon
Nursing Implications Adequately hydrate patients; rapid rebound of serum lead levels can occur; monitor closely
Dosage Forms Capsule: 100 mg

Succinylcholine *(suks in il KOE leen)*

Related Information
　Neuromuscular Blocking Agents Comparison *on page 1508*
U.S. Brand Names Anectine® Chloride; Anectine® Flo-Pack®; Quelicin®
Canadian Brand Names Quelicin®
Synonyms Succinylcholine Chloride; Suxamethonium Chloride

Therapeutic Category Neuromuscular Blocker Agent, Depolarizing; Skeletal Muscle Relaxant

Use Adjunct to general anesthesia to facilitate both rapid sequence and routine endotracheal intubation and to relax skeletal muscles during surgery; to reduce the intensity of muscle contractions of pharmacologically- or electrically-induced convulsions; does not relieve pain or produce sedation

Pregnancy Risk Factor C

Contraindications Hypersensitivity to succinylcholine or any component of the formulation; personal or familial history of malignant hyperthermia; myopathies associated with elevated serum creatine phosphokinase (CPK) values; narrow-angle glaucoma, penetrating eye injuries; disorders of plasma pseudocholinesterase

Warnings/Precautions Use with caution in pediatrics and adolescents secondary to undiagnosed skeletal muscle myopathy and potential for ventricular dysrhythmias and cardiac arrest resulting from hyperkalemia; use with caution in patients with pre-existing hyperkalemia, paraplegia, extensive or severe burns, extensive denervation of skeletal muscle because of disease or injury to the CNS or with degenerative or dystrophic neuromuscular disease; may increase vagal tone

Adverse Reactions

>10%:
Ocular: Increased intraocular pressure
Miscellaneous: Postoperative stiffness

1% to 10%:
Cardiovascular: Bradycardia, hypotension, cardiac arrhythmias, tachycardia
Gastrointestinal: Intragastric pressure, salivation

<1% (Limited to important or life-threatening): Apnea, bronchospasm, circulatory collapse, erythema, hyperkalemia, hypertension, itching, malignant hyperthermia, myalgia, myoglobinuria, rash

Overdosage/Toxicology Symptoms include respiratory paralysis and cardiac arrest. Bradyarrhythmias can often be treated with atropine 0.1 mg (infants). Do not treat with anticholinesterase drugs (eg, neostigmine, physostigmine), since they may worsen toxicity by interfering with succinylcholine metabolism.

Drug Interactions

Increased Effect/Toxicity:

Increased toxicity: Anticholinesterase drugs (neostigmine, physostigmine, or pyridostigmine) in combination with succinylcholine can cause cardiorespiratory collapse; cyclophosphamide, oral contraceptives, lidocaine, thiotepa, pancuronium, lithium, magnesium salts, aprotinin, chloroquine, metoclopramide, terbutaline, and procaine enhance and prolong the effects of succinylcholine

Prolonged neuromuscular blockade: Inhaled anesthetics, local anesthetics, calcium channel blockers, antiarrhythmics (eg, quinidine or procainamide), antibiotics (eg, aminoglycosides, tetracyclines, vancomycin, clindamycin), immunosuppressants (eg, cyclosporine)

Stability
Refrigerate at 2°C to 8°C (36°F to 46°F); however, remains stable for 14 days unrefrigerated; powder form does not require refrigeration
Stability of parenteral admixture at refrigeration temperature (4°C): 24 hours in D_5W or NS
I.V. form is **incompatible** when mixed with sodium bicarbonate, pentobarbital, thiopental

Mechanism of Action Acts similar to acetylcholine, produces depolarization of the motor endplate at the myoneural junction which causes sustained flaccid skeletal muscle paralysis produced by state of accommodation that developes in adjacent excitable muscle membranes

Pharmacodynamics/Kinetics
Onset of action: I.M.: 2-3 minutes; I.V.: Complete muscular relaxation: 30-60 seconds
Duration: I.M.: 10-30 minutes; I.V.: 4-6 minutes with single administration
Metabolism: Rapidly hydrolyzed by plasma pseudocholinesterase

Usual Dosage I.M., I.V.: Dose to effect; doses will vary due to interpatient variability; use ideal body weight for obese patients
I.M.: 2.5-4 mg/kg, total dose should not exceed 150 mg
I.V.:
Children: Initial: 1-2 mg/kg; maintenance: 0.3-0.6 mg/kg every 5-10 minutes as needed; because of the risk of malignant hyperthermia, use of continuous infusions is not recommended in infants and children
Adults: 1-1.5 mg/kg, up to 150 mg total dose
Maintenance: 0.04-0.07 mg/kg every 5-10 minutes as needed
Continuous infusion: 10-100 mcg/kg/minute (or 0.5-10 mg/minute); dilute to concentration of 1-2 mg/mL in D_5W or NS

Note: Initial dose of succinylcholine must be increased when nondepolarizing agent pretreatment used because of the antagonism between succinylcholine and nondepolarizing neuromuscular blocking agents

Dosing adjustment in hepatic impairment: Dose should be decreased in patients with severe liver disease

Administration May be administered by rapid I.V. injection without further dilution; I.M. injections should be made deeply, preferably high into deltoid muscle

Monitoring Parameters Cardiac monitor, blood pressure monitor, and ventilator required during administration; temperature, serum potassium and calcium, assisted ventilator status

Test Interactions ↑ potassium (S)

Dosage Forms
Injection, as chloride: 20 mg/mL (10 mL); 50 mg/mL (10 mL); 100 mg/mL (5 mL, 10 mL, 20 mL)
Powder for injection, as chloride: 500 mg, 1 g

♦ **Succinylcholine Chloride** see Succinylcholine on page 1264

♦ **Sucraid**® see Sacrosidase on page 1218

Sucralfate (soo KRAL fate)

U.S. Brand Names Carafate®

Canadian Brand Names Apo®-Sucralate; Novo-Sucralate; Nu-Sucralate; PMS-Sucralate; Sulcrate®; Sulcrate® Suspension Plus

Synonyms Aluminum Sucrose Sulfate, Basic

Therapeutic Category Gastrointestinal Agent, Miscellaneous

Use Short-term management of duodenal ulcers; maintenance of duodenal ulcers

Unlabeled/Investigational Use Gastric ulcers; suspension may be used topically for treatment of stomatitis due to cancer chemotherapy and other causes of esophageal and gastric erosions; GERD, esophagitis; treatment of NSAID mucosal damage; prevention of stress ulcers; postsclerotherapy for esophageal variceal bleeding

Pregnancy Risk Factor B

Pregnancy/Breast-Feeding Implications

Clinical effects on the fetus: No data available; available evidence suggests safe use during pregnancy and breast-feeding

Breast-feeding/lactation: Compatible with breast-feeding

Contraindications Hypersensitivity to sucralfate or any component of the formulation

Warnings/Precautions Successful therapy with sucralfate should not be expected to alter the posthealing frequency of recurrence or the severity of duodenal ulceration; use with caution in patients with chronic renal failure who have an impaired excretion of absorbed aluminum. Because of the potential for sucralfate to alter the absorption of some drugs, separate administration (take other medication 2 hours before sucralfate) should be considered when alterations in bioavailability are believed to be critical

Adverse Reactions

1% to 10%: Gastrointestinal: Constipation

<1% (Limited to important or life-threatening): Bezoar formation, hypersensitivity (pruritus, urticaria, angioedema), rash

Overdosage/Toxicology Toxicity is minimal. May cause constipation.

Drug Interactions

Decreased Effect: Sucralfate may alter the absorption of digoxin, phenytoin (hydantoins), warfarin, ketoconazole, quinidine, quinolones, tetracycline, theophylline. Because of the potential for sucralfate to alter the absorption of some drugs; separate administration (take other medications at least 2 hours before sucralfate). The potential for decreased absorption should be considered when alterations in bioavailability are believed to be critical.

Ethanol/Nutrition/Herb Interactions Food: Sucralfate may interfere with absorption of vitamin A, vitamin D, vitamin E, and vitamin K.

Stability Suspension: Shake well. Refrigeration is **not** necessary; do **not** freeze.

Mechanism of Action Forms a complex by binding with positively charged proteins in exudates, forming a viscous paste-like, adhesive substance. This selectively forms a protective coating that protects the lining against peptic acid, pepsin, and bile salts.

Pharmacodynamics/Kinetics

Onset of action: Paste formation and ulcer adhesion: 1-2 hours

Duration: Up to 6 hours

Absorption: Oral: <5%

Distribution: Acts locally at ulcer sites; unbound in GI tract to aluminum and sucrose octasulfate

Metabolism: None

Excretion: Urine (small amounts as unchanged compounds)

Usual Dosage Oral:

Children: Dose not established, doses of 40-80 mg/kg/day divided every 6 hours have been used

Stomatitis (unlabeled use): 2.5-5 mL (1 g/10 mL suspension), swish and spit or swish and swallow 4 times/day

Adults:

Stress ulcer prophylaxis: 1 g 4 times/day

Stress ulcer treatment: 1 g every 4 hours

Duodenal ulcer:

Treatment: 1 g 4 times/day on an empty stomach and at bedtime for 4-8 weeks, or alternatively 2 g twice daily; treatment is recommended for 4-8 weeks in adults, the elderly may require 12 weeks

Maintenance: Prophylaxis: 1 g twice daily

Stomatitis (unlabeled use): 1 g/10 mL suspension, swish and spit or swish and swallow 4 times/day

Dosage comment in renal impairment: Aluminum salt is minimally absorbed (<5%), however, may accumulate in renal failure

Dietary Considerations Administer with water on an empty stomach.

Administration Tablet may be broken or dissolved in water before ingestion. Administer with water on an empty stomach.

Patient Information Take before meals or on an empty stomach; do not take antacids 30 minutes before or after taking sucralfate

Nursing Implications Monitor for constipation; administer other medications 2 hours before sucralfate

Dosage Forms

Suspension, oral: 1 g/10 mL (10 mL, 420 mL)

Tablet: 1 g

- ◆ **Sucrets®** [OTC] *see* Dyclonine *on page 455*
- ◆ **Sudafed®** [OTC] *see* Pseudoephedrine *on page 1155*
- ◆ **Sudafed® 12 Hour** [OTC] *see* Pseudoephedrine *on page 1155*
- ◆ **Sudafed® Cold & Allergy** [OTC] *see* Chlorpheniramine and Pseudoephedrine *on page 279*
- ◆ **Sudafed® Cold and Sinus** [OTC] *see* Acetaminophen and Pseudoephedrine *on page 25*

- **Sudafed® Cold & Cough Extra Strength (Can)** *see* Acetaminophen, Dextromethorphan, and Pseudoephedrine *on page 27*
- **Sudafed® Cold & Cough Liquid Caps [OTC]** *see* Guaifenesin, Pseudoephedrine, and Dextromethorphan *on page 648*
- **Sudafed® Decongestant (Can)** *see* Pseudoephedrine *on page 1155*
- **Sudafed® Head Cold and Sinus Extra Strength (Can)** *see* Acetaminophen and Pseudoephedrine *on page 25*
- **Sudafed® Severe Cold [OTC]** *see* Acetaminophen, Dextromethorphan, and Pseudoephedrine *on page 27*
- **Sudafed® Sinus Headache [OTC]** *see* Acetaminophen and Pseudoephedrine *on page 25*
- **Sufenta®** *see* Sufentanil *on page 1267*

Sufentanil (soo FEN ta nil)

Related Information
Narcotic Agonists Comparison *on page 1506*
U.S. Brand Names Sufenta®
Canadian Brand Names Sufenta®
Synonyms Sufentanil Citrate
Therapeutic Category General Anesthetic
Use Analgesic supplement in maintenance of balanced general anesthesia
Restrictions C-II
Pregnancy Risk Factor C
Contraindications Hypersensitivity to sufentanil or any component of the formulation
Warnings/Precautions Sufentanil can cause severely compromised respiratory depression; use with caution in patients with head injuries, hepatic or renal impairment or with pulmonary disease; sufentanil shares the toxic potential of opiate agonists, precaution of opiate agonist therapy should be observed; rapid I.V. infusion may result in skeletal muscle and chest wall rigidity, impaired ventilation, respiratory distress/arrest; inject slowly over 3-5 minutes; nondepolarizing skeletal muscle relaxant may be required

Adverse Reactions
>10%:
  Cardiovascular: Bradycardia, hypotension
  Central nervous system: Somnolence
  Gastrointestinal: Nausea, vomiting
  Respiratory: Respiratory depression
1% to 10%:
  Cardiovascular: Cardiac arrhythmias, orthostatic hypotension
  Central nervous system: CNS depression, confusion
  Gastrointestinal: Biliary spasm
  Ocular: Blurred vision
<1% (Limited to important or life-threatening): Bronchospasm, circulatory depression, convulsions, laryngospasm, mental depression, paradoxical CNS excitation or delirium, physical and psychological dependence with prolonged use, rash, urticaria

Overdosage/Toxicology Treatment consists of naloxone 2 mg I.V. (0.01 mg/kg for children), with repeat administration as necessary, up to a total of 10 mg. Supportive care includes establishment of respiratory change. Naloxone may be used to treat respiratory depression. Muscular rigidity may also respond to opiate antagonist therapy or to neuromuscular blocking agents.

Drug Interactions
Cytochrome P450 Effect: CYP3A3/4 enzyme substrate
Increased Effect/Toxicity: Additive effect/toxicity with CNS depressants or beta-blockers. May increase response to neuromuscular blocking agents.
Mechanism of Action Binds to opioid receptors throughout the CNS. Once receptor binding occurs, effects are exerted by opening K+ channels and inhibiting Ca++ channels. These mechanisms increase pain threshold, alter pain perception, inhibit ascending pain pathways; short-acting narcotic

Pharmacodynamics/Kinetics
Onset of action: 1-3 minutes
Duration: Dose dependent
Metabolism: Primarily hepatic

Usual Dosage
Children 2-12 years: 10-25 mcg/kg (10-15 mcg/kg most common dose) with 100% O_2, maintenance: up to 1-2 mcg/kg total dose

Adults: Dose should be based on body weight. **Note:** In obese patients (ie, >20% above ideal body weight), use lean body weight to determine dosage.
  1-2 mcg/kg with N_2O/O_2 for endotracheal intubation; maintenance: 10-25 mcg as needed
  2-8 mcg/kg with N_2O/O_2 more complicated major surgical procedures; maintenance: 10-50 mcg as needed
  8-30 mcg/kg with 100% O_2 and muscle relaxant produces sleep; at doses ≥8 mcg/kg maintains a deep level of anesthesia; maintenance: 10-50 mcg as needed

Administration Parenteral: I.V.: Slow I.V. injection or by infusion
Nursing Implications Patient may develop rebound respiratory depression postoperatively
Additional Information Short-acting narcotic; sufentanil is 5-10 times more potent than fentanyl. Sufentanil is packaged in the same concentration as fentanyl, 50 mcg/mL. Keep in mind the differences in potency to prevent overdose with sufentanil. May choose to dilute sufentanil to decrease concentration; this will decrease the potential for administering excessive doses.

Dosage Forms Injection, as citrate: 50 mcg/mL (1 mL, 2 mL, 5 mL)

- **Sufentanil Citrate** *see* Sufentanil *on page 1267*
- **Sular®** *see* Nisoldipine *on page 985*
- **Sulbactam and Ampicillin** *see* Ampicillin and Sulbactam *on page 95*

Sulconazole (sul KON a zole)

U.S. Brand Names Exelderm®
Canadian Brand Names Exelderm®
Synonyms Sulconazole Nitrate
Therapeutic Category Antifungal Agent, Imidazole Derivative; Antifungal Agent, Topical
Use Treatment of superficial fungal infections of the skin, including tinea cruris (jock itch), tinea corporis (ringworm), tinea versicolor, and possibly tinea pedis (athlete's foot, cream only)
Pregnancy Risk Factor C
Contraindications Hypersensitivity to sulconazole or any component of the formulation
Warnings/Precautions Use with caution in nursing mothers; for external use only
Adverse Reactions 1% to 10%:
Dermatologic: Itching
Local: Burning, stinging, redness
Mechanism of Action Substituted imidazole derivative which inhibits metabolic reactions necessary for the synthesis of ergosterol, an essential membrane component. The end result is usually fungistatic; however, sulconazole may act as a fungicide in *Candida albicans* and parapsilosis during certain growth phases.
Pharmacodynamics/Kinetics
Absorption: Topical: About 8.7% absorbed percutaneously
Excretion: Primarily urine
Usual Dosage Adults: Topical: Apply a small amount to the affected area and gently massage once or twice daily for 3 weeks (tinea cruris, tinea corporis, tinea versicolor) to 4 weeks (tinea pedis).
Patient Information For external use only; avoid contact with eyes; if burning or irritation develops, notify physician
Dosage Forms
Cream, topical, as nitrate: 1% (15 g, 30 g, 60 g)
Solution, topical, as nitrate: 1% (30 mL)

♦ **Sulconazole Nitrate** *see Sulconazole on page 1268*
♦ **Sulcrate® (Can)** *see Sucralfate on page 1266*
♦ **Sulcrate® Suspension Plus (Can)** *see Sucralfate on page 1266*
♦ **Sulf-10®** *see Sulfacetamide on page 1268*

Sulfabenzamide, Sulfacetamide, and Sulfathiazole

(sul fa BENZ a mide, sul fa SEE ta mide & sul fa THYE a zole)
U.S. Brand Names V.V.S.®
Synonyms Triple Sulfa
Therapeutic Category Antibiotic, Vaginal
Use Treatment of *Haemophilus vaginalis* vaginitis
Pregnancy Risk Factor C (avoid if near term)
Contraindications Hypersensitivity to sulfabenzamide, sulfacetamide, sulfathiazole, or any component of the formulation; renal dysfunction; pregnancy (if near term)
Warnings/Precautions Associated with Stevens-Johnson syndrome; if local irritation or systemic toxicity develops, discontinue therapy
Adverse Reactions Frequency not defined.
Dermatologic: Pruritus, urticaria, Stevens-Johnson syndrome
Local: Local irritation
Miscellaneous: Allergic reactions
Mechanism of Action Interferes with microbial folic acid synthesis and growth via inhibition of para-aminobenzoic acid metabolism
Pharmacodynamics/Kinetics
Absorption: Absorption from vagina is variable and unreliable
Metabolism: Primarily by acetylation
Excretion: Urine
Usual Dosage Intravaginal: Adults:
Cream: Insert one applicatorful into vagina twice daily for 4-6 days; dosage may then be decreased to $\frac{1}{2}$ to $\frac{1}{4}$ of an applicatorful twice daily
Tablet: Insert one intravaginally twice daily for 10 days
Patient Information Complete full course of therapy; notify physician if burning, irritation, or signs of a systemic allergic reaction occur
Dosage Forms
Cream, vaginal: Sulfabenzamide 3.7%, sulfacetamide 2.86%, and sulfathiazole 3.42% (78 g with applicator, 90 g, 120 g)
Tablet, vaginal: Sulfabenzamide 184 mg, sulfacetamide 143.75 mg, and sulfathiazole 172.5 mg (20 tablets/box with vaginal applicator)

Sulfacetamide (sul fa SEE ta mide)

U.S. Brand Names AK-Sulf®; Bleph®-10; Carmol® Scalp; Cetamide®; Klaron®; Ocu-Sul®; Sebizon®; Sodium Sulamyd®; Sulf-10®
Canadian Brand Names Cetamide™; Diosulf™; Sodium Sulamyd®
Synonyms Sodium Sulfacetamide; Sulfacetamide Sodium
Therapeutic Category Antibiotic, Ophthalmic; Antibiotic, Sulfonamide Derivative
Use Treatment and prophylaxis of conjunctivitis due to susceptible organisms; corneal ulcers; adjunctive treatment with systemic sulfonamides for therapy of trachoma; topical application in scaling dermatosis (seborrheic); bacterial infections of the skin
Pregnancy Risk Factor C
Contraindications Hypersensitivity to sulfacetamide or any component of the formulation, sulfonamides; infants <2 months of age
Warnings/Precautions Inactivated by purulent exudates containing PABA; use with caution in severe dry eye; ointment may retard corneal epithelial healing; sulfite in some products may cause hypersensitivity reactions; cross-sensitivity may occur with previous exposure to

other sulfonamides given by other routes. Chemical similarities are present among sulfonamides, sulfonylureas, carbonic anhydrase inhibitors, thiazides, and loop diuretics (except ethacrynic acid). Use in patients with sulfonamide allergy is specifically contraindicated in product labeling, however a risk of cross-reaction exists in patients with allergy to any of these compounds; avoid use when previous reaction has been severe.

Adverse Reactions
1% to 10%: Local: Irritation, stinging, burning
<1% (Limited to important or life-threatening): Exfoliative dermatitis, Stevens-Johnson syndrome, toxic epidermal necrolysis

Drug Interactions
Decreased Effect: Silver containing products are incompatible with sulfacetamide solutions.

Stability Protect from light; discolored solution should not be used; **incompatible** with silver and zinc sulfate; sulfacetamide is inactivated by blood or purulent exudates

Mechanism of Action Interferes with bacterial growth by inhibiting bacterial folic acid synthesis through competitive antagonism of PABA

Pharmacodynamics/Kinetics
Half-life elimination: 7-13 hours
Excretion: When absorbed, primarily urine (as unchanged drug)

Usual Dosage
Children >2 months and Adults: Ophthalmic:
Ointment: Apply to lower conjunctival sac 1-4 times/day and at bedtime
Solution: Instill 1-3 drops several times daily up to every 2-3 hours in lower conjunctival sac during waking hours and less frequently at night
Children >12 years and Adults: Topical:
Seborrheic dermatitis: Apply at bedtime and allow to remain overnight; in severe cases, may apply twice daily
Secondary cutaneous bacterial infections: Apply 2-4 times/day until infection clears

Monitoring Parameters Response to therapy

Patient Information Eye drops will burn upon instillation; wait at least 10 minutes before using another eye preparation; may sting eyes when first applied; do not touch container to eye, ointment will cause blurred vision; notify physician if condition does not improve in 3-4 days; may cause sensitivity to sunlight

Nursing Implications Assess whether patient can adequately instill drops or ointment

Dosage Forms
Lotion, as sodium: 10% (59 mL, 85 g)
Ointment, ophthalmic, as sodium: 10% (3.5 g)
Solution, ophthalmic, as sodium: 10% (1 mL, 2 mL, 2.5 mL, 5 mL, 15 mL); 15% (5 mL, 15 mL); 30% (15 mL)

Sulfacetamide and Prednisolone
(sul fa SEE ta mide SOW dee um & pred NIS oh lone)

U.S. Brand Names AK-Cide®; Blephamide®; Cetapred®; Isopto® Cetapred®; Metimyd®; Vasocidin®

Canadian Brand Names Blephamide®; Dioptimyd®; Vasocidin®

Synonyms Prednisolone and Sulfacetamide

Therapeutic Category Antibiotic, Ophthalmic; Anti-inflammatory Agent, Ophthalmic; Corticosteroid, Ophthalmic

Use Steroid-responsive inflammatory ocular conditions where infection is present or there is a risk of infection; ophthalmic suspension may be used as an otic preparation

Pregnancy Risk Factor C

Usual Dosage Children >2 months and Adults: Ophthalmic:
Ointment: Apply to lower conjunctival sac 1-4 times/day
Solution: Instill 1-3 drops every 2-3 hours while awake

Additional Information Complete prescribing information for this medication should be consulted for additional detail.

Dosage Forms
Ointment, ophthalmic:
AK-Cide®, Metimyd®, Vasocidin®: Sulfacetamide sodium 10% and prednisolone acetate 0.5% (3.5 g)
Blephamide®: Sulfacetamide sodium 10% and prednisolone acetate 0.2% (3.5 g)
Cetapred®: Sulfacetamide sodium 10% and prednisolone acetate 0.25% (3.5 g)
Suspension, ophthalmic: Sulfacetamide sodium 10% and prednisolone sodium phosphate 0.25% (5 mL)
AK-Cide®, Metimyd®: Sulfacetamide sodium 10% and prednisolone acetate 0.5% (5 mL)
Blephamide®: Sulfacetamide sodium 10% and prednisolone acetate 0.2% (2.5 mL, 5 mL, 10 mL)
Isopto® Cetapred®: Sulfacetamide sodium 10% and prednisolone acetate 0.25% (5 mL, 15 mL)
Vasocidin®: Sulfacetamide sodium 10% and prednisolone sodium phosphate: 0.25% (5 mL, 10 mL)

♦ **Sulfacetamide Sodium** *see Sulfacetamide on page 1268*

Sulfacetamide Sodium and Fluorometholone
(sul fa SEE ta mide SOW dee um & flure oh METH oh lone)

U.S. Brand Names FML-S®

Synonyms Fluorometholone and Sulfacetamide

Therapeutic Category Antibiotic/Corticosteroid, Ophthalmic

Use Steroid-responsive inflammatory ocular conditions where infection is present or there is a risk of infection

Pregnancy Risk Factor C

Usual Dosage Children >2 months and Adults: Ophthalmic: Instill 1-3 drops every 2-3 hours while awake
(Continued)

Sulfacetamide Sodium and Fluorometholone *(Continued)*

Additional Information Complete prescribing information for this medication should be consulted for additional detail.

Dosage Forms Suspension, ophthalmic: Sulfacetamide sodium 10% and fluorometholone 0.1% (5 mL, 10 mL)

SulfaDIAZINE *(sul fa DYE a zeen)*

Related Information

Sulfonamide Derivatives *on page 1515*

USPHA/IDSA Guidelines for the Prevention of Opportunistic Infections in Persons With HIV *on page 1574*

Therapeutic Category Antibiotic, Sulfonamide Derivative

Use Treatment of urinary tract infections and nocardiosis, rheumatic fever prophylaxis; adjunctive treatment in toxoplasmosis; uncomplicated attack of malaria

Pregnancy Risk Factor B/D (at term)

Contraindications Hypersensitivity to any sulfa drug or any component of the formulation; porphyria; children <2 months of age unless indicated for the treatment of congenital toxoplasmosis; sunscreens containing PABA; pregnancy (at term)

Warnings/Precautions Use with caution in patients with impaired hepatic function or impaired renal function, G6PD deficiency; dosage modification required in patients with renal impairment; fluid intake should be maintained ≥1500 mL/day, or administer sodium bicarbonate to keep urine alkaline; more likely to cause crystalluria because it is less soluble than other sulfonamides. Chemical similarities are present among sulfonamides, sulfonylureas, carbonic anhydrase inhibitors, thiazides, and loop diuretics (except ethacrynic acid). Use in patients with sulfonamide allergy is specifically contraindicated in product labeling, however a risk of cross-reaction exists in patients with allergy to any of these compounds; avoid use when previous reaction has been severe.

Adverse Reactions Frequency not defined.

Central nervous system: Fever, dizziness, headache

Dermatologic: Lyell's syndrome, Stevens-Johnson syndrome, itching, rash, photosensitivity

Endocrine & metabolic: Thyroid function disturbance

Gastrointestinal: Anorexia, nausea, vomiting, diarrhea

Genitourinary: Crystalluria

Hematologic: Granulocytopenia, leukopenia, thrombocytopenia, aplastic anemia, hemolytic anemia

Hepatic: Hepatitis, jaundice

Renal: Hematuria, acute nephropathy, interstitial nephritis

Miscellaneous: Serum sickness-like reactions

Overdosage/Toxicology Symptoms include drowsiness, dizziness, anorexia, abdominal pain, nausea, vomiting, hemolytic anemia, acidosis, jaundice, fever, and agranulocytosis. Doses of as little as 2-6 g/day in divided doses every 6 hours may produce toxicity. The aniline radical is responsible for hematologic toxicity. High volume diuresis may aid in elimination and prevention of renal failure.

Drug Interactions

Increased Effect/Toxicity: Increased effect of oral anticoagulants and oral hypoglycemic agents.

Decreased Effect: Decreased effect with PABA or PABA metabolites of drugs (eg, procaine, proparacaine, tetracaine, sunblock).

Ethanol/Nutrition/Herb Interactions

Food: Avoid large quantities of vitamin C or acidifying agents (cranberry juice) to prevent crystalluria.

Herb/Nutraceutical: Avoid dong quai, St John's wort (may also cause photosensitization).

Stability Tablets may be crushed to prepare oral suspension of the drug in water or with a sucrose-containing solution; aqueous suspension with concentrations of 100 mg/mL should be stored in the refrigerator and used within 7 days

Mechanism of Action Interferes with bacterial growth by inhibiting bacterial folic acid synthesis through competitive antagonism of PABA

Pharmacodynamics/Kinetics

Absorption: Well absorbed

Distribution: Throughout body tissues and fluids including pleural, peritoneal, synovial, and ocular fluids; throughout total body water; readily diffused into CSF; enters breast milk

Metabolism: By N-acetylation

Half-life elimination: 10 hours

Excretion: Urine (15% to 40% as metabolites, 43% to 60% as unchanged drug)

Usual Dosage Oral:

Asymptomatic meningococcal carriers:

Infants 1-12 months: 500 mg once daily for 2 days

Children 1-12 years: 500 mg twice daily for 2 days

Adults: 1 g twice daily for 2 days

Congenital toxoplasmosis:

Newborns and Children <2 months: 100 mg/kg/day divided every 6 hours in conjunction with pyrimethamine 1 mg/kg/day once daily and supplemental folinic acid 5 mg every 3 days for 6 months

Children >2 months: 25-50 mg/kg/dose 4 times/day

Nocardiosis: 4-8 g/day for a minimum of 6 weeks

Toxoplasmosis:

Children >2 months: Loading dose: 75 mg/kg; maintenance dose: 120-150 mg/kg/day, maximum dose: 6 g/day; divided every 4-6 hours in conjunction with pyrimethamine 2 mg/kg/day divided every 12 hours for 3 days followed by 1 mg/kg/day once daily with supplemental folinic acid

Adults: 2-6 g/day in divided doses every 6 hours in conjunction with pyrimethamine 50-75 mg/day and with supplemental folinic acid

Prevention of recurrent attacks of rheumatic fever:
>30 kg: 1 g/day
<30 kg: 0.5 g/day

Dietary Considerations Supplemental folinic acid should be administered to reverse symptoms or prevent problems due to folic acid deficiency.

Patient Information Drink plenty of fluids; take on an empty stomach; avoid prolonged exposure to sunlight or wear protective clothing and sunscreen; notify physician if rash, difficulty breathing, severe or persistent fever, or sore throat occurs

Nursing Implications Maintain adequate hydration and monitor urine output

Dosage Forms Tablet: 500 mg

Sulfadiazine, Sulfamethazine, and Sulfamerazine
(sul fa DYE a zeen sul fa METH a zeen & sul fa MER a zeen)

Synonyms Multiple Sulfonamides; Trisulfapyrimidines

Therapeutic Category Antibiotic, Sulfonamide Derivative

Use Treatment of toxoplasmosis and other susceptible organisms, however, other agents are preferred

Pregnancy Risk Factor B/D (at term)

Contraindications Hypersensitivity to any sulfa drug or any component of the formulation; porphyria; sulfonamide allergy; pregnancy (at term)

Warnings/Precautions Chemical similarities are present among sulfonamides, sulfonylureas, carbonic anhydrase inhibitors, thiazides, and loop diuretics (except ethacrynic acid). In patients with allergy to one of these compounds, a risk of cross-reaction exists; avoid use when previous reaction has been severe.

Mechanism of Action Interferes with microbial folic acid synthesis and growth via inhibition of para-aminobenzoic acid metabolism

Pharmacodynamics/Kinetics
Metabolism: By acetylation
Excretion: Urine

Usual Dosage Adults: Oral: 2-4 g to start, then 2-4 g/day in 3-6 divided doses

Dietary Considerations Should be taken 1 hour before or 2 hours after a meal on an empty stomach.

Test Interactions Increases cholesterol (S), protein, uric acid (S)

Patient Information Drink plenty of fluids

Dosage Forms Tablet: Sulfadiazine 167 mg, sulfamethazine 167 mg, and sulfamerazine 167 mg

Sulfadoxine and Pyrimethamine (sul fa DOKS een & peer i METH a meen)

U.S. Brand Names Fansidar®

Synonyms Pyrimethamine and Sulfadoxine

Therapeutic Category Antimalarial Agent

Use Treatment of *Plasmodium falciparum* malaria in patients in whom chloroquine resistance is suspected; malaria prophylaxis for travelers to areas where chloroquine-resistant malaria is endemic

Pregnancy Risk Factor C/D (at term)

Contraindications Hypersensitivity to any sulfa drug, pyrimethamine, or any component of the formulation; porphyria, megaloblastic anemia, severe renal insufficiency; children <2 months of age due to competition with bilirubin for protein binding sites; pregnancy (at term)

Warnings/Precautions Use with caution in patients with renal or hepatic impairment, patients with possible folate deficiency, and patients with seizure disorders, increased adverse reactions are seen in patients also receiving chloroquine; fatalities associated with sulfonamides, although rare, have occurred due to severe reactions including Stevens-Johnson syndrome, toxic epidermal necrolysis, hepatic necrosis, agranulocytosis, aplastic anemia and other blood dyscrasias; discontinue use at first sign of rash or any sign of adverse reaction; hemolysis occurs in patients with G6PD deficiency; leucovorin should be administered to reverse signs and symptoms of folic acid deficiency.

Chemical similarities are present among sulfonamides, sulfonylureas, carbonic anhydrase inhibitors, thiazides, and loop diuretics (except ethacrynic acid). Use in patients with sulfonamide allergy is specifically contraindicated in product labeling, however a risk of cross-reaction exists in patients with allergy to any of these compounds; avoid use when previous reaction has been severe.

Adverse Reactions Frequency not defined.
Central nervous system: Ataxia, seizures, headache
Dermatologic: Photosensitivity, Stevens-Johnson syndrome, erythema multiforme, toxic epidermal necrolysis, rash
Endocrine & metabolic: Thyroid function dysfunction
Gastrointestinal: Atrophic glossitis, vomiting, gastritis, anorexia, glossitis
Genitourinary: Crystalluria
Hematologic: Megaloblastic anemia, leukopenia, thrombocytopenia, pancytopenia
Hepatic: Hepatic necrosis, hepatitis
Neuromuscular & skeletal: Tremors
Respiratory: Respiratory failure
Miscellaneous: Hypersensitivity

Overdosage/Toxicology Symptoms include anorexia, vomiting, CNS stimulation including seizures, megaloblastic anemia, leukopenia, thrombocytopenia, and crystalluria. Leucovorin should be administered in a dosage of 3-9 mg/day for 3 days as required to reverse symptoms of folic acid deficiency. Doses of as little as 2-5 g/day may produce toxicity. The aniline radical is responsible for hematologic toxicity. High volume diuresis may aid in elimination and prevention of renal failure. Diazepam can be used to control seizures.

Drug Interactions
Increased Effect/Toxicity: Hydantoin (phenytoin) levels may be increased. Effect of oral hypoglycemics (rare, but severe) may occur. Combination with methenamine may result in
(Continued)

Sulfadoxine and Pyrimethamine *(Continued)*

crystalluria; avoid use. May increase methotrexate-induced bone marrow suppression. NSAIDs and salicylates may increase sulfonamide concentrations. Effect of warfarin may be increased.

Decreased Effect: Cyclosporine concentrations may be decreased; monitor levels and renal function. PABA (para-aminobenzoic acid - may be found in some vitamin supplements): interferes with the antibacterial activity of sulfonamides; avoid concurrent use. Pyrimethamine effectiveness decreased by acid.

Stability Protect from light

Mechanism of Action Sulfadoxine interferes with bacterial folic acid synthesis and growth via competitive inhibition of para-aminiobenzoic acid; pyrimethamine inhibits microbial dihydrofolate reductase, resulting in inhibition of tetrahydrofolic acid synthesis

Pharmacodynamics/Kinetics

Absorption: Well absorbed

Distribution: Sulfadoxine: Well distributed like other sulfonamides; Pyrimethamine: Widely distributed, mainly in blood cells, kidneys, lungs, liver, and spleen

Metabolism: Pyrimethamine: Hepatic; Sulfadoxine: None

Half-life elimination: Pyrimethamine: 80-95 hours; Sulfadoxine: 5-8 days

Time to peak, serum: 2-8 hours

Excretion: Urine (as unchanged drug and several unidentified metabolites)

Usual Dosage Children and Adults: Oral:

Treatment of acute attack of malaria: A single dose of the following number of Fansidar® tablets is used in sequence with quinine or alone:

2-11 months: $1/4$ tablet

1-3 years: $1/2$ tablet

4-8 years: 1 tablet

9-14 years: 2 tablets

>14 years: 3 tablets

Malaria prophylaxis: A single dose should be carried for self-treatment in the event of febrile illness when medical attention is not immediately available:

2-11 months: $1/4$ tablet

1-3 years: $1/2$ tablet

4-8 years: 1 tablet

9-14 years: 2 tablets

>14 years and Adults: 3 tablets

Monitoring Parameters CBC, including platelet counts, and urinalysis should be performed periodically

Patient Information Begin prophylaxis at least 2 days before departure; drink plenty of fluids; avoid prolonged exposure to the sun; notify physician if rash, sore throat, pallor, or glossitis occurs

Dosage Forms Tablet: Sulfadoxine 500 mg and pyrimethamine 25 mg

Sulfamethoxazole *(sul fa meth OKS a zole)*

Related Information

Sulfonamide Derivatives *on page 1515*

U.S. Brand Names Gantanol®

Therapeutic Category Antibiotic, Sulfonamide Derivative

Use Treatment of urinary tract infections, nocardiosis, toxoplasmosis, acute otitis media, and acute exacerbations of chronic bronchitis due to susceptible organisms

Pregnancy Risk Factor B/D (at term)

Contraindications Hypersensitivity to any sulfa drug or any component of the formulation; porphyria; children <2 months of age unless indicated for the treatment of congenital toxoplasmosis; sunscreens containing PABA; pregnancy (at term)

Warnings/Precautions Maintain adequate fluid intake to prevent crystalluria; use with caution in patients with renal or hepatic impairment, and patients with G6PD deficiency; should not be used for group A beta-hemolytic streptococcal infections. Chemical similarities are present among sulfonamides, sulfonylureas, carbonic anhydrase inhibitors, thiazides, and loop diuretics (except ethacrynic acid). Use in patients with sulfonamide allergy is specifically contraindicated in product labeling, however a risk of cross-reaction exists in patients with allergy to any of these compounds; avoid use when previous reaction has been severe.

Adverse Reactions

>10%:

Central nervous system: Fever, dizziness, headache

Dermatologic: Itching, rash, photosensitivity

Gastrointestinal: Anorexia, nausea, vomiting, diarrhea

1% to 10%:

Dermatologic: Lyell's syndrome, Stevens-Johnson syndrome

Hematologic: Granulocytopenia, leukopenia, thrombocytopenia, aplastic anemia, hemolytic anemia

Hepatic: Hepatitis

<1% (Limited to important or life-threatening): Acute nephropathy, hematuria, interstitial nephritis, vasculitis

Overdosage/Toxicology Symptoms include drowsiness, dizziness, anorexia, abdominal pain, nausea, vomiting, hemolytic anemia, acidosis, jaundice, fever, and agranulocytosis. The aniline radical is responsible for hematologic toxicity. High volume diuresis may aid in elimination and prevention of renal failure.

Drug Interactions

Cytochrome P450 Effect: CYP2C9 enzyme inhibitor

Increased Effect/Toxicity: Increased effect of oral anticoagulants, oral hypoglycemic agents, and methotrexate.

Decreased Effect: Decreased effect with PABA or PABA metabolites of drugs (eg, procaine, proparacaine, tetracaine).

Ethanol/Nutrition/Herb Interactions Food: The presence of food delays but does not reduce absorption. Avoid large quantities of vitamin C or acidifying agents (cranberry juice) to prevent crystalluria.

Stability Protect from light

Mechanism of Action Interferes with bacterial growth by inhibiting bacterial folic acid synthesis through competitive antagonism of PABA

Pharmacodynamics/Kinetics

Absorption: 90%

Distribution: Widely into body tissue and fluids (middle ear, prostate, bile, aqueous humor, CSF); crosses placenta; enters breast milk

Protein binding: 70%

Metabolism: Primarily hepatic via N-acetylation and glucuronidation with 10% to 20% as the N-acetylated form in plasma

Half-life elimination: 9-12 hours; prolonged with renal impairment

Time to peak, serum: 1-4 hours

Excretion: Urine (20% as unchanged drug and metabolites)

Usual Dosage Oral:

Children >2 months: 50-60 mg/kg as single dose followed by 50-60 mg/kg/day divided every 12 hours; maximum: 3 g/24 hours or 75 mg/kg/day

Adults: Initial: 2 g, then 1 g 2-3 times/day; maximum: 3 g/24 hours

Dosing adjustment/interval in renal impairment:

Cl_{cr} 10-50 mL/minute: Administer every 12-24 hours

Cl_{cr} <10 mL/minute: Administer every 24 hours

Hemodialysis: Moderately dialyzable (20% to 50%)

Dietary Considerations Should be taken 1 hour before or 2 hours after a meal on an empty stomach.

Administration Administer around-the-clock to promote less variation in peak and trough serum levels

Monitoring Parameters Monitor urine output

Test Interactions May interfere with Jaffé alkaline picrate reaction assay for creatinine resulting in overestimations of ~10% in the range of normal values; decreased effect with PABA or PABA metabolites of drugs (ie, procaine, proparacaine, tetracaine)

Patient Information Drink plenty of fluids; avoid prolonged exposure to sunlight or wear protective clothing; avoid aspirin and vitamin C products, notify physician if rash, unusual bleeding, difficulty breathing, severe or persistent fever, or sore throat occurs

Nursing Implications Maintain adequate hydration

Dosage Forms Tablet: 500 mg

Sulfamethoxazole and Trimethoprim

(sul fa meth OKS a zole & trye METH oh prim)

Related Information

Animal and Human Bites Guidelines *on page 1584*

Antimicrobial Drugs of Choice *on page 1588*

Desensitization Protocols *on page 1525*

USPHA/IDSA Guidelines for the Prevention of Opportunistic Infections in Persons With HIV *on page 1574*

U.S. Brand Names Bactrim™; Bactrim™ DS; Septra®; Septra® DS; Sulfatrim®; Sulfatrim® DS

Canadian Brand Names Apo®-Sulfatrim; Novo-Trimel; Novo-Trimel D.S.; Nu-Cotrimox®; Septra®; Septra® DS; Septra® Injection

Synonyms Co-Trimoxazole; SMZ-TMP; TMP-SMZ; Trimethoprim and Sulfamethoxazole

Therapeutic Category Antibiotic, Sulfonamide Derivative

Use

Oral treatment of urinary tract infections due to *E. coli*, *Klebsiella* and *Enterobacter* sp, *M. morganii*, *P. mirabilis* and *P. vulgaris*; acute otitis media in children and acute exacerbations of chronic bronchitis in adults due to susceptible strains of *H. influenzae* or *S. pneumoniae*; prophylaxis of *Pneumocystis carinii* pneumonitis (PCP), traveler's diarrhea due to enterotoxigenic *E. coli* or *Cyclospora*

I.V. treatment or severe or complicated infections when oral therapy is not feasible, for documented PCP, empiric treatment of PCP in immune compromised patients; treatment of documented or suspected shigellosis, typhoid fever, *Nocardia asteroides* infection, or other infections caused by susceptible bacteria

Unlabeled/Investigational Use Cholera and salmonella-type infections and nocardiosis; chronic prostatitis; as prophylaxis in neutropenic patients with *P. carinii* infections, in leukemics, and in patients following renal transplantation, to decrease incidence of gram-negative rod infections

Pregnancy Risk Factor C/D (at term - expert analysis)

Pregnancy/Breast-Feeding Implications Do not use at term to avoid kernicterus in the newborn and use during pregnancy only if risks outweigh the benefits since folic acid metabolism may be affected

Contraindications Hypersensitivity to any sulfa drug, trimethoprim, or any component of the formulation; porphyria; megaloblastic anemia due to folate deficiency; infants <2 months of age; marked hepatic damage; severe renal disease; pregnancy (at term)

Warnings/Precautions Use with caution in patients with G6PD deficiency, impaired renal or hepatic function or potential folate deficiency (malnourished, chronic anticonvulsant therapy, or elderly); maintain adequate hydration to prevent crystalluria; adjust dosage in patients with renal impairment. Injection vehicle contains benzyl alcohol and sodium metabisulfite.

Chemical similarities are present among sulfonamides, sulfonylureas, carbonic anhydrase inhibitors, thiazides, and loop diuretics (except ethacrynic acid). Use in patients with sulfonamide allergy is specifically contraindicated in product labeling, however a risk of cross-reaction exists in patients with allergy to any of these compounds; avoid use when previous reaction has been severe.

Fatalities associated with severe reactions including Stevens-Johnson syndrome, toxic epidermal necrolysis, hepatic necrosis, agranulocytosis, aplastic anemia and other blood (Continued)

Sulfamethoxazole and Trimethoprim *(Continued)*

dyscrasias; discontinue use at first sign of rash. Elderly patients appear at greater risk for more severe adverse reactions. May cause hypoglycemia, particularly in malnourished, or patients with renal or hepatic impairment. Use with caution in patients with porphyria or thyroid dysfunction. Slow acetylators may be more prone to adverse reactions. Caution in patients with allergies or asthma. May cause hyperkalemia (associated with high doses of trimethoprim). Incidence of adverse effects appears to be increased in patients with AIDS.

Adverse Reactions The most common adverse reactions include gastrointestinal upset (nausea, vomiting, anorexia) and dermatologic reactions (rash or urticaria). Rare, life-threatening reactions have been associated with co-trimoxazole, including severe dermatologic reactions and hepatotoxic reactions. Most other reactions listed are rare, however, frequency cannot be accurately estimated.

Cardiovascular: Allergic myocarditis

Central nervous system: Confusion, depression, hallucinations, seizures, aseptic meningitis, peripheral neuritis, fever, ataxia, kernicterus in neonates

Dermatologic: Rashes, pruritus, urticaria, photosensitivity; rare reactions include erythema multiforme, Stevens-Johnson syndrome, toxic epidermal necrolysis, exfoliative dermatitis, and Henoch-Schönlein purpura

Endocrine & metabolic: Hyperkalemia (generally at high dosages), hyperglycemia

Gastrointestinal: Nausea, vomiting, anorexia, stomatitis, diarrhea, pseudomembranous colitis, pancreatitis

Hematologic: Thrombocytopenia, megaloblastic anemia, granulocytopenia, eosinophilia, pancytopenia, aplastic anemia, methemoglobinemia, hemolysis (with G6PD deficiency), agranulocytosis

Hepatic: Elevated serum transaminases, hepatotoxicity (including hepatitis, cholestasis, and hepatic necrosis), hyperbilirubinemia

Neuromuscular & skeletal: Arthralgia, myalgia, rhabdomyolysis

Renal: Interstitial nephritis, crystalluria, renal failure, nephrotoxicity (in association with cyclosporine), diuresis

Respiratory: Cough, dyspnea, pulmonary infiltrates

Miscellaneous: Serum sickness, angioedema, periarteritis nodosa (rare), systemic lupus erythematosus (rare)

Overdosage/Toxicology Symptoms of acute overdose include nausea, vomiting, GI distress, hematuria, and crystalluria. Following GI decontamination, treatment is supportive. Adequate fluid intake is essential. Peritoneal dialysis is not effective and hemodialysis is only moderately effective in removing sulfamethoxazole and trimethoprim.

Drug Interactions

Cytochrome P450 Effect: CYP2C9 enzyme inhibitor

Increased Effect/Toxicity: Co-trimoxazole may cause an increased effect of sulfonylureas and oral anticoagulants (warfarin). Co-trimoxazole may displace highly protein-bound drugs like methotrexate, phenytoin, or cyclosporine causing increased free serum concentrations, leading to increased toxicity of these agents. May also compete for renal excretion of methotrexate. Co-trimoxazole may enhance the nephrotoxicity of cyclosporine and may increase digoxin concentrations.

Decreased Effect: Co-trimoxazole causes decreased effect of cyclosporines and tricyclic antidepressants. Procaine and indomethacin may cause decreased effect of co-trimoxazole.

Ethanol/Nutrition/Herb Interactions Herb/Nutraceutical: Avoid dong quai, St John's wort (may also cause photosensitization).

Stability Do not refrigerate injection; is less soluble in more alkaline pH; protect from light; do not use NS as a diluent; injection vehicle contains benzyl alcohol and sodium metabisulfite Stability of parenteral admixture at room temperature (25°C):

5 mL/125 mL D_5W = 6 hours
5 mL/100 mL D_5W = 4 hours
5 mL/75 mL D_5W = 2 hours

Mechanism of Action Sulfamethoxazole interferes with bacterial folic acid synthesis and growth via inhibition of dihydrofolic acid formation from para-aminobenzoic acid; trimethoprim inhibits dihydrofolic acid reduction to tetrahydrofolate resulting in sequential inhibition of enzymes of the folic acid pathway

Pharmacodynamics/Kinetics See individual agents.

Usual Dosage Dosage recommendations are based on the trimethoprim component

Children >2 months:

Mild to moderate infections: Oral, I.V.: 8 mg TMP/kg/day in divided doses every 12 hours
Serious infection/*Pneumocystis*: I.V.: 20 mg TMP/kg/day in divided doses every 6 hours
Urinary tract infection prophylaxis: Oral: 2 mg TMP/kg/dose daily
Prophylaxis of *Pneumocystis*: Oral, I.V.: 10 mg TMP/kg/day or 150 mg TMP/m² /day in divided doses every 12 hours for 3 days/week; dose should not exceed 320 mg trimethoprim and 1600 mg sulfamethoxazole 3 days/week
Cholera: Oral, I.V.: 5 mg TMP/kg twice daily for 3 days
Cyclospora: Oral, I.V.: 5 mg TMP/kg twice daily for 7 days

Adults:

Urinary tract infection/chronic bronchitis: Oral: 1 double strength tablet every 12 hours for 10-14 days
Sepsis: I.V.: 20 TMP/kg/day divided every 6 hours
Pneumocystis carinii:
Prophylaxis: Oral: 1 double strength tablet daily or 3 times/week
Treatment: Oral, I.V.: 15-20 mg TMP/kg/day in 3-4 divided doses
Cholera: Oral, I.V.: 160 mg TMP twice daily for 3 days
Cyclospora: Oral, I.V.: 160 mg TMP twice daily for 7 days
Nocardia: Oral, I.V.: 640 mg TMP/day in divided doses for several months (duration is controversial; an average of 7 months has been reported)

Dosing adjustment in renal impairment: Adults:

I.V.:

Cl$_{cr}$ 15-30 mL/minute: Administer 2.5-5 mg/kg every 12 hours

Cl$_{cr}$ <15 mL/minute: Administer 2.5-5 mg/kg every 24 hours

Oral:

Cl$_{cr}$ 15-30 mL/minute: Administer 1 double strength tablet every 24 hours or 1 single strength tablet every 12 hours

Cl$_{cr}$ <15 mL/minute: Not recommended

Dietary Considerations Should be taken with a glass of water on empty stomach.

Administration Infuse over 60-90 minutes, must dilute well before giving; may be given less diluted in a central line; not for I.M. injection; maintain adequate fluid intake to prevent crystalluria

Test Interactions ↑ creatinine (Jaffé alkaline picrate reaction); increased serum methotrexate by dihydrofolate reductase method

Patient Information Take oral medication with 8 oz of water on an empty stomach (1 hour before or 2 hours after meals) for best absorption; report any skin rashes immediately; finish all medication, do not skip doses

Nursing Implications

Maintain adequate fluid intake to prevent crystalluria; infuse I.V. co-trimoxazole over 60-90 minutes; must be further diluted 1:25 (5 mL drug to 125 mL diluent, ie, D$_5$W); in patients who require fluid restriction, a 1:15 dilution (5 mL drug to 75 mL diluent, ie, D$_5$W) or a 1:10 dilution (5 mL drug to 50 mL diluent, ie, D$_5$W) can be administered

Monitor CBC, renal function test, liver function test, urinalysis

Dosage Forms The 5:1 ratio (SMX:TMP) remains constant in all dosage forms:

Injection: Sulfamethoxazole 80 mg and trimethoprim 16 mg per mL (5 mL, 10 mL, 20 mL, 30 mL, 50 mL)

Suspension, oral: Sulfamethoxazole 200 mg and trimethoprim 40 mg per 5 mL (20 mL, 100 mL, 150 mL, 200 mL, 480 mL)

Tablet: Sulfamethoxazole 400 mg and trimethoprim 80 mg

Tablet, double strength: Sulfamethoxazole 800 mg and trimethoprim 160 mg

♦ **Sulfamylon**® *see Mafenide on page 831*

Sulfanilamide (sul fa NIL a mide)

U.S. Brand Names AVC™

Canadian Brand Names AVC®

Therapeutic Category Antifungal Agent, Vaginal

Use Treatment of vulvovaginitis caused by *Candida albicans*

Pregnancy Risk Factor C (avoid use after 7th month)

Contraindications Hypersensitivity to sulfanilamide or any component of the formulation; pregnancy (near term)

Warnings/Precautions Since sulfonamides may be absorbed from vaginal mucosa, the same precaution for oral sulfonamides apply (eg, blood dyscrasias); if a rash develops, terminate therapy immediately. Use vaginal applicators very cautiously after the 7th month of pregnancy.

Adverse Reactions Frequency not defined.

Dermatologic: Stevens-Johnson syndrome (infrequent)

Genitourinary: Burning, increased discomfort, irritation of penis of sexual partner

Miscellaneous: Allergic reactions, systemic reactions (rare)

Mechanism of Action Interferes with microbial folic acid synthesis and growth via inhibition of para-aminiobenzoic acid metabolism; exerts a bacteriostatic action

Usual Dosage Adults: Female: Insert one applicatorful intravaginally once or twice daily continued through 1 complete menstrual cycle or insert one suppository intravaginally once or twice daily for 30 days

Patient Information Complete full course of therapy; notify physician if burning or irritation become severe or persist or if allergic symptoms occur; insert high into vagina; use of an applicator is not recommended during pregnancy; avoid sexual intercourse during treatment

Nursing Implications Avoid excessive exposure to sunlight; complete full course of therapy; notify physician if burning or irritation become severe or persist or if allergic symptoms occur

Dosage Forms

Cream, vaginal: 15% [150 mg/g] (120 g with applicator)

Suppository, vaginal: 1.05 g (16s)

Sulfasalazine (sul fa SAL a zeen)

Related Information

Sulfonamide Derivatives *on page 1515*

U.S. Brand Names Azulfidine®; Azulfidine® EN-tabs®

Canadian Brand Names Alti-Sulfasalazine®; Salazopyrin®; Salazopyrin En-Tabs®; S.A.S.™

Synonyms Salicylazosulfapyridine

Therapeutic Category 5-Aminosalicylic Acid Derivative; Anti-inflammatory Agent

Use Management of ulcerative colitis; enteric coated tablets are also used for rheumatoid arthritis (including juvenile rheumatoid arthritis) in patients who inadequately respond to analgesics and NSAIDs

Unlabeled/Investigational Use Ankylosing spondylitis, collagenous colitis, Crohn's disease, psoriasis, psoriatic arthritis, juvenile chronic arthritis

Pregnancy Risk Factor B/D (at term)

Pregnancy/Breast-Feeding Implications Sulfonamides are excreted in human breast milk and may cause kernicterus in the newborn. Although sulfapyridine has poor bilirubin-displacing ability, use with caution in women who are breast-feeding.

Contraindications Hypersensitivity to sulfasalazine, sulfa drugs, salicylates, or any component of the formulation; porphyria; GI or GU obstruction; children <2 years of age; pregnancy (at term)

(Continued)

Sulfasalazine *(Continued)*

Warnings/Precautions Use with caution in patients with renal impairment; impaired hepatic function or urinary obstruction, blood dyscrasias severe allergies or asthma, or G6PD deficiency; may cause folate deficiency (consider providing 1 mg/day folate supplement). Chemical similarities are present among sulfonamides, sulfonylureas, carbonic anhydrase inhibitors, thiazides, and loop diuretics (except ethacrynic acid). Use in patients with sulfonamide allergy is specifically contraindicated in product labeling, however a risk of cross-reaction exists in patients with allergy to any of these compounds; avoid use when previous reaction has been severe.

Adverse Reactions

>10%:

Central nervous system: Headache (33%)

Dermatologic: Photosensitivity

Gastrointestinal: Anorexia, nausea, vomiting, diarrhea (33%), gastric distress

Genitourinary: Reversible oligospermia (33%)

<3% (Limited to important or life-threatening): Alopecia, anaphylaxis, aplastic anemia, ataxia, crystalluria, depression, exfoliative dermatitis, granulocytopenia, hallucinations, Heinz body anemia, hemolytic anemia, hepatitis, interstitial nephritis, jaundice, leukopenia, Lyell's syndrome, myelodysplastic syndrome, nephropathy (acute), neutropenic enterocolitis, pancreatitis, peripheral neuropathy, photosensitization, pruritus, rhabdomyolysis, seizures, serum sickness-like reactions, skin discoloration, Stevens-Johnson syndrome, thrombocytopenia, thyroid function disturbance, urine discoloration, urticaria, vasculitis, vertigo

Overdosage/Toxicology Symptoms include drowsiness, dizziness, anorexia, abdominal pain, nausea, vomiting, hemolytic anemia, acidosis, jaundice, fever, and agranulocytosis. The aniline radical is responsible for hematologic toxicity. High volume diuresis may aid in elimination and prevention of renal failure, gastric lavage or emesis plus catharsis, alkalinize urine. Dialysis may be helpful.

Drug Interactions

Decreased Effect: Decreased effect with iron, digoxin and PABA or PABA metabolites of drugs (eg, procaine, proparacaine, tetracaine). Decreased effect of oral anticoagulants, methotrexate, and oral hypoglycemic agents.

Ethanol/Nutrition/Herb Interactions

Food: May impair folate absorption.

Herb/Nutraceutical: Avoid dong quai, St John's wort (may also cause photosensitization)

Stability Protect from light; shake suspension well

Mechanism of Action Acts locally in the colon to decrease the inflammatory response and systemically interferes with secretion by inhibiting prostaglandin synthesis

Pharmacodynamics/Kinetics

Absorption: 10% to 15% as unchanged drug from small intestine

Distribution: Small amounts enter feces and breast milk

Metabolism: Via colonic intestinal flora to sulfapyridine and 5-aminosalicylic acid (5-ASA); following absorption, sulfapyridine undergoes N-acetylation and ring hydroxylation while 5-ASA undergoes N-acetylation

Half-life elimination: 5.7-10 hours

Excretion: Primarily urine (as unchanged drug, components, and acetylated metabolites)

Usual Dosage Oral:

Children ≥2 years: Ulcerative colitis: Initial: 40-60 mg/kg/day in 3-6 divided doses; maintenance dose: 20-30 mg/kg/day in 4 divided doses

Children ≥6 years: Juvenile rheumatoid arthritis: 30-50 mg/kg/day in 2 divided doses; Initial: Begin with $1/4$ to $1/3$ of expected maintenance dose; increase weekly; maximum: 2 g/day typically

Adults: Enteric coated tablet:

Ulcerative colitis: Initial: 1 g 3-4 times/day, 2 g/day maintenance in divided doses; may initiate therapy with 0.5-1 g/day

Rheumatoid arthritis: Initial: 0.5-1 g/day; increase weekly to maintenance dose of 2 g/day in 2 divided doses; maximum: 3 g/day (if response to 2 g/day is inadequate after 12 weeks of treatment)

Dosing interval in renal impairment:

Cl_{cr} 10-30 mL/minute: Administer twice daily

Cl_{cr} <10 mL/minute: Administer once daily

Dosing adjustment in hepatic impairment: Avoid use

Dietary Considerations Since sulfasalazine impairs folate absorption, consider providing 1 mg/day folate supplement.

Administration GI intolerance is common during the first few days of therapy (administer with meals)

Patient Information Maintain adequate fluid intake; take after meals; may cause orange-yellow discoloration of urine and skin; take after meals or with food; do not take with antacids; may permanently stain soft contact lenses yellow; avoid prolonged exposure to sunlight; shake well before using

Nursing Implications Drug commonly imparts an orange-yellow discoloration to urine and skin

Dosage Forms

Tablet: 500 mg

Tablet, enteric coated: 500 mg

♦ **Sulfatrim®** *see* Sulfamethoxazole and Trimethoprim *on page 1273*

♦ **Sulfatrim® DS** *see* Sulfamethoxazole and Trimethoprim *on page 1273*

Sulfinpyrazone *(sul fin PEER a zone)*

U.S. Brand Names Anturane®

Canadian Brand Names Apo®-Sulfinpyrazone; Nu-Sulfinpyrazone

Therapeutic Category Uricosuric Agent

Use Treatment of chronic gouty arthritis and intermittent gouty arthritis

Unlabeled/Investigational Use To decrease the incidence of sudden death postmyocardial infarction

Pregnancy Risk Factor C/D (near term - expert analysis)

Contraindications Hypersensitivity to sulfinpyrazone, phenylbutazone, other pyrazoles, or any component of the formulation; active peptic ulcer; GI inflammation; blood dyscrasias; pregnancy (near term)

Warnings/Precautions Safety and efficacy not established in children <18 years of age, use with caution in patients with impaired renal function and urolithiasis

Adverse Reactions Frequency not defined.

Cardiovascular: Flushing

Central nervous system: Dizziness, headache

Dermatologic: Dermatitis, rash

Gastrointestinal (most frequent adverse effects): Nausea, vomiting, stomach pain

Genitourinary: Polyuria

Hematologic: Anemia, leukopenia, increased bleeding time (decreased platelet aggregation)

Hepatic: Hepatic necrosis

Renal: Nephrotic syndrome, uric acid stones

Overdosage/Toxicology Symptoms include drowsiness, dizziness, anorexia, abdominal pain, nausea, vomiting, hemolytic anemia, acidosis, jaundice, fever, and agranulocytosis. The aniline radical is responsible for hematologic toxicity. High volume diuresis may aid in elimination and prevention of renal failure. Leucovorin 5-15 mg/day has been used to speed recovery of bone marrow.

Drug Interactions

Cytochrome P450 Effect: CYP2C and 3A3/4 enzyme inducer; CYP2C9 enzyme inhibitor

Increased Effect/Toxicity: Increased effect of oral hypoglycemics and anticoagulants. Risk of acetaminophen hepatotoxicity is increased, while therapeutic effects may be reduced.

Decreased Effect: Decreased effect/levels of theophylline, verapamil. Decreased uricosuric activity with salicylates, niacins.

Ethanol/Nutrition/Herb Interactions Herb/Nutraceutical: Avoid dong quai, St John's wort (may also cause photosensitization).

Mechanism of Action Acts by increasing the urinary excretion of uric acid, thereby decreasing blood urate levels; this effect is therapeutically useful in treating patients with acute intermittent gout, chronic tophaceous gout, and acts to promote resorption of tophi; also has antithrombic and platelet inhibitory effects

Pharmacodynamics/Kinetics

Absorption: Complete and rapid

Metabolism: Hepatic to two active metabolites

Half-life elimination: 2.7-6 hours

Time to peak, serum: 1.6 hours

Excretion: Urine (22% to 50% as unchanged drug)

Usual Dosage Adults: Oral: 100-200 mg twice daily; maximum daily dose: 800 mg

Dosing adjustment in renal impairment: Cl_{cr} <50 mL/minute: Avoid use

Dietary Considerations Should be taken with food or milk.

Monitoring Parameters Serum and urinary uric acid, CBC

Test Interactions ↓ uric acid (S)

Nursing Implications Monitor serum and urinary uric acid

Dosage Forms

Capsule: 200 mg

Tablet: 100 mg

SulfiSOXAZOLE (sul fi SOKS a zole)

Related Information

Antimicrobial Drugs of Choice *on page 1588*
Sulfonamide Derivatives *on page 1515*

U.S. Brand Names Gantrisin®; Truxazole®

Canadian Brand Names Novo-Soxazole®; Sulfizole®

Synonyms Sulfisoxazole Acetyl; Sulphafurazole

Therapeutic Category Antibiotic, Sulfonamide Derivative

Use Treatment of urinary tract infections, otitis media, *Chlamydia*; nocardiosis; treatment of acute pelvic inflammatory disease in prepubertal children; often used in combination with trimethoprim

Pregnancy Risk Factor B/D (near term)

Contraindications Hypersensitivity to sulfisoxazole, any sulfa drug, or any component of the formulation; porphyria; infants <2 months of age (sulfas compete with bilirubin for protein binding sites); patients with urinary obstruction; sunscreens containing PABA; pregnancy (at term)

Warnings/Precautions Use with caution in patients with G6PD deficiency (hemolysis may occur), hepatic or renal impairment; dosage modification required in patients with renal impairment; risk of crystalluria should be considered in patients with impaired renal function. Chemical similarities are present among sulfonamides, sulfonylureas, carbonic anhydrase inhibitors, thiazides, and loop diuretics (except ethacrynic acid). Use in patients with sulfonamide allergy is specifically contraindicated in product labeling, however a risk of cross-reaction exists in patients with allergy to any of these compounds; avoid use when previous reaction has been severe.

Adverse Reactions Frequency not defined.

Cardiovascular: Vasculitis

Central nervous system: Fever, dizziness, headache

Dermatologic: Itching, rash, photosensitivity, Lyell's syndrome, Stevens-Johnson syndrome

Endocrine & metabolic: Thyroid function disturbance

Gastrointestinal: Anorexia, nausea, vomiting, diarrhea

Genitourinary: Crystalluria, hematuria,

(Continued)

SulfiSOXAZOLE *(Continued)*

Hematologic: Granulocytopenia, leukopenia, thrombocytopenia, aplastic anemia, hemolytic anemia

Hepatic: Jaundice, hepatitis

Renal: Interstitial nephritis

Miscellaneous: Serum sickness-like reactions

Overdosage/Toxicology Symptoms include drowsiness, dizziness, anorexia, abdominal pain, nausea, vomiting, hemolytic anemia, acidosis, jaundice, fever, and agranulocytosis. Doses of as little as 2-5 g/day may produce toxicity. The aniline radical is responsible for hematologic toxicity. High volume diuresis may aid in elimination and prevention of renal failure.

Drug Interactions

Increased Effect/Toxicity: Increased effect of oral anticoagulants, methotrexate, and oral hypoglycemic agents. May increase phenytoin levels. Risk of adverse reactions (thrombocytopenia purpura) may be increased by thiazide.

Decreased Effect: Decreased effect with PABA or PABA metabolites of drugs (eg, procaine, proparacaine, tetracaine), thiopental. May decrease cyclosporine levels.

Ethanol/Nutrition/Herb Interactions

Food: Interferes with folate absorption.

Herb/Nutraceutical: Avoid dong quai, St John's wort (may also cause photosensitization).

Stability Protect from light

Mechanism of Action Interferes with bacterial growth by inhibiting bacterial folic acid synthesis through competitive antagonism of PABA

Pharmacodynamics/Kinetics

Absorption: Sulfisoxazole acetyl is hydrolyzed in GI tract to sulfisoxazole which is readily absorbed

Distribution: Crosses placenta; enters breast milk

CSF:blood level ratio: Normal meninges: 50% to 80%; Inflamed meninges: 80+%

Protein binding: 85% to 88%

Metabolized: Hepatic via acetylation and glucuronide conjugation to inactive compounds

Half-life elimination: 4-7 hours; prolonged with renal impairment

Time to peak, serum: 2-3 hours

Excretion: Primarily urine (95%, 40% to 60% as unchanged drug) within 24 hours

Usual Dosage Oral: Not for use in patients <2 months of age:

Children >2 months: Initial: 75 mg/kg, followed by 120-150 mg/kg/day in divided doses every 4-6 hours; not to exceed 6 g/day

Adults: Initial: 2-4 g, then 4-8 g/day in divided doses every 4-6 hours

Dosing interval in renal impairment:

Cl_{cr} 10-50 mL/minute: Administer every 8-12 hours

Cl_{cr} <10 mL/minute: Administer every 12-24 hours

Hemodialysis: >50% removed by hemodialysis

Dietary Considerations Should be taken with a glass of water on an empty stomach.

Administration Administer around-the-clock to promote less variation in peak and trough serum levels.

Monitoring Parameters CBC, urinalysis, renal function tests, temperature

Test Interactions False-positive protein in urine; false-positive urine glucose with Clinitest®

Patient Information Take with a glass of water on an empty stomach; avoid prolonged exposure to sunlight; report to physician any sore throat, mouth sores, rash, unusual bleeding, or fever; complete full course of therapy

Nursing Implications Maintain adequate fluid intake

Dosage Forms

Suspension, oral, pediatric, as acetyl: 500 mg/5 mL (480 mL) [raspberry flavor]

Tablet: 500 mg

♦ **Sulfisoxazole Acetyl** *see* SulfiSOXAZOLE *on page 1277*

♦ **Sulfisoxazole and Erythromycin** *see* Erythromycin and Sulfisoxazole *on page 485*

♦ **Sulfizole® (Can)** *see* SulfiSOXAZOLE *on page 1277*

♦ **Sulfonamide Derivatives** *see page 1515*

Sulindac *(sul IN dak)*

Related Information

Nonsteroidal Anti-Inflammatory Agents Comparison *on page 1512*

U.S. Brand Names Clinoril®

Canadian Brand Names Apo®-Sulin; Novo-Sundac; Nu-Sundac

Therapeutic Category Analgesic, Nonsteroidal Anti-inflammatory Drug; Anti-inflammatory Agent; Nonsteroidal Anti-inflammatory Drug (NSAID), Oral

Use Management of inflammatory disease, rheumatoid disorders, acute gouty arthritis; structurally similar to indomethacin but acts like aspirin; safest NSAID for use in mild renal impairment

Pregnancy Risk Factor B/D (3rd trimester)

Contraindications Hypersensitivity to sulindac, any component of the formulation, aspirin or other nonsteroidal anti-inflammatory drugs (NSAIDs); pregnancy (3rd trimester)

Warnings/Precautions Use with caution in patients with congestive heart failure, hypertension, dehydration, decreased renal or hepatic function, history of peptic ulcer disease or GI disease (bleeding or ulcers), or those receiving anticoagulants. Elderly are at a high risk for CNS and gastrointestinal adverse effects from nonsteroidal anti-inflammatory agents. As many as 60% of elderly can develop peptic ulceration and/or hemorrhage asymptomatically.

Use lowest effective dose for shortest period possible. Use of NSAIDs can compromise existing renal function especially when Cl_{cr} is <30 mL/minute. Withhold for at least 4-6 half-lives prior to surgical or dental procedures. May have adverse effects on fetus. Use with caution with dehydration. Use in children is not recommended.

Adverse Reactions

1% to 10%:

  Cardiovascular: Edema

  Central nervous system: Dizziness, headache, nervousness

  Dermatologic: Pruritus, rash

  Gastrointestinal: GI pain, heartburn, nausea, vomiting, diarrhea, constipation, flatulence, anorexia, abdominal cramps

  Otic: Tinnitus

<1% (Limited to important or life-threatening): Agranulocytosis, anaphylaxis, angioneurotic edema, aplastic anemia, arrhythmia, aseptic meningitis, bone marrow depression, bronchial spasm, congestive heart failure, crystalluria, depression, dyspnea, erythema multiforme, exfoliative dermatitis, GI bleeding, GI perforation, hemolytic anemia, hepatic failure, hepatitis, hypersensitivity reaction, hypertension, increased prothrombin time, interstitial nephritis, jaundice, leukopenia, nephrotic syndrome, neutropenia, pancreatitis, peptic ulcer, proteinuria, psychosis, renal failure, renal impairment, seizures, Stevens-Johnson syndrome, thrombocytopenia, toxic epidermal necrolysis

Overdosage/Toxicology Symptoms include dizziness, vomiting, nausea, abdominal pain, hypotension, coma, stupor, metabolic acidosis, and renal failure. Management of nonsteroidal anti-inflammatory drug (NSAID) intoxication is primarily supportive and symptomatic. Fluid therapy is commonly effective managing hypotension that may occur following an acute NSAID overdose, except when due to acute blood loss. Seizures tend to be very short-lived and often do not require drug treatment; although, recurrent seizures should be treated with I.V. diazepam.

Drug Interactions

  Cytochrome P450 Effect: CYP2C9 enzyme inhibitor

  Increased Effect/Toxicity: Increased toxicity with probenecid, NSAIDs. Increased toxicity of digoxin, anticoagulants, methotrexate, lithium, aminoglycosides antibiotics (reported in neonates), cyclosporine (increased nephrotoxicity), and potassium-sparing diuretics (hyperkalemia).

  Decreased Effect: Decreased effect of diuretics, beta-blockers, hydralazine, and captopril.

Ethanol/Nutrition/Herb Interactions

  Ethanol: Avoid ethanol (may enhance gastric mucosal irritation).

  Food: Food may decrease the rate but not the extent of oral absorption. The therapeutic effect of sulindac may be decreased if taken with food.

  Herb/Nutraceutical: Avoid cat's claw, dong quai, evening primrose, feverfew, garlic, ginger, ginkgo, red clover, horse chestnut, green tea, ginseng (all have additional antiplatelet activity).

Mechanism of Action Inhibits prostaglandin synthesis by decreasing the activity of the enzyme, cyclo-oxygenase, which results in decreased formation of prostaglandin precursors

Pharmacodynamics/Kinetics

  Onset of action: Analgesic: ~1 hour

  Duration: 12-24 hours

  Absorption: 90%

  Metabolism: Hepatic; sulindac is a prodrug requiring metabolic activation; to sulfide metabolite (active) for therapeutic effects; to sulfone metabolites (inactive)

  Half-life elimination: Parent drug: 7 hours; Active metabolite: 18 hours

  Excretion: Primarily urine (50%); feces (25%)

Usual Dosage Maximum therapeutic response may not be realized for up to 3 weeks

  Oral:

    Children: Dose not established

    Adults: 150-200 mg twice daily or 300-400 mg once daily; not to exceed 400 mg/day

    Dosing adjustment in hepatic impairment: Dose reduction is necessary

Dietary Considerations Drug may cause GI upset, bleeding, ulceration, perforation; take with food or milk to minimize GI upset.

Administration Should be administered with food or milk.

Monitoring Parameters Liver enzymes, BUN, serum creatinine, CBC, blood pressure; signs and symptoms of GI bleeding

Test Interactions ↑ chloride (S), ↑ sodium (S), ↑ bleeding time

Patient Information Take with food or milk; inform dentist or surgeon because of prolonged bleeding time; do not take aspirin; may cause dizziness, drowsiness, impair coordination and judgment

Nursing Implications Observe for edema and fluid retention; monitor blood pressure

Dosage Forms Tablet: 150 mg, 200 mg

Extemporaneous Preparations A suspension of sulindac can be prepared by triturating 1000 mg sulindac (5 x 200 mg tablets) with 50 mg of kelco and 400 mg of Veegum® until a powder mixture is formed; then add 30 mL of sorbitol 35% (prepared from 70% sorbitol) to form a slurry; finally add a sufficient quantity of 35% sorbitol to make a final volume of 100 mL; the final suspension is 10 mg/mL and is stable for 7 days

♦ **Sulphafurazole** *see* SulfiSOXAZOLE *on page 1277*

Sumatriptan Succinate (soo ma TRIP tan SUKS i nate)

Related Information

  Antimigraine Drugs Comparison *on page 1485*

U.S. Brand Names Imitrex®

Canadian Brand Names Imitrex®

Therapeutic Category Antimigraine Agent, Serotonin 5-HT$_{1D}$ Agonist; Serotonin Agonist

Use Acute treatment of migraine with or without aura

  Sumatriptan injection: Acute treatment of cluster headache episodes

Pregnancy Risk Factor C

Pregnancy/Breast-Feeding Implications There are no adequate and well-controlled studies using sumatriptan in pregnant women. Use only if potential benefit to the mother outweighs the potential risk to the fetus. Sumatriptan is excreted in human breast milk. Use caution if administered to a nursing woman.

(Continued)

Sumatriptan Succinate *(Continued)*

Contraindications Hypersensitivity to sumatriptan or any component of the formulation; patients with ischemic heart disease or signs or symptoms of ischemic heart disease (including Prinzmetal's angina, angina pectoris, myocardial infarction, silent myocardial ischemia); cerebrovascular syndromes (including strokes, transient ischemic attacks); peripheral vascular syndromes (including ischemic bowel disease); uncontrolled hypertension; use within 24 hours of ergotamine derivatives; use with in 24 hours of another $5-HT_1$ agonist; concurrent administration or within 2 weeks of discontinuing an MAO inhibitor, specifically MAO type A inhibitors; management of hemiplegic or basilar migraine; prophylactic treatment of migraine; severe hepatic impairment; not for I.V. administration

Warnings/Precautions

Sumatriptan is indicated only in patients ≥18 years of age with a clear diagnosis of migraine or cluster headache

Cardiac events (coronary artery vasospasm, transient ischemia, myocardial infarction, ventricular tachycardia/fibrillation, cardiac arrest and death), cerebral/subarachnoid hemorrhage, and stroke have been reported with $5-HT_1$ agonist administration

Do not give to patients with risk factors for CAD until a cardiovascular evaluation has been performed; if evaluation is satisfactory, the healthcare provider should administer the first dose and cardiovascular status should be periodically evaluated

Significant elevation in blood pressure, including hypertensive crisis, has also been reported on rare occasions in patients with and without a history of hypertension. Vasospasm-related reactions have been reported other than coronary artery vasospasm. Peripheral vascular ischemia and colonic ischemia with abdominal pain and bloody diarrhea have occurred.

Use with caution in patients with a history of seizure disorder; safety and efficacy in pediatric patients have not been established

Adverse Reactions

>10%:

Central nervous system: Dizziness (injection 12%), warm/hot sensation (injection 11%)

Gastrointestinal: Bad taste (nasal spray 13% to 24%), nausea (nasal spray 11% to 13%), vomiting (nasal spray 11% to 13%)

Local: Injection: Pain at the injection site (59%)

Neuromuscular & skeletal: Tingling (injection 13%)

1% to 10%:

Cardiovascular: Chest pain/tightness/heaviness/pressure (injection 2% to 3%, tablet 1% to 2%)

Central nervous system: Burning (injection 7%), dizziness (nasal spray 1% to 2%, tablet >1%), feeling of heaviness (injection 7%), flushing (injection 7%), pressure sensation (injection 7%), feeling of tightness (injection 5%), numbness (injection 5%), drowsiness (injection 3%, tablet >1%), malaise/fatigue (tablet 2% to 3%, injection 1%), feeling strange (injection 2%), headache (injection 2%, tablet >1%), tight feeling in head (injection 2%), nonspecified pain (tablet 1% to 2%, placebo 1%), vertigo (tablet <1% to 2%, nasal spray 1% to 2%), migraine (tablet >1%), sleepiness (tablet >1%), cold sensation (injection 1%), anxiety (injection 1%)

Gastrointestinal: Nausea (tablet >1%), vomiting (tablet >1%), hyposalivation (tablet >1%), abdominal discomfort (injection 1%), dysphagia (injection 1%)

Neuromuscular & skeletal: Neck, throat, and jaw pain/tightness/pressure (injection 2% to 5%, tablet 2% to 3%), mouth/tongue discomfort (injection 5%), paresthesia (tablet 3% to 5%), weakness (injection 5%), myalgia (injection 2%), muscle cramps (injection 1%)

Ocular: Vision alterations (injection 1%)

Respiratory: Nasal disorder/discomfort (nasal spray 2% to 4%, injection 2%), throat discomfort (injection 3%, nasal spray 1% to 2%)

Miscellaneous: Warm/cold sensation (tablet 2% to 3%, placebo 2%), nonspecified pressure/tightness/heaviness (tablet 1% to 3%, placebo 2%), diaphoresis (injection 2%)

<1% (Limited to important or life-threatening): Abdominal aortic aneurysm, acute renal failure, agitation, anaphylactoid reactions, anaphylaxis, angioneurotic edema, arrhythmia, atrial fibrillation, bronchospasm, cerebral ischemia, diarrhea, dysphagia, dystonic reaction, ECG changes, hallucinations, heart block, hematuria, hemolytic anemia, hypersensitivity reactions increased ICP, intestinal obstruction, ischemic colitis, nose/throat hemorrhage, numbness of tongue, pancytopenia, paresthesia, photosensitivity, Prinzmetal's angina, pruritus, psychomotor disorders, pulmonary embolism, rash, Raynaud syndrome, seizures, shock, stroke, subarachnoid hemorrhage, swallowing disorders, syncope, thrombocytopenia, transient myocardial ischemia, visual disturbance (accommodation disorder), xerostomia

Overdosage/Toxicology Single oral doses up to 400 mg, injectable doses up to 16 mg, and nasal doses of 40 mg have been reported without adverse effects. Treatment should be supportive and symptomatic. Monitor for at least 12 hours or until signs and symptoms subside. It is not known if hemodialysis or peritoneal dialysis is effective.

Drug Interactions

Increased Effect/Toxicity: Increased toxicity with ergot-containing drugs, avoid use, wait 24 hours from last ergot containing drug (dihydroergotamine, or methysergide) before administering sumatriptan. MAO inhibitors decrease clearance of sumatriptan increasing the risk of systemic sumatriptan toxic effects. Sumatriptan may enhance CNS toxic effects when taken with selective serotonin reuptake inhibitors (SSRIs) like fluoxetine, fluvoxamine, paroxetine, or sertraline.

Stability Store at 2°C to 20°C (36°F to 86°F); protect from light

Mechanism of Action Selective agonist for serotonin ($5-HT_{1D}$ receptor) in cranial arteries to cause vasoconstriction and reduces sterile inflammation associated with antidromic neuronal transmission correlating with relief of migraine

Pharmacodynamics/Kinetics

Onset of action: ~30 minutes

Distribution: V_d: 2.4 L/kg

Protein binding: 14% to 21%

Bioavailability: 15%

Half-life elimination: Injection, tablet: 2.5 hours; Nasal spray: 2 hours

Time to peak, serum: 5-20 minutes

Excretion:
Injection: Urine (22%) as unchanged drug, (38%) as indole acetic acid metabolite
Nasal spray: Urine (3%) as unchanged drug, (42%) as indole acetic acid metabolite
Tablet: Urine (3% as unchanged drug, 60% as indole acetic acid metabolite); feces (40%)

Usual Dosage Adults:
Oral: A single dose of 25 mg, 50 mg, or 100 mg (taken with fluids). If a satisfactory response has not been obtained at 2 hours, a second dose may be administered. Results from clinical trials show that initial doses of 50 mg and 100 mg are more effective than doses of 25 mg, and that 100 mg doses do not provide a greater effect than 50 mg and may have increased incidence of side effects. Although doses of up to 300 mg/day have been studied, the total daily dose should not exceed 200 mg. The safety of treating an average of >4 headaches in a 30-day period have not been established.

Intranasal: A single dose of 5 mg, 10 mg, or 20 mg administered in one nostril. A 10 mg dose may be achieved by administering a single 5 mg dose in each nostril. If headache returns, the dose may be repeated once after 2 hours, not to exceed a total daily dose of 40 mg. The safety of treating an average of >4 headaches in a 30-day period has not been established.

S.C.: 6 mg; a second injection may be administered at least 1 hour after the initial dose, but not more than 2 injections in a 24-hour period. If side effects are dose-limiting, lower doses may be used.

Dosage adjustment in renal impairment: Dosage adjustment not necessary

Dosage adjustment in hepatic impairment: Bioavailability of oral sumatriptan is increased with liver disease. If treatment is needed, do not exceed single doses of 50 mg. The nasal spray has not been studied in patients with hepatic impairment, however, because the spray does not undergo first-pass metabolism, levels would not be expected to alter. Use of all dosage forms is contraindicated with severe hepatic impairment.

Elderly: Due to increased risk of CAD, decreased hepatic function, and more pronounced blood pressure increases, use of the tablet dosage form in elderly patients is not recommended. Use of the nasal spray has not been studied in the elderly. Pharmacokinetics of injectable sumatriptan in the elderly are similar to healthy patients.

Administration
Oral: Should be taken with fluids as soon as symptoms to appear
Do not administer I.V.; may cause coronary vasospasm

Patient Information Take at first sign of migraine attack. This drug is to be used to relieve your migraine, not to prevent or reduce number of attacks.
Oral: If headache returns or is not fully resolved after first dose, the dose may be repeated after 2 hours. **Do not exceed 200 mg in 24 hours.** Take whole with fluids.
S.C.: If headache returns or is not fully resolved after first dose, the dose may be repeated after 1 hour. **Do not exceed two injections in 24 hours. Do not take within 24 hours of any other migraine medication without first consulting prescriber.**
Nasal: Administer dose into one nostril. If headache returns or is not fully resolved after the first dose, the dose may be repeated after 2 hours. Do not exceed 40 mg in 24 hours.
All dosage forms: Do not take within 24 hours of any other migraine medication without first consulting prescriber. You may experience some dizziness (use caution); hot flashes (cool room may help); nausea or vomiting (frequent small meals, frequent mouth care, sucking lozenges, or chewing gum may help); pain at injection site (lasts about 1 hour, will resolve); or excess sweating (will resolve). Report chest tightness or pain; excessive drowsiness; acute abdominal pain; skin rash or burning sensation; muscle weakness, soreness, or numbness; or respiratory difficulty.

Nursing Implications Pain at injection site lasts <1 hour

Dosage Forms
Injection: 12 mg/mL (0.5 mL, 2 mL)
Solution, intranasal [spray]: 5 mg (100 µL unit dose spray device); 20 mg (100 µL unit dose spray device)
Tablet: 25 mg, 50 mg, 100 mg

TACRINE

- **Synalar®** *see Fluocinolone on page 572*
- **Synalgos®-DC** *see Dihydrocodeine Compound on page 407*
- **Synarel®** *see Nafarelin on page 949*
- **Syn-Diltiazem® (Can)** *see Diltiazem on page 409*
- **Synercid®** *see Quinupristin and Dalfopristin on page 1172*
- **Synflex® (Can)** *see Naproxen on page 958*
- **Synflex® DS (Can)** *see Naproxen on page 958*
- **Synphasic® (Can)** *see Ethinyl Estradiol and Norethindrone on page 522*
- **Synthetic Lung Surfactant** *see Colfosceril Palmitate on page 333*
- **Synthroid®** *see Levothyroxine on page 799*
- **Syntocinon® (Can)** *see Oxytocin on page 1029*
- **Syprine®** *see Trientine on page 1371*
- **Syracol-CF® [OTC]** *see Guaifenesin and Dextromethorphan on page 646*
- **T₃ Sodium** *see Liothyronine on page 808*
- **T₃/T₄ Liotrix** *see Liotrix on page 808*
- **T₄** *see Levothyroxine on page 799*
- **642® Tablet (Can)** *see Propoxyphene on page 1147*
- **Tac™-3** *see Triamcinolone on page 1366*
- **Tac™-40** *see Triamcinolone on page 1366*
- **Tacozin® (Can)** *see Piperacillin and Tazobactam Sodium on page 1091*

Tacrine (TAK reen)

U.S. Brand Names Cognex®
Synonyms Tacrine Hydrochloride; Tetrahydroaminoacrine; THA
Therapeutic Category Acetylcholinesterase Inhibitor; Cholinergic Agent
Use Treatment of mild to moderate dementia of the Alzheimer's type
Pregnancy Risk Factor C
Contraindications Hypersensitivity to tacrine, acridine derivatives, or any component of the formulation; patients previously treated with tacrine who developed jaundice
Warnings/Precautions The use of tacrine has been associated with elevations in serum transaminases; serum transaminases (specifically ALT) must be monitored throughout therapy; use extreme caution in patients with current evidence of a history of abnormal liver function tests; use caution in patients with urinary tract obstruction (bladder outlet obstruction or prostatic hypertrophy), asthma, and sick-sinus syndrome (tacrine may cause bradycardia). Also, patients with cardiovascular disease, asthma, or peptic ulcer should use cautiously. Use with caution in patients with a history of seizures. May cause nausea, vomiting, or loose stools. Abrupt discontinuation or dosage decrease may worsen cognitive function. May be associated with neutropenia.
Adverse Reactions
>10%:
   Central nervous system: Headache, dizziness
   Gastrointestinal: Nausea, vomiting, diarrhea
   Miscellaneous: Elevated transaminases
1% to 10%:
   Cardiovascular: Flushing
   Central nervous system: Confusion, ataxia, insomnia, somnolence, depression, anxiety, fatigue
   Dermatologic: Rash
   Gastrointestinal: Dyspepsia, anorexia, abdominal pain, flatulence, constipation, weight loss
   Neuromuscular & skeletal: Myalgia, tremor
   Respiratory: Rhinitis
Overdosage/Toxicology Symptoms included cholinergic crisis characterized by severe nausea, vomiting, salivation, sweating, bradycardia, hypotension, cardiovascular collapse, and convulsions. Increased muscle weakness is a possibility and may result in death if respiratory muscles are involved. Treatments includes general supportive measures. Tertiary anticholinergics, such as atropine, may be used as an antidote. I.V. atropine sulfate titrated to effect is recommended; initial dose of 1-2 mg I.V. with subsequent doses based upon clinical response. Atypical increases in blood pressure and heart rate have been reported with other cholinomimetics when coadministered with quaternary anticholinergics such as glycopyrrolate.
Drug Interactions
   Cytochrome P450 Effect: CYP1A2 enzyme substrate; CYP1A2 inhibitor
   Increased Effect/Toxicity: Tacrine in combination with other cholinergic agents (eg, ambenonium, edrophonium, neostigmine, pyridostigmine, bethanechol), will likely produce additive cholinergic effects. Tacrine in combination with beta-blockers may produce additive bradycardia. Tacrine may increase the levels/effect of succinylcholine and theophylline. in elevated plasma levels. Fluvoxamine, enoxacin, and cimetidine increase tacrine concentrations via enzyme inhibition (CYP1A2).
   Decreased Effect: Enzyme inducers and cigarette smoking may reduce tacrine plasma levels via enzyme induction (CYP1A2). Tacrine may worsen Parkinson's disease and inhibit the effects of levodopa. Tacrine may antagonize the therapeutic effect of anticholinergic agents (benztropine, trihexphenidyl).
Ethanol/Nutrition/Herb Interactions Food: Food decreases bioavailability.
Mechanism of Action Centrally-acting cholinesterase inhibitor. It elevates acetylcholine in cerebral cortex by slowing the degradation of acetylcholine.
Pharmacodynamics/Kinetics
   Onset of action: May require weeks of treatment
   Time to peak, plasma: 1-2 hours
   Plasma bound: 55%
   Half-life elimination, serum: 2-4 hours, steady-state achieved in 24-36 hours

Usual Dosage Adults: Initial: 10 mg 4 times/day; may increase by 40 mg/day adjusted every 6 weeks; maximum: 160 mg/day; best administered separate from meal times.

Dose adjustment based upon transaminase elevations:

ALT ≤3 x ULN*: Continue titration

ALT >3 to ≤5 x ULN*: Decrease dose by 40 mg/day, resume when ALT returns to normal

ALT >5 x ULN*: Stop treatment, may rechallenge upon return of ALT to normal

*ULN = upper limit of normal

Patients with clinical jaundice confirmed by elevated total bilirubin (>3 mg/dL) should not be rechallenged with tacrine

Dietary Considerations Give with food if GI side effects are intolerable.

Monitoring Parameters ALT (SGPT) levels and other liver enzymes weekly for at least the first 18 weeks, then monitor once every 3 months

Reference Range In clinical trials, serum concentrations >20 ng/mL were associated with a much higher risk of development of symptomatic adverse effects

Patient Information Effect of tacrine therapy is thought to depend upon its administration at regular intervals, as directed; possibility of adverse effects such as those occurring in close temporal association with the initiation of treatment or an increase in dose (ie, nausea, vomiting, loose stools, diarrhea) and those with a delayed onset (ie, rash, jaundice, changes in the color of stool); inform physician of the emergence of new or any increase in the severity of existing adverse effects; abrupt discontinuation of the drug or a large reduction in total daily dose (80 mg/day or more) may cause a decline in cognitive function and behavioral disturbances; unsupervised increases in the dose may also have serious consequences; do not change dose without consulting physician

Nursing Implications Monitor ALT levels and other liver enzymes weekly for at least the first 18 weeks, then monitor once every 3 months

Dosage Forms Capsule, as hydrochloride: 10 mg, 20 mg, 30 mg, 40 mg

♦ **Tacrine Hydrochloride** *see* Tacrine *on page 1282*

Tacrolimus (ta KROE li mus)

U.S. Brand Names Prograf®; Protopic®

Canadian Brand Names Prograf®

Synonyms FK506

Therapeutic Category Immunosuppressant Agent; Topical Skin Product

Use

Oral/injection: Potent immunosuppressive drug used in liver or kidney transplant recipients

Topical: Moderate to severe atopic dermatitis in patients not responsive to conventional therapy or when conventional therapy is not appropriate

Unlabeled/Investigational Use Potent immunosuppressive drug used in heart, lung, small bowel transplant recipients; immunosuppressive drug for peripheral stem cell/bone marrow transplantation

Pregnancy Risk Factor C

Pregnancy/Breast-Feeding Implications

Tacrolimus crosses the placenta and reaches concentrations four times greater than maternal plasma concentrations. Neonatal hyperkalemia and renal dysfunction have been reported.

Concentrations in breast milk are equivalent to plasma concentrations; breast-feeding is not advised

Contraindications Hypersensitivity to tacrolimus or any component of the formulation

Warnings/Precautions

Oral/injection: Insulin-dependent post-transplant diabetes mellitus (PTDM) has been reported (1% to 20%); risk increases in African-American and Hispanic kidney transplant patients. Increased susceptibility to infection and the possible development of lymphoma may occur after administration of tacrolimus. Nephrotoxicity and neurotoxicity have been reported, especially with higher doses; to avoid excess nephrotoxicity do not administer simultaneously with cyclosporine; monitoring of serum concentrations (trough for oral therapy) is essential to prevent organ rejection and reduce drug-related toxicity; tonic clonic seizures may have been triggered by tacrolimus. Use caution in renal or hepatic dysfunction, dosing adjustments may be required. Delay initiation if postoperative oliguria occurs. Myocardial hypertrophy has been reported (rare). Each mL of injection contains polyoxyl 60 hydrogenated castor oil (HCO-60) (200 mg) and dehydrated alcohol USP 80% v/v. Anaphylaxis has been reported with the injection, use should be reserved for those patients not able to take oral medications.

Topical: Infections at the treatment site should be cleared prior to therapy. Patients with atopic dermatitis are predisposed to skin infections, including eczema herpeticum, varicella zoster, and herpes simplex. Discontinue use in patients with unknown cause of lymphadenopathy or acute infectious mononucleosis. Not recommended for use in patients with Netherton's syndrome. Safety not established in patients with generalized erythroderma.

Adverse Reactions

Oral, I.V.:

≥15%:

Cardiovascular: Chest pain, hypertension

Central nervous system: Dizziness, headache, insomnia, tremor (headache and tremor are associated with high whole blood concentrations and may respond to decreased dosage)

Dermatologic: Pruritus, rash

Endocrine & metabolic: Diabetes mellitus, hyperglycemia, hyperkalemia, hyperlipemia, hypomagnesemia, hypophosphatemia

Gastrointestinal: Abdominal pain, constipation, diarrhea, dyspepsia, nausea, vomiting

Genitourinary: Urinary tract infection

Hematologic: Anemia, leukocytosis, thrombocytopenia

Hepatic: Ascites

Neuromuscular & skeletal: Arthralgia, back pain, weakness, paresthesia

(Continued)

Tacrolimus *(Continued)*

Renal: Abnormal kidney function, increased creatinine, oliguria, urinary tract infection, increased BUN

Respiratory: Atelectasis, dyspnea, increased cough

3% to 15% (Limited to important or life-threatening):

Cardiovascular: Abnormal EKG, angina pectoris, deep thrombophlebitis, hemorrhage, hypotension, postural hypotension, thrombosis

Central nervous system: Agitation, amnesia, anxiety, confusion, depression, encephalopathy, hallucinations, psychosis, somnolence

Dermatologic: Acne, alopecia, exfoliative dermatitis, hirsutism, photosensitivity reaction, skin discoloration

Endocrine & metabolic: Cushing's syndrome, decreased bicarbonate, decreased serum iron, diabetes mellitus, hypercalcemia, hypercholesterolemia, hyperphosphatemia

Gastrointestinal: Dysphagia, esophagitis, GI perforation/hemorrhage, ileus

Hematologic: Coagulation disorder, decreased prothrombin, leukopenia

Hepatic: Cholangitis, jaundice, hepatitis

Neuromuscular & skeletal: Incoordination, myasthenia, neuropathy, osteoporosis

Respiratory: Asthma, pneumothorax, pulmonary edema

Miscellaneous: Abscess, allergic reaction, flu-like syndrome, peritonitis, sepsis

Postmarketing and/or case reports (Limited to important or life-threatening): Acute renal failure, anaphylaxis, coma, deafness, delirium, hearing loss, hemolytic-uremic syndrome, leukoencephalopathy, lymphoproliferative disorder (related to EBV), myocardial hypertrophy (associated with ventricular dysfunction), pancreatitis, seizures, Stevens-Johnson syndrome, thrombocytopenic purpura, torsade de pointes

Topical:

\>10%:

Central nervous system: Headache (5% to 20%), fever (1% to 21%)

Dermatologic: Skin burning (43% to 58%), pruritus (41% to 46%), erythema (12% to 28%)

Respiratory: Increased cough (18% children)

Miscellaneous: Flu-like syndrome (23% to 28%), allergic reaction (4% to 12%)

Overdosage/Toxicology Symptoms are extensions of pharmacologic activity and listed adverse effects. Symptomatic and supportive treatment is required. Hemodialysis is not effective.

Drug Interactions

Cytochrome P450 Effect: CYP3A3/4 enzyme substrate

Increased Effect/Toxicity: Amphotericin B and other nephrotoxic antibiotics have the potential to increase tacrolimus-associated nephrotoxicity. Agents which may increase tacrolimus plasma concentrations resulting in toxicity are erythromycin, clarithromycin, clotrimazole, fluconazole, itraconazole, ketoconazole, diltiazem, nicardipine, verapamil, bromocriptine, cimetidine, cisapride, danazol, metoclopramide, methylprednisolone, and cyclosporine (synergistic immunosuppression).

Decreased Effect:

Antacids: Impaired tacrolimus absorption (separate administration by at least 2 hours).

Agents which may decrease tacrolimus plasma concentrations and reduce the therapeutic effect include rifampin, rifabutin, phenytoin, phenobarbital, and carbamazepine.

St John's wort may reduce tacrolimus serum concentrations (avoid concurrent use).

Ethanol/Nutrition/Herb Interactions

Food: Decreases rate and extent of absorption. High-fat meals have most pronounced effect (35% decrease in AUC, 77% decrease in C_{max}). Grapefruit juice, CYP3A3/4 inhibitor, may increase serum level and/or toxicity of tacrolimus; avoid concurrent use.

Herb/Nutraceutical: St John's wort: May reduce tacrolimus serum concentrations (avoid concurrent use).

Stability

Injection: Prior to dilution, store at 5°C to 25°C (41°F to 77°F). Polyvinyl-containing sets (eg, Venoset®, Accuset®) adsorb significant amounts of the drug, and their use may lead to a lower dose being delivered to the patient. FK506 admixtures prepared in 5% dextrose injection or 0.9% sodium chloride injection should be stored in polyolefin containers or glass bottles. Infusion of FK506 through PVC tubings did not result in decreased concentration of the drug, however, loss by absorption may be more important when lower concentrations of FK506 are used. Stable for 24 hours in D_5W or NS in glass or polyolefin containers.

Capsules and ointment: Store at room temperature 25°C (77°F)

Mechanism of Action Suppresses cellular immunity (inhibits T-lymphocyte activation), possibly by binding to an intracellular protein, FKBP-12

Pharmacodynamics/Kinetics

Absorption: Better in resected patients with a closed stoma; unlike cyclosporine, clamping of the T-tube in liver transplant patients does not alter trough concentrations or AUC

Oral: Incomplete and variable; food within 15 minutes of administration decreases absorption (27%)

Topical: Serum concentrations range from undetectable to 20 ng/mL (<5 ng/mL in majority of adult patients studied)

Protein binding: 99%

Metabolism: Extensively hepatic via CYP3A3/4 to eight possible metabolites (major metabolite: 31-demethyl tacrolimus, shows same activity as tacrolimus *in vitro*)

Bioavailability: Oral: Adults: 7% to 28%, Children: 10% to 52%; Topical: <0.5%, absolute bioavailability is unknown

Half-life elimination: Variable, 21-61 hours in healthy volunteers

Time to peak: 0.5-4 hours

Excretion: Feces (~92%); feces/urine (<1% as unchanged drug)

Usual Dosage

Children:

Liver transplant: Patients without pre-existing renal or hepatic dysfunction have required and tolerated higher doses than adults to achieve similar blood concentrations. It is recommended that therapy be initiated at high end of the recommended adult I.V. and oral dosing ranges; dosage adjustments may be required.

Oral: Initial dose: 0.15-0.20 mg/kg/day in 2 divided doses, given every 12 hours; begin oral dose no sooner than 6 hours post-transplant; adjunctive therapy with corticosteroids is recommended; if switching from I.V. to oral, the oral dose should be started 8-12 hours after stopping the infusion

Typical whole blood trough concentrations: Months 1-12: 5-20 ng/mL

I.V.: **Note:** I.V. route should only be used in patients not able to take oral medications, anaphylaxis has been reported. Initial dose: 0.03-0.05 mg/kg/day as a continuous infusion; begin no sooner than 6 hours post-transplant; adjunctive therapy with corticosteroids is recommended; continue only until oral medication can be tolerated

Children ≥2 years: Moderate to severe atopic dermatitis: Topical: Apply 0.03% ointment to affected area twice daily; rub in gently and completely; continue applications for 1 week after symptoms have cleared

Adults:

Kidney transplant:

Oral: Initial dose: 0.2 mg/kg/day in 2 divided doses, given every 12 hours; initial dose may be given within 24 hours of transplant, but should be delayed until renal function has recovered; African-American patients may require larger doses to maintain trough concentration

Typical whole blood trough concentrations: Months 1-3: 7- 20 ng/mL; months 4-12: 5-15 ng/mL

I.V.: **Note:** I.V. route should only be used in patients not able to take oral medications, anaphylaxis has been reported. Initial dose: 0.03-0.05 mg/kg/day as a continuous infusion; begin no sooner than 6 hours post-transplant, starting at lower end of the dosage range; adjunctive therapy with corticosteroids is recommended; continue only until oral medication can be tolerated

Liver transplant:

Oral: Initial dose: 0.1-0.15 mg/kg/day in 2 divided doses, given every 12 hours; begin oral dose no sooner than 6 hours post-transplant; adjunctive therapy with corticosteroids is recommended; if switching from I.V. to oral, the oral dose should be started 8-12 hours after stopping the infusion

Typical whole blood trough concentrations: Months 1-12: 5-20 ng/mL

I.V.: **Note:** I.V. route should only be used in patients not able to take oral medications, anaphylaxis has been reported. Initial dose: 0.03-0.05 mg/kg/day as a continuous infusion; begin no sooner than 6 hours post-transplant starting at lower end of the dosage range; adjunctive therapy with corticosteroids is recommended; continue only until oral medication can be tolerated

Prevention of graft-vs-host disease: I.V.: 0.03 mg/kg/day as continuous infusion

Moderate to severe atopic dermatitis: Topical: Apply 0.03% or 0.1% ointment to affected area twice daily; rub in gently and completely; continue applications for 1 week after symptoms have cleared

Dosing adjustment in renal impairment: Evidence suggests that lower doses should be used; patients should receive doses at the lowest value of the recommended I.V. and oral dosing ranges; further reductions in dose below these ranges may be required

Tacrolimus therapy should usually be delayed up to 48 hours or longer in patients with postoperative oliguria

Hemodialysis: Not removed by hemodialysis; supplemental dose is not necessary

Peritoneal dialysis: Significant drug removal is unlikely based on physiochemical characteristics

Dosing adjustment in hepatic impairment: Use of tacrolimus in liver transplant recipients experiencing post-transplant hepatic impairment may be associated with increased risk of developing renal insufficiency related to high whole blood levels of tacrolimus. The presence of moderate-to-severe hepatic dysfunction (serum bilirubin >2 mg/dL) appears to affect the metabolism of FK506. The half-life of the drug was prolonged and the clearance reduced after I.V. administration. The bioavailability of FK506 was also increased after oral administration. The higher plasma concentrations as determined by ELISA, in patients with severe hepatic dysfunction are probably due to the accumulation of FK506 metabolites of lower activity. These patients should be monitored closely and dosage adjustments should be considered. Some evidence indicates that lower doses could be used in these patients.

Dietary Considerations Capsule: Take on an empty stomach; be consistent with timing and composition of meals if GI intolerance occurs (per manufacturer).

Administration I.V.: Administer by I.V. continuous infusion only (use infusion pump). Dilute with 5% dextrose injection or 0.9% sodium chloride injection to a final concentration between 0.004 mg/mL and 0.02 mg/mL. Use glass or polyethylene containers, do not use PVC containers. Do not use PVC tubing when administering dilute solutions

Monitoring Parameters Renal function, hepatic function, serum electrolytes, glucose and blood pressure, measure 3 times/week for first few weeks, then gradually decrease frequency as patient stabilizes. Whole blood concentrations should be used for monitoring (trough for oral therapy). Signs/symptoms of anaphylactic reactions during infusion should also be monitored.

Reference Range

Liver transplant: Whole blood trough concentration: 5-20 ng/mL

Kidney transplant: whole blood trough concentrations:

Months 1-3: 7-20 ng/mL

Months 4-12: 5-15 ng/mL

Patient Information You will be susceptible to infection (avoid crowds and people with infections or contagious diseases). May lead to diabetes mellitus, notify prescriber if you develop increased urination, increased thirst, or increased hunger. If you are diabetic, monitor glucose levels closely (may alter glucose levels). You may experience nausea, vomiting, loss of appetite (frequent small meals, frequent mouth care may help); diarrhea (boiled milk, yogurt, or buttermilk may help); constipation (increased exercise or dietary fruit, fluid, or fiber may help, if not consult prescriber); muscle or back pain (mild analgesics may be recommended). Report chest pain; acute headache or dizziness; symptoms of respiratory

(Continued)

Tacrolimus *(Continued)*

infection, cough, or difficulty breathing; unresolved gastrointestinal effects; fatigue, chills, fever, unhealed sores, white plaques in mouth, irritation in genital area; unusual bruising or bleeding; pain or irritation on urination or change in urinary patterns; rash or skin irritation; or other unusual effects related to this medication.

Oral: Take as directed, preferably 30 minutes before or 30 minutes after meals. Do not take within 2 hours before or after antacids. Do not alter dose and do not discontinue without consulting prescriber. Maintain adequate hydration (2-3 L/day of fluids unless instructed to restrict fluid intake) during entire course of therapy.

Topical: For external use only. Avoid exposure to sunlight or tanning beds. Apply to clean, dry skin. Do not cover with occlusive dressings. Burning and itching are most common in the first few days of use and improve as atopic dermatitis improves. Wash hands after use, unless hands are an area of treatment.

Nursing Implications

I.V. administration: Tacrolimus is dispensed in a 50 mL glass container or nonpolyvinyl chloride container; it is intended to be infused over at least 12 hours; polyolefin administration sets should be used. Patients should be monitored during the first 30 minutes of the infusion, and frequently thereafter, for signs/symptoms of anaphylactic reactions

Topical: Do not cover with occlusive dressings

Additional Information Additional dosing considerations:

Switch from I.V. to oral therapy: Threefold increase in dose

Pediatric patients: About 2 times higher dose compared to adults

Liver dysfunction: Decrease I.V. dose; decrease oral dose

Renal dysfunction: Does not affect kinetics; decrease dose to decrease levels if renal dysfunction is related to the drug

Dosage Forms

Capsule: 0.5 mg, 1 mg, 5 mg

Injection, with alcohol and surfactant: 5 mg/mL (1 mL)

Ointment, topical: 0.03% (30 g, 60 g); 0.1% (30 g, 60g)

Extemporaneous Preparations Tacrolimus oral suspension can be compounded at a concentration of 0.5 mg/mL; an extemporaneous suspension can be prepared by mixing the contents of six 5-mg tacrolimus capsules with equal amounts of Ora-Plus® and Simple Syrup, N.F., to make a final volume of 60 mL. The Suspension is stable for 56 days at room temperature in glass or plastic amber prescription bottles.

Esquivel C, So S, McDiarmid S, Andrews W, Colombani P. Suggested guidelines for the use of tacrolimus in pediatric liver transplant patients. *Transplantation* 1996, 61(5):847-8.

Foster JA, Jacobson PA, Johnson CE, et al. Stability of tacrolimus in an extemporaneously compounded oral liquid. (Abstract of Meeting Presentation) *American Society of Health-System Pharmacists Annual Meeting* 1996, 53:P-52(E).

♦ **Tagamet**® *see* Cimetidine *on page 293*

♦ **Tagamet**® **HB [OTC]** *see* Cimetidine *on page 293*

♦ **Talwin**® *see* Pentazocine *on page 1057*

♦ **Talwin**® **NX** *see* Pentazocine *on page 1057*

♦ **Tambocor**™ *see* Flecainide *on page 564*

♦ **Tamiflu**™ *see* Oseltamivir *on page 1015*

♦ **Tamofen**® **(Can)** *see* Tamoxifen *on page 1286*

Tamoxifen *(ta MOKS i fen)*

U.S. Brand Names Nolvadex®

Canadian Brand Names Apo®-Tamox; Gen-Tamoxifen; Nolvadex®; Nolvadex®-D; Novo-Tamoxifen; PMS-Tamoxifen; Tamofen®

Synonyms Tamoxifen Citrate

Therapeutic Category Antineoplastic Agent, Hormone Antagonist; Estrogen Receptor Antagonist

Use Palliative or adjunctive treatment of advanced breast cancer; reduce the incidence of breast cancer in women at high risk (taking into account age, number of first-degree relatives with breast cancer, previous breast biopsies, age at first live birth, age at first menstrual period, and a history of lobular carcinoma *in situ*); reduce risk of invasive breast cancer in women with ductal carcinoma *in situ* (DCIS); metastatic male breast cancer

Unlabeled/Investigational Use Treatment of mastalgia, gynecomastia, pancreatic carcinoma, and induction of ovulation. Studies have shown tamoxifen to be effective in the treatment of primary breast cancer in elderly women. Comparative studies with other antineoplastic agents in elderly women with breast cancer had more favorable survival rates with tamoxifen. Initiation of hormone therapy rather than chemotherapy is justified for elderly patients with metastatic breast cancer who are responsive.

Pregnancy Risk Factor D

Contraindications Hypersensitivity to tamoxifen or any component of the formulation; pregnancy

Warnings/Precautions Use with caution in patients with leukopenia, thrombocytopenia, or hyperlipidemias; ovulation may be induced; "hot flashes" may be countered by Bellergal-S® tablets or clonidine; decreased visual acuity, retinopathy and corneal changes have been reported with use for more than 1 year at doses above recommended; hypercalcemia in patients with bone metastasis; hepatocellular carcinomas have been reported in animal studies; endometrial hyperplasia and polyps have occurred

Adverse Reactions

>10%:

Cardiovascular: Flushing (64%)

Endocrine & metabolic: Hot flashes (67%); decreased libido (29%); tumor flare (26%) (with bone pain [5%], tumor pain, erythema)

Gastrointestinal: Mild to moderate nausea (10% to 58%), may be severe in ~3% of patients

Genitourinary: Vaginal bleeding, discharge (18%)

Hematologic: Thrombocytopenia (24% to 28%), leukopenia (28%)

1% to 10%:

Cardiovascular: Arterial and venous thrombosis

Central nervous system: Lightheadedness, depression, dizziness, headache, lassitude, mental confusion

Dermatologic: Skin rash (5%), dry skin (7%)

Endocrine & metabolic: Hypercalcemia, sodium and water retention, edema (8%)

Gastrointestinal: Vomiting

Genitourinary: Pruritus vulvae (2%), endometriosis, priapism

Hematologic: Decreased hemoglobin/hematocrit, anemia

Ocular: Retinopathy, including optic disk swelling, retinal hemorrhage, visual impairment, seen with high (>200 mg/day) doses

<1% (Limited to important or life-threatening): Endometrial and uterine cancers, neutropenia

Overdosage/Toxicology Symptoms include hypercalcemia and edema. Administer general supportive care.

Drug Interactions

Cytochrome P450 Effect: CYP3A3/4 enzyme substrate

Increased Effect/Toxicity: Allopurinol and tamoxifen results in exacerbation of allopurinol-induced hepatotoxicity. Cyclosporine serum levels may be increased when taken with tamoxifen. Significant enhancement of the anticoagulant effects of warfarin may occur with concomitant use of tamoxifen.

Ethanol/Nutrition/Herb Interactions Herb/Nutraceutical: Avoid black cohosh, dong quai in estrogen-dependent tumors.

Stability Tablets are stored at room temperature.

Mechanism of Action Competitively binds to estrogen receptors on tumors and other tissue targets, producing a nuclear complex that decreases DNA synthesis and inhibits estrogen effects; nonsteroidal agent with potent antiestrogenic properties which compete with estrogen for binding sites in breast and other tissues; cells accumulate in the G_0 and G_1 phases; therefore, tamoxifen is cytostatic rather than cytocidal.

Pharmacodynamics/Kinetics

Absorption: Well absorbed

Distribution: High concentrations found in uterus, endometrial and breast tissue

Protein binding: 99%

Metabolism: Hepatic: Major metabolites: Desmethyltamoxifen, 4-hydroxytamoxifen; undergoes enterohepatic recycling

Half-life: Distribution: 7-14 hours; Elimination: >7 days

Time to peak, serum: 4-7 hours

Excretion: Feces (26% to 51%); urine (9% to 13%)

Usual Dosage Oral (refer to individual protocols): Adults:

Breast cancer:

Adjunct to surgery/radiation therapy: 20-40 mg/day; dosages >20 mg/day in divided doses; 20 mg/day is most common

Females >50 years with positive axillary nodes: 10 mg twice daily

Metastatic: 20-40 mg/day; dosages >20 mg/day in divided doses; 20 mg/day is most common

Prevention (in high-risk females): 20 mg/day for 5 years

DCIS: 20 mg once daily for 5 years

Males: 20 mg/day

Higher dosages (up to 700 mg/day) have been investigated for use in modulation of multidrug resistance (MDR), but are not routinely used in clinical practice

Induction of ovulation (unlabeled use): 5-40 mg twice daily for 4 days

Monitoring Parameters Monitor WBC and platelet counts, tumor

Test Interactions T_4 elevations (no clinical evidence of hyperthyroidism)

Patient Information Take as directed, morning and night, and maintain adequate hydration (2-3 L/day of fluids unless instructed to restrict fluid intake). You may experience menstrual irregularities, vaginal bleeding, hot flashes, hair loss, loss of libido (these will subside when treatment is completed). Bone pain may indicate a good therapeutic response (consult prescriber for mild analgesics). For nausea/vomiting, small frequent meals, chewing gum, or sucking lozenges may help. You may experience photosensitivity (use sunscreen, wear protective clothing and eyewear, and avoid direct sunlight). Report unusual bleeding or bruising, severe weakness, sedation, mental changes, swelling or pain in calves, difficulty breathing, or any changes in vision.

Nursing Implications Increase of bone pain usually indicates a good therapeutic response

Additional Information "Hot flashes" may be countered by Bellergal-S® tablets. Oral clonidine is being studied for the treatment of tamoxifen-induced "hot flashes." The tumor flare reaction may indicate a good therapeutic response, and is often considered a good prognostic factor.

Dosage Forms Tablet, as citrate: 10 mg, 20 mg

♦ **Tamoxifen Citrate** *see* Tamoxifen *on page 1286*

Tamsulosin (tam SOO loe sin)

U.S. Brand Names Flomax®

Canadian Brand Names Flomax®

Synonyms Tamsulosin Hydrochloride

Therapeutic Category Alpha-Adrenergic Blocking Agent, Oral

Use Treatment of signs and symptoms of benign prostatic hyperplasia (BPH)

Pregnancy Risk Factor B

Contraindications Hypersensitivity to tamsulosin or any component of the formulation

Warnings/Precautions Not intended for use as an antihypertensive drug. May cause orthostasis, syncope or dizziness. Patients should avoid situations where injury may occur as a (Continued)

Tamsulosin *(Continued)*

result of syncope. Rule out prostatic carcinoma before beginning therapy with tamsulosin. Anticipate a similar effect if therapy is interrupted for a few days, if dosage is rapidly increased, or if another antihypertensive drug is introduced.

Adverse Reactions

Orthostatic hypotension (by testing criteria): First-dose orthostatic hypotension at 4 hours postdose has been observed in 7% of patients following a 0.4 mg dose as compared to 3% in a placebo group. Overall, at least one positive test was observed in 16% of patients receiving 0.4 mg and 19% of patients receiving the 0.8 mg dose as compared to 11% in a placebo group. **Percentages correspond to the 0.4 mg and 0.8 mg doses, respectively.**

>10%:
Central nervous system: Headache (19% to 21%), dizziness (15% to 17%)
Genitourinary: Abnormal ejaculation (8% to 18%)
Respiratory: Rhinitis (13% to 18%)

1% to 10%:
Cardiovascular: Chest pain (~4%)
Central nervous system: Weakness (8% to 9%), somnolence (3% to 4%), insomnia (1% to 2%)
Endocrine & metabolic: Decreased libido (1% to 2%)
Gastrointestinal: Diarrhea (4% to 6%), nausea (3% to 4%), stomach discomfort (2% to 3%), bitter taste (2% to 3%)
Neuromuscular & skeletal: Back pain (7% to 8%)
Ocular: Amblyopia (0.2% to 1%)
Respiratory: Pharyngitis (6% to 5%), cough (3% to 5%), sinusitis (2% to 4%)
Miscellaneous: Infection (9% to 11%), tooth disorder (1% to 2%)

<1% (Limited to important or life-threatening): Allergic reactions (rash, angioedema, pruritus, urticaria), constipation, elevated transaminases (case reports), orthostasis (symptomatic) (0.2% to 0.4%), palpitations, priapism, syncope (0.2% to 0.4%), vertigo (0.6% to 1%), vomiting

Drug Interactions

Cytochrome P450 Effect: Extensive metabolism via CYP isoenzymes, profile not characterized.

Increased Effect/Toxicity: Metabolized by cytochrome P450 isoenzymes. Profile of involved isoenzymes has not been established. Concurrent cimetidine therapy increased AUC of tamsulosin by 44%. Use with caution in patients receiving concurrent warfarin therapy (may increase anticoagulant effect). Do not use in combination with other alpha-blocking drugs.

Decreased Effect: Metabolism by cytochrome P450 isoenzymes may, in theory, be influenced by enzyme-inducing agents, resulting in decreased effects.

Ethanol/Nutrition/Herb Interactions

Food: The time to maximum concentration (T_{max}) is reached by 4-5 hours under fasting conditions and by 6-7 hours when administered with food. Taking it under fasted conditions results in a 30% increase in bioavailability and 40% to 70% increase in peak concentrations (C_{max}) compared to fed conditions.

Herb/Nutraceutical: Avoid saw palmetto (due to limited experience with this combination).

Mechanism of Action An antagonist of alpha$_{1A}$ adrenoreceptors in the prostate. Three subtypes identified: alpha$_{1A}$, alpha$_{1B}$, alpha$_{1D}$ have distribution that differs between human organs and tissue. Approximately 70% of the alpha$_1$-receptors in human prostate are of alpha$_{1A}$ subtype. The symptoms associated with benign prostatic hyperplasia (BPH) are related to bladder outlet obstruction, which is comprised of two underlying components: static and dynamic. Static is related to an increase in prostate size, partially caused by a proliferation of smooth muscle cells in the prostatic stroma. Severity of BPH symptoms and the degree of urethral obstruction do not correlate well with the size of the prostate. Dynamic is a function of an increase in smooth muscle tone in the prostate and bladder neck leading to constriction of the bladder outlet. Smooth muscle tone is mediated by the sympathetic nervous stimulation of alpha$_1$ adrenoreceptors, which are abundant in the prostate, prostatic capsule, prostatic urethra, and bladder neck. Blockade of these adrenoreceptors can cause smooth muscles in the bladder neck and prostate to relax, resulting in an improvement in urine flow rate and a reduction in symptoms of BPH.

Pharmacodynamics/Kinetics

Absorption: >90%
Protein binding: 94% to 99%, primarily to alpha$_1$ acid glycoprotein (AAG); not affected by amitriptyline, diclofenac, glyburide, simvastatin plus simvastatin-hydroxy acid metabolite, warfarin, diazepam, propranolol, trichlormethiazide, or chlormadinone, nor does tamsulosin effect extent of binding of these drugs
Metabolism: Hepatically via CYP450 enzymes; profile of metabolites in humans has not been established; metabolites undergo extensive conjugation to glucuronide or sulfate
Bioavailability: Fasting: 30% increase
Steady-state: By the fifth day of once daily dosing
Half-life elimination: Healthy volunteers: 9-13 hours; Target population: 14-15 hours
Time to peak: C_{max}: Fasting: 40% to 70% increase; T_{max}: Fasting: 4-5 hours; With food: 6-7 hours
Excretion: Urine (<10% as unchanged drug)

Usual Dosage Oral: Adults: 0.4 mg once daily approximately 30 minutes after the same meal each day

Patient Information Symptoms related to postural hypotension (ie, dizziness) may occur; do not drive, operate machinery, or perform hazardous activities; do not crush, chew, or open capsules

Dosage Forms Capsule, as hydrochloride: 0.4 mg

♦ **Tamsulosin Hydrochloride** *see Tamsulosin on page 1287*

♦ **Tanoral**® *see Chlorpheniramine, Pyrilamine, and Phenylephrine on page 282*

- **Tao**® *see* Troleandomycin *on page 1383*
- **Tapazole**® *see* Methimazole *on page 882*
- **Targretin**® *see* Bexarotene *on page 166*
- **Tarka**® *see* Trandolapril and Verapamil *on page 1357*
- **Tarka**® **(Can)** *see* Verapamil *on page 1412*
- **Taro-Carbamazepin (Can)** *see* Carbamazepine *on page 221*
- **Taro-Desoximetasone (Can)** *see* Desoximetasone *on page 380*
- **Taro-Sone**® **(Can)** *see* Betamethasone *on page 161*
- **Taro-Warfarin (Can)** *see* Warfarin *on page 1425*
- **Tasmar**® *see* Tolcapone *on page 1344*
- **TAT** *see* Tetanus Antitoxin *on page 1303*
- **Tavist**® *see* Clemastine *on page 308*
- **Tavist**®**-1 [OTC]** *see* Clemastine *on page 308*
- **Taxol**® *see* Paclitaxel *on page 1030*
- **Taxotere**® *see* Docetaxel *on page 428*

Tazarotene (taz AR oh teen)

U.S. Brand Names Tazorac®

Canadian Brand Names Tazorac™

Therapeutic Category Keratolytic Agent

Use Topical treatment of facial acne vulgaris; topical treatment of stable plaque psoriasis of up to 20% body surface area involvement

Pregnancy Risk Factor X

Pregnancy/Breast-Feeding Implications May cause fetal harm if administered to a pregnant woman. A negative pregnancy test should be obtained 2 weeks prior to treatment; treatment should begin during a normal menstrual period. It is not known if tazarotene is excreted in human breast milk; use caution if administered to a nursing woman.

Contraindications Hypersensitivity to tazarotene, other retinoids or vitamin A derivatives (isotretinoin, tretinoin, etretinate), or any component of the formulation; use in women of childbearing potential who are unable to comply with birth control requirements; pregnancy (negative pregnancy test required)

Warnings/Precautions Women of childbearing potential must use adequate contraceptive measures because of potential teratogenicity. Due to heightened burning susceptibility, exposure to sunlight should be avoided unless deemed medically necessary, and in such cases, exposure should be minimized during use of tazarotene. Administer with caution if the patient is also taking drugs known to be photosensitizers (thiazides, tetracyclines, fluoroquinolones, phenothiazines, sulfonamides) because of the increased possibility of augmented photosensitivity. Patients should be warned to use sunscreens (SPF minimum of 15) and protective clothing when using tazarotene. Application may cause a transitory feeling of burning or stinging. For external use only; avoid contact with eyes, eyelids, and mouth. Do not use on eczematous, broken, or sunburned skin. Avoid application over extensive areas; specifically, safety and efficacy of gel applied over >20% of BSA have not been established. If oral ingestion children <12 years of age for acne and <18 years of age for psoriasis have not been established.

Adverse Reactions Percentage of incidence varies with formulation and/or strength:

>10%: Dermatologic: Burning/stinging, dry skin, erythema, pruritus, skin pain, worsening of psoriasis

1% to 10%: Dermatologic: Contact dermatitis, desquamation, discoloration, fissuring, hypertriglyceridemia, inflammation, localized bleeding, rash

Frequency not defined:
  Dermatologic: Photosensitization
  Neuromuscular & skeletal: Peripheral neuropathy

Overdosage/Toxicology Excessive topical use may lead to marked redness, peeling, or discomfort. Oral ingestion may lead to the same adverse effects as those associated with excessive oral intake of Vitamin A (hypervitaminosis A) or other retinoids. If oral ingestion occurs, monitor the patient and administer appropriate supportive measures as necessary.

Drug Interactions

Increased Effect/Toxicity: Increased toxicity may occur with sulfur, benzoyl peroxide, salicylic acid, resorcinol, or any product with strong drying effects (including alcohol-containing compounds) due to increased drying actions. May augment phototoxicity of sensitizing medications (thiazides, tetracyclines, fluoroquinolones, phenothiazines, sulfonamides).

Stability Store at room temperature of 25°C (77°F), away from heat and direct light; do not freeze.

Mechanism of Action Synthetic, acetylenic retinoid which modulates differentiation and proliferation of epithelial tissue and exerts some degree of anti-inflammatory and immunological activity

Pharmacodynamics/Kinetics

Absorption: Minimal following cutaneous application (≤6% of dose)

Distribution: Retained in skin for prolonged periods after topical application.

Duration: Therapeutic: Psoriasis: ≤3 months after a 3-month course of topical treatment

Protein binding: >99%

Metabolism: Prodrug, rapidly metabolized via esterases to an active metabolite (tazarotenic acid) following topical application and systemic absorption; tazarotenic acid undergoes further hepatic metabolism

Half-life elimination: 18 hours

Excretion: Urine and feces (as metabolites)

Usual Dosage Topical: **Note:** In patients experiencing excessive pruritus, burning, skin redness, or peeling, discontinue until integrity of the skin is restored, or reduce dosing to an interval the patient is able to tolerate.

(Continued)

Tazarotene *(Continued)*

Children ≥12 years and Adults:

Acne: Cream/gel 0.1%: Cleanse the face gently. After the skin is dry, apply a thin film of tazarotene (2 mg/cm^2) once daily, in the evening, to the skin where the acne lesions appear; use enough to cover the entire affected area

Psoriasis: Gel 0.05% or 0.1%: Apply once daily, in the evening, to psoriatic lesions using enough (2 mg/cm^2) to cover only the lesion with a thin film to no more than 20% of body surface area. If a bath or shower is taken prior to application, dry the skin before applying. Unaffected skin may be more susceptible to irritation, avoid application to these areas.

Children ≥18 years and Adults: Cream 0.05% or 0.1%: Apply once daily, in the evening, to psoriatic lesions using enough (2 mg/cm^2) to cover only the lesion with a thin film to no more than 20% of body surface area. If a bath or shower is taken prior to application, dry the skin before applying. Unaffected skin may be more susceptible to irritation, avoid application to these areas.

Elderly: No differences in safety or efficacy were seen when administered to patients >65 years of age; may experience increased sensitivity

Administration Do not apply to eczematous or sunburned skin; apply thin film to affected areas; avoid eyes, eyelids, and mouth

Monitoring Parameters Disease severity in plaque psoriasis during therapy (reduction in erythema, scaling, induration); routine blood chemistries (including transaminases) are suggested during long-term topical therapy; pregnancy test prior to treatment of female patients

Patient Information Do not take this medication if you have had an allergic reaction to tazarotene. Do not use tazarotene if you are pregnant or planning to become pregnant. Tazarotene may cause birth defects or be harmful to an unborn baby if used during pregnancy. This may be more likely if the medicine is used on large areas of skin.

Your physician will tell you how much medicine to use and how often. Do not use more of the medication than your physician ordered. Using too much of the medication can cause red, peeling, or irritated skin. Wash your hands before and after using this medication (unless treating psoriasis lesions on your hands). Use this medication on your skin only. Do not put the medication in your eyes, eyelids, or in your mouth. If you do get the medication in your eyes, rinse them with large amounts of cool water. Tell your physician if you have eye pain or redness that does not go away.

Acne patients: Gently wash and dry your face. Apply a thin layer of medication to cover the acne. Your acne should start to clear up in about 4 weeks.

Psoriasis patients: If using the medication after bathing or showering, make sure your skin is completely dry before applying the medication. Apply a thin layer to lesions.

Wash off any medication that gets on skin areas that do not need to be treated. The medication can irritate skin that does not need treatment. Do not bandage or cover the treated skin. Ask your physician or pharmacist before taking any other medication, including over-the-counter products. Talk with your physician or pharmacist before using medicated cosmetics or shampoos, abrasive soaps or cleansers, products with alcohol, spice, or lime in them, other acne medicines, hair removal products, or products that dry your skin.

This medication may make your skin sensitive to sunlight and cause a rash or sunburn. Avoid spending long periods of time in direct sunlight and protect your skin with clothing and a strong sunscreen when you are outdoors. Do not use a sunlamp or tanning booth. Call your physician if you have blistering or crusting skin, severe redness, pain, or swelling on the areas that you use the medication.

Dosage Forms

Cream, topical: 0.05% (15 g, 30 g, 60 g); 0.1% (15 g, 30 g, 60g)
Gel, topical: 0.05% (30 g, 100 g); 0.1% (30 g, 100 g)

- ◆ **Tazicef**® *see* Ceftazidime *on page 253*
- ◆ **Tazidime**® *see* Ceftazidime *on page 253*
- ◆ **Tazorac**® *see* Tazarotene *on page 1289*
- ◆ **3TC** *see* Lamivudine *on page 771*
- ◆ **3TC, Abacavir, and Zidovudine** *see* Abacavir, Lamivudine, and Zidovudine *on page 17*
- ◆ **T-Cell Growth Factor** *see* Aldesleukin *on page 43*
- ◆ **TCGF** *see* Aldesleukin *on page 43*
- ◆ **TCN** *see* Tetracycline *on page 1306*
- ◆ **Td** *see* Diphtheria and Tetanus Toxoid *on page 417*
- ◆ **TDF** *see* Tenofovir *on page 1296*
- ◆ **Tebrazid**™ **(Can)** *see* Pyrazinamide *on page 1159*
- ◆ **Tecnal**® **(Can)** *see* Butalbital Compound *on page 197*
- ◆ **Tedral**® *see* Theophylline, Ephedrine, and Phenobarbital *on page 1310*
- ◆ **Teejel**® **(Can)** *see* Choline Salicylate *on page 288*
- ◆ **Tegretol**® *see* Carbamazepine *on page 221*
- ◆ **Tegretol**®**-XR** *see* Carbamazepine *on page 221*
- ◆ **Tegrin**®**-HC [OTC]** *see* Hydrocortisone *on page 682*

Telmisartan *(tel mi SAR tan)*

Related Information

Angiotensin Agents Comparison *on page 1473*

U.S. Brand Names Micardis®

Canadian Brand Names Micardis®

Therapeutic Category Angiotensin II Receptor Antagonist (ARB); Antihypertensive Agent

Use Treatment of hypertension; may be used alone or in combination with other antihypertensive agents

Pregnancy Risk Factor C (1st trimester); D (2nd and 3rd trimesters)

Pregnancy/Breast-Feeding Implications Avoid use in the nursing mother, if possible, since telmisartan may be excreted in breast milk. The drug should be discontinued as soon as possible when pregnancy is detected. Drugs which act directly on renin-angiotensin can cause fetal and neonatal morbidity and death.

Contraindications Hypersensitivity to telmisartan or any component of the formulation; hypersensitivity to other A-II receptor antagonists; primary hyperaldosteronism; bilateral renal artery stenosis; pregnancy (2nd and 3rd trimesters)

Warnings/Precautions Avoid use or use a smaller dose in patients who are volume depleted; correct depletion first. Deterioration in renal function can occur with initiation. Use with caution in unilateral renal artery stenosis and pre-existing renal insufficiency; significant aortic/mitral stenosis. Use with caution in patients who have biliary obstructive disorders or hepatic dysfunction.

Adverse Reactions May be associated with worsening of renal function in patients dependent on renin-angiotensin-aldosterone system.

1% to 10%:
Cardiovascular: Hypertension (1%), chest pain (1%), peripheral edema (1%)
Central nervous system: Headache (1%), dizziness (1%), pain (1%), fatigue (1%)
Gastrointestinal: Diarrhea (3%), dyspepsia (1%), nausea (1%), abdominal pain (1%)
Genitourinary: Urinary tract infection (1%)
Neuromuscular & skeletal: Back pain (3%), myalgia (1%)
Respiratory: Upper respiratory infection (7%), sinusitis (3%), pharyngitis (1%), cough (2%)
Miscellaneous: Flu-like syndrome (1%)
<1% (Limited to important or life-threatening): Abnormal vision, allergic reaction, angina, angioedema, depression, dyspnea, epistaxis, gout, impotence, increased serum creatinine and BUN, insomnia, involuntary muscle contractions, migraine, paresthesia, pruritus, rash, somnolence, tinnitus, vertigo

Overdosage/Toxicology Signs and symptoms of overdose include hypotension, dizziness, and tachycardia. Treatment is supportive. Vagal stimulation may result in bradycardia.

Drug Interactions

Cytochrome P450 Effect: CYP2C19 enzyme inhibitor

Increased Effect/Toxicity: Telmisartan may increase serum digoxin concentrations. Potassium salts/supplements, co-trimoxazole (high dose), ACE inhibitors, and potassium-sparing diuretics (amiloride, spironolactone, triamterene) may increase the risk of hyperkalemia with telmisartan.

Decreased Effect: Telmisartan decreased the trough concentrations of warfarin during concurrent therapy, however INR was not changed.

Ethanol/Nutrition/Herb Interactions Herb/Nutraceutical: Avoid dong quai if using for hypertension (has estrogenic activity). Avoid ephedra, yohimbe, ginseng (may worsen hypertension). Avoid garlic (may have increased antihypertensive effect).

Mechanism of Action Angiotensin II acts as a vasoconstrictor. In addition to causing direct vasoconstriction, angiotensin II also stimulates the release of aldosterone. Once aldosterone is released, sodium as well as water are reabsorbed. The end result is an elevation in blood pressure. Telmisartan is a nonpeptide AT1 angiotensin II receptor antagonist. This binding prevents angiotensin II from binding to the receptor thereby blocking the vasoconstriction and the aldosterone secreting effects of angiotensin II.

Pharmacodynamics/Kinetics Orally active, not a prodrug
Onset of action: 1-2 hours
Peak effect: 0.5-1 hours
Duration: Up to 24 hours
Protein binding: >99.5%
Metabolism: Hepatic via conjugation to inactive metabolites; not metabolized via CYP isoenzyme
Bioavailability: 42% to 58% (dose-dependent)
Half-life elimination: Terminal: 24 hours
Excretion: Feces (97%)
Clearance: Total body: 800 mL/minute

Usual Dosage Adults: Oral: Initial: 40 mg once daily; usual maintenance dose range: 20-80 mg/day. Patients with volume depletion should be initiated on the lower dosage with close supervision.

Dosage adjustment in hepatic impairment: Supervise patients closely.

Dietary Considerations May be taken without regard to food.

Monitoring Parameters Supine blood pressure, electrolytes, serum creatinine, BUN, urinalysis, symptomatic hypotension, and tachycardia

Patient Information Patients of childbearing age should be informed about the consequences of 2nd and 3rd trimester exposure to drugs that act on the renin-angiotensin system, and that these consequences do not appear to have resulted from intrauterine drug exposure that has been limited to the 1st trimester. Patients should report pregnancy to their physician as soon as possible.

Dosage Forms Tablet: 20 mg, 40 mg, 80 mg

♦ **Telmisartan and HCTZ** see Telmisartan and Hydrochlorothiazide on page 1291

Telmisartan and Hydrochlorothiazide

(tel mi SAR tan & hye droe klor oh THYE a zide)

U.S. Brand Names Micardis® HCT

Synonyms HCTZ and Telmisartan; Hydrochlorothiazide and Telmisartan; Telmisartan and HCTZ

Therapeutic Category Angiotensin II Antagonist Combination; Antihypertensive Agent, Combination

Use Treatment of hypertension; combination product should not be used for initial therapy

Pregnancy Risk Factor C (1st trimester); D (2nd and 3rd trimesters)

(Continued)

Telmisartan and Hydrochlorothiazide *(Continued)*

Usual Dosage Adults: Oral: Replacement therapy: Combination product can be substituted for individual titrated agents. Initiation of combination therapy when monotherapy has failed to achieve desired effects:

Patients currently on telmisartan: Initial dose if blood pressure is not currently controlled on monotherapy of 80 mg telmisartan: Telmisartan 80 mg/hydrochlorothiazide 12.5 mg once daily; may titrate up to telmisartan 160 mg/hydrochlorothiazide 25 mg if needed

Patients currently on HCTZ: Initial dose if blood pressure is not currently controlled on monotherapy of 25 mg once daily, or is controlled and experiencing hypokalemia: Telmisartan 80 mg/hydrochlorothiazide 12.5 mg once daily; may titrate up to telmisartan 160 mg/hydrochlorothiazide 25 mg if blood pressure remains uncontrolled after 2-4 weeks of therapy

Dosage adjustment in renal impairment:
Cl_{cr} >30 mL/minute: Usual recommended dose
Cl_{cr} <30 mL/minute: Not recommended

Dosage adjustment in hepatic impairment: Dosing should be started at telmisartan 40 mg/hydrochlorothiazide 12.5 mg; do **not** use in patients with severe hepatic impairment
Elderly: No dosing adjustment needed based on age; monitor renal and hepatic function

Additional Information Complete prescribing information for this medication should be consulted for additional detail.

Dosage Forms
Tablet:
Telmisartan 40 mg and hydrochlorothiazide 12.5 mg
Telmisartan 80 mg and hydrochlorothiazide 12.5 mg

Temazepam *(te MAZ e pam)*

Related Information
Antacid Drug Interactions *on page 1477*
Benzodiazepines Comparison *on page 1490*

U.S. Brand Names Restoril®

Canadian Brand Names Apo®-Temazepam; Gen-Temazepam; Novo-Temazepam; Nu-Temazepam; PMS-Temazepam; Restoril®

Therapeutic Category Benzodiazepine; Hypnotic; Sedative

Use Short-term treatment of insomnia

Unlabeled/Investigational Use Treatment of anxiety; adjunct in the treatment of depression; management of panic attacks

Restrictions C-IV

Pregnancy Risk Factor X

Contraindications Hypersensitivity to temazepam or any component of the formulation (cross-sensitivity with other benzodiazepines may exist); narrow-angle glaucoma (not in product labeling, however, benzodiazepines are contraindicated); pregnancy

Warnings/Precautions Should be used only after evaluation of potential causes of sleep disturbance. Failure of sleep disturbance to resolve after 7-10 days may indicate psychiatric or medical illness. A worsening of insomnia or the emergence of new abnormalities of thought or behavior may represent unrecognized psychiatric or medical illness and requires immediate and careful evaluation.

Use with caution in elderly or debilitated patients, patients with hepatic disease (including alcoholics), or renal impairment. Use with caution in patients with respiratory disease, or impaired gag reflex. Avoid use inpatients with sleep apnea.

Causes CNS depression (dose-related) resulting in sedation, dizziness, confusion, or ataxia which may impair physical and mental capabilities. Patients must be cautioned about performing tasks which require mental alertness (ie, operating machinery or driving). Use with caution in patients receiving other CNS depressants or psychoactive agents. Effects with other sedative drugs or ethanol may be potentiated. Benzodiazepines have been associated with falls and traumatic injury and should be used with extreme caution in patients who are at risk of these events (especially the elderly).

Use caution in patients with suicidal risk. Use with caution in patients with a history of drug dependence. Benzodiazepines have been associated with dependence and acute withdrawal symptoms on discontinuation or reduction in dose (may occur after as little as 10 days). Acute withdrawal, including seizures, may be precipitated after administration of flumazenil to patients receiving long-term benzodiazepine therapy.

Benzodiazepines have been associated with anterograde amnesia. Paradoxical reactions, including hyperactive or aggressive behavior, have been reported with benzodiazepines, particularly in adolescent/pediatric or psychiatric patients. Does not have analgesic, antidepressant, or antipsychotic properties.

Adverse Reactions
1% to 10%:
Central nervous system: Confusion, dizziness, drowsiness, fatigue, anxiety, headache, lethargy, hangover, euphoria, vertigo
Dermatologic: Rash
Endocrine & metabolic: Decreased libido
Gastrointestinal: Diarrhea
Neuromuscular & skeletal: Dysarthria, weakness
Otic: Blurred vision
Miscellaneous: Diaphoresis
<1% (Limited to important or life-threatening): Amnesia, ataxia, blood dyscrasias, drug dependence, paradoxical reactions, vomiting

Overdosage/Toxicology Symptoms include somnolence, confusion, coma, hypoactive reflexes, dyspnea, hypotension, slurred speech, and impaired coordination. Treatment for benzodiazepine overdose is supportive. Rarely is mechanical ventilation required. Flumazenil has been shown to selectively block the binding of benzodiazepines to CNS receptors, resulting in reversal of benzodiazepine-induced CNS depression.

Drug Interactions

Cytochrome P450 Effect: CYP3A3/4 enzyme substrate

Increased Effect/Toxicity: Temazepam potentiates the CNS depressant effects of narcotic analgesics, barbiturates, phenothiazines, ethanol, antihistamines, MAO inhibitors, sedative-hypnotics, and cyclic antidepressants. Serum levels of temazepam may be increased by inhibitors of CYP3A3/4, including cimetidine, ciprofloxacin, clarithromycin, clozapine, diltiazem, disulfiram, digoxin, erythromycin, ethanol, fluconazole, fluoxetine, fluvoxamine, grapefruit juice, isoniazid, itraconazole, ketoconazole, labetalol, levodopa, loxapine, metoprolol, metronidazole, miconazole, nefazodone, omeprazole, phenytoin, rifabutin, rifampin, troleandomycin, valproic acid, and verapamil.

Decreased Effect: Oral contraceptives may increase the clearance of temazepam. Temazepam may decrease the antiparkinsonian efficacy of levodopa. Theophylline and other CNS stimulants may antagonize the sedative effects of temazepam. Carbamazepine, rifampin, rifabutin may enhance the metabolism of temazepam and decrease its therapeutic effect.

Ethanol/Nutrition/Herb Interactions

Ethanol: Avoid ethanol (may increase CNS depression).

Food: Serum levels may be increased by grapefruit juice.

Herb/Nutraceutical: St John's wort may decrease temazepam levels. Avoid valerian, St John's wort, kava kava, gotu kola (may increase CNS depression).

Mechanism of Action Binds to stereospecific benzodiazepine receptors on the postsynaptic GABA neuron at several sites within the central nervous system, including the limbic system, reticular formation. Enhancement of the inhibitory effect of GABA on neuronal excitability results by increased neuronal membrane permeability to chloride ions. This shift in chloride ions results in hyperpolarization (a less excitable state) and stabilization.

Pharmacodynamics/Kinetics

Protein binding: 96%

Metabolism: Hepatic

Half-life elimination: 9.5-12.4 hours

Time to peak, serum: 2-3 hours

Excretion: Urine (80% to 90% as inactive metabolites)

Usual Dosage Oral:

Adults: 15-30 mg at bedtime

Elderly or debilitated patients: 15 mg

Monitoring Parameters Respiratory and cardiovascular status

Reference Range Therapeutic: 26 ng/mL after 24 hours

Patient Information Avoid alcohol and other CNS depressants; avoid activities needing good psychomotor coordination until CNS effects are known; drug may cause physical or psychological dependence; avoid abrupt discontinuation after prolonged use

Nursing Implications Provide safety measures (ie, side rails, night light, and call button); remove smoking materials from area; supervise ambulation

Additional Information Abrupt discontinuation after sustained use (generally >10 days) may cause withdrawal symptoms.

Dosage Forms Capsule: 7.5 mg, 15 mg, 30 mg

♦ **Temodal™ (Can)** *see* Temozolomide *on page 1293*

♦ **Temodar®** *see* Temozolomide *on page 1293*

♦ **Temovate®** *see* Clobetasol *on page 311*

Temozolomide (te moe ZOE loe mide)

U.S. Brand Names Temodar®

Canadian Brand Names Temodal™; Tomedar®

Therapeutic Category Antineoplastic Agent, Alkylating Agent

Use Treatment of adult patients with refractory (first relapse) anaplastic astrocytoma who have experienced disease progression on nitrosourea and procarbazine

Unlabeled/Investigational Use Glioma, first relapse/advanced metastatic malignant melanoma

Pregnancy Risk Factor D

Pregnancy/Breast-Feeding Implications May cause fetal harm when administered to pregnant women. Animal studies, at doses less than used in humans, resulted in numerous birth defects. Testicular toxicity was demonstrated in animal studies using smaller doses than recommended for cancer treatment. Male and female patients should avoid pregnancy while receiving drug. It is not known whether temozolomide is excreted in breast milk, but breast-feeding is not recommended.

Contraindications Hypersensitivity to temozolomide or any component of the formulation; hypersensitivity to DTIC (since both drugs are metabolized to MTIC); pregnancy

Warnings/Precautions Prior to dosing, patients must have an absolute neutrophil count (ANC) of ≥1.5 x 10 9/L and a platelet count of ≥100 x 10 9/L. Must have ANC >1,500/μL, platelet count >100,000/μL before starting each cycle. Elderly patients and women have a higher incidence of myelosuppression. Safety/efficacy in pediatrics not established. Use caution in patients with severe hepatic or renal impairment. The U.S. Food and Drug Administration (FDA) currently recommends that procedures for proper handling and disposal of antineoplastic agents be considered.

Adverse Reactions

>10%:

Central nervous system: Headache (41%), fatigue (34%), convulsions (23%), hemiparesis (29%), dizziness (19%), fever (11%), coordination abnormality (11%), amnesia (10%), insomnia (10%), somnolence. In the case of CNS malignancies, it is difficult to distinguish the relative contributions of temozolomide and progressive disease to CNS symptoms.

(Continued)

Temozolomide *(Continued)*

Gastrointestinal: Nausea (53%), vomiting (42%), constipation (33%), diarrhea (16%), anorexia

Hematologic: Neutropenia (grade 3-4, 14%), thrombocytopenia (grade 3-4 19%)

Neuromuscular & skeletal: Weakness (13%)

1% to 10%:

Central nervous system: Ataxia (8%), confusion (5%), anxiety (7%), depression (6%)

Dermatologic: Rash (8%), pruritus (8%)

Gastrointestinal: Dysphagia (7%), abdominal pain (9%)

Hematologic: Anemia (8%; grade 3-4, 4%)

Neuromuscular & skeletal: Paresthesia (9%), back pain (8%), myalgia (5%)

Ocular: Diplopia (5%), vision abnormality (5%)

Overdosage/Toxicology Dose-limiting toxicity is hematological. In the event of an overdose, hematological evaluation is necessary. Treatment is supportive.

Drug Interactions

Decreased Effect: Although valproic acid reduces the clearance of temozolomide by 5%, the clinical significance of this is unknown.

Ethanol/Nutrition/Herb Interactions Food: Food reduces rate and extent of absorption.

Stability Store at controlled room temperature (15°C to 10°C/59°F to 86°F)

Mechanism of Action Like DTIC, temozolomide is converted to the active alkylating metabolite MTIC. Unlike DTIC, however, this conversion is spontaneous, nonenzymatic, and occurs under physiologic conditions in all tissues to which the drug distributes.

Pharmacodynamics/Kinetics

Distribution: V_d: Parent drug: 0.4 L/kg

Protein binding: 15%

Metabolism: Temozolomide (prodrug) is hydrolyzed to the active form, MTIC; MTIC is eventually eliminated as CO_2 and 5-aminoimidazole-4-carboxamide (AIC), a natural constituent in urine

Bioavailability: 100%

Half-life elimination: Mean: Parent drug: 1.8 hours

Time to peak: 1 hour if taken on empty stomach

Excretion: Urine (5% to 7% of total)

Usual Dosage Refer to individual protocols.

Usual dose: Oral: 150-200 mg/m²/day for 5 days; repeat every 28 days.

Dosage is adjusted according to nadir neutrophil and platelet counts of previous cycle and counts at the time of the next cycle

Measure day 22 ANC and platelets. Measure day 29 ANC and platelets. Based on lowest counts at either day 22 or day 29:

On day 22 or day 29, if ANC <1000/µL or the platelet count is <50,000/µL, postpone therapy until ANC >1500/µL and platelet count >100,000/µL. Reduce dose by 50 mg/m² for subsequent cycle.

If ANC 1000-1500/µL or platelets 50,000-100,000/µL, postpone therapy until ANC >1500/µL and platelet count >100,000/µL; maintain initial dose.

If ANC >1500/µL (on day 22 and day 29) and platelet count >100,000/µL, increase dose to, or maintain dose at 200 mg/m²/day for 5 for subsequent cycle.

Temozolomide therapy can be continued until disease progression. Treatment could be continued for a maximum of 2 years in the clinical trial, but the optimum duration of therapy is not known.

Elderly: Patients ≥70 years of age had a higher incidence of grade 4 neutropenia and thrombocytopenia in the first cycle of therapy than patients <70 years of age

Dosage adjustment in renal impairment: No guidelines exist. Caution should be used when administered to patients with severe renal impairment (Cl_{cr} <39 mL/minute).

Dosage adjustment in hepatic impairment: Caution should be used when administering to patients with severe hepatic impairment

Dietary Considerations The incidence of nausea/vomiting is decreased when the drug is taken on an empty stomach.

Administration Capsules should not be opened or chewed but swallowed whole with a glass of water. May be administered on an empty stomach to reduce nausea and vomiting. Bedtime administration may be advised.

Monitoring Parameters A complete blood count on day 22 of cycle or within 48 hours of that day and weekly until the ANC >1500 µL, platelet count >100,000/µL

Patient Information Swallow capsules whole with a glass of water. Take on an empty stomach at similar time each day. If you have nausea and vomiting, contact prescriber for medicine to decrease this. Male and female patients who take temozolomide should protect against pregnancy (use effective contraception). Do not breast-feed while on medicine. Blood work necessary on day 22 and day 29 of each cycle to determine when to start next cycle and how much medicine to give.

Nursing Implications Capsules should not be opened. Educate patients about most frequent side effects and blood work required.

Dosage Forms Capsule: 5 mg, 20 mg, 100 mg, 250 mg

♦ **Tempra® (Can)** *see* Acetaminophen *on page 22*

Tenecteplase *(ten EK te plase)*

U.S. Brand Names TNKase™

Therapeutic Category Fibrinolytic Agent

Use Thrombolytic agent used in the management of acute myocardial infarction for the lysis of thrombi in the coronary vasculature to restore perfusion and reduce mortality.

Pregnancy Risk Factor C

Pregnancy/Breast-Feeding Implications Administer to pregnant women only if the potential benefits justify the risk to the fetus. Exercise caution when administering to a nursing woman.

Contraindications Hypersensitivity to tenecteplase or any component of the formulation; active internal bleeding; history of stroke; intracranial/intraspinal surgery or trauma within 2 months; intracranial neoplasm; arteriovenous malformation or aneurysm; bleeding diathesis; severe uncontrolled hypertension

Warnings/Precautions Stop antiplatelet agents and heparin if serious bleeding occurs. Avoid I.M. injections and nonessential handling of the patient for a few hours after administration. Monitor for bleeding complications. Venipunctures should be performed carefully and only when necessary. If arterial puncture is necessary, then use an upper extremity that can be easily compressed manually. For the following conditions, the risk of bleeding is higher with use of tenecteplase and should be weighed against the benefits: Recent major surgery, cerebrovascular disease, recent GI or GU bleed, recent trauma, uncontrolled hypertension (systolic BP ≥180 mm Hg and/or diastolic BP ≥110 mm Hg), suspected left heart thrombus, acute pericarditis, subacute bacterial endocarditis, hemostatic defects, severe hepatic dysfunction, pregnancy, hemorrhagic diabetic retinopathy or other hemorrhagic ophthalmic conditions, septic thrombophlebitis or occluded arteriovenous cannula at seriously infected site, advanced age (see Usual Dosing, Elderly), anticoagulants, recent administration of GP IIb/IIIa inhibitors. Coronary thrombolysis may result in reperfusion arrhythmias. Caution with readministration of tenecteplase. Safety and efficacy have not been established in pediatric patients. Cholesterol embolism has rarely been reported.

Adverse Reactions As with all drugs which may affect hemostasis, bleeding is the major adverse effect associated with tenecteplase. Hemorrhage may occur at virtually any site. Risk is dependent on multiple variables, including the dosage administered, concurrent use of multiple agents which alter hemostasis, and patient predisposition. Rapid lysis of coronary artery thrombi by thrombolytic agents may be associated with reperfusion-related arterial and/or ventricular arrhythmias.

>10%:
  Local: Hematoma (12% minor)
  Hematologic: Bleeding (22% minor: ASSENT-2 trial)
1% to 10%:
  Central nervous system: Stroke (2%)
  Gastrointestinal: GI hemorrhage (1% major, 2% minor), epistaxis (2% minor)
  Genitourinary: GU bleeding (4% minor)
  Hematologic: Bleeding (5% major; ASSENT-2 trial)
  Local: Bleeding at catheter puncture site (4% minor), hematoma (2% major)
  Respiratory: Pharyngeal (3% minor)
The incidence of stroke and bleeding increase with age above 65 years.
<1% (Limited to important or life-threatening): Anaphylaxis, angioedema, bleeding at catheter puncture site (<1% major), cholesterol embolism (clinical features may include livedo reticularis, "purple toe" syndrome, acute renal failure, gangrenous digits, hypertension, pancreatitis, myocardial infarction, cerebral infarction, spinal cord infarction, retinal artery occlusion, bowel infarction, rhabdomyolysis), GU bleeding (<1% major), intracranial hemorrhage (0.9%), laryngeal edema, rash, respiratory tract bleeding, retroperitoneal bleeding, urticaria
Additional cardiovascular events associated with use in myocardial infarction: Arrhythmias, AV block, cardiac arrest, cardiac tamponade, cardiogenic shock, electromechanical disso-ciation, embolism, fever, heart failure, hypotension, mitral regurgitation, myocardial reinfarction, myocardial rupture, nausea, pericardial effusion, pericarditis, pulmonary edema, recurrent myocardial ischemia, thrombosis, vomiting

Overdosage/Toxicology Symptom include increased incidence of bleeding.

Drug Interactions
  Increased Effect/Toxicity: Drugs which affect platelet function (eg, NSAIDs, dipyridamole, ticlopidine, clopidogrel, IIb/IIIa antagonists) may potentiate the risk of hemorrhage; use with caution.
    Heparin and aspirin: Use with aspirin and heparin may increase bleeding. However, aspirin and heparin were used concomitantly with tenecteplase in the majority of patients in clinical studies.
    Warfarin or oral anticoagulants: Risk of bleeding may be increased during concurrent therapy.
  Decreased Effect: Aminocaproic acid (antifibrinolytic agent) may decrease effectiveness.

Stability Store at room temperature not to exceed 30°C (86°F) or under refrigeration 2°C to 8°C (36°F to 46°F). If reconstituted and not used immediately, store in refrigerator and use within 8 hours.

Mechanism of Action Initiates fibrinolysis by binding to fibrin and converting plasminogen to plasmin.

Pharmacodynamics/Kinetics
  Distribution: V_d is weight related and approximates plasma volume
  Metabolism: Primarily hepatic
  Half-life elimination: 90-130 minutes
  Excretion: Clearance: Plasma: 99-119 mL/minute

Usual Dosage I.V.:
  Adult: Recommended total dose should not exceed 50 mg and is based on patient's weight; administer as a bolus over 5 seconds
    If patient's weight:
      <60 kg, dose: 30 mg
      ≥60 to <70 kg, dose: 35 mg
      ≥70 to <80 kg, dose: 40 mg
      ≥80 to <90 kg, dose: 45 mg
      ≥90 kg, dose: 50 mg
  All patients received 150-325 mg of aspirin as soon as possible and then daily. Intravenous heparin was initiated as soon as possible and aPTT was maintained between 50-70 seconds.
  Dosage adjustment in renal impairment: No formal recommendations for renal impairment
  Dosage adjustment in hepatic impairment: Severe hepatic failure is a relative contraindi-cation. Recommendations were not made for mild to moderate hepatic impairment.
(Continued)

Tenecteplase *(Continued)*

Elderly: Although dosage adjustments are not recommended, the elderly have a higher incidence of morbidity and mortality with the use of tenecteplase. The 30-day mortality in the ASSENT-2 trial was 2.5% for patients <65 years, 8.5% for patients 65-74 years, and 16.2% for patients ≥75 years. The intracranial hemorrhage rate was 0.4% for patients <65, 1.6 % for patients 65-74 years, and 1.7 % for patients ≥75. The risks and benefits of use should be weighted carefully in the elderly.

Administration Tenecteplase should be reconstituted using the supplied 10 cc syringe with TwinPak™ dual cannula device and 10 mL sterile water for injection. Do not shake when reconstituting. Slight foaming is normal and will dissipate if left standing for several minutes. The reconstituted solution is 5 mg/mL. Any unused solution should be discarded. Tenecteplase is **incompatible** with dextrose solutions. Dextrose-containing lines must be flushed with a saline solution before and after administration. Administer as a single I.V. bolus over 5 seconds.

Monitoring Parameters CBC, aPTT, signs and symptoms of bleeding, EKG monitoring

Patient Information This medication can only be administered I.V. You will have a tendency to bleed easily following its use; use caution to prevent injury (use electric razor, soft toothbrush), and use caution when using sharp objects (eg, scissors, knives). Strict bedrest should be maintained to reduce the risk of bleeding. If bleeding occurs, apply pressure to bleeding spot until bleeding stops completely. Report unusual bruising or bleeding; blood in urine, stool, or vomitus; bleeding gums; changes in vision; difficulty breathing; or chest pain/pressure.

Nursing Implications Dextrose-containing lines must be flushed with a saline solution before and after administration. Check frequently for signs of bleeding. Avoid I.M. injections and nonessential handling of patient.

Dosage Forms Powder for injection, lyophilized, recombinant: 50 mg

♦ **Tenex**® *see Guanfacine on page 650*

Teniposide *(ten i POE side)*

U.S. Brand Names Vumon

Canadian Brand Names Vumon®

Synonyms EPT; VM-26

Therapeutic Category Antineoplastic Agent, Miscellaneous

Use Treatment of acute lymphocytic leukemia, small cell lung cancer

Pregnancy Risk Factor D

Usual Dosage I.V.:

Children: 130 mg/m^2/week, increasing to 150 mg/m^2 after 3 weeks and up to 180 mg/m^2 after 6 weeks

Acute lymphoblastic leukemia (ALL): 165 mg/m^2 twice weekly for 8-9 doses **or** 250 mg/m^2 weekly for 4-8 weeks

Adults: 50-180 mg/m^2 once or twice weekly for 4-6 weeks or 20-60 mg/m^2/day for 5 days

Small cell lung cancer: 80-90 mg/m^2/day for 5 days every 4-6 weeks

Dosage adjustment in renal/hepatic impairment: Data is insufficient, but dose adjustments may be necessary in patient with significant renal or hepatic impairment

Dosage adjustment in Down syndrome patients: Reduce initial dosing; administer the first course at half the usual dose. Patients with both Down syndrome and leukemia may be especially sensitive to myelosuppressive chemotherapy.

Additional Information Complete prescribing information for this medication should be consulted for additional detail.

Dosage Forms Injection: 10 mg/mL (5 mL)

♦ **Ten-K**® *see Potassium Chloride on page 1108*

Tenofovir *(te NOE fo veer)*

U.S. Brand Names Viread™

Synonyms PMPA; TDF; Tenofovir Disoproxil Fumarate

Therapeutic Category Antiretroviral Agent, Reverse Transcriptase Inhibitor (Nucleotide)

Use Management of HIV infections in combination with at least two other antiretroviral agents

Pregnancy Risk Factor B

Pregnancy/Breast-Feeding Implications No adequate or well-controlled studies in pregnant women. Use in pregnancy only if clearly needed. Cases of lactic acidosis/hepatic steatosis syndrome have been reported in pregnant women receiving nucleoside analogues. It is not known if pregnancy itself potentiates this known side effect; however, pregnant women may be at increased risk of lactic acidosis and liver damage. Hepatic enzymes and electrolytes should be monitored frequently during the 3rd trimester of pregnancy in women receiving nucleoside analogues. Health professionals are encouraged to contact the Antiretroviral Pregnancy Registry to monitor outcomes of pregnant women exposed to antiretroviral medications (1-800-258-4263).

Contraindications Hypersensitivity to tenofovir or any component of the formulation

Warnings/Precautions Lactic acidosis and severe hepatomegaly with steatosis have been reported with nucleoside analogues, including fatal cases; use with caution in patients with risk factors for liver disease (risk may be increased in obese patients or prolonged exposure) and suspend treatment in any patient who develops clinical or laboratory findings suggestive of lactic acidosis (transaminase elevation may/may not accompany hepatomegaly and steatosis).

Avoid use in patients with renal impairment (Cl$_{cr}$ <60 mL/minute); data to support dosage adjustment not yet available. May have potential to cause osteomalacia and/or renal toxicity (based on preclinical animal studies); monitor renal function and possible bone abnormalities during therapy. Use caution in hepatic impairment. Safety and effectiveness not established in pediatric patients.

Adverse Reactions Clinical trials involved addition to prior antiretroviral therapy. Frequencies listed are treatment-emergent adverse effects noted at higher frequency than in the placebo group.

>10%: Gastrointestinal: Nausea (11%)

1% to 10%:
  Endocrine & metabolic: Glycosuria (3%, frequency equal to placebo); other metabolic effects (hyperglycemia, hypertriglyceridemia) noted at frequencies less than placebo
  Gastrointestinal: Diarrhea (9%), vomiting (5%), flatulence (4%), abdominal pain (3%, frequency equal to placebo), anorexia (3%)
  Hematologic: Neutropenia (1%, frequency equal to placebo)
  Hepatic: Increased transaminases (2% to 4%)
  Neuromuscular & skeletal: Weakness (8%, frequency equal to placebo)

Note: Uncommon, but significant adverse reactions reported with other reverse transcriptase inhibitors include pancreatitis, peripheral neuropathy, and myopathy. These have not been reported in clinical trials with tenofovir prior to marketing approval.

Overdosage/Toxicology Limited experience with overdose. Treatment is supportive.

Drug Interactions
  Cytochrome P450 Effect: CYP1A2 inhibitor (minor)
  Increased Effect/Toxicity: Serum concentrations of didanosine may be increased by tenofovir. Separate administration times (tenofovir should be given 2 hours after or 1 hour before didanosine). Lopinavir/ritonavir may increase serum concentrations of tenofovir.
  Note: Drugs which may compete for renal tubule secretion, including acyclovir, cidofovir, ganciclovir, valacyclovir, valganciclovir, may increase the serum concentrations of tenofovir. Nephrotoxic drugs may also reduce elimination of tenofovir.
  Decreased Effect: Serum levels of lopinavir and/or ritonavir may be decreased by tenofovir.

Ethanol/Nutrition/Herb Interactions Food: Fatty meals may increase the bioavailability of tenofovir. Tenofovir should be taken with food.

Stability Store at 25°C (77°F); excursions permitted to 15°C to 30°C (59°F to 86°F).

Mechanism of Action Tenofovir disoproxil fumarate (TDF) is an analog of adensoine 5'-monophosphate; it interferes with the HIV viral RNA dependent DNA polymerase resulting in inhibition of viral replication. TDF is first converted intracellularly by hydrolysis to tenofovir and subsequently phosphorylated to the active tenofovir diphosphate; nucleotide reverse transcriptase inhibitor.

Pharmacodynamics/Kinetics
  Distribution: 1.2-1.3 L/kg
  Protein binding: Minimal (7% to serum proteins)
  Metabolism: Not metabolized by CYP isoenzymes. Tenofovir disoproxil fumarate is first converted intracellularly by hydrolysis to tenofovir and subsequently phosphorylated to the active tenofovir diphosphate.
  Bioavailability: 25% (fasting); increases ~40% with high-fat meal
  Time to peak: 1 hour (fasting); 2 hours (with food)
  Excretion: In urine (70% to 80%), via filtration and active secretion, primarily as unchanged tenofovir

Usual Dosage Oral: Adults: HIV infection: 300 mg once daily
  Note: When used concurrently with didanosine, tenofovir should be administered at least 2 hours before or 1 hour after didanosine.
  Dosage adjustment in renal impairment: Avoid use in renal impairment (Cl$_{cr}$ <60 mL/minute). No dosage guidelines available.

Dietary Considerations Take with food to increase absorption.

Monitoring Parameters CBC with differential, reticulocyte count, serum creatine kinase, CD4 count, HIV RNA plasma levels, renal and hepatic function tests, bone density (long-term), serum phosphorus

Patient Information Tenofovir is not a cure for AIDS. Take as directed, with a meal. Do not take with other medications. Take precautions to avoid transmission to others. Report unresolved nausea or vomiting; abdominal pain; tingling, numbness, or pain of toes or fingers; skin rash or irritation; or muscle weakness or tremors. Notify prescriber if you are pregnant or plan to be pregnant. HIV infected mothers are discouraged from breast-feeding to prevent potential transmission of HIV.

Additional Information Approval was based on two clinical trials involving patients who were previously treated with antiretrovirals with continued evidence of HIV replication despite therapy. The risk:benefit ratio for untreated patients has not been established (studies currently ongoing), however patients who received tenofovir showed significant decreases in HIV replication as compared to continuation of standard therapy. At the time of approval, there are no long-term trials to demonstrate inhibition of clinical HIV progression by tenofovir.

Dosage Forms Tablet, as disoproxil fumarate: 300 mg [equivalent to 245 mg tenofovir disoproxil]

Terazosin (ter AY zoe sin)

U.S. Brand Names Hytrin®

Canadian Brand Names Alti-Terazosin; Apo®-Terazosin; Hytrin®; Novo-Terazosin; Nu-Terazosin

Therapeutic Category Alpha-Adrenergic Blocking Agent, Oral; Antihypertensive Agent

Use Management of mild to moderate hypertension; alone or in combination with other agents such as diuretics or beta-blockers; benign prostate hyperplasia (BPH)

Pregnancy Risk Factor C

Contraindications Hypersensitivity to quinazolines (doxazosin, prazosin, terazosin) or any component of the formulation

Warnings/Precautions Marked orthostatic hypotension, syncope, and loss of consciousness may occur with first dose ("first dose phenomenon"). This reaction is more likely to occur in patients receiving beta-blockers, diuretics, low sodium diets, or first doses >1 mg/dose in adults; avoid rapid increase in dose; use with caution in patients with renal impairment.

Adverse Reactions Asthenia, postural hypotension, dizziness, somnolence, nasal congestion/rhinitis, and impotence were the only events noted in clinical trials to occur at a frequency significantly greater than placebo (p<0.05).

>10%: Central nervous system: Dizziness, headache, muscle weakness

1% to 10%:
Cardiovascular: Edema, palpitations, chest pain, peripheral edema (3%), orthostatic hypotension (2.7% to 3.9%), tachycardia
Central nervous system: Fatigue, nervousness, drowsiness
Gastrointestinal: Dry mouth
Genitourinary: Urinary incontinence
Ocular: Blurred vision
Respiratory: Dyspnea, nasal congestion

<1% (Limited to important or life-threatening): Allergic reactions, anaphylaxis, atrial fibrillation, priapism, sexual dysfunction, syncope (0.8%), thrombocytopenia

Overdosage/Toxicology Symptoms include hypotension, drowsiness, and shock (but very unusual). Hypotension usually responds to I.V. fluids or Trendelenburg positioning. If unresponsive to these measures, the use of a parenteral vasoconstrictor may be required. Treatment is primarily supportive and symptomatic.

Drug Interactions

Increased Effect/Toxicity: Terazosin's hypotensive effect is increased with beta-blockers, diuretics, ACE inhibitors, calcium channel blockers, and other antihypertensive medications.

Decreased Effect: Decreased antihypertensive response with NSAIDs. Alpha-blockers reduce the response to pressor agents (norepinephrine).

Ethanol/Nutrition/Herb Interactions Herb/Nutraceutical: Avoid dong quai if using for hypertension (has estrogenic activity). Avoid ephedra, yohimbe, ginseng (may worsen hypertension). Avoid saw palmetto. Avoid garlic (may have increased antihypertensive effect).

Mechanism of Action Alpha$_1$-specific blocking agent with minimal alpha$_2$ effects; this allows peripheral postsynaptic blockade, with the resultant decrease in arterial tone, while preserving the negative feedback loop which is mediated by the peripheral presynaptic alpha$_2$-receptors; terazosin relaxes the smooth muscle of the bladder neck, thus reducing bladder outlet obstruction

Pharmacodynamics/Kinetics
Onset of action: 1-2 hours
Absorption: Rapid
Protein binding: 90% to 95%
Metabolism: Extensively hepatic
Half-life elimination: 9.2-12 hours
Time to peak, serum: ~1 hour
Excretion: Primarily feces (60%); urine (40%)

Usual Dosage Oral: Adults:
Hypertension: Initial: 1 mg at bedtime; slowly increase dose to achieve desired blood pressure, up to 20 mg/day; usual dose: 1-5 mg/day
Dosage reduction may be needed when adding a diuretic or other antihypertensive agent; if drug is discontinued for greater than several days, consider beginning with initial dose and retitrate as needed; dosage may be given on a twice daily regimen if response is diminished at 24 hours and hypotensive is observed at 2-4 hours following a dose
Benign prostatic hyperplasia: Initial: 1 mg at bedtime, increasing as needed; most patients require 10 mg day; if no response after 4-6 weeks of 10 mg/day, may increase to 20 mg/day

Dietary Considerations May be taken without regard to meals at the same time each day.

Monitoring Parameters Standing and sitting/supine blood pressure, especially following the initial dose at 2-4 hours following the dose and thereafter at the trough point to ensure adequate control throughout the dosing interval; urinary symptoms

Patient Information Report any gain of body weight or painful, persistent erection; fainting sometimes occurs after the first dose; rise slowly from prolonged sitting or standing

Nursing Implications
Syncope may occur usually within 90 minutes of the initial dose; administer initial dose at bedtime
Monitor blood pressure, standing and sitting/supine

Dosage Forms
Capsule: 1 mg, 2 mg, 5 mg, 10 mg
Tablet: 1 mg, 2 mg, 5 mg, 10 mg

Terbinafine (TER bin a feen)

Related Information
Antifungal Agents Comparison *on page 1484*

U.S. Brand Names Lamisil®; Lamisil® AT™; Lamisil® Dermgel; Lamisil® Solution

Canadian Brand Names Lamisil®; PMS-Terbinafine

Synonyms Terbinafine Hydrochloride

Therapeutic Category Antifungal Agent, Topical

Use Active against most strains of *Trichophyton mentagrophytes*, *Trichophyton rubrum*; may be effective for infections of *Microsporum gypseum* and *M. nanum*, *Trichophyton verrucosum*, *Epidermophyton floccosum*, *Candida albicans*, and *Scopulariopsis brevicaulis*
Oral: Onychomycosis of the toenail or fingernail due to susceptible dermatophytes
Topical: Antifungal for the treatment of tinea pedis (athlete's foot), tinea cruris (jock itch), and tinea corporis (ringworm)

Unlabeled/Investigational Use Topical: Cutaneous candidiasis and pityriasis versicolor

Pregnancy Risk Factor B

Pregnancy/Breast-Feeding Implications
Clinical effects on the fetus: Avoid use in pregnancy since treatment of onychomycosis is postponable
Breast-feeding/lactation: Although minimal concentrations of terbinafine cross into breast milk after topical use, oral or topical treatment during lactation should be avoided

Contraindications Hypersensitivity to terbinafine, naftifine, or any component of the formulation; pre-existing liver or renal disease (≤50 mL/minute GFR)

Warnings/Precautions While rare, the following complications have been reported and may require discontinuation of therapy: Changes in the ocular lens and retina, pancytopenia, neutropenia, Stevens-Johnson syndrome, toxic epidermal necrolysis. Rare cases of hepatic failure (including fatal cases) have been reported following oral treatment of onychomycosis. Not recommended for use in patients with active or chronic liver disease. Discontinue if symptoms or signs of hepatobiliary dysfunction or cholestatic hepatitis develop. If irritation/sensitivity develop with topical use, discontinue therapy. **Use caution in writing and/or filling prescription/orders. Confusion between Lamictal® (lamotrigine) and Lamisil® (terbinafine) has occurred.**

Adverse Reactions
Oral:
1% to 10%:
Central nervous system: Headache, dizziness, vertigo
Dermatologic: Rash, pruritus, and alopecia with oral therapy
Gastrointestinal: Nausea, diarrhea, dyspepsia, abdominal pain, appetite decrease, taste disturbance
Hematologic: Lymphocytopenia
Hepatic: Liver enzyme elevations
Ocular: Visual disturbance
Miscellaneous: Allergic reaction
<1% (Limited to important or life-threatening): Agranulocytosis, allergic reactions, anaphylaxis, hepatic failure, neutropenia, Stevens-Johnson syndrome, taste disturbance (with prolonged recovery and weight loss), thrombocytopenia, toxic epidermal necrolysis; changes in ocular lens and retina have been reported (clinical significance unknown)

Topical: 1% to 10%:
Dermatologic: Pruritus, contact dermatitis, irritation, burning, dryness
Local: Irritation, stinging

Drug Interactions
Cytochrome P450 Effect: CYP2D6 enzyme inhibitor
Increased Effect/Toxicity: Terbinafine clearance is decreased by cimetidine (33%) and terfenadine (16%); caffeine clearance is decreased by terfenadine (19%); effects of drugs metabolized by CYP2D6 (including beta-blockers, SSRIs, MAO inhibitors, tricyclic antidepressants) may be increased; warfarin effects may be increased
Decreased Effect: Cyclosporine clearance is increased (~15%) with concomitant terbinafine; rifampin increases terbinafine clearance (100%); rifampin increases the metabolism of terbinafine (decreases serum concentration)

Stability
Cream: Store at 5°C to 30°C (41°F to 86°F).
Solution: Store at 8°C to 25°C (46°F to 77°F).

Mechanism of Action Synthetic alkylamine derivative which inhibits squalene epoxidase, a key enzyme in sterol biosynthesis in fungi. This results in a deficiency in ergosterol within the fungal cell wall and results in fungal cell death.

Pharmacodynamics/Kinetics
Absorption: Topical: Limited (<5%); Oral: >70%
Distribution: V_d: 2000 L; distributed to sebum and skin predominantly
Protein binding, plasma: >99%
Metabolism: Hepatic; no active metabolites; first-pass effect (40%); little effect on CYP450 isoenzyme of the liver
Bioavailability: Oral: 80%
Half-life elimination: 22-26 hours; very slow release of drug from skin and adipose tissues occurs
Time to peak, plasma: 1-2 hours
Excretion: Oral: Urine (~75%); Topical: Urine and feces (3.5%)

Usual Dosage Adults:
Oral:
Superficial mycoses: Fingernail: 250 mg/day for up to 6 weeks; toenail: 250 mg/day for 12 weeks; doses may be given in two divided doses
Systemic mycosis: 250-500 mg/day for up to 16 months
Topical cream, solution:
Athlete's foot (tinea pedis): Apply to affected area twice daily for at least 1 week, not to exceed 4 weeks
Ringworm (tinea corporis) and jock itch (tinea cruris): Apply cream to affected area once or twice daily for at least 1 week, not to exceed 4 weeks; apply solution once daily for 7 days

(Continued)

Terbinafine *(Continued)*

Topical gel: Tinea versicolor, tinea corporis, and tinea pedis: Apply to affected area once daily for 7 days

Dosing adjustment in renal impairment: Oral administration: Although specific guidelines are not available, dose reduction in significant renal insufficiency (GFR <50 mL/minute) is recommended

Monitoring Parameters CBC and LFTs at baseline and repeated if use is for >6 weeks

Patient Information Topical: Avoid contact with eyes, nose, or mouth during treatment; nursing mothers should not use on breast tissue; advise physician if eyes or skin becomes yellow or if irritation, itching, or burning develops. Do not use occlusive dressings concurrent with therapy. Full clinical effect may require several months due to the time required for a new nail to grow.

Nursing Implications Patients should not be considered therapeutic failures until they have been symptom-free for 2-4 weeks off following a course of treatment; GI complaints usually subside with continued administration

Additional Information Due to potential toxicity, the manufacturer recommends confirmation of diagnosis testing of nail specimens prior to treatment of onychomycosis.

A meta-analysis of efficacy studies for toenail infections revealed that weighted average mycological cure rates for continuous therapy were 36.7% (griseofulvin), 54.7% (itraconazole), and 77% (terbinafine). Cure rate for 4-month pulse therapy for itraconazole and terbinafine were 73.3% and 80%. Additionally, the final outcome measure of final costs per cured infections for continuous therapy was significantly lower for terbinafine.

Dosage Forms
Cream, topical [OTC]: 1% (15 g, 30 g)
Gel, topical: 1% (5 g, 15 g, 30 g)
Solution, topical [spray, OTC]: 1%
Tablet: 250 mg

♦ **Terbinafine Hydrochloride** *see Terbinafine on page 1298*

Terbutaline *(ter BYOO ta leen)*

Related Information
Antacid Drug Interactions *on page 1477*
Bronchodilators, Comparison of Inhaled Sympathomimetics *on page 1493*

U.S. Brand Names Brethaire® [DSC]; Brethine®; Bricanyl® [DSC]

Canadian Brand Names Bricanyl® [DSC]

Therapeutic Category Beta$_2$-Adrenergic Agonist Agent; Bronchodilator; Sympathomimetic; Tocolytic Agent

Use Bronchodilator in reversible airway obstruction and bronchial asthma; tocolytic agent

Unlabeled/Investigational Use Tocolytic agent (management of preterm labor)

Pregnancy Risk Factor B

Contraindications Hypersensitivity to terbutaline or any component of the formulation; cardiac arrhythmias associated with tachycardia; tachycardia caused by digitalis intoxication

Warnings/Precautions Excessive or prolonged use may lead to tolerance. Paradoxical bronchoconstriction may occur with excessive use. If it occurs, discontinue terbutaline immediately. When used for tocolysis, there is some risk of maternal pulmonary edema, which has been associated with the following risk factors, excessive hydration, multiple gestation, occult sepsis and underlying cardiac disease. To reduce risk, limit fluid intake to 2.5-3 L/day, limit sodium intake, maintain maternal pulse to <130 beats/minute.

Adverse Reactions
>10%:
Central nervous system: Nervousness, restlessness
Neuromuscular & skeletal: Trembling
1% to 10%:
Cardiovascular: Tachycardia, hypertension, pounding heartbeat
Central nervous system: Dizziness, lightheadedness, drowsiness, headache, insomnia
Gastrointestinal: Dry mouth, nausea, vomiting, bad taste in mouth
Neuromuscular & skeletal: Muscle cramps, weakness
Miscellaneous: Diaphoresis
<1% (Limited to important or life-threatening): Arrhythmia, chest pain, paradoxical bronchospasm

Overdosage/Toxicology Symptoms include seizures, nausea, vomiting, tachycardia, cardiac dysrhythmias, and hypokalemia. In cases of overdose, supportive therapy should be instituted. Prudent use of a cardioselective beta-adrenergic blocker (eg, atenolol or metoprolol) should be considered, keeping in mind the potential for induction of bronchoconstriction in an asthmatic individual. Dialysis has not been shown to be of value in the treatment of an overdose with this agent.

Drug Interactions
Increased Effect/Toxicity: Increased toxicity with MAO inhibitors, tricyclic antidepressants.
Decreased Effect: Decreased effect with beta-blockers.

Ethanol/Nutrition/Herb Interactions Herb/Nutraceutical: Avoid ephedra, yohimbe (may cause CNS stimulation).

Stability Store injection at room temperature; protect from heat, light, and from freezing; use only clear solutions

Mechanism of Action Relaxes bronchial smooth muscle by action on beta$_2$-receptors with less effect on heart rate

Pharmacodynamics/Kinetics
Onset of action: Oral: 30-45 minutes; S.C.: 6-15 minutes
Protein binding: 25%
Metabolism: Hepatic to inactive sulfate conjugates
Bioavailability: S.C. doses are more bioavailable than oral
Half-life elimination: 11-16 hours

Excretion: Urine

Usual Dosage

Children <12 years: Bronchoconstriction:

Oral: Initial: 0.05 mg/kg/dose 3 times/day, increased gradually as required; maximum: 0.15 mg/kg/dose 3-4 times/day or a total of 5 mg/24 hours

S.C.: 0.005-0.01 mg/kg/dose to a maximum of 0.3 mg/dose every 15-20 minutes for 3 doses

Children >12 years and Adults: Bronchoconstriction:

Oral:

12-15 years: 2.5 mg every 6 hours 3 times/day; not to exceed 7.5 mg in 24 hours

>15 years: 5 mg/dose every 6 hours 3 times/day; if side effects occur, reduce dose to 2.5 mg every 6 hours; not to exceed 15 mg in 24 hours

S.C.: 0.25 mg/dose repeated in 15-30 minutes for one time only; a total dose of 0.5 mg should not be exceeded within a 4-hour period inhalations

Adults: Premature labor (tocolysis; unlabeled use):

Acute: I.V. 2.5-10 mcg/minute; increased gradually every 10-20 minutes; effective maximum dosages from 17.5-30 mcg/minute have been used with caution. Duration of infusion is at least 12 hours.

Maintenance: Oral: 2.5-10 mg every 4-6 hours for as long as necessary to prolong pregnancy depending on patient tolerance

Dosing adjustment/comments in renal impairment:

Cl_{cr} 10-50 mL/minute: Administer at 50% of normal dose

Cl_{cr} <10 mL/minute: Avoid use

Administration

I.V.: Use infusion pump.

Oral: Administer around-the-clock to promote less variation in peak and trough serum levels

Monitoring Parameters Serum potassium, glucose; heart rate, blood pressure, respiratory rate; monitor for signs and symptoms of pulmonary edema

Patient Information Precede administration of aerosol adrenocorticoid by 15 minutes; report any decreased effectiveness of drug; do not exceed recommended dose or frequency; may take last dose at 6 PM to avoid insomnia

Nursing Implications Assess lung sounds, pulse, and blood pressure before administration and during peak of medication; observe patient for wheezing after administration, if this occurs, call physician

Dosage Forms

Injection, as sulfate: 1 mg/mL (1 mL)

Tablet, as sulfate: 2.5 mg, 5 mg

Extemporaneous Preparations A 1 mg/mL suspension made from terbutaline tablets in simple syrup NF is stable 30 days when refrigerated

Horner RK and Johnson CE, "Stability of An Extemporaneously Compounded Terbutaline Sulfate Oral Liquid," *Am J Hosp Pharm*, 1991, 48(2):293-5.

Terconazole (ter KONE a zole)

Related Information

Treatment of Sexually Transmitted Diseases *on page 1609*

U.S. Brand Names Terazol® 3; Terazol® 7

Canadian Brand Names Terazol®

Synonyms Triaconazole

Therapeutic Category Antifungal Agent, Vaginal

Use Local treatment of vulvovaginal candidiasis

Pregnancy Risk Factor C

Contraindications Hypersensitivity to terconazole or any component of the formulation

Warnings/Precautions Should be discontinued if sensitization or irritation occurs. Microbiological studies (KOH smear and/or cultures) should be repeated in patients not responding to terconazole in order to confirm the diagnosis and rule out other other pathogens.

Adverse Reactions

1% to 10%:

Central nervous system; Fever, chills

Gastrointestinal: Abdominal pain

Genitourinary: Vulvar/vaginal burning, dysmenorrhea

<1% (Limited to important or life-threatening): Burning or itching of penis of sexual partner, flu-like syndrome, polyuria; vulvar itching, soreness, edema, or discharge

Stability Store at room temperature of 13°C to 30°C (59°F to 86°F).

Mechanism of Action Triazole ketal antifungal agent; involves inhibition of fungal cytochrome P450. Specifically, terconazole inhibits cytochrome P450-dependent 14-alpha-demethylase which results in accumulation of membrane disturbing 14-alpha-demethylsterols and ergosterol depletion.

Pharmacodynamics/Kinetics Absorption: Extent of systemic absorption after vaginal administration may be dependent on the presence of a uterus; 5% to 8% in women who had a hysterectomy versus 12% to 16% in nonhysterectomy women

Usual Dosage Adults: Female:

Terazol® 3 vaginal cream: Insert 1 applicatorful intravaginally at bedtime for 3 consecutive days

Terazol® 7 vaginal cream: Insert 1 applicatorful intravaginally at bedtime for 7 consecutive days

Terazol® 3 vaginal suppository: Insert 1 suppository intravaginally at bedtime for 3 consecutive days

Patient Information Insert high into vagina; complete full course of therapy; contact physician if itching or burning occurs

Nursing Implications Watch for local irritation; assist patient in administration, if necessary; assess patient's ability to self-administer, may be difficult in patients with arthritis or limited range of motion

(Continued)

Terconazole *(Continued)*

Dosage Forms
Cream, vaginal:
Terazol® 7: 0.4% (45 g)
Terazol® 3: 0.8% (20 g)
Suppository, vaginal (Terazol® 3): 80 mg (3s)

♦ **Terramycin® (Can)** *see* Oxytetracycline *on page 1028*

♦ **Terramycin® I.M.** *see* Oxytetracycline *on page 1028*

♦ **Terramycin® w/Polymyxin B Ophthalmic** *see* Oxytetracycline and Polymyxin B *on page 1029*

♦ **Teslac®** *see* Testolactone *on page 1302*

♦ **TESPA** *see* Thiotepa *on page 1323*

♦ **Tessalon®** *see* Benzonatate *on page 156*

♦ **Testoderm®** *see* Testosterone *on page 1302*

♦ **Testoderm® TTS** *see* Testosterone *on page 1302*

♦ **Testoderm® with Adhesive** *see* Testosterone *on page 1302*

Testolactone *(tes toe LAK tone)*

U.S. Brand Names Teslac®
Canadian Brand Names Teslac®
Therapeutic Category Antineoplastic Agent, Androgen
Use Palliative treatment of advanced disseminated breast carcinoma
Restrictions C-III
Pregnancy Risk Factor C
Usual Dosage Adults: Female: Oral: 250 mg 4 times/day for at least 3 months; desired response may take as long as 3 months
Additional Information Complete prescribing information for this medication should be consulted for additional detail.
Dosage Forms Tablet: 50 mg

♦ **Testopel® Pellet** *see* Testosterone *on page 1302*

Testosterone *(tes TOS ter one)*

U.S. Brand Names Androderm®; AndroGel®; Delatestryl®; Depo®-Testosterone; Testoderm®; Testoderm® TTS; Testoderm® with Adhesive; Testopel® Pellet; Testro® AQ; Testro® LA
Canadian Brand Names Andriol®; Androderm®; Androgel®; Andropository; Delatestryl®; Depotest® 100; Everone® 200; Testoderm®; Virilon® IM
Synonyms Aqueous Testosterone; Testosterone Cypionate; Testosterone Enanthate; Testosterone Propionate
Therapeutic Category Androgen
Use Androgen replacement therapy in the treatment of delayed male puberty; inoperable breast cancer; male hypogonadism
Restrictions C-III
Pregnancy Risk Factor X
Contraindications Hypersensitivity to testosterone or any component of the formulation (including soy); severe renal or cardiac disease; benign prostatic hyperplasia with obstruction; undiagnosed genital bleeding; males with carcinoma of the breast or prostate; pregnancy
Warnings/Precautions Perform radiographic examination of the hand and wrist every 6 months to determine the rate of bone maturation. May accelerate bone maturation without producing compensating gain in linear growth. Has both androgenic and anabolic activity, the anabolic action may enhance hypoglycemia. Prolonged use has been associated with serious hepatic effects (hepatitis, hepatic neoplasms, cholestatic hepatitis, jaundice). May potentiate sleep apnea in some male patients (obesity or chronic lung disease) or exacerbate heart failure due to fluid retention.
Adverse Reactions Frequency not defined.
Cardiovascular: Flushing, edema
Central nervous system: Excitation, aggressive behavior, sleeplessness, anxiety, mental depression, headache
Dermatologic: Hirsutism (increase in pubic hair growth), acne
Endocrine & metabolic: Menstrual problems (amenorrhea), virilism, breast soreness, gynecomastia, hypercalcemia, hypoglycemia
Gastrointestinal: Nausea, vomiting, GI irritation
Genitourinary: Prostatic hyperplasia, prostatic carcinoma, impotence, testicular atrophy, epididymitis, priapism, bladder irritability
Hepatic: Hepatic dysfunction, cholestatic hepatitis, hepatic necrosis
Hematologic: Leukopenia, polycythemia, suppression of clotting factors
Miscellaneous: Hypersensitivity reactions
Drug Interactions
Cytochrome P450 Effect: CYP3A3/4 and 3A5-7 enzyme substrate
Increased Effect/Toxicity: Warfarin and testosterone: Effects of oral anticoagulants may be enhanced. Testosterone may increase levels of oxyphenbutazone. May enhance fluid retention from corticosteroids.
Ethanol/Nutrition/Herb Interactions Herb/Nutraceutical: St John's wort may decrease testosterone levels.
Mechanism of Action Principal endogenous androgen responsible for promoting the growth and development of the male sex organs and maintaining secondary sex characteristics in androgen-deficient males
Pharmacodynamics/Kinetics
Duration: Route- and ester-dependent; I.M.: Cypionate and enanthate esters have longest duration, ≤2-4 weeks

Absorption: Transdermal: ~10% of dose (gel) systemically
Distribution: Crosses placenta; enters breast milk
Protein binding: 98% to transcortin and albumin
Metabolism: Hepatic
Half-life elimination: 10-100 minutes
Excretion: Urine (90%); feces (6%)

Usual Dosage

Children: I.M.:

Male hypogonadism:
Initiation of pubertal growth: 40-50 mg/m^2/dose (cypionate or enanthate ester) monthly until the growth rate falls to prepubertal levels
Terminal growth phase: 100 mg/m^2/dose (cypionate or enanthate ester) monthly until growth ceases
Maintenance virilizing dose: 100 mg/m^2/dose (cypionate or enanthate ester) twice monthly

Delayed puberty: 40-50 mg/m^2/dose monthly (cypionate or enanthate ester) for 6 months

Adults: Inoperable breast cancer: I.M.: 200-400 mg every 2-4 weeks

Male: Short-acting formulations: Testosterone aqueous/testosterone propionate (in oil): I.M.:
Androgen replacement therapy: 10-50 mg 2-3 times/week
Male hypogonadism: 40-50 mg/m^2/dose monthly until the growth rate falls to prepubertal levels (~5 cm/year); during terminal growth phase: 100 mg/m^2/dose monthly until growth ceases; maintenance virilizing dose: 100 mg/m^2/dose twice monthly or 50-400 mg/dose every 2-4 weeks

Male: Long-acting formulations: Testosterone enanthate (in oil)/testosterone cypionate (in oil): I.M.:
Male hypogonadism: 50-400 mg every 2-4 weeks
Male with delayed puberty: 50-200 mg every 2-4 weeks for a limited duration

Male ≥18 years: Transdermal: Primary hypogonadism **or** hypogonadotropic hypogonadism:
Testoderm®: Apply 6 mg patch daily to scrotum (if scrotum is inadequate, use a 4 mg daily system)
Testoderm® TTS: Apply 5 mg patch daily to clean, dry area of skin on the arm, back or upper buttocks. **Do not apply Testoderm® TTS to the scrotum.**
Androderm®: Apply 2 systems nightly to clean, dry area on the back, abdomen, upper arms, or thighs for 24 hours for a total of 5 mg/day
AndroGel®: Male >18 years: 5 g (to deliver 50 mg of testosterone with 5 mg systemically absorbed) applied once daily (preferably in the morning) to clean, dry, intact skin of the shoulder and upper arms and/or abdomen. Upon opening the packet(s), the entire contents should be squeezed into the palm of the hand and immediately applied to the application site(s). Application sites should be allowed to dry for a few minutes prior to dressing. Hands should be washed with soap and water after application. **Do not apply AndroGel® to the genitals.**

Dosing adjustment/comments in hepatic disease: Reduce dose

Monitoring Parameters Periodic liver function tests, radiologic examination of wrist and hand every 6 months (when using in prepubertal children)

Reference Range Testosterone, urine: Male: 100-1500 ng/24 hours; Female: 100-500 ng/24 hours

Test Interactions May cause a decrease in creatinine and creatine excretion and an increase in the excretion of 17-ketosteroids, thyroid function tests

Patient Information Virilization may occur in female patients; report menstrual irregularities; male patients report persistent penile erections; all patients should report persistent GI distress, diarrhea, or jaundice; see Nursing Implications for AndroGel®-specific patient instructions

Nursing Implications Warm injection to room temperature and shaking vial will help redissolve crystals that have formed after storage; administer by deep I.M. injection into the upper outer quadrant of the gluteus maximus. Transdermal system (Testoderm®) should be applied on clean, dry, scrotal skin. Dry-shave scrotal hair for optimal skin contact. Do not use chemical depilatories. Androderm® and Testoderm® TTS should be applied to clean dry area of skin on the arm, back, or upper buttocks.

Dosage Forms

Gel, transdermal (AndroGel®): 1%: 50 mg (5 g gel); 75 mg (7.5 g gel)
Injection, aqueous suspension (Testro® AQ): 25 mg/mL (10 mL, 30 mL); 50 mg/mL (10 mL, 30 mL); 100 mg/mL (10 mL, 30 mL)
Injection, in oil, as cypionate (Depo® Testosterone): 100 mg/mL (1 mL, 10 mL); 200 mg/mL (1 mL, 10 mL)
Injection, in oil, as enanthate (Delatestryl®, Testro® LA): 200 mg/mL (1 mL, 5 mL, 10 mL)
Injection, in oil, as propionate: 100 mg/mL (10 mL)
Pellet (Testopel®): 75 mg (1 pellet per vial)
Transdermal system:
Androderm®: 2.5 mg/day; 5 mg/day
Testoderm®: 4 mg/day; 6 mg/day
Testoderm® TTS: 5 mg/day

♦ **Testosterone and Estradiol** *see* Estradiol and Testosterone *on page 495*
♦ **Testosterone Cypionate** *see* Testosterone *on page 1302*
♦ **Testosterone Enanthate** *see* Testosterone *on page 1302*
♦ **Testosterone Propionate** *see* Testosterone *on page 1302*
♦ **Testred®** *see* MethylTESTOSTERone *on page 898*
♦ **Testro® AQ** *see* Testosterone *on page 1302*
♦ **Testro® LA** *see* Testosterone *on page 1302*
♦ **Tetanus and Diphtheria Toxoid** *see* Diphtheria and Tetanus Toxoid *on page 417*

Tetanus Antitoxin (TET a nus an tee TOKS in)

Synonyms TAT
Therapeutic Category Antitoxin
(Continued)

Tetanus Antitoxin *(Continued)*

Use Tetanus prophylaxis or treatment of active tetanus only when tetanus immune globulin (TIG) is not available; tetanus immune globulin (Hyper-Tet®) is the preferred tetanus immunoglobulin for the treatment of active tetanus; may be given concomitantly with tetanus toxoid adsorbed when immediate treatment is required, but active immunization is desirable

Pregnancy Risk Factor D

Contraindications Hypersensitivity to equine-derived preparations or any component of the formulation

Warnings/Precautions Tetanus antitoxin is not the same as tetanus immune globulin; sensitivity testing should be conducted in all individuals regardless of clinical history; have epinephrine 1:1000 available

Adverse Reactions ≥10%:
Dermatologic: Skin eruptions, urticaria, erythema
Neuromuscular & skeletal: Arthralgia

Stability Refrigerate, do not freeze

Mechanism of Action Provides passive immunization; solution of concentrated globulins containing antitoxic antibodies obtained from horse serum after immunization against tetanus toxin

Usual Dosage
Prophylaxis: I.M., S.C.:
Children <30 kg: 1500 units
Children and Adults ≥30 kg: 3000-5000 units
Treatment: Children and Adults: Inject 10,000-40,000 units into wound; administer 40,000-100,000 units

Nursing Implications All patients should have sensitivity testing prior to starting therapy with tetanus antitoxin

Dosage Forms Injection, equine: Not less than 400 units/mL (12.5 mL, 50 mL)

Tetanus Immune Globulin (Human)

(TET a nus i MYUN GLOB yoo lin HYU man)

Related Information
Adverse Events and Vaccination *on page 1553*
Immunization Recommendations *on page 1538*

U.S. Brand Names BayTet™

Canadian Brand Names BayTet™

Synonyms TIG

Therapeutic Category Immune Globulin

Use Passive immunization against tetanus; tetanus immune globulin is preferred over tetanus antitoxin for treatment of active tetanus; part of the management of an unclean, wound in a person whose history of previous receipt of tetanus toxoid is unknown or who has received less than three doses of tetanus toxoid; elderly may require TIG more often than younger patients with tetanus infection due to declining antibody titers with age

Pregnancy Risk Factor C

Contraindications Hypersensitivity to tetanus immune globulin, thimerosal, or any component of the formulation

Warnings/Precautions Have epinephrine 1:1000 available for anaphylactic reactions. Use caution in patients with isolated immunoglobulin A deficiency or a history of systemic hypersensitivity to human immunoglobulins. As a product of human plasma, this product may potentially transmit disease; screening of donors, as well as testing and/or inactivation of certain viruses reduces this risk. Use caution in patients with thrombocytopenia or coagulation disorders (I.M. injections may be contraindicated). Not for intravenous administration.

Adverse Reactions
>10%: Local: Pain, tenderness, erythema at injection site
1% to 10%:
Central nervous system: Fever (mild)
Dermatologic: Urticaria, angioedema
Neuromuscular & skeletal: Muscle stiffness
Miscellaneous: Anaphylaxis reaction
<1% (Limited to important or life-threatening): Sensitization to repeated injections

Stability Refrigerate

Mechanism of Action Passive immunity toward tetanus

Pharmacodynamics/Kinetics Absorption: Well absorbed

Usual Dosage I.M.:
Prophylaxis of tetanus:
Children: 4 units/kg; some recommend administering 250 units to small children
Adults: 250 units
Treatment of tetanus:
Children: 500-3000 units; some should infiltrate locally around the wound
Adults: 3000-6000 units

Administration Do not administer I.V.; I.M. use only

Additional Information Tetanus immune globulin (TIG) must not contain <50 units/mL. Protein makes up 10% to 18% of TIG preparations. The great majority of this (≥90%) is IgG. TIG has almost no color or odor and it is a sterile, nonpyrogenic, concentrated preparation of immunoglobulins that has been derived from the plasma of adults hyperimmunized with tetanus toxoid. The pooled material from which the immunoglobulin is derived may be from fewer than 1000 donors. This plasma has been shown to be free of hepatitis B surface antigen.

Dosage Forms Injection: 250 units/mL

Tetanus Toxoid (Adsorbed) (TET a nus TOKS oyd, ad SORBED)

Related Information
Adverse Events and Vaccination *on page 1553*

Immunization Recommendations *on page 1538*
Skin Tests *on page 1533*

Therapeutic Category Toxoid

Use Selective induction of active immunity against tetanus in selected patients. **Note:** Tetanus and diphtheria toxoids for adult use (Td) is the preferred immunizing agent for most adults and for children after their seventh birthday. Young children should receive trivalent DTwP or DTaP (diphtheria/tetanus/pertussis - whole cell or acellular), as part of their childhood immunization program, unless pertussis is contraindicated, then TD is warranted.

Pregnancy Risk Factor C

Contraindications Hypersensitivity to tetanus toxoid or any component of the formulation (may use the fluid tetanus toxoid to immunize the rare patient who is hypersensitive to aluminum adjuvant); avoid use with chloramphenicol or if neurological signs or symptoms occurred after prior administration; poliomyelitis outbreaks require deferral of immunizations; acute respiratory infections or other active infections may dictate deferral of administration of routine primary immunizing but not emergency doses

Warnings/Precautions Not equivalent to tetanus toxoid fluid; the tetanus toxoid adsorbed is the preferred toxoid for immunization and Td, TD or DTaP/DTwP are the preferred adsorbed forms; avoid injection into a blood vessel; have epinephrine (1:1000) available; not for use in treatment of tetanus infection nor for immediate prophylaxis of unimmunized individuals; immunosuppressive therapy or other immunodeficiencies may diminish antibody response, however it is recommended for routine immunization of symptomatic and asymptomatic HIV-infected patients; deferral of immunization until immunosuppression is discontinued or administration of an additional dose >1 month after treatment is recommended; allergic reactions may occur; epinephrine 1:1000 must be available; use in pediatrics should be deferred until >1 year of age when a history of a CNS disorder is present; elderly may not mount adequate antibody titers following immunization

Adverse Reactions
>10%: Local: Induration/redness at injection site
1% to 10%:
  Central nervous system: Chills, fever
  Local: Sterile abscess at injection site
  Miscellaneous: Allergic reaction
<1% (Limited to important or life-threatening): Arthus-type hypersensitivity reactions, blistering at injection site, fever >103°F, malaise, neurological disturbances

Stability Refrigerate, do not freeze

Mechanism of Action Tetanus toxoid preparations contain the toxin produced by virulent tetanus bacilli (detoxified growth products of *Clostridium tetani*). The toxin has been modified by treatment with formaldehyde so that it has lost toxicity but still retains ability to act as antigen and produce active immunity; the aluminum salt, a mineral adjuvant, delays the rate of absorption and prolongs and enhances its properties; duration ~10 years.

Pharmacodynamics/Kinetics Duration: Primary immunization: ~10 years

Usual Dosage Adults: I.M.:
Primary immunization: 0.5 mL; repeat 0.5 mL at 4-8 weeks after first dose and at 6-12 months after second dose
Routine booster doses are recommended only every 5-10 years

Administration Inject intramuscularly in the area of the vastus lateralis (midthigh laterally) or deltoid

For patients at risk of hemorrhage following intramuscular injection, the ACIP recommends "it should be administered intramuscularly if, in the opinion of the physician familiar with the patients bleeding risk, the vaccine can be administered with reasonable safety by this route. If the patient receives antihemophilia or other similar therapy, intramuscular vaccination can be scheduled shortly after such therapy is administered. A fine needle (23 gauge or smaller) can be used for the vaccination and firm pressure applied to the site (without rubbing) for at least 2 minutes. The patient should be instructed concerning the risk of hematoma from the injection."

Patient Information A nodule may be palpable at the injection site for a few weeks. DT, Td and T vaccines cause few problems; they may cause mild fever or soreness, swelling, and redness where the shot was given. These problems usually last 1-2 days, but this does not happen nearly as often as with DTP vaccine. Sometimes, adults who get these vaccines can have a lot of soreness and swelling where the shot was given.

Additional Information Federal law requires that the date of administration, the vaccine manufacturer, lot number of vaccine, and the administering person's name, title and address be entered into the patient's permanent medical record.

Dosage Forms
Injection, adsorbed:
  Tetanus 5 Lf units per 0.5 mL dose (0.5 mL, 5 mL)
  Tetanus 10 Lf units per 0.5 mL dose (0.5 mL, 5 mL)

Tetanus Toxoid (Fluid) (TET a nus TOKS oyd FLOO id)

Related Information

Adverse Events and Vaccination *on page 1553*
Immunization Recommendations *on page 1538*
Skin Tests *on page 1533*

Synonyms Tetanus Toxoid Plain

Therapeutic Category Toxoid

Use Detection of delayed hypersensitivity and assessment of cell-mediated immunity; active immunization against tetanus in the rare adult or child who is allergic to the aluminum adjuvant (a product containing adsorbed tetanus toxoid is preferred)

Pregnancy Risk Factor C

Contraindications Hypersensitivity to tetanus toxoid or any component of the formulation

Warnings/Precautions Epinephrine 1:1000 should be readily available; skin test responsiveness may be delayed or reduced in elderly patients

(Continued)

Tetanus Toxoid (Fluid) *(Continued)*

Adverse Reactions Frequency not defined: Very hypersensitive persons may develop a local reaction at the injection site; urticaria, anaphylactic reactions, shock, and death are possible.

Stability Refrigerate

Mechanism of Action Tetanus toxoid preparations contain the toxin produced by virulent tetanus bacilli (detoxified growth products of *Clostridium tetani*). The toxin has been modified by treatment with formaldehyde so that is has lost toxicity but still retains ability to act as antigen and produce active immunity.

Usual Dosage

Anergy testing: Intradermal: 0.1 mL

Primary immunization (**Note:** Td, TD, DTaP/DTwP are recommended): Adults: Inject 3 doses of 0.5 mL I.M. or S.C. at 4- to 8-week intervals; administer fourth dose 6-12 months after third dose

Booster doses: I.M., S.C.: 0.5 mL every 10 years

Administration Must not be used I.V.; for skin testing, use 0.1 mL of 1:100 v/v or 0.02 mL of 1:10 v/v solution

Additional Information Federal law requires that the date of administration, the vaccine manufacturer, lot number of vaccine, and the administering person's name, title and address be entered into the patient's permanent medical record.

Dosage Forms

Injection, fluid:

Tetanus 4 Lf units per 0.5 mL dose (7.5 mL)

Tetanus 5 Lf units per 0.5 mL dose (0.5 mL, 7.5 mL)

♦ **Tetanus Toxoid Plain** *see* Tetanus Toxoid (Fluid) *on page 1305*

Tetracaine *(TET ra kane)*

U.S. Brand Names Pontocaine®

Canadian Brand Names Ametop™; Pontocaine®

Synonyms Amethocaine Hydrochloride; Tetracaine Hydrochloride

Therapeutic Category Local Anesthetic, Ester Derivative; Local Anesthetic, Injectable; Local Anesthetic, Ophthalmic; Local Anesthetic, Oral; Local Anesthetic, Topical

Use Spinal anesthesia; local anesthesia in the eye for various diagnostic and examination purposes; topically applied to nose and throat for various diagnostic procedures; **approximately 10 times more potent than procaine**

Pregnancy Risk Factor C

Usual Dosage Maximum adult dose: 50 mg

Children: Safety and efficacy have not been established

Adults:

Ophthalmic (not for prolonged use):

Ointment: Apply ¹/₂" to 1" to lower conjunctival fornix

Solution: Instill 1-2 drops

Spinal anesthesia:

High, medium, low, and saddle blocks: 0.2% to 0.3% solution

Prolonged (2-3 hours): 1% solution

Subarachnoid injection: 5-20 mg

Saddle block: 2-5 mg; a 1% solution should be diluted with equal volume of CSF before administration

Topical mucous membranes (2% solution): Apply as needed; dose should not exceed 20 mg

Topical for skin: Ointment/cream: Apply to affected areas as needed

Additional Information Complete prescribing information for this medication should be consulted for additional detail.

Dosage Forms

Cream, as hydrochloride: 1% (28 g)

Injection, as hydrochloride: 1% [10 mg/mL] (2 mL)

Injection, with dextrose 6%, as hydrochloride: 0.2% [2 mg/mL] (2 mL); 0.3% [3 mg/mL] (5 mL)

Ointment, ophthalmic, as hydrochloride: 0.5% [5 mg/mL] (3.75 g)

Ointment, topical, as hydrochloride: 0.5% [5 mg/mL] (28 g)

Powder for injection, as hydrochloride: 20 mg

Solution, ophthalmic, as hydrochloride: 0.5% [5 mg/mL] (1 mL, 2 mL, 15 mL, 59 mL)

Solution, topical, as hydrochloride: 2% [20 mg/mL] (30 mL, 118 mL)

♦ **Tetracaine Hydrochloride** *see* Tetracaine *on page 1306*

♦ **Tetracaine Hydrochloride, Benzocaine Butyl Aminobenzoate, and Benzalkonium Chloride** *see* Benzocaine, Butyl Aminobenzoate, Tetracaine, and Benzalkonium Chloride *on page 156*

♦ **TetraCap®** *see* Tetracycline *on page 1306*

♦ **Tetracosactide** *see* Cosyntropin *on page 336*

Tetracycline *(tet ra SYE kleen)*

Related Information

Antacid Drug Interactions *on page 1477*

Antimicrobial Drugs of Choice *on page 1588*

Helicobacter pylori Treatment *on page 1668*

Treatment of Sexually Transmitted Diseases *on page 1609*

U.S. Brand Names Achromycin® [DSC]; Brodspec®; EmTet®; Sumycin®; TetraCap®; Topicycline®; Wesmycin®

Canadian Brand Names Apo®-Tetra; Novo-Tetra; Nu-Tetra

Synonyms TCN; Tetracycline Hydrochloride

Therapeutic Category Acne Products; Antibiotic, Ophthalmic; Antibiotic, Tetracycline Derivative; Antibiotic, Topical

Use Treatment of susceptible bacterial infections of both gram-positive and gram-negative organisms; also infections due to *Mycoplasma*, *Chlamydia*, and *Rickettsia*; indicated for acne, exacerbations of chronic bronchitis, and treatment of gonorrhea and syphilis in patients that are allergic to penicillin; as part of a multidrug regimen for *H. pylori* eradication to reduce the risk of duodenal ulcer recurrence

Pregnancy Risk Factor D (systemic)/B (topical)

Pregnancy/Breast-Feeding Implications Breast-feeding/lactation: Excreted in breast milk; avoid use if possible in lactating mothers

Contraindications Hypersensitivity to tetracycline or any component of the formulation; do not administer to children ≤8 years of age; pregnancy (systemic use)

Warnings/Precautions Use of tetracyclines during tooth development may cause permanent discoloration of the teeth and enamel, hypoplasia and retardation of skeletal development and bone growth with risk being the greatest for children <4 years and those receiving high doses; use with caution in patients with renal or hepatic impairment (eg, elderly) and in pregnancy; dosage modification required in patients with renal impairment since it may increase BUN as an antianabolic agent; pseudotumor cerebri has been reported with tetracycline use (usually resolves with discontinuation); outdated drug can cause nephropathy; superinfection possible; use protective measure to avoid photosensitivity

Adverse Reactions

>10%: Gastrointestinal: Discoloration of teeth and enamel hypoplasia (young children)

1% to 10%:

Dermatologic: Photosensitivity

Gastrointestinal: Nausea, diarrhea

<1% (Limited to important or life-threatening): Acute renal failure, anaphylaxis, bulging fontanels in infants, diabetes insipidus, esophagitis, exfoliative dermatitis, hepatotoxicity, hypersensitivity reactions, increased intracranial pressure, pancreatitis, paresthesia, pericarditis, pigmentation of nails, pruritus, pseudomembranous colitis, pseudotumor cerebri, staphylococcal enterocolitis, superinfection, thrombophlebitis, vomiting

Overdosage/Toxicology Symptoms include nausea, anorexia, and diarrhea. Following GI decontamination, supportive care only.

Drug Interactions

Increased Effect/Toxicity: Methoxyflurane anesthesia when concurrent with tetracycline may cause fatal nephrotoxicity. Warfarin with tetracyclines may cause increased anticoagulation.

Decreased Effect: Calcium, magnesium- or aluminum-containing antacids, iron, zinc, sodium bicarbonate, sucralfate, didanosine, or quinapril may decrease tetracycline absorption. Therapeutic effect of oral contraceptives and penicillins may be reduced with coadministration of tetracycline.

Ethanol/Nutrition/Herb Interactions

Food: Tetracycline serum concentrations may be decreased if taken with dairy products.

Herb/Nutraceutical: Avoid dong quai, St John's wort (may also cause photosensitization)

Stability Outdated tetracyclines have caused a Fanconi-like syndrome; protect oral dosage forms from light

Mechanism of Action Inhibits bacterial protein synthesis by binding with the 30S and possibly the 50S ribosomal subunit(s) of susceptible bacteria; may also cause alterations in the cytoplasmic membrane

Pharmacodynamics/Kinetics

Absorption: Oral: 75%

Distribution: Small amount appears in bile

Relative diffusion from blood into CSF: Good only with inflammation (exceeds usual MICs)

CSF:blood level ratio: Inflamed meninges: 25%

Protein binding: 20% to 60%

Half-life elimination: Normal renal function: 8-11 hours; End-stage renal disease: 57-108 hours

Time to peak, serum: Oral: 2-4 hours

Excretion: Primarily urine (60% as unchanged drug); feces (as active form)

Usual Dosage

Children >8 years: Oral: 25-50 mg/kg/day in divided doses every 6 hours

Children >8 years and Adults:

Ophthalmic:

Ointment: Instill every 2-12 hours

Suspension: Instill 1-2 drops 2-4 times/day or more often as needed

Topical: Apply to affected areas 1-4 times/day

Adults: Oral: 250-500 mg/dose every 6 hours

Helicobacter pylori eradication: 500 mg 2-4 times/day depending on regimen; requires combination therapy with at least one other antibiotic and an acid-suppressing agent (proton pump inhibitor or H_2 blocker)

Dosing interval in renal impairment:

Cl_{cr} 50-80 mL/minute: Administer every 8-12 hours

Cl_{cr} 10-50 mL/minute: Administer every 12-24 hours

Cl_{cr} <10 mL/minute: Administer every 24 hours

Dialysis: Slightly dialyzable (5% to 20%) via hemo- and peritoneal dialysis or via continuous arteriovenous or venovenous hemofiltration; no supplemental dosage necessary

Dosing adjustment in hepatic impairment: Avoid use or maximum dose is 1 g/day

Administration Oral formulation should be administered on an empty stomach (ie, 1 hour prior to, or 2 hours after meals) to increase total absorption. Administer at least 1-2 hours prior to, or 4 hours after antacid because aluminum and magnesium cations may chelate with tetracycline and reduce its total absorption.

Monitoring Parameters Renal, hepatic, and hematologic function test, temperature, WBC, cultures and sensitivity, appetite, mental status

Test Interactions False-negative urine glucose with Clinistix®

Patient Information Take 1 hour before or 2 hours after meals with adequate amounts of fluid; avoid prolonged exposure to sunlight or sunlamps; avoid taking antacids, iron, or dairy products within 2 hours of taking tetracyclines; report persistent nausea, vomiting, yellow coloring of skin or eyes, dark urine, or pale stools; ophthalmic may cause transient burning or itching; topical is for external use only and may stain skin yellow

(Continued)

Tetracycline *(Continued)*

Dosage Forms

Capsule, as hydrochloride: 250 mg, 500 mg
Ointment, ophthalmic: 1% [10 mg/mL] (3.5 g)
Ointment, topical, as hydrochloride: 3% [30 mg/mL] (14.2 g, 30 g)
Solution, topical: 2.2 mg/mL (70 mL)
Suspension, ophthalmic: 1% [10 mg/mL] (0.5 mL, 1 mL, 4 mL)
Suspension, oral, as hydrochloride: 125 mg/5 mL (60 mL, 480 mL)
Tablet, as hydrochloride: 250 mg, 500 mg

♦ **Tetracycline, Bismuth Subsalicylate, and Metronidazole** *see* Bismuth Subsalicylate, Metronidazole, and Tetracycline *on page 172*

♦ **Tetracycline Hydrochloride** *see* Tetracycline *on page 1306*

♦ **Tetracycline, Metronidazole, and Bismuth Subsalicylate** *see* Bismuth Subsalicylate, Metronidazole, and Tetracycline *on page 172*

♦ **Tetrahydroaminoacrine** *see* Tacrine *on page 1282*

♦ **Tetrahydrocannabinol** *see* Dronabinol *on page 450*

♦ **Tetramune® [DSC]** *see* Diphtheria, Tetanus Toxoids, Whole-Cell Pertussis, and *Haemophilus influenzae* Type b Conjugate Vaccines *on page 421*

♦ **Teveten®** *see* Eprosartan *on page 479*

♦ **Texacort®** *see* Hydrocortisone *on page 682*

♦ **TG** *see* Thioguanine *on page 1318*

♦ **6-TG** *see* Thioguanine *on page 1318*

♦ **T-Gesic®** *see* Hydrocodone and Acetaminophen *on page 676*

♦ **THA** *see* Tacrine *on page 1282*

Thalidomide *(tha LI doe mide)*

U.S. Brand Names Thalomid®

Canadian Brand Names Thalomid®

Therapeutic Category Immunosuppressant Agent

Use Treatment and maintenance of cutaneous manifestations of erythema nodosum leprosum
Orphan status: Treatment of Crohn's disease

Unlabeled/Investigational Use Treatment or prevention of graft-versus-host reactions after bone marrow transplantation; AIDS-related aphthous stomatitis; Langerhans cell histiocytosis, Behçet's syndrome; hypnotic agent; also may be effective in rheumatoid arthritis, discoid lupus erythematosus, and erythema multiforme; useful in type 2 lepra reactions, but not type 1; renal cell carcinoma, multiple myeloma, myeloma, Waldenström's macroglobulinemia

Restrictions Thalidomide is approved for marketing only under a special distribution program. This program, called the "System for Thalidomide Education and Prescribing Safety" (STEPS™), has been approved by the FDA. Prescribing and dispensing of thalidomide is restricted to prescribers and pharmacists registered with the program. Prior to dispensing, an authorization number must be obtained (1-888-423-5436) from Celgene (write authorization number on prescription). No more than a 4-week supply should be dispensed. Blister packs should be dispensed intact (do not repackage capsules). Prescriptions must be filled within 7 days.

Pregnancy Risk Factor X

Pregnancy/Breast-Feeding Implications Embryotoxic with limb defects noted from the 27th to 40th gestational day of exposure; all cases of phocomelia occur from the 27th to 42nd gestational day; fetal cardiac, gastrointestinal, and genitourinary tract abnormalities have also been described. Effective contraception must be used for at least 4 weeks before initiating therapy, during therapy, and for 4 weeks following discontinuation of thalidomide. Males (even those vasectomized) must use a latex condom during any sexual contact with women of childbearing age.

Contraindications Hypersensitivity to thalidomide or any component of the formulation; neuropathy (peripheral); pregnancy or women in childbearing years unless alternative therapies are inappropriate and adequate precautions are taken to avoid pregnancy; patient unable to comply with STEPS™ program.

Warnings/Precautions Liver, hepatic, neurological disorders, constipation, congestive heart failure, hypertension; safety and efficacy have not been established in children <12 years of age. Use caution in patients with a history of seizures, receiving concurrent therapy with drugs which alter seizure threshold, or conditions which predispose to seizures.

Adverse Reactions

Controlled clinical trials: ENL:
>10%:
Central nervous system: Somnolence (37.5%), headache (12.5%)
Dermatologic: Rash (20.8%)
1% to 10% (Limited to important or life-threatening):
Dermatologic: Rash (maculopapular) (4.2%)
Genitourinary: Impotence (8.2%)

HIV-seropositive:
General: An increased viral load has been noted in patients treated with thalidomide. This is of uncertain clinical significance - see monitoring
>10%:
Central nervous system: Somnolence (36% to 37%), dizziness (18.7% to 19.4%), fever (19.4% to 21.9%), headache (16.7% to 18.7%)

Dermatologic: Rash (25%), maculopapular rash (16.7% to 18.7%), acne (3.1% to 11.1%)

Gastrointestinal: AST increase (2.8% to 12.5%), diarrhea (11.1% to 18.7%), nausea (≤12.5%), oral moniliasis (6.3% to 11.1%)

Hematologic: Leukopenia (16.7% to 25%), anemia (5.6% to 12.5%)

Neuromuscular & skeletal: Paresthesia (5.6% to 15.6%), weakness (5.6% to 21.9%)

Miscellaneous: Diaphoresis (≤12.5%), lymphadenopathy (5.6% to 12.5%)

1% to 10% (Limited to important or life-threatening): Central nervous system: Agitation (≤9.4%)

Literature reports of other adverse reactions (limited to important or life-threatening): Acute renal failure, bradycardia, chronic myelogenous leukemia (CML), dyspnea, erythema nodosum, Hodgkin's disease, hypersensitivity, hyperthyroidism, lymphopenia, myxedema, orthostatic hypotension, pancytopenia, photosensitivity, Raynaud's syndrome, seizures, Stevens-Johnson syndrome, suicide attempt, toxic epidermal necrolysis

Drug Interactions

Increased Effect/Toxicity: Other medications known to cause peripheral neuropathy should be used with caution in patients receiving thalidomide; thalidomide may enhance the sedative activity of other drugs such as ethanol, barbiturates, reserpine, and chlorpromazine

Ethanol/Nutrition/Herb Interactions

Ethanol: Avoid ethanol (may increase sedation).

Herb/Nutraceutical: Avoid cat's claw (has immunostimulant properties).

Stability Store at 15°C to 30°C (50°F to 86°F). Protect from light. Keep in original package.

Mechanism of Action A derivative of glutethimide; mode of action for immunosuppression is unclear; inhibition of neutrophil chemotaxis and decreased monocyte phagocytosis may occur; may cause 50% to 80% reduction of tumor necrosis factor - alpha

Pharmacodynamics/Kinetics

Distribution: V_d: 120 L

Metabolism: Hepatic

Half-life elimination: 8.7 hours

Time to peak, plasma: 2-6 hours

Usual Dosage Oral:

Cutaneous ENL:

Initiate dosing at 100-300 mg/day taken once daily at bedtime with water (at least 1 hour after evening meal)

Patients weighing <50 kg: Initiate at lower end of the dosing range

Severe cutaneous reaction or previously requiring high dose may be initiated at 400 mg/day; doses may be divided, but taken 1 hour after meals

Dosing should continue until active reaction subsides (usually at least 2 weeks), then tapered in 50 mg decrements every 2-4 weeks

Patients who flare during tapering or with a history or requiring prolonged maintenance should be maintained on the minimum dosage necessary to control the reaction. Efforts to taper should be repeated every 3-6 months, in increments of 50 mg every 2-4 weeks.

Behçet's syndrome (unlabeled use): 100-400 mg/day

Graft-vs-host reactions (unlabeled use): 100-1600 mg/day; usual initial dose: 200 mg 4 times/day for use up to 700 days

AIDS-related aphthous stomatitis (unlabeled use): 200 mg twice daily for 5 days, then 200 mg/day for up to 8 weeks

Discoid lupus erythematosus (unlabeled use): 100-400 mg/day; maintenance dose: 25-50 mg

Dietary Considerations Should be taken at least 1 hour after the evening meal.

Monitoring Parameters Required pregnancy testing, WBC with differential. In HIV-seropositive patients: viral load after 1 and 3 months, then every 3 months. Pregnancy testing is required within 24 hours of initiation of therapy.

Reference Range Therapeutic plasma thalidomide levels in graft-vs-host reactions are 5-8 µg/mL, although it has been suggested that lower plasma levels (0.5-1.5 µg/mL) may be therapeutic; peak serum thalidomide level after a 200 mg dose: 1.2 µg/mL

Dosage Forms Capsule: 50 mg

Theophylline and Guaifenesin (thee OFF i lin & gwye FEN e sin)

U.S. Brand Names Bronchial®; Glycerol-T®; Quibron®; Slo-Phyllin® GG

Synonyms Guaifenesin and Theophylline

Therapeutic Category Theophylline Derivative

Use Symptomatic treatment of bronchospasm associated with bronchial asthma, chronic bronchitis, and pulmonary emphysema

Pregnancy Risk Factor C

Usual Dosage Adults: Oral: 16 mg/kg/day or 400 mg theophylline/day, in divided doses, every 6-8 hours

Additional Information Complete prescribing information for this medication should be consulted for additional detail.

Dosage Forms
Capsule:
   Theophylline 150 mg and guaifenesin 90 mg
   Theophylline 300 mg and guaifenesin 180 mg
Elixir: Theophylline 150 mg and guaifenesin 90 mg per 15 mL (480 mL)

Theophylline, Ephedrine, and Phenobarbital
(thee OFF i lin, e FED rin, & fee noe BAR bi tal)

U.S. Brand Names Tedral®

Synonyms Ephedrine, Theophylline and Phenobarbital

Therapeutic Category Theophylline Derivative

Use Prevention and symptomatic treatment of bronchial asthma; relief of asthmatic bronchitis and other bronchospastic disorders

Pregnancy Risk Factor D

Usual Dosage
Children >60 lb: 1 tablet or 5 mL every 4 hours
Adults: 1-2 tablets or 10-20 mL every 4 hours

Additional Information Complete prescribing information for this medication should be consulted for additional detail.

Dosage Forms
Suspension: Theophylline 65 mg, ephedrine sulfate 12 mg, and phenobarbital 4 mg per 5 mL
Tablet:
   Theophylline 118 mg, ephedrine sulfate 25 mg, and phenobarbital 11 mg
   Theophylline 130 mg, ephedrine sulfate 24 mg, and phenobarbital 8 mg

Theophylline Salts (thee OFF i lin salts)

Related Information
Asthma *on page 1645*

U.S. Brand Names Aerolate®; Aerolate III®; Aerolate JR®; Aerolate SR®; Aminophyllin™; Aquaphyllin®; Asmalix®; Bronkodyl®; Choledyl®; Constant-T®; Duraphyl™; Elixophyllin®; LaBID®; Phyllocontin®; Quibron®-T/SR; Respbid®; Slo-bid™; Slo-Phyllin®; Sustaire®; Theo-24®; Theobid®; Theochron®; Theoclear® L.A.; Theo-Dur®; Theolair™; Theon®; Theospan®-SR; Theovent®; Truphylline®

Synonyms Aminophylline; Choline Theophyllinate; Ethylenediamine; Oxtriphylline; Theophylline

Therapeutic Category Bronchodilator; Theophylline Derivative

Use Bronchodilator in reversible airway obstruction due to asthma, chronic bronchitis, and emphysema; for neonatal apnea/bradycardia

Pregnancy Risk Factor C

Pregnancy/Breast-Feeding Implications
Clinical effects on the fetus: Crosses the placenta. Transient tachycardia, irritability, vomiting in newborn especially if maternal serum concentrations >20 mcg/mL. Apneic spells attributed to withdrawal in newborn exposed throughout gestation period. Available evidence suggests safe use during pregnancy.
Breast-feeding/lactation: Crosses into breast milk
Clinical effects on the infant: Irritability reported in infants. American Academy of Pediatrics considers **compatible** with breast-feeding.

Contraindications Uncontrolled arrhythmias, hyperthyroidism, peptic ulcers, uncontrolled seizure disorders, hypersensitivity to xanthines or any component

Warnings/Precautions Use with caution in patients with peptic ulcer, hyperthyroidism, hypertension, tachyarrhythmias, and patients with compromised cardiac function; do not inject I.V. solution faster than 25 mg/minute; elderly, acutely ill, and patients with severe respiratory problems, pulmonary edema, or liver dysfunction are at greater risk of toxicity because of reduced drug clearance

Although there is a great intersubject variability for half-lives of methylxanthines (2-10 hours), elderly as a group have slower hepatic clearance. Therefore, use lower initial doses and monitor closely for response and adverse reactions. Additionally, elderly are at greater risk for toxicity due to concomitant disease (eg, CHF, arrhythmias), and drug use (eg, cimetidine, ciprofloxacin, etc).

Adverse Reactions See table.

Theophylline Serum Levels (mcg/mL)*	Adverse Reactions
15-25	GI upset, diarrhea, N/V, abdominal pain, nervousness, headache, insomnia, agitation, dizziness, muscle cramp, tremor
25-35	Tachycardia, occasional PVC
>35	Ventricular tachycardia, frequent PVC, seizure

*Adverse effects do not necessarily occur according to serum levels. Arrhythmia and seizure can occur without seeing the other adverse effects.

Uncommon at serum theophylline concentrations ≤20 mcg/mL

1% to 10%:
Cardiovascular: Tachycardia
Central nervous system: Nervousness, restlessness
Gastrointestinal: Nausea, vomiting
<1%: Allergic reactions, gastric irritation, insomnia, irritability, rash, seizures, tremor

Drug Interactions

Cytochrome P450 Effect: CYP1A2 and 3A3/4 enzyme substrate, CYP2E enzyme substrate (minor)

Increased Effect/Toxicity: See table for factors affecting serum levels.

Decreased Effect: Changes in diet may affect the elimination of theophylline; charcoal-broiled foods may increase elimination, reducing half-life by 50%; see table for factors affecting serum levels.

Factors Reported to Affect Theophylline Serum Levels

Decreased Theophylline Level	Increased Theophylline Level
Aminoglutethimide	Allopurinol (>600 mg/d)
Barbiturates	Beta-blockers
Carbamazepine	Calcium channel blockers
Charcoal	Carbamazepine
High protein/low carbohydrate diet	CHF
Hydantoins	Cimetidine
Isoniazid	Ciprofloxacin
I.V. isoproterenol	Cor pulmonale
Ketoconazole	Corticosteroids
Loop diuretics	Disulfiram
Phenobarbital	Ephedrine
Phenytoin	Erythromycin
Rifampin	Fever/viral illness
Smoking (cigarettes, marijuana)	Hepatic cirrhosis
Sulfinpyrazone	Influenza virus vaccine
Sympathomimetics	Interferon
	Isoniazid
	Loop diuretics
	Macrolides
	Mexiletine
	Oral contraceptives
	Propranolol
	Quinolones
	Thiabendazole
	Thyroid hormones
	Troleandomycin
	Zafirlukast
	Zileuton

St John's wort (*Hypericum*) can induce CYP1A2 enzymes and as a result may explain why theophylline serum levels have decreased when given concurrently. Theophylline dosages may need to be increased in patients concurrently receiving theophylline and St John's wort to retain theophylline's clinical efficacy.

Stability

Theophylline injection should be stored at room temperature and protected from freezing

Stability of parenteral admixture at room temperature (25°C): manufacturer expiration dating; out of overwrap stability: 30 days

Standard diluent: 400 mg theophylline/500 mL D$_5$W (premixed); 800 mg theophylline/1000 mL D$_5$W (premixed)

Aminophylline injection [content = 80% theophylline] should be stored at room temperature and protected from freezing and light

Stability of parenteral admixture at room temperature (25°C): 24 hours

Standard diluent: 250 mg aminophylline/100 mL D$_5$W ; 500 mg aminophylline/100 mL D$_5$W

(Continued)

Theophylline Salts *(Continued)*

Mechanism of Action Causes bronchodilatation, diuresis, CNS and cardiac stimulation, and gastric acid secretion by blocking phosphodiesterase which increases tissue concentrations of cyclic adenine monophosphate (cAMP) which in turn promotes catecholamine stimulation of lipolysis, glycogenolysis, and gluconeogenesis and induces release of epinephrine from adrenal medulla cells

Pharmacodynamics/Kinetics

Absorption: Oral: 100% of a dose is absorbed, depending upon the formulation used

Distribution: V_d: 0.45 L/kg; distributes into breast milk (approximates serum concentration); crosses the placenta

Metabolism: In the liver by demethylation and oxidation

Half-life: Highly variable and dependent upon age, liver function, cardiac function, lung disease, and smoking history

Aminophylline

Patient Group	Approximate Half-Life (h)
Neonates	
Premature	30
Normal newborn	24
Infants	
4-52 weeks	4-30
Children/Adolescents	
1-9 years	2-10 (4 avg)
9-16 years	4-16
Adults	
Nonsmoker	4-16 (8.7 avg)
Smoker	4.4
Cardiac compromised, liver failure	20-30

Dosage Form	Time to Peak	Dosing Interval
Uncoated tablet/syrup	2 h	6 h
Enteric coated tablet	5 h	12 h
Chewable tablet	1-1.5 h	6 h
Extended release	4-7 h	12 h
Intravenous	<30 min	

Elimination: In the urine; adults excrete 10% in urine as unchanged drug; neonates excrete a greater percentage of the dose unchanged in the urine (up to 50%)

Usual Dosage Use ideal body weight for obese patients

I.V.: Initial: Maintenance infusion rates:

Infants 6-52 weeks: 0.008 (age in weeks) + 0.21 mg/kg/hour theophylline

Children >1 year and Adults:

Treatment of acute bronchospasm: I.V.: Loading dose (in patients not currently receiving aminophylline or theophylline): 6 mg/kg (based on aminophylline) given I.V. over 20-30 minutes; administration rate should not exceed 25 mg/minute (aminophylline). See table on next page.

Approximate I.V. maintenance dosages are based upon continuous infusions; bolus dosing (often used in children <6 months of age) may be determined by multiplying the hourly infusion rate by 24 hours and dividing by the desired number of doses/day; see table on next page.

Dosage should be adjusted according to serum level measurements during the first 12- to 24-hour period; see table on page 1314.

Oral theophylline: Initial dosage recommendation: Loading dose (to achieve a serum level of about 10 mcg/mL; loading doses should be given using a rapidly absorbed oral product **not** a sustained release product):

If no theophylline has been administered in the previous 24 hours: 4-6 mg/kg theophylline

If theophylline has been administered in the previous 24 hours: administer ½ loading dose or 2-3 mg/kg theophylline can be given in emergencies when serum levels are not available

On the average, for every 1 mg/kg theophylline given, blood levels will rise 2 mcg/mL

Approximate I.V. Theophylline Dosage for Treatment of Acute Bronchospasm

Group	Dosage for Next 12 h*	Dosage After 12 h*
Infants 6 wk - 6 mo	0.5 mg/kg/h	
Children 6 mo - 1 y	0.6-0.7 mg/kg/h	
Children 1-9 y	0.95 mg/kg/h (1.2 mg/kg/h)	0.79 mg/kg/h (1 mg/kg/h)
Children 9-16 y and young adult smokers	0.79 mg/kg/h (1 mg/kg/h)	0.63 mg/kg/h (0.8 mg/kg/h)
Healthy, nonsmoking adults	0.55 mg/kg/h (0.7 mg/kg/h)	0.39 mg/kg/h (0.5 mg/kg/h)
Older patients and patients with cor pulmonale	0.47 mg/kg/h (0.6 mg/kg/h)	0.24 mg/kg/h (0.3 mg/kg/h)
Patients with congestive heart failure or liver failure	0.39 mg/kg/h (0.5 mg/kg/h)	0.08-0.16 mg/kg/h (0.1-0.2 mg/kg/h)

*Equivalent hydrous aminophylline dosage indicated in parentheses.

Maintenance Dose for Acute Symptoms

Population Group	Oral Theophylline (mg/kg/day)	I.V. Aminophylline
Premature infant or newborn - 6 wk (for apnea/bradycardia)	4	5 mg/kg/day
6 wk - 6 mo	10	12 mg/kg/day or continuous I.V. infusion*
Infants 6 mo - 1 y	12-18	15 mg/kg/day or continuous I.V. infusion*
Children 1-9 y	20-24	1 mg/kg/h
Children 9-12 y, and adolescent daily smokers of cigarettes or marijuana, and otherwise healthy adult smokers <50 y	16	0.9 mg/kg/h
Adolescents 12-16 y (nonsmokers)	13	0.7 mg/kg/h
Otherwise healthy nonsmoking adults (including elderly patients)	10 (not to exceed 900 mg/day)	0.5 mg/kg/h
Cardiac decompensation, cor pulmonale and/or liver dysfunction	5 (not to exceed 400 mg/day)	0.25 mg/kg/h

*For continuous I.V. infusion divide total daily dose by 24 = mg/kg/h.

Ideally, defer the loading dose if a serum theophylline concentration can be obtained rapidly. However, if this is not possible, exercise clinical judgment. If the patient is not experiencing theophylline toxicity, this is unlikely to result in dangerous adverse effects.

See table on next page.

Increasing dose: The dosage may be increased in approximately 25% increments at 2- to 3-day intervals so long as the drug is tolerated or until the maximum dose is reached

Maintenance dose: In newborns and infants, a fast-release oral product can be used. The total daily dose can be divided every 12 hours in newborns and every 6-8 hours in infants. In children and healthy adults, a slow-release product can be used. The total daily dose can be divided every 8-12 hours.

These recommendations, based on mean clearance rates for age or risk factors, were calculated to achieve a serum level of 10 mcg/mL (5 mcg/mL for newborns with apnea/bradycardia)

Dosage should be adjusted according to serum level

Oral oxtriphylline:

Children 1-9 years: 6.2 mg/kg/dose every 6 hours

Children 9-16 years and Adult smokers: 4.7 mg/kg/dose every 6 hours

Adult nonsmokers: 4.7 mg/kg/dose every 8 hours

Dose should be further adjusted based on serum levels

Dosing adjustment/comments in hepatic disease: Higher incidence of toxic effects including seizures in cirrhosis; plasma levels should be monitored closely during long-term administration in cirrhosis and during acute hepatitis, with dose adjustment as necessary

Hemodialysis: Administer dose posthemodialysis or administer supplemental 50% dose

Peritoneal dialysis: Supplemental dose is not necessary

Continuous arteriovenous or venovenous hemodiafiltration effects: Supplemental dose is not necessary

(Continued)

Theophylline Salts (Continued)

Dosage Adjustment After Serum Theophylline Measurement

Serum Theophylline		Guidelines
Within normal limits	10-20 mcg/mL	Maintain dosage if tolerated. Recheck serum theophylline concentration at 6- to 12-month intervals.*
Too high	20-25 mcg/mL	Decrease doses by about 10%. Recheck serum theophylline concentration after 3 days and then at 6- to 12-month intervals.*
	25-30 mcg/mL	Skip next dose and decrease subsequent doses by about 25%. Recheck serum theophylline.
	>30 mcg/mL	Skip next 2 doses and decrease subsequent doses by 50%. Recheck serum theophylline.
Too low	7.5-10 mcg/mL	Increase dose by about 25%.† Recheck serum theophylline concentration after 3 days and then at 6- to 12-month intervals.*
	5-7.5 mcg/mL	Increase dose by about 25% to the nearest dose increment† and recheck serum theophylline for guidance in further dosage adjustment (another increase will probably be needed, but this provides a safety check).

*Finer adjustments in dosage may be needed for some patients.

†Dividing the daily dose into 3 doses administered at 8-hour intervals may be indicated if symptoms occur repeatedly at the end of a dosing interval.

From Weinberger M and Hendeles L, "Practical Guide to Using Theophylline," *J Resp Dis*, 1981,2:12-27.

Oral Theophylline Dosage for Bronchial Asthma*

Age	Initial 3 Days	Second 3 Days	Steady-State Maintenance
<1 y	0.2 x (age in weeks) + 5		0.3 x (age in weeks) + 8
1-9 y	16 up to a maximum of 400 mg/ 24 h	20	22
9-12 y	16 up to a maximum of 400 mg/ 24 h	16 up to a maximum of 600 mg/ 24 h	20 up to a maximum of 800 mg/ 24 h
12-16 y	16 up to a maximum of 400 mg/ 24 h	16 up to a maximum of 600 mg/ 24 h	18 up to a maximum of 900 mg/ 24 h
Adults	400 mg/24 h	600 mg/24 h	900 mg/24 h

*Dose in mg/kg/24 hours of theophylline.

Administration Administer oral and I.V. administration around-the-clock to promote less variation in peak and trough serum levels; theophylline injection may be administered by continuous I.V. infusion (requires an infusion pump) or IVPB; maximum rate of I.V. administration of theophylline is 20-25 mg per minute

Monitoring Parameters Heart rate, CNS effects (insomnia, irritability); respiratory rate (COPD patients often have resting controlled respiratory rates in low 20s), serum theophylline level, arterial or capillary blood gases (if applicable)

Reference Range
Sample size: 0.5-1 mL serum (red top tube)
Saliva levels are approximately equal to 60% of plasma levels

Therapeutic levels: 10-20 μg/mL
  Neonatal apnea 6-13 μg/mL
  Pregnancy: 3-12 μg/mL
  Toxic concentration: >20 μg/mL

Timing of serum samples: If toxicity is suspected, draw a level any time during a continuous I.V. infusion, or 2 hours after an oral dose; if lack of therapeutic is effected, draw a trough immediately before the next oral dose; see table.

Guidelines for Drawing Theophylline Serum Levels

Dosage Form	Time to Draw Level
I.V. bolus	30 min after end of 30 min infusion
I.V. continuous infusion	12-24 h after initiation of infusion
P.O. liquid, fast-release tab	Peak: 1 h postdose after at least 1 day of therapy Trough: Just before a dose after at least one day of therapy
P.O. slow-release product	Peak: 4 h postdose after at least 1 day of therapy Trough: Just before a dose after at least one day of therapy

Test Interactions May elevate uric acid levels

Patient Information Oral preparations should be taken with a full glass of water; capsule forms may be opened and sprinkled on soft foods; do not chew beads; notify physician if nausea, vomiting, severe GI pain, restlessness, or irregular heartbeat occurs; do not drink or eat large quantities of caffeine-containing beverages or food (colas, coffee, chocolate); remain in bed for 15-20 minutes after inserting suppository; do not chew or crush enteric coated or sustained release products; take at regular intervals; notify physician if insomnia, nervousness, irritability, palpitations, seizures occur; do not change brands or doses without consulting physician

Nursing Implications Do not crush sustained release drug products; do not crush enteric coated drug product; encourage patient to drink adequate fluids (2 L/day) to decrease mucous viscosity

Additional Information See table for theophylline content.

Salt	% Theophylline Content
Theophylline anhydrous (eg, most oral solids)	100%
Theophylline monohydrate (eg, oral solutions)	91%
Aminophylline (theophylline) (eg, injection)	80% (79% to 86%)
Oxtriphylline (choline theophylline) (eg, Choledyl®)	64%

Dosage Forms
Aminophylline (79% theophylline):
    Injection: 25 mg/mL (10 mL, 20 mL); 250 mg (equivalent to 187 mg theophylline) per 10 mL; 500 mg (equivalent to 394 mg theophylline) per 20 mL
    Liquid, oral: 105 mg (equivalent to 90 mg theophylline) per 5 mL (240 mL, 500 mL)
    Suppository, rectal: 250 mg (equivalent to 198 mg theophylline); 500 mg (equivalent to 395 mg theophylline)
    Tablet: 100 mg (equivalent to 79 mg theophylline); 200 mg (equivalent to 158 mg theophylline)
    Tablet, controlled release: 225 mg (equivalent to 178 mg theophylline)
Oxtriphylline (64% theophylline):
    Elixir: 100 mg (equivalent to 64 mg theophylline)/5 mL (5 mL, 10 mL, 473 mL)
    Syrup: 50 mg (equivalent to 32 mg theophylline)/5 mL (473 mL)
    Tablet: 100 mg (equivalent to 64 mg theophylline); 200 mg (equivalent to 127 mg theophylline)
    Tablet, sustained release: 400 mg (equivalent to 254 mg theophylline); 600 mg (equivalent to 382 mg theophylline)
Theophylline:
    Capsule:
      Immediate release: 100 mg, 200 mg
      Sustained release (8-12 hours): 50 mg, 60 mg, 65 mg, 75 mg, 100 mg, 125 mg, 130 mg, 200 mg, 250 mg, 260 mg, 300 mg
      Timed release (12 hours): 50 mg, 75 mg, 125 mg, 130 mg, 200 mg, 250 mg, 260 mg
      Timed release (24 hours): 100 mg, 200 mg, 300 mg
    Injection: Theophylline in 5% dextrose: 200 mg/container (50 mL, 100 mL); 400 mg/container (100 mL, 250 mL, 500 mL, 1000 mL); 800 mg/container (250 mL, 500 mL, 1000 mL)
    Elixir, oral: 80 mg/15 mL (15 mL, 30 mL, 500 mL, 4000 mL)
    Solution, oral: 80 mg/15 mL (15 mL, 18.75 mL, 30 mL, 120 mL, 500 mL, 4000 mL); 150 mg/15 mL (480 mL)
    Syrup, oral: 80 mg/15 mL (5 mL, 15 mL, 30 mL, 120 mL, 500 mL, 4000 mL); 150 mg/15 mL (480 mL)
    Tablet:
      Immediate release: 100 mg, 125 mg, 200 mg, 250 mg, 300 mg
      Timed release (8-12 hours): 100 mg, 200 mg, 250 mg, 300 mg, 500 mg
      Timed release (8-24 hours): 100 mg, 200 mg, 300 mg, 450 mg
      Timed release (12-24 hours): 100 mg, 200 mg, 300 mg
      Timed release (24 hours): 400 mg

♦ **Theospan®-SR** see Theophylline Salts on page 1310

♦ **Theovent®** see Theophylline Salts on page 1310

♦ **Therabid® [OTC]** see Vitamins (Multiple) on page 1424

♦ **TheraCys®** see BCG Vaccine on page 148

♦ **Thera-Flu® Flu and Cold** see Acetaminophen, Chlorpheniramine, and Pseudoephedrine on page 27

♦ **Thera-Flu® Non-Drowsy Flu, Cold and Cough [OTC]** see Acetaminophen, Dextromethorphan, and Pseudoephedrine on page 27

♦ **Thera-Flur®** see Fluoride on page 574

♦ **Thera-Flur-N®** see Fluoride on page 574

♦ **Theragran® [OTC]** see Vitamins (Multiple) on page 1424

♦ **Theragran® Hematinic®** see Vitamins (Multiple) on page 1424

♦ **Theragran® Liquid [OTC]** see Vitamins (Multiple) on page 1424

♦ **Theragran-M® [OTC]** see Vitamins (Multiple) on page 1424

♦ **Therapeutic Multivitamins** see Vitamins (Multiple) on page 1424

♦ **Thermazene®** see Silver Sulfadiazine on page 1238

Thiabendazole (thye a BEN da zole)

U.S. Brand Names Mintezol®
Canadian Brand Names Mintezol®
Synonyms Tiabendazole
Therapeutic Category Anthelmintic
(Continued)

Thiabendazole *(Continued)*

Use Treatment of strongyloidiasis, cutaneous larva migrans, visceral larva migrans, dracunculiasis, trichinosis, and mixed helminthic infections

Pregnancy Risk Factor C

Contraindications Hypersensitivity to thiabendazole or any component of the formulation

Warnings/Precautions Use with caution in patients with renal or hepatic impairment, malnutrition or anemia, or dehydration

Adverse Reactions Frequency not defined.

Central nervous system: Seizures, hallucinations, delirium, dizziness, drowsiness, headache, chills

Dermatologic: Rash, Stevens-Johnson syndrome, pruritus, angioedema

Endocrine & metabolic: Hyperglycemia

Gastrointestinal: Anorexia, diarrhea, nausea, vomiting, drying of mucous membranes, abdominal pain

Genitourinary: Malodor of urine, hematuria, crystalluria, enuresis

Hematologic: Leukopenia

Hepatic: Jaundice, cholestasis, hepatic failure, hepatotoxicity

Neuromuscular & skeletal: Numbness, incoordination

Ocular: Visual changes, dry eyes, sicca syndrome

Otic: Tinnitus

Renal: Nephrotoxicity

Miscellaneous: Anaphylaxis, hypersensitivity reactions, lymphadenopathy

Overdosage/Toxicology Symptoms include altered mental status and visual problems. Supportive care only following GI decontamination.

Drug Interactions

Increased Effect/Toxicity: Increased levels of theophylline and other xanthines.

Mechanism of Action Inhibits helminth-specific mitochondrial fumarate reductase

Pharmacodynamics/Kinetics

Absorption: Rapid and well absorbed

Metabolism: Rapid

Half-life elimination: 1.2 hours

Excretion: Feces (5%) and urine (87%) primarily as conjugated metabolites

Usual Dosage Purgation is not required prior to use; drinking of fruit juice aids in expulsion of worms by removing the mucous to which the intestinal tapeworms attach themselves.

Children and Adults: Oral: 50 mg/kg/day divided every 12 hours (if >68 kg: 1.5 g/dose); maximum dose: 3 g/day

Treatment duration:

Strongyloidiasis, ascariasis, uncinariasis, trichuriasis: For 2 consecutive days

Cutaneous larva migrans: For 2-5 consecutive days

Visceral larva migrans: For 5-7 consecutive days

Trichinosis: For 2-4 consecutive days

Dracunculosis: 50-75 mg/kg/day divided every 12 hours for 3 days

Dosing comments in renal/hepatic impairment: Use with caution

Patient Information Take after meals, chew chewable tablet well; may decrease alertness, avoid driving or operating machinery; drinking of fruit juice aids in expulsion of worms by removing the mucous to which the intestinal tapeworms attach themselves

Nursing Implications

Purgation is not required prior to use

Monitor periodic renal and hepatic function tests

Dosage Forms

Suspension, oral: 500 mg/5 mL (120 mL)

Tablet, chewable: 500 mg [orange flavor]

♦ **Thiamazole** *see Methimazole on page 882*

♦ **Thiamilate®** *see Thiamine on page 1316*

Thiamine *(THYE a min)*

U.S. Brand Names Thiamilate®

Canadian Brand Names Betaxin®

Synonyms Aneurine Hydrochloride; Thiamine Hydrochloride; Thiaminium Chloride Hydrochloride; Vitamin B_1

Therapeutic Category Vitamin, Water Soluble

Use Treatment of thiamine deficiency including beriberi, Wernicke's encephalopathy syndrome, and peripheral neuritis associated with pellagra, alcoholic patients with altered sensorium; various genetic metabolic disorders

Pregnancy Risk Factor A/C (dose exceeding RDA recommendation)

Contraindications Hypersensitivity to thiamine or any component of the formulation

Warnings/Precautions Use with caution with parenteral route (especially I.V.) of administration

Adverse Reactions <1% (Limited to important or life-threatening): Cardiovascular collapse and death, paresthesia

Ethanol/Nutrition/Herb Interactions Food: High carbohydrate diets may increase thiamine requirement.

Stability Protect oral dosage forms from light; **incompatible** with alkaline or neutral solutions and with oxidizing or reducing agents

Mechanism of Action An essential coenzyme in carbohydrate metabolism by combining with adenosine triphosphate to form thiamine pyrophosphate

Pharmacodynamics/Kinetics

Absorption: Oral: Adequate; I.M.: Rapid and complete

Excretion: Urine (as unchanged drug and as pyrimidine after body storage sites become saturated)

Usual Dosage
Recommended daily allowance:
- <6 months: 0.3 mg
- 6 months to 1 year: 0.4 mg
- 1-3 years: 0.7 mg
- 4-6 years: 0.9 mg
- 7-10 years: 1 mg
- 11-14 years: 1.1-1.3 mg
- >14 years: 1-1.5 mg

Thiamine deficiency (beriberi):
Children: 10-25 mg/dose I.M. or I.V. daily (if critically ill), or 10-50 mg/dose orally every day for 2 weeks, then 5-10 mg/dose orally daily for 1 month
Adults: 5-30 mg/dose I.M. or I.V. 3 times/day (if critically ill); then orally 5-30 mg/day in single or divided doses 3 times/day for 1 month
Wernicke's encephalopathy: Adults: Initial: 100 mg I.V., then 50-100 mg/day I.M. or I.V. until consuming a regular, balanced diet
Dietary supplement (depends on caloric or carbohydrate content of the diet):
- Infants: 0.3-0.5 mg/day
- Children: 0.5-1 mg/day
- Adults: 1-2 mg/day

Note: The above doses can be found in multivitamin preparations
Metabolic disorders: Oral: Adults: 10-20 mg/day (dosages up to 4 g/day in divided doses have been used)

Dietary Considerations Dietary sources include legumes, pork, beef, whole grains, yeast, and fresh vegetables. A deficiency state can occur in as little as 3 weeks following total dietary absence.

Administration Parenteral form may be administered by I.M. or slow I.V. injection

Reference Range Therapeutic: 1.6-4 mg/dL

Test Interactions False-positive for uric acid using the phosphotungstate method and for urobilinogen using the Ehrlich's reagent; large doses may interfere with the spectrophotometric determination of serum theophylline concentration

Patient Information Dietary sources include legumes, pork, beef, whole grains, yeast, fresh vegetables; a deficiency state can occur in as little 3 weeks following total dietary absence

Nursing Implications Single vitamin deficiency is rare; look for other deficiencies

Dosage Forms
Injection, as hydrochloride: 100 mg/mL (1 mL, 2 mL, 10 mL, 30 mL); 200 mg/mL (30 mL)
Tablet, as hydrochloride: 50 mg, 100 mg, 250 mg, 500 mg
Tablet, enteric coated, as hydrochloride (Thiamilate®): 20 mg

- **Thiamine Hydrochloride** see Thiamine on page 1316
- **Thiaminium Chloride Hydrochloride** see Thiamine on page 1316

Thiethylperazine (thye eth il PER a zeen)
Related Information
Antacid Drug Interactions on page 1477
U.S. Brand Names Norzine®; Torecan®
Canadian Brand Names Torecan®
Synonyms Thiethylperazine Maleate
Therapeutic Category Antiemetic; Phenothiazine Derivative
Use Relief of nausea and vomiting
Unlabeled/Investigational Use Treatment of vertigo
Pregnancy Risk Factor X
Contraindications Hypersensitivity to thiethylperazine or any component of the formulation (cross-sensitivity to other phenothiazines may exist); comatose states; pregnancy
Warnings/Precautions Reduce or discontinue if extrapyramidal symptoms occur; safety and efficacy in children <12 years of age have not been established; postural hypotension may occur after I.M. injection; the injectable form contains sulfite which may cause allergic reactions in some patients; use caution in patients with narrow-angle glaucoma

Adverse Reactions
>10%:
Central nervous system: Drowsiness, dizziness
Gastrointestinal: Xerostomia
Respiratory: Dry nose
1% to 10%:
Cardiovascular: Tachycardia, orthostatic hypotension
Central nervous system: Confusion, convulsions, extrapyramidal effects, tardive dyskinesia, fever, headache
Hematologic: Agranulocytosis
Hepatic: Cholestatic jaundice
Otic: Tinnitus

Overdosage/Toxicology Symptoms include deep sleep, coma, extrapyramidal symptoms, abnormal involuntary muscle movements, and hypotension. Following initiation of essential overdose management, toxic symptom treatment and supportive treatment should be initiated. Hypotension usually responds to I.V. fluids or Trendelenburg positioning. If unresponsive to these measures, use of a parenteral inotrope may be required (eg, norepinephrine 0.1-0.2 mcg/kg/minute titrated to response. Avoid epinephrine for thiethylperazine-induced hypotension. Seizures commonly respond to diazepam (I.V. 5-10 mg bolus in adults every 15 minutes, if needed, up to a total of 30 mg; I.V. 0.25-0.4 mg/kg/dose up to a total of 10 mg in children) or to phenytoin or phenobarbital. Critical cardiac arrhythmias often respond to I.V. phenytoin (15 mg/kg up to 1 g), while other antiarrhythmics can be used. Neuroleptics often cause extrapyramidal symptoms (eg, dystonic reactions) requiring management with diphenhydramine 1-2 mg/kg (adults) up to a maximum of 50 mg I.M. or slow I.V. push followed, by a
(Continued)

Thiethylperazine (Continued)

maintenance dose for 48-72 hours. When these reactions are unresponsive to diphenhydramine, anticholinergic agents such as benztropine mesylate I.V. 1-2 mg (adults) may be effective. These agents are generally effective within 2-5 minutes.

Drug Interactions
Increased Effect/Toxicity: Increased effect with CNS depressants (eg, anesthetics, opiates, tranquilizers, alcohol), lithium, atropine, epinephrine, MAO inhibitors, TCAs

Ethanol/Nutrition/Herb Interactions
Ethanol: Avoid ethanol (may increase CNS depression).
Herb/Nutraceutical: Avoid valerian, St John's wort, kava kava, gotu kola (may increase CNS depression).

Stability Store suppositories below 25°C (77°F) in foil

Mechanism of Action Blocks postsynaptic mesolimbic dopaminergic receptors in the brain; exhibits a strong alpha-adrenergic blocking effect and depresses the release of hypothalamic and hypophyseal hormones; acts directly on chemoreceptor trigger zone and vomiting center

Pharmacodynamics/Kinetics
Onset of action: Antiemetic: ~30 minutes
Duration: ~4 hours

Usual Dosage Children >12 years and Adults:
Oral, I.M., rectal: 10 mg 1-3 times/day as needed
I.V. and S.C. routes of administration are not recommended
Hemodialysis: Not dialyzable (0% to 5%)
Dosing comments in hepatic impairment: Use with caution

Administration Inject I.M. deeply into large muscle mass, patient should be lying down and remain so for at least 1 hour after administration

Patient Information May cause drowsiness, impair judgment and coordination; may cause photosensitivity; avoid excessive sunlight; notify physician of involuntary movements or feelings of restlessness

Nursing Implications Assist with ambulation, observe for extrapyramidal symptoms

Dosage Forms
Injection, as maleate: 5 mg/mL (2 mL)
Suppository, rectal, as maleate: 10 mg
Tablet, as maleate: 10 mg

♦ **Thiethylperazine Maleate** see Thiethylperazine on page 1317

Thioguanine (thye oh GWAH neen)

Canadian Brand Names Lanvis®
Synonyms 2-Amino-6-Mercaptopurine; TG; 6-TG; 6-Thioguanine; Tioguanine
Therapeutic Category Antineoplastic Agent, Antimetabolite (Purine)
Use Remission induction, consolidation, and maintenance therapy of acute myelogenous (nonlymphocytic) leukemia; treatment of chronic myelogenous leukemia and granulocytic leukemia

Pregnancy Risk Factor D

Contraindications Hypersensitivity to thioguanine or any component of the formulation; history of previous therapy resistance with either thioguanine or mercaptopurine (there is usually complete cross resistance between these two); pregnancy

Warnings/Precautions The U.S. Food and Drug Administration (FDA) currently recommends that procedures for proper handling and disposal of antineoplastic agents be considered. Use with caution and reduce dose of thioguanine in patients with renal or hepatic impairment; thioguanine is potentially carcinogenic and teratogenic; myelosuppression may be delayed.

Adverse Reactions
>10%:
Hematologic: Leukopenia; Thrombocytopenia; Myelosuppressive:
WBC: Moderate
Platelets: Moderate
Onset: 7-10 days
Nadir: 14 days
Recovery: 21 days
1% to 10%:
Dermatologic: Skin rash
Endocrine & metabolic: Hyperuricemia
Gastrointestinal: Mild nausea or vomiting, anorexia, stomatitis, diarrhea
Emetic potential: Low (<10%)
Neuromuscular & skeletal: Unsteady gait
<1% (Limited to important or life-threatening): Hepatitis, jaundice, neurotoxicity, veno-occlusive hepatic disease

Overdosage/Toxicology Symptoms include bone marrow suppression, nausea, vomiting, malaise, hypertension, and sweating. Treatment is supportive and dialysis is not useful.

Drug Interactions
Increased Effect/Toxicity: Allopurinol can be used in full doses with 6-TG unlike 6-MP. Use with busulfan may cause hepatotoxicity and esophageal varices.

Ethanol/Nutrition/Herb Interactions Food: Enhanced absorption if administered between meals.

Stability The (investigational) parenteral preparation is supplied as a 75 mg vial and should be stored in the refrigerator. It is reconstituted with 5 mL of 0.9% NaCl for injection, providing a concentration of 15 mg/mL, which is stable for at least 24 hours under refrigeration. When this solution is further diluted in 500 mL D_5W or 0.9% NaCl, it is stable for at least 24 hours at room temperature, or under refrigeration of thioguanine (1 vial). The resultant solution is reported to be stable for 8 hours at room temperature or under refrigeration.

Mechanism of Action Purine analog that is incorporated into DNA and RNA resulting in the blockage of synthesis and metabolism of purine nucleotides

Pharmacodynamics/Kinetics
Absorption: 30%
Distribution: Crosses placenta
Metabolism: Rapidly and extensively hepatic to 2-amino-6-methylthioguanine (active) and inactive compounds
Half-life elimination: Terminal: 11 hours
Time to peak, serum: Within 8 hours
Excretion: Urine

Usual Dosage Total daily dose can be given at one time; offers little advantage over mercaptopurine; is sometimes ordered as 6-thioguanine, with 6 being part of the drug name and not a unit or strength

Oral (refer to individual protocols):
Infants and Children <3 years: Combination drug therapy for acute nonlymphocytic leukemia: 3.3 mg/kg/day in divided doses twice daily for 4 days
Children and Adults: 2-3 mg/kg/day calculated to nearest 20 mg or 75-200 mg/m²/day in 1-2 divided doses for 5-7 days or until remission is attained

Dosing comments in renal or hepatic impairment: Reduce dose

Monitoring Parameters CBC with differential and platelet count, liver function tests, hemoglobin, hematocrit, serum uric acid

Patient Information You may experience nausea and vomiting, diarrhea, or loss of appetite (frequent small meals may help/request medication) or weakness or lethargy (use caution when driving or engaging in tasks requiring alertness until response to drug is known). Use good oral care to reduce incidence of mouth sores. Maintain adequate hydration (2-3 L/day of fluids unless instructed to restrict fluid intake). May cause headache (request medication). Report signs or symptoms of infection (eg, fever, chills, sore throat, burning urination, fatigue), bleeding (eg, tarry stools, easy bruising), vision changes, unresolved mouth sores, nausea or vomiting, CNS changes (hallucinations), or respiratory difficulty. Avoid crowds or exposure to infected persons; you will be susceptible to infection. The drug may cause permanent sterility and may cause birth defects. Contraceptive measures should be used during therapy. The drug may be excreted in breast milk; therefore, an alternative form of feeding your baby should be used.

Nursing Implications Monitor CBC with differential and platelet count, liver function tests, hemoglobin, hematocrit, serum uric acid

Dosage Forms Tablet, scored: 40 mg

Extemporaneous Preparations A 40 mg/mL oral suspension compounded from tablets which were crushed, mixed with a volume of Cologel® suspending agent equal to ⅓ the final volume, and brought to the final volume with a 2:1 mixture of simple syrup and cherry syrup was stable for 84 days when stored in an amber bottle at room temperature

Dressman JB and Poust RI, "Stability of Allopurinol and Five Antineoplastics in Suspension," Am J Hosp Pharm, 1983, 40:616-8.

♦ **6-Thioguanine** see Thioguanine on page 1318

Thiopental (thye oh PEN tal)

U.S. Brand Names Pentothal® Sodium
Canadian Brand Names Pentothal®
Synonyms Thiopental Sodium
Therapeutic Category Anticonvulsant; Barbiturate; General Anesthetic; Sedative
Use Induction of anesthesia; adjunct for intubation in head injury patients; control of convulsive states; treatment of elevated intracranial pressure
Restrictions C-III
Pregnancy Risk Factor C
Contraindications Hypersensitivity to thiopental, barbiturates, or any component of the formulation; status asthmaticus; severe cardiovascular disease; porphyria (variegate or acute intermittent); inflammatory bowel disease or lower gastrointestinal neoplasm (rectal gel); should not be administered by intra-arterial injection
Warnings/Precautions Laryngospasm or bronchospasms may occur; use with extreme caution in patients with reactive airway diseases (asthma or COPD). Use with caution when the hypnotic may be prolonged or potentiated (excessive premedication, Addison's disease, hepatic or renal dysfunction, myxedema, increased blood urea, severe anemia, or myasthenia gravis). Potential for drug dependency exists, abrupt cessation may precipitate withdrawal, including status epilepticus in epileptic patients. Use caution in patients with unstable aneurysms, cardiovascular disease, renal impairment, or hepatic disease. Use caution in elderly, debilitated, or pediatric patients. May cause paradoxical responses, including agitation and hyperactivity, particularly in acute pain and pediatric patients. Effects with other sedative drugs or ethanol may be potentiated. May cause respiratory depression or hypotension; use with caution in hemodynamically unstable patients (hypotension or shock) or patients with respiratory disease. Repeated dosing or continuous infusions may cause cumulative effects. Extravasation or intra-arterial injection causes necrosis due to pH of 10.6, ensure patient has intravenous access.
Adverse Reactions Frequency not defined.
Cardiovascular: Bradycardia, hypotension, syncope
Central nervous system: Drowsiness, lethargy, CNS excitation or depression, impaired judgment, "hangover" effect, confusion, somnolence, agitation, hyperkinesia, ataxia, nervousness, headache, insomnia, nightmares, hallucinations, anxiety, dizziness
Dermatologic: Rash, exfoliative dermatitis, Stevens-Johnson syndrome
Gastrointestinal: Nausea, vomiting, constipation
Hematologic: Agranulocytosis, thrombocytopenia, megaloblastic anemia
Local: Pain at injection site, thrombophlebitis with I.V. use
Renal: Oliguria
Respiratory: Laryngospasm, respiratory depression, apnea (especially with rapid I.V. use), hypoventilation, apnea
Miscellaneous: Gangrene with inadvertent intra-arterial injection
(Continued)

Thiopental *(Continued)*

Overdosage/Toxicology Symptoms include respiratory depression, hypotension, shock. Hypotension should respond to I.V. fluids and Trendelenburg positioning. If necessary, pressors such as norepinephrine may be used. Ventilatory support may be required.

Drug Interactions

Increased Effect/Toxicity: In chronic use, barbiturates are potent inducers of CYP isoenzymes resulting in multiple interactions with medication groups. When used for limited periods, thiopental is not likely to interact via this mechanism. Sedative effects and/or respiratory depression with barbiturates may be additive with other CNS depressants; includes ethanol, sedatives, antidepressants, narcotic analgesics, and benzodiazepines. Felbamate may inhibit the metabolism of barbiturates and barbiturates may increase the metabolism of felbamate. Barbiturates may enhance the nephrotoxic effects of methoxyflurane

Stability Reconstituted solutions remain stable for 3 days at room temperature and 7 days when refrigerated; solutions are alkaline and **incompatible** with drugs with acidic pH, such as succinylcholine, atropine sulfate, etc. I.V. form is **incompatible** when mixed with amikacin, benzquinamide, chlorpromazine, codeine, dimenhydrinate, diphenhydramine, glycopyrrolate, hydromorphone, insulin, levorphanol, meperidine, metaraminol, morphine, norepinephrine, penicillin G, prochlorperazine, succinylcholine, tetracycline

Mechanism of Action Short-acting barbiturate with sedative, hypnotic, and anticonvulsant properties. Barbiturates depress the sensory cortex, decrease motor activity, alter cerebellar function, and produce drowsiness, sedation, and hypnosis. In high doses, barbiturates exhibit anticonvulsant activity; barbiturates produce dose-dependent respiratory depression.

Pharmacodynamics/Kinetics

Onset of action: Anesthetic: I.V.: 30-60 seconds

Duration: 5-30 minutes

Distribution: V_d: 1.4 L/kg

Protein binding: 72% to 86%

Metabolism: Hepatic, primarily to inactive metabolites but pentobarbital is also formed

Half-life elimination: 3-11.5 hours, decreased in children

Usual Dosage

I.V.:

Induction anesthesia:

Infants: 5-8 mg/kg

Children 1-12 years: 5-6 mg/kg

Adults: 3-5 mg/kg

Maintenance anesthesia:

Children: 1 mg/kg as needed

Adults: 25-100 mg as needed

Increased intracranial pressure: Children and Adults: 1.5-5 mg/kg/dose; repeat as needed to control intracranial pressure

Seizures:

Children: 2-3 mg/kg/dose; repeat as needed

Adults: 75-250 mg/dose; repeat as needed

Rectal administration (patient should be NPO for no less than 3 hours prior to administration):

Suggested initial doses of thiopental rectal suspension are:

<3 months: 15 mg/kg/dose

>3 months: 25 mg/kg/dose

Note: The age of a premature infant should be adjusted to reflect the age that the infant would have been if full-term (eg, an infant, now age 4 months, who was 2 months premature should be considered to be a 2-month old infant).

Doses should be rounded downward to the nearest 50 mg increment to allow for accurate measurement of the dose

Inactive or debilitated patients and patients recently medicated with other sedatives (eg, chloral hydrate, meperidine, chlorpromazine, and promethazine), may require smaller doses than usual

If the patient is not sedated within 15-20 minutes, a single repeat dose of thiopental can be given. The single repeat doses are:

<3 months: <7.5 mg/kg/dose

>3 months: 15 mg/kg/dose

Children weighing >34 kg should not receive >1 g as a total dose (initial plus repeat doses)

Adults weighing >90 kg should not receive >3 g as a total dose (initial plus repeat doses)

Neither adults nor children should receive more than one course of thiopental rectal suspension (initial dose plus repeat dose) per 24-hour period

Dosing adjustment in renal impairment: Cl_{cr} <10 mL/minute: Administer at 75% of normal dose

Note: Accumulation may occur with chronic dosing due to lipid solubility; prolonged recovery may result from redistribution of thiopental from fat stores

Administration Rapid I.V. injection may cause hypotension or decreased cardiac output

Monitoring Parameters Respiratory rate, heart rate, blood pressure

Reference Range Therapeutic: Hypnotic: 1-5 µg/mL (SI: 4.1-20.7 µmol/L); Coma: 30-100 µg/mL (SI: 124-413 µmol/L); Anesthesia: 7-130 µg/mL (SI: 29-536 µmol/L); Toxic: >10 µg/mL (SI: >41 µmol/L)

Nursing Implications Monitor vital signs every 3-5 minutes; monitor for respiratory distress; place patient in Sim's position if vomiting, to prevent from aspirating vomitus; avoid extravasation, necrosis may occur

Additional Information Sodium content of 1 g (injection): 86.8 mg (3.8 mEq). Thiopental switches from linear to nonlinear pharmacokinetics following prolonged continuous infusions.

Dosage Forms

Injection, as sodium: 250 mg, 400 mg, 500 mg, 1 g, 2.5 g, 5 g

Suspension, rectal, as sodium: 400 mg/g (2 g)

- **Thiopental Sodium** *see* Thiopental *on page 1319*
- **Thiophosphoramide** *see* Thiotepa *on page 1323*
- **Thioplex®** *see* Thiotepa *on page 1323*

Thioridazine (thye oh RID a zeen)

Related Information
Antacid Drug Interactions *on page 1477*
Antipsychotic Agents Comparison *on page 1486*

U.S. Brand Names Mellaril®

Canadian Brand Names Apo®-Thioridazine; Mellaril®

Synonyms Thioridazine Hydrochloride

Therapeutic Category Antipsychotic Agent, Phenothiazine; Phenothiazine Derivative

Use Management of schizophrenic patients who fail to respond adequately to treatment with other antipsychotic drugs, either because of insufficient effectiveness or the inability to achieve an effective dose due to intolerable adverse effects from those medications

Unlabeled/Investigational Use Psychosis

Pregnancy Risk Factor C

Contraindications Hypersensitivity to thioridazine or any component of the formulation (cross-reactivity between phenothiazines may occur); severe CNS depression; circulatory collapse; severe hypotension; bone marrow suppression; blood dyscrasias; coma; in combination with other drugs that are known to prolong the QT_c interval; in patients with congenital long QT syndrome or a history of cardiac arrhythmias; concurrent use with medications that inhibit the metabolism of thioridazine (fluoxetine, paroxetine, fluvoxamine, propranolol, pindolol); patients known to have genetic defect leading to reduced levels of activity of CYP2D6

Warnings/Precautions Oral formulations may cause stomach upset; may cause thermoregulatory changes; use caution in patients with narrow-angle glaucoma; doses of 1 g/day frequently cause pigmentary retinopathy; thioridazine has dose-related effects on ventricular repolarization leading to QT_c prolongation, a potentially life-threatening effect. As a result, it should be reserved for patients whose schizophrenia has failed to respond to adequate trials of other antipsychotic drugs. Use with caution in Parkinson's disease; hemodynamic instability; bone marrow suppression; predisposition to seizures; subcortical brain damage; severe cardiac, hepatic, renal, or respiratory disease. Esophageal dysmotility and aspiration have been associated with antipsychotic use - use with caution in patients at risk of pneumonia (ie, Alzheimer's disease). Caution in breast cancer or other prolactin-dependent tumors (may elevate prolactin levels). May alter temperature regulation or mask toxicity of other drugs due to antiemetic effects.

Phenothiazines may cause anticholinergic effects (confusion, agitation, constipation, dry mouth, blurred vision, urinary retention); therefore, they should be used with caution in patients with decreased gastrointestinal motility, urinary retention, BPH, xerostomia, or visual problems. Conditions which also may be exacerbated by cholinergic blockade include narrow-angle glaucoma (screening is recommended) and worsening of myasthenia gravis. Relative to other neuroleptics, thioridazine has a high potency of cholinergic blockade.

May cause extrapyramidal reactions, including pseudoparkinsonism, acute dystonic reactions, akathisia, and tardive dyskinesia (risk of these reactions is low relative to other neuroleptics). May be associated with neuroleptic malignant syndrome (NMS).

Adverse Reactions Frequency not defined.

Cardiovascular: Hypotension, orthostatic hypotension, peripheral edema, EKG changes

Central nervous system: EPS (pseudoparkinsonism, akathisia, dystonias, tardive dyskinesia), dizziness, drowsiness, neuroleptic malignant syndrome (NMS), impairment of temperature regulation, lowering of seizures threshold

Dermatologic: Increased sensitivity to sun, rash, discoloration of skin (blue-gray)

Endocrine & metabolic: Changes in menstrual cycle, changes in libido, breast pain, galactorrhea, amenorrhea

Gastrointestinal: Constipation, weight gain, nausea, vomiting, stomach pain, xerostomia, nausea, vomiting, diarrhea

Genitourinary: Difficulty in urination, ejaculatory disturbances, urinary retention, priapism

Hematologic: Agranulocytosis, leukopenia

Hepatic: Cholestatic jaundice, hepatotoxicity

Neuromuscular & skeletal: Tremor, seizure

Ocular: Pigmentary retinopathy, blurred vision, cornea and lens changes

Respiratory: Nasal congestion

Overdosage/Toxicology
Symptoms include deep sleep, coma, extrapyramidal symptoms, abnormal involuntary muscle movements, hypotension, and arrhythmias. Immediate cardiovascular monitoring, including continuous EKG monitoring, to detect arrhythmias.

Following initiation of essential overdose management, toxic symptom treatment and supportive treatment should be initiated. **Avoid use of other medications that may also prolong the QT_c interval, such as disopyramide, procainamide and quinidine.** Hypotension usually responds to I.V. fluids or Trendelenburg positioning. If unresponsive to these measures, the use of a parenteral inotrope may be required (eg, norepinephrine 0.1-0.2 mcg/kg/minute titrated to response); do not use epinephrine. Seizures commonly respond to diazepam (I.V. 5-10 mg bolus in adults every 15 minutes if needed up to a total of 30 mg; I.V. 0.25-0.4 mg/kg/dose up to a total of 10 mg in children) or to phenytoin. Neuroleptics often cause extrapyramidal symptoms (eg, dystonic reactions) requiring management with diphenhydramine 1-2 mg/kg (adults) up to a maximum of 50 mg I.M. or slow I.V. push followed by a maintenance dose for 48-72 hours. When these reactions are unresponsive to diphenhydramine, anticholinergic agents such as benztropine mesylate I.V. 1-2 mg (adults) may be effective. These agents are generally effective within 2-5 minutes. Avoid barbiturates; may potentiate respiratory depression.

(Continued)

Thioridazine (Continued)

Drug Interactions

Cytochrome P450 Effect: CYP1A2 and 2D6 enzyme substrate; CYP2D6 enzyme inhibitor

Increased Effect/Toxicity: Concurrent use of phenothiazines with an antihypertensive may produce additive hypotensive effects (particularly orthostasis). Concurrent use of beta-blockers may increase the risk of arrhythmia; propranolol and pindolol are **contraindicated.** Phenothiazines inhibit the ability of bromocriptine to lower serum prolactin concentrations. Serum concentrations of carvedilol or valproic acid may be increased by phenothiazines. The sedative effects of CNS depressants or ethanol may be additive with phenothiazines. Phenothiazines and trazodone may produce additive hypotensive effects Concurrent use of phenothiazines and tricyclic antidepressants may produce increased toxicity or altered therapeutic response.

QT_c-prolonging agents: Effects on QT_c interval may be additive with phenothiazines, increasing the risk of malignant arrhythmias; includes type Ia antiarrhythmics, TCAs, and some quinolone antibiotics (sparfloxacin, moxifloxacin and gatifloxacin). **These agents are contraindicated with thioridazine.** Potassium depleting agents may increase the risk of serious arrhythmias with thioridazine (includes many diuretics, aminoglycosides, and amphotericin).

CYP2D6 inhibitors: Metabolism of phenothiazines may be decreased; increasing clinical effect or toxicity. Inhibitors include amiodarone, cimetidine, delavirdine, fluoxetine, paroxetine, propafenone, quinidine, and ritonavir; monitor for increased effect/toxicity. **Thioridazine is contraindicated with inhibitors of this enzyme, including fluoxetine and paroxetine.** Inhibitors of CYP1A2, including cimetidine, ciprofloxacin, fluvoxamine, isoniazid, ritonavir, and zileuton may also decrease thioridazine metabolism. **Concurrent use with fluvoxamine is contraindicated.**

Phenothiazines may produce neurotoxicity with lithium; this is a rare effect. Rare cases of respiratory paralysis have been reported with concurrent use of phenothiazines and polypeptide antibiotics. Naltrexone in combination with thioridazine has been reported to cause lethargy and somnolence. Phenylpropanolamine has been reported to result in cardiac arrhythmias when combined with thioridazine.

Decreased Effect: Aluminum salts may decrease the absorption of phenothiazines. The efficacy of amphetamines may be diminished by antipsychotics; in addition, amphetamines may increase psychotic symptoms; avoid concurrent use. Anticholinergics may inhibit the therapeutic response to phenothiazines and excess anticholinergic effects may occur (includes benztropine, trihexyphenidyl, biperiden, and drugs with significant anticholinergic activity). Chlorpromazine (and possibly other low potency antipsychotics) may diminish the pressor effects of epinephrine. The antihypertensive effects of guanethidine or guanadrel may be inhibited by phenothiazines. Phenothiazines may inhibit the antiparkinsonian effect of levodopa. Enzyme inducers may enhance the hepatic metabolism of phenothiazines; larger doses may be required; includes rifampin, rifabutin, barbiturates, phenytoin, and cigarette smoking.

Ethanol/Nutrition/Herb Interactions

Ethanol: Avoid ethanol (may increase CNS depression).

Herb/Nutraceutical: Avoid kava kava, valerian, St John's wort, gotu kola (may increase CNS depression). Avoid dong quai, St John's wort (may also cause photosensitization).

Stability Protect all dosage forms from light

Mechanism of Action Blocks postsynaptic mesolimbic dopaminergic receptors in the brain; exhibits a strong alpha-adrenergic blocking effect and depresses the release of hypothalamic and hypophyseal hormones

Pharmacodynamics/Kinetics

Duration: 4-5 days

Half-life elimination: 21-25 hours

Time to peak, serum: ~1 hour

Usual Dosage Oral:

Children >2-12 years: Range: 0.5-3 mg/kg/day in 2-3 divided doses; usual: 1 mg/kg/day; maximum: 3 mg/kg/day

Behavior problems: Initial: 10 mg 2-3 times/day, increase gradually

Severe psychoses: Initial: 25 mg 2-3 times/day, increase gradually

Children >12 years and Adults:

Schizophrenia/psychoses: Initial: 50-100 mg 3 times/day with gradual increments as needed and tolerated; maximum: 800 mg/day in 2-4 divided doses; if >65 years, initial dose: 10 mg 3 times/day

Depressive disorders/dementia: Initial: 25 mg 3 times/day; maintenance dose: 20-200 mg/day

Elderly: Behavioral symptoms associated with dementia: Oral: Initial: 10-25 mg 1-2 times/day; increase at 4- to 7-day intervals by 10-25 mg/day; increase dose intervals (qd, bid, etc) as necessary to control response or side effects. Maximum daily dose: 400 mg; gradual increases (titration) may prevent some side effects or decrease their severity.

Hemodialysis: Not dialyzable (0% to 5%)

Administration Oral concentrate must be diluted in 2-4 oz of liquid (eg, water, fruit juice, carbonated drinks, milk, or pudding) before administration. Do not take antacid within 2 hours of taking drug. Thioridazine concentrate is not compatible with carbamazepine suspension; schedule dosing at least 1-2 hours apart from each other. **Note:** Avoid skin contact with oral suspension or solution; may cause contact dermatitis.

Monitoring Parameters Baseline and periodic EKG and serum potassium; periodic eye exam, CBC with differential, blood pressure, liver enzyme tests; do not initiate if QT_c >450 msec

Reference Range Toxic: >1 mg/mL; lethal: 2-8 mg/dL

Test Interactions False-positives for phenylketonuria, urinary amylase, uroporphyrins, urobilinogen

Patient Information Oral concentrate must be diluted in 2-4 oz of liquid (water, fruit juice, carbonated drinks, milk, or pudding); do not take antacid within 1 hour of taking drug; avoid excess sun exposure; may cause drowsiness, restlessness, avoid alcohol and other CNS depressants; do not alter dosage or discontinue without consulting physician; yearly eye exams are necessary; might discolor urine (pink or reddish brown)

Nursing Implications Avoid skin contact with oral suspension or solution; may cause contact dermatitis

Dosage Forms

Solution, oral concentrate, as hydrochloride: 30 mg/mL (120 mL); 100 mg/mL (3.4 mL, 120 mL)

Tablet, as hydrochloride: 10 mg, 15 mg, 25 mg, 50 mg, 100 mg, 150 mg, 200 mg

♦ **Thioridazine Hydrochloride** *see* Thioridazine *on page 1321*

Thiotepa (thye oh TEP a)

U.S. Brand Names Thioplex®

Synonyms TESPA; Thiophosphoramide; Triethylenethiophosphoramide; TSPA

Therapeutic Category Antineoplastic Agent, Alkylating Agent

Use Treatment of superficial tumors of the bladder; palliative treatment of adenocarcinoma of breast or ovary; lymphomas and sarcomas; controlling intracavitary effusions caused by metastatic tumors; I.T. use: CNS leukemia/lymphoma

Pregnancy Risk Factor D

Contraindications Hypersensitivity to thiotepa or any component of the formulation; severe myelosuppression with leukocyte count <3000/mm^3 or platelet count <150,000 mm^3, except in stem cell transplant; pregnancy

Warnings/Precautions The U.S. Food and Drug Administration (FDA) currently recommends that procedures for proper handling and disposal of antineoplastic agents be considered. The drug is potentially mutagenic, carcinogenic, and teratogenic. Reduce dosage in patients with hepatic, renal, or bone marrow damage.

Adverse Reactions

>10%:

Hematopoietic: Myelosuppression (dose-related and cumulative): Anemia and pancytopenia may become fatal; careful hematologic monitoring is required; intravesical administration may cause bone marrow suppression as well.

Hematologic: Myelosuppressive:

WBC: Moderate

Platelets: Severe

Onset: 7-10 days

Nadir: 14 days

Recovery: 28 days

1% to 10%:

Central nervous system: Dizziness, fever, headache

Dermatologic: Alopecia, rash, pruritus, hyperpigmentation with high-dose therapy

Endocrine & metabolic: Hyperuricemia

Gastrointestinal: Anorexia, nausea and vomiting rarely occur

Emetic potential: Low (<10%)

Genitourinary: Hemorrhagic cystitis

Local: Pain at injection site

Renal: Hematuria

Miscellaneous: Tightness of the throat, allergic reactions

<1% (Limited to important or life-threatening): Carcinogenesis: Like other alkylating agents, this drug is carcinogenic.

BMT:

Central nervous system: Confusion, inappropriate behavior, somnolence

Dermatologic: Hyperpigmentation

Gastrointestinal: Mucositis, mild nausea and vomiting

Hepatic: Serum transaminitis, hyperbilirubinemia

Overdosage/Toxicology Symptoms include nausea, vomiting, precipitation of uric acid in kidney tubules, bone marrow suppression, and bleeding. Therapy is supportive only. Thiotepa is dialyzable. Transfusions of whole blood or platelets have been proven beneficial.

Drug Interactions

Increased Effect/Toxicity: Other alkylating agents or irradiation used concomitantly with thiotepa intensifies toxicity rather than enhancing therapeutic response. Prolonged muscular paralysis and respiratory depression may occur when neuromuscular blocking agents are administered. Succinylcholine and other neuromuscular blocking agents' action can be prolonged due to thiotepa inhibiting plasma pseudocholinesterase.

Ethanol/Nutrition/Herb Interactions

Ethanol: Avoid ethanol (due to GI irritation).

Herb/Nutraceutical: Avoid black cohosh, dong quai in estrogen-dependent tumors.

Stability

Store intact vials under refrigeration (2°C to 8°C) and protect from light. **Not stable** at room temperature for any duration of time.

Dilute powder 1.5 mL SWI to a concentration of 10.4 mg/mL which is stable for 8 hours at refrigeration

Further dilution in NS: Thiotepa is stable for 24 hours at a concentration of 5 mg/mL in NS at 8°C and 23°C; however, stability decreases significantly at concentrations of ≤0.5 mg/mL (<8 hours); concentrations of 1-3 mg/mL are stable 48 hours at 8°C and 24 hours at 23°C

Standard I.V. dilution:

I.V. push: Dose/syringe (concentration = 10 mg/mL)

IVPB: Dose/100-150 mL NS for a final concentration of 1.5-3.5 mg/mL

Standard intravesicular dilution: 60 mg/30-60 mL NS; solution is placed via catheter and retained for two hours for maximum effect.

Standard intrathecal dilution: Intrathecal doses of 1-10 mg/m^2 should be diluted to 1-5 mg/mL in preservative-free NS or LR or 1 mg/mL in preservative-free SWI

ALL solutions should be **prepared fresh** and administered within one hour of preparation

(Continued)

Thiotepa *(Continued)*

Mechanism of Action Alkylating agent that reacts with DNA phosphate groups to produce cross-linking of DNA strands leading to inhibition of DNA, RNA, and protein synthesis; mechanism of action has not been explored as thoroughly as the other alkylating agents, it is presumed that the aziridine rings open and react as nitrogen mustard; reactivity is enhanced at a lower pH

Pharmacodynamics/Kinetics

Absorption: Intracavitary instillation: Unreliable (10% to 100%) through bladder mucosa; I.M.: variable

Metabolism: Extensively hepatic

Half-life elimination: Terminal: 109 minutes with dose-dependent clearance

Excretion: Urine (as metabolites and unchanged drug)

Usual Dosage Refer to individual protocols; dosing must be based on the clinical and hematologic response of the patient

Children: Sarcomas: I.V.: 25-65 mg/m² as a single dose every 21 days

Adults:

I.M., I.V., S.C.: 30-60 mg/m² once per week

I.V. doses of 0.3-0.4 mg/kg by rapid I.V. administration every 1-4 weeks, or 0.2 mg/kg or 6-8 mg/m²/day for 4-5 days every 2-4 weeks

High-dose therapy for bone marrow transplant: I.V.: 500 mg/m²; up to 900 mg/m²

I.M. doses of 15-30 mg in various schedules have been given

Intracavitary: 0.6-0.8 mg/kg

Intrapericardial dose: Usually 15-30 mg

Dosing comments/adjustment in renal impairment: Use with extreme caution, reduced dose may be warranted. Less than 3% of alkylating species are detected in the urine in 24 hours.

Intrathecal: Doses of 1-10 mg/m² administered 1-2 times/week in concentrations of 1 mg/mL diluted with preservative-free sterile water for injection

Intravesical: Used for treatment of carcinoma of the bladder; patients should be dehydrated for 8-12 hours prior to treatment; instill 60 mg (in 30-60 mL of NS) into the bladder and retain for a minimum of 2 hours. Patient should be positioned every 15 minutes for maximal area exposure. Instillations usually once a week for 4 weeks. Monitor for bone marrow suppression.

Intratumor: Use a 22-gauge needle to inject thiotepa directly into the tumor. Initial dose: 0.6-0.8 mg/kg (diluted to 10 mg/mL) are used every 1-4 weeks; maintenance dose: 0.07-0.8 mg/kg are administered at 1- to 4-week intervals

Ophthalmic: 0.05% solution in LR has been instilled into the eye every 3 hours for 6-8 weeks for the prevention of pterygium recurrence

Administration Thiotepa is usually administered intravenously, either as a short bolus or push, or a 1-hour infusion; or as an intravesical infusion. The drug is occasionally administered as intracavitary, intramuscular, or intrathecal injections. Intrathecal doses are usually diluted to a concentration of 1 mg/mL in preservative-free sterile water or normal saline. Bladder irrigations should be diluted in 50-100 mL of sterile water or normal saline, and retained for at least 2 hours. The patient should be repositioned every 15 minutes for maximal exposure.

Monitoring Parameters CBC with differential and platelet count, uric acid, urinalysis

Patient Information This drug can only be administered I.V. You will require regular blood tests to assess response to therapy. Avoid alcohol and aspirin or aspirin-containing medications unless approved by prescriber. Maintain adequate hydration (2-3 L/day of fluids unless instructed to restrict fluid intake) to prevent kidney damage. For nausea and vomiting, small frequent meals, chewing gum, or sucking lozenges may help, antiemetics may be prescribed. You may experience amenorrhea or changed sperm production, rash, hair loss, or loss of appetite (maintaining adequate nutrition is important). You may have increased sensitivity to infection (avoid crowds and infected persons). Report unusual bleeding or bruising, persistent fever or chills, sore throat, sores in mouth or vagina, blackened stool, or difficulty breathing. The drug may cause permanent sterility and may cause birth defects. The drug may be excreted in breast milk, therefore, an alternative form of feeding your baby should be used. Contraceptive measures are recommended during therapy.

Nursing Implications Not a vesicant

Additional Information A 1 mg/mL solution is considered isotonic.

Dosage Forms Powder for injection: 15 mg

Thiothixene *(thye oh THIKS een)*

Related Information

Antacid Drug Interactions *on page 1477*
Antipsychotic Agents Comparison *on page 1486*

U.S. Brand Names Navane®

Canadian Brand Names Navane™

Synonyms Tiotixene

Therapeutic Category Antipsychotic Agent, Miscellaneous; Phenothiazine Derivative

Use Management of schizophrenia

Unlabeled/Investigational Use Psychotic disorders

Pregnancy Risk Factor C

Contraindications Hypersensitivity to thiothixene or any component of the formulation; severe CNS depression; circulatory collapse; blood dyscrasias; coma

Warnings/Precautions When administering I.M. or I.V., watch for hypotension. Safety in children <12 years of age has not been established. May be sedating. Use with caution in Parkinson's disease; hemodynamic instability; predisposition to seizures; subcortical brain damage; bone marrow suppression; severe cardiac, hepatic, renal, or respiratory disease. Esophageal dysmotility and aspiration have been associated with antipsychotic use - use with caution in patients at risk of pneumonia (ie, Alzheimer's disease). Caution in breast cancer or other prolactin-dependent tumors (may elevate prolactin levels). May alter temperature regulation or mask toxicity of other drugs due to antiemetic effects. May alter cardiac conduction - life-threatening arrhythmias have occurred with therapeutic doses of neuroleptics. May cause orthostatic hypotension - use with caution in patients at risk of this effect or those who would tolerate transient hypotensive episodes (cerebrovascular disease, cardiovascular disease, or other medications which may predispose).

Phenothiazines may cause anticholinergic effects (confusion, agitation, constipation, dry mouth, blurred vision, urinary retention); therefore, they should be used with caution in patients with decreased gastrointestinal motility, urinary retention, BPH, xerostomia, or visual problems. Conditions which also may be exacerbated by cholinergic blockade include narrow-angle glaucoma (screening is recommended) and worsening of myasthenia gravis. Relative to other neuroleptics, thiothixene has a low potency of cholinergic blockade.

May cause extrapyramidal reactions, including pseudoparkinsonism, acute dystonic reactions, akathisia, and tardive dyskinesia (risk of these reactions is high relative to other neuroleptics). May be associated with neuroleptic malignant syndrome (NMS) or pigmentary retinopathy.

Adverse Reactions Frequency not defined:
Cardiovascular: Hypotension, tachycardia, syncope, nonspecific EKG changes
Central nervous system: Extrapyramidal symptoms (pseudoparkinsonism, akathisia, dystonias, lightheadedness, tardive dyskinesia), dizziness, drowsiness, restlessness, agitation, insomnia
Dermatologic: Discoloration of skin (blue-gray), rash, pruritus, urticaria, photosensitivity
Endocrine & metabolic: Changes in menstrual cycle, changes in libido, breast pain, galactorrhea, lactation, amenorrhea, gynecomastia, hyperglycemia, hypoglycemia
Gastrointestinal: Weight gain, nausea, vomiting, stomach pain, constipation, xerostomia, increased salivation
Genitourinary: Difficulty in urination, ejaculatory disturbances, impotence
Hematologic: Leukopenia, leukocytes
Neuromuscular & skeletal: Tremors
Ocular: Pigmentary retinopathy, blurred vision
Respiratory: Nasal congestion
Miscellaneous: Diaphoresis

Overdosage/Toxicology Symptoms include muscle twitching, drowsiness, dizziness, rigidity, tremor, hypotension, and cardiac arrhythmias. Following initiation of essential overdose management, toxic symptom treatment and supportive treatment should be initiated. Hypotension usually responds to I.V. fluids or Trendelenburg positioning. If unresponsive to these measures, the use of a parenteral inotrope may be required (eg, norepinephrine 0.1-0.2 mcg/kg/minute titrated to response). Seizures commonly respond to diazepam (I.V. 5-10 mg bolus in adults every 15 minutes if needed up to a total of 30 mg; I.V. 0.25-0.4 mg/kg/dose up to a total of 10 mg in children) or to phenytoin or phenobarbital. Neuroleptics often cause extrapyramidal symptoms (eg, dystonic reactions) requiring management with diphenhydramine 1-2 mg/kg (adults) up to a maximum of 50 mg I.M. or slow I.V. push, followed by a maintenance dose for 48-72 hours. When these reactions are unresponsive to diphenhydramine, anticholinergic agents such as benztropine mesylate I.V. 1-2 mg (adults) may be effective. These agents are generally effective within 2-5 minutes.

Drug Interactions
Cytochrome P450 Effect: CYP1A2 enzyme substrate
Increased Effect/Toxicity: Thiothixene and CNS depressants (ethanol, narcotics) may produce additive CNS depressant effects. Thiothixene may increase the effect/toxicity of antihypertensives, benztropine (and other anticholinergic agents), lithium, trazodone, and TCAs. Thiothixene's concentrations may be increased by chloroquine, sulfadoxine-pyrimethamine, and propranolol.
Decreased Effect: Thiothixene inhibits the activity of guanadrel, guanethidine, levodopa, and bromocriptine. Benztropine (and other anticholinergics) may inhibit the therapeutic response to thiothixene. Barbiturates and cigarette smoking may enhance the hepatic metabolism of thiothixene. Thiothixene and low potency antipsychotics may reverse the pressor effects of epinephrine.

Ethanol/Nutrition/Herb Interactions
Ethanol: Avoid ethanol (may increase CNS depression).
Herb/Nutraceutical: Avoid kava kava, valerian, St John's wort, gotu kola (may increase CNS depression).

Stability Refrigerate powder for injection. Reconstituted powder for injection is stable at room temperature for 48 hours.

Mechanism of Action Elicits antipsychotic activity by postsynaptic blockade of CNS dopamine receptors resulting in inhibition of dopamine-mediated effects; also has alpha-adrenergic blocking activity

Pharmacodynamics/Kinetics
Metabolism: Extensively hepatic
Half-life elimination: >24 hours with chronic use

Usual Dosage
Children <12 years (unlabeled): Schizophrenia/psychoses: Oral: 0.25 mg/kg/24 hours in divided doses (dose not well established; use not recommended)
Children >12 years and Adults: Mild to moderate psychosis:
Oral: 2 mg 3 times/day, up to 20-30 mg/day; more severe psychosis: Initial: 5 mg 2 times/day, may increase gradually, if necessary; maximum: 60 mg/day
I.M.: 4 mg 2-4 times/day, increase dose gradually; usual: 16-20 mg/day; maximum: 30 mg/day; change to oral dose as soon as able
Rapid tranquilization of the agitated patient (administered every 30-60 minutes):
Oral: 5-10 mg
I.M.: 10-20 mg
Average total dose for tranquilization: 15-30 mg
Hemodialysis: Not dialyzable (0% to 5%)

Administration Oral concentration contains 7% alcohol. Dilute immediately before administration with water, fruit juice, milk, etc. **Note:** Avoid skin contact with oral medication; may cause contact dermatitis.
(Continued)

Thiothixene (Continued)

Monitoring Parameters Orthostatic blood pressures; tremors, gait changes, abnormal movement in trunk, neck, buccal area or extremities; monitor target behaviors for which the agent is given

Test Interactions May cause false-positive pregnancy test

Patient Information May cause drowsiness, restlessness, avoid alcohol and other CNS depressants; do not alter dosage or discontinue without consulting physician

Nursing Implications Observe for extrapyramidal symptoms; concentrate should be mixed in juice before administration

Additional Information Coadministration of two or more antipsychotics does not improve clinical response and may increase the potential for adverse effects.

Dosage Forms

Capsule: 1 mg, 2 mg, 5 mg, 10 mg, 20 mg

Powder for injection, as hydrochloride: 5 mg/mL (2 mL)

Solution, oral concentrate, as hydrochloride: 5 mg/mL (30 mL, 120 mL)

- ◆ **Thorazine®** *see* ChlorproMAZINE *on page 282*
- ◆ **Thrombate III™** *see* Antithrombin III *on page 107*
- ◆ **Thymocyte Stimulating Factor** *see* Aldesleukin *on page 43*
- ◆ **Thymoglobulin®** *see* Antithymocyte Globulin (Rabbit) *on page 108*
- ◆ **Thyro-Block® (Can)** *see* Potassium Iodide *on page 1111*
- ◆ **Thyrogen®** *see* Thyrotropin Alpha *on page 1327*

Thyroid (THYE roid)

U.S. Brand Names Armour® Thyroid; Nature-Throid® NT; Westhroid®

Synonyms Desiccated Thyroid; Thyroid Extract; Thyroid USP

Therapeutic Category Thyroid Product

Use Replacement or supplemental therapy in hypothyroidism; pituitary TSH suppressants (thyroid nodules, thyroiditis, multinodular goiter, thyroid cancer), thyrotoxicosis, diagnostic suppression tests

Pregnancy Risk Factor A

Contraindications Hypersensitivity to beef or pork or any component of the formulation; recent myocardial infarction; thyrotoxicosis uncomplicated by hypothyroidism; uncorrected adrenal insufficiency

Warnings/Precautions Ineffective for weight reduction. High doses may produce serious or even life-threatening toxic effects particularly when used with some anorectic drugs. Use cautiously in patients with pre-existing cardiovascular disease (angina, CHD), elderly since they may be more likely to have compromised cardiovascular function. Chronic hypothyroidism predisposes patients to coronary artery disease. Desiccated thyroid contains variable amounts of T_3, T_4, and other triiodothyronine compounds which are more likely to cause cardiac signs or symptoms due to fluctuating levels. Should avoid use in the elderly for this reason. Drug of choice is levothyroxine in the minds of many clinicians.

Adverse Reactions <1% (Limited to important or life-threatening): Alopecia, cardiac arrhythmia, chest pain, dyspnea, excessive bone loss with overtreatment (excess thyroid replacement), hand tremors, myalgia, palpitations, tachycardia, tremor

Drug Interactions

Increased Effect/Toxicity: Thyroid may potentiate the hypoprothrombinemic effect of oral anticoagulants. Tricyclic antidepressants (TAD) coadministered with thyroid hormone may increase potential for toxicity of both drugs.

Decreased Effect: Thyroid hormones increase the therapeutic need for oral hypoglycemics or insulin. Cholestyramine can bind thyroid and reduce its absorption. Phenytoin may decrease thyroxine serum levels. Thyroid hormone may decrease effect of oral sulfonylureas.

Mechanism of Action The primary active compound is T_3 (triiodothyronine), which may be converted from T_4 (thyroxine) and then circulates throughout the body to influence growth and maturation of various tissues; exact mechanism of action is unknown; however, it is believed the thyroid hormone exerts its many metabolic effects through control of DNA transcription and protein synthesis; involved in normal metabolism, growth, and development; promotes gluconeogenesis, increases utilization and mobilization of glycogen stores and stimulates protein synthesis, increases basal metabolic rate

Pharmacodynamics/Kinetics

Absorption: T_4: 48% to 79%; T_3: 95%; desiccated thyroid contains thyroxine, liothyronine, and iodine (primarily bound)

Metabolism: Thyroxine: Largely converted to liothyronine

Half-life elimination, serum: Liothyronine: 1-2 days; Thyroxine: 6-7 days

Usual Dosage Oral:

Children: See table.

Recommended Pediatric Dosage for Congenital Hypothyroidism

Age	Daily Dose (mg)	Daily Dose/kg (mg)
0-6 mo	15-30	4.8-6
6-12 mo	30-45	3.6-4.8
1-5 y	45-60	3-3.6
6-12 y	60-90	2.4-3
>12 y	>90	1.2-1.8

Adults: Initial: 15-30 mg; increase with 15 mg increments every 2-4 weeks; use 15 mg in patients with cardiovascular disease or myxedema. Maintenance dose: Usually 60-120 mg/day; monitor TSH and clinical symptoms.

Thyroid cancer: Requires larger amounts than replacement therapy

Dietary Considerations Should be taken on an empty stomach.

Nursing Implications Monitor T_4, TSH, heart rate, blood pressure, clinical signs of hypo- and hyperthyroidism; in cases when T_4 remains low and TSH is within normal limits, an evaluation of "free" (unbound) T_4 is needed to evaluate further increase in dosage. Thyroid replacement requires periodic assessment of thyroid status; TSH is the most reliable guide for evaluating adequacy of thyroid replacement dosage. TSH may be elevated during the first few months of thyroid replacement despite patients being clinically euthyroid.

Dosage Forms

Capsule, pork source in soybean oil (S-P-T): 60 mg, 120 mg, 180 mg, 300 mg

Tablet:

Armour® Thyroid: 15 mg, 30 mg, 60 mg, 90 mg, 120 mg, 180 mg, 240 mg, 300 mg

Thyroid USP: 15 mg, 30 mg, 60 mg, 120 mg, 180 mg, 300 mg

♦ **Thyroid Extract** *see Thyroid on page 1326*
♦ **Thyroid Stimulating Hormone** *see Thyrotropin on page 1327*
♦ **Thyroid USP** *see Thyroid on page 1326*
♦ **Thyrolar®** *see Liotrix on page 808*
♦ **Thyrotropic Hormone** *see Thyrotropin on page 1327*

Thyrotropin (thye roe TROH pin)

U.S. Brand Names Thytropar®

Synonyms Thyroid Stimulating Hormone; Thyrotropic Hormone; TSH

Therapeutic Category Diagnostic Agent, Hypothyroidism; Diagnostic Agent, Thyroid Function

Use Diagnostic aid to differentiate thyroid failure; diagnosis of decreased thyroid reserve, to differentiate between primary and secondary hypothyroidism and between primary hypothyroidism and euthyroidism in patients receiving thyroid replacement

Pregnancy Risk Factor C

Contraindications Hypersensitivity to thyrotropin or any component of the formulation; coronary thrombosis, untreated Addison's disease

Warnings/Precautions Use with caution in patients with angina pectoris or cardiac failure, patients with hypopituitarism, adrenal cortical suppression as may be seen with corticosteroid therapy; may cause thyroid hyperplasia

Adverse Reactions <1% (Limited to important or life-threatening): Anaphylaxis with repeated administration, fever, tachycardia

Overdosage/Toxicology Symptoms include weight loss, nervousness, sweating, tachycardia, insomnia, heat intolerance, menstrual irregularities, headache, angina pectoris, and CHF. Acute massive overdose may require cardiac glycosides for CHF. Fever should be controlled with the help of acetaminophen. Antiadrenergic agents, particularly propranolol 1-3 mg I.V. every 6 hours or 80-160 mg/day, can be used to treat increased sympathetic activity.

Stability Refrigerate at 2°C to 8°C (36°F to 46°F) after reconstitution; use within 2 weeks

Mechanism of Action Stimulates formation and secretion of thyroid hormone, increases uptake of iodine by thyroid gland

Pharmacodynamics/Kinetics

Half-life elimination: 35 minutes, dependent upon thyroid state

Excretion: Urine

Usual Dosage Adults: I.M., S.C.: 10 units/day for 1-3 days; follow by a radioiodine study 24 hours past last injection, no response in thyroid failure, substantial response in pituitary failure

Dosage Forms Injection: 10 units

Thyrotropin Alpha (thye roe TROH pin AL fa)

U.S. Brand Names Thyrogen®

Synonyms Human Thyroid Stimulating Hormone; TSH

Therapeutic Category Diagnostic Agent

Use As an adjunctive diagnostic tool for serum thyroglobulin (Tg) testing with or without radioiodine imaging in the follow-up of patients with well-differentiated thyroid cancer

Potential clinical use:

1. Patients with an undetectable Tg on thyroid hormone suppressive therapy to exclude the diagnosis of residual or recurrent thyroid cancer
2. Patients requiring serum Tg testing and radioiodine imaging who are unwilling to undergo thyroid hormone withdrawal testing and whose treating physician believes that use of a less sensitive test is justified
3. Patients who are either unable to mount an adequate endogenous TSH response to thyroid hormone withdrawal or in whom withdrawal is medically contraindicated

Pregnancy Risk Factor C

Contraindications Hypersensitivity to thyrotropin alpha or any component of the formulation

Warnings/Precautions Caution should be exercised when administered to patients who have been previously treated with bovine TSH and, in particular, to those patients who have experienced hypersensitivity reactions to bovine TSH

Considerations in the use of Thyrogen®:

1. There remains a meaningful risk of a diagnosis of thyroid cancer or of an underestimating the extent of disease when Thyrogen®-stimulated Tg testing is performed and in combination with radioiodine imaging
2. Thyrogen® Tg levels are generally lower than, and do not correlate with, Tg levels after thyroid hormone withdrawal
3. Newly detectable Tg level or a Tg level rising over time after Thyrogen® or a high index of suspicion of metastatic disease, even in the setting of a negative or low-stage Thyrogen® radioiodine scan, should prompt further evaluation such as thyroid hormone withdrawal to definitively establish the location and extent of thyroid cancer.
4. Decision to perform a Thyrogen® radioiodine scan in conjunction with a Thyrogen® serum Tg test and whether or when to withdraw a patient from thyroid hormones are

(Continued)

Thyrotropin Alpha *(Continued)*

complex. Pertinent factors in this decision include the sensitivity of the Tg assay used, the Thyrogen® Tg level obtained, and the index of suspicion of recurrent or persistent local or metastatic disease.

5. Thyrogen® is not recommended to stimulate radioiodine uptake for the purposes of ablative radiotherapy of thyroid cancer

6. The signs and symptoms of hypothyroidism which accompany thyroid hormone withdrawal are avoided with Thyrogen® use

Adverse Reactions 1% to 10%:

Central nervous system: Headache, chills, fever, dizziness

Gastrointestinal: Nausea, vomiting

Neuromuscular & skeletal: Weakness, paresthesia

Miscellaneous: Flu-like syndrome

Overdosage/Toxicology There has been no reported experience of overdose in humans.

Stability Store intact vials at 2°C to 8°C (36°F to 46°F); reconstitute each vial with 1.2 mL of sterile water for injection - each vial should be reconstituted immediately prior to use with diluent provided. If necessary, the reconstituted solution can be stored for up to 24 hours at 2°C to 8°C.

Mechanism of Action An exogenous source of human TSH that offers an additional diagnostic tool in the follow-up of patients with a history of well-differentiated thyroid cancer. Binding of thyrotropin alpha to TSH receptors on normal thyroid epithelial cells or on well-differentiated thyroid cancer tissue stimulates iodine uptake and organification and synthesis and secretion of thyroglobulin, triiodothyronine, and thyroxine.

Pharmacodynamics/Kinetics

Half-life elimination: 25 ± 10 hours

Time to peak: Mean: 3-24 hours after injection

Usual Dosage Children >16 years and Adults: I.M.: 0.9 mg every 24 hours for 2 doses or every 72 hours for 3 doses

For radioiodine imaging, radioiodine administration should be given 24 hours following the final Thyrogen® injection. Scanning should be performed 48 hours after radioiodine administration (72 hours after the final injection of Thyrogen®).

For serum testing, serum Tg should be obtained 72 hours after final injection.

Administration I.M. injection into the buttock

Dosage Forms Powder for injection [kit]: 1.1 mg vials (>4 int. units) [kit contains two vials of Thyrogen® and two vials of SWFI - 10 mL]

- ♦ **Thyrox®** *see* Levothyroxine *on page 799*
- ♦ **Thytropar®** *see* Thyrotropin *on page 1327*
- ♦ **Tiabendazole** *see* Thiabendazole *on page 1315*

Tiagabine *(tye AG a been)*

Related Information

Anticonvulsants by Seizure Type *on page 1481*

U.S. Brand Names Gabitril®

Canadian Brand Names Gabitril®

Synonyms Tiagabine Hydrochloride

Therapeutic Category Anticonvulsant

Use Adjunctive therapy in adults and children ≥12 years of age in the treatment of partial seizures

Unlabeled/Investigational Use Bipolar disorder

Pregnancy Risk Factor C

Contraindications Hypersensitivity to tiagabine or any component of the formulation

Warnings/Precautions Anticonvulsants should not be discontinued abruptly because of the possibility of increasing seizure frequency; tiagabine should be withdrawn gradually to minimize the potential of increased seizure frequency, unless safety concerns require a more rapid withdrawal. Rarely, nonconvulsive status epilepticus has been reported following abrupt discontinuation or dosage reduction.

Use with caution in patients with hepatic impairment. Experience in patients not receiving enzyme-inducing drugs has been limited - caution should be used in treating any patient who is not receiving one of these medications. Weakness, sedation, and confusion may occur with tiagabine use. Patients must be cautioned about performing tasks which require mental alertness (ie, operating machinery or driving). Effects with other sedative drugs or ethanol may be potentiated. May cause potentially serious rash, including Stevens-Johnson syndrome.

Adverse Reactions

>10%:

Central nervous system: Dizziness, somnolence

Gastrointestinal: Nausea

Neuromuscular & skeletal: Weakness

1% to 10%:

Central nervous system: Nervousness, difficulty with concentration, insomnia, ataxia, confusion, speech disorder, depression, emotional lability, abnormal gait, hostility

Dermatologic: Rash, pruritus

Gastrointestinal: Diarrhea, vomiting, increased appetite

Neuromuscular & skeletal: Tremor, paresthesia

Ocular: Nystagmus

Otic: Hearing impairment

Respiratory: Pharyngitis, cough

Drug Interactions

Cytochrome P450 Effect: CYP2D6 and 3A3/4 enzyme substrate

Increased Effect/Toxicity: Valproate increased free tiagabine concentrations by 40%.

Decreased Effect: Primidone, phenobarbital, phenytoin, and carbamazepine increase tiagabine clearance by 60%.

Ethanol/Nutrition/Herb Interactions

Ethanol: Avoid ethanol (may increase CNS depression).

Food: Food reduces the rate but not the extent of absorption.

Herb/Nutraceutical: St John's wort may decrease tiagabine levels. Avoid valerian, St John's wort, kava kava, gotu kola (may increase CNS depression).

Mechanism of Action The exact mechanism by which tiagabine exerts antiseizure activity is not definitively known; however, in vitro experiments demonstrate that it enhances the activity of gamma aminobutyric acid (GABA), the major neuroinhibitory transmitter in the nervous system; it is thought that binding to the GABA uptake carrier inhibits the uptake of GABA into presynaptic neurons, allowing an increased amount of GABA to be available to postsynaptic neurons; based on in vitro studies, tiagabine does not inhibit the uptake of dopamine, norepinephrine, serotonin, glutamate, or choline

Pharmacodynamics/Kinetics

Absorption: Rapid (within 1 hour); prolonged with food

Protein binding: 96%

Half-life elimination: 6.7 hours

Usual Dosage Oral (administer with food):

Children 12-18 years: 4 mg once daily for 1 week; may increase to 8 mg daily in 2 divided doses for 1 week; then may increase by 4-8 mg weekly to response or up to 32 mg daily in 2-4 divided doses

Adults: 4 mg once daily for 1 week; may increase by 4-8 mg weekly to response or up to 56 mg daily in 2-4 divided doses

Dietary Considerations Take with food.

Monitoring Parameters A reduction in seizure frequency is indicative of therapeutic response to tiagabine in patients with partial seizures; complete blood counts, renal function tests, liver function tests, and routine blood chemistry should be monitored periodically during therapy

Reference Range Maximal plasma level after a 24 mg/dose: 552 ng/mL

Patient Information Use exactly as directed; take orally with food, usually beginning at 4 mg once daily, and usually in addition to other antiepilepsy drugs. The dose will be increased based on age and medical condition, up to 2-4 times/day. Do not interrupt or discontinue treatment without consulting your physician or pharmacist. If told to stop this medication, it should be discontinued gradually.

Dosage Forms Tablet: 2 mg, 4 mg, 12 mg, 16 mg, 20 mg

♦ **Tiagabine Hydrochloride** see Tiagabine on page 1328

♦ **Tiamate®** see Diltiazem on page 409

♦ **Tiamol® (Can)** see Fluocinonide on page 573

♦ **Tiazac®** see Diltiazem on page 409

♦ **Ticar®** see Ticarcillin on page 1329

Ticarcillin (tye kar SIL in)

Related Information

Antimicrobial Drugs of Choice on page 1588

Community-Acquired Pneumonia in Adults on page 1603

U.S. Brand Names Ticar®

Synonyms Ticarcillin Disodium

Therapeutic Category Antibiotic, Penicillin

Use Treatment of susceptible infections such as septicemia, acute and chronic respiratory tract infections, skin and soft tissue infections, and urinary tract infections due to susceptible strains of Pseudomonas, and other gram-negative bacteria

Pregnancy Risk Factor B

Contraindications Hypersensitivity to ticarcillin, any component of the formulation, or penicillins

Warnings/Precautions Due to sodium load and adverse effects (anemia, neuropsychological changes), use with caution and modify dosage in patients with renal impairment; serious and occasionally severe or fatal hypersensitivity (anaphylactoid) reactions have been reported in patients on penicillin therapy (especially with a history of beta-lactam hypersensitivity and/or a history of sensitivity to multiple allergens); use with caution in patients with seizures

Adverse Reactions Frequency not defined.

Central nervous system: Confusion, convulsions, drowsiness, fever, Jarisch-Herxheimer reaction

Dermatologic: Rash

Endocrine & metabolic: Electrolyte imbalance

Gastrointestinal: Clostridium difficile colitis

Hematologic: Bleeding, eosinophilia, hemolytic anemia, leukopenia, neutropenia, positive Coombs' reaction, thrombocytopenia

Hepatic: Hepatotoxicity, jaundice

Local: Thrombophlebitis

Neuromuscular & skeletal: Myoclonus

Renal: Interstitial nephritis (acute)

Miscellaneous: Anaphylaxis, hypersensitivity reactions

Overdosage/Toxicology Symptoms of penicillin overdose include neuromuscular hypersensitivity (agitation, hallucinations, asterixis, encephalopathy, confusion, and seizures) and electrolyte imbalance (with potassium or sodium salts), especially in renal failure. Hemodialysis may be helpful to aid in the removal of the drug from the blood, otherwise most treatment is supportive or symptom directed.

(Continued)

Ticarcillin *(Continued)*

Drug Interactions

Increased Effect/Toxicity: Probenecid may increase penicillin levels. Neuromuscular blockers may have an increased duration of action (neuromuscular blockade).

Decreased Effect: Tetracyclines may decrease penicillin effectiveness. Efficacy of oral contraceptives may be reduced when taken with ticarcillin. Aminoglycosides may cause physical inactivation of aminoglycosides in the presence of high concentrations of ticarcillin and potential toxicity in patients with mild-moderate renal dysfunction.

Stability Reconstituted solution is stable for 72 hours at room temperature and 14 days when refrigerated; for I.V. infusion in NS or D_5W solution is stable for 72 hours at room temperature, 14 days when refrigerated or 30 days when frozen; after freezing, thawed solution is stable for 72 hours at room temperature or 14 days when refrigerated; **incompatible** with aminoglycosides

Mechanism of Action Inhibits bacterial cell wall synthesis by binding to one or more of the penicillin binding proteins (PBPs); which in turn inhibits the final transpeptidation step of peptidoglycan synthesis in bacterial cell walls, thus inhibiting cell wall biosynthesis. Bacteria eventually lyse due to ongoing activity of cell wall autolytic enzymes (autolysins and murein hydrolases) while cell wall assembly is arrested.

Pharmacodynamics/Kinetics

Absorption: I.M.: 86%

Distribution: Blister fluid, lymph tissue, and gallbladder; low concentrations into CSF increasing with inflamed meninges, otherwise widely distributed; crosses placenta; enters breast milk (low concentrations)

Protein binding: 45% to 65%

Half-life elimination:

Neonates: <1 week old: 3.5-5.6 hours; 1-8 weeks old: 1.3-2.2 hours

Children 5-13 years: 0.9 hour

Adults: 66-72 minutes; prolonged with renal and/or hepatic impairment

Time to peak, serum: I.M.: 30-75 minutes

Excretion: Almost entirely urine (as unchanged drug and metabolites); feces (3.5%)

Usual Dosage Ticarcillin is generally given I.V., I.M. injection is only for the treatment of uncomplicated urinary tract infections and dose should not exceed 2 g/injection when administered I.M.

Neonates: I.M., I.V.:

Postnatal age <7 days:

<2000 g: 75 mg/kg/dose every 12 hours

>2000 g: 75 mg/kg/dose every 8 hours

Postnatal age >7 days:

<1200 g: 75 mg/kg/dose every 12 hours

1200-2000 g: 75 mg/kg/dose every 8 hours

>2000 g: 75 mg/kg/dose every 6 hours

Infants and Children:

Systemic infections: I.V.: 200-300 mg/kg/day in divided doses every 4-6 hours

Urinary tract infections: I.M., I.V.: 50-100 mg/kg/day in divided doses every 6-8 hours

Maximum dose: 24 g/day

Adults: I.M., I.V.: 1-4 g every 4-6 hours, usual dose: 3 g I.V. every 4-6 hours

Dosing adjustment in renal impairment: Adults:

Cl_{cr} 30-60 mL/minute: 2 g every 4 hours or 3 g every 8 hours

Cl_{cr} 10-30 mL/minute: 2 g every 8 hours or 3 g every 12 hours

Cl_{cr} <10 mL/minute: 2 g every 12 hours

Moderately dialyzable (20% to 50%)

Continuous arteriovenous or venovenous hemodiafiltration effects: Dose as for Cl_{cr} 10-50 mL/minute

Administration Administer 1 hour apart from aminoglycosides

Monitoring Parameters Serum electrolytes, bleeding time, and periodic tests of renal, hepatic, and hematologic function; monitor for signs of anaphylaxis during first dose

Test Interactions May interfere with urinary glucose tests using cupric sulfate (Benedict's solution, Clinitest®); may inactivate aminoglycosides *in vitro*; false-positive urinary or serum protein

Nursing Implications Draw sample for culture and sensitivity before administering first dose, if possible

Additional Information Sodium content of 1 g: 119.6-149.5 mg (5.2-6.5 mEq)

Dosage Forms Powder for injection, as disodium: 3 g, 20 g

Ticarcillin and Clavulanate Potassium

(tye kar SIL in & klav yoo LAN ate poe TASS ee um)

Related Information

Antimicrobial Drugs of Choice *on page 1588*

Community-Acquired Pneumonia in Adults *on page 1603*

U.S. Brand Names Timentin®

Canadian Brand Names Timentin®

Synonyms Ticarcillin and Clavulanic Acid

Therapeutic Category Antibiotic, Penicillin; Antibiotic, Penicillin & Beta-lactamase Inhibitor

Use Treatment of infections of lower respiratory tract, urinary tract, skin and skin structures, bone and joint, and septicemia caused by susceptible organisms. Clavulanate expands activity of ticarcillin to include beta-lactamase producing strains of *S. aureus, H. influenzae, Bacteroides* species, and some other gram-negative bacilli

Pregnancy Risk Factor B

Contraindications Hypersensitivity to ticarcillin, clavulanate, any penicillin, or any component of the formulation

Warnings/Precautions Not approved for use in children <12 years of age; use with caution and modify dosage in patients with renal impairment; use with caution in patients with a history of allergy to cephalosporins and in patients with CHF due to high sodium load

Adverse Reactions Frequency not defined.

Central nervous system: Confusion, convulsions, drowsiness, fever, Jarisch-Herxheimer reaction

Dermatologic: Rash

Endocrine & metabolic: Electrolyte imbalance

Gastrointestinal: *Clostridium difficile* colitis

Hematologic: Bleeding, hemolytic anemia, leukopenia, neutropenia, positive Coombs' reaction, thrombocytopenia

Hepatic: Hepatotoxicity, jaundice

Local: Thrombophlebitis

Neuromuscular & skeletal: Myoclonus

Renal: Interstitial nephritis (acute)

Miscellaneous: Anaphylaxis, hypersensitivity reactions

Overdosage/Toxicology Symptoms include neuromuscular hypersensitivity and seizures. Many beta-lactam containing antibiotics have the potential to cause neuromuscular hyperirritability or convulsive seizures. Hemodialysis may be helpful to aid in removal of the drug from the blood, otherwise most treatment is supportive or symptom directed.

Drug Interactions

Increased Effect/Toxicity: Probenecid may increase penicillin levels. Neuromuscular blockers may have an increased duration of action (neuromuscular blockade).

Decreased Effect: Tetracyclines may decrease penicillin effectiveness. Efficacy of oral contraceptives may be reduced when taken with ticarcillin and clavulanate potassium. Aminoglycosides may cause physical inactivation of aminoglycosides in the presence of high concentrations of ticarcillin and potential toxicity in patients with mild-moderate renal dysfunction.

Stability Reconstituted solution is stable for 6 hours at room temperature and 72 hours when refrigerated; for I.V. infusion in NS is stable for 24 hours at room temperature, 7 days when refrigerated or 30 days when frozen; after freezing, thawed solution is stable for 8 hours at room temperature; for I.V. infusion in D_5W solution is stable for 24 hours at room temperature, 3 days when refrigerated or 7 days when frozen; after freezing, thawed solution is stable for 8 hours at room temperature; darkening of drug indicates loss of potency of clavulanate potassium; **incompatible** with sodium bicarbonate, aminoglycosides

Mechanism of Action Inhibits bacterial cell wall synthesis by binding to one or more of the penicillin binding proteins (PBPs); which in turn inhibits the final transpeptidation step of peptidoglycan synthesis in bacterial cell walls, thus inhibiting cell wall biosynthesis. Bacteria eventually lyse due to ongoing activity of cell wall autolytic enzymes (autolysins and murein hydrolases) while cell wall assembly is arrested.

Pharmacodynamics/Kinetics

Ticarcillin: See Ticarcillin monograph.

Clavulanic acid:

Protein binding: 9% to 30%

Metabolism: Hepatic

Half-life elimination: 66-90 minutes

Excretion: Urine (45% as unchanged drug)

Clearance: Does not affect clearance of ticarcillin

Usual Dosage I.V.:

Children and Adults <60 kg: 200-300 mg of ticarcillin component/kg/day in divided doses every 4-6 hours

Children >60 kg and Adults: 3.1 g (ticarcillin 3 g plus clavulanic acid 0.1 g) every 4-6 hours; maximum: 24 g/day

Urinary tract infections: 3.1 g every 6-8 hours

Dosing adjustment in renal impairment:

Cl_{cr} 30-60 mL/minute: Administer 2 g every 4 hours or 3.1 g every 8 hours

Cl_{cr} 10-30 mL/minute: Administer 2 g every 8 hours or 3.1 g every 12 hours

Cl_{cr} <10 mL/minute: Administer 2 g every 12 hours

Moderately dialyzable (20% to 50%)

Continuous arteriovenous or venovenous hemodiafiltration effects: Dose as for Cl_{cr} 10-50 mL/minute

Peritoneal dialysis: 3.1 g every 12 hours

Hemodialysis: 2 g every 12 hours; supplemented with 3.1 g after each dialysis

Administration Infuse over 30 minutes; administer 1 hour apart from aminoglycosides

Monitoring Parameters Observe signs and symptoms of anaphylaxis during first dose

Test Interactions Positive Coombs' test, false-positive urinary proteins

Nursing Implications Draw sample for culture and sensitivity prior to first dose if possible

Additional Information Sodium content of 1 g: 4.75 mEq; potassium content of 1 g: 0.15 mEq

Dosage Forms

Infusion [premixed, frozen]: Ticarcillin disodium 3 g and clavulanate potassium 0.1 g (100 mL)

Powder for injection: Ticarcillin disodium 3 g and clavulanate potassium 0.1 g (3.1 g, 31 g)

◆ **Ticarcillin and Clavulanic Acid** *see* Ticarcillin and Clavulanate Potassium *on page 1330*

◆ **Ticarcillin Disodium** *see* Ticarcillin *on page 1329*

◆ **TICE® BCG** *see* BCG Vaccine *on page 148*

◆ **Ticlid®** *see* Ticlopidine *on page 1331*

Ticlopidine (tye KLOE pi deen)

U.S. Brand Names Ticlid®

Canadian Brand Names Alti-Ticlopidine; Apo®-Ticlopidine; Gen-Ticlopidine; Nu-Ticlopidine; Rhoxal-ticlopidine; Ticlid®

Synonyms Ticlopidine Hydrochloride

Therapeutic Category Antiplatelet Agent; Platelet Aggregation Inhibitor

(Continued)

Ticlopidine *(Continued)*

Use Platelet aggregation inhibitor that reduces the risk of thrombotic stroke in patients who have had a stroke or stroke precursors. **Note:** Due to its association with life-threatening hematologic disorders, ticlopidine should be reserved for patients who are intolerant to aspirin, or who have failed aspirin therapy. Adjunctive therapy (with aspirin) following successful coronary stent implantation to reduce the incidence of subacute stent thrombosis.

Unlabeled/Investigational Use Protection of aortocoronary bypass grafts, diabetic microangiopathy, ischemic heart disease, prevention of postoperative DVT, reduction of graft loss following renal transplant

Pregnancy Risk Factor B

Contraindications Hypersensitivity to ticlopidine or any component of the formulation; active pathological bleeding such as PUD or intracranial hemorrhage; severe liver dysfunction; hematopoietic disorders (neutropenia, thrombocytopenia, a past history of TTP)

Warnings/Precautions Use with caution in patients who may be at risk of increased bleeding. Consider discontinuing 10-14 days before elective surgery. Use caution in mixing with other antiplatelet drugs. Use with caution in patients with severe liver disease (experience is limited). May cause life-threatening hematologic reactions, including neutropenia, agranulocytosis, thrombotic thrombocytopenia purpura (TTP), and aplastic anemia. Routine monitoring is required (see Monitoring Parameters). Monitor for signs and symptoms of neutropenia including WBC count. Discontinue if the absolute neutrophil count falls to <1200/mm^3 or if the platelet count falls to <80,000/mm^3.

Adverse Reactions As with all drugs which may affect hemostasis, bleeding is associated with ticlopidine. Hemorrhage may occur at virtually any site. Risk is dependent on multiple variables, including the use of multiple agents which alter hemostasis and patient susceptibility.

>10%:
    Endocrine & metabolic: Increased total cholesterol (increases of ~8% to 10% within 1 month of therapy)
    Gastrointestinal: Diarrhea (13%)
1% to 10%: Central nervous system: Dizziness (1%)
    Dermatologic: Rash (5%), purpura (2%), pruritus (1%)
    Gastrointestinal: Nausea (7%), dyspepsia (7%), gastrointestinal pain (4%), vomiting (2%), flatulence (2%), anorexia (1%)
    Hematologic: Neutropenia (2%)
    Hepatic: Abnormal liver function test (1%)
<1% (Limited to important or life-threatening): Agranulocytosis, anaphylaxis, angioedema, aplastic anemia, arthropathy, bone marrow suppression, bronchiolitis obliterans-organized pneumonia, chronic diarrhea, conjunctival bleeding, eosinophilia, erythema multiforme, erythema nodosum, exfoliative dermatitis, gastrointestinal bleeding, hematuria, hemolytic anemia, hepatic necrosis, hepatitis, hyponatremia, intracranial bleeding (rare), jaundice, maculopapular rash, menorrhagia, myositis, nephrotic syndrome, pancytopenia, peptic ulcer, peripheral neuropathy, pneumonitis (allergic), positive ANA, renal failure, sepsis, serum creatinine increased, serum sickness, Stevens-Johnson syndrome, systemic lupus erythematosus, thrombocytopenia (immune), thrombocytosis, thrombotic thrombocytopenic purpura, urticaria, vasculitis

Overdosage/Toxicology Symptoms include ataxia, seizures, vomiting, abdominal pain, and hematologic abnormalities. Specific treatments are lacking; after decontamination. Treatment is symptomatic and supportive.

Drug Interactions

Cytochrome P450 Effect: CYP3A3/4 enzyme substrate; CYP1A2 (possible), 2C19 (potent), 2D6 (weak) enzyme inhibitor

Increased Effect/Toxicity: Ticlopidine may increase effect/toxicity of aspirin, anticoagulants, theophylline, and NSAIDs. Cimetidine may increase ticlopidine blood levels. Phenytoin blood levels may be increased by ticlopidine (case reports).

Decreased Effect: Decreased effect of ticlopidine with antacids (decreased absorption). Ticlopidine may decrease the effect of digoxin, cyclosporine.

Ethanol/Nutrition/Herb Interactions

Food: Ticlopidine bioavailability may be increased (20%) if taken with food. High-fat meals increase absorption, antacids decrease absorption.

Herb/Nutraceutical: Avoid cat's claw, dong quai, evening primrose, feverfew, garlic, ginkgo, ginger, red clover, horse chestnut, green tea, ginseng (all have additional antiplatelet activity).

Mechanism of Action Ticlopidine is an inhibitor of platelet function with a mechanism which is different from other antiplatelet drugs. The drug significantly increases bleeding time. This effect may not be solely related to ticlopidine's effect on platelets. The prolongation of the bleeding time caused by ticlopidine is further increased by the addition of aspirin in *ex vivo* experiments. Although many metabolites of ticlopidine have been found, none have been shown to account for *in vivo* activity.

Pharmacodynamics/Kinetics

Onset of action: ~6 hours
    Peak effect: 3-5 days; serum levels do not correlate with clinical antiplatelet activity
Metabolism: Extensively hepatic; has at least one active metabolite
Half-life elimination: 24 hours

Usual Dosage Oral: Adults:

Stroke prevention: 250 mg twice daily with food
Coronary artery stenting (initiate after successful implantation): 250 mg twice daily with food (in combination with antiplatelet doses of aspirin) for up to 30 days

Dietary Considerations Should be taken with food to reduce stomach upset.

Administration Oral: Administer with food.

Monitoring Parameters Signs of bleeding; CBC with differential every 2 weeks starting the second week through the third month of treatment; more frequent monitoring is recommended for patients whose absolute neutrophil counts have been consistently declining or are 30% less than baseline values. The peak incidence of TTP occurs between 3-4 weeks, the peak incidence of neutropenia occurs at approximately 4-6 weeks, and the incidence of aplastic anemia peaks after 4-8 weeks of therapy. Few cases have been reported after 3 months of treatment. Liver function tests (alkaline phosphatase and transaminases) should be performed in the first 4 months of therapy if liver dysfunction is suspected.

Test Interactions ↑ cholesterol (S), ↑ alkaline phosphatase, ↑ transaminases (S)

Nursing Implications Monitor bleeding times, platelets, CBC, hemoglobin and hematocrit

Dosage Forms Tablet, as hydrochloride: 250 mg

◆ **Ticlopidine Hydrochloride** see Ticlopidine on page 1331

◆ **TIG** see Tetanus Immune Globulin (Human) on page 1304

◆ **Tigan**® see Trimethobenzamide on page 1375

◆ **Tikosyn**™ see Dofetilide on page 431

◆ **Tilade**® see Nedocromil on page 963

Tiludronate (tye LOO droe nate)

U.S. Brand Names Skelid®

Synonyms Tiludronate Disodium

Therapeutic Category Bisphosphonate Derivative

Use Treatment of Paget's disease of the bone in patients who have a level of serum alkaline phosphatase (SAP) at least twice the upper limit of normal, or who are symptomatic, or who are at risk for future complications of their disease

Pregnancy Risk Factor C

Contraindications Hypersensitivity to biphosphonates or any component of the formulation

Warnings/Precautions Not recommended in patients with severe renal impairment (Cl_{cr} <30 mL/minute). Use with caution in patients with active upper GI problems (eg, dysphagia, symptomatic esophageal diseases, gastritis, duodenitis, ulcers).

Adverse Reactions The following events occurred >2% and at a frequency > placebo:

1% to 10%:
Cardiovascular: Chest pain (2.7%), edema (2.7%)
Central nervous system: Dizziness (4.0%), paresthesia (4.0%)
Dermatologic: Rash (2.7%), skin disorder (2.7%)
Gastrointestinal: Nausea (9.3%), diarrhea (9.3%), heartburn (5.3%), vomiting (4.0%), flatulence (2.7%)
Neuromuscular & skeletal: Arthrosis (2.7%)
Ocular: cataract (2.7%), conjunctivitis (2.7%), glaucoma (2.7%)
Respiratory: Rhinitis (5.3%), sinusitis (5.3%), coughing (2.7%), pharyngitis (2.7%)
<1% (Limited to important or life-threatening): Stevens-Johnson syndrome

Overdosage/Toxicology Hypocalcemia is a potential consequence of tiludronate overdose. No specific information on overdose treatment is available. Dialysis would not be beneficial. Standard medical practices may be used to manage renal insufficiency or hypocalcemia, if signs of these occur.

Drug Interactions
Increased Effect/Toxicity: Administration of indomethacin increases bioavailability of tiludronate two- to fourfold.
Decreased Effect: Concurrent administration of calcium salts, aluminum- or magnesium-containing antacids, and aspirin markedly decrease absorption/bioavailability (by 50% to 60%) of tiludronate if given within 2 hours of a dose.

Ethanol/Nutrition/Herb Interactions Food: In single-dose studies, the bioavailability of tiludronate was reduced by 90% when an oral dose was administered with, or 2 hours after, a standard breakfast compared to the same dose administered after an overnight fast and 4 hours before a standard breakfast.

Stability Do not remove tablets from the foil strips until they are to be used

Mechanism of Action Inhibition of normal and abnormal bone resorption. Inhibits osteoclasts through at least two mechanisms: disruption of the cytoskeletal ring structure, possibly by inhibition of protein-tyrosine-phosphatase, thus leading to the detachment of osteoclasts from the bone surface area and the inhibition of the osteoclast proton pump.

Pharmacodynamics/Kinetics
Onset of action: Delayed, may require several weeks
Metabolism: Little, if any
Bioavailability: 6%; reduced by food
Time to peak, plasma: ~2 hours

Usual Dosage Tiludronate should be taken with 6-8 oz of plain water and not taken within 2 hours of food
Adults: Oral: 400 mg (2 tablets of tiludronic acid) daily for a period of 3 months; allow an interval of 3 months to assess response
Dosing adjustment in renal impairment: Cl_{cr} <30 mL/minute: **Not recommended**
Dosing adjustment in hepatic impairment: Adjustment is not necessary

Dietary Considerations Do not take within 2 hours of food.

Administration Administer as a single oral dose, take with 6-8 oz of plain water. Beverages other than plain water (including mineral water), food, and some medications (see Drug Interactions) are likely to reduce the absorption of tiludronate. Do not take within 2 hours of food. Take calcium or mineral supplements at least 2 hours before or after tiludronate. Take aluminum- or magnesium-containing antacids at least 2 hours after taking tiludronate. Do not take tiludronate within 2 hours of indomethacin.

Patient Information Take tiludronate with 6-8 oz of plain water. Do not take within 2 hours of food. Maintain adequate vitamin D and calcium intake. Do not take calcium supplements, aspirin, and indomethacin within 2 hours before or after tiludronate. Take aluminum- or magnesium-containing antacids, if needed, at least 2 hours after tiludronate.

Dosage Forms Dosage expressed in terms of tiludronic acid
Tablet, as disodium: 240 mg [tiludronic acid 200 mg]

◆ **Tiludronate Disodium** see Tiludronate on page 1333

◆ **Tim-AK (Can)** see Timolol on page 1334

♦ **Timentin**® *see* Ticarcillin and Clavulanate Potassium *on page 1330*

Timolol (TYE moe lole)

Related Information
Beta-Blockers Comparison *on page 1491*
Glaucoma Drug Therapy Comparison *on page 1499*

U.S. Brand Names Betimol®; Blocadren®; Timoptic®; Timoptic® OcuDose®; Timoptic-XE®

Canadian Brand Names Apo®-Timol; Apo®-Timop; Gen-Timolol; Novo-Timol; Nu-Timolol; Phoxal-timolol; PMS-Timolol; Tim-AK; Timoptic®; Timoptic-XE®

Synonyms Timolol Hemihydrate; Timolol Maleate

Therapeutic Category Antianginal Agent; Antihypertensive Agent; Antimigraine Agent; Beta-Adrenergic Blocker; Beta-Adrenergic Blocker, Ophthalmic

Use Ophthalmic dosage form used in treatment of elevated intraocular pressure such as glaucoma or ocular hypertension; oral dosage form used for treatment of hypertension and angina, to reduce mortality following myocardial infarction, and for prophylaxis of migraine

Pregnancy Risk Factor C (manufacturer); D (2nd and 3rd trimesters - expert analysis)

Contraindications Hypersensitivity to timolol or any component of the formulation; sinus bradycardia; sinus node dysfunction; heart block greater than first degree (except in patients with a functioning artificial pacemaker); cardiogenic shock; uncompensated cardiac failure; bronchospastic disease; pregnancy (2nd and 3rd trimesters)

Warnings/Precautions Administer cautiously in compensated heart failure and monitor for a worsening of the condition. Avoid abrupt discontinuation in patients with a history of CAD; slowly wean while monitoring for signs and symptoms of ischemia. Use caution with concurrent use of beta-blockers and either verapamil or diltiazem; bradycardia or heart block can occur. Beta-blockers can aggravate symptoms in patients with PVD. Patients with bronchospastic disease should generally not receive beta-blockers - monitor closely if used in patients with potential risk of bronchospasm. Use cautiously in diabetics because it can mask prominent hypoglycemic symptoms. Can mask signs of thyrotoxicosis. Can cause fetal harm when administered in pregnancy. Use cautiously in severe renal impairment: marked hypotension can occur in patients maintained on hemodialysis. Use care with anesthetic agents which decrease myocardial function. Can worsen myasthenia gravis. Similar reactions found with systemic administration may occur with topical administration.

Adverse Reactions
Ophthalmic:
>10%: Ocular: Conjunctival hyperemia
1% to 10%: Ocular: Anisocoria, corneal punctate keratitis, keratitis, corneal staining, decreased corneal sensitivity, eye pain, vision disturbances
<1% (Limited to important or life-threatening): Systemic allergic reaction (anaphylaxis, angioedema, rash, urticaria)

Systemic:
>10%:
Central nervous system: Drowsiness, insomnia
Endocrine & metabolic: Decreased sexual ability
1% to 10%:
Cardiovascular: Bradycardia, palpitations, edema, congestive heart failure, reduced peripheral circulation
Central nervous system: Mental depression
Gastrointestinal: Diarrhea or constipation, nausea, vomiting, stomach discomfort
Respiratory: Bronchospasm
Miscellaneous: Cold extremities
<1% (Limited to important or life-threatening): Anaphylaxis, angina, arrhythmias, orthostatic hypotension, depression, hallucinations, confusion, thrombocytopenia, leukopenia, dyspnea, nightmares, memory loss, Raynaud's phenomenon, rash, psoriasis

Overdosage/Toxicology Symptoms of intoxication include cardiac disturbances, CNS toxicity, bronchospasm, hypoglycemia, and hyperkalemia. The most common cardiac symptoms include hypotension and bradycardia. Atrioventricular block, intraventricular conduction disturbances, cardiogenic shock, and asystole may occur with severe overdose, especially with membrane-depressant drugs (eg, propranolol). CNS effects include convulsions, coma, and respiratory arrest (commonly seen with propranolol and other membrane-depressant and lipid-soluble drugs). Treatment is symptomatic for seizures, hypotension, hyperkalemia, and hypoglycemia. Bradycardia and hypotension resistant to atropine, isoproterenol or pacing may respond to glucagon. Wide QRS defects caused by membrane-depressant poisoning may respond to hypertonic sodium bicarbonate. Repeat-dose charcoal, hemoperfusion, or hemodialysis may be helpful in removal of only those beta-blockers with a small V_d, long half-life, or low intrinsic clearance (acebutolol, atenolol, nadolol, sotalol).

Drug Interactions
Cytochrome P450 Effect: CYP2D6 enzyme substrate

Increased Effect/Toxicity: The heart rate lowering effects of timolol are additive with other drugs which slow AV conduction (digoxin, verapamil, diltiazem). Reserpine increases the effects of timolol. Concurrent use of timolol may increase the effects of alpha-blockers (prazosin, terazosin), alpha-adrenergic stimulants (epinephrine, phenylephrine), and the vasoconstrictive effects of ergot alkaloids. Timolol may mask the tachycardia from hypoglycemia caused by insulin and oral hypoglycemics. In patients receiving concurrent therapy, the risk of hypertensive crisis is increased when either clonidine or the beta-blocker is withdrawn. Beta-blockers may increase the action or levels of ethanol, disopyramide, nondepolarizing muscle relaxants, and theophylline although the effects are difficult to predict.

Decreased Effect: Decreased effect of timolol with aluminum salts, barbiturates, calcium salts, cholestyramine, colestipol, NSAIDs, penicillins (ampicillin), rifampin, salicylates, and sulfinpyrazone due to decreased bioavailability and plasma levels. Beta-blockers may decrease the effect of sulfonylureas. Beta-blockers may affect the action or levels of ethanol, disopyramide, nondepolarizing muscle relaxants, and theophylline, although the effects are difficult to predict.

Mechanism of Action Blocks both beta$_1$- and beta$_2$-adrenergic receptors, reduces intraocular pressure by reducing aqueous humor production or possibly outflow; reduces blood pressure by blocking adrenergic receptors and decreasing sympathetic outflow, produces a negative chronotropic and inotropic activity through an unknown mechanism

Pharmacodynamics/Kinetics

Onset of action: Hypotensive: Oral: 15-45 minutes

Peak effect: 0.5-2.5 hours

Duration: ~4 hours; Ophthalmic: Intraocular: 24 hours

Protein binding: 60%

Metabolism: Extensively hepatic; extensive first-pass effect

Half-life elimination: 2-2.7 hours; prolonged with reduced renal function

Excretion: Urine (15% to 20% as unchanged drug)

Usual Dosage

Children and Adults: Ophthalmic:

Solution: Initial: 0.25% solution, instill 1 drop twice daily; increase to 0.5% solution if response not adequate; decrease to 1 drop/day if controlled; do not exceed 1 drop twice daily of 0.5% solution

Gel-forming solution (Timoptic-XE®): Instill 1 drop (either 0.25% or 0.5%) once daily

Adults: Oral:

Hypertension: Initial: 10 mg twice daily, increase gradually every 7 days, usual dosage: 20-40 mg/day in 2 divided doses; maximum: 60 mg/day

Prevention of myocardial infarction: 10 mg twice daily initiated within 1-4 weeks after infarction

Migraine headache: Initial: 10 mg twice daily, increase to maximum of 30 mg/day

Dietary Considerations Oral product should be administered with food at the same time each day.

Administration Administer other topically-applied ophthalmic medications at least 10 minutes before Timoptic-XE®; wash hands before use; invert closed bottle and shake once before use; remove cap carefully so that tip does not touch anything; hold bottle between thumb and index finger; use index finger of other hand to pull down the lower eyelid to form a pocket for the eye drop and tilt head back; place the dispenser tip close to the eye and gently squeeze the bottle to administer 1 drop; remove pressure after a single drop has been released; **do not allow the dispenser tip to touch the eye**; replace cap and store bottle in an upright position in a clean area; do **not** enlarge hole of dispenser; do **not** wash tip with water, soap, or any other cleaner

Monitoring Parameters Blood pressure, apical and radial pulses, fluid I & O, daily weight, respirations, mental status, and circulation in extremities before and during therapy

Patient Information Apply gentle pressure to lacrimal sac during and immediately following instillation (1 minute) to avoid systemic absorption; stop drug if breathing difficulty occurs

Nursing Implications Monitor for systemic effect of beta-blockade even when administering ophthalmic product

Dosage Forms

Gel, ophthalmic, as maleate (Timoptic-XE®): 0.25% (2.5 mL, 5 mL); 0.5% (2.5 mL, 5 mL)

Solution, ophthalmic, as hemihydrate (Betimol®): 0.25% (2.5 mL, 5 mL, 10 mL, 15 mL); 0.5% (2.5 mL, 5 mL, 10 mL, 15 mL)

Solution, ophthalmic, as maleate (Timoptic®): 0.25% (2.5 mL, 5 mL, 10 mL, 15 mL); 0.5% (2.5 mL, 5 mL, 10 mL, 15 mL)

Solution, ophthalmic, as maleate [single use] [preservative free] (Timoptic® OcuDose®): 0.25%, 0.5%

Tablet, as maleate (Blocadren®): 5 mg, 10 mg, 20 mg

♦ **Timolol and Dorzolamide** see Dorzolamide and Timolol on page 438

♦ **Timolol Hemihydrate** see Timolol on page 1334

♦ **Timolol Maleate** see Timolol on page 1334

♦ **Timoptic®** see Timolol on page 1334

♦ **Timoptic® OcuDose®** see Timolol on page 1334

♦ **Timoptic-XE®** see Timolol on page 1334

♦ **Tinactin® [OTC]** see Tolnaftate on page 1347

♦ **Tinactin® for Jock Itch [OTC]** see Tolnaftate on page 1347

♦ **Tine Test** see Tuberculin Tests on page 1386

♦ **Tine Test PPD** see Tuberculin Tests on page 1386

♦ **Ting® [OTC]** see Tolnaftate on page 1347

♦ **Tinver®** see Sodium Thiosulfate on page 1250

Tinzaparin (tin ZA pa rin)

U.S. Brand Names Innohep®

Canadian Brand Names Innohep®

Synonyms Tinzaparin Sodium

Therapeutic Category Low Molecular Weight Heparin

Use Treatment of acute symptomatic deep vein thrombosis, with or without pulmonary embolism, in conjunction with warfarin sodium

Pregnancy Risk Factor B

Pregnancy/Breast-Feeding Implications There are no adequate, well-controlled studies in pregnant women. Cases of teratogenic effects and/or fetal death have been reported (relationship to tinzaparin not established). Use during pregnancy only if clearly needed. Pregnant women, or those who become pregnant while receiving tinzaparin, should be informed of the potential risks to the fetus. It is not known if tinzaparin is excreted in human milk. Exercise caution when administering to a breast-feeding woman.

Contraindications Hypersensitivity to tinzaparin sodium, heparin, sulfites, benzyl alcohol, pork products, or any component of the formulation; active major bleeding; heparin-induced thrombocytopenia (current or history of)

(Continued)

Tinzaparin *(Continued)*

Warnings/Precautions

Patients with recent or anticipated neuraxial anesthesia (epidural or spinal anesthesia) are at risk of spinal or epidural hematoma and subsequent paralysis. Consider risk versus benefit prior to neuraxial anesthesia; risk is increased by concomitant agents that may alter hemostasis, as well as traumatic or repeated epidural or spinal puncture, and indwelling epidural catheters. Patient should be observed closely for signs and symptoms of neurological impairment. Not to be used interchangeably (unit for unit) with heparin or any other low molecular weight heparins.

Monitor patient closely for signs or symptoms of bleeding. Certain patients are at increased risk of bleeding. Risk factors include bacterial endocarditis; congenital or acquired bleeding disorders; active ulcerative or angiodysplastic GI diseases; severe uncontrolled hypertension; hemorrhagic stroke; use shortly after brain, spinal, or ophthalmologic surgery; patients treated concomitantly with platelet inhibitors; recent GI bleeding; thrombocytopenia or platelet defects; severe liver disease; hypertensive or diabetic retinopathy; or in patients undergoing invasive procedures.

Safety and efficacy in pediatric patients has not been established. Use with caution in the elderly (delayed elimination may occur). Patients with severe renal impairment may show reduced elimination of tinzaparin

Heparin can cause hyperkalemia by affecting aldosterone; similar reactions could occur with LMWHs. Monitor for hyperkalemia. Discontinue therapy if platelets are <100,000/mm^3. For subcutaneous injection only, do not mix with other injections or infusions. Clinical experience is limited in patients with BMI >40 kg.

Adverse Reactions As with all anticoagulants, bleeding is the major adverse effect of tinzaparin. Hemorrhage may occur at virtually any site. Risk is dependent on multiple variables.

>10%:
Hepatic: Increased ALT (13%)
Local: Injection site hematoma (16%)

1% to 10%:
Cardiovascular: Angina pectoris, chest pain (2%), hypertension, hypotension, tachycardia
Central nervous system: Confusion, dizziness, fever (2%), headache (2%), insomnia, pain (2%)
Dermatologic: Bullous eruption, pruritus, rash (1%), skin disorder
Gastrointestinal: Constipation (1%), dyspepsia, flatulence, nausea (2%), nonspecified gastrointestinal disorder, vomiting (1%)
Genitourinary: Dysuria, urinary retention, urinary tract infection (4%)
Hematologic: Anemia, hematoma, hemorrhage (2%), thrombocytopenia (1%)
Hepatic: Increased AST (9%)
Local: Deep vein thrombosis, injection site hematoma
Neuromuscular & skeletal: Back pain (2%)
Renal: Hematuria (1%)
Respiratory: Dyspnea (1%), epistaxis (2%), pneumonia, pulmonary embolism (2%), respiratory disorder
Miscellaneous: Impaired healing, infection, unclassified reactions

<1% (Limited to important or life-threatening): Agranulocytosis, allergic purpura, allergic reaction, angioedema, arrhythmia, cholestatic hepatitis, epidermal necrolysis, gastrointestinal hemorrhage, granulocytopenia, hemarthrosis, hematoma, hemoptysis, intracranial hemorrhage, ischemic necrosis, major bleeding, myocardial infarction, ocular hemorrhage, pancytopenia, priapism, purpura, rash, retroperitoneal/intra-abdominal bleeding, severe thrombocytopenia, skin necrosis, spinal epidural hematoma, Stevens-Johnson syndrome, urticaria, vaginal hemorrhage

Case reports: The following adverse effects have been reported in infants of women receiving tinzaparin during pregnancy (relationship has not been established): Cleft palate (one report), optic nerve hypoplasia (one report), trisomy 21 (one report), fetal death/miscarriage, fetal distress, neonatal hypotonia, cutis aplasia of the scalp

Overdosage/Toxicology Overdose may lead to bleeding; bleeding may occur at any site. In case of overdose, discontinue medication, apply pressure to the bleeding site if possible, and replace volume and hemostatic blood elements as required. If these measures are ineffective, or if bleeding is severe, protamine sulfate may be administered by slow infusion at 1 mg per every 100 anti-Xa int. units of tinzaparin administered. However, protamine does not completely neutralize tinzaparin anti-Xa activity.

Drug Interactions

Increased Effect/Toxicity: Drugs which affect platelet function (eg, aspirin, NSAIDs, dipyridamole, ticlopidine, clopidogrel, sulfinpyrazone, dextran) may potentiate the risk of hemorrhage. Thrombolytic agents increase the risk of hemorrhage.

Warfarin: Risk of bleeding may be increased during concurrent therapy. Tinzaparin is commonly continued during the initiation of warfarin therapy to assure anticoagulation and to protect against possible transient hypercoagulability

Stability Store at 25°C (77°F); excursions permitted to 15°C to 30°C (59°F to 86°F)

Mechanism of Action Standard heparin consists of components with molecular weights ranging from 4000-30,000 daltons with a mean of 16,000 daltons. Heparin acts as an anticoagulant by enhancing the inhibition rate of clotting proteases by antithrombin III, impairing normal hemostasis and inhibition of factor Xa. Low molecular weight heparins have a small effect on the activated partial thromboplastin time and strongly inhibit factor Xa. The primary inhibitory activity of tinzaparin is through antithrombin. Tinzaparin is derived from porcine heparin that undergoes controlled enzymatic depolymerization. The average molecular weight of tinzaparin ranges between 5500 and 7500 daltons which is distributed as (<10%) 2000 daltons (60% to 72%) 2000-8000 daltons, and (22% to 36%) >8000 daltons. The antifactor Xa activity is approximately 100 int. units/mg.

Pharmacodynamics/Kinetics

Onset of action: 2-3 hours
Distribution: 3-5 L

Half-life elimination: 3-4 hours
Metabolism: Partially metabolized by desulphation and depolymerization
Bioavailability: 87%
Time to peak: 4-5 hours
Excretion: Urine

Usual Dosage S.C.:

Adults: 175 anti-Xa int. units/kg of body weight once daily. Warfarin sodium should be started when appropriate. Administer tinzaparin for at least 6 days and until patient is adequately anticoagulated with warfarin.

Note: To calculate the volume of solution to administer per dose: Volume to be administered (mL) = patient weight (kg) x 0.00875 mL/kg (may be rounded off to the nearest 0.05 mL)

Elderly: No significant differences in safety or response were seen when used in patients ≥65 years of age. However, increased sensitivity to tinzaparin in elderly patients may be possible due to a decline in renal function.

Dosage adjustment in renal impairment: Patients with severe renal impairment had a 24% decrease in clearance, use with caution.

Dosage adjustment in hepatic impairment: No specific dosage adjustment has been recommended.

Administration Patient should be lying down or sitting. Administer by deep S.C. injection, alternating between the left and right anterolateral and left and right posterolateral abdominal wall. Vary site daily. The entire needle should be introduced into the skin fold formed by the thumb and forefinger. Hold the skin fold until injection is complete. To minimize bruising, do not rub the injection site.

Monitoring Parameters CBC including platelet count and hematocrit or hemoglobin, and stool for occult blood; the monitoring of PT and/or aPTT is not necessary. Patients receiving both warfarin and tinzaparin should have their INR drawn just prior to the next scheduled dose of tinzaparin.

Test Interactions Asymptomatic increases in AST (SGOT) (8.8%) and ALT (SGPT) (13%) have been reported. Elevations were >3 times the upper limit of normal and were reversible and rarely associated with increases in bilirubin.

Patient Information This drug can only be administered by S.C. injection. You may have a tendency to bleed easily while taking this drug; brush teeth with soft brush; floss with waxed floss; use electric razor; avoid scissors or sharp knives and potentially harmful activities. Report chest pain; persistent constipation; persistent erection; unusual bleeding or bruising (bleeding gums, nosebleed, blood in urine, dark stool); pain in joints or back; or numbness, tingling, weakness, or pain at injection site.

Nursing Implications Patient should be lying down or sitting. Administer by deep S.C. injection, alternating between the left and right anterolateral and left and right posterolateral abdominal wall. Vary site daily. The entire needle should be introduced into the skin fold formed by the thumb and forefinger. Hold the skin fold until injection is complete. To minimize bruising, do not rub the injection site.

Additional Information Contains sodium metabisulfite and benzyl alcohol, 10 mg/mL

Dosage Forms Injection: 20,000 anti-Xa int. units/mL (2 mL vial)

♦ **Tinzaparin Sodium** *see* Tinzaparin *on page 1335*

Tioconazole (tye oh KONE a zole)

Related Information
Treatment of Sexually Transmitted Diseases *on page 1609*
U.S. Brand Names 1-Day™ [OTC]; Vagistat®-1 [OTC]
Canadian Brand Names GyneCure™; Trosyd™ AF; Trosyd™ J
Therapeutic Category Antifungal Agent, Imidazole Derivative; Antifungal Agent, Vaginal
Use Local treatment of vulvovaginal candidiasis
Pregnancy Risk Factor C
Contraindications Hypersensitivity to tioconazole or any component of the formulation
Warnings/Precautions For vaginal use only. Petrolatum-based vaginal products may damage rubber or latex condoms or diaphragms. Separate use by 3 days.
Adverse Reactions Frequency not defined.
Central nervous system: Headache
Gastrointestinal: Abdominal pain
Dermatologic: Burning, desquamation
Genitourinary: Discharge, dyspareunia, dysuria, irritation, itching, nocturia, vaginal pain, vaginitis, vulvar swelling
Stability Store at room temperature.
Mechanism of Action A 1-substituted imidazole derivative with a broad antifungal spectrum against a wide variety of dermatophytes and yeasts, including *Trichophyton mentagrophytes*, *T. rubrum*, *T. erinacei*, *T. tonsurans*, *Microsporum canis*, *Microsporum gypseum*, and *Candida albicans*. Both agents appear to be similarly effective against *Epidermophyton floccosum*.
Pharmacodynamics/Kinetics
Absorption: Intravaginal: Systemic (small amounts)
Distribution: Vaginal fluid: 24-72 hours
Elimination: Urine and feces
Usual Dosage Adults: Vaginal: Insert 1 applicatorful in vagina, just prior to bedtime, as a single dose
Patient Information Insert high into vagina; contact physician if itching or burning continues; May interact with condoms and vaginal contraceptive diaphragms (ie, weaken latex); do not rely on these products for 3 days following treatment
Nursing Implications Insert high into vagina; contact physician if itching or burning continues
Dosage Forms Ointment, vaginal: 6.5% with applicator (4.6 g)

♦ **Tioguanine** *see* Thioguanine *on page 1318*
♦ **Tiotixene** *see* Thiothixene *on page 1324*

Tirofiban (tye roe FYE ban)

Related Information

Glycoprotein Antagonists *on page 1500*

U.S. Brand Names Aggrastat®

Canadian Brand Names Aggrastat®

Synonyms MK383; Tirofiban Hydrochloride

Therapeutic Category Antiplatelet Agent; Glycoprotein IIb/IIIa Inhibitor; Platelet Aggregation Inhibitor

Use In combination with heparin, is indicated for the treatment of acute coronary syndrome, including patients who are to be managed medically and those undergoing PTCA or atherectomy. In this setting, it has been shown to decrease the rate of a combined endpoint of death, new myocardial infarction or refractory ischemia/repeat cardiac procedure.

Pregnancy Risk Factor B

Contraindications Hypersensitivity to tirofiban or any component of the formulation; active internal bleeding or a history of bleeding diathesis within the previous 30 days; history of intracranial hemorrhage, intracranial neoplasm, arteriovenous malformation, or aneurysm; history of thrombocytopenia following prior exposure; history of CVA within 30 days or any history of hemorrhagic stroke; major surgical procedure or severe physical trauma within the previous month; history, symptoms, or findings suggestive of aortic dissection; severe hypertension (systolic BP >180 mm Hg and/or diastolic BP >1110 mm Hg); concomitant use of another parenteral GP IIb/IIIa inhibitor; acute pericarditis

Warnings/Precautions Bleeding is the most common complication encountered during this therapy; most major bleeding occurs at the arterial access site for cardiac catheterization. Caution in patients with platelets <150,000/mm^3; patients with hemorrhagic retinopathy; chronic dialysis patients; when used in combination with other drugs impacting on coagulation. To minimize bleeding complications, care must be taken in sheath insertion/removal. Sheath hemostasis should be achieved at least 4 hours before hospital discharge. Other trauma and vascular punctures should be minimized. Avoid obtaining vascular access through a noncompressible site (eg, subclavian or jugular vein). Patients with severe renal insufficiency require dosage reduction. Do not administer in the same I.V. line as diazepam.

Adverse Reactions Bleeding is the major drug-related adverse effect. Patients received background treatment with aspirin and heparin. Major bleeding was reported in 1.4% to 2.2%; minor bleeding in 10.5% to 12%; transfusion was required in 4.0% to 4.3%.

>1% (nonbleeding adverse events):
Cardiovascular: Bradycardia (4%), coronary artery dissection (5%), edema (2%)
Central nervous system: Dizziness (3%), fever (>1%), headache (>1%), vasovagal reaction (2%)
Gastrointestinal: Nausea (>1%)
Genitourinary: Pelvic pain (6%)
Hematologic: Thrombocytopenia: <90,000/mm^3 (1.5%), <50,000/mm^3 (0.3%)
Neuromuscular & skeletal: Leg pain (3%)
Miscellaneous: Diaphoresis (2%)

<1% (Limited to important or life-threatening): Acutely decreased platelets in association with fever, anaphylaxis, GI bleeding (0.1% to 0.2%), GU bleeding (0.0% to 0.1%), hemopericardium, intracranial bleeding (0.0% to 0.1%), pulmonary alveolar hemorrhage, rash, retroperitoneal bleeding (0.0% to 0.6%), severe (<10,000/mm^3) thrombocytopenia (rare) urticaria

Overdosage/Toxicology The most frequent manifestation of overdose is bleeding. Treatment is cessation of therapy and assessment of transfusion. Tirofiban has a relatively short half-life and its platelet effects dissipate rather quickly. However, when immediate reversal is required, platelet transfusions can be useful. Tirofiban is dialyzable.

Tirofiban Dosing
(Using 50 mcg/mL Concentration)

Patient Weight (kg)	Patients With Normal Renal Function		Patients With Renal Dysfunction	
	30-Min Loading Infusion Rate (mL/h)	Maintenance Infusion Rate (mL/h)	30-Min Loading Infusion Rate (mL/h)	Maintenance Infusion Rate (mL/h)
30-37	16	4	8	2
38-45	20	5	10	3
46-54	24	6	12	3
55-62	28	7	14	4
63-70	32	8	16	4
71-79	36	9	18	5
80-87	40	10	20	5
88-95	44	11	22	6
96-104	48	12	24	6
105-112	52	13	26	7
113-120	56	14	28	7
121-128	60	15	30	8
128-137	64	16	32	8
138-145	68	17	34	9
146-153	72	18	36	9

Drug Interactions

Increased Effect/Toxicity: Use of tirofiban with aspirin and heparin is associated with an increase in bleeding over aspirin and heparin alone; however, efficacy of tirofiban is improved. Risk of bleeding is increased when used with thrombolytics, oral anticoagulants, nonsteroidal anti-inflammatory drugs, dipyridamole, ticlopidine, and clopidogrel. Avoid concomitant use of other IIb/IIIa antagonists. Cephalosporins which contain the MTT side chain may theoretically increase the risk of hemorrhage.

Decreased Effect: Levothyroxine and omeprazole decrease tirofiban levels; however, the clinical significance of this interaction remains to be demonstrated.

Stability Store at 25°C (77°F); do not freeze. Protect from light during storage. Not compatible with diazepam.

Mechanism of Action A reversible antagonist of fibrinogen binding to the GP IIb/IIIa receptor, the major platelet surface receptor involved in platelet aggregation. When administered intravenously, it inhibits *ex vivo* platelet aggregation in a dose- and concentration-dependent manner. When given according to the recommended regimen, >90% inhibition is attained by the end of the 30-minute infusion. Platelet aggregation inhibition is reversible following cessation of the infusion.

Pharmacodynamics/Kinetics
Distribution: 35% unbound
Metabolism: Minimal
Half-life elimination: 2 hours
Excretion: Urine (65%) and feces (25%) primarily as unchanged drug
Clearance: Elderly: Reduced by 19% to 26%

Usual Dosage Adults: I.V.: Initial rate of 0.4 mcg/kg/minute for 30 minutes and then continued at 0.1 mcg/kg/minute; dosing should be continued through angiography and for 12-24 hours after angioplasty or atherectomy. See table on previous page.

Dosing adjustment in severe renal impairment: Cl_{cr} <30 mL/minute: Reduce dose to 50% of normal rate.

Administration Intended for intravenous delivery using sterile equipment and technique. Do not add other drugs or remove solution directly from the bag with a syringe. Do not use plastic containers in series connections; such use can result in air embolism by drawing air from the first container if it is empty of solution. Discard unused solution 24 hours following the start of infusion. May be administered through the same catheter as heparin. Tirofiban injection must be diluted to a concentration of 50 mcg/mL (premixed solution does not require dilution). Infuse over 30 minutes.

Monitoring Parameters Platelet count. Hemoglobin and hematocrit should be monitored prior to treatment, within 6 hours following loading infusion, and at least daily thereafter during therapy. Platelet count may need to be monitored earlier in patients who received prior glycoprotein IIb/IIIa antagonists. Persistent reductions of platelet counts <90,000/mm³ may require interruption or discontinuation of infusion. Because tirofiban requires concurrent heparin therapy, aPTT levels should also be followed. Monitor vital signs and laboratory results prior to, during, and after therapy. Assess infusion insertion site during and after therapy (every 15 minutes or as institutional policy). Observe and teach patient bleeding precautions (avoid invasive procedures and activities that could result in injury). Monitor closely for signs of unusual or excessive bleeding (eg, CNS changes, blood in urine, stool, or vomitus, unusual bruising or bleeding). Breast-feeding is contraindicated.

Dosage Forms
Injection [premixed] 50 mcg/mL (500 mL)
Injection for solution: 250 mcg/mL (50 mL)

♦ **Tirofiban Hydrochloride** *see* Tirofiban *on page 1338*
♦ **Tisit® [OTC]** *see* Pyrethrins and Piperonyl Butoxide *on page 1160*
♦ **Tisit® Blue Gel [OTC]** *see* Pyrethrins and Piperonyl Butoxide *on page 1160*
♦ **Ti-U-Lac® H (Can)** *see* Urea and Hydrocortisone *on page 1391*

Tizanidine (tye ZAN i deen)

U.S. Brand Names Zanaflex®
Canadian Brand Names Zanaflex®
Synonyms Sirdalud®
Therapeutic Category Alpha$_2$-Adrenergic Agonist Agent
Use Skeletal muscle relaxant used for treatment of muscle spasticity
Unlabeled/Investigational Use Tension headaches, low back pain, and trigeminal neuralgia
Pregnancy Risk Factor C
Contraindications Hypersensitivity to tizanidine or any component of the formulation
Warnings/Precautions Reduce dose in patients with liver or renal disease; use with caution in patients with hypotension or cardiac disease. Tizanidine clearance is reduced by more than 50% in elderly patients with renal insufficiency (Cl_{cr} <25 mL/minute) compared to healthy elderly subjects; this may lead to a longer duration of effects and, therefore, should be used with caution in renally impaired patients.

Adverse Reactions
>10%:
Cardiovascular: Hypotension
Central nervous system: Sedation, daytime drowsiness, somnolence
Gastrointestinal: Xerostomia
1% to 10%:
Cardiovascular: Bradycardia, syncope
Central nervous system: Fatigue, dizziness, anxiety, nervousness, insomnia
Dermatologic: Pruritus, skin rash
Gastrointestinal: Nausea, vomiting, dyspepsia, constipation, diarrhea
Hepatic: Elevation of liver enzymes
Neuromuscular & skeletal: Muscle weakness, tremor
<1% (Limited to important or life-threatening): Delusions, hepatic failure, palpitations, psychotic-like symptoms, ventricular extrasystoles, visual hallucinations

Overdosage/Toxicology Symptoms include dry mouth, bradycardia, and hypotension. Lavage (within 2 hours of ingestion) with activated charcoal; benzodiazepines for seizure control. Atropine can be given for treatment of bradycardia. Flumazenil has been used to (Continued)

Tizanidine *(Continued)*

reverse coma successfully. Forced diuresis is not helpful. Multiple dosing of activated charcoal may be helpful. Following attempts to enhance drug elimination, hypotension should be treated with I.V. fluids and/or Trendelenburg positioning.

Drug Interactions
Increased Effect/Toxicity:
Increased effect: Oral contraceptives

Increased toxicity: Additive hypotensive effects may be seen with diuretics, other alpha adrenergic agonists, or antihypertensives; CNS depression with alcohol, baclofen or other CNS depressants

Ethanol/Nutrition/Herb Interactions
Ethanol: Avoid ethanol (may increase CNS depression).

Food: Increases maximum concentration of tizanidine by 33% and reduces the time to peak by 40 minutes; extent of absorption is unchanged.

Herb/Nutraceutical: Avoid valerian, St John's wort, kava kava, gotu kola (may increase CNS depression).

Mechanism of Action An alpha$_2$-adrenergic agonist agent which decreases excitatory input to alpha motor neurons; an imidazole derivative chemically-related to clonidine, which acts as a centrally acting muscle relaxant with alpha$_2$-adrenergic agonist properties; acts on the level of the spinal cord

Pharmacodynamics/Kinetics
Duration: 3-6 hours

Bioavailability: 40%

Half-life elimination: 2.5 hours

Time to peak, serum: 1-5 hours

Usual Dosage
Adults: 2-4 mg 3 times/day

Usual initial dose: 4 mg, may increase by 2-4 mg as needed for satisfactory reduction of muscle tone every 6-8 hours to a maximum of three doses in any 24 hour period

Maximum dose: 36 mg/day

Dosing adjustment in renal/hepatic impairment: May require dose reductions or less frequent dosing

Monitoring Parameters Monitor liver function (aminotransferases) at baseline, 1, 3, 6 months and then periodically thereafter; monitor ophthalmic function

Dosage Forms Tablet: 2 mg, 4 mg

♦ **TMP** *see* Trimethoprim *on page 1376*

♦ **TMP-SMZ** *see* Sulfamethoxazole and Trimethoprim *on page 1273*

♦ **TNKase™** *see* Tenecteplase *on page 1294*

♦ **TOBI™** *see* Tobramycin *on page 1340*

♦ **TobraDex®** *see* Tobramycin and Dexamethasone *on page 1342*

Tobramycin *(toe bra MYE sin)*

Related Information
Aminoglycoside Dosing and Monitoring *on page 1470*

Antimicrobial Drugs of Choice *on page 1588*

Prevention of Wound Infection & Sepsis in Surgical Patients *on page 1569*

U.S. Brand Names AKTob®; Nebcin®; TOBI™; Tobrex®

Canadian Brand Names Nebcin®; PMS-Tobramycin; TOBI®; Tobrex®; Tomycine™

Synonyms Tobramycin Sulfate

Therapeutic Category Antibiotic, Aminoglycoside; Antibiotic, Ophthalmic

Use Treatment of documented or suspected infections caused by susceptible gram-negative bacilli including *Pseudomonas aeruginosa*; topically used to treat superficial ophthalmic infections caused by susceptible bacteria. Tobramycin solution for inhalation is indicated for the management of cystic fibrosis patients (>6 years of age) with *Pseudomonas aeruginosa*.

Pregnancy Risk Factor C

Contraindications Hypersensitivity to tobramycin, other aminoglycosides, or any component of the formulation

Warnings/Precautions Use with caution in patients with renal impairment; pre-existing auditory or vestibular impairment; and in patients with neuromuscular disorders; dosage modification required in patients with impaired renal function; (I.M. & I.V.) Aminoglycosides are associated with significant nephrotoxicity or ototoxicity; the ototoxicity is directly proportional to the amount of drug given and the duration of treatment; tinnitus or vertigo are indications of vestibular injury; ototoxicity is often irreversible; renal damage is usually reversible

Adverse Reactions
1% to 10%:

Neuromuscular & skeletal: Neurotoxicity (neuromuscular blockade)

Otic: Ototoxicity (auditory), ototoxicity (vestibular)

Renal: Nephrotoxicity

<1% (Limited to important or life-threatening): Anemia, dyspnea, eosinophilia

Overdosage/Toxicology Symptoms include ototoxicity, nephrotoxicity, and neuromuscular toxicity. The treatment of choice following a single acute overdose appears to be the maintenance of urine output of at least 3 mL/kg/hour. Dialysis is of questionable value in the enhancement of aminoglycoside elimination. If required, hemodialysis is preferred over peritoneal dialysis in patients with normal renal function. Careful hydration may be all that is required to promote diuresis and therefore enhance elimination.

Drug Interactions
Increased Effect/Toxicity: Increased antimicrobial effect of tobramycin with extended spectrum penicillins (synergistic). Neuromuscular blockers may have an increased duration of action (neuromuscular blockade). Amphotericin B, cephalosporins, and loop diuretics may increase the risk of nephrotoxicity.

Stability

Tobramycin is stable at room temperature both as the clear, colorless solution and as the dry powder; reconstituted solutions remain stable for 24 hours at room temperature and 96 hours when refrigerated

Stability of parenteral admixture at room temperature (25°C) and at refrigeration temperature (4°C): 48 hours

Standard diluent: Dose/100 mL NS

Minimum volume: 50 mL NS

Incompatible with penicillins

Mechanism of Action Interferes with bacterial protein synthesis by binding to 30S and 50S ribosomal subunits resulting in a defective bacterial cell membrane

Pharmacodynamics/Kinetics

Absorption: I.M.: Rapid and complete

Distribution: V_d: 0.2-0.3 L/kg; Pediatrics: 0.2-0.7 L/kg; to extracellular fluid including serum, abscesses, ascitic, pericardial, pleural, synovial, lymphatic, and peritoneal fluids; crosses placenta; poor penetration into CSF, eye, bone, prostate

Protein binding: <30%

Half-life elimination:

Neonates: ≤1200 g: 11 hours; >1200 g: 2-9 hours

Adults: 2-3 hours; directly dependent upon glomerular filtration rate

Adults with impaired renal function: 5-70 hours

Time to peak, serum: I.M.: 30-60 minutes; I.V.: ~30 minutes

Excretion: Normal renal function: Urine (~90% to 95%) within 24 hours

Usual Dosage Individualization is critical because of the low therapeutic index

Use of ideal body weight (IBW) for determining the mg/kg/dose appears to be more accurate than dosing on the basis of total body weight (TBW)

In morbid obesity, dosage requirement may best be estimated using a dosing weight of IBW + 0.4 (TBW - IBW)

Initial and periodic peak and trough plasma drug levels should be determined, particularly in critically ill patients with serious infections or in disease states known to significantly alter aminoglycoside pharmacokinetics (eg, cystic fibrosis, burns, or major surgery). Two to three serum level measurements should be obtained after the initial dose to measure the half-life in order to determine the frequency of subsequent doses.

Once daily dosing: Higher peak serum drug concentration to MIC ratios, demonstrated aminoglycoside postantibiotic effect, decreased renal cortex drug uptake, and improved cost-time efficiency are supportive reasons for the use of once daily dosing regimens for aminoglycosides. Current research indicates these regimens to be as effective for nonlife-threatening infections, with no higher incidence of nephrotoxicity, than those requiring multiple daily doses. Doses are determined by calculating the entire day's dose via usual multiple dose calculation techniques and administering this quantity as a single dose. Doses are then adjusted to maintain mean serum concentrations above the MIC(s) of the causative organism(s). (Example: 2.5-5 mg/kg as a single dose; expected Cp_{max}: 10-20 mcg/mL and Cp_{min}: <1 mcg/mL). Further research is needed for universal recommendation in all patient populations and gram-negative disease; exceptions may include those with known high clearance (eg, children, patients with cystic fibrosis, or burns who may require shorter dosage intervals) and patients with renal function impairment for whom longer than conventional dosage intervals are usually required.

Some clinicians suggest a daily dose of 4-7 mg/kg for all patients with normal renal function. This dose is at least as efficacious with similar, if not less, toxicity than conventional dosing; see "Aminoglycoside Dosing and Monitoring" *on page 1470* in the Appendix

Infants and Children <5 years: I.M., I.V.: 2.5 mg/kg/dose every 8 hours

Children >5 years: 1.5-2.5 mg/kg/dose every 8 hours

Note: Some patients may require larger or more frequent doses if serum levels document the need (ie, cystic fibrosis or febrile granulocytopenic patients).

Adults: I.M., I.V.:

Severe life-threatening infections: 2-2.5 mg/kg/dose

Urinary tract infection: 1.5 mg/kg/dose

Synergy (for gram-positive infections): 1 mg/kg/dose

Children and Adults: Ophthalmic: Instill 1-2 drops of solution every 4 hours; apply ointment 2-3 times/day; for severe infections apply ointment every 3-4 hours, or solution 2 drops every 30-60 minutes initially, then reduce to less frequent intervals

Inhalation:

Standard aerosolized tobramycin:

Children: 40-80 mg 2-3 times/day

Adults: 60-80 mg 3 times/day

High-dose regimen: Children ≥6 years and Adults: 300 mg every 12 hours (do not administer doses less than 6 hours apart); administer in repeated cycles of 28 days on drug followed by 28 days off drug

Dosing interval in renal impairment:

Cl_{cr} ≥60 mL/minute: Administer every 8 hours

Cl_{cr} 40-60 mL/minute: Administer every 12 hours

Cl_{cr} 20-40 mL/minute: Administer every 24 hours

Cl_{cr} 10-20 mL/minute: Administer every 48 hours

Cl_{cr} <10 mL/minute: Administer every 72 hours

Hemodialysis: Dialyzable; 30% removal of aminoglycosides occurs during 4 hours of HD - administer dose after dialysis and follow levels

Continuous arteriovenous or venovenous hemofiltration: Dose as for Cl_{cr} of 10-40 mL/minute and follow levels

Administration in CAPD fluid:

Gram-negative infection: 4-8 mg/L (4-8 mcg/mL) of CAPD fluid

Gram-positive infection (ie, synergy): 3-4 mg/L (3-4 mcg/mL) of CAPD fluid

Administration IVPB/I.M.: Dose as for Cl_{cr} <10 mL/minute and follow levels

(Continued)

Tobramycin (Continued)

Dosing adjustment/comments in hepatic disease: Monitor plasma concentrations

Dietary Considerations May require supplementation of calcium, magnesium, potassium.

Monitoring Parameters Urinalysis, urine output, BUN, serum creatinine, peak and trough plasma tobramycin levels; be alert to ototoxicity; hearing should be tested before and during treatment

Reference Range

Timing of serum samples: Draw peak 30 minutes after 30-minute infusion has been completed or 1 hour following I.M. injection or beginning of infusion; draw trough immediately before next dose

Therapeutic levels:

Peak:

Serious infections: 6-8 µg/mL (SI: 12-17 mg/L)

Life-threatening infections: 8-10 µg/mL (SI: 17-21 mg/L)

Urinary tract infections: 4-6 µg/mL (SI: 7-12 mg/L)

Synergy against gram-positive organisms: 3-5 µg/mL

Trough:

Serious infections: 0.5-1 µg/mL

Life-threatening infections: 1-2 µg/mL

Monitor serum creatinine and urine output; obtain drug levels after the third dose unless otherwise directed

Patient Information Report symptoms of superinfection; for eye drops - no other eye drops 5-10 minutes before or after tobramycin; report any dizziness or sensations of ringing or fullness in ears

Nursing Implications

Eye solutions: Allow 5 minutes between application of "multiple-drop" therapy

I.M., I.V.: Obtain drug levels after the third dose; peak levels are drawn 30 minutes after the end of a 30-minute infusion or 1 hour after initiation of infusion or I.M. injection; the trough is drawn just before the next dose. Separate administration of extended-spectrum penicillins (eg, carbenicillin, ticarcillin, piperacillin) from tobramycin in patients with severe renal impairment; tobramycin's efficacy may be reduced if given concurrently.

Dosage Forms

Injection, as sulfate (Nebcin®): 10 mg/mL (2 mL, 6 mL, 8 mL); 40 mg/mL (1 mL, 2 mL, 30 mL, 50 mL)

Ointment, ophthalmic (Tobrex®): 0.3% (3.5 g)

Powder for injection (Nebcin®): 40 mg/mL (1.2 g vials)

Solution for nebulization (TOBI™): 60 mg/mL (5 mL)

Solution, ophthalmic: 0.3% (5 mL)

AKTob®, Tobrex®: 0.3% (5 mL)

Tobramycin and Dexamethasone (toe bra MYE sin & deks a METH a sone)

U.S. Brand Names TobraDex®

Canadian Brand Names Tobradex®

Synonyms Dexamethasone and Tobramycin

Therapeutic Category Antibiotic, Ophthalmic; Corticosteroid, Ophthalmic

Use Treatment of external ocular infection caused by susceptible gram-negative bacteria and steroid responsive inflammatory conditions of the palpebral and bulbar conjunctiva, lid, cornea, and anterior segment of the globe

Pregnancy Risk Factor B

Usual Dosage Children and Adults: Ophthalmic: Instill 1-2 drops of solution every 4 hours; apply ointment 2-3 times/day; for severe infections apply ointment every 3-4 hours, or solution 2 drops every 30-60 minutes initially, then reduce to less frequent intervals

Additional Information Complete prescribing information for this medication should be consulted for additional detail.

Dosage Forms

Ointment, ophthalmic: Tobramycin 0.3% and dexamethasone 0.1% (3.5 g)

Suspension, ophthalmic: Tobramycin 0.3% and dexamethasone 0.1% (2.5 mL, 5 mL)

♦ **Tobramycin Sulfate** see Tobramycin on page 1340

♦ **Tobrex®** see Tobramycin on page 1340

Tocainide (toe KAY nide)

Related Information

Antiarrhythmic Drugs Comparison on page 1478

U.S. Brand Names Tonocard®

Canadian Brand Names Tonocard®

Synonyms Tocainide Hydrochloride

Therapeutic Category Antiarrhythmic Agent, Class I-B

Use Suppression and prevention of symptomatic life-threatening ventricular arrhythmias

Unlabeled/Investigational Use Trigeminal neuralgia

Pregnancy Risk Factor C

Contraindications Hypersensitivity to tocainide, any component of the formulation, or any local anesthetics of the amide type; second- or third-degree heart block (except in patients with a functioning artificial pacemaker)

Warnings/Precautions May exacerbate some arrhythmias (ie, atrial fibrillation/flutter); use with caution in CHF patients; administer with caution in patients with pre-existing bone marrow failure, cytopenia, severe renal or hepatic disease; bone marrow depression can rarely occur during the first 3 months of therapy

Adverse Reactions

>10%:

Central nervous system: Dizziness (8% to 15%)

Gastrointestinal: Nausea (14% to 15%)

1% to 10%:
  Cardiovascular: Tachycardia (3%), bradycardia/angina/palpitations (0.5% to 1.8%), hypotension (3%)
  Central nervous system: Nervousness (0.5% to 1.5%), confusion (2% to 3%), headache (4.6%), anxiety, incoordination, giddiness, vertigo
  Dermatologic: Rash (0.5% to 8.4%)
  Gastrointestinal: Vomiting (4.5%), diarrhea (4% to 5%), anorexia (1% to 2%), loss of taste
  Neuromuscular & skeletal: Paresthesia (3.5% to 9%), tremor (dose-related: 2.9% to 8.4%), ataxia (dose-related: 2.9% to 8.4%), hot and cold sensations
  Ocular: Blurred vision (~1.5%), nystagmus (1%)
<1% (Limited to important or life-threatening): Alopecia, angina, AV block, cardiomegaly, cinchonism, coma, convulsions, delirium, depression, diplopia, dysarthria, dysphagia, dyspnea, erythema multiforme, exfoliative dermatitis, fibrosing alveolitis, granulomatous hepatitis, hallucinations, hepatitis, hypersensitivity reactions, immune complex glomerulonephritis, increased ANA, increased QRS duration, interstitial pneumonitis, jaundice, local anesthesia, myasthenia gravis, orthostatic hypotension, pancreatitis, pericarditis, prolonged QT interval, psychic disturbances, psychosis, pulmonary edema, pulmonary fibrosis, respiratory arrest, right bundle branch block, sinoatrial block, sinus arrest, Stevens-Johnson syndrome, syncope, urinary retention, urticaria, vasculitis, vasovagal episodes, xerostomia

Note: Rare, potentially severe hematologic reactions, have occurred (generally within the first 12 weeks of therapy). These may include agranulocytosis, bone marrow depression, aplastic anemia, hypoplastic anemia, hemolytic anemia, anemia, leukopenia, neutropenia, thrombocytopenia, and eosinophilia.

Overdosage/Toxicology Has a narrow therapeutic index. Severe toxicity may occur slightly above the therapeutic range, especially with other antiarrhythmic drugs. Acute ingestion of twice the daily therapeutic dose is potentially life-threatening. Symptoms include sedation, confusion, coma, seizures, respiratory arrest, and cardiac toxicity (sinus arrest, A-V block, asystole, and hypotension). The QRS and QT intervals are usually normal, although they may be prolonged after massive overdose. Other effects include dizziness, paresthesias, tremor, ataxia, and GI disturbance. Treatment is supportive using conventional therapies (fluids, positioning, vasopressors, antiarrhythmics, anticonvulsants). Sodium bicarbonate may reverse QRS prolongation (if present), bradyarrhythmias, and hypotension. Enhanced elimination with dialysis, hemoperfusion, or repeat charcoal is not effective.

Drug Interactions
  Increased Effect/Toxicity: Tocainide may increase serum levels of caffeine and theophylline.
  Decreased Effect: Decreased tocainide plasma levels with cimetidine, phenobarbital, phenytoin, rifampin, and other hepatic enzyme inducers.

Stability Store at 25°C (77°F); excursions permitted to 15°C to 30°C (59°F to 86°F)

Mechanism of Action Class 1B antiarrhythmic agent; suppresses automaticity of conduction tissue, by increasing electrical stimulation threshold of ventricle, HIS-Purkinje system, and spontaneous depolarization of the ventricles during diastole by a direct action on the tissues; blocks both the initiation and conduction of nerve impulses by decreasing the neuronal membrane's permeability to sodium ions, which results in inhibition of depolarization with resultant blockade of conduction

Pharmacodynamics/Kinetics
  Absorption: Oral: 99% to 100%
  Distribution: V_d: 1.62-3.2 L/kg
  Protein binding: 10% to 20%
  Metabolism: Hepatic to inactive metabolites; negligible first-pass effect
  Half-life elimination: 11-14 hours; renal and hepatic impairment: 23-27 hours
  Time to peak, serum: 30-160 minutes
  Excretion: Urine (40% to 50% as unchanged drug)

Usual Dosage Adults: Oral: 1200-1800 mg/day in 3 divided doses, up to 2400 mg/day

  Dosing adjustment in renal impairment: Cl_{cr} <30 mL/minute: Administer 50% of normal dose or 600 mg once daily.
  Hemodialysis: Moderately dialyzable (20% to 50%)
  Dosing adjustment in hepatic impairment: Maximum daily dose: 1200 mg

Dietary Considerations Should be taken with food.

Reference Range Therapeutic: 5-12 µg/mL (SI: 22-52 µmol/L)

Patient Information Report any unusual bleeding, fever, sore throat, or any breathing difficulties; do not discontinue or alter dose without notifying physician; may cause drowsiness, dizziness, impair judgment, and coordination

Nursing Implications Monitor for tremor; titration of dosing and initiation of therapy require cardiac monitoring

Dosage Forms Tablet, as hydrochloride: 400 mg, 600 mg

♦ **Tocainide Hydrochloride** *see* Tocainide *on page 1342*
♦ **Tofranil**® *see* Imipramine *on page 708*
♦ **Tofranil-PM**® *see* Imipramine *on page 708*

TOLAZamide (tole AZ a mide)

Related Information
  Antacid Drug Interactions *on page 1477*
  Hypoglycemic Drugs & Thiazolidinedione Information *on page 1502*
  Sulfonamide Derivatives *on page 1515*

U.S. Brand Names Tolinase®

Canadian Brand Names Tolinase®

Therapeutic Category Antidiabetic Agent, Sulfonylurea; Hypoglycemic Agent, Oral; Sulfonylurea Agent

Use Adjunct to diet for the management of mild to moderately severe, stable, type 2 diabetes mellitus (noninsulin dependent, NIDDM)

(Continued)

TOLAZamide *(Continued)*

Pregnancy Risk Factor D

Usual Dosage Oral (doses >1000 mg/day normally do not improve diabetic control):

Adults:

Initial: 100-250 mg/day with breakfast or the first main meal of the day

Fasting blood sugar <200 mg/dL: 100 mg/day

Fasting blood sugar >200 mg/dL: 250 mg/day

Patient is malnourished, underweight, elderly, or not eating properly: 100 mg/day

Adjust dose in increments of 100-250 mg/day at weekly intervals to response. If >500 mg/day is required, give in divided doses twice daily; maximum daily dose: 1 g (doses >1 g/day are not likely to improve control)

Conversion from insulin → tolazamide

10 units day = 100 mg/day

20-40 units/day = 250 mg/day

>40 units/day = 250 mg/day and 50% of insulin dose

Doses >500 mg/day should be given in 2 divided doses

Dosing adjustment in renal impairment: Conservative initial and maintenance doses are recommended because tolazamide is metabolized to active metabolites, which are eliminated in the urine

Dosing comments in hepatic impairment: Conservative initial and maintenance doses and careful monitoring of blood glucose are recommended

Additional Information Complete prescribing information for this medication should be consulted for additional detail.

Dosage Forms Tablet: 100 mg, 250 mg, 500 mg

Tolazoline *(tole AZ oh leen)*

U.S. Brand Names Priscoline®

Synonyms Benzazoline Hydrochloride; Tolazoline Hydrochloride

Therapeutic Category Alpha-Adrenergic Blocking Agent, Parenteral

Use Treatment of persistent pulmonary vasoconstriction and hypertension of the newborn (persistent fetal circulation), peripheral vasospastic disorders

Pregnancy Risk Factor C

Usual Dosage

Neonates: Initial: I.V.: 1-2 mg/kg over 10-15 minutes via scalp vein or upper extremity; maintenance: 1-2 mg/kg/hour; use lower maintenance doses in patients with decreased renal function. Also used in neonates for acute vasospasm "cath toes" at 0.25 mg/kg/hour (no load); maximum dose: 6-8 mg/kg/hour.

Dosing interval in renal impairment in newborns: Urine output <0.9 mL/kg/hour: Decrease dose to 0.08 mg/kg/hour for every 1 mg/kg of loading dose

Adults: Peripheral vasospastic disorder: I.M., I.V., S.C.: 10-50 mg 4 times/day

Additional Information Complete prescribing information for this medication should be consulted for additional detail.

Dosage Forms Injection, as hydrochloride: 25 mg/mL (4 mL)

♦ **Tolazoline Hydrochloride** *see Tolazoline on page 1344*

TOLBUTamide *(tole BYOO ta mide)*

Related Information

Antacid Drug Interactions *on page 1477*

Hypoglycemic Drugs & Thiazolidinedione Information *on page 1502*

Sulfonamide Derivatives *on page 1515*

U.S. Brand Names Orinase Diagnostic®; Tol-Tab®

Canadian Brand Names Apo®-Tolbutamide

Synonyms Tolbutamide Sodium

Therapeutic Category Antidiabetic Agent, Sulfonylurea; Diagnostic Agent, Hypoglycemia; Diagnostic Agent, Insulinoma; Hypoglycemic Agent, Oral; Sulfonylurea Agent

Use Adjunct to diet for the management of mild to moderately severe, stable, type 2 diabetes mellitus (noninsulin dependent, NIDDM)

Pregnancy Risk Factor D

Usual Dosage Divided doses may increase gastrointestinal side effects

Adults:

Oral: Initial: 1-2 g/day as a single dose in the morning or in divided doses throughout the day. Total doses may be taken in the morning; however, divided doses may allow increased gastrointestinal tolerance. Maintenance dose: 0.25-3 g/day; however, a maintenance dose >2 g/day is seldom required.

I.V. bolus: 1 g over 2-3 minutes

Elderly: Oral: Initial: 250 mg 1-3 times/day; usual: 500-2000 mg; maximum: 3 g/day

Dosing adjustment in renal impairment: Adjustment is not necessary

Hemodialysis: Not dialyzable (0% to 5%)

Dosing adjustment in hepatic impairment: Reduction of dose may be necessary in patients with impaired liver function

Additional Information Complete prescribing information for this medication should be consulted for additional detail.

Dosage Forms

Injection, powder for reconstitution, as sodium (Orinase Diagnostic®): 1 g

Tablet (Tol-Tab®): 500 mg

♦ **Tolbutamide Sodium** *see TOLBUTamide on page 1344*

Tolcapone *(TOLE ka pone)*

Related Information

Parkinson's Agents *on page 1513*

U.S. Brand Names Tasmar®

Therapeutic Category Anti-Parkinson's Agent, COMT Inhibitor; Reverse COMT Inhibitor

Use Adjunct to levodopa and carbidopa for the treatment of signs and symptoms of idiopathic Parkinson's disease

Pregnancy Risk Factor C

Contraindications Hypersensitivity to tolcapone or any component of the formulation

Warnings/Precautions Note: Due to reports of fatal liver injury associated with use of this drug, the manufacturer is advising that tolcapone be reserved for use only in patients who do not have severe movement abnormalities and who do not respond to or who are not appropriate candidates for other available treatments. Before initiating therapy with tolcapone, the risks should be discussed with the patient, and the patient can provide written informed consent (form available from Roche).

It is not recommended that patients receive tolcapone concomitantly with nonselective MAO inhibitors (see Drug Interactions). Selegiline is a selective MAO-B inhibitor and can be taken with tolcapone.

Patients receiving tolcapone are predisposed to orthostatic hypotension, diarrhea (usually within the first 6-12 weeks of therapy), transient hallucinations (most commonly within the first 2 weeks of therapy), and new onset or worsened dyskinesia. Use with caution in patients with severe renal failure. Tolcapone is secreted into maternal milk in rats and may be excreted into human milk; until more is known, tolcapone should be considered **incompatible** with breast-feeding.

Adverse Reactions

>10%:

    Cardiovascular: Orthostatic hypotension

    Central nervous system: Sleep disorder, excessive dreaming, somnolence, headache

    Gastrointestinal: Nausea, diarrhea, anorexia

    Neuromuscular & skeletal: Dyskinesia, dystonia, muscle cramps

1% to 10%:

    Central nervous system: Hallucinations, fatigue, loss of balance, hyperkinesia

    Gastrointestinal: Vomiting, constipation, xerostomia, abdominal pain, flatulence, dyspepsia

    Genitourinary: Urine discoloration

    Neuromuscular & skeletal: Paresthesia, stiffness

    Miscellaneous: Diaphoresis (increased)

Drug Interactions

    Cytochrome P450 Effect: CYP2A6 and 3A3/4 enzyme substrate

    Increased Effect/Toxicity: Tolcapone may increase the effect/levels of methyldopa, dobutamine, apomorphine, and isoproterenol due to inhibition of catechol-O-methyl transferase enzymes (COMT).

Ethanol/Nutrition/Herb Interactions

    Ethanol: Avoid ethanol (may increase CNS depression).

    Food: Tolcapone, taken with food within 1 hour before or 2 hours after the dose, decreases bioavailability by 10% to 20%.

    Avoid valerian, St John's wort, kava kava, gotu kola (may increase CNS depression).

Mechanism of Action Tolcapone is a selective and reversible inhibitor of catechol-o-methyl-transferase (COMT)

Pharmacodynamics/Kinetics

    Absorption: Rapid

    Protein binding: >99.0%

    Metabolism: Glucuronidation

    Bioavailability: 65%

    Half-life elimination: 2-3 hours

    Time to peak: ~2 hours

    Excretion: Urine and feces (40%)

Usual Dosage Adults: Oral: Initial: 100-200 mg 3 times/day; levodopa therapy may need to be decreased upon initiation of tolcapone

Monitoring Parameters Blood pressure, symptoms of Parkinson's disease, liver enzymes at baseline and then every 2 weeks for the first year of therapy, every 4 weeks for the next 6 months, then every 8 weeks thereafter. If the dose is increased to 200 mg 3 times/day, reinitiate LFT monitoring at the previous frequency. Discontinue therapy if the ALT or AST exceeds the upper limit of normal or if the clinical signs and symptoms suggest the onset of liver failure.

Patient Information Take exactly as directed (may be prescribed in conjunction with levodopa/carbidopa); do not change dosage or discontinue without consulting prescriber.

Therapeutic effects may take several weeks or months to achieve and you may need frequent monitoring during first weeks of therapy.

Best to take 2 hours before or after a meal; however, may be taken with meals if GI upset occurs. Take at same time each day. Maintain adequate hydration (2-3 L/day). Do not use alcohol, prescription or OTC sedatives, or CNS depressants without consulting prescriber.

Urine or perspiration may become darker. You may experience drowsiness, dizziness, confusion, or vision changes (use caution when driving, climbing stairs, or engaging in hazardous tasks). Orthostatic hypotension (use caution when changing position - rising to standing from sitting or lying); increased susceptibility to heat stroke, decreased perspiration (use caution in hot weather - maintain adequate fluids and reduce exercise activity); constipation (increased exercise, fluids, or dietary fruit and fiber may help); dry skin or nasal passages (consult prescriber for appropriate relief); nausea, vomiting, loss of appetite, or stomach discomfort (small frequent meals, chewing gum, or sucking on lozenges may help).

Report unresolved constipation or vomiting; chest pain or irregular heartbeat; difficulty breathing; acute headache or dizziness; CNS changes (hallucination, loss of memory, nervousness, etc); painful or difficult urination; abdominal pain or blood in stool; increased muscle spasticity, rigidity, or involuntary movements; skin rash; or significant worsening of condition. Inform prescriber if you are or intend to be pregnant. Do not breast-feed.

Dosage Forms Tablet: 100 mg, 200 mg

♦ **Tolectin**® *see* Tolmetin *on page 1346*

◆ **Tolectin® DS**   *see* Tolmetin *on page 1346*

◆ **Tolinase®**   *see* TOLAZamide *on page 1343*

Tolmetin (TOLE met in)

Related Information
Antacid Drug Interactions *on page 1477*
Nonsteroidal Anti-Inflammatory Agents Comparison *on page 1512*

U.S. Brand Names Tolectin®; Tolectin® DS

Canadian Brand Names Novo-Tolmetin; Tolectin®

Synonyms Tolmetin Sodium

Therapeutic Category Analgesic, Nonsteroidal Anti-inflammatory Drug; Anti-inflammatory Agent; Nonsteroidal Anti-inflammatory Drug (NSAID), Oral

Use Treatment of rheumatoid arthritis and osteoarthritis, juvenile rheumatoid arthritis

Pregnancy Risk Factor C/D (3rd trimester or at term)

Contraindications Hypersensitivity to tolmetin, any component of the formulation, aspirin, or other nonsteroidal anti-inflammatory drugs (NSAIDs); pregnancy (3rd trimester or near term)

Warnings/Precautions Use with caution in patients with upper GI disease, impaired renal function, congestive heart failure, dehydration, hypertension, and patients receiving anticoagulants; if GI upset occurs with tolmetin, take with antacids other than sodium bicarbonate. Withhold for at least 4-6 half-lives prior to surgical or dental procedures.

Adverse Reactions
1% to 10%:
    Cardiovascular: Chest pain, hypertension, edema
    Central nervous system: Headache, dizziness, drowsiness, depression
    Dermatologic: Skin irritation
    Endocrine & metabolic: Weight gain/loss
    Gastrointestinal: Heartburn, abdominal pain, diarrhea, flatulence, vomiting, constipation, gastritis, peptic ulcer, nausea
    Genitourinary: Urinary Tract Infection
    Hematologic: Elevated BUN, transient decreases in hemoglobin/hematocrit
    Ocular: Visual disturbances
    Otic: Tinnitus
<1% (Limited to important or life-threatening): Abnormal LFTs, agranulocytosis, bronchospasm, congestive heart failure, dyspnea, erythema multiforme, GI bleeding, granulocytopenia, hematuria, hemolytic anemia, hepatitis, proteinuria, renal failure, thrombocytopenia, toxic epidermal necrolysis

Overdosage/Toxicology Symptoms include lethargy, mental confusion, dizziness, leukocytosis, and renal failure. Management of nonsteroidal anti-inflammatory drug (NSAID) intoxication is primarily supportive and symptomatic. Fluid therapy is commonly effective in managing hypotension that may occur following an acute NSAID overdose, except when due to acute blood loss. Seizures tend to be very short-lived and often do not require drug treatment; although, recurrent seizures should be treated with I.V. diazepam. Since many of the NSAIDs undergo enterohepatic cycling, multiple doses of charcoal may be needed to reduce the potential for delayed toxicities.

Drug Interactions
Increased Effect/Toxicity: Increased toxicity of digoxin, methotrexate, cyclosporine, lithium, insulin, sulfonylureas, potassium-sparing diuretics, and aspirin.

Decreased Effect: Decreased effect with aspirin. Decreased effect of thiazides and furosemide.

Ethanol/Nutrition/Herb Interactions
Ethanol: Avoid ethanol (may enhance gastric mucosal irritation).
Food: Tolmetin peak serum concentrations may be decreased if taken with food or milk.
Herb/Nutraceutical: Avoid cat's claw, dong quai, evening primrose, feverfew, garlic, ginger, ginkgo, red clover, horse chestnut, green tea, ginseng (all have additional antiplatelet activity).

Mechanism of Action Inhibits prostaglandin synthesis by decreasing the activity of the enzyme, cyclo-oxygenase, which results in decreased formation of prostaglandin precursors

Pharmacodynamics/Kinetics
Onset of action: Analgesic: 1-2 hours; Anti-inflammatory: Days to weeks
Absorption: Well absorbed
Bioavailability: Food/milk decreases total bioavailability by 16%
Time to peak, serum: 30-60 minutes

Usual Dosage Oral:
Children ≥2 years:
    Anti-inflammatory: Initial: 20 mg/kg/day in 3 divided doses, then 15-30 mg/kg/day in 3 divided doses
    Analgesic: 5-7 mg/kg/dose every 6-8 hours
Adults: 400 mg 3 times/day; usual dose: 600 mg to 1.8 g/day; maximum: 2 g/day

Dietary Considerations Should be taken with food, milk, or antacids to decrease GI adverse effects.

Monitoring Parameters Occult blood loss, CBC, liver enzymes, BUN, serum creatinine, periodic liver function test

Patient Information Take with food, milk, or water; may cause drowsiness, impair judgment or coordination

Nursing Implications Monitor occult blood loss, CBC, liver enzymes, BUN, serum creatinine, periodic liver function test

Additional Information Sodium content of 200 mg: 0.8 mEq

Dosage Forms
Capsule, as sodium (Tolectin® DS): 400 mg
Tablet, as sodium (Tolectin®): 200 mg, 600 mg

◆ **Tolmetin Sodium**   *see* Tolmetin *on page 1346*

Tolnaftate (tole NAF tate)

U.S. Brand Names Absorbine® Antifungal [OTC]; Absorbine® Jock Itch [OTC]; Absorbine Jr.® Antifungal [OTC]; Aftate® for Athlete's Foot [OTC]; Aftate® for Jock Itch [OTC]; Blis-To-Sol® [OTC]; Dr Scholl's Athlete's Foot [OTC]; Dr Scholl's Maximum Strength Tritin [OTC]; Genaspor® [OTC]; NP-27® [OTC]; Quinsana Plus® [OTC]; Tinactin® [OTC]; Tinactin® for Jock Itch [OTC]; Ting® [OTC]

Canadian Brand Names Pitrex

Therapeutic Category Antifungal Agent, Topical

Use Treatment of tinea pedis, tinea cruris, tinea corporis, tinea manuum, tinea versicolor infections

Pregnancy Risk Factor C

Contraindications Hypersensitivity to tolnaftate or any component of the formulation; nail and scalp infections

Warnings/Precautions Cream is not recommended for nail or scalp infections; keep from eyes; if no improvement within 4 weeks, treatment should be discontinued. Usually not effective alone for the treatment of infections involving hair follicles or nails.

Adverse Reactions 1% to 10%:
Dermatologic: Pruritus, contact dermatitis
Local: Irritation, stinging

Mechanism of Action Distorts the hyphae and stunts mycelial growth in susceptible fungi

Pharmacodynamics/Kinetics Onset of action: 24-72 hours

Usual Dosage Children and Adults: Topical: Wash and dry affected area; apply 1-3 drops of solution or a small amount of cream or powder and rub into the affected areas 2-3 times/day for 2-4 weeks

Patient Information Avoid contact with the eyes; apply to clean dry area; consult the physician if a skin irritation develops or if the skin infection worsens or does not improve after 10 days of therapy; does not stain skin or clothing

Nursing Implications Itching, burning, and soreness are usually relieved within 24-72 hours

Dosage Forms
Aerosol, liquid, topical: 1% (59.2 mL, 90 mL, 120 mL)
Aerosol, powder, topical: 1% (56.7 g, 100 g, 105 g, 150 g)
Cream, topical: 1% (15 g, 30 g)
Gel, topical: 1% (15 g)
Powder, topical: 1% (45 g, 90 g)
Solution, topical: 1% (10 mL)

♦ **Tol-Tab®** see TOLBUTamide on page 1344

Tolterodine (tole TER oh deen)

U.S. Brand Names Detrol™; Detrol® LA

Canadian Brand Names Detrol™

Synonyms Tolterodine Tartrate

Therapeutic Category Anticholinergic Agent

Use Treatment of patients with an overactive bladder with symptoms of urinary frequency, urgency, or urge incontinence

Pregnancy Risk Factor C

Pregnancy/Breast-Feeding Implications Reproduction studies have not been conducted in pregnant women; use during pregnancy only if the potential benefit to the mother outweighs the possible risk to the fetus

Contraindications Hypersensitivity to tolterodine or any component of the formulation; urinary retention, gastric retention, or uncontrolled narrow-angle glaucoma

Warnings/Precautions Use with caution in patients with bladder flow obstruction, may increase the risk of urinary retention. Use with caution in patients with gastrointestinal obstructive disorders (ie, pyloric stenosis), may increase the risk of gastric retention. Use with caution in patients with controlled (treated) narrow-angle glaucoma; metabolized in the liver and excreted in the urine and feces, dosage adjustment is required for patients with renal or hepatic impairment. Patients on CYP3A4 inhibitors require lower dose. Safety and efficacy in pediatric patients have not been established.

Adverse Reactions As reported with immediate release tablet, unless otherwise specified

>10%: Gastrointestinal: Dry mouth (35%; extended release capsules 23%)

1% to 10%:
Cardiovascular: Chest pain (2%)
Central nervous system: Headache (7%; extended release capsules 6%), somnolence (3%; extended release capsules 3%), fatigue (4%; extended release capsules 2%), dizziness (5%; extended release capsules 2%), anxiety (extended release capsules 1%)
Dermatologic: Dry skin (1%)
Gastrointestinal: Abdominal pain (5%; extended release capsules 4%), constipation (7%; extended release capsules 6%), dyspepsia (4%; extended release capsules 3%), diarrhea (4%), weight gain (1%)
Genitourinary: Dysuria (2%; extended release capsules 1%)
Neuromuscular & skeletal: Arthralgia (2%)
Ocular: Abnormal vision (2%; extended release capsules 1%), dry eyes (3%; extended release capsules 3%)
Respiratory: Bronchitis (2%), sinusitis (extended release capsules 2%)
<1% (Limited to important or life-threatening): Anaphylactoid reactions, peripheral edema, tachycardia

Overdosage/Toxicology Overdosage can potentially result in severe central anticholinergic effects and should be treated accordingly. EKG monitoring is recommended in the event of overdosage.
(Continued)

Tolterodine *(Continued)*

Drug Interactions
  Cytochrome P450 Effect: CYP2D6 and CYP3A3/4 enzyme substrate
  Increased Effect/Toxicity:

  Serum levels and/or toxicity of tolterodine may be increased by drugs which inhibit CYP2D6; effect was seen with fluoxetine. Inhibitors include amiodarone, cimetidine, delavirdine, paroxetine, propafenone, quinidine, and ritonavir. No dosage adjustment was needed in patients coadministered tolterodine and fluoxetine.

  Serum level and/or toxicity of tolterodine may be increased by drugs which inhibit CYP3A3/4, particularly in patients who are poor metabolizers via CYP2D6; effect was seen with ketoconazole. Other inhibitors include amiodarone, cimetidine, clarithromycin, cyclosporine, erythromycin, delavirdine, diltiazem, dirithromycin, disulfiram, fluoxetine, fluvoxamine, grapefruit juice, indinavir, itraconazole, nefazodone, nevirapine, propoxyphene, quinupristin-dalfopristin, ritonavir, saquinavir, verapamil, vinblastine, zafirlukast, zileuton.

Ethanol/Nutrition/Herb Interactions
  Food: Increases bioavailability (~53% increase) of tolterodine tablets, but does not affect the pharmacokinetics of tolterodine extended release capsules; adjustment of dose is not needed. As a CYP3A3/4 inhibitor, grapefruit juice may increase the serum level and/or toxicity of tolterodine, but unlikely secondary to high oral bioavailability.
  Herb/Nutraceutical: St John's wort (*Hypericum*) appears to induce CYP3A enzymes.

Stability Store at room temperature, protect from light

Mechanism of Action Tolterodine is a competitive antagonist of muscarinic receptors. In animal models, tolterodine demonstrates selectivity for urinary bladder receptors over salivary receptors. Urinary bladder contraction is mediated by muscarinic receptors. Tolterodine increases residual urine volume and decreases detrusor muscle pressure.

Pharmacodynamics/Kinetics
  Absorption: Immediate release tablet: Rapid
  Distribution: I.V.: V_d: 113 ± 27 L
  Protein binding: Highly bound to alpha$_1$-acid glycoprotein
  Metabolism: Extensively hepatic primarily via CYP2D6 isoenzyme (some metabolites share activity) and 3A4 usually (minor pathway). In patients with a genetic deficiency of isoenzyme 2D6, metabolism via isoenzyme 3A4 predominates. Forms 3 active metabolites.
  Bioavailability: Immediate release tablet: 77%; food increases bioavailability
  Half-life elimination:
    Immediate release tablet: Extensive metabolizers: ~2 hours; poor metabolizers: ~10 hours
    Extended release capsule: Extensive metabolizers: ~7 hours; poor metabolizers: ~18 hours
  Time to peak: Immediate release tablet: 1-2 hours; Extended release tablet: 2-6 hours
  Excretion: Urine (77% as unchanged drug, 5% to 14% as metabolites, <1% as metabolites in poor metabolizers); feces (17%, <1% as unchanged drug, <2.5% in poor metabolizers)

Usual Dosage
  Children: Safety and efficacy in pediatric patients have not been established
  Adults: Treatment of overactive bladder: Oral:
    Immediate release tablet: 2 mg twice daily; the dose may be lowered to 1 mg twice daily based on individual response and tolerability
      Dosing adjustment in patients concurrently taking CYP3A4 inhibitors: 1 mg twice daily
    Extended release capsule: 4 mg once a day; dose may be lowered to 2 mg daily based on individual response and tolerability
      Dosing adjustment in patients concurrently taking CYP3A4 inhibitors: 2 mg daily
  Elderly: Safety and efficacy in patients >64 years was found to be similar to that in younger patients; no dosage adjustment is needed based on age

  Dosing adjustment in renal impairment: Use with caution (studies conducted in patients with Cl$_{cr}$ 10-30 mL/minute):
    Immediate release tablet: 1 mg twice daily
    Extended release capsule: 2 mg daily

  Dosing adjustment in hepatic impairment:
    Immediate release tablet: 1 mg twice daily
    Extended release capsule: 2 mg daily

Administration Extended release capsule: Swallow whole; do not crush, chew, or open

Patient Information Take as directed, preferably with food. Do not crush, chew, or open extended release capsule; swallow whole. You may experience headache (a mild analgesic may help); blurred vision, dizziness, nervousness, or sleepiness (use caution when driving, climbing stairs, or engaging in tasks requiring alertness until response to drug is known); abdominal discomfort, diarrhea, constipation, nausea or vomiting (small frequent meals, increased exercise, adequate fluid intake may help). Report back pain, muscle spasms, alteration in gait, or numbness of extremities; unresolved or persistent constipation, diarrhea, or vomiting; or symptoms of upper respiratory infection or flu. Report immediately any chest pain or palpitations; difficulty urinating or pain on urination.

Dosage Forms
  Capsule, extended release, as tartrate: 2 mg, 4 mg
  Tablet, as tartrate: 1 mg, 2 mg

♦ **Tolterodine Tartrate** *see* Tolterodine *on page 1347*
♦ **Tolu-Sed® DM [OTC]** *see* Guaifenesin and Dextromethorphan *on page 646*
♦ **Tomedar® (Can)** *see* Temozolomide *on page 1293*
♦ **Tomycine™ (Can)** *see* Tobramycin *on page 1340*
♦ **Tonocard®** *see* Tocainide *on page 1342*
♦ **Topamax®** *see* Topiramate *on page 1349*
♦ **Topicort®** *see* Desoximetasone *on page 380*
♦ **Topicort®-LP** *see* Desoximetasone *on page 380*

♦ **Topicycline**® *see* Tetracycline *on page 1306*
♦ **Topilene**® **(Can)** *see* Betamethasone *on page 161*

Topiramate (toe PYRE a mate)

Related Information
Anticonvulsants by Seizure Type *on page 1481*

U.S. Brand Names Topamax®

Canadian Brand Names Topamax®

Therapeutic Category Anticonvulsant

Use In adults and pediatric patients (ages 2-16 years), adjunctive therapy for partial onset seizures and adjunctive therapy of primary generalized tonic-clonic seizures; treatment of seizures associated with Lennox-Gastaut syndrome in patients ≥2 years of age

Unlabeled/Investigational Use Bipolar disorder, infantile spasms, neuropathic pain

Pregnancy Risk Factor C

Pregnancy/Breast-Feeding Implications No studies in pregnant women; use only if benefit to the mother outweighs the risk to the fetus. Postmarketing experience includes reports of hypospadias following *in vitro* exposure to topiramate.

Contraindications Hypersensitivity to topiramate or any component of the formulation

Warnings/Precautions Avoid abrupt withdrawal of topiramate therapy, it should be withdrawn slowly to minimize the potential of increased seizure frequency; the risk of kidney stones is about 2-4 times that of the untreated population, the risk of this event may be reduced by increasing fluid intake; use cautiously in patients with hepatic or renal impairment and during pregnancy. Has been associated with secondary angle-closure glaucoma in adults and children, typically within 1 month of initiation. Discontinue in patients with acute onset of decreased visual acuity or ocular pain. Safety and efficacy have not been established in children <2 years of age.

Adverse Reactions
>10%:
    Central nervous system: Dizziness, ataxia, somnolence, psychomotor slowing, nervousness, memory difficulties, speech problems, fatigue
    Gastrointestinal: Nausea
    Neuromuscular & skeletal: Paresthesia, tremor
    Ocular: Nystagmus, diplopia, abnormal vision
    Respiratory: Upper respiratory infections
1% to 10%:
    Cardiovascular: Chest pain, edema
    Central nervous system: Language problems, abnormal coordination, confusion, depression, difficulty concentrating, hypoesthesia
    Endocrine & metabolic: Hot flashes
    Gastrointestinal: Dyspepsia, abdominal pain, anorexia, constipation, xerostomia, gingivitis, weight loss
    Neuromuscular & skeletal: Myalgia, weakness, back pain, leg pain, rigors
    Otic: Decreased hearing
    Renal: Nephrolithiasis
    Respiratory: Pharyngitis, sinusitis, epistaxis
    Miscellaneous: Flu-like symptoms
<1% (Limited to important or life-threatening): Apraxia, AV block, bone marrow depression, delirium, dyskinesia, encephalopathy, eosinophilia, granulocytopenia, hepatic failure, hepatitis, manic reaction, neuropathy, pancreatitis, pancytopenia, paranoid reaction, photosensitivity, psychosis, renal calculus, renal tubular acidosis, suicidal behavior, syndrome of acute decreased myopia/secondary angle-closure glaucoma, tinnitus

Overdosage/Toxicology Activated charcoal has not been shown to adsorb topiramate and is, therefore, not recommended. Hemodialysis can remove the drug, however, most cases do not require removal and instead are best treated with supportive measures.

Drug Interactions
Cytochrome P450 Effect: CYP2C19 enzyme substrate; CYP2C19 enzyme inhibitor
Increased Effect/Toxicity: Concomitant administration with other CNS depressants will increase its sedative effects. Coadministration with other carbonic anhydrase inhibitors may increase the chance of nephrolithiasis. Topiramate may increase phenytoin concentration by 25%.
Decreased Effect: Phenytoin can decrease topiramate levels by as much as 48%, carbamazepine reduces it by 40%, and valproic acid reduces topiramate by 14%. Digoxin levels and ethinyl estradiol blood levels are decreased when coadministered with topiramate. Topiramate may decrease valproic acid concentration by 11%.

Ethanol/Nutrition/Herb Interactions
Ethanol: Avoid ethanol (may increase CNS depression).
Herb/Nutraceutical: Avoid evening primrose (seizure threshold decreased).

Stability Store at room temperature; protect capsules from moisture.

Mechanism of Action Mechanism is not fully understood, it is thought to decrease seizure frequency by blocking sodium channels in neurons, enhancing GABA activity and by blocking glutamate activity

Pharmacodynamics/Kinetics
Absorption: Good; unaffected by food
Protein binding: 13% to 17%
Metabolism: Hepatic (minimal) via hydroxylation, hydrolysis, glucuronidation
Metabolism: Minimal
Bioavailability: 80%
Half-life elimination: Mean: Adults: 21 hours in adults; shorter in pediatric patients
Time to peak, serum: ~2-4 hours
Excretion: Primarily urine (~70% as unchanged drug)
Dialyzable: ~30%
(Continued)

Topiramate (Continued)

Usual Dosage Oral:

Children 2-16 years: Partial seizures (adjunctive therapy), primary generalized tonic-clonic seizures (adjunctive therapy), or seizure associated with Lennox-Gastaut syndrome: Initial dose titration should begin at 25 mg (or less, based on a range of 1-3 mg/kg/day) nightly for the first week; dosage may be increased in increments of 1-3 mg/kg/day (administered in 2 divided doses) at 1- or 2-week intervals to a total daily dose of 5-9 mg/kg/day.

Adults: Partial onset seizures (adjunctive therapy), primary generalized tonic-clonic seizures (adjunctive therapy): Initial: 25-50 mg/day; titrate in increments of 25-50 mg per week until an effective daily dose is reached; the daily dose may be increased by 25 mg at weekly intervals for the first 4 weeks; thereafter, the daily dose may be increased by 25-50 mg weekly to an effective daily dose (usually at least 400 mg); usual maximum dose: 1600 mg/day

Note: A more rapid titration schedule has been previously recommended (ie, 50 mg/week), and may be attempted in some clinical situations; however, this may reduce the patient's ability to tolerate topiramate.

Dosing adjustment in renal impairment: Cl_{cr} <70 mL/minute: Administer 50% dose and titrate more slowly

Hemodialysis: Supplemental dose may be needed during hemodialysis

Dosing adjustment in hepatic impairment: Clearance may be reduced

Administration Oral: May be administered without regard to meals

Capsule sprinkles: May be swallowed whole or opened to sprinkle the contents on soft food (drug/food mixture should not be chewed).

Tablet: Because of bitter taste, tablets should not be broken.

Additional Information May be associated with weight loss in some patients

Dosage Forms

Capsule, sprinkle (Topamax®): 15 mg, 25 mg

Tablet (Topamax®): 25 mg, 100 mg, 200 mg

- ♦ **Topisone® (Can)** see Betamethasone on page 161
- ♦ **TOPO** see Topotecan on page 1350
- ♦ **Toposar®** see Etoposide on page 533

Topotecan (toe poe TEE kan)

U.S. Brand Names Hycamtin™

Canadian Brand Names Hycamtin™

Synonyms Hycamptamine; SK and F 104864; SKF 104864; SKF 104864-A; TOPO; Topotecan Hydrochloride; TPT

Therapeutic Category Antineoplastic Agent, Antibiotic

Use Treatment of metastatic carcinoma of the ovary after failure of initial or subsequent chemotherapy; second-line treatment of small cell lung cancer

Unlabeled/Investigational Use Investigational: Treatment of nonsmall cell lung cancer, sarcoma (pediatrics)

Pregnancy Risk Factor D

Contraindications Hypersensitivity to topotecan or any component of the formulation; pregnancy

Warnings/Precautions The U.S. Food and Drug Administration (FDA) currently recommends that procedures for proper handling and disposal of antineoplastic agents be considered; monitor bone marrow function

Adverse Reactions

>10%:

Central nervous system: Headache

Dermatologic: Alopecia (reversible)

Gastrointestinal: Nausea, vomiting, diarrhea

Emetic potential: Moderately low (10% to 30%)

Hematologic: Myelosuppressive: Principle dose-limiting toxicity; white blood cell count nadir is 8-11 days after administration and is more frequent than thrombocytopenia (at lower doses); recover is usually within 21 days and cumulative toxicity has not been noted.

WBC: Mild to severe

Platelets: Mild (at low doses)

Nadir: 8-11 days

Recovery: 14-21 days

1% to 10%:

Neuromuscular & skeletal: Paresthesia

Respiratory: Dyspnea

Drug Interactions

Decreased Effect: Concurrent administration of TPT and G-CSF in clinical trials results in severe myelosuppression. Concurrent in vitro exposure to TPT and the topoisomerase II inhibitor etoposide results in no altered effect; sequential exposure results in potentiation. Concurrent exposure to TPT and 5-azacytidine results in potentiation both in vitro and in vivo. Myelosuppression was more severe when given in combination with cisplatin.

Ethanol/Nutrition/Herb Interactions Ethanol: Avoid ethanol (due to GI irritation).

Stability

Store intact vials of lyophilized powder for injection at room temperature and protected from light. Topotecan should be initially reconstituted with 4 mL SWI. This solution is stable for 24 hours at room temperature. Topotecan should be further diluted in 100 mL D_5W. This solution is stable for 24 hours at room temperature.

Standard I.V. dilution: Dose/100 mL D_5W; stability is pH dependent; although topotecan may be further diluted in 0.9% NaCl, stability is longer in D_5W

Mechanism of Action Inhibits topoisomerase I (an enzyme which relaxes torsionally strained-coiled duplex DNA) to prevent DNA replication and translocation; topotecan acts in S phase

Pharmacodynamics/Kinetics

Absorption: Oral: ~30%

Distribution: V_{dss} of the lactone is high (mean: 87.3 L/mm^2; range: 25.6-186 L/mm^2), suggesting wide distribution and/or tissue sequestering

Protein binding: 35%

Metabolism: Undergoes a rapid, pH-dependent opening of the lactone ring to yield a relatively inactive hydroxy acid in plasma.

Half-life elimination: 3 hours

Excretion: Primarily urine (30%) within 24 hours

Usual Dosage Refer to individual protocols:

Adults:

Metastatic ovarian cancer and small cell lung cancer: IVPB: 1.5 mg/m^2/day for 5 days; repeated every 21 days (neutrophil count should be >1500/mm^3 and platelet count should be >100,000/mm^3)

Dosage adjustment for hematological effects: If neutrophil count <1500/mm^3, reduce dose by 0.25 mg/m^2/day for 5 days for next cycle

Dosing adjustment in renal impairment:

Cl$_{cr}$ 20-39 mL/minute: Administer 50% of normal dose

Cl$_{cr}$ <20 mL/minute: Do not use, insufficient data available

Hemodialysis: Supplemental dose is not necessary

CAPD effects: Unknown

CAVH effects: Unknown

Dosing adjustment in hepatic impairment: Bilirubin 1.5-10 mg/dL: Adjustment is not necessary

Administration Administer lower doses IVPB over 30 minutes

Monitoring Parameters CBC with differential and platelet count and renal function tests

Test Interactions None known

Patient Information This medication can only be administered I.V. and frequent blood tests may be necessary to monitor effects of the drug. Report pain, swelling, or irritation at infusion site. Do not use alcohol, prescription, and/or OTC medications without consulting prescriber. Maintain adequate hydration (2-3 L/day of fluids unless instructed to restrict fluid intake); maintain good oral hygiene (use a soft toothbrush or cotton applicators several times a day and rinse mouth frequently). You may experience nausea, vomiting, or loss of appetite (frequent small meals, frequent mouth care, sucking lozenges, or chewing gum may help, or consult prescriber). Hair loss may occur (reversible). You will be susceptible to infection; avoid crowds and infected persons and do not receive any vaccinations unless approved by prescriber. Report persistent fever or chills, unhealed sores, oral or vaginal sores, foul-smelling urine, painful urination, easy bruising or bleeding, yellowing of eyes or skin, and change in color of urine or stool. The drug may cause permanent sterility and may cause birth defects. Contraceptive measures should be used during therapy. The drug may be excreted in breast milk, therefore, an alternative form of feeding your baby should be used.

Dosage Forms Powder for injection, lyophilized, as hydrochloride: 4 mg (base)

♦ **Topotecan Hydrochloride** *see* Topotecan *on page 1350*

♦ **Toprol XL**® *see* Metoprolol *on page 902*

♦ **Topsyn**® **(Can)** *see* Fluocinonide *on page 573*

♦ **Toradol**® *see* Ketorolac *on page 764*

♦ **Toradol**® **IM (Can)** *see* Ketorolac *on page 764*

♦ **Torecan**® *see* Thiethylperazine *on page 1317*

Toremifene (TORE em i feen)

U.S. Brand Names Fareston®

Canadian Brand Names Fareston®

Synonyms FC1157a; Toremifene Citrate

Therapeutic Category Antineoplastic Agent, Hormone Antagonist; Estrogen Receptor Antagonist

Use Treatment of metastatic breast cancer in postmenopausal women with estrogen-receptor (ER) positive or ER unknown tumors

Pregnancy Risk Factor D

Contraindications Hypersensitivity to toremifene or any component of the formulation; pregnancy

Warnings/Precautions Hypercalcemia and tumor flare have been reported in some breast cancer patients with bone metastases during the first weeks of treatment. Tumor flare is a syndrome of diffuse musculoskeletal pain and erythema with increased size of tumor lesions that later regress. It is often accompanied by hypercalcemia. Tumor flare does not imply treatment failure or represent tumor progression. Institute appropriate measures if hypercalcemia occurs, and if severe, discontinue treatment. Drugs that decrease renal calcium excretion (eg, thiazide diuretics) may increase the risk of hypercalcemia in patients receiving toremifene.

Patients with a history of thromboembolic disease should generally not be treated with toremifene

Adverse Reactions

>10%:

Endocrine & metabolic: Hot flashes (35%), vaginal discharge (13%)

Gastrointestinal: Nausea, vomiting

Emetic potential: Moderate (30% to 40%)

Miscellaneous: Diaphoresis (20%)

1% to 10%:

Cardiovascular: Thromboembolism (venous thrombosis, pulmonary embolism, arterial thrombosis), cardiac failure, myocardial infarction, angina, edema

Central nervous system: Dizziness

Endocrine & metabolic: Hypercalcemia (patients with bone metastases), galactorrhea, vitamin deficiency, menstrual irregularities

(Continued)

Toremifene (Continued)

Gastrointestinal: Elevated transaminase levels

Genitourinary: Vaginal bleeding or discharge, endometriosis, priapism, possible endometrial cancer

Ocular: Ophthalmologic effects (visual acuity changes, cataracts, or retinopathy), corneal opacities, dry eyes, blurred vision

Other events observed with unclear association with toremifene: Alopecia, anorexia, asthenia, dermatitis, dyspnea, jaundice, paresis, pruritus, rigors, skin discoloration, tremor

Overdosage/Toxicology Theoretically, overdose may be manifested as an increase of antiestrogenic effects such as hot flashes; estrogenic effects such as vaginal bleeding; or nervous system disorders such as vertigo, dizziness, ataxia and nausea. No specific antidote exists and treatment is symptomatic.

Drug Interactions

Cytochrome P450 Effect: CYP3A3/4 enzyme substrate

Increased Effect/Toxicity: Enzyme inhibitors (such as ketoconazole or erythromycin) may increase blood levels of toremifene. Concurrent therapy with warfarin results in significant enhancement of anticoagulant effects; has been speculated that a ↓ in antitumor effect of tamoxifen may also occur due to alterations in the percentage of active tamoxifen metabolites.

Decreased Effect: Phenobarbital, phenytoin, and carbamazepine increase the rate of toremifene metabolism and lower blood levels.

Mechanism of Action Nonsteroidal, triphenylethylene derivative. Competitively binds to estrogen receptors on tumors and other tissue targets, producing a nuclear complex that decreases DNA synthesis and inhibits estrogen effects. Nonsteroidal agent with potent antiestrogenic properties which compete with estrogen for binding sites in breast and other tissues; cells accumulate in the G_0 and G_1 phases; therefore, tamoxifen is cytostatic rather than cytocidal.

Pharmacodynamics/Kinetics

Absorption: Well absorbed

Distribution: V_d: 580 L

Protein binding, plasma: >99.5%, mainly to albumin

Metabolism: Extensively, principally by CYP450 3A4 to N-demethyltoremifene, which is also antiestrogenic but with weak *in vivo* antitumor potency

Half-life elimination: ~5 days

Time to peak, serum: ~3 hours

Excretion: Primarily feces; urine (10%) during a 1-week period

Usual Dosage Refer to individual protocols.

Adults: Oral: 60 mg once daily, generally continued until disease progression is observed

Dosage adjustment in renal impairment: No dosage adjustment necessary

Dosage adjustment in hepatic impairment: Toremifene is extensively metabolized in the liver and dosage adjustments may be indicated in patients with liver disease; however, no specific guidelines have been developed

Administration Orally, usually as a single daily dose; occasionally in 2 or 3 divided doses

Monitoring Parameters Obtain periodic complete blood counts, calcium levels, and liver function tests. Closely monitor patients with bone metastases for hypercalcemia during the first few weeks of treatment. Leukopenia and thrombocytopenia have been reported rarely; monitor leukocyte and platelet counts during treatment.

Patient Information Take as directed, without regard to food. You may experience an initial "flare" of this disease (increased bone pain and hot flashes) which will subside with continued use. You may experience nausea, vomiting, or loss of appetite (frequent mouth care, frequent small meals, chewing gum, or sucking lozenges may help); dizziness (use caution when driving, climbing stairs, or engaging in tasks requiring alertness until response to drug is known); or loss of hair (reversible). Report vomiting that occurs immediately after taking medication; chest pain, palpitations or swollen extremities; vaginal bleeding, hot flashes, or excessive perspiration; chest pain, unusual coughing, or difficulty breathing; or any changes in vision or dry eyes.

Nursing Implications Increase of bone pain usually indicates a good therapeutic response

Dosage Forms Tablet, as citrate: 60 mg

♦ **Toremifene Citrate** *see* Toremifene *on page 1351*

♦ **Tornalate®** [DSC] *see* Bitolterol *on page 173*

Torsemide (TORE se mide)

Related Information

Heart Failure *on page 1663*

Sulfonamide Derivatives *on page 1515*

U.S. Brand Names Demadex®

Therapeutic Category Antihypertensive Agent; Diuretic, Loop

Use Management of edema associated with congestive heart failure and hepatic or renal disease; used alone or in combination with antihypertensives in treatment of hypertension; I.V. form is indicated when rapid onset is desired

Pregnancy Risk Factor B

Pregnancy/Breast-Feeding Implications Clinical effect on the fetus: A decrease in fetal weight, an increase in fetal resorption, and delayed fetal ossification has occurred in animal studies

Contraindications Hypersensitivity to torsemide, any component of the formulation, or any sulfonylureas; anuria

Warnings/Precautions Excessive diuresis may result in dehydration, acute hypotensive or thromboembolic episodes and cardiovascular collapse; rapid injection, renal impairment, or excessively large doses may result in ototoxicity; SLE may be exacerbated; sudden alterations in electrolyte balance may precipitate hepatic encephalopathy and coma in patients with hepatic cirrhosis and ascites; monitor carefully for signs of fluid or electrolyte imbalances, especially hypokalemia in patients at risk for such (eg, digitalis therapy, history of ventricular arrhythmias, elderly, etc), hyperuricemia, hypomagnesemia, or hypocalcemia; use caution with exposure to ultraviolet light. Ototoxicity is associated with rapid I.V. administration of other loop diuretics and has been seen with oral torsemide. Do not administer intravenously in less than 2 minutes; single doses should not exceed 200 mg.

Chemical similarities are present among sulfonamides, sulfonylureas, carbonic anhydrase inhibitors, thiazides, and loop diuretics (except ethacrynic acid). Use in patients with sulfonylurea allergy is specifically contraindicated in product labeling, however a risk of cross-reaction exists in patients with allergy to any of these compounds; avoid use when previous reaction has been severe.

Adverse Reactions
1% to 10%:
Cardiovascular: Edema (1.1%), EKG abnormality (2%), chest pain (1.2%)
Central nervous system: Headache (7.3%), dizziness (3.2%), insomnia (1.2%), nervousness (1%)
Endocrine & metabolic: Hyperglycemia, hyperuricemia, hypokalemia
Gastrointestinal: Diarrhea (2%), constipation (1.8%), nausea (1.8%), dyspepsia (1.6%), sore throat (1.6%)
Genitourinary: Excessive urination (6.7%)
Neuromuscular & skeletal: Weakness (2%), arthralgia (1.8%), myalgia (1.6%)
Respiratory: Rhinitis (2.8%), cough increase (2%)
<1% (Limited to important or life-threatening): Angioedema, atrial fibrillation, GI hemorrhage, hypernatremia hypotension, hypovolemia, rash, rectal bleeding, shunt thrombosis, syncope, ventricular tachycardia

Overdosage/Toxicology Symptoms include electrolyte depletion, volume depletion, hypotension, dehydration, and circulatory collapse. Electrolyte depletion may be manifested by weakness, dizziness, mental confusion, anorexia, lethargy, vomiting, and cramps. Following GI decontamination, treatment is supportive. Hypotension responds to fluids and Trendelenburg positioning.

Drug Interactions
Cytochrome P450 Effect: CYP2C9 enzyme substrate
Increased Effect/Toxicity: Torsemide-induced hypokalemia may predispose to digoxin toxicity and may increase the risk of arrhythmia with drugs which may prolong QT interval, including type Ia and type III antiarrhythmic agents, cisapride, terfenadine, and some quinolones (sparfloxacin, gatifloxacin, and moxifloxacin). The risk of toxicity from lithium and salicylates (high dose) may be increased by loop diuretics. Hypotensive effects and/or adverse renal effects of ACE inhibitors and NSAIDs are potentiated by bumetanide-induced hypovolemia. The effects of peripheral adrenergic-blocking drugs or ganglionic blockers may be increased by bumetanide.

Torsemide may increase the risk of ototoxicity with other ototoxic agents (aminoglycosides, cis-platinum), especially in patients with renal dysfunction. Synergistic diuretic effects occur with thiazide-type diuretics. Diuretics tend to be synergistic with other antihypertensive agents, and hypotension may occur.
Decreased Effect: Torsemide efficacy may be decreased with NSAIDs. Torsemide action may be reduced with probenecid. Diuretic action may be impaired in patients with cirrhosis and ascites if used with salicylates. Glucose tolerance may be decreased when used with sulfonylureas.

Ethanol/Nutrition/Herb Interactions Herb/Nutraceutical: Avoid dong quai if using for hypertension (has estrogenic activity). Avoid ephedra, yohimbe, ginseng (may worsen hypertension). Avoid garlic (may have increased antihypertensive effect).

Stability If torsemide is to be administered via continuous infusion, stability has been demonstrated through 24 hours at room temperature in plastic containers for the following fluids and concentrations:
200 mg torsemide (10 mg/mL) added to 250 mL D$_5$W, 250 mL NS or 500 mL 0.45% sodium chloride
50 mg torsemide (10 mg/mL) added to 500 mL D$_5$W, 250 mL NS or 500 mL 0.45% sodium chloride

Mechanism of Action Inhibits reabsorption of sodium and chloride in the ascending loop of Henle and distal renal tubule, interfering with the chloride-binding cotransport system, thus causing increased excretion of water, sodium, chloride, magnesium, and calcium; does not alter GFR, renal plasma flow, or acid-base balance

Pharmacodynamics/Kinetics
Onset of action: Diuresis: 30-60 minutes
Peak effect: 1-4 hours
Duration: ~6 hours
Absorption: Oral: Rapid
Protein binding, plasma: ~97% to 99%
Metabolism: Hepatic (80%) via CYP450
Bioavailability: 80% to 90%
Half-life elimination: 2-4; Cirrhosis: 7-8 hours
Excretion: Urine (20% as unchanged drug)

Usual Dosage Adults: Oral, I.V.:
Congestive heart failure: 10-20 mg once daily; may increase gradually for chronic treatment by doubling dose until the diuretic response is apparent (for acute treatment, I.V. dose may be repeated every 2 hours with double the dose as needed)
Chronic renal failure: 20 mg once daily; increase as described above
Hepatic cirrhosis: 5-10 mg once daily with an aldosterone antagonist or a potassium-sparing diuretic; increase as described above
Hypertension: 5 mg once daily; increase to 10 mg after 4-6 weeks if an adequate hypotensive response is not apparent; if still not effective, an additional antihypertensive agent may be added

Administration I.V. injections should be administered over ≥2 minutes; the oral form may be administered regardless of meal times; patients may be switched from the I.V. form to the oral (Continued)

Torsemide *(Continued)*

and vice-versa with no change in dose; no dosage adjustment is needed in the elderly or patients with hepatic impairment

To administer as a continuous infusion: 50 mg or 200 mg torsemide should be diluted in 250 mL or 500 mL of compatible solution in plastic containers

Monitoring Parameters Renal function, electrolytes, and fluid status (weight and I & O), blood pressure

Patient Information May be taken with food or milk; rise slowly from a lying or sitting position to minimize dizziness, lightheadedness or fainting; also use extra care when exercising, standing for long periods of time, and during hot weather; take dose in the morning or early in the evening to prevent nocturia; use caution with exposure to ultraviolet light

Nursing Implications

Administer the I.V. dose slowly over 2 minutes

Monitor renal function, electrolytes, and fluid states closely including weight and I & O

Additional Information 10-20 mg torsemide is approximately equivalent to furosemide 40 mg or bumetanide 1 mg.

Dosage Forms

Injection: 10 mg/mL (2 mL, 5 mL)

Tablet: 5 mg, 10 mg, 20 mg, 100 mg

- ◆ **Touro Ex**® *see Guaifenesin on page 645*
- ◆ **Touro LA**® *see Guaifenesin and Pseudoephedrine on page 647*
- ◆ **Toxicology Information** *see page 1693*
- ◆ **Toxidromes** *see page 1702*
- ◆ **tPA** *see Alteplase on page 59*
- ◆ **TPT** *see Topotecan on page 1350*
- ◆ **Tracleer**™ *see Bosentan on page 177*
- ◆ **Tracrium**® *see Atracurium on page 130*

Tramadol *(TRA ma dole)*

U.S. Brand Names Ultram®

Canadian Brand Names Ultram®

Synonyms Tramadol Hydrochloride

Therapeutic Category Analgesic, Miscellaneous

Use Relief of moderate to moderately-severe pain

Pregnancy Risk Factor C

Pregnancy/Breast-Feeding Implications Tramadol has been shown to cross the placenta. Postmarketing reports following tramadol use during pregnancy include neonatal seizures, withdrawal syndrome, fetal death and stillbirth. Not recommended for use during labor and delivery.

Contraindications Hypersensitivity to tramadol, opioids, or any component of the formulation; opioid-dependent patients; acute intoxication with alcohol, hypnotics, centrally-acting analgesics, opioids, or psychotropic drugs

Warnings/Precautions Should be used only with extreme caution in patients receiving MAO inhibitors. May cause CNS depression and/or respiratory depression, particularly when combined with other CNS depressants. Use with caution and reduce dosage when administered to patients receiving other CNS depressants. An increased risk of seizures may occur in patients receiving serotonin reuptake inhibitors (SSRIs or anorectics), tricyclic antidepressants, other cyclic compounds (including cyclobenzaprine, promethazine), neuroleptics, MAO inhibitors, or drugs which may lower seizure threshold. Patients with a history of seizures, or with a risk of seizures (head trauma, metabolic disorders, CNS infection, or malignancy, or during ethanol/drug withdrawal) are also at increased risk.

Elderly patients and patients with chronic respiratory disorders may be at greater risk of adverse events. Use with caution in patients with increased intracranial pressure or head injury. Use tramadol with caution and reduce dosage in patients with liver disease or renal dysfunction and in patients with myxedema, hypothyroidism, or hypoadrenalism. Not recommended during pregnancy or in nursing mothers. Tolerance or drug dependence may result from extended use; abrupt discontinuation should be avoided. Safety and efficacy in pediatric patients have not been established.

Adverse Reactions Incidence of some adverse effects may increase over time

>10%:

Central nervous system: Dizziness, headache, somnolence, vertigo

Gastrointestinal: Constipation, nausea

1% to 10%:

Cardiovascular: Vasodilation

Central nervous system: Agitation, anxiety, confusion, coordination impaired, emotional lability, euphoria, hallucinations, malaise, nervousness, sleep disorder, tremor

Dermatologic: Pruritus, rash

Endocrine & metabolic: Menopausal symptoms

Gastrointestinal: Abdominal pain, anorexia, diarrhea, dry mouth, dyspepsia, flatulence, vomiting

Genitourinary: Urinary frequency, urinary retention

Neuromuscular & skeletal: Hypertonia, spasticity, weakness

Ocular: Miosis, visual disturbance

Miscellaneous: Diaphoresis

<1% (Limited to important or life-threatening): Allergic reaction, amnesia, anaphylaxis, angioedema, bronchospasm, cognitive dysfunction, creatinine increased, death, depression, dyspnea, gastrointestinal bleeding, liver failure, seizure, serotonin syndrome, Stevens-Johnson syndrome, suicidal tendency, syncope, toxic epidermal necrolysis, vesicles

Overdosage/Toxicology Symptoms include CNS and respiratory depression, lethargy, coma, seizure, cardiac arrest, and death. Treatment consists of naloxone 2 mg I.V. (0.01 mg/

kg children), with repeat administration as needed up to 18 mg. Naloxone may increase the risk of seizures in tramadol overdose.

Drug Interactions

Cytochrome P450 Effect: CYP2D6 and 3A3/4 (minor) enzyme substrate

Increased Effect/Toxicity: Amphetamines may increase the risk of seizures with tramadol. Cimetidine increases the half-life of tramadol by 20% to 25%. SSRIs may increase the risk of seizures with tramadol. Tricyclic antidepressants may increase the risk of seizures. Linezolid may be associated with increased risk of seizures (due to MAO inhibition). MAO inhibitors may increases the risk of seizures. It is not clear if drugs with selective MAO type B inhibition are safer than nonselective agents. Avoid drugs with MAO activity (ie, linezolid). Naloxone may increase the risk of seizures in tramadol overdose. Neuroleptic agents may increase the risk of tramadol-associated seizures and may have additive CNS depressant effects. Opioids may increase the risk of seizures, and may have additive CNS depressant effects. Quinidine (and other inhibitors of CYP2D6) may increase the tramadol serum concentrations.

Decreased Effect: Carbamazepine may decrease analgesic efficacy of tramadol (half-life decreases 33% to 50%) and may increase the risk of seizures in patients requiring anticonvulsants.

Ethanol/Nutrition/Herb Interactions

Ethanol: Avoid ethanol (may increase CNS depression).

Food: Does not affect the rate or extent of absorption.

Herb/Nutraceutical: Avoid valerian, St John's wort, kava kava, gotu kola (may increase CNS depression).

Stability Store at controlled room temperature of 25°C (77°F).

Mechanism of Action Binds to μ-opiate receptors in the CNS causing inhibition of ascending pain pathways, altering the perception of and response to pain; also inhibits the reuptake of norepinephrine and serotonin, which also modifies the ascending pain pathway

Pharmacodynamics/Kinetics

Onset of action: ~1 hour

Duration of action: 9 hours

Absorption: Rapid and complete

Distribution: V_d: 2.5-3 L/kg

Protein binding, plasma: 20%

Metabolism: Extensively hepatic via demethylation, glucuronidation, and sulfation; has pharmacologically active metabolite formed by CYP2D6

Bioavailability: 75%

Half-life elimination: Tramadol: ~6 hours; Active metabolite: 7 hours; prolonged in elderly, hepatic or renal dysfunction

Time to peak: 2 hours

Excretion: Urine, as metabolites

Usual Dosage Oral:

Adults: Moderate to severe chronic pain: 50-100 mg every 4-6 hours, not to exceed 400 mg/day

For patients not requiring rapid onset of effect, tolerability may be improved by starting dose at 25 mg/day and titrating dose by 25 mg every 3 days, until reaching 25 mg 4 times/day. Dose may then be increased by 50 mg every 3 days as tolerated, to reach dose of 50 mg 4 times/day.

Elderly: >75 years: 50-100 mg every 4-6 hours (not to exceed 300 mg/day); see dosing adjustments for renal and hepatic impairment

Dosing adjustment in renal impairment: Cl_{cr} <30 mL/minute: Administer 50-100 mg dose every 12 hours (maximum: 200 mg/day)

Dosing adjustment in hepatic impairment: Cirrhosis: Recommended dose: 50 mg every 12 hours

Dietary Considerations May be taken with or without food.

Monitoring Parameters Pain relief, respiratory rate, blood pressure, and pulse; signs of tolerance or abuse

Reference Range 100-300 ng/mL; however, serum level monitoring is not required

Patient Information Avoid driving or operating machinery until the effect of drug wears off. Report cravings to your physician immediately

Nursing Implications Driving or operating machinery should be avoided until the effect of drug wears off. Cravings should be reported to physician immediately.

Dosage Forms Tablet, as hydrochloride: 50 mg

- ◆ **Tramadol Hydrochloride** *see* Tramadol *on page 1354*
- ◆ **Tramadol Hydrochloride and Acetaminophen** *see* Acetaminophen and Tramadol *on page 26*
- ◆ **Trandate®** *see* Labetalol *on page 768*

Trandolapril (tran DOE la pril)

Related Information

Angiotensin Agents Comparison *on page 1473*

Heart Failure *on page 1663*

U.S. Brand Names Mavik®

Canadian Brand Names Mavik™

Therapeutic Category Angiotensin-Converting Enzyme (ACE) Inhibitor; Antihypertensive Agent

Use Management of hypertension alone or in combination with other antihypertensive agents; treatment of left ventricular dysfunction after myocardial infarction

Unlabeled/Investigational Use As a class, ACE inhibitors are recommended in the treatment of systolic congestive heart failure

Pregnancy Risk Factor C/D (2nd and 3rd trimesters)

(Continued)

Trandolapril *(Continued)*

Contraindications Hypersensitivity to trandolapril or any component of the formulation; history of angioedema-related to previous treatment with an ACE inhibitor; bilateral renal artery stenosis; primary hyperaldosteronism; pregnancy (2nd and 3rd trimesters)

Warnings/Precautions Neutropenia, agranulocytosis, angioedema, decreased renal function (hypertension, renal artery stenosis, CHF), hepatic dysfunction (elimination, activation), proteinuria, first-dose hypotension (hypovolemia, CHF, dehydrated patients at risk, eg, diuretic use, elderly), elderly (due to renal function changes); use with caution and modify dosage in patients with renal impairment (Cl_{cr} <30 mL/minute); use with caution in patients with collagen vascular disease, CHF, hypovolemia, valvular stenosis, hyperkalemia (>5.7 mEq/L), anesthesia

Patients taking diuretics are at risk for developing hypotension on initial dosing; to prevent this, discontinue diuretics 2-3 days prior to initiating trandolapril; may restart diuretics if blood pressure is not controlled by trandolapril alone

Adverse Reactions Note: Frequency ranges include data from hypertension and heart failure trials. Higher rates of adverse reactions have generally been noted in patients with congestive heart failure. However, the frequency of adverse effects associated with placebo is also increased in this population.

>1%:
   Cardiovascular: Hypotension (<1% to 11%), bradycardia (<1% to 4.7%), intermittent claudication (3.8%), stroke (3.3%)
   Central nervous system: Dizziness (1.3% to 23%), syncope (5.9%), asthenia (3.3%)
   Endocrine & metabolic: Elevated uric acid (15%), hyperkalemia (5.3%), hypocalcemia (4.7%)
   Gastrointestinal: Dyspepsia (6.4%), gastritis (4.2%)
   Neuromuscular & skeletal: Myalgia (4.7%)
   Renal: Elevated BUN (9%), elevated serum creatinine (1.1% to 4.7%) Respiratory: Cough (1.9% to 35%)
   <1% (Limited to important or life-threatening): Angina, angioedema, anxiety, AV block (first-degree), dyspnea, gout, impotence, increased ALT, increased serum creatinine, insomnia, laryngeal edema, muscle pain, neutropenia, pancreatitis, paresthesia, pruritus, rash, symptomatic hypotension, thrombocytopenia, vertigo. Worsening of renal function may occur in patients with bilateral renal artery stenosis or in hypovolemic patients. In addition, a syndrome which may include fever, myalgia, arthralgia, interstitial nephritis, vasculitis, rash, eosinophilia and positive ANA, and elevated ESR has been reported with ACE inhibitors.

Overdosage/Toxicology Symptoms include hypertension, vertigo, and dizziness. Following initiation of essential overdose management, toxic symptom treatment and supportive treatment should be initiated. Hypotension usually responds to I.V. fluids or Trendelenburg positioning. If unresponsive to these measures, the use of a parenteral inotrope may be required (eg, norepinephrine 0.1-0.2 mcg/kg/minute titrated to response). Seizures commonly respond to diazepam (I.V. 5-10 mg bolus in adults every 15 minutes, if needed, up to a total of 30 mg) or to phenytoin or phenobarbital.

Drug Interactions
   Increased Effect/Toxicity: Potassium supplements, co-trimoxazole (high dose), angiotensin II receptor antagonists (candesartan, losartan, irbesartan, etc) or potassium-sparing diuretics (amiloride, spironolactone, triamterene) may result in elevated serum potassium levels when combined with trandolapril. ACE inhibitor effects may be increased by phenothiazines or probenecid (increases levels of captopril). ACE inhibitors may increase serum concentrations/effects of digoxin, lithium, and sulfonlyureas.

   Diuretics have additive hypotensive effects with ACE inhibitors, and hypovolemia increases the potential for adverse renal effects of ACE inhibitors. In patients with compromised renal function, coadministration with nonsteroidal anti-inflammatory drugs may result in further deterioration of renal function. Allopurinol and ACE inhibitors may cause a higher risk of hypersensitivity reaction when taken concurrently.

   Decreased Effect: Aspirin (high dose) may reduce the therapeutic effects of ACE inhibitors; at low dosages this does not appear to be significant. Rifampin may decrease the effect of ACE inhibitors. Antacids may decrease the bioavailability of ACE inhibitors (may be more likely to occur with captopril); separate administration times by 1-2 hours. NSAIDs, specifically indomethacin, may reduce the hypotensive effects of ACE inhibitors. More likely to occur in low renin or volume dependent hypertensive patients.

Ethanol/Nutrition/Herb Interactions Herb/Nutraceutical: Avoid dong quai if using for hypertension (has estrogenic activity). Avoid ephedra, yohimbe, ginseng (may worsen hypertension). Avoid garlic (may have increased antihypertensive effect).

Mechanism of Action Trandolapril is an angiotensin-converting enzyme (ACE) inhibitor which prevents the formation of angiotensin II from angiotensin I. Trandolapril must undergo enzymatic hydrolysis, mainly in liver, to its biologically active metabolite, trandolaprilat. A CNS mechanism may also be involved in the hypotensive effect as angiotensin II increases adrenergic outflow from the CNS. Vasoactive kallikrein's may be decreased in conversion to active hormones by ACE inhibitors, thus, reducing blood pressure.

Pharmacodynamics/Kinetics
   Onset of action: 1-2 hours
      Peak effect: Reduction in blood pressure: 6 hours
   Duration: Prolonged; 72 hours after single dose
   Absorption: Rapid
   Distribution: Trandolaprilat (active metabolite) is very lipophilic in comparison to other ACE inhibitors
   Metabolism: Hydrolyzed hepatically to active metabolite, trandolaprilat
   Half-life elimination:
      Trandolapril: 6 hours; Trandolaprilat: Effective: 10 hours, Terminal: 24 hours
   Elimination: As metabolites in urine;
   Time to peak: Parent: 1 hour; Active metabolite trandolaprilat: 4-10 hours

Excretion: Urine (as metabolites)
  Clearance: Reduce dose in renal failure; creatinine clearances ≤30 mL/minute result in accumulation of active metabolite

Usual Dosage Adults: Oral:

Hypertension: Initial dose in patients not receiving a diuretic: 1 mg/day (2 mg/day in black patients). Adjust dosage according to the blood pressure response. Make dosage adjustments at intervals of ≥1 week. Most patients have required dosages of 2-4 mg/day. There is a little experience with doses >8 mg/day. Patients inadequately treated with once daily dosing at 4 mg may be treated with twice daily dosing. If blood pressure is not adequately controlled with trandolapril monotherapy, a diuretic may be added.

Heart failure postmyocardial infarction or left ventricular dysfunction postmyocardial infarction: Initial: 1 mg/day; titrate patients (as tolerated) towards the target dose of 4 mg/day. If a 4 mg dose is not tolerated, patients can continue therapy with the greatest tolerated dose.

Dosing adjustment in renal impairment: Cl$_{cr}$ ≤30 mL/minute: Recommended starting dose: 0.5 mg/day.

Dosing adjustment in hepatic impairment: Cirrhosis: Recommended starting dose: 0.5 mg/day.

Monitoring Parameters Serum potassium, renal function, serum creatinine, BUN, CBC

Patient Information Do not discontinue medication without advice of physician; notify physician if sore throat, swelling, palpitations, cough, chest pains, difficulty swallowing, swelling of face, eyes, tongue, lips, hoarseness, sweating, vomiting, or diarrhea occurs; may cause dizziness, lightheadedness during first few days; may also cause changes in taste perception; do not use salt substitutes containing potassium without consulting a physician

Nursing Implications May cause depression in some patients; discontinue if angioedema of the face, extremities, lips, tongue, or glottis occurs; watch for hypotensive effects within 1-3 hours of first dose or new higher dose

Dosage Forms Tablet: 1 mg, 2 mg, 4 mg

Trandolapril and Verapamil (tran DOE la pril & ver AP a mil)

U.S. Brand Names Tarka®

Synonyms Verapamil and Trandolapril

Therapeutic Category Angiotensin-Converting Enzyme (ACE) Inhibitor Combination; Antihypertensive Agent, Combination

Use Combination drug for the treatment of hypertension, however, not indicated for initial treatment of hypertension; replacement therapy in patients receiving separate dosage forms (for patient convenience); when monotherapy with one component fails to achieve desired antihypertensive effect, or when dose-limiting adverse effects limit upward titration of monotherapy

Pregnancy Risk Factor C/D (2nd and 3rd trimesters)

Usual Dosage Dose is individualized

Additional Information Complete prescribing information for this medication should be consulted for additional detail.

Dosage Forms
  Tablet, combination (trandolapril component is immediate release, verapamil component is sustained release):
    Trandolapril 1 mg and verapamil hydrochloride 240 mg
    Trandolapril 2 mg and verapamil hydrochloride 180 mg
    Trandolapril 2 mg and verapamil hydrochloride 240 mg
    Trandolapril 4 mg and verapamil hydrochloride 240 mg

Tranexamic Acid (tran eks AM ik AS id)

U.S. Brand Names Cyklokapron®

Canadian Brand Names Cyklokapron®

Therapeutic Category Antihemophilic Agent

Use Short-term use (2-8 days) in hemophilia patients during and following tooth extraction to reduce or prevent hemorrhage

Unlabeled/Investigational Use Has been used as an alternative to aminocaproic acid for subarachnoid hemorrhage

Pregnancy Risk Factor B

Contraindications Acquired defective color vision; active intravascular clotting; subarachnoid hemorrhage; concurrent factor IX complex or anti-inhibitor coagulant concentrates

Warnings/Precautions Dosage modification required in patients with renal impairment; ophthalmic exam before and during therapy required if patient is treated beyond several days; caution in patients with cardiovascular, renal, or cerebrovascular disease; when used for subarachnoid hemorrhage, ischemic complications may occur; history of thrombolism may increase risk for venous or arterial thrombosis

Adverse Reactions
  >10%: Gastrointestinal: Nausea, diarrhea, vomiting
  1% to 10%:
    Cardiovascular: Hypotension, thrombosis
    Ocular: Blurred vision
  <1% (Limited to important or life-threatening): Deep venous thrombosis, pulmonary embolus, renal cortical necrosis, retinal artery obstruction, retinal vein obstruction, unusual menstrual discomfort, ureteral obstruction

Drug Interactions
  Increased Effect/Toxicity: Chlorpromazine may increase cerebral vasospasm and ischemia. Coadministrations of Factor IX complex or anti-inhibitor coagulant concentrates may increase risk of thrombosis.

Stability Incompatible with solutions containing penicillin

Mechanism of Action Forms a reversible complex that displaces plasminogen from fibrin resulting in inhibition of fibrinolysis; it also inhibits the proteolytic activity of plasmin

Pharmacodynamics/Kinetics
  Half-life elimination: 2-10 hours
  (Continued)

Tranexamic Acid *(Continued)*

Excretion: Primarily urine (>90% as unchanged drug)

Usual Dosage Children and Adults: I.V.: 10 mg/kg immediately before surgery, then 25 mg/kg/dose orally 3-4 times/day for 2-8 days

Alternatively:

Oral: 25 mg/kg 3-4 times/day beginning 1 day prior to surgery

I.V.: 10 mg/kg 3-4 times/day in patients who are unable to take oral

Dosing adjustment/interval in renal impairment:

Cl_{cr} 50-80 mL/minute: Administer 50% of normal dose or 10 mg/kg twice daily I.V. or 15 mg/kg twice daily orally

Cl_{cr} 10-50 mL/minute: Administer 25% of normal dose or 10 mg/kg/day I.V. or 15 mg/kg/day orally

Cl_{cr} <10 mL/minute: Administer 10% of normal dose or 10 mg/kg/dose every 48 hours I.V. or 15 mg/kg/dose every 48 hours orally

Administration May be administered by direct I.V. injection at a maximum rate of 100 mg/minute; compatible with dextrose, saline, and electrolyte solutions; use plastic syringe only for I.V. push

Reference Range 5-10 µg/mL is required to decrease fibrinolysis

Patient Information Report any signs of bleeding or myopathy, changes in vision; GI upset usually disappears when dose is reduced

Nursing Implications Dosage modification required in patients with renal impairment

Dosage Forms

Injection: 100 mg/mL (10 mL)

Tablet: 500 mg

- **Transamine Sulphate** *see* Tranylcypromine *on page 1358*
- **Transderm-Nitro®** (Can) *see* Nitroglycerin *on page 989*
- **Transderm-Nitro® Patch** *see* Nitroglycerin *on page 989*
- **Transderm Scōp®** *see* Scopolamine *on page 1225*
- **Transderm-V®** (Can) *see* Scopolamine *on page 1225*
- **trans-Retinoic Acid** *see* Tretinoin (Topical) *on page 1365*
- **Tranxene®** *see* Clorazepate *on page 322*

Tranylcypromine *(tran il SIP roe meen)*

Related Information

Antidepressant Agents Comparison *on page 1482*

Tyramine Content of Foods *on page 1737*

U.S. Brand Names Parnate®

Canadian Brand Names Parnate®

Synonyms Transamine Sulphate; Tranylcypromine Sulfate

Therapeutic Category Antidepressant, Monoamine Oxidase Inhibitor

Use Treatment of major depressive episode without melancholia

Unlabeled/Investigational Use Post-traumatic stress disorder

Pregnancy Risk Factor C

Contraindications Hypersensitivity to tranylcypromine or any component of the formulation; uncontrolled hypertension; pheochromocytoma; hepatic or renal disease; cerebrovascular defect; cardiovascular disease (CHF); concurrent use of sympathomimetics (and related compounds), CNS depressants, ethanol, meperidine, bupropion, buspirone, dexfenfluramine, dextromethorphan, guanethidine, and serotonergic drugs (including SSRIs) - do not use within 5 weeks of fluoxetine discontinuation or 2 weeks of other antidepressant discontinuation; general anesthesia (discontinue 10 days prior to elective surgery); local vasoconstrictors; spinal anesthesia (hypotension may be exaggerated); foods which are high in tyramine, tryptophan, or dopamine, chocolate, or caffeine.

Warnings/Precautions Safety in children <16 years of age has not been established; use with caution in patients who are hyperactive, hyperexcitable, or who have glaucoma, suicidal tendencies, hyperthyroidism, or diabetes; avoid use of meperidine within 2 weeks of phenelzine use. Toxic reactions have occurred with dextromethorphan. Hypertensive crisis may occur with tyramine, tryptophan, or dopamine-containing foods. Should not be used in combination with other antidepressants. Hypotensive effects of antihypertensives (beta-blockers, thiazides) may be exaggerated. Use with caution in depressed patients at risk of suicide. May cause orthostatic hypotension (especially at dosages >30 mg/day) - use with caution in patients with hypotension or patients who would not tolerate transient hypotensive episodes - effects may be additive when used with other agents known to cause orthostasis (phenothiazines). Has been associated with activation of hypomania and/or mania in bipolar patients. May worsen psychotic symptoms in some patients. Use with caution in patients at risk of seizures, or in patients receiving other drugs which may lower seizure threshold. Discontinue at least 48 hours prior to myelography. Use with caution in patients receiving disulfiram. Use with caution in patients with renal impairment.

The MAO inhibitors are effective and generally well tolerated by older patients. It is the potential interactions with tyramine or tryptophan-containing foods and other drugs, and their effects on blood pressure that have limited their use.

Adverse Reactions Frequency not defined.

Cardiovascular: Orthostatic hypotension, edema

Central nervous system: Dizziness, headache, drowsiness, sleep disturbances, fatigue, hyper-reflexia, twitching, ataxia, mania, akinesia, confusion, disorientation, memory loss

Dermatologic: Rash, pruritus, urticaria, localized scleroderma, cystic acne (flare), alopecia

Endocrine & metabolic: Sexual dysfunction (anorgasmia, ejaculatory disturbances, impotence), hypernatremia, hypermetabolic syndrome, SIADH

Gastrointestinal: Xerostomia, constipation, weight gain

Genitourinary: Urinary retention, incontinence

Hematologic: Leukopenia, agranulocytosis

Hepatic: Hepatitis

Neuromuscular & skeletal: Weakness, tremor, myoclonus
Ocular: Blurred vision, glaucoma
Miscellaneous: Diaphoresis

Overdosage/Toxicology Symptoms include tachycardia, palpitations, muscle twitching, seizures, insomnia, transient hypotension, hypertension, hyperpyrexia, and coma. Competent supportive care is the most important treatment for an overdose with a monoamine oxidase (MAO) inhibitor. Both hypertension or hypotension can occur with intoxication. Hypotension may respond to I.V. fluids or vasopressors, and hypertension usually responds to an alpha-adrenergic blocker. While treating hypertension, care is warranted to avoid sudden drops in blood pressure, since this may worsen MAO inhibitor toxicity. Muscle irritability and seizures often respond to diazepam, while hyperthermia is best treated with antipyretics and cooling blankets. Cardiac arrhythmias are best treated with phenytoin or procainamide.

Drug Interactions
Cytochrome P450 Effect: CYP2A6 and 2C19 enzyme inhibitor
Increased Effect/Toxicity: In general, the combined use of tranylcypromine with TCAs, venlafaxine, trazodone, dexfenfluramine, sibutramine, lithium, meperidine, fenfluramine, dextromethorphan, and SSRIs should be avoided due to the potential for severe adverse reactions (serotonin syndrome, death). Tranylcypromine in combination with amphetamines, other stimulants (methylphenidate), levodopa, metaraminol, buspirone, bupropion, reserpine, and decongestants (pseudoephedrine) may result in severe hypertensive reactions. MAO inhibitors (including tranylcypromine) may inhibit the metabolism of barbiturates and prolong their effect. Foods (eg, cheese) and beverages (eg, ethanol) containing tyramine should be avoided; hypertensive crisis may result. Tranylcypromine may increase the pressor response of norepinephrine and may prolong neuromuscular blockade produced by succinylcholine. Tramadol may increase the risk of seizures and serotonin syndrome in patients receiving an MAO inhibitor. Tranylcypromine may produce additive hypoglycemic effect in patients receiving hypoglycemic agents and may produce delirium in patients receiving disulfiram. Tryptophan combined use with an MAO inhibitor has been reported to cause disorientation, confusion, anxiety, delirium, agitation, hypomanic signs, ataxia, and myoclonus; concurrent use is contraindicated.
Decreased Effect: Tranylcypromine inhibits the antihypertensive response to guanadrel or guanethidine.

Ethanol/Nutrition/Herb Interactions
Ethanol: Avoid ethanol (many contain tyramine).
Food: Clinically-severe elevated blood pressure may occur if tranylcypromine is taken with tyramine-containing food. Avoid foods containing tryptophan or dopamine, chocolate or caffeine.
Herb/Nutraceutical: Avoid valerian, St John's wort, SAMe, ginseng. Avoid ginkgo (may lead to MAO inhibitor toxicity). Avoid ephedra, yohimbe (can cause hypertension).

Mechanism of Action Thought to act by increasing endogenous concentrations of epinephrine, norepinephrine, dopamine and serotonin through inhibition of the enzyme (monoamine oxidase) responsible for the breakdown of these neurotransmitters

Pharmacodynamics/Kinetics
Onset of action: Therapeutic: 2-3 weeks continued dosing
Duration: May continue to have a therapeutic effect and interactions 2 weeks after discontinuing therapy
Half-life elimination: 90-190 minutes
Time to peak, serum: ~2 hours
Excretion: Urine

Usual Dosage Adults: Oral: 10 mg twice daily, increase by 10 mg increments at 1- to 3-week intervals; maximum: 60 mg/day
Dosing comments in hepatic impairment: Use with care and monitor plasma levels and patient response closely

Dietary Considerations Avoid food which contains high amounts of tyramine. Avoid foods containing tryptophan or dopamine, including chocolate and caffeine.

Monitoring Parameters Blood pressure, blood glucose

Patient Information Tablets may be crushed; avoid alcohol; do not discontinue abruptly; avoid foods high in tyramine (eg, aged cheeses, Chianti wine, raisins, liver, bananas, chocolate, yogurt, sour cream); discuss list of drugs and foods to avoid with pharmacist or physician; arise slowly from prolonged sitting or lying

Nursing Implications Assist with ambulation during initiation of therapy; monitor blood pressure closely, patients should be cautioned against eating foods high in tyramine or tryptophan (cheese, wine, beer, pickled herring, dry sausage)

Additional Information Tranylcypromine has a more rapid onset of therapeutic effect than other MAO inhibitors, but causes more severe hypertensive reactions.

Dosage Forms Tablet, as sulfate: 10 mg

♦ **Tranylcypromine Sulfate** *see* Tranylcypromine *on page 1358*

Trastuzumab (tras TU zoo mab)

U.S. Brand Names Herceptin®
Canadian Brand Names Herceptin®
Therapeutic Category Antineoplastic Agent, Natural Source (Plant) Derivative; Monoclonal Antibody
Use
Single agent for the treatment of patients with metastatic breast cancer whose tumors overexpress the HER-2/*neu* protein and who have received one or more chemotherapy regimens for their metastatic disease
Combination therapy with paclitaxel for the treatment of patients with metastatic breast cancer whose tumors overexpress the HER-2/*neu* protein and who have not received chemotherapy for their metastatic disease
Note: HER-2/*neu* protein overexpression or amplification has been noted in ovarian, gastric, colorectal, endometrial, lung, bladder, prostate, and salivary gland tumors. It is not yet
(Continued)

Trastuzumab *(Continued)*

known whether trastuzumab may be effective in these other carcinomas which overexpress HER-2/*neu* protein.

Pregnancy Risk Factor B

Pregnancy/Breast-Feeding Implications It is not known whether trastuzumab is secreted in human milk; because many immunoglobulins are secreted in milk, and the potential for serious adverse reactions exists, patients should discontinue nursing during treatment and for 6 months after the last dose

Contraindications No specific contraindications noted in product labeling. However, patients experiencing severe hypersensitivity reactions have been reported to have repeat episodes despite pretreatment with antihistamines and corticosteroids.

Warnings/Precautions Congestive heart failure associated with trastuzumab may be severe and has been associated with disabling cardiac failure, death, mural thrombus, and stroke. Left ventricular function should be evaluated in all patients prior to and during treatment with trastuzumab. Discontinuation should be strongly considered in patients who develop a clinically significant decrease in ejection fraction during therapy. Combination therapy which includes anthracyclines and cyclophosphamide increases the incidence and severity of cardiac dysfunction. Extreme caution should be used when treating patients with pre-existing cardiac disease or dysfunction, and in patients with previous exposure to anthracyclines. Advanced age may also predispose to cardiac toxicity. Hypersensitivity to hamster ovary cell proteins or any component of this product.

Serious adverse events, including hypersensitivity reaction (anaphylaxis), infusion reactions (including fatalities), and pulmonary events (including adult respiratory distress syndrome) have been associated with trastuzumab. Most of these events occur within 24 hours of infusion, however delayed reactions have occurred. Use with caution in pre-existing pulmonary disease. Discontinuation of trastuzumab should be strongly considered in any patient who develops anaphylaxis, angioedema, or acute respiratory distress syndrome. Retreatment of patients who experienced severe hypersensitivity reactions has been attempted (with premedication). Some patients tolerated retreatment, while others experienced a second severe reaction.

Adverse Reactions The most common reactions were infusion-associated, occurring in up to 40% of patients, consisting primarily of fever and/or chills which were mild to moderate in severity. These may be treated with acetaminophen, diphenhydramine, and meperidine with or without reduction of the infusion rate.

>10%:

Central nervous system: Pain (47%), fever (36%), chills (32%), headache (26%)

Dermatologic: Rash (18%)

Gastrointestinal: Nausea (33%), diarrhea (25%), vomiting (23%), abdominal pain (22%), anorexia (14%)

Neuromuscular & skeletal: Weakness (42%), back pain (22%)

Respiratory: Cough (26%), dyspnea (22%), rhinitis (14%), pharyngitis (12%)

Miscellaneous: Infection (20%)

1% to 10%:

Cardiovascular: Peripheral edema (10%), congestive heart failure (7%), tachycardia (5%)

Central nervous system: Insomnia (14%), dizziness (13%), paresthesia (9%), depression (6%), peripheral neuritis (2%), neuropathy (1%)

Dermatologic: Herpes simplex (2%), acne (2%)

Gastrointestinal: Nausea and vomiting (8%)

Genitourinary: Urinary tract infection (5%)

Hematologic: Anemia (4%), leukopenia (3%)

Neuromuscular & skeletal: Bone pain (7%), arthralgia (6%)

Respiratory: Sinusitis (9%)

Miscellaneous: Flu syndrome (10%), accidental injury (6%), allergic reaction (3%)

<1% (Limited to important or life-threatening): Amblyopia, anaphylactoid reaction, arrhythmia, ascites, cardiac arrest, cellulitis, coagulopathy, deafness, esophageal ulcer, hematemesis, hemorrhage, hepatic failure, hepatitis, hydrocephalus, hypotension, hypothyroidism, ileus, intestinal obstruction, pancreatitis, pancytopenia, pericardial effusion, radiation injury, shock, stomatitis, syncope, vascular thrombosis

Overdosage/Toxicology There is no experience with overdosage in human trials. Single doses >500 mg have not been tested.

Drug Interactions

Increased Effect/Toxicity: Paclitaxel may result in a decrease in clearance of trastuzumab, increasing serum concentrations.

Stability Store intact vials under refrigeration (2°C to 8°C/36°F to 46°F) prior to reconstitution. Reconstituted each vial with 20 mL of bacteriostatic sterile water for injection. Do not shake. This solution results in a concentration of 21 mg/mL and is stable for 28 days from the date of reconstitution under refrigeration. If the patient has a known hypersensitivity to benzyl alcohol, trastuzumab may be reconstituted with sterile water for injection which must be used immediately.

Determine the dose of trastuzumab and further dilute to an infusion bag containing 0.9% sodium chloride. **Dextrose 5% solution CANNOT BE used.** This solution is stable for 24 hours at room temperature. However, since diluted trastuzumab contains no effective preservative, the reconstituted and diluted solution should be stored under refrigeration (2°C to 8°C).

Mechanism of Action Trastuzumab is a monoclonal antibody which binds to the extracellular domain of the human epidermal growth factor receptor 2 protein (HER2); it mediates antibody-dependent cellular cytotoxicity against cells which overproduce HER2

Pharmacodynamics/Kinetics

Distribution: V_d: 44 mL/kg

Half-life elimination: Mean: 5.8 days (range: 1-32 days)

Usual Dosage I.V. infusion:

Adults:

Initial loading dose: 4 mg/kg intravenous infusion over 90 minutes

Maintenance dose: 2 mg/kg intravenous infusion over 90 minutes (can be administered over 30 minutes if prior infusions are well tolerated) weekly until disease progression

Dosing adjustment in renal impairment: Data suggest that the disposition of trastuzumab is not altered based on age or serum creatinine (up to 2 mg/dL); however, no formal interaction studies have been performed

Dosing adjustment in hepatic impairment: No data is currently available

Administration Administer initial infusion over 90 minutes. Subsequent weekly infusions may be administered over 30 minutes if prior infusions are well tolerated. During the first infusion with trastuzumab, a complex of symptoms most commonly consisting of chills, and/or fever were observed in ~ 40% of patients. These symptoms were usually mild to moderate in severity and were treated with acetaminophen, diphenhydramine and meperidine (with or without reduction in the rate of trastuzumab infusion). These symptoms occurred infrequently with subsequent trastuzumab infusions.

Monitoring Parameters Signs and symptoms of cardiac dysfunction; monitor vital signs during infusion

Dosage Forms Injection, vial: 440 mg, with vial of bacteriostatic water for injection

♦ **Trasylol**® *see* Aprotinin *on page 111*

♦ **Travatan**™ *see* Travoprost *on page 1361*

Travoprost (TRA voe prost)

Related Information

Glaucoma Drug Therapy Comparison *on page 1499*

U.S. Brand Names Travatan™

Therapeutic Category Prostaglandin, Ophthalmic

Use Reduction of elevated intraocular pressure in patients with open-angle glaucoma or ocular hypertension who are intolerant to the other IOP-lowering medications or insufficiently responsive (failed to achieve target IOP determined after multiple measurements over time) to another IOP-lowering medication

Pregnancy Risk Factor C

Pregnancy/Breast-Feeding Implications May interfere with the maintenance of pregnancy. Do not use during pregnancy or in women attempting to become pregnant. Teratogenic effects in humans are not known. Excretion in breast milk unknown; use caution.

Contraindications Hypersensitivity to travoprost or any component of the formulation; pregnancy

Warnings/Precautions May permanently change/increase brown pigmentation of the iris, the eyelid skin, and eyelashes. In addition, may increase the length and/or number of eyelashes (may vary between eyes); changes occur slowly and may not be noticeable for months or years. Bacterial keratitis, caused by inadvertent contamination of multiple-dose ophthalmic solutions, has been reported. Use caution in patients with intraocular inflammation, aphakic patients, pseudophakic patients with a torn posterior lens capsule, or patients with risk factors for macular edema. Contains benzalkonium chloride which may be adsorbed by contact lenses; remove contacts prior to administration and wait 15 minutes before reinserting. Contact with contents of vial should be avoided in women who are pregnant or attempting to become pregnant; in case of accidental exposure to the skin, wash the exposed area with soap and water immediately. Safety and efficacy for use in patients with renal or hepatic impairment, angle-closure-, inflammatory-, or neovascular glaucoma. Safety and efficacy in pediatric patients have not been established.

Adverse Reactions

>10%: Ocular: Hyperemia (35% to 50%)

5% to 10%: Ocular: Decreased visual acuity, eye discomfort, foreign body sensation, pain, pruritus

1% to 5%:

Cardiovascular: Angina pectoris, bradycardia, hypotension, hypertension

Central nervous system: Depression, pain, anxiety, headache

Endocrine & metabolic: Hypercholesterolemia

Gastrointestinal: Dyspepsia

Genitourinary: Prostate disorder, urinary incontinence

Neuromuscular & skeletal: Arthritis, back pain, chest pain

Ocular (1% to 4%): Abnormal vision, blepharitis, blurred vision, conjunctivitis, dry eye, iris discoloration, keratitis, lid margin crusting, photophobia, subconjunctival hemorrhage, cataract, tearing, periorbital skin discoloration (darkening), eyelash darkening, eyelash growth increased

Respiratory: Bronchitis, sinusitis

Postmarketing and/or case reports: Bacterial keratitis (due to solution contamination)

Stability Store between 2°C to 25°C (36°F to 77°F); discard within 6 weeks of removing from sealed pouch

Mechanism of Action A selective FP prostanoid receptor agonist which lowers intraocular pressure by increasing outflow

Pharmacodynamics/Kinetics

Onset of action: ~2 hours

Peak effect: 12 hours

Duration: Plasma levels decrease to <10 pg/mL within 1 hour

Absorption: Absorbed via cornea

Metabolism: Hydrolyzed by esterases in the cornea to active free acid; systemically; the free acid is metabolized to inactive metabolites

Usual Dosage Ophthalmic: Adults: Glaucoma (open angle) or ocular hypertension: Instill 1 drop into affected eye(s) once daily in the evening; do not exceed once-daily dosing (may decrease IOP-lowering effect). If used with other topical ophthalmic agents, separate administration by at least 5 minutes.

(Continued)

Travoprost *(Continued)*

Administration May be used with other eye drops to lower intraocular pressure. If using more than one ophthalmic product, wait at least 5 minutes in between application of each medication. Remove contact lenses prior to administration and wait 15 minutes before reinserting.

Patient Information Wash hands before instilling. Sit or lie down to instill. Open eye, look at ceiling, and instill prescribed amount of solution. Apply gentle pressure to inner corner of eye. Do not let tip of applicator touch eye; do not contaminate tip of applicator (contamination may cause eye infection leading to possible eye damage or vision loss). Contact prescriber concerning continued use of drops if eye infection develops, trauma occurs to the eye, and prior to eye surgery. This product contains benzalkonium chloride which may be adsorbed by contact lenses; remove contacts prior to administration and wait 15 minutes before reinserting. May cause permanent changes in eye color (increases the amount of brown pigment in the iris), eyelid, and eyelashes. May also increase the length and/or number of eyelashes. Changes may occur slowly (months to years). May be used with other eye drops to lower intraocular pressure. If using more than one eye drop medicine, wait at least 5 minutes in between application of each medication. Notify prescriber if conjunctivitis or eyelid reactions occur with use of this product.

Nursing Implications May be used with other eye drops to lower intraocular pressure. If using more than one ophthalmic product, wait at least 5 minutes in between application of each medication.

Additional Information The IOP-lowering effect was shown to be 7-8 mm Hg in clinical studies. The mean IOP reduction in African-American patients was up to 1.8 mm Hg greater than in non-African-American patients. The reason for this effect is unknown.

Dosage Forms Solution, ophthalmic: 0.004% [contains benzalkonium chloride] (2.5 mL)

Trazodone *(TRAZ oh done)*

Related Information
Antidepressant Agents Comparison *on page 1482*

U.S. Brand Names Desyrel®

Canadian Brand Names Alti-Trazodone Apo®-Trazodone; Apo®-Trazodone D; Desyrel®; Gen-Trazodone; Novo-Trazodone; Nu-Trazodone; PMS-Trazodone; Trazorel

Synonyms Trazodone Hydrochloride

Therapeutic Category Antidepressant, Miscellaneous

Use Treatment of depression

Unlabeled/Investigational Use Potential augmenting agent for antidepressants, hypnotic

Pregnancy Risk Factor C

Contraindications Hypersensitivity to trazodone or any component of the formulation

Warnings/Precautions Safety and efficacy in children <18 years of age have not been established; monitor closely and use with extreme caution in patients with cardiac disease or arrhythmias. Very sedating, but little anticholinergic effects; therapeutic effects may take up to 4 weeks to occur; therapy is normally maintained for several months after optimum response is reached to prevent recurrence of depression.

Adverse Reactions
>10%:
Central nervous system: Dizziness, headache, sedation
Gastrointestinal: Nausea, xerostomia
1% to 10%:
Cardiovascular: Syncope, hypertension, hypotension, edema
Central nervous system: Confusion, decreased concentration, fatigue, incoordination
Gastrointestinal: Diarrhea, constipation, weight gain/loss
Neuromuscular & skeletal: Tremor, myalgia
Ocular: Blurred vision
Respiratory: Nasal congestion
<1% (Limited to important or life-threatening): Agitation, bradycardia, extrapyramidal reactions, hepatitis, priapism, rash, seizures, tachycardia, urinary retention

Overdosage/Toxicology Symptoms include drowsiness, vomiting, hypotension, tachycardia, incontinence, coma, and priapism. Following initiation of essential overdose management, toxic symptoms should be treated. Ventricular arrhythmias often respond to lidocaine 1.5 mg/kg bolus, followed by 2 mg/minute infusion with concurrent systemic alkalinization (sodium bicarbonate 0.5-2 mEq/kg I.V.). Seizures usually respond to diazepam I.V. boluses (5-10 mg for adults up to 30 mg or 0.25-0.4 mg/kg/dose for children up to 10 mg/dose). If seizures are unresponsive or recur, phenytoin or phenobarbital may be required. Hypotension is best treated by I.V. fluids and by Trendelenburg positioning.

Drug Interactions
Cytochrome P450 Effect: CYP2D6 and 3A3/4 enzyme substrate
Increased Effect/Toxicity: Trazodone, in combination with other serotonergic agents (buspirone, MAO inhibitors), may produce additive serotonergic effects, including serotonin syndrome. Trazodone, in combination with other psychotropics (low potency antipsychotics), may result in additional hypotension. Trazodone, in combination with ethanol, may result in additive sedation and impairment of motor skills. Fluoxetine may inhibit the metabolism of trazodone resulting in elevated plasma levels.
Decreased Effect: Trazodone inhibits the hypotensive response to clonidine.

Ethanol/Nutrition/Herb Interactions
Ethanol: Avoid ethanol (may increase CNS depression).
Food: Time to peak serum levels may be increased if trazodone is taken with food.
Herb/Nutraceutical: Avoid valerian, St John's wort, SAMe, kava kava (may increase risk of serotonin syndrome and/or excessive sedation).

Mechanism of Action Inhibits reuptake of serotonin, causes adrenoreceptor subsensitivity, and induces significant changes in 5-HT presynaptic receptor adrenoreceptors. Trazodone also significantly blocks histamine (H_1) and alpha$_1$-adrenergic receptors.

Pharmacodynamics/Kinetics
Onset of action: Therapeutic: 1-3 weeks
Protein binding: 85% to 95%

Metabolism: Hepatic
Half-life elimination: 4-7.5 hours, two compartment kinetics
Time to peak, serum: 30-100 minutes; prolonged in presence of food (up to 2.5 hours)
Excretion: Primarily urine; secondarily feces

Usual Dosage Oral: Therapeutic effects may take up to 6 weeks to occur; therapy is normally maintained for 6-12 months after optimum response is reached to prevent recurrence of depression

Children 6-12 years: Depression: Initial: 1.5-2 mg/kg/day in divided doses; increase gradually every 3-4 days as needed; maximum: 6 mg/kg/day in 3 divided doses

Adolescents: Depression: Initial: 25-50 mg/day; increase to 100-150 mg/day in divided doses

Adults:
  Depression: Initial: 150 mg/day in 3 divided doses (may increase by 50 mg/day every 3-7 days); maximum: 600 mg/day
  Sedation/hypnotic (unlabeled use): 25-50 mg at bedtime (often in combination with daytime SSRIs); may increase up to 200 mg at bedtime

Elderly: 25-50 mg at bedtime with 25-50 mg/day dose increase every 3 days for inpatients and weekly for outpatients, if tolerated; usual dose: 75-150 mg/day

Reference Range
Plasma levels do not always correlate with clinical effectiveness
Therapeutic: 0.5-2.5 µg/mL
Potentially toxic: >2.5 µg/mL
Toxic: >4 µg/mL

Patient Information Take shortly after a meal or light snack, can be given as bedtime dose if drowsiness occurs; avoid alcohol; be aware of possible photosensitivity reaction; report any prolonged or painful erection

Nursing Implications Dosing after meals may decrease lightheadedness and postural hypotension; use side rails on bed if administered to the elderly; observe patient's activity and compare with admission level; assist with ambulation; sitting and standing blood pressure and pulse

Additional Information Therapeutic effect for sleep occurs in 1-3 hours
Dosage Forms Tablet, as hydrochloride: 50 mg, 100 mg, 150 mg, 300 mg

◆ **Trazodone Hydrochloride** *see* Trazodone *on page 1362*
◆ **Trazorel (Can)** *see* Trazodone *on page 1362*
◆ **Treatment of Sexually Transmitted Diseases** *see page 1609*
◆ **Trecator®-SC** *see* Ethionamide *on page 530*
◆ **Trelstar™ Depot** *see* Triptorelin *on page 1381*
◆ **Trelstar™ LA** *see* Triptorelin *on page 1381*
◆ **Trental®** *see* Pentoxifylline *on page 1061*

Tretinoin (Oral) (TRET i noyn, oral)

U.S. Brand Names Vesanoid®
Canadian Brand Names Vesanoid™
Synonyms All-*trans*-Retinoic Acid
Therapeutic Category Antineoplastic Agent, Miscellaneous; Retinoic Acid Derivative; Vitamin A Derivative
Use Acute promyelocytic leukemia (APL): Induction of remission in patients with APL, French American British (FAB) classification M3 (including the M3 variant), characterized by the presence of the t(15;17) translocation or the presence of the PML/RARα gene who are refractory to or who have relapsed from anthracycline chemotherapy, or for whom anthracycline-based chemotherapy is contraindicated. Tretinoin is for the induction of remission only. All patients should receive an accepted form of remission consolidation or maintenance therapy for APL after completion of induction therapy with tretinoin.
Pregnancy Risk Factor D
Contraindications Sensitivity to parabens, vitamin A, other retinoids, or any component of the formulation; pregnancy
Warnings/Precautions Patients with acute promyelocytic leukemia (APL) are at high risk and can have severe adverse reactions to tretinoin. Administer under the supervision of a physician who is experienced in the management of patients with acute leukemia and in a facility with laboratory and supportive services sufficient to monitor drug tolerance and to protect and maintain a patient compromised by drug toxicity, including respiratory compromise.

About 25% of patients with APL, who have been treated with tretinoin, have experienced a syndrome called the retinoic acid-APL (RA-APL) syndrome which is characterized by fever, dyspnea, weight gain, radiographic pulmonary infiltrates and pleural or pericardial effusions. This syndrome has occasionally been accompanied by impaired myocardial contractility and episodic hypotension. It has been observed with or without concomitant leukocytosis. Endotracheal intubation and mechanical ventilation have been required in some cases due to progressive hypoxemia, and several patients have expired with multiorgan failure. The syndrome usually occurs during the first month of treatment, with some cases reported following the first dose.

Management of the syndrome has not been defined, but high-dose steroids given at the first suspicion of RA-APL syndrome appear to reduce morbidity and mortality. At the first signs suggestive of the syndrome, immediately initiate high-dose steroids (dexamethasone 10 mg I.V.) every 12 hours for 3 days or until resolution of symptoms, regardless of the leukocyte count. The majority of patients do not require termination of tretinoin therapy during treatment of the RA-APL syndrome.

During treatment, ~40% of patients will develop rapidly evolving leukocytosis. Rapidly evolving leukocytosis is associated with a higher risk of life-threatening complications.

If signs and symptoms of the RA-APL syndrome are present together with leukocytosis, initiate treatment with high-dose steroids immediately. Consider adding full-dose chemotherapy (including an anthracycline, if not contraindicated) to the tretinoin therapy on day 1 or (Continued)

Tretinoin (Oral) *(Continued)*

2 for patients presenting with a WBC count of >5 x 10^9/L or immediately, for patients presenting with a WBC count of <5 x 10^9/L, if the WBC count reaches ≥6 x 10^9/L by day 5, or ≥10 x 10^9/L by day 10 or ≥15 x 10^9/L by day 28.

Not to be used in women of childbearing potential unless the woman is capable of complying with effective contraceptive measures; therapy is normally begun on the second or third day of next normal menstrual period; two reliable methods of effective contraception must be used during therapy and for 1 month after discontinuation of therapy, unless abstinence is the chosen method. Within one week prior to the institution of tretinoin therapy, the patient should have blood or urine collected for a serum or urine pregnancy test with a sensitivity of at least 50 mIU/L. When possible, delay tretinoin therapy until a negative result from this test is obtained. When a delay is not possible, place the patient on two reliable forms of contraception. Repeat pregnancy testing and contraception counseling monthly throughout the period of treatment.

Initiation of therapy with tretinoin may be based on the morphological diagnosis of APL. Confirm the diagnosis of APL by detection of the t(15;17) genetic marker by cytogenetic studies. If these are negative, PML/RARα fusion should be sought using molecular diagnostic techniques. The response rate of other AML subtypes to tretinoin has not been demonstrated.

Retinoids have been associated with pseudotumor cerebri (benign intracranial hypertension), especially in children. Early signs and symptoms include papilledema, headache, nausea, vomiting and visual disturbances.

Up to 60% of patients experienced hypercholesterolemia or hypertriglyceridemia, which were reversible upon completion of treatment.

Elevated liver function test results occur in 50% to 60% of patients during treatment. Carefully monitor liver function test results during treatment and give consideration to a temporary withdrawal of tretinoin if test results reach >5 times the upper limit of normal.

Adverse Reactions Virtually all patients experience some drug-related toxicity, especially headache, fever, weakness and fatigue. These adverse effects are seldom permanent or irreversible nor do they usually require therapy interruption

About 25% of patients with APL, who have been treated with tretinoin, have experienced a syndrome called the retinoic acid-APL (RA-APL) syndrome (fever, dyspnea, weight gain, pulmonary infiltrates and pleural or pericardial effusions). Occasionally accompanied by impaired myocardial contractility and episodic hypotension, with or without concomitant leukocytosis. High-dose steroids given at the first suspicion of RA-APL syndrome appear to reduce morbidity and mortality (dexamethasone 10 mg I.V. every 12 hours for 3 days or until resolution of symptoms). Many patients do not require termination of tretinoin therapy during treatment of the RA-APL syndrome.

>10%:
- Cardiovascular: Arrhythmias, flushing, hypotension, hypertension, peripheral edema, chest discomfort, edema
- Central nervous system: Dizziness, anxiety, insomnia, depression, confusion, malaise, pain
- Dermatologic: Burning, redness, cheilitis, inflammation of lips, dry skin, pruritus, photosensitivity
- Endocrine & metabolic: Increased triglycerides, increased cholesterol (up to 60%)
- Gastrointestinal: GI hemorrhage, abdominal pain, other GI disorders, diarrhea, constipation, heartburn, abdominal distention, weight gain/loss, anorexia, dry mouth
- Hematologic: Hemorrhage, disseminated intravascular coagulation Hepatic: Increased transaminases (50% to 60%)
- Local: Phlebitis, injection site reactions
- Neuromuscular & skeletal: Bone pain, arthralgia, myalgia, paresthesia
- Ocular: Itching of eye
- Renal: Renal insufficiency
- Respiratory: Upper respiratory tract disorders, dyspnea, respiratory insufficiency, pleural effusion, pneumonia, rales, expiratory wheezing, dry nose
- Miscellaneous: Infections, shivering

1% to 10% (Limited to important or life-threatening):
- Cardiovascular: Cardiac failure, cardiac arrest, myocardial infarction, stroke, myocarditis, pericarditis, pulmonary hypertension, cardiomyopathy, cerebral hemorrhage
- Central nervous system: Intracranial hypertension, agitation, hallucination, aphasia, cerebellar edema, convulsions, coma, CNS depression, encephalopathy, hypotaxia, no light reflex, neurologic reaction, spinal cord disorder, dementia, somnolence, hypothermia
- Dermatologic: Skin peeling on hands or soles of feet, rash, cellulitis
- Hepatic: Ascites, hepatitis
- Neuromuscular & skeletal: Tremor, hyporeflexia, dysarthria, facial paralysis, hemiplegia, asterixis, abnormal gait
- Ocular: Dry eyes, photophobia
- Renal: Acute renal failure, renal tubular necrosis
- Respiratory: Asthma, pulmonary/laryngeal edema

<1% (Limited to important or life-threatening): Alopecia, hepatitis, pseudomotor cerebri

Overdosage/Toxicology The maximum tolerated dose in adult patients with myelodysplastic syndrome in solid tumors was 195 mg/m²/day; the maximum tolerated dose in pediatric patients was lower at 60 mg/m²/day. Overdosage with other retinoids has been associated with transient headache, facial flushing, cheilosis, abdominal pain, dizziness, and ataxia. These symptoms resolved quickly without residual effects.

Drug Interactions

Cytochrome P450 Effect: CYP3A3/4 enzyme substrate

Increased Effect/Toxicity: Ketoconazole increases the mean plasma AUC of tretinoin. Other drugs which inhibit CYP3A4 would be expected to increase tretinoin concentrations, potentially increasing toxicity.

Decreased Effect: Metabolized by the hepatic cytochrome P450 system: All drugs that induce this system would be expected to interact with tretinoin.

Ethanol/Nutrition/Herb Interactions

Ethanol: Avoid ethanol (may increase CNS depression).

Food: Absorption of retinoids has been shown to be enhanced when taken with food.

Herb/Nutraceutical: St John's wort may decrease tretinoin levels. Avoid dong quai, St John's wort (may also cause photosensitization). Avoid additional vitamin A supplementation. May lead to vitamin A toxicity.

Mechanism of Action Retinoid that induces maturation of acute promyelocytic leukemia (APL) cells in cultures; induces cytodifferentiation and decreased proliferation of APL cells

Pharmacodynamics/Kinetics

Protein binding: >95%

Metabolism: Hepatic via CYP450 enzymes

Half-life elimination: Terminal: Parent drug: 0.5-2 hours

Time to peak, serum: 1-2 hours

Excretion: Urine and feces (equal amounts)

Usual Dosage Oral:

Children: There are limited clinical data on the pediatric use of tretinoin. Of 15 pediatric patients (age range: 1-16 years) treated with tretinoin, the incidence of complete remission was 67%. Safety and efficacy in pediatric patients <1 year of age have not been established. Some pediatric patients experience severe headache and pseudotumor cerebri, requiring analgesic treatment and lumbar puncture for relief. Increased caution is recommended. Consider dose reduction in children experiencing serious or intolerable toxicity; however, the efficacy and safety of tretinoin at doses <45 mg/m^2/day have not been evaluated.

Adults: 45 mg/m^2/day administered as two evenly divided doses until complete remission is documented. Discontinue therapy 30 days after achievement of complete remission or after 90 days of treatment, whichever occurs first. If after initiation of treatment the presence of the t(15;17) translocation is not confirmed by cytogenetics or by polymerase chain reaction studies and the patient has not responded to tretinoin, consider alternative therapy.

Note: Tretinoin is for the induction of remission only. Optimal consolidation or maintenance regimens have not been determined. All patients should therefore receive a standard consolidation or maintenance chemotherapy regimen for APL after induction therapy with tretinoin unless otherwise contraindicated.

Monitoring Parameters Monitor the patient's hematologic profile, coagulation profile, liver function test results and triglyceride and cholesterol levels frequently

Patient Information Take with food; do not crush, chew, or dissolve capsules. You will need frequent blood tests while taking this medication. Maintain adequate hydration (2-3 L/day of fluids unless instructed to restrict fluid intake), avoid alcohol and foods containing vitamin A, and foods with high fat content. You may experience lethargy, dizziness, visual changes, confusion, anxiety (avoid driving or engaging in tasks requiring alertness until response to drug is known). For nausea/vomiting, loss of appetite, or dry mouth, small frequent meals, chewing gum, or sucking lozenges may help. You may experience photosensitivity (use sunscreen, wear protective clothing and eyewear, and avoid direct sunlight). You may experience dry, itchy, skin, and dry or irritated eyes (avoid contact lenses). Report persistent vomiting or diarrhea, difficulty breathing, unusual bleeding or bruising, acute GI pain, bone pain, or vision changes immediately.

Dosage Forms Capsule: 10 mg

Tretinoin (Topical) (TRET i noyn, TOP i kal)

U.S. Brand Names Altinac™; Avita®; Renova®; Retin-A®; Retin-A® Micro

Canadian Brand Names Rejuva-A®; Retin-A®; Retinova®

Synonyms Retinoic Acid; trans-Retinoic Acid; Vitamin A Acid

Therapeutic Category Acne Products; Retinoic Acid Derivative; Vitamin A Derivative

Use Treatment of acne vulgaris; photodamaged skin; palliation of fine wrinkles, mottled hyperpigmentation, and tactile roughness of facial skin as part of a comprehensive skin care and sun avoidance program

Unlabeled/Investigational Use Some skin cancers

Pregnancy Risk Factor C

Pregnancy/Breast-Feeding Implications Clinical effects on the fetus: Oral tretinoin is teratogenic and fetotoxic in rats at doses 1000 and 500 times the topical human dose, respectively. Tretinoin does not appear to be teratogenic when used topically since it is rapidly metabolized by the skin; however, there are rare reports of fetal defects. Use for acne only if benefit to mother outweighs potential risk to fetus. During pregnancy, do not use for palliation of fine wrinkles, mottled hyperpigmentation, and tactile roughness of facial skin.

Contraindications Hypersensitivity to tretinoin or any component of the formulation; sunburn

Warnings/Precautions Use with caution in patients with eczema; avoid excessive exposure to sunlight and sunlamps; avoid contact with abraded skin, mucous membranes, eyes, mouth, angles of the nose. Palliation of fine wrinkles, mottled hyperpigmentation, and tactile roughness of facial skin: Do not use the 0.05% cream for longer than 48 weeks or the 0.02% cream for longer than 52 weeks. Not for use on moderate- to heavily-pigmented skin.

Adverse Reactions 1% to 10%:

Cardiovascular: Edema

Dermatologic: Excessive dryness, erythema, scaling of the skin, hyperpigmentation or hypopigmentation, photosensitivity, initial acne flare-up

Local: Stinging, blistering

Overdosage/Toxicology Excessive application may lead to marked redness, peeling or discomfort. Oral ingestion of the topical product may lead to the same adverse reactions seen with excessive vitamin A intake (increased intracranial pressure, jaundice, ascites, cutaneous desquamation; symptoms of acute overdose [12,000 units/kg] include nausea, vomiting, and diarrhea). Toxic signs of an overdose commonly respond to drug discontinuation, and generally return to normal spontaneously within a few days to weeks. When confronted with signs of increased intracranial pressure, treatment with mannitol (0.25 g/kg I.V. up to 1 g/kg/dose (Continued)

Tretinoin (Topical) *(Continued)*

repeated every 5 minutes as needed), dexamethasone (1.5 mg/kg I.V. load followed with 0.375 mg/kg every 6 hours for 5 days), and/or hyperventilation should be employed.

Drug Interactions

Cytochrome P450 Effect: CYP3A3/4 enzyme substrate

Increased Effect/Toxicity: Topical application of sulfur, benzoyl peroxide, salicylic acid, resorcinol, or any product with strong drying effects potentiates adverse reactions with tretinoin.

Photosensitizing medications (thiazides, tetracyclines, fluoroquinolones, phenothiazines, sulfonamides) augment phototoxicity and should not be used when treating palliation of fine wrinkles, mottled hyperpigmentation, and tactile roughness of facial skin.

Ethanol/Nutrition/Herb Interactions

Food: Avoid excessive intake of vitamin A (cod liver oil, halibut fish oil).

Herb/Nutraceutical: Avoid dong quai, St John's wort (may also cause photosensitization). Avoid excessive amounts of vitamin A supplements.

Stability Store at 25°C (77°F); gel is flammable, keep away from heat and flame

Mechanism of Action Keratinocytes in the sebaceous follicle become less adherent which allows for easy removal; inhibits microcomedone formation and eliminates lesions already present

Pharmacodynamics/Kinetics

Absorption: Minimal

Metabolism: Hepatic for the small amount absorbed

Excretion: Urine and feces

Usual Dosage Topical:

Children >12 years and Adults: Acne vulgaris: Begin therapy with a weaker formulation of tretinoin (0.025% cream or 0.01% gel) and increase the concentration as tolerated; apply once daily to acne lesions before retiring or on alternate days; if stinging or irritation develop, decrease frequency of application

Adults ≥18: Palliation of fine wrinkles, mottled hyperpigmentation, and tactile roughness of facial skin: Pea-sized amount of the 0.02% or 0.05% emollient cream applied to entire face once daily in the evening

Elderly: Use of the 0.02% emollient cream in patients 65-71 years of age showed similar improvement in fine wrinkles as seen in patients <65 years. Safety and efficacy of the 0.02% cream have not been established in patients >71 years of age. Safety and efficacy of the 0.05% cream have not been established in patients >50 years of age.

Administration Palliation of fine wrinkles, mottled hyperpigmentation, and tactile roughness of facial skin: Emollient cream: Prior to application, gently wash face with a mild soap. Pat dry. Wait 20-30 minutes to apply cream. Avoid eyes, ears, nostrils, and mouth.

Patient Information For once-daily use, do not overuse. Avoid increased intake of vitamin A. Thoroughly wash hands before applying. Wash area to be treated at least 30 minutes before applying. Do not wash face more frequently than 2-3 times a day. Avoid using topical preparations that contain alcohol or harsh chemicals during treatment. You may experience increased sensitivity to sunlight; protect skin with sunblock (minimum SPF 15), wear protective clothing, or avoid direct sunlight. Stop treatment and inform prescriber if rash, skin irritation, redness, scaling, or excessive dryness occurs. When used for hyperpigmentation and tactile redness of facial skin, wrinkles will not be eliminated. Must be used in combination with a comprehensive skin care program.

Nursing Implications Observe for signs of hypersensitivity, blistering, excessive dryness; do not apply to mucous membranes

Dosage Forms

Cream, topical:

Altinac™: 0.025% (20 g, 45 g); 0.05% (20 g, 45 g); 0.1% (20 g, 45 g)

Avita®: 0.025% (20 g, 45 g)

Retin-A®: 0.025% (20 g, 45 g); 0.05% (20 g, 45 g); 0.1% (20 g, 45 g)

Cream, emollient, topical (Renova®): 0.02% (40 g); 0.05% (20 g, 40 g, 60 g)

Gel, topical:

Retin-A®: 0.01% (15 g, 45 g); 0.025% (15 g, 45 g)

Retin-A® Micro: 0.1% (20 g, 45 g)

Liquid, topical (Retin-A®): 0.05% (28 mL)

♦ **Trexall™** *see Methotrexate on page 884*

♦ **Triacet™** *see Triamcinolone on page 1366*

♦ **Triacetyloleandomycin** *see Troleandomycin on page 1383*

♦ **Triacin® [OTC]** *see Triprolidine and Pseudoephedrine on page 1380*

♦ **Triacin-C®** *see Triprolidine, Pseudoephedrine, and Codeine on page 1381*

♦ **Triaconazole** *see Terconazole on page 1301*

♦ **Triad®** *see Butalbital Compound on page 197*

♦ **Triaderm (Can)** *see Triamcinolone on page 1366*

♦ **Triafed® [OTC]** *see Triprolidine and Pseudoephedrine on page 1380*

♦ **Triam-A®** *see Triamcinolone on page 1366*

Triamcinolone *(trye am SIN oh lone)*

Related Information

Asthma *on page 1645*

Corticosteroids Comparison *on page 1495*

Estimated Clinical Comparability of Doses for Inhaled Corticosteroids *on page 1652*

U.S. Brand Names Amcort®; Aristocort®; Aristocort® A; Aristocort® Forte; Aristocort® Intralesional; Aristospan® Intra-Articular; Aristospan® Intralesional; Atolone®; Azmacort®; Delta-Tritex®; Flutex®; Kenacort®; Kenaject-40®; Kenalog®; Kenalog-10®; Kenalog-40®; Kenalog® H; Kenalog® in Orabase®; Kenonel®; Nasacort®; Nasacort® AQ; Tac™-3; Tac™-40; Triacet™; Triam-A®; Triam Forte®; Triderm®; Tri-Kort®; Trilog®; Trilone®; Tri-Nasal®; Tristoject®

Canadian Brand Names Aristocort®; Aristospan®; Azmacort®; Kenalog®; Kenalog® in Orabase; Nasacort™; Nasacort® AQ; Oracort; Triaderm; Trinasal®

Synonyms Triamcinolone Acetonide, Aerosol; Triamcinolone Acetonide, Parenteral; Triamcinolone Diacetate, Oral; Triamcinolone Diacetate, Parenteral; Triamcinolone Hexacetonide; Triamcinolone, Oral

Therapeutic Category Anti-inflammatory Agent; Anti-inflammatory Agent, Inhalant; Corticosteroid, Inhalant; Corticosteroid, Intranasal; Corticosteroid, Systemic; Corticosteroid, Topical (Medium Potency); Corticosteroid, Topical (High Potency); Glucocorticoid

Use

Inhalation: Control of bronchial asthma and related bronchospastic conditions.

Intranasal: Management of seasonal and perennial allergic rhinitis in patients ≥12 years of age

Systemic: Adrenocortical insufficiency, rheumatic disorders, allergic states, respiratory diseases, systemic lupus erythematosus, and other diseases requiring anti-inflammatory or immunosuppressive effects

Topical: Inflammatory dermatoses responsive to steroids

Pregnancy Risk Factor C

Pregnancy/Breast-Feeding Implications

Clinical effects on the fetus: No data on crossing the placenta or effect on fetus

Breast-feeding/lactation: No data on crossing into breast milk or clinical effects on the infant

Contraindications Hypersensitivity to triamcinolone or any component of the formulation; systemic fungal infections; serious infections (except septic shock or tuberculous meningitis); primary treatment of status asthmaticus

Warnings/Precautions May cause suppression of hypothalamic-pituitary-adrenal (HPA) axis, particularly in younger children or in patients receiving high doses for prolonged periods. Particular care is required when patients are transferred from systemic corticosteroids to inhaled products due to possible adrenal insufficiency or withdrawal from steroids, including an increase in allergic symptoms. Patients receiving 20 mg per day of prednisone (or equivalent) may be most susceptible. Fatalities have occurred due to adrenal insufficiency in asthmatic patients during and after transfer from systemic corticosteroids to aerosol steroids; aerosol steroids do **not** provide the systemic steroid needed to treat patients having trauma, surgery, or infections. Withdrawal and discontinuation of the corticosteroid should be done slowly and carefully

Use with caution in patients with hypothyroidism, cirrhosis, nonspecific ulcerative colitis and patients at increased risk for peptic ulcer disease. Corticosteroids should be used with caution in patients with diabetes, hypertension, osteoporosis, glaucoma, cataracts, or tuberculosis. Use caution in hepatic impairment. Do not use occlusive dressings on weeping or exudative lesions and general caution with occlusive dressings should be observed; discontinue if skin irritation or contact dermatitis should occur; do not use in patients with decreased skin circulation; avoid the use of high potency steroids on the face.

Because of the risk of adverse effects, systemic corticosteroids should be used cautiously in the elderly, in the smallest possible dose, and for the shortest possible time. Azmacort® (metered dose inhaler) comes with its own spacer device attached and may be easier to use in older patients.

Controlled clinical studies have shown that orally-inhaled and intranasal corticosteroids may cause a reduction in growth velocity in pediatric patients. (In studies of orally-inhaled corticosteroids, the mean reduction in growth velocity was approximately 1 centimeter per year [range 0.3-1.8 cm per year] and appears to be related to dose and duration of exposure.) The growth of pediatric patients receiving inhaled corticosteroids, should be monitored routinely (eg, via stadiometry). To minimize the systemic effects of orally-inhaled and intranasal corticosteroids, each patient should be titrated to the lowest effective dose.

May suppress the immune system, patients may be more susceptible to infection. Use with caution in patients with systemic infections or ocular herpes simplex. Avoid exposure to chickenpox and measles.

Adverse Reactions

Systemic:

>10%:

Central nervous system: Insomnia, nervousness

Gastrointestinal: Increased appetite, indigestion

1% to 10%:

Central nervous system: Dizziness or lightheadedness, headache

Dermatologic: Hirsutism, hypopigmentation

Endocrine & metabolic: Diabetes mellitus

Neuromuscular & skeletal: Arthralgia

Ocular: Cataracts, glaucoma

Respiratory: Epistaxis

Miscellaneous: Diaphoresis

<1% (Limited to important or life-threatening): Cushing's syndrome, edema, hypertension, pituitary-adrenal axis suppression, seizures

Topical:

1% to 10%:

Dermatologic: Itching, allergic contact dermatitis, erythema, dryness papular rashes, folliculitis, furunculosis, pustules, pyoderma, vesiculation, hyperesthesia, skin infection (secondary)

Local: Burning, irritation

<1% (Limited to important or life-threatening): Cataracts (posterior subcapsular), gastric ulcer, glaucoma

Overdosage/Toxicology When consumed in excessive quantities, systemic hypercorticism and adrenal suppression may occur; in those cases, discontinuation and withdrawal of the corticosteroid should be done judiciously.

(Continued)

Triamcinolone *(Continued)*

Drug Interactions
Increased Effect/Toxicity: Salicylates or NSAIDs coadministered oral corticosteroids may increase risk of GI ulceration.

Decreased Effect: Decreased effect with barbiturates and phenytoin. Rifampin increased metabolism of triamcinolone. Vaccine and toxoid effects may be reduced.

Ethanol/Nutrition/Herb Interactions
Ethanol: Avoid ethanol (may enhance gastric mucosal irritation).

Food: Triamcinolone interferes with calcium absorption.

Herb/Nutraceutical: Avoid cat's claw, echinacea (have immunostimulant properties).

Mechanism of Action Decreases inflammation by suppression of migration of polymorpho-nuclear leukocytes and reversal of increased capillary permeability; suppresses the immune system by reducing activity and volume of the lymphatic system; suppresses adrenal function at high doses

Pharmacodynamics/Kinetics
Duration: Oral: 8-12 hours

Absorption: Topical: Systemic

Time to peak: I.M.: 8-10 hours

Half-life elimination: Biologic: 18-36 hours

Usual Dosage In general, single I.M. dose of 4-7 times oral dose will control patient from 4-7 days up to 3-4 weeks

Children 6-12 years:

Oral inhalation: 1-2 inhalations 3-4 times/day, not to exceed 12 inhalations/day

I.M. (acetonide or hexacetonide): 0.03-0.2 mg/kg at 1- to 7-day intervals

Intra-articular, intrabursal, or tendon-sheath injection: 2.5-15 mg, repeated as needed

Children >12 years and Adults:

Intranasal: 2 sprays in each nostril once daily; may increase after 4-7 days up to 4 sprays once daily or 1 spray 4 times/day in each nostril

Topical: Apply a thin film 2-3 times/day. Therapy should be discontinued when control is achieved; if no improvement is seen, reassessment of diagnosis may be necessary.

Oral: 4-48 mg/day

Oral inhalation: 2 inhalations 3-4 times/day, not to exceed 16 inhalations/day

Children >12 years and Adults: See table.

Triamcinolone Dosing

	Acetonide	Diacetate	Hexacetonide
Intrasynovial	2.5-40 mg	5-40 mg	
Intralesional	1-30 mg	5-40 mg (not >25 mg per lesion)	Up to 0.5 mg/sq inch affected area
Sublesional	1-30 mg		
Systemic I.M.	2.5-60 mg/dose (usual adult dose: 60 mg)	~40 mg/wk	
Intra-articular	2.5-40 mg	2-40 mg	2-20 mg average
large joints	15-40 mg		10-20 mg
small joints	2.5-10 mg		2-6 mg
Tendon sheaths	2.5-10 mg		
Intradermal	1 mg/site		

Dietary Considerations May be taken with food to decrease GI distress.

Administration
I.M.: Inject deep in large muscle mass, avoid deltoid.

Inhalation: Rinse mouth and throat after using inhaler to prevent candidiasis. Use spacer device provided with Azmacort®.

Oral: Once-daily doses should be given in the morning.

Topical: Apply a thin film sparingly and avoid topical application on the face. Do not use on open skin or wounds. Do not occlude area unless directed.

Patient Information
Inhaler: Rinse mouth and throat after use to prevent candidiasis

Nasal spray: Shake gently before use; use at regular intervals, no more frequently than directed; report unusual cough or spasm, persistent nasal bleeding, burning, or irritation, or worsening of condition

Topical: Apply sparingly to affected area, rub in until drug disappears, do not use on open skin

Report any change in body weight; do not discontinue or decrease the drug without contacting your physician; carry an identification card or bracelet advising that you are on steroids; may take with meals to decrease GI upset

Nursing Implications Once daily doses should be given in the morning; evaluate clinical response and mental status; may mask signs and symptoms of infection; inject I.M. dose deep in large muscle mass, avoid deltoid; avoid S.C. dose; a thin film is effective topically and avoid topical application on the face; do not occlude area unless directed

Additional Information 16 mg triamcinolone is equivalent to 100 mg cortisone (no mineralo-corticoid activity).

Effects of inhaled/intranasal steroids on growth have been observed in the absence of laboratory evidence of HPA axis suppression, suggesting that growth velocity is a more sensitive indicator of systemic corticosteroid exposure in pediatric patients than some commonly used tests of HPA axis function. The long-term effects of this reduction in growth velocity associated with orally-inhaled and intranasal corticosteroids, including the impact on final adult height, are unknown. The potential for "catch up" growth following discontinuation of treatment with inhaled corticosteroids has not been adequately studied.

Dosage Forms

Aerosol for oral inhalation (Azmacort®): 100 mcg/metered spray (20 g)

Aerosol, topical, as acetonide: 0.2 mg/2 second spray (23 g, 63 g)

Cream, topical, as acetonide: 0.025% (15 g, 60 g, 80 g, 240 g, 454 g); 0.1% (15 g, 30 g, 60 g, 80 g, 90 g, 120 g, 240 g); 0.5% (15 g, 20 g, 30 g, 240 g)

Injection, as acetonide: 10 mg/mL (5 mL); 40 mg/mL (1 mL, 5 mL, 10 mL)

Injection, as diacetate: 25 mg/mL (5 mL); 40 mg/mL (1 mL, 5 mL, 10 mL)

Injection, as hexacetonide: 5 mg/mL (5 mL); 20 mg/mL (1 mL, 5 mL)

Lotion, topical, as acetonide: 0.025% (60 mL); 0.1% (15 mL, 60 mL)

Ointment, topical, as acetonide: 0.025% (15 g, 30 g, 60 g, 80 g, 120 g, 454 g); 0.1% (15 g, 30 g, 60 g, 80 g, 120 g, 240 g, 454 g); 0.5% (15 g, 20 g, 30 g, 240 g)

Paste, oral, topical, as acetonide (Kenalog® in Orabase®): 0.1% (5 g)

Suspension, intranasal [spray]:

Nasacort®, Nasacort AQ™: 55 mcg per actuation (15 mL)

Tri-Nasal®: 50 mcg per actuation (15 mL)

Syrup: 2 mg/5 mL (120 mL); 4 mg/5 mL (120 mL)

Tablet: 1 mg, 2 mg, 4 mg, 8 mg

♦ **Triamcinolone Acetonide, Aerosol** see Triamcinolone on page 1366

♦ **Triamcinolone Acetonide, Parenteral** see Triamcinolone on page 1366

♦ **Triamcinolone and Nystatin** see Nystatin and Triamcinolone on page 1002

♦ **Triamcinolone Diacetate, Oral** see Triamcinolone on page 1366

♦ **Triamcinolone Diacetate, Parenteral** see Triamcinolone on page 1366

♦ **Triamcinolone Hexacetonide** see Triamcinolone on page 1366

♦ **Triamcinolone, Oral** see Triamcinolone on page 1366

♦ **Triam Forte®** see Triamcinolone on page 1366

♦ **Triaminic® AM Decongestant Formula [OTC]** see Pseudoephedrine on page 1155

♦ **Triaminic® Infant Decongestant [OTC]** see Pseudoephedrine on page 1155

♦ **Triaminic® Sore Throat Formula [OTC]** see Acetaminophen, Dextromethorphan, and Pseudoephedrine on page 27

Triamterene (trye AM ter een)

Related Information

Heart Failure on page 1663

U.S. Brand Names Dyrenium®

Canadian Brand Names Dyrenium®

Therapeutic Category Antihypertensive Agent; Diuretic, Potassium Sparing

Use Alone or in combination with other diuretics in treatment of edema and hypertension; decreases potassium excretion caused by kaliuretic diuretics

Pregnancy Risk Factor B (manufacturer); D (expert analysis)

Pregnancy/Breast-Feeding Implications

Clinical effects on the fetus: No data available. Generally, use of diuretics during pregnancy is avoided due to risk of decreased placental perfusion.

Breast-feeding/lactation: No data available

Contraindications Hypersensitivity to triamterene or any component of the formulation; patients receiving other potassium-sparing diuretics; anuria; severe hepatic disease; hyperkalemia or history of hyperkalemia; severe or progressive renal disease; pregnancy

Warnings/Precautions Avoid potassium supplements, potassium-containing salt substitutes, a diet rich in potassium, or other drugs that can cause hyperkalemia. Monitor for fluid and electrolyte imbalances. Diuretic therapy should be carefully used in severe hepatic dysfunction; electrolyte and fluid shifts can cause or exacerbate encephalopathy. Use cautiously in patients with history of kidney stones and diabetes. Can cause photosensitivity.

Adverse Reactions

1% to 10%:

Cardiovascular: Bradycardia, congestive heart failure, edema, hypotension

Central nervous system: Dizziness, fatigue, headache

Dermatologic: Rash

Gastrointestinal: Constipation, nausea

Respiratory: Dyspnea

<1% (Limited to important or life-threatening): Dehydration, gynecomastia, impotence, metabolic acidosis, postmenopausal bleeding

Overdosage/Toxicology Symptoms include drowsiness, confusion, clinical signs of dehydration, electrolyte imbalance, and hypotension. Chronic or acute ingestion of large amounts of potassium-sparing diuretics, may result in life-threatening hyperkalemia, especially with decreased renal function. If the EKG shows no widening of the QRS or an arrhythmia, discontinue triamterene and any potassium supplement and substitute a thiazide. Consider Kayexalate® to increase potassium excretion. If an abnormal cardiac status is obvious, treat with calcium or sodium bicarbonates as needed, pacing dialysis and/or Kayexalate®. Infusions of glucose and insulin are also useful.

Drug Interactions

Increased Effect/Toxicity: Angiotensin-converting enzyme inhibitors or spironolactone can cause hyperkalemia, especially in patients with renal impairment, potassium-rich diets, or on other drugs causing hyperkalemia; avoid concurrent use or monitor closely. Potassium supplements may further increase potassium retention and cause hyperkalemia; avoid concurrent use.

Mechanism of Action Interferes with potassium/sodium exchange (active transport) in the distal tubule, cortical collecting tubule and collecting duct by inhibiting sodium, potassium-ATPase; decreases calcium excretion; increases magnesium loss

Pharmacodynamics/Kinetics

Onset of action: Diuresis: 2-4 hours

Duration: 7-9 hours

Absorption: Unreliable

(Continued)

Triamterene (Continued)

Usual Dosage Adults: Oral: 100-300 mg/day in 1-2 divided doses; maximum dose: 300 mg/day

  Dosing comments in renal impairment: Cl_{cr} <10 mL/minute: Avoid use.

  Dosing adjustment in hepatic impairment: Dose reduction is recommended in patients with cirrhosis.

Dietary Considerations May be taken with food.

Monitoring Parameters Blood pressure, serum electrolytes (especially potassium), renal function, weight, I & O

Test Interactions Interferes with fluorometric assay of quinidine

Patient Information Take in the morning; take the last dose of multiple doses no later than 6 PM unless instructed otherwise; take after meals; notify physician if weakness, headache or nausea occurs; avoid excessive ingestion of food high in potassium or use of salt substitute; may increase blood glucose; may impart a blue fluorescence color to urine

Nursing Implications Observe for hyperkalemia; assess weight and I & O daily to determine weight loss; if ordered once daily, dose should be given in the morning

Dosage Forms Capsule: 50 mg, 100 mg

♦ **Triamterene and Hydrochlorothiazide** *see Hydrochlorothiazide and Triamterene on page 675*

♦ **Triapin®** *see Butalbital Compound on page 197*

♦ **Triatec-8 (Can)** *see Acetaminophen and Codeine on page 24*

♦ **Triatec-8 Strong (Can)** *see Acetaminophen and Codeine on page 24*

♦ **Triatec-30 (Can)** *see Acetaminophen and Codeine on page 24*

♦ **Triavil®** *see Amitriptyline and Perphenazine on page 78*

Triazolam (trye AY zoe lam)

Related Information

  Antacid Drug Interactions *on page 1477*

  Benzodiazepines Comparison *on page 1490*

U.S. Brand Names Halcion®

Canadian Brand Names Apo®-Triazo; Gen-Triazolam; Halcion®

Therapeutic Category Benzodiazepine; Hypnotic; Sedative

Use Short-term treatment of insomnia

Restrictions C-IV

Pregnancy Risk Factor X

Contraindications Hypersensitivity to triazolam or any component of the formulation (cross-sensitivity with other benzodiazepines may exist); concurrent therapy with CYP3A3/4 inhibitors (including ketoconazole, itraconazole, and nefazodone); pregnancy

Warnings/Precautions Should be used only after evaluation of potential causes of sleep disturbance. Failure of sleep disturbance to resolve after 7-10 days may indicate psychiatric or medical illness. A worsening of insomnia or the emergence of new abnormalities of thought or behavior may represent unrecognized psychiatric or medical illness and requires immediate and careful evaluation.

An increase in daytime anxiety may occur after as few as 10 days of continuous use, which may be related to withdrawal reaction in some patients. Anterograde amnesia may occur at a higher rate with triazolam than with other benzodiazepines. Use with caution in elderly or debilitated patients, patients with hepatic disease (including alcoholics), or renal impairment. Use with caution in patients with respiratory disease or impaired gag reflex. Avoid use in patients with sleep apnea.

Causes CNS depression (dose-related) resulting in sedation, dizziness, confusion, or ataxia which may impair physical and mental capabilities. Patients must be cautioned about performing tasks which require mental alertness (ie, operating machinery or driving). Use with caution in patients receiving other CNS depressants or psychoactive agents. Effects with other sedative drugs or ethanol may be potentiated. Benzodiazepines have been associated with falls and traumatic injury and should be used with extreme caution in patients who are at risk of these events (especially the elderly).

Use caution in patients with suicidal risk. Use with caution in patients with a history of drug dependence. Benzodiazepines have been associated with dependence and acute withdrawal symptoms on discontinuation or reduction in dose. Acute withdrawal, including seizures, may be precipitated after administration of flumazenil to patients receiving long-term benzodiazepine therapy.

Paradoxical reactions, including hyperactive or aggressive behavior have been reported with benzodiazepines, particularly in adolescent/pediatric or psychiatric patients. Does not have analgesic, antidepressant, or antipsychotic properties.

Adverse Reactions

  >10%: Central nervous system: Drowsiness, anteriograde amnesia

  1% to 10%:

    Central nervous system: Headache, dizziness, nervousness, lightheadedness, ataxia

    Gastrointestinal: Nausea, vomiting

  <1% (Limited to important or life-threatening): Confusion, depression, euphoria, memory impairment

Overdosage/Toxicology Symptoms include somnolence, confusion, coma, diminished reflexes, dyspnea, and hypotension. Treatment for benzodiazepine overdose is supportive. Rarely is mechanical ventilation required. Flumazenil has been shown to selectively block the binding of benzodiazepines to CNS receptors, resulting in reversal of benzodiazepine-induced CNS depression, but not always respiratory depression.

Drug Interactions

  Cytochrome P450 Effect: CYP3A3/4 and 3A5-7 enzyme substrate

  Increased Effect/Toxicity: Triazolam levels may be increased by cimetidine, ciprofloxacin, clarithromycin, clozapine, CNS depressants, diltiazem, disulfiram, digoxin, erythromycin, ethanol, fluconazole, fluoxetine, fluvoxamine, grapefruit juice, isoniazid, itraconazole, keto-conazole, labetalol, levodopa, loxapine, metoprolol, metronidazole, miconazole, nefazodone, omeprazole, phenytoin, rifabutin, rifampin, troleandomycin, valproic acid, and verapamil. Concurrent use of some protease inhibitors (including ritonavir and amprenavir) is contraindicated.

Decreased Effect: Carbamazepine, rifampin, and rifabutin may enhance the metabolism of triazolam and decrease its therapeutic effect.

Ethanol/Nutrition/Herb Interactions
Ethanol: Avoid ethanol (may increase CNS depression).
Food: Food may decrease the rate of absorption. Triazolam serum concentration may be increased by grapefruit juice; avoid concurrent use.
Herb/Nutraceutical: St John's wort may decrease levels. Avoid valerian, St John's wort, kava kava, gotu kola (may increase CNS depression).

Mechanism of Action Binds to stereospecific benzodiazepine receptors on the postsynaptic GABA neuron at several sites within the central nervous system, including the limbic system, reticular formation. Enhancement of the inhibitory effect of GABA on neuronal excitability results by increased neuronal membrane permeability to chloride ions. This shift in chloride ions results in hyperpolarization (a less excitable state) and stabilization.

Pharmacodynamics/Kinetics
Onset of action: Hypnotic: 15-30 minutes
Duration: 6-7 hours
Distribution: V_d: 0.8-1.8 L/kg
Protein binding: 89%
Metabolism: Extensively hepatic
Half-life elimination: 1.7-5 hours
Excretion: Urine as unchanged drug and metabolites

Usual Dosage Oral (onset of action is rapid, patient should be in bed when taking medication):
Children <18 years: Dosage not established
Adults:
Hypnotic: 0.125-0.25 mg at bedtime
Preprocedure sedation (dental): 0.25 mg taken the evening before oral surgery; or 0.25 mg 1 hour before procedure
Dosing adjustment/comments in hepatic impairment: Reduce dose or avoid use in cirrhosis

Monitoring Parameters Respiratory and cardiovascular status

Patient Information Avoid alcohol and other CNS depressants; avoid activities needing good psychomotor coordination until CNS effects are known; drug may cause physical or psychological dependence; avoid abrupt discontinuation after prolonged use

Nursing Implications Patients may require assistance with ambulation; lower doses in the elderly are usually effective; institute safety measures

Additional Information Onset of action is rapid, patient should be in bed when taking medication. Prescription should be written for 7-10 days and should not be prescribed in quantities exceeding a 1-month supply. Abrupt discontinuation after sustained use (generally >10 days) may cause withdrawal symptoms.

Dosage Forms Tablet: 0.125 mg, 0.25 mg

♦ **Tribavirin** see Ribavirin on page 1189
♦ **Trichlorex® (Can)** see Trichlormethiazide on page 1371

Trichlormethiazide (trye klor meth EYE a zide)

Related Information
Sulfonamide Derivatives on page 1515
U.S. Brand Names Metahydrin®; Naqua®
Canadian Brand Names Metahydrin®; Metatensin®; Naqua®; Trichlorex®
Therapeutic Category Antihypertensive Agent; Diuretic, Thiazide
Use Management of mild to moderate hypertension; treatment of edema in congestive heart failure and nephrotic syndrome
Pregnancy Risk Factor D
Usual Dosage Adults: Oral: 1-4 mg/day; initially doses may be given twice daily.
Dosing adjustment in renal impairment: Reduced dosage is necessary.
Additional Information Complete prescribing information for this medication should be consulted for additional detail.
Dosage Forms Tablet: 2 mg, 4 mg

♦ **Trichloroacetaldehyde Monohydrate** see Chloral Hydrate on page 270
♦ **Trichloromonofluoromethane and Dichlorodifluoromethane** see Dichlorodifluoromethane and Trichloromonofluoromethane on page 393
♦ **TriCor®** see Fenofibrate on page 548
♦ **Tricosal®** see Choline Magnesium Trisalicylate on page 287
♦ **Tri-Cyclen® (Can)** see Ethinyl Estradiol and Norgestimate on page 525
♦ **Triderm®** see Triamcinolone on page 1366
♦ **Tridesilon®** see Desonide on page 379
♦ **Tridil®** see Nitroglycerin on page 989

Trientine (TRYE en teen)

U.S. Brand Names Syprine®
Canadian Brand Names Syprine®
Synonyms Trientine Hydrochloride
Therapeutic Category Antidote, Copper Toxicity; Chelating Agent, Oral
Use Treatment of Wilson's disease in patients intolerant to penicillamine
Pregnancy Risk Factor C
Contraindications Hypersensitivity to trientine or any component of the formulation; rheumatoid arthritis, biliary cirrhosis, cystinuria
(Continued)

Trientine *(Continued)*

Warnings/Precautions May cause iron-deficiency anemia; monitor closely; use with caution in patients with reactive airway disease

Adverse Reactions Frequency not defined.
Central nervous system: Dystonia, malaise
Dermatologic: Thickening and fissuring of skin
Endocrine & metabolic: Iron deficiency
Gastrointestinal: Epigastric pain, heartburn
Hematologic: Anemia
Local: Tenderness
Neuromuscular & skeletal: Muscle cramps, muscular spasm, myasthenia gravis
Miscellaneous: Systemic lupus erythematosus

Overdosage/Toxicology Overdosage is unknown. A single 30 g ingestion resulted in no toxicity. Following GI decontamination, treatment is supportive.

Drug Interactions
Decreased Effect: Iron and possibly other mineral supplements may decrease effect.

Mechanism of Action Trientine hydrochloride is an oral chelating agent structurally dissimilar from penicillamine and other available chelating agents; an effective oral chelator of copper used to induce adequate cupriuresis

Usual Dosage Oral (administer on an empty stomach):
Children <12 years: 500-750 mg/day in divided doses 2-4 times/day; maximum: 1.5 g/day
Adults: 750-1250 mg/day in divided doses 2-4 times/day; maximum dose: 2 g/day

Dietary Considerations Should be taken 1 hour before or 2 hours after meals and at least 1 hour apart from any drug, food, or milk.

Patient Information Take 1 hour before or 2 hours after meals and at least 1 hour apart from any drug, food, or milk; do not chew capsule, swallow whole followed by a full glass of water; notify physician of any fever or skin changes; any skin exposed to the contents of a capsule should be promptly washed with water

Nursing Implications Do not chew capsule, swallow whole followed by a full glass of water; notify physician of any fever or skin changes; any skin exposed to the contents of a capsule should be promptly washed with water

Dosage Forms Capsule, as hydrochloride: 250 mg

♦ **Trientine Hydrochloride** *see Trientine on page 1371*

Triethanolamine Polypeptide Oleate-Condensate
(trye eth a NOLE a meen pol i PEP tide OH lee ate-KON den sate)

U.S. Brand Names Cerumenex®

Canadian Brand Names Cerumenex®

Therapeutic Category Otic Agent, Cerumenolytic

Use Removal of ear wax (cerumen)

Pregnancy Risk Factor C

Usual Dosage Children and Adults: Otic: Fill ear canal, insert cotton plug; allow to remain 15-30 minutes; flush ear with lukewarm water as a single treatment; if a second application is needed for unusually hard impactions, repeat the procedure

Additional Information Complete prescribing information for this medication should be consulted for additional detail.

Dosage Forms Solution, otic: 6 mL, 12 mL

♦ **Triethylenethiophosphoramide** *see Thiotepa on page 1323*

♦ **Tri-Fed® [OTC]** *see Triprolidine and Pseudoephedrine on page 1380*

Trifluoperazine (trye floo oh PER a zeen)

Related Information
Antacid Drug Interactions *on page 1477*
Antipsychotic Agents Comparison *on page 1486*

U.S. Brand Names Stelazine®

Canadian Brand Names Apo®-Trifluoperazine; Stelazine®

Synonyms Trifluoperazine Hydrochloride

Therapeutic Category Antianxiety Agent; Antipsychotic Agent, Phenothiazine; Phenothiazine Derivative

Use Treatment of schizophrenia

Unlabeled/Investigational Use Management of psychotic disorders

Pregnancy Risk Factor C

Contraindications Hypersensitivity to trifluoperazine or any component of the formulation (cross-reactivity between phenothiazines may occur); severe CNS depression; bone marrow suppression; blood dyscrasias; severe hepatic disease; coma

Warnings/Precautions Safety in children <6 months of age has not been established; use with caution in patients with cardiovascular disease, seizures, hepatic dysfunction, narrow-angle glaucoma, or bone marrow suppression; watch for hypotension when administering I.M. or I.V.; use with caution in patients with myasthenia gravis or Parkinson's disease

Adverse Reactions Frequency not defined.
Cardiovascular: Hypotension, orthostatic hypotension, cardiac arrest
Central nervous system: Extrapyramidal symptoms (pseudoparkinsonism, akathisia, dystonias, tardive dyskinesia), dizziness, headache, neuroleptic malignant syndrome (NMS), impairment of temperature regulation, lowering of seizures threshold
Dermatologic: Increased sensitivity to sun, rash, discoloration of skin (blue-gray)
Endocrine & metabolic: Changes in menstrual cycle, changes in libido, breast pain, hyperglycemia, hypoglycemia, gynecomastia, lactation, galactorrhea
Gastrointestinal: Constipation, weight gain, nausea, vomiting, stomach pain, xerostomia
Genitourinary: Difficulty in urination, ejaculatory disturbances, urinary retention, priapism
Hematologic: Agranulocytosis, leukopenia, pancytopenia, thrombocytopenic purpura, eosinophilia, hemolytic anemia, aplastic anemia

Hepatic: Cholestatic jaundice, hepatotoxicity

Neuromuscular & skeletal: Tremor

Ocular: Pigmentary retinopathy, cornea and lens changes

Respiratory: Nasal congestion

Overdosage/Toxicology Symptoms include deep sleep, coma, extrapyramidal symptoms, abnormal involuntary muscle movements, hypo- or hypertension, and cardiac arrhythmias. Following initiation of essential overdose management, toxic symptom treatment and supportive treatment should be initiated. Hypotension usually responds to I.V. fluids or Trendelenburg positioning. If unresponsive to these measures, the use of a parenteral inotrope may be required (eg, norepinephrine 0.1-0.2 mcg/kg/minute titrated to response). Seizures commonly respond to diazepam (I.V. 5-10 mg bolus in adults every 15 minutes if needed up to a total of 30 mg; I.V. 0.25-0.4 mg/kg/dose up to a total of 10 mg in children) or to phenytoin or phenobarbital. Neuroleptics often cause extrapyramidal symptoms (eg, dystonic reactions) requiring management with diphenhydramine 1-2 mg/kg (adults) up to a maximum of 50 mg I.M. or slow I.V. push followed by a maintenance dose for 48-72 hours. When these reactions are unresponsive to diphenhydramine, anticholinergic agents such as benztropine mesylate I.V. 1-2 mg (adults) may be effective. These agents are generally effective within 2-5 minutes. Cardiac arrhythmias are treated with lidocaine 1-2 mg/kg bolus followed by a maintenance infusion.

Drug Interactions

Cytochrome P450 Effect: CYP1A2 enzyme substrate

Increased Effect/Toxicity: Trifluoperazine's effects on CNS depression may be additive when trifluoperazine is combined with CNS depressants (narcotic analgesics, ethanol, barbiturates, cyclic antidepressants, antihistamines, or sedative-hypnotics). Trifluoperazine may increase the effects/toxicity of anticholinergics, antihypertensives, lithium (rare neurotoxicity), trazodone, or valproic acid. Concurrent use with TCA may produce increased toxicity or altered therapeutic response. Chloroquine and propranolol may increase trifluoperazine concentrations. Hypotension may occur when trifluoperazine is combined with epinephrine. May increase the risk of arrhythmia when combined with antiarrhythmics, cisapride, pimozide, sparfloxacin, or other drugs which prolong QT interval.

Decreased Effect: Phenothiazines inhibit the effects of levodopa, guanadrel, guanethidine, and bromocriptine. Benztropine (and other anticholinergics) may inhibit the therapeutic response to trifluoperazine and excess anticholinergic effects may occur. Cigarette smoking and barbiturates may enhance the hepatic metabolism of trifluoperazine. Trifluoperazine and possibly other low potency antipsychotics may reverse the pressor effects of epinephrine.

Ethanol/Nutrition/Herb Interactions

Ethanol: Avoid ethanol (may increase CNS depression).

Herb/Nutraceutical: Avoid kava kava, gotu kola, valerian, St John's wort (may increase CNS depression). Avoid dong quai, St John's wort (may also cause photosensitization).

Stability Store injection at room temperature; protect from heat and from freezing; use only clear or slightly yellow solutions

Mechanism of Action Blocks postsynaptic mesolimbic dopaminergic receptors in the brain; exhibits alpha-adrenergic blocking effect and depresses the release of hypothalamic and hypophyseal hormones

Pharmacodynamics/Kinetics

Metabolism: Extensively hepatic

Half-life elimination: >24 hours with chronic use

Usual Dosage

Children 6-12 years: Schizophrenia/psychoses:

Oral: Hospitalized or well-supervised patients: Initial: 1 mg 1-2 times/day, gradually increase until symptoms are controlled or adverse effects become troublesome; maximum: 15 mg/day

I.M.: 1 mg twice daily

Adults:

Schizophrenia/psychoses:

Outpatients: Oral: 1-2 mg twice daily

Hospitalized or well-supervised patients: Initial: 2-5 mg twice daily with optimum response in the 15-20 mg/day range; do not exceed 40 mg/day

I.M.: 1-2 mg every 4-6 hours as needed up to 10 mg/24 hours maximum

Nonpsychotic anxiety: Oral: 1-2 mg twice daily; maximum: 6 mg/day; therapy for anxiety should not exceed 12 weeks; do not exceed 6 mg/day for longer than 12 weeks when treating anxiety; agitation, jitteriness, or insomnia may be confused with original neurotic or psychotic symptoms

Elderly:

Schizophrenia/psychoses:

Oral: Refer to adult dosing. Dose selection should start at the low end of the dosage range and titration must be gradual.

I.M.: Initial: 1 mg every 4-6 hours; increase at 1 mg increments; do not exceed 6 mg/day

Behavioral symptoms associated with dementia behavior: Oral: Initial: 0.5-1 mg 1-2 times/day; increase dose at 4- to 7-day intervals by 0.5-1 mg/day; increase dosing intervals (bid, tid, etc) as necessary to control response or side effects. Maximum daily dose: 40 mg. Gradual increases (titration) may prevent some side effects or decrease their severity.

Hemodialysis: Not dialyzable (0% to 5%)

Dietary Considerations May be taken with food to decrease GI distress.

Administration Administer I.M. injection deep in upper outer quadrant of buttock

Monitoring Parameters Mental status, blood pressure

Reference Range Therapeutic response and blood levels have not been established

Test Interactions False-positive for phenylketonuria

Patient Information This drug usually requires several weeks for a full therapeutic response to be seen. Avoid excessive exposure to sunlight tanning lamps; concentrate must be diluted in 2-4 oz of liquid (water, carbonated drinks, fruit juices, tomato juice, milk, or pudding); wash hands if undiluted concentrate is spilled on skin to prevent contact dermatosis

(Continued)

Trifluoperazine *(Continued)*

Nursing Implications Watch for hypotension when administering I.M. or I.V.; observe for extrapyramidal symptoms

Additional Information Do not exceed 6 mg/day for longer than 12 weeks when treating anxiety. Agitation, jitteriness, or insomnia may be confused with original neurotic or psychotic symptoms.

Dosage Forms
Injection, as hydrochloride: 2 mg/mL (10 mL)
Solution, oral concentrate, as hydrochloride: 10 mg/mL (60 mL)
Tablet, as hydrochloride: 1 mg, 2 mg, 5 mg, 10 mg

- ◆ **Trifluoperazine Hydrochloride** *see Trifluoperazine on page 1372*
- ◆ **Trifluorothymidine** *see Trifluridine on page 1374*

Trifluridine *(trye FLURE i deen)*

U.S. Brand Names Viroptic®

Canadian Brand Names Viroptic®

Synonyms F_3T; Trifluorothymidine

Therapeutic Category Antiviral Agent, Nonantiretroviral; Antiviral Agent, Ophthalmic

Use Treatment of primary keratoconjunctivitis and recurrent epithelial keratitis caused by herpes simplex virus types I and II

Pregnancy Risk Factor C

Contraindications Hypersensitivity to trifluridine or any component of the formulation

Warnings/Precautions Mild local irritation of conjunctiva and cornea may occur when instilled but usually transient effects

Adverse Reactions
>10%: Local: Burning, stinging
<1% (Limited to important or life-threatening): Epithelial keratopathy, increased intraocular pressure, keratitis, palpebral edema, stromal edema

Stability Refrigerate at 2°C to 8°C (36°F to 46°F); storage at room temperature may result in a solution altered pH which could result in ocular discomfort upon administration and/or decreased potency

Mechanism of Action Interferes with viral replication by incorporating into viral DNA in place of thymidine, inhibiting thymidylate synthetase resulting in the formation of defective proteins

Pharmacodynamics/Kinetics Absorption: Ophthalmic: Systemic absorption negligible, corneal penetration adequate

Usual Dosage Adults: Instill 1 drop into affected eye every 2 hours while awake, to a maximum of 9 drops/day, until re-epithelialization of corneal ulcer occurs; then use 1 drop every 4 hours for another 7 days; do **not** exceed 21 days of treatment; if improvement has not taken place in 7-14 days, consider another form of therapy

Patient Information Notify physician if improvement is not seen after 7 days, condition worsens, or if irritation occurs; do not discontinue without notifying the physician, do not exceed recommended dosage

Nursing Implications Monitor ophthalmologic exam (test for corneal staining with fluorescein or rose bengal)

Dosage Forms Solution, ophthalmic: 1% (7.5 mL)

Trihexyphenidyl *(trye heks ee FEN i dil)*

Related Information
Parkinson's Agents *on page 1513*

U.S. Brand Names Artane®

Canadian Brand Names Apo®-Trihex

Synonyms Benzhexol Hydrochloride; Trihexyphenidyl Hydrochloride

Therapeutic Category Anticholinergic Agent; Anti-Parkinson's Agent, Anticholinergic

Use Adjunctive treatment of Parkinson's disease; treatment of drug-induced extrapyramidal symptoms

Pregnancy Risk Factor C

Contraindications Hypersensitivity to trihexyphenidyl or any component of the formulation; narrow-angle glaucoma; pyloric or duodenal obstruction; stenosing peptic ulcers; bladder neck obstructions; achalasia; myasthenia gravis

Warnings/Precautions Use with caution in hot weather or during exercise. Elderly patients require strict dosage regulation. Use with caution in patients with tachycardia, cardiac arrhythmias, hypertension, hypotension, prostatic hyperplasia or any tendency toward urinary retention, liver or kidney disorders, and obstructive disease of the GI or GU tract. May exacerbate mental symptoms when used to treat extrapyramidal symptoms. When given in large doses or to susceptible patients, may cause weakness.

Adverse Reactions Frequency not defined.
Cardiovascular: Tachycardia
Central nervous system: Confusion, agitation, euphoria, drowsiness, headache, dizziness, nervousness, delusions, hallucinations, paranoia
Dermatologic: Dry skin, increased sensitivity to light, rash
Gastrointestinal: Constipation, xerostomia, dry throat, ileus, nausea, vomiting, parotitis
Genitourinary: Urinary retention
Neuromuscular & skeletal: Weakness
Ocular: Blurred vision, mydriasis, increase in intraocular pressure, glaucoma
Respiratory: Dry nose
Miscellaneous: Diaphoresis (decreased)

Overdosage/Toxicology Symptoms include blurred vision, urinary retention, and tachycardia. Anticholinergic toxicity is caused by strong binding of the drug to cholinergic receptors. Anticholinesterase inhibitors reduce acetylcholinesterase. For anticholinergic overdose with severe life-threatening symptoms, physostigmine 1-2 mg (0.5 mg or 0.02 mg/kg for children) S.C. or slow I.V. may be given to reverse these effects.

Drug Interactions

Increased Effect/Toxicity: Central and/or peripheral anticholinergic syndrome can occur when administered with amantadine, rimantadine, narcotic analgesics, phenothiazines and other antipsychotics (especially with high anticholinergic activity), tricyclic antidepressants, quinidine and some other antiarrhythmics, and antihistamines.

Decreased Effect: May increase gastric degradation of levodopa and decrease the amount of levodopa absorbed by delaying gastric emptying; the opposite may be true for digoxin. Therapeutic effects of cholinergic agents (tacrine, donepezil) and neuroleptics may be antagonized.

Ethanol/Nutrition/Herb Interactions Ethanol: Avoid ethanol (may increase CNS depression).

Mechanism of Action Exerts a direct inhibitory effect on the parasympathetic nervous system. It also has a relaxing effect on smooth musculature; exerted both directly on the muscle itself and indirectly through parasympathetic nervous system (inhibitory effect)

Pharmacodynamics/Kinetics

Onset of action: Peak effect: ~1 hour
Half-life elimination: 3.3-4.1 hours
Time to peak, serum: 1-1.5 hours
Excretion: Primarily urine

Usual Dosage Adults: Oral: Initial: 1-2 mg/day, increase by 2 mg increments at intervals of 3-5 days; usual dose: 5-15 mg/day in 3-4 divided doses

Monitoring Parameters IOP monitoring and gonioscopic evaluations should be performed periodically

Patient Information Take after meals or with food if GI upset occurs; do not discontinue drug abruptly; notify physician if adverse GI effects, rapid or pounding heartbeat, confusion, eye pain, rash, fever or heat intolerance occurs. Observe caution when performing hazardous tasks or those that require alertness such as driving, as may cause drowsiness. Avoid alcohol and other CNS depressants. May cause dry mouth - adequate fluid intake or hard sugar free candy may relieve. Difficult urination or constipation may occur - notify physician if effects persist; may increase susceptibility to heat stroke.

Nursing Implications Tolerated best if given in 3 daily doses and with food; high doses may be divided into 4 doses, at meal times and at bedtime

Additional Information Incidence and severity of side effects are dose related. Patients may be switched to sustained-action capsules when stabilized on conventional dosage forms.

Dosage Forms

Elixir, as hydrochloride: 2 mg/5 mL (480 mL)
Tablet, as hydrochloride: 2 mg, 5 mg

Trimethobenzamide (trye meth oh BEN za mide)

U.S. Brand Names Benzacot®; Tigan®
Canadian Brand Names Tigan®
Synonyms Trimethobenzamide Hydrochloride
Therapeutic Category Antiemetic
Use Treatment of postoperative nausea and vomiting; nausea associated with gastroenteritis
Pregnancy Risk Factor C
Contraindications Hypersensitivity to trimethobenzamide, benzocaine, or any component of the formulation; injection contraindicated in children; suppositories contraindicated in premature infants or neonates
Warnings/Precautions May mask emesis due to Reye's syndrome or mimic CNS effects of Reye's syndrome in patients with emesis of other etiologies; use in patients with acute vomiting should be avoided

Adverse Reactions

>10%: Central nervous system: Drowsiness
1% to 10%:
Cardiovascular: Hypotension
Central nervous system: Dizziness, headache
Gastrointestinal: Diarrhea
Neuromuscular & skeletal: Muscle cramps
Ocular: Blurred vision
<1% (Limited to important or life-threatening): Blood dyscrasias, convulsions, extrapyramidal symptoms, hepatic impairment

Overdosage/Toxicology Symptoms include hypotension, seizures, CNS depression, cardiac arrhythmias, disorientation, and confusion. Following initiation of essential overdose management, toxic symptom and supportive treatment should be initiated. Hypotension usually responds to I.V. fluids or Trendelenburg positioning. If unresponsive to these measures, the use of a parenteral inotrope may be required (eg, norepinephrine 0.1-0.2 mcg/kg/minute titrated to response). Seizures commonly respond to diazepam (I.V. 5-10 mg bolus in adults every 15 minutes, if needed, up to a total of 30 mg; I.V. 0.25-0.4 mg/kg/dose up to a total of 10 mg in children) or to phenytoin or phenobarbital. Critical cardiac arrhythmias often respond
(Continued)

Trimethobenzamide (Continued)

to lidocaine 1-2 mg/kg bolus followed by a maintenance infusion. Extrapyramidal symptoms (eg, dystonic reactions) may be managed with diphenhydramine 1-2 mg/kg (adults) up to a maximum of 50 mg I.M. or slow I.V. push followed by a maintenance dose for 48-72 hours. When these reactions are unresponsive to diphenhydramine, anticholinergic agents such as benztropine mesylate I.V. 1-2 mg (adults) may be effective. These agents are generally effective within 2-5 minutes.

Drug Interactions
Decreased Effect: Antagonism of oral anticoagulants may occur.

Stability Store injection at room temperature; protect from heat and from freezing; use only clear solutions

Mechanism of Action Acts centrally to inhibit the medullary chemoreceptor trigger zone

Pharmacodynamics/Kinetics
Onset of action: Antiemetic: Oral: 10-40 minutes; I.M.: 15-35 minutes
Duration: 3-4 hours
Absorption: Rectal: ~60%

Usual Dosage Rectal use is contraindicated in neonates and premature infants
Children:
Rectal: <14 kg: 100 mg 3-4 times/day
Oral, rectal: 14-40 kg: 100-200 mg 3-4 times/day
Adults:
Oral: 250 mg 3-4 times/day
I.M., rectal: 200 mg 3-4 times/day

Administration Administer I.M. only

Patient Information May cause drowsiness, impair judgment and coordination; report any restlessness or involuntary movements to physician

Nursing Implications Use only clear solution; observe for extrapyramidal and anticholinergic effects

Dosage Forms
Capsule, as hydrochloride: 100 mg, 250 mg
Injection, as hydrochloride: 100 mg/mL (2 mL, 20 mL)
Suppository, rectal, as hydrochloride: 100 mg, 200 mg

♦ **Trimethobenzamide Hydrochloride** *see* Trimethobenzamide *on page 1375*

Trimethoprim (trye METH oh prim)

U.S. Brand Names Primsol®; Proloprim®; Trimpex®
Canadian Brand Names Proloprim®
Synonyms TMP
Therapeutic Category Antibiotic, Miscellaneous

Use Treatment of urinary tract infections due to susceptible strains of E. coli, P. mirabilis, K. pneumoniae, Enterobacter sp and coagulase-negative Staphylococcus including S. saprophyticus; acute otitis media in children; acute exacerbations of chronic bronchitis in adults; in combination with other agents for treatment of toxoplasmosis, Pneumocystis carinii; treatment of superficial ocular infections involving the conjunctiva and cornea

Pregnancy Risk Factor C

Contraindications Hypersensitivity to trimethoprim or any component of the formulation; megaloblastic anemia due to folate deficiency

Warnings/Precautions Use with caution in patients with impaired renal or hepatic function or with possible folate deficiency

Adverse Reactions
1% to 10%:
Central nervous system: Headache
Gastrointestinal: Nausea, vomiting, epigastric distress
<1% (Limited to important or life-threatening): Aseptic meningitis, blood dyscrasias, cholestatic jaundice, exfoliative dermatitis, hyperkalemia, hypersensitivity, increased LFTs, methemoglobinemia, rash, Stevens-Johnson syndrome

Overdosage/Toxicology Symptom of acute toxicity includes nausea, vomiting, confusion, and dizziness. Chronic overdose results in bone marrow suppression. Treatment of acute overdose is supportive following GI decontamination. Treatment of chronic overdose includes the use of oral leucovorin 5-15 mg/day.

Drug Interactions
Cytochrome P450 Effect: CYP2C8/9 enzyme inhibitor
Increased Effect/Toxicity: Increased effect/toxicity/levels of phenytoin. Concurrent use with ACE inhibitors increases risk of hyperkalemia. Increased myelosuppression with methotrexate. May increase levels of digoxin. Concurrent use with dapsone may increase levels of dapsone and trimethoprim. Concurrent use with procainamide may increase levels of procainamide and trimethoprim.

Stability Protect the 200 mg tablet from light.

Mechanism of Action Inhibits folic acid reduction to tetrahydrofolate, and thereby inhibits microbial growth

Pharmacodynamics/Kinetics
Absorption: Readily and extensive
Distribution: Widely into body tissues and fluids (middle ear, prostate, bile, aqueous humor, CSF); crosses placenta; enters breast milk
Protein binding: 42% to 46%
Metabolism: Partially hepatic
Half-life elimination: 8-14 hours; prolonged with renal impairment
Time to peak, serum: 1-4 hours
Excretion: Primarily urine (60% to 80%) as unchanged drug

Usual Dosage Oral:
Children: 4 mg/kg/day in divided doses every 12 hours

Adults: 100 mg every 12 hours or 200 mg every 24 hours; in the treatment of *Pneumocystis carinii* pneumonia; dose may be as high as 15-20 mg/kg/day in 3-4 divided doses

Dosing interval in renal impairment: Cl$_{cr}$ 15-30 mL/minute: Administer 50 mg every 12 hours

Hemodialysis: Moderately dialyzable (20% to 50%)

Dietary Considerations May cause folic acid deficiency, supplements may be needed.

Reference Range Therapeutic: Peak: 5-15 mg/L; Trough: 2-8 mg/L

Patient Information Take with milk or food; report any skin rash, persistent or severe fatigue, fever, sore throat, or unusual bleeding or bruising; complete full course of therapy

Nursing Implications Monitor for signs of bone marrow suppression such as fever, sore throat, or bleeding; tablets can be crushed

Dosage Forms
Solution, oral: 50 mg (base)/5 mL
Tablet: 100 mg, 200 mg

Trimethoprim and Polymyxin B (trye METH oh prim & pol i MIKS in bee)

U.S. Brand Names Polytrim®

Canadian Brand Names PMS-Polytrimethoprim; Polytrim™

Synonyms Polymyxin B and Trimethoprim

Therapeutic Category Antibiotic, Ophthalmic

Use Treatment of surface ocular bacterial conjunctivitis and blepharoconjunctivitis

Pregnancy Risk Factor C

Usual Dosage Instill 1-2 drops in eye(s) every 4-6 hours
Elderly: No overall differences observed between elderly and other adults

Additional Information Complete prescribing information for this medication should be consulted for additional detail.

Dosage Forms Solution, ophthalmic: Trimethoprim sulfate 1 mg and polymyxin B sulfate 10,000 units per mL (10 mL)

- **Trimethoprim and Sulfamethoxazole** *see* Sulfamethoxazole and Trimethoprim *on page 1273*
- **Trimethylpsoralen** *see* Trioxsalen *on page 1379*

Trimetrexate Glucuronate (tri me TREKS ate gloo KYOOR oh nate)

U.S. Brand Names Neutrexin®

Therapeutic Category Antineoplastic Agent, Folate Antagonist

Use Alternative therapy for the treatment of moderate-to-severe *Pneumocystis carinii* pneumonia (PCP) in immunocompromised patients, including patients with acquired immunodeficiency syndrome (AIDS), who are intolerant of, or are refractory to, co-trimoxazole therapy or for whom co-trimoxazole and pentamidine are contraindicated. **Concurrent folinic acid (leucovorin) must always be administered.**

Pregnancy Risk Factor D

Contraindications Hypersensitivity to trimetrexate, methotrexate, or any component of the formulation; severe existing myelosuppression; pregnancy

Warnings/Precautions The U.S. Food and Drug Administration (FDA) currently recommends that procedures for proper handling and disposal of antineoplastic agents be considered. Appropriate safety equipment is recommended for preparation, administration, and disposal of antineoplastics. If trimetrexate contacts the skin, immediately wash with soap and water. **Must be administered with concurrent leucovorin to avoid potentially serious or life-threatening toxicities.** Leucovorin therapy must extend for 72 hours past the last dose of trimetrexate. Use with caution in patients with mild myelosuppression, severe hepatic or renal dysfunction, hypoproteinemia, hypoalbuminemia, or previous extensive myelosuppressive therapies.

Adverse Reactions 1% to 10%:
Central nervous system: Seizures, fever
Dermatologic: Rash
Gastrointestinal: Stomatitis, nausea, vomiting
Hematologic: Neutropenia, thrombocytopenia, anemia
Hepatic: Elevated LFTs
Neuromuscular & skeletal: Peripheral neuropathy
Renal: Increased serum creatinine
Miscellaneous: Flu-like illness, hypersensitivity reactions

Drug Interactions
Cytochrome P450 Effect: Metabolized by cytochrome isoenzyme, possibly CYP3A3/4
Increased Effect/Toxicity: Cimetidine, clotrimazole, ketoconazole, and acetaminophen have been shown to decrease clearance of trimetrexate resulting in increased serum levels.
Decreased Effect: Trimetrexate is metabolized by cytochrome P450 enzymes in the liver. Examples of drugs where this interaction may occur are erythromycin, rifampin, rifabutin, ketoconazole, and fluconazole.

Stability Reconstituted I.V. solution is stable for 24 hours at room temperature or 7 days when refrigerated; intact vials should be refrigerated at 2°C to 8°C

Mechanism of Action Exerts an antimicrobial effect through potent inhibition of the enzyme dihydrofolate reductase (DHFR)

Pharmacodynamics/Kinetics
Distribution: V$_d$: 0.62 L/kg
Metabolism: Extensively hepatic
Half-life elimination: 15-17 hours

Usual Dosage Adults: I.V.: 45 mg/m^2 once daily over 60 minutes for 21 days; it is necessary to reduce the dose in patients with liver dysfunction, although no specific recommendations exist; concurrent folinic acid 20 mg/m^2 every 6 hours orally or I.V. for at least 24 hours after the last dose of trimetrexate
(Continued)

Trimetrexate Glucuronate *(Continued)*

Administration Reconstituted solution should be filtered (0.22 μM) prior to further dilution; final solution should be clear, hue will range from colorless to pale yellow; trimetrexate forms a precipitate instantly upon contact with chloride ion or leucovorin; therefore it should not be added to solutions containing sodium chloride or other anions; trimetrexate and leucovorin solutions **must** be administered separately; intravenous lines should be flushed with at least 10 mL of D₅W between trimetrexate and leucovorin

Monitoring Parameters Check and record patient's temperature daily; absolute neutrophil counts (ANC), platelet count, renal function tests (serum creatinine, BUN), hepatic function tests (ALT, AST, alkaline phosphatase)

Patient Information Report promptly any fever, rash, flu-like symptoms, numbness or tingling in the extremities, nausea, vomiting, abdominal pain, mouth sores, increased bruising or bleeding, black tarry stools

Nursing Implications Notify primary physician if there is fever ≥103°F, generalized rash, seizures, bleeding from any site, uncontrolled nausea/vomiting; laboratory abnormalities which warrant dose modification; any other clinical adverse event or laboratory abnormality occurring in therapy which is judged as serious for that patient or which causes unexplained effects or concern; initiate "Bleeding Precautions" for platelet counts ≤50,000/mm³; initiate "Infection Control Measures" for absolute neutrophil counts (ANC) ≤1000/mm³

Must administer folinic acid 20 mg/m² orally or I.V. every 6 hours for 24 days

Additional Information Not a vesicant; methotrexate derivative

Dosage Forms Powder for injection: 25 mg, 200 mg

Trimipramine *(trye MI pra meen)*

Related Information

Antidepressant Agents Comparison *on page 1482*

U.S. Brand Names Surmontil®

Canadian Brand Names Apo®-Trimip; Novo-Tripramine; Nu-Trimipramine; Rhotrimine®; Surmontil®

Synonyms Trimipramine Maleate

Therapeutic Category Antidepressant, Tricyclic

Use Treatment of depression

Pregnancy Risk Factor C

Contraindications Hypersensitivity to trimipramine, any component of the formulation, or other dibenzodiazepines; use of MAO inhibitors within 14 days; use in a patient during the acute recovery phase of MI

Warnings/Precautions Often causes sedation, resulting in impaired performance of tasks requiring alertness (ie, operating machinery or driving). Sedative effects may be additive with other CNS depressants and/or ethanol. The degree of sedation is very high relative to other antidepressants. May worsen psychosis in some patients or precipitate a shift to mania or hypomania in patients with bipolar disease. May increase the risks associated with electro-convulsive therapy. This agent should be discontinued, when possible, prior to elective surgery. Therapy should not be abruptly discontinued in patients receiving high doses for prolonged periods. Use with caution in patients with hepatic or renal dysfunction and in elderly patients.

May cause orthostatic hypotension (risk is high relative to other antidepressants) - use with caution in patients at risk of hypotension or in patients where transient hypotensive episodes would be poorly tolerated (cardiovascular disease or cerebrovascular disease). The degree of anticholinergic blockade produced by this agent is very high relative to other cyclic antide-pressants - use caution in patients with urinary retention, benign prostatic hypertrophy, narrow-angle glaucoma, xerostomia, visual problems, constipation, or history of bowel obstruction. May cause alteration in glucose regulation - use with caution in patients with diabetes.

Use caution in patients with suicidal risk. Use with caution in patients with a history of cardiovascular disease (including previous MI, stroke, tachycardia, or conduction abnormali-ties). The risk conduction abnormalities with this agent is high relative to other antidepres-sants. Use caution in patients with a previous seizure disorder or condition predisposing to seizures such as brain damage, alcoholism, or concurrent therapy with other drugs which lower the seizure threshold. Use with caution in hyperthyroid patients or those receiving thyroid supplementation.

Adverse Reactions Frequency not defined.

Cardiovascular: Arrhythmias, hypotension, hypertension, tachycardia, palpitations, heart block, stroke, myocardial infarction

Central nervous system: Headache, exacerbation of psychosis, confusion, delirium, halluci-nations, nervousness, restlessness, delusions, agitation, insomnia, nightmares, anxiety, seizures, drowsiness

Dermatologic: Photosensitivity, rash, petechiae, itching

Endocrine & metabolic: Sexual dysfunction, breast enlargement, galactorrhea, SIADH

Gastrointestinal: Xerostomia, constipation, increased appetite, nausea, unpleasant taste, weight gain, diarrhea, heartburn, vomiting, anorexia, trouble with gums, decreased lower esophageal sphincter tone may cause GE reflux

Genitourinary: Difficult urination, urinary retention, testicular edema

Hematologic: Agranulocytosis, eosinophilia, purpura, thrombocytopenia

Hepatic: Cholestatic jaundice, increased liver enzymes

Neuromuscular & skeletal: Tremors, numbness, tingling, paresthesia, incoordination, ataxia, peripheral neuropathy, extrapyramidal symptoms

Ocular: Blurred vision, eye pain, disturbances in accommodation, mydriasis, increased intra-ocular pressure

Otic: Tinnitus

Miscellaneous: Allergic reactions

Overdosage/Toxicology Symptoms include agitation, confusion, hallucinations, urinary retention, hypothermia, hypotension, tachycardia, and cardiac arrhythmias. Following initiation of essential overdose management, toxic symptoms should be treated. Sodium bicarbonate is indicated when the QRS interval is >0.10 seconds or the QT$_c$ >0.42 seconds. Ventricular arrhythmias and EKG changes (QRS widening) often respond to systemic alkalinization (sodium bicarbonate 0.5-2 mEq/kg I.V.). Arrhythmias unresponsive to this therapy may respond to lidocaine 1 mg/kg I.V. followed by a titrated infusion. Physostigmine (1-2 mg slow I.V. for adults or 0.5 mg slow I.V. for children) may be indicated in reversing life-threatening cardiac arrhythmias. Seizures usually respond to diazepam I.V. boluses (5-10 mg for adults up to 30 mg or 0.25-0.4 mg/kg/dose for children up to 10 mg/dose). If seizures are unresponsive or recur, phenytoin or phenobarbital may be required.

Drug Interactions

Cytochrome P450 Effect: CYP2D6 enzyme substrate

Increased Effect/Toxicity: Trimipramine increases the effects of amphetamines, anticholinergics, other CNS depressants (sedatives, hypnotics, or ethanol), chlorpropamide, tolazamide, and warfarin. When used with MAO inhibitors, hyperpyrexia, hypertension, tachycardia, confusion, seizures, and **deaths have been reported** (serotonin syndrome). Serotonin syndrome has also been reported with ritonavir (rare). The SSRIs (to varying degrees), cimetidine, grapefruit juice, indinavir, methylphenidate, ritonavir, quinidine, diltiazem, and verapamil inhibit the metabolism of TCAs and clinical toxicity may result. Use of lithium with a TCA may increase the risk for neurotoxicity. Phenothiazines may increase concentration of some TCAs and TCAs may increase concentration of phenothiazines. Pressor response to I.V. epinephrine, norepinephrine, and phenylephrine may be enhanced in patients receiving TCAs (**Note:** Effect is unlikely with epinephrine or levonordefrin dosages typically administered as infiltration in combination with local anesthetics). Combined use of beta-agonists or drugs which prolong QT$_c$ (including quinidine, procainamide, disopyramide, cisapride, sparfloxacin, gatifloxacin, moxifloxacin) with TCAs may predispose patients to cardiac arrhythmias.

Decreased Effect: Carbamazepine, phenobarbital, and rifampin may increase the metabolism of trimipramine resulting in decreased effect of trimipramine. Trimipramine inhibits the antihypertensive response to bethanidine, clonidine, debrisoquin, guanadrel, guanethidine, guanabenz, and guanfacine. Cholestyramine and colestipol may bind TCAs and reduce their absorption; monitor for altered response.

Ethanol/Nutrition/Herb Interactions

Ethanol: Avoid ethanol (may increase CNS depression).

Food: Grapefruit juice may inhibit the metabolism of some TCAs and clinical toxicity may result.

Herb/Nutraceutical: Avoid valerian, St John's wort, SAMe, kava kava (may increase risk of serotonin syndrome and/or excessive sedation).

Stability Solutions stable at a pH of 4-5; turns yellowish or reddish on exposure to light. Slight discoloration does not affect potency; marked discoloration is associated with loss of potency. Capsules stable for 3 years following date of manufacture.

Mechanism of Action Increases the synaptic concentration of serotonin and/or norepinephrine in the central nervous system by inhibition of their reuptake by the presynaptic neuronal membrane

Pharmacodynamics/Kinetics

Onset of action: Therapeutic: >2 weeks

Protein binding: 95%

Metabolism: Hepatic; significant first-pass effect

Half-life elimination: 20-26 hours

Time to peak: ~6 hours

Excretion: Urine

Usual Dosage Oral:

Adults: 50-150 mg/day as a single bedtime dose up to a maximum of 200 mg/day outpatient and 300 mg/day inpatient

Elderly: Adequate studies have not been done in the elderly. In general, dosing should be cautious, starting at the lower end of dosing range.

Monitoring Parameters Blood pressure and pulse rate prior to and during initial therapy; evaluate mental status; monitor weight; EKG in older adults

Patient Information Avoid unnecessary exposure to sunlight; avoid alcohol; do not discontinue medication abruptly; may cause urine to turn blue-green; may cause drowsiness; can use sugarless gum or hard candy for dry mouth; full effect may not occur for 4-6 weeks

Nursing Implications May increase appetite; may cause drowsiness, raise bed rails, institute safety precautions

Additional Information May cause alterations in bleeding time.

Dosage Forms Capsule, as maleate: 25 mg, 50 mg, 100 mg

◆ **Trimipramine Maleate** see Trimipramine on page 1378

◆ **Trimox®** see Amoxicillin on page 84

◆ **Trimpex®** see Trimethoprim on page 1376

◆ **Trinalin®** see Azatadine and Pseudoephedrine on page 136

◆ **Tri-Nasal®** see Triamcinolone on page 1366

◆ **Tri-Norinyl®** see Ethinyl Estradiol and Norethindrone on page 522

◆ **Triostat™** see Liothyronine on page 808

◆ **Triotann®** see Chlorpheniramine, Pyrilamine, and Phenylephrine on page 282

Trioxsalen (trye OKS a len)

U.S. Brand Names Trisoralen®

Synonyms Trimethylpsoralen

Therapeutic Category Psoralen

Use In conjunction with controlled exposure to ultraviolet light or sunlight for repigmentation of idiopathic vitiligo; increasing tolerance to sunlight with albinism; enhance pigmentation

Pregnancy Risk Factor C

(Continued)

Trioxsalen (Continued)

Contraindications Hypersensitivity to psoralens, melanoma, a history of melanoma, or other diseases associated with photosensitivity; porphyria; acute lupus erythematosus; patients <12 years of age

Warnings/Precautions Serious burns from UVA or sunlight can occur if dosage or exposure schedules are exceeded; patients must wear protective eye wear to prevent cataracts; use with caution in patients with severe hepatic or cardiovascular disease

Adverse Reactions

>10%:

Dermatologic: Itching

Gastrointestinal: Nausea

1% to 10%:

Central nervous system: Dizziness, headache, mental depression, insomnia, nervousness

Dermatologic: Severe burns from excessive sunlight or ultraviolet exposure

Gastrointestinal: Gastric discomfort

Mechanism of Action Psoralens are thought to form covalent bonds with pyrimidine bases in DNA which inhibit the synthesis of DNA. This reaction involves excitation of the trioxsalen molecule by radiation in the long-wave ultraviolet light (UVA) resulting in transference of energy to the trioxsalen molecule producing an excited state. Binding of trioxsalen to DNA occurs only in the presence of ultraviolet light. The increase in skin pigmentation produced by trioxsalen and UVA radiation involves multiple changes in melanocytes and interaction between melanocytes and keratinocytes. In general, melanogenesis is stimulated but the size and distribution of melanocytes is unchanged.

Pharmacodynamics/Kinetics

Onset of action: Peak effect: Photosensitivity: 2 hours

Duration: Skin sensitivity to light: 8-12 hours

Absorption: Rapid

Half-life elimination: ~2 hours

Usual Dosage Children >12 years and Adults: Oral: 10 mg/day as a single dose, 2-4 hours before controlled exposure to UVA (for 15-35 minutes) or sunlight; do not continue for longer than 14 days

Patient Information To minimize gastric discomfort, tablets may be taken with milk or after a meal; wear sunglasses during exposure and a light-screening lipstick; do not exceed dose or exposure duration

Nursing Implications To minimize gastric discomfort, tablets may be administered with milk or after a meal; wear sunglasses during exposure and a light-screening lipstick; do not exceed dose or exposure duration

Dosage Forms Tablet: 5 mg

♦ **Tripedia®** see Diphtheria, Tetanus Toxoids, and Acellular Pertussis Vaccine *on page 418*

Tripelennamine (tri pel ENN a meen)

U.S. Brand Names PBZ®; PBZ-SR®

Synonyms Tripelennamine Citrate; Tripelennamine Hydrochloride

Therapeutic Category Antihistamine, H_1 Blocker

Use Perennial and seasonal allergic rhinitis and other allergic symptoms including urticaria

Pregnancy Risk Factor B

Usual Dosage Oral:

Infants and Children: 5 mg/kg/day in 4-6 divided doses, up to 300 mg/day maximum

Adults: 25-50 mg every 4-6 hours, extended release tablets 100 mg morning and evening up to 100 mg every 8 hours

Additional Information Complete prescribing information for this medication should be consulted for additional detail.

Dosage Forms Tablet, as hydrochloride: 50 mg

♦ **Tripelennamine Citrate** see Tripelennamine *on page 1380*

♦ **Tripelennamine Hydrochloride** see Tripelennamine *on page 1380*

♦ **Triphasil®** see Ethinyl Estradiol and Levonorgestrel *on page 518*

♦ **Triphed® [OTC]** see Triprolidine and Pseudoephedrine *on page 1380*

♦ **Triple Antibiotic®** see Bacitracin, Neomycin, and Polymyxin B *on page 143*

♦ **Triple Sulfa** see Sulfabenzamide, Sulfacetamide, and Sulfathiazole *on page 1268*

♦ **Triposed® Tablet [OTC]** see Triprolidine and Pseudoephedrine *on page 1380*

Triprolidine and Pseudoephedrine (trye PROE li deen & soo doe e FED rin)

U.S. Brand Names Act-A-Med® [OTC]; Actanol® [OTC]; Actedril® [OTC]; Actifed® [OTC]; Allerfed® [OTC]; Allerfrim® [OTC]; Allerphed® [OTC]; Altafed® [OTC]; Aphedrid™ [OTC]; Aprodine® [OTC]; Biofed-PE® [OTC]; Cenafed® Plus Tablet [OTC]; Genac® Tablet [OTC]; Histafed® [OTC]; Hista-Tabs® [OTC]; Pseudocot-T® [OTC]; Ridifed® [OTC]; Ritifed® [OTC]; Silafed® [OTC]; Triacin® [OTC]; Triafed® [OTC]; Tri-Fed® [OTC]; Triphed® [OTC]; Triposed® Tablet [OTC]; Tri-Pseudafed® [OTC]; Tri-Pseudo® [OTC]; Tri-Sofed® [OTC]; Trisudex® [OTC]; Tri-Sudo® [OTC]; Uni-Fed® [OTC]; Vi-Sudo® [OTC]

Canadian Brand Names Actifed®

Synonyms Pseudoephedrine and Triprolidine

Therapeutic Category Alpha/Beta Agonist; Antihistamine

Use Temporary relief of nasal congestion, decongest sinus openings, running nose, sneezing, itching of nose or throat and itchy, watery eyes due to common cold, hay fever, or other upper respiratory allergies

Pregnancy Risk Factor C

Usual Dosage Oral:

Children:

Syrup:

4 months to 2 years: 1.25 mL 3-4 times/day

2-4 years: 2.5 mL 3-4 times/day

4-6 years: 3.75 mL 3-4 times/day
6-12 years: 5 mL every 4-6 hours; do not exceed 4 doses in 24 hours
Tablet: ½ every 4-6 hours; do not exceed 4 doses in 24 hours
Children >12 years and Adults:
Syrup: 10 mL every 4-6 hours; do not exceed 4 doses in 24 hours
Tablet: 1 every 4-6 hours; do not exceed 4 doses in 24 hours
Additional Information Complete prescribing information for this medication should be consulted for additional detail.
Dosage Forms
Capsule: Triprolidine hydrochloride 2.5 mg and pseudoephedrine hydrochloride 60 mg
Capsule, extended release: Triprolidine hydrochloride 5 mg and pseudoephedrine hydrochloride 120 mg
Syrup: Triprolidine hydrochloride 1.25 mg and pseudoephedrine hydrochloride 30 mg per 5 mL
Tablet: Triprolidine hydrochloride 2.5 mg and pseudoephedrine hydrochloride 60 mg

♦ **Triprolidine, Codeine, and Pseudoephedrine** *see* Triprolidine, Pseudoephedrine, and Codeine *on page 1381*

Triprolidine, Pseudoephedrine, and Codeine
(trye PROE li deen, soo doe e FED rin, & KOE deen)
U.S. Brand Names Aprodine® w/C; Triacin-C®
Canadian Brand Names CoActifed®
Synonyms Codeine, Pseudoephedrine, and Triprolidine; Pseudoephedrine, Triprolidine, and Codeine Pseudoephedrine, Codeine, and Triprolidine; Triprolidine, Codeine, and Pseudoephedrine; Triprolidine, Pseudoephedrine, and Codeine, Triprolidine, and Pseudoephedrine
Therapeutic Category Antihistamine/Decongestant/Antitussive
Use Symptomatic relief of upper respiratory symptoms and cough
Restrictions C-V
Pregnancy Risk Factor C
Usual Dosage Oral:
Children:
2-6 years: 2.5 mL 4 times/day
7-12 years: 5 mL 4 times/day
Children >12 years and Adults: 10 mL 4 times/day
Additional Information Complete prescribing information for this medication should be consulted for additional detail.
Dosage Forms Syrup: Triprolidine hydrochloride 1.25 mg, pseudoephedrine hydrochloride 30 mg, and codeine phosphate 10 mg per 5 mL with alcohol 4.3%

♦ **Triprolidine, Pseudoephedrine, and Codeine, Triprolidine, and Pseudoephedrine** *see* Triprolidine, Pseudoephedrine, and Codeine *on page 1381*

♦ **Tri-Pseudafed® [OTC]** *see* Triprolidine and Pseudoephedrine *on page 1380*

♦ **Tri-Pseudo® [OTC]** *see* Triprolidine and Pseudoephedrine *on page 1380*

♦ **Triptil® (Can)** *see* Protriptyline *on page 1154*

Triptorelin (trip toe REL in)
U.S. Brand Names Trelstar™ Depot; Trelstar™ LA
Canadian Brand Names Trelstar™ Depot
Synonyms Triptorelin Pamoate
Therapeutic Category Luteinizing Hormone-Releasing Hormone Analog
Use Palliative treatment of advanced prostate cancer as an alternative to orchiectomy or estrogen administration
Pregnancy Risk Factor X
Pregnancy/Breast-Feeding Implications Contraindicated in women who are or may become pregnant.
Contraindications Hypersensitivity to triptorelin or any component of the formulation, other LHRH agonists or LHRH; pregnancy
Warnings/Precautions Transient increases in testosterone can lead to worsening symptoms (bone pain, hematuria, bladder outlet obstruction) of prostate cancer during the first few weeks of therapy. Cases of spinal cord compression have been reported with LHRH agonists. Hypersensitivity reactions including angioedema and anaphylaxis have rarely occurred. Safety and efficacy not established in pediatric population.
Adverse Reactions As reported with Trelstar™ Depot and Trelstar™ LA; frequency of effect may vary by product:

>10%:
Endocrine & metabolic: Hot flashes (59% to 73%), glucose increased, hemoglobin decreased, RBC count decreased
Hepatic: Alkaline phosphatase increased, ALT increased, AST increased
Neuromuscular & skeletal: Skeletal pain (12% to 13%)
Renal: BUN increased
1% to 10%:
Cardiovascular: Leg edema (6%), hypertension (4%), chest pain (2%), peripheral edema (1%)
Central nervous system: Headache (5% to 7%), dizziness (1% to 3%), pain (2% to 3%), emotional lability (1%), fatigue (1%), insomnia (2%)
Dermatologic: Rash (2%), pruritus (1%)
Endocrine & metabolic: Alkaline phosphatase increased (2%), breast pain (2%), gynocomastia (2%), libido decreased (2%)
Gastrointestinal: Nausea (3%), anorexia (2%), constipation (2%), dyspepsia (2%), vomiting (2%), abdominal pain (1%), diarrhea (1%)
Genitourinary: Dysuria (5%), impotence (2% to 7%), urinary retention (1%), urinary tract infection (1%)
Hematologic: Anemia (1%)
(Continued)

Triptorelin *(Continued)*

Local: Injection site pain (4%)

Neuromuscular & skeletal: Leg pain (2% to 5%), back pain (3%), arthralgia (2%), leg cramps (2%), myalgia (1%), weakness (1%)

Ocular: Conjunctivitis (1%), eye pain (1%)

Respiratory: Cough (2%), dyspnea (1%), pharyngitis (1%)

Postmarketing and/or case reports (Limited to important or life-threatening): Anaphylaxis, angioedema, hypersensitivity reactions, renal dysfunction, spinal cord compression

Overdosage/Toxicology Accidental or intentional overdose unlikely. If it were to occur, supportive and symptomatic treatment would be indicated.

Drug Interactions

Increased Effect/Toxicity: Not studied. Hyperprolactinemic drugs (dopamine antagonists such as antipsychotics, and metoclopramide) are contraindicated.

Decreased Effect: Not studied. Hyperprolactinemic drugs (dopamine antagonists such as antipsychotics, and metoclopramide) are contraindicated.

Stability

Trelstar™ Depot: Store at 15°C to 30°C (59°F to 86°F)

Trelstar™ LA: Store at 20°C to 25°C (68°F to 77°F)

Reconstitution: Reconstitute with 2 mL sterile water for injection. Shake well to obtain a uniform suspension. Withdraw the entire contents into the syringe and inject immediately.

Mechanism of Action Causes suppression of ovarian and testicular steroidogenesis due to decreased levels of LH and FSH with subsequent decrease in testosterone (male) and estrogen (female) levels. After chronic and continuous administration, usually 2-4 weeks after initiation, a sustained decrease in LH and FSH secretion occurs.

Pharmacodynamics/Kinetics

Absorption: Oral: Not active

Distribution: V_d: 30-33 L

Protein binding: None

Metabolism: Unknown, unlikely to involve P450 system; no known metabolites

Half-life elimination: 2.8 ± 1.2 hours

Moderate to severe renal impairment: 6.5-7.7 hours

Hepatic impairment: 7.6 hours

Time to peak: 1-3 hours

Excretion: Urine (42% as intact peptide); hepatic

Usual Dosage I.M.: Adults: Prostate cancer:

Trelstar™ Depot: 3.75 mg once every 28 days

Trelstar™ LA: 11.25 mg once every 84 days

Dosage adjustment in renal/hepatic impairment: Patients with renal or hepatic impairment showed two- to fourfold higher exposure than young healthy males. The clinical consequences of this increase, as well as the potential need for dose adjustment, is currently unknown.

Administration Must be administered under the supervision of a physician. Administer by I.M. injection into the buttock; alternate injection sites.

Debioclip™: Follow manufacturer's instructions for mixing prior to use.

Monitoring Parameters Serum testosterone levels, prostate-specific antigen

Test Interactions Pituitary-gonadal function may be suppressed with chronic administration and for up to 8 weeks after triptorelin therapy has been discontinued.

Patient Information Use as directed. Do not miss monthly appointment for injection. You may experience disease flare (increased bone pain), blood in urine, and urinary retention during early treatment (usually resolves within 1 week). Hot flashes are common; you may feel flushed and hot (wearing layers of clothes or summer clothes and cool environment may help). If it becomes annoying and bothersome, let prescriber know. Report irregular or rapid heartbeat, unresolved nausea or vomiting, numbness of extremities, breast swelling or pain, difficulty breathing, or infection at injection sites. Do not get pregnant; females must use barrier contraceptives during and for a time following therapy. Breast-feeding is not recommended.

Nursing Implications Disease flare (increased bone pain, urinary retention) can briefly occur with initiation of therapy.

Dosage Forms Powder for injection, as pamoate:

Trelstar™ Depot: 3.75 mg [also available packaged with Debioclip™, a prefilled syringe containing sterile water]

Trelstar™ LA: 11.25 mg [also available packaged with Debioclip™, a prefilled syringe containing sterile water]

♦ **Triptorelin Pamoate** *see* Triptorelin *on page 1381*

♦ **Triquilar® (Can)** *see* Ethinyl Estradiol and Levonorgestrel *on page 518*

♦ **Tris Buffer** *see* Tromethamine *on page 1383*

♦ **Trisenox™** *see* Arsenic Trioxide *on page 115*

♦ **Tris(hydroxymethyl)aminomethane** *see* Tromethamine *on page 1383*

♦ **Tri-Sofed® [OTC]** *see* Triprolidine and Pseudoephedrine *on page 1380*

♦ **Trisoralen®** *see* Trioxsalen *on page 1379*

♦ **Tristoject®** *see* Triamcinolone *on page 1366*

♦ **Trisudex® [OTC]** *see* Triprolidine and Pseudoephedrine *on page 1380*

♦ **Tri-Sudo® [OTC]** *see* Triprolidine and Pseudoephedrine *on page 1380*

♦ **Trisulfapyrimidines** *see* Sulfadiazine, Sulfamethazine, and Sulfamerazine *on page 1271*

♦ **Tri-Tannate®** *see* Chlorpheniramine, Pyrilamine, and Phenylephrine *on page 282*

♦ **Tri-Tannate Plus® [OTC]** *see* Chlorpheniramine, Ephedrine, Phenylephrine, and Carbetapentane *on page 280*

♦ **Tritec®** *see* Ranitidine Bismuth Citrate *on page 1180*

♦ **Trivagizole 3™** *see* Clotrimazole *on page 323*

♦ **Trivora®** *see* Ethinyl Estradiol and Levonorgestrel *on page 518*

♦ **Trizivir**® *see* Abacavir, Lamivudine, and Zidovudine *on page 17*
♦ **Trobicin**® *see* Spectinomycin *on page 1256*
♦ **Trocaine**® [OTC] *see* Benzocaine *on page 154*

Troleandomycin (troe lee an doe MYE sin)

U.S. Brand Names Tao®
Synonyms Triacetyloleandomycin
Therapeutic Category Antibiotic, Macrolide
Use Adjunct in the treatment of corticosteroid-dependent asthma due to its steroid-sparing properties; antibiotic with spectrum of activity similar to erythromycin
Pregnancy Risk Factor C
Contraindications Hypersensitivity to troleandomycin, other macrolides, or any component of the formulation; concurrent use with cisapride
Warnings/Precautions Use with caution in patients with impaired hepatic function; chronic hepatitis may occur in patients with long or repetitive courses
Adverse Reactions
>10%: Gastrointestinal: Abdominal cramping and discomfort (dose-related)
1% to 10%:
Dermatologic: Urticaria, rashes
Gastrointestinal: Nausea, vomiting, diarrhea
<1% (Limited to important or life-threatening): Cholestatic jaundice, rectal burning
Overdosage/Toxicity Symptoms include nausea, vomiting, diarrhea, and hearing loss. Following GI decontamination, treatment is supportive.
Drug Interactions
Cytochrome P450 Effect: CYP3A3/4 enzyme substrate; CYP3A3/4 and 3A5-7 enzyme inhibitor
Increased Effect/Toxicity: May increase serum concentrations of carbamazepine, ergot alkaloids, methylprednisolone, oral contraceptives, theophylline, and triazolam; contraindicated with terfenadine, astemizole, cisapride, and pimozide due to decreased metabolism of this agent and resultant risk of cardiac arrhythmias and death.
Ethanol/Nutrition/Herb Interactions Food: Presence of food delays absorption, but has no effect on the extent of absorption.
Mechanism of Action Decreases methylprednisolone clearance from a linear first order decline to a nonlinear decline in plasma concentration. Troleandomycin also has an undefined action independent of its effects on steroid elimination. Inhibits RNA-dependent protein synthesis at the chain elongation step; binds to the 50S ribosomal subunit resulting in blockage of transpeptidation.
Pharmacodynamics/Kinetics
Time to peak, serum: ~2 hours
Excretion: Urine (10% to 25% as active drug); feces
Usual Dosage Oral:
Children 7-13 years: 25-40 mg/kg/day divided every 6 hours (125-250 mg every 6 hours)
Adjunct in corticosteroid-dependent asthma: 14 mg/kg/day in divided doses every 6-12 hours not to exceed 250 mg every 6 hours; dose is tapered to once daily then alternate day dosing
Adults: 250-500 mg 4 times/day
Dietary Considerations May be taken with food.
Administration Administer around-the-clock instead of 4 times/day
Monitoring Parameters Hepatic function tests
Patient Information Complete full course of therapy; notify physician if persistent or severe abdominal pain, nausea, vomiting, jaundice, darkened urine, or fever occurs
Nursing Implications Monitor hepatic function tests
Dosage Forms Capsule: 250 mg

♦ **Trombovar**® (Can) *see* Sodium Tetradecyl *on page 1249*

Tromethamine (troe METH a meen)

U.S. Brand Names THAM®
Synonyms Tris Buffer; Tris(hydroxymethyl)aminomethane
Therapeutic Category Alkalinizing Agent, Parenteral
Use Correction of metabolic acidosis associated with cardiac bypass surgery or cardiac arrest; to correct excess acidity of stored blood that is preserved with acid citrate dextrose; to prime the pump-oxygenator during cardiac bypass surgery; indicated in infants needing alkalinization after receiving maximum sodium bicarbonate (8-10 mEq/kg/24 hours); (advantage of THAM® is that it alkalinizes without increasing pCO_2 and sodium)
Pregnancy Risk Factor C
Contraindications Uremia or anuria; chronic respiratory acidosis (neonates); salicylate intoxication (neonates)
Warnings/Precautions Reduce dose and monitor pH carefully in renal impairment; drug should not be given for a period of longer than 24 hours unless for a life-threatening situation
Adverse Reactions
1% to 10%:
Cardiovascular: Venospasm
Local: Tissue irritation, necrosis with extravasation
<1% (Limited to important or life-threatening): Apnea, hyperkalemia, hyperosmolality of serum, hypoglycemia (transient), increased blood coagulation time, infusion via low-lying umbilical venous catheters has been associated with hepatocellular necrosis, liver cell destruction from direct contact with THAM®, respiratory depression
Overdosage/Toxicity Symptoms include alkalosis, hypokalemia, respiratory depression, and hypoglycemia. Supportive therapy is required to correct electrolyte, osmolality, and abnormalities.
Mechanism of Action Acts as a proton acceptor, which combines with hydrogen ions to form bicarbonate buffer, to correct acidosis
(Continued)

Tromethamine (Continued)

Pharmacodynamics/Kinetics
Absorption: 30% of dose is not ionized
Excretion: Urine (>75%) within 3 hours

Usual Dosage
Neonates and Infants: Metabolic acidosis associated with RDS: Initial: Approximately 1 mL/kg for each pH unit below 7.4; additional doses determined by changes in PaO_2, pH, and pCO_2; **Note:** Although THAM® solution does not raise pCO_2 when treating metabolic acidosis with concurrent respiratory acidosis, bicarbonate may be preferred because the osmotic effects of THAM® are greater.

Adults: Dose depends on buffer base deficit; when deficit is known: tromethamine (mL of 0.3 M solution) = body weight (kg) x base deficit (mEq/L); when base deficit is not known: 3-6 mL/kg/dose I.V. (1-2 mEq/kg/dose)
Metabolic acidosis with cardiac arrest:
    I.V.: 3.5-6 mL/kg (1-2 mEq/kg/dose) into large peripheral vein; 500-1000 mL if needed in adults
    I.V. continuous drip: Infuse slowly by syringe pump over 3-6 hours
    Acidosis associated with cardiac bypass surgery: Average dose: 9 mL/kg (2.7 mEq/kg); 500 mL is adequate for most adults; maximum dose: 500 mg/kg in ≤1 hour
    Excess acidity of acid citrate dextrose priming blood: 14-70 mL of 0.3 molar solution added to each 500 mL of blood

Dosing comments in renal impairment: Use with caution and monitor for hyperkalemia and EKG

Administration Maximum concentration: 0.3 molar; infuse slowly over at least 1 hour (THAM-E® requires the reconstitution with 1 L sterile water before use)

Monitoring Parameters Serum electrolytes, arterial blood gases, serum pH, blood sugar, EKG monitoring, renal function tests

Reference Range Blood pH: 7.35-7.45

Nursing Implications If extravasation occurs, aspirate as much fluid as possible, then infiltrate area with procaine 1% to which hyaluronidase has been added

Additional Information 1 mM = 120 mg = 3.3 mL = 1 mEq of THAM®

Dosage Forms Injection (THAM®): 18 g [0.3 molar] (500 mL)

♦ **Tropicacyl®** see Tropicamide on page 1384

Tropicamide (troe PIK a mide)

Related Information
Cycloplegic Mydriatics Comparison on page 1498

U.S. Brand Names Mydriacyl®; Opticyl®; Tropicacyl®

Canadian Brand Names Diotrope®; Mydriacyl®

Synonyms Bistropamide

Therapeutic Category Ophthalmic Agent, Mydriatic

Use Short-acting mydriatic used in diagnostic procedures; as well as preoperatively and postoperatively; treatment of some cases of acute iritis, iridocyclitis, and keratitis

Pregnancy Risk Factor C

Usual Dosage Children and Adults (individuals with heavily pigmented eyes may require larger doses):
Cycloplegia: Instill 1-2 drops (1%); may repeat in 5 minutes
    Exam must be performed within 30 minutes after the repeat dose; if the patient is not examined within 20-30 minutes, instill an additional drop
Mydriasis: Instill 1-2 drops (0.5%) 15-20 minutes before exam; may repeat every 30 minutes as needed

Additional Information Complete prescribing information for this medication should be consulted for additional detail.

Dosage Forms Solution, ophthalmic: 0.5% (2 mL, 15 mL); 1% (2 mL, 3 mL, 15 mL)

♦ **Trosyd™ AF (Can)** see Tioconazole on page 1337
♦ **Trosyd™ J (Can)** see Tioconazole on page 1337

Trovafloxacin (TROE va floks a sin)

Related Information
Antacid Drug Interactions on page 1477

U.S. Brand Names Trovan®

Canadian Brand Names Trovan™

Synonyms Alatrofloxacin Mesylate; CP-99,219-27

Therapeutic Category Antibiotic, Quinolone

Use Should be used only in life- or limb-threatening infections
Treatment of nosocomial pneumonia, community-acquired pneumonia, complicated intra-abdominal infections, gynecologic/pelvic infections, complicated skin and skin structure infections

Pregnancy Risk Factor C

Contraindications History of hypersensitivity to trovafloxacin, alatrofloxacin, quinolone antimicrobial agents, or any component of the formulation

Warnings/Precautions For use only in serious life- or limb-threatening infections. Initiation of therapy must occur in an inpatient healthcare facility. May alter GI flora resulting in pseudomembranous colitis due to *Clostridium difficile*; use with caution in patients with seizure disorders or severe cerebral atherosclerosis; photosensitivity; CNS stimulation may occur which may lead to tremor, restlessness, confusion, hallucinations, paranoia, depression, nightmares, insomnia, or lightheadedness. Hepatic reactions have resulted in death. Risk of hepatotoxicity is increased if therapy exceeds 14 days. Tendon inflammation and/or rupture have been reported with other quinolone antibiotics. Discontinue at first sign of tendon inflammation or pain. Quinolones may exacerbate myasthenia gravis.

Severe hypersensitivity reactions, including anaphylaxis, have occurred with quinolone therapy. If an allergic reaction occurs (itching, urticaria, dyspnea, facial edema, loss of consciousness, tingling, cardiovascular collapse), discontinue drug immediately. Prolonged use may result in superinfection; pseudomembranous colitis may occur and should be considered in all patients who present with diarrhea.

Adverse Reactions Note: Fatalities have occurred in patients developing hepatic necrosis.

1% to 10% (range reported in clinical trials):
    Central nervous system: Dizziness (2% to 11%), lightheadedness (<1% to 4%), headache (1% to 5%)
    Dermatologic: Rash (<1% to 2%), pruritus (<1% to 2%)
    Gastrointestinal: Nausea (4% to 8%), abdominal pain (<1% to 1%), vomiting, diarrhea
    Genitourinary: Vaginitis (<1% to 1%)
    Hepatic: Increased LFTs
    Local: Injection site reaction, pain, or inflammation
<1% (Limited to important or life-threatening): Allergic/anaphylactoid reaction, anaphylaxis, bronchospasm, convulsions, dyskinesia, hepatic necrosis, interstitial nephritis, pancreatitis, phototoxicity, pseudomembranous colitis, Stevens-Johnson syndrome, tendonitis; quinolones have been associated with tendon rupture.

Overdosage/Toxicology Empty the stomach by vomiting or gastric lavage. Observe carefully and give symptomatic and supportive treatment. Maintain adequate hydration.

Drug Interactions
  Decreased Effect: Coadministration with antacids containing aluminum or magnesium, citric acid/sodium citrate, sucralfate, and iron markedly reduces absorption of trovafloxacin. Separate oral administration by at least 2 hours. Coadministration of intravenous morphine also reduces absorption. Separate I.V. morphine by 2 hours (when trovafloxacin is taken in fasting state) or 4 hours (when taken with food). Do not administer multivalent cations (eg, calcium, magnesium) through the same intravenous line.

Ethanol/Nutrition/Herb Interactions
  Food: Dairy products such as milk or yogurt may reduce absorption of oral trovafloxacin; avoid concurrent use. Enteral feedings may also limit absorption.
  Herb/Nutraceutical: Avoid dong quai, St John's wort (may also cause photosensitization).

Stability Store undiluted vials of solution at 15°C to 30°C (50°F to 86°F). Diluted solutions are stable for up to 7 days when refrigerated and up to 3 days at room temperature. Trovan® I.V. should not be diluted with 0.9% sodium chloride injection, USP (normal saline), alone or in combination with other diluents. A precipitate may form under these conditions. In addition, Trovan® I.V. should not be diluted with lactated Ringer's, USP.

Dilute to a concentration of 0.5-2 mg/mL in dextrose 5% in water, 0.45% sodium chloride, dextrose 5% in water and 0.45% sodium chloride, dextrose 5% in water and 0.2% sodium chloride, or lactated Ringer's in dextrose 5% in water.

Mechanism of Action Inhibits DNA-gyrase in susceptible organisms; inhibits relaxation of supercoiled DNA and promotes breakage of double-stranded DNA

Pharmacodynamics/Kinetics
  Distribution: Concentration in most tissues greater than plasma or serum
  Protein binding: 76%
  Metabolism: Hepatic conjugation; glucuronidation 13%, acetylation 9%
  Bioavailability: 88%
  Half-life elimination: 9-12 hours
  Excretion: Feces (43% as unchanged drug); urine (6% as unchanged drug)

Usual Dosage Adults:
  Nosocomial pneumonia: I.V.: 300 mg single dose followed by 200 mg/day orally for a total duration of 10-14 days
  Community-acquired pneumonia: Oral, I.V.: 200 mg/day for 7-14 days
  Complicated intra-abdominal infections, including postsurgical infections/gynecologic and pelvic infections: I.V.: 300 mg as a single dose followed by 200 mg/day orally for a total duration of 7-14 days
  Skin and skin structure infections, complicated, including diabetic foot infections: Oral, I.V.: 200 mg/day for 10-14 days
  Dosage adjustment in renal impairment: No adjustment is necessary
  Dosage adjustment for hemodialysis: None required; trovafloxacin not sufficiently removed by hemodialysis
  Dosage adjustment in hepatic impairment:
    Mild to moderate cirrhosis:
      Initial dose for normal hepatic function: 300 mg I.V.; 200 mg I.V. or oral; 100 mg oral
      Reduced dose: 200 mg I.V.; 100 mg I.V. or oral; 100 mg oral
    Severe cirrhosis: No data available

Administration
  Oral: Administer without regard to meals.
  I.V.: Not for I.M. or S.C.; administer IVPB over 60 minutes

Monitoring Parameters Periodic assessment of liver function tests should be considered

Patient Information Drink fluids liberally; do not take antacids containing magnesium or aluminum or products containing iron or zinc simultaneously or within 4 hours before or 2 hours after taking dose. May cause dizziness or lightheadedness; observe caution while driving or performing other tasks requiring alertness, coordination, or physical dexterity. CNS stimulation may occur (eg, tremor, restlessness, confusion). Avoid excessive sunlight/artificial ultraviolet light; discontinue drug if phototoxicity occurs. Avoid re-exposure to ultraviolet light. Reactions may recur up to several weeks after stopping therapy.

Dosage Forms
  Injection, as mesylate (alatrofloxacin): 5 mg/mL (40 mL, 60 mL)
  Tablet, as mesylate (trovafloxacin): 100 mg, 200 mg

- **Truxazole**® *see* SulfiSOXAZOLE *on page 1277*
- **Truxcillin**® *see* Penicillin V Potassium *on page 1055*

Trypsin, Balsam Peru, and Castor Oil
(TRIP sin, BAL sam pe RUE, & KAS tor oyl)

U.S. Brand Names Granulex

Therapeutic Category Protectant, Topical

Use Treatment of decubitus ulcers, varicose ulcers, debridement of eschar, dehiscent wounds and sunburn

Usual Dosage Apply a minimum of twice daily or as often as necessary

Additional Information Complete prescribing information for this medication should be consulted for additional detail.

Dosage Forms Aerosol, topical: Trypsin 0.1 mg, balsam Peru 72.5 mg, and castor oil 650 mg per 0.82 mL (60 g, 120 g)

- **TSH** *see* Thyrotropin *on page 1327*
- **TSH** *see* Thyrotropin Alpha *on page 1327*
- **TSPA** *see* Thiotepa *on page 1323*
- **TST** *see* Tuberculin Tests *on page 1386*
- **Tuberculin Purified Protein Derivative** *see* Tuberculin Tests *on page 1386*
- **Tuberculin Skin Test** *see* Tuberculin Tests *on page 1386*

Tuberculin Tests (too BER kyoo lin tests)

U.S. Brand Names Aplisol®; Tine Test PPD; Tubersol®

Synonyms Mantoux; PPD; Tine Test; TST; Tuberculin Purified Protein Derivative; Tuberculin Skin Test

Therapeutic Category Diagnostic Agent, Skin Test

Use Skin test in diagnosis of tuberculosis, cell-mediated immunodeficiencies

Pregnancy Risk Factor C

Contraindications 250 TU strength should not be used for initial testing

Warnings/Precautions Do not administer I.V. or S.C.; epinephrine (1:1000) should be available to treat possible allergic reactions

Adverse Reactions Frequency not defined.
Dermatologic: Ulceration, necrosis, vesiculation
Local: Pain at injection site

Stability Refrigerate; Tubersol™ opened vials are stable for up to 24 hours at <75°F

Mechanism of Action Tuberculosis results in individuals becoming sensitized to certain antigenic components of the *M. tuberculosis* organism. Culture extracts called tuberculins are contained in tuberculin skin test preparations. Upon intracutaneous injection of these culture extracts, a classic delayed (cellular) hypersensitivity reaction occurs. This reaction is characteristic of a delayed course (peak occurs >24 hours after injection, induration of the skin secondary to cell infiltration, and occasional vesiculation and necrosis). Delayed hypersensitivity reactions to tuberculin may indicate infection with a variety of nontuberculosis mycobacteria, or vaccination with the live attenuated mycobacterial strain of *M. bovis* vaccine, BCG, in addition to previous natural infection with *M. tuberculosis*.

Pharmacodynamics/Kinetics
Onset of action: Delayed hypersensitivity reactions: 5-6 hours
Peak effect: 48-72 hours
Duration: Reactions subside over a few days

Usual Dosage Children and Adults: Intradermal: 0.1 mL about 4" below elbow; use ¼" to ½" or 26- or 27-gauge needle; significant reactions are ≥5 mm in diameter
Interpretation of induration of tuberculin skin test injections: Positive: ≥10 mm; inconclusive: 5-9 mm; negative: <5 mm
Interpretation of induration of Tine test injections: Positive: >2 mm and vesiculation present; inconclusive: <2 mm (give patient Mantoux test of 5 TU/0.1 mL - base decisions on results of Mantoux test); negative: <2 mm or erythema of any size (no need for retesting unless person is a contact of a patient with tuberculosis or there is clinical evidence suggestive of the disease)

Administration Select a site without acne or hair

Patient Information Return to physician for reaction interpretation at 48-72 hours

Nursing Implications Test dose: 0.1 mL intracutaneously; store in refrigerator; examine site at 48-72 hours after administration; whenever tuberculin is administered, a record should be made of the administration technique (Mantoux method, disposable multiple-puncture device), tuberculin used (OT or PPD), manufacturer and lot number of tuberculin used, date of administration, date of test reading, and the size of the reaction in millimeters (mm).

Dosage Forms
Injection:
First test strength: 1 TU/0.1 mL (1 mL)
Intermediate test strength: 5 TU/0.1 mL (1 mL, 5 mL, 10 mL)
Second test strength: 250 TU/0.1 mL (1 mL)
Tine: 5 TU each test

- **Tuberculosis Prophylaxis** *see page 1572*
- **Tuberculosis Treatment Guidelines** *see page 1612*
- **Tubersol**® *see* Tuberculin Tests *on page 1386*

Tubocurarine (too boe kyoor AR een)

Related Information
Neuromuscular Blocking Agents Comparison *on page 1508*

Synonyms *d*-Tubocurarine Chloride; Tubocurarine Chloride

Therapeutic Category Neuromuscular Blocker Agent, Nondepolarizing; Skeletal Muscle Relaxant

Use Adjunct to general anesthesia to facilitate endotracheal intubation and to relax skeletal muscles during surgery; to facilitate mechanical ventilation in ICU patients; diagnosis of myasthenia gravis; does not relieve pain or produce sedation

Pregnancy Risk Factor C

Usual Dosage I.M., I.V.: Dose to effect; doses will vary due to interpatient variability; use ideal body weight for obese patients

Neonates: Induction and maintenance: 0.3 mg/kg

Children: Induction and maintenance: 0.6 mg/kg

Adults: Neuromuscular blockade: 0.5-0.6 mg/kg or 0.3 mg/kg after initial dose of succinylcholine for intubation; administer maintenance doses every 40-60 minutes as needed

Pretreatment/priming: 10% of intubating dose given 3-5 minutes before initial dose

ICU muscle relaxation: 0.2-0.3 mg/kg every 80 minutes or 0.6-4.2 mcg/kg/minute

Diagnosis of myasthenia gravis: 0.01-0.03 mg/kg

Dosing adjustment/comments in renal impairment: May accumulate with multiple doses and reductions in subsequent doses is recommended

Cl_{cr} 50-80 mL/minute: Administer 75% of normal dose

Cl_{cr} 10-50 mL/minute: Administer 50% of normal dose

Cl_{cr} <10 mL/minute: Avoid use

Dosing comments in hepatic impairment: Larger doses may be necessary

Additional Information Complete prescribing information for this medication should be consulted for additional detail.

Dosage Forms Injection, as chloride: 3 mg/mL [3 units/mL] (5 mL, 10 mL, 20 mL)

Typhoid Vaccine (TYE foid vak SEEN)

Related Information

Immunization Recommendations on page 1538

U.S. Brand Names Typhim Vi®; Vivotif Berna™

Canadian Brand Names Vivotif Berna®

Synonyms Typhoid Vaccine Live Oral Ty21a

Therapeutic Category Vaccine, Inactivated Bacteria

(Continued)

Typhoid Vaccine *(Continued)*

Use Typhoid vaccine: Live, attenuated Ty21a typhoid vaccine should not be administered to immunocompromised persons, including those known to be infected with HIV. Parenteral inactivated vaccine is a theoretically safer alternative for this group.

Parenteral: Promotes active immunity to typhoid fever for patients intimately exposed to a typhoid carrier or foreign travel to a typhoid fever endemic area

Oral: For immunization of children >6 years of age and adults who expect intimate exposure of or household contact with typhoid fever, travelers to areas of world with risk of exposure to typhoid fever, and workers in microbiology laboratories with expected frequent contact with *S. typhi*

Pregnancy Risk Factor C

Contraindications Acute respiratory or other active infections, previous sensitivity to typhoid vaccine, congenital or acquired immunodeficient state, acute febrile illness, acute GI illness, other active infection, persistent diarrhea or vomiting

Warnings/Precautions Postpone use in presence of acute infection; use during pregnancy only when clearly needed, immune deficiency conditions; not all recipients of typhoid vaccine will be fully protected against typhoid fever. Travelers should take all necessary precautions to avoid contact or ingestion of potentially contaminated food or water sources. Unless a complete immunization schedule is followed, an optimum immune response may not be achieved.

Adverse Reactions All serious adverse reactions must be reported to the U.S. Department of Health and Human Services (DHHS) Vaccine Adverse Event Reporting System (VAERS) 1-800-822-7967.

Oral:

1% to 10%:

Dermatologic: Rash

Gastrointestinal: Abdominal discomfort, stomach cramps, diarrhea, nausea, vomiting

<1% (Limited to important or life-threatening): Anaphylactic reaction

Injection:

>10%:

Central nervous system: Headache (9% to 30%), fever

Dermatologic: Local tenderness, erythema, induration (6% to 40%)

Neuromuscular & skeletal: Myalgia (14% to 29%)

<1% (Limited to important or life-threatening): Hypotension

Stability Refrigerate, do not freeze; potency is not harmed if mistakenly placed in freezer; however, remove from freezer as soon as possible and place in refrigerator; can still be used if exposed to temperature ≤80°F

Mechanism of Action Virulent strains of *Salmonella typhi* cause disease by penetrating the intestinal mucosa and entering the systemic circulation via the lymphatic vasculature. One possible mechanism of conferring immunity may be the provocation of a local immune response in the intestinal tract induced by oral ingesting of a live strain with subsequent aborted infection. The ability of *Salmonella typhi* to produce clinical disease (and to elicit an immune response) is dependent on the bacteria having a complete lipopolysaccharide. The live attenuate Ty21a strain lacks the enzyme UDP-4-galactose epimerase so that lipopolysaccharide is only synthesized under conditions that induce bacterial autolysis. Thus, the strain remains avirulent despite the production of sufficient lipopolysaccharide to evoke a protective immune response. Despite low levels of lipopolysaccharide synthesis, cells lyse before gaining a virulent phenotype due to the intracellular accumulation of metabolic intermediates.

Pharmacodynamics/Kinetics

Onset of action: Immunity to *Salmonella typhi*: Oral: ~1 week

Duration: Immunity: Oral: ~5 years; Parenteral: ~3 years

Usual Dosage

S.C. (AKD and H-P):

Children 6 months to 10 years: 0.25 mL; repeat in ≥4 weeks (total immunization is 2 doses)

Children >10 years and Adults: 0.5 mL; repeat dose in ≥4 weeks (total immunization is 2 doses)

Booster: 0.25 mL every 3 years for children 6 months to 10 years and 0.5 mL every 3 years for children >10 years and adults

Oral: Adults:

Primary immunization: 1 capsule on alternate days (day 1, 3, 5, and 7)

Booster immunization: Repeat full course of primary immunization every 5 years

Administration Only the H-P vaccine may be administered intradermally and only for booster doses. The AKD vaccine may be given by jet injection; Typhim Vi® may be given I.M. and is indicated for children ≥2 years of age, give as a single 0.5 mL (25 mcg) injection in deltoid muscle

Patient Information Oral capsule should be taken 1 hour before a meal with cold or lukewarm drink, do not chew, swallow whole; systemic adverse effects may persist for 1-2 days. Take all 4 doses exactly as directed on alternate days to obtain a maximal response.

Nursing Implications The doses of vaccine are different between S.C. and intradermal; S.C. injection only should be used

Additional Information Inactivated bacteria vaccine. Federal law requires that the date of administration, the vaccine manufacturer, lot number of vaccine, and the administering person's name, title, and address be entered into the patient's permanent medical record.

Dosage Forms

Capsule, enteric coated (Vivotif Berna™): Viable *S. typhi* Ty21a colony-forming units 2-6 x 10^9 and nonviable *S. typhi* Ty21a colony-forming units 50 x 10^9 with sucrose, ascorbic acid, amino acid mixture, lactose, and magnesium stearate

Injection, suspension (H-P): Heat- and phenol-inactivated, killed Ty-2 strain of *S. typhi* organisms; provides 8 units/mL, ≤1 billion/mL and ≤35 mcg nitrogen/mL (5 mL, 10 mL)

Injection (Typhim Vi®): Purified Vi capsular polysaccharide 25 mcg/0.5 mL (0.5 mL)

Powder for suspension (AKD): 8 units/mL ≤1 billion/mL, acetone inactivated dried (50 doses)

♦ **Typhoid Vaccine Live Oral Ty21a** *see* Typhoid Vaccine *on page 1387*

+ **Tyramine Content of Foods** *see page 1737*
+ **Tyrodone® Liquid** *see Hydrocodone and Pseudoephedrine on page 681*
+ **U-90152S** *see Delavirdine on page 371*
+ **UAD Otic®** *see Neomycin, Polymyxin B, and Hydrocortisone on page 969*
+ **UCB-P071** *see Cetirizine on page 265*
+ **Ucephan®** *see Sodium Phenylacetate and Sodium Benzoate on page 1248*
+ **UK** *see Urokinase Not Currently Manufactured on page 1392*
+ **UK 92480** *see Sildenafil on page 1236*
+ **Ulcidine® (Can)** *see Famotidine on page 543*
+ **Ultane®** *see Sevoflurane on page 1234*
+ **Ultiva™** *see Remifentanil on page 1182*
+ **Ultracet™** *see Acetaminophen and Tramadol on page 26*
+ **Ultram®** *see Tramadol on page 1354*
+ **Ultra Mide®** *see Urea on page 1391*
+ **UltraMide 25™ (Can)** *see Urea on page 1391*
+ **Ultramop™ (Can)** *see Methoxsalen on page 889*
+ **Ultraquin™ (Can)** *see Hydroquinone on page 686*
+ **Ultrase®** *see Pancrelipase on page 1034*
+ **Ultrase® MT** *see Pancrelipase on page 1034*
+ **Ultravate™** *see Halobetasol on page 653*
+ **Unasyn®** *see Ampicillin and Sulbactam on page 95*
+ **Uni-Bent® Cough Syrup** *see DiphenhydrAMINE on page 414*
+ **Unicap® [OTC]** *see Vitamins (Multiple) on page 1424*
+ **Uni-Fed® [OTC]** *see Triprolidine and Pseudoephedrine on page 1380*
+ **Unipen® (Can)** *see Nafcillin on page 950*
+ **Uniretic™** *see Moexipril and Hydrochlorothiazide on page 931*
+ **Unithroid™** *see Levothyroxine on page 799*
+ **Uni-tussin® [OTC]** *see Guaifenesin on page 645*
+ **Uni-tussin® DM [OTC]** *see Guaifenesin and Dextromethorphan on page 646*
+ **Univasc®** *see Moexipril on page 929*
+ **Univol® (Can)** *see Aluminum Hydroxide and Magnesium Hydroxide on page 64*
+ **Unna's Boot** *see Zinc Gelatin on page 1438*
+ **Unna's Paste** *see Zinc Gelatin on page 1438*

Unoprostone (yoo noe PROS tone)

Related Information
Glaucoma Drug Therapy Comparison *on page 1499*

U.S. Brand Names Rescula®

Synonyms Unoprostone Isopropyl

Therapeutic Category Ophthalmic Agent, Miscellaneous

Use To lower intraocular pressure (IOP) in patients with open-angle glaucoma or ocular hypertension; should be used in patients who are not tolerant of, or failed treatment with other IOP-lowering medications

Pregnancy Risk Factor C

Pregnancy/Breast-Feeding Implications No adequate and well-controlled studies have been conducted in pregnant women. Use during pregnancy only if the potential benefit to the mother outweighs the potential risk to the fetus. It is not known if unoprostone is secreted in human breast milk. Use caution if administering to a nursing woman.

Contraindications Hypersensitivity to unoprostone, benzalkonium chloride, or any component of the formulation

Warnings/Precautions May cause permanent changes in eye color (increases the amount of brown pigment in the iris); long-term consequences and potential injury to eye are not known. Bacterial keratitis, caused by inadvertent contamination of multiple-dose ophthalmic solutions, has been reported. Use caution in patients with intraocular inflammation. Contains benzalkonium chloride which may be adsorbed by contact lenses; remove contacts prior to administration and wait 15 minutes before reinserting. Safety and efficacy have not been determined for use in patients with renal or hepatic impairment, angle closure, inflammatory or neovascular glaucoma. Safety and efficacy in pediatric patients have not been established.

Adverse Reactions

>10%: Ocular: Burning/stinging (10% to 25%), dry eyes (10% to 25%), injection (10% to 25%), ophthalmic itching (10% to 25%), increased length of eyelashes (10% to 14%)

1% to 10%:
  Cardiovascular: Hypertension
  Central nervous system: Dizziness, headache, insomnia, pain
  Endocrine & metabolic: Diabetes mellitus
  Neuromuscular & skeletal: Back pain
  Ocular: Abnormal vision (5% to 10%), eyelid disorder (5% to 10%), foreign body sensation (5% to 10%), lacrimation disorder (5% to 10%), decreased length of eyelashes (7%), blepharitis, cataract, conjunctivitis, corneal lesion, eye discharge, eye hemorrhage, eye pain, irritation, keratitis, photophobia, vitreous disorder
  Respiratory: Bronchitis, increased cough, pharyngitis, rhinitis, sinusitis
  Miscellaneous: Flu-like syndrome (6%), accidental injury, allergic reaction

<1% (Limited to important or life-threatening): Ocular: Acute elevated intraocular pressure, color blindness, corneal deposits, corneal edema, corneal opacity, diplopia, hyperpigmentation of eyelid, increase in number of eyelashes, iris hyperpigmentation, iritis, optic atrophy, ptosis, retinal hemorrhage, visual field defect

Overdosage/Toxicology No data available. If overdose occurs, treatment should be symptomatic.

(Continued)

Unoprostone (Continued)

Drug Interactions
Increased Effect/Toxicity: Specific drug interactions have not been reported. When using more than one ophthalmic product, wait at least 5 minutes between application of each medication.

Stability Store between 2°C to 25°C (36°F to 77°F)

Mechanism of Action The exact mechanism of action is unknown; however, unoprostone decreases IOP by increasing the outflow of aqueous humor. Cardiovascular and pulmonary function were not affected in clinical studies. IOP was decreased by 3-4 mm Hg in patients with a mean baseline IOP of 23 mm Hg.

Pharmacodynamics/Kinetics
Absorption: Through cornea and conjunctival epithelium
Metabolism: Hydrolyzed by esterases to metabolite, unoprostone-free acid
Half-life elimination: 14 minutes
Excretion: Urine (as metabolites)

Usual Dosage Ophthalmic: Adults: Instill 1 drop into affected eye(s) twice daily
Dosage adjustment in renal impairment: Use with caution, no dosing adjustment reported.
Dosage adjustment in hepatic impairment: Use with caution, no dosing adjustment reported.
Elderly: No differences in safety and efficacy have been reported in the elderly.

Administration May be used with other eye drops to lower intraocular pressure; if using more than one product, wait at least 5 minutes between application of each medication. Remove contact lenses prior to administration and wait 15 minutes before reinserting.

Patient Information Wash hands before instilling solution. Sit or lie down to instill. Open eye, look at ceiling, and instill prescribed amount of solution. Apply gentle pressure to inner corner of eye. Do not let tip of applicator touch eye; do not contaminate tip of applicator (contamination may cause eye infection leading to possible eye damage or vision loss). Contact prescriber concerning continued use of drops if eye infection develops, trauma occurs to the eye, and prior to eye surgery. This product contains benzalkonium chloride which may be adsorbed by contact lenses; remove contacts prior to administration and wait 15 minutes before reinserting. May cause permanent changes in eye color (increases the amount of brown pigment in the iris); long-term consequences and potential injury to eye are not known. Changes to eye color may occur slowly (months to years). May be used with other eye drops to lower intraocular pressure; if using more than one product, wait at least 5 minutes between application of each medication. Notify prescriber if conjunctivitis or eyelid reactions occur with use of this product.

Nursing Implications May be used with other eye drops to lower intraocular pressure; if using more than one product, wait at least 5 minutes in between application of each medication.

Additional Information Contains benzalkonium chloride 0.015% as a preservative
Dosage Forms Solution, ophthalmic: 0.15% (5 mL, 7.5 mL)

♦ **Unoprostone Isopropyl** *see Unoprostone on page 1389*

Uracil Mustard (YOOR a sil MUS tard)

Therapeutic Category Antineoplastic Agent, Alkylating Agent; Antineoplastic Agent, Nitrogen Mustard

Use Palliative treatment in symptomatic chronic lymphocytic leukemia; non-Hodgkin's lymphomas, chronic myelocytic leukemia, mycosis fungoides, thrombocytosis, polycythemia vera, ovarian carcinoma

Pregnancy Risk Factor X

Contraindications Hypersensitivity to uracil mustard or any component of the formulation; severe leukopenia, thrombocytopenia, aplastic anemia; patients whose bone marrow is infiltrated with malignant cells; pregnancy

Warnings/Precautions The U.S. Food and Drug Administration (FDA) currently recommends that procedures for proper handling and disposal of antineoplastic agents be considered. Impaired kidney or liver function. The drug should be discontinued if intractable vomiting or diarrhea, precipitous falls in leukocyte or platelet count, or myocardial ischemia occurs. Use with caution in patients who have had high-dose pelvic radiation or previous use of alkylating agents. Patient should be hospitalized during initial course of therapy; may impair fertility in men and women; use with caution in patients with pre-existing marrow suppression.

Adverse Reactions
>10%:
Gastrointestinal: Nausea, vomiting, diarrhea
Emetic potential: Moderate (30% to 60%)
Hematologic: Myelosuppressive; leukopenia and thrombocytopenia nadir: 2-4 weeks, anemia
1% to 10%:
Central nervous system: Mental depression, nervousness
Dermatologic: Hyperpigmentation, alopecia
Endocrine & metabolic: Hyperuricemia
<1% (Limited to important or life-threatening): Hepatotoxicity

Overdosage/Toxicology Symptoms include diarrhea, vomiting, and severe marrow suppression. No specific antidote to marrow toxicity is available.

Mechanism of Action Polyfunctional alkylating agent. The basic reaction of uracil mustard, like that of any alkylating agent, is the replacement of the hydrogen in a reacting chemical with an alkyl group; cell cycle-phase nonspecific antineoplastic agent; exact site of drug action within the cell is not known, but the nucleoproteins of the cell nucleus are believed to be involved.

Pharmacodynamics/Kinetics
Absorption: Oral
Excretion: Urine (<1%)

Usual Dosage Oral (do not administer until 2-3 weeks after maximum effect of any previous x-ray or cytotoxic drug therapy of the bone marrow is obtained):

Children: 0.3 mg/kg in a single weekly dose for 4 weeks
Adults: 0.15 mg/kg in a single weekly dose for 4 weeks
Thrombocytosis: 1-2 mg/day for 14 days

Patient Information This drug may take weeks or months for effectiveness to become apparent. Do not discontinue without consulting prescriber. Maintain adequate hydration (2-3 L/day of fluids unless instructed to restrict fluid intake). For nausea or vomiting, loss of appetite, or dry mouth, small frequent meals, chewing gum, or sucking lozenges may help. You may experience hair loss (reversible); diarrhea (if persistent, consult prescriber); nervousness, irritability, shakiness, amenorrhea, altered sperm production (usually reversible). Report persistent nausea or vomiting, fever, sore throat, chills, unusual bleeding or bruising, consistent feelings of tiredness or weakness, or yellowing of skin or eyes.

Nursing Implications Notify physician of persistent or severe nausea, diarrhea, fever, sore throat, chills, bleeding, or bruising

Dosage Forms Capsule: 1 mg

♦ **Urasal®** (Can) see Methenamine on page 881

Urea (yoor EE a)
U.S. Brand Names Amino-Cerv™ Vaginal Cream; Aquacare® [OTC]; Carmol® [OTC]; Gormel® Creme [OTC]; Lanaphilic® [OTC]; Nutraplus® [OTC]; Rea-Lo® [OTC]; Ultra Mide®; Ureacin®-20 [OTC]; Ureaphil®
Canadian Brand Names UltraMide 25™; Uremol®; Urisec®
Synonyms Carbamide
Therapeutic Category Diuretic, Osmotic; Keratolytic Agent; Topical Skin Product
Use Reduces intracranial pressure and intraocular pressure; topically promotes hydration and removal of excess keratin in hyperkeratotic conditions and dry skin; mild cervicitis
Pregnancy Risk Factor C
Usual Dosage
Children: I.V. slow infusion:
<2 years: 0.1-0.5 g/kg
>2 years: 0.5-1.5 g/kg
Adults:
I.V. infusion: 1-1.5 g/kg by slow infusion (1-2½ hours); maximum: 120 g/24 hours
Topical: Apply 1-3 times/day
Vaginal: Insert 1 applicatorful in vagina at bedtime for 2-4 weeks
Elderly: Start at low end of dosing range; use caution due to greater frequency of renal, hepatic, and cardiac dysfunction
Additional Information Complete prescribing information for this medication should be consulted for additional detail.
Dosage Forms
Cream, topical: 2% [20 mg/mL] (75 g); 10% [100 mg/mL] (75 g, 90 g, 454 g); 20% [200 mg/mL] (45 g, 75 g, 90 g, 454 g); 30% [300 mg/mL] (60 g, 454 g); 40% (30 g)
Cream, vaginal: 8.34% [83.4 mg/g] (82.5 g)
Injection: 40 g/150 mL
Lotion: 2% (240 mL); 10% (180 mL, 240 mL, 480 mL); 15% (120 mL, 480 mL); 25% (180 mL)

Urea and Hydrocortisone (yoor EE a & hye droe KOR ti sone)
U.S. Brand Names Carmol-HC®
Canadian Brand Names Ti-U-Lac® H; Uremol® HC
Synonyms Hydrocortisone and Urea
Therapeutic Category Corticosteroid, Topical (Low Potency)
Use Inflammation of corticosteroid-responsive dermatoses
Pregnancy Risk Factor C
Usual Dosage Apply thin film and rub in well 1-4 times/day. Therapy should be discontinued when control is achieved; if no improvement is seen, reassessment of diagnosis may be necessary.
Additional Information Complete prescribing information for this medication should be consulted for additional detail.
Dosage Forms Cream, topical: Urea 10% and hydrocortisone acetate 1% in a water-washable vanishing cream (30 g)

♦ **Ureacin®-20 [OTC]** see Urea on page 1391
♦ **Urea Peroxide** see Carbamide Peroxide on page 224
♦ **Ureaphil®** see Urea on page 1391
♦ **Urecholine®** see Bethanechol on page 165
♦ **Uremol® (Can)** see Urea on page 1391
♦ **Uremol® HC (Can)** see Urea and Hydrocortisone on page 1391
♦ **Urex®** see Methenamine on page 881
♦ **Urimax™** see Methenamine, Sodium Biphosphate, Phenyl Salicylate, Methylene Blue, and Hyoscyamine on page 882
♦ **Urisec® (Can)** see Urea on page 1391
♦ **Urispas®** see Flavoxate on page 563
♦ **Uristat® [OTC]** see Phenazopyridine on page 1068
♦ **Urodol® [OTC]** see Phenazopyridine on page 1068
♦ **Urofemme® [OTC]** see Phenazopyridine on page 1068
♦ **Urofollitropin** see Follitropins on page 596

Urofollitropin (yoor oh fol li TROE pin)
U.S. Brand Names Fertinex®; Metrodin®
Canadian Brand Names Fertinorm® H.P.
(Continued)

Urofollitropin *(Continued)*

Therapeutic Category Ovulation Stimulator

Use Induction of ovulation in patients with polycystic ovarian disease and to stimulate the development of multiple oocytes

Pregnancy Risk Factor X

Usual Dosage Adults: Female: S.C.: 75 units/day for 7-12 days, used with hCG may repeat course of treatment 2 more times

Additional Information Complete prescribing information for this medication should be consulted for additional detail.

Dosage Forms Injection: 0.83 mg [75 units FSH activity] (2 mL); 1.66 mg [150 units FSH activity]

♦ **Urogesic**® *see Phenazopyridine on page 1068*

Urokinase *Not Currently Manufactured* (yoor oh KIN ase)

U.S. Brand Names Abbokinase®

Synonyms UK

Therapeutic Category Fibrinolytic Agent

Use Thrombolytic agent used in treatment of recent severe or massive deep vein thrombosis, pulmonary emboli, myocardial infarction, and occluded I.V. or dialysis cannulas; more expensive than streptokinase; not useful on thrombi over 1 week old

Note: Not currently being manufactured; contact Abbott Labs (800-615-0187) for further information.

Pregnancy Risk Factor B

Contraindications Hypersensitivity to urokinase or any component of the formulation; active internal bleeding; history of CVA; recent (within 2 months) intracranial or intraspinal surgery or trauma; intracranial neoplasm, arteriovenous malformation, or aneurysm; known bleeding diathesis; severe uncontrolled hypertension

Warnings/Precautions Concurrent heparin anticoagulation can contribute to bleeding; careful attention to all potential bleeding sites. I.M. injections and nonessential handling of the patient should be avoided. Venipunctures should be performed carefully and only when necessary. If arterial puncture is necessary, use an upper extremity vessel that can be manually compressed. If serious bleeding occurs, then the infusion of urokinase and heparin should be stopped.

For the following conditions the risk of bleeding is higher with use of anistreplase and should be weighed against the benefits of therapy: recent (within 10 days) major surgery (eg, CABG, obstetrical delivery, organ biopsy, previous puncture of noncompressible vessels), cerebrovascular disease, recent (within 10 days) gastrointestinal or genitourinary bleeding, recent trauma (within 10 days) including CPR, hypertension (systolic BP >180 mm Hg and/or diastolic BP >110 mm Hg), high likelihood of left heart thrombus (eg, mitral stenosis with atrial fibrillation), acute pericarditis, subacute bacterial endocarditis, hemostatic defects including ones caused by severe renal or hepatic dysfunction, significant hepatic dysfunction, pregnancy, diabetic hemorrhagic retinopathy or other hemorrhagic ophthalmic conditions, septic thrombophlebitis or occluded AV cannula at seriously infected site, advanced age (eg, >75 years), patients receiving oral anticoagulants, any other condition in which bleeding constitutes a significant hazard or would be particularly difficult to manage because of location.

Coronary thrombolysis may result in reperfusion arrhythmias. Follow standard MI management. Rare anaphylactoid reactions can occur. Safety and efficacy in pediatric patients have not been established.

Adverse Reactions As with all drugs which may affect hemostasis, bleeding is the major adverse effect associated with urokinase. Hemorrhage may occur at virtually any site. Risk is dependent on multiple variables, including the dosage administered, concurrent use of multiple agents which alter hemostasis, and patient predisposition. Rapid lysis of coronary artery thrombi by thrombolytic agents may be associated with reperfusion-related atrial and/or ventricular arrhythmias.

>10%: Local: Injection site bleeding

1% to 10%:

    Dermatologic: Bruising

    Gastrointestinal: Gastrointestinal hemorrhage, nausea, vomiting

    Genitourinary: Genitourinary hemorrhage

    Hematologic: Anemia

    Neuromuscular & skeletal: Muscle pain

    Respiratory: Epistaxis

<1% (Limited to important or life-threatening): Allergic reactions, anaphylactoid reactions, anaphylaxis, back pain, bronchospasm, chills, epistaxis, fever, gingival hemorrhage, hypotension, intracranial hemorrhage, pericardial hemorrhage, rash, retroperitoneal hemorrhage, tachycardia, urticaria

Additional cardiovascular events associated with use in myocardial infarction: Asystole, AV block, cardiac arrest, cardiac tamponade, cardiogenic shock, electromechanical dissociation, heart failure, mitral regurgitation, myocardial rupture, pericardial effusion, pericarditis, pulmonary edema, recurrent ischemia/infarction, thromboembolism, ventricular tachycardia

Overdosage/Toxicology Symptoms include epistaxis, bleeding gums, hematoma, spontaneous ecchymoses, and oozing at the catheter site. In case of overdose, stop the infusion reverse bleeding with blood products that contain clotting factors.

Drug Interactions

Increased Effect/Toxicity: Oral anticoagulants (warfarin), heparin, low molecular weight heparins, and drugs which affect platelet function (eg, NSAIDs, dipyridamole, ticlopidine, clopidogrel, IIb/IIIa antagonists) may potentiate the risk of hemorrhage.

Decreased Effect: Aminocaproic acid (an antifibrinolytic agent) may decrease the effectiveness of thrombolytic therapy.

Stability Store in refrigerator; reconstitute by gently rolling and tilting; do not shake; contains no preservatives, should not be reconstituted until immediately before using, discard unused portion; stable at room temperature for 24 hours after reconstitution

Mechanism of Action Promotes thrombolysis by directly activating plasminogen to plasmin, which degrades fibrin, fibrinogen, and other procoagulant plasma proteins

Pharmacodynamics/Kinetics
Onset of action: I.V.: Fibrinolysis occurs rapidly
Duration: ≥4 hours
Half-life elimination: 10-20 minutes
Excretion: Urine and feces (small amounts)

Usual Dosage
Children and Adults: Deep vein thrombosis: I.V.: Loading: 4400 units/kg over 10 minutes, then 4400 units/kg/hour for 12 hours
Adults:
Myocardial infarction: Intracoronary: 750,000 units over 2 hours (6000 units/minute over up to 2 hours)
Occluded I.V. catheters:
5000 units (use only Abbokinase® Open Cath) in each lumen over 1-2 minutes, leave in lumen for 1-4 hours, then aspirate; may repeat with 10,000 units in each lumen if 5000 units fails to clear the catheter; **do not infuse into the patient**; volume to instill into catheter is equal to the volume of the catheter
I.V. infusion: 200 units/kg/hour in each lumen for 12-48 hours at a rate of at least 20 mL/hour
Dialysis patients: 5000 units is administered in each lumen over 1-2 minutes; leave urokinase in lumen for 1-2 days, then aspirate
Clot lysis (large vessel thrombi): Loading: I.V.: 4400 units/kg over 10 minutes, increase to 6000 units/kg/hour; maintenance: 4400-6000 units/kg/hour adjusted to achieve clot lysis or patency of affected vessel; doses up to 50,000 units/kg/hour have been used. **Note:** Therapy should be initiated as soon as possible after diagnosis of thrombi and continued until clot is dissolved (usually 24-72 hours).
Acute pulmonary embolism: Three treatment alternatives: 3 million unit dosage
Alternative 1: 12-hour infusion: 4400 units/kg (2000 units/lb) bolus over 10 minutes followed by 4400 units/kg (2000 units/lb); begin heparin 1000 units/hour approximately 3-4 hours after completion of urokinase infusion or when aPTT is <100 seconds
Alternative 2: 2-hour infusion: 1 million unit bolus over 10 minutes followed by 2 million units over 110 minutes; begin heparin 1000 units/hour approximately 3-4 hours after completion of urokinase infusion or when PTT is <100 seconds
Alternative 3: Bolus dose only: 15,000 units/kg over 10 minutes; begin heparin 1000 units/hour approximately 3-4 hours after completion of urokinase infusion or when PTT is <100 seconds

Administration Use 0.22 or 0.45 micron filter during I.V. therapy

Monitoring Parameters CBC, reticulocyte count, platelet count, DIC panel (fibrinogen, plasminogen, FDP, D-dimer, PT, aPTT), thrombosis panel (AT-III, protein C), urinalysis, ACT

Nursing Implications Use 0.22 or 0.45 micron filter during I.V. systemic therapy; I.V. infusion: Usual concentration: 1250-1500 units/mL; maximum concentration not yet defined

Dosage Forms
Powder for injection: 250,000 units (5 mL)
Powder for injection, catheter clear: 5000 units (1 mL), 9000 units

Ursodiol (ER soe dye ole)

U.S. Brand Names Actigall™; Urso®
Canadian Brand Names Urso®
Synonyms Ursodeoxycholic Acid
Therapeutic Category Gallstone Dissolution Agent
Use Actigall™: Gallbladder stone dissolution; prevention of gallstones in obese patients experiencing rapid weight loss; Urso®: Primary biliary cirrhosis
Unlabeled/Investigational Use Liver transplantation
Pregnancy Risk Factor B
Contraindications Hypersensitivity to ursodiol, bile acids, or any component of the formulation; not to be used with cholesterol, radiopaque, bile pigment stones, or stones >20 mm in diameter; allergy to bile acids
Warnings/Precautions Gallbladder stone dissolution may take several months of therapy; complete dissolution may not occur and recurrence of stones within 5 years has been observed in 50% of patients; use with caution in patients with a nonvisualizing gallbladder and those with chronic liver disease; not recommended for children
Adverse Reactions
>10%:
Central nervous system: Headache (up to 25%), dizziness (up to 17%)
Gastrointestinal: In treatment of primary biliary cirrhosis: Constipation (up to 26%)
1% to 10%:
Dermatologic: Rash (<1% to 3%), alopecia (<1% to 5%)
Gastrointestinal:
In gallstone dissolution: Most GI events (diarrhea, nausea, vomiting) are similar to placebo and attributable to gallstone dissolution.
In treatment of primary biliary cirrhosis: Diarrhea (1%)
Hematologic: Leukopenia (3%)
Miscellaneous: Allergy (5%)
(Continued)

Ursodiol *(Continued)*

<1% (Limited to important or life-threatening): Abdominal pain, biliary pain, fatigue, metallic taste, nausea, pruritus, vomiting

In treatment of primary biliary cirrhosis: Constipation, dyspepsia, headache

Overdosage/Toxicology Symptom include diarrhea. No specific therapy for diarrhea or overdose.

Drug Interactions

Decreased Effect: Decreased effect with aluminum-containing antacids, cholestyramine, colestipol, clofibrate, and oral contraceptives (estrogens).

Stability Do not store above 30°C (86°F)

Mechanism of Action Decreases the cholesterol content of bile and bile stones by reducing the secretion of cholesterol from the liver and the fractional reabsorption of cholesterol by the intestines. Mechanism of action in primary biliary cirrhosis is not clearly defined.

Pharmacodynamics/Kinetics

Metabolism: Undergoes extensive enterohepatic recycling; following hepatic conjugation and biliary secretion, the drug is hydrolyzed to active ursodiol, where it is recycled or transformed to lithocholic acid by colonic microbial flora

Half-life elimination: 100 hours

Excretion: Feces

Usual Dosage Adults: Oral:

Gallstone dissolution: 8-10 mg/kg/day in 2-3 divided doses; use beyond 24 months is not established; obtain ultrasound images at 6-month intervals for the first year of therapy; 30% of patients have stone recurrence after dissolution

Gallstone prevention: 300 mg twice daily

Primary biliary cirrhosis: 13-15 mg/kg/day in 4 divided doses (with food)

Dietary Considerations Urso® should be taken with food.

Monitoring Parameters ALT, AST, sonogram

Patient Information Frequent blood work necessary to follow drug effects; report any persistent nausea, vomiting, abdominal pain

Dosage Forms

Capsule (Actigall™): 300 mg

Tablet, film coated (Urso®): 250 mg

Extemporaneous Preparations A 60 mg/mL ursodiol suspension may be made by opening twelve 300 mg capsules and wetting with sufficient glycerin and triturating to make a fine paste; gradually add 45 mL of simple syrup in three steps:

1. Add 15 mL to paste, triturate well and transfer to 2 oz amber bottle
2. Rinse mortar with 10 mL simple syrup and add to amber bottle
3. Repeat step 2 with sufficient syrup to make 60 mL final volume; label "Shake Well and Store in Refrigerator"; 35-day stability

♦ **USPHA/IDSA Guidelines for the Prevention of Opportunistic Infections in Persons With HIV** *see page 1574*

♦ **Utradol™ (Can)** *see Etodolac on page 532*

♦ **Uvadex®** *see Methoxsalen on page 889*

♦ **Vagifem®** *see Estradiol on page 491*

♦ **Vagistat®-1 [OTC]** *see Tioconazole on page 1337*

Valacyclovir *(val ay SYE kloe veer)*

Related Information

Treatment of Sexually Transmitted Diseases *on page 1609*

U.S. Brand Names Valtrex®

Canadian Brand Names Valtrex®

Synonyms Valacyclovir Hydrochloride

Therapeutic Category Antiviral Agent, Oral

Use Treatment of herpes zoster (shingles) in immunocompetent patients; episodic treatment or prophylaxis of recurrent genital herpes in immunocompetent patients; for first episode genital herpes

Pregnancy Risk Factor B

Pregnancy/Breast-Feeding Implications

Clinical effects on the fetus: Teratogenicity registry has shown no increased rate of birth defects than that of the general population; however, the registry is small and use during pregnancy is only warranted if the potential benefit to the mother justifies the risk of the fetus

Breast-feeding/lactation: Avoid use in breast-feeding, if possible, since the drug distributes in high concentrations in breast milk

Contraindications Hypersensitivity to valacyclovir, acyclovir, or any component of the formulation

Warnings/Precautions Thrombotic thrombocytopenic purpura/hemolytic uremic syndrome has occurred in immunocompromised patients; use caution and adjust the dose in elderly patients or those with renal insufficiency; safety and efficacy in children have not been established

Adverse Reactions

>10%:

Central nervous system: Headache (14% to 38%)

Gastrointestinal: Nausea (11% to 15%)

1% to 10%:

Central nervous system: Dizziness (2% to 4%), depression (0% to 7%)

Endocrine: Dysmenorrhea (≤1% to 8%)

Gastrointestinal: Abdominal pain (2% to 11%), vomiting (<1% to 6%)

Hematologic: Leukopenia (≤1%), thrombocytopenia (≤1%)

Hepatic: AST increased (1% to 4%)

Neuromuscular & skeletal: Arthralgia (≤1 to 6%)

<1% (Limited to important or life-threatening): Acute hypersensitivity reactions, agitation, anaphylaxis, aplastic anemia, auditory hallucinations, coma, confusion, encephalopathy, erythema multiforme, hepatitis, mania, photosensitivity reaction, psychosis, rash, renal failure, thrombotic thrombocytopenic purpura/hemolytic uremic syndrome, visual hallucinations

Overdosage/Toxicology Symptoms include elevated serum creatinine, renal failure, encephalitis, and precipitation in renal tubules. Hemodialysis has resulted in up to 60% reduction in serum acyclovir levels after administration of acyclovir.

Drug Interactions
Increased Effect/Toxicity: Valacyclovir and acyclovir have increased CNS side effects with zidovudine and probenecid.
Decreased Effect: Cimetidine and/or probenecid has decreased the rate but not the extent of valacyclovir conversion to acyclovir leading to decreased effectiveness of valacyclovir.

Stability Store at 15°C to 25°C (59°F to 77°F).

Mechanism of Action Valacyclovir is rapidly and nearly completely converted to acyclovir by intestinal and hepatic metabolism. Acyclovir is converted to acyclovir monophosphate by virus-specific thymidine kinase then further converted to acyclovir triphosphate by other cellular enzymes. Acyclovir triphosphate inhibits DNA synthesis and viral replication by competing with deoxyguanosine triphosphate for viral DNA polymerase and being incorporated into viral DNA.

Pharmacodynamics/Kinetics
Absorption: Rapid
Distribution: Acyclovir is widely distributed throughout the body including brain, kidney, lungs, liver, spleen, muscle, uterus, vagina, and CSF
Protein binding: 13.5% to 17.9%
Metabolism: Hepatic; valacyclovir is rapidly and nearly completely converted to acyclovir and L-valine by first pass intestinal and/or hepatic metabolism; acyclovir is hepatically metabolized to a very small extent by aldehyde oxidase and by alcohol and aldehyde dehydrogenase (inactive metabolites)
Bioavailability: ~55% once converted to acyclovir
Half-life elimination: Normal renal function: Adults: 2.5-3.3 hours (acyclovir), ~30 minutes (valacyclovir); End-stage renal disease: 14-20 hours (acyclovir)
Excretion: Urine: Acyclovir (88%), valacyclovir (46%); feces: Valacyclovir (47%)

Usual Dosage Oral: Adults:
Herpes zoster (shingles): 1 g 3 times/day for 7 days
Genital herpes:
  Initial episode: 1 g 2 times/day for 10 days
  Episodic treatment: 500 mg twice daily for 3 days
  Prophylaxis: 500-1000 mg once daily
Dosing interval in renal impairment:
  Herpes zoster:
    Cl_{cr} 30-49 mL/minute: 1 g every 12 hours
    Cl_{cr} 10-29 mL/minute: 1 g every 24 hours
    Cl_{cr} <10 mL/minute: 500 mg every 24 hours
  Genital herpes:
    Initial episode:
      Cl_{cr} 10-29 mL/minute: 1 g every 24 hours
      Cl_{cr} <10 mL/minute: 500 mg every 24 hours
    Episodic treatment: Cl_{cr} <10-29 mL/minute: 500 mg every 24 hours
    Prophylaxis: Cl_{cr} <10-29 mL/minute:
      For usual dose of 1 g every 24 hours, decrease dose to 500 mg every 24 hours
      For usual dose of 500 mg every 24 hours, decrease dose to 500 mg every 48 hours
Hemodialysis: Dialyzable (~33% removed during 4-hour session); administer dose postdialysis
Chronic ambulatory peritoneal dialysis/continuous arteriovenous hemofiltration dialysis: Pharmacokinetic parameters are similar to those in patients with ESRD; supplemental dose not needed following dialysis

Dietary Considerations May be taken with or without food.
Monitoring Parameters Urinalysis, BUN, serum creatinine, liver enzymes, and CBC
Patient Information Take with plenty of water
Herpes zoster: Therapy is most effective when started within 48 hours of onset of zoster rash
Recurrent genital herpes: Therapy should be initiated within 24 hours after the onset of signs or symptoms
Nursing Implications Observe for CNS changes; avoid dehydration; for episodic treatment of zoster, begin therapy at the earliest sign of infection (within 48 hours of the rash)
Dosage Forms Caplet: 500 mg, 1000 mg

♦ **Valacyclovir Hydrochloride** *see Valacyclovir on page 1394*
♦ **Valcyte™** *see Valganciclovir on page 1397*

Valdecoxib (val de KOKS ib)
U.S. Brand Names Bextra®
Therapeutic Category Analgesic, COX-2 Inhibitor; Nonsteroidal Anti-inflammatory Drug (NSAID), COX-2 Selective
Use Relief of signs and symptoms of osteoarthritis and adult rheumatoid arthritis; treatment of primary dysmenorrhea
Pregnancy Risk Factor C/D (3rd trimester)
Pregnancy/Breast-Feeding Implications Use should be avoided in late pregnancy because it may cause premature closure of the ductus arteriosus. Excretion in breast milk is unknown; breast-feeding is not recommended.
Contraindications Hypersensitivity to valdecoxib or any component of the formulation; patients who have experienced asthma, urticaria, or allergic-type reactions to aspirin or NSAIDs; pregnancy (3rd trimester)
(Continued)

Valdecoxib *(Continued)*

Warnings/Precautions Gastrointestinal irritation, ulceration, bleeding, and perforation may occur with NSAIDs. Use with caution in patients with a history of GI bleeding, ulcers, or risk factor for GI bleeding. Use with caution in patients with decreased renal function, hepatic disease, congestive heart failure, hypertension, dehydration, or asthma. Anaphylactoid reactions may occur. Use caution in patients with known or suspected deficiency of cytochrome P450 isoenzyme 2C9. Use in patients with severe hepatic impairment (Child-Pugh Class C) is not recommended. Safety and efficacy have not been established for patients <18 years of age.

Adverse Reactions <2% (Limited to important or life threatening): Allergy, aneurysm, angina, aortic stenosis, arrhythmia, atrial fibrillation, bradycardia, breast neoplasm, cardiomyopathy, carotid stenosis, colitis, congestive heart failure, convulsion, coronary thrombosis, depression exacerbation, diabetes mellitus, diverticulosis, duodenal ulcer, emphysema, esophageal perforation, facial edema, gastric ulcer, gastroesophageal reflux, gastrointestinal bleeding, gout, heart block, hepatitis, hiatal hernia, hyperlipemia, hyperparathyroidism, hypertension exacerbation, hypertensive encephalopathy, hypotension, impotence, intermittent claudication, liver function tests increased, lymphadenopathy, lymphangitis, lymphopenia, migraine, mitral insufficiency, myocardial infarction, myocardial ischemia, neuropathy, osteoporosis, ovarian cyst (malignant), pericarditis, periorbital swelling, photosensitivity, pneumonia, rash (erythematous, maculopapular, psoriaform), syncope, tachycardia, thrombocytopenia, thrombophlebitis, unstable angina, urinary tract infection, vaginal hemorrhage, ventricular fibrillation, vertigo

Overdosage/Toxicology Symptoms of overdose may include epigastric pain, drowsiness, lethargy, nausea, and vomiting; gastrointestinal bleeding may occur. Rare manifestations include hypertension, respiratory depression, coma, and acute renal failure. Treatment is symptomatic and supportive. Forced diuresis, hemodialysis, hemoperfusion, and/or urinary alkalinization may not be useful.

Drug Interactions

Cytochrome P450 Effect: CYP3A3/4 and 2C9 enzyme substrate; CYP2C9 enzyme inhibitor (weak *in vitro*), 3A3/4 enzyme inhibitor (weak *in vitro*), 2C19 enzyme inhibitor (moderate *in vitro*), 2D6 enzyme inhibitor (weak at supratherapeutic doses)

Increased Effect/Toxicity: Anticoagulants and antiplatelet drugs may increase risk of bleeding. Warfarin efficacy may increase. Corticosteroids may increase risk of GI ulceration. CYP2C9 and 3A3/4 inhibitors may increase valdecoxib levels. Cyclosporine, dextromethorphan, lithium, levels increased.

Decreased Effect: ACE inhibitors, angiotensin II antagonists, hydralazine, loop and thiazide diuretics effects reduced.

Ethanol/Nutrition/Herb Interactions

Ethanol: Avoid ethanol (may enhance gastric mucosal irritation).

Food: Time to peak level is delayed by 1-2 hours when taken with high-fat meal, but other parameters are unaffected.

Herb/Nutraceutical: Avoid cat's claw, dong quai, evening primrose, feverfew, garlic, ginger, ginkgo, red clover, horse chestnut, green tea, ginseng (may cause increased risk of bleeding).

Stability Store at 15°C to 30°C (59°F to 86°F).

Mechanism of Action Inhibits prostaglandin synthesis by decreasing the activity of the enzyme, cyclooxygenase-2 (COX-2), which results in decreased formation of prostaglandin precursors. Does not affect platelet function.

Pharmacodynamics/Kinetics

Onset of action: Dysmenorrhea: 60 minutes

Distribution: V_d: 86 L

Protein binding: 98%

Metabolism: Extensively hepatic via CYP3A3/4 and 2C9; glucuronidation

Bioavailability: 83%

Half-life elimination: 8-11 hours

Time to peak: 2.25-3 hours

Excretion: Primarily urine (as metabolites)

Usual Dosage Oral: Adults:

Osteoarthritis and rheumatoid arthritis: 10 mg once daily; **Note:** No additional benefits seen with 20 mg/day

Primary dysmenorrhea: 20 mg twice daily as needed

Dosage adjustment in renal impairment: Not recommended for use in advanced disease

Dosage adjustment in hepatic impairment: Not recommended for use in advanced liver dysfunction (Child-Pugh Class C)

Dietary Considerations May be taken with or without food.

Administration Avoid dehydration. Encourage patient to drink plenty of fluids.

Monitoring Parameters If used in patients with advanced renal disease, monitor serum creatinine closely; signs and symptoms of GI bleeding

Patient Information Do not take more than recommended dose. May be taken with food to reduce GI upset. Avoid alcohol, aspirin, and OTC medication unless approved by prescriber. Drink plenty of fluids unless advised not to. You may experience dizziness, headache; abdominal pain, nausea, vomiting, gastric distress (small frequent meals, frequent mouth care, sucking lozenges, or chewing gum may help). GI bleeding, ulceration, or perforation can occur with or without pain. Stop taking medication and report immediately stomach pain or cramping, unusual bleeding or bruising, or blood in vomitus, stool, or urine. Report persistent skin rash; unusual fatigue, lethargy, yellowing of skin or eyes, itching, abdominal tenderness, flu-like symptoms, easy bruising or bleeding; sudden weight gain; fluid build up, changes in urination pattern; or respiratory difficulty.

Nursing Implications Avoid use in dehydration. Encourage patient to drink plenty of fluids.

Dosage Forms Tablet: 10 mg, 20 mg

♦ **23-Valent Pneumococcal Polysaccharide Vaccine** *see* Pneumococcal Polysaccharide Vaccine (Polyvalent) *on page 1098*

♦ **Valertest No.1**® *see* Estradiol and Testosterone *on page 495*

Valganciclovir (val gan SYE kloh veer)
U.S. Brand Names Valcyte™

Synonyms Valganciclovir Hydrochloride

Therapeutic Category Antiviral Agent, Oral

Use Treatment of cytomegalovirus (CMV) retinitis in patients with acquired immunodeficiency syndrome (AIDS)

Pregnancy Risk Factor C

Pregnancy/Breast-Feeding Implications Valganciclovir is converted to ganciclovir and shares its reproductive toxicity. Ganciclovir may adversely affect spermatogenesis and fertility; due to its mutagenic potential, contraceptive precautions for female and male patients need to be followed during and for at least 90 days after therapy with this drug. Excretion in breast milk unknown; breast-feeding is contraindicated.

Contraindications Hypersensitivity to valganciclovir, ganciclovir, acyclovir, or any component of the formulation; absolute neutrophil count <500/mm³; platelet count <25,000/mm³; hemoglobin <8 g/dL

Warnings/Precautions Dosage adjustment or interruption of valganciclovir therapy may be necessary in patients with neutropenia and/or thrombocytopenia and patients with impaired renal function. Ganciclovir may adversely affect spermatogenesis and fertility; due to its mutagenic potential, contraceptive precautions for female and male patients need to be followed during and for at least 90 days after therapy with the drug. Due to differences in bioavailability, valganciclovir tablets cannot be substituted for ganciclovir capsules on a one-to-one basis. Safety and efficacy not established in pediatric patients.

Adverse Reactions
>10%:
  Central nervous system: Fever (31%), headache (9% to 22%), insomnia (16%)
  Gastrointestinal: Diarrhea (16% to 41%), nausea (8% to 30%), vomiting (21%), abdominal pain (15%)
  Hematologic: Granulocytopenia (11% to 27%), anemia (8% to 26%)
  Ocular: Retinal detachment (15%)
1% to 10%:
  Central nervous system: Peripheral neuropathy (9%), paresthesia (8%), seizures (<5%), psychosis, hallucinations (<5%), confusion (<5%), agitation (<5%)
  Hematologic: Thrombocytopenia (8%), pancytopenia (<5%), bone marrow depression (<5%), aplastic anemia (<5%), bleeding (potentially life-threatening due to thrombocytopenia <5%)
  Renal: Decreased renal function (<5%)
  Miscellaneous: Local and systemic infections, including sepsis (<5%); allergic reaction (<5%)
<1% (Limited to important or life-threatening): Valganciclovir is expected to share the toxicities which may occur at a low incidence or due to idiosyncratic reactions which have been associated with ganciclovir

Overdosage/Toxicology Symptoms of overdose with ganciclovir include neutropenia, vomiting, hypersalivation, bloody diarrhea, cytopenia, and testicular atrophy. Treatment is supportive. Hemodialysis removes 50% of the drug. Hydration may be of some benefit.

Drug Interactions
  Increased Effect/Toxicity: Reported for ganciclovir: Immunosuppressive agents may increase hematologic toxicity of ganciclovir. Imipenem/cilastatin may increase seizure potential. Oral ganciclovir increases blood levels of zidovudine, although zidovudine decreases steady-state levels of ganciclovir. Since both drugs have the potential to cause neutropenia and anemia, some patients may not tolerate concomitant therapy with these drugs at full dosage. Didanosine levels are increased with concurrent ganciclovir. Other nephrotoxic drugs (eg, amphotericin and cyclosporine) may have additive nephrotoxicity with ganciclovir.
  Decreased Effect: Reported for ganciclovir: A decrease in blood levels of ganciclovir AUC may occur when used with didanosine.

Ethanol/Nutrition/Herb Interactions Food: Coadministration with a high-fat meal increased AUC by 30%.

Stability Store at 25°C (77°F), excursions permitted to 15°C to 30°C (59°F to 86°F).

Mechanism of Action Valganciclovir is rapidly converted to ganciclovir in the body. The bioavailability of ganciclovir from valganciclovir is increased tenfold compared to the oral ganciclovir. A dose of 900 mg achieved systemic exposure of ganciclovir comparable to that achieved with the recommended doses of intravenous ganciclovir of 5 mg/kg. Ganciclovir is phosphorylated to a substrate which competitively inhibits the binding of deoxyguanosine triphosphate to DNA polymerase resulting in inhibition of viral DNA synthesis.

Pharmacodynamics/Kinetics
  Absorption: Well absorbed, high-fat meal increases AUC by 30%
  Distribution: Ganciclovir: V_d: 15.26 L/1.73 m²; widely to all tissues including CSF and ocular tissue
  Metabolism: Valganciclovir is converted to ganciclovir by intestinal mucosal cells and hepatocytes
  Bioavailability: 60% (when administered with food)
  Protein binding: 1% to 2%
  Half-life elimination: Ganciclovir: 4.08 hours; increases with impaired renal function; Severe renal impairment: Up to 68 hours
  Excretion: Urine (primarily as ganciclovir)

Usual Dosage Oral: Adults: CMV retinitis:
  Induction: 900 mg twice daily for 21 days (with food)
  Maintenance: Following induction treatment, or for patients with inactive CMV retinitis who require maintenance therapy: Recommended dose: 900 mg once daily (with food)
  Dosage adjustment in renal impairment:
    Induction dose (for 21 days):
      Cl_{cr} 40-59 mL/minute: 450 mg twice daily
(Continued)

Valganciclovir *(Continued)*

    Cl$_{cr}$ 25-39 mL/minute: 450 mg once daily
    Cl$_{cr}$ 10-24 mL/minute: 450 mg every 2 days
  Maintenance dose:
    Cl$_{cr}$ 40-59 mL/minute: 450 mg once daily
    Cl$_{cr}$ 25-39 mL/minute: 450 mg every 2 days
    Cl$_{cr}$ 10-24 mL/minute: 450 mg twice weekly

  Note: Valganciclovir is not recommended in patients receiving hemodialysis. For patients on hemodialysis (Cl$_{cr}$ <10 mL/minute), it is recommended that ganciclovir be used (dose adjusted as specified for ganciclovir).

Dietary Considerations Should be taken with meals.

Administration Avoid direct contact with broken or crushed tablets. Consideration should be given to handling and disposal according to guidelines issued for antineoplastic drugs. However, there is no consensus on the need for these precautions.

Monitoring Parameters Retinal exam (at least every 4-6 weeks), CBC, platelet counts, serum creatinine

Patient Information Valganciclovir is not a cure for CMV retinitis; for oral administration, take as directed (with food) and maintain adequate hydration (2-3 L/day of fluids unless instructed to restrict fluid intake). Swallow tablets whole, do not break or crush. Avoid handling broken or crushed tablets. Wash area thoroughly if contact occurs. Report fever, chills, unusual bleeding or bruising, infection, or unhealed sores or white plaques in mouth.

Nursing Implications Consideration should be given to handling and disposal according to guidelines issued for antineoplastic drugs. However, there is no consensus on the need for these precautions. Avoid direct contact with crushed or broken tablets.

Dosage Forms Tablet, as hydrochloride: 450 mg [496.3 mg valganciclovir hydrochloride equivalent to 450 mg valganciclovir]

- ◆ **Valganciclovir Hydrochloride** *see Valganciclovir on page 1397*
- ◆ **Valisone® [DSC]** *see Betamethasone on page 161*
- ◆ **Valisone® Scalp Lotion (Can)** *see Betamethasone on page 161*
- ◆ **Valium®** *see Diazepam on page 390*
- ◆ **Valorin [OTC]** *see Acetaminophen on page 22*
- ◆ **Valorin Extra [OTC]** *see Acetaminophen on page 22*
- ◆ **Valproate Semisodium** *see Valproic Acid and Derivatives on page 1398*
- ◆ **Valproate Sodium** *see Valproic Acid and Derivatives on page 1398*
- ◆ **Valproic Acid** *see Valproic Acid and Derivatives on page 1398*

Valproic Acid and Derivatives *(val PROE ik AS id & dah RIV ah tives)*

Related Information
  Anticonvulsants by Seizure Type *on page 1481*
  Epilepsy & Seizure Treatment *on page 1659*
  Febrile Seizures *on page 1660*

U.S. Brand Names Depacon®; Depakene®; Depakote® Delayed Release; Depakote® ER; Depakote® Sprinkle®

Canadian Brand Names Alti-Divalproex; Apo®-Divalproex; Depakene®; Epival® I.V.; Gen-Divalproex; Novo-Divalproex; Nu-Divalproex; PMS-Valproic Acid; PMS-Valproic Acid E.C.; Rhoxal-valproic

Synonyms Dipropylacetic Acid; Divalproex Sodium; DPA; 2-Propylpentanoic Acid; 2-Propylvaleric Acid; Valproate Semisodium; Valproate Sodium; Valproic Acid

Therapeutic Category Anticonvulsant; Antimigraine Agent

Use

Mania associated with bipolar disorder (Depakote®)

Migraine prophylaxis (Depakote®, Depakote® ER)

Monotherapy and adjunctive therapy in the treatment of patients with complex partial seizures that occur either in isolation or in association with other types of seizures (Depacon™, Depakote®)

Sole and adjunctive therapy of simple and complex absence seizures (Depacon™, Depakene®, Depakote®)

Adjunctively in patients with multiple seizure types that include absence seizures (Depacon™, Depakene®)

Unlabeled/Investigational Use Behavior disorders in Alzheimer's disease

Pregnancy Risk Factor D

Pregnancy/Breast-Feeding Implications

Clinical effects on the fetus: Crosses the placenta. Neural tube, cardiac, facial (characteristic pattern of dysmorphic facial features), skeletal, multiple other defects reported. Epilepsy itself, number of medications, genetic factors, or a combination of these probably influence the teratogenicity of anticonvulsant therapy. Risk of neural tube defects with use during first 30 days of pregnancy warrants discontinuation prior to pregnancy and through this period of possible.

Breast-feeding/lactation: Crosses into breast milk. AAP considers **compatible** with breast-feeding.

Contraindications Hypersensitivity to valproic acid, derivatives, or any component of the formulation; hepatic dysfunction; pregnancy

Warnings/Precautions Hepatic failure resulting in fatalities has occurred in patients; children <2 years of age are at considerable risk; other risk factors include organic brain disease, mental retardation with severe seizure disorders, congenital metabolic disorders, and patients on multiple anticonvulsants. Hepatotoxicity has been reported after 3 days to 6 months of therapy. Monitor patients closely for appearance of malaise, weakness, facial edema, anorexia, jaundice, and vomiting; may cause severe thrombocytopenia, inhibition of platelet aggregation and bleeding; tremors may indicate overdosage; use with caution in patients receiving other anticonvulsants.

Cases of life-threatening pancreatitis, occurring at the start of therapy or following years of use, have been reported in adults and children. Some cases have been hemorrhagic with rapid progression of initial symptoms to death. Signs of pancreatitis may include abdominal pain, nausea, vomiting, and/or anorexia. Patients or guardians should be instructed to notify prescriber of these symptoms, and medications should be discontinued if pancreatitis is suspected.

In vitro studies have suggested valproate stimulates the replication of HIV and CMV viruses under experimental conditions. The clinical consequence of this is unknown, but should be considered when monitoring affected patients.

Anticonvulsants should not be discontinued abruptly because of the possibility of increasing seizure frequency; valproate should be withdrawn gradually to minimize the potential of increased seizure frequency, unless safety concerns require a more rapid withdrawal. Concomitant use with clonazepam may induce absence status.

Hyperammonemia may occur, even in the absence of overt liver function abnormalities. Asymptomatic elevations require continued surveillance; symptomatic elevations should prompt modification or discontinuation of valproate therapy. CNS depression may occur with valproate use. Patients must be cautioned about performing tasks which require mental alertness (operating machinery or driving). Effects with other sedative drugs or ethanol may be potentiated.

Adverse Reactions
Adverse reactions reported when used as monotherapy for complex partial seizures:
>10%:
  Central nervous system: Somnolence (18% to 30%), dizziness (13% to 18%), insomnia (9% to 15%), nervousness (7% to 11%)
  Dermatologic: Alopecia (13% to 24%)
  Gastrointestinal: Nausea (26% to 34%), diarrhea (19% to 23%), vomiting (15% to 23%), abdominal pain (9% to 12%), dyspepsia (10% to 11%), anorexia (4% to 11%)
  Hematologic: Thrombocytopenia (1% to 24%)
  Neuromuscular & skeletal: Tremor (19% to 57%), weakness (10% to 21%)
  Respiratory: Respiratory tract infection (13% to 20%), pharyngitis (2% to 8%), dyspnea (1% to 5%)

1% to 10%:
  Cardiovascular: Hypertension, palpitation, peripheral edema (3% to 8%), tachycardia, chest pain
  Central nervous system: Amnesia (4% to 7%), abnormal dreams, anxiety, confusion, depression (4% to 5%), malaise, personality disorder
  Dermatologic: Bruising (4% to 5%), dry skin, petechia, pruritus, rash
  Endocrine & metabolic: Amenorrhea, dysmenorrhea
  Gastrointestinal: Eructation, flatulence, hematemesis, increased appetite, pancreatitis, periodontal abscess, taste perversion, weight gain (4% to 9%)
  Genitourinary: Urinary frequency, urinary incontinence, vaginitis
  Hepatic: Increased AST and ALT
  Neuromuscular & skeletal: Abnormal gait, arthralgia, back pain, hypertonia, incoordination, leg cramps, myalgia, myasthenia, paresthesia, twitching
  Ocular: Amblyopia/blurred vision (4% to 8%), abnormal vision, nystagmus (1% to 7%)
  Otic: Deafness, otitis media, tinnitus (1% to 7%)
  Respiratory: Epistaxis, increased cough, pneumonia, sinusitis

  Additional adverse effects (Limited to important or life-threatening): Anaphylaxis, aplastic anemia, asterixis, ataxia, bone marrow suppression, cerebral atrophy (reversible), cutaneous vasculitis, decreased carnitine, dementia, encephalopathy (rare), eosinophilia, erythema multiforme, Fanconi-like syndrome (rare, in children), hallucinations, hemorrhage, hyperammonemia, hyperglycinemia, hypofibrinogenemia, hyponatremia, inappropriate ADH secretion, incoordination, intermittent porphyria, lupus erythematosus, pancreatitis (rare, may be hemorrhagic/life-threatening), pancytopenia, Parkinsonism, photosensitivity, psychosis, Stevens-Johnson syndrome, toxic epidermal necrolysis (rare), vertigo

Overdosage/Toxicology Symptoms include coma, deep sleep, motor restlessness, and visual hallucinations. Supportive treatment is necessary. Naloxone has been used to reverse CNS depressant effects, but may block the action of other anticonvulsants. In overdose, the fraction of unbound valproate is high. Hemodialysis or tandem hemodialysis plus hemoperfusion may lead to significant removal of the drug.

Drug Interactions
Cytochrome P450 Effect: CYP2C19 enzyme substrate; CYP2C9 and 2D6 enzyme inhibitor, CYP3A3/4 enzyme inhibitor (weak)

Increased Effect/Toxicity: Absence seizures have been reported in patients receiving VPA and clonazepam. Valproic acid may increase, decrease, or have no effect on carbamazepine and phenytoin levels. Valproic acid may increase serum concentrations of carbamazepine - epoxide (active metabolite). Valproic acid may increase serum concentrations of diazepam, lamotrigine, nimodipine, and phenobarbital, and tricyclic antidepressants. Chlorpromazine (and possibly other phenothiazines), macrolide antibiotics (clarithromycin, erythromycin, troleandomycin), felbamate, and isoniazid may inhibit the metabolism of valproic acid. Aspirin or other salicylates may displace valproic acid from protein-binding sites, leading to acute toxicity.
CYP2C18/19 inhibitors: May increase serum concentrations of valproic acid; inhibitors include cimetidine, felbamate, fluoxetine, and fluvoxamine

Decreased Effect: Valproic acid may displace clozapine from protein binding site resulting in decreased clozapine serum concentrations. Carbamazepine, lamotrigine, and phenytoin may induce the metabolism of valproic acid. Cholestyramine (and possibly colestipol) may bind valproic acid in GI tract, decreasing absorption. Acyclovir may reduce valproic acid levels.

Ethanol/Nutrition/Herb Interactions
  Ethanol: Avoid ethanol (may increase CNS depression).
  (Continued)

Valproic Acid and Derivatives *(Continued)*

Food: Food may delay but does not affect the extent of absorption. Valproic acid serum concentrations may be decreased if taken with food. Milk has no effect on absorption.

Herb/Nutraceutical: Avoid evening primrose (seizure threshold decreased)

Stability Injection is physically compatible and chemically stable in D_5W, NS, and LR for at least 24 hours when stored in glass or PVC; store vials at room temperature 15°C to 30°C (59°F to 86°F)

Mechanism of Action Causes increased availability of gamma-aminobutyric acid (GABA), an inhibitory neurotransmitter, to brain neurons or may enhance the action of GABA or mimic its action at postsynaptic receptor sites

Pharmacodynamics/Kinetics

Distribution: Total valproate: 11 L/1.73 m^2; free valproate 92 L/1.73 m^2

Protein binding (dose dependent): 80% to 90%

Metabolism: Extensively hepatic; glucuronide conjugation and mitochondrial beta-oxidation

Bioavailability: Extended release: 90%; Delayed release: 81% to 90%

Half-life elimination: (increased in neonates and with liver disease): Children: 4-14 hours; Adults: 8-17 hours

Time to peak, serum: 1-4 hours; 3-5 hours after divalproex (enteric coated)

Excretion: Urine (30% to 50% as glucuronide conjugate, 3% as unchanged drug)

Usual Dosage

Seizures:

Children >10 years and Adults:

Oral: Initial: 10-15 mg/kg/day in 1-3 divided doses; increase by 5-10 mg/kg/day at weekly intervals until therapeutic levels are achieved; maintenance: 30-60 mg/kg/day in 2-3 divided doses. Adult usual dose: 1000-2500 mg/day

Children receiving more than one anticonvulsant (ie, polytherapy) may require doses up to 100 mg/kg/day in 3-4 divided doses

I.V.: Administer as a 60-minute infusion (≤20 mg/minute) with the same frequency as oral products; switch patient to oral products as soon as possible. Rapid infusions have been given: ≤15 mg/kg over 5-10 minutes. (1.5-3 mg/kg/minute).

Rectal: Dilute syrup 1:1 with water for use as a retention enema; loading dose: 17-20 mg/kg one time; maintenance: 10-15 mg/kg/dose every 8 hours

Mania: Adults: Oral: 750 mg/day in divided doses; dose should be adjusted as rapidly as possible to desired clinical effect; a loading dose of 20 mg/kg may be used; maximum recommended dosage: 60 mg/kg/day

Migraine prophylaxis: Adults: Oral:

Extended release tablets: 500 mg once daily for 7 days, then increase to 1000 mg once daily; adjust dose based on patient response; usual dosage range 500-1000 mg/day

Delayed release tablets: 250 mg twice daily; adjust dose based on patient response, up to 1000 mg/day

Elderly: Elimination is decreased in the elderly. Studies of elderly patients with dementia show a high incidence of somnolence. In some patients, this was associated with weight loss. Starting doses should be lower and increases should be slow, with careful monitoring of nutritional intake and dehydration. Safety and efficacy for use in patients >65 years have not been studied for migraine prophylaxis.

Dosing adjustment in renal impairment: A 27% reduction in clearance of unbound valproate is seen in patients with Cl_{cr} <10 mL/minute. Hemodialysis reduces valproate concentrations by 20%, therefore no dose adjustment is needed in patients with renal failure. Protein binding is reduced, monitoring only total valproate concentrations may be misleading.

Dosing adjustment/comments in hepatic impairment: Reduce dose. Clearance is decreased with liver impairment. Hepatic disease is also associated with increased albumin concentrations and 2- to 2.6-fold increase in the unbound fraction. Free concentrations of valproate may be elevated while total concentrations appear normal.

Dietary Considerations Valproic acid may cause GI upset; take with large amount of water or food to decrease GI upset. May need to split doses to avoid GI upset.

Coated particles of divalproex sodium may be mixed with semisolid food (eg, applesauce or pudding) in patients having difficulty swallowing; particles should be swallowed and not chewed

Valproate sodium oral solution will generate valproic acid in carbonated beverages and may cause mouth and throat irritation; do not mix valproate sodium oral solution with carbonated beverages

Administration

Depakote® ER: Swallow whole, do not crush or chew. Patients who need dose adjustments smaller than 500 mg/day for migraine prophylaxis should be changed to Depakote® delayed release tablets. Sprinkle capsules may be swallowed whole or open cap and sprinkle on small amount (1 teaspoonful) of soft food and use immediately (do not store or chew).

Depacon®: Final concentration: ≤20 mg/minute over 60 minutes; use for longer than 14 days has not been studied. Alternatively, may be administered as a rapid infusion over 5-10 minutes (1.5-3 mg/kg/minute).

Monitoring Parameters Liver enzymes, CBC with platelets

Reference Range

Therapeutic: 50-100 μg/mL (SI: 350-690 μmol/L)

Toxic: >200 μg/mL (SI: >1390 μmol/L)

Seizure control: May improve at levels >100 μg/mL (SI: 690 μmol/L), but toxicity may occur at levels of 100-150 μg/mL (SI: 690-1040 μmol/L)

Mania: Clinical response seen with trough levels between 50-125 μg/mL; risk of toxicity increases at levels >125 μg/mL

Test Interactions False-positive result for urine ketones; accuracy of thyroid function tests

Patient Information When used to treat generalized seizures, patient instructions are determined by patient's condition and ability to understand.

Oral: Take as directed; do not alter dose or timing of medication. Do not increase dose or take more than recommended. Do not crush or chew capsule or enteric-coated pill. While using this medication, do not use alcohol and other prescription or OTC medications (especially pain medications, sedatives, antihistamines, or hypnotics) without consulting prescriber. Maintain adequate hydration (2-3 L/day of fluids unless instructed to restrict fluid intake). Diabetics should monitor serum glucose closely (valproic acid will alter results of urine ketones). Report alterations in menstrual cycle; abdominal cramps, unresolved diarrhea, vomiting, or constipation; skin rash; unusual bruising or bleeding; blood in urine, stool or vomitus; malaise; weakness; facial swelling; yellowing of skin or eyes; excessive sedation; or restlessness.

Do not get pregnant while taking this medication; use appropriate barrier contraceptive measures

Nursing Implications Do not crush enteric coated drug product or capsule; do not crush or chew gelatin capsules or tablet formulations

Additional Information
Sodium content of valproate sodium syrup (5 mL): 23 mg (1 mEq)
Extended release tablets have 10% to 20% less fluctuation in serum concentration than delayed release tablets. Extended release tablets are not bioequivalent to delayed release tablets.

Dosage Forms
Capsule, as valproic acid (Depakene®): 250 mg
Capsule, sprinkles, as divalproex sodium (Depakote® Sprinkle®): 125 mg
Injection, solution, as sodium valproate (Depacon®): 100 mg/mL (5 mL)
Syrup, as sodium valproate: 250 mg/5 mL (5 mL, 480 mL)
  Depakene®: 250 mg/mL (480 mL)
Tablet, delayed release, as divalproex sodium (Depakote®): 125 mg, 250 mg, 500 mg
Tablet, extended release, as divalproex sodium (Depakote® ER): 500 mg

Valrubicin (val ROO bi sin)

U.S. Brand Names Valstar™
Canadian Brand Names Valstar™
Therapeutic Category Antineoplastic Agent, Anthracycline
Use Intravesical therapy of BCG-refractory carcinoma *in situ* of the urinary bladder
Pregnancy Risk Factor C
Pregnancy/Breast-Feeding Implications It is not known whether valrubicin is secreted in human milk. Because many drugs are secreted in milk, and the potential for serious adverse reactions exists, a decision should be made whether to discontinue nursing or discontinue the drug, taking into account the importance of the drug to the mother.
Contraindications Hypersensitivity to anthracyclines, Cremophor® EL, or any component of the formulation; concurrent urinary tract infection or small bladder capacity (unable to tolerate a 75 mL instillation)
Warnings/Precautions Complete response observed in only 1 of 5 patients, delay of cystectomy may lead to development of metastatic bladder cancer, which is lethal. If complete response is not observed after 3 months or disease recurs, cystectomy must be reconsidered. Do not administer if mucosal integrity of bladder has been compromised or bladder perforation is present. Following TURP, status of bladder mucosa should be evaluated prior to initiation of therapy. Administer under the supervision of a physician experienced in the use of intravesical chemotherapy. Aseptic technique must be used during administration. All patients of reproductive age should use an effective method of contraception during the treatment period. Irritable bladder symptoms may occur during instillation and retention. Caution in patients with severe irritable bladder symptoms. Do not clamp urinary catheter. Red-tinged urine is typical for the first 24 hours after instillation. Prolonged symptoms or discoloration should prompt contact with the physician.

Valrubicin preparation should be performed in a class II laminar flow biologic safety cabinet. Personnel should be wearing surgical gloves and a closed front surgical gown with knit cuffs. Appropriate safety equipment is recommended for preparation, administration, and disposal of antineoplastics. If valrubicin contacts the skin, wash and flush thoroughly with water.

Adverse Reactions
>10%: Genitourinary: Frequency (61%), dysuria (56%), urgency (57%), bladder spasm (31%), hematuria (29%), bladder pain (28%), urinary incontinence (22%), cystitis (15%), urinary tract infection (15%)

1% to 10%:
  Cardiovascular: Chest pain (2%), vasodilation (2%), peripheral edema (1%)
  Central nervous system: Headache (4%), malaise (4%), dizziness (3%), fever (2%)
  Dermatologic: Rash (3%)
  Endocrine & metabolic: Hyperglycemia (1%)
  Gastrointestinal: Abdominal pain (5%), nausea (5%), diarrhea (3%), vomiting (2%), flatulence (1%)
  Genitourinary: Nocturia (7%), burning symptoms (5%), urinary retention (4%), urethral pain (3%), pelvic pain (1%), hematuria (microscopic) (3%)
  Hematologic: Anemia (2%)
  Neuromuscular & skeletal: Weakness (4%), back pain (3%), myalgia (1%)
  Respiratory: Pneumonia (1%)
<1% (Limited to important or life-threatening): Decreased urine flow, pruritus, skin irritation, taste disturbance, tenesmus, urethritis

Overdosage/Toxicology Inadvertent paravenous extravasation has not been associated with skin ulceration or necrosis. Myelosuppression is possible following inadvertent systemic administration or following significant systemic absorption from intravesical instillation.

Drug Interactions
Increased Effect/Toxicity: No specific drug interactions studies have been performed. Systemic exposure to valrubicin is negligible, and interactions are unlikely.
Decreased Effect: No specific drug interactions studies have been performed. Systemic exposure to valrubicin is negligible, and interactions are unlikely.

(Continued)

Valrubicin *(Continued)*

Stability Store unopened vials under refrigeration at 2°C to 8°C (36°F to 48°F). Stable for 12 hours when diluted in 0.9% sodium chloride. Withdraw contents of four vials, each containing 200 mg in 5 mL (allowed to warm to room temperature without heating), and dilute with 55 mL of 0.9% sodium chloride injection, USP.

Mechanism of Action Blocks function of DNA topoisomerase II; inhibits DNA synthesis, causes extensive chromosomal damage, and arrests cell development

Pharmacodynamics/Kinetics

Absorption: Well absorbed into bladder tissue, negligible systemic absorption. Trauma to mucosa may increase absorption, and perforation greatly increases absorption with significant systemic myelotoxicity.

Metabolism: Negligible after intravesical instillation and 2 hour retention

Excretion: Urine when expelled from urinary bladder

Usual Dosage Adults: Intravesical: 800 mg once weekly for 6 weeks

Dosing adjustment in renal impairment: No specific adjustment recommended

Dosing adjustment in hepatic impairment: No specific adjustment recommended

Administration Withdraw contents of 4 vials, each containing 200 mg in 5 mL (allowed to warm to room temperature without heating), and dilute with 55 mL of 0.9% sodium chloride injection, USP. Instill slowly via gravity flow through a urinary catheter (following sterile insertion). Withdraw the catheter and allow patient to retain solution for 2 hours. After 2 hours, the patient should void.

Monitoring Parameters Cystoscopy, biopsy, and urine cytology every 3 months for recurrence or progression

Patient Information This medication will be instilled into your bladder through a catheter to be retained for as long as possible. Your urine will be red tinged for the next 24 hours; report promptly if this continues for a longer period. You may experience altered urination patterns (frequency, dysuria, or incontinence), some bladder pain, pain on urination, or pelvic pain; report if these persist. Diabetics should monitor glucose levels closely (may cause hyperglycemia). It is important that you maintain adequate hydration (2-3 L/day of fluids unless instructed to restrict fluid intake). You may experience some dizziness or fatigue (use caution when driving or engaging in tasks requiring alertness until response to drug is known); or nausea, vomiting, or taste disturbance (small frequent meals, frequent mouth care, chewing gum, or sucking lozenges may help). Report chest pain or palpitations; persistent dizziness; swelling of extremities; persistent nausea, vomiting, diarrhea, or abdominal pain; muscle weakness, pain, or tremors; unusual cough or difficulty breathing; or other adverse effects related to this medication. Do not become pregnant or cause pregnancy (males) during treatment. Do not breast-feed during treatment period.

Dosage Forms Injection: 40 mg/mL (5 mL)

Valsartan *(val SAR tan)*

Related Information

Angiotensin Agents Comparison *on page 1473*

U.S. Brand Names Diovan®

Canadian Brand Names Diovan®

Therapeutic Category Angiotensin II Receptor Antagonist (ARB); Antihypertensive Agent

Use Alone or in combination with other antihypertensive agents in treating essential hypertension; may have an advantage over losartan due to minimal metabolism requirements and consequent use in mild to moderate hepatic impairment

Pregnancy Risk Factor C/D (2nd and 3rd trimesters)

Pregnancy/Breast-Feeding Implications Breast-feeding/lactation: Although no human data exist, valsartan is known to be excreted in animal breast milk and should be avoided in lactating mothers if possible

Contraindications Hypersensitivity to valsartan or any component of the formulation; hypersensitivity to other A-II receptor antagonists; primary hyperaldosteronism; bilateral renal artery stenosis; pregnancy (2nd and 3rd trimesters)

Warnings/Precautions Use extreme caution with concurrent administration of potassium-sparing diuretics or potassium supplements, in patients with mild to moderate hepatic dysfunction (adjust dose), in those who may be sodium/water depleted (eg, on high-dose diuretics), and in the elderly; avoid use in patients with congestive heart failure, unilateral renal artery stenosis, aortic/mitral valve stenosis, coronary artery disease, or hypertrophic cardiomyopathy, if possible

Adverse Reactions Similar incidence to placebo; independent of race, age, and gender.

>1%:

Cardiovascular: Hypotension (6.9%)

Central nervous system: Dizziness (2% to 9%), drowsiness(2.1%), ataxia (1.4%), fatigue (2%)

Endocrine & metabolic: Increased serum potassium (4.4%)

Gastrointestinal: Abdominal pain (2%), dysgeusia (1.4%)

Hematologic: Neutropenia (1.9%)

Hepatic: Increased LFTs

Respiratory: Cough (2.9% versus 1.5% in placebo)

Miscellaneous: Viral infection (3%)

<1% (Limited to important or life-threatening): Allergic reactions, alopecia, angioedema, antisynthetase syndrome without myositis, depression, dyspnea, hyperkalemia, impotence, neuralgia, paresthesia, rash, renal function impairment, somnolence, syncope, vertigo

Overdosage/Toxicology Only mild toxicity (hypotension, bradycardia, hyperkalemia) has been reported with large overdoses (up to 5 g of captopril and 300 mg of enalapril). No fatalities have been reported. Treatment is symptomatic (eg, fluids).

Drug Interactions

Increased Effect/Toxicity: Valsartan blood levels may be increased by cimetidine and monoxidine; clinical effect is unknown. Concurrent use of potassium salts/supplements, co-trimoxazole (high dose), ACE inhibitors, and potassium-sparing diuretics (amiloride, spironolactone, triamterene) may increase the risk of hyperkalemia.

Decreased Effect: Phenobarbital, ketoconazole, troleandomycin, sulfaphenazole

Ethanol/Nutrition/Herb Interactions

Food: Decreases rate and extent of absorption by 50% and 40%, respectively.

Herb/Nutraceutical: Avoid dong quai if using for hypertension (has estrogenic activity). Avoid ephedra, yohimbe, ginseng (may worsen hypertension). Avoid garlic (may have increased antihypertensive effect).

Mechanism of Action As a prodrug, valsartan produces direct antagonism of the angiotensin II (AT2) receptors, unlike the angiotensin-converting enzyme inhibitors. It displaces angiotensin II from the AT1 receptor and produces its blood pressure lowering effects by antagonizing AT1-induced vasoconstriction, aldosterone release, catecholamine release, arginine vasopressin release, water intake, and hypertrophic responses. This action results in more efficient blockade of the cardiovascular effects of angiotensin II and fewer side effects than the ACE inhibitors.

Pharmacodynamics/Kinetics

Onset of action: Peak effect: 4-6 hours

Distribution: V_d: 17 L (adults)

Protein binding: 94% to 97%

Metabolism: Metabolized to an inactive metabolite

Bioavailability: 23%

Half-life elimination: 9 hours

Time to peak, serum: 2 hours

Excretion: Urine (13%) and feces (83%) as unchanged drug

Usual Dosage Adults: 80 mg/day; may be increased to 160 mg if needed (maximal effects observed in 4-6 weeks); maximum recommended dose: 320 mg/day

Dosing adjustment in renal impairment: No dosage adjustment necessary if Cl_{cr} >10 mL/minute.

Dosing adjustment in hepatic impairment (mild - moderate): ≤80 mg/day

Dialysis: Not significantly removed

Monitoring Parameters Baseline and periodic electrolyte panels, renal and liver function tests, urinalysis; symptoms of hypotension or hypersensitivity

Patient Information Do not stop taking this medication unless instructed by a physician, do not take this medication during pregnancy or lactation; take a missed dose as soon as possible unless it is almost time for your next dose; call your physician immediately if you have symptoms of allergy or develop side effects including headache and dizziness

Dosage Forms

Capsule: 80 mg, 160 mg, 320 mg [Note: This form to be discontinued]

Tablet: 80 mg, 160 mg, 320 mg

Valsartan and Hydrochlorothiazide

(val SAR tan & hye droe klor oh THYE a zide)

U.S. Brand Names Diovan HCT®

Canadian Brand Names Diovan HCT®

Synonyms Hydrochlorothiazide and Valsartan

Therapeutic Category Angiotensin II Antagonist Combination; Antihypertensive Agent, Combination

Use Treatment of hypertension (not indicated for initial therapy)

Pregnancy Risk Factor C (1st trimester); D (2nd and 3rd trimester)

Usual Dosage Adults: Oral: Dose is individualized

Additional Information Complete prescribing information for this medication should be consulted for additional detail.

Dosage Forms

Tablet:

Valsartan 80 mg and hydrochlorothiazide 12.5 mg

Valsartan 160 mg and hydrochlorothiazide 12.5 mg

Valsartan 160 mg and hydrochlorothiazide 25 mg

- **Valstar™** *see Valrubicin on page 1401*
- **Valtrex®** *see Valacyclovir on page 1394*
- **Vanatrip®** *see Amitriptyline on page 76*
- **Vancenase® (Can)** *see Beclomethasone on page 149*
- **Vancenase® AQ 84 mcg** *see Beclomethasone on page 149*
- **Vancenase® Pockethaler®** *see Beclomethasone on page 149*
- **Vanceril®** *see Beclomethasone on page 149*
- **Vancocin®** *see Vancomycin on page 1403*
- **Vancoled®** *see Vancomycin on page 1403*

Vancomycin (van koe MYE sin)

Related Information

Antibiotic Treatment of Adults With Infective Endocarditis *on page 1585*

Antimicrobial Drugs of Choice *on page 1588*

Community-Acquired Pneumonia in Adults *on page 1603*

Desensitization Protocols *on page 1525*

Prevention of Bacterial Endocarditis *on page 1563*

Prevention of Wound Infection & Sepsis in Surgical Patients *on page 1569*

U.S. Brand Names Lyphocin®; Vancocin®; Vancoled®

Canadian Brand Names Vancocin®

Synonyms Vancomycin Hydrochloride

Therapeutic Category Antibiotic, Miscellaneous

(Continued)

Vancomycin (Continued)

Use Treatment of patients with infections caused by staphylococcal species and streptococcal species; used orally for staphylococcal enterocolitis or for antibiotic-associated pseudomembranous colitis produced by *C. difficile*

Pregnancy Risk Factor C

Contraindications Hypersensitivity to vancomycin or any component of the formulation; avoid in patients with previous severe hearing loss

Warnings/Precautions Use with caution in patients with renal impairment or those receiving other nephrotoxic or ototoxic drugs; dosage modification required in patients with impaired renal function (especially elderly)

Adverse Reactions

Oral:

>10%: Gastrointestinal: Bitter taste, nausea, vomiting, stomatitis

1% to 10%:

Central nervous system: Chills, drug fever

Hematologic: Eosinophilia

<1% (Limited to important or life-threatening): Interstitial nephritis, ototoxicity, renal failure, skin rash, thrombocytopenia, vasculitis

Parenteral:

>10%:

Cardiovascular: Hypotension accompanied by flushing

Dermatologic: Erythematous rash on face and upper body (red neck or red man syndrome)

1% to 10%:

Central nervous system: Chills, drug fever

Hematologic: Eosinophilia

<1% (Limited to important or life-threatening): Ototoxicity, renal failure, thrombocytopenia, vasculitis

Overdosage/Toxicology Symptoms include ototoxicity and nephrotoxicity. There is no specific therapy for vancomycin overdose. Care is symptomatic and supportive. Peritoneal filtration and hemofiltration (not dialysis) have been shown to reduce the serum concentration of vancomycin. High flux dialysis may remove up to 25%.

Drug Interactions

Increased Effect/Toxicity: Increased toxicity with other ototoxic or nephrotoxic drugs. Increased neuromuscular blockade with most neuromuscular blocking agents.

Stability

Vancomycin reconstituted intravenous solutions are stable for 14 days at room temperature or refrigeration

Stability of parenteral admixture at room temperature (25°C) or refrigeration temperature (4°C): 7 days

Standard diluent: 500 mg/150 mL D$_5$W; 750 mg/250 mL D$_5$W; 1 g/250 mL D$_5$W

Minimum volume: Maximum concentration is 5 mg/mL to minimize thrombophlebitis

Incompatible with heparin, phenobarbital

After the oral solution is reconstituted, it should be refrigerated and used within 2 weeks

Mechanism of Action Inhibits bacterial cell wall synthesis by blocking glycopeptide polymerization through binding tightly to D-alanyl-D-alanine portion of cell wall precursor

Pharmacodynamics/Kinetics

Absorption: Oral: Poor; I.M.: Erratic; Intraperitoneal: ~38%

Distribution: Widely in body tissues and fluids. except for CSF

Relative diffusion from blood into CSF: Good only with inflammation (exceeds usual MICs)

CSF:blood level ratio: Normal meninges: Nil; Inflamed meninges: 20% to 30%

Protein binding: 10% to 50%

Half-life elimination: Biphasic: Terminal:

Newborns: 6-10 hours

Infants and Children 3 months to 4 years: 4 hours

Children >3 years: 2.2-3 hours

Adults: 5-11 hours; prolonged significantly with reduced renal function

End-stage renal disease: 200-250 hours

Time to peak, serum: I.V.: 45-65 minutes

Excretion: I.V.: Urine (80% to 90% as unchanged drug); Oral: Primarily feces

Usual Dosage Initial dosage recommendation: I.V.:

Neonates:

Postnatal age ≤7 days:

<1200 g: 15 mg/kg/dose every 24 hours

1200-2000 g: 10 mg/kg/dose every 12 hours

>2000 g: 15 mg/kg/dose every 12 hours

Postnatal age >7 days:

<1200 g: 15 mg/kg/dose every 24 hours

≥1200 g: 10 mg/kg/dose divided every 8 hours

Infants >1 month and Children:

40 mg/kg/day in divided doses every 6 hours

Prophylaxis for bacterial endocarditis:

Dental, oral, or upper respiratory tract surgery: 20 mg/kg 1 hour prior to the procedure

GI/GU procedure: 20 mg/kg plus gentamicin 2 mg/kg 1 hour prior to surgery

Infants >1 month and Children with staphylococcal central nervous system infection: 60 mg/kg/day in divided doses every 6 hours

Adults:

With normal renal function: 1 g **or** 10-15 mg/kg/dose every 12 hours

Prophylaxis for bacterial endocarditis:

Dental, oral, or upper respiratory tract surgery: 1 g 1 hour before surgery

GI/GU procedure: 1 g plus 1.5 mg/kg gentamicin 1 hour prior to surgery

Dosing interval in renal impairment (vancomycin levels should be monitored in patients with any renal impairment):

Cl$_{cr}$ >60 mL/minute: Start with 1 g or 10-15 mg/kg/dose every 12 hours

Cl$_{cr}$ 40-60 mL/minute: Start with 1 g or 10-15 mg/kg/dose every 24 hours

Cl$_{cr}$ <40 mL/minute: Will need longer intervals; determine by serum concentration monitoring

Hemodialysis: Not dialyzable (0% to 5%); generally not removed; exception minimal-moderate removal by some of the newer high-flux filters; dose may need to be administered more frequently; monitor serum concentrations

Continuous ambulatory peritoneal dialysis (CAPD): Not significantly removed; administration via CAPD fluid: 15-30 mg/L (15-30 mcg/mL) of CAPD fluid

Continuous arteriovenous hemofiltration: Dose as for Cl$_{cr}$ 10-40 mL/minute

Antibiotic lock technique (for catheter infections): 2 mg/mL in SWI/NS or D$_5$W; instill 3-5 mL into catheter port as a flush solution instead of heparin lock (**Note:** Do not mix with any other solutions)

Intrathecal: Vancomycin is available as a powder for injection and may be diluted to 1-5 mg/mL concentration in preservative-free 0.9% sodium chloride for administration into the CSF

Neonates: 5-10 mg/day

Children: 5-20 mg/day

Adults: Up to 20 mg/day

Oral: Pseudomembranous colitis produced by *C. difficile*:

Neonates: 10 mg/kg/day in divided doses

Children: 40 mg/kg/day in divided doses, added to fluids

Adults: 125 mg 4 times/day for 10 days

Dietary Considerations May be taken with food.

Monitoring Parameters Periodic renal function tests, urinalysis, serum vancomycin concentrations, WBC, audiogram

Reference Range

Timing of serum samples: Draw peak 1 hour after 1-hour infusion has completed; draw trough just before next dose

Therapeutic levels: Peak: 25-40 µg/mL; Trough: 5-12 µg/mL

Toxic: >80 µg/mL (SI: >54 µmol/L)

Patient Information Report pain at infusion site, dizziness, fullness or ringing in ears with I.V. use; nausea or vomiting with oral use

Nursing Implications Obtain drug levels after the third dose unless otherwise directed; peaks are drawn 1 hour after the completion of a 1- to 2-hour infusion; troughs are obtained just before the next dose; slow I.V. infusion rate if maculopapular rash appears on face, neck, trunk, and upper extremities (Red man reaction)

Additional Information Because of its long half-life, vancomycin should be dosed on an every 12 hour basis; monitoring of peak and trough serum levels is advisable. The "red man syndrome" characterized by skin rash and hypotension is not an allergic reaction but rather is associated with too rapid infusion of the drug. To alleviate or prevent the reaction, infuse vancomycin at a rate of ≥30 minutes for each 500 mg of drug being administered (eg, 1 g over ≥60 minutes); 1.5 g over ≥90 minutes.

Dosage Forms

Capsule, as hydrochloride: 125 mg, 250 mg

Powder for injection, as hydrochloride: 500 mg, 1 g, 2 g, 5 g, 10 g

Powder for oral solution, as hydrochloride: 1 g, 10 g

♦ **Vancomycin Hydrochloride** *see* Vancomycin *on page 1403*

♦ **Vaniqa™** *see* Eflornithine *on page 461*

♦ **Vanoxide-HC®** *see* Benzoyl Peroxide and Hydrocortisone *on page 157*

♦ **Vanquish® Extra Strength Pain Reliever [OTC]** *see* Acetaminophen, Aspirin, and Caffeine *on page 26*

♦ **Vansil™** *see* Oxamniquine *on page 1018*

♦ **Vantin®** *see* Cefpodoxime *on page 251*

♦ **Vaponefrin® (Can)** *see* Epinephrine *on page 470*

♦ **VAQTA®** *see* Hepatitis A Vaccine *on page 660*

Varicella Virus Vaccine (var i SEL a VYE rus vak SEEN)

Related Information

Immunization Recommendations *on page 1538*

Recommendations of the Advisory Committee on Immunization Practices (ACIP) *on page 1540*

Recommended Childhood Immunization Schedule - US - 2002 *on page 1539*

U.S. Brand Names Varivax®

Canadian Brand Names Varivax®

Synonyms Chicken Pox Vaccine; Varicella-Zoster Virus (VZV) Vaccine

Therapeutic Category Vaccine, Live Virus

Use Immunization against varicella in children ≥12 months of age and adults. The American Association of Pediatrics recommends that the chickenpox vaccine should be given to all healthy children between 12 months and 18 years; children between 12 months and 13 years who have not been immunized or who have not had chickenpox should receive 1 vaccination while children 13-18 years of age require 2 vaccinations 4-8 weeks apart; the vaccine has been added to the childhood immunization schedule for infants 12-28 months of age and children 11-12 years of age who have not been vaccinated previously or who have not had the disease; it is recommended to be given with the measles, mumps, and rubella (MMR) vaccine

Pregnancy Risk Factor C

Pregnancy/Breast-Feeding Implications Animal reproduction studies have not been conducted. Varivax® should not be administered to pregnant females and pregnancy should be avoided for 3 months following vaccination. Excretion in breast milk is unknown; use caution in breast-feeding.

Contraindications Hypersensitivity to any component of the vaccine, including gelatin; a history of anaphylactoid reaction to neomycin; individuals with blood dyscrasias, leukemia, lymphomas, or other malignant neoplasms affecting the bone marrow or lymphatic systems; those receiving immunosuppressive therapy; primary and acquired immunodeficiency states; (Continued)

Varicella Virus Vaccine *(Continued)*

a family history of congenital or hereditary immunodeficiency; active untreated tuberculosis; current febrile illness; pregnancy; I.V. injection

Warnings/Precautions Immediate treatment for anaphylactoid reaction should be available during vaccine use; defer vaccination for at least 5 months following blood or plasma transfusions, immune globulin (IgG), or VZIG (avoid IgG or IVIG use for 2 months following vaccination); salicylates should be avoided for 5 weeks after vaccination; vaccinated individuals should not have close association with susceptible high risk individuals (newborns, pregnant women, immunocompromised persons) following vaccination

Adverse Reactions All serious adverse reactions must be reported to the U.S. Department of Health and Human Services (DHHS) Vaccine Adverse Event Reporting System (VAERS) 1-800-822-7967.

As reported in ≥1% of patients, unless otherwise specified:

>10%:
Central nervous system: Fever (10% to 15%)
Local: Injection site reaction (19% to 24%)

1% to 10%:
Central nervous system: Chills, fatigue, headache, irritability, malaise, nervousness, sleep disturbance
Dermatologic: Generalized varicella-like rash (4% to 5%), contact rash, dermatitis, diaper rash, dry skin, eczema, heat rash, itching
Gastrointestinal: Abdominal pain, appetite decreased, cold/canker sore, constipation, nausea, vomiting
Hematologic: Lymphadenopathy
Local: Varicella-like rash at the injection site (3%)
Neuromuscular & skeletal: Arthralgia, myalgia, stiff neck
Otic: Otitis
Respiratory: Cough, lower/upper respiratory illness
Miscellaneous: Allergic reactions, teething

<1% (Limited to important or life-threatening) Anaphylaxis, Bell's palsy, cellulitis, cerebrovascular accident, dizziness, encephalitis, erythema multiforme, febrile seizures, Guillain-Barré syndrome, Henoch-Schönlein purpura, nonfebrile seizures, Stevens-Johnson syndrome, thrombocytopenia, transverse myelitis

Drug Interactions

Increased Effect/Toxicity: Salicylates may increase the risk of Reye's following varicella vaccination (avoid salicylate use for 6 weeks following vaccination).

Decreased Effect: The effect of the vaccine may be decreased and the risk of varicella disease in individuals who are receiving immunosuppressant drugs (including high dose systemic corticosteroids) may be increased. Effect of vaccine may be decreased in given within 5 months of immune globulins. Effectiveness of varicella vaccine may be decreased if given within 30 days of MMR vaccine (effectiveness not decreased when administered simultaneously).

Stability Store powder in freezer at -15°C (5°F), protect from light; store diluent separately at room temperature or in refrigerator. Powder may be stored under refrigeration for up to 72 continuous hours prior to reconstitution; if not used within 72 hours, vaccine should be discarded. Use 0.7 mL of the provided diluent to reconstitute vaccine. Gently agitate to mix thoroughly. (Total volume of reconstituted vaccine will be ~0.5 mL.) Discard if reconstituted vaccine is not used within 30 minutes. Do not freeze reconstituted vaccine.

Mechanism of Action As a live, attenuated vaccine, varicella virus vaccine offers active immunity to disease caused by the varicella-zoster virus

Pharmacodynamics/Kinetics
Onset of action: Seroconversion: ~4-6 weeks
Duration: Lowest breakthrough rates (0.2% to 2.9%) in the first 2 years following postvaccination, slightly higher rates in third through fifth year

Usual Dosage S.C.:
Children 12 months to 12 years: 0.5 mL
Children 12 years to Adults: 2 doses of 0.5 mL separated by 4-8 weeks

Administration Do not administer I.V.; inject S.C. into the outer aspect of the upper arm, if possible. Federal law requires that the date of administration, the vaccine manufacturer, lot number of vaccine, and the administering person's name, title and address be entered into the patient's permanent medical record.

Monitoring Parameters Rash, fever

Patient Information Report any adverse reactions to the prescriber or Vaccine Adverse Event Reporting System (1-800-822-7967). Some side effects may occur 1-6 weeks after the shot. Common side effects include soreness or swelling in the area where the shot is given, mild rash, fever. Do not take aspirin for 6 weeks after getting the vaccine. Do not use in pregnancy and do not get pregnant for 3 months after getting this vaccine.

Nursing Implications Obtain the previous immunization history (including allergic reactions) to previous vaccines; do not inject into a blood vessel; use the supplied diluent only for reconstitution; inject immediately after reconstitution. Federal law requires that the date of administration, the vaccine manufacturer, lot number of vaccine, and the administering person's name, title and address be entered into the patient's permanent medical record.

Dosage Forms Injection, powder for reconstitution [single-dose vial] [preservative free]: 1350 plaque-forming units (PFU)/0.5 mL [contains gelatin and trace amounts of neomycin]

Varicella-Zoster Immune Globulin (Human)

(var i SEL a- ZOS ter i MYUN GLOB yoo lin HYU man)

Related Information
Adverse Events and Vaccination *on page 1553*
Immunization Recommendations *on page 1538*
USPHA/IDSA Guidelines for the Prevention of Opportunistic Infections in Persons With HIV *on page 1574*

Synonyms VZIG

Therapeutic Category Immune Globulin

Use Passive immunization of susceptible immunodeficient patients after exposure to varicella; most effective if begun within 96 hours of exposure; there is no evidence VZIG modifies established varicella-zoster infections.

Restrict administration to those patients meeting the following criteria:
Neoplastic disease (eg, leukemia or lymphoma)
Congenital or acquired immunodeficiency
Immunosuppressive therapy with steroids, antimetabolites or other immunosuppressive treatment regimens
Newborn of mother who had onset of chickenpox within 5 days before delivery or within 48 hours after delivery
Premature (≥28 weeks gestation) whose mother has no history of chickenpox
Premature (<28 weeks gestation or ≤1000 g VZIG) regardless of maternal history

One of the following types of exposure to chickenpox or zoster patient(s) may warrant administration:
Continuous household contact
Playmate contact (>1 hour play indoors)
Hospital contact (in same 2-4 bedroom or adjacent beds in a large ward or prolonged face-to-face contact with an infectious staff member or patient)
Susceptible to varicella-zoster
Age <15 years; administer to immunocompromised adolescents and adults and to other older patients on an individual basis
An acceptable alternative to VZIG prophylaxis is to treat varicella, if it occurs, with high-dose I.V. acyclovir
Age is the most important risk factor for reactivation of varicella zoster; persons <50 years of age have incidence of 2.5 cases per 1000, whereas those 60-79 have 6.5 cases per 1000 and those >80 years have 10 cases per 1000

Pregnancy Risk Factor C

Contraindications **Not** for prophylactic use in immunodeficient patients with history of varicella, unless patient's immunosuppression is associated with bone marrow transplantation; **not** recommended for nonimmunodeficient patients, including pregnant women, because the severity of chickenpox is much less than in immunosuppressed patients; allergic response to gamma globulin or anti-immunoglobulin; sensitivity to thimerosal; persons with IgA deficiency; do not administer to patients with thrombocytopenia or coagulopathies

Warnings/Precautions VZIG is not indicated for prophylaxis or therapy of normal adults who are exposed to or who develop varicella; it is not indicated for treatment of herpes zoster. Do not inject I.V.

Adverse Reactions
1% to 10%: Local: Discomfort at the site of injection (pain, redness, edema)
<1% (Limited to important or life-threatening): Anaphylactic shock, angioedema, GI symptoms, headache, malaise, rash, respiratory symptom

Stability Refrigerate at 2°C to 8°C (36°F to 46°F)

Mechanism of Action The exact mechanism has not been clarified but the antibodies in varicella-zoster immune globulin most likely neutralize the varicella-zoster virus and prevent its pathological actions

Usual Dosage High risk susceptible patients who are exposed again more than 3 weeks after a prior dose of VZIG should receive another full dose; there is no evidence VZIG modifies established varicella-zoster infections.

I.M.: Administer by deep injection in the gluteal muscle or in another large muscle mass. Inject 125 units/10 kg (22 lb); maximum dose: 625 units (5 vials); minimum dose: 125 units; do not administer fractional doses. Do not inject I.V.
VZIG dose based on weight: See table.

VZIG Dose Based on Weight

Weight of Patient		Dose	
kg	lb	Units	No. of Vials
0-10	0-22	125	1
10.1-20	22.1-44	250	2
20.1-30	44.1-66	375	3
30.1-40	66.1-88	500	4
>40	>88	625	5

Administration Do not inject I.V.; administer deep I.M. into the gluteal muscle or other large muscle mass. For patients ≤10 kg, administer 1.25 mL at a single site; for patients >10 kg, administer no more than 2.5 mL at a single site. Administer entire contents of each vial

Nursing Implications Administer as soon as possible after presumed exposure; do not inject I.V.; administer by deep I.M. injection into gluteal muscle or other large muscle; administer contents of each vial

Dosage Forms Injection [single-dose vial]: 125 units of antibody

♦ **Vasocon Regular®** see Naphazoline *on page 957*

♦ **Vasodilan®** see Isoxsuprine *on page 755*

Vasopressin (vay soe PRES in)

U.S. Brand Names Pitressin®

Canadian Brand Names Pressyn®

Synonyms ADH; Antidiuretic Hormone; 8-Arginine Vasopressin; Vasopressin Tannate

Therapeutic Category Antidiuretic Hormone Analog; Hormone, Posterior Pituitary; Vesicant

Use Treatment of diabetes insipidus; prevention and treatment of postoperative abdominal distention; differential diagnosis of diabetes insipidus

Unlabeled/Investigational Use Adjunct in the treatment of GI hemorrhage and esophageal varices; pulseless ventricular tachycardia (VT)/ventricular fibrillation (VF)

Pregnancy Risk Factor B

Contraindications Hypersensitivity to vasopressin or any component of the formulation

Warnings/Precautions Use with caution in patients with seizure disorders, migraine, asthma, vascular disease, renal disease, cardiac disease; chronic nephritis with nitrogen retention. Goiter with cardiac complications, arteriosclerosis; I.V. infiltration may lead to severe vasoconstriction and localized tissue necrosis; also, gangrene of extremities, tongue, and ischemic colitis. Elderly patients should be cautioned not to increase their fluid intake beyond that sufficient to satisfy their thirst in order to avoid water intoxication and hyponatremia; under experimental conditions, the elderly have shown to have a decreased responsiveness to vasopressin with respect to its effects on water homeostasis

Adverse Reactions Frequency not defined.

Cardiovascular: Increased blood pressure, arrhythmias, venous thrombosis, vasoconstriction (with higher doses), chest pain, myocardial infarction

Central nervous system: Pounding in the head, fever, vertigo

Dermatologic: Urticaria, circumoral pallor

Gastrointestinal: Flatulence, abdominal cramps, nausea, vomiting

Genitourinary: Uterine contraction

Neuromuscular & skeletal: Tremor

Respiratory: Bronchial constriction

Miscellaneous: Diaphoresis

Overdosage/Toxicology Symptoms include drowsiness, weight gain, confusion, listlessness, and water intoxication. Water intoxication requires withdrawal of the drug. Severe intoxication may require osmotic diuresis and loop diuretics.

Drug Interactions

Increased Effect/Toxicity: Chlorpropamide, urea, clofibrate, carbamazepine, and fludrocortisone potentiate antidiuretic response.

Decreased Effect: Lithium, epinephrine, demeclocycline, heparin, and ethanol block antidiuretic activity to varying degrees.

Ethanol/Nutrition/Herb Interactions Ethanol: Avoid ethanol (due to effects on ADH).

Stability Store injection at room temperature; protect from heat and from freezing; use only clear solutions

Mechanism of Action Increases cyclic adenosine monophosphate (cAMP) which increases water permeability at the renal tubule resulting in decreased urine volume and increased osmolality; causes peristalsis by directly stimulating the smooth muscle in the GI tract

Pharmacodynamics/Kinetics

Onset of action: Nasal: 1 hour

Duration: Nasal: 3-8 hours; Parenteral: I.M., S.C.: 2-8 hours

Metabolism: Nasal/Parenteral: Hepatic, renal

Half-life elimination: Nasal: 15 minutes; Parenteral: 10-20 minutes

Excretion: Nasal: Urine; Parenteral: S.C. (aqueous): Urine (5% as unchanged drug) after 4 hours

Usual Dosage

Diabetes insipidus (highly variable dosage; titrated based on serum and urine sodium and osmolality in addition to fluid balance and urine output):

I.M., S.C.:

Children: 2.5-10 units 2-4 times/day as needed

Adults: 5-10 units 2-4 times/day as needed (dosage range 5-60 units/day)

Continuous I.V. infusion: Children and Adults: 0.5 milliunit/kg/hour (0.0005 unit/kg/hour); double dosage as needed every 30 minutes to a maximum of 0.01 unit/kg/hour

Intranasal: Administer on cotton pledget or nasal spray

Abdominal distention (aqueous): Adults: I.M.: 5 mg stat, 10 mg every 3-4 hours

GI hemorrhage: I.V. infusion: Dilute aqueous in NS or D_5W to 0.1-1 unit/mL

Children: Initial: 0.002-0.005 units/kg/minute; titrate dose as needed; maximum: 0.01 unit/kg/minute; continue at same dosage (if bleeding stops) for 12 hours, then taper off over 24-48 hours

Adults: Initial: 0.2-0.4 unit/minute, then titrate dose as needed, if bleeding stops; continue at same dose for 12 hours, taper off over 24-48 hours

Pulseless VT/VF (ACLS protocol): Adults: I.V.: 40 int. units (as a single dose only)

Dosing adjustment in hepatic impairment: Some patients respond to much lower doses with cirrhosis

Administration

I.V. infusion administration requires the use of an infusion pump and should be administered in a peripheral line to minimize adverse reactions on coronary arteries

Infusion rates: 100 units (aqueous) in 500 mL D_5W rate

0.1 unit/minute: 30 mL/hour

0.2 unit/minute: 60 mL/hour

0.3 unit/minute: 90 mL/hour

0.4 unit/minute: 120 mL/hour

0.5 unit/minute: 150 mL/hour

0.6 unit/minute: 180 mL/hour

Monitoring Parameters Serum and urine sodium, urine output, fluid input and output, urine specific gravity, urine and serum osmolality

Reference Range Plasma: 0-2 pg/mL (SI: 0-2 ng/L) if osmolality <285 mOsm/L; 2-12 pg/mL (SI: 2-12 ng/L) if osmolality ≥290 mOsm/L

Patient Information Side effects such as abdominal cramps and nausea may be reduced by drinking a glass of water with each dose

Nursing Implications Watch for signs of I.V. infiltration and gangrene; elderly patients should be cautioned not to increase their fluid intake beyond that sufficient to satisfy their thirst in order to avoid water intoxication and hyponatremia; under experimental conditions, the elderly have shown to have a decreased responsiveness to vasopressin with respect to its effects on water homeostasis

Additional Information Vasopressin tannate in oil must not be administered I.V. Vasopressin increases factor VIII levels and may be useful in hemophiliacs.

Dosage Forms Injection, aqueous: 20 vasopressor units/mL (0.5 mL, 1 mL, 10 mL)

♦ **Vasopressin Tannate** see Vasopressin on page 1408
♦ **Vasotec®** see Enalapril on page 462
♦ **Vasotec® I.V.** see Enalapril on page 462
♦ **Vaxigrip® (Can)** see Influenza Virus Vaccine on page 721
♦ **VCR** see VinCRIStine on page 1417
♦ **Vectrin® [DSC]** see Minocycline on page 918

Vecuronium (ve KYOO roe ni um)

Related Information
Neuromuscular Blocking Agents Comparison on page 1508

U.S. Brand Names Norcuron®

Canadian Brand Names Norcuron®

Synonyms ORG NC 45

Therapeutic Category Neuromuscular Blocker Agent, Nondepolarizing; Skeletal Muscle Relaxant

Use Adjunct to general anesthesia to facilitate endotracheal intubation and to relax skeletal muscles during surgery; to facilitate mechanical ventilation in ICU patients; does not relieve pain or produce sedation

Pregnancy Risk Factor C

Pregnancy/Breast-Feeding Implications Use in cesarean section has been reported. Umbilical venous concentrations were 11% of maternal. Excretion in human breast milk is unknown; use caution.

Contraindications Hypersensitivity to vecuronium or any component of the formulation

Warnings/Precautions Ventilation must be supported during neuromuscular blockade; certain clinical conditions may result in potentiation or antagonism of neuromuscular blockade:

Potentiation: Electrolyte abnormalities, severe hyponatremia, severe hypocalcemia, severe hypokalemia, hypermagnesemia, neuromuscular diseases, acidosis, acute intermittent porphyria, renal failure, hepatic failure

Antagonism: Alkalosis, hypercalcemia, demyelinating lesions, peripheral neuropathies, diabetes mellitus

Increased sensitivity in patients with myasthenia gravis, Eaton-Lambert syndrome; resistance in burn patients (>30% of body) for period of 5-70 days postinjury; resistance in patients with muscle trauma, denervation, immobilization, infection; use with caution in patients with hepatic or renal impairment; does not counteract bradycardia produced by anesthetics/vagal stimulation.

Adverse Reactions <1% (Limited to important or life-threatening): Bradycardia, circulatory collapse, edema, flushing, hypersensitivity reaction, hypotension, itching, rash, tachycardia

Overdosage/Toxicology Symptoms include prolonged skeletal muscle weakness, apnea, and cardiovascular collapse. Use neostigmine, edrophonium, or pyridostigmine with atropine to antagonize skeletal muscle relaxation. Mechanical cardiovascular and respiratory support, fluids, and pressors may be necessary.

Drug Interactions

Increased Effect/Toxicity: Increased effects are possible with aminoglycosides, beta-blockers, clindamycin, calcium channel blockers, halogenated anesthetics, imipenem, ketamine, lidocaine, loop diuretics (furosemide), macrolides (case reports), magnesium sulfate, procainamide, quinidine, quinolones, tetracyclines, and vancomycin. May increase risk of myopathy when used with high- dose corticosteroids for extended periods.

Stability Stable for 5 days at room temperature when reconstituted with bacteriostatic water; stable for 24 hours at room temperature when reconstituted with preservative-free sterile water (avoid preservatives in neonates); do not mix with alkaline drugs

Mechanism of Action Blocks acetylcholine from binding to receptors on motor endplate inhibiting depolarization

Pharmacodynamics/Kinetics
Good intubation conditions within 2.5-3 minutes; maximum neuromuscular blockade within 3-5 minutes
Excretion: Primarily feces; urine (as unchanged drug and metabolites)

Usual Dosage Administer I.V.; dose to effect; doses will vary due to interpatient variability; use ideal body weight for obese patients
Surgery:
Neonates: 0.1 mg/kg/dose; maintenance: 0.03-0.15 mg/kg every 1-2 hours as needed
Infants >7 weeks to 1 year: Initial: 0.08-0.1 mg/kg/dose; maintenance: 0.05-0.1 mg/kg every 60 minutes as needed
Children >1 year and Adults: Initial: 0.08-0.1 mg/kg or 0.04-0.06 mg/kg after initial dose of succinylcholine for intubation; maintenance: 0.01-0.015 mg/kg 25-40 minutes after initial dose, then 0.01-0.015 mg/kg every 12-15 minutes (higher doses will allow less frequent maintenance doses); may be administered as a continuous infusion at 0.8-2 mcg/kg/minute

(Continued)

Vecuronium *(Continued)*

Pretreatment/priming: Adults: 10% of intubating dose given 3-5 minutes before initial dose
ICU: Adults: 0.05-0.1 mg/kg bolus followed by 0.8-1.7 mcg/kg/minute once initial recovery from bolus observed or 0.1-0.2 mg/kg/dose every 1 hour

Note: Children (1-10 years) may require slightly higher initial doses and slightly more frequent supplementation; infants >7 weeks to 1 year may be more sensitive to vecuronium and have a longer recovery time

Dosing adjustment in renal impairment: Prolongation of blockade

Dosing adjustment in hepatic impairment: Dose reductions are necessary in patients with cirrhosis or cholestasis

Administration Dilute vial to a maximum concentration of 2 mg/mL and administer by rapid direct injection; for continuous infusion, dilute to a maximum concentration of 1 mg/mL

Monitoring Parameters Blood pressure, heart rate

Nursing Implications Does not alter the patient's state of consciousness; addition of sedation and analgesia are recommended; dilute vial to a maximum concentration of 2 mg/mL and administer by rapid direct injection; for continuous infusion, dilute to a maximum concentration of 1 mg/mL

Additional Information Vecuronium is classified as an intermediate-duration neuromuscular-blocking agent. It produces minimal, if any, histamine release; does not relieve pain or produce sedation. It may produce cumulative effect on duration of blockade.

Dosage Forms Powder for injection: 10 mg (5 mL, 10 mL)

- ◆ **Veetids®** *see Penicillin V Potassium on page 1055*
- ◆ **Velban®** *see VinBLAStine on page 1415*
- ◆ **Velosef®** *see Cephradine on page 263*
- ◆ **Velosulin® BR (Buffered)** *see Insulin Preparations on page 722*

Venlafaxine *(VEN la faks een)*

Related Information
Antidepressant Agents Comparison *on page 1482*

U.S. Brand Names Effexor®; Effexor® XR

Canadian Brand Names Effexor®; Effexor® XR

Therapeutic Category Antidepressant, Miscellaneous

Use Treatment of depression, generalized anxiety disorder (GAD)

Unlabeled/Investigational Use Obsessive-compulsive disorder (OCD), chronic fatigue syndrome; attention-deficit/hyperactivity disorder (ADHD) and autism in children

Pregnancy Risk Factor C

Pregnancy/Breast-Feeding Implications There are no adequate or well-controlled studies in pregnant women. Use only in pregnancy if clearly needed. Venlafaxine is excreted in human milk; breast-feeding is not recommended.

Contraindications Hypersensitivity to venlafaxine or any component of the formulation; use of MAO inhibitors within 14 days; should not initiate MAO inhibitor within 7 days of discontinuing venlafaxine

Warnings/Precautions May cause sustained increase in blood pressure; may cause increase in anxiety, nervousness, insomnia; may cause weight loss (use with caution in patients where weight loss is undesirable). May worsen psychosis in some patients or precipitate a shift to mania or hypomania in patients with bipolar disease. May increase the risks associated with electroconvulsive therapy. Use caution in patients with depression, particularly if suicidal risk may be present. The risks of cognitive or motor impairment, as well as the potential for anticholinergic effects are very low. May cause or exacerbate sexual dysfunction. Abrupt discontinuation or dosage reduction after extended (≥6 weeks) therapy may lead to agitation, dysphoria, nervousness, anxiety, and other symptoms. When discontinuing therapy, dosage should be tapered gradually over at least a 2-week period. Use caution in patients with increased intraocular pressure or at risk of acute narrow-angle glaucoma.

Adverse Reactions

≥10%:
    Central nervous system: Headache (25%), somnolence (23%), dizziness (19%), insomnia (18%), nervousness (13%)
    Gastrointestinal: Nausea (37%), xerostomia (22%), constipation (15%), anorexia (11%)
    Genitourinary: Abnormal ejaculation/orgasm (12%)
    Neuromuscular & skeletal: Weakness (12%)
    Miscellaneous: Diaphoresis (12%)

1% to 10%:
    Cardiovascular: Vasodilation (4%), hypertension (dose-related; 3% in patients receiving <100 mg/day, up to 13% in patients receiving >300 mg/day), tachycardia (2%), chest pain (2%), postural hypotension (1%)
    Central nervous system: Anxiety (6%), abnormal dreams (4%), yawning (3%), agitation (2%), confusion (2%), abnormal thinking (2%), depersonalization (1%), depression (1%)
    Dermatologic: Rash (3%), pruritus (1%)
    Endocrine & metabolic: Decreased libido
    Gastrointestinal: Diarrhea (8%), vomiting (6%), dyspepsia (5%), flatulence (3%), taste perversion (2%), weight loss (1%)
    Genitourinary: Impotence (6%), urinary frequency (3%), impaired urination (2%), orgasm disturbance (2%), urinary retention (1%)
    Neuromuscular & skeletal: Tremor (5%), hypertonia (3%), paresthesia (3%), twitching (1%)
    Ocular: Blurred vision (6%), mydriasis (2%)
    Otic: Tinnitus (2%)
    Miscellaneous: Infection (6%), chills (3%), trauma (2%)

<1% (Limited to important or life-threatening): Agranulocytosis, akathisia, anaphylaxis, aplastic anemia, asthma, catatonia, delirium, dyspnea, epidermal necrolysis, erythema

multiforme, erythema nodosum, exfoliative dermatitis, extrapyramidal symptoms, hallucinations, hemorrhage (including ophthalmic and gastrointestinal), hepatic failure, hepatic necrosis, hirsutism, manic reaction (0.5%), pancreatitis, psychosis, rash (maculopapular, pustular, or vesiculobullous), seizures, serotonin syndrome, SIADH, Stevens-Johnson syndrome, tardive dyskinesia, torticollis, vertigo

Overdosage/Toxicology Symptoms include somnolence and occasionally tachycardia. Most overdoses resolve with only supportive treatment. Use of activated charcoal, inductions of emesis, or gastric lavage should be considered for acute ingestion. Forced diuresis, dialysis, and hemoperfusion are not effective due to the large volume of distribution.

Drug Interactions

Cytochrome P450 Effect: CYP2D6, 2E1, and 3A3/4 enzyme substrate; CYP2D6 enzyme inhibitor (weak)

Increased Effect/Toxicity: Concurrent use of MAO inhibitors (phenelzine, isocarboxazid), or drugs with MAO inhibitor activity (linezolid) may result in serotonin syndrome; should not be used within 2 weeks of each other. Selegiline may have a lower risk of this effect, particularly at low dosages, due to selectivity for MAO type B. In addition, concurrent use of buspirone, lithium, meperidine, nefazodone, selegiline, serotonin agonists (sumatriptan, naratriptan), sibutramine, SSRIs, trazodone, or tricyclic antidepressants may increase the risk of serotonin syndrome. Serum levels of haloperidol may be increased by venlafaxine. Inhibitors of CYP2D6, CYP2E1, or CYP3A3/4 may increase the serum levels and/or toxicity of venlafaxine.

Decreased Effect: Serum levels of indinavir may be reduced be venlafaxine (AUC reduced by 28%) - clinical significance not determined. Enzyme inducers (carbamazepine, phenytoin, phenobarbital) may reduce the serum concentrations of venlafaxine.

Ethanol/Nutrition/Herb Interactions

Ethanol: Avoid ethanol (may increase CNS effects).

Herb/Nutraceutical: Avoid valerian, St John's wort, SAMe, kava kava, tryptophan (may increase risk of serotonin syndrome and/or excessive sedation).

Mechanism of Action Venlafaxine and its active metabolite o-desmethylvenlafaxine (ODV) are potent inhibitors of neuronal serotonin and norepinephrine reuptake and weak inhibitors of dopamine reuptake

Pharmacodynamics/Kinetics

Absorption: Oral: 92% to 100%; food has no significant effect on the absorption of venlafaxine or formation of the active metabolite O-desmethyl-venlafaxine (ODV); absolute bioavailability is ~45%

Distribution: At steady state: Venlafaxine 7.5 ± 3.7 L/kg, ODV 5.7 ± 1.8 L/Kg

Protein binding: Bound to human plasma protein: Venlafaxine 27%, ODV 30%

Metabolism: In the liver by CYP2D6 to active metabolite, O-desmethyl-venlafaxine (ODV); other metabolites include N-desmethylvenlafaxine and N,O-didesmethylvenlafaxine

Half-life: Venlafaxine 3-7 hours; ODV 9-13 hours; steady state concentrations of both venlafaxine and ODV in plasma were attained within 3 days of multiple dose therapy. Half-life is prolonged with cirrhosis (Adults: Venlafaxine ~30%, ODV ~60%) and with dialysis (Adults: Venlafaxine ~180%, ODV ~142%)

Time to peak:

Immediate release: Venlafaxine: 2 hours, ODV: 3 hours

Extended release: Venlafaxine: 5.5 hours, ODV: 9 hours

Excretion: ~87 excreted in urine within 48 hours (5% as unchanged drug, 29% as unconjugated ODV, 26% as conjugated ODV, 27% as minor metabolites)

Clearance at steady state: Venlafaxine: 1.3 ± 0.6 L/hour/kg, ODV 0.4 ± 0.2 L/hour/kg

Clearance decreased with:

Cirrhosis: Adults: Venlafaxine ~50, ODV ~30%

Severe cirrhosis: Adults: Venlafaxine ~90%

Renal impairment (Cl_{cr} 10-70 mL/minute): Adults: Venlafaxine ~24%

Dialysis: Adults: Venlafaxine ~57%, ODV ~56%; due to large volume of distribution, a significant amount of drug is not likely to be removed.

Usual Dosage Oral:

Children and Adolescents:

ADHD (unlabeled use): Initial: 12.5 mg/day

Children <40 kg: Increase by 12.5 mg/week to maximum of 50 mg/day in 2 divided doses

Children ≥40 kg: Increase by 25 mg/week to maximum of 75 mg/day in 3 divided doses.

Mean dose: 60 mg or 1.4 mg/kg administered in 2-3 divided doses

Autism (unlabeled use): Initial: 12.5 mg/day; adjust to 6.25-50 mg/day

Adults:

Immediate-release tablets: 75 mg/day, administered in 2 or 3 divided doses, taken with food; dose may be increased in 75 mg/day increments at intervals of at least 4 days, up to 225-375 mg/day

Extended-release capsules: 75 mg once daily taken with food; for some new patients, it may be desirable to start at 37.5 mg/day for 4-7 days before increasing to 75 mg once daily; dose may be increased by up to 75 mg/day increments every 4 days as tolerated, up to a maximum of 225 mg/day

Note: When discontinuing this medication after more than 1 week of treatment, it is generally recommended that the dose be tapered. If venlafaxine is used for 6 weeks or longer, the dose should be tapered over 2 weeks when discontinuing its use.

Dosing adjustment in renal impairment: Cl_{cr} 10-70 mL/minute: Decrease dose by 25%; decrease total daily dose by 50% if dialysis patients; dialysis patients should receive dosing after completion of dialysis

Dosing adjustment in moderate hepatic impairment: Reduce total daily dosage by 50%

Dietary Considerations Should be taken with food.

Administration Administer with food.

Monitoring Parameters Blood pressure should be regularly monitored, especially in patients with a high baseline blood pressure

Reference Range Peak serum level of 163 ng/mL (325 ng/mL of ODV metabolite) obtained after a 150 mg oral dose

(Continued)

1411

Venlafaxine (Continued)

Patient Information Avoid alcohol; use caution when operating hazardous machinery; if a rash or shortness of breath occurs while using venlafaxine, contact physician immediately

Nursing Implications May cause mean increase in heart rate of 4-9 beats/minute; tapering to minimize symptoms of discontinuation is recommended when the drug is discontinued; tapering should be over a 2-week period if the patient has received it for at least 6 weeks

Dosage Forms
Capsule, extended release (Effexor® XR): 37.5 mg, 75 mg, 150 mg
Tablet (Effexor®): 25 mg, 37.5 mg, 50 mg, 75 mg, 100 mg

♦ **Venoglobulin®-I** *see Immune Globulin (Intravenous) on page 711*

♦ **Venoglobulin®-S** *see Immune Globulin (Intravenous) on page 711*

♦ **Ventolin®** *see Albuterol on page 41*

♦ **Ventolin® HFA** *see Albuterol on page 41*

♦ **Ventolin Rotacaps® [DSC]** *see Albuterol on page 41*

♦ **VePesid®** *see Etoposide on page 533*

♦ **Veralan® (Can)** *see Verapamil on page 1412*

Verapamil *(ver AP a mil)*

Related Information
Adult ACLS Algorithms *on page 1632*
Antiarrhythmic Drugs Comparison *on page 1478*
Calcium Channel Blockers Comparison *on page 1494*
Hypertension *on page 1675*

U.S. Brand Names Calan®; Calan® SR; Covera-HS®; Isoptin®; Isoptin® SR; Verelan®; Verelan® PM

Canadian Brand Names Alti-Verapamil; Apo®-Verap; Calan®; Chronovera®; Covera®; Gen-Verapamil; Gen-Verapamil SR; Isoptin®; Isoptin® I.V.; Isoptin® SR; Novo-Veramil; Novo-Veramil SR; Nu-Verap; Tarka®; Veralan®

Synonyms Iproveratril Hydrochloride; Verapamil Hydrochloride

Therapeutic Category Antianginal Agent; Antiarrhythmic Agent, Class IV; Antihypertensive Agent; Calcium Channel Blocker

Use Orally for treatment of angina pectoris (vasospastic, chronic stable, unstable) and hypertension; I.V. for supraventricular tachyarrhythmias (PSVT, atrial fibrillation, atrial flutter)

Unlabeled/Investigational Use Migraine; hypertrophic cardiomyopathy; bipolar disorder (manic manifestations)

Pregnancy Risk Factor C

Pregnancy/Breast-Feeding Implications
Clinical effects on the fetus: Use in pregnancy only when clearly needed and when the benefits outweigh the potential hazard to the fetus. Crosses the placenta. 1 report of suspected heart block when used to control fetal supraventricular tachycardia. May exhibit tocolytic effects.
Breast-feeding/lactation: Crosses into breast milk. AAP considers **compatible** with breast-feeding.

Contraindications Hypersensitivity to verapamil or any component of the formulation; severe left ventricular dysfunction; hypotension (systolic pressure <90 mm Hg) or cardiogenic shock; sick sinus syndrome (except in patients with a functioning artificial pacemaker); second- or third-degree AV block (except in patients with a functioning artificial pacemaker); atrial flutter or fibrillation and an accessory bypass tract (WPW, Lown-Ganoang-Levine syndrome)

Warnings/Precautions Use with caution in sick-sinus syndrome, severe left ventricular dysfunction, hepatic or renal impairment, hypertrophic cardiomyopathy (especially obstructive), abrupt withdrawal may cause increased duration and frequency of chest pain; avoid I.V. use in neonates and young infants due to severe apnea, bradycardia, or hypotensive reactions; elderly may experience more constipation and hypotension. Monitor EKG and blood pressure closely in patients receiving I.V. therapy particularly in patients with supraventricular tachycardia.

Adverse Reactions
>10%: Gastrointestinal: Gingival hyperplasia (up to 19%), constipation (12% up to 42% in clinical trials)

1% to 10%:
Cardiovascular: Bradycardia (1.2 to 1.4%), first-, second-, or third-degree AV block (1.2%), congestive heart failure (1.8%), peripheral edema (1.9%), hypotension (2.5% to 3%), symptomatic hypotension (1.5% I.V.), severe tachycardia (1%)
Central nervous system: Dizziness (1.2% to 3.3%), fatigue (1.7%), headache (1.2% to 2.2%)
Dermatologic: Rash (1.2%)
Gastrointestinal: Nausea (0.9% to 2.7%)
Respiratory: Dyspnea (1.4%)

<1% (Limited to important or life-threatening): Alopecia, angina, arthralgia, asystole, atrioventricular dissociation, bronchial/laryngeal spasm, cerebrovascular accident, chest pain, claudication, confusion, diarrhea, dry mouth, ecchymosis, electrical mechanical dissociation (EMD), emotional depression, eosinophilia, equilibrium disorders, erythema multiforme, exanthema, exfoliative dermatitis, galactorrhea/hyperprolactinemia, GI obstruction, gingival hyperplasia, gynecomastia, hair color change, impotence, muscle cramps, myocardial infarction, myoclonus, paresthesia, Parkinsonian syndrome, psychotic symptoms, purpura (vasculitis), rash, respiratory failure, rotary nystagmus, shakiness, shock, somnolence, Stevens-Johnson syndrome, syncope, urticaria, ventricular fibrillation, vertigo

Overdosage/Toxicology
Primary cardiac symptoms of calcium blocker overdose include hypotension and bradycardia. Hypotension is caused by peripheral vasodilation, myocardial depression, and bradycardia. Bradycardia results from sinus bradycardia, second- or third-degree atrioventricular block, or sinus arrest with junctional rhythm. Intraventricular conduction is usually not affected, so QRS duration is normal (verapamil prolongs the P-R interval and bepridil

prolongs the QT interval and may cause ventricular arrhythmias, including torsade de pointes).

The noncardiac symptoms include confusion, stupor, nausea, vomiting, metabolic acidosis and hyperglycemia.

Following initial gastric decontamination, if possible, repeated calcium administration may promptly reverse depressed cardiac contractility (but not sinus node depression or peripheral vasodilation). Glucagon, epinephrine, and inamrinone (amrinone) may treat refractory hypotension. Glucagon and epinephrine also increase the heart rate (outside the U.S., 4-aminopyridine may be available as an antidote). Dialysis and hemoperfusion are not effective in enhancing elimination, although repeat-dose activated charcoal may serve as an adjunct with sustained-release preparations.

In a few reported cases, overdose with calcium channel blockers has been associated with hypotension and bradycardia, initially refractory to atropine, but becoming more responsive to this agent when larger doses (approaching 1 g/hour for more than 24 hours) of calcium chloride were administered.

Drug Interactions

Cytochrome P450 Effect: CYP2C8/9 (minor), 2C18 (minor), 3A3/4, and 1A2 enzyme substrate; CYP3A3/4 inhibitor

Increased Effect/Toxicity: Use of verapamil with amiodarone, beta-blockers, or flecainide may lead to bradycardia and decreased cardiac output. Aspirin and concurrent verapamil use may increase bleeding times. Azole antifungals, cimetidine, erythromycin may inhibit verapamil metabolism, increasing serum concentrations/effect of verapamil. Lithium neurotoxicity may result when verapamil is added. Effect of nondepolarizing neuromuscular blocker is prolonged by verapamil. Grapefruit juice may increase verapamil serum concentrations.

Cisapride, astemizole, and terfenadine levels may be increased by verapamil, potentially resulting in life-threatening arrhythmias; avoid concurrent use. Serum concentrations of the following drugs may be increased by verapamil: alfentanil, buspirone, carbamazepine, cyclosporine, digoxin, doxorubicin, ethanol, HMG-CoA reductase inhibitors (atorvastatin, cerivastatin, lovastatin, simvastatin), midazolam, prazosin, quinidine, tacrolimus, and theophylline.

Decreased Effect: Rifampin or phenobarbital may decrease verapamil serum concentrations by increased hepatic metabolism. Lithium levels may be decreased by verapamil. Nafcillin decreases plasma concentration of verapamil.

Ethanol/Nutrition/Herb Interactions

Ethanol: Avoid or limit ethanol (may increase ethanol levels).

Food: Grapefruit juice may increase the serum concentration of verapamil; avoid concurrent use.

Herb/Nutraceutical: St John's wort may decrease levels. Avoid dong quai if using for hypertension (has estrogenic activity). Avoid ephedra, yohimbe, ginseng (may worsen arrhythmia or hypertension). Avoid garlic (may have increased antihypertensive effect).

Stability Store injection at room temperature; protect from heat and from freezing; use only clear solutions; **compatible** in solutions of pH of 3-6, but may precipitate in solutions having a pH ≥6

Mechanism of Action Inhibits calcium ion from entering the "slow channels" or select voltage-sensitive areas of vascular smooth muscle and myocardium during depolarization; produces a relaxation of coronary vascular smooth muscle and coronary vasodilation; increases myocardial oxygen delivery in patients with vasospastic angina; slows automaticity and conduction of AV node.

Pharmacodynamics/Kinetics

Onset of action: Peak effect: Oral: Immediate release: 2 hours; I.V.: 1-5 minutes

Duration: Oral: Immediate release tablets: 6-8 hours; I.V.: 10-20 minutes

Protein binding: 90%

Metabolism: Hepatic via multiple CYP isoenzymes; extensive first-pass effect

Bioavailability: Oral: 20% to 30%

Half-life elimination: Infants: 4.4-6.9 hours; Adults: Single dose: 2-8 hours, increased up to 12 hours with multiple dosing; increased half-life with hepatic cirrhosis

Excretion: Urine (70%, 3% to 4% as unchanged drug); feces (16%)

Usual Dosage

Children: SVT:

I.V.:

<1 year: 0.1-0.2 mg/kg over 2 minutes; repeat every 30 minutes as needed

1-15 years: 0.1-0.3 mg/kg over 2 minutes; maximum: 5 mg/dose, may repeat dose in 15 minutes if adequate response not achieved; maximum for second dose: 10 mg/dose

Oral (dose not well established):

1-5 years: 4-8 mg/kg/day in 3 divided doses **or** 40-80 mg every 8 hours

>5 years: 80 mg every 6-8 hours

Adults:

SVT: I.V.: 2.5-5 mg (over 2 minutes); second dose of 5-10 mg (~0.15 mg/kg) may be given 15-30 minutes after the initial dose if patient tolerates, but does not respond to initial dose; maximum total dose: 20 mg

Angina: Oral: Initial dose: 80-120 mg 3 times/day (elderly or small stature: 40 mg 3 times/day); range: 240-480 mg/day in 3-4 divided doses

Hypertension: Oral: 80 mg 3 times/day or 240 mg/day (sustained release); range: 240-480 mg/day; 120 mg/day in the elderly or small patients (no evidence of additional benefit in doses >360 mg/day)

Note: One time per day dosing is recommended at bedtime with Covera-HS®.

Dosing adjustment in renal impairment: Cl$_{cr}$ <10 mL/minute: Administer at 50% to 75% of normal dose.

Dialysis: Not dialyzable (0% to 5 %) via hemo- or peritoneal dialysis; supplemental dose is not necessary.

Dosing adjustment/comments in hepatic disease: Reduce dose in cirrhosis, reduce dose to 20% to 50% of normal and monitor EKG.

(Continued)

Verapamil *(Continued)*

Dietary Considerations Sustained release product should be administered with food or milk, other formulations may be administered without regard to meals; sprinkling contents of capsule onto food does not affect oral absorption.

Administration

Oral: Administer sustained release product with food or milk; sprinkling contents of capsules onto food does not affect absorption; should be dosed 1-2 times/day; **do not crush sustained release drug product.** Other oral formulations may be given with or without food.

I.V.: Rate of infusion: Over 2 minutes.

Monitoring Parameters Monitor blood pressure closely

Reference Range Therapeutic: 50-200 ng/mL (SI: 100-410 nmol/L) for parent; under normal conditions norverapamil concentration is the same as parent drug. Toxic: >90 µg/mL

Patient Information Sustained release products should be taken with food and not crushed; limit caffeine intake; notify physician if angina pain is not reduced when taking this drug, or if irregular heartbeat or shortness of breath occurs

Nursing Implications Do not crush sustained release drug product

Dosage Forms

Capsule, sustained release, as hydrochloride: 120 mg, 180 mg, 240 mg, 360 mg

Verelan®: 120 mg, 180 mg, 240 mg, 360 mg

Verelan® PM: 100 mg, 200 mg, 300 mg

Injection, as hydrochloride: 2.5 mg/mL (2 mL, 4 mL)

Isoptin®: 2.5 mg/mL (2 mL, 4 mL)

Tablet, as hydrochloride: 40 mg, 80 mg, 120 mg

Calan®, Isoptin®: 40 mg, 80 mg, 120 mg

Tablet, sustained release, as hydrochloride: 180 mg, 240 mg

Calan® SR, Isoptin® SR: 120 mg, 180 mg, 240 mg

Covera-HS®: 180 mg, 240 mg

Extemporaneous Preparations A 50 mg/mL oral suspension may be made using twenty 80 mg verapamil tablets, 3 mL of purified water USP, 8 mL of methylcellulose 1% and simple syrup qs ad to 32 mL; the expected stability is 30 days under refrigeration; shake well before use. A mixture of verapamil 50 mg/mL plus hydrochlorothiazide 5 mg/mL was stable 60 days in refrigerator in a 1:1 preparation of Ora-Sweet® and Ora-Plus®, of Ora-Sweet® SF and Ora-Plus®, and of cherry syrup.

Allen LV and Erickson III MA, "Stability of Labetalol Hydrochloride, Metoprolol Tartrate, Verapamil Hydrochloride, and Spironolactone With Hydrochlorothiazide in Extemporaneously Compounded Oral Liquids," *Am J Health Syst Pharm*, 1996, 53:304-9.

Nahata MC and Hipple TF, *Pediatric Drug Formulations*, 2nd ed, Cincinnati, OH: Harvey Whitney Books Co, 1992.

Vidarabine *(vye DARE a been)*

U.S. Brand Names Vira-A®

Synonyms Adenine Arabinoside; Ara-A; Arabinofuranosyladenine; Vidarabine Monohydrate

Therapeutic Category Antiviral Agent, Nonantiretroviral; Antiviral Agent, Ophthalmic

Use Treatment of acute keratoconjunctivitis and epithelial keratitis due to herpes simplex virus type 1 and 2; superficial keratitis caused by herpes simplex virus

Pregnancy Risk Factor C

Contraindications Hypersensitivity to vidarabine or any component of the formulation; sterile trophic ulcers

Warnings/Precautions Not effective against RNA virus, adenoviral ocular infections, bacterial fungal or chlamydial infections of the cornea, or trophic ulcers; temporary visual haze may be produced; neoplasia has occurred with I.M. vidarabine-treated animals; although *in vitro* studies have been inconclusive, they have shown mutagenesis

Adverse Reactions Frequency not defined: Ocular: Burning eyes, foreign body sensation, keratitis, lacrimation, photophobia, uveitis

Overdosage/Toxicology No untoward effects are anticipated with ingestion.

Drug Interactions

    Increased Effect/Toxicity: Allopurinol (may increase vidarabine levels).

Mechanism of Action Inhibits viral DNA synthesis by blocking DNA polymerase

Usual Dosage Children and Adults: Ophthalmic: Keratoconjunctivitis: Instill ½" of ointment in lower conjunctival sac 5 times/day every 3 hours while awake until complete re-epithelialization has occurred, then twice daily for an additional 7 days

Administration Administer by I.V. infusion over 12 to 24 hours; vidarabine must be filtered with a 0.45 micron or smaller pore size inline filter; administer at a final concentration not to exceed 0.45 mg/mL to prevent precipitation. However, concentrations up to 0.7 mg/mL have been administered to fluid-restricted patients.

Patient Information Do not use eye make-up when on this medication for ophthalmic infection; use sunglasses if photophobic reaction occurs; may cause blurred vision; notify physician if improvement not seen after 7 days or if condition worsens

Dosage Forms Ointment, ophthalmic, as monohydrate: 3% [30 mg/mL = 28 mg/mL base] (3.5 g)

♦ **Vidarabine Monohydrate** see Vidarabine *on page 1414*
♦ **ViDaylin**® see Vitamins (Multiple) *on page 1424*
♦ **Videx**® see Didanosine *on page 397*
♦ **Videx**® **EC** see Didanosine *on page 397*

VinBLAStine (vin BLAS teen)

U.S. Brand Names Alkaban-AQ®; Velban®

Canadian Brand Names Velban®

Synonyms Vinblastine Sulfate; Vincaleukoblastine; VLB

Therapeutic Category Antineoplastic Agent, Vesicant; Antineoplastic Agent, Vinca Alkaloid; Vesicant

Use Treatment of Hodgkin's and non-Hodgkin's lymphoma, testicular, lung, head and neck, breast, and renal carcinomas, Mycosis fungoides, Kaposi's sarcoma, histiocytosis, choriocarcinoma, and idiopathic thrombocytopenic purpura

Pregnancy Risk Factor D

Contraindications For I.V. use only; **I.T. use may result in death**; hypersensitivity to vinblastine or any component of the formulation; severe bone marrow suppression or presence of bacterial infection not under control prior to initiation of therapy; pregnancy

Warnings/Precautions The U.S. Food and Drug Administration (FDA) currently recommends that procedures for proper handling and disposal of antineoplastic agents be considered. Avoid extravasation; discontinue immediately if extravasation occurs (remaining portion of dose to be infused through another vein); dosage modification required in patients with impaired liver function and neurotoxicity. Using small amounts of drug daily for long periods may increase neurotoxicity and is therefore not advised. For I.V. use only. **Intrathecal administration may result in death.** Immediate neurosurgical intervention is required if inadvertent intrathecal administration occurs. Use with caution in patients with cachexia or ulcerated skin; monitor closely for shortness of breath or bronchospasm in patients receiving mitomycin C.

Adverse Reactions

  >10%:

    Dermatologic: Alopecia

    Gastrointestinal: Nausea, vomiting, constipation, diarrhea (less common), stomatitis, abdominal cramps, anorexia, metallic taste

      Emetic potential: Moderate (30% to 60%)

    Hematologic: Leukopenia, severe bone marrow suppression (dose-limiting toxicity - unlike vincristine)

    Myelosuppressive:

      WBC: Moderate - severe

      Platelets: Moderate - severe

      Onset: 4-7 days

      Nadir: 4-10 days

      Recovery: 17 days

  1% to 10%:

    Cardiovascular: Hypertension, Raynaud's phenomenon

    Central nervous system: Depression, malaise, headache, seizures

    Dermatologic: Rash, photosensitivity, dermatitis

    Endocrine & metabolic: Hyperuricemia

    Gastrointestinal: Paralytic ileus, stomatitis

    Genitourinary: Urinary retention

    Local: **Vesicant chemotherapy**

    Neuromuscular & skeletal: Jaw pain, myalgia, paresthesia

    Respiratory: Bronchospasm

  <1% (Limited to important or life-threatening): Hemorrhagic colitis, neurotoxicity (rare; symptoms may include peripheral neuropathy, loss of deep tendon reflexes, headache, weakness, urinary retention, GI symptoms, tachycardia, orthostatic hypotension, convulsions), rectal bleeding

Overdosage/Toxicology Symptoms include bone marrow suppression, mental depression, paresthesias, loss of deep reflexes, and neurotoxicity. There is no information regarding the effectiveness of dialysis. There are no antidotes for vinblastine. Treatment is supportive and (Continued)

VinBLAStine (Continued)

symptomatic, including fluid restriction or administration of hypertonic saline (3% sodium chloride) for drug-induced secretion of inappropriate antidiuretic hormone (SIADH), diazepam or phenytoin for seizures, laxatives for constipation, and antiemetics for toxic emesis. Inadvertent intrathecal administration requires emergent neurosurgical intervention.

Drug Interactions

Cytochrome P450 Effect: CYP3A3/4 and 3A5-7 enzyme substrate; CYP2D6 enzyme inhibitor

Increased Effect/Toxicity: Vinblastine levels may be increased when given with drugs that inhibit cytochrome P450 3A enzyme substrate. Previous or simultaneous use with mitomycin-C has resulted in acute shortness of breath and severe bronchospasm within minutes or several hours after *Vinca* alkaloid injection and may occur up to 2 weeks after the dose of mitomycin. Mitomycin-C in combination with administration of VLB may cause acute shortness of breath and severe bronchospasm, onset may be within minutes or several hours after VLB injection.

Decreased Effect: Phenytoin plasma levels may be reduced with concomitant combination chemotherapy with vinblastine. Alpha-interferon enhances interferon toxicity; phenytoin may ↓ plasma levels.

Ethanol/Nutrition/Herb Interactions Herb/Nutraceutical: St John's wort may decrease vinblastine levels. Avoid black cohosh, dong quai in estrogen-dependent tumors.

Stability

Store intact vials under refrigeration (2°C to 8°C) and protect from light; stable for 24 hours at room temperature

Further dilution in D$_5$W or NS is stable for 21 days at room temperature (25°C) and refrigeration (4°C)

Standard I.V. dilution:
I.V. push: Dose/syringe (concentration = 1 mg/mL)
Maximum syringe size for IVP is a 30 mL syringe and syringe should be ≤75% full
CIV: Dose/250-1000 mL D$_5$W or NS
Protect from light

Note: Must be dispensed in overwrap which bears the statement "Do not remove covering until the moment of injection. Fatal if given intrathecally. For I.V. use only." Syringes should be labeled: "Fatal if given intrathecally. For I.V. use only."

Mechanism of Action VLB binds to tubulin and inhibits microtubule formation, therefore, arresting the cell at metaphase by disrupting the formation of the mitotic spindle; it is specific for the M and S phases; binds to microtubular protein of the mitotic spindle causing metaphase arrest

Pharmacodynamics/Kinetics

Distribution: V$_d$: 27.3 L/kg; binds extensively to tissues; does not penetrate CNS or other fatty tissues; distributes to liver

Protein binding: 99%

Metabolism: Hepatic metabolism to an active metabolite

Half-life elimination: Biphasic: Initial 0.164 hours; Terminal: 25 hours

Excretion: Feces (95%); urine (<1% as unchanged drug)

Usual Dosage Refer to individual protocols. Varies depending upon clinical and hematological response. Give at intervals of at least 14 days and only after leukocyte count has returned to at least 4000/mm^3; maintenance therapy should be titrated according to leukocyte count. Dosage should be reduced in patients with recent exposure to radiation therapy or chemotherapy; single doses in these patients should not exceed 5.5 mg/m^2.

Children and Adults: I.V.: 4-20 mg/m^2 (0.1-0.5 mg/kg) every 7-10 days **or** 5-day continuous infusion of 1.5-2 mg/m^2/day **or** 0.1-0.5 mg/kg/week

Dosing adjustment in hepatic impairment:
Serum bilirubin 1.5-3.0 mg/dL or AST 60-180 units: Administer 50% of normal dose
Serum bilirubin 3.0-5.0 mg/dL: Administer 25% of dose
Serum bilirubin >5.0 mg/dL or AST >180 units: Omit dose

Administration

FATAL IF GIVEN INTRATHECALLY

IVP over at least one minute is desired route of administration because of potential for extravasation. However, has also been administered CIV - **CENTRAL LINE ONLY** for CIV administration. Vinblastine is administered intravenously, usually as a slow (2- to 3-minute) push, or a bolus (5- to 15-minute) infusion. It is occasionally given as a 24-hour continuous infusion.

Avoid extravasation

Protect from light

Monitoring Parameters CBC with differential and platelet count, serum uric acid, hepatic function tests

Patient Information This medication can only be administered by infusion, usually on a cyclic basis. Maintain adequate hydration (2-3 L/day of fluids unless instructed to restrict fluid intake) and nutrition (small frequent meals will help). You will most likely lose your hair (reversible after therapy); experience nausea or vomiting (request antiemetic); photosensitivity (use sunscreen, wear protective clothing and eyewear, and avoid direct sunlight); or feel weak or lethargic (use caution when driving or engaging in tasks requiring alertness until response to drug is known). Use good oral care to reduce incidence of mouth sores. You will be more susceptible to infection; avoid crowds and exposure to infection. Report numbness or tingling in fingers or toes (use care to prevent injury); signs of infection (eg, fever, chills, sore throat, burning urination, fatigue); unusual bleeding (eg, tarry stools, easy bruising, blood in stool, urine, or mouth); unresolved mouth sores; skin rash or itching; or difficulty breathing. The drug may cause permanent sterility and may cause birth defects. Contraceptive measures are recommended during therapy. The drug may be excreted in breast milk, therefore, an alternative form of feeding your baby should be used.

Nursing Implications May be administered by I.V. push or into a free flowing I.V.; monitor for life-threatening bronchospasm (most likely to occur if patient is also taking mitomycin).

Maintain adequate hydration; allopurinol may be given to prevent uric acid nephropathy; may cause sloughing upon extravasation. Discontinue infusion **immediately** if extravasation occurs (remaining portion of dose may be infused via a separate vein).

Extravasation treatment:
Mix 250 units hyaluronidase with 6 mL of NS
Inject the hyaluronidase solution subcutaneously through 6 clockwise injections into the infiltrated area using a 25-gauge needle; change the needle with each new injection
Apply heat immediately for 1 hour; repeat 4 times/day for 3-5 days
Application of cold or hydrocortisone is contraindicated

Dosage Forms
Injection, as sulfate: 1 mg/mL (10 mL)
Powder for injection, as sulfate: 10 mg

♦ **Vinblastine Sulfate** see VinBLAStine on page 1415
♦ **Vincaleukoblastine** see VinBLAStine on page 1415
♦ **Vincasar® PFS™** see VinCRIStine on page 1417

VinCRIStine (vin KRIS teen)
U.S. Brand Names Oncovin®; Vincasar® PFS™
Canadian Brand Names Oncovin®; Vincasar® PFS™
Synonyms LCR; Leurocristine; VCR; Vincristine Sulfate
Therapeutic Category Antineoplastic Agent, Vesicant; Antineoplastic Agent, Vinca Alkaloid; Vesicant
Use Treatment of leukemias, Hodgkin's disease, non-Hodgkin's lymphomas, Wilms' tumor, neuroblastoma, rhabdomyosarcoma
Pregnancy Risk Factor D
Contraindications Hypersensitivity to vincristine or any component of the formulation; **for I.V. use only, fatal if given intrathecally**; patients with demyelinating form of Charcot-Marie-Tooth syndrome; pregnancy
Warnings/Precautions The U.S. Food and Drug Administration (FDA) currently recommends that procedures for proper handling and disposal of antineoplastic agents be considered. Dosage modification required in patients with impaired hepatic function or who have pre-existing neuromuscular disease; avoid extravasation; use with caution in the elderly; avoid eye contamination; observe closely for shortness of breath, bronchospasm, especially in patients treated with mitomycin C. For I.V. use only; **intrathecal administration results in death**; administer allopurinol to prevent uric acid nephropathy; not to be used with radiation.
Adverse Reactions
>10%: Dermatologic: Alopecia occurs in 20% to 70% of patients
1% to 10%:
Cardiovascular: Orthostatic hypotension or hypertension, hypertension, hypotension
Central nervous system: Motor difficulties, seizures, headache, CNS depression, cranial nerve paralysis, fever
Dermatologic: Rash
Endocrine & metabolic: Hyperuricemia
Gastrointestinal: Constipation and possible paralytic ileus secondary to neurologic toxicity; oral ulceration, abdominal cramps, anorexia, metallic taste, bloating, nausea, vomiting, weight loss, diarrhea
Genitourinary: Bladder atony (related to neurotoxicity)
Emetic potential: Low (<10%)
Local: Phlebitis
Vesicant chemotherapy
Neuromuscular & skeletal: Jaw pain, leg pain, myalgia, cramping, numbness, weakness
Peripheral neuropathy: Frequently the dose-limiting toxicity of VCR. Most frequent in patients >40 years of age; occurs usually after an average of 3 weekly doses, but may occur after just one dose. Manifested as loss of the deep tendon reflexes in the lower extremities, numbness, tingling, pain, paresthesias of the fingers and toes (stocking glove sensation), and "foot drop" or "wrist drop"
Ocular: Photophobia
<1% (Limited to important or life-threatening): Mild leukopenia and thrombocytopenia, SIADH (rare, may be related to neurologic toxicity; symptomatic hyponatremia may cause seizures)
Overdosage/Toxicology Symptoms include bone marrow suppression, mental depression, paresthesias, loss of deep reflexes, alopecia, and nausea. Severe symptoms may occur with 3-4 mg/m². There are no antidotes for vincristine. Treatment is supportive and symptomatic, including fluid restriction or administration of hypertonic saline (3% sodium chloride) for drug-induced secretion of inappropriate antidiuretic hormone (SIADH), diazepam or phenytoin for seizures, laxatives for constipation, and antiemetics for toxic emesis. Case reports suggest that folinic acid may be helpful in treating vincristine overdose. It is suggested that 100 mg folinic acid be given I.V. every 3 hours for 24 hours, then every 6 hours for 48 hours; this is in addition to supportive care. The use of pyridoxine, leucovorin factor, cyanocobalamin, or thiamine have been used with little success for drug-induced peripheral neuropathy.
Drug Interactions
Cytochrome P450 Effect: CYP3A3/4 and 3A5-7 enzyme substrate; CYP2D6 enzyme inhibitor
Increased Effect/Toxicity: Vincristine levels may be increased when given with drugs that inhibit cytochrome P450 3A enzyme (itraconazole has been shown to increase onset and severity of neuromuscular adverse effects of vincristine). Digoxin plasma levels and renal excretion may decrease with combination chemotherapy including vincristine. Vincristine should be given 12-24 hours before asparaginase to minimize toxicity (may decrease the hepatic clearance of vincristine). Acute pulmonary reactions may occur with mitomycin-C. Previous or simultaneous use with mitomycin-C has resulted in acute shortness of breath and severe bronchospasm within minutes or several hours after *Vinca* alkaloid injection and may occur up to 2 weeks after the dose of mitomycin.
(Continued)

VinCRIStine *(Continued)*

Decreased Effect: Digoxin and phenytoin levels may decrease with combination chemotherapy.

Ethanol/Nutrition/Herb Interactions Herb/Nutraceutical: St John's wort may decrease vincristine levels.

Stability

Store intact vials at refrigeration (2°C to 8°C); stable for one month at room temperature
Further dilution in NS or D$_5$W is stable for 21 days at room temperature (25°C) and refrigeration (4°C)

Compatible with bleomycin, cytarabine, doxorubicin, fluorouracil, methotrexate, metoclopramide

Standard I.V. dilution:

I.V. push: Dose/syringe (concentration = 1 mg/mL)
Maximum syringe size for IVP is 30 mL syringe and syringe should be ≤75% full
IVPB: Dose/50 mL D$_5$W

Mechanism of Action Binds to microtubular protein of the mitotic spindle causing metaphase arrest; cell-cycle phase specific in the M and S phases

Pharmacodynamics/Kinetics

Absorption: Oral: Poor

Distribution: Poor penetration into CSF; rapidly removed from bloodstream and tightly bound to tissues; penetrates blood-brain barrier poorly

Protein binding: 75%

Metabolism: Extensively hepatic

Half-life elimination: Terminal: 24 hours

Excretion: Primarily feces (~80%); urine (<1% as unchanged drug)

Usual Dosage Refer to individual protocols as dosages vary with protocol used; adjustments are made depending upon clinical and hematological response and upon adverse reactions

Children ≤10 kg or BSA <1 m^2: Initial therapy: 0.05 mg/kg once weekly then titrate dose; maximum single dose: 2 mg

Children >10 kg or BSA ≥1 m^2: 1-2 mg/m^2, may repeat once weekly for 3-6 weeks; maximum single dose: 2 mg

Neuroblastoma: I.V. continuous infusion with doxorubicin: 1 mg/m^2/day for 72 hours

Adults: I.V.: 0.4-1.4 mg/m^2 (up to 2 mg maximum in most patients); may repeat every week

Dosing adjustment in hepatic impairment:

Serum bilirubin 1.5-3.0 mg/dL or AST 60-180 units: Administer 50% of normal dose

Serum bilirubin 3.0-5.0 mg/dL: Administer 25% of dose

Serum bilirubin >5.0 mg/dL or AST >180 units: Omit dose

The average total dose per course of treatment should be around 2-2.5 mg; some recommend capping the dose at 2 mg maximum to reduce toxicity; however, it is felt that this measure can reduce the efficacy of the drug

Administration

FATAL IF GIVEN INTRATHECALLY

IVP over at least one minute is desired route of administration because of potential for extravasation. However, has also been administered IVPB over 15 minutes - **CENTRAL LINE ONLY** for IVPB administration.

Avoid extravasation

Protect from light

Monitoring Parameters Serum electrolytes (sodium), hepatic function tests, neurologic examination, CBC, serum uric acid

Patient Information This medication can only be administered by infusion, usually on a cyclic basis. Maintain adequate hydration (2-3 L/day of fluids unless instructed to restrict fluid intake) and nutrition (small frequent meals will help). You will most likely lose your hair (reversible after therapy); experience constipation (request medication); or feel weak or lethargic (use caution when driving or engaging in tasks requiring alertness until response to drug is known). Use good oral care to reduce incidence of mouth sores. You will be more susceptible to infection; avoid crowds or exposure to infection. Report pain, numbness, tingling in fingers or toes (use care to prevent injury); alterations in mental status (eg, confusion, insomnia, headaches, jaw pain, loss of vision); signs of infection (eg, fever, chills, sore throat, burning urination, fatigue); unusual bleeding (eg, tarry stools, easy bruising, or blood in stool, urine, or mouth), unresolved mouth sores; skin rash or itching; nausea; vomiting; abdominal pain; bloating; or difficulty breathing. Contraceptive measures are recommended during therapy.

Nursing Implications Observe for life-threatening bronchospasm after administration; use of rectal thermometer or rectal tubing should be avoided to prevent injury to rectal mucosa

Extravasation treatment:

Mix 250 units hyaluronidase with 6 mL of NS

Inject the hyaluronidase solution subcutaneously through 6 clockwise injections into the infiltrated area using a 25-gauge needle; change the needle with each new injection

Apply heat immediately for 1 hour; repeat 4 times/day for 3-5 days

Application of cold or hydrocortisone is contraindicated

Dosage Forms Injection, as sulfate: 1 mg/mL (1 mL, 2 mL, 5 mL)

♦ **Vincristine Sulfate** *see VinCRIStine on page 1417*

Vinorelbine *(vi NOR el been)*

U.S. Brand Names Navelbine®

Canadian Brand Names Navelbine®

Synonyms Vinorelbine Tartrate

Therapeutic Category Antineoplastic Agent, Vesicant; Antineoplastic Agent, Vinca Alkaloid; Vesicant

Use Treatment of nonsmall cell lung cancer (as a single agent or in combination with cisplatin)

Unlabeled/Investigational Use Breast cancer, ovarian carcinoma (cisplatin-resistant), Hodgkin's disease

Pregnancy Risk Factor D

Contraindications For I.V. use only; **I.T. use may result in death**; hypersensitivity to vinorelbine or any component of the formulation; severe bone marrow suppression (granulocyte counts <1000 cells/mm^3) or presence of bacterial infection not under control prior to initiation of therapy; pregnancy

Warnings/Precautions The U.S. Food and Drug Administration (FDA) currently recommends that procedures for proper handling and disposal of antineoplastic agents be considered. Avoid extravasation; dosage modification required in patients with impaired liver function and neurotoxicity. Frequently monitor patients for myelosuppression both during and after therapy. Granulocytopenia is dose-limiting. **Intrathecal administration may result in death.** Use with caution in patients with cachexia or ulcerated skin.

Acute shortness of breath and severe bronchospasm have been reported, most commonly when administered with mitomycin. Fatal cases of interstitial pulmonary changes and ARDS have been reported. May cause severe constipation (grade 3-4), paralytic ileus, intestinal obstruction, necrosis, and/or perforation.

Adverse Reactions

>10%:
  Central nervous system: Fatigue (27%)
  Dermatologic: Alopecia (12%)
  Gastrointestinal: Nausea (44%, severe <2%), constipation (35%), vomiting (20%), diarrhea (17%)
    Emetic potential: Moderate (30% to 60%)
  Hematologic: May cause severe bone marrow suppression and is the dose-limiting toxicity of vinorelbine; severe granulocytopenia (90%) may occur following the administration of vinorelbine; leukopenia (92%), anemia (83%)
  Myelosuppressive:
    WBC: Moderate - severe
    Onset: 4-7d days
    Nadir: 7-10 days
    Recovery: 14-21 days
  Hepatic: Elevated SGOT (67%), elevated total bilirubin (13%)
  Local: Injection site reaction (28%), injection site pain (16%)
  Neuromuscular & skeletal: Weakness (36%), peripheral neuropathy (20% to 25%)
1% to 10%:
  Cardiovascular: Chest pain (5%)
  Gastrointestinal: Paralytic ileus (1%)
  Hematologic: Thrombocytopenia (5%)
  Local: Extravasation: Vesicant and can cause tissue irritation and necrosis if infiltrated; if extravasation occurs, follow institutional policy, which may include hyaluronidase and hot compresses; phlebitis (7%)
    Vesicant chemotherapy
  Neuromuscular & skeletal: Mild to moderate peripheral neuropathy manifested by paresthesia and hyperesthesia, loss of deep tendon reflexes (<5%); myalgia (<5%), arthralgia (<5%), jaw pain (<5%)
  Respiratory: Dyspnea (3% to 7%)
<1% (Limited to important or life-threatening): Anaphylaxis, angioedema, deep vein thrombosis, dysphagia, esophagitis, gait instability, hemorrhagic cystitis, pancreatitis, pulmonary edema, pulmonary embolus, radiation recall (dermatitis, esophagitis), severe peripheral neuropathy (generally reversible), SIADH

Overdosage/Toxicology Symptoms include bone marrow suppression, mental depression, paresthesias, loss of deep reflexes, and neurotoxicity. Overdoses involving quantities of up to 10 times the recommended dose (30 mg/m^2) have been reported. The toxicities described were consistent with those listed in the Adverse Reactions section including paralytic ileus, stomatitis, and esophagitis. Bone marrow aplasia, sepsis, and paresis have also been reported. Fatalities have occurred following overdose of vinorelbine. There are no antidotes for vinorelbine. Treatment is supportive and symptomatic, including fluid restriction or administration of hypertonic saline (3% sodium chloride) for drug-induced secretion of inappropriate antidiuretic hormone (SIADH), diazepam or phenytoin for seizures, laxatives for constipation, blood transfusions, growth factors, antibiotics, and antiemetics for toxic emesis.

Drug Interactions

  Cytochrome P450 Effect: CYP2D6 and 3A3/4 enzyme inhibitor

  Increased Effect/Toxicity: Previous or simultaneous use with mitomycin-C has resulted in acute shortness of breath and severe bronchospasm within minutes or several hours after *Vinca* alkaloid injection and may occur up to 2 weeks after the dose of mitomycin.

  Cisplatin: Incidence of granulocytopenia is significantly higher than with single-agent vinorelbine.

Ethanol/Nutrition/Herb Interactions Herb/Nutraceutical: St John's wort may decrease vinorelbine levels.

Stability

  Store intact vials under refrigeration (2°C to 8°C) and protect from light; vials are stable at room temperature for up to 72 hours
  Further dilution in D$_5$W or NS is stable for 24 hours at room temperature

  Standard I.V. dilution:
    I.V. push: Dose/syringe (concentration = 1.5-3 mg/mL)
      Maximum syringe size for IVP is a 30 mL syringe and syringe should be ≤75% full
    IVPB: Dose/50-250 mL D$_5$W or NS (concentration = 0.5-2 mg/mL)
      Solutions are stable for 24 hours at room temperature

Mechanism of Action Semisynthetic vinca alkaloid which binds to tubulin and inhibits microtubule formation, therefore, arresting the cell at metaphase by disrupting the formation of the mitotic spindle; it is specific for the M and S phases; binds to microtubular protein of the mitotic spindle causing metaphase arrest

(Continued)

Vinorelbine *(Continued)*

Pharmacodynamics/Kinetics

Absorption: Unreliable; must be given I.V.

Distribution: V_d: 25.4-40.1 L/kg; binds extensively to human platelets and lymphocytes (79.6% to 91.2%)

Metabolism: Extensively hepatic to two metabolites, deacetylvinorelbine (active) and vinorelbine N-oxide

Half-life elimination: Triphasic: Terminal: 27.7-43.6 hours

Excretion: Feces (46%); urine (18%)

Clearance: Plasma: Mean: 0.97-1.26 L/hour/kg

Usual Dosage
Refer to individual protocols; varies depending upon clinical and hematological response

Adults: I.V.:

Single-agent therapy: 30 mg/m² every 7 days

Combination therapy with cisplatin: 25 mg/m² every 7 days (with cisplatin 100 mg/m² every 4 weeks)

Dosage adjustment in hematological toxicity: Granulocyte counts should be ≥1000 cells/mm³ prior to the administration of vinorelbine. Adjustments in the dosage of vinorelbine should be based on granulocyte counts obtained on the day of treatment as follows:

Granulocytes ≥1500 cells/mm³ on day of treatment: Administer 30 mg/m²

Granulocytes 1000-1499 cells/mm³ on day of treatment: Administer 15 mg/m²

Granulocytes <1000 cells/mm³ on day of treatment: Do not administer. Repeat granulocyte count in one week; if 3 consecutive doses are held because granulocyte count is <1000 cells/mm³, discontinue vinorelbine

For patients who, during treatment, have experienced fever and/or sepsis while granulocytopenic or had 2 consecutive weekly doses held due to granulocytopenia, subsequent doses of vinorelbine should be:

22.5 mg/m² for granulocytes ≥1500 cells/mm³

11.25 mg/m² for granulocytes 1000-1499 cells/mm³

Dosage adjustment in renal impairment: No dose adjustments are required for renal insufficiency. If moderate or severe neurotoxicity develops, discontinue vinorelbine.

Dosing adjustment in hepatic impairment: Vinorelbine should be administered with caution in patients with hepatic insufficiency. In patients who develop hyperbilirubinemia during treatment with vinorelbine, the dose should be adjusted for total bilirubin as follows:

Serum bilirubin ≤2 mg/dL: Administer 30 mg/m²

Serum bilirubin 2.1-3 mg/dL: Administer 15 mg/m²

Serum bilirubin >3 mg/dL: Administer 7.5 mg/m²

Dosing adjustment in patients with concurrent hematologic toxicity and hepatic impairment: Administer the lower doses determined from the above recommendations

Administration

FATAL IF GIVEN INTRATHECALLY

Administer IVPB over 20-30 minutes or as a direct intravenous push or rapid bolus, over 5-10 minutes. Intravenous doses should be followed by 150-250 mL of saline or dextrose to reduce the incidence of phlebitis and inflammation.

CENTRAL LINE ONLY for IVPB administration

Avoid extravasation

Monitoring Parameters
CBC with differential and platelet count, serum uric acid, hepatic function tests

Patient Information
This medication can only be administered by infusion, usually on a cyclic basis. Maintain adequate hydration (2-3 L/day of fluids unless instructed to restrict fluid intake) and nutrition (small frequent meals will help). You will most likely lose your hair (reversible after therapy); experience nausea or vomiting (request medication); feel weak or lethargic (use caution when driving or engaging in tasks requiring alertness until response to drug is known). Use good oral care to reduce incidence of mouth sores. You will be more susceptible to infection; avoid crowds or exposure to infection. Report weakness, skeletal pain, or tremors; signs of infection (eg, fever, chills, sore throat, burning urination, fatigue); unusual bleeding (eg, tarry stools, easy bruising, blood in stool, urine, or mouth); numbness, pain, or tingling of fingers or toes; unresolved mouth sores; skin rash or itching; uncontrolled nausea, vomiting, or abdominal pain; or difficulty breathing. The drug may cause permanent sterility and may cause birth defects. Contraceptive measures are recommended during therapy. The drug is excreted in breast milk, therefore, an alternative form of feeding your baby should be used.

Nursing Implications

Extravasation treatment:

Mix 250 units hyaluronidase with 6 mL of NS

Inject the hyaluronidase solution subcutaneously through 6 clockwise injections into the infiltrated area using a 25-gauge needle; change the needle with each new injection

Apply heat immediately for 1 hour; repeat 4 times/day for 3-5 days

Application of cold or hydrocortisone is contraindicated.

Monitor for life-threatening bronchospasm (most likely to occur if patient is also taking mitomycin). Maintain adequate hydration; allopurinol may be given to prevent uric acid nephropathy; may cause sloughing upon extravasation.

Dosage Forms
Injection, as tartrate: 10 mg/mL (1 mL, 5 mL)

- **Virazole® Aerosol** *see Ribavirin on page 1189*
- **Viread™** *see Tenofovir on page 1296*
- **Virilon®** *see MethylTESTOSTERone on page 898*
- **Virilon® IM (Can)** *see Testosterone on page 1302*
- **Viroptic®** *see Trifluridine on page 1374*
- **Viscoat®** *see Chondroitin Sulfate-Sodium Hyaluronate on page 289*
- **Visken®** *see Pindolol on page 1086*
- **Vistacot®** *see HydrOXYzine on page 691*
- **Vistaril®** *see HydrOXYzine on page 691*
- **Vistide®** *see Cidofovir on page 291*
- **Vi-Sudo® [OTC]** *see Triprolidine and Pseudoephedrine on page 1380*
- **Vita-C® [OTC]** *see Ascorbic Acid on page 116*
- **Vitacarn®** *see Levocarnitine on page 789*

Vitamin A (VYE ta min aye)

U.S. Brand Names Aquasol®; Palmitate-A® [OTC]

Synonyms Oleovitamin A

Therapeutic Category Vitamin, Fat Soluble

Use Treatment and prevention of vitamin A deficiency; parenteral (I.M.) route is indicated when oral administration is not feasible or when absorption is insufficient (malabsorption syndrome)

Pregnancy Risk Factor A/X (dose exceeding RDA recommendation)

Pregnancy/Breast-Feeding Implications Clinical effect on the fetus: Excessive use of vitamin A shortly before and during pregnancy could be harmful to babies

Contraindications Hypersensitivity to vitamin A or any component of the formulation; hypervitaminosis A; pregnancy (dose exceeding RDA)

Warnings/Precautions Evaluate other sources of vitamin A while receiving this product; patients receiving >25,000 units/day should be closely monitored for toxicity. Parenteral vitamin A: In low birth weight infants, polysorbates have been associated with thrombocytopenia, renal dysfunction, hepatomegaly, cholestasis, ascites, hypotension, and metabolic acidosis (E-Ferol syndrome).

Adverse Reactions Systemic: 1% to 10%:

Central nervous system: Irritability, vertigo, lethargy, malaise, fever, headache

Dermatologic: Drying or cracking of skin

Endocrine & metabolic: Hypercalcemia

Gastrointestinal: Weight loss

Ocular: Visual changes

Miscellaneous: Hypervitaminosis A

Overdosage/Toxicology

Toxic manifestations are dependent on age, dose, and duration of administration. General manifestations of hypervitaminosis A syndrome include fatigue, malaise, lethargy, abdominal discomfort, anorexia, and vomiting. Systemic manifestations occurring with plasma levels >1200 units/mL include hepatotoxicity, hypomenorrhea, hepatosplenomegaly, jaundice, and leukopenia. Skeletal, CNS, and dermatologic effects also occur.

Acute toxicity: Single dose of 25,000 units/kg

Chronic toxicity: 4000 units/kg for 6-15 months

Treat intracranial hypertension from chronic exposure, if needed. For acute exposure, use gut decontamination, otherwise treatment is symptomatic and supportive.

Drug Interactions

Increased Effect/Toxicity: Retinoids may have additive adverse effects.

Decreased Effect: Cholestyramine resin decreases absorption of vitamin A. Neomycin and mineral oil may also interfere with vitamin A absorption.

Stability Protect from light

Mechanism of Action Needed for bone development, growth, visual adaptation to darkness, testicular and ovarian function, and as a cofactor in many biochemical processes

Pharmacodynamics/Kinetics

Absorption: Vitamin A in dosages **not** exceeding physiologic replacement is well absorbed after oral administration; water miscible preparations are absorbed more rapidly than oil preparations; large oral doses, conditions of fat malabsorption, low protein intake, or hepatic or pancreatic disease reduces oral absorption

Distribution: Large amounts concentrate for storage in the liver; enters breast milk

Metabolism: Conjugated with glucuronide, undergoes enterohepatic circulation

Excretion: Feces

Usual Dosage

RDA:

<1 year: 375 mcg

1-3 years: 400 mcg

4-6 years: 500 mcg*

7-10 years: 700 mcg*

>10 years: 800-1000 mcg*

Male: 1000 mcg

Female: 800 mcg

* mcg retinol equivalent (0.3 mcg retinol = 1 unit vitamin A)

Vitamin A supplementation in measles (recommendation of the World Health Organization):

Children: Oral: Administer as a single dose; repeat the next day and at 4 weeks for children with ophthalmologic evidence of vitamin A deficiency:

6 months to 1 year: 100,000 units

>1 year: 200,000 units

Note: Use of vitamin A in measles is recommended only for patients 6 months to 2 years of age hospitalized with measles and its complications **or** patients >6 months of age who have any of the following risk factors and who are not already receiving vitamin A: immunodeficiency, ophthalmologic evidence of vitamin A deficiency including night blindness, Bitot's spots or evidence of xerophthalmia, impaired intestinal absorption, moderate to

(Continued)

Vitamin A (Continued)

severe malnutrition including that associated with eating disorders, or recent immigration from areas where high mortality rates from measles have been observed

Note: Monitor patients closely; dosages >25,000 units/kg have been associated with toxicity

Severe deficiency with xerophthalmia: Oral:

Children 1-8 years: 5000-10,000 units/kg/day for 5 days or until recovery occurs

Children >8 years and Adults: 500,000 units/day for 3 days, then 50,000 units/day for 14 days, then 10,000-20,000 units/day for 2 months

Deficiency (without corneal changes): Oral:

Infants <1 year: 100,000 units every 4-6 months

Children 1-8 years: 200,000 units every 4-6 months

Children >8 years and Adults: 100,000 units/day for 3 days then 50,000 units/day for 14 days

Deficiency: I.M.: **Note:** I.M. route is indicated when oral administration is not feasible or when absorption is insufficient (malabsorption syndrome):

Infants: 7500-15,000 units/day for 10 days

Children 1-8 years: 17,500-35,000 units/day for 10 days

Children >8 years and Adults: 100,000 units/day for 3 days, followed by 50,000 units/day for 2 weeks

Note: Follow-up therapy with an oral therapeutic multivitamin (containing additional vitamin A) is recommended:

Low Birth Weight Infants: Additional vitamin A is recommended, however no dosage amount has been established

Children ≤8 years: 5000-10,000 units/day

Children >8 years and Adults: 10,000-20,000 units/day

Malabsorption syndrome (prophylaxis): Children >8 years and Adults: Oral: 10,000-50,000 units/day of water miscible product

Dietary supplement: Oral:

Infants up to 6 months: 1500 units/day

Children:

6 months to 3 years: 1500-2000 units/day

4-6 years: 2500 units/day

7-10 years: 3300-3500 units/day

Children >10 years and Adults: 4000-5000 units/day

Reference Range 1 RE = 1 retinol equivalent; 1 RE = 1 μg retinol or 6 μg beta-carotene; Normal levels of Vitamin A in serum = 80-300 units/mL

Patient Information Avoid use of mineral oil when taking drug; take with food; notify physician if nausea, vomiting, anorexia, malaise, drying or cracking of skin or lips, irritability, headache, or loss of hair occurs

Nursing Implications Do not administer by I.V. push; patients receiving >25,000 units/day should be closely monitored for toxicity

Additional Information 1 mg = 3333 units

Dosage Forms

Capsule: 8000 units, 10,000 units [OTC], 25,000 units, 50,000 units

Injection (Aquasol®-A): 50,000 units/mL (2 mL)

Tablet [OTC]: 5000 units, 10,000 units, 15,000 units

Palmitate-A®: 5000 units, 15,000 units

♦ **Vitamin A Acid** see Tretinoin (Topical) on page 1365

Vitamin A and Vitamin D (VYE ta min aye & VYE ta min dee)

U.S. Brand Names A and D™ Ointment [OTC]

Synonyms Cod Liver Oil

Therapeutic Category Topical Skin Product

Use Temporary relief of discomfort due to chapped skin, diaper rash, minor burns, abrasions, as well as irritations associated with ostomy skin care

Pregnancy Risk Factor B

Usual Dosage Topical: Apply locally with gentle massage as needed

Additional Information Complete prescribing information for this medication should be consulted for additional detail.

Dosage Forms Ointment, topical: In lanolin-petrolatum base (60 g)

♦ **Vitamin B₁** see Thiamine on page 1316

♦ **Vitamin B₂** see Riboflavin on page 1191

♦ **Vitamin B₃** see Niacin on page 974

♦ **Vitamin B₃** see Niacinamide on page 976

♦ **Vitamin B₆** see Pyridoxine on page 1162

♦ **Vitamin B₁₂** see Cyanocobalamin on page 339

♦ **Vitamin B₁₂** see Hydroxocobalamin on page 687

Vitamin B Complex With Vitamin C and Folic Acid

(VYE ta min bee KOM pleks with VYE ta min see & FOE lik AS id)

U.S. Brand Names Berocca®; Nephrocaps®

Therapeutic Category Vitamin, Water Soluble

Use Supportive nutritional supplementation in conditions in which water-soluble vitamins are required like GI disorders, chronic alcoholism, pregnancy, severe burns, and recovery from surgery

Usual Dosage Adults: Oral: 1 every day

Additional Information Complete prescribing information for this medication should be consulted for additional detail.

Dosage Forms Content may vary slightly depending on product used

Capsule/Tablet: Folic acid 0.1-0.4 mg, vitamin B₁ 10-15 mg, vitamin B₂ 10 mg, vitamin B₃ 100 mg, vitamin B₅ 20 mg, vitamin B₆ 2-5 mg, vitamin B₁₂ 6-10 mg, vitamin C 300-500 mg

♦ **Vitamin C** *see Ascorbic Acid on page 116*

♦ **Vitamin D₂** *see Ergocalciferol on page 481*

Vitamin E (VYE ta min ee)

U.S. Brand Names Amino-Opti-E® [OTC]; Aquasol E® [OTC]; E-Complex-600® [OTC]; E-Vitamin® [OTC]; Vita-Plus® E Softgels® [OTC]; Vitec® [OTC]; Vite E® Creme [OTC]

Synonyms *d*-Alpha Tocopherol; *dl*-Alpha Tocopherol

Therapeutic Category Vitamin, Fat Soluble; Vitamin, Topical

Use Prevention and treatment hemolytic anemia secondary to vitamin E deficiency, dietary supplement

Unlabeled/Investigational Use To reduce the risk of bronchopulmonary dysplasia or retro-lental fibroplasia in infants exposed to high concentrations of oxygen; prevention and treatment of tardive dyskinesia and Alzheimer's disease

Pregnancy Risk Factor A/C (dose exceeding RDA recommendation)

Contraindications Hypersensitivity to vitamin E or any component of the formulation; I.V. route

Warnings/Precautions May induce vitamin K deficiency; necrotizing enterocolitis has been associated with oral administration of large dosages (eg, >200 units/day) of a hyperosmolar vitamin E preparation in low birth weight infants

Adverse Reactions <1% (Limited to important or life-threatening): Blurred vision, contact dermatitis with topical preparation, gonadal dysfunction

Drug Interactions

Increased Effect/Toxicity: Vitamin E may alter the effect of vitamin K actions on clotting factors resulting in an increase hypoprothrombinemic response to warfarin; monitor.

Decreased Effect: Vitamin E may impair the hematologic response to iron in children with iron-deficiency anemia; monitor.

Stability Protect from light

Mechanism of Action Prevents oxidation of vitamin A and C; protects polyunsaturated fatty acids in membranes from attack by free radicals and protects red blood cells against hemolysis

Pharmacodynamics/Kinetics

Absorption: Oral: Depends on presence of bile; reduced in conditions of malabsorption, in low birth weight premature infants, and as dosage increases; water miscible preparations are better absorbed than oil preparations

Distribution: To all body tissues, especially adipose tissue, where it is stored

Metabolism: Hepatic to glucuronides

Excretion: Feces

Usual Dosage One unit of vitamin E = 1 mg *dl*-alpha-tocopherol acetate. Oral:

Recommended daily allowance (RDA):

Premature infants ≤3 months: 17 mg (25 units)

Infants:

≤6 months: 3 mg (4.5 units)

7-12 months: 4 mg (6 units)

Children:

1-3 years: 6 mg (9 units); upper limit of intake should not exceed 200 mg/day

4-8 years: 7 mg (10.5 units); upper limit of intake should not exceed 300 mg/day

9-13 years: 11 mg (16.5 units); upper limit of intake should not exceed 600 mg/day

14-18 years: 15 mg (22.5 units); upper limit of intake should not exceed 800 mg/day

Adults: 15 mg (22.5 units); upper limit of intake should not exceed 1000 mg/day

Pregnant female:

≤18 years: 15 mg (22.5 units); upper level of intake should not exceed 800 mg/day

19-50 years: 15 mg (22.5 units); upper level of intake should not exceed 1000 mg/day

Lactating female:

≤18 years: 19 mg (28.5 units); upper level of intake should not exceed 800 mg/day

19-50 years: 19 mg (28.5 units); upper level of intake should not exceed 1000 mg/day

Vitamin E deficiency:

Children (with malabsorption syndrome): 1 unit/kg/day of water miscible vitamin E (to raise plasma tocopherol concentrations to the normal range within 2 months and to maintain normal plasma concentrations)

Adults: 60-75 units/day

Prevention of vitamin E deficiency: Adults: 30 units/day

Prevention of retinopathy of prematurity or BPD secondary to O₂ therapy (AAP considers this use investigational and routine use is not recommended):

Retinopathy prophylaxis: 15-30 units/kg/day to maintain plasma levels between 1.5-2 μg/mL (may need as high as 100 units/kg/day)

Cystic fibrosis, beta-thalassemia, sickle cell anemia may require higher daily maintenance doses:

Children:

Cystic fibrosis: 100-400 units/day

Beta-thalassemia: 750 units/day

Adults:

Sickle cell: 450 units/day

Alzheimer's disease: 1000 units twice daily

Tardive dyskinesia: 1600 units/day

Reference Range Therapeutic: 0.8-1.5 mg/dL (SI: 19-35 μmol/L), some method variation

Patient Information Drops can be placed directly in the mouth or mixed with cereal, fruit juice, or other food; take only the prescribed dose. Vitamin E toxicity appears as blurred vision, diarrhea, dizziness, flu-like symptoms, nausea, headache; swallow capsules whole, do not crush or chew

Nursing Implications Monitor plasma tocopherol concentrations (normal range: 6-14 mcg/mL)

Additional Information 1 mg *dl*-alpha tocopheryl acetate = 1 int. unit

(Continued)

Vitamin E *(Continued)*

Dosage Forms

Capsule: 100 units, 200 units, 400 units, 500 units, 600 units, 1000 units
Capsule, water miscible: 73.5 mg, 147 mg, 165 mg, 330 mg, 400 units
Cream: 50 mg/g (15 g, 30 g, 60 g, 75 g, 120 g, 454 g)
Liquid, oral [drops]: 50 mg/mL (12 mL, 30 mL)
Liquid, topical: 10 mL, 15 mL, 30 mL, 60 mL
Lotion: 120 mL
Oil: 15 mL, 30 mL, 60 mL
Ointment, topical: 30 mg/g (45 g, 60 g)
Tablet: 200 units, 400 units

◆ **Vitamin G** *see* Riboflavin *on page 1191*

◆ **Vitamin K₁** *see* Phytonadione *on page 1082*

◆ **Vitamin K Content in Selected Foods** *see page 1738*

Vitamins (Multiple) *(VYE ta mins, MUL ti pul)*

U.S. Brand Names Becotin® Pulvules®; Cefol® Filmtab®; Eldercaps® [OTC]; NeoVadrin® [OTC]; Niferex®-PN; Secran®; Stresstabs® 600 Advanced Formula [OTC]; Therabid® [OTC]; Theragran® [OTC]; Theragran® Hematinic®; Theragran® Liquid [OTC]; Theragran-M® [OTC]; Unicap® [OTC]; Vicon Forte®; Vicon® Plus [OTC]; ViDaylin®

Synonyms B Complex; B Complex With C; Children's Vitamins; Hexavitamin; Multiple Vitamins; Multivitamins, Fluoride; Parenteral Multiple Vitamins; Prenatal Vitamins; Therapeutic Multivitamins; Vitamins, Multiple (Injectable); Vitamins, Multiple (Oral); Vitamins, Multiple (Pediatric); Vitamins, Multiple (Prenatal); Vitamins, Multiple (Therapeutic); Vitamins, Multiple With Iron

Therapeutic Category Vitamin

Use Dietary supplement

Pregnancy Risk Factor A/C (dose exceeding RDA recommendation)

Contraindications Hypersensitivity to any component of the formulation; pre-existing hypervitaminosis

Warnings/Precautions RDA values are not requirements, but are recommended daily intakes of certain essential nutrients; periodic dental exams should be performed to check for dental fluorosis; use with caution in patients with severe renal or liver failure. Pediatric infusion contains vitamin K (caution in patients receiving coumarin anticoagulants). Additional vitamin A may be required in pediatric patients.

Adverse Reactions

1% to 10%: Hypervitaminosis; refer to individual vitamin entries for individual reactions
<1% (Limited to important or life-threatening): Allergic reactions, anaphylaxis following parenteral administration (rare)
Rare reports following I.V. administration: Agitation, anxiety, diplopia, dizziness, edema (peripheral), erythema, headache, pruritus, rash, urticaria

Drug Interactions

Decreased Effect:

Hydralazine: May decreased the effect of pyridoxine
Isoniazid: May decreased the effect of pyridoxine
Levodopa: Pyridoxine may decrease the effect of levodopa
Methotrexate: Folic acid may decrease response to methotrexate therapy
Phenytoin: Folic acid may lower serum phenytoin concentrations; phenytoin may lower serum folate concentrations
Warfarin: Vitamin K (contained in pediatric infusion) may antagonize the effect of warfarin

Stability Store injection at 2°C to 8°C (36°F to 46°F); some components are light sensitive

Not compatible with alkaline solutions/medications (such as, acetazolamide, chlorothiazide, aminophylline, or bicarbonate); not compatible with ampicillin or fat emulsions

Usual Dosage

Infants 1.5-3 kg: I.V.: 3.25 mL/24 hours (M.V.I.® Pediatric)
Children:
Oral:
≤2 years: Drops: 1 mL/day (premature infants may get 0.5-1 mL/day)
>2 years: Chew 1 tablet/day
≥4 years: 5 mL/day liquid
I.V.: >3 kg and <11 years: 5 mL/24 hours (M.V.I.® Pediatric)
Adults:
Oral: 1 tablet/day or 5 mL/day liquid
I.V.: >11 years: 5 mL of vials 1 and 2 (M.V.I.®-12)/one TPN bag/day
I.V. solutions: 10 mL/24 hours (M.V.I.®-12)

Reference Range Recommended daily allowances are published by Food and Nutrition Board, National Research Council - National Academy of Sciences and are revised periodically. RDA quantities apply only to healthy persons and are not intended to cover therapeutic nutrition requirements in disease or other abnormal states (ie, metabolic disorders, weight reduction, chronic disease, drug therapy).

Test Interactions Ascorbic acid in the urine can cause false negative urine glucose determinations

Patient Information Take only amount prescribed

Nursing Implications Doses may be higher for burn or cystic fibrosis patients

Dosage Forms

Caplet/Tablet (content per caplet/tablet) (Hexavitamin): A 5000 int. units, D 400 int. units, C 75 mg, B_1 2 mg, B_2 3 mg, B_3 20 mg
Injection (content per 5 mL) (M.V.I.®-12): A 3300 int. units, D 200 int. units, E 10 int. units, C 100 mg, FA 0.4 mg, B_1 3 mg, B_2 3.6 mg, B_3 40 mg, B_6 4 mg, B_{12} 5 mcg, B_5 15 mg, biotin 60 mcg
Liquid, oral (content per 5 mL) (Theragran®): A 10,000 int. units, D 400 int. units, C 200 mg, B_1 10 mg, B_2 10 mg, B_3 100 mg, B_6 4.1 mg, B_{12} 5 mcg, B_5 21.4 mg

Liquid, oral [drops] (content per 1 mL):

Vi-Daylin®: A 1500 int. units, D 400 int. units, E 4.1 int. units, C 35 mg, B_1 0.5 mg, B_2 0.6 mg, B_3 8 mg, B_6 0.4 mg, B_{12} 1.5 mcg, alcohol <0.5%

Vi-Daylin® Iron (content per 1 mL): A 1500 int. units, D 400 int. units, E 4.1 int. units, C 35 mg, B_1 0.5 mg, B_2 0.6 mg, B_3 8 mg, B_6 0.4 mg, Fe 10 mg

Powder, pediatric (content per 5 mL) (M.V.I.®): A 2300 int. units, D 400, E 7 int. units, C 80 mg, FA 0.14 mg, B_1 1.2 mg, B_2 1.4 mg, B_3 17 mg, B_6 1 mg, B_{12} 1 mcg, B_5 5 mg, biotin 20 mcg, vitamin K 200 mcg

Tablet (content per tablet):

Albee® with C: C 300 mg, B_1 15 mg, B_2 10.2 mg, B_6 5 mg, niacinamide 50 mg, pantothenic acid 10 mg

Iberet-Folic-500®: C 500 mg, FA 0.8 mg, B_1 6 mg, B_2 6 mg, B_3 30 mg, B_6 5 mg, B_{12} 25 mcg, B_5 10 mg, Fe 105 mg

Stuartnatal® 1+1: A 4000 int. units, D 400 int. units, E 11 int units, C 120 mg, FA 1 mg, B_1 1.5 mg, B_2 3 mg, B_3 20 mg, B_6 10 mg, B_{12} 12 mcg, Cu, Zn 25 mg, Fe 65 mg, Ca 200 mg

Theragran-M®: A 5000 int. units, D 400 int. units, E 30 int. units, C 90 mg, FA 0.4 mg, B_1 3 mg, B_2 3.4 mg, B_3 30 mg, B_6 3 mg, B_{12} 9 mcg, Cl, Cr, I, K, B_5 10 mg, Mg, Mn, Mo, P, Se, Zn 15 mg, Fe 27 mg, biotin 30 mcg, beta-carotene 1250 int. units

Vi-Daylin®: A 2500 int. units, D 400 int. units, E 15 int. units, C 60 mg, FA 0.3 mg, B_1 1.05 mg, B_2 1.2 mg, B_3 13.5 mg, B_6 1.05 mg, B_{12} 4.5 mcg

Vitamin B complex: FA 400 mcg, B_1 1.5 mg, B_2 1.7 mg, B_6 2 mg, B_{12} 6 mcg, niacinamide 20 mg

- ♦ **Vitamins, Multiple (Injectable)** *see* Vitamins (Multiple) *on page 1424*
- ♦ **Vitamins, Multiple (Oral)** *see* Vitamins (Multiple) *on page 1424*
- ♦ **Vitamins, Multiple (Pediatric)** *see* Vitamins (Multiple) *on page 1424*
- ♦ **Vitamins, Multiple (Prenatal)** *see* Vitamins (Multiple) *on page 1424*
- ♦ **Vitamins, Multiple (Therapeutic)** *see* Vitamins (Multiple) *on page 1424*
- ♦ **Vitamins, Multiple With Iron** *see* Vitamins (Multiple) *on page 1424*
- ♦ **Vita-Plus® E Softgels® [OTC]** *see* Vitamin E *on page 1423*
- ♦ **Vitec® [OTC]** *see* Vitamin E *on page 1423*
- ♦ **Vite E® Creme [OTC]** *see* Vitamin E *on page 1423*
- ♦ **Vitrasert®** *see* Ganciclovir *on page 618*
- ♦ **Vitravene™** *see* Fomivirsen *on page 601*
- ♦ **Vivactil®** *see* Protriptyline *on page 1154*
- ♦ **Vivelle®** *see* Estradiol *on page 491*
- ♦ **Vivelle-Dot™** *see* Estradiol *on page 491*
- ♦ **Vivol® (Can)** *see* Diazepam *on page 390*
- ♦ **Vivotif Berna™** *see* Typhoid Vaccine *on page 1387*
- ♦ **VLB** *see* VinBLAStine *on page 1415*
- ♦ **VM-26** *see* Teniposide *on page 1296*
- ♦ **Volmax®** *see* Albuterol *on page 41*
- ♦ **Voltaren®** *see* Diclofenac *on page 393*
- ♦ **Voltaren Ophtha® (Can)** *see* Diclofenac *on page 393*
- ♦ **Voltaren Rapide® (Can)** *see* Diclofenac *on page 393*
- ♦ **Voltaren®-XR** *see* Diclofenac *on page 393*
- ♦ **VōSol®** *see* Acetic Acid *on page 31*
- ♦ **VōSol® HC** *see* Acetic Acid, Propylene Glycol Diacetate, and Hydrocortisone *on page 31*
- ♦ **VP-16** *see* Etoposide *on page 533*
- ♦ **VP-16-213** *see* Etoposide *on page 533*
- ♦ **Vumon** *see* Teniposide *on page 1296*
- ♦ **V.V.S.®** *see* Sulfabenzamide, Sulfacetamide, and Sulfathiazole *on page 1268*
- ♦ **Vytone®** *see* Iodoquinol and Hydrocortisone *on page 738*
- ♦ **VZIG** *see* Varicella-Zoster Immune Globulin (Human) *on page 1406*

Warfarin (WAR far in)

U.S. Brand Names Coumadin®

Canadian Brand Names Coumadin®; Taro-Warfarin

Synonyms Warfarin Sodium

Therapeutic Category Anticoagulant

Use Prophylaxis and treatment of venous thrombosis, pulmonary embolism and thromboembolic disorders; atrial fibrillation with risk of embolism and as an adjunct in the prophylaxis of systemic embolism after myocardial infarction

Unlabeled/Investigational Use Prevention of recurrent transient ischemic attacks and to reduce risk of recurrent myocardial infarction

Pregnancy Risk Factor D

Pregnancy/Breast-Feeding Implications

Clinical effects on the fetus: Oral anticoagulants cross the placenta and produce fetal abnormalities. Warfarin should not be used during pregnancy because of significant risks. Adjusted-dose heparin can be given safely throughout pregnancy in patients with venous thromboembolism.

Breast-feeding/lactation: Warfarin does not pass into breast milk and can be given to nursing mothers

Contraindications Hypersensitivity to warfarin or any component of the formulation; hemorrhagic tendencies; hemophilia; thrombocytopenia purpura; leukemia; recent or potential surgery of the eye or CNS; major regional lumbar block anesthesia or surgery resulting in large, open surfaces; patients bleeding from the GI, respiratory, or GU tract; threatened abortion; aneurysm; ascorbic acid deficiency; history of bleeding diathesis; prostatectomy; continuous tube drainage of the small intestine; polyarthritis; diverticulitis; emaciation; malnutrition; cerebrovascular hemorrhage; eclampsia/pre-eclampsia; blood dyscrasias; severe

(Continued)

Warfarin *(Continued)*

uncontrolled or malignant hypertension; severe hepatic disease; pericarditis or pericardial effusion; subacute bacterial endocarditis; visceral carcinoma; following spinal puncture and other diagnostic or therapeutic procedures with potential for significant bleeding; history of warfarin-induced necrosis; an unreliable, noncompliant patient; alcoholism; patient who has a history of falls or is a significant fall risk; pregnancy

Warnings/Precautions

Do not switch brands once desired therapeutic response has been achieved

Use with caution in patients with active tuberculosis or diabetes

Concomitant use with vitamin K may decrease anticoagulant effect; monitor carefully

Concomitant use with NSAIDs or aspirin may cause severe GI irritation and also increase the risk of bleeding due to impaired platelet function

Salicylates may further increase warfarin's effect by displacing it from plasma protein binding sites

Patients with protein C or S deficiency are at increased risk of skin necrosis syndrome

Before committing an elderly patient to long-term anticoagulation therapy, their risk for bleeding complications secondary to falls, drug interactions, living situation, and cognitive status should be considered. The risk for bleeding complications decreases with the duration of therapy and may increase with advancing age.

If a patient is to undergo an invasive surgical procedure (dental to actual minor/major surgery), warfarin should be stopped 3 days before the scheduled surgery date and the INR/PT should be checked prior to the procedure

Adverse Reactions As with all anticoagulants, bleeding is the major adverse effect of warfarin. Hemorrhage may occur at virtually any site. Risk is dependent on multiple variables, including the intensity of anticoagulation and patient susceptibility.

Additional adverse effects are often related to idiosyncratic reactions, and the frequency cannot be accurately estimated.

Cardiovascular: Vasculitis, edema, hemorrhagic shock

Central nervous system: Fever, lethargy, malaise, asthenia, pain, headache, dizziness, stroke

Dermatologic: Rash, dermatitis, bullous eruptions, urticaria, pruritus, alopecia

Gastrointestinal: Anorexia, nausea, vomiting, stomach cramps, abdominal pain, diarrhea, flatulence, gastrointestinal bleeding, taste disturbance, mouth ulcers

Genitourinary: Priapism, hematuria

Hematologic: Hemorrhage, leukopenia, unrecognized bleeding sites (eg, colon cancer) may be uncovered by anticoagulation, retroperitoneal hematoma, agranulocytosis

Hepatic: Increased transaminases, hepatic injury, jaundice,

Neuromuscular & skeletal: Paresthesia, osteoporosis

Respiratory: Hemoptysis, epistaxis, pulmonary hemorrhage, tracheobronchial calcification

Miscellaneous: Hypersensitivity/allergic reactions

Skin necrosis/gangrene, due to paradoxical local thrombosis, is a known but rare risk of warfarin therapy. Its onset is usually within the first few days of therapy and is frequently localized to the limbs, breast or penis. The risk of this effect is increased in patients with protein C or S deficiency.

"Purple toes syndrome," caused by cholesterol microembolization, also occurs rarely. Typically, this occurs after several weeks of therapy, and may present as a dark, purplish, mottled discoloration of the plantar and lateral surfaces. Other manifestations of cholesterol microembolization may include rash, livedo reticularis, rash, gangrene, abrupt and intense pain in lower extremities, abdominal, flank, or back pain, hematuria, renal insufficiency, hypertension, cerebral ischemia, spinal cord infarction, or other symptom of vascular compromise.

Overdosage/Toxicology See table. Symptoms include internal or external hemorrhage and hematuria. Avoid emesis and lavage to avoid possible trauma and incidental bleeding. When

Management of Elevated INR

INR	Patient Situation	Action
>3 and <5	No bleeding or need for rapid reversal (ie, no need for surgery)	Omit next few warfarin dose and/or restart at lower dose when INR approaches desired range. If only minimally above range, then no dosage reduction may be required.
>5 and <9.0	No bleeding or need for rapid reversal	Omit next 1-2 doses, monitor INR more frequently, and restart at lower dose when INR approaches target range **or** omit dose and give 1-2.5 mg vitamin K orally (use this if patient has risk factors for bleeding).
	No bleeding but reversal needed for surgery or dental extraction within 24 hours	Vitamin K 2-4 mg orally (expected reversal within 24 hours); give additional 1-2 mg if INR remains high at 24 hours.
>9.0 and <20.0	No bleeding	Stop warfarin, give vitamin K 3-5 mg orally; follow INR closely; repeat vitamin K if needed. Reassess need and dose of warfarin when INR approaches desirable range.
Rapid reversal required (ie, INR >20)	Serious bleeding or major warfarin overdose	Stop warfarin, give vitamin K 10 mg by slow I.V. infusion. May repeat vitamin K every 12 hours and give fresh plasma transfusion or prothrombin complex concentrate as needed. When appropriate, heparin can be given until the patient becomes responsive to warfarin.

an overdose occurs, the drug should be immediately discontinued and vitamin K_1 (phytonadione) may be administered, up to 25 mg I.V. for adults. When hemorrhage occurs, fresh frozen plasma transfusions can help control bleeding by replacing clotting factors. In urgent bleeding, prothrombin complex concentrates may be needed.

Drug Interactions
Cytochrome P450 Effect: CYP1A2 enzyme substrate (minor), CYP2C8, 2C9, 2C18, 2C19, and 3A3/4 enzyme substrate; CYP2C9, 2C19 enzyme inhibitor

Increased Effect/Toxicity:

See tables.

Increased Bleeding Tendency

Inhibit Platelet Aggregation	Inhibit Procoagulant Factors	Ulcerogenic Drugs
Cephalosporins Dipyridamole Indomethacin Oxyphenbutazone Penicillin, parenteral Phenylbutazone Salicylates Sulfinpyrazone	Antimetabolites Quinidine Quinine Salicylates	Adrenal corticosteroids Indomethacin Oxyphenbutazone Phenylbutazone Potassium products Salicylates

Use of these agents with oral anticoagulants may increase the chances of hemorrhage.

Enhanced Anticoagulant Effects

Decrease Vitamin K	Displace Anticoagulant	Inhibit Metabolism	Other
Oral antibiotics: Can ↑/↓ INR Check INR 3 days after a patient begins antibiotics to see the INR value and adjust the warfarin dose accordingly	Chloral hydrate Clofibrate Diazoxide Ethacrynic acid Miconazole (including intravaginal use) Nalidixic acid Phenylbutazone Salicylates Sulfonamides Sulfonylureas	Allopurinol Amiodarone Azole antifungals Capecitabine Chloramphenicol Chlorpropamide Cimetidine Ciprofloxacin Co-trimoxazole Disulfiram Ethanol (acute ingestion)* Flutamide Isoniazid Metronidazole Norfloxacin Ofloxacin Omperazole Phenylbutazone Phenytoin Propafenone Propoxyphene Protease inhibitors Quinidine Sulfinpyrazone Sulfonamides Tamoxifen Tolbutamide Zafirlukast Zileuton	Acetaminophen Anabolic steroids Clarithromycin Clofibrate Danazol Erythromycin Gemfibrozil Glucagon Influenza vaccine Propranolol Propylthiouracil Ranitidine SSRIs Sulindac Tetracycline Thyroid drugs Vitamin E (≥400 int. units)

* The hypoprothrombinemic effect of oral anticoagulants has been reported to be both increased and decreased during chronic and excessive alcohol ingestion. Data are insufficient to predict the direction of this interaction in alcoholic patients.

Decreased Effect: See table.

Decreased Anticoagulant Effects

Induction of Enzymes		Increased Procoagulant Factors	Decreased Drug Absorption	Other
Barbiturates Carbamazepine Glutethimide Griseofulvin	Nafcillin Phenytoin Rifampin	Estrogens Oral contraceptives Vitamin K (including nutritional supplements)	Aluminum hydroxide Cholestyramine* Colestipol*	Ethchlorvynol Griseofulvin Spironolactone† Sucralfate

Decreased anticoagulant effect may occur when these drugs are administered with oral anticoagulants.

*Cholestyramine and colestipol may increase the anticoagulant effect by binding vitamin K in the gut; yet, the decreased drug absorption appears to be of more concern.

†Diuretic-induced hemoconcentration with subsequent concentration of clotting factors has been reported to decrease the effects of oral anticoagulants.

Ethanol/Nutrition/Herb Interactions
Ethanol: Avoid ethanol. Acute ethanol ingestion (binge drinking) decreases the metabolism of warfarin and increases PT/INR. Chronic daily ethanol use increases the metabolism of warfarin and decreases PT/INR.

Food: The anticoagulant effects of warfarin may be decreased if taken with foods rich in vitamin K. Vitamin E may increase warfarin effect.

(Continued)

Warfarin *(Continued)*

Herb/Nutraceutical: St John's wort may decrease warfarin levels. Alfalfa contains large amounts of vitamin K as do many enteral products. Coenzyme Q_{10} may decrease response to warfarin. Avoid cat's claw, dong quai, evening primrose, feverfew, red clover, horse chestnut, garlic, green tea, ginseng, ginkgo (all have additional antiplatelet activity).

Stability Protect from light; injection is stable for 4 hours at room temperature after reconstitution with 2.7 mL of sterile water (yields 2 mg/mL solution)

Mechanism of Action Interferes with hepatic synthesis of vitamin K-dependent coagulation factors (II, VII, IX, X)

Pharmacodynamics/Kinetics

Onset of action: Anticoagulation: Oral: 36-72 hours

Peak effect: Full therapeutic effect: 5-7 days; INR may increase in 36-72 hours

Duration: 2-5 days

Absorption: Oral: Rapid

Metabolism: Hepatic

Half-life elimination: 20-60 hours; Mean: 40 hours; highly variable among individuals

Usual Dosage

Oral:

Infants and Children: 0.05-0.34 mg/kg/day; infants <12 months of age may require doses at or near the high end of this range; consistent anticoagulation may be difficult to maintain in children <5 years of age

Adults: Initial dosing must be individualized based upon patient's end organ function, concurrent therapy, and risk of bleeding; ACCP recommendation: 5 mg/day for 2-5 days, then adjust dose according to results of prothrombin time; usual maintenance dose ranges from 2-10 mg/day (selected sensitive patients may require less; resistant patients may require higher dosages).

Note: Lower starting doses may be required for patients with hepatic impairment, poor nutrition, CHF, elderly, or a high risk of bleeding. Higher initial doses may be reasonable in selected patients (ie, receiving enzyme-inducing agents and with low risk of bleeding).

I.V. (administer as a slow bolus injection): 2-5 mg/day

Dosing adjustment/comments in hepatic disease: Monitor effect at usual doses; the response to oral anticoagulants may be markedly enhanced in obstructive jaundice (due to reduced vitamin K absorption) and also in hepatitis and cirrhosis (due to decreased production of vitamin K-dependent clotting factors); prothrombin index should be closely monitored

Dietary Considerations Foods high in vitamin K (eg, beef liver, pork liver, green tea and leafy green vegetables) inhibit anticoagulant effect. Do not change dietary habits once stabilized on warfarin therapy; a balanced diet with a consistent intake of vitamin K is essential; avoid large amounts of alfalfa, asparagus, broccoli, Brussels sprouts, cabbage, cauliflower, green teas, kale, lettuce, spinach, turnip greens, watercress decrease efficacy of warfarin. It is recommended that the diet contain a CONSISTENT vitamin K content of 70-140 mcg/day. Check with healthcare provider before changing diet.

Administration

Oral: Do not take with food. Take at the same time each day.

I.V.: Administer as a slow bolus injection over 1-2 minutes; avoid all I.M. injections

Monitoring Parameters Prothrombin time, hematocrit, INR

Reference Range

Therapeutic: 2-5 µg/mL (SI: 6.5-16.2 µmol/L)

Prothrombin time should be 1½ to 2 times the control or INR should be ↑ 2 to 3 times based upon indication

Normal prothrombin time: 10-13 seconds

INR ranges based upon indication: See table.

INR Ranges Based Upon Indication

Indication	Targeted INR Range	Targeted INR
Acute myocardial infarction with risk factor*	2.0-3.0	2.5
Atrial fibrillation (moderate- to high-risk patients)	2.0-3.0	2.5
Bileaflet or tilting disk mechanical aortic valve (NSR, NL LA)	2.0-3.0	2.5
Bileaflet mechanical aortic valve with atrial fibrillation	2.5-3.5	3
Bileaflet mechanical aortic valve with atrial fibrillation with ASA 80-100 mg/day	2.0-3.0	2.5
Bileaflet or tilting disk mechanical mitral valve	2.5-3.5	3
Bileaflet or tilting disk mechanical mitral valve with ASA 80-100 mg/day	2.0-3.0	2.5
Bioprosthetic mitral or aortic valve†	2.0-3.0	2.5
Bioprosthetic mitral or aortic valve with atrial fibrillation	2.0-3.0	2.5
Cardioembolic cerebral ischemic events	2.0-3.0	2.5
Mechanical heart valve (caged ball, caged disk) with ASA 80-100 mg/day	2.5-3.5	3
Mechanical prosthetic valve with systemic embolism despite adequate anticoagulation‡	2.5-3.5	3
Rheumatic mitral valve disease and NSR (left atrial diameter >5.5 cm)	2.0-3.0	2.5
Venous thromboembolism	2.0-3.0	2.5

*Up to 3 months of therapy following heparin or LMWH in patients with anterior Q-wave infarction, severe left-ventricular dysfunction, mural thrombus on 2D echo, atrial fibrillation, history of systemic or pulmonary embolism, congestive heart failure

†Maintained for 3 months; chronic low-dose aspirin (80 mg/day) after warfarin therapy.

‡Add ASA 80-100 mg/day

For complete discussion, *Chest*, 2001, 119 (Suppl):1S-370S

Warfarin levels are not used for monitoring degree of anticoagulation. They may be useful if a patient with unexplained coagulopathy is using the drug surreptitiously or if it is unclear whether clinical resistance is due to true drug resistance or lack of drug intake.

Normal prothrombin time (PT): 10.9-12.9 seconds. Healthy premature newborns have prolonged coagulation test screening results (eg, PT, aPTT, TT) which return to normal adult values at approximately 6 months of age. Healthy prematures, however, do not develop spontaneous hemorrhage or thrombotic complications because of a balance between procoagulants and inhibitors

The World Health Organization (WHO), in cooperation with other regulatory-advisory bodies, has developed system of standardizing the reporting of PT values through the determination of the International Normalized Ratio (INR). The INR involves the standardization of the PT by the generation of two pieces of information: the PT ratio and the International Sensitivity Index (ISI)

Therapeutic ranges are now available or being developed to assist practicing physicians in their treatment of patients with a wide variety of thrombotic disorders

Test Interactions Warfarin increases aPTT

Patient Information
  Call your physician or nurse immediately if you have any of the following:
    A fever or developing illness, including vomiting, diarrhea, or infection
    Pain, swelling, discomfort or any other unusual symptoms
    Prolonged bleeding from cuts, nosebleeds
    Unusual bleeding from gums when brushing teeth
    Increased menstrual flow or vaginal bleeding
    Red or dark brown urine
    Red or tarry-black stools
    Unusual bruising for unknown reasons
    Pregnancy or planned pregnancy

  Call your physician immediately if you have serious fall or trauma.

  Discuss any new medications with your physician or pharmacist - talk to your physician before starting, changing, or discontinuing any medication (including OTC medications).

  Notify you physician immediately with any severe diarrhea (alters absorption of vitamin K) to discuss the need to check INR.

  Try to keep the same general diet and avoid excessive amounts of alcohol.

  Carry Medi-Alert® ID identifying drug usage.

  If you forget to take a pill one day, let your physician know. DO NOT TAKE ANOTHER PILL TO "CATCH UP".

  Consult physician before undergoing dental work or elective surgery.

  Concomitant use of aspirin or nonsteroidal anti-inflammatory medicine, such as Motrin® or Advil®, is NOT RECOMMENDED unless discussed with your physician.

  It is important to strictly adhere to the prescribed dosing schedule. Dosage is highly individual and may need to be adjusted several times based on lab test results.

Nursing Implications Should not be given in close proximity to other drugs because absorption may be decreased. Administer warfarin at least 1-2 hours prior to, or 6 hours after, cholestyramine or sucralfate, because cholestyramine or sucralfate may bind warfarin and decrease its total absorption; avoid all I.M. injections.

Dosage Forms
  Powder for injection, lyophilized, as sodium: 5 mg
  Tablet, as sodium: 1 mg, 2 mg, 2.5 mg, 3 mg, 4 mg, 5 mg, 6 mg, 7.5 mg, 10 mg

♦ **Yeast-Gard® Medicated Douche [OTC]** *see Povidone-Iodine on page 1114*

Yellow Fever Vaccine (YEL oh FEE ver vak SEEN)

Related Information
Immunization Recommendations *on page 1538*

U.S. Brand Names YF-VAX®

Canadian Brand Names YF-Vax™

Therapeutic Category Vaccine, Live Virus

Use Induction of active immunity against yellow fever virus, primarily among persons traveling or living in areas where yellow fever infection exists. (Some countries require a valid international Certification of Vaccination showing receipt of vaccine; if a pregnant woman is to be vaccinated only to satisfy an international requirement, efforts should be made to obtain a waiver letter.) The WHO requires revaccination every 10 years to maintain traveler's vaccination certificate.

Pregnancy Risk Factor D

Contraindications Hypersensitivity to egg or chick embryo protein, or any component of the formulation; pregnant women, children <6 months of age unless in high risk area

Warnings/Precautions Do not use in immunodeficient persons or patients receiving immunosuppressants (eg, steroids, radiation); have epinephrine available in persons with previous history of egg allergy if the vaccine must be used. Avoid use in infants <6 months and pregnant women unless travel to high-risk areas are unavoidable; avoid use in infants <4 months of age.

Adverse Reactions All serious adverse reactions must be reported to the U.S. Department of Health and Human Services (DHHS) Vaccine Adverse Event Reporting System (VAERS) 1-800-822-7967.
>10%: Central nervous system: Fever, malaise (7-14 days after administration ~10%)
1% to 10%:
 Central nervous system: Headache (2% to 5%)
 Neuromuscular & skeletal: Myalgia (2% to 5%)
<1% (Limited to important or life-threatening): Anaphylaxis, encephalitis in very young infants (rare)

Stability Yellow fever vaccine is shipped with dry ice; do not use vaccine unless shipping case contains some dry ice on arrival; maintain vaccine continuously at a temperature between 0°C to 5°C (32°F to 41°F)

Usual Dosage One dose (0.5 mL) S.C. 10 days to 10 years before travel, booster every 10 years; see Warnings/Precautions

Administration Do not reconstitute the powder for injection with a diluent that has preservatives since they may inactivate the live virus

Patient Information Immunity develops by the tenth day and **WHO** requires revaccination every 10 years to maintain travelers' vaccination certificates

Nursing Implications Sterilize and discard all unused rehydrated vaccine and containers after 1 hour; avoid vigorous shaking

Additional Information Federal law requires that the date of administration, the vaccine manufacturer, lot number of vaccine, and the administering person's name, title, and address be entered into the patient's permanent medical record.

Dosage Forms Injection: Not less than 5.04 Log_{10} plaque-forming units (PFU) per 0.5 mL

♦ **YF-VAX®** *see Yellow Fever Vaccine on page 1430*
♦ **Yodoxin®** *see Iodoquinol on page 738*
♦ **Zaditen® (Can)** *see Ketotifen on page 767*
♦ **Zaditor™** *see Ketotifen on page 767*

Zafirlukast (za FIR loo kast)

Related Information
Asthma *on page 1645*

U.S. Brand Names Accolate®

Canadian Brand Names Accolate®

Synonyms ICI 204, 219

Therapeutic Category Leukotriene Receptor Antagonist

Use Prophylaxis and chronic treatment of asthma in adults and children ≥5 years of age

Pregnancy Risk Factor B

Pregnancy/Breast-Feeding Implications
Clinical effects on the fetus: At 2000 mg/kg/day in rats, maternal toxicity and deaths were seen with increased incidence of early fetal resorption. Spontaneous abortions occurred in cynomolgus monkeys at a maternally toxic dose of 2000 mg/kg/day orally. There are no adequate and well controlled trials in pregnant women.
Breast-feeding/lactation: Zafirlukast is excreted in breast milk; do not administer to nursing women

Contraindications Hypersensitivity to zafirlukast or any component of the formulation

Warnings/Precautions The clearance of zafirlukast is reduced in patients with stable alcoholic cirrhosis such that the C_{max} and AUC are approximately 50% to 60% greater than those of normal adults.

Zafirlukast is not indicated for use in the reversal of bronchospasm in acute asthma attacks, including status asthmaticus. Therapy with zafirlukast can be continued during acute exacerbations of asthma.

An increased proportion of zafirlukast patients >55 years of age reported infections as compared to placebo-treated patients. These infections were mostly mild or moderate in intensity and predominantly affected the respiratory tract. Infections occurred equally in both sexes, were dose-proportional to total milligrams of zafirlukast exposure and were associated with coadministration of inhaled corticosteroids.

Rare hepatic events have been reported, including hepatitis, hyperbilirubinemia, and hepatic failure. Female patients may be at greater risk. Discontinue **immediately** if liver dysfunction is suspected. If hepatic dysfunction is suspected (due to clinical signs/symptoms) liver function tests should be measured immediately. Do not resume or restart if hepatic function tests are consistent with dysfunction.

Rare cases of eosinophilic vasculitis (Churg-Strauss) have been reported in patients receiving zafirlukast (usually, but not always, associated with reduction in concurrent steroid dosage). No causal relationship established.

Adverse Reactions

>10%: Central nervous system: Headache (12.9%)

1% to 10%:

Central nervous system: Dizziness, pain, fever

Gastrointestinal: Nausea, diarrhea, abdominal pain, vomiting, dyspepsia

Hepatic: SGPT elevation

Neuromuscular & skeletal: Back pain, myalgia, weakness

<1% (Limited to important or life-threatening): Agranulocytosis, arthralgia, bleeding, edema, hepatic failure, hepatitis, hyperbilirubinemia, hypersensitivity reactions (urticaria, angioedema, rash), systemic eosinophilia with clinical features of Churg-Strauss syndrome (rare)

Overdosage/Toxicology Ingestions of up to 200 mg have been reported. Rash and upset stomach were the predominant symptoms. Treatment should be symptomatic and supportive.

Drug Interactions

Cytochrome P450 Effect: CYP2C9 enzyme substrate; CYP2C9 and 3A3/4 enzyme inhibitor

Increased Effect/Toxicity: Zafirlukast concentrations are increased by aspirin. Warfarin effect may be increased with zafirlukast. Zafirlukast may increase theophylline levels.

Decreased Effect: Zafirlukast concentrations may be reduced by erythromycin and terfenadine.

Ethanol/Nutrition/Herb Interactions Food: Decreases bioavailability of zafirlukast by 40%.

Stability Store tablets at controlled room temperature (20°C to 25°C; 68°F to 77°F); protect from light and moisture; dispense in original airtight container

Mechanism of Action Zafirlukast is a selectively and competitive leukotriene-receptor antagonist (LTRA) of leukotriene D4 and E4 (LTD4 and LTE4), components of slow-reacting substance of anaphylaxis (SRSA). Cysteinyl leukotriene production and receptor occupation have been correlated with the pathophysiology of asthma, including airway edema, smooth muscle constriction and altered cellular activity associated with the inflammatory process, which contribute to the signs and symptoms of asthma.

Pharmacodynamics/Kinetics

Protein binding: >99%, primarily albumin

Metabolism: Extensively hepatic via CYP450 2C9 enzyme pathway

Bioavailability: Reduced 40% with food

Half-life elimination: 10 hours

Time to peak, serum: 3 hours

Excretion: Urine (10%); feces

Usual Dosage Oral:

Children <5 years: Safety and effectiveness have not been established

Children 5-11 years: 10 mg twice daily

Children ≥12 years and Adults: 20 mg twice daily

Elderly: The mean dose (mg/kg) normalized AUC and C_{max} increase and plasma clearance decreases with increasing age. In patients >65 years of age, there is a two- to threefold greater C_{max} and AUC compared to younger adults.

Dosing adjustment in renal impairment: There are no apparent differences in the pharmacokinetics between renally impaired patients and normal subjects.

Dosing adjustment in hepatic impairment: In patients with hepatic impairment (ie, biopsy-proven cirrhosis), there is a 50% to 60% greater C_{max} and AUC compared to normal subjects.

Dietary Considerations Should be taken on an empty stomach (1 hour before or 2 hours after meals).

Administration Administer at least 1 hour before or 2 hours after a meal

Patient Information Take regularly as prescribed, even during symptom-free periods. This medication should be taken on an empty stomach (1 hour before or 2 hours after meals). Do not use to treat acute episodes of asthma. Do not decrease the dose or stop taking any other antiasthma medications unless instructed by a physician. Nursing women should not take zafirlukast. Contact prescriber immediately if experiencing right upper abdominal pain, nausea, fatigue, itching, flu-like symptoms; swelling of the eyes, face, neck, or throat; worsening of condition or anorexia.

Dosage Forms Tablet: 10 mg, 20 mg

♦ **Zagam**® see Sparfloxacin on page 1255

Zalcitabine (zal SITE a been)

Related Information

Antiretroviral Agents Comparison on page 1488
Antiretroviral Therapy for HIV Infection on page 1595

U.S. Brand Names Hivid®

Canadian Brand Names Hivid®

Synonyms ddC; Dideoxycytidine

Therapeutic Category Antiretroviral Agent, Nucleoside Reverse Transcriptase Inhibitor (NRTI) [Cytadine Analog]

Use In combination with at least two other antiretrovirals in the treatment of patients with HIV infection; it is not recommended that zalcitabine be given in combination with didanosine, stavudine, or lamivudine due to overlapping toxicities, virologic interactions, or lack of clinical data

Pregnancy Risk Factor C

(Continued)

Zalcitabine *(Continued)*

Pregnancy/Breast-Feeding Implications It is not known if zalcitabine crosses the human placenta. Cases of lactic acidosis/hepatic steatosis syndrome have been reported in pregnant women receiving nucleoside analogue drugs. It is not known if pregnancy itself potentiates this known side effect; however, pregnant women may be at increased risk of lactic acidosis and liver damage. Hepatic enzymes and electrolytes should be monitored frequently during the 3rd trimester of pregnancy in women receiving nucleoside analogues. Health professionals are encouraged to contact the antiretroviral pregnancy registry to monitor outcomes of pregnant women exposed to antiretroviral medications (1-800-258-4263).

Contraindications Hypersensitivity to zalcitabine or any component of the formulation

Warnings/Precautions Careful monitoring of pancreatic enzymes and liver function tests in patients with a history of pancreatitis, increased amylase, those on parenteral nutrition or with a history of ethanol abuse; discontinue use immediately if pancreatitis is suspected; lactic acidosis and severe hepatomegaly and failure have rarely occurred with zalcitabine resulting in fatality (stop treatment if lactic acidosis or hepatotoxicity occurs); some cases may possibly be related to underlying hepatitis B; use with caution in patients on digitalis, congestive heart failure, renal failure, hyperphosphatemia; zalcitabine can cause severe peripheral neuropathy; avoid use, if possible, in patients with pre-existing neuropathy

Adverse Reactions

>10%:

Central nervous system: Fever (5% to 17%), malaise (2% to 13%)

Neuromuscular & skeletal: Peripheral neuropathy (28%)

1% to 10%:

Central nervous system: Headache (2%), dizziness (1%), fatigue (4%), seizures (1.3%)

Dermatologic: Rash (2% to 11%), pruritus (3% to 5%)

Endocrine & metabolic: Hypoglycemia (2% to 6%), hyponatremia (4%), hyperglycemia (1% to 6%)

Gastrointestinal: Nausea (3%), dysphagia (1% to 4%), anorexia (4%), abdominal pain (3% to 8%), vomiting (1% to 3%), diarrhea (<1% to 10%), weight loss, oral ulcers (3% to 7%), increased amylase (3% to 8%)

Hematologic: Anemia (occurs as early as 2-4 weeks), granulocytopenia (usually after 6-8 weeks)

Hepatic: Abnormal hepatic function (9%), hyperbilirubinemia (2% to 5%)

Neuromuscular & skeletal: Myalgia (1% to 6%), foot pain

Respiratory: Pharyngitis (2%), cough (6%), nasal discharge (4%)

<1% (Limited to important or life-threatening): Anaphylaxis, atrial fibrillation, constipation, hepatic failure, hepatitis, hypocalcemia, jaundice, lactic acidosis, night sweats, pancreatitis, syncope

Overdosage/Toxicology Symptoms include delayed peripheral neurotoxicity. Following oral decontamination, treatment is supportive.

Drug Interactions

Increased Effect/Toxicity: Amphotericin, foscarnet, and aminoglycosides may potentiate the risk of developing peripheral neuropathy or other toxicities associated with zalcitabine by interfering with the renal elimination of zalcitabine. Other drugs associated with peripheral neuropathy include chloramphenicol, cisplatin, dapsone, disulfiram, ethionamide, glutethimide, gold, hydralazine, iodoquinol, isoniazid, metronidazole, nitrofurantoin, phenytoin, ribavirin, and vincristine. Concomitant use with zalcitabine may increase risk of peripheral neuropathy. Concomitant use of zalcitabine with didanosine is not recommended.

Ethanol/Nutrition/Herb Interactions Food: Food decreases peak plasma concentrations by 39%. Extent and rate of absorption may be decreased with food.

Stability Tablets should be stored in tightly closed bottles at 59°F to 86°F

Mechanism of Action Purine nucleoside analogue, zalcitabine or 2′,3′-dideoxycytidine (ddC) is converted to active metabolite ddCTP; lack the presence of the 3′-hydroxyl group necessary for phosphodiester linkages during DNA replication. As a result viral replication is prematurely terminated. ddCTP acts as a competitor for binding sites on the HIV-RNA dependent DNA polymerase (reverse transcriptase) to further contribute to inhibition of viral replication.

Pharmacodynamics/Kinetics

Absorption: Well, but variable; decreased by 39% with food

Distribution: Minimal data available; variable CSF penetration

Protein binding: <4%

Metabolism: Intracellularly to active triphosphorylated agent

Bioavailability: >80%

Half-life elimination: 2.9 hours; Renal impairment: ≤8.5 hours

Excretion: Urine (>70% as unchanged drug)

Usual Dosage Oral:

Neonates: Dose unknown

Infants and Children <13 years: Safety and efficacy have not been established; suggested usual dose: 0.01 mg/kg every 8 hours; range: 0.005-0.01 mg/kg every 8 hours

Adolescents and Adults: 0.75 mg 3 times/day

Dosing adjustment in renal impairment: Adults:

Cl_{cr} 10-40 mL/minute: 0.75 mg every 12 hours

Cl_{cr} <10 mL/minute: 0.75 mg every 24 hours

Moderately dialyzable (20% to 50%)

Monitoring Parameters Renal function, viral load, liver function tests, CD4 counts, CBC, serum amylase, triglycerides, calcium

Patient Information Zalcitabine is not a cure; if numbness or tingling occurs, or if persistent, severe abdominal pain, nausea, or vomiting occur, notify physician. Women of childbearing age should use effective contraception while on zalcitabine; take on an empty stomach, if possible.

Additional Information Potential compliance problems, frequency of administration and adverse effects should be discussed with patients before initiating therapy to help prevent the emergence of resistance.

Dosage Forms Tablet: 0.375 mg, 0.75 mg

Zaleplon (ZAL e plon)

U.S. Brand Names Sonata®

Canadian Brand Names Sonata®; Starnoc®

Therapeutic Category Hypnotic

Use Short-term (7-10 days) treatment of insomnia (has been demonstrated to be effective for up to 5 weeks in controlled trial)

Restrictions C-IV

Pregnancy Risk Factor C

Pregnancy/Breast-Feeding Implications Not recommended for use during pregnancy

Contraindications Hypersensitivity to zaleplon or any component of the formulation

Warnings/Precautions Symptomatic treatment of insomnia should be initiated only after careful evaluation of potential causes of sleep disturbance. Failure of sleep disturbance to resolve after 7-10 days may indicate psychiatric and/or medical illness.

Use with caution in patients with depression, particularly if suicidal risk may be present. Use with caution in patients with a history of drug dependence. Abrupt discontinuance may lead to withdrawal symptoms. May impair physical and mental capabilities. Patients must be cautioned about performing tasks which require mental alertness (operating machinery or driving). Use with caution in patients receiving other CNS depressants or psychoactive medications. Effects with other sedative drugs or ethanol may be potentiated.

Use with caution in the elderly, those with compromised respiratory function, or renal and hepatic impairment. Because of the rapid onset of action, zaleplon should be administered immediately prior to bedtime or after the patient has gone to bed and is having difficulty falling asleep.

Adverse Reactions
  1% to 10%:
    Cardiovascular: Peripheral edema, chest pain
    Central nervous system: Amnesia, anxiety, depersonalization, dizziness, hallucinations, hypesthesia, somnolence, vertigo, malaise, depression, lightheadedness, impaired coordination, fever, migraine
    Dermatologic: Photosensitivity reaction, rash, pruritus
    Gastrointestinal: Abdominal pain, anorexia, colitis, dyspepsia, nausea, constipation, xerostomia
    Genitourinary: Dysmenorrhea
    Neuromuscular & skeletal: Paresthesia, tremor, myalgia, weakness, back pain, arthralgia
    Ocular: Abnormal vision, eye pain
    Otic: Hyperacusis
    Miscellaneous: Parosmia
  1% (Limited to important or life-threatening): Alopecia, angina, ataxia, bundle branch block, dysarthria, dystonia, eosinophilia, facial paralysis, glaucoma, intestinal obstruction, paresthesia, pericardial effusion, ptosis, pulmonary embolus, syncope, urinary retention, ventricular tachycardia

Overdosage/Toxicology Symptoms include CNS depression, ranging from drowsiness to coma. Mild overdose is associated with drowsiness, confusion, and lethargy. Serious cases may result in ataxia, respiratory depression, hypotension, hypotonia, coma, and rarely death. Treatment is supportive.

Drug Interactions
  Cytochrome P450 Effect: CYP3A3/4 substrate (minor metabolic pathway)
  Increased Effect/Toxicity: Zaleplon potentiates the CNS effects of CNS depressants, including alcohol, imipramine, and thioridazine. Cimetidine increases concentrations of zaleplon. Avoid concurrent use or use 5 mg zaleplon as starting dose in patient receiving cimetidine.
  Decreased Effect: CYP3A4 inducers (eg, phenytoin, carbamazepine, phenobarbital) could lead to ineffectiveness of zaleplon.

Ethanol/Nutrition/Herb Interactions
  Ethanol: Avoid ethanol (may increase CNS depression).
  Food: High fat meal prolonged absorption; delayed t_{max} by 2 hours, and reduced C_{max} by 35%.
  Herb/Nutraceutical: St John's wort may decrease zaleplon levels. Avoid valerian, St John's wort, kava kava, gotu kola (may increase CNS depression).

Stability Store at controlled room temperature of 20°C to 25°C (68°F to 77°F); protect from light

Mechanism of Action Zaleplon is unrelated to benzodiazepines, barbiturates, or other hypnotics. However, it interacts with the benzodiazepine GABA receptor complex. Nonclinical studies have shown that it binds selectively to the brain omega-1 receptor situated on the alpha subunit of the GABA-A receptor complex.

Pharmacodynamics/Kinetics
  Onset of action: Rapid
    Peak effect: ~1 hour
  Duration: 6-8 hours
  Absorption: Rapid and almost complete
  Distribution: V_d: 1.4 L/kg
  Protein binding: 60% ± 15%
  Metabolism: Extensively metabolized; primarily via aldehyde oxidase to form 5-oxo-zaleplon and to a lesser extent by CYP3A4 to desethylzaleplon; all metabolites are pharmacologically inactive
  Bioavailability: 30%
  Half-life elimination: 1 hour
  Time to peak, serum: 1 hour
  Excretion: Urine (primarily metabolites, <1% as unchanged drug)
  (Continued)

Zaleplon (Continued)

Clearance: Plasma: Oral: 3 L/hour/kg

Usual Dosage Oral:

Adults: 10 mg at bedtime (range: 5-20 mg); has been used for up to 5 weeks of treatment in controlled trial setting

Elderly: 5 mg at bedtime

Dosage adjustment in renal impairment: No adjustment for mild to moderate renal impairment; use in severe renal impairment has not been adequately studied

Dosage adjustment in hepatic impairment: Mild to moderate impairment: 5 mg; not recommended for use in patients with severe hepatic impairment

Administration Immediately before bedtime or when the patient is in bed and cannot fall asleep

Patient Information Take exactly as directed; immediately before bedtime, or when you cannot fall asleep. Do not alter dosage or frequency, may be habit forming. Avoid alcohol and other prescription or OTC medications (especially medications to relieve pain, induce sleep, reduce anxiety, treat or prevent cold, coughs, or allergies) unless approved by prescriber. You may experience drowsiness, dizziness, somnolence, vertigo, lightheadedness, blurred vision (avoid driving or engaging in activities that require alertness until response to drug is known); photosensitivity (avoid exposure to direct sunlight, wear protective clothing, and sunscreen); nausea or GI discomfort (small frequent meals, good mouth care, chewing gum, or sucking hard candy may help); constipation (increase exercise or dietary fiber and fluids); menstrual disturbances (reversible when drug is discontinued). Discontinue drug and report any severe CNS disturbances (hallucinations, acute nervousness or anxiety, persistent sleepiness or lethargy, impaired coordination, amnesia, or impaired thought processes); skin rash or irritation; eye pain or major vision changes; difficulty breathing; chest pain; ear pain; muscle weakness or pain.

Additional Information Prescription quantities should not exceed a 1-month supply.

Dosage Forms Capsule: 5 mg, 10 mg

♦ **Zanaflex®** *see* Tizanidine *on page 1339*

Zanamivir (za NA mi veer)

U.S. Brand Names Relenza®

Canadian Brand Names Relenza®

Therapeutic Category Antiviral Agent, Influenza; Antiviral Agent, Inhalation Therapy; Antiviral Agent, Nonantiretroviral; Neuraminidase Inhibitor

Use Treatment of uncomplicated acute illness due to influenza virus in adults and children ≥7 years of age. Treatment should only be initiated in patients who have been symptomatic for no more than 2 days.

Unlabeled/Investigational Use Investigational: Prophylaxis against influenza A/B infections

Pregnancy Risk Factor C

Pregnancy/Breast-Feeding Implications Zanamivir has been shown to cross the placenta in animal models, however, no evidence of fetal malformations has been demonstrated. Zanamivir has been shown to be excreted in the milk of animals, but its excretion in human milk is unknown. Caution should be used when zanamivir is administered to a nursing mother.

Contraindications Hypersensitivity to zanamivir or any component of the formulation

Warnings/Precautions Patients must be instructed in the use of the delivery system. No data are available to support the use of this drug in patients who begin treatment after 48 hours of symptoms, as a prophylactic treatment for influenza, or in patients with significant underlying medical conditions. Not recommended for use in patients with underlying respiratory disease, such as asthma or COPD, due to lack of efficacy and risk of serious adverse effects. Bronchospasm, decreased lung function, and other serious adverse reactions, including those with fatal outcomes, have been reported. For a patient with an underlying airway disease where a medical decision has been made to use zanamivir, a fast-acting bronchodilator should be made available, and used prior to each dose. Not a substitute for the flu shot. Consider primary or concomitant bacterial infections.

Adverse Reactions Most adverse reactions occurred at a frequency which was equal to the control (lactose vehicle).

>1.5%:

Central nervous system: Headache (2%), dizziness (2%)

Gastrointestinal: Nausea (3%), diarrhea (3% adults, 2% children), vomiting (1% adults, 2% children)

Respiratory: Sinusitis (3%), bronchitis (2%), cough (2%), other nasal signs and symptoms (2%), infection (ear, nose, and throat; 2% adults, 5% children)

<1.5% (Limited to important or life-threatening): Allergic or allergic-like reaction (including oropharyngeal edema), arrhythmias, bronchospasm, dyspnea, facial edema, rash (including serious cutaneous reactions), seizures, syncope, urticaria

Overdosage/Toxicology Information is limited, and symptoms appear similar to reported adverse events from clinical studies.

Drug Interactions

Increased Effect/Toxicity: No clinically significant pharmacokinetic interactions are predicted.

Decreased Effect: No clinically significant pharmacokinetic interactions are predicted.

Stability Store at room temperature (25°C) 77°F; do not puncture blister until taking a dose using the Diskhaler®

Mechanism of Action Zanamivir inhibits influenza virus neuraminidase enzymes, potentially altering virus particle aggregation and release.

Pharmacodynamics/Kinetics

Absorption: Inhalation: 4% to 17%

Protein binding, plasma: <10%

Metabolism: None

Half-life elimination, serum: 2.5-5.1 hours

Excretion: Urine (as unchanged drug)

Usual Dosage Children ≥7 years and Adults: 2 inhalations (10 mg total) twice daily for 5 days. Two doses should be taken on the first day of dosing, regardless of interval, while doses should be spaced by approximately 12 hours on subsequent days.

Prophylaxis (investigational use): 2 inhalations (10 mg) once daily for duration of exposure period (6 weeks has been used in clinical trial)

Administration Inhalation: Must be used with Diskhaler® delivery device. Patients who are scheduled to use an inhaled bronchodilator should use their bronchodilator prior to zanamivir.

Patient Information Use delivery device exactly as directed; complete full 5-day regimen, even if symptoms improve sooner. If you have asthma or COPD you may be at risk for bronchospasm; see prescriber for appropriate bronchodilator before using zanamivir. Stop using this medication and contact your physician if you experience shortness of breath, increased wheezing, or other signs of bronchospasm. You may experience dizziness or headache (use caution when driving or engaging in hazardous tasks until response to drug is known). Report unresolved diarrhea, vomiting, or nausea; acute fever or muscle pain; or other acute and persistent adverse effects. **Breast-feeding precautions:** Consult prescriber if breast-feeding.

Additional Information Majority of patients included in clinical trials were infected with influenza A, however a number of patients with influenza B infections were also enrolled. Patients with lower temperature or less severe symptoms appeared to derive less benefit from therapy. No consistent treatment benefit was demonstrated in patients with chronic underlying medical conditions.

Dosage Forms Powder for oral inhalation (Rotadisk®): 5 mg/blister

Zidovudine (zye DOE vyoo deen)

Related Information

Antiretroviral Agents Comparison on page 1488
Antiretroviral Therapy for HIV Infection on page 1595
Management of Healthcare Worker Exposures to HIV, HBV, HCV on page 1555
Prevention of Perinatal HIV Transmission on page 1567

U.S. Brand Names Retrovir®

Canadian Brand Names Apo®-Zidovudine; AZT™; Novo-AZT; Retrovir®

Synonyms Azidothymidine; AZT; Compound S; ZDV

Therapeutic Category Antiretroviral Agent, Nucleoside Reverse Transcriptase Inhibitor (NRTI) [Thymidine Analog]

Use Management of patients with HIV infections in combination with at least two other antiretroviral agents; for prevention of maternal/fetal HIV transmission as monotherapy

Pregnancy Risk Factor C

Pregnancy/Breast-Feeding Implications Zidovudine crosses the placenta. The use of zidovudine reduces the maternal-fetal transmission of HIV by ~70% and should be considered for antenatal and intrapartum therapy whenever possible. In HIV infected mothers not previously on antiretroviral therapy, treatment may be delayed until after 10-12 weeks gestation. Cases of lactic acidosis/hepatic steatosis syndrome have been reported in pregnant women receiving nucleoside analogues. It is not known if pregnancy itself potentiates this known side effect; however, pregnant women may be at increased risk of lactic acidosis and liver damage. Hepatic enzymes and electrolytes should be monitored frequently during the 3rd trimester of pregnancy in women receiving nucleoside analogues. Health professionals are encouraged to contact the antiretroviral pregnancy registry to monitor outcomes of pregnant women exposed to antiretroviral medications (1-800-258-4263).

Contraindications Life-threatening hypersensitivity to zidovudine or any component of the formulation

Warnings/Precautions Associated with hematologic toxicity [granulocytopenia, severe anemia requiring transfusions, or (rarely) pancytopenia]. Use with caution in patients with bone marrow compromise; dosage adjustment may be required in patients who develop anemia or neutropenia. Lactic acidosis and severe hepatomegaly with steatosis have been reported, including fatal cases; use with caution in patients with risk factors for liver disease and suspend treatment in any patient who develops clinical or laboratory findings suggestive of lactic acidosis. Prolonged use has been associated with symptomatic myopathy. Reduce dose in patients with renal impairment.

(Continued)

Zidovudine *(Continued)*

Adverse Reactions

>10%:

Central nervous system: Severe headache (42%), fever (16%)

Dermatologic: Rash (17%)

Gastrointestinal: Nausea (46% to 61%), anorexia (11%), diarrhea (17%), pain (20%), vomiting (6% to 25%)

Hematologic: Anemia (23% in children), leukopenia, granulocytopenia (39% in children)

Neuromuscular & skeletal: Weakness (19%)

1% to 10%:

Central nervous system: Malaise (8%), dizziness (6%), insomnia (5%), somnolence (8%)

Dermatologic: Hyperpigmentation of nails (bluish-brown)

Gastrointestinal: Dyspepsia (5%)

Hematologic: Changes in platelet count

Neuromuscular & skeletal: Paresthesia (6%)

<1% (Limited to important or life-threatening): Bone marrow suppression, cholestatic jaundice, confusion, granulocytopenia, gynecomastia, hepatotoxicity, mania, myopathy, neurotoxicity, oral pigmentation changes, pancytopenia, seizures, tenderness, thrombocytopenia

Overdosage/Toxicology Symptoms include nausea, vomiting, ataxia, and granulocytopenia. Erythropoietin, thymidine, and cyanocobalamin have been used experimentally to treat zidovudine-induced hematopoietic toxicity, yet none are presently specified as the agent of choice. Treatment is supportive.

Drug Interactions

Cytochrome P450 Effect: CYP3A3/4 enzyme substrate

Increased Effect/Toxicity: Coadministration of zidovudine with drugs that are nephrotoxic (amphotericin B), cytotoxic (flucytosine, vincristine, vinblastine, doxorubicin, interferon), inhibit glucuronidation or excretion (acetaminophen, cimetidine, indomethacin, lorazepam, probenecid, aspirin), or interfere with RBC/WBC number or function (acyclovir, ganciclovir, pentamidine, dapsone). Clarithromycin may increase blood levels of zidovudine (although total body exposure was unaffected, peak plasma concentrations were increased). Valproic acid significantly increases zidovudine's blood levels (believed due to inhibition first pass metabolism).

Ethanol/Nutrition/Herb Interactions Food: Administration with a fatty meal decreased zidovudine's AUC and peak plasma concentration.

Stability After dilution to ≤4 mg/mL, the solution is physically and chemically stable for 24 hours at room temperature and 48 hours if refrigerated; attempt to administer diluted solution within 8 hours, if stored at room temperature or 24 hours if refrigerated to minimize potential for microbially contaminated solutions; store undiluted vials at room temperature and protect from light

Mechanism of Action Zidovudine is a thymidine analog which interferes with the HIV viral RNA dependent DNA polymerase resulting in inhibition of viral replication; nucleoside reverse transcriptase inhibitor

Pharmacodynamics/Kinetics

Absorption: Oral: 66% to 70%

Distribution: Significant penetration into the CSF; crosses placenta

Relative diffusion from blood into CSF: Adequate with or without inflammation (exceeds usual MICs)

CSF:blood level ratio: Normal meninges: ~60%

Protein binding: 25% to 38%

Metabolism: Hepatic via glucuronidation to inactive metabolites; extensive first-pass effect

Half-life elimination: Terminal: 60 minutes

Time to peak, serum: 30-90 minutes

Excretion:

Oral: Urine (72% to 74% as metabolites, 14% to 18% as unchanged drug)

I.V.: Urine (45% to 60% as metabolites, 18% to 29% as unchanged drug)

Usual Dosage

Prevention of maternal-fetal HIV transmission:

Neonatal: Oral: 2 mg/kg/dose every 6 hours for 6 weeks beginning 6-12 hours after birth; infants unable to receive oral dosing may receive 1.5 mg/kg I.V. infused over 30 minutes every 6 hours

Maternal (may delay treatment until after 10-12 weeks gestation): Oral (per HIV/ATIS 2001 guidelines): 200 mg 3 times/day or 300 mg twice daily until start of labor

During labor and delivery, administer zidovudine I.V. at 2 mg/kg over 1 hour followed by a continuous I.V. infusion of 1 mg/kg/hour until the umbilical cord is clamped

Children 3 months to 12 years for HIV infection:

Oral: 160 mg/m²/dose every 8 hours; dosage range: 90 mg/m²/dose to 180 mg/m²/dose every 6-8 hours; some Working Group members use a dose of 180 mg/m² every 12 hours when using in drug combinations with other antiretroviral compounds, but data on this dosing in children is limited

I.V. continuous infusion: 20 mg/m²/hour

I.V. intermittent infusion: 120 mg/m²/dose every 6 hours

Adults:

Oral: 300 mg twice daily or 200 mg 3 times/day

I.V.: 1-2 mg/kg/dose (infused over 1 hour) administered every 4 hours around-the-clock (6 doses/day)

Prevention of HIV following needlesticks: 200 mg 3 times/day plus lamivudine 150 mg twice daily; a protease inhibitor (eg, indinavir) may be added for high risk exposures; begin therapy within 2 hours of exposure if possible

Patients should receive I.V. therapy only until oral therapy can be administered

Dosing interval in renal impairment: Cl$_{cr}$ <10 mL/minute: May require minor dose adjustment

Hemodialysis: At least partially removed by hemo- and peritoneal dialysis; administer dose after hemodialysis or administer 100 mg supplemental dose; during CAPD, dose as for Cl$_{cr}$ <10 mL/minute

Continuous arteriovenous or venovenous hemodiafiltration effects: Administer 100 mg every 8 hours

Dosing adjustment in hepatic impairment: Reduce dose by 50% or double dosing interval in patients with cirrhosis

Administration

Oral: Administer around-the-clock to promote less variation in peak and trough serum levels. Oral zidovudine should be administered 1 hour before or 2 hours after a meal with a glass of water.

I.V.: Infuse over 1 hour; avoid rapid infusion or bolus injection

Monitoring Parameters Monitor CBC and platelet count at least every 2 weeks, MCV, serum creatinine kinase, viral load, and CD4 count; observe for appearance of opportunistic infections

Patient Information Zidovudine is not a cure for AIDS. Take as directed, preferably on an empty stomach (1 hour before or 2 hours after meals). Take around-the-clock; do not take with other medications. Take precautions to avoid transmission to others. You may experience headache or insomnia; if these persist notify prescriber. Report unresolved nausea or vomiting; signs of infection (eg, fever, chills, sore throat, burning urination, flu-like symptoms, fatigue); unusual bleeding (eg, tarry stools, easy bruising, or blood in stool, urine, or mouth); pain, tingling, or numbness of toes or fingers; skin rash or irritation; or muscles weakness or tremors.

Nursing Implications Do not administer I.M.; do not administer I.V. push or by rapid infusion; infuse I.V. zidovudine over 1 hour at a final concentration not to exceed 4 mg/mL in D_5W

Additional Information Potential compliance problems, frequency of administration and adverse effects should be discussed with patients before initiating therapy to help prevent the emergence of resistance.

Dosage Forms
Capsule: 100 mg
Injection: 10 mg/mL (20 mL)
Syrup: 50 mg/5 mL (240 mL) [strawberry flavor]
Tablet: 300 mg

◆ Zidovudine, Abacavir, and Lamivudine *see* Abacavir, Lamivudine, and Zidovudine *on page 17*

Zidovudine and Lamivudine (zye DOE vyoo deen & la MI vyoo deen)

Related Information
Antiretroviral Agents Comparison *on page 1488*

U.S. Brand Names Combivir®

Canadian Brand Names Combivir®

Synonyms AZT + 3TC; Lamivudine and Zidovudine

Therapeutic Category Antiretroviral Agent, Reverse Transcriptase Inhibitor (Combination); Reverse Transcriptase Inhibitor

Use Treatment of HIV infection when therapy is warranted based on clinical and/or immunological evidence of disease progression. Combivir® given twice daily, provides an alternative regimen to lamivudine 150 mg twice daily plus zidovudine 600 mg/day in divided doses; this drug form reduces capsule/tablet intake for these two drugs to 2 per day instead of up to 8.

Pregnancy Risk Factor C

Usual Dosage Children >12 years and Adults: Oral: One tablet twice daily

Additional Information Complete prescribing information for this medication should be consulted for additional detail.

Dosage Forms Tablet: Zidovudine 300 mg and lamivudine 150 mg

◆ Zilactin® **(Can)** *see* Lidocaine *on page 801*
◆ Zilactin®-B [OTC] *see* Benzocaine *on page 154*
◆ Zilactin® Baby [OTC] *see* Benzocaine *on page 154*
◆ Zilactin-L® [OTC] *see* Lidocaine *on page 801*

Zileuton (zye LOO ton)

Related Information
Asthma *on page 1645*

U.S. Brand Names Zyflo™

Therapeutic Category 5-Lipoxygenase Inhibitor

Use Prophylaxis and chronic treatment of asthma in children ≥12 years of age and adults

Pregnancy Risk Factor C

Pregnancy/Breast-Feeding Implications
Clinical effects on the fetus: Developmental studies indicated adverse effects (reduced body weight and increased skeletal variations) in rats at an oral dose of 300 mg/kg/day. There are no adequate and well controlled studies in pregnant women.
Breast-feeding/lactation: Zileuton and its metabolites are excreted in rat milk; it is not known if zileuton is excreted in breast milk

Contraindications Hypersensitivity to zileuton or any component of the formulation; active liver disease or transaminase elevations greater than or equal to three times the upper limit of normal (≥3 x ULN)

Warnings/Precautions Elevations of one or more liver function tests may occur during therapy. These laboratory abnormalities may progress, remain unchanged or resolve with continued therapy. Use with caution in patients who consume substantial quantities of ethanol or have a past history of liver disease. Zileuton is not indicated for use in the reversal of bronchospasm in acute asthma attacks, including status asthmaticus. Zileuton can be continued during acute exacerbations of asthma.

Adverse Reactions
>10%:
Central nervous system: Headache (24.6%)
Hepatic: ALT elevation (12%)
(Continued)

Zileuton (Continued)

1% to 10%:
Cardiovascular: Chest pain
Central nervous system: Pain, dizziness, fever, insomnia, malaise, nervousness, somnolence
Gastrointestinal: Dyspepsia, nausea, abdominal pain, constipation, flatulence
Hematologic: Low white blood cell count
Neuromuscular & skeletal: Myalgia, arthralgia, weakness
Ocular: Conjunctivitis
<1% (Limited to important or life-threatening): Rash, urticaria

Overdosage/Toxicology Symptoms of overdose in humans are limited. Oral minimum lethal doses in mice and rats were 500-1000 and 300-1000 mg/kg, respectively (providing >3 and 9 times the systemic exposure achieved at the maximum recommended human daily oral dose, respectively). No deaths occurred, but nephritis was reported in dogs at an oral dose of 1000 mg/kg. Treat symptomatically. Institute supportive measures as required. If indicated, achieve elimination of unabsorbed drug by emesis or gastric lavage. Observe usual precautions to maintain the airway. Zileuton is NOT removed by dialysis.

Drug Interactions
Cytochrome P450 Effect: CYP1A2, 2C9, and 3A3/4 enzyme substrate; CYP1A2 and 3A3/4 enzyme inhibitor
Increased Effect/Toxicity: Zileuton increases concentrations/effects of beta-blockers (propranolol), terfenadine, theophylline, and warfarin. Potentially, it may increase levels of many drugs, including cisapride, due to inhibition of CYP3A4.

Ethanol/Nutrition/Herb Interactions
Ethanol: Avoid ethanol (may increase CNS depression).
Herb/Nutraceutical: St John's wort may decrease zileuton levels.

Mechanism of Action Specific inhibitor of 5-lipoxygenase and thus inhibits leukotriene (LTB1, LTC1, LTD1 and LTE1) formation. Leukotrienes are substances that induce numerous biological effects including augmentation of neutrophil and eosinophil migration, neutrophil and monocyte aggregation, leukocyte adhesion, increased capillary permeability and smooth muscle contraction.

Pharmacodynamics/Kinetics
Absorption: Rapid
Distribution: 1.2 L/kg
Protein binding: 93%
Metabolism: Several metabolites in plasma and urine; metabolized by the CYP450 isoenzymes 1A2, 2C9 and 3A4
Bioavailability: Unknown
Half-life elimination: 2.5 hours
Time to peak, serum: 1.7 hours
Excretion: Urine (~95% primarily as metabolites); feces (~2%)

Usual Dosage Oral:
Children ≥12 years of age and Adults: 600 mg 4 times/day with meals and at bedtime
Elderly: Zileuton pharmacokinetics were similar in healthy elderly subjects (>65 years) compared with healthy younger adults (18-40 years)
Dosing adjustment in renal impairment: Dosing adjustment is not necessary in renal impairment or renal failure (even during dialysis)
Dosing adjustment in hepatic impairment: Contraindicated in patients with active liver disease

Administration May be administered without regard to meals (ie, with or without food)
Monitoring Parameters Evaluate hepatic transaminases at initiation of and during therapy with zileuton. Monitor serum ALT before treatment begins, once-a-month for the first 3 months, every 2-3 months for the remainder of the first year, and periodically thereafter for patients receiving long-term zileuton therapy. If symptoms of liver dysfunction (right upper quadrant pain, nausea, fatigue, lethargy, pruritus, jaundice or "flu-like" symptoms) develop or transaminase elevations >5 times the ULN occur, discontinue therapy and follow transaminase levels until normal.

Patient Information Inform patients that zileuton is indicated for the chronic treatment of asthma and to take regularly as prescribed even during symptom-free periods. Zileuton is not a bronchodilator; do not use to treat acute episodes of asthma. When taking zileuton, do not decrease the dose or stop taking any other antiasthma medications unless instructed by a physician.

While using zileuton, seek medical attention if short-acting bronchodilators are needed more often than usual or if more than the maximum number of inhalations of short-acting bronchodilator treatment prescribed for a 24-period are needed.

The most serious side effect of zileuton is elevation of liver enzyme tests. While taking zileuton, patients must have liver enzyme tests monitored on a regular basis. If patients experience signs or symptoms of liver dysfunction (right upper quadrant pain, nausea, fatigue, lethargy, pruritus, jaundice, or "flu-like" symptoms), contact a physician immediately.

Zileuton can interact with other drugs. While taking zileuton, consult a physician before starting or stopping any prescription or nonprescription medicines.

Dosage Forms Tablet: 600 mg

♦ **Zinacef®** see Cefuroxime on page 258
♦ **Zinca-Pak®** see Zinc Supplements on page 1439
♦ **Zincate®** see Zinc Supplements on page 1439
♦ **Zinc Chloride** see Zinc Supplements on page 1439
♦ **Zincfrin® [OTC]** see Phenylephrine and Zinc Sulfate on page 1077

Zinc Gelatin (zink JEL ah tin)

U.S. Brand Names Gelucast®
Synonyms Dome Paste Bandage; Unna's Boot; Unna's Paste; Zinc Gelatin Boot

Therapeutic Category Topical Skin Product
Use As a protectant and to support varicosities and similar lesions of the lower limbs
Contraindications Hypersensitivity to zinc gelatin or to any component of the formulation
Adverse Reactions 1% to 10%: Local: Irritation
Usual Dosage Apply externally as an occlusive boot
Nursing Implications After a period of about 2 weeks, the dressing is removed by soaking in warm water
Dosage Forms Bandage: 3" x 10 yards; 4" x 10 yards

♦ **Zinc Gelatin Boot** see Zinc Gelatin on page 1438
♦ **Zinc Gluconate** see Zinc Supplements on page 1439

Zinc Oxide, Cod Liver Oil, and Talc (zink OKS ide, kod LIV er oyl, & talk)

U.S. Brand Names Desitin® [OTC]
Therapeutic Category Topical Skin Product
Use Relief of diaper rash, superficial wounds and burns, and other minor skin irritations
Usual Dosage Topical: Apply thin layer as needed
Additional Information Complete prescribing information for this medication should be consulted for additional detail.
Dosage Forms Ointment, topical: Zinc oxide, cod liver oil, and talc in petrolatum and lanolin base (30 g, 60 g, 120 g, 240 g, 270 g)

♦ **Zinc Sulfate** see Zinc Supplements on page 1439
♦ **Zinc Sulfate and Phenylephrine** see Phenylephrine and Zinc Sulfate on page 1077

Zinc Supplements (zink SUP la ments)

U.S. Brand Names Eye-Sed® [OTC]; Orazinc® [OTC]; Verazinc® [OTC]; Zinca-Pak®; Zincate®
Synonyms Zinc Chloride; Zinc Gluconate; Zinc Sulfate
Therapeutic Category Mineral, Oral; Mineral, Parenteral; Trace Element
Use Cofactor for replacement therapy to different enzymes helps maintain normal growth rates, normal skin hydration and senses of taste and smell; zinc supplement (oral and parenteral); may improve wound healing in those who are deficient. May be useful to promote wound healing in patients with pressure sores.
Pregnancy Risk Factor A
Contraindications Hypersensitivity to any component
Warnings/Precautions Do not take undiluted by direct injection into a peripheral vein because of potential for phlebitis, tissue irritation, and potential to increase renal loss of minerals from a bolus injection; administration of zinc in absence of copper may decrease plasma levels; excessive dose may increase HDL and impair immune system function
Adverse Reactions <1%: Hypotension, indigestion, jaundice, leukopenia, nausea, neutropenia, pulmonary edema, vomiting
Drug Interactions
  Decreased Effect: Decreased penicillamine, decreased tetracycline effect reduced, iron decreased uptake of zinc, bran products, dairy products reduce absorption of zinc
Mechanism of Action Provides for normal growth and tissue repair, is a cofactor for more than 70 enzymes; ophthalmic astringent and weak antiseptic due to precipitation of protein and clearing mucus from outer surface of the eye
Pharmacodynamics/Kinetics
  Absorption: Poor from gastrointestinal tract (20% to 30%)
  Elimination: In feces with only traces appearing in urine
Usual Dosage Clinical response may not occur for up to 6-8 weeks
  Zinc sulfate:
    RDA: Oral:
      Birth to 6 months: 3 mg elemental zinc/day
      6-12 months: 5 mg elemental zinc/day
      1-10 years: 10 mg elemental zinc/day (44 mg zinc sulfate)
      ≥11 years: 15 mg elemental zinc/day (65 mg zinc sulfate)
    Zinc deficiency: Oral:
      Infants and Children: 0.5-1 mg elemental zinc/kg/day divided 1-3 times/day; somewhat larger quantities may be needed if there is impaired intestinal absorption or an excessive loss of zinc
      Adults: 110-220 mg zinc sulfate (25-50 mg elemental zinc)/dose 3 times/day
  Parenteral: TPN: I.V. infusion (chloride or sulfate): Supplemental to I.V. solutions (clinical response may not occur for up to 6-8 weeks):
    Premature Infants <1500 g, up to 3 kg: 300 mcg/kg/day
    Full-term Infants and Children ≤5 years: 100 mcg/kg/day
      or
    Premature Infants: 400 mcg/kg/day
    Term <3 months: 250 mcg/kg/day
    Term >3 months: 100 mcg/kg/day
    Children: 50 mcg/kg/day
    Adults:
      Stable with fluid loss from small bowel: 12.2 mg zinc/liter TPN or 17.1 mg zinc/kg (added to 1000 mL I.V. fluids) of stool or ileostomy output
      Metabolically stable: 2.5-4 mg/day, add 2 mg/day for acute catabolic states
Dietary Considerations Food: Avoid foods high in calcium or phosphorus
Administration Administer oral formulation with food if GI upset occurs
Monitoring Parameters Patients on TPN therapy should have periodic serum copper and serum zinc levels, skin integrity
Reference Range
  Serum: 50-150 μg/dL (<20 μg/dL as solid test with dermatitis followed by alopecia)
  Therapeutic: 66-110 μg/dL (SI: 10-16.8 μmol/L)
  (Continued)

Zinc Supplements *(Continued)*

Patient Information Take with food if GI upset occurs, but avoid foods high in calcium, phosphorous, or phytate; do not exceed recommended dose; if irritation persists or continues with ophthalmic use, notify physician

Nursing Implications Do not administer undiluted by direct injection into a peripheral vein because of potential for phlebitis, tissue irritation, and potential to increase renal loss of minerals from a bolus injection

Dosage Forms

Zinc carbonate, complex: Liquid: 15 mg/mL (30 mL)

Zinc chloride: Injection: 1 mg/mL (10 mL)

Zinc gluconate (14.3% zinc): Tablet: 10 mg (elemental zinc 1.4 mg), 15 mg (elemental zinc 2 mg), 50 mg (elemental zinc 7 mg), 78 mg (elemental zinc 11 mg)

Zinc sulfate (23% zinc):

Capsule: 110 mg (elemental zinc 25 mg), 220 mg (elemental zinc 50 mg)

Injection: 1 mg/mL (10 mL, 30 mL); 4 mg/mL (10 mL); 5 mg/mL (5 mL, 10 mL)

Tablet: 66 mg (elemental zinc 15 mg), 110 mg (elemental zinc 25 mg), 200 mg (elemental zinc 45 mg)

♦ **Zinecard®** *see Dexrazoxane on page 385*

Ziprasidone *(zi PRAY si done)*

Related Information

Antipsychotic Agents Comparison *on page 1486*

U.S. Brand Names Geodon®

Synonyms Zeldox; Ziprasidone Hydrochloride

Therapeutic Category Antipsychotic Agent, Atypical

Use Treatment of schizophrenia

Unlabeled/Investigational Use Tourette's syndrome

Pregnancy Risk Factor C

Pregnancy/Breast-Feeding Implications Developmental toxicity demonstrated in animals. There are no adequate and well-controlled studies in pregnant women. Use only if potential benefit justifies risk to the fetus. Excretion in breast milk is unknown; breast-feeding is not recommended.

Contraindications Hypersensitivity to ziprasidone or any component of the formulation; history (or current) prolonged QT; congenital long QT syndrome; recent myocardial infarction; history of arrhythmias; uncompensated heart failure; concurrent use of other QT_c-prolonging agents including amiodarone, arsenic trioxide, chlorpromazine, cisapride, class Ia antiarrhythmics (quinidine, procainamide), dofetilide, dolasetron, droperidol, halofantrine, levomethadyl, mefloquine, mesoridazine, pentamidine, pimozide, some quinolone antibiotics (moxifloxacin, sparfloxacin, gatifloxacin), sotalol, tacrolimus, and thioridazine

Warnings/Precautions May result in QT_c prolongation (dose-related), which has been associated with the development of malignant ventricular arrhythmias (torsade de pointes). Avoid hypokalemia, hypomagnesemia. Use caution in patients with bradycardia. Discontinue in patients found to have persistent QT_c intervals >500 msec. Patients with symptoms of dizziness, palpitations, or syncope should receive further cardiac evaluation. May cause orthostatic hypotension; use with caution in patients at risk of this effect or those who would tolerate transient hypotensive episodes.

May cause extrapyramidal symptoms, including tardive dyskinesia. Disturbances of temperature regulation and/or neuroleptic malignant syndrome (NMS) have been reported with antipsychotics. Use with caution in patients at risk of seizures, including those receiving medications which may lower seizure threshold. Elderly patients may be at increased risk of seizures due to an increased prevalence of predisposing factors.

Cognitive and/or motor impairment (sedation) is common with ziprasidone. Use with caution in disorders where CNS depression is a feature. Use with caution in Parkinson's disease. Esophageal dysmotility and aspiration have been associated with antipsychotic use; use with caution in patients at risk of aspiration pneumonia (ie, Alzheimer's disease). Caution in breast cancer or other prolactin-dependent tumors (may elevate prolactin levels). Ziprasidone has been associated with a fairly high incidence of rash (5%); discontinue if alternative etiology is not identified. Safety and efficacy have not been established in pediatric patients.

Adverse Reactions Note: Although minor QT_c prolongation (mean 10 msec at 160 mg/day) may occur more frequently (incidence not specified), clinically relevant prolongation (>500 msec) was rare (0.06%).

>10%: Central nervous system: Somnolence (14%)

1% to 10%:

Cardiovascular: Tachycardia (2%), postural hypotension (1%)

Central nervous system: Akathisia (8%), dizziness (8%), extrapyramidal symptoms (5%), dystonia (4%), hypertonia (3%)

Dermatologic: Rash (with urticaria, 4% to 5%), fungal dermatitis (2%)

Gastrointestinal: Nausea (10%), constipation (9%), dyspepsia (8%), diarrhea (5%), xerostomia (4%), anorexia (2%), weight gain (10%)

Neuromuscular & skeletal: Weakness (5%), myalgia (1%)

Ocular: Abnormal vision (3%)

Respiratory: Respiratory disorder (8%, primarily cold symptoms, upper respiratory infection), rhinitis (4%), increased cough (3%)

Miscellaneous: Accidental injury (4%)

<1% (Limited to important or life-threatening): Agitation, akinesia, angina, atrial fibrillation, ataxia, AV block (first degree), bundle branch block, cerebral infarction, cholestatic jaundice, choreoathetosis, cogwheel rigidity, delirium, dysarthria, dyskinesia, dysphagia, dyspnea, eosinophilia, exfoliative dermatitis, gout, gynecomastia, hemorrhage, hepatitis, jaundice, myocarditis, neuropathy, oculogyric crisis, opisthotonos, paresthesia, photophobia, photosensitivity reaction, pneumonia, pulmonary embolism, priapism, QT_c prolongation >500 msec (0.06%), seizure (0.4%), sexual dysfunction (male and female), stroke,

syncope (0.6%), tenosynovitis, thrombocytopenia, thyroiditis, torticollis, urinary retention, withdrawal syndrome

Overdosage/Toxicology Reported symptoms include somnolence, slurring of speech, and hypertension. Acute extrapyramidal symptoms may also occur. Treatment is symptom directed and supportive. Not removed by dialysis.

Drug Interactions

Cytochrome P450 Effect: CYP3A3/4 substrate (limited), CYP1A2 substrate (minor)

Increased Effect/Toxicity:

Ketoconazole may increase serum concentrations of ziprasidone. Other CYP3A3/4 inhibitors may share this potential. Inhibitors include amiodarone, clarithromycin, erythromycin, delavirdine, diltiazem, dirithromycin, disulfiram, fluoxetine, fluvoxamine, grapefruit juice, indinavir, itraconazole, ketoconazole, nefazodone, nevirapine, propoxyphene, quinupristin-dalfopristin, ritonavir, saquinavir, verapamil, zafirlukast, zileuton

Concurrent use with QT_c-prolonging agents may result in additive effects on cardiac conduction, potentially resulting in malignant or lethal arrhythmias. Concurrent use is contraindicated. Includes amiodarone, arsenic trioxide, chlorpromazine, cisapride; class Ia antiarrhythmics (quinidine, procainamide); dofetilide, dolasetron, droperidol, halofantrine, levomethadyl, mefloquine, mesoridazine, pentamidine, pimozide, probucol; some quinolone antibiotics (moxifloxacin, sparfloxacin, gatifloxacin); sotalol, tacrolimus, and thioridazine. Potassium- or magnesium-depleting agents (diuretics, aminoglycosides, cyclosporine, and amphotericin B) may increase the risk of QT_c prolongation. Antihypertensive agents may increase the risk of orthostatic hypotension. CNS depressants may increase the degree of sedation caused by ziprasidone.

Decreased Effect: Carbamazepine may decrease serum concentrations of ziprasidone. Other enzyme-inducing agents may share this potential. Amphetamines may decrease the efficacy of ziprasidone. Ziprasidone may inhibit the efficacy of levodopa.

Ethanol/Nutrition/Herb Interactions

Ethanol: Avoid ethanol (may increase CNS depression).

Food: Administration with food increases serum levels twofold. Grapefruit juice may increase serum concentration of ziprasidone.

Herb/Nutraceutical: St John's wort may decrease serum levels of ziprasidone, due to a potential effect on CYP3A3/4. This has not been specifically studied. Avoid kava kava, chamomile (may increase CNS depression).

Stability Store at controlled room temperature of 15°C to 30°C (59°F to 86°F)

Mechanism of Action The exact mechanism of action is unknown. However, *in vitro* radioligand studies show that ziprasidone has high affinity for D_2, 5-HT_{2A}, 5-HT_{1A}, 5-HT_{2C} and 5-HT_{1D}, moderate affinity for alpha$_1$ adrenergic and histamine H_1 receptors, and low affinity for alpha$_2$ adrenergic, beta adrenergic, 5-HT_3, 5-HT_4, cholinergic, mu, sigma, or benzodiazepine receptors. Ziprasidone moderately inhibits the reuptake of serotonin and norepinephrine.

Pharmacodynamics/Kinetics

Absorption: Well absorbed

Distribution: V_d: 1.5 L/kg

Protein binding: 99%, primarily to albumin and alpha-1-acid glycoprotein

Metabolism: Extensively hepatic, primarily via aldehyde oxidase; less than $1/3$ of total metabolism via CYP450 isoenzymes: CYP3A3/4 and CYP1A2 (minor)

Bioavailability: 60% with food (food increases up to twofold)

Half-life elimination: 7 hours

Time to peak: 6-8 hours

Excretion: Feces (66%) and urine (20%) as metabolites; little as unchanged drug (1% urine, 4% feces)

Usual Dosage Oral:

Children and adolescents: Tourette's syndrome (unlabeled use): 5-40 mg/day

Adults: Psychosis: Initial: 20 mg twice daily (with food)

Adjustment: Increases (if indicated) should be made no more frequently than every 2 days; ordinarily patients should be observed for improvement over several weeks before adjusting the dose

Maintenance: Range 20-100 mg twice daily; however, dosages >80 mg twice daily are generally not recommended

Elderly: No dosage adjustment is recommended; consider initiating at a low end of the dosage range, with slower titration

Dosage adjustment in renal impairment: No dosage adjustment is recommended

Dosage adjustment in hepatic impairment: No dosage adjustment is recommended

Administration Administer with food

Monitoring Parameters Serum potassium, magnesium, improvements in symptomatology. The value of routine ECG screening or monitoring has not been established. Potential for extrapyramidal symptoms. Fever, confusion, and/or stiffness should prompt evaluation of possible NMS.

Patient Information Use exactly as directed (do not change dose or frequency). Ziprasidone should be taken with food. It may take 2-3 weeks to achieve desired results; do not discontinue without consulting prescriber. Avoid excess alcohol, caffeine, grapefruit and grapefruit juice, other prescription or OTC medications not approved by prescriber. Maintain adequate hydration (2-3 L/day of fluids unless instructed to restrict fluid intake). You may experience excess sedation, drowsiness, restlessness, dizziness, or blurred vision (use caution driving or when engaging in tasks requiring alertness until response to drug is known); dry mouth, nausea, or GI upset (small frequent meals, frequent mouth care, chewing gum, or sucking lozenges may help); postural hypotension (use caution climbing stairs or when changing position from lying or sitting to standing); or urinary retention (void before taking medication). Report persistent CNS effects (eg, trembling fingers, altered gait or balance, excessive sedation, seizures, unusual muscle or skeletal movements, anxiety, abnormal thoughts, confusion, personality changes); chest pain, palpitations, rapid heartbeat, severe dizziness; swelling or pain in breasts (male and female), altered menstrual pattern, sexual dysfunction; pain or difficulty on urination; vision changes; skin rash or yellowing of skin; difficulty breathing; or worsening of condition.

(Continued)

Ziprasidone *(Continued)*

Additional Information The increased potential to prolong QT$_c$, as compared to other available antipsychotic agents, should be considered in the evaluation of available alternatives.

Dosage Forms Capsule, as hydrochloride: 20 mg, 40 mg, 60 mg, 80 mg

- ◆ **Ziprasidone Hydrochloride** *see Ziprasidone on page 1440*
- ◆ **Zithromax®** *see Azithromycin on page 139*
- ◆ **Zithromax® Z-PAK®** *see Azithromycin on page 139*
- ◆ **Zocor®** *see Simvastatin on page 1238*
- ◆ **Zofran®** *see Ondansetron on page 1009*
- ◆ **Zofran® ODT** *see Ondansetron on page 1009*
- ◆ **Zoladex® (Can)** *see Goserelin on page 641*
- ◆ **Zoladex® Implant** *see Goserelin on page 641*
- ◆ **Zoladex® LA (Can)** *see Goserelin on page 641*
- ◆ **Zoledronate** *see Zoledronic Acid on page 1442*

Zoledronic Acid *(ZOE le dron ik AS id)*

U.S. Brand Names Zometa®

Canadian Brand Names Zometa®

Synonyms CGP-42446; Zoledronate

Therapeutic Category Antidote, Hypercalcemia; Bisphosphonate Derivative

Use Treatment of hypercalcemia of malignancy, multiple myeloma, and bone metastases of solid tumors in conjunction with standard antineoplastic therapy

Pregnancy Risk Factor D

Pregnancy/Breast-Feeding Implications Animal studies resulted in embryotoxicity and losses. May cause fetal harm when administered to a pregnant woman. Use only if the benefit to the mother outweighs the potential risk to the fetus. Excretion in breast milk is unknown; breast-feeding is not recommended.

Contraindications Hypersensitivity to zoledronic acid, other bisphosphonates, or any component of the formulation; pregnancy

Warnings/Precautions Renal toxicity has been reported with doses >4 mg or infusions administered over <15 minutes. Renal function should be assessed prior to and after treatment; if decreased after treatment, additional treatments should be withheld until renal function returns to within 10% of baseline. Use caution in patients with previous renal impairment; adverse reactions may be greater in patients with impaired renal function. Use is not recommended in patients with severe renal impairment (serum creatinine >3 mg/dL) and bone metastases (limited data). Adequate hydration is required during treatment (urine output ~2 L/day); avoid overhydration, especially in patients with heart failure; diuretics should not be used before correcting hypovolemia. Use caution in patients with aspirin-sensitive asthma (may cause bronchoconstriction), hepatic dysfunction, and the elderly. Safety and efficacy in pediatric patients have not been established.

Adverse Reactions

>10%:

Cardiovascular: Leg edema (up to 19%)

Central nervous system: Fever (30% to 44%), headache (18%), insomnia (15%), anxiety (9% to 14%), dizziness (14%), agitation (13%)

Dermatologic: Alopecia (11%)

Endocrine & metabolic: Hypophosphatemia (13%), hypokalemia (12%), dehydration (up to 12%)

Gastrointestinal: Diarrhea (17% to 22%), abdominal pain (12% to 16%)

Genitourinary: Urinary tract infection (11% to 14%)

Hematologic: Anemia (22% to 29%), neutropenia (11%)

Neuromuscular & skeletal: Myalgia (21%), paresthesias (18%), arthralgia (18%) skeletal pain (12%)

Respiratory: Dyspnea (22%), coughing (12% to 19%)

1% to 10%:

Cardiovascular: Hypotension (10%), chest pain

Central nervous system: Hypoesthesia (10%)

Dermatologic: Dermatitis (10%)

Endocrine & metabolic: Hypomagnesemia (up to 10%), hypocalcemia, hypophosphatemia (9%), hypermagnesemia (Grade 3: 2%)

Gastrointestinal: Anorexia (9%), mucositis, dysphagia

Genitourinary: Urinary tract infection (14%)

Hematologic: Thrombocytopenia, pancytopenia

Neuromuscular & skeletal: Arthralgia, rigors (10%)

Renal: Serum creatinine increased

Respiratory: Pleural effusion , upper respiratory tract infection (8%)

<1% (Limited to important or life-threatening): Conjunctivitis, flu-like symptoms, injection site reactions, pruritus, rash

Symptoms of hypercalcemia include polyuria, nephrolithiasis, anorexia, nausea, vomiting, constipation, weakness, fatigue, confusion, stupor, and coma. These may not be drug-related adverse events, but related to the underlying metabolic condition.

Overdosage/Toxicology Clinically significant hypocalcemia, hypophosphatemia, and hypomagnesemia may occur.

Drug Interactions

Increased Effect/Toxicity: Aminoglycosides may also lower serum calcium levels; loop diuretics increase risk of hypocalcemia; thalidomide increases renal toxicity

Stability Prior to dilution, vials should be stored at 25°C (77°F). Reconstitute powder with 5 mL sterile water for injection. Once fully dissolved, further dilute in 100 mL NS or D$_5$W prior to administration. Following final dilution, solution should be used immediately or stored under refrigeration at 2°C to 8°C (36°F to 46°F). Infusion of solution must be completed within 24 hours of initial reconstitution of powder. Not compatible with calcium-containing solutions, such as lactated Ringer's.

Mechanism of Action A bisphosphonate which inhibits bone resorption via actions on osteo-clasts or on osteoclast precursors; inhibits osteoclastic activity and skeletal calcium release induced by tumors.

Pharmacodynamics/Kinetics
Onset of action: Maximum effect may not been seen for 7 days

Distribution: Binds to bone

Protein binding: ~22%

Half-life elimination: Triphasic; Terminal: 167 hours

Excretion: Urine (44% ± 18% as unchanged drug) within 24 hours; feces (<3%)

Usual Dosage I.V.: Adults:
Hypercalcemia of malignancy (albumin-corrected serum calcium ≥12 mg/dL): 4 mg (maximum) given as a single dose infused over **no less than 15 minutes**; patients should be adequately hydrated prior to treatment (restoring urine output to ~2 L/day). Monitor serum calcium and wait at least 7 days before considering retreatment. Dosage adjustment may be needed in patients with decreased renal function following treatment.

Multiple myeloma or metastatic bone lesions from solid tumors: 4 mg given over 15 minutes every 3-4 weeks; duration of treatment ranges from 9-15 months

Note: Patients should receive a daily calcium supplement and multivitamin containing vitamin D

Dosage adjustment in renal impairment: Specific dosing guidelines are not available. Patients with hypercalcemia of malignancy and pretreatment serum creatinine ≥4.5 mg/dL were excluded from clinical trials. Patients with bone metastases and pretreatment serum creatinine >3 mg/dL were excluded from clinical trials.

Dosage adjustment in hepatic impairment: Specific guidelines are not available.

Dosage adjustment for toxicity:

Hypercalcemia of malignancy: Evidence of renal deterioration: Evaluate risk versus benefit.

Bone metastases: Evidence of renal deterioration: Discontinue further dosing until renal function returns to baseline: renal deterioration defined as follows:

Normal baseline creatinine: Increase of 0.5 mg/dL

Abnormal baseline creatinine: Increase of 1 mg/dL

Dietary Considerations Multiple myeloma or metastatic bone lesions from solid tumors: Take daily calcium supplement (500 mg) and daily multivitamin (with 400 int. units vitamin D).

Administration In order to prevent renal toxicity, infuse solution over at least 15 minutes. Infuse in a line separate from other medications. Patients should be appropriately hydrated prior to treatment.

Monitoring Parameters Renal function (output, serum creatinine); serum calcium, phosphate, magnesium, electrolytes; CBC (with differential), hemoglobin, hematocrit

Patient Information This medication can only be administered intravenously. Avoid food high in calcium or vitamins during infusion or for 2-3 hours after completion. You may experience some nausea or vomiting (small frequent meals, good mouth care, sucking lozenges, or chewing gum may help) or recurrent bone pain (consult prescriber for analgesic). Report unusual muscle twitching or spasms, severe diarrhea/constipation, acute bone pain, or other persistent adverse effects. Inform prescriber if you are or intend to get pregnant. Do not get pregnant during therapy. Consult prescriber for instructions on appropriate contraceptive measures. This drug may cause fetal defects. Consult prescriber if breast-feeding.

Dosage Forms Injection, powder for reconstitution: 4 mg [as monohydrate 4.264 mg]

Zolmitriptan (zohl mi TRIP tan)

Related Information
Antimigraine Drugs Comparison *on page 1485*

U.S. Brand Names Zomig®; Zomig-ZMT™

Canadian Brand Names Zomig®

Synonyms 311C90

Therapeutic Category Antimigraine Agent, Serotonin 5-HT$_{1D}$ Agonist; Serotonin Agonist

Use Acute treatment of migraine with or without auras

Pregnancy Risk Factor C

Pregnancy/Breast-Feeding Implications In pregnant animals, zolmitriptan caused embryo-olethality and fetal abnormalities at doses ≥11 times the equivalent human dose.

Contraindications Hypersensitivity to zolmitriptan or any component of the formulation; ischemic heart disease or Prinzmetal's angina; signs or symptoms of ischemic heart disease; uncontrolled hypertension; symptomatic Wolff-Parkinson-White syndrome or arrhythmias associated with other cardiac accessory conduction pathway disorders; use with ergotamine derivatives (within 24 hours of); use within 24 hours of another 5-HT$_1$ agonist; concurrent administration or within 2 weeks of discontinuing an MAO inhibitor; management of hemi-plegic or basilar migraine

Warnings/Precautions Zolmitriptan is indicated only in patient populations with a clear diag-nosis of migraine. Not for prophylactic treatment of migraine headaches. Cardiac events (coronary artery vasospasm, transient ischemia, myocardial infarction, ventricular tachy-cardia/fibrillation, cardiac arrest, and death) have been reported with 5-HT$_1$ agonist adminis-tration. Should not be given to patients who have risk factors for CAD (eg, hypertension, hypercholesterolemia, smoker, obesity, diabetes, strong family history of CAD, menopause, male >40 years of age) without adequate cardiac evaluation. Patients with suspected CAD should have cardiovascular evaluation to rule out CAD before considering zolmitriptan's use; if cardiovascular evaluation negative, first dose would be safest if given in the healthcare provider's office. Periodic evaluation of those without cardiovascular disease, but with continued risk factors should be done. Significant elevation in blood pressure, including hypertensive crisis, has also been reported on rare occasions in patients with and without a history of hypertension. Vasospasm-related reactions have been reported other than coro-nary artery vasospasm. Peripheral vascular ischemia and colonic ischemia with abdominal (Continued)

Zolmitriptan *(Continued)*

pain and bloody diarrhea have occurred. Use with caution in patients with hepatic impairment. Zomig-ZMT™ tablets contain phenylalanine. Safety and efficacy not established in patients <18 years of age.

Adverse Reactions

1% to 10%:

Cardiovascular: Chest pain (2% to 4%), palpitations (up to 2%)

Central nervous system: Dizziness (6% to 10%), somnolence (5% to 8%), pain (2% to 3%), vertigo (≤2%)

Gastrointestinal: Nausea (4% to 9%), xerostomia (3% to 5%), dyspepsia (1% to 3%), dysphagia (≤2%)

Neuromuscular & skeletal: Paresthesia (5% to 9%), weakness (3% to 9%), warm/cold sensation (5% to 7%), hypesthesia (1% to 2%), myalgia (1% to 2%), myasthenia (up to 2%)

Miscellaneous: Neck/throat/jaw pain (4% to 10%), diaphoresis (up to 3%), allergic reaction (up to 1%)

<1% (Limited to important or life-threatening): Angina, apnea, arrhythmia, ataxia, bronchospasm, cerebral ischemia, coronary artery vasospasm, cyanosis, eosinophilia, esophagitis, hallucinations, hematemesis, hypertension, hypertensive crisis, melena, miscarriage, myocardial infarction, myocardial ischemia, pancreatitis, photosensitivity, QT prolongation, rash, syncope, tetany, thrombocytopenia, tinnitus, ulcer, urticaria

Events related to other serotonin 5-HT$_{1D}$ receptor agonists: Cardiac arrest, cerebral hemorrhage, colonic ischemia, peripheral vascular ischemia, stroke, subarachnoid hemorrhage, ventricular fibrillation

Overdosage/Toxicology Treatment is symptom directed and supportive. It is not known if hemodialysis or peritoneal dialysis is effective.

Drug Interactions

Increased Effect/Toxicity: Ergot-containing drugs may lead to vasospasm; cimetidine, MAO inhibitors, oral contraceptives, propranolol increase levels of zolmitriptan; concurrent use with SSRIs and sibutramine may lead to serotonin syndrome.

Ethanol/Nutrition/Herb Interactions Ethanol: Limit use (may have additive CNS toxicity).

Stability Store at 20°C to 25°C (68°F to 77°F); protect from light and moisture

Mechanism of Action Selective agonist for serotonin (5-HT$_{1B}$ and 5-HT$_{1D}$ receptors) in cranial arteries to cause vasoconstriction and reduce sterile inflammation associated with antidromic neuronal transmission correlating with relief of migraine

Pharmacodynamics/Kinetics

Onset of action: 0.5-1 hour

Absorption: Well absorbed

Distribution: V$_d$: 7 L/kg

Protein binding: 25%

Metabolism: Converted to an active N-desmethyl metabolite (2-6 times more potent than zolmitriptan)

Half-life elimination: 2.8-3.7 hours

Bioavailability: 40%

Time to peak, serum: Tablet: 1.5 hours; orally-disintegrating tablet: 3 hours

Excretion: Urine (~60% to 65% total dose); feces (30% to 40%)

Usual Dosage Oral:

Children: Safety and efficacy have not been established

Adults: Migraine:

Tablet: Initial: ≤2.5 mg at the onset of migraine headache; may break 2.5 mg tablet in half

Orally-disintegrating tablet: Initial: 2.5 mg at the onset of migraine headache

Note: Use the lowest possible dose to minimize adverse events. If the headache returns, the dose may be repeated after 2 hours; do not exceed 10 mg within a 24-hour period. Controlled trials have not established the effectiveness of a second dose if the initial one was ineffective

Elderly: No dosage adjustment needed but elderly patients are more likely to have underlying cardiovascular disease and should have careful evaluation of cardiovascular system before prescribing.

Dosage adjustment in renal impairment: No dosage adjustment recommended. There is a 25% reduction in zolmitriptan's clearance in patients with severe renal impairment (Cl$_{cr}$ 5-25 mL/minute)

Dosage adjustment in hepatic impairment: Administer with caution in patients with liver disease, generally using doses <2.5 mg. Patients with moderate-to-severe hepatic impairment may have decreased clearance of zolmitriptan, and significant elevation in blood pressure was observed in some patients.

Administration Administer as soon as migraine headache starts. Tablets may be broken. Orally-disintegrating tablets: Must be taken whole; do not break, crush or chew; place on tongue and allow to dissolve; administration with liquid is not required

Patient Information Take a single dose with fluids as soon as symptoms of migraine appear; a second dose may be taken if symptoms return, but no sooner than 2 hours following the first dose. For a given attack, if there is no response to the first tablet, do not take a second tablet without first consulting a physician. Do not take >10 mg in any 24-hour period.

If the patient has risk factors for heart disease (high blood pressure, high cholesterol, obesity, diabetes, smoking, strong family history of heart disease, postmenopausal woman, or a male >40 years of age), tell physician

This agent is intended to relieve migraine, but not to prevent or reduce the number of attacks. Use only to treat an actual migraine attack.

Do not use this agent if you are pregnant, think you may be pregnant, are trying to become pregnant, or are not using adequate contraception, unless you have discussed this with your physician

If pain or tightness in the chest or throat occurs when using this agent, discuss with physician before using more. If the chest pain is severe or does not go away, call physician immediately. If shortness of breath; wheezing; heart throbbing; swelling of eyelids, face or lips; skin rash, skin lumps or hives occur, tell physician immediately. Do not take any more unless the physician instructs you to do so. If feelings of tingling, heat, flushing (redness of face lasting a short time), heaviness, pressure, drowsiness, dizziness, tiredness, or sickness develop, tell your physician.

Additional Information Not recommended if the patient has risk factors for heart disease (high blood pressure, high cholesterol, obesity, diabetes, smoking, strong family history of heart disease, postmenopausal woman, or a male >40 years of age).

This agent is intended to relieve migraine, but not to prevent or reduce the number of attacks. Use only to treat an actual migraine attack.

Dosage Forms
Tablet (Zomig®): 2.5 mg, 5 mg
Tablet, orally-disintegrating (Zomig-ZMT™): 2.5 mg [contains 2.81 mg phenylalanine] [orange flavor]; 5 mg [contains 5.62 mg phenylalanine] [orange flavor]

◆ **Zoloft®** *see Sertraline on page 1231*

Zolpidem (zole PI dem)

U.S. Brand Names Ambien®
Canadian Brand Names Ambien®
Synonyms Zolpidem Tartrate
Therapeutic Category Hypnotic; Sedative
Use Short-term treatment of insomnia
Restrictions C-IV
Pregnancy Risk Factor B
Contraindications Hypersensitivity to zolpidem or any component of the formulation
Warnings/Precautions Should be used only after evaluation of potential causes of sleep disturbance. Failure of sleep disturbance to resolve after 7-10 days may indicate psychiatric or medical illness. Use with caution in patients with depression. Behavioral changes have been associated with sedative-hypnotics. Causes CNS depression, which may impair physical and mental capabilities. Effects with other sedative drugs or ethanol may be potentiated. Closely monitor elderly or debilitated patients for impaired cognitive or motor performance; not recommended for use in children <18 years of age. Avoid use in patients with sleep apnea or a history of sedative-hypnotic abuse.

Adverse Reactions
1% to 10%:
Cardiovascular: Palpitations
Central nervous system: Headache, drowsiness, dizziness, lethargy, lightheadedness, depression, abnormal dreams, amnesia
Dermatologic: Rash
Gastrointestinal: Nausea, diarrhea, xerostomia, constipation
Respiratory: Sinusitis, pharyngitis
<1% (Limited to important or life-threatening): Confusion, depression, falls, impaired concentration, manic reaction, tremor, vomiting

Overdosage/Toxicology Symptoms include coma and hypotension. Treatment for overdose is supportive. Rarely is mechanical ventilation required. Flumazenil has been shown to selectively block binding to CNS receptors, resulting in reversal of CNS depression but not always respiratory depression.

Drug Interactions
Cytochrome P450 Effect: CYP3A3/4 enzyme substrate
Increased Effect/Toxicity: Use of zolpidem in combination with other centrally-acting drugs may produce additive CNS depression. Concurrent use of drugs which inhibit cytochrome P450 3A3/4 (including erythromycin, clarithromycin, diltiazem, itraconazole, ketoconazole, nefazodone, and verapamil) may increase the levels of zolpidem.
Decreased Effect: Rifampin may reduce levels and effect of zolpidem. Other enzyme inducers may have a similar effect.

Ethanol/Nutrition/Herb Interactions
Ethanol: Avoid ethanol (may increase CNS depression).
Herb/Nutraceutical: St John's wort may decrease zolpidem levels. Avoid valerian, St John's wort, kava kava, gotu kola (may increase CNS depression).

Mechanism of Action Structurally dissimilar to benzodiazepine, however, has much or all of its actions explained by its effects on benzodiazepine (BZD) receptors, especially the omega-1 receptor (with a high affinity ratio of the alpha 1/alpha 5 subunits); retains hypnotic and much of the anxiolytic properties of the BZD, but has reduced effects on skeletal muscle and seizure threshold.

Pharmacodynamics/Kinetics
Onset of action: 30 minutes
Duration: 6-8 hours
Absorption: Rapid
Distribution: Very low amounts enter breast milk
Protein binding: 92%
Metabolism: Hepatic to inactive metabolites
Half-life elimination: 2-2.6 hours; Cirrhosis: Up to 9.9 hours

Usual Dosage Duration of therapy should be limited to 7-10 days
Adults: Oral: 10 mg immediately before bedtime; maximum dose: 10 mg
Elderly: 5 mg immediately before bedtime
Hemodialysis: Not dialyzable
Dosing adjustment in hepatic impairment: Decrease dose to 5 mg
Administration Ingest immediately before bedtime due to rapid onset of action
Monitoring Parameters Daytime alertness; respiratory and cardiac status
Reference Range 80-150 ng/mL
(Continued)

Zolpidem (Continued)

Patient Information Avoid alcohol and other CNS depressants while taking this medication; for fastest onset, take on an empty stomach; may cause drowsiness

Nursing Implications Patients may require assistance with ambulation; lower doses in the elderly are usually effective; institute safety measures

Additional Information Causes less disturbances in sleep stages as compared to benzodiazepines. Time spent in sleep stages 3 and 4 are maintained; decreases sleep latency. Should not be prescribed in quantities exceeding a 1-month supply.

Dosage Forms Tablet, as tartrate: 5 mg, 10 mg

- ◆ **Zolpidem Tartrate** see Zolpidem on page 1445
- ◆ **Zometa®** see Zoledronic Acid on page 1442
- ◆ **Zomig®** see Zolmitriptan on page 1443
- ◆ **Zomig-ZMT™** see Zolmitriptan on page 1443
- ◆ **Zonalon (Can)** see Doxepin on page 440
- ◆ **Zonalon® Cream** see Doxepin on page 440
- ◆ **Zone-A Forte®** see Pramoxine and Hydrocortisone on page 1117
- ◆ **Zonegran™** see Zonisamide on page 1446

Zonisamide (zoe NIS a mide)

Related Information

Anticonvulsants by Seizure Type on page 1481
Epilepsy & Seizure Treatment on page 1659

U.S. Brand Names Zonegran™

Canadian Brand Names Zonegran™

Therapeutic Category Anticonvulsant, Miscellaneous

Use Adjunct treatment of partial seizures in children >16 years of age and adults with epilepsy

Pregnancy Risk Factor C

Pregnancy/Breast-Feeding Implications Fetal abnormalities and death have been reported in animals, however, there are no studies in pregnant women. It is not known if zonisamide is excreted in human milk. Use during pregnancy/lactation only if the potential benefits outweigh the potential risks.

Contraindications Hypersensitivity to zonisamide, sulfonamides, or any component of the formulation

Warnings/Precautions Rare, but potentially fatal sulfonamide reactions have occurred following the use of zonisamide. These reactions include Stevens-Johnson syndrome and toxic epidermal necrolysis, usually appearing within 2-16 weeks of drug initiation. Discontinue zonisamide if rash develops. Chemical similarities are present among sulfonamides, sulfonylureas, carbonic anhydrase inhibitors, thiazides, and loop diuretics (except ethacrynic acid). Use in patients with sulfonamide allergy is specifically contraindicated in product labeling, however a risk of cross-reaction exists in patients with allergy to any of these compounds; avoid use when previous reaction has been severe. Decreased sweating and hyperthermia requiring hospitalization have been reported in children. The safety and efficacy in children <16 years of age have not been established. Discontinue zonisamide in patients who develop acute renal failure or a significant sustained increase in creatinine/BUN concentration. Kidney stones have been reported. Use cautiously in patients with renal or hepatic dysfunction. Do not use if estimated Cl_{cr} <50 mL/min. Significant CNS effects include psychiatric symptoms, psychomotor slowing, and somnolence. Fatigue and somnolence occur within the first month of treatment, most commonly at doses of 300-500 mg/day. Abrupt withdrawal may precipitate seizures; discontinue or reduce doses gradually.

Adverse Reactions Adjunctive Therapy: Frequencies noted in patients receiving other anticonvulsants:

>10%:
Central nervous system: Somnolence (17%), dizziness (13%)
Gastrointestinal: Anorexia (13%)

1% to 10%:
Central nervous system: Headache (10%), agitation/irritability (9%), fatigue (8%), tiredness (7%), ataxia (6%), confusion (6%), decreased concentration (6%), memory impairment (6%), depression (6%), insomnia (6%), speech disorders (5%), mental slowing (4%), anxiety (3%), nervousness (2%), schizophrenic/schizophreniform behavior (2%), difficulty in verbal expression (2%), status epilepticus (1%), tremor (1%), convulsion (1%), hyperesthesia (1%), incoordination (1%)
Dermatologic: Rash (3%), bruising (2%), pruritus (1%)
Gastrointestinal: Nausea (9%), abdominal pain (6%), diarrhea (5%), dyspepsia (3%), weight loss (3%), constipation (2%), dry mouth (2%), taste perversion (2%), vomiting (1%)
Neuromuscular & skeletal: Paresthesia (4%), weakness (1%), abnormal gait (1%)
Ocular: Diplopia (6%), nystagmus (4%), amblyopia (1%)
Otic: Tinnitus (1%)
Respiratory: Rhinitis (2%), pharyngitis (1%), increased cough (1%)
Miscellaneous: Flu-like syndrome (4%) accidental injury (1%)

<1% (Limited to important and/or life threatening symptoms): Agranulocytosis, allergic reaction, alopecia, aplastic anemia, apnea, atrial fibrillation, bladder calculus, cholangitis, cholecystitis, cholestatic jaundice, colitis, deafness, duodenitis, dysarthria, dyskinesia, dyspnea, dystonia, encephalopathy, esophagitis, facial paralysis, gingival hyperplasia, glaucoma, gum hemorrhage, gynecomastia, heart failure, hematemesis, hemoptysis, hirsutism, impotence, leukopenia, lupus erythematosus, menorrhagia, movement disorder, myoclonus, nephrolithiasis, neuropathy, oculogyric crisis, paresthesia, peripheral neuritis, pulmonary embolus, rash, rectal hemorrhage, Stevens-Johnson syndrome, stroke, syncope, thrombocytopenia, toxic epidermal necrolysis, urinary retention, urticaria

Overdosage/Toxicology No specific antidotes are available, experience with doses >800 mg/day are limited. Emesis or gastric lavage, with airway protection, should be done following a recent overdose. General supportive care and close observation are indicated. Renal dialysis may not be effective due to low protein binding (40%).

Drug Interactions

Cytochrome P450 Effect: CYP3A3/4 enzyme substrate

Increased Effect/Toxicity: Sedative effects may be additive with other CNS depressants; monitor for increased effect; includes barbiturates, benzodiazepines, narcotic analgesics, ethanol, and other sedative agents. Serum level and/or toxicity of zonisamide may be increased by CYP3A3/4 inhibitors; inhibitors include amiodarone, cimetidine, clarithromycin, erythromycin, delavirdine, diltiazem, dirithromycin, disulfiram, fluoxetine, fluvoxamine, grapefruit juice, indinavir, itraconazole, ketoconazole, metronidazole, nefazodone, nevirapine, propoxyphene, quinupristin-dalfopristin, ritonavir, saquinavir, verapamil, zafirlukast, zileuton; monitor for increased response.

Decreased Effect:

Note: Zonisamide did NOT affect steady state levels of carbamazepine, phenytoin, or valproate; zonisamide half-life is decreased by carbamazepine, phenytoin, phenobarbital, and valproate

Enzyme inducers: May increase the metabolism of zonisamide, reducing its effectiveness; inducers include phenytoin, carbamazepine, phenobarbital, and rifampin

Ethanol/Nutrition/Herb Interactions

Ethanol: Avoid ethanol (may increase CNS depression).

Food: Food delays time to maximum concentration, but does not affect bioavailability.

Stability Store at controlled room temperature 25°C (77°F). Protect from moisture and light.

Mechanism of Action The exact mechanism of action is not known. May stabilize neuronal membranes and suppress neuronal hypersynchronization through action at sodium and calcium channels. Does not affect GABA activity.

Pharmacodynamics/Kinetics

Distribution: V_d: 1.45 L/kg

Protein binding: 40%

Metabolism: Hepatic (CYP3A4), forms N-acetyl zonisamide and 2-sulfamoylacetyl phenol (SMAP)

Half-life elimination: 63 hours

Time to peak: 2-6 hours

Excretion: Urine (62%, 35% as unchanged drug, 65% as metabolites); feces (3%)

Usual Dosage Oral:

Children >16 years and Adults: Adjunctive treatment of partial seizures: Initial: 100 mg/day; dose may be increased to 200 mg/day after 2 weeks. Further dosage increases to 300 mg/day and 400 mg/day can then be made with a minimum of 2 weeks between adjustments, in order to reach steady state at each dosage level. Doses of up to 600 mg/day have been studied, however, there is no evidence of increased response with doses above 400 mg/day.

Elderly: Data from clinical trials is insufficient for patients >65 years; begin dosing at the low end of the dosing range.

Dosage adjustment in renal/hepatic impairment: Slower titration and frequent monitoring are indicated in patients with renal or hepatic disease. Do not use if Cl_{cr} <50 mL/minute.

Dietary Considerations May be taken with or without food.

Administration Capsules should be swallowed whole. Dose may be administered once or twice daily. Doses of 300 mg/day and higher are associated with increased side effects. Steady-state levels are reached in 14 days.

Monitoring Parameters Monitor BUN and serum creatinine

Patient Information May cause drowsiness, especially at higher doses. Do not drive a car or operate other complex machinery until effects on performance can be determined. Avoid alcohol and other CNS depressants. Contact prescriber immediately if seizures worsen or for any of the following: skin rash; sudden back pain, abdominal pain, blood in the urine; fever, sore throat, oral ulcers or easy bruising. Contact prescriber before becoming pregnant or breast-feeding. Swallow capsules whole, do not bite or break. It is important to drink 6-8 glasses of water each day while using this medication. Do not stop taking this or other seizure medications without talking to your healthcare professional first.

Nursing Implications See Contraindications and Warning/Precautions for use.

Dosage Forms Capsule: 100 mg

APPENDIX TABLE OF CONTENTS

APPENDIX TABLE OF CONTENTS *(Continued)*

ABBREVIATIONS, ACRONYMS, AND SYMBOLS

Abbreviation	Meaning
$\overline{aa}$, aa	of each
AA	Alcoholics Anonymous
ac	before meals or food
ad	to, up to
a.d.	right ear
ADHD	attention-deficit/hyperactivity disorder
ADLs	activities of daily living
ad lib	at pleasure
AIMS	Abnormal Involuntary Movement Scale
a.l.	left ear
AM	morning
amp	ampul
amt	amount
aq	water
aq. dest.	distilled water
ARDS	adult respiratory distress syndrome
a.s.	left ear
ASAP	as soon as possible
a.u.	each ear
AUC	area under the curve
BDI	Beck Depression Inventory
bid	twice daily
bm	bowel movement
bp	blood pressure
BPRS	Brief Psychiatric Rating Scale
BSA	body surface area
c	a gallon
$\overline{c}$	with
cal	calorie
cap	capsule
CBT	cognitive behavioral therapy
cc	cubic centimeter
CGI	Clinical Global Impression
cm	centimeter
CIV	continuous I.V. infusion
comp	compound
cont	continue
CRF	chronic renal failure
CT	computed tomography
d	day
d/c	discontinue
dil	dilute
disp	dispense
div	divide
DSM-IV	Diagnostic and Statistical Manual
DTs	delirium tremens
dtd	give of such a dose
ECT	electroconvulsive therapy
EEG	electroencephalogram
elix, el	elixir
emp	as directed
EPS	extrapyramidal side effects
ESRD	end stage renal disease
et	and
ex aq	in water
f, ft	make, let be made

Abbreviation	Meaning
FDA	Food and Drug Administration
g	gram
GA	Gamblers Anonymous
GAD	generalized anxiety disorder
GAF	Global Assessment of Functioning Scale
GABA	gamma-aminobutyric acid
GERD	gastroesophageal reflux disease
GITS	gastrointestinal therapeutic system
gr	grain
gtt	a drop
GVHD	graft versus host disease
h	hour
HAM-A	Hamilton Anxiety Scale
HAM-D	Hamilton Depression Scale
hs	at bedtime
HSV	herpes simplex virus
I.M.	intramuscular
IU	international unit
I.V.	intravenous
kcal	kilocalorie
kg	kilogram
KIU	kallikrein inhibitor unit
L	liter
LAMM	L-α-acetyl methadol
liq	a liquor, solution
M.	mix; Molar
MADRS	Montgomery Asbery Depression Rating Scale
MAOIs	monamine oxidase inhibitors
mcg	microgram
MDEA	3,4-methylene-dioxy amphetamine
m. dict	as directed
MDMA	3,4-methylene-dioxy methamphetamine
mEq	milliequivalent
mg	milligram
mixt	a mixture
mL	milliliter
mm	millimeter
mM	millimolar
MMSE	Mini-Mental State Examination
MPPP	l-methyl-4-proprionoxy-4-phenyl pyridine
MR	mental retardation
MRI	magnetic resonance imaging
NF	National Formulary
NMS	neuroleptic malignant syndrome
no.	number
noc	in the night
non rep	do not repeat, no refills
NPO	nothing by mouth
O, Oct	a pint
OCD	obsessive-compulsive disorder
o.d.	right eye
o.l.	left eye
o.s.	left eye
o.u.	each eye
PANSS	Positive and Negative Symptom Scale
pc, post cib	after meals
PCP	phencyclidine
per	through or by
PM	afternoon or evening

ABBREVIATIONS, ACRONYMS, AND SYMBOLS *(Continued)*

Abbreviation	Meaning
P.O.	by mouth
P.R.	rectally
prn	as needed
PTSD	post-traumatic stress disorder
pulv	a powder
q	every
qad	every other day
qd	every day
qh	every hour
qid	four times a day
qod	every other day
qs	a sufficient quantity
qs ad	a sufficient quantity to make
qty	quantity
qv	as much as you wish
REM	rapid eye movement
Rx	take, a recipe
rep	let it be repeated
s̄	without
sa	according to art
sat	saturated
S.C.	subcutaneous
sig	label, or let it be printed
sol	solution
solv	dissolve
s̄s̄	one-half
sos	if there is need
SSRIs	selective serotonin reuptake inhibitors
stat	at once, immediately
STD	sexually transmitted disease
supp	suppository
syr	syrup
tab	tablet
tal	such
TCA	tricyclic antidepressant
TD	tardive dyskinesia
tid	three times a day
tr, tinct	tincture
trit	triturate
tsp	teaspoonful
ULN	upper limits of normal
ung	ointment
USAN	United States Adopted Names
USP	United States Pharmacopeia
u.d., ut dict	as directed
v.o.	verbal order
VZV	varicella zoster virus
w.a.	while awake
x3	3 times
x4	4 times
YBOC	Yale Brown Obsessive-Compulsive Scale
YMRS	Young Mania Rating Scale

APOTHECARY/METRIC EQUIVALENTS

Approximate Liquid Measures

Basic equivalent: 1 fluid ounce = 30 mL

Examples:

1 gallon	3800 mL	1 gallon	128 fluid ounces
1 quart	960 mL	1 quart	32 fluid ounces
1 pint	480 mL	1 pint	16 fluid ounces
8 fluid oz	240 mL	15 minims	1 mL
4 fluid oz	120 mL	10 minims	0.6 mL

Approximate Household Equivalents

1 teaspoonful	5 mL	1 tablespoonful	15 mL

Weights

Basic equivalents:

1 oz	30 g	15 gr	1 g

Examples:

4 oz	120 g	1 gr	60 mg
2 oz	60 g	1/100 gr	600 mcg
10 gr	600 mg	1/150 gr	400 mcg
7 1/2 gr	500 mg	1/200 gr	300 mcg
16 oz	1 lb		

Metric Conversions

Basic equivalents:

1 g	1000 mg	1 mg	1000 mcg

Examples:

5 g	5000 mg	5 mg	5000 mcg
0.5 g	500 mg	0.5 g	500 mcg
0.05 g	50 mg	0.05 mg	50 mcg

Exact Equivalents

1 g	= 15.43 gr	0.1 mg	= 1/600 gr
1 mL	= 16.23 minims	0.12 mg	= 1/500 gr
1 minim	= 0.06 mL	0.15 mg	= 1/400 gr
1 gr	= 64.8 mg	0.2 mg	= 1/300 gr
1 pint (pt)	= 473.2 mL	0.3 mg	= 1/200 gr
1 oz	= 28.35 g	0.4 mg	= 1/150 gr
1 lb	= 453.6 g	0.5 mg	= 1/120 gr
1 kg	= 2.2 lbs	0.6 mg	= 1/100 gr
1 qt	= 946.4 mL	0.8 mg	= 1/80 gr
		1 mg	= 1/65 gr

Solids[1]

1/4 grain	=	15 mg
1/2 grain	=	30 mg
1 grain	=	60 mg
1 1/2 grains	=	90 mg
5 grains	=	300 mg
10 grains	=	600 mg

[1]Use exact equivalents for compounding and calculations requiring a high degree of accuracy.

AVERAGE WEIGHTS AND SURFACE AREAS

Average Weight and Surface Area of Preterm Infants, Term Infants, and Children

Age	Average Weight (kg)[1]	Approximate Surface Area (m²)
Weeks Gestation		
26	0.9-1	0.1
30	1.3-1.5	0.12
32	1.6-2	0.15
38	2.9-3	0.2
40 (term infant at birth)	3.1-4	0.25
Months		
3	5	0.29
6	7	0.38
9	8	0.42
Year		
1	10	0.49
2	12	0.55
3	15	0.64
4	17	0.74
5	18	0.76
6	20	0.82
7	23	0.90
8	25	0.95
9	28	1.06
10	33	1.18
11	35	1.23
12	40	1.34
Adults	70	1.73

[1]Weights from age 3 months and older are rounded off to the nearest kilogram.

BODY SURFACE AREA OF ADULTS AND CHILDREN

Calculating Body Surface Area in Children

In a child of average size, find weight and corresponding surface area on the boxed scale to the left; or, use the nomogram to the right. Lay a straightedge on the correct height and weight points for the child, then read the intersecting point on the surface area scale.

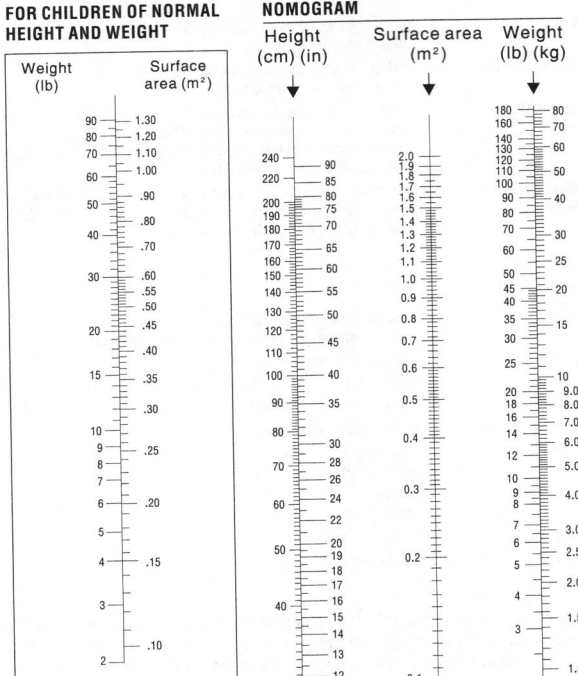

FOR CHILDREN OF NORMAL HEIGHT AND WEIGHT

NOMOGRAM

BODY SURFACE AREA FORMULA
(Adult and Pediatric)

$$\text{BSA (m}^2) = \sqrt{\frac{\text{Ht (in) x Wt (lb)}}{3131}} \quad \text{or, in metric: BSA (m}^2) = \sqrt{\frac{\text{Ht (cm) x Wt (kg)}}{3600}}$$

References
Lam TK and Leung DT, "More on Simplified Calculation of Body Surface Area," *N Engl J Med*, 1988, 318(17):1130 (Letter).
Mosteller RD, "Simplified Calculation of Body Surface Area", *N Engl J Med*, 1987, 317(17):1098 (Letter).

IDEAL BODY WEIGHT CALCULATION

Adults (18 years and older) (IBW is in kg)

    IBW (male) = 50 + (2.3 x height in inches over 5 feet)
    IBW (female) = 45.5 + (2.3 x height in inches over 5 feet)

Children (IBW is in kg; height is in cm)

    a.   1-18 years

$$\text{IBW} = \frac{(\text{height}^2 \times 1.65)}{1000}$$

    b.   5 feet and taller
        IBW (male) = 39 + (2.27 x height in inches over 5 feet)
        IBW (female) = 42.2 + (2.27 x height in inches over 5 feet)

MILLIEQUIVALENT AND MILLIMOLE CALCULATIONS & CONVERSIONS

DEFINITIONS & CALCULATIONS

Definitions

mole	=	gram molecular weight of a substance (aka molar weight)
millimole (mM)	=	milligram molecular weight of a substance (a millimole is 1/1000 of a mole)
equivalent weight	=	gram weight of a substance which will combine with or replace one gram (one mole) of hydrogen; an equivalent weight can be determined by dividing the molar weight of a substance by its ionic valence
milliequivalent (mEq)	=	milligram weight of a substance which will combine with or replace one milligram (one millimole) of hydrogen (a milliequivalent is 1/1000 of an equivalent)

Calculations

moles	=	$\dfrac{\text{weight of a substance (grams)}}{\text{molecular weight of that substance (grams)}}$
millimoles	=	$\dfrac{\text{weight of a substance (milligrams)}}{\text{molecular weight of that substance (milligrams)}}$
equivalents	=	moles x valence of ion
milliequivalents	=	millimoles x valence of ion
moles	=	$\dfrac{\text{equivalents}}{\text{valence of ion}}$
millimoles	=	$\dfrac{\text{milliequivalents}}{\text{valence of ion}}$
millimoles	=	moles x 1000
milliequivalents	=	equivalents x 1000

Note: Use of equivalents and milliequivalents is valid only for those substances which have fixed ionic valences (eg, sodium, potassium, calcium, chlorine, magnesium bromine, etc). For substances with variable ionic valences (eg, phosphorous), a reliable equivalent value cannot be determined. In these instances, one should calculate millimoles (which are fixed and reliable) rather than milliequivalents.

MILLIEQUIVALENT CONVERSIONS

To convert mg/100 mL to mEq/L the following formula may be used:

$$\frac{(\text{mg/100 mL}) \times 10 \times \text{valence}}{\text{atomic weight}} = \text{mEq/L}$$

To convert mEq/L to mg/100 mL the following formula may be used:

$$\frac{(\text{mEq/L}) \times \text{atomic weight}}{10 \times \text{valence}} = \text{mg/100 mL}$$

To convert mEq/L to volume of percent of a gas the following formula may be used:

$$\frac{(\text{mEq/L}) \times 22.4}{10} = \text{volume percent}$$

Valences and Atomic Weights of Selected Ions

Substance	Electrolyte	Valence	Molecular Wt
Calcium	Ca^{++}	2	40
Chloride	Cl^-	1	35.5
Magnesium	Mg^{++}	2	24
Phosphate	HPO_4^{--} (80%)	1.8	96*
pH = 7.4	$H_2PO_4^-$ (20%)	1.8	96*
Potassium	K^+	1	39
Sodium	Na^+	1	23
Sulfate	SO_4^{--}	2	96*

*The molecular weight of phosphorus only is 31, and sulfur only is 32.

Approximate Milliequivalents — Weights of Selected Ions

Salt	mEq/g Salt	Mg Salt/mEq
Calcium carbonate [$CaCO_3$]	20	50
Calcium chloride [$CaCl_2 \cdot 2H_2O$]	14	74
Calcium gluceptate [$Ca(C_7H_{13}O_8)_2$]	4	245
Calcium gluconate [$Ca(C_6H_{11}O_7)_2 \cdot H_2O$]	5	224
Calcium lactate [$Ca(C_3H_5O_3)_2 \cdot 5H_2O$]	7	154
Magnesium gluconate [$Mg(C_6H_{11}O_7)_2 \cdot H_2O$]	5	216
Magnesium oxide [MgO]	50	20
Magnesium sulfate [$MgSO_4$]	17	60
Magnesium sulfate [$MgSO_4 \cdot 7H_2O$]	8	123
Potassium acetate [$K(C_2H_3O_2)$]	10	98
Potassium chloride [KCl]	13	75
Potassium citrate [$K_3(C_6H_5O_7) \cdot H_2O$]	9	108
Potassium iodide [KI]	6	166
Sodium acetate [$Na(C_2H_3O_2)$]	12	82
Sodium acetate [$Na(C_2H_3O_2) \cdot 3H_2O$]	7	136
Sodium bicarbonate [$NaHCO_3$]	12	84
Sodium chloride [$NaCl$]	17	58
Sodium citrate [$Na_3(C_6H_5O_7) \cdot 2H_2O$]	10	98
Sodium iodine [NaI]	7	150
Sodium lactate [$Na(C_3H_5O_3)$]	9	112
Zinc sulfate [$ZnSO_4 \cdot 7H_2O$]	7	144

CORRECTED SODIUM

Corrected Na^+ = measured Na^+ + [1.5 x (glucose − 150 divided by 100)]

Note: Do not correct for glucose <150.

WATER DEFICIT

Water deficit = 0.6 x body weight [1 − (140 divided by Na^+)]

Note: Body weight is estimated weight in kg when fully hydrated; **Na^+** is serum or plasma sodium. Use corrected Na^+ if necessary. Consult medical references for recommendations for replacement of deficit.

TOTAL SERUM CALCIUM CORRECTED FOR ALBUMIN LEVEL

[(Normal albumin − patient's albumin) x 0.8] + patient's measured total calcium

ACID-BASE ASSESSMENT

Henderson-Hasselbalch Equation

$$pH = 6.1 + \log (HCO_3^- / (0.03) (pCO_2))$$

MILLIEQUIVALENT AND MILLIMOLE CALCULATIONS & CONVERSIONS (Continued)

Alveolar Gas Equation

PIO_2 = FiO_2 x (total atmospheric pressure – vapor pressure of H_2O at 37°C)

= FiO_2 x (760 mm Hg – 47 mm Hg)

PAO_2 = PIO_2 – $PACO_2$ / R

Alveolar/arterial oxygen gradient = PAO_2 – PaO_2

Normal ranges:

Children	15-20 mm Hg
Adults	20-25 mm Hg

where:

PIO_2	=	Oxygen partial pressure of inspired gas (mm Hg) (150 mm Hg in room air at sea level)
FiO_2	=	Fractional pressure of oxygen in inspired gas (0.21 in room air)
PAO_2	=	Alveolar oxygen partial pressure
$PACO_2$	=	Alveolar carbon dioxide partial pressure
PaO_2	=	Arterial oxygen partial pressure
R	=	Respiratory exchange quotient (typically 0.8, increases with high carbohydrate diet, decreases with high fat diet)

Acid-Base Disorders

Acute metabolic acidosis (<12 h duration):

$$PaCO_2 \text{ expected} = 1.5 (HCO_3^-) + 8 \pm 2$$
or

expected change in pCO = (1-1.5) x change in HCO_3^-

Acute metabolic alkalosis (<12 h duration):

expected change in pCO_2 = (0.5-1) x change in HCO_3^-

Acute respiratory acidosis (<6 h duration):

expected change in HCO_3^- = 0.1 x pCO_2

Acute respiratory acidosis (>6 h duration):

expected change in HCO_3^- = 0.4 x change in pCO_2

Acute respiratory alkalosis (<6 h duration):

expected change in HCO_3^- = 0.2 x change in pCO_2

Acute respiratory alkalosis (>6 h duration):

expected change in HCO_3^- = 0.5 x change in pCO_2

ACID-BASE EQUATION

H^+ (in mEq/L) = (24 x $PaCO_2$) divided by HCO_3^-

Aa GRADIENT

Aa gradient $[(713)(FiO_2 - (PaCO_2 \text{ divided by } 0.8))] - PaO_2$

Aa gradient	=	alveolar-arterial oxygen gradient
FiO_2	=	inspired oxygen (expressed as a fraction)
$PaCO_2$	=	arterial partial pressure carbon dioxide (mm Hg)
PaO_2	=	arterial partial pressure oxygen (mm Hg)

OSMOLALITY

Definition: The summed concentrations of all osmotically active solute particles.

Predicted serum osmolality =
$$2 Na^+ + glucose (mg/dL) / 18 + BUN (mg/dL) / 2.8$$

The normal range of serum osmolality is 285-295 mOsm/L.

Differential diagnosis of increased serum osmolal gap (>10 mOsm/L)

Medications and toxins
Alcohols (ethanol, methanol, isopropanol, glycerol, ethylene glycol)
Mannitol
Paraldehyde

Calculated Osm

Osmolal gap = measured Osm − calculated Osm

0 to +10: Normal
>10: Abnormal
<0: Probable lab or calculation error

For drugs causing increased osmolar gap, see "Toxicology Information" section in this Appendix.

BICARBONATE DEFICIT

HCO_3^- deficit = (0.4 x wt in kg) x (HCO_3^- desired − HCO_3^- measured)

Note: In clinical practice, the calculated quantity may differ markedly from the actual amount of bicarbonate needed or that which may be safely administered.

ANION GAP

Definition: The difference in concentration between unmeasured cation and anion equivalents in serum.

Anion gap = $Na^+ - (Cl^- + HCO_3^-)$
(The normal anion gap is 10-14 mEq/L)

Differential Diagnosis of Increased Anion Gap Acidosis

Organic anions

Lactate (sepsis, hypovolemia, seizures, large tumor burden)
Pyruvate
Uremia
Ketoacidosis (β-hydroxybutyrate and acetoacetate)
Amino acids and their metabolites
Other organic acids

Inorganic anions

Hyperphosphatemia
Sulfates
Nitrates

Differential Diagnosis of Decreased Anion Gap

Organic cations

Hypergammaglobulinemia

Inorganic cations

Hyperkalemia
Hypercalcemia
Hypermagnesemia

Medications and toxins

Lithium

Hypoalbuminemia

RETICULOCYTE INDEX

(% retic divided by 2) x (patient's Hct divided by normal Hct) or (% retic divided by 2) x (patient's Hgb divided by normal Hgb)

Normal index: 1.0
Good marrow response: 2.0-6.0

PEDIATRIC DOSAGE ESTIMATIONS

Dosage Estimations Based on Weight:

Augsberger's rule:

$$\frac{(1.5 \times \text{weight in kg} + 10)}{\text{\% of adult dose}} = \text{child's approximate dose}$$

Clark's rule:

$$\frac{\text{weight (in pounds)}}{150} \times \text{adult dose} = \text{child's approximate dose}$$

Dosage Estimations Based on Age:

Augsberger's rule:

$$\frac{(4 \times \text{age in years} + 20)}{\text{\% of adult dose}} = \text{child's approximate dose}$$

Bastedo's rule:

$$\frac{\text{age in years} + 3}{30} \times \text{adult dose} = \text{child's approximate dose}$$

Cowling's rule:

$$\frac{\text{age at next birthday (in years)}}{24} \times \text{adult dose} = \text{child's approximate dose}$$

Dilling's rule:

$$\frac{\text{age (in years)}}{20} \times \text{adult dose} = \text{child's approximate dose}$$

Fried's rule for infants (younger than 1 year):

$$\frac{\text{age (in months)}}{150} \times \text{adult dose} = \text{infant's approximate dose}$$

Young's rule:

$$\frac{\text{age (in years)}}{\text{age} + 12} \times \text{adult dose} = \text{child's approximate dose}$$

POUNDS/KILOGRAMS CONVERSION

1 pound = 0.45359 kilograms
1 kilogram = 2.2 pounds

lb	=	kg	lb	=	kg	lb	=	kg
1		0.45	70		31.75	140		63.50
5		2.27	75		34.02	145		65.77
10		4.54	80		36.29	150		68.04
15		6.80	85		38.56	155		70.31
20		9.07	90		40.82	160		72.58
25		11.34	95		43.09	165		74.84
30		13.61	100		45.36	170		77.11
35		15.88	105		47.63	175		79.38
40		18.14	110		49.90	180		81.65
45		20.41	115		52.16	185		83.92
50		22.68	120		54.43	190		86.18
55		24.95	125		56.70	195		88.45
60		27.22	130		58.91	200		90.72
65		29.48	135		61.24			

TEMPERATURE CONVERSION

Celsius to Fahrenheit = ($^\circ$C x 9/5) + 32 = $^\circ$F
Fahrenheit to Celsius = ($^\circ$F − 32) x 5/9 = $^\circ$C

$^\circ$C	=	$^\circ$F	$^\circ$C	=	$^\circ$F	$^\circ$C	=	$^\circ$F
100.0		212.0	39.0		102.2	36.8		98.2
50.0		122.0	38.8		101.8	36.6		97.9
41.0		105.8	38.6		101.5	36.4		97.5
40.8		105.4	38.4		101.1	36.2		97.2
40.6		105.1	38.2		100.8	36.0		96.8
40.4		104.7	38.0		100.4	35.8		96.4
40.2		104.4	37.8		100.1	35.6		96.1
40.0		104.0	37.6		99.7	35.4		95.7
39.8		103.6	37.4		99.3	35.2		95.4
39.6		103.3	37.2		99.0	35.0		95.0
39.4		102.9	37.0		98.6	0		32.0
39.2		102.6						

LIVER DISEASE

Pugh's Modification of Child's Classification for Severity

Parameter	Points for Increasing Abnormality		
	1	2	3
Encephalopathy	None	1 or 2	3 or 4
Ascites	Absent	Slight	Moderate
Bilirubin (mg/dL)	<2.9	2.9-5.8	>5.8
Albumin (g/dL)	>3.5	2.8-3.5	<2.8
Prothrombin time (seconds over control)	1-4	4-6	>6

Scores:

Mild hepatic impairment = <6 points.
Moderate hepatic impairment = 6-10 points.
Severe hepatic impairment = >10 points.

Considerations for Drug Dose Adjustment

Extent of Change in Drug Dose	Conditions or Requirements to Be Satisfied
No or minor change	Mild liver disease
	Extensive elimination of drug by kidneys and no renal dysfunction
	Elimination by pathways of metabolism spared by liver disease
	Drug is enzyme-limited and given acutely
	Drug is flow/enzyme-sensitive and only given acutely by I.V. route
	No alteration in drug sensitivity
Decrease in dose up to 25%	Elimination by the liver does not exceed 40% of the dose; no renal dysfunction
	Drug is flow-limited and given by I.V. route, with no large change in protein binding
	Drug is flow/enzyme-limited and given acutely by oral route
	Drug has a large therapeutic ratio
>25% decrease in dose	Drug metabolism is affected by liver disease; drug administered chronically
	Drug has a narrow therapeutic range; protein binding altered significantly
	Drug is flow-limited and given orally
	Drug is eliminated by kidneys and renal function severely affected
	Altered sensitivity to drug due to liver disease

Reference

Arns PA, Wedlund PJ, and Branch RA, "Adjustment of Medications in Liver Failure," *The Pharmacologic Approach to the Critically Ill Patient*, 2nd ed, Chernow B, ed, Baltimore, MD: Williams & Wilkins, 1988, 85-111.

CREATININE CLEARANCE ESTIMATING METHODS IN PATIENTS WITH STABLE RENAL FUNCTION

These formulas provide an acceptable estimate of the patient's creatinine clearance **except** in the following instances.

- Patient's serum creatinine is changing rapidly (either up or down).

- Patients are markedly emaciated.

In above situations, certain assumptions have to be made.

- In patients with rapidly rising serum creatinines (ie, >0.5-0.7 mg/dL/day), it is best to assume that the patient's creatinine clearance is probably <10 mL/minute.

- In emaciated patients, although their actual creatinine clearance is less than their calculated creatinine clearance (because of decreased creatinine production), it is not possible to easily predict how much less.

Infants

Estimation of creatinine clearance using serum creatinine and body length (to be used when an adequate timed specimen cannot be obtained). **Note:** This formula may not provide an accurate estimation of creatinine clearance for infants younger than 6 months of age and for patients with severe starvation or muscle wasting.

$$Cl_{cr} = K \times L/S_{cr}$$

where:

Cl_{cr} = creatinine clearance in mL/minute/1.73 m^2

K = constant of proportionality that is age specific

Age	K
Low birth weight ≤1 y	0.33
Full-term ≤1 y	0.45
2-12 y	0.55
13-21 y female	0.55
13-21 y male	0.70

L = length in cm

S_{cr} = serum creatinine concentration in mg/dL

Reference

Schwartz GJ, Brion LP, and Spitzer A, "The Use of Plasma Creatinine Concentration for Estimating Glomerular Filtration Rate in Infants, Children and Adolescents," *Ped Clin N Amer*, 1987, 34:571-90.

Children (1-18 years)

Method 1: (Traub SL and Johnson CE, *Am J Hosp Pharm*, 1980, 37:195-201)

Equation:

$$Cl_{cr} = \frac{0.48 \times (height)}{S_{cr}}$$

where

Cl_{cr} = creatinine clearance in mL/min/1.73 m^2

S_{cr} = serum creatinine in mg/dL

Height = height in cm

CREATININE CLEARANCE ESTIMATING METHODS IN PATIENTS WITH STABLE RENAL FUNCTION *(Continued)*

<u>Method 2</u>: Nomogram (Traub SL and Johnson CE, *Am J Hosp Pharm*, 1980, 37:195-201)

Children 1-18 Years

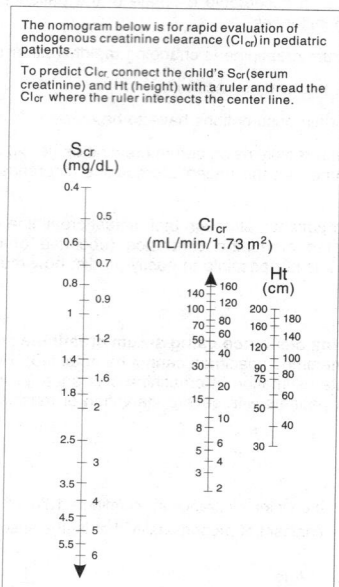

The nomogram below is for rapid evaluation of endogenous creatinine clearance (Cl_{cr}) in pediatric patients.

To predict Cl_{cr} connect the child's S_{cr} (serum creatinine) and Ht (height) with a ruler and read the Cl_{cr} where the ruler intersects the center line.

Adults (18 years and older)

<u>Method 1</u>: (Cockroft DW and Gault MH, *Nephron*, 1976, 16:31-41)

Estimated creatinine clearance (Cl_{cr}) (mL/min):

$$Male = \frac{(140 - age)\ IBW\ (kg)}{72 \times S_{cr}}$$

$$Female = estimated\ Cl_{cr}\ male \times 0.85$$

Note: The use of the patient's ideal body weight (IBW) is recommended for the above formula except when the patient's actual body weight is less than ideal. Use of the IBW is especially important in obese patients.

Method 2: (Jelliffe RW, *Ann Intern Med*, 1973, 79:604)

Estimated creatinine clearance (Cl_{cr}) (mL/min/1.73 m^2):

$$Male = \frac{98 - 0.8\ (age - 20)}{serum\ creatinine}$$

$$Female = Estimated\ Cl_{cr}\ male \times 0.90$$

RENAL FUNCTION TESTS

Endogenous creatinine clearance vs age (timed collection)

Creatinine clearance (mL/min/1.73 m^2) = (Cr_uV/Cr_sT) (1.73/A)

where:

Cr_u	=	urine creatinine concentration (mg/dL)
V	=	total urine collected during sampling period (mL)
Cr_s	=	serum creatinine concentration (mg/dL)
T	=	duration of sampling period (min) (24 h = 1440 min)
A	=	body surface area (m^2)

Age-specific normal values

5-7 d	50.6 ± 5.8 mL/min/1.73 m^2
1-2 mo	64.6 ± 5.8 mL/min/1.73 m^2
5-8 mo	87.7 ± 11.9 mL/min/1.73 m^2
9-12 mo	86.9 ± 8.4 mL/min/1.73 m^2
≥18 mo	
male	124 ± 26 mL/min/1.73 m^2
female	109 ± 13.5 mL/min/1.73 m^2
Adults	
male	105 ± 14 mL/min/1.73 m^2
female	95 ± 18 mL/min/1.73 m^2

Note: In patients with renal failure (creatinine clearance <25 mL/min), creatinine clearance may be elevated over GFR because of tubular secretion of creatinine.

Calculation of Creatinine Clearance From a 24-Hour Urine Collection

Equation 1:

$$Cl_{cr} = \frac{U \times V}{P}$$

where:

Cl_{cr}	=	creatinine clearance
U	=	urine concentration of creatinine
V	=	total urine volume in the collection
P	=	plasma creatinine concentration

Equation 2:

$$Cl_{cr} = \frac{(\text{total urine volume [mL]}) \times (\text{urine Cr concentration [mg/dL]})}{(\text{serum creatinine [mg/dL]}) \times (\text{time of urine collection [minutes]})}$$

Occasionally, a patient will have a 12- or 24-hour urine collection done for direct calculation of creatinine clearance. Although a urine collection for 24 hours is best, it is difficult to do since many urine collections occur for a much shorter period. A 24-hour urine collection is the desired duration of urine collection because the urine excretion of creatinine is diurnal and thus the measured creatinine clearance will vary throughout the day as the creatinine in the urine varies. When the urine collection is less than 24 hours, the total excreted creatinine will be affected by the time of the day during which the collection is performed. A 24-hour urine collection is sufficient to be able to accurately average the diurnal creatinine excretion variations. If a patient has 24 hours of urine collected for creatinine clearance, equation 1 can be used for calculating the creatinine clearance. To use equation 1 to calculate the creatinine clearance, it will be necessary to know the duration of urine collection, the urine collection volume, the urine creatinine concentration, and the serum creatinine value that reflects the urine collection period. In most cases, a serum creatinine concentration is drawn anytime during the day, but it is best to have the value drawn halfway through the collection period.

Amylase/Creatinine Clearance Ratio

$$\frac{\text{Amylase}_u \times \text{creatinine}_p}{\text{Amylase}_p \times \text{creatinine}_u} \times 100$$

u = urine; p = plasma

RENAL FUNCTION TESTS *(Continued)*

Serum BUN/Serum Creatinine Ratio

Serum BUN (mg/dL:serum creatinine (mg/dL))

Normal BUN:creatinine ratio is 10-15

BUN:creatinine ratio >20 suggests prerenal azotemia (also seen with high urea-generation states such as GI bleeding)

BUN:creatinine ratio <5 may be seen with disorders affecting urea biosynthesis such as urea cycle enzyme deficiencies and with hepatitis.

Fractional Sodium Excretion

Fractional sodium secretion (FENa) = $Na_u Cr_s / Na_s Cr_u \times 100\%$

where:

$$
\begin{aligned}
Na_u &= \text{urine sodium (mEq/L)} \\
Na_s &= \text{serum sodium (mEq/L)} \\
Cr_u &= \text{urine creatinine (mg/dL)} \\
Cr_s &= \text{serum creatinine (mg/dL)}
\end{aligned}
$$

FENa <1% suggests prerenal failure

FENa >2% suggest intrinsic renal failure
(for newborns, normal FENa is approximately 2.5%)

Note: Disease states associated with a falsely elevated FENa include severe volume depletion (>10%), early acute tubular necrosis and volume depletion in chronic renal disease. Disorders associated with a lowered FENa include acute glomerulonephritis, hemoglobinuric or myoglobinuric renal failure, nonoliguric acute tubular necrosis and acute urinary tract obstruction. In addition, FENa may be <1% in patients with acute renal failure **and** a second condition predisposing to sodium retention (eg, burns, congestive heart failure, nephrotic syndrome).

Urine Calcium/Urine Creatinine Ratio (spot sample)

Urine calcium (mg/dL): urine creatinine (mg/dL)

Normal values <0.21 (mean values 0.08 males, 0.06 females)

Premature infants show wide variability of calcium:creatinine ratio, and tend to have lower thresholds for calcium loss than older children. Prematures without nephrolithiasis had mean Ca:Cr ratio of 0.75 ± 0.76. Infants with nephrolithiasis had mean Ca:Cr ratio of 1.32 ± 1.03 (Jacinto JS, Modanlou HD, Crade M, et al, "Renal Calcification Incidence in Very Low Birth Weight Infants," *Pediatrics*, 1988, 81:31.)

Urine Protein/Urine Creatinine Ratio (spot sample)

P_u/Cr_u	Total Protein Excretion (mg/m²/d)
0.1	80
1	800
10	8000

where:

P_u = urine protein concentration (mg/dL)
Cr_u = urine creatinine concentration (mg/dL)

ADRENERGIC AGONISTS, CARDIOVASCULAR

Drug	Hemodynamic Effects			
	CO	TPR	Mean BP	Renal Perfusion
Dobutamine (Dobutrex®)	↑	↓	↑	<-->
Dopamine (Intropin®)	↑	+/--[1]	<-->/↑[1]	↑[1]
Epinephrine (Adrenalin®)	↑	↓	↑	↓
Inamrinone (Inocor®)	↑	↓	<-->	↑
Isoproterenol (Isuprel®)	↑	↓	↓	+/--[2]
Metaraminol (Aramine®)	↓	↑	↑	↓
Milrinone (Primacor®)	↑	↓	<-->	↑
Norepinephrine (Levophed®)	<-->/↓	↑	↑	↓
Phenylephrine (Neo-Synephrine®)	↓	↑	↑	↓

↑ = increase ↓ = decrease, <--> = no change.

[1]Dose dependent.

[2]In patients with cardiogenic or septic shock, renal perfusion commonly increases; however, in the normal patient, renal perfusion may be reduced with isoproterenol.

Drug	Hemodynamic Effects			
	α1	β1	β2	Dopamine
Dobutamine	+	++++	++	0
Dopamine	++++	++++	++	++
Epinephrine	++++	++++	++	++
Isoproterenol	0	++++	++++	0
Norepinephrine	++++	++++	0	0

Usual Hemodynamic Effects of Intravenous Agents Commonly Used for the Treatment of Acute/Severe Heart Failure

Drug	Dose	HR	MAP	PCWP	CO	SVR
Dobutamine	2.5-20 mcg/kg/min	0/↑	0/↑	↓	↑	↓
Dopamine	1-3 mcg/kg/min	0	0	0	0/↑	↓
	3-10 mcg/kg/min	↑	↑	0	↑	0
	>10 mcg/kg/min	↑	↑	↑	↑	↑
Furosemide (Lasix®)	20-80 mg, repeated as needed up to 4-6 times/day	0	0	↓	0	0
Inamrinone	5-10 mcg/kg/min	0/↑	0/↓	↓	↑	↓
Milrinone	0.375-0.75 mcg/kg/min	0/↑	0/↓	↓	↑	↓
Nitroglycerin	0.1-2 mcg/kg/min	0/↑	0/↓	↓	0/↑	0/↓
Nitroprusside (Nitropress®)	0.25-3 mcg/kg/min	0/↑	0/↓	↓	↑	↓

HR = heart rate, MAP = mean arterial pressure, PCWP = pulmonary capillary wedge pressure, CO = cardiac output, SVR = systemic vascular resistance

↑ = increase, ↓ = decrease, 0 = no change

AMINOGLYCOSIDE DOSING AND MONITORING

All aminoglycoside therapy should be individualized for specific patients in specific clinical situation. The following are guidelines for initiating therapy.

1. Loading dose based on estimated ideal body weight (IBW). **All patients require a loading dose independent of renal function**.

Agent	Dose
Gentamicin (Garamycin®)	2 mg/kg
Tobramycin (Nebcin®)	2 mg/kg
Amikacin (Amikin®)	7.5 mg/kg

    Significantly higher loading doses may be required in severely ill intensive care unit patients.

2. Initial maintenance doses as a percent of loading dose according to desired dosing interval and creatinine clearance (Cl_{cr}):

    $$\text{Male } Cl_{cr} \text{ (mL/min)} = \frac{(140 - age) \times IBW}{72 \times \text{serum creatinine}}$$

    $$\text{Female} = 0.85 \times Cl_{cr} \text{ males}$$

Cl_{cr} (mL/min)	Dosing Interval (h)		
	8	12	24
90	84%	—	—
80	80%	—	—
70	76%	88%	—
60	—	84%	—
50	—	79%	—
40	—	72%	92%
30	—	—	86%
25	—	—	81%
20	—	—	75%

    Patients >65 years of age should not receive initial aminoglycoside maintenance dosing more often than every 12 hours.

3. Serum concentration monitoring

    a. Serum concentration monitoring is necessary for **safe** and **effective** therapy, particularly in patients with serious infections and those with risk factors for toxicity.

    b. Peak serum concentrations should be drawn 30 minutes after the completion of a 30-minute infusion. Trough serum concentrations should be drawn within 30 minutes prior to the administered dose.

    c. Serum concentrations should be drawn after 5 half-lives, usually around the third dose or thereafter.

4. Desired measured serum concentrations

	Peak (mcg/mL)	Trough (mcg/mL)
Gentamicin	6-10	0.5-2.0
Tobramycin	6-10	0.5-2.0
Amikacin	20-30	<5

5. For patients receiving hemodialysis:

- administer the **same** loading dose
- administer $2/3$ of the loading dose after each dialysis
- **serum concentrations must be monitored**
- watch for ototoxicity from accumulation of drug

6. For individual clinical situations the prescribing physician should feel free to consult Infectious Disease, the Pharmacology Service, or the Pharmacy.

"Once Daily" Aminoglycosides

High dose, "once daily" aminoglycoside therapy for treatment of gram-negative bacterial infections has been studied and remains controversial. The pharmacodynamics of aminoglycosides reveal dose-dependent killing which suggests an efficacy advantage of "high" peak serum concentrations. It is also suggested that allowing troughs to fall to unmeasurable levels decreases the risk of nephrotoxicity without detriment to efficacy. Because of a theoretical saturation of tubular cell uptake of aminoglycosides, decreasing the number of times the drug is administered in a particular time period may play a role in minimizing the risk of nephrotoxicity. Ototoxicity has not been sufficiently formally evaluated through audiometry or vestibular testing comparing "once daily" to standard therapy. Over 100 letters, commentaries, studies and reviews have been published on the topic of "once daily" aminoglycosides with varying dosing regimens, monitoring parameters, inclusion and exclusion criteria, and results (most of which have been favorable for the "once daily" regimens). The caveats of this simplified method of dosing are several, including assurance that creatinine clearances be calculated, that all patients are not candidates and should not be considered for this regimen, and that "once daily" is a semantic misnomer.

Because of the controversial nature of this method, it is beyond the scope of this book to present significant detail and dosing regimen recommendations. Considerable experience with two methods warrants mention. The Hartford Hospital has experience with over 2000 patients utilizing a 7 mg/kg dose, a dosing scheme for various creatinine clearance estimates, and a serum concentration monitoring nomogram.[1] Providence Medical Center utilizes a 5 mg/kg dosing regimen but only in patients with excellent renal function; serum concentrations are monitored 4-6 hours prior to the dose administered.[2] Two excellent reviews discuss the majority of studies and controversies regarding these dosing techniques.[3,4] An editorial accompanies one of the reviews and is worth examination.[5]

"Once daily" dosing may be a safe and effective method of providing aminoglycoside therapy to a large number of patients who require these efficacious yet toxic agents. As with any method of aminoglycoside administration, dosing must be individualized and the caveats of the method considered.

Footnotes

1. Nicolau DP, Freeman CD, Belliveau PP, et al, "Experience With a Once-Daily Aminoglycoside Program Administered to 2,184 Patients," *Antimicrob Agents Chemother*, 1995, 39:650-5.

2. Gilbert DN, "Once-Daily Aminoglycoside Therapy," *Antimicrob Agents Chemother*, 1991, 35:399-405.

3. Preston SL and Briceland LL, "Single Daily Dosing of Aminoglycosides," *Pharmacotherapy*, 1995, 15:297-316.

4. Bates RD and Nahata MC, "Once-Daily Administration of Aminoglycosides," *Ann Pharmacother*, 1994, 28:757-66.

5. Rotschafer JC and Rybak MJ, "Single Daily Dosing of Aminoglycosides: A Commentary," *Ann Pharmacother*, 1994, 28:797-801.

AMINOGLYCOSIDE DOSING AND MONITORING *(Continued)*

Aminoglycoside Penetration Into Various Tissues

Site	Extent of Distribution
Eye	Poor
CNS	Poor (<25%)
Pleural	Excellent
Bronchial secretions	Poor
Sputum	Fair (10%-50%)
Pulmonary tissue	Excellent
Ascitic fluid	Variable (43%-132%)
Peritoneal fluid	Poor
Bile	Variable (25%-90%)
Bile with obstruction	Poor
Synovial fluid	Excellent
Bone	Poor
Prostate	Poor
Urine	Excellent
Renal tissue	Excellent

From Neu HC, "Pharmacology of Aminoglycosides," *The Aminoglycosides*, Whelton E and Neu HC, eds, New York, NY: Marcel Dekker, Inc, 1981.

ANGIOTENSIN AGENTS

Comparisons of Indications and Adult Dosages

Drug	Hypertension	CHF	Renal Dysfunction	Dialyzable	Strengths (mg)
Benazepril (Lotensin®)	20-80 mg qd qd-bid Maximum: 80 mg qd	Not FDA approved	Cl_{cr} <30 mL/min: 5 mg/day initially Maximum: 40 mg qd	Yes	Tablets 5, 10, 20, 40
Candesartan[1] (Atacand®)	8-32 mg qd qd-bid Maximum: 32 mg qd	Not FDA approved	No adjustment necessary	No	Tablets 4, 8, 16, 32
Captopril (Capoten®)	25-150 mg qd bid-tid Maximum: 450 mg qd	6.25-100 mg tid Maximum: 450 mg qd	Cl_{cr} 10-50 mL/min: 75% of usual dose Cl_{cr} <10 mL/min: 50% of usual dose	Yes	Tablets 12.5, 25, 50, 100
Enalapril (Vasotec®)	5-40 mg qd qd-bid Maximum: 40 mg qd	2.5-20 mg bid Maximum: 20 mg bid	Cl_{cr} 30-80 mL/min: 5 mg/day initially Cl_{cr} <30 mL/min: 2.5 mg/day initially	Yes	Tablets 2.5, 5, 10, 20
Enalaprilat[2]	0.625 mg, 1.25 mg, 2.5 mg q6h Maximum: 5 mg q6h	Not FDA approved	Cl_{cr} <30 mL/min: 0.625 mg	Yes	2.5 mg/2 mL vial
Eprosartan[1] (Teveten®)	400-800 mg qd qd-bid	Not FDA approved	No dosage adjustment necessary	Unknown	Tablets 400, 600
Fosinopril (Monopril®)	10-40 mg qd Maximum: 80 mg qd	10-40 mg qd	No dosage reduction necessary	Not well dialyzed	Tablets 10, 20, 40
Irbesartan[1] (Avapro®)	150 mg qd Maximum: 300 mg qd	Not FDA approved	No dosage reduction necessary	No	Tablets 75, 150, 300
Lisinopril (Prinivil®, Zestril®)	10-40 mg qd Maximum: 80 mg qd	5-20 mg qd	Cl_{cr} 10-30 mL/min: 5 mg/day initially Cl_{cr} <10 mL/min: 2.5 mg/day initially	Yes	Tablets 5, 10, 20, 40
Losartan[1] (Cozaar®)	25-100 mg qd or bid	Not FDA approved	No adjustment needed	No	Tablets 25, 50
Moexipril (Univasc®)	7.5-30 mg qd qd-bid Maximum: 30 mg qd	Not FDA approved	Cl_{cr} <30 mL/min: 3.75 mg/day initially Maximum: 15 mg/day	Unknown	Tablets 7.5, 15
Perindopril (Aceon®)	4-16 mg qd	4 mg qd (Not FDA approved)	Cl_{cr} 30-60 mL/min: 2 mg qd Cl_{cr} 15-29 mL/min: 2 mg qod Cl_{cr} <15 mL/min: 2 mg on dialysis days	Yes	Tablets 2, 4, 8
Quinapril (Accupril®)	10-80 mg qd qd-bid	5-20 mg bid	Cl_{cr} 30-60 mL/min: 5 mg/day initially Cl_{cr} <10 mL/min: 2.5 mg qd initially	Not well dialyzed	Tablets 5, 10, 20, 40
Ramipril (Altace™)	2.5-20 mg qd qd-bid	2.5-20 mg qd	Cl_{cr} <40 mL/min: 1.25 mg/day Maximum: 5 mg qd	Unknown	Capsules 1.25, 2.5, 5

ANGIOTENSIN AGENTS (Continued)

Comparisons of Indications and Adult Dosages (continued)

Drug	Hypertension	CHF	Renal Dysfunction	Dialyzable	Strengths (mg)
Telmisartan[1] (Micardis®)	20-80 mg qd	Not FDA approved	No dosage reduction necessary	No	Tablets 20, 40, 80
Trandolapril (Mavik®)	2-4 mg qd maximum: 8 mg/d qd-bid	Not FDA approved	Cl_{cr} <30 mL/min: 0.5 mg/day initially	No	Tablets 1 mg, 2 mg, 4 mg
Valsartan[1] (Diovan®)	80-160 mg qd	Not FDA approved	Decrease dose only if Cl_{cr} <10 mL/minute	No	Tablets 80, 160, 320

Dosage is based on 70 kg adult with normal hepatic and renal function.

[1]Angiotensin II antagonist.

[2]Enalaprilat is the only available ACE inhibitor in a parenteral formulation.

Comparative Pharmacokinetics

Drug	Prodrug	Absorption (%)	Serum t½ (h) Normal Renal Function	Serum Protein Binding (%)	Elimination	Onset of BP Lowering Action (h)	Peak BP Lowering Effects (h)	Duration of BP Lowering Effects (h)
Benazepril	Yes	37		~97	Renal (32%), biliary (~12%)	1	2-4	24
Benazeprilat			10-11 (effective)	~95%				
Captopril	No	60-75 (fasting)	1.9 (elimination)	25-30	Renal	0.25-0.5	1-1.5	~6
Enalapril	Yes	55-75	2	50-60	Renal (60%-80%), fecal	1	4-6	12-24
Enalaprilat			11 (effective)					
Fosinopril		36			Renal (~50%), biliary (~50%)	1		24
Fosinoprilat			12 (effective)	>99				
Moexipril	Yes		1	90	Fecal (53%), renal (8%)		1-2	>24
Moexiprilat			2-10	50				
Perindopril	Yes		1.5-3	60	Renal		3-7	
Perindoprilat			3-10 (effective)	10-20				
Quinapril	Yes	>60	0.8	97	Renal (~60%) as metabolite, fecal	1	2-4	24
Quinaprilat			2					
Ramipril	Yes	50-60	1-2	73	Renal (60%), fecal (40%)	1-2	3-6	24
Ramiprilat			13-17 (effective)	56				
Trandolapril	Yes		6	80	Renal (33%), fecal (66%)	1-2	6	≥24
Trandolaprilat			10	65-94				

ANGIOTENSIN AGENTS (Continued)

Comparative Pharmacokinetics of Angiotensin II Receptor Antagonists

	Candesartan (Atacand®)	Eprosartan (Teveten®)	Irbesartan (Avapro®)	Losartan (Cozaar®)	Telmisartan (Micardis®)	Valsartan (Diovan™)
Prodrug	Yes[1]	No	No	Yes[2]	No	No
Time to peak	3-4 h	1-2 h	1.5-2	1 h / 3-4 h[2]	0.5-1 h	2-4 h
Bioavailability	15%	13%	60%-80%	33%	42%-58%	25%
Food – area-under-the-curve	No effect	No effect	No effect	9% to 10%	9.6% to 20%	9% to 40%
Elimination half-life	9 h	5-9 h	11-15 h	1.5-2 h / 6-9 h[2]	24 h	6 h
Elimination altered in renal dysfunction	Yes[3]	No	No	No	No	No
Precautions in severe renal dysfunction	Yes	Yes	Yes	Yes	Yes	Yes
Elimination altered in hepatic dysfunction	No	No	No	Yes	Yes	Yes
Precautions in hepatic dysfunction	No	Yes	No	No	Yes	No
Protein binding	>99%	98%	90%	~99%	>99.5%	95%

[1]Candesartan cilexetil: Active metabolite candesartan.

[2]Losartan: Active metabolite E-3174.

[3]Dosage adjustments are not necessary.

ANTACID DRUG INTERACTIONS

Drug	Antacid				
	Al Salts	Ca Salts	Mg Salts	NaHCO$_3$	Mg/Al
Allopurinol	↓				
Anorexiants				↑	
Atorvastatin	↓		↓		
Benzodiazepines	↑		↓	↓	↓
Calcitriol			x^1		x^1
Captopril					↓
Cimetidine	↓		↓		↓
Corticosteroids	↓		↓		↓
Digoxin	↓		↓		
Flecainide				↑	
Indomethacin	↓		↓		↓
Iron	↓	↓	↓	↓	↓
Isoniazid	↓				
Itraconazole	↓	↓	↓	↓	↓
Ketoconazole	↓	↓	↓	↓	↓
Levodopa					↑
Lithium				↓	
Mycophenolate	↓		↓		
Naproxen	↑		↑	↓	↑
Nitrofurantoin			↓		
Penicillamine	↓		↓		↓
Phenothiazines	↓		↓		↓
Phenytoin		↓			↓
Quinidine		↑	↑		↑
Quinolones	↓	↓	↓		↓
Ranitidine	↓				↓
Rofecoxib	—	↓	—	—	↓
Salicylates				↓	↓
Sodium polystyrene sulfonate	x^2		x^2		x^2
Sulfonylureas				↑	
Sympathomimetics				↑	
Tetracyclines	↓	↓	↓	↓	↓
Tolmetin				x^3	

Pharmacologic effect increased (↑) or decreased (↓) by antacids.

[1] Concomitant use in patients on chronic renal dialysis may lead to hypermagnesemia.

[2] Concomitant use may cause metabolic alkalosis in patients with renal failure.

[3] Concomitant use not recommended by manufacturer.

ANTIARRHYTHMIC DRUGS

Vaughan Williams Classification of Antiarrhythmic Drugs Based on Cardiac Effects

Type	Drug(s)	Conduction Velocity[1]	Refractory Period	Automaticity
I	Moricizine	↓	↓	↓ (0 on SA node)
Ia	Disopyramide Procainamide Quinidine	↓	↑	↓
Ib	Lidocaine Mexiletine Tocainide	0/↓	↓	↓
Ic	Flecainide Indecainide Propafenone[2]	↓↓	0	↓
II	Beta-blockers	0	0	↓
III	Amiodarone Bretylium Dofetilide Ibutilide Sotalol[2]	0	↑↑	0
IV	Diltiazem Verapamil[3]	↓	↑	↓

[1]Variables for normal tissue models in ventricular tissue.

[2]Also has type II, beta-blocking action.

[3]Variables for SA and AV nodal tissue only.

Vaughan Williams Classification of Antiarrhythmic Agents and Their Indications/Adverse Effects

Type	Drug(s)	Indication	Route of Administration	Adverse Effects
I	Moricizine	VT	P.O.	Dizziness, nausea, rash, seizures
Ia	Disopyramide	AF, VT	P.O.	Anticholinergic effects, CHF
	Procainamide	AF, VT, WPW	P.O./I.V.	GI, CNS, lupus, fever, hematological, anticholinergic effects
	Quinidine	AF, PSVT, VT, WPW	P.O./I.V.	Hypotension, GI, thrombocytopenia, cinchonism
Ib	Lidocaine	VT, VF, PVC	I.V.	CNS, GI
	Mexiletine	VT	P.O.	GI, CNS
	Tocainide	VT	P.O.	GI, CNS, pulmonary, agranulocytosis
Ic	Flecainide	VT	P.O.	CHF, GI, CNS, blurred vision
	Propafenone	VT	P.O.	GI, blurred vision, dizziness
II	Esmolol	VT, SVT	I.V.	CHF, CNS, lupus-like syndrome, hypotension, bradycardia, bronchospasm
	Propranolol	SVT, VT, PVC, digoxin toxicity	P.O./I.V.	CHF, bradycardia, hypotension, CNS, fatigue
III	Amiodarone	VT	P.O.	CNS, GI, thyroid, pulmonary fibrosis, liver, corneal deposits
	Bretylium	VT, VF	I.V.	GI, orthostatic hypotension, CNS
	Dofetilide	AF	P.O.	Headache, dizziness, VT, torsade de pointes
	Ibutilide	AF	I.V.	Torsade de pointes, hypotension, branch bundle block, AV block, nausea, headache
	Sotalol	AF, VT	P.O.	Bradycardia, hypotension, CHF, CNS, fatigue
IV	Diltiazem	AF, PSVT	P.O./I.V.	Hypotension, GI, liver
	Verapamil	AF, PSVT	P.O./I.V.	Hypotension, CHF, bradycardia, vertigo, constipation
Miscellaneous	Adenosine	SVT, PSVT	I.V.	Flushing, dizziness, bradycardia, syncope
	Digoxin	AF, PSVT	P.O./I.V.	GI, CNS, arrhythmias
	Magnesium	VT, VF	I.V.	Hypotension, CNS, hypothermia, myocardial depression

AF = atrial fibrillation; PSVT = paroxysmal supraventricular tachycardia; VT = ventricular tachycardia; WPW = Wolf-Parkinson-White arrhythmias; VF = ventricular fibrillation; SVT = supraventricular tachycardia.

ANTIARRHYTHMIC DRUGS (Continued)

Comparative Pharmacokinetic Properties of Antiarrhythmic Agents

Type	Drug(s)	Bioavailability (%)	Primary Route of Elimination	Volume of Distribution (L/kg)	Protein Binding (%)	Half-Life	Therapeutic Range (mcg/mL)
I	Moricizine	34-38	Hepatic	6-11	92-95	1-6 h	—
Ia	Disopyramide	70-95	Hepatic/Renal	0.8-2	50-80	4-8 h	2-6
	Procainamide	75-95	Hepatic/Renal	1.5-3	10-20	2.5-5 h	4-15
	Quinidine	70-80	Hepatic	2-3.5	80-90	5-9 h	2-6
Ib	Lidocaine	20-40	Hepatic	1-2	65-75	60-180 min	1.5-5
	Mexiletine	80-95	Hepatic	5-12	60-75	6-12 h	0.75-2
	Tocainide	90-95	Hepatic	1.5-3	10-30	12-15 h	4-10
Ic	Flecainide	90-95	Hepatic/Renal	8-10	35-45	12-30 h	0.3-2.5
	Propafenone[1]	11-39	Hepatic	2.5-4	85-95	12-32 h / 2-10 h	—
II	Esmolol			Refer to Beta-Blocker Comparison Chart			
	Propranolol			Refer to Beta-Blocker Comparison Chart			
III	Amiodarone	22-28	Hepatic	70-150	95-97	15-100 d	1-2.5
	Bretylium	15-20	Renal	4-8	Negligible	5-10 h	0.5-2
	Dofetilide	>90%	Renal	3 L/kg	60-70	10 h	—
	Ibutilide	NA	Hepatic	11	40	2-12 h	—
	Sotalol	90-95	Renal	1.6-2.4	Negligible	12-15 h	—
IV	Diltiazem	80-90	Hepatic/Renal	1.7	77-85	4-6 h	0.05-0.2
	Verapamil	20-40	Hepatic	1.5-5	95-99	4-12 h	>50 ng/mL

[1]Top numbers reflect **poor** metabolizers and **bottom** numbers reflect **extensive** metabolizers.

ANTICONVULSANTS BY SEIZURE TYPE

Seizure Type	Age	Commonly Used	Alternatives
Primary generalized tonic-clonic	1 mo - 6 y	Carbamazepine, phenytoin, phenobarbital	Valproate
	6-11 y	Carbamazepine	Valproate, phenytoin, phenobarbital, lamotrigine, primidone
Primary generalized tonic-clonic with absence or with myoclonic	1 mo - 18 y	Valproate	Phenytoin, phenobarbital, carbamazepine, primidone
Partial seizures (with or without secondary generalization)	1-12 mo	Phenobarbital	Carbamazepine, phenytoin
	1-6 y	Carbamazepine	Phenytoin, phenobarbital, valproate, lamotrigine, gabapentin, oxcarbazepine (>4 y), primidone
	>6 y	Carbamazepine	Lamotrigine, levetiracetam, oxcarbazepine, phenytoin, phenobarbital, tiagabine, topiramate, valproate, primidone, zonisamide (>16 y)
Absence seizures	<10 y	Ethosuximide, valproate	Clonazepam, acetazolamide, lamotrigine
	>10 y	Valproate	Ethosuximide, acetazolamide, clonazepam
Juvenile myoclonic		Valproate	Phenobarbital, primidone, clonazepam; consider: carbamazepine, phenytoin, acetazolamide
Progressive myoclonic		Valproate	Valproate plus clonazepam, phenobarbital
Lennox-Gastaut and related syndromes		Valproate	lamotrigine, phenobarbital, clonazepam, ethosuximide; consider: steroids, ketogenic diet
Infantile spasms		ACTH, steroids	Valproate; consider: clonazepam, vigabatrin, pyridoxine
Neonatal seizures		Phenobarbital	Phenytoin; consider: clonazepam, primidone, valproate, pyridoxine

ANTIDEPRESSANT AGENTS

Comparison of Usual Dosage, Mechanism of Action, and Adverse Effects

Drug	Initial Dose	Usual Dosage (mg/d)	Dosage Forms	ACH	Drowsiness	Orthostatic Hypotension[1]	Cardiac Arrhythmias	GI Distress	Weight Gain	Comments
Tricyclic Antidepressants & Related Compounds[1]										
Amitriptyline (Elavil®, Vanatrip®)	25–75 mg qhs	100–300	T, I	4+	4+	4+	3+	1	4+	Also used in chronic pain, migraine, and as a hypnotic; contraindicated with cisapride
Amoxapine (Asendin®)	50 mg bid	100–400	T	2+	2+	2+	2+	0	2+	May cause extrapyramidal symptom (EPS)
Clomipramine[2] (Anafranil®)	25–75 mg qhs	100–250	C	4+	4+	2+	3+	1+	4+	Approved for OCD
Desipramine (Norpramin®)	25–75 mg qhs	100–300	T	1+	2+	2+	2+	0	1+	Blood levels useful for therapeutic monitoring
Doxepin (Sinequan®, Zonalon®)	25–75 mg qhs	100–300	C, L	3+	4+	2+	2+	0	4+	
Imipramine (Tofranil®)	25–75 mg qhs	100–300	T, C	3+	3+	4+	3+	1+	4+	Blood levels useful for therapeutic monitoring
Maprotiline (Ludiomil®)	25–75 mg qhs	100–225	T	2+	3+	2+	2+	0	2+	
Nortriptyline (Aventyl®, Pamelor®)	25–50 mg qhs	50–150	C, L	2+	2+	1+	2+	0	1+	Blood levels useful for therapeutic monitoring
Protriptyline (Vivactil®)	15 mg qAM	15–60	T	2+	1+	3+	3+	1+	1+	
Trimipramine (Surmontil®)	25–75 mg qhs	100–300	C	4+	4+	3+	3+	0	4+	
Selective Serotonin Reuptake Inhibitors[3]										
Citalopram (Celexa™)	20 mg qAM	20–60	T	0	0	0	0	3+–4	1+	CYP2D6 inhibitor (weak)
Fluoxetine (Prozac®, Sarafem™)	10–20 mg qAM	20–80	C, L, T	0	0	0	0	3+–4	1+	CYP2D6, 2C19, and 3A3/4 inhibitor
Fluvoxamine (Luvox®)[1]	50 mg qhs	100–300	T	0	0	0	0	3+–4	1+	Contraindicated with pimozide, thioridazine, mesoridazine, CYP1A2, 2C19, and 3A3/4 inhibitors
Paroxetine (Paxil®)	10–20 mg qAM	20–50	T, L	1+	1+	0	0	3+–4	2+	CYP2D6 inhibitor
Sertraline (Zoloft®)	25–50 mg qAM	50–200	T	0	0	0	0	3+–4	1+	CYP2D6 inhibitor (weak)
Dopamine-Reuptake Blocking Compounds										
Bupropion (Wellbutrin®, Wellbutrin SR®, Zyban™)	100 mg bid-tid IR[5] 150 mg qAM-bid SR[6]	300–450[7]	T	0	0	0	1+	1+	0	Contraindicated with seizures, bulimia, and anorexia; low incidence of sexual dysfunction IR: 6 h dosing interval preferred SR: 8 h dosing interval

1482

Comparison of Usual Dosage, Mechanism of Action, and Adverse Effects *(continued)*

Drug	Initial Dose	Usual Dosage (mg/d)	Dosage Forms	ACH	Drowsiness	Orthostatic Hypotension	Cardiac Arrhythmias	GI Distress	Weight Gain	Comments
						Adverse Effects				
					Serotonin/Norepinephrine Reuptake Inhibitors[8]					
Venlafaxine (Effexor®, Effexor®-XR)	25 mg bid-tid IR 37.5 mg qd XR	75–375	T	1+	1+	0	1+	3+[4]	0	High-dose is useful to treat refractory depression
					5HT2 Receptor Antagonist Properties					
Nefazodone (Serzone®)	100 mg bid	300–600	T	1+	1+	0	0	1+	0	Contraindicated with carbamazepine, pimozide, astemizole, cisapride, and terfenadine; caution with triazolam and alprazolam; low incidence of sexual dysfunction
Trazodone (Desyrel®)	50 mg tid	150–600	T	0	4+	3+	1+	1+	2+	
					Noradrenergic Antagonist					
Mirtazapine (Remeron®)	15 mg qhs	15–45	T	1+	3+	0	0	0	3+	Dose >15 mg/d less sedating, low incidence of sexual dysfunction
					Monoamine Oxidase Inhibitors					
Phenelzine (Nardil®)	15 mg tid	15–90	T	2+	2+	2+	1+	1+	3+	Diet must be low in tyramine; contraindicated with sympathomimetics and other antidepressants
Tranylcypromine (Parnate®)	10 mg bid	10–60	T	2+	1+	2+	1+	1+	2+	

Key: ACH = anticholinergic effects (dry mouth, blurred vision, urinary retention, constipation); 0 - 4+ = absent or rare - relatively common. T = tablet, L = liquid, I = injectable, C = capsule; IR = immediate release, SR = sustained release.

[1]**Important note:** A 1-week supply taken all at once in a patient receiving the maximum dose can be fatal.

[2]Not approved by FDA for depression. Approved for OCD.

[3]Flat dose response curve, headache, nausea, and sexual dysfunction are common side effects for SSRIs.

[4]Nausea is usually mild and transient.

[5]IR: 100 mg bid, may be increased to 100 mg tid no sooner than 3 days after beginning therapy.

[6]SR: 150 mg qAM, may be increased to 150 mg bid as early as day 4 of dosing.

[7]Not to exceed 150 mg/dose seizure risk for IR and 200 mg/dose for SR.

[8]Do not use with sibutramine; relatively safe in overdose.

ANTIFUNGAL AGENTS

Activities of Various Agents Against Specific Fungi

Fungus	Amphotericin B	Caspofungin	Fluconazole	Flucytosine
Aspergillus	x	x	?	—
Blastomyces	x	?	?	—
Candida	x	x	x	x
Chromomycosis	—	?	?	—
Coccidioides	x	?	x	—
Cryptococcus	x	—	x	x
Epidermophyton	—	?	—	—
Histoplasma	x	?	x	—
Microsporum	—	?	—	—
Mucor	x	—	—	—
Paracoccidioides	—	?	—	—
Phialophora	—	?	—	—
Pseudoallescheria	—	?	—	—
Rhodotorula	x	?	—	—
Sporothrix	x	?	?	—
Trichophyton	—	?	—	—

Fungus	Griseofulvin	Itraconazole	Ketoconazole
Aspergillus	—	x	—
Blastomyces	—	x	x
Candida	—	x	x
Chromomycosis	—	x	—
Coccidioides	—	x	x
Cryptococcus	—	x	x
Epidermophyton	x	—	x
Histoplasma	—	x	x
Microsporum	x	—	x
Mucor	—	—	—
Paracoccidioides	—	—	x
Phialophora	—	—	x
Pseudoallescheria	—	—	—
Rhodotorula	—	—	—
Sporothrix	—	x	—
Trichophyton	x	x	x

Fungus	Miconazole	Nystatin	Terbinafine
Aspergillus	—	—	—
Blastomyces	—	—	—
Candida	x	x	x
Chromomycosis	—	—	—
Coccidioides	x	—	—
Cryptococcus	x	—	—
Epidermophyton	—	—	x
Histoplasma	—	—	—
Microsporum	—	—	x
Mucor	—	—	—
Paracoccidioides	x	—	—
Phialophora	—	—	—
Pseudoallescheria	x	—	—
Rhodotorula	—	—	—
Sporothrix	—	—	—
Trichophyton	—	—	x

ANTIMIGRAINE DRUGS

5-HT$_1$ Receptor Agonists: Pharmacokinetic Differences

Pharmacokinetic Parameter	Almotriptan (Axert™) Oral (6.25 mg)	Frovatriptan (Frova™) Oral	Naratriptan (Amerge®) Oral	Rizatriptan (Maxalt®, Maxalt-MLT™) Tablets	Disintegrating Tablets	Sumatriptan (Imitrex®) S.C. (6 mg)	Oral (100 mg)	Nasal (20 mg)	Zolmitriptan (Zomig®, Zomig-ZMT™) Oral (5 mg)	Oral (10 mg)
Onset	<60 min	<2 h	1-3 h	30-120 min	30-120 min	10 min	30-60 min	<60 min	45 min	
Duration	Short	Long	Long	Short	Short	Short	Short	Short	Short	
Time to peak serum concentration (h)	1-3	2-4	2-4	1-1.5	1.6-2.5	5-20	1.5-2.5	1	1.5	2-3.5
Average bioavailability (%)	70	20-30	70	45	—	96	14	17	40-46	46-49
Volume of distribution (L)	180-200	210-280	170	110-140	110-140	170	170	NA	—	402
Half-life (h)	3-4	26	6	2-3	2-3	2	2-2.5[1]	2	2.8-3.4	2.5-3.7
Fraction excreted unchanged in urine (%)	40	32	50	14	14	22	22	—	8	8

[1]With extended dosing the half-life extends to 7 hours.

ANTIPSYCHOTIC AGENTS

Antipsychotic Agent	Dosage Forms	I.M./P.O. Potency	Equiv. Dosages (approx) (mg)	Usual Adult Daily Maint. Dose (mg)	Sedation (Incidence)	Extrapyramidal Side Effects	Anticholinergic Side Effects	Cardiovascular Side Effects	Comments
Chlorpromazine (Thorazine®)	Cap, Conc, Inj, Supp, Syr, Tab	4:1	100	200-1000	High	Moderate	Moderate	Moderate/High	
Clozapine (Clozaril®)	Tab		50	75-900	High	Very Low	High	High	~1% incidence of agranulocytosis; weekly-biweekly CBC required
Fluphenazine (Prolixin®, Permitil®)	Conc, Elix, Inj, Tab	2:1	2	0.5-40	Low	High	Low	Low	
Haloperidol (Haldol®)	Conc, Inj, Tab	2:1	2	1-15	Low	High	Low	Low	
Loxapine (Loxitane®)	Cap, Conc, Inj		10	25-250	Moderate	Moderate	Low	Low	
Mesoridazine (Serentil®)	Inj, Liq, Tab	3:1	50	30-400	High	Low	High	Moderate	Prolongs QTc
Molindone (Moban®)	Conc, Tab		15	15-225	Low	Moderate	Low	Low	May cause less weight gain
Olanzapine (Zyprexa™)	Tab		4	5-20	Moderate/High	Low	Moderate	Moderate	Potential for weight gain, lipid abnormalities, diabetes
Perphenazine (Trilafon®)	Conc, Inj, Tab		10	16-64	Low	Moderate	Low	Low	
Pimozide (Orap™)	Tab		2	1-20	Moderate	High	Moderate	Low	Contraindicated with CYP3A inhibitors
Promazine (Sparine®)	Inj, Tab		200	40-1000	Moderate	Moderate	High	Moderate	
Quetiapine (Seroquel®)	Tab		80	75-750	Moderate	Very Low	Moderate	Moderate	Low weight gain
Risperidone (Risperdal®)	Sol, Tab		1	0.5-6	Low/Moderate	Low	Low	Low/Moderate	Target dose: ≤6 mg/d; low weight gain
Thioridazine (Mellaril®)	Conc, Susp, Tab		100	200-800	High	Low	High	Moderate/High	May cause irreversible retinitis pigmentosa at doses >800 mg/d

Antipsychotic Agent	Dosage Forms	I.M./P.O. Potency	Equiv. Dosages (approx) (mg)	Usual Adult Daily Maint. Dose (mg)	Sedation (Incidence)	Extrapyramidal Side Effects	Anticholinergic Side Effects	Cardiovascular Side Effects	Comments
Thiothixene (Navane®)	Cap, Conc, Inj, Powder for Inj	4:1	4	5-40	Low	High	Low	Low/Moderate	
Trifluoperazine (Stelazine®)	Conc, Inj, Tab		5	2-40	Low	High	Low	Low	
Ziprasidone (Geodon®)	Cap	2:1	40	40-160	Low/Moderate	Low	Low	Low/Moderate	Low weight gain; contraindicated with QTc-prolonging agents

ANTIRETROVIRAL AGENTS

Renal Dosing Adjustment, Dosage Forms, and Adverse Reactions

Chemical and Generic Names	Brand Name	Renal Dosing Adjustment	Dosage Forms	Selected Adverse Reaction
		NRTIs (Nucleoside Reverse Transcriptase Inhibitors)		
Abacavir	Ziagen® (Glaxo-Wellcome)	300 mg bid	Tablet: 300 mg Solution, oral: 20 mg/mL (240 mL)	Hypersensitivity syndrome (fever, fatigue, GI symptoms, ±rash); **do not restart abacavir in patients who have experienced this**; GI symptoms
Didanosine (ddI)	Videx® (Bristol-Myers Squibb)	≥60 kg: 200 mg bid on empty stomach <60 kg: 125 mg bid (adjust for CL_{cr} <60) Renal adjustment varies by dosage form and renal function. Consult additional references/ product labeling.	Tablet, chewable: 25 mg, 50 mg, 100 mg, 150 mg Powder, oral: 100 mg, 167 mg, 250 mg, 375 mg Powder, pediatric: 2 g, 4 g Capsule, sustained release: 125 mg, 200 mg, 250 mg, 400 mg	Peripheral neuropathy, pancreatitis, abdominal pain, nausea, diarrhea, retinal depigmentation, anxiety, insomnia
Lamivudine (3TC)	Epivir® (Glaxo-Wellcome)	CL_{cr} 30-49: 150 mg qd CL_{cr} 15-29: 150 mg first dose, then 100 mg qd CL_{cr} 5-14: 150 mg first dose, then 50 mg qd CL_{cr} <5: 50 mg first dose, then 25 mg qd	Tablet: 100 mg, 150 mg Solution, oral: 5 mg/mL (240 mL); 10 mg/ mL (240 mL)	Headache, insomnia, nausea, vomiting, diarrhea, abdominal pain, myalgia, arthralgia, pancreatitis in children
Stavudine (d4T)	Zerit® (Bristol-Myers Squibb)	CL_{cr} >50: ≥60 kg: 40 mg bid <60 kg: 30 mg bid CL_{cr} 26-50: ≥60 kg: 20 mg bid <60 kg: 15 mg bid	Capsule: 15 mg, 20 mg, 30 mg, 40 mg Solution, oral: 1 mg/mL (200 mL)	Peripheral neuropathy, headache, abdominal or back pain, asthenia, nausea, vomiting, diarrhea, myalgia, anxiety, depression, pancreatitis, less frequently hepatotoxicity
Zalcitabine (ddC)	Hivid® (Roche)	CL_{cr} 10-40: 0.75 mg bid CL_{cr} <10: 0.75 mg qd	Tablet: 0.375 mg, 0.75 mg	Peripheral neuropathy, oral/esophageal ulceration, rash, nausea, vomiting, diarrhea, abdominal pain, myalgia, pancreatitis
Zidovudine (AZT)	Retrovir® (Glaxo-Wellcome)	200 mg tid or 300 mg bid on empty stomach (ESRD: 100 mg q6-8 h)	Tablet: 300 mg Capsule: 100 mg Syrup: 50 mg/5 mL (240 mL) Injection: 10 mg/mL (20 mL)	Anemia, neutropenia, thrombocytopenia, headache, nausea, vomiting, myopathy, hepatitis, hyperpigmentation of nails
Zidovudine/ lamivudine	Combivir® (Glaxo-Wellcome)	1 tablet bid (see lamivudine for dose adjustment)	Tablet: 300 mg zidovudine and 150 mg lamivudine	See individual agents

Renal Dosing Adjustment, Dosage Forms, and Adverse Reactions *(continued)*

Chemical and Generic Names	Brand Name	Renal Dosing Adjustment	Dosage Forms	Selected Adverse Reaction
NNRTIs (Non-nucleoside Reverse Transcriptase Inhibitors)				
Delavirdine	Rescriptor® (Pharmacia/Upjohn)	400 mg tid	Tablet: 100 mg Capsule: 200 mg	Rash
Efavirenz	Sustiva™ (DuPont)	600 mg qd	Capsule: 50 mg, 100 mg, 200 mg	Dizziness, psychiatric symptoms (hallucinations, confusion, depersonalization, others), agitation, vivid dreams, rash, GI intolerance
Nevirapine	Viramune® (Roxane)	200 mg qd for 14 days, then 200 mg bid	Tablet: 200 mg Suspension, oral: 50 mg/5 mL (240 mL)	Rash (severe), abnormal liver function tests, fever, nausea, headache
PIs (Protease Inhibitors)				
Amprenavir	Agenerase™ (Glaxo-Wellcome)	1200 mg bid (avoid high fat meal)	Capsule: 50 mg, 150 mg Solution, oral: 15 mg/mL (240 mL)	Rash (life-threatening), paresthesias (perioral), depression, nausea, diarrhea, vomiting, hyperglycemia (and sometimes diabetes), dyslipidemia including fat redistribution ("buffalo hump," "protease paunch"), hyperlipidemia, hypercholesterolemia
Indinavir	Crixivan® (Merck)	800 mg q8h with water (Hepatic insufficiency: 600 mg tid)	Capsule: 200 mg, 333 mg, 400 mg	Hyperbilirubinemia, nephrolithiasis, elevated AST/ALT, abdominal pain, nausea, vomiting, diarrhea, taste perversion, hyperglycemia (and sometimes diabetes), dyslipidemia including fat redistribution ("buffalo hump," "protease paunch"), hyperlipidemia, hypercholesterolemia
Lopinavir and Ritonavir	Kaletra™ (Abbott)	400 mg lopinavir/100 mg ritonavir bid	Capsule: Lopinavir 133.3 mg and ritonavir 33.3 mg Solution, oral: Lopinavir 80 mg and ritonavir 20 mg per mL	Asthenia, nausea, diarrhea, vomiting, anorexia, abdominal pain, circumoral and peripheral paresthesia, taste perversion, headache, hyperglycemia (and sometimes diabetes), dyslipidemia including fat redistribution ("buffalo hump," "protease paunch"), hyperlipidemia, hypercholesterolemia
Nelfinavir	Viracept® (Agouron)	750 mg tid with food	Tablet: 250 mg Powder, oral: 50 mg/g	Diarrhea, nausea, hyperglycemia (and sometimes diabetes), dyslipidemia including fat redistribution ("buffalo hump," "protease paunch"), hyperlipidemia, hypercholesterolemia
Ritonavir	Norvir® (Abbott)	600 mg bid with food (titrate)	Capsule: 100 mg Solution, oral: 80 mg/mL (240 mL)	Asthenia, nausea, diarrhea, vomiting, anorexia, abdominal pain, circumoral and peripheral paresthesia, taste perversion, headache, hyperglycemia (and sometimes diabetes), dyslipidemia including fat redistribution ("buffalo hump," "protease paunch"), hyperlipidemia, hypercholesterolemia
Saquinavir	Invirase®, Fortovase® (Roche)	600 mg tid with a full meal 1200 mg tid with a full meal	Capsule: 200 mg Gelcap: 200 mg	Diarrhea, abdominal discomfort, nausea, headache, hyperglycemia (and sometimes diabetes), dyslipidemia including fat redistribution ("buffalo hump," "protease paunch"), hyperlipidemia, hypercholesterolemia

NOTE: **Tenofovir** (Viread™) is a new nucleotide reverse transcriptase inhibitor. Use should be avoided in renal impairment (Cl$_{Cr}$ <60 mL/min); Tablet: 300 mg; Adverse reactions: Nausea, vomiting, diarrhea, flatulence, increased CPK, increased transaminases.

BENZODIAZEPINES

Agent	Dosage Forms	Relative Potency	Peak Blood Levels (oral) (h)	Protein Binding (%)	Volume of Distribution (L/kg)	Major Active Metabolite	Half-Life (parent) (h)	Half-Life[1] (metabolite) (h)	Usual Initial Dose	Adult Oral Dosage Range
Anxiolytic										
Alprazolam (Xanax®)	Tab	0.5	1-2	80	0.9-1.2	No	12-15	—	0.25-0.5 tid	0.75-4 mg/d
Chlordiazepoxide (Librium®)	Cap, Powd for inj, Tab	10	2-4	90-98	0.3	Yes	5-30	24-96	5-25 mg tid-qid	15-100 mg/d
Diazepam (Valium®)	Gel, Inj, Sol, Tab	5	0.5-2	98	1.1	Yes	20-80	50-100	2-10 mg bid-qid	4-40 mg/d
Halazepam (Paxipam®)	Tab	20	1-6	88-92	1.3	Yes	14	50-100	20-40 mg tid-qid	80-160 mg/d
Lorazepam (Ativan®)[2]	Inj, Sol, Tab	1	1-6	88-92	1.3	No	10-20	—	0.5-2 mg tid-qid	2-4 mg/d
Oxazepam (Serax®)	Cap, Tab	15-30	2-4	86-99	0.6-2	No	5-20	—	10-30 mg tid-qid	30-120 mg/d
Prazepam[3] (Centrax®)	Cap, Tab	10				Yes	1.2	30-100	10 mg tid	30 mg/d
Sedative/Hypnotic										
Estazolam (ProSom™)	Tab	0.3	2	93	—	No	10-24	—	1 mg qhs	1-2 mg
Flurazepam (Dalmane®)	Cap	5	0.5-2	97	—	Yes	Not significant	40-114	15 mg qhs	15-60 mg
Quazepam (Doral®)	Tab	5	2	95	5	Yes	25-41	28-114	15 mg qhs	7.5-15 mg
Temazepam (Restoril®)	Cap	5	2-3	96	1.4	No	10-40	—	15-30 mg qhs	15-30 mg
Triazolam (Halcion®)	Tab	0.1	1	89-94	0.8-1.3	No	2.3	—	0.125-0.25 qhs	0.125-0.25 mg
Miscellaneous										
Clonazepam (Klonopin™)	Tab	0.25-0.5	1-2	86	1.8-4	No	18-50 h	—	0.5 mg tid	1.5-20 mg/d
Clorazepate (Tranxene®)	Cap, Tab	7.5	1-2	80-95	—	Yes	Not significant	50-100 h	7.5-15 mg bid-qid	15-60 mg
Midazolam (Versed®)	Inj		0.4-0.7[4]	95	0.8-6.6	No	2-5 h	—	NA	

[1]Significant metabolite.

[2]Reliable bioavailability when given I.M.

[3]Not available in U.S.

[4]I.V. only.

NA = not available.

BETA-BLOCKERS

Agent	Adrenergic Receptor Blocking Activity	Lipid Solubility	Protein Bound (%)	Half-Life (h)	Bioavailability (%)	Primary (Secondary) Route of Elimination	Indications	Usual Dosage
Acebutolol (Sectral®)	beta$_1$	Low	15-25	3-4	40 7-fold[1]	Hepatic (renal)	Hypertension, arrhythmias	P.O.: 400-1200 mg/d
Atenolol (Tenormin®)	beta$_1$	Low	<5-10	6-9[2]	50-60 4-fold[1]	Renal (hepatic)	Hypertension, angina pectoris, acute MI	P.O.: 50-200 mg/d I.V.: 5 mg x 2 doses
Betaxolol (Kerlone®)	beta$_1$	Low	50-55	14-22	84-94	Hepatic (renal)	Hypertension	P.O.: 10-20 mg/d
Bisoprolol (Zebeta™)	beta$_1$	Low	26-33	9-12	80	Renal (hepatic)	Hypertension, heart failure	P.O.: 2.5-5 mg
Carteolol (Cartrol®)	beta$_1$ beta$_2$	Low	20-30	6	80-85	Renal	Hypertension	P.O.: 2.5-10 mg/d
Carvedilol (Coreg™)				7-10	25-35	Bile into feces	Hypertension, heart failure (mild to severe)	P.O.: 6.25 mg twice daily
Esmolol (Brevibloc®)	beta$_1$	Low	55	0.15	NA 5-fold[1]	Red blood cell	Supraventricular tachycardia, sinus tachycardia	I.V. infusion: 25-300 mcg/kg/min
Labetalol (Normodyne®, Trandate®)	alpha$_1$ beta$_1$ beta$_2$	Moderate	50	5.5-8	18-30 10-fold[1]	Renal (hepatic)	Hypertension	P.O.: 200-2400 mg/d I.V.: 20-80 mg at 10-min intervals up to a maximum of 300 mg or continuous infusion of 2 mg/min
Metoprolol (Lopressor®, Toprol XL®)	beta$_1$	Moderate	10-12	3-7	50 10-fold[1] (Toprol XL®: 77)	Hepatic/renal	Hypertension, angina pectoris, acute MI, heart failure (mild to moderate, XL formulation only)	P.O.: 100-450 mg/d I.V.: Post-MI 15 mg Angina: 15 mg then 2-5 mg/hour Arrhythmias: 0.2 mg/kg
Nadolol (Corgard®)	beta$_1$ beta$_2$	Low	25-30	20-24	30 5-8 fold[1]	Renal	Hypertension, angina pectoris	P.O.: 40-320 mg/d
Penbutolol (Levatol™)	beta$_1$ beta$_2$	High	80-98	5	≅100	Hepatic (renal)	Hypertension	P.O.: 20-80 mg/d
Pindolol (Visken®)	beta$_1$ beta$_2$	Moderate	57	3-4[2]	90 4-fold[1]	Hepatic (renal)	Hypertension	P.O.: 20-60 mg/d
Propranolol (Inderal® various)	beta$_1$ beta$_2$	High	90	3-5[2]	30 20-fold[1]	Hepatic	Hypertension, angina pectoris, arrhythmias	P.O.: 40-480 mg/d I.V.: Reflex tachycardia 1-10 mg
Propranolol long-acting (Inderal-LA®)	beta$_1$ beta$_2$	High	90	9-18	20-30 fold[1]	Hepatic	Hypertrophic subaortic stenosis, prophylaxis (post-MI)	P.O.: 180-240 mg/d

BETA-BLOCKERS *(Continued)*

Agent	Adrenergic Receptor Blocking Activity	Lipid Solubility	Protein Bound (%)	Half-Life (h)	Bioavail-ability (%)	Primary (Secondary) Route of Elimination	Indications	Usual Dosage
Sotalol (Betapace®, Betapace AF™, Sorine®)	beta$_1$ beta$_2$	Low	0	12	90-100	Renal	Ventricular arrhythmias/ tachyarrhythmias	P.O. 160-320 mg/d
Timolol (Blocadren®)	beta$_1$ beta$_2$	Low to moderate	<10	4	75 7-fold[1]	Hepatic (renal)	Hypertension, prophylaxis (post-MI)	P.O.: 20-60 mg/d P.O.: 20 mg/d

Dosage is based on 70 kg adult with normal hepatic and renal function.

Note: All beta$_1$-selective agents will inhibit beta$_2$ receptors at higher doses.

[1]Interpatient variations in plasma levels.

[2]Half-life increased to 16-27 h in creatinine clearance of 15-35 mL/min and >27 h in creatinine clearance <15 mL/min.

BRONCHODILATORS

Comparison of Inhaled Sympathomimetic Bronchodilators

Drug	Adrenergic Receptor	Onset (min)	Duration Activity (h)
Albuterol (Airet®, Proventil®, Ventolin®)	Beta$_1$ < Beta$_2$	<5	3-8
Bitolterol (Tornalate®)	Beta$_1$ < Beta$_2$	3-4	5 > 8
Epinephrine (various)	Alpha and Beta$_1$ and Beta$_2$	1-5	1-3
Formoterol (Foradil®)	Beta$_1$ < Beta$_2$	3-5	12
Isoetharine (various)	Beta$_1$ < Beta$_2$	<5	1-3
Isoproterenol (Isuprel®)	Beta$_1$ and Beta$_2$	2-5	0.5-2
Levalbuterol (Xopenex™)	Beta$_1$ < Beta$_2$	10-17	5-6
Metaproterenol (Alupent®)	Beta$_1$ < Beta$_2$	5-30	2-6
Pirbuterol (Maxair®)	Beta$_1$ < Beta$_2$	<5	5
Salmeterol (Serevent®)	Beta$_1$ < Beta$_2$	5-14	12
Terbutaline (Brethaire®, Brethine®)	Beta$_1$ < Beta$_2$	5-30	3-6

CALCIUM CHANNEL BLOCKERS

Comparative Pharmacokinetics

Agent	Bioavailability (%)	Protein Binding (%)	Onset (min)	Peak (h)	Half-Life (h)	Volume of Distribution	Route of Metabolism	Route of Excretion
Dihydropyridines								
Nifedipine (prototype) (Adalat® CC, Procardia®/Procardia XL®)	Immediate/sustained release 45-70/86	92-98	20	Immediate/sustained release 0.5/6	2-5	ND	Liver, inactive metabolites	60%-80% urine, feces, bile
Amlodipine (Norvasc®)	52-88	97	6 h	6-9	33.8	21 L/kg	Liver, inactive metabolites, not a significant first-pass metabolism/presystemic metabolism	Bile, gut wall
Felodipine (Plendil®)	10-25	>99	3-5 h	2.5-5	10-36	10.3 L/kg	Liver, inactive metabolites, extensive metabolism by several pathways including cytochrome P-450, extensive first-pass metabolism/presystemic metabolism	70% urine, 10% feces
Isradipine (DynaCirc®)	15-24	97	120	0.5-2.5	8	2.9 L/kg	Liver, inactive metabolites, extensive first-pass metabolism	90% urine, 10% feces
Nicardipine (Cardene®)	35	>95	20	0.5-2	2-4	ND	Liver, saturable first-pass metabolism	60% urine, 35% feces
Nimodipine (Nimotop®)	13	>95	ND	≤1	1-2	0.43 L/kg	Liver, inactive metabolites, high first-pass metabolism	Urine
Nisoldipine (Sular®)	4-8	>99	ND	6-12	7-12	4-5 L/kg	Liver, 1 active metabolite (10%), presystemic metabolism	70%-75% kidney, 6%-12% feces
Phenylalkylamines								
Verapamil (prototype) (Calan®, Isoptin®)	20-35	83-92	30	1-2.2	3-7	4.5-7 L/kg	Liver	70% urine, 16% feces
Benzothiazepines								
Diltiazem (prototype) (Cardizem®/Cardizem® CD, Dilacor® XR)	40-67	70-80	30-60	Immediate/sustained release 2-3/6-11	Immediate/sustained release 3.5-6/5-7	ND	Liver, drugs which inhibit/induce hepatic microsomal enzymes may alter disposition	Urine
Miscellaneous								
Bepridil (Vascor®)	59	>99	60	2-3	24	ND	Liver	70% urine, 22% feces

CORTICOSTEROIDS

Corticosteroids, Systemic Equivalencies

Glucocorticoid	Pregnancy Category	Approximate Equivalent Dose (mg)	Routes of Administration	Relative Anti-inflammatory Potency	Relative Mineralocorticoid Potency	Protein Binding (%)	Half-life Plasma (min)	Half-life Biologic (h)
Short-Acting								
Cortisone	D	25	P.O., I.M.	0.8	2	90	30	8-12
Hydrocortisone	C	20	I.M., I.V.	1	2	90	80-118	8-12
Intermediate-Acting								
Methylprednisolone[1]	—	4	P.O., I.M., I.V.	5	0	—	78-188	18-36
Prednisolone	B	5	P.O., I.M., I.V., intra-articular, intradermal, soft tissue injection	4	1	90-95	115-212	18-36
Prednisone	B	5	P.O.	4	1	70	60	18-36
Triamcinolone[1]	C	4	P.O., I.M. intra-articular, intradermal, intrasynovial, soft tissue injection	5	0	—	200+	18-36
Long-Acting								
Betamethasone	C	0.6-0.75	P.O., I.M., intra-articular, intradermal, intrasynovial, soft tissue injection	25	0	64	300+	36-54
Dexamethasone	C	0.75	P.O., I.M., I.V., intra-articular, intradermal, soft tissue injection	25-30	0	—	110-210	36-54
Mineralocorticoids								
Fludrocortisone	C	—	P.O.	10	125	42	210+	18-36

[1]May contain propylene glyco[l] as an excipient in injectable forms.

CORTICOSTEROIDS *(Continued)*

GUIDELINES FOR SELECTION AND USE OF TOPICAL CORTICOSTEROIDS

The quantity prescribed and the frequency of refills should be monitored to reduce the risk of adrenal suppression. In general, short courses of high-potency agents are preferable to prolonged use of low potency. After control is achieved, control should be maintained with a low potency preparation.

1. Low-to-medium potency agents are usually effective for treating thin, acute, inflammatory skin lesions; whereas, high or super-potent agents are often required for treating chronic, hyperkeratotic, or lichenified lesions.

2. Since the stratum corneum is thin on the face and intertriginous areas, low-potency agents are preferred but a higher potency agent may be used for 2 weeks.

3. Because the palms and sole shave a thick stratum corneum, high or super-potent agents are frequently required.

4. Low potency agents are preferred for infants and the elderly. Infants have a high body surface area to weight ratio; elderly patients have thin, fragile skin.

5. The vehicle in which the topical corticosteroid is formulated influences the absorption and potency of the drug. Ointment bases are preferred for thick, lichenified lesions; they enhance penetration of the drug. Creams are preferred for acute and subacute dermatoses; they may be used on moist skin areas or intertriginous areas. Solutions, gels, and sprays are preferred for the scalp or for areas where a nonoil-based vehicle is needed.

6. In general, super-potent agents should not be used for longer than 3 weeks unless the lesion is limited to a small body area. Medium-to-high potency agents usually cause only rare adverse effects when treatment is limited to 3 months or less, and use on the face and intertriginous areas are avoided. If long-term treatment is needed, intermittent vs continued treatment is recommended.

7. Most preparations are applied once or twice daily. More frequent application may be necessary for the palms or soles because the preparation is easily removed by normal activity and penetration is poor due to a thick stratum corneum. Every-other-day or weekend-only application may be effective for treating some chronic conditions.

Corticosteroids, Topical

Steroid		Vehicle
Very High Potency		
0.05%	Augmented betamethasone dipropionate	Ointment
0.05%	Clobetasol propionate	Cream, ointment
0.05%	Diflorasone diacetate	Ointment
0.05%	Halobetasol propionate	Cream, ointment
High Potency		
0.1%	Amcinonide	Cream, ointment, lotion
0.05%	Betamethasone dipropionate, augmented	Cream
0.05%	Betamethasone dipropionate	Cream, ointment
0.1%	Betamethasone valerate	Ointment
0.05%	Desoximetasone	Gel
0.25%	Desoximetasone	Cream, ointment
0.05%	Diflorasone diacetate	Cream, ointment
0.2%	Fluocinolone acetonide	Cream
0.05%	Fluocinonide	Cream, ointment, gel
0.1%	Halcinonide	Cream, ointment
0.5%	Triamcinolone acetonide	Cream, ointment
Intermediate Potency		
0.025%	Betamethasone benzoate	Cream, gel, lotion
0.05%	Betamethasone dipropionate	Lotion
0.1%	Betamethasone valerate	Cream
0.1%	Clocortolone pivalate	Cream
0.05%	Desoximetasone	Cream
0.025%	Fluocinolone acetonide	Cream, ointment
0.05%	Flurandrenolide	Cream, ointment, lotion, tape
0.005%	Fluticasone propionate	Ointment
0.05%	Fluticasone propionate	Cream

Corticosteroids, Topical *(continued)*

Steroid		Vehicle
0.1%	Hydrocortisone butyrate[1]	Ointment, solution
0.2%	Hydrocortisone valerate[1]	Cream, ointment
0.1%	Mometasone furoate[1]	Cream, ointment, lotion
0.1%	Prednicarbate	Cream, ointment
0.025%	Triamcinolone acetonide	Cream, ointment, lotion
0.1%	Triamcinolone acetonide	Cream, ointment, lotion
Low Potency		
0.05%	Alclometasone dipropionate[1]	Cream, ointment
0.05%	Desonide	Cream
0.01%	Dexamethasone	Aerosol
0.04%	Dexamethasone	Aerosol
0.1%	Dexamethasone sodium phosphate	Cream
0.01%	Fluocinolone acetonide	Cream, solution
0.25%	Hydrocortisone[1]	Lotion
0.5%	Hydrocortisone[1]	Cream, ointment, lotion, aerosol
0.5%	Hydrocortisone acetate[1]	Cream, ointment
1%	Hydrocortisone acetate[1]	Cream, ointment
1%	Hydrocortisone	Cream, ointment, lotion, solution
2.5%	Hydrocortisone	Cream, ointment, lotion

[1] Not fluorinated.

CYCLOPLEGIC MYDRIATICS

Agent	Peak Mydriasis	Peak Cycloplegia	Time to Recovery
Atropine	30-40 min	1-3 h	>14 d
Cyclopentolate	25-75 min	25-75 min	24 h
Homatropine	30-90 min	30-90 min	6 h-4 d
Scopolamine	20-30 min	30 min-1 h	5-7 d
Tropicamide	20-40 min	20-35 min	1-6 h

FOSPHENYTOIN AND PHENYTOIN

Comparison of Parenteral Fosphenytoin and Phenytoin

	Fosphenytoin (Cerebyx®)	Phenytoin (Dilantin®)
Parenteral dosage forms available	50 mg PE/mL in 2 mL and 10 mL vials	50 mg phenytoin sodium/mL in 2 mL and 5 mL vials
Intravenous Administration	Recommended	Recommended
Loading dose	10-20 mg PE[1]/kg	10-15 mg/kg
Maintenance dose	4-7 mg/kg/day	100 mg I.V. q6-8h (oral form available)
Maximum infusion rate	Up to 150 mg PE/min	Up to 50 mg/min
Minimum infusion time for 1000 mg	6.7 min	20 min
Compatible with saline	Yes	Yes
Compatible with D_5W	Yes	No
Saline flush recommended after infusion	No	Yes
Intramuscular Administration	Recommended	Not recommended
Loading dose	10-20 mg PE/kg	10-15 mg/kg
Maintenance dose	4-7 mg/kg	Not recommended

[1]PE = phenytoin equivalents. See Fosphenytoin monograph for more details.

GLAUCOMA DRUG THERAPY

Ophthalmic Agent (Brand)	Reduces Aqueous Humor Production	Increases Aqueous Humor Outflow[1]	Average Duration of Action	Strengths Available
Cholinesterase Inhibitors[1]				
Demecarium (Humorsol®)	No data	Significant	7 d	0.125% to 0.25%
Echothiophate (Phospholine Iodide®)	No data	Significant	2 wk	0.03% to 0.25%
Isoflurophate (Floropryl®)	No data	Significant	2 wk	0.025%
Physostigmine (Antilirium®)	No data	Significant	24 h	0.25%
Direct-Acting Cholinergic Miotics				
Carbachol (Carbastat®, Epitol®)	Some activity	Significant	8 h	0.75% to 3%
Pilocarpine (various)	Some activity	Significant	5 h	0.5%, 1%, 2%, 3%, 4%
Sympathomimetics				
Brimonidine (Alphagan®, Alphagan® P)	Moderate	Moderate	12 h	0.2%
Dipivefrin (AKPro®, Propine®)	Some activity	Moderate	12 h	0.1%
Epinephrine (Epinal®, Epifrin®, Glaucon®)	Some activity	Moderate	18 h	0.25% to 2%
Beta-Blockers				
Betaxolol (Betoptic®, Betoptic® S)	Significant	Some activity	12 h	0.5%
Carteolol (Ocupress®)	Yes	No	12 h	1%
Levobetaxolol (Betaxon®)	Significant	No data	12 h	0.5%
Levobunolol (Betagan®)	Significant	Some activity	18 h	0.5%
Metipranolol (OptiPranolol®)	Significant	Some activity	18 h	0.3%
Timolol (Betimol®, Timoptic®)	Significant	Some activity	18 h	0.25%, 0.5%
Carbonic Anhydrase Inhibitors				
Acetazolamide (Diamox®)	Significant	No data	10 h	250 mg tab; 500 mg cap
Brinzolamide (Azopt®)	Yes	No data	8 h	1%
Dorzolamide (Trusopt®)	Yes	No	8 h	2%
Methazolamide (Neptazane®)	Significant	No data	14 h	50 mg
Prostaglandin Agonists				
Bimatoprost (Lumigan™)		Yes	≥24 h	0.03%
Latanoprost (Xalatan®)		Yes	≥24 h	0.005%
Travoprost (Travatan™)		Yes	20 h	0.004%
Unoprostone (Rescula®)		Yes	12 h	0.15%

[1] All miotic drugs significantly affect accommodation.

GLYCOPROTEIN ANTAGONISTS

Comparison of Glycoprotein IIb/IIIa Receptor Antagonists

	Abciximab (ReoPro®)	Tirofiban (Aggrastat®)	Eptifibatide (Integrelin®)
Type	Monoclonal antibody	Nonpeptide	Peptide
Mechanism of action	Steric hindrance and conformational changes	Mimics native protein sequence in receptor	Mimics native protein sequence in receptor
Biologic half-life	12-24 h	4-8 h	4-8 h
Reversible with platelet infusions	Yes	No (effect dissipates within 4-8 h)	No (effect dissipates within 4-8 h)
Speed of reversibility (return of platelet function)	Slow (>48 h)	Fast (2 h)	Fast (2 h)
Vitronectin activity	Yes	No	No
FDA-approved labeling			
Percutaneous coronary intervention (PCI)	Yes	No	Yes
Coronary stents	Yes	No	No
Unstable angina pre-PCI	When PCI planned	When PCI planned	When PCI planned
Unstable angina, medical stabilization	No	Yes	Yes
FDA-approved dosing for percutaneous coronary intervention	0.25 mg/kg bolus followed by 0.125 mcg/kg/min infusion (max: 10 mcg/min) x 12 h	Not approved for use in planned PCI	135 mcg/kg bolus followed by 0.5 mcg/kg/min infusion for 20-24 h
FDA-approved dosing for unstable angina stabilization	0.25 mg/kg bolus followed by 10 mcg/min infusion x 18-24 h, concluding 1 h post-PCI	0.4 mcg/kg/min x 30 min followed by 0.1 mcg/kg/min infusion through angiography or 12-24 h after subsequent PCI	180 mcg/kg/bolus followed by 2 mcg/kg/min infusion until discharge, CABG procedure or up to 72 h
How supplied – volume of injectable (total drug contents/vial)	5 mL vial (10 mg)	50 mL vial (12.5 mg) 500 mL premixed solution (25 mg)	10 mL vial (20 mg) 100 mL vial (75 mg)
Storage requirements	Refrigerate, do not freeze and do not shake	Can store at room temperature, do not freeze, protect from light during storage	Refrigerate and protect from light until administered

HEPARINS

Name	Type	Limitation	Dose (S.C. unless otherwise noted)	Average MW (in daltons)
Low Molecular Weight Heparins				
Dalteparin (Fragmin®)	Prophylaxis	Abdominal surgery[1] Abdominal surgery[2]	2500 units/d 5000 units/d	4000-6000
		Hip surgery[1]	5000 units/d postoperatively	
	Treatment	DVT[3]	100 units/kg bid 200 units/kg qd	4000-6000
		Unstable[4] angina Non-Q-wave MI	120 units/kg (max: 10,000 units) q12h for 5-8 d	
Enoxaparin (Lovenox®)	Prophylaxis	Hip or knee replacement	30 mg twice daily[5]	3500-5500
		High-risk hip replacement or abdominal surgery	40 mg once daily	
	Treatment	DVT or PE	1 mg/kg q12h	
		Acute coronary	1 mg/kg q12h	
Tinzaparin (Innohep®)	Treatment	DVT or PE	175 anti-Xa int. units/ kg/day	5500-7500
Heparin				
Heparin (Hep-Lock®)	Prophylaxis	Risk of thromboembolic disease	5000 units q8-12h	3000-30,000
	Treatment	Thrombosis or embolization	80 units/kg IVP then 20,000-40,000 units daily as continuous I.V. infusion	
	Treatment[3]	Unstable angina[3]	80 units/kg IVP then 20,000-40,000 units daily as continuous I.V. infusion	
Heparinoid				
Danaparoid (Orgaran®)	Prophylaxis	Hip replacement	750 units bid	6500
	Treatment[3]		2000 units q12h	

[1]Patients with low risk of DVT.

[2]Patients with high risk of DVT.

[3]Not FDA approved.

[4]Patients >60 years of age may require a lower dose of heparin.

[5]Patients weighing <100 lb or ≥65 years of age may receive 0.5 mg/kg/dose every 12 hours.

HYPOGLYCEMIC DRUGS & THIAZOLIDINEDIONE INFORMATION

Contraindications to Therapy and Potential Adverse Effects of Oral Antidiabetic Agents

	Sulfonylureas/ Meglitinide	Metformin (Glucophage®)	Acarbose (Precose®)/ Miglitol (Glyset™)	Pioglitazone (Actos™)/ Rosiglitazone (Avandia®)
Contraindications				
Insulin dependency	A	A	A*	
Pregnancy/lactation	A	A	A	
Hypersensitivity to the agent	A	A	A	A
Hepatic impairment	R	A	R	A
Renal impairment	R	A	R	
Congestive heart failure		A		R
Chronic lung disease		A		
Peripheral vascular disease		A		
Steroid-induced diabetes	R	R		
Inflammatory bowel disease		A	A	
Major recurrent illness	R	A		
Surgery	R	A		
Alcoholism	R	A		A
Adverse Effects				
Hypoglycemia	Yes	No	No	No
Body weight gain	Yes	No	No	Yes
Hypersensitivity	Yes	No	No	No
Drug interactions	Yes	No	No	Yes/No
Lactic acidosis	No	Yes	No	No
Gastrointestinal disturbances	No	Yes	No	No

*Can be used in conjunction with insulin. A = absolute; R = relative.

Comparative Pharmacokinetics

Drug	Duration of Action (h)	Daily Dose and Frequency (mg)	Metabolism
First Generation Sulfonylurea Agents			
Acetohexamide (Dymelor®)	12-24	250-1500 bid	Hepatic (60%) with active metabolite
Chlorpropamide (Diabinese®)	24-72	100-500 qd	Renal excretion (30%) and hepatic metabolism with active metabolites
Tolazamide (Tolinase®)	10-24	100-1000 qd or bid	Hepatic with active metabolites
Tolbutamide (Orinase®)	6-24	500-3000 qd-tid	Hepatic
Second Generation Sulfonylurea Agents			
Glimepiride (Amaryl®)	24	1-4 mg qd	Hepatic
Glipizide (Glucotrol®)	12-24	2.5-40 mg qd or bid	Hepatic
Glipizide GITS	24	5-10 qd	Hepatic
Glyburide (DiaBeta®, Glynase™, Micronase®)	16-24	1.25-20 qd or bid	Hepatic with active metabolites
Biguanine			
Metformin (Glucophage®)	12-24	1000-2550 mg/day bid or tid	None; excreted unchanged in urine
Alpha-Glucosidase Inhibitors			
Acarbose (Precose®)	8-12	150-300 mg/day tid	GI tract
Miglitol (Glyset™)	8	50 mg 3 times/day	Renal excretion
Meglitinides			
Nateglinide (Starlix®)	<4	120 mg 3 times/day before meals	Hepatic with active metabolites
Repaglinide (Prandin®)	<4 (single dose)	0.4-4 mg administered with meals 2, 3, or 4 times/day	Hepatic to inactive metabolites

Comparative Thiazolidinedione Pharmacokinetics

Parameter	Pioglitazone (Actos®)	Rosiglitazone (Avandia®)
Absorption	Food slightly delays but does not alter the extent of absorption	Absolute bioavailability is 99% Food ↓ C_{max} and delays T_{max}, but not change in AUC
C_{max}	156-342 ng/mL	–
T_{max}	2 hours	1 hour
Distribution	0.63 ± 0.41 L/kg	17.6 L
Plasma protein binding	>99% to serum albumin	99.8% to serum albumin
Metabolism	Extensive liver metabolism by hydroxylation and oxidation. Some metabolites are pharmacologically active. CYP2C8 and CYP3A4 metabolism	Extensive metabolism via N-demethylation and hydroxylation with no unchanged drug excreted in the urine CYP2C8 and some CYP2C9 metabolism
Excretion	Urine (15% to 30%) and bile	Urine (64%) and feces (23%)
Half-life	3-6 hours (pioglitazone) 16-24 hours (pioglitazone and metabolites)	3.15-3.59 hours
Effect of hemodialysis	Not removed	Not removed

(Package inserts: Actos®, 1999; Avandia®, 1999; Plosker, 1999.)

Approved Indications for Thiazolidinedione Derivatives

Indication	Pioglitazone (Actos™)	Rosiglitazone (Avandia®)
Monotherapy	x	x
Combination Therapy – Dual Therapy		
Combination with sulfonylureas	x	x
Combination therapy with Glucophage® (metformin)	x	x
Combination therapy with insulin	x	–
Combination Therapy – Triple Therapy		
Combination therapy with sulfonylureas and Glucophage® (metformin)	–	–

(Package inserts: Actos®, 1999; Avandia®, 1999.)

Comparative Lipid Effects

Parameter	Pioglitazone (Actos®)	Rosiglitazone (Avandia®)
LDL	No significant change	↑ up to 12.1%
HDL	↑ up to 13%	↑ up to 18.5%
Total cholesterol	No significant change	↑
Total cholesterol/HDL ratio	–	–
LDL/HDL ratio	–	No change
Triglycerides	↓ up to 28%	Variable effects

(Package inserts: Actos®, 1999; Avandia®, 1999; Plosker, 1999.)

LAXATIVES, CLASSIFICATION AND PROPERTIES

Laxative	Onset of Action	Site of Action	Mechanism of Action
Saline			
Magnesium citrate (Citroma®) Magnesium hydroxide (Milk of Magnesia)	30 min to 3 h	Small and large intestine	Attract/retain water in intestinal lumen increasing intraluminal pressure; cholecystokinin release
Sodium phosphate/ biphosphate enema (Fleet® Enema)	2-15 min	Colon	
Irritant/Stimulant			
Cascara Casanthranol Senna (Senokot®)	6-10 h	Colon	Direct action on intestinal mucosa; stimulate myenteric plexus; alter water and electrolyte secretion
Bisacodyl (Dulcolax®) tablets, suppositories	15 min to 1 h	Colon	
Castor oil	2-6 h	Small intestine	
Cascara aromatic fluid extract	6-10 h	Colon	
Bulk-Producing			
Methylcellulose (Citrucel®) Psyllium (Metamucil®) Malt soup extract (Maltsupex®) Calcium polycarbophil (Mitrolan®, FiberCon®)	12-24 h (up to 72 h)	Small and large intestine	Holds water in stool; mechanical distention; malt soup extract reduces fecal pH
Lubricant			
Mineral oil	6-8 h	Colon	Lubricates intestine; retards colonic absorption of fecal water; softens stool
Surfactants / Stool Softener			
Docusate sodium (Colace®) Docusate calcium (Surfak®) Docusate potassium (Dialose®)	24-72 h	Small and large intestine	Detergent activity; facilitates admixture of fat and water to soften stool
Miscellaneous and Combination Laxatives			
Glycerin suppository	15-30 min	Colon	Local irritation; hyperosmotic action
Lactulose (Cephulac®)	24-48 h	Colon	Delivers osmotically active molecules to colon
Docusate/casanthranol (Peri-Colace®)	8-12 h	Small and large intestine	Casanthranol – mild stimulant; docusate – stool softener
Polyethylene glycol-electrolyte solution (GoLYTELY®)	30-60 min	Small and large intestine	Nonabsorbable solution which acts as an osmotic agent
Sorbitol 70%	24-48 h	Colon	Delivers osmotically active molecules to colon

LIPID-LOWERING AGENTS

Effects on Lipoproteins

Drug	Total Cholesterol (%)	LDLC (%)	HDLC (%)	TG (%)
Bile-acid resins	↓20-25	↓20-35	→	↑5-20
Fibric acid derivatives	↓10	↓10 (↑)	↑10-25	↓40-55
HMG-CoA RI (statins)	↓15-35	↓20-40	↑2-15	↓7-25
Nicotinic acid	↓25	↓20	↑20	↓40
Probucol	↓10-15	↓<10	↓30	→

Comparative Dosages of Agents Used to Treat Hyperlipidemia

Antilipemic Agent	Usual Daily Dose*	Average Dosing Interval
Fibric Acid Derivatives		
Clofibrate (Atromid-S®)	2000 mg	qid
Fenofibrate (TriCor®)	67-200 mg	qd
Gemfibrozil (Lopid®)	1200 mg	bid
Miscellaneous Agents		
Niacin (various)	6 g	tid
Bile Acid Sequestrants		
Colestipol (Colestid®)	max: 30 g	bid
Colesevelam (WelChol™)	max: 3.75-4.375 g	qd-bid
Cholestyramine (LoCHOLEST®, Prevalite®, Questran®)	max: 24 g	tid-qid

*Dosage is based on 70 kg adult with normal hepatic and renal function.

Recommended Liver Function Monitoring for HMG-CoA Reductase Inhibitors

Agent	Initial and After Elevation in Dose	6 Weeks*	12 Weeks*	Semiannually
Atorvastatin (Lipitor®)	x	x	x	x
Fluvastatin (Lescol®)	x	x	x	x
Lovastatin (Mevacor®)	x	x	x	x
Pravastatin (Pravachol®)	x		x	
Simvastatin (Zocor®)	x			x

*After initiation of therapy or any elevation in dose.

Dose-Related Reduction of LDL-Cholesterol With Statins

Agent	Daily Dose (mg)	% Reduction
Atorvastatin	10	39
	20	43
	40	50
	80	60
Fluvastatin	20	22
	40	25
	80	36
Lovastatin	20	27
	40	32
	80	42
Pravastatin	10	22
	20	32
	40	34
Simvastatin	5	26
	10	30
	20	38
	40	41
	80	47

NARCOTIC AGONISTS

Comparative Pharmacokinetics

Drug	Onset (min)	Peak (h)	Duration (h)	Half-Life (h)	Average Dosing Interval (h)	Equianalgesic Doses[1] (mg) I.M.	Equianalgesic Doses[1] (mg) Oral
Alfentanil	Immediate	ND	ND	1-2	—	ND	NA
Buprenorphine	15	1	4-8	2-3	—	0.4	—
Butorphanol	I.M.: 30-60; I.V.: 4-5	0.5-1	3-5	2.5-3.5	3 (3-6)	2	—
Codeine	P.O.: 30-60; I.M.: 10-30	0.5-1	4-6	3-4	3 (3-6)	120	200
Fentanyl	I.M.: 7-15 I.V.: Immediate	ND	1-2	1.5-6	1 (0.5-2)	0.1	NA
Hydrocodone	ND	ND	4-8	3.3-4.4	6 (4-8)	ND	ND
Hydromorphone	P.O.: 15-30	0.5-1	4-6	2-4	4 (3-6)	1.5	7.5
Levorphanol	P.O.: 10-60	0.5-1	4-8	12-16	6 (6-24)	2 (A) 1 (C)	4 (A) 1 (C)
Meperidine	P.O./I.M./S.C.: 10-15 I.V.: ≤5	0.5-1	2-4	3-4	3 (2-4)	75	300
Methadone	P.O.: 30-60; I.V.: 10-20	0.5-1	4-6 (acute); >8 (chronic)	15-30	8 (6-12)	10 (A) 2-4 (C)	20 (A) 2-4 (C)
Morphine	P.O.: 15-60 I.V.: ≤5	P.O./I.M./S.C.: 0.5-1; I.V.: 0.3	3-6	2-4	4 (3-6)	10	60[2] (A) 30 (C)
Nalbuphine	I.M.: 30; I.V.: 1-3	1	3-6	5	—	10	—
Oxycodone	P.O.: 10-15	0.5-1	4-6	3-4	4 (3-6)	NA	20
Oxymorphone	5-15	0.5-1	3-6	—	—	1	10[3]
Pentazocine	15-20	0.25-1	3-4	2-3	3 (3-6)	—	—
Propoxyphene	P.O.: 30-60	2-2.5	4-6	3.5-15	6 (4-8)	ND	130[4]-200[5]
Remifentanil	1-3	<0.3	0.1-0.2	0.15-0.3	—	ND	ND
Sufentanil	1.3-3	ND	ND	2.5-3	—	0.02	NA

ND = no data available. NA = not applicable. (A) = acute, (C) = chronic.

[1] Based on acute, short-term use. Chronic administration may alter pharmacokinetics and decrease the oral parenteral dose ratio. The morphine oral-parenteral ratio decreases to ~1.5-2.5:1 upon chronic dosing.

[2] Extensive survey data suggest that the relative potency of I.M.:P.O. morphine of 1:6 changes to 1:2-3 with chronic dosing.

[3] Rectal

[4] HCl salt

[5] Napsylate salt

Adapted from *Principles of Analgesic Use in the Treatment of Acute Pain and Cancer Pain*, 4th ed, Skokie, IL: The American Pain Society, 1999.

Comparative Pharmacology

Drug	Analgesic	Antitussive	Constipation	Respiratory Depression	Sedation	Emesis
Phenanthrenes						
Codeine	+	++	+	+	+	+
Hydrocodone	+	+++		+		
Hydromorphone	++	+++	+	++	+	+
Levorphanol	++	++	++	++	++	+
Morphine	++	+++	++	++	++	++
Oxycodone	++	+++	++	++	++	++
Oxymorphone	++	+	++	+++		+++
Phenylpiperidines						
Alfentanil	++			+		
Fentanyl	++			++		+
Meperidine	++	+	+	++	+	
Remifentanil	++			++	+++	++
Sufentanil	+++					
Diphenylheptanes						
Methadone	++	++	++	++	+	+
Propoxyphene	+			+	+	+
Agonist/Antagonist						
Buprenorphine	++	N/A	+++	+++	++	++
Butorphanol	++	N/A	+++	+++	++	+
Dezocine	++		+	++	+	++
Nalbuphine	++	N/A	+++	+++	++	++
Pentazocine	++	N/A	+	++	++ or stimulation	++

NEUROMUSCULAR BLOCKING AGENTS

Suggested Dosing Guidelines for the Use of Neuromuscular Blocking Agents in the Intensive Care Unit

Agent	Intermittent Injection	Continuous Infusion
Short Duration		
Mivacurium (Mivacron®)	0.15-0.25 mg/kg followed by 0.1 mg/kg every 15 minutes	1-15 mcg/kg/min
Intermediate Duration		
Atracurium (Tracrium®)	0.4-0.5 mg/kg every 25-35 minutes	0.4-1 mg/kg/h
Cisatracurium (Nimbex®)	0.15-0.2 mg/kg every 40-60 minutes	0.03-0.6 mg/kg/h
Rocuronium (Zemuron™)	0.6 mg/kg every 30 minutes	0.6 mg/kg/h
Vecuronium (Norcuron®)	0.1 mg/kg every 35-45 minutes	0.05-0.1 mg/kg/h
Long Duration		
Doxacurium (Nuromax®)	0.025 mg/kg every 2-3 hours	0.015-0.045 mg/kg/h
Metocurine (Metubine®)	0.3-0.35 mg/kg every 70-90 minutes	0.1-0.25 mg/kg/h
Pancuronium (Pavulon®)	0.1 mg/kg every 90-100 minutes	0.05-0.1 mg/kg/h
Pipecuronium (Arduan®)	0.085-0.1 mg/kg every 90-100 minutes	0.03-0.12 mg/kg/h
Tubocurarine	0.2-0.3 mg/kg every 80 minutes	0.04-0.25 mg/kg/h

Pharmacokinetic and Pharmacodynamic Properties of Neuromuscular Blocking Agents

Agent	Clearance (mL/kg/min)	V_{dss} (L/kg)	Half-life (min)	ED95[1] (mg/kg)	Initial Adult Dose[2,3] (mg/kg)	Onset (min)	Clinical Duration of Action of Initial Dose (min)	Administration as an Intraoperative Infusion (mcg/kg/min)
Ultra-Short Duration								
Succinylcholine	Unknown	Unknown	Unknown	0.2	1-1.5	0.5-1	4-8	10-100
Short Duration								
Mivacurium	50-100[2]	0.2	2[4]	0.07	0.15-0.25	1.5-3	12-20	1-15
Intermediate Duration								
Atracurium	5-7	0.2	20	0.2	0.4-0.5	2-3	20-45	4-12
Cisatracurium	4.6	0.15	22-29	0.05	0.15-0.2	2-3	40-60	1-3
Rocuronium	4	0.17-0.29	60-70	0.3	0.6-1.2	1-1.5	31-67	4-16
Vecuronium	4.5	0.16-0.27	51-80	0.05	0.08-0.1	2-3	20-40	0.8-2
Long Duration								
Doxacurium	1-2.5	0.2	100-200	0.025	0.05-0.08	4-6	100-160	n/a
Gallamine	1.2	0.2	135	3	3-4	3-5	60-100	n/a
Metocurine	1-2	0.4	80-120	0.28	0.4-0.5	3-5	60-100	n/a
Pancuronium	1-2	0.18-0.26	107-169	0.07	0.08-0.1	3-5	60-100	n/a
Pipecuronium	2.4	0.3	120-180	0.05	0.07-0.085	3-5	60-120	n/a
Tubocurarine	1-2	0.3-0.6	100-120	0.51	0.5-0.6	3-5	60-90	n/a

[1]ED95: Effective dose causing 95% blockade.

[2]Initial dose (intubation dose) is usually 2 × ED95 with the exception of cisatracurium where the recommended initial dose is 3-4 × ED95.

[3]Prior administration of succinylcholine generally enhances the magnitude and duration of nondepolarizing NMB agents; initial doses should be lower.

[4]Values reflect contribution of cis-trans and trans-trans isomers only.

NICOTINE PRODUCTS

Dosage Form	Brand Name	Dosing	Recommended Treatment Duration	Strengths Available
Chewing gum	Nicorette® (OTC)	Chew 1 piece q1-2h for 6 wk, then decrease to 1 piece q2-4h for 3 wk, then 1 piece q4-8h for 3 wk, then discontinue	~12 wk	2 mg, 4 mg
Transdermal	Habitrol® (OTC)	One 21 mg/d patch qd for 4-8 wk, then one 14 mg/d patch qd for 2-4 wk, then one 7 mg/d patch qd for 2-4 wk, then discontinue Low-dose regimen[1]: One 14 mg/d patch qd for 6 wk, then one 7 mg/d patch qd for 2-4 wk, then discontinue	~12 wk	Patch: 21 mg/d 14 mg/d 7 mg/d
	Nicoderm CQ® (OTC)	One 21 mg/d patch qd for 6 wk, then one 14 mg/d patch qd for 2 wk, then one 7 mg/d patch qd for 2 wk, then discontinue Low-dose regimen[1]: One 14 mg/d patch qd for 6 wk, then one 7 mg/d patch qd for 2 wk, then discontinue	~10 wk	Patch: 21 mg/d 14 mg/d 7 mg/d
	Nicotrol®	One 15 mg patch qd, worn for 16 h/d and removed for 8 h/d for a total of 6 wk, then discontinue	~6 wk	15 mg/16 h patch
	ProStep®	One 22 mg patch qd for 6 wks If patient smokes ≤15 cigarettes/day, start one 11 mg patch qd for 6 wks	~6 wk	Patch: 22 mg/d 11 mg/d
Nasal spray	Nicotrol® NS	One dose is 2 sprays (1 spray in each nostril) Initial dose: 1-2 sprays q1h, should not exceed 10 sprays (5 doses)/h or 80 sprays (40 doses)/d	~12 wk	10 mL spray 0.5/mg spray (200 actuations)
Inhaler	Nicotrol®	Inhaler releases 4 mg nicotine (the equivalent of 2 cigarettes smoked) for 20 min of active inhaler puffing Usual dose: 6-16 cartridges/ d for up to 12 wk, then reduce dose gradually over ensuing 12 wk, then discontinue	~18-24 wk	10 mg/ cartridge: releases 4 mg/ cartridge

[1]Transdermal low-dose regimens are intended for patients <100 lb, smoke <10 cigarettes/day, and/or have a history of cardiovascular disease.

NITRATES

Nitrates[1]	Dosage Form	Onset (min)	Duration
Nitroglycerin	I.V.	1-2	3-5 min
	Sublingual	1-3	30-60 min
	Translingual spray	2	30-60 min
	Oral, sustained release	40	4-8 h
	Topical ointment	20-60	2-12 h
	Transdermal	40-60	18-24 h
Isosorbide dinitrate	Sublingual and chewable	2-5	1-2 h
	Oral	20-40	4-6 h
	Oral, sustained release	Slow	8-12 h
Isosorbide mononitrate	Oral	60-120	5-12 h

[1]Hemodynamic and antianginal tolerance often develops within 24-48 hours of continuous nitrate administration.

Adapted from Corwin S and Reiffel JA, "Nitrate Therapy for Angina Pectoris," *Arch Intern Med*, 1985, 145:538-43 and Franciosa JA, "Nitroglycerin and Nitrates in Congestive Heart Failure," *Heart and Lung*, 1980, 9(5):873-82.

NONSTEROIDAL ANTI-INFLAMMATORY AGENTS

Comparative Dosages and Pharmacokinetics

Drug	Maximum Recommended Daily Dose (mg)	Time to Peak Levels (h)[1]	Half-life (h)
Propionic Acids			
Fenoprofen (Nalfon®)	3200	1-2	2-3
Flurbiprofen (Ansaid®)	300	1.5	5.7
Ibuprofen (various)	3200	1-2	1.8-2.5
Ketoprofen (Orudis®, others)	300	0.5-2	2-4
Naproxen (Naprosyn®)	1500	2-4	12-15
Naproxen sodium (Anaprox®, others)	1375	1-2	12-13
Oxaprozin (Daypro™)	1800	3-5	42-50
Acetic Acids			
Diclofenac sodium delayed release (Voltaren®)	225	2-3	1-2
Diclofenac potassium immediate release (Cataflam®)	200	1	1-2
Etodolac (Lodine®)	1200	1-2	7.3
Indomethacin (Indocin®)	200	1-2	4.5
Indomethacin SR	150	2-4	4.5-6
Ketorolac (Toradol®)	I.M.: 120[2] P.O.: 40	0.5-1	3.8-8.6
Sulindac (Clinoril®)	400	2-4	7.8 (16.4)[3]
Tolmetin (Tolectin®)	2000	0.5-1	1-1.5
Fenamates (Anthranilic Acids)			
Meclofenamate	400	0.5-1	2 (3.3)[4]
Mefenamic acid (Ponstel®)	1000	2-4	2-4
Nonacidic Agent			
Nabumetone (Relafen®)	2000	3-6	24
Salicylic Acid Derivative			
Diflunisal (Dolobid®)	1500	2-3	8-12
Oxicam			
Meloxicam (MOBIC®)	15	5-10	15-20
Piroxicam (Feldene®)	20	3-5	30-86
COX-2 Inhibitors			
Celecoxib (Celebrex®)	400	3	11
Rofecoxib (Vioxx®)	50	2-3	17
Valdecoxib (Bextra®)	40	2.25-3	8-11

Dosage is based on 70 kg adult with normal hepatic and renal function.

[1] Food decreases the rate of absorption and may delay the time to peak levels.

[2] 150 mg on the first day.

[3] Half-life of active sulfide metabolite.

[4] Half-life with multiple doses.

PARKINSON'S AGENTS

Drugs Used for the Treatment of Parkinson's Disease

Drug	Receptor Affinity	Initial Dose	Titration Schedule	Usual Daily Dosage Range	Recommended Dosing Schedule
Amantadine (Symadine®, Symmetrel®)	NMDA receptor antagonist and inhibits neuronal reuptake of dopamine	100 mg every other day	100 mg/dose every week, up to 300 mg 3 times/d	100-200 mg	Twice daily
Benztropine (Cogentin®)	Cholinergic receptors, also has antihistamine effects	0.5-2 mg/d in 1-4 divided doses	0.5 mg/dose every 5-6 d	2-6 mg	1-2 times/d
Bromocriptine (Parlodel®)	Moderate affinity for D_2 and D_3 dopamine receptors	1.25 mg twice daily	2.5 mg/d every 2-4 wk	2.5-100 mg	3 times/d
Cabergoline (Dostinex®)[1]	Selective to D_2 dopamine receptors	0.5 mg once daily	0.25-0.5 mg/d every 4 wk	0.5-5 mg	Once daily
Entacapone (Comtan®)	COMT enzyme inhibitor	200 mg 3 times/d	Titrate down the doses of levodopa/carbidopa as required	600-1600 mg	3 times/d; up to 8 times/d
Levodopa/carbidopa (Sinemet® CR)	Converts to dopamine; binds to all CNS dopamine receptors	10-25/100 mg 2-4 times/d	0.5-1 tablet (10 or 25/100 mg) every 1-2 d	50/200 to 200/2000 mg (3-8 tablets)	3 times/d or twice daily (for controlled release)
Pergolide (Permax®)	Low affinity for D_1 and maximal affinity for D_2 and D_3 dopamine receptors	0.05 mg/night	0.1-0.15 mg/d every 3 d for 12 d, then 0.25 mg/d every 3 d	0.05-5 mg	3 times/d
Pramipexole (Mirapex®)	High affinity for D_2 and D_3 dopamine receptors	0.125 mg 3 times/d	0.125 mg/dose every 5-7 d	1.5-4.5 mg	3 times/d
Ropinirole (Requip®)	High affinity for D_2 and D_3 dopamine receptors	0.25 mg 3 times/d	0.25 mg/dose weekly for 4 wk, then 1.5 mg/d every week up to 9 mg/d; 3 mg/d up to a max of 24 mg/d	0.75-24 mg	3 times/d
Selegiline (Atapryl®, Eldepryl®, Selpak®)	No receptor effects, inhibits monoamine oxidase	5-10 mg twice daily	Titrate down the doses of levodopa/carbidopa as required	5-10 mg	Twice daily
Tolcapone (Tasmar®)	COMT enzyme inhibitor	100 mg 3 times/d	Titrate down the doses of levodopa/carbidopa as required	300-600 mg	3 times/d
Trihexyphenidyl (Artane®)	Cholinergic receptors; also some direct effect	1-2 mg/d	2 mg/d at intervals of 3-5 d	5-15 mg	3-4 times/d

[1]Cabergoline is not FDA approved for the treatment of Parkinson's disease.

SELECTIVE SEROTONIN REUPTAKE INHIBITORS (SSRIs) PHARMACOKINETICS

SSRI	Half-life (h)	Metabolite Half-life	Peak Plasma Level (h)	% Protein Bound	Bioavailability (%)	Initial Dose
Citalopram (Celexa™)	35	N/A	4	80	80	20 mg qAM
Fluoxetine (Prozac®)	Initial: 24-72 Chronic: 96-144	Norfluoxetine: 4-16 d	6-8	95	72	10-20 mg qAM
Fluvoxamine (Luvox®)	16	N/A	3	80	53	50 mg qhs
Paroxetine (Paxil®)	21	N/A	5	95	>90	10-20 mg qAM
Sertraline (Zoloft®)	26	N-desmethyl-sertraline: 2-4 d	5-8	98	—	25-50 qAM

SULFONAMIDE DERIVATIVES

The following table lists commonly prescribed drugs which are either sulfonamide derivatives or are structurally similar to sulfonamides. Please note that the list may not be all inclusive.

Commonly Prescribed Drugs

Classification	Specific Drugs
Antimicrobial Agents	Mafenide acetate (Sulfamylon®) Silver sulfadiazine (Silvadene®) Sodium sulfacetamide (Sodium Sulamyd®) Sulfadiazine Sulfamethizole Sulfamethoxazole (ie, Bactrim™ and co-trimoxazole) Sulfisoxazole (Gantrisin®)
Diuretics, Carbonic Anhydrase Inhibitors	Acetazolamide (Diamox®) Dichlorphenamide (Daranide®) Methazolamide (Neptazane®)
Diuretics, Loop	Bumetanide (Bumex®) Furosemide (Lasix®) Torsemide (Demadex®)
Diuretics, Thiazide	Bendroflumethiazide (Naturetin®) Benzthiazide (Exna®) Chlorothiazide (Diuril®) Chlorthalidone (Thalitone®) Cyclothiazide (Anhydron®) Hydrochlorothiazide (various and combinations, eg, Dyazide®, Maxzide®) Indapamide (Lozol®) Methyclothiazide (Enduron®) Metolazone (Mykrox®, Zaroxolyn®) Polythiazide (Renese®) Quinethazone (Hydromox®) Trichlormethiazide (Metahydrin®, Naqua®)
Hypoglycemic Agents, Oral	Acetohexamide (Dymelor®) Chlorpropamide (Diabinese®) Glimepiride (Amaryl®) Glipizide (Glucotrol®) Glyburide (DiaBeta®, Glynase™, Micronase®) Tolazamide (Tolinase®) Tolbutamide (Orinase®, Tol-Tab®)
Other Agents	Celecoxib (Celebrex®) Sulfasalazine (Azulfidine®)

CYTOCHROME P450 ENZYMES AND DRUG METABOLISM

Background

There are five distinct groups of drug metabolizing enzymes which account for the majority of drug metabolism in humans. These enzyme "families", known as isoenzymes, are localized primarily in the liver. The nomenclature of this system has been standardized. Isoenzyme families are identified as a cytochrome (CYP prefix), followed by their numerical designation (eg, 1A2).

Enzymes may be inhibited (slowing metabolism through this pathway) or induced (increased in activity or number). Individual drugs metabolized by a specific enzyme are identified as substrates for the isoenzyme. Considerable effort has been expended in recent years to classify drugs metabolized by this system as either an inhibitor, inducer, or substrate of a specific isoenzyme. It should be noted that a drug may demonstrate complex activity within this scheme, acting as an inhibitor of one isoenzyme while serving as a substrate for another.

By recognizing that a substrate's metabolism may be dramatically altered by concurrent therapy with either an inducer or inhibitor, potential interactions may be identified and addressed. For example, a drug which inhibits CYP1A2 is likely to block metabolism of theophylline (a substrate for this isoenzyme). Because of this interaction, the dose of theophylline required to maintain a consistent level in the patient should be reduced when an inhibitor is added. Failure to make this adjustment may lead to supratherapeutic theophylline concentrations and potential toxicity.

This approach does have limitations. For example, the metabolism of specific drugs may have primary and secondary pathways. The contribution of secondary pathways to the overall metabolism may limit the impact of any given inhibitor. In addition, there may be up to a tenfold variation in the concentration of an isoenzyme across the broad population. In fact, a complete absence of an isoenzyme may occur in some genetic subgroups. Finally, the relative potency of inhibition, relative to the affinity of the enzyme for its substrate, demonstrates a high degree of variability. These issues make it difficult to anticipate whether a theoretical interaction will have a clinically relevant impact in a specific patient.

The details of this enzyme system continue to be investigated, and information is expanding daily. However, to be complete, it should be noted that other enzyme systems also influence a drug's pharmacokinetic profile. For example, a key enzyme system regulating the absorption of drugs is the p-glycoprotein system. Recent evidence suggests that some interaction originally attributed to the cytochrome system may, in fact, have been the result of inhibition of this enzyme.

The following tables represent an attempt to detail the available information with respect to isoenzyme activities. Within certain limits, they may be used to identify potential interactions. Of particular note, an effort has been made in each drug monograph to identify involvement of a particular isoenzyme in the drug's metabolism. These tables are intended to supplement the limited space available to list drug interactions in the monograph. Consequently, they may be used to define a greater range of both actual and potential drug interactions.

CYTOCHROME P450 ENZYMES AND RESPECTIVE METABOLIZED DRUGS

CYP1A2

Substrates

Acetaminophen
Acetanilid
Alosetron
Aminophylline
Amitriptyline (demethylation)
Antipyrine
Apomorphine
Betaxolol
Caffeine
Chlorpromazine
Clomipramine (demethylation)
Clozapine
Cyclobenzaprine (demethylation)
Desipramine (demethylation)
Estradiol
Estradiol and medroxyprogesterone
Fluvoxamine
Frovatriptan
Haloperidol (minor)
Imipramine (demethylation)
Levobupivacaine
Levomepromazine
Lidocaine
Maprotiline
Methadone
Metoclopramide
Mirtazapine (hydroxylation)
Nordiazepam
Nortriptyline
Olanzapine (demethylation, hydroxylation)
Ondansetron
Phenacetin
Phenothiazines
Pimozide (minor)
Propafenone
Propranolol
Riluzole
Ritonavir
Ropinirole
Ropivacaine
Tacrine
Theophylline
Thioridazine
Thiothixene
Trifluoperazine
Verapamil
Warfarin (R-warfarin, minor pathway)
Zileuton
Ziprasidone (minor)
Zopiclone

Inducers

Carbamazepine
Charbroiled foods
Cigarette smoke
Cruciferous vegetables (cabbage, brussels sprouts, broccoli, cauliflower)
Griseofulvin
Modafinil (weak)
Nicotine
Omeprazole
Phenobarbital
Phenytoin
Primidone
Rifampin
Ritonavir

Inhibitors

Albendazole (weak)
Anastrozole
Cimetidine
Ciprofloxacin
Citalopram (weak)
Clarithromycin
Diethyldithiocarbamate
Diltiazem
Enoxacin
Entacapone (high dose)
Erythromycin
Ethinyl estradiol
Estradiol
Fluvoxamine
Fluoxetine (high dose)
Grapefruit juice
Isoniazid
Ketoconazole
Lidocaine
Mexiletine
Mibefradil
Moricizine (possible)
Norfloxacin
Paroxetine (high dose)(weak)
Ritonavir
Sertraline (weak)
Tacrine
Tertiary TCAs
Ticlopidine (possible)
Tenofovir (minor)
Zileuton

CYTOCHROME P450 ENZYMES AND DRUG METABOLISM
(Continued)

CYP2A6

Substrates

Acetaminophen
Dexmedetomidine
Letrozole
Montelukast

Nicotine
Ritonavir
Tolcapone

Inducers

Barbiturates

Inhibitors

Diethyldithiocarbamate
Entacapone (high dose)
Letrozole

Methoxsalen
Ritonavir
Tranylcypromine

CYP2B6

Substrates

Antipyrine
Bupropion (hydroxylation)
Cyclophosphamide
Diazepam

Ifosfamide
Lidocaine
Nicotine
Orphenadrine

Inducers

Modafinil (weak)
Phenobarbital

Phenytoin
Primidone

Inhibitors

Diethyldithiocarbamate

Orphenadrine

CYP2C
(Specific isozyme has not been identified)

Substrates

Antipyrine
Carvedilol
Clozapine (minor)

Mestranol
Mephobarbital
Ticrynafen

Inducers

Carbamazepine
Phenobarbital
Phenytoin

Primidone
Rifampin
Sulfinpyrazone

Inhibitors

Isoniazid
Ketoconazole

Ketoprofen

CYP2C8

Substrates

Carbamazepine
Diazepam
Diclofenac
Ibuprofen
Mephobarbital
Naproxen (5-hydroxylation)
Omeprazole

Paclitaxel
Pioglitazone
Retinoic acid
Rifampin
Rosiglitazone
Tolbutamide
Warfarin (S-warfarin)

Inducers

Carbamazepine
Phenobarbital
Phenytoin

Primidone
Rifampin
Rifapentine

Inhibitors

Anastrozole
Nicardipine

Omeprazole
Trimethoprim

CYP2C9

Substrates

Acetaminophen
Alosetron
Amitriptyline (demethylation)
Amoxapine
Bosentan
Carvedilol
Celecoxib
Dapsone
Desogestrel
Diazepam
Diclofenac
Flurbiprofen
Fluvastatin
Glimepiride
Hexobarbital
Ibuprofen
Imipramine (demethylation)
Indomethacin
Irbesartan
Losartan
Mefenamic acid
Mestranol
Metronidazole

Mirtazapine
Montelukast
Naproxen (5-hydroxylation)
Nateglinide
Omeprazole
Phenytoin
Piroxicam
Quetiapine (minor pathway)
Repaglinide
Rifampin
Ritonavir
Rosiglitazone (minor)
Sildenafil citrate (minor pathway)
Tamoxifen
Tenoxicam
Tetrahydrocannabinol
Tolbutamide
Torsemide
Valdecoxib
Warfarin (S-warfarin)
Zafirlukast (hydroxylation)
Zileuton

Inducers

Bosentan
Carbamazepine
Fluconazole
Fluoxetine

Phenobarbital
Phenytoin
Rifampin
Rifapentine

Inhibitors

Amiodarone
Anastrozole
Chloramphenicol
Cimetidine
Clopidogrel (high conc - *in vitro*)
Co-trimoxazole
Diclofenac
Disulfiram
Drospirenone
Entacapone (high dose)
Flurbiprofen
Fluconazole
Fluoxetine
Fluvastatin
Fluvoxamine (potent)
Imatinib
Isoniazid
Ketoconazole (weak)
Ketoprofen
Leflunomide (*in vitro* only)

Metronidazole
Miconazole
Nateglinide
Nicardipine
Omeprazole
Phenylbutazone
Propoxyphene
Ritonavir
Sertraline
Sulfamethoxazole-trimethoprim
Sulfaphenazole
Sulfinpyrazone
Sulfonamides
Sulindac
Trimethoprim
Troglitazone
Valdecoxib (weak *in vitro*)
Valproic acid
Warfarin (R-warfarin)
Zafirlukast

CYTOCHROME P450 ENZYMES AND DRUG METABOLISM
(Continued)

CYP2C18

Substrates

Dronabinol
Naproxen
Omeprazole
Piroxicam
Proguanil

Propranolol
Retinoic acid
Tolbutamide
Warfarin

Inducers

Carbamazepine
Phenobarbital

Phenytoin
Rifampin

Inhibitors

Cimetidine
Fluconazole

Fluvastatin
Isoniazid

CYP2C19

Substrates

Amitriptyline (demethylation)
Amoxapine
Apomorphine
Barbiturates
Carisoprodol
Cilostazol (minor)
Citalopram
Clomipramine (demethylation)
Desmethyldiazepam
Desogestrel
Diazepam (N-demethylation, minor pathway)
Divalproex sodium
Esomeprazole
Hexobarbital
Imipramine (demethylation)
Lansoprazole

Mephenytoin
Mephobarbital
Moclobemide
Olanzapine (minor)
Omeprazole
Pantoprazole
Pentamidine
Phenytoin
Progesterone
Proguanil
Propranolol
Ritonavir
Tolbutamide
Topiramate
Valproic acid
Warfarin (R-warfarin)

Inducers

Carbamazepine
Phenobarbital

Phenytoin
Rifampin

Inhibitors

Cimetidine
Citalopram (weak)
Diazepam
Disulfiram
Drospirenone
Entacapone (high conc)
Ethinyl estradiol
Felbamate
Fluconazole
Fluoxetine
Fluvastatin
Fluvoxamine
Isoniazid
Ketoconazole (weak)
Letrozole
Modafinil

Nicardipine
Omeprazole
Oxcarbazepine
Proguanil
Ritonavir
Sertraline
Telmisartan
Teniposide
Ticlopidine (potent)
Tolbutamide
Topiramate
Tranylcypromine
Troglitazone
Valdecoxib (moderate *in vitro*)
Warfarin (R-warfarin)

CYP2D6

Substrates

Acetaminophen
Almotriptan
Amitriptyline (hydroxylation)
Amoxapine
Amphetamine
Betaxolol
Bisoprolol
Brofaromine
Bufuronol
Captopril
Carvedilol
Cevimeline
Chlorpheniramine
Chlorpromazine
Cinnarizine
Clomipramine (hydroxylation)
Clozapine (minor pathway)

Codeine (hydroxylation, o-demethylation)
Cyclobenzaprine (hydroxylation)
Cyclophosphamide
Debrisoquin
Delavirdine
Desipramine
Dexfenfluramine
Dextromethorphan (o-demethylation)
Dihydrocodeine
Diphenhydramine
Dolasetron
Donepezil
Doxepin
Encainide
Ethylmorphine
Fenfluramine
Flecainide

Fluoxetine (minor pathway)
Fluphenazine
Galantamine
Halofantrine
Haloperidol (minor pathway)
Hydrocodone
Hydrocortisone
Hydroxyamphetamine
Imipramine (hydroxylation)
Labetalol
Lidocaine
Loratadine
Maprotiline
m-Chlorophenylpiperazine (m-CPP)
Meperidine
Methadone
Methamphetamine
Metoclopramide
Metoprolol
Mexiletine
Mianserin
Mirtazapine (hydroxylation)
Molindone
Morphine
Nortriptyline (hydroxylation)
Olanzapine (minor, hydroxymethylation)
Ondansetron
Orphenadrine
Oxycodone
Papaverine

Paroxetine (minor pathway)
Penbutolol
Pentazocine
Perhexiline
Perphenazine
Phenformin
Pindolol
Promethazine
Propafenone
Propranolol
Quetiapine (minor pathway)
Remoxipride
Risperidone
Ritonavir (minor)
Ropivacaine
Selegiline
Sertindole
Sertraline (minor pathway)
Sparteine
Tamoxifen
Thioridazine[1]
Tiagabine
Timolol
Tolterodine
Tramadol
Trazodone
Trimipramine
Tropisetron
Venlafaxine (o-desmethylation)
Yohimbine

Inducers

Rifampin

Inhibitors

Amiodarone
Celecoxib
Chloroquine
Chlorpromazine
Cimetidine
Citalopram
Clomipramine
Codeine
Delavirdine
Desipramine
Dextropropoxyphene
Diltiazem
Doxorubicin
Entacapone (high dose)
Fexofenadine (weak)
Fluoxetine
Fluphenazine
Fluvoxamine
Haloperidol
Imatinib
Labetalol
Lobeline
Lomustine
Methadone
Mibefradil

Moclobemide
Nicardipine
Norfluoxetine
Paroxetine
Perphenazine
Primaquine
Propafenone
Propoxyphene
Quinacrine
Quinidine (potent)
Ranitidine
Risperidone (weak)
Ritonavir
Sertindole
Sertraline (weak)
Thioridazine
Ticlopidine (weak)
Valdecoxib (weak at supratherapeutic doses)
Valproic acid
Venlafaxine (weak)
Vinblastine
Vincristine
Vinorelbine
Yohimbine

CYP2E1

Substrates

Acetaminophen
Acetone
Aniline
Benzene
Caffeine
Chloral hydrate
Chlorzoxazone
Clozapine
Dapsone
Dextromethorphan
Enflurane
Ethanol
Halothane

Isoflurane
Isoniazid
Methoxyflurane
Nitrosamine
Ondansetron
Phenol
Ritonavir
Sevoflurane
Styrene
Tamoxifen
Theophylline (minor pathway)
Venlafaxine

Inducers

Ethanol
Isoniazid

Mitoxantrone (weak)

Inhibitors

Diethyldithiocarbamate (disulfiram metabolite)
Dimethyl sulfoxide
Disulfiram

Entacapone (high dose)
Ritonavir

CYTOCHROME P450 ENZYMES AND DRUG METABOLISM
(Continued)

CYP3A3/4

Substrates

Acetaminophen
Alfentanil
Almotriptan
Alosetron
Alprazolam[1]
Amiodarone
Amitriptyline (minor)
Amlodipine
Amoxapine
Amprenavir
Anastrozole
Androsterone
Antipyrine
Apomorphine
Astemizole[1]
Atorvastatin
Benzphetamine
Bepridil
Bexarotene
Bosentan
Bromazepam
Bromocriptine
Budesonide
Buprenorphine HCl
Bupropion (minor)
Buspirone
Busulfan
Caffeine
Cannabinoids
Carbamazepine
Cevimeline
Chlordiazepoxide
Chlorpromazine
Cilostazol (major)
Cimetidine
Cisapride[1]
Citalopram
Clarithromycin
Clindamycin
Clofibrate
Clomipramine
Clonazepam
Clorazepate
Clozapine
Cocaine
Codeine (demethylation)
Cortisol
Cortisone
Cyclobenzaprine (demethylation)
Cyclophosphamide
Cyclosporine
Dapsone
Dehydroepiandrostendione
Delavirdine
Desmethyldiazepam
Dexamethasone
Dextromethorphan (minor, N-demethylation)
Diazepam (minor; hydroxylation, N-demethylation)
Digitoxin
Diltiazem
Disopyramide
Docetaxel
Dofetilide (minor)
Dolasetron
Donepezil
Doxorubicin
Doxycycline
Dronabinol
Drospirenone
Dutasteride
Enalapril
Erythromycin
Esomeprazole
Estradiol
Estradiol and medroxyprogesterone
Ethinyl estradiol
Ethosuximide

Etonogestrel
Etoposide
Exemestane
Felodipine
Fentanyl
Fexofenadine
Finasteride
Fluoxetine
Flutamide
Fluticasone
Galantamine
Gemfibrozil
Glyburide
Granisetron
Halofantrine
Haloperidol
Hydrocortisone
Hydroxyarginine
Ifosfamide
Imatinib
Imipramine
Indinavir
Isradipine
Itraconazole
Ketoconazole
Lansoprazole (minor)
Letrozole
Levobupivacaine
Levomethadyl acetate hydrochloride
Levonorgestrel
Lidocaine
Loratadine
Losartan
Lovastatin
Methadone
Mibefradil
Miconazole
Midazolam
Mifepristone
Mirtazapine (N-demethylation)
Modafinil
Montelukast
Nateglinide
Navelbine
Nefazodone
Nelfinavir[1]
Nevirapine
Nicardipine
Nifedipine
Niludipine
Nimodipine
Nisoldipine
Nitrendipine
Norgestrel
Omeprazole (sulfonation)
Ondansetron
Oral contraceptives
Orphenadrine
Paclitaxel
Pantoprazole
Pimecrolimus (only if significantly absorbed)
Pimozide[1]
Pioglitazone
Pravastatin
Prednisone
Progesterone
Proguanil
Propafenone
Quercetin
Quetiapine
Quinidine
Quinine
Repaglinide
Retinoic acid
Rifampin (major)
Risperidone
Ritonavir[1]
Salmeterol

Saquinavir
Sertindole
Sertraline
Sibutramine[2]
Sildenafil citrate
Simvastatin
Sirolimus
Sufentanil
Tacrolimus
Tamoxifen
Temazepam
Teniposide
Terfenadine[1]
Testosterone
Tetrahydrocannabinol
Theophylline
Tiagabine
Ticlopidine
Tolcapone
Tolterodine
Toremifene

Tramadol
Trazodone
Tretinoin
Triazolam[1]
Troglitazone
Troleandomycin
Valdecoxib
Venlafaxine (N-demethylation)
Verapamil
Vinblastine
Vincristine
Warfarin (R-warfarin)
Yohimbine
Zaleplon (minor pathway)
Zatosetron
Zidovudine
Zileuton
Ziprasidone
Zolpidem[1]
Zonisamide

Inducers

Bosentan
Carbamazepine
Dexamethasone
Ethosuximide
Glucocorticoids
Nafcillin
Nelfinavir
Nevirapine
Oxcarbazepine
Phenobarbital
Phenylbutazone

Phenytoin
Primidone
Rifabutin
Rifapentine
Rifampin
Rofecoxib (mild)
St John's wort
Sulfadimidine
Sulfinpyrazone
Troglitazone

Inhibitors

Amiodarone
Amprenavir
Anastrozole (high conc)
Cannabinoids
Cimetidine
Clarithromycin[1]
Clotrimazole
Cyclosporine
Danazol
Delavirdine
Dexamethasone
Diethyldithiocarbamate
Diazepam
Diltiazem
Dirithromycin
Disulfiram (and metabolite
    diethyldithiocarbamate
Drospirenone (weak)
Entacapone (high dose)
Erythromycin[1]
Ethinyl estradiol (weak)
Fluconazole (weak)
Fluoxetine
Fluvoxamine[1]
Gestodene
Grapefruit juice
Imatinib (potent)
Indinavir
Isoniazid
Itraconazole[1]
Ketoconazole[1]
Lopinavir and Ritonavir

Metronidazole
Mibefradil[1]
Miconazole (moderate)
Mifepristone
Modafinil (minor)
Nefazodone[1]
Nelfinavir
Nevirapine
Nicardipine
Norfloxacin
Norfluoxetine
Omeprazole (weak)
Oxiconazole
Paroxetine (weak)
Propoxyphene
Quinidine (weak)
Quinine[1]
Quinupristin and dalfopristin
Ranitidine
Ritonavir[1]
Saquinavir
Sertindole
Sertraline
Troglitazone
Troleandomycin
Valdecoxib (weak in vitro)
Valproic acid (weak)
Verapamil
Vinorelbine
Zafirlukast
Zileuton

CYP3A4/5

Substrate

Argatroban (minor)

Progesterone

Inducer

Oxcarbazepine

CYTOCHROME P450 ENZYMES AND DRUG METABOLISM
(Continued)

CYP3A5-7

Substrates

Cortisol	Terfenadine
Diazepam	Testosterone
Estradiol and medroxyprogesterone	Triazolam
Ethinyl estradiol	Vinblastine
Nifedipine	Vincristine

Inducers

Phenobarbital	Primidone
Phenytoin	Rifampin

Inhibitors

Clotrimazole	Propoxyphene
Ketoconazole	Troleandomycin
Metronidazole	

[1]**Contraindications:**

Terfenadine, astemizole, cisapride, and triazolam contraindicated with nefazodone

Pimozide contraindicated with CYP3A3/4 inhibitors

Alprazolam and triazolam contraindicated with ketoconazole and itraconazole

Terfenadine, astemizole, and cisapride contraindicated with fluvoxamine

Terfenadine contraindicated with mibefradil, ketoconazole, erythromycin, clarithromycin, troleandomycin

Thioridazine contraindicated with CYP2D6 inhibitors

Ritonavir contraindicated with triazolam, zolpidem, astemizole, rifabutin, quinine, clarithromycin, troleandomycin

Mibefradil contraindicated with astemizole

Nelfinavir contraindicated with rifabutin

[2]Do not use with SSRIs, sumatriptan, lithium, meperidine, fentanyl, dextromethorphan, or pentazocine within 2 weeks of an MAOI.

References

Baker GB, Urichuk CJ, and Coutts RT, "Drug Metabolism and Metabolic Drug-Drug Interactions in Psychiatry," *Child Adolescent Psychopharm News (Suppl).*

DeVane CL, "Pharmacogenetics and Drug Metabolism of Newer Antidepressant Agents," *J Clin Psychiatry*, 1994, 55(Suppl 12):38-45.

Drug Interactions Analysis and Management. Cytochrome (CYP) 450 Isozyme Drug Interactions, Vancouver, WA: Applied Therapeutics, Inc, 523-7.

Ereshefsky L, "Drug-Drug Interactions Involving Antidepressants: Focus on Venlafaxine," *J Clin Psychopharmacol*, 1996, 16(3 Suppl 2):375-535.

Ereshefsky L, *Psychiatr Annal*, 1996, 26:342-50.

Fleishaker JC and Hulst LK, "A Pharmacokinetic and Pharmacodynamic Evaluation of the Combined Administration of Alprazolam and Fluvoxamine," *Eur J Clin Pharmacol*, 1994, 46(1):35-9.

Flockhart DA, et al, *Clin Pharmacol Ther*, 1996, 59:189.

Ketter TA, Flockhart DA, Post RM, et al, "The Emerging Role of Cytochrome P450 3A in Psychopharmacology," *J Clin Psychopharmacol*, 1995, 15(6):387-98.

Michalets EL, "Update: Clinically Significant Cytochrome P450 Drug Interactions," *Pharmacotherapy*, 1998, 18(1):84-112.

Nemeroff CB, DeVane CL, and Pollock BG, "Newer Antidepressants and the Cytochrome P450 System," *Am J Psychiatry*, 1996, 153(3):311-20.

Pollock BG, "Recent Developments in Drug Metabolism of Relevance to Psychiatrists," *Harv Rev Psychiatry*, 1994, 2(4):204-13.

Richelson E, "Pharmacokinetic Drug Interactions of New Antidepressants: A Review of the Effects on the Metabolism of Other Drugs," *Mayo Clin Proc*, 1997, 72(9):835-47.

Riesenman C, "Antidepressant Drug Interactions and the Cytochrome P450 System: A Critical Appraisal," *Pharmacotherapy*, 1995, 15(6 Pt 2):84S-99S.

Schmider J, Greenblatt DJ, von Moltke LL, et al, "Relationship of *In Vitro* Data on Drug Metabolism to *In Vivo* Pharmacokinetics and Drug Interactions: Implications for Diazepam Disposition in Humans," *J Clin Psychopharmacol*, 1996, 16(4):267-72.

Slaughter RL, *Pharm Times*, 1996, 7:6-16.

Watkins PB, "Role of Cytochrome P450 in Drug Metabolism and Hepatotoxicity," *Semin Liver Dis*, 1990, 10(4):235-50.

DESENSITIZATION PROTOCOLS

PENICILLIN DESENSITIZATION PROTOCOL: MUST BE DONE BY PHYSICIAN!

Acute penicillin desensitization should only be performed in an intensive care setting. Any remedial risk factor should be corrected. All β-adrenergic antagonists such as propranolol or even timolol ophthalmic drops should be discontinued. Asthmatic patients should be under optimal control. An intravenous line should be established, baseline electrocardiogram (EKG) and spirometry should be performed, and continuous EKG monitoring should be instituted. Premedication with antihistamines or steroids is not recommended, as these drugs have not proven effective in suppressing severe reactions but may mask early signs of reactivity that would otherwise result in a modification of the protocol.

Protocols have been developed for penicillin desensitization using both the oral and parenteral route. As of 1987 there were 93 reported cases of oral desensitization, 74 of which were done by Sullivan and his collaborators. Of these 74 patients, 32% experienced a transient allergic reaction either during desensitization (one-third) or during penicillin treatment after desensitization (two-thirds). These reactions were usually mild and self-limited in nature. Only one IgE-mediated reaction (wheezing and bronchospasm) required discontinuation of the procedure before desensitization could be completed. It has been argued that oral desensitization may be safer than parenteral desensitization, but most patients can also be safely desensitized by parenteral route.

During desensitization any dose that causes mild systemic reactions such as pruritus, fleeting urticaria, rhinitis, or mild wheezing should be repeated until the patient tolerates the dose without systemic symptoms or signs. More serious reactions such as hypotension, laryngeal edema, or asthma require appropriate treatment, and if desensitization is continued, the dose should be decreased by at least 10-fold and withheld until the patient is stable.

Once desensitized, the patient's treatment with penicillin must not lapse or the risk of an allergic reaction increases. If the patient requires a β-lactam antibiotic in the future and still remains skin test-positive to penicillin reagents, desensitization would be required again.

Several patients have been maintained on long-term, low-dose penicillin therapy (usually bid-tid) to sustain a chronic state of desensitization. Such individuals usually require chronic desensitization because of continuous occupationally related exposure to β-lactam drugs.

Order for placement/availability at the bedside in the event of a hypersensitivity reaction during scratch/skin testing and desensitization:

Hydrocortisone: 100 mg IVP
Diphenhydramine: 50 mg IVP
Epinephrine: 1:1000 S.C.

Several investigators have demonstrated that penicillin can be administered to history positive, skin test positive patients if initially small but gradually increasing doses are given. However, patients with a history of exfoliative dermatitis secondary to penicillin should not be re-exposed to the drug, even by desensitization.

Desensitization is a potentially dangerous procedure and should be only performed in an area where immediate access to emergency drugs and equipment can be assured.

Begin between 8-10 AM in the morning.

Follow desensitization as indicated for penicillin G or ampicillin.

AMPICILLIN
Oral Desensitization Protocol

1. Begin 0.03 mg of ampicillin
2. Double the dose administered every 30 minutes until complete
3. Example of oral dosing regimen:

Dose #	Ampicillin (mg)
1	0.03
2	0.06
3	0.12
4	0.23
5	0.47
6	0.94
7	1.87
8	3.75
9	7.5
10	15
11	30
12	60
13	125
14	250
15	500

DESENSITIZATION PROTOCOLS *(Continued)*

PENICILLIN G PARENTERAL
Desensitization Protocol: Typical Schedule

Injection No.	Benzylpenicillin Concentration (units/mL)	Volume and Route (mL)*
1†	100	0.1 I.D.
2	↓	0.2 S.C.
3		0.4 S.C.
4		0.8 S.C.
5†	1,000	0.1 I.D.
6	↓	0.3 S.C.
7		0.6 S.C.
8†	10,000	0.1 I.D.
9	↓	0.2 S.C.
10		0.4 S.C.
11		0.8 S.C.
12†	100,000	0.1 I.D.
13	↓	0.3 S.C.
14		0.6 S.C.
15†	1,000,000	0.1 I.D.
16	↓	0.2 S.C.
17		0.2 I.M.
18		0.4 I.M.
19	Continuous I.V. infusion (1,000,000 units/h)	

*Administer progressive doses at intervals of not less than 20 minutes.

†Observe and record skin wheal and flare response to intradermal dose.

Abbreviations: I.D. = intradermal, S.C. = subcutaneous, I.M. = intramuscular, I.V. = intravenous.

PENICILLIN
Oral Desensitization Protocol

Step*	Phenoxymethyl Penicillin (units/mL)	Amount (mL)	Dose (units)	Cumulative Dosage (units)
1	1000	0.1	100	100
2	1000	0.2	200	300
3	1000	0.4	400	700
4	1000	0.8	800	1500
5	1000	1.6	1600	3100
6	1000	3.2	3200	6300
7	1000	6.4	6400	12,700
8	10,000	1.2	12,000	24,700
9	10,000	2.4	24,000	48,700
10	10,000	4.8	48,000	96,700
11	80,000	1	80,000	176,700
12	80,000	2	160,000	336,700
13	80,000	4	320,000	656,700
14	80,000	8	640,000	1,296,700
	Observe patient for 30 minutes			
Change to benzylpenicillin G I.V.				
15	500,000	0.25	125,000	
16	500,000	0.50	250,000	
17	500,000	1	500,000	
18	500,000	2.25	1,125,000	

*Interval between steps, 15 min

ALLOPURINOL
Successful Desensitization for Treatment of a Fixed Drug Eruption

	Oral Dose of Allopurinol
Days 1-3	50 mcg/day
Days 4-6	100 mcg/day
Days 7-9	200 mcg/day
Days 10-12	500 mcg/day
Days 13-15	1 mg/day
Days 16-18	5 mg/day
Days 19-21	10 mg/day
Days 22-24	25 mg/day
Days 25-27	50 mg/day
Day 28	100 mg/day

Prednisone 10 mg/day through desensitization and 1 month after reaching dose of 100 mg allopurinol

Modified from *J Allergy Clin Immunol*, 1996, 97:1171-2.

AMPHOTERICIN B

Challenge and Desensitization Protocol

1. Procedure supervised by physician

2. Epinephrine, 1:1000 wt/vol, multidose vial at bedside

3. Premixed albuterol solution at bedside for nebulization

4. Endotracheal intubation supplies at bedside with anesthesiologist on standby

5. Continuous cardiac telemetry with electronic monitoring of blood pressure

6. Continuous pulse oximetry

7. Premedication with methylprednisolone, 60 mg, I.V. and diphenhydramine, 25 mg I.V.

8. Amphotericin B (Fungizone®)* administration schedule

   a. 10^{-6} dilution, infused over 10 minutes

   b. 10^{-5} dilution, infused over 10 minutes

   c. 10^{-4} dilution, infused over 10 minutes

   d. 10^{-3} dilution, infused over 10 minutes

   e. 10^{-2} dilution, infused over 10 minutes

   f. 10^{-1} dilution (1 mg), infused over 30 minutes

   g. 30 mg in 250 mL 5% dextrose, infused over 4 hours

From Kemp SF and Lockey RF, "Amphotericin B: Emergency Challenge in a Neutropenic, Asthmatic Patient With Fungal Sepsis," *J Allergy Clin Immunol*, 1995, 96(3):425-7.

*Mixtures were prepared in 10 mL 5% dextrose by hospital intensive care unit pharmacy, unless otherwise noted.

BACTRIM™ ORAL DESENSITIZATION PROTOCOL

(Adapted from Gluckstein D and Ruskin J, "Rapid Oral Desensitization to Trimethoprim-Sulfa-methoxazole (TMP-SMZ): Use in Prophylaxis for *Pneumocystis carinii* Pneumonia in Patients With AIDS Who Were Previously Intolerant to TMP-SMZ," *Clin Infect Dis*, 1995, 20:849-53.)

Please read the directions carefully before starting the protocol!

1. There must be a clear cut need for a sulfa drug or a sulfa drug combination product such as Bactrim™. The decision to use sulfa must be made prior to skin testing.

2. Informed consent from the patient or an appropriate relative must have been obtained.

3. A trained individual, physician, nurse, or aide, **must be with the patient** at all times.

4. A physician **must** be on the floor at all times.

5. Injectable epinephrine 0.3 mL 1:1000, diphenhydramine (Benadryl®) 50 mg, corticosteroids and oral ibuprofen 400 mg solution should be drawn up and available at the bedside.

6. Appropriate resuscitative equipment must be available.

7. All dilution of oral Bactrim™ should be made up prior to beginning procedure.

8. Patient should drink 180 mL of water after each Bactrim™ dose.

Dilution for Bactrim™ Desensitization

Final Concentration	Bottle #	Procedure
Oral Bactrim™ 40/200 mg/5 mL	A	Conventional oral Bactrim™ suspension 5 mL = 40/200 mg
Oral Bactrim™ 0.4/2 mg/mL	B	1. Add 5 mL conventional oral Bactrim™ suspension or A (concentration = 40/200 mg/5 mL) to 95 mL of sterile water 2. Shake well. This will give 100 mL of 40/200 mg Bactrim™; each mL = 0.4/2 mg Bactrim™. 3. Dispense 20 mL for use
Oral Bactrim™ 0.004/0.02 mg/mL	C	1. Add 1 mL of the 0.4/2 mg/mL Bactrim™ or B to 99 mL of sterile water 2. Shake well. This will give 100 mL of 0.4/2 mg Bactrim™; each mL = 0.004/0.02 mg Bactrim™. 3. Dispense 20 mL for use

Adverse Reactions and Response During the Protocol

Types of Reactions	Alteration of Protocol
Mild reactions (rash, fever, nausea)	I.V. diphenhydramine (Benadryl®) 50 mg and oral ibuprofen suspension 400 mg
Urticaria, dyspnea, severe vomiting, or hypotension	**STOP** the protocol IMMEDIATELY

- If patient tolerates up to Bactrim™ DS, he/she is desensitized.
- Assuming that there were no complications, the procedure will take up to 6 hours.

DESENSITIZATION PROTOCOLS (Continued)

Sample Bactrim™ Desensitization Flow Sheet

Patient Name _____ Age _____ Gender _____ Hospital # _____

Diagnosis _____ Physician _____ Pager _____ History of sulfa reaction _____

# Hour	Actual Time	Suggested Dose	Form	Suggested Volume	Actual Dose	Form	Actual Volume	Reaction/ Notes	Initial
0		Bactrim™ 0.004/0.02 mg (use **0.004/0.02 mg/mL** bottle or bottle C)	Susp (C)	1 mL					
1		Bactrim™ 0.04/0.2 mg (use 0.004/0.02 mg/mL bottle or bottle C)	Susp (C)	10 mL					
2		Bactrim™ 0.4/2 mg (use **0.4/2 mg/mL bottle** or bottle B)	Susp (B)	1 mL					
3		Bactrim™ 4/20 mg (use 0.4/2 mg/mL bottle or bottle B)	Susp (B)	10 mL					
4		Bactrim™ 40/200 mg (use **40/200 mg/5 mL unit dose** Bactrim™ or A)	Susp (A)	5 mL					
5		Bactrim™ 80/400 mg (use 40/200 mg/5 mL unit dose Bactrim™ or A)	Susp (A)	10 mL					
6		Bactrim™ DS tablet	Tablet	1 DS pill					

Note: Drink 180 mL of water after each Bactrim™ dose.

VANCOMYCIN DESENSITIZATION PROTOCOL

(Adapted from Wong JT, Ripple RE, MacLean JA, et al, "Vancomycin Hypersensitivity: Synergism with Narcotics and Desensitization by a Rapid Continuous Intravenous Protocol," *J Allergy Clin Immunol*, 1994, 94(2 Pt 1):189-94.)

Please read the directions carefully before starting the protocol!

1. Vancomycin desensitization is indicated only for cases with a definitive need for vancomycin and persistent allergic reaction despiting slowing of infusion rate and the addition of Benadryl® or cases with reported vancomycin anaphylactic reactions.

2. Informed consent from the patient or an appropriate relative must have been obtained.

3. A trained individual, physician, nurse, or aide, **must be with the patient** at all times.

4. A physician **must** be on the floor at all times.

5. Injectable epinephrine 0.3 mL 1:1000, diphenhydramine (Benadryl®) 50 mg, corticosteroids and oral ibuprofen 400 mg solution should be drawn up and available at the bedside.

6. Appropriate resuscitative equipment must be available.

7. All dilution of I.V. vancomycin should be made up prior to beginning procedure.

8. All patients are pretreated with 25-50 mg Benadryl®.

9. Infusion rates are to be tightly regulated with **syringe pump**.

Dilution for Vancomycin Desensitization

Final Concentration	Bottle #	Procedure
10 mg/mL	A	1. Dilute 1 g of vancomycin in 10 mL of sterile water 2. Shake well until the drug is completely dissolved 3. Add 2 mL of solution to 18 mL of 0.9% normal saline 4. Mix well 5. This will give 20 mL of 10 mg/mL concentration of vancomycin or (Bottle A) 6. Dispense 10-15 mL in a syringe for syringe pump. Label the syringe as "SYR A: conc = 10 mg/mL" with patient's name, ID, room number, date, and dispensor's initial/pharmacist's initial.
1 mg/mL	B	1. Add 2 mL of bottle A vancomycin (10 mg/mL) to 18 mL of 0.9% normal saline 2. Mix well 3. This will give 20 mL of 1 mg/mL concentration vancomycin or (Bottle B) 4. Dispense 10-15 mL in a syringe for syringe pump. Label the syringe as "SYR B: conc = 1 mg/mL" with patient's name, ID, room number, date, and dispensor's initial/pharmacist's initial.
0.1 mg/mL	C	1. Add 2 mL of Bottle B vancomycin (1 mg/mL) to 18 mL of 0.9% normal saline 2. Mix well 3. This will give 20 mL of 0.1 mg/mL concentration vancomycin or (Bottle C) 4. Dispense 10-15 mL in a syringe for syringe pump. Label the syringe as "SYR C: conc = 0.1 mg/mL" with patient's name, ID, room number, date, and dispensor's initial/pharmacist's initial.
0.01 mg/mL	D	1. Add 2 mL of Bottle C vancomycin (0.1 mg/mL) to 18 mL of 0.9% normal saline 2. Mix well 3. This will give 20 mL of 0.01 mg/mL concentration vancomycin or (Bottle D) 4. Dispense 10-15 mL in a syringe for syringe pump. Label the syringe as "SYR D: conc = 0.01 mg/mL" with patient's name, ID, room number, date, and dispensor's initial/pharmacist's initial.
0.001 mg/mL	E	1. Add 2 mL of Bottle D vancomycin (0.01 mg/mL) to 18 mL of 0.9% normal saline 2. Mix well 3. This will give 20 mL of 0.001 mg/mL concentration vancomycin or (Bottle E) 4. Dispense 10-15 mL in a syringe for syringe pump. Label the syringe as "SYR E: conc = 0.001 mg/mL" with patient's name, ID, room number, date, and dispensor's initial/pharmacist's initial.
0.0001 mg/mL	F	1. Add 2 mL of Bottle E vancomycin (0.001 mg/mL) to 18 mL of 0.9% normal saline 2. Mix well 3. This will give 20 mL of 0.0001 mg/mL concentration vancomycin or (Bottle F) 4. Dispense 10-15 mL in a syringe for syringe pump. Label the syringe as "SYR F: conc = 0.0001 mg/mL" with patient's name, ID, room number, date, and dispensor's initial/pharmacist's initial.

DESENSITIZATION PROTOCOLS (Continued)

Sample Vancomycin Desensitization Flow Sheet

Patient Name _____ Age _____ Gender _____ Hospital # _____

Diagnosis _____ Physician _____ Pager _____ History of vancomycin reaction _____

Time (h/min)	Actual Time	Vancomycin concentration (mg/mL)	Syr #	Fluid infusion rate (mL/min)	VIR (mg/min)	Actual concentration (mg/mL)	Syr #	Infusion rate (mL/min)	Reaction/Notes	Initial
0:00		0.0001	F	1	0.0001					
0:10		0.001	E	0.33	0.00033					
0:20		0.001	E	1.0	0.001					
0:30		0.01	D	0.33	0.0033					
0:40		0.01	D	1.0	0.010					
0:50		0.1	C	0.33	0.033					
1:00		0.1	C	0.33	0.033					
1:10		1.0	B	0.33	0.33					
1:20		1.0	B	1	1					
1:30		10.0	A	0.22	2.2*					
1:30		10.0	A	0.44	4.4*					

* After a VIR of 2.2 to 4.4 mg/min is achieved, full dose of vancomycin can be administered at the VIR for the first day. The rate can be gradually advanced over the next few days as tolerated. Patients in whom a VIR of 2.2 to 4.4 mg/min cannot be achieved, continue to receive vancomycin at the highest tolerated infusion rate for the first day. The rate is to be gradually advanced over the next few days as tolerated.

CIPROFLOXACIN

Modified from *J Allergy Clin Immunol*, 1996, 97:1426-7.

Premedicated with diphenhydramine hydrochloride, ranitidine, and prednisone 1 hour before the desensitization.

The individual doses were administered at 15-minute intervals. Because the patient was intubated in the intensive care unit, vital signs were continually monitored. The patient's skin was inspected for development of urticaria, and his chest was auscultated for wheezing every 10 minutes. No rash, hypotension, or wheezing developed during desensitization. The procedure took 4 hours, and once finished, the patient had received an equivalent to his first scheduled dose (400 mg twice daily). The second dose was given 4 hours later, followed by routine administration of 400 mg every 12 hours, with a small dose (25 mg intravenously) between therapeutic doses to maintain a drug level in the blood. The patient subsequently received 4 weeks of ciprofloxacin treatment without difficulty.

Desensitization Regimen for Ciprofloxacin

Ciprofloxacin Concentration (mg/mL)	Volume Given (mL)	Absolute Amount (mg)	Cumulative Total Dose (mg)
0.1	0.1	0.01	0.01
0.1	0.2	0.02	0.03
0.1	0.4	0.04	0.07
0.1	0.8	0.08	0.15
1	0.16	0.16	0.31
1	0.32	0.32	0.63
1	0.64	0.64	1.27
2	0.6	1.2	2.47
2	1.2	2.4	4.87
2	2.4	4.8	9.67
2	5	10	19.67
2	10	20	39.67
2	20	40	79.67
2	40	80	159.67
2	120	240	399.67

Drug volumes <1 mL were mixed with normal saline solution to a final volume of 3 mL and then slowly infused; the other doses were administered over 10 minutes, except the last dose (240 mg in 120 mL), which was given with an infusion pump over 20 minutes.

DESENSITIZATION PROTOCOLS *(Continued)*

INSULIN

Lilly's appropriate diluting fluid, sterile saline, or distilled water, to which 1 mL of the patient's blood or the addition of 1 mL of 1% serum albumin (making a 0.1% solution) for each 10 mL of stock diluent, is a satisfactory diluent. The albumin in the blood or serum albumin solution is necessary to retain the integrity of the higher dilutions by preventing adsorption to glass or plastic. Dilution is stable 30 days under refrigeration or room temperature, but should be used within 24 hours due to a lack of preservative.

1.   Make a 1:1 dilution of single species (beef, pork, or human) insulin (50 units/mL).

2.   Add 0.5 mL of the above dilution to 4.5 mL of diluent (5 units/mL).

3.   Add 0.5 mL of the 5 units/mL dilution to 4.5 mL of diluent (0.5 unit/mL).

4.   Add 0.5 mL of the 0.5 unit/mL dilution to 4.5 mL of diluent (0.05 unit/mL).

5.   Add 0.5 mL of the 0.05 unit/mL dilution to 4.5 mL of diluent (0.005 unit/mL).

The 5 vials containing 50, 5, 0.5, 0.05, and 0.005 units/mL are ready for skin testing or desensitization procedures.

One may start desensitization by giving 0.02 mL of 0.05 unit/mL concentration (1/1000 unit) intradermally. If no reaction occurs, administer 0.04 and 0.08 mL of the same concentration at 30-minute intervals.

The procedure continues proceeding to the next greater concentration (0.5 unit/mL) and giving 0.02, 0.04, and 0.08 mL at 30-minute intervals.

In the same manner proceed through the 5 units/mL and 50 units/mL concentrations with the exception that these injections should be given subcutaneously.

Note: If a reaction is noted, back up 2 steps and try to proceed forward again.

If the patient reacts to the initial injection, it will be necessary to utilize the lower concentration (0.005 units/mL) to initiate the procedure.

It is essential that manifestations of allergic reactions not be obscured. Therefore, antihistamines or steroids should not be used during desensitization except to treat severe allergic reactions. The use of these agents may obscure mild to moderate reactions to the lower doses and result in more severe reactions as doses increase, leading to failure of the desensitization program.

RIFAMPIN and ETHAMBUTOL
Oral Desensitization in Mycobacterial Disease

Time from Start (h:min)	Rifampin (mg)	Ethambutol (mg)
0	0.1	0.1
00:45	0.5	0.5
01:30	1	1
02:15	2	2
03:00	4	4
03:45	8	8
04:30	16	16
05:15	32	32
06:00	50	50
06:45	100	100
07:30	150	200
11:00	300	400
Next day		
6:30 AM	300 twice daily	400 three times/day

From *Am J Respir Crit Care Med*, 1994, 149:815-7.

SKIN TESTS

Delayed Hypersensitivity (Anergy)

Delayed cutaneous hypersensitivity (DCH) is a cell-mediated immunological response which has been used diagnostically to assess previous infection (eg, purified protein derivative (PPD), histoplasmin, and coccidioidin) or as an indicator of the status of the immune system by using mumps, *Candida*, tetanus toxoid, or trichophyton to test for anergy. Anergy is a defect in cell-mediated immunity that is characterized by an impaired response, or lack of a response to DCH testing with injected antigens. Anergy has been associated with several disease states, malnutrition, and immunosuppressive therapy, and has been correlated with increased risk of infection, morbidity, and mortality.

Many of the skin test antigens have not been approved by the FDA as tests for anergy, and so the directions for use and interpretation of reactions to these products may differ from that of the product labeling. There is also disagreement in the published literature as to the selection and interpretation of these tests for anergy assessment, leading to different recommendations for use of these products.

General Guidelines

Read these guidelines before using any skin test.

Administration

1. Use a separate sterile TB syringe for each antigen. Immediately after the antigen is drawn up, make the injection intradermally in the flexor surface of the forearm.
2. A small bleb 6-10 mm in diameter will form if the injection is made at the correct depth. If a bleb does not form or if the antigen solution leaks from the site, the injection must be repeated.
3. When applying more than one skin test, make the injections at least 5 cm apart.
4. Do any serologic blood tests before testing or wait 48-96 hours.

Reading

1. Read all tests at 24, 48, and 72 hours. Reactions occurring before 24 hours are indicative of an immediate rather than a delayed hypersensitivity.
2. Measure the diameter of the induration in two directions (at right angles) with a ruler and record each diameter in millimeters. Ballpoint pen method of measurement is the most accurate.
3. Test results should be recorded by the nurse in the Physician's Progress Notes section of the chart, and should include the millimeters of induration present, and a picture of the arm showing the location of the test(s).

Factors Causing False-Negative Reactions

1. Improper administration, interpretation, or use of outdated antigen
2. Test is applied too soon after exposure to the antigen (DCH takes 2-20 weeks to develop)
3. Concurrent viral illnesses (eg, rubeola, influenza, mumps, and probably others) or recent administration of live attenuated virus vaccines (eg, measles)
4. Anergy may be associated with:
    a. Immune suppressing chronic illnesses such as diabetes, uremia, sarcoidosis, metastatic carcinomas, Hodgkin's, acute lymphocytic leukemia, hypothyroidism, chronic hepatitis, and cirrhosis.
    b. Some antineoplastic agents, radiation therapy, and corticosteroids. If possible, discontinue steroids at least 48 hours prior to DCH skin testing.
    c. Congenital immune deficiencies.
    d. Malnutrition, shock, severe burns, and trauma.
    e. Severe disseminated infections (miliary or cavitary TB, cocci granuloma, and other disseminated mycotic infections, gram-negative bacillary septicemia).
    f. Leukocytosis (>15,000 cells/mm^3).

Factors Causing False-Positive Reactions

1. Improper interpretation
2. Patient sensitivity to minor ingredients in the antigen solutions such as the phenol or thimerosal preservatives
3. Cross-reactions between similar antigens

Candida 1:1000
Dose = 0.1 mL intradermally (30% of children <18 months of age and 50% >18 months of age respond)
Can be used as a control antigen

Coccidioidin 1:1000
Dose = 0.1 mL intradermally (apply with PPD **and** a control antigen)
Mercury derivative used as a preservative for spherulin.

Histoplasmin 1:1000
Dose = 0.1 mL intradermally (yeast derived)

Multitest CMI (*Candida*, diphtheria toxoid, tetanus toxoid, *Streptococcus*, old tuberculin, *Trichophyton*, *Proteus* antigen, and negative control)
Press loaded unit into the skin with sufficient pressure to puncture the skin and allow adequate penetration of all points.

SKIN TESTS *(Continued)*

Mumps 40 cfu/mL

Dose = 0.1 mL intradermally (contraindicated in patients allergic to eggs, egg products, or thimerosal)

Dosage as Part of Disease Diagnosis

Tuberculin Testing

Purified Protein Derivative (PPD)

Preparation	Dilution	Units/0.1 mL
First strength	1:10,000	1
Intermediate strength	1:2000	5
Second strength	1:100	250

The usual initial dose is 0.1 mL of the intermediate strength. The first strength should be used in the individuals suspected of being highly sensitive. The second strength is used only for individuals who fail to respond to a previous injection of the first or intermediate strengths.

A positive reaction is ≥10 mm induration except in HIV-infected individuals where a positive reaction is ≥5 mm of induration.

Adverse Reactions

In patients who are highly sensitive, or when higher than recommended doses are used, exaggerated local reactions may occur, including erythema, pain, blisters, necrosis, and scarring. Although systemic reactions are rare, a few cases of lymph node enlargement, fever, malaise, and fatigue have been reported.

To prevent severe local reactions, never use second test strengths as the initial agent. Use diluted first strengths in patients with known or suspected hypersensitivity to the antigen.

Have epinephrine and antihistamines on hand to treat severe allergic reactions that may occur.

Treatment of Adverse Reactions

Severe reactions to intradermal skin tests are rare and treatment consists of symptomatic care.

Skin Testing

All skin tests are given intradermally into the flexor surface of one arm.

Purified protein derivative (PPD) is used most often in the diagnosis of tuberculosis. *Candida*, *Trichophyton*, and mumps skin tests are used most often as controls for anergy.

Dose: The usual skin test dose is as follows:

Antigen		Standard Dose	Concentration
PPD	1 TU	0.1 mL	1 TU — highly sensitive patients
	5 TU	0.1 mL	5 TU — standard dose
	250 TU	0.1 mL	250 TU — anergic patients in whom TB is suspected
Candida		0.02 mL	
Histoplasmin		0.1 mL	Seldom used. Serology is preferred method to diagnose histoplasmosis.
Mumps		0.1 mL	
Trichophyton		0.02 mL	

Interpretation:

Skin Test	Reading Time	Positive Reaction
PPD	48-72 h	**≥5 mm considered positive for:** • close contacts to an infectious case • persons with abnormal chest x-ray indicating old healed TB • persons with known or suspected HIV infection **≥10 mm considered positive for:** • other medical risk factors • foreign born from high prevalence areas • medically underserved, low income populations • alcoholics and intravenous drug users • residents of long-term care facilities (including correctional facilities and nursing homes) • staff in settings where disease would pose a hazard to large number of susceptible persons **≥15 mm considered positive for:** • persons without risk factors for TB
Candida	24-72 h	≥5 mm induration
Histoplasmin	24-72 h	≥5 mm
Mumps	24-36 h	≥5 mm
Trichophyton	24-72 h	≥5 mm induration

Recommended Interpretation of Skin Test Reactions

Reaction	Local Reaction	
	After Intradermal Injections of Antigens	**After Dinitrochlorobenzene**
1+	Erythema >10 mm and/ or induration >1-5 mm	Erythema and/or induration covering <$\frac{1}{2}$ area of dose site
2+	Induration 6-10 mm	Induration covering >$\frac{1}{2}$ area of dose site
3+	Induration 11-20 mm	Vesiculation and induration at dose site or spontaneous flare at days 7-14 at the site
4+	Induration >20 mm	Bulla or ulceration at dose site or spontaneous flare at days 7-14 at the site

Penicillin Allergy

The recommended battery of major and minor determinants used in penicillin skin testing will disclose those individuals with circulating IgE antibodies. This procedure is therefore useful to identify patients at risk for immediate or accelerated reactions. Skin tests are of no value in predicting the occurrence of non-IgE-mediated hypersensitivity reactions to penicillin such as delayed exanthem, drug fever, hemolytic anemia, interstitial nephritis, or exfoliative dermatitis. Based on large scale trials, skin testing solutions have been standardized.

Antihistamines, tricyclic antidepressants, and adrenergic drugs, all of which may inhibit skin test results, should be discontinued at least 24 hours prior to skin testing. Antihistamines with long half-lives (hydroxyzine, terfenadine, astemizole, etc) may attenuate skin test results up to a week, or longer after discontinuation.

When properly performed with due consideration for preliminary scratch tests and appropriate dilutions, skin testing with penicillin reagents can almost always be safely accomplished. Systemic reactions accompany about 1% of positive skin tests; these are usually mild but can be serious. **Therefore skin tests should be done in the presence of a physician and with immediate access to medications and equipment needed to treat anaphylaxis.**

SKIN TESTS *(Continued)*

History of Penicillin Allergy

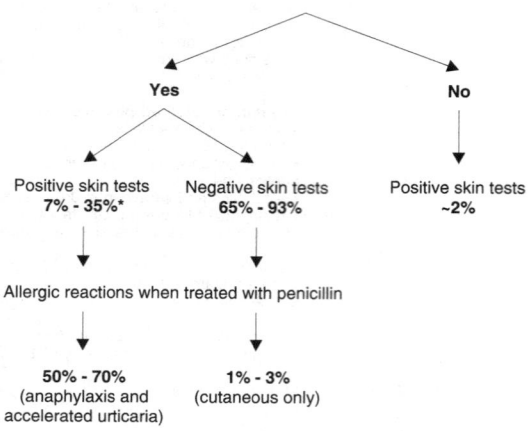

*One study found 65% positive.

Prevalence of positive and negative skin tests and subsequent allergic reactions in patients treated with penicillin (based on studies using both penicilloyl-polylysine and minor determinant mixture as skin test reagents).

Penicillin Skin Testing Protocol

Skin tests evaluate the patient for the presence of penicillin IgE — sensitive mast cells which are responsible for anaphylaxis and other immediate hypersensitivity reactions. Local or systemic allergic reactions rarely occur due to skin testing, therefore, a tourniquet, I.V., and epinephrine should be at the bedside. The breakdown products of penicillin provide the antigen which is responsible for the allergy. Testing is performed with benzylpenicilloyl-polylysine (Pre-Pen®), the major determinant, penicillin G which provides the minor determinants and the actual penicillin which will be administered.

Controls are important if the patient is extremely ill or is taking antihistamines, codeine, or morphine. Normal saline is the negative control. Morphine sulfate, a mast cell degranulator, can be used as a positive control, if the patient is not on morphine or codeine. Histamine is the preferred positive control, however, is not manufactured in a pharmaceutical formulation anymore. A false-positive or false-negative will make further skin testing invalid.

Control Solutions

Normal saline = negative control
Morphine sulfate (10 mg/100 mL 0.9% NaCl, 0.1 mg/mL) = positive control

Test Solutions

Order the necessary solutions as 0.5 mL in a tuberculin syringe. **Note:** May need to order 2 syringes of each — one for scratch testing and one for intradermal skin testing.

I. **Pre-Pen®: Benzylpenicilloyl-polylysine (0.25 mL ampul) = MAJOR DETERMINANT**
    A. Undiluted Pre-Pen®
    B. 1:100 concentration
       To make: Dilute 0.1 mL of Pre-Pen® in 10 mL of 0.9% NaCl
    C. 1:10,000 concentration
       (Only necessary in patients with a history of anaphylaxis)
       To make: Dilute 1 mL of the 1:100 solution in 100 mL of 0.9% NaCl

II. **Penicillin G sodium/potassium = MINOR DETERMINANT**
    A. 5000 units/mL concentration
    B. 5 units/mL concentration
       (Only necessary in patients with a history of anaphylaxis)
       To make: Dilute 0.1 mL of a 5000 units/mL solution in 100 mL of 0.9% NaCl

III. **Penicillin product to be administered — if not penicillin G**
    A. **Ampicillin** 2.5 mg/mL concentration
       To make: Dilute 250 mg in 100 mL of 0.9% NaCl
    B. **Nafcillin** 2.5 mg/mL concentration
       To make: Dilute 250 mg in 100 mL of 0.9% NaCl

Order for placement/availability at the bedside in the event of a hypersensitivity reaction during scratch/skin testing and desensitization:

Hydrocortisone: 100 mg IVP
Diphenhydramine: 50 mg IVP
Epinephrine: 1:1000 S.C.

Scratch/Skin Testing Protocol: Must Be Done by Physician!

1. Begin with the control solutions (ie, normal saline and morphine).

2. Administer **scratch tests** in the following order (beginning with the most dilute solution):

Pre-Pen®	Syringes: C,B,A
Penicillin G	Syringes: E,D
Ampicillin/Nafcillin	Syringe: F

    The inner volar surface of the forearm is usually used.

    A nonbleeding scratch of 3-5 mm in length is made in the epidermis with a 20-gauge needle.

    If bleeding occurs, another site should be selected and another scratch made using less pressure.

    A small drop of the test solution is then applied and rubbed gently into the scratch using an applicator, toothpick, or the side of the needle.

    The scratch test site should be observed for the appearance of a wheal, erythema, and pruritis.

    A positive reaction is signified by the appearance within 15 minutes of a pale wheal (usually with pseudopods) ranging from 5-15 mm or more in diameter.

    As soon as a positive response is elicited, or 15 minutes has elapsed, the solution should be wiped off the scratch.

    If the scratch test is negative or equivocal (ie, a wheal of <5 mm in diameter with little or no erythema or itching appears), an intradermal test may be performed.

    If significant reaction, treat and proceed to desensitization.

3. Administer **intradermal tests** in the following order (beginning with the most dilute solution):

Pre-Pen®	Syringes: C,B,A
Penicillin G	Syringes: E,D
Ampicillin/Nafcillin	Syringe: F

    Intradermal tests are usually performed on a sterilized area of the upper outer arm at a sufficient distance below the deltoid muscle to permit proximal application of a tourniquet if a severe reaction occurs.

    Using a tuberculin syringe with a $^3/_8$-$^5/_8$ inch 26- to 30-gauge needle, an amount of each test solution sufficient to raise the smallest perceptible bleb (usually 0.01-0.02 mL) is injected immediately under the surface of the skin.

    A separate needle and syringe must be used for each solution.

    Each test and control site should be at least 15 cm apart.

    Positive reactions are manifested as a wheal at the test site with a diameter at least 5 mm larger than the saline control, often accompanied by itching and a marked increase in the size of the bleb.

    Skin responses to penicillin testing will develop within 15 minutes.

    If no significant reaction, may challenge patient with reduced dosage of the penicillin to be administered.

    Physician should be at the bedside during this challenge dose!

    If significant reaction, treat and begin desensitization.

IMMUNIZATION RECOMMENDATIONS

Standards for Pediatric Immunization Practices

Standard 1.	Immunization services are readily available.
Standard 2.	There are no barriers or unnecessary prerequisites to the receipt of vaccines.
Standard 3.	Immunization services are available free or for a minimal fee.
Standard 4.	Providers utilize all clinical encounters to screen and, when indicated, immunize children.
Standard 5.	Providers educate parents and guardians about immunizations in general terms.
Standard 6.	Providers question parents or guardians about contraindications and, before immunizing a child, inform them in specific terms about the risks and benefits of the immunizations their child is to receive.
Standard 7.	Providers follow only true contraindications.
Standard 8.	Providers administer simultaneously all vaccine doses for which a child is eligible at the time of each visit.
Standard 9.	Providers use accurate and complete recording procedures.
Standard 10.	Providers co-schedule immunization appointments in conjunction with appointments for other child health services.
Standard 11.	Providers report adverse events following immunization promptly, accurately, and completely.
Standard 12.	Providers operate a tracking system.
Standard 13.	Providers adhere to appropriate procedures for vaccine management.
Standard 14.	Providers conduct semiannual audits to assess immunization coverage levels and to review immunization records in the patient populations they serve.
Standard 15.	Providers maintain up-to-date, easily retrievable medical protocols at all locations where vaccines are administered.
Standard 16.	Providers operate with patient-oriented and community-based approaches.
Standard 17.	Vaccines are administered by properly trained individuals.
Standard 18.	Providers receive ongoing education and training on current immunization recommendations.

Recommended by the National Vaccine Advisory Committee, April 1992.
Approved by the United States Public Health Service, May 1992.
Endorsed by the American Academy of Pediatrics, May 1992.

The Standards represent the consensus of the National Vaccine Advisory Committee (NVAC) and of a broad group of medical and public health experts about what constitutes the most desirable immunization practices. It is recognized by the NVAC that not all of the current immunization practices of public and private providers are in compliance with the Standards. Nevertheless, the Standards are expected to be useful as a means of helping providers to identify needed changes, to obtain resources if necessary, and to actually implement the desirable immunization practices in the future.

Recommended Childhood Immunization Schedule
United States, 2002

	Range of Recommended Ages								Catch-up Vaccination			Preadolescent Assessment	

Age ▶ Vaccine ▼	Birth	1 mo	2 mo	4 mo	6 mo	12 mo	15 mo	18 mo	24 mo	4-6 y	11-12 y	13-18 y
Hepatitis B[1]	Hep B #1	only if mother HB$_s$Ag(-)										
		Hep B #2			Hep B #3					Hep B series		
Diphtheria, tetanus, pertussis[2]			DTaP	DTaP	DTaP		DTaP			DTaP	Td	
H. influenzae type b[3]			Hib	Hib	Hib	Hib						
Inactivated polio[4]			IPV	IPV	IPV					IPV		
Measles, mumps, rubella[5]						MMR #1				MMR #2	MMR #2	
Varicella[6]						Varicella				Varicella		
Pneumococcal[7]			PCV	PCV	PCV	PCV				PCV	PPV	
Hepatitis A[8]										Hepatitis A series		
Influenza[9]						Influenza (yearly)						

Vaccines below this line are for selected populations

This schedule indicates the recommended ages for routine administration of currently licensed childhood vaccines, as of December 1, 2001, for children through 18 years of age. Any dose not given at the recommended age should be given at any subsequent visit when indicated and feasible. ▓▓▓ Indicates age groups that warrant special effort to administer those vaccines not previously given. Additional vaccines may be licensed and recommended during the year. Licensed combination vaccines may be used whenever any components of the combination are indicated and the vaccine's other components are not contraindicated. Providers should consult the manufacturers' package inserts for detailed recommendations.

1 All infants should receive the first dose of **hepatitis B vaccine (Hep B)** soon after birth and before hospital discharge; the 1st dose may also be given by 2 months of age if the infant's mother is HB$_s$Ag-negative. Only monovalent hepatitis B vaccine can be used for the birth dose. Monovalent or combination vaccine containing Hep B may be used to complete the series; four doses of vaccine may be administered if combination vaccine is used. The 2nd dose should be given at least 4 weeks after the 1st dose, except for Hib-containing vaccine which cannot be administered before 6 months of age. The 3rd dose should be given at least 16 weeks after the 1st dose and at least 8 weeks after the 2nd dose. The last dose in the vaccination series (3rd or 4th dose) should not be administered before 6 months of age.

Infants born to HB$_s$Ag-positive mothers should receive hepatitis B vaccine and 0.5 mL hepatitis B immune globulin (HBIG) within 12 hours of birth at separate sites. The 2nd dose is recommended at 1-2 months of age and the vaccination series should be completed (3rd or 4th dose) at 6 months of age.

Infants born to mothers whose HB$_s$Ag status is unknown should receive the 1st dose of the hepatitis B vaccine series within 12 hours of birth. Maternal blood should be drawn at the time of delivery to determine the mother's HB$_s$Ag status; if the HB$_s$Ag test is positive, the infant should receive HBIG as soon as possible (no later than 1 week of age).

2 **Diphtheria and tetanus toxoids and acellular pertussis vaccine (DTaP).** The 4th dose of DTaP may be administered as early as 12 months of age, provided 6 months have elapsed since the 3rd dose and the child is unlikely to return at 15-18 months of age. **Tetanus and diphtheria toxoids (Td)** is recommended at 11-12 years of age if at least 5 years have elapsed since the last dose of tetanus and diphtheria toxoid-containing vaccine. Subsequent routine Td boosters are recommended every 10 years.

3 *Haemophilus influenzae* **type b (Hib) conjugate vaccines.** Three Hib conjugate vaccines are licensed for infant use. If PRP-OMP (PedvaxHIB® or ComVax® [Merck]) is administered at 2 and 4 months of age, a dose at 6 months of age is not required. DTaP/Hib combination products should not be used for primary immunization in infants at 2, 4, or 6 months of age, but can be used as boosters following any Hib vaccine.

4 **Inactivated polio vaccine (IPV).** An all-IPV schedule is recommended for routine childhood polio vaccination in the United States. All children should receive four doses of IPV at 2 months, 4 months, 6-18 months, and 4-6 years of age.

5 **Measles, mumps, and rubella vaccine (MMR).** The 2nd dose of MMR is recommended routinely at 4-6 years of age but may be administered during any visit, provided at least 4 weeks have elapsed since the 1st dose and that both doses are administered beginning at or after 12 months of age. Those who have not previously received the 2nd dose should complete the schedule by the 11- to 12-year old visit.

6 **Varicella vaccine** is recommended at any visit at or after 12 months of age for susceptible children (ie, those who lack a reliable history of chickenpox). Susceptible persons >13 years of age should receive 2 doses, given at least 4 weeks apart.

7 The heptavalent **pneumococcal conjugate vaccine (PCV)** is recommended for all children 2-23 months of age. It is also recommended for certain children 24-59 months of age. **Pneumococcal polysaccharide vaccine (PPV)** is recommended in addition to PCV for certain high-risk groups. See *MMWR Morb Mortal Wkly Rep*, 2000, 49(RR-9),1-35.

8 **Hepatitis A vaccine** is recommended for use in selected states and regions, and for certain high-risk groups; consult your local public health authority. See *MMWR Morb Mortal Wkly Rep*, 1999, 48(RR-12): 1-37.

9 **Influenza vaccine** is recommended annually for children >6 months of age with certain risk factors (including but not limited to asthma, cardiac disease, sickle cell disease, HIV, diabetes (see *MMWR Morb Mortal Wkly Rep*, 2001, 50(RR-4):1-44), and can be administered to all others wishing to obtain immunity. Children ≤12 years of age should receive vaccine in a dosage appropriate for their age (0.25 mL if 6-35 months of age or 0.5 mL if ≥3 years of age). Children ≤8 years of age who are receiving influenza vaccine for the first time should receive two doses separated by at least 4 weeks.

Approved by the Advisory Committee on Immunization Practices (*www.cdc.gov/nip/acip*), the American Academy of Pediatrics (*www.aap.org*), and the American Academy of Family Physicians (www.aafp.org).

For additional information about the vaccines, vaccine supply, and contraindications for immunization, please visit the National Immunization Program web site at *www.cdc.gov/nip* or call the National Immunization Hotline at (800) 232-2522 (English) or (800) 232-0233 (Spanish).

IMMUNIZATION RECOMMENDATIONS *(Continued)*

RECOMMENDATIONS OF THE ADVISORY COMMITTEE ON IMMUNIZATION PRACTICES (ACIP)

Recommended Poliovirus Vaccination Schedules for Children

Vaccine	Child's Age			
	2 mo	4 mo	12-18 mo	4-6 y
Sequential IPV [1]/OPV[1]/OPV[2]	IPV	IPV	OPV	OPV
OPV[1]	OPV	OPV	OPV[3]	OPV
IPV[2]	IPV	IPV	IPV	OPV

[1]Inactivated poliovirus vaccine.

[2]Live, oral poliovirus vaccine.

[3]For children who receive only OPV, the third dose of OPV may be administered as early as 6 months of age.

Adapted from "Poliomyelitis Prevention in the United States: Introduction of a Sequential Vaccination Schedule of Inactivated Poliovirus Vaccine Followed by Oral Poliovirus Vaccine" *MMWR Morb Mortal Wkly Rep*, 1997, 46(RR-3).

Recommendations for Measles Immunization[1]

Category	Recommendations
Unvaccinated, no history of measles (12-15 mo)	A 2-dose schedule (with MMR) is recommended if born after 1956. The first dose is recommended at 12-15 mo; the second is recommended at 4-6 y
Children 6-11 mo in epidemic situations	Immunize (with monovalent measles vaccine or, if not available, MMR); reimmunization (with MMR) at 12-15 mo is necessary, and a third dose is indicated at 4-6 y
Children 4-12 y who have received 1 dose of measles vaccine at ≥12 mo	Reimmunize (1 dose)
Students in college and other post-high school institutions who have received 1 dose of measles vaccine at ≥12 mo	Reimmunize (1 dose)
History of vaccination before the first birthday	Consider susceptible and immunize (2 doses)
Unknown vaccine, 1963-1967	Consider susceptible and immunize (2 doses)
Further attenuated or unknown vaccine given with IG	Consider susceptible and immunize (2 doses)
Egg allergy	Immunize; no reactions likely
Neomycin allergy, nonanaphylactic	Immunize; no reactions likely
Tuberculosis	Immunize; vaccine does not exacerbate infection
Measles exposure	Immunize and/or give IG, depending on circumstances
HIV-infected	Immunize (2 doses) unless severely immunocompromised
Immunoglobulin or blood	Immunize at the appropriate interval

[1] MMR = measles-mumps-rubella vaccine; IG = immune globulin; HIV = human immunodeficiency virus.

Adapted from "Report of the Committee on Infectious Diseases," *2000 Red Book*®, 25th ed, 391.

Recommended Immunization Schedules for Children Not Immunized in the First Year of Life*

Recommended Time/Age	Immunization(s)[1,2,3]	Comments
Younger Than 7 Years		
First visit	DTaP (or DTP), Hib, HBV, MMR, OPV[3]	If indicated, tuberculin testing may be done at same visit.
		If child is ≥5 y of age, Hib is not indicated in most circumstances.
Interval after first visit		
1 mo (4 wk)	DTaP (or DTP), HBV, Var[4]	The second dose of OPV may be given if accelerated poliomyelitis vaccination is necessary, such as for travelers to areas where polio is endemic.
2 mo	DTaP (or DTP), Hib, OPV[3]	Second dose of Hib is indicated only if the first dose was received when <15 mo.
≥8 mo	DTaP (or DTP), HBV, OPV[3]	OPV and HBV are not given if the third doses were given earlier.
Age 4-6 y (at or before school entry)	DTaP (or DTP), OPV,[3] MMR[5]	DTaP (or DTP) is not necessary if the fourth dose was given after the fourth birthday; OPV is not necessary if the third dose was given after the fourth birthday.
Age 11-12 y	See Childhood Immunization Schedule	
7-12 Years		
First visit	HBV, MMR, Td, OPV[3]	
Interval after first visit		
2 mo (8 wk)	HBV, MMR,[5] Var,[4] Td, OPV[3]	OPV also may be given 1 mo after the first visit if accelerated poliomyelitis vaccination is necessary.
8-14 mo	HBV,[6] Td, OPV[3]	OPV is not given if the third dose was given earlier.
Age 11-12 y	See Childhood Immunization Schedule	

*Table is not completely consistent with all package inserts. For products used, also consult manufacturer's package insert for instructions on storage, handling, dosage, and administration. Biologics prepared by different manufacturers may vary, and package inserts of the same manufacturer may change from time to time. Therefore, the physician should be aware of the contents of the current package insert.

Vaccine abbreviations: HBV indicates hepatitis B virus vaccine; Var, varicella vaccine; DTP, diphtheria and tetanus toxoids and pertussis vaccine; DTaP, diphtheria and tetanus toxoids and acellular pertussis vaccine; Hib, *Haemophilus influenzae* type b conjugate vaccine; OPV, oral poliovirus vaccine; IPV, inactivated poliovirus vaccine; MMR, live measles-mumps-rubella vaccine; Td, adult tetanus toxoid (full dose) and diphtheria toxoid (reduced dose), for children ≥7 years and adults.

[1]If all needed vaccines cannot be administered simultaneously, priority should be given to protecting the child against those diseases that pose the greatest immediate risk. In the United States, these diseases for children <2 years usually are measles and *Haemophilus influenzae* type b infection; for children >7 years, they are measles, mumps, and rubella. Before 13 years of age, immunity against hepatitis B and varicella should be ensured.

[2]DTaP, HBV, Hib, MMR, and Var can be given simultaneously at separate sites if failure of the patient to return for future immunizations is a concern.

[3]IPV is also acceptable. However, for infants and children starting vaccination late (ie, after 6 months of age), OPV is preferred in order to complete an accelerated schedule with a minimum number of injections.

[4]Varicella vaccine can be administered to susceptible children any time after 12 months of age. Unvaccinated children who lack a reliable history of chickenpox should be vaccinated before their 13th birthday.

[5]Minimal interval between doses of MMR is 1 month (4 weeks).

[6]HBV may be given earlier in a 0-, 2-, and 4-month schedule.

Adapted from "Report of the Committee on Infectious Diseases," *1997 Red Book*®, 24th ed.

IMMUNIZATION RECOMMENDATIONS *(Continued)*

Minimum Age for Initial Vaccination and Minimum Interval Between Vaccine Doses, by Type of Vaccine

Vaccine	Minimum[1] *Age* for First Dose	Minimum[1] *Interval* From Dose 1 to 2	Minimum[1] *Interval* From Dose 2 to 3	Minimum[1] *Interval* From Dose 3 to 4
DTP (DT)[2]	6 wk[3]	4 wk	4 wk	6 mo
Combined DTP-Hib	6 wk	1 mo	1 mo	6 mo
DTaP[1]	6 wk			6 mo
Hib (primary series)				
HbOC	6 wk	1 mo	1 mo	[4]
PRP-T	6 wk	1 mo	1 mo	[4]
PRP-OMP	6 wk	1 mo	[4]	
OPV			6 wk	
IPV[5]	6 wk	4 wk	6 mo[6]	
MMR	12 mo[7]	1 mo		
Hepatitis B	Birth	1 mo	2 mo[8]	
Varicella-zoster	12 mo	4 wk		

DTP = diphtheria-tetanus-pertussis.

DTaP = diphtheria-tetanus-acellular pertussis.

Hib = *Haemophilus influenzae* type b conjugate.

IPV = inactivated poliovirus vaccine.

MMR = measles-mumps-rubella.

OPV = poliovirus vaccine, live oral, trivalent.

[1]These minimum acceptable ages and intervals may not correspond with the optimal recommended ages and intervals for vaccination. See tables for the current recommended routine and accelerated vaccination schedules.

[2]DTaP can be used in place of the fourth (and fifth) dose of DTP for children who are at least 15 months of age. Children who have received all four primary vaccination doses before their fourth birthday should receive a fifth dose of DTP (DT) or DTaP at 4-6 years of age before entering kindergarten or elementary school **and** at least 6 months after the fourth dose. The total number of doses of diphtheria and tetanus toxoids should not exceed six each before the seventh birthday.

[3]The American Academy of Pediatrics permits DTP to be administered as early as 4 weeks of age in areas with high endemicity and during outbreaks.

[4]The booster dose of Hib vaccine which is recommended following the primary vaccination series should be administered no earlier than 12 months of age **and** at least 2 months after the previous dose of Hib vaccine.

[5]See text to differentiate conventional inactivated poliovirus vaccine from enhanced-potency IPV.

[6]For unvaccinated adults at increased risk of exposure to poliovirus with <3 months but >2 months available before protection is needed, three doses of IPV should be administered at least 1 month apart.

[7]Although the age for measles vaccination may be as young as 6 months in outbreak areas where cases are occurring in children <1 year of age, children initially vaccinated before the first birthday should be revaccinated at 12-15 months of age and an additional dose of vaccine should be administered at the time of school entry or according to local policy. Doses of MMR or other measles-containing vaccines should be separated by at least 1 month.

[8]This final dose is recommended no earlier than 4 months of age.

Modified from *MMWR Morb Mortal Wkly Rep*, 1994, 43(RR-1).

Recommended Immunization Schedule For HIV-Infected Children[1]

Age ▶ Vaccine ▼	Birth	1 mo	2 mos	4 mos	6 mos	12 mos	15 mos	18 mos	24 mos	4-6 yrs	11-12 yrs	14-16 yrs
Recommendations for these vaccines are the same as those for immunocompetent children												
Hepatitis B[2]	Hep B-1											
		Hep B-2			Hep B-3					Hep B[3]	
Diphtheria, Tetanus, Pertussis[4]			DTaP	DTaP	DTaP		DTaP			DTaP	Td	
Haemophilus influenzae type b[5]			Hib	Hib	Hib	Hib						
Recommendations for these vaccines differ from those for immunocompetent children												
Polio[6]			IPV	IPV		IPV				IPV		
Measles, Mumps, Rubella[7]	Do not give to severely immunosuppressed (Category 3) children.					MMR			MMR			
Influenza[8]					Influenza (a dose is required every year)						
Streptococcus pneumoniae[9]									pneumo-coccal		
Varicella[10]	Give only to asymptomatic nonimmunosuppressed (Category 1) children. CONTRAINDICATED in all other HIV-infected children.					Varicella						

Note: Modified from the immunization schedule for immunocompetent children. This schedule also applies to children born to HIV-infected mothers whose HIV infection status has not been determined. Once a child is known not to be HIV-infected, the schedule for immunocompetent children applies. This schedule indicates the recommended age for routine administration of currently licensed childhood vaccines. Some combination vaccines are available and may be used whenever administration of all componeents of the vaccine is indicated. Providers should consult the manufacturers' package inserts for detailed recommendations.

1   Vaccines are listed under the routinely recommended ages. Bars indicate range of acceptable ages for vaccination. Shaded bars indicate catch-up vaccination: at 11-12 years of age, hepatitis B vaccine should be administered to children not previously vaccinated.

2   *Infants born to HBsAg-negative mothers* should receive 2.5 mcg of Merch vaccine (Recombivax HB®) or 10 mcg of Smith Kline Beecham (SB) vaccine (Engerix-B®). The 2nd dose should be administered >1 mo after the 1st dose.

   Infants born to HBsAg-positive mothers should receive 0.5 mL of hepatitis B immune globulin (HBIG) within 12 h of birth and either 5 mcg of Merck vaccine (Recombivax HB®) or 10 mcg of SB vaccine (Engerix-B®) at a separate site. The 2nd dose is recommended at 1-2 months of age and the 3rd dose at 6 months of age.

   Infants born to mothers whose HBsAg status is unknown should receive either 5 mcg of Merck vaccine (Recombivax HB®) or 10 mcg of SB vaccine (Engerix-B®) within 12 h of birth. The 2nd dose of vaccine is recommended at 1 month of age and the 3rd dose at 6 of age. Blood should be drawn at the time of delivery to determine the mother's HBsAg status; if it is positive, the infant should receive HBIG as soon as possible (no later than 1 week of age). The dosage and timing of subsequent vaccine doses should be based upon the mother's HBsAg status.

3   Children and adolescents who have not been vaccinated against hepatitis B in infancy can begin the series during any childhood visit. Those who have not previously received 3 doses of hepatitis B vaccine should initiate or complete the series during the 11 to 12 year old visit. The 2nd dose should be administered at least 1 month after the 1st dose, and the 3rd dose should be administered at least 4 mos after the 1st dose and at 2 mos after 2nd dose.

4   DTaP (diphtheria and tetanus toxoids and acellular pertusssis vaccine) is the preferred vaccine for all doses in the vaccination series, including copletion of the series in children who have received >1 dose of whole-cell DtP vaccine. The 4th dose of DTaP may be administered as early as 12 months of age, provided 6 months have elapsed since the 3rd dose, and if the child is considered unlikely to return at 15-18 months of age. Td (tetanus and diphtheria toxoids, absorbed for adult use) is recommended at 11-12 years of age if at least 5 years have elapsed since the last dose of DTaP or DT. Subsequent routine Td boosters are recommended every 10 years.

5   Three H. influenzae type b (Hib) conjugate vaccines are licensed for infant use. If PRP-OMP (PedvaxHIB® [Merck]) is administered at 2 and 4 months of age, a dose at 6 months is not required. After the primary series has been completed, any Hib conjugate vaccine may be used as a booster.

6   Inactivated poliovirus vaccine (IPV) is the only polio vaccine recommended for HIV-infected persons and their household contacts. Although the third dose fo IPV is generally administered at 12-18 months, the 3rd dose of IPV has been approved to be administered as early as 6 months of age. Oral poliovirus vaccine (OPV) should NOT be administered to HIV-infected persons or their household contacts.

7   MMR should not be administered to severely immunocompromised children. HIV-infected children without severe immunosuppression should routinely receive their first dose of MMR as soon as possible upon reaching the first birthday. Consideration should be given to administering the 2nd dose of MMR vaccine as soon as one month (ie, minimum 28 days) after the 1st dose, rather than waiting until school entry.

8   Influenza virus vaccine should be administered to all HIV-infected children >6 months of age each year. Children aged 6 months to 8 years who are receiving influenza vaccine for the first time should receive two doses of split virus vaccine separated by at least one month. In subsequent years, a single dose of vaccine (split virus for persons ≥12 y of age, whole or split virus for persons >12 y of age) should be administered each year. The dose of vaccine for children aged 6-35 months is 0.25 mL: the dose for children aged ≥3 years is 0.5 mL.

9   The 23-valent pneumococcal vaccine should be administered to HIV-infected children at 24 months of age. Revaccination should generally be offered to HIV-infected children vaccinated 3-5 years (children aged ≤10 years) or >5 years (children aged >10 years) earlier.

10 Varicella zoster virus vaccine, 0.5 mL, is given as a subcutaneous dose between 12 mos and 12 y of age; a second dose should be given 3 mos later. The vaccine should be given only to asymptomatic, nonimmunosuppressed children.

Adapted from the American Academy of Pediatrics and American Academy of Family Practice Physicians, Advisory Committee on Immunization Practices and the Centers for Disease Control.

IMMUNIZATION RECOMMENDATIONS (Continued)

Vaccines Licensed in the United States and Their Routes of Administration

Vaccine[1]	Type	Route
Adenovirus[2]	Live virus	Oral
Anthrax[3]	Inactivated bacteria	S.C.
BCG	Live bacteria	I.D. (preferred) or S.C.
Cholera	Inactivated bacteria	S.C., I.M., or I.D.
Diphtheria-tetanus (dT, DT)	Toxoids	I.M.
DTP	Toxoids and inactivated bacteria	I.M.
DTaP	Toxoids and inactivated bacterial components	I.M.
Hepatitis A	Inactivated viral antigen	I.M.
Hepatitis B	Inactivated viral antigen	I.M.
Hib conjugates	Polysaccharide-protein conjugate	I.M.
Hib conjugate-DTP (HbOC-DTP and PRP-T reconstituted with DTP)	Polysaccharide-protein conjugate with toxoids and inactivated bacteria	I.M.
Hib conjugate-DTaP (PRP-T reconstituted with DTaP)	Polysaccharide-protein conjugate with toxoids and inactivated bacterial components	I.M.
Hib conjugate (PRP-OMP)-hepatitis B	Polysaccharide-protein conjugate with inactivated virus	I.M.
Influenza	Inactivated virus (whole virus), viral components	I.M.
Japanese encephalitis	Inactivated virus	S.C.
Lyme disease	Inactivated protein	I.M.
Measles	Live virus	S.C.
MMR	Live viruses	S.C.
Measles-rubella	Live viruses	S.C.
Meningococcal	Polysaccharide	S.C.
Mumps	Live virus	S.C.
Pertussis[3]	Inactivated bacteria	I.M.
Plague	Inactivated bacteria	I.M.
Pneumococcal	Polysaccharide	I.M. or S.C.
Poliovirus		
IPV	Inactivated virus	S.C.
OPV	Live virus	Oral
Rabies	Inactivated virus	I.M. or I.D.[4]
Rubella	Live virus	S.C.
Tetanus	Toxoid	I.M.
Typhoid		
Parenteral	Inactivated bacteria	S.C.
Parenteral	Capsular polysaccharide	S.C. (boosters may be I.D.)
Oral	Live bacteria	Oral
Varicella	Live virus	S.C.
Yellow fever	Live virus	S.C.

[1]BCG = bacillus Calmette-Guérin; DTP = diphtheria and tetanus toxoids and pertussis, adsorbed; DTaP = diphtheria and tetanus toxoids and acellular pertussis, adsorbed; Hib = *Haemophilus influenzae* type b; MMR = live measles-mumps-rubella viruses; OPV = oral poliovirus; IPV = inactivated poliovirus; dT = diphtheria and tetanus toxoids (for children ≥7 years of age and adults); DT = diphtheria and tetanus toxoids (for children <7 years of age).

[2]Available only to the U.S. Armed Forces. No longer being manufactured; existing supplies continue to be used.

[3]Distributed by Bio Port Corporation, Lansing, MI.

[4]Human diploid cell rabies vaccine for intradermal use is different in constitution and potency from the I.M. vaccine; it should be used for pre-exposure immunization only. Rabies vaccine adsorbed and RabAvert should not be given intradermally.

Adapted from "Report of the Committee on Infectious Diseases," *2000 Red Book*®, 25th ed, 7-8.

Recommendations for Pneumococcal Conjugate Vaccine Use Among Healthy Children During Moderate and Severe Shortages

Age at First Vaccination (mo)	No Shortage[1]	Moderate Shortage	Severe Shortage
<6	2, 4, 6, and 12-15 months	2, 4, and 6 months (defer fourth dose)	2 doses at 2-month interval in first 6 months of life (defer third and fourth doses)
7-11	2 doses at 2-month interval; 12-15 month dose	2 doses at 2-month interval; 12-15-month dose	2 doses at 2-month interval (defer third dose)
12-23	2 doses at 2-month interval	2 doses at 2-month interval	1 dose (defer second dose)
>24	1 dose should be considered	No vaccination	No vaccination
Reduction in vaccine doses used[2]		21%	46%

[1]The vaccine schedule for no shortage is included as a reference. Providers should not use the no shortage schedule regardless of their vaccine supply until the national shortage is resolved.

[2]Assumes that approximately 85% of vaccine is administered to healthy infants beginning at age <7 months; approximately 5% is administered to high-risk infants beginning at age <7 months; and approximately 10% is administered to healthy children beginning at age 7-24 months. Actual vaccine savings will depend on a provider's vaccine use.

Adapted from the Advisory Committee on Immunization Practices, "Updated Recommendations on Use of Pneumococcal Conjugate Vaccine in a Setting of Vaccine Shortage," *MMWR Morb Mortal Wkly Rep*, 2001, 50(50):1140-2.

Immune Globulins and Antitoxins[1] Available in the United States, by Type of Antibodies and Indications for Use

Immunobiologic	Type	Indication(s)
C. botulinum antitoxin	Specific equine antibodies	Treatment of botulism
Cytomegalovirus immune globulin, intravenous (CMV-IGIV)	Specific human antibodies	Prophylaxis for bone marrow and kidney transplant recipients
Diphtheria antitoxin	Specific equine antibodies	Treatment of respiratory diphtheria
Immune globulin (IG)	Pooled human antibodies	Hepatitis A pre- and postexposure prophylaxis; measles postexposure prophylaxis
Immune globulin, intravenous (IGIV)	Pooled human antibodies	Replacement therapy for antibody deficiency disorders; immune thrombocytopenic purpura (ITP); hypogammaglobulinemia in chronic lymphocytic leukemia; Kawasaki disease
Hepatitis B immune globulin (HBIG)	Specific human antibodies	Hepatitis B postexposure prophylaxis
Rabies immune globulin (HRIG)[2]	Specific human antibodies	Rabies postexposure management of persons not previously immunized with rabies vaccine
Tetanus immune globulin (TIG)	Specific human antibodies	Tetanus treatment; postexposure prophylaxis of persons not adequately immunized with tetanus toxoid
Vaccinia immune globulin (VIG)	Specific human antibodies	Treatment of eczema vaccinatum, vaccinia necrosum, and ocular vaccinia
Varicella-zoster immune globulin (VZIG)	Specific human antibodies	Postexposure prophylaxis of susceptible immunocompromised persons, certain susceptible pregnant women, and perinatally exposed newborn infants

[1]Immune globulin preparations and antitoxins are administered intramuscularly unless otherwise indicated.

[2]HRIG is administered around the wounds in addition to the intramuscular injection.

Modified from *MMWR Morb Mortal Wkly Rep*, 1994, 43(RR-1).

IMMUNIZATION RECOMMENDATIONS *(Continued)*

Suggested Intervals Between Immunoglobulin Administration and Measles Immunization (MMR or Monovalent Measles Vaccine)[1]

Indication for Immunoglobulin	Dose	(mg IgG/kg)	Interval (mo)[2]
Tetanus (TIG)	I.M.: 250 units	~10	3
Hepatitis A prophylaxis (IG)			
Contact prophylaxis	I.M.: 0.02 mL/kg	3.3	3
International travel	I.M.: 0.06 mL/kg	10	3
Hepatitis B prophylaxis (HBIG)	I.M.: 0.06 mL/kg	10	3
Rabies prophylaxis (RIG)	I.M.: 20 IU/kg	22	4
Measles prophylaxis (IG)			
Standard	I.M.: 0.25 mL/kg	40	5
Immunocompromised host	I.M.: 0.50 mL/kg	80	6
Varicella prophylaxis (VZIG)	I.M.: 125 units/10 kg (max: 625 units)	20-39	5
Blood transfusion			
Washed RBCs	I.V.: 10 mL/kg	Negligible	0
RBCs, adenine-saline added	I.V.: 10 mL/kg	10	3
Packed RBCs	I.V.: 10 mL/kg	20-60	5
Whole blood cells	I.V.: 10 mL/kg	80-100	6
Plasma or platelet products	I.V.: 10 mL/kg	160	7
Replacement (or therapy) of immune deficiencies	I.V.:	300-400	8
ITP (IGIV)	I.V.	400	8
IRSV-IGIV	I.V.	750	9
ITP	I.V.	1000	10
ITP or Kawasaki disease	I.V.	1600-2000	11

[1]MMR = measles-mumps-rubella; IgG = immunoglobulin G; IG = immune globulin; TIG = tetanus IG; HBIG = hepatitis B IG; RIG = rabies IG; VZIG = varicella-zoster IG; RBC = red blood cell; IGIV = IG intravenous; ITP = immune (formerly termed "idiopathic") thrombocytopenic purpura; RSV-IGIV = respiratory syncytial virus IGIV.

[2]These intervals should provide sufficient time for decreases in passive antibodies in all children to allow for an adequate response to measles vaccine. Physicians should not assume that children are fully protected against measles during these intervals. Additional doses of IG or measles vaccine may be indicated after exposure to measles.

Adapted from "Report of the Committee on Infectious Diseases," *2000 Red Book*®, 25th ed, 390.

HAEMOPHILUS INFLUENZAE VACCINATION

Currently Recommended Regimens for Routine *Haemophilus influenzae* Type b Conjugate Immunization for Children Immunized Beginning at 2-6 Months of Age[1]

Vaccine Product at Initiation	Total No. of Doses to Be Administered	Recommended Regimens
HbOC or PRP-T	4	3 doses at 2-month intervals initially; fourth dose at 12-15 months of age; any conjugate vaccine for dose 4[2]
PRP-OMP	3	2 doses at 2-month intervals initially; when feasible, same vaccine for doses 1 and 2; third dose at 12-15 months of age; any conjugate vaccine for dose 3[2]

[1]These vaccines may be given in combination products or as reconstituted products with DTaP or DTP, provided the combination or reconstituted vaccine is approved by the U.S. Food and Drug Administration for the child's age and the administration of the other vaccine component(s) also is justified.

[2]The safety and efficacy of PRP-OMP, PRP-T, HbOC, and PRP-D are likely to be equivalent for children ≥12 months of age. If a different product is given for dose 2, then the recommendations for that product (eg, HbOC or PRP-T) apply.

Adapted from "Report of the Committee on Infectious Diseases," *2000 Red Book*®, 25th ed, 268.

Recommendations for *Haemophilus influenzae* Type b Conjugate Immunization for Children in Whom Initial Immunization Is Delayed Until 7 Months of Age or Older[1]

Age at Initiation of Immunization (mo)	Vaccine Product at Initiation	Total No. of Doses to Be Administered	Recommended Vaccine Regimens
7-11	HbOC, PRP-T, or PRP-OMP	3	2 doses at 2-month intervals; third dose at 12-15 months, given at 2 months after dose 2; any conjugate vaccine for dose 3[2]
12-14	HbOC, PRP-T, PRP-OMP, or PRP-D	2	2-month interval between doses
15-59	HbOC, PRP-T, PRP-OMP, or PRP-D	1[3]	Any conjugate vaccine
60 and older[4]	HbOC, PRP-T, PRP-OMP, or PRP-D	1 or 2[3]	Any conjugate vaccine

[1]These vaccines may be given in combination products or as reconstituted products with DTaP or DTP, provided the combination or reconstituted vaccine is approved by the U.S. Food and Drug Administration for the child's age and administration of the other vaccine component(s) also is justified.

[2]The safety and efficacy of PRP-OMP, PRP-T, HbOC, or PRP-D are likely to be equivalent for use as a booster dose for children 12 months or older.

[3]Two doses separated by 2 months are recommended by some experts for children with certain underlying diseases associated with increased risk of disease and impaired antibody responses to *H. influenzae* type conjugate vaccination.

[4]Only for children with chronic illness known to be associated with an increased risk for *H. influenzae* type b disease.

Adapted from "Report of the Committee on Infectious Diseases," *2000 Red Book®*, 25th ed, 269.

Recommendations for *Haemophilus influenzae* Type b Conjugate Immunization in Children With a Lapse in Vaccination[1]

Age at Presentation (mo)	Previous Immunization History	Recommended Regimen
7-11	1 dose of HbOC or PRP-T	1 or 2 doses of conjugate vaccine at 7-11 months of age (depending on age), with a booster dose given at least 2 months later, at 12-15 months of age
	2 doses of HbOC or PRP-T or 1 dose of PRP-OMP	1 dose of conjugate vaccine at 7-11 months of age with a booster dose given at least 2 months later at 12-15 month of age
12-14	2 doses before 12 months[2]	A single dose of any licensed conjugate vaccine[3]
	1 dose before 12 months[2]	2 additional doses of any licensed conjugate vaccine, separated by 2 months[3]
15-59	Any incomplete schedule	A single dose of any licensed conjugate[3]

[1]These vaccines may be given in combination products or as reconstituted products with DTaP or DTP, provided the combination or reconstituted vaccine is approved by the U.S. Food and Drug Administration for the child's age and the administration of the other vaccine component(s) also is justified.

[2]PRP-OMP, PRP-T, or HbOC.

[3]The safety and efficacy of PRP-OMP, PRP-T, HbOC, or PRP-D are likely to be equivalent for children ≥12 months of age.

Adapted from "Report of the Committee on Infectious Diseases," *2000 Red Book®*, 25th ed, 271.

IMMUNIZATION RECOMMENDATIONS *(Continued)*

LYME DISEASE VACCINE GUIDELINES

**Recommendations for Use of Recombinant Outer-Surface Protein A Vaccine for the Prevention of Lyme Disease
(Advisory Committee on Immunization Practices, 1999)**

	Vaccination Recommendation
Persons who reside, work, or recreate in areas of high or moderate risk	
Persons 15-70 years of age whose exposure to tick-infested habitat is frequent or prolonged	Should be considered
Persons 15-70 years of age who are exposed to tick-infested habitat, but whose exposure is not frequent or prolonged	May be considered
Persons whose exposure to tick-infested habitat is minimal or none	Not recommended
Persons who reside, work, or recreate in areas of low or no risk	Not recommended
Travelers to areas of high or moderate risk	
Travelers 15-70 years of age whose exposure to tick-infested habitat is frequent or prolonged	Should be considered
Children <15 years of age	Not recommended
Pregnant women	
Healthcare providers are encouraged to register vaccinations of pregnant women by calling SmithKline Beecham, toll free, at (800) 366-8900, ext 5231	Not recommended
Persons with immunodeficiency	No available data
Persons with musculoskeletal disease	Limited data available
Persons with previous history of Lyme disease	
Persons 15-70 years of age with previous uncomplicated Lyme disease who are at continued high risk	Should be considered
Persons with treatment-resistant Lyme arthritis	Not recommended
Persons with chronic joint or neurologic illness related to Lyme disease and persons with second or third degree atrioventricular block	No available data
Other Recommendations	
Vaccine schedule	
Three doses administered by intramuscular infection as follows:	
Initial dose, followed by a second dose 1 month later, followed by a third dose 12 months after the first dose	
Second dose (year 1) and third dose (year 2) administered several weeks before the beginning of the disease-transmission season, which is usually April	
Boosters	
Existing data indicate that boosters might be needed, but additional data are required before recommendations can be made regarding booster schedules	
Simultaneous administration with other vaccines	
Additional data needed	
If simultaneous administration is necessary, use separate syringes and separate injection sites	

From "Recommendations for the Use of Lyme Disease Vaccine. Recommendations of the Advisory Committee on Immunization Practices (ACIP)," *MMWR Morb Mortal Wkly Rep*, 1999, 48(RR-7):25.

POSTEXPOSURE PROPHYLAXIS FOR HEPATITIS B[1]

Exposure	Hepatitis B Immune Globulin	Hepatitis B Vaccine
Perinatal	0.5 mL I.M. within 12 h of birth	0.5 mL[2] I.M. within 12 h of birth (no later than 7 d), and at 1 and 6 mo[3]; test for HB_sAg and anti-HB_s at 12-15 mo
Sexual	0.06 mL/kg I.M. within 14 d of sexual contact; a second dose should be given if the index patient remains HB_sAg-positive after 3 mo and hepatitis B vaccine was not given initially	1 mL I.M. at 0, 1, and 6 mo for homosexual and bisexual men and regular sexual contacts of persons with acute and chronic hepatitis B
Percutaneous; exposed person unvaccinated		
Source known HB_sAg-positive	0.06 mL/kg I.M. within 24 h	1 mL I.M. within 7 d, and at 1 and 6 mo[4]
Source known, HB_sAg status not known	Test source for HB_sAg; if source is positive, give exposed person 0.06 mL/kg I.M. once within 7 d	1 mL I.M. within 7 d, and at 1 and 6 mo[4]
Source not tested or unknown	Nothing required	1 mL I.M. within 7 d, and at 1 and 6 mo
Percutaneous; exposed person vaccinated		
Source known HB_sAg-positive	Test exposed person for anti-HB_s.[5] If titer is protective, nothing is required; if titer is not protective, give 0.06 mL/kg within 24 h.	Review vaccination status[6]
Source known, HB_sAg status not known	Test source for HB_sAg and exposed person for anti-HB_s. If source is HB_sAg-negative, or if source is HB_sAg-positive but anti-HB_s titer is protective, nothing is required. If source is HB_sAg-positive and anti-HB_s titer is not protective or if exposed person is a known nonresponder, give 0.06 mL/kg I.M. within 24 h. A second dose of hepatitis B immune globulin can be given 1 mo later if a booster dose of hepatitis B vaccine is not given.	Review vaccination status[6]
Source not tested or unknown	Test exposed person for anti-HB_s. If anti-HB_s titer is protective, nothing is required. If anti-HB_s titer is not protective, 0.06 mL/kg may be given along with a booster dose of hepatitis B vaccine.	Review vaccination status[6]

[1]HB_sAg = hepatitis B surface antigen; anti-HB_s = antibody to hepatitis B surface antigen; I.M. = intramuscularly; SRU = standard ratio units.
[2]Each 0.5 mL dose of plasma-derived hepatitis B vaccine contains 10 mcg of HB_sAg; each 0.5 mL dose of recombinant hepatitis B vaccine contains 5 mcg (Merck Sharp & Dohme) or 10 mcg (SmithKline Beecham) of HB_sAg.
[3]If hepatitis B immune globulin and hepatitis B vaccine are given simultaneously, they should be given at separate sites.
[4]If hepatitis B vaccine is not given, a second dose of hepatitis B immune globulin should be given 1 month later.
[5]Anti-HB_s titers <10 SRU by radioimmunoassay or negative by enzyme immunoassay indicate lack of protection. Testing the exposed person for anti-HB_s is not necessary if a protective level of antibody has been shown within the previous 24 months.
[6]If the exposed person has not completed a three-dose series of hepatitis B vaccine, the series should be completed. Test the exposed person for anti-HB_s. If the antibody level is protective, nothing is required. If an adequate antibody response in the past is shown on retesting to have declined to an inadequate level, a booster dose (1 mL) of hepatitis B vaccine should be given. If the exposed person has inadequate antibody or is a known nonresponder to vaccination, a booster dose can be given along with one dose of hepatitis B immune globulin.

IMMUNIZATION RECOMMENDATIONS *(Continued)*

PREVENTION OF HEPATITIS A THROUGH ACTIVE OR PASSIVE IMMUNIZATION

Recommendations of the Advisory Committee on Immunization Practices (ACIP)

PROPHYLAXIS AGAINST HEPATITIS A VIRUS INFECTION

Recommended Doses of Immune Globulin (IG) for Hepatitis A Pre-exposure and Postexposure Prophylaxis

Setting	Duration of Coverage	IG Dose[1]
Pre-exposure	Short-term (1-2 months)	0.02 mL/kg
	Long-term (3-5 months)	0.06 mL/kg[2]
Postexposure	—	0.02 mL/kg

[1]IG should be administered by intramuscular injection into either the deltoid or gluteal muscle. For children <24 months of age, IG can be administered in the anterolateral thigh muscle.

[2]Repeat every 5 months if continued exposure to HAV occurs.

Recommended Dosages of Havrix®[1]

Vaccinee's Age (y)	Dose (EL.U.)[2]	Volume (mL)	No. Doses	Schedule (mo)[3]
2-18	720	0.5	2	0, 6-12
>18	1440	1.0	2	0, 6-12

[1]Hepatitis A vaccine, inactivated, SmithKline Beecham Biologicals.

[2]ELISA units.

[3]0 months represents timing of the initial dose; subsequent numbers represent months after the initial dose.

Recommended Dosages of VAQTA®[1]

Vaccinee's Age (y)	Dose (units)	Volume (mL)	No. Doses	Schedule (mo)[2]
2-17	25	0.5	2	0, 6-18
>17	50	1.0	2	0, 6

[1]Hepatitis A vaccine, inactivated, Merck & Company, Inc.

[2]0 months represents timing of the initial dose; subsequent numbers represent months after the initial dose.

From *MMWR Morb Mortal Wkly Rep*, 1996, 45(RR-15).

RECOMMENDATIONS FOR TRAVELERS

Recommended Immunizations for Travelers to Developing Countries[1]

Immunizations	Length of Travel		
	Brief, <2 wk	Intermediate, 2 wk - 3 mo	Long-term Residential, >3 mo
Review and complete age-appropriate childhood schedule	+	+	+
• DTaP; poliovirus vaccine, and *H. influenzae* type b vaccine may be given at 4 wk intervals if necessary to complete the recommended schedule before departure			
• Measles: 2 additional doses given if younger than 12 mo of age at first dose			
• Varicella			
• Hepatitis B[2]			
Yellow fever[3]	+	+	+
Hepatitis A[4]	+	+	+
Typhoid fever[4]	±	+	+
Meningococcal disease[5]	±	±	±
Rabies[6]	±	+	+
Japanese encephalitis[3]	±	±	+

[1] + = recommended; ± = consider.
[2] If insufficient time to complete 6-month primary series, accelerated series can be given.
[3] For endemic regions, see *Health Information for International Travel* in *Red Book®*. For high-risk activities in areas experiencing outbreaks, vaccine is recommended even for brief travel.
[4] Indicated for travelers who will consume food and liquids in areas of poor sanitation.
[5] For endemic regions of Africa, during local epidemics, and travel to Saudi Arabia for the Hajj.
[6] Indicated for person with high risk of animal exposure, and for travelers to endemic countries.
Adapted from "Report of the Committee on Infectious Diseases," *2000 Red Book®*, 25th ed, 78.

Recommendations for Pre-exposure Immunoprophylaxis of Hepatitis A Virus Infection for Travelers[1]

Age (y)	Likely Exposure (mo)	Recommended Prophylaxis
<2	<3	IG 0.02 mL/kg[2]
	3-5	IG 0.06 mL/kg[2]
	Long-term	IG 0.06 mL/kg at departure and every 5 mo if exposure to HAV continues[2]
≥2	<3[3]	HAV vaccine[4,5] **or**
	3-5[3]	HAV vaccine[4,5] **or** IG 0.06 mL/kg[2]
	Long-term	HAV vaccine[4,5]

[1] IG = immune globulin; HAV= hepatitis A virus.
[2] IG should be administered deep into a large muscle mass. Ordinarily, no more than 5 mL should be administered in one site in an adult or large child; lesser amounts (maximum 3 mL) should be given to small children and infants.
[3] Vaccine is preferable, but IG is an acceptable alternative.
[4] To ensure protection in travelers whose departure is imminent, IG also may be given.
[5] Dose and schedule of hepatitis A vaccine as recommended according to age.
Adapted from "Report of the Committee on Infectious Diseases," *2000 Red Book®*, 25th ed, 282.

IMMUNIZATION RECOMMENDATIONS *(Continued)*

Prevention of Malaria[1]

Drug	Adult Dosage	Pediatric Dosage
Chloroquine-Sensitive Areas		
Chloroquine phosphate[2,3]	500 mg (300 mg base), once/week[4]	5 mg/kg base once/week, up to adult dose of 300 mg base[4]
Chloroquine-Resistant Areas		
Mefloquine[3,5]	250 mg once/week[4]	<15 kg: 5 mg/kg[4] 15-19 kg: 1/4 tablet[4] 20-30 kg: 1/2 tablet[4] 31-45 kg: 3/4 tablet[4] >45 kg: 1 tablet[4]
Doxycycline[3]	100 mg/d[6]	2 mg/kg/d, up to 100 mg/d[6]
Atovaquone/Proguanil	250 mg/100 mg (1 tablet) daily[7]	11-20 kg: 62.5 mg/25 mg[7] 21-30 kg: 125 mg/50 mg[7] 31-40 kg: 187.5 mg/75 mg[7]
Alternative:		
Primaquine[8]	30 mg base daily	0.5 mg/kg base daily
Chloroquine phosphate[3] **plus**	Same as above	Same as above
pyrimethamine-sulfadoxine for presumptive treatment[9]	Carry a single dose (3 tablets) for self-treatment of febrile illness when medical care is not immediately available	<1 y: 1/4 tablet 1-3 y: 1/2 tablet 4-8 y: 1 tablet 9-14 y: 2 tablets
or plus		
proguanil[10]	200 mg daily	<2 y: 50 mg daily 2-6 y: 100 mg 7-10 y: 150 mg >10 y: 200 mg

[1]No drug regimen guarantees protection against malaria. If fever develops within a year (particularly within the first 2 months) after travel to malarious areas, travelers should be advised to seek medical attention. Insect repellents, insecticide-impregnated bed nets, and proper clothing are important adjuncts for malaria prophylaxis.

[2]In pregnancy, chloroquine prophylaxis has been used extensively and safely.

[3]For prevention of attack after departure from areas where *P. vivax* and *P. ovale* are endemic, which includes almost all areas where malaria is found (except Haiti), some experts prescribe in addition primaquine phosphate 15 mg base (26.3 mg)/d or, for children, 0.3 mg base/kg/d during the last 2 weeks of prophylaxis. Others prefer to avoid the toxicity of primaquine and rely on surveillance to detect cases when they occur; particularly when exposure was limited or doubtful.

[4]Beginning 1-2 weeks before travel and continuing weekly for the duration of stay and for 4 weeks after leaving.

[5]The pediatric dosage has not been approved by the FDA, and the drug has not been approved for use during pregnancy; however, it has been reported to be safe for prophylactic use during the second or third trimester of pregnancy and possibly during early pregnancy as well (CDC Health Information for International Travel, 1999-2000, page 120; Smoak BL, et al, *J Infect Dis*, 1997, 176:831). Mefloquine is not recommended for patients with cardiac conduction abnormalities. Patients with a history of seizures or psychiatric disorders should avoid mefloquine (*Medical Letter*, 1990, 32:13). Resistance to mefloquine has been reported in some areas, such as Thailand; in these areas, doxycycline should be used for prophylaxis. In children <8 years of age, proguanil plus sulfisoxazole has been used (Suh KN and Keystone JS, *Infect Dis Clin Pract*, 1996, 5:541).

[6]Beginning 1-2 days before travel and continuing for the duration of stay and for 4 weeks after leaving. Use of tetracyclines is contraindicated in pregnancy and in children <8 years old. Doxycycline can cause gastrointestinal disturbances, vaginal moniliasis, and photosensitivity reactions.

[7]Shanks GE et al, *Clin Infect Dis*, 1998, 27:494; Lell B et al, *Lancet*, 1998, 351:709. Beginning 1-2 days before travel and continuing for the duration of stay and for 1 week after leaving.

[8]Several studies have shown that daily primaquine, beginning 1 day before departure and continued until 2 days after leaving the malaria area, provides effective prophylaxis against chloroquine-resistant *P. falciparum* (Schwartz E and Regev-Yochay G, *Clin Infect Dis*, 1999, 29:1502). Some studies have shown less efficacy against *P. vivax*.

[9]In areas with strains resistant to pyrimethamine-sulfadoxine, atovaquone/proguanil or atovaquone plus doxycycline can also be used for presumptive treatment.

[10]Proguanil (Paludrine – Wyeth Ayerst, Canada; Zeneca, United Kingdom), which is not available alone in the U.S.A. but is widely available in Canada and overseas, is recommended mainly for use in Africa south of the Sahara. Prophylaxis is recommended during exposure and for 4 weeks afterwards. Proguanil has been used in pregnancy without evidence of toxicity (Phillips-Howard PA and Wood D, *Drug Saf*, 1996, 14:131).

Adapted from "Report of the Committee on Infectious Diseases," *2000 Red Book®*, 25th ed, 709-10.

ADVERSE EVENTS AND VACCINATION

Reportable Events Following Vaccination[1]

These events are reportable by law to the Vaccine Adverse Event Reporting System (VAERS) (1-800-822-7967). In addition, individuals are encouraged to report any clinically significant or unexpected events (even if uncertain whether the vaccine caused the event) for any vaccine, whether or not it is listed in the table. Manufacturers also are required to report to the VAERS program all adverse events made known to them for any vaccine.

Vaccine		Adverse Event	Interval From Vaccination to Onset of Event for Reporting[2]
Tetanus toxoid-containing vaccines (eg, DTaP, DTP, DTP-Hib; DT; dT or TT)	A.	Anaphylaxis or anaphylactic shock	0-7 d
	B.	Brachial neuritis	0-28 d
	C.	Any acute complication or sequela (including death) of above events	No limit
	D.	Events described in manufacturer's package insert as contraindications to additional doses of vaccine	No limit
Pertussis antigen-containing vaccines (eg, DTaP, DTP, P, DTP-Hib)	A.	Anaphylaxis or anaphylactic shock	0-7 d
	B.	Encephalopathy (or encephalitis)	0-7 d
	C.	Any acute complication or sequela (including death) of above events	No limit
	D.	Events described in manufacturer's package insert as contraindications to additional doses of vaccine	No limit
Measles, mumps, and rubella virus-containing vaccines in any combination (eg, MMR, MR, M, R)	A.	Anaphylaxis or anaphylactic shock	0-7 d
	B.	Encephalopathy (or encephalitis)	0-15 d
	C.	Any acute complication or sequela (including death) of above events	No limit
	D.	Events described in manufacturer's package insert as contraindications to additional doses of vaccine	No limit
Rubella virus-containing vaccines (eg, MMR, MR, R)	A.	Chronic arthritis	0-42 d
	B.	Any acute complication or sequela (including death) of above events	No limit
	C.	Events described in manufacturer's package insert as contraindications to additional doses of vaccine	No limit
Measles virus-containing vaccines (eg, MMR, MR, M)	A.	Thrombocytopenic purpura	0-30 d
	B.	Vaccine-strain measles viral infection in an immunodeficient recipient	0-6 mo
	C.	Any acute complication or sequela (including death) of above events	No limit
	D.	Events described in manufacturer's package insert as contraindications to additional doses of vaccine	No limit
Live poliovirus-containing vaccines (OPV)	A.	Paralytic polio	
		• in a nonimmunodeficient recipient	0-30 d
		• in an immunodeficient recipient	0-6 mo
		• in a vaccine-associated community case	No limit
	B.	Vaccine-strain polio viral infection	
		• in a nonimmunodeficient recipient	0-30 d
		• in an immunodeficient recipient	0-6 mo
		• in a vaccine-associated community case	No limit
	C.	Any acute complication or sequela (including death) of above events	No limit
	D.	Events described in manufacturer's package insert as contraindications to additional doses of vaccine	No limit
Polio inactivated	A.	Anaphylaxis or anaphylactic shock	0-7 d
	B.	Any acute complication or sequela (including death) of above events	No limit
	C.	Events described in manufacturer's package insert as contraindications to additional doses of vaccine	No limit
Hepatitis B	A.	Anaphylaxis or anaphylactic shock	0-7 d
	B.	Any acute complication or sequela (including death) of above events	No limit
	C.	Events described in manufacturer's package insert as contraindications to additional doses of vaccine	No limit
Haemophilus influenzae type b polysaccharide vaccines (unconjugated, PRP vaccines)	A.	Early onset Hib disease	0-7 d
	B.	Any acute complication or sequela (including death) of above events	No limit
	C.	Events described in manufacturer's package insert as contraindications to additional doses of vaccine	No limit
Haemophilus influenzae type b polysaccharide conjugate vaccines	A.	No condition specified for compensation	Not applicable
	B.	Events described in manufacturer's package insert as contraindications to additional doses of vaccine	No limit
Varicella virus-containing vaccine	A.	No condition specified for compensation	Not applicable
	B.	Events described in manufacturer's package insert as contraindications to additional doses of vaccine	No limit

IMMUNIZATION RECOMMENDATIONS *(Continued)*

Vaccine		Adverse Event	Interval From Vaccination to Onset of Event for Reporting[2]
Any new vaccine recommended by the CDC for routine administration to children, after publication by Secretary, HHS of a notice of coverage	A.	No condition specified for compensation	
	B.	Events described in manufacturer's package insert as contraindications to additional doses of vaccine	

[1]Effective October 22, 1998.

[2]Taken from the Reportable Events Table (RET), which lists conditions reportable by law (42 USC §300aa-25) to the Vaccine Adverse Event Reporting System (VAERS), including conditions found in the manufacturer's package insert. In addition, physicians are encouraged to report **ANY** clinically significant or unexpected events (even if you are not certain the vaccine caused the event) for **ANY** vaccine, whether or not it is listed on the RET. Manufacturers also are required by regulation (21 CFR§600.80) to report to the VAERS program all adverse events made known to them for any vaccine. VAERS reporting forms and information can be obtained by calling 1-800-822-7967 or from the Web site (http://www.fda.gov/cber/vaers/report.htm).

Adapted from "Report of the Committee on Infectious Diseases," *2000 Red Book®*, 25th ed, 760-2.

MANAGEMENT OF HEALTHCARE WORKER EXPOSURES TO HIV, HBV, HCV

Adapted from "U.S. Public Health Service Guidelines for the Management of Occupational Exposures to HBV, HCV, and HIV and Recommendations for Postexposure Prophylaxis," *MMWR Morb Mortal Wkly Rep*, 2001, 50(RR-11).

Factors to Consider in Assessing the Need for Follow-up of Occupational Exposures

- **Type of exposure**
    - Percutaneous injury
    - Mucous membrane exposure
    - Nonintact skin exposure
    - Bites resulting in blood exposure to either person involved
- **Type and amount of fluid/tissue**
    - Blood
    - Fluids containing blood
    - Potentially infectious fluid or tissue (semen; vaginal secretions; and cerebrospinal, synovial, pleural, peritoneal, pericardial, and amniotic fluids)
    - Direct contact with concentrated virus
- **Infectious status of source**
    - Presence of HB$_s$Ag
    - Presence of HCV antibody
    - Presence of HIV antibody
- **Susceptibility of exposed person**
    - Hepatitis B vaccine and vaccine response status
    - HBV, HCV, HIV immune status

Evaluation of Occupational Exposure Sources

Known sources

- Test known sources for HB$_s$Ag, anti-HCV, and HIV antibody
    - Direct virus assays for routine screening of source patients are **not** recommended
    - Consider using a rapid HIV-antibody test
    - If the source person is **not** infected with a bloodborne pathogen, baseline testing or further follow-up of the exposed person is **not** necessary
- For sources whose infection status remains unknown (eg, the source person refuses testing), consider medical diagnoses, clinical symptoms, and history of risk behaviors
- Do not test discarded needles for bloodborne pathogens

Unknown sources

- For unknown sources, evaluate the likelihood of exposure to a source at high risk for infection
    - Consider the likelihood of bloodborne pathogen infection among patients in the exposure setting

MANAGEMENT OF HEALTHCARE WORKER EXPOSURES TO HIV, HBV, HCV *(Continued)*

Recommended Postexposure Prophylaxis for Exposure to Hepatitis B Virus

Vaccination and Antibody Response Status of Exposed Workers[1]	Treatment		
	Source HB_sAg[2]-Positive	Source HB_sAg[2]-Negative	Source Unknown or Not Available for Testing
Unvaccinated	HBIG[3] x 1 and initiate HB vaccine series[4]	Initiate HB vaccine series	Initiate HB vaccine series
Previously vaticinated			
Known responder[5]	No treatment	No treatment	No treatment
Known nonresponder[6]	HBIG x 1 and initiate revaccination or HBIG x 2[7]	No treatment	If known high risk source, treat as if source was HB_sAg-positive
Antibody response unknown	Test exposed person for anti-HB_s[8] 1. If adequate,[5] no treatment is necessary 2. If inadequate,[6] administer HBIG x 1 and vaccine booster	No treatment	Test exposed person for anti-HB_s 1. If adequate,[4] no treatment is necessary 2. If inadequate,[4] administer vaccine booster and recheck titer in 1-2 months

[1]Persons who have previously been infected with HBV are immune to reinfection and do not require postexposure prophylaxis.

[2]Hepatitis B surface antigen.

[3]Hepatitis B immune globulin; dose is 0.06 mL/kg intramuscularly.

[4]Hepatitis B vaccine.

[5]A responder is a person with adequate levels of serum antibody to HB_sAg (ie, anti-HB_s ≥10 mIU/mL).

[6]A nonresponder is a person with inadequate response to vaccination (ie, serum anti-HB_s <10 mIU/mL).

[7]The option of giving one dose of HBIG and reinitiating the vaccine series is preferred for nonresponders who have not completed a second 3-dose vaccine series. For persons who previously completed a second vaccine series but failed to respond, two doses of HBIG are preferred.

[8]Antibody to HB_sAg.

Recommended HIV Postexposure Prophylaxis for Percutaneous Injuries

Exposure Type	Infection Status of Source			
	HIV-Positive Class 1[1]	HIV-Positive Class 2[1]	Unknown HIV Status[2]	Unknown Source[3]	HIV-Negative
Less severe[4]	Recommend basic 2-drug PEP	Recommend expanded 3-drug PEP	Generally, no PEP warranted; however, consider basic 2-drug PEP[5] for source with HIV risk factors[6]	Generally, no PEP warranted; however, consider basic 2 drug PEP[5] in settings where exposure to HIV-infected persons is likely	No PEP warranted
More severe[7]	Recommend expanded 3-drug PEP	Recommend expanded 3-drug PEP	Generally, no PEP warranted; however consider basic 2-drug PEP[5] for source with HIV risk factors[6]	Generally, no PEP warranted; however, consider basic 2 drug PEP[5] in settings where exposure to HIV-infected persons is likely	No PEP warranted

[1]HIV-Positive, Class 1 – asymptomatic HIV infection or known low viral load (eg, <1500 RNA copies/mL). HIV-Positive Class 2 – symptomatic HIV infection, AIDS, acute seroconversion, or known high viral load. If drug resistance is a concern, obtain expert consultation. Initiation of postexposure prophylaxis (PEP) should not be delayed pending expert consultation, and, because expert consultation alone cannot substitute for face-to-face counseling, resources should be available to provide immediate evaluation and follow-up care for all exposures.

[2]Source of unknown HIV status (eg, deceased source person with no samples available for HIV testing).

[3]Unknown source (eg, a needle from a sharps disposal container).

[4]Less severe (eg, solid needle and superficial injury).

[5]The designation "consider PEP" indicates the PEP is optional and should be based on an individualized decision between the exposed person and the treating clinician.

[6]If PEP is offered and taken and the source is later determined to be HIV-negative, PEP should be discontinued.

[7]More severe (eg, large-bore hollow needle, deep puncture, visible blood on device, or needle used in patient's artery or vein).

MANAGEMENT OF HEALTHCARE WORKER EXPOSURES TO HIV, HBV, HCV (Continued)

Recommended HIV Postexposure Prophylaxis for Mucous Membrane Exposures and Nonintact Skin[1] Exposures

Exposure Type	HIV-Positive Class 1[2]	HIV-Positive Class 2[2]	Infection Status of Source Unknown HIV Status[3]	Unknown Source[4]	HIV-Negative
Small volume[5]	Consider basic 2-drug PEP[6]	Recommend basic 2-drug PEP	Generally, no PEP warranted; however, consider basic 2-drug PEP[6] for source with HIV risk factors[7]	Generally, no PEP warranted; however, consider basic 2-drug PEP[6] in settings where exposure to HIV-infected persons is likely	No PEP warranted
Large volume[8]	Recommend basic 2-drug PE	Recommend expanded 3-drug PEP	Generally, no PEP warranted; however consider basic 2-drug PEP[6] for source with HIV risk factors[7]	Generally, no PEP warranted; however, consider basic 2-drug PEP[6] in settings where exposure to HIV-infected persons is likely	No PEP warranted

[1]For skin exposures, follow-up is indicated only if there is evidence of compromised skin integrity (eg, dermatitis, abrasion, or open wound).

[2]HIV-Positive, Class 1 – asymptomatic HIV infection or known low viral load (eg, <1500 RNA copies/mL). HIV-Positive Class 2 – symptomatic HIV infection, AIDS, acute seroconversion, or known high viral load. If drug resistance is a concern, obtain expert consultation. Initiation of postexposure prophylaxis (PEP) should not be delayed pending expert consultation, and, because expert consultation alone cannot substitute for face-to-face counseling, resources should be available to provide immediate evaluation and follow-up care for all exposures.

[3]Source of unknown HIV status (eg, deceased source person with no samples available for HIV testing).

[4]Unknown source (eg, splash from inappropriately disposed blood).

[5]Small volume (eg, a few drops).

[6]The designation "consider PEP" indicates the PEP is optional and should be based on an individualized decision between the exposed person and the treating clinician.

[7]If PEP is offered and taken and the source is later determined to be HIV-negative, PEP should be discontinued.

[8]Large volume (eg, major blood splash).

Situations for Which Expert[1] Consultation for HIV Postexposure Prophylaxis Is Advised

- **Delayed (ie, later than 24-36 hours) exposure report**
  - The interval after which there is no benefit from postexposure prophylaxis (PEP) is undefined

- **Unknown source (eg, needle in sharps disposal container or laundry)**
  - Decide use of PEP on a case-by-case basis
  - Consider the severity of the exposure and the epidemiologic likelihood of HIV exposure
  - Do not test needles or sharp instruments for HIV

- **Known or suspected pregnancy in the exposed person**
  - Does not preclude the use of optimal PEP regimens
  - Do not deny PEP solely on the basis of pregnancy

- **Resistance of the source virus to antiretroviral agents**
  - Influence of drug resistance on transmission risk is unknown
  - Selection of drugs to which the source person's virus is unlikely to be resistant is recommended, if the source person's virus is unknown or suspected to be resistant to ≥1 of the drugs considered for the PEP regimen
  - Resistance testing of the source person's virus at the time of the exposure is not recommended

- **Toxicity of the initial PEP regimen**
  - Adverse symptoms, such as nausea and diarrhea, are common with PEP
  - Symptoms can often be managed without changing the PEP regimen by prescribing antimotility and/or antiemetic agents
  - Modification of dose intervals (ie, administering a lower dose of drug more frequently throughout the day, as recommended by the manufacturer), in other situations, might help alleviate symptoms

[1]Local experts and/or the National Clinicians' Postexposure Prophylaxis Hotline (PEPline 1-888-448-4911).

MANAGEMENT OF HEALTHCARE WORKER EXPOSURES TO HIV, HBV, HCV *(Continued)*

Occupational Exposure Management Resources

National Clinicians' Postexposure Prophylaxis Hotline (PEPline)
Run by University of California-San Francisco/San Francisco General Hospital staff; supported by the Health Resources and Services Administration Ryan White CARE Act, HIV/AIDS Bureau, AIDS Education and Training Centers, and CDC

Phone: (888) 448-4911
Internet: http://www.ucsf.edu/hivcntr

Needlestick!
A website to help clinicians manage and document occupational blood and body fluid exposures. Developed and maintained by the University of California, Los Angeles (UCLA), Emergency Medicine Center, UCLA School of Medicine, and funded in part by CDC and the Agency for Healthcare Research and Quality.

Internet: http://www.needlestick.mednet.ucla.edu

Hepatitis Hotline

Phone: (888) 443-7232
Internet: http://www.cdc.gov/hepatitis

Reporting to CDC:
Occupationally acquired HIV infections and failures of PEP

Phone: (800) 893-0485

HIV Antiretroviral Pregnancy Registry

Phone: (800) 258-4263
Fax: (800) 800-1052
Address: 1410 Commonwealth Drive, Suite 215
Wilmington, NC 28405
Internet: http://www.glaxowellcome.com/preg_reg/antiretroviral

Food and Drug Administration
Report unusual or severe toxicity to antiretroviral agents

Phone: (800) 332-1088
Address: MedWatch
HF-2, FDA
5600 Fishers Lane
Rockville, MD 20857
Internet: http://www.fda.gov/medwatch

HIV/AIDS Treatment Information Service

Internet: http://www.hivatis.org

Management of Occupational Blood Exposures

Provide immediate care to the exposure site

- Wash wounds and skin with soap and water
- Flush mucous membranes with water

Determine risk associated with exposure by:

- Type of fluid (eg, blood, visibly bloody fluid, other potentially infectious fluid or tissue, and concentrated virus)
- Type of exposure (ie, percutaneous injury, mucous membrane or nonintact skin exposure, and bites resulting in blood exposure)

Evaluate exposure source

- Assess the risk of infection using available information
- Test known sources for HB_sAg, anti-HCV, and HIV antibody (consider using rapid testing)
- For unknown sources, assess risk of exposure to HBV, HCV, or HIV infection
- Do not test discarded needle or syringes for virus contamination

Evaluate the exposed person

- Assess immune status for HBV infection (ie, by history of hepatitis B vaccination and vaccine response)

Give PEP for exposures posing risk of infection transmission

- HBV: See Recommended Postexposure Prophylaxis for Exposure to Hepatitis B Virus Table
- HCV: PEP not recommended
- HIV: See Recommended HIV Postexposure Prophylaxis for Percutaneous Injuries Table and Recommended HIV Postexposure Prophylaxis for Mucous Membrane Exposures and Nonintact Skin Exposures Table

  - Initiate PEP as soon as possible, preferably within hours of exposure
  - Offer pregnancy testing to all women of childbearing age not known to be pregnant
  - Seek expert consultation if viral resistance is suspected
  - Administer PEP for 4 weeks if tolerated

Perform follow-up testing and provide counseling

- Advise exposed persons to seek medical evaluation for any acute illness occurring during follow-up

HBV exposures

- Perform follow-up anti-HB_s testing in persons who receive hepatitis B vaccine

  - Test for anti-HB_s 1-2 months after last dose of vaccine
  - Anti-HB_s response to vaccine cannot be ascertained if HBIG was received in the previous 3-4 months

HCV exposures

- Perform baseline and follow-up testing for anti-HCV and alanine aminotransferase (ALT) 4-6 months after exposures
- Perform HCV RNA at 4-6 months if earlier diagnosis of HCV infection is desired
- Confirm repeatedly reactive anti-HCV enzyme immunoassays (EIAs) with supplemental tests

HIV exposures

- Perform HIV antibody testing for at least 6 months postexposure (eg, at baseline, 6 weeks, 3 months, and 6 months)
- Perform HIV antibody testing if illness compatible with an acute retroviral syndrome occurs
- Advise exposed persons to use precautions to prevent secondary transmission during the follow-up period
- Evaluate exposed persons taking PEP within 72 hours after exposure and monitor for drug toxicity for at least 2 weeks

MANAGEMENT OF HEALTHCARE WORKER EXPOSURES TO HIV, HBV, HCV *(Continued)*

Basic and Expanded HIV Postexposure Prophylaxis Regimens

Basic Regimens
- Zidovudine (Retrovir™; ZDV; AZT) + Lamivudine (Epivir™; 3TC); available as Combivir™
  - ZDV: 600 mg daily, in two or three divided doses, and
  - 3TC: 150 mg twice daily

Alternative Basic Regimens
- Lamivudine (3TC) + Stavudine (Zerit™; d4T)
  - 3TC: 150 mg twice daily, and
  - d4t: 40 mg twice daily (if body weight is <60 kg, 30 mg twice daily)
- Didanosine (Videx™, chewable/dispersible buffered tablet; Videx™ EC, delayed-release capsule; ddI) + Stavudine (d4T)
  - ddI: 400 mg daily on an empty stomach (if body weight is <60 kg, 125 mg twice daily)
  - d4t: 40 mg twice daily (if body weight is <60 kg, 30 mg twice daily)

Expanded Regimen
Basic regimen plus one of the following:
- Indinavir (Crixivan™; IDV)
  - 800 mg every 8 hours, on an empty stomach
- Nelfinavir (Viracept™; NFV)
  - 750 mg three times daily, with meals or snack, or
  - 1250 mg twice daily, with meals or snack
- Efavirenz (Sustiva™; EFV)
  - 600 mg daily, at bedtime
  - Should not be used during pregnancy because of concerns about teratogenicity
- Abacavir (Ziagen™; ABC); available at Trizivir™, a combination of ZDV, 3TC, and ABC
  - 300 mg twice daily

Antiretroviral Agents for Use at PEP Only With Expert Consultation
- Ritonavir (Norvir™; RTV)
- Amprenavir (Agenerase™; AMP)
- Delavirdine (Rescriptor™; DLV)
- Lopinavir/Ritonavir (Kaletra™)
  - 400/100 mg twice daily

Antiretroviral Agents Generally Not Recommended For Use as PEP
- Nevirapine (Viramune™; NVP)
  - 200 mg daily for 2 weeks, then 200 mg twice daily

PREVENTION OF BACTERIAL ENDOCARDITIS

Recommendations by the American Heart Association
(*JAMA*, 1997, 277:1794-801)

Consensus Process - The recommendations were formulated by the writing group after specific therapeutic regimens were discussed. The consensus statement was subsequently reviewed by outside experts not affiliated with the writing group and by the Science Advisory and Coordinating Committee of the American Heart Association. These guidelines are meant to aid practitioners but are not intended as the standard of care or as a substitute for clinical judgment.

Table 1. Cardiac Conditions[1]

Endocarditis Prophylaxis Recommended

High-Risk Category

    Prosthetic cardiac valves, including bioprosthetic and homograft valves

    Previous bacterial endocarditis

    Complex cyanotic congenital heart disease (eg, single ventricle states, transposition of the great arteries, tetralogy of Fallot)

    Surgically constructed systemic pulmonary shunts or conduits

Moderate-Risk Category

    Most other congenital cardiac malformations (other than above and below)

    Acquired valvar dysfunction (eg, rheumatic heart disease)

    Hypertrophic cardiomyopathy

    Mitral valve prolapse with valvar regurgitation and/or thickened leaflets

Endocarditis Prophylaxis Not Recommended

Negligible-Risk Category (no greater risk than the general population)

    Isolated secundum atrial septal defect

    Surgical repair of atrial septal defect, ventricular septal defect, or patent ductus arteriosus (without residua beyond 6 months)

    Previous coronary artery bypass graft surgery

    Mitral valve prolapse without valvar regurgitation

    Physiologic, functional, or innocent heart murmurs

    Previous Kawasaki disease without valvar dysfunction

    Previous rheumatic fever without valvar dysfunction

    Cardiac pacemakers (intravascular and epicardial) and implanted defibrillators

[1]This table lists selected conditions but is not meant to be all-inclusive.

PREVENTION OF BACTERIAL ENDOCARDITIS *(Continued)*

Patient With Suspected Mitral Valve Prolapse

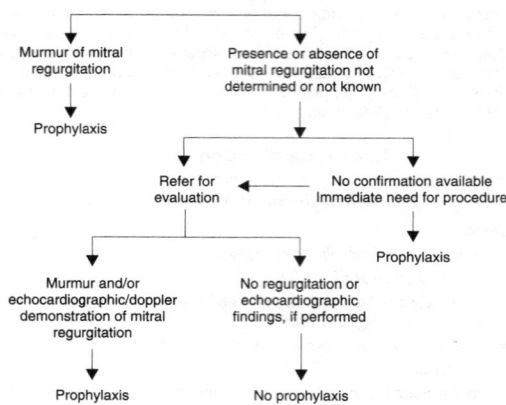

Table 2. Dental Procedures and Endocarditis Prophylaxis

Endocarditis Prophylaxis Recommended[1]

Dental extractions

Periodontal procedures including surgery, scaling and root planing, probing, and recall maintenance

Dental implant placement and reimplantation of avulsed teeth

Endodontic (root canal) instrumentation or surgery only beyond the apex

Subgingival placement of antibiotic fibers or strips

Initial placement of orthodontic bands but not brackets

Intraligamentary local anesthetic injections

Prophylactic cleaning of teeth or implants where bleeding is anticipated

Endocarditis Prophylaxis Not Recommended

Restorative dentistry[2] (operative and prosthodontic) with or without retraction cord[3]

Local anesthetic injections (nonintraligamentary)

Intracanal endodontic treatment; post placement and buildup[3]

Placement of rubber dams[3]

Postoperative suture removal

Placement of removable prosthodontic or orthodontic appliances

Taking of oral impressions[3]

Fluoride treatments

Taking of oral radiographs

Orthodontic appliance adjustment

Shedding of primary teeth

[1]Prophylaxis is recommended for patients with high- and moderate-risk cardiac conditions.

[2]This includes restoration of decayed teeth (filling cavities) and replacement of missing teeth.

[3]Clinical judgment may indicate antibiotic use in selected circumstances that may create significant bleeding.

Table 3. Recommended Standard Prophylactic Regimen for Dental, Oral, or Upper Respiratory Tract Procedures in Patients Who Are at Risk

Endocarditis Prophylaxis Recommended

Respiratory Tract
  Tonsillectomy and/or adenoidectomy
  Surgical operations that involve respiratory mucosa
  Bronchoscopy with a rigid bronchoscope
Gastrointestinal Tract[1]
  Sclerotherapy for esophageal varices
  Esophageal stricture dilation
  Endoscopic retrograde cholangiography with biliary obstruction
  Biliary tract surgery
  Surgical operations that involve intestinal mucosa
Genitourinary Tract
  Prostatic surgery
  Cystoscopy
  Urethral dilation

Endocarditis Prophylaxis Not Recommended

Respiratory Tract
  Endotracheal intubation
  Bronchoscopy with a flexible bronchoscope, with or without biopsy[2]
  Tympanostomy tube insertion
Gastrointestinal Tract
  Transesophageal echocardiography[2]
  Endoscopy with or without gastrointestinal biopsy[2]
Genitourinary Tract
  Vaginal hysterectomy[2]
  Vaginal delivery[2]
  Cesarean section
  In uninfected tissues:
    Urethral catheterization
    Uterine dilatation and curettage
    Therapeutic abortion
    Sterilization procedures
    Insertion or removal of intrauterine devices
Other
  Cardiac catheterization, including balloon angioplasty
  Implanted cardiac pacemakers, implanted defibrillators, and coronary stents
  Incision or biopsy or surgically scrubbed skin
  Circumcision

[1]Prophylaxis is recommended for high-risk patients, optional for medium-risk patients.
[2]Prophylaxis is optional for high-risk patients.

PREVENTION OF BACTERIAL ENDOCARDITIS *(Continued)*

Table 4. Prophylactic Regimens for Dental, Oral, Respiratory Tract, or Esophageal Procedures

Situation	Agent	Regimen[1]	
		Adults	Children
Standard general prophylaxis	Amoxicillin	2 g P.O. 1 h before procedure	50 mg/kg P.O. 1 h before procedure
Unable to take oral medications	Ampicillin	2 g I.M./I.V. within 30 min before procedure	50 mg/kg I.M./I.V. within 30 min before procedure
Allergic to penicillin	Clindamycin or	600 mg P.O. 1 h before procedure	20 mg/kg P.O. 1 h before procedure
	Cephalexin[2] or cefadroxil[2] or	2 g P.O 1 h before procedure	50 mg/kg P.O. 1 h before procedure
	Azithromycin or clarithromycin	500 mg P.O. 1 h before procedure	15 mg/kg P.O. 1 h before procedure
Allergic to penicillin and unable to take oral medications	Clindamycin or	600 mg I.V. within 30 min before procedure	20 mg/kg I.V. within 30 min before procedure
	Cefazolin[2]	1 g I.M./I.V. within 30 min before procedure	25 mg/kg I.M./I.V. within 30 min before procedure

[1]Total children's dose should not exceed adult dose.

[2]Cephalosporins should not be used in individuals with immediate-type hypersensitivity reaction (urticaria, angioedema, or anaphylaxis) to penicillins.

Table 5. Prophylactic Regimens for Genitourinary/Gastrointestinal (Excluding Esophageal) Procedures

Situation	Agents	Regimen[1,2]	
		Adults	Children
High-risk[3] patients	Ampicillin plus gentamicin	Ampicillin 2 g I.M. or I.V. plus gentamicin 1.5 mg/kg (not to exceed 120 mg) within 30 min of starting the procedure; 6 h later, ampicillin 1 g I.M./I.V. or amoxicillin 1 g orally	Ampicillin 50 mg/kg I.M./I.V. (not to exceed 2 g) plus gentamicin 1.5 mg/kg within 30 min of starting the procedure; 6 h later, ampicillin 25 mg/kg I.M./I.V. or amoxicillin 25 mg/kg orally
High-risk[3] patients allergic to ampicillin/ amoxicillin	Vancomycin plus gentamicin	Vancomycin 1 g I.V. over 1-2 h plus gentamicin 1.5 mg/kg I.M./I.V. (not to exceed 120 mg); complete injection/infusion within 30 min of starting the procedure	Vancomycin 20 mg/kg I.V. over 1-2 h plus gentamicin 1.5 mg/kg I.M./I.V.; complete injection/infusion within 30 min of starting the procedure
Moderate-risk[4] patients	Amoxicillin or ampicillin	Amoxicillin 2 g orally 1 h before procedure, or ampicillin 2 g I.M./I.V within 30 min of starting the procedure	Amoxicillin 50 mg/kg orally 1 h before procedure, or ampicillin 50 mg/kg I.M./I.V. within 30 min of starting the procedure
Moderate-risk[4] patients allergic to ampicillin/amoxicillin	Vancomycin	Vancomycin 1 g I.V. over 1-2 h; complete infusion within 30 min of starting the procedure	Vancomycin 20 mg/kg I.V. over 1-2 h; complete infusion within 30 min of starting the procedure

[1]Total children's dose should not exceed adult dose.

[2]No second dose of vancomycin or gentamicin is recommended.

[3]High-risk: Patients are those who have prosthetic valves, a previous history of endocarditis (even in the absence of other heart disease, complex cyanotic congenital heart disease, or surgically constructed systemic pulmonary shunts or conduits).

[4]Moderate-risk: Individuals with certain other underlying cardiac defects. Congenital cardiac conditions include the following uncorrected conditions: Patent ductus arteriosus, ventricular septal defect, ostium primum atrial septal defect, coarctation of the aorta, and bicuspid aortic valve. Acquired valvar dysfunction and hypertrophic cardiomyopathy are also moderate risk conditions.

PREVENTION OF PERINATAL HIV TRANSMISSION

Updated March, 2002 from website
www.hivatis.org/guidelines/perinatal/Feb4_02/Perin.pdf

Pediatric AIDS Clinical Trials Group (PACTG) 076 Zidovudine (ZDV) Regimen

Time of ZDV Administration	Regimen
Antepartum	Oral administration of 100 mg ZDV 5 times/day,[1] initiated at 14-34 weeks gestation and continued throughout the pregnancy
Intrapartum	During labor, intravenous administration of ZDV in a 1-hour initial dose of 2 mg/kg body weight, followed by a continuous infusion of 1 mg/kg body weight/hour delivery
Postpartum	Oral administration of ZDV to the newborn (ZDV syrup at 2 mg/kg body weight/dose every 6 hours) for the first 6 weeks of life, beginning at 8-12 hours after birth. **Note:** Intravenous dosage for infants who cannot tolerate oral intake is 1.5 mg/kg body weight intravenously every 6 hours.

[1]Oral ZDV administered as 200 mg 3 times/day or 300 mg bid is currently used in general clinical practice and is an acceptable alternative regimen to 100 mg orally 5 times/day.

Clinical Scenarios and Recommendations for the Use of Antiretroviral Drugs to Reduce Perinatal Human Immunodeficiency Virus (HIV) Transmission

SCENARIO #1
HIV-infected pregnant women who have not received prior antiretroviral therapy

- Pregnant women with HIV infection must receive standard clinical, immunologic, and virologic evaluation. Recommendations for initiation and choice of antiretroviral therapy should be based on the same parameters used for persons who are not pregnant, although the known and unknown risks and benefits of such therapy during pregnancy must be considered and discussed.

- The three-part ZDV chemoprophylaxis regimen, initiated after the first trimester, should be recommended for all HIV-infected pregnant women regardless of antenatal HIV RNA copy number to reduce the risk for perinatal transmission.

- The combination of ZDV chemoprophylaxis with additional antiretroviral drugs for treatment of HIV infection is recommended for infected women whose clinical, immunologic, or virologic status requires treatment or who have HIV RNA over 1000 copies/mL regardless of clinical or immunologic status.

- Women who are in the first trimester of pregnancy may consider delaying initiation of therapy until after 10-12 weeks gestation.

SCENARIO #2
HIV-infected women receiving antiretroviral therapy during the current pregnancy

- HIV-1-infected women receiving antiretroviral therapy in whom pregnancy is identified after the first trimester should continue therapy. ZDV should be a component of the antenatal antiretroviral treatment regimen after the first trimester whenever possible, although this may not always be feasible.

- For women receiving antiretroviral therapy in whom pregnancy is recognized during the first trimester, the woman should be counseled regarding the benefits and potential risks of antiretroviral administration during this period, and continuation of therapy should be considered. If therapy is discontinued during the first trimester, all drugs should be stopped and reintroduced simultaneously to avoid the development of drug resistance.

- Regardless of the antepartum antiretroviral regimen, ZDV administration is recommended during the intrapartum period and for the newborn.

PREVENTION OF PERINATAL HIV TRANSMISSION *(Continued)*

SCENARIO #3
HIV-infected women in labor who have had no prior therapy

Several effective regimens are available. These include:

- single-dose nevirapine at the onset of labor followed by a single dose of nevirapine for the newborn at age 48 hours

- oral ZDV and 3TC during labor, followed by 1 week of oral ZDV/3TC for the newborn

- intrapartum intravenous ZDV followed by 6 weeks of ZDV for the newborn

- two-dose nevirapine regimen combined with intrapartum intravenous ZDV and 6-week ZDV for the newborn

In the immediate postpartum period, the woman should have appropriate assessments (eg, CD4$^+$ count and HIV-1 RNA copy number) to determine whether antiretroviral therapy is recommended for her own health.

SCENARIO #4
Infants born to mothers who have received no antiretroviral therapy during pregnancy or intrapartum

- The 6-week neonatal ZDV component of the ZDV chemoprophylactic regimen should be discussed with the mother and offered for the newborn.

- ZDV should be initiated as soon as possible after delivery – preferably within 6-12 hours of birth.

- Some clinicians may choose to use ZDV in combination with other antiretroviral drugs, particularly if the mother is known or suspected to have ZDV-resistant virus. However, the efficacy of this approach for prevention of transmission is unknown, and appropriate dosing regimens for neonates are incompletely defined.

- In the immediate postpartum period, the woman should undergo appropriate assessments (eg, CD4$^+$ count and HIV-1 RNA copy number) to determine whether antiretroviral therapy is required for her own health. The infant should undergo early diagnostic testing so that if HIV-infected, treatment can be initiated as soon as possible.

Note: Discussion of treatment options and recommendations should be noncoercive, and the final decision regarding the use of antiretroviral drugs is the responsibility of the woman. A decision to not accept treatment with ZDV or other drugs should not result in punitive action or denial of care. Use of ZDV should not be denied to a woman who wishes to minimize exposure of the fetus to other antiretroviral drugs and who, therefore, chooses to receive only ZDV during pregnancy to reduce the risk for perinatal transmission.

PREVENTION OF WOUND INFECTION & SEPSIS IN SURGICAL PATIENTS

Nature of Operation	Likely Pathogens	Recommended Drugs	Adult Dosage Before Surgery[1]
Cardiac			
Prosthetic valve, coronary artery bypass, other open-heart surgery, pacemaker or defibrillator implant	S. epidermidis, S. aureus, Corynebacterium, enteric gram-negative bacilli	Cefazolin	1-2 g I.V.[2]
		or cefuroxime	1-2 g I.V.[2]
		or vancomycin[3]	1 g I.V.
Gastrointestinal			
Esophageal, gastroduodenal	Enteric gram-negative bacilli, gram-positive cocci	High risk[4] only: cefazolin	1-2 g I.V.
Biliary tract	Enteric gram-negative bacilli, enterococci, clostridia	High risk[5] only: cefazolin	1-2 g I.V.
Colorectal	Enteric gram-negative bacilli, anaerobes, enterococci	Oral: neomycin + erythromycin base[6]	1-2 g I.V.
		Parenteral:	
		Cefoxitin	1-2 g I.V.
		or cefotetan	1-2 g I.V.
Appendectomy, nonperforated	Enteric gram-negative bacilli, anaerobes, enterococci	Cefoxitin	1-2 g I.V.
		or cefotetan	1-2 g I.V.
Genitourinary	Enteric gram-negative bacilli, enterococci	High risk[7] only: Ciprofloxacin	500 mg P.O. or 400 mg I.V.
Gynecologic and Obstetric			
Vaginal or abdominal hysterectomy	Enteric gram-negatives, anaerobes, group B streptococci, enterococci	Cefazolin	1-2 g I.V.
		or cefotetan	1-2 g I.V.
		or cefoxitin	1 g I.V.
Cesarean section	Same as for hysterectomy	High risk[8] only: Cefazolin	1 g I.V. after cord clamping
Abortion	Same as for hysterectomy	First trimester, high-risk[9] only: Aqueous penicillin G	2 mill units I.V.
		or doxycycline	300 mg P.O.[10]
		Second trimester: Cefazolin	1 g I.V.
Head and Neck			
Entering oral cavity or pharynx	S. aureus, streptococci, oral anaerobes	Cefazolin	1-2 g I.V.
		or clindamycin	600-900 mg I.V.
		± gentamicin	1.5 mg/kg I.V.
Neurosurgery			
Craniotomy	S. aureus, S. epidermidis	Cefazolin	1-2 g I.V.
		or vancomycin[3]	1 g I.V.
Ophthalmic	S. aureus, S. epidermidis, streptococci, enteric gram-negative bacilli, Pseudomonas	Gentamicin or tobramycin or neomycin-gramicidin-polymyxin B	Multiple drops topically over 2-24 h
		Cefazolin	100 mg subconjunctivally at end of procedure
Orthopedic			
Total joint replacement, internal fixation of fractures	S. aureus, S. epidermidis	Cefazolin	1-2 g I.V.
		or vancomycin[3]	1 g I.V.
Thoracic (Noncardiac)	S. aureus, S. epidermidis, streptococci, enteric gram-negative bacilli	Cefazolin	1-2 g I.V.
		or cefuroxime	1-2 g I.V.
		or vancomycin[3]	1 g I.V.
Vascular			
Arterial surgery involving the abdominal aorta, a prosthesis, or a groin incision	S. aureus, S. epidermidis, enteric gram-negative bacilli	Cefazolin	1-2 g I.V.
		or vancomycin[3]	1 g I.V.

PREVENTION OF WOUND INFECTION & SEPSIS IN SURGICAL PATIENTS *(Continued)*

Nature of Operation	Likely Pathogens	Recommended Drugs	Adult Dosage Before Surgery[1]
Lower extremity amputation for ischemia	*S. aureus, S. epidermidis,* enteric gram-negative bacilli, clostridia	Cefazolin	1-2 g I.V.
		or vancomycin[3]	1 g I.V.
CONTAMINATED SURGERY[11]			
Ruptured viscus	Enteric gram-negative bacilli, anaerobes, enterococci	Cefoxitin	1-2 g I.V. q6h
		or cefotetan	1-2 g I.V. q12h
		± gentamicin	1.5 mg/kg I.V. q8h
		or clindamycin	600 mg I.V. q6h
		+ gentamicin	1.5 mg/kg I.V. q8h
Traumatic wound	*S. aureus,* Group A strep, clostridia	Cefazolin[12]	1-2 g I.V. q8h

[1]Parenteral prophylactic antimicrobials can be given as a single intravenous dose just before the operation. For prolonged operations, additional intraoperative doses should be given every 4-8 hours for the duration of the procedure.

[2]Some consultants recommend an additional dose when patients are removed from bypass during open-heart surgery.

[3]For hospitals in which methicillin-resistant *S. aureus* and *S. epidermidis* are a frequent cause of postoperative wound infection, or for patients allergic to penicillins or cephalosporin. Rapid I.V. administration may cause hypotension, which could be especially dangerous during induction of anesthesia. Even if the drug is given over 60 minutes, hypotension may occur; treatment with diphenhydramine (Benadryl® and others) and further slowing of the infusion rate may be helpful (Maki DG et al, *J Thorac Cardiovasc Surg*, 1992, 104:1423). For procedures in which enteric gram-negative bacilli are likely pathogens, such as vascular surgery involving a groin incision, cefazolin should be included in the prophylaxis regimen for patients not allergic to cephalosporins.

[4]Morbid obesity, esophageal obstruction, decreased gastric acidity or gastrointestinal motility.

[5]Age >70 years, acute cholecystitis, nonfunctioning gall bladder, obstructive jaundice or common duct stones.

[6]After appropriate diet and catharsis, 1 g of each at 1 PM, 2 PM, and 11 PM the day before an 8 AM operation.

[7]Urine culture positive or unavailable, preoperative catheter.

[8]Active labor or premature rupture of membranes.

[9]Patients with previous pelvic inflammatory disease, previous gonorrhea or multiple sex partners.

[10]Divided into 100 mg one hour before the abortion and 200 mg one half hour after.

[11]For contaminated or "dirty" surgery, therapy should usually be continued for about 5 days.

[12]For bite wounds, in which likely pathogens may also include oral anaerobes, *Eikenella corrodens* (human) and *Pasteurella multocida* (dog and cat), some *Medical Letter* consultants recommend use of amoxicillin/clavulanic acid (Augmentin®) or ampicillin/sulbactam (Unasyn®)

Adapted with permission from *The Medical Letter*, 1997, 39(Issue 1012).

POSTEXPOSURE PROPHYLAXIS FOR HEPATITIS B[1]

Exposure	Hepatitis B Immune Globulin	Hepatitis B Vaccine
Perinatal	0.5 mL I.M. within 12 h of birth	0.5 mL[2] I.M. within 12 h of birth (no later than 7 d), and at 1 and 6 mo[3]; test for HBₛAg and anti-HBₛ at 12-15 mo
Sexual	0.06 mL/kg I.M. within 14 d of sexual contact; a second dose should be given if the index patient remains HBₛAg-positive after 3 mo and hepatitis B vaccine was not given initially	1 mL I.M. at 0, 1, and 6 mo for homosexual and bisexual men and regular sexual contacts of persons with acute and chronic hepatitis B
Percutaneous; exposed person unvaccinated		
Source known HBₛAg-positive	0.06 mL/kg I.M. within 24 h	1 mL I.M. within 7 d, and at 1 and 6 mo[4]
Source known, HBₛAg status not known	Test source for HBₛAg; if source is positive, give exposed person 0.06 mL/kg I.M. once within 7 d	1 mL I.M. within 7 d, and at 1 and 6 mo[4]
Source not tested or unknown	Nothing required	1 mL I.M. within 7 d, and at 1 and 6 mo
Percutaneous; exposed person vaccinated		
Source known HBₛAg-positive	Test exposed person for anti-HBₛ.[5] If titer is protective, nothing is required; if titer is not protective, give 0.06 mL/kg within 24 h	Review vaccination status[6]
Source known, HBₛAg status not known	Test source for HBₛAg and exposed person for anti-HBₛ. If source is HBₛAg-negative, or if source is HBₛAg-positive but anti-HBₛ titer is protective, nothing is required. If source is HBₛAg-positive and anti-HBₛ titer is not protective or if exposed person is a known nonresponder, give 0.06 mL/kg I.M. within 24 h. A second dose of hepatitis B immune globulin can be given 1 mo later if a booster dose of hepatitis B vaccine is not given.	Review vaccination status[6]
Source not tested or unknown	Test exposed person for anti-HBₛ. If anti-HBₛ titer is protective, nothing is required. If anti-HBₛ titer is not protective, 0.06 mL/kg may be given along with a booster dose of hepatitis B vaccine	Review vaccination status[6]

[1]HBₛAg = hepatitis B surface antigen; anti-HBₛ = antibody to hepatitis B surface antigen; I.M. = intramuscularly; SRU = standard ratio units.
[2]Each 0.5 mL dose of plasma-derived hepatitis B vaccine contains 10 mcg of HBₛAg; each 0.5 mL dose of recombinant hepatitis B vaccine contains 5 mcg (Merck Sharp & Dohme) or 10 mcg (SmithKline Beecham) of HBₛAg.
[3]If hepatitis B immune globulin and hepatitis B vaccine are given simultaneously, they should be given at separate sites.
[4]If hepatitis B vaccine is not given, a second dose of hepatitis B immune globulin should be given 1 month later.
[5]Anti-HBₛ titers <10 SRU by radioimmunoassay or negative by enzyme immunoassay indicate lack of protection. Testing the exposed person for anti-HBₛ is not necessary if a protective level of antibody has been shown within the previous 24 months.
[6]If the exposed person has not completed a three-dose series of hepatitis B vaccine, the series should be completed. Test the exposed person for anti-HBₛ. If the antibody level is protective, nothing is required. If an adequate antibody response in the past is shown on retesting to have declined to an inadequate level, a booster dose (1 mL) of hepatitis B vaccine should be given. If the exposed person has inadequate antibody or is a known nonresponder to vaccination, a booster dose can be given along with one dose of hepatitis B immune globulin.

TUBERCULOSIS

Tuberculin Skin Test Recommendations[1]

Children for whom immediate skin testing is indicated:

- Contacts of persons with confirmed or suspected infectious tuberculosis (contact investigation); this includes children identified as contacts of family members or associates in jail or prison in the last 5 years

- Children with radiographic or clinical findings suggesting tuberculosis

- Children immigrating from endemic countries (eg, Asia, Middle East, Africa, Latin America)

- Children with travel histories to endemic countries and/or significant contact with indigenous persons from such countries

Children who should be tested annually for tuberculosis[2]:

- Children infected with HIV or living in household with HIV-infected persons

- Incarcerated adolescents

Children who should be tested every 2-3 years[2]:

- Children exposed to the following individuals: HIV-infected, homeless, residents of nursing homes, institutionalized adolescents or adults, users of illicit drugs, incarcerated adolescents or adults, and migrant farm workers. Foster children with exposure to adults in the preceding high-risk groups are included.

Children who should be considered for tuberculin skin testing at ages 4-6 and 11-16 years:

- Children whose parents immigrated (with unknown tuberculin skin test status) from regions of the world with high prevalence of tuberculosis; continued potential exposure by travel to the endemic areas and/or household contact with persons from the endemic areas (with unknown tuberculin skin test status) should be an indication for repeat tuberculin skin testing

- Children without specific risk factors who reside in high-prevalence areas; in general, a high-risk neighborhood or community does not mean an entire city is at high risk; rates in any area of the city may vary by neighborhood, or even from block to block; physicians should be aware of these patterns in determining the likelihood of exposure; public health officials or local tuberculosis experts should help clinicians identify areas that have appreciable tuberculosis rates

Children at increased risk of progression of infection to disease: Those with other medical risk factors, including diabetes mellitus, chronic renal failure, malnutrition, and congenital or acquired immunodeficiencies deserve special consideration. Without recent exposure, these persons are not at increased risk of acquiring tuberculosis infection. Underlying immune deficiencies associated with these conditions theoretically would enhance the possibility for progression to severe disease. Initial histories of potential exposure to tuberculosis should be included on all of these patients. If these histories or local epidemiologic factors suggest a possibility of exposure, immediate and periodic tuberculin skin testing should be considered. An initial Mantoux tuberculin skin test should be performed before initiation of immunosuppressive therapy in any child with an underlying condition that necessitates immunosuppressive therapy.

---

[1]BCG immunization is not a contraindication to tuberculin skin testing.

[2]Initial tuberculin skin testing is at the time of diagnosis or circumstance, beginning as early as at age 3 months.

Tuberculosis Prophylaxis

Specific Circumstances/ Organism	Comments	Regimen
Category I. Exposure		
(Household members and other close contacts of potentially infectious cases) (Exposee tuberculin test negative)[1]		
Neonate	Rx essential	INH (10 mg/kg/d) for 3 months, then repeat tuberculin test (TBnT). If mother's smear negative and infant's TBnT negative and chest x-ray (CXR) are normal, stop INH. In the United Kingdom, BCG is then given (*Lancet*, 1990, 2:1479), unless mother is HIV-positive. If infants repeat TBnT is positive and/or CXR abnormal (hilar adenopathy and/or infiltrate), administer INH + RIF (10-20 mg/kg/d) (or streptomycin) for a total of 6 months. If mother is being treated, separation from mother is not indicated.
Children <5 y	Rx indicated	As for neonate first 3 months. If repeat TBnT is negative, stop. If repeat TBnT is positive, continue INH for a total of 9 months. If INH is not given initially, repeat TBnT at 3 months; if positive, treat with INH for 9 months (see Category II below).
Older children and adults	No Rx	Repeat TBnT at 3 months, if positive, treat with INH for 6 months (see Category II below)
Category II. Infection Without Disease		
(Positive tuberculin test)[1]		
Regardless of age (see INH Preventive Therapy)	Rx indicated	INH (5 mg/kg/d, maximum: 300 mg/d for adults, 10 mg/kg/d not to exceed 300 mg/d for children). Results with 6 months of treatment are nearly as effective as 12 months (65% vs 75% reduction in disease). *Am Thoracic Society* (6 months), *Am Acad Pediatrics*, 1991 (9 months). If CXR is abnormal, treat for 12 months. In HIV-positive patient, treatment for a minimum of 12 months, some suggest longer. Monitor transaminases monthly (*MMWR Morb Mortal Wkly Rep* 1989, 38:247).
Age <35 y	Rx indicated	Reanalysis of earlier studies favors INH prophylaxis for 6 months (if INH-related hepatitis case fatality rate is <1% and TB case fatality is ≥6.7%, which appears to be the case, monitor transaminases monthly (*Arch Int Med*, 1990, 150:2517).
INH-resistant organisms likely	Rx indicated	Data on efficacy of alternative regimens is currently lacking. Regimens include ETB + RIF daily for 6 months. PZA + RIF daily for 2 months, then INH + RIF daily until sensitivities from index case (if available) known, then if INH-CR, discontinue INH and continue RIF for 9 months, otherwise INH + RIF for 9 months (this latter is *Am Acad Pediatrics*, 1991 recommendation).
INH + RIF resistant organisms likely	Rx indicated	Efficacy of alternative regimens is unknown; PZA (25-30 mg/kg P.O.) + ETB (15-25 mg/kg P.O.) (at 25 mg/kg ETB, monitoring for retrobulbar neuritis required), for 6 months unless HIV-positive, then 12 months; PZA + ciprofloxacin (750 mg P.O. bid) or ofloxacin (400 mg P.O. bid) x 6-12 months (*MMWR Morb Mortal Wkly Rep*, 1992, 41(RR11):68).

INH = isoniazid; RIF = rifampin; KM = kanamycin; ETB = ethambutol
SM = streptomycin; CXR = chest x-ray; Rx = treatment
See also guidelines for interpreting PPD in "Skin Testing for Delayed Hypersensitivity."
[1]Tuberculin test (TBnT). The standard is the Mantoux test, 5 TU PPD in 0.1 mL diluent stabilized with Tween 80. Read at 48-72 hours measuring maximum diameter of induration. A reaction ≥5 mm is defined as positive in the following: positive HIV or risk factors, recent close case contacts, CXR consistent with healed TBc. ≥10 mm is positive in foreign-born in countries of high prevalence, injection drug users, low income populations, nursing home residents, patients with medical conditions which increase risk (see above, preventive treatment). ≥15 mm is positive in all others (*Am Rev Resp Dis*, 1990, 142:725). Two-stage TBnT: Use in individuals to be tested regularly (ie, healthcare workers). TBn reactivity may decrease over time but be boosted by skin testing. If unrecognized, individual may be incorrectly diagnosed as recent converter. If first TBnT is reactive but <10 mm, repeat 5 TU in 1 week, if then ≥10 mm = positive, not recent conversion (*Am Rev Resp Dis*, 1979, 119:587).

USPHS / IDSA GUIDELINES FOR THE PREVENTION OF OPPORTUNISTIC INFECTIONS IN PERSONS INFECTED WITH HIV

Adapted from "2001 USPHS/IDSA Guidelines for the Prevention of Opportunistic Infections in Persons Infected With Human Immunodeficiency Virus. USPHS/IDSA Prevention of Opportunistic Infections Working Group" (www.hivatis.org)

DRUG REGIMENS FOR ADULTS AND ADOLESCENTS

Prophylaxis to Prevent First Episode of Opportunistic Disease in HIV-Infected Adults and Adolescents

Pathogen	Indication	Preventive Regimens	
		First Choice	Alternatives
I. Strongly Recommended as Standard of Care			
Pneumocystis carinii[1]	CD4+ count <200/µL or oropharyngeal candidiasis	TMP-SMZ, 1 DS P.O. every day; TMP-SMZ, 1 SS P.O. every day	Dapsone, 50 mg P.O. twice daily *or* 100 mg P.O. every day; dapsone, 50 mg P.O. every day *plus* pyrimethamine, 50 mg P.O. weekly *plus* leucovorin, 25 mg P.O. weekly; dapsone, 200 mg P.O. *plus* pyrimethamine, 75 mg P.O. *plus* leucovorin, 25 mg P.O. weekly; aerosolized pentamidine, 300 mg monthly via Respirgard II™ nebulizer; atovaquone, 1500 mg P.O. every day; TMP-SMZ, 1 DS P.O. 3 times/week
Mycobacterium tuberculosis			
Isoniazid-sensitive[2]	TST reaction ≥5 mm *or* prior positive TST result without treatment or contact with case of active tuberculosis **regardless of TST result**	Isoniazid, 300 mg P.O. *plus* pyridoxine, 50 mg P.O. every day x 9 months or isoniazid, 900 mg P.O. *plus* pyridoxine, 100 mg P.O. twice a week x 9 months	Rifampin, 600 mg P.O. every day x 4 months or rifabutin, 300 mg P.O. every day x 4 months; Pyrazinamide, 15-20 mg/kg P.O. every day x 2 months *plus* either rifampin, 600 mg P.O. every day x 2 months or rifabutin, 300 mg P.O. every day x 2 months
Isoniazid-resistant	Same as above; high probability of exposure to isoniazid-resistant tuberculosis	Rifampin, 600 mg P.O. or rifabutin, 300 mg P.O. every day x 4 months	Pyrazinamide, 15-20 mg/kg P.O. every day *plus* either rifampin, 600 mg P.O. or rifabutin, 300 mg P.O. every day x 2 months
Multidrug (isoniazid and rifampin)-resistant	Same as above; high probability of exposure to multidrug-resistant tuberculosis	Choice of drugs requires consultation with public health authorities. **Depends on susceptibility of isolate from source patient.**	None
Toxoplasma gondii[3]	IgG antibody to *Toxoplasma* and CD4+ count <100/µL	TMP-SMZ, 1 DS P.O. every day	TMP-SMZ, 1 SS P.O. every day; dapsone, 50 mg P.O. every day *plus* pyrimethamine, 50 mg P.O. once weekly *plus* leucovorin, 25 mg P.O. weekly; dapsone, 200 mg P.O. *plus* pyrimethamine, 75 mg P.O. *plus* leucovorin, 25 mg P.O. weekly; atovaquone, 1500 mg P.O. every day with or without pyrimethamine, 25 mg P.O. every day *plus* leucovorin, 10 mg P.O. every day
Mycobacterium avium complex	CD4+ count <50/µL	Azithromycin, 1200 mg P.O. weekly or clarithromycin,[4] 500 mg P.O. twice daily	Rifabutin, 300 mg P.O. every day; azithromycin, 1200 mg P.O. weekly *plus* rifabutin, 300 mg P.O. every day

Prophylaxis to Prevent First Episode of Opportunistic Disease in HIV-Infected Adults and Adolescents *(continued)*

Pathogen	Indication	Preventive Regimens	
		First Choice	Alternatives
Varicella zoster virus (VZV)	Significant exposure to chickenpox or shingles for patients who have no history of either condition or, if available, negative antibody to VZV	Varicella zoster immune globulin (VZIG), 5 vials (1.25 mL each) I.M., administered ≤96 hours after exposure, ideally within 48 hours	
II. Generally Recommended			
Streptococcus pneumoniae[5]	CD4+ count ≥200/μL	23 valent polysaccharide vaccine, 0.5 mL I.M.	None
Hepatitis B virus[6,7]	All susceptible (anti-HB$_c$-negative) patients	Hepatitis B vaccine: 3 doses	None
Influenza virus[6,8]	All patients (annually, before influenza season)	Inactivated trivalent influenza virus vaccine: One annual dose (0.5 mL) I.M.	Oseltamivir, 75 mg P.O. every day (influenza A or B); rimantadine, 100 mg P.O. twice daily, or amantadine, 100 mg P.O. twice daily (influenza A only)
Hepatitis A virus[6,7]	All susceptible (anti-HAV-negative) patients at increased risk for HAV infection (eg, illicit drug users, men who have sex with men, hemophiliacs) or with chronic liver disease, including chronic hepatitis B or hepatitis C	Hepatitis A vaccine: 2 doses	None
III. Evidence for Efficacy but Not Routinely Indicated			
Bacteria	Neutropenia	Granulocyte-colony-stimulating factor (G-CSF), 5-10 mcg/kg S.C. every day x 2-4 weeks or granulocyte-macrophage colony-stimulating factor (GM-CSF), 250 mcg/m^2 S.C., I.V. x 2-4 weeks	None
Cryptococcus neoformans	CD4+ count <50/μL	Fluconazole, 100-200 mg P.O. every day	Itraconazole capsule, 200 mg P.O. every day
Histoplasma capsulatum[9]	CD4+ count <100/μL, endemic geographic area	Itraconazole capsule, 200 mg P.O. every day	None
Cytomegalovirus (CMV)[10]	CD4+ count <50/μL and CMV antibody positivity	Oral ganciclovir, 1 g P.O. 3 times/day	None

Note: Information included in these guidelines may not represent Food and Drug Administration (FDA) approval or approved labeling for the particular products or indications in question. Specifically, the terms "safe" and "effective" may not be synonymous with the FDA-defined legal standards for product approval.

Abbreviations: Anti-HB$_c$ = antibody to hepatitis B core antigen; CMV = cytomegalovirus; DS = double-strength tablet; HAART = highly active antiretroviral therapy; HAV = hepatitis A virus; SS = single-strength tablet; TMP-SMZ = trimethoprim-sulfamethoxazole; and TST = tuberculin skin test. The Respirgard II™ nebulizer is manufactured by Marquest, Englewood, CO.

[1]Prophylaxis should also be considered for persons with a CD4+ percentage <14%, for persons with a history of an AIDS-defining illness, and possibly for those with CD4+ count >200 but <250 cells/μL. TMP-SMZ also reduces the frequency of toxoplasmosis and some bacterial infections. Patients receiving dapsone should be tested for glucose-6-phosphate dehydrogenase deficiency. A dosage of 50 mg every day is probably less effective than 100 mg every day. The efficacy of parenteral pentamidine (eg, 4 mg/kg/month) is uncertain. Fansidar® (sulfadoxine-pyrimethamine) is rarely used because of severe hypersensitivity reactions. Patients who are being administered therapy for toxoplasmosis with sulfadiazine-pyrimethamine are protected against *Pneumocystis carinii* pneumonia and do not need additional prophylaxis against PCP.

[2]Directly observed therapy is recommended for isoniazid (eg, 900 mg twice weekly); INH regimens should include pyridoxine to prevent peripheral neuropathy. If rifampin or rifabutin are administered concurrently with protease inhibitors or non-nucleoside reverse transcriptase inhibitors, careful consideration should be given to potential pharmacokinetic interactions. There have been reports of fatal and severe liver injury associated with the treatment of latent TB infection in HIV-uninfected persons treated with the 2 month regimen of daily rifampin and pyrazinamide; therefore it may be prudent to use regimens that do not contain pyrazinamide in HIV-infected persons whose completion of treatment can be assured (CDC. "Update: Fatal and Severe Liver Injuries Associated with Rafampin and Pyrazinamide

USPHS / IDSA GUIDELINES FOR THE PREVENTION OF OPPORTUNISTIC INFECTIONS IN PERSONS INFECTED WITH HIV *(Continued)*

for Latent Tuberculosis Infection and Revisions in American Thoracic Society/CDC Recommendations, United States 2001," *MMWR*, 2001, 50(34). Exposure to multidrug-resistant tuberculosis might require prophylaxis with two drugs; consult public health authorities. Possible regimens include pyrazinamide plus either ethambutol or a fluoroquinolone.

[3]Protection against toxoplasmosis is provided by TMP-SMZ, dapsone plus pyrimethamine, and possibly by atovaquone. Atovaquone may be used with or without pyrimethamine. Pyrimethamine alone probably provides little, if any, protection.

[4]**During pregnancy, azithromycin is preferred over clarithromycin because of the teratogenicity in animals of clarithromycin.**

[5]Vaccination **may** be offered to persons who have a CD4[+] T-lymphocyte count <200 cells/μL, although the efficacy **is likely to** be diminished. Revaccination 5 years after the first dose or sooner if the initial immunization was given when the CD4[+] count was <200 cells/μL and if the CD4[+] count has increased to >200 cells/μL on HAART is considered optional. Some authorities are concerned that immunizations may stimulate the replication of HIV.

[6]Although data demonstrating clinical benefit of these vaccines in HIV-infected persons are not available, it is logical to assume that those patients who develop antibody responses will derive some protection. Some authorities are concerned that immunizations may stimulate HIV replication, although for influenza vaccination, a large observational study of HIV-infected persons in clinical care showed no adverse effect of this vaccine, including multiple doses, on patient survival (J. Ward, CDC, personal communication). Also, this concern may be less relevant in the setting of HAART. However, because of the theoretical concern that increases in HIV plasma RNA following vaccination during pregnancy might increase the risk of perinatal transmission of HIV, providers may wish to defer vaccination for such patients until after HAART is initiated.

[7]Hepatitis B vaccine has been recommended for all children and adolescents and for all adults with risk factors for hepatitis B virus (HBV). For persons requiring vaccination against both hepatitis A and hepatitis B, a combination vaccine is now available. For additional information regarding vaccination against hepatitis A and B, see CDC, "Hepatitis B Virus: A Comprehensive Strategy for Eliminating Transmission in the United States Through Universal Childhood Vaccination. Recommendations of the Advisory Committee on Immunization Practices (ACIP)," *MMWR Morb Mortal Wkly Rep*, 1991, 40(RR13).

[8]Oseltamivir is appropriate during outbreaks of either influenza A or influenza B. Rimantadine or amantadine are appropriate during outbreaks of influenza A (although neither rimantadine nor amantadine is recommended during pregnancy). Dosage reduction for antiviral chemoprophylaxis against influenza might be indicated for decreased renal or hepatic function, and for persons with seizure disorders. Physicians should consult the drug package inserts and the annual CDC influenza guidelines for more specific information about adverse effects and dosage adjustments. For additional information about vaccinations, antiviral chemoprophylaxis, and therapy against influenza, see CDC, "Prevention and Control of Influenza: Recommendations of the Advisory Committee on Immunization Practices (ACIP)," *MMWR Morb Mortal Wkly Rep*, 2001, 50(RR-4).

[9]In a few unusual occupational or other circumstances, prophylaxis should be considered; consult a specialist.

[10]Acyclovir is not protective against CMV. Valacyclovir is not recommended because of an unexplained trend toward increased mortality observed in persons with AIDS who were being administered this drug for prevention of CMV disease.

Prophylaxis to Prevent Recurrence of Opportunistic Disease (After Chemotherapy for Acute Disease) in HIV-Infected Adults and Adolescents

Pathogen	Indication	Preventive Regimens	
		First Choice	Alternatives
I. Recommended as Standard of Care			
Pneumocystis carinii	Prior P. carinii pneumonia	TMP-SMZ, 1 DS P.O. every day; TMP-SMZ, 1 SS P.O. every day	Dapsone, 50 mg P.O. twice daily or 100 mg P.O. every day; dapsone, 50 mg P.O. every day plus pyrimethamine, 50 mg P.O. weekly plus leucovorin, 25 mg P.O. weekly; dapsone, 200 mg P.O. plus pyrimethamine, 75 mg P.O. plus leucovorin, 25 mg P.O. weekly; aerosolized pentamidine, 300 mg monthly via Respirgard II™ nebulizer; atovaquone, 1500 mg P.O. every day; TMP-SMZ, 1 DS P.O. 3 times/week
Toxoplasma gondii[1]	Prior toxoplasmic encephalitis	Sulfadiazine, 500-1000 mg P.O. 4 times/day plus pyrimethamine 25-50 mg P.O. every day plus leucovorin, 10-25 mg P.O. every day	Clindamycin, 300-450 mg P.O. every 6-8 hours plus pyrimethamine, 25-50 mg P.O. every day plus leucovorin, 10-25 mg P.O. every day; atovaquone, 750 mg P.O. every 6-12 hours with or without pyrimethamine, 25 mg P.O. every day plus leucovorin 10 mg P.O. every day
Mycobacterium avium complex[2]	Documented disseminated disease	Clarithromycin,[2] 500 mg P.O. twice daily plus ethambutol, 15 mg/kg P.O. every day; with or without rifabutin, 300 mg P.O. every day	Azithromycin, 500 mg P.O. every day plus ethambutol, 15 mg/kg P.O. every day; with or without rifabutin, 300 mg P.O. every day
Cytomegalovirus	Prior end-organ disease	Ganciclovir, 5-6 mg/kg I.V. 5-7 days/week or 1000 mg P.O. 3 times/day; or foscarnet, 90-120 mg/kg I.V. every day; or (for retinitis) ganciclovir sustained-release implant, every 6-9 months plus ganciclovir, 1-1.5 g P.O. 3 times/day	Cidofovir, 5 mg/kg I.V. every other week with probenecid 2 g P.O. 3 hours before the dose followed by 1 g P.O. given 2 hours after the dose, and 1 g P.O. 8 hours after the dose (total of 4 g); fomivirsen, 1 vial (330 mcg) injected into the vitreous, then repeated every 2-4 weeks; valganciclovir 900 mg P.O. every day
Cryptococcus neoformans	Documented disease	Fluconazole, 200 mg P.O. every day	Amphotericin B, 0.6-1 mg/kg I.V. weekly to 3 times/week; itraconazole capsule, 200 mg P.O. every day
Histoplasma capsulatum	Documented disease	Itraconazole capsule, 200 mg P.O. twice daily	Amphotericin B, 1 mg/kg I.V. weekly
Coccidioides immitis	Documented disease	Fluconazole, 400 mg P.O. every day	Amphotericin B, 1 mg/kg I.V. weekly; itraconazole capsule, 200 mg P.O. twice daily
Salmonella species (non-typhi)[3]	Bacteremia	Ciprofloxacin, 500 mg P.O. twice daily for several months	Antibiotic chemoprophylaxis with another active agent
II. Recommended Only if Subsequent Episodes Are Frequent or Severe			
Herpes simplex virus	Frequent/severe recurrences	Acyclovir, 200 mg P.O. 3 times/day or 400 mg P.O. twice daily; famciclovir, 250 mg P.O. twice daily	Valacyclovir, 500 mg P.O. twice daily
Candida (oropharyngeal or vaginal)	Frequent/severe recurrences	Fluconazole, 100-200 mg P.O. every day	Itraconazole solution, 200 mg P.O. every day

USPHS / IDSA GUIDELINES FOR THE PREVENTION OF OPPORTUNISTIC INFECTIONS IN PERSONS INFECTED WITH HIV *(Continued)*

Prophylaxis to Prevent Recurrence of Opportunistic Disease (After Chemotherapy for Acute Disease) in HIV-Infected Adults and Adolescents *(continued)*

Pathogen	Indication	Preventive Regimens	
		First Choice	Alternatives
Candida (esophageal)	Frequent/ severe recurrences	Fluconazole, 100-200 mg P.O. every day	Itraconazole solution, 200 mg P.O. every day

Note: Information included in these guidelines may not represent Food and Drug Administration (FDA) approval or approved labeling for the particular products or indications in question. Specifically, the terms "safe" and "effective" may not be synonymous with the FDA-defined legal standards for product approval.

DS = double-strength tablet; SS = single-strength tablet; and TMP-SMZ = trimethoprim-sulfamethoxazole. The Respirgard II™ nebulizer is manufactured by Marquest, Englewood, CO.

[1]Pyrimethamine/sulfadiazine confers protection against PCP as well as toxoplasmosis; clindamycin-pyrimethamine does **not offer protection against PCP**.

[2]Many multiple-drug regimens are poorly tolerated. Drug interactions (eg, those seen with clarithromycin/rifabutin) can be problematic; rifabutin has been associated with uveitis, especially when administered at daily doses of >300 mg or concurrently with fluconazole or clarithromycin. **During pregnancy, azithromycin is recommended instead of clarithromycin because clarithromycin is teratogenic in animals**.

[3]Efficacy of eradication of *Salmonella* has been demonstrated only for ciprofloxacin.

Effects of Food on Drugs Used to Prevent Opportunistic Infections

Drug	Food Effect	Recommendation
Atovaquone	Bioavailability increased up to threefold with high-fat meal	Administer with food
Ganciclovir (capsules)	High-fat meal results in 22% (GCV) or 30% (VGCV) increase in AUC	High fat meal may increase toxicity of valganciclovir
Itraconazole	Grapefruit juice results in 30% decrease in AUC	Avoid concurrent grapefruit juice
Itraconazole (capsules)	Significant increase in bioavailability when taken with a full meal	Administer with food
Itraconazole (solution)	31% increase in AUC when taken under fasting conditions	Take without food if possible

Criteria for Starting, Discontinuing, and Restarting Opportunistic Infection Prophylaxis for Adult Patients With HIV Infection[1]

Opportunistic Illness	Criteria for Initiating Primary Prophylaxis	Criteria for Discontinuing Primary Prophylaxis	Criteria for Restarting Primary Prophylaxis	Criteria for Initiating Secondary Prophylaxis	Criteria for Discontinuing Secondary Prophylaxis	Criteria for Restarting Secondary Prophylaxis
Pneumocystis carinii pneumonia	CD4+ >200 cells/μL or oropharyngeal candidiasis	CD4+ >200 cells/μL for ≥3 months	CD4+ <200 cells/μL	Prior *Pneumocystis carinii* pneumonia	CD4+ >200 cells/μL for ≥3 months	CD4+ <200 cells/μL
Toxoplasmosis	IgG antibody to *Toxoplasma* and CD4+ <100 cells/μL	CD4+ >200 cells/μL for ≥3 months	CD4+ <100-200 cells/μL	Prior toxoplasmic encephalitis	CD4+ >200 cells/μL sustained (eg, ≥6 months) and completed initial therapy, and asymptomatic for toxoplasmosis	CD4+ <200 cells/μL
Disseminated *Mycobacterium avium* complex	CD4+ <50 cells/μL	CD4+ >100 cells/μL for ≥3 months	CD4+ <50-100 cells/μL	Documented disseminated disease	CD4+ >100 cells/μL sustained (eg, ≥6 months) and completed 12 months of MAC therapy, and asymptomatic for MAC	CD4+ <100 cells/μL
Cryptococcosis	None	Not applicable	Not applicable	Documented disease	CD4+ >100-200 cells/μL sustained (eg, ≥6 months) and completed initial therapy, and asymptomatic for cryptococcosis	CD4+ <100-200 cells/μL
Histoplasmosis	None	Not applicable	Not applicable	Documented disease	No criteria recommended for stopping	Not applicable
Coccidioidomycosis	None	Not applicable	Not applicable	Documented disease	No criteria recommended for stopping	Not applicable
Cytomegalovirus retinitis	None	Not applicable	Not applicable	Documented end-organ disease	CD4+ >100-150 cells/μL sustained (eg, ≥6 months) and no evidence of active disease, and regular ophthalmic examination	CD4+ <100-150 cells/μL

[1]The safety of discontinuing prophylaxis in children whose CD4+ counts have increased in response to HAART has not been studied.

USPHS / IDSA GUIDELINES FOR THE PREVENTION OF OPPORTUNISTIC INFECTIONS IN PERSONS INFECTED WITH HIV *(Continued)*

DRUG REGIMENS FOR INFANTS AND CHILDREN

Prophylaxis to Prevent First Episode of Opportunistic Disease in HIV-Infected Infants and Children

Pathogen	Indication	Preventive Regimens	
		First Choice	Alternatives
I. Strongly Recommended as Standard of Care			
Pneumocystis carinii[1]	HIV-infected or HIV-indeterminate infants 1-12 mo of age HIV-infected children 1-5 y of age with CD4+ count <500/μL or CD4+ percentage <15% HIV-infected children 6-12 y of age with CD4+ count <200/μL or CD4+ percentage <15%	TMP-SMZ, 150/750 mg/m²/day in 2 divided doses P.O. 3 times/week on consecutive days Acceptable alternative dosage schedules: • Single dose P.O. 3 times/week on consecutive days • 2 divided doses P.O. every day; 2 divided doses P.O. 3 times/week on alternate days	Dapsone (children ≥1 mo), 2 mg/kg (max: 100 mg) P.O. every day or 4 mg/kg (max: 200 mg) P.O. once weekly) Aerosolized pentamidine (children ≥5 y), 300 mg/mo via Respirgard II™ nebulizer Atovaquone (1-3 mo and >24 mo, 30 mg/kg P.O. every day; 4-24 mo, 45 mg/kg P.O. every day)
Mycobacterium tuberculosis[2]			
Isoniazid-sensitive	TST reaction, ≥5 mm *or* prior positive TST result without treatment **or contact** with any case of active tuberculosis **regardless of TST result**	Isoniazid, 10-15 mg/kg (max: 300 mg) P.O. every day x 9 mo or 20-30 mg/kg (max: 900 mg) P.O. twice weekly x 9 mo	Rifampin, 10-20 mg/kg (max: 600 mg) P.O. every day x 4-6 mo
Isoniazid-resistant	Same as above; high probability of exposure to isoniazid-resistant tuberculosis	Rifampin, 10-20 mg/kg (max: 600 mg) P.O. every day x 4-6 mo	Uncertain
Multidrug (isoniazid and rifampin)-resistant	Same as above; high probability of exposure to multidrug-resistant tuberculosis	Choice of drug requires consultation with public health authorities and depends on susceptibility of isolate from source patient	
Mycobacterium avium complex[2]	For children ≥6 y, CD4+ count <50/μL; 2-6 y, CD4+ count <75/μL; 1-2 y, CD4+ count <500/μL; <1 y, CD4+ count <750/μL	Clarithromycin, 7.5 mg/kg (max: 500 mg) P.O. twice daily, or azithromycin, 20 mg/kg (max: 1200 mg) P.O. weekly	Azithromycin, 5 mg/kg (max: 250 mg) P.O. every day; children ≥6 y, rifabutin, 300 mg P.O. every day
Varicella zoster virus[3]	Significant exposure to varicella or shingles with no history of chickenpox or shingles	Varicella zoster immune globulin (VZIG), 1 vial (1.25 mL)/10 kg (max: 5 vials) I.M., administered ≤96 hours after exposure, ideally within 48 hours	None
Vaccine-preventable pathogens[4]	HIV exposure/infection	Routine immunizations	None
II. Generally Recommended			
Influenza virus	All patients (annually, before influenza season)	Inactivated split trivalent influenza vaccine	Oseltamivir (during outbreaks of influenza A or B) for children ≥13 y, 75 mg P.O. every day; rimantadine or amantadine (during outbreaks of influenza A); 1-9 y, 5 mg/kg/day P.O. in 2 divided doses (max: 150 mg/day); ≥10 y, use adult doses
Varicella zoster virus	HIV-infected children who are asymptomatic and not immunosuppressed	Varicella zoster vaccine	None

Prophylaxis to Prevent First Episode of Opportunistic Disease in HIV-Infected Infants and Children (continued)

Pathogen	Indication	Preventive Regimens	
		First Choice	Alternatives
Toxoplasma gondii[5]	IgG antibody to Toxoplasma and severe immunosuppression	TMP-SMZ, 150/750 mg/m²/d in 2 divided doses P.O. every day	Dapsone (≥1 mo of age), 2 mg/kg or 15 mg/m² (max: 25 mg) P.O. every day *plus* pyrimethamine, 1 mg/kg P.O. every day *plus* leucovorin, 5 mg P.O. every 3 days
			Atovaquone (aged 1-3 mo and >24 mo, 30 mg/kg P.O. every day; aged 14-24 mo, 45 mg/kg P.O. every day)

III. Not Recommended for Most Children; Indicated for Use Only in Unusual Circumstances

Pathogen	Indication	First Choice	Alternatives
Invasive bacterial infections[6]	Hypogamma-globulinemia (ie, IgG <400 mg/dL)	IVIG (400 mg/kg every 2-4 weeks)	None
Cryptococcus neoformans	Severe immunosuppression	Fluconazole, 3-6 mg/kg P.O. every day	Itraconazole, 2-5 mg/kg P.O. every 12-24 hours
Histoplasma capsulatum	Severe immunosuppression, endemic geographic area	Itraconazole, 2-5 mg/kg P.O. every 12-24 hours	None
Cytomegalovirus (CMV)[7]	CMV antibody positivity and severe immunosuppression	Oral ganciclovir 30 mg/kg P.O. 3 times/day	None

Note: Information included in these guidelines may not represent FDA approval or approved labeling for the particular products or indications in question. Specifically, the terms "safe" and "effective" may not be synonymous with the FDA-defined legal standards for product approval. CMV = cytomegalovirus; IVIG = intravenous immune globulin; TMP-SMZ = trimethoprim-sulfamethoxazole; and VZIG = varicella zoster immune globulin. The Respirgard II™ nebulizer is manufactured by Marquest, Englewood, CO.

Daily TMP-SMZ reduces frequency of some bacterial infections. TMP-SMZ, dapsone-pyrimethamine, and possibly atovaquone (with or without pyrimethamine) appear to protect against toxoplasmosis, although data have not been prospectively collected. When compared with weekly dapsone, daily dapsone is associated with lower incidence of *Pneumocystis carinii* pneumonia (PCP) but higher hematologic toxicity and mortality (McIntosh K, Cooper E, Xu J, et al, "Toxicity and Efficacy of Daily vs Weekly Dapsone for Prevention of *Pneumocystis carinii* Pneumonia in Children Infected With HIV," *Ped Infect Dis J* 1999, 18:432-9.). Efficacy of parenteral pentamidine (eg, 4 mg/kg/every 2-4 weeks) is controversial. Patients receiving therapy for toxoplasmosis with sulfadiazine-pyrimethamine are protected against PCP and do not need TMP-SMZ.

[2]Significant drug interactions may occur between rifamycins (rifampin and rifabutin) and protease inhibitors, and non-nucleoside reverse transcriptase inhibitors. Consult a specialist.

[3]Children routinely being administered intravenous immune globulin (IVIG) should receive VZIG if the last dose of IVIG was administered >21 days before exposure.

[4]HIV-infected and HIV-exposed children should be immunized according to the childhood immunization schedule, which has been adapted from the January-December 2001 schedule recommended for immunocompetent children by the Advisory Committee on Immunization Practices, the American Academy of Pediatrics, and the American Academy of Family Physicians. This schedule differs from that for immunocompetent children in that both the conjugate pneumococcal vaccine (PCV-7) and the pneumococcal polysaccharide vaccine (PPV-23) are recommended and vaccination against influenza should be offered. MMR should not be administered to severely immunocompromised children. Vaccination against varicella is indicated only for asymptomatic nonimmunosuppressed children. Once an HIV-exposed child is determined not to be HIV infected, the schedule for immunocompetent children applies.

[5]Protection against toxoplasmosis is provided by the preferred antipneumocystis regimens and possibly by atovaquone. Atovaquone may be used with or without pyrimethamine. Pyrimethamine alone probably provides little, if any, protection.

[6]If available, respiratory syncytial virus (RSV) IVIG (750 mg/kg), not monoclonal RSV antibody, may be substituted for IVIG during RSV season to provide broad anti-infective protection.

[7]Oral ganciclovir and perhaps valganciclovir results in reduced CMV shedding in CMV-infected children. Acyclovir is not protective against CMV.

USPHS / IDSA GUIDELINES FOR THE PREVENTION OF OPPORTUNISTIC INFECTIONS IN PERSONS INFECTED WITH HIV *(Continued)*

Prophylaxis to Prevent Recurrence of Opportunistic Disease (After Chemotherapy for Acute Disease) in HIV-Infected Infants and Children

Pathogen	Indication	Preventive Regimens	
		First Choice	Alternatives
I. Recommended for Life as Standard of Care			
Pneumocystis carinii	Prior *P. carinii* pneumonia	TMP-SMZ, 150/750 mg/m^2/d in 2 divided doses P.O. 3 times/week on consecutive days Acceptable alternative schedules for same dosage Single dose P.O. 3 times/week on consecutive days; 2 divided doses P.O. daily; 2 divided doses P.O. 3 times/week on alternate days	Dapsone (children ≥1 mo of age), 2 mg/kg (max: 100 mg) P.O. once daily *or* 4 mg/kg (max: 200 mg) P.O. weekly; aerosolized pentamidine (children ≥5 y of age), 300 mg monthly via Respirgard II™ nebulizer; atovaquone (children 1-3 mo and >24 mo of age, 30 mg/kg P.O. every day; children 4-24 mo, 45 mg/kg P.O. every day)
Toxoplasma gondii[1]	Prior toxoplasmic encephalitis	Sulfadiazine, 85-120 mg/kg/d in 2-4 divided doses P.O. daily *plus* pyrimethamine, 1 mg/kg *or* 15 mg/m^2 (max: 25 mg) P.O. every day *plus* leucovorin, 5 mg P.O. every 3 days	Clindamycin, 20-30 mg/kg/d in 4 divided doses P.O. every day *plus* pyrimethamine, 1 mg/kg P.O. every day *plus* leucovorin, 5 mg P.O. every 3 days
Mycobacterium avium complex[2]	Prior disease	Clarithromycin, 7.5 mg/kg (max: 500 mg) P.O. twice daily *plus* ethambutol, 15 mg/kg (max: 900 mg) P.O. every day; with or without rifabutin, 5 mg/kg (max: 300 mg) P.O. once daily	Azithromycin, 5 mg/kg (max: 250 mg) P.O. every day *plus* ethambutol, 15 mg/kg (max: 900 mg) P.O. every day; with or without rifabutin, 5 mg/kg (max: 300 mg) P.O. once daily
Cryptococcus neoformans	Documented disease	Fluconazole, 3-6 mg/kg P.O. every day	Amphotericin B, 0.5-1 mg/kg I.V. 1-3 times/ week; itraconazole, 2-5 mg/kg P.O. every 12-24 hours
Histoplasma capsulatum	Documented disease	Itraconazole, 2-5 mg/kg P.O. every 12-48 hours	Amphotericin B, 1 mg/kg I.V. weekly
Coccidioides immitis	Documented disease	Fluconazole, 6 mg/kg P.O. every day	Amphotericin B, 1 mg/kg I.V. weekly; itraconazole, 2-5 mg/ kg P.O. every 12-48 hours
Cytomegalovirus	Prior end-organ disease	Ganciclovir, 5 mg/kg I.V. every day, *or* foscarnet, 90-120 mg/kg I.V. every day	(For retinitis) — ganciclovir sustained-release implant, every 6-9 mo *plus* ganciclovir, 30 mg/kg P.O. 3 times/d
Salmonella species (non-*typhi*)[3]	Bacteremia	TMP-SMZ, 150/750 mg/m^2 in 2 divided doses P.O. every day for several months	Antibiotic chemoprophylaxis with another active agent
II. Recommended Only if Subsequent Episodes Are Frequent or Severe			
Invasive bacterial infections[4]	>2 infections in 1-year period	TMP-SMZ, 150/750 mg/m^2 in 2 divided doses P.O. every day; *or* IVIG, 400 mg/kg every 2-4 weeks	Antibiotic chemoprophylaxis with another active agent
Herpes simplex virus	Frequent/ severe recurrences	Acyclovir, 80 mg/kg/d in 3-4 divided doses P.O. daily	
Candida (oropharyngeal)	Frequent/ severe recurrences	Fluconazole, 3-6 mg/kg P.O. every day	

Prophylaxis to Prevent Recurrence of Opportunistic Disease (After Chemotherapy for Acute Disease) in HIV-Infected Infants and Children (continued)

Pathogen	Indication	Preventive Regimens	
		First Choice	Alternatives
Candida (esophageal)	Frequent/ severe recurrences	Fluconazole, 3-6 mg/kg P.O. every day	Itraconazole solution, 5 mg/kg P.O. every day; ketoconazole, 5-10 mg/kg P.O. every 12-24 hours

Note: Information included in these guidelines may not represent Food and Drug Administration (FDA) approval or approved labeling for the particular products or indications in question. Specifically, the terms "safe" and "effective" may not be synonymous with the FDA-defined legal standards for product approval. IVIG = intravenous immune globulin and TMP-SMZ = trimethoprim-sulfamethoxazole. The Respirgard II™ nebulizer is manufactured by Marquest, Englewood, CO.

[1]Only pyrimethamine plus sulfadiazine confers protection against PCP as well as toxoplasmosis. Although the clindamycin plus pyrimethamine regimen is the preferred alternative in adults, it has not been tested in children. However, these drugs are safe and are used for other infections.

[2]Significant drug interactions may occur between rifabutin and protease inhibitors and non-nucleoside reverse transcriptase inhibitors. Consult an expert.

[3]Drug should be determined by susceptibilities of the organism isolated. Alternatives to TMP-SMZ include ampicillin, chloramphenicol, or ciprofloxacin. However, ciprofloxacin is not approved for use in persons aged <18 years; therefore, it should be used in children with caution and only if no alternatives exist.

[4]Antimicrobial prophylaxis should be chosen based on the microorganism and antibiotic sensitivities. TMP-SMZ, if used, should be administered daily. Providers should be cautious about using antibiotics solely for this purpose because of the potential for development of drug-resistant microorganisms. IVIG may not provide additional benefit to children receiving daily TMP-SMZ, but may be considered for children who have recurrent bacterial infections despite TMP-SMZ prophylaxis. Choice of antibiotic prophylaxis vs IVIG should also involve consideration of adherence, ease of intravenous access, and cost. If IVIG is used, RSV-IVIG (750 mg/kg), not monoclonal RSV antibody, may be substituted for IVIG during the RSV season to provide broad anti-infective protection, if this product is available.

ANIMAL AND HUMAN BITES

Bite Wound Antibiotic Regimens

	Dog Bite	Cat Bite	Human Bite
Prophylactic Antibiotics			
Prophylaxis	No routine prophylaxis, consider if involves face or hand, or immunosuppressed or asplenic patients	Routine prophylaxis	Routine prophylaxis
Prophylactic antibiotic	Amoxicillin	Amoxicillin	Amoxicillin
Penicillin allergy	Doxycycline if >10 y or co-trimoxazole	Doxycycline if >10 y or co-trimoxazole	Doxycycline if >10 y or erythromycin and cephalexin[1]
Outpatient Oral Antibiotic Treatment (mild to moderate infection)			
Established infection	Amoxicillin and clavulanic acid	Amoxicillin and clavulanic acid	Amoxicillin and clavulanic acid
Penicillin allergy (mild infection only)	Doxycycline if >10 y	Doxycycline if >10 y	Cephalexin[1] or clindamycin
Outpatient Parenteral Antibiotic Treatment (moderate infections – single drug regimens)			
	Ceftriaxone	Ceftriaxone	Cefotetan
Inpatient Parenteral Antibiotic Treatment			
Established infection	Ampicillin + cefazolin	Ampicillin + cefazolin	Ampicillin + clindamycin
Penicillin allergy	Cefazolin[1]	Ceftriaxone[1]	Cefotetan[1] or imipenem
Duration of Prophylactic and Treatment Regimens			
Prophylaxis: 5 days			
Treatment: 10-14 days			

[1]Contraindicated if history of immediate hypersensitivity reaction (anaphylaxis) to penicillin.

ANTIBIOTIC TREATMENT OF ADULTS WITH INFECTIVE ENDOCARDITIS

Table 1. Suggested Regimens for Therapy of Native Valve Endocarditis Due to Penicillin-Susceptible Viridans Streptococci and *Streptococcus bovis* (Minimum Inhibitory Concentration ≤0.1 mcg/mL)[1]

Antibiotic	Dosage and Route	Duration (wk)	Comments
Aqueous crystalline penicillin G sodium or	12-18 million units/24 h I.V. either continuously or in 6 equally divided doses	4	Preferred in most patients older than 65 y and in those with impairment of the eighth nerve or renal function
Ceftriaxone sodium	2 g once daily I.V. or I.M.[2]	4	
Aqueous crystalline penicillin G sodium	12-18 million units/24 h I.V. either continuously or in 6 equally divided doses	2	When obtained 1 hour after a 20- to 30-minute I.V. infusion or I.M. injection, serum concentration of gentamicin of approximately 3 mcg/mL is desirable; trough concentration should be <1 mcg/mL
With gentamicin sulfate[3]	1 mg/kg I.M. or I.V. every 8 hours	2	
Vancomycin hydrochloride[4]	30 mg/kg/24 h I.V. in 2 equally divided doses, not to exceed 2 g/ 24 h unless serum levels are monitored	4	Vancomycin therapy is recommended for patients allergic to β-lactams; peak serum concentrations of vancomycin should be obtained 1 h after completion of the infusion and should be in the range of 30-45 mcg/mL for twice-daily dosing

[1]Dosages recommended are for patients with normal renal function. For nutritionally variant streptococci, see Table 3. I.V. indicates intravenous; I.M., intramuscular.

[2]Patients should be informed that I.M. injection of ceftriaxone is painful.

[3]Dosing of gentamicin on a mg/kg basis will produce higher serum concentrations in obese patients than in lean patients. Therefore, in obese patients, dosing should be based on ideal body weight. (Ideal body weight for men is 50 kg + 2.3 kg per inch over 5 feet, and ideal body weight for women is 45.5 kg + 2.3 kg per inch over 5 feet.) Relative contraindications to the use of gentamicin are age >65 years, renal impairment, or impairment of the eighth nerve. Other potentially nephrotoxic agents (eg, nonsteroidal anti-inflammatory drugs) should be used cautiously in patients receiving gentamicin.

[4]Vancomycin dosage should be reduced in patients with impaired renal function. Vancomycin given on a mg/kg basis will produce higher serum concentrations in obese patients than in lean patients. Therefore, in obese patients, dosing should be based on ideal body weight. Each dose of vancomycin should be infused over at least 1 hour to reduce the risk of the histamine-release "red man" syndrome.

Table 2. Therapy for Native Valve Endocarditis Due to Strains of Viridans Streptococci and *Streptococcus bovis* Relatively Resistant to Penicillin G (Minimum Inhibitory Concentration >0.1 mcg/mL and <0.5 mcg/mL)[1]

Antibiotic	Dosage and Route	Duration (wk)	Comments
Aqueous crystalline penicillin G sodium	18 million units/24 h I.V. either continuously or in 6 equally divided doses	4	Cefazolin or other first-generation cephalosporins may be substituted for penicillin in patients whose penicillin hypersensitivity is not of the immediate type.
With gentamicin sulfate[2]	1 mg/kg I.M. or I.V. every 8 h	2	
Vancomycin hydrochloride[3]	30 mg/kg/24 h I.V. in 2 equally divided doses, not to exceed 2 g/ 24 h unless serum levels are monitored	4	Vancomycin therapy is recommended for patients allergic to β-lactams

[1]Dosages recommended are for patients with normal renal function. I.V. indicates intravenous; I.M., intramuscular.

[2]For specific dosing adjustment and issues concerning gentamicin (obese patients, relative contraindications), see Table 1 footnotes.

[3]For specific dosing adjustment and issues concerning vancomycin (obese patients, length of infusion), see Table 1 footnotes.

ANTIBIOTIC TREATMENT OF ADULTS WITH INFECTIVE ENDOCARDITIS *(Continued)*

Table 3. Standard Therapy for Endocarditis Due to Enterococci[1]

Antibiotic	Dosage and Route	Duration (wk)	Comments
Aqueous crystalline penicillin G sodium	18-30 million units/24 h I.V. either continuously or in 6 equally divided doses	4-6	4-week therapy recommended for patients with symptoms <3 months in duration; 6-week therapy recommended for patients with symptoms >3 months in duration.
With gentamicin sulfate[2]	1 mg/kg I.M. or I.V. every 8 h	4-6	
Ampicillin sodium	12 g/24 h I.V. either continuously or in 6 equally divided doses	4-6	
With gentamicin sulfate[2]	1 mg/kg I.M. or I.V. every 8 hours	4-6	
Vancomycin hydrochloride[2,3]	30 mg/kg/24 h I.V. in 2 equally divided doses, not to exceed 2 g/24 h unless serum levels are monitored	4-6	Vancomycin therapy is recommended for patients allergic to β-lactams; cephalosporins are not acceptable alternatives for patients allergic to penicillin
With gentamicin sulfate[2]	1 mg/kg I.M. or I.V. every 8 h	4-6	

[1]All enterococci causing endocarditis must be tested for antimicrobial susceptibility in order to select optimal therapy. This table is for endocarditis due to gentamicin- or vancomycin-susceptible enterococci, viridans streptococci with a minimum inhibitory concentration of >0.5 mcg/mL, nutritionally variant viridans streptococci, or prosthetic valve endocarditis caused by viridans streptococci or *Streptococcus bovis.* Antibiotic dosages are for patients with normal renal function. I.V. indicates intravenous; I.M., intramuscular.

[2]For specific dosing adjustment and issues concerning gentamicin (obese patients, relative contraindications), see Table 1 footnotes.

[3]For specific dosing adjustment and issues concerning vancomycin (obese patients, length of infusion), see Table 1 footnotes.

Table 4. Therapy for Endocarditis Due to *Staphylococcus* in the Absence of Prosthetic Material[1]

Antibiotic	Dosage and Route	Duration	Comments
Methicillin-Susceptible Staphylococci			
Regimens for non-β-lactam-allergic patients			
Nafcillin sodium or oxacillin sodium	2 g I.V. every 4 h	4-6 wk	Benefit of additional aminoglycosides has not been established
With optional addition of gentamicin sulfate[2]	1 mg/kg I.M. or I.V. every 8 h	3-5 d	
Regimens for β-lactam-allergic patients			
Cefazolin (or other first-generation cephalosporins in equivalent dosages)	2 g I.V. every 8 h	4-6 wk	Cephalosporins should be avoided in patients with immediate-type hypersensitivity to penicillin
With optional addition of gentamicin[2]	1 mg/kg I.M. or I.V. every 8 hours	3-5 d	
Vancomycin hydrochloride[3]	30 mg/kg/24 h I.V. in 2 equally divided doses, not to exceed 2 g/24 h unless serum levels are monitored	4-6 wk	Recommended for patients allergic to penicillin
Methicillin-Resistant Staphylococci			
Vancomycin hydrochloride[3]	30 mg/kg/24 h I.V. in 2 equally divided doses; not to exceed 2 g/24 h unless serum levels are monitored	4-6 wk	

[1]For treatment of endocarditis due to penicillin-susceptible staphylococci (minimum inhibitory concentration ≤0.1 mcg/mL), aqueous crystalline penicillin G sodium (Table 1, first regimen) can be used for 4-6 weeks instead of nafcillin or oxacillin. Shorter antibiotic courses have been effective in some drug addicts with right-sided endocarditis due to *Staphylococcus aureus.* I.V. indicates intravenous; I.M., intramuscular.

[2]For specific dosing adjustment and issues concerning gentamicin (obese patients, relative contraindications), see Table 1 footnotes.

[3]For specific dosing adjustment and issues concerning vancomycin (obese patients, length of infusion), see Table 1 footnotes.

Table 5. Treatment of Staphylococcal Endocarditis in the Presence of a Prosthetic Valve or Other Prosthetic Material[1]

Antibiotic	Dosage and Route	Duration (wk)	Comments
Regimen for Methicillin-Resistant Staphylococci			
Vancomycin hydrochloride[2]	30 mg/kg/24 h I.V. in 2 or 4 equally divided doses, not to exceed 2 g/24 h unless serum levels are monitored	≥6	
With rifampin[3]	300 mg orally every 8 h	≥6	Rifampin increases the amount of warfarin sodium required for antithrombotic therapy.
And with gentamicin sulfate[4,5]	1 mg/kg I.M. or I.V. every 8 h	2	
Regimen for Methicillin-Susceptible Staphylococci			
Nafcillin sodium or oxacillin sodium	2 g I.V. every 4 h	≥6	First-generation cephalosporins or vancomycin should be used in patients allergic to β-lactam. Cephalosporins should be avoided in patients with immediate-type hypersensitivity to penicillin or with methicillin-resistant staphylococci.
With rifampin[3]	300 mg orally every 8 h	≥6	
And with gentamicin sulfate[4,5]	1 mg/kg I.M. or I.V. every 8 h	2	

[1]Dosages recommended are for patients with normal renal function. I.V. indicates intravenous; I.M., intramuscular.

[2]For specific dosing adjustment and issues concerning vancomycin (obese patients, relative contraindications), see Table 1 footnotes.

[3]Rifampin plays a unique role in the eradication of staphylococcal infection involving prosthetic material; combination therapy is essential to prevent emergence of rifampin resistance.

[4]For a specific dosing adjustment and issues concerning gentamicin (obese patients, relative contraindications), see Table 1 footnotes.

[5]Use during initial 2 weeks.

Table 6. Therapy for Endocarditis Due to HACEK Microorganisms (*Haemophilus parainfluenzae, Haemophilus aphrophilus, Actinobacillus actinomycetemcomitans, Cardiobacterium hominus, Eikenella corrodens,* and *Kingella kingae*)[1]

Antibiotic	Dosage and Route	Duration (wk)	Comments
Ceftriaxone sodium[2]	2 g once daily I.V. or I.M.[2]	4	Cefotaxime sodium or other third-generation cephalosporins may be substituted
Ampicillin sodium[3]	12 g/24 h I.V. either continuously or in 6 equally divided doses	4	
With gentamicin sulfate[4]	1 mg/kg I.M. or I.V. every 6 h	4	

[1]Antibiotic dosages are for patients with normal renal function. I.V. indicates intravenous; I.M. intramuscular.

[2]Patients should be informed that I.M. injection of ceftriaxone is painful.

[3]Ampicillin should not be used if laboratory tests show β-lactamase production.

[4]For specific dosing adjustment and issues concerning gentamicin (obese patients, relative contraindications), see Table 1 footnotes.

Note: Tables 1-6 are from Wilson WR, Karchmer AW, Dajani AS, et al, "Antibiotic Treatment of Adults With Infective Endocarditis Due to Streptococci, Enterococci, Staphylococci, and HACEK Microorganisms," *JAMA*, 1995, 274(21):1706-13, with permission.

ANTIMICROBIAL DRUGS OF CHOICE

The following table lists the antibacterial drugs of choice for various infecting organisms. This table is reprinted with permission from *The Medical Letter*, 2001, 43(1111-1112):69-78. Users should not assume that all antibiotics which are appropriate for a given organism are listed or that those not listed are inappropriate. The infection caused by the organism may encompass varying degrees of severity, and since the antibiotics listed may not be appropriate for the differing degrees of severity, or because of other patient-related factors, it cannot be assumed that the antibiotics listed for any specific organism are interchangeable. This table should not be used by itself without first referring to *The Medical Letter*, an infectious disease manual, or the infectious disease department. Therefore, only use this table as a tool for obtaining more information about the therapies available.

Infecting Organism	Drug of First Choice	Alternative Drugs
GRAM-POSITIVE COCCI		
Enterococcus[1]		
endocarditis or other severe infection	Penicillin G or ampicillin + gentamicin or streptomycin[2]	Vancomycin + gentamicin or streptomycin[2]; linezolid; quinupristin/dalfopristin
uncomplicated urinary tract infection	Ampicillin or amoxicillin	Nitrofurantoin; a fluoroquinolone[3]; fosfomycin
Staphylococcus aureus or *epidermidis*		
methicillin-sensitive	A penicillinase-resistant penicillin[4]	A cephalosporin[5,6]; vancomycin; amoxicillin/clavulanic acid; ticarcillin/clavulanic acid; piperacillin/tazobactam; ampicillin/sulbactam; imipenem or meropenem; clindamycin; a fluoroquinolone[3]
methicillin-resistant[7]	Vancomycin ± gentamicin ± rifampin	Linezolid; quinupristin/dalfopristin; a fluoroquinolone[3]; a tetracycline[8]; trimethoprim-sulfamethoxazole
Streptococcus pyogenes (group A[9]) and groups C and G	Penicillin G or V[10]	Clindamycin; erythromycin; a cephalosporin[5,6]; vancomycin; clarithromycin[11]; azithromycin
Streptococcus, group B	Penicillin G or ampicillin	A cephalosporin[5,6]; vancomycin; erythromycin
Streptococcus, viridans group[1]	Penicillin G ± gentamicin	A cephalosporin[5,6]; vancomycin
Streptococcus bovis	Penicillin G	A cephalosporin[5,6]; vancomycin
Streptococcus, anaerobic or *Peptostreptococcus*	Penicillin G	Clindamycin; a cephalosporin[5,6]; vancomycin
Streptococcus pneumoniae[12] (pneumococcus), penicillin-susceptible (MIC <0.1 mcg/mL)	Penicillin G or V[10]; amoxicillin	A cephalosporin[5,6]; erythromycin; azithromycin; clarithromycin[11]; levofloxacin[13]; gatifloxacin[13] or moxifloxacin[13]; meropenem; imipenem; trimethoprim-sulfamethoxazole; clindamycin; a tetracycline[8]
penicillin-intermediate resistance (MIC 0.1-≤2 mcg/mL)	Penicillin G I.V. (12 million units/day for adults); ceftriaxone or cefotaxime	Levofloxacin[13]; gatifloxacin[13] or moxifloxacin[13]; vancomycin; clindamycin
penicillin-high level resistance (MIC ≥2 mcg/mL)	**Meningitis:** Vancomycin + ceftriaxone or cefotaxime ± rifampin	Meropenem; imipenem
	Other Infections: Vancomycin + ceftriaxone or cefotaxime; or levofloxacin,[13] gatifloxacin[13] or moxifloxacin[13]	Linezolid; quinupristin/dalfopristin
GRAM-NEGATIVE COCCI		
Moraxella (Branhamella) catarrhalis	Cefuroxime[5]; a fluoroquinolone[3]	Trimethoprim-sulfamethoxazole; amoxicillin/clavulanic acid; erythromycin; a tetracycline[8]; cefotaxime[5]; ceftizoxime[5]; ceftriaxone[5]; cefuroxime axetil[5]; cefixime[5]; cefpodoxime[5]; clarithromycin[11]; azithromycin

Infecting Organism	Drug of First Choice	Alternative Drugs
Neisseria gonorrhoeae (gonococcus)[14]	Ceftriaxone[5] or cefixime[5]; or ciprofloxacin,[13] gatifloxacin[13] or ofloxacin[13]	Cefotaxime[5]; penicillin G
Neisseria meningitidis[15] (meningococcus)	Penicillin G	Cefotaxime[5]; ceftizoxime[5]; ceftriaxone[5]; chloramphenicol[16]; a sulfonamide[17]; a fluoroquinolone[3]

GRAM-POSITIVE BACILLI

Bacillus anthracis (anthrax)	Penicillin G	Ciprofloxacin[13]; erythromycin; a tetracycline[8]
Bacillus cereus, subtilis	Vancomycin	Imipenem or meropenem; clindamycin
Clostridium perfringens[18]	Penicillin G; clindamycin	Metronidazole; imipenem or meropenem; chloramphenicol[16]
Clostridium tetani[19]	Metronidazole	Penicillin G; a tetracycline[8]
Clostridium difficile[20]	Metronidazole	Vancomycin (oral)
Corynebacterium diphtheriae[21]	Erythromycin	Penicillin G
Corynebacterium, JK group	Vancomycin	Penicillin G + gentamicin; erythromycin
Erysipelothrix rhusiopethiae	Penicillin G	Erythromycin, a cephalosporin[5,6]; a fluoroquinolone[3]
Listeria monocytogenes	Ampicillin ± gentamicin	Trimethoprim-sulfamethoxazole

ENTERIC GRAM-NEGATIVE BACILLI

Bacteroides	Metronidazole or clindamycin	Imipenem or meropenem; amoxicillin/clavulanic acid; ticarcillin/clavulanic acid; piperacillin/tazobactam; ampicillin/sulbactam; cefoxitin[5]; cefotetan[5]; chloramphenicol[16]; cefmetazole[5]; penicillin G; gatifloxacin[13] or moxifloxacin[13]
Campylobacter fetus	Imipenem or meropenem	Gentamicin
Campylobacter jejuni	Erythromycin or azithromycin	A fluoroquinolone[2]; a tetracycline[8]; gentamicin
Citrobacter freundii	Imipenem or meropenem[22]	A fluoroquinolone[3]; amikacin; a tetracycline[8]; trimethoprim-sulfamethoxazole; cefotaxime[5,22]; ceftizoxime[5,22]; ceftriaxone[5,22]; cefepime[5,22] or ceftazidime[5,22]
Enterobacter	Imipenem or meropenem[22]	Gentamicin, tobramycin or amikacin; trimethoprim-sulfamethoxazole; ciprofloxacin[13]; ticarcillin[23]; mezlocillin[23] or piperacillin[23]; aztreonam[22]; cefotaxime[5,22]; ceftizoxime[5,22]; ceftriaxone[5,22]; cefepime[5,22] or ceftazidime[5,22]
Escherichia coli[24]	Cefotaxime, ceftizoxime, ceftriaxone, cefepime or ceftazidime[5,22]	Ampicillin ± gentamicin, tobramycin or amikacin; carbenicillin[23]; ticarcillin[23]; mezlocillin[23] or piperacillin[23]; gentamicin, tobramycin or amikacin; amoxicillin/clavulanic acid[22]; ticarcillin/clavulanic acid[23]; piperacillin/tazobactam[23]; ampicillin/sulbactam[22]; trimethoprim/sulfamethoxazole; imipenem or meropenem[22]; aztreonam[22]; a fluoroquinolone[3]; another cephalosporin[5,6]
Helicobacter pylori[25]	Omeprazole + amoxicillin + clarithromycin; or tetracycline HCl[8] + metronidazole + bismuth subsalicylate	Tetracycline HCl[8] + clarithromycin[11] + bismuth subsalicylate; amoxicillin + metronidazole + bismuth subsalicylate; amoxicillin + clarithromycin[11]

ANTIMICROBIAL DRUGS OF CHOICE (Continued)

Infecting Organism	Drug of First Choice	Alternative Drugs
*Klebsiella pneumoniae[24]	Cefotaxime, ceftizoxime, ceftriaxone, cefepime or ceftazidime[5,22]	Imipenem or meropenem[22]; gentamicin, tobramycin or amikacin; amoxicillin/clavulanic acid[22]; ticarcillin/clavulanic acid[23]; piperacillin/tazobactam[23]; ampicillin sulbactam[22]; trimethoprim-sulfamethoxazole; aztreonam[22]; a fluoroquinolone[3]; mezlocillin[23] or piperacillin[23]; another cephalosporin[5,6]
*Proteus mirabilis[24]	Ampicillin[26]	A cephalosporin[5,6,22]; ticarcillin[23]; mezlocillin[23] or piperacillin[23]; gentamicin, tobramycin, or amikacin; trimethoprim-sulfamethoxazole; imipenem or meropenem[22]; aztreonam[23]; a fluoroquinolone[3]; chloramphenicol[16]
Proteus, indole-positive (including Providencia rettgeri, Morganella morganii, and Proteus vulgaris)	Cefotaxime, ceftizoxime, ceftriaxone, cefepime, or ceftazidime[5,22]	Imipenem or meropenem[22]; gentamicin, tobramycin, or amikacin; carbenicillin[23]; ticarcillin[23]; mezlocillin[23] or piperacillin[23]; amoxicillin/clavulanic acid[22]; ticarcillin/clavulanic acid[23]; piperacillin/tazobactam[23]; ampicillin/sulbactam[22]; aztreonam[22]; trimethoprim-sulfamethoxazole; a fluoroquinolone[3]
*Providencia stuartii	Cefotaxime, ceftizoxime, ceftriaxone, cefepime, or ceftazidime[5,22]	Imipenem or meropenem[22]; ticarcillin/clavulanic acid[23]; piperacillin/tazobactam[23]; gentamicin, tobramycin, or amikacin; carbenicillin[23]; ticarcillin,[23] mezlocillin,[23] or piperacillin[23]; aztreonam[22]; trimethoprim-sulfamethoxazole; a fluoroquinolone[3]
*Salmonella typhi[27] (typhoid fever)	A fluoroquinolone[3] or ceftriaxone[5]	Chloramphenicol[16]; trimethoprim-sulfamethoxazole; ampicillin; amoxicillin; azithromycin[28]
*other Salmonella[29]	Cefotaxime[5] or ceftriaxone[5] or a fluoroquinolone[3]	Ampicillin or amoxicillin; trimethoprim-sulfamethoxazole; chloramphenicol[16]
*Serratia	Imipenem or meropenem[22]	Gentamicin or amikacin; cefotaxime, ceftizoxime, ceftriaxone, cefepime, or ceftazidime[5,22]; aztreonam[22]; trimethoprim-sulfamethoxazole; carbenicillin[30], ticarcillin[30], mezlocillin[30] or piperacillin[30]; a fluoroquinolone[3]
*Shigella	A fluoroquinolone[3]	Azithromycin; trimethoprim-sulfamethoxazole; ampicillin; ceftriaxone[5]
*Yersinia enterocolitica	Trimethoprim-sulfamethoxazole	A fluoroquinolone[3]; gentamicin, tobramycin, or amikacin; cefotaxime or ceftizoxime[5]

OTHER GRAM-NEGATIVE BACILLI

Infecting Organism	Drug of First Choice	Alternative Drugs
*Acinetobacter	Imipenem or meropenem[22]	An aminoglycoside; ciprofloxacin[13]; trimethoprim-sulfamethoxazole; ticarcillin,[23] mezlocillin[23], or piperacillin[23]; ceftazidime[22]; minocycline[8]; doxycycline[8]; sulbactam[31]; polymyxin
*Aeromonas	Trimethoprim-sulfamethoxazole	Gentamicin or tobramycin; imipenem; a fluoroquinolone[3]
Bartonella henselae or quintana (bacillary angiomatosis)	Erythromycin	Doxycycline[8]; azithromycin
Bartonella henselae[32] (cat scratch bacillus)	Azithromycin	Ciprofloxacin[13]; erythromycin; trimethoprim-sulfamethoxazole; gentamicin; rifampin
Bordetella pertussis (whooping cough)	Erythromycin	Azithromycin or clarithromycin[11]; trimethoprim-sulfamethoxazole
*Brucella	A tetracycline[8] + rifampin	A tetracycline[8] + streptomycin or gentamicin; chloramphenicol[16] ± streptomycin; trimethoprim-sulfamethoxazole ± gentamicin; ciprofloxacin[13] + rifampin

Infecting Organism	Drug of First Choice	Alternative Drugs
*Burkholderia cepacia	Trimethoprim-sulfamethoxazole	Ceftazidime[5]; chloramphenicol[16]; imipenem
Burkholderia (Pseudomonas) mallei (glanders)	Streptomycin + a tetracycline[8]	Streptomycin + chloramphenicol[16]; imipenem
*Burkholderia (Pseudomonas) pseudomallei (melioidosis)	Imipenem; ceftazidime[5]	Meropenem; chloramphenicol[16] + doxycycline[8] + trimethoprim-sulfamethoxazole; amoxicillin/clavulanic acid
Calymmatobacterium granulomatis (granuloma inguinale)	Trimethoprim-sulfamethoxazole	Doxycycline[8] or ciprofloxacin[13] ± gentamicin
Capnocytophaga canimorsus[33]	Penicillin G	Cefotaxime[5]; ceftizoxime[5]; ceftriaxone[5]; imipenem or meropenem; vancomycin; a fluoroquinolone[3]; clindamycin
*Eikenella corrodens	Ampicillin	An erythromycin; a tetracycline[8]; amoxicillin/clavulanic acid; ampicillin/sulbactam; ceftriaxone[5]
*Francisella tularensis (tularemia)	Streptomycin	Gentamicin; a tetracycline[8]; chloramphenicol[16]; ciprofloxacin[13]
*Fusobacterium	Penicillin G	Metronidazole; clindamycin; cefoxitin[5]; chloramphenicol[16]
Gardnerella vaginalis (bacterial vaginosis)	Oral metronidazole[34]	Topical clindamycin or metronidazole; oral clindamycin
*Haemophilus ducreyi (chancroid)	Azithromycin or ceftriaxone	Ciprofloxacin[13] or erythromycin
*Haemophilus influenzae		
meningitis, epiglottitis, arthritis, and other serious infections	Cefotaxime or ceftriaxone	Cefuroxime[5] (not for meningitis); chloramphenicol[16]; meropenem
upper respiratory infections and bronchitis	Trimethoprim-sulfamethoxazole	Cefuroxime[5]; amoxicillin/clavulanic acid; cefuroxime axetil[5]; cefpodoxime[5]; cefaclor[5]; cefotaxime[5]; ceftizoxime[5]; ceftriaxone[5]; cefixime[5]; a tetracycline[8]; clarithromycin[11]; azithromycin; a fluoroquinolone[3]; ampicillin or amoxicillin
Legionella species	Azithromycin or a fluoroquinolone[3] ± rifampin	Doxycycline[8] ± rifampin; trimethoprim-sulfamethoxazole; erythromycin
Leptotrichia buccalis	Penicillin G	A tetracycline[8]; clindamycin; erythromycin
Pasteurella multocida	Penicillin G	A tetracycline[8]; a cephalosporin[5,6]; amoxicillin/clavulanic acid; ampicillin/sulbactam
*Pseudomonas aeruginosa		
urinary tract infection	Ciprofloxacin[13]	Levofloxacin[13]; carbenicillin, ticarcillin, piperacillin, or mezlocillin; ceftazidime[5]; cefepime[5]; imipenem or meropenem; aztreonam; tobramycin; gentamicin; amikacin
other infections	Ticarcillin, mezlocillin, or piperacillin + tobramycin, gentamicin, or amikacin[35]	Ceftazidime[5], imipenem, meropenem, aztreonam, cefepime[5] + tobramycin, gentamicin, or amikacin; ciprofloxacin[13]
Spirillum minus (rat bite fever)	Penicillin G	A tetracycline[8]; streptomycin
*Stenotrophomonas maltophilia	Trimethoprim-sulfamethoxazole	Minocycline[8]; a fluoroquinolone[3]
Streptobacillus moniliformis (rat bite fever, Haverhill fever)	Penicillin G	A tetracycline[8]; streptomycin
Vibrio cholerae (cholera)[36]	A tetracycline[8]	A fluoroquinolone[3]; trimethoprim-sulfamethoxazole
Vibrio vulnificus	A tetracycline[8]	Cefotaxime[5]
Yersinia pestis (plague)	Streptomycin ± a tetracycline[8]	Chloramphenicol[16]; gentamicin; trimethoprim-sulfamethoxazole
ACID-FAST BACILLI		
*Mycobacterium tuberculosis	Isoniazid + rifampin + pyrazinamide ± ethambutol or streptomycin[16]	A fluoroquinolone[3]; cycloserine[16]; capreomycin[16] or kanamycin[16] or amikacin[16]; ethionamide[16]; para-aminosalicylic acid[16]; ± clofazimine[16]

ANTIMICROBIAL DRUGS OF CHOICE *(Continued)*

Infecting Organism	Drug of First Choice	Alternative Drugs
Mycobacterium kansasii	Isoniazid + rifampin ± ethambutol or streptomycin[16]	Clarithromycin[11] or azithromycin; ethionamide[16]; cycloserine[16]
Mycobacterium avium complex	Clarithromycin[11] or azithromycin + ethambutol ± rifabutin	Ciprofloxacin[13]; amikacin[16]
prophylaxis	Clarithromycin[11] or azithromycin ± rifabutin	
Mycobacterium fortuitum/ chelonae complex	Amikacin + clarithromycin[11]	Cefoxitin[5]; rifampin; a sulfonamide; doxycycline[8]; ethambutol; linezolid
Mycobacterium marinum (balnei)[37]	Minocycline[8]	Trimethoprim-sulfamethoxazole; rifampin; clarithromycin[11]; doxycycline[8]
Mycobacterium leprae (leprosy)	Dapsone + rifampin ± clofazimine	Minocycline[8]; ofloxacin[13]; sparfloxacin[13]; clarithromycin[11]

ACTINOMYCETES

Infecting Organism	Drug of First Choice	Alternative Drugs
Actinomyces israelii (actinomycosis)	Penicillin G	A tetracycline[8]; erythromycin; clindamycin
Nocardia	Trimethoprim-sulfamethoxazole	Sulfisoxazole; amikacin[16]; a tetracycline[8]; imipenem or meropenem; cycloserine[16]; linezolid
Rhodococcus equi	Vancomycin ± a fluoroquinolone[3], rifampin, imipenem or meropenem; amikacin	Erythromycin
Tropheryma whippelii (agent of Whipple's disease)	Trimethoprim-sulfamethoxazole	Penicillin G; a tetracycline[8]

CHLAMYDIAE

Infecting Organism	Drug of First Choice	Alternative Drugs
Chlamydia psittaci (psittacosis, ornithosis)	A tetracycline[8]	Chloramphenicol[16]
Chlamydia trachomatis		
(trachoma)	Azithromycin	A tetracycline[8] (topical plus oral); a sulfonamide (topical plus oral)
(inclusion conjunctivitis)	Erythromycin (oral or I.V.)	A sulfonamide
(pneumonia)	Erythromycin	A sulfonamide
(urethritis, cervicitis)	Azithromycin or doxycycline[8]	Erythromycin; ofloxacin[13]; amoxicillin
(lymphogranuloma venereum)	A tetracycline[8]	Erythromycin
Chlamydia pneumoniae (TWAR strain)	Erythromycin; a tetracycline[8]; clarithromycin[11] or azithromycin	A fluoroquinolone[3]

EHRLICHIA

Infecting Organism	Drug of First Choice	Alternative Drugs
Ehrlichia chaffeensis	Doxycycline[8]	Chloramphenicol[16]
Ehrlichia ewingii	Doxycycline[8]	
Ehrlichia phagocytophila	Doxycycline[8]	Rifampin

MYCOPLASMA

Infecting Organism	Drug of First Choice	Alternative Drugs
Mycoplasma pneumoniae	Erythromycin; a tetracycline[8]; clarithromycin[11] or azithromycin	A fluoroquinolone[3]
Ureaplasma urealyticum	Erythromycin	A tetracycline[8]; clarithromycin[11]; azithromycin; ofloxacin[13]
RICKETTSIA – Rocky Mountain spotted fever, endemic typhus (murine), epidemic typhus (louse-borne), scrub typhus (*Orientia tsutsugamushi*), trench fever, Q fever	Doxycycline[8]	Chloramphenicol[16]; a fluoroquinolone[3]; rifampin

Infecting Organism	Drug of First Choice	Alternative Drugs
SPIROCHETES		
Borrelia burgdorferi (Lyme disease)[36]	Doxycycline[8]; amoxicillin; cefuroxime axetil[5]	Ceftriaxone[5]; cefotaxime[5]; penicillin G; azithromycin; clarithromycin[11]
Borrelia recurrentis (relapsing fever)	A tetracycline[8]	Penicillin G
Leptospira	Penicillin G	A tetracycline[8]
Treponema pallidum (syphilis)	Penicillin G[10]	A tetracycline[8]; ceftriaxone[5]
Treponema pertenue (yaws)	Penicillin G	A tetracycline[8]

*Resistance may be a problem; susceptibility tests should be used to guide therapy.

[1]Disk sensitivity testing may not provide adequate information; beta-lactamase assays, "E" tests, and dilution tests for susceptibility should be used in serious infections.

[2]Aminoglycoside resistance is increasingly common among enterococci; treatment options include ampicillin 2 g I.V. q4h, continuous infusion of ampicillin, a combination of ampicillin plus a fluoroquinolone, or a combination of ampicillin, imipenem, and vancomycin.

[3]Among the fluoroquinolones, levofloxacin, gatifloxacin, and moxifloxacin have excellent *in vitro* activity against *S. pneumoniae*, including penicillin- and cephalosporin-resistant strains. Levofloxacin, gatifloxacin, and moxifloxacin also have good activity against many strains of *S. aureus*, but resistance has become frequent among methicillin-resistant strains. Ciprofloxacin has the greatest activity against *Pseudomonas aeruginosa*. For urinary tract infections, norfloxacin, lomefloxacin, or enoxacin can be used. For tuberculosis, levofloxacin, ofloxacin, ciprofloxacin, gatifloxacin, or moxifloxacin could be used. Ciprofloxacin, ofloxacin, levofloxacin, and gatifloxacin are available for intravenous use. None of these agents are recommended for children or pregnant women.

[4]For oral use against staphylococci, cloxacillin or dicloxacillin is preferred; for severe infections, a parenteral formulation of nafcillin or oxacillin should be used. Ampicillin, amoxicillin, carbenicillin, ticarcillin, and piperacillin are not effective against penicillinase-producing staphylococci. The combinations of clavulanic acid with amoxicillin or ticarcillin, sulbactam with ampicillin, and tazobactam with piperacillin may be active against these organisms.

[5]The cephalosporins have been used as alternatives to penicillins in patients allergic to penicillins, but such patients may also have allergic reactions to cephalosporins.

[6]For parenteral treatment of staphylococcal or nonenterococcal streptococcal infections, a first-generation cephalosporin such as cefazolin can be used. For oral therapy, cephalexin or cephradine can be used. The second-generation cephalosporins cefamandole, cefprozil, cefuroxime, cefonicid, cefotetan, cefmetazole, cefoxitin, and loracarbef are more active than the first-generation drugs against gram-negative bacteria. Cefuroxime is active against ampicillin-resistant strains of *H. influenzae*. Cefoxitin, cefotetan, and cefmetazole are the most active of the cephalosporins against *B. fragilis*, but cefotetan and cefmetazole have been associated with prothrombin deficiency. The third-generation cephalosporins cefotaxime, cefoperazone, ceftizoxime, ceftriaxone, and ceftazidime, and the "fourth-generation" cefepime have greater activity than the second-generation drugs against enteric gram-negative bacilli. Ceftazidime has poor activity against many gram-positive cocci and anaerobes, and ceftizoxime has poor activity against penicillin-resistant *S. pneumoniae*. Cefepime has *in vitro* activity against gram-positive cocci similar to cefotaxime and ceftriaxone and somewhat greater activity against enteric gram-negative bacilli. The activity of cefepime against *Pseudomonas aeruginosa* is similar to that of ceftazidime. Cefixime, cefpodoxime, cefdinir, and ceftibuten are oral cephalosporins with more activity than second-generation cephalosporins against facultative gram-negative bacilli; they have no useful activity against anaerobes or *P. aeruginosa*, and cefixime and ceftibuten have no useful activity against staphylococci. With the exception of cefoperazone (which, like cefamandole, can cause bleeding), ceftazidime and cefepime, the activity of all currently available cephalosporins against *P. aeruginosa* is poor or inconsistent.

[7]Many strains of coagulase-positive staphylococci and coagulase-negative staphylococci are resistant to penicillinase-resistant penicillins; these strains are also resistant to cephalosporins, imipenem, and meropenem, and are often resistant to fluoroquinolones, trimethoprim/sulfamethoxazole, and clindamycin.

[8]Tetracyclines are generally not recommended for pregnant women or children younger than 8 years old.

[9]For serious soft-tissue infection due to group A streptococci, clindamycin may be more effective than penicillin. Group A streptococci may, however, be resistant to clindamycin; therefore, some *Medical Letter* consultants suggest using both clindamycin and penicillin, with or without I.V. immune globulin, to treat serious soft-tissue infections. Group A streptococci may also be resistant to erythromycin, azithromycin, and clarithromycin.

[10]Penicillin V (or amoxicillin) is preferred for oral treatment of infections caused by nonpenicillinase-producing streptococci. For initial therapy of severe infections, penicillin G, administered parenterally, is first choice. For somewhat longer action in less severe infections due to group A streptococci, pneumococci or *Treponema pallidum*, procaine penicillin G, an intramuscular formulation, can be given once or twice daily, but is seldom used now. Benzathine penicillin G, a slowly absorbed preparation, is usually given in a single monthly injection for prophylaxis of rheumatic fever, once for treatment of group A streptococcal pharyngitis and once or more for treatment of syphilis.

[11]Not recommended for use in pregnancy.

[12]Some strains of *S. pneumoniae* are resistant to erythromycin, clindamycin, trimethoprim-sulfamethoxazole, clarithromycin, azithromycin and chloramphenicol, and resistance to the newer fluoroquinolones is increasing. Nearly all strains tested so far are susceptible to linezolid and quinupristin/dalfopristin *in vitro* (Patel R, Rouse MS, Piper KE, et al, "*In Vitro* Activity of Linezolid Against Vancomycin-Resistant Enterococci, Methicillin-Resistant *Staphylococcus aureus* and Penicillin-Resistant *Streptococcus pneumoniae*," *Diagn Microbiol Infect Dis*, 1999, 34(2):119-22; Verhaegen J and Verbist L, "*In Vitro* Activities of 16 Non-beta-lactam Antibiotics Against Penicillin-Susceptible and Penicillin-Resistant *Streptococcus pneumoniae*," *J Antimicrob Chemother*, 1999, 43(4):563-7.

[13]Usually not recommended for use in children or pregnant women.

[14]Patients with gonorrhea should be treated presumptively for coinfection with *C. trachomatis* with azithromycin or doxycycline.

[15]Rare strains of *N. meningitidis* are resistant or relatively resistant to penicillin. A fluoroquinolone or rifampin is recommended for prophylaxis after close contact with infected patients.

[16]Because of the possibility of serious adverse effects, this drug should be used only for severe infections when less hazardous drugs are ineffective.

[17]Sulfonamide-resistant strains are frequent in the U.S.A; sulfonamides should be used only when susceptibility is established by susceptibility tests.

ANTIMICROBIAL DRUGS OF CHOICE *(Continued)*

[18]Debridement is primary. Large doses of penicillin G are required. Hyperbaric oxygen therapy may be a useful adjunct to surgical debridement in management of the spreading, necrotizing type of infection.

[19]For prophylaxis, a tetanus toxoid booster and, for some patients, tetanus immune globulin (human) are required.

[20]In order to decrease the emergence of vancomycin-resistant enterococci in hospitals and to reduce costs, most clinicians now recommend use of metronidazole first in treatment of patients with *C. difficile* colitis, with oral vancomycin used only for seriously ill patients or those who do not respond to metronidazole.

[21]Antitoxin is primary; antimicrobials are used only to halt further toxin production and to prevent the carrier state.

[22]In severely ill patients, most *Medical Letter* consultants would add gentamicin, tobramycin, or amikacin.

[23]In severely ill patients, most *Medical Letter* consultants would add gentamicin, tobramycin, or amikacin (but see footnote 35).

[24]For an acute, uncomplicated urinary tract infection, before the infecting organism is known, the drug of first choice is trimethoprim-sulfamethoxazole.

[25]Eradication of *H. pylori* with various antibacterial combinations, given concurrently with an H_2-receptor blocker or proton pump inhibitor, has led to rapid healing of active peptic ulcers and low recurrence rates (Mégraud F and Marshall BJ, "How to Treat *Helicobacter pylori*. First-line, Second-line, and Future Therapies," *Gastroenterol Clin North Am*, 2000, 29(4):759-73.

[26]Large doses (6 g or more daily) are usually necessary for systemic infections. In severely ill patients, some *Medical Letter* consultants would add gentamicin, tobramycin, or amikacin.

[27]A fluoroquinolone or amoxicillin is the drug of choice for *S. typhi* carriers.

[28]Frenck RW Jr, Nakhla I, Sultan Y, et al, "Azithromycin Versus Ceftriaxone for the Treatment of Uncomplicated Typhoid Fever in Children," *Clin Infect Dis*, 2000, 31(5):1134-8.

[29]Most cases of *Salmonella* gastroenteritis subside spontaneously without antimicrobial therapy. Immunosuppressed patients, young children, and the elderly may benefit the most from antibacterials.

[30]In severely ill patients, most *Medical Letter* consultants would add gentamicin or amikacin (but see footnote 35).

[31]Sulbactam may be useful to treat multidrug resistant *Acinetobacter*. It is only available in combination with ampicillin as Unasyn®. *Medical Letter* consultants recommend 3 g I.V. q4h.

[32]Role of antibiotics is not clear (Conrad DA, "Treatment of Cat-Scratch Disease," *Curr Opin Pediatr*, 2001, 13(1):56-9.

[33]Pers C, Gahrn-Hansen B, Frederiksen W, et al, "*Capnocytophaga canimorsus* Septicemia in Denmark, 1982-1995: Review of 39 Cases," *Clin Infect Dis*, 1996, 23(1):71-5.

[34]Metronidazole is effective for bacterial vaginosis even though it is not usually active *in vitro* against *Gardnerella*.

[35]Neither gentamicin, tobramycin, netilmicin, or amikacin should be mixed in the same bottle with carbenicillin, ticarcillin, mezlocillin, or piperacillin for intravenous administration. When used in high doses or in patients with renal impairment, these penicillins may inactivate the aminoglycosides.

[36]Antibiotic therapy is an adjunct to and not a substitute for prompt fluid and electrolyte replacement.

[37]Most infections are self-limited without drug treatment.

[38]For treatment of erythema migrans, facial nerve palsy, mild cardiac disease, and some cases of arthritis, oral therapy is satisfactory; for more serious neurologic or cardiac disease or arthritis, parenteral therapy with ceftriaxone, cefotaxime, or penicillin G is recommended (*Medical Letter*, 2000, 42:37).

ANTIRETROVIRAL THERAPY FOR HIV INFECTION

Report of the NIH Panel to Define Principles of Therapy of HIV Infection

GUIDELINES FOR THE USE OF ANTIRETROVIRAL AGENTS IN HIV-INFECTED ADULTS AND ADOLESCENTS

Adapted from *MMWR Morb Mortal Wkly Rep*, 1998, 47(RR-5)
and *JAMA*, 1998, 280:78-86.
(Updated March 2001 from www.hivatis.org)

Indications for Plasma HIV RNA Testing[1]

Clinical Indication	Information	Use
Syndrome consistent with acute HIV infection	Establishes diagnosis when HIV antibody test is negative or indeterminate	Diagnosis[2]
Initial evaluation of newly diagnosed HIV infection	Baseline viral load "set point"	Decision to start or defer therapy
Every 3-4 months in patients not on therapy	Changes in viral load	Decision to start therapy
2-8 weeks after initiation of antiretroviral therapy	Initial assessment of drug efficacy	Decision to continue or change therapy
3-4 months after start of therapy	Maximal effect of therapy	Decision to continue or change therapy
Every 3-4 months in patients on therapy	Durability of antiretroviral effect	Decision to continue or change therapy
Clinical event or significant decline in CD4+ T cells	Association with changing or stable viral load	Decision to continue, initiate, or change therapy

[1]Acute illness (eg, bacterial pneumonia, tuberculosis, HSV, PCP) and immunizations can cause increases in plasma HIV RNA for 2-4 weeks; viral load testing should not be performed during this time. Plasma HIV RNA results should usually be verified with a repeat determination before starting or making changes in therapy.

[2]Diagnosis of HIV infection determined by HIV RNA testing should be confirmed by standard methods (eg, Western blot serology) performed 2-4 months after the initial indeterminate or negative test.

Risks and Benefits of Delayed Initiation of Therapy and of Early Therapy in the Asymptomatic HIV-Infected Patient

Risks and Benefits of Delayed Therapy[1]

Benefits of Delayed Therapy
- Avoid negative effects on quality of life (ie, inconvenience)
- Avoid drug-related adverse events
- Delay in development of drug resistance
- Preserve maximum number of available and future drug options when HIV disease risk is highest

Risks of Delayed Therapy
- Possible risk of irreversible immune system depletion
- Possible greater difficulty in suppressing viral replication
- Possible increased risk of HIV transmission

Risks and Benefits of Early Therapy[1]

Benefits of Early Therapy
- Control of viral replication easier to achieve and maintain
- Delay or prevention of immune system compromise
- Lower risk of resistance with complete viral suppression
- Possible decreased risk of HIV transmission[2]

Risks of Early Therapy
- Drug-related reduction in quality of life
- Greater cumulative drug-related adverse events
- Earlier development of drug resistance, if viral suppression is suboptimal
- Limitation of future antiretroviral treatment options

[1]See table, "Indications for the Initiation of Antiretroviral Therapy in the Chronically HIV-1 Infected Patient," for consensus recommendations regarding when to initiate therapy.

[2]The risk of viral transmission still exists; antiretroviral therapy cannot substitute for primary HIV prevention measures (eg, use of condoms and safer sex practices).

ANTIRETROVIRAL THERAPY FOR HIV INFECTION *(Continued)*

Indications for the Initiation of Antiretroviral Therapy in the Chronically HIV-1 Infected Patient

The optimal time to initiate therapy in asymptomatic individuals with >200 CD4$^+$ T cells is not known. This table provides general guidance rather than absolute recommendations for an individual patient. All decisions to initiate therapy should be based on prognosis as determined by the CD4$^+$ T cell count and level of plasma HIV RNA, the potential benefits and risks of therapy, and the willingness of the patient to accept therapy.

Clinical Category	CD4$^+$ T Cell Count	Plasma HIV RNA	Recommendation
Symptomatic (AIDS, severe symptoms)	Any value	Any value	Treat
Asymptomatic, AIDS	CD4$^+$ T cells <200/mm^3	Any value	Treat
Asymptomatic	CD4$^+$ T cells >200/mm^3 but <350/mm^3	Any value	Treatment should generally be offered, though controversy exists.[1]
Asymptomatic	CD4$^+$ T cells >350/mm^3	>55,000 (by bDNA) **or** RT-PCR)[2]	Some experts would recommend initiating therapy, recognizing that the 3-year risk of developing AIDS in untreated patients is >30% and some would defer therapy and monitor CD4$^+$ T cell counts more frequently.
Asymptomatic	CD4$^+$ T cells >350/mm^3	<55,000 (by bDNA) **or** RT-PCR)[2]	Many experts would defer therapy and observe, recognizing that the 3-year risk of developing AIDS in untreated patients is <15%.

[1]Clinical benefit has been demonstrated in controlled trials only for patients with CD4$^+$ T cells <200/mm^3. However, most experts would offer therapy at a CD4$^+$ T cell threshold <350/mm^3. A recent evaluation of data from the MACS cohort of 231 individuals with CD4$^+$ T cell counts >200 and <350 cells/mm^3 demonstrated that of 40 (17%) individuals with plasma HIV RNA <10,000 copies/mL, none progressed to AIDS by 3 years (Alvaro Munoz, personal communication). Of 28 individuals (29%) with plasma viremia of 10,000-20,000 copies/mL, 4% and 11% progressed to AIDS at 2 and 3 years respectively. Plasma HIV RNA was calculated as RT-PCR values from measured bDNA values.

[2]Although there was a 2- to 2.5-fold difference between RT-PCR and the first bDNA assay (version 2.0), with the current bDNA assay (version 3.0), values obtained by bDNA and RT-PCR are similar except at the lower end of the linear range (<1500 copies/mL).

Recommended Antiretroviral Agents for Initial Treatment of Established HIV Infection

This table provides a guide to the use of available treatment regimens for individuals with no prior or limited experience on HIV therapy. In accordance with the established goals of HIV therapy, priority is given to regimens in which clinical trials data suggest sustained suppression of HIV plasma RNA (particularly in patients with high baseline viral load) and sustained increase in CD4$^+$ T cell count (in most cases over 48 weeks), and favorable clinical outcome (ie, delayed progression to AIDS and death). Particular emphasis is given to regimens that have been compared directly with other regimens that perform sufficiently well with regard to these parameters to be included in the "Strongly Recommended" category. Additional consideration is given to the regimen's pill burden, dosing frequency, food requirements, convenience, toxicity, and drug interaction profile compared with other regimens.

Note: All antiretroviral agents, including those in the "Strongly Recommended" category, have potentially serious toxic and adverse events associated with their use.

Antiretroviral drug regimens are comprised of one choice each from column A and column B. Drugs are listed in alphabetical, not priority, order:

	Column A	Column B
Strongly Recommended	Efavirenz Indinavir Nelfinavir Ritonavir + Indinavir[1] Ritonavir + Lopinavir[2] Ritonavir + Saquinavir (SGC[3] or HGC[3])	Didanosine + Lamivudine Stavudine + Didanosine[4] Stavudine + Lamivudine Zidovudine + Didanosine Zidovudine + Lamivudine
Recommended as Alternatives	Abacavir Amprenavir Delavirdine Nelfinavir + Saquinavir-SGC Nevirapine Ritonavir Saquinavir-SGC	Zidovudine + Zalcitabine

	Column A	Column B
No Recommendation; Insufficient Data[5]	Hydroxyurea in combination with antiretroviral drugs Ritonavir + Amprenavir Ritonavir + Nelfinavir	
Not Recommended; Should Not Be Offered (All monotherapies, whether from column A or B[6])	Saquinavir-HGC[7]	Stavudine + Zidovudine Zalcitabine + Didanosine Zalcitabine + Lamivudine Zalcitabine + Stavudine

[1]Based on expert opinion.

[2]Co-formulated as Kaletra®.

[3]Saquinavir-SGC, soft-gel capsule (Fortovase®); Saquinavir-HGC, hard-gel capsule (Invirase®).

[4]Pregnant women may be at increased risk for lactic acidosis and liver damage when treated with the combination of stavudine and didanosine. This combination should be used in pregnant women only when the potential benefit clearly outweighs the potential risk.

[5]This category includes drugs or combinations for which information is too limited to allow a recommendation for or against use.

[6]Zidovudine monotherapy may be considered for prophylactic use in pregnant women with low viral load and high CD4+ T cell counts to prevent perinatal transmission.

[7]Use of saquinavir-HGC (Invirase®) is not recommended, except in combination with ritonavir.

Goals of HIV Therapy and Tools to Achieve Them

Goals of Therapy

Maximal and durable suppression of viral load

Restoration and/or preservation of immunologic function

Improvement of quality of life

Reduction of HIV-related morbidity and mortality

Tools to Achieve Goals of Therapy

Maximize adherence to the antiretroviral regimen

Rational sequencing of drugs

Preservation of future treatment options

Use of resistance testing in selected clinical settings

GUIDELINES FOR THE USE OF ANTIRETROVIRAL AGENTS IN PEDIATRIC HIV INFECTION

Adapted from *MMWR Morb Mort Wkly Rep*, 1998, 47(RR-4).

(Updated March 2000 from www.hivatis.org)

1994 Revised Human Immunodeficiency Virus Pediatric Classification System: Immune Categories Based on Age-specific CD4+ T-lymphocyte and Percentage[1]

Immune Category	<12 (mo)		1-5 (y)		6-12 (y)	
	No./μL	%	No./μL	%	No./μL	%
Category 1 (no suppression)	≥1500	≥25	≥1000	≥25	≥500	≥25
Category 2 (moderate suppression)	750-1499	15-24	500-999	15-24	200-499	15-24
Category 3 (severe suppression)	<750	<15	<500	<15	<200	<15

[1]Modified from CDC, 1994 Revised Classification System for Human Immunodeficiency Virus Infection in Children Less Than 13 Years of Age, *MMWR Morb Mort Wkly Rep*, 1994, 43(RR-12):1-10.

ANTIRETROVIRAL THERAPY FOR HIV INFECTION *(Continued)*

1994 Revised Human Immunodeficiency Virus Pediatric Classification System: Clinical Categories[1]

Category N: Not Symptomatic

Children who have no signs or symptoms considered to be the result of HIV infection or who have only **one** of the conditions listed in category A

Category A: Mildly Symptomatic

Children with **two** or more of the following conditions, but none of the conditions listed in categories B and C:

- Lymphadenopathy (≥0.5 cm at more than two sites; bilateral = one site)
- Hepatomegaly
- Splenomegaly
- Dermatitis
- Parotitis
- Recurrent or persistent upper respiratory infection, sinusitis, or otitis media

Category B: Moderately Symptomatic

Children who have symptomatic conditions other than those listed for category A or category C that are attributed to HIV infection. Examples of conditions in clinical category B include, but are not limited to, the following:

- Anemia (<8 g/dL), neutropenia (<1000/mm^3), or thrombocytopenia (<100,000/mm^3) persisting ≥30 days
- Bacterial meningitis, pneumonia, or sepsis (single episode)
- Candidiasis, oropharyngeal (ie, thrush) persisting for >2 months in children aged >6 months
- Cardiomyopathy
- Cytomegalovirus infection with onset before age 1 month
- Diarrhea, recurrent or chronic
- Hepatitis
- Herpes simplex virus (HSV) stomatitis, recurrent (ie, more than two episodes within 1 year)
- HSV bronchitis, pneumonitis, or esophagitis with onset before age 1 month
- Herpes zoster (ie, shingles) involving at least two distinct episodes or more than one dermatome
- Leiomyosarcoma
- Lymphoid interstitial pneumonia (LIP) or pulmonary lymphoid hyperplasia complex
- Nephropathy
- Nocardiosis
- Fever lasting >1 month
- Toxoplasmosis with onset before age 1 month
- Varicella, disseminated (ie, complicated chickenpox)

Category C: Severely Symptomatic

Children who have any condition listed in the 1987 surveillance case definition for acquired immunodeficiency syndrome, with the exception of LIP (which is a category B condition).

[1]Modified from CDC, 1994 Revised Classification System for Human Immunodeficiency Virus Infection in Children Less Than 13 Years of Age, *MMWR Morb Mort Wkly Rep*, 1994, 43(RR-12):1-10.

Association of Baseline CD4+ T-lymphocyte Percentage With Long-Term Risk for Death in Human Immunodeficiency Virus (HIV)-Infected Children[1]

Baseline (%)	No. Patients[2]	Deaths[3]	
		No.	%
<5	33	32	97
5-9	29	22	76
10-14	30	13	43
15-19	41	18	44
20-24	52	13	25
25-29	49	15	31
30-34	48	5	10
≥35	92	30	33

[1]Data from the National Institute of Child Health and Human Development Intravenous Immunoglobulin Clinical Trial.

[2]Includes 374 patients for whom baseline CD4+ T-lymphocyte percentage data were available.

[3]Mean follow-up: 5.1 years.

Adapted from Mofenson L, Korelitz J, Meyer WA, et al, "The Relationship Between Serum Human Immunodeficiency Virus Type 1 (HIV-1) RNA Level, CD4 Lymphocyte Percent and Long-Term Mortality Risk in HIV-1 Infected Children," *J Infect Dis*, 1997, 175:1029-38.

Indications for Initiation of Antiretroviral Therapy in Children With Human Immunodeficiency Virus (HIV) Infection[1]

- Clinical symptoms associated with HIV infection (clinical categories A, B, or C)
- Evidence of immune suppression, indicated by CD4+ T-cell absolute number or percentage (ie, immune category 2 or 3)
- Age <12 months – regardless of clinical, immunologic, or virologic status[2]
- For asymptomatic children ≥1 year of age with normal immune status, two options can be considered:

  Option 1: Initiate therapy regardless of age or symptom status

  Option 2: Defer treatment in situations in which the risk for clinical disease progression is low and other factors (ie, concern for the durability of response, safety, and adherence) favor postponing treatment. In such cases, the healthcare provider should regularly monitor virologic, immunologic, and clinical status. Factors to be considered in deciding to initiate therapy include the following:

  - High or increasing HIV RNA copy number
  - Rapidly declining CD4+ T-cell number or percentage to values approaching those indicative of moderate immune suppression (ie, immune category 2)
  - Development of clinical symptoms

[1]Indications for initiation of antiretroviral therapy need to address issues of adherence. Postpubertal adolescents should follow the Guidelines for the Use of Antiretroviral Agents in Adults and Adolescents (http://www.hivatis.org).

[2]The Working Group recognizes that clinical trial data documenting therapeutic benefit from this approach are not currently available, and information on pharmacokinetics in infants <3-6 months is limited. This recommendation is based on expert opinion. Issues associated with adherence should be fully assessed, discussed, and addressed with the HIV-infected infant's caregivers before the decision to initiate therapy is made.

Recommended Antiretroviral Regimens for Initial Therapy for Human Immunodeficiency Virus (HIV) Infection in Children

Strongly Recommended

Clinical trial evidence of clinical benefit and/or sustained suppression of HIV replication in adults and/or children.

- One highly active protease inhibitors (nelfinavir or ritonavir) plus two nucleoside analogue reverse transcriptase inhibitors

  - Recommended dual NRTI combinations: the most data on use in children are available for the combinations of *zidovudine (ZDV)* and *dideoxyinosine (ddl)*, ZDV and *lamivudine (3TC)*, and *stavudine (d4T)* and *ddl*. More limited data is available for the combinations of *d4T* and *3TC*, and ZDV and *zalcitabine (ddC)*[1]

- For children who can swallow capsules: the non-nucleoside reverse transcriptase inhibitor (NNRTI) efavirenz (Sustiva®)[2] plus 2 NRTIs, or efavirenz (Sustiva®) plus nelfinavir and 1 NRTI

ANTIRETROVIRAL THERAPY FOR HIV INFECTION *(Continued)*

Recommended as an Alternative

Clinical trial evidence of suppression of HIV replication, but 1) durability may be less in adults and/or children than with strongly recommended regimens or may not yet be defined; or 2) evidence of efficacy may not outweigh potential adverse consequences (ie, toxicity, drug interactions, cost, etc); 3) experience in infants and children is limited.

- Nevirapine (NVP) and two NRTIs
- Abacavir (ABC) in combination with ZDV and 3TC
- Lopinavir/ritonavir with two NRTIs or one NRTI and NNRTI[3]
- IDV or SQV soft gel capsule with two NRTIs for children who can swallow capsules

Offered Only in Special Circumstances

Clinical trial evidence of either 1) virologic suppression that is less durable than for the Strongly Recommended or Alternative regimens; or 2) data are preliminary or inconclusive for use as initial therapy but may be reasonably offered in special circumstances.

- Two NRTIs
- Amprenavir in combination with 2 NRTIs or abacavir

Not Recommended

Evidence against use because 1) overlapping toxicity may occur; and/or 2) use may be virologically undesirable

- Any monotherapy[4]
- d4T and ZDV
- ddC[1] and ddI
- ddC[1] and d4T
- ddC[1] and 3TC

[1]ddC is not available commercially in a liquid preparation; although, a liquid formulation is available through a compassionate use program of the manufacturer (Hoffman-LaRoche Inc, (http://www.rocheusa.com), Nutley, New Jersey). ZDV and ddC is a less preferred choice for use in combination with a protease inhibitor.

[2]Efavirenz is currently available only in capsule form, although a liquid formulation is available through an expanded access program of the manufacturer (Bristol-Myers Squibb Company (http://www.bms.com). There are currently no data on appropriate dosage of efavirenz in children <3 years of age.

[3]The data presented to the Food and Drug Administration for review during the drug approval process provided significant data on the pharmacokinetics and safety in children receiving lopinavir/ritonavir (Kaletra™) for 24 weeks. The combination of lopinavir/ritonavir with either two NRTIs or one NRTI and an NNRTI may be moved up to the Strongly Recommended category as experience with this drug is gained by U.S. investigators.

[4]Except for ZDV, chemoprophylaxis administered to HIV-exposed infants during the first 6 weeks of life to prevent perinatal HIV transmission; if an infant is confirmed as HIV-infected while receiving ZDV prophylaxis, therapy should be changed to a combination antiretroviral drug regimen.

Considerations for Changing Antiretroviral Therapy for Human Immunodeficiency Virus (HIV)-Infected Children

Virologic Considerations[1]

- Less than a minimally acceptable virologic response after 8-12 weeks of therapy; for children receiving antiretroviral therapy with two nucleoside analogue reverse transcriptase inhibitors (NRTIs) and a protease inhibitor, such a response is defined as a <10-fold (1.0 $\log_{10}$) decrease from baseline HIV RNA levels; for children who are receiving less potent antiretroviral therapy (ie, dual NRTI combinations), an insufficient response is defined as a <5-fold (0.7 $\log_{10}$) decrease in HIV RNA levels from baseline
- HIV RNA not suppressed to undetectable levels after 4-6 months of antiretroviral therapy[2]
- Repeated detection of HIV RNA in children who initially responded to antiretroviral therapy with undetectable levels[3]
- A reproducible increase in HIV RNA copy number among children who have had a substantial HIV RNA response, but still have low levels of detectable HIV RNA; such an increase would warrant change in therapy if, after initiation of the therapeutic regimen, a >3-fold (0.5 $\log_{10}$) increase in copy number for children ≥2 years of age and a >5-fold (0.7 $\log_{10}$) increase is observed for children <2 years of age

Immunologic Considerations[1]

- Change in immunologic classification[4]
- For children with CD4+ T-lymphocyte percentages of <15% (ie, those in immune category 3), a persistent decline of five percentiles or more in CD4+ cell percentage (eg, from 15% to 10%)
- A rapid and substantial decrease in absolute CD4+ T-lymphocyte count (eg, a >30% decline in <6 months)

Clinical Considerations

- Progressive neurodevelopmental deterioration

- Growth failure defined as persistent decline in weight-growth velocity despite adequate nutritional support and without other explanation

- Disease progression defined as advancement from one pediatric clinical category to another (eg, from clinical category A to clinical category B)[5]

---

[1]At least two measurements (taken 1 week apart) should be performed before considering a change in therapy.

[2]The initial HIV RNA level of the child at the start of therapy and the level achieved with therapy should be considered when contemplating potential drug changes. For example, an immediate change in therapy may not be warranted if there is a sustained 1.5-2.0 $\log_{10}$ decrease in HIV RNA copy number, even if RNA remains detectable at low levels.

[3]More frequent evaluation of HIV RNA levels should be considered if the HIV RNA increase is limited (eg, if when using an HIV RNA assay with a lower limit of detection of 1000 copies/mL, there is a ≤0.7 $\log_{10}$ increase from undetectable to approximately 5000 copies/mL in an infant <2 years of age).

[4]Minimal changes in CD4+ T-lymphocyte percentile that may result in change in immunologic category (eg, from 26% to 24%, or 16% to 14%) may not be as concerning as a rapid substantial change in CD4+ percentile within the same immunologic category (eg, a drop from 35% to 25%).

[5]In patients with stable immunologic and virologic parameters, progression from one clinical category to another may not represent an indication to change therapy. Thus, in patients whose disease progression is not associated with neurologic deterioration or growth failure, virologic and immunologic considerations are important in deciding whether to change therapy.

Guidelines for Changing an Antiretroviral Regimen for Suspected Drug Failure

- Criteria for changing therapy include a suboptimal reduction in plasma viremia after initiation of therapy, reappearance of viremia after suppression to undetectable, significant increases in plasma viremia from the nadir of suppression, and declining CD4+ T cell numbers.

- When the decision to change therapy is based on viral load determination, it is preferable to confirm with a second viral load test.

- Distinguish between the need to change a regimen because of drug intolerance or inability to comply with the regimen versus failure to achieve the goal of sustained viral suppression; single agents can be changed in the event of drug intolerance.

- In general, do not change a single drug or add a single drug to a failing regimen; it is important to use at least two new drugs and preferably to use an entirely new regimen with at least three new drugs. If susceptibility testing indicates resistance to only one agent in a combination regimen, it may be possible to replace only that drug; however, this approach requires clinical validation.

- Many patients have limited options for new regimens of desired potency; in some of these cases, it is rational to continue the prior regimen if partial viral suppression was achieved.

- In some cases, regimens identified as suboptimal for initial therapy are rational due to limitations imposed by toxicity, intolerance, or nonadherence. This especially applies in late-stage disease. For patients with no rational alternative options who have virologic failure with return of viral load to baseline (pretreatment levels) and a declining CD4+ T cell count, there should be consideration for discontinuation of antiretroviral therapy.

- Experience is limited with regimens using combinations of two protease inhibitors or combinations of protease inhibitors with NNRTIs; for patients with limited options due to drug intolerance or suspected resistance, these regimens provide possible alternative treatment options.

  There is limited information about the value of restarting a drug that the patient has previously received. Susceptibility testing may be useful in this situation if clinical evidence suggestive of the emergence of resistance is observed. However, testing for phenotypic or genotypic resistance in peripheral blood virus may fail to detect minor resistant variants. Thus, the presence of resistance is more useful information in altering treatment strategies than the absence of detectable resistance.

- Avoid changing from ritonavir to indinavir or vice versa for drug failure, because high-level cross-resistance is likely.

- Avoid changing among NNRTIs for drug failure, since high-level cross-resistance is likely.

- The decision to change therapy and the choice of a new regimen requires that the clinician have considerable expertise in the care of persons living with HIV. Physicians who are less experienced in the care of persons with HIV infection are strongly encouraged to obtain assistance through consultation with or referral to a clinician who has considerable expertise in the care of HIV-infected patients.

ANTIRETROVIRAL THERAPY FOR HIV INFECTION *(Continued)*

Zidovudine Perinatal Transmission Prophylaxis Regimen

Antepartum	Initiation at 14-34 weeks gestation and continued throughout pregnancy
	A. PACTG 076 regimen: ZDV 100 mg 5 times/day
	B. Acceptable alternative regimen:
	ZDV 200 mg 3 times/day
	or
	ZDV 300 mg twice daily
Intrapartum	During labor, ZDV 2 mg/kg I.V. over 1 hour, followed by a continuous infusion of 1 mg/kg I.V. until delivery
Postpartum	Oral administration of ZDV to the newborn (ZDV syrup, 2 mg/kg every 6 hours) for the first 6 weeks of life, beginning at 8-12 hours after birth

COMMUNITY-ACQUIRED PNEUMONIA IN ADULTS

GUIDELINES FOR MANAGEMENT

Algorithm

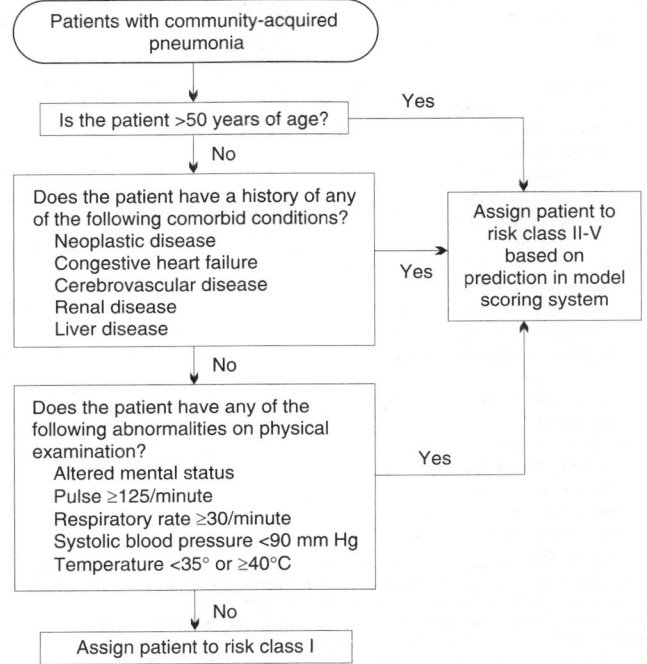

Stratification of Risk Score

Risk	Risk Class	Based on
	I	Algorithm
Low	II	≤70 total points
	III	71-90 total points
Moderate	IV	91-130 total points
High	V	>130 total points

COMMUNITY-ACQUIRED PNEUMONIA IN ADULTS *(Continued)*

The table below is the prediction model for identification of patient risk for persons with community-acquired pneumonia. This model may be used to help guide the initial decision on site of care; however, its use may not be appropriate for all patients with this illness and, therefore, should be applied in conjunction with physician judgment.

Scoring System: Assignment to Risk Classes II-V

Patient Characteristic	Points Assigned[1]
Demographic factors	
Age	
Male	No. of years
Female	No. of years -10
Nursing home resident	+10
Comorbid illnesses	
Neoplastic disease[2]	+30
Liver disease[3]	+20
Congestive heart failure[4]	+10
Cerebrovascular disease[5]	+10
Renal disease[6]	+10
Physical examination findings	
Altered mental status[7]	+20
Respiratory rate >30 breaths/minute	+20
Systolic blood pressure <90 mm Hg	+20
Temperature <35°C or >40°C	+15
Pulse >125 beats/minute	+10
Laboratory or radiographic findings	
Arterial pH <7.35	+30
BUN >30 mg/dL	+20
Sodium <130 mEq/L	+20
Glucose >250 mg/dL	+10
Hematocrit <30%	+10
pO_2 <60 mm Hg[8]	+10
Pleural effusion	+10

[1]A total point score for a given patient is obtained by adding the patient's age in years (age -10, for females) and the points for each applicable patient characteristic.

[2]Any cancer except basal or squamous cell cancer of the skin that was active at the time of presentation or diagnosed within 1 year of presentation.

[3]A clinical or histologic diagnosis of cirrhosis or other form of chronic liver disease such as chronic active hepatitis.

[4]Systolic or diastolic ventricular dysfunction documented by history and physical examination, as well as chest radiography, echocardiography, Muga scanning, or left ventriculography.

[5]A clinical diagnosis of stroke, transient ischemic attack, or stroke documented by MRI or computed axial tomography.

[6]A history of chronic renal disease or abnormal blood urea nitrogen (BUN) and creatinine values documented in the medical record.

[7]Disorientation (to person, place, or time, not known to be chronic), stupor, or coma.

[8]In the Pneumonia Patient Outcome Research Team cohort study, an oxygen saturation value <90% on pulse oximetry or intubation before admission was also considered abnormal.

Risk-Class Mortality Rates for Patients With Pneumonia

Risk Class	Validation Cohort			Recommended Site of Care
	No. of Points	No. of Patients	Mortality (%)	
I	No predictors	3034	0.1	Outpatient
II	≤70	5778	0.6	Outpatient
III	71-90	6790	2.8	Outpatient or brief inpatient
IV	91-130	13,104	8.2	Inpatient
V	>130	9333	29.2	Inpatient

Pathogen-Directed Antimicrobial Therapy for Community-Acquired Pneumonia

Organism	Preferred Antimicrobial	Alternative Antimicrobial
Streptococcus pneumoniae		
Penicillin susceptible (MIC, <2 mcg/mL)	Penicillin G, amoxicillin	Cephalosporins (cefazolin, cefuroxime, cefotaxime, ceftriaxone, or cefepime), oral cephalosporins (cefpodoxime, cefprozil, or cefuroxime), imipenem or meropenem, macrolides,[1] clindamycin, fluoroquinolone,[2] doxycycline, ampicillin ± sulbactam or piperacillin ± tazobactam
Penicillin resistant (MIC, ≥2 mcg/mL)	Agents based on *in vitro* susceptibility tests, including cefotaxime and ceftriaxone, fluoroquinolone,[2] vancomycin	—
Haemophilus influenzae	Cephalosporins (2nd or 3rd generation), doxycycline, beta-lactam/beta-lactamase inhibitor, azithromycin, TMP-SMZ	Fluoroquinolone,[2] clarithromycin
Moraxella catarrhalis	Cephalosporin (2nd or 3rd generation), TMP-SMZ, macrolide, beta-lactam/beta-lactamase inhibitor	Fluoroquinolone[2]
Anaerobe	Beta-lactam/beta-lactamase inhibitor, clindamycin	Imipenem
Staphylococcus aureus[3]		
Methicillin-susceptible	Nafcillin/oxacillin ± rifampin or gentamicin[3]	Cefazolin or cefuroxime, vancomycin, clindamycin, TMP-SMZ
Methicillin-resistant	Vancomycin ± rifampin or gentamicin	Linezolid
Enterobacteriaceae (coliforms: *Escherichia coli, Klebsiella, Proteus, Enterobacter*)	Cephalosporin (3rd generation) ± aminoglycoside, carbapenem	Aztreonam, beta-lactam/beta-lactamase inhibitor, fluoroquinolone[2]
Pseudomonas aeruginosa[3]	Aminoglycoside + antipseudomonal beta-lactam: ticarcillin, piperacillin, mezlocillin, ceftazidime, cefepime, aztreonam, or carbapenem	Aminoglycoside + ciprofloxacin, ciprofloxacin + antipseudomonal beta-lactam
Legionella	Macrolide[1] ± rifampin, fluoroquinolone[2] (including ciprofloxacin)	Doxycycline ± rifampin
Mycoplasma pneumoniae	Doxycycline, macrolide[1]	Fluoroquinolone[2]
Chlamydia pneumoniae	Doxycycline, macrolide[1]	Fluoroquinolone[2]
Chlamydia psittaci	Doxycycline	Erythromycin, chloramphenicol
Nocardia	TMP-SMZ, sulfonamide ± minocycline or amikacin	Imipenem ± amikacin, doxycycline or minocycline
Coxiella burnetii (Q fever)	Tetracycline	Chloramphenicol
Influenza virus	Amantadine or rimantadine (influenza A), zanamivir or oseltamivir (influenza A or B)	—
Hantavirus	Supportive care	—

Note: TMP-SMZ = trimethoprim-sulfamethoxazole.
[1]Erythromycin, clarithromycin, azithromycin, or dirithromycin; *S. pneumoniae*, especially strains with reduced susceptibility to penicillin, should have verified *in vitro* susceptibility.
[2]Levofloxacin, gatifloxacin, moxifloxacin, trovafloxacin, or other fluoroquinolone with enhanced activity against *S. pneumoniae*; ciprofloxacin is appropriate for *Legionella, C. pneumoniae*, fluoroquinolone-susceptible *S. aureus*, and most gram-negative bacilli; ciprofloxacin may not be as effective as other quinolones against *S. pneumoniae*.
[3]*In vitro* susceptibility tests are required for optimal treatment; against *Enterobacter* species, the preferred antibiotics are fluoroquinolones and carbapenems.

COMMUNITY-ACQUIRED PNEUMONIA IN ADULTS *(Continued)*

Empirical Selection of Antimicrobial Agents for Treating Patients With Community-Acquired Pneumonia

Outpatients

Generally preferred (not in any particular order): Doxycycline, a macrolide, or a fluoroquinolone

Selection considerations

These agents have activity against the most likely pathogens in this setting, which include *Streptococcus pneumoniae*, *Mycoplasma pneumoniae*, and *Chlamydia pneumoniae*

Selection should be influenced by regional antibiotic susceptibility patterns for *S. pneumoniae* and the presence of other risk factors for drug-resistant *S. pneumoniae*

Penicillin-resistant pneumococci may be resistant to macrolides and/or doxycycline

For older patients or those with underlying disease, a fluoroquinolone may be a preferred choice; some authorities prefer to reserve fluoroquinolones for such patients

Hospitalized Patients

General medical ward

Generally preferred: An extended-spectrum cephalosporin combined with a macrolide or a beta-lactam/beta-lactamase inhibitor combined with a macrolide or a fluoroquinolone (alone)

Intensive care unit

Generally preferred: An extended-spectrum cephalosporin or beta-lactam/beta-lactamase inhibitor plus either fluoroquinolone or macrolide

Alternatives or modifying factors

Structural lung disease: Antipseudomonal agents (piperacillin, piperacillin-tazobactam, carbapenem, or cefepime) plus a fluoroquinolone (including high-dose ciprofloxacin)

Beta-lactam allergy: Fluoroquinolone ± clindamycin

Suspected aspiration: Fluoroquinolone ± clindamycin, metronidazole, or a beta-lactam/beta-lactamase inhibitor

Note:

Beta-lactam/beta-lactamase inhibitor: Ampicillin-sulbactam or piperacillin-tazobactam.

Extended-spectrum cephalosporin: Cefotaxime or ceftriaxone.

Fluoroquinolone: Gatifloxacin, levofloxacin, moxifloxacin, or other fluoroquinolone with enhanced activity against *S. pneumoniae* (for aspiration pneumonia, some fluoroquinolones show *in vitro* activity against anaerobic pulmonary pathogens, although there are no clinical studies to verify activity *in vivo*).

Macrolide: Azithromycin, clarithromycin, or erythromycin.

References

Bartlett JG, Breiman RF, Mandell LA, et al, "Community-Acquired Pneumonia in Adults: Guidelines for Management. The Infectious Diseases Society of America," *Clin Infect Dis*, 1998, 26(4):811-38.

Bartlett JG, Dowell SF, Mandell LA, et al, "Practice Guidelines for the Management of Community-Acquired Pneumonia in Adults. The Infectious Diseases Society of America," *Clin Infect Dis*, 2000, 31(2):347-82.

MALARIA TREATMENT

Drug of Choice	Adult Dosage	Pediatric Dosage
Chloroquine-Resistance *Plasmodium falciparum*[1]		
ORAL		
Quinine sulfate	650 mg q8h x 3-7 d[2]	25 mg/kg/d in 3 doses x 3-7 d[2]
plus doxycycline	100 mg bid x 7 d	2 mg/kg/d x 7 d
or plus tetracycline	250 mg qid x 7 d	6.25 mg/kg qid x 7 d
or plus pyrimethamine-sulfadoxine[3]	3 tablets at once on last day of quinine	<1 y: ¼ tablet 1-3 y: ½ tablet 4-8 y: 1 tablet 9-14 y: 2 tablets
or plus clindamycin[4]	900 mg tid x 5 d	20-40 mg/kg/d in 3 doses x 5 d
Alternatives:[5]		
Mefloquine[6,7]	750 mg followed by 500 mg 12 h later	15 mg/kg followed by 10 mg/kg 8-12 h later (<45 kg)
Halofantrine[8]	500 mg q6h x 3 doses; repeat in 1 week[9]	8 mg/kg q6h x 3 doses (<40 kg); repeat in 1 week[9]
Atovaquone[10]	500 mg bid x 3 d	11-20 kg: 125 mg bid x 3 d 21-30 kg: 250 mg bid x 3 d 31-40 kg: 375 mg bid x 3 d
plus proguanil	200 mg bid x 3 d	11-20 kg: 50 mg bid x 3 d 21-30 kg: 100 mg bid x 3 d 31-40 kg: 150 mg bid x 3 d
or plus doxycycline	100 mg bid x 3 d	2 mg/kg/d x 3 d
Artesunate*	4 mg/kg/d x 3 d	
plus mefloquine[6,7]	750 mg followed by 500 mg 12 h later	15 mg/kg followed 8-12 h later by 10 mg/kg
Chloroquine-Resistant *P. vivax*[11]		
Quinine sulfate	650 mg q8h x 3-7 d[2]	25 mg/kg/d in 3 doses x 3-7 d[2]
plus doxycycline	100 mg bid x 7 d	2 mg/kg/d x 7 d
or plus pyrimethamine-sulfadoxine[3]	3 tablets at once on last day of quinine	<1 y: ¼ tablet 1-3 y: ½ tablet 4-8 y: 1 tablet 9-14 y: 2 tablets
OR		
Mefloquine	750 mg followed by 500 mg 12 h later	15 mg/kg followed 8-12 h later by 10 mg/kg
Alternatives:		
Halofantrine[8,12*]	500 mg q6h x 3 doses	8 mg/kg q6h x 3 doses
Chloroquine **plus**	25 mg base/kg in 3 doses over 48 h	
primaquine[13]	2.5 mg base/kg in 3 doses over 48 h	
All *Plasmodium* Except Chloroquine-Resistant *P. falciparum*[1] and Chloroquine-Resistant *P. vivax*[11]		
ORAL		
Chloroquine phosphate[14]	1 g (600 mg base), then 500 mg (300 mg base) 6 h later, then 500 mg (300 mg base) at 24 and 48 h	10 mg base/kg (max 600 mg base), then 5 mg base/kg 6 h later, then 5 mg base/kg at 24 and 48 h
All *Plasmodium*[15]		
PARENTERAL		
Quinidine gluconate[16,17]	10 mg/kg loading dose (max 600 mg) in normal saline slowly over 1-2 h, followed by continuous infusion of 0.02 mg/kg/min until oral therapy can be started	Same as adult dose
OR		
Quinine dihydrochloride[16,17]	20 mg/kg loading dose I.V. in 5% dextrose over 4 h, followed by 10 mg/kg over 2-4 h q8h (max 1800 mg/d) until oral therapy can be started	Same as adult dose
Alternative		
Artemether[18*]	3.2 mg/kg I.M., then 1.6 mg/kg daily x 5-7 d	Same as adult dose
Prevention of Relapses: *P. vivax* and *P. ovale* Only		
Primaquine phosphate[13,19]	26.3 mg (15 mg base)/d x 14 d or 79 mg (45 mg base)/wk x 8 wk	0.3 mg base/kg/d x 14 d

*Availability problems.

[1]Chloroquine-resistant *P. falciparum* occur in all malarious areas except Central America west of the Panama Canal Zone, Mexico, Haiti, the Dominican Republic, and most of the Middle East (chloroquine resistance has been reported in Yemen, Oman, Saudi Arabia, and Iran).

[2]In Southeast Asia, relative resistance to quinine has increased and the treatment should be continued for 7 days.

MALARIA TREATMENT *(Continued)*

[3]Fansidar® tablets contain 25 mg pyrimethamine and 500 mg sulfadoxine. Resistance to pyrimethamine-sulfadoxine has been reported from Southeast Asia, the Amazon Basin, sub-Saharan Africa, Bangladesh, and Oceania.

[4]For use in pregnancy.

[5]For treatment of multiple-drug-resistant *P. falciparum* in Southeast Asia, especially Thailand, where resistance to mefloquine and halofantrine is frequent, a 7-day course of quinine and tetracycline is recommended (Watt G, Loesuttivibool L, Shanks GD, et al, "Quinine with Tetracycline for the Treatment of Drug-Resistant *Falciparum malariae* in Thailand," *Am J Trop Med Hyg*, 1992, 47(1):108-11). Artesunate plus mefloquine (Luxemburger C, ter Kuile FO, Nosten F, et al, "Single Day Mefloquine-Artesunate Combination in the Treatment of Multi-drug Resistant *Falciparum malariae*, *Trans R Soc Trop Med Hyg*, 1994, 88(2):213-7), artemether plus mefloquine (Karbwang J et al, *Trans R Soc Trop Med Hyg*, 1995, 89:296), or mefloquine plus doxycycline are also used to treat multiple-drug-resistant *P. falciparum*.

[6]At this dosage, adverse effects including nausea, vomiting, diarrhea, dizziness, disturbed sense of balance, toxic psychosis, and seizures can occur. Mefloquine is teratogenic in animals and should not be used for treatment of malaria in pregnancy. It should not be given together with quinine, quinidine, or halofantrine, and caution is required in using quinine, quinidine, or halofantrine to treat patients with malaria who have taken mefloquine for prophylaxis. The pediatric dosage has not been approved by the FDA. Resistance to mefloquine has been reported in some areas, such as the Thailand-Myanmar and Cambodia borders and in the Amazon, where 25 mg/kg should be used.

[7]In the U.S.A., a 250 mg tablet of mefloquine contains 228 mg mefloquine base. Outside the U.S.A., each 275 mg tablet contains 250 mg base.

[8]May be effective in multiple-drug-resistant *P. falciparum* malaria, but treatment failures and resistance have been reported, and the drug has caused lengthening of the PR and QTc intervals and fatal cardiac arrhythmias. It should not be used for patients with cardiac conduction defects or with other drugs that may affect the QT interval, such as quinine, quinidine, and mefloquine. Cardiac monitoring is recommended. Variability in absorption is a problem; halofantrine should not be taken 1 hour before to 2 hours after meals because food increases its absorption. It should not be used in pregnancy.

[9]A single 250 mg dose can be used for repeat treatment in mild to moderate infections (Touze JE, Perret JL, Nicolas X, et al, "Efficacy of Low-Dose Halofantrine for Second Treatment of Uncomplicated *P. falciparum* malaria," *Lancet*, 1997, 25:349(9047):255-6.

[10]Atovaquone plus proguanil is marketed as a combination tablet in many countries and will soon be available in the United States (250 mg atovaquone/100 mg proguanil as Malarone™ – Glaxo Wellcome and 62.5 mg atovaquone/25 mg proguanil as Malarone™ Pediatric). The combination should be used only for acute uncomplicated malaria caused by *P. falciparum*. The dose of Malarone™ for 3-day treatment of malaria is 4 tablets/day in adults; 3 adult tablets/day for children 31-40 kg; 2 adult tablets/day for children 21-30 kg; and 1 adult tablet/day for children 11-20 kg. To enhance absorption, it should be taken within 45 minutes after eating (Looareesuwan S, Chulay JD, Canfield CJ, "Malarone™ (Atovaquone and proguanil hydrochloride): A Review of Its Clinical Development for Treatment of Malaria," Malarone Clinical Trials Study Group, *Am J Trop Med Hyg*, 1999, 60(4):533-41). Although approved for once daily dosing, to decrease nausea and vomiting the dose can be divided in two.

[11]*P. vivax* with decreased susceptibility to chloroquine is a significant problem in Papua-New Guinea and Indonesia. There are also a few reports of resistance from Myanmar, India, Thailand, the Solomon Islands, Vanuatu, Guyana, Brazil, and Peru.

[12]Baird JK, Basri H, Subianto B, et al, "Treatment of Chloroquine-Resistant *Plasmodium vivax* With Chloroquine and Primaquine or Halofantrine., *J Infect Dis*, 1995, 171(6):1678-82.

[13]Primaquine phosphate can cause hemolytic anemia, especially in patients whose red cells are deficient in glucose-6-phosphate dehydrogenase. This deficiency is most common in African, Asian, and Mediterranean peoples. Patients should be screened for G-6-PD deficiency before treatment. Primaquine should not be used during pregnancy.

[14]If chloroquine phosphate is not available, hydroxychloroquine sulfate is as effective; 400 mg of hydroxychloroquine sulfate is equivalent to 500 mg of chloroquine phosphate.

[15]Exchange transfusion has been helpful for some patients with high-density (>10%) parasitemia, altered mental status, pulmonary edema, or renal complications (Miller KD, Greenberg AE, and Campbell CC, "Treatment of Severe Malaria in the United States With a Continuous Infusion of Quinidine Gluconate and Exchange Transfusion, *N Engl J Med.*, 1989, 321(2):65-7).

[16]Continuous EKG, blood pressure and glucose monitoring are recommended, especially in pregnant women and young children.

[17]Quinidine may have greater antimalarial activity then quinine. The loading dose should be decreased or omitted in those patients who have received quinine or mefloquine. If more than 48 hours of parenteral treatment is required, the quinine or quinidine dose should be reduced by 1/3 to 1/2.

[18]White NJ, "The Treatment of Malaria," *N Engl J Med*, 1996, 335(11):800-6. Not available in the United States.

[19]Relapses have been reported with this regimen, and should be treated with a second 14-day course of 30 mg base/day.

Adapted from "Report of the Committee on Infectious Diseases," *2000, Red Book®*, 25th ed, 705-8.

TREATMENT OF SEXUALLY TRANSMITTED DISEASES

Type or Stage	Drug of Choice	Alternatives
CHLAMYDIAL INFECTION AND RELATED CLINICAL SYNDROMES[1]		
Urethritis, cervicitis, conjunctivitis, or proctitis (except lymphogranuloma venereum)		
	Azithromycin 1 g oral once **OR** Doxycycline[2,3] 100 mg oral bid x 7 d	Ofloxacin[3] 300 mg oral bid x 7 d **OR** Erythromycin[4] 500 mg oral qid x 7 d
Recurrent/persistent		
	Metronidazole 2 g oral **plus** Erythromycin 500 mg oral qid x 7 d	
Infection in pregnancy		
	Amoxicillin 500 mg oral tid x 10 d **OR** Erythromycin[4] 500 mg oral qid x 7 d	Azithromycin[5] 1 g oral once **OR** Erythromycin base 250 mg oral qid x 14 d **OR** Erythromycin ethylsuccinate 800 mg oral qid x 7 d **OR** Erythromycin ethylsuccinate 400 mg oral qid x 14 d
Neonatal		
Ophthalmia	Erythromycin 12.5 mg/kg oral qid x 10-14 d	
Pneumonia	Erythromycin 12.5 mg/kg oral or I.V. qid x 14 d	
Lymphogranuloma venereum		
	Doxycycline[2,3] 100 mg oral bid x 21 d	Erythromycin[4] 500 mg oral qid x 21 d
GONORRHEA[6]		
Urethral, cervical, rectal, or pharyngeal		
	Cefixime 400 mg oral once **OR** Ceftriaxone 125 mg I.M. once **OR** Ciprofloxacin[3] 500 mg oral once **OR** Ofloxacin[3] 400 mg oral once **plus** Azithromycin 1 g oral once **OR** Doxycycline 100 mg oral bid x 7 d	Spectinomycin 2 g I.M. once[7] **OR** Lomefloxacin 400 mg oral once **OR** Norfloxacin 800 mg oral once
Disseminated gonococcal infection		
	Ceftriaxone 1 g I.M. or I.V. q24h	Cefotaxime 1 g I.V. q8h **OR** Ceftizoxime 1 g I.V. q8h **OR** **For persons allergic to β-lactam drugs:** Ciprofloxacin 500 mg I.V. q12h **OR** Ofloxacin 400 mg I.V. q12h **OR** Spectinomycin 2 g I.M. q12h All regimens should be continued for 24-48 hours after improvement begins, at which time therapy may be switched to one of the following regimens to complete a full week of antimicrobial therapy: Cefixime 400 mg oral bid **OR** Ciprofloxacin 500 mg oral bid **OR** Ofloxacin 400 mg oral bid
Gonococcal meningitis and endocarditis		
	Ceftriaxone 1-2 g I.V. q12h	
EPIDIDYMITIS		
Most likely caused by enteric organisms, or in patients allergic to cephalosporins and/or tetracyclines		
	Ofloxacin 300 mg bid x 10 d	
Most likely caused by gonococcal or chlamydial infection		
	Ceftriaxone 250 mg I.M. once **followed by** Doxycycline[2] 100 mg oral bid x 10 d	

TREATMENT OF SEXUALLY TRANSMITTED DISEASES
(Continued)

Type or Stage	Drug of Choice	Alternatives
PELVIC INFLAMMATORY DISEASE		
– Inpatients	Cefotetan 2 g I.V. q12h **OR** Cefoxitin 2 g I.V. q6h **plus** Doxycycline 100 mg I.V. or oral q12h, until improved **followed by** Doxycycline[3] 100 mg oral bid to complete 14 days **OR** Clindamycin 900 mg I.V. q8h **plus** Gentamicin 2 mg/kg I.V. once, then 1.5 mg/kg I.V. q8h, until improved **followed by** Doxycycline[3] 100 mg oral bid to complete 14 days	Ofloxacin 400 mg I.V. q12h **plus** Metronidazole 500 mg I.V. q8h Ampicillin/sulbactam 3 g I.V. q6h **plus** Doxycycline[3] 100 mg oral or I.V. q12h Ciprofloxacin 200 mg I.V. q12h **plus** Doxycycline[3] 100 mg I.V. q12h **plus** Metronidazole 500 mg I.V. q8h All continued until improved, then followed by doxycycline[3] 100 mg oral bid to complete 14 d[8]
– Outpatients	Ofloxacin[3] 400 mg oral bid x 14 d **plus** Metronidazole 500 mg oral bid x 14 d **OR** Ceftriaxone 250 mg I.M. once **OR** Cefoxitin 2 g I.M. once **plus** Probenecid 1 g oral once **OR** Other parenteral 3rd generation cephalosporin (ceftizoxime or cefotaxime) **OR** Any cephalosporin **followed by** Doxycycline[3,9] 100 mg oral bid x 14 d	
VAGINAL INFECTION		
Trichomoniasis	Metronidazole 2 g oral once	Metronidazole 375 mg or 500 mg oral bid x 7 d
Bacterial vaginosis	Metronidazole 500 mg oral bid x 7 d **OR** Metronidazole gel 0.75% 5 g intravaginally once or twice daily x 5 d **OR** Clindamycin 2% cream 5 g intravaginally qhs x 3-7 d	Metronidazole 250 mg oral tid x 7 d **OR** Clindamycin 300 mg oral bid x 7 d **OR** Metronidazole 2 g oral once[10]
Vulvovaginal candidiasis	Intravaginal butoconazole, clotrimazole, miconazole, terconazole, or tioconazole[11] **OR** Fluconazole 150 mg oral once	Nystatin 100,000 unit vaginal tablet once daily x 14 d
SYPHILIS		
Early (primary, secondary, or latent <1 y)	Penicillin G benzathine 2.4 million units I.M. once[12]	Doxycycline[3] 100 mg oral bid x 14 d **OR** Tetracycline 500 mg oral qid x 24 d
Late (>1 year's duration, cardiovascular, gumma, late-latent)	Penicillin G benzathine 2.4 million units I.M. weekly x 3 wk	Doxycycline[3] 100 mg oral bid x 4 wk
Neurosyphilis[13]	Penicillin G 3-4 million units I.V. q4h x 10-14 d	Penicillin G procaine 2.4 million units I.M. daily, **plus** Probenecid 500 mg qid oral, both x 10-14 d
Congenital	Penicillin G 50,000 units/kg I.V. q8-12h (q12h during first 7 d of life, then q8h for total of 10 d) **OR** Penicillin G procaine 50,000 units/kg I.M. daily for 10 d	

Type or Stage	Drug of Choice	Alternatives
CHANCROID[14]	Azithromycin 1 g oral once **OR** Ceftriaxone 250 mg I.M. once **OR** Ciprofloxacin[3] 500 mg oral bid x 3 d **OR** Erythromycin[4] 500 mg oral qid x 7 d	
GENITAL HERPES		
First episode	Acyclovir 400 mg oral tid x 7-10 d[15] **OR** Famciclovir 250 mg oral tid x 7-10 d **OR** Valacyclovir 1 g oral bid x 7-10 d	Acyclovir 200 mg oral 5 times/d x 7-10 d[15]
Recurrent[16]	Acyclovir 400 mg oral tid x 5 d **OR** Famciclovir 125 mg oral bid x 5 d **OR** Valacyclovir 500 mg oral bid x 5 d	Acyclovir 200 mg orally 5 times/day for 5 d **OR** Acyclovir 800 mg oral bid x 5 d
Severe (hospitalized patients)	Acyclovir 5-10 mg/kg I.V. q8h x 5-7 d	
Suppression of recurrence[17]	Valacyclovir 500 mg - 1 g once daily[18] **OR** Acyclovir 400 mg oral bid **OR** Famciclovir 250 mg oral bid	
GRANULOMA INGUINALE	TMP-SMZ 1 double-strength tablet oral bid for a minimum of 3 wk **OR** Doxycycline 100 oral bid for a minimum of 3 wk	Ciprofloxacin 750 mg oral bid for a minimum of 3 wk **OR** Erythromycin base 500 mg oral qid for a minimum of 3 wk

[1]Related clinical syndromes include nonchlamydial nongonococcal urethritis and cervicitis.
[2]Or tetracycline 500 mg oral qid or minocycline 100 mg oral bid.
[3]Contraindicated in pregnancy.
[4]Erythromycin estolate is contraindicated in pregnancy.
[5]Safety in pregnancy not established.
[6]All patients should also receive a course of treatment effective for *Chlamydia*.
[7]Recommended only for use during pregnancy in patients allergic to beta-lactams. Not effective for pharyngeal infection.
[8]Or clindamycin 450 mg oral qid to complete 14 days.
[9]Some experts would add metronidazole 500 mg bid.
[10]Higher relapse rate with single dose, but useful for patients who may not comply with multiple-dose therapy.
[11]For preparations and dosage of topical products, see *Medical Letter*, 36:81,1994; single-dose therapy is not recommended.
[12]Some experts recommend repeating this regimen after 7 days, especially in patients with HIV infection.
[13]Patients allergic to penicillin should be desensitized.
[14]All regimens, especially single-dose ceftriaxone, are less effective in HIV-infected patients.
[15]For first-episode proctitis, use acyclovir 800 mg oral tid or 400 mg oral 5 times/day.
[16]Antiviral therapy is variably effective for treatment of recurrences; only effective if started early.
[17]Preventive treatment should be discontinued for 1-2 months once a year to reassess the frequency of recurrence.
[18]Use 500 mg qd in patients with <10 recurrences per year and 500 mg bid or 1 g daily in patients with ≥10 recurrences per year.

Adapted from "1998 Guidelines for Treatment of Sexually Transmitted Diseases," *MMWR Morb Mortal Wkly Rep*, 1998, 47(RR-1).

TUBERCULOSIS TREATMENT GUIDELINES

Recommended Treatment Regimens for Drug-Susceptible Tuberculosis in Infants, Children, and Adolescents

Infection or Disease Category	Regimen	Remarks
Latent tuberculosis infection (positive skin test, no disease):		If daily therapy is not possible, therapy twice a week directly observed therapy may be used for 9 months. HIV-infected children should be treated for 9-12 months.
• Isoniazid-susceptible	9 months of isoniazid once a day	
• Isoniazid-resistant	6 months of rifampin once a day	
• Isoniazid-rifampin-resistant[1]	Consult a tuberculosis specialist	
Pulmonary	**6-Month Regimens** 2 months of isoniazid, rifampin, and pyrazinamide once a day, followed by 4 months of isoniazid and rifampin daily	If possible drug resistance is a concern, another drug (ethambutol or streptomycin) is added to the initial 3-drug therapy until drug susceptibilities are determined.
	OR	
	2 months of isoniazid, rifampin, and pyrazinamide daily, followed by 4 months of isoniazid and rifampin twice a week	Drugs can be given 2 or 3 times per week under direct observation in the initial phase if nonadherence is likely.
	9-Month Alternative Regimens (for hilar adenopathy only) 9 months of isoniazid and rifampin once a day **OR** 1 month of isoniazid and rifampin once a day, followed by 8 months of isoniazid and rifampin twice a week	Regimens consisting of 6 months of isoniazid and rifampin once a day, and 1 month of isoniazid and rifampin once a day, followed by 5 months of isoniazid and rifampin directly observed therapy twice a week, have been successful in areas where drug resistance is rare.
Extrapulmonary meningitis, disseminated (miliary), bone/joint disease	2 months of isoniazid, rifampin, pyrazinamide, and streptomycin once a day, followed by 7-10 months of isoniazid and rifampin once a day (9-12 months total)	Streptomycin is given with initial therapy until drug susceptibility is known.
	OR	
	2 months of isoniazid, rifampin, pyrazinamide, and streptomycin once a day, followed by 7-10 months of isoniazid and rifampin twice a week (9-12 months total)	For patients who may have acquired tuberculosis in geographic areas where resistance to streptomycin is common, capreomycin (15-30 mg/kg/d) or kanamycin (15-30 mg/kg/d) may be used instead of streptomycin.
Other (eg, cervical lymphadenopathy)	Same as for pulmonary disease	See Pulmonary.

[1]Duration of therapy is longer in HIV-infected persons and additional drugs may be indicated.

Adapted from "Report of the Committee on Infectious Diseases," *2000 Red Book®*, 25th ed.

Commonly Used Drugs for the Treatment of Tuberculosis in Infants, Children, and Adolescents

Drugs	Dosage Forms	Daily Dose (mg/kg/d)	Twice a Week Dose (mg/kg per dose)	Maximum Dose	Adverse Reactions
Ethambutol	Tablets 100 mg 400 mg	15-25	50	2.5 g	Optic neuritis (usually reversible), decreased visual acuity, decreased red-green color discrimination, gastrointestinal disturbances, hypersensitivity
Isoniazid[1]	Scored tablets 100 mg 300 mg Syrup 10 mg/mL	10-15[2]	20-30	Daily, 300 mg Twice a week, 900 mg	Mild hepatic enzyme elevation, hepatitis,[2] peripheral neuritis, hypersensitivity
Pyrazinamide[1]	Scored tablets 500 mg	20-40	50	2 g	Hepatotoxicity, hyperuricemia
Rifampin[1]	Capsules 150 mg 300 mg Syrup formulated in syrup from capsules	10-20	10-20	600 mg	Orange discoloration of secretions/urine, staining contact lenses, vomiting, hepatitis, flu-like reaction, and thrombocytopenia; may render birth-control pills ineffective
Streptomycin (I.M. administration)	Vials 1 g 4 g	20-40	20-40	1 g	Auditory and vestibular toxicity, nephrotoxicity, rash

[1]Rifamate® is a capsule containing 150 mg of isoniazid and 300 mg of rifampin. Two capsules provide the usual adult (>50 kg body weight) daily doses of each drug. Rifater® is a capsule containing 50 mg of isoniazid, 120 mg of rifampin, and 300 mg of pyrazinamide.

[2]When isoniazid in a dosage exceeding 10 mg/kg/day is used in combination with rifampin, the incidence of hepatotoxicity may be increased.

Adapted from "Report of the Committee on Infectious Diseases," *2000 Red Book®*, 25th ed.

Rifampin is a bactericidal agent. It is metabolized by the liver and affects the pharmacokinetics of many other drugs, affecting their serum concentrations. Mycobacterium tuberculosis, initially resistant to rifampin, remains relatively uncommon in most areas of the United States. Rifampin is excreted in bile and urine and can cause orange urine, sweat and tears. It can also cause discoloration of soft contact lenses and render oral contraceptives ineffective. Hepatotoxicity occurs rarely. Blood dyscrasia accompanied by influenza-like symptoms can occur if doses are taken sporadically.

TUBERCULOSIS TREATMENT GUIDELINES *(Continued)*

Less Commonly Used Drugs for Treatment of Drug-Resistant Tuberculosis in Infants, Children, and Adolescents[1]

Drugs	Dosage Forms	Daily Dose (mg/kg/d)	Maximum Dose	Adverse Reactions
Capreomycin	Vials 1 g	15-30 I.M.	1 g	Ototoxicity, nephrotoxicity
Ciprofloxacin[2]	Tablets 250 mg 500 mg 750 mg	Adults 500-1500 mg total per day (twice daily)	1.5 g	Theoretical effect on growing cartilage, gastrointestinal tract disturbances, rash, headache
Cycloserine	Capsules 250 mg	10-20	1 g	Psychosis, personality changes, seizures, rash
Ethionamide	Tablets 250 mg	15-20 given in 2-3 divided doses	1 g	Gastrointestinal tract disturbances, hepatotoxicity, hypersensitive reactions
Kanamycin	Vials 75 mg/2 mL 500 mg/2 mL 1 g/3 mL	15-30 I.M.	1 g	Auditory and vestibular toxic effects, nephrotoxicity
Levofloxacin[2]	Tablets 250 mg 500 mg Vials 25 mg/mL	Adults 500-1000 mg once daily	1 g	Theoretical effect on growing cartilage, gastrointestinal tract disturbances, rash, headache
Ofloxacin[2]	Tablets 200 mg 300 mg 400 mg	Adults 400-800 mg total per day (twice daily)	0.8 g	Theoretical effect on growing cartilage, gastrointestinal tract disturbances, rash, headache
Para-amino salicylic acid (PAS)	Tablets 500 mg	200-300 (3-4 times/day)	10 g	Gastrointestinal tract disturbances, hypersensitivity, hepatotoxicity

[1]These drugs should be used in consultation with a specialist in tuberculosis.

[2]Fluoroquinolones are not currently approved for use in persons <18 years; their use in younger patients necessitates assessment of the potential risks and benefits.

Adapted from "Report of the Committee on Infectious Diseases," *2000 Red Book®*, 25th ed.

TB Drugs in Special Situations

Drug	Pregnancy	CNS TB Disease	Renal Insufficiency
Isoniazid	Safe	Good penetration	Normal clearance
Rifampin	Safe	Fair penetration Penetrates inflamed meninges (10% to 20%)	Normal clearance
Pyrazinamide	Avoid	Good penetration	Clearance reduced Decrease dose or prolong interval
Ethambutol	Safe	Penetrates inflamed meninges only (4% to 64%)	Clearance reduced Decrease dose or prolong interval
Streptomycin	Avoid	Penetrates inflamed meninges only	Clearance reduced Decrease dose or prolong interval
Capreomycin	Avoid	Penetrates inflamed meninges only	Clearance reduced Decrease dose or prolong interval
Kanamycin	Avoid	Penetrates inflamed meninges only	Clearance reduced Decrease dose or prolong interval
Ethionamide	Do not use	Good penetration	Normal clearance
Para-aminosalicylic acid	Safe	Penetrates inflamed meninges only (10% to 50%)	Incomplete data on clearance
Cycloserine	Avoid	Good penetration	Clearance reduced Decrease dose or prolong interval
Ciprofloxacin	Do not use	Fair penetration (5% to 10%) Penetrates inflamed meninges (50% to 90%)	Clearance reduced Decrease dose or prolong interval
Ofloxacin	Do not use	Fair penetration (5% to 10%) Penetrates inflamed meninges (50% to 90%)	Clearance reduced Decrease dose or prolong interval
Amikacin	Avoid	Penetrates inflamed meninges only	Clearance reduced Decrease dose or prolong interval
Clofazimine	Avoid	Penetration unknown	Clearance probably normal

Safe = the drug has not been demonstrated to have teratogenic effects.

Avoid = data on the drug's safety are limited, or the drug is associated with mild malformations (as in the aminoglycosides).

Do not use = studies show an association between the drug and premature labor, congenital malformations, or teratogenicity.

TUBERCULOSIS TREATMENT GUIDELINES *(Continued)*

Recommendations for Coadministering Different Antiretroviral Drugs With the Antimycobacterial Drugs Rifabutin and Rifampin

Antiretroviral	Use in Combination with Rifabutin	Use in Combination with Rifampin	Comments
Saquinavir[1] Hard-gel capsules (HGC)	Possibly[2], if antiretroviral regimen also includes ritonavir	Possibly, if antiretroviral regimen also includes ritonavir	Coadministration of saquinavir SGC with usual-dose rifabutin (300 mg/day or 2-3 times/week) is a possibility. However, the pharmacokinetic data and clinical experience for this combination are limited.
Soft-gel capsules (SGC)	Probably[3]	Possibly, if antiretroviral regimen also includes ritonavir	The combination of saquinavir SGC or saquinavir HGC and ritonavir, coadministered with 1) usual-dose rifampin (600 mg/day or 2-3 times/week), or 2) reduced-dose rifabutin (150 mg 2-3 times/week) is a possibility. However, the pharmacokinetic data and clinical experience for these combinations are limited. Coadministration of saquinavir or saquinavir SGC with rifampin is not recommended because rifampin markedly decreases concentrations of saquinavir.
Ritonavir	Probably	Probably	If the combination of ritonavir and rifabutin is used, then a substantially reduced-dose rifabutin regimen (150 mg 2-3 times/week) is recommended. Coadministration of ritonavir with usual-dose rifampin (600 mg/day or 2-3 times/week) is a possibility, though pharmacokinetic data and clinical experience are limited.
Indinavir	Yes	No	There is limited, but favorable, clinical experience with coadministration of indinavir[4] with a reduced daily dose of rifabutin (150 mg) or with the usual dose of rifabutin (300 mg 2-3 times/week). Coadministration of indinavir with rifampin is not recommended because rifampin markedly decreases concentrations of indinavir.
Nelfinavir	Yes	No	There is limited, but favorable, clinical experience with coadministration of nelfinavir[5] with a reduced daily dose of rifabutin (150 mg) or with the usual dose of rifabutin (300 mg 2-3 times/week). Coadministration of nelfinavir with rifampin is not recommended because rifampin markedly decreases concentrations of nelfinavir.
Amprenavir	Yes	No	Coadministration of amprenavir with a reduced daily dose of rifabutin (150 mg) or with the usual dose of rifabutin (300 mg 2-3 times/week) is a possibility, but there is no published clinical experience. Coadministration of amprenavir with rifampin is not recommended because rifampin markedly decreases concentrations of amprenavir.
Nevirapine	Yes	Possibly	Coadministration of nevirapine with usual-dose rifabutin (300 mg/day or 2-3 times/week) is a possibility based on pharmacokinetic study data. However, there is no published clinical experience for this combination. Data are insufficient to assess whether dose adjustments are necessary when rifampin is coadministered with nevirapine. Therefore, rifampin and nevirapine should be used only in combination if clearly indicated and with careful monitoring.

Recommendations for Coadministering Different Antiretroviral Drugs With the Antimycobacterial Drugs Rifabutin and Rifampin

(continued)

Antiretroviral	Use in Combination with Rifabutin	Use in Combination with Rifampin	Comments
Delavirdine	No	No	Contraindicated because of the marked decrease in concentrations of delavirdine when administered with either rifabutin or rifampin.
Efavirenz	Probably	Probably	Coadministration of efavirenz with increased-dose rifabutin (450 mg/day or 600 mg/day, or 600 mg 2-3 times/week) is a possibility, though there is no published clinical experience. Coadministration of efavirenz[6] with usual-dose rifampin (600 mg/day or 2-3 times/week) is a possibility, though there is no published clinical experience.

[1]Usual recommended doses are 400 mg twice daily for each of these protease inhibitors and 400 mg of ritonavir.

[2]Despite limited data and clinical experience, the use of this combination is potentially successful.

[3]Based on available data and clinical experience, the successful use of this combination is likely.

[4] Usual recommended dose is 800 mg every 8 hours; some experts recommend increasing the indinavir dose to 1000 mg every 8 hours if indinavir is used in combination with rifabutin.

[5]Usual recommended dose is 750 mg 3 times/day or 1250 mg twice daily; some experts recommend increasing the nelfinavir dose to 1000 mg if the 3-times/day dosing is used and nelfinavir is used in combination with rifabutin.

[6]Usual recommended dose is 600 mg/day; some experts recommend increasing the efavirenz dose to 800 mg/day if efavirenz is used in combination with rifampin.

Updated March 2000 from www.hivatis.org -"Updated Guidelines for the Use of Rifabutin or Rifampin for the Treatment and Prevention of Tuberculosis Among HIV-Infected Patients Taking Protease Inhibitors or Nonnucleoside Reverse Transcriptase Inhibitors," *MMWR,* March 10, 2000, 49(09):185-9.

Changes From Prior Recommendations on Tuberculin Testing and Treatment of Latent Tuberculosis Infection (LTBI)

Tuberculin Testing

- Emphasis on targeted tuberculin testing among persons at high risk for recent LTBI or with clinical conditions that increase the risk for tuberculosis (TB), regardless of age; testing is discouraged among persons at lower risk.
- For patients with organ transplant and other immunosuppressed patients (eg, persons receiving the equivalent of ≥15 mg/day prednisone for 1 month or more), 5 mm of induration rather than 10 mm of induration as a cut-off level for tuberculin positivity.
- A tuberculin skin test conversion is defined as an increase of ≥10 mm of induration within a 2-year period, regardless of age.

Treatment of Latent Tuberculosis Infection

- For HIV-negative persons, isoniazid given for 9 months is preferred over 6-month regimens.
- For HIV-positive persons and those with fibrotic lesions on chest x-ray consistent with previous TB, isoniazid should be given for 9 months instead of 12 months.
- For HIV-negative and HIV-positive persons, rifampin and pyrazinamide should be given for 2 months.
- For HIV-negative and HIV-positive persons, rifampin should be given for 4 months.

Clinical and Laboratory Monitoring

- Routine baseline and follow-up laboratory monitoring can be eliminated in most persons with LTBI, except for those with HIV infection, pregnant women (or those in the immediate postpartum period), and persons with chronic liver disease or those who use alcohol regularly.
- Emphasis on clinical monitoring for signs and symptoms of possible adverse effects, with prompt evaluation and changes in treatment, as indicated.

Modified from *MMWR Morb Mortal Wkly Rep,* 2000, 49(RR-6).

TUBERCULOSIS TREATMENT GUIDELINES *(Continued)*

Criteria for Tuberculin Positivity, by Risk Group

Reaction ≥5 mm of Induration	Reaction ≥10 mm of Induration	Reaction ≥15 mm of Induration
HIV-positive persons	Recent immigrants (ie, within the last 5 years) from high prevalence countries	Persons with no risk factors for TB
Recent contacts of tuberculosis (TB) case patients	Injection drug users	
Fibrotic changes on chest radiograph consistent with prior TB	Residents and employees[1] of the following high risk congregate settings: prisons and jails, nursing homes and other long-term facilities for the elderly, hospitals and other healthcare facilities, residential facilities for patients with AIDS, and homeless shelters	
Patients with organ transplant and other immunosuppressed patients (receiving the equivalent of ≥15 mg/day of prednisone for 1 month of more)[2]	Mycobacteriology laboratory personnel	
	Persons with the following clinical conditions that place them at high risk: silicosis, diabetes mellitus, chronic renal failure, some hematologic disorders (eg, leukemias and lymphomas), other specific malignancies (eg, carcinoma of the head or neck and lung), weight loss of ≥10% of ideal body weight, gastrectomy, and jejunoileal bypass	
	Children <4 years of age or infants, children, and adolescents exposed to adults at high-risk	

[1]For persons who are otherwise at low risk and are tested at the start of employment, a reaction of ≥15 mm induration is considered positive.

[2]Risk of TB in patients treated with corticosteroids increases with higher dose and longer duration.

Modified from *MMWR Morb Mortal Wkly Rep*, 2000, 49(RR-6).

Recommended Drug Regimens for Treatment of Latent Tuberculosis (TB) Infection in Adults

Drug	Interval and Duration	Comments	Rating[1] (Evidence)[2] HIV⁻	HIV⁺
Isoniazid	Daily for 9 months[3,4]	In HIV-infected patients, isoniazid may be administered concurrently with nucleoside reverse transcriptase inhibitors (NRTIs), protease inhibitors, or non-nucleoside reverse transcriptase inhibitors (NNRTIs)	A (II)	A (II)
	Twice weekly for 9 months[3,4]	Directly observed therapy (DOT) must be used with twice-weekly dosing	B (II)	B (II)
Isoniazid	Daily for 6 months[4]	Not indicated for HIV-infected persons, those with fibrotic lesions on chest radiographs, or children	B (I)	C (I)
	Twice weekly for 6 months[4]	DOT must be used with twice-weekly dosing	B (II)	C (I)
Rifampin plus pyrazinamide	Daily for 2 months	May also be offered to persons who are contacts of pyrazinamide patients with isoniazid-resistant, rifampin-susceptible TB	B (II)	A (II)
		In HIV-infected persons, protease inhibitors or NNRTIs should generally not be administered concurrently with rifampin; rifabutin can be used as an alternative for patients treated with indinavir, nelfinavir, amprenivir, ritonavir, or efavirenz, and possibly with nevirapine or soft-gel saquinavir[5]		
	Twice weekly for 2-3 months	DOT must be used with twice-weekly dosing	C (II)	C (I)
Rifampin	Daily for 4 months	For persons who cannot tolerate pyrazinamide	B (II)	B (III)
		For persons who are contacts of patients with isoniazid-resistant rifampin-susceptible TB who cannot tolerate pyrazinamide		

[1]Strength of recommendation: A = preferred; B = acceptable alternative; C = offer when A and B cannot be given.

[2]Quality of evidence: I = randomized clinical trial data; II = data from clinical trials that are not randomized or were conducted in other populations; III = expert opinion.

[3]Recommended regimen for children <18 years of age.

[4]Recommended regimens for pregnant women. Some experts would use rifampin and pyrazinamide for 2 months as an alternative regimen for HIV-infected pregnant women, although pyrazinamide should be avoided during the first trimester.

[5]Rifabutin should not be used with hard-gel saquinavir or delavirdine. When used with other protease inhibitors or NNRTIs, dose adjustment of rifabutin may be required.

Modified from *MMWR Morb Mortal Wkly Rep*, 2000, 49(RR-6).

Chemistry *(continued)*

Uric acid	Male	3-7 mg/dL
	Female	2-6 mg/dL

ENZYMES

Alanine aminotransferase (ALT)	0-2 mo	8-78 units/L
(SGPT)	>2 mo	8-36 units/L
Alkaline phosphatase (ALKP)	Newborns	60-130 units/L
	0-16 y	85-400 units/L
	>16 y	30-115 units/L
Aspartate aminotransferase (AST)	Infants	18-74 units/L
(SGOT)	Children	15-46 units/L
	Adults	5-35 units/L
Creatine kinase (CK)	Infants	20-200 units/L
	Children	10-90 units/L
	Adult male	0-206 units/L
	Adult female	0-175 units/L
Lactate dehydrogenase (LDH)	Newborns	290-501 units/L
	1 mo to 2 y	110-144 units/L
	>16 y	60-170 units/L

BLOOD GASES

	Arterial	Capillary	Venous
pH	7.35-7.45	7.35-7.45	7.32-7.42
pCO_2 (mm Hg)	35-45	35-45	38-52
pO_2 (mm Hg)	70-100	60-80	24-48
HCO_3 (mEq/L)	19-25	19-25	19-25
TCO_2 (mEq/L)	19-29	19-29	23-33
O_2 saturation (%)	90-95	90-95	40-70
Base excess (mEq/L)	-5 to +5	-5 to +5	-5 to +5

THYROID FUNCTION TESTS

T_4 (thyroxine)	1-7 d	10.1-20.9 µg/dL
	8-14 d	9.8-16.6 µg/dL
	1 mo to 1 y	5.5-16.0 µg/dL
	>1 y	4-12 µg/dL
FTI	1-3 d	9.3-26.6
	1-4 wks	7.6-20.8
	1-4 mo	7.4-17.9
	4-12 mo	5.1-14.5
	1-6 y	5.7-13.3
	>6 y	4.8-14.0
T_3 by RIA	Newborns	100-470 ng/dL
	1-5 y	100-260 ng/dL
	5-10 y	90-240 ng/dL
	10 y to adult	70-210 ng/dL
T_3 uptake		35%-45%
TSH	Cord	3-22 µU/mL
	1-3 d	<40 µU/mL
	3-7 d	<25 µU/mL
	>7 d	0-10 µU/mL

REFERENCE VALUES FOR ADULTS

Automated Chemistry (CHEMISTRY A)

Test	Values	Remarks
SERUM PLASMA		
Acetone	Negative	
Albumin	3.2-5 g/dL	
Alcohol, ethyl	Negative	
Aldolase	1.2-7.6 IU/L	
Ammonia	20-70 mcg/dL	Specimen to be placed on ice as soon as collected
Amylase	30-110 units/L	
Bilirubin, direct	0-0.3 mg/dL	
Bilirubin, total	0.1-1.2 mg/dL	
Calcium	8.6-10.3 mg/dL	
Calcium, ionized	2.24-2.46 mEq/L	
Chloride	95-108 mEq/L	
Cholesterol, total	≤220 mg/dL	Fasted blood required – normal value affected by dietary habits. This reference range is for a general adult population
HDL cholesterol	40-60 mg/dL	Fasted blood required – normal value affected by dietary habits
LDL cholesterol	65-170 mg/dL	LDLC calculated by Friewald formula... which has certain inaccuracies and is invalid at trig levels >300 mg/dL
CO_2	23-30 mEq/L	
Creatine kinase (CK) isoenzymes		
CK-BB	0%	
CK-MB (cardiac)	0%-3.9%	
CK-MM (muscle)	96%-100%	
CK-MB levels must be both ≥4% and 10 IU/L to meet diagnostic criteria for CK-MB positive result consistent with myocardial injury.		
Creatine phosphokinase (CPK)	8-150 IU/L	
Creatinine	0.5-1.4 mg/dL	
Ferritin	13-300 ng/mL	
Folate	3.6-20.0 ng/mL	
GGT (gamma-glutamyltranspeptidase)		
male	11-63 IU/L	
female	8-35 IU/L	
GLDH	To be determined	
Glucose (2-h postprandial)	Up to 140 mg/dL	
Glucose, fasting	60-110 mg/dL	
Glucose, nonfasting (2-h postprandial)	60-140 mg/dL	
Hemoglobin A_{1c}	8	
Hemoglobin, plasma free	<2.5 mg/100 mL	
Hemoglobin, total glycosylated (Hb A_1)	4%-8%	
Iron	65-150 mcg/dL	
Iron binding capacity, total (TIBC)	250-420 mcg/dL	
Lactic acid	0.7-2.1 mEq/L	Specimen to be kept on ice and sent to lab as soon as possible
Lactate dehydrogenase (LDH)	56-194 IU/L	
Lactate dehydrogenase (LDH) isoenzymes		
LD_1	20%-34%	
LD_2	29%-41%	
LD_3	15%-25%	
LD_4	1%-12%	
LD_5	1%-15%	
Flipped LD_1/LD_2 ratios (>1 may be consistent with myocardial injury) particularly when considered in combination with a recent CK-MB positive result		
Lipase	23-208 units/L	
Magnesium	1.6-2.5 mg/dL	Increased by slight hemolysis
Osmolality	289-308 mOsm/kg	
Phosphatase, alkaline		
adults 25-60 y	33-131 IU/L	
adults 61 y or older	51-153 IU/L	

Automated Chemistry (CHEMISTRY A) *(continued)*

Test	Values	Remarks
infancy-adolescence	Values range up to 3-5 times higher than adults	
Phosphate, inorganic	2.8-4.2 mg/dL	
Potassium	3.5-5.2 mEq/L	Increased by slight hemolysis
Prealbumin	>15 mg/dL	
Protein, total	6.5-7.9 g/dL	
SGOT (AST)	<35 IU/L (20-48)	
SGPT (ALT) (10-35)	<35 IU/L	
Sodium	134-149 mEq/L	
Transferrin	>200 mg/dL	
Triglycerides	45-155 mg/dL	Fasted blood required
Urea nitrogen (BUN)	7-20 mg/dL	
Uric acid		
male	2.0-8.0 mg/dL	
female	2.0-7.5 mg/dL	

CEREBROSPINAL FLUID

Test	Values	Remarks
Glucose	50-70 mg/dL	
Protein		
adults and children	15-45 mg/dL	CSF obtained by lumbar puncture
newborn infants	60-90 mg/dL	

On CSF obtained by cisternal puncture: About 25 mg/dL
On CSF obtained by ventricular puncture: About 10 mg/dL
Note: Bloody specimen gives erroneously high value due to contamination with blood proteins

URINE
(24-hour specimen is required for all these tests unless specified)

Test	Values	Remarks
Amylase	32-641 units/L	The value is in units/L and **not** calculated for total volume
Amylase, fluid (random samples)		Interpretation of value left for physician, depends on the nature of fluid
Calcium	Depends upon dietary intake	
Creatine		
male	150 mg/24 h	Higher value on children and during pregnancy
female	250 mg/24 h	
Creatinine	1000-2000 mg/24 h	
Creatinine clearance (endogenous)		
male	85-125 mL/min	A blood sample must accompany urine specimen
female	75-115 mL/min	
Glucose	1 g/24 h	
5-hydroxyindoleacetic acid	2-8 mg/24 h	
Iron	0.15 mg/24 h	Acid washed container required
Magnesium	146-209 mg/24 h	
Osmolality	500-800 mOsm/kg	With normal fluid intake
Oxalate	10-40 mg/24 h	
Phosphate	400-1300 mg/24 h	
Potassium	25-120 mEq/24 h	Varies with diet; the interpretation of urine electrolytes and osmolality should be left for the physician
Sodium	40-220 mEq/24 h	
Porphobilinogen, qualitative	Negative	
Porphyrins, qualitative	Negative	
Proteins	0.05-0.1 g/24 h	
Salicylate	Negative	
Urea clearance	60-95 mL/min	A blood sample must accompany specimen
Urea N	10-40 g/24 h	Dependent on protein intake
Uric acid	250-750 mg/24 h	Dependent on diet and therapy
Urobilinogen	0.5-3.5 mg/24 h	For qualitative determination on random urine, send sample to urinalysis section in Hematology Lab

REFERENCE VALUES FOR ADULTS *(Continued)*

Automated Chemistry (CHEMISTRY A) *(continued)*

Test	Values	Remarks
Xylose absorption test		
children	16%-33% of ingested xylose	
adults	>4 g in 5 h	
FECES		
Fat, 3-day collection	<5 g/d	Value depends on fat intake of 100 g/d for 3 days preceding and during collection
GASTRIC ACIDITY		
Acidity, total, 12 h	10-60 mEq/L	Titrated at pH 7

BLOOD GASES

	Arterial	Capillary	Venous
pH	7.35-7.45	7.35-7.45	7.32-7.42
pCO_2 (mm Hg)	35-45	35-45	38-52
pO_2 (mm Hg)	70-100	60-80	24-48
HCO_3 (mEq/L)	19-25	19-25	19-25
TCO_2 (mEq/L)	19-29	19-29	23-33
O_2 saturation (%)	90-95	90-95	40-70
Base excess (mEq/L)	-5 to +5	-5 to +5	-5 to +5

HEMATOLOGY

Complete Blood Count

Age	Hgb (g/dL)	Hct (%)	RBC (mill/mm³)	RDW
0-3 d	15.0-20.0	45-61	4.0-5.9	<18
1-2 wk	12.5-18.5	39-57	3.6-5.5	<17
1-6 mo	10.0-13.0	29-42	3.1-4.3	<16.5
7 mo to 2 y	10.5-13.0	33-38	3.7-4.9	<16
2-5 y	11.5-13.0	34-39	3.9-5.0	<15
5-8 y	11.5-14.5	35-42	4.0-4.9	<15
13-18 y	12.0-15.2	36-47	4.5-5.1	<14.5
Adult male	13.5-16.5	41-50	4.5-5.5	<14.5
Adult female	12.0-15.0	36-44	4.0-4.9	<14.5

Age	MCV (fL)	MCH (pg)	MCHC (%)	Plts (x 10³/mm³)
0-3 d	95-115	31-37	29-37	250-450
1-2 wk	86-110	28-36	28-38	250-450
1-6 mo	74-96	25-35	30-36	300-700
7 mo to 2 y	70-84	23-30	31-37	250-600
2-5 y	75-87	24-30	31-37	250-550
5-8 y	77-95	25-33	31-37	250-550
13-18 y	78-96	25-35	31-37	150-450
Adult male	80-100	26-34	31-37	150-450
Adult female	80-100	26-34	31-37	150-450

WBC and Diff

Age	WBC (x 10^3/mm^3)	Segs	Bands	Lymphs	Monos
0-3 d	9.0-35.0	32-62	10-18	19-29	5-7
1-2 wk	5.0-20.0	14-34	6-14	36-45	6-10
1-6 mo	6.0-17.5	13-33	4-12	41-71	4-7
7 mo to 2 y	6.0-17.0	15-35	5-11	45-76	3-6
2-5 y	5.5-15.5	23-45	5-11	35-65	3-6
5-8 y	5.0-14.5	32-54	5-11	28-48	3-6
13-18 y	4.5-13.0	34-64	5-11	25-45	3-6
Adults	4.5-11.0	35-66	5-11	24-44	3-6

Age	Eosinophils	Basophils	Atypical Lymphs	No. of NRBCs
0-3 d	0-2	0-1	0-8	0-2
1-2 wk	0-2	0-1	0-8	0
1-6 mo	0-3	0-1	0-8	0
7 mo to 2 y	0-3	0-1	0-8	0
2-5 y	0-3	0-1	0-8	0
5-8 y	0-3	0-1	0-8	0
13-18 y	0-3	0-1	0-8	0
Adults	0-3	0-1	0-8	0

Segs = segmented neutrophils
Bands = band neutrophils

Lymphs = lymphocytes
Monos = monocytes

Erythrocyte Sedimentation Rates and Reticulocyte Counts

Sedimentation rate, Westergren	Children	0-20 mm/hour
	Adult male	0-15 mm/hour
	Adult female	0-20 mm/hour
Sedimentation rate, Wintrobe	Children	0-13 mm/hour
	Adult male	0-10 mm/hour
	Adult female	0-15 mm/hour
Reticulocyte count	Newborns	2%-6%
	1-6 mo	0%-2.8%
	Adults	0.5%-1.5%

CALCULATIONS FOR TOTAL PARENTERAL NUTRITION THERAPY – ADULT PATIENTS

Condition	Calorie Requirement (kcal/kg/d)	Protein Requirement (g/kg/d)
Resting state (adult medical patient)	20-30	0.8-1
Uncomplicated postop patients	25-35	1-1.3
Depleted patients	30-40	1.3-1.7
Hypermetabolic patients (trauma, sepsis, burns)	35-45	1.5-2

1 g protein yields 4 kcal/g
1 g fat yields 9 kcal/g
1 g dextrose yields 3.4 kcal/g
1 g nitrogen = 6.25 g protein

Electrolytes Required/Day

	mEq/d
Sodium	60-120
Potassium	60-120
Chloride	100-150
Magnesium	10-24
Calcium	10-20
Phosphate	20-50 mmol/d
Sulfate	10-24
Acetate	60-150
Bicarbonate	Should not be added

Estimated Energy Requirements

Basal Energy Expenditure (BEE)	
Harris Benedict equation	
males	$BEE_{mal} = 66.67 + (13.75 \times kg) + (5 \times cm) - (6.76 \times y)$
females	$BEE_{fem} = 665.1 + (9.56 \times kg) + (1.85 \times cm) - (4.68 \times y)$
Total daily energy expenditure (TDE)	**TDE = BEE x activity factor x injury factor**
Activity factor	Confined to bed = 1.2
	Out of bed = 1.3
Injury factor	Surgery: Minor operations = 1-1.1 Major operations = 1.1-1.2
	Infection: Mild = 1-1.2 Moderate = 1.2-1.4 Severe = 1.4-1.6
	Skeletal trauma = 1.2-1.35
	Head injury (treated with corticosteroids) = 1.6
	Blunt trauma = 1.15-1.35
	Burns ≤20% body surface area (BSA) = 2 20%-30% BSA = 2-2.2 >30% BSA = 2.2

Estimated Fluid Requirements

30-35 mL/kg/d
or
mL/d = 1500 mL for first 20 kg of body weight + 20 mL/kg for body weight >20 kg

MEDIAN HEIGHTS AND WEIGHTS AND RECOMMENDED ENERGY INTAKE[1]

Age (y) or Condition	Weight (kg)	Weight (lb)	Height (cm)	Height (in)	REE[2] (kcal/d)	Average Energy Allowance (kcal)[3] Multiples of REE	/kg	/d[4]
Infants								
0-0.5	6	13	60	24	320		108	650
0.5-1	9	20	71	28	500		98	850
Children								
1-3	13	29	90	35	740		102	1300
4-6	20	44	112	44	950		90	1800
7-10	28	62	132	52	1130		70	2000
Male								
11-14	45	99	157	62	1440	1.70	55	2500
15-18	66	145	176	69	1760	1.67	45	3000
19-24	72	160	177	70	1780	1.67	40	2900
25-50	79	174	176	70	1800	1.60	37	2900
51+	77	170	173	68	1530	1.50	30	2300
Female								
11-14	46	101	157	62	1310	1.67	47	2200
15-18	55	120	163	64	1370	1.60	40	2200
19-24	58	128	164	65	1350	1.60	38	2200
25-50	63	138	163	64	1380	1.55	36	2200
51+	65	143	160	63	1280	1.50	30	1900
Pregnant								+0
1st trimester								+300
2nd trimester								+300
3rd trimester								+300
Lactating								
1st 6 months								+500
2nd 6 months								+500

[1]From *Recommended Dietary Allowances*, 10th ed, Washington, DC: National Academy Press, 1989.
[2]Calculation based on FAO equations, then rounded.
[3]In the range of light to moderate activity, the coefficient of variation is ±20%.
[4]Figure is rounded.

PEDIATRIC ALS ALGORITHMS
PALS Bradycardia Algorithm

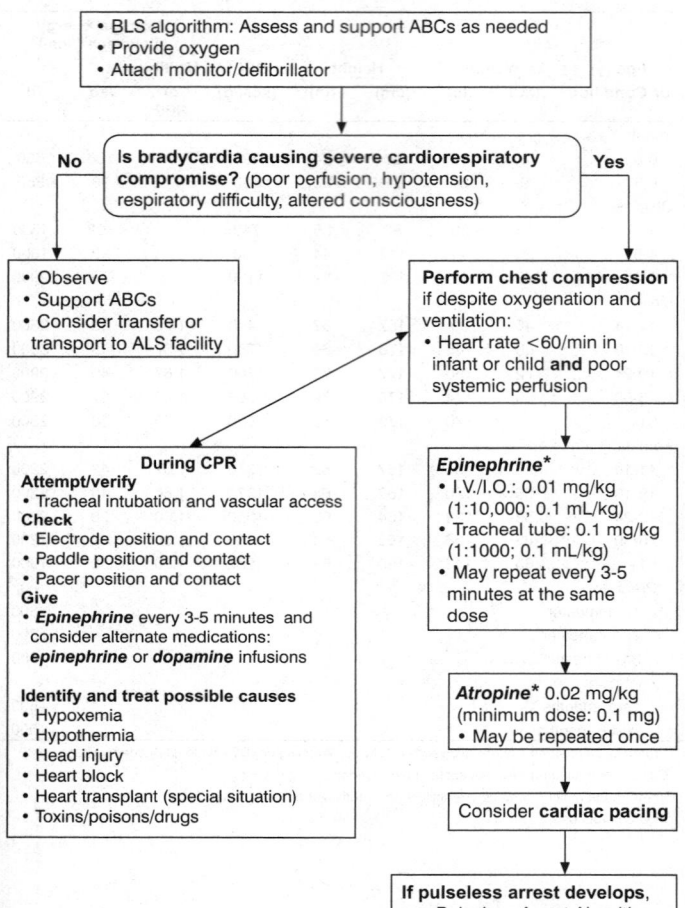

* BLS algorithm: Assess and support ABCs as needed
* Provide oxygen
* Attach monitor/defibrillator

No   **Is bradycardia causing severe cardiorespiratory compromise?** (poor perfusion, hypotension, respiratory difficulty, altered consciousness)   **Yes**

* Observe
* Support ABCs
* Consider transfer or transport to ALS facility

Perform chest compression if despite oxygenation and ventilation:
* Heart rate <60/min in infant or child **and** poor systemic perfusion

During CPR
Attempt/verify
* Tracheal intubation and vascular access
Check
* Electrode position and contact
* Paddle position and contact
* Pacer position and contact
Give
* *Epinephrine* every 3-5 minutes and consider alternate medications: *epinephrine* or *dopamine* infusions

Identify and treat possible causes
* Hypoxemia
* Hypothermia
* Head injury
* Heart block
* Heart transplant (special situation)
* Toxins/poisons/drugs

Epinephrine*
* I.V./I.O.: 0.01 mg/kg (1:10,000; 0.1 mL/kg)
* Tracheal tube: 0.1 mg/kg (1:1000; 0.1 mL/kg)
* May repeat every 3-5 minutes at the same dose

Atropine* 0.02 mg/kg (minimum dose: 0.1 mg)
* May be repeated once

Consider **cardiac pacing**

If pulseless arrest develops, *see* Pulseless Arrest Algorithm

*Give atropine first for bradycardia due to suspected increased vagal tone or primary AV block.

Adapted with permission of Lippincott Williams & Wilkins, "Guidelines 2000 for Cardiopulmonary Resuscitation and Emergency Cardiovascular Care, Part 10: Pediatric Advanced Life Support, The American Heart Association in Collaboration With the International Liaison Committee on Resuscitation," *Circulation*, 2000, 102(8 Suppl):I313.

PALS Pulseless Arrest Algorithm

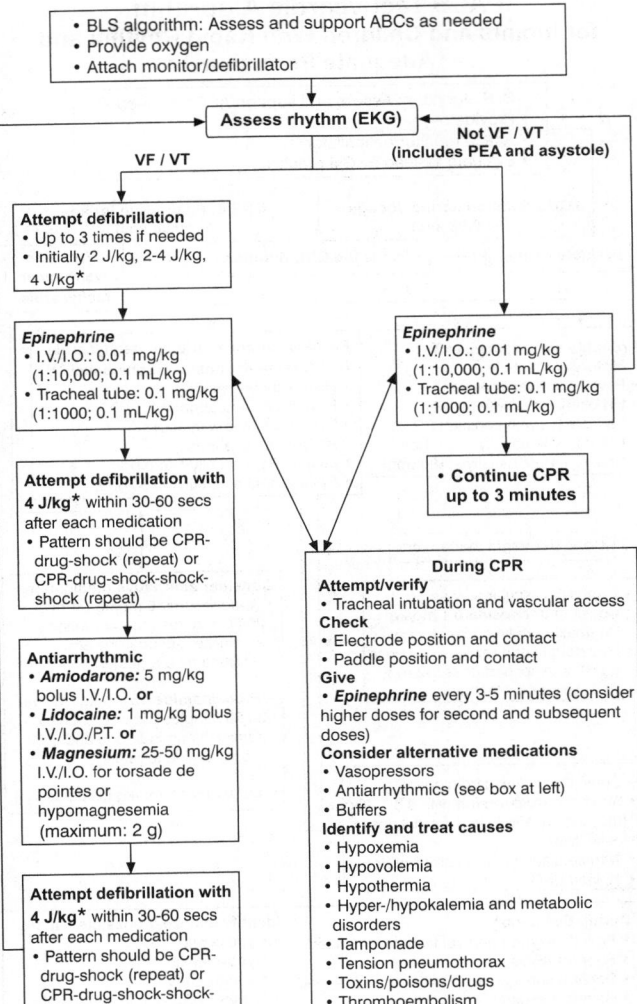

• BLS algorithm: Assess and support ABCs as needed
• Provide oxygen
• Attach monitor/defibrillator

Assess rhythm (EKG)

VF / VT

Not VF / VT
(includes PEA and asystole)

Attempt defibrillation
• Up to 3 times if needed
• Initially 2 J/kg, 2-4 J/kg, 4 J/kg*

Epinephrine
• I.V./I.O.: 0.01 mg/kg
  (1:10,000; 0.1 mL/kg)
• Tracheal tube: 0.1 mg/kg
  (1:1000; 0.1 mL/kg)

Epinephrine
• I.V./I.O.: 0.01 mg/kg
  (1:10,000; 0.1 mL/kg)
• Tracheal tube: 0.1 mg/kg
  (1:1000; 0.1 mL/kg)

Attempt defibrillation with 4 J/kg* within 30-60 secs after each medication
• Pattern should be CPR-drug-shock (repeat) or CPR-drug-shock-shock-shock (repeat)

• **Continue CPR up to 3 minutes**

Antiarrhythmic
• *Amiodarone:* 5 mg/kg bolus I.V./I.O. **or**
• *Lidocaine:* 1 mg/kg bolus I.V./I.O./P.T. **or**
• *Magnesium:* 25-50 mg/kg I.V./I.O. for torsade de pointes or hypomagnesemia (maximum: 2 g)

During CPR
Attempt/verify
• Tracheal intubation and vascular access
Check
• Electrode position and contact
• Paddle position and contact
Give
• *Epinephrine* every 3-5 minutes (consider higher doses for second and subsequent doses)
Consider alternative medications
• Vasopressors
• Antiarrhythmics (see box at left)
• Buffers
Identify and treat causes
• Hypoxemia
• Hypovolemia
• Hypothermia
• Hyper-/hypokalemia and metabolic disorders
• Tamponade
• Tension pneumothorax
• Toxins/poisons/drugs
• Thromboembolism

Attempt defibrillation with 4 J/kg* within 30-60 secs after each medication
• Pattern should be CPR-drug-shock (repeat) or CPR-drug-shock-shock-shock (repeat)

*Alternative waveforms and higher doses are Class Indeterminate for children.

Adapted with permission of Lippincott Williams & Wilkins, "Guidelines 2000 for Cardiopulmonary Resuscitation and Emergency Cardiovascular Care, Part 10: Pediatric Advanced Life Support, The American Heart Association in Collaboration With the International Liaison Committee on Resuscitation," *Circulation*, 2000, 102(8 Suppl):I311.

PEDIATRIC ALS ALGORITHMS *(Continued)*

PALS Tachycardia Algorithm
for Infants and Children With Rapid Rhythm and Adequate Perfusion

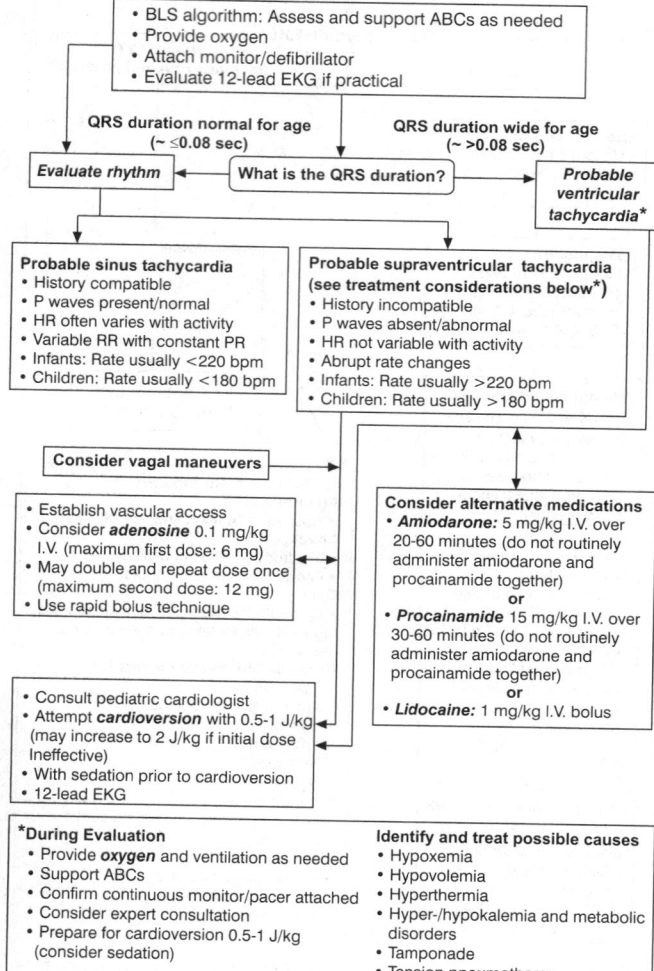

- BLS algorithm: Assess and support ABCs as needed
- Provide oxygen
- Attach monitor/defibrillator
- Evaluate 12-lead EKG if practical

QRS duration normal for age (~ ≤0.08 sec)

QRS duration wide for age (~ >0.08 sec)

Evaluate rhythm ← **What is the QRS duration?** → *Probable ventricular tachycardia**

Probable sinus tachycardia
- History compatible
- P waves present/normal
- HR often varies with activity
- Variable RR with constant PR
- Infants: Rate usually <220 bpm
- Children: Rate usually <180 bpm

Probable supraventricular tachycardia (see treatment considerations below*)
- History incompatible
- P waves absent/abnormal
- HR not variable with activity
- Abrupt rate changes
- Infants: Rate usually >220 bpm
- Children: Rate usually >180 bpm

Consider vagal maneuvers

- Establish vascular access
- Consider *adenosine* 0.1 mg/kg I.V. (maximum first dose: 6 mg)
- May double and repeat dose once (maximum second dose: 12 mg)
- Use rapid bolus technique

Consider alternative medications
- *Amiodarone:* 5 mg/kg I.V. over 20-60 minutes (do not routinely administer amiodarone and procainamide together)
  or
- *Procainamide* 15 mg/kg I.V. over 30-60 minutes (do not routinely administer amiodarone and procainamide together)
  or
- *Lidocaine:* 1 mg/kg I.V. bolus

- Consult pediatric cardiologist
- Attempt *cardioversion* with 0.5-1 J/kg (may increase to 2 J/kg if initial dose Ineffective)
- With sedation prior to cardioversion
- 12-lead EKG

*During Evaluation
- Provide *oxygen* and ventilation as needed
- Support ABCs
- Confirm continuous monitor/pacer attached
- Consider expert consultation
- Prepare for cardioversion 0.5-1 J/kg (consider sedation)

Identify and treat possible causes
- Hypoxemia
- Hypovolemia
- Hyperthermia
- Hyper-/hypokalemia and metabolic disorders
- Tamponade
- Tension pneumothorax
- Toxins/poisons/drugs
- Thromboembolism
- Pain

Adapted with permission of Lippincott Williams & Wilkins, "Guidelines 2000 for Cardiopulmonary Resuscitation and Emergency Cardiovascular Care, Part 10: Pediatric Advanced Life Support, The American Heart Association in Collaboration With the International Liaison Committee on Resuscitation," *Circulation*, 2000, 102(8 Suppl):I315.

PALS Tachycardia Algorithm
for Infants and Children With Rapid Rhythm and Evidence of Poor Perfusion

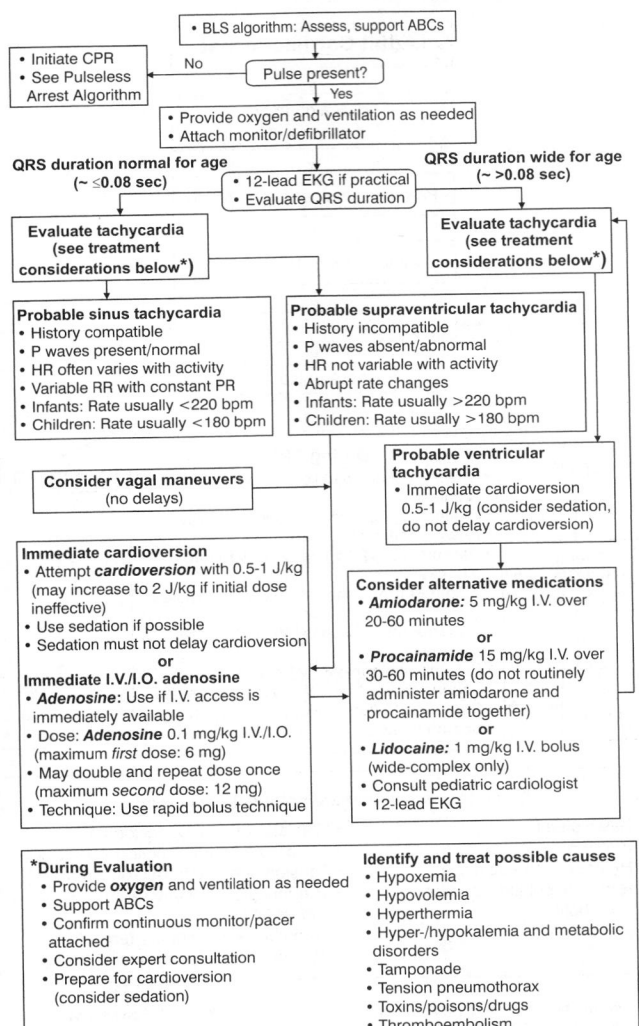

Adapted with permission of Lippincott Williams & Wilkins, "Guidelines 2000 for Cardiopulmonar Resuscitation and Emergency Cardiovascular Care, Part 10: Pediatric Advanced Life Support, The American Heart Association in Collaboration With the International Liaison Committee on Resuscitation," *Circulation*, 2000, 102(8 Suppl):I316.

ADULT ACLS ALGORITHMS
ILCOR Universal / International ACLS Algorithm

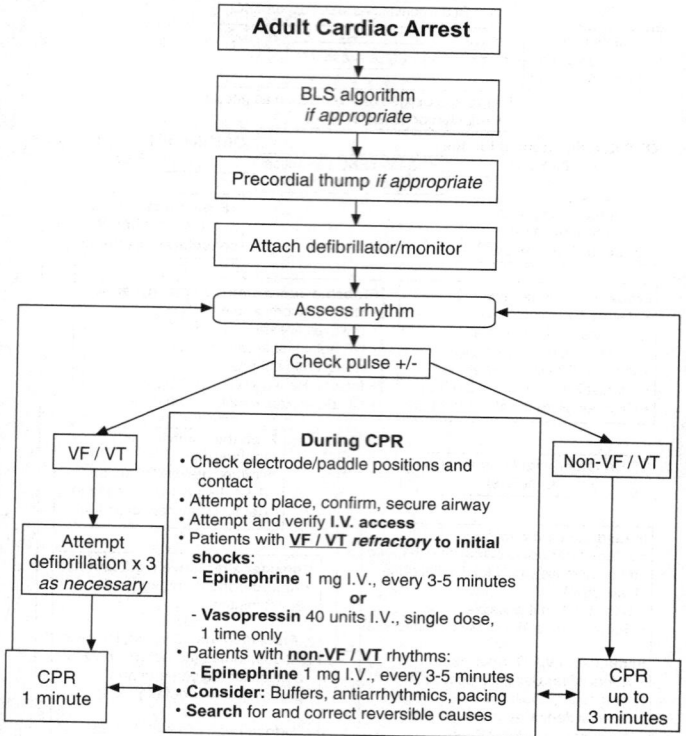

Consider causes that are potentially reversible

- Hypovolemia
- Hypoxia
- Hydrogen ion - acidosis
- Hyper-/hypokalemia, other metabolic
- Hypothermia

- "Tablets" (drug OD, accidents)
- Tamponade, cardiac (pericardiocentesis)
- Tension pneumothorax (decompress)
- Thrombosis, coronary (ACS); (fibrinolytics)
- Thrombosis, pulmonary (embolism, fibrinolytics, surgical evacuation)

Adapted with permission of Lippincott Williams & Wilkins, "Guidelines 2000 for Cardiopulmonary Resuscitation and Emergency Cardiovascular Care, Part 6: Advanced Cardiovascular Life Support, The American Heart Association in Collaboration With the International Liaison Committee on Resuscitation," *Circulation*, 2000, 102(8 Suppl):I143.

Comprehensive ECC Algorithm

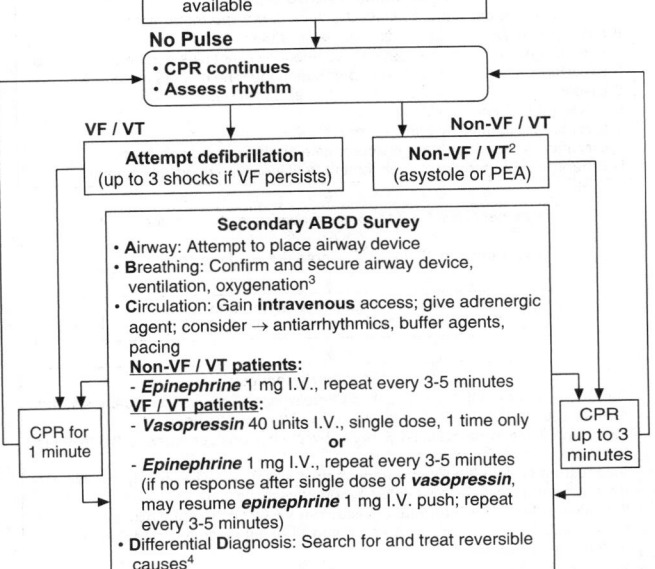

- Person collapses
- Possible cardiac arrest
- *Assess responsiveness*

Unresponsive ↓

Begin Primary ABCD Survey[1]
(Begin BLS Algorithm)
- Activate emergency response system
- Call for defibrillator
- **A** Assess breathing (open airway,
  look, listen, and feel)

Not Breathing ↓

- **B** Give 2 slow breaths
- **C** Assess pulse, if no pulse →
- **C** Start chest compressions
- **D** Attach monitor / defibrillator when
  available

No Pulse ↓

- CPR continues
- Assess rhythm

VF / VT   Non-VF / VT

Attempt defibrillation
(up to 3 shocks if VF persists)

Non-VF / VT[2]
(asystole or PEA)

Secondary ABCD Survey
- **A**irway: Attempt to place airway device
- **B**reathing: Confirm and secure airway device,
  ventilation, oxygenation[3]
- **C**irculation: Gain **intravenous** access; give adrenergic
  agent; consider → antiarrhythmics, buffer agents,
  pacing
  Non-VF / VT patients:
  - *Epinephrine* 1 mg I.V., repeat every 3-5 minutes
  VF / VT patients:
  - *Vasopressin* 40 units I.V., single dose, 1 time only
    or
  - *Epinephrine* 1 mg I.V., repeat every 3-5 minutes
    (if no response after single dose of *vasopressin*,
    may resume *epinephrine* 1 mg I.V. push; repeat
    every 3-5 minutes)
- **D**ifferential Diagnosis: Search for and treat reversible
  causes[4]

CPR for 1 minute

CPR up to 3 minutes

[1]Do not attempt resuscitation if any objective indicators of DNAR status or clinical
indicators that resuscitation attempts are not indicated (eg, signs of death).
[2]Recommendation is to consider non-VF / VT rhythms as one rthythm when the patient
is in cardiac arrest.
[3]Use 2 methods to confirm tube placement: Primary physical examination criteria plus a
secondary device (qualitative and quantitative measures of end-tidal CO_2).
[4]Reversible causes: See ILCOR Universal / International ACLS Algorithm.

Adapted with permission of Lippincott Williams & Wilkins, "Guidelines 2000 for Cardiopulmonary
Resuscitation and Emergency Cardiovascular Care, Part 6: Advanced Cardiovascular Life
Support, The American Heart Association in Collaboration With the International Liaison
Committee on Resuscitation," *Circulation*, 2000, 102(8 Suppl):I144.

ADULT ACLS ALGORITHMS *(Continued)*

Ventricular Fibrillation / Pulseless VT Algorithm

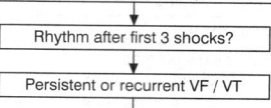

Primary ABCD Survey[1]
Focus: Basic CPR and defibrillation
- **Check** responsiveness
- **Activate** emergency response system
- **Call** for defibrillator

A Airway: Open the airway
B Breathing: Provide positive-pressure ventilations
C Circulation: Give chest compressions
D Defibrillation: Assess for and shock VF / pulseless VT, up to 3 times (200 J, 200-300 J, 360 J, or equivalent *biphasic*) if necessary

↓

Rhythm after first 3 shocks?

↓

Persistent or recurrent VF / VT

↓

Secondary ABCD Survey
Focus: More advanced assessments and treatments
A Airway: Place airway device as soon as possible
B Breathing: Confirm airway device placement by exam plus confirmation device[2]
B Breathing: Secure airway device; purpose-made tube holders preferred[3]
B Breathing: Confirm effective oxygenation and ventilation[4]
C Circulation: Establish I.V. access
C Circulation: Identify rhythm → monitor
C Circulation: Administer drugs appropriate for rhythm and condition
D Differential Diagnosis: Search for and treat identified reversible causes

↓

- *Epinephrine* 1 mg I.V. push, repeat every 3-5 minutes[5]
or
- *Vasopressin* 40 units I.V., **single dose**, 1 time only[6]

↓

Resume attempts to defibrillate
1 × 360 J (or equivalent *biphasic*) within 30-60 seconds

↓

Consider antiarrhythmics:[7]
Amiodarone (IIb): 300 mg I.V. push. If VF/pulseless VT recurs, consider a second dose of 150 mg (maximum cumulative dose: 2.2 g over 24 hours)
Lidocaine (indeterminate): 1-1.5 mg/kg I.V. push. Consider repeat in 3-5 minutes to maximum cumulative dose of 3 mg/kg
Magnesium sulfate (IIb if hypomagnesemic state): 1-2 g I.V. in polymorphic VT (torsade de pointes) and suspected hypomagnesemic state
Procainamide (IIb for intermittent/recurrent VF / VT): 30 mg/min in refractory VF (maximum total dose: 17 mg/kg) - acceptable but not recommended due to prolonged administration time
Consider buffers

↓

Resume attempts to defibrillate

[1]Do not attempt resuscitation if any objective indicators of DNAR status or clinical indicators that resuscitation attempts are not indicated (eg, signs of death).
[2]Consider continuous qualitative end-tidal CO_2 monitor (Class IIa - acceptable, probably effective).
[3]Commercial purpose-made tracheal tube holders recommended (Class IIb - acceptable, possibly effective).
[4]End-tidal CO_2 monitor and oxygen saturation monitor.
[5]If this fails, higher doses of epinephrine (up to 0.2 mg/kg) are acceptable (growing evidence of potential harm).
[6]No evidence about value of repeat vasopressin doses.
[7]Numbers in parentheses represent strength of recommendation (Class IIb - acceptable, possibly effective).

Adapted with permission of Lippincott Williams & Wilkins, "Guidelines 2000 for Cardiopulmonary Resuscitation and Emergency Cardiovascular Care, Part 6: Advanced Cardiovascular Life Support, The American Heart Association in Collaboration With the International Liaison Committee on Resuscitation," *Circulation*, 2000, 102(8 Suppl):I147.

Pulseless Electrical Activity Algorithm

(PEA = rhythm on monitor, without detectable pulse)

Primary ABCD Survey[1]
Focus: Basic CPR and defibrillation

- **Check** responsiveness
- **Activate** emergency response system
- **Call** for defibrillator

A Airway: Open the airway
B Breathing: Provide positive-pressure ventilations
C Circulation: Give chest compressions
D Defibrillation: Assess for and shock VF / pulseless VT

↓

Secondary ABCD Survey
Focus: More advanced assessments and treatments

A Airway: Place airway device as soon as possible
B Breathing: Confirm airway device placement by exam plus confirmation device[2]
B Breathing: Secure airway device; purpose-made tube holders preferred[3]
B Breathing: Confirm effective oxygenation and ventilation[4]
C Circulation: Establish I.V. access
C Circulation: Identify rhythm → monitor
C Circulation: Administer drugs appropriate for rhythm and condition
C Circulation: Assess for occult blood flow ("pseudo-EMT")
D Differential Diagnosis: Search for and treat identified reversible causes

↓

Review for most frequent causes[5]

- Hypovolemia
- Hypoxia
- Hydrogen ion - acidosis
- Hyper-/hypokalemia
- Hypothermia

- "Tablets" (drug OD, accidents)
- Tamponade, cardiac
- Tension pneumothorax
- Thrombosis, coronary (ACS)
- Thrombosis, pulmonary (embolism)

↓

- ***Epinephrine*** 1 mg I.V. push, repeat every 3-5 minutes[6]

↓

- ***Atropine*** 1 mg I.V. (if PEA rate is **slow**), repeat every 3-5 minutes as needed, to a total dose of 0.04 mg/kg

[1]Do not attempt resuscitation if any objective indicators of DNAR status or clinical indicators that resuscitation attempts are not indicated (eg, signs of death).
[2]Consider continuous qualitative end-tidal CO_2 monitor (Class IIa - acceptable, probably effective).
[3]Commercial purpose-made tracheal tube holders recommended (Class IIb - acceptable, possibly effective).
[4]End-tidal CO_2 monitor and oxygen saturation monitor.
[5]Sodium bicarbonate 1 mEq/kg recommended in the following:
    Class I: If patient has known, preexisting hyperkalemia
    Class IIa: If known, preexisting bicarbonate-responsive acidosis
    Class IIb: In intubated and ventilated patients with a long arrest interval
    On return of circulation after a long arrest interval
    TCA overdose
    To alkalinize urine (eg, ASA overdose)
[6]If this fails, higher doses of epinephrine (up to 0.2 mg/kg) are acceptable (growing evidence of potential harm).

Adapted with permission of Lippincott Williams & Wilkins, "Guidelines 2000 for Cardiopulmonary Resuscitation and Emergency Cardiovascular Care, Part 6: Advanced Cardiovascular Life Support, The American Heart Association in Collaboration With the International Liaison Committee on Resuscitation," *Circulation*, 2000, 102(8 Suppl):I151.

ADULT ACLS ALGORITHMS *(Continued)*

Asystole: The Silent Heart Algorithm

Primary ABCD Survey[1]
Focus: Basic CPR and defibrillation

- **Check** responsiveness
- **Activate** emergency response system
- **Call** for defibrillator

A **Airway:** Open the airway
B **Breathing:** Provide positive-pressure ventilations
C **Circulation:** Give chest compressions
C **Confirm** true asystole
D **Defibrillation:** Assess for VF / pulseless VT; shock if indicated

Rapid scene survey: Any evidence personnel should **not** attempt resuscitation?

Secondary ABCD Survey[2,3]
Focus: More advanced assessments and treatments

A **Airway:** Place airway device as soon as possible
B **Breathing:** Confirm airway device placement by exam plus confirmation device
B **Breathing:** Secure airway device; purpose-made tube holders preferred[4]
B **Breathing:** Confirm effective oxygenation and ventilation[5]
C **Circulation:** Confirm true asystole
C **Circulation:** Establish I.V. access
C **Circulation:** Identify rhythm → monitor
C **Circulation:** Administer drugs appropriate for rhythm and condition
C **Circulation:** Give medications appropriate for rhythm and condition
D **Differential Diagnosis:** Search for and treat identified reversible causes

---

Transcutaneous pacing
If considered, perform immediately

- **Epinephrine** 1 mg I.V. push, repeat every 3-5 minutes[6]

- **Atropine** 1 mg I.V., repeat every 3-5 minutes up to a total of 0.04 mg/kg

---

Asystole persists
Withhold or cease resuscitation efforts?
- Consider quality of resuscitation?
- Atypical clinical features present?
- Support for cease-efforts protocols in place?

---

[1] Do not attempt resuscitation if any objective indicators of DNAR status or clinical indicators that resuscitation attempts are not indicated (eg, signs of death).
[2] Confirm true asystole.
[3] Sodium bicarbonate 1 mEq/kg indicated for patients with tracheal intubation plus long arrest intervals; on return of spontaneous circulation if long arrest interval. **Note:** Ineffective or harmful in hypercarbic acidosis.
[4] Commercial purpose-made tracheal tube holders recommended (Class IIb - acceptable, possibly effective).
[5] End-tidal CO_2 monitor and oxygen saturation monitor
[6] If this fails, higher doses of epinephrine (up to 0.2 mg/kg) are acceptable (growing evidence of potential harm).

Adapted with permission of Lippincott Williams & Wilkins, "Guidelines 2000 for Cardiopulmonary Resuscitation and Emergency Cardiovascular Care, Part 6: Advanced Cardiovascular Life Support, The American Heart Association in Collaboration With the International Liaison Committee on Resuscitation," *Circulation*, 2000, 102(8 Suppl):I153.

Bradycardia Algorithm

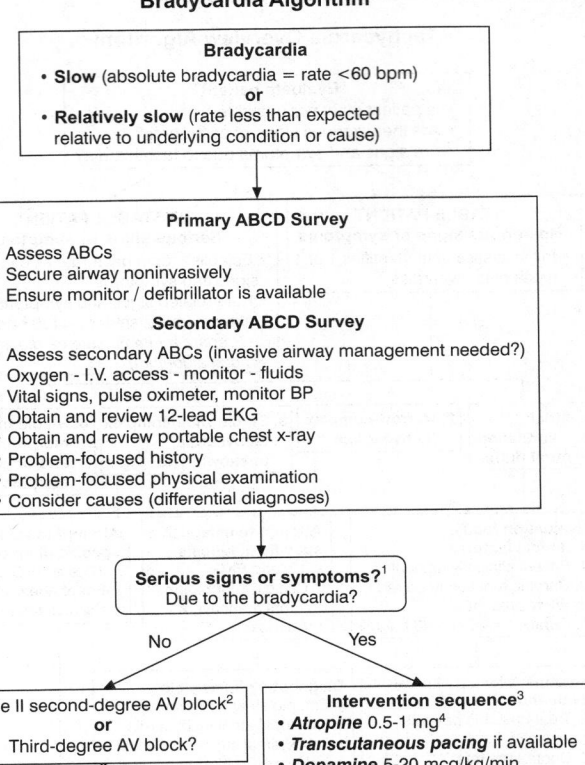

Bradycardia
- **Slow** (absolute bradycardia = rate <60 bpm)

or

- **Relatively slow** (rate less than expected relative to underlying condition or cause)

Primary ABCD Survey
- Assess ABCs
- Secure airway noninvasively
- Ensure monitor / defibrillator is available

Secondary ABCD Survey
- Assess secondary ABCs (invasive airway management needed?)
- Oxygen - I.V. access - monitor - fluids
- Vital signs, pulse oximeter, monitor BP
- Obtain and review 12-lead EKG
- Obtain and review portable chest x-ray
- Problem-focused history
- Problem-focused physical examination
- Consider causes (differential diagnoses)

Serious signs or symptoms?[1]
Due to the bradycardia?

No / Yes

Type II second-degree AV block[2]
or
Third-degree AV block?

No / Yes

Intervention sequence[3]
- *Atropine* 0.5-1 mg[4]
- *Transcutaneous pacing* if available
- *Dopamine* 5-20 mcg/kg/min
- *Epinephrine* 2-10 mcg/min

Observe

- Prepare for transvenous pacer[5]
- If symptoms develop, use transcutaneous pacemaker until transvenous pacer placed

[1]Signs/symptoms must be attributable to slow rate. Manifestations include chest pain, shortness of breath, decreased LOC, hypotension, shock, CHF, pulmonary congestion.
[2]Never treat combination of third-degree heart block and ventricular escape beats with lidocaine (or any agent which suppresses ventricular escape rhythms).
[3]Denervated transplanted hearts will not respond to atropine - go directly to catecholamine infusion or pacing.
[4]Atropine should be repeated every 3-5 minutes up to 0.03-0.04 mg/kg total dose.
[5]Verify patient tolerance and mechanical capture. Use analgesia and sedation as needed.

Adapted with permission of Lippincott Williams & Wilkins, "Guidelines 2000 for Cardiopulmonary Resuscitation and Emergency Cardiovascular Care, Part 6: Advanced Cardiovascular Life Support, The American Heart Association in Collaboration With the International Liaison Committee on Resuscitation," *Circulation*, 2000, 102(8 Suppl):I156.

ADULT ACLS ALGORITHMS *(Continued)*

Tachycardia Overview Algorithm

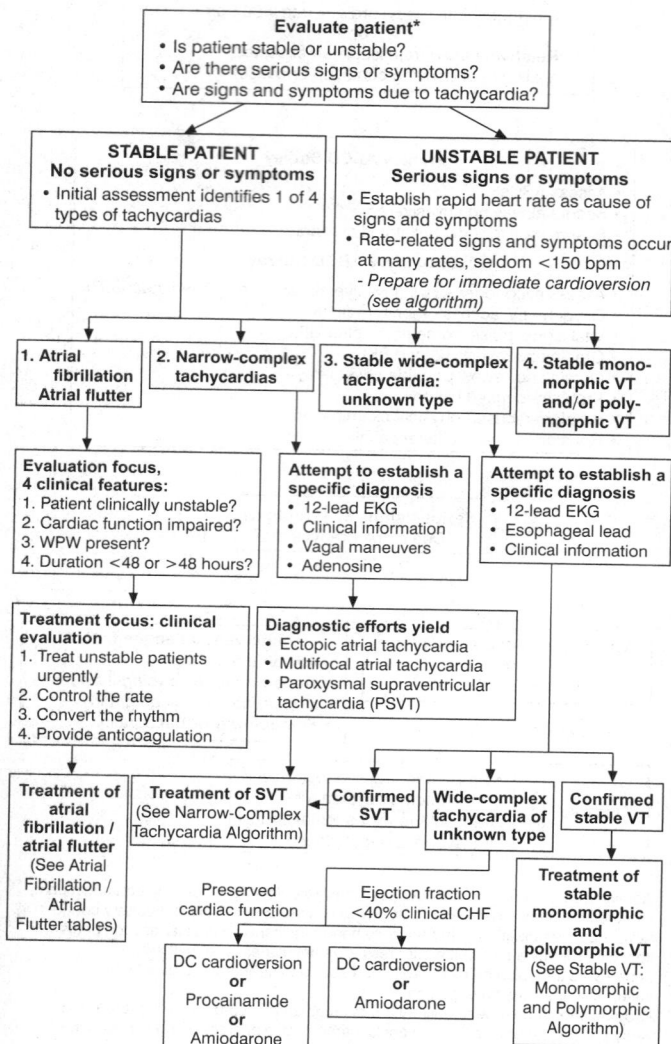

*Unstable condition must be related to the tachycardia. Signs and symptoms may include chest pain, shortness of breath, decreased LOC, hypotension, shock, pulmonary congestion, CHF, and AMI.

Adapted with permission of Lippincott Williams & Wilkins, "Guidelines 2000 for Cardiopulmonary Resuscitation and Emergency Cardiovascular Care, Part 6: Advanced Cardiovascular Life Support, The American Heart Association in Collaboration With the International Liaison Committee on Resuscitation," Circulation, 2000, 102(8 Suppl):I159.

Narrow-Complex Supraventricular Tachycardia Algorithm

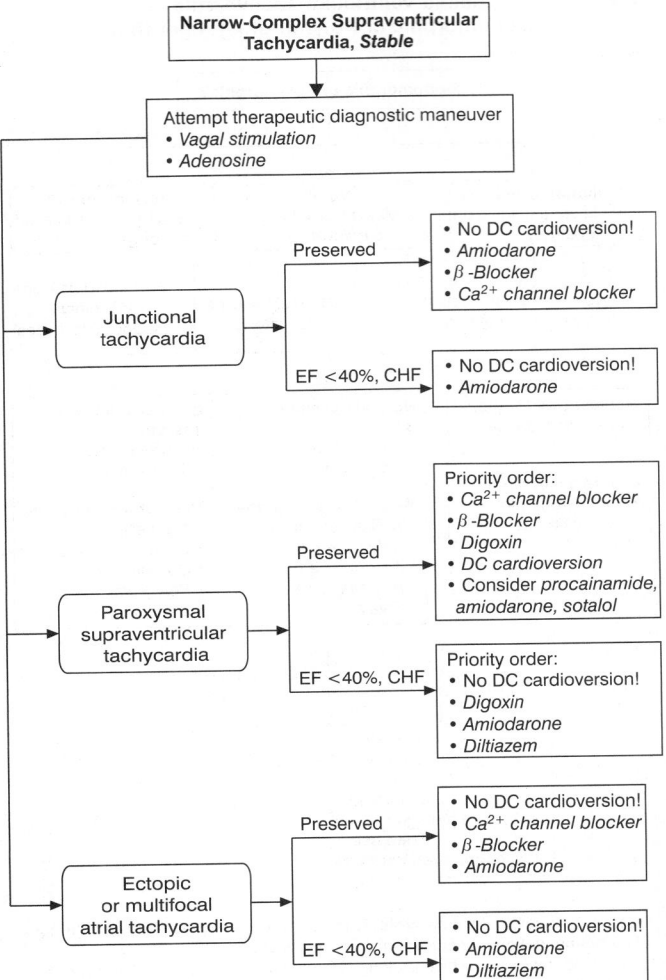

ADULT ACLS ALGORITHMS *(Continued)*

Stable Ventricular Tachycardia (Monomorphic or Polymorphic) Algorithm

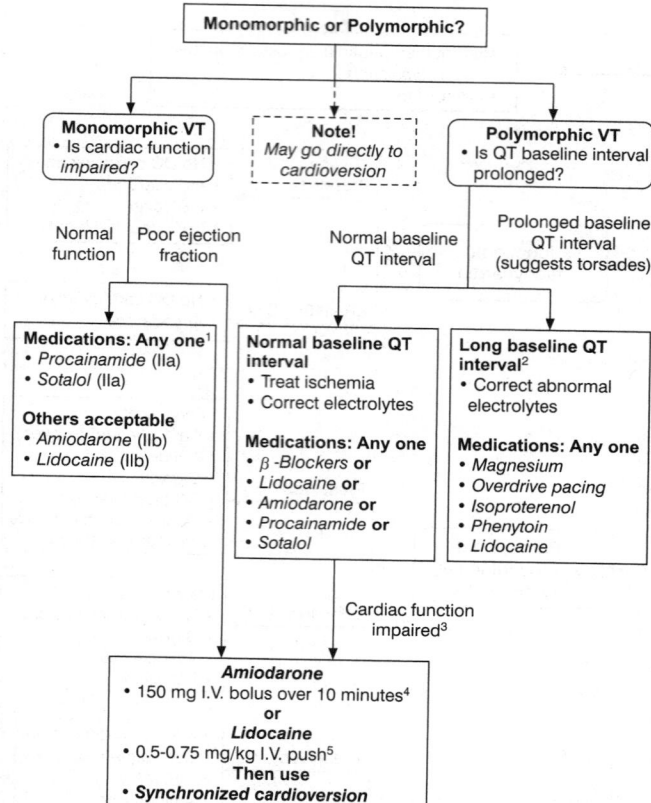

¹Use just one agent at a time. **Note:** Numbers in parentheses represent strength of recommendation, not antiarrhythmic classification.

²Stop/avoid treatments which prolong QT. Identify and treat any electrolyte abnormalities.

³Clinical signs suggestive of impaired LV function.

⁴Repeat 150 mg I.V. over 10 minutes every 10-15 minutes as needed. Alternative infusion: 360 mg over 6 hours, then 540 mg over the remaining 18 hours. Maximum total dose: 2.2 g in 24 hours.

⁵Repeat every 5-10 minutes, then infuse 1-4 mg/min. Maximum total dose: 3 mg/kg (or 300 mg) over 1 hour.

Note: Class IIa recommendation: Acceptable, probably effective;
Class IIb: Acceptable, possibly effective.

Adapted with permission of Lippincott Williams & Wilkins, "Guidelines 2000 for Cardiopulmonary Resuscitation and Emergency Cardiovascular Care, Part 6: Advanced Cardiovascular Life Support, The American Heart Association in Collaboration With the International Liaison Committee on Resuscitation," *Circulation*, 2000, 102(8 Suppl):I163.

Synchronized Cardioversion Algorithm

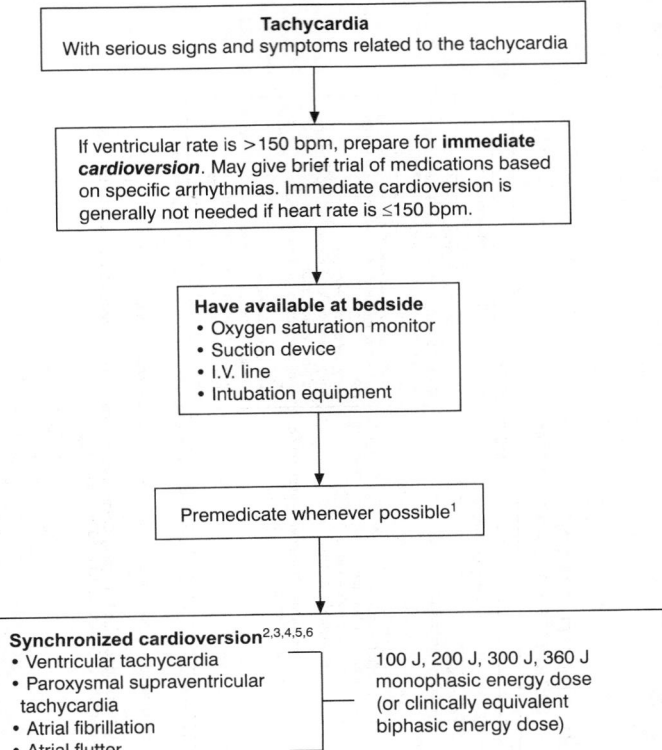

[1]Effective regimens have included a sedative (eg, *diazepam*, *midazolam*, *barbiturates*, *etomidate*, *ketamine*, *methohexital*) with or without an analgesic agent (eg, *fentanyl*, *morphine*, *meperidine*). Many experts recommend anesthesia if service is readily available.

[2]Both monophasic and biphasic waveforms are acceptable if documented as clinically equivalent to reports of monophasic shock success.

[3]Note possible need to resynchronize after each cardioversion.

[4]If delays in synchronization occur and clinical condition is critical, go immediately to unsynchronized shocks.

[5]Treat polymorphic ventricular tachycardia (irregular form and rate) like ventricular fibrillation: see ventricular fibrillation/pulseless ventricular tachycardia algorithm.

[6]Paroxysmal supraventricular tachycardia and atrial flutter often respond to lower energy levels (start with 50 J).

Adapted with permission of Lippincott Williams & Wilkins, "Guidelines 2000 for Cardiopulmonary Resuscitation and Emergency Cardiovascular Care, Part 6: Advanced Cardiovascular Life Support, The American Heart Association in Collaboration With the International Liaison Committee on Resuscitation," *Circulation*, 2000, 102(8 Suppl):I164.

ATRIAL FIBRILLATION / ATRIAL FLUTTER

ATRIAL FIBRILLATION / ATRIAL FLUTTER IN
NORMAL CARDIAC FUNCTION — CONTROL OF RATE AND RHYTHM

Control Rate		Convert Rhythm	
Heart Function Preserved	Impaired Heart Function EF <40% or CHF	Duration <48 Hours	Duration >48 Hours or Unknown
Note: AF >48-hours duration: Use agents to convert rhythm with extreme caution in patient not receiving adequate anticoagulation because of possible embolic complications Use only one of the following agents:[1] • Calcium channel blocker (Class I) • Beta blocker (Class I) • Other drugs (class IIb recommendations) eg, digoxin, amiodarone	Not applicable	**Consider:** • DC cardioversion Use only one of the following agents:[1] • Amiodarone (Class IIa) • Ibutilide (Class IIa) • Flecainide (Class IIa) • Propafenone (Class IIa) • Procainamide (Class IIa) • Other drugs (class IIb recommendations) eg. sotalol, disopyramide	**NO DC CARDIOVERSION!** **Note:** Conversion of AF to NSR with drugs or shock may cause embolization of atrial thrombi unless patient has adequate anticoagulation. Use antiarrhythmic agents with extreme caution (see Note above) if AF is >48-hours duration **OR** ***Delayed cardioversion*** Anticoagulation for 3 weeks at proper levels • Cardioversion, ***then*** • Anticoagulation for 4 more weeks **OR** ***Early cardioversion*** • Begin I.V. heparin at once • TEE to exclude atrial clot, ***then*** • Cardioversion within 24 hours, ***then*** • Anticoagulation for 4 more weeks

Legend: AF: Atrial fibrillation; Class I: Acceptable, definitely effective; Class IIa: Acceptable, probably effective; Class IIb: Acceptable, possibly effective; Class III: Not indicated, may be harmful; EF: Ejection fraction; NSR: Normal sinus rhythm; TEE: Transesophageal echocardiogram

[1]Occasionally, two of the named antiarrhythmic agents may be used, but use of these agents in combination may have proarrhythmic potential; classes listed represent the *Class of Recommendation* rather than the Vaughn-Williams classification of antiarrhythmics.

Adapted with permission from Lippincott Williams & Wilkins, "Guidelines 2000 for Cardiopulmonary Resuscitation and Emergency Cardiovascular Care. Part 6: Advanced Cardiovascular Life Support. The American Heart Association in Collaboration With the International Liaison Committee on Resuscitation," *Circulation*, 2000, 102(8 Suppl), I160-1.

ATRIAL FIBRILLATION / ATRIAL FLUTTER IN
IMPAIRED HEART FUNCTION (EF <40% or CHF) — CONTROL OF RATE AND RHYTHM

	Control Rate	Convert Rhythm	
	Impaired Heart Function EF <40% or CHF	Duration <48 Hours	Duration >48 Hours or Unknown
Heart Function Preserved			
Not applicable	**Note:** AF >48-hours duration: Use agents to convert rhythm with extreme caution in patient not receiving adequate anticoagulation because of possible embolic complications Use only one of the following agents:[1] • Digoxin (Class IIb) • Diltiazem (Class IIb) • Amiodarone (Class IIb)	**Consider:** • DC cardioversion **OR** • Amiodarone (Class IIb)	• **Anticoagulation** (as described in "Control of Rate and Rhythm - Normal Cardiac Function"), followed by • **DC Cardioversion**

Legend: AF: Atrial fibrillation; Class I: Acceptable, definitely effective; Class IIa: Acceptable, probably effective; Class IIb: Acceptable, possibly effective; Class III: Not indicated, may be harmful; EF: Ejection fraction; NSR: Normal sinus rhythm; TEE: Transesophageal echocardiogram

[1]Occasionally, two of the named antiarrhythmic agents may be used, but use of these agents in combination may have proarrhythmic potential; classes listed represent the *Class of Recommendation* rather than the Vaughn-Williams classification of antiarrhythmics.

Adapted with permission from Lippincott Williams & Wilkins, "Guidelines 2000 for Cardiopulmonary Resuscitation and Emergency Cardiovascular Care. Part 6: Advanced Cardiovascular Life Support. The American Heart Association in Collaboration With the International Liaison Committee on Resuscitation," *Circulation*, 2000, 102(8 Suppl), I160-1.

ATRIAL FIBRILLATION / ATRIAL FLUTTER IN
WOLFF-PARKINSON-WHITE SYNDROME — CONTROL OF RATE AND RHYTHM

Control Rate		Convert Rhythm	
Heart Function Preserved	Impaired Heart Function EF <40% or CHF	Duration <48 Hours	Duration >48 Hours or Unknown
Note: AF >48-hours duration: Use agents to convert rhythm in patient not receiving adequate anticoagulation because of possible embolic complications • DC Cardioversion **OR** • **Primary antiarrhythmic agents** Use only one of the following agents:[1] • Amiodarone (Class IIb) • Flecainide (Class IIb) • Procainamide (Class IIb) • Propafenone (Class IIb) • Sotalol (Class IIb) • **Class III (can be harmful)** • Adenosine • Beta-blockers • Calcium channel blockers • Digoxin	**Note:** AF >48-hours duration: Use agents to convert rhythm with extreme caution in patient not receiving adequate anticoagulation because of possible embolic complications • DC Cardioversion **OR** • Amiodarone (Class IIb)	• DC Cardioversion **OR** • **Primary antiarrhythmic agents** Use only one of the following agents:[1] • Amiodarone (Class IIb) • Flecainide (Class IIb) • Procainamide (Class IIb) • Propafenone (Class IIb) • Sotalol (Class IIb) • **Class III (can be harmful)** • Adenosine • Beta-blockers • Calcium channel blockers • Digoxin	• **Anticoagulation** (as described in "Control of Rate and Rhythm - Normal Cardiac Function"), followed by • **DC Cardioversion**

Legend: AF: Atrial fibrillation; Class I: Acceptable, definitely effective; Class IIa: Acceptable, probably effective; Class IIb: Acceptable, possibly effective; Class III: Not indicated, may be harmful; EF: Ejection fraction; NSR: Normal sinus rhythm; TEE: Transesophageal echocardiogram

[1]Occasionally, two of the named antiarrhythmic agents may be used, but use of these agents in combination may have proarrhythmic potential; classes listed represent the *Class of Recommendation* rather than the Vaughn-Williams classification of antiarrhythmics.

Adapted with permission from Lippincott Williams & Wilkins, "Guidelines 2000 for Cardiopulmonary Resuscitation and Emergency Cardiovascular Care. Part 6: Advanced Cardiovascular Life Support. The American Heart Association in Collaboration With the International Liaison Committee on Resuscitation," *Circulation*, 2000, 102(8 Suppl), I160-1.

ASTHMA

NATIONAL ASTHMA EDUCATION AND PREVENTION PROGRAM

EXPERT PANEL REPORT II:
GUIDELINES FOR THE DIAGNOSIS AND MANAGEMENT OF ASTHMA

February 1997

Stepwise Approach for Managing Asthma in Adults and Children >5 Years of Age: Classify Severity

Goals of Asthma Treatment

- Prevent chronic and troublesome symptoms (eg, coughing or breathlessness in the night, in the early morning, or after exertion)
- Maintain (near) "normal" pulmonary function
- Maintain normal activity levels (including exercise and other physical activity)
- Prevent recurrent exacerbations of asthma and minimize the need for emergency department visits or hospitalizations
- Provide optimal pharmacotherapy with minimal or no adverse effects
- Meet patients' and families' expectations of and satisfaction with asthma care

Clinical Features Before Treatment*

Symptoms**	Nighttime Symptoms	Lung Function
STEP 4: Severe Persistent		
• Continual symptoms • Limited physical activity • Frequent exacerbations	Frequent	• FEV_1/PEF ≤60% predicted • PEF variability >30%
STEP 3: Moderate Persistent		
• Daily symptoms • Daily use of inhaled short-acting beta$_2$-agonist • Exacerbations affect activity • Exacerbations ≥2 times/week; may last days	>1 time/week	• FEV_1/PEF >60% - 80% predicted • PEF variability >30%
STEP 2: Mild Persistent		
• Symptoms >2 times/week but <1 time/day • Exacerbations may affect activity	>2 times/month	• FEV_1/PEF ≥80% predicted • PEF variability 20% - 30%
STEP 1: Mild Intermittent		
• Symptoms ≤2 times/week • Asymptomatic and normal PEF between exacerbations • Exacerbations brief (from a few hours to a few days); intensity may vary	≤2 times/month	• FEV_1/PEF ≥80% predicted • PEF variability ≤20%

*The presence of one of the features of severity is sufficient to place a patient in that category. An individual should be assigned to the most severe grade in which any feature occurs. The characteristics noted in this figure are general and may overlap because asthma is highly variable. Furthermore, an individual's classification may change over time.

**Patients at any level of severity can have mild, moderate, or severe exacerbations. Some patients with intermittent asthma experience severe and life-threatening exacerbations separated by long periods of normal lung function and no symptoms.

ASTHMA *(Continued)*

Stepwise Approach for Managing Asthma in Adults and Children >5 Years of Age: Treatment

(Preferred treatments are in **bold** print)

Long-Term Control	Quick Relief	Education
STEP 4: Severe Persistent		
Daily medications: • **Anti-inflammatory: Inhaled corticosteroid (high dose)** AND • Long-acting bronchodilator: Either **long-acting inhaled beta₂-agonist**, sustained-release theophylline, or long-acting beta₂-agonist tablets AND • Corticosteroid tablets or syrup long term (2 mg/kg/day, generally do not exceed 60 mg per day).	• Short-acting bronchodilator: **Inhaled beta₂-agonists** as needed for symptoms. • Intensity of treatment will depend on severity of exacerbation; see "Managing Exacerbations" • Use of short-acting inhaled beta₂-agonists on a daily basis, or increasing use, indicates the need for additional long-term control therapy.	Steps 2 and 3 actions plus: • Refer to individual education/counseling
STEP 3: Moderate Persistent		
Daily medication: • Either — **Anti-inflammatory: Inhaled corticosteroid (medium dose)** OR — **Inhaled corticosteroid (low-medium dose)** and add a long-acting bronchodilator, especially for nighttime symptoms: Either **long-acting inhaled beta₂-agonist**, sustained-release theophylline, or long-acting beta₂-agonist tablets. • If needed — Anti-inflammatory: **Inhaled corticosteroids (medium-high dose) AND** — **Long-acting bronchodilator,** especially for nighttime symptoms; either **long-acting inhaled beta₂-agonist,** sustained-release theophylline, or long-acting beta₂-agonist tablets.	• Short-acting bronchodilator: **Inhaled beta₂-agonists** as needed for symptoms. • Intensity of treatment will depend on severity of exacerbation; see "Managing Exacerbations." • Use of short-acting inhaled beta₂-agonists on a daily basis, or increasing use, indicates the need for additional long-term control therapy.	Step 1 actions plus: • Teach self-monitoring • Refer to group education if available • Review and update self-management plan
STEP 2: Mild Persistent		
One daily medication: • **Anti-inflammatory:** Either **inhaled corticosteroid (low doses) or cromolyn or nedocromil** (children usually begin with a trial of cromolyn or nedocromil). • Sustained-release theophylline to serum concentration of 5-15 mcg/mL is an alternative, but not preferred, therapy. Zafirlukast or zileuton may also be considered for patients ≥12 years of age, although their position in therapy is not fully established.	• Short-acting bronchodilator: **Inhaled beta₂-agonists** as needed for symptoms. • Intensity of treatment will depend on severity of exacerbation; see "Managing Exacerbations." • Use of short-acting inhaled beta₂-agonists on a daily basis, or increasing use, indicates the need for additional long-term control therapy.	Step 1 actions plus: • Teach self-monitoring • Refer to group education if available • Review and update self-management plan
STEP 1: Mild Intermittent		
No daily medication needed.	• Short-acting bronchodilator: **Inhaled beta₂-agonists** as needed for symptoms. • Intensity of treatment will depend on severity of exacerbation; see "Managing Exacerbations." • Use of short-acting inhaled beta₂-agonists more than 2 times/week may indicate the need to initiate long-term control therapy	• Teach basic facts about asthma • Teach inhaler/spacer/holding chamber technique • Discuss roles of medications • Develop self-management plan • Develop action plan for when and how to take rescue actions, especially for patients with a history of severe exacerbations • Discuss appropriate environmental control measures to avoid exposure to known allergens and irritants

↓ **Step down**
Review treatment every 1-6 months; a gradual stepwise reduction in treatment may be possible.

↑**Step up**
If control is not maintained, consider step up. First, review patient medication technique, adherence, and environmental control (avoidance of allergens or other factors that contribute to asthma severity.)

Notes:

- The stepwise approach presents general guidelines to assist clinical decision making; it is not intended to be a specific prescription. Asthma is highly variable; clinicians should tailor specific medication plans to the needs and circumstances of individual patients.

- Gain control as quickly as possible; then decrease treatment to the least medication necessary to maintain control. Gaining control may be accomplished by either starting treatment at the step most appropriate to the initial severity of the condition or starting at a higher level of therapy (eg, a course of systemic corticosteroids or higher dose of inhaled corticosteroids).

- A rescue course of systemic corticosteroids may be needed at any time and at any step.

- Some patients with intermittent asthma experience severe and life-threatening exacerbations separated by long periods of normal lung function and no symptoms. This may be especially common with exacerbations provoked by respiratory infections. A short course of systemic corticosteroids is recommended.

- At each step, patients should control their environment to avoid or control factors that make their asthma worse (eg, allergens, irritants); this requires specific diagnosis and education.

Stepwise Approach for Managing Infants and Young Children (≤5 Years of Age) With Acute or Chronic Asthma Symptoms

Long-Term Control	Quick Relief
STEP 4: Severe Persistent	
Daily anti-inflammatory medicine • High-dose inhaled corticosteroid with spacer/holding chamber and face mask • If needed, add systemic corticosteroids 2 mg/kg/day and reduce to lowest daily or alternate-day dose that stabilizes symptoms	•Bronchodilator as needed for symptoms (see step 1) up to 3 times/day
STEP 3: Moderate Persistent	
Daily anti-inflammatory medication. Either: • Medium-dose inhaled corticosteroid with spacer/holding chamber and face mask OR Once control is established: • Medium-dose inhaled corticosteroid and nedocromil OR • Medium-dose inhaled corticosteroid and long-acting bronchodilator (theophylline)	• Bronchodilator as needed for symptoms (see step 1) up to 3 times/day
STEP 2: Mild Persistent	
Daily anti-inflammatory medication. Either: • Cromolyn (nebulizer is preferred; or MDI) or nedocromil (MDI only) tid-qid • Infants and young children usually begin with a trial of cromolyn or nedocromil OR • Low-dose inhaled corticosteroid with spacer/holding chamber and face mask	• Bronchodilator as needed for symptoms (see step 1)
STEP 1: Mild Intermittent	
No daily medication needed	• Bronchodilator as needed for symptoms <2 times/week. Intensity of treatment will depend upon severity of exacerbation (see "Managing Exacerbations"). Either: — Inhaled short-acting beta$_2$-agonist by nebulizer or face mask and spacer/holding chamber OR — Oral beta$_2$-agonist for symptoms • With viral respiratory infection: — Bronchodilator q4-6h up to 24 hours (longer with physician consult) but, in general, repeat no more than once every 6 weeks — Consider systemic corticosteroid if current exacerbation is severe OR Patient has history of previous severe exacerbations

ASTHMA *(Continued)*

↓ **Step Down**
Review treatment every 1-6 months. If control is sustained for at least 3 months, a gradual stepwise reduction in treatment may be possible.

↑ **Step Up**
If control is not achieved, consider step up. But first: review patient medication technique, adherence, and environmental control (avoidance of allergens or other precipitant factors)

Notes:

- **The stepwise approach presents guidelines to assist clinical decision making. Asthma is highly variable; clinicians should tailor specific medication plans to the needs and circumstances of individual patients.**

- Gain control as quickly as possible; then decrease treatment to the least medication necessary to maintain control. Gaining control may be accomplished by either starting treatment at the step most appropriate to the initial severity of their condition or by starting at a higher level of therapy (eg, a course of systemic corticosteroids or higher dose of inhaled corticosteroids).

- A rescue course of systemic corticosteroid (prednisolone) may be needed at any time and step.

- In general, use of short-acting beta$_2$-agonist on a daily basis indicates the need for additional long-term control therapy.

- It is important to remember that there are very few studies on asthma therapy for infants.

- Consultation with an asthma specialist is recommended for patients with moderate or severe persistent asthma in this age group. Consultation should be considered for all patients with mild persistent asthma.

Management of Asthma Exacerbations: Home Treatment*

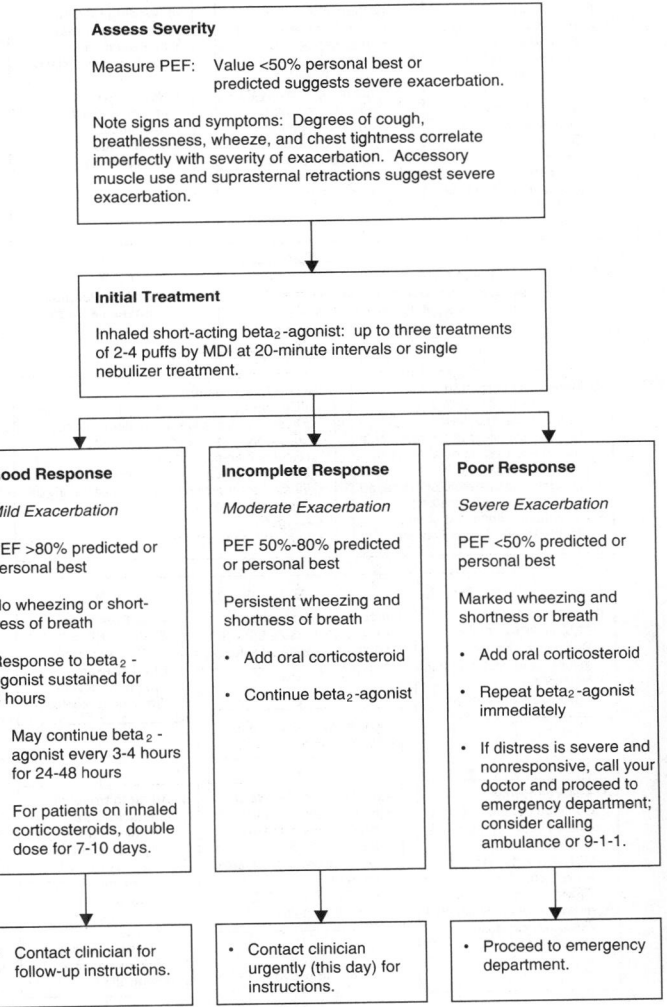

Assess Severity

Measure PEF: Value <50% personal best or predicted suggests severe exacerbation.

Note signs and symptoms: Degrees of cough, breathlessness, wheeze, and chest tightness correlate imperfectly with severity of exacerbation. Accessory muscle use and suprasternal retractions suggest severe exacerbation.

Initial Treatment

Inhaled short-acting beta$_2$-agonist: up to three treatments of 2-4 puffs by MDI at 20-minute intervals or single nebulizer treatment.

Good Response

Mild Exacerbation

PEF >80% predicted or personal best

No wheezing or shortness of breath

Response to beta$_2$-agonist sustained for 4 hours

- May continue beta$_2$-agonist every 3-4 hours for 24-48 hours

- For patients on inhaled corticosteroids, double dose for 7-10 days.

- Contact clinician for follow-up instructions.

Incomplete Response

Moderate Exacerbation

PEF 50%-80% predicted or personal best

Persistent wheezing and shortness of breath

- Add oral corticosteroid

- Continue beta$_2$-agonist

- Contact clinician urgently (this day) for instructions.

Poor Response

Severe Exacerbation

PEF <50% predicted or personal best

Marked wheezing and shortness or breath

- Add oral corticosteroid

- Repeat beta$_2$-agonist immediately

- If distress is severe and nonresponsive, call your doctor and proceed to emergency department; consider calling ambulance or 9-1-1.

- Proceed to emergency department.

*Patients at high risk of asthma-related death should receive immediate clinical attention after initial treatment. Additional therapy may be required.

ASTHMA (Continued)

Management of Asthma Exacerbations: Emergency Department and Hospital-Based Care

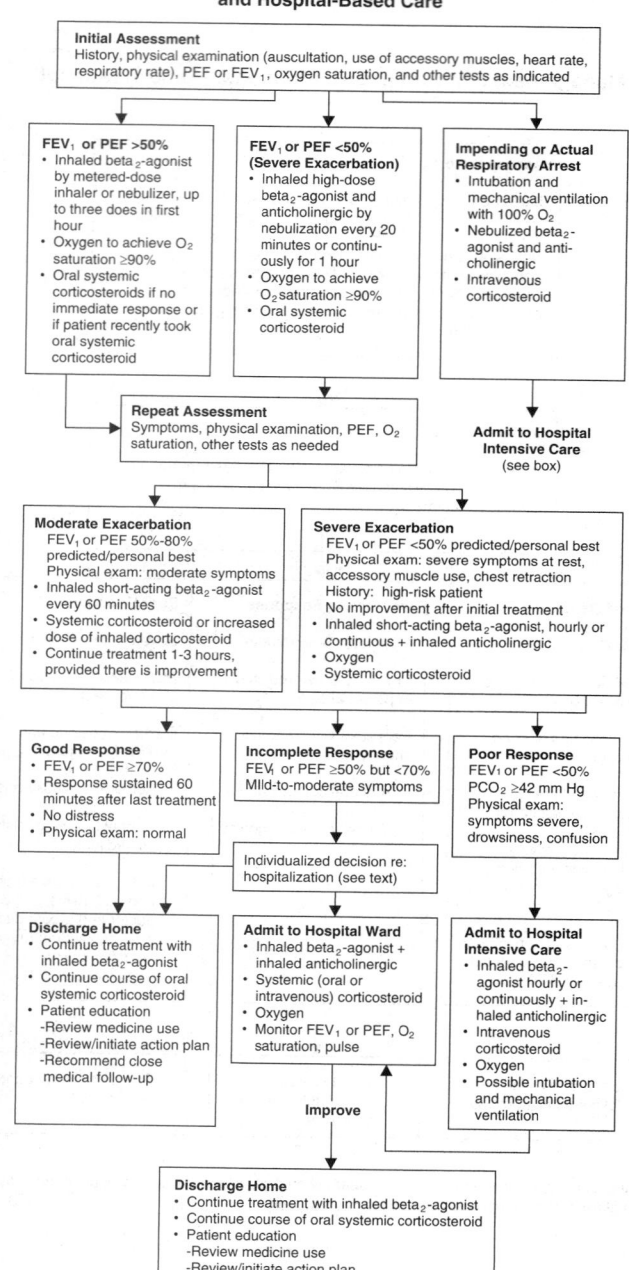

Initial Assessment
History, physical examination (auscultation, use of accessory muscles, heart rate, respiratory rate), PEF or FEV_1, oxygen saturation, and other tests as indicated

FEV_1 or PEF >50%
- Inhaled beta$_2$-agonist by metered-dose inhaler or nebulizer, up to three does in first hour
- Oxygen to achieve O$_2$ saturation ≥90%
- Oral systemic corticosteroids if no immediate response or if patient recently took oral systemic corticosteroid

FEV_1 or PEF <50% (Severe Exacerbation)
- Inhaled high-dose beta$_2$-agonist and anticholinergic by nebulization every 20 minutes or continuously for 1 hour
- Oxygen to achieve O$_2$ saturation ≥90%
- Oral systemic corticosteroid

Impending or Actual Respiratory Arrest
- Intubation and mechanical ventilation with 100% O$_2$
- Nebulized beta$_2$-agonist and anticholinergic
- Intravenous corticosteroid

Repeat Assessment
Symptoms, physical examination, PEF, O$_2$ saturation, other tests as needed

Admit to Hospital Intensive Care
(see box)

Moderate Exacerbation
FEV_1 or PEF 50%-80% predicted/personal best
Physical exam: moderate symptoms
- Inhaled short-acting beta$_2$-agonist every 60 minutes
- Systemic corticosteroid or increased dose of inhaled corticosteroid
- Continue treatment 1-3 hours, provided there is improvement

Severe Exacerbation
FEV_1 or PEF <50% predicted/personal best
Physical exam: severe symptoms at rest, accessory muscle use, chest retraction
History: high-risk patient
No improvement after initial treatment
- Inhaled short-acting beta$_2$-agonist, hourly or continuous + inhaled anticholinergic
- Oxygen
- Systemic corticosteroid

Good Response
- FEV_1 or PEF ≥70%
- Response sustained 60 minutes after last treatment
- No distress
- Physical exam: normal

Incomplete Response
FEV_1 or PEF ≥50% but <70%
Mlld-to-moderate symptoms

Poor Response
FEV_1 or PEF <50%
PCO_2 ≥42 mm Hg
Physical exam: symptoms severe, drowsiness, confusion

Individualized decision re: hospitalization (see text)

Discharge Home
- Continue treatment with inhaled beta$_2$-agonist
- Continue course of oral systemic corticosteroid
- Patient education
  -Review medicine use
  -Review/initiate action plan
  -Recommend close medical follow-up

Admit to Hospital Ward
- Inhaled beta$_2$-agonist + inhaled anticholinergic
- Systemic (oral or intravenous) corticosteroid
- Oxygen
- Monitor FEV_1 or PEF, O$_2$ saturation, pulse

Admit to Hospital Intensive Care
- Inhaled beta$_2$-agonist hourly or continuously + inhaled anticholinergic
- Intravenous corticosteroid
- Oxygen
- Possible intubation and mechanical ventilation

Improve

Discharge Home
- Continue treatment with inhaled beta$_2$-agonist
- Continue course of oral systemic corticosteroid
- Patient education
  -Review medicine use
  -Review/initiate action plan
  -Recommend close medical follow-up

ESTIMATED COMPARATIVE DAILY DOSAGES FOR INHALED CORTICOSTEROIDS

Adults

Drug	Low Dose	Medium Dose	High Dose
Beclomethasone dipropionate	168-504 mcg	504-840 mcg	>840 mcg
42 mcg/puff	(4-12 puffs — 42 mcg)	(12-20 puffs — 42 mcg)	(>20 puffs — 42 mcg)
84 mcg/puff	(2-6 puffs — 84 mcg)	(6-10 puffs — 84 mcg)	(>10 puffs — 84 mcg)
Budesonide Turbuhaler	200-400 mcg	400-600 mcg	>600 mcg
200 mcg/dose	(1-2 inhalations)	(2-3 inhalations)	(>3 inhalations)
Flunisolide	500-1000 mcg	1000-2000 mcg	>2000 mcg
250 mcg/puff	(2-4 puffs)	(4-8 puffs)	(>8 puffs)
Fluticasone	88-264 mcg	264-660 mcg	>660 mcg
MDI: 44, 110, 220 mcg/puff	(2-6 puffs — 44 mcg)	(2-6 puffs — 110 mcg)	(>6 puffs — 110 mcg)
	or		or
	(2 puffs — 110 mcg)		(>3 puffs — 220 mcg)
DPI: 50, 100, 250 mcg/dose	(2-6 inhalations — 50 mcg)	(3-6 inhalations — 100 mcg)	(>6 inhalations — 100 mcg)
Triamcinolone acetonide	400-1000 mcg	1000-2000 mcg	>2000 mcg
100 mcg/puff	(4-10 puffs)	(10-20 puffs)	(>20 puffs)

Children

Drug	Low Dose	Medium Dose	High Dose
Beclomethasone dipropionate	84-336 mcg	336-672 mcg	>672 mcg
42 mcg/puff 84 mcg/puff	(2-8 puffs)	(8-16 puffs)	(>16 puffs)
Budesonide Turbuhaler	100-200 mcg	200-400 mcg	>400 mcg
200 mcg/dose		(1-2 inhalations — 200 mcg)	(>2 inhalations — 200 mcg)
Flunisolide	500-750 mcg	1000-1250 mcg	>1250 mcg
250 mcg/puff	(2-3 puffs)	(4-5 puffs)	(>5 puffs)
Fluticasone	88-176 mcg	176-440 mcg	>440 mcg
MDI: 44, 110, 220 mcg/puff	(2-4 puffs — 44 mcg)	(4-10 puffs — 44 mcg)	(>4 puffs — 110 mcg)
		or	
		(2-4 puffs — 110 mcg)	
DPI: 50, 100, 250 mcg/dose	(2-4 inhalations — 50 mcg)	(2-4 inhalations — 100 mcg)	(>4 inhalations — 100 mcg)
Triamcinolone acetonide	400-800 mcg	800-1200 mcg	>1200 mcg
100 mcg/puff	(4-8 puffs)	(8-12 puffs)	(>12 puffs)

Notes:

- **The most important determinant of appropriate dosing is the clinician's judgment of the patient's response to therapy.** The clinician must monitor the patient's response on several clinical parameters and adjust the dose accordingly. The stepwise approach to therapy emphasizes that once control of asthma is achieved, the dose of mediation should be carefully titrated to the minimum dose required to maintain control, thus reducing the potential for adverse effect.

- The reference point for the range in the dosages for children is data on the safety on inhaled corticosteroids in children, which, in general, suggest that the dose ranges are equivalent to beclomethasone dipropionate 200-400 mcg/day (low dose), 400-800 mcg/day (medium dose), and >800 mcg/day (high dose).

- Some dosages may be outside package labeling.

- Metered-dose inhaler (MDI) dosages are expressed as the actuator dose (the amount of drug leaving the actuator and delivered to the patient), which is the labeling required in the United States. This is different from the dosage expressed as the valve dose (the amount of drug leaving the valve, all of which is not available to the patient), which is used in many European countries and in some of the scientific literature. Dry powder inhaler (DPI) doses (eg, Turbuhaler) are expressed as the amount of drug in the inhaler following activation.

ASTHMA (Continued)

ESTIMATED CLINICAL COMPARABILITY OF DOSES FOR INHALED CORTICOSTEROIDS

Data from *in vitro* and in clinical trials suggest that the different inhaled corticosteroid preparations are not equivalent on a per puff or microgram basis. However, it is not entirely clear what implications these differences have for dosing recommendations in clinical practice because there are few data directly comparing the preparations. Relative dosing for clinical comparability is affected by differences in topical potency, clinical effects at different doses, delivery device, and bioavailability. The Expert Panel developed recommended dose ranges for different preparations based on available data and the following assumptions and cautions about estimating relative doses needed to achieve comparable clinical effect.

- **Relative topical potency using human skin blanching**

    - The standard test for determining relative topical anti-inflammatory potency is the topical vasoconstriction (MacKenzie skin blanching) test.

    - The MacKenzie topical skin blanching test correlates with binding affinities and binding half-lives for human lung corticosteroid receptors (see table below) (Dahlberg, et al, 1984; Hogger and Rohdewald 1994).

    - The relationship between relative topical anti-inflammatory effect and clinical comparability in asthma management is not certain. However, recent clinical trials suggest that different in vitro measures of anti-inflammatory effect is not certain. However, recent clinical trials suggest that different in vitro measures of anti-inflammatory effect correlate with clinical efficacy (Barnes and Pedersen 1993; Johnson 1996; Kamada, et al, 1996; Ebden, et al, 1986; Leblanc, et al, 1994; Gustaffson, et al, 1993; Lundback, et al, 1993; Barnes, et al, 1993; Fabbri, et al, 1993; Langdon and Capsey, 1994; Ayres, et al, 1995; Rafferty, et al, 1985; Bjorkander, et al, 1982, Stiksa, et al, 1982; Willey, et al, 1982.)

Medication	Topical Potency (Skin Blanching)*	Corticosteroid Receptor Binding Half-Life	Receptor Binding Affinity
Beclomethasone dipropionate (BDP)	600	7.5 hours	13.5
Budesonide (BUD)	980	5.1 hours	9.4
Flunisolide (FLU)	330	3.5 hours	1.8
Fluticasone propionate (FP)	1200	10.5 hours	18.0
Triamcinolone acetonide (TAA)	330	3.9 hours	3.6

*Numbers are assigned in reference to dexamethasone, which has a value of "1" in the MacKenzie test.

- **Relative doses to achieve similar clinical effects**

    - Clinical effects are evaluated by a number of outcome parameters (eg, changes in spirometry, peak flow rates, symptom scores, quick-relief beta$_2$-agonist use, frequency of exacerbations, airway responsiveness).

    - The daily dose and duration of treatment may affect these outcome parameters differently (eg, symptoms and peak flow may improve at lower doses and over a shorter treatment time than bronchial reactivity) (van Essen-Zandvliet, et al, 1992; Haahtela, et al, 1991)

    - Delivery systems influence comparability. For example, the delivery device for budesonide (Turbuhaler) delivers approximately twice the amount of drug to the airway as the MDI, thus enhancing the clinical effect (Thorsson, et al, 1994); Agertoft and Pedersen, 1993).

    - Individual patients may respond differently to different preparations, as noted by clinical experience.

    - Clinical trials comparing effects in reducing symptoms and improving peak expiratory flow demonstrate:

    - BDP and BUD achieved comparable effects at similar microgram doses by MDI (Bjorkander, et al, 1982; Ebden, et al, 1986; Rafferty, et al, 1985).

    - BDP achieved effects similar to twice the dose of TAA on a microgram basis.

CONTRAST MEDIA REACTIONS, PREMEDICATION FOR PROPHYLAXIS

American College of Radiology Guidelines for Use of Nonionic Contrast Media

is estimated that approximately 5% to 10% of patients will experience adverse reactions to administration of contrast dye (less for nonionic contrast). In approximately 000-2000 administrations, a life-threatening reaction will occur.

variety of premedication regimens have been proposed, both for pretreatment of "at sk" patients who require contrast media and before the routine administration of the travenous high osmolar contrast media. Such regimens have been shown in clinical ials to decrease the frequency of all forms of contrast medium reactions. Pretreatment ith a 2-dose regimen of methylprednisolone 32 mg, 12 and 2 hours prior to intrave- ous administration of HOCM (ionic), has been shown to decrease mild, moderate, and evere reactions in patients at increased risk and perhaps in patients without risk actors. Logistical and feasibility problems may preclude adequate premedication with his or any regimen for all patients. It is unclear at this time that steroid pretreatment rior to administration of ionic contrast media reduces the incidence of reactions to the ame extent or less than that achieved with the use of nonionic contrast media alone. nformation about the efficacy of nonionic contrast media combined with a premedica- on strategy, including steroids, is preliminary or not yet currently available. For high- isk patients (ie, previous contrast reactors), the combination of a pretreatment regimen vith nonionic contrast media has empirical merit and may warrant consideration. Oral dministration of steroids appears preferable to intravascular routes, and the drug may e prednisone or methylprednisolone. Supplemental administration of H_1 and H_2 anti- istamine therapies, orally or intravenously, may reduce the frequency of urticaria, ngioedema, and respiratory symptoms. Additionally, ephedrine administration has een suggested to decrease the frequency of contrast reactions, but caution is advised n patients with cardiac disease, hypertension, or hyperthyroidism. No premedication strategy should be a substitute for the ABC approach to preadministration prepared- ess listed above. Contrast reactions do occur despite any and all premedication prophylaxis. The incidence can be decreased, however, in some categories of "at risk" patients receiving high osmolar contrast media plus a medication regimen. For patients with previous contrast medium reactions, there is a slight chance that recurrence may e more severe or the same as the prior reaction, however, it is more likely that there will be no recurrence.

A general premedication regimen is

Methylprednisolone	32 mg orally at 12 and 2 hours prior to procedure
Diphenhydramine	50 mg orally 1 hour prior to the procedure

An alternative premedication regimen is

Prednisone	50 mg orally 13, 7, and 1 hour before the procedure
Diphenhydramine	50 mg orally 1 hour before the procedure
Ephedrine	25 mg orally 1 hour before the procedure (except when contraindicated)

Investigational (nephroprotective)

N-acetylcysteine, P.O.	600 mg orally twice daily on the day before and the day of the scan in addition to hydration with 0.45% saline intravenously
Fenoldopam, I.V.	Continuous infusion starting at 2 hours preprocedure and maintained until at least 4 hours postprocedure. Initiate dose at 0.1 mcg/kg/minute and titrate to a maximum dose 0.5 mg/kg/minute at increments of 0.1 mg/kg/minute if systolic blood pressure is >100 mm Hg and diastolic blood pressure is within 20 mm Hg of baseline; intravenous saline can be given for hydration prior to contrast administration.

CONTRAST MEDIA REACTIONS, PREMEDICATION FOR PROPHYLAXIS *(Continued)*

Indication for nonionic contrast are

Previous reaction to contrast — premedicate[1]
Known allergy to iodine or shellfish
Asthma, especially if on medication
Myocardial instability or CHF
Risk for aspiration or severe nausea and vomiting
Difficulty communicating or inability to give history
Patients taking beta-blockers
Small children at risk for electrolyte imbalance or extravasation
Renal failure with diabetes, sickle cell disease, or myeloma
At physician or patient request

[1]Life-threatening reactions (throat swelling, laryngeal edema, etc), consider omitting the intravenous contrast.

DEPRESSION

Criteria for Major Depressive Episode

A. Five (or more) of the following symptoms have been present during the same 2-week period and represent a change from previous functioning; at least one of the symptoms is either (1) depressed mood or (2) loss of interest or pleasure.

1. Depressed mood most of the day, nearly every day

2. Marked diminished interest or pleasure in all, or almost all, activities

3. Significant weight loss (not dieting) or weight gain, or decrease or increase in appetite nearly every day

4. Insomnia or hypersomnia nearly every day

5. Psychomotor agitation or retardation nearly every day

6. Fatigue or loss of energy nearly every day

7. Feelings of worthlessness or excessive or inappropriate guilt (may be delusional) nearly every day

8. Diminished ability to think or concentrate, or indecisiveness

9. Recurrent thoughts of death, recurrent suicidal ideation without a specific plan, or a suicide attempt or a specific suicide plan

B. The symptoms cause clinically significant distress or impairment in social, occupational or other important areas of functioning.

C. The symptoms are not due to the direct physiologic effects of a substance or a general medical condition (eg, hypothyroidism).

Medications That May Precipitate Depression

Anticancer agents	Vinblastine, vincristine, interferon, procarbazine, asparaginase, tamoxifen, cyproterone
Anti-inflammatory & analgesic agents	Indomethacin, pentazocine, phenacetin, phenylbutazone
Antimicrobial agents	Cycloserine, ethambutol, sulfonamides, select gram-negative antibiotics
Cardiovascular/ antihypertensive agents	Clonidine, digitalis, diuretics, guanethidine, hydralazine, indapamide, methyldopa, prazosin, procainamide, propranolol, reserpine
CNS agents	Alcohol, amantadine, amphetamine & derivatives, barbiturates, benzodiazepines, chloral hydrate, carbamazepine, cocaine, haloperidol, L-dopa, phenothiazines, succinimide derivatives
Hormonal agents	ACTH, corticosteroids, estrogen, melatonin, oral contraceptives, progesterone
Miscellaneous	Cimetidine, disulfiram, organic pesticides, physostigmine

Medical Disorders & Psychiatric Disorders Associated With Depression

Endocrine diseases	Acromegaly, Addison's disease, Cushing's disease, diabetes mellitus, hyperparathyroidism, hypoparathyroidism, hyperthyroidism, hypothyroidism, insulinoma, pheochromocytoma, pituitary dysfunction
Deficiency states	Pernicious anemia, severe anemia, Wernicke's encephalopathy
Infections	Encephalitis, fungal infections, meningitis, neurosyphilis, influenza, mononucleosis, tuberculosis, AIDS
Collagen disorders	Rheumatoid arthritis
Systemic lupus erythematosus	
Metabolic disorders	Electrolyte imbalance, hypokalemia, hyponatremia, hepatic encephalopathy, Pick's disease, uremia, Wilson's disease
Cardiovascular disease	Cerebral arteriosclerosis, chronic bronchitis, congestive heart failure, emphysema, myocardial infarction, paroxysmal dysrhythmia, pneumonia
Neurologic disorders	Alzheimer's disease, amyotrophic lateral sclerosis, brain tumors, chronic pain syndrome, Creutzfeldt-Jakob disease, Huntington's disease, multiple sclerosis, myasthenia gravis, Parkinson's disease, poststroke, trauma (postconcussion)
Malignant disease	Breast, gastrointestinal, lung, pancreas, prostate
Psychiatric disorders	Alcoholism, anxiety disorders, eating disorders, schizophrenia

DEPRESSION (Continued)

Somatic Treatments of Depression in the Patient With Medical Illness

Condition	First Choice	Second-Line Options	Alternatives
Thyroid			
Hypothyroid	Thyroid (T)	T_4 or T_3 + antidepressant (SSRIs , TCAs, new generation agents)	ECT, other antidepressants psychostimulants
Hyperthyroid	Antidepressant and antihyperthyroid medications	Select a different group of antidepressants	
Diabetes mellitus	SSRIs, other new generation antidepressants	TCAs (second amine or low-dose tertiary amine) MAOIs	ECT, buspirone, psychostimulants, thyroid supplements, mood stabilizers
Cardiovascular disorders	SSRIs, bupropion	ECT, psychostimulants B-blockers, buspirone	ECT, TCAs, MAOIs, mood stabilizers
Renal disease	Fluoxetine, sertraline	TCAs, other new generation antidepressants, psychostimulants	ECT, anticonvulsants, lithium (if dialysis or CLOSELY monitored)
Hepatic disease (reduced dose ALL)	Sertraline	Other new generation antidepressants, TCAs-secondary amines	TCAs-tertiary amines
HIV	Bupropion, SSRIs, psychostimulants	TCAs	ECT
Transplant	**Closely monitor.** See cardiovascular, renal, liver, pulmonary, new antidepressant agents, TCAs-secondary amines		
Neurologic	Newer generation antidepressants, TCAs-secondary amines	Selegiline, anticonvulsants	Bromocriptine
Malignancy	Newer generation antidepressants, TCAs-secondary amines psychostimulants	TCAs-tertiary amines of pain MAOIs	ECT
Respiratory	Activating antidepressants, buspirone		More sedating antidepressants, ECT
Gastrointestinal	TCAs-secondary amines, new generation antidepressants	TCAs-tertiary amines	ECT

DIABETES MELLITUS TREATMENT

INSULIN-DEPENDENT DIABETES MELLITUS

Treatment goals that emphasize glycemic control have been recommended by the American Diabetes Association.

Glycemic Control for People With Diabetes

Biochemical Index	Nondiabetic	Goal	Action Suggested
Preprandial glucose	<115	80-120	<80 >140
Bedtime glucose (mg/dL)	<120	100-140	<100 >160
Hb A$_{1C}$ (%)	<8	<7	>8

These values are for nonpregnant individuals. Action suggested depends on individual patient circumstances, Hb A$_{1c}$ referenced to a nondiabetic range of 4% to 6% (mean 5%, SD 0.5%).

Effect on Glycemic Control of Oral Hypoglycemic Agents as Monotherapy

Agent	Fasting Blood Glucose	Postprandial Blood Glucose	Hb A$_{1c}$
Precose® (acarbose) 25-100 mg 3 times/day	-25 mg/dL	-49 mg/dL	-0.44% to -0.74%
Glucophage® (metformin) Up to 2500 mg/day	-52 mg/dL	–	-1.4%
Amaryl® (glimepiride) 1-8 mg/day			
Diaβeta/Micronase (glyburide) 1.25-20 mg/day	-60 mg/dL	–	-1.5% to 2%
Glynase PresTab® (glyburide) 0.75-12 mg/day			
Prandin® (repaglinide) 0.25-4 mg 3 times/day	-31 to -82 mg/dL	-48 mg/dL	-0.6% to -1.9%
Glyset™ (miglitol) 25-50 mg 3 times/day	–	-35 to -60 mg/dL	-0.3% to -0.82%
Starlix® (nateglinide) 60-120 mg 3 times/day	–	–	-0.3% to -0.5%

(Package inserts: Diaβeta®, 1997; Glynase PresTab®, 1999; Micronase®, 1999; Prandin®, 1997; Glyset™, 2001; Starlix®, 2000; Goldberg, 1999)

DIABETES MELLITUS TREATMENT *(Continued)*

Pharmacological Algorithm for Treatment of Type 2 Diabetes
(Patients inadequately controlled with diet and exercise)

Education
Nutrition
Exercise
Home Blood Glucose Monitoring
Goal:
FPG <126 mg/dL
Hb A$_{1c}$ <7.0%

Continue if initial intervention is effective; follow-up every 3 months

Usual Monotherapy
If FPG ≥126 mg/dL and/or Hb A$_{1c}$ ≥7.0% after 4-8 weeks, *start therapy with sulfonylureas or metformin*. (Metformin is preferred if patient is obese or dyslipidemic.)
Other monotherapy options:
Insulin
Precose® (acarbose)
Prandin™ (repaglinide)

Monotherapy Adequate
(FPG <126 mg/dL and Hb A$_{1c}$ <7.0%)
Continue therapy

Monotherapy Inadequate
after 4-8 weeks
(FPG ≥126 mg/dL or Hb A$_{1c}$ ≥7.0%),
add second oral agent

Other option:
Add bedtime insulin

Combination Therapy Adequate
(FPG <126 mg/dL and Hb A$_{1c}$ <7.0%)
Continue therapy

Combination Therapy Inadequate
(FPG ≥126 mg/dL or Hb A$_{1c}$ ≥7.0%)
• Add bedtime insulin
• Add third oral agent
• Switch to insulin monotherapy
• Consider referral to specialist

Modified from DeFronzo RA, "Pharmacological Treatment for Type 2 Diabetes Mellitus," *Ann Intern Med,* 1999, 131:281-303.

EPILEPSY

Antiepileptic Drugs for Children and Adolescents by Seizure Type and Epilepsy Syndrome

Seizure Type or Epilepsy Syndrome	First Line Therapy	Alternatives
Partial seizures (with or without secondary generalization)	Carbamazepine	Valproate, phenytoin, gabapentin, lamotrigine, vigabatrin, phenobarbital, primidone; consider clonazepam, clorazepate, acetazolamide, oxcarbazepine
Generalized tonic-clonic seizures	Valproate or carbamazepine	Phenytoin, phenobarbital, primidone; consider clonazepam
Childhood absence epilepsy		
Before 10 years of age	Ethosuximide or valproate	Methsuximide, acetazolamide, clonazepam, lamotrigine
After 10 years of age	Valproate	Ethosuximide, methsuximide, acetazolamide, clonazepam, lamotrigine; consider adding carbamazepine, phenytoin, or phenobarbital for generalized tonic-clonic seizures if valproate not tolerated
Juvenile myoclonic epilepsy	Valproate	Phenobarbital, primidone, clonazepam; consider carbamazepine, phenytoin, methsuximide, acetazolamide
Progressive myoclonic epilepsy	Valproate	Valproate plus clonazepam, phenobarbital
Lennox-Gastaut and related syndromes	Valproate	Clonazepam, phenobarbital, lamotrigine, ethosuximide, felbamate; consider methsuximide, ACTH or steroids, pyridoxine, ketogenic diet, topiramate
Infantile spasms	ACTH or steroids	Valproate; consider clonazepam, vigabatrin (especially with tuberous sclerosis), pyridoxine
Benign epilepsy of childhood with centrotemporal spikes	Carbamazepine or valproate	Phenytoin; consider phenobarbital, primidone
Neonatal seizures	Phenobarbital	Phenytoin; consider clonazepam, primidone, valproate, pyridoxine

Adapted from Bourgeois BFD, "Antiepileptic Drugs in Pediatric Practice," *Epilepsia*, 1995, 36(Suppl 2):S34-S45.

EPILEPSY *(Continued)*

FEBRILE SEIZURES

A febrile seizure is defined as a seizure occurring for no reason other than an elevated temperature. It does not have an infectious or metabolic origin within the CNS (ie, it is not caused by meningitis or encephalitis). Fever is usually >102°F rectally, but the more rapid the rise in temperature, the more likely a febrile seizure may occur. About 4% of children develop febrile seizures at one time of their life, usually occurring between 3 months and 5 years of age with the majority occurring at 6 months to 3 years of age. There are 3 types of febrile seizures:

1. **Simple** febrile seizures are nonfocal febrile seizures of less than 15 minutes duration. They do not occur in multiples.

2. **Complex** febrile seizures are febrile seizures that are either focal, have a focal component, are longer than 15 minutes in duration, or are multiple febrile seizures that occur within 30 minutes.

3. **Febrile status epilepticus** is a febrile seizure that is a generalized tonic-clonic seizure lasting longer than 30 minutes.

Note: Febrile seizures should not be confused with true epileptic seizures associated with fever or "seizure with fever." "Seizure with fever" includes seizures associated with acute neurologic illnesses (ie, meningitis, encephalitis).

Long-term prophylaxis with phenobarbital may reduce the risk of subsequent febrile seizures. The 1980 NIH Consensus paper stated that after the first febrile seizure, long-term prophylaxis should be considered under any of the following:

1. Presence of abnormal neurological development or abnormal neurological exam

2. Febrile seizure was complex in nature: duration >15 minutes focal febrile seizure followed by transient or persistent neurological abnormalities

3. Positive family history of afebrile seizures (epilepsy)

Also consider long-term prophylaxis in certain cases if:

1. the child has multiple febrile seizures

2. the child is <12 months of age

Anticonvulsant prophylaxis is usually continued for 2 years or 1 year after the last seizure, whichever is longer. With the identification of phenobarbital's adverse effects on learning and cognitive function, many physicians will not start long-term phenobarbital prophylaxis after the first febrile seizure unless the patient has more than one of the above risk factors. Most physicians would start long-term prophylaxis if the patient has a second febrile seizure.

Daily administration of phenobarbital and therapeutic phenobarbital serum concentrations ≥15 mcg/mL decrease recurrence rates of febrile seizures. Valproic acid is also effective in preventing recurrences of febrile seizures, but is usually reserved for patients who have significant adverse effects to phenobarbital. The administration of rectal diazepam (as a solution or suppository) at the time of the febrile illness has been shown to be as effective as daily phenobarbital in preventing recurrences of febrile seizures. However, these rectal dosage forms are not available in the United States. Some centers in the USA are using the injectable form of diazepam rectally. The solution for injection is filtered prior to use if drawn from an ampul. A recent study suggests that oral diazepam, 0.33 mg/kg/dose given every 8 hours only when the child has a fever, may reduce the risk of recurrent febrile seizures (see Rosman, et al). **Note**: A more recent study by Uhari (1995) showed that lower doses of diazepam, 0.2 mg/kg/dose, were not effective.) Carbamazepine and phenytoin are not effective in preventing febrile seizures.

References

Berg AT, Shinnar S, Hauser WA, et al, "Predictors of Recurrent Febrile Seizures: A Meta-Analytic Review," *J Pediatr*, 1990, 116 (3):329-37.

Camfield PR, Camfield CS, Gordon K, et al, "Prevention of Recurrent Febrile Seizures," *J Pediatr*, 1995, 126 (6):929-30.

NIH Consensus Statement, "Febrile Seizures: A Consensus of Their Significance, Evaluation and Treatment," *Pediatrics*, 1980, 66 (6):1009-12.

Rosman NP, Colton T, Labazzo J, et al, "A Controlled Trial of Diazepam Administration During Febrile Illnesses to Prevent Recurrence of Febrile Seizures," *N Engl J Med*, 1993, 329 (2):79-84.

Uhari M, Rantala H, Vainionpaa L, et al, "Effects of Acetaminophen and of Low Intermittent Doses of Diazepam on Prevention of Recurrences of Febrile Seizures," *J Pediatr*, 1995, 126(6):991-5.

CONVULSIVE STATUS EPILEPTICUS

Recommendations of the Epilepsy Foundation of America's Working Group on Status Epilepticus

(*JAMA*, 1993, 270:854-9)

Convulsive status epilepticus is an emergency that is associated with high morbidity and mortality. The outcome largely depends on etiology, but prompt and appropriate pharmacological therapy can reduce morbidity and mortality. Etiology varies in children and adults and reflects the distribution of disease in these age groups. Antiepileptic drug administration should be initiated whenever a seizure has lasted 10 minutes. Immediate concerns include supporting respiration, maintaining blood pressure, gaining intravenous access, and identifying and treating the underlying cause. Initial therapeutic and diagnostic measures are conducted simultaneously. The goal of therapy is rapid termination of clinical and electrical seizure activity; the longer a seizure continues, the greater the likelihood of an adverse outcome. Several drug protocols now in use will terminate status epilepticus. Common to all patients is the need for a clear plan, prompt administration of appropriate drugs in adequate doses, and attention to the possibility of apnea, hypoventilation, or other metabolic abnormalities.

Figure 1. Algorithm for the Initial Management of Status Epilepticus

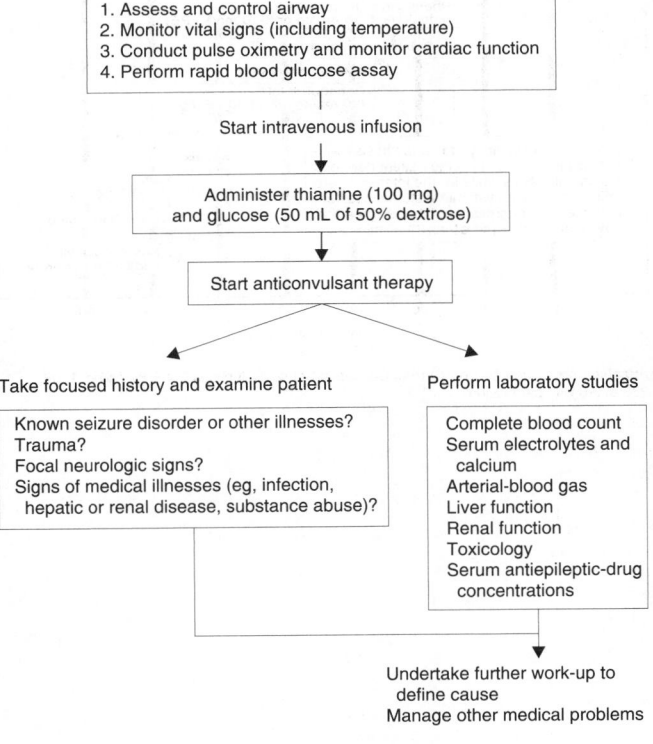

Adapted from Lowenstein A, "Current Concepts: Status Epilepticus," *N Engl J Med*, 1998, 338:970-6 with permission.

EPILEPSY *(Continued)*

Figure 2. Antiepileptic Drug Therapy for Status Epilepticus

I.V. denotes intravenous and PE denoted phenytoin equivalents. The horizontal bars indicate the approximate duration of drug infusions

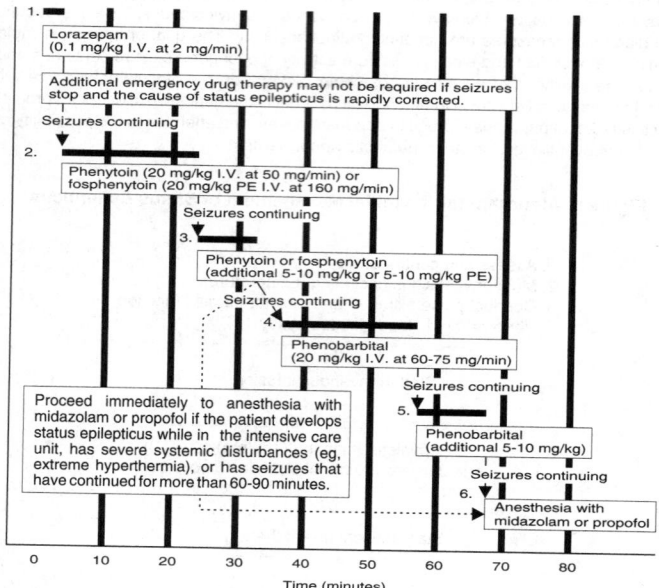

Adapted from Lowenstein A, "Current Concepts: Status Epilepticus," *N Engl J Med*, 1998, 338:970-6 with permission.

HEART FAILURE

This appendix piece outlines a general approach to treatment of chronic systolic heart failure and highlights various aspects of drug therapy in this population. Patient assessment, management, and select drug therapies for heart failure are listed (see following table), followed by general considerations for each class of drugs. Detailed consensus recommendations for the management of chronic heart failure are published (http://www.acc.org/clinical/guidelines/failure/hf_index.htm and *J Heart Lung Transplant*, 2002, 21(2):189-203.

Drug Therapy for Systolic Heart Failure

Drug Therapy[1]	Role	Benefit	Comment
Routine Use			
ACEI	Standard therapy for patients with asymptomatic and symptomatic heart failure (NYHA class I-IV)	Improves morbidity and mortality	– Achieve target or maximum tolerated dose – Optimize diuretic therapy, if needed, prior to initiating ACEI therapy – Ramipril may improve cardiovascular morbidity and mortality in high-risk patients without heart failure
Beta-blockers	Standard therapy for patients with **stable** NYHA class II-III heart failure	Improves morbidity and mortality	– Beneficial effects specific to individual agents – Need close patient contact / follow-up
Diuretics	Standard therapy for the treatment of symptoms of heart failure	Improves symptoms; spironolactone improves mortality in severe (NYHA class IV) heart failure	– Achieve and maintain euvolemia – Combine with standard therapy – Consider spironolactone in severe heart failure
Digoxin	Patients with symptoms despite optimal standard therapy	Improves symptoms and frequency of hospitalizations for heart failure	– No beneficial impact on mortality – No therapeutic range for efficacy (toxicity >2 ng/mL) – Potential for drug interactions
Selected Patients			
Aldosterone antagonist	Recent or current symptoms at rest despite digoxin, diuretics, ACEI and (usually) a beta-blocker	May reduce morbidity and mortality	– Initiate only in patients with S$_{cr}$ <2.5 mg/dL and serum potassium <5.0 mmol/L
Angiotensin-II receptor blockers	Patients intolerant to ACEI	Very limited data showing similar improvements in morbidity and mortality compared to ACEI	– Mechanistically similar to ACEI – Should not be considered equivalent or superior to ACEI
Hydralazine/ISDN	Patients intolerant to ACEI	Improves mortality	– Requires frequent daily dosing – No outcome data for combined therapy with standard therapy

[1]See following information and also individual monographs.

DRUG THERAPY

Angiotensin-Converting Enzyme Inhibitors (ACEI)

ACEI improve morbidity and mortality and are "standard therapy" for the treatment of systolic heart failure. All patients with symptomatic or asymptomatic systolic heart failure (NYHA class I-IV) should be on ACEI therapy unless contraindicated. Therapy should be initiated and titrated to the established target dose (see the following table) or to the maximum tolerated dose. Therapy should be continued long-term unless the patient cannot tolerate or develops a contraindication.

Contraindications for therapy include hypotension (systolic pressure <90 mm Hg; diastolic pressure <60 mm Hg), shock, angioedema, anuric renal failure, pregnancy, significant hyperkalemia, and bilateral renal artery stenosis. Patients on diuretic therapy or those with asymptomatic low blood pressure should be monitored more closely for signs of symptomatic hypotension with initiation of ACEI therapy. ACEIs should not be

HEART FAILURE *(Continued)*

used to treat hemodynamically unstable heart failure. See specific ACEI monographs for drug and dosing information.

Dosing of ACEIs in Heart Failure[1]

ACEI	Initial Dose	Maximum Dose
Captopril	6.25-12.5 mg tid	50 mg tid
Enalapril	2.5 mg bid	10-20 mg bid
Fosinopril	5-10 mg daily	40 mg daily
Lisinopril	2.5-5 mg daily	20-40 mg daily
Quinapril	10 mg bid	40 mg bid
Ramipril	1.25-2.5 mg bid	10 mg daily
Trandolapril	1 mg daily	4 mg daily

[1]Doses are based on Clinical Trials and National Guidelines.

Beta-Blockers

Carvedilol, sustained release metoprolol (CR/XL), and bisoprolol have demonstrated in clinical trials to decrease morbidity and mortality in patients with mild to moderate heart failure (NYHA class II-III) when combined with standard therapy (target doses of ACEI, diuretics, ± digoxin). Other beta-blockers (eg, bucindolol and celiprolol) have no benefit or may tend to increase mortality. Only carvedilol is FDA approved for the treatment of heart failure. (See individual drug monographs for carvedilol, metoprolol, and bisoprolol.)

All patients on standard therapy with **stable** NYHA class II-III systolic heart failure should be on beta-blocker therapy. Beta-blocker therapy may be considered for patients on standard therapy with mild systolic heart failure (NYHA class I). Patients with sympathetic nervous system activation (eg, heart rate >85 beats/minute) may derive greatest benefit. Beta-blocker therapy is not recommended for patients with unstable heart failure and in those that cannot tolerate therapy or where therapy is contraindicated.

Contraindications to beta blockade include bradycardia, 2nd or 3rd degree AV block, hypotension (systolic pressure <90 mm Hg/diastolic pressure <60 mm Hg), decompensated heart failure, and noncompliance. Special consideration should be given in evaluating the risk versus benefit for beta blockade in patients with coexisting conditions, including poorly controlled diabetes, severe COPD, and severe reactive airway disease. These patients should be followed more frequently if beta-blocker therapy is prescribed.

In general, beta-blocker therapy should be initiated at low dose and titrated slowly, no faster than doubling the dose at weekly intervals to tolerated or target doses (see following table). Therapy should be initiated and titrated by practitioners or clinics with experience and capabilities for close patient contact and follow-up.

During the initiation and titration of beta-blocker therapy it is imperative that patients be frequently monitored for signs of worsening heart failure. Significant weight gain, increasing shortness of breath, edema, paroxysmal nocturnal dyspnea, and dyspnea on exertion may necessitate slowing or decreasing the dose of beta-blocker with dose adjustment of ACEI and diuretic therapies. Patients should be well educated on the potential signs of worsening heart failure, importance of diet and drug compliance, and the need to notify the practitioner or clinic immediately if symptoms of worsening heart failure occur.

Initial and Target Doses for Beta-Blocker Therapy in Heart Failure[1]

Beta-Blocker	Starting Dose	Target Dose	Comment
Bisoprolol	1.25 mg/day	10 mg/day	– β_1-selective: possible benefit in patients with reactive airway disease – Inconvenient dosage forms for initial dose titration
Carvedilol	3.125 mg twice daily	25-50 mg twice daily	– FDA approved for heart failure – Nonselective beta-blocker/α_1-blocker – Possible greater reduction in blood pressure (α-blocking effects) – Convenient dosages
Metoprolol XL/CR	12.5-25 mg/day	200 mg/day	– Compelling data for mortality benefit – β_1-selective: possible benefit in patients with reactive airway disease – Inconvenient dosage forms for initial dose titration – Less potential to decrease blood pressure (no α-blocking properties)

[1]Doses are those used in clinical trials.

Digoxin

Digoxin improves symptoms of heart failure and decreases hospitalizations for heart failure, but does not improve mortality. Digoxin should be used in patients who have symptoms despite optimal standard therapy (ACEIs, diuretics, beta-blocker). There is no compelling evidence for a target therapeutic serum level for digoxin in the treatment of heart failure.

Digoxin should be avoided in patients with sinus and AV block. Caution should be used with digoxin in patients with potential drug interactions, unstable renal function, hypokalemia, and hypomagnesemia.

Diuretics

Therapy should be initiated immediately in patients with heart failure who have signs of volume overload. Patients with mild volume overload can be managed adequately on thiazide diuretics. Patients with more severe volume overload, particularly in patients with a creatinine clearance <30 mL/minute should be started on a loop diuretic. Diuretic therapy should eliminate symptoms of heart failure (eg, edema) and may be monitored and dosed by changes in body weight. Resistance to therapy, as is seen in severe heart failure, may necessitate intravenous diuretic therapy or the use of more than one diuretic. See monographs for individual diuretics.

HEART FAILURE *(Continued)*

Diuretic Therapy for Heart Failure

Diuretic	Initial Dose (mg)	Target Dose (mg)	Recommended Maximal Dose (mg)	Comment
Thiazide Diuretics				
Chlorthalidone Hydrochlorothiazide	25 qd	As needed	50 qd	– Postural hypotension, hypokalemia, hyperglycemia, hyperuricemia, rash; rare severe reaction includes pancreatitis, bone marrow suppression, and anaphylaxis
Loop Diuretics				
Bumetanide Furosemide Torsemide	0.5-1 qd-bid 10-40 qd-bid 10-20 mg qd-bid	As needed	10 qd 240 bid 200 mg qd	– Same as thiazide diuretics
Thiazide-Related Diuretic				
Metolazone	2.5[1]	As needed	10 qd	– Same as thiazide diuretics
Potassium-Sparing Diuretics				
Amiloride Triamterene	5 qd 50 qd	As needed	40 qd 100 bid	– Hyperkalemia (especially if administered with ACEI), rash
Aldosterone Antagonist				
Spironolactone	25 qd	As needed	50 qd	– Hyperkalemia (especially if administered with ACEI), gynecomastia – Decreases mortality in severe heart failure (initiate only in patients with S_{cr} <2.5 mg/dL and serum potassium <5.0 mmol/L)

[1]Given as a single test dose initially.

Adapted from U.S. Department of Health & Human Services, the Agency for Healthcare Policy and Research (ACHPR) Publication No. 94-0613, June, 1994

Hydralazine/Isosorbide Dinitrate (ISDN)

The combination of hydralazine (initial dose 10 mg qid up to 75 mg qid) and isosorbide dinitrate (initial dose 5 mg tid up to 40 mg tid), has been shown to improve mortality in patients with heart failure not on ACEI therapy. ACEI therapy is superior compared to hydralazine/ISDN in improving mortality.

The combination of hydralazine/ISDN may be considered in patients intolerant to ACEI therapy. The combination is sometimes added to standard therapy if symptoms or fatigue persist. However, there is little data to suggest that the addition of hydralazine/ISDN to standard therapy further improves morbidity and mortality.

The chronic use of other direct vasodilators may increase morbidity and mortality in this population.

Angiotensin II Receptor Blockers (ARBs)

The renin-angiotensin-aldosterone system plays a key role in the progression of heart failure. For this reason, the role of ARBs in this patient population is being extensively evaluated. Mechanistically, angiotensin II is also produced through non-ACE systems and heart failure patients have "escape" of angiotensin II levels with chronic ACEI therapy. For these reasons, ARB therapy may confer a positive impact on morbidity and mortality by directly blocking the detrimental affects of angiotensin II. It is not established if ARB therapy provides similar mortality benefits as ACEIs or if there is an added benefit in combining an ABR to standard (ACEI) therapy.

In the Evaluation of Losartan in the Elderly (ELITE) trial, losartan and captopril therapy produced similar effects on renal function (primary study endpoint). The risk for cardiovascular events (secondary study endpoint) were significantly decreased in those treated with losartan. A follow-up study (ELITE-II) showed similar cardiovascular events and no differences in hospitalization rates between patients randomized to captopril or losartan. In another ARB trial (RESOLVD), candesartan and enalapril therapy alone and the combination of these two agents were evaluated. The findings of this trial showed no difference in clinical effects overall and a trend for improved left ventricular structure with ARB and ACEI combination therapy. The addition of ARBs to ACEI therapy (as well as other heart failure treatment) did not result in a decrease in mortality, although hospitalization was significantly reduced (ValHeFT) and the combined endpoint of mortality and morbidity was reduced. In a subgroup analysis, patients taking both an ACEI and a beta-blocker at baseline had a higher mortality after valsartan was added. Ongoing studies will give more data on the potential role of ARBs in the treatment of heart failure.

Current recommendations for ARB therapy is in those heart failure patients who are intolerant of ACEI therapy (see drug monographs).

Aldosterone Antagonists

In the RALES study, a large, long-term trial (*N Engl J Med*, 1999, 341:709-17), low-dose spironolactone, when added to prior ACEI therapy in patients with recent or current Class IV symptoms, resulted in a reduced risk of hospitalization and death. Patients who were also receiving digitalis and beta-blockers appeared to demonstrate the most marked effect. Therapy should only be initiated in patients with a serum potassium <5.0 mmol/L and a serum creatinine <2.5 mg/dL. Close monitoring of serum potassium is required.

Resources

Guidelines

Hung SA, Baker DW, Chin MH, et al, "ACC/AHA Guidelines for the Evaluation and Management of Chronic Heart Failure in the Adult: A Report of the American College of Cardiology/American Heart Association Task Force on Practice Guidelines (Committee to Revise the 1995 Guidelines for the Evaluation and Management of Heart Failure)," 2001.), *J Heart Lung Transplant*, 2002, 21(2):189-203. American College of Cardiology Web site available at http://www.acc.org/clinical/guidelines/failure/hf_index.htm.

HELICOBACTER PYLORI TREATMENT

Multiple Drug Regimens for the Treatment of H. pylori Infection

Drug	Dosages	Duration of Therapy
H₂-receptor antagonist[1]	Any one given at appropriate dose	4 weeks
plus		
Bismuth subsalicylate	525 mg 4 times/day	2 weeks
plus		
Metronidazole	250 mg 4 times/day	2 weeks
plus		
Tetracycline	500 mg 4 times/day	2 weeks
Ranitidine bismuth citrate	400 mg twice daily	2 weeks
plus		
Clarithromycin	500 mg twice daily	2 weeks
plus		
Amoxicillin	1000 mg twice daily	2 weeks
Ranitidine bismuth citrate	400 mg twice daily	2 weeks
plus		
Clarithromycin	500 mg twice daily	2 weeks
plus		
Metronidazole	500 mg twice daily	2 weeks
Ranitidine bismuth citrate	400 mg twice daily	2 weeks
plus		
Clarithromycin	500 mg twice daily	2 weeks
plus		
Tetracycline	500 mg twice daily	2 weeks
Proton pump inhibitor[1]	Esomeprazole 40 mg once daily	10 days
plus		
Clarithromycin	500 mg twice daily	10 days
plus		
Amoxicillin	1000 mg twice daily	10 days
Proton pump inhibitor[1]	Lansoprazole 30 mg twice daily Omeprazole 20 mg twice daily	10-14 days
plus		
Clarithromycin	500 mg twice daily	10-14 days
plus		
Amoxicillin	1000 mg twice daily	10-14 days
Proton pump inhibitor	Lansoprazole 30 mg twice daily Omeprazole 20 mg twice daily	2 weeks
plus		
Clarithromycin	500 mg twice daily	2 weeks
plus		
Metronidazole	500 mg twice daily	2 weeks
Proton pump inhibitor	Lansoprazole 30 mg once daily Omeprazole 20 mg once daily	2 weeks
plus		
Bismuth	525 mg 4 times/day	2 weeks
plus		
Metronidazole	500 mg 3 times/day	2 weeks
plus		
Tetracycline	500 mg 4 times/day	2 weeks

[1]FDA-approved regimen

Modified from Howden CS and Hunt RH, "Guidelines for the Management of Helicobacter pylori Infection," AJG, 1998, 93:2336.

HYPERGLYCEMIA- OR HYPOGLYCEMIA-CAUSING DRUGS

Hyperglycemia	Hypoglycemia	Hyperglycemia or Hypoglycemia
Caffeine	Anabolic steroids	Beta-blockers (also may mask symptoms of hypoglycemia)
Calcitonin	ACE inhibitors	Alcohol
Corticosteroids	Chloramphenicol	Lithium
Diltiazem	Clofibrate	Phenothiazines
Estrogens	Disopyramide	Rifampin
Isoniazid	MAO inhibitors	Octreotide
Morphine	Miconazole (oral form)	Fluoxetine
Nifedipine	Probenecid	
Nicotine	Pyridoxine	
Nicotinic acid	Salicylates	
Oral contraceptives	Sulfonamides	
Phenytoin	Tetracycline	
Sympathomimetic amines	Verapamil	
Theophylline	Warfarin	
Thiazide diuretics		
Thyroid products		

Adapted from American Association of Diabetes Educators, *A Core Curriculum for Diabetes Education*, 3rd ed, Vol 10, Chicago, IL, 1998, 338-41.

HYPERLIPIDEMIA MANAGEMENT

MORTALITY

There is a strong link between serum cholesterol and cardiovascular mortality. This association becomes stronger in patients with established coronary artery disease. Lipid-lowering trials show that reductions in LDL cholesterol are followed by reductions in mortality. In general, each 1% fall in LDL cholesterol confers a 2% reduction in cardiovascular events. The aim of therapy for hyperlipidemia is to decrease cardiovascular morbidity and mortality by lowering cholesterol to a target level using safe and cost-effective treatment modalities. The target LDL cholesterol is determined by the number of patient risk factors (see the following Risk Factors and Goal LDL Cholesterol tables). The goal is achieved through diet, lifestyle modification, and drug therapy. The basis for these recommendations is provided by longitudinal interventional studies demonstrating that lipid-lowering in patients with prior cardiovascular events (secondary prevention) and in patients with hyperlipidemia but no prior cardiac event (primary prevention) lowers the occurrence of future cardiovascular events, including stroke. In a recent randomized study of relatively low-risk patients with LDLs ≥115 mg/dL, who were referred for revascularization (angioplasty), those assigned to aggressive lipid-lowering therapy were at the same or lower risk for subsequent ischemic events than those who underwent angioplasty (*N Engl J Med*, 1999, 341:170-6).

Major Risk Factors That Modify LDL Goals

Positive risk factors	Male ≥45 years
	Female ≥55 years
	Family history of premature coronary heart disease, defined as CHD in male first-degree relative <55 years; CHD in female first-degree relative <65 years
	Cigarette smoking
	Hypertension (blood pressure ≥140/90 mm Hg) or taking antihypertensive medication
	Low HDL (<40 mg/dL / 1.03 mmol/L)
Negative risk factors	High HDL (≥60 mg/dL / 1.6 mmol/L)[1]

[1]If HDL is ≥60 mg/dL, may subtract one positive risk factor.

Treatment Goals for LDL Cholesterol

Risk Factors	Target LDL Cholesterol	Target Non-HDL Cholesterol[1]
0-1 risk factor	<160 mg/dL	<190 mg/dL
Multiple (2+) risk factors	<130 mg/dL	<160 mg/dL
CHD or CHD risk equivalents[2]	<100 mg/dL	<130 mg/dL
Diabetes (with or without established coronary artery disease)	<100 mg/dL	<130 mg/dL

[1]Non-HDL cholesterol = total cholesterol minus HDL; for use in patients with serum triglyceride ≥200 mg/dL

[2]CHD risk equivalent: Other form of atherosclerotic disease (peripheral arterial disease, abdominal aortic aneurysm, and symptomatic carotid artery disease).

Any person with elevated LDL cholesterol or other form of hyperlipidemia should undergo evaluation to rule out secondary dyslipidemia. Causes of secondary dyslipidemia include diabetes, hypothyroidism, obstructive liver disease, chronic renal failure, and drugs that increase LDL and decrease HDL (progestins, anabolic steroids, corticosteroids).

Elevated Serum Triglyceride Levels

Elevated serum triglyceride levels may be an independent risk factor for coronary heart disease. Factors that contribute to hypertriglyceridemia include obesity, inactivity, cigarette smoking, excess alcohol intake, high carbohydrate diets (>60% of energy intake), type 2 diabetes, chronic renal failure, nephrotic syndrome, certain medications (corticosteroids, estrogens, retinoids, higher doses of beta-blockers), and genetic disorders. Non-HDL cholesterol (total cholesterol minus HDL cholesterol) is a secondary focus for clinicians treating patients with high serum triglyceride levels (≥200 mg/dL). The goal for non-HDL cholesterol in patients with high serum triglyceride levels can be set 30 mg/dL higher than usual LDL cholesterol goals. Patients with serum triglyceride levels <200 mg/dL should aim for the target LDL cholesterol goal.

ATP classification of serum triglyceride levels:

- – Normal triglycerides: <150 mg/dL
- – Borderline-high: 150-199 mg/dL
- – High: 200-499 mg/dL
- – Very high: ≥500 mg/dL

NONDRUG THERAPY

Dietary therapy and lifestyle modifications should be individualized for each patient. A total lifestyle change is recommended for all patients. Dietary and lifestyle modifications should be tried for 3 months, if deemed appropriate. Nondrug and drug therapy should be initiated simultaneously in patients with highly elevated cholesterol (see LDL Cholesterol Goals and Cutpoints for Therapeutic Lifestyle Changes and Drug Therapy in Different Risk Categories table). Increasing physical activity and smoking cessation will aid in the treatment of hyperlipidemia and improve cardiovascular health.

Note: Refer to the National Cholesterol Education Program reference for details concerning the calculation of 10-year risk of CHD using Framingham risk scoring. Risk assessment tool is available online at http://hin.nhlbi.nih.gov/atpiii/calculator.asp?usertype=prof, last accessed March 14, 2002.

Total Lifestyle Change (TLC) Diet

	Recommended Intake
Total fat	25%-35% of total calories
Saturated fat[1]	<7% of total calories
Polyunsaturated fat	≤10% of total calories
Monounsaturated fat	≤20% of total calories
Carbohydrates[2]	50%-60% of total calories
Fiber	20-30 g/day
Protein	~15% of total calories
Cholesterol	<200 mg/day
Total calories[3]	Balance energy intake and expenditure to maintain desirable body weight/prevent weight gain

[1] *Trans* fatty acids (partially hydrogenated oils) intake should be kept low. These are found in potato chips, other snack foods, margarines and shortenings, and fast-foods.

[2] Complex carbohydrates including grains (especially whole grains, fruits, and vegetables).

[3] Daily energy expenditure should include at least moderate physical activity.

LDL Cholesterol Goals and Cutpoints for Therapeutic Lifestyle Changes (TLC) and Drug Therapy in Different Risk Categories

Risk Category	LDL-C Goal	LDL Level at Which to Initiate TLC	LDL Level at Which to Consider Drug Therapy
CHD or CHD risk equivalents (10-year risk >20%)	<100 mg/dL	≥100 mg/dL	≥130 mg/dL (100-129 mg/dL: drug optional)[1]
2+ risk factors (10-year risk ≤20%)	<130 mg/dL	≥130 mg/dL	10-year risk 10%-20%: ≥130 mg/dL
			10-year risk <10%: ≥160 mg/dL
0-1 risk factor[2]	<160 mg/dL	≥160 mg/dL	≥190 mg/dL (160-189 mg/dL: drug optional)

[1] Some authorities recommend use of LDL-lowering drugs in this category if an LDL cholesterol <100 mg/dL cannot be achieved by therapeutic lifestyle changes. Others prefer use of drugs that primarily modify triglycerides and HDL (eg, nicotinic acid or fibrate). Clinical judgment also may call for deferring drug therapy in this subcategory.

[2] Almost all people with 0-1 risk factor have a 10-year risk <10%, thus 10-year risk assessment in people with 0-1 risk factor is not necessary.

HYPERLIPIDEMIA MANAGEMENT *(Continued)*

DRUG THERAPY

Drug therapy should be selected based on the patient's lipid profile, concomitant disease states, and the cost of therapy. The following table lists specific advantages and disadvantages for various classes of lipid-lowering medications. The cost and expected reduction in lipids with therapy are listed in the Lipid-Lowering Agents table. Refer to individual drug monographs for detailed information.

Advantages and Disadvantages of Specific Lipid-Lowering Therapies

	Advantages	Disadvantages
Bile acid sequestrants	Good choice for ↑ LDL, especially when combined with a statin (↓ LDL ≤50%); low potential for systemic side effects; good choice for younger patients	May increase triglycerides; higher incidence of adverse effects; moderately expensive; drug interactions; inconvenient dosing
Niacin	Good choice for almost any lipid abnormality; inexpensive; greatest increase in HDL	High incidence of adverse effects; may adversely affect NIDDM and gout; sustained release niacin may decrease the incidence of flushing and circumvent the need for multiple daily dosing; sustained release niacin may not increase HDL cholesterol or decrease triglycerides as well as immediate release niacin
HMG-CoA reductase inhibitors	Produces greatest ↓ in LDL; generally well-tolerated; convenient once-daily dosing; proven decrease in mortality	Expensive
Gemfibrozil	Good choice in patients with ↑ triglycerides where niacin is contraindicated or not well-tolerated; gemfibrozil is well tolerated	Variable effects on LDL

Lipid-Lowering Agents

Drug	Dose/Day	Effect on LDL (%)	Effect on HDL (%)	Effect on TG (%)	Avg Wholesale Price/Mo ($)
HMG-CoA Reductase Inhibitors					
Atorvastatin	10 mg	-38	+6	-13	62
	20 mg	-46	+5	-20	93
	40 mg	-51	+5	-32	105
	80 mg	-54	+5	-37	105
Fluvastatin	20 mg	-17	+2	-5	42
	40 mg	-23	+3	-12	42
	40 mg bid	-32	+4	-12	84
Lovastatin	20 mg	-29	+7	-8	42
	40 mg	-31	+5	-2	75
	80 mg	-48	+8	-13	135
Pravastatin	10 mg	-20	+5	-3	67
	20 mg	-24	+3	-15	72
	40 mg	-34	+6	-10	118
Simvastatin	10 mg	-28	+7	-12	68
	20 mg	-35	+5	-17	119
	40 mg	-41	+10	-15	119
	80 mg	-47	+8	-24	119
Bile Acid Sequestrants					
Cholestyramine	8-24 g/day	-15 to -30	+3 to +5	+0 to +20	82-246
Colesevelam	3.8-4.4 g/day	-15 to -18	+3	+0 to +10	140-163
Colestipol	10-20 g/day	-15 to -30	+3 to +5	+0 to +20	132-260
Gemfibrozil	600 mg bid	-5 to -10*	+10 to +20	-40 to -60	11
Fenofibrate	67-201 mg/day	-20 to -25	+1 to -34	-30 to -50	24-72
Niacin	2-3 g/day	-21 to -27	+10 to +35	-10 to -50	4-8

*May increase LDL in some patients.

Recommended Liver Function Monitoring for HMG-CoA Reductase Inhibitors

Agent	Initial and After Increase in Dose	6 Weeks[1]	12 Weeks[1]	Semiannually
Atorvastatin	x	x	x	x
Fluvastatin	x	x	x	x
Lovastatin	x	x	x	x
Pravastatin	x		x	
Simvastatin	x			x

[1]After initiation of therapy or any increase in dose.

Progression of Drug Therapy in Primary Prevention

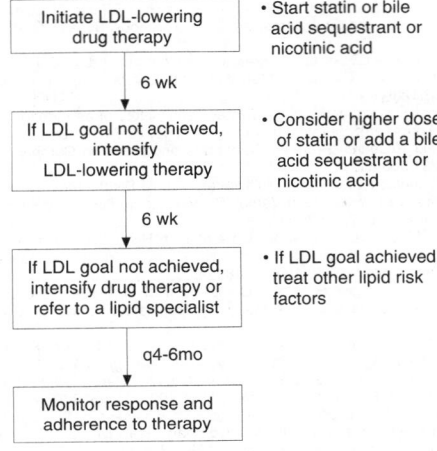

Initiate LDL-lowering drug therapy	• Start statin or bile acid sequestrant or nicotinic acid

↓ 6 wk

If LDL goal not achieved, intensify LDL-lowering therapy	• Consider higher dose of statin or add a bile acid sequestrant or nicotinic acid

↓ 6 wk

If LDL goal not achieved, intensify drug therapy or refer to a lipid specialist	• If LDL goal achieved, treat other lipid risk factors

↓ q4-6mo

Monitor response and adherence to therapy

DRUG SELECTION

Lipid Profile	Monotherapy	Combination Therapies
Increased LDL with normal HDL and triglycerides (TG)	Resin Niacin[1] Statin	Resin plus niacin[1] or statin Statin plus niacin[1,2]
Increased LDL and increased TG (200-499 mg/dL)[2]	Intensify LDL-lowering therapy	Statin plus niacin[1,3] Statin plus fibrate[3]
Increased LDL and increased TG (≥500 mg/dL)[2]	Consider combination therapy (niacin,[1] fibrates, statin)	
Increased TG	Niacin[1] Fibrates	Niacin[1] plus fibrates
Increased LDL and low HDL	Niacin[1] Statin	Statin plus niacin[1,2]

[1] Avoid in diabetics.

[2] Emphasize weight reduction and increased physical activity.

[3] Risk of myopathy with combination.

Resins = bile acid sequestrants; statins = HMG-CoA reductase inhibitors; fibrates = fibric acid derivatives (eg, gemfibrozil, fenofibrate).

COMBINATION DRUG THERAPY

If after at least 6 weeks of therapy at the maximum recommended or tolerated dose, the patient's LDL cholesterol is not at target, consider optimizing nondrug measures, prescribing a higher dose of current lipid-lowering drug, or adding another lipid-lowering medication to the current therapy. Successful drug combinations include statin and niacin, statin and bile acid sequestrant, or niacin and bile acid sequestrant. At maximum recommended doses, LDL cholesterol may be decreased by 50% to 60% with combination therapy. This is the same reduction achieved by atorvastatin 40 mg twice daily. If a bile acid sequestrant is used with other lipid-lowering agents, space doses 1 hour before or 4 hours after the bile acid sequestrant administration. Statins combined with either fenofibrate, clofibrate, gemfibrozil, or niacin increase the risk of rhabdomyolysis. In this situation, patient education (muscle pain/weakness) and careful follow-up are warranted.

References

Guidelines

Gavin JR, Alberti KGMM, Davidson MB, et al, for the Members of the Expert Committee on the Diagnosis and Classification of Diabetes Mellitus, "American Diabetes Association: Clinical Practice Recommendations," *Diabetes Care*, 1999, 22(Suppl 1):S1-S114.

National Cholesterol Education Program, "Third Report of the Expert Panel on Detection, Evaluation, and Treatment of High Blood Cholesterol in Adults (Adult Treatment Panel III)," *JAMA*, 2001, 285:2486-97.

Others

Berthold HK, Sudhop T, and von Bergmann K, "Effect of a Garlic Oil Preparation on Serum Lipoproteins and Cholesterol Metabolism: A Randomized Controlled Trial," *JAMA*, 1998, 279:1900-2.

HYPERLIPIDEMIA MANAGEMENT *(Continued)*

Bertolini S, Bon GB, Campbell LM, et al, "Efficacy and Safety of Atorvastatin Compared to Pravastatin in Patients With Hypercholesterolemia," *Atherosclerosis*, 1997, 130:191-7.

Blankenhorn DH, Nessim SA, Johnson RL, et al, "Beneficial Effects of Combined Colestipol Niacin Therapy on Coronary Atherosclerosis and Venous Bypass Grafts," *JAMA*, 1987 257:3233-40.

Brown G, Albers JJ, Fisher LD, et al, "Regression of Coronary Artery Disease as a Result of Intensive Lipid-Lowering Therapy in Men With High Levels of Apolipoprotein B," *N Engl J Med*, 1990, 323:1289-98.

Capuzzi DM, Guyton JR, Morgan JM, et al, "Efficacy and Safety of an Extended-Release Niacin (Niaspan®): A Long-Term Study," *Am J Cardiol*, 1998, 82:74U-81U.

Coronary Drug Project Research Program, "Clofibrate and Niacin in Coronary Heart Disease," *JAMA*, 1975, 231:360-81.

Dart A, Jerums G, Nicholson G, et al, "A Multicenter, Double-Blind, One-Year Study Comparing Safety and Efficacy of Atorvastatin Versus Simvastatin in Patients With Hypercholesterolemia," *Am J Cardiol*, 1997, 80:39-44.

Davidson MH, Dillon MA, Gordon B, et al, "Colesevelam Hydrochloride (Cholestagel): A New Potent Bile Acid Sequestrant Associated With a Low Incidence of Gastrointestinal Side Effects," *Arch Intern Med*, 1999, 159(16):1893-900.

Davidson M, McKenney J, Stein E, et al, "Comparison of One-Year Efficacy and Safety of Atorvastatin Versus Lovastatin in Primary Hypercholesterolemia," *Am J Cardiol*, 1997, 79:1475-81.

Frick MH, Heinonen OP, Huttunen JK, et al, "Helsinki Heart Study: Primary-Prevention Trial With Gemfibrozil in Middle-Aged Men With Dyslipidemia," *N Engl J Med*, 1987, 317:1237-45.

Garber AM, Browner WS, and Hulley SB, "Clinical Guideline, Part 2: Cholesterol Screening in Asymptomatic Adults, Revisited," *Ann Intern Med*, 1995, 124:518-31.

Johannesson M, Jonsson B, Kjekshus J, et al, "Cost-Effectiveness of Simvastatin Treatment to Lower Cholesterol Levels in Patients With Coronary Heart Disease. Scandinavian Simvastatin Survival Study Group," *N Engl N Med*, 1997, 336:332-6.

Jones P, Kafonek S, Laurora I, et al, "Comparative Dose Efficacy Study of Atorvastatin Versus Simvastatin, Pravastatin, Lovastatin, and Fluvastatin in Patients With Hypercholesterolemia," *Am J Cardiol*, 1998, 81:582-7.

Kasiske BL, Ma JZ, Kalil RS, et al, "Effects of Antihypertensive Therapy on Serum Lipids," *Ann Intern Med*, 1995, 133-41.

Lipid Research Clinics Program, "The Lipid Research Clinics Coronary Primary Prevention Trial Results: I. Reduction in Incidence of Coronary Heart Disease," *JAMA*, 1984, 251:351-64.

Multiple Risk Factor Intervention Trial Research Group, "Multiple Risk Factor Intervention Trial: Risk Factor Changes and Mortality Results," *JAMA*, 1982, 248:1465-77.

Pitt B, Waters D, Brown WV, et al, "Aggressive Lipid-Lowering Therapy Compared With Angioplasty in Stable Coronary Artery Disease. Atorvastatin Versus Revascularization Treatment Investigators," *N Engl J Med*, 1999, 341(2):70-6.

Ross SD, Allen IE, Connelly JE, et al, "Clinical Outcomes in Statin Treatment Trials: A Meta-Analysis," *Arch Intern Med*, 1999, 159:1793-802.

Sacks FM, Pfeffer MA, Moye LA, et al, "The Effect of Pravastatin on Coronary Events After Myocardial Infarction in Patients With Average Cholesterol Levels," *N Engl J Med*, 1996, 335:1001-9.

Scandinavian Simvastatin Survival Study, "Randomized Trial of Cholesterol Lowering in 4444 Patients With Coronary Heart Disease: The Scandinavian Simvastatin Survival Study (4S)," *Lancet*, 1994, 344:1383-9.

Schrott HG, Bittner V, Vittinghoff E, et al, "Adherence to National Cholesterol Education Program Treatment Goals in Postmenopausal Women With Heart Disease. The Heart and Estrogen/Progestin Replacement Study (HERS)," *JAMA*, 1997, 277:1281-6.

Shepherd J, Cobbe SM, Ford I, et al, "Prevention of Coronary Heart Disease With Pravastatin in Men With Hypercholesterolemia, The West of Scotland Coronary Prevention Study Group," *N Engl J Med*, 1995, 333:1301-7.

Stein EA, Davidson MH, Dobs AS, et al, "Efficacy and Safety of Simvastatin 80 mg/day in Hypercholesterolemic Patients. The Expanded Dose Simvastatin U.S. Study Group," *Am J Cardiol*, 1998, 82:311-6.

HYPERTENSION

The optimal blood pressure for adults is <120/80 mm Hg. Consistent systolic pressure ≥140 mm Hg or a diastolic pressure ≥90 mm Hg, in the absence of a secondary cause, define hypertension. Hypertension affects approximately 25% (50 million people) of the United States population. Of those patients on antihypertensive medication, only one in four patients have their blood pressure controlled (<140/90 mm Hg). Recent mortality rates for stroke and heart disease, in which hypertension is an antecedent, remain unchanged. The prevention, detection, evaluation, and treatment of high blood pressure is therefore paramount for each person and for all healthcare providers.

The Sixth Report of the Joint National Committee (JNC VI) is an excellent reference and guide for the treatment of hypertension (*Arch Intern Med*, 1997, 157:2413-46). For adults, hypertension is classified in stages (see Table 1).

Table 1. Adult Classification of Blood Pressure

Category	Systolic (mm Hg)		Diastolic (mm Hg)
Optimal	<120	and	<80
Normal	<130	and	<85
High normal	130-139	or	85-89
Hypertension			
Stage 1	140-159	or	90-99
Stage 2	160-179	or	100-109
Stage 3	≥180	or	≥110
Isolated systolic	≥140		<90

Adapted from the Sixth Report of the Joint National Committee on Prevention, Detection, Evaluation, and Treatment of High Blood Pressure, NIH Publication No. 98-4080, November 1997.

Table 2. Normal Blood Pressure in Children

Age (y)	Girls' SBP/DBP (mm Hg)		Boys' SBP/DBP (mm Hg)	
	50th Percentile for Height	75th Percentile for Height	50th Percentile for Height	75th Percentile for Height
1	104/58	105/59	102/57	104/58
6	111/73	112/73	114/74	115/75
12	123/80	124/81	123/81	125/82
17	129/84	130/85	136/87	138/88

SBP = systolic blood pressure.

DBP = diastolic blood pressure.

Adapted from the report by the NHBPEP Working Group on Hypertension Control in Children and Adolescents, *Pediatrics*, 1996, 98(4 Pt 1):649-58.

Initial follow up of adult patients is based on office blood pressure recordings (see Table 3).

Table 3. Blood Pressure Screening and Follow-up

Initial Screening BP (mm Hg)		Follow-up Recommended
Systolic	Diastolic	
<130	<85	Recheck in 2 years
130-139	85-89	Recheck in 1 year
140-159	90-99	Confirm within 2 months
160-179	100-109	Evaluate/treatment within 1 month
≥180	≥110	Evaluate/treatment immediately or within 1 week

Adapted from the Sixth Report of the Joint National Committee on Prevention, Detection, Evaluation, and Treatment of High Blood Pressure, NIH Publication No. 98-4080, November 1997.

Based on these initial assessments, treatment strategies for patients with hypertension are stratified based on their blood pressure and their risk group classification (see Table 4).

HYPERTENSION *(Continued)*

Table 4. Blood Pressure and Risk Stratification

Blood Pressure Stages	Risk Group A (no RF or TOD)	Risk Group B (≥1 RF, not including diabetes, no TOD)	Risk Group C (TOD and/or diabetes regardless of RF)
High normal (130-139/85-89 mm Hg)	Lifestyle modification	Lifestyle modification	Drug therapy[1] and lifestyle modification
Stage 1 (140-159/90-99 mm Hg)	Lifestyle modification (up to 12 mo)	Lifestyle modification (up to 6 mo)[2]	Drug therapy and lifestyle modification
Stages 2 and 3 (≥160/≥100 mm Hg)	Drug therapy and lifestyle modification	Drug therapy and lifestyle modification	Drug therapy and lifestyle modification

[1]For those with heart failure, renal insufficiency, or diabetes.

[2]For patients with multiple risk factors, consider starting both drug and lifestyle modification together.

RF = risk factor.

TOD = target-organ disease.

Adapted from the Sixth Report of the Joint National Committee on Prevention, Detection, Evaluation, and Treatment of High Blood Pressure, NIH Publication No. 98-4080, November 1997.

Patients in Risk **Group A** have no risk factors; **Group B**, at least one risk factor (other than diabetes), and no cardiovascular disease or target-organ disease (see Table 5); **Group C**, have cardiovascular disease or diabetes or target-organ disease (see Table 5). Risk factors include smoking, dyslipidemia, diabetes, age >60 years, male gender, postmenopausal women, and family history of cardiovascular disease (cardiovascular event in first degree female relatives <65 years and in first degree male relatives <55 years).

Table 5. Target-Organ Disease

Organ System	Manifestation
Cardiac	Clinical, EKG, or radiologic evidence of coronary artery disease; prior MI, angina, post-CABG; left ventricular hypertrophy (LVH); left ventricular dysfunction or cardiac failure
Cerebrovascular	Transient ischemic attack or stroke
Peripheral vascular	Absence of pulses in extremities (except dorsalis pedis), claudication, aneurysm
Renal	Serum creatinine ≥130 μmol/L (1.5 mg/dL); proteinuria (≥1+); microalbuminuria
Retinopathy	Hemorrhages or exudates, with or without papilledema

Adapted from the Sixth Report of the Joint National Committee on Prevention, Detection, Evaluation, and Treatment of High Blood Pressure, NIH Publication No. 98-4080, November 1997.

Treatment of hypertension should be individualized. Lower blood pressures should be achieved in patients with diabetes or renal disease. A Hypertension Treatment Algorithm (see following page) may be used to select specific antihypertensives based on specific or compelling indications. Special consideration for starting combination therapy should be made in each patient. Starting drug therapy at a low dose and titrating upward if blood pressure is not controlled is recommended. The benefit of these strategies is to minimize the occurrence of adverse effects while achieving optimal blood pressure control. One caveat for starting at a low dose and then titrating upward is that patients and clinicians must commit to well-timed follow-up so that blood pressure is controlled in a timely manner. Lifestyle modification and risk reduction should be initiated and continued throughout treatment.

Hypertension Treatment Algorithm

Begin or continue lifestyle modifications

↓

Not at goal blood pressure (<140/90 mm Hg)
Lower goals for patients with diabetes or renal disease

↓

Initial Drug Choice
(Unless contraindicated. ACE indicates angiotensin-converting enzyme; ISA, intrinsic sympathomimetic activity. Based on randomized controlled trials.)

Uncomplicated hypertension
Diuretics
Beta-blockers

Specific Indications for the following drugs
ACE inhibitors
Angiotensin II receptor blockers
Alpha-blockers
Alpha-beta-blockers
Beta-blockers
Calcium antagonists
Diuretics

Compelling Indications
Diabetes mellitus (type 1) with proteinuria
• ACE inhibitors
Heart failure
• ACE inhibitors
• Diuretics
Isolated systolic hypertension (older persons)
• Diuretics **preferred**
• Long-acting dihydropyridine calcium antagonists
Myocardial infarction
• Beta-blockers (non-ISA)
• ACE inhibitors (with systolic dysfunction)

• Start with a low dose of a long-acting once-daily drug, and **titrate dose.**
• Low-dose combinations may be appropriate.

↓

Not at goal blood pressure

↓

No response or troublesome side effects

↓

Substitute another drug from a different class.

Inadequate response but well tolerated

↓

Add a second agent from a different class (diuretic if not already used).

↓

Not at goal blood pressure

↓

Continue adding agents from other classes.
Consider referral to a hypertension specialist.

HYPERTENSION *(Continued)*

COMBINATION THERAPY IN THE TREATMENT OF HYPERTENSION

Important concerns in treating hypertension are the efficacy and side effects of therapy. In the past, progressive increases in dosage of a single drug were used to improve blood pressure control. Historically (based on the Joint National Committee [JNC] recommendations), the maximum doses of recommended drugs have decreased from those proposed in earlier JNC reports.

More recently, the concept of combination therapy has begun to gain increasing favor. This is reflected most clearly in the report of the Sixth Joint National Committee on Detection, Evaluation, and Treatment of High Blood Pressure (JNC VI). Specifically, JNC VI endorses the use of low doses of two antihypertensive drugs in fixed-dose combinations as a possible route for initial treatment of hypertension. This recommendation extends earlier JNC V recognition that combining drugs with different modes of action may allow smaller doses of drugs to be used to achieve control, and minimize the potential for dose-dependent side effects.

Combination therapy thus constitutes the use of an additional antihypertensive medication before the first therapeutic agent is necessarily at maximum dose, or the use of two agents in low doses at the onset of antihypertensive treatment. The rationale, background, and experience with combination therapy are nicely reviewed in Kaplan NM and Sever PS, "Combination Therapy: A Key to Comprehensive Patient Care," *Am J Hyperten*, 1997, 10(7 part 2):127S and by Moser M and Black HR, "The Role of Combination Therapy in the Treatment of Hypertension," *Am J Hyperten*, 11:73S-8S).

Fundamental to the combination therapy approach are the following considerations.

- Drugs with different and complementary mechanisms of action may often produce synergistic reductions in blood pressure, classically evident in the use of diuretics and ACE inhibitors.

- Low doses of a single drug are less likely to induce side effects.

- More than 50% of all hypertensive patients will need more than one drug to achieve blood pressure control.

In effect, this therapeutic strategy allows exploitation of the steepest part of the antihypertensive dose response curve, achieving synergistic or additive therapeutic benefit while limiting potential for side effects. Disadvantages include first, the need to take two drugs, often resulting in taking two separate tablets. It is important to ensure that both therapeutic preparations have equivalent durations of action. Second, the cost of separate products may exceed that of increased doses of a single medication.

In mitigation, fixed-dose combinations of antihypertensive preparations are available with recent options, including Lexxel™ (calcium channel blocker and ACE inhibitor), Hyzaar® (angiotensin receptor blocker and hydrochlorothiazide), Capozide® (ACE inhibitor and hydrochlorothiazide), and Ziac™ (beta-blocker and hydrochlorothiazide). These combinations help address cost and convenience issues in combination therapy.

COMPELLING INDICATIONS FOR SPECIFIC THERAPIES

Indication	Drug Therapy
COMPELLING INDICATIONS UNLESS CONTRAINDICATED	
Diabetes mellitus (type I) with proteinuria	ACEI
Heart failure	ACEI, diuretics, beta-blockers (carvedilol, metoprolol XL/CR, bisoprolol, hydralazine + isosorbide dinitrate)
Isolated systolic hypertension (older patients)	Diuretics (preferred), CCB (long-acting)
Myocardial infarction	Beta-blockers (non-ISA), ACEI (with systolic dysfunction)
High-risk patients (CVD plus risk factors)	ACEI (ramipril)
MAY HAVE FAVORABLE EFFECTS ON COMORBID CONDITIONS	
Angina	Beta-blockers, CCB (long-acting)
Atrial tachycardia and fibrillation	Beta-blockers, CCB (non-DHP)
Cyclosporine-induced hypertension (caution with the dose of cyclosporine)	CCB
Diabetes mellitus (types I and II) with proteinuria	ACEI (preferred), CCB
Diabetes mellitus (type II)	Low-dose diuretics (≤25 mg HCTZ)
Dyslipidemia	Alpha-blockers
Essential tremor	Beta-blockers (noncardioselective)
Heart failure	Losartan, candesartan
Hyperthyroidism	Beta-blockers
Migraine	Beta-blockers (noncardioselective), CCB (long-acting) (non-DHP)
Myocardial infarction (non-Q-wave with normal systolic function and no edema)	Diltiazem, verapamil (long-acting)
Osteoporosis	Thiazides
Preoperative hypertension	Beta-blockers
Prostatism (BPH)	Alpha-blockers
Renal insufficiency (caution in renovascular hypertension and creatinine ≥265.2 mmol/L [3 mg/dL])	ACEI
MAY HAVE UNFAVORABLE EFFECTS ON COMORBID CONDITIONS[1]	
Bronchospastic disease	Beta-blockers[2]
Depression	Beta-blockers, central alpha-agonists, reserpine[2]
Diabetes mellitus (types I and II)	Beta-blockers, high-dose diuretics
Dyslipidemia	Beta-blockers (non-ISA), diuretics (high-dose)
Gout	Diuretics
Second or third degree heart block	Beta-blockers,[2] CCB (non-DHP)[2]
Heart failure	Beta-blockers (with high ISA), CCB (except amlodipine, felodipine)
Liver disease	Labetalol hydrochloride, methyldopa[2]
Peripheral vascular disease	Beta-blockers
Pregnancy	ACEI,[2] angiotensin II receptor blockers[2]
Renal insufficiency	Potassium-sparing agents
Renovascular disease	ACEI, angiotensin II receptor blockers

ACEI = angiotensin-converting enzyme inhibitors; BPH = benign prostatic hyperplasia; CCB = calcium antagonists; CVD = cardiovascular disease; DHP = dihydropyridine; HCTZ = hydrochlorothiazide; ISA = intrinsic sympathomimetic activity; MI = myocardial infarction; and non-CS = noncardioselective.

Conditions and drugs are listed in alphabetical order.

[1]These drugs may be used with special monitoring unless contraindicated.

[2]Contraindicated.

HYPERTENSION *(Continued)*

HYPERTENSION AND PREGNANCY

The report of the NHBPEP Working Group on High Blood Pressure in Pregnancy permits continuation of drug therapy in women with chronic hypertension (**except for ACE inhibitors**). In addition, angiotensin II receptor blockers should not be used during pregnancy. In women with chronic hypertension with diastolic levels ≥100 mm Hg (lower when end organ damage or underlying renal disease is present) and in women with acute hypertension when levels are ≥105 mm Hg, the following agents are suggested (see table).

Suggested Drug	Comments
Central alpha-agonists	Methyldopa (C) is the drug of choice recommended by the NHBPEP Working Group.
Beta-blockers	Atenolol (C) and metoprolol (C) appear to be safe and effective in late pregnancy. Labetalol (C) also appears to be effective (alpha- and beta-blockers).
Calcium antagonists	Potential synergism with magnesium sulfate may lead to precipitous hypotension. (C)
ACE inhibitors, angiotensin II receptor blockers	Fetal abnormalities, including death, can be caused, and these drugs **should not** be used in pregnancy. (D)
Diuretics	Diuretics (C) are recommended for chronic hypertension if prescribed before gestation or if patients appear to be salt-sensitive. They are not recommended in pre-eclampsia.
Direct vasodilators	Hydralazine (C) is the parenteral drug of choice based on its long history of safety and efficacy. (C)

Adapted from Sibai and Lindheimer. There are several other antihypertensive drugs for which there are very limited data. The U.S. Food and Drug Administration classifies pregnancy risk as follows: C = adverse effects in animals; no controlled trials in humans; use if risk appears justified; D = positive evidence of fetal risk. ACE = angiotensin-converting enzyme.

HYPERTENSIVE EMERGENCIES AND URGENCIES

General Treatment Principles in the Treatment of Hypertensive Emergencies

Principle	Considerations
Admit the patient to the hospital, preferably in the ICU. Monitor vital signs appropriately.	Establish I.V. access and place patient on a cardiac monitor. Place a femoral intra-arterial line and pulmonary arterial catheter, if indicated, to assess cardiopulmonary function and intravascular volume status.
Perform rapid but thorough history and physical examination.	Determine cause of, or precipitating factors to, hypertensive crisis if possible (remember to obtain a medication history including Rx, OTC, and illicit drugs). Obtain details regarding any prior history of hypertension (severity, duration, treatment), as well as other coexisting illnesses. Assess the extent of hypertensive end organ damage. Determine if a hypertensive urgency or emergency exists.
Determine goal blood pressure based on premorbid level, duration, severity and rapidity of increase of blood pressure, concomitant medical conditions, race, and age.	Acute decreases in blood pressure to normal or subnormal levels during the initial treatment period may reduce perfusion to the brain, heart, and kidneys, and must be avoided except in specific instances (ie, dissecting aortic aneurysm). Gradually establish a normal (or reasonable) blood pressure over the next 1-2 weeks.
Select an appropriate antihypertensive regimen depending on the individual patient and clinical setting.	Initiate a controlled decrease in blood pressure. Avoid concomitant administration of multiple agents that may cause precipitous falls in blood pressure. Select the agent with the best hemodynamic profile based on the primary treatment goal. Avoid diuretics and sodium restriction during the initial treatment period unless there is a clear clinical indication (ie, CHF, pulmonary edema). Avoid sedating antihypertensives in patients with hypertensive encephalopathy, CVA, or other CNS disorders in whom mental status must be monitored. Use caution with direct vasodilating agents that induce reflex tachycardia or increase cardiac output in patients with coronary heart disease, history of angina or myocardial infarction, or dissecting aortic aneurysm. Preferably choose an agent that does not adversely affect glomerular filtration rate or renal blood flow and also agents that have favorable effects on cerebral blood flow and its autoregulation, especially for patients with hypertensive encephalopathy or CVAs. Select the most efficacious agent with the fewest adverse effects based on the underlying cause of the hypertensive crisis and other individual patient factors.
Initiate a chronic antihypertensive regimen after the patient's blood pressure is stabilized	Begin oral antihypertensive therapy once goal blood pressure is achieved before gradually tapering parenteral medications. Select the best oral regimen based on cost, ease of administration, adverse effect profile, and concomitant medical conditions.

Oral Agents Used in the Treatment of Hypertensive Urgencies and Emergencies

Drug	Dose	Onset	Cautions
Captopril[1]	P.O.: 25 mg, repeat as required	15-30 min	Hypotension, renal failure in bilateral renal artery stenosis
Clonidine	P.O.: 0.1-0.2 mg, repeated every hour as needed to a total dose of 0.6 mg	30-60 min	Hypotension, drowsiness, dry mouth
Labetalol	P.O.: 200-400 mg, repeat every 2-3 h	30 min to 2 h	Bronchoconstriction, heart block, orthostatic hypotension

[1]There is no clearly defined clinical advantage in the use of sublingual over oral routes of administration with these agents.

Recommendations for the Use of Intravenous Antihypertensive Drugs in Selected Hypertensive Emergencies

Condition	Agent(s) of Choice	Agent(s) to Avoid or Use With Caution	General Treatment Principles
Hypertensive encephalopathy	Nitroprusside, labetalol, diazoxide	Methyldopa, reserpine	Avoid drugs with CNS-sedating effects
Acute intracranial or subarachnoid hemorrhage	Nicardipine,[1] nitroprusside, trimethaphan	Beta-blockers	Careful titration with a short-acting agent
Cerebral infarction	Nicardipine,[1] nitroprusside, labetalol, trimethaphan	Beta-blockers, minoxidil, diazoxide	Careful titration with a short-acting agent. Avoid agents that may decrease cerebral blood flow.
Head trauma	Esmolol, labetalol	Methyldopa, reserpine, nitroprusside, nitroglycerin, hydralazine	Avoid drugs with CNS-sedating effects, or those that may increase intracranial pressure
Acute myocardial infarction, myocardial ischemia	Nitroglycerin, nicardipine[1] (calcium channel blockers), labetalol	Hydralazine, diazoxide, minoxidil	Avoid drugs which cause reflex tachycardia and increased myocardial oxygen consumption
Acute pulmonary edema	Nitroprusside, nitroglycerin, loop diuretics	Beta-blockers (labetalol), minoxidil, methyldopa	Avoid drugs which may cause sodium and water retention and edema exacerbation
Renal dysfunction	Hydralazine, calcium channel blockers	Nitroprusside, ACE inhibitors, beta-blockers (labetalol)	Avoid drugs with increased toxicity in renal failure and those that may cause decreased renal blood flow.
Eclampsia	Hydralazine, labetalol, nitroprusside[2]	Trimethaphan, diuretics, diazoxide (diazoxide may cause cessation of labor)	Avoid drugs that may cause adverse fetal effects, compromise placental circulation, or decrease cardiac output.
Pheochromocytoma	Phentolamine, nitroprusside, beta-blockers (eg, esmolol) only after alpha blockade (phentolamine)	Beta-blockers in the absence of alpha blockade, methyldopa, minoxidil	Use drugs of proven efficacy and specificity. Unopposed beta blockade may exacerbate hypertension.
Dissecting aortic aneurysm	Nitroprusside and beta blockade, trimethaphan	Hydralazine, diazoxide, minoxidil	Avoid drugs which may increase cardiac output.
Postoperative hypertension	Nitroprusside, nicardipine,[1] labetalol	Trimethaphan	Avoid drugs which may exacerbate postoperative ileus.

[1]The use of nicardipine in these situations is by the recommendation of the author based on a review of the literature.

[2]Reserve nitroprusside for eclamptic patients with life-threatening hypertension unresponsive to other agents due to the potential risk to the fetus (cyanide and thiocyanate metabolites may cross the placenta).

HYPERTENSION *(Continued)*

Selected Intravenous Agents for Hypertensive Emergencies

Drug	Dose[1]	Onset of Action	Duration of Action	Adverse Effects[2]	Special Indications
Vasodilators					
Sodium nitroprusside	0.25-10 mcg/kg/min as I.V. infusion[3] (max: 10 min only)	Immediate	1-2 min	Nausea, vomiting, muscle twitching, sweating, thiocyanate and cyanide intoxication	Most hypertensive emergencies; caution with high intracranial pressure or azotemia
Nicardipine hydrochloride	5-15 mg/h I.V.	5-10 min	1-4 h	Tachycardia, headache, flushing, local phlebitis	Most hypertensive emergencies except acute heart failure; caution with coronary ischemia
Fenoldopam mesylate	0.1-0.3 mcg/kg/min I.V. infusion	<5 min	30 min	Tachycardia, headache, nausea, flushing	Most hypertensive emergencies; caution with glaucoma
Nitroglycerin	5-100 mcg/min as I.V. infusion[3]	2-5 min	3-5 min	Headache, vomiting, methemoglobinemia, tolerance with prolonged use	Coronary ischemia
Enalaprilat	1.25-5 mg every 6 hours I.V.	15-30 min	6 h	Precipitous fall in pressure in high-renin states; response variable	Acute left ventricular failure; avoid in acute myocardial infarction
Hydralazine hydrochloride	10-20 mg I.V. 10-50 mg I.M.	10-20 min 20-30 min	3-8 h	Tachycardia, flushing, headache, vomiting, aggravation of angina	Eclampsia
Diazoxide	50-100 mg I.V. bolus repeated, or 15-30 mg/min infusion	2-4 min	6-12 h	Nausea, flushing, tachycardia, chest pain	Now obsolete; when no intensive monitoring available
Adrenergic Inhibitors					
Labetalol hydrochloride	20-80 mg I.V. bolus every 10 min; 0.5-2 mg/min I.V. infusion	5-10 min	3-6 h	Vomiting, scalp tingling, burning in throat, dizziness, nausea, heart block, orthostatic hypotension	Most hypertensive emergencies except acute heart failure
Esmolol hydrochloride	250-500 mcg/kg/min for 1 min, then 50-100 mcg/kg/min for 4 min; may repeat	1-2 min	10-20 min	Hypotension, nausea	Aortic dissection, perioperative
Phentolamine	5-15 mg I.V.	1-2 min	3-10 min	Tachycardia, flushing, headache	Catecholamine excess

[1]These doses may vary from those in the *Physicians' Desk Reference* (51st edition).

[2]Hypotension may occur with all agents.

[3]Require special delivery system.

Resources

Guidelines

1999 World Health Organization-International Society of Hypertension Guidelines for the Management of Hypertension. Guidelines Subcommittee, *J Hypertens*, 1999, 17:151-83.

National High Blood Pressure Education Program Working Group on Hypertension Control in Children and Adolescents. Update on the 1987 Task Force Report on High Blood Pressure in Children and Adolescents: A Working Group Report From the National High Blood Pressure Education Program, *Pediatrics*, 1996, 98(4 Pt 1):649-58.

National High Blood Pressure Education Program Working Group. 1995 Update of the Working Group Reports on Chronic Renal Failure and Renovascular Hypertension, *Arch Intern Med*, 1996, 156:1938-47.

"The Sixth Report of the National Committee on Detection, Evaluation, and Treatment of High Blood Pressure (JNC-VI)," *Arch Intern Med*, 1997, 157:2413-46.

Others

Appel LJ, Moore TJ, Obarzanek E, et al, "A Clinical Trial of the Effect of Dietary Patterns on Blood Pressure. The DASH Collaborative Research Group," *N Engl J Med*, 1997, 336:1117-24.

Epstein M and Bakris G, "Newer Approaches to Antihypertensive Therapy: Use of Fixed-Dose Combination Therapy," *Arch Intern Med*, 1996, 156:1969-78.

Estacio RO and Schrier RW, "Antihypertensive Therapy in Type II Diabetes: Implications of the Appropriate Blood Pressure Control in Diabetes (ABCD) Trial," *Am J Cardiol*, 1998, 82:9R-14R.

Flack JM, Neaton J, Grimm RJ, et al, "Blood Pressure and Mortality Among Men With Prior Myocardial Infarction. The Multiple Risk Factor Intervention Trial Research Group," *Circulation*, 1995, 92:2437-45.

Frishman WH, Bryzinski BS, Coulson LR, et al, "A Multifactorial Trial Design to Assess Combination Therapy in Hypertension: Treatment With Bisoprolol and Hydrochlorothiazide," *Arch Intern Med*, 1994, 154:1461-8.

Furberg CD, Psaty BM, and Meyer JV, "Nifedipine: Dose-Related Increase in Mortality in Patients With Coronary Heart Disease," *Circulation*, 1995, 92:1326-31.

Glynn RJ, Brock DB, Harris T, et al, "Use of Antihypertensive Drugs and Trends in Blood Pressure in the Elderly," *Arch Intern Med*, 1995, 155:1855-60.

Gradman AH, Cutler NR, Davis PJ, et al, "Combined Enalapril and Felodipine Extended Release (ER) for Systemic Hypertension. The Enalapril-Felodipine ER Factorial Study Group," *Am J Cardiol*, 1997, 79:431-5.

Grim RH Jr, Flack JM, Grandits GA, et al, "Long-Term Effects on Plasma Lipids of Diet and Drugs to Treat Hypertension. The Treatment of Mild Hypertension Study (TOMHS) Research Group," *JAMA*, 1996, 275:1549-56.

Grim RH Jr, Grandits GA, Cutler JA, et al, "Relationships of Quality-of-Life Measures to Long-Term Lifestyle and Drug Treatment in the Treatment of Mild Hypertension Study. The TOMHS Research Group," *Arch Intern Med*, 1997, 157:638-48.

Grossman E, Messerli FH, Grodzicki T, et al, "Should a Moratorium Be Placed on Sublingual Nifedipine Capsules Given for Hypertensive Emergencies and Pseudoemergencies?" *JAMA*, 1996, 276:1328-31.

Hansson L, Zanchetti A, Carruthers SG, et al, "Effects of Intensive Blood Pressure Lowering and Low-Dose Aspirin in Patients With Hypertension: Principal Results of the Hypertension Optimal Treatment (HOT) Randomized Trial. HOT Study Group," *Lancet*, 1998, 351:1755-62.

Kaplan NM and Gifford RW Jr, "Choice of Initial Therapy for Hypertension," *JAMA*, 1996, 275:1577-80.

Kasiske BL, Ma JZ, Kalil RSN, et al, "Effects of Antihypertensive Therapy in Serum Lipids," *Ann Intern Med*, 1995, 122:133-41.

Kostis JB, Davis BR, Cutler J, et al, "Prevention of Heart Failure by Antihypertensive Drug Treatment in Older Persons With Isolated Systolic Hypertension. SHEP Cooperative Research Group," *JAMA*, 1997, 278:212-6.

Lazarus JM, Bourgoignie JJ, Buckalew VM, et al, "Achievement and Safety of a Low Blood Pressure Goal in Chronic Renal Disease: The Modification of Diet in Renal Disease Study Group," *Hypertension*, 1997, 29:641-50.

Lindheimer MD, "Hypertension in Pregnancy," *Hypertension*, 1993, 22:127-37.

Materson BJ, Reda DJ, Cushman WC, et al, "Single-Drug Therapy for Hypertension in Men: A Comparison of Six Antihypertensive Agents With Placebo. The Department of Veterans Affairs Cooperative Study Group on Antihypertensive Agents," *N Engl J Med*, 1993, 328:914-21.

Miller NH, Hill M, Kottke T, et al, "The Multi-Level Compliance Challenge: Recommendations for a Call to Action; A Statement for Healthcare Professionals," *Circulation*, 1997, 95:1085-90.

Neaton JD and Wentworth D, "Serum Cholesterol, Blood Pressure, Cigarette Smoking, and Death From Coronary Heart Disease: Overall Findings and Differences by Age for 316,099 White Men. The Multiple Risk Factor Intervention Trial Research Group," *Arch Intern Med*, 1992, 152:56-64.

Neaton JD, Grim RH, Prineas RJ, et al, "Treatment of Mild Hypertension Study (TOHMS). Final Results," *JAMA*, 1993, 270:721-31.

Oparil S, Levine JH, Zuschke CA, et al, "Effects of Candesartan Cilexetil in Patients With Severe Systemic Hypertension," *Am J Cardiol*, 1999, 84:289-93.

Perloff D, Grim C, Flack J, et al, "Human Blood Pressure Determination by Sphygmomanometry," *Circulation*, 1993, 88:2460-7.

Perry HM Jr, Bingham S, Horney A, et al, "Antihypertensive Efficacy of Treatment Regimens Used in Veterans Administration Hypertension Clinics. Department of Veterans Affairs Cooperative Study Group on Antihypertensive Agents," *Hypertension*, 1998, 31:771-9.

Preston RA, Materson BJ, Reda DJ, et al, "Age-Race Subgroup Compared With Renin Profile as Predictors of Blood Pressure Response to Antihypertensive Therapy," *JAMA*, 1998, 280:1168-72.

Psaty BM, Smith NL, Siscovick DS, et al, "Health Outcomes Associated With Antihypertensive Therapies Used as First-Line Agents. A Systemic Review and Meta-analysis," *JAMA*, 1997, 277:739-45.

HYPERTENSION (Continued)

Radevski IV, Valtchanova SP, Candy GP, et al, "Comparison of Acebutolol With and Without Hydrochlorothiazide Versus Carvedilol With and Without Hydrochlorothiazide in Black Patients With Mild to Moderate Systemic Hypertension," *Am J Cardiol*, 1999, 84(1):70-5.

Setaro JF and Black HR, "Refractory Hypertension," *N Engl J Med*, 1992, 327:543-7.

SHEP Cooperative Research Group, "Prevention of Stroke by Antihypertensive Drug Treatment in Older Persons With Isolated Systolic Hypertension: Final Results of the Systolic Hypertension in the Elderly Program (SHEP)," *JAMA*, 1991, 265:3255-64.

Sibai BM, "Treatment of Hypertension in Pregnant Women," *N Engl J Med*, 1996, 335:257-65.

Sowers JR, "Comorbidity of Hypertension and Diabetes: The Fosinopril Versus Amlodipine Cardiovascular Events Trial," *Am J Cardiol*, 1998, 82:15R-19R.

Sternberg H, Rosenthal T, Shamiss A, et al, "Altered Circadian Rhythm of Blood Pressure in Shift Workers," *J Hum Hypertens*, 1995, 9:349-53.

"The Hypertension Prevention Trial: Three-Year Effects of Dietary Changes on Blood Pressure. Hypertension Prevention Trial Research Group," *Arch Intern Med*, 1990, 150:153-62.

Trials of Hypertension Prevention Collaborative Research Group, "Effects of Weight Loss and Sodium Reduction Intervention on Blood Pressure and Hypertension Incidence in Overweight People With High-Normal Blood Pressure: The Trials of Hypertension Prevention, Phase II," *Arch Intern Med*, 1997, 157:657-67.

Tuomilehto J, Rastenyte D, Birkenhager WH, et al, "Effects of Calcium Channel Blockade in Older Patients With Diabetes and Systolic Hypertension," *N Engl J Med*, 1999, 340:677-84.

Veelken R and Schmieder RE, "Overview of Alpha-1 Adrenoceptor Antagonism and Recent Advances in Hypertensive Therapy," *Am J Hypertens*, 1996, 9:139S-49S.

White WB, Black HR, Weber MA, et al, "Comparison of Effects of Controlled Onset Extended Release Verapamil at Bedtime and Nifedipine Gastrointestinal Therapeutic System on Arising on Early Morning Blood Pressure, Heart Rate, and the Heart Rate-Blood Pressure Product," *Am J Cardiol*, 1998, 81:424-31.

OBESITY TREATMENT GUIDELINES FOR ADULTS

Summary of Clinical Practice Guidelines

National Heart, Lung, and Blood Institute, June 1998

Note: Weight loss treatment for children and adolescents are not covered by these guidelines.

ASSESSMENT

Assessment of weight involves evaluating body mass index, waist circumference, and the patient's risk factors

A. Body mass Index (BMI)

1. BMI should be calculated for all adults (see table). Those with normal BMI should be reassessed in 2 years. A very muscular person may have a high BMI without the additional health risks.

2. Overweight is defined as a BMI of 25-29.9 kg/m^2

3. Obesity is defined as a BMI of ≥30 kg/m^2

B. Abdominal Fat

1. Excess abdominal fat, not proportional to total body fat, is an independent predictor for risk and morbidity

2. Waist circumference for men >40 inches or women >35 inches is an increased risk for those with a BMI of 25-34.9

C. Risk Factors

1. Coronary heart disease or other atherosclerotic diseases, type 2 diabetes, and sleep apnea are factors associated with a very high risk of developing disease complications and mortality

2. Other obesity-associated diseases: Gynecological abnormalities, osteoarthritis, gallstones, stress incontinence

3. Cardiovascular risk factors: Cigarette smoking, hypertension, high-risk LDL-cholesterol, low HDL-cholesterol, impaired fasting glucose, family history of premature CHD

4. Other risk factors: Physical inactivity, high serum triglycerides

Weight loss is recommended for those who are obese and for those who are classified as overweight or have a high waist circumference and two or more risk factors

Body Mass Index (BMI), kg/m^2
Height (feet, inches)

Weight (lb)	5'0"	5'3"	5'6"	5'9"	6'0"	6'3"
140	27	25	23	21	19	18
150	29	27	24	22	20	19
160	31	28	26	24	22	20
170	33	30	28	25	23	21
180	35	32	29	27	25	23
190	37	34	31	28	26	24
200	39	36	32	30	27	25
210	41	37	34	31	29	26
220	43	39	36	33	30	28
230	45	41	37	34	31	29
240	47	43	39	36	33	30
250	49	44	40	37	34	31

OBESITY TREATMENT GUIDELINES FOR ADULTS *(Continued)*

TREATMENT

Patients who are overweight or obese, but are not candidates for weight loss or do not wish to lose weight, should be counseled to avoid further weight gain

A. Goals of Treatment

1. Prevent further weight gain

2. Reduce body weight. The initial goal is to reduce body weight by 10% from baseline over the suggested time period of 6 months

3. Maintain a lower body weight, long term

B. Nonpharmacologic treatment should include:

1. An individually-planned diet which includes a decrease in fat as well as total calories

2. An increase in physical activity. Physical activity should be gradually increased to a goal of 30 minutes per day of moderate-intensity activity

3. Behavior therapy, which should include tools to help overcome individual barriers to weight loss

    Nonpharmacologic treatment should be tried for 6 months before starting physician-prescribed drug therapy

C. Drug Therapy

    In select patients with BMI ≥30, or BMI ≥27 with 2 or more risk factors, who did not lose weight or maintain weight loss, drug therapy can be started along with dietary therapy and physical activity

D. Surgery

    Patients with severe clinical obesity, BMI ≥40 or BMI ≥35 with coexisting conditions, can be considered for weight loss surgery when other methods have failed. Lifelong surveillance after surgery is necessary

Medications for the Treatment of Obesity

Generic (Trade) Name	Therapeutic Category / Mechanism of Action	Usual Adult Dosage
Orlistat (Xenical®)	Lipase inhibitor; a reversible inhibitor of gastric and pancreatic lipases thus inhibiting absorption of dietary fats by 30% (at doses of 120 mg 3 times/day)	120 mg 3 times/day with each main meal containing fat (during or up to 1 hour after the meal); omit dose if meal is occasionally missed or contains no fat.
Amphetamine	The amphetamines are noncatecholamine sympathomimetic amines with CNS stimulant activity. The anorexigenic effect is probably secondary to the CNS-stimulating effect; the site of action is probably the hypothalamic feeding center.	Long-acting capsule: 10 or 15 mg/day, up to 30 mg/day; Immediate release tablets: 5-30 mg/day in divided doses
Benzphetamine (Didrex®)	Anorexiant; noncatechol sympathomimetic amines with pharmacologic actions similar to ephedrine; anorexigenic effect is probably secondary to the CNS-stimulating effect; the site of action is probably the hypothalamic feeding center	25-50 mg 2-3 times/day, preferably twice daily (midmorning and midafternoon); maximum dose: 50 mg 3 times/day
Diethylpropion (Tenuate®; Tenuate® Dospan®)	Anorexiant; pharmacological and chemical properties similar to those of amphetamines. The mechanism of action of diethylpropion in reducing appetite appears to be secondary to CNS effects, specifically stimulation of the hypothalamus to release catecholamines into the central nervous system; anorexiant effects are mediated via norepinephrine and dopamine metabolism. An increase in physical activity and metabolic effects (inhibition of lipogenesis and enhancement of lipolysis) may also contribute to weight loss.	Tablet: 25 mg 3 times/day before meals or food Tablet, controlled release: 75 mg at midmorning

Medications for the Treatment of Obesity *(continued)*

Generic (Trade) Name	Therapeutic Category / Mechanism of Action	Usual Adult Dosage
Mazindol (Mazanor®, Sanorex®)	Anorexiant; an isoindole with pharmacologic activity similar to amphetamine; produces CNS stimulation in humans and animals and appears to work primarily in the limbic system	Initial dose: 1 mg once daily and adjust to patient response; usual dose: 1 mg 3 times/day, 1 hour before meals, or 2 mg once daily, 1 hour before lunch; take with meals to avoid GI discomfort
Methamphetamine (Desoxyn®)	A sympathomimetic amine related to ephedrine and amphetamine with CNS stimulant activity	5 mg, 30 minutes before each meal; long-acting formulation: 10-15 mg in morning; treatment duration should not exceed a few weeks
Phentermine (Adipex-P®, Fastin®, Ionamin®, Zantryl®)	Anorexiant; structurally similar to dextroamphetamine and is comparable to dextroamphetamine as an appetite suppressant, but is generally associated with a lower incidence and severity of CNS side effects. Stimulates the hypothalamus to result in decreased appetite; anorexiant effects are most likely mediated via norepinephrine and dopamine metabolism. However, other CNS effects or metabolic effects may be involved.	8 mg 3 times/day 30 minutes before meals or food or 15-37.5 mg/day before breakfast or 10-14 hours before retiring
Sibutramine (Meridia™)	Anorexiant; blocks the neuronal uptake of norepinephrine and, to a lesser extent, serotonin and dopamine	Initial: 10 mg once daily; after 4 weeks may titrate up to 15 mg once daily as needed and tolerated

MANAGEMENT OF OVERDOSAGES

Antidote	Poison/Drug	Indications	Dosage	Comments
Acetylcysteine (Mucomyst®)	Acetaminophen	Unknown quantity ingested and <24 hours have elapsed since the time of ingestion or unable to obtain serum acetaminophen levels within 12 hours of ingestion. >7.5 g acetaminophen acutely ingested. Serum acetaminophen level >140 mcg/mL at 4 hours postingestion. Ingested dose >140 mg/kg.	Dilute to 5% solutions with carbonated beverage, fruit juice, or water and administer orally. **Loading:** 140 mg/kg for 1 dose **Maintenance:** 70 mg/kg for 17 doses, starting 4 hours after the loading dose and given every 4 hours	SGOT, SGPT, bilirubin, prothrombin time, creatinine, BUN, blood sugar, and electrolytes should be obtained daily if a toxic serum acetaminophen level has been determined. **Note:** Activated charcoal has been shown to absorb acetylcysteine *in vitro* and may do so in patients. Serum acetaminophen levels may not peak until 4 hours postingestion, and therefore, serum levels should not be drawn earlier.
Amyl nitrate, sodium nitrate, sodium thiosulfate (cyanide antidote package)	Cyanide	Begin treatment at the first sign of toxicity if exposure is known or strongly expected.	Break ampul of amyl nitrate and allow patient to inhale for 15 seconds, then take away for 15 seconds. Use a fresh ampul every 3 minutes. Continue until injection of sodium nitrate (3% solution) 300 mg (0.15-0.33 mL/kg over 5 minutes in pediatric patients) can be injected at 2.5-5 mL/min. Then immediately inject 12.5 g 25% sodium thiosulfate, slow I.V. (1.65 mL/kg in children).	If symptoms return, treatment may be repeated at half the normal dosages. For pediatric dosing see package insert. Do **not** use methylene blue to reduce elevated methemoglobin. Oxygen therapy may be useful when combined with sodium thiosulfate therapy.
Antivenin (*Crotalidae*) polyvalent (equine origin)	Pit viper bites (rattlesnakes, cotton-mouths, copperheads)	Mild, moderate, or severe symptoms and history of envenomation by a pit viper **Mild:** Local swelling (progressive), pain, no systemic systems **Moderate:** Ecchymosis and swelling beyond the bite site, some systemic symptoms and/or lab changes **Severe:** Profound edema involving entire extremity, cyanosis, serious systemic involvement, significant lab changes	**Mild:** 3-5 vials of antivenin in 250-500 mL NS **Moderate:** 6-10 vials of antivenin in 500 mL NS **Severe:** Minimum of 10 vials in 500-1000 mL NS Administer over 4-6 hours. Additional antivenin should be given on the basis of clinical response and continuing assessment of severity of the poisoning.	Draw blood for type and crossmatch, hematocrit, BUN, electrolytes, CBC, platelets, coagulation profile. Do **not** administer heparin for possible allergic reaction. A tetanus shot should also be given.

Antidote	Poison/Drug	Indications	Dosage	Comments
Atropine	Organophosphate and carbamate insecticides, mushrooms containing muscarine (inocybe or clitocybe)	Myoclonic seizures, severe hallucinations, weakness, arrhythmias, excessive salivation, involuntary urination, and defecation	**Children:** I.V.: 0.05 mg/kg **Adults:** I.V.: 1-2 mg Repeat dosage every 10 minutes until patient is atropinized (normal pulse, dilated pupils, absence of rales, dry mouth)	Caution should be used in patients with narrow-angle glaucoma, cardiovascular disease, or pregnancy. Plasma and/or erythrocyte cholinesterase levels will be depressed from normal. Atropine should only be used when indicated; otherwise, use may result in anticholinergic poisoning. For organophosphate poisoning, large doses of atropine may be required.
Calcium EDTA (calcium disodium versenate)	Lead	Symptomatic patients or asymptomatic children with blood levels >50 mcg/dL	50-75 mg/kg/day deep I.M. or slow I.V. infusion in 3-6 divided doses for up to 5 days	If urine flow is not established, hemodialysis must accompany calcium EDTA dosing. In most cases, the I.M. route is preferred.
Calcium gluconate	Hydrofluoric acid (HF), magnesium	Calcium gluconate gel 2.5% for dermal exposures of HF <20% concentration. S.C. injections of calcium gluconate for dermal exposures of HF in >20% concentration or failure to respond to calcium gluconate gel.	Massage 2.5% gel into exposed area for 15 minutes. Infiltrate each square centimeter of exposed area with 0.5 mL of 10% calcium gluconate S.C. using a 30-gauge needle. 1 mL/kg I.V. of a 10% solution for magnesium toxicity (intra-arterial injection).	Injections of calcium gluconate should not be used in digital area. With exposures to dilute concentrations of HF, symptoms may take several hours to develop. Calcium gluconate gel is not currently available. Contact your regional poison control center for compounding instructions.
Deferoxamine (Desferal®)	Iron	Serum iron >350 mcg/dL. Inability to obtain serum iron in a reasonable time and patient is symptomatic.	**Mild symptoms:** I.M.: 10 mg/kg up to 1 g every 8 hours **Severe symptoms:** I.V.: 10-15 mg/kg/hour not to exceed 6 g in 24 hours; rates up to 35 mg/kg have been given.	Passing of vin rose-colored urine indicates free iron was present. Therapy should be discontinued when urine returns to normal color. Monitor for hypotension, especially when giving deferoxamine I.V.
Digoxin immune fab (ovine), (Digibind®)	Digoxin, digitoxin, oleander, foxglove, lily-of-the-valley (?), red squill (?)	Life-threatening cardiac arrhythmias, progressive bradyarrhythmias, second or third degree heart block unresponsive to atropine, serum digoxin level >5 ng/mL, potassium levels >5 mEq/L, or ingestion >10 mg in adults (or 4 mg in children).	Multiply serum digoxin concentration at steady-state level by 5.6 and multiply the result by the patient's weight in kilograms, divide this by 1000 and divide the result by 0.6. This gives the dose in number of vials to use. For other dosing methods, see package insert.	Monitor potassium levels, continuous EKG. **Note:** Digibind® interferes with serum digoxin/digitoxin levels.

MANAGEMENT OF OVERDOSAGES (Continued)

Antidote	Poison/Drug	Indications	Dosage	Comments
Dimercaprol (BAL in oil)	Arsenic, lead, mercury, gold, trivalent antimony, methyl bromide, methyl iodide	Any symptoms due to arsenic exposure. All patients with symptoms or asymptomatic children with blood levels >70 mcg/dL. Any symptoms due to mercury and patient unable to take D-penicillamine.	3-5 mg/kg/dose deep I.M. every 4 hours until GI symptoms subside and patient switched to D-penicillamine. 3-5 mg/kg/dose deep I.M. every 4 hours for 2 days then every 4-12 hours for up to 7 additional days. 3-5 mg/kg/dose deep I.M. every 4 hours for 48 hours, then 3 mg/kg/dose every 6 hours, then 3 mg/kg/dose every 12 hours for 7 more days.	Patients receiving dimercaprol should be monitored for hypertension, tachycardia, hyperpyrexia, and urticaria. Used in conjunction with calcium EDTA in lead poisoning.
Ethanol	Ethylene glycol or methanol	Ethylene glycol or methanol blood levels >20 mg/dL. Blood levels not readily available and suspected ingestion of toxic amounts. Any symptomatic patient with a history of ethylene glycol or methanol ingestion.	**Loading dose:** I.V.: 7.5-10 mL/kg 10% ethanol in D_5W over 1 hour. **Maintenance dose:** I.V.: 1.4 mL/kg/hour of 10% ethanol in D_5W. Maintain blood ethanol level of 100-200 mg/dL.	Monitor blood glucose, especially in children, as ethanol may cause hypoglycemia. Do not use 5% ethanol in D_5W as excessive amounts of fluid would be required to maintain adequate ethanol blood levels. If dialysis is performed, adjustment of ethanol dosing is required.
Flumazenil (Romazicon®)	Benzodiazepine	As adjunct to conventional management/diagnosis of benzodiazepine overdose.	I.V.: 0.2 mg over 30 seconds; wait another 30 seconds, and then give an additional 0.3 mg over 30 seconds. Additional doses of 0.5 mg over 30 seconds at 1-minute intervals up to a cumulative dose of 3 mg.	Onset of reversal usually within 1-2 minutes. Contraindicated in patients with epilepsy, increased intracranial pressure, or coingestion of seizuregenic agents (ie, cyclic antidepressant).
Glucagon	Propranolol: Hypoglycemic agents	Propranolol-induced cardiac dysfunction. Treatment of hypoglycemia.	S.C., I.M., or I.V.: 0.5-1 mg. May repeat after 15 minutes.	Requires liver glycogen stores for hyperglycemic response. Intravenous glucose must also be given in treatment of hypoglycemia.
Leucovorin (citrovorum factor, folinic acid)	Methotrexate, trimethoprim, pyrimethamine, methanol, trimetrexate	Methotrexate-induced bone marrow depression (methotrexate serum level >1 x 10^{-5} mmol/L); may also be useful in pyrimethamine-trimethoprim bone marrow depression	Dose should be equal to or greater than the dose of methotrexate ingested. Usually 10-100 mg/m^2 is given I.V. or orally every 6 hours for 72 hours.	Most effective if given within 1 hour after exposure. May not be effective to prevent liver toxicity. Monitor methotrexate levels. May enhance the toxicity of fluorouracil.
Methylene blue	Methemoglobin inducers (ie, nitrites, phenazopyridine)	Cyanosis. Methemoglobin level >30% in an asymptomatic patient	I.V.: 1-2 mg/kg (0.1-0.2 mL/kg) per dose over 2-3 minutes. May repeat doses as needed clinically. Injection can be given as 1% solution or diluted in normal saline.	Treatment can result in falsely elevated methemoglobin levels when measured by a co-oximeter. Large doses (>15 mg/kg) may cause hemolysis.
Naloxone (Narcan®)	Opiates (eg, heroin, morphine, codeine)	Coma or respiratory depression from unknown cause or from opiate overdose	Give 0.4-2.0 mg I.V. bolus. Doses may be repeated if there is no response, up to 10 mg.	For prolonged intoxication, a continuous infusion may be used.

Antidote	Poison/Drug	Indications	Dosage	Comments
D-penicillamine (Cuprimine®)	Arsenic, lead, mercury	Following BAL therapy in symptomatic acutely poisoned patients. Asymptomatic patients with excess lead burden. Patient symptomatic from mercury exposure or excessive levels	100 mg/kg/day up to 2 g in 4 divided doses for 5 days. 1-2 g/day in 4 divided doses for 5 days. **Children:** 100 mg/kg/day up to 1 g/day in 4 divided doses. Given for 3-10 days. **Adults:** P.O.: 250 mg 4 times/day	Possible contraindication for patients with penicillin allergy. Monitor heavy metal levels daily in severely poisoned patients. Monitor CBC and renal function in patients receiving chronic D-penicillamine therapy. Dosages given are for short-term acute therapy only.
Physostigmine salicylate (Antilirium®)	Atropine and anticholinergic agents, cyclic antidepressants, intrathecal baclofen	Myoclonic seizures, severe arrhythmias. Refractory seizures or arrhythmias unresponsive to conventional therapies	**Children:** Slow I.V. push: 0.5 mg. Repeat as required for life-threatening symptoms. **Adults:** Slow I.V. push: 0.5-2 mg. Same as above	Dramatic reversal of anticholinergic symptoms after I.V. use. Should not be used just to keep patient awake. **Contraindications:** Asthma, gangrene; physostigmine use in cyclic antidepressant-induced cardiac toxicity it controversial. **Extreme caution** is advised — should be considered only in the presence of life-threatening anticholinergic symptoms.
Pralidoxime (2-PAM, Protopam®)	Organophosphate, insecticides, tacrine	An adjunct to atropine therapy for treatment of profound muscle weakness, respiratory depression, muscle twitching	**Children:** 25-50 mg/kg in 250 mL saline over 30 minutes. **Adults:** I.V.: 2 g at 0.5 g/minute or infused in 250 mL NS over 30 minutes	Most effective when used in initial 24-36 hours after the exposure. Dosage may be repeated in 1 hour followed by every 8 hours if indicated.
Phytonadione (vitamin K₁)	Coumarin derivatives, indandione derivatives	Large acute ingestion of warfarin rodenticides; chronic exposure or greater than normal prothrombin time	**Children:** I.M.: 1-5 mg. With severe toxicity, vitamin K₁ may be given I.V. **Adults:** I.M.: 10 mg	Vitamin K therapy is relatively contraindicated for patients with prosthetic heart valves unless toxicity is life-threatening.
Protamine sulfate	Heparin	Severe hemorrhage	Maximum rate of 5 mg/minute up to a total dose of 200 mg in 2 hours. 1 mg of protamine neutralizes 90 units of beef lung heparin or 115 units of pork intestinal heparin.	Monitor partial thromboplastin time or activated coagulation time. Effect may be immediate and can last for 2 hours. Monitor for hypotension.
Pyridoxine (vitamin B₆)	Isoniazid monomethyl-hydrazine-containing mushrooms (Gyromitra); acrylamide, hydrazine	Unknown overdose or ingested isoniazid (INH) amount >80 mg/kg	I.V. pyridoxine in the amount of INH ingested or 5 g if amount is unknown given over 30-60 minutes.	Cumulative dose of pyridoxine is arbitrarily limited to 40 g in adults and 20 g in children.
Succimer (Chemet®)	Lead, arsenic, mercury	Asymptomatic children with venous blood lead 45-69 mcg/dL. Not FDA approved for adult lead exposure or other metals.	P.O.: 10 mg/kg or 350 mg/m² every 8 hours for 5 days. Reduce to 10 mg/kg or 350 mg/m² every 12 hours for an additional 2 weeks.	Monitor liver function; emits "rotten egg" sulfur odor.

From Rush Poison Control Center, Rush-Presbyterian-St Luke's Medical Center, Chicago, IL 60612.

SALICYLATES

Toxic Symptoms	Treatment
Overdose	Induce emesis with ipecac, and/or lavage with saline, followed with activated charcoal
Dehydration	I.V. fluids with KCl (no D_5W only)
Metabolic acidosis (must be treated)	Sodium bicarbonate
Hyperthermia	Cooling blankets or sponge baths
Coagulopathy/hemorrhage	Vitamin K I.V.
Hypoglycemia (with coma, seizures, or change in mental status)	Dextrose 25 g I.V.
Seizures	Diazepam 5-10 mg I.V.

TOXICOLOGY INFORMATION

Initial Stabilization of the Patients

The recommended treatment plan for the poisoned patient is not unlike general treatment plans taught in advanced cardiac life support (ACLS) or advanced trauma life support (ATLS) courses. In this manner, the initial approach to the poisoned patient should be essentially similar in every case, irrespective of the toxin ingested, just as the initial approach to the trauma patient is the same irrespective of the mechanism of injury. This approach, which can be termed as routine poison management, essentially includes the following aspects.

- Stabilization: ABCs (airway, breathing, circulation; administration of glucose, thiamine, oxygen, and naloxone
- History, physical examination leading toward the identification of class of toxin (toxidrome recognition)
- Prevention of absorption (decontamination)
- Specific antidote, if available
- Removal of absorbed toxin (enhancing excretion)
- Support and monitoring for adverse effects

Drug	Effect	Comment
25-50 g **dextrose** ($D_{50}W$) intravenously to reverse the effects of drug-induced hypoglycemia (adult) 1 mL/kg $D_{50}W$ diluted 1:1 (child)	This can be especially effective in patients with limited glycogen stores (ie, neonates and patients with cirrhosis)	Extravasation into the extremity of this hyperosmolar solution can cause Volkmann's contractures
50-100 mg intravenous **thiamine**	Prevent Wernicke's encephalopathy	A water-soluble vitamin with low toxicity; rare anaphylactoid reactions have been reported
Initial dosage of **naloxone** should be 2 mg in adult patients preferably by the intravenous route, although intramuscular, subcutaneous, intralingual, and endotracheal routes may also be utilized. Pediatric dose is 0.1 mg/kg from birth until 5 years of age	Specific opioid antagonist without any agent properties	It should be noted that some semisynthetic opiates (such as meperidine or propoxyphene) may require higher initial doses for reversal, so that a total dose of 6-10 mg is not unusual for the adults. If the patient responds to a bolus dose and then relapses to a lethargic or comatose state, a naloxone drip can be considered. This can be accomplished by administering two-thirds of the bolus dose that revives the patient per hour or injecting 4 mg naloxone in 1 L crystalloid solution and administering at a rate of 100 mL/hour 0.4 mg/hour)
Oxygen, utilized in 100% concentration	Useful for carbon monoxide, hydrogen, sulfide, and asphyxiants	While oxygen is antidotal for carbon monoxide intoxication, the only relative toxic contraindication is in paraquat intoxication (in that it can promote pulmonary fibrosis)
Flumazenil	Benzodiazepine antagonist	Not routinely recommended due to increased risk of seizures

TOXICOLOGY INFORMATION *(Continued)*

Laboratory Evaluation of Overdose

Unknown ingestion: Electrolytes, anion gap, serum osmolality, arterial blood gases, serum drug concentration

Known ingestion: Labs tailored to agent

Toxins Affecting the Anion Gap

Drugs Causing Increased Anion Gap (>12 mEq/L)

<u>Nonacidotic</u>

Carbenicillin

Sodium salts

<u>Metabolic Acidosis</u>

Acetaminophen
(ingestion >75-100 g)

Acetazolamide

Amiloride

Ascorbic acid

Benzalkonium chloride

Benzyl alcohol

Beta-adrenergic drugs

Bialaphos

2-butanone

Carbon monoxide

Centrimonium bromide

Chloramphenicol

Colchicine

Cyanide

Dapsone

Dimethyl sulfate

Dinitrophenol

Endosulfan

Epinephrine (I.V. overdose)

Ethanol

Ethylene dibromide

Ethylene glycol

Fenoprofen

Fluoroacetate

Formaldehyde

Fructose (I.V.)

Glycol ethers

Hydrogen sulfide

Ibuprofen (ingestion >300 mg/kg)

Inorganic acid

Iodine

Iron

Isoniazid

Ketamine

Ketoprofen

Metaldehyde

Metformin

Methanol

Methenamine mandelate

Monochloracetic acid

Nalidixic acid

Naproxen

Niacin

Papaverine

Paraldehyde

Pennyroyal oil

Pentachlorophenol

Phenelzine

Phenformin (off the market)

Phenol

Phenylbutazone

Phosphoric acid

Potassium chloroplatinite

Propylene glycol

Salicylates

Sorbitol (I.V.)

Strychnine

Surfactant herbicide

Tetracycline (outdated)

Theophylline

Tienilic acid

Toluene

Tranylcypromine

Vacor

Verapamil

Drugs Causing Decreased Anion Gap (<6 mEq/L)

<u>Acidosis</u>

Ammonium chloride

Bromide

Iodide

Lithium

Polymyxin B

Tromethamine

Drugs Causing Increased Osmolar Gap

(by freezing-point depression, gap is >10 mOsm)

Ethanol[1]
Ethylene glycol[1]
Glycerol
Hypermagnesemia (>9.5 mEq/L)
Isopropanol[1] (acetone)
Iodine (questionable)

Mannitol
Methanol[1]
Propylene glycol
Severe alcoholic ketoacidosis or
    lactic acidosis
Sorbitol[1]

[1]Toxins increasing both anion and osmolar gap.

Toxins Associated With Oxygen Saturation Gap

(>5% difference between measured and calculated value)

Carbon monoxide
Cyanide (questionable)

Hydrogen sulfide (possible)
Methemoglobin

Acetaminophen Toxicity

The Toxicology Laboratory is also very useful for determining levels of toxin in body fluids. Often these drug levels will guide therapy. For example, use of the Rumack-Matthew nomogram for acute acetaminophen poisoning can direct N-acetylcysteine therapy if the serum acetaminophen level falls above the treatment line.

Acetaminophen Toxicity Nomogram

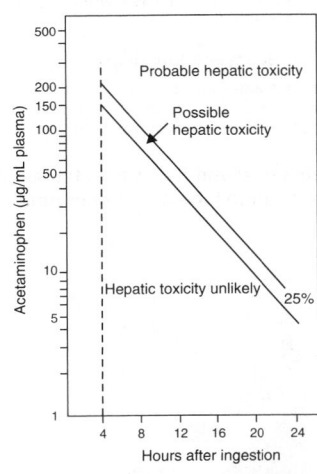

The Rumack-Matthew nomogram, relating expected severity of liver toxicity to serum acetaminophen concentrations.

From Smilkstein MJ, Bronstein AC, Linden C, et al, "Acetaminophen Overdose: A 48-Hour Intravenous N-Acetylcysteine Treatment Protocol," *Ann Emerg Med*, 1991, 20(10):1058, with permission.

TOXICOLOGY INFORMATION *(Continued)*

Ibuprofen Toxicity Nomogram

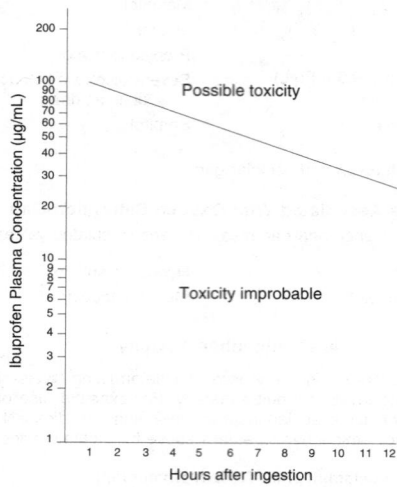

Adapted from Hall AH, Smolinske SC, Stover B, et al, "Ibuprofen Overdose in Adults," *J Toxicol Clin Toxicol*, 1992, 30:34.

Serum Salicylate Intoxication

Similarly, the Done nomogram is somewhat useful in predicting salicylate toxicity in pediatric patients. Neither nomogram should be utilized with chronic ingestions. Recently, a nomogram has been devised for theophylline ingestion; see the following nomogram.

Serum Salicylate Level and Severity of Intoxication
Single Dose Acute Ingestion Nomogram

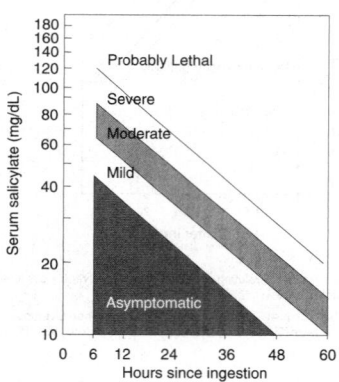

Done nomogram for salicylate poisoning. Note that this nomogram is not accurate for chronic ingestions nor for acute ingestions with enteric coated tabs. Clinical laboratory signs and symptoms are best indicators for assessments. (From Done AK, "Salicylate Intoxication: Significance of Measurements of Salicylate in Blood in Cases of Acute Ingestions," *Pediatrics*, 1960, 26:800; copyright American Academy of Pediatrics, 1960.)

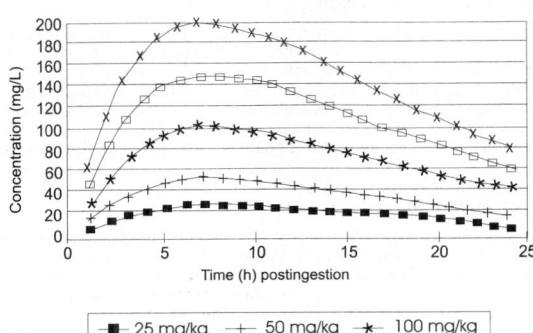

Serum Theophylline Overdose

Nonsmokers

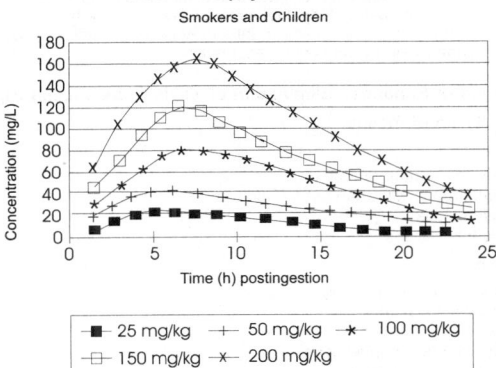

Serum Theophylline Overdose

Smokers and Children

Nomogram for overdose of sustained-release theophylline in 1) nonsmoking adults, and 2) smokers and children. (Courtesy of Frank Paloucek, PharmD, College of Pharmacy, University of Illinois, Chicago.)

TOXICOLOGY INFORMATION *(Continued)*

History and Physical Examination

While the history and physical examination is the cornerstone of clinical patient management, it takes on special meaning with regard to the toxic patient. While taking a history may be a more direct method of the determination of the toxin, quite often is is not reliable. Information obtained may prove minimal in some cases and could be considered partial or inaccurate in suicide gestures and addicts. A quick physical examination often leads to important clues about the nature of the toxin. These clues can be specific symptom complexes associated with certain toxins and can be referred to as "toxidromes".

Prevention of Absorption

Toxic substances can enter the body through the dermal, ocular, pulmonary, parenteral, and gastrointestinal routes. The basic principle of decontamination involves appropriate copious irrigation of the toxic substances relatable to the route of exposure. For example, with ocular exposure, this can be done with normal saline for 30-40 minutes through a Morgan therapeutic lens. With alkali exposures, the pH should be checked until the runoff of the solution is either neutral or slightly acidic. Skin decontamination involves removal of the toxin with nonabrasive soap. This should especially be considered for organophosphates, methylene chloride, dioxin, radiation, hydrocarbons, and herbicide exposure. Separate drainage areas should be obtained for the contaminated runoff.

Since >80% of incidents of accidental poisoning in children occur through the gastrointestinal tract, a thorough knowledge of gastric decontamination is essential. There are essentially four modes of gastric decontamination, of which three are physical removal (emesis, gastric lavage, and whole bowel irrigation). Activated charcoal associated with a cathartic is the fourth mode for preventing absorption.

Methods of Enhanced Elimination of Toxic Substances/Drugs

Emesis with Syrup of Ipecac

Indications

- Use within 1 hour of ingestion
- Hydrocarbons with "dangerous additives"
- Heavy metals
- Toxic insecticides

Contraindications

- Children <6 months of age
- Nontoxic ingestion
- Lack of gag reflex
- Caustic/corrosive ingestions
- Hemorrhagic diathesis
- Sharp object ingestion
- Prior vomiting
- Ingestion of pure petroleum distillate

Dose: + 15 mL H_2O

Children:	6-12 months: 10 mL
	1-5 years: 15 mL
	>5 years: 30 mL
Adults:	30 mL

Note: Ipecac use is becoming less frequently recommended since <30% of the stomach is usually emptied and its use may delay the use of activated charcoal.

Gastric Lavage

Indications

- Use within 1 hour of ingestion
- Comatose patient with significant ingestion without contraindications
- Failure to respond to ipecac
- Large quantities of toxins

Contraindications

- Seizures
- Nontoxic ingestion
- Significant hemorrhagic diathesis
- Caustic ingestions, hydrocarbons
- Usually unable to use large enough tube in children <12 years of age

Note: Lavage is not routinely recommended except for recent and very large ingestions of noncontraindicated toxins since it is believed to actually push a significant portion of drug into the intestine and may delay administration of activated charcoal.

Enhancement of Elimination

Only recently has this aspect of poison management received more than cursory attention in practice and in the literature. The standard practice for enhancement of elimination consisted primarily of forced diuresis in order to excrete the toxin. However, the past 10 years experience has produced a radical change in the approach to this and therefore, a more focused methodology to eliminating absorbed toxins. Essentially, there are three methods by which absorbed toxins may be eliminated: recurrent adsorption with multiple dosings of activated charcoal, use of forced diuresis in combination with possible alkalinization of the urine, and use of dialysis or charcoal hemoperfusion.

Activated Charcoal Indications

Indications

- Single dose for agents known to be bound

- Multiple dose for drugs with favorable characteristics: Small volume of distribution (<1 L/kg), low plasma protein binding, biliary or gastric secretion, active metabolites that recirculate, drugs that exhibit a large free fraction (eg, dapsone, carbamazepine, digitalis, methotrexate, phenobarbital, salicylates, theophylline, tricyclic antidepressants), unchanged, lipophilic, long half-life

Recently, multiple dosing of activated charcoal ("pulse dosing") has been advocated as a method for removal of absorbed drug. This procedure has been demonstrated to be efficacious in drugs that re-enter the gastrointestinal tract through enterohepatic circulation (ie, digitoxin, carbamazepine, glutethimide) and with drugs that diffuse from the systemic circulation into the gastrointestinal tract due to formation of a concentration gradient ("the infinite sink" hypothesis).

Toxins Eliminated by Multiple Dosing of Activated Charcoal (MDAC)

Acetaminophen	Meprobamate
Amitriptyline	Methotrexate
Amoxapine	Methyprylon
Baclofen (?)	Nadolol
Benzodiazepines (?)	Nortriptyline
Bupropion (?)	Phencyclidine
Carbamazepine[1]	Phenobarbital[1]
Chlordecone	Phenylbutazone
Cyclosporine	Phenytoin (?)
Dapsone	Piroxicam
Diazepam	Propoxyphene
Digoxin	Propranolol
Disopyramide	Salicylates (?)[1]
Glutethimide	Theophylline[1]
Maprotiline	Valproic acid[1]

[1] Only agents routinely recommended for removal with MDAC.

Contraindications

- Absence of hypoactive bowel sounds
- Caustic ingestions
- Drugs without effect: Acids, alkalis, alcohols, boric acid, cyanide, iron, heavy metals, lithium, insecticides

Dose

Children and Adults: 50-100 g initially or 1 g/kg weight; repeat doses of 25 g or 0.5 g/kg every 2-4 hours

Most effective at 1-hour postingestion but can remove at >1-hour postingestion

Doses subsequent to first may be admixed with water rather than a cathartic such as sorbitol to avoid diarrhea and consequent electrolyte disturbances.

TOXICOLOGY INFORMATION *(Continued)*

Whole Bowel Irrigation – propylene glycol based solutions

Initial dose of charcoal is necessary prior to use. Avoid pretreatment with ipecac.

Indications

- Iron, lead, lithium
- Agents not bound by charcoal
- Modified or sustained release dosage forms
- Body packers

Contraindications

- Bowel perforation
- Obstruction
- Ileus
- Gastrointestinal bleed

Dose

Maximum: 5-10 L
Toddlers/preschool: 250-500 mL/hour or 35 mL/kg
Adults: 1-2 L/hour
Terminate when rectal effluent = infusate = clear

Urinary Ion Trapping – to alkalinize the urine

Indications

- Salicylates
- Phenobarbital

Toxins Eliminated by Forced Saline Diuretics	Toxins Eliminated by Alkaline Diuresis
Bromidex	2,4-D chlorphenoxyacetic acid
Chromium	Fluoride
Cimetidine (?)	Isoniazid (?)
Cis-platinum	Mephobarbital
Cyclophosphamide	Methotrexate
Hydrazine	Phenobarbital
Iodide	Primidone
Iodine	Quinolones antibiotic
Isoniazid (?)	Salicylates
Lithium	Uranium
Methyl iodide	
Potassium chloroplatinite	
Thallium	

Dose

Sodium bicarbonate 1-2 mEq/kg every 3-4 hours or 100 mEq $NaHCO_3$ in 1 L $D_5\frac{1}{4}NS$ at 200 mL/hour (desired urine pH: 7.6-7.8)

A urine flow of 3-5 mL/kg/hour should be achieved with a combination of isotonic fluids or diuretics. Although several drugs can exhibit enhanced elimination through an acidic urine (quinine, amphetamines, PCP, nicotine, bismuth, ephedrine, flecainide), the practice of acidifying the urine should be discouraged in that it can produce metabolic acidosis and promote renal failure in the presence of rhabdomyolysis. **Note:** Use caution in alkalinizing urine of children to avoid fluid overdose.

Hemodialysis

Indications

Drugs with favorable characteristics

- Low molecular weight (<500 daltons)
- Ionically charged
- H_2O soluble
- Low plasma protein binding (<70%-80%)
- Small volume of distribution (<1 L/kg)
- Low tissue binding
- Methanol, ethylene glycol, boric acid

Drugs and Toxins Removed by Hemodialysis

Acetaminophen
Acyclovir
Amanita phalloides (?)
Amantadine (?)
Ammonium chloride
Amphetamine
Anilines
Atenolol
Boric acid
Bromides
Bromisoval
Calcium
Captopril (?)
Carbromal
Carisoprodol
Chloral hydrate
Chlorpropamide
Chromium
Cimetidine (?)
Cyclophosphamide
Dapsone
Disopyramide
Enalapril (?)
Ethanol
Ethylene glycol
Famotidine (?)
Fluoride
Folic acid
Formaldehyde
Foscarnet sodium
Gabapentin
Glycol ethers
Hydrazine (?)
Hydrochlorothiazide

Iodides
Isoniazid
Isopropanol
Ketoprofen
Lithium
Magnesium
Meprobamate
Metal-chelate compounds
Metformin (?)
Methanol
Methaqualone
Methotrexate
Methyldopa
Methylprylone
Monochloroacetic acid
Nadolol
Oxalic acid
Paraldehyde
Phenelzine (?)
Phenobarbital
Phosphoric acid
Potassium
Procainamide
Quinidine
Ranitidine (?)
Rifabutin
Salicylates
Sotalol
Strychnine
Thallium
Theophylline
Thiocyanates
Tranylcypromine sulfate (?)
Verapamil (?)

Hemoperfusion

Indications

Drugs with favorable characteristics:

- Affinity for activated charcoal
- Tissue binding
- High rate of equilibration from peripheral tissues to blood

Examples: Barbiturates, carbamazepine, ethchlorvynol, methotrexate, phenytoin, theophylline

Drugs and Toxins Removed by Hemoperfusion (Charcoal)

Aconitine
Amanita phalloides (?)
Atenolol (?)
Bromisoval
Bromoethylbutyramide
Caffeine
Carbamazepine
Carbon tetrachloride (?)
Carbromal
Chloral hydrate (trichloroethanol)
Chloramphenicol
Chlorpropamide
Colchicine (?)
Creosote (?)
Dapsone
Diltiazem (?)
Disopyramide
Ethchlorvynol
Ethylene oxide
Glutethimide
Lindane

Meprobamate
Methaqualone
Methotrexate
Methsuximide
Methyprylon (?)
Metoprolol (?)
Nadolol (?)
Oxalic acid (?)
Paraquat
Phenelzine (?)
Phenobarbital
Phenytoin
Podophyllin (?)
Procainamide (?)
Quinidine (?)
Rifabutin (?)
Sotalol (?)
Thallium
Theophylline
Verapamil (?)

Exchange transfusion is another mode of extracorporeal removal of toxins that can be utilized in neonatal infant drug toxicity. It may be especially useful for barbiturate, iron, caffeine, sodium nitrite, or theophylline overdose.

TOXIDROMES

Overdose Signs and Symptoms

Toxin	Vital Signs	Mental Status	Symptoms	Physical Exam	Laboratories
Acetaminophen	Normal	Normal	Anorexia, nausea, vomiting	RUQ tenderness, jaundice	Elevated LFTs
Cocaine	Hypertension, tachycardia, hyperthermia	Anxiety, agitation, delirium	Hallucinations	Mydriasis, tremor, diaphoresis, seizures, perforated nasal septum	EKG abnormalities, increased CPK
Cyclic antidepressants	Tachycardia, hypotension, hyperthermia	Decreased, including coma	Confusion, dizziness	Mydriasis, dry mucous membranes, distended bladder, decreased bowel sounds, flushed, seizures	Long QRS complex, cardiac dysrhythmias
Iron	Early: Normal Late: Hypotension, tachycardia	Normal; lethargic if hypotensive	Nausea, vomiting, diarrhea, abdominal pain, hematemesis	Abdominal tenderness	Heme + stool and vomit, metabolic acidosis, EKG and x-ray findings, elevated serum iron (early); child: hyperglycemia, leukocytosis
Opioids	Hypotension, bradycardia, hypoventilation, hypothermia	Decreased, including coma	Intoxication	Miosis, absent bowel sounds	Abnormal ABGs
Salicylates	Hyperventilation, hyperthermia	Agitation; lethargy; including coma	Tinnitus, nausea, vomiting, confusion	Diaphoresis, tender abdomen	Anion gap metabolic acidosis, respiratory alkalosis, abnormal LFTs, and coagulation studies
Theophylline	Tachycardia, hypotension, hyperventilation, hyperthermia	Agitation, lethargy, including coma	Nausea, vomiting, diaphoresis, tremor, confusion	Seizures, arrhythmias	Hypokalemia, hyperglycemia, metabolic acidosis, abnormal EKG

Examples of Toxidromes

Toxidromes	Pattern	Example of Drugs	Treatment Approach
Anticholinergic	Fever, ileus, flushing, tachycardia, urinary retention, inability to sweat, visual blurring, and mydriasis. Central manifestations include myoclonus, choreoathetosis, toxic psychosis with lilliputian hallucinations, seizures, and coma.	Antihistamines Baclofen Benztropine Jimson weed Methylpyroline Phenothiazines Propantheline Tricyclic antidepressants	Physostigmine for life-threatening symptoms only; may predispose to arrhythmias[1]
Cholinergic	Characterized by salivation, lacrimation, urination, defecation, gastrointestinal cramps, and emesis ("sludge"). Bradycardia and bronchoconstriction may also be seen.	Carbamate Organophosphates Pilocarpine	• Atropine[1] • Pralidoxime for organophosphate insecticides[1]
Extrapyramidal	Choreoathetosis, hyperreflexia, trismus, opisthotonos, rigidity, and tremor	Haloperidol Phenothiazines	• Diphenhydramine • Benztropine
Hallucinogenic	Perceptual distortions, synthesis, depersonalization, and derealization	Amphetamines Cannabinoids Cocaine Indole alkaloids Phencyclidine	Benzodiazepine
Narcotic	Altered mental status, unresponsiveness, shallow respirations, slow respiratory rate or periodic breathing, miosis, bradycardia, hypothermia	Opiates Dextromethorphan Pentazocine Propoxyphene	Naloxone[1]

TOXIDROMES *(Continued)*

Examples of Toxidromes *(continued)*

Toxidromes	Pattern	Example of Drugs	Treatment Approach
Sedative/Hypnotic	Manifested by sedation with progressive deterioration of central nervous system function. Coma, stupor, confusion, apnea, delirium, or hallucinations may accompany this pattern.	Anticonvulsants Antipsychotics Barbiturates Benzodiazepines Ethanol Ethchlorvynol Fentanyl Glutethimide Meprobamate Methadone Methocarbamol Opiates Quinazolines Propoxyphene Tricyclic antidepressants	• Naloxone[1] • Flumazenil; usually not recommended due to increased risk of seizures[1] • Urinary alkalinization (barbiturates)
Seizuregenic	May mimic stimulant pattern with hyperthermia, hyperreflexia, and tremors being prominent signs	Anticholinergics Camphor Chlorinated hydrocarbons Cocaine Isoniazid Lidocaine Lindane Nicotine Phencyclidine Strychnine Xanthines	• Antiseizure medications • Pyridoxine for isoniazid[1] • Extracorporeal removal of drug (ie, lindane, camphor, xanthines) • Physostigmine for anticholinergic agents[1]

Examples of Toxidromes *(continued)*

Toxidromes	Pattern	Example of Drugs	Treatment Approach
Serotonin	Confusion, myoclonus, hyperreflexia, diaphoresis, tremor, facial flushing, diarrhea, fever, trismus	Clomipramine Fluoxetine Isoniazid L-tryptophan Paroxetine Phenelzine Sertraline Tranylcypromine Drug combinations include: • MAO inhibitors with L-tryptophan • Fluoxetine or meperidine • Fluoxetine with carbamazepine or sertraline • Clomipramine and meclobemide • Trazadol and buspirone • Paroxetine and dextromethorphan	Withdrawal of drug/benzodiazepine
Solvent	Lethargy, confusion, dizziness, headache, restlessness, incoordination, derealization, depersonalization	Acetone Chlorinated hydrocarbons Hydrocarbons Naphthalene Trichloroethane Toluene	Avoid catecholamines
Stimulant	Restlessness, excessive speech and motor activity, tachycardia, tremor, and insomnia — may progress to seizure. Other effects noted include euphoria, mydriasis, anorexia, and paranoia.	Amphetamines Caffeine (xanthines) Cocaine Ephedrine/pseudoephedrine Methylphenidate Nicotine Phencyclidine	Benzodiazepines

TOXIDROMES *(Continued)*

Examples of Toxidromes *(continued)*

Toxidromes	Pattern	Example of Drugs	Treatment Approach
Uncoupling of oxidative phosphorylation	Hyperthermia, tachypnea, diaphoresis, metabolic acidosis (usually)	Aluminum phosphide Aspirin/salicylates 2,4-Dichlorophenol Di-n-Butyl phthalate Dinitrophenols Dinitro-o-cresols Hexachlorobutadiene Phosphorus Pentachlorophenol Tin (?) Zinc phosphide	Sodium bicarbonate to treat metabolic acidosis; patient cooling techniques; avoidance of atropine or salicylate agents; hemodialysis may be required for acidosis treatment

¹See the Poison Control Center Antidote Chart.

From Nice A, Leikin JB, Maturen A, et al, "Toxidrome Recognition to Improve Efficiency of Emergency Urine Drug Screens," *Ann Emerg Med*, 1988, 17:676-80.

ADVERSE HEMATOLOGIC EFFECTS, DRUGS ASSOCIATED WITH

Drug	Red Cell Aplasia	Thrombo-cytopenia	Neutro-penia	Pancyto-penia	Hemolysis
Acetazolamide		+	+	+	
Allopurinol			+		
Amiodarone	+				
Amphotericin B				+	
Amrinone		++			
Asparaginase		+++	+++	+++	++
Barbiturates		+		+	
Benzocaine					++
Captopril			++		+
Carbamazepine		++	+		
Cephalosporins			+		++
Chloramphenicol		+	++	+++	
Chlordiazepoxide			+	+	
Chloroquine		+			
Chlorothiazides		++			
Chlorpropamide	+	++	+	++	+
Chlortetracycline				+	
Chlorthalidone			+		
Cimetidine		+	++	+	
Codeine		+			
Colchicine				+	
Cyclophosphamide		+++	+++	+++	+
Dapsone					+++
Desipramine		++			
Digitalis		+			
Digitoxin		++			
Erythromycin		+			
Estrogen		+		+	
Ethacrynic acid			+		
Fluorouracil		+++	+++	+++	+
Furosemide		+	+		
Gold salts	+	+++	+++	+++	
Heparin		++		+	
Ibuprofen			+		+
Imipramine			++		
Indomethacin		+	++	+	
Isoniazid		+		+	
Isosorbide dinitrate					+
Levodopa					++
Linezolid		+++	++	++	
Meperidine		+			
Meprobamate		+	+	+	
Methimazole			++		
Methyldopa		++			+++
Methotrexate		+++	+++	+++	++
Methylene blue					+
Metronidazole			+		
Nalidixic acid					+
Naproxen				+	
Nitrofurantoin			++		+
Nitroglycerine		+			
Penicillamine		++	+		
Penicillins		+	++	+	+++
Phenazopyridine					+++
Phenothiazines		+	++	+++	+

ADVERSE HEMATOLOGIC EFFECTS, DRUGS ASSOCIATED WITH (Continued)

Drug	Red Cell Aplasia	Thrombo-cytopenia	Neutro-penia	Pancyto-penia	Hemolysis
Phenylbutazone		+	++	+++	+
Phenytoin		++	++	++	+
Potassium iodide		+			
Prednisone		+			
Primaquine					+++
Procainamide			+		
Procarbazine		+	++	++	+
Propylthiouracil		+	++	+	+
Quinidine		+++	+		
Quinine		+++	+		
Reserpine		+			
Rifampicin		++	+		+++
Spironolactone			+		
Streptomycin		+		+	
Sulfamethoxazole with trimethoprim			+		
Sulfonamides	+	++	++	++	++
Sulindac	+	+	+	+	
Tetracyclines		+			+
Thioridazine			++		
Tolbutamide		++	+	++	
Triamterene					+
Valproate	+				
Vancomycin			+		

+ = rare or single reports.

++ = occasional reports.

+++ = substantial number of reports.

Adapted from D'Arcy PF and Griffin JP, eds, *Iatrogenic Diseases*, New York, NY: Oxford University Press, 1986, 128-30.

BREAST-FEEDING AND DRUGS

Prior to recommending or prescribing medications to a lactating woman, the following should be considered:

- Is drug therapy necessary?
- Can drug exposure to the infant be minimized? (Using a different route of administration, timing of the dose in relation to breast-feeding, length of therapy, using breast milk stored prior to treatment, etc)
- The infants age and health status (their own ability to metabolize the medication)
- The pharmacokinetics of the drug
- Will the drug interact with a medication the infant is prescribed?
- If medications must be used, pick the safest drug possible.
- In situations where the only drug available may have adverse effects in the nursing infant, consider measuring the infants blood levels.

The tables presented below have been adapted from the American Academy of Pediatrics Committee on Drugs report "Transfer of Drugs and Other Chemicals Into Human Milk," September 2001. It should not be inferred that if a medication is not in the tables it is considered safe for administration to a lactating woman; only that published reports concerning their use were not available at the time the report was published.

Table 1. Cytotoxic Drugs

Cyclophosphamide	Doxorubicin
Cyclosporine	Methotrexate

These are medications thought to interfere with cellular metabolism in the nursing infant. Immune suppression may be possible; effects on growth or carcinogenesis are not known. In addition, doxorubicin is concentrated in human milk; methotrexate is associated with neutropenia in the nursing infant.

Table 2. Drugs of Abuse

Amphetamine	Marijuana
Cocaine	Phencyclidine
Heroin	

Drugs of abuse are not only dangerous to the nursing infant, but also to the mother. Women should be encouraged to avoid their use completely. Effects to the infant reported with amphetamine use in the mother include irritability and poor sleeping; it is also a substance that is concentrated in human milk. Cocaine may cause irritability, vomiting, diarrhea, tremors, or seizures in the infant. Heroin may also cause tremors as well as restlessness, vomiting, and poor feeding.

Nicotine, which was previously on this list, is associated with decreased milk production, decreased weight gain in the infant, and possible increased respiratory illness in the infant. Although there are still questions outstanding regarding smoking and breast-feeding, women should be counseled on the possible effects to their infants and offered aid to smoking cessation if appropriate.

BREAST-FEEDING AND DRUGS *(Continued)*

Table 3. Radioactive Compounds That Require Temporary Cessation of Breast-Feeding

Drug	Recommended Time for Cessation of Breast-Feeding
Copper 64 (^{64}Cu)	Radioactivity in milk present at 50 h
Gallium 67 (^{67}Ga)	Radioactivity in milk present for 2 wk
Indium 111 (^{111}In)	Very small amount present at 20 h
Iodine 123 (^{123}I)	Radioactivity in milk present up to 36 h
Iodine 125 (^{125}I)	Radioactivity in milk present for 12 d
Iodine 131 (^{131}I)	Radioactivity in milk present 2-14 d, depending on study
Iodine^{131}	If used for thyroid cancer, high radioactivity may prolong exposure to infant
Radioactive sodium	Radioactivity in milk present 96 h
Technetium-99m (^{99m}Tc), ^{99m}Tc macroaggregates, ^{99m}Tc O4	Radioactivity in milk present 15 h to 3 d

Consider pumping and storing milk prior to study for use during the radioactive period. Pumping should continue after the study to maintain milk production; however, this milk should be discarded until radioactivity is gone. Notify nuclear medicine physician prior to study that the mother is breast-feeding; a short-acting radionuclide may be appropriate. Contact Radiology Department after testing is complete to screen milk samples before resuming feeding.

Table 4a. Psychotropic Drugs Whose Effect on Nursing Infants Is Unknown But May Be of Concern

Antianxiety	Antidepressant	Antipsychotic
Alprazolam	Amitriptyline	Chlorpromazine
Diazepam	Amoxapine	Chlorprothixene
Lorazepam	Bupropion	Clozapine[1]
Midazolam	Clomipramine	Haloperidol
Perphenazine	Desipramine	Mesoridazine
Prazepam[1]	Dothiepin	Trifluoperazine
Quazepam	Doxepin	
Temazepam	Fluoxetine	
	Fluvoxamine	
	Imipramine	
	Nortriptyline	
	Paroxetine	
	Sertraline[1]	
	Trazodone	

[1]Drug is concentrated in human milk.

Psychotropic medications usually appear in the breast milk in low concentrations. Although adverse effects in the infant may be limited to a few case reports, the long half-life of these medications and their metabolites should be considered. In addition, measurable amounts may be found in the infants plasma and also brain tissue. Long-term effects are not known. Colic, irritability, feeding and sleep disorders, and slow weight gain are effects reported with fluoxetine. Chlorpromazine may cause galactorrhea in the mother, while drowsiness and lethargy have been reported in the nursing infant. A decline in developmental scores has been reported with chlorpromazine and haloperidol.

Table 4b. Additional Drugs Whose Effect on Nursing Infants Is Unknown But May Be of Concern

Drug	Reported Effect in Nursing Infant
Amiodarone	Hypothyroidism
Chloramphenicol	Idiosyncratic bone marrow suppression
Clofazimine	Increase in skin pigmentation; high transfer of mothers dose to infant is possible
Lamotrigine	Therapeutic serum concentrations in infant
Metoclopramide[1]	
Metronidazole	
Tinidazole	

[1]Drug is concentrated in human milk.

No adverse effects to the infant have been reported for metoclopramide; however, it should be recognized that it is a dopaminergic agent. Metronidazole and tinidazole are *in vitro* mutagenic agents. In cases where single dose therapy is appropriate for the mother, breast-feeding may be discontinued for 12-24 hours to allow excretion of the medication.

Table 5. Drugs That Have Been Associated With Significant Effects on Some Nursing Infants and Should Be Given to Nursing Mothers With Caution[1]

Drug	Reported Effect
Acebutolol	Hypotension, bradycardia, tachypnea
5-Aminosalicylic acid	Diarrhea (one case)
Atenolol	Cyanosis, bradycardia
Bromocriptine	Suppresses lactation; may be hazardous to the mother
Aspirin (salicylates)	Metabolic acidosis (one case)
Clemastine	Drowsiness, irritability, refusal to feed, high-pitched cry, neck stiffness (one case)
Ergotamine	Vomiting, diarrhea, convulsions (doses used in migraine medications
Lithium	One-third to one-half therapeutic blood concentration in infants
Phenindone	Anticoagulant: increased prothrombin and partial thromboplastin time in one infant; not used in the United States
Phenobarbital	Sedation; infantile spasms after weaning from milk-containing phenobarbital, methemoglobinemia (one case)
Primidone	Sedation, feeding problems
Sulfasalazine (salicylazosulfapyridine)	Bloody diarrhea (one case)

[1]Blood concentration in the infant may be of clinical importance; measure when possible.

BREAST-FEEDING AND DRUGS *(Continued)*

Table 6. Maternal Medication Usually Compatible With Breast-Feeding

Drug	Reported Effect
Acetaminophen	
Acetazolamide	
Acitretin[1]	
Acyclovir[1]	
Alcohol (ethanol)	Large amounts may lead to drowsiness, diaphoresis, deep sleep, weakness, decreased linear growth, and/or abnormal weight gain. Ingestion of 1 g/kg/d decreases mothers milk ejection reflex.
Allopurinol	
Amoxicillin	
Antimony	
Atropine	
Azapropazone (apazone)	
Aztreonam	
B₁ (thiamine)	
B₆ (pyridoxine)	
B₁₂	
Baclofen	
Barbiturate	Refer to Table 5
Bendroflumethiazide	Lactation suppressed
Bishydroxycoumarin (Dicumarol®)	
Bromide	Rash, weakness, absence of cry with maternal intake of 5.4 g/d
Butorphanol	
Caffeine	Irritability and poor sleep may be seen with >2-3 cups/d; excreted slowly
Captopril	
Carbamazepine	
Carbetocin	
Carbimazole	Goiter
Cascara	
Cefadroxil	
Cefazolin	
Cefotaxime	
Cefoxitin	
Cefprozil	
Ceftazidime	
Ceftriaxone	
Chloral hydrate	Sleepiness
Chloroform	
Chloroquine	
Chlorothiazide	
Chlorthalidone	Slow excretion
Cimetidine[1]	
Ciprofloxacin	Theoretically, may affect cartilage in weight-bearing joints; pseudomembranous colitis reported in one infant
Cisapride	
Cisplatin	Not found in milk
Clindamycin	
Clogestone	
Codeine	
Colchicine	
Contraceptive pill with estrogen and progesterone	Breast enlargement (rare), decreased milk production and protein count (unconfirmed)
Cycloserine	
D (vitamin)	Infant calcium levels should be monitored if mother receives pharmacologic doses
Danthron	Bowel activity increased
Dapsone	No effects reported, but sulfonamide detected in infants urine

Table 6. Maternal Medication Usually Compatible With Breast-Feeding *(continued)*

Drug	Reported Effect
Dexbrompheniramine maleate with d-isoephedrine	Crying, poor sleeping patterns, irritability
Diatrizoate	
Digoxin	
Diltiazem	
Dipyrone	
Disopyramide	
Domperidone	
Dyphylline[1]	
Enalapril	
Erythromycin[1]	
Estradiol	Withdrawal, vaginal bleeding
Ethambutol	
Ethanol	See alcohol
Ethosuximide	No effects reported, but detected in infants urine
Fentanyl	
Fexofenadine	
Flecainide	
Fleroxacin	In one report, a single 400 mg dose was administered to the mother and breast milk not given to infant for 48 hours
Fluconazole	
Flufenamic acid	
Fluorescein	
Folic acid	
Gadopentetic (Gadolinium)	
Gentamicin	
Gold salts	
Halothane	
Hydralazine	
Hydrochlorothiazide	
Hydroxychloroquine[1]	
Ibuprofen	
Indomethacin	Seizure (one case)
Iodides	May affect thyroid activity; see Iodine
Iodine	Goiter
Iodine (povidone-iodine/vaginal douche)	Increased iodine levels in breast milk; iodine odor on infants skin
Iohexol	
Iopanoic acid	
Isoniazid	Metabolite secreted in breast milk; no hepatotoxicity reported in infant
Interferon alfa	
Ivermectin	
K_1 (vitamin)	
Kanamycin	
Ketoconazole	
Ketorolac	
Labetalol	
Levonorgestrel	
Levothyroxine	
Lidocaine	
Loperamide	
Loratadine	
Magnesium sulfate	
Medroxyprogesterone	
Mefenamic acid	
Meperidine	
Methadone	
Methimazole (active metabolite of carbimazole)	
Methyldopa	

BREAST-FEEDING AND DRUGS *(Continued)*

Table 6. Maternal Medication Usually Compatible With Breast-Feeding *(continued)*

Drug	Reported Effect
Methprylon	Drowsiness
Metoprolol[1]	
Metrizamide	
Metrizoate	
Mexiletine	
Minoxidil	
Morphine	No effects reported but found in infants serum
Moxalactam	
Nadolol[1]	
Nalidixic acid	Hemolysis reported in infant with glucose-g-phosphate dehydrogenase deficiency
Naproxen	
Nefopam	
Nifedipine	
Nitrofurantoin	Hemolysis reported in infant with G6PD deficiency
Norethynodrel	
Norsteroids	
Noscapine	
Ofloxacin	Theoretically, may affect cartilage in weight-bearing joints
Oxprenolol	
Phenylbutazone	
Phenytoin	
Piroxicam	
Prednisolone	
Prednisone	
Procainamide	
Progesterone	
Propoxyphene	
Propranolol	
Propylthiouracil	
Pseudoephedrine[1]	
Pyridostigmine	
Pyrimethamine	
Quinidine	
Quinine	
Riboflavin	
Rifampin	
Scopolamine	
Secobarbital	
Senna	
Sotalol	
Spironolactone	
Streptomycin	
Sulbactam	
Sulfapyridine	Use with caution in infants with G6PD deficiency and in ill, stressed, or premature infants
Sulfisoxazole	Use with caution in infants with G6PD deficiency and in ill, stressed, or premature infants
Sumatriptan	
Suprofen	
Terbutaline	
Terfenadine	
Tetracycline	Negligible absorption by infant; potential to stain infants unerupted teeth
Theophylline	Irritability
Thiopental	
Thiouracil	
Ticarcillin	
Timolol	

Table 6. Maternal Medication Usually Compatible With Breast-Feeding *(continued)*

Drug	Reported Effect
Tolbutamide	Jaundice is possible
Tolmetin	
Trimethoprim and sulfamethoxazole	
Triprolidine	
Valproic acid	
Verapamil	
Vitamin (see individual entries, eg, B₁, B₆, B₁₂, D, K)	
Warfarin	
Zolpidem	

¹Drug is concentrated in human milk.

Table 7. Selected Food and Environmental Agents

Agent	Effect Related to Breast-Feeding
Aspartame	Use with caution if mother or infant has phenylketonuria
Chocolate	Irritability or increased bowel activity observed in infant when >16 oz/d consumed by mother
Fava beans	Hemolysis reported in infant with G6PD deficiency
Hexachlorobenzene	Skin rash, diarrhea, vomiting, dark urine, neurotoxicity, death
Hexachlorophene	No effects reported; however, possibility of milk contamination following nipple washing
Lead	Neurotoxicity possible
Mercury, methylmercury	Possible effects on neurodevelopment
Silicone breast implants	Breast-feeding not contraindicated
Vegetarian diet	B₁₂ deficiency

References

American Academy of Pediatrics Committee on Drugs, "Transfer of Drugs and Other Chemicals Into Human Milk," *Pediatrics*, 2001, 108(3): 776-89.
2000 Red Book: Report of the Committee on Infectious Diseases, 25th ed, Elk Grove Village, IL: American Academy of Pediatrics, 2000, 98-104.

DISCOLORATION OF FECES DUE TO DRUGS

Black
Acetazolamide
Alcohols
Alkalies
Aluminum hydroxide
Aminophylline
Aminosalicylic acid
Amphetamine
Amphotericin
Antacids
Anticoagulants
Aspirin
Betamethasone
Bismuth
Charcoal
Chloramphenicol
Chlorpropamide
Clindamycin
Corticosteroids
Cortisone
Cyclophosphamide
Cytarabine
Dicumarol
Digitalis
Ethacrynic acid
Ferrous salts
Floxuridine
Fluorides
Fluorouracil
Halothane
Heparin
Hydralazine
Hydrocortisone
Ibuprofen
Indomethacin
Iodine drugs
Iron salts
Levarterenol
Levodopa
Manganese
Melphalan
Methylprednisolone

Methotrexate
Methylene blue
Oxyphenbutazone
Paraldehyde
Phenacetin
Phenolphthalein
Phenylbutazone
Phenylephrine
Phosphorous
Potassium salts
Prednisolone
Procarbazine
Pyrvinium
Reserpine
Salicylates
Sulfonamides
Tetracycline
Theophylline
Thiotepa
Triamcinolone
Warfarin

Blue
Chloramphenicol
Methylene blue

Dark Brown
Dexamethasone

Gray
Colchicine

Green
Indomethacin
Iron
Medroxyprogesterone

Greenish Gray
Oral antibiotics
Oxyphenbutazone
Phenylbutazone

Light Brown
Anticoagulants

Orange-Red
Phenazopyridine
Rifampin

Pink
Anticoagulants
Aspirin
Heparin
Oxyphenbutazone
Phenylbutazone
Salicylates

Red
Anticoagulants
Aspirin
Heparin
Oxyphenbutazone
Phenolphthalein
Phenylbutazone
Pyrvinium
Salicylates
Tetracycline syrup

Red-Brown
Oxyphenbutazone
Phenylbutazone
Rifampin

Tarry
Ergot preparations
Ibuprofen
Salicylates
Warfarin

White/Speckling
Aluminum hydroxide
Antibiotics (oral)
Indocyanine green

Yellow
Senna

Yellow-Green
Senna

Adapted from Drugdex® — Drug Consults, Micromedex, Vol 62, Denver, CO: Rocky Mountain Drug Consultation Center, 1998.

DISCOLORATION OF URINE
DUE TO DRUGS

Black
Cascara
Cotrimoxazole
Ferrous salts
Iron dextran
Levodopa
Methocarbamol
Methyldopa
Naphthalene
Pamaquine
Phenacetin
Phenols
Quinine
Sulfonamides

Blue
Anthraquinone
DeWitt's pills
Indigo blue
Indigo carmine
Methocarbamol
Methylene blue
Mitoxantrone
Nitrofurans
Resorcinol
Triamterene

Blue-Green
Amitriptyline
Anthraquinone
DeWitt's pills
Doan's® pills
Indigo blue
Indigo carmine
Magnesium salicylate
Methylene blue
Resorcinol

Brown
Anthraquinone dyes
Cascara
Chloroquine
Hydroquinone
Levodopa
Methocarbamol
Methyldopa
Metronidazole
Nitrofurans
Nitrofurantoin
Pamaquine
Phenacetin
Phenols
Primaquine
Quinine
Rifabutin
Rifampin
Senna
Sodium diatrizoate
Sulfonamides

Brown-Black
Isosorbide mono- or
  dinitrate
Methyldopa
Metronidazole
Nitrates
Nitrofurans
Phenacetin
Povidone iodine
Quinine
Senna

Dark
p-Aminosalicylic acid
Cascara
Levodopa
Metronidazole
Nitrites
Phenacetin
Phenol
Primaquine
Quinine
Resorcinol
Riboflavin
Senna

Green
Amitriptyline
Anthraquinone
DeWitt's pills
Indigo blue
Indigo carmine
Indomethacin
Methocarbamol
Methylene blue
Nitrofurans
Phenols
Propofol
Resorcinol
Suprofen

Green-Yellow
DeWitt's pills
Methylene blue

Milky
Phosphates

Orange
Chlorzoxazone
Dihydroergotamine
  mesylate
Heparin sodium
Phenazopyridine
Phenindione
Rifabutin
Rifampin
Sulfasalazine
Warfarin

Orange-Red-Brown
Chlorzoxazone
Doxidan
Phenazopyridine
Rifampin
Warfarin

Orange-Yellow
Fluorescein sodium
Rifampin
Sulfasalazine

Pink
Aminopyrine
Anthraquinone dyes
Aspirin
Cascara
Danthron
Deferoxamine
Merbromin
Methyldopa
Phenazopyridone
Phenolphthalein
Phenothiazines
Phenytoin
Salicylates
Senna

Purple
Phenolphthalein

Red
Anthraquinone
Cascara
Chlorpromazine
Daunorubicin
Deferoxamine
Dihydroergotamine
  mesylate
Dimethyl sulfoxide
DMSO
Doxorubicin
Heparin
Ibuprofen
Methyldopa
Oxyphenbutazone
Phenacetin
Phenazopyridine
Phenolphthalein
Phenothiazines
Phensuximide
Phenylbutazone
Phenytoin
Rifampin
Senna

Red-Brown
Cascara
Deferoxamine
Methyldopa
Oxyphenbutazone
Pamaquine
Phenacetin
Phenazopyridine
Phenolphthalein
Phenothiazines
Phenylbutazone
Phenytoin
Quinine
Senna

Red-Purple
Chlorzoxazone
Ibuprofen
Phenacetin
Senna

DISCOLORATION OF URINE DUE TO DRUGS *(Continued)*

Rust
Cascara
Chloroquine
Metronidazole
Nitrofurantoin
Pamaquine
Phenacetin
Quinacrine
Riboflavin
Senna
Sulfonamides

Yellow
Nitrofurantoin
Phenacetin
Quinacrine
Riboflavin
Sulfasalazine

Yellow-Brown
Aminosalicylate acid
Bismuth
Cascara
Chloroquine
DeWitt's pills
Methylene blue
Metronidazole
Nitrofurantoin
Pamaquine
Primaquine
Quinacrine
Senna
Sulfonamides

Yellow-Pink
Cascara
Senna

Adapted from Drugdex® — Drug Consults, Micromedex, Vol 62, Denver, CO: Rocky Mountain Drug Consultation Center, 1998.

FEVER DUE TO DRUGS

Most Common		Less Common
Cephalosporins	Allopurinol	Hydralazine
Iodides	Antihistamines	Hydroxyurea
Isoniazid	Azathioprine	Ibuprofen
Methyldopa	Barbiturates	Mercaptopurine
Penicillins	Bleomycin	Nitrofurantoin
Phenytoin	Carbamazepine	Para-aminosalicylic acid
Procainamide	Cimetidine	Pentazocine
Quinidine	Cisplatin	Procarbazine
Streptomycin	Clofibrate	Propylthiouracil
Sulfas	Colistimethate	Sulindac
Vancomycin	Diazoxide	Streptozocin
	Folic acid	Triamterene

Drug Intell Clin Pharm, Table 2, "Drugs Implicated in Causing a Fever," 1986, 20:416.

DRUGS IN PREGNANCY

Medications Known to Be Teratogens

Alcohol	Isotretinoin
Androgens	Lithium
Anticonvulsants	Live vaccines
Antineoplastics	Methimazole
Cocaine	Penicillamine
Diethylstilbestrol	Tetracyclines
Etretinate	Warfarin
Iodides (including radioactive iodine)	

Medications Suspected to Be Teratogens

ACE inhibitors	Oral hypoglycemic drugs
Benzodiazepines	Progestogens
Estrogens	Quinolones

Medications With No Known Teratogenic Effects[1]

Acetaminophen	Narcotic analgesics
Cephalosporins	Penicillins
Corticosteroids	Phenothiazines
Docusate sodium	Thyroid hormones
Erythromycin	Tricyclic antidepressants
Multiple vitamins	

[1]No drug is absolutely without risk during pregnancy. These drugs appear to have a minimal risk when used judiciously in usual doses under the supervision of a medical professional.

Medications With Nonteratogenic Adverse Effects in Pregnancy

Antithyroid drugs	Diuretics
Aminoglycosides	Isoniazid
Aspirin	Narcotic analgesics (chronic use)
Barbiturates (chronic use)	Nicotine
Benzodiazepines	Nonsteroidal anti-inflammatory agents
Beta-blockers	Oral hypoglycemic agents
Caffeine	Propylthiouracil
Chloramphenicol	Sulfonamides
Cocaine	

Adapted from DiPiro JT, Talbert RL, Hayes PE, et al, "Therapeutic Considerations During Pregnancy and Lactation," *Pharmacotherapy: A Pathophysiologic Approach*, 4th ed, Stamford, CT: Appleton & Lange, 1999.

MATERNAL/FETAL MEDICATIONS

Adapted from Briggs GG, "Medication Use During the Perinatal Period,"
J Am Pharm Assoc, 1998, 38:717-27.

Antibiotics in Pregnancy

Antibiotics Which Are Generally Regarded as Safe	
Antibiotic	**Comments**
Aminoglycosides (limited use)	
Penicillins	
Cephalosporins	
Clindamycin	
Erythromycin	
Antibiotics to Be Avoided	
Tetracyclines	Staining of deciduous teeth (4th month through term)
Aminoglycosides (prolonged use)	Eighth cranial nerve damage (hearing loss, vestibulotoxicity)
Fluoroquinolones	Potentially mutagenic, cartilage damage, arthropathy, and teratogenicity
Erythromycin estolate	Hepatotoxic in mother
Ribavirin	Possibly fetotoxic

Treatment and Prevention of Infection

Prophylaxis	
Preterm premature rupture of membranes	Ampicillin, amoxicillin, cefazolin, amoxicillin/clavulanate, ampicillin/sulbactam, erythromycin
Prevention of bacterial endocarditis	Ampicillin 2 g and gentamicin 1.5 mg/kg (max: 120 mg) within 30 min of delivery, followed by 1 g ampicillin (I.V.) or amoxicillin (oral) 6 hours later
Cesarean section	Cefazolin (I.V. or uterine irrigation) or clindamycin/gentamicin
Treatment	
Bacterial vaginosis	Clindamycin (oral or gel) in first trimester (gel has been associated with higher rate of preterm deliveries) Metronidazole (oral) for 7 days or gel for 5 days (after first trimester)
Chorioamnionitis	Ampicillin plus gentamicin (clindamycin, erythromycin, or vancomycin if PCN allergic)
Genital herpes	First episode: Oral acyclovir Near term treatment may reduce Cesarian sections I.V. therapy for disseminated infection
Group B streptococci	Penicillin G 5 million units once, then 2.5 million units q4h Ampicillin 2 g once, then 1 g q4h Clindamycin or erythromycin if PCN allergic
HIV	Zidovudine (limits maternal-fetal transmission) Oral dosing during pregnancy/I.V. prior to delivery Other antiretroviral agents - effects unknown Lamivudine during labor used in combination with zidovudine in women who have not received prior antiretroviral therapy
Postpartum endometritis	Ampicillin (vancomycin if PCN allergic) plus clindamycin (or metronidazole) plus gentamicin until afebrile
Pyelonephritis	Ampicillin-gentamicin Cefazolin Co-trimoxazole
Urinary tract infection	Amoxicillin/ampicillin (resistance has increased) Co-trimoxazole Nitrofurantoin Cephalexin
Vaginal candidiasis	Buconizole for 7 days Clotrimazole for 7 days Miconazole for 7 days Terconazole for 7 days

DRUGS IN PREGNANCY (Continued)

Preterm Labor: Tocolytic Agents

Drug Class	Route	Fetal/Neonatal Toxicities	Maternal Toxicities
Beta-adrenergic agonists			
Ritodrine, terbutaline	Oral, I.V., S.C.	Fetal tachycardia, intraventricular septal hypertrophy, neonatal hyperinsulinemia/hypoglycemia	Pulmonary, edema, myocardial infarction, hypokalemia, hypotension, hyperglycemia, tachycardia
Magnesium	I.V.	Neurologic depression in newborn (loss of reflexes, hypotonia, respiratory depression); fetal hypocalcemia and hypercalcuria; abnormal fetal bone mineralization and enamel hypoplasia	Hypotension, respiratory depression, ileus/constipation, hypocalcemia, pulmonary edema, hypotension, headache/dizziness
NSAIDs			
Indomethacin	Oral, P.R.	Ductus arteriosis: premature closure, ricuspid regurgitation, primary pulmonary hypertension of the newborn, PDA; intraventricular hemorrhage, necrotizing enterocolitis, renal failure	GI bleeding, oligohydramnios, pulmonary edema, acute renal failure
Calcium channel blockers			
Nifedipine	Oral	Hypoxia secondary to maternal hypotension	Hypotension, flushing, tachycardia, headache
Nitrates			
Nitroglycerin	I.V./S.L.	Hypoxia secondary to maternal hypotension	Hypotension, headache, dizziness

Pregnancy-Induced Hypertension[1]

Drug Class	Maternal/Fetal Effects
Antihypertensives Contraindicated in PIH	
Diuretics	Reduction of maternal plasma volume exacerbates disease; use in chronic hypertension acceptable (if no superimposed pregnancy-induced hypertension)
ACE-inhibitors	Teratogenic in second and third trimester; fetal/newborn anuria and hypotension, fetal oligohydramnios; neonatal death (congenital abnormalities of skull and renal failure)
Hypertension Treatment[2]	
Central-acting	
Methyldopa	Relatively safe in second/third trimester
Beta-blockers	
Acebutolol, atenolol, metoprolol, pindolol, propranolol	Increased risk of IUGR
Alpha-/beta-blocking	
Labetolol	See beta-blockers
Vasodilators	
Hydralazine	Relatively safe in second/third trimester
Nitrates	
Nitroglycerin	Relatively safe in second/third trimester
Calcium channel blockers	
Nifedipine	Relatively safe in second/third trimester

[1]Includes management of pre-eclampsia/eclampsia and HELLP syndrome. **Note:** Prevention may include low-dose aspirin (81 mg/day) or calcium supplementation (2 g/day).

[2]All agents must be carefully titrated to avoid fetal hypoxia.

HERB – DRUG INTERACTIONS / CAUTIONS

Herb	Drug Interaction / Caution
Acidophilus / bifidobacterium	Antibiotics (oral)
Activated charcoal	Vitamins or oral medications may be adsorbed
Alfalfa	Do not use with lupus due to amino acid L-canavanine; causes pancytopenia at high doses; warfarin (alfalfa contains a large amount of vitamin K)
Aloe vera	Caution in pregnancy, may cause uterine contractions; digoxin, diuretics (hypokalemia)
Ashwagandha	May cause sedation and other CNS effects
Asparagus root	Causes diuresis
Barberry	Normal metabolism of vitamin B may be altered with high doses
Birch	If taking a diuretic, drink plenty of fluids
Black cohosh	Estrogen-like component; pregnant and nursing women should probably avoid this herb; also women with estrogen-dependent cancer and women who are taking birth control pills or estrogen supplements after menopause; caution also in people taking sedatives or blood pressure medications
Black haw	Do not give to children <6 years of age (salicin content) with flu or chickenpox due to potential Reye's syndrome; do not take if allergic to aspirin
Black pepper (*Piper nigrum*)	Antiasthmatic drugs (decreases metabolism)
Black tea	May inhibit body's utilization of thiamine
Blessed thistle	Do not use with gastritis, ulcers, or hyperacidity since herb stimulates gastric juices
Blood root	Large doses can cause nausea, vomiting, CNS sedation, low BP, shock, coma, and death
Broom (*Cytisus scoparius*)	MAO inhibitors lead to sudden blood pressure changes
Bugleweed (*Lycopus virginicus*)	May interfere with nuclear imaging studies of the thyroid gland (thyroid uptake scan)
Cat's claw (*Uncaria tomentosa*)	Avoid in organ transplant patients or patients on ulcer medications, antiplatelet drugs, NSAIDs, anticoagulants, immunosuppressive therapy, intravenous immunoglobulin therapy
Chaste tree berry (*Vitex agnus-castus*)	Interferes with actions of oral contraceptives, HRT, and other endocrine therapies; may interfere with metabolism of dopamine-receptor antagonists
Chicory (*Cichorium intybus*)	Avoid with gallstones due to bile-stimulating properties
Chlorella (*Chlorella vulgaris*)	Contains significant amounts of vitamin K
Chromium picolinate	Picolinic acid causes notable changes in brain chemicals (serotonin, dopamine, norepinephrine); do not use if patient has behavioral disorders or diabetes
Cinnabar root (*Salviae miltiorrhizae*)	Warfarin (increases INR)
Deadly nightshade (*Atropa belladonna*)	Contains atropine
Dong quai	Warfarin (increases INR), estrogens, oral contraceptives, photosensitizing drugs, histamine replacement therapy, anticoagulants, antiplatelet drugs, antihypertensives
Echinacea	Caution with other immunosuppressive therapies; stimulates TNF and interferons
Ephedra	Avoid with blood pressure medications, antidepressants, and MAOIs
Evening primrose oil	May lower seizure threshold; do not combine with anticonvulsants or phenothiazines
Fennel	Do not use in women who have had breast cancer or who have been told not to take birth control pills

HERB – DRUG INTERACTIONS / CAUTIONS *(Continued)*

Herb	Drug Interaction / Caution
Fenugreek	Practice moderation in patients on diabetes drugs, MAO inhibitors, cardiovascular agents, hormonal medicines, or warfarin due to the many components of fenugreek
Feverfew	Antiplatelets, anticoagulants, NSAIDs
Forskolin, coleonol	This herb lowers blood pressure (vasodilator) and is a bronchodilator and increases the contractility of the heart, inhibits platelet aggregation, and increases gastric acid secretion
Foxglove	Digitalis-containing herb
Garlic	Blood sugar-lowering medications, warfarin, and aspirin at medicinal doses of garlic
Ginger	May inhibit platelet aggregation by inhibiting thromboxane synthetase at large doses; *in vitro* and animal studies indicate that ginger may interfere with diabetics; has anticoagulant effect, so avoid in medicinal amounts in patients on warfarin or heart medicines
Ginkgo biloba	Warfarin (ginkgo decreases blood clotting rate); NSAIDs, MAO inhibitors
Ginseng	Blood sugar-lowering medications (additive effects) and other stimulants
Ginseng (American, Korean)	Furosemide (decreases efficacy)
Ginseng (Siberian)	Digoxin (increases digoxin level)
Glucomannan	Diabetics (herb delays absorption of glucose from intestines, decreasing mean fasting sugar levels)
Goldenrod	Diuretics (additive properties)
Gymnema	Blood sugar-lowering medications (additive effects)
Hawthorn	Digoxin or other heart medications (herb dilates coronary vessels and other blood vessels, also inotropic)
Hibiscus	Chloroquine (reduced effectiveness of chloroquine)
Hops	Those with estrogen-dependent breast cancer should not take hops (contains estrogen-like chemicals); patients with depression (accentuate symptoms); alcohol or sedative (additive effects)
Horehound	May cause arrhythmias at high doses
Horseradish	In medicinal amounts with thyroid medications
Kava	CNS depressants (additive effects, eg, alcohol, barbiturates, etc); benzodiazepines
Kelp	Thyroid medications (additive effects or opposite effects by negative feedback); kelp contains a high amount of sodium
Labrador tea	Plant has narcotic properties, possible additive effects with other CNS depressants
Lemon balm	Do not use with Graves disease since it inhibits certain thyroid hormones
Licorice	Acts as a corticosteroid at high doses (about 1.5 lbs candy in 9 days) which can lead to hypertension, edema, hypernatremia, and hypokalemia (pseudoaldosteronism); do not use in persons with hypertension, glaucoma, diabetes, kidney or liver disease, or those on hormonal therapy; may interact with digitalis (due to hypokalemia)
Lobelia	Contains lobeline which has nicotinic activity; may mask withdrawal symptoms from nicotine; it can act as a polarizing neuromuscular blocker
Lovage	Is a diuretic
Ma huang	MAO inhibitors, digoxin, beta-blockers, methyldopa, caffeine, theophylline, decongestants (increases toxicity)
Marshmallow	May delay absorption of other drugs taken at the same time; may interfere with treatments of lowering blood sugar
Meadowsweet	Contains salicylates

Herb	Drug Interaction / Caution
Melatonin	Acts as contraceptive at high doses; antidepressants (decreases efficacy)
Mistletoe	May interfere with medications for blood pressure, depression, and heart disease
L-phenylalanine	MAO inhibitors
Pleurisy root	Digoxin (plant contains cardiac glycosides); also contains estrogen-like compounds; may alter amine concentrations in the brain and interact with antidepressants
Prickly ash (Northern)	Contains coumarin-like compounds
Prickly ash (Southern)	Contains neuromuscular blockers
Psyllium	Digoxin (decreases absorption)
Quassia	High doses may complicate heart or blood-thinning treatments (quassia may be inotropic)
Red clover	May have estrogen-like actions; avoid when taking birth control pills, HRT, people with heart disease or at risk for blood clots, patients who suffer from estrogen-dependent cancer; do not take with warfarin
Red pepper	May increase liver metabolism of other medications and may interfere with high blood pressure medications or MAO inhibitors
Rhubarb, Chinese	Do not use with digoxin (enhanced effects)
St John's wort	Indinavir, cyclosporine, SSRIs or any antidepressants, tetracycline (increases sun sensitivity); digoxin (decreases digoxin concentration); may also interact with diltiazem, nicardipine, verapamil, etoposide, paclitaxel, vinblastine, vincristine, glucocorticoids, cyclosporine, dextromethorphan, ephedrine, lithium, meperidine, pseudoephedrine, selegiline, yohimbine, ACE inhibitors (serotonin syndrome, hypertension, possible exacerbation of allergic reaction)
Saw palmetto	Acts an antiandrogen; do not take with prostate medicines or HRT
Squill	Digoxin or persons with potassium deficiency; also not with quinidine, calcium, laxatives, saluretics, prednisone (long-term)
Tonka bean	Contains coumarin, interacts with warfarin
Vervain	Avoid large amounts of herb with blood pressure medications or HRT
Wild Oregon grape	High doses may alter metabolism of vitamin B
Wild yam	May interfere with hormone precursors
Wintergreen	Warfarin, increased bleeding
Sweet woodruff	Contains coumarin
Yarrow	Interferes with anticoagulants and blood pressure medications
Yohimbe	Do not consume tyramine-rich foods; do not take with nasal decongestants, PPA-containing diet aids, antidepressants, or mood-altering drugs

LABORATORY DETECTION OF DRUGS

Agent	Time Detectable in Urine[1]
Alcohol	12-24 h
Amobarbital	2-4 d
Amphetamine	2-4 d
Butalbital	2-4 d
Cannabinoids	
Occasional use	2-7 d
Regular use	30 d
Cocaine (benzoylecgonine)	12-72 h
Codeine	2-4 d
Chlordiazepoxide	30 d
Diazepam	30 d
Dilaudid®	2-4 d
Ethanol	12-24 h
Heroin (morphine)	2-4 d
Hydromorphone	2-4 d
Librium®	30 d
Marijuana	
Occasional use	2-7 d
Regular use	30 d
Methamphetamine	2-4 d
Methaqualone	2-4 d
Morphine	2-4 d
Pentobarbital	2-4 d
Phencyclidine (PCP)	
Occasional use	2-7 d
Regular use	30 d
Phenobarbital	30 d
Quaalude®	2-4 d
Secobarbital	2-4 d
Valium®	30 d

Chang JY, "Drug Testing and Interpretation of Results," *Pharmchem Newsletter*, 1989, 17:1.

[1]The periods of detection for the various abused drugs listed above should be taken as estimates since the actual figures will vary due to metabolism, user, laboratory, and excretion.

LOW POTASSIUM DIET

Potassium is a mineral found in most all foods except sugar and lard. It plays a role in maintaining normal muscle activity and helps to keep body fluids in balance. Too much potassium in the blood can lead to changes in heartbeat and can lead to muscle weakness. The kidneys normally help to keep blood potassium controlled, but in kidney disease or when certain drugs are taken, dietary potassium must be limited to maintain a normal level of potassium in the blood.

The following guideline includes 2-3 g of potassium per day.

1. **Milk Group:** Limit to one cup serving of milk or milk product (yogurt, cottage cheese, ice cream, pudding).

2. **Fruit Group:** Limit to two servings daily from the low potassium choices. Watch serving sizes. Avoid the high potassium choices.

> **Low Potassium**
> Apple, 1 small
> Apple juice, applesauce $\frac{1}{2}$ cup
> Apricot, 1 medium or $\frac{1}{2}$ cup canned in syrup
> Blueberries, $\frac{1}{2}$ cup
> Cherries, canned in syrup $\frac{1}{3}$ cup
> Cranberries, cranberry juice $\frac{1}{2}$ cup
> Fruit cocktail, canned in syrup $\frac{1}{2}$ cup
> Grapes, 10 fresh
> Lemon, lime 1 fresh
> Mandarin orange, canned in syrup $\frac{1}{2}$ cup
> Nectar: apricot, pear, peach $\frac{1}{2}$ cup
> Peach, 1 small or $\frac{1}{2}$ cup canned with syrup
> Pear, 1 small or $\frac{1}{2}$ cup canned with syrup
> Pineapple, $\frac{1}{2}$ cup raw or canned with syrup
> Plums, 1 small or $\frac{1}{2}$ cup canned with syrup
> Tangerine, 1 small
> Watermelon, $\frac{1}{2}$ cup
>
> **High Potassium**
> Avocado
> Banana
> Cantaloupe
> Cherries, fresh
> Dried fruits
> Grapefruit, fresh and juice
> Honeydew melon
> Kiwi
> Mango
> Nectarine
> Orange, fresh and juice
> Papaya
> Prunes, prune juice
> Raisins

3. Avoid use of the following salt substitutes due to their high potassium contents: Adolph's, Lawry's Season Salt Substitute, No Salt, Morton Season Salt Free, Nu Salt, Papa Dash, and Morton Lite Salt.

ORAL DOSAGES THAT SHOULD NOT BE CRUSHED

There are a variety of reasons for crushing tablets or capsule contents prior to administering to the patient. Patients may have nasogastric tubes which do not permit the administration of tablets or capsules; an oral solution for a particular medication may not be available from the manufacturer or readily prepared by pharmacy; patients may have difficulty swallowing capsules or tablets; or mixing of powdered medication with food or drink may make the drug more palatable.

Generally, medications which should not be crushed fall into one of the following categories:

- **Extended-Release Products**. The formulation of some tablets is specialized as to allow the medication within it to be slowly released into the body. This is sometimes accomplished by centering the drug within the core of the tablet, with a subsequent shedding of multiple layers around the core. Wax melts in the GI tract. Slow-K® is an example of this. Capsules may contain beads which have multiple layers which are slowly dissolved with time.

- **Medications Which Are Irritating to the Stomach**. Tablets which are irritating to the stomach may be enteric coated which delays release of the drug until the time when it reaches the small intestine. Enteric-coated aspirin is an example of this.

- **Foul Tasting Medication**. Some drugs are quite unpleasant in their taste and the manufacturer, to increase their palatability will coat the tablet in a sugar coating. By crushing the tablet, this sugar coating is lost and the patient tastes the unpleasant tasting medication.

- **Sublingual Medication**. Medication intended for use under the tongue should not be crushed. While it appears to be obvious, it is not always easy to determine if a medication is to be used sublingually. Sublingual medications should indicate on the package that they are intended for sublingual use.

- **Effervescent Tablets**. These are tablets which, when dropped into a liquid, quickly dissolve to yield a solution. Many effervescent tablets, when crushed, lose their ability to quickly dissolve.

Recommendations

1. It is not advisable to crush certain medications.

2. Consult individual monographs prior to crushing capsule or tablet.

3. If crushing a tablet or capsule is contraindicated, consult with your pharmacist to determine whether an oral solution exists or can be compounded.

4. Refer to individual drug monograph for crushing information.

Summary of Drug Formulations That Preclude Crushing

Type	Reason(s) for the Formulation
Enteric-coated	Designed to pass through the stomach intact with drug released in the intestines to: • prevent destruction of drug by stomach acids • prevent stomach irritation • delay onset of action
Extended release	Designed to release drug over an extended period of time. Such products include: • multiple layered tablets releasing drug as each layer is dissolved • mixed release pellets that dissolve at different time intervals • special matrixes that are themselves inert but slowly release drug from the matrix
Sublingual buccal	Designed to dissolve quickly in oral fluids for rapid absorption by the abundant blood supply of the mouth
Miscellaneous	Drugs that: • produce oral mucosa irritation • are extremely bitter • contain dyes or inherently could stain teeth and mucosal tissue

OVER-THE-COUNTER PRODUCTS[1]

Generic Name	Brand Name	Comments
Analgesics		
Acetaminophen and aspirin (caffeine in all products)	Excedrin® Extra Strength Tablet; Gelpirin® Geltabs; Goody's® Headache Powders	Relief of mild to moderate pain or fever; avoid alcoholic beverages; take with food or a full glass of water
Acetaminophen and diphenhydramine	Anacin® PM; Legatrin PM® Caplet; Tylenol® PM	Relief of mild to moderate pain or sinus headache
Acetaminophen and phenyltolaxamine	Percogesic® Tablet	Relief of mild to moderate pain
Capsaicin	Capsin®; Zostrix®; Zostrix®-HP	FDA approved for the topical treatment of pain associated with postherpetic neuralgia, rheumatoid arthritis, osteoarthritis, diabetic neuropathy, and postsurgical pain. Unlabeled use: Treatment of pain associated with psoriasis, chronic neuralgias unresponsive to other forms of therapy, and intractable pruritis.
Choline salicylate	Arthropan®	Temporary relief of pain of rheumatoid arthritis, rheumatic fever, osteoarthritis, and other conditions for which oral salicylates are recommended; useful in patients in which there is difficulty in administering doses in a tablet or capsule dosage form because of the liquid dosage form
Trolamine salicylate	Myoflex® Cream	Relief of pain of muscular aches, rheumatism, neuralgia, sprains, arthritis on intact skin
Antacids, Antiflatulents, or Antiemetics		
Aluminum carbonate	Basaljel®	Hyperacidity; hyperphosphatemia
Aluminum hydroxide and magnesium carbonate	Gaviscon® Liquid	Temporary relief of symptoms associated with gastric acidity
Aluminum hydroxide and magnesium hydroxide	Maalox®; Maalox® Therapeutic Concentrate; Mylanta® Night	Antacid; used to treat hyperphosphatemia in renal failure
Aluminum hydroxide and magnesium trisilicate		Temporary relief of hyperacidity
Aluminum hydroxide, magnesium hydroxide, and simethicone	Di-Gel®; Maalox® Extra; Mylanta®; Mylanta® Double Strength	Temporary relief of hyperacidity associated with gas; may be used for indications associated with other antacids
Calcium carbonate and magnesium carbonate		Relief of hyperacidity
Calcium carbonate and simethicone	Gas-Ban®; Titralac® Plus	Relief of acid indigestion, heartburn, peptic esophagitis, hiatal hernia, and gas
Dimenhydrinate	Calm-X® Oral; Dramamine® Oral; TripTone® Caplets®	Treatment and prevention of nausea, vertigo, and vomiting associated with motion sickness
Magaldrate and simethicone	Riopan Plus ®	Relief of hyperacidity associated with peptic ulcer, gastritis, peptic esophagitis, and hiatal hernia

OVER-THE-COUNTER PRODUCTS[1] (Continued)

Generic Name	Brand Name	Comments
Phosphorated carbohydrate solution	Emetrol® Liquid; Nausetrol® Liquid	Relief of nausea associated with upset stomach that occurs with intestinal flu, pregnancy, food indiscretions, and emotional upsets
Simethicone	Gas-X®; Maalox Anti-Gas®; Mylanta Gas®; Mylicon®; Phazyme®	Relieves flatulence and functional gastric bloating, and postoperative gas pains
Antidiarrheals and Laxatives		
Attapulgite	Children's Kaopectate®; Diasorb®; Donnagel®; Kaopectate® Advanced Formula	Symptomatic treatment of diarrhea
Bisacodyl	Bisac-Evac®; Bisacodyl Uniserts®; Bisco-Lax®; Dulcolax®; Fleet® Laxative	Treatment of constipation; colonic evacuation prior to procedures or examination
Calcium polycarbophil	Equalactin® Chewable Tablet; Fiberall® Chewable Tablet; FiberCon® Tablet; Fiber-Lax® Tablet; Mitrolan® Chewable Tablet	Treatment of constipation or diarrhea by restoring a more normal moisture level and providing bulk in the patient's intestinal tract; calcium polycarbophil is supplied as the approved substitute whenever a bulk-forming laxative is ordered in a tablet, capsule, wafer, or other oral solid dosage form
Castor oil	Emulsoil®; Neoloid®; Purge®	Preparation for rectal or bowel examination or surgery; rarely used to relieve constipation; also applied to skin as emollient and protectant
Docusate and casanthranol	Diocto C®; D-S-S Plus®; Genasoft® Plus; Peri-Colace®; Silace-C®	Treatment of constipation generally associated with dry, hard stools and decreased intestinal motility
Glycerin	Fleet® Babylax® Rectal; Sani-Supp® Suppository	Constipation
Kaolin and pectin	Kao-Spen®; Kapectolin®	Treatment of uncomplicated diarrhea
Lactase enzyme	Dairy Ease®; Lactaid®; Lactrase®	Helps to digest lactose in milk for patients with lactose intolerance; may be administered with meals
Magnesium hydroxide and mineral oil emulsion	Haley's M-O® Oral Suspension	Short-term treatment of occasional constipation
Malt soup extract	Maltsuprex®	Short-term treatment of constipation
Methylcellulose	Citrucel® Powder	Adjunct in treatment of constipation
Mineral oil	Fleet® Mineral Oil Enema; Kondremul®	Temporary relief of constipation; relieve fecal impaction; preparation for bowel studies or surgery
Senna	Black Draught®; Senokot®; X-Prep® Liquid	Short-term treatment of constipation; evacuate the colon for bowel or rectal examinations; liquid may be administered with fruit juice or milk to mask taste
Sodium phosphate	Fleet® Enema; Fleet® Phospho®-Soda	Short-term treatment of constipation; evacuation of the colon for rectal and bowel exams; source of sodium and phosphorus; treatment and prevention of hypophosphatemia

Generic Name	Brand Name	Comments
Cough/Cold or Allergy		
Acetaminophen and pseudoephedrine	Allerest® No Drowsiness; Coldrine®; Dristan® Cold Caplets; Ornex® No Drowsiness; Sine-Aid®, Maximum Strength; Sine-Off® Maximum Strength No Drowsiness Formula; Tylenol® Sinus	Temporary relief of sinus symptoms with no drowsiness
Acetaminophen, chlorpheniramine, and pseudoephedrine	Comtrex®; Sine-Off®; Sinutab® Tablet; Tylenol® Allergy Sinus; Theraflu® Flu & Cold	Temporary relief of sinus symptoms
Acetaminophen, dextromethorphan, and pseudoephedrine	Sudafed® Severe Cold; Theraflu® Non-Drowsy Formula Maximum Strength; Tylenol® Cold No Drowsiness; Tylenol® Flu Maximum Strength; Vicks® DayQuil®	Relief of cold and flu symptoms with no drowsiness
Brompheniramine	Dimetapp® (4 mg tablet/capsule); Nasahist B®; ND-Stat®	Treatment of seasonal and perennial allergic rhinitis and other allergic symptoms including urticaria
Brompheniramine and pseudoephedrine	Brofed® Elixir; Bromfed®; Bromfed® PD; Bromfenex®; Bromfenex® PD; Dallergy® JR	Temporary relief of symptoms of seasonal and perennial allergic rhinitis, and vasomotor rhinitis, including nasal obstruction
Chlorpheniramine	Aller-Chlor®; Chlor-Trimeton®; Efidac 24®	Relief of perennial and seasonal allergic rhinitis and other allergic symptoms including urticaria
Chlorpheniramine and acetaminophen	Coricidin® Tablet	Symptomatic relief of congestion, headache, aches, and pains of colds and flu
Chlorpheniramine and phenylephrine	Ed A-Hist® Liquid; Histatab® Plus Tablet; Novahistine® Elixir	Temporary relief of nasal congestion and eustachian tube congestion as well as runny nose, sneezing, itching of nose or throat, itchy and watery eyes
Chlorpheniramine and pseudoephedrine	Allerest® Maximum Strength; Anamine® Syrup; Deconamine® SR; Deconamine® Syrup ; Deconamine® Tablet; Hayfebrol® Liquid; Rhinosyn® Liquid; Rhinosyn-PD® Liquid; Ryna® Liquid; Sudafed Plus® Tablet	Relief of nasal congestion associated with the common cold, hay fever, and other allergies, sinusitis, eustachian tube blockage, and vasomotor and allergic rhinitis
Chlorpheniramine, phenylephrine, and dextromethorphan	Norel DM™	Temporary relief of cough due to minor throat and bronchial irritation; relief of nasal congestion, runny nose, and sneezing
Dexbrompheniramine and pseudoephedrine	Disobrom®; Disophrol® Chronotabs®; Disophrol® Tablet; Drixomed®; Drixoral®	Relief of symptoms of upper respiratory mucosal congestion in seasonal and perennial nasal allergies, acute rhinitis, rhinosinusitis, and eustachian tube blockage
Dextromethorphan	Benylin® Adult Formula; Creo-Terpin®; Delsym®; Hold® DM; Pertussin® CS; Pertussin® DM; Robitussin® Cough Calmers; Robitussin® Pediatric; Scot-Tussin DM® Cough Chasers; Silphen DM®; St. Joseph® Cough Suppressant; Sucrets® Cough Calmers; Suppress®; Trocal®; Vicks Formula 44®; Vicks Formula 44® Pediatric Formula	Symptomatic relief of coughs caused by minor viral upper respiratory tract infections or inhaled irritants; most effective for a chronic nonproductive cough
Diphenhydramine and pseudoephedrine	Benadryl® Decongestant Allergy Tablet; Benylin® Multi-Symptom	Relief of symptoms of upper respiratory mucosal congestion in seasonal and perennial nasal allergies, acute rhinitis, rhinosinusitis, and eustachian tube blockage
Guaifenesin and pseudoephedrine	Congestac®; Guiatuss® PE; Robitussin-PE®; Robitussin® Severe Congestion Liqui-Gels	Enhances output of respiratory tract fluid and reduces mucosal congestion and edema in nasal passage
Guaifenesin, pseudoephedrine, and dextromethorphan	Novahistine® DMX; Rhinosyn-X® Liquid; Ru-Tuss® Expectorant	Relief of nasal congestion and cough

OVER-THE-COUNTER PRODUCTS[1] *(Continued)*

Generic Name	Brand Name	Comments
Oxymetazoline	Afrin® Children's Nose Drops; Afrin® Nasal Solution; Duramist® Plus®; Duration® Nasal Solution; Neo-Synephrine® 12-Hour Nasal Solution; Nostrilla®; OcuClear® Ophthalmic; Sinarest® 12 Hour Nasal Solution; Visine® L.R. Ophthalmic; 4-Way® Long Acting Nasal Solution	Symptomatic relief of nasal mucosal congestion and adjunctive therapy of middle ear infections associated with acute or chronic rhinitis, the common cold, sinusitis, hay fever, or other allergies; relief of redness of eye due to minor eye irritations
Phenindamine	Nolahist®	Treatment of perennial and seasonal allergic rhinitis and chronic urticaria
Propylhexedrine	Benzedrex® Inhaler	Topical nasal decongestant
Pseudoephedrine and dextromethorphan	PediaCare® Decongestant Plus Cough; Robitussin® Cold & Cough; Triaminic® AM Cough & Decongestant Formula; Vicks® 44D Cough & Head Congestion Capsule; Vicks® 44D Non-Drowsy Cold & Cough Liqui-Caps	Temporary symptomatic relief of nasal congestion due to the common cold, upper respiratory allergies, and sinusitis; promotes nasal or sinus drainage; symptomatic relief of coughs caused by minor viral upper respiratory tract infections or inhaled irritants; most effective for a chronic nonproductive cough
Pseudoephedrine and ibuprofen	Advil® Cold & Sinus Caplets; Dristan® Sinus Caplets; Motrin® Cold & Flu; Motrin® Cold Children's Suspension; Motrin® Sinus Headache; Vicks® DayQuil® Sinus & Pain	Temporary symptomatic relief of nasal congestion due to the common cold, upper respiratory allergies, and sinusitis; promotes nasal or sinus drainage; relief of sinus headaches and pains
Terpin hydrate		Symptomatic relief of cough; contains 42% ethyl alcohol
Triprolidine and pseudoephedrine	Actifed®; Allerfrin® Syrup; Allerfrin® Tablet; Allerphed Syrup; Aprodine® Syrup; Aprodine® Tablet; Genac® Tablet; Silafed® Syrup; Triposed® Syrup; Triposed® Tablet	Temporary relief of nasal congestion; decongest sinus openings, runny nose, sneezing, itching of nose or throat, and itchy watery eyes due to common cold, hay fever, or other upper respiratory allergies; may cause drowsiness
Xylometazoline	Otrivin® Nasal	Symptomatic relief of nasal and nasopharyngeal mucosal congestion; use with caution in patients with hypertension, diabetes, cardiovascular or coronary artery disease; do not use for more than 4 days
Dermatologics		
Aluminum sulfate and calcium acetate	Bluboro®; Domeboro® Topical; Pedi-Boro®	Astringent wet dressing for relief of inflammatory conditions of the skin and used to reduce weeping that may occur in dermatitis
Bacitracin, neomycin, polymyxin B, and lidocaine	Clomycin®	Prevent and treat susceptible superficial topical infections
Benzoin	TinBen®	Protective application for irritations of the skin; sometimes used in boiling water as steam inhalants for their expectorant and soothing action
Benzoyl peroxide	Advanced Formula Oxy® Sensitive Gel; Benoxyl®; Del Aqua-5® Gel; Fostex® 10% BPO Gel; Fostex® 10% Wash; Fostex® Bar; Loroxide® Neutrogena® Acne Mask; PanOxyl® Bar	Adjunctive treatment of mild to moderate acne vulgaris acne rosacea

Generic Name	Brand Name	Comments
Camphor and phenol	Campho-Phenique® Liquid	Relief of pain and for minor infections
Chlorophyll	Nullo®	Topically promotes normal healing; relief of pain and inflammation; reduce malodors in wounds, burns, surface ulcers, abrasions, and skin irritations; used orally to control fecal and urinary odors in colostomy, ileostomy, or incontinence
Chloroxine	Capitrol® Shampoo	Treatment of dandruff or seborrheic dermatitis of the scalp
Coal tar	Denorex®; DHS® Tar; Duplex® T; Estar®; Fototar®; Neutrogena® T/Derm; Oxipor® VHC; Pentrax®; Polytar®; psoriGel®; T/Gel®; Zetar®	Topically for controlling dandruff, seborrheic dermatitis, or psoriasis
Coal tar and salicylic acid	Ionil T®; X-seb® T Shampoo	Control seborrheal dermatitis, dandruff
Coal tar, lanolin, and mineral oil	Balnetar® Bath Oil	Control psoriasis, seborrheal dermatitis, atopic dermatitis, eczematoid dermatitis
Dibucaine	Nupercainal®	Fast, temporary relief of pain and itching due to hemorrhoids, minor burns, or other minor skin conditions (amide derivative local anesthetic)
Glycerin, lanolin, and peanut oil	Massé® Breast Cream	Nipple care of pregnant and nursing women
Lactic acid	LactiCare® Lotion	Lubricate and moisturize the skin counteracting dryness and itching
Ammonium lactate	Lac-Hydrin® Lotion	Treatment of moderate to severe xerosis and ichthyosis vulgaris
Lanolin, cetyl alcohol, glycerin, and petrolatum	Lubriderm® Lotion	Treatment of dry skin
Merbromin	Mercurochrome® Topical Solution	Topical antiseptic
Methoxycinnamate and oxybenzone	Ti-Screen®	Reduce the chance of premature aging of the skin and skin cancer from overexposure to the sun
Nonoxynol 9	Delfen®; Emko®; Encare®; Gynol II®; Semicid®; Shur-Seal®	Spermatocide in contraception
Povidone-iodine	Betadine®; Betadine® 5% Sterile Ophthalmic Prep Solution; Massengil® Medicated Douche w/ Cepticin; Minidyne®; Polydine®; Summer's Eve® Medicated Douche	External antiseptic with broad microbicidal spectrum against bacteria, fungi, viruses, protozoa, and yeasts
Pyrithione zinc	DHS Zinc®; Sebulon®; Theraplex Z®; Zincon® Shampoo; ZNP® Bar	Relief of itching, irritation, and scalp flaking associated with dandruff and/or seborrheal dermatitis of the scalp
Salicylic acid	Compound W®; DuoFilm®; DuoPlant® Gel; Freezone® Solution; Gordofilm® Liquid; Keralyt® Gel; Mediplast® Plaster; Mosco® Liquid; Occlusal-HP Liquid; Sal-Acid® Plaster; Salactic® Film; Sal-Plant® Gel; Trans-Ver-Sal® AdultPatch; Trans-Ver-Sal® PediaPatch; Trans-Ver-Sal® PlantarPatch; Wart-Off®;	Topically used for its keratolytic effect in controlling seborrheic dermatitis or psoriasis of body and scalp, dandruff, and other scaling dermatoses; remove warts, corns, and calluses
Sulfur and salicylic acid	Fostex®; Sebulex®	Therapeutic shampoo for dandruff and seborrheal dermatitis; acne skin cleanser
Thimerosal	Mersol®; Merthiolate®	Organomercurial antiseptic with sustained bacteriostatic and fungistatic activity
Triacetin	Myco-Nail	Fungistat for athlete's foot and other superficial fungal infections

OVER-THE-COUNTER PRODUCTS[1] *(Continued)*

Generic Name	Brand Name	Comments
Undecyclenic acid and derivatives	Caldesene® Topical	Treatment of athlete's foot, ringworm, prickly heat, jock itch, diaper rash, and other minor skin irritations
Vitamin A and vitamin D	A and D™ Ointment	Temporary relief of discomfort due to chapped skin, diaper rash, minor burns, abrasions, as well as irritations associated with ostomy skin care
Zinc oxide	Balmex®; Desitin®; Diaparene Diaper Rash; Vicon-C®	Protective coating for mild skin irritations and abrasions; soothing and protective ointment to promote healing of chapped skin, diaper rash; if irritation develops, discontinue use and consult a physician; paste is easily removed with mineral oil; for external use only; do not use in eyes
Dietary Supplements		
Calcium citrate	Citracal®	Adjunct in prevention of postmenopausal osteoporosis; treatment and prevention of calcium depletion
Calcium lactate		Adjunct in prevention of postmenopausal osteoporosis; treatment and prevention of calcium depletion
Calcium phosphate, dibasic	Posture®	Adjunct in prevention of postmenopausal osteoporosis; treatment and prevention of calcium depletion
Ferrous salt and ascorbic acid	Fero-Grad 500®	Treatment of iron deficiency in nonpregnant or pregnant adults
Ferrous sulfate, ascorbic acid, and vitamin B complex	Iberet®-Liquid	Treatment of conditions of iron deficiency with an increased need for B complex vitamins and vitamin C; should be administered with water or juice on an empty stomach; may be administered with food to prevent irritation, however, not with cereals, dietary fiber, tea, coffee, eggs, or milk
Glucose, instant	B-D Glucose®; Glutose®; Insta-Glucose®	Management of hypoglycemia
Glucose polymers	Moducal®; Polycose®; Sumacal®	Supplies calories for those persons not able to meet the caloric requirement with usual food intake
Magnesium chloride	Slow-Mag®	Correct or prevent hypomagnesemia
Magnesium gluconate	Magonate®	Dietary supplement for treatment of magnesium deficiencies
Medium chain triglycerides	MCT Oil®	Dietary supplement for those who cannot digest long chain fats; malabsorption associated with disorders such as pancreatic insufficiency, bile salt deficiency, and bacterial overgrowth of the small bowel; induce ketosis as a prevention for seizures (akinetic, clonic, and petit mal)
Polysaccharide-iron complex	Hytinic®; Niferex®; Nu-Iron®	Prevention and treatment of iron deficiency anemias

Generic Name	Brand Name	Comments
Vitamin B complex	Apatate®; MegaB®; Orexin®	Prevention and treatment of B complex vitamin deficiency
Vitamin B complex with vitamin C	Allbee® With C; Surbex-T® Filmtabs®; Surbex® With C Filmtabs®; Vicon-C®	Supportive nutritional supplementation in conditions in which water-soluble vitamins are required like GI disorders, chronic alcoholism, pregnancy, severe burns, and recovery from surgery
Vitamin B complex with vitamin C and folic acid	Berocca®; Nephrocaps®	Supportive nutritional supplementation in conditions in which water-soluble vitamins are required like GI disorders, chronic alcoholism, pregnancy, severe burns, and recovery from surgery
Zinc sulfate	Eye-Sed® Ophthalmic; Orazinc® Oral	Zinc supplement (oral and parenteral); may improve wound healing in those who are deficient
Hemorrhoidal Preparations		
Pramoxine	Proctofoam® NS; Tronolane®	Temporary relief of pain and itching associated with anogenital pruritus or irritation; treatment of dermatosis, minor burns, or hemorrhoids
Witch hazel	Tucks® Cream/Gel/Pads	After-stool wipe to remove most causes of local irritation; temporary management of vulvitis, pruritus ani, and vulva; help relieve the discomfort of simple hemorrhoids, anorectal surgical wounds, and episiotomies
Ophthalmics		
Artificial tears	Akwa Tears® Solution; AquaSite® Ophthalmic Solution; Bion® Tears Solution; Dakrina® Ophthalmic Solution; Dry Eye® Therapy Solution; Dry Eyes® Solution; Dwelle® Ophthalmic Solution; HypoTears PF Solution; HypoTears Solution; Isopto® Plain Solution; Isopto® Tears Solution; Liquifilm® Forte Solution; Moisture® Ophthalmic Drops; Murine® Solution; Murocel® Ophthalmic Solution; Nature's Tears® Solution; Nu-Tears® Solution; Nu-Tears® II Solution; OcuCoat® Ophthalmic Solution; OcuCoat® PF Ophthalmic Solution; Puralube® Tears Solution; Refresh® Ophthalmic Solution; Refresh® Plus Ophthalmic Solution; Teargen® Ophthalmic Solution; Tearisol® Solution; Tears Naturale® Free Solution; Tears Naturale® II Solution; Tears Naturale® Solution; Tears Plus® Solution; Tears Renewed® Solution; Ultra Tears® Solution; Viva-Drops® Solution	Ophthalmic lubricant; relief of dry eyes and eye irritation
Balanced salt solution	BSS® Ophthalmic	Intraocular irrigating solution; used to soothe and cleanse the eye in conjunction with hard contact lenses
Benzalkonium chloride	Benza®; Zephiran®	Surface antiseptic and germicidal preservative
Carboxymethylcellulose sodium	Celluvisc® Ophthalmic Solution	Preservative-free artificial tear substitute
Glycerin	Ophthalgan® Ophthalmic; Osmoglyn® Ophthalmic	Reduction of intraocular pressure; reduction of corneal edema; glycerin had been administered orally to reduce intracranial pressure

OVER-THE-COUNTER PRODUCTS[1] *(Continued)*

Generic Name	Brand Name	Comments
Naphazoline	AK-Con® Ophthalmic; Albalon® Liquifilm® Ophthalmic; Clear Eyes®; Estivin® II Ophthalmic; Nafazair® Ophthalmic; Naphcon Forte® Ophthalmic; Naphcon® Ophthalmic; Privine® Nasal; VasoClear® Ophthalmic; Vasocon Regular® Ophthalmic	Topical ocular vasoconstrictor; will temporarily relieve congestion, itching, and minor irritation; control hyperemia in patients with superficial corneal vascularity
Naphazoline and antazoline	Vasocon-A® Ophthalmic Solution	Topical ocular congestion, irritation, and itching; use with caution in patients with cardiovascular disease
Naphazoline and pheniramine	Naphcon-A® Ophthalmic Solution; Opcon A®; Visine® A	Topical ocular vasoconstrictor; use with caution in patients with cardiovascular disease
Phenylephrine and zinc sulfate	Zincfrin® Ophthalmic	Soothe, moisturize, and remove redness due to minor eye irritation; discontinue use if ocular pain or visual changes are present after 3 days
Tetrahydrozoline	Eyesine® Ophthalmic; Geneye® Ophthalmic; Murine® Plus Ophthalmic; Tetrasine® Extra Ophthalmic; Tetrasine® Ophthalmic; Tyzine® Nasal; Visine® Extra Ophthalmic	Symptomatic relief of nasal congestion and conjunctival congestion
Oral		
Benzocaine, gelatin, pectin, and sodium carboxymethylcellulose	Orabase® With Benzocaine Paste	Topical anesthetic and emollient for oral lesions
Cetylpyridinium	Cêpacol® Troches	Temporary relief of sore throat
Cetylpyridinium and benzocaine	Cylex®; Mycinette®	Symptomatic relief of sore throat
Gelatin, pectin, and methylcellulose	Orabase® Plain	Temporary relief from minor oral irritations
Phenol	Ulcerease®	Relief of sore throat pain and mouth, gum, and throat irritations
Saliva substitute	Moi-Stir®	Relief of dry mouth and throat in xerostomia
Otic		
Boric acid	Borofax® Topical	Ophthalmic: Mild antiseptic used for inflamed eyelids. Otic: Prophylaxis of swimmer's ear. Topical ointment: Temporary relief of chapped, chafed, or dry skin; diaper rash; abrasions; minor burns; sunburn; insect bites; and other skin irritations.
Miscellaneous or Multiple Use		
Sodium chloride	Adsorbonac® Ophthalmic; AK-NaCl®; Ayr® Saline; Breathe Free®; HuMist® Nasal Mist; Muro 128® Ophthalmic; NaSal™; Nasal Moist®; Ocean Nasal Mist; Pretz®; SalineX®; SeaMist®	Prevention of muscle cramps and heat prostration; restoration of sodium ion in hyponatremia; induce abortion; restore moisture to nasal membranes; GU irrigant; reduction of corneal edema; source of electrolytes and water for expansion of the extracellular fluid compartment

[1]On November 6, 2000, the FDA issued a publich health advisory concerning the risk of hemorrhagic stroke associated with the use of phenylpropanolamine hydrochloride (PPA). An increased risk of hemorrhagic stroke has been identified in women following the first dose of PPA when used as an appetite suppressant, and within the first 3 days of use when used as a decongestant. Men may also be at risk. The FDA has asked all drug companies to discontinue the marketing of products containing PPA.

TYRAMINE CONTENT OF FOODS

Food	Allowed	Minimize Intake	Not Allowed
Beverages	Milk, decaffeinated coffee, tea, soda	Chocolate beverage, caffeine-containing drinks, clear spirits	Acidophilus milk, beer, ale, wine, malted beverages
Breads/cereals	All except those containing cheese	None	Cheese bread and crackers
Dairy products	Cottage cheese, farmers or pot cheese, cream cheese, ricotta cheese, all milk, eggs, ice cream, pudding (except chocolate)	Yogurt (limit to 4 oz per day)	All other cheeses (aged cheese, American, Camembert, cheddar, Gouda, gruyere, mozzarella, parmesan, provolone, romano, Roquefort, stilton)
Meat, fish, and poultry	All fresh or frozen	Aged meats, hot dogs, canned fish and meat	Chicken and beef liver, dried and pickled fish, summer or dry sausage, pepperoni, dried meats, meat extracts, bologna, liverwurst
Starches — potatoes/rice	All	None	Soybean (including paste)
Vegetables	All fresh, frozen, canned, or dried vegetable juices except those not allowed	Chili peppers, Chinese pea pods	Fava beans, sauerkraut, pickles, olives, Italian broad beans
Fruit	Fresh, frozen, or canned fruits and fruit juices	Avocado, banana, raspberries, figs	Banana peel extract
Soups	All soups not listed to limit or avoid	Commercially canned soups	Soups which contain broad beans, fava beans, cheese, beer, wine, any made with flavor cubes or meat extract, miso soup
Fats	All except fermented	Sour cream	Packaged gravy
Sweets	Sugar, hard candy, honey, molasses, syrups	Chocolate candies	None
Desserts	Cakes, cookies, gelatin, pastries, sherbets, sorbets	Chocolate desserts	Cheese-filled desserts
Miscellaneous	Salt, nuts, spices, herbs, flavorings, Worcestershire sauce	Soy sauce, peanuts	Brewer's yeast, yeast concentrates, all aged and fermented products, monosodium glutamate, vitamins with Brewer's yeast

VITAMIN K CONTENT IN SELECTED FOODS

The following lists describe the relative amounts of vitamin K in selected foods. The abbreviations for vitamin K is "H" for high amounts, "M" for medium amounts, and "L" for low amounts.

Foods[1]	Portion Size†	Vitamin K Content
Coffee brewed	10 cups	L
Cola, regular and diet	3½ fl oz	L
Fruit juices, assorted types	3½ fl oz	L
Milk	3½ fl oz	L
Tea, black, brewed	3½ fl oz	L
Bread, assorted types	4 slices	L
Cereal, assorted types	3½ oz	L
Flour, assorted types	1 cup	L
Oatmeal, instant, dry	1 cup	L
Rice, white	½ cup	L
Spaghetti, dry	3½ oz	L
Butter	6 Tbsp	L
Cheddar cheese	3½ oz	L
Eggs	2 large	L
Margarine	7 Tbsp	M
Mayonnaise	7 Tbsp	H
Oils		
Canola, salad, soybean	7 Tbsp	H
Olive	7 Tbsp	M
Corn, peanut, safflower, sesame, sunflower	7 Tbsp	L
Sour cream	8 Tbsp	L
Yogurt	3½ oz	L
Apple	1 medium	L
Banana	1 medium	L
Blueberries	⅔ cup	L
Cantaloupe pieces	⅔ cup	L
Grapes	1 cup	L
Grapefruit	½ medium	L
Lemon	2 medium	L
Orange	1 medium	L
Peach	1 medium	L
Abalone	3½ oz	L
Beef, ground	3½ oz	L
Chicken	3½ oz	L
Mackerel	3½ oz	L
Meatloaf	3½ oz	L
Pork, meat	3½ oz	L
Tuna	3½ oz	L
Turkey, meat	3½ oz	L
Asparagus, raw	7 spears	M
Avocado, peeled	1 small	M
Beans, pod, raw	1 cup	M
Broccoli, raw and cooked	½ cup	H
Brussel sprout, sprout and top leaf	5 sprouts	H
Cabbage, raw	1½ cups shredded	H
Cabbage, red, raw	1½ cups shredded	M
Carrot	⅔ cup	L
Cauliflower	1 cup	L
Celery	2½ stalks	L
Coleslaw	¾ cup	M
Collard greens	½ cup chopped	H
Cucumber peel, raw	1 cup	H

Foods[1]	Portion Size†	Vitamin K Content
Cucumber, peel removed	1 cup	L
Eggplant	1¼ cups pieces	L
Endive, raw	2 cups chopped	H
Green scallion, raw	⅔ cup chopped	H
Kale, raw leaf	¾ cup	H
Lettuce, raw, heading, bib, red leaf	1¾ cups shredded	H
Mushroom	1½ cups	L
Mustard greens, raw	1½ cups	H
Onion, white	⅔ cup chopped	L
Parsley, raw and cooked	1½ cups chopped	H
Peas, green, cooked	⅔ cup	M
Pepper, green, raw	1 cup chopped	L
Potato	1 medium	L
Pumpkin	½ cup	L
Spinach, raw leaf	1½ cups	H
Tomato	1 medium	L
Turnip greens, raw	1½ cups chopped	H
Watercress, raw	3 cups chopped	H
Honey	5 Tbsp	L
Jell-O® Gelatin	⅓ cup	L
Peanut butter	6 Tbsp	L
Pickle, dill	1 medium	M
Sauerkraut	1 cup	M
Soybean, dry	½ cup	M

[1]This list is a partial listing of foods. For more complete information, refer to references 1-2.

†Portions in chart are calculated from estimated portions provided in reference 4.

References

Booth SL, Sadowski JA, Weihrauch JL, et al, "Vitamin K₁ (Phylloquinone) Content of Foods a Provisional Table," *J Food Comp Anal*, 1993, 6:109-20.

Ferland G, MacDonald DL, and Sadowski JA, "Development of a Diet Low in Vitamin K₁ (Phylloquinone)," *J Am Diet Assoc*, 1992, 92, 593-7.

Hogan RP, "Hemorrhagic Diathesis Caused by Drinking an Herbal Tea," *JAMA*, 1983, 249:2679-80.

Pennington JA, *Bowes and Church's Food Values of Portions Commonly Used*, 15th ed, JP Lippincott Co, 1985.

THERAPEUTIC CATEGORY & KEY WORD INDEX

NOTES

NOTES

NOTES

NOTES

NOTES

NOTES

NOTES

Other titles offered by

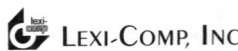 LEXI-COMP, INC

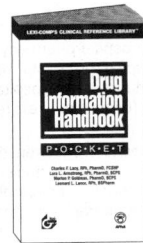
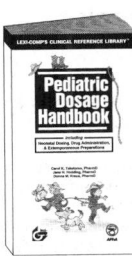
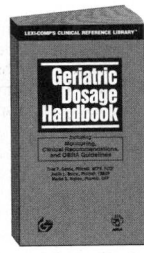

Other titles offered by

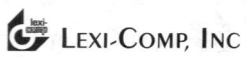 LEXI-COMP, INC

DRUG INFORMATION HANDBOOK FOR THE ALLIED HEALTH PROFESSIONAL
by Leonard L. Lance, RPh, BSPharm; Charles Lacy, RPh, PharmD, FCSHP; Lora L. Armstrong, RPh, PharmD, BCPS; and Morton P. Goldman, PharmD, BCPS

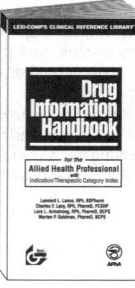

Working with clinical pharmacists, hospital pharmacy and therapeutics committees, and hospital drug information centers, the authors have assisted hundreds of hospitals in developing institution-specific formulary reference documentation.

The most current basic drug and medication data from those clinical settings have been reviewed, coalesced, and cross referenced to create this unique handbook. The handbook offers quick access to abbreviated monographs for generic drugs.

This is a great tool for physician assistants, medical records personnel, medical transcriptionists and secretaries, pharmacy technicians, and other allied health professionals.

DRUG-INDUCED NUTRIENT DEPLETION HANDBOOK
by Ross Pelton, RPh, PhD, CCN; James B. LaValle, RPh, DHM, NMD, CCN; Ernest B. Hawkins, RPh, MS; Daniel L. Krinsky, RPh, MS

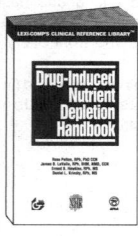

A complete and up-to-date listing of all drugs known to deplete the body of nutritional compounds.

This book is alphabetically organized and provides extensive cross-referencing to related information in the various sections of the book. Drug monographs identify the nutrients depleted and provide cross-references to the nutrient monographs for more detailed information on Effects of Depletion, Biological Function & Effect, Side Effects & Toxicity, RDA, Dosage Range, and Dietary Sources. This book also contains a Studies & Abstracts section, a valuable Appendix, and Alphabetical & Pharmacological Indexes.

NATURAL THERAPEUTICS POCKET GUIDE
by James B. LaValle, RPh, DHM, NMD, CCN; Daniel L. Krinsky, RPh, MS; Ernest B. Hawkins, RPh, MS; Ross Pelton, RPh, PhD, CCN; Nancy Ashbrook Willis, BA, JD

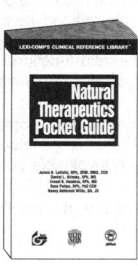

Provides condition-specific information on common uses of natural therapies. Each condition discussed includes the following: review of condition, decision tree, list of commonly recommended herbals, nutritional supplements, homeopathic remedies, lifestyle modifications, and special considerations.

Provides herbal/nutritional/nutraceutical monographs with over 10 fields including references, reported uses, dosage, pharmacology, toxicity, warnings & interactions, and cautions & contraindications.

The Appendix includes: drug-nutrient depletion, herb-drug interactions, drug-nutrient interaction, herbal medicine use in pediatrics, unsafe herbs, and reference of top herbals.

To order call toll free anywhere in the U.S.: 1-800-837-LEXI (5394)
Outside of the U.S. call: 330-650-6506 or online at www.lexi.com

Other titles offered by

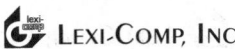
LEXI-COMP, INC

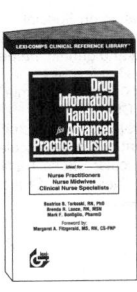
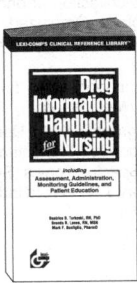
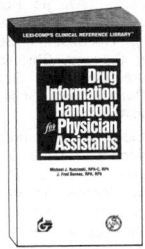

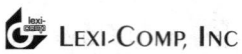
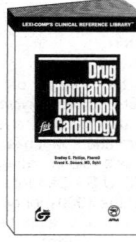
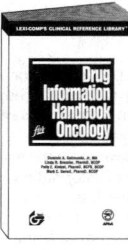
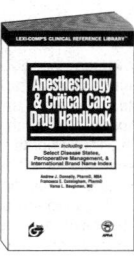

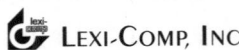
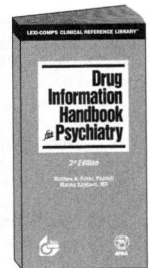
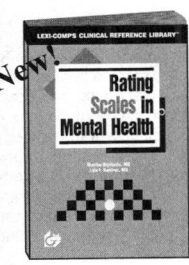
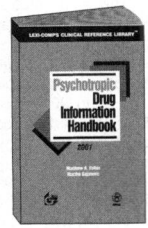

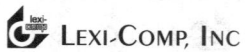
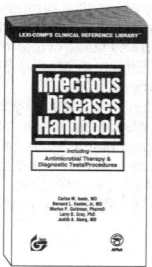
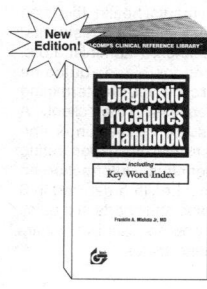
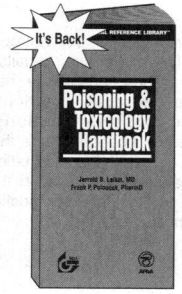

Other titles offered by

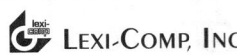
LEXI-COMP, INC

CLINICIAN'S GUIDE TO DIAGNOSIS—A Practical Approach
by Samir Desai, MD

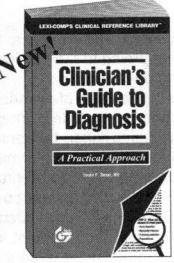

Symptoms are what prompt patients to seek medical care. In the evaluation of a patient's symptom, it is not unusual for healthcare professionals to ask "What do I do next?" This is precisely the question for which the *Clinician's Guide to Diagnosis: A Practical Approach* provides the answer. It will lead you from symptom to diagnosis through a series of steps designed to mimic the logical thought processes of seasoned clinicians. For the young clinician, this is an ideal book to help bridge the gap between the classroom and actual patient care. For the experienced clinician, this concise handbook offers rapid answers to the questions that are commonly encountered on a day-to-day basis. Let this guide become your companion, providing you with the tools necessary to tackle even the most challenging symptoms.

CLINICIAN'S GUIDE TO LABORATORY MEDICINE—A Practical Approach
by Samir P. Desai, MD and Sana Isa-Pratt, MD

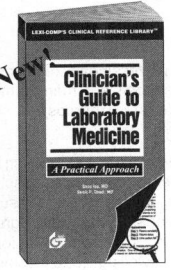

When faced with the patient presenting with abnormal laboratory tests, the clinician can now turn to the *Clinician's Guide to Laboratory Medicine: A Practical Approach*. This source is unique in its ability to lead the clinician from laboratory test abnormality to clinical diagnosis. Written for the busy clinician, this concise handbook will provide rapid answers to the questions that busy clinicians face in the care of their patients. No longer does the clinician have to struggle in an effort to find this information - *it's all here.*

LABORATORY TEST HANDBOOK & CONCISE version
by David S. Jacobs MD, FACP; Wayne R. DeMott, MD, FACP; and Dwight K. Oxley, MD, FACP

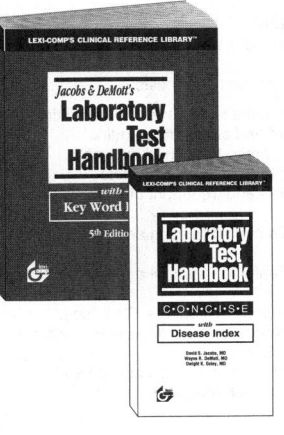

Contains over 900 clinical laboratory tests and is an excellent source of laboratory information for physicians of all specialties, nurses, laboratory professionals, students, medical personnel, or anyone who needs quick access to most routine and many of the more specialized testing procedures available in today's clinical laboratory.

Each monograph contains test name, synonyms, patient care, specimen requirements, reference ranges, and interpretive information with footnotes, references, and selected websites.

The *Laboratory Test Handbook Concise* is a portable, abridged (800 tests) version and is an ideal, quick reference for anyone requiring information concerning patient preparation, specimen collection and handling, and test result interpretation.

To order call toll free anywhere in the U.S.: 1-800-837-LEXI (5394)
Outside of the U.S. call: 330-650-6506 or online at www.lexi.com

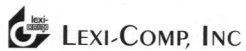
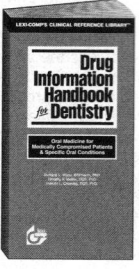
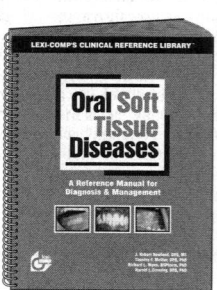
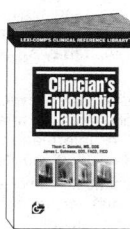

Other titles offered by

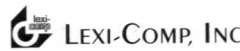
DENTAL OFFICE MEDICAL EMERGENCIES
by Timothy F. Meiller, DDS, PhD; Richard L. Wynn, BSPharm, PhD; Ann Marie McMullin, MD; Cynthia Biron, RDH, EMT, MA; and Harold L. Crossley, DDS, PhD

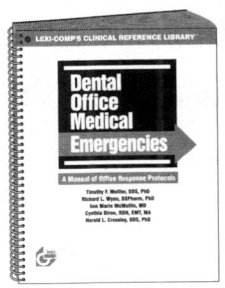

Designed specifically for general dentists during times of emergency. A tabbed paging system allows for quick access to specific crisis events. Created with urgency in mind, it is spiral bound and drilled with a hole for hanging purposes.

* Basic Action Plan for Stabilization
* Allergic / Drug Reactions
* Loss of Consciousness / Respiratory Distress / Chest Pain
* Altered Sensation / Changes in Affect
* Management of Acute Bleeding
* Office Preparedness / Procedures and Protocols
* Automated External Defibrillator (AED)
* Oxygen Delivery

POISONING & TOXICOLOGY COMPENDIUM
by Jerrold B. Leikin, MD and Frank P. Paloucek, PharmD

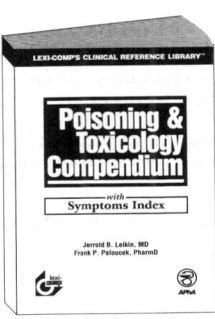

A six-in-one reference wherein each major entry contains information relative to one or more of the other sections. This compendium offers comprehensive, concisely-stated monographs covering 645 medicinal agents, 256 nonmedicinal agents, 273 biological agents, 49 herbal agents, 254 laboratory tests, 79 antidotes, and 222 pages of exceptionally useful appendix material.

A truly unique reference that presents signs and symptoms of acute overdose along with considerations for overdose treatment. Ideal reference for emergency situations.

DRUG INFORMATION HANDBOOK FOR THE CRIMINAL JUSTICE PROFESSIONAL
by Marcelline Burns, PhD; Thomas E. Page, MA; and Jerrold B. Leikin, MD

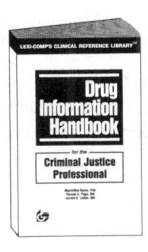

Compiled and designed for police officers, law enforcement officials, and legal professionals who are in need of a reference which relates to information on drugs, chemical substances, and other agents that have abuse and/or impairment potential. Contains over 450 medications, agents, and substances. Contains up to 33 fields of information including Scientific Name, Commonly Found In, Abuse Potential, Impairment Potential, Use, When to Admit to Hospital, Mechanism of Toxic Action, Signs & Symptoms of Acute Overdose, Drug Interactions, Reference Range, and Warnings/Precautions. There is a glossary of medical terms for the layman along with a slang street drug listing and an Appendix includes Chemical, Bacteriologic, and Radiologic Agents - Effects and Treatment; Controlled Substances - Uses and Effects; Medical Examiner Data; Federal Trafficking Penalties, *and much more.*

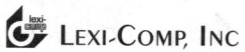
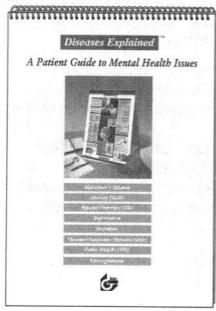
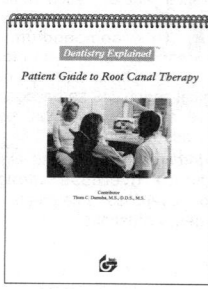
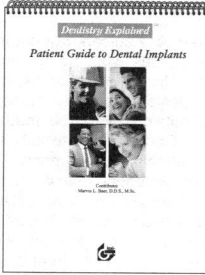

Introducing . . . Diseases Explained™

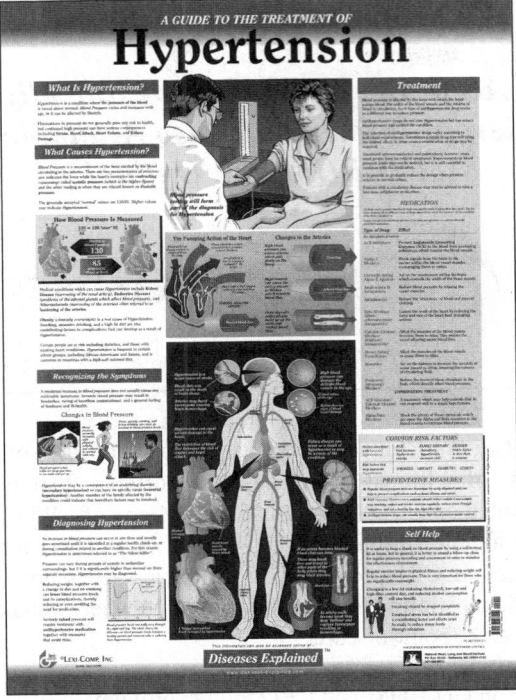

A GUIDE TO THE TREATMENT OF
Hypertension

Lexi-Comp is proud to introduce Diseases Explained™, our new series of patient education material. Written in a language a patient can easily understand, each product will help the healthcare professional explain to patients about their specific medical condition.

Available now in a wall chart format and soon to be released as booklets, leaflets, and desk flip charts, this series will help you educate the patient about the cause, symptoms, diagnosis, treatment, and self-help concerning their condition.

Available now:

- Alzheimer's Disease
- Anemia
- Angina
- Asthma
- Anxiety
- Cholesterol
- COPD
- Depression
- Diabetes
- Enlarged Prostate

- Epilepsy
- Essential Tremor
- Glaucoma
- Heart Attack
- Hypertension
- Incontinence
- Insomnia
- Irritable Bowel Syndrome
- Menopause
- Migraine

- Multiple Sclerosis
- Obsessive-Compulsive Disorder
- Osteoporosis
- Otitis
- Panic Disorder
- Parkinson's Disease
- Schizophrenia
- Spasticity
- Stroke
- Thyroid Disease

Visit www.diseases-explained.com/catalog for an updated list of products or for more information call toll free: 1-877-837-5394

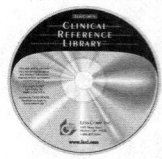 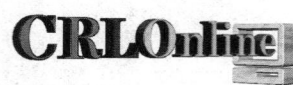